THE NEUROLOGY OF AIDS

THE NEUROLOGY OF AIDS

THIRD EDITION

EDITED BY

Howard E. Gendelman, MD

PROFESSOR AND CHAIR
DEPARTMENT OF PHARMACOLOGY AND
EXPERIMENTAL NEUROSCIENCE
UNIVERSITY OF NEBRASKA MEDICAL CENTER
OMAHA, NE

Igor Grant, MD

DISTINGUISHED PROFESSOR OF PSYCHIATRY
DIRECTOR, HIV NEUROBEHAVIORAL
RESEARCH PROGRAM
UNIVERSITY OF CALIFORNIA-SAN DIEGO
LA JOLLA, CA

Ian Paul Everall, MD, PhD

PROFESSOR OF PSYCHIATRY AND
HEAD OF DEPARTMENT
UNIVERSITY OF MELBOURNE
VICTORIA, AUSTRALIA

Howard S. Fox, MD, PhD

PROFESSOR
DEPARTMENT OF PHARMACOLOGY AND
EXPERIMENTAL NEUROSCIENCE
UNIVERSITY OF NEBRASKA MEDICAL CENTER
OMAHA, NE

Harris A. Gelbard, MD, PhD

DIRECTOR OF THE CENTER FOR NEURAL
DEVELOPMENT AND DISEASE
PROFESSOR OF NEUROLOGY, PEDIATRICS,
MICROBIOLOGY AND IMMUNOLOGY
UNIVERSITY OF ROCHESTER MEDICAL CENTER
ROCHESTER, NY

Stuart A. Lipton, MD, PhD

PROFESSOR AND SCIENTIFIC DIRECTOR
SANFORD-BURNHAM MEDICAL RESEARCH INSTITUTE
ADJUNCT PROFESSOR OF NEUROSCIENCES,
UNIVERSITY OF CALIFORNIA-SAN DIEGO
ADJUNCT PROFESSOR, THE SALK INSTITUTE
FOR BIOLOGICAL STUDIES AND
THE SCRIPPS RESEARCH INSTITUTE
LA JOLLA, CA

Susan Swindells, MBBS

PROFESSOR OF MEDICINE
DEPARTMENT OF INTERNAL MEDICINE
UNIVERSITY OF NEBRASKA MEDICAL CENTER
OMAHA, NE

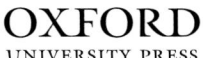

OXFORD
UNIVERSITY PRESS

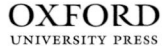

OXFORD
UNIVERSITY PRESS

Oxford University Press, Inc., publishes works that further Oxford University's objective of excellence in research, scholarship, and education.

Oxford   New York
Auckland   Cape Town   Dar es Salaam   Hong Kong   Karachi   Kuala Lumpur
Madrid   Melbourne   Mexico City   Nairobi   New Delhi   Shanghai   Taipei   Toronto

With offices in
Argentina   Austria   Brazil   Chile   Czech Republic   France   Greece   Guatemala   Hungary   Italy
Japan   Poland   Portugal   Singapore   South Korea   Switzerland   Thailand   Turkey   Ukraine   Vietnam

Library of Congress Cataloging-in-Publication Data
The neurology of AIDS / edited by Howard E. Gendelman ... [et al.]. — 3rd ed.
      p. ; cm.
   Includes bibliographical references and index.
   ISBN 978-0-19-539934-9 (hardcover) 1. AIDS (Disease) 2. Neurology. I. Gendelman, Howard E., 1954-
   [DNLM: 1. Acquired Immunodeficiency Syndrome—complications. 2. Central Nervous System Diseases—etiology.
   3. Neurologic Manifestations. WC 503.5]
   RC359.5.N48 2012
   616.97'9207—dc22   2010053537

9 8 7 6 5 4 3 2 1

Printed in China on acid-free paper

With gratitude to Bonnie, Lisa, Nora, Wendy, Emily and Charlie, who are our greatest supporters.

To our students, fellows, colleagues and mentors, who teach, guide and inspire us.

To our patients, who provide our research focus and make our efforts meaningful.

FOREWORD TO THE SECOND EDITION

The Neurology of AIDS is both a well-crafted and timely offering. The book will broadly appeal to the medical community through its thorough evaluation of basic and applied research targeting cognitive, behavioral and mental health issues facing so many HIV-infected people. This book will certainly also be valuable to students, scientists, and health care providers who are involved in research or in the clinical care of people with HIV/AIDS. The contributors are well-respected leaders in AIDS research and clinical care, some of whom have benefitted, in part, from the vision and financial support offered by the American Foundation for AIDS Research (amfAR). We were touched that for this reason and to acknowledge the contributions of amfAR to the fight against AIDS, we were asked to write this dedication.

It is profoundly gratifying to us to see not only the publication of an updated second edition of the encyclopedic text on AIDS neurology reflecting extensive new information collected in the past half-decade, but also to see the contribution we made to it, however modest, so genuinely appreciated.

It is difficult to condense in a few lines how our individual concerns for the people afflicted with HIV/AIDS, and our indignation at the gross prejudices and the many injustices they have had to suffer in addition to their disease, brought the three of us together. It is even more difficult to recount how a myriad of heartbreaks, struggles, disappointments, frustrations and shattered hopes did not destroy our faith in either the power of modern biomedical science or the decency and generosity of spirit of most Americans. In the early 80s, two of us (Mathilde Krim and Elizabeth Taylor) were already deeply concerned by the emergence of a new deadly disease whose epidemic spread appeared so eminently predictable. We were appalled by the failure of our health authorities and elected officials to promptly institute prevention programs in the communities at risk and to provide adequate federal funds for critical research work. We had soon reached the conclusion that the independent nonprofit sector had to step in and start assuming a significant part of these tasks. We proposed that two preexisting organizations (the AIDS Medical Foundation, founded in New York in 1983, and the National AIDS Research Foundation, founded in 1985 in Los Angeles with a substantial gift from the dying Rock Hudson) had to unify their operations and form a single, truly national nonprofit organization. This was done and this larger organization has operated ever since under the name of American Foundation for AIDS Research (amfAR). The third signatory to this dedication (Sharon Stone) became deeply involved somewhat later but with equal determination after the shattering personal experience of losing a close and important friend to the epidemic.

Since its inception, amfAR's mission has been to foster and support biomedical research on the prevention, pathogenesis, and treatment of HIV infection and AIDS, as well as to conduct public education and advocacy efforts on behalf of all people with HIV disease or at high risk for it, so that their civil rights are protected, and their rights to dignity, care, and privacy respected. Much progress was made in these regards through the early and sustained efforts of amfAR.

The support of AIDS-relevant basic biomedical research has always been at the core of amfAR's mission. As do all responsible grant-making agencies, amfAR selects its grantees through stringent peer review. For this, it has enlisted the services of more than 100 volunteer professionals, who are experts in the Foundation's diverse programmatic areas. The senior editor of *The Neurology of AIDS*, Dr. Howard E. Gendelman, is a dedicated member of amfAR's Scientific Advisory Committee (SAC), as are many of this book's contributing authors. For its granting decisions, amfAR relies on its SAC's recommendations. These are based on the originality, promise, and technical excellence of the research proposed in the grant applications it reviews as well as the skills, facilities, and financial needs of the applicants. As an independent foundation, amfAR can respond to funding requests with greater speed and flexibility than government agencies; and it can narrowly focus its funding on HIV/AIDS-relevant proposals. Fields of work to which *The Neurology of AIDS* pays particular attention—innovative treatment strategies, emerging opportunistic infections, disease trends, anti-retroviral drugs, health care delivery, psychosocial aspects of disease, and strategies in vaccine research—all are major concerns of amfAR.

As a research-centered organization, amfAR has helped achieve substantial scientific and medical advances and, in certain instances, it has opened important new avenues to scientific inquiry. This includes the very early studies of Dr. Nancy T. Chang on HIV's protease that spurred the development of protease inhibitors, the drugs that have so dramatically improved the treatment of people with HIV/AIDS in recent years. And, amfAR funded Dr. Ruth M. Ruprecht's preclinical studies in the use of zidovudine for the prevention of vertical retrovirus transmission. Her experiments proved successful and they provided the scientific and ethical rationale for a National Institutes of Health trial in pregnant women that succeeded in "markedly reducing" mother to infant HIV transmission. Another exciting result of amfAR support was the first demonstrations by Dr. Stephen A. Johnston that "naked DNA" can induce humoral and cellular immunity which opened the novel field of "genetic immunization." In 1992, Dr. Carl Wild, an amfAR Fellow, first synthesized and characterized the anti-HIV activity of the peptide T-20 that the Food and Drug Administration approved for marketing in March 2003. T-20, now called Fuzeon, is the first of a class of drugs known as "entry inhibitors." More recently, in 1996, Dr. Nathaniel R. Landau discovered the CCR5 HIV co-receptor with a grant from amfAR, making it now possible to design drugs to block that receptor to prevent infection.

As early as 1986, amfAR's public education and advocacy efforts had started to impact very significantly on AIDS-related policy decision-making at the federal, state, and municipal levels. This Foundation has, in addition, provided substantial support to community-based clinical research groups. And, after a $30 million amfAR investment over several years in the creation and training of 24 such groups, their nationwide network had become capable of operating independently of amfAR. Its successful completion of a number of amfAR- and industry-sponsored clinical studies has produced important results that have helped improve the medical management of HIV disease. In prevention, innovative, and comprehensive approaches (including syringe exchange programs) were funded and continue to be funded and evaluated.

Our goals remain to contribute significantly to: (1) the control of HIV disease until it is fully medically manageable, and (2) the worldwide control of HIV's epidemic spread, which must include safe and highly effective immunization. To date, amfAR has invested over $220 million in its programs, primarily in grants to more than 2,000 research teams worldwide.

The second edition of *The Neurology of AIDS* provides an important glimpse into how far we have come to a better understanding of how HIV infection can damage the nervous system and, even more importantly, how this damage can be prevented. Fresh perspectives are provided in this second edition on viral infection and opportunistic diseases of the brain, spinal cord, and peripheral nerves, which are among AIDS research's most difficult frontiers.

As did its first edition, this book offers a most comprehensive and well-organized description, in both format and style, of some of the most devastating complications of HIV infection. Topics covered span from a basic science review—the structure and function of HIV genes and gene products—to neurobiology, clinical disease manifestations and diagnosis, pathological outcomes of viral infection, and therapeutics. Recent scientific advances are newly included, such as chemokine receptor expression in brain cells and stem cells; brain immunity in health and disease; common disease mechanisms of neurodegenerative disorders; neuroimaging; and molecular markers. All are discussed in some detail. In addition, this book informatively addresses the psychiatric manifestations of HIV disease and its complications, including its psychological impact on the patients themselves as well as their caregivers and the legal implications of such disease manifestations. Several clinical chapters written by patients themselves—an unusual occurrence in the medical literature—provide unique and very moving insights into the torments of both people living with HIV and their caregivers. Importantly, this book also reports on, and discusses, the extraordinary progress afforded by both highly active antiretroviral and adjunctive therapies that can, in no small measure, reverse the neurological and psychiatric manifestations of nervous system involvement in HIV infection. As HIV disease can be made to change from an acute to a more chronic illness, it is important that state-of-the-art therapeutic approaches be described and discussed in some detail. Altogether, we have here a quite monumental undertaking that offers a view of singular breadth and depth on manifestations of HIV disease that have long appeared mysterious and intractable.

Of course, many unresolved questions remain and research in this important field must continue unabated. But this book can be a solid basis of enlightenment for all those interested in the neurological aspects of HIV/AIDS, and we wholeheartedly congratulate the book's many contributing authors and its editors, for an outstanding achievement.

Mathilde Krim, PhD
Founding Chairman and
Chairman of the Board
American Foundation for
AIDS Research (amfAR)

Dame Elizabeth Taylor
Founding International Chairman
American Foundation for
AIDS Research (amfAR)

Sharon Stone
Chairman, Campaign for
AIDS Research
American Foundation for
AIDS Research (amfAR)

PREFACE

The Neurology of AIDS is a comprehensive treatise on the neurological, behavioral, motor, sensory, cognitive, psychiatric, developmental, and basic research of human immunodeficiency virus (HIV) infection. Since the start of the epidemic, neurological disorders emerged rapidly as the most feared and significant complication of progressive HIV infection. Despite considerable advances in combination active antiretroviral therapy (cART), these disorders continue, albeit at a chronic level. The disorders include peripheral neuropathy; myopathy; myelopathy; and, most significantly, HIV-associated neurocognitive disorders (HAND), comprising cognitive, motor, and behavior abnormalities.

The mechanisms by which the virus invades the nervous system and induces neurological disorders are complex. They give rise to novel pathological processes and, when understood correctly, point to therapeutic interventions that are relevant to many neurodegenerative disorders. The neurological disorders are becoming an even more important component of the HIV epidemic, as patients live longer and increasingly productive lives. Accordingly, separate chapters on aging and on linkages between HAND and other neurodegenerative disorders are included in the text. This third edition expresses our collective vision and our collective hope to move research even faster from laboratory bench to patient bedside. With continued new insights emerging for disease causation, considerable emphasis was placed on basic science at the molecular, cellular, animal, and applied human levels. With a focus on genomics, we redoubled our efforts to tie this work to an understanding of host antiretroviral immunity and to include discussions of both the positive potential and the possible pitfalls in vaccine developments. The text goes on to provide thorough and updated reviews of the epidemiological, psychological, and psychiatric aspects of HAND. One unique aspect of the text lies in the section on clinical and personal perspectives. Based on the popularity of this section, the chapters were expanded, and now include a broader disease view from infected patients, who describe their life journey living with HIV/AIDS in their own terms and in their own way. Personal experiences are provided on what it is like living daily with the challenges and difficulties of peripheral neuropathy, sexual dysfunction, substance abuse, anxiety, and depression. These patient perspectives supplement the descriptions written by physicians and scientists. The emerging fields of stem cell biology, proteomics, and adjunctive therapies serve to define how host factors affect active viral replication and neurodegenerative events—and some of the discoveries from these fields are harnessed as biomarkers to improve diagnosis and therapeutic monitoring.

The ultimate goal will be to use combined approaches to prevent or reverse disease by positively affecting the processes of neuronal injury and death. Such information, we believe, will serve to define HIV neurology. The advances reflected in this text have already aided in developing new therapeutics for many neurodegenerative disorders, including but not limited to Alzheimer's and Parkinson's disease, amyotrophic lateral sclerosis, and Huntington's disease.

Overall, significant advances in cART have reduced the incidence of HIV-1-associated dementia, while peripheral neuropathy remains common. Neuropsychological tests to monitor cognitive impairments are now more precise, and as patients continue to live longer, more subtle neurological dysfunctions are now the most common disease features. Advances in studies of viral neuropathogenesis, diagnostics, and therapeutics for HAND are provided. A panel discussion by internationally recognized authorities in HIV biology and HAND, including some of the editors, addresses timely questions on neurovirulence, cellular factors influencing viral replication, therapeutic challenges, and the constantly changing epidemiological patterns of disease.

Since the first edition, the book has evolved from 4 to now 12 major sections. The dedication is provided by scientific and public leaders. We acknowledge their contributions, insights, and support for the three decades of the epidemic. Clearly, the merger of efforts between community leaders, scientists, physicians, and policy makers has enabled sustained success in both biomedical research and patient care. Discussion of HAND in the developing world, including links to new research efforts, is provided throughout this volume.

The basic science components of the text were once again revamped considerably from the prior edition. Comprehensive reviews are provided into the molecular and cellular biology, immunology, and neuroscience of HIV infection and into host genomics. A novice reader who picks up the book for the first time can gain a broad understanding of the basic aspects of HIV/AIDS, and its relationships to neurological disease manifestations, without having to refer to other information sources. The next section then focuses on the innate and adaptive immune systems and how they affect the pathogenesis of other neurodegenerative disorders and can be used to develop protective vaccines. A significant feature of the neurological disease complex involves disorders of the blood-brain barrier. Discussions of this barrier's structure and function are provided, as are discussions of mechanisms of viral and cell entry into the brain at both the organ and cellular level. One of the most critical aspects of HIV disease is the disordered regulation of glial function. The section on this topic was expanded substantively, as deficits in innate glial immunity often underlie the pathogenesis of HIV infection and peripheral neuropathy. Adjunctive medicines that target glial secretory functions, including agents that deactivate microglial responses, can affect both productive viral replication and neurotoxic activities. The means to deliver adjunctive medicines, as well as ART, now have expanded into the field of nanomedicine. Neurotoxicity may manifest through both cellular and viral products and can affect neurogenesis and cellular functions. These neurotoxic products are covered in greater depth, both at the molecular and cellular levels, with viral targets described in relationship to progenitor cells, mononuclear phagocytes, and astrocytes. Animal model systems remain pivotal for studies of viral pathogenesis and developmental therapeutics, and for developing vaccine approaches to prevent disease. As most lentiviral infections show prominent neurological manifestations, a range of infectious disorders is covered, including the simian and feline immunodeficiency viruses, caprine arthritis-encephalitis, and visna-maedi infections of goats and sheep, as well as the more recently developed murine viral systems for HAND, including transgenic and immunodeficient systems. Several chapters discussing the role of drugs of abuse in the disease process are provided. These chapters look at the interrelationships, as observed both in the laboratory and at the patient bedside, among virus, immunity, and drugs of abuse as they pertain to disease progression and protection.

Subsequent sections and chapters provide a "bread and butter" description of the clinical and pathological aspects of disease. These cover features of dementia, neuropathology, drug abuse, spinal cord disease, peripheral neuropathy, myopathy, neoplasms, opportunistic infections including hepatitis C, and psychiatric disorders.

Significant progress has been made in methods for diagnosing and monitoring cognitive function following HIV infection. These methods are now reviewed in chapters on structural brain imaging, magnetic resonance spectroscopy, evoked potentials, neuropsychological assessments, and measures of cellular and viral products as molecular markers of disease and disease progression.

The section on pediatric manifestations of HIV disease was expanded once again to include clinical and neuropathological features along with evaluation of neurodevelopmental deficits and psychosocial aspects. The severity of neurological disease in children is more significant than observed in adults and often devastating. The breakthroughs of ART for children and for prevention of maternal-fetal transmission are also discussed; these breakthroughs have altered markedly the natural history and severity of disease.

A complete section is provided on new treatment paradigms for opportunistic infections. This section should provide the clinician with a comprehensive set of up-to-date management paradigms as well as an understanding of future prospects for adjunctive therapies that target specific disease pathways and mechanisms. The book concludes with a prospectus on changes in HIV epidemiology and the evolution of the disease complex. The clinical and neuropathological aspects of disease in the cART era provide new perspectives for disease and the changing outcomes for neurological impairments that are being developed.

We suspect that the reader, whether a student, researcher, or health care provider, will find this book an important resource and reference on the neurological aspects of HIV infection. Synthesizing in one text contributions from patients, activists, health care providers, scientists, and clinicians proved to be a fascinating undertaking. On reflection, this synthesis provides a unique perspective not only on HIV neurology but on the field of HIV/AIDS as a whole—and on the continued positive prospects for the future.

Howard E. Gendelman, MD
Igor Grant, MD
Ian Paul Everall, MD
Howard S. Fox, MD, PhD
Harris A. Gelbard, MD, PhD
Stuart A. Lipton, MD, PhD
Susan Swindells, MD

ACKNOWLEDGMENTS

Craig Panner and Kathryn Winder of Oxford University Press provided invaluable guidance, administrative, logistic, and editorial support. No task ever seemed too difficult, too challenging, or beyond the scope of their competences. It was a simple pleasure working with such a talented and dedicated group of people.

This comprehensive work was made possible, in large measure, by the often thankless and tireless efforts of one single person, Ms. Lana Reichardt. Lana remains forever a special and talented individual. Her selfless professionalism and her dauntless encouragement of me enabled the completion of this book. Her organizational abilities, expressed in a quiet and thoughtful manner, proved exceptional. These abilities, together with a personal friendship forged, made many difficult issues pass with ease. A simple thank you seems inadequate.

The untimely deaths of Al Kerza-Kwiatecki, Anthony Johnson, and Opendra (Bill) Narayan are noted with both sadness and life's celebration. Their lives are a tattooed imprint towards friendship, thoughtfulness, unbridled life determination, inspiration, kindness, and scientific rigor.

To Carol Swarts, a friend, guide, and fellow journeyperson; a thank you for who you are is offered, and also a prayer that you never change.

To John Gollan, Harold M. and Beverly Maurer, Rodney Markin, Michael McGlade, Fran and Louie Blumkin, Harriet Singer, and Brian and Laura Lauer—who have played and continue to play many diverse and important roles in support of our research and in my own life journey —a sincere thank you is offered. Gratitude is extending for allowing our work to prosper continuously at the highest levels.

To our administrators, assistants, leaders, and cheerleaders Robin Taylor, Julie Ditter, Johna Belling, and Amy Volk, who place their fingers on our research and oftentimes our life pursuits.

To Anindita Sengupta and Karen Kwak, a special thank you to acknowledge their dedication, resourcefulness, and a job very well done.

With appreciation to Benjamin Abelow, our new colleague and literary assistant, this book should be only our beginning.

To Soffia Gendelman, who taught me perseverance and understanding, and to Bonnie Bloch, who as my life's partner is also my best friend and guide to self-improvement each and every day.

To my children and grandchild Lesley, Sierra, Jason, Adam, and Emma, my windows for each today.

Howard E. Gendelman, MD
Editor-in-Chief

SHORT CONTENTS

CONTENTS

CONTRIBUTORS

Lauren Abrey
Department of Neurology
Memorial Sloan Kettering Cancer Center
New York, NY

Shaona Acharjee
Division of Neurology
University of Alberta, Edmonton
Department of Microbiology and Infectious Diseases
University of Calgary
Calgary, Alberta, Canada

Cristian L. Achim
HIV Neurobehavioral Research Program
Department of Psychiatry
University of California, San Diego
La Jolla, CA

Sunil K. Ahuja
Departments of Medicine and
   Microbiology/Immunology
Veterans Administration Research Center for
   AIDS and HIV Infection
University of Texas Health Science Center
San Antonio, TX

Lisa N. Akhtar
Department of Cell Biology
The University of Alabama at Birmingham
Birmingham, AL

Ibolya E. András
Molecular Neuroscience and
   Vascular Biology Laboratory
Department of Neurosurgery
University of Kentucky Medical Center
Lexington, KY

Valgerdur Andrésdóttir
Institute for Experimental Pathology
University of Iceland
Keldur v/Vesturlandsveg, Iceland

Sarah L. Archibald
Laboratory of Cognitive Imaging
Department of Psychiatry
University of California, San Diego
La Jolla, CA

J. Hampton Atkinson
Department of Psychiatry
University of California, San Diego
La Jolla, CA

Brandi J. Baker
Spain Rehabilitation Center
Department of Physical Medicine
   and Rehabilitation
The University of Alabama at Birmingham
Birmingham, AL

Shantanu Balkundi
Department of Pharmacology
   and Experimental Neuroscience
University of Nebraska Medical Center
Omaha, NE

William A. Banks
GRECC, Veterans Affairs Puget
   Sound Health Care System
University of Washington School of Medicine
Division of Gerontology and Geriatric Medicine
Department of Internal Medicine
Seattle, WA

Eric J. Benner
Department of Pediatrics
Duke University Medical Center
Durham, NC

Etty N. Benveniste
Department of Cell Biology
Comprehensive Cancer Center
University of Alabama Birmingham
Birmingham, AL

Joseph R. Berger
Departments of Neurology and Internal Medicine
University of Kentucky Medical Center
Lexington, KY

Joan W. Berman
Departments of Pathology and
   Microbiology and Immunology
Albert Einstein College of Medicine
Bronx, NY

Brookie M. Best
Pediatric Pharmacology Research Unit
University of California, San Diego
La Jolla, CA

Ruth Brack-Werner
Institute of Virology
Helmholtz Zentrum München
German Research Center for Environmental Health
Neuherberg, Germany

Jessica Breslow
Department of Microbiology and Immunology
Center for Substance Abuse Research
Temple University School of Medicine
Philadelphia, PA

Bruce J. Brew
Department of Neurology and St Vincent's Centre for
    Applied Medical Research
St Vincent's Hospital and University of
    New South Wales
Sydney, Australia

R. Douglas Bruce
Yale University AIDS Program
New Haven, CT

Shilpa Buch
Department of Pharmacology and Experimental
    Neuroscience
University of Nebraska Medical Center
Omaha, NE

Michael Bukrinsky
Department of Microbiology
Immunology and Tropical Medicine
George Washington University
Washington, DC

Tricia H. Burdo
Department of Biology
Boston College
Chestnut Hill, MA

Guy A. Cabral
Department of Microbiology and Immunology
Virginia Commonwealth
    University School of Medicine
Richmond, VA

Shannon Callen
Department of Pharmacology and Experimental
    Neuroscience
University of Nebraska Medical Center
Omaha, NE

Edmund V. Capparelli
Pediatric Pharmacology Research Unit
University of California, San Diego
La Jolla, CA

Jordan Elizabeth Cattie
Joint Doctoral Program in Clinical Psychology
San Diego State University
University of California
San Diego, CA

Linda Chang
Department of Medicine
University of Hawaii at Manoa
The Queen's Medical Center
Honolulu, HI

Sulie L. Chang
Department of Biological Sciences
Institute of NeuroImmune Pharmacology
The College of Arts and Science
Seton Hall University
South Orange, NJ

Qiang Chen
Department of Pharmacology and
    Experimental Neuroscience
University of Nebraska Medical Center
Omaha, NE

Paul Cheney
Department of Molecular and Integrative Physiology
University of Kansas Medical Center
Kansas City, KS

Sumedha Chugh
Fels Institute for Cancer Research and Molecular Biology
Temple University School of Medicine
Philadelphia, PA

Pawel Ciborowski
Department of Pharmacology and
    Experimental Neuroscience
University of Nebraska Medical Center
Omaha, NE

Lucy A. Civitello
Departments of Neurology
George Washington University
Children's National Medical Center
Washington, DC

Janice E. Clements
Molecular and Comparative Pathobiology
The Johns Hopkins University School of Medicine
Baltimore, MD

David B. Clifford
Department of Neurology
Washington University School of Medicine
Saint Louis, MO

Bruce A. Cohen
Department of Neurology
Feinberg School of Medicine
Northwestern University
Chicago, IL

Denise R. Cook
Department of Neurology
Department of Neuroscience Graduate Group
University of Pennsylvania School of Medicine
Philadelphia, PA

William D. Cornwell
Fels Institute for Cancer Research
    and Molecular Biology
Temple University School of Medicine
Philadelphia, PA

Stephanie A. Cross
Department of Neurology
Department of Neuroscience Graduate Group
University of Pennsylvania School of Medicine
Philadelphia, PA

Nicholas W.S. Davies
Department of Neurology
Chelsea and Westminster Hospital
London, UK

Shirley F. Delair
Department of Pediatrics
University of Nebraska Medical Center
Omaha, NE

Alexis Demopoulos
Tisch Cancer Institute
Mount Sinai Medical Center
New York, NY

Krishnakumar Devadas
Laboratory of Molecular Virology
Division of Emerging and Transfusion Transmitted Diseases
Center for Biologics Evaluation and Research
Food and Drug Administration
Rockville, MD

Subhash Dhawan
Viral Immunology Section
Laboratory of Molecular Virology
Division of Emerging and Transfusion Transmitted Diseases
Center for Biologics Evaluation and Research
Food and Drug Administration
Rockville, MD

Anna Dow
Department of Epidemiology
University of North Carolina School
    of Global Public Health
The University of North Caroline at Chapel Hill
Chapel Hill, NC

Nichole A. Duarte
HIV Neurobehavioral Research Center
University of California, San Diego
San Diego, CA

Gigi Ebenezer
SOM Neuro Neuroimmunology
The Johns Hopkins University
Baltimore, MD

Toby K. Eisenstein
Center for Substance Abuse Research
Department of Microbiology and Immunology
Temple University School of Medicine
Philadelphia, PA

Kathryn J. Elliott
Department of Neurology
Mount Sinai School of Medicine
New York, NY

Ronald J. Ellis
Department of Neurosciences
HIV Neurobehavioral Research Center
University of California, San Diego
San Diego, CA

Thomas M. Ernst
Department of Medicine
John A. Burns School of Medicine
University of Hawaii at Manoa
The Queen's Medical Center
Honolulu, HI

Eliseo A. Eugenin
Department of Pathology
Albert Einstein College of Medicine
Bronx, NY

Ian Paul Everall
Department of Psychiatry
Faculty of Medicine, Dentistry and Health Sciences
The University of Melbourne
Melbourne, Australia

Ute Feger
Department of Medicine
John A. Burns School of Medicine
University of Hawaii at Manoa
The Queen's Medical Center
Honolulu, HI

Christine Fennema-Notestine
Departments of Psychiatry and Radiology
University of California, San Diego
La Jolla, CA

Matthew J. Finley
Fels Institute for Cancer Research and Molecular Biology
Temple University School of Medicine
Philadelphia, PA

Howard S. Fox
Department of Pharmacology
    and Experimental Neuroscience
University of Nebraska Medical Center
Omaha, NE

Kenneth A. Fox
Department of Neurology
San Francisco Medical Center
San Francisco, CA

Lucio Gama
Department of Molecular and Comparative Pathobiology
The Johns Hopkins University School of Medicine
Baltimore, MD

Harris A. Gelbard
Center for Neural Development and Disease
Departments of Neurology
Pediatrics and Microbiology
    and Immunology
University of Rochester Medical Center
Rochester, NY

Benjamin B. Gelman
Texas NeuroAIDS Research Center
Departments of Pathology and Neuroscience & Cell Biology
University of Texas Medical Branch
Galveston, TX

Howard E. Gendelman
Department of Pharmacology
    and Experimental Neuroscience
Center for Neurodegenerative Disorders
University of Nebraska Medical Center
Omaha, NE

Gudmundur Georgsson
Institute for Experimental Pathology
University of Iceland
Keldur v/Vesturlandsveg
Reykjavik, Iceland

M. John Gill
Department of Medicine
Division of Infectious Diseases
University of Calgary
Calgary, Alberta, Canada

Eric M. Glare
Speaker and Volunteer
Positive Speakers Bureau
People Living with HIV/AIDS
Victoria, Australia

Raul Gonzalez
Department of Psychiatry
University of Illinois at Chicago
Chicago, IL

R. Gilberto González
Radiology-Massachusetts General Hospital
Neuroradiology Division and the A.A.
    Martinos Center for Biomedical Imaging
Massachusetts General Hospital
    and Harvard Medical School
Boston, MA

David R. Graham
Department of Molecular and Comparative
    Pathobiology
The Johns Hopkins University School
    of Medicine
Baltimore, MD

Igor Grant
Department of Psychiatry
HIV Neurobehavioral Research Center
Translational Methamphetamine AIDS Research Center
University of California, San Diego
La Jolla, CA

Weijing He
Veterans Administration Research Center for AIDS and
    HIV-1 Infection
South Texas Veterans Health Care System
Department of Medicine
University of Texas Health Science Center
San Antonio, TX

Robert K. Heaton
Department of Psychiatry
HIV Neurobehavioral Research Center
University of California, San Diego
San Diego, CA

William F. Hickey
Department of Pathology and Microbiology/Immunology
Dartmouth Medical School
Lebanon, NH

Charles H. Hinkin
University of California Los Angeles
Department of Psychiatry and Biobehavioral Sciences
Veterans Administration Greater Los Angeles
    Healthcare System
Los Angeles, CA

Wenzhe Ho
Departments of Pathology and Laboratory
    Medicine and Anatomy and Cell Biology
Temple University School of Medicine
Philadelphia, PA

Adelina Holguin
Nebraska Center for Virology
University of Nebraska
Lincoln, NE

Yunlong Huang
Laboratory of Neuroimmunology and Regenerative Therapy
Department of Pharmacology and Experimental Neuroscience
University of Nebraska Medical Center
Omaha, NE

Jessica A. L. Hutter-Saunders
Department of Pharmacology and Experimental
    Neuroscience
University of Nebraska Medical Center
Omaha, NE

Sergey Iordanskiy
George Washington University
Department of Microbiology
Immunology and Tropical Medicine
Washington, DC

Terry L. Jernigan
Center for Human Development
Laboratory of Cognitive Imaging
Departments of Cognitive SciencePsychiatry and Radiology
University of California, San Diego
La Jolla, CA

Darren Kane
Positive Speakers Bureau
Melbourne
People Living with HIV/AIDS
Victoria, Australia

Georgette D. Kanmogne
Department of Pharmacology and Experimental Neuroscience
University of Nebraska Medical Center
Omaha, NE

Karen
A woman living with AIDS
Omaha, NE

Marley D. Kass
Institute of NeuroImmune Pharmacology
Seton Hall University
South Orange, NJ

Marcus Kaul
Infectious and Inflammatory Disease Center
Sanford-Burnham Medical Research Institute
Department of Psychiatry
University of California, San Diego
La Jolla, CA

Dennis L. Kolson
Department of Neurology
University of Pennsylvania School of Medicine
Philadelphia, PA

Max V. Kuenstling
Department of Pharmacology and Experimental
    Neuroscience
Center for Neurodegenerative Disorders
University of Nebraska Medical Center
Omaha, NE

Anil Kumar
Division of Pharmacology and Toxicology
School of Pharmacy
University of Missouri-Kansas City
    School of Medicine
Kansas City, MO

Victoria A. Laast
Department of Molecular and
    Comparative Pathobiology
The Johns Hopkins University School of Medicine
Baltimore, MD

T. Dianne Langford
Department of Neuroscience
Temple University School of Medicine
Philadelphia, PA

Sunhee C. Lee
Department of Pathology
Albert Einstein College of Medicine
Bronx, NY

Margaret R. Lentz
Neuroradiology Division
Radiology-Massachusetts General Hospital
The A.A. Martinos Center for Biomedical Imaging
Harvard Medical School
Massachusetts General Hospital
Charlestown, MA

Scott L. Letendre
Department of Medicine
HIV Neurobehavioral Research Center
University of California, San Diego
San Diego, CA

Andrew J. Levine
Department of Neurology
University of California, Los Angeles
Los Angeles, CA

Guanhan Li
Section of Infections of the Nervous System
National Institute of Neurological Disorders and Stroke
National Institutes of Health
Bethesda, MD

Wenxue Li
Section of Infections of the Nervous System
National Institute of Neurological Disorders and Stroke
National Institutes of Health
Bethesda, MD

Kevin J. Liner
Department of Neurology
University of North Carolina at Chapel Hill
Chapel Hill, NC

Stuart A. Lipton
Del E. Webb Center for Neuroscience
    Aging, and Stem Cell Research
Sanford-Burnham Medical Research Institute
Salk Institute for Biological Studies
The Scripps Research Institute
Departments Neurosciences and Psychiatry
University of California, San Diego
La Jolla, CA

Eugene O. Major
Laboratory of Molecular Medicine and Neuroscience
Division of Intramural Research
National Institute of Neurological
    Disorders and Stroke
National Institutes of Health
Bethesda, MD

Joseph L. Mankowski
Department of Molecular and
    Comparative Pathobiology
The Johns Hopkins University School of Medicine
Baltimore, MD

Thomas D. Marcotte
Department of Psychiatry
HIV Neurobehavioral Research Center
University of California, San Diego
San Diego, CA

Christina M. Marra
Department of Neurology
University of Washington School of Medicine
Harborview Medical Center
Seattle, WA

Eileen M. Martin
Department of Psychiatry
University of Illinois at Chicago
Chicago, IL

Andrea Martinez-Skinner
Department of Pharmacology
    and Experimental Neuroscience
University of Nebraska Medical Center
Omaha, NE

Eliezer Masliah
Departments of Pathology and Neurosciences
University of California, San Diego
La Jolla, CA

James May
Positive Speakers Bureau
Melbourne, Australia

Justin C. McArthur
Department of Neurology
Molecular & Comparative
    Pathobiology and Pathology
The Johns Hopkins University
SOM Comp Med Retrovirus Bio Laboratory
Baltimore, MD

Jennifer A. McCombe
Department of Medicine (Neurology)
University of Alberta
Edmonton, Alberta, Canada
Department of Medicine (Infectious Diseases)
    University of Calgary
Calgary, Alberta, Canada

J. Allen McCutchan
Department of Medicine
University of California, San Diego
HIV Neurobehavioral Research Center (HNRC)
San Diego, CA

JoEllyn M. McMillan
Department of Pharmacology and Experimental Neuroscience
University of Nebraska Medical Center
Omaha, NE

Rick B. Meeker
Department of Neurology
University of North Carolina
Chapel Hill, NC

Manja Meggendorfer
Institute of Virology
Helmholtz Zentrum München
German Research Center for Environmental Health
Neuherberg, Germany

Joseph J. Meissler
Department of Microbiology and Immunology
Center for Substance Abuse Research
Temple University School of Medicine
Philadelphia, PA

Claude Mellins
National Cancer Institute
National Institutes of Health
Bethesda, MD

Richard J. Miller
Department of Molecular Pharmacology
   and Biological Chemistry
Northwestern University
Feinberg School of Medicine
Chicago, IL

Mark Mintz
The Center for Neurological and
   Neurodevelopmental Health, and
The Clinical Research Center of New Jersey
Gibbsboro, NJ

Maria G. Chiara
Laboratory of Molecular Medicine
   and Neuroscience
Division of Intramural Research
National Institute of Neurological Disorder and Stroke
National Institutes of Health
Bethesda, MD

David J. Moore
Department of Psychiatry
University of California, San Diego
HIV Neurobehavioral Research Center (HNRC)
San Diego, CA

Susan Morgello
Department of Pathology and Neuroscience
Mount Sinai Medical Center
New York, NY

R. Lee Mosley
Department of Pharmacology and Experimental
   Neuroscience
Center for Neurodegenerative Disorders
University of Nebraska Medical Center
Omaha, NE

Srinivas Mummidi
University of Texas Health Science Center at San Antonio
South Texas Veterans Health Care System and
VA Research Center for AIDS and HIV-1 Infection
San Antonio, TX

Madhavan P.N. Nair
Department of Immunology
Institute of Neuroimmune Pharmacology
Herbert Wertheim College of Medicine
Florida International University
Miami, FL

Shinsuke Nakagawa
Molecular Neuroscience and Vascular
   Biology Laboratory
Department of Neurosurgery
University of Kentucky Medical Center
Lexington, KY

Avindra Nath
Section of Infections of the Nervous System
National Institute of Neurological Disorders
   and Stroke
National Institutes of Health
Bethesda, MD

Timothy B. Nguyen
Department of Psychiatry
Faculty of Medicine Dentistry and Health Sciences
The University of Melbourne
Royal Melbourne Hospital
Victoria, Australia

Ari S. Nowacek
Department of Pharmacology and
   Experimental Neuroscience
University of Nebraska Medical Center
Omaha, NE

Shu-ichi Okamoto
Del E. Webb Center for Neuroscience,
   Aging, and Stem Cell Research
Sanford-Burnham Medical Research Institute
La Jolla, CA

Jason F. Okulicz
Infectious Disease Service
Department of Internal Medicine
Uniformed Services University of the Health Sciences
Brooke Army Medical Center
Fort Sam Houston, TX

David G. Ostrow
Ogburn-Stouffer Center for Social
   Organizational Research
National Opinion Research Center (NORC)
University of Chicago and Multicenter
   AIDS Cohort Study (MACS)
Northwestern University
Chicago, IL

Susan Paxton
Positive Speakers Bureau
Melbourne;
People Living with HIV/AIDS
Victoria, Australia

Hui Peng
Laboratory of Neuroimmunology and Regenerative Therapy
Department of Pharmacology and Experimental
    Neuroscience
University of Nebraska Medical Center
Omaha, NE

Yuri Persidsky
Department of Pathology and Laboratory Medicine
Temple University School of Medicine
Philadelphia, PA

Larisa Y. Poluektova
Department of Pharmacology and Experimental
    Neuroscience
University of Nebraska Medical Center
Omaha, NE

Gwenael Pottiez
Department of Pharmacology and
    Experimental Neuroscience
University of Nebraska Medical Center
Omaha, NE

Christopher Power
Canada Research Chair (Tier 1) in Neurological
    Infection and Immunity
Departments of Medicine
Medical Microbiology and Immunology
University of Alberta
Edmonton, Canada

Michael C. Previti
Forsyth Medical Center
Winston-Salem, NC

Richard W. Price
Department of Neurology
University of California, San Francisco
San Francisco General Hospital
San Francisco, CA

Erinn S. Raborn
Department of Microbiology and Immunology
Virginia Commonwealth University
School of Medicine
Richmond, VA

Servio H. Ramirez
Department of Pathology and Laboratory Medicine
Temple University School of Medicine
Philadelphia, PA

Cetewayo S. Rashid
Molecular Neuroscience and Vascular
    Biology Laboratory
Department of Neurosurgery
University of Kentucky Medical Center
Lexington, KY

Eva-Maria Ratai
Radiology-Massachusetts General Hospital
Neuroradiology Division
The A.A. Martinos Center
    for Biomedical Imaging
Harvard Medical School
Boston, MA

James B. Reinecke
Laboratory of Neuroimmunology
    and Regenerative Therapy
Department of Pharmacology
    and Experimental Neuroscience
University of Nebraska Medical Center
Omaha, NE

Michelle Ro
Department of Neurology
University of North Carolina at Chapel Hill
Chapel Hill, NC

Kevin R. Robertson
Department of Neurology
University of North Carolina at Chapel Hill
Chapel Hill, NC

Jessica Robinson-Papp
Department of Neurology
Mount Sinai Medical Center
New York, NY

Thomas J. Rogers
Center for Inflammation
Translational and Clinical Lung Research
Department of Pharmacology
Fels Institute for Cancer Research
    and Molecular Biology
Center for Substance Abuse Research
Temple University School of Medicine
Philadelphia, PA

Ina Rothenaigner
Institute of Virology
Helmholtz Zentrum München
German Research Center for
    Environmental Health
Neuherberg, Germany

Sabita Roy
Division of Infection
Inflammation and Vascular Biology
Department of Surgery and Pharmacology
University of Minnesota
Minneapolis, MN

Upal Roy
Department of Pharmacology and
    Experimental Neuroscience
University of Nebraska Medical Center
Omaha, NE

Ned Sacktor
The Johns Hopkins Bayview Medical Center
Johns Hopkins Medical Institutions
SOM Neuro Bay Neuroimmunology
Baltimore, MD

Zainulabedin M. Saiyed
Department of Immunology
Institute of Neuroimmune Pharmacology
Herbert Wertheim College of Medicine
Florida International University
Miami, FL

Uriel Sandkovsky
Department of Internal Medicine
University of Nebraska Medical Center
Omaha, NE

Lynnae Schwartz
The Children's Hospital of Philadelphia
Abramson Research Center
Philadelphia, PA

J. Cobb Scott
HIV Neurobehavioral Research Center
Department of Psychiatry
University of California, San Diego
San Diego, CA

Leslie K. Serchuck
Department of Pediatrics
University of Pennsylvania School of Medicine
Philadelphia, PA

Leroy R. Sharer
Department of Pathology & Laboratory Medicine
University of Medicine and Dentistry of New Jersey
New Jersey Medical School
Newark, NJ

David M. Simpson
Department of Neurology
Mount Sinai Medical Center
New York, NY

Davey M. Smith
Division of Infectious Diseases
Department of Neuroscience
University of California, San Diego
La Jolla, CA

Samantha S. Soldan
Department of Neurology
University of Pennsylvania School of Medicine
Philadelphia, PA

Changcheng Song
Temple University School of Medicine
Fels Institute for Cancer Research and Molecular Biology
Philadelphia, PA

Virawudh Soontornniyomkij
HIV Neurobehavioral Research Program
Department of Psychiatry
University of California, San Diego
San Diego, CA

Caroline Soulas
Department of Biology
Boston College
Chestnut Hill, MA

Serena S. Spudich
Department of Neurology
Yale University School of Medicine
New Haven, CT

Joseph Steiner
Department of Neuroscience
The Johns Hopkins University School of Medicine
Baltimore, MD

Susan Swindells
HIV Clinic
Department of Internal Medicine
University of Nebraska Medical Center
Omaha, NE

Bianca Tigges
Institute of Virology
Helmholtz Zentrum München
German Research Center for
    Environmental Health
Neuherberg, Germany

Michal Toborek
Department of Neurosurgery
Molecular Neuroscience and Vascular Biology Laboratory
University of Kentucky Medical Center
Lexington, KY

Sigurbjörg Torsteinsdóttir
Institute for Experimental Pathology
University of Iceland
Keldur v/Vesturlandsveg
Reykjavik, Iceland

Glenn J. Treisman
Department of Psychiatry and Behavioral Sciences
The Johns Hopkins University Medical Center
Baltimore, MD

Warren B. Treisman
The Law Office of Warren Treisman, ALC
San Diego, CA

Damien C. Tully
Nebraska Center for Virology
University of Nebraska
Lincoln, NE

Annelies Van Rie
Department of Epidermiology
University of North Carolina School
    of Global Public Health
The University of North Caroline at Chapel Hill
Chapel Hill, NC

Michelle Vincendeau
Institute of Virology
Helmholtz Zentrum München
German Research Center for Environmental Health
Neuherberg, Germany

Jayme Wiederin
Department of Pharmacology and Experimental Neuroscience
University of Nebraska Medical Center
Omaha, NE

Lori Wiener
National Cancer Institute
National Institutes of Health
Bethesda, MD

Kenneth C. Williams
Department of Biology
Boston College
Chestnut Hill, MA

Charles Wood
Nebraska Center for Virology
School of Biological Sciences
University of Nebraska
Lincoln, NE

Steven Paul Woods
HIV Neurobehavioral Research Center
Translational Methamphetamine AIDS Research Center
University of California, San Diego
San Diego, CA

Edwina J. Wright
Infectious Diseases
The Alfred Hospital;
The Burnet Institute
Melbourne, Victoria, Australia
Departments of Medicine
Nursing Health Sciences
Monash University, Clayton
Victoria, Australia

Honghong Yao
Department of Pharmacology and Experimental
    Neuroscience
University of Nebraska Medical Center
Omaha, NE

Li Ye
Department of Pathology and Laboratory Medicine
Temple University School of Medicine
Philadelphia, PA

Jialin C. Zheng
Laboratory of Neuroimmunology and
    Regenerative Therapy
Department of Pharmacology and Experimental
    Neuroscience
University of Nebraska Medical Center
Omaha, NE

Yu Zhong
Molecular Neuroscience and Vascular
    Biology Laboratory
Department of Neurosurgery
University of Kentucky Medical Center
Lexington, KY

M. Christine Zink
Department of Molecular and
    Comparative Pathobiology
The Johns Hopkins University School of Medicine
Baltimore, MD

INTERACTIVE TOPICAL DISCUSSION ON AIDS NEUROLOGY

PAST, PRESENT, AND FUTURE

Moderator: Howard E. Gendelman

Participants: Roger J. Bedimo, Linda Chang, Ian Paul Everall, Howard S. Fox, Harris A. Gelbard, Igor Grant, Scott L. Letendre, Stuart A. Lipton, Eliezer Masliah, Susan Swindells, and Babafemi Taiwo

The authors thank Ms. Lana J. Reichardt for her organizational, literary, and transcriptional skills, which proved invaluable for this teleconference discussion.

INTRODUCTION

While the pages of our book offer the reader a comprehensive review of the neurological, behavioral, motor, sensory, cognitive, psychiatric, developmental, and basic research performed on HIV-1 infection of the nervous system, a frank discussion of the field, its future direction, and needs was lacking. To this end, our faculty (the editors, with assistance of other chosen clinician-scientists) used a platform of an interactive conference to discuss what we considered to be the timely questions facing the field. The listed contributors are active investigators and authorities on HIV/AIDS. Particular emphasis is placed within this discussion on current thinking about disease pathogenesis, patient care, and the evolution of these areas for the future. Each question posed to the expert panel is followed by several responses. Each response is preceded by the speaker's last name.

QUESTION 1

"What is the evidence that there are pathobiological and clinical manifestations of human immunodeficiency virus (HIV) infection on the central nervous system (CNS) for the period immediately following the viral seroconversion reaction? What are the mechanisms for such effects and could early intervention attenuate the development of HIV-associated neurocognitive disorders (HAND)?"

Grant: I think that the evidence for early neurocognitive impairment and clinical neurological symptoms in the acute phase of infection remains controversial. There are certainly people who develop early seroconversion illness with neurological symptoms but I think this is not really what we are focusing on here in this discussion. The question is whether the neurocognitive complications, that is, HAND, begin early.

There is some evidence that that may be true. For example, Dr. Serena Spudich and colleagues reported on changes in cerebrospinal fluid (CSF) profiles in relationship to systemic infection and antiretroviral treatment early in the course of infections that were also linked to molecular measures of HIV-1 variants (Spudich et al., 2005; Schnell et al., 2009). Recently, our group completed some work that showed that from a neurocognitive standpoint people with acute and early infection scored intermediate between noninfected controls and people with established infection, but the changes were very subtle. So I think it remains an open question. The other point I would make is that there are quite a few data now that suggest that having experienced a very low CD4+ T cell count, that is, a low nadir, predisposes to neurocognitive complications later. And so the question arises whether preventing low CD4 during the acute phase could spare the brain from injury.

Fox: I would like to speak on the mechanism since, as Dr. Grant said, we do not know the cause. What we do know about the early infection period is that there is consistent evidence for early infection of the CNS during this acute period (Chakrabarti et al., 1991; Davis et al., 1992; Lane et al., 1996; Pilcher et al., 2001; Roberts et al., 2004). This evidence is derived from studies on the brain and cerebrospinal fluid in nonhuman primates and people. So certainly, there are early events that affect the brain. This is seen with reactions of both the innate as well as the adaptive immune response in the CNS. Early treatment in the SIV-monkey model revealed a decrease in functional (neurophysiological) CNS abnormalities and a decrease in brain viral load, potentially pointing to a role for early antiviral intervention (Marcondes et al., 2009).

Letendre: I will just add a point that was made about the low nadir CD4 count and what impact that may have on the nervous system. Dr. Ronald Ellis saw a patient in the hospital recently along with our infectious disease team at the University of California-San Diego. The person presented with acute encephalitis and coma and had no infections other than acute HIV infection and had 10 million copies per cubic millimeter of HIV-1 RNA in cerebrospinal fluid (CSF) and with only 1 million copies per cubic millimeter of virus in his plasma. While this is an extreme case, I think that it is a very clear example that HIV along with the attendant immune response can result in altered sensorium. It may be that there is substantial migration of immune cells in response to new infection and that the damage caused by these cells could account for the cognitive decline that has been described. If this is true, then this damage could potentially be prevented or treated by antiretroviral therapy.

Swindells: The treatment of acute or early or primary HIV infection remains controversial from the clinician perspective. It is unclear really whether we are benefiting people in the long run by starting treatment acutely, and if you do should it then be interrupted? But I think the ongoing debate of when to start antiretroviral therapy is informed to a degree by concern about neurological damage. Concerns exist about virus-induced end organ damage that may be irreversible even if subtle, and there are observational data that support the idea that earlier initiation of therapy may help to prevent neurologic disease from the HIV that develops significantly later on in the course of viral infection (Ellis et al., 2010; CROI abstract 429).

QUESTION 2

What is the importance of combination antiretroviral therapy (cART) for treatment or prevention of HAND? Is the CNS effectiveness of ART important in managing HAND or in preventing it?

Letendre: The data have been accumulating in recent years to support the idea that better-penetrating antiretroviral regimens better reduce HIV in the nervous system. Most—but not all—of the studies that have been performed looking at cognitive performance support the idea that better-penetrating therapy improves impaired performance or maintains normal performance. However, there are no controlled trials. The field has moved from performing cross-sectional analyses to prospective observational uncontrolled studies, but randomized clinical trials have not yet been completed. Dr. Ronald Ellis is leading a randomized controlled clinical trial for treatment of HAND; randomizing people to better-penetrating or worse-penetrating therapy. I am here in Beijing now setting up our new NIH-funded randomized clinical trial of better-penetrating versus worse-penetrating therapy for the prevention of HAND. We need the data from these trials for the field to move forward, particularly since not all the observational data have been supportive. In the last two years there have been a couple of publications that have indicated that antiretroviral therapy could be neurotoxic, at least under certain circumstances. These data highlight the need for randomized clinical trials and tell us that certain drugs with neurotoxic potential may have to be used with caution because they could either cause mild impairment or could limit recovery from impaired neuropsychological performance.

Taiwo: I would just like to add that one of the most important things that we are able to do is to help prevent the neurological consequences of HIV infection that clearly persist despite ART. There is very strong evidence that the longer you wait to start therapy the worse the outcome will likely be. But I think for us to really know how best to intervene we have to understand better the mechanisms of injury to the CNS. As had been said, perhaps it is cryptic viral replication, or maybe persistent immune activation or irreversible neuronal injury from these mechanisms, that plays the dominant role. Immune reconstitution from treatment and direct adverse effects of ART are potential pathways for neurological injury as well. Currently, the field suffers from limited understanding of the relative contribution of these potential mechanisms. So, it is still very difficult to say how best to intervene and in the same vein to define which ART regimen will be most beneficial because there may be subtle differences in their effects. For example, it is unknown if CCR5 inhibition will lead to differential neurological effects. This is one of the important areas for future inquiry.

Lipton: Obviously, with effective ART, the disease has changed. It is a more mild disease, but that said, and this will be brought up in subsequent questions, the prevalence particularly of more mild cases of HAND is still increasing. So, clearly we are not getting to all of the infection or its consequences in the brain. That still needs to be addressed with improved treatments.

Bedimo: Dr. Scott Letendre has done more work on this but I would also like to add that there is not as close a correlation between the viral load in the CNS and the clinical signs of HAND as there is between immune activation and neuronal damage (Kelder, Arthur, Nance-Sproson, McClernon, & Griffin, 1998). In fact, treatment discontinuation in stable patients has recently been shown to be associated with improved cognitive function (Robertson et al., 2010). This suggests that HIV invasion of the CNS might not be sufficient, but other mechanisms might be necessary to cause HAND. So I guess that brings up the next question that you are going to ask about adjunctive therapies. Maybe getting a handle on the mechanisms of HAND will be required in order to evaluate the potential role of adjunctive therapies, and for clinicians to be able to decide whether they're likely to benefit an individual patient.

Swindells: I think from where I sit, the jury is still out on whether clinicians should include CNS antiretroviral penetrance in decision making about choices of antiviral therapy. And it is certainly something we think about and talk about. At the moment, our "go-to" combination for treatment-naïve patients is the simplest: three drugs in one pill—a combination consisting of emtricitabine, tenofovir, and efavirenz—the elements of which do have reasonable penetrance. But there may be patients for whom a different regimen might be preferable for brain-protective effect or for trying to reverse neuronal damage from untreated HIV disease. As Scott mentioned, I think results of randomized controlled clinical trials would be really helpful in informing the field and changing treatment guidelines. So for now, the guidelines don't include this piece and perhaps in the future they will.

Everall: While we still have a long way to go in terms of collecting information regarding efficacy of treating and preventing HAND, as Scott and Susan have just commented on, I think we still have to remember that we have come such a long way since the era when we had no treatment to now having treatment and we have to sort out which is the best regimen (Everall et al., 2009). I was reminded of just how far we have come a few weeks ago when I saw a patient with the most severe HIV-associated dementia (HAD) that I've seen in 15 years. The patient knew that he was living with HIV for 20 years but refused all treatment and antiretroviral drugs so I saw almost a historical presentation of the HIV dementia complex. So, as I say, we have come a very long way.

QUESTION 3

"What is the place for adjunctive therapies for neuroAIDS? How should it or they be utilized? What is the best developmental scheme?"

Gelbard: I think that after my comments Dr. Stuart Lipton's insights would nicely dovetail for this discussion. I obviously share previously mentioned viewpoints that infection of the CNS happens early with HIV-1, with subsequent events that presumably result in an altered homeostasis between immune effector cells and normal synaptic function. And I believe that normalization of immune indices, particularly those that reflect peripheral immune function, do not adequately reflect the environment that continues to exist in the CNS. I think that even with "perfect" control of viral load, or near-perfect control (currently below 50 copies/mL), we will continue to have CNS disease, and thus we will need adjunctive therapy (Gelbard et al., 2010). The problems with adjunctive therapy in the past have been largely due to limited choice of a single agent with variable pharmocodynamic and pharmocokinetic characteristics that might hinder optimal concentrations in brain regions that are most vulnerable to damage by the virus. The fact remains that many of the same principles that have guided combination chemotherapy for the virus also can and likely should be applied to the adjunctive therapies. By that, I specifically mean because this loss of homoeostasis between the peripheral immune system and cells in the CNS, particularly with respect to normal synaptic function, involves more than one target, it is likely that we need more than one agent at a time to best effect neuroprotection or neurorestoration with adjunctive therapy.

Lipton: I agree with my colleague Dr. Harris Gelbard that there are many cases of HAND even when cART has been optimized. So, clearly, adjunct therapy or better antiretrovirals are needed. I think today, however, the studies with these secondary agents just have not been innovative enough or careful enough. Dr. Gelbard indicated many of the reasons and we need more of an innovative approach to neuroprotection in the brain. We also have to pay more attention to the absorption, distribution, metabolism, excretion, and toxicity (ADME/T) of drugs to insure that they get into the brain adequately, and, unfortunately, many scientists are not remaining aware of these factors in their efforts to make a feasible drug. In the brain a lot of things have to happen for a drug to work and to avoid intolerable side effects. So I think we need a better system of communication between academic institutions and pharmaceutical companies in order to attack this problem in a more coherent manner and produce better neuroprotective agents.

Bedimo: I would like to say as a clinician that the best developmental scheme would be translating currently available information on potential pathogenic mechanisms into clinical trials evaluating therapies that are likely to address those mechanisms. As far as we understand now, potential pathogenic mechanisms leading to HAND include inflammation, excitotoxicity, and oxidative stress. AIDS Clinical Trials Group (ACTG) 5235 is a study that it is focusing on the anti-inflammatory effect of minocycline for the management of HAND and I am not exactly sure of how that study has progressed. Memantine has also been used as a neuroprotective agent to counter the excitotoxicity leading to HAND. To my knowledge, all the adjunctive therapies have yet to yield any positive outcomes.

Lipton: I am involved with the drug memantine as the inventor listed on worldwide patents and I just want to disclose this fact. That said, many of these studies with memantine and other drugs have been ill conceived, and the large variability in the placebo group was belied by the power analysis. At the end of the day, we have found that with several studies either there were not sufficient patients entered or the study was not long enough to allow a real test of efficacy. Then a type II statistical error can be made in which we determine that a drug is not effective, but in fact it might have been had the proper trial be carried out. Having run some of these trials myself, I know that clinical studies are difficult to perform well. Patients are demented, forget to take their medicines, may share medicines between the active group and the placebo group, and I think we need to take better care of exactly how we perform trials. Results can be biased for technical reasons that change the outcome and determine whether the trial was successful or failed for essentially trivial reasons.

Fox: That is a very good point, Dr. Lipton. And let me add, as you and others mentioned, that the clinical presentation is certainly different from severe dementia seen previously. And my question is whether the mechanism is the same, and so, as to the last part of this question, what type of drug should be developed? How much are we using what we have known from the excellent studies on dementia and HIV encephalitis, and how much is due to what we know about the pathogenesis of HAND in its current presentation? I will just leave that as an open question.

Everall: I would like to make one response. I think that the assessment and measurement of neuropsychological outcomes is a critical issue to advising the effectiveness of ARVs and how to treat people with HAND. Let's remember that we still don't have any actual documented guidelines that treatment of HAND with antiretrovirals by themselves improves cognition. I think that maybe we need to have treatment guidelines established that will then help guide us in terms of the use of potential adjunctive therapies as well.

Gendelman: I will add one point. It is clear that HAND in its current form, while mild, remains a persistent problem. It is also clear, despite cART and its therapeutic efficacy in reducing viral load and while significant and confers positive benefits in ameliorating disease severity and comorbid conditions, that adjunctive therapies will likely be needed. The search for new pathways and new means to alter the pathobiological responses that remain even following effective therapy will be a continued mainstay for the future treatment of HAND (reviewed by Kraft-Terry, Buch, Fox, & Gendelman, 2009; Kraft-Terry, Stothert, Buch, & Gendelman, 2010).

QUESTION 4

"What are the most useful animal model systems for neuroAIDS? How should they be used and do they have a role in studies of disease, pathogenesis, and developmental therapeutics?"

Masliah: Although the simian models and rodent models expressing the HIV genome have demonstrated to be highly useful for studies of pathogenesis and therapeutic development, models over-expressing HIV-1 proteins such as gp120, tat, and vpr have demonstrated to be of interest in terms of uncovering the mechanisms of neurotoxicity. For example, studies in GFAP-gp120 tg mice have shown that selectively neuronal populations including glutaminergic pyramidal neurons are more susceptible via activation of the CDK/cyclin signaling pathway, in contrast, over-expression of Tat under the GFAP promoter has shown activation of other pathways of neurodegeneration such as the GSK3 signaling pathway. This is also of interest because such models could allow us to screen in a rapid manner for compounds with therapeutic potential that selectively target these signaling pathways, such as roscovitine and lithium, respectively.

Fox: One principle advantage of nonhuman primates is that they enable the study of the CNS and immune and other organ systems together, with parameters that are the closest to people. Differences in brain structure and function between rodents and primates are well known, and differences in the immune system are becoming increasingly recognized. Significant attention is now being paid to the relatively poor translatability of rodent studies to humans (Davis, 2008; Schnabel, 2008). While they are more difficult to work with, monkeys have great translatability. One excellent example is the role of the gastrointestinal tract in HIV pathogenesis, discovered in monkeys (Veazey et al., 1998), leading to a wealth of findings in people, including a link between GI microbial translocation and HIV dementia (Ancuta et al., 2008). Other examples are the studies on early viral entry into the CNS (referred to above) and the state of the CNS during stable chronic (non-end stage) infection in the absence or presence of treatment (Roberts et al., 2006; Zink et al., 2010). That said, measuring some of the effects manifest in HAND, in particular the cognitive effects, is difficult. It was much easier in the pretreatment era when people and monkeys got more severe neurologic disease. It is now difficult to measure the finer nuances of cognitive dysfunction in monkeys and correlate those with the current functional findings in people. Still, SIV-infected monkeys are an excellent model for studying a variety of molecular, immune, viral, neuronal, and neurophysiologic properties of the brain due to chronic infection and even with antiretroviral therapy or any adjunctive or other therapy on top of this, with the realization that your group size and number of groups that you can study will be smaller than other lower animal model systems. One has to then balance the translatability with the ability to examine more hypotheses and perform larger studies, uncovering mechanisms that can then be examined in monkeys and people.

Everall: I would also like to say that the primate model has actually provided insights into human disease and especially in the simulation of disease progression. But those experiments take a long time and they obviously cannot be easily repeated due to costs and access. For quicker experiments to generate informative data, you can actually use rodent models. We have been using one of those models and have actually found it very useful in terms in elucidating certain mechanisms of neurotoxicity as well as neuroprotection and they are especially useful in assessing agents and potential agents. A clear experimental path can be to take experiments from tissue cultures through to rodent animal models and then through clinical trial. So while there are limitations with the rodent model, I think this model certainly helped us progress understanding in the field.

Lipton: I would like to say this before giving Dr. Howard Gendelman the floor: I had the great privilege of seeing the data compiled from his new rodent model, which I believe will be revolutionary. It is a new rodent model for neuroAIDS. Many of you know about it but I want to make it clear for our readers; it involved reconstitution of the mouse with a human immune system, allowing HIV infection in the brain, and it is from Dr. Howard Gendelman's laboratory done with several of his colleagues. I really think it is the first time that a mouse model has recapitulated many of the features of HAND, and particularly in its most severe form, HAD. I think this mouse will provide a tremendous advantage to the entire field in elucidating the pathophysiology and in testing drugs before we go into people in clinical trials. With that I would like to hand the floor to Howard so he can tell us a little bit more about this new model.

Gendelman: Thank you, Dr. Stuart Lipton. I would just like to review very briefly the path that led us to these new studies (Dash et al., 2011; Gorantla et al., 2010). There were limited model systems available during the 20 years when we first were involved in developing early systems. Preceding this model were the HIV-1gp120 and viral gene systems, including other transgenic models where HIV subgenomic fragments were put under the control of robust promoters to elicit histopathologic correlates of human disease, along with a broad range of human-cell–mouse-brain reconstitutions and viral chimeras (Toggas et al., 1994; Zou et al., 2007; Potash et al., 2005; Gorantla et al., 2007; Tyor, Power, Gendelman, & Markham, 1993; Persidsky et al., 1996; Avgeropoulos et al., 1998). We have recapitulated human disease components of neuroAIDS, which centered on neuroinflammation as well as the mechanisms of neuronal destruction. These animal model systems have yielded a tremendous amount of data not only on pathobiology but also in many of the developmental adjunctive therapies that have come forward, although none has made it as yet into the drug combination therapies commonly used in patients. These models nonetheless taught us a lot about mechanisms of neuronal destruction and likely built a foundation for the future for new successful therapies that are in the pipeline today. In recent years, our labs and others have begun to use immunodeficient mice that were reconstituted with HIV-infected cells. In the early stages these were HIV-infected monocyte-derived macrophages, and this model was an encephalitis model where an acute intracranial injection of infected macrophages induces a robust inflammatory process and encephalitis with neuronal dropout and mimics a florid macrophage-induced neuronal and glial process. Following that model system was the reconstitution of human leukocytes of the use of chimeric recombinant viruses that allowed *de novo* infection of murine cells. This model allowed investigators to study and begin to unravel the role of adaptive immune function and that consisted of CD4-positive T cell subsets and CD8 cells in disease, surveillance, and progression. In the last three years, my lab, in collaboration with Drs. Harris Gelbard and Larisa Poluektova, has begun to reconstitute essentially performing bone marrow transplants in immunodeficient animals in generating, with C34-positive human stem cells, a true humanized mouse where the bone marrow progenitor cells are human and the reconstitution of the immune system is human in a homeostatic environment. These are not activated T cells; these are immunocytes that will survive over a year and will respond to a number of antigenic stimuli, including viral infection. These animals can be infected for many months, and about a year and a half ago we began to see results that excited us in the field of neuroAIDS. About 50% of the animals, spontaneously after four, five, or six months of viral infection, would develop a mingle encephalitis, meningitis, or low-level nervous system disease. There was then the characterization of the system demonstrating infiltration and infection of human macrophages in perivascular distribution with low level of innate astrocyte and microglial responses. In 10% of the animals, there was the development of a florid encephalitis. Eight months ago, and in conjunction with other studies,we began to monitor the development of neuronal aberrations, and with support from Dr. Harris Gelbard we began to show changes in neuronal responses. We prospectively monitored these animals by spectroscopy and diffusion tense imaging. This was done by Dr. Michael Boska, who showed very focal changes in N-acetyl aspartate levels in areas that are most affected in humans, so we saw those areas in the cortex and subcortex as well, and they progressed. The animals were sacrificed after several months and these animals showed very significant histopathological correlates of disease, including changes in the neurofilament, which mapped to the same areas of the brain shown to be abnormal by spectroscopy and diffusion tensor imaging techniques. We hope that in conjunction with our own works and works of others that these will be used not only for studies of antiretroviral therapy and combination therapy, but also for adjunctive therapies to combat human disease.

QUESTION 5

"Do drugs of abuse affect the progression of HIV/AIDS and/or neuroAIDS? If so, under what sets of circumstances and which drugs?"

Chang: Regarding the question as to whether drugs of abuse affect the progression of HIV and if so, under what sets of circumstances and which drugs: The published data have shown that additive or interactive effects of neurotoxicity can occur in individuals with HIV who are drug users. For example, neurotoxicity has been shown in HIV patients who use methamphetamine additively (Chang, Ernst, Speck, & Grob, 2005; Alicata, Chang, Cloak, Abe, & Ernst, 2009) or interactively (Jernigan et al., 2005). Our neuroimaging studies that used magnetic resonance spectroscopy to measure N-acetyl-asprate (NAA) and other metabolites showed additional decreased NAA or further elevation of choline or myo-inositol, which is indicative of neurodegeneration and astrogliosis, especially in the subcortical brain regions and notably the basal ganglia (Chang et al., 2005). However, instead of seeing an additive effect, you might actually see an interactive effect, such as in the work done by Dr. Terry Jernigan's group where they saw enlarged subcortical brain structural changes in methamphetamine users but smaller subcortical volumes in HIV-infected people (Jernigan et al., 2005). However, in the HIV subjects who used methamphetamine, they found relatively normal basal ganglia structures (Jernigan et al., 2009). Hence, the different imaging techniques demonstrate different brain changes that are associated with the combined effects of HIV and drugs of abuse. For instance, the interactive effect of HIV and marijuana use on brain glutamate also was documented using MR spectroscopy techniques (Chang, Cloak, Yakupov, & Ernst, 2006). There are other neuroimaging techniques such as PET imaging, which found that HIV patients who used cocaine had additional decreases in the brain dopamine transporters (Chang et al., 2008). The dopamine receptors were also found to be decreased, especially in the HIV+ cocaine users, but the effects on the receptors were primarily related to nicotine use, which is quite prevalent in both the HIV-infected population and amongst drug users. So there are really many examples of human studies as well as animal studies that have actually shown an accelerated disease progression of HIV associated with drug use. For example, both cocaine and methamphetamine can enhance viral replication which can lead to further neurotoxicity.

Everall: This is a very complex issue and the interaction of drugs of abuse with HIV occur at many different levels that could be biological, behavioral, personality, and so on. At the biological level, some studies have shown that drugs such as opiates, through binding at the u-opioid receptor, increase viral replication, which is obviously going to have an effect on progression of HIV disease. With regard to stimulants, such as methamphetamine, I would like to mention the neuropathological findings from the work done by Dr. Eliezer Masliah and myself, that has demonstrated a selective degeneration of calbindin-expressing GABAnergic inter-neurons that results in more severe memory deficits in HIV-infected methamphetmaine users. In addition to the biological mechanisms, there is also the issue of behavior. Drug-using individuals may well be prone to impulsive or sensation-seeking behavior, which puts themselves and others they interact with at risk of infection. It is also known that individuals who regularly take drugs of abuse may well have personality issues and more chaotic lifestyles, which means that they are much less likely to engage and retain in HIV mental health services and be less adherent to any antiretroviral medication, which again is going to have a negative impact upon their well-being and possibly increase the progression of the HIV disease and/or development of HAND.

Grant: I think Linda and Ian have covered a lot of the issues and I would like to underscore a couple and then add a couple of more. One is that these drugs, some of them like methamphetamine and alcohol and central nervous system depressants, can independently cause neurocognitive impairment. That impairment is probably most likely to be seen in connection with length of abstinence, in other words, in most cases as people refrain from drug abuse their cognitive disturbance relative to drugs decreases. So part of the issue of the interaction between HIV and drugs needs to be seen within a timeframe of detoxification as well. The second point is that not all drugs are alike; so methamphetamine has been mentioned by Linda and Ian as neurotoxic, but, for example, drugs like marijuana are really not known to independently produce substantial neurocognitive changes in the long run in people who are abstinent. And, in fact, some studies suggest that concurrent use of marijuana and meth actually confers a better neuropsychological outcome than using meth alone, perhaps suggesting a neuroprotective action of the cannabinoids. The third point I would make is that substance abusers are also more likely to have dual HIV infection or HCV infections that also can affect neurological function. The final point would be that this has been really a relatively understudied area in the context of large clinical trials such as those being conducted by ACTGs and HPTNs and so forth. Historically, substance users are either excluded or not properly diagnosed in these settings and that is a situation that needs to be corrected if we are really to understand the long-term neurological effects of these drugs in relation to HIV and HIV treatments.

Fox: Dr. Grant nicely raised the issues of different effects of different drugs, and certainly when it comes to people the predominant case is poly drug abuse. It is rare that a drug user uses only one substance, and as pointed out, these may have the opposite effects of different drugs on HIV and the brain. The sum of the data on human drug abusers reveals that there is not a profound effect. People just don't show dramatic changes, and often the apparent effects of drug abuse can be attributed to other factors such as access to health care, medication compliance, and so on. (Ellis et al., 2003; King, Alicata, Cloak, & Chang, 2009). The concept of protection, while seemingly counterintuitive, can arise from the effects drugs have on their receptors not only in the brain but also the immune system. In addition to the human studies with cannabinoids that Dr. Grant refers to, Dr. Robert Donahoe performed a study in SIV-infected monkeys revealing that constant doses of opiates leads to improved survival (Donahoe et al., 2009). But of course human opiate abusers don't have regular supplies of drugs taken on regular schedules. But it serves as an example that, for the true sense of effects of drugs of abuse on infection, they certainly are not dramatic nor always adverse. We did try to mimic human abuse patterns in our studies on the effects of methamphetamine on SIV in monkeys. In the time period that we examined, there was not an effect on progression of disease nor on peripheral viral

perimeters; however, we did see increased virus in the brain and effects on macrophages and natural killer cells (Marcondes, Alicata, Cloak, & Chang, 2010). So, I think the results of the drugs may be subtle and require very careful control to get around issues such as poly drug abuse, compliance, co-infections, and other comorbidities. So, I agree with Igor that it is an open question and more studies need to be done but the variables and confounds may be large.

Lipton: Because of drug abuse in humans, the situation is very different from that seen in animal models of HAND, which is much cleaner. Human drug abusers usually bring a whole set of other comorbidities, including head injuries, abuse histories, and so on. Hence, further studies are necessary to look at the effect of interaction of comorbidity, drugs, and HIV.

Everall: I would just like to make an additional comment to Igor's very important point about the potential protection of cannabis. Clinically, my role is a psychiatrist and we know that the more potent forms of cannabis are associated with an increased risk for psychosis. There are a number of active ingredients in cannabis and we need to clarify which ingredients are associated with neuroprotection and which exacerbate psychosis.

QUESTION 6

"How significant is HAND in the cART era? What need clinicians be mindful of?"

Swindells: We have already had some discussion from contributors on the conference call that the overall incidence of what is considered classic AIDS dementia has decreased. Thanks in large part to the availability of effective antiretroviral therapy, this is something we see rarely now in the clinic. However, there are subtle impairments that are still present, and particularly in untreated patients, which are worse with more advanced disease. But, you also have to look for it. Occasionally, it will be obvious, but diagnosis requires careful attention to cognitive impairment and that is difficult in the context of a busy HIV clinic. However, there are some tools that are available that do not require extensive formal neuropsychological testing (Power et al., 1995). There are tools that take a few minutes to apply and we in fact use those in screening and they are extremely helpful for us in terms of assessing severity of impairment and also monitoring progressively to see whether patients make a full or partial recovery neurologically.

Grant: I think this is an important question, as Dr. Swindells mentioned. It is a real challenge in clinics: how to ascertain and monitor these complications. Just to remind readers, we do see at least mild neurocognitive impairment in anywhere from one-third to over one-half of people with HIV disease, most of whom are well treated on cART. So this is a problem that persists. It is important to the patient because it affects their everyday functioning, in some instances including ability to continue with their regular work, may affect driving skills, adherence to complex medical regimens, and other life activities. So, it is not a trivial issue even though the impairments can be considered mild. As to how to monitor this, it is a bit of a dilemma. As with any complex medical problem, such as for example the diagnosis of mild heart disease, it is not easy to do this at the bedside. It does require specialized evaluations, and so what is then also needed is a high index of suspicion as to the possibility a person may be experiencing neurocognitive decline. Some points to alert the clinician to someone at greater risk would be the patient who has had a low nadir CD4, the patient who has continued viremia despite treatment, and of course patients who complain of memory and other cognitive problems. However, self-report of cognitive difficulties can also be increased when the patient is depressed. Dr. Swindells mentioned that there are brief neurocognitive screens, and they should be employed routinely in the monitoring of persons with HIV, but they do have their limitations, unfortunately. To diagnose mild forms of impairment there is no getting around performing more comprehensive neuropsychological testing whenever the clinician suspects that neurocognitive change may be occurring. Examples of test batteries that are sensitive to neurocognitive complications of HIV can be found in the publication describing the Frascati Criteria for HAND (Antinori, et al., 2007), and in the CHARTER Study report (Heaton et al., 2010).

Chang: In the clinical setting, the scales that are developed to assess HIV-1-associated dementia or HAND are better than the traditional clinical examinations, such as the HIV dementia scale instead of the MMSE (which is more useful for assessing Alzheimer's disease but not too sensitive for detecting HIV-associated dementia or HAND). Another major issue is that it is often difficult to diagnose the comorbid conditions that Igor mentioned and that we discussed earlier, such as, the comorbid effects of substance abuse can additionally impact the cognitive dysfunction. Lastly, in the era of cART, some of the antiretroviral medications themselves may be neurotoxic and may lead to additional brain abnormalities that can be assessed with neuroimaging techniques (Schweinsburg et al., 2005; Chang et al., 2008), and so some of the cognitive deficits you are seeing may not be due to HIV directly, but to the treatment. There are many issues that we don't have complete understanding of and how much of each component contributes to the cognitive dysfunction, and it would be wise to do more research in these areas.

Bedimo: I just wanted to add for the readers one good reference on the incidence and determinants of HAND: the CASCADE cohort (Bhaskaran et al., 2008). They were able to show that compared to the pre-HAART era, the incidence of HAND has decreased about tenfold in the later part of the HAART era (2003–2006). I believe it has also been shown that the prevalence of HAND has not decreased and may in fact be increasing, especially as we are getting better at detecting the more subtle forms of the disorder. A few years ago there was an international HIV dementia scale published that looked at three areas—memory, psychomotor skills, and motor speed (Sacktor et al., 2005). This tool might be more useful at differentiating HIV-1-associated dementia from other forms of dementia in the aging HIV population, given the psychomotor slowing accompanying memory deficits and the accumulation of intraneuronal amyloid beta and alpha synuclein in the former (Achim, Adame, Dumaop, Everall, &

Masliah, 2009; Khanlou et al., 2009). And also one thing that I have seen and am not sure what others think about it, it is said that there is significant olfactory deficits in HAND and this might be clinically useful to test (Zucco & Ingegneri, 2004).

Gendelman: Hepatitis C and neuroAIDS in resource-limited settings. Dr. Letendre, if you can respond in order to provide a broad clinical perspective, this would balance the discussion.

Letendre: I want to quickly support what has recently been said, which is that HAND in the clinic has to be interpreted in the context of other complications, which has been termed either multimorbidity or polypathology, depending on which term you prefer. What is clear is that there are several factors that increase with time including age, duration of HIV infection, duration of treatment, the number of comorbidities, and the number of concomitant medications. Those morbidities not only include cardiovascular disease, bone loss, and renal disease, but chronic co-infections, such as the viral hepatitides. I think it is clear that hepatitis C does affect the brain either by infecting glial cells—and I think there is very strong evidence that supports that—or by other mechanisms such as an indirect effect from liver disease. I think this is going to become increasingly important in the next few years because of the new hepatitis C treatments that are going to be moving into the clinic. With these new treatments, many of the issues that we have dealt with in terms of penetration into the brain of antiretrovirals may now also apply to penetration of these new protease and polymerase inhibitor drugs for hepatitis C. In terms of the international setting, I think the comment that was just made about the international HIV scale is good. Of course, we need geographically and culturally relevant screening instruments to use in the clinic everywhere and the international HIV dementia scale promises to do that, but I am not certain that it always succeeds. We must ensure that we screen for the comorbidities that are relevant in each setting and account for them in our assessments. I just want to quickly add there may also be an impact in differences in host genetics. Gene frequencies of several polymorphisms and copy number variants differ by geographical region. Subtypes of HIV also differ geographically and may also be important to account for since subtype C HIV may be less neurovirulent and subtype D may be more neurovirulent, at least in adults.

Gendelman: We should address survival at this point in time, as people live longer and complications of other neurodegenerative disorders or comorbidity conditions related to Alzheimer's, Parkinson's, or other diseases. What do we think of its importance of comorbid neurodegenerative diseases and in HIV-infected patients? Is this going to be a problem? Is this something we need to be mindful of and what might do we do for the future?

Swindells: The short answer to your question is that it is extremely important and an area of great interest from the affected community and the research institutes and foundations. There are often aging-related complications that appear to occur prematurely in people who are infected with HIV and this is not restricted only to neurological disease, but we see this with cardiovascular disease, bone disease, and overall frailty, and so this is an area of active ongoing investigation. My prediction is the more that we look for premature brain aging; the more likely we are to find it. There is evidence now from cardiovascular studies, which in some ways are a little easier to implement and interpret, that patients with HIV disease may have a heart of someone ten years older than them. And I think that is a reasonable analogy that also may be applied to brain disease. Lastly, there is some early but concerning signal that other neurodegenerative diseases such as Alzheimer's disease may be becoming more common going forward as the population living with HIV ages.

Lipton: Just to follow up on what has been said by other people, the interplay of HIV infection and aging on neurocognitive effects and structural brain imaging are very complex and merit further study. In part, chronicity of infection, as I believe Dr. Ian Everall mentioned, and the treatment, which itself can be neurotoxic, plus the development of other systemic complications linked to inflammation can all affect cognitive functioning. So, I think that the manifestations of HAND in the elderly may appear somewhat different, both neuropathologically and neurocognitively, than HAND in younger people. That is yet to be determined, but something worthy of study. Finally, there may also be an important impact of mild cases of HAND in elderly persons who may already have had some cerebral compromise, such as a stroke or vascular disease, and this could play out with more severe effects on activities of daily living, including driving, and so forth, so this will need to be addressed.

Chang: I just had this thought when we were talking about the neurodegenerative diseases in the aging HIV population. We really don't know what the prevalence is of comorbid Alzheimer's disease, Parkinson's disease, or other diseases that might affect the HIV-infected population as they get older. They should at least have the same prevalence as uninfected individuals. One way to possibly track something like that is to maybe create a registry so that everyone could then log onto to the database and record comorbid conditions, including AD, PD, or other degenerative conditions. This would be similar to how we track other neurological conditions or treatment effects, for example, if we were looking for a new pattern of toxicity associated with a new drug, we would form a registry and everyone would log in and report on that. Perhaps something like that could facilitate and allow us to get a handle on the prevalence of comorbid neurodegenerative conditions. For example, I am especially concerned about Parkinson's disease because HIV-infected patients already have a subcortical type of dementia and they have motor slowing or dysfunction, so perhaps that could hasten the development of Parkinson's disease, and their prematurely aging brains also might lead them to be more vulnerable for Alzheimer's disease; both are diseases of aging.

Lipton: This is often a bit difficult to assess because many young patients with HIV have Parkinson's symptoms because of the involvement of HIV in the striatum. This form of parkinsonism in HIV, as opposed to Parkinson's disease, which is really a progressive neurodegenerative disorder, needs to be discerned.

Chang: That is right, but that is why it is somewhat different because PD is a progressive disease whereas parkinsonism in

HIV can be rather static and I think most neurologists can tell the difference. HIV patients come into the clinic with a broad range of brain disorders.

Lipton: Sometimes it can be difficult to tell the difference, particularly early on in the symptomatology.

QUESTION 7

"What is the 'true' neuropathology of HAND in the cART era?"

Masliah: I appreciate the comments of Dr. Lipton crediting our studies of neurodegeneration in the brains of patients with HIV and in animal models. In the cART era, we have noted that HIV encephalitis has gone from a sub-acute neuro-inflammatory disorder to a protected chronic condition accompanied by astrogliosis, microgliosis, and lower levels of HIV, but more widespread degeneration accompanied on several occasions by accumulation of misfolded proteins such as Abeta, Tau, and alpha-synuclein. It appears that in aged HIV-positive individuals, mechanisms of aggregated protein clearance failed and in combination with HIV trigger more widespread neurodegeneration. Other comorbidities that contribute to the neurodegenerative process in patients with HIV include HCV infection, drug abuse, psychiatric conditions, immunological reconstitution syndromes, and toxicity of antiretrovirals.

Everall: Assessment of the "true" neuropathology in HAND is somewhat complicated by the dramatic effectiveness of cART in significantly reducing mortality, thereby limiting the number of brains that we can assess at autopsy. With those brains we do have access to I think that pathologic changes still do exist. We do not see the multinucleated giant cells any longer but we certainly see viral infection in the brain by either immunohistochemistry for viral proteins or by RNA as a measure of brain viral load. We recently published a paper assessing neuropathological changes in a large brain cohort of individuals who were recruited by the National NeuroAIDS Tissue Consortium with advanced HIV disease. We observed high rates of HIV encephalitis and other pathological changes. In addition, there were high rates of clinical cognitive impairment during life in this cohort so it was not possible to assess whether the HIV encephalitis predicted cognitive impairment. In a separate study assessing the brains of individuals with HIV aged 55 years and older, we noted high rates of deposition of a-synuclein and b-catenin, which are markers of Parkinson's disease and Alzheimer's disease, respectively. So, we are now worried that the "true" neuropathology has extended to other neurodegenerative disorders.

Gelbard: I think I would just add that we should emphasize in the future investigation of mechanisms that may underlie impaired homeostasis between immune effector cells and synaptic architecture as opposed to sole focus on viral load because in gaining an equally deep understanding of the biologic substrates for multiple clinical entities that comprise HAND, I think that this body of knowledge will help advance us toward a more informative use of biomarkers and a greater understanding of key molecular targets for the development of new drugs. That may be the next generation of adjunctive therapy.

Chang: A quick comment regarding the value of in vivo neuroimaging studies. In general, when we evaluate neuropathology, we are waiting until the patients have died, and by then many of them might have suffered severe end-stage AIDS or some other kinds of peri-mortem complications. So, being able to assess in vivo living pathology is important; the work we do with neuroimaging is important and can allow us to assess the severity and progression of HIV-associated brain injury, and all the comorbid conditions in the living patients.

Lipton: I wanted to follow up on something that Dr. Gelbard said. I think that Dr. Eliezer Masliah deserves a lot of credit for looking at HAND in terms of a chronic neurodegenerative condition that affects synaptic function. This is why I think we need to look at neurodegenerative diseases in a broader context. I think it is becoming increasingly clear that virtually every neurodegenerative disorder, including cognitive dysfunction in HAND and particularly in HAD, is probably closely correlated with synaptic damage. Protecting the synapse seems to be the real disease modification that is needed, not only in HAD but probably also in Alzheimer's disease and other forms of dementia. The synaptic damage may occur in different areas of the brain for reasons that are still unclear even after all these years, but as Dr. Gelbard said, it is going to be very important to afford neuroprotection at the synapse, and it is going to be critical that our future therapeutic approaches look at this issue very carefully. Certainly, microglial infection leads to the production of toxins, is going to become a dominant way that we need to interfere with the disease in order to affect neuroprotection or prevent neuroinflammation, or both, as Dr. Gelbard stated earlier.

This is why we need to look at neurodegenerative diseases more broadly. It is becoming increasingly clear that nearly that every virtually every neurodegenerative disorders, including cognitive dysfunction in HAND and particularly in HAD, is probably closely correlated with synaptic damage. Protecting the synapse seems to be the real disease modification that is needed, not only in HAD but also in Alzheimer's disease and other forms of dementia. The synaptic damage make occur in different areas of the brain for reasons that are still unclear even after all these years, but as Dr. Gelbard said, it is going to be very important to afford neuroprotection at the synapse, and it is going to be critical that our future therapeutic approaches look at this issue very carefully. Recent papers show that microglia can affect the syanpse. I think that microglia infection, as well as immune stimulation of microglia to produce toxins, are going to become a dominant way that we need to interfere with the disease in order to effect neuroprotection or prevent neuroinflammation, or both, as Dr. Gelbard stated earlier.

Everall: We became interested in looking at whether HIV was also disrupting emerging mechanisms that regulate the translation of mRNA into protein. We assessed specifically the expression of microRNA (miRNA). Micro RNAs are noncoding RNAs that regulate whether the mRNAs become translated into proteins. So we looked at the expression of micro RNAs in the brain in individuals with HIV and compared those with HIV in individuals that had also had a recent documented episode of majoremajor depressive disorder (MDD) (Tatro et al., 2010). We found that there were in fact a two separate signatures of microRNA dysregulation in the brains of individuals who had HIV and HIV with MDD. This may be another mechanisms by which HIV is disrupting the function of the brain during advanced HIV disease.

Letendre: Another broad area that deserves attention is the role of neural progenitor cells in the brains of patients with HAND. I think there is mounting evidence from a number of groups that progenitor cells may be important in the recovery of the brain from injury. Relevant to HIV disease, neural progenitor cells express CXCR4, one of the entry receptors used by virus. Since infection or injury of neural progenitor cells by HIV may limit recovery from nervous system injury, this is a potentially fruitful area for future research.

Gendelman: In closing, let me acknowledge the outstanding support we received from our Oxford colleagues and notably Craig Panner and Kathryn Winder who made this teleconference and other unique aspects of this book possible. Lana Reichardt's organizational and transcriptional skills are appreciated beyond any thank you. The impetus for this teleconference and the book itself rests with our patients and students, who are our singular driver towards excellence in all we do. The neurological complications of HIV-1 infection have continued and will certainly do so until a protective vaccine or a better means to eliminate viral sanctuaries is realized. We are dedicated to seeing the dream of viral eradication, whatever the means, turned into reality. Until this is realized, a thorough means to understand the disease process, the means to best diagnose and stage it, and pathways towards suitable therapeutics as presented herein serves to best address our patients' needs.

REFERENCES

Achim, C. L., Adame, A., Dumaop, W., Everall, I. P., & Masliah, E.; Neurobehavioral Research Center. (2009). Increased accumulation of intraneuronal amyloid beta in HIV-infected patients. *J Neuroimmune Pharmacol, 4*(2), 190–9.

Alicata, D., Chang, L., Cloak, C., Abe, K., & Ernst, T. (2009). Higher diffusion in striatum and lower fractional anisotropy in white matter of methamphetamine users. *Psychiatry Res, 174*(1), 1–8.

Ancuta, P., Kamat, A., Kunstman, K. J., Kim, E. Y., Autissier, P., Wurcel, A., et al. (2008). Microbial translocation is associated with increased monocyte activation and dementia in AIDS patients. *PLoS One, 3,* e2516.

Antinori, A., Arendt, G., Becker, J. T., Brew, B. J., Byrd, D. A., Cherner, M., et al. (2007). Updated research nosology for HIV-associated neurocognitive disorders. *Neurology, 69*(18), 1789–1799.

Bhaskaran, K., Mussini, C., Antinori, A., Walker, A. S., Dorrucci, M., Sabin, C., et al.; CASCADE Collaboration. (2008). Changes in the incidence and predictors of human immunodeficiency virus-associated dementia in the era of highly active antiretroviral therapy. *Ann Neurol, 63*(2), 213–21.

Chakrabarti, L., Hurtrel, M., Maire, M. A., Vazeux, R., Dormont, D., Montagnier, L., et al. (1991). Early viral replication in the brain of SIV-infected rhesus monkeys. *Am J Pathol, 139,* 1273–1280.

Chang, L., Ernst, T., Speck, O., & Grob, C. S. (2005). Additive effects of HIV and chronic methamphetamine use on brain metabolite abnormalities. *American Journal of Psychiatry, 162*(2), 361–369.

Chang, L., Cloak, C., Yakupov, R., & Ernst, T. (2006). Combined and independent effects of chronic marijuana use and HIV on brain metabolites. *Journal of Neuroimmune Pharmacology, 1,* 65–76.

Chang, L., Wang, G. J., Volkow, N. D., Ernst, T., Telang, F., Logan, J., et al. (2008). Decreased brain dopamine transporters are related to cognitive deficits in HIV patients with or without cocaine abuse. *Neuroimage*, 42(2), 869–78.

Chang, L., Yakupov, R., Nakama, H., Stokes, B., & Ernst, T. (2008). Antiretroviral treatment is associated with increased attentional load-dependent brain activation in HIV patients. *J Neuroimmune Pharmacol*, 3(2), 95–104.

Crews, L., Patrick, C., Achim, C. L., Everall, I. P., & Masliah, E. (2009). Molecular pathology of neuroAIDS (CNS-HIV). *Int J Mol Sci*, 10(3), 1045–63

Dash, P., Gorantla, S., Gendelman, H. E., Makarov, E., Finke-Dwyer, J., Castanedo, A., et al. (2010). Links between progressive HIV-1 infection of humanized mice and viral neuropathogenesis. *J Neurosci*.

Davis, L. E., Hjelle, B. L., Miller, V. E., Palmer, D. L., Llewellyn, A. L., Merlin, T. L., et al. (1992). Early viral brain invasion in iatrogenic human immunodeficiency virus infection. *Neurology*, 42, 1736–9.

Davis, M. M. (2008). A prescription for human immunology. *Immunity*, 29, 835–8.

Donahoe, R. M., O'Neil, S. P., Marsteller, F. A., Novembre, F. J., Anderson, D. C., Lankford-Turner, P., et al. (2009). Probable deceleration of progression of Simian AIDS affected by opiate dependency: Studies with a rhesus macaque/SIVsmm9 model. *J Acquir Immune Defic Syndr*, 50, 241–9.

Ellis, R. J., Childers, M. E., Cherner, M., Lazzaretto, D., Letendre, S., & Grant, I: (2003). Increased human immunodeficiency virus loads in active methamphetamine users are explained by reduced effectiveness of antiretroviral therapy. *J Infect Dis*, 188, 1820–1826

Everall, I., Vaida, F., Khanlou, N., Lazzaretto, D., Achim, C., Letendre, S., et al.; National NeuroAIDS Tissue Consortium (NNTC). (2009). Cliniconeuropathologic correlates of human immunodeficiency virus in the era of antiretroviral therapy. *J Neurovirol*, 15(5–6), 360–70.

Gelbard, H. A., Dewhurst, S., Maggirwar, S. B., Kiebala, M., Polesskaya, O., & Gendelman, H. E. (2010). Rebuilding synaptic architecture in HIV-1 associated neurocognitive disease: A therapeutic strategy based on modulation of mixed lineage kinase. *Neurotherapeutics*, 7(4), 392–8.

Gorantla, S., Makarov, E., Finke-Dwyer, J., Castanedo, A., Holguin, A., Gebhart, C. L., et al. (2010). Links between progressive HIV-1 infection of humanized mice and viral neuropathogenesis. *Am J Pathol*.

Gorantla, S., Liu, J., Sneller, H., Dou, H., Holguin, A., Smith, L., et al. (2007). Copolymer-1 induces adaptive immune anti-inflammatory glial and neuroprotective responses in a murine model of HIV-1 encephalitis. *J Immunol*, 179(7), 4345–56.

Heaton, R. K., Clifford, D. B., Franklin, Jr. D. R., Woods, S. P., Ake, C., Vaida, F., et al., the CHARTER Group. (in press). HIV-associated neurocognitive disorders persist in the era of potent antiretroviral therapy. *Neurology*.

Jernigan, T. L., Gamst, A. C., Archibald, S. L., Fennema-Notestine, C., Mindt, M. R., Marcotte, T. D., et al. (2009). Effects of methamphetamine dependence and HIV infection on cerebral morphology. *J Affect Disord*, 119(1–3), 84–91.

Jernigan, T. L., Gamst, A. C., Archibald, S. L., Fennema-Notestine, C., Mindt, M. R., Marcotte, T. D., et al. (2005). Effects of methamphetamine dependence and HIV infection on cerebral morphology. *Am J Psychiatry*, 162(8), 1461–1472.

Kelder, W., McArthur, J. C., Nance-Sproson, T., McClernon, D., & Griffin, D. E. (1998). Beta-chemokines MCP-1 and RANTES are selectively increased in cerebrospinal fluid of patients with human immunodeficiency virus-associated dementia. *Ann Neurol*, 44(5), 831–5.

Khanlou, N., Moore, D. J., Chana, G., Cherner, M., Lazzaretto, D., Dawes, S., et al.; HNRC Group. (2009). Increased frequency of alpha-synuclein in the substantia nigra in human immunodeficiency virus infection. *J Neurovirol*, 15(2), 131–8.

King, G., Alicata, D., Cloak, C., & Chang, L. (2010). Neuropsychological deficits in adolescent methamphetamine abusers. *Psychopharmacology (Berl)*, 212(2), 243–9.

King, W. D., Larkins, S., Hucks-Ortiz, C., Wang, P. C., Gorbach, P. M., Veniegas, R., et al. (2009). Factors associated with HIV viral load in a respondent-driven sample in Los Angeles. *AIDS Behav*, 13, 145–153.

Kraft-Terry, S. D., Buch, S. J., Fox, H. S., & Gendelman, H. E. (2009). A coat of many colors: Neuroimmune crosstalk in human immunodeficiency virus infection. *Neuron*, 64(1), 133–45.

Kraft-Terry, S. D., Stothert, A. R., Buch, S., & Gendelman, H. E. (2010). HIV-1 neuroimmunity in the era of antiretroviral therapy. *Neurobiol Dis*, 37(3), 542–8.

Lane, J. H., Sasseville, V. G., Smith, M. O., Vogel, P., Pauley, D. R., Heyes, M. P., et al. (1996). Neuroinvasion by simian immunodeficiency virus coincides with increased numbers of perivascular macrophages/microglia and intrathecal immune activation. *J Neurovirol*, 2, 423–432.

Marcondes, M. C., Flynn, C., Huitron-Rezendiz, S., Watry, D. D., Zandonatti, M., & Fox, H. S. (2009). Early antiretroviral treatment prevents the development of central nervous system abnormalities in simian immunodeficiency virus-infected rhesus monkeys. *AIDS*, 23, 1187–95.

Marcondes, M. C., Flynn, C., Watry, D. D., Zandonatti, M., & Fox, H. S. (2010). Methamphetamine increases brain viral load and activates natural killer cells in simian immunodeficiency virus-infected monkeys. *Am J Pathol*, 177, 355–61.

Persidsky, Y., Limoges, J., McComb, R., Bock, P., Baldwin, T., Tyor, W., et al. (1996). Human immunodeficiency virus encephalitis in SCID mice. *Am J Pathol*, 149(3), 1027–53.

Pilcher, C. D., Shugars, D. C., Fiscus, S. A., Miller, W. C., Menezes, P., Giner, J., et al. (2001). HIV in body fluids during primary HIV infection: Implications for pathogenesis, treatment and public health. *AIDS*, 15, 837–45.

Potash, M. J., Chao, W., Bentsman, G., Paris, N., Saini, M., Nitkiewicz, J., et al. (2005). A mouse model for study of systemic HIV-1 infection, antiviral immune responses, and neuroinvasiveness. *Proc Natl Acad Sci USA*, 102(10), 3760–5.

Roberts, E. S., Burudi, E. M., Flynn, C., Madden, L. J., Roinick, K. L., Watry, D. D., et al. (2004). Acute SIV infection of the brain leads to upregulation of IL6 and interferon-regulated genes: Expression patterns throughout disease progression and impact on neuroAIDS. *J Neuroimmunol*, 157, 81–92.

Roberts, E. S., Huitron-Resendiz, S., Taffe, M. A., Marcondes, M. C., Flynn, C. T., Lanigan, C. M., et al. (2006). Host response and dysfunction in the CNS during chronic simian immunodeficiency virus infection. *J Neurosci*, 26, 4577–85.

Robertson, K. R., Su, Z., Margolis, D. M., Krambrink, A., Havlir, D. V., et al.; A5170 Study Team. (2010). Neurocognitive effects of treatment interruption in stable HIV-positive patients in an observational cohort. *Neurology*, 74(16), 1260–6.

Sacktor, N. C., Wong, M., Nakasujja, N., Skolasky, R. L., Selnes, O. A., Musisi, S., et al. (2005). The International HIV Dementia Scale: A new rapid screening test for HIV dementia. *AIDS*, 19(13), 1367–74

Schnabel, J. (2008). Neuroscience: Standard model. *Nature*, 454, 682–5.

Schnell, G., Price, R. W., Swanstrom, R., & Spudich, S. (2010). Compartmentalization and clonal amplification of HIV-1 variants in t he cerebrospinal fluid during primary infection. *J Virol*, 84(5), 2395–407.

Schweinsburg, B. C., Taylor, M. J., Alhassoon, O. M., Gonzalez, R., Brown, G. G., et al.; HNRC Group. (2005). Brain mitochondrial injury in human immunodeficiency virus-seropositive (HIV+) individuals taking nucleoside reverse transcriptase inhibitors. *J Neurovirology*, 11(4), 356–64.

Spudich, S. S., Nilsson, A. C., Lollo, N. D., Liegler, T. J., Petropoulos, C. J., Deeks, S. G., et al. (2005). Cerebrospinal fluid HIV infection and pleocytosis: Relation to systemic infection and antiretroviral treatment. *BMC Infect Dis*.

Tatro, E. T., Scott, E. R., Nguyen, T. B., Salaria, S., Banerjee, S., Moore, D/ J., et al. (2010). Evidence for alteration of gene regulatory networks through microRNAs of the HIV-infected brain: Novel analysis of retrospective cases. *PLoS One*, 5(4), e10337.

Veazey, R. S., DeMaria, M., Chalifoux, L. V., Shvetz, D. E., Pauley, D. R., Knight, H. L., et al. (1998). Gastrointestinal tract as a major site of CD4+ T cell depletion and viral replication in SIV infection. *Science*, 280, 427–31.

Toggas, S. M., Masliah, E., Rockenstein, E. M., Rall, G. F., Abraham, C. R., & Mucke, L. (1994). Central nervous system damage produced by expression of the HIV-1 coat protein gp120 in transgenic mice. *Nature*, *367*(6459), 188–93.

Tyor, W. R., Power, C., Gendelman, H. E., & Markham, R. B. (1993). A model of human immunodeficiency virus encephalitis in SCID mice. *Proc Natl Acad Sci USA*, *90*(18), 8658–62.

Zink, M. C., Brice, A. K., Kelly, K. M., Queen, S. E., Gama, L., Li, M., et al. (2010). Simian immunodeficiency virus-infected macaques treated with highly active antiretroviral therapy have reduced central nervous system viral replication and inflammation but persistence of viral DNA. *J Infect Dis*, *202*, 161–70.

Zou, W., Kim, B. O., Zhou, B. Y., Liu, Y., Messing, A., & He, J. J. (2007). Protection against human immunodeficiency virus type 1 Tat neurotoxicity by Ginkgo biloba extract EGb 761 involving glial fibrillary acidic protein. *Am J Pathol*, *171*(6), 1923–35.

Zucco, G. M. & Ingegneri, G. (2004). Olfactory deficits in HIV-infected patients with and without AIDS dementia complex. *Physiol Behav*, *80*, 669–674.

SECTION 1

HIV-1 BIOLOGY AND IMMUNOLOGY

Harris A. Gelbard

1.1

HIV-1 BIOLOGY

Sergey Iordanskiy and Michael Bukrinsky

Viral determinants necessary for efficient human immuno-deficiency virus (HIV) infection of cells of the central nervous system (CNS) parallel those of the immune system. Factors that regulate viral infection of its host and instigate specific pathogenic outcomes are often a combination of host and virus-specific products. Any understanding of how HIV affects the CNS must first start with a thorough analysis of functional and molecular properties of the virus. This chapter serves this stated purpose.

OVERVIEW

Many patients infected with human immunodeficiency virus type 1 (HIV-1) develop a syndrome of neurologic deteriora-tion known as HIV-1-associated neurocognitive disorders (HAND); the most severe form is HIV-associated dementia (HAD). Well-accepted neuropathologic correlates of HAD include encephalitis, increased numbers of macrophages in the brain, and the presence of HIV antigen-positive micro-glial cells (for a recent review see Kaul, 2009). Neurons are not productively infected by HIV-1; thus, the mechanism of HIV-induced neuronal injury is most likely indirect. It is gen-erally accepted that the primary host cells for productive HIV infection within the brain are cells of the macrophage lineage, such as perivascular macrophages and microglial cells, point-ing to a pivotal role for the macrophage in the development of HAND. The most likely mechanisms for HIV-induced central nervous system (CNS) injuries is neuronal apoptosis. Microglial and glial activation, directly or indirectly related to HIV infection, plays a major role in neuronal death, pos-sibly through the mediation of oxidative stress (Turchan et al., 2003; Gray et al., 2001; Louboutin, Agrawal, Reyes, Van Bockstaele, & Strayer, 2007).

HIV neurotropism does not always correlate with neuro-virulence, as some patients do not show signs of neuronal damage despite the presence of replicating HIV-1 in the brain (Gorry et al., 2001). Prototype HIV-1 isolates from the CNS are macrophage (M)-tropic, non-syncytia-inducing (NSI), and use CCR5 for entry (R5 strains). However, in vitro stud-ies have shown that X4 viruses induce neuronal apoptosis more frequently than R5 viruses (Ohagen et al., 1999; Zheng et al., 1999), and highly neurovirulent X4 strains can be iso-lated from the CNS (Yi et al., 2003; Zheng et al., 1999). Interestingly, despite X4 tropism, these viruses effectively replicate in macrophages. Similarly, X4 viruses are generally more cytopathic than R5 viruses for cells of the immune system.

In this chapter, which will overview the molecular biology of HIV, we will focus on those aspects of HIV biology that are important for replication of this virus within cells of the CNS.

HIV-1 GENOMIC ELEMENTS AND PROTEINS

HIV-1 belongs to the group of complex retroviruses whose replication is controlled by several regulatory and accessory proteins that are expressed in addition to classical retroviral structural proteins and enzymes encoded by *gag*, *pol*, and *env* genes. The nucleotide sequencing of the original HIV-1 isolates revealed multiple overlapping open reading frames (ORFs) in addition to these archetypal retroviral genes (Figure 1.1.1).

HIV-1 LONG TERMINAL REPEAT (LTR)

The LTRs are two identical regions at the ends of viral DNA that are generated during the process of reverse transcription. In the integrated proviral DNA, the LTRs serve as the main function of regulating viral RNA synthesis. The highly com-plex structure of the LTR contains important regulatory regions for transcription initiation and polyadenylation. The 630 bp-long HIV-1 LTR is functionally divided into three regions. The R (repeat) region of the LTR corresponds to a 92 nucleotide repeat located at both termini of the HIV-1 genomic RNA. The U5 region is an 84 nucleotide sequence located at the 5' end of the viral genome; it is positioned immediately downstream of the R region in the LTR. The U3 segment (454 nucleotides) corresponding to the sequence at the 3' end of the viral genome is located 5' to the R region in the LTR. Thus, the overall arrangement in the LTR is 5'-U3-R-U5-3'. The U3 region of the LTR also harbors part of the *nef* ORF, which contributes to the larger size of HIV-1 U3 as compared to other retroviruses.

During replication, LTR sequences serve additional functions (beyond regulation of transcription), both at the DNA and RNA levels. DNA and RNA sequences in the R region of LTR participate in the formation of DNA–RNA hybrids in an early step of reverse transcription (first tem-plate switch). During integration, LTR sequences (*att*) at the

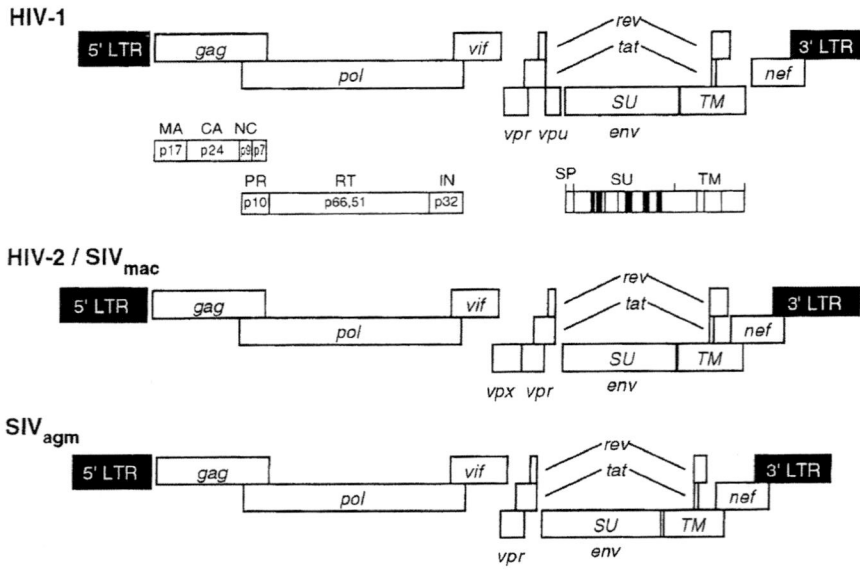

Figure 1.1.1 Genomic maps of HIV-1, HIV-2, and SIV. The provirus genomic organization is shown.

termini of the full-length linear DNA mediate insertion into the host cell genome (Masuda, Kuroda, & Harada, 1998). Sequences in the U5 RNA are involved in the packaging of the progeny HIV-1 RNA genome during viral assembly.

Since the main function of the LTR is to serve as a promoter region, it contains several elements that facilitate Pol II activity on an HIV-1 template. These include a variety of general transcription factors, such as TFIID, that bind to the TATA elements upstream of the transcription initiation site (Baltimore, 1970), thus setting the stage for the assembly of the transcription complex. Other transcription factors that bind to HIV-1 LTR include Sp1, NF-κB, NRE, Ap-3-like, DBF-1 (Pereira, Bentley, Peeters, Churchill, & Deacon, 2000). The HIV-1 genome codes for three factors that can modulate 5′-LTR transcription - Nef, Vpr, and Tat (see below). In addition, chromatin structure associated with the LTR contributes to the activation and repression of the LTR in response to external stimuli (He, Ylisastigui, & Margolis, 2002; Blazkova et al., 2009; Holmes, Knudsen, Key-Cushman, & Su, 2007). Regulation of the HIV-1 genome expression plays a pivotal role in the replication and pathogenesis of this virus and the LTR is central to these events.

TAT RESPONSIVE ELEMENT (TAR)

TAR, or the target sequence for viral transactivation, is the binding site for the viral transactivating protein, Tat, and its partner cellular proteins involved in HIV-1 transcription. TAR RNA forms a hairpin stem-loop structure 59 nucleotides long in HIV-1 and 100 nucleotides long in HIV-2 and simian immunodeficiency virus [SIV]) with a side bulge. The bulge is necessary for Tat binding and function. The minimal TAR element maps between bases +19 and +43 and contains three important components: a base-paired stem, a trinucleotide

bulge that contains UCU at positions +23 to +25 and a hexa-nucleotide G-rich loop (Greenbaum, 1996). TAR functions as an RNA element that recruits cellular RNA polymerase machinery to the HIV-1 promoter, thus stimulating viral transcription.

REV RESPONSIVE ELEMENT (RRE)

RRE is a cis-acting RNA element present in all unspliced and partially spliced viral mRNAs. It consists of approximately 200 nucleotides (positions 7327 to 7530 from the transcription start in HIV-1, spanning the border of gp120 and gp41). It has a complex secondary structure containing several stem-loop arrangements branching from a large central bubble (Grate & Wilson, 1997). The RRE is a binding site for Rev, a viral protein regulating nuclear export of viral intron-containing RNAs (e.g., Gag, Env, and genomic RNAs). Other lentiviruses (HIV-2, SIV, visna) have similar RRE elements in similar locations within *env*.

STRUCTURAL PROTEINS (GAG, POL, ENV)

Gag

Gag is the genomic region encoding group-specific antigens. Gag proteins are necessary and sufficient for the formation of noninfectious, virus-like particles. Retroviral Gag proteins are synthesized as a polyprotein precursor (Figure 1.1.2) containing the p55 myristylated protein (Pr55 Gag), which is processed to p17 (MAtrix), p24 (CApsid), p7 (NucleoCapsid), and p6 proteins by the viral protease during virus maturation, which occurs after budding of the nascent virions from the infected cell. Gag associates with the cholesterol- and sphingomyelin-enriched lipid raft regions of the plasma membrane, where virus assembly takes place. This association is determined by membrane-targeting signals within the MA portion of the Pr55 Gag (see below).

Matrix Antigen (MA)

The MA domain is located at the N-terminal end of the Gag precursor and plays several important roles during viral life cycle. During the assembly step, it directs Pr55 Gag to the plasma membrane via membrane-binding signals. The affinity towards membrane is provided by the myristoylation of the N-terminal glycine residue of p17 (Morikawa, Hockley, Nermut, & Jones, 2000). Another MA feature responsible for interaction with the membrane is a patch of basic amino acid residues that can interact with the negatively charged phospholipids on the inner surface of the plasma membrane (Ono & Freed, 1999). Specific targeting of Pr55 to lipid rafts is determined by phosphatidylinositol-(4,5)-bisphosphate, a phospholipid that is enriched in lipid rafts and can specifically interact with the MA globular domain (Ono, Ablan, Lockett, Nagashima, & Freed, 2004; Saad, Miller, Tai, Kim, Ghanam, & Summers, 2006; Chukkapalli, Hogue, Boyko, Hu, & Ono, 2008). Thus, matrix plays an important role in the trafficking of Gag to the plasma membrane and participates in assembly of the viral particles.

It has been suggested that matrix participates in early events following fusion between the viral and cellular membranes. Mutations in the matrix protein have been shown to impair viral reverse transcription (Kiernan, Ono, Englund, & Freed, 1998). This effect is supposedly due to an inability of the mutant matrix to disengage from the lipid bilayer resulting in an uncoating defect and failure to form a functional reverse transcription complex (Koh et al., 2000).

One of the properties of matrix that is of special interest to this chapter is its activity in the HIV-1 infection of nondividing cells, in particular, macrophages. The basic domains located in the N-terminal part of matrix resemble nuclear localization signals of cellular nuclear proteins and were proposed to play a role in translocating the viral preintegration complex to the nucleus (Bukrinsky et al., 1993; Haffar et al., 2000). This interesting step of the HIV-1 life cycle is discussed later in this chapter.

Capsid Antigen (CA)

The CA protein also functions in the early and the late stages of the viral replication. It contains two structural and functional domains. The N-terminal portion forms the core domain and the C-terminal is the dimerization domain (Freed, 2001). The core domain is a helical structure and has the cyclophilin A (CypA)–binding loop (Luban, Bossolt, Franke, Kalpana, & Goff, 1993). Incorporated CypA is required during an early post-entry step of de novo infection (Braaten & Luban, 2001), likely by protecting the incoming HIV from a host restriction factor (Sokolskaja & Luban, 2006), but exact mechanisms of this activity are still debated.

Nucleocapsid (NC)

The NC is involved in the specific encapsidation of full-length, unspliced genomic RNA into virions. HIV-1 NC

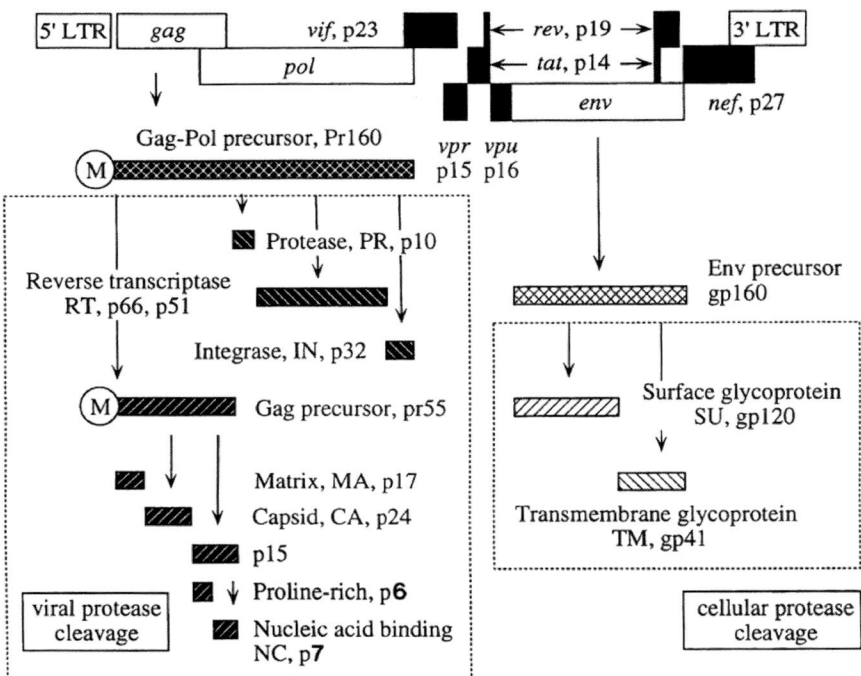

Figure 1.1.2 HIV-1 protein processing. The Gag-Pol precursor of 160 kDa (Pr160) is processed by the viral (aspartyl) protease into seven proteins, which include four Gag proteins (MA, p17; CA, p24; proline—rich, p6; NC, p9), protease (PR, p10), reverse transcriptase (RT, p66/p51) and integrase (IN, p32). The Env precursor (gp160) is processed by a cellular protease into the surface glycoprotein (SU, gp120) and the transmembrane glycoprotein (TM, gp41). Viral regulatory and accessory proteins, which include Tat (p14), Rev (p19), Nef (p27), Vif (p23), Vpr (p15), and Vpu (p16), are not processed. M, myristoylated (Figure courtesy of J. Levy).

protein contains two zinc-finger motifs, which can bind zinc strongly in virions and in vitro (Feng et al., 1996). Mutations or drugs that eliminate zinc-binding capacity of NC greatly diminish viral infectivity (McDonnell, De Guzman, Rice, Turpin, & Summers, 1997). The specificity of HIV genome encapsidation is based on the interaction between NC and a 120-nucleotide sequence located between the 5'-LTR and the Gag initiation codon. Thus, this sequence is called packaging signal, encapsidation element, or ψ-site (Lawrence, Stover, Noznitsky, Wu, & Summers, 2003).

NC is also required for efficient reverse transcription and initial integration processes in a target cell (Buckman, Bosche, & Gorelick, 2003). This NC activity also involves the zinc fingers and appears to be mediated by a protective effect of NC on the full-length viral DNA.

p6 Protein

Retroviral *gag* genes encode a variety of additional ORFs that are generally unique to particular genera of retroviruses. HIV-1 has a proline-rich 6 kD protein, called p6, at the C-terminus of the Pr55 Gag. The p6 region of p55 is responsible for incorporation into virions of another viral protein, Vpr (Checroune, Yao, Gottlinger, Bergeron, & Cohen, 1995). P6 also contains specific sequences, YPLTSL and PTAP, called the late domains, which bind cellular proteins normally functioning as part of the endosomal sorting complexes required for transport (ESCRT) machinery (Garrus et al., 2001). The ESCRT machinery normally mediates the budding of vesicles into the late endosomal lumen, and by recruiting this machinery HIV achieves separation of the budding virions from the membrane of a producer cell (Bieniasz, 2006; Morita & Sundquist, 2004). Thus, PTAP binds Tsg101 (a component of ESCRT-I) and YPLTSL binds ALIX (an ESCRT-I- and ESCRT-III-binding protein). Mutations in late domain sequences lead to inefficient release of the virions, which accumulate at the plasma membrane.

Pol

The *pol* gene represents the genomic region encoding the viral enzymes protease (PR), reverse transcriptase (RT) and integrase (IN). These enzymes are produced as a Gag-Pol precursor polyprotein, Gag-Pol Pr160, which is processed by the viral protease. The Gag-Pol precursor is produced by ribosome frameshifting at the C-terminus of the *gag* gene, thus allowing the ribosomes to avoid the Gag termination codon and fusing the Gag and Pol reading frames (Figure 1.1.2). The *pol* gene is the most conserved region of HIV-1. The *pol*-encoded viral enzymes are targets for currently used anti-HIV drugs.

Protease

The HIV-1 protease plays a critical role in late stages of the viral life cycle. It mediates the production of mature, infectious virions by cleaving the Gag Pr55 and Gag-Pol Pr160. This proteolytic digestion is mandatory for viral infectivity. Retroviral proteases are related to pepsin and similar "aspartic" proteases (Dunn, Goodenow, Gustchina, & Wlodawer,

2002). Interestingly, while the primary sequences of retroviral proteases are highly divergent, their tertiary structures are remarkably similar. The HIV-1 protease functions as a dimer, which carries flexible overhangs that cover the binding site (Dunn et al., 2002). Introduction of protease inhibitors into anti-retroviral drug cocktails has revolutionized the efficacy of anti-HIV therapy.

Reverse Transcriptase (RT)

The retrovirus nomenclature is consistent with the properties of this enzyme. By definition, the replication cycle of all retroviruses includes a step of reverse transcriptase (RNA-dependent DNA polymerase) mediated conversion of the RNA genome into a DNA copy. RT directs synthesis of both minus and plus strands of viral DNA and also degrades the tRNA primer and genomic RNA present in the RNA-DNA hybrid intermediates with its RNAse H activity. Reverse transcription of the HIV-1 RNA genome is a complex process completed via multiple steps (Jonckheere, Anne, & De Clercq, 2000). A plethora of RT inhibitors have been developed and are currently used in highly active antiretroviral therapy (HAART).

Integrase (IN)

Retroviruses insert their full-length genome into the host cell genome via activity of the integrase. Integrase is a 32 kDa protein generated by the viral protease-mediated cleavage of the C-terminal portion of the HIV-1 Gag-Pol polyprotein precursor. Integrase inhibitors potently suppress HIV replication and represent a recent advance in anti-HIV therapy (Marchand, Maddali, Metifiot, & Pommier, 2009).

Envelope (Env)

Viral envelope glycoproteins are produced as a heavily glycosylated precursor protein (gp160). At a late stage of synthesis, most probably in the trans-Golgi network, gp160 is cleaved by furin or other related subtilisin-like proteases into the surface (SU; gp120) and transmembrane (TM; gp41) subunits (Moulard & Decroly, 2000). The gp120 and gp41 proteins then remain noncovalently associated, forming the functional, native trimeric gp120-gp41 complex (Figure 1.1.3), which is delivered to the plasma membrane via the endoplasmic reticulum network (Chen, Lee, & Wang, 2001; Ou & Silver, 2005; Bultmann, Muranyi, Seed, & Haas, 2001; Leung et al., 2008). Since the noncovalent interaction between gp120 and gp41 is weak, a substantial amount of gp120 can be released in the medium. The gp120 is the major antigenic determinant of HIV-1 that triggers a potent antibody response in infected individuals. The viral Env glycoproteins play a major role in viral entry into target cells. Gp120 contains the binding sites for the CD4 receptor and the chemokine co-receptor that serve as attachment sites for HIV-1, whereas gp41 mediates fusion between the viral and target cell membranes (Melikyan, 2008). Interestingly, virus-cell fusion occurs not at the cell surface, as was surmised for a long time, but inside the cell, after endocytosis of the virus-receptor complex (Miyauchi, Kim, Latinovic, Morozov, & Melikyan, 2009).

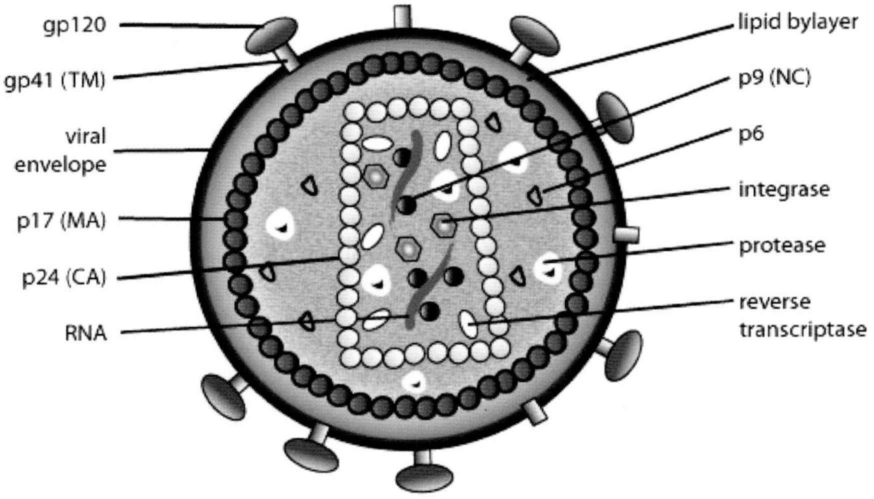

Human Immunodeficiency Virus Structure

Figure 1.1.3 Schematic representation of the mature virion. This schematic representation of the virus shows the relative locations of the structures and proteins. The virion proteins that make up the envelope (each knob represents trimeric gp120 non-covalently attached to trimeric gp41) and nucleocapsid (p24, p17, p9, p7) are noted. The genome consists of diploid RNA associated with reverse transcriptase and integrase.

Regulatory Proteins (Tat, Rev)

HIV-1 encodes two essential regulatory proteins, Tat and Rev. The Tat protein interacts with the regulatory element TAR and Rev interacts with RRE. They both modulate transcriptional (Tat) and posttranscriptional (Rev) steps of viral gene expression.

TransActivator of Transcription (Tat)

The HIV Tat increases the steady-state levels of viral RNA several hundred fold (Marcello, Zoppe, & Giacca, 2001). HIV-1 Tat is a nuclear protein containing 101 amino acids encoded by two exons. It acts by binding to the TAR RNA element and activates transcription elongation by recruiting to the HIV-1 transcription unit the pTEFb factor, which phosphorylates the C-terminal domain of RNA polymerase II, thus increasing its processivity (Liang & Wainberg, 2002). It is the first eukaryotic transcription factor known to interact with RNA rather than DNA and may have similarities with prokaryotic anti-termination factors. Tat is also found in the extracellular milieu and can be taken up by cells in culture to activate LTR-driven transcription.

Regulator for Expression of Viral Proteins (Rev)

For HIV progeny to be produced, unspliced HIV-1 Gag-Pol encoding RNA and partially spliced Env-encoding RNA need to exit the nucleus to associate with ribosomes for translation. However, cellular nuclear export machinery does not support export of unspliced or incompletely spliced RNAs. To circumvent this limitation, HIV-1 relies on Rev. Rev is a 19 kDa phosphoprotein localized primarily in the nucleolus/nucleus. It binds to the RRE sequence present in viral Gag, Gag-Pol, and Env mRNAs and promotes their nuclear export by connecting them to the cellular exportin protein, CRM1, which is responsible for nuclear export of cellular messenger RNAs (Cullen, 1998). In addition, Rev regulates HIV splicing by engaging a number of cellular cofactors, such as eIF5a, hRIP, Sam68 and RNA helicases (Suhasini & Reddy, 2009).

Accessory/Auxiliary Proteins (Vif, Vpr, Vpu, Nef)

HIV-1 encodes four additional virion- and non-virion-associated proteins, Vif, Vpr, Vpu and Nef. They are referred to as accessory or auxiliary proteins as early evidence suggested that their presence was not essential for HIV-1 replication. However, later studies demonstrated that these proteins are highly conserved in viral isolates and play important roles in viral replication in vivo. The mechanisms of their activity are actively investigated, and current evidence suggests that the role of these HIV proteins is to either counteract intrinsic cellular anti-viral activities termed restriction factors (Bieniasz, 2004) or down-regulate cellular proteins that inadvertently interfere with HIV replication.

Viral Infectivity Factor (Vif)

Vif is a basic 192 amino acid protein with the molecular mass of 23 kDa, which promotes the infectivity of HIV-1 without affecting production of viral particles. Vif is essential for viral replication in HIV natural targets, primary CD4+ T cells and macrophages. Certain cell lines support replication of *vif*-deficient viruses, and cell fusion experiments indicated that such cells lack expression of inhibitory factor(s) that naturally block viral replication when Vif is absent (reviewed in Malim & Emerman, 2008). Analysis of mRNA expression profiles in cells restrictive for replication of Vif-deficient HIV-1 identified *APOBEC3G* (*A3G*) as a cellular anti-HIV inhibitory factor targeted by Vif (Sheehy, Gaddis, Choi, & Malim, 2002). This protein is a member of the APOBEC family of editing deaminases, and its activity leads to deamination of the cytidine (C) to uridine (U) in the first newly synthesized DNA strand of HIV-1 cDNA, resulting in massive guanosine (G)-to-adenosine (A) transitions in the complementary strand (Zennou, Perez-Caballero, Gottlinger, & Bieniasz, 2004). In the absence of Vif, host cellular A3G is packaged into budding viral particles through interactions with viral RNA and Gag (Bogerd & Cullen, 2008; Soros, Yonemoto, & Greene, 2007) and consequently carried forward to newly infected cells where it impairs viral reverse transcription (Harris & Liddament, 2004). About 10% of G residues can be mutated to A as a result of this process, which is sufficient to stop further viral spread through the gross loss of genetic integrity (Malim & Emerman, 2008).

Vif effectively antagonizes the antiviral effects of A3G through induction of polyubiquitylation and subsequent degradation of A3G (Conticello, Harris, & Neuberger, 2003; Mehle et al., 2004). By eliminating A3G from virus-producing cells, Vif allows progeny viral particles to be free of A3G. It should be noted here that *A3G* is one of a family of seven cytidine deaminase genes encoded in human genome (Holmes, Malim, & Bishop, 2007b); another member of this family, A3F, is also active in restricting replication of Vif-deficient HIV-1, and Vif induces its polyubiquitylation and degradation (Liu et al., 2005).

Viral Protein R (Vpr)

Vpr is a 96-amino acid (14 kDa) accessory protein, highly conserved among primate lentiviruses (Tristem, Purvis, & Quicke, 1998). Vpr is incorporated into the virion due to interaction with the NC p7 and p6 portions of Pr55 Gag precursor (Lavallee et al., 1994; de Rocquigny et al., 1997). Proposed activities of Vpr include the nuclear import of the viral pre-integration complexes, growth arrest of target cells in the G2 phase, induction of apoptosis in infected cells, and transactivation of viral genes (Bukrinsky & Adzhubei, 1999; Planelles & Benichou, 2010). The ability to cause cell cycle blockade is conserved among Vpr proteins from different isolates and thus is important for HIV-1 infection. A likely reason for this is that G_2 arrest may promote optimal transcription from the LTR and an increase in viral output (Goh et al., 1998; Hrimech, Yao, Bachand, Rougeau, & Cohen, 1999; Andersen, Le, & Planelles, 2008). Data about proapoptotic activity of Vpr and association of the Vpr-induced apoptosis with cell-cycle arrest are still controversial. Some studies suggest that Vpr-induced apoptosis of infected cells is linked to the pathway leading to G2 arrest (Andersen et al., 2006). However, other evidence suggests that cell cycle blockade and cytopathicity are independent functions, at least in CD4+ T (Chen et al., 1999; Nishizawa, Kamata, Mojin, Nakai, & Aida, 2000; Bolton & Lenardo, 2007). Moreover, some reports indicate that the cytostatic effect of Vpr serves to prevent cell death and, by some accounts, protects against apoptotic stimuli ((Bartz, Rogel, & Emerman, 1996; Conti et al., 1998). The reason for this controversy is likely due to the different experimental conditions used in different studies, and in particular the level of Vpr expression. It is possible that low levels of Vpr expression protect cells from apoptosis, whereas high expression promotes cell death. Notably, some

of these activities, and in particular the G2 arrest, depend on association of Vpr with DCAF1/VprBP (Le et al., 2007). DCAF1 bridges Vpr to DDB1, a core subunit of Cul4 E3 ubiquitin ligases, which are involved in regulation of protein degradation by proteasomes.

Intriguingly, Vpr activity is much more pronounced in macrophages than in CD4+ T cells (Subbramanian et al., 1998). Initially, this finding was explained by the role of Vpr in HIV nuclear import, which was considered to be required for viral replication in non-dividing, but not in proliferating cells. However, later studies demonstrated that travel through the nuclear pore is a necessary step in HIV replication in both dividing and non-dividing cells (Bukrinsky, 2004; Yamashita & Emerman, 2006; Riviere, Darlix, & Cimarelli, 2010). Recent evidence suggests that a close relative of Vpr, the Vpx protein found in SIV and HIV-2, functions to counteract an as yet unidentified cellular restriction factor that limits viral replication in macrophages (Sharova et al., 2008; Srivastava et al., 2008). This activity of Vpx depends on interaction with DDB1-Cul4 E3, the same ubiquitin ligase that interacts with Vpr (Bergamaschi et al., 2009; Gramberg et al., 2010; Sharova et al., 2008; Srivastava et al., 2008). Nevertheless, Vpr appears not to target this hypothetical restriction factor, as Vpx potently stimulates replication in macrophages of a Vpr-positive HIV-1 (Sharova et al., 2008). Therefore, either Vpr is a weaker inhibitor of a Vpx-targeted restriction factor, or Vpr's target is different from that of Vpx. Vpr and Vpx may both work in concert with an ubiquitin-proteasome system to limit cellular factor(s) restricting HIV replication in macrophages, and additional factors determine the target of this activity.

Viral Protein U (Vpu)

Vpu is unique to HIV-1 and SIVcpz, a close relative of HIV-1. There is no similar gene in HIV-2 or other SIVs. Vpu is a 16-kDa (81-amino acid) type I integral membrane protein with at least two biological activities: (a) degradation of CD4 in the endoplasmic reticulum, and (b) virion release from the plasma membrane. Vpu is not incorporated into virions, and its function is essential in virus-producing cells. The effect of Vpu on CD4 disrupts the complex between nascent gp120 and CD4 formed in the endoplasmic reticulum and allows delivery of Env proteins to the plasma membrane. The effect on virus release is due to ability of Vpu to counteract activity of a cellular interferon-induced restriction factor called B cell stromal factor 2 (BST-2), also known as CD317 or tetherin. This factor prevents release of enveloped viruses, including retroviruses, from the plasma membrane (Neil, Zang, & Bieniasz, 2008; Neil, Sandrin, Sundquist, & Bieniasz, 2007; Van Damme et al., 2008). Since HIV-1, as many other enveloped viruses, is known to accumulate and bud from lipid raft regions of the plasma membrane, tetherin may form connections between lipid rafts on plasma and viral membranes and thereby physically tether virions to cells (Perez-Caballero et al., 2009). As a result, viral particles made in the absence of Vpu in tetherin-expressing cells fail to detach from the plasma membrane and are transported to endosomes and degraded (Malim & Emerman, 2008). It is still not clear how Vpu counteracts tetherin activity. It may directly target tetherin for proteasomal degradation (Neil et al., 2008) or reduce the surface expression of tetherin (Van Damme et al., 2008). Interestingly, macrophages express higher levels of tetherin than CD4+ T cells, explaining ability of viruses carrying certain Vpu mutations to replicate in T cells but not in macrophages (Schindler et al., 2010).

Negative Factor (Nef)

Nef is a multifunctional 27-kDa myristoylated protein produced by an open reading frame located at the 3'-end of the HIV-1 or SIV genome. It is an early protein abundantly expressed at all stages of infection. Nef is predominantly distributed in cytoplasm but can associate with the plasma membrane via the myristyl residue linked to the conserved second amino acid (Gly). One of the first HIV proteins to be produced in infected cells, Nef is the most immunogenic of the accessory proteins. Despite its original misleading name—the "negative factor," attributed to dispensability of Nef for in vitro infection—Nef in HIV and SIV is essential for efficient viral spread and disease progression in natural infections of different species of primates (Schindler et al., 2006). Viruses with defective Nef have been found in some HIV-1-infected long-term non-progressors (Dyer et al., 1997). Nef downregulates CD4 and MHC class I molecules, and these functions map to different parts of the protein (Geyer, Fackler, & Peterlin, 2001).

Interaction of Nef with the cytoplasmic tail of CD4 accelerates endocytosis of CD4 from the surface of infected cells with subsequent internalization through clathrin-coated pits, with transport to endosomes, and then lysosomes for degradation (Chaudhuri, Lindwasser, Smith, Hurley, & Bonifacino, 2007). Nef performs this function synergistically with another accessory protein, Vpu (described in the previous section). Downregulation of MHC I by Nef proceeds through a different, endocytosis-independent mechanism. Instead, Nef-induced MHC-I downregulation depends on PACS-1 (phosphofurin acidic cluster sorting protein-1) to sort and sequester MHC-I to the trans-Golgi network (Piguet et al., 2000; Crump et al., 2001). Suppression of MHC class I function blunts cytotoxic T cell (CTL) recognition of infected cells and provides a selective advantage to the virus (Malim & Emerman, 2008). Nef also downregulates CD28, a major co-stimulatory receptor that mediates effective T-cell activation (Swigut et al., 2001). In addition, Nef interacts with components of host cell signal transduction and clathrin-dependent protein sorting pathways (Fackler & Baur, 2002). Nef also is a major regulator of viral cholesterol, as it targets the cellular cholesterol transporter ABCA1, which reduces the amount of cholesterol delivered to assembling virions (Mujawar et al., 2006). Nef is incorporated into HIV virions and stimulates early post-entry steps of HIV replication through the interaction with proteins involved in the rearrangements of actin filaments to penetrate the cortical actin network, a known barrier for intracellular parasitic organisms (Campbell, Nunez, & Hope, 2004; Pizzato et al., 2007). In summary, most Nef activities are associated with modulation of cellular proteins in the infected cell to provide optimal conditions for viral propagation.

HIV-1 REPLICATION IN CELLS OF THE MONOCYTE/MACROPHAGE LINEAGE

It is generally accepted that the primary host cells for productive HIV infection within the brain are cells of the macrophage lineage, such as perivascular macrophages and microglial cells. Therefore, in this section we will focus on peculiarities of HIV-1 infection of macrophages as compared to infection of another susceptible cell type, CD4+ T lymphocyte. The differences in HIV-1 replication between these two types of susceptible cells provide an understanding of what viral features define the neurotropism of HIV-1.

HIV-1 ENTRY/TROPISM

Since identification of CD4 as an essential component of HIV-1 receptor, it has been appreciated that additional molecules are required for the entry of HIV-1 into target cells. This idea came from experiments with several nonhuman cell lines, which remain resistant to HIV infection even when engineered to express human CD4. The nature of additional co-receptors remained elusive for many years, until the breakthrough report from Berger's group (reviewed in Berger, 1998). Using expression cloning, these authors identified an orphan 7-transmembrane domain G protein-coupled receptor (which they named fusin) as a co-receptor for T cell line-adapted HIV-1 strains. This co-receptor was later identified as a receptor for chemokine SDF-1α and renamed CXCR4. Following this report, another chemokine receptor, CCR5, was described by several groups as the main co-receptor for primary, macrophage-tropic HIV-1 isolates (Alkhatib et al., 1996; Deng et al., 1996; Dragic et al., 1996). The importance of CCR5 for HIV-1 transmission is underscored by the finding that individuals homozygous for a defective CCR5 allele (a 32 base pair deletion in the gene encoding CCR5 resulting in truncation of the receptor and its retention in the endoplasmic reticulum) are almost completely protected from HIV-1 infection (Liu et al., 1996). Transmitted HIV-1 strains are almost uniformly CCR5-tropic, but later in disease X4 strains may evolve. Emergence of X4 viruses is usually associated with rapid development of immunodeficiency and poor clinical prognosis (Casper et al., 2002).

In addition to promoting virus entry, interaction with chemokine co-receptor also contributes to post-entry steps of HIV replication by initiating signal transduction (Davis et al., 1997; Yoder et al., 2008). The signaling induced by gp120-CCR5 or CXCR4 interaction might facilitate various stages of the HIV replicative cycle, such as trafficking of the RTC through the cytoplasm, reverse transcription, and integration (Yoder et al., 2008; Lin et al., 2002). A correlation between the capacity of R5 HIV-1 strains to signal through CCR5 and to replicate in macrophages has been reported (Arthos et al., 2000). These data are consistent with a model of M-tropism in which early events in HIV replication in macrophages, in particular reverse transcription, are facilitated by signaling initiated by envelope-CCR5 interaction. Intriguingly, replication in macrophages of some primary X4 isolates could be enhanced by addition of CC chemokines (Arthos et al., 2000).

This observation indicates that signaling through CC chemokine receptors may promote the replication in macrophages of some primary CXCR4-utilizing isolates.

The mechanism by which envelope or CC chemokine signaling promotes HIV-1 replication in MDMs may involve changes in the cytoskeleton. Bukrinskaya et al. demonstrated that after viral entry, reverse transcription complexes rapidly localize to the cytoskeletal compartment (Bukrinskaya et al., 1998). In addition, they showed that actin polymerization is a prerequisite for efficient reverse transcription. CCR5 stimulation by CC chemokines promotes actin polymerization (Premack & Schall, 1996). Because M-tropic envelopes share with CC chemokines the ability to transduce signals through CCR5, it appears likely that CCR5-utilizing envelopes may also induce actin polymerization. This hypothesis is supported by our observation that heterologous desensitization of CCR5 by the B-oligomer of the pertussis toxin blocks gp120-induced capping of CD4 and CCR5, a process dependent on actin polymerization (Alfano, Schmidtmayerova, Amella, Pushkarsky, & Bukrinsky, 1999). A recent report indicated that signaling through CXCR4 activates a cellular actin depolymerization factor, cofilin, to promote the cortical actin dynamics that are critical for viral intracellular migration across the cortical actin barrier (Yoder et al., 2008). While this effect has been described for infection of T cells (Wu et al., 2008), it remains to be determined whether similar activities can be found in macrophages.

Molecular studies of viral sequences found in the brain underscore the critical role of macrophages and macrophage-tropic viruses in CNS disease. While an early report suggested that CCR3 (a receptor for chemokine eotaxin [CCL11]) may function as an HIV-1 co-receptor for infection of microglial cells (He et al., 1997), later studies demonstrated that CCR5 is the major co-receptor for HIV-1 infection of macrophages and microglia (Gabuzda & Wang, 1999). Furthermore, CCR5 is the principal co-receptor used by HIV-1 viruses isolated from the brain (Smit, et al., 2001; Li et al., 1999). However, CCR5 usage by primary brain-derived HIV-1 isolates is neither necessary nor sufficient for neurotropism (defined as the ability of viruses to replicate in microglia), as infection of microglial cells by some isolates occurs via the CXCR4 co-receptor (Gorry et al., 2001; Yi et al., 2003). Importantly, some R5 isolates described in the Gorry et al. study did not replicate in macrophages due to a block to virus entry, indicating that additional factors, beside co-receptors, are involved in regulating macrophage- and neuro-tropism.

One such factor may be CD4 density on the surface of macrophages. Studies in rhesus macaques demonstrated that low levels of CD4 on macrophages account for the lack of infection by M-tropic HIV-1 or T-tropic SIV strains (Bannert, Schenten, Craig, & Sodroski, 2000; Mori et al., 2000). Indeed, CD4 expression levels on macrophages are lower than on T lymphocytes, and this difference might explain in part low efficiency of entry into macrophages of X4 strains (Dimitrov et al., 1999). It may also restrict entry of some R5 viruses (Platt, Wehrly, Kuhmann, Chesebro, & Kabat, 1998). Other possible factors affecting macrophage tropism are affinity of the interaction between gp120 and the co-receptor (CCR5 or CXCR4) and the exposure of the co-receptor binding site on gp120 (Doms, 2000).

Overall, macrophage (M)-tropism appears to fully determine the capacity of an HIV or SIV isolate to replicate in the CNS. Macrophage tropism is necessary for the virus to remain in the CNS and for the development of encephalitis.

REVERSE TRANSCRIPTION

Following HIV-1 entry into a target cell, viral RNA genome is converted to a DNA form by the viral RNA-dependent DNA polymerase, reverse transcriptase. While reverse transcription is completed intracellularly, it may be initiated within virions outside the cell ("endogenous" reverse transcription); and this capacity may contribute to efficiency of HIV infection process (Zhang, Dornadula, & Pomerantz, 1998; 1996). Intracellular reverse transcription of HIV-1 entirely depends on the cellular dNTP pool. Treatment with hydroxyurea, which blocks de novo dNTP synthesis, has been shown to inhibit HIV-1 replication in acutely infected peripheral blood mononuclear cells (PBMC) and primary macrophages (Lori et al., 1994). The observed low dNTP pools in quiescent T cells and macrophages might explain the slow rate of reverse transcription in these cells as compared to activated T lymphocytes (Meyerhans et al., 1994; O'Brien et al., 1994; Collin & Gordon, 1994; Zack et al., 1990). Indeed, activated T cells reverse transcription is completed within 6 hours, while in macrophages it can take as long as 36–48 hours (O'Brien et al., 1994). However, in contrast to quiescent T lymphocytes, where inefficient reverse transcription is one of the main blocks to HIV replication (Zack et al., 1990), substrate limitations in mononuclear phagocytes slow but do not arrest HIV-1 reverse transcription. As a result, virus replicates efficiently in macrophages, albeit with slower kinetics.

Interestingly, the effects of cell activation on the fate of the virus are opposite in T cells and macrophages. While activated T cells are highly susceptible to HIV-1 infection, in part due to high efficiency of viral reverse transcription in such cells, activated macrophages are resistant to infection by HIV-1 (Zybarth et al., 1999; Pushkarsky et al., 2001). This resistance probably stems from increased degradation of the viral RNA, which is not compensated by an increased efficiency of reverse transcription in activated macrophages.

One characteristic feature of the genome of HIV-1 and other lentiviruses is the presence of two additional *cis*-acting sequences, the central polypurine tract (cPPT) and the central termination sequence (CTS). The effect of these sequences on reverse transcription is formation of a three-stranded DNA structure, the central DNA flap, which is essential for viral replication (Charneau, Alizon, & Clavel, 1992; Charneau et al., 1994; Arhel et al., 2006). This central DNA flap contributes to PIC (pre-integration complex) nuclear import (Zennou et al., 2000), likely by promoting uncoating (loss of CA p24) of the RTC at the nuclear membrane, thus preparing the RTC for translocation through the nuclear pore (Arhel et al., 2007).

NUCLEAR IMPORT

A crucial factor in HIV-1 replication in macrophages is the capacity of this virus to transport its reverse transcribed genome through the intact nuclear membrane. Although one report suggested that macrophage infection occurs during rare cell division events, possibly during monocyte-to-macrophage maturation process (Schuitemaker et al., 1994), an overwhelming evidence supports the notion that HIV-1 can infect terminally differentiated, non-dividing macrophages (Weinberg, Matthews, Cullen, & Malim, 1991; Schmidtmayerova et al., 1997; and reviewed in Stevenson & Gendelman, 1994). To be able to replicate in such cells, a mechanism for nuclear importation through intact nuclear membrane of the viral pre-integration complex (PIC) carrying HIV-1 genome is required. Inability to cross the nuclear membrane of the interphase cell is the main barrier that restricts replication of simple retroviruses to proliferating cells (Roe, Reynolds, Yu, & Brown, 1993).

The journey of the HIV-1 PIC to the cell's nucleus is comprised of several distinct steps. To deliver its PIC through the cytoplasm and into the nucleus, HIV-1 relies on the cellular machinery. Following the fusion of the viral and cell membranes, the HIV-1 nucleocapsid is released into the cytoplasm. This process is accompanied by partial dissociation of the capsid shell composed of the CA p24 (uncoating) and the formation of a reverse transcription complex (RTC) (step 1 in Fig. 1.1.4).

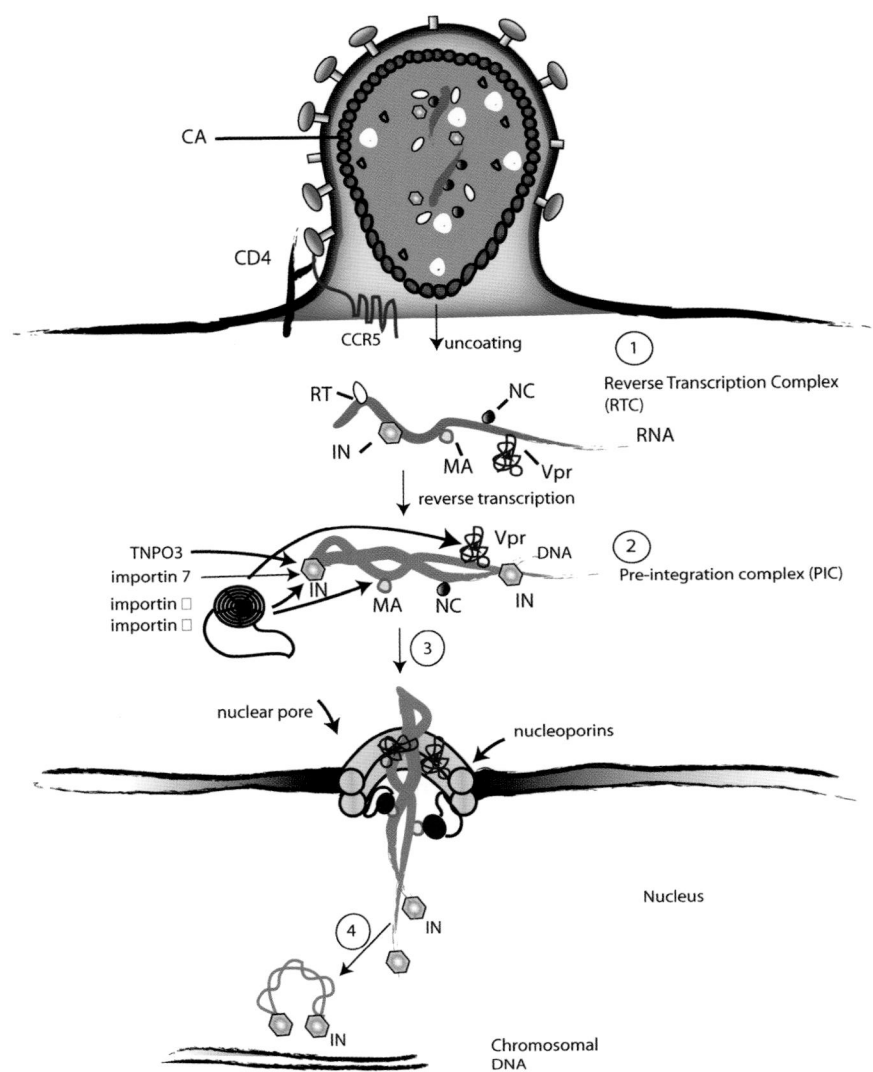

Figure 1.1.4 A model of HIV-1 nuclear translocation. Following binding to cell-surface receptors (CD4 and CCR5 or CXCR4), HIV-1 fuses with the cellular membrane resulting in the entry of the viral core into the cytosol. Entry is accompanied by initiation of a poorly defined step termed *uncoating*, the most characteristic feature of which is dissociation of the capsid shell made of capsid antigen (CA) and the formation of a reverse transcription complex (RTC) (step 1). Of note, uncoating continues along the translocation of the RTC through the cytoplasm and is completed at the nuclear membrane. Upon reverse transcription of the viral genomic RNA, the complex becomes competent for integration and is termed pre-integration complex (PIC) (step 2). Several cellular nuclear transport proteins, including importins α and β, bind to karyophilic proteins within the PIC, such as Vpr, MA, and IN, and target the complex to the nuclear pore (step 3). Importin β and Vpr mediate the interaction between the PIC and the nuclear pore proteins (nucleoporins). Transfer of the PIC through the nuclear pore is likely accompanied by dissociation of MA, Vpr, and NC proteins (step 4), leaving IN, which mediates integration of the viral genome into the host cell DNA.

Uncoating is likely a gradual process which proceeds in parallel to reverse transcription and the movement of the RTC through the cytoplasm, with final steps occurring at the nuclear membrane (Arhel et al., 2007). Because of the high viscosity of the cytoplasm, movement of RTCs by diffusion is likely to be very limited, especially considering the size of the HIV-1 RTC, which has been estimated to be at least 50 nm in diameter (Miller, Farnet, & Bushman, 1997). To overcome this obstacle, HIV-1 utilizes the cellular cytoskeleton. Initial movements of the virus within the peripheral regions of the cell cytoplasm occur in association with the actin cytoskeleton (Bukrinskaya et al., 1998). However, subsequent translocation of the HIV-1 pre-integration complex towards the nucleus takes place along the microtubule network (McDonald et al., 2002). Transfer from the actin to the microtubule network is consistent with the evidence that actin can be used to gain access to tubulin (Taunton, 2001). The structural basis for interaction of the RTC and microtubules remains to be determined. This interaction likely engages a cellular dynein-dependent motor complex, which has both minus end (towards the microtubule-organizing center located close to the nucleus)- and plus end (towards cell periphery)–directed motor activities. A similar mechanism is used by herpes simplex virus (HSV)-1 (Sodeik, Ebersold, & Helenius, 1997) and adenovirus (Suomalainen et al., 1999) for intracellular transport.

Reverse transcription occurs during this translocation converting the HIV-1 RTC to an integration competent pre-integration complex (PIC) (step 2 in Fig. 1.1.4). Once near the nuclear membrane, HIV-1 most likely relies on the cellular nuclear import proteins to pass through the nuclear pore (step 3 in Figure 1.1.4), although other mechanisms, such as entry through reversible ruptures of the nuclear membrane made by the Vpr protein (de Noronha et al., 2001), might contribute to this process.

Cellular Nuclear Import Machinery

Nuclear transport of macromolecules occurs through the nuclear pore complexes and is controlled by nuclear localization signals (NLSs). The most common type of NLS is a short stretch of basic amino acids introducing an overall net positive charge crucial for the nuclear targeting properties of these sequences (reviewed in Dingwall & Laskey, 1991). Import of NLS-containing proteins across the nuclear pore complex is mediated by karyopherin α/β heterodimers (also termed NLS receptor/importin), which bind NLS-containing proteins in the cytosol and target them to the nucleus (Mattaj & Englmeier, 1998). Karyopherin α affinity for the NLS is enhanced by karyopherin β. Karyopherin β also mediates docking of karyopherin-NLS protein complexes to nucleoporins (a collective term for nuclear pore complex proteins) containing FG peptide repeats (Terry & Wente, 2009; Moroianu et al., 1995; Rexach & Blobel, 1995). Some NLSs interact with karyopherin β directly, without engaging the adapter protein karyopherin α (Barry & Wente, 2000). The small guanosine 5'-triphosphate (GTP) binding protein, Ran (Moore & Blobel, 1993; Melchior, Paschal, Evans, & Gerace, 1993), is a key regulator of the import process. Ran switches between the guanosine 5'-diphosphate (GDP) and GTP-bound states by nucleotide exchange and GTP hydrolysis. The concentration of Ran-GTP is high in the nucleus and low in the cytoplasm. It is believed that this gradient is used to provide direction to the nucleo-cytoplasmic exchange. In particular, by directly binding to karyopherin β: in the nucleoplasm, Ran-GTP disassembles the import complex and thus terminates the import process (Gorlich et al., 1996). It also stimulates assembly of the karyopherin α complex with cellular apoptosis susceptibility (CAS) factor, a protein originally implicated in apoptosis and cell proliferation but then rediscovered as an export factor (Kutay, Bischoff, Kostka, Kraft, & Gorlich, 1997). CAS promotes re-export of karyopherin α into the cytoplasm for recycling.

Nuclear Entry of the HIV-1 PIC

The model favored by investigators working in the area of HIV nuclear import is that the PIC itself is nucleophilic. This implies that a component or components of the complex contain targeting signals that direct the PIC to the nucleus. The most likely candidates for this role are viral proteins associated with the PIC (see below), although they can do it indirectly by binding to karyophilic cellular proteins (Gupta, Ott, Hope, Siliciano, & Boeke, 2000). Nuclear import of HIV PIC requires timely uncoating to expose the complex to cellular nuclear targeting machinery, so it is not surprising that mutations that accelerate or delay uncoating impair nuclear translocation and replication of HIV (Yamashita, Perez, Hope, & Emerman, 2007; Yamashita & Emerman, 2006). Several karyopherins/importins, including importins α and β (Hearps & Jans, 2006; Nitahara-Kasahara et al., 2007), importin 7 (Fassati, Gorlich, Harrison, Zaytseva, & Mingot, 2003), and TNPO3/transportin-SR2 (Christ et al., 2008) have been implicated in nuclear targeting of the HIV-1 PIC. TNPO3 was also identified in genome-wide screens for factors essential for HIV-1 replication, which used proliferating cells to monitor HIV replication, indicating that this importin, and by extension the process of nuclear import, is critical for HIV replication regardless of cellular proliferation status (Goff, 2008; Riviere, Darlix, & Cimarelli, 2010).

Role of MA, IN, and Vpr in HIV Nuclear Import

MA was the first protein implicated in HIV-1 nuclear import (Bukrinsky et al., 1993). However, later studies questioned this role of MA (Fouchier et al., 1997; Freed, Englund, & Martin, 1995). It appears that HIV-1 MA carries functional, yet rather weak, NLSs whose activity may be enhanced by Vpr (Haffar et al., 2000). While MA is clearly required for efficient nuclear import of the HIV-1 PIC, its role is most likely nonessential (Reil, Bukovsky, Gelderblom, & Gottlinger, 1998).

Gallay and coworkers have proposed a role for IN in HIV-1 nuclear import (Gallay, Hope, Chin, & Trono et al., 1997). They demonstrated that IN associates with karyopherin α and can target a fusion GST-IN protein into the nucleus of microinjected cells. A report from Malim's group (Bouyac-Bertoia et al., 2001) extended this observation. This group identified an unusual NLS spanning residues 161–173 within the central core domain of IN and demonstrated that certain mutations within this NLS, such as V165A or R166A, disrupt nuclear import of the viral PIC but do not affect IN catalytic activity. However, these results could not be reproduced in later studies demonstrating that the mutations described by Bouyac-Bertoia and colleagues primarily affected integration and not the PIC nuclear import (Bouyac-Bertoia et al., 2001; Limon, Nakajima, Lu, Ghory, & Engelman, 2002). IN was also reported to interact with lens epithelium-derived growth factor/p75 (LEDGF/p75), which is a karyophilic protein that may facilitate nuclear localization of IN and PIC (Maertens, Cherepanov, Debyser, Engelborghs, & Engelman, 2004). HIV-1 IN is likely an important factor in HIV-1 nuclear import (Woodward, Prakobwanakit, Mosessian, & Chow, 2009; Levin et al., 2009).

Vpr is another important contributor to HIV-1 nuclear import (Nie et al., 1998; Popov, Rexach, Ratner, Blobel, & Bukrinsky, 1998a; Popov et al., 1998b; Vodicka, Koepp, Silver, & Emerman, 1998). Three hypotheses (not necessarily mutually exclusive) for the mode of action of Vpr have been proposed: i) Vpr targets the HIV-1 PIC to the nucleus via a distinct, karyopherin α/β-independent pathway (Gallay, Stitt, Mundy, Oettinger, & Trono, 1996; de Noronha et al., 2001; Jenkins, McEntee, Weis, & Greene, 1998); ii) Vpr-mediated import requires karyopherin α, but not β (Vodicka et al., 1998); and iii) Vpr modifies cellular karyopherin α/β-dependent import machinery (Popov et al., 1998a; Popov et al., 1998b). The first model is based on the observation that in an in vitro nuclear import assay Vpr can enter nuclei in the absence of soluble import factors (Jenkins et al., 1998). Later, the same group reported that Vpr induces dynamic disruptions in nuclear envelope integrity, which may serve as entry points for large complexes such as HIV-1 PIC (de Noronha et al., 2001; Segura-Totten & Wilson, 2001). However, this latter assumption has not been tested experimentally. In addition, the effect of Vpr on the nuclear envelope was demonstrated in HeLa cells, where HIV-1 replication is Vpr-independent (Gallay et al., 1997). The second hypothesis relies on the ability of Vpr to bind nucleoporins (Fouchier et al., 1998; Popov et al., 1998a) and proposes that nuclear translocation of the HIV-1 PIC is mediated by direct binding of Vpr to the nuclear pore. The third model is based on findings that Vpr binds to karyopherin α (Popov et al., 1998b; Vodicka et al., 1998) and changes its affinity for the nuclear localization signal (NLS) (Popov et al., 1998b), and that nuclear import and docking of the HIV-1 pre-integration complex to nucleoporins are inhibited by antibodies to karyopherin β (Popov et al., 1998a). Most of the experimental data supporting these models have been obtained using individually expressed Vpr. The actual mechanism for Vpr activity in the nuclear importation of the HIV-1 PIC remains unresolved. In any case, Vpr is definitely involved in the process of HIV-1 nuclear import in macrophages. However, its role is not strictly essential, as viruses lacking Vpr can still replicate in macrophages, albeit with reduced efficiency (Heinzinger et al., 1994).

How could all these seemingly conflicting results be assembled into a unified model? One likely possibility is that all the mentioned constituents contribute to HIV-1 nuclear import in a redundant manner. Such redundancy would ensure the efficiency of this extremely important step for the virus. It is also possible that HIV-1 uses different pathways for the nuclear import, depending on the cell type and the activation state of the target cell (Lee et al., 2010; discussed in Levin, Loyter, & Bukrinsky, 2010). Such flexible use of the nuclear import machinery would employ different viral proteins under different conditions. Based on studies with HIV and other viruses replicating in the nucleus, it appears safe to assume that the HIV-1 PIC is delivered to the nuclear envelope along the microtubule network and enters the nucleoplasm through the nuclear pore. The simplified model depicting the main steps in the process of nuclear translocation of the HIV genome is shown in Figure 1.1.4. During the passage through the nuclear pore or shortly after entering the nucleus, the PIC likely undergoes additional disassembly, getting rid of the factors unnecessary for integration, such as MA and Vpr (step 4 in Fig. 1.1.4). The detailed mechanisms responsible for the steps shown in Figure 1.1.4 await their resolution.

INTEGRATION

Integration of the HIV-1 DNA into the host-cell genome, catalyzed by the integrase (IN) protein, is a prerequisite for viral replication in both T cells and macrophages. Integrase is a recombinase responsible for the cutting-and-joining reaction that leads to the covalent ligation of the viral genome with the cellular DNA and the formation of the provirus. Integration usually proceeds in multiple steps (Pluymers, De Clercq, & Debyser, 2001). First, two to three nucleotides from the initially blunt 3' ends of the viral DNA are removed to form a preintegration substrate. This step presumably occurs in the cytoplasm (Kulkosky & Skalka, 1994). Second, in the nucleus, integrase catalyzes a staggered cleavage of the cellular target DNA. Third, the cellular DNA repair machinery repairs the gaps and ligates the 3' recessed ends to the 5' overhangs. The integrated viral DNA is called provirus and is retained in the host genome throughout the life of the infected cell. Some low-level replication in macrophages of an integrase-defective HIV-1 mutant has been described (Cara, Guarnaccia, Reitz, Gallo, & Lori, 1995). However, replication of this mutant virus was inefficient and self-limiting. While extra-chromosomal circular forms of viral DNA are produced in both peripheral blood lymphocytes (PBLs) and macrophages, they cannot sustain viral replication, despite their reported stability, at least in T cells (Pierson et al., 2002).

Studies using integration in vitro have clarified factors influencing integration site selection in simplified models. Access of integration complexes to target DNA can be obstructed by DNA binding proteins bound at or near the integration sites (Pryciak & Varmus, 1992). In contrast, proteins that induce DNA bending, such as nucleosomal histones, can actually promote integration (Pryciak & Varmus, 1992; Pruss, Reeves, Bushman, & Wolffe, 1994b; Pruss, Bushman, & Wolffe, 1994a). In vivo, nucleosomal DNA is assembled into higher-order chromatin. A recent analysis of HIV-1 integration sites in vivo using genomics approaches revealed that genes were clearly preferential integration targets in vivo but not in vitro (Schroder et al., 2002). Transcriptional profiling revealed a strong correlation between gene activity and integration targeting. In addition, hotspots for integration were detected, for example, a 2.5 kb region that contained 1% of all integration events (Schroder et al., 2002). Therefore, there is a certain degree of specificity in the integration targeting by HIV.

How can this specificity be accomplished? Obviously, cellular proteins must be involved, as integration in vitro is random. Search for cellular proteins interacting with HIV-1 integrase produced a number of candidates, including LEDGF/p75, transportin-SR2 (TNPO3), von Hippel-Lindau binding protein 1 (VBP1), and sucrose non-fermenting 5 (SNF5) (Rain, Cribier, Gerard, Emiliani, & Benarous, 2009). Further studies are required to determine the role of these factors in HIV-1 integration.

Efficiency of HIV-1 integration in CD4$^+$ T cells and macrophages appears to be influenced by the activation state of the target cell. HIV gp120 induces multiple cellular signaling pathways, including the phosphatidylinositol 3-kinase (PI3-kinase) pathway. The PI3-kinase inhibitor LY294002 inhibited infection of CD4$^+$ T cells and macrophages with X4 and R5 HIV-1 strains (Francois & Klotman, 2003). The inhibition of the PI3-kinase signaling pathway suppressed virus infection post-entry and post-reverse transcription but prior to HIV gene expression, suggesting an effect at the step of integration. So far, there is no indication in the literature that differences exist between T cells and macrophages with regard to the mechanism of HIV-1 integration.

TRANSCRIPTION

Despite some evidence that unintegrated HIV-1 DNA can be transcribed (Poon & Chen, 2003; Wu & Marsh, 2003), the vast majority of HIV-1 transcription occurs from integrated proviral DNA. Main elements of HIV transcriptional control are located in the 5'-LTR. Transcriptional regulation depends on the recognition of *cis* regulatory regions in the 5'-LTR by a set of transcription factors which interact with the basal transcriptional complex (reviewed in Cullen, 1991). A TATA box, which recruits host cell RNA polymerase II, three Sp1 sites, and a strong enhancer composed of two NF-κB sites are located in the U3 region (Nabel & Baltimore, 1987). Additional binding sites for transcriptional regulatory proteins have been identified 5' to the NF-κB enhancer, in the so-called NRE of the HIV-1 LTR. The NRE includes binding sites for USF, AP1, LEF, NF-AT, and ETS transcription factors (Naghavi et al., 2001, and references therein). Inducible activation of the viral LTR appears to depend principally on the generation of a functional NF-κB complex and requires a trans-activating protein, Tat, to interact with a trans-activating responsive element, TAR. NF-κB defines a family of transcription factors composed by members of the NF-κB/Rel family, namely NF-κB1 (p50), NF-κB2 (p52), RelA (p65), RelB, v-Rel, and c-Rel, all sharing a sequence homology over a 300 amino acids ("rel homology domain") (Siebenlist, Franzoso, & Brown, 1994). NF-κB proteins form homo- or heterodimers that bind with different affinities to the NF-κB enhancer of HIV-1.

Transcription and splicing of HIV mRNAs is a complex process, in which the viral regulatory proteins Tat and Rev play essential roles. HIV-1 genes are expressed through the complex splicing of a single mRNA precursor, leading to three major classes of transcripts: unspliced (US), singly spliced (SS), and multiply spliced (MS) mRNAs. In vitro, reactivation of latent HIV-1 infection is characterized by an early increase in MS transcripts, followed by a rise in SS and US viral mRNA (Cullen & Greene, 1989). Thus, early in the infection only MS transcripts are produced, which encode the regulatory proteins Tat, Rev, and Nef. Accumulation of Tat and Rev has profound effects on viral transcription. Tat greatly enhances the processivity of transcription from the HIV LTR, while Rev is essential for the export of SS and US viral transcripts from the nucleus into the cytoplasm. Together, these regulatory proteins ensure accumulation of the viral structural proteins required for efficient production of new viral particles. Interestingly, HIV infection of macrophages in vitro is characterized by a dramatic reduction of Tat expression following the peak of productive infection, perhaps accounting for the slower non-cytopathic infection of cells of the macrophage lineage (Sonza et al., 2002).

VIRUS PARTICLE ASSEMBLY

The final steps of the viral life cycle include assembly of an immature viral particle on the cytoplasmic face of a cell membrane, encapsidation of the viral RNA, viral budding and release of the viral particles from the infected cell, and proteolytic processing of Gag and Gag-Pol polyprotein-precursors resulting in formation of infectious virions. These steps are controlled by Gag polyproteins, Pr55 Gag and Pr160 GagPol synthesized from unspliced genomic RNA. Gag itself is enough for a formation and budding of virus-like particles (VLP) independently of an active viral encoded protease (PR) (Klein, Reed, & Lingappa, 2007). The assembly process is driven primarily by elements within Gag, such as the N-terminal membrane-targeting domain (M), central Gag-Gag interaction domain (I), the NC (nucleocapsid) domain which binds RNA enabling packaging of the viral genome, and a C-terminal proline-rich late assembly (L) domain located in the p6 region of Gag, which is required for separation of the virion from the host cell membrane (Pincetic & Leis, 2009; Bieniasz, 2009).

HIV assembly begins with Gag precursor molecules coming into close contact with each other to form a Gag protein sphere within a lipid bilayer envelope (Hermida-Matsumoto & Resh, 2000). Gag localization in the cell membrane is not uniform and seems to be concentrated in lipid rafts (the membrane areas highly enriched in cholesterol, sphingolipids, and glycosylphosphatidylinositol-linked proteins) (Ono & Freed, 2001) where the Env complexes are also preferentially accumulated. Some data provide evidence that HIV-1 Gag monomers might multimerize and associate with viral RNA in the cytoplasm prior to arriving to the membrane and then diffuse through the cytoplasm to sites of assembly on cell membranes (Yuan, Yu, Lee, & Essex, 1993; Gomez & Hope, 2006). Other observations suggest that Gag remains entirely monomeric or forms low-order multimers in the cytoplasm and Gag oligomerization occurs only at the cell membrane (Datta et al., 2007).

Interestingly, studies in macrophages initially contradicted the model of HIV particle assembly at the inner face of plasma membrane, as considerable amounts of HIV-1 Gag protein and/or mature virion particles were detected in late endosomes (Nydegger, Foti, Derdowski, Spearman, & Thali, 2003; Sherer et al., 2003; Pelchen-Matthews, Kramer, & Marsh, 2003). These findings suggested that at least in macrophages Gag was initially targeted to late endosomal membranes, virions were formed by budding into the endosomal lumen, and extracellular particles were liberated via an endosome-based secretory pathway (Nguyen, Booth, Gould, & Hildreth, 2003). Consistent with this view, virion budding requires the ESCRT proteins, which normally mediate the budding of vesicles into the late endosomal lumen (Bieniasz, 2006). However, later studies demonstrated that in this cell type, productive HIV-1 assembly occurs at the plasma membrane (Jouvenet et al., 2006). Large areas of the macrophage plasma membrane are sequestered within the cell, forming invaginations that have the appearance of an intracellular compartment. However, this "compartment" is bounded by a plasma membrane that is continuous with the conventional plasma membrane. Virions assembled in these intracellular pseudo-compartments bounded by the plasma membrane become trapped and accumulate therein, presenting an impression of enriched production at intracellular sites as compared to the conventional plasma membrane upon ultrastructural analysis. These intracellular pseudo-compartments may represent favored sites for HIV-1 assembly in macrophages, but it is not currently clear whether they are static or dynamic or whether they represent exocytic, endocytic, or phagocytic intermediates (Bieniasz, 2009).

HIV-1 genomic RNA is brought to the site of aggregation of Gag, GagPol, and Env complexes through an interaction between the *cis*-acting region of the viral RNA, RNA packaging (psi) sequence, and the zinc fingers of the Gag precursor NC domain (Cimarelli, Sandin, Hoglund, & Luban, 2000). The psi region consists of four stem-loop structures (SL1, SL2, SL3, and SL4) and is located between the 5'-LTR and the Gag initiation site (Lever, 2000). The NC domain also facilitates dimerization of the viral RNA, a process, which seems to be important for RNA packaging (Sakuragi, Ueda, Iwamoto, & Shioda, 2003). Once delivered to the plasma membrane, Gag, GagPol, and Env complexes start to interact and initiate encapsidation of two copies of viral genomic RNA and Lysine tRNA, which serves as a primer for reverse transcription.

The L domains of HIV-1 and other retroviruses bind directly or indirectly to components of the ESCRT pathway in order to complete assembly and separate the nascent virion envelope from cell membranes (Bieniasz, 2006; Morita & Sundquist, 2004). The HIV-1 L domains consist of peptide sequences PTAP and YPLTSL, which bind Tsg101

(a component of ESCRT-I) and ALIX (an ESCRT-I- and ESCRT-III-binding protein), respectively (Garrus et al., 2001; Bieniasz, 2006; Morita & Sundquist, 2004; Bieniasz, 2009). The ESCRT pathway is normally implicated in (1) selection of ubiquitin-tagged transmembrane protein cargos and their sorting into specified areas of endosomal membranes, (2) induction of membrane invagination away from the cytoplasm and toward the endosomal lumen, and (3) fusion of the neck of the induced membrane invagination to generate a vesicle within the endosomal lumen (Bieniasz, 2009). The model of recruitment of the ESCRT machinery components by the retroviruses to build a budding complex for particle release includes the following steps (reviewed in Pincetic & Leis, 2009). (1) The PTAP L domain of HIV-1 binds to Tsg101. Whether this initial interaction takes place in the cytosol or at the plasma membrane remains to be defined. (2) The Gag polyprotein is ubiquitylated by an unidentified E3 ubiquitin ligase. Some evidence suggests that Nedd4L may play a role since its over-expression rescues budding of HIV-1 Gag/ΔPTAP. (3) Gag oligomerization in the cytosol increases membrane avidity and rapidly targets Gag to sites of assembly/budding on the plasma membrane. (4) During the budding process, Gag may recruit additional ESCRT factors eventually leading to ESCRT-III polymerization at the base of a budding particle. (5) ESCRT-III subunits recruit the AAA ATPase, Vps4, to mediate the disassembly of membrane-bound ESCRT complexes and to provide the energy for membrane fission. (6) Immature viral particles are released from cellular membranes.

During or shortly after the budding of immature viral particles from the host cell, the noninfectious virions with a spherical core composed of Pr55^{Gag} and Pr160^{GagPol} polyproteins are transformed to infectious virions during a step termed maturation. During maturation, the *pol*-encoded HIV protease processes itself from GagPol precursor, forms homodimers and then cleaves the Gag of Pr55 and Pr160 polyprotein precursors into three major proteins (matrix, capsid, and nucleocapsid) and three polypeptides (p6, p2, and p1), and the Pol domain of the GagPol Pr160 precursor into the p51 and p66 subunits of reverse transcriptase and the integrase. These events lead to reorganization of the internal virion structure characterized by formation of conical-shaped cores (Gross et al., 2000). Gag cleavage and maturation are essential for infectivity.

CONCLUSION

Understanding of the mechanisms governing HIV-1 replication has lead to development of effective antiretroviral agents and is expected to provide new therapeutic leads in the future. Introduction of highly active antiretroviral therapy (HAART) dramatically improved patients' survival; however, its impact on the prevalence and the course of HAD and HAND remains debatable. While multiple studies suggest that the incidence rates of HAD and CNS opportunistic infections are decreasing, some research indicates that the prevalence of HAND is rising as people with HIV live longer (Kaul, 2009).

Since the introduction of HAART in 1996, the incidence of HAD has decreased by approximately 50%. However, as resistance of the virus to antiretroviral drugs develops and CD4 cell counts decline, the incidence of HAD may begin to rise again. Poor CNS penetration of many antiretroviral agents contributes to persistence of HIV-1 in the brain and explains, at least in part, the sanctuary status of the CNS for the ancestral viral variants (Van Marle et al., 2002; Nowacek & Gendelman, 2009; Liu et al., 2000). It is clear that new drugs, especially those that can cross the blood-brain barrier and are tailored to inhibit HIV-1 replication in macrophages, will be needed to eliminate HAND from the list of diseases associated with HIV infection.

REFERENCES

Alfano, M., Schmidtmayerova, H., Amella, C. A., Pushkarsky, T., & Bukrinsky, M. (1999). The B-oligomer of pertussis toxin deactivates CC chemokine receptor 5 and blocks entry of M-tropic HIV-1 strains. *J Exp Med*, *190*, 597–606.

Alkhatib, G., Combadiere, C., Broder, C. C., Feng, Y., Kennedy, P. E., Murphy, P. M., et al. (1996). CC CKR5: A RANTES, MIP-1alpha, MIP-1beta receptor as a fusion cofactor for macrophage-tropic HIV-1. *Science*, *272*, 1955–1958.

Andersen, J. L., DeHart, J. L., Zimmerman, E. S., Ardon, O., Kim, B., Jacquot, G., et al. (2006). HIV-1 Vpr-induced apoptosis is cell cycle dependent and requires Bax but not ANT. *PLoS Pathog*, *2*, e127.

Andersen, J. L., Le, R. E., & Planelles, V. (2008). HIV-1 Vpr: Mechanisms of G2 arrest and apoptosis. *Exp Mol Pathol*, *85*, 2–10.

Arhel, N., Munier, S., Souque, P., Mollier, K., & Charneau, P. (2006). Nuclear import defect of human immunodeficiency virus type 1 DNA flap mutants is not dependent on the viral strain or target cell type. *J Virol*, *80*, 10262–10269.

Arhel, N. J., Souquere-Besse, S., Munier, S., Souque, P., Guadagnini, S., Rutherford, S., et al. (2007). HIV-1 DNA flap formation promotes uncoating of the pre-integration complex at the nuclear pore. *EMBO J*, *26*, 3025–3037.

Arthos, J., Rubbert, A., Rabin, R. L., Cicala, C., Machado, E., Wildt, K., et al. (2000). CCR5 signal transduction in macrophages by human immunodeficiency virus and simian immunodeficiency virus envelopes. *J Virol*, *74*, 6418–6424.

Baltimore, D. (1970). RNA-dependent DNA polymerase in virions of RNA tumour viruses. *Nature*, *226*, 1209–1211.

Bannert, N., Schenten, D., Craig, S., & Sodroski, J. (2000). The level of CD4 expression limits infection of primary rhesus monkey macrophages by a T-tropic simian immunodeficiency virus and macrophagetropic human immunodeficiency viruses. *J Virol*, *74*, 10984–10993.

Barry, D. M. & Wente, S. R. (2000). Nuclear transport: Never-ending cycles of signals and receptors. *Essays Biochem*, *36*, 89–103.

Bartz, S. R., Rogel, M. E., & Emerman, M. (1996). Human immunodeficiency virus type 1 cell cycle control: Vpr is cytostatic and mediates G2 accumulation by a mechanism which differs from DNA damage checkpoint control. *J Virol*, *70*, 2324–2331.

Bergamaschi, A., Ayinde, D., David, A., Le, R. E., Morel, M., Collin, G., et al. (2009). The human immunodeficiency virus type 2 Vpx protein usurps the CUL4A-DDB1 DCAF1 ubiquitin ligase to overcome a postentry block in macrophage infection. *J Virol*, *83*, 4854–4860.

Berger, E. A. (1998). HIV entry and tropism. When one receptor is not enough. *Adv Exp Med Biol*, *452*:151–7, 151–157.

Bieniasz, P. D. (2004). Intrinsic immunity: Afront-line defense against viral attack. *Nat Immunol*, *5*, 1109–1115.

Bieniasz, P. D. (2006). Late budding domains and host proteins in enveloped virus release. *Virology*, *344*, 55–63.

Bieniasz, P. D. (2009). The cell biology of HIV-1 virion genesis. *Cell Host Microbe*, *5*, 550–558.

Blazkova, J., Trejbalova, K., Gondois-Rey, F., Halfon, P., Philibert, P., Guiguen, A., et al. (2009). CpG methylation controls reactivation of HIV from latency. *PLoS Pathog*, *5*, e1000554.

Bogerd, H. P. & Cullen, B. R. (2008). Single-stranded RNA facilitates nucleocapsid: APOBEC3G complex formation. *RNA*, *14*, 1228–1236.

Bolton, D. L. & Lenardo, M. J. (2007). Vpr cytopathicity independent of G2/M cell cycle arrest in human immunodeficiency virus type 1-infected CD4+ T cells. *J Virol*, *81*, 8878–8890.

Bouyac-Bertoia, M., Dvorin, J. D., Fouchier, R. A., Jenkins, Y., Meyer, B. E., Wu, L. I., et al. (2001). Hiv-1 infection requires a functional integrase nls. *Mol Cell*, *7*, 1025–1035.

Braaten, D. & Luban, J. (2001). Cyclophilin A regulates HIV-1 infectivity, as demonstrated by gene targeting in human T cells. *EMBO J*, *20*, 1300–1309.

Buckman, J. S., Bosche, W. J., & Gorelick, R. J. (2003). Human immunodeficiency virus type 1 nucleocapsid zn(2+) fingers are required for efficient reverse transcription, initial integration processes, and protection of newly synthesized viral DNA. *J Virol*, *77*, 1469–1480.

Bukrinskaya, A., Brichacek, B., Mann, A., & Stevenson, M. (1998). Establishment of a functional human immunodeficiency virus type 1 (HIV-1) reverse transcription complex involves the cytoskeleton. *J Exp Med*, *188*, 2113–2125.

Bukrinsky, M. (2004). A hard way to the nucleus. *Mol Med*, *10*, 1–5.

Bukrinsky, M. & Adzhubei, A. (1999). Viral protein R of HIV-1. *Rev Med Virol*, *9*, 39–49.

Bukrinsky, M. I., Haggerty, S., Dempsey, M. P., Sharova, N., Adzhubel, A., Spitz, L., et al. (1993). A nuclear localization signal within HIV-1 matrix protein that governs infection of non-dividing cells. *Nature*, *365*, 666–669.

Bultmann, A., Muranyi, W., Seed, B., & Haas, J. (2001). Identification of two sequences in the cytoplasmic tail of the human immunodeficiency virus type 1 envelope glycoprotein that inhibit cell surface expression. *J Virol*, *75*, 5263–5276.

Campbell, E. M., Nunez, R., & Hope, T. J. (2004). Disruption of the actin cytoskeleton can complement the ability of Nef to enhance human immunodeficiency virus type 1 infectivity. *J Virol*, *78*, 5745–5755.

Cara, A., Guarnaccia, F., Reitz, M. S., Gallo, R. C., & Lori, F. (1995). Self-limiting, cell type-dependent replication of an integrase-defective human immunodeficiency virus type 1 in human primary macrophages but not T lymphocytes. *Virology*, *208*, 242–248.

Casper, C., Naver, L., Clevestig, P., Belfrage, E., Leitner, T., Albert, J., et al. (2002). Coreceptor change appears after immune deficiency is established in children infected with different HIV-1 subtypes. *AIDS Res Hum Retroviruses*, *18*, 343–352.

Charneau, P., Alizon, M., & Clavel, F. (1992). A second origin of DNA plus-strand synthesis is required for optimal human immunodeficiency virus replication. *J Virol*, *66*, 2814–2820.

Charneau, P., Mirambeau, G., Roux, P., Paulous, S., Buc, H., & Clavel, F. (1994). HIV-1 reverse transcription. A termination step at the center of the genome. *J Mol Biol*, *241*, 651–662.

Chaudhuri, R., Lindwasser, O. W., Smith, W. J., Hurley, J. H., & Bonifacino, J. S. (2007). Downregulation of CD4 by human immunodeficiency virus type 1 Nef is dependent on clathrin and involves direct interaction of Nef with the AP2 clathrin adaptor. *J Virol*, *81*, 3877–3890.

Checroune, F., Yao, X. J., Gottlinger, H. G., Bergeron, D., & Cohen, E. A. (1995). Incorporation of Vpr into human immunodeficiency virus type 1: Role of conserved regions within the P6 domain of Pr55gag. *J Acquir Immune Defic Syndr Hum Retrovirol*, *10*, 1–7.

Chen, M., Elder, R. T., Yu, M., O'Gorman, M. G., Selig, L., Benarous, R., et al. (1999). Mutational analysis of Vpr-induced G2 arrest, nuclear localization, and cell death in fission yeast. *J Virol*, *73*, 3236–3245.

Chen, S. S., Lee, S. F., & Wang, C. T. (2001). Cellular membrane-binding ability of the C-terminal cytoplasmic domain of human immunodeficiency virus type 1 envelope transmembrane protein gp41. *J Virol*, *75*, 9925–9938.

Christ, F., Thys, W., De, R. J., Gijsbers, R., Albanese, A., Arosio, D., et al. (2008). Transportin-SR2 imports HIV into the nucleus. *Curr Biol*, *18*, 1192–1202.

Chukkapalli, V., Hogue, I. B., Boyko, V., Hu, W. S., & Ono, A. (2008). Interaction between the human immunodeficiency virus type 1 Gag matrix domain and phosphatidylinositol-(4,5)-bisphosphate is essential for efficient gag membrane binding. *J Virol, 82*, 2405–2417.

Cimarelli, A., Sandin, S., Hoglund, S., & Luban, J. (2000). Rescue of multiple viral functions by a second-site suppressor of a human immunodeficiency virus type 1 nucleocapsid mutation. *J Virol, 74*, 4273–4283.

Collin, M. & Gordon, S. (1994). The kinetics of human immunodeficiency virus reverse transcription are slower in primary human macrophages than in a lymphoid cell line. *Virology, 200*, 114–120.

Conti, L., Rainaldi, G., Matarrese, P., Varano, B., Rivabene, R., Columba, S., et al. (1998). The HIV-1 vpr protein acts as a negative regulator of apoptosis in a human lymphoblastoid T cell line: Possible implications for the pathogenesis of *AIDS J Exp Med, 187*, 403–413.

Conticello, S. G., Harris, R. S., & Neuberger, M. S. (2003). The Vif protein of HIV triggers degradation of the human antiretroviral DNA deaminase APOBEC3G. *Curr Biol, 13*, 2009–2013.

Crump, C. M., Xiang, Y., Thomas, L., Gu, F., Austin, C., Tooze, S. A., et al. (2001). PACS-1 binding to adaptors is required for acidic cluster motif-mediated protein traffic. *EMBO J, 20*, 2191–2201.

Cullen, B. R. (1991). Regulation of HIV-1 gene expression. *FASEB J, 5*, 2361–2368.

Cullen, B. R. (1998). Retroviruses as model systems for the study of nuclear RNA export pathways. *Virology, 249*, 203–210.

Cullen, B. R. & Greene, W. C. (1989). Regulatory pathways governing HIV-1 replication. *Cell, 58*, 423–426.

Datta, S. A., Zhao, Z., Clark, P. K., Tarasov, S., Alexandratos, J. N., Campbell, S. J., et al. (2007). Interactions between HIV-1 Gag molecules in solution: An inositol phosphate-mediated switch. *J Mol Biol, 365*, 799–811.

Davis, C. B., Dikic, I., Unutmaz, D., Hill, C. M., Arthos, J., Siani, M. A., et al. (1997). Signal transduction due to HIV-1 envelope interactions with chemokine receptors CXCR4 or CCR5. *J Exp Med, 186*, 1793–1798.

de Noronha, C. M., Sherman, M. P., Lin, H. W., Cavrois, M. V., Moir, R. D., Goldman, R. D., et al. (2001). Dynamic disruptions in nuclear envelope architecture and integrity induced by HIV-1 Vpr. *Science, 294*, 1105–1108.

de Rocquigny, H., Petitjean, P., Tanchou, V., Decimo, D., Drouot, L., Delaunay, T., et al. (1997). The zinc fingers of HIV nucleocapsid protein NCp7 direct interactions with the viral regulatory protein Vpr. *J Biol Chem, 272*, 30753–30759.

Deng, H., Liu, R., Ellmeier, W., Choe, S., Unutmaz, D., Burkhart, M., et al. (1996). Identification of a major co-receptor for primary isolates of HIV-1. *Nature, 381*, 661–666.

Dimitrov, D. S., Norwood, D., Stantchev, T. S., Feng, Y., Xiao, X., & Broder, C. C. (1999). A mechanism of resistance to HIV-1 entry: Inefficient interactions of CXCR4 with CD4 and gp120 in macrophages. *Virology, 259*, 1–6.

Dingwall, C. & Laskey, R. A. (1991). Nuclear targeting sequences—a consensus? *Trends Biochem Sci, 16*, 478–481.

Doms, R. W. (2000). Beyond receptor expression: The influence of receptor conformation, density, and affinity in HIV-1 infection. *Virology, 276*, 229–237.

Dragic, T., Litwin, V., Allaway, G. P., Martin, S. R., Huang, Y., Nagashima, K. A., et al. (1996). HIV-1 entry into CD4+ cells is mediated by the chemokine receptor CC- CKR-5. *Nature, 381*, 667–673.

Dunn, B. M., Goodenow, M. M., Gustchina, A., & Wlodawer, A. (2002). Retroviral proteases. *Genome Biol, 3*, REVIEWS3006.

Dyer, W. B., Geczy, A. F., Kent, S. J., McIntyre, L. B., Blasdall, S. A., Learmont, J. C., et al. (1997). Lymphoproliferative immune function in the Sydney Blood Bank Cohort, infected with natural nef/long terminal repeat mutants, and in other long-term survivors of transfusion-acquired HIV-1 infection. *AIDS, 11*, 1565–1574.

Fackler, O. T. & Baur, A. S. (2002). Live and let die: Nef functions beyond HIV replication. *Immunity. 16*, 493–497.

Fassati, A., Gorlich, D., Harrison, I., Zaytseva, L., & Mingot, J. M. (2003). Nuclear import of HIV-1 intracellular reverse transcription complexes is mediated by importin 7. *EMBO J, 22*, 3675–3685.

Feng, Y. X., Copeland, T. D., Henderson, L. E., Gorelick, R. J., Bosche, W. J., Levin, J. G., et al. (1996). HIV-1 nucleocapsid protein induces "maturation" of dimeric retroviral RNA in vitro. *Proc Natl Acad Sci USA, 93*, 7577–7581.

Fouchier, R. A., Meyer, B. E., Simon, J. H., Fischer, U., Albright, A. V., Gonzalez-Scarano, F., et al. (1998). Interaction of the human immunodeficiency virus type 1 Vpr protein with the nuclear pore complex. *J Virol, 72*, 6004–6013.

Fouchier, R. A., Meyer, B. E., Simon, J. H., Fischer, U., & Malim, M. H. (1997). HIV-1 infection of non-dividing cells: Evidence that the amino-terminal basic region of the viral matrix protein is important for Gag processing but not for post-entry nuclear import. *EMBO J, 16*, 4531–4539.

Francois, F. & Klotman, M. E. (2003). Phosphatidylinositol 3-kinase regulates human immunodeficiency virus type 1 replication following viral entry in primary CD4(+) T lymphocytes and macrophages. *J Virol, 77*, 2539–2549.

Freed, E. O. (2001). HIV-1 replication. *Somat Cell Mol Genet, 26*, 13–33.

Freed, E. O., Englund, G., & Martin, M. A. (1995). Role of the basic domain of human immunodeficiency virus type 1 matrix in macrophage infection. *J Virol, 69*, 3949–3954.

Gabuzda, D. & Wang, J. (1999). Chemokine receptors and virus entry in the central nervous system. *J Neurovirol, 5*, 643–658.

Gallay, P., Hope, T., Chin, D., & Trono, D. (1997). HIV-1 infection of nondividing cells through the recognition of integrase by the importin/karyopherin pathway. *Proc Natl Acad Sci USA, 94*, 9825–9830.

Gallay, P., Stitt, V., Mundy, C., Oettinger, M., & Trono, D. (1996). Role of the karyopherin pathway in human immunodeficiency virus type 1 nuclear import. *J Virol, 70*, 1027–1032.

Garrus, J. E., von Schwedler, U. K., Pornillos, O. W., Morham, S. G., Zavitz, K. H., Wang, H. E., et al. (2001). Tsg101 and the vacuolar protein sorting pathway are essential for HIV-1 budding. *Cell, 107*, 55–65.

Geyer, M., Fackler, O. T., & Peterlin, B. M. (2001). Structure—function relationships in HIV-1 Nef. *EMBO Rep, 2*, 580–585.

Goff, S. P. (2008). Knockdown screens to knockout HIV-1. *Cell, 135*, 417–420.

Goh, W. C., Rogel, M. E., Kinsey, C. M., Michael, S. F., Fultz, P. N., Nowak, M. A., et al. (1998). HIV-1 Vpr increases viral expression by manipulation of the cell cycle: A mechanism for selection of Vpr in vivo. *Nat Med, 4*, 65–71.

Gomez, C. Y. & Hope, T. J. (2006). Mobility of human immunodeficiency virus type 1 Pr55Gag in living cells. *J Virol, 80*, 8796–8806.

Gorlich, D., Pante, N., Kutay, U., Aebi, U., & Bischoff, F. R. (1996). Identification of different roles for RanGDP and RanGTP in nuclear protein import. *EMBO J, 15*, 5584–5594.

Gorry, P. R., Bristol, G., Zack, J. A., Ritola, K., Swanstrom, R., Birch, C. J., et al. (2001). Macrophage tropism of human immunodeficiency virus type 1 isolates from brain and lymphoid tissues predicts neurotropism independent of coreceptor specificity. *J Virol, 75*, 10073–10089.

Gramberg, T., Sunseri, N., & Landau, N. R. (2010). Evidence for an activation domain at the amino terminus of simian immunodeficiency virus Vpx. *J Virol, 84*, 1387–1396.

Grate, D. & Wilson, C. (1997). Role REVersal: understanding how RRE RNA binds its peptide ligand. *Structure, 5*, 7–11.

Gray, F., Adle-Biassette, H., Chretien, F., Lorin, d. l. G., Force, G., & Keohane, C. (2001). Neuropathology and neurodegeneration in human immunodeficiency virus infection. Pathogenesis of HIV-induced lesions of the brain, correlations with HIV-associated disorders and modifications according to treatments. *Clin Neuropathol, 20*, 146–155.

Greenbaum, N. L. (1996). How Tat targets TAR: Structure of the BIV peptide-RNA complex. *Structure, 4*, 5–9.

Gross, I., Hohenberg, H., Wilk, T., Wiegers, K., Grattinger, M., Muller, B., et al. (2000). A conformational switch controlling HIV-1 morphogenesis. *EMBO J, 19*, 103–113.

Gupta, K., Ott, D., Hope, T. J., Siliciano, R. F., & Boeke, J. D. (2000). A human nuclear shuttling protein that interacts with human immunodeficiency virus type 1 matrix is packaged into virions. *J Virol, 74*, 11811–11824.

Haffar, O. K., Popov, S., Dubrovsky, L., Agostini, I., Tang, H., Pushkarsky, T., et al. (2000). Two nuclear localization signals in the HIV-1 matrix protein regulate nuclear import of the HIV-1 pre-integration complex. *J Mol Biol, 299,* 359–368.

Harris, R. S. & Liddament, M. T. (2004). Retroviral restriction by APOBEC proteins. *Nat Rev Immunol, 4,* 868–877.

He, G., Ylisastigui, L., & Margolis, D. M. (2002). The regulation of HIV-1 gene expression: The emerging role of chromatin. *DNA Cell Biol, 21,* 697–705.

He, J., Chen, Y., Farzan, M., Choe, H., Ohagen, A., Gartner, S., et al. (1997). CCR3 and CCR5 are co-receptors for HIV-1 infection of microglia. *Nature, 385,* 645–649.

Hearps, A. C. & Jans, D. A. (2006). HIV-1 integrase is capable of targeting DNA to the nucleus via an Importin alpha/beta-dependent mechanism. *Biochem J, 398,* 475–484.

Heinzinger, N. K., Bukrinsky, M. I., Haggerty, S. A., Ragland, A. M., Kewalramani, V., Lee, M. et al. (1994). The Vpr protein of human immunodeficiency virus type 1 influences nuclear localization of viral nucleic acids in nondividing host cells. *Proc Natl Acad Sci USA, 91,* 7311–7315.

Hermida-Matsumoto, L. & Resh, M. D. (2000). Localization of human immunodeficiency virus type 1 Gag and Env at the plasma membrane by confocal imaging. *J Virol, 74,* 8670–8679.

Holmes, D., Knudsen, G., key-Cushman, S., & Su, L. (2007). FoxP3 enhances HIV-1 gene expression by modulating NFkappaB occupancy at the long terminal repeat in human T cells. *J Biol Chem, 282,* 15973–15980.

Holmes, R. K., Malim, M. H., & Bishop, K. N. (2007). APOBEC-mediated viral restriction: Not simply editing? *Trends Biochem Sci, 32,* 118–128.

Hrimech, M., Yao, X. J., Bachand, F., Rougeau, N., & Cohen, E. A. (1999). Human immunodeficiency virus type 1 (HIV-1) Vpr functions as an immediate-early protein during HIV-1 infection. *J Virol, 73,* 4101–4109.

Jenkins, Y., McEntee, M., Weis, K., & Greene, W. C. (1998). Characterization of HIV-1 vpr nuclear import: Analysis of signals and pathways. *J Cell Biol, 143,* 875–885.

Jonckheere, H., Anne, J., & De Clercq, E. (2000). The HIV-1 reverse transcription (RT) process as target for RT inhibitors. *Med Res Rev, 20,* 129–154.

Jouvenet, N., Neil, S. J., Bess, C., Johnson, M. C., Virgen, C. A., Simon, S. M., et al. (2006). Plasma membrane is the site of productive HIV-1 particle assembly. *PLoS Biol, 4,* e435.

Kaul, M. (2009). HIV-1 associated dementia: Update on pathological mechanisms and therapeutic approaches. *Curr Opin Neurol, 22,* 315–320.

Kiernan, R. E., Ono, A., Englund, G., & Freed, E. O. (1998). Role of matrix in an early postentry step in the human immunodeficiency virus type 1 life cycle. *J Virol, 72,* 4116–4126.

Klein, K. C., Reed, J. C., & Lingappa, J. R. (2007). Intracellular destinies: Degradation, targeting, assembly, and endocytosis of HIV Gag. *AIDS Rev, 9,* 150–161.

Koh, K., Miyaura, M., Yoshida, A., Sakurai, A., Fujita, M., & Adachi, A. (2000). Cell-dependent gag mutants of HIV-1 are crucially defective at the stage of uncoating/reverse transcription in non-permissive cells. *Microbes Infect, 2,* 1419–1423.

Kulkosky, J. & Skalka, A. M. (1994). Molecular mechanism of retroviral DNA integration. *Pharmacol Ther, 61,* 185–203.

Kutay, U., Bischoff, F. R., Kostka, S., Kraft, R., & Gorlich, D. (1997). Export of importin alpha from the nucleus is mediated by a specific nuclear transport factor. *Cell, 90,* 1061–1071.

Lavallee, C., Yao, X. J., Ladha, A., Gottlinger, H., Haseltine, W. A., & Cohen, E. A. (1994). Requirement of the Pr55gag precursor for incorporation of the Vpr product into human immunodeficiency virus type 1 viral particles. *J Virol, 68,* 1926–1934.

Lawrence, D. C., Stover, C. C., Noznitsky, J., Wu, Z., & Summers, M. F. (2003). Structure of the intact stem and bulge of HIV-1 Psi-RNA stem-loop SL1. *J Mol Biol, 326,* 529–542.

Le, R. E., Belaidouni, N., Estrabaud, E., Morel, M., Rain, J. C., Transy, C., et al. (2007). HIV1 Vpr arrests the cell cycle by recruiting DCAF1/ VprBP, a receptor of the Cul4-DDB1 ubiquitin ligase. *Cell Cycle, 6,* 182–188.

Lee, K., Ambrose, Z., Martin, T. D., Oztop, I., Mulky, A., Julias, J. G., et al. (2010). Flexible use of nuclear import pathways by HIV-1. *Cell Host Microbe, 7,* 221–233.

Leung, K., Kim, J. O., Ganesh, L., Kabat, J., Schwartz, O., & Nabel, G. J. (2008). HIV-1 assembly: Viral glycoproteins segregate quantally to lipid rafts that associate individually with HIV-1 capsids and virions. *Cell Host Microbe, 3,* 285–292.

Lever, A. M. (2000). HIV RNA packaging and lentivirus-based vectors. *Adv Pharmacol, 48,* 1–28.

Levin, A., Loyter, A., & Bukrinsky, M. I. (2010). Strategies to inhibit viral protein nuclear import: HIV-1 as a target. *Biochim Biophys Acta* (in press).

Levin, A., rmon-Omer, A., Rosenbluh, J., Melamed-Book, N., Graessmann, A., Waigmann, E., et al. (2009). Inhibition of HIV-1 integrase nuclear import and replication by a peptide bearing integrase putative nuclear localization signal. *Retrovirology, 6,* 112.

Li, S., Juarez, J., Alali, M., Dwyer, D., Collman, R., Cunningham, A., et al. (1999). Persistent CCR5 utilization and enhanced macrophage tropism by primary blood human immunodeficiency virus type 1 isolates from advanced stages of disease and comparison to tissue-derived isolates. *J Virol, 73,* 9741–9755.

Liang, C. & Wainberg, M. A. (2002). The role of Tat in HIV-1 replication: An activator and/or a suppressor? *AIDS Rev, 4,* 41–49.

Limon, A., Nakajima, N., Lu, R., Ghory, H. Z., & Engelman, A. (2002). Wild-type levels of nuclear localization and human immunodeficiency virus type 1 replication in the absence of the central DNA flap. *J Virol, 76,* 12078–12086.

Lin, Y. L., Mettling, C., Portales, P., Reynes, J., Clot, J., & Corbeau, P. (2002). Cell surface CCR5 density determines the post-entry efficiency of R5 HIV-1 infection. *Proc Natl Acad Sci USA, 99,* 15590–15595.

Liu, B., Sarkis, P. T., Luo, K., Yu, Y., & Yu, X. F. (2005). Regulation of Apobec3F and human immunodeficiency virus type 1 Vif by Vif-Cul5-ElonB/C E3 ubiquitin ligase. *J Virol, 79,* 9579–9587.

Liu, R., Paxton, W. A., Choe, S., Ceradini, D., Martin, S. R., Horuk, R., et al. (1996). Homozygous defect in HIV-1 coreceptor accounts for resistance of some multiply-exposed individuals to HIV-1 infection. *Cell, 86,* 367–377.

Liu, Y., Tang, X. P., McArthur, J. C., Scott, J., & Gartner, S. (2000). Analysis of human immunodeficiency virus type 1 gp160 sequences from a patient with HIV dementia: Evidence for monocyte trafficking into brain. *J Neurovirol, 6 Suppl 1,* S70–S81.

Lori, F., Malykh, A., Cara, A., Sun, D., Weinstein, J. N., Lisziewicz, J., &. (1994). Hydroxyurea as an inhibitor of human immunodeficiency virus-type 1 replication. *Science, 266,* 801–805.

Louboutin, J. P., Agrawal, L., Reyes, B. A., Van Bockstaele, E. J., & Strayer, D. S. (2007). Protecting neurons from HIV-1 gp120-induced oxidant stress using both localized intracerebral and generalized intraventricular administration of antioxidant enzymes delivered by SV40-derived vectors. *Gene Ther, 14,* 1650–1661.

Luban, J., Bossolt, K. L., Franke, E. K., Kalpana, G. V., & Goff, S. P. (1993). Human immunodeficiency virus type 1 Gag protein binds to cyclophilins A and B. *Cell, 73,* 1067–1078.

Maertens, G., Cherepanov, P., Debyser, Z., Engelborghs, Y., & Engelman, A. (2004). Identification and characterization of a functional nuclear localization signal in the HIV-1 integrase interactor LEDGF/p75. *J Biol Chem, 279,* 33421–33429.

Malim, M. H. & Emerman, M. (2008). HIV-1 accessory proteins—ensuring viral survival in a hostile environment. *Cell Host Microbe, 3,* 388–398.

Marcello, A., Zoppe, M., & Giacca, M. (2001). Multiple modes of transcriptional regulation by the HIV-1 Tat transactivator. *IUBMB Life, 51,* 175–181.

Marchand, C., Maddali, K., Metifiot, M., & Pommier, Y. (2009). HIV-1 IN inhibitors: 2010 update and perspectives. *Curr Top Med Chem, 9,* 1016–1037.

Masuda, T., Kuroda, M. J., & Harada, S. (1998). Specific and independent recognition of U3 and U5 att sites by human immunodeficiency virus type 1 integrase in vivo. *J Virol, 72,* 8396–8402.

Mattaj, I. W. & Englmeier, L. (1998). Nucleocytoplasmic transport: The soluble phase. *Annu Rev Biochem, 67,* 265–306.

McDonald, D., Vodicka, M. A., Lucero, G., Svitkina, T. M., Borisy, G. G., Emerman, M., et al. (2002). Visualization of the intracellular behavior of HIV in living cells. *J Cell Biol, 159,* 441–452.

McDonnell, N. B., De Guzman, R. N., Rice, W. G., Turpin, J. A., & Summers, M. F. (1997). Zinc ejection as a new rationale for the use of cystamine and related disulfide-containing antiviral agents in the treatment of AIDS. *J Med Chem, 40,* 1969–1976.

Mehle, A., Strack, B., Ancuta, P., Zhang, C., McPike, M., & Gabuzda, D. (2004). Vif overcomes the innate antiviral activity of APOBEC3G by promoting its degradation in the ubiquitin-proteasome pathway. *J Biol Chem, 279,* 7792–7798.

Melchior, F., Paschal, B., Evans, J., & Gerace, L. (1993). Inhibition of nuclear protein import by nonhydrolyzable analogues of GTP and identification of the small GTPase Ran/TC4 as an essential transport factor. *J Cell Biol, 123,* 1649–1659.

Melikyan, G. B. (2008). Common principles and intermediates of viral protein-mediated fusion: The HIV-1 paradigm. *Retrovirology, 5,* 111.

Meyerhans, A., Vartanian, J. P., Hultgren, C., Plikat, U., Karlsson, A., Wang, L., et al. (1994). Restriction and enhancement of human immunodeficiency virus type 1 replication by modulation of intracellular deoxynucleoside triphosphate pools. *J Virol, 68,* 535–540.

Miller, M. D., Farnet, C. M., & Bushman, F. D. (1997). Human immunodeficiency virus type 1 preintegration complexes: Studies of organization and composition. *J Virol, 71,* 5382–5390.

Miyauchi, K., Kim, Y., Latinovic, O., Morozov, V., & Melikyan, G. B. (2009). HIV enters cells via endocytosis and dynamin-dependent fusion with endosomes. *Cell, 137,* 433–444.

Moore, M. S. & Blobel, G. (1993). The GTP-binding protein Ran/TC4 is required for protein import into the nucleus. *Nature, 365,* 661–663.

Mori, K., Rosenzweig, M., & Desrosiers, R. C. (2000). Mechanisms for adaptation of simian immunodeficiency virus to replication in alveolar macrophages. *J Virol, 74,* 10852–10859.

Morikawa, Y., Hockley, D. J., Nermut, M. V., & Jones, I. M. (2000). Roles of matrix, p2, and N-terminal myristoylation in human immunodeficiency virus type 1 Gag assembly. *J Virol, 74,* 16–23.

Morita, E. & Sundquist, W. I. (2004). Retrovirus budding. *Annu Rev Cell Dev Biol, 20,* 395–425.

Moroianu, J., Blobel, G., & Radu, A. (1995). Previously identified protein of uncertain function is karyopherin alpha and together with karyopherin beta docks import substrate at nuclear pore complexes. *Proc Natl Acad Sci USA, 92,* 2008–2011.

Moulard, M. & Decroly, E. (2000). Maturation of HIV envelope glycoprotein precursors by cellular endoproteases. *Biochim Biophys Acta, 1469,* 121–132.

Mujawar, Z., Rose, H., Morrow, M. P., Pushkarsky, T., Dubrovsky, L., Mukhamedova, N., et al. (2006). Human immunodeficiency virus impairs reverse cholesterol transport from macrophages. *PLoS Biol, 4,* e365.

Nabel, G. & Baltimore, D. (1987). An inducible transcription factor activates expression of human immunodeficiency virus in T cells. *Nature, 326,* 711–713.

Naghavi, M. H., Estable, M. C., Schwartz, S., Roeder, R. G., & Vahlne, A. (2001). Upstream stimulating factor affects human immunodeficiency virus type 1 (HIV-1) long terminal repeat-directed transcription in a cell-specific manner, independently of the HIV-1 subtype and the core-negative regulatory element. *J Gen Virol, 82,* 547–559.

Neil, S. J., Sandrin, V., Sundquist, W. I., & Bieniasz, P. D. (2007). An interferon-alpha-induced tethering mechanism inhibits HIV-1 and Ebola virus particle release but is counteracted by the HIV-1 Vpu protein. *Cell Host Microbe, 2,* 193–203.

Neil, S. J., Zang, T., & Bieniasz, P. D. (2008). Tetherin inhibits retrovirus release and is antagonized by HIV-1 Vpu. *Nature, 451,* 425–430.

Nguyen, D. G., Booth, A., Gould, S. J., & Hildreth, J. E. (2003). Evidence that HIV budding in primary macrophages occurs through the exosome release pathway. *J Biol Chem, 278,* 52347–52354.

Nie, Z., Bergeron, D., Subbramanian, R. A., Yao, X. J., Checroune, F., Rougeau, N., et al. (1998). The putative alpha helix 2 of human immunodeficiency virus type 1 Vpr contains a determinant which is responsible for the nuclear translocation of proviral DNA in growth-arrested cells. *J Virol, 72,* 4104–4115.

Nishizawa, M., Kamata, M., Mojin, T., Nakai, Y., & Aida, Y. (2000). Induction of apoptosis by the Vpr protein of human immunodeficiency virus type 1 occurs independently of G(2) arrest of the cell cycle. *Virology, 276,* 16–26.

Nitahara-Kasahara, Y., Kamata, M., Yamamoto, T., Zhang, X., Miyamoto, Y., Muneta, K., et al. (2007). Novel nuclear import of Vpr promoted by importin alpha is crucial for human immunodeficiency virus type 1 replication in macrophages. *J Virol, 81,* 5284–5293.

Nowacek, A. & Gendelman, H. E. (2009). NanoART, neuroAIDS and CNS drug delivery. *Nanomed, 4,* 557–574.

Nydegger, S., Foti, M., Derdowski, A., Spearman, P., & Thali, M. (2003). HIV-1 egress is gated through late endosomal membranes. *Traffic, 4,* 902–910.

O'Brien, W. A., Namazi, A., Kalhor, H., Mao, S. H., Zack, J. A., & Chen, I. S. (1994). Kinetics of human immunodeficiency virus type 1 reverse transcription in blood mononuclear phagocytes are slowed by limitations of nucleotide precursors. *J Virol, 68,* 1258–1263.

Ohagen, A., Ghosh, S., He, J., Huang, K., Chen, Y., Yuan, M., et al. (1999). Apoptosis induced by infection of primary brain cultures with diverse human immunodeficiency virus type 1 isolates: Evidence for a role of the envelope. *J Virol, 73,* 897–906.

Ono, A., Ablan, S. D., Lockett, S. J., Nagashima, K., & Freed, E. O. (2004). Phosphatidylinositol (4,5) bisphosphate regulates HIV-1 Gag targeting to the plasma membrane. *Proc Natl Acad Sci USA, 101,* 14889–14894.

Ono, A. & Freed, E. O. (1999). Binding of human immunodeficiency virus type 1 Gag to membrane: Role of the matrix amino terminus. *J Virol, 73,* 4136–4144.

Ono, A. & Freed, E. O. (2001). Plasma membrane rafts play a critical role in HIV-1 assembly and release. *Proc Natl Acad Sci USA, 98,* 13925–13930.

Ou, W. & Silver, J. (2005). Efficient trapping of HIV-1 envelope protein by hetero-oligomerization with an N-helix chimera. *Retrovirology, 2,* 51.

Pelchen-Matthews, A., Kramer, B., & Marsh, M. (2003). Infectious HIV-1 assembles in late endosomes in primary macrophages. *J Cell Biol, 162,* 443–455.

Pereira, L. A., Bentley, K., Peeters, A., Churchill, M. J., & Deacon, N. J. (2000). A compilation of cellular transcription factor interactions with the HIV-1 LTR promoter. *Nucleic Acids Res, 28,* 663–668.

Perez-Caballero, D., Zang, T., Ebrahimi, A., McNatt, M. W., Gregory, D. A., Johnson, M. C., et al. (2009). Tetherin inhibits HIV-1 release by directly tethering virions to cells. *Cell, 139,* 499–511.

Pierson, T. C., Kieffer, T. L., Ruff, C. T., Buck, C., Gange, S. J., & Siliciano, R. F. (2002). Intrinsic stability of episomal circles formed during human immunodeficiency virus type 1 replication. *J Virol, 76,* 4138–4144.

Piguet, V., Wan, L., Borel, C., Mangasarian, A., Demaurex, N., Thomas, G., et al. (2000). HIV-1 Nef protein binds to the cellular protein PACS-1 to downregulate class I major histocompatibility complexes. *Nat Cell Biol, 2,* 163–167.

Pincetic, A. & Leis, J. (2009). The mechanism of budding of retroviruses from cell membranes. *Adv Virol, 2009,* 6239691–6239699.

Pizzato, M., Helander, A., Popova, E., Calistri, A., Zamborlini, A., Palu, G., et al. (2007). Dynamin 2 is required for the enhancement of HIV-1 infectivity by Nef. *Proc Natl Acad Sci USA, 104,* 6812–6817.

Planelles, V. & Benichou, S. (2010). Vpr and its interactions with cellular proteins. *Curr Top Microbiol Immunol, 339,* 177–200.

Platt, E. J., Wehrly, K., Kuhmann, S. E., Chesebro, B., & Kabat, D. (1998). Effects of CCR5 and CD4 cell surface concentrations on infections by macrophagetropic isolates of human immunodeficiency virus type 1. *J Virol, 72,* 2855–2864.

Pluymers, W., De Clercq, E., & Debyser, Z. (2001). HIV-1 integration as a target for antiretroviral therapy: A review. *Curr Drug Targets Infect Disord, 1,* 133–149.

Poon, B. & Chen, I. S. (2003). Human immunodeficiency virus type 1 (HIV-1) Vpr enhances expression from unintegrated HIV-1 DNA. *J Virol, 77,* 3962–3972.

Popov, S., Rexach, M., Ratner, L., Blobel, G., & Bukrinsky, M. (1998a). Viral protein R regulates docking of the HIV-1 preintegration complex to the nuclear pore complex. *J Biol Chem, 273*, 13347–13352.

Popov, S., Rexach, M., Zybarth, G., Reiling, N., Lee, M. A., Ratner, L., et al. (1998b). Viral protein R regulates nuclear import of the HIV-1 pre-integration complex. *EMBO J, 17*, 909–917.

Premack, B. A. & Schall, T. J. (1996). Chemokine receptors: Gateways to inflammation and infection. *Nat Med, 2*, 1174–1178.

Pruss, D., Bushman, F. D., & Wolffe, A. P. (1994a). Human immunodeficiency virus integrase directs integration to sites of severe DNA distortion within the nucleosome core. *Proc Natl Acad Sci USA, 91*, 5913–5917.

Pruss, D., Reeves, R., Bushman, F. D., & Wolffe, A. P. (1994b). The influence of DNA and nucleosome structure on integration events directed by HIV integrase. *J Biol Chem, 269*, 25031–25041.

Pryciak, P. M. & Varmus, H. E. (1992). Nucleosomes, DNA-binding proteins, and DNA sequence modulate retroviral integration target site selection. *Cell, 69*, 769–780.

Pushkarsky, T., Dubrovsky, L., & Bukrinsky, M. (2001). Lipopolysaccharide stimulates HIV-1 entry and degradation in human macrophages. *J Endotoxin Res, 7*, 271–276.

Rain, J. C., Cribier, A., Gerard, A., Emiliani, S., & Benarous, R. (2009). Yeast two-hybrid detection of integrase-host factor interactions. *Methods, 47*, 291–297.

Reil, H., Bukovsky, A. A., Gelderblom, H. R., & Gottlinger, H. G. (1998). Efficient HIV-1 replication can occur in the absence of the viral matrix protein. *EMBO J, 17*, 2699–2708.

Rexach, M. & Blobel, G. (1995). Protein import into nuclei: Association and dissociation reactions involving transport substrate, transport factors, and nucleoporins. *Cell, 83*, 683–692.

Riviere, L., Darlix, J. L., & Cimarelli, A. (2010). Analysis of the viral elements required in the nuclear import of HIV-1 DNA. *J Virol, 84*, 729–739.

Roe, T., Reynolds, T. C., Yu, G., & Brown, P. O. (1993). Integration of murine leukemia virus DNA depends on mitosis. *EMBO J, 12*, 2099–2108.

Saad, J. S., Miller, J., Tai, J., Kim, A., Ghanam, R. H., & Summers, M. F. (2006). Structural basis for targeting HIV-1 Gag proteins to the plasma membrane for virus assembly. *Proc Natl Acad Sci USA, 103*, 11364–11369.

Sakuragi, J. I., Ueda, S., Iwamoto, A., & Shioda, T. (2003). Possible role of dimerization in human immunodeficiency virus type 1 genome RNA packaging. *J Virol, 77*, 4060–4069.

Schindler, M., Munch, J., Kutsch, O., Li, H., Santiago, M. L., Bibollet-Ruche, F., et al. (2006). Nef-mediated suppression of T cell activation was lost in a lentiviral lineage that gave rise to HIV-1. *Cell, 125*, 1055–1067.

Schindler, M., Rajan, D., Banning, C., Wimmer, P., Koppensteiner, H., Iwanski, A., et al. (2010). Vpu serine 52 dependent counteraction of tetherin is required for HIV-1 replication in macrophages, but not in ex vivo human lymphoid tissue. *Retrovirology, 7*, 1.

Schmidtmayerova, H., Nuovo, G. J., & Bukrinsky, M. (1997). Cell proliferation is not required for productive HIV-1 infection of macrophages. *Virology, 232*, 379–384.

Schroder, A. R., Shinn, P., Chen, H., Berry, C., Ecker, J. R., & Bushman, F. (2002). HIV-1 integration in the human genome favors active genes and local hotspots. *Cell, 110*, 521–529.

Schuitemaker, H., Kootstra, N. A., Fouchier, R. A., Hooibrink, B., & Miedema, F. (1994). Productive HIV-1 infection of macrophages restricted to the cell fraction with proliferative capacity. *EMBO J, 13*, 5929–5936.

Segura-Totten, M. & Wilson, K. L. (2001). Virology. HIV—breaking the rules for nuclear entry. *Science, 294*, 1016–1017.

Sharova, N., Wu, Y., Zhu, X., Stranska, R., Kaushik, R., Sharkey, M., et al. (2008). Primate lentiviral Vpx commandeers DDB1 to counteract a macrophage restriction. *PLoS Pathogens, 4*, e1000057.

Sheehy, A. M., Gaddis, N. C., Choi, J. D., & Malim, M. H. (2002). Isolation of a human gene that inhibits HIV-1 infection and is suppressed by the viral Vif protein. *Nature, 418*, 646–650.

Sherer, N. M., Lehmann, M. J., Jimenez-Soto, L. F., Ingmundson, A., Horner, S. M., Cicchetti, G., et al. (2003). Visualization of retroviral replication in living cells reveals budding into multivesicular bodies. *Traffic, 4*, 785–801.

Siebenlist, U., Franzoso, G., & Brown, K. (1994). Structure, regulation and function of NF-kappa B. *Annu Rev Cell Biol, 10*, 405–455.

Smit, T. K., Wang, B., Ng, T., Osborne, R., Brew, B., & Saksena, N. K. (2001). Varied tropism of HIV-1 isolates derived from different regions of adult brain cortex discriminate between patients with and without AIDS dementia complex (ADC): Evidence for neurotropic HIV variants. *Virology, 279*, 509–526.

Sodeik, B., Ebersold, M. W., & Helenius, A. (1997). Microtubule-mediated transport of incoming herpes simplex virus 1 capsids to the nucleus. *J Cell Biol, 136*, 1007–1021.

Sokolskaja, E. & Luban, J. (2006). Cyclophilin, TRIM5, and innate immunity to HIV-1. *Curr Opin Microbiol, 9*, 404–408.

Sonza, S., Mutimer, H. P., O'Brien, K., Ellery, P., Howard, J. L., Axelrod, J. H., et al. (2002). Selectively reduced tat mRNA heralds the decline in productive human immunodeficiency virus type 1 infection in monocyte-derived macrophages. *J Virol, 76*, 12611–12621.

Soros, V. B., Yonemoto, W., & Greene, W. C. (2007). Newly synthesized APOBEC3G is incorporated into HIV virions, inhibited by HIV RNA, and subsequently activated by RNase H. *PLoS Pathog, 3*, e15.

Srivastava, S., Swanson, S. K., Manel, N., Florens, L., Washburn, M. P., & Skowronski, J. (2008). Lentiviral Vpx accessory factor targets VprBP/DCAF1 substrate adaptor for cullin 4 E3 ubiquitin ligase to enable macrophage infection. *PLoS Pathog, 4*, e1000059.

Stevenson, M. & Gendelman, H. E. (1994). Cellular and viral determinants that regulate HIV-1 infection in macrophages. *J Leukoc Biol, 56*, 278–288.

Subbramanian, R. A., Kessous-Elbaz, A., Lodge, R., Forget, J., Yao, X. J., Bergeron, D., et al. (1998). Human immunodeficiency virus type 1 Vpr is a positive regulator of viral transcription and infectivity in primary human macrophages. *J Exp Med, 187*, 1103–1111.

Suhasini, M. & Reddy, T. R. (2009). Cellular proteins and HIV-1 Rev function. *Curr HIV Res, 7*, 91–100.

Suomalainen, M., Nakano, M. Y., Keller, S., Boucke, K., Stidwill, R. P., & Greber, U. F. (1999). Microtubule-dependent plus- and minus end-directed motilities are competing processes for nuclear targeting of adenovirus. *J Cell Biol, 144*, 657–672.

Swigut, T., Shohdy, N., & Skowronski, J. (2001). Mechanism for down-regulation of CD28 by Nef. *EMBO J, 20*, 1593–1604.

Taunton, J. (2001). Actin filament nucleation by endosomes, lysosomes and secretory vesicles. *Curr Opin Cell Biol, 13*, 85–91.

Terry, L. J. & Wente, S. R. (2009). Flexible gates: Dynamic topologies and functions for FG nucleoporins in nucleocytoplasmic transport. *Eukaryot Cell, 8*, 1814–1827.

Tristem, M., Purvis, A., & Quicke, D. L. (1998). Complex evolutionary history of primate lentiviral vpr genes. *Virology, 240*, 232–237.

Turchan, J., Pocernich, C. B., Gairola, C., Chauhan, A., Schifitto, G., Butterfield, D. A., et al. (2003). Oxidative stress in HIV demented patients and protection ex vivo with novel antioxidants. *Neurology, 60*, 307–314.

Van Damme, N., Goff, D., Katsura, C., Jorgenson, R. L., Mitchell, R., Johnson, M. C., et al. (2008). The interferon-induced protein BST-2 restricts HIV-1 release and is downregulated from the cell surface by the viral Vpu protein. *Cell Host Microbe, 3*, 245–252.

Van Marle, G., Rourke, S. B., Zhang, K., Silva, C., Ethier, J., Gill, M. J., et al. (2002). HIV dementia patients exhibit reduced viral neutralization and increased envelope sequence diversity in blood and brain. *AIDS, 16*, 1905–1914.

Vodicka, M. A., Koepp, D. M., Silver, P. A., & Emerman, M. (1998). HIV-1 Vpr interacts with the nuclear transport pathway to promote macrophage infection. *Genes Dev, 12*, 175–185.

Weinberg, J. B., Matthews, T. J., Cullen, B. R., & Malim, M. H. (1991). Productive human immunodeficiency virus type 1 (HIV-1) infection of nonproliferating human monocytes. *J Exp Med, 174*, 1477–1482.

Woodward, C. L., Prakobwanakit, S., Mosessian, S., & Chow, S. A. (2009). Integrase interacts with nucleoporin NUP153 to mediate the nuclear import of human immunodeficiency virus type 1. *J Virol*, *83*, 6522–6533.

Wu, Y. & Marsh, J. W. (2003). Early transcription from nonintegrated DNA in human immunodeficiency virus infection. *J Virol*, *77*, 10376–10382.

Wu, Y., Yoder, A., Yu, D., Wang, W., Liu, J., Barrett, T., et al. (2008). Cofilin activation in peripheral CD4 T cells of HIV-1 infected patients: A pilot study. *Retrovirology*, *5*, 95.

Yamashita, M. & Emerman, M. (2006). Retroviral infection of non-dividing cells: Old and new perspectives. *Virology*, *344*, 88–93.

Yamashita, M., Perez, O., Hope, T. J., & Emerman, M. (2007). Evidence for direct involvement of the capsid protein in HIV infection of non-dividing cells. *PLoS Pathog*, *3*, 1502–1510.

Yi, Y., Chen, W., Frank, I., Cutilli, J., Singh, A., Starr-Spires, L.,et al. (2003). An unusual syncytia-inducing human immunodeficiency virus type 1 primary isolate from the central nervous system that is restricted to CXCR4, replicates efficiently in macrophages, and induces neuronal apoptosis. *J Neurovirol*, *9*, 432–441.

Yoder, A., Yu, D., Dong, L., Iyer, S. R., Xu, X., Kelly, J., et al. (2008). HIV Envelope-CXCR4 signaling activates cofilin to overcome cortical actin restriction in resting CD4 T cells. *Cell*, *134*, 782–792.

Yuan, X., Yu, X., Lee, T. H., & Essex, M. (1993). Mutations in the N-terminal region of human immunodeficiency virus type 1 matrix protein block intracellular transport of the Gag precursor. *J Virol*, *67*, 6387–6394.

Zack, J. A., Arrigo, S. J., Weitsman, S. R., Go, A. S., Haislip, A., & Chen, I. S. (1990). HIV-1 entry into quiescent primary lymphocytes: Molecular analysis reveals a labile, latent viral structure. *Cell*, *61*, 213–222.

Zennou, V., Perez-Caballero, D., Gottlinger, H., & Bieniasz, P. D. (2004). APOBEC3G incorporation into human immunodeficiency virus type 1 particles. *J Virol*, *78*, 12058–12061.

Zennou, V., Petit, C., Guetard, D., Nerhbass, U., Montagnier, L., & Charneau, P. (2000). HIV-1 genome nuclear import is mediated by a central DNA flap. *Cell*, *101*, 173–185.

Zhang, H., Dornadula, G., & Pomerantz, R. J. (1996). Endogenous reverse transcription of human immunodeficiency virus type 1 in physiological microenviroments: An important stage for viral infection of nondividing cells. *J Virol*, *70*, 2809–2824.

Zhang, H., Dornadula, G., & Pomerantz, R. J. (1998). Natural endogenous reverse transcription of HIV type 1. *AIDS Res Hum Retroviruses*, *14 Suppl 1*:S93–5, S93–S95.

Zheng, J., Thylin, M. R., Ghorpade, A., Xiong, H., Persidsky, Y., Cotter, R., et al. (1999). Intracellular CXCR4 signaling, neuronal apoptosis and neuropathogenic mechanisms of HIV-1-associated dementia. *J Neuroimmunol*, *98*, 185–200.

Zybarth, G., Reiling, N., Schmidtmayerova, H., Sherry, B., & Bukrinsky, M. (1999). Activation-induced resistance of human macrophages to HIV-1 infection in vitro. *J Immunol*, *162*, 400–406.

1.2

HIV-1 IMMUNOLOGY

Sabita Roy, Krishnakumar Devadas, Subhash Dhawan, and Shilpa Buch

This chapter serves as a bridge between the molecular and structural biology of the human immunodeficiency virus type one (HIV-1) and the immunological consequences that viral infection produces. The innate and adaptive immune systems and their responses play a critical role in the control of HIV replication. Unfortunately, immune dysfunction is common in HIV-infected individuals and the virus as well is capable of developing strategies to evade host defenses. Thus, in most untreated individuals, if viral replication is not fully contained, persistent viremia is sustained, eventually resulting in progressive disease and the development of acquired immunodeficiency syndrome (AIDS).

GENETIC ORGANIZATION OF HIV-1

HIV primarily targets the immune system and therefore the clinical consequences are manifested because of immune dysfunction and depletion. HIV-1 is a member of the primate lentivirus subgroup of retroviruses (Weiss et al., 1986, 2008; Burton & Weiss, 2010 Kellam & Weiss, 2006), and is a close relative of HIV-2 and simian immunodeficiency viruses (SIV). The HIV-1 particle is composed of two identical (+) strand RNA copies of the viral genome (Weiss et al., 1986, 2009). Following infection of host cell, the RNA genome is reversed transcribed into DNA or a provirus. The 5' and the 3' ends of the provirus contain 634 nucleotides of long terminal repeat structures (Figure 1.2.1). While the 5' LTR regulates the initiation of RNA transcription, the 3' LTR regulates RNA termination and polyadenylation. Gag and env genes encode the structural protein of the virus particle. Virus entry is regulated by the envelope proteins which are embedded in the lipid bilayer and mediate receptor binding and membrane fusion. The pol gene encodes the viral protease, reverse transcriptase, ribonuclease H, and integrase. The regulatory proteins Tat and Rev influence the replication of HIV by mediating their effects through the Tat response element and the Rev response element (RRE), respectively. Accessory proteins, which are at least partially dispensable for virus replication in vitro, are encoded by Vif, Vpr, Vpu, and Nef. Vif, a virion infectivity factor, promotes infectivity of virus particles but is not packaged to a significant extent in the virus particle. Vpr, a viral protein R, is homologous to Vpx, a viral protein X, of HIV-2 and SIVs, and is packaged into the virus particle, but its function is incompletely described. Vpu, viral protein U, is required for efficient virus budding and

CD4 downregulation. Nef, that is, "negative factor," has multiple effects on virus replication and T cell activation. The envelope proteins play an important role in interactions with cellular receptor membrane, in membrane fusion effects, and in initiation of signal transduction into cells. The presentation of viral proteins to T cells is a critical early step in the immune response to HIV-1. Class 1 and class II restricted epitopes are located throughout the HIV-1 env protein. Analysis of these epitopes has provided new insights into antigen processing pathways and vaccine design strategies.

EARLY EVENTS FOLLOWING HIV-1 INFECTION

Attachment of the virus particle to the cell surface is the initial step in the infection process. Fusion of the viral and cellular membranes allows for the delivery of the viral core into the cytoplasm of the cell. The process of attachment and fusion is mediated by the interaction of viral glycoprotein spikes with cell surface receptors. HIV-1 glycoprotein spikes specifically interact with the CD4 receptor and a seven-trans-membrane G-protein coupled co-receptor on the cell surface. There is 1:1 binding stoichiometry of a monomer of gp120 with CD4. The binding of one CD4 molecule by a single gp120 in the trimeric spike is sufficient to induce conformational changes in all three glycoprotein subunits of the trimer (Salzwedel & Berger, 2000). The interaction of CD4 and co-receptor with the gp120 causes a rearrangement in gp41

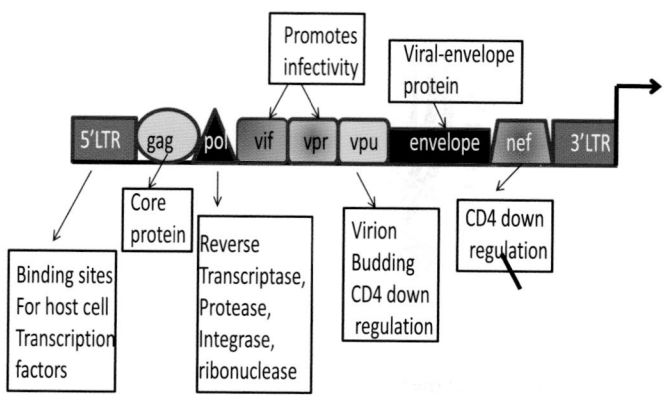

Figure 1.2.1 Genetic organization of the HIV-1 genome. Location of each gene are shown together with their function.

exposing the hydrophobic fusion domain, which then comes in contact with the cell membrane and becomes embedded into it, leading to viral entry (Figure 1.2.2).

During the viral entry process, the viral envelope disassociates from the virion, initiating the process of uncoating. Once inside the cell, further uncoating involves the disintegration of the viral capsid core and shedding of the capsid proteins (Figure 1.2.3).

The uncoating process involves the cellular protein cyclophilin A, which interacts with HIV-1 Gag polyprotein and is incorporated into the virion prior to reverse transcription (Franke, Yuan, & Luban, 1994; Thali, Bukovsky, & Kondo, 1994; Braaten, Franke, & Luban, 1996). The main early event in the life cycle of HIV-l is the reverse transcription of viral RNA into double-stranded DNA. This is catalyzed in the cytoplasm of the infected cell by the virus-encoded reverse transcriptase through the use of a cellular lysine tRNA molecule as a primer (Cen et al., 2001). Several viral and cellular factors are involved in the formation of the replication complex. The replication complex consists of the viral DNA/RNA, reverse transcriptase, integrase, viral matrix protein p17, viral protease, the accessory protein Vpr, and cellular histones and non-histone proteins. During the formation of the replication complex, various core viral proteins are lost. This replication complex, also termed the pre-integration complex, is subsequently transported into the nucleus.

The entry of the HIV-l pre-integration complex into the nucleus is mediated by the interaction between the cellular receptor karyopherin alpha and the nuclear localization signals (NLS) present on viral proteins, matrix, and integrase (Bukrinsky & Haffar, 1999). The viral protein Vpr increases the affinity of interaction between the viral NLS and the cellular receptor karyopherin alpha, facilitating nuclear

transport of the pre-integration complex (Popov et al., 1998). Additional factors contribute to the nuclear transport of the pre-integration complex, including a triple-stranded intermediate produced during reverse transcription, called the DNA flap (Sherman & Greene, 2002). The viral integrase then catalyzes a series of reactions whereby the intact viral DNA is inserted into the cellular chromosomal DNA forming the provirus. The first step of the integration process is the removal of two nucleotides from the 3' ends of the viral DNA. In the second step, the host chromosome is randomly cut producing a 5-base staggered cut. This is followed by the insertion of the viral DNA. The third and final step consists of removal of unpaired bases at the 5' end of viral DNA, gap filling, and ligation. The first two steps are catalyzed by integrase, but the repair and ligation steps are thought to be mediated by cellular enzymes (Craigie, 2001).

The early phase of the viral replication cycle ends following DNA integration and the virus enters the late phase of its life cycle and begins to multiply. The provirus is far more efficient in transcription of viral RNA than the free unintegrated HIV-1 viral DNA. The provirus produces multiple copies of the progeny viral RNA and mRNAs that are later translated into viral proteins. HIV-1 proviral transcription is greatly influenced by the activation state of the host cell and is regulated by sequences in the 5' long terminal repeat (LTR) of the viral genome. A large number of these regulatory sequences are able to specifically bind cellular transcription factors, thus enabling the HIV-1 provirus to use the cellular transcription machinery to replicate.

The HIV-1 primary transcript is the 9.2 kb mRNA, which is the full-length transcript encoding the Gag and Pol proteins. Translation initiation starts with the Gag open reading frame. The major translation product is the Gag polyprotein (p55), which is first translated as a precursor polyprotein and later cleaved by the viral protease. The Gag precursor polyprotein (p55) is also modified by myristoylation. The mature proteins derived from the gag precursor polyprotein consist of the matrix protein (MA) p17, the capsid protein (CA) p24, the nucleocapsid protein (NC) p7, and the p6 protein that binds to the Vpr protein. The minor translation product is the Gag-Pol precursor p160. The Pol gene products derived from the Gag-Pol polyprotein are the viral protease (Pr) p11, reverse transcriptase (RT) p66, and integrase (IN) p31. The primary transcript also serves as genomic RNA for the production of progeny virions after being capped at the 5' end and polyadenylated at the 3' end. The 4 kb transcript contains mRNAs encoding the Env proteins, Vif, Vpr, and Vpu proteins, as well as mRNAs for the minor forms of the Tat protein. The 4 kb transcript coding for the envelope proteins is first translated as a polyprotein and subsequently glycosylated. The glycosylated precursor polyprotein (gp160) is transported to the rough endoplasmic reticulum where it forms oligomers and enters the secretory pathway. A cellular enzyme in the Golgi apparatus then cleaves these oligomers to produce the surface glycoprotein (gp120) and the transmembrane glycoprotein (gp4l). The oligomeric forms of gp120 and gp41 are finally transported to the plasma membrane. The 2 kb transcript contains mRNAs encoding Nef, Rev, and the major forms of Tat proteins

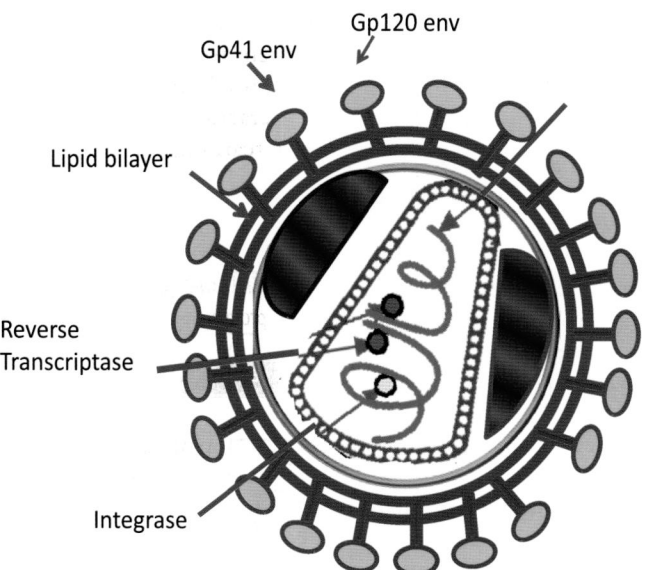

Figure 1.2.2 Structure of the HIV-1 virion. The envelope subunit proteins (gp41 and gp120), matrix protein (p18), viral capsid protein (p24), viral genomic RNA (RNA), and the reverse transcriptase enzyme CRT) are illustrated.

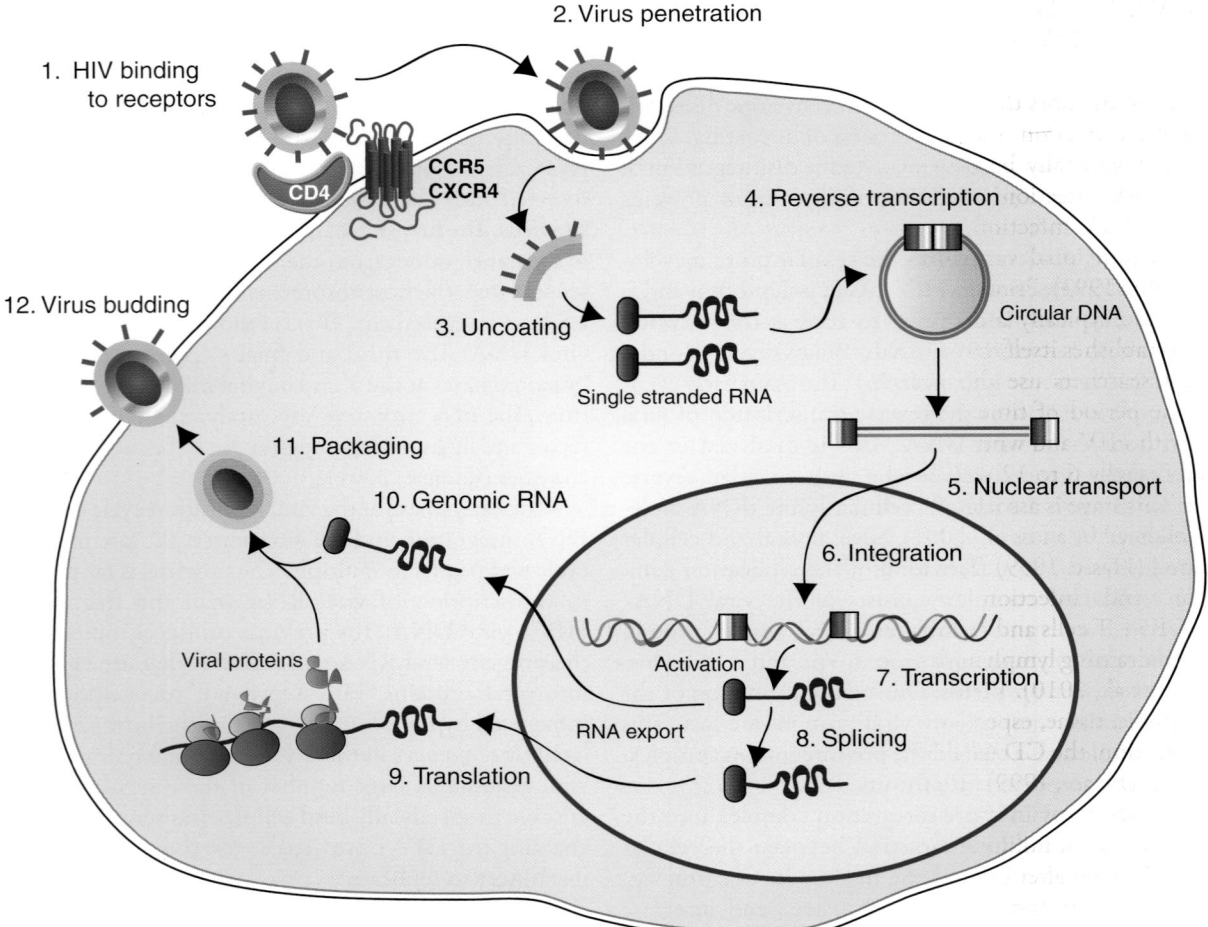

Figure 1.2.3 The replication cycle of the HIV-1 virion. HIV binds to CD4 receptors on the surface of T cells or macrophages and to one of two co-receptors, CCR5 and CXCR4. The next event involves the fusion of the viral protein gp41 to the host cell membranes. After the fusion event, the virus capsid is partially uncoated to form a ribonucleoprotein complex capable of reverse transcription. Viral genomic RNA is reverse transcribed to yield double stranded viral DNA. Viral DNA forms the pre-integration complex and is transported to the cell nucleus where it is integrated in to the cellular chromosome to form the provirus. From the provirus, the viral RNAs and proteins are expressed. Viral assembly and budding occur at the cell membrane forming the progeny virus.

(Purcell & Martin, 1993). All HIV-l RNA transcripts contain a transcription regulation sequence called TAR (transactivation-responsive or Tat-activation responsive) sequence. The 9 kb and 4 kb HIV-l RNA transcripts also contain a post-transcription regulatory sequence called an RRE (Rev-responsive element) sequence. These sequences are involved in the activation and regulation of viral RNA expression through interactions with the viral regulatory proteins Tat and Rev.

The exact mechanism of viral assembly and maturation is poorly understood. Viral assembly is energy dependent and probably involves unidentified cellular factors (Treitel & Resh, 2001). Viral assembly involves the transportation of the Gag and Gag-Pol precursor polyproteins and the envelope glycoproteins to the plasma membrane followed by the assembly of the viral capsid proteins and finally the packaging of HIV-l genomic RNA. Budding, the final stage of progeny virus production, is by the process of exocytosis. The Gag precursor proteins and viral components form the major components of the budding

virus. In addition, cellular components including tRNAs and proteins are also incorporated into the budding virions.

Viral budding occurs at the plasma membrane of infected T cells, whereas in infected macrophages budding occurs at intracellular membrane sites, forming vacuoles containing the viral progeny (Gelderblom, 1991). During the maturation stage, the Gag and Gag-Pol precursor polyproteins are cleaved to yield mature viral proteins, the capsid core is formed, and the dimerization of viral RNA takes place. These events are believed to occur after budding has taken place.

An alternate route of HIV-l infection is by cell-to-cell transmission. One mechanism is the fusion of HIV-l infected cells with uninfected susceptible cells. The fusion event brings the infectious viral components into the uninfected cell, forming multinucleated giant cells (syncytia). This process is very efficient and does not involve cell-free virus. The other mechanism involves the unidirectional budding of HIV-l at the site of cell-to-cell contact.

IMMUNE RESPONSE FOLLOWING HIV-1 INFECTION

HIV infection disrupts the immune system through generalized immune activation and CD4+ T cell depletion. HIV infection can generally be broken down into four distinct stages: primary infection, a clinically asymptomatic stage, symptomatic HIV infection, and progression from HIV to AIDS, with individual variation in length, symptoms, and severity (Fauci, 1993). Primary HIV infection is the first stage of HIV disease, typically lasting only a week or two, when the virus first establishes itself in the body (Figure 1.2.4).

Some researchers use the term acute HIV infection to describe the period of time between when a person is first infected with HIV and when antibodies against the virus are produced (usually 6 to 12 weeks) and can be detected by an HIV test. This stage is associated with high levels of viral replication followed by a loss of CD4+ T cells in the gut and later in the blood (Hasse, 1999). This phase is characterized by the replication and infection of cells that express both CD4+CCR5+ T cells and remains localized in genital/rectal mucosa and draining lymph nodes (Gasper-Smith et. al, 2008; McMichael et al., 2010). Virus then spreads via the blood to other lymphoid tissue, especially in the gut. Even at an early stage of infection, the CD 4+T lymphocytes appear to be the major targets (Haase, 1999). There, it replicates profusely and the level of free virus in the blood rises exponentially and reaches a peak, often millions of virus copies per milliliter of plasma, 21–28 days after infection. Virus population doubles every 6 to 10 hours and the infected cell can productively infect 20 new cells (Nowak et al., 1997; Little, McLean, Spina, Richman, & Havlir, 1999). Virus levels then fall, rapidly at first, until a stable level is reached. This high level of viremia at the primary stage may be responsible for the systemic infection of the peripheral lymphoid organs. Within a few weeks of the initial viremia, the level of the virus decreases in the blood. This decrease coincides with the development of an immune response to HIV-l. Virus-specific cytolytic T lymphocytes (CTL) appear early and may play an important role in down-regulation of virus replication (Borrow et al., 1991 Pantaleo et al., 1994; Schmitz et al., 1999). HIV-1 infection may go undetected for long periods due to the nonspecific nature of the symptoms (Weber, 2001). Early CD8+ T cell responses are generally credited for controlling the initial peak of viral replication and establishment of a viral set point and partial recovery of CD4+ T cells in the periphery (Koup, Safrit, & Cao, 1994; Goonetilleke et al., 2009; Almeida et al., 2007). When CD4+ T cell numbers decline to critical levels, cell-mediated immunity is compromised, and the patient develops AIDS.

It is uncertain how the peak viremia of acute HIV-1 infection is controlled. Some mathematical models (Phillips, 1996; Davenport et al., 2007; Petravic, 2008) suggest that the rampant early infection results in the massive destruction of CD4+ T cells in the gut (Brenchley, 2004; Guadalupe et al., 2003) and elsewhere such that the cell substrate becomes limiting. However, studies in rhesus macaques infected with simian immunodeficiency virus (SIV) show that reduction of peak viremia is dependent on the presence of CD8+ cells (Schmitz et al., 1999) and either T or NK cells, or both. In HIV-1 infection, virus-specific CD8+ T cells first appear in the blood just before the viremia peaks and then expand and contract as virus load falls (Borrow et al., 1991 Koup, Safrit, & Cao, 1994; Wilson et al., 2000). HIV-1–specific CD8+ T cells are detectable before the development of detectable specific antibodies to HIV-1 and long before neutralizing antibodies (Huber & Trkola, 2007) are detected.

Three mechanisms are proposed by which CD8+ T cells suppress viral replication. In the first mechanism, IFN-gamma, an antiviral cytokine, is produced, which in turn inhibits HIV-1 replication (Meylan, Guatelli, Munis, Richman, & Kornbluth, 1993; Emilie, Maillot, Nicholas, Fior, & Galanaud, 1992). In addition, the chemokines MIP-1 -alpha, MIP-1 beta, and RANTES are secreted to suppress HIV-1 replication by competing or downregulating the cellular co-receptor CCR5. Downregulation of the co-receptor protects uninfected cells by limiting the availability of virus co-receptor (Wagner, Yang, & Garcia-Zepeda, 1998; Price et al., 1998). The second mechanism involves the lysis of virus-infected 'target' cells via Fas–FasL interaction, and FAS mediated apoptosis. Inhibition of HIV-1 replication in the third mechanism involves lysis of the cell through secretion of perforins and granzymes (Kagi, Seiler, & Pavlovic, 1995). CD8+ CTLs recognize viral antigens that have been intracellularly processed into peptides. These viral peptides, which are typically 8–11 amino acids in length, are presented on the infected cell together with a class I major histocompatibility complex (MHC) molecule and β2 microglobulin. The receptor on the CD8+ T cells recognizes the MHC class I molecule, β2 microglobulin, and the viral peptide complex. This recognition by the CTLs triggers the lysis of the infected cells. Cultured HIV-1 specific CTLs have been shown to lyse CD8+ CTL

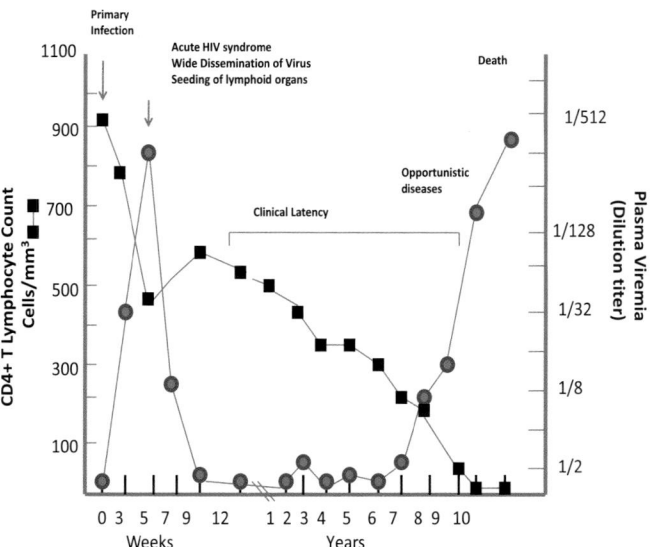

Figure 1.2.4 Time course of HIV-1 infection (redrawn from Pantaleo et al., 1993, with permission).

cells in vitro (Yang, Kalams, & Rosenzweig, 1996). The virus-specific CD8+ T-cell responses are narrowly directed against a limited number of CTL epitopes despite exposure to a high level of viral antigens (Yu et al., 2002). The most frequently recognized viral epitopes are derived from the Gag, Pol, Env, and Nef proteins (Goulder et al 1996). Interestingly, epitopes derived from Tat, Rev, and Vif proteins are encountered at a lower frequency (Lamhamedi-Cherradi, Culman-Penciolelli, & Guy, 1995). In addition, viral replication is downregulated by the expression of membrane-bound Fas ligands that induce apoptosis in Fas-expressing cells (Kagi et al., 1995).

In addition to the CTL responses, cellular immune response consists of specific CD4+ T helper (Th-I) cell responses. Viral proteins that are endocytosed by antigen-presenting cells are cleaved into peptide antigens triggering the CD4+ T cell response. The antigens that are presented on the surface of the antigen-presenting cells, together with the MHC class II molecules are recognized by the CD4+ T cell receptor, which triggers the activation and differentiation of the CD4+T cells. Activated Th-1 cells produce cytokines such as interleukin-2 (IL-2) and IFN-γ (Th-1 response), which help to sustain the CTL response. Th-2 effector T cells secrete interleukins IL-4, IL-5, IL-6 and IL-1 0, which help in promoting B-cell responses to infection. In addition, the Th-1 cells activate antigen-presenting cells, such as dendritic cells, which further promote an effective immune response.

The combined effects of CTL and other elements of immune response cause the viral load in blood to decrease drastically. The cellular immune response is followed by an effective humoral response (Koup, Safrit, & Cao, 1994). In the primary acute phase of HIV-1 infection, partial viral clearance occurs before the specific antibody response is generated. Despite the early appearance of a vigorous immune response, this response ultimately fails to eliminate the virus. Several virological characteristics, such as the replication and mutation rate, proviral latency, and sequestration of viral reservoirs, play an important role in the immune evasion of HIV-1 (McMichael & Rowland-Jones, 2001). Transition of virus from R5 to X4 type, when the co-receptor requirement is changed from CCR5 to CXCR4 makes the virus resistant to inhibition by chemokines released by activated T cells. Other factors, like the downregulation of MHC molecules (Collins et al., 1998) and the upregulation of Fas ligands (Xu et al., 1999), contribute to the immune evasion and persistence of HIV-1 infection leading to disease progression.

The second phase of HIV-1 infection is the long asymptomatic period between the acute primary infection phase and the development of clinical immunodeficiency (AIDS). During this stage, HIV-1 continuously replicates in the infected cells and can be readily detected in the lymphoid tissues. This persistent viral replication and the associated chronic immune stimulation have been proposed to be responsible for the progressive destruction of lymphoid tissue and deterioration of the immune system. The immunological hallmark of this asymptomatic period leading to progression of AIDS is the gradual *loss* of CD4+T cells. The rate of CD4+ T-cell loss correlates with the level of ongoing viral replication; however, the exact mechanism by which HIV-I causes the depletion of CD4+ T cells is not known. There is increasing evidence that T cell activation, accelerated cell turnover, and imbalance of cytokines induces "cell cycle dysregulation" (CCD), which can result in the depletion of both CD4+ and CD8+ uninfected T cells (Gallati & Bocchino, 2007). A series of recent studies have proposed that the depletion of CD4+ T cells is more rapid and severe at the level of gut-associated lymphoid tissue than in peripheral blood and secondary lymphoid organs (i.e., lymph nodes and spleen) (Haase, 2005; Paiardini, Frank, Pandrea, Apetrei, & Silvestri, 2008). Identifying distinctions between pathogenic HIV and simian immunodeficiency virus (SIV) infections and nonprogressive SIV in natural African primate hosts might provide key insights into HIV pathogenesis. Similar to pathogenic HIV infection in humans, natural SIV infections result in high viral replication and massive acute depletion of mucosal CD4+ T cells. A key distinction of natural SIV infections is a rapidly developing anti-inflammatory milieu that prevents chronic activation, apoptosis, and proliferation of T cells, and preserves the function of other immune cell subsets, thus contributing to the integrity of the mucosal barrier and the lack of microbial translocation from the gut to the peritoneum. Immunologic features observed during natural SIV infections suggest approaches for designing new strategies for producing novel second-generation vaccines and therapeutic approaches to inhibit disease progression in HIV-infected humans (Pandrea et al., 2008).

More recently, the FOXP3(+)/CD8(+) T (Treg) population has been implicated to play a key role in controlling the magnitude and duration of adaptive immune responses through suppression of T cell activation (Torheim et al., 2009). A rapid expansion of CD25(+)/FOXP3(+)/CD8(+) regulatory T cells (Tregs) in the blood, lymphoid and colorectal mucosal tissues, preferential sites of virus replication, has been demonstrated following a pathogenic SIV infection in rhesus macaques (Nigam et al., 2010). Expression of molecules associated with immune suppressor function such as CTLA-4 and CD39 were associated with these Tregs with suppressed proliferation of SIV-specific T cells in vitro. These also express low levels of granzyme B and perforin, suggesting that these cells do not possess killing potential. Expansion of CD8+ Tregs correlated directly with acute phase viremia and inversely with the magnitude of antiviral T cell response. Expansion was observed in HIV-infected humans but not in SIV-infected sooty mangabeys with high viremia, suggesting a direct role for hyperimmune activation and an indirect role for viremia in the induction of these cells. These results suggest an important but previously unappreciated role for CD8+ Tregs in suppressing antiviral immunity during immunodeficiency virus infections. These results also suggest that CD8+ Tregs expand in pathogenic immunodeficiency virus infections in the non-natural hosts and that therapeutic strategies that prevent expansion of these cells may enhance control of HIV infection.

The final phase of infection (symptomatic HIV infection, and progression from HIV to AIDS) is characterized by the onset of clinical immunodeficiency commonly known as acquired immunodeficiency syndrome (AIDS). Prior to the onset of clinical immunodeficiency, there is a rapid decline in CD4+ T cell count and an overall increase in viral load (Connor, Mohri, Cao, & Ho, 1993). Viral replication occurs in many sites in addition to the lymphoid tissue (Reinhart et al., 1997). When the CD4+ T cell counts fall below 200 cells/ml, opportunistic infections begin to surface. The average period for the development of AIDS after initial infection varies among infected individuals. Prospective studies involving large cohorts of HIV-infected individuals clearly indicate that while some individuals remain asymptomatic for as long as 10 years after initial infection (long-term non-progressors; LTNPs), others develop AIDS within 24 months (rapid progressors; RPs). Among these individuals are some who progress to AIDS similarly to rapid progressors, but in whom both clinical and laboratory parameters remain stable for an unusually long period of time once the disease progression has occurred (slow progressors; SPs).

Between the multitude of factors that govern the natural history and pathogenesis of HIV-1 infection, viral and host factors and their complex interactions are considered crucial determinants of disease outcome (Fauci, 1993; Schnittman & Fauci, 1994; Pantaleo, Graziosi, & Fauci, 1997; Burinsky, Stanwick, & Dempsey, 1991; Wahl & Orenstein, 1997; Haynes, 1996; McCune, 1995;; Pantaleo & Fauci, 1994). For instance, LTNPs appear to have predominantly Th1 -T cell profiles, strong CD8+ lymphocyte antiviral responses, absence of enhancing antibodies, low viral loads, and predominantly non-syncytium-inducing (NSI) viral phenotypes, whereas RPs have high viral loads and predominantly syncytium-inducing (S1) viral phenotypes. RPs are believed to be infected with more rapidly replicating virulent HIV strains, whereas NPs may be infected with less pathogenic HIV variants. Thus, preservation of immune function and low viral replication are common findings in HIV-infected subjects with non-progressive disease, whereas loss of immune function and high viremia are characteristic features for rapid progression (Haynes et al., 1996). However, with the advent of combination antiretroviral therapies, there are some changes in the natural history of HIV disease (Feinberg & McLean, 1997).

CLINICAL PROFILE OF HIV-1 INFECTION

Acute HIV-l infection is symptomatic in 90% of the infected individuals (Bell et al., 2010). The clinical manifestations of acute HIV-l infection appear in some cases within days, but most often 2–6 weeks after exposure to the virus. The period of illness associated with the acute phase is generally 10 days, but may also vary from 3 to 25 days (Pedersen, Lindhardt, & Jensen, 1989). The symptoms commonly include fever, night sweats, fatigue, headache, weight loss, and a mononucleosis-like illness consisting of fever, pharyngitis, and adenopathy. In addition, an erythematous, maculopapular, non-pruritic rash distributed on the face and trunks may also be evident. In general, oral candidiasis is not seen in patients with acute infection, but it can occur as a manifestation of initial infection. Oral or genital lesions may also occur. The central nervous system (CNS) may also manifest symptoms resembling a syndrome of meningoencephalitis (Tambussi et al., 2000). Laboratory findings in patients with acute HIV-l infection may include thrombocytopenia, leukopenia, and elevated liver enzyme values; however, none of these are diagnostic. During this early symptomatic phase, antibodies are not yet generated and a standard diagnostic test based on antibody reactivity will be negative (Busch & Satten, 1997). However, plasma viral RNA detection methods and assays detecting the p24 antigen in plasma, in general, give positive results during this symptomatic early phase of infection (Bollinger, Brookmeyer, & Mehendale, 1997). Since none of the clinical or laboratory findings are distinctive for the acute retroviral syndrome, the main factor that facilitates diagnosis is a history of exposure. All patients who present with a compatible syndrome should be questioned about their risk for HIV-l infection and, if suspicion is high, a presumptive diagnosis can be made. During the chronic asymptomatic phase of HIV-l infection, persistent generalized lymphadenopathy is observed in individuals who are otherwise well. HIV-l-related lymphadenopathy persists for at least 3 months. The progression of HIV-l infection is a result of a decline in immunocompetence that occurs due to increased replication of HIV-l from previously latent sites.

As the disease progresses, infected individuals may suffer from constitutional symptoms, such as weight loss, nausea and vomiting, and hematological disorders. Administering antiretroviral drugs, which can abrogate viral replication, can control or reverse these symptoms of disease.

Initial disease symptoms that follow the asymptomatic period are a sudden and unexplained loss in body weight, also known as wasting syndrome, usually accompanied by diarrhea; persistence of generalized lymphadenopathy; and the onset of neurological disease. The infected individual also suffers from dangerously high fevers, causing night sweats. Furthermore, HIV can spread to the brain and cause neurological damage by itself or by creating an immunocompromised environment that is permissive for other opportunistic infectious agents. About one-third of all AIDS patients exhibit some form of the following neurological symptoms: dementia caused by brain damage leading to loss of mental function; myelopathy leading to the weakness of limbs or paralysis; and a sensory neuropathy causing numbness, especially in the feet, and sensations of burning or stinging in the hands or feet.

As the disease progresses into the symptomatic phase, the immune system is severely compromised, resulting in a wide range of adverse immunological clinical conditions. The two major consequences of immunological damage are the occurrence of opportunistic infections, caused by infectious agents that seldom cause disease in healthy individuals, and the development of cancers.

INNATE IMMUNE RESPONSES FOLLOWING HIV-1 INFECTION

The early immune response to HIV-1 infection is an important factor in determining the clinical course of disease. The innate immune system is the first line of defense against invading organisms that rapidly functions to limit bacterial and viral infection before the activation of the adaptive immune system can occur. The elements of the innate (non-specific) immune system include anatomical barriers, secretory molecules, and cellular components. Among the mechanical anatomical barriers are the skin and internal epithelial layers, the movement of the intestines, and the oscillation of bronchopulmonary cilia. Associated with these protective surfaces are chemical and biological agents. The anatomical barriers are very effective in preventing colonization of tissues by microorganisms. However, when there is damage to tissues the anatomical barriers are breached and infection ensues. Both soluble and cellular components contribute to the innate immune response. Dendritic cells, macrophages, interferon-producing cells, natural killer (NK) cells, neutrophils, eosinophils, γδ T cells, NK T cells, CD8+ T cells with non-cytotoxic antiviral activity, and B 1 cells are the cellular components of the innate immune system (Levy, 2001). These cells are normally rapidly recruited and/or activated at the site of virus infection. The key soluble molecules of innate immunity include cytokines, chemokines, complement, defensins, acute phase reactants, mannan-binding lectins, and C-reactive proteins (Levy, 2001). HIV-1 infection causes a wide range of abnormalities in the innate immune system, contributing to the lung pathology observed in HIV-l-infected individuals (McMichael et al., 2010; Hewson et al., 1999; Agostini & Semenzato, 1996), downregulation of the normal continuous production of nitric oxide (NO) by the lung epithelium, upregulation of NO production by tissue macrophages, aberrations in systemic and pulmonary glutathione metabolism, and alteration in macrophage function. (Voelkel et al 2008 Adams et al., 1993).

Neutrophils, DCs, NK cells, NK T cells, γδ T cells, CD8+ T cells, and B1 cells are the other important cellular components of the innate immune system. Neutrophils are rapidly recruited to the site of viral infection by chemokines secreted by activated macrophages and virus-infected cells (Chang and Altfeld 2010). Neutrophils release proteins and inflammatory cytokines that help in controlling infection by pathogens. HIV-1 infection can cause a decrease in neutrophil function (Szelc, McMicheltree, Roberts, & Stiehm, 1992). Dendritic cells are highly specialized in capturing and presenting antigens to T cells and stimulating the differentiation and proliferation of B cells (Banchereau & Steinman, 2007;). They are thought to be key modulators of adaptive immune response during viral infections. Upon activation, dendritic cells are known to secrete a number of antiviral and immunoregulatory cytokines such as interferons; tumor necrosis factor alpha (TNF-α); and interleukins IL-l, IL-6, IL-12 and IL-18 (Stockwin, McGonagle, Martin, & Blair, 2000). DCs express chemokine receptors used for HIV-1 entry. Chemokine receptors facilitate the migration of DCs to areas of inflammation where they can secrete cytokines and type II interferons, which can suppress HIV-l infection. In addition, the NK cells can be rapidly recruited into infected organs and tissues by chemoattractant factors produced by virally infected cells and activated macrophages. NK cells can eliminate HIV-l-infected cells by cell-dependent cytolysis and secreted cytokines such as IFN-α, TNF-alpha, granulocyte-macrophage colony-stimulating factor (GM-CSF), and β-chemokines. The γδ T cells generally present in mucosal surfaces exhibit a more restricted repertoire compared with that of αβ T cells. These cells interact directly with non-peptide antigens or cellular stress proteins and serve as a link between innate and adaptive immune systems (Medzhitov & Janeway, 2000). Furthermore, these cells have the ability to lyse HIV-1 infected cells (Wallace et al., 1996). Monocytes from infected individuals exhibit decreased phagocytosis, chemotaxis, intracellular killing, and cytokine expression. Similarly, the granulocyte subset of neutrophils exhibit decreased phagocytosis and intracellular killing.

Mannose-binding lectins and complement are among the soluble components of innate immunity that exhibit anti HIV-1 activity. These soluble products can bind to HIV-1 and bring about the lysis of the virus or help macrophages to efficiently engulf them by phagocytosis (Sato et al., 2011). Studies have shown that individuals with low levels of circulating mannose-binding lectins are more susceptible to HIV-l infection and enhanced disease progression (Garred, Madsen, & Balslev, 1997). Complement can also cause the rapid clearance and destruction of HIV-l. It has been shown that complement lyses HIV-l in the presence of antiviral antibodies (Sullivan et al., 1996). In addition, it also serves as an opsonin for phagocytosis of HIV-1 virus (Spear, Sullivan, Landay, & Lint, 1990). Thus, the complement system is involved in both the innate immune system and the adaptive immune system. Other soluble components of the innate immune system such as cytokines and chemokines are released following interaction of pathogens with cells. Cytokines like IL-4, IL-6 and IL-12 secreted by the innate immune response can determine whether a Th-I or Th2-type adaptive immunity prevails. Furthermore, other cytokines like TNF-α and interferons can modulate HIV-l replication. Similarly, the production of chemokines can function as chemoattractants recruiting NK cells, T cells, and macrophages to sites of infection.

T CELL RESPONSES FOLLOWING HIV-1 INFECTION

CD4 + T cells are the major reservoirs of both actively replicating and latent HIV-1 throughout the course of disease. While both naive and memory T cells have the capacity to be infected with HIV-l, only activated memory T cells preferentially replicate virus (Woods, Roberts, Butera, & Follzs, 1997; Chun et al., 1995). Naive T cells do not have the ability to replicate HIV-l, even after activation (Roederer et al., 1997). These data lend support to the theory that antigen-specific interactions between infected macrophage or dendritic cells and uninfected memory CD4+ T cells leads to dissemination of HIV-1 and explain, in part, why chronic immune activation in the context of antigen presentation and cell activation such as seen in people from sub-Saharan Africa, may accelerate HIV-l disease progression.

T-cell abnormalities such as CD4+ T cell lymphopenia, characterized by decreased lymphoproliferation and a decreased number of cells having naive phenotype, are seen in HIV-1-infected individuals. In addition, infected individuals demonstrate a decreased delayed hypersensitivity skin test response to recall antigens. CD8+ T cells exhibit impaired cytokine production and cytolysis. Other viral immunomodulation strategies by the virus include chemokine and cytokine modulation, inhibition of apoptosis, inhibition of NK cell activity, and interference with MHC class I and class II antigen presentation.

The acute primary HIV-1 infection is characterized by a TH 1 profile including the secretion of pro-inflammatory cytokines IL-l, IL-2, IL-6, TNF-α, IFN-gamma (Graziosi et al., 1996; Rinaldo et al., 1990), as well as the other cytokines IL-4, IL-7, IL-l0, IL-12 and IL-13 (Chehimi, Starr, & Frank, 1994; Chehimi et al., 1996; Than et al., 1997; Patella, Florio, Petraroli, & Marone, 2000). Several viral proteins, such as gp120, Tat, Nef, and Vpr, are able to induce the secretion of a number of cytokines. The Th-1 type cytokines help to induce the strong cellular response that is responsible for the initial control of viremia. The progression of disease in HIV-1-infected individuals is associated with the switch of cytokine response from Th-1 to Th-2. The exact mechanism that causes this shift during AIDS progression is not known. However, reports suggest that HIV-1 viral proteins may contribute to the shift in Th-2 immune response. The viral protein Nef has been reported to decrease the production of IFN-gamma and IL-2 (Collette et al., 1996) and impair the signaling of Th-1 cytokines (Collette, Dutartre, Benziane, & Olive, 1997). In addition, Tat induces the expression of the IL 4 receptor alpha chain (Husain, Leland, Aggarwal, & Puri et al., 1996) and inhibits IL-2 production (Ito, Ishida, & He, 1998). These functions of the HIV-1 proteins may contribute to the shift in cytokine profile as the infection progresses.

A major host defense against viruses is induction of apoptosis of infected cells. However, many viruses can counteract these cellular responses by targeting specific stages of the downstream apoptotic pathways by using proteins that often mimic or counteract host cell functions. While apoptosis plays an important role in the destruction of HIV-1-infected T cells, other cell types such as myeloid cells become chronically or latently infected and serve as reservoirs for HIV-1. Anti-apoptotic pathways are likely to play an important role in the establishment and maintenance of latency by preventing infected cells from being rapidly killed. HIV-1 can inhibit TNF-alpha-mediated apoptosis by using mechanisms that persistently activate NF-κB, thus protecting myeloid cells from destruction (DeLuca, Kwon, Pelletier, Wainberg, & Hiscott, 1998). In addition, HIV-1 Tat protein can apparently upregulate cellular Bcl-2 in different cell types, and Vpr protein can inhibit NF-κB activation leading to suppression of T-cell receptor (TCR)-mediated apoptosis in resting T cells (Roulston, Marcellus, & Branton, 1999).

HIV-1 expresses two proteins, Nef and Vpu, that have been shown to downregulate the expression of surface MHC class I molecule (Piguet et al., 1999). HIV-1 glycoprotein, Nef, downregulates the expression of class I HLA -A2 protein on the surface of infected cells. Vpu prevents the cell surface expression of class I molecules by interfering with the processing of these molecules and destabilizing them (Kerkau, Bacik, & Bennink, 1997). This downregulation of the MHC class I molecule protects HIV-I infected cells from NK-cell-mediated lysis (Collins et al., 1998).

Although HIV-1 does not directly reduce expression of MHC class II molecules in infected cells, it can markedly impair MHC class II antigen-specific pathways. HIV-I viral proteins, Vpu, Env, and Nef, cooperate in the degradation of CD4, leading to a significant reduction of CD4 expression on T cells (Aiken, Konner, Landau, Lenburg, & Trono, 1994; Anderson, Lenburg, Landau, & Garcia, 1994; Fujita, Omura, & Silver, 1997). CD4 serves as a co-receptor during antigen recognition by the TCR on T cells, and ligation of CD4 increases the sensitivity of a T cell antigen presented by MHC class II molecules. The reduction of CD4 expression on T cells contributes to the gradual loss of responsiveness of T lymphocytes to MHC class II-restricted antigens (Louie, Wahl, Hewlett, Epstein, & Dhawan, 1996).

B CELL RESPONSES IN HIV-1 INFECTION

Although HIV-1 does not replicate in B cells, it produces severe B-cell abnormalities eventually leading to B-cell depletion (Patke & Shearer, 2000; Rodriguez, Thomas, O'Rourke, Stiehm, & Plaeger, 1996). The B-cell abnormalities detected in HIV-1 infected individuals are a decrease in B-cell number, detection of circulating immune complexes, elevated levels of autoantibodies, and increased production of nonspecific immunoglobulins G, A and M. Impaired production of specific antibodies to new and recall antigens is also seen. This includes both T-dependent and -independent antigens (Shirai, Cosentino, Leitman-Klinman, & Klinman, 1992; Yarchoan, Redfield, & Broder, 1986; Borkowsky et al., 1992; Gibb et al., 1995). Recent reports have identified a subpopulation of B cells with low CD21 expression in high viremia patients. These cells, which are poor antibody responders and low secretors of immunoglobulins, could be partly responsible for causing the humoral defects seen in HIV-1-infected individuals (Moir, Malaspina, & Ogwaro, 2001). Furthermore, HIV-1 gene products like gp120 can modulate B-cell function apparently by binding to the VB3 domain of membrane immunoglobulin (Goodglick, Zevit, Neshat, & Braun, 1995).

HIV-1 activates complement through alternative and classic pathways (Montefiori, Robinson, & Mitchell, 1989). Although there is deposition of C3 on viral surfaces, there is decreased activity of the complement C5-C9 membrane attack complex. In addition, HIV-I downregulates cell surface complement receptors after infection (Munson, Scott, Landay, & Spear, 1995). HIV-1 infection decreases CRI expression on B cells and erythrocytes by proteolytic cleavage of the receptor (Jouvi, Rozenbaum, Russo, & Kazatchkine, 1987). HIV-1 infection also downregulates CR2 expression by altered transcription (Larcher, Schultz, & Hofbauer, 1990). HIV-1 gp120 decreases

C5a receptor expression and thus impairs the chemotatic response of monocytes to inflammatory stimuli (Wahl et al., 1989). In some cases, HIV-1 may infect cells using complement receptors. Villous processes of follicular dendritic cells expressing high levels of complement receptors and Fc receptors trap numerous particles of opsonized HIV-1 virus particles that are highly infectious (Heath, Tew, Szakal, & Burton, 1995).

ROLE OF CHEMOKINES HIV-1 PATHOGENESIS

Chemokines and their receptors play a critical role in HIV-1 infection and disease pathogenesis (reviewed in Reinhart et al., 2009). The seven transmembrane G-protein coupled receptors CXCR4 and CCR5 act as coreceptors for HIV-1 entry into immune cells (Feng, Broder, Kennedy, & Berger, 1996, Deng et al., 1996). Interestingly, SIVs predominantly use CCR5 for entry (Edinger et al., 1997). Deletion in CCR5 is associated with increased protection from both acquisition of HIV-1 and subsequent disease. Secondary lymphoid tissues are critical sites of soluble and cell-associated antigen sampling of peripheral tissues, and they are key compartments for the generation of cellular and humoral immune responses. Chemokines are major mediators of cell trafficking during immune inductive and effector activities, and changes in their expression patterns in lymphoid tissues could contribute to the pathogenesis of HIV-1 and SIV in multiple ways. Infection of rhesus macaques with pathogenic SIV leads to the induction of multiple inflammatory chemokines in lymph nodes and spleen including: CXCL8, CXCL9, CXCL10, and CXCL11, CCL3, CCL4, CCL5, CCL2 CCL19 and CCL20. In a study of host responses to oral transmission of SIV, high CXCL9 and CXCL10 levels in lymph nodes after infection were associated with rapid progression of disease, whereas high levels of these chemokines in the oral mucosa were associated with slow progression of disease (Milush et al., 2007). When chemokine expression in peripheral blood mononuclear cells (PBMCs) were examined from SIV- or SHIV-infected nonhuman primates, CCL3, CCL4 and CCL5 were found to be upregulated (reviewed in Reinhart et al., 2009). In contrast, the homeostatic lymphoid chemokine CCL21 and the Th2 recruiting chemokines CCL17 and CCL22 and the anti-apoptotic chemokines CCL25 and CXCL12 chemokines are downregulated during SIV infection. The overall implications of the findings regarding chemokine expression associated with lymphoid tissues from SIV-infected macaques suggest that SIV infection leads to development of a Th-1 polarized, inflammatory milieu. These modified environments in lymphoid tissues are polarized toward type 1, IFN-gamma production due to increased recruitment of T cells expressing CCR5 and CXCR3, which are found predominantly on Th-1 cells and due to decreased recruitment of T cells expressing CCR4, which is found predominantly on Th-2 T cells and Tregs. Although it would be reasonable to expect that increased local expression of CCR5 ligands would decrease viral replication, this does not appear to be the case in these tissues.

NEUROPATHOGENESIS IN HIV-1 INFECTION—ROLE OF PERIPHERAL IMMUNE CELLS

HIV-1-associated dementia (HIV-D) is a syndrome of motor and cognitive dysfunction observed in approximately 5% to 10% of patients infected with HIV-1 (McArthur et al., 1993; Sacktor et al., 2010). Although the neuropathogenesis of HIV-D is not completely understood, the role of immune cells in its manifestation is well demonstrated (Fischer-Smith, Bell, Croul, Lewis, & Rappaport, 2008). CNS infection of HIV-1 has been shown early during the acute phase of infection; however, the action of cytotoxic T cells eliminates productively infected cells. At later phase of the disease, productive infection of the CNS sets in, with the concomitant development of CNS disease (Fischer-Smith & Rappaport, 2008). The source and mechanism of this latter infection of the CNS has been a matter of considerable debate, with two divergent models. In the first model, the re-emergence of the virus from a latent reservoir (Trojan horse model) is thought to be the mechanism for the productive infection. In the second model, new invasion of the CNS with virus-infected cells (late invasion model; Fischer-Smith & Rappaport, 2008) is proposed to be the causative factor. In the Trojan horse model, it is proposed that the virus enters the CNS early, and replicates at low levels as a reservoir separated from the periphery. During the course of the disease, a more virulent CNS phenotype of the virus emerges, leading to the manifestation of disease pathogenesis. In support of the Trojan horse model, several studies suggest CNS compartmentalization of the HIV virus through comparisons of viral quasispecies found in the plasma compared with those virus found in cerebrospinal fluid (CSF) (Clements et al., 2005, 2008; Cunningham, 2000; Stingele et al., 2001; Strain et al., 2005; Tashima et al., 2002). These studies demonstrate suppression of virus replication in the CNS as early as 21 days, without loss of CNS viral DNA (Barber, 2004). However, macrophage trafficking is also observed in this model, negating microglial activation as the sole contributor to CNS disease. Although these studies do not preclude the contribution of infiltrating macrophages, the constant level of viral DNA in CNS suggested a latent CNS reservoir as a major contributor.

Despite the early viral entry, several lines of evidence also support the late invasion model. According to this model, virus entry into the CNS is due largely to the trafficking of HIV-1–infected monocytes/macrophages from the systemic circulation into the CNS (Meltzer et al., 1990). The number of total brain macrophages is dramatically increased in HIV encephalopathy (HIVE), the pathogenic manifestation of HIV, without additional evidence of local proliferation of these cells (Fischer-Smith et al., 2004;). Additional studies have shown that macrophage/microglia represent the principle productive reservoir of HIV-1 infection in the CNS (Kure et al., 1991; Porwit et al.,1989;). The contribution of infected macrophage and microglial cells to neuronal injury through secretion of viral and host factors has been the subject of numerous reviews (Fischer-Smith & Rappaport, 2005; Gonzalez-Scarano & Martin-Garcia, 2005).

The late invasion model proposes that the peripheral immune compartment plays a prominent role and contributes to the development of CNS disease. Previous studies comparing HIV-1 gp120 sequences have demonstrated the greatest similarity between envelope sequences derived from the brain with those derived from bone marrow and blood (Gartner et al., 1997)). The role of monocytes/macrophage trafficking from the periphery into the CNS is further supported by the beneficial effects of highly active antiretroviral therapy (HAART) despite poor CNS penetration of most of these antiretroviral compounds (Vehmas et al., 2004). Although conclusively discriminating between resident microglia and perivascular macrophages is difficult, combined CD markers have been used to make this distinction. The combination of antigenic markers for perivascular macrophage positive for CD14 (lipopolysaccharide [LPS] receptor) and CD45 (leukocyte common antigen [LCA]), neither of which are expressed on microglia, has been used to identify two populations of activated macrophages in the CNS of patients with HIVE (Fischer-Smith et al., 2001). Macrophages accumulating perivascularly with a CD14+/CD45(LCA)+/CD16+ (FcγIII receptor) phenotype appear to be the principal reservoir of productive HIV-1 infection in the CNS. Similar observations were also reported in SIVE (Williams et al., 2001. Importantly, CD16+ monocytes preferentially harbor HIV in vivo, are more permissive to HIV infection than CD16− monocytes, and are likely important as reservoirs of infection and tissue dissemination (Ellery et al., 2007; Joworoski et al., 2007). In support of the latter hypothesis, the increase in total brain macrophages that bear antigenic markers of the peripheral compartment appears to be due to trafficking of monocytes/macrophage into the CNS from the periphery, rather than local microglial proliferation (Fischer-Smith et al., 2004).

The passage of monocyte and leukocyte into the CNS would not occur without the complex chemokine gradient that is established during HIV-1 infection. Chemokine involvement in HIV-1 neuropathogenesis is well recognized because of their abilities to: (i) recruit HIV-1-infected immune cells into the brain, (ii) serve as mediators for inflammatory responses, and (iii) serve as ligands for HIV-1 coreceptors, specifically CXCR4 and CCR5 (Hesselgesser et al., 1998). CCL2 is considered to be a critical factor involved in the infiltration of monocytes and lymphocytes across the BBB during CNS inflammation. Numerous studies strongly suggest that increased CCL2 expression in the CNS is associated with enhanced progression of HIVE (Dhillon et al., 2008). Chemokines can also promote virus replication and contribute to injury and eventual loss of neurons (Asensio & Campbell, 1999; Miller & Meucci, 1999). In addition to CCL2, another chemokine, CXCL10 (interferon 1-inducible peptide) has also been detected in the CSF of individuals with HIV-1 infection (Kolb et al., 1999). Understanding the underlying mechanisms that lead to the migration of HIV-1-infected monocytes from the periphery into the CNS are

important future directions in therapeutic strategies (Kraft-Terry et al., 2009).

CONCLUSION

The complete eradication of HIV-1 from infected patients remains problematic, although the use of HAART has improved the prognosis of patients who are HIV-positive. A major obstacle to total viral eradication is the persistence of viral reservoirs and continuous rounds of de novo virus infection of host cells with rapid turnover of both free virus and virus-producing cells. It is likely that various immune activation stimuli, including most pathogens, can potentially affect the infectivity, transmissibility and pathogenesis of HIV by influencing several aspects of HIV biology. First, infection of monocytes/macrophages by many pathogens can induce immune activation of monocytes and T lymphocytes, thus increasing the infectivity of these cells to HIV. Second, these infections can also promote disease progression by creating a cytokine environment that favors faster replication of HIV. Third, these infectious agents can modulate the expression of coreceptors on the surfaces of permissive cellular targets, thus altering the cellular tropism. Such immune pressures can lead to emergence of viral variants that not only use multiple coreceptors, but also are more virulent. Collectively, all these factors are likely to increase HIV pathogenesis.

REFERENCES

Almeida, J. R., Price, D. A., Papagno, L., Arkoub, Z. A., Sauce, D., Bornstein, E., et al. (2007). Superior control of HIV-1 replication by CD8+ T cells is reflected by their avidity, polyfunctionality, and clonal turnover. *J Exp Med, 204*(10), 2473–85.

Aiken, C., Konner, J., Landau, N., Lenburg, M., & Trono, D. (1994). Nef induces CD4 endocytosis: Requirement for a critical dileucine motif in the membrane-proximal CD4 cytoplasmic domain. *Cell, 76*, 853–64.

Agostini C, Semenzato G. (1996). Immunologic effects of HIV in the lung. *Clin Chest Med.* 1996 Dec;17(4):633–45.

Anderson, S., Lenburg, M., Landau, N., & Garcia, J. (1994). 111e cytoplasmic domain of CD4 is sufficient for its down-regulation from the cell surface by human immunodeficiency virus type I Nef *J Virol, 68*, 3092–101.

Asensio, V. C. & Campbell, I. L. (1999). Chemokines in the CNS: Plurifunctional mediators in 501 diverse states. *Trends Neurosci, 22*, 504–512.

Barber, C. G. (2004). CCR5 antagonists for the treatment of HIV. *Curr Opin Investig Drugs, 8*, 851–61. Review.

Bell, S. K., Little, S. J., Rosenberg, E. S. (2010). Clinical management of acute HIV infection: best practice remains unknown. *J Infect Dis.* 202 Suppl 2:S278–88. Review.

Bollinger, R. C., Brookmeyer, R. S., & Mehendale, S. (1997). Risk factors and clinical presentation of acute primary HIV infection in India. *J Am Med Ass, 278*, 2085.

Bonavia, R., Bajello, A., Barbero, S., Albini, A., Noonan, D. M., & Schettini, G. (2001). HIV-1 Tat causes apoptotic death and calcium homeostasis alterations in rat neurons. *Biochem Biophys Res Comm, 288*, 301–8.

Borkowsky, W., Rigaud M., Krasinski, K., Moore, T., Lawrence, R. & Pollack H. (1992). Cell-mediated and humoral immune responses in children infected with human immunodeficiency virus during the first 4 years of life. *J Pediatr, 120*, 371–5.

Borrow, P., Lewicki, H., Hahn, B.1-I., Shaw, G. M., & Oldstone M. (1991). Virus-specific C8+ cytotoxic T-Iymphocyte activity associated with control of viremia in primary human immunodeficiency virus type j infection. *J Virol, 68*, 6103–6110.

Braaten, D., Franke, E. K., & Luban, J. (1996). Cyclophillin A is required for an early step in the life cycle of human immunodeficiency virus type I before initiation of reverse transcription. *J Virol, 70*, 3551–60.

Brenchley, J. M., Schacker, T. W., Ruff, L. E., Price, D. A., Taylor, J. H. Beilman, G. J., et al. (2004). CD4+ T cell depletion during all stages of HIV disease occurs predominantly in the gastrointestinal tract. *J Exp Med, 200*, 749–759.

Bukrinsky, M. I., Stanwick, T. L., & Dempsey, M. P. (1991). Quiescent T lymphocytes as an inducible virus reservoir in HIV-l infection. *Science, 254*, 423–7.

Burton, D. R., Weiss, R. A. (2010). AIDS/HIV. A boost for HIV vaccine design. *Science.* 13;329(5993):770–3.

Busch, M. P., Satten G. A. (1997) Time course of viremia and antibody seroconversion following human immunodeficiency virus exposure. *Am J Med.*;102(5B):117–24; discussion 125–6.

Cen, S., Khorchid, A., Lavanbakht, 1-1., Gabor, J., Stello, T, & Shiba, K. (2001). Incorporation of lysyl-tRNA synthethase into human immunodeficiency virus type I. *J Virol, 75*, 5043–8.

Chang, J.J., Altfeld, M. (2010). Innate immune activation in primary HIV-1 infection. *J Infect Dis.* Oct 15;202 Suppl 2:S297–301.

Chehimi, J., Ma, X., Chouaib, S., et al. (1996). Differential production of interleukin-10 during human immunodeficiency virus infection. *AIDS Res Human Retroviruses, 12*, 4053–61.

Chehimi, J., Starr, S.E., & Frank, I. (1994). Impaired interleukin-12 production in human immunodeficiency virus-infected patients. *J Exp Med, 141*, 99–104.

Chun, T.-W., Finzi, D., Margolick, J., Chadwick, K., Schwartz, D., & Siliciano, R. F. (1995). The in vivo fate of HIV-I-infected T cells: Quantitative analysis of the transition to stable latency. *Nat Med, I*, 1284–90.

Chun, T. W., Chadwick, K., Margolick, J., & Siliciano, R. F. (1970). Differential susceptibility of naive and memory CD4+ T cells to the cytopathic effects of infection with human immunodeficiency virus type I strain. *J Virol, 71*, 4436–44.

Clements, J. E., Mankowski, J. L., Gama, L., & Zink, M. C. (2008). The accelerated simian immunodeficiency virus macaque model of human immunodeficiency virus-associated neurological disease: From mechanism to treatment. *J Neurovirol, 14*(4), 309–17. Review.

Clements, J. E., Li, M., Gama, L., Bullock, B., Carruth, L. M., Mankowski, J. L., et al. (2005). The central nervous system is a viral reservoir in simian immunodeficiency virus—infected macaques on combined antiretroviral therapy: A model for human immunodeficiency virus patients on highly active antiretroviral therapy. *J Neurovirol, 11*(2), 180–9.

Cunningham A. (2000). African Americans and AIDS: highlights of 2nd annual Washington conference. *AIDS Treat News, 17*(339), 8.

Collette, Y., Chang, H. L., & Cerdan, H., et al. (1996). Specific Thl cytokine down-regulation associated with primary clinically derived human immunodeficiency virus type I Nef gene-induced expression. *J Immunol, 156*, 360–70.

Collette, Y., Dutartre, H., Benziane, A., & Olive, D. (1997). The role of HIV-2 Nef in T-cell activation: Nef impairs induction of Th I cytokines and interacts with Src family tyrosine kinase Lck. *Res Virol, 148*, 52–8.

Collins, K. L., Chen, B. K., Kalams, S. A., Walker, B. D., & Baltimore D. (1998). HIV-I Nef protein protects infected primary cells against killing by cytotoxic T lymphocytes. *Nature, 391*, 397–401.

Connor, R. I., Mohri, H., Cao, Y., & Ho, D. D. (1993). Increased viral burden and cytopathicity correlate temporally with CD4+ T-Iymphocyte decline and clinical progression in human immunodeficiency virus type I-infected individuals. *J Virol, 67*, 1772–7.

Connor, R. I., Sheridan, I. C. E., Ceradini, D., Choe, S., & Landau, N. R. (1997). Change in coreceptor use correlates with disease progression in HIV-I infected individuals. *J Exp Med, 185*, 621–8.

Craigie, R. (200l). HIV integrase, a brief overview from chemistry to therapeutics. *J BiolChem, 266*, 23213–16.

Davenport, M. P., Ribeiro, R. M., Zhang, L., Wilson, D. P., & Perelson A. S. (2007). Understanding the mechanisms and limitations of immune control of HIV. *Immunol Rev, 216*, 164–175.

DeLuca, C., Kwon, H., Pelletier, N., Wainberg, M., & Hiscott, J. (1998). NF-KB protects HIV-I infected myeloid cells from apoptosis. *Virology, 244*, 27–38.

Deng, H., Liu, R., Ellmeier, W., et al. (1996). Identification of a major coreceptor for primary isolates of HIV-1. *Nature, 381*, 661–6.

Dhillon, N. K., et al. (2008). Roles of MCP-1 in development of HIV-dementia. *Front Biosci, 560 13*, 3913–3918.

Ellery, P. J., Tippett, E., Chiu, Y. L., Paukovics G., Cameron, P. U., Solomon, A., Lewin, S. R., Gorry, P. R., Jaworowski, A., Greene, W. C., Sonza, S., Crowe, S.M. (2007). The CD16+ monocyte subset is more permissive to infection and preferentially harbors HIV-1 in vivo. *J Immunol.* 178(10):6581–9.

Edinger, A. L., Amedee, A., Miller, K., et al. (1997). Differential utilization of CCR5 by macrophage and T cell tropic simian immunodeficiency virus strains. *Proc Natl Acad Sci USA, 94*, 4005–10.

Emilie, D., Maillot, M. C., Nicholas, J. E, Fior, R., & Galanaud P. (1992). Antagonistic effect of interferon gamma on Tat-induced transactivation of HIV long terminal repeats. *J BioI Chem, 267*, 20565–70.

Fauci, A. S. (1993). Multifactorial nature of human immunodeficiency virus disease: Implication for therapy. *Science, 262*, 1011–18.

Feinberg, M. B., McLean, A. R. (1997). AIDS: decline and fall of immune surveillance? *Curr Biol.*7(3):R136–40. Review.

Feng, Y., Broder, C. C., Kennedy, P. E., & Berger, E. A. (1996). HIV-1 entry cofactor: Functional cDNA cloning of a seven-transmembrane, G protein- coupled receptor. *Science, 272*, 872–7.

Fischer-Smith, T, Croul S, Adeniyi A, Rybicka K, Morgello S, Khalili K, Rappaport J. (2004). Macrophage/microglial accumulation and proliferating cell nuclear antigen expression in the central nervous system in human immunodeficiency virus encephalopathy. *Am J Pathol.* 164(6):2089–99.

Fischer-Smith, T, Rappaport J. (2005). Evolving paradigms in the pathogenesis of HIV-1-associated dementia. *Expert Rev Mol Med.* 7(27): 1–26.

Fischer-Smith, T., Bell, C., Croul, S., Lewis, M., & Rappaport, J. (2008). Monocyte/macrophage trafficking in acquired immunodeficiency syndrome encephalitis: Lessons from human and nonhuman primate studies. *J Neurovirol, 14*(4), 318–26. Review.

Fischer-Smith, T., Tedaldi, E. M., & Rappaport, J. (2008). CD163/CD16 co-expression by circulating monocytes/macrophages in HIV: Potential biomarkers for HIV infection and AIDS progression. *AIDS Res Hum Retroviruses, 24*(3), 417–21.

Franke, E. K., Yuan, H. E. H., & Luban, J. (1994). Specific incorporation of cyclophilin A into HIV-1 virion. *Nature, 372*, 359–62.

Fujita, K., Omura, S., & Silver, J. (1997). Rapid degradation of CD4 in cells expressing human immunodeficiency virus type I Env and Vpu is blocked by proteasome inhibitors. *J Gen Virol, 78*, 619–725.

Galati D, Bocchino M. (2007). New insights on the perturbations of T cell cycle during HIV infection. *Curr Med Chem.*, 14(18):1920–4. Review.

Garred, P., Madsen, H. O., & Balslev, U (1997). Susceptibility of HIV infection and progression of AIDS in relation to variant alleles of mannose-binding lectin. *Lancet, 349*, 236–40.

Gartner S, McDonald RA, Hunter EA, Bouwman F, Liu Y, Popovic M. (1997). Gp120 sequence variation in brain and in T-lymphocyte human immunodeficiency virus type 1 primary isolates. *J Hum Virol.* Nov-Dec;1(1):3–18.

Gasper-Smith N, Crossman D. M., Whitesides, J. F., Mensali, N., Ottinger J. S., Plonk SG, et al. (2008). Induction of plasma (TRAIL), TNFR-2, Fas ligand, and plasma microparticles after human immunodeficiency virus type 1 (HIV-1) transmission: Implications for HIV-1 vaccine design. *J Virol.*;82(15):7700–10.

Gelderblom, H. R. (1991). Assembly and morphology of HIV: potential effect of structure on viral function. *AIDS.* 5(6):617–37.

Gibb, D., Spoulou, V., Giacomelli, A., Griffiths, H., Masters, J., & Misbah, S. (1995). Antibody response to *Haemophilus inlfluenzae* type b and

Streptoccocus pneumoniae vaccines in children with human immunodeficiency virus infection. *Ped Inect Dis J, 14*, 129–35.

Glass, W. G., McDermott, D. H., Lim, J. K., Lekhong, S., Yu, S. F., Frank, W. A., et al. (2006). CCR5 deficiency increases risk of symptomatic West Nile virus infection. *J Exp Med, 203*(1), 35–40.

Goodglick, L., Zevit, N., Neshat, M., & Braun, J. (1995). Mapping the Ig super-antigen-binding site of HIV gp120. *J Immunol, 155*, 5151–9.

González-Scarano, F. & Martín-García, J. (2005). The neuropathogenesis of AIDS. *Nat Rev Immunol, 5*(1), 69–81. Review.

Goonetilleke, N., Liu, M. K., Salazar-Gonzalez, J. F., Ferrari, G., Giorgi, E., Ganusov, V. V., et al. (2009). The first T cell response to transmitted/founder virus contributes to the control of acute viremia in HIV-1 infection. *J Exp Med, 206*(6), 1253–72.

Goulder PJ, Bunce M, Krausa P, McIntyre K, Crowley S, Morgan B, Edwards A, Giangrande P, Phillips RE, McMichael AJ. (1996) Novel, cross-restricted, conserved, and immunodominant cytotoxic T lymphocyte epitopes in slow progressors in HIV type 1 infection. *AIDS Res Hum Retroviruses*. 12(18):1691–8.

Graziosi C, Gantt KR, Vaccarezza M, Demarest JF, Daucher M, et al (1996). Kinetics of cytokine expression during primary human immunodeficiency virus type 1 infection. Proc Natl Acad Sci U S A. 1996 Apr 30;93(9):4386–91.

Guadalupe, M., Reay, E., Sankaran, S., Prindiville, T., Flamm, J., McNeil, A., et al. (2003). Severe CD4+ T-cell depletion in gut lymphoid tissue during primary human immunodeficiency virus type 1 infection and substantial delay in restoration following highly active antiretroviral therapy. *J Virol, 77*, 11708–11717.

Haase, A. T. (1999). Population biology of HIV-I infection: Viral demographics and dynamics in lymphatic tissues. *Ann Rev Immunol Rev, 17*, 625–56.

Haase, A. T., Henry, K., Zupancic, M., et al. (1996). Quantitative image analysis of HIV-I infection in lymphoid tissue. *Science, 274*, 985–9.

Haase, A. (2005). Pencil at mucosal front lines for HIV and SIV and their hosts. *Nat Rev Immunol, 5*, 783–89.

Heath, S. L., Tew, J. G., Szakal, A. K., & Burton, G. E (1995). Follicular dendritic cells and human immunodeficiency virus infectivity. *Nature, 377*, 740–4.

Hesselgesser, J., et al. (1998). Identification and characterization of the CXCR4 chemokine 614 receptor in human T cell lines: Ligand binding, biological activity, and HIV-1 615 infectivity. *J Immunol, 160*, 877–883.

Haynes, B. F. (1996). HIV vaccines: Where we are and where we are going. *Lancet, 348*(9032), 933–7. Review.

Huber, M. & Trkola, A. (2007). Humoral immunity to HIV-1: Neutralization and beyond. *J Intern Med, 262*, 5–25.

Husain, S. R., Leland, P., Aggarwal, B. B, & Puri, R. K. (1996). Transcriptional upregulation of interleukin 4 receptors by human immunodeficiency virus type I Tat gene. *AIDS Res Hum Retroviruses, 12*, 1349–59.

Ito, M., Ishida, T., & He, L. (1998). HIV-I type 1 TAT protein inhibits interleukin•12 production by human peripheral blood mononuclear cells. *AIDS Res Hum Retrovirus, 14*, 845–9.

Jaworowski A, Kamwendo DD, Ellery P, Sonza S, Mwapasa V, Tadesse E, Molyneux ME, Rogerson SJ, Meshnick SR, Crowe SM. (2007). CD16+ monocyte subset preferentially harbors HIV-1 and is expanded in pregnant Malawian women with Plasmodium falciparum malaria and HIV-1 infection. *J Infect Dis*. 196(1):38–42.

Jouvin, M. H., Rozenbaum, R., Russo, & Kazatchkine, M. D. (1987). Decreased expression of C3b/C4b complement receptor (CRI) in AIDS and AIDS-related syndromes correlates with clinical subpopulations of patients with HIV-1 infection. *AIDS, 1*, 89–94.

Kagi, D., Seiler, P., & Pavlovic, I., (1995). The roles of perforin and Fas-dependent cytotoxicity in protection against cytopathic and non-cytopathic viruses. *Eur J Immunol, 25*, 3256–62.

Kellam P, Weiss R. A. (2006). Infectogenomics: insights from the host genome into infectious diseases. Cell. 2006 Feb 24;124(4): 695–7.

Kerkau, L., Bacik, I., & Bennink, I. R. (1997). The human immunodeficiency virus type 1 (HIV-I) Vpu protein interferes with an early step in

the biosynthesis of major histocompatibility. (MHC) class I molecules. *J Exp Med, 185*, 1295–305.

Kolb, S. A., et al. (1999). Identification of a T cell chemotactic factor in the cerebrospinal fluid of HIV-1-infected individuals as interferon-gamma inducible protein. *J Neuroimmunol, 93*, 172.

Koup, R. A, Safrit, J. A., & Cao, Y., (1994). Temporal association of cellular immune responses with the initial control of viremia in primary human immunodeficiency virus type I syndrome. *J Immunol. 68*, 4650–5.

Kraft-Terry, S. D., Stothert, A. R., Buch, S., & Gendelman, H. E. (2010). HIV-1 neuroimmunity in the era of antiretroviral therapy, *Neurobiol Dis*.

Kraft-Terry, S. D., Buch, S. J., Fox, H. S., & Gendelman, H. E. (2009). A coat of many colors: Neuroimmune crosstalk in human immunodeficiency virus infection. *Neuron, 64*, 33–45.

Kure, K., Llena, J. F., Lyman, W. D., Soeiro, R., Weidenheim, K. M., Hirano, A., et al. (1991). Human immunodeficiency virus-1 infection of the nervous system: An autopsy study of 268 adult, pediatric, and fetal brains. *Hum Pathol, 22*(7), 700–10.

Lamhamedi-Cherradi, S., Culman-Penciolelli, B., & Guy, B. (1995). Different patterns of HIV-I specific cytotoxic T-lymphocyte activity after primary infection. *AIDS, 9*, 421–6.

Larcher, C., Schultz, T. E., & Hofbauer, P. (1990). Expression of the OC// EBV receptor and of' other cell membrane surface markers is altered upon HIV-I infection of myeloid T and B cells. *J Acq Immune Defic Syndrome, 3*, 103–8.

Levy, I. A. (2001). The importance of the innate immune system in controlling HIV infection and disease. *Trends Immunol, 22*, 312–I5.

Levy, I. A., Mackewicz, C. E., & Barker, E. (1996). Controlling HIV-1 pathogenesis: The role of noncytotoxic anti-HIV activity of' CD8+ cells. *Immunol Today, 17*, 217–24

Little, S. J., McLean, A. F., Spina, C. F, Richman, D. D., & Havlir D. V. (1999). Viral dynamics of acute HIV-I infection. *J Exp Med, 190*, 841–50.

Li, Qingsheng, et al. (2009). Microarray analysis of lymphatic tissue reveals stage-specific, gene expression signatures in HIV-1 infection. *J Immunol, 183*(3), 1975–1982.

Louie, A. T., Wahl, L. M., Hewlett, J. K., Epstein, I., & Dhawan, S. (1996). Impaired antigen presentation to CD4+ T-cells by HIV-infected monocytes is related to down-modulation of CD 4 expression on helper T cells: Possible involvement of H1V-induced cellular factors. *FEBS Lett, 398*, 1–6.

McArthur, J. C., Hoover, D. R., Bacellar, H., Miller, E. N., Cohen, B. A., Becker, J. T., et al. (1993). Dementia in AIDS patients: Incidence and risk factors. Multicenter AIDS Cohort Study. *Neurology, 43*(11), 2245–52.

McCune, J. M. (1995). Viral latency in HIV diseases. *Cell, 82*, 183–8.

McMichael, A. J. & Rowland-Jones, S. L. (2001). Cellular immune responses to HIV-1. *Nature, 10*, 980–7.

McMichael, A. J. & Walker, D. B. (1991). Cytotoxic T lymphocyte epitopes: Implications of rHIV vaccines. *AIDS, 8*(suppI), Suppl-73.

McMichael AJ, Borrow P, Tomaras GD, Goonetilleke N, Haynes BF. (2010) The immune response during acute HIV-1 infection: clues for vaccine development. *Nat Rev Immunol,10*(1):11–23.

Medzhitov, R. & Janeway, C. (l998). Innate immune recognition and control of adaptive immune responses. *Scand Immunol, 10*, 351–3.

Medzhitov, R. & Janeway, C. (2000). Innate immunity. *New Eng J Med, 343*, 338–44.

Meltzer, M. S., Nakamura, M., Hansen, B. D., Turpin, J. A., Kalter, D. C., & Gendelman, H. E. (1990). Macrophages as susceptible targets for HIV infection, persistent viral reservoirs in tissue, and key immunoregulatory cells that control levels of virus replication and extent of disease. *AIDS Res Hum Retroviruses, 6*(8), 967–71. Review.

Meucci, O., et al. (1998). Chemokines regulate hippocampal neuronal signaling and gp120 neurotoxicity. *Proc Natl Acad Sci USA, 95*, 14500–14505.

Meucci, O., et al. (2000). Expression of CX3CR1 chemokine receptors on neurons and their role in neuronal survival. *Proc Natl Acad Sci USA, 97*, 8075–8080.

Meylan, P. R., Guatelli, J. C., Munis, J. R., Richman, D. D., & Kornbluth, H. S. (1993). lvlechanisms for the inhibition of HIV replication by interferons-alpha., beta, gamma primary human macrophages. *Virology*, 193, 138–48.

Milush, J. M., Stefano-Cole, K., Schmidt, K., Durudas, A., Pandrea, I., & Sodora, D. L. (2007). Mucosal innate immune response associated with a timely humoral immune response and slower disease progression after oral transmission of simian immunodeficiency virus to rhesus macaques. *J Virol*, 81, 6175–86.

Miller RJ, Meucci O. (1999) AIDS and the brain: is there a chemokine connection? *Trends Neurosci.*, 22(10):471–9.

Moir, S., Malaspina, A., & Ogwaro, K. M. (2001). HIV-l induced phenotypic and functional perturbations of B-cells in chronically infected individuals. *Proc Natl Acad Sci USA*, 98, 10362–7.

Montefiori, D. C., Robinson, W. E., & Mitchell, W. M. (1989). Antibody independent, complement-mediated enhancement of HIV-l infection by mannosidase I and II inhibitors. *Antiviral Res*, 11, 137–46.

Munson, L. G., Scott, M. E., Landay, A. L., & Spear, G. T. (1995). Decreased levels of complement receptor 1 (CD35) on B lymphocytes in persons with HIV infection. *Clin Immunol Immunopath*, 75, 20–5.

Nigam, P., Velu, V., Kannanganat, S., Chennareddi, L., Kwa, S., Siddiqui, M., et al. (2010). Expansion of FOXP3+ CD8 T cells with suppressive potential in colorectal mucosa following a pathogenic simian immunodeficiency virus infection correlates with diminished antiviral T cell response and viral control. *J Immunol*, 184(4), 1690–701. Epub 2010 Jan 6.

Nowak, M. A., Bonhoeffer, S., Shaw, G. M., May, R. M. (1997) Anti-viral drug treatment: dynamics of resistance in free virus and infected cell populations. *J Theor Biol*. 21;184(2):203–17.

Pandrea, I., Sodora, D. L., Silvestri, G., Apetrei, C. (2008) Into the wild: simian immunodeficiency virus (SIV) infection in natural hosts. *Trends Immunol*. 2008 Sep;29(9):419–28. Review.

Pantaleo, G. & Fauci, A. S. (1994). Tracking HIV during disease progression. *Curr Opin Immunol*, 6, 600–64.

Pantaleo, G., Demarest, J. E, Soudeyns, H., et al. (1994). Major expansion of CD8+ T cells with a predominant VB during the primary immune response to HIV. *Nature*, 370, 463–7.

Pantaleo, G., Graziosi, C., & Demarest, J. F. (1993). HIV infection is active and progressive in lymphoid tissue during the clinically latent stage of disease. *Nature*, 362, 355–8.

Pantaleo, G., Graziosi, E., & Fauci, A. S. (1997). Virologic and immunologic events in primary HIV infection. *Springer Seminal Immunopathol*, 18, 257–66.

Pascual, M., Danielsson, C., Steiger, G., & Schifferli, J. A. (1994). Proteolytic cleavage of CR1 on human erythrocytes in vivo: Evidence for enhanced cleavage in AIDS. *Eur J Immunol*, 24, 702–8.

Pastinen, T., Liitsola, K., Niini, P., Salminen, M., & Syvanen, A. C. (1998). Contribution of the CCR5 and MBL genes to susceptibility to HIV type I infection in the Finnish population. *AIDS Res HIV Retroviruses*, 14, 695–8.

Patella, V., Florio, G., Petraroli, A., & Marone, G. (2000). HIV-1 gp120 induces IL-1 and IL-13 release from human FcgR1+ cells through interaction with the VH3 region of IgE. *J Immunol*, 164, 589–95.

Patke, C. L. & Shearer, W. T. (2000). Gp120 and TNF-alpha-induced modulation of human II cell function: Proliferation, cyclic AMP generation, IgG production, and B cell receptor expression. *J Allergy Clin Immunol*, 105, 975–82.

Patterson, S., English, N. R., Longhurst, H., et al. (1998). Analysis of human immunodeficiency virus type 1 (HIV-1) variants and levels of infection in dendritic and T cells from symptomatic HIV-1 infected patients. *J Gen Virol*, 79, 247–57.

Pedersen, C., Lindhardt, B. O., & Jensen, B. L. (1989). Clinical course of primary HIV infection: Consequences for subsequent course of infection. *Br Med J*, 299, 154–7.

Pereira, L., Bentley, K., Peeters, A., Churchill, M. J., & Deacon, N. (2000). A compilation of cellular transcription factor interactions with the HIV-I LTR promoter. *Nucleic Acids Res*, 28, 663–8.

Petravic, J., Loh, L., Kent, S. J., & Davenport, M. P. (2008). CD4+ target cell availability determines the dynamics of immune escape and reversion in vivo. *J Virol*, 82, 4091–4101.

Phillips, A. N. (1996). Reduction of HIV concentration during acute infection: Independence from a specific immune response. *Science*, 271, 497–499.

Piguet, V., Schwartz, O., Le Gall, S., & Trono, D. (1999). The downregulation of CD4 and MHC-l by primate lentiviruses: A paradigm for the modulation of cell surface receptors. *Immunol Rev*, 168, 51–63.

Pleskoff, O., Sol, N., & Labrosse, B. (1997a). Human immunodeficiency virus strains differ in their ability to infect CD4+ cells expressing the rat homolog of CXCR-4 (Fusin). *J Virol*, 71, 3259–62.

Pleskoff, O., Treboute, C., & Brelot, A. (1997b). Identification of a chemokine receptor encoded by human cytomegalovirus as a cofactor for HIV-l entry. *Science*, 276, 1874–8.

Poccia, F., Battistini, L., Cipriani, B., Mancino, G., Martini, F., Gougeon, M. L., et al. (1999). Phosphoantigen-reactive Vgamma9Vdelta2 T lymphocytes suppress in vitro human immunodeficiency virus type 1 replication by cell-released antiviral factors including CC chemokines. *J Infect Dis*, 180(3), 858–61.

Poli, G., Bressler, P., & Kinter, E. (1990a). Interleukin-6 induces human immunodeficiency virus expression in infected monocytes alone and in synergy with tumor necrosis factor alpha by transcriptional and post-transcriptional mechanisms. *J Exp Med*, 172, 253–6.

Popov, S., Rexach, M., & Zybarth, G. (1998). Viral protein R regulates nuclear import of the HIV-l preintegration complex. *EMBO J*, 17, 909–17.

Porwit, A., Böttiger, B., Pallesen, G., Bodner, A., & Biberfeld, P. (1989a). Follicular involution in HIV lymphadenopathy. A morphometric study. *APMIS* 97(2), 153–65.

Porwit, A., Parravicini, C., Petren, A. L., Barkhem, T., Costanzi, G., Josephs, S., et al. (1989b). Cell association of HIV in AIDS-related encephalopathy and dementia. *APMIS* 97(1), 79–90.

Price, D. A., Sewell, A. K., Dong, T., et al. (1998). Antigen-specific release of beta-chemokines by anti-HIV-I cytotoxic T-Iymphocytes. *Curro Biol*, 8, 355–8.

Paiardini, M., Frank, I., Pandrea, I., Apetrei, C., & Silvestri, G. (2008). Mucosal immune dysfunction in AIDS pathogenesis *AIDS Review*, 10, 36–46, 4.

Reinhart, T. A., Rogan, M. J., Huddleston, D., Rausch, D. M., Eiden, L. E., & Haase, A. T. (1997). Sinlian immunodeficiency virus burden in tissues and cellular compartments during cellular latency and AIDS. *J Infect Dis*, 176, 1198–208.

Reinhart, T. A., Qin, S., & Sui, Y. (2009). Multiple roles for chemokines in the pathogenesis of SIV infection. *Curr HIV Res*, 7(1), 73–82. Review.

Rinaldo, C. R. Jr., Armstrong, J. A., Kingsley, L. A., Zhou, S., & Ho, M. (1990). Relation of alpha and gamma interferon levels to development of AIDS in homosexual men. *J Exp Pathol*, 5, 127–32.

Roederer M, Raju PA, Mitra DK, Herzenberg LA, Herzenberg LA. (1997) HIV does not replicate in naive CD4 T cells stimulated with CD3/CD28. *J Clin Invest*. 99(7):1555–64.

Rodriguez, C., Thomas, J. K., O'Rourke, S., Stiehm, E. R., & Plaeger, S. (1996). HIV disease in children is associated with selective decrease in CD23 and CD62L B-cells. *Clin Immunol Immunopathol*, 81, 191–9.

Roulston, A., Lin, R., Beuparlant, P., Weinberger, M. A., & Hiscott, J. (1995). Regulation of human immunodeficiency virus type I and cytokine gene expression in myeloid cells by NF-κB/Rel transcription factors. *Microbiol Rev*, 59, 481–505.

Roulston, A., Marcellus, R. C., & Branton, P. E. (1999). Viruses and apoptosis. *Annu Rev Microbiol*, 11, 578–608.

Sacktor N, Skolasky RL, Cox C, Selnes O, Becker JT, Cohen B, Martin E, Miller EN; Multicenter AIDS Cohort Study (MACS). (2010) Longitudinal psychomotor speed performance in human immunodeficiency virus-seropositive individuals: impact of age and serostatus. *J Neurovirol*, 16(5):335–41.

Salzwedel, K. & Berger, E. A. (2000). Cooperative subunit interactions within the oligomeric envelope glycoproteins of HIV-l: Functional complementation of specific defects in gp120 and gp41. *Proc Natl Acad Sci USA*, 97, 12794–9.

Sato, Y., Hirayama, M., Morimoto, K., Yamamoto, N., Okuyama, S., Hori, K. (2011), High mannose-binding lectin with preference for the cluster of {alpha}1-2 mannose from the green alga Boodlea coacta is a potent entry inhibitor of HIV-1 and influenza viruses. *J Biol Chem*, 2011 Apr 1.

Schmitz, J. E., Kuroda, M. J., Santra, S. Sasseville, V. G., Simon, M. A., Lifton, P., et al. (1999). Control of viremia in simian immunodeficiency virus infection by CD8+ lymphocytes. *Science, 283*, 857–860.

Schnittman, S. M. & Fauci, A. S. (1994). Human immunodeficiency virus and acquired immunodeficiency syndrome: An update. *Adv Intern Med, 39*, 305–55.

Sherman, M. P. & Greene, W. C. (2002). Slipping through the door: HIV entry into the nucleus. *Microbes Infection, 4*, 67–73.

Shirai, A, Cosentino, M., Leitman-Klinman, S., & Klinman, D. (1992). Human immunodeficiency virus infection induces both polyclonal and virus specific B-cell activation. *J Clin Invest, 89*, 561–6.

Spear, T, Sullivan, B. L., Landay, A. L., & Lint, T. F. (1990). Neutralization of human immunodeficiency virus type 1 by complement occurs by viral lysis. *J Virol, 64*, 5869–73.

Spira, A. I., Marx, P. A., & Patterson, B. K. (1996). Cellular targets of infection and route of viral dissemination after an intravaginal inoculation of simian immunodeficiency virus into rhesus macaques. *J Exp Med, 183*, 215–25.

Steinman, R. M. (1991). The dendritic cell system and its role in immunogenicity. *Annu Rev Immunol, 9*, 271–96.

Steinman RM, Banchereau J. (2007) Taking dendritic cells into medicine. Nature. 27;449(7161):419–26.

Stevenson M, Gendelman HE. (1994) Cellular and viral determinants that regulate HIV-1 infection in macrophages. *J Leukoc Biol.* 56(3):278–88.

Stockwin, L. H, McGonagle, D., Martin, I. G., & Blair, G. E. (2000). Dendritic cells: Immunological sentinels with a central role in health and disease. *Immunol Cell Biol, 78*, 91–102.

Stingele, K., Haas, J., Zimmermann, T., Stingele, R., Hübsch-Müller, C., Freitag, M., et al. (2001). Independent HIV replication in paired CSF and blood viral isolates during antiretroviral therapy. *Neurology, 56*(3), 355–61.

Strain, M. C., Letendre, S., Pillai, S. K., Russell, T., Ignacio, C. C., Günthard, H. F., et al. (2005). Genetic composition of human immunodeficiency virus type 1 in cerebrospinal fluid and blood without treatment and during failing antiretroviral therapy. *J Virol, 79*(3), 1772–88.

Sullivan, B. L., Knopoff, E. J., Saifuddin, M., et al. (1996). Susceptibility of HIV-1 plasma virus to complement-mediated lysis. *J Immunol, 157*, 1791–98.

Szelc, E. M., McMicheltree, E., Roberts, R. L., & Stiehm, E. R. (1992). Deficient polymorphonuclear cell and mononuclear cell antibody-dependent cellular cytotoxicity in pediatric and adult human immunodeficiency virus infection. *J Infect Dis, 166*, 486–93.

Tambussi, G., Gori, A., Capiluppi, B., et al. (2000). Neurological symptoms during primary human immunodeficiency virus infection correlate with high levels of HN RNA in cerebrospinal fluid. *Clin Infect Dis, 20*, 962–5.

Tashima, K. T., Flanigan, T. P., Kurpewski, J., Melanson, S. M., & Skolnik, P. R. (2002). Discordant human immunodeficiency virus type 1 drug resistance mutations, including K103N, observed in cerebrospinal fluid and plasma. *Clin Infect Dis, 35*(1), 82–3.

Thali, M., Bukovsky, A., & Kondo, E. (1994). Functional association of cyclophilin A with HIV virions. *Nature, 372*, 363–5.

Than, S., Hu, R., Oyaizu, N., et al. (1997). Cytokine pattern in relation to disease progression in human immunodeficiency virus-infected children. *J Infect Dis, 179*, 47–56.

Torheim, E. A., et al. (2009). Interleukin-10-secreting T cells defines a suppressive subset 748 within the HIV-1-specific T-cell population. *Eur J Immunol, 39*, 1280–1287.

Treitel, M. & Resh, M. D. (2001). The late stage of immunodeficiency virus type 1 assembly is an energy dependent process. *J Virol, 75*, 5473–81.

Vehmas A, Lieu J, Pardo CA, McArthur JC, Gartner S. (2004). Amyloid precursor protein expression in circulating monocytes and brain macrophages from patients with HIV-associated cognitive impairment. *J Neuroimmunol.* 157(1–2):99–110.

Voelkel, N. F., Cool, C. D., Flores, S. (2008) From viral infection to pulmonary arterial hypertension: a role for viral proteins? *AIDS.* Suppl 3:S49–53.

Wagner, L., Yang, O. O., & Garcia-Zepeda, E. A. (1998). B-chemokines are released from HIV-1 specific cytolytic T-cell granules complexed to proteglycans. *Nature, 391*, 1811–15.

Wahl, S. M. & Orenstein, J. M. (1997). Immune stimulation and HIV-1 viral replication. *J Leuco Biol, 62*, 67–71.

Wahl, S. M., Allen, J. B., Gartner, S., et al. (1989). HN-1 and its envelope glycoproteins downregulate chemotatic ligand receptors and chemotatic function of peripheral blood monocytes. *J Immunol, 142*, 3553–9.

Walker, C. M., Moody, D. J., Stites, D. P., & Levy J. A. (1986). CD8+ lymphocytes can control HN infection in vitro by suppressing virus replication. *Science, 234*, 1563–66.

Wallace, M., Bartz, S. R., Chang, W. L., Mackenzie, D. A., Pauza, C. D., & Malkovsky, M. (1996). gd T lymphocyte responses to HIV. *Clin Exp Immunol, 103*, 177–84.

Weber, R., Bossart, W., Cone, R., Luethy, R., Moelling, K. (2001) Phase I clinical trial with HIV-1 gp160 plasmid vaccine in HIV-1-infected asymptomatic subjects. *Eur J Clin Microbiol Infect Dis.* 20(11):800–3.

Wei, X., Gosh, S., & Taylor, M (1995). Viral dynamics in human immunodeficiency virus type 1 infection. *Nature, 373*, 117–22.

Weichold, E. F., Zelia, D., & Barabitskaja, O. (1998). Neither human immunodeficiency virus-1 (HIV-1) nor HIV-2 infects most-primitive human hematopoietic stem cells as assessed in long-term bone marrow cultures. *Blood, 91*, 907–15.

Weiss, R. A. (2008). On viruses, discovery, and recognition. *Cell, 135*(6), 983–6.

Weiss, R. A (1996). HIV receptors and the pathogenesis of AIDS. *Science, 272*, 1885–6.

Weiss, R. A. & Clapham, P. R. (1996). AIDS: Hot fusion of HIV-1. *Nature, 381*, 647–8.

Weiss, R. A., Clapham, P., Nagy, I. C., & Hosino, H. (1990). Oligomeric organization of gp120 on infectious human immunodeficiency virus type 1 particles. *J Virol, 64*, 5674–7.

Weiss, R. A., Clapham, P. R., Weber, J. N., Dalgleish, A. G., Lasky, L. A., & Berman, P. W. (1986). Variable and conserved neutralization antigens of human immunodeficiency virus. *Nature, 324*(6097), 572–5.

Williams KC, Corey S, Westmoreland SV, Pauley D, Knight H, deBakker C, Alvarez X, Lackner AA. (2001) Perivascular macrophages are the primary cell type productively infected by simian immunodeficiency virus in the brains of macaques: implications for the neuropathogenesis of AIDS. *J Exp Med.* 193(8):905–15.

Wilson, J. D., Ogg, G. S., Allen, R. L., Davis, C., Shaunak, S., Downie, J., et al. (2000). Direct visualization of HIV-1-specific cytotoxic T lymphocytes during primary infection. *AIDS, 14*, 225–233.

Woods, T. E., Roberts, B. D., Butera, S. T., & Follzs, T. M. (1997). Loss of inducible virus in CD45RA naive cells after human immunodeficiency virus-1 entry accounts for preferential viral replication in CD45RO memory cells. *Blood, 89*, 1635–41.

Wyatt, R. & Sodroski, J. (1998). The HIV-1 envelope glycoproteins: Fusogens, antigens, and immunogens. *Science, 280*, 1884–8.

Xu, X. N., Laffert, B., Screaton, G. R., et al. (1999). Induction of Fas ligand expression by HIV-1 involves the interaction of Nef with the T cell receptor zeta chain. *J Exp Med, 189*, 1489–96.

Yang, O. O, Kalams, S. A., & Rosenzweig, M. (1996). Efficient lysis of human immunodeficiency virus type I-infected cells by cytotoxic T lymphocytes. *J Virol, 70*, 5799–806.

Yang, X. & Gabuzda, D. (1999). Regulation of human immunodeficiency virus type-1 infectivity by the ERK mitogen-activated protein kinase signaling pathway. *J Virol, 73*, 3460–6.

Yarchoan, R., Redfield, R., & Broder, S. (1986). Mechanism of cell activation in patients with acquired immunodeficiency syndrome and related disorders. *J Clin Invest, 78*, 439–47.

Yu, X. G., Addo, M. M., Rosenberg, E. S., et al. (2002). Consistent patterns in the development and immunodominance of human immunodeficiency virus -1 (HIV-1)-specific CD8+ T-cell responses following acute HIV-1 infection. *J Virol, 76*, 8690–701.

1.3

CHEMOKINES

Richard J. Miller

HIV-1-related central and peripheral nervous system problems are highly prevalent but the details of their pathogenesis are poorly understood. A widely held hypothesis is that infected cells in the nervous system secrete neurotoxins that exert direct and indirect deleterious effects. Candidate neurotoxins include excitotoxins, inflammatory mediators, and HIV-1 viral proteins. There is evidence that chemokines and chemokine receptors, which are expressed in all major cell types in the brain, may play pivotal roles in many of these diverse neurotoxic processes. This chapter explores these possible roles. Close attention is paid to a several proposed mechanisms, including those involving the CXCR4 chemokine receptor and the HIV gp120 protein, whose effects may be partly mediated by cytokine-related processes. To help provide a framework for understanding these complex pathogenic phenomena, the role of chemokines and chemokine receptors in normal development and function is discussed.

INTRODUCTION

It is a truth, universally acknowledged, that the consequences of HIV-1 infection encompass not only the immune system but the nervous system as well. The majority of individuals infected by HIV-1 display neurological symptoms and associated neuropathology involving both the central (CNS) and peripheral (PNS) nervous systems. (Kaul, Garden, & Lipton, 2001; Kolson & Gonzales-Scarano, 2001). The serious and incapacitating nature of these syndromes means that neurological problems make a significant contribution to the overall clinical picture in AIDS.

In spite of the fact that HIV-1-related neurological problems are so prevalent, there is little real understanding as to the mechanisms underlying HIV-1-related damage to the nervous system. Indeed, in many respects the situation is less straightforward than that associated with HIV-1-related problems with the immune system. The destruction of leukocytes by HIV-1 is associated with infection of these cells by the virus and its subsequent replication. On the other hand, this is not the case for HIV-1-related neuropathology (Kaul et al., 2001; Kolson & Gonzales-Scarano, 2001). The brains of HIV-1-infected individuals exhibit morphological changes to microglia, astrocytes, and neuronal populations, although it is widely believed that the virus only productively infects microglia (Gabuzda & Wang, 2000; Garden, 2002; Kaul et al., 2001; Kolson & Gonzales-Scarano, 2001). It is therefore not at all obvious how such widespread neuropathology might be produced. A generally held hypothesis suggests that infected cells in the nervous system such as microglia must secrete one or more neurotoxins that elicit a cascade of deleterious effects (Kaul et al., 2001). Although such an idea seems reasonable, the precise nature of these secondary neurotoxins remains obscure, even though there is a long list of possibilities. Indeed, it is likely that HIV-1-related neuropathology stems from more than one process. For example, problems resulting from the presence of inflammatory reactions in the brain (HIV encephalitis, HIVE) or from opportunistic infections may be important (Williams & Hickey, 2002). However, other mechanisms directly related to the effects of the virus within the nervous system should also be considered.

In order to understand how HIV-1 compromises the nervous system, it is useful to first examine its mechanism of action in the immune system. HIV-1 infects target cells by binding to receptors expressed in their membranes. The major coat protein of the virus, gp120, binds with high affinity to one of the chemokine receptors, usually in conjunction with the hCD4 molecule (Rossi & Zlotnik, 2000). Conformational changes ensuing from this interaction allow the virus to fuse its membrane with that of its target and insert its DNA into the host cell. However, as we shall discuss, chemokine receptors normally function as important signaling elements in cells. Indeed, an increasing number of papers have now reported that binding of HIV-1 to these receptors may do more than just allow fusion of the virus with its target and may also elicit important signaling events that regulate the fate of target cells (Davis et al., 1997; Gabuzda & Wang, 2000). Are these observations relevant for attempts to explain HIV-1-related neuropathology? It is now clear that all of the major cell types in the brain are capable of expressing both chemokines and chemokine receptors, including those chemokine receptors like CXCR4 that normally act as binding sites for HIV-1 (Bajetto et al., 2001; Bajetto, Bonavia, Barbero, & Schettini, 2002; Kolson & Gonzalez-Scarano, 2001; Martin-Garcia et al., 2002). An important question, therefore, is whether, as in the immune system, chemokine receptors in the brain are important for HIV-1-related neuropathology and, if so, which chemokine receptors and why.

CHEMOKINES AND THEIR RECEPTORS

In order to be able to answer such questions, we should discuss the nature of chemokines and their receptors as well as their normal functions in the brain. Chemokines (the name is a contraction of the words CHEMOtactic cytoKINE) are a family of small proteins, originally shown to play a pivotal role in the control of leukocyte trafficking (Rossi & Zlotnik, 2000). Although this is still their best-studied function, chemokines have now been shown to be of key importance in the overall organization of the entire hematopoietic/lymphopoietic system, including the regulation of stem cell maturation, the formation of secondary lymphoid tissues, and angiogenesis (Ma, Jones, & Springer, 1999; Schwartz & Farber, 2002; Szekanecz & Koch, 2001; Nagasawa et al., 1996). Moreover, because chemokines and their receptors are also intimately involved in the orchestration of inflammatory responses and in the pathogenesis of AIDS (Berger, Murphy, & Farber, 1999), they are considered to be important potential therapeutic targets in these diseases (Proudfoot, 2002). Based on recent findings that chemokines and their receptors are involved in controlling organogenesis, as well the maturation and migration of different types of stem cells (Knaut, Werz, Gelser, & Nusslein-Volhard, 2002; Doitsidou et al., 2002; McGrath, Koniski, Maltby, McGann, & Palis, 1999; Braun et al., 2002; Moepps et al., 2000; Tachibana et al., 1998), it is now becoming clear that chemokine-mediated signaling may have a far wider influence than originally anticipated. Thus, aside from the hematopoietic/lymphopoietic system, chemokines probably have important roles to play in the development and homeostasis of all tissues.

What then, if anything, do chemokines have to do with the nervous system? It is well known that chemokines and their receptors have an important part to play in neuroinflammatory disease (DeGroot & Woodroofe, 2001). In keeping with their traditionally defined roles as organizers of the immune system, chemokines produced by resident brain cells have been shown to be of central importance in guiding leukocytes to sites of inflammation within the brain. In addition, however, recent work has established that all of the major cell types in the brain, including microglia, glia, neurons and neural stem cells, can express different chemokine receptors, making them all potential targets for the actions of chemokines. Furthermore, it is known that these different cell types are capable of synthesizing chemokines, suggesting that a complete chemokine ligand/receptor system exists independently within the brain. Thus, it now appears that chemokines may play a much more complex role in the nervous system, extending far beyond their known role as local mediators of immune and inflammatory responses.

Although these observations are intriguing, they also raise many questions. For instance, do the effects of chemokines in the brain merely recapitulate their well-established effects on leukocytes or is something else afoot? Indeed, we now know that chemokines and their receptors participate in the development of the cerebellum, hippocampus, and many other parts of the nervous system; regulate oligodendrocyte maturation and myelination in the spinal cord; and influence axonal growth, neuronal survival, and a host of other interesting phenomena. Many of the effects described so far have involved the CXCR4 chemokine receptor and its unique ligand, the chemokine CXCL12/SDF-1. However, there are numerous

indications that other chemokines and their receptors are important as well.

Over 50 chemokines have been identified to date (Berger, Murphy, & Farber, 1999; Murphy et al., 2000; Murphy, 2002). All of these molecules share certain similarities in their primary sequences and, more importantly, a similar overall tertiary structure (Proudfoot, 2002). Chemokines can be tentatively grouped into subfamilies according to different structural criteria, particularly the position of a pair of cysteines located near the N terminal of each protein (Rossi & Zlotnik, 2000; Proudfoot, 2002; Proudfoot, Shaw, Power, & Wells, 2002). If a single amino acid separates the two cysteines the chemokine is designated an α-chemokine. If the two cysteines directly follow one another, then the chemokine is designated a β-chemokine. Moreover, the presence of only a single cysteine residue, such as in lymphotactin, places the chemokine in the δ-chemokine family, whereas two cysteines separated by three amino acids as in the case of fractalkine, places it in the γ-chemokine family. The majority of chemokines are in the α or β families. There is only one member in the γ and δ-families known at this time. In general, chemokines are secreted from cells. However in rare cases, such as the δ-chemokine fractalkine and CXCL16, the unique ligand for the CXCR6 receptor, the chemokine moiety is found tethered to a transmembrane mucin–like stalk. Fractalkine can act in this tethered mode or else be cleaved from its mucin stalk and act at remote targets. Each chemokine possesses a "trivial" name, such as stromal cell-derived factor 1 (SDF-1), as well as a systematic name, such as CXCL12. In this chapter I will generally use the trivial name.

All of the known effects of chemokines are transduced through the activation of G-protein-coupled receptors (GPCRs), whereby 6 GPCRs mediate the effects of α- and 10 GPCRs mediate the effects of β-chemokines. As for the γ-and δ-chemokines, their effects are mediated by only one GPCR. Two major patterns of chemokine/receptor selectivity are apparent: Some chemokine receptors can be activated by multiple chemokines, whereas others, such as the CXCR4 receptor, have only one known agonist, in this case the chemokine SDF-1. Recently, a second receptor for SDF-1 has been identified and named CXCR7 (Thelen & Thelen, 2008). This receptor, which is widely expressed in the developing and adult nervous systems (Fig 1.3.1), also recognizes CXCL11/ITAC (Interferon-inducible T-cell Alpha Chemoattractant). This is a very interesting receptor as although it has a typical GPCR structure it does not seem to signal in a typical GPCR manner. Thus, rather than activating a G-protein, signaling resulting from the activation of CXCR7 receptors appears to exclusively utilize the β-arrestin signaling pathway (Rajagopal et al., 2010). How CXCR7 contributes to the biological effects of SDF-1 is not yet understood. However, the phenotype of CXCR7 knockout mice is clearly not identical to that of CXCR4 knockout mice. Indeed the former are viable whereas the latter die during embryogenesis (Sierro et al., 2007). Hence, it is clear that CXCR4 and CXCR7 must have predominantly separate functions.

Although a rapid expansion in the number of chemokines and their receptors is phylogenetically associated with the

CXCR7 -EGFP expression pattern in the hippocampus

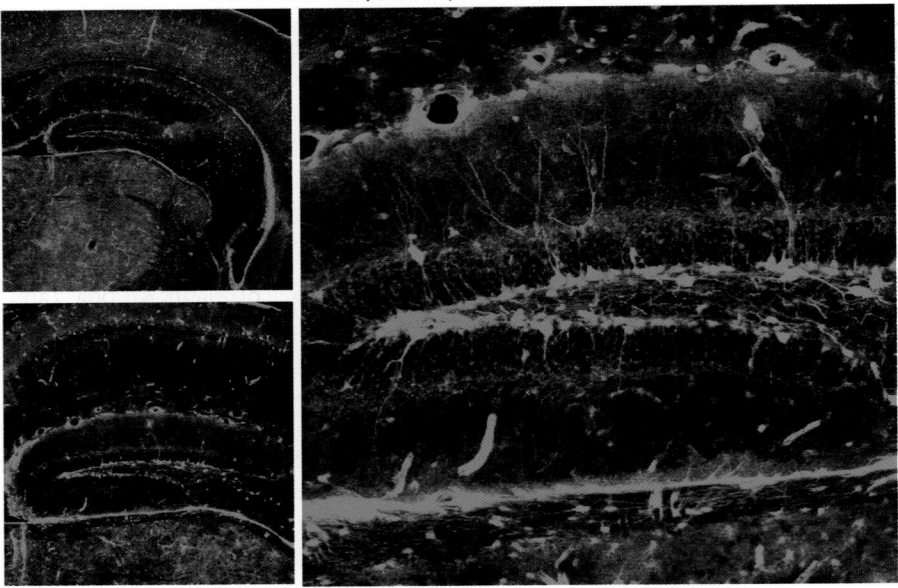

Figure 1.3.1 Expression of CXCR7 receptors in the hippocampus of a 6 week old CXCR7-EGFP transgenic mouse. Note the expression of CXCR7 by numerous blood vessels and neurons (unpublished observations).

development of vertebrates, homologues of these molecules have been identified in simpler systems. For instance the genomes of several viruses encode chemokines and their receptors, and these genes are of importance for viral pathogenesis (Proudfoot et al., 2002). An observation of considerable significance was the finding that certain chemokine receptors, particularly CCR5 and CXCR4, are used by HIV-1 to infect target cells, as discussed above (Berger et al., 1999). Because the sequence of the HIV-1 coat protein gp120 varies with each viral strain, different viruses exhibit greater affinity for either CCR5 or CXCR4 receptors, which are predominantly expressed by different subsets of leukocytes. Hence, these observations also help to explain HIV-1 tropism—the reason why different viral strains selectively infect different types of cells.

BRAIN CHEMOKINE RECEPTORS IN HIV-1-RELATED DEMENTIA

As discussed above, the view is widely held that HIV-1-related neuropathology results from the secretion of toxic factors from infected cells in the brain. The infected cells might be microglia or other macrophage-like cells (perivascular macrophages) that enter the brain in association with HIVE. Furthermore, it is quite possible that more than one type of neurotoxin might be involved. There has been no shortage of suggestions as to the nature of these secreted toxins. For example, glutamate-induced excitotoxicity has long been thought to play a role in HIV-1-related effects in the brain and drugs that block glutamate receptors have been suggested as potential therapeutic agents in HAD (Kaul, Garden, & Lipton, 2001; Kolson & Gonzalez-Scarano, 2001). Inflammatory

cytokines, such as TNF-α, IL-1, and IL-6 have also been frequently suggested as playing an important role (Kaul et al., 2001; Kolson & Gonzalez-Scarano, 2001). Finally, it is also widely believed that viral proteins, shed from replicating viruses in microglia or other cells, may act as toxins in the brain. These could be proteins such as gp120, the HIV-1 coat protein, or other viral proteins such as Tat. Indeed, there is evidence suggesting a role for many of these proteins as potential neurotoxins (Kaul et al., 2001; Kolson & Gonzalez-Scarano, 2001; Nath, 2002). The participation of gp120 has been the focus of considerable attention. The idea that gp120 could be an endogenous neurotoxin in HAD comes from a variety of sources. For example, purified gp120 injected into the brains of rodents (Corasaniti, 2001), or incubated with neurons in culture, clearly induces neuronal death as well as activation of microglia and astrocytes, indicating that the protein could be directly toxic to neurons or kill neurons by inducing the release of toxins from cells such as microglia and astrocytes (Kaul et al., 2001; Garden, 2002; Meucci et al., 1998; Meucci & Miller, 1996). Furthermore, transgenic mice which overexpress gp120 develop pathological signs that are reminiscent of those in HAD. (Toggas et al., 1994) If, as these data suggest, gp120 is a significant participant in HIV-1 related events in the brain, then this raises the issue of how it produces its effects. As we know that chemokine receptors are the major binding sites for gp120, one would imagine that these receptors in the brain would mediate the effects of the protein. One consideration is that although many types of chemokine receptors are expressed by cells in the brain, not all of these are susceptible to interactions with gp120. The major receptors of importance are likely to be CXCR4 and CCR5 receptors and possibly CCR3 receptors that are known to be highly expressed by microglia. Neural stem cells in neurogenic regions of the adult brain and some neurons also express CXCR4 receptors (Bhattacharrya et al., 2008; Tran, Ren, Chenn, & Miller, 2007). It is therefore interesting to examine data on which strains of the HIV-1 virus are most likely to be associated with HAD. The development of HIV-1 in the brain occurs separately from virus in the periphery. Currently, it is thought that viruses with selectivity for the CXCR4 receptor or those able to bind to both CXCR4 and CCR5 are the most likely to produce neurological symptoms (Gorry et al., 2001). Such selectivity is only part of the story, as some brain-derived viruses with selectivity for CXCR4 do not produce neuronal apoptosis when tested in vitro (Gorry et al., 2001). Nevertheless, binding of virus/gp120 to the CXCR4 receptor would seem to be an important factor in the genesis of HAD. It should be noted in passing that many of the studies that have demonstrated the neurotoxic potential of gp120 have been performed in rodents (Meucci et al., 1998; Meucci & Miller, 1996; Toggas et al., 1994; Corasaniti et al., 2001). Given the fact that interactions of gp120 with chemokine receptors normally require the participation of the human (rodent won't do) CD4 molecule (Berger et al., 1999), one may wonder how this is achieved. Several studies have demonstrated that gp120s of various types can interact with neurons and other cells in the nervous system in a "CD4 independent manner" (Hesselgesser et al., 1998). How this occurs is not at all clear at this time. One possibility is that these cells express a molecule that can be used as a co-receptor instead of the CD4 molecule. Alternatively, much of the HIV-1-related neuropathology may involve the action of the virus at sites such as Toll-like receptors (Heil et al., 2004).

THE NORMAL FUNCTIONS OF BRAIN CHEMOKINE RECEPTORS

Prior to examining the role of chemokine receptors in the nervous system in the neuropathological aspects of HIV-1 infection, it is important to understand the normal functions of these receptors in the nervous system. Thus, if CXCR4 and CCR5 play important roles in the normal physiology of the nervous system it would be quite possible that these might be disrupted by HIV-1. The first papers demonstrating that neurons and other types of resident brain cells normally express chemokine receptors began to appear around 1997. Subsequently, several studies have been published describing the detailed distribution of certain chemokine receptors in the nervous system (Jazin, Soderstrom, Ebendal, & Larhammer, 1997; Lavi et al., 1997; Moepps, Frodl, Rodewald, Bagglioni, & Gierschik, 1997; Horuk et al., 1997; reviewed in Bajetto, Bonavia, Barbero, & Schettini, 2002; Bajetto et al., 2001). In those instances where the question has been examined, it appears that individual neurons can express complex combinations of different chemokine receptors (Meucci et al., 1998; Oh et al., 2001; Gillard, Mastracci, & Miller, 2001). Although the significance of this diversity of chemokine receptor expression is not fully understood, specific functions for particular chemokine receptors in the nervous system have now been clearly identified. In particular, the CXCR4 receptor and its sole known ligand SDF-1 are extensively expressed in the developing embryo from very early times, including at very high levels in the developing nervous system (McGrath et al., 1999; Braun et al., 2002; Moepps et al., 2000; Jazin et al., 1997). Patterns of CXCR4/SDF-1 expression are complementary and dynamic throughout embryogenesis, suggesting that CXCR4 receptors might be important in the development of the nervous system. This possibility was confirmed in 1998 when two groups described the phenotypes of mice in which the genes for the CXCR4 receptor or SDF-1 had been deleted (Zou, Kottmann, Kuroda, Taniuchi, & Littman, 1998, Ma et al., 1998). These mutant mice usually die around the time of birth and display various defects in organogenesis, including significant alterations in the development of the brain (Tachibana et al., 1998, Zou et al., 1998, Ma et al., 1998). The first neurological problem to be described concerned the cerebellum. During the normal course of cerebellar development, precursors for cerebellar granule neurons proliferate extensively during the early postnatal period (approx 4 weeks in rodents and 2 years in man) in a specialized zone known as the external granule layer (EGL). The EGL lies immediately beneath a layer of externally situated meningeal cells (pia mater), localized on the cerebellar surface. Following proliferation, postmitotic immature granule cells move to the inner aspect of the EGL and then migrate inwards along the processes of Bergmann glial cells to form the internal granule layer (IGL), consisting of mature granule cells. This orderly process was shown to be disrupted in the cerebella of CXCR4 and SDF-1 knockout (ko) mice. It was observed that the cerebella from mutant embryos contained groups of ectopically situated granule neurons within or beneath the Purkinje cell layer, suggesting aberrant early migration of granule cells and/or their precursors out of the EGL. However, other aspects of cerebellar development appeared to be normal. These results make perfect sense when one considers the normal spatial and temporal expression patterns of CXCR4 receptors and SDF-1 in the cerebellum at this time. (Klein et al., 2001, Reiss, Mentlein, Sievers, & Hartmann, 2002) SDF-1 is not expressed by cerebellar neurons, but is strongly expressed by the meningeal cells in the external pial layer. In contrast, CXCR4 receptors are expressed by dividing cells, presumably granule cell progenitors, in the EGL. Moreover, it had been previously demonstrated that the normal development of the IGL was dependent on the integrity of the pial layer and it had been suggested that these cells secreted some factor that regulated granule cell migration by attracting as well as maintaining granule cell progenitors within the EGL (Hartmann, Schulze, & Sievers, 1998). Indeed, the role of SDF-1 in this regard has now been demonstrated by showing that isolated granule cell progenitors or progenitors within EGL explants will migrate toward a source of exogenously provided SDF-1 (Klein et al., 2001, Zou et al., 1998). Furthermore, the observations that granule cell progenitors will normally migrate toward cerebellar meningeal cells (Klein et al., 2001, Reiss et al., 2002, Hartmann et al., 1998, Zhu et al., 2002), and that this migration is impeded in SDF-1 ko mice indicates that SDF-1 is the only, or at least the major, factor that maintains granule cell progenitors within the EGL (Zhu et al., 2002). Thus, granule progenitors are maintained in the proliferative environment of the EGL through the chemoattractant effects of SDF-1 secreted from the overlying pia mater. Moreover, as demonstrated by Klein et al. (2001), SDF-1 not only serves to localize progenitors within the EGL, but also plays a role in ensuring their proliferation through facilitatory interactions with sonic hedgehog (SHH), an important mitogen for granule cell precursors also found within the EGL. Although the synthesis of SDF-1 is maintained during development, at some point, perhaps because of interactions with other receptor signaling systems, granule cell progenitors downregulate CXCR4 expression and/or signaling and stop dividing. They move to the inner aspect of the EGL and then migrate to the IGL, presumably attracted there by other chemo attractants such as BDNF (Borghesani et al., 2002). An echo of these observations can be found in the known role of CXCR4/SDF-1 signaling in lymphocyte development. SDF-1 is expressed by cells in secondary lymphoid organs and serves to attract and maintain CXCR4 expressing precursor cells in this proliferative environment (Bleul, Schultze, & Springer, 1998). Moreover, deletion of the genes for SDF-1 or CXCR4 results in inappropriate redistribution of stem cells into the circulation prior to their maturation (Nagasawa et al., 1996, Zou et al., 1998, Ma et al., 1998).

When one examines the properties of embryonic cerebellar neurons, it is clear that they express many types of chemokine receptors (Gillard et al., 2001), suggesting that in addition to SDF-1, other chemokines and their receptors may also play distinct roles in cerebellar development. In support of this contention, a recent study has described the changing expression pattern of CCR1 receptors, as well as the CCR1 activating chemokine MIP-1α, during the development of the cerebellum (Cowell & Silverstein, 2003). It was observed that during the first three weeks after birth, CCR1 receptors are transiently expressed by all of the major cell types in the cerebellum, including granule cells, Purkinje and Golgi neurons, astrocytes, Bergmann glia, and microglia. However, the times at which all of these cell types express CCR1 receptors differ. Interestingly, during the times of peak receptor expression each cell type exhibits close interactions with Purkinje cells. Furthermore, the Purkinje cells themselves appear to synthesize the chemokine MIP-1α, a major ligand for CCR1 receptors. It has therefore been suggested that MIP-1α/CCR1 signaling may be of importance in the maturation of neurites and synapse formation during this crucial period of cerebellar development (Cowell & Silverstein 2003). Indeed, chemokines and their receptors may play a widespread role in the regulation of axonal growth. A recent study has demonstrated that SDF-1 can either attract or repel the growth cones of developing cerebellar granule neurons or Xenopus spinal neurons in culture, depending on the circumstances (Xiang et al., 2002). When levels of cGMP are low, SDF-1 produces growth cone repulsion, but this is transformed into attraction when the levels of this cyclic nucleotide are high. Thus, it is possible that CCR1 receptor signaling may play a role of this kind in the cerebellum.

In addition to the cerebellum, the widespread expression pattern for SDF-1/CXCR4 in the embryonic nervous system (McGrath et al., 1999) suggests that chemokine signaling may be important in the development of other brain areas as well. Indeed, it has now been demonstrated that CXCR4 receptors play an essential role in the development of the hippocampal dentate gyrus. Studies conducted by Lu et al. (2002) and Bagri et al. (2002) have shown that in CXCR4 KO mice the granule cell layer of the dentate gyrus fails to develop properly. Normally, precursors that are destined to form these granule cells originate in the dentate neuroepithelium (Altman & Bayer, 1990, Sievers, Hartmann, Pehlemann, & Berry, 1992). As they migrate away from this proliferative zone ("primary germinal matrix"), they form a stream of migratory cells that continue to proliferate (secondary germinal matrix), and which eventually populate the developing blades of the dentate gyrus, producing its typical V-shaped pattern. Subsequently, precursor cells continue to proliferate within the hilar region of the dentate gyrus (tertiary germinal matrix), producing very large numbers of dentate granule neurons in the early postnatal period. Eventually, reduced numbers of granule cell precursors settle in a narrow region between the granule cell layer and the hilus, and these precursors continue to generate new neurons throughout adult life. Adult neurogenesis in the hippocampal dentate gyrus is thought to be of great importance for the consolidation of memories, and disruption of this process may also be a key event in the generation of seizures and other abnormal brain activity (Gould & Gross, 2002). Thus, a clear understanding of the molecular events that underlie the formation and maintenance of the dentate gyrus has many important implications. Using a variety of molecular markers, cells that can be identified as dentate granule neurons can be observed in CXCR4 ko mice, although they appear to occur in reduced numbers (Lu, Grove, & Miller, 2002; Bagri et al., 2002). This implies that, as in the case of the cerebellum, SDF-1 may have proliferative effects on dentate granule cell precursors. Moreover, those granule cells that do occur are mostly found localized ectopically within the migratory stream. In other words, it appears as if reduced numbers of dentate granule cells can go through their normal developmental program, but do so without ever reaching their normal destination. As in the case of the cerebellum, these results can be understood by considering the normal localization of CXCR4\SDF-1 in the developing hippocampus (Fig 1.3.2) (Lu et al., 2002; Bagri et al., 2002). During embryogenesis in rodents, from around E14 until birth, SDF-1 is highly expressed in the meninges overlying the hippocampus as well as in Cajal-Retzius cells. These latter cells also express the molecule reelin, which has been shown to play a critical role in dentate granule cell migration. In contrast to the expression of SDF-1, CXCR4 receptors are strongly expressed over the same time period, but by cells in the migratory stream as well as the developing dentate gyrus, presumably immature granule cells and their precursors. (Fig 1.3.2) Thus, SDF-1 secreted by meningeal cells is in an excellent position to provide a guiding chemoattractant cue for CXCR4-expressing cells as they migrate towards the dentate gyrus. Therefore, in many respects, this situation represents an inversion of that in the developing cerebellum, where SDF-1 serves to maintain precursors in the EGL prior to migration. It is interesting to note that in adult

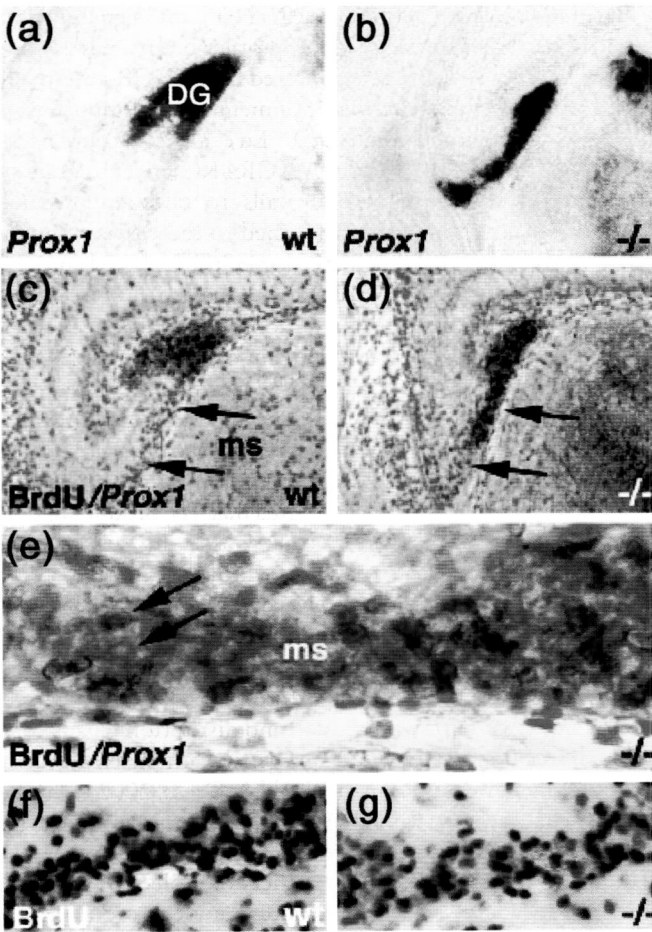

Figure 1.3.2 Defects in secondary proliferative cell population that forms the dentate gyrus (DG). (A-D) Coronal sections through the E18.5 hippocampus of wild type (A and C) ir CXCR4 mutant mice (B and D), processed to show expression of Prox1 blue or Prox1 together with BrdUrd-labeled dividing cells (orange). In the wild type mouse, Prox1 is expressed the forming dg (A and C). By contrast, in the mutant, Prox1 is expressed in the vestigal DG but also along the migratory stream (ms) (arrows in D) of dividing cells running along the ventral surface of the hippocampus into the dg. BrdUrd-labeled cells of the ms can be stream of cells shown in D. Numerous blue, Prox1-expressing appear among the brown, BrdUrd-labeled cells, but the populations appear largely distinct. (E) Higher magnification views of BrdUrd-labeled dividing cells (dark Blue) coursing through the ms in a wild-type (F) and a CXCR4 mutant mouse (G). About 30% fewer BrdUrd-labeled cells appear in the mutant (G) than in the wild type (F). From Lu et al., 2002.

animals, SDF-1 and CXCR4 continue to be expressed in the dentate gyrus, but by granule neurons and progenitor cells in the intragranular zone respectively. This suggests that CXCR4 signaling may be of continued importance in the production of new dentate granule neurons throughout life (Lu et al., 2002). SDF-1 is also produced by meningeal cells covering the surface of the entire cortex and might therefore be expected to play a role in cortical development as well. Intriguingly, many types of lissencephalic disease (i.e. neuronal migrational defects that lead to abnormal sulci in the cerebral cortex) are associated with hypertrophy of the meningeal layer and abnormal "overmigration" of developing cortical neurons,

consistent with some chemoattractant role for SDF-1 in the migration of these cells (Hartmann et al., 1999). Meningeal expression of CXCL12 controls positioning and migration of Cajal-Retzius cells via CXCR4 signaling (Borrell & Marin, 2006; Paredes, Li, Berger, Baraban, & Pleasure, 2006). Furthermore, SDF-1/CXCR4 signaling controls cortical interneuron migration by focusing the cells within migratory streams and controlling their position within the cortical plate (Li et al., 2008; Lopez-Bendito et al., 2008; Stumm et al., 2003; Tiveron et al., 2006).

In summary, therefore, there is good evidence for both chemotactic and proliferative effects of chemokine signaling, particularly through the CXCR4 receptor, in association with several important aspects of neuronal development. Additional studies have indicated that different chemokines may act as chemotactic cues for other neuronal populations, (Bolin et al., 1998) so a widespread role for chemokines in the orchestration of neuronal development is certainly possible.

Aside from neurons, chemokine receptor signaling also appears to be important in the development of glia. Signaling via CXCR2 receptors, which are also widely expressed in the nervous system throughout embryogenesis (Luan, Furuta, Du, & Richmond, 2001), has been shown to direct the development of oligodendrocytes and myelination in the spinal cord (Tsai et al., 2002; Robinson et al., 1998; Wu, Miller, Ransohoff, Robinson, & Nishayama, 2000). In the first week after birth, oligodendrocyte precursor cells (OPCs) develop in the ventral ventricular zone of the embryonic spinal cord and these cells express CXCR2 receptors. At the same time, the chemokine GRO-α, which acts as an agonist at CXCR2 receptors, is synthesized by astrocytes in this region. GRO-α has two effects on OPCs. First, somewhat surprisingly for a chemokine, it inhibits their migration. This effect is achieved by enhancing adhesive interactions between OPCs and the extra cellular matrix. Secondly, GRO-α cooperates with platelet-derived growth factor (PDGF), a widely expressed mitogen for OPCs, which enhances proliferation of OPCs in the ventral cord. These cells subsequently differentiate and myelinate axons in this part of the cord. At later times the synthesis of GRO-α in the ventral cord wanes, and as a result the migration of OPCs is no longer inhibited, allowing OPCs to migrate into the dorsal portion of the cord. Simultaneously, the synthesis of GRO-α by astrocytes in the dorsal cord is upregulated. Thus, the proliferation of OPCs is now stimulated in the dorsal cord and myelination of axons in this region of cord can proceed. In addition to CXCR2, it has also been reported that oligodendrocyte progenitors express CXCR4 receptors and that interference with SDF-1/CXCR4 signaling may disrupt the development of oligodendrocytes in the spinal cord. Hence, the development of oligodendrocytes may be under the control of several chemokine signaling systems.

Chemokine receptors may also play a key role in the control of myelination in the peripheral nervous system (Kury, Greiner-Petter, Cornely, Jurgens, & Muller, 2002). Following peripheral nerve injury, axons distal to the lesion degenerate and are broken down in a process known as Wallerian degeneration. As a result, new axons can now regenerate from the remaining stump. During the process of nerve regeneration,

Schwann cells, the glial cells that are responsible for myelination in the peripheral nervous system, actively proliferate, and it has been demonstrated that these cells express the β helix-loop-helix transcription factor, Mash2. Furthermore, this transcription factor is downregulated after peripheral nerve injury and appears to be a negative regulator of Schwann cell proliferation. Interestingly, two of the genes that are downstream of Mash2 are the chemokine Mob-1 (the mouse homologue of the chemokine IP-10) and the CXCR4 receptor. It is interesting to note that Schwann cells in adult peripheral nerve have been shown to co-express Mash2 and CXCR4 receptors. Because these cells also express SDF-1, it seems highly likely that SDF-1 is involved in the paracrine regulation of Schwann cell development.

In summary, two major themes emerge from the reported effects of chemokines in the developing nervous system. The first is that chemokines are clearly important in directing the movement of progenitor cells to different locales—something that one might expect based on their well-established chemoattractant effects on leukocytes. Interestingly, however, there appear to be multiple variations on this theme, with chemokines acting as either "stop" or "go" signals depending on the circumstances. The second major theme to emerge is the apparent role of chemokines in ensuring the continued proliferation of progenitor cell populations, something that has been observed in the cerebellum, hippocampus, and spinal cord. In such cases, chemokines usually seem to play the role of facilitating the effects of another major mitogen such as SHH or PDGF. Thus, chemokines may act as generally important regulators of neural progenitor cell development—something that is clearly worth investigating further. It is an intriguing possibility that interference of some of the developmentally important functions of CXCR4 receptors by HIV-1 could contribute to its neuropathological effects.

CHEMOKINE RECEPTOR FUNCTION IN ADULT NEURONS

As we have discussed, many of the effects of chemokines that have been described in the developing nervous system are analogous to those observed in the developing hematopoietic/lymphopoietic system. According to some reports, chemokine receptors are also widely expressed in the adult nervous system by neurons, glia, and microglia. Data from several species, including rodents and primates, have demonstrated expression of many types of chemokine receptors by different subsets of mature neurons and glia under normal conditions (reviewed in Bajetto et al., 2002; Bajetto et al., 2001; Oh et al., 2001). Intriguingly, many of these receptors are up- or down-regulated under pathological conditions as well as in response to stressful stimuli (Bajetto et al., 2002; Bajetto et al., 2001; Oh et al., 2001). However, roles for chemokine receptor signaling in adult neurons have not been completely defined at this time, although the data so far suggests some strong possibilities.

GPCRs are extremely versatile molecules and can signal in a wide variety of modes (Pierce et al., 2002). Classically, receptor activation affords signaling through the subunits of heterotrimeric G protein. In addition, however, activation of GPCRs can also lead to signaling through several other pathways. For example, the recruitment of members of the family of β-arrestin scaffolding proteins to GPCRs can produce downstream activation of src, the MAP kinases as well as many other pathways that are associated with cell survival and differentiation. Indeed, as discussed above, the CXCR7 receptor may signal exclusively through this pathway (Rajagopal et al., 2010). The consequences of activating GPCRs in neurons have been extensively studied. It has been demonstrated that activation of heterotrimeric G protein can produce rapid effects on neuronal ion channels that result in changes in neuronal excitability and synaptic communication (Miller, 1998). In addition, activation of GPCRs can also produce long-term effects on the survival of neurons and other types of cells (e.g., Molina-Holgado et al., 2002; Yan, Lin, Irwin, & Paul, 1995; Vaudry et al., 2002). Evidence is accumulating that chemokines can produce both rapid and long-term effects on neurons through the direct activation of neuronally expressed chemokine receptors. For example, presynaptically localized GPCRs often function to reduce evoked transmitter release through the modulation of Ca and/or K channels, resulting in the subsequent inhibition of depolarization-induced Ca entry into nerve terminals (Miller, 1998). Experiments using heterologous expression systems have demonstrated that chemokine receptors can effectively signal to voltage-dependent Ca and K channels (Madani, Kozak, Kavanaugh, & Kabat, 1998; Oh et al., 2002). In keeping with these observations, activation of chemokine receptors expressed by neurons has been shown to alter Ca^{+2} influx as well as synaptic communication in the cerebellum (Ragozzino et al., 2002; Limatola et al., 2000; Ragozzino et al., 1998; Giovannelli et al., 1998), hippocampus (Meucci et al., 1998), and septum (Puma et al., 2001). Activation of CXCR4 receptors in cerebellar slices produces presynaptic inhibition of glutamate release at parallel fiber synapses (Ragozzino et al., 2002). In addition, activation of CXCR4, as well as several other types of chemokine receptors, has been shown to decrease excitatory transmission between hippocampal neurons in culture (Meucci et al., 1998) and activation of CXCR2 receptors can inhibit voltage-sensitive Ca^{+2} influx into acutely isolated septal neurons (Puma et al., 2001). Thus, as is the case with many other types of GPCRs, activation of presynaptically situated chemokine receptors may regulate transmitter release throughout the brain. Moreover, chemokines may also produce other types of electrophysiological effects resulting from activation of alternative signaling pathways. For example, activation of CXCR2 receptors in cerebellar slices produced Ca^{+2} mobilization, resulting in enhanced spontaneous transmitter release from granule and Purkinje cells (Ragozzino et al., 1998). In the peripheral nervous system, chemokine receptors have been shown to be expressed by sensory neurons, particularly small diameter nociceptors (Oh et al., 2001; Bolin et al., 1998). It was observed that activation of these receptors by chemokines or gp120, the coat protein of HIV-1, produced powerful excitatory effects reminiscent of those produced by pain-producing agents such as bradykinin or capsaicin. Such effects could be of significance for our understanding of increased pain sensitivity associated with inflammation or with HIV-1 infection.

In addition to rapid regulation of neuronal excitability and synaptic transmission, there is also evidence that neuronal chemokine receptors can produce important effects on neuronal survival. Several reports have demonstrated the survival-promoting actions of chemokines on hippocampal and cerebellar granule neurons in culture (Meucci et al., 1998; Limatola et al., 2000; Araujo & Cotman, 1993; Meucci et al., 2000; Kaul et al., 1999; Tong et al., 2000), and it was observed that activation of neuronal chemokine receptors could inhibit neuronal death produced by a variety of pro-apoptotic stimuli. Furthermore, in keeping with the observation that different neurons express multiple types of chemokine receptors, several different types of chemokines seem to promote neuronal survival depending on the neuronal population under consideration. The signaling pathways through which chemokines enhance survival appear to involve activation of ERK and Akt (Meucci et al., 1998; Meucci et al., 2000; Lazarini et al., 2000; Xia et al., 2002; Xia et al., 2000), pathways that have frequently been linked to pro-survival responses. For example, it has been shown that the ability of fractalkine to enhance the survival of hippocampal neurons in culture depends on the activation of Akt (Meucci et al., 2000). However, it is interesting to note that in some reports SDF-1 actually produces neuronal death rather than increasing neuronal survival (Kaul & Lipton, 1999; Hesselgesser et al., 1998). Consistent with this, it has been shown that stimulation of CXCR4 receptors expressed by neuronal and non-neuronal cells can simultaneously produce activation of multiple members of the MAP kinase pathway, including those such as p38 that are associated with increased apoptosis (Kaul & Lipton, 1999; Vlahakis et al., 2002). Thus, the ultimate cellular response to activation of some chemokine receptors may depend on a balance between several different competing outputs—something that might change according to circumstances.

These data also raise questions about the circumstances under which the observed effects of chemokines might be physiologically relevant. For instance, what are the normal sources of chemokines that might activate these receptors and when is chemokine signaling normally utilized in the adult brain? Based on examination of the distribution of chemokine receptors and their potential ligands, it seems that, in addition to glia and microglia, neurons may also be the source of chemokines in some instances (e.g., Cowell & Silverstein, 2003; Xia et al., 2002; Harori, Nagai, Heisel, Ryu, & Kim, 2002; Schreiber et al., 2001; Meng, Oka, & Takashima, 1999). This can be illustrated by recent detailed reports on the distribution of SDF-1 and CXCR4 receptors in the brains of rodents and other species (Stumm et al., 2002; Banisadr et al., 2002; Cheng et al., 2000; Banisadr et al., 2000; Gleichmann et al., 2000; Tham et al., 2001; Van der Meer, Ulrich, Gonzalez-Scarano, & Lavi, 2000; Westmoreland et al., 2002), whereby SDF-1 is clearly expressed by the granule neurons of the

dentate gyrus as well as neurons in the entorhinal cortex. In contrast, CXCR4 receptors are expressed by numerous neurons located in the lacunosum molecular layer of the hippocampus as well as in the hilar and molecular layers of the dentate gyrus. Based on what is known about the neuroanatomy of this part of the brain, synaptic contacts between SDF-1-expressing and CXCR4-expressing neurons are likely to occur. Whether SDF-1 is actually released from neurons and exactly what controls the secretion of chemokines in such cases is currently unknown. However, it has been reported that SDF-1 is tonically released from dentate granule neurons and that this downregulates the expression of CXCR4 receptors in this area of the brain (Kolodziej et al., 2008).

Neural stem cells in the subgranular zone of the dentate gyrus that participate in adult neurogenesis also express CXCR4 receptors (Bhattacharrya et al., 2008; Tran et al., 2007). SDF-1-expressing neurons and SDF-1-expressing endothelial cells in blood vessels are observed in close proximity to CXCR4-expressing neural stem cells, suggesting that SDF-1 might influence the development of these cells. It is known that the first synapses that contact developing neural stem cells are GABA mediated. The high Cl^- concentration found in neural stem cells means that activation of GABA-A receptors expressed by these cells results in an excitatory current due to the efflux of Cl^-. Prior to the establishment of *bona fide* synaptic connections, release of GABA from presynaptic neurons binds to high affinity GABA-A receptors to produce a tonic inward current. The presence of this current can be revealed by a GABA-A antagonist such as bicuculline, which blocks the tonic effects of GABA and therefore produces an outward current (Ge et al., 2007). Once GABAergic synapses are formed, GABA-mediated postsynaptic currents (PSCs) are also observed. When recording such GABA-mediated currents from DG neural stem cells, Bhattacharrya et al. (2008) observed that the effects of GABA were greatly enhanced by the addition of SDF-1. Like bicuculline, AMD3100 produced an outward current indicating that it contributed to the tonic inward current that can be observed in these cells. These data indicate that both GABA and SDF-1 are released in the DG and collaborate in producing excitatory inputs to neural stem cells. Thus, the neuroanatomical localization of SDF-1/CXCR4 together with the electrophysiological data indicate that, as in the original development of the DG discussed above, CXCR4 signaling is also important in the regulation of adult neurogenesis. However, the source of SDF-1 changes from the meninges (embryo/newborn) to DG interneurons (adult). Needless to say, the role of CXCR4 signaling we have demonstrated clearly indicates that adult neurogenesis may be a target for T-tropic HIV-1 strains in the brain.

In other circumstances, particularly in association with brain disease, it has been shown that chemokine synthesis and release can be upregulated by astrocytes or microglia (DeGroot & Woodroofe, 2001). Chemokines secreted from these cells might then act upon neuronal chemokine receptors and given the survival promoting effects of chemokines, it is possible that this might represent a survival strategy in the face of stressful stimuli.

CHEMOKINE-MEDIATED SIGNALING IN NEURONS

The effects produced by chemokines in the developing and adult nervous systems take place over vastly different time courses and presumably require the deployment of a wide range of signal transduction options. There are now several indications as to how this can be achieved. Interestingly, because of the versatility of chemokine receptors, it is possible that they can extend their signaling range through interactions with several other signaling systems. These signaling pathways may be blocked or inappropriately activated by HIV-1/gp120 leading to the resulting neuropathology.

As discussed above, all chemokine receptors are members of the extended family of GPCRs, and stimulation of these receptors will produce activated G protein subunits, which can then mediate different types of signaling. The vast majority of effects produced by chemokines in the hematopoietic/lymphopoietic system are blocked by pertussis toxin (PTX), indicating that chemokine receptors signal through activation of the Gi/o subfamily of Gprotein (Rossi & Zlotnik, 2000). In contrast, the PTX sensitivity of chemokine-mediated signaling in neurons is not always apparent (Gillard et al., 2001; Limatola et al., 2000; Xia et al., 2002). However, this may indicate that chemokine receptors in neurons sometimes signal through the non-PTX-sensitive Gz, which is highly expressed in neurons and is structurally related to Gi/o. Subsequently, activated G protein subunits may then mediate the rapid effects of chemokines on neuronal ion channels and synaptic communication. Furthermore, as with other GPCRs, chemokine receptors can also undergo cycles of desensitization, endocytosis, and resensitization in response to agonists (Cheng et al., 2000), and this phenomenon is associated with the binding of members of the arrestin family of scaffold proteins to the C terminal of the receptor (Perry & Lefkowitz, 2002). Binding of arrestins can then divert chemokine signaling into the MAP kinase pathway, something that might be important for the survival-promoting effects of chemokines, as discussed above. In addition, chemokine receptors may also exist as higher order structures, a phenomenon that appears to be common with GPCRs, and may even hetero-oligomerize with other closely related members of the chemokine receptor family (Rodriguez-Frade, Mellado, & Martinez, 2001; Issafras et al., 2002; Babcock, Farzan, & Sodroski, 2003). Indeed, one current model of chemokine receptor function suggests that receptor oligomerization is a *sine quae non* for all chemokine receptor signaling. It has also been suggested that chemokine receptors bind JAK kinases, which can then trans-phosphorylate tyrosine residues on chemokine receptor subunits following dimerization, in a manner similar to traditional cytokine receptors. As a result, these phosphotyrosines then act as docking sites for downstream signaling molecules including, in this case, a G protein (Rodriguez-Frade et al., 2001). In support of such an idea, a role for JAK signaling has been demonstrated in mediating certain effects of chemokines on leukocytes (Zhang et al., 2001). Presumably JAK-mediated signaling might also mediate some of the effects of chemokines in the nervous system.

What mechanisms might explain the different effects of chemokines observed during brain development? In both the cerebellum and dentate gyrus it has been shown that chemokines can produce proliferative as well as chemotactic effects (Klein et al., 2001; Lu et al., 2002; Bagri et al., 2002). However, it was observed that SDF-1 itself does not directly have proliferative effects on cerebellar granule cell progenitors, but rather it facilitates the effects of SHH (Klein et al., 2001). As it is well known that SHH signaling is inhibited by cAMP it has been suggested that inhibition of adenylate cyclase by SDF-1 could underlie the observed facilitation of SHH-induced proliferation. Subsequently, following an extended period of proliferation, postmitotic granule cell progenitors move to the inner aspect of the EGL and then migrate through the Purkinje cell layer to the IGL. The signals that terminate granule cell precursor proliferation and their SDF-1-mediated localization in the EGL are unknown, but since SDF-1 synthesis is maintained during this period, its influence must somehow be attenuated or overcome. According to one scenario, CXCR4 receptor expression by postmitotic granule cells is actually reduced (Reiss et al., 2002). However, two other interesting possibilities have also been suggested. One of these involves reverse signaling via ephrin-b, the ligand for the eph-b receptor. Both ephrin-b and its receptor are transmembrane-signaling molecules. Lu et al. (2001) demonstrated that expression of ephrin-b is upregulated in the EGL in the early postnatal period when granule cell migration is about to commence. Furthermore, these authors also showed that the cytoplasmic region of ephrin-b can bind a novel RGS (Regulator of Gprotein Signaling) protein, PDZ-RGS3, through interactions with its PDZ domain. Normally, RGS proteins act as GAP proteins that down-regulate GPCR signaling by accelerating the GTPase activity of the α-subunits of heterotrimeric G protein. In this case, it is possible that clustering or activation of ephrin-b by eph receptors would activate PDZ-RGS3, resulting in the termination of SDF-1-mediated signaling via CXCR4 receptors in the same cells. A further possibility is that GPCRs localized in the internal aspect of the EGL might antagonize SDF-1-mediated signaling. For example, it has been shown that receptors for pituitary adenylate cyclase activating protein (PACAP), a widely expressed neuropeptide, are localized postnatally in the EGL (Nicot et al., 2002). Activation of these receptors is linked to Gs as well as increases in cAMP. Given the known ability of cAMP to antagonize SHH-mediated signaling, these effects would oppose the faciliatory actions of SDF-1. Moreover, PACAP receptor activation also produces transactivation of TrkB neurotrophin receptors (Lee, Rajagopal, Kim, Chang, & Chao, 2002). Interestingly, TrkB receptors are not only localized on pre-migratory granule cells but it was observed that their activation by the neurotrophin BDNF may be a major chemotactic influence on granule cell migration to the IGL (Borghesani et al., 2002). Thus, PACAP receptor activation could simultaneously down-regulate SDF-1 signaling as it up-regulates BDNF signaling, two effects that would prime granule cell precursors for inward migration. In summary, therefore, there are a number of ways in which SDF-1/CXCR4 signaling might produce diverse effects on granule cell development through interactions with other signaling pathways.

Further unique influences on chemokine-mediated signaling that may be important during development have recently been demonstrated. Several families of molecules that act as axon guidance cues have been defined, including molecules of the Slit and netrin families. Typically Slit, acting via its receptor roundabout (Robo), acts as an axonal repellent (Brose & Tessier-Lavigne, 2000). It has recently been shown that Slit/Robo are also expressed by leukocytes (Wu et al., 2001), whereby activation of Robo-opposed SDF-1-mediated leukocyte chemotaxis. Although this type of interaction has not yet been demonstrated in the nervous system, it seems likely that it would occur, since Slit/Robo and SDF-1/CXCR4 are certainly both expressed in similar regions of the developing nervous system. Furthermore, because the interaction between Slit and SDF-1 can be recapitulated in a heterologous expression system, this clearly indicates that the interaction between these two factors is not cell specific.

As discussed above, the recent identifications of a new receptor for SDF-1 named CXCR7 has suggested that SDF-1 signaling may have another dimension (Thelen & Thelen, 2008). However, it has been difficult to understand the signaling significance of SDF-1 binding to CXCR7. Reports have indicated that no detectable signaling occurs and that CXCR7 may just function as a "decoy" receptor or that CXCR7 may function through the formation of hetero-oligomers with CXCR4. However, SDF-1 does produce CXCR7 endocytosis and recent reports suggest that this may be coupled to activation of the β-arrestin signaling pathway. CXCR7 receptors are highly expressed by neurons and blood vessels in the developing and adult brains and so may play several important roles in mediating chemokine signaling in the nervous system.

HIV-1 ASSOCIATED NEUROPATHOLOGY

Considering the widespread expression of CXCR4 and other chemokine receptors in the nervous system, we should now consider how these are important in the neuropathogenesis of HAD. One important question is to define which population of cells in the brain is the most important in terms of their interactions with HIV-1/gp120. First we should consider the receptors that are expressed by neurons themselves. It is certainly clear that purified gp120 can be neurotoxic in vivo and in vitro (Corasaniti et al., 2001; Meucci & Miller, 1996). Interpretation of this data has not been entirely straightforward, however, as it is not clear whether gp120 can be directly toxic to neurons, or whether this can only occur in the context of other types of cells such as microglia and or astrocytes (Bezzi et al., 2001; Kaul et al., 2001). Another complication concerns the effects of the unique CXCR4 ligand SDF-1 on neurons. Here some reports suggest that SDF-1 has a survival-promoting effect on neurons, as do other chemokines (Meucci et al., 1998), whereas other reports suggest that SDF-1 has a uniquely pro-apoptotic effect (Hesselgesser et al., 1998). At any rate one possibility is that gp120 might interact directly with CXCR4 receptors expressed by neurons to produce

neurotoxicity. One way this might happen is if gp120 acts to antagonize the survival-promoting effects of SDF-1 through competition for the same binding site. Alternatively, it appears that under some circumstances gp120 can not only bind to chemokine receptors but also elicit signaling through them (Davis et al., 1997). It is possible, therefore, that aberrant signaling elicited in this way might also be pro-apoptotic. As discussed above it has been demonstrated that activation of the CXCR4 receptor by SDF-1 may also result in pro- or anti-apoptotic signaling through p38 or ERK activation, respectively (Vlahakis et al., 2002). Thus, it is conceivable that the overall balance between these diverse outputs may determine the extent of gp120 or SDF-1-induced neuronal death or survival. In keeping with this possibility, blockers of different members of the MAP kinase pathway have been shown to ameliorate gp120-induced toxicity. For example, blockade of signaling via the JNK pathway inhibits gp120-induced neurotoxicity of cultured hippocampal neurons (Bodner et al., 2002). Inhibition of the enzyme MLK3, which is an upstream activator of JNK, blocks gp120-induced apoptosis of hippocampal neurons in culture, raising the possibility that this might be a therapeutic possibility in HAD. Activation of neuronal chemokine receptors aside from CXCR4 may also be important in HAD. Chemokines that activated these receptors have been widely reported to have anti-apoptotic/survival-promoting effects. Indeed, activation of receptors such as CX3CR1 with fractalkine can inhibit gp120-induced apoptosis (Meucci et al., 2000). The signaling pathways that mediate these effects include activation of the Akt pathway, which has been widely associated with anti-apoptotic actions.

Although the direct effects of gp120/chemokines on neurons may be of importance in deciphering the molecular basis of HAD, the contribution to gp120 neurotoxicity of chemokine receptors expressed by glia or microglia has also been considered (Bezzi et al., 2001), and one model suggests that activation of glial CXCR4 receptors by gp120 causes them to release glutamate which might then produce excitotoxic effects. Alternatively, it has been suggested that gp120 blocks the uptake of glutamate by neurons and/or glia, something that would also promote excitotoxicity (Vesce et al., 1997). Indeed, considering the fact that receptors such as CXCR4 are expressed on all types of brain cells, it is quite possible that several cellular/molecular mechanisms may contribute to HAD.

In this context one should consider the effects of HIV-1 on cells in the brain such as microglia, astrocytes, and endothelial cells that result in the upregulated expression of multiple inflammatory cytokines and chemokines that may then compromise the function of the brain through their actions. Thus it is becoming quite clear that HIV-1 infection produces the increased expression of numerous chemokines by these cells which can alter the permeability of the blood brain barrier (BBB) resulting in the influx of numerous leukocytes. As these cells also express chemokines and their receptors, including CXCR4/CCR5 receptors, they are a secondary source of HIV-1 as well as inflammatory cytokines of various types. For example, it is clear that HIV-1-infected microglia can up-regulate their expression of the chemokine MCP-1/CCL2. This chemokine can increase the permeability of the BBB and attract different classes of leukocytes into the brain. The precise mechanism through which HIV-1 produces up-regulated chemokine synthesis by microglia and other cell types is not known. However, in addition to binding to chemokine receptors through their envelope protein gp120, it should also be recognized that other HIV-1-associated proteins and nucleic acid may also activate receptors that are responsible for these effects. One should consider, for example, Toll-like receptors (e.g., TLR7) which act as part of the brain's innate immune response and can be activated by HIV-1(Heil et al., 2004). Hence, a scenario for the effects of HIV-1 in the CNS may be as follows: HIV-1 enters the brain early in infection by a Trojan horse mechanism within leukocytes involved in immune surveillance. HIV-1 infects microglia (and possibly astrocytes) via binding to chemokine receptors expressed by these cells. Infected cells produce a variety of chemokines and cytokines and shed HIV-1-related proteins. These cytokines and proteins then have a number of secondary effects on the BBB and other structures in the brain leading to the influx of further infected leukocytes. Infiltrating leukocytes may then produce neurotoxic, anti-neurogenic, and other effects due to their elaboration of inflammatory chemokines and cytokines.

Currently, the cellular and molecular bases for HIV-1-induced syndromes in the PNS are also unknown. These syndromes constitute a group of painful neuropathies and related problems that can be produced by the virus or by antiretroviral drugs used to treat HIV-1 infection. It is known that pain-transmitting small sensory nociceptors do express chemokine receptors and that activation of these receptors can produce excitation through a variety of mechanisms including the transactivation of TRP channels expressed by nociceptors (Oh et al., 2001). As with neurons in the CNS, long-term exposure of sensory neurons to gp120 also produces neuronal apoptosis (unpublished observations). Thus, it is quite possible that gp120 might produce HIV-1-related allodynia and sensory neuropathies through direct interactions with chemokine receptors expressed by these neurons. In addition, however, the effects of HIV-1 in the peripheral nervous system may involve a scenario similar to that described above for the CNS. Thus, HIV-1 infection may trigger the up-regulated expression of chemokines and their receptors in the dorsal root ganglion (DRG), peripheral nerve, and spinal cord. These chemokines may then produce pro-algesic effects leading to chronic pain behaviors. In particular, HIV-1-related proteins such as gp120 or NRTIs can produce the up-regulation of chemokine expression by DRG neurons, satellite glial cells, and endoneurial fibroblasts in the peripheral nerve. In association with these effects, chemokine receptor expression is upregulated by DRG neurons, including nociceptors. As described above, the direct effects of chemokines on DRG nociceptors is to produce excitation. Hence, up-regulated chemokine signaling in these nerves is inherently pro-algesic. Hence, there appears to be two main ways in which chemokine signaling may contribute to HIV-1-related pain syndromes. The first of these is by direct binding of gp120 to CXCR4 receptors expressed by DRG nociceptors and the second is by

the up-regulation of chemokine and chemokine receptor expression by cells in the DRG and peripheral nerve, which may also result in increased excitatory chemokine signaling in nociceptors.

REFERENCES

Altman, J. & Bayer, S. A. (1990a). Mosaic organization of the hippocampal neuroepithelium and the multiple germinal sources of dentate granule cells. *J Comp Neurol, 301,* 325–342.

Altman, J. & Bayer, S. A. (1990b). Migration and distribution of two populations of hippocampal granule cell precursors during the perinatal and postnatal periods. *J Comp Neurol, 301,* 365–381.

Arujo, D. M. & Cotman, C. (1993). Trophic effects of interleukin-4, -7, and-8 on hippocampal neuronal cultures: Potential involvement of glial-derived factors. *Brain Res, 600,* 49–55.

Babcock, G. J., Farzan, M., & Sodroski, J. (2003). Ligand-independent dimerization of CXCR4, a principal HIV-1 coreceptor. *J Biol Chem, 278,* 3378–3383.

Bagri, A., Gurney, T., He, X., Zou, Y. R., Littman, D. R., Tessier-Lavigne, M., et al. (2002). The chemokine SDF-1 regulates migration of dentate granule cells. *Development, 129,* 4249–4260.

Bajetto, A., Bonavia, R., Barbero, S., & Schettini, G. (2002). Characterization of chemokines and their receptors in the central nervous system: Physiopathological implications. *J Neurochem, 82,* 1311–1329.

Bajetto, A., Bonavia, R., Barbero, S., Florio, T., & Schettini, G. (2001). Chemokines and their receptors in the central nervous system. *Front Neuroendocrinol, 22,* 147–184.

Banisadr, G., Dicou, E., Berbar, T., Rostène, W., Lombet, A., Haour, F. (2000). Characterization and visualization of [125I] stromal cell-derived factor-1alpha binding to CXCR4 receptors in rat brain and human neuroblastoma cells. *J Neuroimmunol, 2;*110(1–2):151–60.

Banisadr, G., Fontanges, P., Haour, F., Kitabgi, P., Rostene, W. & Parsadaniantz, S. M. (2002). Neuroanatomical distribution of CXCR4 in adult rat brain and its localization in cholinergic and dopaminergic neurons. *Eur J Neurosci, 16,* 1661–1671.

Berger, E. A., Murphy, P. M., & Farber, J. M. (1999). Chemokine receptors as HIV-1 receptors: Roles in viral entry, tropism, and disease. *Ann Rev Immunol, 17,* 657–700.

Bezzi, P., Domercq, M., Brambilla, L., Galli, R., Schols, D., De Clercq, E., et al. (2001). CXCR4-activated astrocyte glutamate release via TNFalpha: Amplification by microglia triggers neurotoxicity. *Nat Neurosci, 4,* 702–10.

Bhattacharyya, B. J., Banisadr, G., Jung, H., Ren, D., Cronshaw, D. G., Zou, Y., et al. (2008). The chemokine stromal cell-derived factor-1 regulates GABAergic inputs to neural progenitors in the postnatal dentate gyrus. *J Neurosci, 28,* 6720–30.

Bleul, C., Schultze, J. L., & Springer, T. A. (1998). B lymphocyte chemotaxis regulated in association with microanatomic localization, differentiation state and B cell receptor engagement. *J Exp Med, 187,* 753–762.

Bodner, A., Maroney, A. C., Finn, J. P., Ghadge, G., Roos, R., & Miller, R. J. (2002). Mixed lineage kinase 3 mediates gp120IIIB-induced neurotoxicity. *J Neurochem, 82,* 1424–34.

Bolin, L. M., Murray, R., Lukacs, N. W., Strieter, R. M., Kunkel, S. L., Schall, T. J. et al. (1998). Primary sensory neurons migrate in response to the chemokine RANTES. *J Neuroimmunol, 81,* 49–57.

Borghesani, P. R., Peyrin, J. M., Klein, R., Rubin, J., Carter, A. R., Schwartz, P. M., et al. (2002). BDNF stimulates migration of cerebellar granule cells. *Development, 129,* 1435–42.

Borrell V. & Marín O. (2006). Meninges control tangential migration of hem-derived Cajal-Retzius cells via CXCL12/CXCR4 signaling. *Nat Neurosci, 9,* 1284–93.

Braun, M., Wunderlin, M., Spieth, K., Knochel, W., Gierschik, P., & Moepps, B. (2002). Xenopus laevis Stromal cell-derived factor 1:

Conservation of structure and function during vertebrate development. *J Immunol, 168,* 2340–7.

Brose, K. & Tessier-Lavigne, M. (2000). Slit proteins: Key regulators of axon guidance, axonal branching and cell migration. *Curr Opinion Neurobiol, 10,* 95–102.

Cheng, Z. J., Zhao, J., Sun, Y., Hu, W., Wu, Y. L., Cen, B., et al. (2000). Beta-arrestin differentially regulates the chemokine receptor CXCR4-mediated signaling and receptor internalization, and this implicates multiple interaction sites between β-arrestin and CXCR4. *J Biol Chem, 275,* 2479–85.

Corasaniti, M. T., Maccarrone, M., Nistico, R., Malorni, W., Rotiroti, D., & Bagetta, G. (2001). Exploitation of the HIV-1 coat glycoprotein, gp120, in neurodegenerative studies in vivo. *J Neurochem, 79,* 1–8.

Cowell, R. M. & Silverstein, F. S. (2003). Developmental changes in the expression of chemokine receptor CCR1 in the rat cerebellum. *J Comp Neurol, 457,* 7–23.

Davis, C. B., Dikic, I., Unutmaz, D., Hill, C. M., Arthos, J., Siani, M.A., et al. (1997). Signal transduction due to HIV-1 envelope interactions with chemokine receptors CXCR4 or CCR5. *J Exp Med, 186,* 1793–8.

DeGroot, C. J. A. & Woodroofe, M. N. (2001). The role of chemokines and chemokine receptors in CNS inflammation. *Prog in Brain Res, 132,* 533–544.

Doitsidou, M., Reichman-Fried, M., Stebler, J., Koprunner, M., Dorries, J., Meyer, D., et al. (2002). Guidance of primordial germ cell migration by the chemokine SDF-1. *Cell, 111,* 647–659.

Gabuzda, D. & Wang, J. (2000). Chemokine receptors and mechanisms of cell death in HIV neuropathogenesis. *J Neurovirol, 6* Suppl 1, S24–32.

Garden, G. A. (2002). Microglia in human immunodeficiency virus associated neurodegeneration. *Glia, 40,* 240–251.

Ge, S., Pradhan, D. A., Ming, G. L., & Song, H. (2007). GABA sets the tempo for activity-dependent adult neurogenesis. *Trends Neurosci, 30,* 1–8.

Gillard, S. E., Mastracci, R. M., & Miller, R. J. (2001). Expression of functional chemokine receptors by cerebellar neurons. *J Neuroimmunol, 124,* 16–28.

Giovannelli, A., Limatola, C., Ragozzino, D., Mileo, A. M., Ruggieri, A., Ciotti, M. T., et al. (1998). CXC chemokines interleukin-8 (IL-8) and growth-related gene product alpha (GRO-α) modulate Purkinje neuron activity in mouse cerebellum. *J Neuroimmunol, 92,* 122–32.

Gleichmann, M., Gillen, C., Czardybon, M., Bosse, F., Greiner-Petter, R., Auer, J. et al. (2000). Cloning and characterization of SDF-1γ, a novel SDF-1 chemokine transcript with developmentally regulated expression in the nervous system. *Eur J Neurosci, 12,* 1857–1866.

Gorry, P. R., Bristol, G., Zack. J. A., Ritola, K., Swanstrom, R., Birch, C. J., et al. (2001). Macrophage tropism of human immunodeficiency virus type 1 isolates from brain and lymphoid tissues predicts neurotropism independent of coreceptor specificity. *J Virol, 75,* 10073–89.

Gould, E. & Gross, C. G. (2002). Neurogenesis in adult mammals: Some progress and problems. *J Neurosci, 22,* 619–23.

Harori, K., Nagai, A., Heisel, R., Ryu, J. K. & Kim, S. U. (2002). Fractalkine and fractalkine receptors in human neurons and glial cells. *J Neurosci Res, 69,* 418–426.

Hartmann, D., Schulze, M., & Sievers, J. (1998). Meningeal cells stimulate and direct the migration of cerebellar external granule cells in vitro. *J Neurocytol, 27,* 395–409.

Hartmann, D., De Strooper, B., & Saftig, P. (1999). Presenilin-1 deficiency leads to loss of Cajal-Retzius neurons and cortical dysplasia similar to human type 2 lissencephaly. *Current Biol, 9,* 719–727.

Heil, F., Hemmi, H., Hochrein, H., Ampenberger, F., Kirschning, C., Akira, S., et al. (2004). Species-specific recognition of single-stranded RNA via toll-like receptor 7 and 8. *Science, 303,* 1526–9.

Hesselgesser, J., Taub, D., Baskar, P., Greenberg, M., Hoxie, J., Kolson, D. L., et al. (1998). Neuronal apoptosis induced by HIV-1 gp120 and the chemokine SDF-1α is mediated by the chemokine receptor CXCR4. *Curr Biol, 8,* 595–8.

Horuk, R., Martin, A. W., Wang, Z., Schweitzer, L., Gerassimides, A., Guo, H., et al. (1997). Expression of chemokine receptors by subsets of neurons in the central nervous system. *J Immunol, 158,* 2882–2890.

Issafras, H., Angers, S., Bulenger, S., Blanpain, C., Parmentier, M., Labbe-Jullie, C., et al. (2002). Constitutive agonist-independent CCR5 oligomerization and antibody-mediated clustering occurring at physiological levels of receptors. *J Biol Chem, 277,* 34666–73.

Jazin, E. E., Soderstrom, S., Ebendal, T., & Larhammer, D. (1997). Embryonic expression of the mRNA for the rat homologue of the fusin/CXCR4 HIV-1 co-receptor. *J Neuroimmunol, 79,* 148–154.

Kaul, M. & Lipton, S. A. (1999). Chemokines and activated macrophages in HIV-1 and gp120-induced neuronal apoptosis. *Proc Natl Acad Sci, 96,* 8212–6.

Kaul, M., Garden, G. A., & Lipton, S. A. (2001). Pathways to neuronal injury and apoptosis in HIV associated dementia. *Nature, 410,* 988–994.

Klein, R. S., Rubin, J. B., Gibson, H. D., DeHaan, E. N., Alvarez-Hernandez, X., Segal, R. A. et al. (2001). SDF-1α induces chemotaxis and enhances sonic hedgehog induced proliferation of cerebellar granule cells. *Development, 128,* 1971–1981.

Knaut, H., Werz, C., Gelser, R., & Nusslein-Volhard, C. (2002). A zebrafish homologue of the chemokine receptor CXCR4 is a germ-cell guidance receptor. *Nature,* published online Dec 18, 2002.

Kolodziej, A., Schulz, S., Guyon, A., Wu, D. F., Pfeiffer, M., Odemis, V., et al. (2008). Tonic activation of CXC chemokine receptor 4 in immature granule cells supports neurogenesis in the adult dentate gyrus. *J Neurosci, 28,* 4488–500.

Kolson, D.L. & Gonzalez-Scarano, F. (2001). HIV-associated neuropathies: Role of HIV-1, CMV, and other viruses. *J Peripher Nerv Syst, 6,* 2–7.

Kury, P., Greiner-Petter, R., Cornely, C., Jurgens, T., & Muller, H. W. (2002). Mammalian Achaete Scute homolog 2 is expressed in the adult sciatic nerve and regulates the expression of Krox 24, Mob-1, CXCR4 and p57kip2 in Schwann cells. *J Neurosci, 22,* 7586–7595.

Lavi, E., Strizki, J. M., Ulrich, A. M., Zhang, W., Fu, L., Wang, Q., et al. (1997). CXCR4 (Fusin), a co-receptor for the type I human immunodeficiency virus (HIV-1), is expressed in the human brain in a variety of cell types, including microglia and neurons. *Am J Pathol, 151,* 1035–1042.

Lazarini, F., Casanova, P., Tham, T. N., De Clercq, E., Arenzana-Seisdedos, F., Baleux, F. et al. (2000). Differential signaling of the chemokine receptor CXCR4 by stromal cell-derived factor 1 and the HIV glycoprotein in rat neurons and astrocytes. *Eur J Neurosci, 12,* 117–25.

Lee, F. S., Rajagopal, R., Kim, A. H., Chang, P. C., & Chao, M. V. (2002). Activation of Trk neurotrophin receptor signaling by pituitary adenylate cyclase-activating polypeptides. *J Biol Chem, 277,* 9096–102.

Li, G., Adesnik, H., Li, J., Long, J., Nicoll, R. A., Rubenstein, J. L., et al. (2008). Regional distribution of cortical interneurons and development of inhibitory tone are regulated by Cxcl12/Cxcr4 signaling. *J Neurosci, 28,* 1085–1098.

Limatola, C., Giovannelli, A., Maggi, L., Ragozzino, D., Castellani, L., Ciotti, M. T., et al. (2000). SDF-1α-mediated modulation of synaptic transmission in rat cerebellum. *Eur J Neurosci, 12,* 2497–504.

Limatola, C., Ciotti, M. T., Mercanti, D., Vacca, F., Ragozzino, D., Giovannelli, A., et al. (2000). The chemokine growth-related gene product β protects rat cerebellar granule cells from apoptotic cell death through α-amino-3-hydroxy-5-methyl-4-isoxazolepropionate receptors. *Proc Natl Acad Sci USA, 97,* 6197–201.

Lopez-Bendito, G., Sanchez-Alcaniz, J. A., Pla, R., Borrell, V., Pico, E., Valdeolmillos, M., et al. (2008). Chemokine signaling controls intracortical migration and final distribution of GABAergic interneurons. *J Neurosci, 28,* 1613–1624.

Lu, Q., Sun, E. E., Klein, R. S. & Flanagan, J. G. (2001). Ephrin-B reverse signaling is mediated by a novel PDZ-RGS protein and selectively inhibits G protein coupled chemoattraction. *Cell, 105,* 69–79.

Lu, M., Grove, E. A., & Miller, R. J. (2002). Abnormal development of the hippocampal dentate gyrus in mice lacking the CXCR4 chemokine receptor. *Proc Natl Acad Sci, 99,* 7090–7095.

Luan, J., Furuta, Y., Du, J., & Richmond, A. (2001). Developmental expression of two CXC chemokines, MIP-2 and KC, and their receptors. *Cytokine, 14,* 253–63.

Ma, Q., Jones, D., Borghesani, P. R., Segal, R. A., Nagasawa, T, Kishimoto, T., et al. (1998). Impaired B lymphopoiesis, myelopoiesis, and derailed cerebellar neuronal migration in CXCR4 and SDF-1 deficient mice. *Proc Natl Acad Sci, 95,* 9448–9453.

Ma, Q., Jones, D., & Springer, T. A. (1999). The chemokine receptor CXCR4 is required for the retention of B lineage and granulocytic precursors within the bone marrow microenvironment. *Immunity, 10,* 463–471.

Madani, N., Kozak, S. L., Kavanaugh, M. P., & Kabat, D. (1998). gp120 envelope glycoproteins of human immunodeficiency viruses competitively antagonize signaling by coreceptors CXCR4 and CCR5. *Proc Nat'l Acad Sci USA, 95,* 8005–8010.

Martin-Garcia, J., Kolson, D. L., & Gozalez-Scarano, F. (2002). Chemokine receptors in the brain: Their role in HIV infection and pathogenesis. *AIDS, 16,* 1709–1730.

McGrath, K. E., Koniski, A. D., Maltby, K. M., McGann, J. K., & Palis, J. (1999). Embryonic expression and function of the chemokine SDF-1 and its receptor, CXCR4. *Dev Biol, 213,* 442–56.

Meng, S. Z., Oka, A., & Takashima, S. (1999). Development expression of monocyte chemoattractant protein–1 in the human cerebellum and brainstem. *Brain Dev, 21,* 30–35.

Meucci, O. & Miller, R. J. (1996). gp120-induced neurotoxicity in hippocampal pyramidal neuron cultures: Protective action of TGF-β1. *J Neurosci, 16,* 4080–8.

Meucci, O., Fatatis, A., Simen, A., Bushell, T. J., Gray, P. W., & Miller, R. J. (1998). Chemokines regulate hippocampal neuronal signaling and gp120 neurotoxicity. *Proc Natl Acad Sci, 95,* 14500–14505.

Meucci, O., Fatatis, A., Simen, A. A., & Miller, R. J. (2000). Expression of CX3CR1 chemokine receptors on neurons and their role in neuronal survival. *Proc Natl Acad Sci, 97,* 8075–80.

Miller, R. J. (1998). Presynaptic receptors. *Ann Rev of Pharmacol and Toxicol, 38,* 201–227.

Moepps, B., Frodl, R., Rodewald, H. R., Bagglioni, M., & Gierschik, P. (1997). Two murine homologues of the human chemokine receptor CXCR4 mediating stromal cell derived factor–1-alpha activation of Gi2 are differentially expressed in vivo. *Eur J Immunol, 27,* 2102–2112.

Moepps, B., Braun, M., Knopfle, K., Dillinger, K., Knochel, W., & Gierschik, P. (2000). Characterization of a Xenopus laevis CXC chemokine receptor 4: Implications for hematopoietic cell development in the vertebrate embryo. *Eur J Immunol, 30,* 2924–34.

Molina-Holgado, E., Vela, J. M., Arevalo-Martin, A., Almazan, G., Molina-Holgado, F., Borrell, J. et al. (2002). Cannabinoids promote oligodendrocyte progenitor survival: Involvement of cannabinoid receptors and phosphatidylinositol-3 kinase/Akt signaling. *J. Neurosci, 22,* 9742–53.

Murphy, P. M., Baggiolini, M., Charo, I. F., Hebert, C. A., Horuk, R., Matsushima, K., et al. (2000). International union of pharmacology. XXII. Nomenclature: Chemokine receptors. *Pharmacol. Review, 52,* 145–76.

Murphy, P. M. (2002). International Union of Pharmacology. Update on chemokine receptor nomenclature. *Pharmacol. Review, 54,* 227–9.

Nagasawa, T., Hirota, S., Tachibana, K., Takakura, N., Nishikawa, S., Kitamura, Y., et al. (1996). Defects of B-cell lymphopoiesis and bone marrow myelopoiesis in mice lacking the CXC chemokine PBSF/SDF-1. *Nature, 382,* 635–8.

Nath, A, (2002). Human immunodeficiency virus (HIV) proteins in the neuropathogenesis of HIV dementia. *J Infect Dis, 186* (suppl2), S193–198.

Nicot, A., Lelievre, V., Tam, J., Waschek, J. A., & DiCicco-Bloom, E. (2002). Pituitary adenylate cyclase activating polypeptide and sonic hedgehog interact to control cerebellar granule precursor cell proliferation. *J Neurosci, 22,* 9244–9254.

Oh, S. B., Tran, P. B., Gillard, S. E., Hurley, R. W. Hammond, D. L., & Miller, R. J. (2001). Chemokines and gp120 produce pain hypersensitivity by directly exciting polymodal nociceptors. *J Neurosci, 21,* 5027–5035.

Oh, S. B., Endoh, T., Simen, A. A., Ren, D., & Miller, R. J. (2002). Regulation of calcium currents by chemokines and their receptors. *J Neuroimmunol, 123,* 66–75.

Paredes, M. F., Li, G., Berger, O., Baraban, S. C., & Pleasure, S. J. (2006). Stromalderived factor-1 (CXCL12) regulates laminar position of Cajal-Retzius cells in normal and dysplastic brains. *J Neurosci, 26,* 9404–9412.

Perry, S. J. & Lefkowitz, R. J. (2002). Arresting developments in heptahelical receptor signaling and regulation. *Trends Cell Biol, 12,* 130–8.

Proudfoot, A. E. I. (2002). Chemokine receptors: Multifaceted therapeutic targets. *Nature Reviews Immunol, 2,* 106–115.

Proudfoot, A. E. I., Shaw, J. P., Power, C. A., & Wells, T. N. C. (2002). Chemokines. In R. M. Ransohoff, K. Suzuki, A. E. I. Proudfoot, W. F. Hickey, & J. K. Harrison, (Ed.). *Universes in delicate balance: Chemokines and the nervous system* (p. 65–85). Philadelphia; Elsevier.

Puma, C., Danik, M., Quirion, R., Ramon, F., & Williams, S. (2001). The chemokine interleukin-8 acutely reduces Ca(2+) currents in identified cholinergic septal neurons expressing CXCR1 and CXCR2 receptor mRNAs. *J Neurochem, 78,* 960–71.

Rajagopal, S., Kim, J., Ahn, S., Craig, S., Lam, C. M., Gerard, N. P., et al. (2010). Beta-arrestin- but not G protein-mediated signaling by the "decoy" receptor CXCR7. *Proc Natl Acad Sci USA, 107,* 628–32.

Ragozzino, D., Giovannelli, A., Mileo, A. M., Limatola, C., Santoni, A., & Eusebi, F. (1998). Modulation of the neurotransmitter release in rat cerebellar neurons by GRO -β. *Neuroreport, 9,* 3601–6.

Ragozzino, D., Renzi, M., Giovannelli, A., & Eusebi, F. (2002). Stimulation of chemokine CXC receptor 4 induces synaptic depression of evoked parallel fibers inputs onto Purkinje neurons in mouse cerebellum. *Neuroimmunol, 127,* 30–6.

Reiss, K., Mentlein, R., Sievers, J., & Hartmann, D. (2002). Stromal cell derived factor 1 is secreted by meningeal cells and acts as chemotactic factor on neuronal stem cells of the cerebellar external granule layer. *Neurosci, 115,* 295–305.

Robinson, S., Tani, M., Streiter, R. M., Ransohoff, R. M., & Miller, R. H. (1998). The chemokine growth related oncogene–α promotes spinal cord precursor proliferation. *J Neurosci, 18,* 10457–10463.

Rodriguez-Frade, J. M., Mellado, M., & Martinez, A. C. (2001). Chemokine receptor dimerization: Two are better than one. *Trends in Immunol, 22,* 612–7.

Rossi, D. & Zlotnik, A. (2000). The biology of chemokines and their receptors. *Ann Rev Immunol, 18,* 217–242.

Schreiber, R. C., Krivacic, K., Kirby, B., Vaccariello, S. A., Wei, T., Ransohoff, R. M., Zigmond, R. E. (2001). Monocyte chemoattractant protein (MCP)-1 is rapidly expressed by sympathetic ganglion neurons following axonal injury. *Neuroreport, 5;12(3):601–6.*

Schwartz, G. N. & Farber, J. M. (2002). Development and function of the hematopoietic-lymphopoietic system. In R. M. Ransohoff, K. Suzuki, A. E. I. Proudfoot, W. F. Hickey, & J. K. Harrison, (Ed.). *Universes in delicate balance: Chemokines and the nervous system* (p. 65–85). Philadelphia; Elsevier.

Schönemeier, B., Kolodziej, A., Schulz, S., Jacobs, S., Hoellt, V., & Stumm, R. (2008). Regional and cellular localization of the CXCl12/SDF-1 chemokine receptor CXCR7 in the developing and adult rat brain. *J Comp Neurol, 510,* 207–20.

Sievers, J., Hartmann, D., Pehlemann, F. W., & Berry, M. (1992). Development of astroglial cells in the proliferative matrices, the granule cell layer and the hippocampal fissure of the hamster dentate gyrus. *J Comp Neurol, 320,* 1–32.

Sierro, F., Biben, C., Martínez-Muñoz, L., Mellado, M., Ransohoff, R. M., Li, M., et al. (2007). Disrupted cardiac development but normal hematopoiesis in mice deficient in the second CXCL12/SDF-1 receptor, CXCR7. *Proc Natl Acad Sci USA, 104,* 14759–64.

Stumm, R. K., Rummel, J., Junker, V., Culmsee, C., Pfeiffer, M., Krieglstein, J., et al. (2002). A dual role for the SDF-1/CXCR4 chemokine receptor system in adult brain: Isoform selective regulation of SDF-1 expression modulates CXCR4 dependent neuronal plasticity and cerebral leukocyte recruitment after focal ischemia *J Neurosci, 22,* 5865–5878.

Stumm, R. K., Zhou, C., Ara, T., Lazarini, F., Dubois-Dalcq, M., Nagasawa, T., et al. (2003). CXCR4 regulates interneuron migration in the developing neocortex. *J Neurosci, 23,* 5123–5130.

Szekanecz, Z. & Koch, A. E. (2001). Chemokines and angiogenesis. *Current Opinion Rheumatol*, *13*, 202–8.

Tachibana, K., Hirota, S., Iizasa, H., Yoshida, H., Kawabata, K., Kataoka, Y., et al. (1998). The chemokine receptor CXCR4 is essential for vascularization of the gastrointestinal tract. *Nature*, *393*, 591–4.

Tham, T. N., Lazarini, F., Francheschini, I. A., Lachapelle, F., Amara, A., & Dubois-Dalcq, M. (2001). Developmental pattern of expression of the alpha chemokine stromal cell derived factor 1 in the rat central nervous system. *Eur J Neurosci*, *13*, 845–856.

Thelen, M. & Thelen, S. (2008). CXCR7, CXCR4, and CXCL12: An eccentric trio? *J Neuroimmunol*, *198*, 9–13.

Tiveron, M. C., Rossel, M., Moepps, B., Zhang, Y. L., Seidenfaden, R., Favor, J., et al. (2006). Molecular interaction between projection neuron precursors and invading interneurons via stromal-derived factor 1 (CXCL12)/CXCR4 signaling in the cortical subventricular zone/intermediate zone. *J Neurosci*, *26*, 13273–13278.

Toggas, S. M., Masliah, E., Rockenstein, E. M., Rall, G. F., Abraham, C. R., & Mucke L. (1994). Central nervous system damage produced by expression of the HIV-1 coat protein gp120 in transgenic mice. *Nature*, *367*, 188–93.

Tong, N., Perry, S. W., Zhang, Q., James, H. J., Guo, H., Brooks, A., et al. (2000). Neuronal fractalkine expression in HIV-1 encephalitis: Roles for macrophage recruitment and neuroprotection in the central nervous system. *J Immunol*, *164*, 1333–9.

Tran, P. B., Ren, D., Chenn, A., & Miller, R. J. (2007). Chemokine receptor expression by neural progenitor cells in neurogenic regions of mouse brain. *J Comp Neurol*, *500*, 1007–33.

Tsai, H. H., Frost, E., To, V., Robinson, S., French-Constant, C., Geertman, R., et al. (2002). The chemokine receptor CXCR2 controls positioning of oligodendrocyte precursors in developing spinal cord by arresting their migration. *Cell*, *110*, 373–383.

Van der Meer, P., Ulrich, A. M., Gonzalez-Scarano, F., & Lavi, E. (2000). Immunohistochemical analysis of CCR2, CCR3, CCR5 and CXCR4 in the human brain: Potential mechanisms for HIV dementia. *Exp and Mol Pathol*, *69*, 192–201.

Vaudry, D., Pamantung, T. F., Basille, M., Rousselle, C., Fournier, A. Vaudry, H., et al. (2002). PACAP protects cerebellar granule neurons against oxidative stress induced apoptosis. *Eur J Neurosci*, *15*, 1451–60.

Vlahakis, S. R., Villasis-Keever, A., Gomez, T., Vanegas, M., Vlahakis, N. and Paya, C. V. (2002). Gprotein coupled chemokine receptors induce both survival and apoptotic signaling pathways. *J Immunol*, *169*, 5546–5554.

Vesce, S., Bezzi, P., Rossi, D., Meldolesi, J., & Volterra, A. (1997). HIV-1 gp120 glycoprotein affects the astrocyte control of extracellular glutamate by both inhibiting the uptake and stimulating the release of the amino acid. *FEBS Lett*, *411*, 107–9.

Westmoreland, S. V., Alvarez, X., deBakker, C., Aye, P., Wilson, M. L., Williams, K. C., et al. (2002). Developmental expression of CCR5 and CXCR4 in the rhesus macaque brain. *J Neuroimmunol*, *122*, 146–158.

Williams, K. C. & Hickey, W. F. (2002). Central nervous system damage, monocytes and macrophages, and neurological disorders in AIDS. *Ann Rev Neurosci*, 2537–562.

Wu, Q., Miller, R. H., Ransohoff, R. M., Robinson, S., & Nishayama, A. (2000). Elevated levels of the chemokine GRO-1 correlate with elevated oligodendrocyte progenitor proliferation in the jimpy mutant. *J Neurosci*, *20*, 2609–2617.

Wu, J. Y, Feng, L., Park, H. T., Havlioglu, N., Wen, L., Tang, H., et al. (2001). The neuronal repellent Slit inhibits leukocyte chemotaxis induced by chemotactic factors. *Nature*, *410*, 948–952.

Xia, M. & Hyman, B. T. (2002). GROalpha/KC, a chemokine receptor CXCR2 ligand, can be a potent trigger for neuronal ERK1/2 and PI-3 kinase pathways and for tau hyperphosphorylation-a role in Alzheimer's disease? *J Neuroimmunol*, *122*, 55–64.

Xia, M. Q., Bacskai, B. J., Knowles, R. B., Qin, S. X., & Hyman, B. T. (2000). Expression of the chemokine receptor CXCR3 on neurons and the elevated expression of its ligand IP-10 in reactive astrocytes: In vitro ERK1/2 activation and role in Alzheimer's disease. *J Neuroimmunol*, *108*, 227–35.

Xiang, Y., Li, Y., Zhang, Z., Cui, K., Wang, S., Yuan, X., et al. (2002). Nerve growth cone guidance mediated by Gprotein coupled receptors. *Nature Neurosci*, *5*, 843–848.

Yan, G. M., Lin, S. Z., Irwin, R. P., & Paul, S. M. (1995). Activation of muscarinic cholinergic receptors blocks apoptosis of cultured cerebellar granule neurons. *Mol Pharmacol*, *47*, 248–57.

Zhang, X. F., Wang, J. F., Matczak, E., Proper, J. A., & Groopman, J. E. (2001). Janus kinase 2 is involved in stromal cell-derived factor-1alpha-induced tyrosine phosphorylation of focal adhesion proteins and migration of hematopoietic progenitor cells. *Blood*, *97*, 3342–8.

Zhu, Y., Yu, T., Zhang, X. C., Nagasawa, T., Wu, J. Y., & Rao, Y. (2002). Role of the chemokine SDF-1 as the meningeal attractant for embryonic cerebellar neurons. *Nature Neurosci*, *5*, 719–720.

Zou, Y. R., Kottmann, A. H., Kuroda, M., Taniuchi, I., & Littman, D. R. (1998). Function of chemokine receptor CXCR4 in haematopoiesis and in cerebellar development. *Nature*, *393*, 595–599.

1.4

VIRAL AND HOST GENETIC FACTORS

Jennifer A. McCombe, Shaona Acharjee, M. John Gill, and Christopher Power

Neurological disorders caused by HIV-1 infection are common and diverse. In the present chapter we highlight both host and viral genetic determinants of HIV-induced neuropathogenesis in the central and peripheral nervous systems. The key properties of neuropathogenesis including neuroinvasion, neurotropism, neurovirulence and neurosusceptibility are used as guidelines to the discussion.

INTRODUCTION

Human immunodeficiency virus type 1 (HIV-1) causes a broad spectrum of neurological disorders that constitute a substantial source of morbidity and mortality. HIV-1 infects cells within the central nervous system (CNS) soon after primary infection (Davis et al., 1992; Sasseville & Lackner, 1997; Poli et al., 1990) although not all individuals with HIV/AIDS develop clinically detectable neurological disease (Power & Johnson, 2001). This raises the question of why some individuals develop clinically apparent neurological disease while others do not.

In this chapter, we will discuss both host and viral genetic factors that contribute to HIV neuropathogenesis. HIV neuropathogenesis can be subdivided into stages including *neuroinvasion* (entry of the virus into nervous system tissues and cells without multiplication of the virus), *neurotropism* (infection of cells of the nervous system), and *neurovirulence* (ability to cause neurological dysfunction). In the case of the CNS, neurovirulence has been applied chiefly to impaired neurocognitive performance including HIV-associated dementia (HAD) and its often antecedent disorder, minor neurocognitive disorder (MND); more recent studies group these two conditions under the neuropsychological term, HIV-associated neurocognitive disorders (HAND). In the peripheral nervous system (PNS), the occurrence of distal sensory polyneuropathy (DSP) is the chief neurological disorder assumed to be caused directly by HIV infection with or without exacerbation by specific antiretroviral drugs. We will outline various viral and host factors which contribute to each stage of neuropathogenesis. It can be difficult to separate viral from host pathogenic factors as they interact, but ultimately neural cell loss or dysfunction, presumably caused by a combination of toxic viral proteins and host inflammatory molecules, are usually the convergent end points (Rumbaugh & Nath, 2006).

Other non-genetic host factors also affect an individual's *neurosusceptibility* (Patrick, Johnston, & Power, 2002), including age; immune status; availability and compliance with medications; concurrent infections including hepatitis C; illicit drug use; and nutritional status (reviewed in Jayadev & Garden, 2009); however, we will not discuss these latter factors in this chapter. There is also increasing evidence that drug selection may contribute to the development of neurological disease (Cysique & Brew, 2009); this latter issue requires further study. Herein, we focus on the genetic determinants of the host and virus which contribute to the development of neurological disease.

HOST DETERMINANTS OF HIV-1 NEUROPATHOGENESIS

Neuropathogenesis is influenced by several host factors which both increase and decrease neurosusceptibility. We will discuss how host genetic differences have been demonstrated to contribute to neuroinvasion, neurotropism, and neurovirulence. In addition, we will briefly review how gender and ethnicity might contribute to genetic differences observed. Finally, we will examine host genetic factors that contribute to the response to and side effects of antiretroviral drugs, as they relate to neurological disease and the development of immune reconstitution inflammatory syndrome (IRIS) and opportunistic infections of the nervous system. Important host genes and genetic polymorphisms in HIV neuropathogenesis are summarized in table 1.4.1.

NEUROINVASION

There are five possible mechanisms by which HIV might enter the brain (first four reviewed in Buckner et al., 2006). The first mechanism involves infected macrophages and lymphocytes entering the CNS with subsequent spread of virus to resident cells. This process involves leukocyte recruitment and adhesion, with subsequent migration across the blood-brain barrier, and has been termed the *Trojan horse* mechanism (Peluso, Haase, Stowring, Edwards, & Ventura, 1985). These processes are mediated by adhesion molecules found on leukocytes and the endothelial cells of the blood-brain barrier. There is evidence of upregulation of adhesion molecules in patients with HIV infection and associated neurological disease (Heidenreich, Arendt, Jander, Jablonowski,

& Stoll, 1994; Nottet et al., 1996). There are also reports of increased expression of monocyte chemoattractants expressed in the HIV-infected brain (reviewed in Dunfee et al., 2006); however, the precise mechanisms by which they ultimately contribute to the development of neurological disease have yet to be elucidated.

The second potential mechanism by which HIV enters the CNS involves direct infection of the cells of the blood-brain barrier by cell-free HIV (Buckner et al., 2006). Although endothelial cells do not express the primary HIV-1 receptor, CD4, it appears that HIV interacts with endothelial cell surface proteoglycans through gp120 (Bobardt et al., 2004; Argyris et al., 2003), although this mechanism has not been convincingly demonstrated in vivo to date. The third mechanism involves endocytosis of the HIV virion by endothelial cells and/or astrocytic foot processes (Buckner et al., 2006). A fourth mechanism involves cell-free HIV entering the brain directly by passing through a disrupted blood-brain barrier. There are many studies supporting disruption of the blood-brain barrier during HIV infection (reviewed in Toborek et al., 2005), lending credibility to the notion that circulating free virus might access the brain via a more permeable blood-brain barrier. Finally, HIV infection of the choroid plexus might also serve as a portal of entry for the virus into the brain (Falangola, Hanly, Galvao-Castro, & Petito, 1995; Petito et al., 1999). Again, it remains unclear which, if any, host genetic factors contribute to these mechanisms.

NEUROTROPISM

In terms of host factors, neurotropism is determined by individual cell types in the CNS permissive to viral entry and replication as well as expression of individual receptor molecules that mediate cellular entry by the virus. The cells productively infected by HIV-1 in the CNS are of macrophage and microglial (myeloid) lineage. Astrocytes are also infected by HIV-1, resulting in the expression of viral proteins with minimal replication of the viral genome (Saito et al., 1994; Gorry et al., 1999; Messam & Major, 2000; Neumann et al., 1995; Churchill et al., 2009). Although there is significant neuronal loss and injury, neurons per se are not infected to any extent, as determined by viral genome and antigen detection. There is no compelling evidence for in vivo infection of oligodendrocytes or brain endothelial cells (reviewed in Gonzalez-Scarano & Martin-Garcia 2005).

The HIV-1 envelope glycoprotein is responsible for viral binding and entry into the cell. Apart from using CD4 as the primary receptor, HIV-1 also requires chemokine receptors such as CCR5, CXCR4, CCR2b, and CCR3 to act as co-receptors (reviewed in Berger et al., 1999; Choe et al., 1996; Doranz et al., 1996). Cells of macrophage and microglial lineage express CCR5 and CCR3, together with CD4 (He et al., 1997; Bagasra et al., 1996; Nuovo, Gallery, MacConnell, & Braum, 1994). Microglia and invading macrophages are considered the principal reservoir for active viral replication in the brain (Clements & Zink, 1996; Narayan, Joag, & Stephens, 1995). Astrocytes express both CXCR4 and CCR5 but not CD4, limiting infection in these cell types

(Saito et al., 1994; Gorry et al., 1999; Messam & Major, 2000; Neumann et al., 1995).

Several chemokine receptor polymorphisms have been described that correlate with differences in HIV-1 disease progression and survival prognosis (reviewed in Piacentini, Biasin, Fenizia, & Clerici, 2009). The most familiar of these is the Δ32 variant of the CCR5 co-receptor. Homozygotes for this allele exhibit a significantly diminished susceptibility to HIV-1 infection (Samson et al., 1996; Liu et al., 1996). Heterozygous individuals demonstrate delayed progression of disease (Dean et al., 1996; Meyer et al., 1997; Stewart et al., 1997). Heterozygotes have also been noted to be less represented among patients with neurological disease (Boven, van der Bruggen, van Asbeck, Marx, & Nottet, 1999; van Rij et al., 1999, Singh et al., 2003). Allelic variants in the CCR5 promoter region as well as other co-receptor variants have also been described and are associated with variable progression (reviewed in Piacentini et al., 2009). There is some suggestion that the CCR5–59353 variant found in the promoter region may confer protection in terms of neurological impairment (Singh et al., 2003).

In addition to selective infection of specific cell types, there also appear to be specific regions within the brain that are differentially permissive to infection; white matter and subcortical grey matter are apparently more permissive to infection, perhaps due to the increased abundance of myeloid cells in these regions. It has also been reported that viral envelope sequences cluster together by brain region based on phylogenetic analyses (Chang et al., 1998; Shapshak et al., 1999). Based on pathological studies, the basal ganglia and hippocampus appear to be preferentially affected in terms of neuronal loss (Masliah, Ge, Achim, Hansen, & Wiley, 1992; Reyes et al., 1991) with proportionally more gp41 immunoreactivity detected in these same regions (Kure et al., 1991). Other brain regions including cerebral cortex and brainstem are affected to varying degrees (Everall et al., 1999; Wiley et al., 1991), which may reflect the relative abundance of susceptible resident cells including perivascular macrophages and microglia in a given anatomical site.

NEUROVIRULENCE

There are multiple host characteristics correlated with the occurrence and severity of HIV-associated neurological disease. These include specific host niche genes and variants thereof. Socio-demographic aspects and co-morbidities, although not necessarily shown to be causative, likely also modulate the severity of HIV-1 neurovirulence.

Host Inflammatory Response

Inflammation and immune activation are pivotal contributors to HIV neurovirulence (reviewed in Gonzalez-Scarano & Martin-Garcia 2005). In fact, activated macrophages and multinucleated giant cells are among the as the most robust pathological correlates of HIV neurocognitive impairment (Glass, Fedor, Wesselingh, & McArthur, 1995). Inflammatory indices associated with HIV neurological disease include pro-inflammatory cytokines and chemokines, such as interleukin-1β (Williams & Hickey, 2002; Gartner, 2000; Tyor et al., 1992), tumor necrosis factor-α (Sippy, Hofman, Wallach, & Hinton, 1995; Achim, Heyes, & Wiley, 1993; Wesselingh et al., 1993; Gelbard et al., 1994), interferon-α (Sas et al., 2009), normal T-cell expressed and secreted (RANTES)/CCL5 (Kelder et al., 1998), and CCL2 (monocyte chemoattractant protein) (Monteiro de Almeida, 2006). Many of these important mediators of inflammation are upregulated in the brains or cerebrospinal fluid (CSF) of individuals with HIV-associated dementia. Proteases are another group of molecules contributing to HIV neurovirulence, as exemplified by the conversion of the chemokine CXCL12 to a highly neurotoxic protein through its proteolytic cleavage by matrix metalloproteinase (MMP)-2 (Zhang et al., 2003; Vergote et al., 2006). However, very recent data from our group indicate host-encoded microRNAs are selectively suppressed in the brains of HIV/AIDS patients (Noorbakhsh et al., 2010). This mechanism and many of the above, however, have not been definitively associated with individual genetic polymorphisms. Nonetheless, genetic polymorphisms resulting in gene induction or upregulation have been clearly documented for the chemokines CCL2 (Gonzalez et al., 2002), CCL5–403A, -28G (Guerini et al., 2008; Kelder et al., 1998; Letendre, Lanier, & McCutchan, 1999), CXCL12–3'A (Winkler et al., 1998; Singh et al., 2003), and the cytokine, tumor necrosis factor (TNF)-α (Quasney et al., 2001, Pemberton, Stone, Price, van Bockxmeer, & Brew, 2008); these will be discussed in further detail below. Most of the host genes described above are principally induced in monocyte/macrophage cells, and perhaps, astrocytes, but the contributions of different T lymphocyte subsets to neurovirulence remain largely unexplored. However, it is during HIV infection that different populations of T cells infiltrate the brain and dorsal root ganglia and in some instances exert pathogenic effects (Wesselingh et al., 1993; Zhu et al., 2005).

TUMOR NECROSIS FACTOR-A

TNF-α is upregulated in the brains and CSF of patients with HIV-associated dementia, and increased TNF-α mRNA levels in HAD patients is correlated with dementia severity (Achim et al., 1993; Wesselingh et al., 1993; Gelbard et al., 1994; Tyor et al., 1992). The genetic polymorphism TNF-α-308A has been observed more frequently among HAD patients (Quasney et al., 2001). Located in the promoter region, this polymorphism causes increased TNF-α production. TNF-α can cause direct neuronal damage and induces quinolinic acid production (Pemberton et al., 1997), which likewise causes neuronal damage and has been found in higher concentrations in patients with HAD (Achim et al., 1993).

MONOCYTE CHEMOATTRACTANT PROTEIN-1/CCL2

Increased CCL2 expression has been correlated with an increased risk of accelerated systemic disease progression and the development of HAD. The 2578G variant is associated with increased CCL2 production, presumably resulting in increased infiltration of monocytes (Gonzales et al., 2002). Interestingly, homozygotes for the 2578G allele have a decreased risk of acquiring HIV; however, following infection with HIV-1, accelerated disease progression occurs as described above (Gonzales et al., 2002).

NORMAL T-CELL EXPRESSED AND SECRETED (RANTES)/CCL5–403A, -28G

The CCL5–28G mutation has been shown to increase CCL5 expression in HIV-infected individuals, which reduces CD4+ T lymphocyte depletion rates, thus delaying the progression of disease (Liu et al., 1999). Despite this effect, neurocognitive impairment has been associated with higher levels of CCL5 (Letendre et al., 1999). It has been speculated that CCL5 may stimulate HIV-replication in the CSF (Letendre et al., 1999). Furthermore, an increased rate of the CCL5–403 G/A polymorphism has been documented in patients with "non-determined leukoencephalopathy" compared to HIV seropositive controls (see below for details) (Guerini et al., 2008).

CXCL12/STROMAL CELL-DERIVED FACTOR-1

The chemokine CXCL12/SDF-1 is the cognate ligand for CXCR4, and has been reported to exhibit a genetic polymorphism which contributes to disease progression (Winkler et al., 1998, van Rij et al., 1998). The polymorphism CXCL12–3'A has been shown to both delay and accelerate the progression to AIDS (Winkler et al., 1998, van Rij et al., 1998). In addition, it has also been shown to increase perinatal transmission of HIV-1 (John et al., 2000). In a meta-analysis, however, no significant difference between homozygotes, heterozygotes, and wild-type was noted (Ioannidis et al., 2003). In a subsequent study, CXCL12–3'A was found to be associated with more rapid disease progression, and increased development of neurocognitive impairment in children (Singh et al., 2003).

APOLIPOPROTEIN (APO) E

ApoE functions in cholesterol transport (Mahley & Rall Jr., 2000), and is produced in the CNS by glia, macrophages, and neurons (Boyles, Pitas, Wilson, Mahley, & Taylor, 1985; Pitas, Boyles, Lee, Hui, & Weisgraber, 1987; Han et al., 1994). The role of ApoE in the pathogenesis of HIV-associated dementia remains unclear; studies report conflicting results. It has been reported that HIV-infected patients carrying an ApoE-ε4 allele have a higher frequency of neurological disease (Corder et al., 1998). HAD patients with the ApoE-ε4 allele have also been shown to have dysregulated sterol and lipid metabolism (Cutler et al., 2004). Other studies, however, have found no statistically significant difference between the presence of any ApoE alleles and HIV dementia (Dunlop et al., 1997; Pemberton et al., 2008; Diaz-Arrastia, Gong, Kelly, & Gelman, 2004).

High Throughput Analyses of Host Genes

With the advent of high throughput technologies, including genomics and proteomics, several host genes have been highlighted in HIV neuropathogenesis using brain tissues and cerebrospinal fluid. A seminal study of brain transcriptomics in HIV/AIDS patients with and without HAD revealed substantial dysregulation of ion channel expression that was, in some cases, directly linked to glutamate receptors (Gelman et al., 2004). Similarly, transcriptomic analyses of HIV-1 *tat*-transfected cells, using a brain-derived Tat sequence from a person with HAD, disclosed induction of an enzyme mediating heparan sulphate synthesis, HS3ST3B1, which was also found to be increased in the brains of patients with HAD (Boven et al., 2007). Similarly, transcriptomic analyses of astrocytes transduced by HIV-1 revealed upregulation of interferon-mediated antiviral responses (OAS1, IFIT1), intercellular contacts (SH3, glia-derived nexin), cell homing/adhesion (matrix metalloproteinases), and cell-cell signaling (neuropilin 1 and 2) (Borjabad, Brooks, & Volsky, 2010). Proteomic studies have reported multiple results including increased heat shock protein 70, heme oxygenase-1, and inducible nitric oxide synthase in HIV *tat*-transfected cells (Pocernich, Sultana, Mohmmad-Abdul, Nath, & Butterfield, 2005). Similarly, diverse findings have been reported for proteomic analyses including monocytes derived from patients with HIV infection (Luo et al., 2003). Very recently, we reported that microRNA profiling in brains from persons with and without HIV infection revealed that microRNAs targeting caspase 6 were markedly suppressed in HIV-infected brains (Noorbakhsh et al., 2010). Other high throughput technologies including deep sequencing will reveal new aspects of gene expression and regulation contributing to neurovirulence in HIV infection but will require analyses based on substantial bioinformatics capacity and application of a systems biology approach (Noorbakhsh et al., 2009).

Gender

Gender differences in HIV-1 seropositive patients have been described in association with drug abuse, with a more frequent history of drug abuse in females compared to males (Mason et al., 1998; Metsch et al., 1998); socioeconomic status and education, with lower levels noted in females (Ickovics & Rodin, 1992; Stern, Silva, Chaisson, & Evans, 1996); psychiatric co-morbidities, with greater psychiatric disease described in female patients (Melnick et al., 1994); as well as mortality rates, with higher rates described in females (Melnick et al., 1994). Studies examining differences in neuropsychological profiles, however, have shown conflicting results. Several studies have identified differences in neuropsychological performance (Failde-Garrido, Alvarez, & Simon-Lopez, 2008), while others have not (Tozzi et al., 2007; Pereda et al., 2000; Rabkin et al., 2000). Failde-Garrido et al. (2008) demonstrated different impairment patterns between genders, with greater deficits in visual memory, attention, psychomotor speed, and abstract reasoning noted in men while women displayed greater deficits in attention, psychomotor speed, and verbal memory.

In another study investigating a variety of neurologic syndromes in HIV-seropositive patients, Lopez et al. did not find differences in the presence of these neurological syndromes in females compared to males (Lopez et al., 1999). Similarly, a prospective study found no difference in the development of neurological symptoms and signs over time in females compared to males (Robertson et al., 2004).

Ethnicity

Many of the aforementioned genetic polymorphisms associated with varying degrees of neurological disease in HIV are found at varying frequencies worldwide (Voevodin, Samilchuk, & Dashti, 1998; Su et al., 1999; Martinson et al., 1997; Su et al., 2000; Martinson et al., 2000). For example, the CCR5-Δ32 allele is frequently found in European populations but is rare in the Middle East, Asia, and Africa (Voevodin et al., 1998; Martinson et al., 1997). Numerous studies looking at specific allele frequencies such as CCR5-Δ32, CCL2–2518GG, and TNFα-308 in particular ethnic groups demonstrate variable frequencies of genetic polymorphisms (Pemberton et al., 2008; Parczewski et al., 2009; Vilades et al., 2007).

HLA Subtypes

Multiple studies have demonstrated an association between HLA subtypes and susceptibility to HIV-1 infection and immune control of the virus (de Sorrentino et al., 2000; Fabio et al., 1990; Goulder & Watkins, 2008; MacDonald et al., 2000; Telenti, 2005). Genetic polymorphisms in the MHC region may account for as much as 15% of the variability seen in indices of immune control such as viral load (Fellay et al., 2007). It is reasonable to assume that improved immune control might lead to a reduced incidence of neurological disease in these patients. Interestingly, it has been found that HLA-DQB*0402 and DRB1*08 alleles are associated with a higher likelihood of developing toxoplasmic encephalitis in the setting of HIV (de Sorrentino et al., 2000). In addition, our clinical observations imply that HIV seropositive individuals of aboriginal (North American Indian) origin do not develop neurological disease as often as Caucasians or other ethnic groups (Power and Gill, unpublished); this may reflect differences in HLA background, as reported for the same ethnic groups who develop the neuromyelitis phenotype of multiple sclerosis (Mirsattari et al., 2001).

Response to Antiretroviral Therapy

Host genetic polymorphisms have been suggested as contributors to the efficacy of selected antiretrovirals in addition to their side-effects. In terms of efficacy, genetic differences in drug transport, metabolism, and clearance have all been described (reviewed in Phillips & Mallal, 2008). An intensively

Table 1.4.1 IMPORTANT HOST GENES AND GENETIC POLYMORPHISMS IN HIV NEUROPATHOGENESIS

GENETIC POLYMORPHISM	EFFECT	REFERENCES
Neurotropism		
Δ32 variant of the CCR5 co-receptor	Diminished neurological disease	Boven et al., 1999; van Rij et al., 1999, Singh et al., 2003
CCR5–59353 variant (in promoter region)	Protection from neurological impairment	Singh et al., 2003
Neurovirulence		
TNF-α-308A	Observed more frequently among HAD patients	Quasney et al., 2001
2578G variant of CCL2	Correlated with the development of HAD	Gonzales et al., 2002
CCL5–28G mutation	Associated with neurocognitive impairment	Letendre et al., 1999
CCL5–403 G/A polymorphism	Non-determined leukoencephalopathy	Guerini et al., 2008
CXCL12–3'A polymorphism	Increased development of neurocognitive impairment in children	Singh et al., 2003
Other		
ApoE-ε4 allele	Conflicting results	Corder et al., 1998; Dunlop et al., 1997; Pemberton et al., 2008; Diaz-Arrastia et al., 2004
HLA-DQB*0402 and DRB1*08 alleles	Higher likelihood of developing toxoplasmic encephalitis in the setting of HIV	de Sorrentino et al., 2000
Mitochondrial 4917G polymorphism of haplotype T	Higher incidence of peripheral neuropathy in NRTI-exposed patients	Hulgan et al., 2005; Canter et al., 2008
TNF-α-1031*2	Higher incidence of peripheral neuropathy in NRTI-exposed patients	Cherry et al., 2008
IL-12B (3_ UTR)*2	Lower incidence of peripheral neuropathy in NRTI-exposed patients	Cherry et al., 2008
Polymorphism in the gene encoding for the hepatic enzyme CYP2B6	Greater incidence of neurological side-effects with Efavirenz	Haas et al., 2004
HLA-B44 and HLA-A2, B44 DR4	More common in patients who experience neuroIRIS in the form of CMV retinitis and/or encephalomyelitis	Price et al., 2001

studied example of this phenomenon is the P-glycoprotein drug transporter in which genetic polymorphisms are known to affect the bioavailability of protease inhibitors and may also influence viral replication (reviewed in Owen, Chandler, & Back, 2005). In addition, many of the genetic polymorphisms mentioned previously in this chapter have also been studied in patients receiving antiretroviral therapy (Hendrickson et al., 2008). In particular, it has been observed that the polymorphisms CCR5-Δ32, CX3CR1-V249I, and CCL5 haplotype H1 all decreased time to viral suppression, whereas the CCR5 P1 haplotype, CXCL12–3'A, and two CCCL5 haplotypes were associated with delayed viral suppression (Hendrickson et al., 2008). It is conceivable these polymorphisms might also lead to variable outcomes in the development of neurological disease.

Multiple studies have demonstrated how genetic polymorphisms contribute to the development of neurological side effects associated with antiretroviral therapies. Nucleoside reverse transcriptase inhibitors (NRTIs) were a frequent cause of distal sensory polyneuropathy in HIV-seropositive patients although recently these drugs have been used less frequently as a result of this off-target effect. The putative mechanism involves mitochondrial injury resulting in peripheral neuropathy (Cui, Locatelli, Xie, & Sommadossi, 1997; Dalakas, Semino-Mora, & Leon-Monzon, 2001, Zhu et al., 2007). One group has demonstrated that the mitochondrial haplotype T is associated with a higher incidence of peripheral neuropathy in NRTI-exposed patients (Hulgan et al., 2005). This same group has demonstrated that it is the mitochondrial 4917G polymorphism of haplotype T which is associated with peripheral neuropathy (Canter et al., 2008). In addition, it has been demonstrated that specific genetic polymorphisms in inflammatory cytokines are also associated with increased and decreased incidence of peripheral neuropathy, suggesting a role for inflammation in the pathophysiology of NRTI-associated peripheral neuropathy (Cherry et al., 2008). Specifically, TNF-α-1031*2 was positively associated with the development of neuropathy while IL-12B (3_ UTR)*2 appeared to be protective.

Efavirenz, a non-nucleoside reverse transcriptase inhibitor, is commonly associated with neurological side effects including dizziness, concentration difficulties, somnolence or difficulty sleeping, and vividly abnormal dreams (Marzolini et al., 2001). A polymorphism in the gene encoding for the hepatic enzyme CYP2B6 has been associated with a greater incidence of neurological side effects (Haas et al., 2004), and this genotype has also been associated with a higher plasma level of the drug suggesting that the increased side effects represent a dose-response effect. Interestingly, in this study, all of the patients developed tolerance to these side effects over time.

Differences in the development of hyperlipidemia and hypertriglyceridemia have also been described among HIV seropositive patients receiving protease inhibitors (Chang et al., 2009; Tarr et al., 2005; Fauvel et al., 2001; Foulkes et al., 2006). Dyslipidemia contributes to cardiovascular disease and increased risk of cardiovascular disease in patients with HIV (reviewed in Anuurad, Semrad, & Berglund, 2009).

Immune Reconstitution Inflammatory Syndrome

There is evidence that genetic factors might participate in the development of neurological immune reconstitution inflammatory syndrome (neuroIRIS). One study has shown that HLA-B44 and HLA-A2, B44 DR4 are more common in patients who experience neuroIRIS in the form of CMV retinitis and/or encephalomyelitis (Price, Keane, Stone, Cheong, & French, 2001). This same group has demonstrated that IRIS appears to be associated with polymorphisms in the TNF-α, IL-12B, and IL-6 genes (Price et al., 2002). Another study examined the frequency of genetic polymorphisms observed in the CCR5, CCL5, CCR2, and CXL12 genes among patients with HIV-related progressive multifocal leukoencephalopathy (PML) or an entity termed "non-determined leukoencephalopathy" (Guerini et al., 2008). Guerini et al.'s term, "non-determined leukoencephalopathy," describes a PML-like leukoencephalopathy, which occurs after initiation of antiretroviral therapy in the absence of detectable JC virus in the CSF, and resembles, in many ways, neuroIRIS. In the latter study, the investigators reported no differences in the distribution of the mutations of CCR5, CCR2, or CXCL in the populations studied; however, they did observe a statistically significant increased rate of the CCL5–403 G/A polymorphism in the non-determined leukoencephalopathy group compared with HIV seropositive controls with neurological disease.

VIRUS-ENCODED DETERMINANTS OF HIV-1 NEUROPATHOGENESIS

In addition to differences in host factors, neuropathogenesis is also affected by a variety of viral factors which contribute to neuroinvasion, neurotropism, and neurovirulence. We will discuss how different viral proteins and genetic polymorphisms thereof contribute to differences in these aspects of neuropathogenesis. We will also address these issues in direct relation to clade differences and in the relative occurrence of shared genetic differences between clades.

NEUROINVASION AND NEUROTROPISM

Several mechanisms of neuroinvasion have been highlighted above although the principal route of viral entry into the CNS remains unclear. For example, a low CD4 T cell nadir, indicative of marked immunosuppression in the peripheral circulation at the time of HIV-1 seroconversion, confers a greater risk of developing subsequent neurological disease. By inference, HIV-1 strains, which replicate efficiently in blood as a quasi-species by causing early immunosuppression, are more likely to enter the nervous system and eventually cause disease, as suggested by studies of simian immunodeficiency virus (SIV) infections (van Marle & Power, 2005). What viral factors determine the relative success in terms of brain entry remain obscure to date; although, it is evident most viral strains entering the CNS are macrophage-tropic while both macrophage- and dual-tropic strains are present in the PNS (Jones et al., 2005). The brain and peripheral nerve microenvironments are distinct from the peripheral circulation in terms of immunological surveillance, cytokine milieu, and target cell characteristics. This uniqueness in the CNS environment can contribute to the variation of viral genotypic characteristics. Analysis of viral isolates from different brain regions of HIV-infected patients revealed the predominance of CCR5 co-receptor usage for entry and macrophage tropism (Albright et al., 1999; Gorry et al., 2001; Ohagen et al., 2003; Power et al., 1998). The different viral genotypes residing in diverse areas of the brain combined with their differential tropism and co-receptor use suggest that neurotropic variants exist that may be governing the neurological manifestations of HIV disease in infected patients (Smit et al., 2001). In this section, the role of different viral proteins and their genetic variations related to neurotropism will be discussed (Table 1.4.2).

Viral Differences in Receptor Usage

As previously discussed, in the nervous system, productive HIV infection is limited to macrophages and microglia. The CD4 molecule expressed by microglial cells binds to the viral envelope glycoprotein, gp120, and initiates viral entry. This binding induces a conformational change and allows subsequent interaction with a chemokine receptor, usually CCR5 or CXCR4, leading to fusion of viral and target cell membrane (Deng et al., 1996; Dragic et al., 1996; Wu et al., 1996). The viral strains that are macrophage-tropic (R5) tend to use the CCR5 co-receptor while the CXCR4 co-receptor is used principally by the lymphotropic (X4) virus strains. There are some viral strains that are dual-tropic (X4R5) and infect both the macrophages and lymphocytes. In fact, dual-tropic strains have been described in both the peripheral and central nervous systems (Choe et al., 1996). Several viruses also engage different sets of co-receptors, including CCR3 and CCR2b (Choe et al., 1996). CCR5 is chiefly used as the co-receptor in the CNS, and macrophage tropism is essential for CNS HIV infection (Albright et al., 1999; Gorry et al., 2001; Ohagen et al., 2003;

Power et al., 1998). Macrophages and microglia express CCR5 and CCR3 together with lower levels of CD4 compared with CD4+ T cells (Bannert, Schenten, Craig, & Sodroski, 2000). Several brain-derived HIV strains have been identified in patients with HAD that replicate efficiently in macrophages and microglia yet have reduced dependence on CD4 and CCR5 receptors (Gorry et al., 2002). Reduced CD4 viral dependence on CD4 has been associated with increased macrophage tropism (Thomas et al., 2007).

Env

The *env* gene of the HIV genome encodes the viral envelope protein gp160, which is subsequently cleaved into two proteins: gp120 and gp41. During HIV infection, the envelope protein gp120 binds to the CD4 receptor on susceptible cells resulting in viral entry (Wyatt & Sodroski, 1998). The protein gp120 is detectable in the autopsied brains of HIV-infected patients (Jones, Bell, & Nath, 2000). It can disrupt blood-brain barrier integrity and enhance monocyte migration, thereby enhancing viral entry into the brain (Kanmogne et al., 2007). Mutations in gp120, especially in the hypervariable V3, V4, and V5 domains, are distinct in the brain compared to other tissues (Dunfee et al., 2007; Shimizu, Shimizu, Takeuchi, & Hoshino, 1994; Gartner et al., 1997). Analysis of V3 region sequences of the *env* gene from the brains of HIV-infected patients with and without dementia showed predominant CCR5 use. Given that macrophages are the chief cells infected in the CNS, the prevalence of CCR5 use in brain-derived HIV strains from patients with and without dementia may have important clinical implications (Shah et al., 2006). Phylogenetic analyses of full length viral sequences isolated from blood plasma and CSF of infected individuals showed clustering of sequences by compartment (Pond et al., 2008). Mutations in positions 5, 9, 13, and 19 of the V3 loop have been demonstrated as signatures for brain-derived HIV strains. Particularly, proline at position 13 is the most significant marker for compartmentalized HIV strain (in contrast to histidine in HIV strains found in the periphery) (Power et al., 1994; Pillai et al., 2006), even though this substitution is not thought to influence macrophage tropism (Thomas et al., 2007). Moreover, the V4 and V5 regions appear to be important for neurotropism (Gartner et al., 1997). On the other hand, a variant in the CD4-binding site of HIV gp120, Asn 283 (N283), has been identified at high frequency in the brain from patients with HAD. N283 increases gp120's affinity for CD4, enhancing the capacity of the HIV envelope to use low levels of CD4 and increasing viral replication in macrophages and microglia (Dunfee et al., 2006). The envelope from a neurovirulent SIV strain interacts with CCR5 in a CD4-independent manner similar to that of the neurotropic HIV-1 strain (Bonavia, Bullock, Gisselman, Margulies, & Clements, 2005). Additionally, there is significant sequence diversity in the V1-V2 loop among demented and nondemented groups in brain-derived *env* sequences showing distinct phylogenetic clustering (Power et al., 1994; Power et al., 1998).

In the peripheral nervous system, analysis of the C2V3 nucleotide sequences of the *env* gene from patients with and without sensory neuropathy showed no distinct clustering. The charge and amino acid composition of the V3 loop isolated from the peripheral nervous system suggests some CCR5 dependence as opposed to seemingly exclusive CCR5 dependence as observed in the CNS (Jones et al., 2005).

Nef

Nef is a 27KDa accessory HIV-1 protein synthesized early in the viral cycle. It interacts with various host proteins and plays a key role in CD4 downregulation and viral infectivity (reviewed in Foster & Garcia, 2008). Although it is not essential for viral infection and replication, it has been observed that *nef*-deleted strains of HIV have lower infectivity (Messmer, Ignatius, Santisteban, Steinman, & Pope, 2000). In the CNS, *nef* mRNA and protein has been detected in the astrocytes of brain autopsies of HIV-infected individuals (Saito et al., 1994; Tornatore, Chandra, Berger, & Major, 1994). In vitro infection of microglia cells infected with *nef*-expressing viral strains induced higher p24 levels compared with *nef*-null strains, indicating its role in infecting the macrophage (Si et al., 2002). *Nef* also increases blood-brain barrier permeability (Sporer et al., 2000) and recruits leukocytes into the CNS (Koedel et al., 1999), perhaps resulting in increased viral entry. Sequence analysis of *nef* reveals that the gene is more conserved in the brains of patients with dementia, possibly as a consequence of positive selection pressure(s) (van Marle et al., 2004).

LTR

The long terminal repeats (LTRs) within the HIV genome are important for viral replication, playing an important role in viral integration and acting as promoters/enhancers. The LTR contains three regions: U5, R, and U3; the U3 region of the promoter is comprised of the promoter, enhancer, and modulatory regions. The LTR relies on various viral and host transcription factors for its activity. These host factors include NFκB, Sp, ATF/CREB, and members of the C/EBP (Kilareski, Shah, Nonnemacher, & Wigdahl, 2009). Of interest, Nef/LTR-deleted SIV strains fail to infect the CNS because it has diminished neurotropism or inefficient viral entry (Thompson et al., 2003). The LTR is essential for HIV infection in the CNS; diversity in its sequence has been reported within and between different regions of the brain and the majority of these variations is located in the region upstream from the NF-kβ sites (Kilareski et al., 2009).

LTR has three C/EBP binding sites upstream of the transcriptional start site that play a crucial role in viral transcription in macrophage-monocyte cells. Brain-derived LTRs possess a 6G configuration (where T is substituted by G at position 6) at C/EBP site I. This mutation is present mainly in the mid-frontal gyrus of the brains of patients with dementia and is associated with a high affinity for the C/EBP factor resulting in a higher rate of viral replication. Conversely, a mutation (4C) in the C/EBP site II, found predominantly in the cerebellum of patients with HAD, is associated with lower rates of viral replication (Ross et al., 2001; Burdo,

Gartner, Mauger, & Wigdahl, 2004). The high affinity of C/EBP binding may be associated with the maintenance and pathogenesis of HIV-1 in the brain, while the low affinity binding may be required for sustaining a reservoir for HIV infection (Kilareski et al., 2009).

Tat

Tat is a basic protein of 104 amino acids encoded by HIV-1 that binds to the transactivation region (TAR) segment of the LTR and regulates transcription. It is the first protein produced during viral replication and is involved in the assembly of the pre-initiation complex during viral transcription (Brady & Kashanchi, 2005). Tat activity is limited in the undifferentiated monocyte as there is a lack of cyclinT1, a molecule through which Tat exerts its actions on viral replication. However, differentiation of monocytes into macrophages increases cyclinT1 expression in the cell and results in greater Tat activity (Yu, Wang, Shaw, Qin, & Rice, 2006). Cooperative interaction can occur among Tat, Vpr, and CyclinT1, leading to upregulated transcription of the viral genome (Sawaya, Khalili, Gordon, Taube, & Amini, 2000). Distinct functional and sequence variation is observed in Tat between brain and periphery. Comparison of matched brain- and spleen-derived *tat* sequences indicates that similarity among brain-derived clones was greater than that between the brain- and spleen-derived clones, perhaps stemming from different selective pressure between the organs (Mayne et al., 1998). Tat-mediated LTR transactivation in astrocytes is unique, and involves complex interplay between viral and cellular transcription factors (Coyle-Rink et al., 2002). In certain CNS-derived cells, Tat is capable of activating HIV-1 in a TAR-independent pathway (Taylor et al., 1992). *Tat* clones derived from patients with HAD also show different functional properties compared to those derived from nondemented HIV-infected patients; analyses of brain-derived *tat* sequences showed distinct clustering between HAD and nondemented subjects (Bratanich et al., 1998). For example, LTR transactivation is decreased while

the pro-apoptotic gene, PDCD7, is upregulated by *tat* cloned from individuals with HAD (Boven et al., 2007). Remarkably, brain-derived *tat* sequences are heterogeneous in regions which influence viral replication and intracellular transport (Bratanich et al., 1998).

Pol

HIV-1 *pol* encodes a polyprotein of 1447 amino acids which is cleaved into several functional proteins including reverse transcriptase (RT), protease, RNAse H, and integrase. Like the other viral proteins discussed before, distinct sequence variation for the *pol* region is found in the CNS. Different patterns of RT and protease mutations develop in systemic infection compared to the CNS (Caragounis et al., 2008). However, unlike *tat* and *env*, phylogenetic clustering or distinct polymorphisms were not observed within brain-derived RT sequences from HIV/AIDS patients with or without HAD (Bratanich et al., 1998). Many of the mutations in RT sequences are within the active sites of the enzyme, possibly leading to positive selection pressure (Huang, Alter, & Wooley, 2002). These findings are complemented by previous observations that drug-resistant mutations found in the brain and CSF differ from those detected in the periphery (Cunningham et al., 2000; Venturi et al., 2000).

NEUROVIRULENCE

Several experimental approaches have been utilized to delineate the contributions of different HIV-1 genes and regions to neurovirulence including in vitro and in vivo models. Furthermore, clinically-derived HIV-1 sequences, largely derived from the brain, have also been informative. Recombinant viral proteins can be applied, or vectors containing the viral gene of interest can be transfected into monocytoid (macrophage/microglia) or astrocytic cells. However, it should be kept in mind that the effects of the proteins vary depending on the mode of delivery and give rise

Table 1.4.2 ROLE OF VIRAL PROTEINS IN NEUROTROPISM

Env	• Disrupts BBB and mediates viral entry into the brain • Brain-derived *envs* have mutations in the V3, V4, and V5 that are associated with increased macrophage tropismIncreases blood-brain barrier permeability • Increases viral infectivity in macrophages and microglia	• Kanmogne et al., 2007 • Dunfee et al., 2007; Shimizu et al., 1994; Shah et al., 2006
Nef	• Increases blood-brain barrier permeability • Increases viral infectivity in macrophages and microglia	• Sporer et al., 2000 • Si et al., 2002
LTR	• Essential for viral infection of CNS • Diversity in LTR sequence within and between different regions of the brain is associated with effective viral infection	• Thompson et al., 2003 • Kilareski et al., 2009
Pol	• Distinct sequence variations in the RT sequence are found in the CNS, many of the which occur within the active sites of the enzyme leading to positive selection pressure	• Huang et al., 2002
Tat	• Exhibits distinct functional and sequence variation between brain and periphery perhaps stemming from different selective pressure between the organs • Mediates LTR transactivation in astrocytes in an unique manner involving complex interplay between viral and cellular transcription factors • Capable of activating HIV-1 in a TAR-independent pathway	• Mayne et al., 1998 • Coyle-Rink et al., 2002 • Taylor et al., 1992

to contradictory results. Similarly, HIV-1 gp120 has been transgenically expressed in mice using a GFAP promoter that limits its expression largely to the CNS (Toggas et al., 1994) and PNS (Keswani, Jack, Zhou, & Hoke, 2006). A *vpr* transgenic animal expresses Vpr only in monocytoid cell lines (Jones et al. 2007) while transgenic animals for *nef*, *tat*, and LTR express the transgene in T cells (Brady, Pennington, Miles, & Dzierzak, 1993; Lindemann et al., 1994; Brady et al. 1995). This section summarizes the role of different viral proteins in neurovirulence based on the *ex vivo* and in vivo data (Table 1.4.3).

Envelope Proteins

Gp120 mediates its neurotoxic effects by direct action on the neurons or indirectly by activating macrophages, microglia, and astrocytes (Lipton, Sucher, Kaiser, & Dreyer, 1991; Lipton, 1992; Lannuzel, Lledo, Lamghitnia, Vincent, & Tardieu, 1995). Gp120 might elicit oxidative stress in neurons and astrocytes through calcium signal dysregulation, although neurons are more susceptible to injury (Haughey & Mattson, 2002; Mattson, Haughey, & Nath, 2005). An anti-oxidant enzyme, Mn-superoxide dismutase, is reported to be downregulated in neurons and upregulated in astrocytes by gp120, rendering differential effects on astrocytes and neurons (Saha & Pahan, 2007). The interaction of gp120 with the chemokine receptors CXCR4 and CCR5 activates intracellular pathways leading to neuronal apoptosis (Kaul et al., 2005). This action is mediated by a number of downstream molecules including RNA-activated protein kinase (Alirezaei et al., 2007), p38, and mitogen-activated protein kinase (Singh et al., 2005). Gp120 can also induce host molecules, including MMPs (Russo et al., 2007), IL-1β (Cheung et al., 2008), and TNF-α (Buriani et al., 1999).

Gp120 induces excitotoxicity by suppressing the expression of the glutamate transporter gene, EAAT2 (Wang et al., 2003), or by activating NMDA receptors. The V3 region within gp120 binds to the NMDA receptor at the glycine binding site and stimulates glutamate release (Pattarini et al., 1998). However, NMDA receptor antagonists have not been able to reverse gp120-mediated neurotoxicity (Alessia & Italo, 2004). Dopaminergic neurons also appear to be vulnerable to gp120-mediated injury (Bennett, Rusyniak, & Hollingsworth, 1995). Gp120 can act synergistically with some drugs of abuse including methamphetamine and cocaine that also damage the dopaminergic system (Nath et al., 2000).

Gp41 has been readily detected in the autopsied brains of patients (Kure et al., 1990). It induces NOS2 production, resulting in neurotoxicity mediated by the N-terminal domain of the protein (Adamson et al., 1996; Adamson, Kopnisky, Dawson, & Dawson, 1999). Gp41 might also be involved in increasing excitotoxicity by eliciting the release of glutamate and noradrenaline (Wang & White, 2000).

HIV-1 gp120 also participates in the pathogenesis of peripheral neuropathy. It can exert axonal toxicity directly resulting in "dying back" of axons and nerve damage (reviewed in Cornblath & Hoke, 2006). Gp120 is also involved in eliciting peripheral pain responses (Milligan et al., 2000;

Herzberg & Sagen, 2001), and perineural HIV-1 gp120 exposure induces a persistent mechanical hypersensitivity (Wallace et al., 2007). Gp120 may also act through its interaction with the CCR2 or CXCR4 receptors on Schwann cells, leading to the release of toxic cytokines and subsequent neuronal injury (Bhangoo, Ripsch, Buchanan, Miller, & White, 2009).

Transgenic mice expressing gp120 under control of the GFAP promoter, permitting expression in astrocytes, exhibit features which are reminiscent of HIV-associated dementia, including neuronal injury and glial activation. Moreover, these same animals show neurobehavioral deficits. Likewise, transgenic expression of g120 in the PNS is limited to Schwann cells without an apparent neurobehavioral or neuropathological phenotype. However, if these animals are exposed to neurotoxic antiretroviral drugs, they exhibit features of peripheral neuropathy (Toggas et al., 1994; Keswani et al., 2006).

Importantly, many of the studies described above use gp120 genes or proteins derived from representative HIV-1 sequences, including viruses from patients with HIV-associated dementia. However, there are multiple studies indicating that HIV-1 gp120, particularly from brain-derived sequences, contains mutations highly associated with the development of dementia (Power et al., 1998). Several of these mutations have been shown to influence in vitro neurovirulence but none have been expressed in vivo in transgenic mice or in other in vivo models (Bonavia et al., 2005).

Vpr

HIV-1 Vpr is a 96 amino acid (14KDa) accessory viral protein synthesized late in the viral life cycle (Schwartz et al., 1991) and it is essential for infection of macrophages and monocytes. Vpr is a soluble protein that is released by infected cells although the conditions governing its release remain unclear despite its potent extracellular actions. Vpr plays an important role in different cellular functions, including cell cycle arrest in the G_2 phase, induction of apoptosis, and nuclear import of viral DNA into macrophages and other nondividing cells (Ayyavoo et al., 1997). It is detectable in CSF and brain tissue from HIV-infected subjects (Levy, Refaeli, MacGregor, & Weiner, 1994; Jones et al., 2007). Vpr can bind to the LTR sequence of HIV-1 and contributes to viral production. A substantial proportion of patients with HAD exhibits a particular sequence at the C/EBP binding site I in the LTR derived from the brain allowing Vpr to bind with high affinity to the C/EBP binding site, thereby influencing viral replication (Burdo, Gartner, Mauger, & Wigdahl, 2004). Vpr expression in microglia induces chemoattractant CCL5, which is essential for viral infection (Si et al., 2002). Application of recombinant Vpr (rVpr) as well as intracellular Vpr expression induces neuronal apoptosis through caspase-9 activation (Patel, Mukhtar, & Pomerantz, 2000; Patel, Mukhtar, Harley, Kulkosky, & Pomerantz, 2002; Cheng et al., 2007; Jones et al., 2007). rVpr also inhibits axonal outgrowth in neurons through induction of mitochondrial dysfunction; however, point mutations of arginine residues at sites 73, 77, or 80 can render soluble rVpr incapable of causing axonal damage (Kitayama et al., 2008). Of interest, a similar point mutation (R77Q) in blood-derived HIV-1 stains has been associated with long-term nonprogressive HIV infection (Lum et al., 2003; Mologni et al., 2006). Vpr induces H_2O_2 and mitochondrial ROS (reactive oxygen species) production in the microglia, underscoring its role in generating oxidative stress in the brain (Rom et al., 2009; Deshmane et al., 2009); although, neuroinflammation is not a feature of Vpr's pathogenic actions unlike gp120 and Tat. HIV-1 Vpr has also been proposed to form ion channels within the plasma membrane (Piller, Ewart, Premkumar, Cox, & Gage, 1996; Piller, Ewart, Jans, Gage, & Cox, 1999). This proposed channel-forming property has been attributed to the N-terminal of the peptide, and the channels are thought to be open at negative potentials. Vpr can also alter membrane properties by inducing rapid changes in neuronal membrane currents by inhibiting voltage-dependent potassium channels (Jones et al., 2007).

Recent findings suggest that Vpr can exert its actions directly on astrocytes and microglia. Exposure to Vpr diminishes expression of astrocyte-specific markers and causes caspase-6 mediated apoptosis (Noorbakhsh et al., 2010). Vpr also drives the expression of HIF-1α in microglia cells, which can lead to oxidative stress (Deshmane et al., 2009). Induction of calcium signal by Vpr has been observed in astrocytes and neurons (Rom et al., 2009; Noorbakhsh et al., 2010), and can cause dysregulation of intracellular signaling pathways. Alteration or dysfunction of astrocytes and glial cells, in turn, can cause neuronal damage.

Studies from our group indicate that Vpr is expressed in the PNS of HIV-infected persons and indeed, a transgenic mouse expressing Vpr in the PNS exhibits mechanical allodynia with evidence of dorsal root neuronal injury (Acharjee et al., 2009).

Nef

Nef appears to play an important albeit undefined role in HIV neuropathogenesis. Nef has an N-terminal myristoylation site which is co-translationally modified (Hammes, Dixon, Malim, Cullen, & Greene, 1989) and associates with the plasma membrane (Bentham, Mazaleyrat, & Harris, 2006). Recent studies also indicate that Nef may be secreted (Campbell et al., 2008); antibodies to Nef have been detected in the serum in a large proportion of HIV-infected individuals, suggesting Nef is secreted extracellularly (Ameisen et al., 1989; Cheingsong-Popov et al., 1990). Nevertheless, the presence of extracellular Nef remains controversial. Recombinant Nef (rNef) is cytotoxic to neurons and glial cell culture (Trillo-Pazos, McFarlane-Abdulla, Campbell, Pilkington, & Everall, 2000). HIV-1 Nef might contribute directly to neuropathogenesis by causing astrocyte death together with indirect neuronal death through the cytotoxic actions of induced IP-10 on neurons (van Marle et al., 2004). Grafting of Nef-transduced macrophages into the rat hippocampus induced monocyte/macrophage recruitment, expression of TNF-alpha, astrogliosis, and behavior changes in rats (Mordelet et al., 2004). Nef is also shown to induce quinolinic acid production in macrophages (Smith et al., 2001). Quinolinic acid is a neurotoxic molecule, and indeed, it is elevated in the brains of HIV-demented individuals (Heyes et al., 1991). Nef has sequence and structural similarity to a neurotoxic scorpion peptide and also shares some of its functional properties (Werner et al., 1991). Nef induces a range of host genes including MMP-9, MCP-1, IL-6, TNF-α, IFN-γ, and CCL5 in the CNS which can influence neuronal viability (Koedel et al., 1999; Sporer et al., 2000; Si et al., 2002). Transgenic expression of *nef* under the control of the LTR did not exhibit neuropathogenic effects despite its immunosuppressive phenotype (Hanna et al., 2009).

Tat

Tat is a secreted viral protein with diverse effects on neural cells in the CNS (Li et al., 2009). Tat causes neuronal damage by acting directly on neurons or indirectly by activating glial cells. Tat-induced neuronal injury occurs through multiple cellular pathways; Tat induces neuronal apoptosis through mitochondrial dysfunction and caspase activation (Kruman, Nath, & Mattson, 1998). Several types of neurons in the dentate gyrus, striatum, and the CA3 region of the hippocampus are more vulnerable to Tat (Rappaport et al., 1999; Maragos et al., 2003; Li et al., 2009). In vivo and in vitro studies have shown that Tat can affect dopaminergic neuron function (Zauli et al., 2000; Ferris, Frederick-Duus, Fadel, Mactutus, & Booze, 2009; Zhu et al., 2009). Tat induces cytosolic calcium in neuronal cells using extracellular sources and IP₃ sensitive intracellular stores of the cell (Haughey, Holden, Nath, & Geiger, 1999). Tat also activates ryanodine receptors in the endoplasmic reticulum, inducing an unfolded protein response and mitochondrial hyperpolarization (Norman et al., 2008). Mitochondrial hyperpolarization leads to generation of ROS, activation of caspases, and ultimately, apoptosis (Kruman et al., 1998; Singh et al., 2004). Amino acids 31–61 of Tat are thought to be the active region that is involved in electrophysiological changes, specifically, by depolarizing the membrane (Magnuson et al., 1995; Nath et al., 1996; Cheng et al., 1997), increasing the whole-cell inward current and decreasing membrane resistance (Brailoiu, Brailoiu, Chang, & Dun, 2008). Tat interacts with neurons through at least two receptors, heparan sulfate and lipoprotein receptor associate protein (LRP) (Liu et al., 2000). Heparan sulfate helps Tat to localize to the cell membrane while LRP helps to internalize it through endocytosis. Tat can also bind to the NR1 subunit of the NMDA receptor (Li et al., 2008). Tat's interaction with NMDA receptors is yet another way by which it exerts its effects. Tat induces calcium entry through NMDA receptors and causes synaptic loss in neuronal cultures (Kim et al., 2008). LRP, an NMDA receptor and the post-synaptic density protein-95 (PSD-95) form a complex and Tat stimulates this complex leading to neuronal injury (Eugenin et al., 2007). Tat might also cause synaptic dysfunction by upregulating mir-128, which is a neuron-encoded microRNA involved in regulating SNAP25 expression. Tat can also act synergistically with other toxic molecules, like gp120, (Bansal et al., 2000; Nath et al., 2000a) and substances of abuse (Nath et al. 2002), resulting in exacerbation of neuronal dysfunction.

In addition to direct toxicity, Tat acts on the glial cells causing them to release host toxic molecules. Tat stimulates production of a multitude of host cytokines and chemokines, including TNF-α, CCL2, CCL5, CXCL10, and SDF-1 (Li et al., 2009). MMPs (Johnston et al., 2001), NOS2 (Polazzi, Levi, & Minghetti, 1999), and quinolic acid (Smith et al., 2001) expression are induced by Tat, all of which can result in neurotoxicity. Sequence variation in Tat is linked to differences in neurotoxic potential. For example, clade B Tat is more neurotoxic compared with clade C Tat, and alteration in a dicysteine motif within the neurotoxic region of clade B Tat is associated with this difference (Mishra, Vetrivel, Siddappa, Ranga, & Seth, 2008).

Virus-encoded microRNAs

MicroRNAs (miRNA) are small RNA molecules encoded from the genomic (host or viral) DNA in the same manner as RNA. The hairpin secondary structure in the RNA is recognized and cleaved sequentially by the action of two enzymes, Dicer and Drosha, giving rise to an miRNA which is a duplex of two RNA strands approximately 22 nucleotides long (Yeung, Bennasser, Le, & Jeang, 2005). The microRNA binds to the 3' UTR with imperfect complementarity and functions as a transcription repressor. There is growing evidence that many viruses express miRNA and regulate their replication and host response (Klase et al., 2007; Klase et al., 2009). Recent studies show that HIV also encodes microRNAs through processing of the HIV-1 TAR element by the Dicer enzyme (Klase et al., 2007). This viral miRNA is detectable in infected cells and appears to contribute to viral latency and alters cellular function (Klase et al., 2007; Klase et al., 2009). Further research may elucidate the role of miRNA and differential Dicer enzyme expression in HIV replication in the CNS.

Table 1.4.3 ROLE OF VIRAL PROTEINS IN NEUROVIRULENCE

GENE	FUNCTION	REFERENCE
Env	• Elicit oxidative stress in neurons and astrocytes • Induce neuronal apoptosis • Cause glutamate excitotoxicity by suppressing the expression of glutamate transporter gene, EAAT2 or by activating NMDA receptors • Induces painful peripheral neuropathy	• Haughey et al., 2002; Mattson, 2005 • Kaul et al., 2005 • Pattarini et al., 1998; Wang et al., 2003 • Reviewed in Cornblath & Hoke, 2006; Wallace, 2007; Bhangoo et al., 2009
Nef	• *nef* sequence is more conserved in the brains of patients with dementia, possibly as a consequence of positive selection pressure(s) • Causes astrogliosis and astrocyte death • Mediates behavior changes in rats • Induces quinolinic acid production in macrophages • Activates host genes including MMP-9, MCP-1, IL-6, TNF-α, IFN-γ, and CCL5 in the CNS which can influence neuronal viability	• van Marle et al., 2004 • Mordelet et al., 2004 • Smith et al., 2001 • Koedel et al., 1999; Sporer et al., 2000; Si et al., 2002
Vpr	• Expression in microglia induces chemoattractant CCL5, which is essential for viral infection • Expression induces neuronal apoptosis through caspase-9 activation • Inhibits axonal outgrowth in neurons through induction of mitochondrial dysfunction • Induces H_2O_2 and mitochondrial ROS production in the microglia, underscoring its role in generating oxidative stress in the brain • Alters neuronal membrane properties • Causes astrogliosis and causes caspase-6-mediated apoptosis • Can cause peripheral neuropathy	• Si et al., 2002 • Patel et al., 2000; Patel et al., 2002; Cheng et al., 2007; Jones et al., 2007 • Kitayama et al., 2008 • Rom et al., 2009; Deshmane et al., 2009 • Piller et al., 1996; Piller et al., 1999; Jones et al., 2007 • Noorbakhsh et al., 2010 • Acharjee et al., 2009
Tat	• Induces neuronal apoptosis through mitochondrial dysfunction and caspase activation • Causes cytosolic calcium influx in neuronal cells • Induces unfolded protein response, mitochondrial hyperpolarization, generation of ROS, activation of caspases, and ultimately, apoptosis • Alters neuronal membrane properties by inducing membrane depolarization, increasing whole-cell inward current, and decreasing membrane resistance • Affects dopaminergic neuron function • Activates NMDA receptor and causes neuronal injury • Causes synaptic dysfunction by upregulating mir-128 which is a neuron-encoded microRNA involved in regulating SNAP25 expression • Acts synergistically with other toxic molecules, like gp120, and substances of abuse resulting in exacerbation of neuronal dysfunction • Stimulates production of a multitude of host toxic molecules including TNF-α, CCL2, CCL5, CXCL10, and SDF-1, MMP, iNOS, and quinolic acid which can result in neurotoxicity	• Kruman et al., 1998 • Haughey et al., 1999 • Norman et al., 2008; Kruman et al., 1998; Singh et al., 2004 • Magnuson et al., 1995; Nath et al., 1996; Cheng et al., 1997; Brailoiu et al., 2008 • Zauli et al., 2000; Ferris et al., 2009; Zhu et al., 2009. • Li et al., 2008; Kim et al., 2008 • Eletto et al., 2008 • Bansal et al., 2000; Nath et al., 2000a; Nath et al., 2002 • Li et al., 2009, Johnston et al., 2001, Polazzi et al., 1999, Smith et al., 2001

HIV-1 CLADE-RELATED NEUROPATHOGENESIS

There are four genetic groups of HIV-1 virus recognized worldwide: group M (major), group O (outlier), group N (new, non-M, non-O) (Hemelaar, Gouws, Ghys, & Osmanov, 2006), and group P (Plantier et al., 2009). Group M accounts for the vast majority of cases and is subdivided into nine major subtypes or clades (Hemelaar et al., 2006). Clade C accounts for 50% of cases worldwide, followed by clades A (12%), B (10%), G (6%), and D (3%) (Hemelaar et al., 2006). Clade B is the subtype most frequently encountered in North America and Europe (Hemelaar et al., 2006) and is therefore the clade which has been the most studied in the clinic. Prevalence of subtypes differs markedly throughout the world with the largest variability in clade prevalence in Africa (Hemelaar et al., 2006). The classification system was initially based on the *env* sequence but applies to all regions of the viral genome (Hemelaar et al., 2006). Of interest, we reported that molecular diversity in brain-derived HIV-1 A and D clade *env* sequences displayed greater evolutionary distance than B clade brain-derived viruses (Zhang et al., 2001). Similarly, molecular diversity between matched brain and spleen *env* clones was clade-dependent and concentrated in the hypervariable V4 region (Zhang et al., 2001).

Whether HIV clade contributes to pathogenesis, progression to AIDS, mortality, drug resistance, or neuropathogenesis remains a topic of ongoing debate and research (Hemelaar et al., 2006; Liner, Hall, & Robertson, 2007). There is evidence supporting differences in disease progression comparing different subtypes in isolated populations (Kiwanuka et al., 2008; Kaleebu et al., 2002; Vasan et al., 2006). There have also been several studies highlighting possible differences in neurological complications comparing different subtypes. This topic was reviewed by Liner and colleagues (Liner et al., 2007). Previously, it was believed that the prevalence of HIV-associated dementia was rare in clade C-seropositive patients (Teja, Talasila, & Vemu, 2005; Wadia et al., 2001). This notion is also supported by the observation that the pathological changes seen within brains from HIV-1 clade C-infected patients are different from those described in clade B patients with the striking absence of multifocal microglial nodules and multinucleated giant cells (Mahadevan et al., 2007). More recently however, Gupta and colleagues found a prevalence of 60.5% of mild to moderate cognitive impairment among a group of HIV-1 clade C-seropositive adults from South India, which is similar to reports of prevalence in clade B infection. No cases of severe cognitive impairment were identified in this cohort (Gupta et al., 2007). In a prospective study completed in South Africa, Modi and colleagues reported a 38% prevalence of HAD, similar to that reported in clade B infection (Modi, Hari, Modi, & Mochan, 2007). Significant differences in the frequency of HAD comparing HIV-1 clade D and clade A have also been reported (Sacktor et al., 2009). It appears as though conflicting evidence regarding prevalence of various neurological complications among HIV-1 clades exists and further study is therefore warranted.

Possible mechanisms have also been explored for viral subtype differences in disease progression. One postulated mechanism relates to subtype differences in viral tropism related to differences in the use of chemokine receptors by different virus subtypes. CCR5 is the co-receptor used by non-syncytium-inducing variants for viral entry and CXCR4 is the co-receptor most commonly used by syncytium-inducing variants (Peeters et al., 1999; Kaleebu et al., 2007; Zhang et al., 1996; Tscherning et al., 1998). Strains utilizing the CXCR4 co-receptor replicate more quickly which is correlated with faster disease progression (Peeters et al., 1999; Tscherning et al., 1998). Many HIV-1 strains also change co-receptor usage as the disease progresses with higher frequency of co-receptor CXCR4 use later in the disease during the rapidly progressing end-stage (Kaleebu et al., 2007). There also appears to be an earlier shift to CXCR4 co-receptor use from CCR5 co-receptor use in clade D compared to clade A, which has been postulated as a reason for increased systemic pathogenicity seen in clade D (Kaleebu et al., 2007). In the CNS, however, macrophage tropism and use of CCR5 as co-receptor for viral entry appear to be important prerequisites for infection (Power et al., 1998; Reddy et al., 1996; Gorry et al., 2001; Albright et al., 1999; Chan et al., 1999). CXCR4-dependent viruses and dual tropic viruses are infrequently found in the CNS (Reddy et al., 1996; Gorry et al., 2001), and although these differences in co-receptor use may prove to be important when considering differences in disease progression, it seems unlikely that these differences explain the variation seen in neurological disease among subtypes.

One possible mechanism for subtype difference relates to the Tat protein and excitotoxicity. HIV-infected macrophages can cause neuronal injury through the extracellular release of Tat protein (Magnuson et al., 1995). Tat activates the NMDA receptor (Song, Nath, Geiger, Moore, & Hochman, 2003), resulting in excitotoxicity. It appears as though this activation occurs through the direct binding of Tat protein to the NMDA receptor and the resulting neurotoxic response is clade specific (Li et al., 2008; Mishra, Vetrivel, Siddappa, Ranga, & Seth, 2008). When comparing clades B and C, it appears as though there is an equal amount of Tat protein released; however, the Tat released from clade C results in significantly lower toxicity (Li et al., 2008; Mishra et al., 2008). It is thought that the Cys31Ser mutation in clade C Tat may be critical for activation of the NMDA receptor with resultant excitotoxicity without affecting the binding of Tat to the NMDA receptor (Li et al., 2008).

Differences between clades B and C have also been demonstrated using the SCID mouse HIV encephalitis model (Rao et al., 2008). Clade B infected mice develop more severe neurobehavioral deficits as compared to clade C infected mice with similar brain viral loads. Mice infected with clade C, however, showed decreased pathology and reduced monocyte chemotaxis (Rao et al., 2008). It appears as though chemotaxis is induced by macrophages through the release of Tat (Rao et al., 2008), which also results in the release of CCL2 by astrocytes and monocytes (Conant et al., 1998; Weiss et al., 1999; D'Aversa, Yu, & Berman, 2004). It appears as though there is reduced release of CCL2 chemokine with infection by clade C virus, resulting in reduced monocyte chemotaxis.

Another possible mechanism involves differences in the V3 loop of the envelope glycoprotein, gp120, between subtypes, which also may affect neurovirulence (Liner et al., 2007; De Jong et al., 1992; Zhong et al., 1995). Clade D strains appear to have a more variable pattern of the V3 loop as compared to clade C, and in particular, this variability has been shown in HIV entry into the CD4 cell (Hwang, Boyle, Lyerly, & Cullen, 1991; Zhang et al., 2001). Similar types of viral envelope diversity have also been shown to affect the progression of neurological disease in other retroviruses (Johnston et al., 2000; Mankowski et al., 1997). The V3 region of the envelope has been shown to influence the release of neurotoxins from macrophages and has been postulated to be directly neurotoxic (Liner et al., 2007; Kaul et al., 1999; Kong et al., 1996; Power et al., 1998; Yeung, Pulliam, & Lau, 1995; Zhao, Kim, Morgello, & Lee, 2001).

FUTURE PERSPECTIVES

Most of the studies described herein have been performed using the models of HIV-infected brain cells or using brain tissues from patients with or without HAD from HIV-1 clade B-infected persons. The full spectrum of non-clade B virus-related neurological disease remains unknown. With increasing migration, there is growing viral subtype diversity globally, which may impact on care and provides increasing impetus for the further study of all viral subtypes (Krentz et al., 2009). Similarly, the contributions of viral and host genetic diversity to the occurrence of HIV-associated neurological disease and/ or neurodevelopment in children remains unclear to date.

In addition, genome-wide scans of different populations infected by HIV will likely highlight new susceptibility loci or mutations for HIV-related neurological disorders. Comprehensive molecular studies of peripheral neuropathy are lacking and it is plausible individual differences in the development of HIV DSP and other peripheral nervous system manifestations of HIV infection may also be, in part, affected by viral and host genetic differences. Moreover, the impact of antiretroviral therapy and ensuing drug resistance mutations on the neurological disease phenotypes and response to treatments remains to be defined. The increasing use of advanced technologies such as pyrosequencing as well as verifiable clinical and epidemiological data are imperative for the ongoing understanding of HIV/AIDS neuropathogenesis, permitting the development of new diagnostic and therapeutic options for this broad group of disabling neurological disorders.

ACKNOWLEDGMENTS

We thank Krista Nelles for assistance with manuscript preparation. JAM is a University of Alberta Clinical Scholar. CP is an AHFMR Senior Scholar and holds a Canada Research Chair in Neurological Infection and Immunity.

REFERENCES

Acharjee, S., Zhu, Y., Noorbakhsh, F., Stemkowski, P., Olechowski, C., Cohen, E., et al. (2009). Human immunodeficiency virus-1 vpr expression in the peripheral nervous system: Evidence for neuronal injury and neuropathic pain. *Abstract SfN 2009, 561*.13/DD11

Achim, C. L., Heyes, M. P., & Wiley, C. A. (1993). Quantitation of human immunodeficiency virus, immune activation factors, and quinolinic acid in AIDS brains. *Journal of Clinical Investigation, 91*(6), 2769–2775.

Adamson, D. C., Kopnisky, K. L., Dawson, T. M., & Dawson, V. L. (1999). Mechanisms and structural determinants of HIV-1 coat protein, gp41-induced neurotoxicity. *J Neurosci, 19*(1), 64–71.

Adamson, D., Wildemann, B., Sasaki, M., Glass, J., McArthur, J., Christov, V., et al. (1996). Immunologic NO synthase: Elevation in severe AIDS dementia and induction by HIV-1 gp41. *Science, 274*(5294), 1917–21; 1917.

Albright, A. V., Shieh, J. T., Itoh, T., Lee, B., Pleasure, D., O'Connor, M. J., et al. (1999). Microglia express CCR5, CXCR4, and CCR3, but of these, CCR5 is the principal coreceptor for human immunodeficiency virus type 1 dementia isolates. *Journal of Virology, 73*(1), 205–213.

Alessia, B. & Italo, M. (2004). The chemokine receptor CXCR4 and not the N-methyl-D-aspartate receptor mediates gp120 neurotoxicity in cerebellar granule cells. *Journal of Neuroscience Research, 75*(1), 75–82.

Alirezaei, M., Watry, D. D., Flynn, C. F., Kiosses, W. B., Masliah, E., Williams, B. R. G., et al. (2007). Human immunodeficiency virus-1/ Surface glycoprotein 120 induces apoptosis through RNA-activated protein kinase signaling in neurons. *J Neurosci, 27*(41), 11047–11055.

Ameisen, J., Guy, B., Chamaret, S., Loche, M., Mouton, Y., Neyrinck, J., et al. (1989). Antibodies to the nef protein and to nef peptides in HIV-1â€"Infected seronegative individuals. *AIDS Research and Human Retroviruses, 5*(1), 279–291.

Anuurad, E., Semrad, A., & Berglund, L. (2009). Human immunodeficiency virus and highly active antiretroviral therapy-associated metabolic disorders and risk factors for cardiovascular disease. *Metabolic Syndrome & Related Disorders, 7*(5), 401–410.

Argyris, E. G., Acheampong, E., Nunnari, G., Mukhtar, M., Williams, K. J., & Pomerantz, R. J. (2003). Human immunodeficiency virus type 1 enters primary human brain microvascular endothelial cells by a mechanism involving cell surface proteoglycans independent of lipid rafts. *Journal of Virology, 77*(22), 12140–12151.

Ayyavoo, V., Mahalingam, S., Rafaeli, Y., Kudchodkar, S., Chang, D., Nagashunmugam, T., et al. (1997). HIV-1 viral protein R (vpr) regulates viral replication and cellular proliferation in T cells and monocytoid cells in vitro. *J Leukoc Biol, 62*(1), 93–99.

Bagasra, O., Lavi, E., Bobroski, L., Khalili, K., Pestaner, J. P., Tawadros, R., et al. (1996). Cellular reservoirs of HIV-1 in the central nervous system of infected individuals: Identification by the combination of in situ polymerase chain reaction and immunohistochemistry. *AIDS, 10*(6), 573–585.

Bannert, N., Schenten, D., Craig, S., & Sodroski, J. (2000). The level of CD4 expression limits infection of primary rhesus monkey macrophages by a T-tropic simian immunodeficiency virus and macrophagetropic human immunodeficiency viruses. *Journal of Virology, 74*(23), 10984–10993.

Bansal, A. K., Mactutus, C. F., Nath, A., Maragos, W., Hauser, K. F., & Booze, R. M. (2000). Neurotoxicity of HIV-1 proteins gp120 and tat in the rat striatum. *Brain Research, 879*(1–2), 42–49.

Bennett, B. A., Rusyniak, D. E., & Hollingsworth, C. K. (1995). HIV-1 gp120-induced neurotoxicity to midbrain dopamine cultures. *Brain Research, 705*(1–2), 168–176.

Bentham, M., Mazaleyrat, S., & Harris, M. (2006). Role of myristoylation and N-terminal basic residues in membrane association of the human immunodeficiency virus type 1 nef protein. *J Gen Virol, 87*(3), 563–571.

Berger, E. A., Murphy, P. M., & Farber, J. M. (1999). Chemokine receptors as HIV-1 coreceptors: Roles in viral entry, tropism, and disease. *Annual Review of Immunology, 17*, 657–700.

Bhangoo, S., Ripsch, M., Buchanan, D., Miller, R., & White, F. (2009). Increased chemokine signaling in a model of HIV1-associated peripheral neuropathy. *Molecular Pain, 5*(1), 48.

Bobardt, M. D., Salmon, P., Wang, L., Esko, J. D., Gabuzda, D., Fiala, M., et al. (2004). Contribution of proteoglycans to human immunodeficiency virus type 1 brain invasion. *Journal of Virology, 78*(12), 6567–6584.

Bonavia, A., Bullock, B. T., Gisselman, K. M., Margulies, B. J., & Clements, J. E. (2005). A single amino acid change and truncated TM are sufficient for simian immunodeficiency virus to enter cells using CCR5 in a CD4-independent pathway. *Virology, 341*(1), 12–23.

Borjabad, A., Brooks, A. I., & Volsky, D. J. (2010). Gene expression profiles of HIV-1-infected glia and brain: Toward better understanding of the role of astrocytes in HIV-1-associated neurocognitive disorders. *Journal of Neuroimmune Pharmacology: The Official Journal of the Society on NeuroImmune Pharmacology, 5*(1), 44–62.

Boven, L. A., van der Bruggen, T., van Asbeck, B. S., Marx, J. J., & Nottet, H. S. (1999). Potential role of CCR5 polymorphism in the development of AIDS dementia complex. *FEMS Immunology & Medical Microbiology, 26*(3–4), 243–247.

Boven, L. A., Noorbakhsh, F., Bouma, G., van der Zee, R., Vargas, D. L., Pardo, C., et al. (2007). Brain-derived human immunodeficiency virus-1 tat exerts differential effects on LTR transactivation and neuroimmune activation. *Journal of Neurovirology, 13*(2), 173–184.

Boyles, J. K., Pitas, R. E., Wilson, E., Mahley, R. W., & Taylor, J. M. (1985). Apolipoprotein E associated with astrocytic glia of the central nervous system and with nonmyelinating glia of the peripheral nervous system. *Journal of Clinical Investigation, 76*(4), 1501–1513.

Brady, H. J., Abraham, D. J., Pennington, D. J., Miles, C. G., Jenkins, S., & Dzierzak, E. A. (1995). Altered cytokine expression in T lymphocytes from human immunodeficiency virus tat transgenic mice. *Journal of Virology, 69*(12), 7622–7629.

Brady, H. J., Pennington, D. J., Miles, C. G., & Dzierzak, E. A. (1993). CD4 cell surface downregulation in HIV-1 nef transgenic mice is a consequence of intracellular sequestration. *EMBO Journal, 12*(13), 4923–4932.

Brady, J. & Kashanchi, F. (2005). Tat gets the "green" light on transcription initiation. *Retrovirology, 2*(1), 69.

Brailoiu, G. C., Brailoiu, E., Chang, J. K., & Dun, N. J. (2008). Excitatory effects of human immunodeficiency virus 1 tat on cultured rat cerebral cortical neurons. *Neuroscience, 151*(3), 701–710.

Bratanich, A., Liu, C., McArthur, J., Fudyk, T., Glass, J., Mittoo, S., et al. (1998). Brain-derived HIV-1 tat sequences from AIDS patients with dementia show increased molecular heterogeneity. *J Neurovirol, 4*, 387–393.

Buckner, C. M., Luers, A. J., Calderon, T. M., Eugenin, E. A., & Berman, J. W. (2006). Neuroimmunity and the blood-brain barrier: Molecular regulation of leukocyte transmigration and viral entry into the nervous system with a focus on neuroAIDS. *Journal of Neuroimmune Pharmacology: The Official Journal of the Society on NeuroImmune Pharmacology, 1*(2), 160–181.

Burdo, T. H., Gartner, S., Mauger, D., & Wigdahl, B. (2004). Region-specific distribution of human immunodeficiency virus type 1 long terminal repeats containing specific configurations of CCAAT/enhancer-binding protein site II in brains derived from demented and nondemented patients. *Journal of Neurovirology, 10*(Suppl 1), 7–14.

Burdo, T. H., Nonnemacher, M., Irish, B. P., Choi, C. H., Krebs, F. C., Gartner, S., et al. (2004). High-affinity interaction between HIV-1 vpr and specific sequences that span the C/EBP and adjacent NF-kappaB sites within the HIV-1 LTR correlate with HIV-1-associated dementia. *DNA Cell Biol, 23*, 261–269.

Buriani, A., Petrelli, L., Facci, L., Romano, P., Dal Tosso, R., Leon, A., et al. (1999). Human immunodeficiency virus type 1 envelope glycoprotein gp120 induces tumor necrosis factor-alpha in astrocytes. *J NeuroAIDS, 2*(2), 1–13.

Campbell, T., Khan, M., Huang, M., Bond, V., & Powell, M. (2008). HIV-1 nef protein is secreted into vesicles that can fuse with target cells and virions. *Ethn Dis, 18*(2 Suppl 2), 14–9.

Canter, J. A., Haas, D. W., Kallianpur, A. R., Ritchie, M. D., Robbins, G. K., Shafer, R. W., et al. (2008). The mitochondrial pharmacogenomics of haplogroup T: MTND2*LHON4917G and antiretroviral therapy-associated peripheral neuropathy. *Pharmacogenomics Journal, 8*(1), 71–77.

Caragounis, E. C., Gisslén, M., Lindh, M., Nordborg, C., Westergren, S., Hagberg, L., et al. (2008). Comparison of HIV-1 pol and env sequences of blood, CSF, brain and spleen isolates collected ante-mortem and post-mortem. *Acta Neurologica Scandinavica, 117*(2), 108–116.

Carlum, S., Elisabeth, B., Francescopaolo Di, C., Hee Jung, C., & Monique, S. (2007). HIV-1 gp120 as well as alcohol affect blood–brain barrier permeability and stress fiber formation: Involvement of reactive oxygen species. *Alcoholism: Clinical and Experimental Research, 31*(1), 130–137.

Chan, S. Y., Speck, R. F., Power, C., Gaffen, S. L., Chesebro, B., & Goldsmith, M. A. (1999). V3 recombinants indicate a central role for CCR5 as a coreceptor in tissue infection by human immunodeficiency virus type 1. *Journal of Virology, 73*(3), 2350–2358.

Chang, J., Jozwiak, R., Wang, B., Ng, T., Ge, Y. C., Bolton, W., et al. (1998). Unique HIV type 1 V3 region sequences derived from six different regions of brain: Region-specific evolution within host-determined quasispecies. *AIDS Research & Human Retroviruses, 14*(1), 25–30.

Chang, S. Y., Ko, W. S., Kao, J. T., Chang, L. Y., Sun, H. Y., Chen, M. Y., et al. (2009). Association of single-nucleotide polymorphism 3 and c.553G>T of APOA5 with hypertriglyceridemia after treatmennt with highly active antiretroviral therapy containing protease inhibitors in HIV-infected individuals in Taiwan. *Clinical Infectious Diseases, 48*(6), 832–835.

Cheingsong-Popov, R., Panagiotidi, C., Ali, M., Bowcock, S., Watkins, P., Aronstam, A., et al. (1990). Antibodies to HIV-1 nef(p27): Prevalence, significance, and relationship to seroconversion. *AIDS Research and Human Retroviruses, 6*(9), 1099–1105.

Cheng, J., Nath, A., Knudsen, B., Hochman, S., Geiger, J. D., Ma, M., et al. (1997). Neuronal excitatory properties of human immunodeficiency virus type 1 tat protein. *Neuroscience, 82*(1), 97–106.

Cheng, X., Mukhtar, M., Acheampong, E. A., Srinivasan, A., Rafi, M., Pomerantz, R. J., et al. (2007). HIV-1 vpr potently induces programmed cell death in the CNS in vivo. *DNA & Cell Biology, 26*(2), 116–131.

Cherry, C. L., Rosenow, A., Affandi, J. S., McArthur, J. C., Wesselingh, S. L., & Price, P. (2008). Cytokine genotype suggests a role for inflammation in nucleoside analog-associated sensory neuropathy (NRTI-SN) and predicts an individual's NRTI-SN risk. *AIDS Research & Human Retroviruses, 24*(2), 117–123.

Cheung, R., Ravyn, V., Wang, L., Ptasznik, A., & Collman, R. G. (2008). Signaling mechanism of HIV-1 gp120 and virion-induced IL-1{beta} release in primary human macrophages. *J Immunol, 180*(10), 6675–6684.

Choe, H., Farzan, M., Sun, Y., Sullivan, N., Rollins, B., Ponath, P. D., et al. (1996). The beta-chemokine receptors CCR3 and CCR5 facilitate infection by primary HIV-1 isolates. *Cell, 85*(7), 1135–1148.

Churchill, M. J., Wesselingh, S. L., Cowley, D., Pardo, C. A., McArthur, J. C., Brew, B. J., et al. (2009). Extensive astrocyte infection is prominent in human immunodeficiency virus-associated dementia. *Annals of Neurology, 66*(2), 253–258.

Clements, J. E. & Zink, M. C. (1996). Molecular biology and pathogenesis of animal lentivirus infections. *Clinical Microbiology Reviews, 9*(1), 100–117.

Conant, K., Garzino-Demo, A., Nath, A., McArthur, J. C., Halliday, W., Power, C., et al. (1998). Induction of monocyte chemoattractant protein-1 in HIV-1 tat-stimulated astrocytes and elevation in AIDS dementia. *Proceedings of the National Academy of Sciences of the United States of America, 95*(6), 3117–3121.

Corder, E. H., Robertson, K., Lannfelt, L., Bogdanovic, N., Eggertsen, G., Wilkins, J., et al. (1998). HIV-infected subjects with the E4 allele for APOE have excess dementia and peripheral neuropathy. *Nature Medicine, 4*(10), 1182–1184.

Cornblath, D. R. & Hoke, A. (2006). Recent advances in HIV neuropathy. *Current Opinion in Neurology, 19*(5), 446–450.

Coyle-Rink, J., Sweet, T. M., Abraham, S., Sawaya, B. E., Batuman, O., Khalili, K., et al. (2002). Interaction between TGF[beta] signaling proteins and C/EBP controls basal and tat-mediated transcription of HIV-1 LTR in astrocytes. *Virology, 299*(2), 240–247.

Cui, L., Locatelli, L., Xie, M. Y., & Sommadossi, J. P. (1997). Effect of nucleoside analogs on neurite regeneration and mitochondrial DNA synthesis in PC-12 cells. *Journal of Pharmacology & Experimental Therapeutics, 280*(3), 1228–1234.

Cunningham, P. H., Smith, D. G., Satchell, C., Cooper, D. A., & Brew, B. (2000). Evidence for independent development of resistance to HIV-1 reverse transcriptase inhibitors in the cerebrospinal fluid. *AIDS, 14*(13), 1949–1954.

Cutler, R. G., Haughey, N. J., Tammara, A., McArthur, J. C., Nath, A., Reid, R., et al. (2004). Dysregulation of sphingolipid and sterol metabolism by ApoE4 in HIV dementia. *Neurology, 63*(4), 626–630.

Cysique, L. A. & Brew, B. J. (2009). Neuropsychological functioning and antiretroviral treatment in HIV/AIDS: A review. *Neuropsychology Review, 19*(2), 169–185.

Dalakas, M. C., Semino-Mora, C., & Leon-Monzon, M. (2001). Mitochondrial alterations with mitochondrial DNA depletion in the nerves of AIDS patients with peripheral neuropathy induced by 2'3'-dideoxycytidine (ddC). *Laboratory Investigation, 81*(11), 1537–1544.

D'Aversa, T. G., Yu, K. O., & Berman, J. W. (2004). Expression of chemokines by human fetal microglia after treatment with the human immunodeficiency virus type 1 protein tat. *Journal of Neurovirology, 10*(2), 86–97.

Davis, L. E., Hjelle, B. L., Miller, V. E., Palmer, D. L., Llewellyn, A. L., Merlin, T. L., et al. (1992). Early viral brain invasion in iatrogenic human immunodeficiency virus infection. *Neurology, 42*(9), 1736–1739.

De Jong, J. J., De Ronde, A., Keulen, W., Tersmette, M., & Goudsmit, J. (1992). Minimal requirements for the human immunodeficiency virus type 1 V3 domain to support the syncytium-inducing phenotype: Analysis by single amino acid substitution. *Journal of Virology, 66*(11), 6777–6780.

de Sorrentino, A. H., Marinic, K., Motta, P., Sorrentino, A., Lopez, R., & Illiovich, E. (2000). HLA class I alleles associated with susceptibility or resistance to human immunodeficiency virus type 1 infection among a population in Chaco Province, Argentina. *Journal of Infectious Diseases, 182*(5), 1523–1526.

Dean, M., Carrington, M., Winkler, C., Huttley, G. A., Smith, M. W., Allikmets, R., et al. (1996). Genetic restriction of HIV-1 infection and progression to AIDS by a deletion allele of the CKR5 structural gene. hemophilia growth and development study, multicenter AIDS cohort study, multicenter hemophilia cohort study, San Francisco city cohort, ALIVE study. *Science, 273*(5283), 1856–1862.

Deng, H. K., Liu, R., Ellmeier, W., Choe, S., Unutmaz, D., Burkhart, M., et al. (1996). Identification of a major co-receptor for primary isolates of HIV-1. *Nature, 381*, 661.

Deshmane, S. L., Mukerjee, R., Fan, S., Del Valle, L., Michiels, C., Sweet, T., et al. (2009). Activation of the oxidative stress pathway by HIV-1 vpr leads to induction of hypoxia-inducible factor 1α expression. *Journal of Biological Chemistry, 284*(17), 11364–11373.

Diaz-Arrastia, R., Gong, Y., Kelly, C. J., & Gelman, B. B. (2004). Host genetic polymorphisms in human immunodeficiency virus-related neurologic disease. *Journal of Neurovirology, 10*(Suppl 1), 67–73.

Doranz, B. J., Rucker, J., Yi, Y., Smyth, R. J., Samson, M., Peiper, S. C., et al. (1996). A dual-tropic primary HIV-1 isolate that uses fusin and the beta-chemokine receptors CKR-5, CKR-3, and CKR-2b as fusion cofactors. *Cell, 85*(7), 1149–1158.

Dragic, T., Litwin, V., Allaway, G. P., Martin, S. R., Huang, Y. X., Nagashima, K. A., et al. (1996). HIV-1 entry into CD4+ cells is mediated by the chemokine receptor CC-CKR-5. *Nature, 381*, 667.

Dunfee, R., Thomas, E. R., Gorry, P. R., Wang, J., Ancuta, P., & Gabuzda, D. (2006). Mechanisms of HIV-1 neurotropism. *Current HIV Research, 4*(3), 267–278.

Dunfee, R. L., Thomas, E. R., Wang, J., Kunstman, K., Wolinsky, S. M., & Gabuzda, D. (2007). Loss of the N-linked glycosylation site at position 386 in the HIV envelope V4 region enhances macrophage tropism and is associated with dementia. *Virology, 367*(1), 222–234.

Dunfee, R. L., Thomas, E. R., Gorry, P. R., Wang, J., Taylor, J., Kunstman, K., et al. (2006). The HIV env variant N283 enhances macrophage tropism and is associated with brain infection and dementia. *Proceedings of the National Academy of Sciences, 103*(41), 15160–15165.

Dunlop, O., Goplen, A. K., Liestol, K., Myrvang, B., Rootwelt, H., Christophersen, B., et al. (1997). HIV dementia and apolipoprotein E. *Acta Neurologica Scandinavica, 95*(5), 315–318.

Eletto, D., Russo, G., Passiatore, G., Del Valle, L., Giordano, A., Khalili, K., et al. (2008). Inhibition of SNAP25 expression by HIV-1 tat involves the activity of mir-128a. *Journal of Cellular Physiology, 216*(3), 764–770.

Eugenin, E. A., King, J. E., Nath, A., Calderon, T. M., Zukin, R. S., Bennett, M. V. L., et al. (2007). HIV-tat induces formation of an LRP–PSD-95–NMDAR–nNOS complex that promotes apoptosis in neurons and astrocytes. *Proceedings of the National Academy of Sciences, 104*(9), 3438–3443.

Everall, I. P., Heaton, R. K., Marcotte, T. D., Ellis, R. J., McCutchan, J. A., Atkinson, J. H., et al. (1999). Cortical synaptic density is reduced in mild to moderate human immunodeficiency virus neurocognitive disorder. HNRC group. HIV Neurobehavioral Research Center. *Brain Pathology, 9*(2), 209–217.

Fabio, G., Smeraldi, R. S., Gringeri, A., Marchini, M., Bonara, P., & Mannucci, P. M. (1990). Susceptibility to HIV infection and AIDS in Italian haemophiliacs is HLA associated. *British Journal of Haematology, 75*(4), 531–536.

Failde-Garrido, J. M., Alvarez, M. R., & Simon-Lopez, M. A. (2008). Neuropsychological impairment and gender differences in HIV-1 infection. *Psychiatry & Clinical Neurosciences, 62*(5), 494–502.

Falangola, M. F., Hanly, A., Galvao-Castro, B., & Petito, C. K. (1995). HIV infection of human choroid plexus: A possible mechanism of viral entry into the CNS. *Journal of Neuropathology & Experimental Neurology, 54*(4), 497–503.

Fauvel, J., Bonnet, E., Ruidavets, J. B., Ferrieres, J., Toffoletti, A., Massip, P., et al. (2001). An interaction between apo C-III variants and protease inhibitors contributes to high triglyceride/low HDL levels in treated HIV patients. *AIDS, 15*(18), 2397–2406.

Fellay, J., Shianna, K. V., Ge, D., Colombo, S., Ledergerber, B., Weale, M., et al. (2007). A whole-genome association study of major determinants for host control of HIV-1. *Science, 317*(5840), 944–947.

Ferris, M., Frederick-Duus, D., Fadel, J., Mactutus, C., & Booze, R. (2009). In vivo microdialysis in awake, freely moving rats demonstrates HIV-1 tat-induced alterations in dopamine transmission. *Synapse, 63*, 181–185.

Foster, J., & Garcia, J. V. (2008). HIV-1 nef: At the crossroads. *Retrovirology, 5*(1), 84.

Foulkes, A. S., Wohl, D. A., Frank, I., Puleo, E., Restine, S., Wolfe, M. L., et al. (2006). Associations among race/ethnicity, ApoC-III genotypes, and lipids in HIV-1-infected individuals on antiretroviral therapy. *PLoS Medicine/Public Library of Science, 3*(3), e52.

Gartner, S. (2000). HIV infection and dementia. *Science, 287*(5453), 602–604.

Gartner, S., McDonald, R., Hunter, E., Bouwman, F., Liu, Y., & Popovic, M. (1997). Gp120 sequence variation in brain and in T-lymphocyte human immunodeficiency virus type 1 primary isolates. *J Hum Virol, 1*(1), 3–18.

Gelbard, H. A., Nottet, H. S., Swindells, S., Jett, M., Dzenko, K. A., Genis, P., et al. (1994). Platelet-activating factor: A candidate human immunodeficiency virus type 1-induced neurotoxin. *Journal of Virology, 68*(7), 4628–4635.

Gelman, B. B., Soukup, V. M., Schuenke, K. W., Keherly, M. J., Holzer, C.,3rd, Richey, F. J., et al. (2004). Acquired neuronal channelopathies in HIV-associated dementia. *Journal of Neuroimmunology, 157*(1–2), 111–119.

Glass, J. D., Fedor, H., Wesselingh, S. L., & McArthur, J. C. (1995). Immunocytochemical quantitation of human immunodeficiency virus in the brain: Correlations with dementia. *Annals of Neurology, 38*(5), 755–762.

Gonzalez, E., Rovin, B. H., Sen, L., Cooke, G., Dhanda, R., Mummidi, S., et al. (2002). HIV-1 infection and AIDS dementia are influenced by a mutant MCP-1 allele linked to increased monocyte infiltration of tissues and MCP-1 levels. *Proceedings of the National Academy of Sciences of the United States of America, 99*(21), 13795–13800.

Gonzalez-Scarano, F., & Martin-Garcia, J. (2005). The neuropathogenesis of AIDS. *Nature Reviews Immunology, 5*(1), 69–81.

Gorry, P. R., Bristol, G., Zack, J. A., Ritola, K., Swanstrom, R., Birch, C. J., et al. (2001). Macrophage tropism of human immunodeficiency virus type 1 isolates from brain and lymphoid tissues predicts neurotropism independent of coreceptor specificity. *Journal of Virology, 75*(21), 10073–10089.

Gorry, P. R., Howard, J. L., Churchill, M. J., Anderson, J. L., Cunningham, A., Adrian, D., et al. (1999). Diminished production of human immunodeficiency virus type 1 in astrocytes results from inefficient translation of gag, env, and nef mRNAs despite efficient expression of tat and rev. *Journal of Virology, 73*(1), 352–361.

Gorry, P. R., Taylor, J., Holm, G. H., Mehle, A., Morgan, T., Cayabyab, M., et al. (2002). Increased CCR5 affinity and reduced CCR5/CD4 dependence of a neurovirulent primary human immunodeficiency virus type 1 isolate. *Journal of Virology, 76*(12), 6277–6292.

Goulder, P. J., & Watkins, D. I. (2008). Impact of MHC class I diversity on immune control of immunodeficiency virus replication. *Nature Reviews Immunology, 8*(8), 619–630.

Guerini, F. R., Delbue, S., Zanzottera, M., Agliardi, C., Saresella, M., Mancuso, R., et al. (2008). Analysis of CCR5, CCR2, SDF1 and RANTES gene polymorphisms in subjects with HIV-related PML and not determined leukoencephalopathy. *Biomedicine & Pharmacotherapy, 62*(1), 26–30.

Gupta, J. D., Satishchandra, P., Gopukumar, K., Wilkie, F., Waldrop-Valverde, D., Ellis, R., et al. (2007). Neuropsychological deficits in human immunodeficiency virus type 1 clade C-seropositive adults from south India. *Journal of Neurovirology, 13*(3), 195–202.

Haas, D. W., Ribaudo, H. J., Kim, R. B., Tierney, C., Wilkinson, G. R., Gulick, R. M., et al. (2004). Pharmacogenetics of efavirenz and central nervous system side effects: An adult AIDS clinical trials group study. *AIDS, 18*(18), 2391–2400.

Habegger de Sorrentino, A., Lopez, R., Motta, P., Marinic, K., Sorrentino, A., Iliovich, E., et al. (2005). HLA class II involvement in HIV-associated toxoplasmic encephalitis development. *Clinical Immunology, 115*(2), 133–137.

Hammes, S. R., Dixon, E. P., Malim, M. H., Cullen, B. R., & Greene, W. C. (1989). Nef protein of human immunodeficiency virus type 1: Evidence against its role as a transcriptional inhibitor. *Proceedings of the National Academy of Sciences of the United States of America, 86*(23), 9549–9553.

Han, S. H., Einstein, G., Weisgraber, K. H., Strittmatter, W. J., Saunders, A. M., Pericak-Vance, M., et al. (1994). Apolipoprotein E is localized to the cytoplasm of human cortical neurons: A light and electron microscopic study. *Journal of Neuropathology & Experimental Neurology, 53*(5), 535–544.

Hanna, Z., Priceputu, E., Chrobak, P., Hu, C., Dugas, V., Goupil, M., et al. (2009). Selective expression of human immunodeficiency virus nef in specific immune cell populations of transgenic mice is associated with distinct AIDS-like phenotypes. *Journal of Virology, 83*(19), 9743–9758.

Haughey, N. J., Holden, C. P., Nath, A., & Geiger, J. D. (1999). Involvement of inositol 1,4,5-trisphosphate-regulated stores of intracellular calcium in calcium dysregulation and neuron cell death caused by HIV-1 protein tat. *Journal of Neurochemistry, 73*(4), 1363–1374.

Haughey, N. J., & Mattson, M. P. (2002). Calcium dysregulation and neuronal apoptosis by the HIV-1 proteins tat and gp120. *Journal of Acquired Immune Deficiency Syndromes: JAIDS, 31*(Suppl 2), S55–61.

He, J., Chen, Y., Farzan, M., Choe, H., Ohagen, A., Gartner, S., et al. (1997). CCR3 and CCR5 are co-receptors for HIV-1 infection of microglia. *Nature, 385*(6617), 645–649.

Heidenreich, F., Arendt, G., Jander, S., Jablonowski, H., & Stoll, G. (1994). Serum and cerebrospinal fluid levels of soluble intercellular adhesion molecule 1 (sICAM-1) in patients with HIV-1 associated neurological diseases. *Journal of Neuroimmunology, 52*(2), 117–126.

Hemelaar, J., Gouws, E., Ghys, P. D., & Osmanov, S. (2006). Global and regional distribution of HIV-1 genetic subtypes and recombinants in 2004. *AIDS, 20*(16), W13–23.

Hendrickson, S. L., Jacobson, L. P., Nelson, G. W., Phair, J. P., Lautenberger, J., Johnson, R. C., et al. (2008). Host genetic influences on highly active antiretroviral therapy efficacy and AIDS-free survival. *Journal of Acquired Immune Deficiency Syndromes: JAIDS, 48*(3), 263–271.

Herzberg, U. & Sagen, J. (2001). Peripheral nerve exposure to HIV viral envelope protein gp120 induces neuropathic pain and spinal gliosis. *Journal of Neuroimmunology, 116*(1), 29–39.

Heyes, M., Brew, B., Martin, A., Price, R., Salazar, A., Sidtis, J., et al. (1991). Quinolinic acid in cerebrospinal fluid and serum in HIV-1 infection: Relationship to clinical and neurological status. *Annals of Neurology, 29*(2), 202–9; 202.

Huang, K. J., Alter, G. M., & Wooley, D. P. (2002). The reverse transcriptase sequence of human immunodeficiency virus type 1 is under positive evolutionary selection within the central nervous system. *Journal of Neurovirology, 8*(4), 281–294.

Hulgan, T., Haas, D. W., Haines, J. L., Ritchie, M. D., Robbins, G. K., Shafer, R. W., et al. (2005). Mitochondrial haplogroups and peripheral neuropathy during antiretroviral therapy: An adult AIDS clinical trials group study. *AIDS, 19*(13), 1341–1349.

Hwang, S. S., Boyle, T. J., Lyerly, H. K., & Cullen, B. R. (1991). Identification of the envelope V3 loop as the primary determinant of cell tropism in HIV-1. *Science, 253*(5015), 71–74.

Ickovics, J. R., & Rodin, J. (1992). Women and AIDS in the United States: Epidemiology, natural history, and mediating mechanisms. *Health Psychology, 11*(1), 1–16.

Ioannidis, J. P., Contopoulos-Ioannidis, D. G., Rosenberg, P. S., Goedert, J. J., De Rossi, A., Espanol, T., et al. (2003). Effects of CCR5-delta32 and CCR2-64I alleles on disease progression of perinatally HIV-1-infected children: An international meta-analysis. *AIDS, 17*(11), 1631–1638.

Jayadev, S. & Garden, G. A. (2009). Host and viral factors influencing the pathogenesis of HIV-associated neurocognitive disorders. *Journal of Neuroimmune Pharmacology: The Official Journal of the Society on NeuroImmune Pharmacology, 4*(2), 175–189.

John, G. C., Rousseau, C., Dong, T., Rowland-Jones, S., Nduati, R., Mbori-Ngacha, D., et al. (2000). Maternal SDF1 3'A polymorphism is associated with increased perinatal human immunodeficiency virus type 1 transmission. *Journal of Virology, 74*(12), 5736–5739.

Johnston, J. B., Jiang, Y., van Marle, G., Mayne, M. B., Ni, W., Holden, J., et al. (2000). Lentivirus infection in the brain induces matrix metalloproteinase expression: Role of envelope diversity. *Journal of Virology, 74*(16), 7211–7220.

Johnston, J., Zhang, K., Silva, C., Shalinsky, D., Conant, K., Ni, W., et al. (2001). HIV-1 tat neurotoxicity is prevented by matrix metalloproteinase inhibitors. *Annals of Neurology, 49*(2), 230–241.

Jones, G. J., Barsby, N. L., Cohen, E. A., Holden, J., Harris, K., Dickie, P., et al. (2007). HIV-1 vpr causes neuronal apoptosis and in vivo neurodegeneration. *J Neurosci, 27*(14), 3703–3711.

Jones, G., Zhu, Y., Silva, C., Tsutsui, S., Pardo, C. A., Keppler, O. T., et al. (2005). Peripheral nerve-derived HIV-1 is predominantly CCR5-dependent and causes neuronal degeneration and neuroinflammation. *Virology, 334*(2), 178–193.

Jones, M. V., Bell, J. E., & Nath, A. (2000). Immunolocalization of HIV envelope gp120 in HIV encephalitis with dementia. *AIDS, 14*(17), 2709–2713.

Kaleebu, P., French, N., Mahe, C., Yirrell, D., Watera, C., Lyagoba, F., et al. (2002). Effect of human immunodeficiency virus (HIV) type 1 envelope subtypes A and D on disease progression in a large cohort of HIV-1-positive persons in Uganda. *Journal of Infectious Diseases, 185*(9), 1244–1250.

Kaleebu, P., Nankya, I. L., Yirrell, D. L., Shafer, L. A., Kyosiimire-Lugemwa, J., Lule, D. B., et al. (2007). Relation between chemokine receptor use, disease stage, and HIV-1 subtypes A and D: Results from a rural Ugandan cohort. *Journal of Acquired Immune Deficiency Syndromes: JAIDS, 45*(1), 28–33.

Kanmogne, G. D., Schall, K., Leibhart, J., Knipe, B., Gendelman, H. E., & Persidsky, Y. (2007). HIV-1 gp120 compromises blood-brain barrier integrity and enhances monocyte migration across blood-brain barrier: Implication for viral neuropathogenesis. *Journal of Cerebral Blood Flow & Metabolism, 27*(1), 123–134.

Kaul, M. & Lipton, S. A. (1999). Chemokines and activated macrophages in HIV gp120-induced neuronal apoptosis. *Proceedings of the National Academy of Sciences of the United States of America, 96*(14), 8212–8216.

Kaul, M., Zheng, J., Okamoto, S., Gendelman, H. E., & Lipton, S. A. (2005). HIV-1 infection and AIDS: Consequences for the central nervous system. *Cell Death & Differentiation, 12*(Suppl 1), 878–892.

Kelder, W., McArthur, J. C., Nance-Sproson, T., McClernon, D., & Griffin, D. E. (1998). Beta-chemokines MCP-1 and RANTES are selectively increased in cerebrospinal fluid of patients with human immunodeficiency virus-associated dementia. *Annals of Neurology, 44*(5), 831–835.

Keswani, S. C., Jack, C., Zhou, C., & Hoke, A. (2006). Establishment of a rodent model of HIV-associated sensory neuropathy. *Journal of Neuroscience, 26*(40), 10299–10304.

Kilareski, E., Shah, S., Nonnemacher, M., & Wigdahl, B. (2009). Regulation of HIV-1 transcription in cells of the monocyte-macrophage lineage. *Retrovirology, 6*(1), 118.

Kim, H. J., Martemyanov, K. A., & Thayer, S. A. (2008). Human immunodeficiency virus protein tat induces synapse loss via a reversible process that is distinct from cell death. *J. Neurosci., 28*(48), 12604–12613.

Kitayama, H., Miura, Y., Ando, Y., Hoshino, S., Ishizaka, Y., & Koyanagi, Y. (2008). Human immunodeficiency virus type 1 vpr inhibits axonal outgrowth through induction of mitochondrial dysfunction. *J. Virol., 82*(5), 2528–2542.

Kiwanuka, N., Laeyendecker, O., Robb, M., Kigozi, G., Arroyo, M., McCutchan, F., et al. (2008). Effect of human immunodeficiency virus type 1 (HIV-1) subtype on disease progression in persons from Rakai, Uganda, with incident HIV-1 infection. *Journal of Infectious Diseases, 197*(5), 707–713.

Klase, Z., Kale, P., Winograd, R., Gupta, M. V., Heydarian, M., Berro, R., et al. (2007). HIV-1 TAR element is processed by dicer to yield a viral micro-RNA involved in chromatin remodeling of the viral LTR. *BMC Mol Biol, 8*, 63.

Klase, Z., Winograd, R., Davis, J., Carpio, L., Hildreth, R., Heydarian, M., et al. (2009). HIV-1 TAR miRNA protects against apoptosis by altering cellular gene expression. *Retrovirology, 6*(1), 18.

Koedel, U., Kohleisen, B., Sporer, B., Lahrtz, F., Ovod, V., Fontana, A., et al. (1999). HIV type 1 nef protein is a viral factor for leukocyte recruitment into the central nervous system. *J Immunol, 163*(3), 1237–1245.

Kong, L. Y., Wilson, B. C., McMillian, M. K., Bing, G., Hudson, P. M., & Hong, J. S. (1996). The effects of the HIV-1 envelope protein gp120 on the production of nitric oxide and proinflammatory cytokines in mixed glial cell cultures. *Cellular Immunology, 172*(1), 77–83.

Krentz, H., & Gill, M. J. (2009). The five-year impact of an evolving global epidemic, changing migration patterns, and policy changes in a regional canadian HIV population. *Health Policy, 90*(2–3), 296–302.

Kruman, I., Nath, A., & Mattson, M. (1998). HIV protein tat induces apoptosis by a mechanism involving mitochondrial calcium overload and caspase activation. *Exp Neurol, 154*, 276–288.

Kure, K., Llena, J. F., Lyman, W. D., Soeiro, R., Weidenheim, K. M., Hirano, A., et al. (1991). Human immunodeficiency virus-1 infection of the nervous system: An autopsy study of 268 adult, pediatric, and fetal brains. *Human Pathology, 22*(7), 700–710.

Kure, K., Lyman, W. D., Weidenheim, K. M., & Dickson, D. W. (1990). Cellular localization of an HIV-1 antigen in subacute AIDS encephalitis using an improved double-labeling immunohistochemical method. *Am J Pathol, 136*(5), 1085–1092.

Lannuzel, A., Lledo, P., Lamghitnia, H. O., Vincent, J., & Tardieu, M. (1995). HIV-1 envelope proteins gp120 and gp160 potentiate NMDA-induced [Ca2+]i increase, alter [Ca2+]i homeostasis and induce neurotoxicity in human embryonic neurons. *European Journal of Neuroscience, 7*(11), 2285–93; 2285.

Letendre, S. L., Lanier, E. R., & McCutchan, J. A. (1999). Cerebrospinal fluid beta chemokine concentrations in neurocognitively impaired individuals infected with human immunodeficiency virus type 1. *Journal of Infectious Diseases, 180*(2), 310–319.

Levy, D. N., Refaeli, Y., MacGregor, R. R., & Weiner, D. B. (1994). Serum vpr regulates productive infection and latency of human immunodeficiency virus type 1. *Proc Natl Acad Sci U S A, 91*, 10873–10877.

Li, W., Huang, Y., Reid, R., Steiner, J., Malpica-Llanos, T., Darden, T. A., et al. (2008). NMDA receptor activation by HIV-tat protein is clade dependent. *Journal of Neuroscience, 28*(47), 12190–12198.

Li, W., Li, G., Steiner, J., & Nath, A. (2009). Role of tat protein in HIV neuropathogenesis. *Neurotoxicity Research, 16*(3), 205–220.

Lindemann, D., Wilhelm, R., Renard, P., Althage, A., Zinkernagel, R., & Mous, J. (1994). Severe immunodeficiency associated with a human immunodeficiency virus 1 NEF/3'-long terminal repeat transgene. *Journal of Experimental Medicine, 179*(3), 797–807.

Liner, K. J., 2nd, Hall, C. D., & Robertson, K. R. (2007). Impact of human immunodeficiency virus (HIV) subtypes on HIV-associated neurological disease. *Journal of Neurovirology, 13*(4), 291–304.

Lipton, S. A. (1992). Requirement for macrophages in neuronal injury induced by HIV envelope protein gp120. *NeuroReport, 3*, 913–915.

Lipton, S. A., Sucher, N. J., Kaiser, P. K., & Dreyer, E. B. (1991). Synergistic effects of HIV coat protein and NMDA receptor-mediated neurotoxicity. *Neuron, 7*(1), 111–118.

Liu, H., Chao, D., Nakayama, E. E., Taguchi, H., Goto, M., Xin, X., et al. (1999). Polymorphism in RANTES chemokine promoter affects HIV-1 disease progression. *Proceedings of the National Academy of Sciences of the United States of America, 96*(8), 4581–4585.

Liu, R., Paxton, W. A., Choe, S., Ceradini, D., Martin, S. R., Horuk, R., et al. (1996). Homozygous defect in HIV-1 coreceptor accounts for resistance of some multiply-exposed individuals to HIV-1 infection. *Cell, 86*(3), 367–377.

Liu, Y., Jones, M., Hingtgen, C., Bu, G., Laribee, N., Tanzi, R., et al. (2000). Uptake of HIV-1 tat proteinmediated by low density lipoprotein receptor-related protein disrupts the neuronal metabolic balance of the receptor ligands. *Nature Medicine, 6*, 1380–1387.

Lopez, O. L., Wess, J., Sanchez, J., Dew, M. A., & Becker, J. T. (1999). Neurological characteristics of HIV-infected men and women seeking primary medical care. *European Journal of Neurology, 6*(2), 205–209.

Lum, J. J., Cohen, O. J., Nie, Z., Weaver, J. G., Gomez, T. S., Yao, X. J., et al. (2003). Vpr R77Q is associated with long-term nonprogressive HIV infection and impaired induction of apoptosis. *J Clin Invest, 111*, 1547–1554.

Luo, X., Carlson, K. A., Wojna, V., Mayo, R., Biskup, T. M., Stoner, J., et al. (2003). Macrophage proteomic fingerprinting predicts HIV-1-associated cognitive impairment. *Neurology, 60*(12), 1931–1937.

MacDonald, K. S., Fowke, K. R., Kimani, J., Dunand, V. A., Nagelkerke, N. J., Ball, T. B., et al. (2000). Influence of HLA supertypes on susceptibility and resistance to human immunodeficiency virus type 1 infection. *Journal of Infectious Diseases, 181*(5), 1581–1589.

Magnuson, D., Knudsen, B., Geiger, J., Brownstone, R., & Nath, A. (1995). Human immunodeficiency virus type 1 tat activates non-N-methyl-D-aspartate excitatory amino acid receptors and causes neurotoxicity. *Annals of Neurology, 37*(3), 373–80.

Mahadevan, A., Shankar, S. K., Satishchandra, P., Ranga, U., Chickabasaviah, Y. T., Santosh, V., et al. (2007). Characterization of human immunodeficiency virus (HIV)-infected cells in infiltrates associated with CNS opportunistic infections in patients with HIV clade C infection. *Journal of Neuropathology & Experimental Neurology, 66*(9), 799–808.

Mahley, R. W. & Rall, S. C., Jr. (2000). Apolipoprotein E: Far more than a lipid transport protein. *Annual Review of Genomics & Human Genetics, 1*, 507–537.

Mankowski, J. L., Flaherty, M. T., Spelman, J. P., Hauer, D. A., Didier, P. J., Amedee, A. M., et al. (1997). Pathogenesis of simian immunodeficiency virus encephalitis: Viral determinants of neurovirulence. *Journal of Virology, 71*(8), 6055–6060.

Maragos, W. F., Tillman, P., Jones, M., Bruce-Keller, A. J., Roth, S., Bell, J. E., et al. (2003). Neuronal injury in hippocampus with human immunodeficiency virus transactivating protein, tat. *Neuroscience*, *117*(1), 43–53.

Martinson, J. J., Chapman, N. H., Rees, D. C., Liu, Y. T., & Clegg, J. B. (1997). Global distribution of the CCR5 gene 32-basepair deletion. *Nature Genetics*, *16*(1), 100–103.

Martinson, J. J., Hong, L., Karanicolas, R., Moore, J. P., & Kostrikis, L. G. (2000). Global distribution of the CCR2–64I/CCR5–59653T HIV-1 disease-protective haplotype. *AIDS*, *14*(5), 483–489.

Marzolini, C., Telenti, A., Decosterd, L. A., Greub, G., Biollaz, J., & Buclin, T. (2001). Efavirenz plasma levels can predict treatment failure and central nervous system side effects in HIV-1-infected patients. *AIDS*, *15*(1), 71–75.

Masliah, E., Ge, N., Achim, C. L., Hansen, L. A., & Wiley, C. A. (1992). Selective neuronal vulnerability in HIV encephalitis. *Journal of Neuropathology & Experimental Neurology*, *51*(6), 585–593.

Mason, K. I., Campbell, A., Hawkins, P., Madhere, S., Johnson, K., & Takushi-Chinen, R. (1998). Neuropsychological functioning in HIV-positive African-American women with a history of drug use. *Journal of the National Medical Association*, *90*(11), 665–674.

Mattson, M. P., Haughey, N. J., & Nath, A. (2005). Cell death in HIV dementia. *Cell Death & Differentiation*, *12*(Suppl 1), 893–904.

Mayne, M., Bratanich, A. C., Chen, P., Rana, F., Nath, A., & Power, C. (1998). HIV-1 tat molecular diversity and induction of TNF-α: Implications for HIV-induced neurological disease. *Neuroimmunomodulation*, *5*, 184–192.

Melnick, S. L., Sherer, R., Louis, T. A., Hillman, D., Rodriguez, E. M., Lackman, C., et al. (1994). Survival and disease progression according to gender of patients with HIV infection. The Terry Beirn Community Programs for Clinical Research on AIDS. *JAMA*, *272*(24), 1915–1921.

Messam, C. A. & Major, E. O. (2000). Stages of restricted HIV-1 infection in astrocyte cultures derived from human fetal brain tissue. *Journal of Neurovirology*, *6*(Suppl 1), S90–4.

Messmer, D., Ignatius, R., Santisteban, C., Steinman, R. M., & Pope, M. (2000). The decreased replicative capacity of simian immunodeficiency virus SIVmac239Delta nef is manifest in cultures of immature dendritic cells and T cells. *J. Virol.*, *74*(5), 2406–2413.

Metsch, L. R., McCoy, C. B., McCoy, H. V., Shultz, J., Inciardi, J., Wolfe, H., et al. (1998). Social influences: Living arrangements of drug using women at risk for HIV infection. *Women & Health*, *27*(1–2), 123–136.

Meyer, L., Magierowska, M., Hubert, J. B., Rouzioux, C., Deveau, C., Sanson, F., et al. (1997). Early protective effect of CCR-5 delta 32 heterozygosity on HIV-1 disease progression: Relationship with viral load. The SEROCO study group. *AIDS*, *11*(11), F73–8.

Milligan, E. D., Mehmert, K. K., Hinde, J. L., Harvey, L. O., Martin, D., Tracey, K. J., et al. (2000). Thermal hyperalgesia and mechanical allodynia produced by intrathecal administration of the human immunodeficiency virus-1 (HIV-1) envelope glycoprotein, gp120. *Brain Research*, *861*(1), 105–116.

Mirsattari, S. M., Johnston, J. B., McKenna, R., Del Bigio, M. R., Orr, P., Ross, R. T., et al. (2001). Aboriginals with multiple sclerosis: HLA types and predominance of neuromyelitis optica. *Neurology*, *56*(3), 317–323.

Mishra, M., Vetrivel, S., Siddappa, N., Ranga, U., & Seth, P. (2008). Clade-specific differences in neurotoxicity of human immunodeficiency virus-1 B and C tat of human neurons: Significance of dicysteine C30C31 motif. *Annals of Neurology*, *63*(3), 366–376.

Modi, G., Hari, K., Modi, M., & Mochan, A. (2007). The frequency and profile of neurology in black South African HIV-infected (clade C) patients—a hospital-based prospective audit. *Journal of the Neurological Sciences*, *254*(1–2), 60–64.

Mologni, D., Citterio, P., Menzaghi, B., Poma, B. Z., Riva, C., Broggini, V., et al. (2006). Vpr and HIV-1 disease progression: R77Q mutation is associated with long-term control of HIV-1 infection in different groups of patients. *AIDS*, *20*(4), 567–574.

Monteiro de Almeida, S., Letendre, S., Zimmerman, J., Kolakowski, S., Lazzaretto, D., McCutchan, J. A., et al. (2006). Relationship of CSF leukocytosis to compartmentalized changes in MCP-1/CCL2 in the CSF of HIV-infected patients undergoing interruption of antiretroviral therapy. *Journal of Neuroimmunology*, *179*(1–2), 180–185.

Mordelet, E., Kissa, K., Cressant, A., Gray, F., Ozden, S., Vidal, C., et al. (2004). Histopathological and cognitive defects induced by nef in the brain. *FASEB J.*, *18*(15), 1851–1861.

Na, H., Acharjee, S., Jones, G., Vivithanaporn, P., Noorbakhsh, F., et al. (2011). Interactions between human immunodeficiency virus (HIV)-1 Vpr expression and innate immunity influence neurovirulence. *Retrovirology*, *8*, 44–61.

Narayan, O., Joag, S. V., & Stephens, E. B. (1995). Selected models of HIV-induced neurological disease. *Current Topics in Microbiology & Immunology*, *202*, 151–166.

Nath, A., Haughey, N., Jones, M., Anderson, C., Bell, J., & Geiger, J. (2000). Synergistic neurotoxicity by human immunodeficiency virus proteins tat and gp120: Protection by memantine. *Annals of Neurology*, *47*, 186–194.

Nath, A., Psooy, K., Martin, C., Knudsen, B., Magnuson, D. S., Haughey, N., et al. (1996). Identification of a human immunodeficiency virus type 1 tat epitope that is neuroexcitatory and neurotoxic. *J. Virol.*, *70*(3), 1475–1480.

Nath, A., Hauser, K. F., Wojna, V., Booze, R. M., Maragos, W., Prendergast, M., et al. (2002). Molecular basis for interactions of HIV and drugs of abuse. *JAIDS: Journal of Acquired Immune Deficiency Syndromes*, *31* Supplement(2), S62–S69.

Nath, A., Anderson, C., Jones, M., Maragos, W., Booze, R., Mactutus, C., et al. (2000). Neurotoxicity and dysfunction of dopaminergic systems associated with AIDS dementia. *J Psychopharmacol*, *14*(3), 222–227.

Neumann, M., Felber, B. K., Kleinschmidt, A., Froese, B., Erfle, V., Pavlakis, G. N., et al. (1995). Restriction of human immunodeficiency virus type 1 production in a human astrocytoma cell line is associated with a cellular block in rev function. *Journal of Virology*, *69*(4), 2159–2167.

Noorbakhsh, F., Overall, C. M., & Power, C. (2009). Deciphering complex mechanisms in neurodegenerative diseases: The advent of systems biology. *Trends in Neurosciences*, *32*(2), 88–100.

Noorbakhsh, F., Ramachandran, R., Barsby, N., Ellestad, K. K., LeBlanc, A., Dickie, P., et al. (2010). MicroRNA profiling reveals new aspects of HIV neurodegeneration: Caspase-6 regulates astrocyte survival. *FASEB J*, fj. 09–147819.

Norman, J. P., Perry, S. W., Reynolds, H. M., Kiebala, M., De Mesy Bentley, K. L., Trejo, M., et al. (2008). HIV-1 tat activates neuronal ryanodine receptors with rapid induction of the unfolded protein response and mitochondrial hyperpolarization. *PLoS ONE*, *3*(11), e3731.

Nottet, H. S., Persidsky, Y., Sasseville, V. G., Nukuna, A. N., Bock, P., Zhai, Q. H., et al. (1996). Mechanisms for the transendothelial migration of HIV-1-infected monocytes into brain. *Journal of Immunology*, *156*(3), 1284–1295.

Nuovo, G. J., Gallery, F., MacConnell, P., & Braun, A. (1994). In situ detection of polymerase chain reaction-amplified HIV-1 nucleic acids and tumor necrosis factor-alpha RNA in the central nervous system. *American Journal of Pathology*, *144*(4), 659–666.

Ohagen, A., Devitt, A., Kunstman, K. J., Gorry, P. R., Rose, P. P., Korber, B., et al. (2003). Genetic and functional analysis of full-length human immunodeficiency virus type 1 env genes derived from brain and blood of patients with AIDS. *Journal of Virology*, *77*(22), 12336–12345.

Owen, A., Chandler, B., & Back, D. J. (2005). The implications of P-glycoprotein in HIV: Friend or foe? *Fundamental & Clinical Pharmacology*, *19*(3), 283–296.

Parczewski, M., Leszczyszyn-Pynka, M., Kaczmarczyk, M., Adler, G., Binczak-Kuleta, A., Loniewska, B., et al. (2009). Sequence variants of chemokine receptor genes and susceptibility to HIV-1 infection. *Journal of Applied Genetics*, *50*(2), 159–166.

Patel, C. A., Mukhtar, M., Harley, S., Kulkosky, J., & Pomerantz, R. J. (2002). Lentiviral expression of HIV-1 vpr induces apoptosis in human neurons. *J Neurovirol*, *8*, 86–99.

Patel, C. A., Mukhtar, M., & Pomerantz, R. J. (2000). Human immunodeficiency virus type 1 vpr induces apoptosis in human neuronal cells. *J Virol*, *74*, 9717–9726.

Patrick, M. K., Johnston, J. B., & Power, C. (2002). Lentiviral neuropatho-genesis: Comparative neuroinvasion, neurotropism, neurovirulence, and host neurosusceptibility. *Journal of Virology, 76*(16), 7923–7931.

Pattarini, R., Pittaluga, A., & Raiteri, M. (1998). The human immunodefi-ciency virus-1 envelope protein gp120 binds through its V3 sequence to the glycine site of N-methyl—aspartate receptors mediating noradrenaline release in the hippocampus. *Neuroscience, 87*(1), 147–157.

Peeters, M., Vincent, R., Perret, J. L., Lasky, M., Patrel, D., Liegeois, F., et al. (1999). Evidence for differences in MT2 cell tropism according to genetic subtypes of HIV-1: Syncytium-inducing variants seem rare among subtype C HIV-1 viruses. *Journal of Acquired Immune Deficiency Syndromes & Human Retrovirology, 20*(2), 115–121.

Peluso, R., Haase, A., Stowring, L., Edwards, M., & Ventura, P. (1985). A Trojan horse mechanism for the spread of visna virus in monocytes. *Virology, 147*(1), 231–236.

Pemberton, L. A., Kerr, S. J., Smythe, G., & Brew, B. J. (1997). Quinolinic acid production by macrophages stimulated with IFN-gamma, TNF-alpha, and IFN-alpha. *Journal of Interferon & Cytokine Research, 17*(10), 589–595.

Pemberton, L. A., Stone, E., Price, P., van Bockxmeer, F., & Brew, B. J. (2008). The relationship between ApoE, TNFA, IL1a, IL1b and IL12b genes and HIV-1-associated dementia. *HIV Medicine, 9*(8), 677–680.

Pereda, M., Ayuso-Mateos, J. L., Gomez Del Barrio, A., Echevarria, S., Farinas, M. C., Garcia Palomo, D., et al. (2000). Factors associated with neuropsychological performance in HIV-seropositive subjects without AIDS. *Psychological Medicine, 30*(1), 205–217.

Petito, C. K., Chen, H., Mastri, A. R., Torres-Munoz, J., Roberts, B., & Wood, C. (1999). HIV infection of choroid plexus in AIDS and asymptomatic HIV-infected patients suggests that the choroid plexus may be a reservoir of productive infection. *Journal of Neurovirology, 5*(6), 670–677.

Phillips, E. J., & Mallal, S. A. (2008). Pharmacogenetics and the potential for the individualization of antiretroviral therapy. *Current Opinion in Infectious Diseases, 21*(1), 16–24.

Piacentini, L., Biasin, M., Fenizia, C., & Clerici, M. (2009). Genetic cor-relates of protection against HIV infection: The ally within. *Journal of Internal Medicine, 265*(1), 110–124.

Pillai, S. K., Pond, S. L. K., Liu, Y., Good, B. M., Strain, M. C., Ellis, R. J., et al. (2006). Genetic attributes of cerebrospinal fluid-derived HIV-1 env. *Brain, 129*(7), 1872–1883.

Piller, S. C., Ewart, G. D., Jans, D. A., Gage, P. W., & Cox, G. B. (1999). The amino-terminal region of vpr from human immunodeficiency virus type 1 forms ion channels and kills neurons. *J Virol, 73,* 4230–4238.

Piller, S. C., Ewart, G. D., Premkumar, A., Cox, G. B., & Gage, P. W. (1996). Vpr protein of human immunodeficiency virus type 1 forms cation-selective channels in planar lipid bilayers. *Proc Natl Acad Sci U S A, 93,* 111–115.

Pitas, R. E., Boyles, J. K., Lee, S. H., Hui, D., & Weisgraber, K. H. (1987). Lipoproteins and their receptors in the central nervous system. Characterization of the lipoproteins in cerebrospinal fluid and identi-fication of apolipoprotein B,E(LDL) receptors in the brain. *Journal of Biological Chemistry, 262*(29), 14352–14360.

Plantier, J. C., Leoz, M., Dickerson, J. E., De Oliveira, F., Cordonnier, F., Lemee, V., et al. (2009). A new human immunodeficiency virus derived from gorillas. *Nature Medicine, 15*(8), 871–872.

Pocernich, C. B., Sultana, R., Mohmmad-Abdul, H., Nath, A., & Butterfield, D. A. (2005). HIV-dementia, tat-induced oxidative stress, and antioxidant therapeutic considerations. *Brain Research - Brain Research Reviews, 50*(1), 14–26.

Polazzi, E., Levi, G., & Minghetti, L. (1999). Human immunodeficiency virus type 1 tat protein stimulates inducible nitric oxide synthase expression and nitric oxide production in microglial cultures. *J Neuropathol Exp Neurol, 58*(8), 825–31.

Poli, G., Kinter, A., Justement, J. S., Kehrl, J. H., Bressler, P., Stanley, S., et al. (1990). Tumor necrosis factor alpha functions in an autocrine manner in the induction of human immunodeficiency virus expres-sion. *Proceedings of the National Academy of Sciences of the United States of America, 87*(2), 782–785.

Pond, S. L. K., Poon, A. F. Y., Zárate, S., Smith, D. M., Little, S. J., Pillai, S. K., et al. (2008). Estimating selection pressures on HIV-1 using phylo-genetic likelihood models. *Statistics in Medicine, 27*(23), 4779–4789.

Power, C., Gill, M., & Johnson, R. (2002). Progress in Clinical Neurosciences: The neuropathogenesis of HIV infection: Host-virus interaction and the impact of therapy. *The Canadian Journal of Neurological Sciences, 29*(1), 19–32.

Power, C. & Johnson, R. T. (2001). Neuroimmune and neurovirological aspects of human immunodeficiency virus infection. *Advances in Virus Research, 56,* 389–433.

Power, C., McArthur, J. C., Johnson, R. T., Griffin, D. E., Glass, J. D., Perryman, S., et al. (1994). Demented and nondemented patients with AIDS differ in brain-derived human immunodeficiency virus type 1 envelope sequences. *J Virol, 68*(7), 4643–4649.

Power, C., McArthur, J. C., Nath, A., Wehrly, K., Mayne, M., Nishio, J., et al. (1998). Neuronal death induced by brain-derived human immu-nodeficiency virus type 1 envelope genes differs between demented and nondemented AIDS patients. *Journal of Virology, 72*(11), 9045–9053.

Price, P., Keane, N. M., Stone, S. F., Cheong, K. Y., & French, M. A. (2001). MHC haplotypes affect the expression of opportunistic infec-tions in HIV patients. *Human Immunology, 62*(2), 157–164.

Price, P., Morahan, G., Huang, D., Stone, E., Cheong, K. Y., Castley, A., et al. (2002). Polymorphisms in cytokine genes define subpopulations of HIV-1 patients who experienced immune restoration diseases. *AIDS, 16*(15), 2043–2047.

Quasney, M. W., Zhang, Q., Sargent, S., Mynatt, M., Glass, J., & McArthur, J. (2001). Increased frequency of the tumor necrosis factor-alpha-308 A allele in adults with human immunodeficiency virus dementia. *Annals of Neurology, 50*(2), 157–162.

Rabkin, J. G., Ferrando, S. J., van Gorp, W., Rieppi, R., McElhiney, M., & Sewell, M. (2000). Relationships among apathy, depression, and cogni-tive impairment in HIV/AIDS. *Journal of Neuropsychiatry & Clinical Neurosciences, 12*(4), 451–457.

Rao, V. R., Sas, A. R., Eugenin, E. A., Siddappa, N. B., Bimonte-Nelson, H., Berman, J. W., et al. (2008). HIV-1 clade-specific differences in the induction of neuropathogenesis. *Journal of Neuroscience, 28*(40), 10010–10016.

Rappaport, J., Joseph, J., Croul, S., Alexander, G., Del Valle, L., Amini, S., et al. (1999). Molecular pathway involved in HIV-1-induced CNS pathology: Role of viral regulatory protein, tat. *J Leukocyte Biol, 65*(458–465).

Reddy, R. T., Achim, C. L., Sirko, D. A., Tehranchi, S., Kraus, F. G., Wong-Staal, F., et al. (1996). Sequence analysis of the V3 loop in brain and spleen of patients with HIV encephalitis. *AIDS Research & Human Retroviruses, 12*(6), 477–482.

Reyes, M. G., Faraldi, F., Senseng, C. S., Flowers, C., & Fariello, R. (1991). Nigral degeneration in acquired immune deficiency syndrome (AIDS). *Acta Neuropathologica, 82*(1), 39–44.

Robertson, K. R., Kapoor, C., Robertson, W. T., Fiscus, S., Ford, S., & Hall, C. D. (2004). No gender differences in the progression of ner-vous system disease in HIV infection. *Journal of Acquired Immune Deficiency Syndromes: JAIDS, 36*(3), 817–822.

Rom, I., Deshmane, S. L., Mukerjee, R., Khalili, K., Amini, S., & Sawaya, B. E. (2009). HIV-1 vpr deregulates calcium secretion in neural cells. *Brain Research, 1275,* 81–86.

Ross, H. L., Gartner, S., McArthur, J. C., Corboy, J. R., McAllister, J. J., Millhouse, S., et al. (2001). HIV-1 LTR C/EBP binding site sequence configurations preferentially encountered in brain lead to enhanced C/EBP factor binding and increased LTR-specific activity. *Journal of Neurovirology, 7*(3), 235–249.

Rumbaugh, J. A. & Nath, A. (2006). Developments in HIV neuropatho-genesis. *Current Pharmaceutical Design, 12*(9), 1023–1044.

Russo, R., Siviglia, E., Gliozzi, M., Amantea, D., Paoletti, A., Berliocchi, L., et al. (2007). Evidence implicating matrix metalloproteinases in the mechanism underlying accumulation of IL-1β and neuronal apoptosis in the neocortex of HIV/gp120-exposed rats. *International Review of Neurobiology* (pp. 407–421). Academic Press.

Sacktor, N., Nakasujja, N., Skolasky, R. L., Rezapour, M., Robertson, K., Musisi, S., et al. (2009). HIV subtype D is associated with dementia, compared with subtype A, in immunosuppressed individuals at risk of cognitive impairment in Kampala, Uganda. *Clinical Infectious Diseases*, 49(5), 780–786.

Saha, R. N. & Pahan, K. (2007). Differential regulation of mn-superoxide dismutase in neurons and astroglia by HIV-1 gp120: Implications for HIV-associated dementia. *Free Radical Biology and Medicine*, 42(12), 1866–1878.

Saito, Y., Sharer, L. R., Epstein, L. G., Michaels, J., Mintz, M., Louder, M., et al. (1994). Overexpression of nef as a marker for restricted HIV-1 infection of astrocytes in postmortem pediatric central nervous tissues. *Neurology*, 44(3 Pt 1), 474–481.

Samson, M., Libert, F., Doranz, B. J., Rucker, J., Liesnard, C., Farber, C. M., et al. (1996). Resistance to HIV-1 infection in Caucasian individuals bearing mutant alleles of the CCR-5 chemokine receptor gene. *Nature*, 382(6593), 722–725.

Sas, A. R., Bimonte-Nelson, H., Smothers, C. T., Woodward, J., & Tyor, W. R. (2009). Interferon-alpha causes neuronal dysfunction in encephalitis. *Journal of Neuroscience*, 29(12), 3948–3955.

Sasseville, V. G., & Lackner, A. A. (1997). Neuropathogenesis of simian immunodeficiency virus infection in macaque monkeys. *Journal of Neurovirology*, 3(1), 1–9.

Sawaya, B. E., Khalili, K., Gordon, J., Taube, R., & Amini, S. (2000). Cooperative interaction between HIV-1 regulatory proteins tat and vpr modulates transcription of the viral genome. *J Biol Chem*, 275, 35209–35214.

Schwartz, S., Felber, B. K., & Pavlakis, G. N. (1991). Expression of human immunodeficiency virus type 1 vif and vpr mRNAs is rev-dependent and regulated by splicing. *Virology*, 183(2), 677–686.

Shah, M., Smit, T. K., Morgello, S., Tourtellotte, W., Gelman, B., Brew, B. J., et al. (2006). Env gp120 sequence analysis of HIV type 1 strains from diverse areas of the brain shows preponderance of CCR5 usage. *AIDS Research and Human Retroviruses*, 22(2), 177–181.

Shapshak, P., Segal, D. M., Crandall, K. A., Fujimura, R. K., Zhang, B. T., Xin, K. Q., et al. (1999). Independent evolution of HIV type 1 in different brain regions. *AIDS Research & Human Retroviruses*, 15(9), 811–820.

Shimizu, N. S., Shimizu, N. G., Takeuchi, Y., & Hoshino, H. (1994). Isolation and characterization of human immunodeficiency virus type 1 variants infectious to brain-derived cells: Detection of common point mutations in the V3 region of the env gene of the variants. *Journal of Virology*, 68(9), 6130–6135.

Si, Q., Kim, M., Zhao, M., Landau, N. R., Goldstein, H., & Lee, S. C. (2002). Vpr- and nef-dependent induction of RANTES/CCL5 in microglial cells. *Virology*, 301(2), 342–353.

Singh, I. N., El-Hage, N., Campbell, M. E., Lutz, S. E., Knapp, P. E., Nath, A., et al. (2005). Differential involvement of p38 and JNK MAP kinases in HIV-1 tat and gp120-induced apoptosis and neurite degeneration in striatal neurons. *Neuroscience*, 135(3), 781–790.

Singh, I. N., Goody, R. J., Dean, C., Ahmad, N. M., Lutz, S. E., Knapp, P. E., et al. (2004). Apoptotic death of striatal neurons induced by human immunodeficiency virus-1 tat and gp120: Differential involvement of caspase-3 and endonuclease G. *Journal of Neurovirology*, 10(3), 141–151.

Singh, K. K., Barroga, C. F., Hughes, M. D., Chen, J., Raskino, C., McKinney, R. E., et al. (2003). Genetic influence of CCR5, CCR2, and SDF1 variants on human immunodeficiency virus 1 (HIV-1)-related disease progression and neurological impairment, in children with symptomatic HIV-1 infection. *Journal of Infectious Diseases*, 188(10), 1461–1472.

Sippy, B. D., Hofman, F. M., Wallach, D., & Hinton, D. R. (1995). Increased expression of tumor necrosis factor-alpha receptors in the brains of patients with AIDS. *Journal of Acquired Immune Deficiency Syndromes & Human Retrovirology*, 10(5), 511–521.

Smit, T. K., Wang, B., Ng, T., Osborne, R., Brew, B., & Saksena, N. K. (2001). Varied tropism of HIV-1 isolates derived from different regions of adult brain cortex discriminate between patients with and without AIDS dementia complex (ADC): Evidence for neurotropic HIV variants. *Virology*, 279(2), 509–526.

Smith, D., Guillemin, G., Pemberton, L., Kerr, S., Nath, A., Smythe, G., et al. (2001). Quinolinic acid is produced by macrophages stimulated by platelet-activating factor, nef and tat. *Journal of Neurovirology*, 7(1), 56–60.

Song, L., Nath, A., Geiger, J. D., Moore, A., & Hochman, S. (2003). Human immunodeficiency virus type 1 tat protein directly activates neuronal N-methyl-D-aspartate receptors at an allosteric zinc-sensitive site. *Journal of Neurovirology*, 9(3), 399–403.

Sporer, B., Koedel, U., Paul, R., Kohleisen, B., Erfle, V., Fontana, A., et al. (2000). Human immunodeficiency virus type-1 nef protein induces blood-brain barrier disruption in the rat: Role of matrix metalloproteinase-9. *Journal of Neuroimmunology*, 102(2), 125–130.

Stern, R. A., Silva, S. G., Chaisson, N., & Evans, D. L. (1996). Influence of cognitive reserve on neuropsychological functioning in asymptomatic human immunodeficiency virus-1 infection. *Archives of Neurology*, 53(2), 148–153.

Stewart, G. J., Ashton, L. J., Biti, R. A., Ffrench, R. A., Bennetts, B. H., Newcombe, N. R., et al. (1997). Increased frequency of CCR-5 delta 32 heterozygotes among long-term non-progressors with HIV-1 infection. The Australian Long-term Non-progressor Study Group. *AIDS*, 11(15), 1833–1838.

Su, B., Jin, L., Hu, F., Xiao, J., Luo, J., Lu, D., et al. (1999). Distribution of two HIV-1-resistant polymorphisms (SDF1-3'A and CCR2-64I) in East Asian and world populations and its implication in AIDS epidemiology. *American Journal of Human Genetics*, 65(4), 1047–1053.

Su, B., Sun, G., Lu, D., Xiao, J., Hu, F., Chakraborty, R., et al. (2000). Distribution of three HIV-1 resistance-conferring polymorphisms (SDF1-3'A, CCR2-641, and CCR5-delta32) in global populations. *European Journal of Human Genetics*, 8(12), 975–979.

Tarr, P. E., Taffe, P., Bleiber, G., Furrer, H., Rotger, M., Martinez, R., et al. (2005). Modeling the influence of APOC3, APOE, and TNF polymorphisms on the risk of antiretroviral therapy-associated lipid disorders. *Journal of Infectious Diseases*, 191(9), 1419–1426.

Taylor, J., Pomerantz, R., Bagasra, O., & Amini, S. (1992). TAR-independent transactivation by tat in cells derived from the CNS: A novel mechanism of HIV-1 gene regulation. *EMBO J*, 11(9), 3395–403.

Teja, V. D., Talasila, S. R., & Vemu, L. (2005). Neurologic manifestations of HIV infection: An Indian hospital-based study. *AIDS Reader*, 15(3), 139–143.

Telenti, A. (2005). Adaptation, co-evolution, and human susceptibility to HIV-1 infection. *Infection, Genetics & Evolution*, 5(4), 327–334.

Thomas, E. R., Dunfee, R. L., Stanton, J., Bogdan, D., Taylor, J., Kunstman, K., et al. (2007). Macrophage entry mediated by HIV envs from brain and lymphoid tissues is determined by the capacity to use low CD4 levels and overall efficiency of fusion. *Virology*, 360(1), 105–119.

Thompson, K. A., Kent, S. J., Gahan, M. E., Purcell, D. F., McLean, C. A., Preiss, S., et al. (2003). Decreased neurotropism of nef long terminal repeat (nef/LTR)-deleted simian immunodeficiency virus. *Journal of Neurovirology*, 9(4), 442–451; 442.

Toborek, M., Lee, Y. W., Flora, G., Pu, H., András, I. E., Wylegala, E., et al. (2005). Mechanisms of the blood-brain barrier disruption in HIV-1 infection. *Cellular & Molecular Neurobiology*, 25(1), 181–199.

Toggas, S. M., Masliah, E., Rockenstein, E. M., Rall, G. F., Abraham, C. R., & Mucke, L. (1994). Central nervous system damage produced by expression of the HIV-1 coat protein gp120 in transgenic mice. *Nature*, 367(6459), 188–193.

Tornatore, C., Chandra, R., Berger, J., & Major, E. (1994). HIV-1 infection of subcortical astrocytes in the pediatric central nervous system. *Neurology*, 44, 481–87.

Tozzi, V., Balestra, P., Bellagamba, R., Corpolongo, A., Salvatori, M. F., Visco-Comandini, U., et al. (2007). Persistence of neuropsychologic deficits despite long-term highly active antiretroviral therapy in patients with HIV-related neurocognitive impairment: Prevalence and risk factors. *Journal of Acquired Immune Deficiency Syndromes: JAIDS*, 45(2), 174–182.

Trillo-Pazos, G., McFarlane-Abdulla, E., Campbell, I. C., Pilkington, G. J., & Everall, I. P. (2000). Recombinant nef HIV-IIIB protein is toxic to human neurons in culture. *Brain Research*, 864(2), 315–326.

Tscherning, C., Alaeus, A., Fredriksson, R., Bjorndal, A., Deng, H., Littman, D. R., et al. (1998). Differences in chemokine coreceptor usage between genetic subtypes of HIV-1. *Virology*, 241(2), 181–188.

Tyor, W. R., Glass, J. D., Griffin, J. W., Becker, P. S., McArthur, J. C., Bezman, L., et al. (1992). Cytokine expression in the brain during the acquired immunodeficiency syndrome. *Annals of Neurology, 31*(4), 349–360.

van Marle, G., Henry, S., Todoruk, T., Sullivan, A., Silva, C., Rourke, S. B., et al. (2004). Human immunodeficiency virus type 1 nef protein mediates neural cell death: A neurotoxic role for IP-10. *Virology, 329*(2), 302–318.

van Marle, G., & Power, C. (2005). Human immunodeficiency virus type 1 genetic diversity in the nervous system: Evolutionary epiphenomenon or disease determinant? *Journal of Neurovirology, 11*(2), 107–128.

van Rij, R. P., Broersen, S., Goudsmit, J., Coutinho, R. A., & Schuitemaker, H. (1998). The role of a stromal cell-derived factor-1 chemokine gene variant in the clinical course of HIV-1 infection. *AIDS, 12*(9), F85–90.

van Rij, R. P., Portegies, P., Hallaby, T., Lange, J. M., Visser, J., de Roda Husman, A. M., et al. (1999). Reduced prevalence of the CCR5 delta32 heterozygous genotype in human immunodeficiency virus-infected individuals with AIDS dementia complex. *Journal of Infectious Diseases, 180*(3), 854–857.

Vasan, A., Renjifo, B., Hertzmark, E., Chaplin, B., Msamanga, G., Essex, M., et al. (2006). Different rates of disease progression of HIV type 1 infection in Tanzania based on infecting subtype. *Clinical Infectious Diseases, 42*(6), 843–852.

Venturi, G., Catucci, M., Romano, L., Corsi, P., Leoncini, F., Valensin, P., et al. (2000). Antiretroviral resistance mutations in human immunodeficiency virus type 1 reverse transcriptase and protease from paired cerebrospinal fluid and plasma samples. *The Journal of Infectious Diseases, 181*(2), 740–745.

Vergote, D., Butler, G. S., Ooms, M., Cox, J. H., Silva, C., Hollenberg, M. D., et al. (2006). Proteolytic processing of SDF-1alpha reveals a change in receptor specificity mediating HIV-associated neurodegeneration. *Proceedings of the National Academy of Sciences of the United States of America, 103*(50), 19182–19187.

Vilades, C., Broch, M., Plana, M., Domingo, P., Alonso-Villaverde, C., Pedrol, E., et al. (2007). Effect of genetic variants of CCR2 and CCL2 on the natural history of HIV-1 infection: CCL2-2518GG is overrepresented in a cohort of spanish HIV-1-infected subjects. *Journal of Acquired Immune Deficiency Syndromes: JAIDS, 44*(2), 132–138.

Voevodin, A., Samilchuk, E., & Dashti, S. (1998). A survey for 32 nucleotide deletion in the CCR-5 chemokine receptor gene (deltaccr-5) conferring resistance to human immunodeficiency virus type 1 in different ethnic groups and in chimpanzees. *Journal of Medical Virology, 55*(2), 147–151.

Wadia, R. S., Pujari, S. N., Kothari, S., Udhar, M., Kulkarni, S., Bhagat, S., et al. (2001). Neurological manifestations of HIV disease. *Journal of the Association of Physicians of India, 49*, 343–348.

Wallace, V. C. J., Blackbeard, J., Pheby, T., Segerdahl, A. R., Davies, M., Hasnie, F., et al. (2007). Pharmacological, behavioural and mechanistic analysis of HIV-1 gp120 induced painful neuropathy. *Pain, 133*(1–3), 47–63.

Wang, Y. S. & White, T. D. (2000). The HIV glycoproteins gp41 and gp120 cause rapid excitation in rat cortical slices. *Neuroscience Letters, 291*(1), 13–16.

Wang, Z., Pekarskaya, O., Bencheikh, M., Chao, W., Gelbard, H. A., Ghorpade, A., et al. (2003). Reduced expression of glutamate transporter EAAT2 and impaired glutamate transport in human primary astrocytes exposed to HIV-1 or gp120. *Virology, 312*(1), 60–73.

Weiss, J. M., Nath, A., Major, E. O., & Berman, J. W. (1999). HIV-1 tat induces monocyte chemoattractant protein-1-mediated monocyte transmigration across a model of the human blood-brain barrier and up-regulates CCR5 expression on human monocytes. *Journal of Immunology, 163*(5), 2953–2959.

Werner, T., Ferroni, S., Saermark, T., Brack-Werner, R., Banati, R. B., Mager, R., et al. (1991). HIV-1 nef protein exhibits structural and functional similarity to scorpion peptides interacting with K+ channels. *AIDS, 5*(11), 1301–1308; 1301.

Wesselingh, S. L., Power, C., Glass, J. D., Tyor, W. R., McArthur, J. C., Farber, J. M., et al. (1993). Intracerebral cytokine messenger RNA expression in acquired immunodeficiency syndrome dementia. *Annals of Neurology, 33*(6), 576–582.

Wiley, C. A., Masliah, E., Morey, M., Lemere, C., DeTeresa, R., Grafe, M., et al. (1991). Neocortical damage during HIV infection. *Annals of Neurology, 29*(6), 651–657.

Williams, K. C., & Hickey, W. F. (2002). Central nervous system damage, monocytes and macrophages, and neurological disorders in AIDS. *Annual Review of Neuroscience, 25*, 537–562.

Winkler, C., Modi, W., Smith, M. W., Nelson, G. W., Wu, X., Carrington, M., et al. (1998). Genetic restriction of AIDS pathogenesis by an SDF-1 chemokine gene variant. ALIVE study, Hemophilia Growth and Development study (HGDS), Multicenter AIDS Cohort study (MACS), Multicenter Hemophilia Cohort study (MHCS), San Francisco city cohort (SFCC). *Science, 279*(5349), 389–393.

Wu, L., Gerard, N. P., Wyatt, R., Choe, H., Parolin, C., Ruffing, N., et al. (1996). CD4-induced interaction of primary HIV-1 gp120 glycoproteins with the chemokine receptor CCR-5. *Nature, 384*, 179.

Wyatt, R. & Sodroski, J. (1998). The HIV-1 envelope glycoproteins: Fusogens, antigens, and immunogens. *Science, 280*(5371), 1884–1888.

Yeung, M. C., Pulliam, L., & Lau, A. S. (1995). The HIV envelope protein gp120 is toxic to human brain-cell cultures through the induction of interleukin-6 and tumor necrosis factor-alpha. *AIDS, 9*(2), 137–143.

Yeung, M. L., Bennasser, Y., Le, S. Y., & Jeang, K. T. (2005). siRNA, miRNA and HIV: Promises and challenges. *Cell Res, 15*(11–12), 935–946.

Yu, W., Wang, Y., Shaw, C. A., Qin, X. F., & Rice, A. P. (2006). Induction of the HIV-1 tat co-factor cyclin T1 during monocyte differentiation is required for the regulated expression of a large portion of cellular mRNAs. *Retrovirology, 3*, 32.

Zauli, G., Secchiero, P., Rodella, L., Gibellini, D., Mirandola, P., Mazzoni, M., et al. (2000). HIV-1 tat-mediated inhibition of the tyrosine hydroxylase gene expression in dopaminergic neuronal cells. *Journal of Biological Chemistry, 275*(6), 4159–4165.

Zhang, K., Hawken, M., Rana, F., Welte, F. J., Gartner, S., Goldsmith, M. A., et al. (2001). Human immunodeficiency virus type 1 clade A and D neurotropism: Molecular evolution, recombination, and coreceptor use. *Virology, 283*(1), 19–30.

Zhang, K., McQuibban, G. A., Silva, C., Butler, G. S., Johnston, J. B., Holden, J., et al. (2003). HIV-induced metalloproteinase processing of the chemokine stromal cell derived factor-1 causes neurodegeneration. *Nature Neuroscience, 6*(10), 1064–1071.

Zhang, L., Huang, Y., He, T., Cao, Y., & Ho, D. D. (1996). HIV-1 subtype and second-receptor use. *Nature, 383*(6603), 768.

Zhao, M. L., Kim, M. O., Morgello, S., & Lee, S. C. (2001). Expression of inducible nitric oxide synthase, interleukin-1 and caspase-1 in HIV-1 encephalitis. *Journal of Neuroimmunology, 115*(1–2), 182–191.

Zhong, P., Peeters, M., Janssens, W., Fransen, K., Heyndrickx, L., Vanham, G., et al. (1995). Correlation between genetic and biological properties of biologically cloned HIV type 1 viruses representing subtypes A, B, and D. *AIDS Research & Human Retroviruses, 11*(2), 239–248.

Zhu, J., Mactutus, C. F., Wallace, D. R., & Booze, R. M. (2009). HIV-1 tat protein-induced rapid and reversible decrease in [3H]dopamine uptake: Dissociation of [3H]dopamine uptake and [3H]2Î²-carbomethoxy-3-Î²-(4-fluorophenyl)tropane (WIN 35,428) binding in rat striatal synaptosomes. *Journal of Pharmacology and Experimental Therapeutics, 329*(3), 1071–1083.

Zhu, Y., Antony, J. M., Martinez, J. A., Glerum, D. M., Brussee, V., Hoke, A., et al. (2007). Didanosine causes sensory neuropathy in an HIV/AIDS animal model: Impaired mitochondrial and neurotrophic factor gene expression. *Brain, 130*(Pt 8), 2011–2023.

Zhu, Y., Jones, G., Tsutsui, S., Opii, W., Liu, S., Silva, C., et al. (2005). Lentivirus infection causes neuroinflammation and neuronal injury in dorsal root ganglia: Pathogenic effects of STAT-1 and inducible nitric oxide synthase. *Journal of Immunology, 175*(2), 1118–1126.

1.5

GENETIC SUSCEPTIBILITIES FOR NEUROAIDS

Srinivas Mummidi, Jason F. Okulicz, Edwina J. Wright, Weijing He, and Sunil K. Ahuja

Among HIV-1 infected patients, clinical involvement of the central and peripheral nervous systems is widespread but far from universal, even among untreated patients. The precise basis for differences among individuals in the natural history of HIV-1 disease is largely unknown. Conceptually, these differences may be attributed to environmental, viral, host, and other factors. This chapter focuses specifically on host genetic polymorphisms that influence susceptibility to the spectrum of HIV-1 associated neurological disorders, peripheral neuropathies, and central nervous system (CNS) opportunistic infections. Particular attention is paid to polymorphisms for cytokines, chemokines and their receptors, and a number of other cellular products (apolipoprotein E, mannose-binding lectin). Also discussed are polymorphic determinants of drug-related CNS effects (efavirenz) and of progressive multifocal leukoencephalopathy and nondetermined leukoencephalopathy.

INTRODUCTION

One of the hallmarks of HIV infection is the involvement of the central and peripheral nervous systems. Approximately one-third of patients with advanced, untreated HIV disease develop neurological disorders, including central nervous system (CNS) opportunistic infections (OIs); HIV-1-associated neurocognitive disorders (HAND), including the most severe form, HIV-associated dementia (HAD); and HIV-related distal sensory peripheral neuropathy (SN).

The advent of highly active antiretroviral therapy (HAART) in 1996 afforded a highly salutary increase in patient survival and decrease in the incidence of CNS disorders including CNS OIs and HAD (Bhaskaran et al., 2008; Dore et al., 1999). However, the availability of HAART has attenuated but not extinguished disorders of the CNS: In HIV-infected patients receiving long-term HAART, milder HIV-associated neurocognitive disorders remain present in up to 40% of patients (Cysique & Brew, 2009; Sacktor et al., 2002); SN remains prevalent in patients in both resource-poor (Wright, 2009) and -rich countries (Ellis et al., 2010) as a consequence of HAART toxicity. Additionally, CNS immune restoration disease (IRD) occurs in up to 20% of patients initiating HAART in the setting of CNS opportunistic infections (Muller et al., 2010). Hence, neurological disorders remain an ongoing challenge for HIV-infected patients and their treating clinicians.

The precise basis for the inter-subject differences in the prevalence of CNS disorders during HIV infection is unknown. Conceptually, these differences may be due to inter-subject differences in environmental (e.g., co-infections), viral (e.g., neurotropism of infecting strain), and host (e.g., genetic polymorphisms) determinants as well as other comorbid conditions such as Alzheimer's Disease (AD) or Parkinson's Disease (PD). There is increasing evidence that genetic variations in human genes may predispose individuals to neurological disorders such as Alzheimer's disease (Bras & Singleton, 2009; Brouwers, Sleegers, & Van Broeckhoven, 2008; Cacabelos, 2009; Pardo & van Duijn, 2005; Pinholt, Frederiksen, & Christiansen, 2006; Rademakers, Cruts, & Van Broeckhoven, 2003; Rademakers & Rovelet-Lecrux, 2009; Tsuang & Bird, 2002) neurodevelopmental and peripheral nerve disorders (Baloh, 2008; Stankiewicz & Lupski, 2010; Verhoeven et al., 2006; Verpoorten, De Jonghe, & Timmerman, 2006), and epilepsy (de Kovel et al., 2010). As a corollary, there has been increasing emphasis on evaluating the role of host genetics in the pathogenesis of viral infections of the nervous system and studies have focused mainly on infections with HSV-1 (Hill, Bhattacharjee, & Neumann, 2007), West Nile virus (Ahuja & He, 2010; Glass et al., 2006; Lim et al., 2009; Lim et al., 2008; Lim et al., 2010), tick-borne encephalitis (Kindberg et al., 2008), and HIV-1 (reviewed in Hill, 2006). In this chapter, we have reviewed the host genetic polymorphisms that influence pathogenesis of HAND, including HIV-1-associated dementia, peripheral neuropathies, CNS opportunistic infections, and drug metabolism relevant to CNS disorders.

HIV-1-ASSOCIATED NEUROCOGNITIVE DISORDERS

The term HIV-associated neurocognitive disorders is an umbrella term used to describe asymptomatic neurocognitive impairment, mild neurocognitive disorder, and HAD (Antinori et al., 2007). Asymptomatic neurocognitive impairment occurs in at least 15% of patients (Antinori et al., 2007; Wojna et al., 2006) and is characterized by abnormal performance on neuropsychological testing. However, this abnormal performance is not reflected in the patients' day-to-day lives, whereby patients are asymptomatic and fully functional. Mild neurocognitive disorders occur in up to 40% of patients (Robertson et al., 2007) and are characterized by abnormal neurocognitive performance and mild interference in performance of activities of work and daily living.

HIV-1-ASSOCIATED DEMENTIA

HIV-1-associated dementia (HAD) is one of the leading causes of dementia in young adults worldwide (Sacktor et al., 2001). Before the introduction of HAART, 15–20% of patients with advanced untreated HIV disease developed HAD. In the pre- and post-HAART eras the estimated incidence of HAD is 6.49 and 0.66 per 1000 person years, respectively (Bhaskaran et al., 2008). HAD is a subcortical dementia characterized by the triumvirate of severe cognitive impairment, psychomotor slowing, and behavioral disturbance that significantly interfere with a patient's activities of daily living and the capacity to work. HAD lies at the severe end of the spectrum of HAND. Approximately half of HIV-infected individuals with HAD had neuropathological changes at postmortem, discovered during autopsy, and a quarter had a triad of clinical cognitive, behavioral, and motor abnormalities ranging from mild motor/cognitive deficits to overt dementia (Gendelman et al., 1997; McArthur et al., 1993). The introduction of HAART has considerably reduced the incidence of HAD (Bhaskaran et al., 2008; Dore et al., 1999).

However, due to increased longevity associated with HAART there has been a significant increase in other clinical manifestations of HAND. For example, Sacktor et al. compared HIV-associated cognitive impairment before and after the advent of HAART, and found that though HAART had reduced the incidence of HIV dementia, HIV-associated cognitive impairment continued to be prevalent in patients receiving HAART (Sacktor et al., 2001). Similar findings were noted in an Australian study by Cysique et al. (2004). Recently, the prevalence rate for HAND was found to be approximately 50% in HIV-1-infected individuals from the United States (McArthur & Brew, 2010). Furthermore, additional factors such as age (Cherner et al., 2004), and comorbid conditions including co-infection with hepatitis C virus (Cherner et al., 2005), vascular disease (Becker et al., 2009; Wright et al., 2010), and substance use (Rippeth et al., 2004) are thought to contribute to the development of cognitive disorders in HIV-infected patients. Furthermore, there is evidence to suggest that neurodegenerative diseases, notably AD and PD are occurring with increased frequency in HIV-infected patients receiving antiretroviral therapy (Brew et al., 2009; Tisch & Brew, 2009). Brew et al. have hypothesized that there are pathways common to aging, HIV infection, and neurodegenerative diseases that may afford this accelerated neurodegeneration and that host factors and antiretroviral toxicity may contribute to this process (Brew et al., 2009). To support this, recent data show an overlap between protein expression from the frontal lobes of patients with AD and patients with HAD (Zhou et al., 2010).

The greater life expectancy of HIV-1-infected individuals in the HAART era coupled with the increasing age of HIV-positive populations (Murray, McDonald, & Law, 2009) suggests that the current prevalence of HAND, albeit compounded or modified by the above-mentioned factors, may persist or rise over the next decade. A proportional increase in HAD compared with other AIDS-defining illnesses and a marked increase in the median CD4 cell count at HAD diagnosis have occurred since the introduction of HAART (Dore et al., 1999). Furthermore, several recent studies suggest that HANDs are prevalent in persistently treated aviremic patients (recently reviewed by McArthur et al., 2010). It should also be noted that in resource-poor countries, the prevalence of HAD is high (Riedel et al., 2006) and hence likely has a negative impact upon the workforce and hence the social and economic framework of these countries.

Surprisingly, there is discordance between the manifested neurocognitive disorders and characteristics related to HIV, including plasma viral load, host immune status, and disease progression rates. HIV-induced neuropathology has been often linked to infiltration of mononuclear phagocytes (MP) from the periphery and inflammatory mediators produced during HIV encephalitis. Clinical disease is often, but not always, correlated with neuropathologic features of HIV-induced encephalitis (HIVE). HAD is a subcortical dementia that traditionally affects the basal ganglia and deep white matter. It is characterized by productive infection of brain macrophages and microglia, giant cell formation, macrophage infiltration into the brain, and neocortical atrophy (neuronal loss, dendritic arbor damage, and spatial neuron alterations) (Asare et al., 1996; Everall et al., 1999; Masliah et al., 1997). Glass et al. demonstrated that the best histopathologic correlate of HAD is the number of inflammatory MPs in the CNS (Glass et al., 1993). Interestingly, most patients with HIVE have HAD, but not all HAD patients have HIVE. Even minimal increases in the numbers and, perhaps even more importantly, the state of MP immune activation could be sufficient to cause neurological dysfunction. Activated MPs produce a variety of neurotoxins including arachidonic acid and its metabolites, platelet-activating factor, pro-inflammatory cytokines, quinolinic acid, neurotoxic amines and nitric oxide (Achim, Heyes, & Wiley, 1993; Adamson et al., 1996; Bukrinsky et al., 1995; Garden et al., 2002; Gelbard et al., 1994; Genis et al., 1992; Giulian et al., 1996; Grimaldi et al., 1991; Heyes et al., 2001; Nottet et al., 1995). Viral proteins such as gp120, gp41, and Tat or virions binding to chemokine receptors expressed on neurons can also affect neuronal viability and/or function. Indeed, there is widespread microglial activation and accompanying reactive astrogliosis in the areas with pronounced dendritic damage (Adle-Biassette et al., 1999; Giometto et al., 1997). Thus, the initial events that lead to entry of the virus into the brain culminate in neurodegenerative changes that manifest as neurocognitive disorders and MPs likely play an important role in both of these processes.

On the basis of the aforementioned, it can be envisaged that polymorphisms that impact on the expression of genes encoding inflammatory mediators can lead to inter-individual differences in MP recruitment and activation, and in turn influence susceptibility to developing the full spectrum of HAND. However, the precise repertoire of host genetic factors/networks that influence HAD/HAND pathogenesis remains largely unknown. Polymorphisms in genes other than those classically involved in inflammatory response have also been implicated in HAND susceptibility (e.g., APOE alleles). Furthermore, host genetic polymorphisms have been found to be involved in CNS side effects resulting from antiretroviral therapies and have provided impetus to develop personalized therapeutic regimens as discussed in the later sections of this chapter. For example, a powerful and an exciting example of use of personalized genetics in clinical therapy is screening for patients for HLA subtype B*5701 allele, as this was found to be associated with hypersensitivity to abacavir (Mallal et al., 2008).

HOST GENETIC VARIATIONS RELATED TO HAND

Overview

Before discussing individual genes that have been implicated in the genetic susceptibility to HAND, we will provide a brief overview on the role of various cytokines and chemokines in HIV-1-induced neuroinflammation. HIV is thought to enter the CNS during very early stages of infection. It has been proposed that there is continuous recruitment of

Table 1.5.1 POLYMORPHISMS ASSOCIATED WITH HIV-ASSOCIATED NEUROCOGNITIVE DISORDERS AND NEUROPATHIES.[a]

NAME	GENETIC VARIATION	MECHANISMS	EFFECT ON HAND AND/OR PERIPHERAL NEUROPATHIES	REFERENCES
Chemokine Receptors				
CCR5	*CCR5 Δ32* (rs333) *CCR5 −2135*[#] T > C (rs1799988)	Truncated CCR5 protein Increased CCR5 expression	Δ32/+ genotype associated with significantly delayed disease progression, including less neurocognitive impairment and low risk of onset of AIDS dementia complex. *59353* C/C genotype associated with CNS abnormalities	Singh, 2003 Boven, 1999 van Rij, 1999 Singh, 2003
CCR2	CCR2–p.Val64Ile [†] (rs1799864)	Linkage disequilibrium with *CCR5* variants; heterologous receptor desensitization of CCR5 and CXCR4	The CCR2 64I bearing allele was associated with faster rate of progression to neuropsychological impairment in HIV-1-infected adults	Singh, 2004
CX3CR1	CX3CR1-p.Val249Ile (rs3732379); CX3CR1p.Thr280Met(rs3732378)	Presence of 280Met reduces receptor expression and binding of the cognate ligand CX3CL1(fractalkine) while 249Val-280Thr does the opposite	Children with 249Ile in homozygous state experienced accelerated disease progression and a trend toward greater CNS impairment; Children with 249Val-280Thr bearing haplotype experienced significantly less disease progression and CNS impairment	Singh, 2005
DARC	*DARC −46T>C* (rs2814778)	Regulate circulating chemokine levels; influences binding of HIV-1 and transinfection of HIV target cells; in linkage disequilibrium with p.Asp42Gly which associates with serum levels of CCL2, CCL5 and CXCL8.	−46C/C protected against the rate of progression of neurocognitive deficits to HAD	He, 2008
Chemokines				
CCL3L1	*CCL3L1* low copies plus detrimental *CCR5* genotypes	Modulation of CCR5 expression levels; HIV-1 suppression	Accelerated rate of disease progression to HAD	Gonzalez, 2005
CCL3 (MIP-1α)	rs1130371	Possible linkage disequilibrium with variation in CCL3, CCL4 or CCL18	TT genotype for the *CCL3* rs1130371 was associated with a twofold increase in risk for HAD	Levine, 2009
CCL5 (RANTES)	*CCL5−403G>A* (rs2107538)	−403A associated with increased CCL5 expression	*CCL5* −403 G/A polymorphism was significantly associated with PML-like leukoencephalopathy, known as nondetermined leukoencephalopathy (NDLE)	Guerini, 2008
CXCL12 (SDF-1)	c.*519G>A (rs1801157) Other Names: *(SDF1–3′-A)*	Increased levels of CXCL12 mRNA and enhanced mRNA stability	Children with the *SDF1–3′A/A* genotype had a faster decline in neurocognitive faculties	Singh, 2003

(*Continues*)

Table 1.5.1 (CONTINUED)

NAME	GENETIC VARIATION	MECHANISMS	EFFECT ON HAND AND/OR PERIPHERAL NEUROPATHIES	REFERENCES
CCL2 (MCP-1)	*CCL2 −2578 A>G* (rs1024611) Other Names: *CCL2 −2518A>G*	*CCL2 −2578G* allele associated with increased transcription, protein production and monocyte recruitment. It is also associated with elevated CCL2 levels in CSF.	*CCL2−2578G* homozygosity was associated with a 50% reduction in the risk of acquiring HIV-1 but accelerated disease progression and a 4.5-fold increased risk of HAD. *CCL2−2518G* allele was marginally associated with central nervous system (CNS) impairment in HIV-infected children	Gonzalez, 2002 Singh, 2006
		Cytokines		
TNF-α	*TNF−A −308G>A* (rs1800629) Other Names: *TNFA2* *TNFA −1031C>T* (rs1799964) Other Names: -1031*2	*TNFA −308A* is associated with increased production of TNF-α. Possible LD with SNPs in other genes involved in inflammation NA	*TNFA −308A* was more common in AIDS dementia complex (HAD) compared to HIV-negative controls. High risk of HAD in African American individuals with −308A. Carriage of *TNFA −1031*2* is associated with highest risk for nucleoside analog-associated sensory neuropathy (NRTI-SN).	Pemberton, 2008 Quasney, 2001 Peterson, 2004
IL-12 (p40)	*IL12B* (c.*159A>C) (rs3212227) Other Names: 3'UTR (+1188 A>C) IL12B (3' UTR)*2	Increased expression? Conflicting reports.	Carriage of *IL12B* (3' UTR)*2 is protective for nucleoside analog-associated sensory neuropathy (NRTI-SN).	Cherry, 2008
IL-1β	*IL1B 3954C>T* (rs1143634) Other Names: 3953C>T	*IL1B 3954T* allele is associated with increased IL-1β expression	*IL1B* 3954C>T polymorphism was less frequent in patients with lipodystrophic syndrome compared with those without; absence of the 3954T allele was significantly associated with lipodystrophic syndrome.	Asensi, 2008
		Others		
MBL2	*MBL-2 O/O* genotype (rs5030737; rs1800450; rs1800451)	Low plasma concentration and structural damage of MBL	*MBL-2* O/O genotypes associate with more rapid HIV-1-related disease progression and CNS impairment, predominantly in children younger than 2 years	Catano, 2008 Spector, 2010
APOE	*APOE ε2, APOE ε3, APOE ε4* alleles (rs429358; rs7412)	apoE4 enhances HIV cell entry in vitro .	*APOE ε4* allele is associated with HAND but not in all cohorts. May be age dependent.	Burt, 2008 Corder, 1993 Spector, 2010
CYP2B6	*CYP2B6 516G>T* (rs3745274)	Efavirenz metabolism; higher plasma levels of efavirenz lead to CNS side effects	The CYP2B6 G/T and T/T genotypes were associated with greater severity of CNS symptoms	Haas, 2005 Rotger, 2005
Mitochondrial DNA	*m.4917A>G* Haplogroup T	Asparagine to aspartic acid change in the ND2 subunit of Complex I. Oxidative phosphorylation?	The mitochondrial 4917G polymorphism may increase susceptibility to antiretroviral therapy-associated peripheral neuropathy This is a common European mitochondrial haplogroup that may predict NRTI-associated peripheral neuropathy	Canter, 2008 Hulgan, 2005

NOTES: ª Studies that showed positive associations with HAND or other neuropathies are shown. Please refer to the text for additional references.
CCR5 polymorphism nomenclature is according to Mummidi et al. (2000).
† Abbreviations used: p, protein; c, coding DNA; m, mitochondrial DNA; LD, linkage disequilibrium.

monocyte-macrophage lineage cells into the brain. The predominant cell type that is recruited is the CD16+ activated macrophage. The CD16+ monocytes are expanded following HIV-1 infection and are elevated in patients with dementia when compared to patients without dementia (Pulliam et al., 1997). The recruitment of CD16+ cells is probably mediated through the soluble form of CX3CL1 (fractalkine) that is physiologically expressed by brain tissue (Ancuta et al., 2003). Of note, the CD16+ fraction of the monocytes express high levels of the fractalkine receptor, CX3CR1 (Ancuta et al., 2003). HIV-1 preferentially infects CD16+ cells and probably gains entry to the CNS through this physiological recruitment (the "Trojan horse" hypothesis). In addition, CD16+ monocytes may serve as latent reservoirs of the virus in vivo (Ellery et al., 2007). The initial recruitment of HIV-1 infected CD16+ monocyte/macrophages into the brain is likely to trigger the inflammatory response leading to the expression of cytokines and chemokines. Two key pro-inflammatory cytokines, TNF-α and IL-1β, are thought to be involved in initiating the inflammatory pathways leading to neuronal injury. In addition to having direct effects on blood-brain barrier permeability as well as the viability of the neuronal cells, TNF-α and IL-1β upregulate expression of several neurotoxic as well as neuroprotective molecules. One of the predominant chemokines that is released by the infected macrophages and the activated astrocytes is CCL2 (MCP-1) which leads to recruitment of CD16- and CC chemokine receptor 2 (CCR2)+ monocytes to the brain. An excellent review of the mechanisms involved in neuroinvasion by HIV-1 has been recently published (Gras & Kaul, 2010). Below, we review the genotype-HAND associations described for polymorphisms in genes that encode proteins that have been implicated in HAND pathogenesis (summarized in Table 1.5.1). The major categories are: I. Cytokines; II. Chemokines and their receptors; III. Other genes.

CYTOKINE GENES

Tumor Necrosis Factor –α

As discussed above, TNF-α that is released by infected microglia may play a key role in neuronal injury following HIV-1 infection (reviewed in (Brabers & Nottet, 2006; Saha & Pahan, 2003)). However, its exact role in the pathogenesis is controversial as it has been implicated in both neurodegeneration as well as neuroprotection. Activated macrophages in HAD show increased expression of TNF-α (Wesselingh et al., 1997) and TNF receptors. The temporal expression of TNF-α was found to correlate with dementia progression and severity (Wesselingh et al., 1993). While the key role of TNF-α in the pathogenesis of HAD and other cognitive disorders is undisputed, its role may be dependent on several factors such as TNF-receptor usage, its known role in induction of beta chemokines, effects on blood-brain barrier, potentiation of toxic effects of other neuroinflammatory molecules, and monocyte trafficking (reviewed in Saha & Pahan, 2003).

The *TNFA* gene is located in the major histocompatability complex (MHC) and polymorphic variation in its regulatory regions has been implicated in a variety of diseases. Of note, a G to A transition in the promoter region at position -308 (TNF-308A, rs1800629 G>A) is associated with increased TNF-α expression and increased susceptibility to several infectious diseases (Elahi et al., 2009). However, *TNFA* gene is proximal to several inflammatory genes such as lymphotoxin, and polymorphisms in this region exhibit strong linkage disequilibrium (linked polymorphisms). Thus, disease associations may not be ascribed a single marker or gene in this locus. Several studies have examined the association between the -308 polymorphism and HAD/HIVE. Two studies have found no association between HIV-1 encephalitis and/or dementia (Diaz-Arrastia et al., 2004; Sato-Matsumura et al., 1998); however, this may be ascribed to low patient numbers in these studies. By contrast, Quasney et al. found that *TNFA2*

allele (i.e., those bearing -308A) was found to be overrepresented in adults with HAD when compared to adults without dementia (Quasney et al., 2001). Similarly, Pemberton et al. also found that *TNFA2* allele was present at increased frequency in patients with HAD when compared to both HIV-1-infected patients who did not develop symptoms of dementia as well as HIV-1-negative controls (Pemberton et al., 2008). The latter study is a meta-analysis and included data from studies conducted by Quasney et al. (2001) and Diaz-Arrastia et al. (2004).

Interleukin-1 (IL-1)

Similar to TNF-α, IL-1 is a pluripotent cytokine and has powerful inflammatory and immunomodulatory effects. Comparative studies on human brain samples from HIV-1 patients with and without HAD initially showed that there was no increase in IL-1 expression during HAD (Wesselingh et al., 1993). However in a subsequent study, Zhao et al, showed that IL-1β expression was significantly higher in brain tissues from patients with HAD when compared to HIV-1-positive patients without dementia and high expression was detected in macrophages, microglia, and multinucleated giant cells (Zhao et al., 2001). IL-1β has pleiotropic effects and modulates expression of several genes that have been implicated in neuronal injury as well as neuroprotection (reviewed in Brabers & Nottet, 2006). Both *IL1A* and *IL1B* genes are polymorphic and may be associated with altered gene expression (Pociot et al., 1992). Pemberton et al. evaluated the role of *IL1A* −889 (C>T; rs1800587) and *IL1B* 3953 (C>T; rs11143634) polymorphisms in HIV-1-infected patients and found no difference between patients with HAD and HIV-positive and HIV-negative controls (Pemberton et al., 2008).

CHEMOKINES AND THEIR RECEPTORS

CC Chemokine Receptor 5 (CCR5)

CCR5 serves as the major co-receptor for the entry of macrophage-tropic HIV-1 (R5) strains into cells of monocyte macrophage lineage as well as memory T cells (Alkhatib et al., 1996; Berger, Murphy, & Farber, 1999; Deng et al., 1996; Samson et al., 1996). A 32-bp deletion mutation (Δ32; rs333) in the *CCR5* open reading frame leads to formation of truncated protein which fails to get expressed on cell surface. Homozygosity for this mutation confers almost an absolute protection against HIV-1 infection (Berger, Murphy, & Farber, 1999; Liu et al., 1996). It also has a protective phenotype in heterozygous state and is associated with decreased surface expression and delayed disease progression (de Roda Husman et al., 1997; Gonzalez et al., 1999; Huang et al., 1996; Ioannidis et al., 2001; Mummidi et al., 1998; Zimmerman et al., 1997), although the level of protection may be determined by the partner CCR5 allele (Gonzalez et al., 1999; Hladik et al., 2005; Mangano et al., 2001; Salkowitz et al., 2003) and was not consistent in all cohorts examined (Eskild et al., 1998; Wilkinson et al., 1998).

Microglia express relatively high levels of CCR5 when compared to CCR3 and CXCR4 (Albright et al., 1999) and CCR5 is the predominant co-receptor used by the HIV-1 dementia isolates for entry into microglia (Albright et al., 1999; Shieh et al., 1998). While the role of Δ32 heterozygosity in HIV-1 dementia is not extensively documented, several studies have shown that its protective effect also extends to HAD and other HIV-1-related neurocognitive disorders (Boven et al., 1999; Singh et al., 2003; van Rij et al., 1999). Van Rij et al. showed that in a cohort of HIV-1-positive individuals, the CCR5-Δ32 allele was less prevalent in patients with AIDS dementia complex. They found that only 4.1% of the AIDS patients with HAD were heterozygous for the Δ32 allele, whereas 14.5% of the AIDS patients in their cohort without HAD were heterozygous for this allele (van Rij et al., 1999). In a small group of HAD patients (n=9), Boven et al. observed no heterozygotes, suggesting that Δ32 may be conferring a protective effect (Boven et al., 1999). Interestingly, they also demonstrated that there is decreased viral replication in monocyte-derived macrophages derived from CCR5-Δ32 heterozygous donors. Singh et al. examined CCR5-Δ32 heterozygosity in 1049 HIV-1-infected children and found it to be protective in neurocognitive disorders (Singh et al., 2003).

In addition to the CCR5-Δ32 allele, polymorphisms in the regulatory regions of CCR5 also influence the expression levels of CCR5 (Hladik et al., 2005; Kawamura et al., 2003; McDermott et al., 1998; Mummidi et al., 2000; Salkowitz et al., 2003; Shieh et al., 2000; Thomas et al., 2006). Mummidi et al. organized the polymorphisms in the CCR2-CCR5 locus into distinct haplotypes and have shown that the CCR5 haplotypes influence its transcriptional activity (Mummidi et al., 2000). Several other studies have reaffirmed the critical role played by CCR5 cis-regulatory polymorphisms and haplotypes in CCR5 expression and HIV-1 pathogenesis (Carrington et al., 1999a; Catano et al., 2008; Gonzalez et al., 1999; Kawamura et al., 2003; Knudsen et al., 2001; Kostrikis et al., 1999; Martin et al., 1998; McDermott et al., 1998; Mummidi et al., 1998; Mummidi et al., 2000; Ometto et al., 2001; Salkowitz et al., 2003; Shieh et al., 2000). Singh et al. have examined the association of various promoter polymorphisms with CNS abnormalities and found that the proportion of children with the CCR5–59353-C/C genotype (rs1799988) who had a CNS abnormality (33%) was higher than that of children with either the CCR5–59353-T/C genotype (25%) or the CCR5–59353-T/T genotype (28%) (Singh et al., 2003).

From these associations, the following mechanistic possibilities may be considered. (1) Polymorphisms that associate with higher CCR5 expression promote viral entry and by extension HIV-1 viral load. This in turn, may correlate with increased risk of HAND. (2) Higher expression of CCR5 may associate with increased recruitment of MP to CNS, promoting HAND. However, studies by Dolan et al. have suggested that CCR5 may also influence HIV pathogenesis by impacting on parameters that are independent of viral load (e.g., cell-mediated immunity) (Dolan et al., 2007). The latter may also play a role in the differential susceptibility to HAND associated with CCR5 polymorphisms. Nevertheless, as a general rule, those CCR5 variations that associated with a faster rate of disease progression to AIDS are also associated with a high risk of HIV-1-associated neurocognitive disorders.

CCR5 ligands

CCR5 serves as the receptor for several chemokine ligands including CCL3 (MIP-1α), CCL3L1, CCL4 (MIP-1β), as well as RANTES (CCL5). The expression of these chemokines is elevated in the CNS of HIV-1-infected patients and several studies have shown that polymorphisms in these genes may influence HAND susceptibility. Levine et al. examined the role of seven distinct cytokine polymorphisms in 143 HIV-infected individuals enrolled in the National NeuroAIDS Tissue Consortium and found that a SNP localized to CCL3 and designated as rs1130371 was associated with a twofold increase in risk for HAD (Levine et al., 2009). While this polymorphism is present in the coding region of CCL3, it does not lead to changes in the open reading frame. However, it is in linkage disequilibrium with several other single nucleotide polymorphisms (SNPs) in the CCL3-CCL18 locus on chromosome 17 (Levine et al., 2009) and additional studies are needed to decipher whether this association is due to this SNP in CCL3 or linked polymorphisms. Of note, in the same study, no association with HAD was noted with the SNP designated as rs1719130 which localizes to the CCL5 gene (Levine et al., 2009).

Gonzalez et al. have examined the role of segmental duplications in chromosome 17q (a region that contains several chemokine genes including ligands of CCR5) on HIV-1 disease susceptibility, disease progression, as well as HAD susceptibility (Gonzalez et al., 2005). The segmental duplication in this region leads to inter-individual variation in the gene copy number of the chemokine CCL3L1, such that individuals may possess varying numbers of CCL3L1 gene-containing segmental duplications (range: 0–12). This variation in copy number may play an important role in HIV pathogenesis because CCL3L1 is the most potent ligand for CCR5, influences its expression levels, and exhibits potent HIV-1 suppressive properties (Menten, Wuyts, & Van Damme, 2002). The variability in the copy number of the CCL3L1 gene-containing segmental duplication is population specific and the median copy number varies based on the race, with individuals of African ancestry possessing a higher copy number relative to those of European ancestry (Gonzalez et al., 2005). Of note, lower CCL3L1 copy number is associated with lower gene expression levels (Gonzalez et al., 2005). Gonzalez et al. demonstrated that possession of a low copy number of the CCL3L1 gene-containing segmental duplication relative to the population median was associated with an increased risk of acquiring HIV-1 and rapid progression to AIDS (Gonzalez et al., 2005) and these observations were subsequently confirmed in independent cohorts (reviewed in Colobran et al., 2010). Gonzalez et al. also evaluated the combined effect of CCR5 haplotypes and copy number of the CCL3L1 gene-containing segmental duplication (CCL3L/CCR5 genetic risk groups or GRGs, Gonzalez et al., 2005). They found that possession of detrimental CCR5 haplotypes and a lower copy number of the *CCL3L1* gene-containing segmental duplication was associated with a threefold increase in risk to HAD development (Gonzalez et al., 2005). Taken together, the aforementioned studies suggest that polymorphisms (e.g., *CCL3)* and structural variations (e.g., *CCL3L1)* in genes encoding CCR5 ligands may play an influential role in determining the disease outcomes in HIV-1 infection and associated neurocognitive disorders.

CC Chemokine Ligand 2 (CCL2)

CCL2 is the first human chemokine to be characterized and is the most potent inducer of monocyte chemotaxis (Deshmane et al., 2009). Multiple lines of evidence suggest a critical role of this chemokine in the pathogenesis of HAD and other neurocognitive diseases (reviewed in Dhillon et al., 2008). First, CCL2 expression has been consistently associated with HAD in HIV-1-infected patients as well as in simian models of HAD (Cinque et al., 1998; Kelder et al., 1998; Zink et al., 2001). Second, CCL2 may enhance HIV spread/replication and therefore could play a role in the early MP-mediated events necessary for the establishment and spread of infection (Hirsch et al., 1998). Third, CCL2 can inhibit HIV-1 infection in vitro, although it remains unclear whether these effects are direct, that is, blockade of HIV-1 entry via its receptor CCR2 or indirect, that is, by inducing receptor-mediated heterologous desensitization of the major HIV-1 co-receptors CCR5 and/or CXCR4 (Berger et al., 1999; Frade et al., 1997; Lee et al., 1998). Fourth, CCL2 may influence the blood-brain barrier permeability and therefore facilitate transmigration of leukocytes into the brain (Eugenin et al., 2006). Of note, the CSF levels of CCL2 were predictive of dementia in simian immunodeficiency virus encephalitis (Zink et al., 2005), providing further links between CCL2 expression and HAND pathogenesis. However, recent studies have also indicated that CCL2 may have a protective effect on neurons from HIV-1 Tat-induced apoptosis (Eugenin et al., 2003). In the intact CNS, the primary sources of CCL2 are the parenchymal astrocytes and neurons (Deshmane et al., 2009; Dhillon et al., 2008). Under inflammatory conditions, CCL2 is also released by the infiltrating macrophages (Deshmane et al., 2009).

Two SNPs in the *CCL2* promoter region were described by Rovin et al. and their positions relative to the adenine in ATG are −2578 and −2136 (Rovin, Lu, & Saxena, 1999). −2578G homozygosity is always linked to −2136A homozygosity, whereas −2136T homozygosity is linked to −2578A homozygosity. Thus, the SNPs at −2578 and −2136 defined three *CCL2* haplotypes, designated as AA (the ancestral haplotype), GA, and AT (Gonzalez et al., 2002). The polymorphism at −2578 position (rs 1024611) has been associated with striking in vitro and in vivo biological effects including increased CCL2 production from stimulated peripheral blood mononuclear cells, higher serum and CSF CCL2 levels, and increased leukocyte trafficking (Gonzalez et al., 2002; Rovin, Lu, & Saxena, 1999). This polymorphism has been linked to increased transcriptional activity, but subsequent studies could not confirm the same (Rovin, Lu, & Saxena, 1999; Wright et al., 2008). It has also been linked to

differential transcription factor binding; however, additional confirmatory functional studies are awaited (Gonzalez et al., 2002; Wright et al., 2008). Gonzalez et al. examined the role of this polymorphism in a large cohort of HIV-1-infected patients and found that possession of the *CCL2*−2578G SNP is associated with more rapid rate of progression to AIDS and death in European Americans and a higher likelihood of developing HAD. This association remained significant even after adjusting for the year in which HAD developed ($P = 0.048$, odds ratio = 3.69, confidence interval (CI) = 1.01–12.45), suggesting that the administration of new classes of antiretroviral agents did not mitigate the increased susceptibility of individuals with this polymorphism for HAD (Gonzalez et al., 2002). The effects of *CCL2* GA/GA haplotype pair were also specifically associated with an increased risk for HAD and infection with *Mycobacterium avium* complex (MAC), and an association was not detected for more common AIDS-defining illnesses such as *Pneumocystis carinii* pneumonia (PCP), cytomegalovirus infection, or Kaposi's sarcoma. Furthermore, compared with the ancestral haplotype pair AA/AA, possession of GA/GA was associated with accelerated progression to HAD and MAC infection, but not to other common AIDS-defining illnesses such as PCP.

Singh et al. examined the role of *CCL2*−2578G in a smaller cohort of adults and found that this polymorphism had no influence on HIV-1 disease progression (p = 0.70, n = 216) and HIV-1-related neuropsychological impairment (p = 0.90) (Singh et al., 2004). In another study involving a large cohort of HIV-1-infected children, the possession of the −2578G allele did not have an impact upon HIV disease progression or neurocognitive impairment (Singh et al., 2006). Whether these differences associated with the *CCL2*−2578G-bearing allele in children versus adults relates to distinct pathogenesis of HAND in these two groups of HIV-infected individuals is unknown.

CC Chemokine Receptor 2 (CCR2)

CCR2 is a CC chemokine receptor that is the primary receptor for CCL2 and is expressed mainly by monocytes and a subset of T cells (Boring et al., 1997; Charo et al., 1994). In the brain it is also expressed in neurons as well as glial cells (van der Meer et al., 2000). As shown in several brain inflammatory models, the CCR2-CCL2 axis mediates leukocyte recruitment to the brain. In vitro CCR2 can serve as a minor co-receptor for HIV-1 cellular entry; however, its in vivo role in HIV-1 infection is not clear (Atchison et al., 1996; Frade et al., 1997). A G to A transition in the CCR2 coding region (190G>A; rs1799864) leads to replacement of valine by isoleucine at amino acid position 64 (V64I) in the encoded protein and the presence of this polymorphism has been associated with delayed disease progression in HIV-1-infected adults, although this finding has not been consistent across different cohorts (Kostrikis et al., 1998; Michael et al., 1997; Mummidi et al., 1998; Smith et al., 1997). The mechanism by which the CCR2 V64I polymorphism influences HIV-1 disease progression is unclear. Both forms of the protein (CCR2 with 64V or CCR2 with 64I) function equally well as HIV-1 co-receptors and no differences in expression levels have been noted (Lee et al., 1998; Mariani et al., 1999; Mummidi et al., 1998). CCR2 may be involved in heterologous receptor desensitization of CCR5 and CXCR4, which might explain some of the protective effects associated with CCL2 (Lee et al., 1998). Further adding to this complexity, the CCR2 64I is in linkage disequilibrium with a genetic variant in intron 2 of *CCR5* (Kostrikis et al., 1998; Mummidi et al., 1998), which suggests that the biological outcomes associated with the *CCR2* polymorphism may in fact be indirect effects of the linked *CCR5* SNP.

Singh et al. examined the role of CCR2 V64I polymorphism in HIV-1-infected adults and found that the carriers of CCR2–64I allele were at a higher risk of developing neuropsychological complications (Singh et al., 2004). This is an unexpected result in view of the protective effect of this polymorphism observed in several studies on HIV-1 disease progression. The authors posit that frailty or lead time bias which may be due to selective loss of CCR2–64V carriers may not be influencing their results (Singh et al., 2004). Further, these findings were independent of serum or CSF plasma viral levels, suggesting that CCR2 may be mediating its effects by modulating the CNS inflammatory pathways. However, these findings need to be confirmed in cohorts with well-documented dates of HIV seroconversion. Singh et al. also evaluated the role of CCR2 64 V/I polymorphism in a pediatric cohort in conjunction with the *CCL2* −2578A/G polymorphism and did not detect an association with HIV-1 disease progression or CNS impairment (Singh et al., 2006). Thus, further studies are required to clarify further the role of the CCR2 V64I polymorphism in HAND pathogenesis.

CXC Chemokine Ligand 12 (CXCL12)

CXCL12 or stromal-cell-derived factor (SDF)-1 serves as the exclusive ligand for CXCR4, which serves as a major co-receptor for HIV-1 entry. SDF-1/CXCR4 axis is involved in neuronal migration and maturation. CXCR4 is also expressed in the dendritic processes and axons of the neurons and may play a key role in neuron-glial communication. SDF-1 may competitively inhibit HIV-1 binding to CXCR4 and may in fact downregulate its expression. In an initial study, Winkler et al. reported that homozygosity for a polymorphism in the SDF 3'UTR (SDF1–3′-A; rs1801157) associates with delayed progression to AIDS (Winkler et al., 1998). However, several of subsequent studies failed to detect this association (Meyer et al., 1999; Mummidi et al., 1998; van Rij et al., 1998) and in two of these studies SDF1–3′-A was associated with a faster progression to AIDS (Mummidi et al., 1998; van Rij et al., 1998). Singh et al. examined the role of this polymorphism in a cohort of HIV-1-positive children and found that this SNP is associated with faster disease progression and decreased neurocognitive ability (Singh et al., 2003).

CX3C Chemokine Receptor 1 (CX3CR1)

Both CX3CR1 and its ligand fractalkine (CX3CL1) play a key role in the recruitment of monocytes to the brain as well

as trafficking of the cells of myeloid lineage into the brain parenchyma. Both fractalkine as well as CX3CR1 are expressed at high levels in the brain and HIV-1 infection leads to their increased expression (Tong et al., 2000). The coding region of the CX3CR1 is polymorphic and genetic variation leads to nonsynonymous amino acid substitutions leading to structural changes in the protein and differences in ligand recognition (Faure et al., 2000). A G to A transition at nt 745 (rs3732379) leads to a valine to isoleucine substitution at aa 249 (V249I) in the sixth transmembrane domain of the CX3CR1 protein. A C to T polymorphism at nt 849 (rs3732378) changes threonine to methionine at aa 280 (T280M) in the seventh transmembrane domain. Faure et al. reported that fractalkine binding affinity was greatest when the receptor contained V249 and T280 relative to those variants that contained I249-T280 and I249-M280 amino acid substitutions (Faure et al., 2000).

There are conflicting data in several cohorts with regards to the associations of the CX3CR1 polymorphisms on HIV-1 disease progression. The initial report by Faure et al. showed that the individuals who were homozygous for the 249I-280M haplotype progressed to AIDS more rapidly than did those with other haplotypes (Faure et al., 2000). Supporting these studies, Singh et al. demonstrated that children with the 249I/249I genotype experienced more rapid HIV disease progression (Singh et al., 2005). They also found that children with this particular genotype also showed a trend (although not statistically significant) towards CNS impairment. Further, supporting their analyses, children with the 249V-280T haplotype had half the risk of developing CNS disease when compared to children who had other CX3CR1 haplotypes (Singh et al., 2005). In contrast to the aforementioned studies, both McDermott et al. and Kwa et al. showed that CX3CR1 polymorphisms had a minimal role in HIV-1 disease pathogenesis (Kwa, Boeser-Nunnink, & Schuitemaker, 2003; McDermott et al., 2000).

Duffy Antigen Receptor for Chemokines (DARC)

DARC is a promiscuous receptor for chemokines including the CCR5 ligand CCL5 and such binding is thought to be a mechanism to regulate the inflammatory response by reducing the levels of plasma chemokines (Horne & Woolley, 2009). DARC is mainly expressed on red blood cells (RBC) as well as on some endothelial and neuronal cells (Hadley & Peiper, 1997). Although DARC does not function as an HIV-1 co-receptor, it may serve to sequester HIV-1 and was shown to have the ability to transfer HIV bound to RBC to its target cells (He et al., 2008; Lachgar et al., 1998). DARC is not expressed uniformly in all populations. A mutation in the consensus GATA1 binding site at −46 position (T>C; rs2814778) in the promoter leads to loss of DARC expression on RBC in the majority of West African individuals and this mutation in homozygous condition confers complete resistance to *Plasmodium vivax* infection (Tournamille et al., 1995). Cohort studies by He et al. suggest that DARC-null individuals associate with increased susceptibility to HIV infection, but slower HIV disease progression once infected. In addition, the presence of this polymorphism also conferred a strong protection against development of HAD (He et al., 2008). While the mechanism for these findings is not clear, the contrasting effect of the DARC effect on acquisition and disease progression may contribute to the higher prevalence of HIV in Africa as the infected individuals with longer survival times may have more chances to pass the virus to others (He et al., 2008; Kulkarni et al., 2009). It is notable that the DARC-null state on RBC is strongly ascribed to be a causal factor for low WBC and neutrophil counts observed in persons of African ancestry (benign ethnic leukopenia/neutropenia (Nalls et al., 2008; Reich et al., 2009)) and Kulkarni et al. found that the association of this genetic state with slow disease course was observed only in HIV-infected African Americans who were also leukopenic (Kulkarni et al., 2009).

As the promoter polymorphism leads to loss of DARC expression only on erythrocytes but not neurons, its impact on HAD is less likely to be due to this polymorphism itself, but due to its role in regulating chemokine levels. In support of this hypothesis, it was found that the *DARC* coding region polymorphism (p.Asp42Gly, rs12075), which is in high linkage disequilibrium with the promoter polymorphism, was highly associated with serum level of CCL2, CCL5, and CXCL8 levels (Schnabel et al., 2010).

OTHER GENES

Apolipoprotein E (APOE)

ApoE is a 34kDa protein that serves as major receptor for LDL and LDL-receptor-related proteins and also binds heparin sulfate proteoglycans (Mahley & Rall, 2000; Mahley, Weisgraber, & Huang, 2009). Its main function in the body is plasma clearance of triglycerides and cholesterol-rich glycoproteins (Mahley, 1988; Mahley & Rall, 2000). The human *APOE* gene is encoded on chromosome 19 and has several coding region polymorphisms that alter the protein sequence (Strittmatter et al., 1993). The three most common protein isoforms are prevalent, namely, apoE2, apoE3, and apoE4, which differ from each other based on the presence of either cysteine or arginine residues at amino acid positions 112 (rs429358) and 158 (rs7412) (Strittmatter & Bova Hill, 2002). APOE ε3 allele is the most frequent allele (65–70%) followed by APOE ε4 (15–20%), and APOE ε2 (5–10%). The amino acid changes were found to have direct structural effects on the different isoforms (Raffai et al., 2001; Strittmatter & Bova Hill, 2002). For example, the protein domains of the APOE4 isoform have relatively weaker interaction when compared to other isoforms and the protein itself is relatively unstable (Gregg et al., 1986; Mahley, Weisgraber, & Huang, 2009). This leads to preferential degradation of this isoform as well as lower expression levels in animal models. ApoE is expressed at high levels in the brain and is synthesized by astrocytes, stressed neurons, and infiltrating macrophages. Homozygosity for APOE ε4 allele is a strong genetic risk factor for late-onset Alzheimer's disease (Corder et al., 1993).

Several mechanisms can be envisaged to explain how ApoE may influence HIV-1 pathogenesis (Mahley, Weisgraber, & Huang, 2009). Firstly, cells that express APOE4 appear to be more susceptible to HIV-1 infection when compared to cells that express APOE3. Secondly, the amphipathic helices of APOE may promote HIV-1 fusion by interacting with gp41 (Martin et al., 1992). Thirdly, APOE also plays a key role in cholesterol delivery in the CNS and given the critical role played by cholesterol-rich lipid rafts in the HIV-1 replication cycle (Waheed & Freed, 2009) it is plausible that this may be another mechanism by which APOE isoforms influence HAND susceptibility.

A study by Corder et al. found that a group of HIV-1-infected patients lacking the APOE ε4 allele had twice the number of demented patients when compared to a group possessing the APOE ε4 allele (Corder et al., 1998). In a subsequent study, Valcour et al. have shown that possession of the APOE ε4 allele conferred a greater risk of developing HAD in patients over the age of 50 (Valcour et al., 2004). Here the authors determined APOE genotype in 182 participants who were enrolled in the Hawaii Aging with HIV Cohort. After adjusting for age and diabetes status, they found that the presence of APOE ε4 allele was associated with detrimental effects (for HAND) in older patients but not in younger patients. Burt et al. analyzed a large cohort of 1,267 HIV-infected patients and found that APOE ε4 homozygosity was associated with a faster rate of disease progression (Burt et al., 2008). However, in this cohort the APOE ε4 genotype did not influence the risk of developing HAD. The latter observation may reflect the fact that in the cohort evaluated by Burt et al, HAD and not HAND was the major phenotypic endpoint and patients were not evaluated for milder HIV-associated neurocognitive disorders. In a recent study, Spector et al. determined the role of APOE genetic variants in 201 HIV-1-positive patients of Chinese origin (Spector et al., 2010). In this cohort they found that 58% of the individuals with APOE ε4 allele were cognitively impaired compared with 31% of the individuals without the allele (P = 0.001, odds ratio 3.09, 95% confidence interval 1.54–6.18).

A number of reasons could contribute to the variable associations with APOE and HIV disease among different cohorts. In addition to the demographics as well as the size of the cohorts studied, the age of subjects studied may have significantly influenced the associations detected as age is an independent risk factor of HAD. Valcour et al. only found a positive association of APOE ε4 allele with HAD risk in patients over the age of 50 (Valcour et al., 2004), while the negative association by Burt et al. is from subjects of younger age (mean age, 30 years old (Burt et al., 2008)). These findings suggest the deleterious CNS effects of the APOE ε4 allele in individuals with HIV-1 infection may be age-dependent (Pomara, Belzer, & Sidtis, 2008).

Mannose Binding Lectin (MBL)

MBL is a C-type protein synthesized by the liver that circulates predominantly as a serum form (Turner & Hamvas, 2000). MBL participates in innate immunity and binds glycans from a broad variety of pathogens and effector molecules through pattern-recognition motifs (Presanis, Kojima, & Sim, 2003). MBL binds C1q, thus initiating complement activation (Thiel et al., 2000) and also triggers opsonization and subsequent phagocytosis (Ip et al., 2009; Zhang & Ali, 2008). *MBL2* is a highly variable gene with polymorphisms identified in both the coding and promoter regions. Three variations in the coding region at codons 52 (rs5030737), 54 (rs1800450), and 57 (rs1800451) discriminate the alleles D, B, and C respectively. The absence of mutation in all three positions defined the "A allele," whereas the presence of polymorphisms in the coding sequence (B, C, and D alleles) are collectively designated as the "O allele" (Garred, 2008). Genetic variations in the coding sequence alter the structural integrity of MBL (Larsen et al., 2004), and may result in dramatic reductions in circulating MBL levels and defective opsonization of pathogens (Super et al., 1989). Polymorphisms in the promoter region were also found to influence MBL levels (Madsen et al., 1995). For example, the −221C polymorphism in the *MBL2* promoter (designated the "X allele") is associated with significantly lower levels of the structurally intact MBL protein. Thus, coding region and regulatory region polymorphisms in *MBL2* provide, in part, a genetic basis for the wide range of circulating MBL levels (Garred, 2008).

Catano et al. examined the role of the MBL polymorphisms in a large cohort of HIV-1-positive patients and found that heterozygosity for polymorphisms that alter the structural integrity of MBL (i.e., the A/O genotype) is associated with disease-retarding effects (Catano et al., 2008), suggesting a heterozygosity advantage similar to the heterozygosity advantage observed for HLA alleles (Carrington et al., 1999b). In addition, Catano et al. also found that homozygosity for the promoter X allele, which results in a structurally intact protein but markedly reduced levels of MBL, is associated with disease-accelerating effects. Additional analyses in the same cohort using MBL genotypic groups and in the context of CCL3L1-CCR5 genetic risk groups, suggested that *MBL* genotype 3 increased the risk of rapid progression to HAD (Catano et al., 2008). These effects were later confirmed by Mangano et al. in a population of HIV-1 perinatally exposed children from Argentina (Mangano et al., 2008). They reported that the genotype XA/XA was associated with an eightfold increased risk of acquiring HIV-1 and almost a threefold risk of progression to pediatric AIDS. An independent positive correlation between the rate of AIDS progression and MBL plasma concentration was also found in this study (Mangano et al., 2008). However, neurological end points were not evaluated in later study. Spector et al. examined the loss of neurocognitive skills associated with different MBL alleles in a cohort of Chinese adults after one year follow-up and found that individuals possessing MBL O/O genotype had an increased risk of decline in cognitive function when compared to those possessing MBL A/A genotype (Spector et al., 2010). Singh et al. evaluated the role of *MBL* alleles in HIV-1-positive children and found that children with *MBL2* O/O alleles rapidly progressed to CNS impairment predominantly in those who are less than 2 years old (Singh et al., 2008). Collectively, these results suggest that MBL may play an influential role in HIV pathogenesis including neurological impairment.

HOST GENETICS RELATED TO HIV-1-ASSOCIATED DISTAL SENSORY POLYNEUROPATHY

Distal sensory polyneuropathy (DSP) is characterized by distal, symmetric anesthesia in a stocking-glove distribution with or without painful dysesthesia. Symptomatic DSP remains a very common neurologic complication and occurs in up to 40% of HIV-infected individuals (Ellis et al., 2010). DSP can be subcategorized as occurring secondary to HIV infection or due to drug toxicity of certain antiretrovirals, although the clinical features are identical.

DSP has been associated with use of the nucleoside reverse transcriptase inhibitors (NRTIs) didanosine (ddI), stavudine (d4T), and zalcitabine (ddC) (collectively denoted as dNRTI). Symptoms commonly occur within the first year of treatment or in patients with pre-existing peripheral neuropathy (Lichtenstein et al., 2005). In patients with DSP due to untreated HIV infection, a sudden worsening of symptoms may occur upon initiation of dNRTI therapy. Although the mechanism of dNRTI-associated DSP is unknown, studies suggest mitochondrial dysfunction may be the principal pathway. As a requirement for both activity and toxicity, NRTIs must first undergo intracellular phosphorylation. Long-term toxicity may be related to excessive activation of intracellular phosphorylation and/or to the inhibition of mitochondrial DNA polymerase-gamma by the dNRTI (Anderson, Kakuda, & Lichtenstein, 2004; Keswani et al., 2002). An increase in abnormal mitochondria in neuronal axons and Schwann cells as well as a depletion of mitochondrial DNA polymerase-gamma has been demonstrated in DSP associated with ddC (Dalakas, Semino-Mora, & Leon-Monzon, 2001).

Over approximately the last 150,000 years, the divergence of human mitochondrial genomes due to human migration and natural selection has led to many distinct patterns of single-nucleotide polymorphisms in mitochondrial DNA, termed haplotypes (Anderson et al., 1981; DiMauro & Schon, 2003; Herrnstadt & Howell, 2004; Torroni et al., 1996; Wallace, 1999; Wallace, Brown, & Lott, 1999). With the increased recognition of an association between mitochondrial haplotypes and neurodegenerative disorders such as Parkinson's disease, Hulgan et al. studied European mitochondrial haplotypes in patients treated with dNRTIs (Hulgan et al., 2005). They found that mitochondrial haplotype T, defined by point mutation 7028C>T, 10398G>A, and 13368G>A, was associated with DSP. Among the 137 subjects randomized to receive ddI + d4T, haplotype T was associated with 20.8% of those who developed DSP compared to 4.5% among controls (OR 5.4; 95% CI 1.4–25.1). These findings were also supported by Canter et al. who studied two non-synonymous mitochondrial DNA polymorphisms found in haplotype T, 4216C and 4917G, in 250 HIV-infected individuals treated with dNRTIs (Canter et al., 2008). Both polymorphisms were more frequently identified in patients with

DSP, and these polymorphisms were independently associated with DSP after adjustment for age, baseline CD4 cell count, plasma viral load, and drug exposure. The association with 4216C was no longer observed when 4917G individuals were excluded from the analysis, suggesting that the 4917G polymorphism may increase susceptibility to DSP during dNRTI therapy.

In several neurodegenerative disorders that involve mitochondrial dysfunction, a dysregulation in neuronal iron metabolism has been described (Atamna, 2004; Sadrzadeh & Saffari, 2004; Thomas & Jankovic, 2004). Hemochromatosis is a multisystem iron-overload disorder characterized by increased absorption of dietary iron and pathologic iron deposition in various organs (Pietrangelo, 2004). Since iron is essential for mitochondrial function and deficiency in iron is associated with several types of peripheral neuropathy, Kallianpur et al. investigated a possible link between hemochromatosis gene (HFE) mutations and DSP associated with dNRTI therapy (Kallianpur et al., 2006). They found that patients with HFE 845G>A, resulting in C282Y substitution, developed DSP less often than C282Y noncarriers. These results suggest that iron-loading hemochromatosis mutations, such as C282Y, may protect against DSP. This association remains controversial, however, since no relationship between HFE mutations and DSP was observed in a case-control study of 57 HIV patients with electromyography-confirmed DSP compared to 57 HIV-positive controls (Costarelli et al., 2007). The HFE gene is located on chromosome 6 and may be in linkage disequilibrium with other MHC alleles. This may explain the C282Y association with DSP in that a number of cytokine-related genes in this region have been associated with toxic neuropathy (Cherry et al., 2008).

In HIV-associated DSP, the host inflammatory response has been shown to have a significant role in the disease. For example, one study showed increased levels of TNF-α and reduced IL-4 in peripheral nerves in patients with HIV-associated DSP (Tyor et al., 1995). Since HIV- and dNRTI-associated DSP are phenotypically similar, Cherry at al. studied the role of inflammation in patients with DSP after initiation of NRTIs (Cherry et al., 2008). Of 16 Australian patients with onset of DSP in the first 6 months of dNRTI therapy, 13 (81%) carried the polymorphism TNFA- 1031*2 (rs1799964). This polymorphism was significantly lower in control subjects (24 of 79; 33%). Similarly, a study in Indonesia found that DSP following d4T exposure was associated with increasing age, increasing patient height, and presence of TNFA -1031*2 in a multivariate model (Affandi et al., 2008). Whether carriage of this allele affects TNF-α production is unclear. However, TNFA -1031*2 occurs in a TNFA haplotype associated with Behcet's disease, a syndrome associated with increased local production of TNF-α (Ahn et al., 2006; Park et al., 2006).

DSP as a complication of dNRTI therapy has been linked also to mitochondrial dysfunction in HIV-infected patients. Polymorphisms in the mitochondrial genome, specifically with haplotype T, have been associated with DSP (Canter et al., 2008; Hulgan et al., 2005). Mutations in the HFE gene may also be involved, but this association is less clear due to

conflicting studies (Costarelli et al., 2007; Kallianpur et al., 2006). In addition, the host inflammatory response to HIV and dNRTI therapy may also play a role as the TNFA-1031*2 polymorphism has also been associated with DSP in several studies. Additional studies are required to further identify the host genetic variants associated with DSP.

HOST GENETIC DETERMINANTS OF PROGRESSIVE MULTIFOCAL LEUKOENCEPHALOPATHY AND NONDETERMINED LEUKOENCEPHALOPATHY

Progressive multifocal leukoencephalopathy (PML) results from destruction of oligodendrocytes and myelin processes secondary to infection of the CNS by the polyomavirus JC virus (JCV) (Cinque et al., 2009). Although rare, PML develops most commonly in patients with advanced HIV infection; however, the disease has also been associated with other conditions resulting in compromised immunity, such as hematologic malignancies, as well as in patients treated with immunosuppressive agents (Garcia-Suarez et al., 2005; Richardson, 1961). In the HAART era, the frequency of PML has not declined in contrast to other opportunistic infections. More recently, a PML-like leukoencephalopathy termed nondetermined leukoencephalopathy (NDLE) has been described. NDLE is characterized by demyelinating lesions on MRI with milder clinical features resembling PML, but with the absence of JCV by cerebrospinal fluid analysis (Langford et al., 2003).

Although the genetic determinants of PML and NDLE risk and subsequent disease course have not been extensively explored, several genetic associations have been described. A study by Guerini et al. examined gene polymorphisms in CCR5, CCL5, CCR2, and CXCL12 genes in HAART-treated subjects with or without PML or NDLE (Guerini et al., 2008). The results showed that SDF1–3'G/A and A/A genotypes were more frequent in patients with PML while the CCL5—403 G/A polymorphism was significantly associated with NDLE. Polymorphisms in the p53 gene may also contribute to disease since PML lesions have demonstrated increased expression of p53 (Ariza et al., 1996). By sequencing the p53 gene in a population-based analysis of PML, Power et al. showed that arginine-proline heterozygosity at codon 72 of exon 4 was present in five of six evaluable patients (Power et al., 2000). Polymorphisms in the same site have also been associated with increased frequency of cervical cancer caused by a virus related to JCV, human papilloma virus, which suggests that polymorphisms in this position may affect multiple diseases (Storey et al., 1998).

PML is typically fatal within 1 year of diagnosis; however, approximately 10% of patients can exhibit a more protracted clinical course with prolonged survival (Berger et al., 1998). Koralnik et al. showed that having detectable cytotoxic CD8+ T lymphocytes against an epitope of the JCV VP1 protein is associated with a prolonged survival of HIV-positive individuals possessing the HLA-A2 serological allele with leukoencephalopathy (Koralnik et al., 2002). Thus, a JCV-specific cellular immune response may be an important factor in the containment of PML.

HOST GENETICS RELATED TO EFAVIRENZ CNS EFFECTS AND METABOLISM

The NRTI efavirenz is commonly recommended as a component of initial HAART regimens in most treatment guidelines. CNS and neuropsychiatric adverse effects occur in approximately 25–70% of patients, including abnormal dreams, dizziness, headache, confusion, impaired concentration, agitation, amnesia, psychotic symptoms, sleep abnormalities, and insomnia (Fumaz et al., 2002; Haas et al., 2004; Hawkins et al., 2005; Perez-Molina, 2002; Staszewski et al., 1999). These symptoms are typically noted in the first several days of therapy; however, the prevalence of most neuropsychiatric symptoms declines within a few weeks if treatment is continued (Arendt et al., 2007; Fumaz et al., 2002; Perez-Molina, 2002; Staszewski et al., 1999). In a minority of patients treated with efavirenz, however, neuropsychiatric disturbances may persist for several months or longer (Arendt et al., 2007; Munoz-Moreno et al., 2009).

Increased levels of efavirenz in the plasma can contribute CNS side effects, which are associated with a greater risk of virologic failure (Marzolini et al., 2001). Efavirenz is converted to inactive metabolites by the cytochrome P450 system, mainly via the CYP2B6 isozyme (Ward et al., 2003). The expression and function of CYP2B6 can vary amongst individuals and between certain ethnic groups. A study by Haas et al. examined the effect of $CYP2B6G>T$ polymorphisms in patients receiving efavirenz (Haas et al., 2004). They showed that $CYP2B6\ T/T$ genotype at position 516 was associated with higher plasma levels of efavirenz. Median values for area under the concentration-time curve between 0 and 24 hours were 44, 60, and 130 ug · h/mL according to G/G, G/T, and T/T genotypes, respectively ($P<0.0001$). G/T and T/T genotypes were associated with greater severity in CNS symptoms at week 1. Rotger et al. also reported a strong association between $CYP2B6\ 516\ T/T$ genotype and both higher plasma efavirenz levels and greater CNS toxicity (Rotger et al., 2005). Similarly, the association between $CYP2B6\ G516T$ polymorphisms and oral clearance of efavirenz was also confirmed in HIV-infected children (Saitoh et al., 2007).

To expand on these findings, Rotger et al. assessed the relationship between 15 single nucleotide polymorphisms of the CYP2B6 gene and efavirenz pharmacokinetics (Rotger et al., 2007). Subjects with a CYP2B6 poor metabolizer genotype had a greater risk for achieving very high plasma efavirenz levels. Similarly, patients homozygous for the CYP2B6*6 allele containing both $516G>T$ and $785A>G$ polymorphisms were shown to have higher plasma levels of efavirenz compared to heterozygous patients, or those without the CYP2B6 allele (Tsuchiya et al., 2004). Moreover, the CYP2B6*16 allele has also been associated with higher efavirenz levels when the $983T>C$ and $785A>G$ polymorphisms are present (Wang et al., 2006). Due to the considerably longer half-life of efavirenz compared to co-administered NRTIs and the low genetic barrier to resistance for efavirenz, a poor metabolizer genotype may have a higher rate of efavirenz resistance after cessation of HAART. After withdrawal of an efavirenz-plus-two NRTI regimen, elevated plasma concentrations of efavirenz were predicted to occur for at least 21 days in half of the patients with the CYP2B6 516 T/T genotype (Ribaudo et al., 2006).

With the growing body of evidence demonstrating increased plasma exposure to efavirenz and CNS side effects with certain CYP2B6 polymorphisms, research in individualizing efavirenz dosing based on CYP2B6 genotype has been ongoing. A study by Gatanaga et al. in 456 patients with CYP2B6 genotyping and treatment with efavirenz showed that all CYP2B6 *6/*6 and *6/*26 carriers had extremely elevated plasma levels (>6000 ng/mL) while receiving the standard 600 mg daily dose of efavirenz (Gatanaga et al., 2007). The dose was subsequently reduced to 400 mg and 200 mg in 11 and 7 patients, respectively, with persistently suppressed viral loads. Similar findings were demonstrated by Torno et al. (Torno et al., 2008). Further studies are needed to assess the utility of this approach before CYP2B6 genotyping can be recommended for widespread use in clinical practice.

The drug transponder P-gp affects oral absorption and tissue penetration of NNRTIs. Since P-gp is encoded by MDR1, several groups have studied polymorphisms in this gene, albeit with conflicting results. Allelic variants of MDR1 and several other genes were analyzed for their association with plasma efavirenz levels by Fellay et al. (Fellay et al., 2002). They found that median efavirenz concentrations were significantly different between patients with MDR1 3435 TT, CT, and CC genotypes reflecting the 30th, 50th, and 75th percentiles, respectively. They also noted that patients with MDR1 3435 TT genotype had a greater CD4+ T cell reconstitution 6 months after starting therapy. Neither of these findings, however, was confirmed in studies by Winzer et al. (Winzer et al., 2003; Winzer et al., 2005). Another study investigated polymorphisms in CYP2B6 and MDR1 in patients taking efavirenz. While the association between CYP2B6 516 TT polymorphism and greater efavirenz plasma levels was in agreement with results from other studies, the MDR1 3435 TT genotype was found to have a lower likelihood of virologic failure and decreased emergence of efavirenz resistance (Haas et al., 2005). Thus, the findings related to MDR1 polymorphisms remain controversial.

There is evidence that multi-locus genetic interactions between variant drug metabolism and transporter may be predictive of efavirenz pharmacokinetics and toxicity. In a single locus model involving $CYP2B6\ 516G>T$, the association with higher plasma levels of efavirenz was observed with an accuracy of 73% ($P<0.001$) (Motsinger et al., 2006). This model was also found to most accurately fit data in the African-American population with 69% accuracy ($P<0.001$). The best model to describe efavirenz pharmacokinetic data in Caucasians, however, involved a gene-gene interaction between $CYP2B6$ $516G>T$ and $ABCB1\ 2677G>T$ with a 65% accuracy ($P<0.001$). Overall, toxicity was best predicted by another two-locus interaction between $ABCB1\ 2677G>T$ and $ABCB1$ $3435C>T$ with a 71% accuracy ($P<0.001$).

FUTURE PERSPECTIVES

As reviewed above, the role of genetic variability in genes involved in neuroinflammation in susceptibility to HANDs is well documented. However, it is plausible that such variation in genes encoding neurophysiological and neurotransmitter factors may also influence HAND susceptibility. Candidate genes for such studies include Catechol-*O*-methyltransferase (*COMT*), dopamine transporter (*DAT*), dopamine receptor (*DRD*), dopamine-beta-hydroxylase (*DBH*) and brain-derived neurotrophic factor (*BDNF*) (Levine, Singer, & Shapshak, 2009). Another understudied area is the role of genetics at the interface of alcohol and substance abuse and HAND susceptibility. In addition, recent studies have illuminated the role of structural variation in genome (e.g., copy number variation) in CNS diseases such as schizophrenia and thus it is conceivable that these variants may also influence HAND susceptibility. Another major development is the increasing recognition of the role of epigenetics and epigenetic variation in disease pathogenesis; consequently, inter-individual differences in histone profiles and methylation signatures may correlate with risk to develop HANDs. There has been a recent explosion of genome-wide association studies for unbiased identification of protective loci for complex diseases. We can envisage such studies being extended to identify markers that are associated with HAND susceptibility, although one limiting factor is the large numbers of well-characterized subjects needed to accomplish such studies.

ACKNOWLEDGMENTS

We thank Gabriel Catano for helpful advice. This work was supported by the VA HIV/AIDS Center of the South Texas Veterans Health Care System, NIH (R37046326), and the Doris Duke Distinguished Clinical Scientist Award to S.K.A. S.K.A. is also supported by a VA MERIT Review award and the Burroughs Wellcome Clinical Scientist Award in Translational Research. S.M. is supported by a Department of Veterans Affairs MERIT Review award.

REFERENCES

Achim, C. L., Heyes, M. P., & Wiley, C. A. (1993). Quantitation of human immunodeficiency virus, immune activation factors, and quinolinic acid in AIDS brains. *J Clin Invest*, 91(6), 2769–75.

Adamson, D. C., Wildemann, B., Sasaki, M., Glass, J. D., McArthur, J. C., Christov, V. I., et al. (1996). Immunologic NO synthase: Elevation in severe AIDS dementia and induction by HIV-1 gp41. *Science*, 274(5294), 1917–21.

Adle-Biassette, H., Chretien, F., Wingertsmann, L., Hery, C., Ereau, T., Scaravilli, F., et al. (1999). Neuronal apoptosis does not correlate with dementia in HIV infection but is related to microglial activation and axonal damage. *Neuropathol Appl Neurobiol*, 25(2), 123–33.

Affandi, J. S., Price, P., Imran, D., Yunihastuti, E., Djauzi, S., & Cherry, C. L. (2008). Can we predict neuropathy risk before stavudine prescription in a resource-limited setting? *AIDS Res Hum Retroviruses*, 24(10), 1281–4.

Ahn, J. K., Yu, H. G., Chung, H., & Park, Y. G. (2006). Intraocular cytokine environment in active Behcet uveitis. *Am J Ophthalmol*, 142(3), 429–34.

Ahuja, S. K. & He, W. (2010). Double-edged genetic swords and immunity: Lesson from CCR5 and beyond. *J Infect Dis*, 201(2), 171–4.

Albright, A. V., Shieh, J. T., Itoh, T., Lee, B., Pleasure, D., O'Connor, M. J., et al. (1999). Microglia express CCR5, CXCR4, and CCR3, but of these, CCR5 is the principal co-receptor for human immunodeficiency virus type 1 dementia isolates. *J Virol*, 73(1), 205–13.

Alkhatib, G., Combadiere, C., Broder, C. C., Feng, Y., Kennedy, P. E., Murphy, P. M., et al. (1996). CC CKR5: A RANTES, MIP-1alpha, MIP-1beta receptor as a fusion cofactor for macrophage-tropic HIV-1. *Science*, 272(5270), 1955–8.

Ancuta, P., Rao, R., Moses, A., Mehle, A., Shaw, S. K., Luscinskas, F. W., et al. (2003). Fractalkine preferentially mediates arrest and migration of CD16+ monocytes. *J Exp Med*, 197(12), 1701–7.

Anderson, P. L., Kakuda, T. N., & Lichtenstein, K. A. (2004). The cellular pharmacology of nucleoside- and nucleotide-analogue reverse-transcriptase inhibitors and its relationship to clinical toxicities. *Clin Infect Dis*, 38(5), 743–53.

Anderson, S., Bankier, A. T., Barrell, B. G., de Bruijn, M. H., Coulson, A. R., Drouin, J., et al. (1981). Sequence and organization of the human mitochondrial genome. *Nature*, 290(5806), 457–65.

Antinori, A., Arendt, G., Becker, J. T., Brew, B. J., Byrd, D. A., Cherner, M., et al. (2007). Updated research nosology for HIV-associated neurocognitive disorders. *Neurology*, 69(18), 1789–99.

Arendt, G., de Nocker, D., von Giesen, H. J., & Nolting, T. (2007). Neuropsychiatric side effects of efavirenz therapy. *Expert Opin Drug Saf*, 6(2), 147–54.

Ariza, A., von Uexkull-Guldeband, C., Mate, J. L., Isamat, M., Aracil, C., Cruz-Sanchez, F. F., et al. (1996). Accumulation of wild-type p53 protein in progressive multifocal leukoencephalopathy: A flow of cytometry and DNA sequencing study. *J Neuropathol Exp Neurol*, 55(2), 144–9.

Asare, E., Dunn, G., Glass, J., McArthur, J., Luthert, P., Lantos, P., et al. (1996). Neuronal pattern correlates with the severity of human immunodeficiency virus-associated dementia complex. Usefulness of spatial pattern analysis in clinicopathological studies. *Am J Pathol*, 148(1), 31–8.

Atamna, H. (2004). Heme, iron, and the mitochondrial decay of ageing. *Ageing Res Rev*, 3(3), 303–18.

Atchison, R. E., Gosling, J., Monteclaro, F. S., Franci, C., Digilio, L., Charo, I. F., et al. (1996). Multiple extracellular elements of CCR5 and HIV-1 entry: Dissociation from response to chemokines. *Science*, 274(5294), 1924–6.

Baloh, R. H. (2008). Mitochondrial dynamics and peripheral neuropathy. *Neuroscientist*, 14(1), 12–8.

Becker, J. T., Kingsley, L., Mullen, J., Cohen, B., Martin, E., Miller, E. N., et al. (2009). Vascular risk factors, HIV serostatus, and cognitive dysfunction in gay and bisexual men. *Neurology*, 73(16), 1292–9.

Berger, E. A., Murphy, P. M., & Farber, J. M. (1999). Chemokine receptors as HIV-1 co-receptors: Roles in viral entry, tropism, and disease. *Annu Rev Immunol*, 17, 657–700.

Berger, J. R., Levy, R. M., Flomenhoft, D., & Dobbs, M. (1998). Predictive factors for prolonged survival in acquired immunodeficiency syndrome-associated progressive multifocal leukoencephalopathy. *Ann Neurol*, 44(3), 341–9.

Berger, O., Gan, X., Gujuluva, C., Burns, A. R., Sulur, G., Stins, M., et al. (1999). CXC and CC chemokine receptors on coronary and brain endothelia. *Mol Med*, 5(12), 795–805.

Bhaskaran, K., Mussini, C., Antinori, A., Walker, A. S., Dorrucci, M., Sabin, C., et al. (2008). Changes in the incidence and predictors of human immunodeficiency virus-associated dementia in the era of highly active antiretroviral therapy. *Ann Neurol*, 63(2), 213–21.

Boring, L., Gosling, J., Chensue, S. W., Kunkel, S. L., Farese, R. V., Jr., Broxmeyer, H. E., et al. (1997). Impaired monocyte migration and reduced type 1 (Th1) cytokine responses in C-C chemokine receptor 2 knockout mice. *J Clin Invest*, 100(10), 2552–61.

Boven, L. A., van der Bruggen, T., van Asbeck, B. S., Marx, J. J., & Nottet, H. S. (1999). Potential role of CCR5 polymorphism in the development of AIDS dementia complex. *FEMS Immunol Med Microbiol*, 26(3–4), 243–7.

Brabers, N. A., & Nottet, H. S. (2006). Role of the pro-inflammatory cytokines TNF-alpha and IL-1beta in HIV-associated dementia. *Eur J Clin Invest*, 36(7), 447–58.

Bras, J. M. & Singleton, A. (2009). Genetic susceptibility in Parkinson's disease. *Biochim Biophys Acta*, 1792(7), 597–603.

Brew, B. J., Crowe, S. M., Landay, A., Cysique, L. A., & Guillemin, G. (2009). Neurodegeneration and ageing in the HAART era. *J Neuroimmune Pharmacol*, 4(2), 163–74.

Brouwers, N., Sleegers, K., & Van Broeckhoven, C. (2008). Molecular genetics of Alzheimer's disease: An update. *Ann Med*, 40(8), 562–83.

Bukrinsky, M. I., Nottet, H. S., Schmidtmayerova, H., Dubrovsky, L., Flanagan, C. R., Mullins, M. E., et al. (1995). Regulation of nitric oxide synthase activity in human immunodeficiency virus type 1 (HIV-1)-infected monocytes: Implications for HIV-associated neurological disease. *J Exp Med*, 181(2), 735–45.

Burt, T. D., Agan, B. K., Marconi, V. C., He, W., Kulkarni, H., Mold, J. E., et al. (2008). Apolipoprotein (apo) E4 enhances HIV-1 cell entry in vitro, and the APOE epsilon4/epsilon4 genotype accelerates HIV disease progression. *Proc Natl Acad Sci USA*, 105(25), 8718–23.

Cacabelos, R. (2009). Pharmacogenomics and therapeutic strategies for dementia. *Expert Rev Mol Diagn*, 9(6), 567–611.

Canter, J. A., Haas, D. W., Kallianpur, A. R., Ritchie, M. D., Robbins, G. K., Shafer, R. W., et al. (2008). The mitochondrial pharmacogenomics of haplogroup T: MTND2*LHON4917G and antiretroviral therapy-associated peripheral neuropathy. *Pharmacogenomics J*, 8(1), 71–7.

Carrington, M., Dean, M., Martin, M. P., & O'Brien, S. J. (1999a). Genetics of HIV-1 infection: Chemokine receptor CCR5 polymorphism and its consequences. *Hum Mol Genet*, 8(10), 1939–45.

Carrington, M., Nelson, G. W., Martin, M. P., Kissner, T., Vlahov, D., Goedert, J. J., et al. (1999b). HLA and HIV-1: Heterozygote advantage and B*35-Cw*04 disadvantage. *Science*, 283(5408), 1748–52.

Catano, G., Agan, B. K., Kulkarni, H., Telles, V., Marconi, V. C., Dolan, M. J., et al. (2008). Independent effects of genetic variations in mannose-binding lectin influence the course of HIV disease: The advantage of heterozygosity for coding mutations. *J Infect Dis*, 198(1), 72–80.

Charo, I. F., Myers, S. J., Herman, A., Franci, C., Connolly, A. J., & Coughlin, S. R. (1994). Molecular cloning and functional expression of two monocyte chemoattractant protein 1 receptors reveals alternative splicing of the carboxyl-terminal tails. *Proc Natl Acad Sci USA*, 91(7), 2752–6.

Cherner, M., Ellis, R. J., Lazzaretto, D., Young, C., Mindt, M. R., Atkinson, J. H., et al. (2004). Effects of HIV-1 infection and aging on neurobehavioral functioning: Preliminary findings. *AIDS*, 18 Suppl 1, S27–34.

Cherner, M., Letendre, S., Heaton, R. K., Durelle, J., Marquie-Beck, J., Gragg, B., et al. (2005). Hepatitis C augments cognitive deficits associated with HIV infection and methamphetamine. *Neurology*, 64(8), 1343–7.

Cherry, C. L., Rosenow, A., Affandi, J. S., McArthur, J. C., Wesselingh, S. L., & Price, P. (2008). Cytokine genotype suggests a role for inflammation in nucleoside analog-associated sensory neuropathy (NRTI-SN) and predicts an individual's NRTI-SN risk. *AIDS Res Hum Retroviruses*, 24(2), 117–23.

Cinque, P., Koralnik, I. J., Gerevini, S., Miro, J. M., & Price, R. W. (2009). Progressive multifocal leukoencephalopathy in HIV-1 infection. *Lancet Infect Dis*, 9(10), 625–36.

Cinque, P., Vago, L., Mengozzi, M., Torri, V., Ceresa, D., Vicenzi, E., et al. (1998). Elevated cerebrospinal fluid levels of monocyte chemotactic protein-1 correlate with HIV-1 encephalitis and local viral replication. *AIDS*, 12(11), 1327–32.

Colobran, R., Pedrosa, E., Carretero-Iglesia, L., & Juan, M. (2010). Copy number variation in chemokine superfamily: The complex scene of CCL3L-CCL4L genes in health and disease. *Clin Exp Immunol*, 162(1), 41–52.

Corder, E. H., Robertson, K., Lannfelt, L., Bogdanovic, N., Eggertsen, G., Wilkins, J., et al. (1998). HIV-infected subjects with the E4 allele for APOE have excess dementia and peripheral neuropathy. *Nat Med*, 4(10), 1182–4.

Corder, E. H., Saunders, A. M., Strittmatter, W. J., Schmechel, D. E., Gaskell, P. C., Small, G. W., et al. (1993). Gene dose of apolipoprotein E type 4 allele and the risk of Alzheimer's disease in late onset families. *Science*, 261(5123), 921–3.

Costarelli, S., Torti, C., Gatta, L. B., Tinelli, C., Lapadula, G., Quiros-Roldan, E., et al. (2007). No evidence of relation between peripheral neuropathy and presence of hemochromatosis gene mutations in HIV-1-positive patients. *J Acquir Immune Defic Syndr*, 46(2), 255–6.

Cysique, L. A. & Brew, B. J. (2009). Neuropsychological functioning and antiretroviral treatment in HIV/AIDS: A review. *Neuropsychol Rev*, 19(2), 169–85.

Cysique, L. A., Maruff, P., & Brew, B. J. (2004). Prevalence and pattern of neuropsychological impairment in human immunodeficiency virus-infected/acquired immunodeficiency syndrome (HIV/AIDS) patients across pre- and post-highly active antiretroviral therapy eras: A combined study of two cohorts. *J Neurovirol*, 10(6), 350–7.

Dalakas, M. C., Semino-Mora, C., & Leon-Monzon, M. (2001). Mitochondrial alterations with mitochondrial DNA depletion in the nerves of AIDS patients with peripheral neuropathy induced by 2'3'-dideoxycytidine (ddC). *Lab Invest*, 81(11), 1537–44.

de Kovel, C. G., Pinto, D., Tauer, U., Lorenz, S., Muhle, H., Leu, C., et al. (2010). Whole-genome linkage scan for epilepsy-related photosensitivity: A mega-analysis. *Epilepsy Res*, 89(2–3), 286–94.

de Roda Husman, A. M., Koot, M., Cornelissen, M., Keet, I. P., Brouwer, M., Broersen, S. M., et al. (1997). Association between CCR5 genotype and the clinical course of HIV-1 infection. *Ann Intern Med*, 127(10), 882–90.

Deng, H., Liu, R., Ellmeier, W., Choe, S., Unutmaz, D., Burkhart, M., et al. (1996). Identification of a major co-receptor for primary isolates of HIV-1. *Nature*, 381(6584), 661–6.

Deshmane, S. L., Kremlev, S., Amini, S., & Sawaya, B. E. (2009). Monocyte chemoattractant protein-1 (MCP-1): An overview. *J Interferon Cytokine Res*, 29(6), 313–26.

Dhillon, N. K., Williams, R., Callen, S., Zien, C., Narayan, O., & Buch, S. (2008). Roles of MCP-1 in development of HIV-dementia. *Front Biosci*, 13, 3913–8.

Diaz-Arrastia, R., Gong, Y., Kelly, C. J., & Gelman, B. B. (2004). Host genetic polymorphisms in human immunodeficiency virus-related neurologic disease. *J Neurovirol*, 10 Suppl 1, 67–73.

DiMauro, S. & Schon, E. A. (2003). Mitochondrial respiratory-chain diseases. *N Engl J Med*, 348(26), 2656–68.

Dolan, M. J., Kulkarni, H., Camargo, J. F., He, W., Smith, A., Anaya, J. M., et al. (2007). CCL3L1 and CCR5 influence cell-mediated immunity and affect HIV-AIDS pathogenesis via viral entry-independent mechanisms. *Nat Immunol*, 8(12), 1324–36.

Dore, G. J., Correll, P. K., Li, Y., Kaldor, J. M., Cooper, D. A., & Brew, B. J. (1999). Changes to AIDS dementia complex in the era of highly active antiretroviral therapy. *AIDS*, 13(10), 1249–53.

Elahi, M. M., Asotra, K., Matata, B. M., & Mastana, S. S. (2009). Tumor necrosis factor alpha-308 gene locus promoter polymorphism: An analysis of association with health and disease. *Biochim Biophys Acta*.

Ellery, P. J., Tippett, E., Chiu, Y. L., Paukovics, G., Cameron, P. U., Solomon, A., et al. (2007). The CD16+ monocyte subset is more permissive to infection and preferentially harbors HIV-1 in vivo. *J Immunol*, 178(10), 6581–9.

Ellis, R. J., Rosario, D., Clifford, D. B., McArthur, J. C., Simpson, D., Alexander, T., et al. (2010). Continued high prevalence and adverse clinical impact of human immunodeficiency virus-associated sensory neuropathy in the era of combination antiretroviral therapy: the CHARTER Study. *Arch Neurol*, 67(5), 552–8.

Eskild, A., Jonassen, T. O., Heger, B., Samuelsen, S. O., & Grinde, B. (1998). The estimated impact of the CCR-5 delta32 gene deletion on HIV disease progression varies with study design. Oslo HIV Cohort Study Group. *AIDS*, 12(17), 2271–4.

Eugenin, E. A., D'Aversa, T. G., Lopez, L., Calderon, T. M., & Berman, J. W. (2003). MCP-1 (CCL2) protects human neurons and astrocytes from NMDA or HIV-tat-induced apoptosis. *J Neurochem*, 85(5), 1299–311.

Eugenin, E. A., Osiecki, K., Lopez, L., Goldstein, H., Calderon, T. M., & Berman, J. W. (2006). CCL2/monocyte chemoattractant protein-1 mediates enhanced transmigration of human immunodeficiency virus (HIV)-infected leukocytes across the blood-brain barrier: A potential mechanism of HIV-CNS invasion and neuroAIDS. *J Neurosci, 26*(4), 1098–106.

Everall, I. P., Heaton, R. K., Marcotte, T. D., Ellis, R. J., McCutchan, J. A., Atkinson, J. H., et al. (1999). Cortical synaptic density is reduced in mild to moderate human immunodeficiency virus neurocognitive disorder. HNRC Group. HIV Neurobehavioral Research Center. *Brain Pathol, 9*(2), 209–17.

Faure, S., Meyer, L., Costagliola, D., Vaneensberghe, C., Genin, E., Autran, B., et al. (2000). Rapid progression to AIDS in HIV+ individuals with a structural variant of the chemokine receptor CX3CR1. *Science, 287*(5461), 2274–7.

Fellay, J., Marzolini, C., Meaden, E. R., Back, D. J., Buclin, T., Chave, J. P., et al. (2002). Response to antiretroviral treatment in HIV-1-infected individuals with allelic variants of the multidrug resistance transporter 1: A pharmacogenetics study. *Lancet, 359*(9300), 30–6.

Frade, J. M., Llorente, M., Mellado, M., Alcami, J., Gutierrez-Ramos, J. C., Zaballos, A., et al. (1997). The amino-terminal domain of the CCR2 chemokine receptor acts as co-receptor for HIV-1 infection. *J Clin Invest, 100*(3), 497–502.

Fumaz, C. R., Tuldra, A., Ferrer, M. J., Paredes, R., Bonjoch, A., Jou, T., et al. (2002). Quality of life, emotional status, and adherence of HIV-1-infected patients treated with efavirenz versus protease inhibitor-containing regimens. *J Acquir Immune Defic Syndr, 29*(3), 244–53.

Garcia-Suarez, J., de Miguel, D., Krsnik, I., Banas, H., Arribas, I., & Burgaleta, C. (2005). Changes in the natural history of progressive multifocal leukoencephalopathy in HIV-negative lymphoproliferative disorders: Impact of novel therapies. *Am J Hematol, 80*(4), 271–81.

Garden, G. A., Budd, S. L., Tsai, E., Hanson, L., Kaul, M., D'Emilia, D. M., et al. (2002). Caspase cascades in human immunodeficiency virus-associated neurodegeneration. *J Neurosci, 22*(10), 4015–24.

Garred, P. (2008). Mannose-binding lectin genetics: from A to Z. *Biochem Soc Trans, 36*(Pt 6), 1461–6.

Gatanaga, H., Hayashida, T., Tsuchiya, K., Yoshino, M., Kuwahara, T., Tsukada, H., et al. (2007). Successful efavirenz dose reduction in HIV type 1-infected individuals with cytochrome P450 2B6 *6 and *26. *Clin Infect Dis, 45*(9), 1230–7.

Gelbard, H. A., Nottet, H. S., Swindells, S., Jett, M., Dzenko, K. A., Genis, P., et al. (1994). Platelet-activating factor: A candidate human immunodeficiency virus type 1-induced neurotoxin. *J Virol, 68*(7), 4628–35.

Gendelman, H. E., Persidsky, Y., Ghorpade, A., Limoges, J., Stins, M., Fiala, M., et al. (1997). The neuropathogenesis of the AIDS dementia complex. *AIDS, 11* Suppl A, S35–45.

Genis, P., Jett, M., Bernton, E. W., Boyle, T., Gelbard, H. A., Dzenko, K., et al. (1992). Cytokines and arachidonic metabolites produced during human immunodeficiency virus (HIV)-infected macrophage-astroglia interactions: Implications for the neuropathogenesis of HIV disease. *J Exp Med, 176*(6), 1703–18.

Giometto, B., An, S. F., Groves, M., Scaravilli, T., Geddes, J. F., Miller, R., et al. (1997). Accumulation of beta-amyloid precursor protein in HIV encephalitis: Relationship with neuropsychological abnormalities. *Ann Neurol, 42*(1), 34–40.

Giulian, D., Yu, J., Li, X., Tom, D., Li, J., Wendt, E., et al. (1996). Study of receptor-mediated neurotoxins released by HIV-1-infected mononuclear phagocytes found in human brain. *J Neurosci, 16*(10), 3139–53.

Glass, J. D., Wesselingh, S. L., Selnes, O. A., & McArthur, J. C. (1993). Clinical-neuropathologic correlation in HIV-associated dementia. *Neurology, 43*(11), 2230–7.

Glass, W. G., McDermott, D. H., Lim, J. K., Lekhong, S., Yu, S. F., Frank, W. A., et al. (2006). CCR5 deficiency increases risk of symptomatic West Nile virus infection. *J Exp Med, 203*(1), 35–40.

Gonzalez, E., Bamshad, M., Sato, N., Mummidi, S., Dhanda, R., Catano, G., et al. (1999). Race-specific HIV-1 disease-modifying effects associated with CCR5 haplotypes. *Proc Natl Acad Sci USA, 96*(21), 12004–9.

Gonzalez, E., Kulkarni, H., Bolivar, H., Mangano, A., Sanchez, R., Catano, G., et al. (2005). The influence of CCL3L1 gene-containing segmental duplications on HIV-1/AIDS susceptibility. *Science, 307*(5714), 1434–40.

Gonzalez, E., Rovin, B. H., Sen, L., Cooke, G., Dhanda, R., Mummidi, S., et al. (2002). HIV-1 infection and AIDS dementia are influenced by a mutant MCP-1 allele linked to increased monocyte infiltration of tissues and MCP-1 levels. *Proc Natl Acad Sci USA, 99*(21), 13795–800.

Gras, G. & Kaul, M. (2010). Molecular mechanisms of neuroinvasion by monocytes-macrophages in HIV-1 infection. *Retrovirology, 7*, 30.

Gregg, R. E., Zech, L. A., Schaefer, E. J., Stark, D., Wilson, D., & Brewer, H. B., Jr. (1986). Abnormal in vivo metabolism of apolipoprotein E4 in humans. *J Clin Invest, 78*(3), 815–21.

Grimaldi, L. M., Martino, G. V., Franciotta, D. M., Brustia, R., Castagna, A., Pristera, R., et al. (1991). Elevated alpha-tumor necrosis factor levels in spinal fluid from HIV-1-infected patients with central nervous system involvement. *Ann Neurol, 29*(1), 21–5.

Guerini, F. R., Delbue, S., Zanzottera, M., Agliardi, C., Saresella, M., Mancuso, R., et al. (2008). Analysis of CCR5, CCR2, SDF1 and RANTES gene polymorphisms in subjects with HIV-related PML and not determined leukoencephalopathy. *Biomed Pharmacother, 62*(1), 26–30.

Haas, D. W., Ribaudo, H. J., Kim, R. B., Tierney, C., Wilkinson, G. R., Gulick, R. M., et al. (2004). Pharmacogenetics of efavirenz and central nervous system side effects: an Adult AIDS Clinical Trials Group study. *AIDS, 18*(18), 2391–400.

Haas, D. W., Smeaton, L. M., Shafer, R. W., Robbins, G. K., Morse, G. D., Labbe, L., et al. (2005). Pharmacogenetics of long-term responses to antiretroviral regimens containing Efavirenz and/or Nelfinavir: An Adult Aids Clinical Trials Group Study. *J Infect Dis, 192*(11), 1931–42.

Hadley, T. J. & Peiper, S. C. (1997). From malaria to chemokine receptor: The emerging physiologic role of the Duffy blood group antigen. *Blood, 89*(9), 3077–91.

Hawkins, T., Geist, C., Young, B., Giblin, A., Mercier, R. C., Thornton, K., et al. (2005). Comparison of neuropsychiatric side effects in an observational cohort of efavirenz- and protease inhibitor-treated patients. *HIV Clin Trials, 6*(4), 187–96.

He, W., Neil, S., Kulkarni, H., Wright, E., Agan, B. K., Marconi, V. C., et al. (2008). Duffy antigen receptor for chemokines mediates trans-infection of HIV-1 from red blood cells to target cells and affects HIV-AIDS susceptibility. *Cell Host Microbe, 4*(1), 52–62.

Herrnstadt, C. & Howell, N. (2004). An evolutionary perspective on pathogenic mtDNA mutations: Haplogroup associations of clinical disorders. *Mitochondrion, 4*(5–6), 791–8.

Heyes, M. P., Ellis, R. J., Ryan, L., Childers, M. E., Grant, I., Wolfson, T., et al. (2001). Elevated cerebrospinal fluid quinolinic acid levels are associated with region-specific cerebral volume loss in HIV infection. *Brain, 124*(Pt 5), 1033–42.

Hill, A. V. (2006). Aspects of genetic susceptibility to human infectious diseases. *Annu Rev Genet, 40*, 469–86.

Hill, J. M., Bhattacharjee, P. S., & Neumann, D. M. (2007). Apolipoprotein E alleles can contribute to the pathogenesis of numerous clinical conditions including HSV-1 corneal disease. *Exp Eye Res, 84*(5), 801–11.

Hirsch, V. M., Sharkey, M. E., Brown, C. R., Brichacek, B., Goldstein, S., Wakefield, J., et al. (1998). Vpx is required for dissemination and pathogenesis of SIV(SM) PBj: Evidence of macrophage-dependent viral amplification. *Nat Med, 4*(12), 1401–8.

Hladik, F., Liu, H., Speelmon, E., Livingston-Rosanoff, D., Wilson, S., Sakchalathorn, P., et al. (2005). Combined effect of CCR5-Delta32 heterozygosity and the CCR5 promoter polymorphism -2459 A/G on CCR5 expression and resistance to human immunodeficiency virus type 1 transmission. *J Virol, 79*(18), 11677–84.

Horne, K. & Woolley, I. J. (2009). Shedding light on DARC: The role of the Duffy antigen/receptor for chemokines in inflammation, infection and malignancy. *Inflamm Res, 58*(8), 431–5.

Huang, Y., Paxton, W. A., Wolinsky, S. M., Neumann, A. U., Zhang, L., He, T., et al. (1996). The role of a mutant CCR5 allele in HIV-1 transmission and disease progression. *Nat Med, 2*(11), 1240–3.

Hulgan, T., Haas, D. W., Haines, J. L., Ritchie, M. D., Robbins, G. K., Shafer, R. W., et al. (2005). Mitochondrial haplogroups and peripheral neuropathy during antiretroviral therapy: An adult AIDS clinical trials group study. *AIDS*, *19*(13), 1341–9.

Ioannidis, J. P., Rosenberg, P. S., Goedert, J. J., Ashton, L. J., Benfield, T. L., Buchbinder, S. P., et al. (2001). Effects of CCR5-Delta32, CCR2-64I, and SDF-1 3'A alleles on HIV-1 disease progression: An international meta-analysis of individual-patient data. *Ann Intern Med*, *135*(9), 782–95.

Ip, W. K., Takahashi, K., Ezekowitz, R. A., & Stuart, L. M. (2009). Mannose-binding lectin and innate immunity. *Immunol Rev*, *230*(1), 9–21.

Kallianpur, A. R., Hulgan, T., Canter, J. A., Ritchie, M. D., Haines, J. L., Robbins, G. K., et al. (2006). Hemochromatosis (HFE) gene mutations and peripheral neuropathy during antiretroviral therapy. *AIDS*, *20*(11), 1503–13.

Kawamura, T., Gulden, F. O., Sugaya, M., McNamara, D. T., Borris, D. L., Lederman, M. M., et al. (2003). R5 HIV productively infects Langerhans cells, and infection levels are regulated by compound CCR5 polymorphisms. *Proc Natl Acad Sci USA*, *100*(14), 8401–6.

Kelder, W., McArthur, J. C., Nance-Sproson, T., McClernon, D., & Griffin, D. E. (1998). Beta-chemokines MCP-1 and RANTES are selectively increased in cerebrospinal fluid of patients with human immunodeficiency virus-associated dementia. *Ann Neurol*, *44*(5), 831–5.

Keswani, S. C., Pardo, C. A., Cherry, C. L., Hoke, A., & McArthur, J. C. (2002). HIV-associated sensory neuropathies. *AIDS*, *16*(16), 2105–17.

Kindberg, E., Mickiene, A., Ax, C., Akerlind, B., Vene, S., Lindquist, L., et al. (2008). A deletion in the chemokine receptor 5 (CCR5) gene is associated with tickborne encephalitis. *J Infect Dis*, *197*(2), 266–9.

Knudsen, T. B., Kristiansen, T. B., Katzenstein, T. L., & Eugen-Olsen, J. (2001). Adverse effect of the CCR5 promoter -2459A allele on HIV-1 disease progression. *J Med Virol*, *65*(3), 441–4.

Koralnik, I. J., Du Pasquier, R. A., Kuroda, M. J., Schmitz, J. E., Dang, X., Zheng, Y., et al. (2002). Association of prolonged survival in HLA-A2+ progressive multifocal leukoencephalopathy patients with a CTL response specific for a commonly recognized JC virus epitope. *J Immunol*, *168*(1), 499–504.

Kostrikis, L. G., Huang, Y., Moore, J. P., Wolinsky, S. M., Zhang, L., Guo, Y., et al. (1998). A chemokine receptor CCR2 allele delays HIV-1 disease progression and is associated with a CCR5 promoter mutation. *Nat Med*, *4*(3), 350–3.

Kostrikis, L. G., Neumann, A. U., Thomson, B., Korber, B. T., McHardy, P., Karanicolas, R., et al. (1999). A polymorphism in the regulatory region of the CC-chemokine receptor 5 gene influences perinatal transmission of human immunodeficiency virus type 1 to African-American infants. *J Virol*, *73*(12), 10264–71.

Kulkarni, H., Marconi, V. C., He, W., Landrum, M. L., Okulicz, J. F., Delmar, J., et al. (2009). The Duffy-null state is associated with a survival advantage in leukopenic HIV-infected persons of African ancestry. *Blood*, *114*(13), 2783–92.

Kwa, D., Boeser-Nunnink, B., & Schuitemaker, H. (2003). Lack of evidence for an association between a polymorphism in CX3CR1 and the clinical course of HIV infection or virus phenotype evolution. *AIDS*, *17*(5), 759–61.

Lachgar, A., Jaureguiberry, G., Le Buenac, H., Bizzini, B., Zagury, J. F., Rappaport, J., et al. (1998). Binding of HIV-1 to RBCs involves the Duffy antigen receptors for chemokines (DARC). *Biomed Pharmacother*, *52*(10), 436–9.

Langford, T. D., Letendre, S. L., Larrea, G. J., & Masliah, E. (2003). Changing patterns in the neuropathogenesis of HIV during the HAART era. *Brain Pathol*, *13*(2), 195–210.

Larsen, F., Madsen, H. O., Sim, R. B., Koch, C., & Garred, P. (2004). Disease-associated mutations in human mannose-binding lectin compromise oligomerization and activity of the final protein. *J Biol Chem*, *279*(20), 21302–11.

Lee, B., Doranz, B. J., Rana, S., Yi, Y., Mellado, M., Frade, J. M., Martinez, A. C., et al. (1998). Influence of the CCR2-V64I polymorphism on human immunodeficiency virus type 1 co-receptor activity and on chemokine receptor function of CCR2b, CCR3, CCR5, and CXCR4. *J Virol*, *72*(9), 7450–8.

Levine, A. J., Singer, E. J., & Shapshak, P. (2009). The role of host genetics in the susceptibility for HIV-associated neurocognitive disorders. *AIDS Behav*, *13*(1), 118–32.

Levine, A. J., Singer, E. J., Sinsheimer, J. S., Hinkin, C. H., Papp, J., Dandekar, S., et al. (2009). CCL3 genotype and current depression increase risk of HIV-associated dementia. *Neurobehav HIV Med*, *1*, 1–7.

Lichtenstein, K. A., Armon, C., Baron, A., Moorman, A. C., Wood, K. C., & Holmberg, S. D. (2005). Modification of the incidence of drug-associated symmetrical peripheral neuropathy by host and disease factors in the HIV outpatient study cohort. *Clin Infect Dis*, *40*(1), 148–57.

Lim, J. K., Lisco, A., McDermott, D. H., Huynh, L., Ward, J. M., Johnson, B., et al. (2009). Genetic variation in OAS1 is a risk factor for initial infection with West Nile virus in man. *PLoS Pathog*, *5*(2), e1000321.

Lim, J. K., Louie, C. Y., Glaser, C., Jean, C., Johnson, B., Johnson, H., et al. (2008). Genetic deficiency of chemokine receptor CCR5 is a strong risk factor for symptomatic West Nile virus infection: A meta-analysis of 4 cohorts in the US epidemic. *J Infect Dis*, *197*(2), 262–5.

Lim, J. K., McDermott, D. H., Lisco, A., Foster, G. A., Krysztof, D., Follmann, D., et al. (2010). CCR5 deficiency is a risk factor for early clinical manifestations of West Nile virus infection but not for viral transmission. *J Infect Dis*, *201*(2), 178–85.

Liu, R., Paxton, W. A., Choe, S., Ceradini, D., Martin, S. R., Horuk, R., et al. (1996). Homozygous defect in HIV-1 co-receptor accounts for resistance of some multiply-exposed individuals to HIV-1 infection. *Cell*, *86*(3), 367–77.

Madsen, H. O., Garred, P., Thiel, S., Kurtzhals, J. A., Lamm, L. U., Ryder, L. P., et al. (1995). Interplay between promoter and structural gene variants control basal serum level of mannan-binding protein. *J Immunol*, *155*(6), 3013–20.

Mahley, R. W. (1988). Apolipoprotein E: Cholesterol transport protein with expanding role in cell biology. *Science*, *240*(4852), 622–30.

Mahley, R. W. & Rall, S. C., Jr. (2000). Apolipoprotein E: Far more than a lipid transport protein. *Annu Rev Genomics Hum Genet*, *1*, 507–37.

Mahley, R. W., Weisgraber, K. H., & Huang, Y. (2009). Apolipoprotein E: structure determines function, from atherosclerosis to Alzheimer's disease to AIDS. *J Lipid Res*, *50* Suppl, S183–8.

Mallal, S., Phillips, E., Carosi, G., Molina, J. M., Workman, C., Tomazic, J., et al. (2008). HLA-B*5701 screening for hypersensitivity to abacavir. *N Engl J Med*, *358*(6), 568–79.

Mangano, A., Gonzalez, E., Dhanda, R., Catano, G., Bamshad, M., Bock, A., et al. (2001). Concordance between the CC chemokine receptor 5 genetic determinants that alter risks of transmission and disease progression in children exposed perinatally to human immunodeficiency virus. *J Infect Dis*, *183*(11), 1574–85.

Mangano, A., Rocco, C., Marino, S. M., Mecikovsky, D., Genre, F., Aulicino, P., et al. (2008). Detrimental effects of mannose-binding lectin (MBL2) promoter genotype XA/XA on HIV-1 vertical transmission and AIDS progression. *J Infect Dis*, *198*(5), 694–700.

Mariani, R., Wong, S., Mulder, L. C., Wilkinson, D. A., Reinhart, A. L., LaRosa, G., et al. (1999). CCR2–64I polymorphism is not associated with altered CCR5 expression or co-receptor function. *J Virol*, *73*(3), 2450–9.

Martin, I., Dubois, M. C., Saermark, T., & Ruysschaert, J. M. (1992). Apolipoprotein A-1 interacts with the N-terminal fusogenic domains of SIV (simian immunodeficiency virus) GP32 and HIV (human immunodeficiency virus) GP41: Implications in viral entry. *Biochem Biophys Res Commun*, *186*(1), 95–101.

Martin, M. P., Dean, M., Smith, M. W., Winkler, C., Gerrard, B., Michael, N. L., et al. (1998). Genetic acceleration of AIDS progression by a promoter variant of CCR5. *Science*, *282*(5395), 1907–11.

Marzolini, C., Telenti, A., Decosterd, L. A., Greub, G., Biollaz, J., & Buclin, T. (2001). Efavirenz plasma levels can predict treatment failure and central nervous system side effects in HIV-1-infected patients. *AIDS*, *15*(1), 71–5.

Masliah, E., Heaton, R. K., Marcotte, T. D., Ellis, R. J., Wiley, C. A., Mallory, M., et al. (1997). Dendritic injury is a pathological substrate for human immunodeficiency virus-related cognitive disorders. HNRC Group. The HIV Neurobehavioral Research Center. *Ann Neurol, 42*(6), 963–72.

McArthur, J. C. & Brew, B. J. (2010). HIV-associated neurocognitive disorders: Is there a hidden epidemic? *AIDS, 24*(9), 1367–70.

McArthur, J. C., Hoover, D. R., Bacellar, H., Miller, E. N., Cohen, B. A., Becker, J. T., et al. (1993). Dementia in AIDS patients: Incidence and risk factors. Multicenter AIDS Cohort Study. *Neurology, 43*(11), 2245–52.

McArthur, J. C., Steiner, J., Sacktor, N., & Nath, A. (2010). Human immunodeficiency virus-associated neurocognitive disorders: Mind the gap. *Ann Neurol, 67*(6), 699–714.

McDermott, D. H., Colla, J. S., Kleeberger, C. A., Plankey, M., Rosenberg, P. S., Smith, E. D., et al. (2000). Genetic polymorphism in CX3CR1 and risk of HIV disease. *Science, 290*(5499), 2031.

McDermott, D. H., Zimmerman, P. A., Guignard, F., Kleeberger, C. A., Leitman, S. F., & Murphy, P. M. (1998). CCR5 promoter polymorphism and HIV-1 disease progression. Multicenter AIDS Cohort Study (MACS). *Lancet, 352*(9131), 866–70.

Menten, P., Wuyts, A., & Van Damme, J. (2002). Macrophage inflammatory protein-1. *Cytokine Growth Factor Rev, 13*(6), 455–81.

Meyer, L., Magierowska, M., Hubert, J. B., Theodorou, I., van Rij, R., Prins, M., et al. (1999). CC-chemokine receptor variants, SDF-1 polymorphism, and disease progression in 720 HIV-infected patients. SEROCO Cohort. Amsterdam Cohort Studies on AIDS. *AIDS, 13*(5), 624–6.

Michael, N. L., Louie, L. G., Rohrbaugh, A. L., Schultz, K. A., Dayhoff, D. E., Wang, C. E., et al. (1997). The role of CCR5 and CCR2 polymorphisms in HIV-1 transmission and disease progression. *Nat Med, 3*(10), 1160–2.

Motsinger, A. A., Ritchie, M. D., Shafer, R. W., Robbins, G. K., Morse, G. D., Labbe, L., et al. (2006). Multilocus genetic interactions and response to efavirenz-containing regimens: An adult AIDS clinical trials group study. *Pharmacogenet Genomics, 16*(11), 837–45.

Muller, M., Wandel, S., Colebunders, R., Attia, S., Furrer, H., & Egger, M. (2010). Immune reconstitution inflammatory syndrome in patients starting antiretroviral therapy for HIV infection: A systematic review and meta-analysis. *Lancet Infect Dis, 10*(4), 251–61.

Mummidi, S., Ahuja, S. S., Gonzalez, E., Anderson, S. A., Santiago, E. N., Stephan, K. T., et al. (1998). Genealogy of the CCR5 locus and chemokine system gene variants associated with altered rates of HIV-1 disease progression. *Nat Med, 4*(7), 786–93.

Mummidi, S., Bamshad, M., Ahuja, S. S., Gonzalez, E., Feuillet, P. M., Begum, K., et al. (2000). Evolution of human and non-human primate CC chemokine receptor 5 gene and mRNA. Potential roles for haplotype and mRNA diversity, differential haplotype-specific transcriptional activity, and altered transcription factor binding to polymorphic nucleotides in the pathogenesis of HIV-1 and simian immunodeficiency virus. *J Biol Chem, 275*(25), 18946–61.

Munoz-Moreno, J. A., Fumaz, C. R., Ferrer, M. J., Gonzalez-Garcia, M., Molto, J., Negredo, E., et al. (2009). Neuropsychiatric symptoms associated with efavirenz: prevalence, correlates, and management. A neurobehavioral review. *AIDS Rev, 11*(2), 103–9.

Murray, J. M., McDonald, A. M., & Law, M. G. (2009). Rapidly ageing HIV epidemic among men who have sex with men in Australia. *Sex Health, 6*(1), 83–6.

Nalls, M. A., Wilson, J. G., Patterson, N. J., Tandon, A., Zmuda, J. M., Huntsman, S., et al. (2008). Admixture mapping of white cell count: Genetic locus responsible for lower white blood cell count in the Health ABC and Jackson Heart studies. *Am J Hum Genet, 82*(1), 81–7.

Nottet, H. S., Jett, M., Flanagan, C. R., Zhai, Q. H., Persidsky, Y., Rizzino, A., et al. (1995). A regulatory role for astrocytes in HIV-1 encephalitis. An overexpression of eicosanoids, platelet-activating factor, and tumor necrosis factor-alpha by activated HIV-1-infected monocytes is attenuated by primary human astrocytes. *J Immunol, 154*(7), 3567–81.

Ometto, L., Bertorelle, R., Mainardi, M., Zanchetta, M., Tognazzo, S., Rampon, O., et al. (2001). Polymorphisms in the CCR5 promoter region influence disease progression in perinatally human immunodeficiency virus type 1-infected children. *J Infect Dis, 183*(5), 814–8.

Pardo, L. M., & van Duijn, C. M. (2005). In search of genes involved in neurodegenerative disorders. *Mutat Res, 592*(1–2), 89–101.

Park, K., Kim, N., Nam, J., Bang, D., & Lee, E. S. (2006). Association of TNFA promoter region haplotype in Behcet's Disease. *J Korean Med Sci, 21*(4), 596–601.

Pemberton, L. A., Stone, E., Price, P., van Bockxmeer, F., & Brew, B. J. (2008). The relationship between ApoE, TNFA, IL1a, IL1b and IL12b genes and HIV-1-associated dementia. *HIV Med, 9*(8), 677–80.

Perez-Molina, J. A. (2002). Safety and tolerance of efavirenz in different antiretroviral regimens: Results from a national multicenter prospective study in 1,033 HIV-infected patients. *HIV Clin Trials, 3*(4), 279–86.

Pietrangelo, A. (2004). Hereditary hemochromatosis—a new look at an old disease. *N Engl J Med, 350*(23), 2383–97.

Pinholt, M., Frederiksen, J. L., & Christiansen, M. (2006). The association between apolipoprotein E and multiple sclerosis. *Eur J Neurol, 13*(6), 573–80.

Pociot, F., Molvig, J., Wogensen, L., Worsaae, H., & Nerup, J. (1992). A TaqI polymorphism in the human interleukin-1 beta (IL-1 beta) gene correlates with IL-1 beta secretion in vitro. *Eur J Clin Invest, 22*(6), 396–402.

Pomara, N., Belzer, K., & Sidtis, J. J. (2008). Deleterious CNS effects of the APOE epsilon4 allele in individuals with HIV-1 infection may be age-dependent. *Proc Natl Acad Sci USA, 105*(41), E65; author reply E67–8.

Power, C., Gladden, J. G., Halliday, W., Del Bigio, M. R., Nath, A., Ni, W., et al. (2000). AIDS- and non-AIDS-related PML association with distinct p53 polymorphism. *Neurology, 54*(3), 743–6.

Presanis, J. S., Kojima, M., & Sim, R. B. (2003). Biochemistry and genetics of mannan-binding lectin (MBL). *Biochem Soc Trans, 31*(Pt 4), 748–52.

Pulliam, L., Gascon, R., Stubblebine, M., McGuire, D., & McGrath, M. S. (1997). Unique monocyte subset in patients with AIDS dementia. *Lancet, 349*(9053), 692–5.

Quasney, M. W., Zhang, Q., Sargent, S., Mynatt, M., Glass, J., & McArthur, J. (2001). Increased frequency of the tumor necrosis factor-alpha-308 A allele in adults with human immunodeficiency virus dementia. *Ann Neurol, 50*(2), 157–62.

Rademakers, R., Cruts, M., & Van Broeckhoven, C. (2003). Genetics of early-onset Alzheimer dementia. *Scientific World Journal, 3*, 497–519.

Rademakers, R. & Rovelet-Lecrux, A. (2009). Recent insights into the molecular genetics of dementia. *Trends Neurosci, 32*(8), 451–61.

Raffai, R. L., Dong, L. M., Farese, R. V., Jr., & Weisgraber, K. H. (2001). Introduction of human apolipoprotein E4 "domain interaction" into mouse apolipoprotein E. *Proc Natl Acad Sci USA, 98*(20), 11587–91.

Reich, D., Nalls, M. A., Kao, W. H., Akylbekova, E. L., Tandon, A., Patterson, N., et al. (2009). Reduced neutrophil count in people of African descent is due to a regulatory variant in the Duffy antigen receptor for chemokines gene. *PLoS Genet, 5*(1), e1000360.

Ribaudo, H. J., Haas, D. W., Tierney, C., Kim, R. B., Wilkinson, G. R., Gulick, R. M., et al. (2006). Pharmacogenetics of plasma efavirenz exposure after treatment discontinuation: An Adult AIDS Clinical Trials Group Study. *Clin Infect Dis, 42*(3), 401–7.

Richardson, E. P., Jr. (1961). Progressive multifocal leukoencephalopathy. *N Engl J Med, 265*, 815–23.

Riedel, D. J., Pardo, C. A., McArthur, J., & Nath, A. (2006). Therapy Insight: CNS manifestations of HIV-associated immune reconstitution inflammatory syndrome. *Nat Clin Pract Neurol, 2*(10), 557–65.

Rippeth, J. D., Heaton, R. K., Carey, C. L., Marcotte, T. D., Moore, D. J., Gonzalez, R., et al. (2004). Methamphetamine dependence increases risk of neuropsychological impairment in HIV infected persons. *J Int Neuropsychol Soc, 10*(1), 1–14.

Robertson, K. R., Smurzynski, M., Parsons, T. D., Wu, K., Bosch, R. J., Wu, J., et al. (2007). The prevalence and incidence of neurocognitive impairment in the HAART era. *AIDS, 21*(14), 1915–21.

Rotger, M., Colombo, S., Furrer, H., Bleiber, G., Buclin, T., Lee, B. L., et al. (2005). Influence of CYP2B6 polymorphism on plasma and intracellular concentrations and toxicity of efavirenz and nevirapine in HIV-infected patients. *Pharmacogenet Genomics, 15*(1), 1–5.

Rotger, M., Tegude, H., Colombo, S., Cavassini, M., Furrer, H., Decosterd, L., et al. (2007). Predictive value of known and novel alleles of CYP2B6 for efavirenz plasma concentrations in HIV-infected individuals. *Clin Pharmacol Ther*, 81(4), 557–66.

Rovin, B. H., Lu, L., & Saxena, R. (1999). A novel polymorphism in the MCP-1 gene regulatory region that influences MCP-1 expression. *Biochem Biophys Res Commun*, 259(2), 344–8.

Sacktor, N., Lyles, R. H., Skolasky, R., Kleeberger, C., Selnes, O. A., Miller, E. N., et al. (2001). HIV-associated neurologic disease incidence changes: Multicenter AIDS Cohort Study, 1990–1998. *Neurology*, 56(2), 257–60.

Sacktor, N., McDermott, M. P., Marder, K., Schifitto, G., Selnes, O. A., McArthur, J. C., et al. (2002). HIV-associated cognitive impairment before and after the advent of combination therapy. *J Neurovirol*, 8(2), 136–42.

Sadrzadeh, S. M. & Saffari, Y. (2004). Iron and brain disorders. *Am J Clin Pathol*, 121 Suppl, S64–70.

Saha, R. N. & Pahan, K. (2003). Tumor necrosis factor-alpha at the crossroads of neuronal life and death during HIV-associated dementia. *J Neurochem*, 86(5), 1057–71.

Saitoh, A., Fletcher, C. V., Brundage, R., Alvero, C., Fenton, T., Hsia, K., et al. (2007). Efavirenz pharmacokinetics in HIV-1-infected children are associated with CYP2B6-G516T polymorphism. *J Acquir Immune Defic Syndr*, 45(3), 280–5.

Salkowitz, J. R., Bruse, S. E., Meyerson, H., Valdez, H., Mosier, D. E., Harding, C. V., et al. (2003). CCR5 promoter polymorphism determines macrophage CCR5 density and magnitude of HIV-1 propagation in vitro. *Clin Immunol*, 108(3), 234–40.

Samson, M., Libert, F., Doranz, B. J., Rucker, J., Liesnard, C., Farber, C. M., et al. (1996). Resistance to HIV-1 infection in Caucasian individuals bearing mutant alleles of the CCR-5 chemokine receptor gene. *Nature*, 382(6593), 722–5.

Sato-Matsumura, K. C., Berger, J., Hainfellner, J. A., Mazal, P., & Budka, H. (1998). Development of HIV encephalitis in AIDS and TNF-alpha regulatory elements. *J Neuroimmunol*, 91(1–2), 89–92.

Schnabel, R. B., Baumert, J., Barbalic, M., Dupuis, J., Ellinor, P. T., Durda, P., et al. (2010). Duffy antigen receptor for chemokines (Darc) polymorphism regulates circulating concentrations of monocyte chemoattractant protein-1 and other inflammatory mediators. *Blood*, 115(26), 5289–99.

Shieh, B., Liau, Y. E., Hsieh, P. S., Yan, Y. P., Wang, S. T., & Li, C. (2000). Influence of nucleotide polymorphisms in the CCR2 gene and the CCR5 promoter on the expression of cell surface CCR5 and CXCR4. *Int Immunol*, 12(9), 1311–8.

Shieh, J. T., Albright, A. V., Sharron, M., Gartner, S., Strizki, J., Doms, R. W., et al. (1998). Chemokine receptor utilization by human immunodeficiency virus type 1 isolates that replicate in microglia. *J Virol*, 72(5), 4243–9.

Singh, K. K., Barroga, C. F., Hughes, M. D., Chen, J., Raskino, C., McKinney, R. E., et al. (2003). Genetic influence of CCR5, CCR2, and SDF1 variants on human immunodeficiency virus 1 (HIV-1)-related disease progression and neurological impairment, in children with symptomatic HIV-1 infection. *J Infect Dis*, 188(10), 1461–72.

Singh, K. K., Ellis, R. J., Marquie-Beck, J., Letendre, S., Heaton, R. K., Grant, I., et al. (2004). CCR2 polymorphisms affect neuropsychological impairment in HIV-1-infected adults. *J Neuroimmunol*, 157(1–2), 185–92.

Singh, K. K., Hughes, M. D., Chen, J., & Spector, S. A. (2005). Genetic polymorphisms in CX3CR1 predict HIV-1 disease progression in children independently of CD4+ lymphocyte count and HIV-1 RNA load. *J Infect Dis*, 191(11), 1971–80.

Singh, K. K., Hughes, M. D., Chen, J., & Spector, S. A. (2006). Impact of MCP-1-2518-G allele on the HIV-1 disease of children in the United States. *AIDS*, 20(3), 475–8.

Singh, K. K., Lieser, A., Ruan, P. K., Fenton, T., & Spector, S. A. (2008). An age-dependent association of mannose-binding lectin-2 genetic variants on HIV-1-related disease in children. *J Allergy Clin Immunol*, 122(1), 173–80, 180 e1–2.

Smith, M. W., Dean, M., Carrington, M., Winkler, C., Huttley, G. A., Lomb, D. A., et al. (1997). Contrasting genetic influence of CCR2 and CCR5 variants on HIV-1 infection and disease progression. Hemophilia Growth and Development Study (HGDS), Multicenter AIDS Cohort Study (MACS), Multicenter Hemophilia Cohort Study (MHCS), San Francisco City Cohort (SFCC), ALIVE Study. *Science*, 277(5328), 959–65.

Spector, S. A., Singh, K. K., Gupta, S., Cystique, L. A., Jin, H., Letendre, S., et al. (2010). APOE epsilon4 and MBL-2 O/O genotypes are associated with neurocognitive impairment in HIV-infected plasma donors. *AIDS*, 24(10), 1471–9.

Stankiewicz, P. & Lupski, J. R. (2010). Structural variation in the human genome and its role in disease. *Annu Rev Med*, 61, 437–55.

Staszewski, S., Morales-Ramirez, J., Tashima, K. T., Rachlis, A., Skiest, D., Stanford, J., et al. (1999). Efavirenz plus zidovudine and lamivudine, efavirenz plus indinavir, and indinavir plus zidovudine and lamivudine in the treatment of HIV-1 infection in adults. Study 006 Team. *N Engl J Med*, 341(25), 1865–73.

Storey, A., Thomas, M., Kalita, A., Harwood, C., Gardiol, D., Mantovani, F., et al. (1998). Role of a p53 polymorphism in the development of human papillomavirus-associated cancer. *Nature*, 393(6682), 229–34.

Strittmatter, W. J. & Bova Hill, C. (2002). Molecular biology of apolipoprotein E. *Curr Opin Lipidol*, 13(2), 119–23.

Strittmatter, W. J., Saunders, A. M., Schmechel, D., Pericak-Vance, M., Enghild, J., Salvesen, G. S., et al. (1993). Apolipoprotein E: High-avidity binding to beta-amyloid and increased frequency of type 4 allele in late-onset familial Alzheimer disease. *Proc Natl Acad Sci USA*, 90(5), 1977–81.

Super, M., Thiel, S., Lu, J., Levinsky, R. J., & Turner, M. W. (1989). Association of low levels of mannan-binding protein with a common defect of opsonisation. *Lancet*, 2(8674), 1236–9.

Thiel, S., Petersen, S. V., Vorup-Jensen, T., Matsushita, M., Fujita, T., Stover, C. M., et al. (2000). Interaction of C1q and mannan-binding lectin (MBL) with C1r, C1s, MBL-associated serine proteases 1 and 2, and the MBL-associated protein MAp19. *J Immunol*, 165(2), 878–87.

Thomas, M. & Jankovic, J. (2004). Neurodegenerative disease and iron storage in the brain. *Curr Opin Neurol*, 17(4), 437–42.

Thomas, S. M., Tse, D. B., Ketner, D. S., Rochford, G., Meyer, D. A., Zade, D. D., et al. (2006). CCR5 expression and duration of high risk sexual activity among HIV-seronegative men who have sex with men. *AIDS*, 20(14), 1879–83.

Tisch, S. & Brew, B. (2009). Parkinsonism in HIV-infected patients on highly active antiretroviral therapy. *Neurology*, 73(5), 401–3.

Tong, N., Perry, S. W., Zhang, Q., James, H. J., Guo, H., Brooks, A., et al. (2000). Neuronal fractalkine expression in HIV-1 encephalitis: roles for macrophage recruitment and neuroprotection in the central nervous system. *J Immunol*, 164(3), 1333–9.

Torno, M. S., Witt, M. D., Saitoh, A., & Fletcher, C. V. (2008). Successful use of reduced-dose efavirenz in a patient with human immunodeficiency virus infection: Case report and review of the literature. *Pharmacotherapy*, 28(6), 782–7.

Torroni, A., Huoponen, K., Francalacci, P., Petrozzi, M., Morelli, L., Scozzari, R., et al. (1996). Classification of European mtDNAs from an analysis of three European populations. *Genetics*, 144(4), 1835–50.

Tournamille, C., Colin, Y., Cartron, J. P., & Le Van Kim, C. (1995). Disruption of a GATA motif in the Duffy gene promoter abolishes erythroid gene expression in Duffy-negative individuals. *Nat Genet*, 10(2), 224–8.

Tsuang, D. W. & Bird, T. D. (2002). Genetics of dementia. *Med Clin North Am*, 86(3), 591–614.

Tsuchiya, K., Gatanaga, H., Tachikawa, N., Teruya, K., Kikuchi, Y., Yoshino, M., et al. (2004). Homozygous CYP2B6 *6 (Q172H and K262R) correlates with high plasma efavirenz concentrations in HIV-1 patients treated with standard efavirenz-containing regimens. *Biochem Biophys Res Commun*, 319(4), 1322–6.

Turner, M. W. & Hamvas, R. M. (2000). Mannose-binding lectin: Structure, function, genetics and disease associations. *Rev Immunogenet*, 2(3), 305–22.

Tyor, W. R., Wesselingh, S. L., Griffin, J. W., McArthur, J. C., & Griffin, D. E. (1995). Unifying hypothesis for the pathogenesis of HIV-associated dementia complex, vacuolar myelopathy, and sensory neuropathy. *J Acquir Immune Defic Syndr Hum Retrovirol, 9*(4), 379–88.

Valcour, V., Shikuma, C., Shiramizu, B., Watters, M., Poff, P., Selnes, O. A., et al. (2004). Age, apolipoprotein E4, and the risk of HIV dementia: The Hawaii Aging with HIV Cohort. *J Neuroimmunol, 157*(1–2), 197–202.

van der Meer, P., Ulrich, A. M., Gonzalez-Scarano, F., & Lavi, E. (2000). Immunohistochemical analysis of CCR2, CCR3, CCR5, and CXCR4 in the human brain: Potential mechanisms for HIV dementia. *Exp Mol Pathol, 69*(3), 192–201.

van Rij, R. P., Broersen, S., Goudsmit, J., Coutinho, R. A., & Schuitemaker, H. (1998). The role of a stromal cell-derived factor-1 chemokine gene variant in the clinical course of HIV-1 infection. *AIDS, 12*(9), F85–90.

van Rij, R. P., Portegies, P., Hallaby, T., Lange, J. M., Visser, J., de Roda Husman, A. M., et al. (1999). Reduced prevalence of the CCR5 delta32 heterozygous genotype in human immunodeficiency virus-infected individuals with AIDS dementia complex. *J Infect Dis, 180*(3), 854–7.

Verhoeven, K., Timmerman, V., Mauko, B., Pieber, T. R., De Jonghe, P., & Auer-Grumbach, M. (2006). Recent advances in hereditary sensory and autonomic neuropathies. *Curr Opin Neurol, 19*(5), 474–80.

Verpoorten, N., De Jonghe, P., & Timmerman, V. (2006). Disease mechanisms in hereditary sensory and autonomic neuropathies. *Neurobiol Dis, 21*(2), 247–55.

Waheed, A. A., & Freed, E. O. (2009). Lipids and membrane microdomains in HIV-1 replication. *Virus Res, 143*(2), 162–76.

Wallace, D. C. (1999). Mitochondrial diseases in man and mouse. *Science, 283*(5407), 1482–8.

Wallace, D. C., Brown, M. D., & Lott, M. T. (1999). Mitochondrial DNA variation in human evolution and disease. *Gene, 238*(1), 211–30.

Wang, J., Sonnerborg, A., Rane, A., Josephson, F., Lundgren, S., Stahle, L., et al. (2006). Identification of a novel specific CYP2B6 allele in Africans causing impaired metabolism of the HIV drug efavirenz. *Pharmacogenet Genomics, 16*(3), 191–8.

Ward, B. A., Gorski, J. C., Jones, D. R., Hall, S. D., Flockhart, D. A., & Desta, Z. (2003). The cytochrome P450 2B6 (CYP2B6) is the main catalyst of efavirenz primary and secondary metabolism: Implication for HIV/AIDS therapy and utility of efavirenz as a substrate marker of CYP2B6 catalytic activity. *J Pharmacol Exp Ther, 306*(1), 287–300.

Wesselingh, S. L., Power, C., Glass, J. D., Tyor, W. R., McArthur, J. C., Farber, J. M., et al. (1993). Intracerebral cytokine messenger RNA expression in acquired immunodeficiency syndrome dementia. *Ann Neurol, 33*(6), 576–82.

Wesselingh, S. L., Takahashi, K., Glass, J. D., McArthur, J. C., Griffin, J. W., & Griffin, D. E. (1997). Cellular localization of tumor necrosis factor mRNA in neurological tissue from HIV-infected patients by combined reverse transcriptase/polymerase chain reaction in situ hybridization and immunohistochemistry. *J Neuroimmunol, 74*(1–2), 1–8.

Wilkinson, D. A., Operskalski, E. A., Busch, M. P., Mosley, J. W., & Koup, R. A. (1998). A 32-bp deletion within the CCR5 locus protects against transmission of parenterally acquired human immunodeficiency virus but does not affect progression to AIDS-defining illness. *J Infect Dis, 178*(4), 1163–6.

Winkler, C., Modi, W., Smith, M. W., Nelson, G. W., Wu, X., Carrington, M., et al. (1998). Genetic restriction of AIDS pathogenesis by an SDF-1 chemokine gene variant. ALIVE Study, Hemophilia Growth and Development Study (HGDS), Multicenter AIDS Cohort Study (MACS), Multicenter Hemophilia Cohort Study (MHCS), San Francisco City Cohort (SFCC). *Science, 279*(5349), 389–93.

Winzer, R., Langmann, P., Zilly, M., Tollmann, F., Schubert, J., Klinker, H., et al. (2003). No influence of the P-glycoprotein genotype (MDR1 C3435T) on plasma levels of lopinavir and efavirenz during antiretroviral treatment. *Eur J Med Res, 8*(12), 531–4.

Winzer, R., Langmann, P., Zilly, M., Tollmann, F., Schubert, J., Klinker, H., et al. (2005). No influence of the P-glycoprotein polymorphisms MDR1 G2677T/A and C3435T on the virological and immunological response in treatment-naive HIV-positive patients. *Ann Clin Microbiol Antimicrob, 4*, 3.

Wojna, V., Skolasky, R. L., Hechavarria, R., Mayo, R., Selnes, O., McArthur, J. C., et al. (2006). Prevalence of human immunodeficiency virus-associated cognitive impairment in a group of Hispanic women at risk for neurological impairment. *J Neurovirol, 12*(5), 356–64.

Wright, E. J. (2009). Neurological disease: The effects of HIV and antiretroviral therapy and the implications for early antiretroviral therapy initiation. *Curr Opin HIV AIDS, 4*(5), 447–52.

Wright, E. J., Grund, B., Robertson, K., Brew, B. J., Roediger, M., Bain, M. P., et al. (2010). Cardiovascular risk factors associated with lower baseline cognitive performance in HIV-positive persons. *Neurology.*

Wright, E. K., Jr., Page, S. H., Barber, S. A., & Clements, J. E. (2008). Prep1/Pbx2 complexes regulate CCL2 expression through the -2578 guanine polymorphism. *Genes Immun, 9*(5), 419–30.

Zhang, X. L. & Ali, M. A. (2008). Ficolins: Structure, function and associated diseases. *Adv Exp Med Biol, 632*, 105–15.

Zhao, M. L., Kim, M. O., Morgello, S., & Lee, S. C. (2001). Expression of inducible nitric oxide synthase, interleukin-1 and caspase-1 in HIV-1 encephalitis. *J Neuroimmunol, 115*(1–2), 182–91.

Zhou, L., Diefenbach, E., Crossett, B., Tran, S. L., Ng, T., Rizos, H., et al. (2010). First evidence of overlaps between HIV-associated dementia (HAD) and non-viral neurodegenerative diseases: Proteomic analysis of the frontal cortex from HIV+ patients with and without dementia. *Mol Neurodegener, 5*, 27.

Zimmerman, P. A., Buckler-White, A., Alkhatib, G., Spalding, T., Kubofcik, J., Combadiere, C., et al. (1997). Inherited resistance to HIV-1 conferred by an inactivating mutation in CC chemokine receptor 5: Studies in populations with contrasting clinical phenotypes, defined racial background, and quantified risk. *Mol Med, 3*(1), 23–36.

Zink, M. C., Coleman, G. D., Mankowski, J. L., Adams, R. J., Tarwater, P. M., Fox, K., et al. (2001). Increased macrophage chemoattractant protein-1 in cerebrospinal fluid precedes and predicts simian immunodeficiency virus encephalitis. *J Infect Dis, 184*(8), 1015–21.

Zink, M. C., Uhrlaub, J., DeWitt, J., Voelker, T., Bullock, B., Mankowski, J., et al. (2005). Neuroprotective and anti-human immunodeficiency virus activity of minocycline. *JAMA, 293*(16), 2003–11.

SECTION 2

INNATE AND CELLULAR IMMUNITY AND NEUROGENESIS

Howard E. Gendelman

2.1

MONONUCLEAR PHAGOCYTES

Kenneth C. Williams, William F. Hickey, Tricia H. Burdo, and Caroline Soulas

Due to the presence of the blood-brain barrier, the central nervous system (CNS) had long been considered "immune privileged," that is, insulated with respect to the extra-CNS immune system. It is now clear that this privileging is relative, not absolute, and breaks down under a variety of circumstances. In fact, with respect to HIV-1 infection, it has been hypothesized that latently infected immune cells may themselves provide the primary mechanism for infecting the brain. This has been hypothesized to occur via entry into the CNS of immune-activated mononuclear phagocyte (MP) cells that harbor HIV-1 provirus in their genomes (the "Trojan horse" phenomenon). Furthermore, it is clear that immunocompetent cells of the MP system are the principal CNS cells infected by HIV-1. This chapter focuses on those MP activities and susceptibilities that may help explain the onset, maintenance, and propagation of HIV-1 infection in the CNS. Specific areas of focus are the heterogeneity of CNS MP cells, the turnover kinetics of these cells, their susceptibility to HIV-1 infection, and the spread of infection from outside to inside the CNS. The correlation of systemic (specifically, bone marrow) monocytic expansion with the clinical severity of HIV and SIV disease is also discussed, as is the composition of HIV- and SIV-encephalitis lesions from three cell groups of macrophage lineage.

INTRODUCTION

Interest in the immune competence of the central nervous system (CNS) has grown during the past century. Supporting the notion of "immunological privilege" of the CNS were absence of cellular elements of the immune system in healthy individuals, constitutively undetectable (major histocompatibility complex (MHC) molecule expression and the presence of a blood-brain barrier (BBB) that excludes serum proteins, including antibodies, complement, and coagulation factors (Barker & Billingham, 1977; Wekerle, Linnington, Lassmann, & Meyermann, 1986; Hauser et al., 1983). More recently, our understanding of the BBB has evolved to include a selective capillary barrier for solutes and a mechanism for regulating the recruitment of leukocytes in response to ongoing pathologies. This recruitment mechanism involves several differentially regulated steps, including control of cell passage across postcapillary venules into the perivascular space and, the regulated passage of cells through the glial limitans to the parenchyma. (Bechmann, Galea, & Perry, 2007; Galea, Bechmann, & Perry, 2007). Related to our changed view of

the BBB, our understanding of the immune privileged status of the CNS has evolved. This privileging is now recognized to be relative and compartmentalized, as opposed to absolute and anatomically homogeneous, and to be directionally specific, involving differences between the efferent arm (entry of lymphocytes, monocytes, and antibodies) and afferent arms (exit of dendritic cells, soluble CNS antigens and viruses, and monocyte/macrophages) (Bechmann, Galea, & Perry, 2007; Galea, Bechmann, & Perry, 2007). We now understand that in many conditions, including viral infection, "immune privilege" vanishes and immunocompetent cells enter the CNS with alacrity (Williams & Hickey, 1995a; Williams & Hickey, 1995b; Achim, Schrier, & Wiley, 1991; Tyor, Moench, & Griffin, 1989; Oldstone & Southern, 1993; Griffin, Levine, Tyor, & Irani, 1992; Cserr & Knopf, 1992).

Few conditions rival HIV-associated neurological diseases in demonstrating the complex interplay between the immune and nervous systems. With HIV infection, both early and with the development of AIDS, changes outside the brain include bone marrow hyperplasia, translocation of LPS across the gastrointestinal barrier, expansion of activated monocytes and maturation of these cells in the vasculature, and monocyte/macrophage traffic to the CNS. To add to the complexity, it is important to understand the roles of CNS macrophages, some of which are extra-parenchymal and therefore sensitive to non-CNS immune interactions, and others that are intra-parenchymal within the confines of the relative CNS immune control. All of these macrophage populations will be discussed in this chapter with regard to their biology of HIV infection. While cells of the immune system are considered the principle targets of HIV infection, the effects of virus on the nervous system are protean and potentially devastating.

Macrophages, CD4[+] T cells, and in some instances dendritic cells (DC) are targets of HIV infection and sources of viral particles that infect other cells (Pantaleo et al., 1993; Massari et al., 1990; Fauci, 1988a; Fauci, 1988b). Each of these cell populations can be productively infected, producing viral protein and RNA; also, importantly, the cells can be latently infected and thus serve as a potential viral reservoir. Following infection with virus, cells of the immune system can become highly activated, and release numerous soluble factors that can result in tissue damage and endothelial cell activation (Pantaleo & Fauci, 1994; Pantaleo et al., 1994). This spread of retrovirus and infected cells through the body ultimately destroys the immune system and produces a variety of

HIV-associated diseases. After the immune system, it appears that the CNS is the most adversely affected organ in the body. Why?

Outside of the CNS, the major cell types studied with regard to HIV infection are monocytes, macrophages, and DC and CD4[+] T cells (Pantaleo et al., 1994; Orenstein, 2001; Pope et al.1994; Rosenberg & Fauci, 1989; Meltzer et al., 1990). Infection of bone marrow cells, potentially including infection of bone marrow hematopoietic progenitor cells and thus the precursors of some or all of the monocyte subtypes, has been described in early simian immunodeficiency virus (SIV) and HIV infection (Kitagawa, Lackner, Martfeld, Gardner, & Dandekar, 1991; Gartner, 2000; Thiele et al., 1986; Folks et al., 1988; Stanley et al., 1992; Gendelman et al., 1985; Mandell, Jain, Miller, & Dandekar, 1995; Alexaki & Wigdahl, 2008; Alexaki, Liu, & Wigdahl, 2008). A hypothesis in HIV viral infection is that virus enters the CNS as provirus via monocyte/macrophages (the "Trojan horse" phenomenon) (Gartner, 2000; Peluso, Haase, Stowring, Edwards, & Ventura, 1985; Dickson et al., 1991). Macrophages and microglia are the major CNS cell types infected by HIV (Gartner, 2000; Gendelman, Lipton, Tardieu, Bukrinsky, & Nottet, 1994; Fischer-Smith et al., 2001; Williams & Hickey, 2002; Gonzalez-Scarano & Baltuch, 1999; Price et al., 1988; Koenig et al., 1986); astrocytes and possibly endothelial cells have also been reported as being infected, although productive infection of these cells is seldom observed (Tornatore, Nath, Amemiya, & Major, 1991; Tornatore, Chandra, Berger, & Major, 1994; Gabuzda et al., 1986; Wiley, Schrier, Nelson, Lampert, & Oldstone, 1986). Yet, there is no question that human immunodeficiency virus encephalitis (HIVE), HIV-associated neurocognitive disorders (HAND), and vacuolar myelopathy are a result of CNS infection by HIV (Dickson et al., 1991; Gonzalez-Scarano & Baltuch, 1999; Kure, Lyman, Weidenheim, & Dickson, 1990). In fact, the pathological diagnosis of HIVE includes the presence of HIV-laden perivascular cells, virus in the CNS, and multinucleated giant cells (MNGC). In addition, before the era of antiretroviral therapy, the number of inflammatory macrophages was a histopathologic correlate of neurologic disease (Achim et al., 1991; Dickson et al., 1991; Budka, 1986; Budka, 1991). To date, there is an absence of conclusive data specifying the exact mechanism(s) for establishing HIV infection in the CNS (Williams & Hickey, 1995b; Achim et al., 1991; Gartner, 2000; Dickson et al., 1991; Williams & Hickey, 2002; Gonzalez-Scarano & Baltuch, 1999). In order to define the pathogenic mechanisms active in HIV-associated CNS disease, several questions must be addressed: How does the virus enter the CNS? How and where does retroviral infection of the CNS persist? What changes are produced that result in neurological disease?

While circulating monocytic cells and macrophages were not initially considered to be a significant target of productive infection by HIV, they are recognized as a cell type whose precursors may be infected in the bone marrow, and a potential reservoir in blood. Once they enter the circulation, following maturation, they likely become a source of virus in multiple tissues including the gut, lungs, and brain (Gendelman et al., 1985; Williams et al., 2002: Stevenson & Gendelman, 1994; Bissel et al., 2008; Naif et al., 1997). These same cells have been identified as reservoirs of HIV in individuals undergoing anti-retroviral therapy, who have low-to-nondetectable free virus in plasma or cerebrospinal fluid (CSF) (Sonza et al. 2004; Igarashi et al., 2001; Crowe, Zhu, & Muller, 2003). Thus, they represent a cell family, which can harbor HIV for extended periods (Sonza et al. 2001; Schrager & D'Souza, 1998). In many species including humans, hematogenously derived monocyte/macrophages express the CD4 molecule and the specific chemokine receptors including CCR5 and CXCR4 required for infection by different viral strains (Meltzer et al., 1990; Gartner, 2000; Dickson et al., 1991; Lavi et al., 1997; He et al., 1997; Jordan, Watkins, Kufta, & Dublois-Dalcq, 1991; Crocker et al., 1987; Naif et al., 1998; Embretson et al., 1993). CD4 and CCR5 are detectable on perivascular cells and upon microglial cells in the neural parenchyma when they are stimulated. Indeed the microglia, macrophages and perivascular cells are the principal cells infected in the CNS (Price et al., 1988; Koenig et al., 1986; Kure et al., 1990; Navia, Cho, Pettito, & Price, 1986) (Figure 2.1.1). While macrophages in the choroid plexus and meninges are probably infected during early HIV-associated aseptic meningitis (Harouse et al., 1989), perivascular and parenchymal microglia also harbor the virus, albeit later in disease evolution (Kure et al., 1990; Williams et al., 2001; Kure, Weidenheim, Lyman, & Dickson, 1990). It is interesting to note that most of the virus strains cloned from the CNS of HIV-infected humans, and SIV-infected nonhuman primates, are thought to be strains that infect cells in a CD4-independent manner. Whether such CD4-independent infection occurs outside of the CNS or in the CNS is not determined. Overall, careful consideration of this entire group of CNS resident mononuclear cells is warranted.

MACROPHAGE/MONOCYTE HETEROGENEITY IN THE CENTRAL NERVOUS SYSTEM

Historically, it has been commonplace to consider monocytes and macrophages as a relatively short-lived, homogeneous group of hematogenous elements having a limited functional repertoire. This view has been dramatically altered by studies of myeloid lineage cells in the CNS performed under a variety of experimental conditions. In the past, a large panel of monoclonal antibodies from mice hyperimmunized with living, cultured rat microglial cells failed to produce a unique marker specific for this CNS resident cell (Flaris, Densmore, Molleston, & Hickey, 1993). All monoclonal antibodies, which recognize any of the monocyte/macrophage family members residing in the CNS, also identify subsets of monocytoid cells in tissues of the immune system (Flaris et al., 1993; Dijkstra, Dopp, Joling, & Kraal, 1985; Sminia et al., 1987). Nevertheless, the studies resulting from that work and from the efforts of many others (themselves making antibodies against rodent monocyte/macrophages, or using established commercially available

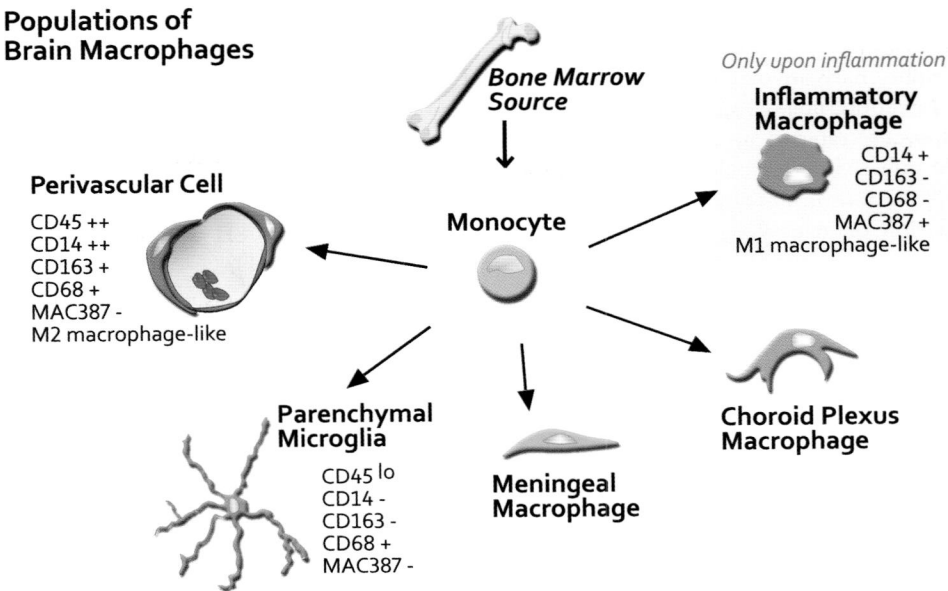

Figure 2.1.1 Brain macrophage populations in HIV and SIV encephalitis with distinguishing myeloid markers.

antibodies with defined CD specificity; Dijkstra et al., 1985; Sminia et al., 1987; Perry, 1994) also demonstrate the heterogeneity of cells of macrophage/monocyte origin found in the brain. All of the cell types noted below are linked together by a number of features: They express leukocyte common antigen (LCA, CD45) and CD11b/CD18 (CR3) constitutively. In addition, most of the macrophage populations in the CNS also express CD markers found on monocytes, including CD14, a receptor for LPS; CD16, an Fc gamma receptor type III with a low affinity for immunoglobulin; and the hemoglobin-haptoglobin receptor CD163—all of which are important to differentiate monocyte subpopulations (Williams et al., 2001; Fabriek et al., 2005; Kim, Corey, Alvarez, & Williams, 2003). In addition to these myeloid lineage markers, brain macrophages share critical chemokine and cell-trafficking receptors, including CCR2, CX3CR1, CXCR4, and CCR5, that differentiate between classic versus inflammatory monocytes, and likely macrophage populations in the CNS (Zou et al., 1998; Geissmann, Jung, & Littman, 2003; Kim et al., 2010; Fischer-Smith, Tedaldi, & Rappaport, 2008; Serbina & Pamer, 2006; Strauss-Ayali, Conrad, & Mosser, 2007). Lastly, both monocytes and brain macrophages express varying levels of Toll-like receptors TLR2 and TLR4, which effectively link the innate and adaptive immune responses with the CNS (Sato & Iwasaki, 2004; Iwasaki & Medzhitov, 2004). Interestingly, brain macrophages do not possess any markers common to glial or neuronal lineage.

In the CNS alone, a variety of morphologically and phenotypically distinct macrophage/monocyte family members exist. At least four types can be identified: meningeal macrophages, perivascular cells, choroid plexus macrophages, and parenchymal microglial cells (Williams & Hickey, 1995b; Williams & Hickey, 2002; Williams et al., 2001; Hickey & Kimura, 1988; Hickey, Vass, & Lassmann, 1992). Studies in

rodent systems have elucidated these various subtypes of myeloid cells, and various experimental manipulations have demonstrated their unique capacities to function in distinct ways (Flaris et al., 1993; Perry, 1994).

MENINGEAL MACROPHAGES

Morphologically normal tissue macrophages can be recognized in the arachnoid and pial membranes. These cells constitutively express low levels of MHC class I and II molecules and have CD4 (in rats and humans) on their membranes (Honda, Kimura, Silvers, & Rostami, 1990). Moreover, they have a low but constitutive expression of a variety of adhesion molecules (e.g., ICAM-1). It is probable that their role is predominantly that of a tissue phagocyte. While it has long been known that they become activated and dramatically increase in number during meningeal inflammatory processes, especially those producing chronic inflammation, such as *M. tuberculosis* and *Cryptococcus*, their function in normal homeostasis is undefined. This macrophage type is influenced by events in the immune system because of these macrophages' association with the CNS vasculature.

Macrophages of the Virchow-Robins space appear to be closely related to the meningeal macrophages, although they are not identical. Morphologically, they resemble their meningeal counterparts at the light microscopic and ultrastructural level; however, they do not express detectable levels of MHC class II or CD4 in the normal state (Honda et al., 1990; Esiri & Gay, 1990). They may represent the same cell type as the meningeal macrophage, but they are a subgroup that has to a greater extent come under the immunoinhibitory influence of the neural parenchyma. To date, no specific or unique function has been attributable to macrophages of the Virchow-Robins space of which meningeal macrophages are not capable. Thus, they are distinct as a macrophage subclass for two major reasons: their different pattern of cell surface molecule expression and the different kinetics of their turnover rate (see below). Early involvement of meninges in HIV and SIV brain infection suggests that infection of meningeal macrophages occurs rapidly and is followed by the slower appearance of infected perivascular cells in the CNS. With established CNS lesions in SIV and HIV encephalitis, there is an accumulation of macrophages in the Virchow-Robins space.

PERIVASCULAR CELLS AND CHOROID PLEXUS MACROPHAGES

The next two cell types are possibly closely related, although they differ in location and morphology to some extent. There are the perivascular cells (a.k.a. perivascular microglial cells, perivascular macrophages) and the choroid plexus macrophages. Both of these cell types are situated adjacent to the endothelial cells immediately beyond the basement membrane around small CNS parenchymal vessels for the former and capillaries and in the choroid plexus for the latter. These cell types are located in the perivascular space wherein they extend long, branching tendrils along and to some extent wrapped around the small vessel to which they are apposed (Hickey & Kimura, 1988; Hickey et al., 1992; Williams, Alvarez, & Lackner, 2001; Streit & Graeber, 1993; Graeber, Streit, & Buringer, 1992) (Figure 2.1.1). Being closely associated with a blood vessel, they are thus ideally situated to sense changes in the endothelium, in BBB permeability, and to encounter cells crossing into the tissue from the blood.

In rats, humans, and nonhuman primates, the perivascular cells have been shown to be phenotypically distinct from regular histiocytes, and are capable of performing specific immunological functions. In studies using rat irradiation bone marrow chimeras (a system in which the immune function of cells derived from the bone marrow can be selectively exploited if they express a critical MHC molecule that the native host's cells lack), the perivascular cells (and possibly meningeal macrophages) functioned as fully competent antigen-presenting cells (APCs) for pathogenic T cells (Hickey & Kimura, 1988). Likewise, isolated choroid plexus macrophages have been demonstrated to be competent APCs in vitro (Nathanson & Chun, 1989). In mice, rats, and humans, reports differ about which cell surface molecules these cells express constitutively or can be induced to elaborate (Perry, 1994; Lassmann, Zimprich, Rossler, & Vass, 1991; Perry & Gordon, 1987; Perry & Gordon, 1988; Vass & Lassmann, 1990). The cells certainly can express MHC antigens, CD4, and a variety of adhesion molecules if the stimuli are appropriate (Perry & Gordon, 1988; Vass & Lassmann, 1990; Hickey & Kimura, 1987). These cells express MHC molecules and the CD4 antigen in normal adult brains (Honda et al., 1990; Perry & Gordon, 1987; Peudenier, Hery, & Montagnier, 1991; Mittelbronn et al., 2001). They also express CD14 in human and nonhuman primate brains. In HIV and SIV infection, CD14 and CD163 can differentiate perivascular cells from parenchymal microglia, further supporting the monocytic origin of perivascular cells (Fischer-Smith et al., 2001; Williams et al.,

2001; Kim et al., 2006; Roberts, Masliah, & Fox, 2004). The majority of CD14+ cells are also CD16+, CD163, and/or CD45+, many of which are retrovirus-infected (Figure 2.1.1). Thus, in HIV the infected cells in the perivascular region appear to be due to, or directly derived from, the transvascular spread of peripherally infected monocytes. It is principally members of this cell group that are suspected of serving as "Trojan horses" for HIV-1 and possibly other CNS viruses (Dickson et al., 1991).

PARENCHYMAL MICROGLIAL CELLS

These cells may be the most complex cells in the CNS. Certainly, in this book the number of chapters concentrating on them attests to their potential importance. These cells constitute up to 10% of the CNS parenchymal cells in some brain areas. They are found in both white and gray matter where they set up non-overlapping areas, the arborizing processes of one extending out to touch the dendritic tips of the adjacent microglia, thereby establishing a continuous web that invests the whole CNS (Perry, 1994; Perry, Andersson, & Gordon, 1993; Nimmerjahn, Kirchhoff, & Helmchen, 2005). In addition, these cells form part of the *glia limitans*, the true boundary of the CNS parenchyma. Ultrastructural and immunohistochemical analyses of the CNS have demonstrated that between 5% and 13% of the foot processes extending from the CNS parenchyma to abut on CNS vessels are microglial derived (Williams et al., 2001; Lassmann, Zimprich, Vass, & Hickey, 1991). Thus, a subset of these cells, so-called juxtavascular microglia, is also immediately available to any cell or material crossing the BBB from the circulation.

It appears that these cells, in distinction to their perivascular cousins, are relatively poor antigen-presenting cells, at least when freshly isolated from the adult rat CNS (Lassmann et al., 1991). In mammals, parenchymal microglial cells can be distinguished from the perivascular cells and other hematogenously derived leukocytes by their level of CD45 (Sedgwick et al., 1991; Ford et al., 1995). These CD45 negative or "low" cells do possess some antigen processing and presenting functions, but they appear defective when compared to the perivascular cells (Figure 2.1.1). Their role may be more of an immunoprotective one rather than pro-inflammatory (Ford et al., 1995). Work by Williams and colleagues (Ulvestad et al., 1994; Williams, Ulvestad, & Antel, 1994a; Williams, Ulvestad, & Antel, 1994b) has demonstrated that in vitro adult parenchymal microglial cells are immunologically competent, and they can be induced to express the critical co-stimulatory molecules necessary to effectively present antigens and stimulate T cells.

In healthy animals and humans, these parenchymal cells are very quiescent immunologically. They express no detectable MHC molecules, low or no adhesion molecules, and their CD4 expression is not detectable (Hauser et al., 1983; Flaris et al., 1993; Perry & Gordon, 1987; Hickey & Kimura, 1987; Mittelbronn et al., 2001; Lampson & Hickey, 1986). However, in a state of activation, as would occur following cytokine exposure or in a zone of inflammation, they rapidly become positive for several of these molecules (Perry, 1994;

Hickey et al., 1992; Vass & Lassmann, 1990). Additionally, though CD4 is not readily detected on human brain-derived parenchymal microglia, they appear to be infected, in vitro, in a manner that is CD4-dependent (Watkins et al., 1990).

Parenchymal microglial cells have one ability that it appears the previous cell types do not: They can become fully competent macrophages. This transforming ability was detailed over half a century ago by del Rio-Hortega in his famous treatise on this cell type (del Rio Hortega, 1932). In areas of inflammation associated with the autoimmune condition experimental allergic encephalomyelitis (EAE), they convert from their ramified state to reactive microglia that engulf tissue debris (Bauer, Siminia, Wouterlood, & Dijkstra, 1994; Rinner et al., 1995; Lassmann, & Hickey, 1993; Lassmann, Schmied, Vass, & Hickey, 1993). Also, at the edge of CNS infarctions or traumatic contusions, some microglia are induced to become macrophages also to remove necrotic and injured tissue, a phenomenon that is at least mediated by ATP at the injury site and is dependent on ATP gradients (Davalos et al., 2005). Yet, in injury, EAE, or infarction, the bulk of the macrophages, which appear in the area of reaction, are not derived from microglia; they are freshly recruited hematogenous cells of the monocyte/macrophage group (Bauer et al., 1994; Rinner et al., 1995; Lassmann, & Hickey, 1993; Lassmann et al., 1993). In encephalitic lesions with HIV and SIV infection, there are classically described "microglial nodules," but also an accumulation of infiltrating hematogenous cells. These macrophages appear to be a mix, depending on the "age" and the inflammatory activity of the lesion, of recently recruited MAC387+ monocyte/macrophages, perivascular cells, and parenchymal microglia (discussed below). These cell types can be distinguished using immunohistochemistry and combinations of MAC387 for recently recruited monocyte/macrophages, CD14 and/or CD163 for perivascular cells, and CD68 and HAM56 for parenchymal microglia (Soulas, et al., 2011). Examination of such diverse CNS injuries as stab wound, Wallerian degeneration, abscess formation (a neutrophil, plasma cell, macrophage reaction), and EAE (a T-cell-mediated inflammation) reveal that parenchymal microglial cells possess a range of response potentials, which are not necessarily stereotypic or uniform (Flaris et al., 1993).

Between these populations of monocyte/macrophage derivatives, there appears to be very little interconversion. Microglial cells can become macrophages, but there is no evidence that the reverse is possible. Investigations in chimeric rats have shown that macrophages responding to an inflammatory focus in the CNS do not remain after the inflammation subsides (Rinner et al., 1995; Lassmann et al., 1993). Moreover, these cells certainly do not remain and assume the morphology of parenchymal microglial cells. Interestingly, the perivascular cells (which in the rat CNS are the only parenchymal monocytic cells identified by the monoclonal antibodies ED-2 which is thought to be a homologue of CD163 in humans and nonhuman primates; Sminia et al., 1987; Perry, 1994) do not become either parenchymal microglial cells nor do they become fully active macrophages in areas of inflammation (Bauer et al., 1994; Rinner et al., 1995;

Lassmann, & Hickey, 1993; Lassmann et al., 1993). Thus, this cell type appears to be distinct and subject to a narrowly defined repertoire, which does not overlap with other CNS resident members of this family. How much interconversion actually does occur between specific CNS macrophage/monocyte cell phenotypes remains to be fully elucidated; however, the data to date suggests that these conversions might be very limited and governed by factors unknown at this time.

KINETICS OF MONOCYTE LINEAGE TURNOVER IN THE CENTRAL NERVOUS SYSTEM

Not all cells of the CNS are permanent residents. A number of studies in rodent bone-marrow chimeras (Hickey & Kimura, 1988; Hickey et al., 1992; Rinner et al., 1995; Lassmann, & Hickey, 1993; Lassmann et al., 1993; Priller et al., 2001; Flugel et al., 2001; Bechmann et al., 2001; Kennedy & Abkowitz, 1997; Lawson, Perry, & Gordon, 1992; Ajami et al., 2007; Vallieres & Sawchenko, 2003), monkeys receiving autologous CD34+ hematopoetic stem cells (Soulas et al., 2009), and humans receiving partially nonidentical allogeneic bone-marrow transplants (Unger et al., 1993) have documented the dynamic nature of these populations of cells. Interestingly, it seems that the pace at which their members turn over is quite distinct. One fact that has emerged from these many studies is that all of the CNS resident cell types noted above are derived ultimately from the bone marrow and *can* be replaced from that source during adult life (Figure 2.1.2).

The meningeal macrophages are a transient, rapidly cycling group. In the healthy rodent CNS, 50%–60% of these cells will be replaced from the bone marrow withintwo to three months (Hickey et al., 1992). In that same period of time, only about 30% of the perivascular cells and choroid plexus cells will be replaced. Macrophages of the Virchow-Robins space are replaced more slowly from the bone marrow than are meningeal macrophages, but more rapidly than

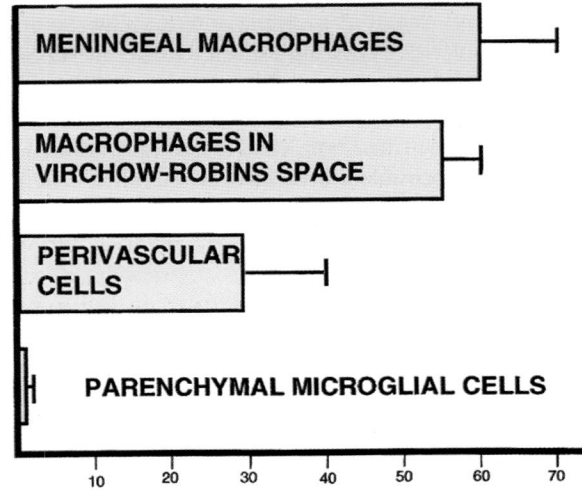

Figure 2.1.2 Relative rates of replacement of the major types CNS resident monocyte lineage cells from the bone marrow in adult rodents.

perivascular cells. Since little is known about the migratory capacity of these macrophage subsets from the perivascular zones around the venules and capillaries deep in the brain to the meningeal surface, the Virchow-Robins space macrophages could represent a combination of meningeal macrophages and perivascular cells.

The parenchymal microglial cells are distinct from the other monocytic cells in the CNS in their repopulation rate. In adult rodents (Hickey et al., 1992; Lawson, Perry, & Gordon, 1992) and in humans (Unger et al., 1993), these cells are replaced from the bone marrow at a very low rate. In rats and mice (Fabriek et al., 2005; Hickey et al., 1992; Unger et al., 1993) the repopulation occurs at less than 1% in 90 days, and even after a year of bone marrow chimerism in the rat, the microglial cells of bone marrow origin amount only to a few percent of the total microglial population. While this might ultimately permit a total turnover of these CNS resident cells, such replacement must require many years. Therefore, it may be noteworthy that these quiescent cells, in addition to neurons, are one of the few cell types in the CNS to express bcl-2 (Merry et al., 1994; Hockenberry et al., 1991), bespeaking their apparently great longevity. Currently, microglial cells are believed to enter the CNS during fetal life. Initially they are phagocyte-like cells, which become more ramified and quiescent as the BBB becomes established and they are isolated in the privileged environment of the CNS, away from the disturbances occurring in tissues of the immune system or in the circulation.

When considering the turnover of these monocyte-related cells in the CNS, it must be borne in mind that the traffic described above occurs as part of normal physiology. Members of the greater monocyte family are continuously entering the normal CNS to take up their assigned position and fully differentiate into their ultimate phenotype. It is unknown whether this continuous reseeding of the CNS from the marrow compartment reflects (a) the activity of numerous, semi-differentiated stem cells, each repopulating the CNS with an already distinct cell type having a unique set of kinetics and potentials; or (b) a simple, common progenitor cell providing the blood with one relatively undifferentiated cell type that realizes one of its multiple potentials by responding to certain chemokines, entering a specific tissue, and taking up residence in a location wherein the environment provides the final differentiating stimuli. Are these marrow-derived monocytoid cells "predestined" or "environmentally influenced"? (Of course, it is possible a little of both might be true.) The importance of this question for the spread of HIV-1 to the CNS, and possibly for the clinical picture that ultimately emerges, is obvious.

As noted above, in the rapid pace of inflammatory processes, CNS resident monocytes and macrophages do not exhibit much interconversion of phenotype. Yet, it cannot be determined given the available data if this occurs on a larger time scale. It appears that this CNS group is not totally sessile, and some movement within the CNS occurs. One of the most interesting aspects of this movement might be the departure of CNS monocyte family members to return to the blood and the tissues of the immune system.

In a study of neural grafting in which tissue from the forebrain of a neonatal Lewis rat was placed in the frontal lobe of an MHC-mismatched BN rat, evidence for traffic of this type appeared (Broadwell, Baker, Ebert, & Hickey, 1994). A few days after graft placement, the recipient animal was killed and its cervical lymph nodes and spleen were extensively examined for cells bearing the donor MHC molecules. Such cells were found in both locations, although they were rare. Since they are almost exclusively members of the monocyte/macrophage family, which can express MHC molecules in CNS tissue, and since the grafts contained no meninges (hence no meningeal macrophages), the cells found in the recipient's immune tissue were most probably derived from either parenchymal microglial cells or perivascular cells. While this experiment cannot be said to replicate the physiological condition, it does bespeak a potential two-way traffic of monocytic cells into and out of the CNS. In addition, it suggests an answer to the question concerning what happens to the meningeal and perivascular cells as they are replaced from the bone marrow. In other experiments in our laboratory, we have used dextran dyes, injected into the CNS, to study the dynamics of perivascular macrophage turnover in normal and SIV-infected monkeys. In these studies, using combinations of dextran dyes with different fluorescence tags injected into the third ventricle on days 1, 7, and 8, we found perivascular cells that were labeled with all dyes, as well as some that were labeled only with the last dye, indicating that the cells had entered the CNS at the time of the last injection (Kim et al., 2006). More recently, we injected fluorescently labeled superparamagnetic iron oxide nanoparticles (SPIONS) into the CSF, from where the particles are taken up by macrophages, and found macrophages infiltrating different regions of the CNS 1, 3, 7, and 21 days after injection, but also exiting the CNS, in some cases with SIV-p28 immune reactivity, via the cribriform plate, cranial nerve roots, and the optic nerve. Amazingly, we found significant accumulations of these cells in dorsal root ganglia (DRG), cervical draining lymph nodes (LN), and the spleen and thymus, underscoring a significant ability of macrophages to leave the CNS, in some instances as infected cells (Alvarez, Lackner, Williams, unpublished). Unfortunately, this gives basis to the fear that anti-HIV therapies, which succeed in eliminating the virus from the peripheral immune system, might be subverted by a long, slow re-infection emanating from reservoirs in the CNS that are relatively resistant to most antiretroviral formulations.

It is likely that HIV infection enhances or in some manner alters traffic from the blood into the neural parenchyma. HIV *tat* protein induces the types of adhesion molecules on endothelial cells utilized for transendothelial traffic (Hoffman et al., 1994) and the presence of a focus of inflammation, all too common in AIDS patients, induces endothelial cell expression of adhesion molecules (Sasseville et al., 1994; Sasseville et al., 1996; Rinaldo, 1994; Pober et al., 1987; Lassmann et al., 1991). With HIV and SIV infections, adhesion molecule expression by CNS endothelial cells can resemble that of high endothelial vessels (Sasseville et al., 1994; Sasseville et al., 1996; Lassmann et al., 1991; Tyor et al., 1992;

Persidsky et al., 2000; Nottet et al., 1996; Sobel, Mitchell, & Fondren, 1990; Deckert-Schluter et al., 1994). In addition to the upregulation of adhesion molecules, abnormal BBB permeability has been demonstrated in HIV infection. This BBB breakdown has been correlated with the diffuse "demyelination" or myelin pallor found in some cases of HIVE and HAND (Smith et al., 1990; Power & Johnson, 1995; Power et al., 1993; Rhodes, 1991; Rhodes, 1993). Morphological, vascular changes in HIV-infected CNS include increased vessel wall cellularity, mural thickenings, and enlargement of endothelial cells (Smith et al., 1990). The observation of deposited serum proteins, IgG, and complement associated with neurons and glial cells are also suggestive of loss of BBB integrity (Smith et al., 1990; Power & Johnson, 1995; Power et al., 1993; Rhodes, 1991; Rhodes, 1993). Complement deposition has also been noted in the choroid plexus, hinting at an abnormal permeability of that structure also (Falangola, Castro-Filho, & Petito, 1994). It has been postulated that a compromised BBB, measured by IgG and serum deposition, is part of the central pathogenetic mechanism in HAND (Power et al., 1993; Rhodes, 1991). Thus, the normal traffic from the bone marrow to the CNS as well as normal BBB integrity may be dramatically augmented or distorted in HIV-1-infected individuals (Persidsky et al., 2000; Nottet et al., 1996). Even during the era of combination ART, issues of monocyte traffic and viral entry to the CNS as a source of long-term infection are still relevant. HIV-infected monocytes are found in patients on ART and proviral DNA can be measured in monocytes despite nondetectable plasma virus (Sonza et al., 2001; Harrold et al., 2002; Zhu et al., 2002; Perno et al., 2006). It has also been demonstrated in vitro that reverse transcriptase inhibitors, although effective on acutely infected monocyte/macrophages, had little effect on chronically infected monocyte/macrophages (when HIV-DNA is already integrated). Protease inhibitors appeared to be the only drugs able to reduce replication in chronically infected monocyte/macrophages (Perno et al., 2006). Moreover, once macrophages in the CNS are infected, ART is less effective on them, due in part to low CNS penetration of these agents (Langford et al., 2006).

MACROPHAGES AND MICROGLIAL CELLS AS HIV TARGETS

Many studies have sought to localize the HIV-1 virus to specific types of resident cells in the CNS. Three cell types infected with HIV-1 are readily identified in the brains of individuals afflicted with HIVE and HAND: meningeal macrophages, perivascular cells, and multinucleated giant cells (Fischer-Smith et al., 2001; Koenig et al., 1986; Kure et al., 1990; Budka, 1986; Budka, 1991; Kure, Weidenheim et al., 1990; Dickson et al., 1993). Occasionally, but not consistently, parenchymal microglial cells are found to harbor virus (Kure et al., 1990; Budka, 1991). In vitro studies examining the HIV infectability of such cells demonstrate that macrophages and microglial cells (presumably, a small subset of parenchymal microglial cells) are both capable of becoming infected

(He et al., 1997; Watkins et al., 1990; Ghorpade et al., 1998; Strizki et al., 1996; Boche et al., 1995; Sharpless et al., 1992). A past report documenting recovery of HIV-1 from cells of the choroid plexus (Harouse et al., 1989) may reflect infection of resident macrophages in that location. No data exist that pertain to the perivascular cell specifically relative to this parameter; however, in HIVE, the most frequently encountered cells in which virus can be demonstrated are clusters of perivascular cells. In these cells the virus can reach high concentration so that it is easily demonstrable with antibodies against specific HIV-encoded protein antigens. Moreover, the formation of giant cells, a hallmark of HIVE, is a property of stimulated macrophages. These cells also are frequently located in the perivascular area around small venules and capillaries. Based upon both the expression of perivascular cell surface markers such as CD4, CD14, and CD45, CD163 and their frequent location in close association with the vasculature it is possible that these giant cells might be considered to originate from the fusion of HIV-infected perivascular cells (Williams et al., 2001).

It is probable that all of these cell types can and do become infected by the retrovirus during the spread of HIV-1 through the body. One highly probable scenario is that some precursors of selected members of all the macrophage/monocyte residents in the CNS become infected in the bone marrow and blood and enter the brain and spinal cord carrying provirus, although this remains to be experimentally proven in the SIV system or demonstrated in patients. Since the subpopulation of CD14+CD16+ monocytes is expanding in AIDS—especially with AIDS dementia pre-highly active antiretroviral treatment (HAART) (Pulliam et al., 1997; Thieblemont et al., 1995)—and since these cells co-localized with HIV (Fischer-Smith et al., 2001) or SIV (Williams et al., 2001), it seems logical to conclude that there is a slow, relentless passage of such cells from the marrow into the CNS over years before AIDS becomes clinically apparent. In fact, it might even account for the evolution of some HIV-associated syndromes (Gartner, 2000).

The meningeal macrophages are the most rapidly changing population of these cells. In many individuals infected with the virus, a picture of aseptic meningitis appears within a few months of contracting the infection. Virus can be demonstrated at that time in the CSF. The appearance of such a syndrome is not dependent on any comorbidity existing in the nervous system; it occurs in the absence of other neurological dysfunction or infections. This may indicate the arrival of disease macrophages in the pia and arachnoid. If this is true, then it follows that the macrophages that are coming to the meninges bearing the virus are severely dysfunctional, and themselves are releasing substances that produce the meningitis-like picture. Alternatively, it is possible that the macrophages are not themselves dysregulated, but because of their viral load they may be serving as the targets of a futile attack by the immune system, which is trying to eliminate the pathogen (Williams & Hickey, 2002; Kim et al., 2004).

It may be important to note in passing that in the peripheral nervous system, especially in the dorsal root and autonomic ganglia, a population of monocytic phagocytes normally reside immediately adjacent to neurons (Vass et al., 1993). These cells have the same immunophenotype as perivascular cells of the CNS. Moreover, they are physiologically replaced from the bone marrow (Vass et al., 1993), like CNS monocytic cells, and could arrive at their station infected with virus and potentially dysfunctional so that they perturb the normal ganglionic milieu. Such cells are readily demonstrated to be productively infected by SIV (Williams, Alvarez et al., 2001). The painful sensory neuropathies and autonomic problems experienced by some HIV-1-infected individuals, in addition to being caused by anti-HIV drug therapies, could possibly be attributed to these cells (Pardo, McArthur, & Griffin, 2001; Dalakas, 2001; Kolson & Gonzalez-Scarano, 2001; Brinley, Pardo, & Verma, 2001).

SPREAD OF HIV TO THE CENTRAL NERVOUS SYSTEM

Given the complexity of the macrophage/monocyte system in the brain and spinal cord, we wonder which cells are responsible for carrying and maintaining the virus therein. After considering the above data on the traffic of monocytic phagocytes and T cells into the nervous system, it is difficult to identify a "Trojan horse"—it appears that the CNS of an HIV-infected individual is actually confronted with a "Trojan herd." Multiple mechanisms experimentally documented to occur would permit HIV-infected monocytic cells or T cells behind the BBB in a position to spread the virus to resident CNS cells with which they make contact. Despite this abundance of potential suspects, there are reasons to most strongly suspect the perivascular cell of the CNS as being the principle culprit in the carriage of HIV into the nervous system. First, their kinetics of replacement is sufficiently frequent that it would permit a significant number of viral-laden cells to enter the brain or spinal cord over a few years. Second, immunohistological examination of brains from HIVE patients most frequently demonstrates virus in perivascular cells; in many instances these cells have accumulated in that area and are strongly positive for virus. Third, these cells are in prolonged, intimate contact with parenchymal microglial cells through the foot-processes of the latter; thus they could pass virus to them when the microglial cell entered a susceptible, stimulated state. Fourth, perivascular cells are the only CNS resident macrophage type demonstrated in vivo to be an antigen-presenting cell for T cells. Therefore, they must regularly make intimate contact with transiting T cells, increasing their own chance of becoming HIV infected. And finally, in patients with HIV-associated CNS syndromes attributable to neural dysfunction, there is BBB breakdown. The perivascular cells are in close apposition to the endothelial cells, ideally situated to disturb their normal functioning. However, with so many possible cells types that could carry and maintain HIV-1 in the nervous system and whose dysfunction could disturb that organ's normal homeostasis, it is likely that all of the mononuclear phagocyte types have a role in some HIV-associated syndrome's pathogenesis.

MONOCYTE EXPANSION FROM BONE MARROW CORRELATES WITH DEVELOPMENT OF AIDS AND SEVERITY OF SIV ENCEPHALITIS

It has become increasingly clear that monocyte expansion from the bone marrow into the blood occurs with HIV infection and contributes to increased traffic of monocyte/macrophages to tissues. Monocytes of bone marrow origin are circulating precursors that give rise to and replenish some macrophage populations in tissues, including the brain (Soulas et al., 2009). Monocytes that originate from hematopoietic stem cells in bone marrow undergo three stages of differentiation, from monoblasts to promonocytes to monocytes, which are released into the circulation (Gonzalez-Mejia & Doseff, 2009; van Furth, 1989; Tushinski et al., 1982). Thus, monocytes exit the bone marrow, transit through the blood and enter the CNS. This occurs in normal conditions and is accelerated with viral infection, such as HIV and SIV. It is not surprising then that there is an increased exchange of monocytes in the brain associated with HIV infection, and in fact changes in bone marrow as well as in blood monocyte populations are correlated with the development of AIDS, AIDS dementia, and CNS neuropathogenesis.

Recent radiologic reports have demonstrated bone marrow diffusion, investigating clivial and calvarial marrow of the skull, which account for approximately 13% of red marrow in adults, correlated with severity of dementia in HIV patients (Ragin et al, 2006). Similarly, anemia before the onset of AIDS is predictive of HIV neuropathogenesis (Ragin et al, 2006; Williams & Hickey, 2002; McArthur et al., 1993). In addition, thrombocytopenia also has been shown to correlate with the development of HAD, underscoring the notion that events in the bone marrow are associated with and may potentially predict HAD development (Wachtman et al., 2006).

Expanded numbers and relative percentages of select monocyte subsets occur early with HIV infection, with peak plasma virus and then again with the development of AIDS. Thus, monocyte expansion, likely a result of viremia, microbial products translocating across the gut, and in response to dying macrophages in lymph nodes, is critical in HIV pathogenesis (Fischer-Smith et al., 2001; Crowe et al., 2003; Kim et al., 2003; Kim, Alvarez & Williams, 2005; Marcondes et al., 2008). Thus, expansion in the absolute number or relative percentage of activated, pro-inflammatory CD14^{low}CD16+ monocytes correlate with the incidence of HIV dementia and accumulation of monocyte/macrophages in the brain (Fischer-Smith et al., 2001; Pulliam et al., 1997; Thieblemont et al., 1995). In an elegant experiment in monkeys, leukocytes were labeled ex vivo with fluorescent dyes and reinfused in infected animals and CD68+CD16+ monocyte/macrophages were detected in the choroid plexus and perivascular spaces (Clary et al., 2007). Our laboratory has shown a biphasic increase in percentage and absolute number of CD14^{low}CD16+ monocytes occurring first with viremia and then with development of AIDS in SIV-infected monkeys (Williams et al., 2001; Williams, Schwartz, et al., 2001; Williams et al., 2005). Whether or not this increase of cells with infection was truly from bone marrow was not directly demonstrated.

Recently, we and others performed studies to determine the role of turnover and release of monocytes from bone marrow, quantified using bromodeoxyuridine (BrdU) as a marker for monocytes newly released into blood (Burdo et al., 2010; Wang et al., 2008; Shih et al., 2005; Brown, Wijewardana, Liu, & Barratt-Boyes, 2009; Hasegawa et al., 2009; Goto et al, 2003). Using this method, we showed a massive turnover of peripheral monocytes that was associated with apoptotic macrophages in lymph nodes. The percentage of BrdU+ monocytes increased with acute and chronic SIV infection within animals that developed and died of AIDS (Hasegawa et al., 2009). In fact, the increased percentage of BrdU+ monocytes correlated with AIDS development more so than CD4+ T lymphocyte loss or viral load (Hasegawa et al., 2009; Kuroda, 2010). More recently, we demonstrated in a rapid model of SIV-induced AIDS that the magnitude of BrdU+ monocytes in blood, as early as 21 days post infection, correlates with rapid AIDS progression and the severity of SIV encephalitis (SIVE) (Burdo et al., 2010). These data together underscore the importance of monocyte activation and augmented turnover from bone marrow to the brain in SIV neuropathogenesis.

Interestingly, we found that the percentage of BrdU+ monocytes correlated with the level of a monocyte/macrophage-specific soluble protein, sCD163, in plasma. In vitro and in vivo studies have shown that CD163 expression on monocytes inversely correlated with sCD163 in tissue culture media or plasma, directly linking sCD163 to monocyte activation Weaver et al., 2007; Weaver et al., 2006; Moller et al., 2002; Davis & Zarev, 2005). In our studies, increased monocyte turnover correlated with high levels of sCD163 in plasma, where the initial spike in sCD163 was detected in the first few weeks post infection, prior to development of AIDS (Burdo et al., 2010). Thus, it would seem that this critical marker unique to monocyte/macrophages, and expressed and likely shed from perivascular cells in the brain, is telling us something important about AIDS pathogenesis. It is of interest that sCD163 has known anti-inflammatory properties (Moestrup & Moller, 2004) when shed from alternatively activated macrophages (Komohara et al., 2006). It might be that sCD163 dampens ongoing immune activation and at the same time monocytes expand in blood and traffic to the CNS. It is clear that there is an accumulation of macrophages in the CNS with pathology in AIDS, and the majority of these cells have been recruited from the bone marrow and blood (Dickson et al., 1991; Williams et al., 2002; Williams & Hickey, 2002). It is noteworthy that we find BrdU+ monocyte/macrophages in the meninges, perivascular cuffs, and SIVE lesions of the CNS parenchyma of the animals described above. Moreover, the majority of the BrdU+ cells are MAC387+, which is an early marker of newly recruited monocyte/macrophages (Otani et al., 1998) and consistent with lesions in neuroAIDS as ongoing, active, and dynamic processes. In this regard, we consider as our last topic, monocyte/macrophage populations in SIV and HIV encephalitic lesions.

SIV AND HIV ENCEPHALITIS LESIONS ARE COMPOSED OF AT LEAST THREE MACROPHAGE POPULATIONS—NOTES ON IMMUNE REGULATION

Historically, HIV and SIV encephalitis lesions are considered to compriseat least two main macrophage populations: the resident parenchymal microglia and perivascular cells. As discussed, these had been originally differentiated initially based on morphology and more recently using expression levels of CD14 and CD45, both of which are easily detected on perivascular cells. To this list, we add the multinucleated giant cells, which are likely fused monocyte/macrophages or perivascular cells (Fischer-Smith et al., 2001; Williams et al., 2001). In addition to CD14 and CD45 as markers to differentiate perivascular cells from parenchymal microglia, we and others also use CD163 that readily identifies perivascular cells in the noninfected brain, as well as HIV and SIV lesions (Roberts, Masliah, & Fox, 2004; Kim et al., 2005) (Figure 2.1.1). Traditionally, markers used for "resident macrophages" in HIVE lesions include CD68 and HAM-56, both of which identify mature resident macrophages in tissues and whose numbers in the CNS positively correlate with the severity of encephalitis (O'Neil et al.2004; Adamson et al., 1999). CD68 can be used to detect both perivascular cells and parenchymal microglia while HAM-56 primarily identifies the latter. Recent work by our laboratory has identified another critical monocyte/macrophage population sometimes found in the CNS of monkeys (21 days post infection) and consistently found in chronically infected monkeys and humans with AIDS and encephalitis: a MAC387+ monocyte/macrophage (Soulas et al., 2011). In contrast to the CD68+, HAM-56+ parenchymal microglia, and CD163+ perivascular cells that can be productively infected, the MAC387+ cells are not. Additionally, they are CD163, with few or none expressing CD68. The MAC387 antibody primarily recognizes the myeloid-related protein MRP14 and, to a lesser extent, a heterocomplex comprised of MRP8 and MRP14, also known as S100A8/S100A9 or calprotectin (Goebeler et al., 1984; Guignard, Mauel, & Markert, 1996; Flavel, Jones, & Wright, 1987). MAC387, MRP8, and MRP8/MRP14 immune reactivity on monocyte/macrophages generally distinguishes stages of inflammation and more particularly activation states of neurologic disorders including multiple sclerosis, HTLV-1-associated myelopathy, autoimmune neuropathies, and traumatic brain injury, where in each case detection of macrophages with these antigens has been interpretive as a marker of active, ongoing lesion activity (Beschorner et al., 2002; Kiefer et al., 1998; Abe et al., 1999; Merkler et al., 2006).

We have identified few scattered MAC387+ cells in animals sacrificed 21 days post infection, similar to the number of macrophages accumulating in the perivascular space. With AIDS, we detect larger numbers of MAC387+ cells in both monkey and human brains almost exclusively accumulated within encephalitic lesions. Interestingly, within the CNS of uninfected macaques whose CNS had been repopulated four years after EGFP+ autologous hematopoietic stem cell transplantation, a large number of CD163+ cells were renewed by

CD34+ stem cells, but none of these cells were MAC387+ (Soulas et al., 2009). This is because there was no active inflammation in the CNS of animals receiving transplanted stem cells. In contrast, in animals with AIDS that had BrdU administered early in infection, or late, or at both time points, the majority of BrdU+ cells in the CNS lesions were MAC387+ cells (Burdo et al., 2010; Soulas et al., 2011, Am J Pathol, in press). It is important to note that within the SIVE and HIVE lesions we examined, there are differing numbers of accumulated MAC387+ cells, as well as CD163+ perivascular cells and CD68+ resident macrophages which are all likely indicative of the "relative activity" of each lesion, and indeed CNS pathogenesis. Calprotectin, which is recognized by the MAC387 antibody, is significantly elevated in serum of HIV patients and in patients with active multiple sclerosis and rheumatoid arthritis (Frosch et al., 2000; Bogumil et al., 1998; Strasser, Gowland, & Ruef, 1997; Muller et al., 1994). It is thought to amplify pro-inflammatory responses via autocrine and paracrine mechanisms in phagocytes and endothelial cells, leading to increased extravasation (Foell, Wittkowski, Vogl, & Roth, 2007; Eue et al., 2000).

Thus, SIV and HIV encephalitis lesions are composed of productively infected perivascular cells, which are CD14+CD16+CD45+CD163+ cells, parenchymal microglia that are CD68 and HAM56 positive and in some cases CD163+ and infected, and lastly recently recruited MAC387+ monocyte/macrophages (Figure 2.1.3). It would seem that there is an early accumulation of CD14+CD163+ perivascular cells and some MAC387+ cells in the CNS just after infection, and significant accumulation of all these cell types with active, severe lesions with AIDS. It is tempting to hypothesize that each macrophage type functions to amplify or, alternatively, to dampen and perhaps contain the CNS lesions. In this scenario, MAC387+ cells that are only present within active, ongoing lesions are consistent with immune expanders or inflammatory M1-type macrophages. In contrast, the CD163+ perivascular cells that are clearly activated and contribute to immune reactivity in the CNS may also by virtue of their CD163 expression be regulatory M2-type macrophages that are attempting to wall off the lesion, isolating it from the rest of the noninfected tissues. A similar scenario has been hypothesized in a brain abscess model where the early lesions in the abscess are surrounded by ED-2-positive macrophages, which are eventually replaced by myofibroblasts and a scar, separating the abscess from the rest of the brain (Flaris et al., 1993; Flaris & Hickey, 1992).

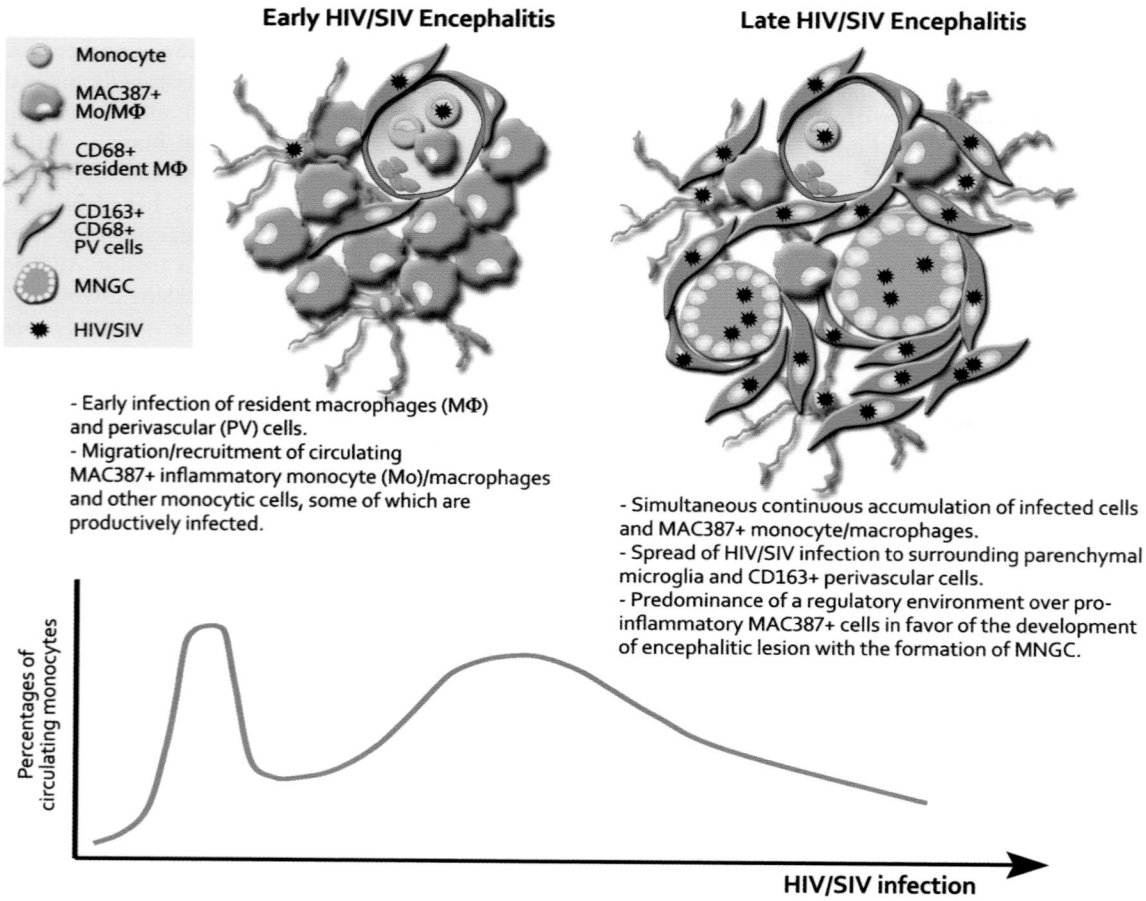

Figure 2.1.3 Hypothetical contribution of MAC387+ monocyte/macrophages, CD163+ perivascular cells, and parenchymal microglia in early and late HIV and SIV encephalitis lesions. Proposed role of MAC387+ cells as regulator M1 macrophages and CD163+ perivascular cells as regulatory M2 macrophages.

SUMMARY

The spread of HIV-1 into the CNS is known to occur early in the course of the infection. However, besides the early HIV-associated meningitis, most nervous system complications of HIV in the CNS take years to appear. As noted in prior chapters, these syndromes are highly variable and it seems impossible to tie all of them together with a single thread.

Despite this, over the past decade the belief has emerged that cells of the monocyte/macrophage family resident in the CNS play a critical role in some if not most of these HIV-related diseases. This chapter has attempted to demonstrate that the biology and function of these types of cells are very complex. It must be kept in mind that these cells are not a homogeneous group and they do not necessarily respond to stimuli in a stereotypical manner. The opposite is true; they are very heterogeneous, and even a single cell type has a considerable repertoire of functional responses available to it. Thus, it seems less amazing that a specific virus, which can infect them, has the ability to induce a wide variety of clinical illnesses. Perhaps some of the distinct clinical syndromes are attributable to a major or selective infection of only one or two of these monocyte subtypes.

While this survey has concentrated on monocytic phagocytes, it has omitted any mention of the interactions of such cells with other neuroglial elements. Obviously, such interactions are most probably critical in the pathogenesis of some of the disorders induced by HIV in the nervous system. However, at this point in time, available data from human patients and experimental models suggest that members of the monocyte family play an early, major, and central role in the neurological diseases associated with HIV-1 infection. This is a strong stimulus for urging a more complete understanding of their physiology and pathogenic potential.

ACKNOWLEDGMENT

Supported in part by awards from the NIH, NINDS R01's NS37654 (KW) NS40237 (KW).

REFERENCES

Abe, M., Umehara, F., Kubota, R., Moritoyo, T., Izumo, S., & Osame, M. (1999). Activation of macrophages/microglia with the calcium-binding proteins MRP14 and MRP8 is related to the lesional activities in the spinal cord of HTLV-I associated myelopathy. *J Neurol*, 246(5), 358–64.

Achim, C. L., Schrier, R. D., & Wiley, C. A. (1991). Immunopathogenesis of HIV encephalitis. *Brain Pathol*, 1, 177–84.

Adamson, D. C., McArthur, J. C., Dawson, T. M., & Dawson, V. L. (1999). Rate and severity of HIV-associated dementia (HAD): Correlations with Gp41 and iNOS. *Mol Med*, 5(2), 98–109.

Ajami, B., Bennett, J. L., Krieger, C., Tetzlaff, W., & Rossi, F. M. (2007). Local self-renewal can sustain CNS microglia maintenance and function throughout adult life. *Nat Neurosci*, 10(12), 1538–43.

Alexaki, A. & Wigdahl, B. (2008). HIV-1 infection of bone marrow hematopoietic progenitor cells and their role in trafficking and viral dissemination. *PLoS Pathog*, 4(12), e1000215.

Alexaki, A., Liu, Y., & Wigdahl, B. (2008). Cellular reservoirs of HIV-1 and their role in viral persistence. *Curr HIV Res*, 6(5), 388–400.

Barker, C. F. & Billingham, R. E. (1977). Immunologically privileged sites. *Adv Immunol*, 25, 1–6.

Bauer, J., Siminia, T., Wouterlood, F. G., & Dijkstra, C. D. (1994). Phagocytic activity of macrophages and microglial cells during the course of allergic encephalymyelitis. *J Immunol*, 126, 365–75.

Bechmann, I., Galea, I., & Perry, V. H. (2007). What is the blood-brain barrier (not)? *Trends Immunol*, 28(1), 5–11.

Bechmann, I., Kwidzinski, E., Kovac, A. D., Simburger, E., Horvath, T., Gimsa, U., et al. (2001). Turnover of rat brain perivascular cells. *Exp Neurol*, 168(2), 242–9.

Beschorner, R., Nguyen, T. D., Gozalan, F., Pedal, I., Mattern, R., Schluesener, H. J., et al. (2002). CD14 expression by activated parenchymal microglia/macrophages and infiltrating monocytes following human traumatic brain injury. *Acta Neuropathol*, 103(6), 541–9.

Bissel, S. J., Wang, G., Bonneh-Barkay, D., Starkey, A., Trichel, A. M., Murphey-Corb, M., et al. (2008). Systemic and brain macrophage infections in relation to the development of simian immunodeficiency virus encephalitis. *J Virol*, 82(10), 5031–42.

Boche, D., Gray, F., Chakrabarti, L., Hurtrel, M., Montagnier, L., & Hurtrel, B. (1995). Low susceptibility of resident microglia to simian immunodeficiency virus replication during the early stages of infection. *Neuropathol Appl Neurobiol*, 21(6), 535–9.

Bogumil, T., Rieckmann, P., Kubuschok, B., Felgenhauer, K., & Bruck, W. (1998). Serum levels of macrophage-derived protein MRP-8/14 are elevated in active multiple sclerosis. *Neurosci Lett*, 247(2–3), 195–7.

Brinley, F. J., Pardo, C., & Verma, A. (2001). Human immunodeficiency virus and the peripheral nervous system workshop. *Arch Neurol*, 58, 1561–1566.

Broadwell, R. D., Baker, B. J., Ebert, P. S., & Hickey, W. F. (1994). Allografts of CNS tissue possess a blood-brain barrier: III. Neuropathological, methodological, and immunological considerations. *Microsc Res Tech*, 27(6), 471–94.

Brown, K. N., Wijewardana, V., Liu, X., & Barratt-Boyes, S. M. (2009). Rapid influx and death of plasmacytoid dendritic cells in lymph nodes mediate depletion in acute simian immunodeficiency virus infection. *PLoS Pathog*, 5(5), e1000413.

Budka, H. (1986). Multinucleated giant cells in brain: A hallmark of the acquired immune deficiency syndrome (AIDS). *Acta Neuropathol*, 69(3-4), 253–8.

Budka, H. (1991). Neuropathology of human immunodeficiency virus infection. *Brain Pathol*, 163–75.

Burdo, T. H., Soulas, C., Orzechowski, K., Button, J., Krishnan, A., Sugimoto, C., et al. (2010). Increased monocyte turnover from bone marrow correlates with severity of SIV encephalitis and CD163 levels in plasma. *PLoS Pathog*, 6(4), e1000842.

Clay, C. C., Rodrigues, D. S., Ho, Y. S., Fallert, B. A., Janatpour, K., Reinhart, T. A., et al. (2007). Neuroinvasion of fluorescein-positive monocytes in acute simian immunodeficiency virus infection. *J Virol*, 81(21), 12040–8.

Crocker, P. R., Jeffries, W. A., Clark, S. J., Chung, L. P., & Gordon, S. (1987). Species heterogeneity in macrophage expression of the CD4 antigen. *J Exp Med*, 166, 613–8.

Crowe, S., Zhu, T., & Muller, W. A. (2003). The contribution of monocyte infection and trafficking to viral persistence, and maintenance of the viral reservoir in HIV infection. *J Leukoc Biol*, 74(5), 635–41.

Cserr, H. F. & Knopf, P. M. (1992). Cervical lymphatics, the blood-brain barrier and the immunoactivity of the brain: A new view. *Immunol Today*, 13, 507–12.

Dalakas, M. C. (2001). Peripheral neuropathy and retroviral drugs. *J Peripher Nerv Syst*, 6, 14–20.

Davalos, D., Grutzendler, J., Yang, G., Kim, J. V., Zuo, Y., Jung, S., et al. (2005). ATP mediates rapid microglial response to local brain injury in vivo. *Nat Neurosci*, 8(6), 752–8.

Davis, B. H. & Zarev, P. V. (2005). Human monocyte CD163 expression inversely correlates with soluble CD163 plasma levels. *Cytometry B Clin Cytom*, 63(1), 16–22.

Deckert-Schluter, M., Schluter, D., Hof, H., Wiestler, O. D., & Lassmann, H. (1994). Differential expression of ICAM-1, VCAM-1 and their ligands LFA-1, Mac- 1, CD43, VLA-4, and MHC class II antigens in murine Toxoplasma encephalitis: A light microscopic and ultrastructural immunohistochemical study. *J Neuropathol Exp Neurol, 53*(5), 457–68.

del rio Hortega, P. (1932). *Cytology and cellular pathology of the nervous system*. W. Penfield, (Ed.). New York: Hoeber.

Dickson, D. W., Lee, S. C., Mattiace, L. A., Yen, S. H-C., & Brosnan, C. (1993). Microglia and cytokines in neurological disease, with special reference to AIDS and Alzheimer's disease. *Glia, 7*(1), 75–83.

Dickson, D. W., Mattiace, L. A., Kure, K., Hutchins, K., Lyman, W. D., & Brosnan, C. F. (1991). Microglia in human disease, with an emphasis on acquired immune deficiency syndrome. *Lab Invest, 64*(2), 135–56.

Dijkstra, C. D., Dopp, E. A., Joling, P., & Kraal, G. (1985). The heterogeneity of mononuclear phagocytes in lymphoid organs: Distinct macrophage subpopulations in the rat recognized by monoclonal antibodies ED1, ED2, and ED3. *Immunology, 54*(3), 589–599.

Embretson, J., Zupancic, M., Ribas, J. L., Burke, A., Racz, P., Tenner-Racz, K., et al. (1993). Massive covert infection of helper T lymphocytes and macrophages by HIV during the incubation period of AIDS. *Nature, 362*(6418), 359–362.

Esiri, M. M. & Gay, D. (1990). Immunological and neuropathological significance of the Virchow-Robin space. *J Neurol Sci, 100*(1–2), 3–8.

Eue, I., Pietz, B., Storck, J., Klempt, M., & Sorg, C. (2000). Transendothelial migration of 27E10+ human monocytes. *Int Immunol, 12*(11), 1593–604.

Fabriek, B. O., Van Haastert, E. S., Galea, I., Polfliet, M. M., Dopp, E. D., Van Den Heuvel, M. M., et al. (2005). CD163-positive perivascular macrophages in the human CNS express molecules for antigen recognition and presentation. *Glia, 51*(4), 297–305.

Falangola, M. F., Castro-Filho, B. G., & Petito, C. K. (1994). Immune complex deposition in the choroid plexus of patients with acquired immunodeficiency syndrome. *Ann Neurol, 36*, 437–40.

Fauci, A. S. (1988a). The human immunodeficiency syndrome. *Ann Neurol, 36*:437–440.

Fauci, A. S. (1988b). The human immunodeficiency virus: Infectivity and mechanisms of pathogenesis. *Science, 239*, 617–622.

Fischer-Smith, T., Tedaldi, E. M., & Rappaport, J. (2008). CD163/CD16 coexpression by circulating monocytes/macrophages in HIV: Potential biomarkers for HIV infection and AIDS progression. *AIDS Res Hum Retroviruses, 24*(3), 417–21.

Fischer-Smith, T., Croul, S., Sverstiuk, A. E., Capini, C., L'Heureux, D., Regulier, E. G., et al. (2001). CNS invasion by CD14+/CD16+ peripheral blood-derived monocytes in HIV dementia: Perivascular accumulation and reservoir of HIV infection. *J Neurovirol, 7*(6), 528–41.

Flaris, N. A. & Hickey, W. F. (1992). Development and characterization of an experimental model of brain abscess in the rat. *Am J Pathol, 141*(6), 1299–307.

Flaris, N. A., Densmore, T. L., Molleston, M. C., & Hickey, W. F. (1993). Characterization of microglia and macrophages in the central nervous system of rats: Definition of the differential expression of molecules using standard and novel monoclonal antibodies in normal CNS and in four models of parenchymal reaction. *Glia, 7*(1), 34–40.

Flavell, D. J., Jones, D. B., & Wright, D. H. (1987). Identification of tissue histiocytes on paraffin sections by a new monoclonal antibody. *J Histochem Cytochem, 35*(11), 1217–26.

Flugel, A., Bradl, M., Kreutzberg, G. W., & Graeber, M. B. (2001). Transformation of donor-derived bone marrow precursors into host microglia during autoimmune CNS inflammation and during the retrograde response to axotomy. *J Neurosci Res, 66*(1), 74–82.

Foell, D., Wittkowski, H., Vogl, T., & Roth, J. (2007). S100 proteins expressed in phagocytes: A novel group of damage-associated molecular pattern molecules. *J Leukoc Biol, 81*(1), 28–37.

Folks, T. M., Kessler, S. W., Orenstein, J. M., Justement, J. S., Jaffe, E. S., & Fauci, A. S. (1988). Infection and replication of HIV-1 in purified progenitor cells of normal human bone marrow. *Science, 242*(4880), 919–22.

Ford, A. L., Goodsall, A. L., Hickey, W. F., & Sedgwick, J. D. (1995). Normal adult rat microglia seperated from other CNS macrophages by flow cytomteric sorting: Phenotypic differences defined and direct ex vivo antigen presentation to myelin basic protein reactive CD4 cells compared. *J Immunol, 154*, 4309–21.

Frosch, M., Strey, A., Vogl, T., Wulffraat, N. M., Kuis, W., Sunderkotter, C., et al. (2000). Myeloid-related proteins 8 and 14 are specifically secreted during interaction of phagocytes and activated endothelium and are useful markers for monitoring disease activity in pauciarticular-onset juvenile rheumatoid arthritis. *Arthritis Rheum, 43*(3), 628–37.

Gabuzda, D. H., Ho, D. D., de la Monte, S., Hirsch, M. S., Rota, T. R., & Sobel, R. A. (1986). Immunohistochemical identification of HTLV-III antigen in brains of patients with AIDS. *Ann Neurol, 20*, 289–95.

Galea, I., Bechmann, I., & Perry, V. H. (2007). What is immune privilege (not)? *Trends Immunol, 28*(1), 12–8.

Gartner, S. (2000). HIV infection and dementia. *Science, 287*(5453), 602–4.

Geissmann, F., Jung, S., & Littman, D. R. (2003). Blood monocytes consist of two principal subsets with distinct migratory properties. *Immunity, 19*(1), 71–82.

Gendelman, H. E., Lipton, S. A., Tardieu, M., Bukrinsky, M. I., & Nottet, H. S. (1994). The neuropathogenesis of HIV-1 infection. *J Leukoc Biol, 56*(3), 389–98.

Gendelman, H. E., Narayan, O., Molineaux, S., Clements, J. E., & Ghotbi, Z. (1985). Slow, persistent replication of lentiviruses: role of tissue macrophages and macrophage precursors in bone marrow. *Proc Natl Acad Sci USA, 82*(20), 7086–90.

Ghorpade, A., Nukuna, A., Che, M., Haggerty, S., Persidsky, Y., Carter, E., et al. (1998). Human immunodeficiency virus neurotropism: An analysis of viral replication and cytopathicity for divergent strains in monocytes and microglia. *J Virol, 72*(4), 3340–50.

Goebeler, M., Roth, J., Teigelkamp, S., & Sorg, C. (1994). The monoclonal antibody MAC387 detects an epitope on the calcium-binding protein MRP14. *J Leukoc Biol, 55*(2), 259–61.

Gonzalez-Mejia, M. E. & Doseff, A. I. (2009). Regulation of monocytes and macrophages cell fate. *Front Biosci, 14*, 2413–2431.

Gonzalez-Scarano, F. & Baltuch, G. (1999). Microglia as mediators of inflammatory and degenerative diseases. *Annu Rev Neurosci, 22*, 219–40.

Goto, Y., Hogg, J. C., Suwa, T., Quinlan, K. B., & van Eeden, S. F. (2003). A novel method to quantify the turnover and release of monocytes from the bone marrow using the thymidine analog 5'-bromo-2'-deoxyuridine. *Am J Physiol Cell Physiol, 285*(2), C253–9.

Graeber, M. B., Streit, W. J., & Buringer, D. (1992). Ultrastructural location of major histocompatibility complex (MHC) class II positive perivascular cells in histologically normal human brain. *J Neuropath Exp Neurol, 51*, 303–11.

Griffin, D. E., Levine, B., Tyor, W. R., & Irani, D. N. (1992). The immune response in viral encephalitis. *Sem Immunol, 4*, 111–9.

Guignard, F., Mauel, J., & Markert, M. (1996). The monoclonal antibody Mac 387 recognizes three S100 proteins in human neutrophils. *Immunol Cell Biol, 74*(1), 105–7.

Harouse, J. M., Wroblewsha, Z., Laughlin, M. A., Hickey, W. F., Schonwetter, B. S., & Gonzalez-Scarano, F. (1989). Human choroid plexus cells can be latently infected with human immunodeficiency virus. *Ann Neurol, 4*, 406–11.

Harrold, S. M., Wang, G., McMahon, D. K., Riddler, S. A., Mellors, J. W., Becker, J. T., et al. (2002). Recovery of replication-competent HIV type 1-infected circulating monocytes from individuals receiving antiretroviral therapy. *AIDS Res Hum Retroviruses, 18*(6), 427–34.

Hasegawa, A., Liu, H., Ling, B., Borda, J. T., Alvarez, X., Sugimoto, C., et al. (2009). The level of monocyte turnover predicts disease progression in the macaque model of AIDS. *Blood, 114*(14), 2917–25.

Hauser, S. L., Bhan, A. K., Gilles, F. H., Hoban, C. J., Reinherz, E. L., & Weiner, H. L. (1983). Immunohistochemical staining of human brain with monoclonal antibodies that identify lymphocytes, monocytes and the Ia antigen. *J Immunol, 5*, 197–205.

He, J., Chen, Y., Farzan, M., Choe, H., Ohagen, A., Gartner, S., et al. (1997). CCR3 and CCR5 are co-receptors for HIV-1 infection of microglia. *Nature*, 385, 645–9.

Hickey, W. F. & Kimura, H. (1987). Graft-vs.-host disease elicits expression of class I and class II histocompatibility antigens and the presence of scattered T lymphocytes in rat central nervous system. *Proc Natl Acad Sci USA*, 84(7), 2082–6.

Hickey, W. F. & Kimura, H. (1988). Perivascular microglial cells of the CNS are bone marrow-derived and present antigen in vivo. *Science*, 239(4837), 290–2.

Hickey, W. F., Vass, K., & Lassmann, H. (1992). Bone marrow-derived elements in the central nervous system: An immunohistochemical and ultrastructural survey of rat chimeras. *J Neuropath Exp Neurol*, 5, 246–56.

Hockenberry, D. M., Zutter, M., Hickey, W. F., & Korsemeyer, S. J. (1991). BCL-2 protein is topographically restricted to long lived and proliferating cells in tissues characterized by apoptotic cell death. *Clin Res*, 39, 339.

Hoffman, F. M., Dohadwala, M. M., Wright, A. D., Hinton, D. R., & Walker, S. M. (1994). Exogenous tat protein activates central nervous system-derived endothelial cells. *J Neuroimmumol*, 54, 19–28.

Honda, H., Kimura, H., Silvers, W. K., & Rostami, A. (1990). Perivascular location and phenotypic heterogeneity of microglial cells in the rat brain. *J Neuroimmunol*, 29(1–3), 183–91.

Igarashi, T., Brown, C. R., Endo, Y., Buckler-White, A., Plishka, R., Bischofberger, N., et al. (2001). Macrophage are the principal reservoir and sustain high virus loads in rhesus macaques after the depletion of CD4+ T cells by a highly pathogenic simian immunodeficiency virus/HIV type 1 chimera (SHIV): Implications for HIV-1 infections of humans. *Proc Natl Acad Sci USA*, 98(2), 658–63.

Iwasaki, A. & Medzhitov, R. (2004). Toll-like receptor control of the adaptive immune responses. *Nat Immunol*, 5(10), 987–95.

Jordan, C. A., Watkins, B. A., Kufta, C., & Dublois-Dalcq. (1991). Infection of brain microglial cells by human immunodeficiency virus type 1 is CD4 dependent. *J Virol*, 65, 736–42.

Kennedy, D. W. & Abkowitz, J. L. (1997). Kinetics of central nervous system microglial and macrophage engraftment: Analysis using a transgenic bone marrow transplantation model. *Blood*, 90(3), 986–93.

Kiefer, R., Kieseier, B. C., Bruck, W., Hartung, H. P., & Toyka, K. V. (1998). Macrophage differentiation antigens in acute and chronic autoimmune polyneuropathies. *Brain*, 121(Pt 3), 469–79.

Kim, W. K., Avarez, X., & Williams, K. (2005). The role of monocytes and perivascular macrophages in HIV and SIV neuropathogenesis: Information from non-human primate models. *Neurotox Res*, 8(1–2), 107–15.

Kim, W. K., Alvarez, X., Fisher, J., Bronfin, B., Westmoreland, S., McLaurin, J., et al. (2006). CD163 identifies perivascular macrophages in normal and viral encephalitic brains and potential precursors to perivascular macrophages in blood. *Am J Pathol*, 168(3), 822–34.

Kim, W. K., Corey, S., Alvarez, X., & Williams, K. (2003). Monocyte/macrophage traffic in HIV and SIV encephalitis. *J Leukoc Biol*, Aug 1.

Kim, W. K., Corey, S., Chesney, G., Knight, H., Klumpp, S., Wuthrich, C., et al. (2004). Identification of T lymphocytes in simian immunodeficiency virus encephalitis: Distribution of CD8+ T cells in association with central nervous system vessels and virus. *J Neurovirol*, 10(5), 315–25.

Kim, W. K., Sun, Y., Do, H., Autissier, P., Halpern, E. F., Piatak, M., Jr., et al. (2010). Monocyte heterogeneity underlying phenotypic changes in monocytes according to SIV disease stage. *J Leukoc Biol*, 87(4), 557–67.

Kitagawa, M., Lackner, A. A., Martfeld, D. J., Gardner, M. B., & Dandekar, S. (1991). Simian immunodeficiency virus infection of bone marrow: Correlation of viral infection with disease progression and hematologic abnormalities. *Am J Pathol*, 138, 921–30.

Koenig, S., Gendelman, H. E., Orenstein, J. M., Dal Canto, M. C., Pezeshkpour, G. H., Yungbluth, P., et al. (1986). Detection of AIDS virus in macrophages in brain tissue from AIDS patients with encephalopathy. *Science*, 233, 1089–93.

Kolson, D. L. & Gonzalez-Scarano, F. (2001). HIV-associated neuropathies: Role of HIV-1, CMS, and other viruses. *J Peripher Nerv Syst*, 6, 2–7.

Komohara, Y., Hirahara, J., Horikawa, T., Kawamura, K., Kiyota, E., Sakashita, N., et al. (2006). AM-3K, an anti-macrophage antibody, recognizes CD163, a molecule associated with an anti-inflammatory macrophage phenotype. *J Histochem Cytochem*, 54(7), 763–71.

Kure, K., Lyman, W. D., Weidenheim, K., & Dickson, D. W. (1990). Cellular localization of an HIV-1 antigen in subacute AIDS encephalitis using an improved double-labeling immunohistochemical method. *Am J Pathol*, 136, 1085–92.

Kure, K., Weidenheim, K. M., Lyman, W. D., & Dickson, D. W. (1990). Morphology and distribution of HIV-1 gp41-positive microglia in subacute AIDS encephalitis. Pattern of involvement resembling a multisystem degeneration. *Acta Neuropathol*, 80(4), 393–400.

Kuroda, M. J. (2010). Macrophages: Do they impact AIDS progression more than CD4 T cells? *J Leukoc Biol*, 87(4), 569–73.

Lampson, L. A. & Hickey, W. F. (1986). Monoclonal antibody analysis of MHC expression in histologically normal glioma containing human brain biopsies. *J Immunol*, 136, 4054–62.

Langford, D., Marquie-Beck, J., de Almeida, S., Lazzaretto, D., Letendre, S., Grant, I., et al. (2006). Relationship of antiretroviral treatment to postmortem brain tissue viral load in human immunodeficiency virus-infected patients. *J Neurovirol*, 12(2), 100–7.

Lassmann, H. & Hickey, W. F. (1993). Radiation bone marrow chimeras as a tool to study microglia turnover in normal brain and inflammation. *Clin Neuropath*, 12, 284–5.

Lassmann, H., Rossler, K., Zimprich, F., & Vass, K. (1991). Expression of adhesion molecules and histocompatibility antigens at the blood-brain barrier. *Brain Pathol*, 1(2), 115–23.

Lassmann, H., Schmied, M., Vass, K., & Hickey, W. F. (1993). Bone marrow derived elements and resident microglia in brain inflammation. *Glia*, 7(1), 19–24.

Lassmann, H., Zimprich, F., Rossler, K., & Vass, K. (1991). Inflammation in the nervous system. Basic mechanisms and immunological concepts. *Rev Neurol*, 147(12), 763–81.

Lassmann, H., Zimprich, F., Vass, K., & Hickey, W. F. (1991). Microglial cells are a component of the perivascular glia limitans. *J Neurosci Res*, 28(2), 236–43.

Lawson, L. J., Perry, V. H., & Gordon, S. (1992). Turnover of resident microglia in the normal adult mouse brain. *Neuroscience*, 48, 405–15.

Lavi, E., Strizki, J. M., Ulrich, A. M., Zhang, W., Fu, L., Wang, Q., et al. (1997). CXCR-4 (fusin), a co-receptor for the type 1 human immunodeficiency virus (HIV-1), is expressed in the human brain in a variety of cell types, including microglia and neurons. *Am J Pathol*, 151, 1035–42.

Mandell, C. P., Jain, N. C., Miller, C. J., & Dandekar, S. (1995). Bone marrow monocyte/macrophages are an early cellular target of pathogenic and nonpathogenic isolates of simian immunodeficiency virus (SIVmac) in rhesus macaques. *Lab Invest*, 72(3), 323–333.

Marcondes, M. C., Lanigan, C. M., Burdo, T. H., Watry, D. D., & Fox, H. S. (2008). Increased expression of monocyte CD44v6 correlates with the deveopment of encephalitis in rhesus macaques infected with simian immunodeficiency virus. *J Infect Dis*, 197(11): 1567–76.

Massari, F. E., Poli, G., Schnittman, S. M., Psalliuopoulos, M. C., Davey, V., & Fauci, A S. (1990). T lymphocyte origin of macrophage tropic strains of HIV: Role of monocytes during in vitro isolation and in vivo infection. *J Immunol*, 144, 4628–1432.

McArthur, J. C., Hoover, D. R., Bacellar, H., Miller, E. N., Cohen, B. A., Becker, J. T., et al. (1993). Dementia in AIDS patients: Incidence and risk factors. *Neurology*, 43(11), 2245–52.

Meltzer, M. S., Skillman, D. R., Gomatos, P. J., Kalter, D. C., & Gendelman, H. E. (1990). Role of mononuclear phagocytes in the pathogenesis of human immunodeficiency virus infection. *Annu Rev Immunol*, 8, 169–94.

Merkler, D., Boscke, R., Schmelting, B., Czeh, B., Fuchs, E., & Bruck, W., et al. (2006). Differential macrophage/microglia activation in neocortical EAE lesions in the marmoset monkey. *Brain Pathol*, 16(2), 117–23.

Merry, D. E., Veis, D. J., Hickey, W. F., & Korsmeyer, S. J. (1994). bcl-2 protein expression is widespread in the developing nervous system and retained in the adult PNS. *Development*, 120(2), 301–11.

Mittelbronn, M., Dietz, K., Schluesener, H. J, & Meyermann, R. (2001). Local distribution of microglia in the normal adult human central nervous system differs by up to one order of magnitude. *Acta Neuropathol (Berl)*, 101(3), 249–55.

Moestrup, S. K. & Moller, H. J. (2004). CD163: A regulated hemoglobin scavenger receptor with a role in the anti-inflammatory response. *Ann Med*, 36(5), 347–54.

Moller, H. J., Peterslund, N. A., Graversen, J. H., & Moestrup, S. K. (2002). Identification of the hemoglobin scavenger receptor/CD163 as a natural soluble protein in plasma. *Blood*, 99(1), 378–80.

Muller, F., Froland, S. S., Aukrust, P., & Fagerhol, M. K. (1994). Elevated serum calprotectin levels in HIV-infected patients: The calprotectin response during ZDV treatment is associated with clinical events. *J Acquir Immune Defic Syndr*, 7(9), 931–9.

Naif, H. M., Li, S., Alali, M., Sloane, A., Wu, L., Kelly, M., et al. (1998). CCR5 expression correlates with susceptibility of maturing monocytes to human immunodeficiency virus type 1 infection. *J Virol*, 72(1), 830–6.

Naif, H. M., Li, S., Ho-Shon, M., Mathijs, J. M., Williamson, P., & Cunningham, A. L. (1997). The state of maturation of monocytes into macrophages determines the effects of IL-4 and IL-13 on HIV replication. *J Immunol*, 158(1), 501–11.

Nathanson, J. A. & Chun, L. L. (1989). Immunological function of the blood-cerebrospinal fluid barrier. *Proc Natl Acad Sci USA*, 86, 1684–8.

Navia, B. A., Cho, E-S., Pettito, C. K., & Price, R. W. (1986). The AIDS dementia complex: II. Neuropathology. *Ann Neurol*, 19, 525–35.

Nimmerjahn, A., Kirchhoff, F., & Helmchen, F. (2005). Resting microglial cells are highly dynamic surveillants of brain parenchyma in vivo. *Science*, 308(5726), 1314–8.

Nottet, H. S. L. M., Persidsky, Y., Sasseville, V. G., Nakuna, A. N., Bock, P., Zhai, Q., et al. (1996). Mechanisms for the transendothelial migration of HIV-1-infected monocytes into brain. *J Immunol*, 156, 1284–95.

Oldstone, M. B. A. & Southern, P. J. (1993). Trafficking of activated cytotoxic T lymphocytes into the central nervous system: Use of a transgenic model. *J Neuroimmunol*, 46, 25–32.

O'Neil, S. P., Suwyn, C., Anderson, D. C., Niedziela, G., Bradley, J., Novembre, F. J., et al. (2004) Correlation of acute humoral response with brain virus burden and survival time in pig-tailed macaques infected with the neurovirulent simian immunodeficiency virus SIVsmmFGb. *Am J Pathol*, 164(4), 1157–72.

Orenstein, J. M. (2001). The macrophage in HIV infection. *Immunobiology*, 204, 598–602.

Otani, I., Akari, H., Nam, K. H., Mori, K., Suzuki, E., Shibata, H., et al. (1998). Phenotypic changes in peripheral blood monocytes of cynomolgus monkeys acutely infected with simian immunodeficiency virus. *AIDS Res Hum Retroviruses*, 14, 1181–6.

Pantaleo, G. & Fauci, A. S. (1994). Tracking HIV during disease progression. *Curr Opin Immunol*, 6(4), 600–604.

Pantaleo, G., Graziosi, C., Demarest, J. F., Butini, L., Montroni, M., Fox, C. H., et al. (1993). HIV infection is active and progressive in lymphoid tissue during the clinically latent stage of disease. *Nature*, 362(6418), 355–8.

Pantaleo, G., Graziosi, C., Demarest, J. F., Cohen, O. J., Vaccarezza, M., Gantt, K., et al. (1994). Role of lymphoid organs in the pathogenesis of human immunodeficiency virus (HIV) infection. *Immunol Rev*, 140, 104–29.

Pardo, C., McArthur, J. C., & Griffin, J. W. (2001). HIV neuropathy: Insights in the pathology of HIV peripheral nerve disease. *J Peripher Nerv Syst*, 6, 21–7.

Peluso, R., Haase, A., Stowring, L., Edwards, M., & Ventura, P. (1985). A Trojan horse mechanism for the spread of visna virus in monocytes. *Virology*, 147, 231–6.

Perno, C. F., Svicher, V., Schols, D., Pollicita, M., Balzarini, J., & Aquaro, S. (2006). Therapeutic strategies towards HIV-1 infection in macrophages. *Antiviral Res*, 71(2–3):293–300.

Perry, V. H. (1994). *Macrophages and the nervous system*. Austin: CRC Press.

Perry, V. H. & Gordon, S. (1987). Modulation of CD4 antigens on macrophages and microglia in rat brain. *J Exp Med*, 166, 1138–43.

Perry, V. H. & Gordon, S. (1988). Macrophages and microglia in the nervous system. *Trends Neurosci*, 11, 273–5.

Perry, V. H., Andersson, P. B, & Gordon, S. (1993). Macrophages and inflammation in the central nervous system. *TINS*, 16, 268–73.

Persidsky, Y., Zheng, J., Miller, D., & Gendelman, H. E. (2000). Mononuclear phagocytes mediate blood-brain barrier compromise and neuronal injury during HIV-1-associated dementia. *J Leukoc Biol*, 68(3), 413–22.

Peudenier, S., Hery, C., & Montagnier, T. M. (1991). Human microglial cells: Characterization in cerebral tissue and in primary culture, and study of their susceptibility to HIV-1 infection. *Ann Neurol*, 29, 152–61.

Pober, J. S., Lapierre, L. A., Stolpen, A. H., Brock, R., Springer, T. A., Fiers, W., et al. (1987). Activation of cultured human endothelial cells by recombinant lymphotoxin: Comparison with tumor necrosis factor and interleukin-1 species. *J Immunol*, 138, 3319–224.

Pope, M., Betjes, M. G. H., Romani, N., Hirmand, H., Cameron, P. U., Hoffman, L., et al. (1994) Conjugates of dendritic cells and memmory T lymphocytes from skin facilitate productive infection with HIV-1. *Cell*, 78, 389–98.

Power, C. & Johnson, R. T. (1995). HIV-1 associated dementia: Clinical features and pathogenesis. *Can J Neurol Sci*, 22, 92–100.

Power, C., Kong, P-A., Crawford, T. O., Wesselingh, S., Glass, J. D., McArthur, J. C., et al. (1993). Cerebral white matter changes in acquired immunodeficiency syndrome dementia: Alterations of the blood-brain barrier. *Ann Neurol*, 34, 339–50.

Price, R. W., Brew, B., Sidtis, J., Rosenblum, M., Scheck, A. C., & Cleary, P. (1988). The brain in AIDS: Central nervous system HIV-1 infection and AIDS dementia complex. *Science*, 239, 586–92.

Priller, J., Flugel, A., Wehner, T., Boentert, M., Haas, C. A., Prinz, M., et al. (2001). Targeting gene-modified hematopoietic cells to the central nervous system: Use of green fluorescent protein uncovers microglial engraftment. *Nat Med*, 7(12), 1356–61.

Pulliam, L., Gascon, R., Stubblebine, M., McGuire, D., & McGrath, M. S. (1997). Unique monocyte subset in patients with AIDS dementia. *Lancet*, 349, 692–5.

Ragin, A. B., Wu, Y., Storey, P., Cohen, B. A., Edelman, R. R., Epstein, L. G., et al. (2006). Bone marrow diffusion measures correlate with dementia severity in HIV patients. *AJNR Am J Neuroradiol*, 27(3), 589–92.

Rhodes, R. H. (1991). Evidence of serum-protein leakage across the blood-brain barrier in the acquired immunodeficiency syndrome. *J Neuropath Exp Neurol*, 50, 171–83.

Rhodes, R. H. (1993). Histopathologic features in the central nervous system of 400 acquired immunodeficiency syndrome cases: Implications of rates of occurrence. *Human Pathol*, 24(11), 1189–98.

Rinaldo, C. R. (1994). Modulation of major histocompatibility complex antigen expression by viral infection. *Am J Pathol*, 144, 637–650.

Rinner, W. A., Bauer, J., Schmidts, M., Lassmann, H., & Hickey, W. F. (1995). Resident microglia and hematogenous macrophages as phagocytes in adoptively transfered EAE: An investigation using rat radiation bone marrow chimeras. *Glia*, 14, 257–66.

Roberts, E. S., Masliah, E., & Fox, H. S. (2004). CD163 identifies a unique population of ramified microglia in HIV encephalitis (HIVE). *J Neuropathol Exp Neurol*, 63(12), 1255–64.

Rosenberg, Z. F. & Fauci, A. S. (1989). The immunopathogenesis of HIV infection. *Adv Immunol*, 47, 377–431.

Sasseville, V. G., Newman, W., Brodie, S. J., Hesterberg, P., Pauley, D., & Ringler, D. J. (1994). Monocyte adhesion to endothelium in simian immunodeficiency virus-induced AIDS encephalitis is mediated by vascular cell adhesion molecule-1/a4b1 integrin interactions. *Am J Pathol*, 144, 27–40.

Sasseville, V. G., Newman, W., Lackner, A. A., Smith, M. O., Lausen, N. C. G., Beall, D., et al. (1992). Elevated vascular cell adhesion molecule-1 in AIDS encephalitis induced by simian immunodeficiency virus. *Am J Pathol*, 141, 1021–130.

Sato, A. & Iwasaki, A. (2004). Induction of antiviral immunity requires Toll-like receptor signaling in both stromal and dendritic cell compartments. *Proc Natl Acad Sci USA*, 101(46), 16274–9.

Schrager, L. K. & D'Souza, M. P. (1998). Cellular and anatomical reservoirs of HIV-1 in patients receiving potent antiretroviral combination therapy. *JAMA*, 280(1), 67–71.

Sedgwick, J. D., Schender, S., Imrich, H., Dorries, R., Butcher, G. W., & ter Meulen, V. (1991). Isolation and direct characterization of resident microglial cells from the normal and inflamed central nervous system. *Proc Natl Acad Sci*, 88, 7438–42.

Serbina, N. V. & Pamer, E. G. (2006). Monocyte emigration from bone marrow during bacterial infection requires signals mediated by chemokine receptor CCR2. *Nat Immunol*, 7(3), 311–7.

Sharpless, N., Gilbert, D., Vandercam, B., Zhou, J. M., Verdin, E., Ronnett, G., et al. (1992). The restricted nature of HIV-1 tropism for cultured neural cells. *Virol*, 191, 813–25.

Shih, C. H., van Eeden, S. F., Goto, Y., & Hogg, J. C. (2005). CCL23/myeloid progenitor inhibitory factor-1 inhibits production and release of polymorphonuclear leukocytes and monocytes from the bone marrow. *Exp Hematol*, 33(10), 1101–8.

Sminia, T., de Groot, C. J., Dijkstra, C. D., Koetsier, J. C., & Polman, C. H. (1987). Macrophages in the central nervous system of the rat. *Immunobiology*, 54, 43–52.

Smith, T. W., DeGirolami, U., Henin, D., Bolgert, F., & Hauw, J-J. (1990). Human immunodeficiency virus (HIV) leukoencephalopathy and the microcirculation. 49, 357–70.

Sobel, R. A., Mitchell, M. E., & Fondren, G. (1990). Intercellular adhesion molecule-1 (ICAM-1) in cellular immune reactions in the human central nervous system. *Am J Pathol*, 136, 1309–1316.

Sonza, S., Mutimer, H. P., Oelrichs, R., Jardine, D., Harvey, K., Dunne, A., et al. (2001). Monocytes harbour replication-competent, non-latent HIV-1 in patients on highly active antiretroviral therapy. *AIDS*, 15(1), 17–22.

Soulas, C., Donahue, R. E., Dunbar, C. E., Persons, D. A., Alvarez, X., & Williams, K. C. (2009). Genetically modified CD34+ hematopoietic stem cells contribute to turnover of brain perivascular macrophages in long-term repopulated primates. *Am J Pathol*, 174(5), 1808–17.

Soulas, C., Conerly, C., Kim, W. K., Burdo,T. H., Alvarez, X, Lackner, A. A., Williams, K. C. (2011). Recently infiltrating MAC387(+) monocytes/macrophages a third macrophage population involved in SIV and HIV encephalitic lesion formation. *Am J Pathol*, 178(5), 2121–35.

Stanley, S. K., Kessler, S. W., Justement, J. S., Schnittman, S. M., Greenhouse, J. J., Brown, C. C., et al. (1992). CD34+ bone marrow cells are infected with HIV in a subset of seropositive individuals. *J Immunol*, 149(2), 689–97.

Stevenson, M. & Gendelman, H. E. (1994). Cellular and viral determinants that regulate HIV-1 infection in macrophages. *J Leukoc Biol*, 56(3), 278–88.

Strasser, F., Gowland, P. L., & Ruef, C. (1997). Elevated serum macrophage inhibitory protein (MRP) 8/14 levels in advanced HIV infection and during disease exacerbation. *J Acquir Immune Defic Syndr Hum Retrovirol*, 16(4), 230–8.

Strauss-Ayali, D., Conrad, S. M., & Mosser, D. M. (2007). Monocyte subpopulations and their differentiation patterns during infection. *J Leukoc Biol*, 82(2), 244–52.

Streit, W. J. & Graeber, M. B. (1993). Heterogeneity of microglial and perivascular cell populations: insights gained from the facial nucleus paradigm. *Glia*, 7(1), 68–74.

Strizki, J. M., Albright, A. V., O'Conner, M., Perrin, L., Gonzalez-Scarano, F. (1996). Infection of primary human microglia and monocyte-derived macrophages with human immunodeficiency virus type 1 isolates: Evidence of differential tropism. *J Virol*, 70, 7654–62.

Thieblemont, N., Weiss, L., Sadeghi, H. M., Estcourt, C., & Haeffner-Cavaillon, N. (1995). CD14lowCD16high: A cytokine-producing monocyte subset which expands during human immunodeficiency virus infection. *Eur J Immunol*, 25(12), 3418–24.

Thiele, J., Zirbes, T. K., Bertsch, H. P., Titius, B. R., Lorenzen, J., & Fischer, R. (1996). AIDS-related bone marrow lesions—myelodysplastic features or predominant inflammatory-reactive changes (HIV-myelopathy)? A comparative morphometric study by immunohistochemistry with special emphasis on apoptosis and PCNA-labeling. *Anal Cell Pathol*, 11(3), 141–57.

Tornatore, C., Chandra, R., Berger, J. R., & Major, E. O. (1994). HIV-1 infection of subcortical astrocytes in the pediatric central nervous system. *Neurology*, 44(3 Pt 1), 481–7.

Tornatore, C., Nath, A., Amemiya, K., & Major, E. O. (1991). Persistent human immunodeficiency virus type 1 infection in human fetal glial cells reactivated by T cell factors or by the cytokines tumor necrosis factor alpha and interleukin-1 beta. *J Virol*, 65, 6094–100.

Tushinski, R. J., Oliver, I. T., Guilbert, L. J., Tynan, P. W., Warner, J. R., & Stanley, E. R. (1982). Survival of mononuclear phagocytes depends on a lineage-specific growth factor that the differentiated cells selectively destroy. *Cell*, 28(1), 71–81.

Tyor, W. R., Glass, J. D., Griffin, J. W., Becker, P. S., McArthur, J. C., Bezman, L., et al. (1992). Cytokine expression in the brain during the acquired immunodeficiency syndrome. *Ann Neurol*, 31(4), 349–60.

Tyor, W. R., Moench, T. R., & Griffin, D. E. (1989). Characterization of the local and systemic B cell response of normal and athymic nude mice with sindbis virus encephalitis. *J Neuroimmunol*, 24, 207–15.

Ulvestad, E., Williams, K., Bjerkvig, R., Tiekotter, K., Antel, J., & Matre, R. (1994). Human microglial cells have phenotypic and functional characteristics in common with both macrophages and dendritic antigen-presenting cells. *J Leukoc Biol*, 56, 732–40.

Unger, E. R., Sung, J. H., Manivel, J. C., Chenggis, M. L., Blazar, B. R., & Krivit, W. (1993). Male donor-derived cells in the brains of female sex-mismatched bone marrow transplant recipients: A Y chromosome specific in situ hybridization study. *J Neuropathol Exp Neurol*, 52, 460–70.

Vallieres, L. & Sawchenko, P. E. (2003). Bone marrow-derived cells that populate the adult mouse brain preserve their hematopoietic identity. *J Neurosci*, 23(12), 5197–207.

van Furth, R. (1989). Origin and turnover of monocytes and macrophages. *Curr Top Pathol*, 79, 125–50.

Vass, K. & Lassmann, H. (1990). Intrathecal application of interferon gamma. Progressive appearance of MHC antigens within the rat nervous system. *Am J Pathol*, 137(4), 789–800.

Vass, K., Hickey, W. F., Schmidt, R. E., & Lassmann, H. (1993). Bone marrow-derived elements in the peripheral nervous system. An immunohistochemical and ultrastructural investigation in chimeric rats. *Lab Invest*, 69(3), 275–82.

Wachtman, L. M., Tarwater, P. M., Queen, S. E., Adams, R. J., & Mankowski, J. L. (2006). Platelet decline: An early predictive hematologic marker of simian immunodeficiency virus central nervous system disease. *J Neurovirol*, 12(1), 25–33.

Watkins, B. A., Dorn, H. H., Kelly, W. B., Armstrong, R. C., Potts, B. J., Michaels, F., et al. (1990). Specific tropism of HIV-1 for microglial cells in primary human brain cultures. *Science*, 249, 549–53.

Wang, X., Das, A., Lackner, A. A., Veazey, R. S., & Pahar, B. (2008). Intestinal double-positive CD4+CD8+ T cells of neonatal rhesus macaques are proliferating, activated memory cells and primary targets for SIVMAC251 infection. *Blood*, 112(13), 4981–90.

Weaver, L. K., Pioli, P. A., Wardwell, K., Vogel, S. N., & Guyre, P. M. (2007). Up-regulation of human monocyte CD163 upon activation of cell-surface Toll-like receptors. *J Leukoc Biol*, 81(3), 663–71.

Weaver, L. K., Hintz-Goldstein, K. A., Pioli, P. A., Wardwell, K., Qureshi, N., Vogel, S. N., et al. (2006). Pivotal advance: Activation of cell surface Toll-like receptors causes shedding of the hemoglobin scavenger receptor CD163. *J Leukoc Biol*, 80(1), 26–35.

Wekerle, H., Linnington, C., Lassmann, H., & Meyermann, R. (1986). Cellular immune reactivity within the CNS. *Trends Neurosci*, 9, 271–7.

Wiley, C. A., Schrier, R. D., Nelson, J. A., Lampert, P. W., Oldstone, M. B. A. (1986). Cellular localization of human immunodeficiency virus infection within the brains of acquired immunodeficiency syndrome patients. *Proc Natl Acad Sci, USA*, 83, 7089–93.

Williams, K. & Hickey, W. F. (1995). Traffic of lymphocytes into the CNS during inflammation and HIV infection. *J Neuro-AIDS*, 1, 31–55.

Williams, K. & Hickey, W. F. (1995). Traffic of hematogenous cells through the central nervous system. *Curr Top Micro Immunol, 202,* 221–45.

Williams, K. & Hickey, W. F. (2002). Central nervous system damage, monocytes and macrophages, and neurological disorders in AIDS. *Ann Rev Neurosci, 25,* 537–62.

Williams, K., Alvarez, X., & Lackner, A. A. (2001). Central nervous system perivascular cells are immunoregulatory cells that connect the CNS with the peripheral immune system. *Glia, 36*(2), 156–64.

Williams, K., Ulvestad, E., & Antel, J. (1994). Immune regulatory and effector properties of human adult microglia studies in vitro and in situ. *Adv Neuroimmunol, 4*(3), 273–81.

Williams, K., Ulvestad, E., & Antel, J. P. (1994). B7/BB-1 expression on adult human microglia studied in vitro and in situ. *Eur J Immunol, 24,* 3031–7.

Williams, K. C., Corey, S., Westmoreland, S. V., Pauley, D., Knight, H., deBakker, C., et al. (2001). Perivascular macrophages are the primary cell type productively infected by simian immunodeficiency virus in the brains of macaques: Implications for the neuropathogenesis of AIDS. *J Exp Med, 193*(8), 905–15.

Williams, K., Schwartz, A., Corey, S., Orandle, M., Kennedy, W., Thompson, B., et al. (2001). Proliferating cellular nuclear antigen (PCNA) expression as a marker of perivascular macrophages in SIV encephalitis. *Am J Pathol, 161,* 575–85.

Williams, K., Schwartz, A., Corey, S., Orandle, M., Kennedy, W., Thompson, B., et al. (2002). Proliferating cellular nuclear antigen expression as a marker of perivascular macrophages in simian immunodeficiency virus encephalitis. *Am J Pathol, 161*(2), 575–85.

Williams, K., Westmoreland, S., Greco, J., Ratai, E., Lentz, M., Kim, W. K., et al. (2005). Magnetic resonance spectroscopy reveals that activated monocytes contribute to neuronal injury in SIV neuroAIDS. *J Clin Invest, 115*(9), 2534–45.

Wong-Ki, K., Alvarez, A., Fisher, J., Bronfin, B., Westmoreland, S., McLaurin, J., et al. (2005). CD163 identifies perivascular macrophages in normal and viral encephalitic brains and potential precursors to perivascular macrophages in blood. *Am J Pathol,* In press.

Zhu, T., Muthui, D., Holte, S., Nickle, D., Feng, F., Brodie, S., et al. (2002). Evidence for human immunodeficiency virus type 1 replication in vivo in CD14(+) monocytes and its potential role as a source of virus in patients on highly active antiretroviral therapy. *J Virol, 76*(2), 707–16.

Zou, Y. R., Kottmann, A. H., Kuroda, M., Taniuchi, I., & Littman, D. R. (1998). Function of the chemokine receptor CXCR4 in haematopoiesis and in cerebellar development. *Nature, 393*(6685), 595–9.

2.2

MICROGLIA

Sunhee C. Lee

Microglia, which are the resident macrophages of the brain, become "activated" in response to immunological challenges. Specifically, the microglia change their cell morphology, upregulate surface antigens and receptors, and produce soluble mediators such as interferons, cytokines, and chemokines. Through the secretion of these soluble mediators, unopposed microglial activation can initiate an inflammatory cascade by activating other glial cells and by recruiting systemic inflammatory cells into the central nervous system (CNS). Microglial activation, which when occurring on a wide scale is referred to as "reactive gliosis," accompanies CNS disorders and is an important feature of neuroAIDS. Although generalized glial activation has traditionally been viewed as deleterious to neuronal function and survival, the prevailing view now is that, depending on the context, activated glia can also function to downmodulate the immune response and promote repair through production of anti-inflammatory cytokines, neurotrophins, and other growth factors. In this chapter, we consider the properties of microglia that are relevant to an understanding of HIV diseases. To that end, we also discuss recent advances in microglial biology that provide clues to how microglial responses might be modulated and harnessed for the benefit of patients with HIV.

INTRODUCTION

Microglia react to insults in several ways: by changing their cell morphology in ways that alter their interactions with adjacent cell populations, by up-regulating surface antigens and receptors that modulate responses to the surrounding environment, and by producing soluble mediators such as cytokines and chemokines that activate a range of downstream signaling cascades. Microglia, the resident macrophages of the brain, play a central role in this response through the expression of a wide range of cell-surface receptors, such as the toll-like receptors and other innate immune receptors that enable a rapid response to invading microbial pathogens. Innate immunity is characterized by the de novo production of mediators that directly contribute to antimicrobial activity or set off secondary inflammatory cascades that could ultimately result in inflammation and host injury. Some of the best characterized gene products that are induced as a result of the innate immune response are interferons, chemokines, and cytokines. The products of unopposed activated microglia can initiate an inflammatory cascade by activating other glial cells and by recruiting systemic inflammatory cells into the CNS.

Microglial alterations accompany CNS disorders including neuroAIDS, a response that is collectively referred to as a reactive gliosis. Although reactive glia have traditionally been viewed as being deleterious to neuronal function and survival, the prevailing view now is that depending on the context, the "activated" glia can also function to downmodulate the immune response and promote repair through production of anti-inflammatory cytokines, neurotrophins, and other growth factors. In this chapter, the properties of microglia that contribute to these processes during HIV diseases will be examined, along with the recent advances in microglial biology that provide clues suggesting that these properties could be harnessed to the benefit of the host.

BIOLOGY OF MICROGLIA

MICROGLIA IN NORMAL CNS

It is now firmly established that microglia are bone marrow-derived mesodermal cells that invade the brain during fetal development, in contrast to all other CNS resident cells that are neuroectodermal in origin (neurons, astrocytes, oligodendrocytes, and ependymal cells). Upon entering the brain through a highly specialized interaction with blood vessels, they migrate into the brain parenchyma and undergo a series of morphological and antigenic changes, a process that can be characterized as immune downregulation or "calming." Microglia eventually populate the entire brain as highly ramified cells with low to undetectable levels of monocyte surface antigens. This low expression of cell surface markers has long hampered visualization of "resting" microglia in the normal brain. However, recent studies have revealed a few microglial-specific proteins that are constitutively expressed in the normal state.

One such example is the receptor for the chemokine fractalkine (CX_3CR1) in normal microglia. Mice in which the CX_3CR1 gene was replaced with a green fluorescent protein (GFP) reporter gene showed GFP+, highly ramified microglia without impairment of microglial function (Jung et al., 2000). Two-photon imaging of the superficial cortex of these (live) mice show that "resting" microglial cells are highly active, continually surveying their microenvironment with extremely motile processes (Nimmerjahn, Kirchhoff, & Helmchen, 2005; Davalos et al., 2005). Blood-brain barrier (BBB) disruption or trauma in these animals provoked immediate focal activation of microglia and shielding of the injured site. Davalos et al. further found that both the rapid chemotactic and the baseline motility of microglial processes are regulated by extracellular ATP, presumably released from the damaged tissue or from astrocytes. Together, these studies showed that "resting" microglia are busily involved in sensing and sampling of their local surroundings and that upon injury, microglia are the first line of cells called to action to protect the neuropil.

Numerous studies have now shown that there are opposing forces in action in maintaining microglial balance (Figure 2.2.1). Although most microglial activating signals produce "reactive" states, there are many examples of microglial receptors and antigens the engagement of which result in an inhibited state of the cell ("calming" effect) (Hanisch & Kettenmann, 2007). The examples of the latter are numerous. For example, the transmembrane antigen CD45 in the mouse and in human microglia contributes to the downregulated state of microglia (Tan, Town, & Mullan, 2000; Suh, Kim, & Lee, 2005; Kim, Suh, Si, Terman, & Lee, 2006). The fractalkine receptor has been shown to function to protect the nervous system from damage (Cardona et al., 2006). CD200R (expressed in microglia) and CD200 (expressed in neurons) in the mouse is another example in which neuron-microglia interactions maintain the immune downregulated state of the CNS (Hoek et al., 2000; Lyons et al., 2007). Triggered receptor expressed on myeloid cells-2 (TREM-2) on microglia is yet another example (Klesney-Tait, Turnbull, & Colonna, 2006; Piccio et al., 2008).

There are microglial antigens that are expressed at high levels in the normal state which then diminish following cell activation. Examples of the latter are rare but include the recently described purinergic receptor P2Y12 in the mouse (but not in humans: unpublished observations) (Haynes et al., 2006). TREM-2 is also thought to be another example

(Schmid et al., 2002). However, in human microglia we find this not to be the case since exposure to toll-like receptor (TLR) ligands *increases* the expression of TREM-2 (unpublished observations).

There is evidence not only that normal brain homeostasis is maintained through an active process of reinforcing the calming signals, but that these forces are also operative when microglial cells are activated during injury. In fact, a microglial reactive state could be viewed as a failure of this normal balancing act. Much effort is now devoted to understanding the nature and regulation of the "calming" signals in order to harness brain inflammation (see below). In addition to immune receptors and antigens on microglia, a whole host of neural molecules (neurotransmitters, for example) and neural activity typically exert immune downmodulatory effects on microglia, as well as other glial cells, contributing to the "immune-privileged" state of the normal brain (Lee, Collins, Vanguri, & Shin, 1992; Neumann, Misgeld, Matsumuro, & Wekerle, 1998; Neumann, Boucraut, Hahnel, Misgeld, & Wekerle, 1996). In addition, astrocytes provide signals that are downmodulatory to microglia through multiple mechanisms (Liu, Brosnan, Dickson, & Lee, 1994; Wang et al., 2008).

MICROGLIA IN DISEASE AND THEIR RELATIONSHIP TO BLOOD-DERIVED MACROPHAGES

Upon various insults to the brain, microglia undergo characteristic morphologic and antigenic changes unique to each disease process. At the same time, depending on the nature and the tempo of the injury, monocytes can cross the BBB to enter the brain. Monocyte infiltration occurs in the setting of obvious BBB breakdown, such as in stroke or in multiple sclerosis, as well as in subacute HIV encephalitis, but typically not in chronic neurodegenerative diseases such as Alzheimer's disease. Determining the relative contribution of monocyte-derived macrophages and intrinsic microglia to the disease process, while conceptually important, is hampered by the fact that no single surface marker reliably differentiates intrinsic microglia from blood-borne monocytes (Dickson & Lee, 1997). Bone marrow chimerism in combination with the gene knockout or knock-in strategies in the mouse has contributed significantly to an understanding of microglial cell biology.

The bone marrow chimera studies by Hickey and colleagues provided the first evidence that perivascular microglia (macrophages) in the normal brain are a distinct population of CNS macrophages, different from parenchymal microglia. Perivascular macrophages turn over more rapidly, and they are capable of presenting antigen in immune response reactions, while intrinsic microglia represent a stable population with limited antigen-presenting potential (Hickey & Kimura, 1988). In addition to "perivascular" microglia, "juxtavascular" microglia are probably an important intrinsic microglial population that has received little attention. Juxtavascular microglia are characterized by the parenchymal location of the cell body, ramified cell processes, and direct contact with the

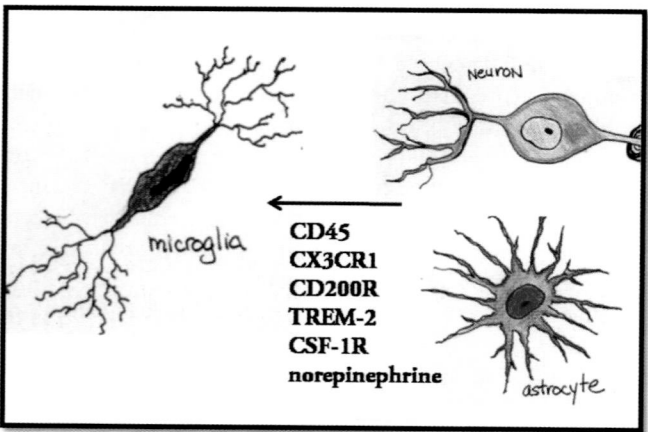

Figure 2.2.1 Microglial "resting" states are maintained by calming forces that are operative in normal brain. Neurons and astrocytes contribute significantly to this. Examples include neuronal electrical conductivity, neurotransmitters, astrocyte-derived microglial growth factor, neuronally derived ligands (fractalkine, CD200) that bind to microglial calming receptors (fractalkine receptor, CD200R), as well as unknown ligands that bind to microglial CD45 or TREM-2.

basal lamina of blood vessels by the cell processes. According to Dailey and colleagues, approximately 10% to 30% of total brain microglia in the rat hippocampus belongs to this population (Grossmann et al., 2002). The authors identified them as a mobile subpopulation of parenchymal microglia that activate rapidly and that are preferentially recruited to the surfaces of blood vessels following brain tissue injury. As such, this particular subpopulation of microglia may represent cells specialized to facilitate signaling between the injured brain parenchyma and components of the blood-brain barrier in vivo. For example, it is now clear that the microglia described in the study of Nimmerjahn et al. (see above) following BBB injury are almost certainly juxtavascular microglia (Nimmerjahn et al., 2005).

With the invention of the green fluorescence protein+ (GFP+) mice and their use as donor cell sources, there have been serious efforts to understand the origin of CNS mononuclear phagocytes in normal and diseased brains. When bone marrow stem cells expressing GFP are transplanted into the systemic circulation of irradiated mice, a range of CNS engraftment by donor GFP$^+$ cells has been reported. One group has reported these cells becoming predominantly perivascular macrophages (Vallieres & Sawchenko, 2003), similar to the original study by Hickey and Kimura. Others have found that a significant portion (~ a quarter) of microglia being donor-derived (Priller et al., 2001), and yet another group found nearly all of the infiltrating cells becoming highly ramified microglia (Simard & Rivest, 2004). The reasons for the highly variable results obtained by various investigators using very similar bone marrow chimeric models are not entirely clear. Information regarding donor cell engraftment of CNS in humans is limited, but an earlier study of human subjects with sex-mismatched bone marrow transplantation showed only rare donor-derived cells entering the normal-appearing brains to become perivascular cells (Unger et al., 1993).

All of the aforementioned bone marrow chimera studies have used lethal total body irradiation of the recipient mice. However, irradiation changes the local tissue environment, renders the BBB leaky, and induces local cytokine production. Therefore, it is questionable how well the irradiation models mimic the normal situation. To address this issue, Mildner et al. studied the effect of head shielding during lethal irradiation of the mice. They found that in brain pathologies not associated with overt BBB disruption, head irradiation was required for brain engraftment by donor GFP+ cells (Mildner et al., 2007). They also found that not all monocytes are equally capable of entering the brain. Rather, a specific subset of monocytes bearing the markers Ly-6C^{hi} CCR2$^+$ (corresponding to the CD14^{hi} CD16^{lo} subset in humans) are preferentially recruited to the brain. Curiously, the subset of monocytes that are assumed to accumulate in the brains of HIV encephalitis patients correspond to the CD14^{lo}CD16^{hi} subset rather than CD14^{hi} CD16^{lo} subset (Pulliam, Gascon, Stubblebine, McGuire, & McGrath, 1997; Fischer-Smith et al., 2001), posing questions regarding potential species differences, disease-specific monocyte recruitment, or other unexplained possibilities.

In another bone marrow transplantation study, chimerism was established by bypassing irradiation altogether. Ajami et al. adopted temporary surgical joining (parabiosis) of the recipient (GFP-) and donor (GFP+) mice to create chimeric animals. When they then induced CNS insults such as facial axotomy or amyotrophic lateral sclerosis (a genetic model), they also found no evidence for CNS engraftment by donor cells (Ajami, Bennett, Krieger, Tetzlaff, & Rossi, 2007). These studies using novel approaches to examine the contribution of peripherally derived monocytes to microglial population in the adult reinforce the original observation of Hickey and Kimura that the resident CNS microglia constitute a mononuclear phagocyte pool separate from the systemic population.

EXPERIMENTAL MODELS TO STUDY MICROGLIAL FUNCTIONS

Regardless of their ontogeny and relationship to blood-borne monocytes, it is well established that microglial cells are capable of mounting various reactive and reparative responses. Using the rat facial nerve axotomy model, Kreutzberg and colleagues have elegantly illustrated the various cellular and molecular changes that occur in microglial cells within the degenerating facial nucleus (Kreutzberg, 1996). They demonstrated that microglial activation is a key factor in the defense of the neural parenchyma against various insults, and showed that microglia function as scavenger cells, as well as in tissue repair and neural regeneration, ultimately facilitating the return to tissue homeostasis.

Ablation of a selective cell population is a useful way of exploring the function of the cell population in the brain. For example, using a cell-specific promoter (glial fibrillary acidic protein or S-100β for astrocytes) to drive expression of a "suicide gene" (mutant Herpes simplex thymidine kinase gene) enabled killing of a specific cell population (astrocytes, in this case) upon treatment with the antiviral agent, ganciclovir. Of note, unlike gene deletion strategies (GFAP knockout, for example), the suicide gene approach only ablates the proliferating cell population, not the entire population expressing the cell-specific promoter. Lalancette-Hebert et al. attempted the suicide gene expression under the CD11b promoter in order to study the role of proliferating microglia in ischemic stroke. Surprisingly, selective ablation of proliferating microglia was associated with a significant increase in infarct size accompanied by an alteration in proinflammatory cytokine expression (Lalancette-Hebert, Gowing, Simard, Weng, & Kriz, 2007). The proliferating microglia in control mice (that were killed following ganciclovir treatment) were also positive for insulin-like growth factor 1 (IGF-1), suggesting a neuroprotective role for microglia in this model. This study also showed that the resident microglia express a unique antigen Mac-2 and were separate from the monocyte-derived (GFP+) macrophages that infiltrated the brain following ischemic injury. These studies are unique in that they invoke the idea that there are indeed different microglial populations that may contribute to neuroprotection (see below).

MICROGLIA, HIV AND INNATE IMMUNITY

MICROGLIA AND INNATE IMMUNE RESPONSES

The early phase of an effective immune response to invading pathogens is essential for the survival of organisms and is known as the innate immune response. It is a type of immunity that is not dependent on T cells or B cells but is dependent on myeloid (neutrophils, monocytes, macrophages, microglia, and dendritic cells) or NK cells and their secretory products. The microglial phenotypic change and associated functional change (implied in most cases) that occur in brain disorders have been referred to as "neuroinflammation" and have been compared to innate immunity. The innate immune response can be driven through specific recognition systems, the best examples being the interactions between microbial components (termed "pathogen-associated molecular patterns," PAMPs) and toll-like receptors (TLR). In the CNS, the cells that bear the appropriate receptors to interact with these microbial components are monocyte-derived macrophages and resident brain microglia. The presence of abundant cell surface receptors renders microglia highly reactive to a variety of innate and adaptive immunological stimuli. For example, microglia are exquisitely sensitive to the TLR4 ligand, lipopolysaccharide (LPS), a component of the cell wall of gram-negative bacteria, and are likely the only cell type that can effectively respond to LPS in the CNS (Laflamme & Rivest, 2001). Recent studies also showed that significant levels of plasma LPS exist in HIV+ individuals (Brenchley et al., 2006) and that the levels of plasma LPS correlate with the degree of monocyte activation and dementia (Ancuta et al., 2008). These studies suggest that LPS might be a significant modifier of the HIV diseases and that HIV-infected individuals are at risk for "activating" peripheral and brain macrophages through TLR4. In addition to TLR4, TLR3 is also shown to be expressed in macrophages and microglia (but not in monocytes) (Jack et al., 2005; Muzio et al., 2000). Furthermore, endogenous host brain molecules are being increasingly recognized as ligands for TLR, in addition to pathogen components. These findings suggest that TLRs might be involved in the innate response in noninfectious settings as well.

MICROGLIAL ALTERNATIONS IN HIV/AIDS

There is a considerable variation in the type and degree of microglial involvement in HIV diseases. Prior to the introduction of combination anti-retroviral therapy (cART), approximately one-third of individuals with HIV developed HIV encephalitis characterized by productive infection of microglia and macrophages, activation of microglia and astrocytes, and varying degrees of degeneration of neuronal elements. Many individuals with HIV encephalitis develop neurologic impairments characterized by cognitive, motor, and behavioral abnormalities, termed HIV-associated dementia (HAD). However, in the post-cART era, CNS changes associated with HIV/AIDS have become much more subtle and diverse in etiology and nature. These reflect the effectiveness of cART in lessening the systemic and CNS viral burdens, as well as the toxicity and complications of cART (such as immune reconstitution inflammatory syndrome: IRIS). A large percentage of these individuals also exhibit confounding comorbidities such as hepatitis virus C infection or substance use. The neuropsychiatric disorders in individuals with HIV are now termed HIV-associated neurocognitive disorder (HAND). Readers are referred to other sections of this book for the clinical and neuropathologic aspects of HAND.

TLRs and viral infections: The TLRs that recognize viral pathogen-associated molecular patterns (PAMPs) are TLR3 (recognizes double stranded RNA: dsRNA), TLR7/8 (recognizes single stranded RNA: ssRNA), and TLR9 (recognizes viral DNA) (Kawai & Akira, 2007). TLR3 can also be activated by synthetic dsRNA, poly-riboinosinic-ribocytidylic acid (poly IC), a viral mimic. Of the 11 TLRs involved in the innate immune response, TLR3 and TLR4 are unique in that they can transmit signals through the MyD88-independent, toll/interleukin-1 receptor domain-containing adaptor protein inducing IFNβ (TRIF)-dependent pathway, resulting in activation of interferon regulatory factor 3 (IRF3) and subsequent IFNβ gene expression (Figure 2.2.2). Activation of IRF3 and induction of IFNβ is a critical component of innate antiviral immune signaling (see below). Of the CNS cells, microglia express all known TLRs and respond robustly to both poly IC (TLR3 ligand) and LPS (TLR4 ligand) (Suh, Brosnan, & Lee, 2009a). In addition to microglia, astrocytes also expressed

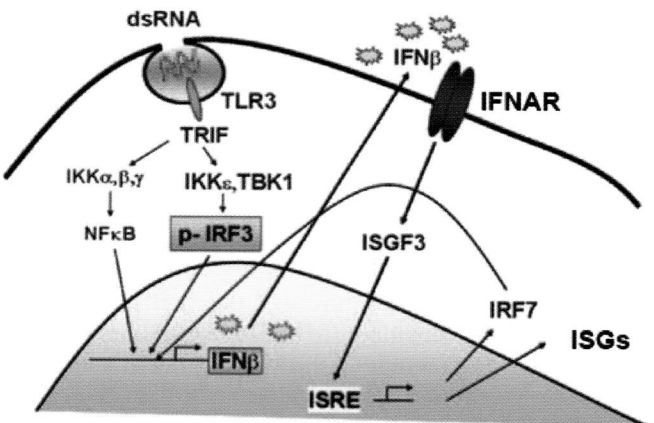

Figure 2.2.2 Effective innate antiviral immune signaling in microglia involves activation of the IRF3-IFNβ axis through several mechanisms. Shown here is an example of TLR3. In addition, TLR4 and the cytosolic RIG-like receptors can also activate the IRF3-IFNβ axis. dsRNA binding of endosomally located TLR3 activates the adaptor protein TRIF. TRIF then phosphorylates IRF3 through kinases such as IKKε or TANK-binding kinase 1 (TBK1). In addition, the canonical IKK (α, β, γ) necessary for NF-κB are also activated. Together, they elicit IFNβ transcription (primary response gene). The secreted IFNβ then acts on the cell's receptor (type I interferon receptor: IFNAR) to stimulate ISGF3 (Stat1, Stat2, IRF9) which then activate IFN-stimulated response elements (ISRE) on many IFN-stimulated genes (ISGs: secondary response genes). Several of the ISGs are also involved in positive feedback response amplifying the IFN cascades. IRF7 is shown for example. Modified from Suh et al., *J Virol*, 2007.

certain TLRs, with TLR3 being the predominant TLR on astrocytes (Farina et al., 2005). Although astrocytes express TLR4, due to the lack of the LPS binding receptor (CD14), they do not respond to LPS to a significant degree (Lee, Dickson, & Brosnan, 1995). In both microglia and astrocytes, poly IC activates IRF3 and type I interferons and other antiviral response genes, resulting in effective antiviral responses. Of note, in addition to TLR4 and TLR3 that are located on the cell membrane, cytosolic dsRNA receptors called "RIG-like helicases" or "RIG-like receptors (RLR)" constitute the third known pathway of IRF3 activation in cells (Hiscott, Lin, Nakhaei, & Paz, 2006; Sen & Sarkar, 2005). Importantly, gene deletion studies in mice have shown that most viral dsRNA activate host antiviral response through the cytosolic RIG-like receptors rather than TLR3 (Kato et al., 2005).

More intriguing responses are obtained with IL-1β, which shares the TLR signaling pathway through the common receptor domain called TIR (TLR and interleukin-1 receptor domain) and activation of the MyD88 pathway. Although IL-1β does induce IFNβ in astrocytes through IRF3 activation, IL-1β does not trigger antiviral activity against intracellular HIV or CMV (Rivieccio et al., 2005; Rivieccio et al., 2006; Suh et al., 2007). We also found that astrocytes stimulated with poly IC or IL-1β show differential activation of antiviral and inflammatory cytokine genes, suggesting that the small amount of phospho-IRF3 induced by IL-1β does not provide significant antiviral activity against intracellular pathogens (Rivieccio et al., 2006). These results emphasize the importance of the relative strengths of cell signals that may govern the ultimate functional outcomes.

DOES HIV ACTIVATE TLR?

The ability of HIV to induce type I interferons (IFNα or IFNβ) has been demonstrated in experimental and clinical settings, including in the macaque models of SIV encephalitis (Voth et al., 1990; Barber, Herbst, Bullock, Gama, & Clements, 2004). Therefore, it is of interest to determine whether HIV has the ability to trigger TLRs. Studies in peripheral macrophages and dendritic cells have demonstrated that HIV does activate the cells via ssRNA receptors (TLR7 or TLR8) resulting in type I interferon production (Heil et al., 2004). In microglia, we have examined whether HIV can activate the antiviral transcription factor IRF3 and its downstream antiviral genes (Suh et al., 2009b). Gene profiling studies have shown that while poly IC and LPS potently induced many ISGs, only a small number of ISGs were induced by HIV in microglia. Further examination of HIV-infected microglia demonstrated that while many of the cell activation pathways were preserved, the level of IRF3 protein was reduced, similar to that shown for Sendai virus-infected cells (Okumura et al., 2008). These results together suggest that HIV does not stimulate dsRNA receptors and that it lacks the ability to induce IRF3-dependent antiviral immune response in microglia. Furthermore, HIV might interfere with innate antiviral mechanisms by degrading transcription factors critical in antiviral immune responses. The type I interferon response demonstrated following HIV/SIV infection of macrophages and microglia, although very limited (Gendelman et al., 1990), is most probably mediated by viral sensors such as TLR7/8, or indirectly through other cytokines.

TLRs AND CYTOKINES IN MICROGLIAL ANTI-HIV ACTIVITY

In human microglia productively infected by HIV, both the TLR3 and the TLR4 ligands have potent anti-HIV activity (Suh et al., 2009b). This was shown in the acute spreading infection model using regular HIV as well as the single cycle infection model using env-pseudotyped HIV. The anti-HIV activity mediated by TLR ligands was IRF3-dependent. These results in microglia were somewhat surprising given the generally believed notion that unlike interferons (known antiviral agents), LPS and proinflammatory cytokines are activators of HIV infection (Osiecki et al., 2005; Folks et al., 1989; Rosenberg & Fauci, 1990). However, much of these data were derived from cell lines or cells with stably integrated HIV proviruses, such as U1 cells (monocytic), ACH-2 cells (T cell line), or HIV-transgenic murine macrophages (Sun, Zheng, Zhao, Lee, & Goldstein, 2008; Equils et al., 2003). Indeed, when the chronic latent infection model (U1 cells) was compared with primary microglial cultures side by side, we find that LPS as well as proinflammatory cytokines IL-1, TNFα, and IL-6 (all downstream products of TLR activation) have opposing effects in the two systems (i.e., they inhibit acute infection but activate latent infection). These results with the TLR ligands corroborate earlier results obtained in microglia treated with cytokines (Lokensgard et al., 1997) (and our unpublished data), suggesting that the role of inflammatory mediators in HIV expression are suppressive in primary macrophages and microglia. Indeed, several TLRs including TLR3, TLR7/8, and TLR9 have all been shown to enhance HIV/SIV in chronically-infected cell lines, whereas their effects are inhibitory in acute infection models (Scheller et al., 2004; Schlaepfer, Audige, Joller, & Speck, 2006; Schlaepfer et al., 2004; Equils et al., 2003; Sanghavi & Reinhart, 2005). These results together show that proinflammatory cytokines and TLR ligands play different roles in HIV replication depending on the types of infection, and call for caution in extrapolating data from different infection models. These findings are also relevant to the viral eradication strategies for HIV+ individuals on antiretroviral therapy, in which activation of latent infection from the viral reservoirs simultaneously with suppression of acute (new) infection is desired.

NEUROINFLAMMATION, CYTOKINES, AND NEURODEGENERATION

In viral encephalitides, activation of innate immune receptors in microglia and macrophages is essential for efficient antiviral immunity, but the inevitable consequences are that chronic inflammatory activation will occur as a result of TLR signaling in the CNS, leading to neurodegeneration. These findings suggest that while it would be desirable to activate the innate immune response through microglial immune receptors, it would also be necessary to suppress the proinflammatory activity induced by sustained signaling. Since TLR ligands are being actively considered for antiviral and adjuvant therapy, this will be an important issue to address in the context of the CNS environment.

MICROGLIAL ACTIVATION PHENOTYPE: BENEFICIAL OR DELETERIOUS?

Although microglial "activation" has been seen in almost all neurological diseases with various etiologies, microglial activation does not always lead to neurodegeneration, as microglia can also generate anti-inflammatory cytokines and growth factors that can contribute to neuroprotection (Block, Zecca, & Hong, 2007; Gordon, 2003; Hanisch & Kettenmann, 2007; Schwartz, Butovsky, Bruck, & Hanisch, 2006; Martinez, Helming, & Gordon, 2009). Therefore, much effort has been made in the past several years to examine the characteristics of microglial activation that contribute to either the beneficial or the deleterious outcome in neuroinflammatory conditions.

Similar to the T cells that differentiate along the Th1 or Th2 phenotype (and now Th17 and Treg [regulatory T cells] are added to this list), it is now widely accepted that monocytes, macrophages, and microglia may also have different activation phenotypes. In particular, it has been recognized that in addition to classical activation (M1), characterized by expression of proinflammatory cytokines, iNOS, and reactive oxygen species (ROS), a pathway to alternative activation (M2) also exists. Although the strict criteria and definition for the M1 and M2 classification can be debated, it is generally accepted that M2 microglia have anti-inflammatory and growth-promoting properties, including enhanced phagocytic activity. It is also important to recognize that the M1 and M2 distinction does not refer to intrinsic differences or heterogeneity of microglia (unlike T cells), but rather to differences in their functional and gene expression profiles. Therefore, the M1 and M2 phenotypes should also be reversible to a certain extent. It is also important to recognize that under most circumstances it is not the expression of a single molecule that will signify either the M1 or the M2 status. Rather, it is the relative expression (balance) of a group of inflammatory mediators that will determine the phenotype. Thus, the M1 phenotype is characterized by preferential expression of proinflammatory cytokines (IL-1, TNFα) or cytokines that induce Th1 or Th17 differentiation of T cells (IL-12, IL-23), and the M2 phenotype is characterized by anti-inflammatory cytokines (IL-1ra, IL-10) or cytokines that induce Th2 or Treg differentiation (IL-13, TGFβ, IL-6, IL-10). The exact types of cytokines that are expressed by M1 or M2 microglia will likely depend on the specific inflammatory environment to which they are exposed. In addition, species-dependent differences also exist; for example, in the mouse, inducible nitric oxide synthase (iNOS) is a marker of M1 microglia, whereas in humans, astrocytes rather than microglia express iNOS (Lee, Dickson, Liu, & Brosnan, 1993; Liu, Zhao, Brosnan, & Lee, 1996). In addition, human macrophages or microglia do not express the murine M2 markers (Ym1/2, FIZZ1). Contrary to the findings of some articles that report microglial expression of what are otherwise known as T cell cytokines (see Kavanagh, Lonergan, & Lynch, 2004, for example), human microglia (or astrocytes, for that matter) do not express IFNγ, IL-4, or IL-2. It is the author's opinion that there is a rather strict division between systemic inflammatory cells and endogenous brain cells when it comes to certain cytokines.

CYTOKINES AND NEURODEGENERATION

Much of the data in the literature suggest that proinflammatory cytokines such as IL-1 or TNFα are associated with deleterious effects in the brain, while anti-inflammatory cytokines such as IL-1ra and IL-10 have been associated with beneficial effects. The two major "proinflammatory" cytokines, IL-1 and TNFα, share many properties. They are induced very early in brain lesion formation, primarily by intrinsic microglia and later by infiltrating macrophages. For example, the widespread induction of IL-1 in microglia early in the course of lesion formation has been demonstrated for Alzheimer's disease, multiple sclerosis, ischemic stroke, traumatic brain injury, and HIV encephalitis, and in animal models of inflammatory and neurodegenerative diseases (Griffin & Mrak, 2002; Liu, Zhao, Brosnan, & Lee, 2001; Simi, Tsakiri, Wang, & Rothwell, 2007; Zhao, Kim, Morgello, & Lee, 2001; Perry, Cunningham, & Holmes, 2007; Cunningham, Wilcockson, Campion, Lunnon, & Perry, 2005; Cardona et al., 2006). A number of in vitro and in vivo studies have demonstrated their potency in inducing cell signaling that results in the activation of cytokine cascades in the brain. In addition, their ability to induce cell death, particularly in neurons (Downen, Amaral, Hua, Zhao, & Lee, 1999) and oligodendrocytes, and damage to their processes, has been repeatedly documented.

In spite of these similarities, TNFα differs from IL-1 in several respects. For example, microglia appear to be the primary source of IL-1 (and IL-1 ra) whereas TNFα can be induced by astrocytes and endothelial cells, in addition to microglia. TNFα cannot replace IL-1 as an inducing signal for human iNOS or its neurotoxic role in human neuronal cultures (Lee et al., 1995; Lee, Cosenza, Si, Rivieccio, & Brosnan, 2005; John, Lee, Song, Rivieccio, & Brosnan, 2005; Downen et al., 1999). While IL-1 is an IFNβ-repressible gene, and IL-1ra is an IFNβ-stimulated gene, IFNβ can either repress or stimulate TNFα production depending on the cell type and the cell stimulus applied (Suh et al., 2009b; Rani et al., 2007; Steinman, 2008b; Tarassishin & Lee, unpublished observations).

In addition, the IL-1 system is unique in that it is equipped with a naturally occurring cytokine inhibitor, IL-1 receptor antagonist (IL-1ra). Similar to IL-1, IL-1ra is produced primarily by microglia and macrophages in response to the same stimuli that elicit IL-1 production. The importance of balancing agonists and antagonists of the IL-1 system in fighting disease has been elucidated in very recent human studies of an inflammatory disease caused by homozygous deletion/mutations of the IL1RN locus (Aksentijevich et al., 2009; Dinarello, 2009; Reddy et al., 2009). The term "DIRA" (deficiency of the

IL-1ra) has been proposed to denote this autoinflammatory disease caused by unopposed action of IL-1, resulting in life-threatening systemic inflammation. In addition, there are numerous accounts of animal studies in which IL-1 blockade or administration of IL-1ra have been shown to be beneficial in acute as well as chronic CNS conditions. These include ischemic stroke, trauma, and chronic neurodegenerative diseases such as amyotrophic lateral sclerosis (Rothwell, 2003; Cardona et al., 2006).

ANTI-INFLAMMATORY STRATEGIES FOR CNS DISEASES

Based on the number of studies implicating toxic roles for inflammatory cytokines, cytokine blockade therapies have been tested in animal models of CNS diseases, and some have been carried to human clinical trials. The results of these experiments and trials are not always straightforward, showing surprising results. For example, despite cumulative evidence pointing to the toxic role of TNFα in the pathogenesis of multiple sclerosis (MS), TNFα blockade therapy in MS patients resulted in worsening of the disease (Steinman, 2008b). In Alzheimer's disease, microglial IL-1 was believed to take part in a vicious cycle of inflammation and neuropathology, yet a recent animal study surprisingly found that IL-1 transgene expression actually helped to reduce the amyloid plaque burden (Shaftel et al., 2007). Extrapolating animal data to humans is complicated by the fact that animal models only partially recapitulate the human illness. For example, amyloid precursor protein (APP) transgenic mice hardly ever show neuronal loss, and there is no correlation between β-amyloid accumulation and cognitive dysfunction in humans. Another example of a cytokine with paradoxical effects is the Th1 cytokine IFNγ. Although earlier clinical trials have clearly shown that IFNγ is deleterious in MS, IFNγ deletion worsens the disease in mice with experimental autoimmune encephalomyelitis (EAE), an animal model for MS (Steinman, 2008a).

A NEED FOR THERAPIES THAT WILL REBALANCE THE INFLAMMATORY RESPONSE

What is intriguing from the "inflammatory cytokine cascades" point of view is that the two accepted therapies for multiple sclerosis, IFNβ and glatiramer acetate, are both known to induce differential regulation of proinflammatory and anti-inflammatory cytokines. Take, for example, the IL-1 axis. IFNβ not only suppresses IL-1 production, it also induces IL-1ra in both CNS microglia (Liu, Amaral, Brosnan, & Lee, 1998) and peripheral mononuclear cells (Rani et al., 2007). Glatiramer acetate has also been found to induce IL-1ra and decrease IL-1 levels from monocytes and in MS patients (Burger et al., 2009). Furthermore, the list of IFNβ-induced genes in peripheral mononuclear cells includes IL-10, while that of IFNβ-repressed genes (IRGs) includes the CXC chemokine GROα and IL-8. In fact, in human microglia expressing the IRF3 transgene (Suh et al., 2009b; Tarassishin & Lee, unpublished observations), the list of

stimulated and repressed genes resembles that found in PBMCs from MS patients immediately following IFNβ administration. Furthermore, IFNβ mimics or antagonizes IFNγ (Th1 cytokine), depending on the cell context (such as the presence or absence of the MyD88 signal) (Hua et al., 2002). These are all desirable aspects of a potential immune therapy for CNS diseases. Together, these results strongly suggest that in human microglia and macrophages, IRF3 gene therapy or IFNβ administration can switch their activation phenotype from M1 to M2 (Figure 2.2.3).

Additional examples of modulation of neuroinflammation and neuroprotection by IFNβ and glatiramer acetate can be found in experimental models of stroke (Marsh et al., 2009) and Alzheimer's disease (Butovsky et al., 2006). Marsh et al. have shown that pretreatment of mice with LPS before stroke ("preconditioning") reduces infarct size and this neuroprotective effect of LPS is attributable to the activation of the innate immune response through the transcription factor IRF3. The authors have demonstrated that systemic LPS administration reprograms brain signaling in subsequent ischemic injury such that there was over-expression of type I IFN and IFN-inducible genes accompanying LPS's neuroprotective effects. They further observed that intracerebroventricular injection of IFNβ produced the same beneficial effect, and LPS preconditioning had no protective effect in IRF3-deficient mice. These studies support the idea that IFNβ, when administered in the right context, might produce neuroprotective effects in neurological diseases in addition to MS that are characterized by microglial activation and neuroinflammation.

Given the beneficial effects of IFNβ in a number of neurological diseases, it is important to determine which cells are the cytokine target. The cell-type dependent activity of IFNβ (type I IFN) has been examined in detail in a recent study of EAE (Prinz et al., 2008). When the type I IFN receptor (IFNAR, common to both IFNα and IFNβ) gene was

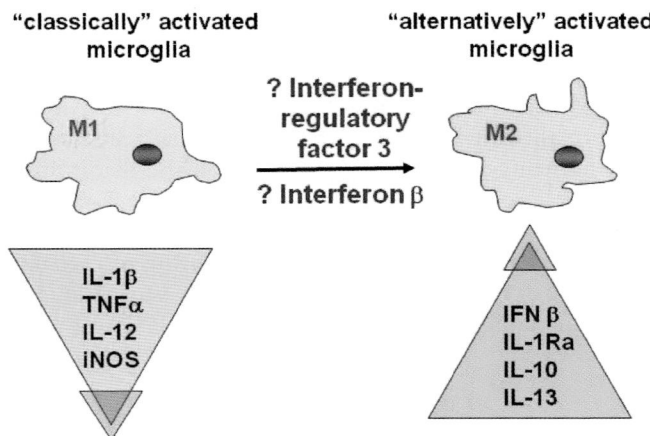

The goal of Immune Therapy

Figure 2.2.3 Effective immune therapies for neuroinflammatory diseases should aim for rebalancing of microglial and macrophage activation in favor of M2 over M1 phenotype. Activation of the transcription factor IRF3 or administration of IFNβ might be ideal candidates to achieve this balance in neuroAIDS.

deleted in a cell-lineage specific manner, it was found that it was myeloid cells (macrophages and microglia) that mediated the beneficial effects of endogenous IFNα/β, and not neuroepithelial cells (neurons, astrocytes, or oligodendrocytes) or lymphocytes (T cells and B cells). IFNAR signaling was critical in the effector phase rather than in the early adaptive immune phase. Furthermore, in IFNβ-stimulated microglia, the gene expression profile indicated its activity on the innate immune response rather than the adaptive immune response. These results together suggest that in EAE, microglia and macrophages play a crucial role in immune modulation by type I IFN. They also provide further examples of how myeloid cells can function to protect the nervous system (M2 activation).

Study of cytokine biology and immune contribution in the context of HIV infection is hampered by the fact that there are no small animal models that reasonably well recapitulate the human disease (see other chapters in this book for review of animal models). The primary reason is the species-specificity of HIV (infects only human cells). For CNS manifestations of HIV/AIDS in which both viral infection and microglial activation play significant pathogenetic roles, a therapy aiming at both the antiviral immunity and M2 activation might be of paramount importance. As such, targeting the IRF3-IFNβ axis as described above might hold promise as an immune therapy for HIV-associated neurological disorders.

CONCLUDING REMARKS

Substantial progress has been made in recent years in the identification of several key mechanisms that are involved in neuroinflammation. The availability of high throughput technologies and systems biology approaches have aided our understanding of innate immune signaling, cytokine biology, and neuroinflammation. We are now more mindful of the presence of the complex, interconnected biological networks triggered by experimental or therapeutic manipulations. We are also aware of the paradoxical effects of certain cytokines in their CNS protective and antiviral activities. These provide cautionary tales for future explorations of immune-based therapies of viral infections and other CNS disorders. Evidence supports the conclusion that activated microglia are not uniform in their gene expression and function and that it might be possible to influence the microglial activation program towards an "alternatively" activated phenotype. A switch of the microglial phenotype through rebalancing of cytokines might be key to immune therapy, and a promising avenue for neuroAIDS might be activation of the IRF3-IFNβ axis.

ACKNOWLEDGMENT

The author is indebted to many of her former and present colleagues and trainees for their collaboration, assistance and support. The author is especially grateful to Dr. Celia F. Brosnan who kindly read the manuscript and provided helpful discussions. Drs. Judy S. Liu, Hyeon-Sook Suh, and Leonid Tarassishin contributed the figures. Due to the space limitation, many of the previously published works relevant to this chapter could not be cited. This work was supported by NIH RO1 MH55477 and the Einstein CFAR P30 AI051519.

REFERENCES

Ajami, B., Bennett, J. L., Krieger, C., Tetzlaff, W., & Rossi, F. M. (2007). Local self-renewal can sustain CNS microglia maintenance and function throughout adult life. *Nat Neurosci, 10*, 1538–1543.

Aksentijevich, I., et al. (2009). An autoinflammatory disease with deficiency of the interleukin-1-receptor antagonist. *N Engl J Med, 360*, 2426–2437.

Ancuta, P., Kamat, A., Kunstman, K. J., Kim, E. Y., Autissier, P., Wurcel, A., et al. (2008). Microbial translocation is associated with increased monocyte activation and dementia in AIDS patients. *PLoS ONE, 3*, e2516.

Barber, S. A., Herbst, D. S., Bullock, B. T., Gama, L., & Clements, J. E. (2004). Innate immune responses and control of acute simian immunodeficiency virus replication in the central nervous system. *J Neurovirol, 10* Suppl 1, 15–20.

Block, M. L., Zecca, L., & Hong, J. S. (2007). Microglia-mediated neurotoxicity: Uncovering the molecular mechanisms. *Nat Rev Neurosci, 8*, 57–69.

Brenchley, J. M., Price, D. A., Schacker, T. W., Asher, T. E., Silvestri, G., Rao, S., et al. (2006). Microbial translocation is a cause of systemic immune activation in chronic HIV infection. *Nat Med, 12*, 1365–1371.

Burger, D., Molnarfi, N., Weber, M. S., Brandt, K. J., Benkhoucha, M., Gruaz, L., et al. (2009). Glatiramer acetate increases IL-1 receptor antagonist but decreases T cell-induced IL-1beta in human monocytes and multiple sclerosis. *Proc Natl Acad Sci USA, 106*, 4355–4359.

Butovsky, O., Koronyo-Hamaoui, M., Kunis, G., Ophir, E., Landa, G., Cohen, H., et al. (2006). Glatiramer acetate fights against Alzheimer's disease by inducing dendritic-like microglia expressing insulin-like growth factor 1. *Proc Natl Acad Sci USA, 103*, 11784–11789.

Cardona, A. E., Pioro, E. P., Sasse, M. E., Kostenko, V., Cardona, S. M., Dijkstra, I. M., et al. (2006). Control of microglial neurotoxicity by the fractalkine receptor. *Nat Neurosci, 9*, 917–924.

Cunningham, C., Wilcockson, D. C., Campion, S., Lunnon, K., & Perry, V. H. (2005). Central and systemic endotoxin challenges exacerbate the local inflammatory response and increase neuronal death during chronic neurodegeneration. *J Neurosci, 25*, 9275–9284.

Davalos, D., Grutzendler, J., Yang, G., Kim, J. V., Zuo, Y., Jung, S., et al. (2005). ATP mediates rapid microglial response to local brain injury in vivo. *Nat Neurosci, 8*, 752–758.

Dickson, D. W. & Lee, S. C. (1997). Microglia. In R. L. Davis & D. M. Robertson (Eds.). *Textbook of neuropathology*, pp 165–205. Baltimore: Williams & Wilkins.

Dinarello, C. A. (2009). Interleukin-1beta and the autoinflammatory diseases. *N Engl J Med, 360*, 2467–2470.

Downen, M., Amaral, T. D., Hua, L. L., Zhao, M. L., & Lee, S. C. (1999). Neuronal death in cytokine-activated primary human brain cell culture: Role of tumor necrosis factor-alpha. *Glia, 28*, 114–127.

Equils, O., Schito, M. L., Karahashi, H., Madak, Z., Yarali, A., Michelsen, K. S., et al. (2003). Toll-like receptor 2 (TLR2) and TLR9 signaling results in HIV-long terminal repeat trans-activation and HIV replication in HIV-1 transgenic mouse spleen cells: Implications of simultaneous activation of TLRs on HIV replication. *J Immunol, 170*, 5159–5164.

Farina, C., Krumbholz, M., Giese, T., Hartmann, G., Aloisi, F., & Meinl, E. (2005). Preferential expression and function of Toll-like receptor 3 in human astrocytes. *J Neuroimmunol, 159*, 12–19.

Fischer-Smith, T., Croul, S., Sverstiuk, A. E., Capini, C., L'Heureux, D., Regulier, E. G., et al. (2001). CNS invasion by CD14+/CD16+

peripheral blood-derived monocytes in HIV dementia: Perivascular accumulation and reservoir of HIV infection. *J Neurovirol, 7*, 528–541.

Folks, T. M., Clouse, K. A., Justement, J., Rabson, A., Duh, E., Kehrl, J. H., et al. (1989). Tumor necrosis factor alpha induces expression of human immunodeficiency virus in a chronically infected T-cell clone. *Proc Natl Acad Sci USA, 86*, 2365–2368.

Gendelman, H. E., Friedman, R. M., Joe, S., Baca, L. M., Turpin, J. A., Dveksler, G., et al. (1990) A selective defect of interferon alpha production in human immunodeficiency virus-infected monocytes. *J Exp Med, 172*, 1433–1442.

Gordon, S. (2003). Alternative activation of macrophages. *Nat Rev Immunol, 3*, 23–35.

Griffin, W. S. & Mrak, R. E. (2002). Interleukin-1 in the genesis and progression of and risk for development of neuronal degeneration in Alzheimer's disease. *J Leukoc Biol, 72*, 233–238.

Grossmann, R., Stence, N., Carr, J., Fuller, L., Waite, M., & Dailey, M. E. (2002). Juxtavascular microglia migrate along brain microvessels following activation during early postnatal development. *Glia, 37*, 229–240.

Hanisch, U. K. & Kettenmann, H. (2007). Microglia: Active sensor and versatile effector cells in the normal and pathologic brain. *Nat Neurosci, 10*, 1387–1394.

Haynes, S. E., Hollopeter, G., Yang, G., Kurpius, D., Dailey, M. E., Gan, W. B., et al. (2006). The P2Y12 receptor regulates microglial activation by extracellular nucleotides. *Nat Neurosci, 9*, 1512–1519.

Heil, F., Hemmi, H., Hochrein, H., Ampenberger, F., Kirschning, C., Akira, S., et al. (2004). Species-specific recognition of single-stranded RNA via toll-like receptor 7 and 8. *Science, 303*, 1526–1529.

Hickey, W. F. & Kimura, H. (1988). Perivascular microglial cells of the CNS are bone marrow-derived and present antigen in vivo. *Science, 239*, 290–292.

Hiscott, J., Lin, R., Nakhaei, P., & Paz, S. (2006). MasterCARD: A priceless link to innate immunity. *Trends Mol Med, 12*, 53–56.

Hoek, R. M., Ruuls, S. R., Murphy, C. A., Wright, G. J., Goddard, R., Zurawski, S. M., et al. (2000). Down-regulation of the macrophage lineage through interaction with OX2 (CD200). *Science, 290*, 1768–1771.

Hua, L. L., Kim, M. O., Brosnan, C. F., Lee, S. C. (2002). Modulation of astrocyte inducible nitric oxide synthase and cytokine expression by interferon beta is associated with induction and inhibition of interferon gamma-activated sequence binding activity. *J Neurochem, 83*, 1120–1128.

Jack, C. S., Arbour, N., Manusow, J., Montgrain, V., Blain, M., McCrea, E., et al. (2005) TLR signaling tailors innate immune responses in human microglia and astrocytes. *J Immunol, 175*, 4320–4330.

John, G. R., Lee, S. C., Song, X., Rivieccio, M., & Brosnan, C. F. (2005). IL-1-regulated responses in astrocytes: Relevance to injury and recovery. *Glia, 49*, 161–176.

Jung, S., Aliberti, J., Graemmel, P., Sunshine, M. J., Kreutzberg, G. W., Sher, A., et al. (2000). Analysis of fractalkine receptor CX(3)CR1 function by targeted deletion and green fluorescent protein reporter gene insertion. *Mol Cell Biol, 20*, 4106–4114.

Kato, H., Sato, S., Yoneyama, M., Yamamoto, M., Uematsu, S., Matsui, K., et al. (2005). Cell type-specific involvement of RIG-I in antiviral response. *Immunity, 23*, 19–28.

Kavanagh, T., Lonergan, P. E., & Lynch, M. A. (2004). Eicosapentaenoic acid and gamma-linolenic acid increase hippocampal concentrations of IL-4 and IL-10 and abrogate lipopolysaccharide-induced inhibition of long-term potentiation. *Prostaglandins Leukot Essent Fatty Acids, 70*, 391–397.

Kawai, T. & Akira, S. (2007). Antiviral signaling through pattern recognition receptors. *J Biochem, 141*, 137–145.

Kim, M. O., Suh, H. S., Si, Q., Terman, B. I., & Lee, S. C. (2006). Anti-CD45RO suppresses human immunodeficiency virus type 1 replication in microglia: Role of Hck tyrosine kinase and implications for AIDS dementia. *J Virol, 80*, 62–72.

Klesney-Tait, J., Turnbull, I. R., & Colonna, M. (2006). The TREM receptor family and signal integration. *Nat Immunol, 7*, 1266–1273.

Kreutzberg, G. W. (1996). Microglia: A sensor for pathological events in the CNS. *Trends Neurosci, 19*, 312–318.

Laflamme, N. & Rivest, S. (2001). Toll-like receptor 4: The missing link of the cerebral innate immune response triggered by circulating gram-negative bacterial cell wall components. *FASEB J, 15*, 155–163.

Lalancette-Hebert, M., Gowing, G., Simard, A., Weng, Y. C., & Kriz, J. (2007). Selective ablation of proliferating microglial cells exacerbates ischemic injury in the brain. *J Neurosci, 27*, 2596–2605.

Lee, S. C., Collins, M., Vanguri, P., & Shin, M. L. (1992). Glutamate differentially inhibits the expression of class II MHC antigens on astrocytes and microglia. *J Immunol, 148*, 3391–3397.

Lee, S. C., Cosenza, M. A., Si, Q., Rivieccio, M., & Brosnan, C. F. (2005). The CNS: Cells, tissues, and reactions to insult. In R. M. Ransohoff & E. N. Benveniste (Eds.). *Cytokines and the CNS*. Boca Raton, FL: CRC Press.

Lee, S. C., Dickson, D. W., & Brosnan, C. F. (1995). Interleukin-1, nitric oxide and reactive astrocytes. *Brain, Behavior, and Immunity, 9*, 345–354.

Lee, S. C., Dickson, D. W., Liu, W., & Brosnan, C. F. (1993). Induction of nitric oxide synthase activity in human astrocytes by IL-1b and IFN-g. *J Neuroimmunol, 46*, 19–24.

Liu, J., Zhao, M-L., Brosnan, C. F., & Lee, S. C. (1996). Expression of type II nitric oxide synthase in primary human astrocytes and microglia: Role of IL-1b and IL-1 receptor antagonist. *J Immunol, 157*, 3569–3576.

Liu, J. S., Amaral, T. D., Brosnan, C. F., & Lee, S. C. (1998). IFNs are critical regulators of IL-1 receptor antagonist and IL-1 expression in human microglia. *J Immunol, 161*, 1989–1996.

Liu, J. S. H., Zhao, M. L., Brosnan, C. F., & Lee, S. C. (2001). Expression of inducible nitric oxide synthase and nitrotyrosine in multiple sclerosis lesions. *Am J Pathol, 158*, 2057–2066.

Liu, W., Brosnan, C. F., Dickson, D. W., & Lee, S. C. (1994). Macrophage colony stimulating factor mediates astrocyte-induced microglial ramification in human fetal CNS culture. *Am J Pathol, 145*, 48–53.

Lokensgard, J. R., Gekker, G., Ehrlich, L. C., Hu, S., Chao, C. C., & Peterson, P. K. (1997). Proinflammatory cytokines inhibit HIV-1(SF162) expression in acutely infected human brain cell cultures. *J Immunol, 158*, 2449–2455.

Lyons, A., Downer, E. J., Crotty, S., Nolan, Y. M., Mills, K. H., Lynch MA (2007). CD200 ligand receptor interaction modulates microglial activation in vivo and in vitro: A role for IL-4. *J Neurosci, 27*, 8309–8313.

Marsh, B., Stevens, S. L., Packard, A. E., Gopalan, B., Hunter, B., Leung, P. Y., et al. (2009). Systemic lipopolysaccharide protects the brain from ischemic injury by reprogramming the response of the brain to stroke: A critical role for IRF3. *J Neurosci, 29*, 9839–9849.

Martinez, F. O., Helming, L., & Gordon, S. (2009). Alternative activation of macrophages: An immunologic functional perspective. *Annu Rev Immunol, 27*, 451–483.

Mildner, A., Schmidt, H., Nitsche, M., Merkler, D., Hanisch, U. K., Mack, M., et al. (2007). Microglia in the adult brain arise from Ly-6ChiCCR2+ monocytes only under defined host conditions. *Nat Neurosci, 10*, 1544–1553.

Muzio, M., Bosisio, D., Polentarutti, N., D'amico, G., Stoppacciaro, A., Mancinelli, R., et al. (2000). Differential expression and regulation of toll-like receptors (TLR) in human leukocytes: Selective expression of TLR3 in dendritic cells. *J Immunol, 164*, 5998–6004.

Neumann, H., Boucraut, J., Hahnel, C., Misgeld, T., & Wekerle, H. (1996). Neuronal control of MHC class II inducibility in rat astrocytes and microglia. *Eur J Neurosci, 8*, 2582–2590.

Neumann, H., Misgeld, T., Matsumuro, K., & Wekerle, H. (1998). Neurotrophins inhibit major histocompatibility class II inducibility of microglia: Involvement of the p75 neurotrophin receptor. *Proc Natl Acad Sci USA, 95*, 5779–5784.

Nimmerjahn, A., Kirchhoff, F., & Helmchen, F. (2005). Resting microglial cells are highly dynamic surveillants of brain parenchyma in vivo. *Science, 308*, 1314–1318.

Okumura, A., Alce, T., Lubyova, B., Ezelle, H., Strebel, K., & Pitha, P. M. (2008). HIV-1 accessory proteins VPR and Vif modulate antiviral response by targeting IRF-3 for degradation. *Virology, 373*, 85–97.

Osiecki, K., Xie, L., Zheng, J. H., Squires, R., Pettoello-Mantovani, M., & Goldstein, H. (2005). Identification of granulocyte-macrophage colony-stimulating factor and lipopolysaccharide-induced signal transduction pathways that synergize to stimulate HIV type 1 production by monocytes from HIV type 1 transgenic mice. *AIDS Res Hum Retroviruses, 21,* 125–139.

Perry, V. H., Cunningham, C., & Holmes, C. (2007). Systemic infections and inflammation affect chronic neurodegeneration. *Nat Rev Immunol, 7,* 161–167.

Piccio, L., Buonsanti, C., Cella, M., Tassi, I., Schmidt, R. E., Fenoglio, C., et al. (2008). Identification of soluble TREM-2 in the cerebrospinal fluid and its association with multiple sclerosis and CNS inflammation. *Brain, 131,* 3081–3091.

Priller, J., Flugel, A., Wehner, T., Boentert, M., Haas, C. A., Prinz, M., et al. (2001). Targeting gene-modified hematopoietic cells to the central nervous system: Use of green fluorescent protein uncovers microglial engraftment. *Nat Med, 7,* 1356–1361.

Prinz, M., Schmidt, H., Mildner, A., Knobeloch, K. P., Hanisch, U. K., Raasch, J., et al. (2008). Distinct and nonredundant in vivo functions of IFNAR on myeloid cells limit autoimmunity in the central nervous system. *Immunity, 28,* 675–686.

Pulliam, L., Gascon, R., Stubblebine, M., McGuire, D., & McGrath, M. S. (1997). Unique monocyte subset in patients with AIDS dementia. *Lancet, 349,* 692–695.

Rani, M. R., Shrock, J., Appachi, S., Rudick, R. A., Williams, B. R., & Ransohoff, R. M. (2007). Novel interferon-beta-induced gene expression in peripheral blood cells. *J Leukoc Biol, 82,* 1353–1360.

Reddy, S., Jia, S., Geoffrey, R., Lorier, R., Suchi, M., Broeckel, U., et al. (2009). An autoinflammatory disease due to homozygous deletion of the IL1RN locus. *N Engl J Med, 360,* 2438–2444.

Rivieccio, M. A., John, G. R., Song, X., Suh, H. S., Zhao, Y., Lee, S. C., et al. (2005). The cytokine IL-1beta activates IFN response factor 3 in human fetal astrocytes in culture. *J Immunol, 174,* 3719–3726.

Rivieccio, M. A., Suh, H. S., Zhao, Y., Zhao, M. L., Chin, K. C., Lee, S. C., et al. (2006). TLR3 ligation activates an antiviral response in human fetal astrocytes: A role for viperin/cig5. *J Immunol, 177,* 4735–4741.

Rosenberg, Z. F. & Fauci, A. S. (1990). Immunopathogenic mechanisms of HIV infection: Cytokine induction of HIV expression. *Immunol Today, 11,* 176–180.

Rothwell, N. (2003). Interleukin-1 and neuronal injury: Mechanisms, modification, and therapeutic potential. *Brain Behav Immun, 17,* 152–157.

Sanghavi, S. K. & Reinhart, T. A. (2005). Increased expression of TLR3 in lymph nodes during simian immunodeficiency virus infection: Implications for inflammation and immunodeficiency. *J Immunol, 175,* 5314–5323.

Scheller, C., Ullrich, A., McPherson, K., Hefele, B., Knoferle, J., Lamla, S., et al. (2004). CpG oligodeoxynucleotides activate HIV replication in latently infected human T cells. *J Biol Chem, 279,* 21897–21902.

Schlaepfer, E., Audige, A., Joller, H., & Speck, R. F. (2006). TLR7/8 triggering exerts opposing effects in acute versus latent HIV infection. *J Immunol, 176,* 2888–2895.

Schlaepfer, E., Audige, A., von, B. B., Manolova, V., Weber, M., Joller, H., et al. (2004). CpG oligodeoxynucleotides block human immunodeficiency virus type 1 replication in human lymphoid tissue infected ex vivo. *J Virol, 78,* 12344–12354.

Schmid CD, Sautkulis LN, Danielson PE, Cooper J, Hasel KW, Hilbush BS, et al. (2002) Heterogeneous expression of the triggering receptor expressed on myeloid cells-2 on adult murine microglia. *J Neurochem, 83,* 1309–1320.

Schwartz, M., Butovsky, O., Bruck, W., & Hanisch, U. K. (2006). Microglial phenotype: Is the commitment reversible? *Trends Neurosci, 29,* 68–74.

Sen, G. C. & Sarkar, S. N. (2005). Hitching RIG to action. *Nat Immunol, 6,* 1074–1076.

Shaftel, S. S., Kyrkanides, S., Olschowka, J. A., Miller, J. N., Johnson, R. E., & O'Banion, M. K. (2007). Sustained hippocampal IL-1 beta overexpression mediates chronic neuroinflammation and ameliorates Alzheimer plaque pathology. *J Clin Invest, 117,* 1595–1604.

Simard, A. R. & Rivest, S. (2004). Bone marrow stem cells have the ability to populate the entire central nervous system into fully differentiated parenchymal microglia. *FASEB J.*

Simi, A., Tsakiri, N., Wang, P., & Rothwell, N. J. (2007). Interleukin-1 and inflammatory neurodegeneration. *Biochem Soc Trans, 35,* 1122–1126.

Steinman, L. (2008a). A rush to judgment on Th17. *J Exp Med, 205,* 1517–1522.

Steinman, L. (2008b). Nuanced roles of cytokines in three major human brain disorders. *J Clin Invest, 118,* 3557–3563.

Suh, H. S., Brosnan, C. F., & Lee, S. C. (2009a). Toll-like receptors in CNS viral infections. *Curr Top Microbiol Immunol, 336,* 63–81.

Suh, H. S., Kim, M. O., & Lee, S. C. (2005). Inhibition of granulocyte-macrophage colony-stimulating factor signaling and microglial proliferation by anti-CD45RO: Role of Hck tyrosine kinase and phosphatidylinositol 3-kinase/Akt. *J Immunol, 174,* 2712–2719.

Suh, H. S., Zhao, M. L., Choi, N., Belbin, T. J., Brosnan, C. F., Lee, S. C. (2009b). TLR3 and TLR4 are innate antiviral immune receptors in human microglia: Role of IRF3 in modulating antiviral and inflammatory response in the CNS. *Virology.*

Suh, H. S., Zhao, M. L., Rivieccio, M., Choi, S., Connolly, E., Zhao, Y., et al. (2007) Astrocyte indoleamine 2, 3 dioxygenase (IDO) is induced by the TLR3 ligand poly IC: mechanism of induction and role in antiviral response. *J Virol, 81,* 9838–9850.

Sun, J., Zheng, J. H., Zhao, M., Lee, S., & Goldstein, H. (2008). Increased in vivo activation of microglia and astrocytes in the brains of mice transgenic for an infectious R5 human immunodeficiency virus type 1 provirus and for CD4-specific expression of human cyclin T1 in response to stimulation by lipopolysaccharides. *J Virol, 82,* 5562–5572.

Tan, J., Town, T., & Mullan, M. (2000). CD45 inhibits CD40L-induced microglial activation via negative regulation of the Src/p44/42 MAPK pathway. *J Biol Chem, 275,* 37224–37231.

Unger, E. R., Sung, J. H., Manivel, J. C., Chenggis, M. L., Blazar, B. R., & Krivit, W. (1993). Male donor-derived cells in the brains of female sex-mismatched bone marrow transplant recipients: A Y-chromosome specific in situ hybridization study. *J Neuropathol Exp Neurol, 52,* 460–470.

Vallieres, L. & Sawchenko, P. E. (2003). Bone marrow-derived cells that populate the adult mouse brain preserve their hematopoietic identity. *J Neurosci, 23,* 5197–5207.

Voth, R., Rossol, S., Klein, K., Hess, G., Schutt, K. H., Schroder, H. C., et al. (1990). Differential gene expression of IFN-alpha and tumor necrosis factor-alpha in peripheral blood mononuclear cells from patients with AIDS related complex and AIDS. *J Immunol, 144,* 970–975.

Wang, T., Gong, N., Liu, J., Kadiu, I., Kraft-Terry, S. D., Mosley, R. L., et al. (2008). Proteomic modeling for HIV-1 infected microglia-astrocyte crosstalk. *PLoS ONE, 3,* e2507.

Zhao, M. L., Kim, M. O., Morgello, S., & Lee, S. C. (2001). Expression of inducible nitric oxide synthase, interleukin-1 and caspase-1 in HIV-1 encephalitis. *J Neuroimmunol, 115,* 182–191.

2.3

ASTROCYTES

Etty N. Benveniste, Lisa N. Akhtar, and Brandi J. Baker

Astrocytes are the most abundant glial cell type in the CNS and represent a diverse population of cells. In the past, the direct role of astrocytes in HIV-1-associated neurocognitive disorders (HAND) has been controversial, due to the belief that HIV-1 infection of astrocytes was relatively rare. Convincing data now exist that astrocyte infection can be widespread, especially in HIV-associated dementia. When latently infected with HIV-1, astrocytes release toxic mediators that cause apoptosis in uninfected astrocytes and neurons. In fact, a strong association exists between astrocyte apoptosis and rapid progression of dementia. Furthermore, HIV-1-infected astrocytes produce high levels of CCL2 and glutamate, which play an important role in HAND. These and other findings implicate HIV-1-infected astrocytes in HAND pathogenesis. This chapter discusses the normal functioning of astrocytes and, in particular, how this function becomes perturbed during HIV-1 disease.

INTRODUCTION

HIV-1-ASSOCIATED NEUROCOGNITIVE DISORDERS (HAND)

The brain is a major target organ for HIV-1 infection, resulting in significant neuropathological changes in most HIV-infected patients, and a wide range of neurological symptoms including cognitive, behavioral, and motor dysfunction, and this has been characterized as a subcortical dementia (Boisse, Gill, & Power, 2008; Kaul, 2009; Nath et al., 2008; Anthony & Bell, 2008). Although the use of highly active antiretroviral therapy (HAART) has led to a decline in the incidence of HAND, the prevalence has actually risen due to the increasing number of HIV-1-infected patients and increased life expectancy (McCombe, Noorbakhsh, Buchholz, Trew, & Power, 2009; Power, Boisse, Rourke, & Gill, 2009). HIV-1 infection has significant effects on the nervous system as the virus both infects and affects the brain. Furthermore, the brain is recognized as a viral sanctuary that requires additional therapeutic efforts, given the low CNS penetrance of most HAART regimens (Kraft-Terry, Buch, Fox, & Gendelman, 2009; Kaul, Zheng, Okamoto, Gendelman, & Lipton, 2005). HAND defines three categories of disorders according to standardized measures of dysfunction: asymptomatic neurocognitive impairment (ANI), HIV-associated mild cognitive motor disorder (MND), and the most severe disease of HIV-associated dementia (HAD) (Kaul,

2009; Kraft-Terry, Buch, Fox, & Gendelman, 2009; Hult, Chana, Masliah, & Everall, 2008). The incident of dementia as an AIDS-defining illness has increased in recent years as HIV patients live longer, and HAND remains a significant independent risk factor for death due to AIDS. In the current era of HAART, HIV-associated CNS disease presents with more subtle neuropathological changes and is likely associated with synaptodendritic damage (Kraft-Terry, Buch, Fox, & Gendelman, 2009; Ellis, Langford, & Masliah, 2007).

HIV enters the brain early after infection while viremia is still high by a mechanism known as the "Trojan horse," whereby HIV-1-infected monocytes/macrophages are attracted to the brain by a chemokine gradient and penetrate the blood-brain barrier (BBB). This infiltration of peripheral immune cells then allows viral dissemination within the brain to the endogenous glial cells, predominantly microglia and astrocytes (Kraft-Terry, Buch, Fox, & Gendelman, 2009; Kaul, Zheng, Okamoto, Gendelman, & Lipton, 2005; Clay et al., 2007). Of importance, macrophages and microglia can support a productive HIV infection in the absence of cellular activation, and are not killed by infection, making them a long-lasting and efficient viral reservoir. Virus localizes predominantly to subcortical regions of the brain including the basal ganglia and deep white matter, which likely reflects the increased presence of perivascular macrophages in these locations. Because the brain typically lacks a fully functional immune response to viral infection (Speth, Dierich, & Sopper, 2005), the result is a sequestered infection that is not self-limited by cell death. In addition, the low penetrance of most HAART regimens into the brain hinders even therapeutic control of viral replication. Many investigators have suggested that this difficult-to-target population of infected cells may be responsible for reseeding of virus back into the systemic population, making this an important viral reservoir in the context of overall infection.

Neuroinflammation ensues, which increases as infected individuals progress from the asymptomatic stage of AIDS to HAND. The presence of activated endogenous microglia and infiltrating macrophages, together with reduced synaptic and dendritic density and neuronal loss, are in fact the best neuropathological correlates of HAND (Kaul, 2009; Kaul & Lipton, 2006). One mechanism contributing to HAND is neurotoxicity as a consequence of either direct exposure to HIV-1 or its viral proteins, or indirect injury through neurotoxins released by infected or immune-stimulated inflammatory microglia and macrophages in the brain (Figure 2.3.1). Although neurons are not infected with HIV-1, HIV replication within CNS macrophages results in the production of viral proteins and activation-induced cytokines and chemokines which can be damaging, if not directly toxic, to neurons. The HIV protein gp120 has been shown to interact with CXCR4 to induce neuronal apoptosis (Corasaniti et al., 2001), while the HIV protein Tat, which can be secreted from infected cells (Chang, Samaniego, Nair, Buonaguro, & Ensoli, 1997), has been shown to induce neuronal excitotoxicity either through interactions with nonNMDA or NMDA receptors (Magnuson et al., 1995). In addition, neurons are injured by virus-induced neurotoxins produced by microglia and macrophages (Kraft-Terry, Buch, Fox, & Gendelman, 2009; Wang et al., 2008). Cytokines and chemokines produced by activated macrophages and microglia (TNF-α, IL-1β, IL-6, IL-8, IL-12, MCP-1 (CCL2), IP-10 (CXCL10), TGF-β, nitric oxide (NO)) can also facilitate disease progression (Kraft-Terry, Buch, Fox, & Gendelman, 2009). Some of these mediators, such as TNF-α, NO, and CXCL10, are directly neurotoxic (Sui et al., 2004).

THE ASTROCYTE

ASTROCYTE FUNCTIONS AND INVOLVEMENT IN HAND

Astrocytes are the most abundant glial cell type in the CNS, and represent a diverse population of cells that co-exist with different molecular identities and specialized functions, based on the microenvironment. Their direct role in HAND has been controversial in the past due to the premise that HIV-1 infection of astrocytes is a very rare event (1–3% of astrocytes). There are now convincing data that astrocyte infection is extensive in patients with HAD, occurring in up to 19% of GFAP+ cells (Churchill et al., 2009). In conjunction with the view of astrocytes as "amplifers" in HAND, we must also consider their direct involvement (Figure 2.3.1). To appreciate fully the functional involvement of the astrocyte in HAND, it is instructive to first discuss some of the important physiological properties as they relate to CNS homeostasis. Astrocytes affect neuronal function by the release of neurotrophic factors, guide neuronal development, contribute to the metabolism of neurotransmitters, and regulate extracellular concentrations

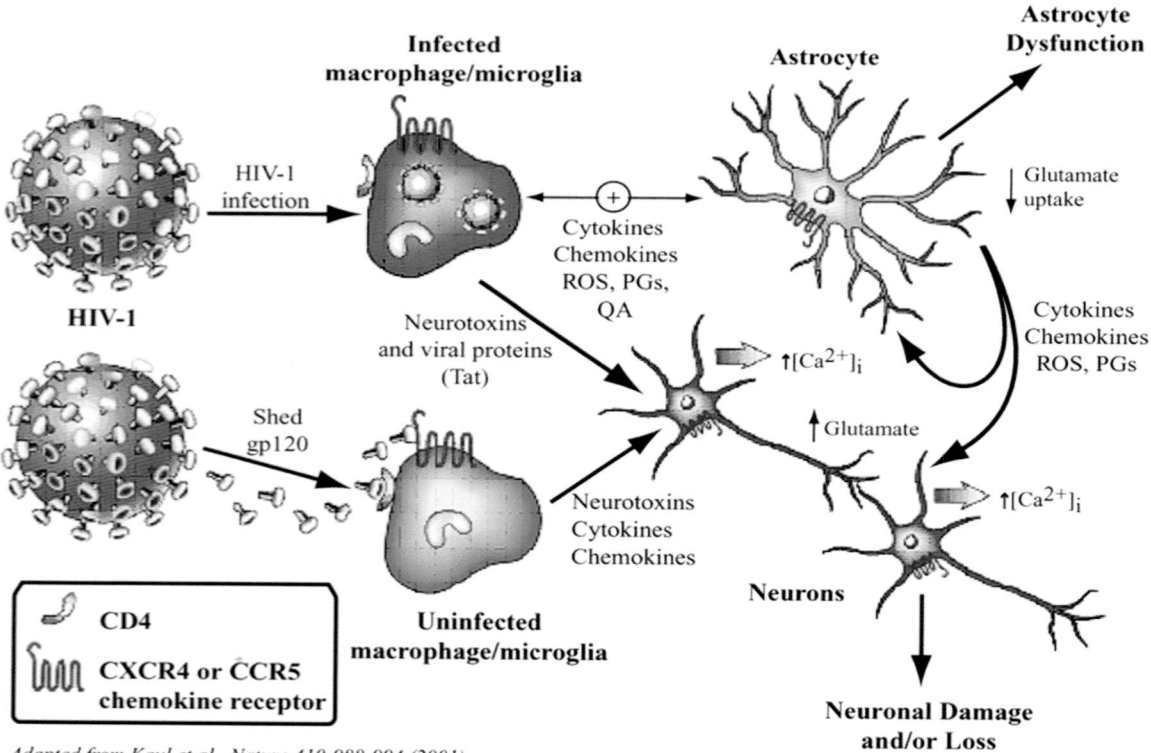

Adapted from Kaul et al., Nature 410:988–994 (2001)

Figure 2.3.1 Model of HIV-1 Induced Changes in Astrocytic Functions Leading to Neuronal Damage. Infected and/or activated macrophages and microglia release viral proteins such as gp120 and Tat, cytokines such as IL-1, IL-6 and TNF-α, chemokines, prostaglandins (PGs) quinolinic acid (QA), and reactive oxygen species (ROS). All these soluble mediators can directly affect neurons, as well as affect astrocytic functions. Activated astrocytes in turn produce a wide array of cytokines, chemokines (CCL2, CCL20, CXCL10, etc.), PGs and ROS that impact neuronal functioning. As well, gp120 and TNF-α also affect the ability of astrocytes to take up glutamate, resulting in increased extracellular glutamate levels, and ultimately excitotoxicity. Astrocytes are influenced by cytokines/chemokines to undergo astrocytosis. Astrocytes are also infected with HIV-1, which leads to production of soluble mediators that promote apoptosis of uninfected astrocytes and neurons. Cell-cell signaling between macrophages, microglia, astrocytes, and neurons is intimately involved in contributing to the neurotoxicity that is an important hallmark of HAND. Adapted from Kaul et al., *Nature* 4 10, 988–994 (2001).

of ions and metabolites (Table 2.3.1) (Dong & Benveniste, 2001; Farina, Aloisi, & Meinl, 2007). Accordingly, impairment in these astrocytic functions during HAND can significantly influence neuronal function and/or survival (Kaul, Garden, & Lipton, 2001). In addition to providing structural and trophic support to neurons, astrocytes modulate synaptic activity through the release and uptake of chemical transmitters, such as glutamate (Perea & Araque, 2007). Astrocytes have a critical role in HIV-1-induced CNS damage through contributing to glutamate excitotoxicity due to impaired glutamate uptake (Benos et al., 1994; Benos, McPherson, Hahn, Chaikin, & Benveniste, 1994). Astrocytes also release D-serine, a co-agonist of glutamate at the NMDA receptor, suggesting that astrocytes can directly modulate synaptic transmission (Barres, 2008). Astrocytes also produce factors that induce synaptic remodeling. One example is secretion of thrombospondins by astrocytes that promotes synaptogenesis (Barres, 2008). On the other hand, astrocytes can induce neurons to secrete the complement protein C1q that activates the complement cascade, leading to the elimination of inappropriate synapses. Thus, astrocytes play a fundamental role in the modulation of synaptic transmission and neuronal function, a process termed "gliotransmission" (Haydon, 2000). In response to synaptic activity, astrocytes bind extracellular glutamate, which induces the generation of $Ca^{2}+$ waves that are propagated throughout local networks of glial cells to enhance blood flow and nutrients to active brain regions.

Astrocytes critically influence the formation and maintenance of the BBB, a structure that serves to limit entry of blood-borne elements in the CNS. In vivo, astrocyte foot processes (endfeet) are in close apposition to the abluminal surface of the microvascular endothelium of the BBB; thus, astrocytes contribute to both the structural and functional integrity of the BBB (Wolburg & Risau, 1995). Derangement of the BBB has been implicated in the pathophysiology of HAND. A compromised BBB is thought to contribute to entry of HIV-infected macrophages into the CNS, leading to mononuclear giant cell formation, viral spread, and subsequent neurologic dysfunction. In support of this, Petito et al. (1992) have

documented the presence of serum proteins in the brains of AIDS patients, indicating that the BBB is altered in HIV infection. Furthermore, Power et al. (1993) have shown a strong correlation between disruption of the BBB and the presentation of HAND. Extravasation of HIV-infected cells across the BBB is likely to be facilitated by the production of chemokines by astrocytes, including CCL2 and CXCL10 (Eugenin et al., 2006; Thompson, McArthur, & Wesselingh, 2001). This will be discussed in more detail below.

HIV-1 INFECTION OF ASTROCYTES

Utilizing highly sensitive PCR for detection of HIV DNA in microdissected astrocytes, Churchill et al. (2009) have recently shown that up to 19% of astrocytes are infected in patients with HAD, which correlates with the severity of neuropathological changes and proximity to activated macrophages. Because of their large numbers in the CNS, the astrocyte may serve as another potential reservoir of HIV-1 in the CNS. In contrast to macrophages/microglia, which are productively infected with HIV-1, astrocytes are latently infected, and produce few new virus particles. This leads to the accumulation of multiply spliced mRNAs (Tat, Rev, and Nef), and translation of proteins, particularly Nef (Sabri, Titanji, De Milito, & Chiodi, 2003). However, this latent infection undoubtedly affects a variety of astrocytic functions. One example is that HIV-1-infected astrocytes produce toxic signals that are transmitted to uninfected astrocytes by gap junctions (Eugenin & Berman, 2007). This leads to significant apoptosis of uninfected astrocytes, as well as apoptosis of uninfected neurons. In this regard, there is a strong association of astrocyte apoptosis in patients with rapidly progressing dementia (Thompson, McArthur, & Wesselingh, 2001). Furthermore, HIV-1-infected astrocytes produce high levels of CCL2 and glutamate (Eugenin & Berman, 2007), key factors involved in HAND. These findings collectively implicate HIV-1 infected astrocytes in contributing to HAND pathogenesis and the cognitive impairment which is evident in many HIV-infected patients (Figure 2.3.1).

CYTOKINE/CHEMOKINE PRODUCTION BY ASTROCYTES

Astrocytes are intimately involved in immunological and inflammatory events occurring in the CNS, due to their ability to secrete and respond to a large number of immunoregulatory cytokines/chemokines including IL-1β, IL-6, IL-8, IL-10, IL-17, IL-27, TNF-α, TGF-β, IFN-γ, IFN-β, CCL2, CCL3, CCL5, CCL20, CXCL10, CXCL12, and oncostatin M (OSM) (Farina, Aloisi, & Meinl, 2007; Benveniste, 1998; Bajetto, Bonavia, Barbero, & Schettini, 2002; John, Lee, & Brosnan, 2003); (Table 2.3.1). Although expression of cytokines and chemokines is limited in the normal CNS, expression of these proteins, as seen in disease entities such as HAND, contributes to the development of inflammation and progression to disease. On the other hand, astrocyte production of growth factors such as insulin-like growth factor-I (IGF-I),

---

Table 2.3.1 **FUNCTIONS OF ASTROCYTES**

- Metabolic support of neurons; glycogen storage and export of lactate
- Uptake of neurotransmitters, including glutamate
- Production of neurotrophic factors (NGF, CNTF, BDNF, LIF, IGF-1) and gliotransmitters (ATP, Adenosine, D-serine, Eicosinoids)
- Ion homeostasis (i.e., potassium uptake)
- Participate in synaptic plasticity, synapse formation, and stabilization
- Control of cerebral blood flow
- Blood-brain barrier induction and maintenance
- Scar formation and tissue repair
- Regulation of immune and inflammatory responses in the CNS by production of cytokines and chemokines (IL-6, TNF-α, IFN-β, TGF-β, IL-8, IL-10, CCL2, CCL3, CCL5, CCL20, CXCL10, CXCL12)

leukemia inhibitory factor (LIF), and ciliary neurotrophic factor (CNTF) serve neuroprotective functions by promoting neuronal survival, oligodendrocyte maturation, and remyelination (Bauer, Kerr, & Patterson, 2007). As a potent source of cytokines, chemokines, and growth factors, astrocytes play a pivotal role in the type and extent of neuroinflammatory responses. As examples that are relevant to HAND, the role of IL-6 family members (IL-6, OSM) will be discussed in detail below.

IL-6

IL-6 is the prototypic member of the IL-6 family of cytokines, which includes IL-6, IL-11, OSM, LIF, CNTF, cardiotrophin-1 (CT-1), and cardiotrophin-like cytokine (Naka, Nishimoto, & Kishimoto, 2002; Van Wagoner & Benveniste, 1999). These cytokines play pivotal roles in immune, hematopoietic, nervous, cardiovascular, and endocrine systems, and also function in bone metabolism, inflammation, and acute-phase responses. IL-6 family members exert their diverse biological effects by the formation of high affinity transmembrane receptor complexes that are characterized by the presence of the shared 130 kDa receptor subunit, gp130, which is ubiquitously expressed. IL-6 requires a ligand-specific receptor, which is found in both membrane-associated and soluble forms. Interestingly, the IL-6 soluble receptor (sIL-6R) functions as an agonist of IL-6 (Rose-John, Ehlers, Grötzinger, Müllberg, 1995). This process, called "trans-signaling," makes cells expressing gp130, but not the membrane-bound form of the IL-6R, responsive upon addition of the sIL-6R. IL-6 acts on target cells through a receptor complex composed of IL-6, either membrane-bound IL-6R or the sIL-6R, and gp130. Receptor activation requires formation of a hexameric complex composed of two each of the above-mentioned proteins. This event leads to activation of gp130-associated Janus kinases (JAKs). Although IL-6 has been shown to activate JAK1, JAK2, and TYK2, JAK1 is most important for signaling through gp130 (Rodig et al., 1998). JAK activation leads to the tyrosine phosphorylation of STATs (signal transducer and activator of transcription). The cytoplasmic domain of gp130 contains STAT recruitment motifs that become phosphorylated by JAKs upon receptor oligomerization, allowing for the interaction of STAT proteins, predominantly STAT-3, and to a lesser extent, STAT-1. Upon tyrosine phosphorylation, STAT-3 dimers translocate to the nucleus, and activate transcription from IL-6 target gene promoters. It has been demonstrated that serine phosphorylation is required for optimal transcriptional activation by STAT-3 (Wen & Darnell, 1997). IL-6 signaling also activates the mitogen-activated protein kinase (MAPK) pathway, which activates a number of transcription factors responsible for IL-6-mediated effects.

IL-6 PRODUCTION BY ASTROCYTES

Astrocytes are the most potent producers of IL-6 in the diseased CNS, and elevated IL-6 levels have been detected in patients with HAND (Van Wagoner & Benveniste, 1999). Astrocytes can be induced to express IL-6 by a wide array of stimuli. Some of these include; LPS, IL-1, TNF-α, OSM, TGF-β, PGE$_2$, norepinephrine, substance P, vasoactive intestinal peptide, complement components (C3a and C5a), histamine, hypoxia, viral infection (measles, hepatitis), and of relevance to HAND, by the HIV-1 viral proteins gp120 and Tat (Van Wagoner & Benveniste, 1999). Thus, numerous factors including HIV-1 viral proteins can induce IL-6 expression by astrocytes. Of importance is the fact that many of these stimuli can synergize with each other, that is, OSM, IL-1, and TNF-α, leading to high levels of IL-6 expression.

ASTROCYTE RESPONSIVENESS TO IL-6

Do astrocytes have the ability to respond to IL-6, as well as produce it? We have demonstrated that astrocytes can not respond directly to IL-6 stimulation, because they lack the membrane-associated form of the IL-6 receptor (Van Wagoner, Oh, Repovic, & Benveniste, 1999). However, treatment of astrocytes with IL-6 and the sIL-6R results in the production of IL-6, suggesting an autocrine pathway for regulation of IL-6 expression by these cells (Van Wagoner, Oh, Repovic, & Benveniste, 1999). IL-6 has recently received much attention as a critical regulator of the CD4+ Th17 cell lineage, and production of IL-17, the signature cytokine produced by Th17 cells. IL-17 plays important roles in host defense against extracellular bacterial infections, and contributes to the pathogenesis of several autoimmune diseases, including collagen-induced arthritis, inflammatory bowel disease, and experimental autoimmune encephalomyelitis (EAE), an animal model of MS (Bettelli, Oukka, & Kuchroo, 2007; Weaver et al., 2006; Steinman, 2010; Qian, Kang, Liu, & Li, 2010). IL-17 is a proinflammatory cytokine that activates T cells and other immune cells to produce a variety of cytokines, chemokines, and cell adhesion molecules (Gaffen, 2009). IL-6 activation of STAT-3 induces the expression of IL-17, a STAT-3 target gene (Mathur et al., 2007). In turn, IL-17 signals through the NF-κB pathway, and one of its downstream target genes is IL-6 (Gaffen, 2009), thereby establishing a positive, autocrine loop for IL-6 and IL-17 gene expression.

With respect to HIV-1, CD4+ Th17 cells can be infected with the virus, as well as SIV, and are found at lower frequency at mucosal and systemic sites within a few weeks after infection (Cecchinato et al., 2008). Because Th17 cells play a critical role in controlling commensal bacteria, it has been proposed that lack of IL-17 expressing cells may contribute to the chronic enteropathy in HIV/SIV infection (Cecchinato et al., 2008; Campillo-Gimenez et al., 2010). There is little known about Th17 cells and IL-17 in the context of HAND. However, the role of Th17 cells/IL-17 has been extensively studied in EAE and patients with MS, which may provide clues to potential functions in HAND. First of all, IL-17 has the capacity to disrupt the BBB (Huppert et al., 2010). In patients with MS, IL-17 mRNA and protein are increased in both brain lesions and mononuclear cells isolated from blood and cerebrospinal fluid (Graber et al., 2008; Tzartos et al., 2008). Furthermore, the accumulation of Th17 cells in CNS MS lesions has been demonstrated. EAE is significantly suppressed in IL-17$^{-/-}$ mice; these animals exhibit a delay in disease onset, reduced maximum severity scores, ameliorated histological changes, and early recovery (Bettelli, Oukka, & Kuchroo, 2007; Langrish et al., 2005). More importantly, IL-17 signaling in astrocytes is critical for EAE disease induction. Kang et al. (2010) recently demonstrated that targeted deletion in astrocytes of the Act1 adaptor protein, which is essential for IL-17 signaling, impaired IL-17-mediated inflammatory gene induction, and rendered mice resistant to EAE. We have shown that astrocytes express the receptors for IL-17, IL-17RA, and IL-17RC, and respond to IL-17 treatment by activation of the NF-κB and MAPK signaling pathways (Ma et al., 2010), indicating astrocytes are a cellular CNS target for IL-17. Furthermore, IL-17 functions in a synergistic manner with IL-6 and the soluble IL-6R to further amplify IL-6 production by astrocytes (Ma et al., 2010). In addition, the combination of IL-6/sIL-6R plus IL-17 induces the expression of CCL20 by astrocytes, which is a potent chemoattractant for Th17 cells (Ransohoff, 2009). IL-17 also functions in a synergistic manner with TNF-α for expression of CXCL1, CXCL2, and CCL20 in astrocytes (Kang et al., 2010). CD4+T cells accumulate in the brains of patients with progressive HIV-1 infection (Petito, 2004); it will be of interest to determine if CD4+ Th17 cells are part of this inflammatory T-cell infiltrate, and whether IL-17 is detected in the HAND brain. This would establish a positive feedback loop in which naïve CD4+ T cells can differentiate into Th17 cells in the presence of IL-6 secreted by astrocytes. IL-17 in conjunction with IL-6/sIL-6R triggers a positive feed-forward loop of IL-6 expression in astrocytes, which will then continue to influence Th17 cell differentiation, resulting in the amplification of neuroinflammatory responses within the CNS (Figure 2.3.2). This appears to be the case in the disease of MS, and whether this is true for HAND remains to be determined. One recent study suggests this scenerio is relevant to HAND. Liu et al., (2009) demonstrated that adoptive transfer of CD4+ T effector cells (which comprise both Th1 and Th17 cells) into a mouse model of HAND promoted astrogliosis, microglial activation and increased TNF-α production. Whether IL-17 was involved in this response was not examined.

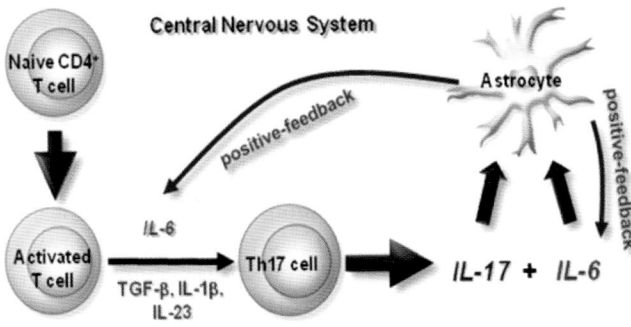

Figure 2.3.2 Model of IL-17 Enhancement of the IL-6 Signaling Cascade in Astrocytes. Naive CD4+ T cells, upon activation by signaling through the TCR and costimulatory molecules, can differentiate into Th17 cells in the presence of IL-6, TGF-β, IL-1, and IL-23. IL-17 together with IL-6/R triggers a positive feed-forward loop of IL-6 expression in astrocytes, which may also influence Th17 cell differentiation.

IL-6 also promotes astrocyte proliferation, and is believed to be involved in astrogliosis, one of the distinguishing features of HAND. IL-6-deficient mice exhibit depressed astrogliosis after focal cryo-injury compared with IL-6 wild-type mice (Penkowa et al., 1999). Interestingly, the IL-6-deficient mice had reduced numbers of activated brain macrophages associated with the lesion, suggesting that IL-6 is important for neuroinflammation. Conversely, IL-6/sIL-6R double transgenic mice exhibit massive reactive gliosis (Brunello et al., 2000). Transgenic mice in which IL-6 is expressed under the control of the astrocyte-specific GFAP promoter display neurodegeneration, breakdown of the BBB, CNS inflammation, angiogenesis, increased expression of complement proteins, and impaired learning (Barnum, Jones, Müller-Ladner, Samimi, & Campbell, 1996; Campbell et al., 1993; Heyser, Masliah, Samimi, Campbell, & Gold, 1997). This neuropathology is reminiscent of that seen in HAND. Another important consequence of IL-6 overexpression in the CNS is the induction of cytokines such as IL-1 and TNF-α (Santo et al., 1996; Santo et al., 1997), which in general have proinflammatory properties and are also overexpressed in the HAND brain (Wesselingh et al., 1993; Wilt et al., 1995; Griffin, 1997).

ONCOSTATIN M

OSM is another member of the IL-6 family of cytokines, and was identified originally for its inhibitory activity of tumor cell growth (Zarling et al., 1986). It is now appreciated that OSM has wide-ranging functions including the maintenance of embryonic stem cells, and growth stimulation of Kaposi's sarcoma cells. In human cells, OSM signals through two different receptor complexes: a gp130/LIFR complex (type I) or an OSMRβ/gp130 complex (type II). In murine cells, OSM signals exclusively through the type II receptor complex (Tanaka et al., 1999). OSM binds the OSMRβ with low affinity, but binds the OSMRβ/gp130 complex with high affinity (Tanaka et al., 1999). OSMRβ knock-out mice are viable but display defects in hematopoiesis and liver regeneration (Tanaka et al., 2003). Binding of OSM to the OSM receptor complex activates a number of signaling cascades including the JAK/STAT, MAPK, and NF-κB pathways to induce gene expression (Figure 2.3.3) (Chen & Benveniste, 2004). The identity and degree of pathway activation is cell-type specific.

Activation of the JAK/STAT pathway is achieved by OSM binding to the gp130 subunit and subsequent recruitment of either the LIFR or OSMRβ subunit, resulting in dimerization of the receptor. STAT-1 and STAT-3 are the predominant proteins recruited to the OSM receptor complex. Activated STAT-1 and/or STAT-3 proteins dissociate from the receptor and form homo- or hetero-dimeric complexes, which then translocate to the nucleus to activate transcription of genes that have STAT-responsive elements in their promoters (Shuai & Liu, 2003). OSM can also activate the MAPK pathways, which include the ERK, JNK, and p38 pathways. Activation of the MAPK pathways by OSM is mediated through the recruitment of the tyrosine phosphatase SHP-2 to the gp130 receptor, or recruitment of the adaptor protein Shc to the OSMRβ subunit (Hermanns, Radtke, Schaper, Heinrich, &

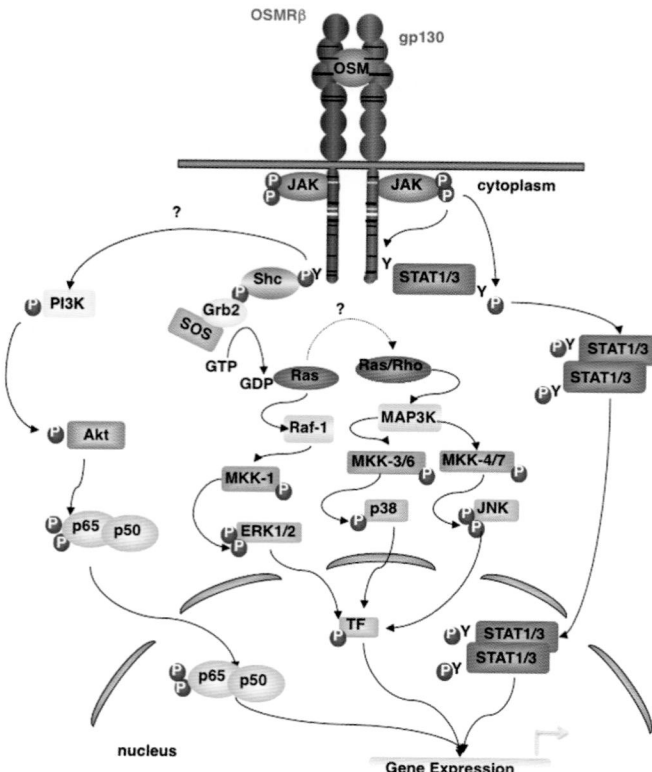

Figure 2.3.3 OSM Activation of the JAK/STAT, NF-κB and MAPK Pathways. OSM binding to the gp130/OSMRβ complex leads to the tyrosine phosphorylation of gp130 and OSMRβ by JAKs. Recruited STAT-1 and/or -3 are tyrosine phosphorylated. The STATs then dimerize and translocate to the nucleus to activate gene expression. The adaptor protein Shc is recruited to phosphotyrosine residues on the OSMRβ to activate the MAPK pathway. It is not clear how OSM activates the NF-κB pathway, although activation through the PI3K/Akt pathway is one possibility. Activation of the MAPK and NF-κB pathways then leads to phosphorylation of transcription factors (TF) and NF-κB (p65/p50) to modulate gene expression.

Yamamoto, & Wang, 2004). Some of the NF-κB-regulated genes include IL-8, IL-1β, TNF-α, IL-6, iNOS, and CD40.

OSM PRODUCTION IN THE CNS

What is the biological source(s) of OSM within the CNS? To date, the most frequently reported sources of OSM have been monocytes and macrophages. OSM production by these cells is induced by a number of stimuli, such as IL-3 and GM-CSF (Ma, Streiff, Liu, Spence, & Vestal, 1992), PMA and cisplatin (Sodhi, Shishodia, & Shrivastava, 1997), and HIV-1 infection (Ensoli et al., 1999). We have recently shown that microglia, the resident macrophages of the brain, produce OSM (Repovic & Benveniste, 2002). In this context, PGE$_2$ served as a novel inducer of OSM, and involved cooperation between astrocytes and microglia. In this system, inflammatory mediators such as IL-1 or TNF-α stimulated PGE$_2$ production by astrocytes, and this PGE$_2$ induced microglia to produce OSM (Repovic & Benveniste, 2002). PGE$_2$ induction of OSM occurred via Gs-protein-coupled receptors, adenylate cyclase, cAMP, and PKA, indicating that OSM is a cAMP-responsive gene. Accordingly, other activators of cAMP signaling such as norepinephrine and PGE$_1$ also induced OSM expression (Repovic & Benveniste, 2002). OSM expression is induced by other factors such as complement component C5a, IL-1β, and TNF-α (Repovic & Benveniste, 2002; Kastl et al., 2009). Elevated levels of OSM expression have been shown in inflammatory brain lesions, lesions of MS patients, HAND, and gliomas, as well as in mouse models of epilepsy and MS (Ensoli et al., 1999; Ensoli et al., 2002; Vecchiet et al., 2003). In MS lesions, OSM staining was most prominent in microglial cells, while no OSM expression was observed in normal brain and noninflammatory neurological disease controls (Ruprecht et al., 2001).

OSM EFFECTS ON CELLS OF THE CNS

OSM has been shown to induce the expression of a number of pro-inflammatory molecules including PGE$_2$, IL-6, TNF-α, iNOS, IL-1β, CCL2, COX-2, VEGF, matrix metalloproteinase-1 (MMP-1), MMP-3, ICAM-1, and VCAM-1 in a number of cell types including astrocytes and cerebral endothelial cells (Chen & Benveniste, 2004; Repovic, Fears, Gladson, & Benveniste, 2003; Korzus, Nagase, Rydell, & Travis, 1997). The OSM-induction of VEGF in astrocytes is STAT-3 dependent, as overexpression of a STAT-3 dominant-negative construct attenuates this response (Repovic, Fears, Gladson, & Benveniste, 2003). Plasminogen activator inhibitor-1 and urokinase-type plasminogen activator, proteins involved in tissue remodeling and cell invasion, are also induced by OSM in astrocytes (Kasza et al., 2002). Similarly, human astrocytes are activated by OSM to express α1-antichymotrypsin, an acute phase response protein. This protein is associated with amyloid deposits in the brains of Alzheimer's disease patients (Kordula et al., 1998). Furthermore, OSM regulates the differentiation of astrocytes (Yanagisawa, Nakashima, & Taga, 1999; Yanagisawa et al., 2001). In a model of HIV-1-associated neurodegeneration, OSM induced neuronal damage, likely through an apoptotic process (Ensoli et al., 1999). OSM was

Behrmann, 2000). In general, downstream phosphorylation of MKK1 leads to activation of the ERK pathway; phosphorylation of MKK4 and MKK7 activates the JNK pathway; and phosphorylation of MKK3 and MKK6 activates the p38 pathway (Weston & Davis, 2002). Signaling through the MAPK pathways regulates chromatin remodeling, and induces changes in the expression of genes involved in mitosis, migration, and programmed cell death (Hazzalin & Mahadevan, 2002). The upstream kinases linking OSM receptor activation to downstream activation of the NF-κB pathway have not been identified, although Akt is one candidate. In general, cytokine-mediated activation of the NF-κB pathway is achieved by downstream activation of the inhibitor of NF-κB kinase (IKK) complex. Upon activation, the IKK complex phosphorylates an inhibitory molecule bound to the NF-κB dimer, termed inhibitor of NF-κB (IκB). Phosphorylation of IκB targets it for proteosomal degradation, releasing the NF-κB dimers, which then translocate to the nucleus, bind to κB elements in the promoters of target genes, and activate gene expression (Karin, 2009; Karin, also shown to decrease transendothelial resistance of brain capillary endothelial cells by disrupting the tight junctions between these cells, suggesting that the expression of OSM may compromise the integrity of the BBB (Takata et al., 2008). These studies collectively suggest detrimental influences of OSM in the context of neuroinflammation. However, protective effects of OSM have also been observed. An anti-inflammatory effect of OSM was observed in EAE, where administration of OSM suppressed the inflammatory response and tissue damage in the CNS that is characteristic of this model (Wallace et al., 1999). The authors suggest that the anti-inflammatory effect of OSM may be due to its ability to inhibit TNF-α production. Another study showed that OSM injection into the striatum was protective in an NMDA-mediated mouse model of excitotoxicity (Weiss et al., 2006). This protection occurred via OSM-mediated downregulation of the NMDA receptor subunit NR2C. Another intriguing feature of OSM is a strong promyelinating effect on oligodendrocytes via activation of the gp130-JAK-STAT pathway (Stankoff et al., 2002). This effect was also observed using CNTF, LIF, and cardiotrophin-1, but not by IL-11 or IL-6 (Stankoff et al., 2002). Thus, the ultimate response to OSM, either pro-or anti-inflammatory, may be cell-type specific.

THE SOCS FAMILY

The two cytokines highlighted above, IL-6 and OSM, predominantly utilize the JAK-STAT pathway for signal transduction. Dysregulation of the JAK-STAT pathway has pathological implications, particularly in cancer and autoimmune diseases (Shuai & Liu, 2003). A number of mechanisms have evolved that negatively regulate the JAK-STAT signaling pathway, thereby attenuating biological responses. Control via a negative feedback loop is one of the major mechanisms to inhibit signal transduction, which is accomplished by suppressors of cytokine signaling (SOCS) proteins (Kubo, Hanada, & Yoshimura, 2003; Campbell, 2005; Alexander, & Hilton, 2004). This family contains eight members: cytokine-inducible SH2 domain-containing protein (CIS) and SOCS1 through SOCS7 (Figure 2.3.4). Each has a central SH2 domain; an N-terminal domain of variable length; and a C-terminal 40 amino acid module called the SOCS box. In addition, a small kinase inhibitory region (KIR) found in the N-terminal domain of SOCS1 and SOCS3 inhibits the activity of JAKs by acting as a pseudosubstrate. The central SH2 domain determines the target of each SOCS protein by binding specific phosphorylated tyrosine residues within the JAK-STAT signaling receptor complex. Once bound, SOCS can inhibit JAK-STAT signaling through a domain in its N-terminal region, or by the general use of its SOCS box which functions as an E3 ubiquitin to target both SOCS and their associated proteins for ubiquitination and degradation by the proteosome. Therefore, SOCS proteins combine specific inhibition of JAK activity with a generic mechanism of targeting interacting proteins for proteosomal degradation, via their SOCS box. SOCS proteins regulate the

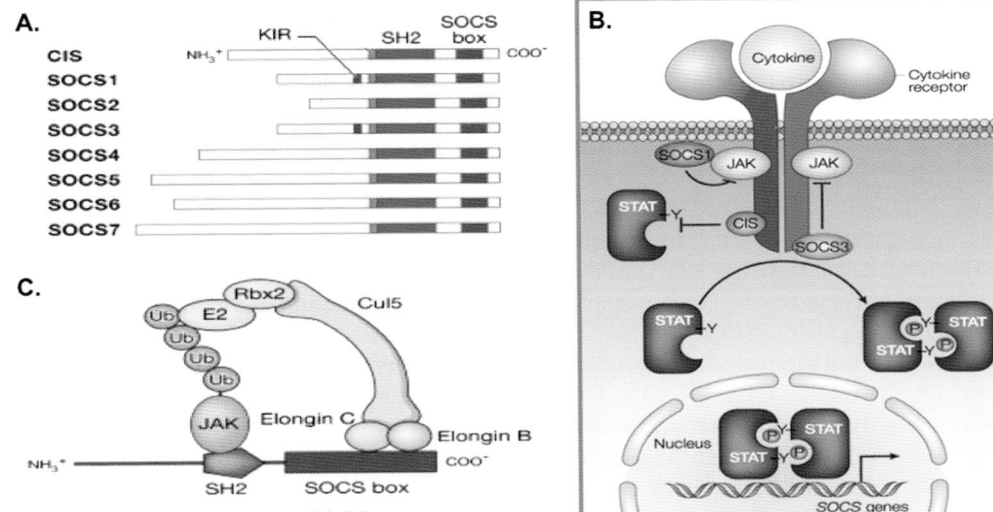

Figure 2.3.4 *SOCS Protein Structure and Function.* (A) The Suppressor of Cytokine Signaling (SOCS) family consists of eight members. Each contain a central SH2 domain, a C-terminal SOCS box, and an N-terminal domain of varying length and structure. SOCS1 and SOCS3 posses a kinase inhibitory region (KIR) in their N-terminus that serves as a pseudo-substrate for JAKs, thereby inhibiting JAK function. (B) SOCS proteins inhibit the JAK-STAT signaling pathway through different mechanisms. Each bind distinct sites within the JAK-STAT signaling receptor complex, and subsequently terminate pathway activation through inhibition of JAK activity, competition with STATs for receptor docking sites, or proteosomal degradation of receptor complex components. (C) The SOCS box interacts with Elongin B and C, Cullin-5 (Cul5), and RING-box-2 (Rbx2), to form an E3 ubiquitin ligase. The central SH2 domain binds target proteins, such as JAKs, bringing them into close proximity with the E2 and E3 ubiquitinating machinery. Ubiquitination of target proteins marks them for degradation via the proteosome. Adapted from Shuai and Liu, 2003, *Nature Reviews Immunology*, 3, p. 909. Copyright 2003 by Nature Publishing Group; and from Palmer and Restifo, 2009, *Trends Immunology*, 30, p. 592. Copyright 2009 by Elsevier. Adapted with permission.

half-life of a wide range of proteins including JAKs, the TEL-JAK2 oncogene, CD33, Siglec 7, the guanine nucleotide exchange factor Vav, the TLR adapter protein Mal, the E7 protein of human papilloma viruses, and focal adhesion kinase, to name a few (Piessevaux, Lavens, Peelman, & Tavernier, 2008). Most of these effects have been ascribed to SOCS1 and/or SOCS3, while less is known about the other SOCS family members. Importantly, SOCS3 has been shown to associate with tyrosine 757 in the gp130 receptor subunit, which allows SOCS3 to inhibit signaling by the IL-6 family of cytokines. Although initially identified for their ability to inhibit JAK-STAT signaling, SOCS proteins have broader effects by inhibiting signaling of other stimuli such as LPS, type I and type II interferons, IL-2, IL-12, IL-17, and IL-21. In addition, SOCS1 and SOCS3 inhibit the NF-κB pathway and cAMP-mediated signaling, while enhancing signaling through the Ras pathway (Baker, Akhtar, & Benveniste, 2009). Thus, SOCS proteins are involved in regulating a wide range of cellular processes including innate and adaptive immune responses, growth and differentiation of lymphoid cells, and responses to bacterial and viral infections.

SOCS1/SOCS3 EXPRESSION AND FUNCTION IN THE CNS

SOCS proteins can be induced by a broad range of stimuli (Baker, Akhtar, & Benveniste, 2009). In primary astrocytes, OSM, IL-6, IFN-γ, IFN-β, IL-17, IL-10, and peroxisome proliferator-activated receptor (PPAR)-γ agonists such as 15d-PGJ$_2$ and rosiglitazone induce the expression of SOCS1 and/or SOCS3 (Qin, Wilson, Lee, & Benveniste, 2006; Stark, Lyons, & Cross, 2004; Park, Park, Joe, & Jou, 2003; Dalpke, Opper, Zimmermann, & Heeg, 2001). Induction of SOCS proteins by interferons IL-10 and IL-6 occurs in a JAK/STAT-dependent manner (Quinn et al., 2006; Niemand et al., 2003), while SOCS expression in response to OSM and LPS involves both the JAK/STAT and MAPK pathways (Baker, Qin, & Benveniste, 2008; Qin et al., 2007). With respect to astrocytes, we have identified both SOCS1 and SOCS3 as attenuators of inflammatory responses in these cells. SOCS1 and SOCS3 are induced in astrocytes by a variety of stimuli in a transient manner. Specific small interfering RNA inhibition of SOCS1 and SOCS3 in astrocytes led to enhancement of STAT1 and STAT3 signaling, enhanced their proinflammatory responses to IFN-β stimulation, such as heightened expression of the chemokines CCL2, CCL3, CCL4, CCL5, and CXCL10, and promoted enhanced chemotaxis of macrophages and CD4$^+$ T cells (Qin, Niyongere, Lee, Baker, & Benveniste, 2008). These results indicate that SOCS1 and SOCS3 in primary astrocytes function to attenuate their own chemokine-related inflammation in the CNS. In addition, SOCS3 expression in astrocytes serves to inhibit IL-6/sIL-6R plus IL-17 induction of IL-6 (Ma et al., 2010). In these studies, both siRNA knockdown of SOCS3 and the use of SOCS3-deficient astrocytes led to enhanced activation of the NF-κB, p38 MAPK, and JNK MAPK pathways, indicating that SOCS3 negatively regulates the expression of IL-6 via inhibition of these pathways. Collectively, SOCS1 and SOCS3

regulate numerous signaling pathways of importance in astrocyte biology, such as the JAK-STAT, NF-κB, and MAPK pathways.

Within the CNS, SOCS3 has been shown to elicit a wide range of functions depending on the disease context and cell type. In a mouse model of SCI, SOCS3 inhibits astrocyte scar formation, leading to prolonged inflammatory cell infiltration and limited functional recovery (Herrman et al., 2008; Okada et al., 2006). In this system, STAT3 signaling in astrocytes is beneficial, thus SOCS3 expression worsened the clinical features of SCI. By contrast, SOCS-3 was shown to be protective in a model of stroke (Baker et al., 2009), although the mechanism was not elucidated. In a cuprizone model of demyelination, the IL-6 family member LIF protects against demyelination. In this model, SOCS3 expression in oligodendrocytes was shown to limit the protective effect of LIF (Emery, Butzkueven, Snell, Binder, & Kilpatrick, 2006; Emery et al., 2006). Therefore, inhibition of SOCS3 in the context of demyelination might enable greater LIF-mediated protection. Lastly, HIV-1, by means of its regulatory protein Tat, can induce SOCS proteins to evade innate immune responses. We have recently shown that SOCS3 is elevated in an SIV/macaque model of HAD, and that the pattern of SOCS3 expression correlates with recurrance of SIV replication and onset of CNS disease (Akhtar et al., 2010). HIV-1 Tat induces the selective expression of SOCS3 in macrophages and microglia, with little induction of SOCS1 or SOCS2. Interestingly, Tat did not induce expression of SOCS proteins in either astrocytes or neurons, although these cells are capable of expressing SOCS3 in response to other stimuli, and have been previously shown to respond functionally to Tat (Nath, Chen, Scott, & Major, 1999; Kutsch, Oh, Nath, & Benveniste, 2000). These results indicate that Tat-induced SOCS3 expression is restricted to cells of macrophage lineage within the CNS. SOCS3 inhibits the response of macrophages/microglia to IFN-β at the level of STAT activation and downstream antiviral gene expression (PKR, ISG20, APOBEC3G). Most importantly, SOCS3 is able to suppress the inhibitory effect of IFN-β on HIV-1 replication, leading to an enhancement of HIV-1 replication in macrophages. Thus, we propose that SOCS3, a molecular inhibitor of cytokine signaling, serves as a host cell factor that allows HIV-1 to evade innate immunity within the CNS. It is also relevant to discuss SOCS3 in relationship to hepatitis C virus (HCV). While HCV is primarily hepatotropic, there is evidence of neuroinvasion and infection of macrophages and microglia in the CNS (Wilkinson, Radkowski, & Laskus, 2009; Radkowski et al., 2002). These findings imply that HCV and HIV-1 replicate in the same cells in the CNS, that is, macrophages/microglia, which raises the possibility of direct interactions between these pathogens. The prevalence of HIV-HCV co-infection is ~33% in HIV-1 infected patients in the United States, and may increase to 80–90% when HIV-1 patients are drug abusers. Patients co-infected with HIV and HCV present with worse cognitive dysfunction than patients mono-infected with HIV or HCV (Letendre et al., 2005). The HCV core protein was shown to induce SOCS3 expression in HepG2 cells, which correlated with an inhibition of IFN-α-induced STAT1 activation and enhancement of viral replication (Bode et al., 2003). Our preliminary results indicate that HCV core protein induces very strong expression of SOCS3 mRNA in macrophages. Of interest is that inclusion of the P6 compound, a pharmacologic inhibitor of JAKs, abrogated SOCS3 expression, suggesting that HCV core protein induction of SOCS3 occurs through activation of the JAK-STAT pathway. Thus, viral induction of SOCS3 in macrophages has the potential to enhance both HIV-1 and HCV replication, contributing to aspects of HAND (Akhtar & Benveniste, 2011).

SUMMARY AND PROSPECTUS

Astrocytes play a pivotal role in CNS development, biology, and the pathophysiology of numerous CNS diseases (Table 2.3.2). Not only do they serve numerous critical functions within the brain such as maintenance of extracellular ionic concentrations, guiding neuronal development, modulating synaptic activity, neurotransmitter uptake and metabolism, and maintenance of BBB integrity, they function as a bridge between the CNS and immune system. In particular, astrocytes produce a wide array of cytokines and chemokines that act as immune mediators in the CNS in response to traumatic injury and invasion by foreign pathogens (i.e., viruses such as HIV). Although expression of cytokines/chemokines is restricted under normal conditions, during CNS diseases such as HAND, expression is enhanced and thus contributes directly to brain inflammation, neuronal damage, and disease progression.

Table 2.3.2 AASTROCYTE INVOLVEMENT IN DISEASE STATES

HIV-1 Associated Neurocognitive Disorders	Indirect mechanism: amplified glutamate and cytokine release from astrocytes, resulting in neuronal apoptosis Direct mechanism: HIV-1 infection of astrocytes leads to production of neurotoxic factors
Alzheimer's Disease	Promote Aβ accumulation and plaque formation; enhanced calcium transients in astrocytes
Amyotrophic Lateral Sclerosis	Release toxic signal(s) that kills motor neurons; focal degeneration of subset of neurons; control microglial activation
Spinal Cord Injury	Form glial scar that acts as a barrier to regeneration of damaged axons
Glioblastoma (GBM)	Derived from malignant transformation of astrocytes. Aberrant glutamate signaling promotes glioma growth and invasiveness
Rett Syndrome	Aberrant secretion of soluble factor(s) that causes neuronal damage
Multiple Sclerosis	Inflammatory signaling in astrocytes is detrimental in EAE model. Inhibition of the NF-κB pathway in astrocytes ameliorates EAE by decreasing expression of cytokines, chemokines and adhesion molecules. Also, leads to neuroprotective effects such as preservation of axons and synapses

In addition, the appreciation that astrocytes are infected with HIV-1 and may serve as another viral reservoir in the CNS elevates their importance in the pathogenesis of HAND. The physiological effects of cytokines/chemokines on astrocytes as well as other CNS cells such as microglia, neurons, and oligodendrocytes are complex, and mediated by numerous signaling cascades. Many responses, that is, pro- or anti-inflammatory, are cell-type specific. The situation is made even more complicated by the fact that many different cytokines/chemokines that are elevated in HAND work either synergistically or antagonistically. A major challenge is to integrate data on signaling molecules and signaling pathway interactions, and understand it in the broader context of disease development, progression, and subsequent cognitive, sensory, and motor abnormalities associated with HAND. Our emerging knowledge of endogenous regulators of these pathways, such as SOCS proteins, protein inhibitors of activated STATs (PIAS) proteins, and protein tyrosine phosphatases (PTPs) (Shuai, 2006; Yoshimura, Naka, & Kubo, 2007) adds to the complexity of regulating signal transduction. There is growing interest in SOCS proteins, particularly SOCS1 and SOCS3, as therapeutic targets in a variety of cancers and autoimmune diseases, and mimetics/antagonists are currently being tested in preclinical models (Akhtar & Benveniste, 2011; Jo, Liu, Yao, Collins, & Hawiger, 2005; Ahmed et al., 2010; Ahmed et al., 2009; Flowers et al., 2004; Flowers, Subramaniam, & Johnson, 2005;. Frey et al., 2009; Mujtaba et al., 2005; Waiboci et al., 2007; Fletcher, Digiandomenico, & Hawiger, 2010). Such approaches may be considered in murine and simian models of HAND.

ACKNOWLEDGMENTS

This work was supported in part by grants from the National Institutes of Health and the National Multiple Sclerosis Society, to E.N.B. L.N.A. was supported by the University of Alabama at Birmingham Medical Scientist Training Program, and by NIH Grants T32-AI-07493 and F30-NS-65600, and B.J.B was supported by NIH Grant T32-NS-48039. The authors thank Cheryl Lyles for excellent editorial assistance.

REFERENCES

Ahmed, C. M., Dabelic, R., Martin, J. P., Jager, L. D., Haider, S. M., & Johnson, H. M. (2010). Enhancement of antiviral immunity by small molecule antagonist of suppressor of cytokine signaling. *J Immunol*, *185*, 1103.

Ahmed, C. M., Dabelic, R., Waiboci, L. W., Jager, L. D., Heron, L. L., & Johnson, H. M. (2009). SOCS-1 mimetics protect mice against lethal poxvirus infection: Identification of a novel endogenous antiviral system. *J Virol*, *83*, 1402.

Akhtar, L.N., & Benveniste, E.N. (2011). Viral exploitation of host SOCS protein functions. *J Virol*, *85*, 1912.

Akhtar, L. N., Qin, H., Muldowney, M. T., Yanagisawa, L. L., Kutsch, O., Clemens, J. E., et al. (2010). Suppressor of cytokine signaling 3 inhibits antiviral IFN-β signaling to enhance HIV-1 replication in macrophages. *J Immunol*, *185*, 2393.

Alexander, W. S. & Hilton, D. J. (2004). The role of suppressors of cytokine signaling (SOCS) proteins in regulation of the immune response. *Annu Rev Immunol*, *22*, 503.

Anthony, I. C. & Bell, J. E. (2008). The neuropathology of HIV/AIDS. *International Review of Psychiatry, 20*, 15.

Bajetto, A., Bonavia, R., Barbero, S., & Schettini, G. (2002). Characterization of chemokines and their receptors in the central nervous system: Physiopathological implications. *J Neurochem, 82*, 1311.

Baker, B. J., Akhtar, L. N., & Benveniste, E. N. (2009). SOCS1 and SOCS3 in the control of CNS immunity. *Trends Immunol. 30l*, 392.

Baker, B. J., Qin, H., & Benveniste, E. N. (2008). Molecular basis of oncostatin M-induced SOCS-3 expression in astrocytes. *Glia, 56*, 1250.

Barnum, S. R., Jones, J. L., Müller-Ladner, U., Samimi, A., & Campbell, I. L. (1996). Chronic complement C3 gene expression in the CNS of transgenic mice with astrocyte-targeted interleukin-6 expression. *Glia, 18*, 107.

Barres, B. A. (2008). The mystery and magic of glia: A perspective on their roles in health and disease. *Neuron, 60*, 430.

Bauer, S., Kerr, B. J., & Patterson, P. H. (2007). The neuropoietic cytokine family in development, plasticity, disease and injury. *Nat Rev Neurosci, 8*, 221.

Benos, D. J., Hahn, B. H., Bubien, J. K., Ghosh, S. K., Mashburn, N. A., Chaikin, M. A., et al. (1994). Envelope glycoprotein gp120 of human immunodeficiency virus type 1 alters ion transport in astrocytes: Implications for AIDS dementia complex. *Proc Natl Acad Sci USA, 91*, 494.

Benos, D. J., McPherson, S., Hahn, B. H., Chaikin, M. A., & Benveniste, E. N. (1994). Cytokines and HIV envelope glycoprotein gp120 stimulate Na+/H+ exchange in astrocytes. *J Biol Chem, 269*, 13811.

Benveniste, E. N. (1998). Cytokine actions in the central nervous system. *Cytokine and Growth Factor Rev, 9*, 259.

Bettelli, E., Oukka, M., & Kuchroo, V. K. (2007). TH-17 cells in the circle of immunity and autoimmunity. *Nat Immunol, 8*, 345.

Bode, J. G., Ludwig, S., Ehrhardt, C., Albrecht, U., Erhardt, A., Schaper, F., et al. (2003). IFN-α antagonistic activity of HCV core protein involves induction of suppressor of cytokine signaling-3. *Faseb J, 17*, 488.

Boisse, L., Gill, M. J., & Power, C. (2008). HIV infection of the central nervous system: Clinical features and neuropathogenesis. *Neurol Clin, 26*, 799.

Brunello, A. G., Weissenberger, J., Kappeler, A., Vallan, C., Peters, M., Rose-John, S., et al. (2000). Astrocytic alterations in interleukin-6/soluble interleukin-6 receptor a double-transgenic mice. *Am J Pathol, 157*, 1485.

Campbell, I. L. (2005). Cytokine-mediated inflammation, tumorigenesis, and disease-associated JAK/STAT/SOCS signaling circuits in the CNS. *Brain Res Brain Res Rev, 48*, 166.

Campbell, I. L., Abraham, C. R., Masliah, E., Kemper, P., Inglis, J. D., Oldstone, M. B. A., et al. (1993). Neurologic disease induced in transgenic mice by cerebral overexpression of interleukin 6. *Proc Natl Acad Sci USA, 90*, 10061.

Campillo-Gimenez, L., Cumont, M. C., Fay, M., Kared, H., Monceaux, V., Diop, O., et al. (2010). AIDS progression is associated with the emergence of IL-17-producing cells early after simian immunodeficiency virus infection. *J Immunol, 184*, 984.

Cecchinato, V., Trindade, C. J., Laurence, A., Heraud, J. M., Brenchley, J. M., Ferrari, M. G., et al. (2008). Altered balance between Th17 and Th1 cells at mucosal sites predicts AIDS progression in simian immunodeficiency virus-infected macaques. *Mucosal Immunol, 1*, 279.

Chang, H. C., Samaniego, F., Nair, B. C., Buonaguro, L., & Ensoli, B. (1997). HIV-1 Tat protein exits from cells via a leaderless secretory pathway and binds to extracellular matrix-associated heparan sulfate proteoglycans through its basic region. *AIDS, 11*, 1421.

Chen, S.-H. & Benveniste, E. N. (2004). Oncostatin M: A pleiotropic cytokine in the central nervous system. *Cytokine & Growth Factor Reviews, 15*, 379.

Churchill, M. J., Wesselingh, S. L., Cowley, D., Pardo, C. A., McArthur, J. C., Brew, B. J., et al. (2009). Extensive astrocyte infection is prominent in human immunodeficiency virus-associated dementia. *Ann Neurol, 66*, 253.

Clay, C. C., Rodrigues, D. S., Ho, Y. S., Fallert, B. A., Janatpour, K., Reinhart, T. A., et al. (2007). Neuroinvasion of fluorescein-positive monocytes in acute simian immunodeficiency virus infection. *J Virol, 81*, 12040.

Corasaniti, M. T., Piccirilli, S., Paoletti, A., Nistico, R., Stringaro, A., Malorni, W., et al. (2001). Evidence that the HIV-1 coat protein gp120 causes neuronal apoptosis in the neocortex of rat via a mechanism involving CXCR4 chemokine receptor. *Neurosci Lett, 312*, 67.

Dalpke, A. H., Opper, S., Zimmermann, S., & Heeg, K. (2001). Suppressors of cytokine signaling (SOCS)-1 and SOCS-3 are induced by CpG-DNA and modulate cytokine responses in APCs. *J Immunol, 166*, 7082.

Dong, Y. & Benveniste, E. N. (2001). Immune function of astrocytes. Glia, 36, 180.

Ellis, R., Langford, D., & Masliah, E. (2007). HIV and antiretroviral therapy in the brain: Neuronal injury and repair. *Nat Rev Neurosci, 8*, 33.

Emery, B., Butzkueven, H., Snell, C., Binder, M., & Kilpatrick, T. J. (2006). Oligodendrocytes exhibit selective expression of suppressor of cytokine signaling genes and signal transducer and activator of transcription 1 independent inhibition of interferon-γ-induced toxicity in response to leukemia inhibitory factor. *Neuroscience, 137*, 463.

Emery, B., Cate, H. S., Marriott, M., Merson, T., Binder, M. D., Snell, C., et al. (2006). Suppressor of cytokine signaling 3 limits protection of leukemia inhibitory factor receptor signaling against central demyelination. *Proc Natl Acad Sci USA, 103*, 7859.

Ensoli, F., Fiorelli, V., DeCristofaro, M., Muratori, D. S., Novi, A., Vannelli, B., et al. (1999). Inflammatory cytokines and HIV-1 associated neurodegeneration: oncostatin-M produced by mononuclear cells from HIV-1 infected individuals induces apoptosis of primary neurons. *J Immunol, 162*, 6268.

Ensoli, F., Fiorelli, V., Lugaresi, A., Farina, D., De Cristofaro, M., Collacchi, B., et al. (2002). Lymphomononuclear cells from multiple sclerosis patients spontaneously produce high levels of oncostatin M, tumor necrosis factors α and β, and interferon γ. *Mult Scler 8*, 284.

Eugenin, E. A. & Berman, J. W. (2007). Gap junctions mediate human immunodeficiency virus-bystander killing in astrocytes. *J Neurosci, 27*, 12844.

Eugenin, E. A., Osiecki, K., Lopez, L., Goldstein, H., Calderon, T. M., & Berman. J. W. (2006). CCL2/monocyte chemoattractant protein-1 mediates enhanced transmigration of human immunodeficiency virus (HIV)-infected leukocytes across the blood-brain barrier: A potential mechanism of HIV-CNS invasion and neuroAIDS. *J Neurosci, 26*, 1098.

Farina, C., Aloisi, F., & Meinl, E. (2007). Astrocytes are active players in cerebral innate immunity. *Trends Immunol, 28*, 138.

Fletcher, T. C., Digiandomenico, A., & Hawiger, J. (2010). Extended anti-inflammatory action of a degradation-resistant mutant of cell-penetrating suppressor of cytokine signaling 3. *J Biol Chem, 285*, 18727.

Flowers, L. O., Johnson, H. M., Mujtaba, M. G., Ellis, M. R., Haider, S. M., & Subramaniam, P. S. (2004). Characterization of a peptide inhibitor of Janus kinase 2 that mimics suppressor of cytokine signaling 1 function. *J Immunol, 172*, 7510.

Flowers, L. O., Subramaniam, P. S., & Johnson, H. M. (2005). A SOCS-1 peptide mimetic inhibits both constitutive and IL-6 induced activation of STAT3 in prostate cancer cells. *Oncogene, 24*, 2114.

Frey, K. G., Ahmed, C. M., Dabelic, R., Jager, L. D., Noon-Song, E. N., Haider, S. M., et al. (2009). HSV-1-induced SOCS-1 expression in keratinocytes: use of a SOCS-1 antagonist to block a novel mechanism of viral immune evasion. *J Immunol, 183*, 1253.

Gaffen, S. L. (2009). Structure and signalling in the IL-17 receptor family. *Nat Rev Immunol, 9*, 556.

Graber, J. J., Allie, S. R., Mullen, K. M., Jones, M. V., Wang, T., Krishnan, C., et al. (2008). Interleukin-17 in transverse myelitis and multiple sclerosis. *J Neuroimmunol, 196*, 124.

Griffin, D. E. (1997). Perspectives Series: Cytokines and the brain. Cytokines in the brain during viral infection: Clues to HIV-associated dementia. *J Clin Invest, 100*, 2948.

Haydon, P. G. (2000). Neuroglial networks: Neurons and glia talk to each other. *Curr Biol, 10*, R712.

Hazzalin, C. A. & Mahadevan, L. C. (2002). MAPK-regulated transcription: A continuously variable gene switch? *Nat Rev Mol Cell Biol, 3*, 30.

Herrman, J., Imura, T., Song, B., Qi, J., Yan, A., Nguyen, T., et al. (2008). STAT3 is a critical regulator of astrogliosis and scar formation after spinal cord injury. *J Neurosci, 28,* 7231.

Hermanns, H. M., Radtke, S., Schaper, F., Heinrich, P. C., & Behrmann, I. (2000). Non-redundant signal transduction of interleukin-6-type cytokines. *J Biol Chem, 275,* 40742.

Heyser, C. J., Masliah, E., Samimi, A., Campbell, I. L., & Gold, L. H. (1997). Progressive decline in avoidance learning paralleled by inflammatory neurodegeneration in transgenic mice expressing interleukin 6 in the brain. *Proc Natl Acad Sci USA, 94,*1500.

Hult, B., Chana, G., Masliah, E., & Everall, I. (2008). Neurobiology of HIV. *International Review of Psychiatry, 20,* 3.

Huppert, J., Closhen, D., Croxford, A., White, R., Kulig, P., Pietrowski, E., et al. (2010). Cellular mechanisms of IL-17-induced blood-brain barrier disruption. *Faseb J, 24,* 1023.

Jo, D., Liu, D., Yao, S., Collins, R. D., & Hawiger, J. (2005). Intracellular protein therapy with SOCS3 inhibits inflammation and apoptosis. *Nat Med, 11,* 892.

John, G. R., Lee, S. C., & Brosnan, C. F. (2003). Cytokines: Powerful regulators of glial cell activation. *Neuroscientist, 9,* 10.

Kang, Z., Altuntas, C. Z., Gulen, M. F., Liu, C., Giltiay, N., Qin, H., et al. (2010). Astrocyte-restricted ablation of Interleukin-17-induced Act1-mediated signaling ameliorates autoimmune encephalomyelitis. *Immunity, 32,* 414.

Karin, M. (2009). NF-κB as a critical link between inflammation and cancer. *Cold Spring Harb Perspect Biol, 1,* 141.

Karin, M., Yamamoto, Y., & Wang, Q. M. (2004). The IKK NF-κB System: A treasure trove for drug development. *Nature Rev, 3,* 17.

Kastl, S. P., Speidl, W. S., Katsaros, K. M., Kaun, C., Rega, G., Assadian, A., et al. (2009). Thrombin induces the expression of oncostatin M via AP-1 activation in human macrophages: A link between coagulation and inflammation. *Blood, 114,* 2812.

Kasza, A., Kiss, D. L., Gopalan, S., Xu, W., Rydel, R. E., Koj, A., et al. (2002). Mechanism of plasminogen activator inhibitor-1 regulation by oncostatin M and interleukin-1 in human astrocytes. *J Neurochem, 83,* 696.

Kaul, M. (2009). HIV-1 associated dementia: Update on pathological mechanisms and therapeutic approaches. *Curr Opin Neurol, 22,* 315.

Kaul, M., Garden, G. A., & Lipton, S. A. (2001). Pathways to neuronal injury and apoptosis in HIV-associated dementia. *Nature, 410,* 988.

Kaul, M., & Lipton, S. A. (2006). Mechanisms of neuronal injury and death in HIV-1 associated dementia. *Curr HIV Res, 4,* 307.

Kaul, M., Zheng, J., Okamoto, S., Gendelman, H. E., & Lipton, S. A. (2005). HIV-1 infection and AIDS: Consequences for the central nervous system. *Cell Death Differ, 12,* 878.

Kordula, T., Rydel, R. E., Brigham, E. F., Horn, F., Heinrich, P. C., & Travis, J. (1998). Oncostatin M and the interleukin-6 and soluble interleukin-6 receptor complex regulate a1-antichymotrypsin expression in human cortical astrocytes. *J Biol Chem, 273,* 4112.

Korzus, E., Nagase, H., Rydell, R., & Travis, J. (1997). The mitogen-activated protein kinase and JAK-STAT signaling pathways are required for an oncostatin M-responsive element-mediated activation of matrix metalloproteinase 1 gene expression. *J Biol Chem, 272,* 1188.

Kraft-Terry, S. D., Buch, S. J., Fox, H. S., & Gendelman, H. E. (2009). A coat of many colors: Neuroimmune crosstalk in human immunodeficiency virus infection. *Neuron, 64,* 133.

Kubo, M., Hanada, T., & Yoshimura, A. (2003). Suppressors of cytokine signaling and immunity. *Nat Immunol, 4,* 1169.

Kutsch, O., Oh, J-W., Nath, A., & Benveniste, E. N. (2000). Induction of the chemokines interleukin-8 and IP-10 by human immunodeficiency virus type 1 Tat in astrocytes. *J Virol, 74,* 9214.

Langrish, C. L., Chen, Y., Blumenschein, W. M., Mattson, J., Basham, B., Sedgwick, J. D., et al. (2005). IL-23 drives a pathogenic T cell population that induces autoimmune inflammation. *J Exp Med, 201,* 233.

Letendre, S. L., Cherner, M., Ellis, R. J., Marquie-Beck, J., Gragg, B., Marcotte, T., et al. (2005). The effects of hepatitis C, HIV, and methamphetamine dependence on neuropsychological performance: Biological correlates of disease. *AIDS, 19,* Suppl 3, S72.

Liu, J., Gong, N., Huang, X., Reynolds, A. D., Mosley, R. L., & Gendelman, H. E. (2009). Neuromodulatory activities of CD4+CD25+ regulatory T cells in a murine model of HIV-1-associated neurodegeneration. *J Immunol, 182,* 3855.

Ma, X., Reynolds, S. L., Baker, B. J., Li, X., Benveniste, E. N., & Qin, H. (2010). IL-17 enhancement of the IL-6 signaling cascade in astrocytes. *J Immunol, 184,* 4898.

Ma, Y., Streiff, R. J., Liu, J., Spence, M. J., & Vestal, R. E. (1999). Cloning and characterization of human oncostatin M promoter. *Nucleic Acids Res, 27,* 4649.

Magnuson, D. S. K., Knudsen, B. E., Geiger, J. D., Brownstone, R. M., & Nath, A. (1995). Human immunodeficiency virus type 1 tat activates non-N-methyl-D-aspartate excitatory amino acid receptors and causes neurotoxicity. *Ann Neurol, 37,* 373.

Mathur, A. N., Chang, H. C., Zisoulis, D. G., Stritesky, G. L., Yu, Q., O'Malley, T., et al. (2007). STAT-3 and STAT4 direct development of IL-17-secreting Th cells. *J Immunol, 178,* 4901.

McCombe, J. A., Noorbakhsh, F., Buchholz, C., Trew, M., & Power, C. (2009). NeuroAIDS: A watershed for mental health and nervous system disorders. *J Psychiatry Neurosci, 34,* 83.

Mujtaba, M. G., Flowers, L. O., Patel, C. B., Patel, R. A., Haider, M. I., & Johnson, H. M. (2005). Treatment of mice with the suppressor of cytokine signaling-1 mimetic peptide, tyrosine kinase inhibitor peptide, prevents development of the acute form of experimental allergic encephalomyelitis and induces stable remission in the chronic relapsing/remitting form. *J Immunol, 175,* 5077.

Naka, T., Nishimoto, N., & Kishimoto, T. (2002). The paradigm of IL-6: From basic science to medicine. *Arthritis Res, 4* Suppl 3, S233.

Nath, A., Chen, P., Scott, C., & Major, E. O. (1999). Transient exposure to HIV-1 Tat protein results in cytokine production in macrophages and astrocytes. A hit and run phenomenon. *J Biol Chem, 274,* 17098.

Nath, A., Schiess, N., Venkatesan, A., Rumbaugh, J., Sacktor, N., & McArthur, J. (2008). Evolution of HIV dementia with HIV infection. *International Review of Psychiatry, 20,* 25.

Niemand, C., Nimmesgern, A., Haan, S., Fischer, P., Schaper, F., Rossaint, R., et al. (2003). Activation of STAT3 by IL-6 and IL-10 in primary human macrophages is differentially modulated by suppressor of cytokine signaling 3. *J Immunol, 170,* 3263.

Okada, S., Nakamura, M., Katoh, H., Miyao, T., Shimazaki, T., Ishii, K., et al. (2006). Conditional ablation of Stat3 or Socs3 discloses a dual role for reactive astrocytes after spinal cord injury. *Nat Med, 12,* 829.

Park, E. J., Park, S. Y., Joe, E. H., & Jou, I. (2003). 15d-PGJ2 and rosiglitazone suppress Janus kinase-STAT inflammatory signaling through induction of suppressor of cytokine signaling 1 (SOCS1) and SOCS3 in glia. *J Biol Chem, 278,* 14747.

Penkowa, M., Moos, T., Carrasco, J., Hadberg, H., Molinero, A., Bluethmann, H., et al. (1999). Strongly compromised inflammatory response to brain injury in interleukin-6-deficient mice. *Glia, 25,* 343.

Perea, G. & Araque, A. (2007). Astrocytes potentiate transmitter release at single hippocampal synapses. *Science, 317,* 1083.

Petito, C. K. (2004). Human immunodeficiency virus type 1 compartmentalization in the central nervous system. *J Neurovirol, 10* Suppl 1, 21.

Petito, C. K. & Cash, K. S. (1992). Blood-brain barrier abnormalities in the acquired immunodeficiency syndrome: Immunohistochemical localization of serum proteins in postmortem brain. *Ann Neurol, 32,* 658.

Piessevaux, J., Lavens, D., Peelman, F., & Tavernier, J. (2008). The many faces of the SOCS box. *Cytokine Growth Factor Rev, 19,* 371.

Power, C., Boisse, L., Rourke, & Gill, M. J. (2009). NeuroAIDS: An evolving epidemic. *Can J Neurol Sci, 36,* 285.

Power, C., Kong, P. A., Crawford, T. O., Wesselingh, S., Glass, J. D., McArthur, J. C., et al. (1993). Cerebral white matter changes in acquired immunodeficiency syndrome dementia: Alterations of the blood-brain barrier. *Ann Neurol, 34,* 339.

Qian, Y., Kang, Z., Liu, C., & Li, X. (2010). IL-17 signaling in host defense and inflammatory diseases. *Cell Mol Immunol, 7,* 328.

Qin, H., Niyongere, S. A., Lee, S. J., Baker, B. J., & Benveniste, E. N. (2008). Expression and functional significance of SOCS-1 and SOCS-3 in astrocytes. *J Immunol, 181,* 3167.

Qin, H., Roberts, K. L., Niyongere, S. A., Cong, Y., Elson, C. O., & Benveniste. E. N. (2007). Molecular mechanism of lipopolysaccharide-Induced SOCS-3 gene expression in macrophages and microglia. *J Immunol*, *179*, 5966.

Qin, H., Wilson, C., Lee, S. J., & Benveniste, E. N. (2006). IFN-β induced SOCS-1 negatively regulates CD40 gene expression in macrophages and microglia. *FASEB J*, *20*, 985.

Radkowski, M., Wilkinson, J., Nowicki, M., Adair, D., Vargas, H., Ingui, C., et al. (2002). Search for hepatitis C virus negative-strand RNA sequences and analysis of viral sequences in the central nervous system: Evidence of replication. *J Virol*, *76*, 600.

Ransohoff, R. M. (2009). Chemokines and chemokine receptors: Standing at the crossroads of immunobiology and neurobiology. *Immunity*, *31*, 711.

Repovic, P. & Benveniste, E. N. (2002). Prostaglandin E2 is a novel inducer of oncostatin-M expression in macrophages and microglia. *J Neurosci*, *22*, 5334.

Repovic, P., Fears, C. Y., Gladson, C. L., & Benveniste, E. N. (2003). Oncostatin-M induction of vascular endothelial growth factor expression in astroglioma cells. *Oncogene*, *22*, 8117.

Rodig, S. J., Meraz, M. A., White, J. M., Lampe, P. A., Riley, J. K., Arthur, C. D., et al. (1998). Disruption of the JAK1 gene demonstrates obligatory and nonredundant roles of the JAKs in cytokine-induced biologic responses. *Cell*, *93*, 373.

Rose-John, S., Ehlers, M., Grötzinger, J., Müllberg, J. (1995). The soluble interleukin-6 receptor. *Ann NY Acad Sci*, *762*, 207.

Ruprecht, K., Kuhlmann, T., Seif, F., Hummel, V., Kruse, N., Bruck, W., et al. (2001). Effects of oncostatin M on human cerebral endothelial cells and expression in inflammatory brain lesions. *J Neuropathol Exp Neurol*, *60*, 1087.

Sabri, F., Titanji, K., De Milito, A., & Chiodi, F. (2003). Astrocyte activation and apoptosis: Their roles in the neuropathology of HIV infection. *Brain Pathol*, *13*, 84.

Santo, E., Alonzi, T., Fattori, E., Poli, V., Ciliberto, G., Sironi, M., et al. (1996). Overexpression of interleukin-6 in the central nervous system of transgenic mice increases central but not systemic proinflammatory cytokine production. *Brain Res*, *740*, 239.

Santo, E., Alonzi, T., Poli, V., Fattori, E., Toniatti, C., Sironi, M., et al. (1997). Differential effects of IL-6 on systemic and central production of TNF: A study with IL-6-deficient mice. *Cytokine*, *9*, 300.

Shuai, K. (2006). Regulation of cytokine signaling pathways by PIAS proteins. Cell Res, 16, 196.

Shuai, K. & Liu, B. (2003). Regulation of JAK-STAT signalling in the immune system. *Nat Rev Immunol*, *3*, 900.

Sodhi, A., Shishodia, S., & Shrivastava, A. (1997). Cisplatin-stimulated murine bone marrow-derived macrophages secrete oncostatin M. Immunol, *Cell Biol*, *75*, 492.

Speth, C., Dierich, M. P., & Sopper, S. (2005). HIV-infection of the central nervous system: The tightrope walk of innate immunity. *Mol Immunol*, *42*, 213.

Stankoff, B., Aigrot, M-S., Noël, F., Wattilliaux, A., Zalc, B., & Lubetzki, C. (2002). Ciliary neurotrophic factor (CNTF) enhances myelin formation: A novel role for CNTF and CNTF-related molecules. *J Neurosci*, *22*, 9221.

Stark, J. L., Lyons, J. A., & Cross, A. H. (2004). Interferon-γ produced by encephalitogenic cells induces suppressors of cytokine signaling in primary murine astrocytes. *J Neuroimmunol*, *151*, 195.

Steinman, L. (2010). Mixed results with modulation of TH-17 cells in human autoimmune diseases. *Nat Immunol*, *11*, 41.

Sui, Y., Potula, R., Dhillon, N., Pinson, D., Li, S., Nath, A., et al. (2004). Neuronal apoptosis is mediated by CXCL10 overexpression in simian human immunodeficiency virus encephalitis. *Am J Pathol*, *164*, 1557.

Takata, F., Sumi, N., Nishioku, T., Harada, E., Wakigawa, T., Shuto, H., et al. (2008). Oncostatin M induces functional and structural impairment of blood-brain barriers comprised of rat brain capillary endothelial cells. *Neurosci Lett*, *441*, 163.

Tanaka, M., Hara, T., Copeland, N. G., Gilbert, D. J., Jenkins, N. A., & Miyajima, A. (1999). Reconstitution of the functional mouse oncostain M (OSM) receptor: Molecular cloning of the mouse OSM receptor b subunit. *Blood*, *93*, 804.

Tanaka, M., Hirabayashi, Y., Sekiguchi, T., Inoue, T., Katsuki, M., & Miyajima, A. (2003). Targeted disruption of Oncostatin M receptor results in altered hematopoiesis. *Blood*, *102*, 3154.

Thompson, K. A., McArthur, J. C., & Wesselingh, S. L. (2001). Correlation between neurological progression and astrocyte apoptosis in HIV-associated dementia. *Ann Neurol*, *49*, 745.

Tzartos, J. S., Friese, M. A., Craner, M. J., Palace, J., Newcombe, J., Esiri, M. M., et al. (2008). Interleukin-17 production in central nervous system-infiltrating T cells and glial cells is associated with active disease in multiple sclerosis. *Am J Pathol*, *172*, 146.

Van Wagoner, N. J. & Benveniste, E. N. (1999). Interleukin-6 expression and regulation in astrocytes. *J Neuroimmunol*, *100*, 124.

Van Wagoner, N., Oh, J. W., Repovic, P., & Benveniste, E. N. (1999). IL-6 production by astrocytes: Autocrine regulation by IL-6 and the soluble IL-6 receptor. *J Neurosci*, *19*, 5236.

Vecchiet, J., Dalessandro, M., Falasca, K., Di Iorio, A., Travasi, F., Zingariello, P., et al. (2003). Increased production of oncostatin-M by lymphomononuclear cells from HIV-1-infected patients with neuroAIDS. *J Acquir Immune Defic Syndr*, *32*, 464.

Waiboci, L. W., Ahmed, C. M., Mujtaba, M. G., Flowers, L. O., Martin, J. P., Haider, M. I., et al. (2007). Both the suppressor of cytokine signaling 1 (SOCS-1) kinase inhibitory region and SOCS-1 mimetic bind to JAK2 autophosphorylation site: Implications for the development of a SOCS-1 antagonist. *J Immunol*, *178*, 5058.

Wallace, P. M., MacMaster, J. F., Rouleau, K. A., Brown, T. J., Loy, J. K., Donaldson, K. L., et al. (1999). Regulation of inflammatory responses by oncostatin M. *J Immunol*, *162*, 5547.

Wang, T., Gong, N., Liu, J., Kadiu, I., Kraft-Terry, S. D., Mosley, R. L., et al. (2008). Proteomic modeling for HIV-1 infected microglia-astrocyte crosstalk. *PLoS ONE*, *3*, e2507.

Weaver, C. T., Harrington, L. E., Mangan, P. R., Gavrieli, M., & Murphy, K. M. (2006). Th 17: An effector CD4 T cell lineage with regulatory T cell ties. *Immunity*, *24*, 677.

Weiss, T. W., Samson, A. L., Niego, B., Daniel, P. B., & Medcalf, R. L. (2006). Oncostatin M is a neuroprotective cytokine that inhibits excitotoxic injury in vitro and in vivo. *FASEB J*, *20*, 2369.

Wen, Z. & Darnell, J. E., Jr. (1997). Mapping of Stat3 serine phosphorylation to a single residue (727) and evidence that serine phosphorylation has no influence on DNA binding of Stat1 and Stat3. *Nucleic Acids Res*, *25*, 2062.

Wesselingh, S. L., Power, C., Glass, J., Tyor, W. R., McArthur, J. C., Farber, J. M., et al. (1993). Intracerebral cytokine mRNA expression in AIDS dementia. Ann Neurol, 33, 576.

Weston, C. R. & Davis, R. J. (2002). The JNK signal transduction pathway. *Curr Opin Genet Dev*, *12*.

Wilkinson, J., Radkowski, M., & Laskus, T. (2009). Hepatitis C virus neuroinvasion: identification of infected cells. *J Virol*, *83*, 1312.

Wilt, S. G., Milward, E., Zhou, J. M., Nagasato, K., Patton, H., Rusten, R., et al. (1995). In vitro evidence for a dual role of tumor necrosis factor-a in human immunodeficiency virus type 1 encephalopathy. *Ann Neurol*, *37*, 381.

Wolburg, H. & Risau, W. (1995). Formation of the blood-brain barrier. In B. R. Ransom & H. Kettenmann, (Eds.). *Neuroglia*, p. 763. New York: Oxford University Press.

Yanagisawa, M., Nakashima, K., & Taga, T. (1999). STAT3-mediated astrocyte differentiation from mouse fetal neuroepithelial cells by mouse oncostatin M., *Neurosci Lett 269*, 169.

Yanagisawa, M., Nakashima, K., Takizawa, T., Ochiai, W., Arakawa, H., & Taga, T. (2001). Signaling crosstalk underlying synergistic induction of astrocyte differentiation by BMPs and IL-6 family of cytokines. *FEBS Lett*, *489*, 139.

Yoshimura, A., Naka, T., & Kubo, M. (2007). SOCS proteins, cytokine signalling and immune regulation. *Nat Rev Immunol*, *7*, 454.

Zarling, J. M., Shoyab, M., Marquardt, H., Hanson, M. B., Lioubin, M. N., & Todaro, G. J. (1986). Oncostatin M: A growth regulator produced by differentiated histiocytic lymphoma cells. *Proc Natl Acad Sci USA*, *83*, 9739.

2.4

ADAPTIVE IMMUNITY

Jessica A. L. Hutter-Saunders, Larisa Y. Poluektova, Subhash Dhawan, and Howard E. Gendelman

Innate and adaptive immune responses against human immunodeficiency virus type one (HIV-1) infection parallel those seen against misfolded, aggregated, and nitrated proteins during neurodegenerative diseases. These include, but are not limited to, amyloid beta and alpha synuclein for Alzheimer's and Parkinson's diseases, respectively. The altered protein structures engage microglial activities and lead to robust and specific adaptive immune responses that affect the tempo and progression of neurodegenerative processes. Similar responses are also operative in neuroAIDS where the target is HIV-1. This chapter serves to discuss then dissect how microbes and aberrant proteins similarly serve as immune triggers for nervous system diseases. To this end, we first introduce the reader to the workings of the adaptive immune system, discuss the host's responses to infection, and describe how the host response affects neurologic diseases. We then explore how the adaptive immune response can lead to progressive neurodegeneration and ultimately be harnessed for neural repair.

OVERVIEW OF THE IMMUNE SYSTEM

INNATE AND ADAPTIVE IMMUNITY

A host's immune response consists of the innate and the adaptive immune systems. The innate immune system is present before birth, and its mechanisms of host protection are well conserved and lack immunological memory. It is considered a host's first line of defense and consists of physical barriers such as skin, and chemicals such as lysozyme; it functions to clear pathogens and debris though phagocytosis mediated by mononuclear phagocytes and neutrophils. The innate immune system also recruits cells of the adaptive immune system by establishing chemokine gradients and activates these cells by providing the "second signal" during antigen presentation. In contrast, the adaptive immune system develops with the host's postnatal exposure to non-self antigens and has the capacity to recognize billions of epitopes, recall them, and respond quickly and with force during re-exposures. While differences in innate and adaptive immunity allow for convenient categorization of cell types and immune responses, in real-time the two systems work in concert to protect the host, and loss of either system proves detrimental (reviewed in detail in Janeway et al., 2001).

Upon encounter of a non-self antigen by the innate immune system, antigen-presenting cells (APC) process and then present specific peptides in the context of major histocompatibility complex (MHC) to T cells. When T cells recognize foreign peptides presented by the APC as non-self and are given the appropriate co-stimulatory signals (CD86/B7 - CD28), T cells are activated (Linsley et al., 1990). These activated T cells proliferate and secrete cytokines and chemokines to attract more lymphocytes to the site of insult or injury. Before discussing the role of the adaptive immune system in HIV-1 and neurodegenerative diseases, we will first introduce the adaptive immune response, the major players of the adaptive immune system, and their general functions and interactions with other cells of both the innate and adaptive immune systems.

ADAPTIVE IMMUNE COMPOSITION AND FUNCTION

B Lymphocytes

B cells are so named because they were first discovered in the bursa of Frabricius of the chicken, where B cells mature (Cooper et al., 1984). In mammals, bone marrow is the site of hematopoiesis, and development of B cells occurs in the bone marrow, spleen, and fetal liver. Like macrophages and dendritic cells of the innate immune system, B cells are APCs, which phagosytose, process, and present antigen in the context of MHC II to T cells, thereby activating the T cells. However, unlike the innate immune system's APCs, B cells are also capable of manufacturing antibodies. Upon activation, B cells undergo class switching, clonal expansion, and differentiation into plasma B cells, which produce antigen-specific antibodies. Antibodies may be membrane-bound or secreted; they clear pathogens and debris by binding to them, increasing opsonization, activation of complement, and preventing adherence of bacteria. Most antigens do not produce a strong enough signal to activate the B cell alone; mature T helper type 2 (Th2) cells are needed to co-stimulate B cells by the secretion of cytokines and by interaction between CD40 and CD40L cell surface molecules. This is called T cell-dependent activation (Andersson et al., 1980). However, there are some antigens that are capable of inducing T cell-independent activation of B cells. This occurs without co-stimulation when cross-linking of their membrane-bound immunoglobulin M (mIgM) occurs (Maino et al., 1975). In both instances, activated B cells undergo class switching and proliferate in secondary lymphoid tissues and terminally differentiate into plasma cells.

T Lymphocytes

Like B cells, T cells develop in the bone marrow from a common lymphoid progenitor, but T cells leave the bone marrow and migrate to the thymus, from which T cells derive their name. In the thymus, T cell precursors undergo positive and negative selection to select T cells that recognize self-MHC and eliminate auto-reactive T cells. Most T cells undergo apoptosis during this process, and only about 2–4% of thymocytes leave the thymus as mature T cells (Janeway et al., 2001; Joel et al., 1977). Mature T cells leaving the thymus can be categorized into two major classes based on surface expression of the co-receptors CD4 and CD8.

CD4-positive T cells are MHC class II restricted, meaning they only recognize antigen presented by an APC in the context of MHC II (Shevach & Rosenthal, 1973; Katz et al., 1973). MHC II molecules present peptides from pathogens that have been phagocytosed and processed in the endocytic pathway. If the peptide is recognized by the CD4 T cell as non-self, an adaptive immune response ensues; the CD4 T cell responds by making interleukin 2 (IL-2) among other cytokines, facilitating their differentiation, and proliferative capacity. CD4-positive T cells can differentiate into T helper 1 (Th1), T helper 2 (Th2), T helper 17 (Th17), or regulatory T cells (Treg) (Janeway & Medzhitov, 1998). The type of adaptive immune response that follows activation depends on the microenvironment (cytokines) and the nature of the MHC:peptide complex, and it can play an important role in the outcome of disease. Differentiation into Th1 type leads to cell-mediated immunity (activation of macrophages), while the Th2 type leads to humoral immunity (activation of B cells). According to the Th1/Th2 paradigm, Th1 cells, which produce IL-2, interferon gamma (IFN-γ), and tumor necrosis factor (TNF-α are pro-inflammatory and induce neurotoxic microglial release of reactive oxygen species (ROS) and nitric oxide (NO), while Th2 cells that produce IL-4, IL-5, and IL-13 are more anti-inflammatory and enhance microglial-mediated neuroprotective activities (Weiner, 2008).

CD8-positive T cells, often called cytotoxic T lymphocytes (CTL), are MHC class I restricted (Zinkernagel & Doherty, 1974, 1979). MHC I molecules are expressed on all nucleated cells and present peptides from intracellular pathogens such as viruses and some bacteria to CD8+ T cells. The CD8+ CTL will be activated if it recognizes the peptide presented by MHC I as non-self and will then kill the infected cell via cytolysis (release of perforin and granzyme) or by inducing apoptosis (Fas/FasL engagement) (Ju et al., 1994).

Natural Killer (NK) Cells

Due to their lack of antigen-specific receptors, NK cells are traditionally considered cells of the innate immune system. However, NK cells have many functions similar to those of lymphocytes of the adaptive immune system, and they are from the same common lymphoid progenitor as T and B cells and thus are often considered to be the third major lymphocyte population (Yokoyama, 1999). While NK cells do not have the same immunological specificity and memory of T cells, they are able to detect the presence or absence of MHC I molecules, which is normally expressed on all nucleated cells (Piontek et al., 1985; Quillet et al., 1988; Franksson et al., 1993; Salcedo et al., 1994). When a cell is virally infected or is a tumor cell, MHC I is downregulated to decrease presentation of viral or tumor antigens to CD8+ T cells. When an NK cell detects the absence of MHC I, it is activated and kills the cell using the same cytotoxic mechanism as CTLs (perforin and granzyme release) (Lowin et al., 1994). Granules in the cytoplasm of activated NK cells contain perforin and granzyme. When NK cells come in contact with an infected cell, the granules fuse with the NK cell's membrane, and its contents are released in the direction of the cell to be killed. Perforin creates a hole in the membrane of the cell, and the granzyme then enters the cell and induces apoptosis.

NEUROIMMUNITY

THE CENTRAL NERVOUS SYSTEM (CNS) AND ADAPTIVE IMMUNITY

It was once thought that the CNS was an immune privileged site, in which immune cells of the periphery could not enter or rarely entered and thus the two systems had little to no interaction. This hypothesis was supported by the early observation that tissue grafts in the eye or brain survived longer than grafts in other areas of the body (Medawar, 1948). However, today, evidence for the interaction of the adaptive immune system and the CNS is well recognized. The CNS is capable of influencing the response of the immune system to pathogens in the periphery though the neuroendocrine system, and the immune system is not only charged with protecting the CNS from pathogens and injury but is also capable of affecting the functions and homeostasis of the resident CNS cells, for better or worse. Furthermore, researchers are beginning to harness the neurotrophic effects of the immune system to aid in repair and regeneration in the CNS. William Hickey once wrote, "vertebrates possess two bodily systems capable of learning and remembering: the nervous system and the immune system" (Hickey, 2001; Weiner, 2008). Here, we will discuss the interactions of these two remarkable systems with focus on HIV-1, Alzheimer's disease (AD), and Parkinson's disease (PD).

It is now known that even under normal conditions, activated T and B lymphocytes patrol the CNS in low numbers while naïve lymphocytes are excluded (Engelhardt &

Ransohoff, 2005; Hickey, 1999; Togo et al., 2002), and fewer activated T cells infiltrate the normal CNS than other tissues (Yeager et al., 2000). This may be due to the low level of adhesion molecules expressed on CNS endothelial cells under normal conditions (Hickey, 2001). When cytokines such as IL-1 and TNF-α are secreted by activated glia in the brain, permeability of the blood-brain barrier (BBB) is increased and the expression of cellular adhesion molecules (such as E-selectin) on microvascular endothelial cells is upregulated (Wong et al., 1999). Activated T cells and B cells are then able to extravasate and migrate to the site of neuronal injury in increased numbers (Olson & Miller, 2004; Aloisi et al., 1999; McGeer & McGeer, 2003). Indeed, abnormalities in the BBB have been found, and T cell infiltration occurs, in several neurodegenerative diseases, such as HIV-1 (Petito & Cash, 1992; Petito et al., 2003), AD (Desai et al., 2007; Rogers et al., 1988; Togo et al., 2002), and PD (Farkas et al., 2000). Furthermore, while the CNS lacks a defined lymphatic system, antigens do exit the CNS and enter the lymph via arachnoid villi, cranial nerves, and spinal nerve root ganglia (Cserr & Knopf, 1992). Once in the lymph, these antigens may be taken up by dendritic cells and presented to T and B cells to mobilize an adaptive immune response to the CNS. While acute neuroinflammation is beneficial to regaining homeostasis and normal function of the CNS after injury or infection, chronic inflammation is damaging to the CNS and may contribute to the neurodegeneration seen in HIV-1, AD, and PD.

HIV-1 INFECTION OF THE BRAIN

HIV-1 infection of the brain underlies the development of HIV-1-associated neurological disorders (Nottet & Gendelman, 1995; Kraft-Terry, Stothert, Buch, & Gendelman, 2010). Infection of CNS occurs shortly after peripheral infection (Maslin, Kedzierska, Webster, Muller, & Crowe, 2005). The selective localization of HIV-1 into brain mononuclear phagocytes (blood borne macrophages and microglia) requires penetration of infected cells across the BBB, which normally restricts the free diffusion of circulating molecules and cells into brain interstitial spaces. The BBB consists of epithelial-like, high-resistance tight junctions that fuse brain capillary endothelia together into a continuous cellular layer that separates blood and cerebrospinal fluid from brain interstitial space (Sharpless et al., 1992). The tight junctions of the BBB, although impermeable to systemically produced neurotransmitters, efficiently regulate the movement of ions from blood to brain for optimal function of the CNS. Thus, to enter the brain from the periphery, HIV-1 must travel either as cell-free virus between endothelial cells or by infected monocyte-macrophages as they circulate through the brain (reviewed in Kraft-Terry et al., 2010).

Although HIV-1 could infect brain microvascular endothelial cells, which would subsequently release virus to brain macrophages, there is no evidence for such infection or mode of viral spread (Sharpless et al., 1992; Dhawan et al., 1995). Indeed, HIV-1 selectively infects and replicates within brain perivascular and parenchymal blood-derived macrophages and microglia (Glass, Fedor, Wesselingh, & McArthur, 1995; Ghorpade et al., 1998). These findings support productive HIV-1 replication in the CNS and further suggest that HIV-1 gains entry into the brain via infected macrophages. Transport of virus into the CNS is a complex process and requires diapedesis of HIV-1-infected monocytes across the BBB, a process that begins with the adhesion of monocytes to the vascular endothelium (Maslin et al., 2005). Adhesion of monocytes is mediated by interactions between specific adhesive receptors, expressed on the monocyte surface, and counter-receptors expressed on endothelial cells. HIV-1 infection upregulates the expression of adhesion molecules on monocytes (Lafrenie et al., 1996), thereby promoting the extravasation of HIV-1-infected monocytes into brain parenchyma. After penetrating the BBB, although HIV-1 does not directly infect neurons, it activates the surrounding cells and releases soluble factors that affect the function of neurons.

HIV-1-induced alterations in macrophage function might underlie early viral entry into the CNS during the acute phase of HIV-1 infection and explain how HIV-1-infected macrophages can serve as viral reservoirs inside tissue compartments. Indeed, it is known that viral replication is inhibited by IFN-β early in disease (Kornbluth, Oh, Munis, Cleveland, & Richman, 1990), which may allow HIV-1 to evade adaptive immune surveillance in the brain, and may explain why neurological symptoms do not occur until later in disease (McArthur, Brew, & Nath, 2005). However, it was recently shown that an inhibitor of IFN-β signaling, suppressor of cytokine signaling (SOCS)3, is elevated during recurrence of viral replication in the SIV/macaque model of HIV encephalitis (HIV-e)-related dementia, and this may decrease the response of the innate immune system to HIV-1 replication and allow progression toward HIV-1-associated dementia (HAD) (Akhtar et al., 2010).

ADAPTIVE IMMUNITY AND NEUROAIDS

HIV-1 infection in the CNS is not classically characterized as "neurodegenerative." Etymologically, this word is composed of the prefix "neuro-," which designates neurons, and "degeneration," which refers to the process of losing structure or function (reviewed in Przedborski et al., 2003). While direct neurotoxicity by HIV-1-related viral proteins is a cause of neuronal dysfunction and loss of structural neuronal elements, this toxicity is not the sole pathogenic mode for neuronal loss, just as it is not the sole pathogenic mode in simian immunodeficiency virus (SIV) infection or HIV (reviewed in Kraft-Terry et al., 2009; Abel, 2009; Jones & Power, 2006; Anderson et al., 2002). The causes of CNS functional and structural changes are more precisely related to the increase in BBB permeability, which allows HIV-1 virus, carried by cells of the mononuclear phagocyte (MP) lineage, to enter the brain and contact neurons; viral products also contribute to neuronal loss.

The peripheral immune cells, which pass through the BBB and migrate through the brain parenchyma (white matter tracts) or become entrapped in perivascular spaces, can activate microglial cells, and activated microglia can persistently contribute to the loss of neuronal function, with or without productive HIV-1-infection. Microglial cells are the major sensor of the neuronal microenvironment and respond to neuronal dysfunction by multiple mechanisms. Activation of microglial cells by CNS-infiltrating activated immune cells has been observed in many types of neurodegenerative disorders. The ability of activated lymphocytes—primarily functionally mature CD4 T helper 1 (Th1) T cells and CD8+ cytotoxic lymphocytes, NK (Sadagopal et al., 2008; Bissel et al., 2008; Mankowski et al., 2002; Shieh et al., 2001), and to a lesser extent in HIV-1/SIV brain infection, NK T cells, and γδ T cells—to prime microglial cells via IFN-γ is part of the cascade of cytokines and events associated with the adaptive immune response.

IFN-γ is particularly effective as an inducer of MHC class II proteins by microglia, which are essential to elicit an adaptive immune response (Aloisi et al., 1999). Activated microglia can stimulate naïve T cells though cell-cell interaction and by IL-23 secretion (Louis et al.); they can elicit differentiation into Th17 (IL17, IL-21, and IFN-γ-producing cells), which contribute to inflammation in the brain (Gottfried-Blackmore et al., 2009; Goverman, 2009); and they play a significant role in protecting the host from opportunistic bacterial infections (Jin et al., 2004; Riol-Blanco et al., 2010; Khader et al., 2005; Meeks et al., 2009; Martin et al., 2009; Dietlin et al., 2009; Desvignes & Ernst, 2009). The profound decline in gut-associated CD4+ IL-17 producing cells (Th17 cells) in HIV-1/SIV infection, and the increased susceptibility to peripheral opportunistic infections, may not correlate with the amount of brain tissue-affiliated Th17 cells (Prendergast et al.). The decline of protective HIV-1-specific CD4+ cells due to HIV-1 infection may be associated with increased migration and local CNS expansion of antiviral/antibacterial T cells, which produce IL-17 and IFN-γ in response to damage signals, and destroy infected cells by MHC-independent mechanisms (Fenoglio et al., 2009). The presence and dynamics of these cell populations (NK T cells and T cells) in the brain during HIV-1/SIV infection has not been vigorously investigated. Moreover, in the brain, the balance between effector and regulatory CD4+ cells, which are susceptible to HIV-1 infection and could contribute to the brain inflammatory responses (Nistala & Wedderburn, 2009), is unknown.

In the majority of natural and experimental HIV-1 infection cases, except highly pathogenic SIV infection, adaptive immunity contributes significantly, and for prolonged periods, to the control of HIV/SIV replication in the brain. However, the adaptive immune response is not sufficient to eradicate HIV-1 infection in the CNS, and there are still no strong correlates for protection or evidence that such protection is possible (Pantaleo & Koup, 2004).

The productive infection of brain macrophages/microglia attracts effector immune cells from the periphery and generates a second wave of local expansion of HIV-1-specific T and B cells, which represent the adaptive immune response related to antiviral defense. Unfortunately, this second wave

of the adaptive immune response brings cells susceptible to HIV-1 into the brain, which significantly accelerates HIV-1 replication, and leads to development of HIV-1 encephalitis. Often, this cascade coincides with secondary opportunistic infections.

Evidence of the increase in activated immune cells and virus-specific antibodies in the CNS has been collected from the time that HIV-1 infection was discovered in the brain (Elovaara & Muller, 1993; Michaels et al., 1988; Ljunggren et al., 1989; Lucey et al., 1993; An & Scaravilli, 1997; Sadagopal et al., 2008; Spudich et al., 2005), and development of experimental SIV models has also increased the knowledge of HIV-1 CNS infection (Smith et al., 1994; Sopper et al., 1998; Marcondes et al., 2001; Mankowski et al., 2002; Dean et al., 1993).

The broad spectrum of cytokines, chemokines, oxidative stress-related enzymes, and their byproducts have been attributed to neurologic dysfunction during chronic HIV-1/SIV infection (Orandle et al., 2002; Burudi et al., 2002; Kaul & Lipton, 2006; Brabers & Nottet, 2006; Yadav & Collman, 2009; Tran & Miller, 2005; Li et al., 2005b; Navia & Rostasy, 2005; Konsman et al., 2007). In relation to adaptive immune responses, associated regulatory intracellular signaling pathways are most interesting. How are the processes of synaptic stability, repulsion, and attraction, which represent basic mechanisms for memory formation and cognition, connected with adaptive immunity and IFN-γ? Receptors for IFN-γ are present on all types of cells, including neurons (Yang et al., 2006; Rose et al., 2007). Adaptive immune responses are based on cellular processing, expression, and recognition of viral, bacterial, and self-modified proteins. The two main systems involved in the cellular mechanisms of processing and presentation of antigens in immune and target-infected cells are the proteasomal (Tanaka & Kasahara, 1998; Liu, 2004) and lysosomal systems (Schmidt et al., 2005; Gannage & Munz, 2009; Munz, 2009). The same intracellular compartments (proteasome and lysosome) are the basic structures for the control of synaptic plasticity and neurodegeneration (McNaught et al., 2010; Kim et al., 2008; Korolchuk et al., 2008; Korolchuk et al., 2010; Garcia-Arencibia et al., 2010; Whatley et al., 2008; Staal et al., 2009).

IFN-γ function is related to stimulation of both the proteasomal and the lysosomal protein degradation pathways. In immune (antigen-presenting dendritic cells) and nonimmune cell types, stimulation with IFN-γ has two features. First, it induces the expression of three new proteasome β subunits that are preferentially incorporated into new proteasomes ("immunoproteasomes") and alter their pattern of peptidase activities to enhance the yield of peptides for presentation in MHC class I context (Bauer et al., 1998; York et al., 1999; Rock & Goldberg, 1999; Sigal et al., 1999). Second, IFN-γ downregulates the expression of a metalloproteinase, thimet oligopeptidase and others that actively destroy many antigenic and non-antigenic self-recycling proteins and peptides (Ma et al., 2001; Ho et al., 2008). Thus, IFN-γ appears to increase the supply of peptides by stimulating their generation and decreasing their destruction. In the case of β-amyloid processing in neurons and astrocytes, stimulation with IFN-γ leads to plaque formation and memory decline in transgenic IFN-γ receptor knockout mice (Yamamoto et al., 2007; Xu & Ikezu, 2009) by changing the activity of membrane-associated protease BACE1 (Cho et al., 2007). A variety of other intracellular protein-processing enzymes involved in synaptic plasticity also could be affected (Ferri et al., 2008; Lin et al., 2005).

The accumulation of abnormal proteins (Kim et al., 2008; An et al., 1997; Giometto et al., 1997) and persistent changes in protein-processing machinery in synaptic terminals could be associated with IFN-γ-related adaptive immunity. The appearance of immuno-proteasomes instead of proteasomes in synaptic regions, as a result of inflammatory responses, correlates with the degree of neurocognitive disturbances in HIV-1-infected patients (Gelman & Nguyen, 2010; Nguyen et al., 2010; Aprea et al., 2006). The decrease of postsynaptic dopamine receptor type 2 (D(2)R) with preferential loss of the alternatively spliced long isoform of D(2)R relative to the short isoform with decline of neurocognitive performance was documented for HIV-1-infected patients (Gelman et al., 2006; Chang et al., 2008).

IFN-γ is the major player in MHC class II-related protein-processing machinery that is associated with the lysosomal processing of modified cellular "self" proteins, viral and bacterial proteins, and apoptotic and necrotic cellular debris (Li et al., 2005a). There is a significant overlap between immune cell MHC II-associated mechanisms of protein processing and non-immune cell machinery, even with the neuronal cells that do not express MHC II molecules on the surface (Kennedy & Gairns, 1992; Wong et al., 1984; Caplazi & Ehrensperger, 1998).

It has been shown that fasting stimulates a mild cellular stress and provides protection against different types of damage to neurons via stimulation of IFN-γ expression (Lee et al., 2006). It is well known that fasting is a powerful inducer of autophagy and is protective in neurodegeneration (Rami, 2009; Munz, 2009). IFN-γ-stimulated autophagy is a powerful mechanism for killing intracellular pathogens (Zhao et al., 2008; Huang et al., 2009; Halonen, 2009; Al-Zeer et al., 2009). The signaling and response proteins involved in neuronal autophagy and antibacterial protection may have significant overlap, and it is reasonable to investigate this in HIV-1/SIV-associated neurocognitive complications. Decreased neuronal autophagy by infected microglial cells has also been found in HIV-1/SIV infections, and this finding supports the idea that there is a tight link between neuronal function and adaptive immunity (Alirezaei et al., 2008).

The complex mechanisms of anti-HIV-1 protection in the brain are associated with immune activation. Such activation leads to a prolonged period of suppressed viral replication in the brain. However, such suppression might cause structural and functional changes associated with IFN-γ signaling pathways. Even the pattern of immune activation is affected by the host immune response or by antiretroviral treatment. Nonetheless, viral replication continues to persist despite such strong control (Abdulle et al., 2005; Yilmaz et al., 2006; Price & Spudich, 2008; Hagberg et al., 1992). During the later stages of disease, the re-activation of viral

replication and the elimination of local protective mechanisms will lead not only to the appearance of opportunistic infections, but to cognitive decline, known as HIV-1-associated neurocognitive disorder (Kraft-Terry et al., 2009).

NEURODEGENERATIVE DISORDERS AND ADAPTIVE IMMUNITY

ALZHEIMER'S DISEASE

Alzheimer's disease (AD) is the most common neurodegenerative disorder. One in ten persons over the age of 65 and nearly half of those over the age of 85 are affected with AD, and there is no cure (Evans et al., 1989; von Strauss et al., 1999; Hall & Yao, 2005). The highest incidence of sporadic AD is in people over the age of 65, and with the American population living longer, the U.S. Census Bureau predicts that AD will affect over 14 million Americans by 2050. AD patients become increasingly difficult to care for due to losses in cognitive function caused by disease progression in the hippocampus and neocortex. AD patients begin to show shortened attention spans and lose short-term memory function, language skills, visual-spatial orientation, abstract thinking ability, and judgment (Katzman, 1976).

The two pathological hallmarks of AD are extracellular amyloid plaques and intracellular neurofibrillary tangles, which are accompanied by a diffuse loss of neurons (Gorevic et al., 1986). Amyloid plaques are composed of the amyloid β (Aβ) peptide (Glenner, Wong, Quaranta, & Eanes, 1984; Masters et al., 1985a; Joachim, Duffy, Morris, & Selkoe, 1988), which is a product of the amyloid precursor protein (APP), a normal transmembrane glycoprotein (Selkoe, 2001; Sisodia, 2002). When APP is successively cleaved by β/γ-secretases, the Aβ peptide that is formed is between 40 and 42 amino acids long, with the most common form in diseased brains being 42 amino acids long (Aβ42) (reviewed in Selkoe, 1998). Accumulation of Aβ peptides in AD is thought to be caused in part by the overproduction of APP and impaired clearance of Aβ peptides (Hardy & Higgins, 1992). APP is normally produced at low levels, but in AD, activated microglia secrete pro-inflammatory cytokines that cause neurons to increase the synthesis of APP, which is secreted and processed into Aβ peptides by secretases (Goldgaber et al., 1989). The Aβ peptides aggregate to form the fibrils found in senile plaques, and activated microglia are associated with these plaques (Crystal et al., 1988). In fact, Aβ has been shown to activate microglia and complement, perpetuating the inflammatory process (Dickson et al., 1993a). These observations led to the amyloid cascade theory, which posits that the accumulation of Aβ protein activates microglia and may initiate the inflammatory disease process (Hardy & Higgins, 1992; Meda et al., 1995; Meda et al., 2001).

Neurofibrillary tangles (NFTs) are composed of the microtubule-associated protein tau, which normally functions to promote and stabilize microtubule polymerization. Since senile plaques are seen before the formation of neurofibrillary tangles, it has been hypothesized that the accumulation of senile plaques in the extracellular milieu initiates an inflammatory cascade that perpetuates the disease and leads to the accumulation of neurofibrillary tangles through a mechanism involving cytokine and chemokine secretion by activated microglia (Hardy & Selkoe, 2002; Hinkin et al., 2002; Hardy, 2006). In aged patients, it is thought that abnormal kinase and phosphatase activities cause the normal intracellular tau protein to become abnormally hyper-phosphorylated at serine and threonine residues (Masters et al., 1985b). These phosphorylations allow the tau protein to form paired helical filaments (PHFs), which then aggregate to form NFTs inside neuron somas and dendrites. Aggregation of the PHFs is accelerated by inflammation, oxidative stress, and some genetic factors such as ApoE E4 expression (Bales et al., 1997; Bales et al., 1999). The aggregated tau proteins lose their normal function, causing microtubule dysfunction that leads to neuronal synaptic dysfunction and eventually to neuronal cell death and the cognitive and memory impairments seen in AD patients.

The innate immune response in the AD brain has been well studied, but the adaptive immune response is less well characterized. While microglia have both neurotrophic and neurotoxic roles, it is hypothesized that the damaging neurotoxic effects of the activated microglia eventually predominate over the neurotrophic effects (Rock et al., 2004). Activated microglia are associated with amyloid plaques (Dickson et al., 1988; Mattiace et al., 1990). Early in disease, microglia phagocytose Aβ protein, but cytokines secreted by activated microglia increase production of ROS and APP in nearby neurons, which ultimately leads to increased accumulation and decreased clearance of Aβ (Goldgaber et al., 1989).

As mentioned above, microglial cells secrete both anti- and pro-inflammatory cytokines; T cells also secret many of these molecules. Altered levels of cytokines and chemokines have been found in the brains, cerebral spinal fluid (CSF), and peripheral blood of AD patients. AD brains have elevated levels of cytokines such as TGF-β, IL-1α/β, IL-6, IL-10, IL-12, IL-23, and TNF-α many chemokines such as RANTES/CCL5, MCP-1/CCL2, and IP-10/CXCL10; proteolytic enzymes; matrix metalloproteinases; complement factors; growth factors; and glutamate and chemokines that are secreted by activated microglia (Moore & Thanos, 1996; Griffin et al., 1989; Dickson et al., 1993b; Qiu et al., 1997). Together, these molecules increase permeability of the BBB and increase homing, extravasation, and activation of lymphocytes, as well as increasing the transport of Aβ from the CNS to the periphery.

Most notably of the anti-inflammatory cytokines, TGF-β has been shown to contribute to the anti-inflammatory response during brain injury (Finch et al., 1993), and increased immunoreactivity of TGF-β 1, 2, and 3 have been found in the brains of AD patients (Flanders et al., 1995; Peress & Perrilo, 1995), as well as in the CSF and serum of AD patients before and after death (Chao et al., 1994). These studies suggest that TGF-β levels may represent a protective host response to neuronal damage (Chao et al., 1994). However, TGF-β released from the AD brain microvasculature may actually contribute to inflammation by increasing expression of IL-1β and TNF-α by brain endothelial cells (Grammas & Ovase, 2001).

Cytokine and chemokine levels in the CSF and peripheral blood are also altered in AD patients. Increased levels of IL-1β and IL-6, (Cacabelos et al., 1991; Blum-Degen et al., 1995a), which increase fas (Apo-1) levels (Martinez et al., 2000), have been found in the CFS of AD patients. However, soluble IL-6 receptor (sIL-6R), a potent enhancer of IL-6, has been shown to be decreased in AD CSF, suggesting either lower biological efficacy of IL-6 or increased accumulation of sIL-6R in the brain, which would increase the biological efficacy of IL-6 in the brain (Hampel et al., 1998). IL-1 and IL-6 are also elevated in the peripheral blood of AD patients (Licastro et al., 2000), and another study found that serum levels of IL-6 correlate with the severity of dementia in Down's syndrome and AD (Kalman et al., 1997).

Numerous studies have observed increased numbers of T cells in AD brains. Increased numbers of CD4+ T cells and CD8+ T cells have been found at sites of gliosis in the AD brain (Itagaki et al., 1988; Fiala et al., 2002). These cells are also increased in peripheral blood (Schindowski et al., 2007), and CSF of AD patients has increased numbers of activated T cells (Robinson Agramonte et al., 2001). Interestingly, one study found that APP peptides could induce proliferation of T cells from normal donors but not AD donors (Trieb et al., 1996). However, T cells from AD donors still elicited increased expression of IL-2 receptor when stimulated with APP peptides, and they were responsive to anti-CD3, suggesting that the lack of a proliferative response to APP peptides was not due to apoptosis but to anergy (Trieb et al., 1996). Auto-reactive T cells induce clearance of Aβ (Monsonego & Weiner, 2003) and in AD patients this response may be deficient. A decrease in Aβ-specific T cells in AD patients could decrease the humoral response to Aβ; without helper T cells, B cells would not produce antibody to Aβ and clearance would be decreased. More recently, adoptive transfer of Aβ-specific T cells was shown to reverse cognitive decline and synaptic loss while increasing Aβ clearance in the brains of APP + PS1 mice (Ethell et al., 2006). The benefits of adoptive transfer of T cells could be due to several mechanisms, including an increase in the humoral B-cell response, suppression of the pro-neurotoxic microglial response, and/or increased production of neurotrophic factors (Ethell et al., 2006).

ADAPTIVE IMMUNITY AND PARKINSON'S DISEASE

Parkinson's disease (PD) is the second most common neurodegenerative disorder, and an estimated 1.5 million Americans currently suffer from this debilitating disease. Like Alzheimer's disease, PD is a neurodegenerative disease characterized by the presence of protein plaques in the brain. PD can be pathologically characterized by the cytoplasmic accumulation of proteinaceous aggregates called Lewy bodies (LB), which are mainly comprised of the α-synuclein (α-syn) protein and ubiquitin (Spillantini et al., 1997; Spillantini et al., 1998). Progressive degeneration of dopaminergic (DAergic) neurons in the substantia nigra pars compacta and their projections into the caudate nucleus lead to a substantial decrease in dopamine levels, which manifest as resting tremor, bradykinesia, rigidity, and gait dysfunction (Hornykiewicz & Kish, 1987; Dauer & Przedborski, 2003; Olanow et al., 2009). While the etiology of PD remains unknown, numerous studies implicate immune system abnormalities and CNS inflammation in the pathobiology of PD (Hisanaga et al., 2001; Mozley et al., 2000; McGeer et al., 1988a; McGeer et al., 1988c, Barker & Cahn, 1988; Fiszer et al., 1994; Pouplard & Emile, 1984; Rentzos et al., 2009).

Inflammation, oxidative stress, and diminished neurotrophic support occur in PD; activated microglia are known to precipitate neurotoxic activities (Mosley et al., 2006). There are approximately three times more glial cells than neurons in the brain, and the concentration of microglia (one of the three types of glial cells) varies by brain region (Lawson et al., 1990). For example, notable for PD, the substantia nigra has a high density of microglia (Kim et al., 2000) and may contribute to the region-specific neurodegeneration seen in PD. In 1988, McGeer and colleagues found human leukocyte antigen (HLA)-DR positive (activated) microglia phagocytosing free neuromelanin in post-mortem PD substantia nigra (McGeer et al., 1988b); others have shown higher HLA-DR expression on CSF monocytes in PD patients (Fiszer et al., 1994). As in HIV-1 and AD, activated microglia and monocytes in PD brains and CFS secrete pro-inflammatory and neurotoxic cytokines and chemokines that disrupt the BBB and attract lymphocytes to the site of neuronal injury. Indeed, levels of IL-1β, IL-6, and TNF-α are elevated in the CFS of PD patients (Blum-Degen et al., 1995b; Gonzalez-Scarano & Baltuch, 1999), and intercellular adhesion molecule-1 (ICAM-1)-positive glia are also increased in the substantia nigra of PD brains (Miklossy et al., 2006). Together, these data support the hypothesis that activation of cells of the innate immune system, such as microglia and monocytes, directly contribute to the pathobiology of PD. Furthermore, it has been shown that these cells are activated by overexpression of α-syn or aberrant forms of TNF-α syn. Aberrant posttranslational modifications of α-syn, such as nitration (N-α-syn) can be found in LB inclusions in PD brains (Giasson et al., 2000) and cause the protein to aggregate more readily (Uversky et al., 2005). Aggregated α-syn activates microglia (Zhang et al., 2005), which have been shown to produce nitric oxide (NO) and superoxide in mice and inducible nitric oxide synthase (iNOS) in humans, all of which nitrate α-syn, perpetuating the pro-inflammatory innate immune response in PD (Gao et al., 2008; Hunot et al., 1996).

While it was shown in 1988 that auto-antibodies against dopamine neuron antigens are present in the CSF of PD patients (McRae-Degueurce et al., 1988), the role of the adaptive immune system in PD has only recently been investigated in depth. Several changes in the adaptive immune response have been found in the peripheral blood of PD patients and in the CNS. Decreased naïve (CD4+CD45RA+) T cells and increased memory (CD4+ CD45RO+) T cells (Fiszer et al., 1994), increased activated CD4+ T cells expressing Fas (Hisanaga et al., 2001) and increased IFN-γ-producing Th1 cells, decreased IL-4-producing Th2 cells, and a decrease in CD4+CD25+ T cells (Baba et al., 2005) have been found in the peripheral blood of PD patients. Also, circulating IL-15,

RANTES, and IL-10 are significantly elevated in PD compared to controls (Rentzos et al., 2007; Rentzos et al., 2009). In the CNS, CD4+ and CD8+ T cells can be found near DAergic neurons in PD patients and in MPTP (1-methyl-4-phenyl-1,2,3,6-tetrahydropyridine) mice (Brochard et al., 2009). One way in which the adaptive immune system could be mobilized to infiltrate the CNS during PD is though the drainage of aberrant forms of α-syn into the lymphatic system where the protein could activate lymphocytes. Indeed, in MPTP-intoxicated mice, α-syn drains to cervical lymph nodes where it activates T cells (Benner et al., 2008). An influx of α-syn-specific lymphocytes into the brain could increase the pro-inflammatory phenotype and neurotoxic response of microglia near DAergic neurons by increasing the concentration of pro-inflammatory molecules within the substantia nigra.

HARNESSING THE ADAPTIVE IMMUNE RESPONSE FOR THERAPEUTIC GAIN

Similarities abound in the adaptive immune system's response to CNS in AD, PD, and HIV-1. Each disease has a substantive inflammatory component that is linked to neuronal impairment and loss leading to neurologic deficits and disease. Thus, therapeutic strategies aimed at modulating the immune response during disease may be applicable to several neurodegenerative diseases. Here, we will discuss recent therapeutic approaches to modulating the adaptive immune system.

REGULATORY T CELLS IN NEUROAIDS AND PARKINSON'S DISEASE

Regulatory T cells (Treg) are an important subset of CD4+ helper T cells that are known to maintain self-tolerance, prevent autoimmunity, and maintain immune homeostasis by attenuating excessive inflammation caused by pathogens or injury (Sakaguchi et al., 1995; Sakaguchi et al., 2003; Sakaguchi, 2004; Kim et al., 2007; Coombes et al., 2005; Bourreau et al., 2009; Cederbom et al., 2000; Kipnis et al., 2002). These cells are identified by the expression of CD4 and CD25 cell surface markers and by the transcription factor forkhead box P3 (FoxP3) in mice (Fontenot et al., 2003; Hall et al.,1990; Hori et al., 2003), and the expression of FoxP3, CD4, CD25, CD39, CD49d 53, and a lack of CD127 in humans (Fletcher et al., 2009; Kleinewietfeld et al., 2009). While naturally occurring Treg mature in the thymus, naïve CD4+-stimulated T cells in the periphery can be polarized into the inducible Treg (iTreg) phenotype under certain conditions. For example, TGF-β, IL-2, IL-10, and all-trans retinoic acid are known to polarize T cells to the iTreg phenotype (Lee et al., 2009; Khattar et al., 2009; Zheng et al., 2008; Zheng et al., 2007), and histone deacetylase inhibitors are known to increase proliferation and suppressor activity of Treg (Johnson et al., 2008; Lucas et al., 2009; Saouaf et al., 2009; Tao et al., 2007). In vitro studies have shown that Treg can suppress effector T cell (Teff) responses via cell-to-cell contact (Cederbom et al., 2000) and soluble factors (Wahl et al., 2004;). Treg can also inhibit the adaptive immune system indirectly by affecting antigen presentation by APCs (Maloy et al., 2003). In the brain, Treg promote neurotrophic support by inducing astrocytes to increase expression of brain-derived neurotrophic factor (BDNF) and glial-cell-derived neurotrophic factor (GDNF) (Reynolds et al., 2007b; Benner et al., 2004) and may promote glutamate clearance (Garg et al., 2008). Dysfunctional and reduced frequencies of Treg are associated with several autoimmune diseases (Costantino et al., 2008), including multiple sclerosis (MS) (Fletcher et al., 2009; Royal, Mia, Li, & Naunton, 2009 ; Koen, 2010 ; Venken et al., 2008a ; Venken et al., 2008b), type I diabetes (Glisic et al., 2009), inflammatory skin disorders (Fujimura et al., 2008), autoimmune myasthenia gravis (Mu et al., 2009), and rheumatoid arthritis (Cao et al., 2003), as well as chronic inflammatory diseases such as systemic lupus erythematosus (Barreto et al., 2009; Horwitz, 2008; Venigalla et al., 2008), asthma (Xue, Zhou, Xiong, Xiong, & Tang, 2007), inflammatory bowel disease (Bourreau et al., 2009), and immune dysregulation polyendocrinopathy enteropathy X-linked (IPEX) syndrome, which is caused by a genetic mutation in the transcription factor FoxP3 (Bennett et al., 2001). Furthermore, Treg are being investigated for therapeutic use in several of these diseases (Putnam et al., 2009; Brusko et al., 2008; Gonzalez-Rey et al., 2006; Haas et al., 2009; Vandenbark et al., 2009) and may be applicable to HIV-1 neurodegeneration, PD, and AD.

Indeed, Treg have been shown to migrate from the periphery to the site of HIV-1-induced neuroinflammation in a mouse model of HIV-1 encephalitis (unpublished observations), and adoptive transfer of Treg in a mouse model of human HIV-1 encephalitis is neuroprotective (Liu et al., 2009). This study showed that adoptively transferred Treg attenuated microgliosis and astrogliosis, increased expression of BDNF and GDNF, downregulated expression of proinflammatory cytokines, and decreased oxidative stress and viral replication, while effector CD4+ T cells sped histopathological manifestations for disease (Liu et al., 2009). Another recent study showed that in vitro, human Treg inhibit release of viral particles from HIV-1-infected human MP, kill infected MP, and induce phenotypic changes in MP. Upregulation of the antiviral ubiquitin-like protein, interferon stimulated gene 15, was concordant with the decrease in viral release from MP cells. This study also implicated caspase-3 and granzyme/perforin pathways in the killing of MP cells. Finally, it was shown that Treg could induce the phenotypic switch of MP from the neurotoxic M1 phenotype to the more neurotrophic M2 phenotype with the downregulation of iNOS and upregulation of arginase 1 (Huang et al., 2010).

It has also been demonstrated in the MPTP mouse model of PD that Treg control microglia function by suppressing ROS production and NF-κB activation through mechanisms that modulate redox enzymes, cell migration, and phagocytosis (Reynolds et al., 2007b; Reynolds et al., 2010; Reynolds et al., 2009; Reynolds et al., 2007a). Furthermore, the adoptive transfer of Treg leads to greater than 90% protection of the nigrostriatal system, while adoptive transfer of Th1 or Th17 cells exacerbates neuronal degeneration (Reynolds et al.,

2010). Together, these data suggest that Treg may be used to suppress the activity of the innate and adaptive immune responses operative in HIV-1 neurodegeneration and PD pathogenesis by modulating the neurotoxic phenotype of activated microglia, Th1 and Th17 cells.

SUMMARY AND CONCLUSIONS

The adaptive immune system is a complex system designed to protect the host from infection and injury. However, when an adaptive immune response continues unchecked in the CNS, the pro-inflammatory microglial responses are enhanced and lead to increases in neurotoxins and neurodegeneration. While the antigen driving HIV-1-associated neurodegeneration is a virus and in AD and PD are aberrant self-proteins, the adaptive immune response in these diseases within the CNS is remarkably similar. Ingress of lymphocytes and chronic activation of glial cells are directly related to neurodegeneration. With an understanding of the interplay between the immune system and neurodegeneration, new therapies aimed at modulating the adaptive immune system's response during diseases will lead to decreased neuronal loss and effect improvements in a range of neurologic deficits seen in what were previously considered divergent disorders of the CNS.

ACKNOWLEDGMENTS

This work was supported by NIH grants P01 NS043985, P20 RR15635, 2R37 NS36126, PO1 NS31492, 2R01 NS034239, and P01MH64570.

REFERENCES

Abdulle, S., Hagberg, L., & Gisslen, M. (2005). Effects of antiretroviral treatment on blood-brain barrier integrity and intrathecal immunoglobulin production in neuroasymptomatic HIV-1-infected patients. *HIV Med, 6,* 164–9.

Abel, K. (2009). The rhesus macaque pediatric SIV infection model—a valuable tool in understanding infant HIV-1 pathogenesis and for designing pediatric HIV-1 prevention strategies. *Curr HIV Res, 7,* 2–11.

Akhtar, L. N., Qin, H., Muldowney, M. T., Yanagisawa, L. L., Kutsch, O., Clements, J. E. et al. (2010). Suppressor of cytokine signaling 3 inhibits antiviral IFN-{beta} signaling to enhance HIV-1 replication in macrophages. *J Immunol.*

Al-zeer, M. A., Al-younes, H. M., Braun, P. R., Zerrahn, J., & Meyer, T. F. (2009). IFN-gamma-inducible Irga6 mediates host resistance against *Chlamydia trachomatis* via autophagy. *PLoS One, 4,* e4588.

Alirezaei, M., Kiosses, W. B., Flynn, C. T., Brady, N. R., & Fox, H. S. (2008). Disruption of neuronal autophagy by infected microglia results in neurodegeneration. *PLoS ONE, 3,* e2906.

Aloisi, F., Ria, F., Columba-Cabezas, S., Hess, H., Penna, G., & Adorini, L. (1999). Relative efficiency of microglia, astrocytes, dendritic cells and B cells in naive CD4+ T cell priming and Th1/Th2 cell restimulation. *Eur J Immunol, 29,* 2705–14.

An, S. F., Giometto, B., Groves, M., Miller, R. F., Beckett, A. A., Gray, F., et al. (1997). Axonal damage revealed by accumulation of beta-APP in HIV-positive individuals without AIDS. *J Neuropathol Exp Neurol, 56,* 1262–8.

An, S. F. & Scaravilli, F. (1997). Early HIV-1 infection of the central nervous system. *Arch Anat Cytol Pathol*, 45, 94–105.

Anderson, E., Zink, W., Xiong, H., & Gendelman, H. E. (2002). HIV-1-associated dementia: A metabolic encephalopathy perpetrated by virus-infected and immune-competent mononuclear phagocytes. *J Acquir Immune Defic Syndr*, 31 Suppl 2, S43–54.

Andersson, J., Schreier, M. H., & Melchers, F. (1980). T-cell-dependent B-cell stimulation is H-2 restricted and antigen dependent only at the resting B-cell level. *Proc Natl Acad Sci USA*, 77, 1612–6.

Aprea, S., Del Valle, L., Mameli, G., Sawaya, B. E., Khalili, K., & Peruzzi, F. (2006). Tubulin-mediated binding of human immunodeficiency virus-1 Tat to the cytoskeleton causes proteasomal-dependent degradation of microtubule-associated protein 2 and neuronal damage. *J Neurosci*, 26, 4054–62.

Baba, Y., Kuroiwa, A., Uitti, R. J., Wszolek, Z. K., & Yamada, T. (2005). Alterations of T-lymphocyte populations in Parkinson disease. *Parkinsonism Relat Disord*, 11, 493–8.

Bales, K. R., Verina, T., Cummins, D. J., Du, Y., Dodel, R. C., Saura, J., et al. (1999). Apolipoprotein E is essential for amyloid deposition in the APP(V717F) transgenic mouse model of Alzheimer's disease. *Proc Natl Acad Sci USA*, 96, 15233–15238.

Bales, K. R., Verina, T., Dodel, R. C., Du, Y., Alstiel, L., Bender, M., et al. (1997). Lack of apolipoprotein E dramatically reduces amyloid beta-peptide deposition. *Nature genetics*, 17, 263–264.

Barker, R. A. & Cahn, A. P. (1988). Parkinson's disease: An autoimmune process. *Int J Neurosci*, 43, 1–7.

Barreto, M., Ferreira, R. C., Lourenco, L., Moraes-Fontes, M. F., Santos, E., Alves, M., et al. (2009). Low frequency of CD4+CD25+ Treg in SLE patients: A heritable trait associated with CTLA4 and TGFbeta gene variants. *BMC Immunology*, 10, 5–5.

Bauer, S., Willie, S. T., Spies, T., & Stron, R. K. (1998). Expression, purification, crystallization and crystallographic characterization of the human MHC class I related protein MICA. *Acta Crystallogr D Biol Crystallogr*, 54, 451–3.

Benner, E. J., Banerjee, R., Reynolds, A. D., Sherman, S., Pisarev, V. M., Tsiperson, V., et al. (2008). Nitrated alpha-synuclein immunity accelerates degeneration of nigral dopaminergic neurons. *PLoS ONE*, 3, e1376.

Benner, E. J., Mosley, R. L., Destache, C. J., Lewis, T. B., Jackson-Lewis, V., Gorantla, S., et al. (2004). Therapeutic immunization protects dopaminergic neurons in a mouse model of Parkinson's disease. *Proc Natl Acad Sci USA*, 101, 9435–9440.

Bennett, C. L., Christie, J., Ramsdell, F., Brunkow, M. E., Ferguson, P. J., Whitesell, L., et al. (2001). The immune dysregulation, polyendocrinopathy, enteropathy, X-linked syndrome (IPEX) is caused by mutations of FOXP3. *Nature genetics*, 27, 20–21.

Bissel, S. J., Wang, G., Bonneh-Barkay, D., Starkey, A., Trichel, A. M., Murphey-Corb, M., et al. (2008). Systemic and brain macrophage infections in relation to the development of simian immunodeficiency virus encephalitis. *J Virol*, 82, 5031–42.

Blum-Degen, D., Frolich, L., Hoyer, S., & Riederer, P. (1995a). Altered regulation of brain glucose metabolism as a cause of neurodegenerative disorders? *J Neural Transm Suppl*, 46, 139–47.

Blum-Degen, D., Muller, T., Kuhn, W., Gerlach, M., Pruzuntek, H., & Riederer, P. (1995b). Interleukin-1 beta and interleukin-6 are elevated in the cerebrospinal fluid of Alzheimer's and de novo Parkinson's disease patients. *Neurosci Lett*, 202, 17–20.

Bourreau, E., Ronet, C., Darcissac, E., Lise, M. C., Sainte Marie, D., Clity, E., et al. (2009). Intralesional regulatory T-cell suppressive function during human acute and chronic cutaneous leishmaniasis due to Leishmania guyanensis. *Infection and immunity*, 77, 1465–1474.

Brabers, N. A. & Nottet, H. S. (2006). Role of the pro-inflammatory cytokines TNF-alpha and IL-1beta in HIV-associated dementia. *Eur J Clin Invest*, 36, 447–58.

Brochard, V., Combadiere, B., Prigent, A., Laouar, Y., Perrin, A., Beray-Berthat, V., et al. (2009). Infiltration of CD4+ lymphocytes into the brain contributes to neurodegeneration in a mouse model of Parkinson disease. *J Clin Invest*, 119, 182–92.

Brusko, T. M., Putnam, A. L., & Bluestone, J. A. (2008). Human regulatory T cells: Role in autoimmune disease and therapeutic opportunities. *Immunological reviews*, 223, 371–390.

Burudi, E. M., Marcondes, M. C., Watry, D. D., Zandonatti, M., Taffe, M. A., & Fox, H. S. (2002). Regulation of indoleamine 2,3-dioxygenase expression in simian immunodeficiency virus-infected monkey brains. *J Virol*, 76, 12233–41.

Cacabelos, R., Barquero, M., Garcia, P., Alvarez, X. A., & Varela de Seijas, E. (1991). Cerebrospinal fluid interleukin-1 beta (IL-1 beta) in Alzheimer's disease and neurological disorders. *Methods Find Exp Clin Pharmacol*, 13, 455–8.

Cao, D., Malmstrom, V., Baecher-Allan, C., Hafler, D., Klareskog, L., & Trollmo, C. (2003). Isolation and functional characterization of regulatory CD25brightCD4+ T cells from the target organ of patients with rheumatoid arthritis. *European journal of immunology*, 33, 215–223.

Caplazi, P. & Ehrensperger, F. (1998). Spontaneous Borna disease in sheep and horses: Immunophenotyping of inflammatory cells and detection of MHC-I and MHC-II antigen expression in Borna encephalitis lesions. *Vet Immunol Immunopathol*, 61, 203–20.

Cederbom, L., Hall, H., & Ivars, F. (2000). CD4+CD25+ regulatory T cells down-regulate co-stimulatory molecules on antigen-presenting cells. *European Journal of Immunology*, 30, 1538–1543.

Chang, L., Yakupov, R., Nakama, H., Stokes, B., & Ernst, T. (2008). Antiretroviral treatment is associated with increased attentional load-dependent brain activation in HIV patients. *J Neuroimmune Pharmacol*, 3, 95–104.

Chao, C. C., Hu, S., Kravitz, F. H., Tsang, M., Anderson, W. R., & Peterson, P. K. (1994). Transforming growth factor-b protects human neurons against b-amyloid-induced injury. *Molec Chem Neuropathol.*, 23, 159–178.

Cho, H. J., Kim, S. K., Jin, S. M., Hwang, E. M., Kim, Y. S., Huh, K., et al. (2007). IFN-gamma-induced BACE1 expression is mediated by activation of JAK2 and ERK1/2 signaling pathways and direct binding of STAT1 to BACE1 promoter in astrocytes. *Glia*, 55, 253–62.

Coombes, J. L., Robinson, N. J., Maloy, K. J., Uhlig, H. H., & Powrie, F. (2005). Regulatory T cells and intestinal homeostasis. *Immunological Reviews*, 204, 184–194.

Cooper, M. D., Kearney, J., & Scher, I. (1984). B lymphocytes. In W. E. Paul. (Ed.). *Fundamental immunology*. New York: Raven.

Costantino, C. M., Baecher-Allan, C. M., & Hafler, D. A. 2008. Human regulatory T cells and autoimmunity. *European Journal of Immunology*, 38, 921–924.

Crystal, H., Dickson, D., Fuld, P., Masur, D., Scott, R., Mehler, M., et al. (1988). Clinico-pathologic studies in dementia: Nondemented subjects with pathologically confirmed Alzheimer's disease. *Neurology*, 38, 1682–7.

Cserr, H. F. & Knopf, P. M. (1992). Cervical lymphatics, the blood-brain barrier and the immunoreactivity of the brain: A new view. *Immunol Today*, 13, 507–12.

Dauer, W. & Przedborski, S. (2003). Parkinson's disease: Mechanisms and models. *Neuron*, 39, 889–909.

Dean, A. F., Montgomery, M., Baskerville, A., Cook, R. W., Cranage, M. P., Sharpe, S. A., et al. (1993). Different patterns of neuropathological disease in rhesus monkeys infected by simian immunodeficiency virus, and their relation to the humoral immune response. *Neuropathol Appl Neurobiol*, 19, 336–45.

Desai, B. S., Monahan, A. J., Carvey, P. M., & Hendey, B. (2007). Blood-brain barrier pathology in Alzheimer's and Parkinson's disease: Implications for drug therapy. *Cell Transplant*, 16, 285–99.

Desvignes, L. & Ernst, J. D. (2009). Interferon-[gamma]-responsive non-hematopoietic cells regulate the immune response to Mycobacterium tuberculosis. *Immunity*, 31, 974–985.

Dhawan, S., Weeks, B. S., Soderland, C., Schnaper, H. W., TORO, L. A., Asthana, S. P., et al. (1995). HIV-1 infection alters monocyte interactions with human microvascular endothelial cells. *Journal of Immunology*, 154, 422–432.

Dickson, D., Lee, S., Mattiace, L., Yen, S., & Brosnan, C. (1993a). Microglia and cytokines in neurological disease, with special reference to AIDS and Alzheimer's disease. *Glia*, 7, 75–83.

Dickson, D. W., Lee, S. C., Mattiace, L. A., Yen, S. H., & Brosnan, C. (1993b). Microglia and cytokines in neurological disease, with special reference to AIDS and Alzheimer's disease. *Glia*, 7, 75–83.

Dickson, D. W., Farlo, J., Davies, P., Crystal, H., Fuld, P. & Yen, S. H. (1988). Alzheimer's disease. A double-labeling immunohistochemical study of senile plaques. *The American journal of pathology, 132*, 86–101.

Dietlin, T. A., Cua, D. J., Burke, K. A., Lund, B. T., & Van der Veen, R. C. (2009). Role of IL-23 in mobilization of immunoregulatory nitric oxide- or superoxide-producing Gr-1+ cells from bone marrow. *Free Radical Biology and Medicine, 47*, 357–363.

Elovaara, I. & Muller, K. M. (1993). Cytoimmunological abnormalities in cerebrospinal fluid in early stages of HIV-1 infection often precede changes in blood. *J Neuroimmunol, 44*, 199–204.

Engelhardt, B. & Ransohoff, R. M. (2005). The ins and outs of T-lymphocyte trafficking to the CNS: Anatomical sites and molecular mechanisms. *Trends Immunol, 26*, 485–95.

Ethell, D. W., Shippy, D., Cao, C., Cracchiolo, J. R., Rrunfeldt, M., Blake, B., et al. (2006). Abeta-specific T-cells reverse cognitive decline and synaptic loss in Alzheimer's mice. *Neurobiol Dis, 23*, 351–61.

Evans, D., Funkenstein, H., Albert, M., & Al., E. (1989). Prevalence of Alzheimer's disease in a community population higher than previously reported. *JAMA, 262*, 2551–2556.

Farkas, E., De Jong, G. I., Apro, E., De Vos, R. A., Steur, E. N., & Luiten, P. G. (2000). Similar ultrastructural breakdown of cerebrocortical capillaries in Alzheimer's disease, Parkinson's disease, and experimental hypertension. What is the functional link? *Ann N Y Acad Sci, 903*, 72–82.

Fenoglio, D., Poggi, A., Catellani, S., Battaglia, F., Ferrera, A., Setti, M., et al. (2009). Vdelta1 T lymphocytes producing IFN-gamma and IL-17 are expanded in HIV-1-infected patients and respond to Candida albicans. *Blood, 113*, 6611–8.

Ferri, A., Nencini, M., Cozzolino, M., Carrara, P., Moreno, S., & Carri, M. T. (2008). Inflammatory cytokines increase mitochondrial damage in motoneuronal cells expressing mutant SOD1. *Neurobiol Dis, 32*, 454–60.

Fiala, M., Liu, Q. N., Sayre, J., Pop, V., Brahmandam, V., Graves, M. C., et al. (2002). Cyclooxygenase-2-positive macrophages infiltrate the Alzheimer's disease brain and damage the blood-brain barrier. *Eur J Clin Invest, 32*, 360–71.

Finch, C. E., Laping, N. J., Morgan, T. E., Nichols, N. R., & Pasinetti, G. M. (1993). TGF-beta 1 is an organizer of responses to neurodegeneration. *J Cell Biochem, 53*, 314–22.

Fiszer, U., Mix, E., Fredrikson, S., Kostulas, V., & Link, H. (1994). Parkinson's disease and immunological abnormalities: Increase of HLA-DR expression on monocytes in cerebrospinal fluid and of CD45RO+ T cells in peripheral blood. *Acta Neurol Scand, 90*, 160–6.

Flanders, K., Lippa, C., Smith, T., Pollen, D., & Sorn, M. 1995. Altered expression oftransforming growth factor-b in Alzheimer's disease. *Neurol, 45*, 1561–1569.

Fletcher, J. M., Lonergan, R., Costelloe, L., Kinsella, K., Moran, B., O'Farrelly, C., et al. (2009). CD39+Foxp3+ regulatory T Cells suppress pathogenic Th17 cells and are impaired in multiple sclerosis. *Journal of Immunology, 183*, 7602–7610.

Fontenot, J. D., Gavin, M. A., & Rudensky, A. Y. (2003). Foxp3 programs the development and function of CD4+CD25+ regulatory T cells. *Nature immunology, 4*, 330–336.

Franksson, L., George, E., Powis, S., Butcher, G., Howard, J., & Karre, K. (1993). Tumorigenicity conferred to lymphoma mutant by major histocompatibility complex-encoded transporter gene. *J Exp Med, 177*, 201–5.

Fujimura, T., Okuyama, R., Ito, Y., & Aiba, S. (2008). Profiles of Foxp3+ regulatory T cells in eczematous dermatitis, psoriasis vulgaris and mycosis fungoides. *The British Journal of Dermatology, 158*, 1256–1263.

Gannage, M. & Munz, C. (2009). Macroautophagy in immunity and tolerance. *Traffic, 10*, 615–20.

Gao, H. M., Kotzbauer, P. T., Uryu, K., Leight, S., Trojanowski, J. Q., & Lee, V. M. (2008). Neuroinflammation and oxidation/nitration of alpha-synuclein linked to dopaminergic neurodegeneration. *J Neurosci, 28*, 7687–98.

Garcia-Arencibia, M., Hochfeld, W. E., Toh, P. P., & Rubinsztein, D. C. (2010). Autophagy, a guardian against neurodegeneration. *Semin Cell Dev Biol*.

Garg, S. K., Banerjee, R., & Kipnis, J. (2008). Neuroprotective immunity: T cell-derived glutamate endows astrocytes with a neuroprotective phenotype. *Journal of Immunology, 180*, 3866–3873.

Gelman, B. B. & Nguyen, T. P. (2010). Synaptic proteins linked to HIV-1 infection and immunoproteasome induction: Proteomic analysis of human synaptosomes. *J Neuroimmune Pharmacol, 5*, 92–102.

Gelman, B. B., Spencer, J. A., Holzer, C. E., 3rd., & Soukup, V. M. (2006). Abnormal striatal dopaminergic synapses in National NeuroAIDS Tissue Consortium subjects with HIV encephalitis. *J Neuroimmune Pharmacol, 1*, 410–20.

Ghorpade, A., Nukuna, A., Che, M., Haggerty, S., Persidsky, Y., Carter, E., et al. (1998). Human immunodeficiency virus neurotropism: An analysis of viral replication and cytopathicity for divergent strains in monocytes and microglia. *Journal of Virology, 72*, 3340–3350.

Giasson, B. I., Duda, J. E., Murray, I. V., Chen, Q., Souza, J. M., Hurtig, H. I., et al. (2000). Oxidative damage linked to neurodegeneration by selective alpha-synuclein nitration in synucleinopathy lesions. *Science, 290*, 985–9.

Giometto, B., An, S. F., Groves, M., Scaravilli, T., Geddes, J. F., Miller, R., et al. (1997). Accumulation of beta-amyloid precursor protein in HIV encephalitis: Relationship with neuropsychological abnormalities. *Ann Neurol, 42*, 34–40.

Glass, J. D., Fedor, H., Wesselingh, S. L., & McArthur, J. C. (1995). Immunocytochemical quantitation of human immunodeficiency virus in the brain: Correlations with dementia. *Annals of Neurology, 38*, 755–762.

Glenner, G. G., Wong, C. W., Quaranta, V., & Eanes, E. D. (1984). The amyloid deposits in Alzheimer's disease: Their nature and pathogenesis. *Appl Pathol, 2*, 357–69.

Glisic, S., Klinker, M., Waukau, J., Jailwala, P., Jana, S., Basken, J., et al. (2009). Genetic association of HLA DQB1 with CD4+CD25+(high) T-cell apoptosis in type 1 diabetes. *Genes and Immunity, 10*, 334–340.

Goldgaber, D., Harris, H., Hla, T., Maciag, T., Donnelly, R., Jacobsen, J., et al. (1989). IL-1 regulates synthesis of amyloid beta-protein precursor mRNA in human endothelial cells. *Proc Natl Acad Sci USA, 86*, 7606–7610.

Gonzalez-Rey, E., Fernandez-Martin, A., Chorny, A., & Delgado, M. (2006). Vasoactive intestinal peptide induces CD4+, CD25+ T regulatory cells with therapeutic effect in collagen-induced arthritis. *Arthritis and Rheumatism, 54*, 864–876.

Gonzalez-Scarano, F. & Baltuch, G. (1999). Microglia as mediators of inflammatory and degenerative diseases. *Annu Rev Neurosci, 22*, 219–40.

Gorevic, P. D., Goni, F., Pons-Estel, B., Alvarez, F., Peress, N. S., & Frangione, B. (1986). Isolation and partial characterization of neurofibrillary tangles and amyloid plaque core in Alzheimer's disease: Immunohistological studies. *Journal of Neuropathology and Experimental Neurology, 45*, 647–664.

Gottfried-Blackmore, A., Kaunzner, U. W., Idoyaga, J., Felger, J. C., Mcewen, B. S., & Bulloch, K. (2009). Acute in vivo exposure to interferon-{gamma} enables resident brain dendritic cells to become effective antigen presenting cells. *Proc Natl Acad Sci USA*.

Goverman, J. (2009). Autoimmune T cell responses in the central nervous system. *Nat Rev Immunol, 9*, 393–407.

Grammas, P. & Ovase, R. (2001). Inflammatory factors are elevated in brain microvessels in Alzheimer's disease. *Neurobiol Aging, 22*, 837–42.

Griffin, W. S., Stanley, L. C., Ling, C., White, L., MacLeod, V., Perrot, L. J., et al. (1989). Brain interleukin 1 and S-100 immunoreactivity are elevated in Down syndrome and Alzheimer disease. *Proc Natl Acad Sci USA, 86*, 7611–5.

Haas, J., Korporal, M., Balint, B., Fritzsching, B., Schwarz, A., & Wildemann, B. (2009). Glatiramer acetate improves regulatory T-cell function by expansion of naive CD4(+)CD25(+)FOXP3(+) CD31(+) T-cells in patients with multiple sclerosis. *Journal of Neuroimmunology, 216*, 113–117.

Hagberg, L., Norkkans, G., Andersson, M., Wachter, H., & Fuchs, D. (1992). Cerebrospinal fluid neopterin and beta 2-microglobulin levels in neurologically asymptomatic HIV-infected patients before and after initiation of zidovudine treatment. *Infection, 20*, 313–5.

Hall, B. M., Pearce, N. W., Gurley, K. E., & Dorsch, S. E. (1990). Specific unresponsiveness in rats with prolonged cardiac allograft survival after treatment with cyclosporine. III. Further characterization of the CD4+ suppressor cell and its mechanisms of action. *The Journal of Experimental Medicine, 171*, 141–157.

Hall, G. F. & Yao, J. (2005). Modeling tauopathy: A range of complementary approaches. *Biochim Biophys Acta, 1739*, 224–39.

Halonen, S. K. (2009). Role of autophagy in the host defense against *Toxoplasma gondii* in astrocytes. *Autophagy, 5*, 268–9.

Hampel, H., Sunderland, T., Kotter, H. U., Schneider, C., Teipel, S. J., Padberg, F., et al. (1998). Decreased soluble interleukin-6 receptor in cerebrospinal fluid of patients with Alzheimer's disease. *Brain Res, 780*, 356–9.

Hardy, J. (2006). Has the amyloid cascade hypothesis for Alzheimer's disease been proved? *Curr Alzheimer Res, 3*, 71–3.

Hardy, J. & Selkoe, D. J. (2002). The amyloid hypothesis of Alzheimer's disease: progress and problems on the road to therapeutics. *Science, 297*, 353–6.

Hardy, J. A. & Higgins, G. A. (1992). Alzheimer's disease: The amyloid cascade hypothesis. *Science, 256*, 184–5.

Hickey, W. F. (1999). Leukocyte traffic in the central nervous system: The participants and their roles. *Semin Immunol, 11*, 125–37.

Hickey, W. F. (2001). Basic principles of immunological surveillance of the normal central nervous system. *Glia, 36*, 118–24.

Hinkin, C. H., Castellon, S. A., Durvasula, R. S., Hardy, D. J., Lam, M. N., Mason, K. I., et al. (2002). Medication adherence among HIV+ adults: Effects of cognitive dysfunction and regimen complexity. *Neurology, 59*, 1944–50.

Hisanaga, K., Asagi, M., Itoyama, Y., & Iwasaki, Y. (2001). Increase in peripheral CD4 bright+ CD8 dull+ T cells in Parkinson disease. *Arch Neurol, 58*, 1580–3.

Ho, H. H., Antoniv, T. T., Ji, J. D., & Ivashkiv, L. B. (2008). Lipopolysaccharide-induced expression of matrix metalloproteinases in human monocytes is suppressed by IFN-gamma via superinduction of ATF-3 and suppression of AP-1. *J Immunol, 181*, 5089–97.

Hori, S., Nomura, T., & Sakaguchi, S. (2003). Control of regulatory T cell development by the transcription factor Foxp3. *Science, 299*, 1057–1061.

Hornykiewicz, O. & Kish, S. J. (1987). Biochemical pathophysiology of Parkinson's disease. *Advances in Neurology, 45*, 19–34.

Horwitz, D. A. (2008). Regulatory T cells in systemic lupus erythematosus: Past, present and future. *Arthritis Research & Therapy, 10*, 227.

Huang, J., Canadien, V., Lam, G. Y., Steinberg, B. E., Dinauer, M. C., Magalhaes, M. A., et al. (2009). Activation of antibacterial autophagy by NADPH oxidases. *Proc Natl Acad Sci USA, 106*, 6226–31.

Huang, X., Stone, D.K., Yu, F., Zeng, Y., Gendelman, H.E. (2010). Functional proteomic analysis for regulatory T cell surveillance of the HIV-1-infected macrophage. *Journal of Proteome Research, 9*, 6759–73.

Hunot, S., Boissiere, F., Faucheux, B., Brugg, B., Mouatt-Prigent, A., Agid, Y. et al. (1996). Nitric oxide synthase and neuronal vulnerability in Parkinson's disease. *Neuroscience, 72*, 355–63.

Itagaki, S., McGeer, P. L., & Akiyama, H. (1988). Presence of T-cytotoxic suppressor and leucocyte common antigen positive cells in Alzheimer's disease brain tissue. *Neurosci Lett, 91*, 259–64.

Janeway, C. A., JR. & Medzhitov, R. (1998). Introduction: The role of innate immunity in the adaptive immune response. *Semin Immunol, 10*, 349–50.

Janeway, C. A. J., Travers, P., Walport, M., & Shlomchik, M. (2001). *Immunobiology: The immune system in health and disease, Fifth edition*, New York: Garland Science.

Jin, H., Carrio, R., Yu, A., & Malek, T. R. (2004). Distinct activation signals determine whether IL-21 induces B cell costimulation, growth arrest, or Bim-dependent apoptosis. *J Immunol, 173*, 657–65.

Joachim, C. L., Duffy, L. K., Morris, J. H., & Selkoe, D. J. (1988). Protein chemical and immunocytochemical studies of meningovascular beta-amyloid protein in Alzheimer's disease and normal aging. *Brain Res, 474*, 100–11.

Joel, D. D., Chanana, A. D., Cottier, H., Cronkite, E. P., & Laissue, J. A. (1977). Fate of thymocytes: Studies with 125I-iododeoxyuridine and 3H-thymidine in mice. *Cell Tissue Kinet, 10*, 57–69.

Johnson, J., Pahuja, A., Graham, M., Hering, B., Hancock, W. W., & Bansal-Pakala, P. (2008). Effects of histone deacetylase inhibitor SAHA on effector and FOXP3+regulatory T cells in rhesus macaques. *Transplantation Proceedings, 40*, 459–461.

Jones, G. & Power, C. (2006). Regulation of neural cell survival by HIV-1 infection. *Neurobiol Dis, 21*, 1–17.

Ju, S. T., Cui, H., Panka, D. J., Ettinger, R., & Marshak-Rothstein, A. (1994). Participation of target Fas protein in apoptosis pathway induced by CD4+ Th1 and CD8+ cytotoxic T cells. *Proc Natl Acad Sci USA, 91*, 4185–9.

Kalman, J., Juhasz, A., Laird, G., Dickens, P., Jardanhazy, T., Rimanoczy, A., et al. (1997). Serum interleukin-6 levels correlate with the severity of dementia in Down syndrome and in Alzheimer's disease. *Acta Neurol Scand, 96*, 236–40.

Katz, D. H., Paul, W. E., & Benacerraf, B. (1973). Carrier function in anti-hapten antibody responses. VI. Establishment of experimental conditions for either inhibitory or enhancing influences of carrier-specific cells on antibody production. *J Immunol, 110*, 107–17.

Katzman, R. (1976). Editorial: The prevalence and malignancy of Alzheimer disease. A major killer. *Arch Neurol, 33*, 217–8.

Kaul, M. & Lipton, S. A. (2006). Mechanisms of neuronal injury and death in HIV-1 associated dementia. *Curr HIV Res, 4*, 307–18.

Kennedy, P. G. & Gairns, J. (1992). Major histocompatibility complex (MHC) antigen expression in HIV encephalitis [published erratum appears in Neuropathol Appl Neurobiol 1992 Dec;18(6):627]. *Neuropathol Appl Neurobiol, 18*, 515–22.

Khader, S. A., Pearl, J. E., Sakamoto, K., Gilmartin, L., Bell, G. K., Jelley-Gibbs, D. M., et al. (2005). IL-23 compensates for the absence of IL-12p70 and is essential for the IL-17 response during tuberculosis but is dispensable for protection and antigen-specific IFN-gamma responses if IL-12p70 is available. *J Immunol, 175*, 788–95.

Khattar, M., Chen, W., & Stepkowski, S. M. (2009). Expanding and converting regulatory T cells: A horizon for immunotherapy. *Archivum Immunologiae et Therapiae Experimentalis, 57*, 199–204.

Kim, J. M., Rasmussen, J. P., & Rudensky, A. Y. (2007). Regulatory T cells prevent catastrophic autoimmunity throughout the lifespan of mice. *Nature Immunology, 8*, 191–197.

Kim, P. K., Hailey, D. W., Mullen, R. T., & Lippincott-Schwartz, J. (2008). Ubiquitin signals autophagic degradation of cytosolic proteins and peroxisomes. *Proc Natl Acad Sci USA, 105*, 20567–74.

Kim, W. G., Mohney, R. P., Wilson, B., Jeohn, G. H., Liu, B., & Hong, J. S. (2000). Regional difference in susceptibility to lipopolysaccharide-induced neurotoxicity in the rat brain: Role of microglia. *J Neurosci, 20*, 6309–16.

Kipnis, J., Mizrahi, T., Hauben, E., Shaked, I., Shevach, E., & Schwartz, M. (2002). Neuroprotective autoimmunity: Naturally occurring CD4+CD25+ regulatory T cells suppress the ability to withstand injury to the central nervous system. *Proceedings of the National Academy of Sciences of the USA, 99*, 15620–15625.

Kleinewietfeld, M., Starke, M., Di Mitri, D., Borsellino, G., Battistini, L., Rotzschke, O. et al. (2009). CD49d provides access to "untouched" human Foxp3+ Treg free of contaminating effector cells. *Blood, 113*, 827–836.

Koen, V. (2010). Disturbed regulatory T cell homeostasis in multiple sclerosis. *Trends in Molecular Medicine, 16*, 58.

Konsman, J. P., Drukarch, B., & Van Dam, A. M. (2007). (Peri)vascular production and action of pro-inflammatory cytokines in brain pathology. *Clin Sci (Lond), 112*, 1–25.

Kornbluth, R. S., Oh, P. S., Munis, J. R., Cleveland, P. H., & Richman, D. D. (1990). The role of interferons in the control of HIV replication in macrophages. *Clin Immunol Immunopathol, 54*, 200–19.

Korolchuk, V. I., Mansilla, A., Menzies, F. M., & Rubinsztein, D. C. (2009). Autophagy inhibition compromises degradation of ubiquitin-proteasome pathway substrates. *Mol Cell, 33*, 517–27.

Korolchuk, V. I., Menzies, F. M., & Rubinsztein, D. C. (2010). Mechanisms of cross-talk between the ubiquitin-proteasome and autophagy-lysosome systems. *FEBS Lett, 584*, 1393–8.

Kraft-Terry, S. D., Buch, S. J., Fox, H. S., & Gendelman, H. E. (2009). A coat of many colors: Neuroimmune crosstalk in human immunodeficiency virus infection. *Neuron, 64*, 133–45.

Kraft-Terry, S. D., Stothert, A. R., Buch, S., & Gendelman, H. E. (2010). HIV-1 neuroimmunity in the era of antiretroviral therapy. *Neurobiol Dis*, 37, 542–8.

Lafrenie, R. M., Wahl, L. M., Epstein, J. S., Hewlett, I. K., Yamada, K. M., & Dhawan, S. (1996). HIV-1-Tat protein promotes chemotaxis and invasive behavior by monocytes. *Journal of Immunology*, 157, 974–977.

Lawson, L. J., Perry, V. H., Dri, P., & Gordon, S. (1990). Heterogeneity in the distribution and morphology of microglia in the normal adult mouse brain. *Neuroscience*, 39, 151–70.

Lee, J., Kim, S. J., Son, T. G., Chan, S. L., & Mattson, M. P. (2006). Interferon-gamma is up-regulated in the hippocampus in response to intermittent fasting and protects hippocampal neurons against excitotoxicity. *J Neurosci Res*, 83, 1552–7.

Lee, Y. K., Mukasa, R., Hatton, R. D., & Weaver, C. T. (2009). Developmental plasticity of Th17 and Treg cells. *Current Opinion in Immunology*, 21, 274–280.

Li, P., Gregg, J. L., Wang, N., Zhou, D., O'Donnell, P., Blum, J. S. et al. (2005a). Compartmentalization of class II antigen presentation: contribution of cytoplasmic and endosomal processing. *Immunol Rev*, 207, 206–17.

Li, W., Galey, D., Mattson, M. P., & Nath, A. (2005b). Molecular and cellular mechanisms of neuronal cell death in HIV dementia. *Neurotox Res*, 8, 119–34.

Licastro, F., Masliah, E., Pedrini, S., & Thal, L. J. (2000). Blood levels of alpha-1-antichymotrypsin and risk factors for Alzheimer's disease: Effects of gender and apolipoprotein E genotype. *Dement Geriatr Cogn Disord*, 11, 25–8.

Lin, W. L., Fincke, J. E., Sharer, L. R., Monos, D. S., Lu, S., Gaughan, J., et al. (2005). Oligoclonal T cells are infiltrating the brains of children with AIDS: Sequence analysis reveals high proportions of identical beta-chain T-cell receptor transcripts. *Clin Exp Immunol*, 141, 338–56.

Linsely, P. S., Clark, E. A., & Ledbetter, J. A. (1990). T-cell antigen CD28 mediates adhesion with B cells by interacting with activation antigen B7/BB-1. *Proc Natl Acad Sci USA*, 87, 5031–5.

Liu, J., Gong, N., Huang, X., Rerynolds, A. D., Mosley, R. L., & Gendelman, H. E. (2009). Neuromodulatory activities of CD4+CD25+ regulatory T cells in a murine model of HIV-1-associated neurodegeneration. *J Immunol*, 182, 3855–65.

Liu, Y. C. (2004). Ubiquitin ligases and the immune response. *Annu Rev Immunol*, 22, 81–127.

Ljunggren, K., Chiodi, F., Broliden, P. A., Albert, J., Norkrans, G., Hagberg, L., et al. (1989). HIV-1-specific antibodies in cerebrospinal fluid mediate cellular cytotoxicity and neutralization. *AIDS Res Hum Retroviruses*, 5, 629–38.

Louis, S., Dutertre, C.-A., Vimeux, L., Fery, L., Henno, L., Diocou, S., et al. IL-23 and IL-12p70 production by monocytes and dendritic cells in primary HIV-1 infection. *J Leukoc Biol*, jlb.1009684.

Lowin, B., Beermann, F., Schmidt, A., & Tschopp, J. (1994). A null mutation in the perforin gene impairs cytolytic T lymphocyte- and natural killer cell-mediated cytotoxicity. *Proc Natl Acad Sci USA*, 91, 11571–5.

Lucas, J. L., Mirshahpanah, P., Haas-Stapleton, E., Asadullah, K., Zollner, T. M., & Numerof, R. P. (2009). Induction of Foxp3+ regulatory T cells with histone deacetylase inhibitors. *Cellular Immunology*, 257, 97–104.

Lucey, D. R., McGuire, S. A., Abbadessa, S., Hall, K., Woolford, B., Valtier, S., et al. (1993). Cerebrospinal fluid neopterin levels in 159 neurologically asymptomatic persons infected with the human immunodeficiency virus (HIV-1): relationship to immune status. *Viral Immunol*, 6, 267–72.

Ma, Z., Qin, H., & Benveniste, E. N. (2001). Transcriptional suppression of matrix metalloproteinase-9 gene expression by IFN-gamma and IFN-beta: Critical role of STAT-1alpha. *J Immunol*, 167, 5150–9.

Maino, V. C., Hayman, M. J., & Crumpton, M. J. (1975). Relationship between enhanced turnover of phosphatidylinositol and lymphocyte activation by mitogens. *Biochem J*, 146, 247–52.

Maloy, K. J., Salaun, L., Cahill, R., Dougan, G., Saunders, N. J., & Powrie, F. (2003). CD4+CD25+ T(R) cells suppress innate immune pathology through cytokine-dependent mechanisms. *The Journal of Experimental Medicine*, 197, 111–119.

Mankowski, J. L., Clements, J. E., & Zink, M. C. (2002). Searching for clues: Tracking the pathogenesis of human immunodeficiency virus central nervous system disease by use of an accelerated, consistent simian immunodeficiency virus macaque model. *J Infect Dis*, 186 Suppl 2, S199–208.

Marcondes, M. C. G., Burudi, E. M. E., Huitron-Resendiz, S., Sanchez-Alavez, M., Watry, D., Zandonatti, M., et al. (2001). Highly activated CD8+ T cells in the brain correlate with early central nervous system dysfunction in simian immunodeficiency virus infection. *J Immunol*, 167, 5429–5438.

Martin, B., Hirota, K., Cua, D. J., Stockinger, B., & Veldhoen, M. (2009). Interleukin-17-producing [gamma][delta] T cells selectively expand in response to pathogen products and environmental signals. *Immunity*, 31, 321–330.

Martinez, M., Fernandez-Vivancos, E., Frank, A., De La Fuente, M., & Hernanz, A. (2000). Increased cerebrospinal fluid fas (Apo-1) levels in Alzheimer's disease. Relationship with IL-6 concentrations. *Brain Res*, 869, 216–9.

Maslin, C. L., Kedzierska, K., Webster, N. L., Muller, W. A., & Crowe, S. M. (2005). Transendothelial migration of monocytes: The underlying molecular mechanisms and consequences of HIV-1 infection. *Curr HIV Res*, 3, 303–17.

Masters, C. L., Multhaup, G., Simms, G., Pottgiesser, J., Martins, R. N., & Beyreuther, K. (1985a). Neuronal origin of a cerebral amyloid: Neurofibrillary tangles of Alzheimer's disease contain the same protein as the amyloid of plaque cores and blood vessels. *EMBO J*, 4, 2757–63.

Masters, C. L., Simms, G., Weinman, N. A., Multhaup, G., McDonald, B. L., & Beyreuther, K. (1985b). Amyloid plaque core protein in Alzheimer disease and Down syndrome. *Proc Natl Acad Sci USA*, 82, 4245–9.

Mattiace, L. A., Davies, P., Yen, S. H., & Dickson, D. W. (1990). Microglia in cerebellar plaques in Alzheimer's disease. *Acta Neuropathol*, 80, 493–8.

McArthur, J. C., Brew, B. J., & Nath, A. (2005). Neurological complications of HIV infection. *Lancet Neurol*, 4, 543–55.

McGeer, E. G. & McGeer, P. L. (2003). Inflammatory processes in Alzheimer's disease. *Prog Neuropsychopharmacol Biol Psychiatry*, 27, 741–9.

McGeer, E. G., Singh, E. A., & McGeer, P. L. (1988a). Peripheral-type benzodiazepine binding in Alzheimer disease. *Alzheimer Dis Assoc Disord*, 2, 331–6.

McGeer, P. L., Itagaki, S., Akiyama, H., & McGeer, E. G. (1988b). Rate of cell death in parkinsonism indicates active neuropathological process. *Ann Neurol*, 24, 574–6.

McGeer, P. L., Itagaki, S., Boyes, B. E., & McGeer, E. G. (1988c). Reactive microglia are positive for HLA-DR in the substantia nigra of Parkinson's and Alzheimer's disease brains. *Neurology*, 38, 1285–91.

McNaught, K. S., Jonbaptiste, R., Jackson, T., & Jengelley, T. A. (2010). The pattern of neuronal loss and survival may reflect differential expression of proteasome activators in Parkinson's disease. *Synapse*, 64, 241–50.

McRae-Degueurce, A., Rosengren, L., Haglid, K., Booj, S., Gottfries, C. G., Granerus, A. C., et al. (1988). Immunocytochemical investigations on the presence of neuron-specific antibodies in the CSF of Parkinson's disease cases. *Neurochem Res*, 13, 679–84.

Meda, L., Baron, P., & Scarlato, G. (2001). Glial activation in Alzheimer's disease: The role of Abeta and its associated proteins. *Neurobiol Aging*, 22, 885–93.

Meda, L., Cassatella, M. A., Szendrei, G. I., Otvos, L. Jr., Baron, P., Villalba, M., et al. (1995). Activation of microglial cells by b-amyloid protein and interferon-g. *Nature*, 374, 647–650.

Medawar, P. B. (1948). Immunity to homologous grafted skin; the fate of skin homografts transplanted to the brain, to subcutaneous tissue, and to the anterior chamber of the eye. *Br J Exp Pathol*, 29, 58–69.

Meeks, K. D., Sieve, A. N., Kolls, J. K., Ghilardi, N., & Berg, R. E. (2009). IL-23 is required for protection against systemic infection with Listeria monocytogenes. *J Immunol*, 183, 8026–34.

Michaels, J., Sharer, L. R., & Epstein, L. G. (1988). Human immunodeficiency virus type 1 (HIV-1) infection of the nervous system: A review. *Immunodefic Rev*, 1, 71–104.

Miklossy, J., Doudet, D. D., Schwab, C., Yu, S., McGeer, E. G., & McGeer, P. L. (2006). Role of ICAM-1 in persisting inflammation in Parkinson disease and MPTP monkeys. *Exp Neurol*, 197, 275–83.

Monsonego, A. & Weiner, H. L. (2003). Immunotherapeutic approaches to Alzheimer's disease. *Science*, 302, 834–8.

Moore, S. & Thanos, S. (1996). The concept of microglia in relation to central nervous system disease and regeneration. *Progress in Neurobiology*, 48, 441–460.

Mosley, R. L., Benner, E. J., Kadiu, I., Thomas, M., Boska, M. D., Hasan, K., et a l. (2006). Neuroinflammation, oxidative stress and the pathogenesis of Parkinson's disease. *Clin Neurosci Res*, 6, 261–281.

Mozley, P. D., Schneider, J. S., Acton, P. D., Plossl, K., Stern, M. B., Siderowf, A., et al. (2000). Binding of [99mTc]TRODAT-1 to dopamine transporters in patients with Parkinson's disease and in healthy volunteers. *J Nucl Med*, 41, 584–9.

Mu, L., Sun, B., Kong, Q., Wang, J., Wang, G., Zhang, S., et al. (2009). Disequilibrium of T helper type 1, 2 and 17 cells and regulatory T cells during the development of experimental autoimmune myasthenia gravis. *Immunology*, 128, e826–36.

Munz, C. (2009). Enhancing immunity through autophagy. *Annu Rev Immunol*, 27, 423–49.

Navia, B. A. & Rostasy, K. (2005). The AIDS dementia complex: Clinical and basic neuroscience with implications for novel molecular therapies. *Neurotox Res*, 8, 3–24.

Nguyen, T. P., Soukup, V. M., & Gelman, B. B. (2010). Persistent hijacking of brain proteasomes in HIV-associated dementia. *Am J Pathol*, 176, 893–902.

Nistala, K. & Wedderburn, L. R. (2009). Th17 and regulatory T cells: Rebalancing pro- and anti-inflammatory forces in autoimmune arthritis. *Rheumatology* (*Oxford*), 48, 602–6.

Nottet, H. S. & Gendelman, H. E. (1995). Unraveling the neuroimmune mechanisms for the HIV-1-associated cognitive/motor complex. *Immunology Today*, 16, 441–448.

Olanow, C. W., Stern, M. B., & Sethi, K. (2009). The scientific and clinical basis for the treatment of Parkinson disease (2009). *Neurology*, 72, S1–136.

Olson, J. K. & Miller, S. D. (2004). Microglia initiate central nervous system innate and adaptive immune responses through multiple TLRs. *J Immunol*, 173, 3916–24.

Orandle, M. S., MacLean, A. G., Sasseville, V. G., Alvarez, X., & Lackner, A. A. (2002). Enhanced expression of proinflammatory cytokines in the central nervous system is associated with neuroinvasion by simian immunodeficiency virus and the development of encephalitis. *J Virol*, 76, 5797–802.

Pantaleo, G. & Koup, R. A. (2004). Correlates of immune protection in HIV-1 infection: What we know, what we don't know, what we should know. *Nat Med*, 10, 806–10.

Peress, N. & Perrilo, E. (1995). Different expression of TGF-b1, 2 and 3 isotypes in Alzheimer's disease: A comparative immunocytochemical study with cerebral infarction, aged human, and mouse control brains. *Exp Neurol*, 54, 802–811.

Petito, C. K., Adkins, B., McCarthy, M., Roberts, B., & Khamis, I. (2003). CD4+ and CD8+ cells accumulate in the brains of acquired immunodeficiency syndrome patients with human immunodeficiency virus encephalitis. *J Neurovirol*, 9, 36–44.

Petito, C. K. & Cash, K. S. (1992). Blood-brain barrier abnormalities in the acquired immunodeficiency syndrome: Immunohistochemical localization of serum proteins in postmortem brain. *Ann. Neurol.*, 32, 658–666.

Piontek, G. E., Taniguchi, K., Ljunggren, H. G., Gronberg, A., Kiessling, R., Klein, G. et al. (1985). YAC-1 MHC class I variants reveal an association between decreased NK sensitivity and increased H-2 expression after interferon treatment or in vivo passage. *J Immunol*, 135, 4281–8.

Pouplard, A. & Emile, J. (1984). Autoimmunity in Parkinson's disease. *Adv Neurol*, 40, 307–13.

Prendergast, A., Prado, J. G., Kang, Y. H., Chen, F., Riddell, L. A., Luzzi, G., et al. HIV-1 infection is characterized by profound depletion of CD161+ Th17 cells and gradual decline in regulatory T cells. *AIDS*, 24, 491–502.

Price, R. W. & Spudich, S. (2008). Antiretroviral therapy and central nervous system HIV type 1 infection. *J Infect Dis*, 197 Suppl 3, S294–306.

Przedborski, S., Vila, M., & Jackson-Lewis, V. (2003). Neurodegeneration: What is it and where are we? *J Clin Invest*, 111, 3–10.

Putnam, A. L., Brusko, T. M., Lee, M. R., Liu, W., Szot, G. L., Ghosh, T., et al. (2009). Expansion of human regulatory T-cells from patients with type 1 diabetes. *Diabetes*, 58, 652–662.

Qiu, W. Q., Ye, Z., Kholodenko, D., Seubert, P., & Selkoe, D. J. (1997). Degradation of amyloid beta-protein by a metalloprotease secreted by microglia and other neural and non-neural cells. *J Biol Chem*, 272, 6641–6.

Quillet, A., Presse, F., Marchiol-Fournigault, C., Harel-Bellan, A., Benbunan, M., Ploegh, H. et al. (1988). Increased resistance to non-MHC-restricted cytotoxicity related to HLA A, B expression. Direct demonstration using beta 2-microglobulin-transfected Daudi cells. *J Immunol*, 141, 17–20.

Rami, A. (2009). Review: Autophagy in neurodegeneration: firefighter and/or incendiarist? *Neuropathol Appl Neurobiol*, 35, 449–61.

Renna, M., Jimenez-Sanchez, M., Sarkar, S., & Rubinsztein, D. C. (2010). Chemical inducers of autophagy that enhance the clearance of mutant proteins in neurodegenerative diseases. *J Biol Chem*, 285, 11061–7.

Rentzos, M., Nikolaou, C., Andreadou, E., Paraskevas, G. P., Rombos, A., Zoga, M., et al. (2007). Circulating interleukin-15 and RANTES chemokine in Parkinson's disease. *Acta Neurol Scand*, 116, 374–9.

Rentzos, M., Nikolaou, C., Andreadou, E., Paraskevas, G. P., Rombos, A., Zoga, M., et al. (2009). Circulating interleukin-10 and interleukin-12 in Parkinson's disease. *Acta Neurol Scand*, 119, 332–7.

Reynolds, A., Laurie, C., Mosley, R. L., & Gendelman, H. E. (2007a). Oxidative stress and the pathogenesis of neurodegenerative disorders. *International Review of Neurobiology*, 82, 297–325.

Reynolds, A. D., Banerjee, R., Liu, J., Gendelman, H. E., & Mosley, R. L. (2007b). Neuroprotective activities of CD4+CD25+ regulatory T cells in an animal model of Parkinson's disease. *Journal of Leukocyte Biology*, 82, 1083–1094.

Reynolds, A. D., Stone, D. K., Hutter, J. A., Benner, E. J., MOSLEY, R. L. & Gendelman, H. E. (2010). Regulatory T cells attenuate th17 cell-mediated nigrostriatal dopaminergic neurodegeneration in a model of Parkinson's disease. *Journal of Immunology*, 184, 2261–2271.

Reynolds, A. D., Stone, D. K., Mosley, R. L., & Gendelman, H. E. (2009). Proteomic studies of nitrated alpha-synuclein microglia regulation by CD4+CD25+ T cells. *Journal of Proteome Research*, 8, 3497–3511.

Riol-Blanco, L., Lazarevic, V., Awasthi, A., Mitsdoerffer, M., Wilson, B. S., Croxford, A., et al. (2010). IL-23 receptor regulates unconventional IL-17-producing T cells that control bacterial infections. *J Immunol*, 184, 1710–20.

Robinson Agramonte, M., Dorta-Contreras, A. J., & Lorigados Pedre, L. (2001). [Immune events in central nervous system of early and late onset Alzheimer's disease patients]. *Rev Neurol*, 32, 901–4.

Rock, K. L. & Goldberg, A. L. (1999). Degradation of cell proteins and the generation of MHC class I-presented peptides. *Annu Rev Immunol*, 17, 739–79.

Rcok, R. B., Gekker, G., Hu, S., Sheng, W. S., Cheeran, M., Lokensgard, J. R., et al. (2004). Role of microglia in central nervous system infections. *Clinical Microbiology Reviews*, 17, 942–64.

Rogers, J., Luber-Narod, J., Styren, S. D., & Civin, W. H. (1988). Expression of immune system-associated antigens by cells of the human central nervous system: Relationship to the pathology of Alzheimer's disease. *Neurobiol Aging*, 9, 339–49.

Rose, R. W., Vorobyeva, A. G., Skipworth, J. D., Nicolas, E., & Rall, G. F. (2007). Altered levels of STAT1 and STAT3 influence the neuronal response to interferon gamma. *J Neuroimmunol*, 192, 145–56.

Royal, W., 3rd, Mia, Y., Li, H., & Naunton, K. (2009). Peripheral blood regulatory T cell measurements correlate with serum vitamin D levels in patients with multiple sclerosis. *Journal of Neuroimmunology*, 213, 135–141.

Sadagopal, S., Lorey, S. L., Barnett, L., Basham, R., Lebo, L., Erdem, H., et al. (2008). Enhancement of human immunodeficiency virus (HIV)-specific CD8+ T cells in cerebrospinal fluid compared to those in blood among antiretroviral therapy-naive HIV-positive subjects. *J Virol*, 82, 10418–28.

Sakaguchi, S. (2004). Naturally arising CD4+ regulatory t cells for immunologic self-tolerance and negative control of immune responses. *Annual Review of Immunology*, 22, 531–562.

Sakaguchi, S., Hori, S., Fukui, Y., Sasazuki, T., Sakaguchi, N., & Takahashi, T. (2003). Thymic generation and selection of CD25+CD4+ regulatory T cells: Implications of their broad repertoire and high self-reactivity for the maintenance of immunological self-tolerance. *Novartis Foundation Symposium*, 252, 6–16; discussion 16–23, 106–14.

Sakaguchi, S., Sakaguchi, N., Asano, M., Itoh, M., & Toda, M. (1995). Immunologic self-tolerance maintained by activated T cells expressing IL-2 receptor alpha-chains (CD25). Breakdown of a single mechanism of self-tolerance causes various autoimmune diseases. *Journal of Immunology*, 155, 1151–1164.

Salcedo, M., Momburg, F., Hammerling, G. J., & Ljunggren, H. G. (1994). Resistance to natural killer cell lysis conferred by TAP1/2 genes in human antigen-processing mutant cells. *J Immunol*, 152, 1702–8.

Saouaf, S. J., Li, B., Zhang, G., Shen, Y., Furuuchi, N., Hancock, W. W., et al. (2009). Deacetylase inhibition increases regulatory T cell function and decreases incidence and severity of collagen-induced arthritis. *Experimental and Molecular Pathology*, 87, 99–104.

Schindowski, K., Eckert, A., Peters, J., Gorriz, C., Schramm, U., Weinandi, T., et al. (2007). Increased T-cell reactivity and elevated levels of CD8+ memory T-cells in Alzheimer's disease-patients and T-cell hyporeactivity in an Alzheimer's disease-mouse model: Implications for immunotherapy. *Neuromolecular Med*, 9, 340–54.

Schmidt, M., Hanna, J., Elsasser, S., & Finley, D. (2005). Proteasome-associated proteins: Regulation of a proteolytic machine. *Biol Chem*, 386, 725–37.

Selkoe, D. J. (1998). The cell biology of beta-amyloid precursor protein and presenilin in Alzheimer's disease. *Trends Cell Biol*, 8, 447–53.

Selkoe, D. J. 2001. Alzheimer's disease results from the cerebral accumulation and cytotoxicity of amyloid beta-protein. *J Alzheimers Dis*, 3, 75–80.

Sharpless, N. E., O'Brien, W. A., Verdin, E., Kufta, C. V., Chen, I. S., & Dubois-Dalcq, M. (1992). Human immunodeficiency virus type 1 tropism for brain microglial cells is determined by a region of the env glycoprotein that also controls macrophage tropism. *Journal of Virology*, 66, 2588–2593.

Shevach, E. M. & Rosenthal, A. S. (1973). Function of macrophages in antigen recognition by guinea pig T lymphocytes. II. Role of the macrophage in the regulation of genetic control of the immune response. *J Exp Med*, 138, 1213–29.

Shieh, T. M., Carter, D. L., Blosser, R. L., Mankowski, J. L., Zink, M. C., & Clements, J. E. (2001). Functional analyses of natural killer cells in macaques infected with neurovirulent simian immunodeficiency virus. *J Neurovirol*, 7, 11–24.

Sigal, L. J., Crotty, S., Andino, R., & Rock, K. L. (1999). Cytotoxic T-cell immunity to virus-infected non-haematopoietic cells requires presentation of exogenous antigen. *Nature*, 398, 77–80.

Sisodia, S. S. (2002). Biomedicine. A cargo receptor mystery APParently solved? *Science*, 295, 805–7.

Smith, C., Farrah, T., & Goodwin, R. (1994). The TNF receptor superfamily of cellular and viral proteins: Activation, costimulation, and death. *Cell*, 76, 959–962.

Sopper, S., Sauer, U., Hemm, S., Demuth, M., Muller, J., Stahl-Hennig, C., et al. (1998). Protective role of the virus-specific immune response for development of severe neurologic signs in simian immunodeficiency virus-infected macaques. *J Virol*, 72, 9940–7.

Spillantini, M. G., Crowther, R. A., Jakes, R., Hasegawa, M., & Goedert, M. (1998). alpha-Synuclein in filamentous inclusions of Lewy bodies from Parkinson's disease and dementia with lewy bodies. *Proc Natl Acad Sci USA*, 95, 6469–6473.

Spillantini, M. G., Schmidt, M. L., Lee, V. M., Trojanowski, J. Q., Jakes, R., & Goedert, M. (1997). Alpha-synuclein in Lewy bodies. *Nature*, 388, 839–840.

Spudich, S. S., Nilsson, A. C., Lollo, N. D., Liegler, T. J., Petropoulos, C. J., Deeks, S. G., et al. (2005). Cerebrospinal fluid HIV infection and pleocytosis: Relation to systemic infection and antiretroviral treatment. *BMC Infect Dis*, 5, 98.

Staal, J. A., Dickson, T. C., Chung, R. S., & Vickers, J. C. (2009). Disruption of the ubiquitin proteasome system following axonal stretch injury accelerates progression to secondary axotomy. *J Neurotrauma*, 26, 781–8.

Tanaka, K. & Kasahara, M. (1998). The MHC class I ligand-generating system: Roles of immunoproteasomes and the interferon-gamma-inducible proteasome activator PA28. *Immunol Rev*, 163, 161–76.

Tao, R., De Zoeten, E. F., Ozkaynak, E., Wang, L., Li, B., Greene, M. I., et al. (2007). Histone deacetylase inhibitors and transplantation. *Current Opinion in Immunology*, 19, 589–595.

Togo, T., Akiyama, H., Iseki, E., Kondo, H., Ikeda, K., Kato, M., et al. (2002). Occurrence of T cells in the brain of Alzheimer's disease and other neurological diseases. *J Neuroimmunol*, 124, 83–92.

Tran, P. B. & Miller, R. J. (2005). HIV-1, chemokines and neurogenesis. *Neurotox Res*, 8, 149–58.

Trieb, K., Ransmayr, G., Sgonc, R., Lassmann, H., & Grubeck-Loebenstein, B. (1996). APP peptides stimulate lymphocyte proliferation in normals, but not in patients with Alzheimer's disease. *Neurobiol Aging*, 17, 541–7.

Uversky, V. N., Yamin, G., Munishkina, L. A., Karymov, M. A., Millet, I. S., Doniach, S., et al. (2005). Effects of nitration on the structure and aggregation of alpha-synuclein. *Brain Res Mol Brain Res*, 134, 84–102.

Vandenbark, A. A., Huan, J., Agotsch, M., La Tocha, D., Goelz, S., Offner, H., et al. (2009). Interferon-beta-1a treatment increases CD56bright natural killer cells and CD4+CD25+ Foxp3 expression in subjects with multiple sclerosis. *Journal of Neuroimmunology*, 215, 125–128.

Venigalla, R. K., Tretter, T., Krienke, S., Max, R., Eckstein, V., Blank, N., et al. (2008). Reduced CD4+,CD25- T cell sensitivity to the suppressive function of CD4+,CD25high,CD127 -/low regulatory T cells in patients with active systemic lupus erythematosus. *Arthritis and Rheumatism*, 58, 2120–2130.

Venken, K., Hellings, N., Broekmans, T., Hensen, K., Rummens, J. L., & Stinissen, P. (2008a). Natural naive CD4+CD25+CD127 low regulatory T cell (Treg) development and function are disturbed in multiple sclerosis patients: Recovery of memory Treg homeostasis during disease progression. *Journal of Immunology*, 180, 6411–6420.

Venken, K., Hellings, N., Thewissen, M., Somers, V., Hensen, K., Rummens, J.-L., et al. (2008b). Compromised CD4+ CD25high regulatory T-cell function in patients with relapsing-remitting multiple sclerosis is correlated with a reduced frequency of FOXP3-positive cells and reduced FOXP3 expression at the single-cell level. *Immunology*, 123, 79–89.

Von Strauss, E., Viitanen, M., De Ronchi, D., Winblad, B., & Fratiglioni, L. (1999). Aging and the occurrence of dementia: Findings from a population-based cohort with a large sample of nonagenarians. *Arch Neurol*, 56, 587–92.

Wahl, S. M., Swisher, J., McCartney-Francis, N., & Chen, W. (2004). TGF-beta: The perpetrator of immune suppression by regulatory T cells and suicidal T cells. *Journal of Leukocyte Biology*, 76, 15–24.

Weiner, H. L. (2008). A shift from adaptive to innate immunity: A potential mechanism of disease progression in multiple sclerosis. *J Neurol*, 255 Suppl 1, 3–11.

Whatley, B. R., Li, L., & Chin, L. S. (2008). The ubiquitin-proteasome system in spongiform degenerative disorders. *Biochim Biophys Acta*, 1782, 700–12.

Wong, D., Prameya, R., & Dorovini-Zis, K. (1999). In vitro adhesion and migration of T lymphocytes across monolayers of human brain microvessel endothelial cells: Regulation by ICAM-1, VCAM-1, E-selectin and PECAM-1. *J Neuropathol Exp Neurol*, 58, 138–52.

Wong, G. H., Bartlett, P. F., Clark-Lewis, I., Battye, F., & Schrader, J. W. (1984). Inducible expression of H-2 and Ia antigens on brain cells. *Nature*, 310, 688–91.

Xu, J. & Ikezu, T. (2009). The comorbidity of HIV-associated neurocognitive disorders and Alzheimer's disease: A foreseeable medical challenge in post-HAART era. *J Neuroimmune Pharmacol*, 4, 200–12.

Xue, K., Zhou, Y., Xiong, S., Xiong, W., & Tang, T. (2007). Analysis of CD4+ CD25+ regulatory T cells and Foxp3 mRNA in the peripheral blood of patients with asthma. *Journal of Huazhong University of Science and Technology. Medical Sciences = Hua zhong ke ji da xue xue bao.Yi xue Ying De wen ban = Huazhong keji daxue xuebao. Yixue Yingdewen ban, 27,* 31–33.

Yadav, A. & Collman, R. G. (2009). CNS inflammation and macrophage/microglial biology associated with HIV-1 infection. *J Neuroimmune Pharmacol, 4,* 430–47.

Yamamoto, M., Kiyota, T., Horiba, M., Buescher, J. L., Walsh, S. M., Gendelman, H. E., et al. (2007). Interferon-gamma and tumor necrosis factor-alpha regulate amyloid-beta plaque deposition and beta-secretase expression in Swedish mutant APP transgenic mice. *Am J Pathol, 170,* 680–92.

Yang, J., Tugal, D., & Reiss, C. S. (2006). The role of the proteasome-ubiquitin pathway in regulation of the IFN-gamma mediated anti-VSV response in neurons. *J Neuroimmunol, 181,* 34–45.

Yeager, M. P., Deleo, J. A., Hoopes, P. J., Hartov, A., Hildebrandt, L., & Hickey, W. F. (2000). Trauma and inflammation modulate lymphocyte localization in vivo: Quantitation of tissue entry and retention using indium-111-labeled lymphocytes. *Crit Care Med, 28,* 1477–82.

Yilmaz, A., Fuchs, D., Hagberg, L., Nillroth, U., Stahle, L., Svensson, J. O., et al. (2006). Cerebrospinal fluid HIV-1 RNA, intrathecal immunoactivation, and drug concentrations after treatment with a combination of saquinavir, nelfinavir, and two nucleoside analogues: The M61022 study. *BMC Infect Dis, 6,* 63.

Yokoyama, A. (1999). Natural killer cells. In E., P. W. (ed.) *Fundamental immunology.* 4th ed. Philadelphia: Lippincott-Raven.

York, I. A., Goldberg, A. L., Mo, X. Y., & Rock, K. L. (1999). Proteolysis and class I major histocompatibility complex antigen presentation. *Immunol Rev, 172,* 49–66.

Zhang, W., Wang, T., Pei, Z., Miller, D. S., Wu, X., Block, M. L., et al. (2005). Aggregated alpha-synuclein activates microglia: A process leading to disease progression in Parkinson's disease. *FASEB J, 19,* 533–42.

Zhao, Z., Fux, B., Goodwin, M., Dunay, I. R., Strong, D., Miller, B. C., et al. (2008). Autophagosome-independent essential function for the autophagy protein Atg5 in cellular immunity to intracellular pathogens. *Cell Host Microbe, 4,* 458–69.

Zheng, S. G., Wang, J., & Horwitz, D. A. (2008). Cutting edge: Foxp3+CD4+CD25+ regulatory T cells induced by IL-2 and TGF-beta are resistant to Th17 conversion by IL-6. *Journal of Immunology, 180,* 7112–7116.

Zheng, S. G., Wang, J., Wang, P., Gray, J. D., & Horwitz, D. A. (2007). IL-2 is essential for TGF-beta to convert naive CD4+CD25- cells to CD25+Foxp3+ regulatory T cells and for expansion of these cells. *Journal of Immunology, 178,* 2018–2027.

Zinkernagel, R. M. & Doherty, P. C. (1974). Restriction of in vitro T cell-mediated cytotoxicity in lymphocytic choriomeningitis within a syngeneic or semiallogeneic system. *Nature, 248,* 701–2.

Zinkernagel, R. M. & Doherty, P. C. (1979). MHC-restricted cytotoxic T cells: Studies on the biological role of polymorphic major transplantation antigens determining T-cell restriction-specificity, function, and responsiveness. *Adv Immunol, 27,* 51–177.

2.5

VACCINES

Max V. Kuenstling, Eric J. Benner, and R. Lee Mosley

The ultimate goal of vaccination is to deliver effective immunity that, following microbial exposure, either prevents infection or allows rapid clearance of infected cells. However, developing an effective vaccine for HIV-1 is fraught with difficulties. A major challenge is the speed with which HIV-1 incorporates its genomic information into host DNA in the form of a relatively inaccessible provirus. Other challenges include the inability of vaccines to elicit adequate neutralizing antibodies; difficulties in finding adequate small-animal models for vaccine research; and the threat that an otherwise-effective vaccine would, by stimulating an immune response in the brain, itself exacerbates the inflammatory response. The latter appears to play a central role in the neuropathogenesis of HIV-1 infection. This chapter aims to provide an understanding of the challenges that have impeded the development of a successful HIV vaccine, and to describe some potentially effective strategies that may ultimately provide vaccine protection. As part of the presentation, the results of clinical vaccine trials are discussed.

THE SEARCH FOR AN HIV-1 VACCINE: RAISON D'ETRE

HIV-1-COMPROMISED IMMUNE SYSTEM

The global scale of the human immunodeficiency virus (HIV) pandemic has warranted an urgent need to develop an effective vaccine. The current repertoire of infectious disease vaccines, most of which were developed during the latter half of the 20th century and directed against a number of viral pathogens, have played a major role in eradicating life-threatening diseases, especially for children, limiting morbidity, and extending lifetimes among most of the world's population. Such vaccines have provided exceptional improvements in health with respect to infectious diseases that ravaged large populations during epidemics and pandemics. Certainly, vaccinated individuals are not only protected from the consequences of infection, but also the incidence of transmission is drastically reduced, thus diminishing the possibility of epidemic spread.

The ultimate goal of vaccination is to deliver effective immunity that, under conditions of exposure, either prevents further infection or allows rapid clearance of infected cells. However, this objective, which is seen by some as the only solution, is fraught with pitfalls, especially for HIV-1-infected individuals. Challenges that preclude efficacious vaccine

strategies include the extensive diversity of the viral sequences among viral clades, multiple variants within the same clade, and some variants within different tissue reservoirs in the same individual. Indeed, accumulated evidence of viral persistence suggests that viral reservoirs established soon after initial infection by HIV-1 may be sufficient to thwart efficacious therapeutic vaccination. Although, whereas no current prophylactic vaccine for other viral pathogens has been shown to fully prevent primary infection, most efficacious vaccines diminish viral replication and dissemination below the threshold of clinical disease until an adequate memory immune response is mounted. The speed and efficiency by which HIV-1 incorporates into the genome and establishes latency present a huge obstacle that vaccine-induced immune responses must surmount. The inability to elicit robust, reactive neutralizing antibodies in humans and the lack of animal models (especially smaller animal models) that effectively translate to human disease, further slow vaccine progress. Thus, a more realistic goal for HIV-1 vaccine development may be to lessen the initial viremia and maintain low viral loads that prevent progression to acquired immune deficiency syndrome (AIDS), as well as prevent viral transmission.

Through the advent of antiretroviral therapy (ART), the number of HIV-infected individuals progressing towards AIDS has diminished. While ART decreases plasma and tissue levels of virus below clinical detection, depots of virus remain contained within cellular reservoirs. Many cell sources from numerous anatomical sites have been identified as HIV-1 reservoirs (Blankson, Persaud, & Siliciano, 2002; Pierson, McArthur, & Siliciano, 2000). CD4$^+$ T cells represent a primary latent reservoir. Although activated CD4$^+$ T cells are preferentially infected by HIV-1 (Margolick et al., 1987) with subsequent rapid progression through the viral life cycle, many are eliminated either by viral-induced cytotoxicity or by various host immune mechanisms. However, viruses within activated CD4$^+$ T cells which survive infection and clearance and revert to memory T cells, attain a more stable form of latency that establishes an integrated form of the pro-virus in a potentially long-lived cell (Chun et al., 1997; Chun et al., 1995). Indeed, the majority of CD4$^+$ T cells from which integrated HIV-1 can be detected are memory T cells that express CD62L and CD45RO (Chun et al., 1997; Ostrowski et al., 1999; Pierson et al., 2000; Schnittman et al., 1990; Sleasman et al., 1996). HIV-1 gene expression and progeny virus production are regulated by the HIV-1 long terminal repeat (LTR), which in turn is regulated by HIV-1 tat and T cell activation factors that are typically downregulated in memory T cells. HIV-1 is thus restricted by the host until reactivation occurs in response to antigen (Duh et al., 1989; Nabel & Baltimore, 1987). Additionally, naïve CD4$^+$ T cells also harbor latent HIV-1 (Blaak et al., 2000; Ostrowski et al., 1999), although this population upon activation produces significantly less virus than memory CD4$^+$ T cells (Ostrowski et al., 1999). Nonetheless, the total resting CD4$^+$ T cell population represents a significant reservoir for HIV-1, the extent of which has come to realization with the advent of ART. The half-life of this reservoir in patients on ART is prolonged and has been estimated at > 44 months (Finzi et al., 1999; Siliciano et al., 2003). The finding that the number of latently infected cells after prolonged ART was indistinguishable from those before therapy suggests that the reservoir(s) of HIV continues to evade therapy, and thus exists for extended periods, perhaps for more than 5 years (Blankson, Persaud, & Siliciano, 2002). The resting CD4$^+$ T cells, particularly memory T cells, containing integrated HIV-1 comprise the ideal viral reservoir. Studies show that discontinuation of ART correlates with virus reemergence throughout the body from CD4$^+$ T cell reservoirs (Joos et al., 2008), thus underscoring the need for a vaccine to interdict infection before reservoir formation.

A specific subset of CD4$^+$ T cells has come to light in recent years, which may also play a role in HIV-1 infection. Regulatory T cells (Tregs), characterized as CD4$^+$CD25^{hi}CD127^{lo}FoxP3$^+$, play a large role in maintaining homeostasis of the immune system, primarily via regulation of effector T cell (Teff) activation (Curotto de Lafaille & Lafaille, 2009). While their primary role is to prevent autoimmunity via peripheral tolerance to self antigens, Tregs also regulate inflammation to reduce potential damage done if inflammatory responses towards infectious agents go unchecked (Vignali, Collison, & Workman, 2008). Initially, the susceptibility of Tregs to HIV-1 infection was questioned (Chase et al., 2008; Dunham et al., 2008; Tran et al., 2008). However, more recent findings showed that Tregs are susceptible to HIV-1 infection, but susceptibility varies depending on host factors and viral strain (Moreno-Fernandez et al., 2009). During infection, conventional CD4$^+$ T cell numbers are reduced during the early acute phase and slowly decrease during the chronic phase, which if left unchecked leads to increased risk of infection and AIDS onset (Mehandru et al., 2004). Conversely, Tregs appear to follow a different distribution pattern that shows an initial increase in Treg numbers during early infection, followed by a substantial decrease in circulating Tregs during chronic infection (Cao et al., 2009; Jiao et al., 2009). In the acute phase, increased Treg levels potentially could suppress activation of CD4$^+$ T cells as well as diminish function of antiviral CD8$^+$ cytotoxic T cells, thereby preventing effective virus clearance and permitting a more persistent infection (Kinter et al., 2007). Gradual decline in Treg numbers during chronic infection would reduce Treg-mediated immunosuppression, thereby leading to increased immune activation and disease progression (Prendergast et al., 2010). Chronic immune activation via the loss of Treg

numbers eventually leads to a decline of CD4$^+$ T cells (Eggena et al., 2005), but may boost disease progression by facilitating increased immune activation, viremia, and further CD4$^+$ decline due to cytopathology. These findings are supported from elite suppressors (untreated HIV-1-infected individuals that have viral loads below detectable levels and normal CD4$^+$ T cell counts) who maintain high levels of Tregs, whereas Tregs are typically depleted in ART-treated patients (Chase et al., 2008). A recent study in asymptomatic patients indicated that Teffs are more sensitive to Treg-mediated suppression during HIV-1 infection, thus compensating for reduced Treg frequencies, and suggests that elevated Treg-induced suppression might be a natural host response to fight chronic viral infection (Thorborn et al., 2010). In relation to HIV-1 vaccine research, a recent trial showed a therapeutic vaccine provided slight increases in Treg number and substantial increases in HIV-specific Treg suppression after immunization (Macatangay et al., 2010), suggesting that the role of vaccine-induced effects on Treg number and function should be of considerable interest in future HIV-1 vaccine strategies.

HIV-1-infected monocytes and macrophages represent another significant and more long-lived HIV-1 reservoir. Although rarer than infected CD4$^+$ T lymphocytes in lymphoid tissues (Chun et al., 1997), infected macrophages have long been appreciated as sources of infectious virus from many tissues and as a reservoir (Koenig et al., 1986; McElrath, Pruett, & Cohn, 1989; Meltzer et al., 1990; Tschachler et al., 1987). Monocytes, the circulating precursors of tissue macrophages, also express low levels of CD4 and co-receptors necessary for infection, but were thought limited in their abilities to allow completion of the viral life cycle due to their short half-life (measured as a few days) and the requirement for cell differentiation that is necessary prior to productive viral replication (Finzi & Siliciano, 1998; Schnittman et al., 1989). However, more rigorous inspection of virus-monocyte interactions has shown that blood monocytes express low amounts of viral nucleic acids and proteins, and produce replication competent progeny virus (Innocenti et al., 1992; Lambotte et al., 2000; Sharkey et al., 2000; Sonza et al., 2001; Williams et al., 2001; Zhu, 2000). With T cells, the viral replication cycle is very rapid and typically cytopathic; however, macrophages are able to survive for long periods and develop vacuoles containing large amounts of viral particles (Sharova et al., 2005). HIV-infected macrophages can enter the central nervous system (CNS) and establish viral reservoirs that are most likely culpable for disorders observed in neuroAIDS (Gonzalez-Scarano & Martin-Garcia, 2005).

Another reservoir within secondary lymphoid tissue is contained within the follicular dendritic cells (FDC). Reports demonstrate that FDC can retain for up to 9 months, greater than 10^8 copies of HIV-1 per gram of tissue, and that association with trapped, concentrated HIV-1 within the germinal center affects viral dissemination. Moreover, HIV-1-infected FDC have been shown to induce the upregulation of the viral co-receptor CXCR4 by CD4$^+$CD57$^+$ T cells through cell contact-dependent mechanisms. These interactions facilitate binding and entry of HIV-1 CXCR4-trophic strains into CD4$^+$ T cells within the surrounding germinal center (Burton et al., 1997; Cavert et al., 1997; Embretson et al., 1993; Estes et al., 2002; Fox et al., 1991; Pantaleo et al., 1993; Racz, 1988; Racz et al., 1990; Smith et al., 2001). FDC can effectively activate HIV-1 replication in latent-infected monocytes and macrophages via juxtracrine signaling through the interaction of P-selectin and the P-selectin glycoprotein ligand 1 (Ohba et al., 2009). In addition, FDC co-cultured with HIV-infected CD4+ T cells can induce twofold increases in the virus transcription rates and fourfold more virus than T cells cultured in the absence of FDC; possibly acting via a TNF-α-mediated mechanism (Thacker et al. 2009). Thus, not only do FDC provide a reservoir for HIV, they also aid in increasing viral production to create a microenvironment sufficient to amplify the expression and transmission of HIV-1 by infected cells.

Although distinct from FDC, blood dendritic cells (DC), including both plasmacytoid (pDC) and myeloid (mDC) cell types, also can serve as reservoirs of HIV-1 as evidenced by their ability to transmit bound HIV-1 to CD4+ T cells during antigen presentation and T cell activation (Cameron et al., 1992; Frankel et al., 1996; Pope et al., 1994). In fact, under conditions of rapid turnover, HIV-1 replication in T cells was observed in the presence of immature DC that express the cellular lectin, DC-specific intracellular adhesion molecule 3 [ICAM-3]-grabbing nonintegrin (DC-SIGN). Transfer of virus from DC to lymphocytes is presumed via lectin-ICAM-3 interactions of virus presenting DC and CD4+ T cells (Geijtenbeek et al., 2000; Gummuluru, KewalRamani, & Emerman, 2002). Interestingly, whereas only CCR5-tropic viral strains can replicate in macrophages, infection and replication by CCR5- and CXCR4-trophic viral strains are permissive in immature DC, but not in LPS-stimulated and matured DC. Moreover, viral infection in DC was shown to be enhanced in the presence of activated T cells, demonstrating the capacity of immature DC to function as an HIV-1 reservoir (MacDougall et al., 2002).

During HIV-1 infection, circulating pDC produce high levels of interferon alpha (IFN-α) even though the number of pDC decreases during infection (Lehmann et al., 2010). IFN-α is associated with HIV-1 disease progression and is thought to function by inhibition of cell proliferation and immune response activation. Therefore, increased production and secretion of IFN-α may have a large effect on nearby CD4+ T cells, preventing their differentiation and decreasing their immune function, thereby leading to higher disease pathogenesis and shorter progression to AIDS. Most recently, the importance of DC as initiators of immunity and the mechanism by which HIV-1 infection interferes with immune activation was realized. As natural killer T cells (NKT) interact with surface CD1d expressed by DC, which allow activation of both cell types to initiate an immune response, HIV-1 infection reduces or inhibits CD1d expression by DC, thus preventing DC interaction and activation of NKT cells (Moll et al., 2010) and demonstrating another mechanism by which HIV-1 evades cellular immune responses.

Other cell types that support HIV-1 replication have also been suggested. Several studies have demonstrated that CD8+ T cells provide another reservoir of HIV-1, indicating a much broader tropism than previously described (Chun et al., 2002; Flamand et al., 1998; Imlach et al., 2001; Kitchen et al., 1998; Kitchen et al., 2002; Livingstone et al., 1996; Mercure, Phaneuf, & Wainberg, 1993; Saha et al., 2001; Yang et al., 1998). In one study, CD8+ T cells accounted for up to 97% of the proviral load among peripheral blood mononuclear cells from late-stage patients (< 200 CD4+ T cells/μl) (Livingstone et al., 1996). The mechanism by which CD8+ T cells become susceptible to HIV-1 infection is thought to be via activation-induced upregulation of surface CD4 and co-receptors, allowing a permissive state for infection, integration, and viral production (Flamand et al., 1998; Kitchen et al., 1998; Yang et al., 1998). The frequency of infection in CD8+ T cells is estimated to include 30–1400 proviral copies per 10^6 CD8+CD45RA+ T cells and 70–260 copies per 10^6 CD8+CD45RO+ T cells (Imlach et al., 2001). Importantly, viruses produced from CD8+ T cells are capable of infecting both CD4+ and CD8+ T cells (Saha et al., 2001).

Evidence that infectious virions isolated from B cells strongly implicated those cells as another potential HIV-1 reservoir (Fritsch et al., 1998; Gras et al., 1993; Lapointe, Lemieux, & Darveau, 1996; Moir et al., 1999). However, findings that the infectious virions were only strongly bound to surface of B cells by CD21 and immune complexes, and could be released by protease treatment, suggested a more limited role for B cells as long-term reservoirs for infectious viral progeny (Jakubik et al., 2000; Moir et al., 2000). Nevertheless, evidence that B cell lines and activated B cells can be infected with HIV-1 (De Silva et al., 2001; Titti et al., 2002), and that viral variants from B and T cells of peripheral blood and lymph nodes from chronically infected patients that do not differ significantly by genetic sequence analysis suggest that viremia characteristic of late stage HIV disease originates from cells other than CD4+ T cells (Malaspina et al., 2002).

A recent area of interest involves infection of mucosal tissues and their associated reservoirs. The mucosa represents one of the more common sites of initial HIV-1 infection, during which viral particles quickly move to the lamina propria and likely form numerous reservoirs of infected cells. Thus, the mucosa provides a rich source of lymphocytes, dendritic cells, and macrophages within the genitourinary and gastrointestinal tracts that are infected early and allow rapid HIV-1 replication (Smith et al., 2003). Preventing infection by any vaccine approach necessitates the consideration not only of virus complexities, but also unique host cell and reservoir interactions. To efficiently eliminate HIV-1 infection, the potent suppression of viral replication within cellular compartments wherein the virus enters early and resides is vital. To thwart the initial infection and inhibit HIV-1 reservoir formation, while daunting, would provide the most efficacious vaccine strategy. Thus, vaccine studies should focus on preventing the development of HIV-1 reservoirs within the mucosal immune system early in the course of infection.

HIV VACCINE STRATEGIES

Current vaccine strategies for HIV-1 infection and progression into AIDS are numerous and varied. Initially, traditional vaccine strategies were based primarily on those successfully utilized for other viral vaccines. These traditional strategies included using inactivated virus for influenza; live attenuated viruses for polio, measles, and smallpox; and more recently, recombinant protein strategies for hepatitis B. However, traditional strategies used to derive most successful viral vaccines have yet to provide adequate protective immunity to HIV-1.

While some strategies using inactivated or attenuated virus have been tested in simian immunodeficiency virus (SIV)-infected nonhuman primates, little hope is rendered that a vaccine of this type could provide efficient, long-lasting protection in humans (Lifson et al., 2004). Moreover, use of a live-attenuated virus with a potential for reversion after vaccine administration, may possess the capacity to become infectious and eventually progress to AIDS. One study called into question the safety of using attenuated HIV-1 after finding faltering T cell counts and disease progression in a number of vaccinated patients. A group of eight subjects were infected via a blood sample containing a strain of HIV-1 with a deleted *nef* gene. The subjects were initially deemed free of disease, but ultimately progressed to AIDS (Learmont et al., 1999). Similar examples have dampened vaccine strategies utilizing attenuated virus and are not currently pursued with great enthusiasm.

Initial vaccine attempts using traditional strategies that have failed have not been in vain since data have directed a reexamination of problems leading to the formulation of novel approaches. For instance, studies of live virions and chemically attenuated virions begot current studies focused on noninfectious virus-like particles. These particles are safer than inactivated virus and are easier to manipulate (Zhang et al., 2010). Similarly, currently used naked DNA or plasmid-based strategies are safer and more useful than attenuated viruses. While DNA vaccines in combination with live recombinant vaccines have not yielded efficacious prophylaxis, they may provide control over viral replication and load, decrease the chance of viral transmission, and provide a competent therapeutic strategy (Sauter, Rahman, & Muralidhar, 2005). Thus, with the emergence of newer technologies, better targeted and more efficacious vaccine strategies may be developed that can better thwart the HIV-1 pandemic.

Initial HIV-1 vaccine strategies favored the induction of humoral immune responses as protective measures characterized by the presence of neutralizing antibodies, in large measure, within the V3 loop of the viral envelope. The first phase I trials began in 1987, less than 5 years after the virus identification protocol, and utilized a gp160 recombinant protein (Dolin et al., 1991). This strategy proved to be well-tolerated and safe, and after administration of the third and fourth doses, resulted in a high conversion rate of antibody response as determined by Western blot analysis. Additionally, serum-neutralizing activity and complement-mediated antibody-dependent enhancement of cytotoxicity in some subjects were generated after the fourth dose. Several other protocols that followed also used the envelope gp120 or the full-length gp160 as viral antigens, but were produced in different cell systems (Bojak, Deml, & Wagner, 2002). However, the limiting factor with these strategies was the inability to induce levels of antibodies capable of neutralizing primary and diverse isolates of HIV-1 (Mascola, Louder et al., 1996; Moore et al., 2002). Although no correlation between HIV-1 subtypes and virus neutralization has been shown, cross-clade neutralization has been described (Moore et al., 2002), suggesting the existence of common antibody epitopes, at least among some HIV-1 subtypes. Broad neutralizing capacity represents a pivotal hurdle that must be overcome to achieve an effective HIV-1 vaccine. Interestingly, the first HIV-1 vaccine in phase III clinical trials reflected this concept (Francis et al., 1998). Results from phase I and phase II trials indicated that all recipients developed substantial antibody responses, including neutralizing antibody responses that peaked after a 12-month boost, thus elevating AIDSVAX to phase III trials. The results of the phase III trial, sponsored by vaccine developer VAXGEN (San Francisco, CA) tested the AIDSVAX B/B product or placebo in 3,330 North American and European volunteers that were at high risk of contracting HIV-1. Of the 1,651 volunteers who received the vaccine, only 5.7% contracted HIV, while 5.8% of placebo-vaccinated subjects contracted the virus (Check, 2003). A parallel trial using AIDSVAX B/E, formulated for HIV clades that exist in Asia, showed similar results. Of the 1,017 persons receiving the vaccine, 8.4% acquired HIV-1 infections, while virus was detected in 8.3% of the 1,013 placebo-treated subjects (Pitisuttithum et al., 2006). Although unsuccessful, these trials demonstrated that antibodies directed at gp160 are not efficacious as prophylactic measures for HIV-1 infection and suggested that vaccine strategies targeting other viral products or inducing alternative immune responses may be necessary.

A relevant observation described by many research groups showed an inverse association between the presence of HIV-1-specific CD8+ cytotoxic T lymphocytes (CTL) and the decrease of plasma viral loads in HIV infection (Brander & Walker, 1999). Indeed, a negative correlation was demonstrated between the frequency of CTL and progression to disease in HIV-infected individuals (Klein et al., 1995; Musey et al., 1997). Also, dramatic increases in viral loads were observed in SIV-infected macaques subsequent to depletion of CD8+ T cells, while viral loads coincidentally decreased with the reappearance of CD8+ cells (Jin et al., 1999; Schmitz et al., 1999). These findings strengthen the importance of cell-mediated immunity in the control of HIV-1 infection and disease progression, and redirected vaccine development to utilize live vectors in an attempt to target HIV-1 specific antigens to the MHC class I pathway with more efficient presentation to CD8+ T-lymphocytes. Furthermore, broad cross-reactive CTL recognition has been demonstrated in relation to the CTL epitopes located in very conserved regions of HIV-1 genome among several HIV-1 subtypes (Cao et al., 1997; Ferrari et al., 1997; McAdam et al., 1998), although higher magnitude responses have been described for subtype-specific CTL responses (Cao et al., 2000; Novitsky et al., 2001; Rowland-Jones et al., 1998). Indeed, one study showed positive correlations between polymorphisms in certain residues of the viral amino acid sequence and expression of specific MHC class I molecules (Moore et al., 2002). More recent studies have revealed that CD8+ T cell epitopes are a common and significant factor in the diversity of both SIV and HIV viral sequences, most likely due to viral escape mechanisms (Allen et al., 2005; O'Connor et al., 2004). Moreover, if specific CTL responses were observed in volunteers vaccinated against HIV-1, while only limited neutralizing antibody responses were generated, the likelihood of success may be considerably narrow. This phenomenon was observed when recombinant pox virus vaccines were administered alone in human vaccine trials (Mulligan & Weber, 1999). Considering the relevance of both humoral and cell-mediated immunity for HIV-1 control, more promising vaccine approaches were proposed that used prime-boost regimens with complementary immunogenic profiles and multi-antigen components of selected HIV-1 structural, as well as regulatory, protein-encoding genes. Together, these vaccine approaches aim to amplify the immune response to the virus by inducing multi-specific, long-lasting humoral responses *and* cell-mediated immunity that are able to reduce initial HIV-1 infection and suppress viral loads.

Since the first human trial of an HIV-1 vaccine, over 30 different candidate vaccines have been tested in more than 200 phase I/II/III clinical trials including 170 phase I trials, 16 phase I/II, 15 phase II, and only 3 phase III efficacy trials. Databases and listings for clinical trials of candidate vaccines are maintained at the following sites:

AIDS Vaccine Evaluation Group: (http://scharp.org/public/redbook/protocol/table1.htm);

HIV Vaccine Trials Network: (http://www.hvtn.org/);

HIV/SIV Vaccine Trials Database: (http://www.hiv.lanl.gov/content/vaccine/home.html);

International AIDS Vaccine Initiative (IAVI) Database of AIDS Vaccines in Human Trials: (http://www.iavireport.org/trials-db/Pages/default.aspx);

National Institutes of Health (NIH) Database of Clinical Trials: (http://www.clinicaltrials.gov/ct2/results?term="hiv+ vaccine");

AIDS Vaccine Advocacy Coalition: (http://www.avac.org/trials).

CLINICAL TRIALS OF CANDIDATE HIV-1 VACCINES

ENVELOPE PROTEIN-BASED VACCINE STRATEGIES

Since envelope proteins were perceived as the most prominent target of neutralizing antibodies, early vaccine trial strategies included full-length recombinant HIV-1 *env*-based proteins (Table 2.5.1). In 1987, the first HIV-1 vaccine candidate to undergo phase I clinical trials was initiated by MicroGeneSys (Meriden, CT) using the full-length recombinant *env* gene product, rgp160 (Dolin et al., 1991; Keefer et al., 1994; Kovacs

et al., 1993). Since then, gp120 and gp160 envelope preparations derived from mammalian cells, insect cells, and yeast have been combined with adjuvants, primarily $Al(OH)_3$ and MF59, to enhance neutralizing antibody responses. While all full-length recombinant preparations were found to induce antigen-specific proliferative responses among $CD4^+$ T cells, the highest levels of neutralizing antibodies were induced by Chinese hamster ovary (CHO) cell-derived rgp120 preparations. However, none of the preparations induced high levels of HIV-1 specific CTL (Belshe et al., 1994; Dolin et al., 1991; Graham et al., 1996; Keefer et al., 1996; Stanhope, Clements, & Siliciano, 1993). Although relatively high titers of neutralizing antibodies are attainable with these vaccine preparations, the neutralizing capacity of virus-specific antibodies was restricted primarily to T cell line-adapted viruses and some primary strains of syncytia-inducing strains, while having little capability to neutralize nonsyncytia-inducing strains (Mascola, Snyder et al., 1996). This restriction was associated with the utilization of laboratory-adapted, clade B HIV-1 strains (LAI, MN, and SF-2 for rpg160, and IIIB for rgp120) as sources for recombinant proteins. Three rgp120 preparations from CHO cells (rgp120 SF-2, rgp120 MN, and rgp120 SF-2/CM235) were evaluated in phase II trials. One study, wherein rgp120 SF-2 and rgp120 MN were tested, found that 87% of 241 vaccinated subjects developed neutralizing antibodies that persisted for over 2 years in 59% of the subjects (McElrath et al., 2000). Gp120-specific lymphoproliferation to homologous and heterologous antigens peaked after one boost and also persisted for up to 2 years. Additionally, 54% of vaccinated subjects displayed gp120-specfic recall delayed-type hypersensitivity (DTH) responses 4 years after immunization. Unfortunately, CTL responses were not reported. Two bivalent gp120 vaccine preparations (AIDSVAX gp120 B/B and AIDSVAX gp120 B/E) derived from laboratory clade B strains and a primary clade E isolate entered phase III clinical trials in the United States and Thailand, respectively (Berman et al., 1999). Initial results of one 4-year trial with over 5,000 participants, of which 67% received at least three doses of the AIDSVAX gp120 B/B and 34% received placebo, showed no detectable differences in the percentages of HIV-1 infected individuals among vaccinated (5.8%) and control (5.7%) groups. However, stratification of the participants by race indicated that the percentage of infected participants were significantly less among vaccinated Blacks (2.0%), Asians (3.8%), and other minorities (8.5%), as well as combined minorities (3.7%) compared to placebo treated controls (8.1%, 10.0%, 15.0%, and 9.9%, respectively) (Cohen, 2003). Enthusiasm for this initial analysis diminished after adjustment for subgroup analysis demonstrated that significances between groups disappeared and after the disclosure that infected vaccinated participants had not controlled the virus any better than infected placebo-treated participants (Cohen, 2003). Interestingly, females and Black males had higher levels of HIV-specific antibodies than White males, and molecular analysis of infecting HIV-1 strains indicated substantial differences from the vaccine strain. Although AIDSVAX as a single entity was not protective, a prime-boost strategy combined with another nonefficacious immunogen increased the protective capacity compared with control treatment (*vide infra*, RV144 study) (Rerks-Ngarm et al., 2009).

In addition to recombinant Env variants, the efficacy of several other recombinant viral proteins, such as p24 and Tat, have been evaluated in phase I clinical trials (Cafaro et al., 1999; Martin et al., 1993). Of 16 volunteers receiving p24, 75% demonstrated significant p24-specific proliferative responses with good correlation between proliferation and production of p24-specific antibodies. In infected patients

Table 2.5.1 CLINICAL TRIALS OF ENVELOPE PROTEIN-BASED VACCINE STRATEGIES

TRIAL START	VACCINE CANDIDATE (HIV STRAIN)	ADJUVANT	VACCINE DEVELOPER	TRIAL ID
Envelope Proteins (Phase I Studies)				
1987	gp160 Envelope Protein	Alum	NIH, National Institute of Allergy and Infectious Diseases (NIAID)[1]	87 I-114
1988	VaxSyn gp160 Vaccine, MicroGeneSys	Alum	NIAID	AVEG 003
1990	gp160 Vaccine, Immuno-AG	Alum	NIAID	AVEG 004
1990	VaxSyn gp160 Vaccine, MicroGeneSys	Alum	NIAID	AVEG 003A
1990	VaxSyn gp160 Vaccine, MicroGeneSys	Alum	NIAID	AVEG 003B
1991	Env 2–3	MTP-PE/MF59	NIAID	AVEG 005A/B
1991	Env 2–3	MF59	NIAID	AVEG 005C
1991	gp160 Vaccine, Immuno-AG	Alum	NIAID	AVEG 004B
1991	rgp120 (MN)	Alum	NIAID	AVEG 006X, VEU 006
1991	rgp120/HIV-1 SF-2	MF59 or MTP-PE/MF59	NIAID	AVEG 007A/B
1992	gp160 Vaccine, Immuno-AG	Alum	NIAID	AVEG 004A
1992	rgp120 (MN)	Alum	NIAID	AVEG 009
1992	rgp120/HIV-1 SF-2	MF59	NIAID	AVEG 007C
1993	gp160 Vaccine, Immuno-AG	Alum	NIAID	AVEG 013A
1993	rgp120 (MN)	Alum	NIAID	AVEG 016
1993	rgp120/HIV-1 SF-2	Alum, MPA, liposome-encapsulated MPA, MF59, MTP-PE + MF59, SAF/2, SAF/2 + threonyl MDP	NIAID	AVEG 015
1994	rgp120 (MN)	QS-21, Alum	NIAID	AVEG 016A
1995	gp160 Vaccine, Immuno-AG	Alum	NIAID	AVEG 013B
1995	rgp120 (w61d)	Alum	Merck[2]	MRC V001
1995	rgp120/HIV-1 SF-2	MF59	NIAID	AVEG 024
1996	rgp120 (MN)	QS-21, Alum	NIAID	AVEG 016B
1998	rgp120 (SF-2)	MF59	NIAID	ACTG 233
1999	AIDSVAX B/E/rgp120/HIV-1 SF-2	MF59	NIAID	ACTG 230
1999	rsgp120 (MN)	Alum or QS-21	NIAID	ACTG 279
2000	gp160 Vaccine	Alum	NIAID, Immuno-AG[3], MicroGeneSys[4]	ACTG 221
2000	rgp120 (IIIB/MN/SF-2), Env 2–3	Alum, MF59	NIAID	ACTG 214
2000	rgp120 (MN)	Alum	NIAID	ACTG 235, AVEG 104
2001	gp160 Vaccine	Alum	NIAID, Protein Sciences Co.[5]	ACTG 137
2001	gp160 Vaccine	Alum	NIAID, MicroGeneSys	ACTG 148
2001	rgp120 (MN) + Ritonavir/ Stavudine/Didanosine	Alum	NIAID, Immuno-US[6], Bristol-Myers Squibb[7]	ACTG 246/946

(*Continued*)

Table 2.5.1 (CONTINUED)

TRIAL START	VACCINE CANDIDATE (HIV STRAIN)	ADJUVANT	VACCINE DEVELOPER	TRIAL ID
2001	rgp120 (MN/SF-2)	Alum	NIAID, Genetech[8]	ACTG 218
2002	gp160 Vaccine	Alum	NIAID, MicroGeneSys	ACTG 234
2002	rgp120w61d	AS202A	HIV Vaccine Trials Network (HVTN)[9]	HVTN 041
2003	EnvPro	Alum	St. Jude Children's Research Hospital[10], NIH[11]	EnvPro
2003	gp160 (MN/LAI)	DC-Chol	Agence Nationale de Recherche sur le Sida (ANRS)[12], Sanofi-Pasteur[13]	ANRS VAC 14
2003	rgp120 (MN)	Alum	NIAID, Genetech, GlaxoSmithKline[14]	ACTG 209
Envelope Proteins (Phase II Studies)				
1992	rgp120/HIV-1 SF-2/MN rgp120		NIAID	AVEG 201
1997	AIDSVAX B/B/AIDSVAX B/E	Alum	VaxGen[15]	VAX 002
	F4/AS01	Alum	GlaxoSmithKline	F4/AS01
Envelope Proteins (Phase III Studies)				
1998	AIDSVAX B/B	Alum	VaxGen	VAX 004
1999	AIDSVAX B/E	Alum	VaxGen	VAX 003
Non-Envelope Proteins (Phase I Studies)				
1999	HGP-30	Alum	Cel-Sci[16]	HGP-30 memory responses
2001	HIV p24/MF59 Vaccine	MF59	Chiron[17]	V24P1
2004	LFn-p24	Alum	Walter Reed Army Institute of Research (WRAIR)[18], NIAID	LFn-p24 vaccine
2004	LFn-p24	Alum	U.S. Military HIV Research Program (USMHRP)[19]	RV 151/WRAIR 984
2006	HIV gp140 ZM96	Labile Toxin mutant LTK63	St. George's University of London[20], Richmond Pharmacology Ltd[21], Novartis[22]	C86P1
2007	HIV gp140 ZM96	Alum	St George's University of London	SG06RS02
2009	GTU-MultiHIV B clade vaccine	IL-2, GM-CSF	Medical Research Council[23], Imperial College London[24]	CRO930

Vaccine candidates and corresponding data can be found in the IAVI AIDS Vaccine Trials Database (www.iavireport.org/Trials-db/) and the NIH Clinical Trials Database (www.clinicaltrials.gov)
[1]Bethesda, MD; [2]Whitehouse Station, NJ; [3]Vienna, Austria; [4]Meriden, CT; [5]Meriden, CT; [6]Deerfield, IL; [7]New York, NY; [8]San Francisco, CA; [9]Seattle, WA; [10]Memphis, TN; [11]Bethesda, MD; [12]Paris, France; [13]Bridgewater, NJ; [14]Brentford, Middlesex UK; [15]Brisbane, CA; [16]Vienna, VA; [17]Emeryville, CA; [18]Silver Spring, MD; [19]Rockville, MD; [20]London, UK; [21]London, UK; [22]St. Louis, MO; [23]London, UK; [24]London, UK.

receiving as many as eight injections of recombinant Tat, no untoward clinical side effects were observed and all patients exhibited antibody responses to Tat, while some exhibited increased cell-mediated immunity as evaluated by skin tests for DTH and peripheral blood lymphocyte proliferation (Gringeri et al., 1998). In two trials using p17/p24:Ty virus-like particles (p24-VLP) that produced Gag-specific antibodies, proliferative responses to p17 and p24, as well as Gag-specific CD8+ CTL, levels of serum viral loads did not differ between treated and control groups and did not slow HIV disease progression to AIDS (Klein et al., 1997; Lindenburg et al., 2002). To date, trials involving p24 or Tat have not progressed to phase II.

PEPTIDE-BASED VACCINE STRATEGIES

The promise of enhanced immune responses with greater specificity was the basis for utilization of defined B cell and T cell epitopes from HIV-1 in peptide-based vaccine candidates (Table 2.5.2). Clinical trials of an octamer V3 MN strain-based peptide in alum were conducted by United Biomedical (Hauppauge, NY) in seronegative volunteers (Kelleher et al., 1997). Vaccine dosages ranging from 20–500 μg were delivered at 0, 1, and 6 months. The vaccine was well tolerated without clinical abnormalities and stimulated significant lymphocyte proliferation in 75% of the subjects. Although neutralizing antibodies were also induced in 60–90% of the volunteers, only homologous, laboratory-adapted isolates, but not primary isolates were susceptible to neutralization. Additionally, subcutaneous administration of this vaccine also was found to be safe, but did not result in uniform or robust immunological responses; therefore, this vaccine candidate has not progressed to further trials.

Other clinical trials using multivalent chimeric peptides have been derived from diverse HIV-1 proteins. A lipopeptide vaccine with six peptides from Nef, Gag, and Env proteins was administered to HIV-1-seronegative volunteers in three injections containing 100 µg, 250 µg, or 500 µg of each lipopeptide with or without QS21 adjuvant (Gahery-Segard et al., 2000). This lipopeptide vaccine elicited strong B- and T-cell responses. After two injections, vaccinated individuals developed specific IgG antibodies that recognized Nef and Gag proteins, and

Table 2.5.2 CLINICAL TRIALS OF PEPTIDE-BASED VACCINE STRATEGIES

TRIAL START	VACCINE CANDIDATE (HIV STRAIN)	ADJUVANT	VACCINE DEVELOPER	TRIAL ID
Peptides (Phase I Studies)				
1992	rgp 160 + peptide V3 ANRS VAC 02	Alum	ANRS, Sanofi-Pasteur	ANRS VAC 02
1993	UBI HIV-1 Peptide Immunogen, Multivalent	Alum	NIAID	AVEG 011
1993	UBI HIV-1 Peptide Immunogen, Multivalent	Alum	United Biomedical Inc (UBI)[1]	UBI HIV-1 MN China
1994	UBI HIV-1 Peptide Vaccine, Microparticulate Monovalent	Alum	NIAID	AVEG 017
1994	UBI HIV-1 Peptide Vaccine, Microparticulate Monovalent	Alum	NIAID	AVEG 018
1995	P3C541b Lipopeptide	Alum	NIAID	AVEG 021
1995	UBI HIV-1 Peptide Immunogen, Multivalent	Alum	NIAID	AVEG 023
1996	LIPO-6	QS-21	ANRS	ANRS VAC 04
1996	TAB9	Alum	Instituto de Medicina Tropical[2]	TAB9
1997	gp120 C4-V3	IFA	NIAID	AVEG 020
1998	C4-V3 Polyvalent Peptide Vaccine	IL-12	NIAID	ACTG A5049
1998	LIPO-6	QS-21	ANRS	ANRS VAC 04 bis
1998	MN rgp120/AIDSVAX B/E	QS-21, QS-21/ Alum	NIAID	AVEG 036
1999	C4-V3 Polyvalent Peptide	IFA	NIAID, Lederle-Praxis Biologicals[3]	DATRI 010
1999	gp160 + Hepatitis B Vaccine	Alum	NIAID, Immuno-US	ACTG 205, AVEG 101
1999	MTP-PE, Env 2–3	MF59	NIAID, Biocine[4]	AVEG 103
2000	Dendritic Cells Pulsed with HIV antigens		NIAID	R01AI44628
2001	LPHIV1	Alum	ANRS, Biovector Therapeutics[5]	ANRS VAC 12
2002	EP HIV-1090	Alum	NIAID	IPCP 01
2003	Autologous Dendritic Cell with Synthetic HIV Particles		NIAID	P01AI43664–04
2003	Recombinant HIV-1 Tat protein	Alum	Instituto Superiore di Sanità[6]	ISS T-001
2003	Tat vaccine	Alum	Instituto Superiore di Sanità	ISS P-001
2004	LIPO-6	Alum	ANRS	ANRS VAC 17
2004	LPHIV1	Alum	ANRS	ANRS VAC 16
2004	MEP	RC529-SE or GM-CSF/RC529-SE	NIAID, HVTN, Wyeth[7]	HVTN 056
2005	gp120/Nef Tat Vaccine	AS02A	GlaxoSmithKline	PARC001
2006	EP HIV-1043/EP HIV-1090		NIAID, HVTN, Pharmexa-Epimmune[8]	HVTN 064
2006	Vichrepol	Polyoxidonium	Moscow Institute of Immunology[9]	HVRF-380–131004
2010	PENNVAX™-B, Gag, Pol, Env	IL-12, IL-15	VGX Pharmaceuticals[10]	HIV-001
Peptides (Phase II Studies)				
1993	UBI HIV-1 Peptide Immunogen, Multivalent	Alum	UBI	UBI HIV-1MN octameric - Australia study

(Continued)

Table 2.5.2 (CONTINUED)

TRIAL START	VACCINE CANDIDATE (HIV STRAIN)	ADJUVANT	VACCINE DEVELOPER	TRIAL ID
1999	UBI HIV-1 Peptide Vaccine, Microparticulate Monovalent	Alum	UBI	UBI V106
2004	LIPO-5	Alum	ANRS, Sanofi-Pasteur	ANRS VAC 18
2007	MVA-mBN32 + peptides	Alum	NIH, Bavarian Nordic[11]	HIV-POL-002
2008	Tat protein	Alum	Instituto Superiore di Sanità	ISS T-002

Vaccine candidates and corresponding data can be found in the IAVI AIDS Vaccine Trials Database (www.iavireport.org/Trials-db/) and the NIH Clinical Trials Database (www.clinicaltrials.gov)
[1] Hauppauge, NY; [2]Lisboa, Portugal; [3]West Henrieta, NY; [4]Emeryville, CA; [5]Labege, France; [6]Rome, Italy; [7]Madison, NJ; [8]San Diego, CA; [9]Moscow, Russia; [10]Blue Bell, PA; [11]Kvistgaard, Denmark.

after a second boost, strong helper CD4[+] and cytotoxic CD8[+] T cell responses were also detected; the latter as specific IFN-γ secreting cells that recognized naturally processed viral proteins. Further enhancements to peptide chains or immunization routes could provide a more efficient vehicle for inducing selective immunity against multiple targets. Another lipopeptide vaccine with a mixture of Nef, Gag, and Env was tested on 24 patients at 0, 3, and 6 weeks (Gahery et al., 2006). The 6-week boost produced new antigen-specific CD4[+] and CD8[+] T cell responses in over 70% of patients. Another study testing the safety and efficacy of intramuscular and intradermal routes for the vaccine found no serious adverse affects (Launay et al., 2007). However, while local pain was more common after intramuscular injection, a local inflammatory reaction was observed more often with the intradermal routes; the latter regimen inducing similar HIV-specific T cell responses, while requiring only one-fifth of the intramuscular dose. In a study testing the lipopeptide strategy as a therapeutic vaccine, HIV-infected, ART-treated patients were vaccinated at 0, 3, and 6 weeks and at week 24, followed by discontinuation of ART (Pialoux, Quercia et al., 2008). Of the 21 patients evaluated, 13 resumed ART by 60 weeks after immunization when plasma viral load reached 3×10^4 copies/ml, but 8 patients were still ART-free at 96 weeks. Unfortunately, the absence of a control arm will necessitate a follow-up study for efficacy evaluation.

DNA VACCINE STRATEGIES

Intramuscular or gene-gun delivery of naked or formulated DNA plasmids that imitate a natural viral infection represent a novel immunization strategy to induce both humoral and cellular responses (Donnelly et al., 1997); therefore, numerous vaccine strategies utilize both DNA alone or are combined with other strategies (Table 2.5.3). After delivery, DNA is taken up and expressed by somatic and/or immune cells. Expressed peptides are either released from cells to initiate immune responses or degraded by the proteasome and shuttled into the class I pathway or cross-presented in class II molecules. Thus, DNA vaccination has the potential capacity to engage both arms of the immune system. A phase I clinical trial in asymptomatic HIV-1 patients to assess a therapeutic DNA vaccine encoding Env and Rev with dose escalations of 30 μg, 100 μg, and 300 μg every 10 weeks demonstrated that the vaccine was tolerated and no patient developed anti-DNA antibodies or abnormal muscle enzyme levels (Boyer et al., 2000; Hanke & McMichael, 2000; MacGregor et al., 1998; Weber et al., 2001). While having no effects on CD4[+] T lymphocyte levels or disease progression in any of the vaccinated groups, modest increases in T cell proliferative and CTL responses were detected to gp160 and anti-gp120 serum antibody titers increased in groups receiving the higher two doses. HIV-1-seronegative individuals who received 300 μg of the DNA vaccine at 0, 4, 8, and 24 weeks exhibited antigen-specific production of IFN-γ and the β-chemokines MIP-1α, MIP-1β, and RANTES (Hanke & McMichael, 2000). Moreover, 4/5 of the subjects responded to both Rev and Env, and by increasing the dosage to 1000 μg of DNA, significant numbers of IFN-γ-secreting cells were detectable by ELISPOT assay (MacGregor et al., 2002).

In an attempt to increase post-injection expression of DNA vaccines, plasmids have been re-engineered by modifying viral genes to conform to codon utilization that matches highly expressed human genes, as well as removing residual inhibitory sequences to optimize codon utilization. This strategy increases expression by 300- to 900-fold (Haas, Park, & Seed, 1996; zur Megede et al., 2000) and permits the incorporation of multicomponent genes into the vector. In one study, optimized constructs for pGag and pEnv, which expressed 20–100 fold greater product than first generation vectors and included genes encoding B7 co-stimulatory molecules (CD80 and CD86), IL-12, and IL-15 were shown to significantly increase CD8 effector function (Boyer et al., 2002). One phase I clinical trial assessed a codon-optimized DNA plasmid vaccine containing genes encoding HIV-1 clade B Gag that proved efficacious in rhesus macaques (Caulfield et al., 2002). A total of 54 subjects with chronic HIV infection were assessed for frequency and magnitude of cell-mediated immune responses towards HIV antigens, including Gag, Pol, Nef, Rev, and Tat (Fu et al., 2007). Results indicated that Gag, Pol, and Nef were the most common targets among T cell responses, but no significant associations with viral loads and T cell immune responses were shown. However, in nonvaccinated patients, viral loads were positively correlated with T cell responses to Gag and Pol, suggesting that high levels of T cell responses were reflective of a persistent viral infection.

Table 2.5.3 CLINICAL TRIALS OF DNA AND COMBINED DNA VACCINE STRATEGIES

TRIAL START	VACCINE CANDIDATE (HIV STRAIN)	ADJUVANT	VACCINE DEVELOPER	TRIAL ID
			DNA (Phase I Studies)	
1996	APL 400–003 GENEVAX-HIV		NIAID	96-I-0050
2000	APL 400–003 GENEVAX-HIV		Wyeth, Lederle-Praxis Biologicals	04/400–003-04
2000	DNA.HIVA		MRC/Oxford[1], International AIDS Vaccine Initiative (IAVI)[2]	IAVI 001
2001	DNA.HIVA		Kenya AIDS Vaccine Initiative (KAVI)[3], IAVI	IAVI 002
2001	VRC4302, Gag/Pol		NIAID	01-I-0079
2002	GTU-Nef		FIT Biotech[4]	FIT Biotech
2002	VRC-HIVDNA009–00-VP		NIAID, NIH Vaccine Research Center (VRC)[5]	VRC 004 (03-I-0022)
2003	ADVAX		Aaron Diamond AIDS Research Center (ADARC)[6], IAVI	IAVI C001
2003	EP HIV-1090		HVTN	HVTN 048
2003	pGA2/JS7 DNA		HVTN	HVTN 045
2003	VRC-HIVDNA009–00-VP	IL-2	NIAID, HVTN	HVTN 044
2003	VRC-HIVDNA009–00-VP		NIAID, HVTN	HVTN 052
2004	VRC-HIVDNA016–00-VP		NIAID, VRC	VRC 007 (04-I-0254)
2005	Chinese DNA		Changchun BCHT[7], Guangxi CD[8]	Guangxi CDC DNA vaccine
2005	EnvDNA		St. Jude Children's Research Hospital, NIH	EnvDNA
2005	HIV-1 gag DNA	RC529-SE, GM-CSF	NIAID, HVTN, Profectus BioSciences[9]	HVTN 060
2005	HIV-1 gag DNA	IL-12, IL-15, RC529-SE, GM-CSF	NIAID, HVTN, Wyeth, Profectus	HVTN 063
2005	HIVIS-DNA	GM-CSF	Karolinska Institute[10], Swedish Institute for Infectious Disease Control (SMI)[11], Vecura[12]	HIVIS 01
2005	VRC-HIVDNA009–00-VP		NIAID, HVTN, VRC, USMHRP	RV 156
2007	ADVAX		ADARC, Ichor Medical Systems Inc[13], IAVI	IAVI C004/DHO-614
2007	PENNVAX-B	IL-12, IL-15	NIAID, HVTN, University of Pennsylvania[14], Wyeth	HVTN 070
2009	PENNVAX-B	IL-12	HVTN, VGX Pharmaceuticals	HVTN 080
			DNA (Phase II Studies)	
2004	GTU-MultiHIV		FIT Biotech	C060301
2006	LC002		NIAID	ACTG A5176
2007	VRC-HIVDNA009–00-VP		NIAID	ACTG A5187
			Combination: DNA and Protein (Phase I Studies)	
2003	Gag and Env DNA/PLG microparticles/Oligomeric gp140/MF59	MF59	NIAID, HVTN	HVTN 049
2004	DP6/u8722 001 DNA/DP6 protein		Advanced BioScience Laboratories[15]	DP6/uc0/u8722 001
2007	EnvDNA/EnvPro/PolyEnv1	Alum	St. Jude Children's Research Hospital	DVP-1
			Combination: DNA and Viral Vector—Adeno (Phase I Studies)	
2004	VRC-HIVDNA009–00-VP/VRC-HIVADV014–00-VP		NIAID, HVTN, VRC	HVTN 057
2005	VRC-HIVDNA009–00-VP/VRC-HIVADV014–00-VP		NIAID, VRC	VRC 009 (05-I-0081)
2005	VRC-HIVDNA016–00-VP/VRC-HIVADV014–00-VP		NIAID, IAVI, VRC	IAVI V001
2005	VRC-HIVDNA016–00-VP/VRC-HIVADV014–00-VP		NIAID, VRC	VRC 008 (05-I-0148)
2006	VRC-HIVDNA009–00-VP/VRC-HIVADV014–00-VP		NIAID, HVTN, VRC	HVTN 069

(Continued)

Table 2.5.3 (CONTINUED)

2006	VRC-HIVDNA016–00-VP/VRC-HIVADV014–00-VP	NIAID, VRC	VRC 011(06-I-0149)
2007	VRC-HIVDNA009–00-VP/VRC-HIVADV014–00-VP	VRC, WRAIR	RV 156A
2007	VRC-HIVDNA044–00-VP/VRC-HIVADV027–00-VP/ VRC-HIVADV038–00-VP	NIAID, HVTN, VRC	HVTN 072
2010	VRC-HIVDNA016–00-VP/VRC-HIVADV014–00-VP	NIAID, HVTN	HVTN 082

Combination: DNA and Viral Vector—Adeno (Phase II Studies

2005	VRC-HIVDNA016–00-VP/VRC-HIVADV014–00-VP	NIAID, HVTN, VRC	HVTN 204
2005	VRC-HIVDNA016–00-VP/VRC-HIVADV014–00-VP	USMHRP, NIAID	RV 172
2006	VRC-HIVDNA016–00-VP/VRC-HIVADV014–00-VP	NIAID, IAVI	IAVI V002
2007	VRC-HIVDNA016–00-VP/VRC-HIVADV014–00-VP	IAVI, NIAID, CDC[16], HVTN, USMHRP	PAVE100
2009	VRC-HIVDNA016–00-VP/VRC-HIVADV014–00-VP	NIAID, HVTN	HVTN 505

Combination: DNA and Viral Vector—Pox (Phase I Studies)

1997	APL 400–047/ALVAC-HIV MN120TMG strain (vCP205)	NIAID	AVEG 031
2001	DNA.HIVA/MVA.HIVA	MRC/Oxford, IAVI	IAVI 005
2003	DNA.HIVA/MVA.HIVA	IAVI	IAVI 009
2006	pGA2/JS7 DNA/MVA/HIV62	NIAID, HVTN, Geovax[17]	HVTN 065
2007	EP-1233/MVA-mBN32	NIAID, HVTN, Epimmune, Bavarian Nordic	HVTN 067
2008	ADVAX/TBC-M4	IAVI	IAVI P002
2009	ADVAX/TBC-M4	ADARC, IAVI	IAVI P001
2009	Chinese DNA/Tiantian vaccinia	Changchun BCHT, Guangxi CDC	Tiantian vaccinia HIV Vaccine
2009	HIVIS-DNA/MVA-CMDR	SMI	HIVIS 05
2009	pGA2/JS7 DNA/MVA/HIV62	NIAID, HVTN, Geovax	HVTN 908
2009	SAAVI DNA-C2/SAAVI MVA-C	South African AIDS Vaccine Initiative (SAAVI)[18], HVTN	HVTN 073

Combination: DNA and Viral Vector—Pox (Phase II Studies)

2002	DNA.HIVA/MVA.HIVA	MRC/Oxford, IAVI	IAVI 006
2003	DNA.HIVA/MVA.HIVA	IAVI, SAAVI	IAVI 010
2006	HIVIS-DNA/MVA-CMDR	Muhimbili University[19], SMI, Vecura, USMHRP	HIVIS 03
2007	DNA-C/NYVAC-C	ANRS, EuroVacc[20]	EV02
2007	DNA-C/NYVAC-C	ANRS, EuroVacc	EV03/ANRSVAC20
2007	pHIS-HIV-AE/rFPV-HIV-AE	The National Centre in HIV Epidemiology and Clinical Research[21]	NCHECR-AE1
2009	pGA2/JS7 DNA/MVA/HIV62	GeoVax, HVTN	HVTN 205

Vaccine candidates and corresponding data can be found in the IAVI AIDS Vaccine Trials Database (www.iavireport.org/Trials-db/) and the NIH Clinical Trials Database (www.clinicaltrials.gov)

[1] Oxford, UK; [2]New York, NY; [3]Nairobi, Africa; [4]Tampere, Finland; [5]Bethesda, MD; [6]New York, NY; [7]Changchun, Jilin China; [8]Guangxi, China; [9]Baltimore, MD; [10]Stockholm, Sweden; [11]Stockholm, Sweden; [12]Stockholm, Sweden; [13]San Diego, CA; [14]Philadelphia, PA; [15]Kensington, MD; [16]Atlanta, GA; [17]Smyrna, Georgia; [18]Cape Town, Africa; [19]Dar es Salaam, Tanzania; [20]Lausanne, Swizerland; [21]Darlinghurst, Australia.

In a phase I trial, a polyvalent, multi-gene DNA vaccine was administered in a DNA prime-protein boost regimen to non-infected volunteers (Wang et al., 2008). Strong HIV-specific T cell responses were observed, with considerable titers of antibodies specific for a wide range of HIV Env epitopes. These results showed that a DNA prime-protein boost strategy is feasible to elicit not only cell-mediated immunity, but also humoral responses. Moreover, using a polyvalent formulation of Env sequences may create broad immune response against other strains of HIV viruses.

The use of vaccine cocktails has proven successful in combating a number of other pathogens; therefore, research efforts increased to develop an HIV-1 antigen cocktail that induces broad immune specificity which could protect against diverse HIV-1 forms. An ongoing clinical trial utilized a cocktail vaccine that contains dozens of envelope sequences delivered in a variety of ways, including recombinant DNA, vaccinia virus, and protein (Sealy et al., 2009). Major adverse effects have not been detected; and although not complete, preliminary results show the multi-envelope vaccine also capable of inducing neutralizing antibody responses to diverse HIV-1 strains. In yet another study to test the efficacy of a therapeutic vaccine to delay or eliminate the need for ART, 20 HIV-1-infected ART-treated subjects were randomly split into vaccine or control groups and given either an HIV-1 DNA vaccine (VRC-HVDNA 009–00-VP) or a placebo, respectively, then ART was discontinued (Rosenberg et al., 2010). While the vaccine proved safe, it was poorly immunogenic in ART-treated patients with acute or early HIV-1 infection and produced no change in HIV-1 viral load or CD4[+] T cell counts after treatment was discontinued.

RECOMBINANT VIRAL VECTORS AND COMBINED VACCINE STRATEGIES

To induce more potent immune responses that enhance the cell-mediated arm, multiple delivery systems and vaccination strategies utilizing recombinant viral vectors have been developed that often employ a prime-boost strategy (Table 2.5.4). Most of these strategies utilize recombinant delivery vectors as nonpathogenic virus constructs containing several HIV-1 genes; however, the use of several different viral vectors may be necessary for this strategy since initial vaccination may limit efficacy of subsequent boosts with the same vector.

Table 2.5.4 CLINICAL TRIALS OF RECOMBINANT VIRAL VECTOR AND OTHER VACCINE STRATEGIES

TRIAL START	VACCINE CANDIDATE (HIV STRAIN)	ADJUVANT	VACCINE DEVELOPER	TRIAL ID
Adeno Virus Vector Recombinants/Combinations (Phase I Studies)				
2003	MRK Ad5/ALVAC-HIV MN120TMG strain (vCP205)		Merck, Sanofi-Pasteur	MRKAd5 + ALVAC
2003	MRKAd5 HIV-1 gag		NIAID, HVTN, Merck	HVTN 050/Merck 018
2003	tgAAC09		IAVI, Targeted Genetics[1]	IAVI A001
2004	Ad-5 HIV-1 gag		Merck	MRK Ad5
2004	VRC-HIVADV014–00-VP		NIAID, VRC	VRC 006 (04-I-0172)
2005	MRKAd5 HIV-1 gag/pol/nef/MRKAd6/MRKAd5+6 HIV-1		Merck	V526–001 MRKAd5 and MRKAd6 HIV-1 Trigene Vaccines
2005	VRC-HIVADV014–00-VP		NIAID, HVTN, VRC	HVTN 054
2007	MRK Ad5		NIAID, HVTN	HVTN 071
2007	VRC-HIVADV027–00-VP/VRC-HIVADV038–00-VP		NIAID, VRC	VRC 012 (07-I-0167)
2008	Ad26.EnvA-01		NIAID	Ad26.ENVA.01
2008	VRC-HIVADV014–00-VP		NIAID, VRC	VRC 015 (08-I-0171)
2009	Ad35-GRIN/ENV/Ad35-GRIN/ENV		ADARC, IAVI	IAVI B001
2009	Ad5HVR48.ENVA.01		NIAID	Ad5HVR48.ENVA.01
2009	VRC-HIVADV027–00-VP/VRC-HIVADV038–00-VP/VRC-HIVDNA044–00-VP		NIAID, HVTN	HVTN 077
Adeno Virus Vector Recombinants/Combinations (Phase II Studies)				
2005	MRKAd5 HIV-1 gag/pol/nef		Merck, HVTN	HVTN 502/Merck 023 (Step Study)
2005	tgAAC09		University of Rochester[2], IAVI	IAVI A002
2006	VRC-HIVADV014–00-VP/VRC-HIVADV014–00-VP		NIAID, HVTN, VRC	HVTN 068
2007	MRKAd5 HIV-1 gag/pol/nef		NIAID, HVTN, Merck	HVTN 503 (Phambili)
Alphavirus Vector Recombinants/Combinations (Phase I Studies)				
2003	AVX101		NIAID, HVTN, SAAVI	HVTN 040
2004	AVX101		NIAID, HVTN, AlphaVax[3]	HVTN 059
Pox Virus Vector Recombinants/Combinations (Phase I Studies)				
1988	HIVAC-1e/gp160 MN/LAI		NIAID	AVEG 002
1991	HIVAC-1e		NIAID	AVEG 002A
1991	HIVAC-1e/VaxSyn gp160 Vaccine, MicroGeneSys		NIAID	AVEG 002B

(Continued)

Table 2.5.4 (CONTINUED)

TRIAL START	VACCINE CANDIDATE (HIV STRAIN)	ADJUVANT	VACCINE DEVELOPER	TRIAL ID
1992	ALVAC vCP125/gp160 Vaccine, Immuno-AG		ANRS	ANRS VAC 01
1992	HIVAC-1e		NIAID	AVEG 008
1992	HIVAC-1e/rgp120/HIV-1 SF-2/MN rgp120		NIAID	AVEG 010
1993	ALVAC vCP125		NIAID	AVEG 012A/B
1993	TBC-3B/MN rgp120	Alum	NIAID	AVEG 014C
1994	ALVAC-HIV MN120TMG strain (vCP205)/ CLTB-36 (gp24E-V3 MN)		ANRS	ANRS VAC 03
1994	TBC-3B		NIAID	AVEG 014A/B
1995	ALVAC vCP125/ALVAC (vCP rage)		ANRS	ANRS VAC 05
1995	ALVAC vCP125/ALVAC (vCP rage)		ANRS	ANRS VAC 06
1995	ALVAC vCP300		ANRS	ANRS VAC 07
1995	ALVAC-HIV MN120TMG strain (vCP205)		ANRS	ANRS VAC 08
1995	ALVAC-HIV MN120TMG strain (vCP205)		NIAID	AVEG 022
1996	ALVAC vCP300/rgp120/HIV-1 SF-2		NIAID	AVEG 026
1996	ALVAC-HIV MN120TMG strain (vCP205)/ rgp120/HIV-1 SF-2		NIAID	AVEG 022A
1996	ALVAC-HIV MN120TMG strain (vCP205)/ rgp120/HIV-1 SF-2		NIAID	AVEG 029
1997	PolyEnv1	Alum	St. Jude Children's Research Hospital	PolyEnv1
1998	ALVAC vCP1433/ALVAC vCP1452/ALVAC-HIV MN120TMG strain (vCP205)		NIAID	AVEG 034/034A
1998	ALVAC-HIV MN120TMG strain (vCP205)	GM-CSF	NIAID	AVEG 033
1998	ALVAC-HIV MN120TMG strain, (vCP205)/ gp160MN/LAI-2		WRAIR	RV 124
1999	ALVAC vCP1452/LIPO-6T/LIPO-5		ANRS	ANRS VAC 10
1999	ALVAC-HIV MN120TMG strain (vCP205)		NIAID	AVEG 027
1999	ALVAC-HIV MN120TMG strain (vCP205)		NIAID	HIVNET 007
1999	ALVAC-HIV MN120TMG strain (vCP205)/ rgp120/HIV-1 SF-2	MF59	NIAID	AVEG 032
2000	ALVAC-HIV MN120TMG strain (vCP205)	MF59 or Alum	NIAID	AVEG 038
2001	ALVAC vCP1452		NIAID, HVTN	HVTN 039
2001	MVA.HIVA		MRC/Oxford, IAVI	IAVI 003
2002	MVA.HIVA		KAVI, IAVI	IAVI 004
2002	TBC-3B		NIAID, University of California: Los Angeles (UCLA)[4]	UCLA MIG-001
2003	ALVAC-HIV MN120TMG strain (vCP205)		NIAID, UCLA	UCLA MIG-003
2003	MVA.HIVA		Uganda Virus Research Institute[5], IAVI	IAVI 008
2003	MVA.HIVA		IAVI	IAVI 011
2003	NYVAC-C		Imperial College London, EuroVacc	EV01 (EuroVacc 01)
2004	ALVAC(2)120(B,MN)GNP (vCP1452)		NIAID	ACTG A5058s
2004	MVA.HIVA/DNA.HIVA/MVA.HIVA		IAVI	IAVI 016
2004	TBC-M335/TBC-M358/TBC-F357		NIAID, HVTN, Therion[6]	HVTN 055
2005	ADMVA		ADARC, IAVI	IAVI C002
2005	MVA-CMDR		USMHRP, WRAIR	RV 158
2005	TBC-M4		IAVI, Therion	IAVI D001
2005	VRC-HIVADV014–00-VP		NIAID, VRC	VRC 010 (05-I-0140)

Table 2.5.4 (CONTINUED)

TRIAL START	VACCINE CANDIDATE (HIV STRAIN)	ADJUVANT	VACCINE DEVELOPER	TRIAL ID
2006	ADMVA		ADARC, IAVI	IAVI C003
2006	ALVAC-HIV MN120TMG strain (vCP205)		WRAIR	RV 138; B011
2006	ALVAC-HIV vCP1521		NIAID, Sanofi-Pasteur	HPTN 027
2006	MVA-CMDR		Karolinska Institute, SMI, USMHRP	HIVIS 02
2006	MVA-mBN32		Bavarian Nordic	HIV-POL-001
2009	MVA.HIVA		Medical Research Council	PedVacc001 & PedVacc002
2009	NYVAC-B/VRC-HIVADV038–00-VP		NIAID, HVTN, EuroVacc	HVTN 078

Pox Virus Vector Recombinants/Combinations (Phase II Studies)

1997	ALVAC vCP1452/AIDSVAX B/B		NIAID	ACTG 326; PACTG 326
1997	ALVAC-HIV MN120TMG strain (vCP205)/ rgp120/HIV-1 SF-2	MF59	NIAID	AVEG 202/HIVNET 014
2000	ALVAC vCP1452/AIDSVAX B/B	Alum	NIAID, HVTN	HVTN 203
2000	ALVAC vCP1452/MN rgp120	Alum	NIAID	HIVNET 026
2000	ALVAC-HIV vCP1521/gp120 C4-V3		WRAIR	RV 135
2000	ALVAC-HIV vCP1521/gp160 THO23/ LAI-DID/rgp120/HIV-1 SF-2		WRAIR	RV 132
2002	ALVAC HIV vaccine (vCP1452)	IL-2	NIAID	1R01AI51181–01A1
2003	ALVAC(2)120(B,MN)GNP (vCP1452)		NIAID	B012, 0900–397
2004	ALVAC vCP1452/LIPO-5		NIAID, ANRS, HVTN	HVTN 042/ANRS VAC 19
2005	ALVAC(2)120(B,MN)GNP (vCP1452)		NIAID	ACTG A5068
2006	ALVAC(2)120(B,MN)GNP (vCP1452)	IL-2	NIAID	ACTG A5024

Pox Virus Vector Recombinants/Combinations (Phase III Study)

2003	ALVAC-HIV vCP1521/AIDSVAX gp120 B/E		DoD, Thailand MOPH[8], NIAID, Thai AIDS Vaccine Evaluation Group (TAVEG)[9], Sanofi, VaxGen	RV 144

Bacterium + gp120/Protein (Phase I Study)

1997	Salmonella typhi CVD 908-HIV-1 LAI gp 120/ MN rgp120	MF59	NIAID	AVEG 028

T Cell Vaccine (Phase I Study)

2009	WT-gag-TCR or α/6-gag-TCR modified T cells		University of Pennsylvania	810108

T Cell Vaccine (Phase II Study)

2006	Autologous CD4 reactive T cells		Soroka University[10]	sor444006ctil

Virus-Like-Particles (Phase I Study)

1995	p17/p24:Ty- VLP	Alum	NIAID	AVEG 019

Vaccine candidates and corresponding data can be found in the IAVI AIDS Vaccine Trials Database (www.iavireport.org/Trials-db/) and the NIH Clinical Trials Database (www.clinicaltrials.gov)
[1] Seattle, WA; [2]Rochester, NY; [3]Research Triangle Park, NC; [4]Los Angeles, CA; [5]Entebbe, Uganda; [6]Hauppauge, NY; [7]Washington, DC; [8]Nonthaburi, Thailand; [9]Thailand; [10]New York, NY.

Additionally, antibody titers to particular viral vectors may deleteriously affect vaccine efficacies.

In a series of phase I trials, the HIV-1 gp160 envelope protein from strain IIIB was assessed as a recombinant vaccinia virus construct and a baculovirus-derived recombinant protein (Clements-Mann et al., 1998; Cooney et al., 1993; Graham et al., 1993). In the initial study, priming with either the vaccinia vector or recombinant protein induced low and transient T cell and antibody responses. However, priming with gp160 vaccinia virus and subsequent boost with recombinant protein resulted in sustained responses in 75% of the volunteers. These responses were detectable beyond 18 months post-boost; were three- to tenfold higher than single moiety priming; and consisted of significant CTL responses and anti-gp160 antibody titers in excess of 1:800. More importantly, 7 of 13 subjects developed neutralizing antibodies. In another trial, both neutralizing and fusion inhibitory activities to homologous virus were demonstrated in 8/12 and 5/12 volunteers, respectively, as well as cross-reactive neutralizing activity to strain MN (Graham et al., 1993). In another trial using an HIV-1 LAI gp160/vaccinia virus prime and boost with recombinant gp120SF-2, gp120LAI, gp120MN, or gp160MN, significantly higher levels of homologous and heterologous viral neutralization and inhibitory activities were induced with gp120 boosts than with boosts using gp160 in all subjects, and were detectable for an excess of 6 months in 91% of the subjects (Gorse et al., 1998). Taken together, these studies demonstrated the potential of a vector prime-protein boost vaccine strategy; however, the potential for pathogenic reversion by vaccinia virus vectors represents a major concern. To address this concern, vaccinia vectors have been altered by genetic engineering or serial passage in chicken fibroblasts to further attenuate the virus (Hanke & McMichael, 2000; Sutter & Moss, 1992; Tartaglia et al., 1998). The attenuated virus was used in a phase I/II clinical trial in healthy adults adopting a prime-boost strategy with two initial doses of an HIV-1 clade A DNA vaccine followed by a boosting dose of HIV-1 clade A-modified vaccinia Ankara (MVA) vaccine. The vaccine was shown to be safe and well tolerated, and elicited HIV-1-specific CTL responses in vaccinated individuals (Guimaraes-Walker et al., 2008). Clinical trials to test safety and immunogenicity of HIV-1 modified MVA candidates in infected and uninfected adults, as well as infants born to uninfected and infected mothers are planned within the next 2 years (studies HIV-CORE001, HIV-CORE002, PV001, and PV002 at ClinicalTrials.gov).

Other nonpathogenic recombinant vectors have undergone clinical trials. Canarypox virus vectors, such as ALVAC, represent the utilization of vectors that are replication-restricted to avian tissues and are nonpermissive in mammalian cells (Tartaglia et al., 1998). In an initial phase I study, volunteers were primed and boosted at 1 month with gp160 (strain MN) canarypox vector (ALVAC) and boosted with recombinant gp160 formulated in alum or incomplete Freund's adjuvant. Priming failed to induce significant antibody responses; however, after a first and second gp160 boost, 65% and 90% of subjects, respectively, developed neutralizing antibody responses to homologous virus. These responses were retained in 55% of subjects after more than 6 months and no differences in immune responses were detected regardless of adjuvant formulation. Only the highest titered antisera maintained the capacity for neutralization of SF2 isolates, but none neutralized LAI or primary isolates. All subjects exhibited antigen-specific T cell proliferation after the first gp160 boost, while MHC-restricted cytotoxic CD8$^+$ T cell activity was detected in 39% of the volunteers and was retained in 10% of the subjects after 2 years (Fleury et al., 1996; Pialoux et al., 1995).

In another study, volunteers were primed once with either 10^6 or 10^7 TCID$_{50}$ of ALVAC/gp160 (strain MN) or recombinant rabies glycoprotein canarypox vector, and boosted with recombinant gp120 (strain SF2), while others were primed and boosted with gp120. Neutralizing activity to strains MN and SF2 were detected in 100% of subjects immunized with ALVAC-gp160 and gp120, compared to 65% and 89% of those immunized with only ALVAC-gp160 or gp120, respectively. Also, those that received an ALVAC/gp120 prime/boost regimen exhibited greater levels of fusion-inhibitory, lymphoproliferative, and CD8$^+$ CTL activities than those that received either vaccine alone. Additionally, no significant differences in responses were afforded by different doses of priming vaccine (Clements-Mann et al., 1998).

In an attempt to induce CTL activity along with neutralizing antibody, volunteers were primed with an ALVAC vaccine constructed with genes encoding for gp120, transmembrane gp41, Gag, protease (PR) and CTL epitopes from Nef and Pol, and boosted or primed simultaneously with gp120 (strain SF2). CD8$^+$ CTL activity was detected in 61% of the subjects. Simultaneous immunization with ALVAC and gp120 induced earlier antibody responses than later boosting (Evans et al., 1999). After boosting with a second gp120, all subjects developed neutralizing antibody against several laboratory-maintained isolates, and 88% of subjects' sera could neutralize the laboratory isolate, but none of eight other primary isolates (Belshe et al., 1998). In another study, volunteers were immunized with ALVAC canarypox expressing gp120 (MN), transmembrane gp41, Gag, and PR (all from LAI strain), and boosted with the ALVAC vector or with a p24E-V3 synthetic peptide (CLTB-36). Neutralizing antibodies to HIV-1 MN were induced in 33% of the subjects immunized and boosted with the ALVAC vector; however, no neutralizing antibodies were detected to a nonsyncytial clade B primary isolate (Bx08). After a fourth injection of the ALVAC vector, 33% of the subjects exhibited CTL activity to Env, Gag, and Pol, which was mediated by both CD8$^+$ and CD4$^+$ T cell subsets. Boosting with CLTB-36 induced no detectable CTL or neutralizing antibodies suggesting that in this regimen the synthetic peptide boost strategy was poorly immunogenic (Salmon-Ceron et al., 1999).

In a study to assess CD4$^+$ helper T cell responses to ALVAC vaccination, Env-specific T cell lines were generated from three groups of volunteers immunized with ALVAC encoded for Env, Gag, and PR (vCP205); gp160 (MN and LAI strains) using 15 overlapping amino acid peptides spanning the entire gp160 moiety; or vCP205 and boosted with the gp160 (Ratto-Kim et al., 2003). T cell lines from vCP205-primed, gp160-boosted subjects afforded strong reactivity that spanned the entire HIV-1 Env sequence; however, T cell lines from the other two groups reacted to only a few epitopes. In the first preventative clinical trial to be carried out in Africa, Ugandan volunteers received at 0, 1, 3, and 6 months, a canarypox vector encoding genes for gp120 (strain MN) linked to the transmembrane portion of gp41 (strain LAI) and genes for the entire gag and pol regions (ALVAC-HIV, clade B), control vector containing the rabies virus glycoprotein G gene (ALVAC-RG), or saline placebo. Detectable CTL responses to either Gag or Env antigens from clades A, B, and D were generated in 20% of the ALVAC-HIV recipients and 45%

developed CD8[+] T cell responses as evaluated by IFN-γ ELISPOT assay. Only 5% of the control group exhibited vaccine-specific T cell responses. Neutralizing antibodies against HIV-1 clade B strains were detected in 15% of vaccine recipients, but responses against clades A and D were not detected (Cao et al., 2003). In a retrospective study to determine the frequency of subjects that developed antigen-specific antibody responses among trial participants and to identify any factors associated with these results, serum samples were tested with six serologic screening tests and reactive specimens were confirmed by Western blot. Of 490 serum specimens, 100 (20.4%) were reactive for at least one serologic test, and 65 (13%) were positive by Western blot assay. All sera deemed positive by Western blot were from individuals vaccinated with vaccinia or canarypox vectors with or without gp120 or gp160 boosts; however, antibody reactivity by Western blot analysis could not be detected in sera obtained from subjects vaccinated with gp120 moieties (Ackers et al., 2003).

As mentioned previously, vaccine efficacy of 31.2% was achieved with an ALVAC prime then boost with AIDSVAX recombinant gp120 subunit (Rerks-Ngarm et al., 2009). The resulting successful vaccine formed by the marriage of two non-efficacious regimens underscores the importance of combined vaccine strategies. The first statistically beneficial vaccine trial (RV144) utilized two immunogens, AIDSVAX and ALVAC; both deemed to have little efficacy as individual monotherapies. From various communities in Thailand, 16,395 subjects considered at high risk for HIV-1 exposure were randomized to receive either placebo or four injections of the ALVAC-HIV ([vCP1521) encoding for gp120, gp41, Gag, and PR at weeks 0, 4, 12, and 24, and two booster injections of AIDSVAX gp120 at weeks 12 and 24. From the final 12,542 subjects analyzed, HIV infection occurred in 51 patients who received the vaccine, while 74 subjects were infected from those receiving placebo, yielding a 31.2% vaccine efficacy. The protective effect was significant but modest (P = 0.04) and did not alter viral loads or CD4[+] T cell count in vaccinated compared with control group. Although resulting in a slight benefit, the study provides a starting point from which to base future HIV-1 vaccine research.

In addition to the aforementioned strategies, alternative vectors have been devised for HIV-1 vaccines including recombinant viral vectors based on poliovirus, adenovirus, herpesviruses, and Venezuelan equine encephalitis (VEE) virus, as well as vectors based on attenuated bacteria such as Bacille Calmette-Guerin (BCG), *Salmonella*, and *Shigella* (Wu et al., 1997). Of these, some of the most promising, yet plagued during clinical trials, have been those using recombinant adenoviruses (rAd). Initial studies in nonhuman primates compared, either alone or in combination, three different formulations: a plasmid DNA vector, a modified vaccinia Ankara (MVA) virus, and a replication incompetent adenovirus type 5 (Ad5) vector (Shiver et al., 2002). The best responses were supported using the Ad5 vector both alone and as a booster after DNA vector priming, providing the longest attenuation of viral infection after challenge by HIV-SIV hybrid virus (SHIV). Following these positive initial results, an early clinical trial looked at the safety and possible efficacy

of several dosage levels of rAd serotype 5 (rAd5) vectors that expressed a Gag-Pol fusion protein, as well as Env (Catanzaro et al., 2006). The vaccine proved to be safe, inducing both antigen-specific T cell and antibody responses, but neutralizing antibodies were not detected. These results supported a phase I clinical trial involving a multi-clade implementation of this vaccine strategy. In the study, 217 subjects received a three-dose prime-boost regimen of a trivalent rAd5 vaccine encoding Gag, Nef, and Pol developed by Merck (Whitehouse Station, NJ, US) at 0, 4, and 26 weeks (Priddy et al., 2008). Adverse events were not reported by participants and induced a cellular immune response in greater than 60% of subjects.

From these results, two phase IIb "proof-of-concept" trials were initiated by Merck and the NIH to assess whether the vaccine would prevent initial HIV infection, or at least would reduce viral loads after initial infection, and included 3,000 subjects from the Americas and Australia with another 3,000 from South Africa, (Steinbrook, 2007). The trial was stopped prematurely after statistical evidence revealed that the vaccine neither prevented infection nor diminished plasma virus levels compared to controls. In addition, an unexpected and troubling result indicated that compared with the placebo-treated group, a larger number of HIV-1 infections occurred in those receiving the vaccine, chiefly in those who had pre-existing titers of Ad5-neutralizing antibodies (Buchbinder et al., 2008). Although not yet fully understood, these results highlight the lack of knowledge about factors that determine HIV-1 susceptibility. Moreover, this suggests the necessity to exclude in future trials those individuals with pre-existing neutralizing antibodies to adenoviral vectors when utilized in vaccine regimens, despite the fact that 30–40% of the United States and European population, as well as 80–90% of southern Africans, have pre-existing Ad5-specific neutralizing antibodies (Abbink et al., 2007). Thus, future viral vector-based vaccine studies will likely only move to clinical trials upon convincing superiority of the vaccine candidate compared to non-efficacious strategies.

MUCOSAL VACCINE STRATEGIES

In light of the fact that rectal and vaginal sites represent primary HIV-1 entry and infection foci, induction of anti-HIV-1 immunoglobulin A (IgA) antibodies, especially secretory IgA (s-IgA), within mucosal tissues early after exposure may be imperative for an efficacious response to the virus (Brenchley et al., 2004). A vaccine that forms a robust pre-infection immune response in mucosal-associated lymphoid tissue (MALT) may suppress HIV-1 infection by providing a strong defense at sites of entry and primary infection (Stevceva & Strober, 2004). The strategy for protective immunity is to inoculate at a mucosal site with the intent to induce both mucosal and systemic protection from all other sites by distribution of plasma cells and/or T cells.

Immunity at mucosal sites during early HIV-1 infection is critical as virus can form reservoirs within infected tissues, as well as damage multiple cellular elements of the immune system. Early during infection, HIV-1 virus particles quickly move to the lamina propria, likely forming reservoirs within infected lamina propria lymphoid cells. Within the gastrointestinal trac, the lamina propria provides a source rich in activated CD4$^+$ T cells and dendritic cells that, in part due to expression of CCR5 and CXCR4, become infected early and allow rapid HIV-1 replication (Smith et al., 2003). In addition to reservoir formation, the mucosal immune system sustains permanent localized damage as early as the first week after infection (Mehandru et al., 2004). Over 50% of memory CD4$^+$T cells throughout the host quickly become infected, leading to elimination of the majority of infected cells after 10 days due to cytolysis or other immune-mediated mechanisms (Mattapallil et al., 2005). These observations seemingly correlate with epidemiological findings which support the significance of protective anti-HIV-1 IgA responses and reduced HIV-1 susceptibility. In a study of high-risk Kenyan sex workers, many of whom were repeatedly exposed to HIV-seropositive persons, but never contracted HIV, genital HIV-neutralizing IgA was directly correlated with reduced HIV acquisition and viral proliferation (Hirbod et al., 2008). Still other studies point to the possibility that mucosal protection may be due in part to increased mucosal levels of innate immune proteins that have anti-HIV-1 properties, such as secretory leukocyte protease inhibitor (SLPI) and trappin-2 (Iqbal & Kaul, 2008). As a protease inhibitor, trappin-2 inhibits HIV-1 viral infection in vitro (Iqbal et al., 2005). Additionally, proteomic analysis revealed that elevated levels of trappin-2 represent a major difference in vaginal tissues from high-risk sex workers compared to low-risk females. Similarly, increased levels of SLPI in vaginal tissues are correlated with reduced vertical HIV-1 transmission; however, the effect of SLPI on sexual transmission is not yet fully understood (Pillay et al., 2001). Further investigations into these findings may prove useful in the mechanism by which a strong mucosal immune response to HIV-1 correlates with protective immunity.

Although the route of inoculation is thought to be of vital significance to induce a functional mucosal immune response, conflicting results exist as to whether mucosal immunization is necessary. Attempts at mucosal inoculation have been widely explored via genital, rectal, nasal, and oral delivery of HIV immunogens. One consensus is that only a mucosal vaccine could induce migration of CD8$^+$ T cells into mucosal tissues, whereas traditional systemic vaccinations would induce T cells to migrate into peripheral and lymphoid tissues (Kivisakk et al., 2006). However, a recent study using intramuscular inoculation of nonhuman primates with recombinant adenovirus serotype 5 (rAd5)-encoded immunogens, stimulated a large number of CD8$^+$ and CD4$^+$ T cells in mucosal tissues localized mainly to the colon (Sun et al., 2009).

Genital delivery has proven difficult, not only due to the patient misgivings, but also to the idea that the vagina serves as a less than ideal location for vaccine delivery (Mestecky, Moldoveanu, & Russell, 2005). Vaccine administration via the male genital track is thought too impractical for clinical utility. Vaginal administration of antigens primarily develops antibodies in secretions localized to sites of administration and typically has not provided systemic distribution or to other mucosal tissues. However, with newer formulations a vaginal

vaccination route is not without hope. Rheologically structured vehicle (RSV) gels have been used to release the envelope glycoprotein into vaginal mucosal tissue. Using the HIV-1 gp140 as immunogen, a RSV gel formulation included a vaginal fluid-absorbing polymer, as well as a mucoadhesive (Curran et al., 2009). In rabbits, this system elicited serum IgG, as well as mucosal IgG and IgA, in genital secretions that were specific for gp140. As multiple vaginal gels used for drug delivery currently exist, mostly as microbiocidal formulations, future studies using RSV gels as a vaginal vaccination delivery system may prove beneficial for inducing both mucosal and systemic immunity.

Nasal delivery systems have been studied extensively with successful antiviral vaccination strategies applicable for influenza, rubella, and other viral pathogens. Clinical studies have shown that intranasal delivery (via sprays or drops) induces immunity in the nasal mucosa and lung, as well as remote vaginal tissue in females (Durrani et al., 1998). Other advantages of nasal delivery include ease of vaccine delivery compared to delivery to other mucosal sites, needleless administration, smaller doses of antigen, and antibody titers equivalent to those afforded by vaginal administration (Vajdy & Singh, 2006); however, multiple side effects represent significant drawbacks with this strategy. In addition to potential damage to nasal epithelium and olfactory nervous system, Bell's palsy (idiopathic facial paralysis) can develop as demonstrated in multiple cases using bacterial toxins as antigens (Lewis et al., 2009) and in initial studies of the intranasal influenza vaccine (Mutsch et al., 2004). While numerous clinical trials using intranasal antigens for other viruses have provided promising results, only few trials have assessed nasal delivery for HIV-1. A phase I trial was performed on 34 randomized females receiving either nasal or vaginal vaccines containing recombinant HIV gp160 with or without an adjuvant (Pialoux, Hocini et al., 2008). The vaccine produced no adverse effects; however, IgA against the envelope protein was neither detected in sera nor in vaginal and nasal secretions. Although the vaccine was shown to be safe, no benefit was realized and has not progressed to further trials. Two recent intranasal vaccine trials (NCT00122564 and NCT00369031) utilizing gp160 and gp140, respectively, have been terminated, one due to safety issues. Another phase I trial (NCT010843430) utilizing HIV-1 and influenza peptide combinations was recently initiated to test the combination of intramuscular prime and intranasal boost on systemic and mucosal antibody production, but has not been completed.

Strategies for rectal vaccination also face challenges. Most studies show moderate levels of localized IgG and IgA at immunization sites, but low serum IgG titers (Holmgren & Czerkinsky, 2005). In one of the few clinical trials, participants were given an initial inoculation intramuscularly containing HIV-1 p17/p24 in a viral-like particle (VLP) formulation with subsequent rectal boosts. Neither humoral nor cellular immune responses were observed (Lindenburg et al., 2002). In addition to little or no systemic immune responses to rectal vaccination, accurate and sensitive measures of immune responses in human colorectal tissues are poorly developed. Thus, major obstacles in clinical practicality and patient acceptance impose challenges that seemingly outweigh the benefits for this strategy and render its future development unlikely.

Oral HIV-1 vaccination could provide a feasible method to induce systemic and mucosal protective immunity similar to that observed with oral polio vaccines. Like other mucosal strategies, the vaccine, adjuvant, formulation, tolerance induction, and harsh GI conditions leading to degradation of vaccine components represent formidable challenges for an oral vaccine strategy (Czerkinsky & Holmgren, 2009). If surmountable, a safe, easy, and needleless route of administration coupled with a nonrefrigerated product would provide a practical mucosal vaccine, as well as potentially beneficial for developing countries where medical care and necessary resources are scarce. To overcome degradation by GI conditions, formulations will need to protect vaccine components for successful delivery of immunogens to antigen-presenting cells by slow and steady release (Misumi et al., 2009). One formulation is a combined lipid-bile vesicle system, a bilosome, with improved chemical stability using bile salts that allow creation of more stable structures compared to liposomes (Mann et al., 2006). These vaccine formulations resist harsh conditions of the stomach and intestines, with slow release and increased immunogen absorption to the mucosal tissues. Clinical trials of oral vaccines have been limited and have yet to progress past phase I studies. One study used a polymerized HIV-1 peptide packaged into biodegradable microspheres and administered via oral doses to 33 volunteers (seronegative for HIV). After two boosts, no T cell or antibody responses in any mucosal site were detectable (Lambert et al., 2001). In another study, 18 individuals were vaccinated with one dose of a live *S. typhimurium* bacterial vector that expressed the HIV-1 Gag (Kotton et al., 2006). Although responses to *Salmonella* LPS and flagella were detectable, serum antibodies to Gag were not, but up to 40% of individuals showed increased numbers of cytokine-producing cells in response to Gag by ELISPOT analysis. More effective means of delivery through the GI tract while retaining structural integrity of the immunogens will be vital for an orally administered vaccine.

Given the success of the oral polio vaccine and the routes of entry of the HIV-1 virus, one can easily appreciate a vaccine that triggers a strong mucosal immune response should be a major focus of HIV-1 vaccine investigations, yet only a small number of vaccines have yet to address this concept and move into clinical trials. Indeed, special challenges exist exclusively to mucosal tissues that will need to be overcome for a safe efficacious mucosal vaccine.

NANOTECHNOLOGY-BASED VACCINE STRATEGIES

As many past HIV-1 vaccine strategies have failed to prove beneficial outcomes, future research strategies may need to be more outside the box. One promising novel approach is the use of nanotechnology, defined as the use of structures that measure 1–100 nanometers in at least one dimension, but may be up to a few hundred nanometers in other directions (Farokhzad, 2008). Nanotechnology in therapeutic or diagnostic uses has been successfully applied in many areas, especially cancer therapies and detection strategies (Zhang et al., 2008) and thus has increased the plausibility that nanotechnology can be transferred to other strategies for therapeutic modalities in infectious diseases. This approach is at an early stage in the area of HIV-1 treatment and prevention, but has enjoyed an increased focus as therapeutic HIV-1 strategies utilizing nanotechnology are currently being explored.

Nanotechnology has been used to improve current therapeutic treatments for HIV-1, as well as creating more efficient means of delivering gene therapy or "jump-starting" the immune response to HIV-1 via immunotherapeutic strategies. Major problems with gene therapy approaches involve the successful delivery using viral vectors of RNAi systems to target tissues. Thus nanotechnology may yield more effective and safer delivery vehicles than viral vectors (Rossi, June, & Kohn, 2007). More recently, strategies using immune cells as natural drug carriers to areas of inflammation have been explored. Nanoformulated antiretroviral drugs taken up by monocyte-derived macrophages which are systemically administered have afforded delayed and consistent drug release for weeks instead of hours with inhibition of HIV-1 replication (Nowacek et al., 2010). While these strategies provide major improvements in the treatment of HIV-1, the ultimate goal remains to prevent viral transmission. Properly nanoformulated vaccines that target augmented absorption of immunogen resulting in increased processing and presentation by dendritic and macrophage antigen-presenting cells, could lead to augmented immune responses and more efficacious vaccines (Pett, 2009).

Nanoparticles show great potential for use in developing HIV-1 vaccines. Employed either as an adjuvant or as a delivery system, nanoformulated vaccines would allow controlled release of antigen, protect antigens from degradation, and consequently allow stronger and extended immune responses. Vaccines can be formulated to accommodate a variety of inoculation routes such that while most vaccines are given intramuscularly, vaccines using nanoparticles could be given intranasally, orally, mucosally, or even intravenously to home to particular targeted afferent lymphoid tissues with the capacity to induce both systemic and mucosal immunity (Csaba, Garcia-Fuentes, & Alonso, 2009). Antigen delivery to targeted tissues or cell types is possible through directed formulation of nanovaccines with surface-optimized ligands that only antigen-presenting cells can recognize with cell-specific cognate receptors (Fahmy et al., 2008). Nanovaccines may either contain the antigens in their core or present them on their surface, allowing the potential to elicit cellular or humoral immune responses by presentation directly to B cells with surface epitopes exposed or indirectly to dendritic cells after phagocytosis, processing, and presentation by MHC molecules. For an efficacious vaccine, the combined efforts of both cellular- and antibody-mediated responses may necessitate using nanovaccines designed with both surface and core antigens.

Various nanoformulated vaccine strategies have been studied in vitro and in vivo in mice, rabbits, and nonhuman primates; however, to date, no clinical trials have been initiated. One study targeted dendritic cells with liposome formulated CpG oligonucleotides, which bind toll-like receptor (TLR)-9 and stimulate dendritic cell maturation to a higher response-initiating potential (Takeda, Kaisho, & Akira, 2003). In rhesus macaques, this strategy induced more robust SIV-specific T and B cell responses compared to controls (Fairman et al., 2009). Nanosized adjuvants, such as MF59, an oil-in-water nanoemulsion of squalene, polysorbate 80, and sorbitan trioleate, have been developed to augment and protect immunizing agents or vectors. Baboons primed and boosted with *env* and *gag* DNA plasmids and then boosted with Env/MF59 nanoemulsion produced higher antibody titers and stronger T cell proliferative responses compared with those treated with multiple DNA boosts (Leung et al., 2004). Similarly, mice primed with DNA plasmids encoding gp140, Gag, and Tat, and then boosted with corresponding proteins emulsified in MF59 were completely protected against challenge with HIV-1/murine leukemia virus (MuLV)-infected cells compared with only partial protection in mice primed with recombinant proteins and boosted with proteins formulated in MF59 nanoemulsion (Brave et al., 2007). Targeting specific cells with controlled-release of antigenic epitopes by nanoformulating vaccines will afford investigators better tools with which to fine-tune the immune response of choice and better dissect which immune response(s) will best provide protective immunity against HIV-1 infection.

VACCINE STRATEGIES FOR HIV-1-MEDIATED NEUROINFLAMMATION AND NEURODEGENERATION

With the advent of ART, fulminate HIV-1 infections of CNS tissues have sharply diminished in frequency and magnitude. Nevertheless, while HIV-1 persists, albeit at small levels in the body and in the CNS, the infection and resulting neurotoxins continue to assault neurons to the extent that the prevalence of HIV-1-associated neurocognitive disorder (HAND) is increasing. Neurotoxins, including viral products such as Tat and gp120, initiate a cascade of cytokines, chemokines, and biochemical reactions that exacerbate inflammatory responses and increase oxidative stress. This cascade results in increased neuronal death and vasculature dysfunction in the brain, both of which ultimately lead to gross neurological dysfunction, including atrophy of brain tissue, diminished architectural structure, and dysregulated function. With forms ranging from asymptomatic to fulminant dementia, over half of the AIDS patients are believed to suffer from some form of cognitive or motor impairment.

In more subtle forms, HAND and other inflammation-mediated neurodegenerative disorders, anti-inflammatory therapeutics can have profound beneficial effects; however, chronically administered, anti-inflammatory drugs typically lose effectiveness due to issues of drug-refractory disease progression, regimen compliance, and untoward GI side effects. Alternative anti-inflammatory strategies that can attenuate neuroinflammation, yet preclude the impediments associated with long-term pharmaceutical administration include immunotherapeutic approaches and vaccine strategies

which, unlike all aforementioned vaccines that target HIV-1 or HIV-1-infected cells, target neuroinflammation.

Controlling neuroinflammation through immunoregulation has been wrought with similar difficulties in developing an efficacious vaccine for neurodegenerative disorders including HAND. Traditional vaccine strategies have proved ineffective, and although clinical trials of vaccines for neurodegeneration have been limited, preclinical evidence has shown a need for finding more novel approaches. There have been a large number of clinical trials addressing vaccine strategies for Alzheimer's disease or multiple sclerosis (MS), but few have assessed other neurodegenerative disorders, such as Parkinson's disease (PD) or HAND. Although a vaccine that targets neurodegeneration has yet to reach a level of preparedness for clinical trials, substantial pre-clinical evidence has shown the utility of a potential strategy for clinical translation.

A potential vaccine strategy for Alzheimer's disease (AD) using aggregated human amyloid-beta (Aβ) peptide with QS21 adjuvant (AN1792) to target plaque levels showed promise in preclinical mouse models and in phase I clinical trials with no harmful effects (Schenk, 2002). Significant antibody titers were seen in 24% of 80 AD patients, without notable adverse effects (Bayer et al., 2005). However, the phase IIa trial with 372 patients was halted after two months due to reported meningoencephalitis in 6% of the immunized patients (Nicoll et al., 2003). Although halted, CSF tau levels were reduced in patients who generated antibody responses compared to placebo controls (Gilman et al., 2005). Examinations of brain tissue from patients who have since died of causes unrelated to the vaccine showed significant reduction of plaque deposits (Masliah, Hansen et al., 2005). However, some patients with very few plaques still exhibited severe and progressive dementia in the years before death (Holmes et al., 2008), suggesting that plaque clearance could not reverse neuronal loss and thus underscores the need for vaccine intervention before onset of symptoms. A completed phase IIa trial using passive immunization with bapineuzimab, a humanized monoclonal antibody that binds the amino terminus of Aβ, showed trends of cognitive stabilization but did not meet efficacy end points (Grundman & Black, 2008). Another candidate, solanezumab, an antibody that recognizes a region in the middle of Aβ, has progressed through clinical trials and is currently in two phase III studies with 2,000 AD patients (Lemere & Masliah, 2010). While passive immunization strategies show promise, development of an effective form of active immunotherapy is believed to be more cost-effective, require fewer clinical follow-up visits, and impart a greater and longer-lived immunoprotective effect. Thus, active immunization strategies with Aβ peptides modified from those used in the AN1792 trial have proven safe in phase I trials and have progressed to a current phase II trial (Boche et al., 2010).

Most immunotherapeutic strategies for MS attempt to modulate encephalitogenic autoimmune T cells responsible for directing neuroinflammation and neurodegeneration resulting in disease progression. One immunomodulatory strategy utilizes glatiramer acetate (GA, Copaxone), a synthetic copolymer randomly synthesized from four amino acids: alanine, lysine, glutamic acid, and tyrosine (Teitelbaum et al., 1971). GA suppresses experimental autoimmune encephalomyelitis (EAE) and is FDA approved for use in relapsing-remitting MS (Arnon, Sela, & Teitelbaum, 1996). GA modulates immune responses on many different levels, including 1) cross-reaction with myelin basic protein (MBP) and competition for inclusion in MHC class II molecules to inhibit MBP presentation (Teitelbaum, Arnon, & Sela, 1999); 2) competition of MHC II-T cell receptor (TCR) recognition resulting in TCR antagonism or anergy induction (Brenner et al., 2001); 3) induction of specific regulatory T cells and Th2 cells that secrete anti-inflammatory cytokines (Aharoni et al., 2000); 4) modulation of monocyte/macrophage activation shifting to an M2 phenotype (Weber et al., 2004; Weber et al., 2007); and 5) secretion of neurotrophic factors, such as the brain-derived neurotrophic factor (BDNF), glial-cell-derived neurotrophic factor (GDNF), and neurotrophin 3 (NT3) (Ziemssen et al., 2002; Kerschensteiner, Meinl, & Hohlfeld, 2009). More recent strategies in modulating the immune response in MS patients involve the use of T cell vaccine (TCV) approaches utilizing attenuated T cells or T cell receptors with specificities for myelin peptides, such as MBP or myelin oligodendrocyte glycoprotein (MOG) (Hellings, Raus, & Stinissen, 2006). Initial TCV studies showed that vaccination with irradiated autologous anti-myelin T cells induced two subsets of regulatory T cells that inhibited anti-myelin-reactive T cells; one subset expressing high levels of FoxP3, IFN-γ, and IL-10, the other subset expressing low levels of FoxP3 and predominately only IL-10 (Hong et al., 2006). A number of early-stage clinical trials using TCV have been completed, many of which show improved clinical outcomes (Correale, Farez, & Gilmore 2008). In one study wherein 20 MS patients, nonresponsive to traditional therapies, were primed and boosted with three separate doses of attenuated T cells specific for MBP and MOG peptides, reduced annual relapse rates and the number and activity of MRI lesions (Achiron et al., 2004). A dose escalation study using myelin-reactive, attenuated T cells selected with six separate myelin peptides from MBP, PLP, and MOG found reductions in myelin-reactive T cells, relapses, and MRI detectable lesions, as well as improved clinical evaluations (Loftus et al., 2009). A similar study observed twofold decreases in serum levels of IFN-γ as well as threefold increases of IL-4 at 2 years post-vaccination, suggesting the potential for prolonged protective effects with this therapeutic vaccine strategy (Ivanova et al., 2008).

Whereas vaccine-focused clinical trials have yet to be realized in PD, preclinical investigations suggest the utility of a vaccine strategy that targets the neuroinflammatory component believed associated with subsequent dopaminergic neurodegeneration in PD. Studies addressing alpha-synuclein (α-syn) aggregates and fibrils which lead to neurodegeneration, Lewy body formation, and neuroinflammation have shown that after vaccination with human α-syn, mice produce high titers of antibodies with decreased accumulation of aggregated α-syn and reduced neurodegeneration (Masliah, Rockenstein et al., 2005). Several studies have shown that immunization with MBP cross-reactive copolymer-1 (Cop-1, GA, Copaxone) induces CD4+ T cells that attenuate neuroinflammation and subsequent dopaminergic neurodegeneration in 1-methyl-4-phenyl-1,2,3,6-tetrahydropyridine (MPTP)-intoxicated mice (Benner et al., 2004; Laurie et al., 2007). These studies suggested a possible role for regulatory T cells which comprise a subset of the neuroprotective CD4+ T cells and a vaccine strategy that beneficially boosts their number or activity. Indeed, isolation and adoptive transfer of natural CD4+CD25+FoxP3+ Tregs, those responsible for maintaining tolerance to self, attenuate MPTP-induced neuroinflammation and neurodegeneration, as well as suppress microglial activation, pro-inflammatory cytokine production, and oxidative stress (Reynolds et al., 2007; Reynolds et al., 2009). Contrastingly, nitrated α-syn (N-α-syn) drains from the CNS, activates antigen-presenting cells, and induces Teffs that ultimately exacerbate MPTP-induced neuroinflammation and increase dopaminergic neurodegeneration (Benner et al., 2008). Moreover, recent studies indicated that MPTP-induced dopaminergic neurodegeneration requires a functional cell-mediated immune system with CD4+ T cells providing a necessary component (Benner et al., 2008; Brochard et al., 2009). Furthermore, the efficacy of Tregs is augmented in the presence of Teffs (Reynolds et al., 2010). Taken together, these data suggested that during the asymptomatic phase of PD, Tregs control Teff- and microglia-mediated exacerbation of neurodegenerative processes; however, with age and diminished Treg numbers or activity, neuroinflammation and neurodegeneration increases, leading to increased CNS protein aggregation and accelerated disease progression. Thus, a vaccine strategy for PD could target not only α-syn aggregates with anti-α-syn antibodies, but also boost natural or α-syn-induced Treg number or activity to attenuate Teff- and microglia-mediated neuroinflammation and subsequent neurodegeneration.

Immunotherapeutic studies for intervention of neurodegenerative disorders such as AD and PD provide novel vaccine strategies for neuroAIDS and HAND since HIV-1-associated neuropathology is, in part, attributable to neuroinflammation, pro-inflammatory cytokines, and neurotoxic oxidative stress. Thus, a vaccine that attenuates inflammation would decrease pro-inflammatory cytokines and diminish oxidative stress to afford potential clinical benefits for patients suffering from HAND. In support of this strategy, administration of GA in models of HIV-1 encephalitis led to anti-inflammatory and neuroprotective responses as demonstrated by reduction of activated microglia and astrocytes, downregulation of inducible nitric oxide synthase (iNOS), increased ingress of Foxp3+ regulatory T cells, increased expression of IL-4, IL-10, and BDNF, conservation of NeuN/MAP-2 levels, and restoration of hippocampal neurogenesis (Gorantla et al., 2008; Gorantla et al., 2007). However, this strategy may be a double-edged sword since vaccines that downregulate pro-inflammatory processes in the CNS, particularly via Treg-mediated mechanisms, may negatively impact vaccine strategies that target upregulation of CD4+ Th1 and CD8+ cytotoxic T cells believed necessary to eliminate HIV-1-infected cells in the periphery.

CONCLUSION

While the ultimate goal for an HIV-1 vaccine strategy is to elicit specific sterilizing immunity, preferably in a prophylactic fashion, the reality of rapid integration and latency of HIV-1 renders sterilizing immunity, and thus prophylactic vaccine strategies, unlikely to attain fruition. Although traditional and early novel HIV-1 vaccine strategies have yet to attain robust protection from HIV-1 infection, studies have provided necessary information to change approaches that are beginning to target immune components which afford better protective immune responses for controlling HIV-1-infected cells in the periphery. However, in the face of incomplete viral elimination from the host, an appropriately honed immune response, combined with ART that minimizes systemic spread of the virus, may be a more realistic strategy. Thus, the more plausible goal may utilize a therapeutic vaccine approach that produces broadly reactive neutralizing antibodies, both serum IgG and mucosal IgA, as well as robust central memory helper and cytotoxic T cell responses to immunodominant epitopes covering a greater breadth of viral diversity. Affording both humoral and cell-mediated immunity, this strategy would reduce viral transmission and prolong disease-free periods, which would benefit the individual, as well as slow the pandemic.

Unfortunately, immune responses designed to afford protection from HIV-1 infection and diminish viral reservoirs, may have profound untoward effects in the CNS. To be effective, not only would peripheral HIV-1 infections need to be controlled, but infections and reservoirs within the brain would most likely also need to be diminished. As such, permissive entry into the brain of some vaccine-induced immune components could exacerbate neuroinflammation, increase neuropathology, and thus amplify HAND in the wake of anti-HIV-1 immune responses. Anti-HIV-1 antibodies may activate complement to yield complement-derived peptides, C3a and C5a, which in turn could induce inflammatory responses leading to increased inflammation. Helper T cells that produce cytokines, such as IFN-γ, TNF-α, and IL-17 will most likely increase inflammatory responses. Killing HIV-1 infected T cells, monocytes, and microglia by cytotoxic T cells plausibly will induce higher levels of activated microglia, leading to exacerbated inflammation. In turn, increased inflammation and oxidative stress within the brain may increase the migration of infected macrophages into inflammatory foci and propagate HIV-1 infection and HAND. Thus, for neuroAIDS, a vaccine strategy that targets not only viral infection and HIV-1 reservoirs, but also the inflammatory and neuropathological processes within the CNS may be necessary for an efficacious therapeutic HIV-1 vaccine.

REFERENCES

Abbink, P., Lemckert, A. A., Ewald, B. A., Lynch, D. M., Denholtz, M., Smits, S., et al. (2007). Comparative seroprevalence and immunogenicity of six rare serotype recombinant adenovirus vaccine vectors from subgroups B and D. *J Virol*, 81 (9), 4654–63.

Achiron, A., Lavie, G., Kishner, I., Stern, Y., Sarova-Pinhas, I., Ben-Aharon, T., et al. (2004). T cell vaccination in multiple sclerosis relapsing-remitting nonresponders patients. *Clin Immunol*, 113 (2), 155–60.

Ackers, M-L., Parekh, B., Evans, T. G., Berman, P., Phillips, S., Allen, M., et al. (2003). Human immunodeficiency virus (HIV) seropositivity among uninfected HIV vaccine recipients. *J Infect Dis*, 187(6), 879–86.

Aharoni, R., Teitelbaum, D., Leitner, O., Meshorer, A., Sela, M., & Arnon, R. (2000). Specific Th2 cells accumulate in the central nervous system of mice protected against experimental autoimmune encephalomyelitis by copolymer 1. *Proc Natl Acad Sci USA*, 97(21), 11472–7.

Allen, T. M., Altfeld, M., Geer, S. C., Kalife, E. T., Moore, C., M. O'Sullivan M., et al. (2005). Selective escape from CD8+ T-cell responses represents a major driving force of human immunodeficiency virus type 1 (HIV-1) sequence diversity and reveals constraints on HIV-1 evolution. *J Virol*, 79(21), 13239–49.

Arnon, R., Sela, M., & Teitelbaum, D. (1996). New insights into the mechanism of action of copolymer 1 in experimental allergic encephalomyelitis and multiple sclerosis. *J Neurol*, 243(4 Suppl 1), S8–13.

Bayer, A. J., Bullock, Jones, R. W., Wilkinson, D., Paterson, K. R., Jenkins, L., et al. (2005). Evaluation of the safety and immunogenicity of synthetic Abeta42 (AN1792) in patients with AD. *Neurology*, 64(1), 94–101.

Belshe, R. B., Gorse, G. Mulligan, M. J., Evans, T. G., Keefer, M. C., Excler, J. L., et al. (1998). Induction of immune responses to HIV-1 by canarypox virus (ALVAC) HIV-1 and gp120 SF-2 recombinant vaccines in uninfected volunteers. NIAID AIDS Vaccine Evaluation Group. *AIDS*, 12(18), 2407–15.

Belshe, R. B., Graham, B. S., Keefer, M. C., Gorse, G. J., Wright, P., R. Dolin, R., et al. (1994). Neutralizing antibodies to HIV-1 in seronegative volunteers immunized with recombinant gp120 from the MN strain of HIV-1. NIAID AIDS Vaccine Clinical Trials Network. *JAMA*, 272(6), 475–80.

Benner, E. J., Banerjee, R., Reynolds, A. D., Sherman, S., Pisarev, V. M., Tsiperson, V., et al. (2008). Nitrated alpha-synuclein immunity accelerates degeneration of nigral dopaminergic neurons. *PLoS One*, 3(1), e1376.

Benner, E. J., Mosley, R. L., Destache, C. J., Lewis, T. B., V. Jackson-Lewis, V., Gorantla, S., et al. (2004). Therapeutic immunization protects dopaminergic neurons in a mouse model of Parkinson's disease. *Proc Natl Acad Sci USA*, 101(25), 9435–40.

Berman, P. W., Huang, W., Riddle, L., Gray, A. M., Wrin, T., Vennari, J., et al. (1999). Development of bivalent (B/E) vaccines able to neutralize CCR5-dependent viruses from the United States and Thailand. *Virology*, 265(1), 1–9.

Blaak, H., van't Wout, A. B., Brouwer, M., Hooibrink, B., Hovenkamp, E., & Schuitemaker, H. (2000). In vivo HIV-1 infection of CD45RA(+) CD4(+) T cells is established primarily by syncytium-inducing variants and correlates with the rate of CD4(+) T cell decline. *Proc Natl Acad Sci USA*, 97(3), 1269–74.

Blankson, J. N., Persaud, D., & Siliciano, R. F. (2002). The challenge of viral reservoirs in HIV-1 infection. *Annu Rev Med*, 53, 557–93.

Boche, D., Denham, N., Holmes, C., & Nicoll, J. A. (2010). Neuropathology after active Abeta42 immunotherapy: Implications for Alzheimer's disease pathogenesis. *Acta Neuropathol*, 120(3), 369–84.

Bojak, A., Deml, L., & Wagner, R. (2002). The past, present and future of HIV-vaccine development: A critical view. *Drug Discov Today*, 7(1), 36–46.

Boyer, J. D., Chattergoon, M., Muthumani, K., Kudchodkar, S., Kim, J., Bagarazzi, M., et al. (2002). Next generation DNA vaccines for HIV-1. *J Liposome Res*, 12(1–2), 137–42.

Boyer, J. D., Cohen, A. D., Vogt, S., Schumann, K., Nath, B., Ahn, L., et al. (2000). Vaccination of seronegative volunteers with a human immunodeficiency virus type 1 env/rev DNA vaccine induces antigen-specific proliferation and lymphocyte production of beta-chemokines. *J Infect Dis*, 181(2), 476–83.

Brander, C. & Walker, B. D. (1999). T lymphocyte responses in HIV-1 infection: Implications for vaccine development. *Curr Opin Immunol*, 11(4), 451–9.

Brave, A., Hinkula, J., Cafaro, A., Eriksson, L. E., Srivastava, I. K. Magnani, M., et al. (2007). Candidate HIV-1 gp140DeltaV2, Gag and Tat vaccines protect against experimental HIV-1/MuLV challenge. *Vaccine*, 25(39–40), 6882–90.

Brenchley, J. M., Schacker, T. W., Ruff, L. E. Price, D. A., Taylor, J. H., Beilman, G. J., et al. (2004). CD4+ T cell depletion during all stages of HIV disease occurs predominantly in the gastrointestinal tract. *J Exp Med*, 200(6), 749–59.

Brenner, T., Arnon, R., Sela, M., Abramsky, O., Meiner, Z., Riven-Kreitman, R., et al. (2001). Humoral and cellular immune responses to Copolymer 1 in multiple sclerosis patients treated with Copaxone. *J Neuroimmunol*, 115(1–2), 152–60.

Brochard, V., Combadiere, B., Prigent, A., Laouar, Y., Perrin, A., Beray-Berthat, V., et al. (2009). Infiltration of CD4+ lymphocytes into the brain contributes to neurodegeneration in a mouse model of Parkinson disease. *J Clin Invest*, 119(1), 182–92.

Buchbinder, S. P., Mehrotra, D. V., Duerr, A., Fitzgerald, D. W., Mogg, R., D. Li, D., et al. (2008). Efficacy assessment of a cell-mediated immunity HIV-1 vaccine (the Step Study): A double-blind, randomised, placebo-controlled, test-of-concept trial. *Lancet*, 372(9653), 1881–93.

Burton, G. F., Masuda, A., Heath, S. L., Smith, B. A., Tew, J. G., & Szakal, A. K. (1997). Follicular dendritic cells (FDC) in retroviral infection: Host/pathogen perspectives. *Immunol Rev*, 156, 185–97.

Cafaro, A., Caputo, A., Fracasso, C., Maggiorella, M. T., Goletti, D., Baroncelli, S., et al. (1999). Control of SHIV-89.6P-infection of cynomolgus monkeys by HIV-1 Tat protein vaccine. *Nat Med*, 5(6), 643–50.

Cameron, P. U., Freudenthal, P. S., Barker, J. M., Gezelter, S., Inaba, K., & Steinman, R. M. (1992). Dendritic cells exposed to human immuno-deficiency virus type-1 transmit a vigorous cytopathic infection to CD4+ T cells. *Science*, 257(5068), 383–7.

Cao, H., Kaleebu, P., Hom, D., Flores, J., Agrawal, D., Jones, N., et al. (2003). Immunogenicity of a recombinant human immunodeficiency virus (HIV)-canarypox vaccine in HIV-seronegative Ugandan volunteers: Results of the HIV Network for Prevention Trials 007 Vaccine Study. *J Infect Dis*, 187(6), 887–95.

Cao, H., Kanki, P., Sankale, J. L., Dieng-Sarr, A., Mazzara, G. P., Kalams, S. A., et al. (1997). Cytotoxic T-lymphocyte cross-reactivity among different human immunodeficiency virus type 1 clades: Implications for vaccine development. *J Virol*, 71(11), 8615–23.

Cao, H., Mani, I., Vincent, R., Mugerwa, R., Mugyenyi, P., Kanki, P., et al. (2000). Cellular immunity to human immunodeficiency virus type 1 (HIV-1) clades: relevance to HIV-1 vaccine trials in Uganda. *J Infect Dis*, 182(5), 1350–56.

Cao, W., Jamieson, B. D., Hultin, L. E., Hultin, P. M., & Detels, R. (2009). Regulatory T cell expansion and immune activation during untreated HIV type 1 infection are associated with disease progression. *AIDS Res Hum Retroviruses*, 25(2), 183–91.

Catanzaro, A. T., Koup, R. A., Roederer, M., Bailer, R. T., Enama, M. E., Moodie, Z. et al. (2006). Phase 1 safety and immunogenicity evaluation of a multiclade HIV-1 candidate vaccine delivered by a replication-defective recombinant adenovirus vector. *J Infect Dis*, 194(12), 1638–49.

Caulfield, M. J., Wang, S., Smith, J. G., Tobery, T. W., Liu, X., Davies, M-E., et al. (2002). Sustained peptide-specific gamma interferon T-cell response in rhesus macaques immunized with human immunodeficiency virus gag DNA vaccines. *J Virol*, 76(19), 10038–43.

Cavert, W., D. W. Notermans, K. Staskus, S. W. Wietgrefe, M. Zupancic, K. Gebhard, K. et al. (1997). Kinetics of response in lymphoid tissues to antiretroviral therapy of HIV-1 infection. *Science*, 276(5314), 960–4.

Chase, A. J., Yang, H. C., Zhang, H., Blankson, J. N., & Siliciano, R. F. (2008). Preservation of FoxP3+ regulatory T cells in the peripheral blood of human immunodeficiency virus type 1-infected elite suppressors correlates with low CD4+ T-cell activation. *J Virol*, 82(17), 8307–15.

Check, E. (2003). AIDS vaccines: back to "plan A." *Nature*, 423(6943), 912–4.

Chun, T. W., Carruth, L., Finzi, D., Shen, X., DiGiuseppe, J. A., Taylor, H., et al. (1997). Quantification of latent tissue reservoirs and total body viral load in HIV-1 infection. *Nature*, 387(6629), 183–8.

Chun, T. W., Finzi, D., Margolick, J., Chadwick, K., Schwartz, D., & Siliciano. (1995). In vivo fate of HIV-1-infected T cells: Quantitative analysis of the transition to stable latency. *Nat Med*, 1(12), 1284–90.

Chun, T., J., Justement, S., Pandya, P., Hallahan, C. W., McLaughlin, M., Liu, S., et al. (2002). Relationship between the size of the human immunodeficiency virus type 1 (HIV-1) reservoir in peripheral blood CD4+ T cells and CD4+:CD8+ T cell ratios in aviremic HIV-1-infected individuals receiving long-term highly active antiretroviral therapy. *J Infect Dis*, 185(11), 1672–76.

Clements-Mann, M. L., Weinhold, K., Matthews, T. J., Graham, B. S., Gorse, G. J., Keefer, M. C., et al. (1998). Immune responses to human immunodeficiency virus (HIV) type 1 induced by canarypox expressing HIV-1MN gp120, HIV-1SF2 recombinant gp120, or both vaccines in seronegative adults. NIAID AIDS Vaccine Evaluation Group. *J Infect Dis*, 177(5), 1230–46.

Cohen, J. (2003). Clinical research. AIDS vaccine results draw investor lawsuits. *Science*, 299(5615), 1965.

Cooney, E. L., McElrath, M. J., Corey, L., Hu, S. L., Collier, A. C., Arditti, D., et al. (1993). Enhanced immunity to human immunodeficiency virus (HIV) envelope elicited by a combined vaccine regimen consisting of priming with a vaccinia recombinant expressing HIV envelope and boosting with gp160 protein. *Proc Natl Acad Sci USA*, 90(5), 1882–86.

Correale, J., Farez, M., & Gilmore, W. (2008). Vaccines for multiple sclerosis: Progress to date. *CNS Drugs*, 22(3), 175–98.

Csaba, N., Garcia-Fuentes, M., & Alonso, M. J. (2009). Nanoparticles for nasal vaccination. *Adv Drug Deliv Rev*, 61(2), 140–57.

Curotto de Lafaille, M. A. & Lafaille, J. J. (2009). Natural and adaptive foxp3+ regulatory T cells: More of the same or a division of labor? *Immunity*, 30(5), 626–35.

Curran, R. M., Donnelly, L., Morrow, R. J., Fraser, C., Andrews, G., Cranage, M., et al. (2009). Vaginal delivery of the recombinant HIV-1 clade-C trimeric gp140 envelope protein CN54gp140 within novel rheologically structured vehicles elicits specific immune responses. *Vaccine*, 27(48), 6791–8.

Czerkinsky, C. & Holmgren, J. (2009). Enteric vaccines for the developing world: A challenge for mucosal immunology. *Mucosal Immunol*, 2(4), 284–7.

De Silva, F. S., Venturini, D. S., Wagner, E., Shank, P. R., & Sharma, S. (2001). CD4-independent infection of human B cells with HIV type 1: Detection of unintegrated viral DNA. *AIDS Res Hum Retroviruses*, 17(17), 1585–98.

Dolin, R., Graham, B. S., Greenberg, S. B., Tacket, C. O., Belshe, R. B., Midthun, K., et al. (1991). The safety and immunogenicity of a human immunodeficiency virus type 1 (HIV-1) recombinant gp160 candidate vaccine in humans. NIAID AIDS Vaccine Clinical Trials Network. *Ann Intern Med*, 114(2), 119–27.

Donnelly, J. J., Ulmer, J. B., Shiver, J. W., & Liu, M. A. (1997). DNA vaccines. *Annu Rev Immunol*, 15, 617–48.

Duh, E. J., Maury, W. J., Folks, T. M., Fauci, A. S., & Rabson, A. B. (1989). Tumor necrosis factor alpha activates human immunodeficiency virus type 1 through induction of nuclear factor binding to the NF-kappa B sites in the long terminal repeat. *Proc Natl Acad Sci USA*, 86(15), 5974–78.

Dunham, R. M., Cervasi, B., Brenchley, J. M., Albrecht, H., Weintrob, A., Sumpter, B., et al. (2008). CD127 and CD25 expression defines CD4+ T cell subsets that are differentially depleted during HIV infection. *J Immunol*, 180(8), 5582–92.

Durrani, Z., McInerney, T. L., McLain, L., Jones, T., Bellaby, T., Brennan, F. R., et al. (1998). Intranasal immunization with a plant virus expressing a peptide from HIV-1 gp41 stimulates better mucosal and systemic HIV-1-specific IgA and IgG than oral immunization. *J Immunol Methods*, 220(1–2), 93–103.

Eggena, M. P., Barugahare, B., Jones, N., Okello, M., Mutalya, S., Kityo, C., et al. (2005). Depletion of regulatory T cells in HIV infection is associated with immune activation. *J Immunol*, 174(7), 4407–14.

Embretson, J., Zupancic, M., Ribas, J. L., Burke, A., Racz, P., Tenner-Racz, K., et al. (1993). Massive covert infection of helper T lymphocytes and macrophages by HIV during the incubation period of AIDS. *Nature*, 362(6418), 359–62.

Estes, J. D., Keele, B. F., Tenner-Racz, K., Racz, P., Redd, M. A., Thacker, T. C., et al. (2002). Follicular dendritic cell-mediated up-regulation of CXCR4 expression on CD4 T cells and HIV pathogenesis. *J Immunol*, 169(5), 2313–22.

Evans, T. G., Keefer, M. C., Weinhold, K. J., Wolff, M., Montefiori, D., Gorse, G. J., et al. (1999). A canarypox vaccine expressing multiple human immunodeficiency virus type 1 genes given alone or with rgp120 elicits broad and durable CD8+ cytotoxic T lymphocyte responses in seronegative volunteers. *J Infect Dis*, 180(2), 290–8.

Fahmy, T. M., Demento, S. L., Caplan, M. J., Mellman, I., & Saltzman, W. M. (2008). Design opportunities for actively targeted nanoparticle vaccines. *Nanomedicine (Lond)*, 3(3), 343–55.

Fairman, J., Moore, J., Lemieux, M., Van Rompay, K., Geng, Y., Warner, J., et al. (2009). Enhanced in vivo immunogenicity of SIV vaccine candidates with cationic liposome-DNA complexes in a rhesus macaque pilot study. *Hum Vaccin*, 5(3), 141–50.

Farokhzad, O. C. (2008). Nanotechnology for drug delivery: The perfect partnership. *Expert Opin Drug Deliv*, 5(9), 927–9.

Ferrari, G., Humphrey, W., McElrath, M. J., Excler, J. L., Duliege, A. M., Clements, et al. (1997). Clade B-based HIV-1 vaccines elicit cross-clade cytotoxic T lymphocyte reactivities in uninfected volunteers. *Proc Natl Acad Sci USA*, 94(4), 1396–1401.

Finzi, D., Blankson, J., Siliciano, J. D., Margolick, J. B., Chadwick, K., Pierson, T., et al. (1999). Latent infection of CD4+ T cells provides a mechanism for lifelong persistence of HIV-1, even in patients on effective combination therapy. *Nat Med*, 5(5), 512–7.

Finzi, D. & Siliciano, R. F. (1998). Viral dynamics in HIV-1 infection. *Cell*, 93(5), 665–71.

Flamand, L., Crowley, R. W., Lusso, P., Colombini-Hatch, S., Margolis, D. M., &Gallo, R. C. (1998). Activation of CD8+ T lymphocytes through the T cell receptor turns on CD4 gene expression: Implications for HIV pathogenesis. *Proc Natl Acad Sci USA*, 95(6), 3111–6.

Fleury, B., Janvier, G., Pialoux, G., Buseyne, F., Robertson, M. N., Tartaglia, J., et al. (1996). Memory cytotoxic T lymphocyte responses in human immunodeficiency virus type 1 (HIV-1)-negative volunteers immunized with a recombinant canarypox expressing gp 160 of HIV-1 and boosted with a recombinant gp160. *J Infect Dis*, 174 (4), 734–8.

Fox, C. H., Tenner-Racz, K., Racz, P., Firpo, A., Pizzo, P. A., & Fauci, A. S. (1991). Lymphoid germinal centers are reservoirs of human immunodeficiency virus type 1 RNA. *J Infect Dis*, 164 (6), 1051–7.

Francis, D. P., Gregory, T., McElrath, M. J., Belshe, R. B., Gorse, G. J., Migasena, S., et al. (1998). Advancing AIDSVAX to phase 3. Safety, immunogenicity, and plans for phase 3. *AIDS Res Hum Retroviruses*, 14 Suppl 3, 325–31.

Frankel, S. S., Wenig, B. M., Burke, A. P., Mannan, P., Thompson, L., D., Abbondanzo, S. L., et al. (1996). Replication of HIV-1 in dendritic cell-derived syncytia at the mucosal surface of the adenoid. *Science*, 272 (5258), 115–7.

Fritsch, L., Marechal, V., Schneider, V., Barthet, C., Rozenbaum, W., Moisan-Coppey, M., et al. (1998). Production of HIV-1 by human B cells infected in vitro: Characterization of an EBV genome-negative B cell line chronically synthetizing a low level of HIV-1 after infection. *Virology*, 244 (2), 542–51.

Fu, T. M., Dubey, S. A., Mehrotra, D. V., Freed, D. C., Trigona, W. L., Adams-Muhler, L., et al. (2007). Evaluation of cellular immune responses in subjects chronically infected with HIV type 1. *AIDS Res Hum Retroviruses*, 23 (1), 67–76.

Gahery-Segard, H., Pialoux, G., Charmeteau, B., Sermet, S., Poncelet, H., Raux, M., et al. (2000). Multiepitopic B- and T-cell responses induced in humans by a human immunodeficiency virus type 1 lipopeptide vaccine. *J Virol*, 74 (4), 1694–1703.

Gahery, H., Daniel, N., Charmeteau, B., Ourth, L., Jackson, A., Andrieu, M., et al. (2006). New CD4+ and CD8+ T cell responses induced in chronically HIV type-1-infected patients after immunizations with an HIV type 1 lipopeptide vaccine. *AIDS Res Hum Retroviruses*, 22 (7), 684–94.

Geijtenbeek, T. B., Kwon, D. S., Torensma, R., van Vliet, S. J., van Duijnhoven, G. C., Middel, J., et al. (2000). DC-SIGN, a dendritic cell-specific HIV-1-binding protein that enhances trans-infection of T cells. *Cell*, 100 (5), 587–97.

Gilman, S., Koller, M., Black, R. S., Jenkins, L., Griffith, S. G., Fox, N. C., et al. (2005). Clinical effects of Abeta immunization (AN1792) in patients with AD in an interrupted trial. *Neurology*, 64 (9), 1553–62.

Gonzalez-Scarano, F. & Martin-Garcia, J. (2005). The neuropathogenesis of AIDS. *Nat Rev Immunol*, 5 (1), 69–81.

Gorantla, S., Liu, J., Sneller, H., Dou, H., Holguin, A., Smith, L., (2007). Copolymer-1 induces adaptive immune anti-inflammatory glial and neuroprotective responses in a murine model of HIV-1 encephalitis. *J Immunol*, 179 (7), 4345–56.

Gorantla, S., Liu, J., Wang, T., Holguin, A., Sneller, H. M., Dou, H. (2008). Modulation of innate immunity by copolymer-1 leads to neuroprotection in murine HIV-1 encephalitis. *Glia*, 56 (2), 223–32.

Gorse, G. J., McElrath, M. J., Matthews, T. J., Hsieh, R. H., Belshe, R. B., Corey, L., et al. (1998). Modulation of immunologic responses to HIV-1MN recombinant gp160 vaccine by dose and schedule of administration. National Institute of Allergy and Infectious Diseases AIDS Vaccine Evaluation Group. *Vaccine*, 16 (5), 493–506.

Graham, B. S., Keefer, M. C., McElrath, M. J., Gorse, G. J., Schwartz, D. H., Weinhold, K., et al. (1996). Safety and immunogenicity of a candidate HIV-1 vaccine in healthy adults: recombinant glycoprotein (rgp) 120. A randomized, double-blind trial. NIAID AIDS Vaccine Evaluation Group. *Ann Intern Med*, 125 (4), 270–9.

Graham, B. S., Matthews, T. J., Belshe, R. B., Clements, M. L., Dolin, R., Wright, P. F., et al. (1993). Augmentation of human immunodeficiency virus type 1 neutralizing antibody by priming with gp160 recombinant vaccinia and boosting with rgp160 in vaccinia-naive adults. The NIAID AIDS Vaccine Clinical Trials Network. *J Infect Dis*, 167(3), 533–537.

Gras, G., Richard, Y., Roques, P., Olivier, R., & Dormont, D. (1993). Complement and virus-specific antibody-dependent infection of normal B lymphocytes by human immunodeficiency virus type 1. *Blood*, 81 (7), 1808–18.

Gringeri, A., Santagostino, E., Muca-Perja, M., Mannucci, P. M., Zagury, J. F., Bizzini, B/, et al. (1998). Safety and immunogenicity of HIV-1 Tat toxoid in immunocompromised HIV-1-infected patients. *J Hum Virol*, 1 (4), 293–98.

Grundman, M. & Black, R. (2008). Clinical trials of bapineuzumab, a beta-amyloid-targeted immunotherapy in patients with mild to moderate Alzheimer's disease [abstract]. *Alzheimers Dementia*, 4 (T166).

Guimaraes-Walker, A., Mackie, N., McCormack, S., Hanke, T., Schmidt, C., Gilmour, J., et al. (2008). Lessons from IAVI-006, a phase I clinical trial to evaluate the safety and immunogenicity of the pTHr.HIVA DNA and MVA.HIVA vaccines in a prime-boost strategy to induce HIV-1 specific T-cell responses in healthy volunteers. *Vaccine*, 26(51), 6671–7.

Gummuluru, S., KewalRamani, V. N., & Emerman, M. (2002). Dendritic cell-mediated viral transfer to T cells is required for human immunodeficiency virus type 1 persistence in the face of rapid cell turnover. *J Virol* 76 (21):10692–701.

Haas, J., Park, E. C., & Seed, B. (1996). Codon usage limitation in the expression of HIV-1 envelope glycoprotein. *Curr Biol*, 6 (3), 315–324.

Hanke, T., & McMichael, A. J. (2000). Design and construction of an experimental HIV-1 vaccine for a year-2000 clinical trial in Kenya. *Nat Med*, 6 (9), 951–55.

Hellings, N., Raus, J., & Stinissen, P. (2006). T-cell-based immunotherapy in multiple sclerosis: Induction of regulatory immune networks by T-cell vaccination. *Expert Rev Clin Immunol*, 2 (5), 705–16.

Hirbod, T., Kaul, R., Reichard, C., Kimani, J., Ngugi, E., Bwayo, J. J., et al. (2008). HIV-neutralizing immunoglobulin A and HIV-specific proliferation are independently associated with reduced HIV acquisition in Kenyan sex workers. *AIDS*, 22 (6), 727–35.

Holmes, C., Boche, D., Wilkinson, D., Yadegarfar, G., Hopkins, V., Bayer, A., et al. (2008). Long-term effects of Abeta42 immunisation in

Alzheimer's disease: Follow-up of a randomised, placebo-controlled phase I trial. *Lancet*, 372 (9634), 216–23.

Holmgren, J. & Czerkinsky, C. (2005). Mucosal immunity and vaccines. *Nat Med*, 11 (4 Suppl), S45–53.

Hong, J., Zang, Y. C., Nie, H., & Zhang, J. Z. (2006). CD4+ regulatory T cell responses induced by T cell vaccination in patients with multiple sclerosis. *Proc Natl Acad Sci USA*, 103 (13), 5024–9.

Imlach, S., McBreen, S., Shirafuji, T., Leen, C., Bell, J. E., & Simmonds, P. (2001). Activated peripheral CD8 lymphocytes express CD4 in vivo and are targets for infection by human immunodeficiency virus type 1. *J Virol*, 75 (23), 11555–64.

Innocenti, P., Ottmann, M., Morand, P., Leclercq, P., & Seigneurin, J. M. (1992). HIV-1 in blood monocytes: Frequency of detection of proviral DNA using PCR and comparison with the total CD4 count. *AIDS Res Hum Retroviruses*, 8 (2), 261–68.

Iqbal, S. M., Ball, T. B., Kimani, J., Kiama, P., Thottingal, P., Embree, J. E., et al. (2005). Elevated T cell counts and RANTES expression in the genital mucosa of HIV-1-resistant Kenyan commercial sex workers. *J Infect Dis*, 192 (5), 728–38.

Iqbal, S. M., & Kaul, R. (2008). Mucosal innate immunity as a determinant of HIV susceptibility. *Am J Reprod Immunol*, 59 (1), 44–54.

Ivanova, I. P., Seledtsov, V. I., Seledtsova, G. V., Mamaev, S. V., Potyemkin, A. V., Seledtsov, D. V., et al. (2008). Induction of antiidiotypic immune response with autologous T-cell vaccine in patients with multiple sclerosis. *Bull Exp Biol Med*, 146 (1), 133–8.

Jakubik, J. J., Saifuddin, M., Takefman, D. M., & Spear, G. T. (2000). Immune complexes containing human immunodeficiency virus type 1 primary isolates bind to lymphoid tissue B lymphocytes and are infectious for T lymphocytes. *J Virol*, 74 (1), 552–5.

Jiao, Y., Fu, J., Xing, S., Fu, B., Zhang, Z., Shi, M., et al. (2009). The decrease of regulatory T cells correlates with excessive activation and apoptosis of CD8+ T cells in HIV-1-infected typical progressors, but not in long-term non-progressors. *Immunology*, 128 (1 Suppl), e366–75.

Jin, X., Bauer, D. E., Tuttleton, S. E., Lewin, S., Gettie, A., Blanchard, J., et al. (1999). Dramatic rise in plasma viremia after CD8(+) T cell depletion in simian immunodeficiency virus-infected macaques. *J Exp Med*, 189 (6), 991–8.

Joos, B., Fischer, M., Kuster, H., Pillai, S. K., Wong, J. K., Boni, J., et al. (2008). HIV rebounds from latently infected cells, rather than from continuing low-level replication. *Proc Natl Acad Sci U S A*, 105 (43):16725–30.

Keefer, M. C., Graham, B. S., Belshe, R. B., Schwartz, D., Corey, L., Bolognesi, D. P., et al. (1994). Studies of high doses of a human immunodeficiency virus type 1 recombinant glycoprotein 160 candidate vaccine in HIV type 1-seronegative humans. The AIDS Vaccine Clinical Trials Network. *AIDS Res Hum Retroviruses*, 10 (12): 1713–23.

Keefer, M. C., Graham, B. S., McElrath, M. J., Matthews, T. J., Stablein, D. M., Corey, L., et al. (1996). Safety and immunogenicity of Env 2–3, a human immunodeficiency virus type 1 candidate vaccine, in combination with a novel adjuvant, MTP-PE/MF59. NIAID AIDS Vaccine Evaluation Group. *AIDS Res Hum Retroviruses* 12 (8):683–93.

Kelleher, A. D., Emery, S., Cunningham, P., Duncombe, C., Carr, A., Golding, H., et al. (1997). Safety and immunogenicity of UBI HIV-1MN octameric V3 peptide vaccine administered by subcutaneous injection. *AIDS Res Hum Retroviruses*, 13 (1):29–32.

Kerschensteiner, M., Meinl, E., & Hohlfeld, R. (2009). Neuro-immune crosstalk in CNS diseases. *Neuroscience*, 158 (3):1122–32.

Kinter, A. L., Horak, R., Sion, M., Riggin, L., McNally, J., Lin, Y., et al. (2007). CD25+ regulatory T cells isolated from HIV-infected individuals suppress the cytolytic and nonlytic antiviral activity of HIV-specific CD8+ T cells in vitro. *AIDS Res Hum Retroviruses*, 23 (3):438–50.

Kitchen, S. G., Korin, Y. D., Roth, M. D., Landay, A., & Zack, J. A. (1998). Costimulation of naive CD8(+) lymphocytes induces CD4 expression and allows human immunodeficiency virus type 1 infection. *J Virol*, 72 (11):9054–60.

Kitchen, S. G., LaForge, S., Patel, V. P., Kitchen, C. M., Miceli, M. C., & Zack, J. A. (2002). Activation of CD8 T cells induces expression of CD4, which functions as a chemotactic receptor. *Blood*, 99 (1): 207–12.

Kivisakk, P., Tucky, B., Wei, T., Campbell, J. J., & Ransohoff, R. M. (2006). Human cerebrospinal fluid contains CD4+ memory T cells expressing gut- or skin-specific trafficking determinants: Relevance for immunotherapy. *BMC Immunol*, 7:14.

Klein, M. R., van Baalen, C. A., Holwerda, A. M., Kerkhof Garde, S. R., Bende, R. J., Keet, I. P., et al. (1995). Kinetics of Gag-specific cytotoxic T lymphocyte responses during the clinical course of HIV-1 infection: A longitudinal analysis of rapid progressors and long-term asymptomatics. *J Exp Med*, 181 (4), 1365–72.

Klein, M. R., Veenstra, J., Holwerda, A. M., Roos, M. T., Gow, I., Patou, G., et al. (1997). Gag-specific immune responses after immunization with p17/p24:Ty virus-like particles in HIV type 1-seropositive individuals. *AIDS Res Hum Retroviruses*, 13 (5), 393–9.

Koenig, S., Gendelman, H. E., Orenstein, J. M., Dal Canto, M. C., Pezeshkpour, G. H., Yungbluth, M., et al. (1986). Detection of AIDS virus in macrophages in brain tissue from AIDS patients with encephalopathy. *Science*, 233 (4768), 1089–93.

Kotton, C. N., Lankowski, A. J., Scott, N., Sisul, D., Chen, L. M., Raschke, K., et al. (2006). Safety and immunogenicity of attenuated Salmonella enterica serovar Typhimurium delivering an HIV-1 Gag antigen via the Salmonella Type III secretion system. *Vaccine*, 24 (37–39):6216–24.

Kovacs, J. A., Vasudevachari, M. B., Easter, M., Davey, R. T., Falloon, J., Polis, M. A., et al. (1993). Induction of humoral and cell-mediated anti-human immunodeficiency virus (HIV) responses in HIV seronegative volunteers by immunization with recombinant gp160. *J Clin Invest*, 92 (2):919–28.

Lambert, J. S., Keefer, M., Mulligan, M. J., Schwartz, D., Mestecky, J., Weinhold, K., et al. (2001). A Phase I safety and immunogenicity trial of UBI microparticulate monovalent HIV-1 MN oral peptide immunogen with parenteral boost in HIV-1 seronegative human subjects. *Vaccine*, 19 (23–24):3033–42.

Lambotte, O., Taoufik, Y., de Goer, M. G., Wallon, C., Goujard, C., & Delfraissy, J. F. (2000). Detection of infectious HIV in circulating monocytes from patients on prolonged highly active antiretroviral therapy. *J Acquir Immune Defic Syndr*, 23 (2):114–9.

Lapointe, R., Lemieux, R., & Darveau, A. (1996). HIV-1 LTR activity in human CD40-activated B lymphocytes is dependent on NF-kappaB. *Biochem Biophys Res Commun*, 229 (3), 959–64.

Launay, O., Durier, C., Desaint, C., Silbermann, B., Jackson, A., Pialoux, G., et al. (2007). Cellular immune responses induced with dose-sparing intradermal administration of HIV vaccine to HIV-uninfected volunteers in the ANRS VAC16 trial. *PLoS One*, 2 (1):e725.

Laurie, C., Reynolds, A., Coskun, O., Bowman, E., Gendelman, H. E., & Mosley, R. L. (2007). CD4+ T cells from Copolymer-1 immunized mice protect dopaminergic neurons in the 1-methyl-4-phenyl-1,2,3,6-tetrahydropyridine model of Parkinson's disease. *J Neuroimmunol*, 183 (1–2):60–8.

Learmont, J. C., Geczy, A. F., Mills, J., Ashton, L. J., Raynes-Greenow, C. H., Garsia, R. J., . (1999). Immunologic and virologic status after 14 to 18 years of infection with an attenuated strain of HIV-1. A report from the Sydney Blood Bank Cohort. *N Engl J Med*, 340 (22):1715–22.

Lehmann, C., Lafferty, M., Garzino-Demo, A., Jung, N., Hartmann, P., Fatkenheuer, G., et al. (2010). Plasmacytoid dendritic cells accumulate and secrete interferon alpha in lymph nodes of HIV-1 patients. *PLoS One*, 5 (6):e11110.

Lemere, C. A. & Masliah, E. (2010). Can Alzheimer disease be prevented by amyloid-beta immunotherapy? *Nat Rev Neurol*, 6 (2):108–19.

Leung, L., Srivastava, I. K., Kan, E., Legg, H., Sun, Y., Greer, C., et al. (2004). Immunogenicity of HIV-1 Env and Gag in baboons using a DNA prime/protein boost regimen. *AIDS*, 18 (7):991–01.

Lewis, D. J., Huo, Z., Barnett, S., Kromann, I., Giemza, R., Galiza, E., et al. (2009). Transient facial nerve paralysis (Bell's palsy) following intranasal delivery of a genetically detoxified mutant of Escherichia coli heat labile toxin. *PLoS One* 4 (9):e6999.

Lifson, J. D., Rossio, J. L., Piatak, M. Jr., Bess, J. Jr., Chertova, E., Schneider, D. K., et al. (2004). Evaluation of the safety, immunogenicity, and protective efficacy of whole inactivated simian immunodeficiency virus

(SIV) vaccines with conformationally and functionally intact envelope glycoproteins. *AIDS Res Hum Retroviruses*, 20 (7), 772–87.

Lindenburg, C. E., Stolte, I., Langendam, M. W., Miedema, F., Williams, I. G., Colebunders, R., et al. (2002). Long-term follow-up: no effect of therapeutic vaccination with HIV-1 p17/p24:Ty virus-like particles on HIV-1 disease progression. *Vaccine*, 20 (17–18), 2343–7.

Livingstone, W. J., Moore, M., Innes, D., Bell, J. E., & Simmonds, P. (1996). Frequent infection of peripheral blood CD8-positive T-lymphocytes with HIV-1. Edinburgh Heterosexual Transmission Study Group. *Lancet*, 348 (9028), 649–54.

Loftus, B., Newsom, B., Montgomery, M., Von Gynz-Rekowski, K., Riser, M., Inman, S., et al. (2009). Autologous attenuated T-cell vaccine (Tovaxin) dose escalation in multiple sclerosis relapsing-remitting and secondary progressive patients nonresponsive to approved immunomodulatory therapies. *Clin Immunol*, 131 (2), 202–15.

Macatangay, B. J., Szajnik, M. E., Whiteside, T. L., Riddler, S. A., & Rinaldo, C. R. (2010). Regulatory T cell suppression of Gag-specific CD8 T cell polyfunctional response after therapeutic vaccination of HIV-1-infected patients on ART. *PLoS One*, 5 (3), e9852.

MacDougall, T. H. J., Shattock, R. J., Madsen, C., Chain, B. M., & Katz, D. R. (2002). Regulation of primary HIV-1 isolate replication in dendritic cells. *Clin Exp Immunol*, 127 (1), 66–71.

MacGregor, R. R., Boyer, J. D., Ugen, K. E., Lacy, K. E., Gluckman, S. J., Bagarazzi, M. L., et al. (1998). First human trial of a DNA-based vaccine for treatment of human immunodeficiency virus type 1 infection: Safety and host response. *J Infect Dis*, 178 (1), 92–100.

MacGregor, R.R., Ginsberg, R., Ugen, K. E., Baine, Y., Kang, C. U., et al. (2002). T-cell responses induced in normal volunteers immunized with a DNA-based vaccine containing HIV-1 env and rev. *AIDS*, 16 (16), 2137–43.

Malaspina, A., Moir, S., Nickle, D. C., Donoghue, E. T., Ogwaro, K. M., Ehler, L. A., et al. (2002). Human immunodeficiency virus type 1 bound to B cells: Relationship to virus replicating in CD4+ T cells and circulating in plasma. *J Virol*, 76 (17), 8855–63.

Mann, J. F., Scales, H. E., Shakir, E., Alexander, J., Carter, K. C., Mullen, A. B., et al. (2006). Oral delivery of tetanus toxoid using vesicles containing bile salts (bilosomes) induces significant systemic and mucosal immunity. *Methods*, 38 (2), 90–5.

Margolick, J. B., Volkman, D. J., Folks, T. M., & Fauci, A. S. (1987). Amplification of HTLV-III/LAV infection by antigen-induced activation of T cells and direct suppression by virus of lymphocyte blastogenic responses. *J Immunol*, 138 (6), 1719–23.

Martin, S. J., Vyakarnam, A., Cheingsong-Popov, R., Callow, D., Jones, K. L., Senior, J. M., et al. (1993). Immunization of human HIV-seronegative volunteers with recombinant p17/p24:Ty virus-like particles elicits HIV-1 p24-specific cellular and humoral immune responses. *AIDS*, 7 (10), 1315–23.

Mascola, J. R., Louder, M. K., Surman, S. R., Vancott, T. C., Yu, X. F., Bradac, J., et al. (1996). Human immunodeficiency virus type 1 neutralizing antibody serotyping using serum pools and an infectivity reduction assay. *AIDS Res Hum Retroviruses*, 12 (14), 1319–28.

Mascola, J. R., Snyder, S. W., Weislow, O. S., Belay, S. M., Belshe, R. B., Schwartz, D. H., et al. (1996). Immunization with envelope subunit vaccine products elicits neutralizing antibodies against laboratory-adapted but not primary isolates of human immunodeficiency virus type 1. The National Institute of Allergy and Infectious Diseases AIDS Vaccine Evaluation Group. *J Infect Dis*, 173 (2), 340–48.

Masliah, E., Hansen, L., Adame, A., Crews, L., Bard, F., Lee, C., et al. (2005). Abeta vaccination effects on plaque pathology in the absence of encephalitis in Alzheimer disease. *Neurology*, 64 (1), 129–31.

Masliah, E., Rockenstein, E., Adame, A., Alford, M., Crews, L., Hashimoto, M., et al. (2005). Effects of alpha-synuclein immunization in a mouse model of Parkinson's disease. *Neuron*, 46 (6), 857–68.

Mattapallil, J. J., Douek, D. C., Hill, B., Nishimura, Y., Martin, M., & Roederer, M. (2005). Massive infection and loss of memory CD4+ T cells in multiple tissues during acute SIV infection. *Nature*, 434 (7037), 1093–7.

McAdam, S., Kaleebu, P., Krausa, P., Goulder, P., French, N., Collin, B., et al. (1998). Cross-clade recognition of p55 by cytotoxic T lymphocytes in HIV-1 infection. *AIDS*, 12 (6), 571–79.

McElrath, M. J., Corey, L., Montefiori, D., Wolff, M., Schwartz, D., Keefer, M., et al. (2000). A phase II study of two HIV type 1 envelope vaccines, comparing their immunogenicity in populations at risk for acquiring HIV type 1 infection. AIDS Vaccine Evaluation Group. *AIDS Res Hum Retroviruses*, 16 (9), 907–19.

McElrath, M. J., Pruett, J. E., & Cohn, Z. A. (1989). Mononuclear phagocytes of blood and bone marrow: Comparative roles as viral reservoirs in human immunodeficiency virus type 1 infections. *Proc Natl Acad Sci U S A*, 86 (2), 675–79.

Mehandru, S., Poles, M. A., Tenner-Racz, K., Horowitz, A., Hurley, A., Hogan, C., et al. (2004). Primary HIV-1 infection is associated with preferential depletion of CD4+ T lymphocytes from effector sites in the gastrointestinal tract. *J Exp Med*, 200 (6), 761–70.

Meltzer, M. S., Nakamura, M., Hansen, B. D., Turpin, J. A., Kalter, D. C., & Gendelman, H. E. (1990). Macrophages as susceptible targets for HIV infection, persistent viral reservoirs in tissue, and key immunoregulatory cells that control levels of virus replication and extent of disease. *AIDS Res Hum Retroviruses*, 6 (8), 967–71.

Mercure, L., Phaneuf, D., & Wainberg, M. A. (1993). Detection of unintegrated human immunodeficiency virus type 1 DNA in persistently infected CD8+ cells. *J Gen Virol*, 74 (Pt 10), 2077–83.

Mestecky, J., Moldoveanu, Z., & Russell, M. W. (2005). Immunologic uniqueness of the genital tract: challenge for vaccine development. *Am J Reprod Immunol*, 53 (5), 208–14.

Misumi, S., Masuyama, M., Takamune, N., Nakayama, D., Mitsumata, R., Matsumoto, H., et al. (2009). Targeted delivery of immunogen to primate m cells with tetragalloyl lysine dendrimer. *J Immunol*, 182 (10), 6061–70.

Moir, S., Lapointe, R., Malaspina, A., Ostrowski, M., Cole, C. E., Chun, T. W., et al. (1999). CD40-mediated induction of CD4 and CXCR4 on B lymphocytes correlates with restricted susceptibility to human immunodeficiency virus type 1 infection: potential role of B lymphocytes as a viral reservoir. *J Virol*, 73 (10), 7972–80.

Moir, S., Malaspina, A., Li, Y., Chun, T. W., Lowe, T., Adelsberger, J., et al. (2000). B cells of HIV-1-infected patients bind virions through CD21-complement interactions and transmit infectious virus to activated T cells. *J Exp Med*, 192 (5), 637–46.

Moll, M., Andersson, S. K., Smed-Sorensen, A., & Sandberg, J. K. (2010). Inhibition of lipid antigen presentation in dendritic cells by HIV-1 Vpu interference with CD1d recycling from endosomal compartments. *Blood*, 116 (11), 1876–84.

Moore, C. B., John, M., James, I. R., Christiansen, F. T., Witt, C. S., & Mallal, S. A. (2002). Evidence of HIV-1 adaptation to HLA-restricted immune responses at a population level. *Science*, 296 (5572), 1439–43.

Moreno-Fernandez, M. E., Zapata, W., Blackard, J. T., Franchini, G., & Chougnet, C. A. (2009). Human regulatory T cells are targets for human immunodeficiency Virus (HIV) infection, and their susceptibility differs depending on the HIV type 1 strain. *J Virol*, 83 (24), 12925–33.

Mulligan, M. J. & Weber, J. (1999). Human trials of HIV-1 vaccines. *AIDS*, 13 Suppl A:105–112.

Musey, L., Hughes, J., Schacker, T., Shea, T., Corey, L., & McElrath, M. J. (1997). Cytotoxic-T-cell responses, viral load, and disease progression in early human immunodeficiency virus type 1 infection. *N Engl J Med*, 337 (18), 1267–74.

Mutsch, M., Zhou, W., Rhodes, P., Bopp, M., Chen, R. T., Linder, T., et al. (2004). Use of the inactivated intranasal influenza vaccine and the risk of Bell's palsy in Switzerland. *N Engl J Med*, 350 (9), 896–903.

Nabel, G. & Baltimore, D. (1987). An inducible transcription factor activates expression of human immunodeficiency virus in T cells. *Nature*, 326 (6114), 711–3.

Nicoll, J. A., Wilkinson, D., Holmes, C., Steart, P., Markham, H., & Weller, R. O. (2003). Neuropathology of human Alzheimer disease after immunization with amyloid-beta peptide: A case report. *Nat Med*, 9 (4), 448–52.

Novitsky, V., Rybak, N., McLane, M. F., Gilbert, P., Chigwedere, P., Klein, I., et al. (2001). Identification of human immunodeficiency virus 1 subtype C Gag-, Tat-, Rev-, and Nef-specific elispot-based cytotoxic T-lymphocyte responses for AIDS vaccine design. *J Virol*, 75 (19), 9210–28.

Nowacek, A. S., McMillan, J., Miller, R., Anderson, A., Rabinow, B., & Gendelman, H. E. (2010). Nanoformulated antiretroviral drug combinations extend drug release and antiretroviral responses in HIV-1-infected macrophages: Implications for neuroAIDS therapeutics. *J Neuroimmune Pharmacol*, 5 (4), 592–601.

O'Connor, D. H., McDermott, A. B., Krebs, K. C., Dodds, E. J., Miller, J. E., et al. (2004). A dominant role for CD8+-T-lymphocyte selection in simian immunodeficiency virus sequence variation. *J Virol*, 78 (24), 14012–22.

Ohba, K., Ryo, A., Dewan, M. Z., Nishi, M., Naito, T., Qi, X., et al. (2009). Follicular dendritic cells activate HIV-1 replication in monocytes/macrophages through a juxtacrine mechanism mediated by P-selectin glycoprotein ligand 1. *J Immunol*, 183 (1), 524–32.

Ostrowski, M. A., Chun, T. W., Justement, S. J., Motola, I., Spinelli, M. A., Adelsberger, J., et al. (1999). Both memory and CD45RA+/CD62L+ naive CD4(+) T cells are infected in human immunodeficiency virus type 1-infected individuals. *J Virol*, 73 (8), 6430–35.

Pantaleo, G., Graziosi, C., Demarest, J. F., Butini, L., Montroni, M., Fox, C. H., . (1993). HIV infection is active and progressive in lymphoid tissue during the clinically latent stage of disease. *Nature*, 362 (6418), 355–58.

Pett, S. L. (2009). Immunotherapies in HIV-1 infection. *Curr Opin HIV AIDS*, 4 (3), 188–93.

Pialoux, G., Excler, J. L., Riviere, Y., Gonzalez-Canali, G., Feuillie, V., Coulaud, P., et al. (1995). A prime-boost approach to HIV preventive vaccine using a recombinant canarypox virus expressing glycoprotein 160 (MN) followed by a recombinant glycoprotein 160 (MN/LAI). The AGIS Group, and l'Agence Nationale de Recherche sur le SIDA. *AIDS Res Hum Retroviruses*, 11 (3), 373–81.

Pialoux, G., Hocini, H., Perusat, S., Silberman, B., Salmon-Ceron, D., Slama, L., et al. (2008). Phase I study of a candidate vaccine based on recombinant HIV-1 gp160 (MN/LAI) administered by the mucosal route to HIV-seronegative volunteers: The ANRS VAC14 study. *Vaccine*, 26 (21):2657–66.

Pialoux, G., Quercia, R. P., Gahery, H., Daniel, N., Slama, L., Girard, P. M., et al. (2008). Immunological responses and long-term treatment interruption after human immunodeficiency virus type 1 (HIV-1) lipopeptide immunization of HIV-1-infected patients: The LIPTHERA study. *Clin Vaccine Immunol*, 15 (3), 562–8.

Pierson, T., Hoffman, T. L., Blankson, J., Finzi, D., Chadwick, K., Margolick, J. B., et al. (2000). Characterization of chemokine receptor utilization of viruses in the latent reservoir for human immunodeficiency virus type 1. *J Virol*, 74 (17), 7824–33.

Pierson, T., McArthur, J., & Siliciano, R. F. (2000). Reservoirs for HIV-1: mechanisms for viral persistence in the presence of antiviral immune responses and antiretroviral therapy. *Annu Rev Immunol*, 18, 665–708.

Pillay, K., Coutsoudis, A., Agadzi-Naqvi, A. K., Kuhn, L., Coovadia, H. M., & Janoff, E. N. (2001). Secretory leukocyte protease inhibitor in vaginal fluids and perinatal human immunodeficiency virus type 1 transmission. *J Infect Dis*, 183 (4), 653–6.

Pitisuttithum, P., Gilbert, P., Gurwith, M., Heyward, W., Martin, M., an Griensven, F., et al. (2006). Randomized, double-blind, placebo-controlled efficacy trial of a bivalent recombinant glycoprotein 120 HIV-1 vaccine among injection drug users in Bangkok, Thailand. *J Infect Dis*, 194 (12), 1661–71.

Pope, M., Betjes, M. G., Romani, N., Hirmand, H., Cameron, P. U., Hoffman, L., et al. (1994). Conjugates of dendritic cells and memory T lymphocytes from skin facilitate productive infection with HIV-1. *Cell*, 78 (3), 389–98.

Prendergast, A., Prado, J. G., Kang, Y. H., Chen, F., Riddell, L. A., Luzzi, G., et al. (2010). HIV-1 infection is characterized by profound depletion of CD161+ Th17 cells and gradual decline in regulatory T cells. *AIDS*, 24 (4), 491–502.

Priddy, F. H., Brown, D., Kublin, J., Monahan, K., Wright, D. P., Lalezari, J., et al. (2008). Safety and immunogenicity of a replication-incompetent adenovirus type 5 HIV-1 clade B gag/pol/nef vaccine in healthy adults. *Clin Infect Dis*, 46 (11), 1769–81.

Racz, P. (1988). Molecular, biologic, immunohistochemical, and ultrastructural aspects of lymphatic spread of the human immunodeficiency virus. *Lymphology*, 21 (1), 28–35.

Racz, P., Tenner-Racz, K., van Vloten, F., Schmidt, H., Dietrich, M., Gluckman, J. C., et al. (1990). Lymphatic tissue changes in AIDS and other retrovirus infections: Tools and insights. *Lymphology* 23 (2), 85–91.

Ratto-Kim, S., Loomis-Price, L. D., Aronson, N., Grimes, J., Hill, C., Williams, C., et al. (2003). Comparison between env-specific T-cell epitopic responses in HIV-1-uninfected adults immunized with combination of ALVAC-HIV(vCP205) plus or minus rgp160MN/LAI-2 and HIV-1-infected adults. *J Acquir Immune Defic Syndr*, 32 (1), 9–17.

Rerks-Ngarm, S., Pitisuttithum, P., Nitayaphan, S., Kaewkungwal, J., Chiu, J., Paris, R., et al. (2009). Vaccination with ALVAC and AIDSVAX to prevent HIV-1 infection in Thailand. *N Engl J Med*, 361 (23), 2209–20.

Reynolds, A. D., Banerjee, R., Liu, J., Gendelman, H. E., & Mosley, R. L. (2007). Neuroprotective activities of CD4+CD25+ regulatory T cells in an animal model of Parkinson's disease. *J Leukoc Biol*, 82 (5), 1083–94.

Reynolds, A. D., Stone, D. K., Hutter, J. A., Benner, E. J., Mosley, R. L., & Gendelman, H. E. (2010). Regulatory T cells attenuate Th17 cell-mediated nigrostriatal dopaminergic neurodegeneration in a model of Parkinson's disease. *J Immunol*, 184 (5), 2261–71.

Reynolds, A. D., Stone, D. K., Mosley, R. L., & Gendelman, H. E. (2009). Nitrated {alpha}-synuclein-induced alterations in microglial immunity are regulated by CD4+ T cell subsets. *J Immunol*, 182 (7), 4137–49.

Rosenberg, E. S., Graham, B. S., Chan, E. S., Bosch, R. J., Stocker, V., Maenza, J., et al. (2010). Safety and immunogenicity of therapeutic DNA vaccination in individuals treated with antiretroviral therapy during acute/early HIV-1 infection. *PLoS One*, 5 (5), e10555.

Rossi, J. J., June, C. H., & Kohn, D. B. (2007). Genetic therapies against HIV. *Nat Biotechnol*, 25 (12), 1444–54.

Rowland-Jones, S. L., Dong, T., Fowke, K. R., Kimani, J., Krausa, P., Newell, H., et al. (1998). Cytotoxic T cell responses to multiple conserved HIV epitopes in HIV-resistant prostitutes in Nairobi. *J Clin Invest*, 102 (9), 1758–65.

Saha, K., Zhang, J., Gupta, A., Dave, R., Yimen, M., & Zerhouni, B. (2001). Isolation of primary HIV-1 that target CD8+ T lymphocytes using CD8 as a receptor. *Nat Med*, 7 (1), 65–72.

Salmon-Ceron, D., Excler, J. L., Finkielsztejn, L., Autran, B., Gluckman, J. C., Sicard, D., et al. (1999). Safety and immunogenicity of a live recombinant canarypox virus expressing HIV type 1 gp120 MN MN tm/gag/protease LAI (ALVAC-HIV, vCP205) followed by a p24E-V3 MN synthetic peptide (CLTB-36) administered in healthy volunteers at low risk for HIV infection. AGIS Group and L'Agence Nationale de Recherches sur Le Sida. *AIDS Res Hum Retroviruses*, 15 (7), 633–45.

Sauter, S. L., Rahman, A., & Muralidhar, G. (2005). Non-replicating viral vector-based AIDS vaccines: Interplay between viral vectors and the immune system. *Curr HIV Res*, 3 (2), 157–81.

Schenk, D. (2002). Amyloid-beta immunotherapy for Alzheimer's disease: The end of the beginning. *Nat Rev Neurosci*, 3 (10), 824–8.

Schmitz, J. E., Kuroda, M. J., Santra, S., Sasseville, V. G., Simon, M. A., Lifton, M. A., et al. (1999). Control of viremia in simian immunodeficiency virus infection by CD8+ lymphocytes. *Science*, 283 (5403), 857–60.

Schnittman, S. M., Lane, H. C., Greenhouse, J., Justement, J. S., Baseler, M., & Fauci, A. S. (1990). Preferential infection of CD4+ memory T cells by human immunodeficiency virus type 1: Evidence for a role in the selective T-cell functional defects observed in infected individuals. *Proc Natl Acad Sci U S A*, 87 (16), 6058–62.

Schnittman, S. M., Psallidopoulos, M. C., Lane, H. C., Thompson, L., Baseler, M., Massari, F., et al. (1989). The reservoir for HIV-1 in human peripheral blood is a T cell that maintains expression of CD4. *Science*, 245 (4915), 305–8.

Sealy, R., Slobod, K. S., Flynn, P., Branum, K., Surman, S., Jones, B., et al. (2009). Preclinical and clinical development of a multi-envelope, DNA-virus-protein (D-V-P) HIV-1 vaccine. *Int Rev Immunol*, 28 (1), 49–68.

Sharkey, M. E., Teo, I., Greenough, T., Sharova, N., Luzuriaga, K., Sullivan, J. L., et al. (2000). Persistence of episomal HIV-1 infection intermediates in patients on highly active anti-retroviral therapy. *Nat Med*, 6 (1), 76–81.

Sharova, N., Swingler, C., Sharkey, M., & Stevenson, M. (2005). Macrophages archive HIV-1 virions for dissemination in trans. *EMBO J*, 24 (13), 2481–9.

Shiver, J. W., Fu, T. M., Chen, L., Casimiro, D. R., Davies, M. E., Evans, R. K., et al. (2002). Replication-incompetent adenoviral vaccine vector elicits effective anti-immunodeficiency-virus immunity. *Nature*, 415 (6869), 331–5.

Siliciano, J. D., Kajdas, J., Finzi, D., Quinn, T. C., Chadwick, K., Margolick, J. B., et al. (2003). Long-term follow-up studies confirm the stability of the latent reservoir for HIV-1 in resting CD4+ T cells. *Nat Med*, 9 (6), 727–8.

Sleasman, J. W., Aleixo, L. F., Morton, A., Skoda-Smith, S., & Goodenow, M. M. (1996). CD4+ memory T cells are the predominant population of HIV-1-infected lymphocytes in neonates and children. *AIDS*, 10 (13), 1477–84.

Smith, B. A., Gartner, S., Liu, Y., Perelson, A. S., Stilianakis, N. I., Keele, B. F.,et al. (2001). Persistence of infectious HIV on follicular dendritic cells. *J Immunol*, 166 (1), 690–6.

Smith, P. D., Meng, G., Salazar-Gonzalez, J. F., & Shaw, G. M. (2003). Macrophage HIV-1 infection and the gastrointestinal tract reservoir. *J Leukoc Biol*, 74 (5), 642–9.

Sonza, S., Mutimer, H. P., Oelrichs, R., Jardine, D., Harvey, K., Dunne, A., et al. (2001). Monocytes harbour replication-competent, non-latent HIV-1 in patients on highly active antiretroviral therapy. *AIDS*, 15 (1), 17–22.

Stanhope, P. E., Clements, M. L., & Siliciano, R. F. (1993). Human CD4+ cytolytic T lymphocyte responses to a human immunodeficiency virus type 1 gp160 subunit vaccine. *J Infect Dis*, 168 (1), 92–100.

Steinbrook, R. (2007). One step forward, two steps back—will there ever be an AIDS vaccine? *N Engl J Med*, 357 (26), 2653–5.

Stevceva, L. & Strober, W. (2004). Mucosal HIV vaccines: Where are we now? *Curr HIV Res*, 2 (1), 1–10.

Sun, Y., Bailer, R. T., Rao, S. S., Mascola, J. R., Nabel, G. J., Koup, R. A., et al. (2009). Systemic and mucosal T-lymphocyte activation induced by recombinant adenovirus vaccines in rhesus monkeys. *J Virol*, 83 (20), 10596–604.

Sutter, G. & Moss, B. (1992). Nonreplicating vaccinia vector efficiently expresses recombinant genes. *Proc Natl Acad Sci U S A*, 89(22), 10847–51.

Takeda, K., Kaisho, T., & Akira, S. (2003). Toll-like receptors. *Annu Rev Immunol*, 21, 335–76.

Tartaglia, J., Excler, J. L., El Habib, R., Limbach, K., Meignier, B., Plotkin, S., et al. (1998). Canarypox virus-based vaccines: Prime-boost strategies to induce cell-mediated and humoral immunity against HIV. *AIDS Res Hum Retroviruses*, 14 Suppl 3, 291–98.

Teitelbaum, D., Arnon, R., & Sela, M. (1999). Immunomodulation of experimental autoimmune encephalomyelitis by oral administration of copolymer 1. *Proc Natl Acad Sci U S A*, 96 (7), 3842–7.

Teitelbaum, D., Meshorer, A., Hirshfeld, T., Arnon, R., & Sela, M. (1971). Suppression of experimental allergic encephalomyelitis by a synthetic polypeptide. *Eur J Immunol*, 1 (4), 242–8.

Thacker, T. C., Zhou, X., Estes, J. D., Jiang, Y., Keele, B. F., Elton, T. S., et al. (2009). Follicular dendritic cells and human immunodeficiency virus type 1 transcription in CD4+ T cells. *J Virol*, 83 (1), 150–8.

Thorborn, G., Pomeroy, L., Isohanni, H., Perry, M., Peters, B., & Vyakarnam, A. (2010). Increased sensitivity of CD4+ T-effector cells to CD4+CD25+ Treg suppression compensates for reduced Treg number in asymptomatic HIV-1 infection. *PLoS One*, 5 (2), e9254.

Titti, F., Zamarchi, R., Maggiorella, M. T., Sernicola, L., Geraci, A., Negri, D. R. M., et al. (2002). Infection of simian B lymphoblastoid cells with simian immunodeficiency virus is associated with upregulation of CD23 and CD40 cell surface markers. *J Med Virol*, 68 (1), 129–40.

Tran, T. A., de Goer de Herve, M. G., Hendel-Chavez, H., Dembele, B., Le Nevot, E., . (2008). Resting regulatory CD4 T cells: A site of HIV persistence in patients on long-term effective antiretroviral therapy. *PLoS One*, 3 (10), e3305.

Tschachler, E., Groh, V., Popovic, M., Mann, D. L., Konrad, K., Safai, B., et al. (1987). Epidermal Langerhans cells—a target for HTLV-III/LAV infection. *J Invest Dermatol*, 88 (2), 233–7.

Vajdy, M. & Singh, S. (2006). Intranasal delivery of vaccines against HIV. *Expert Opin Drug Deliv*, 3 (2), 247–59.

Vignali, D. A., Collison, L. W., & Workman, C. J. (2008). How regulatory T cells work. *Nat Rev Immunol*, 8(7), 523–32.

Wang, S., Kennedy, J. S., West, K., Montefiori, D. C., Coley, S., Lawrence, J., et al. (2008). Cross-subtype antibody and cellular immune responses induced by a polyvalent DNA prime-protein boost HIV-1 vaccine in healthy human volunteers. *Vaccine*, 26(8), 1098–110.

Weber, M. S., Prod'homme, T., Youssef, S., Dunn, S. E., Rundle, C. D., Lee, L., et al. (2007). Type II monocytes modulate T cell-mediated central nervous system autoimmune disease. *Nat Med*, 13 (8), 935–43.

Weber, M. S., Starck, M., Wagenpfeil, S., Meinl, E., Hohlfeld, R., & Farina, C. (2004). Multiple sclerosis: Glatiramer acetate inhibits monocyte reactivity in vitro and in vivo. *Brain*, 127(Pt 6), 1370–8.

Weber, R., Bossart, W., Cone, R., Luethy, R., & Moelling, K. (2001). Phase I clinical trial with HIV-1 gp160 plasmid vaccine in HIV-1-infected asymptomatic subjects. *Eur J Clin Microbiol Infect Dis*, 20(11), 800–3.

Williams, K. C., Corey, S., Westmoreland, S. V., Pauley, D., Knight, H., deBakker, C., et al. (2001). Perivascular macrophages are the primary cell type productively infected by simian immunodeficiency virus in the brains of macaques: Implications for the neuropathogenesis of AIDS. *J Exp Med*, 193(8), 905–15.

Wu, S., Pascual, D. W., Lewis, G. K., & Hone, D. M. (1997). Induction of mucosal and systemic responses against human immunodeficiency virus type 1 glycoprotein 120 in mice after oral immunization with a single dose of a Salmonella-HIV vector. *AIDS Res Hum Retroviruses*, 13(14), 1187–94.

Yang, L. P., Riley, J. L., Carroll, R. G., June, C. H., Hoxie, J., Patterson, B. K., et al. (1998). Productive infection of neonatal CD8+ T lymphocytes by HIV-1. *J Exp Med*, 187(7), 1139–44.

Zhang, L., Gu, F. X., Chan, J. M., Wang, A. Z., Langer, R. S., & Farokhzad, O. C. (2008). Nanoparticles in medicine: Therapeutic applications and developments. *Clin Pharmacol Ther*, 83 (5), 761–9.

Zhang, R., Zhang, S., Li, M., Chen, C., & Yao, Q. (2010). Incorporation of CD40 ligand into SHIV virus-like particles (VLP) enhances SHIV-VLP-induced dendritic cell activation and boosts immune responses against HIV. *Vaccine*, 28 (31), 5114–27.

Zhu, T. (2000). HIV-1 genotypes in peripheral blood monocytes. *J Leukoc Biol*, 68(3), 338–44.

Ziemssen, T., Kumpfel, T., Klinkert, W. E., Neuhaus, O., & Hohlfeld, R. (2002). Glatiramer acetate-specific T-helper 1- and 2-type cell lines produce BDNF: Implications for multiple sclerosis therapy. Brain-derived neurotrophic factor. *Brain*, 125(Pt 11), 2381–91.

zur Megede, J., Chen, M. C., Doe, B., Schaefer, M., Greer, C. E., Selby, M., et al. (2000). Increased expression and immunogenicity of sequence-modified human immunodeficiency virus type 1 gag gene. *J Virol*, 74(6), 2628–35.

2.6

NEUROGENESIS

James B. Reinecke, Hui Peng, Yunlong Huang, Qiang Chen, and Jialin C. Zheng

Neurogenesis is a highly regulated process responsible for the generation of new neurons, astrocytes, and oligodendrocytes from neural stem cells. Previously, neurogenesis was thought to be a prenatal phenomenon, halting shortly after birth. Intense investigation over the past decade and a half has reversed that theory. It is now widely accepted that neurogenesis persists into adulthood and may play a crucial role in complicated behaviors such as learning and memory. Consequently, accumulating evidence suggests that impaired neurogenesis may contribute to the pathogenesis of several brain disorders. The purpose of this chapter is three-fold. First, to describe the process of developmental and adult neurogenesis. Second, to extensively review the relationship between brain disorders and neurogenesis, emphasizing how brain inflammation may influence the pathogenesis of neurodegenerative diseases such as HIV-1-associated neurocognitive disorders. Third, to explore how new advances in stem cell biology may lead to exciting new therapies for the treatment of neurodegenerative disorders.

INTRODUCTION

In the early 1900s, prominent neuroscientist Ramon y Cajal stated that:

> "In the adult centers, the nerve paths are something fixed, ended, and immutable. Everything may die, nothing may be regenerated. It is for the science of the future to change, if possible, this harsh decree."
>
> (RAMÓN Y CAJAL ET AL., 1991; MA ET AL., 2009)

For decades this statement was held as dogma. In the late twentieth century, investigators were able to show that neural stem cells could be isolated from postnatal rodent brains and cultured in vitro (Reynolds & Weiss, 1992; Gage, 2000). Adult neural stem cells (aNSC) cultured as aggregated cells known as neurospheres, are capable of self-renewal over many passages and have the ability to differentiate into the three neuronal lineages (neuron, astrocyte, oligodendrocyte).

In the mammalian brain, aNSC are found in the subventricular zone (SVZ) of the lateral wall of the lateral ventricles as well as in the subgranular zone (SGZ) in the dentate gyrus of the hippocampus (Jordan et al., 2007; Basak & Taylor, 2009; Ma et al., 2009). aNSC in the SVZ migrate along the rostral migratory stream to the olfactory bulb where they then differentiate into mature, functional interneurons. aNSC found within the SGZ differentiate into glutamatergic dentate granule cells.

Adult neurogenesis is a three-step process involving aNSC proliferation and maintenance of the stem cell population, directed migration, and differentiation into functional neurons that integrate into the local neuronal circuitry (Gage, 2000). While the exact function of neurogenesis within the adult brain is not fully understood, recent studies in rodent models suggest that aNSC, specifically within the SGZ, may be crucial to learning and memory. One such study found that genetic disruption of aNSC proliferation causes profound deficits in spatial learning (Zhang et al., 2008). A second possible function of aNSC is to respond to brain injury by generating new neurons to replace damaged ones. During brain injury, such as status epilepticus or stroke, signals sent from the injury site induce aNSC in both the SVZ and SGZ to proliferate and migrate to the site of the injury and undergo differentiation (Bengzon et al., 1997; Arvidsson et al., 2002; Ekdahl et al., 2009).

While some disease states such as stroke or seizure may provoke increased neurogenesis, accumulating evidence suggests that decreased neurogenesis may be central to the pathogenesis of many neurodegenerative disorders. HIV-1 infection can lead to several neurocognitive disruptions, collectively named HIV-1-associated neurocognitive disorders (HAND) (Boisse et al., 2008). The most severe form of HAND, HIV-1-associated dementia (HAD), causes a number of cognitive, behavioral, and motor abnormalities (Epstein and Gelbard 1999; McArthur et al., 1999) The pathological correlate of HAD, HIV-1 encephalitis (HIVE), is characterized by the presence of HIV-infected and immune-activated mononuclear phagocytes (MP, monocytes, macrophages, and microglia). Activated MPs release a plethora of pro-inflammatory cytokines and chemokines. The effects of these cytokines and chemokines on neurogenesis, and the possible roles they play in the pathogenesis of neuroinflammatory diseases such as HAND, has been an area of intense focus over the last decade.

Although the advent of highly active anti-retroviral therapy (HAART) has dramatically increased the lifespan of HIV-infected individuals, the number of HIV-related neurocognitive cases continues to rise despite lower plasma viral loads and higher CD4 counts (Liner et al., 2008; Kaul, 2009). Therefore, it is of paramount importance that the underlying pathological mechanisms leading to HAND are delineated so that treatment options can be synthesized to specifically target the disastrous effects of HIV within the central nervous system (CNS). The purpose of this chapter will be to: 1) define stem cells and introduce developmental and adult neurogenesis; 2) describe how neurogenesis may be affected by different pathophysiological states, specifically brain inflammation and HAND (both pediatric and adult cases); 3) propose how recent advances in stem cell biology provide possible avenues for the treatment of neurodegenerative diseases.

STEM CELLS, NEURAL STEM CELLS, AND PROGENITOR CELLS

Stem cells are a unique group of cells that have the ability to both continually self-renew and differentiate into several types of specialized cells. Stem cell cell-division can occur in two ways. In symmetric cell division, a stem cell will divide to produce two identical stem cell progeny. In asymmetric cell division, a stem cell will divide into one stem cell and one progenitor cell. The progenitor cell, while still mitotic, is restricted to a certain lineage of cells. The progenitor continually divides to produce a pool of progenitors that will eventually give rise to highly specialized terminally differentiated cells.

The capacity for a stem cell to differentiate into different lineages of cells is dependent on its potency. Pluripotent cells, such as embryonic stem cells (ESC), are capable of differentiating into all three germ layers (endoderm, ectoderm, mesoderm). Multipotent stem cells, such as NSC, are capable of differentiating into any neuroectoderm-derived cell (neuron, astrocyte, and oligodendrocyte). Thus, multipotent stem cells are restricted based on the tissue in which they are located. Unipotent progenitor cells on the other hand, are tightly restricted to one type of cell. In the case of the CNS, an oligodendrocyte progenitor cell will only produce oligodendrocytes.

ESCs are derived from the inner cell mass of the blastocyst. In the laboratory, ESCs can be maintained in an undifferentiated state and, once exposed to differentiation conditions, can differentiate into cells of all three germ layers. Much work has gone into understanding the complicated transcriptional and epigenetic regulatory mechanisms involved in ESC self-renewal, maintenance, proliferation, survival, and differentiation. The ability to manipulate ESCs to become a certain type of cell is crucial for the use of ESCs in cellular replacement therapy for the treatment of conditions such as neurodegenerative diseases.

As development progresses, pluripotent stem cells give rise to tissue-specific multipotent stem cells that are responsible for organogenesis. After birth, some populations of stem cells persist into adult life and reside within special microenvironments known as "niches." Adult stem cells contained within niches have been identified in tissues such as the skin, intestine, bone marrow, and brain and thus are found in tissues derived from all three germ layers. While the structure of each stem cell niche is unique, one common attribute of each niche is to regulate the function of the stem cell residing within the niche. As to be expected, each niche is comprised of highly complex signals that control the stem cell's fate. Adult stem cells play a crucial role in tissue homeostasis by supporting tissue regeneration, replacing dead cells, and responding to tissue injury (Li & Xie, 2005). Neurogenic regions of the adult CNS are composed of aNSC within highly complex cellular niches. The aNSC niche will be discussed in detail later in the chapter.

Neural stem cells (NSC) are capable of generating all cell types of neuroectodermal origin. Neural progenitor cells (NPC), while still mitotic, can differentiate into neurons or astrocytes but lose the ability to differentiate into oligodendrocytes. Some NPCs are unipotent and produce cells of only one lineage. The next two sections will explain the progression of NSC to functional cells in both the embryonic and adult mammalian brain. An introduction to the cell biological and molecular traits of embryonic and adult NSC is crucial. Only once the traits of NSC are understood can investigators address the question, "How does HIV-1 infection within the brain disrupt neurogenesis?"

NEUROGENESIS DURING DEVELOPMENT

The development of the human brain has fascinated scientists for many years. Understanding the molecular and cell biological mechanisms responsible for the formation of the mammalian adult brain is one of science's great questions and is relevant for those interested in HAND, for several reasons. First, a recent focus in using cellular therapy for the treatment of neurodegenerative diseases, such as HAND, has centered on grasping the pathways responsible for direct differentiation of stem cells towards a certain neuronal type. In order to accomplish this, scientists must understand the developmental mechanisms responsible for generating these specific neuronal sub-types. Second, manipulation of endogenous aNSC may also be of potential benefit for treating brain injury. As will be discussed below, eNSC and aNSC share a number of molecular and cell biological traits. Lastly, infants infected with HIV either peri- or postnatally display a number of deficits, largely due to the malformation of the hippocampus. Thus, understanding brain development and how it might be impacted by maternal HIV infection will hopefully allow for potential treatments that could prevent offspring brain malformation. In this section, we will provide an introductory understanding of the molecular and cellular basis of embryonic neurogenesis. We will highlight the role of CXCL12/CXCR4 in brain development, as HIV interaction with CXCR4 and its effect on CXCL12 regulation and CXCL12/CXCR4 signaling may explain some of the developmental abnormalities seen in pediatric cases of HIV infection (Zheng et al., 1999; Tran et al., 2007; Li & Ransohoff, 2008; Miller et al., 2008; Moll et al., 2009; Ransohoff, 2009).

NEURULATION AND EMBRYONIC NSC

As the embryo forms, its overall structural pattern is determined by the establishment of the anterior-posterior (head-tail), dorsal-ventral (back-belly), and left-right axes.

Neural tissue is formed after the generation of the three primary germ layers: the endoderm, mesoderm, and ectoderm. The endoderm generates tissues of the gut; the mesoderm generates tissues such as connective tissue, musculature, and vasculature; and the ectoderm gives rise to the skin and nervous system. Neural differentiation from ectoderm tissue occurs in response to interactions between signals secreted by the mesoderm and ectoderm. Signals such as chordin, secreted by the mesodermally derived notocord, suppress ectodermal bone morphogenetic protein (BMP) signaling (Levine & Brivanlou, 2007). The binding of BMP to its receptor leads to the activation of intracellular SMAD proteins. Several of the activated SMADs form a complex that, upon translocation into the nucleus, initiates changes in gene expression (Chen et al., 2004). The inhibition of BMP signaling within the early ectoderm leads to neural differentiation. After neural differentiation, neuroepithelial (NE) cells form along the dorsal axis of the embryo. This flat sheet of pseudostratified columnar epithelium is known as the neural plate. Neurulation occurs as the neural plate invaginates ventrally and then closes dorsally, forming the neural tube. The neural tube, which extends along the anterior-posterior axis of the embryo, consists of a fluid-filled center that eventually develops into the ventricular system and the spinal canal. The relation of neural tissue to the ventricular system, especially when discussing NSC in both the embryonic and adult CNS, is an important consideration. For the purpose of this chapter, the layer closest to the ventricles is known as the apical or ventricular surface. The surface furthest away from the ventricles is the pial or basal surface.

While the nucleus of NE cells is found on the ventricular surface of the neural tube, NE cells extend cellular processes that contact both the ventricular and pial surface. After the closure of the neural tube, NE cells undergo symmetric cell divisions in order to increase the pool of NE cells (McConnell, 1995). As neurogenesis begins, there is some controversy over whether or not NE cells divide to produce radial glial cells (RGC), a distinct type of NSC, or directly transform into RGC (Gotz & Huttner, 2005; Merkle & Alvarez-Buylla, 2006; Farkas & Huttner, 2008). Given the number of molecular and morphological characteristics shared between NE cells and RGC (see below), it is probable that NE cells transform into RGC directly, although it must be pointed out that this remains an unresolved issue. Radial glial cells (RGC), also found within the ventricular zone, divide either symmetrically or asymmetrically (Huttner & Kosodo, 2005; Zhong & Chia, 2008). Asymmetric RGC cell division produces one RGC progeny and one non-stem-cell progeny. The potency of RGC is also a matter of uncertainty. Several lines of evidence suggest that RGC can give rise to only one lineage of cells and have varying levels of neurogenesis potential depending on their location in the developing CNS (Malatesta et al., 2003; Gotz & Huttner, 2005), while other studies suggest that RGC have a wider developmental potential (Anthony et al., 2004; Ever & Gaiano, 2005; Casper & McCarthy, 2006). For clarity, we will consider the non-stem-cell progeny to be a neuronal intermediate progenitor. The intermediate progenitor migrates into the zone just above the ventricular zone, the subventricular zone, undergoes symmetric division, and differentiates

into two neuronal precursors known as neuroblasts. The neuroblast then migrates along the RGC basal projection before differentiating into a neuron. An exhaustive discussion of the progression from NE→RGC→intermediate precursors is not within the scope of this chapter; however, it is important to note the properties and location of embryonic NSC in order to compare them to aNSC. NE and RGC share a number of morphological and molecular features. However, RGC are also similar to astrocytes. Interestingly, aNSC share many characteristics with RGCs. Thus, we will briefly consider the cell biological and molecular characteristics of the NE, RGC, and astrocyte in order to properly frame the discussion of aNSC in the next section.

NE cells display characteristics typical of epithelial cells such as tight junctions and adherens junctions, are polarized along their apical-basal axis, and display interkinetic nuclear migration (INM) during the cell cycle (Gotz & Huttner, 2005; Farkas & Huttner, 2008). During INM, the nucleus of the NE cell migrates along the entire apical-basal axis. NE cells express markers such as membrane marker prominin-1 (CD-133), the transcription factor Sox2, and the intermediate filament protein nestin. RGC are also polarized along their apical-basal axis, display INM (restricted to the basal-most end of ventricular zone), contain adherens junctions (but not tight junctions), and retain expression of the NE markers prominin-1, Sox2, and nestin (Aaku-Saraste et al., 1997; Chenn et al., 1998; Hartfuss et al., 2001). However, RGCs also express astroglial markers (Kriegstein & Gotz, 2003), including but not limited to glial fibrillary acidic protein (GFAP) and astrocyte specific glutamate transporter (GLAST). Taken together, RGC exhibit characteristics of NE cells and astrocytes. Although not well delineated, the traits shared between these cells are probably crucial to their function in neurogenesis.

NEURAL PATTERNING AND THE GENERATION OF NEURONAL SUB-TYPES

Two distinct programs along the dorsoventral axis and the rostrocaudal axis of the neural tube control neural patterning, or the generation of neural subtypes. Signaling along the rostrocaudal axis leads to the generation of four subdivisions of the developing CNS: spinal cord, hindbrain, midbrain, and forebrain (arranged caudal-rostral). The interaction between secreted molecules derived from both neural and non-neural tissue influence gene expression programs in neural progenitor cells along the length of the neural tube to promote regionalization (Vieira et al., 2010).

Dorsoventral specification is achieved by secretion of sonic hedgehog (Shh) from the notocord and BMP secreted by overlying non-neural ectoderm. Shh and BMP are examples of morphogens. Morphogens are secreted molecules that exert their effect on a concentration-dependent basis. Shh, a small cholesterol-modified protein, binds to the patched (Ptc) receptor and prevents Ptc-mediated inhibition of smoothened (Smo). Activation of Smo eventually leads to changes in gene expression mediated by the Gli family of transcription factors (Jiang & Hui, 2008). Thus, the generation of neuronal subtypes on the dorsoventral axis is dependent upon concentration gradients of ventrally derived Shh and dorsally derived BMP.

While dorsoventral patterning is generally consistent along the length of the neural tube, several organizer regions along the rostral-caudal axis achieve rostrocaudal specification. Each of these organizer regions secretes specific molecules that direct nearby neural progenitor cells to differentiate into a certain lineage of cells (Vieira et al., 2010). Although a comprehensive overview of rostrocaudal patterning is not within the scope of this chapter, one example will be provided as an introduction to how differential expression of secreted molecules promotes the necessary molecular changes that are responsible for regionalization.

The isthmus, located at the midbrain-hindbrain junction, is required for the specification of the adjacent regions (Partanen, 2007). The isthmus secretes fibroblast growth factor 8 (FGF8). FGF8 binds to its associated fibroblast growth factor receptor and initiates a signaling cascade mediated by receptor tyrosine kinases. Activation of the phosphatidylinositol-3 kinase (PI3K) and Ras-Erk pathways promotes the expression of molecules responsible for regulating cell fate and survival (Martin, 1998; Tsang & Dawid, 2004). Similar to the Shh gradients set up along the ventral axis, rostrocaudal FGF8 concentration gradients within the midbrain-hindbrain junction initiate different gene expression profiles as the distance from the isthmus increases. Interestingly, Shh and FGF8 signaling cascades work in concert to promote the generation of ventral midbrain dopaminergic neurons (Prakash, Brodski et al., 2006; Prakash & Wurst, 2006). Chemokines such as CXCL12 and its receptor CXCR4 have well-delineated roles in the immune system. Interestingly, recent works have begun to show that chemokines like CXCL12/CXCR4 play important roles in brain development, specifically in regulating NPC and neural precursor migration and proliferation. Given the relationship between CXCR4 and HIV, we will briefly discuss the role of CXCL12/CXCR4 in the developing nervous system; disruption of this axis may explain some of the brain abnormalities seen in pediatric cases of HIV infection (see below).

CXCL12/CXCR4 SIGNALING AND THE ROLE OF CXCL12 AND CXCR4 IN NEUROGENESIS

The binding of CXCL12 to CXCR4 activates several heterotrimeric G-proteins, mainly $G\alpha_i$ and $G\alpha_q$ (Ganju et al., 1998; Wu & Yoder, 2009). $G\alpha_i$ inactivates adenyl cyclase, leading to decreased levels of cytosolic 3'-5'-cyclic adenosine monophosphate (cAMP) and activation of PI3K (Zheng et al. 1999; Peng et al. 2004). Activation of PI3K mediates several downstream effector pathways that promote gene transcription, cell survival, and cell migration (Sotsios et al., 1999; Vicente-Manzanares et al., 1999). $G\alpha_q$ activates phospholipase C-γ (PLC-γ), which then hydrolyzes phosphatidylinositol-4, 5-bisphosphase into diacylglycerol (DAG) and inositol triphosphate (IP3). DAG activates protein kinase C (PKC) while IP3 opens calcium channels present on the endoplasmic reticulum causing a rise in intracellular calcium and activation of calcium/calmodulin. The $G\alpha_q$ pathway is crucial for CXCL12-mediated chemotaxis (Petit et al., 2005; Shahabi et al., 2008; Wu & Yoder, 2009).

CXCR4, which is expressed constitutively in the CNS on neurons, astrocytes, and microglia, as well as macrophages, is a co-receptor for HIV (Berson et al., 1996; Brelot et al., 1997; Youn et al., 2000). Similarly, CXCR4 is also highly expressed during development in the cerebellum, hippocampus, and neocortex and is constitutively expressed in the brain during adulthood (Jazin et al., 1997; Ma et al., 1998; Zou et al., 1998; Lu et al., 2001; Stumm et al., 2003). Recent studies suggest that CXCL12 and CXCR4 play important roles in neuronal development and CNS homeostasis (Jazin et al., 1997; Ma et al., 1998; Zou et al., 1998; Bagri et al., 2002; Lu et al., 2002; Stumm et al., 2003). Indeed, deletion of the genes encoding for CXCL12 or CXCR4 is lethal for mice soon after birth, with severe abnormalities affecting neuronal precursor migration in the cerebellum (Ma et al., 1998; Zou et al., 1998), hippocampal dentate gyrus (Lu et al., 2001; Bagri et al., 2002), and neocortex (Stumm et al., 2003). In the case of the cerebellum, CXCL12 has been shown to be highly expressed in the leptomeninx and the major attractant for external germinal layer cells in the developing cerebellum (Klein et al., 2001; Zhu et al., 2002). In mice lacking CXCL12 or CXCR4, migration of granule cell precursors out of the external germinal layer occurs prematurely, resulting in abnormal development of the cerebellum (Ma et al., 1998). Comparatively, CXCR4 mRNA is expressed at sites of neuronal and progenitor cell migration in the hippocampus at late embryonic and early postnatal ages. The absence of CXCR4 shows a reduction in the number of dividing cells in the migratory stream and in the dentate gyrus itself. In addition, neurons appear to differentiate prematurely before reaching their target (Lu et al., 2001; Bagri et al., 2002). In the cortex, it has been recently demonstrated that CXCL12 is highly expressed in the embryonic leptomeninx and is a potent chemo-attractant for isolated striatal precursors, while CXCR4 is present in early generated Cajal-Retzius cells of the cortical marginal zone (Stumm et al., 2003). Mice with a null mutation in CXCR4 or CXCL12 show severe disruption of interneuron placement and proliferation, while the submeningeal positioning of Cajal-Retzius cells remains unaffected (Stumm et al., 2003). Together, these reports suggest that CXCL12 and CXCR4 interaction is required for both proper progenitor cell mitosis and neural precursor cell migration throughout the brain, most prominently in the cerebellum, hippocampus, and cortex regions.

While it might be tempting to speculate that neurogenesis concludes soon after birth, work over the last decade and a half has shown that neurogenesis persists into adult life and is important for normal brain function. The NSC found within the adult brain share many characteristics with their eNSC counterparts. Dysfunction of aNSC may underlie the pathogenesis of neurodegenerative diseases such as HAND. Also, stimulation of neurogenesis via manipulation of endogenous aNSC provides a possible avenue for treatment of brain injury. Thus, we will now turn our attention towards aNSC and their role in the adult brain.

NEUROGENESIS IN THE ADULT BRAIN

Evidence suggesting that new neurons are born in the adult CNS first arose in the 1960s (Altman & Das, 1965; Altman & Das, 1965). However, before the mid-1990s, many scientists believed, as Cajal believed, that the adult CNS was incapable of creating new neurons. Thirty years after the first evidence of adult neurogenesis, Reynolds and Weiss were able to show that NSC-like cells could be isolated from the adult rodent brain and cultured in vitro. These potential aNSC formed aggregates of cells known as neurospheres, were capable of self-renewal, and displayed the ability to differentiate into neurons, astrocytes, and oligodendrocytes (Reynolds & Weiss, 1992). With the improvement of culture conditions, the neurosphere assay has become an invaluable tool for delineating the pathways responsible for controlling aNSC fate (Deleyrolle & Reynolds, 2009). Evidence of aNSC in vivo followed soon after the discovery that aNSC could be cultured in vitro (Morshead et al., 1994; Eriksson et al., 1998; Doetsch et al., 1999). While it is now generally accepted that the adult CNS contains NSC, the identity, properties, and function of aNSC in vivo are incompletely understood.

ADULT NSC AND THE NEUROGENIC NICHE

Even though there is evidence that several brain regions are capable of neurogenesis, the two primary neurogenic regions within the adult CNS are the SVZ of the lateral wall of the lateral ventricle and the SGZ of the hippocampal dentate gyrus (Jordan et al., 2007; Basak & Taylor, 2009; Ma et al., 2009). As stated in the previous section, aNSC share a number of similarities with embryonic RGC and astrocytes. For instance, immunohistochemical studies have shown that aNSC express prominin-1, GFAP, Sox2, and nestin very similar to RGC (Kawaguchi et al., 2001; Morshead et al., 2003; Ellis et al., 2004; Coskun et al., 2008). Indeed, the results of several studies suggest that aNSC are direct descendents of RGC (Alvarez-Buylla et al., 2001; Tramontin et al., 2003; Merkle et al., 2004). Unlike eNSC, which are present in the cellular lining of the ventricles, aNSC are housed one layer above the ependymal epithelium of the ventricles. Putative NSC in the SVZ and SGZ are located within stem cell niches consisting of a very diverse population of cells. The complex cytoarchitecture of the adult neurogenic niche has been extensively studied in recent years. These important studies revealed that the aNSC niche, much like other adult stem cell niches, is crucial for regulating aNSC function.

While the aNSC niches within the SVZ and SGZ are distinct, there are five core cellular components shared in both niches: astrocytes, ependyma, endothelial cells, NSC progeny, and mature neurons (Jordan et al., 2007; Ma et al., 2009). Insights into unique structure of the aNSC niche have resulted from the use of whole-mount preparations of the lateral wall of the lateral ventricles. Much like eNSC, aNSC maintain apical-basal polarity. The aNSC niche is a pinwheel-like structure with the NSC sending two apical processes to the ventricular layer and one basal process to nearby vasculature (Mirzadeh et al., 2008).

Each of the cellular components of the niche has been shown to regulate aNSC function via a variety of mechanisms. For instance, non-neurogenic astrocytes within the SVZ niche express large amounts of fibroblast growth factor 2 (FGF2) (Mudo et al., 2009). FGF2 is required for the successful culture of neurospheres. Also, co-culture and transplantation experiments have shown that astrocytes derived from neurogenic regions, but not from non-neurogenic regions, promote aNSC proliferation and neuronal differentiation (Song et al., 2002; Jiao & Chen, 2008). Recent studies have also demonstrated the importance of the vasculature in maintaining NSC identity. An elegant whole-mount confocal microscopy study combined with 3D reconstruction illustrated that aNSC are found in close proximity to the vasculature and that contact with blood vessels is crucial for aNSC self-renewal (Shen et al., 2008). Co-culture experiments with aNSC and endothelial cells provide evidence that endothelial cells promote aNSC self-renewal and neurogenesis (Leventhal et al., 1999; Shen et al., 2004). Interestingly, the blood-brain barrier within the aNSC niche is much more permeable than non-neurogenic regions, suggesting that cues within the blood stream may impact aNSC. Taken together, it is apparent that non-NSC cells within the niche are specialized cells that play invaluable roles in regulating aNSC self-renewal, proliferation, and differentiation.

FUNCTION OF ANSC AND REGULATION OF ADULT NEUROGENESIS

The function of adult neurogenesis under normal physiological states is uncertain. However, some studies provide clues as to the role of aNSC within the adult brain based on observed behavioral deficits after ablation of NSC. Ablation of nestin-positive cells in the post-natal brain leads to decreased hippocampal volume and impairments of spatial learning and memory (Imayoshi et al., 2008). Genetic disruption of TLX (*tailless*), an important transcription factor in NSC, in the postnatal brain significantly impaired aNSC proliferation. As a result, mice displayed deficits in spatial learning, which is a hippocampal task, but not in contextual fear learning, a task accomplished primarily through the amygdala (Zhang et al., 2008). Physiologically speaking, newborn neurons from SGZ neural stem cells portray high amounts of synaptic plasticity and are preferentially incorporated into spatial memory networks within the dentate gyrus (Ge et al., 2007; Kee et al., 2007; Ma et al., 2009). Increased numbers of newborn neurons are observed in the olfactory bulb in response to novel odorants, suggesting that SVZ neurogenesis is involved in odor learning (Rochefort et al., 2002). While the exact function of aNSC within the adult brain is not well understood, the phenotypes derived from inhibiting neurogenesis in the adult brain strongly suggest that incorporation of adult born neurons is crucial for brain function, especially in learning and memory.

The adult NSC niche is an intricate structure composed of cellular and molecular components that regulate aNSC function. Increasing evidence from in vitro and in vivo studies suggest that neurogenesis within the adult brain is tightly controlled by both extracellular and intracellular factors. Intracellular or cell-intrinsic factors, often influenced by signals coming from the cell exterior, influence gene transcription programs that direct the NSC to self-renew, proliferate, or differentiate (Qu & Shi, 2009).

The nuclear receptor TLX (NR2E1) is a transcription factor that is highly expressed in aNSC and is essential for aNSC self-renewal and maintenance (Shi et al., 2004). TLX promotes NSC proliferation and self-renewal by interacting with histone deacetylases (HDAC). By binding to HDAC, TLX represses expression of genes that promote cell-cycle exit (Sun et al., 2007).

Sox2 (sex-determining region of Y chromosome-related high mobility group box 2) is also expressed highly in aNSC (Ferri et al., 2004; Episkopou, 2005). Sox2 is crucial for the maintenance of NSC identity; loss of Sox2 leads to neuronal differentiation at the expense of NSC self-renewal. Sox2 promotes expression of the Hes family members (see below), which in turn inhibit proneural genes (Bani-Yaghoub et al., 2006).

Neural differentiation from NSC is dependent upon the expression of basic helix-loop-helix (bHLH) transcription factors. Suppression of bHLH genes is required for maintaining NSC identity and suppressing neural differentiation. The Hes family members are transcriptional repressors of the bHLH transcription factors and are expressed in both embryonic and adult NSC (Kageyama et al., 2008). A wide range of brain defects occur in the absence of Hes family members as eNSC prematurely undergo neuronal differentiation (Hatakeyama et al., 2004). The suppression of neurogenesis by the Hes family of transcription factors is an important event, as it allows proliferation of NSC to occur in sufficient quality, ensuring that there will be enough NSC to generate the nervous system. Once sufficient numbers have been generated, proneuronal bHLH proteins will act to stimulate NSC towards neurogenesis. Examples of such transcription factors include Mash1, Math, and neurogenin (Kageyama et al., 2005).

Unlike the previous two factors, the tumor suppressor phosphatase Pten (phosphatase and tensin homolog deleted on chromosome 10) is important for negatively regulating NSC proliferation (Groszer et al., 2001). Pten suppresses the expression of several cyclin proteins required for cell-cycle progression (Groszer et al., 2006). Interestingly, Pten is negatively regulated by TLX, suggesting that there is a delicate balance between enhancing and suppressing NSC renewal or proliferation (Sun et al., 2007).

Although TLX, Sox2, and Pten are a small sample of intracellular regulators of NSC function in the embryonic and adult brain, they serve as examples of the complexity of the network responsible for controlling NSC function. As stated previously, many of the intracellular factors are influenced by signals coming from the cell exterior. For instance, Shh signaling via Gli2 promotes expression of Sox2, thus linking Sox2-Hes with the Shh-Ptc-Gli2 pathway (Takanaga et al., 2009). Many other extracellular factors found within the aNSC microenvironment regulate NSC fate. Factors such as Notch (Androutsellis-Theotokis et al., 2006), FGF2 (Yoshimura et al., 2001), BMP inhibitors (Bonaguidi et al., 2008), and vascular-derived endothelial growth factor (Jin et al., 2002) have all been found to influence aNSC. Given the importance of the extracellular and intracellular environments in controlling and regulating adult neurogenesis, and the role of adult neurogenesis in normal brain function, disruption of the signaling pathways that regulate aNSC may underlie the pathogenesis of diseases such as HAD.

During pathological states such as stroke or in brain inflammatory states such as HAND, activated MP cells secrete cytokines and chemokines such as CXCL12 and other cytokines in order to promote increased NPC proliferation and migration. In addition to CXCL12/CXCR4, monocyte chemoattractant protein 1 (MCP-1)/CCR2 promotes NPC migration in response to inflammation, including inflammation caused by the HIV-1 coat protein gp120 (Belmadani et al., 2006). MCP-1 also promotes migration of SVZ-derived neural precursors into the striatum after striatal damage (Gordon et al., 2009). Conversely, some disease states have

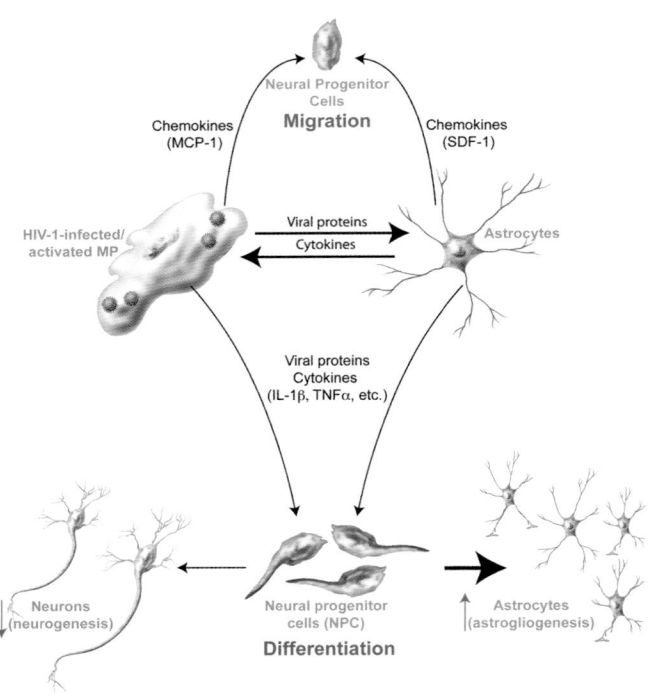

Figure 2.6.1 A proposed mechanism for the simulation of neurogenesis during brain injury and neurodegenerative disorders. During neuronal injury, neurons produce chemokines, which recruit mononuclear phagocytes (MP) into the brain and to the site of injury. As these MP enter an environment of injury or inflammation, they become activated, subsequently releasing factors that might promote neurogenesis. These factors include but are not limited to neurotrophins, which may act directly to enhance the survival and proliferation of neural progenitor cells (NPCs), and cytokines that might activate astrocytes. These activated astrocytes produce chemokines that could promote the migration of NPCs to the site of injury and they can release neurotrophins that can promote neuronal survival. Once the NPCs receive these migratory and neurotrophic signals, the NPCs can migrate, proliferate, and differentiate into neuronal or astrocyte precursors, which then mature into neurons and astrocytes that may integrate into the CNS circuitry.

been shown to negatively impact neurogenesis. In the following section, we will examine how neurogenesis is impacted during brain injury and inflammation, specifically focusing on the roles of pro-inflammatory cytokines.

HAND: THE ROLES OF INFLAMMATION AND NEUROGENESIS

The pathogenesis of HAND is not well understood. The HIV-1 viral coat protein gp120 has been shown to be neurotoxic, inducing apoptosis in neuronal cells (Hayward, 2004; Kaul et al., 2007). In addition, considerable evidence supports neuroinflammation as a key regulator of HIV-related neuropathology. In this model, peripherally located HIV-infected macrophages migrate into the CNS and secrete molecules which activate resident microglia and astrocytes, which, in turn, release many types of pro-inflammatory cytokines, chemokines, and neurotoxins (Pulliam et al., 1991; Gendelman et al., 1994; Minagar et al., 2002; Crews et al., 2008). The chronic release and increasing amounts of these molecules within the CNS promotes neuronal cell death and injury (Pulliam et al., 1994; Meucci et al., 1998; Kaul & Lipton, 1999). The effect of HIV-1-mediated neuroinflammation on neurogenesis is a topic of intense investigation. Recent discoveries from patient data, animal models, and cell culture experiments strongly suggest that neurogenesis is both negatively and positively affected by inflammation. In the following section, we will discuss these recent findings, which strongly support the hypothesis that neurogenesis is affected by neuroinflammatory states, specifically those caused by HIV-1 infection.

HAND AND NEUROGENESIS: CLINICAL EVIDENCE

Although there is no causative data linking aberrant neurogenesis to the pathogenesis of HAND or other HIV-1-mediated neurological disorders, several interesting pathological correlates from HIV-1-infected patients endorse the idea that improper neurogenesis during HIV-1 infection may play a substantial role in the promotion of neurological deficits seen in infected patients, especially in the pediatric population. Disease adversely affecting neurogenesis is not unprecedented, as decreased neurogenesis is an emerging culprit in the progression of major depression (Kempermann & Kronenberg, 2003). Indeed, hippocampal volume and the level of hippocampal neurogenesis have been linked, respectively, to the progression of major depression and the response to antidepressant medication (Schwartz & Major, 2006; Warner-Schmidt & Duman, 2006). Interestingly, a recent cohort study found that major depression and other mood disorders are highly prevalent in HIV-1-infected adults despite HAART treatment (Gibbie et al., 2006). Immunohistochemical studies of hippocampal tissue at autopsy further suggest that neurogenesis is affected in HAD, as the number of proliferating cells in HAD patients is drastically lower than in HAD-negative patients (both HIV-infected patients and non-infected control) (Krathwohl &

Kaiser, 2004). This landmark study, which underscores the effect of HIV on human neurogenesis, will be discussed in detail later in this section. The effects of HIV-1 infection on neurogenesis are thought to be a secondary effect, as microglia and invading peripheral macrophages are the prevalent cells within the brain infected with HIV-1 (Gorry et al., 2003; Aquaro et al., 2005). However, a recent paper found that HIV could directly infect nestin-positive cells neuronal precursors in pediatric patients (Schwartz et al., 2007). The relevance of this finding, and the consequence of direct infection of neural progenitors, remain unknown. It should be noted that, at present, this is probably a pediatric phenomenon, as there is no evidence that HIV-1 can directly infect adult neural progenitors. Pediatric HIV-1-infected patients show dramatically lower hippocampal volumes than noninfected controls (Keller et al. 2004; Schwartz and Major 2006) again suggesting that HIV-1, either directly or indirectly, can negatively affect neurogenesis. Taken together, cases from both HIV-1-infected adult and children strongly promote the theory that neurogenesis plays an important role in the progression of HIV-1-mediated neurological disorders. Work completed in animal and cellular models suggest that both the HIV-1 virus itself, as well as cyto/chemokines secreted by activated cells within the CNS, affect neurogenesis.

HIV INFECTION AND NEUROINFLAMMATION: CYTOKINES AND CHEMOKINES

Recent discoveries have revealed potential mechanisms by which HIV could influence neurogenesis. Some studies provide evidence that components of the virus are directly responsible, while other studies demonstrate that neuroinflammation resulting from HIV-1 infection seems to be the cause. As stated previously, CXCR4 and CXCL12 are crucial for the development of the dentate gyrus and cerebellum. Also, CXCR4 is a co-receptor for HIV and, together with CD4, binds to the viral envelope protein gp120 and promotes entry of the HIV virus into CD4+ T-cells. Binding of gp120 to CXCR4 inhibits CXCL12-induced migration of cultured human fetal NPC (Ni et al., 2004). Interestingly, gp120 was shown not to act in an antagonistic manner as several of the downstream components of the CXCL12/CXCR4 pathway were activated. gp120 has also been shown to decrease aNSC proliferation in vitro and in vivo by causing cell-cycle withdrawal mediated by the p38 MAPK-MAPKAPK2-Cdc25B/C pathway (Okamoto et al., 2007). Another similar study found that HIV coat proteins promote human NPC quiescence by upregulating the expression of cell-cycle inhibitors such as p21 and p27 and downregulating the activity of ERK, a pathway that promotes NPC proliferation (Krathwohl & Kaiser, 2004). This study also found that cerebrospinal fluid isolated from HAD patients, but not from seronegative control patients or HIV-infected patients without dementia, caused quiescence in both cultured human NPC and human hippocampal brain slices isolated from patients undergoing corrective surgery for seizures. This is especially noteworthy, as it suggests that the progression from

HIV infection without dementia to HAND and HAD may be partially due to a currently unknown secreted factor that decreases neurogenesis and promotes NPC quiescence. Krathwohl and Kaiser's data demonstrate that it is likely HIV coat proteins acting through the chemokine receptors CXCR4 and CCR3. However, they also point out that there could be additional factors responsible, as the viral load within the CSF isolated from HAD patients was not significantly higher than in HIV-infected patients without dementia. Chemokines like CXCL12/CXCR4 and MCP-1, as well as pro-inflammatory cytokines such as tumor necrosis factor alpha (TNFα) and interleukin-1 (IL-1), have recently been shown to play an important role in neurogenesis, specifically during neuroinflammatory states. Because an effect of HIV on neurogenesis is still a rather novel concept, many studies analyzing the impact of inflammation, cytokines, and chemokines on neurogenesis have been done in a non-HIV context. Therefore, we will provide evidence that supports the notion that HIV-1 infection affects neurogenesis through the action of these molecules and focus the in-depth discussion on studies that were completed in an inflammatory state that may or may not be specific to HIV-1 infection.

The effect on neurogenesis of pro-inflammatory cytokines released in response to HIV infection is complex. Tumor necrosis factor α (TNFα) is a potent pro-inflammatory cytokine (Park & Bowers, 2010). TNFα exists either as a transmembrane protein or a soluble protein that binds to its cognate receptors p55 (TNF-R1) or p85 (TNF-RII), leading to the activation of several distinct intracellular pathways including induction of apoptosis, activation of the nuclear factor kappa-B pathway, or activation of the JNK signaling pathway (Chen & Goeddel, 2002). Studies using human HIV-infected macrophages show that secretion of TNFα promotes proliferation in cultured human fetal NPC (Peng et al., 2008). However, while TNFα was found to promote NPC proliferation, it did not promote neurogenesis. Instead, TNFα caused increased astrocytic differentiation. In agreement with these findings, other investigators have shown that TNFα treatment during in vitro differentiation of NPC significantly increased astrogliogenesis and decreased neurogenesis by enhancing the expression of Hes-1, a bHLH transcription factor that negatively regulates neurogenesis (Keohane et al., 2010). Contrary to these findings, others have shown that TNFα promotes neurogenesis at relatively low concentrations while excessive levels of TNFα actually caused cell death via apoptosis (Bernardino et al., 2008). It should be noted that each of the studies presented above used different techniques and NSC populations; thus, the discrepancies between the studies may be explained by differences in experimental protocol. The apparent discord between the studies may also be explained by the hypothesis that the effects of TNFα can be modulated by the nearby microenvironment, the concentration of TNFα, the duration of TNFα exposure to NPCs, the expression and activation of different TNFR, as well as a number of other factors. If in fact TNFα does promote the generation of astrocytes at the expense of new neurons in places such as the dentate gyrus of the hippocampus, it is tempting to speculate that this phenomenon may explain the cognitive decline

observed in patients with HAND. Observations from mouse genetic studies found that TNFα knock-out mice have enhanced hippocampal-dependent learning while transgenic mice over-expressing TNFα have impaired hippocampal memory compared to wild-type or TNF null mice (Fiore et al., 2000; Golan et al., 2004). Currently, there is little evidence in vivo to suggest that decreased hippocampal neurogenesis caused by increased TNFα levels is responsible for memory impairment seen in patients with HAND. Besides TNFα, IL-1 is another example of a pro-inflammatory cytokine that has been shown to affect neurogenesis.

Many of the IL-1 family members, such as IL-1α and IL-1β and their associated receptor IL-1R, are expressed in the brain, albeit at low levels under normal physiological conditions (Basu et al., 2004). IL-1 is important as a pro-inflammatory molecule both during innate immunity (Weber et al., 2010) and during CNS injury and neurodegeneration (Basu et al., 2004). Binding of IL-1 to IL-1R leads to the induction of a myriad of intracellular protein kinase cascades, ultimately leading to the activation of pathways such as NFκB, JNK, and p38 MAPK (Weber et al., 2010). IL-1, much like TNFα, has recently been shown to affect neurogenesis (Mathieu et al., 2010). For instance, injection of IL-1β into the dentate gyrus has been shown to reduce NSC proliferation within the SGZ (Duman et al. 2008). As expected, other researchers found that exogenous IL-1β can block memory formation (C. R. Pugh et al. 1999; K. R. Pugh et al. 2001). Taken together, there are several bodies of preliminary evidence that suggest neuroinflammatory states involving increases in IL-1 have drastic effects on neurogenesis. Future work will undoubtedly uncover the magnitude of IL-1 influences on neurogenesis, as well as how the action of IL-1 promotes the progression of diseases such as HAND where neurogenesis is thought to be a critical underlying factor mediating the observed clinical symptoms.

In total, while TNFα and IL-1 are just two examples of many pro-inflammatory molecules found during CNS injury and disease, their effects on neurogenesis are relatively well understood. Our understanding of how neurogenesis is affected during disease states such as Alzheimer's disease (AD), Parkinson's disease (PD), and HAND is limited. Indeed, there is much work supporting the view that neurogenesis is either disrupted or enhanced during these disease states. It seems that during CNS injury and neurodegeneration, the amount of pro-inflammatory molecules markedly increases. Connecting the effects of inflammatory molecules on neurogenesis to the progression of neurodegenerative diseases underscores one of the primary goals of neuroimmunologists. Understanding the molecular pathways involved in neurogenesis, and how these pathways are disrupted or enhanced by inflammatory molecules, will hopefully lead to the development of therapeutics that will either slow the progression of these horrible neurodegenerative states, by protecting endogenous NSC, or facilitate the transplantation of exogenous stem cells. Stem cell therapy represents the bright hope for the treatment of neurodegenerative diseases. In the final section, we will discuss different stem cell populations that show promise for use in cellular therapy.

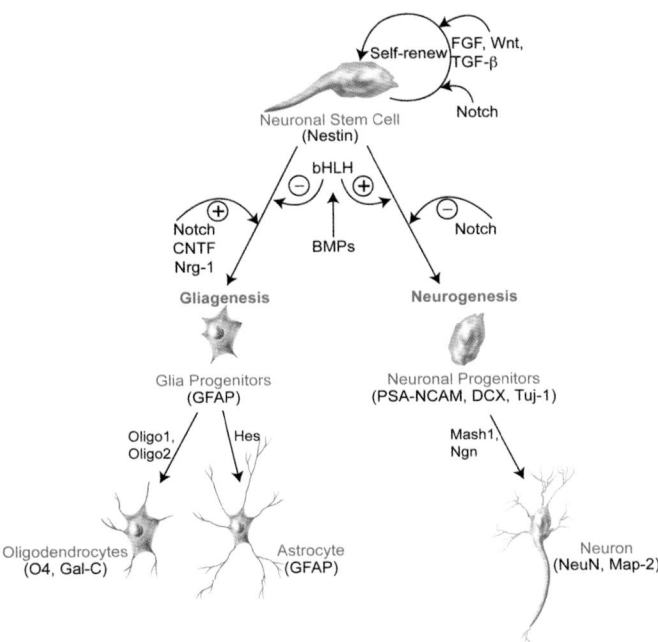

Figure 2.6.2 A proposed mechanism for a select number of factors that regulate self-renew and differentiation of neural stem cells (NSCs) and neural progenitor cells. Factors that promote self-renewal include but are not limited to fibroblast growth factor (FGF), the transforming growth factor-β (TGF-β), Wnt signaling, and Notch signaling. NSCs are directed towards differentiating along the neuronal lineage by a decrease in Notch signaling and an increase in basic helix-loop-helix (bHLH) transcription factors. As these immature neurons mature they express activator-type bHLH genes *Mash1, Math* and *Ngn*. NSCs are directed towards the glial lineage by a low level of bHLH and a higher level of factors such as Notch, ciliary neurotrophic factor (CNTF), and Nrg-1. As these glial progenitors mature to astrocytes they express *Hes* and as they differentiate into oligodendrocytes they express *Oligo1* and *Oligo 2*. Specific cell markers can identify each of these cell types. Nestin and GFAP are expressed by NSC, PSA-NCAM, DCX, and Tuj-1are expressed by neural progenitors, NeuN and Map-2 are expressed by maturing neurons, GFAP is expressed by glial progenitors and astrocytes, and O4 and Gal-C are expressed by oligodendrocytes.

STEM CELL THERAPY AND NEURODEGENERATIVE DISEASES

Neurodegenerative diseases such as HAND, AD, PD, and others are all generally characterized by loss/damage of neuronal tissue. As affected areas of the brain degenerate, patients suffering from these devastating disorders are overcome by debilitating symptoms that severely reduce their quality of life. Currently, most treatments approved for use address only the symptoms of the disease as opposed to curing the underlying pathology responsible for the neurodegeneration. While the mechanisms responsible for nearly all neurodegenerative disorders remain a mystery, recent work dedicated to understanding the biology of stem cells has excited many, as stem cells capable of differentiating into new neurons provide a possible means to replace dead neurons. However, while stem cell therapy remains a bright hope for many as a treatment for neurodegenerative diseases (as well as other non-neurological diseases), it must be noted that we are only

starting to appreciate both the complexity of stem cell biology and the molecular pathways responsible for the differentiation of stem cells into cells of interest. Given the importance of stem cells and their potential for the treatment of neurodegenerative diseases, including HAND, we will finish this chapter with a discussion dedicated to introducing pluripotent stem cells and the latest research which demonstrates their usefulness in treating neurological disorders.

EMBRYONIC STEM CELLS

ESC, as discussed previously, are pluripotent stem cells derived from the inner cell mass of a pre-implantation embryo. Because ESC retain the ability to self-renew and differentiate into each of the three germ layers while being cultured in vitro, they represent an attractive source of unlimited cells to be used for cellular therapy. However, the molecular mechanisms responsible for controlling their self-renewal, as well as the factors required for controlled differentiation, must be well understood before ESC can be responsibly utilized in a clinical setting, as implantation of undifferentiated cells into a patient could lead to tumor formation.

Several important factors regulating ESC self-renewal have been uncovered in the past decade (Bosnali et al., 2009). Transcription factors such as Oct4 (octamer-binding transcription factor 4), Sox2, and Nanog are crucial for the maintenance of ESC in an undifferentiated state. Interestingly, extrinsic factors such as the cytokine leukemia inhibitor factor (LIF) are also required for ESC maintenance (Pan & Thomson, 2007). LIF signaling activates the signal transducer and activator of transcription 3 (STAT3), which dimerizes and translocates to the nucleus in order to activate transcription. Without LIF, ESC in culture differentiate; however, addition of constitutively active Nanog allows for LIF-independent self-renewal and maintenance (Takahashi, 2010). Each of these four transcription factors act cooperatively and also independently to activate gene transcription profiles that are necessary for ESC self-renewal and maintenance. The complexity of this transcriptional network is a topic of intense interest to stem cell biologists. While the maintenance and propagation of ESC is an important consideration, neuroscientists and clinicians alike are more concerned with how ESC can be directed to differentiate into specific neuronal cell types that can be used for treatment of neurological disorders. In recent years, scientists have begun to discover how ESC can be directed to differentiate into different neuronal and glial populations by following the developmental pathways introduced earlier in the chapter.

A chemically defined protocol for directing ESC to the neuronal lineage was first described early in the 21st century (Zhang et al., 2001). Addition of FGF-2 to ESC grown in suspension for a week as aggregated cells known as embryoid bodies led to the formation of neuroepithelial-like structures termed "neural rosettes" that morphologically resemble the neural tube. These neural rosettes stain positive for many of the markers of NE, including nestin. Zhang et al. were able to show that neural precursors derived from human ESC were able to migrate, differentiate, and integrate into existing neuronal circuitry in vivo. This important study paved the way for future studies dedicated to understanding how specific neuronal cells and glia can be obtained from ESC-derived neural precursors. For example, Zhang and colleagues were able to show that treatment of neural rosettes with retinoic acid (RA) and Shh resulted in spinal motor neuron differentiation in a time course that mirrors that of embryonic development (Li, Du et al., 2005; Hu & Zhang, 2009). Other neural subtypes, such as midbrain dopaminergic neurons, can also be derived from neural precursors obtained from ESC by addition of FGF8 and Shh (Zhang & Zhang, 2010). Furthermore, oligodendrocytes can be obtained by temporal addition of RA, Shh, and FGF2 (Hu et al., 2009). Again, following a timeline that mimics embryological development, neural rosettes form pre-oligodendrocyte precursors followed by oligodendrocyte precursors capable of producing myelin. The implications of being able to generate spinal motor neurons, dopaminergic neurons, and oligodendrocytes are vast for diseases such as spinal muscular atrophy (SMA), PD, and ALS respectively.

While ESC show vast potential for use in cellular therapy, several important considerations must be analyzed. The use of human embryonic tissue is fraught with ethical concerns. In addition, without extremely efficient differentiation protocols, lingering undifferentiated ESC contained among differentiated cells used for transplantation could lead to tumor formation. Also, host rejection of transplanted ESC derived is a possibility. Among these concerns, the ethical dilemma and possibility of rejection associated with ESC pose as the major barriers for use of ESC in the clinical setting. However, in 2006, Takahasi and Yamanaka made one of the most important discoveries in recent memory. These scientists, for the first time, were able to show that mouse somatic cells could be transformed into pluripotent embryonic stem cell-like cells by viral transduction with several of the aforementioned transcription factors responsible for ESC maintenance (Takahashi & Yamanaka, 2006). However, these pluripotent stem cells, known as induced pluripotent stem cells (iPSC) come with their share of problems. The generation of iPSC and their potential use in cellular therapy is discussed below.

INDUCED PLURIPOTENT STEM CELLS AND CELL THERAPY

Takahasi and Yamanaka found that mouse embryonic and adult fibroblasts could be reprogrammed into embryonic stem cell-like cells by the addition of four factors including: Oct4, c-MYC, Sox2, and KlF4. These four transcription factors were identified from a list of 24 candidate factors. iPSC appeared morphologically indistinguishable from ESC and generated teratomas after injection into nude mice, demonstrating that they are capable of differentiating into all three germ layers. At the molecular level, iPSC portrayed gene expression and epigenetic profiles that were similar to those of ESC. Others found that mouse iPSC transplanted into blastocysts could give rise to chimeric adult progeny capable of germline transmission (Maherali et al., 2007; Okita et al.,

2007; Wernig et al., 2007). Shortly after this discovery, Yamanaka and colleagues and Thomson and colleagues independently found that iPSC could be generated from human somatic cells (Takahashi et al., 2007; Yu et al., 2007). In contrast to Yamanaka's group, Lu et al. found that human somatic cells could be reprogrammed by a different cocktail of factors (Oct4, Sox2, Nanog, and Lin28). The ability to generate human iPSC not only alleviates some of the problems associated with ESC but also provides a potential human in vitro model for drug discovery and disease research.

After the finding that human somatic cells could be reprogrammed into ESC-like cells, many investigators explored whether or not iPSC behaved like ESC in relation to directed-differentiation capacity. As expected, it has been found that iPSC exhibit the capacity for directed differentiation with protocols identical to those used for ESC. For instance, Hu and Zhang found that spinal motor neurons could be generated from human iPSC in a manner identical to the protocol used for directing ESC (Li et al., 2005; Hu & Zhang, 2009). Dopaminergic neurons can also be derived from human iPSC following ESC protocol. Furthermore, these dopaminergic neurons are functional and capable of improving behavioral deficits in a rat model of PD following transplantation into the lesioned brain. Interestingly, dopaminergic neurons derived from ESC and iPSC displayed similar (but not identical) gene expression profiles, indicating that there could be a difference in differentiation capacity (Swistowski et al., 2010). As alluded to above, iPSC are exciting not only for their capacity to be used in cellular therapy, but also for their potential as in vitro models of human diseases.

The ability to generate patient-specific iPSC is a potentially great opportunity to model human diseases in vitro. Assays involving disease-specific cells would provide excellent platforms for drug discovery and for determining the cellular and molecular mechanisms underlying specific pathologies. From a neurodegenerative standpoint, iPSC have recently been derived from patients suffering from PD and SMA. Dermal fibroblasts isolated from PD patients were capable of generating iPSC. More importantly, these iPSC were successfully differentiated into dopaminergic neurons (Soldner et al., 2009). Similarly, fibroblasts isolated from a child suffering from SMA were capable of being reprogrammed to iPSC (Ebert et al., 2009). While this study is unique in that motor neurons were derived from a patient with SMA, it is perhaps even more unique given that motor neurons derived from the affected child displayed deficits compared to motor neurons derived from iPSC generated from the unaffected mother. Furthermore, Ebert et al. demonstrated that treatment of SMA-derived motor neurons with valproic acid and tobramycin increased levels of survival motor neuron 1 protein (typically downregulated in SMA patients), indicating that patient-derived, disease-specific cell types can be used for drug discovery. While there is obviously much excitement surrounding the use of iPSC for cellular therapy, drug discovery, and disease modeling, scientists and clinicians must exercise caution moving forward as iPSC are not without their limitations.

While iPSC solve the ethical dilemma and rejection issues involved with the use of ESC, they do present their own unique difficulties (Maherali & Hochedlinger, 2008; Cox & Rizzino, 2010) While a detailed analysis of the technical challenges presented by iPSC are not within the scope of this chapter, we will briefly introduce several unique challenges confronting iPSC use. First, the generation of iPSC from somatic cells is typically inefficient; interestingly, efficiency can be dependent on the type of cell used for reprogramming. Secondly, the use of viral vectors for delivery of transgenes that integrate into the genome can lead to insertional mutagenesis. Thirdly, reactivation of transgenes such as c-MYC can lead to tumor formation. Many studies now focus on experimental protocols that aim to rectify some of these hindrances. For instance, Soldner et al. created iPSC from PD patients free of viral reprogramming factors by taking advantage of the Cre-Lox system (Soldner et al., 2009). The use of the Cre-Lox system allowed for the excision of the viral transgenes. Interestingly, they demonstrated that human iPSC free of transgenes more closely resemble human ESC than iPSC containing the transgenes, again emphasizing the importance of removing the transgenes. Other methods involving small molecules, transient transfection, doxycycline inducible transgenes, and adenovirus (non-genomic integrating) all aim to alleviate the dependency on using viral-mediated reprogramming methods that require genomic insertion and leave the cell susceptible to transgene reactivation.

In total, both human ESC and iPSC present exciting avenues to study human disease as well as to be used for cell therapy. As indicated above, while there are still technical and ethical dilemmas that must be resolved, there is still a great need to understand the molecular pathways responsible for directed differentiation. Also, for stem cell therapy to be feasible, the cell type required for transplantation must be identified. In other words, we first need to understand the pathology underlying these devastating degenerative diseases before we insert cells into the damaged brain. In the case of HAND and neuroinflammation, there is a need to comprehend the effects of brain inflammation on neurogenesis. For instance, if neuronal precursors or differentiated cells derived from iPSC or ESC are injected into an inflamed brain, will the cells survive or die? Will pro-inflammatory cytokines cause an over-proliferation of engrafted cells leading to tumor formation? These questions and others must be answered before cell therapy can become a reality.

ACKNOWLEDGMENTS

We kindly acknowledge Li Wu, Beibei Jia, and Lijun Sun who provided technical support for this work. Ms. Julie Ditter, Johna Belling, Robin Taylor, Myhanh Che, Na Ly, and Emilie Scoggins provided outstanding administrative support. Ms. Robin Taylor provided exceptional art illustration support for the figures. This work was supported in part by research grants by the National Institutes of Health: R01 NS41858, R01NS61642, R21MH83525, P01NS43985 and NCRR COBRE grant RR15635 to JZ.

REFERENCES

Aaku-Saraste, E., Oback, B., et al. (1997). Neuroepithelial cells downregulate their plasma membrane polarity prior to neural tube closure and neurogenesis. *Mech Dev, 69*(1–2), 71–81.

Altman, J. & Das, G. D. (1965a). Autoradiographic and histological evidence of postnatal hippocampal neurogenesis in rats. *J Comp Neurol, 124*(3), 319–335.

Altman, J. & Das, G. D. (1965b). Post-natal origin of microneurones in the rat brain. *Nature, 207*(5000), 953–956.

Alvarez-Buylla, A., Garcia-Verdugo, J. M., et al. (2001). A unified hypothesis on the lineage of neural stem cells. *Nat Rev Neurosci, 2*(4), 287–293.

Androutsellis-Theotokis, A., Leker, R. R., et al. (2006). Notch signalling regulates stem cell numbers in vitro and in vivo. *Nature, 442*(7104), 823–826.

Anthony, T. E., Klein, C., et al. (2004). Radial glia serve as neuronal progenitors in all regions of the central nervous system. *Neuron, 41*(6), 881–890.

Aquaro, S., Ronga, L., et al. (2005). Human immunodeficiency virus infection and acquired immunodeficiency syndrome dementia complex: Role of cells of monocyte-macrophage lineage. *J Neurovirol, 11* Suppl 3, 58–66.

Arvidsson, A., Collin, T., et al. (2002). Neuronal replacement from endogenous precursors in the adult brain after stroke. *Nat Med, 8*(9), 963–970.

Bagri, A., Gurney, T., et al. (2002). The chemokine SDF1 regulates migration of dentate granule cells. *Development, 129*(18), 4249–4260.

Bani-Yaghoub, M., Tremblay, R. G., et al. (2006). Role of Sox2 in the development of the mouse neocortex. *Dev Biol, 295*(1), 52–66.

Basak, O. & Taylor, V. (2009). Stem cells of the adult mammalian brain and their niche. *Cell Mol Life Sci, 66*(6), 1057–1072.

Basu, A., Krady, J. K., et al. (2004). Interleukin-1: a master regulator of neuroinflammation. *J Neurosci Res, 78*(2), 151–156.

Belmadani, A., Tran, P. B., et al. (2006). Chemokines regulate the migration of neural progenitors to sites of neuroinflammation. *J Neurosci, 26*(12), 3182–3191.

Bengzon, J., Kokaia, Z., et al. (1997). Apoptosis and proliferation of dentate gyrus neurons after single and intermittent limbic seizures. *Proc Natl Acad Sci USA, 94*(19), 10432–10437.

Bernardino, L., Agasse, F., et al. (2008). Tumor necrosis factor-alpha modulates survival, proliferation, and neuronal differentiation in neonatal subventricular zone cell cultures. *Stem Cells, 26*(9), 2361–2371.

Berson, J. F., Long, D., et al. (1996). A seven-transmembrane domain receptor involved in fusion and entry of T- cell-tropic human immunodeficiency virus type 1 strains. *J Virol, 70*(9), 6288–6295.

Boisse, L., Gill, M. J., et al. (2008). HIV infection of the central nervous system: Clinical features and neuropathogenesis. *Neurol Clin, 26*(3), 799–819.

Bonaguidi, M. A., Peng, C. Y., et al. (2008). Noggin expands neural stem cells in the adult hippocampus. *J Neurosci, 28*(37), 9194–9204.

Bosnali, M., Munst, B., et al. (2009). Deciphering the stem cell machinery as a basis for understanding the molecular mechanism underlying reprogramming. *Cell Mol Life Sci, 66*(21), 3403–3420.

Brelot, A., Heveker, N., et al. (1997). Role of the first and third extracellular domains of CXCR-4 in human immunodeficiency virus coreceptor activity. *J Virol, 71*(6), 4744–4751.

Casper, K. B. & McCarthy, K. D. (2006). GFAP-positive progenitor cells produce neurons and oligodendrocytes throughout the CNS. *Mol Cell Neurosci, 31*(4), 676–684.

Chen, D., Zhao, M., et al. (2004). Bone morphogenetic proteins. *Growth Factors, 22*(4), 233–241.

Chen, G. & Goeddel, D. V. (2002). TNF-R1 signaling: A beautiful pathway. *Science, 296*(5573), 1634–1635.

Chenn, A., Zhang, Y. A., et al. (1998). Intrinsic polarity of mammalian neuroepithelial cells. *Mol Cell Neurosci, 11*(4), 183–193.

Coskun, V., Wu, H., et al. (2008). CD133+ neural stem cells in the ependyma of mammalian postnatal forebrain. *Proc Natl Acad Sci USA, 105*(3), 1026–1031.

Cox, J. L. & Rizzino, A. (2010). Induced pluripotent stem cells: What lies beyond the paradigm shift. *Exp Biol Med (Maywood), 235*(2), 148–158.

Crews, L., Lentz, M. R., et al. (2008). Neuronal injury in simian immunodeficiency virus and other animal models of neuroAIDS. *J Neurovirol, 14*(4), 327–339.

Deleyrolle, L. P. & Reynolds, B. A. (2009). Isolation, expansion, and differentiation of adult mammalian neural stem and progenitor cells using the neurosphere assay. *Methods Mol Biol, 549*, 91–101.

Doetsch, F., Caille, I., et al. (1999). Subventricular zone astrocytes are neural stem cells in the adult mammalian brain. *Cell, 97*(6), 703–716.

Duman, K., et al. (2008). Incidence of auditory neuropathy among the deaf school students. *Int J Pediatr Otorhinolaryngol, 72* (7), 1091–5.

Ebert, A. D., Yu, J., et al. (2009). Induced pluripotent stem cells from a spinal muscular atrophy patient. *Nature, 457*(7227), 277–280.

Ekdahl, C. T., Kokaia, Z., et al. (2009). Brain inflammation and adult neurogenesis: The dual role of microglia. *Neuroscience, 158*(3), 1021–1029.

Ellis, P., Fagan, B. M., et al. (2004). SOX2, a persistent marker for multipotential neural stem cells derived from embryonic stem cells, the embryo or the adult. *Dev Neurosci, 26*(2–4), 148–165.

Episkopou, V. (2005). SOX2 functions in adult neural stem cells. *Trends Neurosci, 28*(5), 219–221.

Epstein, L. G. and Gelbard, H. A. (1999). HIV-1-induced neuronal injury in the developing brain. *J Leukoc Biol* 65 (4), 453–7

Eriksson, P. S., Perfilieva, E., et al. (1998). Neurogenesis in the adult human hippocampus. *Nat Med, 4*(11), 1313–1317.

Ever, L. & Gaiano, N. (2005). Radial 'glial' progenitors: Neurogenesis and signaling. *Curr Opin Neurobiol, 15*(1), 29–33.

Farkas, L. M. & Huttner, W. B. (2008). The cell biology of neural stem and progenitor cells and its significance for their proliferation versus differentiation during mammalian brain development. *Curr Opin Cell Biol, 20*(6), 707–715.

Ferri, A. L., Cavallaro, M., et al. (2004). Sox2 deficiency causes neurodegeneration and impaired neurogenesis in the adult mouse brain. *Development, 131*(15), 3805–3819.

Fiore, M., Angelucci, F., et al. (2000). Learning performances, brain NGF distribution and NPY levels in transgenic mice expressing TNF-alpha. *Behav Brain Res, 112*(1–2), 165–175.

Gage, F. H. (2000). Mammalian neural stem cells. *Science, 287*(5457), 1433–1438.

Ganju, R. K., Brubaker, S. A., et al. (1998). The alpha-chemokine, stromal cell-derived factor-1alpha, binds to the transmembrane G-protein-coupled CXCR-4 receptor and activates multiple signal transduction pathways. *J Biol Chem, 273*(36), 23169–23175.

Ge, S., Yang, C. H., et al. (2007). A critical period for enhanced synaptic plasticity in newly generated neurons of the adult brain. *Neuron, 54*(4), 559–566.

Gendelman, H. E., Lipton, S. A., et al. (1994). The neuropathogenesis of HIV-1 infection. *J Leukoc Biol, 56*(3), 389–398.

Gibbie, T., Mijch, A., et al. (2006). Depression and neurocognitive performance in individuals with HIV/AIDS: 2-year follow-up. *HIV Med, 7*(2), 112–121.

Golan, H., Levav, T., et al. (2004). Involvement of tumor necrosis factor alpha in hippocampal development and function. *Cereb Cortex, 14*(1), 97–105.

Gordon, R. J., McGregor, A. L., et al. (2009). Chemokines direct neural progenitor cell migration following striatal cell loss. *Mol Cell Neurosci, 41*(2), 219–232.

Gorry, P. R., Ong, C., et al. (2003). Astrocyte infection by HIV-1: Mechanisms of restricted virus replication, and role in the pathogenesis of HIV-1-associated dementia. *Curr HIV Res, 1*(4), 463–473.

Gotz, M. & Huttner, W. B. (2005). The cell biology of neurogenesis. *Nat Rev Mol Cell Biol, 6*(10), 777–788.

Groszer, M., Erickson, R., et al. (2006). PTEN negatively regulates neural stem cell self-renewal by modulating G0-G1 cell cycle entry. *Proc Natl Acad Sci USA, 103*(1), 111–116.

Groszer, M., Erickson, R., et al. (2001). Negative regulation of neural stem/progenitor cell proliferation by the Pten tumor suppressor gene in vivo. *Science, 294*(5549), 2186–2189.

Hartfuss, E., Galli, R., et al. (2001). Characterization of CNS precursor subtypes and radial glia. *Dev Biol, 229*(1), 15–30.

Hatakeyama, J., Bessho, Y., et al. (2004). Hes genes regulate size, shape and histogenesis of the nervous system by control of the timing of neural stem cell differentiation. *Development, 131*(22), 5539–5550.

Hayward, P. (2004). Viral proteins cause cell death in HIV-associated dementia. *Lancet Neurol, 3*(6), 325.

Hu, B. Y., Du, Z. W., et al. (2009). Differentiation of human oligodendrocytes from pluripotent stem cells. *Nat Protoc, 4*(11), 1614–1622.

Hu, B. Y. & Zhang, S. C. (2009). Differentiation of spinal motor neurons from pluripotent human stem cells. *Nat Protoc, 4*(9), 1295–1304.

Huttner, W. B. & Kosodo, Y. (2005). Symmetric versus asymmetric cell division during neurogenesis in the developing vertebrate central nervous system. *Curr Opin Cell Biol, 17*(6), 648–657.

Imayoshi, I., Sakamoto, M., et al. (2008). Roles of continuous neurogenesis in the structural and functional integrity of the adult forebrain. *Nat Neurosci, 11*(10), 1153–1161.

Jazin, E., Soderstrom, S., et al. (1997). Embryonic expression of the mRNA for the rat homologue of the fusin/CXCR4 HIV-1 co-receptor. *J Neuroimmunol, 79*, 148–154.

Jiang, J. & Hui, C. C. (2008). Hedgehog signaling in development and cancer. *Dev Cell, 15*(6), 801–812.

Jiao, J. & Chen, D. F. (2008). Induction of neurogenesis in nonconventional neurogenic regions of the adult central nervous system by niche astrocyte-produced signals. *Stem Cells, 26*(5), 1221–1230.

Jin, K., Zhu, Y., et al. (2002). Vascular endothelial growth factor (VEGF) stimulates neurogenesis in vitro and in vivo. *Proc Natl Acad Sci USA, 99*(18), 11946–11950.

Jordan, J. D., Ma, D. K., et al. (2007). Cellular niches for endogenous neural stem cells in the adult brain. *CNS Neurol Disord Drug Targets, 6*(5), 336–341.

Kageyama, R., Ohtsuka, T., et al. (2005). Roles of bHLH genes in neural stem cell differentiation. *Exp Cell Res, 306*(2), 343–348.

Kageyama, R., Ohtsuka, T., et al. (2008). Roles of Hes genes in neural development. *Dev Growth Differ, 50* Suppl 1, S97–103.

Kaul, M. (2009). HIV-1 associated dementia: Update on pathological mechanisms and therapeutic approaches. *Curr Opin Neurol, 22*(3), 315–320.

Kaul, M. & Lipton, S. A. (1999). Chemokines and activated macrophages in HIV gp120-induced neuronal apoptosis. *Proc Natl Acad Sci USA, 96*(14), 8212–8216.

Kaul, M., Ma, Q., et al. (2007). HIV-1 coreceptors CCR5 and CXCR4 both mediate neuronal cell death but CCR5 paradoxically can also contribute to protection. *Cell Death Differ, 14*(2), 296–305.

Kawaguchi, A., Miyata, T., et al. (2001). Nestin-EGFP transgenic mice: visualization of the self-renewal and multipotency of CNS stem cells. *Mol Cell Neurosci, 17*(2), 259–273.

Kee, N., Teixeira, C. M., et al. (2007). Preferential incorporation of adult-generated granule cells into spatial memory networks in the dentate gyrus. *Nat Neurosci, 10*(3), 355–362.

Kempermann, G. & Kronenberg, G. (2003). Depressed new neurons—adult hippocampal neurogenesis and a cellular plasticity hypothesis of major depression. *Biol Psychiatry, 54*(5), 499–503.

Keller, M. A., et al. (2004). Altered neurometabolite development in HIV-infected children: correlation with neuropsychological tests. *Neurology, 62* (10), 1810–7.

Keohane, A., Ryan, S., et al. (2010). Tumour necrosis factor-alpha impairs neuronal differentiation but not proliferation of hippocampal neural precursor cells: Role of Hes1. *Mol Cell Neurosci, 43*(1), 127–135.

Klein, R. S., Rubin, J. B., et al. (2001). SDF-1 alpha induces chemotaxis and enhances sonic hedgehog-induced proliferation of cerebellar granule cells. *Development, 128*(11), 1971–1981.

Krathwohl, M. D. & Kaiser, J. L. (2004). HIV-1 promotes quiescence in human neural progenitor cells. *J Infect Dis, 190*(2), 216–226.

Kriegstein, A. R. & Gotz, M. (2003). Radial glia diversity: A matter of cell fate. *Glia, 43*(1), 37–43.

Leventhal, C., Rafii, S., et al. (1999). Endothelial trophic support of neuronal production and recruitment from the adult mammalian subependyma. *Mol Cell Neurosci, 13*(6), 450–464.

Levine, A. J. & Brivanlou, A. H. (2007). Proposal of a model of mammalian neural induction. *Dev Biol*, 308(2), 247–256.

Li, L. & Xie, T. (2005). Stem cell niche: structure and function. *Annu Rev Cell Dev Biol*, 21, 605–631.

Li, M. & Ransohoff, R. M. (2008). Multiple roles of chemokine CXCL12 in the central nervous system: A migration from immunology to neurobiology. *Prog Neurobiol*, 84(2), 116–131.

Li, X. J., Du, Z. W., et al. (2005). Specification of motoneurons from human embryonic stem cells. *Nat Biotechnol*, 23(2), 215–221.

Liner, K. J., 2nd, Hall, C. D., et al. (2008). Effects of antiretroviral therapy on cognitive impairment. *Curr HIV/AIDS Rep*, 5(2), 64–71.

Lu, L., Su, W. J., et al. (2001). Attenuation of morphine dependence and withdrawal in rats by venlafaxine, a serotonin and noradrenaline reuptake inhibitor. *Life Sci*, 69(1), 37–46.

Lu, M., Grove, E. A., et al. (2002). Abnormal development of the hippocampal dentate gyrus in mice lacking the CXCR4 chemokine receptor. *Proc Natl Acad Sci USA*, 99(10), 7090–7095.

Ma, D. K., Bonaguidi, M. A., et al. (2009). Adult neural stem cells in the mammalian central nervous system. *Cell Res*, 19(6), 672–682.

Ma, Q., Jones, D., et al. (1998). Impaired B -lymphopoiesis, myelopoiesis, and derailed cerebellar neuron migration in CXCR4 and SDF 1 deficient mice. *Proc Natl Acad Sci*, 95, 9448–9453.

Maherali, N. & Hochedlinger, K. (2008). Guidelines and techniques for the generation of induced pluripotent stem cells. *Cell Stem Cell*, 3(6), 595–605.

Maherali, N., Sridharan, R., et al. (2007). Directly reprogrammed fibroblasts show global epigenetic remodeling and widespread tissue contribution. *Cell Stem Cell*, 1(1), 55–70.

Malatesta, P., Hack, M. A., et al. (2003). Neuronal or glial progeny: Regional differences in radial glia fate. *Neuron*, 37(5), 751–764.

Martin, G. R. (1998). The roles of FGFs in the early development of vertebrate limbs. *Genes Dev*, 12(11), 1571–1586.

Mathieu, P., Battista, D., et al. (2010). The more you have, the less you get: The functional role of inflammation on neuronal differentiation of endogenous and transplanted neural stem cells in the adult brain. *J Neurochem*, 112(6), 1368–1385.

McArthur, J. C., Sacktor, N., and Selnes, O. (1999). Human immunodeficiency virus-associated dementia. *Semin Neurol*, 19 (2), 129–50.

McConnell, S. K. (1995). Constructing the cerebral cortex: Neurogenesis and fate determination. *Neuron*, 15(4), 761–768.

Merkle, F. T. & Alvarez-Buylla, A. (2006). Neural stem cells in mammalian development. *Curr Opin Cell Biol*, 18(6), 704–709.

Merkle, F. T., Tramontin, A. D., et al. (2004). Radial glia give rise to adult neural stem cells in the subventricular zone. *Proc Natl Acad Sci USA*, 101(50), 17528–17532.

Meucci, O., Fatatis, A., et al. (1998). Chemokines regulate hippocampal neuronal signaling and gp120 neurotoxicity. *Proc Natl Acad Sci USA*, 95(24), 14500–14505.

Miller, R. J., Rostene, W., et al. (2008). Chemokine action in the nervous system. *J Neurosci*, 28(46), 11792–11795.

Minagar, A., Shapshak, P., et al. (2002). The role of macrophage/microglia and astrocytes in the pathogenesis of three neurologic disorders: HIV-associated dementia, Alzheimer disease, and multiple sclerosis. *J Neurol Sci*, 202(1–2), 13–23.

Mirzadeh, Z., Merkle, F. T., et al. (2008). Neural stem cells confer unique pinwheel architecture to the ventricular surface in neurogenic regions of the adult brain. *Cell Stem Cell*, 3(3), 265–278.

Moll, N. M., Cossoy, M. B., et al. (2009). Imaging correlates of leukocyte accumulation and CXCR4/CXCL12 in multiple sclerosis. *Arch Neurol*, 66(1) 44–53.

Morshead, C. M., Garcia, A. D., et al. (2003). The ablation of glial fibrillary acidic protein-positive cells from the adult central nervous system results in the loss of forebrain neural stem cells but not retinal stem cells. *Eur J Neurosci*, 18(1), 76–84.

Morshead, C. M., Reynolds, B. A., et al. (1994). Neural stem cells in the adult mammalian forebrain: A relatively quiescent subpopulation of subependymal cells. *Neuron*, 13(5), 1071–1082.

Mudo, G., Bonomo, A., et al. (2009). The FGF-2/FGFRs neurotrophic system promotes neurogenesis in the adult brain. *J Neural Transm*, 116(8), 995–1005.

Ni, H. T., Hu, S., et al. (2004). High-level expression of functional chemokine receptor CXCR4 on human neural precursor cells. *Brain Res Dev Brain Res*, 152(2), 159–169.

Okamoto, S., Kang, Y. J., et al. (2007). HIV/gp120 decreases adult neural progenitor cell proliferation via checkpoint kinase-mediated cell-cycle withdrawal and G1 arrest. *Cell Stem Cell*, 1(2): 230–236.

Okita, K., Ichisaka, T., et al. (2007). Generation of germline-competent induced pluripotent stem cells. *Nature*, 448(7151), 313–317.

Pan, G. & Thomson, J. A. (2007). Nanog and transcriptional networks in embryonic stem cell pluripotency. *Cell Res*, 17(1), 42–49.

Park, K. M. & Bowers, W. J. (2010). Tumor necrosis factor-alpha mediated signaling in neuronal homeostasis and dysfunction. *Cell Signal*, 22(7), 977–983.

Partanen, J. (2007). FGF signalling pathways in development of the midbrain and anterior hindbrain. *J Neurochem*, 101(5), 1185–1193.

Peng, H., Huang, Y., et al. (2004). Stromal cell-derived factor 1-mediated CXCR4 signaling in rat and human cortical neural progenitor cells. *J Neurosci Res*, 76(1), 35–50.

Peng, H., Whitney, N., et al. (2008). HIV-1-infected and/or immune-activated macrophage-secreted TNF-alpha affects human fetal cortical neural progenitor cell proliferation and differentiation. *Glia*, 56(8), 903–916.

Petit, I., Goichberg, P., et al. (2005). Atypical PKC-zeta regulates SDF-1-mediated migration and development of human CD34+ progenitor cells. *J Clin Invest*, 115(1), 168–176.

Prakash, N., Brodski, C., et al. (2006). A Wnt1-regulated genetic network controls the identity and fate of midbrain-dopaminergic progenitors in vivo. Development, 133(1), 89–98.

Prakash, N. & Wurst (2006). Genetic networks controlling the development of midbrain dopaminergic neurons. J Physiol, 575(Pt 2), 403–410.

Pugh, C. R., et al. (1999). Role of interleukin-1 beta in impairment of contextual fear conditioning caused by social isolation. *Behav Brain Res*, 106 (1-2), 109–18.

Pugh, K. R., et al. (2001). Neurobiological studies of reading and reading disability. *J Commun Disord*, 34 (6), 479–92.

Pulliam, L., Clarke, J. A., et al. (1994). Investigation of HIV-infected macrophage neurotoxin production from patients with AIDS dementia. *Adv Neuroimmunol*, 4(3), 195–198.

Pulliam, L., Herndier, B. G., et al. (1991). Human immunodeficiency virus-infected macrophages produce soluble factors that cause histological and neurochemical alterations in cultured human brains. *J Clin Invest*, 87(2), 503–512.

Qu, Q. & Shi, Y. (2009). Neural stem cells in the developing and adult brains. *J Cell Physiol*, 221(1), 5–9.

Ramón y Cajal, S., DeFelipe, J., et al. (1991). *Cajal's degeneration and regeneration of the nervous system*. New York: Oxford University Press.

Ransohoff, R. M. (2009). Chemokines and chemokine receptors: Standing at the crossroads of immunobiology and neurobiology. *Immunity*, 31(5), 711–721.

Reynolds, B. A. & Weiss, S. (1992). Generation of neurons and astrocytes from isolated cells of the adult mammalian central nervous system. *Science*, 255(5052), 1707–1710.

Rochefort, C., Gheusi, G., et al. (2002). Enriched odor exposure increases the number of newborn neurons in the adult olfactory bulb and improves odor memory. *J Neurosci*, 22(7), 2679–2689.

Schwartz, L., Civitello, L., et al. (2007). Evidence of human immunodeficiency virus type 1 infection of nestin-positive neural progenitors in archival pediatric brain tissue. *J Neurovirol*, 13(3), 274–283.

Schwartz, L. & Major, E. O. (2006). Neural progenitors and HIV-1-associated central nervous system disease in adults and children. *Curr HIV Res*, 4(3), 319–327.

Shahabi, N. A., McAllen, K., et al. (2008). Stromal cell-derived factor 1-alpha (SDF)-induced human T cell chemotaxis becomes phosphoinositide 3-kinase (PI3K)-independent: role of PKC-theta. *J Leukoc Biol*, 83(3), 663–671.

Shen, Q., Goderie, S. K., et al. (2004). Endothelial cells stimulate self-renewal and expand neurogenesis of neural stem cells. *Science*, 304(5675), 1338–1340.

Shen, Q., Wang, Y., et al. (2008). Adult SVZ stem cells lie in a vascular niche: A quantitative analysis of niche cell-cell interactions. Cell Stem Cell, 3(3), 289–300.

Shi, Y., Chichung Lie, D., et al. (2004). Expression and function of orphan nuclear receptor TLX in adult neural stem cells. *Nature*, *427*(6969), 78–83.

Soldner, F., Hockemeyer, D., et al. (2009). Parkinson's disease patient-derived induced pluripotent stem cells free of viral reprogramming factors. *Cell*, *136*(5), 964–977.

Song, H., Stevens, C. F., et al. (2002). Astroglia induce neurogenesis from adult neural stem cells. *Nature*, *417*(6884), 39–44.

Sotsios, Y., Whittaker, G. C., et al. (1999). The CXC chemokine stromal cell-derived factor activates a Gi-coupled phosphoinositide 3-kinase in T lymphocytes. *J Immunol*, *163*(11), 5954–5963.

Stumm, R. K., Zhou, C., et al. (2003). CXCR4 regulates interneuron migration in the developing neocortex. *J Neurosci*, *23*(12), 5123–5130.

Sun, G., Yu, R. T., et al. (2007). Orphan nuclear receptor TLX recruits histone deacetylases to repress transcription and regulate neural stem cell proliferation. *Proc Natl Acad Sci USA*, *104*(39), 15282–15287.

Swistowski, A., Peng, J., et al. (2010). Efficient generation of functional dopaminergic neurons from human-induced pluripotent stem cells under defined conditions. *Stem Cells*.

Takahashi, K. (2010). Direct reprogramming 101. *Dev Growth Differ*, *52*(3), 319–333.

Takahashi, K., Tanabe, K., et al. (2007). Induction of pluripotent stem cells from adult human fibroblasts by defined factors. *Cell*, *131*(5), 861–872.

Takahashi, K. & Yamanaka, S. (2006). Induction of pluripotent stem cells from mouse embryonic and adult fibroblast cultures by defined factors. *Cell*, *126*(4), 663–676.

Takanaga, H., Tsuchida-Straeten, N., et al. (2009). Gli2 is a novel regulator of sox2 expression in telencephalic neuroepithelial cells. *Stem Cells*, *27*(1), 165–174.

Tramontin, A. D., Garcia-Verdugo, J. M., et al. (2003). Postnatal development of radial glia and the ventricular zone (VZ): A continuum of the neural stem cell compartment. *Cereb Cortex*, *13*(6), 580–587.

Tran, P. B., Banisadr, G., et al. (2007). Chemokine receptor expression by neural progenitor cells in neurogenic regions of mouse brain. *J Comp Neurol*, *500*(6), 1007–1033.

Tsang, M. & Dawid, I. B. (2004). Promotion and attenuation of FGF signaling through the Ras-MAPK pathway. *Sci STKE*, *2004*(228), pe17.

Vicente-Manzanares, M., Rey, M., et al. (1999). Involvement of phosphatidylinositol 3-kinase in stromal cell-derived factor-1 alpha-induced lymphocyte polarization and chemotaxis. *J Immunol*, *163*(7), 4001–4012.

Vieira, C., Pombero, A., et al. (2010). Molecular mechanisms controlling brain development: An overview of neuroepithelial secondary organizers. *Int J Dev Biol*, *54*(1), 7–20.

Warner-Schmidt, J. L. & Duman, R. S. (2006). Hippocampal neurogenesis: Opposing effects of stress and antidepressant treatment. *Hippocampus*, *16*(3), 239–249.

Weber, A., Wasiliew, P., et al. (2010). Interleukin-1 (IL-1) pathway. *Sci Signal*, *3*(105), cm1.

Wernig, M., Meissner, A., et al. (2007). In vitro reprogramming of fibroblasts into a pluripotent ES-cell-like state. *Nature*, *448*(7151), 318–324.

Wu, Y. & Yoder, A. (2009). Chemokine coreceptor signaling in HIV-1 infection and pathogenesis. *PLoS Pathog*, *5*(12), e1000520.

Yoshimura, S., Takagi, Y., et al. (2001). FGF-2 regulation of neurogenesis in adult hippocampus after brain injury. *Proc Natl Acad Sci USA*, *98*(10), 5874–5879.

Youn, B. S., Mantel, C., et al. (2000). Chemokines, chemokine receptors and hematopoiesis. *Immunol Rev*, *177*, 150–174.

Yu, J., Vodyanik, M. A., et al. (2007). Induced pluripotent stem cell lines derived from human somatic cells. *Science*, *318*(5858), 1917–1920.

Zhang, C. L., Zou, Y., et al. (2008). A role for adult TLX-positive neural stem cells in learning and behaviour. *Nature*, *451*(7181), 1004–1007.

Zhang, S. C., Wernig, M., et al. (2001). In vitro differentiation of transplantable neural precursors from human embryonic stem cells. *Nat Biotechnol*, *19*(12), 1129–1133.

Zhang, X. Q. & Zhang, S. C. (2010). Differentiation of neural precursors and dopaminergic neurons from human embryonic stem cells. *Methods Mol Biol*, *584*, 355–366.

Zheng, J., Thylin, M., et al. (1999). Intracellular CXCR4 signaling, neuronal apoptosis and neuropathogenic mechanisms of HIV-1-associated dementia. *J Neuroimmunol*, *98*(2), 185–200.

Zhong, W. & Chia, W. (2008). Neurogenesis and asymmetric cell division. *Curr Opin Neurobiol*, *18*(1), 4–11.

Zhu, Y., Yu, T., et al. (2002). Role of the chemokine SDF-1 as the meningeal attractant for embryonic cerebellar neurons. *Nat Neurosci*, *5*(8), 719–720.

Zou, Y. R., Kottmann, A. H., et al. (1998). Function of the chemokine receptor CXCR4 in haematopoiesis and in cerebellar development. *Nature*, *393*, 595–599.

SECTION 3

BLOOD-BRAIN BARRIER AND HIV CNS ENTRY

Howard S. Fox

3.1

BLOOD-BRAIN BARRIER

STRUCTURE AND FUNCTION

William A. Banks

The blood-brain barrier (BBB) consists of several relatively distinct barriers, operating in parallel to one another in different anatomical regions. These barriers restrict and regulate the passage of materials between the peripheral and cerebrospinal compartments. The best studied and most important of the barriers are the vascular barrier and the choroid plexus. Barrier function arises through mechanisms associated primarily with endothelial cells (tight junctions, infrequent fenestrations, reduced pinocytosis) but also involve the capillary basement membrane, pericytes, and astrocytes. BBB function responds dynamically to the needs of the central nervous system (CNS) and for this reason the BBB is sometimes thought of as a "slave" of the CNS. The BBB communicates with microglia, neurons, and other cells, and it responds to a wide range of soluble factors released by these cells. Multiple transport processes, both passive and active, carry materials into and out of (efflux) the cerebrospinal fluid. Efflux mechanisms help explain why some drugs fail to reach therapeutic concentrations in the CNS; and inter-individual variations in efflux mechanisms can explain why some people are more sensitive or less sensitive to the therapeutic effects or side effects of particular CNS medications. Immune cells, once thought to be excluded from the CNS except under conditions of brain infection, are now recognized to patrol the normal CNS; and a major type of brain cell, the microglia, is derived from peripheral macrophages and may exist in some (as-yet poorly defined) equilibrium with the peripheral macrophage pool. This chapter presents these varied aspects of BBB structure and function in some detail, then builds on that fundamental understanding to discuss the BBB's role in neuroimmune interactions in both health and disease, including in HIV-1 disease.

DEVELOPMENT AND STRUCTURE OF THE BLOOD-BRAIN BARRIER

Evidence for a barrier between the circulation and the central nervous system (CNS) dates back to the end of the 19th century (Bradbury, 1979). The best known of those early studies was done by a young Paul Erlich, who found that some dyes did not stain the brain after their peripheral injection. Erlich concluded erroneously that the lack of staining was because these dyes did not bind to brain tissue. Several decades later, Goldmann, a student of Erlich's, found

that these dyes could stain the brain when injected directly into the brain. Thus, these dye studies were reinterpreted as evidence in favor of some sort of barrier between the CNS and blood.

The location and nature of that barrier was controversial through much of the 20th century. Elegant studies by Davson and colleagues identified the barrier at the vascular level. However, alternative opinions were held until Reese and coworkers conducted classic studies with the electron microscope in the late 1960s (Reese & Karnovsky, 1967; Brightman & Reese, 1969). Previous work had shown no difference between vascular beds of peripheral tissues and the CNS when studied grossly or at the light microscope level. However, Reese and coworkers found numerous ultrastructural differences. These included a much reduced rate of pinocytosis and an absence of intracellular fenestrations. Currently, the most widely discussed finding is the presence of tight junctions between adjacent endothelial cells. The tight junctions, low rate of pinocytosis, and low number of intracellular fenestrations effectively eliminate intercellular and intracellular gaps and pores. This, in turn, essentially eliminates the production of a plasma-derived ultrafiltrate and hence the leakage of serum proteins into the brain.

From this single change of the lack of a production of an ultrafiltrate evolves a large number of consequences for CNS function. Obviously, it is the basis of the restriction of protein access which first defined the BBB in the late 19th century. The need for an efficient lymphatic system is eliminated, but the lack of a lymphatic system means that the CNS needs other methods to rid itself of the free water and wastes produced by metabolism and the secretions of the choroid plexus. Without production of an ultrafiltrate, the CNS depends on other mechanisms to extract nourishment from the blood. The BBB addresses this need with a large number of selective transporters for substances from glucose to electrolytes to regulatory proteins (Davson & Segal, 1996a; 1996b). Because the CNS is not equipped to handle an ultrafiltrate, its reintroduction, as with hypertensive crisis, can result in increased intracranial pressure and encephalopathy (Al-Sarraf & Phillip, 2003; Johansson, 1989; Mayhan & Heistad, 1985). This yin and yang of the BBB, a near absolute elimination of nonspecific leakage counterpointed to highly selective transporters addressing the specific needs of the CNS, complemented by other features means that the BBB functions more as a regulatory interface between the blood and brain than as just a barrier.

COMPONENTS OF THE BLOOD-BRAIN BARRIER

The BBB is not a single barrier, but several barriers which are in parallel. This contrasts with the testis-blood barrier, which consists of several barriers in series (Holash, Harik, Perry, & Stewart, 1993; Neaves, 1977). The most studied of these barriers are the vascular barrier and the choroid plexus. Often, the terms BBB and blood-cerebrospinal fluid (CSF) barrier are used to refer specifically to the vascular barrier and the barrier formed at the choroid plexus, respectively. Less studied barriers are the barriers formed by tanycytes at the circumventricular organs (CVO) and other specialized neural barriers, such as the blood-retinal barrier (Neuwelt et al., 2008).

Vascular Blood-Brain Barrier

The vascular BBB occurs because of the modifications noted by Reese and co-workers in the endothelial cells which comprise the capillary bed and line the venules and arterioles of the CNS. It is likely that these three regions are highly specialized. For example, immune cells primarily cross at the venules, whereas many of the classic transporters are located at the capillaries (Engelhardt & Wolburg, 2004). No CNS cell is more than about 40 microns from a capillary. This means that a substance which can cross the vascular BBB can immediately access the entire CNS. Substances which cross the vascular BBB can be either flow-dependent or not dependent on flow rate. A flow-dependent substance is one in which the BBB extracts from the blood nearly the maximal amount possible (Kety, 1987). The only way to increase the amount of the substance entering the brain is to increase the flow rate to the brain. Glucose is an example of a flow-dependent substance (Rapoport, Ohata, & London, 1981). A brain region which is particularly active has its increased demand for glucose met by an increase in regional blood flow. In contrast, transport of many regulatory substances, such as the cytokine tumor necrosis factor (TNF), is not flow dependent. Only a small percentage of the TNF in blood is extracted by brain via the saturable BBB transporter for TNF (Gutierrez, Banks, & Kastin, 1993). As a result, alterations of blood flow within physiological limits do not alter the uptake of TNF from blood by brain. However, extreme changes in the rate of blood flow or capillary tortuosity can result in rheological changes, such as the loss of laminar flow. Such alterations likely occur in stroke, AIDS, and Alzheimer's disease (de la Torre & Mussivand, 1993; Nelson, Masters, Zagzag, & Kelly, 1999). This may result in impaired permeation of both flow-dependent and flow-independent substances.

The vascular BBB has regional variations in terms of function and susceptibilities to disease. Huber et al. noted that some regions of the brain suffer larger and earlier disruptions to their barriers during diabetes mellitus than others (Huber, VanGilder, & Houser, 2006; Huber, 2008). Many peptides and regulatory substances have unique regional variations in their transport rates across the BBB (Banks & Kastin, 1998; Banks, Kastin, Huang, Jaspan, & Maness, 1996). It is assumed that these reflect on brain functions and needs. For example, the brain region with the highest rate of transport of leptin is the region of the arcuate nucleus, an area important in leptin-mediated control of feeding (Banks et al., 1996; Schwartz, Woods, Porte, Seeley, & Baskin, 2000).

Choroid Plexus

The choroid plexus are bags composed of epithelial cells which project into the ventricles and contain a capillary plexus (Johanson, 1988). The capillaries do not have barrier function and so produce an ultrafiltrate which fills the bag. The epithelial cells have tight junctions and so possess barrier function, thus preventing the ultrafiltrate from entering the ventricular space. Unlike the capillaries, the epithelial cells of the choroid plexus have a high rate of vesicular turnover which is responsible for the production of the CSF. However, the CSF is not an ultrafiltrate, but a secretion. The choroid plexus also has many selective transport systems, some of which are specific to it or are enriched in comparison to the vascular BBB.

Barriers at Circumventricular Organs

The CNS of mammals contains seven regions of the brain where the vasculature does not fully participate in a BBB (Gross & Weindl, 1987). These regions have at least one side which interfaces with a ventricle and so are termed circumventricular organs (CVOs). Together, they comprise about 0.5% of the brain by weight. Their capillaries allow the production of an ultrafiltrate and so their cells are in more intimate contact with the circulation. They are known to play vital roles as sensing organs for critical peripheral events; for example, they act as emetic centers and are important in blood pressure modulation (Johnson & Gross, 1993; Ferguson, 1991). They can relay their signals to the rest of the brain by neurons which project from them to distant brain regions or project to them from other brain regions. However, the mixing of their interstitial fluids with that of adjacent brain tissue or CSF has been shown to be limited in most studies (Peruzzo et al., 2000; Plotkin, Banks, & Kastin, 1996; Rethelyi, 1984). Diffusion through brain tissue is poor and this alone would tend to produce a limit to mixing within a few hundred microns of the CVO (Cserr & Berman, 1978; de Lange et al., 1995). However, the major factor preventing leakage of substances from the CVO into the adjacent CSF and brain tissue is a physical barrier to diffusion. The epithelial cells which line the ventricles form tight junctions when they are over CVOs, thus limiting CVO-to-CSF diffusion. A functional barrier formed by bands of tanycytes prevents the diffusion of substances from the CVO to the adjacent brain region (Peruzzo et al., 2000; Plotkin et al., 1996; Rethelyi, 1984). A recent review by Rodriguez et al. (2010) has explored the various aspects of the CVO barriers.

Other Specialized Neural Barriers

These barriers include the blood-retinal barrier, blood-spinal cord barrier, and blood-nerve barriers (for a more extensive list see Neuwelt et al., 2008). These barriers generally include tight junctions participating in a vascular barrier (the choroid plexus being an exception), but exhibit varying degrees of leakiness. They can also vary markedly in transporter activity from the vascular BBB both during health and in response to disease (Pan & Kastin, 2008; Pan, Zhang, Liao, Csernus, & Kastin, 2003a; Prockop, Naidu, Binard, & Ransohoff, 1996).

PERINATAL DEVELOPMENT AND SPECIAL CHARACTERISTICS OF THE NEONATAL BLOOD-BRAIN BARRIER

The idea that the rodent perinatal BBB is not developed has been extensively revised over the last few decades (Davson & Segal, 1996c). In retrospect, the idea that the neonatal BBB was immature arose because in an early study in which so much dye was administered to neonates that the binding capacity of albumin was saturated. This resulted in unbound dye in the circulation, which readily crosses the BBB. Subsequent dye, ultrastructure, and pharmacokinetic studies all agree that the perinatal BBB is intact to serum proteins (Dobbing, 1968; Dziegielewska et al., 1988; Moos & Mollgard, 1993; Vorbrodt & Dobrogowska, 1994). As reviewed elsewhere (Urayama, Grubb, Sly, & Banks, 2004), work by several other laboratories has shown that the vascular space is smaller per g of brain in the neonate and some evidence suggests that the barrier may be more leaky to much smaller molecules such as sucrose.

Many of the differences in the BBB of developing and adult animals which were ascribed to an immature brain are now known to be adaptations to the altered demands of the CNS. For example, some amino acids enter the CNS of neonates more rapidly than the CNS of adults not because the BBB is leaky, but because the BBB amino acid transporter is altered to favor their transport. The BBB is slave to the CNS and so the reason the BBB transports them more avidly is because they are in greater demand by a developing CNS. Most of these adaptations involve the transporter mechanisms. In comparison, non-saturable passage is not altered with development (Cornford, Braun, Oldendorf, & Hill, 1982).

This theme of the BBB adjusting its transporter capabilities to serve the CNS is repeated throughout development, probably also with aging, and even in disease conditions. One of the most dramatic examples is the developmental loss of the mannose 6-phosphate receptor, which transports the enzyme ß-glucuronidase across the BBB. Transport function is very robust in neonates but is absent in adult animals (Urayama et al., 2004). Transgenic mice which do not produce ß-glucuronidase develop a muccopolysachharidosis which recapitulates Sly's disease (a heritable mucopolysaccharide storage disorder; Sands et al., 1994). Because of the developmental differences in the BBB expression of the mannose 6-phosphate receptor, the brain disease of neonates but not of adults responds to the peripheral administration of glucuronidase (Vogler et al., 1999). Interestingly, this transporter can be induced in the adult BBB by administration of epinephrine (Urayama, Grubb, Banks, & Sly, 2007).

There are other aspects of barrier function which also change with development. The tanycytic barrier between the median eminence and the arcuate nucleus develops after birth in the rodent (Peruzzo et al., 2000). This means the arcuate nucleus is very vulnerable to circulating neurotoxins during the neonatal period. For example, monosodium glutamate destroys the arcuate nucleus with resulting obesity when given intravenously to a neonate, but not an adult. The epithelial cells which line the ventricles of the brain have tight junctions even over non-CVO sites in neonates, but not adults. Thus, neonates have a CSF-brain barrier which limits the diffusion of substances between brain tissue and CSF and so this arm of the BBB system is less leaky in the neonate than in the adult.

CONCEPT OF THE NEUROVASCULAR UNIT AND COMPARISON TO PERIPHERAL VASCULAR BEDS

The endothelial cell is the anatomical site of vascular barrier function and of most of the saturable transporters (Figure 3.1.1). Capillary beds from peripheral tissues have numerous intracellular and intercellular pores and fenestrations and high rates of pinocytosis that account for their leakiness. The brain endothelial cell engages in comparatively little pinocytosis, has few intracellular pores or fenestrations, and intercellular pores or gaps are eliminated because of tight junctions.

However, the brain endothelial cell does not function in isolation. The abluminal (brain side) of the capillary is encased in a basement membrane 40–80 nm thick. This membrane does not act as a barrier to molecules but may restrict viral-sized particles (Muldoon et al., 1999). It also holds pericytes in close approximation to the endothelial cell (Balabanov & Dore-Duffy, 1998). The pericyte is a pluripotent cell and a modulator of BBB function (Deli, Abraham, Kataoka, & Niwa, 2005; Dore-Duffy, 2008; Dore-Duffy, Katychev, Wang, & Van Buren, 2006). Astrocytes project end-feet, which surround the capillary in what looks at the ultrastructural level like a mesh or netting (Abbott, Ronnback, & Hansson, 2006). Astrocytes secrete substances which tend to encourage tight junction formation. All three of these cell types (pericytes, astrocytes, and endothelial cells) secrete a variety of substances, including cytokines, into their local environment (Fabry et al., 1993). Pericytes and astrocytes play interrelated but distinct roles in BBB function. For example, pericytes are the primary protectors of the blood-retinal and blood-brain barriers during glycemic stress (Romeo, Liu, Asnaghi, Kern, & Lorenzi, 2002; Nakaoke, Verma, Niwa, Dohgu, & Banks, 2007).

This greater BBB complex is in further communication with other cell types in the CNS, most notably pericytes, microglia, and neurons. The microglia may, in turn, be at equilibrium with circulating macrophages (Williams & Hickey 1995). Other immune cells also enter and exit the CNS at unknown rates and frequencies as influenced by yet to be determined factors. Clearly, secretions of prostaglandins,

The Brain Endothelial Cell

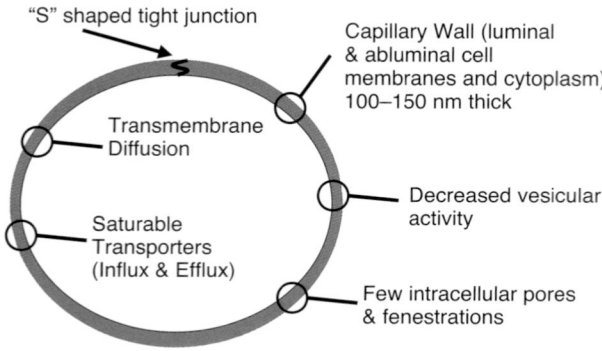

"S" shaped tight junction

Transmembrane Diffusion

Saturable Transporters (Influx & Efflux)

Capillary Wall (luminal & abluminal cell membranes and cytoplasm) 100–150 nm thick

Decreased vesicular activity

Few intracellular pores & fenestrations

A BBB Complex

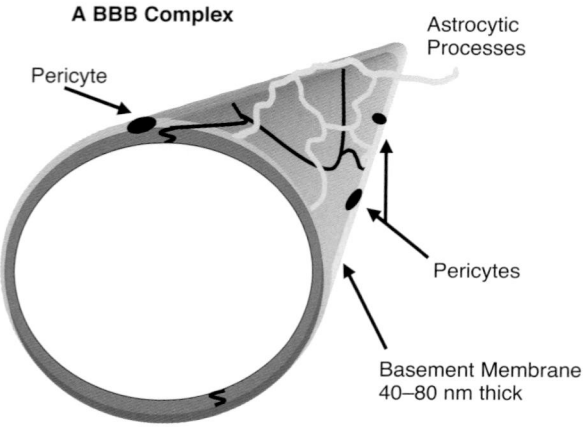

Pericyte

Astrocytic Processes

Pericytes

Basement Membrane 40–80 nm thick

The Neurovascular Unit

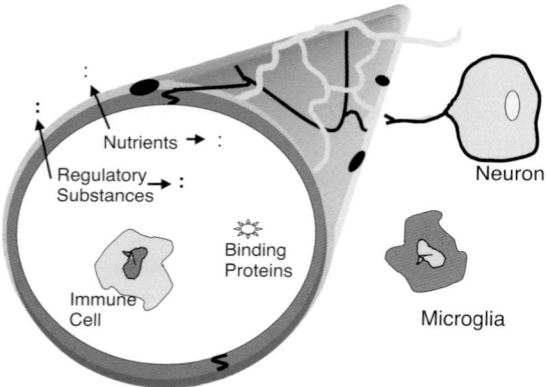

Nutrients →

Regulatory Substances

Binding Proteins

Immune Cell

Neuron

Microglia

Figure 3.1.1. *The Vascular Blood-Brain Barrier: Three Levels of Complexity.* The upper panel illustrates the brain endothelial cell. This is the functional and anatomical site of both barrier function and of saturable and non-saturable mechanisms of passage. The major modifications allowing both barrier function and selective penetration of substances are indicated. The middle panel illustrates other cell types and structures important in BBB function. Pericytes are embedded in a basement membrane and astrocytes form a net-like structure over the capillary bed. Both cell types are in paracellular communication with the brain endothelial cells. The lower panel illustrates the neurovascular unit, a concept which emphasizes integration of peripheral, BBB, and central interactions.

nitric oxide, and cytokines from each of these cells are important for intercellular communication and can influence endothelial cell permeability (Chao et al., 1994; Nath et al., 1999; Shafer & Murphy, 1997).

The concept of the neurovascular unit (NVU) emphasizes the interactive role that cells and events within the CNS and in the circulation play on BBB permeability, as well as the role that the consequences of BBB permeability play on them. The concept of the NVU includes other factors long known to influence the penetration of substances across the BBB, such as degradation, sequestration, and serum protein binding. The encompassing concept of the NVU is particularly useful when considering the next section, the mechanisms of transport across the BBB.

MECHANISMS OF TRANSPORT ACROSS THE BLOOD-BRAIN BARRIER

Substances can enter or exit the CNS by a variety of mechanisms. Some of these mechanisms are operational in both the blood-to-brain (influx) and the brain-to-blood (efflux) directions, whereas others are unidirectional.

BLOOD TO CENTRAL NERVOUS SYSTEM

Saturable and nonsaturable modes predominate influx. Within each of these categories are a diverse number of mechanisms. These different mechanisms tend to favor certain groups or types of substances.

Nonsaturable Passage

The hallmark of nonsaturable passage is that the percent of material crossing into the CNS is not affected by the amount of material available for transport. The two main mechanisms of nonsaturable passage are transmembrane diffusion and the extracellular pathways. The former is much better studied and its principles have been widely applied by industry for the development of CNS drugs; the latter has received much less attention.

Transmembrane Diffusion

The most studied nonsaturable mechanism by which small molecules cross the BBB is by membrane or transmembrane diffusion (Rapoport, 1976). The major determinant of passage is the degree to which the substance is lipid soluble. A substance which is too lipid soluble will be unable to repartition into the brain's interstitial fluid and so become trapped in the cell membranes of the BBB. A ratio of about 10:1 in favor of lipid versus aqueous solubility is near ideal for maximal passage across the BBB. The second most important determinant is molecular weight with passage being favored for smaller molecules. Other physicochemical determinants, such as charge, can occasionally become dominant for specific compounds. Work by Lipinksi in Caco-2 cells, an immortalized cell line derived from a gastrointestinal cancer, clearly shows that smaller, less charged, more lipid soluble drugs are favored in transmembrane diffusion (Lipinski, Lombardo,

Dominy, & Feeney, 1997). Many exogenous substances, including many drugs with CNS activity, enter the brain predominantly by way of transmembrane diffusion. Morphine and ethanol are prime examples of common substances which cross the BBB by this mechanism (Oldendorf, 1974).

Although a higher molecular weight impedes transmembrane diffusion at the BBB, there seems to be no absolute molecular weight (MW) cut-off. A previous study which had thought to define such an absolute limit had discovered, in retrospect, early evidence for an efflux system (Levin, 1980). The largest substance to date noted to have a measurable uptake by brain by way of transmembrane diffusion is cytokine-induced neutrophil chemoattractant-1 (CINC1), with a MW of about 7.8 kDa (Pan & Kastin, 2001a). A surprisingly large number of small, lipid-soluble compounds cross the BBB at a rate which is considerably greater or lesser than that predicted by their physicochemical characteristics (Oldendorf, 1971; 1974). Binding to serum proteins and efflux systems are the major factors which decrease influx and the presence of a saturable transporter is the major factor which increases influx.

Extracellular Pathways

Albumin derived from serum is present in small amounts in the CSF, showing that the BBB is not absolute. The amount of protein in CSF, however, is very small, being about 0.5%, or 1/200th, of that in plasma. The CSF is not an ultrafiltrate, but a secreted fluid. This means that the relative and absolute concentrations of proteins, electrolytes, minerals, and other substances can differ tremendously to that of plasma. The extracelluar pathways are another avenue by which substances can enter the CNS (Balin, Broadwell, Salcman, & el-Kalliny, 1986; Broadwell & Sofroniew, 1993). These represent what have sometimes been termed "functional leaks" at discreet areas of the brain, including the large vessels of the pial surface and subarachnoid space, the circumventricular organs, the nasal epithelium, the sensory ganglia of spinal and cranial nerves, and some deep brain regions such as possibly the nucleus tractus solitarius (Broadwell & Banks, 1993).

The amount of a substance which can enter the brain by the extracellular pathways is small. However, this route may be therapeutically relevant for compounds which have favorable peripheral pharmacokinetics, such as a long serum half-life and a small volume of distribution (Banks, 2004). Antibodies, erythropoietin, and enzymes can access the brain by way of the extracellular pathways (Banks, Jumbe, Farrell, Niehoff, & Heatherington, 2004a; Lyle, Kincaid, Bryant, Prince, & MeGehee, 2001; Banks, Pagliari, Nakaoke, & Morley, 2005a; Kozlowski, Sterzl, & Nilaver, 1992; Banks et al., 2007) and this may underlie their therapeutic benefits when given in high doses (Alafaci et al., 2000; Ehrenreich et al., 2002; Erbyraktar et al., 2003; Morgan et al., 2000; Janus et al., 2000; DeMattos, Bales, Cummins, Paul, & Holtzman, 2002; Farr et al., 2003; Hock et al., 2003).

Receptor-Mediated and Other Saturable Transporters

Saturable processes represent a diverse group of mechanisms. Included in this group for purposes of discussion are two processes which share some characteristics with the saturable systems: diapedesis and adsorptive endocytosis/transcytosis.

Active Transport versus Facilitated Diffusion

Saturable transporters (Yeagle, 1987) can be divided into those which require energy (active transport) and those which do not (facilitated diffusion). Both are dependent on a protein which acts as the transporter, may have co-factors, and be modulated by physiologic and disease processes. Energy requiring systems can be unidirectional; that is, they may have only an influx or efflux component. Non-energy requiring saturable transport (facilitated diffusion) is bidirectional; that is, it transports substances in both directions with net flux being from the side of higher concentration to the side of lower concentration.

Most known saturable transporters at the BBB are facilitated diffusion systems (Kaur, Jaswal, Nagpaul, & Mahmood, 1992). For example, GLUT-1, the transporter for glucose, is a facilitated diffusion transporter. If the level of glucose is artificially raised above that of serum (or if radioactive glucose is introduced into the CNS, but not the serum), efflux of glucose can be shown.

Transcytotic versus Transmembrane Transport

Saturable transporters can also be categorized based on whether they use pores/channels or vesicles to transport their ligands across the BBB. In the pore system, the molecule crosses from one side of the cell membrane to the other by passing through a cavity in the transporter protein. The substance is thus transported either into or out of the cytoplasm of the BBB cell; a second set of transporters on the opposing cell membrane completes the transfer across the BBB or the substance can rely on transmembrane diffusion. With vesicular transport, the transported substance adheres to a binding site, usually a glycoprotein. Invagination then produces a vesicle that is then routed to the opposite membrane, and the contents of the vesicle are released from the cell surface. A specificity of transport distinguishes these vesicles from the macropinocytosis whose reduction is a defining characteristic of the BBB (Reese & Karnovsky, 1967).

Most small molecules, such as glucose, electrolytes, and amino acids, use pores or channels. Pore systems may be either active or facilitated diffusion systems. Vesicular transporters, however, are energy requiring and so are characterized by unidirectional transport. The best described class of these vesicular dependent systems is receptor-mediated transcytosis and is characterized by clathrin and transglutaminase dependence (Davies et al., 1980). However, non-clathrin-dependent vesicles, such as podocytes, are also likely active at the BBB.

It is reasonable to assume that very large molecules would be required to use vesicles rather than pores and channels to cross, but the molecular weight at which vesicles would be requisite is not known. It has been proposed that interleukin-2 (IL-2) is transported (Drach et al., 1996) by p-glycoprotein (P-gp). As P-gp is a pore system (Begley, 2004), IL-2 would be the largest substance currently known to be transported by a pore system. Peptides much smaller than IL-2 are known to cross by vesicular dependent pathways (Shimura, Tabata,

Ohnishi, Terasaki, & Tsuji, 1991; Terasaki et al., 1992). It is clear, then, that the size of the ligand alone does not dictate the need for vesicular transport.

Diapedesis of Immune Cells

A major shift in thinking about the relation of immune cells to the CNS and BBB has occurred over the last few decades. The CNS was once viewed as separate from the immune system and sterile in terms of immune cell occupancy except under conditions of brain infection. It is now clear that immune cells patrol the normal CNS, although the rate at which they enter and exit is not known. A major type of brain cell, the microglia, are known to be derived from peripheral macrophages, although the extent to which the pools of peripheral macrophages and microglia mix in the normal postnatal condition is unknown.

Adsorptive Endo- and Trans- cytosis

Adsorptive endocytosis occurs when a glycoprotein on the brain's endothelial surface binds another glycoprotein in lectin-like fashion (Broadwell, Balin, & Salcman, 1988; Broadwell, 1989). This second glycoprotein (the ligand) may be free or attached to the surface of a virus or immune cell (Mellman, Fuchs, & Helenius, 1986). The binding can initiate endocytosis with the subsequent vesicle having several potential fates (Banks & Broadwell 1994). In some cases, the vesicle is routed to lysosomes, the glycoprotein destroyed, and the vesicle rerouted to the endothelial cell surface for discharge of contents. In other cases, the vesicle can be routed to the Golgi complex and endoplasmic reticulum. In still other cases, the vesicle can be discharged at the endothelial cell surface opposite to that of uptake. In this case, the vesicle has crossed the width of the endothelial cell, and hence crossed the BBB, in a transcytotic event. What determines the fate and trafficking routes of these vesicles is largely unknown, but at least some vesicles can engage in more than one fate (Broadwell, 1993). It may be that binding of a large amount of glycoprotein to the endothelial cell can overwhelm the lysosomal pathway and result in the vesicles being routed to the trancytotic or Golgi complex pathways.

Several principles of adsorptive endocytosis and transcytosis are clear. Many of the glycoprotein ligands are toxic and endocytosis may represent a mechanism to rejuvenate or repair the membrane (Raub & Audus, 1990; Vorbrodt & Trowbridge, 1991; Westergren & Johansson, 1993). Many viruses co-opt adsorptive endocytosis mechanisms to invade and infect brain endothelial cells and adsorptive transcytosis to invade the brain (Marsh, 1984; Chou & Dix, 1989; Schweighardt & Atwood, 2001). These processes may also be related to diapedesis as many of the events of immune cell passage across the BBB resemble these endocytic mechanisms. For example, both LFA-1 and ICAM, important to immune cell passage across the BBB, are glycoproteins. Although adsorptive endocytosis is in some sense saturable because of a finite amount of any single glycoprotein on a cell surface, it is not easy to demonstrate classical saturable kinetics for this process. In fact, excess glycoprotein can sometimes further stimulate endocytosis and so lead to a paradoxical increase,

rather than decrease, in the rate of passage across the BBB (Banks, Kastin, & Akerstrom, 1997). Glycoprotein distribution on brain endothelial cells is polarized; that is, a glycoprotein may be enriched on either the luminal or abluminal membrane (Vorbrodt, 1994; Zambenedetti, Giordano, & Zatta, 1996). The tight junctions act as a "fence" to keep the glycoproteins confined to their respective sides of the endothelial cell (Deli et al., 2005). This means that the movement of a glycoprotein molecule (or a virus whose coat displays that glycoprotein) can be unidirectional as its transcytosis can only be initiated from the side of the brain endothelial cell that contains the ligand's complementary glycoprotein (Villegas & Broadwell, 1993; Broadwell, 1989). The possession and distribution of glycoproteins similarly dictate which viruses can invade the brain; neurovirulent viruses which invade the brain as free virus (as opposed to entering in Trojan horse fashion inside an infected immune cell) can do so because they possess a glycoprotein ligand capable of binding to the BBB.

CENTRAL NERVOUS SYSTEM TO BLOOD

Traditionally, passage in the brain-to-blood direction (efflux) has been neglected. However, efflux often accounts for the inability of otherwise effective drugs to accumulate in the CNS. Pharmacogenomic studies have suggested that the individual variation in efflux mechanisms may explain why some individuals are less sensitive to the CNS effects of drugs or more sensitive to their toxicities (Löscher & Potschka, 2002; Fellay et al., 2002). Efflux mechanisms are important to the homeostasis of the CNS, ridding the brain of toxins (Taylor, 2002). The rate of efflux can be, in addition to synthesis and degradation, an important determinant of the level of a substance produced within the CNS (Chen, Castro, Chow, & Reichlin, 1997; Chen & Reichlin, 1998; Maness, Kastin, Farrell, & Banks, 1998).

Nonsaturable

Efflux, like influx, has both saturable and non-saturable mechanisms of entry. Transmembrane diffusion occurs for both influx and efflux. Other mechanisms, such as bulk flow, are unique for efflux.

Transmembrane Diffusion

Many of the principles that govern influx by transmembrane diffusion are also important in efflux. The dramatic role that efflux by transmembrane diffusion can play can be illustrated by comparing the fate of small, lipid-soluble molecules to that of a protein after intrathecal administration. Intrathecal application of small, lipid-soluble molecules, such as anesthetics, can have a local effect on spinal cord function but have little or no effect on the brain (Bernards, 1999). These substances readily cross the brain endothelial cell by transmembrane diffusion and do this as easily in the brain-to-blood direction as in the blood-to-brain direction. Therefore, they are cleared from the CSF before they are able to reach the brain (McQuay, Sullivan, Smallman, & Dickenson, 1989).

In contrast, proteins such as leptin are too large and water soluble to undergo much transmembrane diffusion (LeBel, 1999; McCarthy et al., 2002). Leptin can reach the brain after intrathecal administration in amounts sufficient to produce effects on feeding through the hypothalamus (McCarthy et al., 2002; Shyng, Huber, & Harris, 1993).

Efflux by transmembrane diffusion can also contribute to the poor diffusion of substances within brain parenchyma. Diffusion within the interstitial space of the brain is dependent on Brownian motion and the production of metabolic free water as driving forces and so is very slow (Cserr, 1984; Cserr & Berman, 1978). However, efflux by non-saturable (and saturable) mechanisms can further reduce the distance a substance will ultimately diffuse. For example, the less lipid-soluble drug atenolol can diffuse about three times further into brain tissue than can the more lipid-soluble drug acetaminophen (de Lange et al., 1993).

Bulk Flow and Cerebrospinal Fluid Lymphatic Drainage

Bulk flow refers to the reabsoption of CSF into the blood at the arachnoid villi (Davson & Segal, 1996d). Any substance dissolved in CSF will enter the blood by this mechanism (Jones & Robinson, 1982; Pollay & Davson, 1963). In some cases, the levels of a substance in blood achieved after injection into the CSF can be sustained longer and at higher levels than after an intravenous bolus (Maness et al., 1998; Chen & Reichlin, 1998; Chen et al., 1997). This is because the central injection acts similarly to an intravenous infusion, slowly delivering drug to the blood. CSF drains from the brain at the level of the cribriform plate into the cervical lymphatic system (Widner et al., 1987; Yamada, DePasquale, Patlak, & Cserr, 1991). This may be the dominant route for CSF drainage at normal CSF pressures (Boulton et al., 1999). This can provide a direct route from the CNS to the cervical lymphatics (Oehmichen, Gruninger, Wietholter, & Gencic, 1979), as has been illustrated for gp120, the glycoprotein of the human immunodeficiency virus, HIV-1 (Cashion, Banks, Bost, & Kastin, 1999). This route to the lymphatics may explain why substances injected into the brain can produce a different immune response than when the substance is injected peripherally (Cserr & Knopf, 1992; Knopf, Cserr, Nolan, Wu, & Harling-Berg, 1995).

Saturable Transport

The last decade has seen a huge increase in the interest of efflux by saturable mechanisms. Just as efflux by transmembrane diffusion can limit diffusion of a substance within the CNS, so can the presence of a saturable efflux transporter (Blasberg, 1977). Much of this interest centers on the multidrug efflux transport systems (Begley, 2004), most notably p-glycoprotein (P-gp). However, other efflux transporters for peptides, proteins, endogenous substances, and drugs are known to play important roles in physiology and disease (Drion, Lemaire, Lefauconnier, & Scherrmann, 1996; Martins, Banks, & Kastin, 1997; Mealey, Bentjen, Gay, & Cantor, 2001). For example, peptide transport system-1 is a major regulator of brain levels of methionine enkephalin, an endogenous

opiate which suppresses voluntary ethanol drinking (Plotkin, Banks, & Kastin, 1998). Depression and recovery of peptide transport systems-1 with ethanol drinking may relate to alcohol withdrawal seizures (Banks & Kastin, 1994; 1989). IL-2 is currently the only cytokine known to be transported by a saturable efflux system; some have postulated this transporter may be P-gp. Poor accumulation of protease inhibitors, antibiotics, AZT, anti-cancer drugs, and many other substances occurs because of efflux systems (Fellay et al., 2002; Glynn & Yazdanian, 1998; King, Su, Chang, Zuckerman, & Pasternak, 2001; Lee et al., 1998; Löscher & Potschka, 2002; Masereeuw, Jaehde, Langemeijer, De Boer, & Breimer, 1994; Spector & Lorenzo, 1974). Impaired efflux of amyloid ß protein, the protein believed to cause Alzheimer's disease, develops with aging in mice which overexpress amyloid precursor protein, thus promoting further accumulation of amyloid ß protein within the brain (Ghersi-Egea et al., 1996; Banks, Robinson, Verma, & Morley, 2003; Deane et al., 2004). Evidence suggests that impaired transport develops in humans as well and so may be a major mechanism for induction of Alzheimer's disease (Tanzi, Moir, & Wagner, 2004; Shibata et al., 2000).

NEUROIMMUNE INTERACTIONS

The above discussion of BBB fundamentals is tailored towards understanding the role of the BBB in neuroimmune interactions. Below are specific examples of how the BBB is involved in neuroimmune interactions.

RECEPTORS THAT ARE EXPRESSED ON THE BLOOD-BRAIN BARRIER FOR RECEPTOR:LIGAND INTERACTIONS

An important distinction for understanding the function of the BBB is that of receptors versus transporters. The term "receptor" has undergone a transformation of its usage since its introduction in the late 19th century when it was first used to denote some physiological function. Eventually, the term receptor was used to denote a physical binding site through which a drug or hormone could exert its effects on a cell. In the 1980s, a distinction was made between receptor and binding site, the former being coupled to intracellular machinery that translated its binding into a cellular effect. Binding sites on the brain endothelial cell can represent transporters, but they can also represent traditional receptors, that is, binding sites coupled to intracellular machinery. For example, brain endothelial cells have both insulin receptors and transporters. As a result, insulin is transported across the BBB to exert effects inside the CNS, but insulin also alters a number of functions of the brain endothelial cell. As examples of the latter, insulin alters the BBB transport of AZT (Ayre, Skaletski, & Mosnaim, 1989), tryptophan (Cangiano et al., 1983), and leptin (Kastin & Akerstrom, 2001) and alters brain endothelial cell alkaline phosphatase activity (Catalan et al., 1988). Many in vitro BBB studies have assumed that a binding site represents transporter function and many in vivo studies are so designed as to not consider whether receptors as well as transporters may exist at the BBB. However, a great deal of indirect evidence and some direct evidence indicates that the vascular BBB and the choroid plexus probably possess a large variety of receptors which can alter BBB functions. Besides insulin, substances which bind to and alter the function of brain endothelial cells include mu opiate receptor ligands (Baba, Oishi, & Saeki, 1988; Vidal, Patel, Wu, Fiala, & Chang, 1998; Chang, Felix, Jiang, & Fiala, 2001), cytokines (Ban et al., 1991; Cunningham et al., 1992; van Dam et al., 1996; Vidal et al., 1998; Moser, Reindl, Blasig, & Humpel, 2004; Khan, DiCello, Nath, & Kim, 2003), leptin (Kastin, Akerstrom, & Pan, 2000; Bjorbaek et al., 1998), acetylcholine (Grammas & Caspers, 1991), adrenergics (Walsh, Slaby, & Posner, 1987; Kalaria & Harik, 1989), glutamate (Koenig, Trout, Goldstone, & Lu, 1992; Krizbai et al., 1998), and chemokines (Sanders et al., 1998).

PERMEABILITY TO CYTOKINES AND RELATED SUBSTANCES

The BBB is known to transport several cytokines in the blood-to-brain direction. For example, the BBB transports the IL-1's, IL-6, and TNF by three separate transport systems. Additionally, nerve growth factor, brain-derived neurotrophic factor, interferons, neurotrophins, and leukemia inhibitory factor (Poduslo & Curran, 1996; Pan, Banks, & Kastin, 1997a; Pan, Banks, & Kastin, 1998a; Pan, Banks, Fasold, Bluth, & Kastin, 1998b) are also transported across the BBB. In some cases, the same gene which gives rise to a cytokine's receptor also produces the cytokine's transporter, whereas in other cases the receptor and transporter are immunologically distinct proteins (Banks & Kastin, 1992; Pan & Kastin, 2002). Recently, the BBB transporter for pituitary adenylate cyclase activating polypeptide (PACAP) was found to be the same protein which acts as a neuronal receptor for enterostatin, but not for PACAP, and acts as a lipid transporter in liver (Martinez et al., 2003; Park et al., 2004; Dogrukol-Ak et al., 2009). In general, transporters occur throughout the CNS, including the spinal cord, although the transport rate can vary greatly among CNS regions (Pan et al., 1998a; Pan, Cornelissen, Halberg, & Kastin, 2002; Banks, Kastin, & Ehrensing, 1994; McLay, Kimura, Banks, & Kastin, 1997). Enough cytokine is transported into the brain to affect CNS function. For example, IL-1 alpha crosses the BBB at the posterior division of the septum where it mediates cognitive impairments (Banks, Farr, La Scola, & Morley, 2001). Similarly, serum TNF crosses the BBB to stimulate release of TNF from CNS stores which in turn can induce apoptosis in the substantia nigra (Qin et al., 2007).

The cytokine transporters are not static but respond to physiological and pathological events. The transport rates of IL-1 and TNF each show diurnal variations (Pan et al., 2002; Banks et al., 1998a). The transport rate of TNF is altered in animals with experimental allergic encephalomyelitis (EAE), spinal cord injury, or blunt trauma to the brain (Pan, Banks, Kennedy, Gutierrez, & Kastin, 1996; Pan, Banks, & Kastin, 1997b; Pan & Kastin, 2001b; Pan, Kastin, Rigai, McLay, & Pick, 2003b).

PERMEABILITY TO OTHER NEUROIMMUNE SUBSTANCES

Other substances with neuroimmune actions are handled by the BBB in a variety of ways. Monoamines are largely excluded by the BBB (Hardebo & Owman, 1990; Kalaria, Mitchell, & Harik, 1987) and opiates and opiate peptides as a rule enter the brain by transmembrane diffusion but are transported by saturable systems in the brain-to-blood direction (King et al., 2001; Elferink & Zadina, 2001; Banks & Kastin, 1990). Pituitary adenylate cyclase activating peptide, a member of the VIP/secretin/PACAP family, has immune functions (Arimura, 1992). Transport of its two major forms across the BBB is complex, involving both brain-to-blood and blood-to-brain components (Banks, Kastin, Komaki, & Arimura, 1993). Its blood-to-brain transport is altered with brain injury (Somogyvari-Vigh, Pan, Reglodi, Kastin, & Arimura, 2000). Some of the other immune active substances whose passage across the BBB has been investigated are melanocyte-stimulating hormone (Wilson, Anderson, Snook, & Llewellyn, 1984), corticotrophin-releasing hormone (Martins, Kastin, & Banks, 1996), and enkephalins (Banks et al., 1986; Elferink & Zadina, 2001).

PERMEABILITY TO IMMUNE CELLS

As discussed above, immune cells cross the BBB by the highly regulated process of diapedesis. The mechanism by which immune cells cross the BBB has also been greatly clarified by recent work. Two major assumptions about how immune cells would enter the CNS have not withstood investigation. The first assumption was that immune cells would enter the CNS by leaking across a disrupted BBB. However, disruptions to the BBB are usually mediated by increased vesicular activity in the endothelial cells (Vorbrodt, Dobrogowska, Ueno, & Lossinsky, 1995; Lossinsky, Vorbrodt, & Wisniewski, 1983; Mayhan & Heistad, 1985). These vesicles of 100 nm or so could not accommodate the passage of an immune cell 10,000 nm in diameter. Even in diseases where there is both increased immune cell trafficking into the CNS and a disrupted BBB, there is often a mismatch between the site of immune cell entry and BBB disruption (Engelhardt & Wolburg, 2004).

The second major assumption is that immune cells would cross between opposing endothelial cells taking the "paracellular route." However, evidence shows that a transcellular route is favored by many immune cells. In brief, immune cells tunnel through venular endothelial cells leaving the intercellular tight junctions intact (Wolburg, Wolburg-Buchholz, & Engelhardt, 2005; Engelhardt, 2008). This tunneling process is complex and is initiated when LFA-1 on an immune cell binds to ICAM on the brain endothelial cell. Other paracellular messengers, which likely include cytokines, are then released (Male, 1995; Persidsky et al., 1997). Protrusions and invaginations of the endothelial cell and protrusions of the immune cell occur, with the immune cell possibly using the tight junction as an initial anchoring site (Lossinsky et al., 1991). Other ligands which have been postulated to play a role in this transcytotic process include PECAM, VE-cadherin, members of the JAM family, and CD99 (Engelhardt &

Wolburg, 2004). Some plasma inevitably accompanies the passage of the immune cell, which can give the appearance of a disrupted BBB (Greenwood, Bamforth, Wang, & Devine, 1995; Avison et al., 2004; Persidsky et al., 2000).

PERMEABILITY TO VIRUSES

Whether a virus is neurovirulent or not depends largely on its ability to cross the BBB (Chou & Dix, 1989). This should not necessarily be assumed, as viruses could induce neurotoxicity without themselves crossing the BBB by several mechanisms. For example, shed viral proteins might cross the BBB, as could circulating cytokines whose release from peripheral sources was induced by the virus. However, most neurovirulent viruses seem to do their major damage directly after entering and replicating within the CNS. Some viruses can replicate within brain endothelial cells and are subsequently shed into the CNS (Cosby & Brankin, 1995). Other viruses invade the CNS by crossing the BBB (Nakaoke, Ryerse, Niwa, & Banks, 2005). Initial uptake by either route involves events reminiscent of adsorptive endocytosis as discussed above. Viral glycoproteins bind to brain endothelial cell (or choroid plexus) glycoproteins to initiate endocytosis. As with adsorptive endocytosis, the virus-containing vesicle is subsequently routed to various membrane systems which can include discharge to the original luminal membrane (recycling) or to the abluminal membrane (transcytosis). Sialic acid and heparan sulfate are common components of the glycoproteins involved in viral uptake by the BBB (Schweighardt & Atwood, 2001; Banks et al., 2004b). In some cases, the functional glycoprotein is known. For example, rabies can bind to acetylcholine and nerve growth factor receptors (Schweighardt & Atwood, 2001). Without an appropriate luminal or basal glycoprotein with which to bind to the BBB cell, the virus is largely excluded from the CNS.

SECRETION OF NEUROIMMUNE-ACTIVE SUBSTANCES

The brain endothelial cells and the epithelial cells of the choroid plexus are capable of secreting a large number of neuroimmune active substances. These include interleukins (Fabry et al., 1993; Hofman, Chen, Incardona, Zidovetzki, & Hinton, 1999; Reyes, Fabry, & Coe, 1999), TNF (Lee et al., 2001), nerve growth factor (Moser et al., 2004), endothelin (Didier, Banks, Creminon, Dereuddre-Bosquet, & Mabondzo, 2002), monocyte chemoattractant peptide (Chen et al., 2001), nitric oxide (Mandi et al., 1998), RANTES (Simpson, Newcombe, Cuzner, & Woodrofe, 1998), and prostacyclin (Faraci & Heistad, 1998). Some of these substances are secreted spontaneously, and many of them can be stimulated with immunoactive substances such as lipopolysaccharide (LPS), bacteria, or viral proteins (Reyes et al., 1999; Vadeboncoeur, Segura, Al-Numani, Vanier, & Gottschalk, 2003; Hofman et al., 1999). The unique, polarized architecture of the BBB that divides its cell membrane into luminal (blood side) and abluminal (brain side) surfaces allows it to receive input from one of its surfaces and to secrete substances into the other.

For example, LPS applied to the abluminal surface of brain endothelial cells in monolayer cultures will enhance release of IL-6 from the luminal surface (Verma, Nakaoke, Dohgu, & Banks, 2006). Secretion of cytokines from brain endothelial cells can be modified by substances such as adiponectin (Spranger et al., 2006).

MODULATION OF BLOOD-BRAIN BARRIER FUNCTION BY NEUROIMMUNE SUBSTANCES

Traditionally, neuroimmune modulation has been thought of in terms of disruption of the BBB. However, as the review above indicates, transporter functions are also vulnerable to manipulation by neuroimmune elements. Alterations in transport function are likely to be a more common event than disruption, as the latter is likely seen only with extreme pathology, whereas the former is likely a physiological, as well as a pathological, aspect of neuroimmune regulation. Other functions of the BBB such as brain endothelial cell secretions are also clearly affected by neuroimmune events.

Agents that Increase Permeability through the Blood-Brain Barrier

Disruption was the first BBB function noted to be perturbed in neuroimmune disease. However, the review above makes it clear that an increase in the BBB permeability can be induced for specific agents by increasing their blood-to-brain transport rate or inhibiting their brain-to-blood efflux rate.

Regulation of Blood-Brain Barrier Integrity and Tight Junction Function

The classic example of BBB disruption is that seen in multiple sclerosis and the animal model of that disease, experimental autoimmune encephalomyelitis (EAE) (Pozzilli et al., 1988; Butter, Baker, O'Neill, & Turk, 1991; Juhler et al., 1984). LPS and treatment with cytokines such as TNF have also been shown to induce BBB disruption (Megyeri et al., 1992). As discussed above, paracellular (through tight junctions) and transcellular mechanisms of transport exist. Although either can underlie BBB disruption, classic studies have shown that the major cause of increased protein leakage across the BBB for almost every kind of insult to the BBB or to the CNS is mediated by transcytotic mechanisms (Lossinsky et al., 1983; Vorbrodt et al., 1995). Nevertheless, recent advances in understanding tight junction assembly and regulation have encouraged many to investigate paracellular mechanisms. Both tight junction function and transcytosis are regulated events, although it is unclear to what extent protein leakage into the brain may be altered under physiological conditions. To some extent, paracellular and transcytotic routes likely involve some of the same cellular machinery, such as the cytoskeleton. TNF is known to induce rearrangements in cytoskeletal architecture. Additionally, cerebral ischemia, diabetes mellitus, and even intense pain are associated with alterations in the expression and cellular distribution tight junction proteins and opening of the BBB (Brown & Davis, 2002; Chehade, Hass, & Mooradian, 2002; Huber et al., 2002). The importance of regulatory processes in BBB disruption is vividly illustrated by the paradoxic finding that maximal disruption does not occur at the time of the CNS injury, even when the event is traumatic, but hours or days later (Baldwin, Fugaccia, Brown, Brown, & Scheff, 1996). It is thought that it is the peripheral and central immune responses, such as cytokine release, to CNS injury rather than the CNS injury itself which results in BBB disruption.

Regulation of Saturable Transporters

Regulation of both influx and efflux transporters are influenced by neuroimmune events. Additionally, cytokine transporters are also affected by various CNS events.

LPS and Blood-to-Brain Transporters

LPS increases the transport of cisplatin, insulin, and the HIV-1 viral coat glycoprotein gp120, but not of TNF or pituitary adenylate cyclase-activating polypeptide (Banks, Kastin, Brennan, & Vallance, 1999; Minami et al., 1998; Nonaka, Shioda, & Banks, 2005; Osburg et al., 2002; Xaio, Banks, Niehoff, & Morley, 2001). LPS affects leptin transport (Nonaka, Hileman, Shioda, Vo, & Banks, 2004) through peripheral mechanisms and increases pituitary adenylate cylcase-activating polypeptide binding to receptors on the BBB but does not alter transport. CNS injuries such as ischemia or trauma to the spinal cord induce a cascade of events which can affect the transport of neuroimmune substances across the BBB as discussed below.

LPS, Cytokines, and Brain-to-Blood (Efflux) Transporters

Efflux systems are also altered by immune modulators. In vitro studies show that LPS, TNF, and interferon gamma regulate P-gp (Theron et al., 2003; Stein, Walther, & Shoemaker, 1996; Bauer, Hartz, & Miller, 2007; Hartz, Bauer, Fricker, & Miller, 2006; Yu et al., 2007). More recently, in vivo studies have shown that LPS downregulates P-gp function at the BBB (Salkeni, Lynch, Price, & Banks, 2009). Interestingly, IL-2 appears to be both a substrate for P-gp and a modulator of its activity (Bonhomme-Faivre et al., 2002; Castagne et al., 2004; Drach et al. 1996). Because P-gp regulates the brain concentration of so many drugs and endogenous substances, immunomodulation could affect many other responses. For example, brain levels of exogenous opiate drugs such as morphine (King et al., 2001), endogenous opiates such as ß-endorphin (Kastin, Fasold, & Zadina, 2002), and neurotoxins such as cyclosporine (Sakata et al., 1994) would all be expected to be increased in patients given IL-2. Immunomodulation of efflux systems, therefore, could have a major effect on CNS metabolism and the response to drugs.

Activity of low density lipoprotein receptor-related protein-1 (LRP-1) is also modulated by LPS. LRP-1 at the BBB acts as an efflux pump to amyloid beta protein (Deane, Sagare, & Zlokovic, 2008), the substance associated causally with Alzheimer's disease. The neurovascular hypothesis states that decreases in LRP-1 activity at the BBB contributes to loss of clearance of amyloid beta protein from the brain and so promotes Alzheimer's disease (Zlokovic, 2005). Inhibition of LRP-1 activity leads to decreased efflux of amyloid beta protein, increased levels of amyloid beta protein in the brain, and cognitive impairment (Jaeger, Dohgu, Lynch, Fleegal-DeMotta, & Banks, 2009a). Mice treated with LPS have decreased efflux of amyloid beta protein, providing a mechanism for connection between inflammatory processes and Alzheimer's disease (Jaeger et al., 2009b).

ROLE OF BLOOD-BRAIN BARRIER IN NEUROIMMUNE DISEASES

The above review has emphasized BBB/neuroimmune interactions under normal physiological conditions. However, the BBB is intimately involved in neuroimmune diseases as well. The BBB can be a target of such disease, its functions may be adaptive to disease, or it can be a contributor to the disease process. Below are some examples of the ways in which the BBB is altered in diseases with neuroimmune processes.

TNF TRANSPORT AND EAE

TNF has a biphasic effect on many neuroimmune processes, with too little or too much producing harmful effects (Pan et al., 1997c). TNF mediates many of its pathological effects through its central receptors and transport of circulating TNF is one source of CNS TNF (Gutierrez et al., 1993; Osburg et al., 2002; Pan & Kastin, 2002). Induction of EAE is partially dependent on TNF and IL-1 (Schiffenbauer et al., 2000). Immune cell invasion in general and during EAE in particular is dependent on TNF-modulated expression of ICAM and VCAM on brain endothelial cells and of LFA-1 on immunocytes (Male, 1995; Barten & Ruddle, 1994). Finally, the saturable transport across the BBB of TNF itself is greatly increased in EAE (Pan et al., 1996).

CNS INJURIES AND CYTOKINE TRANSPORT

As noted above, CNS injuries can produce a disruption of the BBB, but this disruption is temporally dissociated from the injury (Pan et al., 1997b; Baldwin, Fugaccia, Brown, Brown, & Scheff, 1996; Banks, Kastin, & Arimura, 1998b). This dissociation is because the disruption is the consequence of the reactions to injury rather than to injury itself. Not surprisingly, then, CNS injuries can also produce complex alterations in the BBB transport of cytokines. Besides the example of TNF in EAE given above, TNF transport is also increased in spinal cord injury (Pan et al., 1997b; Pan et al., 2003a; Pan & Kastin, 2001b). This increase is not confined to the site of injury, not homogeneous through out the CNS, and not related to the disruption pattern of the BBB (Pan, Kastin, & Pick, 2005; Pan et al., 1997b; Pan & Kastin, 2001b). It is also temporally and regionally independent of the changes in BBB transport rates of other cytokines and immunoactive substances whose transport rates are also altered with CNS injury

ANTI-RETROVIRALS AND THE BLOOD-BRAIN BARRIER

A major problem in treating viruses which can invade the CNS, such as HIV-1, is that antiretrovirals often cross the BBB poorly (Thomas, 2004). The major problem, however, is not that these substances are especially limited by their rate of transmembrane diffusion, but that they are nearly all substrates for efflux systems. For example, AZT is 16 times more lipid soluble than sucrose and so should cross much more rapidly, but actually crosses at the same rate (Wu et al., 1998). AZT is a ligand for at least two efflux systems (Masereeuw et al., 1994; Takasawa, Terasaki, Suzuki, & Sugiyama, 1997; Wang & Sawchuck 1995). Similar problems of penetration exist for the protease inhibitors, which are all substrates for P-gp (Lee et al., 1998). P-gp is expressed by immune and other cells as well with three major phenotypic clusters in humans. Those with higher expression of P-gp, and therefore less able to accumulate protease inhibitors in tissues, are more resistant to treatment for HIV-1 (Fellay et al., 2002).

IMMUNE CELL INVASION

Immune-cell trafficking into the CNS is important in mediating neuroimmune diseases. Immune-cell invasion is an early event in multiple sclerosis and EAE (Wolburg et al., 2005). Infected immune cells are a mechanism by which HIV-1 (Koyanagi et al., 1997; Nottet et al., 1996) and perhaps prions (Klein et al., 1997) invade the CNS.

Immune cell passage across the BBB is, in turn, affected by immune modulators. LPS and the HIV-1 immunoactive protein Tat increase expression by brain endothelial cells of ICAM and VCAM (Pu et al., 2003; Nottet et al., 1996) and monocytes treated with LPS have an increased rate of passage across the BBB (Persidsky et al., 1997). In vitro studies suggest that these events may be mediated through IL-1ß and IL-6 (De Vries et al., 1994).

EFFLUX OF NEUROAIDS-RELATED PROTEINS AND CYTOKINES

Because the BBB prevents the effective accumulation of many of the antivirals, the CNS can act as a reservoir of virus. This reservoir could potentially reinfect the peripheral tissues. The CNS-to-blood movement of HIV-1 has not been investigated, but movement of two of its proteins has. The coat glycoprotein gp120 is cleared by nonsaturable mechanisms (Cashion et al., 1999). However, it has a propensity to be reabsorbed predominately by nasal drainage. As a result, it drains by way of lymphatic vessels directly to the cervical lymphatic nodes. If whole virus also takes this route, then that means that lymph nodes could be directly reinfected without the virus having to enter the circulation where it could be exposed to antiviral agents.

A CNS reservoir of virus could affect the peripheral immune system by a mechanism which does not involve reinfection of peripheral tissues. Tat, like gp120, is also reabsorbed with the CSF into the blood by a nonsaturable mechanism (Banks et al., 2005b). Proteins which are enzymatically resistant in blood, such as Tat, gp120, and cytokines, can achieve high levels in blood even when their only source is the CSF. Production of these proteins within the CNS with subsequent reabsorption with the CSF into blood could be a way in which CNS virus produces toxic effects at peripheral tissues.

To date, IL-2 is the only cytokine known to be transported from the brain to the blood by a saturable transporter (Banks, Niehoff, & Zalcman, 2004c). This transporter, along with binding to plasma proteins and robust degradation by the BBB or CNS, effectively prevents much IL-2 from entering the brain. Evidence suggests that this transporter is likely P-gp. P-gp activity is decreased with HIV encephalitis (Persidsky, Zheng, Miller, & Gendelman, 2000) and this could lead to blood-borne IL-2 entering the CNS. Chronic IL-2 administration induces stereotypic behaviors and is used in an animal model of schizophrenia (Zalcman, 2001; Zalcman, 2002). Therefore, an enhanced entry of IL-2 is one mechanism by which HIV-1 could induce behavioral changes.

SUMMARY

The BBB intimately interacts with cells and their secretions which are in both the CNS and periphery. Some neuroimmune substances, exemplified by cytokines, can cross the BBB directly and also have direct effects on the BBB. The BBB is itself a source of neuroimmune substances and can receive signals from one side, for example the brain side, and release substances in response to that signal from its other side. The passage of immune cells across the BBB is a highly regulated event as is the passage of viruses and viral particles. Overall, the BBB is an important component of the neuroimmune axis and the only component which is simultaneously physically in both the peripheral and central compartments of the neuroimmune system.

REFERENCES

Abbott, N. J., Ronnback, L., & Hansson, E. (2006). Astrocyte-endothelial interactions at the blood-brain barrier. *Nature Reviews, 7,* 41–53.

Al-Sarraf, H. & Phillip, L. (2003). Effect of hypertension on the integrity of blood brain and blood CSF barriers, cerebral blood flow and CSF secretion in the rat. *Brain Res, 975,* 179–188.

Alafaci, C., Salpietro, G., Grasso, G., Sfacteria, A., Passalacqua, M., Morabito, A., et al. (2000). Effect of recombinant human erythropoietin on cerebral ischemia following experimental subarachnoid hemorrhage. *Eur J Pharmacol, 406,* 219–225.

Arimura, A. (1992). Pituitary adenylate cyclase activating polypeptide (PACAP): Discovery and current status of research. *Regul Pept, 37,* 287–303.

Avison, M. J., Nath, A., Greene-Avison, R., Schmitt, F. A., Bales, R. A., Ethisham, A., et al. (2004). Inflammatory changes and breakdown of microvascular integrity in early human immunodeficiency virus dementia. *Journal of Neurovirology, 10,* 223–232.

Ayre, S. G., Skaletski, B., & Mosnaim, A. D. (1989). Blood-brain barrier passage of azidothymidine in rats: Effect of insulin. *Res Comm Chem Path Pharmacol, 63,* 45–52.

Baba, M., Oishi, R., & Saeki, K. (1988). Enhancement of blood-brain barrier permeability to sodium fluorescein by stimulation of mu opioid receptors in mice. *Naunyn-Schmied Arch Pharmacol*, 37, 423–428.

Balabanov, R. & Dore-Duffy, P. (1998). Role of the CNS microvascular pericyte in the blood-brain barrier. *J Neurosci Res*, 53, 637–644.

Baldwin, S. A., Fugaccia, I., Brown, D. R., Brown, L. V., & Scheff, S. W. (1996). Blood-brain barrier breach following cortical contusion in the rat. *J Neurosurg*, 85, 476–481.

Balin, B. J., Broadwell, R. D., Salcman, M., & el-Kalliny, M. (1986). Avenues for entry of peripherally administered protein to the central nervous system in mouse, rat, and squirrel monkey. *J Comp Neurol*, 251, 260–280.

Ban, E., Milon, G., Prudhomme, N., Fillion, G., & Haour, F. (1991). Receptors for interleukin-1 (α and β) in mouse brain: Mapping and neuronal localization in hippocampus. *Neuroscience*, 43, 21–30.

Banks, W. A. (2004). Are the extracellular pathways a conduit for the delivery of therapeutics to the brain? *Current Pharmaceutical Design*, 10, 1365–1370.

Banks, W. A. & Broadwell, R. D. (1994). Blood-to-brain and brain-to-blood passage of native horseradish peroxidase, wheat germ agglutinin and albumin: Pharmacokinetic and morphological assessments. *J Neurochem*, 62, 2404–2419.

Banks, W. A., Farr, S. A., La Scola, M. E., & Morley, J. E. (2001). Intravenous human interleukin-1α impairs memory processing in mice: Dependence on blood-brain barrier transport into posterior division of the septum. *J Pharmacol Exp Ther*, 299, 536–541.

Banks, W. A., Farr, S. A., Morley, J. E., Wolf, K. M., Geylis, V., & Steinitz, M. (2007). Anti-amyloid beta protein antibody passage across the blood-brain barrier in the SAMP8 mouse model of Alzheimer's disease: An age related selective uptake with reversal of learning impairment. *Exp Neurol*, 206, 248–256.

Banks, W. A., Jumbe, N. L., Farrell, C. L., Niehoff, M. L., & Heatherington, A. (2004a). Passage of erythropoietic agents across the blood-brain barrier: A comparison of human and murine erythropoietin and the analog Darbopoetin alpha. *Eur J Pharmacol*, 505, 93–101.

Banks, W. A. & Kastin, A. J. (1989). Inhibition of the brain to blood transport system for enkephalins and Tyr-MIF-1 in mice addicted or genetically predisposed to drinking ethanol. *Alcohol*, 6, 53–57.

Banks, W. A. & Kastin, A. J. (1990). Editorial review: Peptide transport systems for opiates across the blood-brain barrier. *Am J Physiol*, 259, E1–E10.

Banks, W. A. & Kastin, A. J. (1992). The interleukins -1α, -1β, and -2 do not disrupt the murine blood-brain barrier. *Int J Immunopharmac*, 14, 629–636.

Banks, W. A. & Kastin, A. J. (1994). Brain-to-blood transport of peptides and the alcohol withdrawal syndrome. In: F. L. Strand, B. Beckwith, B. Chronwall, C. A. Sandman (Eds.). *Models of neuropeptide action*, pp. 108–118. New York: New York Academy of Sciences.

Banks, W. A. & Kastin, A. J. (1998). Differential permeability of the blood-brain barrier to two pancreatic peptides: Insulin and amylin. *Peptides*, 19, 883–889.

Banks, W. A., Kastin, A. J., & Akerstrom, V. (1997). HIV-1 protein gp120 crosses the blood-brain barrier: Role of adsorptive endocytosis. *Life Sci*, 61, L119–L125.

Banks, W. A., Kastin, A. J., & Arimura, A. (1998b). Effect of spinal cord injury on the permeability of the blood-brain and blood-spinal cord barriers to the neurotropin PACAP. *Exp Neurol*, 151,116–123.

Banks, W. A., Kastin, A. J., Brennan, J. M., & Vallance, K. L. (1999). Adsorptive endocytosis of HIV-1gp120 by blood-brain barrier is enhanced by lipopolysaccharide. *Exp Neurol*, 156, 165–171.

Banks, W. A., Kastin, A. J., & Ehrensing, C. A. (1994). Transport of blood-borne interleukin-1α across the endothelial blood-spinal cord barrier of mice. *J Physiol (London)*, 479, 257–264.

Banks, W. A., Kastin, A. J., & Ehrensing, C. A. (1998a). Diurnal uptake of circulating interleukin-1α by brain, spinal cord, testis and muscle. *NIM*, 5, 36–41.

Banks, W. A., Kastin, A. J., Fischman, A. J., Coy, D. H., & Strauss, S. L. (1986). Carrier-mediated transport of enkephalins and N-Tyr-MIF-1 across blood-brain barrier. *Am J Physiol*, 251, E477–E482.

Banks, W. A., Kastin, A. J., Huang, W., Jaspan, J. B., & Maness, L. M. (1996). Leptin enters the brain by a saturable system independent of insulin. *Peptides*, 17, 305–311.

Banks, W. A., Kastin, A. J., Komaki, G., & Arimura, A. (1993). Passage of pituitary adenylate cyclase activating polypeptide₁₋₂₇ and pituitary adenylate cyclase activating polypeptide₁₋₃₈ across the blood-brain barrier. *J Pharmacol Exp Ther*, 267, 690–696.

Banks, W. A., Niehoff, M. L., & Zalcman, S (2004c). Permeability of the mouse blood-brain barrier to murine interleukin-2: Predominance of a saturable efflux system. *Brain, Behavior, and Immunity*, 18, 434–442.

Banks, W. A., Pagliari, P., Nakaoke, R., & Morley, J. E. (2005a). Effects of a behaviorally active antibody on the brain uptake and clearance of amyloid beta proteins. *Peptides*, 26, 287–294.

Banks, W. A., Robinson, S. M., & Nath, A. (2005b). Permeability of the blood-brain barrier to HIV-1 Tat. *Exp Neurol*, 193, 218–227.

Banks, W. A., Robinson, S. M., Verma, S., & Morley, J. E. (2003). Efflux of human and mouse amyloid ß proteins 1–40 and 1–42 from brain: Impairment in a mouse model of Alzheimer's disease. *Neuroscience*, 121, 487–492.

Banks, W. A., Robinson, S. M., Wolf, K. M., Bess, J. W., Jr., & Arthur, L. O. (2004b). Binding, internalization, and membrane incorporation of human immunodeficiency virus-1 at the blood-brain barrier is differentially regulated. *Neuroscience*, 128, 143–153.

Barten, D. M. & Ruddle, N. H. (1994). Vascular cell adhesion molecule-1 modulation by tumor necrosis factor in experimental allergic encephalomyelitis. *J Neuroimmunol*, 51, 123–133.

Bauer, B., Hartz, A. M. S., & Miller, D. S. (2007). Tumor necorsis factor alpha and endothelin-1 increase P-glycoprotein expression and transport activity at the blood-brain barrier. *Molecular Pharmacology*, 71, 667–675.

Begley, D. J. (2004). ABC transporters and the blood-brain barrier. *Current Pharmaceutical Design*, 10, 1295–1312.

Bernards, C. M. (1999). Epidural and intrathecal drug movement. In: T. L. Yaksh (Ed.). *Spinal drug delivery*, pp. 239–252. New York: Elsevier.

Bjorbaek, C., Elmquist, J. K., Michl, P., Ahima, R. S., van Beuren, A., McCall, A. L., et al. (1998). Expression of leptin receptor isoforms in rat brain microvessels. *Endocrinology*, 139, 3485–3491.

Blasberg, R. G. (1977). Methotrexate, cytosine arabinoside, and BCNU concentration in brain after ventriculocisternal perfusion. *Cancer Treatment Reports*, 61, 625–631.

Bonhomme-Faivre, L., Pelloquin, A., Tardivel, S., Urien, S., Mathieu, M. C., Castagne, V., et al. (2002). Recombinant interleukin-2 treatment decreases P-glycoprotein activity and paclitaxel metabolism in mice. *Anti-Cancer Drugs*, 13, 51–57.

Boulton, M., Flessner, M., Armstrong, D., Mohamed, R., Hay, J., & Johnston, M. (1999). Contribution of extracranial lymphatics and arachnoid villi to the clearance of a CSF tracer in the rat. *Am J Physiology*, 276, R818–R823.

Bradbury, M. (1979). *The concept of a blood-brain barrier*. New York: John Wiley and Sons Ltd.

Brightman, M. W. & Reese, T. S. (1969). Junctions between intimately apposed cell membranes in the vertebrate brain. *J Cell Biol*, 40, 648–677.

Broadwell, R. D. (1989). Transcytosis of macromolecules through the blood-brain barrier: A cell biological perspective and critical appraisal. *Acta Neuropathol (Berl)*, 79, 117–128

Broadwell, R. D. (1993). Endothelial cell biology and the enigma of transcytosis through the blood-brain barrier. *Adv Exp Med Biol*, 331, 137–141.

Broadwell, R. D., Balin, B. J., & Salcman, M. (1988). Transcytotic pathway for blood-borne protein through the blood-brain barrier. *Proc Natl Acad Sci USA*, 85, 632–636

Broadwell, R. D. & Banks, W. A. (1993). Cell biological perspective for the transcytosis of peptides and proteins through the mammalian blood-brain fluid barriers. In: W. M. Pardridge (Ed.). *The blood-brain barrier*, pp. 165–199. New York: Raven Press, Ltd.

Broadwell, R. D. & Sofroniew, M. V. (1993). Serum proteins bypass the blood-brain barrier for extracellular entry to the central nervous system. *Exp Neurol*, 120, 245–263.

Brown, R. C. & Davis, T. P. (2002). Calcium modulation of adherens tight junction function: A potential mechanism for blood-brain barrier disruption after stroke. *Stroke, 33*,1706–1711.

Butter, C., Baker, D., O'Neill, J. K., & Turk, J. L. (1991). Mononuclear cell trafficking and plasma protein extravasation into the CNS during chronic relapsing experimental allergic encephalomyelitis in Biozzi AB/H mice. *J Neurol Sci, 104*, 9–12.

Cangiano, C., Cardelli-Cangiano, P., Cascino, A., Patrizi, M. A., Barberini, F., Rossi, F., et al. (1983). On the stimulation by insulin of tryptophan transport across the blood-brain barrier. *Biochemistry International, 7*, 617–627.

Cashion, M. F., Banks, W. A., Bost, K. L., & Kastin, A. J. (1999). Transmission routes of HIV-1 gp120 from brain to lymphoid tissues. *Brain Res, 822*, 26–33.

Castagne, V., Bonhomme-Faivre, L., Urien, S., Reguiga, M. D., Soursac, M., Gimenez, F., et al. (2004). Effect of recombinant interleukin-2 pretreatment on oral and intravenous digoxin pharmacokinetics and P-glycoprotein activity in mice. *Drug Metab Dispos, 32*, 168–171.

Catalan, R. E., Martinez, A. M., Aragones, M. D., Miguel, B. G., & Robles, A. (1988). Insulin action on brain microvessels: Effect on alkaline phosphatase. *Biochem Biophys Res Commun, 150*, 583–590.

Chang, S. L., Felix, B., Jiang, Y., & Fiala, M. (2001). Actions of endotoxin and morphine. *Adv Exp Med Biol, 493*, 187–196.

Chao, C. C., Gekker, G., Sheng, W. S., Hu, S., Tsang, M., & Peterson, P. K. (1994). Priming effect of morphine on the production of tumor necrosis factor-alpha by microglia: Implications in respiratory burst activity and human immunodeficiency virus-1 expression. *J Pharmacol Exp Ther, 269*, 198–203.

Chehade, J. M., Hass, M. J., & Mooradian, A. D. (2002). Diabetes-related changes in rat cerebral occlusin and zonula occludens-1 (ZO-1) expression. *Neurochem Res, 27*, 249–252.

Chen, G., Castro, W. L., Chow, H. H., & Reichlin, S. (1997). Clearance of ^{125}I-labelled interleukin-6 from brain into blood following intracerebroventricular injection in rats. *Endocrinology, 138*, 4830–4836.

Chen, G. & Reichlin, S. (1998). Clearance of [125I]-tumor necrosis factor-α from the brain into the blood after intracerebroventricular injection into rats. *NIM, 5*, 261–269.

Chen, P., Shibata, M., Zidovetzki, R., Fisher, M., Zlokovic, B. V., & Hofman, F. M. (2001). Endothelin-1 and monocyte chemoattractant protein-1 modulation in ischemia and human brain-derived endothelial cell cultures. *J Neuroimmunol, 116*, 62–73.

Chou, S. & Dix, R. D. (1989). Viral infections and the blood-brain barrier. In: E. A. Neuwelt (Ed.). *Implications of the blood-brain barrier and its manipulation*, Volume 2: Clinical aspects, pp. 449–468. New York: Plenum Publishing Corporation.

Cornford, E. M., Braun, L. D., Oldendorf, W. H., & Hill, M. A. (1982). Comparison of lipid-mediated blood-brain-barrier penetrability in neonates and adults. *Am J Physiol, 243*, C161–C168.

Cosby, S. L. & Brankin, B. (1995). Measles virus infection of cerebral endothelial cells and effect on their adhesive properties. *Veterinary Microbiology, 44*, 135–139.

Cserr, H. F. (1984). Convection of brain interstitial fluid. In: K. Shapiro, A. Marmarou, H. Portnoy (Eds.). *Hydrocephalus*, pp. 59–68. New York: Raven Press.

Cserr, H. F. & Berman, B. J. (1978). Iodide and thiocyanate efflux from brain following injection into rat caudate nucleus. *Am J Physiol, 4*, F331–F337.

Cserr, H. F. & Knopf, P. M. (1992). Cervical lymphatics, the blood-brain barrier, and the immunoreactivity of the brain: A new view. *Immunol Today, 13*, 507–512.

Cunningham, E. T., Jr., Wada, E., Carter, D. B., Tracey, D. E., Battey, J. F., & De Souza, E. B. (1992). In situ histochemical localization of type I interleukin-1 receptor messenger RNA in the central nervous system, pituitary, and adrenal gland of the mouse. *J Neurosci, 12*, 1101–1114.

Davies, P. J. A., Davies, D. R., Levitzki, A., Moxfield, F. R., Milhaud, P., Willingman, M. C., et al. (1980). Transglutaminase is essential in receptor-mediated endocytosis of α-macroglobulin and polypeptide hormones. *Nature, 283*, 162–167.

Davson, H. & Segal, M. B. (1996d). Blood-brain-CSF relations. *Physiology of the CSF and blood-brain barriers*, pp. 257–302. Boca Raton, FL: CRC Press.

Davson, H. & Segal, M. B. (1996c). Ontogenetic aspects of the cerebrospinal system. *Physiology of the CSF and blood-brain barriers*, pp. 607–662. Boca Raton, FL: CRC Press, Inc.

Davson, H. & Segal, M. B. (1996b). Special aspects of the blood-brain barrier. *Physiology of the CSF and blood-brain barriers*, pp. 303–485. Boca Raton, FL: CRC Press.

Davson, H. & Segal, M. B. (1996a). The proteins and other macromolecules of the CSF. *Physiology of the CSF and the blood-brain barrier*, pp. 573–606. Boca Raton, FL: CRC Press.

de la Torre, J. C. & Mussivand, T. (1993). Can disturbed brain microcirculation cause Alzheimer's disease? *Neurological Research, 15*, 146–153.

de Lange, E. C., Bouw, M. R., Mandema, J. W., Danhof, M., De Boer, A. G., & Breimer, D. D. (1995). Application of intracerebral microdialysis to study regional distribution kinetics of drug in rat brain. *Br J Pharmacol, 116*, 2538–2544.

de Lange, E. C. M., Bouw, M. R., Danhof, M., De Boer, A. G., & Breimer, D. D. (1993). Application of intracerebral microdialysis to study regional distribution kinetics of atenolol and acetaminophen in rat brain. *The Use of Intracerebral Microdialysis to Study the Blood-Brain Barrier Transport Characteristics of Drugs* (thesis, Leiden/Amsterdam Center for Drug Research), pp. 93–106. Sinteur, Leiden.

De Vries, H. E., Moor, A. C., Blom-Roosemalen, M. C., De Boer, A. G., Breimer, D. D., van Berkel, T. J., et al. (1994). Lymphocyte adhesion to brain capillary endothelial cells in vitro. J Neuroimmunol, 52, 1–8.

Deane, R., Sagare, A., & Zlokovic, B. (2008). The role of the cell surface LRP and soluble LRP in blood-brain barrier Aß clearance in Alzheimer's disease. *Current Pharmaceutical Design, 14*, 1601–1605.

Deane R, Wu Z, Sagare A, Davis J, Du Yan S, Hamm K, et al. (2004). LRP/amyloid beta-peptide interaction mediates differential brain efflux of Abeta isoforms. *Neuron, 43*, 333–344.

Deli, M. A., Abraham, C. R., Kataoka, Y., & Niwa, M. (2005). Permeability studies on in vitro blood-brain barrier models: physiology, pathology, and pharmacology. *Cell Mol Neurobiol, 25*, 59–127.

DeMattos, R. B., Bales, K. R., Cummins, D. J., Paul, S. M., & Holtzman, D. M. (2002). Brain to plasma amyloid-ß efflux: A measure of brain amyloid burden in a mouse model of Alzheimer's disease. *Science, 295*, 2264.

Didier, N., Banks, W. A., Creminon, C., Dereuddre-Bosquet, N., & Mabondzo, A. (2002). HIV-1-induced production of endothelin-1 in an in vitro model of the human blood-brain barrier. *Neuroreport, 13*, 1179–1183.

Dobbing, J. (1968). The development of the blood-brain barrier. *Prog Brain Res, 29*, 417–427.

Dogrukol-Ak, D., Kumar, V. B., Ryerse, J. S., Farr, S. A., Verma, S., Nonaka, K., et al. (2009). Isolation of peptide transport system-6 from brain endothelial cells: Therapeutic effects with antisense inhibition in Alzheimer's and stroke models. *J Cereb Blood Flow Metab, 29*, 411–422.

Dore-Duffy, P. (2008). Pericytes: Pluripotent cells of the blood brain barrier. *Current Pharmaceutical Design, 14*, 1581–1593.

Dore-Duffy, P., Katychev, A., Wang, X., & Van Buren, E. (2006). CNS microvascular pericytes exhibit multipotential stem cell activity. *J Cereb Blood Flow Metab, 26*, 613–624.

Drach, J., Gsur, A., Hamilton, G., Zhao, S., Angerler, J., Fiegl, M., et al. (1996). Involvement of P-glycoprotein in the transmembrane transport of interleukin-2 (IL-2), IL-4, and interferon-gamma in normal human T lymphocytes. *Blood, 88*, 1747–1754.

Drion, N., Lemaire, M., Lefauconnier, J. M., & Scherrmann, J. M. (1996). Role of p-glycoprotein in the blood-brain transport of colchicine and vinblastine. *J Neurochem, 67*, 1688–1693.

Dziegielewska, K. M., Hinds, L. A., Mollgard, K., Reynolds, M. L., & Saunders, N. R. (1988). Blood-brain, blood-cerebrospinal fluid and cerebrospinal fluid-brain barriers in a marsupial (*Macropus eugenii*) during development. *J Physiol, 403*, 307–388.

Ehrenreich, H., Hasselblatt, M., Dembowski, C., Depek, L., Lewczuk, P., Stiefel, M., et al. (2002). Erythropoietin therapy for acute stroke is both safe and beneficial. Molecular *Medicine, 8*, 495–505.

Elferink, R. P. J. O. & Zadina, J. E. (2001). MDR1 P-glycoprotein transports endogenous opioid peptides. *Peptides, 22,* 2015–2020.

Engelhardt, B. (2008). The blood-central nervous system barriers actively control immune cell entry into the central nervous system. *Current Pharmaceutical Design, 14,* 1555–1565.

Engelhardt, B. & Wolburg, H. (2004). Minireview: Transendothelial migration of leukocytes: Through the front door or around the side of the house? *Eur J Pharmacol, 34,* 2955–2963.

Erbyraktar, S., Grasso, G., Sfacteria, A., Xie, Q. W., Coleman, T., Kreilgaard, M., et al. (2003). Asialoerythropoietin is a nonerythropoietic cytokine with broad neuroprotective activity in vivo. *Proc Natl Acad Sci USA, 100,* 6741–6746.

Fabry, Z., Fitzsimmons, K. M., Herlein, J. A., Moninger, T. O., Dobbs, M. B., & Hart, M. N. (1993). Production of the cytokines interleukin 1 and 6 by murine brain microvessel endothelium and smooth muscle pericytes. *J Neuroimmunol, 47,* 23–34.

Faraci, F. M. & Heistad, D. D. (1998). Regulation of the cerebral circulation: Role of endothelium and potassium channels. *Physiol Rev, 78,* 53–97.

Farr, S. A., Banks, W. A., Uezu, K., Sano, A., Gaskin, F. S., & Morley, J. E. (2003). Antibody to beta-amyloid protein increases acetylcholine in the hippocampus of 12 month SAMP8 male mice. *Life Sci, 73,* 555–562.

Fellay, J., Marzolini, C., Meaden, E. R., Black, D. J., Buclin, T., Chave, J-P., et al. (2002). Response of antiretroviral treatment in HIV-1 infected individuals with allelic variants of the multidrug resistance transporter 1: A pharmacogenetic study. *Lancet, 359,* 30–36.

Ferguson, A. V. (1991). The area postrema: A cardiovascular control centre at the blood-brain interface? *Canadian Journal of Physiology & Pharmacology, 69,* 1026–1034.

Ghersi-Egea, J. F., Gorevic, P. D., Ghiso, J., Frangione, B., Patlak, C. S., & Fenstermacher, J. D. (1996). Fate of cerebrospinal fluid-borne amyloid β-peptide: Rapid clearance into blood and appreciable accumulation by cerebral arteries. *J Neurochem, 67,* 880–883.

Glynn, S. L. & Yazdanian, M. (1998). In vitro blood-brain barrier permeability of nevirapine compared to other HIV antiretroviral agents. *J Pharm Sci, 87,* 306–310.

Grammas, P. & Caspers, M. L. (1991). The effect of aluminum on muscarinic receptors in isolated cerebral microvessels. *Res Comm Chem Path Pharmacol, 72,* 69–79.

Greenwood, J., Bamforth, S., Wang, Y., & Devine, L. (1995). The blood-retinal barrier in immune-mediated diseases of the retina. In: J. Greenwood, D. J. Begley, & M. B. Segal (Eds.). *New concepts of a blood-brain barrier,* pp. 315–326. New York: Plenum Press.

Gross, P. M. & Weindl, A. (1987). Peering through the windows of the brain. *J Cereb Blood Flow Metab, 7,* 663–672.

Gutierrez, E. G., Banks, W. A., & Kastin, A. J. (1993). Murine tumor necrosis factor alpha is transported from blood to brain in the mouse. *J Neuroimmunol, 47,* 169–176.

Hardebo, J. E. & Owman, C. (1990). Enzymatic barrier mechanisms for neurotransmitter monoamines and their precursors at the blood-brain barrier. In: B. B. Johansson, C. Owman, & H. Widner (Eds.). *Pathophysiology of the blood-brain barrier,* pp. 41–55. Amsterdam: Elsevier.

Hartz, A. M. S., Bauer, B., Fricker, G., & Miller, D. S. (2006). Rapid modulation of P-glycoprotein-mediated transport at the blood-brain barrier by tumor necrosis factor-alpha and lipopolysaccharide. *Molecular Pharmacology, 69,* 462–470.

Hock, C., Konietzko, U., Streffer, J. R., Tracy, J., Signorell, A., Muller-Tillmanns, B., et al. (2003). Antibodies against beta-amyloid slow cognitive decline in Alzheimer's disease. *Neuron, 38,* 547–554.

Hofman, F., Chen, P., Incardona, F., Zidovetzki, R., & Hinton, D. R. (1999). HIV-tat protein induces the production of interleukin-8 by human brain-derived endothelial cells. *J Neuroimmunol, 94,* 28–39.

Holash, J. A., Harik, S. I., Perry, G., & Stewart, P. A. (1993). Barrier properties of testis microvessels. *Proc Natl Acad Sci USA, 90,* 11069–11073.

Huber, J. D. (2008). Diabetes, cognitive function, and the blood-brain barrier. *Current Pharmaceutical Design, 14,* 1594–1600.

Huber, J. D., Hau, V. S., Borg, L., Campos, C. R., Egleton, R. D., & Davis, T. P. (2002). Blood-brain barrier tight junctions are altered during a 72-h exposure to lamba-carrageenan-induced inflammatory pain. *Am J Physiol, 283,* H1531–H1537.

Huber, J. D., VanGilder, R. L., & Houser, K. A. (2006). Streptozotocin-induced diabetes progressively increases blood-brain barrier permeability in specific brain regions in rats. *Am J Physiol, 291,* H2660–H2668.

Jaeger, J. B., Dohgu, S., Hwang, M. C., Farr, S. A., Murphy, M. P., Fleegal-DeMotta, M. A., et al. (2009a). Testing the neurovascular hypothesis of Alzheimer's disease: LRP-1 antisense reduced blood-brain barrier clearance, increases brain levels of amyloid beta protein, and impairs cognition. *J Alz Dis, 17,* 553–570.

Jaeger, L. B., Dohgu, S., Lynch, J. L., Fleegal-DeMotta, M. A., & Banks, W. A. (2009b). Effects of lipopolysaccharide on the blood-brain barrier transport of amyloid bea protein: A mechanism for inflammation in the progression of Alzheimer's disease. *Brain, Behavior, and Immunity.*

Janus, C., Pearson, J., McLaurin, J., Mathews, P. M., Jiang, Y., Schmidt, S. D., et al. (2000). Aβ peptide immunization reduces behavioral impairment and plaques in a model of Alzheimer's disease. *Nature, 408,* 979–982.

Johanson, C. E. (1988). The choroid plexus-arachnoid membrane-cerebrospinal fluid system. In: A. A. Boulton, G. B. Baker, & W. Walz (Eds.). *Neuromethods; The neuronal microenvironment,* pp 33–104. Clifton, NJ: The Humana Press.

Johansson, B. B. (1989). Hypertension and the blood-brain barrier. In: E. A. Neuwelt (Ed.). *Implications of the blood-brain barrier and its manipulation.* Vol 2. Clinical aspects, pp. 389–410. New York: Plenum Publishing Co.

Johnson, A. K. & Gross, P. M. (1993). Sensory circumventricular organs and brain homeostatic pathways. *FASEB J, 7,* 678–686.

Jones, P. M. & Robinson, I. C. A. F. (1982). Differential clearance of neurophysin and neurohypophysial peptides from the cerebrospinal fluid in conscious guinea pigs. *Neuroendocrinology, 34,* 297–302.

Juhler, M., Barry, D. I., Offner, H., Konat, G., Klinken, L., & Paulson, O. B. (1984). Blood-brain and blood-spinal cord barrier permeability during the course of experimental allergic encephalomyelitis in the rat. *Brain Res, 302,* 347–355.

Kalaria, R. N. & Harik, S. I. (1989). Increased alpha 2- and beta 2-adrenergic receptors in cerebral microvessels in Alzheimer disease. *Neurosci Lett, 106,* 233–238.

Kalaria, R. N., Mitchell, M. J., & Harik, S. I. (1987). Correlation of 1-methyl-4-phenyl-1,2,3,6-tetrahydropyridine neurotoxicity with blood-brain barrier monoamine oxidase activity. *Proc Natl Acad Sci USA, 84,* 3521–3525.

Kastin, A. J. & Akerstrom, V. (2001). Glucose and insulin increase the transport of leptin through the blood-brain barrier in normal mice but not in streptozotocin-diabetic mice. *Neuroendocrinology, 73,* 237–242.

Kastin, A. J., Akerstrom, V., & Pan, W. (2000). Activation of urocortin transport into brain by leptin. *Peptides, 21,* 1811–1817.

Kastin, A. J., Fasold, M. B., & Zadina, J. E. (2002). Endomorphins, Met-enkephalin, Tyr-MIF-1 and the P-glycoprotein efflux system. *Drug Metab Dispos, 30,* 231–234.

Kaur, J., Jaswal, V. M., Nagpaul, J. P., & Mahmood, A. (1992). Chronic ethanol feeding and microvillus membrane glycosylation in normal and protein-malnourished rat intestine. *Nutrition, 8,* 338–342.

Kety, S. S. (1987). Cerebral circulation and its measurement by inert diffusible tracers. In: G. Adelman (Ed.). *Encyclopedia of neuroscience,* Volume I, pp. 206–208. Boston: Birkh.

Khan, N. A., DiCello, F., Nath, A., & Kim, K. S. (2003). Human immunodeficiency virus type 1 tat-mediated cytotoxicity of human brain microvascular endothelial cells. *J Neurovirology, 9,* 584–593.

King, M., Su, W., Chang, A., Zuckerman, A., & Pasternak, G. W. (2001). Transport of opioids from the brain to the periphery by P-glycoprotein: Peripheral actions of central drugs. *Nature Neuroscience, 4,* 221–222.

Klein, M. A., Frigg, R., Flechsig, E., Raeber, A. J., Kalinke, U., Bluethmann, H., et al. (1997). A crucial role for B cells in neuroinvasive scrapie. *Nature, 390,* 687–690.

Knopf, P. M., Cserr, H. F., Nolan, S. C., Wu, T. Y., & Harling-Berg, C. J. (1995). Physiology and immunology of lymphatic drainage of interstitial and cerebrospinal fluid from the brain. *Neuropathology and Applied Neurobiology, 21,* 175–180.

Koenig, H., Trout, J. J., Goldstone, A. D., & Lu, C. Y. (1992). Capillary NMDA receptors regulate blood-brain barrier function and breakdown. *Brain Res, 588,* 297–303.

Koyanagi, Y., Tanaka, Y., Kira, J., Ito, M., Hioki, K., Misawa, N., et al. (1997). Primary human immunodeficiency virus type 1 viremia and central nervous system invasion in a novel hu-PBL-immunodeficient mouse strain. *J Virol, 71,* 2417–2424.

Kozlowski, G. P., Sterzl, I., & Nilaver, G. (1992). Localization patterns for immunoglobulins and albumins in the brain suggest diverse mechanisms for their transport across the blood-brain barrier (BBB). In: A. Ermisch, R., Landgraf, H. J. Rühle (Eds.). *Progress in brain research,* pp. 149–154. Amsterdam: Elsevier.

Krizbai, I. A., Deli, M. A., Pestenacz, A., Siklose, L., Szabo, C. A., et al. (1998). Expression of glutamate receptors on cultured cerebral endothelial cells. *J Neurosci Res, 54,* 814–819.

LeBel, C. P. (1999). Spinal delivery of neurotrophins and related molecules. In: T. L. Yaksh (Ed.). *Spinal drug delivery,* pp 543–554. Amsterdam: Elsevier.

Lee, C. G. L., Gottesman, M. M., Cardarelli, C. O., Ramachandra, M., Jeang, K. T., Ambudkar, S. V., et al. (1998). HIV-1 protease inhibitors are substrates for the MDR1 multidrug transporter. *Biochemistry, 37,* 3594–3601.

Lee, Y. W., Hennig, B., Fiala, M., Kim, K. S., & Toborek, M. (2001). Cocaine activates redox-regulated transcription factors and induces TNF-alpha expression in human brain endothelial cells. *Brain Res, 920,* 125–133.

Levin, V. A. (1980). Relationship of octanol/water partition coefficient and molecular weight to rat brain capillary permeability. *Journal of Medicinal Chemistry, 23,* 682–684.

Lipinski, C. A., Lombardo, F., Dominy, B. W., & Feeney, P. J. (1997). Experimental and computational approaches to estimate solubility and permeability in drug discovery and developmental settings. *Advanced Drug Delivery Reviews, 23,* 3–25.

Lossinsky, A. S., Pluta, R., Song, M. J., Badmajew, V., Moretz, R. C., & Wisniewski, H. M. (1991). Mechanisms of inflammatory cell attachment in chronic relapsing experimental allergic encephalomyelitis: A scanning and high-voltage electron microscopic study of the injured mouse blood-brain barrier. *Microvasc Res, 41,* 299–310.

Lossinsky, A. S., Vorbrodt, A. W., & Wisniewski, H. M. (1983). Ultracytochemical studies of vesicular and canalicular transport structures in the injured mammalian blood-brain barrier. *Acta Neuropathol (Berl), 61,* 239–245.

Löscher, W. & Potschka, H. (2002). Role of multidrug transporters in pharmacoresistance to antiepileptic drugs. *J Pharmacol Exp Ther, 30,* 7–14.

Lyle, R. E., Kincaid, S. C., Bryant, J. C., Prince, A. M., & MeGehee, R. E. (2001). Human milk contains detectable levels of immunoreactive leptin. *Adv Exp Med Biol, 501,* 87–92.

Male, D. (1995). The blood-brain barrier—No barrier to a determined lymphocyte. In: J. Greenwood, D. J. Begley, M. B. Segal (Eds.). *New concepts of a blood-brain barrier,* pp. 311–314. New York: Plenum Press.

Mandi, Y., Ocsovszki, I., Szabo, D., Nagy, Z., Nelson, J., & Molnar, J. (1998). Nitric oxide production and MDR expression by human brain endothelial cells. *Anticancer Research, 18,* 3049–3052.

Maness, L. M., Kastin, A. J., Farrell, C. L., & Banks, W. A. (1998). Fate of leptin after intracerebroventricular injection into the mouse brain. *Endocrinology, 139,* 4556–4562.

Marsh, M. (1984). The entry of enveloped viruses into cells by endocytosis. *Biochem J, 218,* 1–10.

Martinez, L. O., Jacquet, S., Esteve, J-P., Rolland, C., Cabezon, E., Champagne, E., et al. (2003). Ectopic ß-chain of ATP synthase is an apolipoprotein A-1 receptor in hepatic HDL endocytosis. *Nature, 421,* 75–79.

Martins, J. M., Banks, W. A., & Kastin, A. J. (1997). Acute modulation of the active carrier-mediated brain to blood transport of corticotropin-releasing hormone. *Am J Physiol, 272,* E312–E319.

Martins, J. M., Kastin, A. J., & Banks, W. A. (1996). Unidirectional specific and modulated brain to blood transport of corticotropin-releasing hormone. *Neuroendocrinology, 63,* 338–348.

Masereeuw, R., Jaehde, U., Langemeijer, M. W. E., De Boer, A. G., & Breimer, D. D. (1994). *In vivo* and *in vitro* transport of zidovudine (AZT) across the blood-brain barrier and the effects of transport inhibitors. Pharm Res, 11, 324–330.

Mayhan, W. G. & Heistad, D. D. (1985). Permeability of blood-brain barrier to various sized molecules. *Am J Physiology, 248,* H712–H718.

McCarthy, T. J., Banks, W. A., Farrell, C. L., Adamu, S., Derdeyn, C. P., Snyder, A. Z., et al. (2002) Positron emission tomography shows that intrathecal leptin reaches the hypothalamus in baboons. *J Pharmacol Exp Ther, 307,* 878–883.

McLay, R. N., Kimura, M., Banks, W. A., & Kastin, A. J. (1997). Granulocyte-macrophage colony-stimulating factor crosses the blood-brain and blood-spinal cord barriers. *Brain, 120,* 2083–2091.

McQuay, H. J., Sullivan, A. F., Smallman, K., & Dickenson, A. H. (1989). Intrathecal opioids, potency and lipophilicity. *Pain, 36,* 111–115.

Mealey, K. L., Bentjen, S. A., Gay, J. M., & Cantor, G. H. (2001). Ivermectin sensitivity is associated with a deletion mutation of the mdr1 gene. *Pharmacogenetics, 11,* 727–733.

Megyeri, P., Abraham, C. S., Temesvari, P., Kovacs, J., Vas, T., & Speer, C. P. (1992). Recombinant human tumor necrosis factor alpha constricts pial arterioles and increases blood-brain barrier permeability in newborn piglets. *Neurosci Lett, 148,* 137–140.

Mellman, I., Fuchs, R., & Helenius, A. (1986). Acidification of the endocytic and exocytic pathways. *Ann Rev Biochem, 55,* 663–700.

Minami, T., Okazaki, J., Kawabata, A., Kuroda, R., & Okazaki, Y. (1998). Penetration of cisplatin into mouse brain by lipopolysccharide. *Toxicology, 130,* 107–113.

Moos, T. & Mollgard, K. (1993). Cerebrovascular permeability to azo dyes and plasma proteins in rodents of different ages. *Neuropathology and Applied Neurobiology, 19,* 120–127.

Morgan, D., Diamond, D. M., Gottschall, P. E., Ugen, K. E., Dickey, C., Hardy, J., et al. (2000). Aβ peptide vaccination prevents memory loss in an animal model of Alzheimer's disease. *Nature, 408,* 982–985.

Moser, K. V., Reindl, M., Blasig, I., & Humpel, C. (2004). Brain capillary endothelial cells proliferate in response to NGF, express NGF receptors and secrete NGF after inflammatiion. *Brain Res, 1017,* 53–60.

Muldoon, L. L., Pagel, M. A., Kroll, R. A., Roman-Goldstein, S., Jones, R. S., & Neuwelt, E. A. (1999). A physiological barrier distal to the anatomical blood-brain barrier in a model of transvascular delivery. *American Journal of Neuroradiology, 20,* 217–222.

Nakaoke, R., Ryerse, J. S., Niwa, M., & Banks, W. A. (2005). Human immunodeficiency virus type 1 transport across the in vitro mouse brain endothelial cell monolayer. *Exp Neurol, 193,* 101–109.

Nakaoke, R., Verma, S., Niwa, M., Dohgu, S., & Banks, W. A. (2007). Glucose-regulated blood-brain barrier transport of insulin: Pericyte-astrocyte-endothelial cell cross talk. *International Journal of Neuroprotection and Neuroregeneration, 3,* 195–200.

Nath, A., Conant, K., Chen, P., Scott, C., & Major, E. O. (1999). Transient exposure to HIV-1 Tat protein results in cytokine production in macrophages and astrocytes: A hit and run phenomenon. *J Biol Chem, 274,* 17098–17102.

Neaves, W. B. (1977). The blood-testis barrier. In: A. D. Johnson & W. R. Gomes (Eds.). *The testis,* pp. 125–162. New York: Academic Press.

Nelson, P. K., Masters, L. T., Zagzag, D., & Kelly, P. J. (1999). Angiographic abnormalities in progressive multifocal leukoencephalopathy: An explanation based on neuropathologic findings. *American Journal of Neuroradiology, 20,* 487–494.

Neuwelt, E., Abbott, N. J., Abrey, L., Banks, W. A., Blakley, B., Davis, T., et al.(2008). Strategies to advance translational research into brain barriers. *Lancet Neurology, 7,* 84–96.

Nonaka, N., Hileman, S. M., Shioda, S., Vo, P., & Banks, W. A. (2004). Effects of lipopolysaccharide on leptin transport across the blood-brain barrier. *Brain Res, 1016,* 58–65.

Nonaka, N., Shioda, S., & Banks, W. A. (2005). Effect of lipopolysaccharide on the transport of pituitary adenylate cyclase activating polypeptide across the blood-brain barrier. *Exp Neurol, 191,* 137–144.

Nottet, H. S., Persidsky, Y., Sasseville, V. G., Nukuna, A. N., Bock, P., Zhai, Q. H., et al. (1996). Mechanisms for the transendothelial migration of HIV-1-infected monocytes into brain. *J Immunol, 156,* 1284–1295.

Oehmichen, M., Gruninger, H., Wietholter, H., & Gencic, M. (1979). Lymphatic efflux of intracerebrally injected cells. *Acta Neuropathol, 45,* 61–65.

Oldendorf, W. H. (1971). Brain uptake of radio-labelled amino acids, amines and hexoses after arterial injection. *Am J Physiol, 221,* 1629–1639.

Oldendorf, W. H. (1974). Lipid solubility and drug penetration of the blood-brain barrier. *Proc Soc Exp Biol Med, 147,* 813–816.

Osburg, B., Peiser, C., Domling, D., Schomburg, L., Ko, Y. T., Voight, K., et al. (2002). Effect of endotoxin on expression of TNF receptors and transport of TNF-alpha at the blood-brain barrier of the rat. *Am J Physiol, 283,* E899–E908.

Pan, W., Banks, W. A., Fasold, M. B., Bluth, J., & Kastin, A. J. (1998b). Transport of brain-derived neurotrophic factor across the blood-brain barrier. *Neuropharmacology, 37,* 1553–1561.

Pan, W., Banks, W. A., & Kastin, A. J. (1997b). BBB permeability to ebiratide and TNF in acute spinal cord injury. *Exp Neurol, 146,* 367–373.

Pan, W., Banks, W. A., & Kastin, A. J. (1997a). Permeability of the blood-brain barrier and blood-spinal cord barriers to interferons. *J Neuroimmunol, 76,* 105–111

Pan, W., Banks, W. A., & Kastin, A. J. (1998a). Permeability of the blood-brain barrier to neurotrophins. *Brain Res, 788,* 87–94.

Pan, W., Banks, W. A., Kennedy, M. K., Gutierrez, E. G., & Kastin, A. J. (1996). Differential permeability of the BBB in acute EAE: Enhanced transport of TNF-α. *Am J Physiol, 271,* E636–E642.

Pan, W., Cornelissen, G., Halberg, F., & Kastin, A. J. (2002). Selected contributions: Circadian rhythm of tumor necrosis factor-alpha uptake into mouse spinal cord. *J Appl Physiol, 92,* 1357–1362.

Pan, W. & Kastin, A. J. (2001a). Changing the chemokine gradient: CINC1 crosses the blood-brain barrier. *J Neuroimmunol, 115,* 64–70.

Pan, W. & Kastin, A. J. (2001b). Increase in TNF alpha transport after SCI is specific for time, region, and type of lesion. *Exp Neurol, 170,* 357–363.

Pan, W. & Kastin, A. J. (2002). TNF alpha transport across the blood-brain barrier is abolished in receptor knockout mice. *Exp Neurol, 174,* 193–200.

Pan, W. & Kastin, A. J. (2008). Cytokine transport across the injured blood-spinal cord barrier. *Current Pharmaceutical Design, 14,* 1620–1624.

Pan, W., Kastin, A. J., & Pick, C. G. (2005). The staircase test in mice after spinal cord injury. *International Journal of Neuroprotection and Neuroregeneration, 1,* 32–37.

Pan, W., Kastin, A. J., Rigai, T., McLay, R., & Pick, C. G. (2003b). Increased hippocampal uptake of tumor necrosis factor alpha and behavioral changes in mice. *Exp Brain Res, 149,* 195–199.

Pan, W., Zadina, J. E., Harlan, R. E., Weber, J. T., Banks, W. A., & Kastin, A. J. (1997c). Tumor necrosis factor-alpha: A neuromodulator in the CNS. *Neurosci Biobehav Rev, 21,* 603–613.

Pan, W., Zhang, L., Liao, J., Csernus, B., & Kastin, A. J. (2003a). Selective increase in TNF alpha permeation across the blood-spinal cord barrier after SCI. *J Neuroimmunol, 134,* 111–117.

Park, M., Lin, L., Thomas, S., Braymer, H. D., Smith, P. M., Harrison, D. H. T., et al. (2004). The $F_{1-ATPase}$ ß-subunit is the putative enterostatin receptor. *Peptides, 25,* 2127–2133.

Persidsky, Y., Stins, M., Way, D., Witte, M. H., Weinand, M., Kim, K. S., et al. (1997). A model for monocyte migration through the blood-brain barrier during HIV-1 encephalitis. *J Immunol, 158,* 3499–3510.

Persidsky, Y., Zheng, J., Miller, D., & Gendelman, H. E. (2000). Mononuclear phagocytes mediate blood-brain barrier compromise and neuronal injury during HIV-1-associated dementia. *J Leukoc Biol, 68,* 413–422.

Peruzzo, B., Pastor, F. E., Blazquez, J. L., Schobitz, K., Pelaez, B., Amat, P., et al;. (2000). A second look at the barriers of the medial basal hypothalamus. *Exp Brain Res, 132,* 10–26.

Plotkin, S. R., Banks, W. A., & Kastin, A. J. (1996). Comparison of saturable transport and extracellular pathways in the passage of interleukin-1α across the blood-brain barrier. *J Neuroimmunol, 67,* 41–47.

Plotkin, S. R., Banks, W. A., & Kastin, A. J. (1998). Enkephalin, PPE, mRNA, and PTS-1 in alcohol withdrawal seizure-prone and -resistant mice. *Alcohol, 15,* 25–31.

Poduslo, J. F. & Curran, G. L. (1996). Permeability at the blood-brain barrier and blood-nerve barriers of the neurotrophic factors: NGF, CNTF, NT-3, BDNF. *Mol Brain Res, 36,* 280–286.

Pollay, M. & Davson, H. (1963). The passage of certain substances out of the cerebrospinal fluid. *Brain, 86,* 137–150.

Pozzilli, C., Bernardi, S., Mansi, L., Picozzi, P., Iannotti, F., Alfano, B., et al. (1988). Quantitative assessment of the blood-brain barrier permeability in multiple sclerosis using 68-Ga-EDTA and positron emission tomography. *J Neurol Neurosurg Psych, 51,* 1058–1062.

Prockop, L. D., Naidu, K. A., Binard, J. E., & Ransohoff, J. (1996). Selective permeability of [³H]-D-mannitol and [¹⁴C]-carboxyl-inulin across the blood-brain barrier and blood-spinal cord barrier in the rabbit. *The Journal of Spinal Cord Medicine, 18,* 221–226.

Pu, H., Tian, J., Flora, G., Lee, Y. W., Nath, A., Hennig, B., et al. (2003). HIV-1 Tat protein upregulates inflammatory mediators and induces monocyte invasion into the brain. *Molecular and Cellular Neurosciences, 24,* 224–237.

Qin, L., Wu, X., Block, M. L., Liu, Y., Breese, G. R., Hong, J. S., et al. (2007). Systemic LPS causes chronic neuroinflammation and progressive neurodegeneration. *Glia, 55,* 453–462.

Rapoport, S. I. (1976). *Blood-brain barrier in physiology and medicine.* New York: Raven Press.

Rapoport, S. I., Ohata, M., & London, E. D. (1981). Cerebral blood flow and glucose utilization following opening of the blood-brain barrier and during maturation of the rat brain. *Fed Proc, 40,* 2322–2325.

Raub, T. J. & Audus, K. L. (1990). Adsorptive endocytosis and membrane recycling by cultured primary bovine brain microvessel endothelial cell monolayers. *J Cell Sci, 97,* 127–138.

Reese, T. S. & Karnovsky, M. J. (1967). Fine structural localization of a blood-brain barrier to exogenous peroxidase. *J Cell Biol, 34,* 207–217.

Rethelyi, M. (1984). Diffusional barrier around the hypothalamic arcuate nucleus in the rat. *Brain Res, 307,* 355–358.

Reyes, T. M., Fabry, Z., & Coe, C. L. (1999). Brain endothelial cell production of a neuroprotective cytokine, interleukin-6, in response to noxious stimuli. *Brain Res, 851,* 215–220.

Rodriguez, D. M., Blazquez, J. L., & Guerra, M. (2010). The design in the hypothalamus allows the median eminence and the arcuate nucleus to enjoy private milieus: The former opens to the portal blood and the latter to the cerebrospinal fluid. *Peptides, 31,* 757–76.

Romeo, G., Liu, W. H., Asnaghi, V., Kern, T. S., & Lorenzi, M. (2002). Activation of nuclear factor-kappaB induced by diabetes and high glucose regulates a proapoptotic program in retinal pericytes. *Diabetes, 51,* 2241–2248.

Sakata, A., Tamai, I., Kawazu, K., Deguchi, Y., Ohnishi, T., Saheki, A., et al. (1994). *In vivo* evidence for ATP-dependent and p-glycoprotein-mediated transport of cyclosporin A at the blood-brain barrier. *Biochem Pharmacol, 48,* 1989–1992.

Salkeni, M. A., Lynch, J. L., Price, T. O., & Banks, W. A. (2009). Lipopolysaccharide impairs blood-brain barrier P-glycoprotein function in mice through prostaglandin- and nitric oxide-independent pathways and nitric oxide-independent pathways. *J Neuroimmune Pharmacology, 4,* 276–282.

Sanders, V. J., Pittman, C. A., White, M. G., Wang, G., Wiley, C. A., & Achim, C. L. (1998). Chemokines and receptors in HIV encephalitis. *AIDS, 12,* 1021–1026.

Sands, M. S., Vogler, C., Kyle, J. W., Grubb, J. H., Levy, B., Galvin, N., et al. (1994). Enzyme replacement therapy for murine mucopolysaccharidosis type VII. *J Clin Invest, 93,* 2324–2331.

Schiffenbauer, J., Streit, W. J., Butfiloski, E., LaBow, M., Edward, C., & Moldawer, 3rd. L. L. (2000). The induction of EAE is only partially dependent on TNF receptor signaling but requires the IL-1 type 1 receptor. *Clin Immunol, 95,* 117–125.

Schwartz, M. W., Woods, S. C., Porte, D., Jr., Seeley, R. J., & Baskin, D. G. (2000). Central nervous system control of food intake. *Nature, 404,* 661–671.

Schweighardt, B. & Atwood, W. J. (2001). Virus receptors in the human central nervous system. *Journal of Neurovirology, 7,* 187–195.

Shafer, R. A. & Murphy, S. (1997). Activated astrocytes induce nitric oxide synthase-2 in cerebral endothelium via tumor necrosis factor alpha. *GLIA, 21,* 370–379.

Shibata, M., Yamada, S., Kumar, S. R., Calero, M., Bading, J., Frangione, B., et al. (2000). Clearance of Alzheimer's amyloid-β_{1-40} peptide from brain by LDL receptor-related protein-1 at the blood-brain barrier. *J Clin Invest, 106,* 1489–1499

Shimura, T., Tabata, S., Ohnishi, T., Terasaki, T., & Tsuji, A. (1991). Transport mechanism of a new behaviorally highly potent adrenocorticotropic hormone (ACTH) analog, ebiratide, through the blood-brain barrier. *J Pharmacol Exp Ther, 258,* 459–465.

Shyng, S. L., Huber, M. T., & Harris, E. C. (1993). A prion protein cycles between the cell surface and an endocytic compartment in cultured neoroblastome cells. *Biol Chem, 268,* 15922–15928.

Simpson, J. E., Newcombe, J., Cuzner, M. L., & Woodrofe, M. N. (1998). Expression of monocyte chemoattractant protein-1 and other beta-chemokines by resident glia and inflammatory cells in multiple sclerosis. *J Neuroimmunol, 84,* 238–249.

Somogyvari-Vigh, A., Pan, W., Reglodi, D., Kastin, A. J., & Arimura, A. (2000). Effect of middle cerebral artery occulsion on the passage of pituitary adenylate cyclase activating polypeptide across the blood-brain barrier in the rat. *Regul Pept, 91,* 89–95.

Spector, R. & Lorenzo, A. V. (1974). The effects of salicylate and probenecid on the cerebrospinal fluid transport of penicillin, aminosalicylic acid, and iodide. *J Pharmacol Exp Ther, 188,* 55–65.

Spranger, J., Verma, S., Gohring, I., Bobbert, T., Seifert, J., Sindler, A. L., et al. (2006) Adiponectin does not cross the blood-brain barrier, but modifies cytokine expression of brain endothelial cells. *Diabetes, 55,* 141–147.

Stein, U., Walther, W., & Shoemaker, R. H. (1996). Modulation of mdr1 expression by cytokines in human colon carcinoma cells: an approach for reversal of multidrug resistance. *British Journal of Cancer, 74,* 1384–1391.

Takasawa, M., Terasaki, T., Suzuki, H., & Sugiyama, Y. (1997). In vivo evidence for carrier-mediated efflux transport of 3'azido-3'deoxythymidine and 2',3'-dideoxyinosine across the blood-brain barrier via a probenecid-sensitive transport system. *J Pharmacol Exp Ther, 281,* 369–375.

Tanzi, R. E., Moir, R. D., & Wagner, S. L. (2004). Clearance of Alzheimer's Abeta peptide: The many roads to perdition. *Neuron, 43,* 608–608.

Taylor, E. M. (2002). The impact of efflux transporters in the brain on the development of drugs for CNS disorders. *Clinical Pharmacokinetics, 41,* 81–92.

Terasaki, T., Takakuwa, S., Saheki, A., Moritani, S., Shimura, T., Tabata, S., et al. (1992). Absorptive-mediated endocytosis of an adrenocorticotropic hormone (ACTH) analogue, ebiratide, into the blood-brain barrier: Studies with monolayers of primary cultured bovine brain capillary endothelial cells. *Pharm Res, 9,* 529–534.

Theron, D., de Lagerie, S. B., Tardivel, S., Pelerin, H., Demeuse, P., Mercier, C., et al. (2003). Influence of tumor necrosis factor-alpha on the expression and function of P-glycoprotein in an immortalized rat brain capillary endothelial cell line, GPNT. *Biochem Pharmacol, 66,* 579–587.

Thomas, S. A. (2004). Anti-HIV drug distribution to the central nervous system. *Current Pharmaceutical Design, 10,* 1313–1324.

Urayama, A., Grubb, J. H., Banks, W. A., & Sly, W. S. (2007). Epinephrine enhances lysosomal enzyme delivery across the blood-brain barrier by up-regulation of the mannos 6-phosphate receptor. *Proc Natl Acad Sci USA, 31,* 12873–12878.

Urayama, A., Grubb, J. H., Sly, W. S., & Banks, W. A. (2004). Developmentally regulated mannose 6-phosphate receptor-mediated transport of a lysosomal enzyme across the blood-brain barrier. *Proc Natl Acad Sci USA, 101,* 12658–12663.

Vadeboncoeur, N., Segura, M., Al-Numani, D., Vanier, G., & Gottschalk, M. (2003). Proinflammatory cytokine and chemokine release by human brain microvascular endothelial cells stimulated by *Streptococcus suis* serotype 2. FEMS *Immunology and Medical Microbiology, 35,* 49–58.

van Dam, A. M., De Vries, H. E., Kuiper, J., Zijlstra, F. J., De Boer, A. G., Tilders, F. J. H., et al. (1996). Interleukin-1 receptors on rat brain endothelial cells: A role in neuroimmune interaction? *FASEB J, 10,* 351–356.

Verma, S., Nakaoke, R., Dohgu, S., & Banks, W. A. (2006). Release of cytokines by brain endothelial cells: a polarized response to lipopolysaccharide. *Brain, Behavior, and Immunity, 20,* 449–455.

Vidal, E. L., Patel, N. A., Wu, G., Fiala, M., & Chang, S. L. (1998). Interleukin-1 induces the expression of mu-opioid receptors in endothelial cells. *Immunopharmacology, 38,* 261–266.

Villegas, J. C. & Broadwell, R. D. (1993). Transcytosis of protein through the mammalian cerebral epithelium and endothelium: II. Adsorptive transcytosis of WGA-HRP and the blood-brain and brain-blood barriers. *J Neurocytol, 22,* 67–80.

Vogler, C., Levy, B., Galvin, N. J., Thorpe, C., Sands, M. S., Barker, J. E., et al. (1999). Enzyme replacement in murine mucopolysaccharidosis type VII: Neuronal and glial response to beta-glucuronidase requires early initiation of enzyme replacement therapy. *Pediatric Research, 45,* 838–844.

Vorbrodt, A. W. (1994). Glycoconjugates and anionic sites in the blood-brain barrier. In: M. Nicolini & P. F. Zatta (Eds.). *Glycobiology and the brain,* pp. 37–62. Oxford: Pergamon Press.

Vorbrodt, A. W. & Dobrogowska, D. H. (1994). Immunocytochemical evaluation of blood-brain barrier to endogenous albumin in adult, newborn, and aged mice. *Folia Histochemica et Cytobiologica, 32,* 63–70.

Vorbrodt, A. W., Dobrogowska, D. H., Ueno, M., & Lossinsky, A. S. (1995). Immunocytochemical studies of protamine-induced blood-brain barrier opening to endogenous albumin. *Acta Neuropathol (Berl), 89,* 491–499.

Vorbrodt, A. W. & Trowbridge, R. S. (1991). Ultrastructural study of transcellular transport of native and cationized albumin in cultured sheep brain microvascular endothelium. *J Neurocytol, 20,* 998–1006.

Walsh, R. J., Slaby, F. J., & Posner, B. I. (1987). A receptor-mediated mechanism for the transport of prolactin from blood to cerebrospinal fluid. *Endocrinology, 120,* 1846–1850.

Wang, Y. & Sawchuck, R. J. (1995). Zidovudine transport in the rabbit brain during intravenous and intracerebroventricular infusion. *J Pharm Sci, 7,* 871–876.

Westergren, I. & Johansson, B. B. (1993). Altering the blood-brain barrier in the rat by intracarotid infusion of polycations: A comparison between protamine, poly-L-lysine and poly-L-arginine. *Acta Physiol Scand, 149,* 99–104.

Widner, H., Jonsson, B. A., Hallstadius, L., Wingardh, K., Strand, S. E., & Johansson, B. B. (1987). Scintigraphic method to quantify the passage from brain parenchyma to the deep cervical lymph nodes in the rat. *European Journal of Nuclear Medicine, 13,* 456–461.

Williams, K. C. & Hickey, W. F. (1995). Traffic of hematogenous cells through the central nervous system. *Current Topics in Microbiology and Immunology, 202,* 221–245.

Wilson, J. F., Anderson, S., Snook, G., & Llewellyn, K. D. (1984). Quantification of the permeability of the blood-CSF barrier to α–MSH in the rat. *Peptides, 5,* 681–685.

Wolburg, H., Wolburg-Buchholz, K., & Engelhardt, B. (2005). Diapedesis of mononuclear cells across cerebral venules during experimental autoimmune encephalomyelitis leaves tight junctions intact. *Acta Neuropathol, 109,* 181–190.

Wu, D., Clement, J. G., & Pardridge, W. M. (1998). Low blood-brain barrier permeability to azidothymidine (AZT), 3TC, and thymidine in the rat. *Brain Res, 791,* 313–316.

Xaio, H., Banks, W. A., Niehoff, M. L., & Morley, J. E. (2001). Effect of LPS on the permeability of the blood-brain barrier to insulin. *Brain Res, 896,* 36–42.

Yamada, S., DePasquale, M., Patlak, C. S., & Cserr, H. F. (1991). Albumin outflow into deep cervical lymph from different regions of rabbit brain. *Am J Physiol, 261,* H1197–H1204.

Yeagle, P. (1987). Transport. *The membranes of cells*, pp. 191–215. Orlando, FL: Academic Press, Inc.,

Yu, C., Kastin, A. J., Tu, H., Waters, S., & Pan, W. (2007). TNF activates P-glycoprotein in cerebral microvascular endothelial cells. *Cell Physiol Biochem, 20*, 853–858.

Zalcman, S. S. (2001). Interleukin-2 potentiates novelty—and GBR 12909-induced exploratory activity. *Brain Res, 899*, 1–9.

Zalcman, S. S. (2002). Interleukin-2-induced increases in climbing behavior: inhibition by dopamine D-1 and D-2 receptor antagonists. *Brain Res, 944*, 157–164.

Zambenedetti, P. Giordano, R., & Zatta, P. (1996). Indentification of lectin binding sites in the rat brain. *Glycoconjugate Journal, 13*, 341–346.

Zlokovic, B. V. (2005). Neurovascular mechanisms of Alzheimer's neuro-degeneration. *Trends Neurosci, 28*, 202–208.

3.2

ENDOTHELIAL CELL BIOLOGY AND HIV-1 INFECTION

Michal Toborek, Ibolya E. András, Cetewayo S. Rashid,
Yu Zhong, and Shinsuke Nakagawa

An understanding of endothelial cell function both systemically and in the central nervous system is relevant to many aspects of HIV-1-associated disease. Endothelial cells produce a variety of biologically active factors (e.g., nitric oxide, prostacyclin, chemokines) that control vascular permeability, vessel tone, coagulation, fibrinolysis, and inflammatory responses. These factors can be generated by other vascular cells, as well as nonvascular cells. Alterations of normal endothelial cell biology have critical significance in the development of vascular and neurovascular pathology during HIV-1 infection. For example, such alterations can contribute to disruption of the blood-brain barrier (BBB), to HIV-1 entry into the brain, to the development of vasculopathies, and to atherosclerosis. The underlying mechanisms appear to be related to induction of oxidative stress and alterations of redox-related signaling. Vascular toxicity may be induced by HIV-1 itself or it can be mediated by a variety of HIV-1-specific proteins, as well as by antiretroviral drugs.

INTRODUCTION

The endothelium separates the blood elements from the extravascular tissues. Such a position at the interface between the bloodstream and interstitial fluid is chiefly responsible for the strategic functions of the vascular endothelium in the entry of HIV-1 from the bloodstream into the underlying tissues and for the development of vascular pathology associated with HIV-1 infection. Endothelial cells express an apical-basal polarity with specific composition of the luminal and abluminal sites. The luminal membrane is negatively charged due to a cover by a complex cell coat that consists of glycoproteins, glycolipids, and proteoglycans. The cell coat can bind enzymes, such as lipoprotein lipase and angiotensin-converting enzymes, which are synthesized at different locations and secondarily attached to the endothelium. The enrichment of the luminal membranes with oligosaccharide moieties allows maintaining a nonthrombogenic surface. The luminal site of endothelial cells also contains numerous receptors. Specific for brain microvascular endothelial cells (BMEC) is the polarity in localization of efflux transporters. BMEC closely interact with astrocytes, pericytes, and neurons to create a complex structure of cell-cell interactions called a neurovascular unit (Figure 3.2.1), which is responsible for the integrity of the blood-brain barrier (Abbott, Ronnback, & Hansson, 2006).

The vascular endothelium is a critical structure that regulates blood-interstitial fluid exchange of molecules and vascular permeability. In addition, the endothelium is involved in regulation of vascular tone, coagulation and fibrinolysis, and inflammatory responses (Miller, Budzyn, & Sobey, 2010; Toborek & Kaiser, 1999). Both the peripheral and brain endothelium are targets for HIV-1 (Crowe et al., 2010; Persidsky, Ramirez, Haorah, & Kanmogne, 2006b; Roberts, Buckner, & Berman, 2010; Toborek et al., 2005). In the present chapter, we describe the changes in the biology of the vascular endothelium relevant to HIV-1 infection.

HIV-1-ASSOCIATED VASCULOPATHIES

The association of HIV-1 infection with brain and peripheral vascular diseases is well documented. HIV-1 vasculopathy can be manifested by a variety of syndromes that depend on the affected vascular beds. Morphologically, HIV-1-induced vasculopathy is characterized by small vessel thickening, dilatation of the perivascular space, infiltration with inflammatory cells, and mineralization of the vessel wall. However, HIV-1 infection can also affect larger vessels and thus contribute to the development of atherosclerosis and coronary heart disease. HIV-1 can also infect human arterial smooth muscle, further contributing to the development of vasculopathy of large vessels (Eugenin et al., 2008).

Intracranial aneurysms have been reported primarily in pediatric cases of HIV-1 infection, although recently they have also been described in adult cases. The literature on this subject appears to be limited to 30 case reports in the pediatric literature and 12 adult cases. Pediatric cases revealed fusiform aneurysmal dilation of large arteries of the circle of Willis. Adults with HIV-1-associated intracranial aneurysms are usually significantly immunosuppressed with CD4 count below 200 cells/mm^3 and viral load greater than 100,000 copies/ml. The underlying pathology is unknown; however, HIV-1-mediated activation of inflammatory mediators (discussed later in this chapter) may lead to vascular remodeling resulting in aneurysm formation. HIV-1 sequences in the intracerebral artery were detected in a pediatric case of intracranial aneurysm (Goldstein, Timpone, & Cupps, 2010).

Vasculitis is another vasculopathy associated with HIV-1 infection. It occurs in approximately 1% of infected patients, although one study reported the frequency of vasculitis at

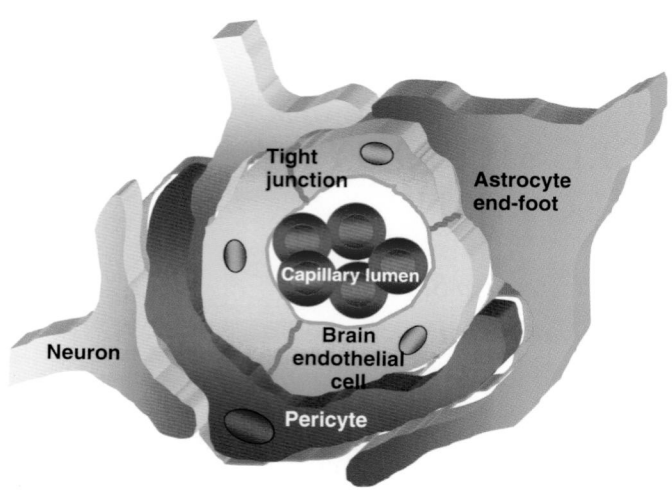

Figure 3.2.1 Schematic diagram of the neurovascular unit. Brain microvascular endothelial cells (colored in yellow) are sealed together by tight junctions and remain in close contact with pericytes (blue), astrocytes (green), and neurons (pink).

23% of HIV-1-positive individuals. The most affected vascular beds are those located in the brain, skin, and neuromuscular tissues. Nevertheless, several other sites, such as the lung, gastrointestinal tract, oropharynx, and kidney can also be affected. The development of vasculitis has been linked directly to the influence of HIV-1 as well as co-infections with cytomegalovirus, Epstein-Barr virus, herpes simplex virus, toxoplasmosis, pneumocystis, salmonella, and Mycobacterium tuberculosis (Chetty, 2001). Vasculitis of the cerebral vessels can result in the opening of the BBB, providing the entry of HIV-1 into the central nervous system.

The direct association of HIV-1 infection with the development of stroke is difficult to establish because no HIV-1 or viral products were detected in the cerebral arteries of stroke patients. The prevalence of stroke in HIV-1-positive individuals of age 15–44 was estimated between 9–12%. In children, the incidence of stroke is approximately 1.3% per year. In a large population of stroke patients, 6% were found to be HIV-1 positive (Nagel, Mahalingam, Cohrs, & Gilden, 2010).

Other vasculopathies associated with HIV-1 infection include coronary vasculopathy, endocarditis, and pulmonary hypertension (Sudano et al., 2006). Retinovascular changes are common during HIV-1 infection with the common changes including the loss of the retinal endothelium and focal occlusions. In addition, retinal endothelial cells were shown to support productive HIV-1 infection (Holland, 2008).

INTERACTION OF HIV-1 AND HIV-1 PROTEINS WITH ENDOTHELIAL CELLS

There are conflicting data whether endothelial cells can be infected by HIV-1. Because no CD4 receptors or galactosylceramide binding sites are present on the vascular endothelium, nonconventional pathways have been considered to participate in the interaction between HIV-1 and vascular endothelial cells.

The consensus appears to be that HIV-1 does not productively infect endothelial cells; nevertheless, small amounts of HIV-1 can be taken up by endothelial cells via a transcellular route that involves lipid rafts and/or heparan sulfate proteoglycans (Argyris et al., 2003; Banks, Ercal, & Price, 2006). Cholesterol depletion, inhibition of micropinocytosis, heparin, and inhibition of mitogen-activated protein kinase (MAPK) signaling pathway can block HIV-1 uptake by endothelial cells. Infection of endothelial cells by HIV-1 is noncytopathic and noncytolytic. One of the possible outcomes of HIV-1 entry into endothelial cells is fusion with lysosomes, followed by lysis of the virus. Nevertheless, it was also demonstrated that HIV-1 can be transported from luminal side to basolateral space of endothelial cells. It was hypothesized that adsorptive endocytosis by BMEC may contribute to the entry of HIV-1 into the brain (Banks et al., 2006) (Figure 3.2.2).

The severity of AIDS pathology and HIV-1 infection often does not correlate directly with viral titers. This fact drove the hypothesis that the effects of HIV-1 infection may be mediated by soluble viral proteins, such as Tat protein, that are released from the infected cells. Tat plays a critical role in viral gene expression and replication. However, having a highly positively charged cell attachment domain, it is able to cross cell membranes and induce a variety of cellular effects. Tat mRNA and protein levels were detected in the brains of AIDS patients, which support a neuropathological significance of this protein (Hudson et al., 2000). It is believed that the interactions between HIV-1 proteins and the vascular endothelium have a major impact on the vascular pathogenesis associated with HIV-1 infection.

The mechanisms underlying the binding of Tat with the cell surface are far from being completely understood; however, lipid rafts and caveolae appear to play an important role in this process (Figure 3.2.2). They are cholesterol- and sphingomyelin-rich membrane microdomains that are believed to be critical in signal transduction by providing important platforms for signaling molecules. Caveolae represent a special group of lipid rafts that is abundant in vascular endothelial cells and believed to play a regulatory role in endothelial functions. The main proteins of caveolae are caveolins, 21–24-kDa integral membrane proteins (Xu, Buikema, van Gilst, & Henning, 2008).

Tat was shown to interact with cell surface and caveolae-localized receptors, such as chemokine receptors CCR2, CCR3, CXCR4, vascular endothelial growth factor receptor-1 (VEGFR-1), and VEGFR-2 (reviewed in Toborek et al., 2005). Tat can enter the cells through the interaction of its basic domain with cell-surface heparan-sulfate proteoglycans (Rusnati et al., 1999). Tat fusion proteins can also be taken up by caveolar endocytosis via a lipid raft-dependent process (Fittipaldi et al., 2003). Finally, it was shown that Tat can mimic extracellular matrix proteins and bind to $\alpha v \beta 3$ and $\alpha 5 \beta 1$ integrins through the arginine-glycine-aspartic domain (Toschi et al., 2006) (Figure 3.2.2).

In addition to Tat, several other HIV-1 proteins were also demonstrated to interact with lipid rafts and/or endothelial cells. The HIV-1 envelope glycoprotein is synthesized as a precursor protein (gp160), which is cleaved into the surface

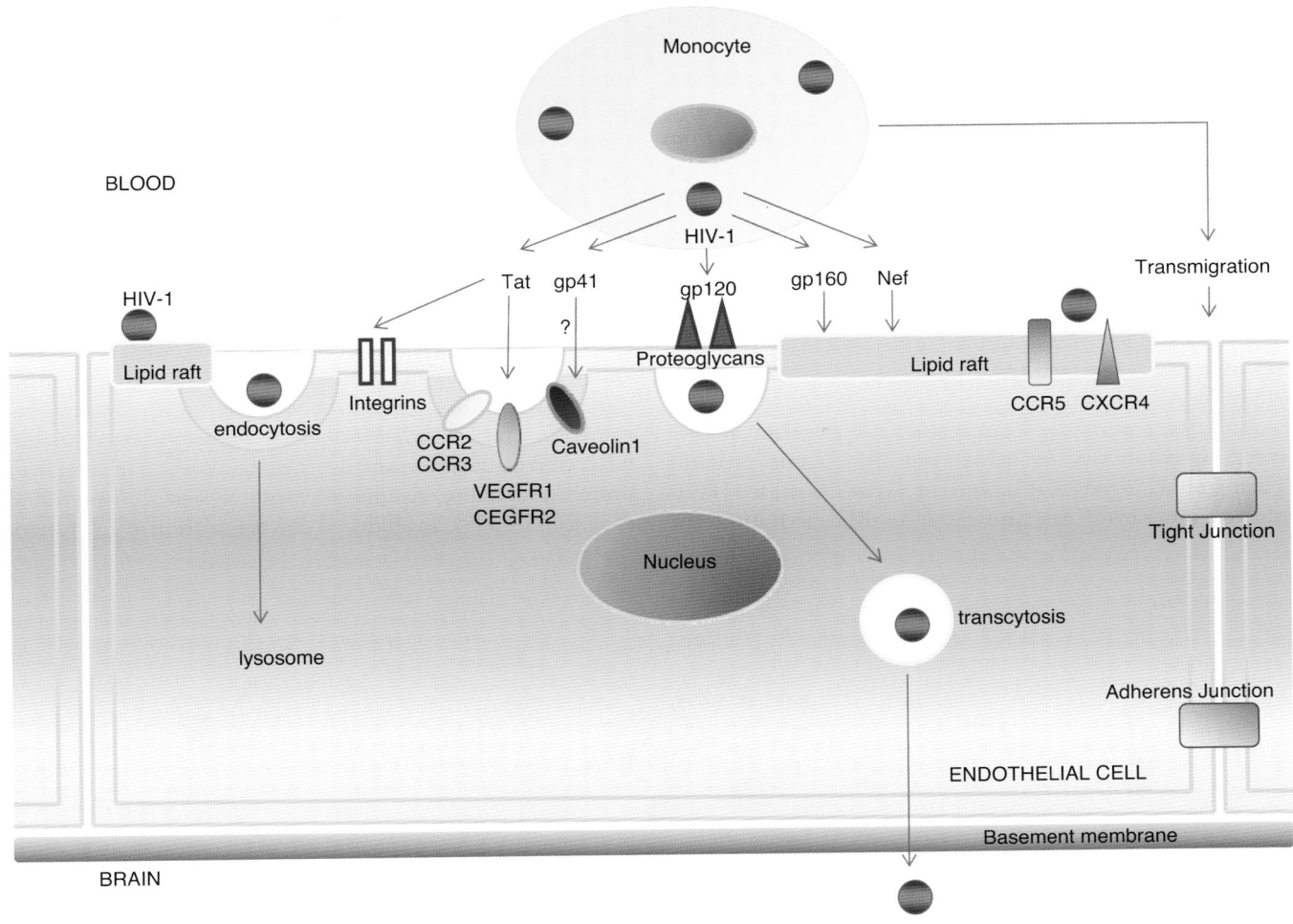

Figure 3.2.2 Interaction of HIV-1 and HIV-1 proteins with endothelial cells. Adsorptive endocytosis may contribute to the uptake of HIV-1 by endothelial cells via a transcellular route that involves lipid rafts/caveolae and/or heparan sulfate proteoglycans. HIV-1 can either cross the endothelial monolayer to be transferred into the brain or be degraded in lysosomes. HIV-1 proteins, such as Tat, gp41, gp120, gp160, or Nef, may interact with integrins, chemokine receptors (CCR2, CCR3, CCR5, CXCR4), and lipid raft/caveolae-localized receptors (e.g., vascular endothelial growth factor receptor-2 [VEGFR2]).

glycoprotein (gp120) and the transmembrane protein (gp41). A recent report demonstrated and characterized the binding of gp140 to chemokine receptor CXCR4 in human brain microvascular endothelial cells (HBMEC) (Mendu, Katinger, Sodroski, & Kim, 2007). In addition, several biological effects of Nef appeared to be associated with lipid rafts (Wang, Kiyokawa, Verdin, & Trono, 2000); however, none of these studies involved vascular endothelial cells.

HIV-1-INDUCED ALTERATIONS OF ENDOTHELIAL BARRIER FUNCTION AND TIGHT JUNCTION INTEGRITY

Regulation of endothelial permeability is one of the main biological functions of the vascular endothelium. Tight junctions (TJs) between endothelial cells represent the morphological basis of the vascular integrity. Well-developed TJs are characteristic of the brain endothelium, where they play a major role in brain homeostasis by restricting paracellular flux

and permeability across the brain endothelium. Transmembrane TJ proteins, such as occludin, claudins, and junctional adhesion molecules (JAMs) are responsible for sealing together BMEC. Transmembrane proteins are linked to the actin cytoskeleton by TJ accessory proteins, such as zonula occludens (ZO)-1, ZO-2, and ZO-3 (Abbott et al., 2006) (Figure 3.2.3).

There is strong evidence of BBB alterations in HIV-1 infection. In AIDS patients, cortical vessels are enlarged with thinning of the basal lamina, decreased collagen IV, and loss of glycoproteins from the endothelial cell surface. Pathological evidence, CSF data, and dynamic magnetic resonance imaging all support the notion of BBB damage in HIV-1 infection. It was also noticed that BBB changes are more frequent in HIV-1-infected patients with dementia as compared to nondemented HIV-1-positive individuals (reviewed in Toborek et al, 2005). Changes in brain permeability in HIV-1-infected brains are accompanied by disruption of TJs. Fragmentation of occludin, claudin-5, and ZO-1 immunoreactivity is observed in human brain tissues with HIV-1-associated encephalitis or dementia (Chaudhuri, Yang, Gendelman, Persidsky, &

Kanmogne, 2008; Dallasta et al., 1999; Persidsky et al., 2006a). Loss of ZO-1 immunoreactivity appears to be correlated with monocyte infiltration and the degree of dementia (Boven, Middel, Verhoef, De Groot, & Nottet, 2000).

Experimental research fully confirms the deleterious effects of HIV-1 on endothelial integrity. Exposure of HBMEC to HIV-1-infected leukocytes evoked reduction in expression of several TJ proteins and increased transendothelial migration of infected leukocytes (Chaudhuri et al., 2008; Eugenin et al., 2006; Huang, Eum, Andras, Hennig, & Toborek, 2009). These changes were associated with increased expression of matrix metalloproteinase (MMP)-2 and MMP-9 and were prevented by STAT1 inhibition (Chaudhuri et al., 2008). Research from our laboratory demonstrated that HIV-1-induced alterations of TJ protein expression can be protected by inhibition of MMP and proteasome activities (Huang et al., 2009). Co-culture of HBMEC with HIV-1-infected monocytes can also result in Rho activation and

Rho-dependent phosphorylation of occludin and claudin-5 (Persidsky et al., 2006a). Phosphorylated occludin and claudin-5 were detected at cell borders of BMEC in a mouse model of HIV-1-associated encephalitis, supporting the notion that changes in TJ phosphorylation might contribute to the BBB pathology during HIV-1 infection (Yamamoto et al., 2008).

Extensive research has been devoted to evaluate the effects of HIV-1 proteins Tat and gp120 on the expression of TJ proteins and transendothelial migration of monocytes (Figure 3.2.3). Experimental evidence indicates that exposure to Tat can increase endothelial permeability via tyrosine kinase and MAPK pathways (Oshima et al., 2000) and evoke recruitment and transmigration of monocytes across an in vitro BBB model (Weiss, Nath, Major, & Berman, 1999). The mechanisms of increased endothelial permeability are related to Tat-induced redistribution and decreased expression of several TJ proteins, including claudin-5, claudin-1, and ZO-2 (Andras et al., 2003, 2005). Tat-induced downregulation of TJ proteins

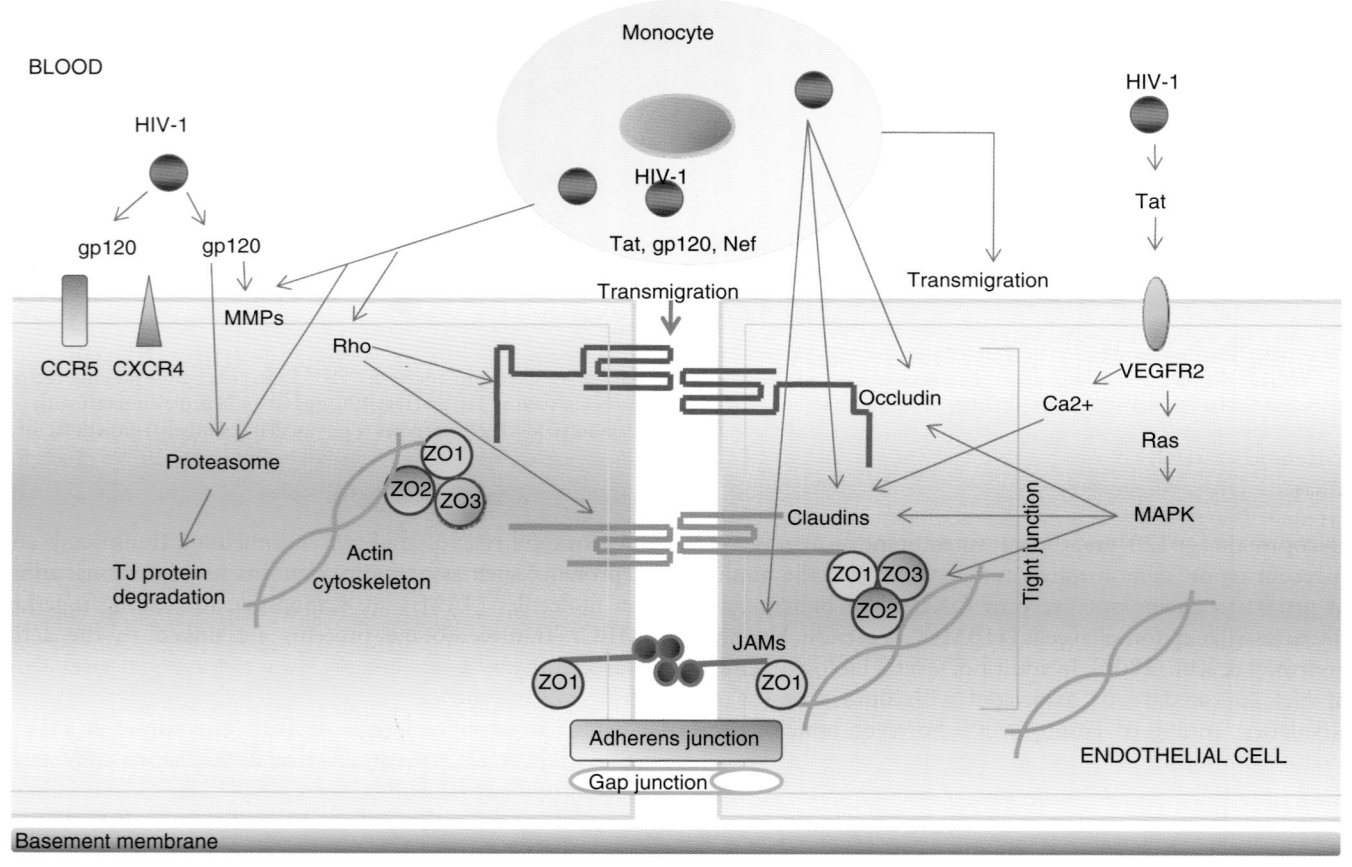

Figure 3.2.3 HIV-1-induced alterations of endothelial barrier function and tight junction integrity. Occludin, claudins, and junctional adhesion molecules (JAMs) are transmembrane tight junction (TJ) proteins. Zonula occludens (ZO)-1, ZO-2, and ZO-3 are TJ-associated proteins that link the transmembrane TJ proteins with actin cytoskeleton. TJs, adherens junctions, and gap junctions can all interact with each other and share the scaffold ZO-1 protein. Exposure of brain endothelial cells to HIV-1-infected monocytes or HIV-1-specific proteins (e.g., Tat, gp120, or Nef) can alter the expression of TJ proteins and promote transendothelial migration of infected monocytes. Degradation of TJ proteins by matrix metalloproteinases (MMPs) and/or proteasome may participate in this process. Rho-dependent phosphorylation of TJ proteins and activation of other redox-regulated signal transduction pathways (e.g., Ras or mitogen-activated protein kinase [MAPK]) also contributes to the altered endothelial permeability. Several Tat-mediated effects may be mediated by activation of vascular endothelial growth factor receptor-2 (VEGFR2). Gp120 interacts with endothelial cells via CCR5 and CXCR4 chemokine receptors.

appears to be regulated at the transcriptional level (Andras et al., 2005) via activation of VEGFR-2 and multiple redox-regulated signal transduction pathways that include the MAPK and phosphoinositide-3-kinase (PI3K) signaling (Andras et al., 2005). These results are supported by the observations that injections of Tat into the hippocampus or into the bloodstream result in a decrease of ZO-1 expression and are associated with inflammatory cell invasion in brain tissue in mice (Pu et al., 2005, 2007). ZO-1 alterations are diminished by the inhibition of the MAPK signaling and by treatment with antioxidant N-acetylcysteine (NAC) (Pu et al., 2005).

Recent studies indicated also the role of caveolae in Tat-induced disruption of endothelial permeability (Figure 3.2.3). Exposure to Tat diminished the expression of occludin, ZO-1, and ZO-2 mainly in the caveolar fraction of HBMEC. These alterations were diminished by pharmacological inhibition of the caveolae-associated Ras signaling and by silencing of caveolin-1 (Zhong et al., 2008). Another mechanism of Tat-induced alterations of endothelial permeability may involve activation of focal adhesion kinase (FAK), followed by the rearrangement of cytoskeletal organization (Avraham, Jiang, Lee, Prakash, & Avraham, 2004).

Recently, the effects of Tat derived from HIV-1 clade B and clade C were investigated using an in vitro co-culture model of primary HBMEC with astrocytes. Exposure to Tat B damaged the integrity of endothelial monolayers to a higher extent than treatment with Tat C. These effects were accompanied by increased transendothelial migration of monocytes. Thus, Tat B and C may contribute differently to HIV-1-associated neurological disorders (Gandhi et al., 2010).

Several reports demonstrated that exposure to gp120 can disrupt endothelial integrity in vitro (Kanmogne et al., 2007; Nakamuta et al., 2008) and in vivo in gp120-overexpressing mice (Cioni & Annunziata, 2002), resulting in enhanced monocyte migration (Figure 3.2.3). The involvement of endothelial receptors CCR5 and CXCR4, myosin light chain kinase, and protein kinase C (PKC) was demonstrated in these events. The gp120-induced intracellular calcium release appeared to be CCR5- and partly CXCR4-dependent. Thus, exposure to gp120 can cause alterations of the BBB through the PKC pathway and receptor-mediated intracellular calcium release, followed by cytoskeletal changes associated with increased monocyte transmigration. Gp120-induced disruption of endothelial permeability was also associated with alterations of TJ protein expression. Finally, the mechanisms of gp120-induced loss of endothelial integrity may include degradation of TJ proteins by the proteasome (Nakamuta et al., 2008) or MMP-9 (Louboutin, Agrawal, Reyes, Van Bockstaele, & Strayer, 2010).

HIV-1-INDUCED ALTERATIONS OF ADHERENS AND GAP JUNCTIONS AND CELL-CELL COMMUNICATION IN THE VASCULAR ENDOTHELIUM

In addition to TJs, plasma membranes of adjacent endothelial cells form complex junctional structures called adherens junctions and gap junctions (Figure 3.2.3). Adherens junctions consist of transmembrane cadherins and cytoplasmic attached α-catenins and β-catenins assembled together into a multiprotein complex. This complex organization of cadherin-catenins and the cytoskeleton strengthens cell-cell adhesion and has a role in signal transduction. Gap junctions, composed of integral membrane proteins from the connexin family, are intercellular channels that connect the cytoplasm of neighboring cells allowing the diffusional exchange of small metabolites, second messengers, ions, and other molecules of molecular weight lower than 1 kDa (Giepmans, 2004). Gap junctions play a prominent role in cell-cell communication. There is relatively little information available on the effects of HIV-1 infection on adherens and gap junctions (Eugenin & Berman, 2007; Salim et al., 2008).

Indirect evidence suggests that adherens and gap junctions may be involved in HIV-1-induced dysfunction of the vascular endothelium. It is known that TJs, adherens junctions, and gap junctions can all interact with each other (Giepmans, 2004). In addition, they share the scaffold ZO-1 protein, which is one of the targets of HIV-1-induced alteration of BMEC. In addition, leukocytes can communicate with endothelial cells via adherens and gap junctions (Véliz, González, Duling, Sáez, & Boric, 2008). Treatment with a gap junction blocker was shown to reduce monocyte/macrophage transmigration across a BBB model. The generation of inflammatory mediators may also be regulated by gap junction communication (Eugenin & Berman, 2007). These facts raise the possibility that adherens and gap junctions may play a role in the inflammatory processes induced by HIV-1 in the vascular endothelium.

HIV-1-INDUCED INFLAMMATORY REACTIONS IN THE VASCULAR ENDOTHELIUM

The development of inflammatory reactions within the vascular endothelium is a normal defense mechanism in response to injury or activation of the vessel wall. The physiologic significance of such reactions is to maintain and repair normal structure and function of the vessel wall. On the other hand, abundant inflammatory reactions with the subsequent and disconcerted self-perpetuating inflammatory pathology can expedite disease progression and lead to vascular pathology (Hansson, 2005). Endothelial cells actively produce chemokines (e.g., CCL2, also called monocyte chemoattractant protein-1 [MCP-1]), adhesion molecules of the selectin family (P-selectin, E-selectin or L-selectin), adhesion molecules of the immunoglobulin superfamily (e.g., intercellular adhesion molecule-1 [ICAM-1], vascular cell adhesion molecule-1 [VCAM-1], and platelet-endothelial cell adhesion molecule-1 [PECAM-1]), and also a wide spectrum of cytokines, including tumor necrosis factor-α (TNFα), interleukin (IL)-1β, IL-6, and IL-8 (reviewed in Toborek & Kaiser, 1999). During HIV-1 infection, inflammatory reactions that involve the vascular endothelium can lead to the loss of endothelial barrier function and/or the development of HIV-1-associated vasculopathies. In the central nervous system,

HIV-1-induced endothelial dysfunction results in disruption of the BBB and virus entry into the brain. One of the consequences of HIV-1-induced dysfunction of peripheral endothelial cells is accelerated atherosclerosis, which appears to be independent on dyslipoproteinemia caused by protease inhibitors.

Endothelial cell dysfunction that occurs in HIV-1-infected patients appears to result from the direct cytopathic effects of viral infection and/or the effects of viral proteins on uninfected bystander endothelial cells. AIDS patients also have major morphological changes of the aortic endothelium. Specific changes include an irregular architecture of the endothelial cell layer, small denuded areas of the endothelium, and abnormal shape and size of endothelial cells with some nuclei being pyknotic. In addition, leukocyte adherence to the aortic endothelium is increased significantly. These changes are accompanied by a marked upregulation of the VCAM-1 and E-selectin. In fact, more than 50% of HIV-1-infected patients display increased immunopositive staining for these adhesion molecules. The endothelium turnover is increased and approximately one half of the HIV-1-infected patients exhibit HLA-DR (major histocompatibility complex class II) antigen in the aortic endothelium (Zietz et al., 1996).

HIV-1-infected patients are in a state of persistent oxidative stress that results in chronic inflammation (Gil et al., 2003; Melendez, McNurlan, Mynarcik, Khan, & Gelato, 2008;

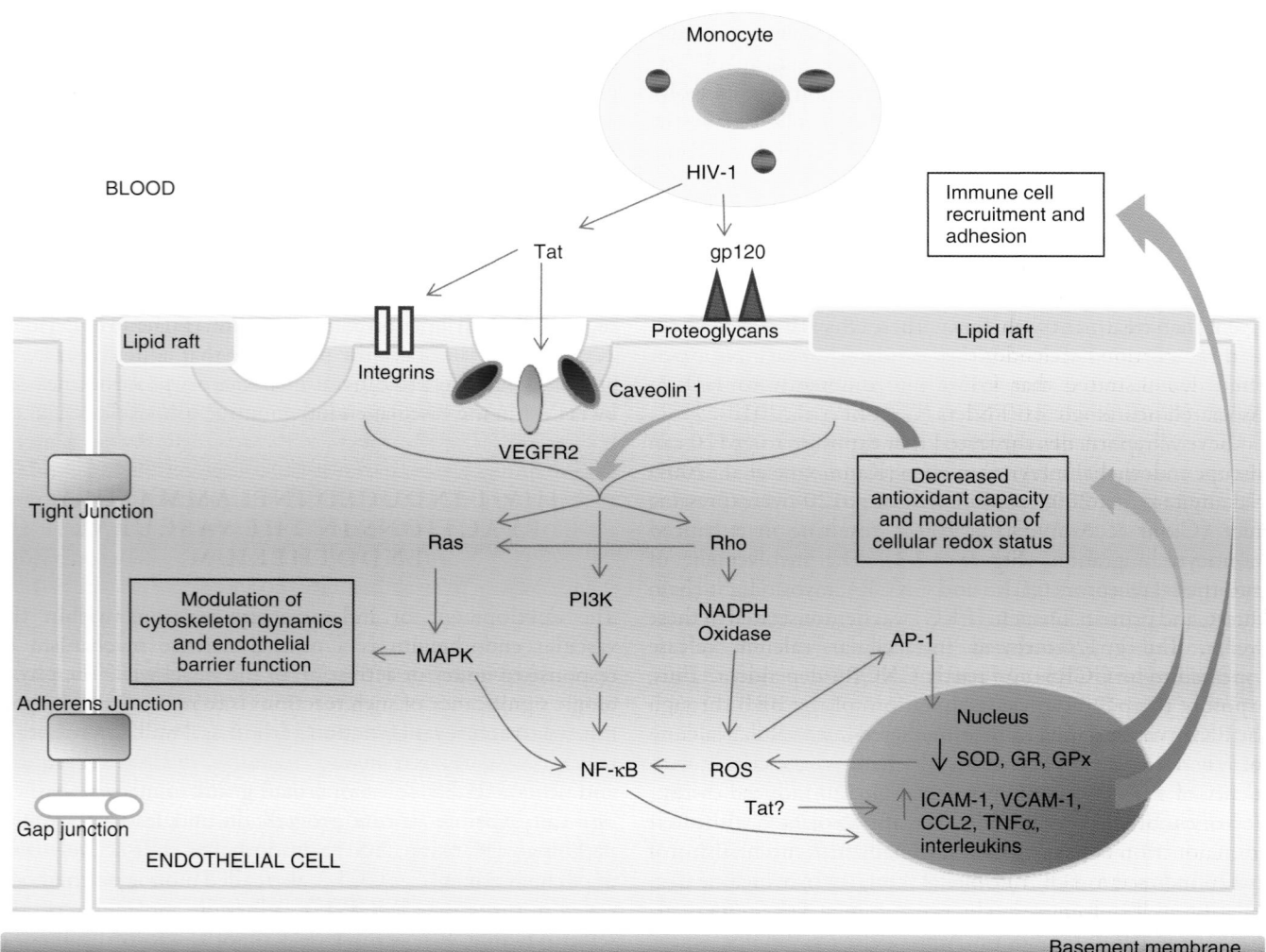

Figure 3.2.4 HIV-1-induced alterations of endothelial cell redox status and induction of inflammatory responses in the vascular endothelium. Exposure to HIV-1 and HIV-1 proteins (e.g., Tat or gp120) can simulate specific cellular receptors (e.g., VEGFR2) and caveolae-associated signaling molecules, such as the Ras and Rho subfamily of small monomeric G proteins or phosphoinositide-3-kinase (PI3K). Stimulation of NADPH oxidase contributes to the induction of cellular oxidative stress. Attenuation of antioxidant capacity due to downregulation of antioxidant enzymes (e.g., SOD, GPx, or GR) further propagates alteration of redox status and the subsequent activation of transcription factors (e.g., STAT1, NF-κB, and AP-1) that are involved in stimulation of inflammatory genes (CAM, CCL-2, TNFα, and/or inflammatory cytokines). Abbreviations: AP-1, activator protein-1; GPx, glutathione peroxidase; GR, glutathione reductase; ICAM-1, intercellular adhesion molecule-1; NF-κB, nuclear factor-κB; SOD, superoxide dismutase; VCAM-1, vascular cell adhesion molecule-1; VEGFR, vascular endothelial growth factor receptor.

Suresh, Annam, Pratibha, & Prasad, 2009) (Figure 3.2.4). Oxidative stress is defined as an imbalance of pro-oxidant production of reactive oxygen species (ROS) including superoxide, hydroxyl radicals, peroxynitrite, and hydrogen peroxide, and the antioxidant activities responsible for their removal, such as superoxide dismutases, catalase, glutathione, or glutathione peroxidase. Imbalanced oxidant production modifies proteins, membrane lipids, and DNA, thereby compromising cellular, tissue, and whole body function. Both HIV-1 asymptomatic and symptomatic patients have elevated serum levels of malondialdehyde (MDA), a product of lipid peroxidation and a marker of oxidative stress. Elevated levels of MDA are associated with reduced serum superoxide dismutase activity, reduced levels of vitamins C and E, and decreased total antioxidant capacity (Gil et al., 2003; Suresh et al., 2009). These clinical data are supported by in vivo experiments based on the HIV transgenic rat model. Increased oxidative stress in vascular tissues was demonstrated in these animals by increased dihydroethidium staining in aortic slices and elevated levels of superoxide as measured by electron spin resonance (Kline et al., 2008).

Compelling evidence indicates that the vascular endothelium is susceptible to HIV-1-induced oxidative stress and alterations of tissue redox status (Figure 3.2.4). For example, HIV-1-infected individuals have elevated serum levels of soluble ICAM-1, VCAM-1, and tumor necrosis factor receptor type 2 (sTNFR2), all of which are markers of peripheral vascular inflammation (Melendez et al., 2008). A different clinical study demonstrated that HIV-1 patients have significantly higher plasma levels of TNFα, IL-6, and von Willebrand factor (vWF). Notably, the levels of vWF and tissue-type plasminogen activator (t-PA), that is, the markers of endothelial dysfunction, were higher in AIDS patients as compared to HIV-1 infected nonAIDS patients. Furthermore, vWF and t-PA levels correlated with IL-6 and viral load, with vWF showing significant negative correlation with CD4 count (de Larrañaga, Petroni, Deluchi, Alonso, & Benetucci, 2003).

Because HIV-1 proteins and HIV-1-induced cytokines and chemokines coexist spatially and temporally, it is often difficult to ascribe an endothelial cell effect or pathology to the virion, a particular viral protein, or to an induced inflammatory mediator. Therefore, extensive research was devoted to evaluate the effects of HIV-1 proteins on endothelial cell inflammatory responses. BMEC stimulated with Tat showed a dose-dependent induction of cellular oxidative stress measured as 2′,7′-dichlorofluorescein (DCF) fluorescence, which mirrored a dose-dependent decrease in glutathione levels indicating alteration of cellular redox status. Exposure to Tat also activated redox-sensitive transcription factors nuclear factor-κB (NF-κB) and activator protein-1 (AP-1) (Toborek et al., 2003). These results are important because these transcription factors regulate induction of genes involved in inflammation including chemokines, inflammatory cytokines, and adhesion molecules.

HIV-1-induced dysfunction of peripheral endothelial cells may also be attributed to the interaction of HIV-1 viral proteins with the vascular endothelium (Figure 3.2.4). Experimental studies have demonstrated a direct impact of HIV-1 proteins gp120 and Tat on disruption of integrity of peripheral endothelium and induced expression of endothelial adhesion molecules ICAM-1 and VCAM-1, followed by transendothelial migration of monocytes (Kanmogne et al., 2007). In addition, Tat-induced endothelial cell augmentation of adhesion molecule expression and leukocyte adhesion was further enhanced by a co-treatment with TNFα, demonstrating interplay between HIV-1 proteins and cytokines in induction of inflammatory responses in vascular endothelial cells (Jiang et al., 2010).

In agreement with cell culture studies, injection of Tat into the mouse hippocampus resulted in elevated levels of CCL2, VCAM-1, ICAM-1, and TNFα mRNA in the hippocampus, frontal cortex, and corpus striatum. Immunohistochemical staining revealed increased immunoreactivity of CCL2 and VCAM-1, but not TNFα or ICAM-1 in endothelial cells of cerebral vessels. Tat exposure also increased infiltration of the brain with monocytes, implicating the enhanced recruitment and adhesion of peripheral blood mononuclear cells into activated brain endothelium (Pu et al., 2003).

Activation of the Rho family GTPases is also involved in inflammatory responses induced by HIV-1 and HIV-1 proteins (Figure 3.2.4). Exposure to Tat results in a rapid activation of RhoA, Rac1, and Cdc42. Rho activation has been ascribed to mediate the disruption of endothelial integrity, permitting transendothelial migration of HIV-1-infected monocytes. Tat and gp120 can also activate the Ras signaling cascade, leading to activation of the MAPK pathway and contributing to endothelial barrier disruption (Andras et al., 2005; Persidsky et al., 2006a; Ramirez et al., 2008; Zhong et al., 2008, Zhong, Hennig, & Toborek, 2010).

Evidence from clinical, animal, and cell culture studies indicates that HIV-1 infection attenuates antioxidant capacity. The diminished antioxidant capacity creates an imbalanced redox status and stimulates activation of redox-sensitive signaling pathways, specifically the Ras and Rho subfamilies of monomeric G proteins, which then stimulate ROS production by NADPH oxidases, leading to the activation of redox-responsive transcription factors (Wu, Ma, Myers, & Terada, 2007). Upregulation of inflammatory mediators, such as adhesion molecules, chemokines, and inflammatory cytokines, mediate the subsequent adherence and transendothelial migration of inflammatory cells (Figure 3.2.4).

HIV-1-MEDIATED ALTERATIONS OF VESSEL TONE

The peripheral endothelium plays a dual role in the regulation of the vasomotor tone by producing and releasing both relaxing and constricting factors. Normally, the biological effects of vasorelaxing factors predominate over the effects of vasoconstrictive substances. HIV-1-induced alterations of endothelial cell-mediated production of vasorelaxing factors gained significance in recent years in the context of accelerated vasculitis, atherosclerosis, stroke, and pulmonary hypertension in HIV-1 patients that develop in the absence of traditional risk factors.

It appears that impaired endothelium-dependent vasorelaxation is mainly responsible for HIV-1-associated alterations of vessel tone.

HIV-1 DECREASES NITRIC OXIDE BIOAVAILABILITY

The basal secretion of nitric oxide (NO) by endothelial cells is chiefly responsible for the active vasodilator tone of vessels. When produced by endothelial cells, NO easily diffuses into underlying tissues and penetrates to smooth muscle cells, activating their soluble guanylate cyclase and increasing cGMP. Elevation of cGMP results in the inhibition of contractile mechanisms of smooth muscle cells, leading to vasorelaxation. In addition, endothelial cells release NO into the bloodstream; therefore, plasma levels of NO or nitrite can serve as biomarkers of NO bioavailability. However, the role of NO is not only limited to the regulation of the vascular tone. NO can decrease endothelial expression of cellular adhesion molecules, inhibit smooth muscle cell proliferation, and decrease leukocyte adherence (Chen, Pittman, & Popel, 2008). These facts implicate decreased NO levels and its related signal transduction and effector functions in the vascular pathology seen in the HIV-1-infected population.

Comprehensive studies were performed to determine NO bioavailability in a model of HIV-1 transgenic rats. NO-hemoglobin, serum nitrite, S-nitrosothiol, and basal NO levels were significantly decreased in aortic tissue of the transgenic rats compared to their wild type controls, indicating a systemic and vascular deficiency of NO. Indeed, acetylcholine-induced, but not sodium nitroprusside-induced, vasorelaxation was impaired in HIV-1 transgenic rats, suggesting endothelial dysfunction as the culprit of the depleted NO availability. These alterations were related to chronic oxidative stress because feeding with glutathione precursor procysteine restored NO levels along with endothelium-dependent vasorelaxation (Kline et al., 2008).

The role of specific HIV-1 proteins in the regulation of vessel tone was also demonstrated. Nef has been detected in vascular cells of patients with HIV-1-associated pulmonary artery hypertension (Marecki et al., 2006). Nef was shown to impair both endothelium-dependent contraction and relaxation in porcine pulmonary artery rings without affecting endothelial-independent relaxation. These effects were associated with decreased levels of endothelial nitric oxidase synthase (eNOS) mRNA and nitrite levels. Treatment with superoxide dismutase mimetic MnTBAP attenuated the Nef-induced alterations of vascular tone, further indicating the role of oxidative stress in HIV-1-induced endothelial impairment (Duffy, Wang, Lin, Yao, & Chen, 2009).

Gp120 in the presence of TNFα was also shown to impair endothelium-dependent vasorelaxation without affecting contraction and endothelium-independent relaxation. Porcine coronary artery rings and human coronary artery endothelial cells exposed to gp120 after pretreatment with TNFα diminished eNOS mRNA and protein levels. Importantly, neutralizing antibody against ICAM-1 or gp120 protected against these effects (Jiang et al., 2010).

THE EFFECTS OF HIV-1 ON PROSTACYCLIN, THROMBOXANE, AND OTHER EICOSANOIDS

The term "eicosanoids" is a collective name for prostaglandins (PGs), prostacyclin (PGI$_2$), thromboxanes (TXs), leukotrienes (LTs), and hydroxyeicosatetraenoic acids (HETEs), which can be formed from different polyunsaturated 20-carbon fatty acids. Because arachidonic acid (AA; 5,8,11,14-eicosatetraenoic acid) is the most prominent 20-carbon fatty acid, its derivatives are the most common and biologically important eicosanoids. AA is a normal component of the phospholipids of cellular membranes and becomes available for eicosanoid synthesis only after it is released from phospholipid moieties. Although release of AA can be mediated by several phospholipases or lipases, phospholipase A$_2$ plays a critical role in this process. Released AA can be metabolized by either cyclooxygenases (COX-1 and COX-2), lipoxygenases (5-, 12-, or 15-lipoxygenase), or cytochrome P450-dependent enzymes. Both COX-1 and COX-2 catalyze conversion of AA to PGH$_2$. While COX-1 is constitutively expressed in the majority of tissue, expression of COX-2 can be markedly enhanced upon cell activation, such as in an inflammatory response. PGH$_2$, which causes vasoconstriction, has a half-life of approximately 5 min and is further enzymatically transformed to several prostaglandins as well as PGI$_2$ and TXA$_2$. Endothelial cells contain a high activity of PGI-synthase, which metabolizes PGH$_2$ to PGI$_2$ resulting in vasodilatation and inhibition of platelet aggregation (Toborek & Kaiser, 1999).

HIV-1 and viral factors can markedly affect eicosanoid balance and metabolism. Strong evidence indicates that COX-2 is upregulated in HIV-1-infected patients. For example, infiltrates of macrophages overexpressing COX-2 are found in HIV-1 myocarditis (Liu et al., 2001), and elevated levels of PGE$_2$ are frequently detected in HIV-1-infected patients. COX-2 and PGE synthase are also highly expressed in perivascular monocytes and cells of the BBB (Teather & Wurtman, 2003).

Research from our laboratory provided evidence that exposure to Tat can upregulate COX-2 in brain tissue (Pu et al., 2007). However, COX-2 immunoreactivity was primarily localized in microglial cells and astrocytes (Flora, Pu, Hennig, & Toborek, 2006). The underlying mechanisms of this effect are not fully understood; however, they may be related to Tat-mediated induction of cellular oxidative stress and activation of redox-regulated transcription factors. For example, Tat can stimulate protein kinase C and the MAPK pathway (Andras et al., 2005), which were demonstrated to induce transcription of COX-2. The COX-2 gene promoter contains several enhancer elements which are sensitive to cellular redox balance. These elements include cAMP response element (CRE), the AP-1 binding site, C/EBP element, and two separate κB enhancer elements. These transcription factors are upregulated in response to HIV-1 or Tat exposure. For example, Tat is a strong inducer of NF-κB as demonstrated in several cell types, including BMEC, astrocytes, and microglia. In addition, Tat was shown to activate and interact with C/EBPβ, as well as stimulate CREB, and AP-1 (reviewed in Toborek et al., 2005). Inhibition of COX-2 partially attenuated Tat-induced loss of TJ proteins. However, COX-2 did not appear to be responsible for Tat-induced disruption of the BBB integrity (Pu et al., 2007).

HIV-1-MEDIATED CHANGES IN EXPRESSION OF ENDOTHELINS AND OTHER VASOCONSTRICTORS

Endothelins are vasoconstrictor polypeptides produced by different tissues as three different isoforms, namely, endothelin (ET)-1, ET-2, and ET-3. Endothelial cells can synthesize only ET-1. ET-1 was first discovered in 1988 when it was isolated from the conditioned medium of cultured endothelial cells. ET-1 is the most potent currently known vasoconstrictor, being approximately 100 times more potent than angiotensin II. The half-life of ET-1 is 4–7 min. The primary sites of the vasoconstrictive effects of ET-1 are on small vessels (Thorin et al., 2010).

The majority of ET-1 (approximately 75%) synthesized by endothelial cells is secreted abluminally, that is, towards smooth muscle cells, while the remaining portion of ET-1 is released luminally to the plasma. Although ET-1 present in plasma most likely does not contribute to the contractile function of this peptide, its level in plasma can serve as an important marker of overall ET-1 production (Toborek & Kaiser, 1999). Increased production and/or activity of ET-1 have been implicated in several pathological states related to the dysfunction of the endothelium. For example, elevated ET-1 levels were observed in the plasma of HIV-1-infected individuals and in the cerebrovascular fluid of HIV-1-associated encephalopathy (Rolinski et al., 1999). Importantly, increased ET-1 levels were detected in HIV-1-associated pulmonary hypertension (Degano, Sitbon, & Simonneau, 2009). Mechanistically, it was demonstrated that exposure to HIV-1 proteins, such as gp120, can induce production of ET-1 in BMEC (Kanmogne et al., 2005).

Compelling evidence indicates the role of the renin-angiotensin system in the development of HIV-1-associated nephropathy (Mikulak et al., 2010). Several elements of this system are localized to endothelium and other elements of the vessel wall. Under the conditions of oxidative stress, superoxide anions can also contribute to endothelium-dependent contractions via inactivation of NO (Vanhoutte, Feletou, & Taddei, 2005). The reaction between NO and superoxide anions can lead to the formation of peroxynitrite. Thus, as a result of this reaction, not only bioavailability of NO is diminished but also a potent form of free radicals is formed.

HIV-1-MEDIATED ALTERATIONS OF HEMOSTATIC AND FIBRINOLYTIC FUNCTIONS OF ENDOTHELIAL CELLS

Maintaining the non-thrombogenic blood-tissue interface is another major function of the vascular endothelium that is affected in HIV-1 infection. Indeed, HIV-1 infection is associated with increased risk of the developing arterial and venous thrombosis. Recent literature indicates thromboembolic complications in HIV-1 patients at the range of 0.26–7.6% (Shen & Frenkel, 2004). Higher incidents of thrombosis are observed in patients with other HIV-1 complications, such as opportunistic infections and malignancies. The thromboembolic events appear to occur more frequently in patients on antiretroviral therapy.

The fundamental mechanism of stable hemostatic clot formation is the polymerization of fibrinogen into fibrin, catalyzed by thrombin, which also activates factor V, factor XIII, platelets, and endothelial cells (Figure 3.2.5). In addition, thrombin induces platelet adhesion and aggregation, increases endothelial permeability, and stimulates adhesion molecule expression on the surface of endothelial cells (Borissoff, Spronk, Heeneman, & ten Cate, 2009). One of the main

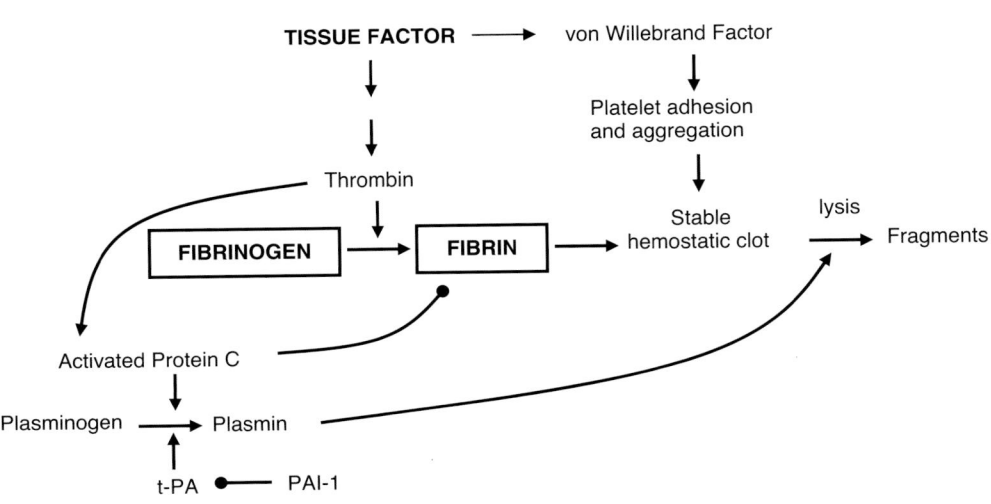

Figure 3.2.5 Simplified mechanisms of coagulation and fibrinolysis. Abbreviations: PAI-1, plasminogen activator inhibitor type 1; tPA, tissue-type plasminogen activator.

endothelial-derived initiators of coagulation is tissue factor (TF), an integral membrane glycoprotein whose extracellular domain functions as the receptor for factor VII/VIIa. The TF promoter has binding sites for several transcription factors, including Spl, Egr-1, NF-κB, and AP-1, which regulate both basal and inducible expression of TF, and are responsible for upregulation of TF expression under conditions of altered redox status (Kretz, Vaezzadeh, & Gross, 2010). Elevated monocyte levels of TF in HIV-1 infection were recently reported (Funderburg et al., 2010).

Binding of thrombin to thrombomodulin activates protein C, which then inhibits coagulation by degradation of factor Va and VIIIa (Figure 3.2.5). In addition, activated protein C stimulates the fibrinolytic pathway by inactivating plasminogen activator inhibitor type 1 (PAI-1). Through inhibition of thrombin, thrombomodulin is a critical regulator of the anti-thrombogenic functions of vascular endothelium. Thrombomodulin is synthesized by endothelial cells and is present on the luminal surface of the endothelium of different vessels, including capillaries, arteries, veins, and lymphatic vessels (Tanaka, Key, & Levy, 2009).

Endothelial cells can regulate platelet activation by production and release of the platelet-activating factor (PAF) (Figure 3.2.5). However, PAF is also produced by neutrophils, monocytes, macrophages, basophils, eosinophils, and mast cells. In addition to stimulatory effects on platelet activation, PAF is a strong proinflammatory agent that is involved in HIV-1-induced pathology. For example, Tat can stimulate PAF production via activation of VEGFR1. PAF stimulates recruitment of lymphomononuclear cells and endothelial hyperpermeability. Importantly, PAF can enhance replication of HIV-1. Based on this complex mechanism of action, it was proposed that PAF antagonists may serve as an adjunctive therapy for HIV-1-associated neurocognitive disorders (Eggert et al., 2009).

Fibrinolysis is primarily mediated by plasmin, an active protease formed from its precursor, plasminogen, upon stimulation by t-PA (Figure 3.2.5). Thus, proper fibrinolysis depends primarily on the balance between t-PA and PAI-1. Both these factors are produced and secreted by endothelial cells; however, in normal conditions, PAI-1 is produced in excess. PAI-1 and t-PA levels are elevated in HIV-1-infected patients, indicating endothelial dysfunction (Kristoffersen et al., 2009; Masiá et al., 2010).

COMBINATION ANTIRETROVIRAL THERAPY (cART) AND ALTERATIONS OF ENDOTHELIAL CELL FUNCTIONS

Antiretroviral drugs, especially protease inhibitors, have been associated with increased cardiovascular events and worsening the risk factors for coronary heart disease, such as dyslipidemia, insulin resistance, and endothelial dysfunction. Currently used antiretroviral drugs are mechanistically divided into five classes: nucleoside reverse transcriptase inhibitors (NRTIs), nonnucleoside reverse transcriptase inhibitors (NNRTIs), protease inhibitors (PIs), integrase inhibitors, and entry inhibitors (EIs). The recommended initial combination therapy consists of two NRTIs with either one or two PIs or one NNRTI. In most cases, NRTIs constitute the backbone of antiretroviral treatment strategies.

Introduction of antiretroviral therapy to HIV-1-infected individuals usually results in initially improved endothelial functions. The decrease in plasma HIV RNA is associated with greater brachial artery flow-mediated dilation (FMD) (Torriani et al., 2008), and a significant reduction in plasma levels of markers of endothelial cell dysfunction, such as E-selectin, soluble ICAM-1, and soluble VCAM-1 (Kristoffersen et al., 2009). Despite this short-term improvement, clinical and experimental evidence strongly indicate that long-term antiretroviral therapy results in endothelial toxicity and vascular dysfunction. Epidemiological studies have linked the use of NRTIs and PIs with a higher risk of coronary heart disease. Nevertheless, there appear to be individual differences in vascular toxicity among specific antiretroviral drugs. For example, most PIs, with the exception of atazanavir, are associated with elevations in the levels of total cholesterol, triglycerides, and LDL cholesterol (Wohl et al., 2006). NNRTIs produce similar metabolic changes; however, epidemiological studies suggest that they are not associated with higher risk of coronary heart disease. Indeed, endothelial functions, and inflammatory and metabolic markers are not affected by NNRTIs (Murphy et al. 2010). In addition, EIs are the class of therapeutics that does not induce vascular toxicity.

Clinical investigations indicate that intima-media thickness (IMT) is elevated in patients receiving protease inhibitors, in current smokers, and in patients with cART-induced dyslipidemia (Depairon et al., 2001). Furthermore, duration of antiretroviral therapy, protease inhibitor use, and nucleoside analogue use were each associated with thicker IMT. These relationships remained significant after adjustment for traditional cardiac risk factors and the duration of HIV-1 diagnosis (Hsue et al., 2009a).

Assessment of FMD of the brachial artery also revealed endothelial cell dysfunction in HIV-1-infected patients, with abacavir further affecting the FMD values. Surprisingly, duration of therapy and CD4 cell count were not associated with reduced FMD. This finding suggests that endothelial dysfunction, a central mechanism in atherosclerosis and a marker of cardiovascular risk, is impaired among antiretroviral-treated patients with undetectable viral load (Hsue et al., 2009b). Similar results were also reported in children infected with HIV-1 on antiretroviral therapy (Charakida et al., 2005).

The mechanisms of antiretroviral drug-induced endothelial cell dysfunction are not fully understood. However, mitochondrial dysfunction with a concomitant increase in mitochondria-derived ROS production appears to be critical for endothelial toxicity of specific PIs (Jiang et al., 2007). For example, it was shown that exposure to indinavir and/or AZT can induce endothelial mitochondrial dysfunction, stimulate oxidative stress, release ET-1, and ultimately, induce proliferation of smooth muscle cells (Hebert, Crenshaw, Romanoff, Ekshyyan, & Dugas, 2004). Furthermore, exposure to saquinavir was demonstrated to induce endothelial cell apoptosis; the effect that was attenuated by the antioxidant N-acetylcysteine (Baliga, Liu, Hoyt, Chaves, & Bauer, 2004).

On the other hand, it was demonstrated that the protease inhibitor ritonavir can decrease the development of atherosclerosis in APOE*3-Leiden transgenic mice despite inducing hypertriglyceridemia (den Boer et al. 2010). Ritonavir has been shown to increase peroxisome proliferator-activated receptor-γ (PPARγ) expression, which may be responsible for its anti-atherogenic effects.

CONCLUSION

Endothelial cells regulate vital functions of the vessel wall. They produce a spectrum of biologically active factors to control vascular permeability, vessel tone, coagulation, fibrinolysis, and inflammatory responses. Some of these factors, such as junctional proteins or adhesion molecules, are integral parts of endothelial cell structure. Others, such as NO, prostacyclin, chemokines, or factors involved in coagulation and fibrinolysis, are produced and then released by endothelial cells either luminally or abluminally. These biologically active factors can frequently be generated not only by endothelial cells but also by other vascular or even nonvascular cells. Thus, endothelial cells are a part of a larger network which preserves the normal vessel wall metabolism. Alterations of the normal endothelial cell biology have critical significance in the development of vascular and neurovascular pathology during HIV-1 infection. For example, they can contribute to the disruption of the BBB, HIV-1 entry into the brain, the development of vasculopathies, and atherosclerosis. The underlying mechanisms appear to be related to induction of oxidative stress and alterations of redox-related signaling. Vascular toxicity may be induced by HIV-1 itself or it can be mediated by a variety of HIV-1-specific proteins. In addition, antiretroviral drugs may induce dysfunction of the vascular endothelium.

REFERENCES

Abbott, N. J., Ronnback, L., & Hansson, E. (2006). Astrocyte-endothelial interactions at the blood-brain barrier. *Nat Rev Neurosci, 7,* 41–53.

Andras, I. E., Pu, H., Deli, M. A., Nath, A., Hennig, B., & Toborek, M. (2003). HIV-1 Tat protein alters tight junction protein expression and distribution in cultured brain endothelial cells. *J Neurosci Res, 74,* 255–65.

Andras, I. E., Pu, H., Tian, J., Deli, M. A., Nath, A., Hennig, B., et al. (2005). Signaling mechanisms of HIV-1 Tat-induced alterations of claudin-5 expression in brain endothelial cells. *J Cereb Blood Flow Metab, 25,* 1159–70.

Argyris, E. G., Acheampong, E., Nunnari, G., Mukhtar, M., Williams, K. J., & Pomerantz, R. J. (2003). Human immunodeficiency virus type 1 enters primary human brain microvascular endothelial cells by a mechanism involving cell surface proteoglycans independent of lipid rafts. *J Virol, 77,* 12140–51.

Avraham, H. K., Jiang, S., Lee, T. H., Prakash, O., & Avraham, S. (2004). HIV-1 Tat-mediated effects on focal adhesion assembly and permeability in brain microvascular endothelial cells. *J Immunol, 173,* 6228–33.

Baliga, R. S., Liu, C., Hoyt, D. G., Chaves, A. A., & Bauer, J. A. (2004). Vascular endothelial toxicity induced by HIV protease inhibitor: Evidence of oxidant-related dysfunction and apoptosis. *Cardiovasc Toxicol, 4,* 199–206.

Banks, W. A., Ercal, N., & Price, T. O. (2006). The blood-brain barrier in neuroAIDS. *Curr HIV Res, 4,* 259–66.

Borisoff, J. I., Spronk, H. M., Heeneman, S., & ten Cate, H. (2009). Is thrombin a key player in the "coagulation-atherogenesis" maze? *Cardiovasc Res, 82,* 392–403.

Boven, L. A., Middel, J., Verhoef, J., De Groot, C. J., & Nottet, H. S. (2000). Monocyte infiltration is highly associated with loss of the tight junction protein zonula occludens in HIV-1-associated dementia. *Neuropathol Appl Neurobiol, 26,* 356–60.

Charakida, M., Donald, A. E., Green, H., Storry, C., Clapson, M., Caslake, M., et al. (2005). Early structural and functional changes of the vasculature in HIV-infected children: Impact of disease and antiretroviral therapy. *Circulation, 112,* 103–9.

Chaudhuri, A., Yang, B., Gendelman, H. E., Persidsky, Y., & Kanmogne, G. D. (2008). STAT1 signaling modulates HIV-1-induced inflammatory responses and leukocyte transmigration across the blood-brain barrier. *Blood, 111,* 2062–72.

Chen, K., Pittman, R. N., & Popel, A. S. (2008). Nitric oxide in the vasculature: Where does it come from and where does it go? A quantitative perspective. *Antioxid Redox Signal, 10,* 1185–98.

Chetty, R. (2001). Vasculitides associated with HIV infection. *J Clin Pathol, 54,* 275–8.

Cioni, C. & Annunziata, P. (2002). Circulating gp120 alters the blood-brain barrier permeability in HIV-1 gp120 transgenic mice. *Neurosci Lett, 330,* 299–301.

Crowe, S. M., Westhorpe, C. L., Mukhamedova, N., Jaworowski, A., Sviridov, D., & Bukrinsky, M. (2010). The macrophage: The intersection between HIV infection and atherosclerosis. *J Leukoc Biol, 87,* 589–98.

Dallasta, L. M., Pisarov, L. A., Esplen, J. E., Werley, J. V., Moses, A. V., Nelson, J. A., et al. (1999). Blood-brain barrier tight junction disruption in human immunodeficiency virus-1 encephalitis. *Am J Pathol, 155,* 1915–27.

Degano, B., Sitbon, O., & Simonneau, G. (2009). Pulmonary arterial hypertension and HIV infection. *Semin Respir Crit Care Med, 30,* 440–7.

de Larrañaga, G. F., Petroni, A., Deluchi, G., Alonso, B. S., & Benetucci, J. A. (2003). Viral load and disease progression as responsible for endothelial activation and/or injury in human immunodeficiency virus-1-infected patients. *Blood Coagul Fibrinolysis, 14,* 15–8.

den Boer, M. A., Westerterp, M., de Vries-van der Weij, J., Wang, Y., Hu, L., Espirito Santo, S. M., et al. (2010). Ritonavir protects against the development of atherosclerosis in APOE*3-Leiden mice. *Atherosclerosis, 210,* 381–7.

Depairon, M., Chessex, S., Sudre, P., Rodondi, N., Doser, N., Chave, J. P., et al. (2001). Premature atherosclerosis in HIV-infected individuals—focus on protease inhibitor therapy. *AIDS, 15,* 329–34.

Duffy, P., Wang, X., Lin, P. H., Yao, Q., & Chen, C. (2009). HIV Nef protein causes endothelial dysfunction in porcine pulmonary arteries and human pulmonary artery endothelial cells. *J Surg Res, 156,* 257–64.

Eggert, D., Dash, P. K., Serradji, N., Dong, C. Z., Clayette, P., Heymans, F., et al. (2009). Development of a platelet-activating factor antagonist for HIV-1 associated neurocognitive disorders. *J Neuroimmunol, 213,* 47–59.

Eugenin, E. A. & Berman, J. W. (2007). Gap junctions mediate human immunodeficiency virus-bystander killing in astrocytes. *J Neurosci, 27,* 12844–50.

Eugenin, E. A., Morgello, S., Klotman, M. E., Mosoian, A., Lento, P. A., Berman, J. W., et al. (2008). Human immunodeficiency virus (HIV) infects human arterial smooth muscle cells in vivo and in vitro: Implications for the pathogenesis of HIV-mediated vascular disease. *Am J Pathol, 172,* 1100–11.

Eugenin, E. A., Osiecki, K., Lopez, L., Goldstein, H., Calderon, T. M., et al. (2006). CCL2/monocyte chemoattractant protein-1 mediates enhanced transmigration of human immunodeficiency virus (HIV)-infected leukocytes across the blood-brain barrier: A potential mechanism of HIV-CNS invasion and neuroAIDS. *J Neurosci, 26,* 1098–106.

Fittipaldi, A., Ferrari, A., Zoppe, M., Arcangeli, C., Pellegrini, V., Beltram, F., et al. (2003). Cell membrane lipid rafts mediate caveolar endocytosis of HIV-1 Tat fusion proteins. *J Biol Chem, 278,* 34141–9.

Flora, G., Pu, H., Hennig, B., & Toborek, M. (2006). Cyclooxygenase-2 is involved in HIV-1 Tat-induced inflammatory responses in the brain. *Neuromolecular Med, 8,* 337–52.

Funderburg, N. T., Mayne, E., Sieg, S. F., Asaad, R., Jiang, W., Kalinowska, M., et al. (2010). Increased tissue factor expression on circulating monocytes in chronic HIV infection: Relationship to in vivo coagulation and immune activation. *Blood, 115,* 161–7.

Gandhi, N., Saiyed, Z. M., Napuri, J., Samikkannu, T., Reddy, P. V., Agudelo, M., et al. (2010). Interactive role of human immunodeficiency virus type 1 (HIV-1) clade-specific Tat protein and cocaine in blood-brain barrier dysfunction: Implications for HIV-1-associated neurocognitive disorder. *J Neurovirol, 16,* 294–305.

Giepmans, B. N. (2004). Gap junctions and connexin-interacting proteins. *Cardiovasc Res, 62,* 233–45.

Gil, L., Martínez, G., González, I., Tarinas, A., Alvarez, A., Giuliani, A., et al. (2003). Contribution to characterization of oxidative stress in HIV/AIDS patients. *Pharmacol Res, 47,* 217–24.

Goldstein, D. A., Timpone, J., & Cupps, T. R. (2010). HIV-associated intracranial aneurysmal vasculopathy in adults. *J Rheumatol, 37,* 226–33.

Hansson, G. K. (2005). Inflammation, atherosclerosis, and coronary artery disease. *N Engl J Med, 352,* 1685–95.

Hebert, V. Y., Crenshaw, B. L., Romanoff, R. L., Ekshyyan, V. P., & Dugas, T. R. (2004). Effects of HIV drug combinations on endothelin-1 and vascular cell proliferation. *Cardiovasc Toxicol, 4,* 117–31.

Holland, G. N. (2008). AIDS and ophthalmology: The first quarter century. *Am J Ophthalmol, 145,* 397–408.

Hsue, P. Y., Hunt, P. W., Schnell, A., Kalapus, S. C., Hoh, R., Ganz, P., et al. (2009a). Role of viral replication, antiretroviral therapy, and immunodeficiency in HIV-associated atherosclerosis. *AIDS, 23,* 1059–67.

Hsue, P. Y., Hunt, P. W., Wu, Y., Schnell, A., Ho, J. E., Hatano, H., et al. (2009b). Association of abacavir and impaired endothelial function in treated and suppressed HIV-infected patients. *AIDS, 23,* 2021–7.

Huang, W., Eum, S. Y., Andras, I. E., Hennig, B., & Toborek, M. (2009). PPARalpha and PPARgamma attenuate HIV-induced dysregulation of tight junction proteins by modulations of matrix metalloproteinase and proteasome activities. *FASEB J, 23,* 1596–606.

Hudson, L., Liu, J., Nath, A., Jones, M., Raghavan, R., Narayan, O., et al. (2000). Detection of the human immunodeficiency virus regulatory protein tat in CNS tissues. *J Neurovirol, 6,* 145–55.

Jiang, B., Hebert, V. Y., Li, Y., Mathis, J. M., Alexander, J. S., & Dugas, T. R. (2007). HIV antiretroviral drug combination induces endothelial mitochondrial dysfunction and reactive oxygen species production, but not apoptosis. *Toxicol Appl Pharmacol, 224,* 60–71.

Jiang, J., Fu, W., Wang, X., Lin, P. H., Yao, Q., & Chen, C. (2010). HIV gp120 induces endothelial dysfunction in tumour necrosis factor-alpha-activated porcine and human endothelial cells. *Cardiovasc Res, 87,* 366–74.

Kanmogne, G. D., Primeaux, C., & Grammas, P. (2005). Induction of apoptosis and endothelin-1 secretion in primary human lung endothelial cells by HIV-1 gp120 proteins. *Biochem Biophys Res Commun, 333,* 1107–15.

Kanmogne, G. D., Schall, K., Leibhart, J., Knipe, B., Gendelman, H. E., & Persidsky, Y. (2007). HIV-1 gp120 compromises blood-brain barrier integrity and enhances monocyte migration across blood-brain barrier: Implication for viral neuropathogenesis. *J Cereb Blood Flow Metab, 27,* 123–34.

Kline, E. R., Kleinhenz, D. J., Liang, B., Dikalov, S., Guidot, D. M., Hart, C. M., et al. (2008). Vascular oxidative stress and nitric oxide depletion in HIV-1 transgenic rats are reversed by glutathione restoration. *Am J Physiol Heart Circ Physiol, 294,* H2792–804.

Kretz, C. A., Vaezzadeh, N., & Gross, P. L. (2010). Tissue factor and thrombosis models. *Arterioscler Thromb Vasc Biol, 30,* 900–8.

Kristoffersen, U. S., Kofoed, K., Kronborg, G., Giger, A. K., Kjaer, A., & Lebech, A. M. (2009). Reduction in circulating markers of endothelial dysfunction in HIV-infected patients during antiretroviral therapy. *HIV Med, 10,* 79–87.

Liu, Q. N., Reddy, S., Sayre, J. W., Pop, V., Graves, M. C., & Fiala, M. (2001). Essential role of HIV type 1-infected and cyclooxygenase 2-activated macrophages and T cells in HIV type 1 myocarditis. *AIDS Res Hum Retroviruses, 17,* 1423–33.

Louboutin, J. P., Agrawal, L., Reyes, B. A., Van Bockstaele, E. J., & Strayer, D. S. (2010). HIV-1 gp120-induced injury to the blood-brain barrier: Role of metalloproteinases 2 and 9 and relationship to oxidative stress. *J Neuropathol Exp Neurol, 69,* 801–16.

Marecki, J. C., Cool, C. D., Parr, J. E., Beckey, V. E., Luciw, P. A., Tarantal, A. F., et al. (2006). HIV-1 Nef is associated with complex pulmonary vascular lesions in SHIV-nef-infected macaques. *Am J Respir Crit Care Med, 174,* 437–45.

Masiá, M., Padilla, S., García, N., Jarrin, I., Bernal, E., López, N., et al. (2010). Endothelial function is impaired in HIV-infected patients with lipodystrophy. *Antivir Ther, 15,* 101–10.

Melendez, M. M., McNurlan, M. A., Mynarcik, D. C., Khan, S., & Gelato, M. C. (2008). Endothelial adhesion molecules are associated with inflammation in subjects with HIV disease. *Clin Infect Dis, 46,* 775–80.

Mendu, D. R., Katinger, H., Sodroski, J., & Kim, K. S. (2007). HIV-1 envelope protein gp140 binding studies to human brain microvascular endothelial cells. *Biochem Biophys Res Commun, 363,* 466–71.

Mikulak, J. & Singhal, P. C. (2010). HIV-1 and kidney cells: Better understanding of viral interaction. *Nephron Exp Nephrol, 115,* e15–21.

Miller, A. A., Budzyn, K., & Sobey, C. G. (2010). Vascular dysfunction in cerebrovascular disease: mechanisms and therapeutic intervention. *Clin Sci (Lond), 119,* 1–17.

Murphy, R. L., Berzins, B., Zala, C., Fichtenbaum, C., Dube, M. P., Guaraldi, G., et al. Change to atazanavir/ritonavir treatment improves lipids but not endothelial function in patients on stable antiretroviral therapy. *AIDS, 24,* 885–90.

Nagel, M. A., Mahalingam, R., Cohrs, R. J., & Gilden, D. (2010). Virus vasculopathy and stroke: An under-recognized cause and treatment target. *Infect Disord Drug Targets, 10,* 105–11.

Nakamuta, S., Endo, H., Higashi, Y., Kousaka, A., Yamada, H., Yano, M., et al. (2008). Human immunodeficiency virus type 1 gp120-mediated disruption of tight junction proteins by induction of proteasome-mediated degradation of zonula occludens-1 and -2 in human brain microvascular endothelial cells. *J Neurovirol, 14,* 186–195.

Oshima, T., Flores, S. C., Vaitaitis, G., Coe, L. L., Joh, T., Park, J. H., et al. (2000). HIV-1 Tat increases endothelial solute permeability through tyrosine kinase and mitogen-activated protein kinase-dependent pathways. *AIDS, 14,* 475–82.

Persidsky, Y., Heilman, D., Haorah, J., Zelivyanskaya, M., Persidsky, R., Weber, G. A., et al. (2006a). Rho-mediated regulation of tight junctions during monocyte migration across the blood-brain barrier in HIV-1 encephalitis (HIVE). *Blood, 107,* 4770–80.

Persidsky, Y., Ramirez, S. H., Haorah, J., & Kanmogne, G. D. (2006b). Blood-brain barrier: Structural components and function under physiologic and pathologic conditions. *J Neuroimmune Pharmacol, 1,* 223–36.

Pu, H., Hayashi, K., Andras, I. E., Eum, S. Y., Hennig, B., & Toborek, M. (2007). Limited role of COX-2 in HIV Tat-induced alterations of tight junction protein expression and disruption of the blood-brain barrier. *Brain Res, 1* 184, 333–44.

Pu, H., Tian, .J, Andras, I. E., Hayashi, K., Flora, G., Hennig, B., et al. (2005). HIV-1 Tat protein-induced alterations of ZO-1 expression are mediated by redox-regulated ERK 1/2 activation. *J Cereb Blood Flow Metab, 25,* 1325–35.

Pu, H., Tian, J., Flora, G., Lee, Y. W., Nath, A., Hennig, B., et al. (2003). HIV-1 Tat protein upregulates inflammatory mediators and induces monocyte invasion into the brain. *Mol Cell Neurosci, 24,* 224–37.

Ramirez, S. H., Heilman, D., Morsey, B., Potula, R., Haorah, J., & Persidsky, Y. (2008). Activation of peroxisome proliferator-activated receptor gamma (PPARgamma) suppresses Rho GTPases in human brain microvascular endothelial cells and inhibits adhesion and transendothelial migration of HIV-1 infected monocytes. *J Immunol, 180,* 1854–65.

Roberts, T. K., Buckner, C. M., & Berman, J. W. (2010). Leukocyte transmigration across the blood-brain barrier: Perspectives on neuroAIDS. *Front Biosci, 15,* 478–536.

Rolinski, B., Heigermoser, A., Lederer, E., Bogner, J. R., Loch, O., & Goebel, F. D. (1999). Endothelin-1 is elevated in the cerebrospinal fluid of HIV-infected patients with encephalopathy. *Infection, 27,* 244–7.

Rusnati, M., Tulipano, G., Spillmann, D., Tanghetti, E., Oreste, P., Zoppetti, G., et al. (1999). Multiple interactions of HIV-I Tat protein with size-defined heparin oligosaccharides. *J Biol Chem, 274,* 28198–205.

Salim, A. & Ratner, L. (2008). Modulation of beta-catenin and E-cadherin interaction by Vpu increases human immunodeficiency virus type 1 particle release. *J Virol, 82,* 3932–8.

Shen, Y. M. & Frenkel, E. P. (2004). Thrombosis and a hypercoagulable state in HIV-infected patients. *Clin Appl Thromb Hemost, 10,* 277–80.

Sudano, I., Spieker, L. E., Noll, G., Corti, R., Weber, R., & Lüscher, T. F. (2006). Cardiovascular disease in HIV infection. *Am Heart J, 151,* 1147–55.

Suresh, D. R., Annam, V., Pratibha, K., & Prasad, B. V. (2009). Total antioxidant capacity—a novel early bio-chemical marker of oxidative stress in HIV infected individuals. *J Biomed Sci, 16,* 61.

Tanaka, K. A., Key, N. S., & Levy, J. H. (2009). Blood coagulation: Hemostasis and thrombin regulation. *Anesth Analg, 108,* 1433–46.

Teather, L. A. & Wurtman, R. J. (2003). Cyclooxygenase-2 mediates platelet-activating factor-induced prostaglandin E2 release from rat primary astrocytes. *Neurosci Lett, 340,* 177–80.

Thorin, E. & Webb, D. J. (2010). Endothelium-derived endothelin-1. *Pflugers Arch, 459,* 951–8.

Toborek, M. & Kaiser, S. (1999). Endothelial cell functions. Relationship to atherogenesis. *Basic Res Cardiol, 94,* 295–314.

Toborek, M., Lee, Y. W., Flora, G., Pu, H., Andras, I. E., Wylegala, E., et al. (2005). Mechanisms of the blood-brain barrier disruption in HIV-1 infection. *Cell Mol Neurobiol, 25,* 181–99.

Toborek, M., Lee, Y. W., Pu, H., Malecki, A., Flora, G., Garrido, R., et al. (2003). HIV-Tat protein induces oxidative and inflammatory pathways in brain endothelium. *J Neurochem, 84,* 169–79.

Torriani, F. J., Komarow, L., Parker, R. A., Cotter, B. R., Currier, J. S., Dubé, M. P., et al. (2008). Endothelial function in human immunodeficiency virus-infected antiretroviral-naive subjects before and after starting potent antiretroviral therapy: The ACTG (AIDS Clinical Trials Group) Study 5152s. *J Am Coll Cardiol, 52,* 569–76.

Toschi, E., Bacigalupo, I., Strippoli, R., Chiozzini, C., Cereseto, A., Falchi, M., et al. (2006). HIV-1 Tat regulates endothelial cell cycle progression via activation of the Ras/ERK MAPK signaling pathway. *Mol Biol Cell, 17,* 1985–94.

Vanhoutte, P. M., Feletou, M., & Taddei, S. (2005). Endothelium-dependent contractions in hypertension. *Br J Pharmacol, 144,* 449–58.

Véliz, L. P., González, F. G., Duling, B. R., Sáez, J. C., & Boric, M. P. (2008). Functional role of gap junctions in cytokine-induced leukocyte adhesion to endothelium in vivo. *Am J Physiol Heart Circ Physiol, 295,* H1056–66.

Wang, J. K., Kiyokawa, E., Verdin, E., & Trono, D. (2000). The Nef protein of HIV-1 associates with rafts and primes T cells for activation. *Proc Natl Acad Sci USA, 97,* 394–9.

Weiss, J. M., Nath, A., Major, E. O., & Berman, J. W. (1999). HIV-1 Tat induces monocyte chemoattractant protein-1-mediated monocyte transmigration across a model of the human blood-brain barrier and up-regulates CCR5 expression on human monocytes. *J Immunol, 163,* 2953–9.

Wohl, D. A., McComsey, G., Tebas, P., Brown, T. T., Glesby, M. J., Reeds, D., et al. (2006). Current concepts in the diagnosis and management of metabolic complications of HIV infection and its therapy. *Clin Infect Dis, 43,* 645–53.

Wu, R. F., Ma, Z., Myers, D. P., & Terada, L. S. (2007). HIV-1 Tat activates dual Nox pathways leading to independent activation of ERK and JNK MAP kinases. *J Biol Chem, 282,* 37412–9.

Xu, Y., Buikema, H., van Gilst, W. H., & Henning, R. H. (2008). Caveolae and endothelial dysfunction: Filling the caves in cardiovascular disease. *Eur J Pharmacol, 585,* 256–60.

Yamamoto, M., Ramirez, S. H., Sato, S., Kiyota, T., Cerny, R. L., Kaibuchi, K., et al. (2008). Phosphorylation of claudin-5 and occludin by rho kinase in brain endothelial cells. *Am J Pathol, 172,* 521–33.

Zhong, Y., Smart, E. J., Weksler, B., Couraud, P. O., Hennig, B., & Toborek, M. (2008). Caveolin-1 regulates human immunodeficiency virus-1 Tat-induced alterations of tight junction protein expression via modulation of the Ras signaling. *J Neurosci, 28,* 7788–96.

Zhong, Y., Hennig, B., & Toborek, M. (2010). Intact lipid rafts regulate HIV-1 Tat protein-induced activation of the Rho signaling and upregulation of P-glycoprotein in brain endothelial cells. *J Cereb Blood Flow Metab, 30,* 522–33.

Zietz, C., Hotz, B., Stürzl, M., Rauch, E., Penning, R., & Löhrs, U. (1996). Aortic endothelium in HIV-1 infection: Chronic injury, activation, and increased leukocyte adherence. *Am J Pathol, 149,* 1887–98.

3.3

BLOOD-BRAIN BARRIER DURING NEUROINFLAMMATION

Yuri Persidsky and Servio H. Ramirez

The blood-brain barrier (BBB) shields the brain from the free entry of many toxins and immune cells, thereby providing a specialized environment for neurons and glial cells. In addition, the BBB plays an important role in the regulation and delivery of nutrients to the central nervous system (CNS). During inflammation, many aspects of BBB function are altered. For example, the overproduction of pro-inflammatory molecules by inflammatory and endothelial cells alters BBB transporter functions and thereby increases BBB permeability to neurotoxins and other substances. Inflammation also disrupts junction complexes between brain microvascular endothelial cells, and alters mediators of leukocyte adhesion to endothelial cells, thereby facilitating entry of leukocytes into the brain parenchyma. This chapter explores BBB function in the setting of neuroinflammation. The chapter is organized around the following broad areas, all with a focus on the impact of inflammation: signaling mechanisms regulating BBB permeability, endothelial efflux transporters, BBB impairment in neuropathologic conditions, and therapeutic approaches to limiting neruoinflammation. The discussion of therapeutic approaches includes agents that target GSK3β, peroxisome proliferator-activated receptors, progesterone, and statins.

INTRODUCTION

The blood-brain barrier (BBB) serves as shield from toxins and immune cells, providing a unique environment for normal function of neurons and glial cells. In addition to its protective function, the BBB plays an important "nurturing" role since numerous transporters deliver necessary nutrients to the central nervous system (CNS). Under inflammatory conditions, these homeostatic functions of the BBB are affected due to overproduction of pro-inflammatory molecules by inflammatory cells and endothelium (Neuwelt et al., 2008), upregulation of inflammation-driven pathways in brain endothelial cells and adjacent CNS cells, and leukocyte endothelial cell engagement (including leukocyte adhesion and transendothelial migration). All these factors and cell-cell interactions result in BBB dysfunction (increased permeability, diminished shield function against neurotoxins, and dysregulated expression/function of transporters).

Tissue leukocyte migration is an important event in immune surveillance, acute self-limiting inflammation, and

antigen recognition. Enhanced transendothelial migration and accumulation of leukocytes in tissues is a sign of chronic pathologic inflammatory processes (like multiple sclerosis [MS], encephalitis). BBB injury in neuroinflammation is believed to result from disruption of junction complexes between brain microvascular endothelial cells (BMVEC) facilitating entry of leukocytes into the brain parenchyma. While other pathways for leukocyte migration have been proposed (e.g. transcytosis), both experimental and clinical observations point to the importance of the paracellular route in leukocyte entry across the BBB during CNS inflammation (Schenkel et al., 2004). Adhesion and migration are mediated by leukocyte-endothelial cell (through integrins, intercellular adhesion molecules [ICAM], vascular cell adhesion molecule [VCAM]) and endothelial-endothelial cell interactions (via various small GTPases) where endothelial cells are active participants and regulators of this process (Cullere et al., 2005; Yang et al., 2005).

BMVEC-leukocyte engagement via adhesion molecules and their leukocyte ligands results in activation of small GTPases and subsequent modification of junctions. BMVEC are connected by tight junctions (TJ) and adherent junctions (AJ), and modifications of TJ/AJ complexes are required during paracellular leukocyte migration. Rho GTPases are potent modulators of the actin cytoskeleton and BMVEC adhesion (Burridge & Wennerberg, 2004). The following section describes signaling events associated with BMVEC-leukocyte interactions that destabilize the TJ directly or via cytoskeletal reorganization.

SIGNALING MECHANISMS REGULATING BLOOD-BRAIN BARRIER PERMEABILITY DURING INFLAMMATION

Various pro-inflammatory insults can trigger signaling mechanisms at the brain endothelial cell that can impact permeability of the BBB. As mentioned earlier, the BBB is not a static structure, but one of great complexity responding to cellular insults coming from the basal (CNS) and luminal (blood) side of the barrier. Therefore, in terms of neuroinflammation, the BBB can be under attack from either side of the barrier. Although compensatory mechanisms are in place, it is not precisely known what signaling thresholds need to be reached or at what point the BBB looses integrity in situations of disease. The most observable dysfunction of the BBB is that of increased permeability and enhanced surface and secreted inflammatory mediators that lead to immune infiltration of the CNS. On both counts, the TJ are greatly involved and are endpoint targets of complex intracellular signaling mechanisms. Multiple pathways have been associated with the disruption of member proteins of the TJ complex with crosstalk signaling that differs temporally (in time of initiation and range of duration) and spatially (i.e., compartmentalized signaling). The pathways that affect TJ proteins during inflammation can result in any of the following outcomes: sub-cellular re-distribution, change in expression and post-translational modification that affect protein half-life, and protein-protein interactions. The following section examines signaling pathways known to act on the tight junction complex.

The cytokine MCP-1/CCL2 is a pro-inflammatory chemoattractant of critical importance for neuroinflammation including the neuropathogenesis of HIV-1 (Persidsky, Ghorpade et al., 1999; Gonzalez et al., 2002; Eugenin et al., 2006). During neuroinflammation, MCP-1/CCL2 can originate from activated astrocytes, microglia, and endothelial cells creating a chemoattractant gradient for infected monocytes in the CNS (Ge et al., 2009). A secondary role of MCP-1/CCL2, upon binding to CCR2, is the stimulation of the opening of the barrier (Dimitrijevic et al., 2005). This interendothelial opening of the BBB occurs by effects on the actin cytoskeleton and TJ proteins, occludin and claudin-5 (Hirase et al., 2001; Stamatovic et al., 2009). MCP-1/CCL2 enhances permeability of the barrier by internalization of both occludin and claudin-5 (subcellular redistribution) into recycling endosomes (Stamatovic et al., 2009). Recycling of the TJ protein can rapidly re-seal the barrier after leukocyte CNS entry, exemplifying the dynamic nature of the TJ (Stamatovic et al., 2009). MCP-1/CCL2-mediated TJ protein internalization has also been shown to be lipid raft/caveolae and caveolin-1 dependent, distinguished from clathrin-mediated endocytosis by strategies that deplete cholesterol and disrupt the lipid raft (Song et al., 2007; Stamatovic et al., 2009). Interestingly, siRNA or gene deletion has shown that loss of caveolin results in hyperpermeability and abnormal TJ protein profile (Jasmin et al., 2007; Lin et al., 2007; Song et al., 2007). Additionally, the effects of MCP-1/CCL2 on the endothelial cell are augmented by reduced caveolin resulting in higher transendothelial migration (Song et al., 2007). As such, this suggests the possibility of non-caveolin-dependent pathways in MCP-1/CCL2 modulation of the BBB. Indeed, MCP-1/CCL2 signaling has been mapped to act on the cytoskeleton-modifying Rho GTPases and Rho kinase pathway (Stamatovic et al., 2006). The contribution of signaling that acts on the Rho family of GTPases is of central importance since TJ proteins are ultrastructurally connected to the cytoskeleton of the endothelial cell (Vandenbroucke et al., 2008). It is thought that one possible mechanism of interendothelial BBB opening comes from cytoskeletal contractile forces that retract the TJ complex and generate a "leakier" barrier. The Rho family of GTPases, RhoA, Rac1, and Cdc42 (the ones most studied in brain endothelial cells) are activated states during TJ

disassembly, which increase permeability (Matter & Balda, 2003). The G-protein-coupled receptor CCR2, upon binding to MCP-1/CCL2, triggers signals that activate RhoA, inducing the subsequent activation of Rho-associated kinase, which then phosphorylates myosin light chain (MLC) allowing actin-myosin interactions (Wettschureck & Offermanns, 2002). Actin and myosin induces stress fiber formation that pulls and retracts the TJ complex. Alternatively activated RhoA and via Rho kinase can also promote phosphorylation of occludin proteins at the C-terminus leading to permeability (Persidsky, Heilman et al., 2006). MCP-1/CCL2 signaling to the RhoA-Rho kinase pathway was determined from studies with the RhoA and the Rho kinase inhibitors (Stamatovic et al., 2003). The addition of Rho pathway inhibitors resulted in complete abrogation of the permeability and TJ protein changes brought by MCP-1/CCL2. As it is often the case in inflammatory signaling, the involvement of not one but multiple pathways can be observed. Like inflammatory activators, such as phorbol esters, bradykinin, and platelet-activating factor, MCP-1/CCL2 can bifurcate the stimulation of endothelial Ca^{2+} and PKC signaling (Hawkins & Davis, 2005; Stamatovic et al., 2006). Ca^{2+} induction and binding to calmodulin activates MLC kinase, which phosphorylates MLC, leading to stress fiber formation. Furthermore, PKC (PKCα and PKCζ)-dependent mechanisms act directly on the TJ proteins via serine/threonine phosphorylation of ZO-1, ZO-2, and on the cytoskeletal actin by MLC phosphorylation. Whereas Rho inhibition eliminates the MCP-1/CCL2 effects on the TJ, inhibition of PKC provides partial inhibition of these effects.

In addition to soluble pro-inflammatory factors, endothelial-immune cell interaction strongly signals to the TJ complex as a priming event for TJ disassembly and immune cell migration. During the course of brain endothelial activation, the surface expression of adhesion molecules such as ICAM-1 and VCAM-1 increases, engaging these adhesion molecules by complementary integrin clusters with the adhesion molecules and signaling is initiated (Etienne et al., 1998). Clustering of ICAM-1 and VCAM-1 triggers Rac-1 and RhoA-Rho kinase activation that lead to BBB opening by phosphorylation of TJ proteins (Persidsky, et al., 2006). In vitro experiments, using peptide mapping, have revealed that Rho kinase directly phosphorylates the C-terminus of occludin (T382 and S507) as well as the C-terminus of claudin-5 (T207) (Yamamoto et al., 2008). Furthermore, antibodies generated to recognize specifically these sites showed high immunoreactivity in human brain vessels of patients affected by HIV-1 encephalitis (HIVE) and in a mouse model for HIVE (Yamamoto et al., 2008). Whether in cytokine activation, as in the case with MCP-1/CCl2, or immune engagement, the Rho pathway in the brain endothelial funnels signaling mechanisms to modulate the TJ dynamically.

Metalloproteinases (MMPs) are also involved in BBB permeability. The MMPs at the BBB have been studied in various settings of neuroinflammation, including hemorrhage/stroke, MS, and Alzheimer's disease (AD) (Candelario-Jalil et al., 2009). MMPs are zinc-dependent endopeptidases that once cleaved to the active form and degrade nearly all components of the basal lamina extracellular matrix, like collagen type IV, fibronectin, and laminins (Hu et al., 2007). The result is a focal weakening in the anchoring of the vessel wall, which disrupts the BBB. In cerebral ischemia and in both acute and chronic brain inflammation, the upregulated and active forms of MMP-2 (activated earlier) and MMP -9 (later) are major contributors of BBB breakdown and neuronal damage. MMP activity has also been implicated in aiding leukocyte trafficking by not only disrupting the BBB, but also the glia limitans, to finally gain access to the CNS (Carvey et al., 2009). Aside from degradation of the basement membrane, the MMPs can also target degradation of TJ proteins occludin and claudin 5 (Reijerkerk et al., 2006). Occludin has a putative MMP cleavage site on its first extracellular loop. Recent studies have shown that the process of diapedesis of monocytes across brain endothelial monolayers use MMPs as means to break down occludin and permit passage (Reijerkerk et al., 2006; Rosenberg & Yang, 2007). It is known that depending on the inflammatory condition the source of MMPs can be immune cells (such monocytes and neutrophils) or endothelial cells. Indeed, dexamethasone tightening of the barrier in brain endothelial cultures was linked to reduction in MMP activity (Harkness et al., 2000). The role of MMPs in BBB integrity will continue to be defined, although it appears that MMPs may be an endpoint part of various pathways that signal to regulate the BBB.

The Wnt signaling pathway is known to play important roles in development and in many biological processes involved in differentiation, cell fate, proliferation, and morphology (Chien & Moon, 2007) recently has been recognized as central to BBB regulation. The canonical WNT signaling pathway is initiated by WNT ligand (i.e., WNT1 and WNT3a) binding to Frizzled (FZD) receptors and lipoprotein receptor-related protein 5 (LRP5) or LRP6 co-receptors (McNeill & Woodgett, 2010). Axin and glycogen synthase kinase (GSK) 3β in the absence of WNT activation induces the degradation of β-catenin; however, binding of WNT ligand to FZD/LRP recruits axin and GSK3β away from β-catenin freeing β-catenin to translocate to the nucleus where it binds to TCF/LEF and mediates transcription of target genes. WNT signaling has been placed at the center of BBB formation during development (Liebner et al., 2008). In vivo analyses showed high activation of the WNT pathway during prenatal development of the brain vasculature. In contrast, monitoring of WNT activation in postnatal and the adult brain vasculature showed significant decrease (former) and near absence (later) of signaling. Inactivation of β-catenin during BBB development resulted in hyperpermeability and increased immunolabeling of the TJ claudin-3. Introduction of condition media containing WNT3a ligand to endothelial cultures upregulated claudin-3, but interestingly ZO-1, claudin-5, or occludin did not (Liebner et al., 2008). Given that β-catenin associates with the TJ complex, it was discerned that it is the transcriptional role of β-catenin rather than the TJ-associated role that was important for increased claudin-3 expression. Another means of affecting β-catenin stabilization is by inhibition of GSK3β; it is still not entirely clear whether the role of β-catenin on TJ protein expression via WNT could be bypassed by this

inhibition. Previous experiments give some validity to the notion of tightening of the barrier by inhibition of GSK3β without the involvement of WNT (Liu et al., 2002). Studies with hepatocyte growth factor, which signals to AKT and subsequently inhibits GSK3β, resulted in higher transendothelial electrical resistance (TEER) on endothelial cells. Besides the effects of GSK3β on barrier integrity, a consequence of GSK3β inhibition on human brain endothelial cells is the potent attenuation of endothelial inflammatory responses (Ramirez et al.). Therefore, WNT ligands and GSK3β pharmacological inhibitors hold promise in protecting the barrier in two ways, by 1) improving barrier integrity and 2) inhibiting endothelial activation.

ENDOTHELIAL ABC EFFLUX TRANSPORTER FUNCTION IN NEUROINFLAMMATION

While TJ provide the structural integrity of the BBB, transport systems and drug-metabolizing enzymes are responsible for an enzymatic barrier (Leslie et al., 2005) restricting penetration of xenobiotics into the brain. BBB transporters belong to the ATP-binding cassette (ABC) super family of proteins that mediates cellular extrusion of many therapeutic agents of diverse origin and clinical applications. BMVEC uniquely express so-called multi-drug resistance (MDR) proteins in a highly polarized fashion. Two major transporters expressed in BMVEC are P-glycoprotein (P-gp), first detected in chemotherapy-resistant cancer cells that over-expressed several efflux transporters (Schinkel & Jonker, 2003), and breast cancer resistance protein (BCRP, also known as ABCG2) (Zhang et al., 2003; Cisternino et al., 2004). Their expression in the blood (luminal) plasma membrane of BMVEC hampers the passage of drugs and toxins across the BBB into the brain and can facilitate their transport from brain to blood (Fricker & Miller, 2004). Diminished expression of BCRP (Persidsky et al., 2006) and P-gp on BMVEC was found in human brain tissues affected by HIVE, indicating that the combination of inflammatory responses and viral infection could result in BBB dysfunction (Persidsky & Gendelman, 2003; Langford et al., 2004) and subsequent neurodegeneration.

There is some controversy regarding the effects of cytokines on the expression of the mRNAs and of the protein for transporters documenting increase, no change, or decrease in mRNAs or protein levels (reviewed in Fernandez et al., 2004). Published results are more unanimous pointing to diminished transporter function after TNF-α treatment (Mandi et al., 1998; Zhao et al., 2002; Theron et al., 2003) or to an LPS-induced inflammation model (Goralski et al., 2003). Poller et al. (Poller, Drewe et al.) investigated the effect of the pro-inflammatory cytokines (IL-1β, IL-6, and TNF-α) on the expression and activity of BCRP and P-gp in a human brain microvascular cell line (hCMEC/D3). BCRP mRNA levels were significantly reduced by all cytokines, and the most prominent suppression of the BCRP protein was detected after IL-1β application. All three cytokines also reduced the BCRP activity (assessed by uptake of the specific substrate, mitoxantrone). Interestingly, P-gp mRNA levels were slightly reduced by IL-6, but significantly increased after TNF-α treatment. TNF-α also increased P-gp protein expression, but the cytokines did not affect uptake the P-gp substrate, rhodamine 123.

Very little is known regarding the mechanisms of P-gp or BCRP modulation by cytokines, as very few have investigated the regulatory mechanisms involved at the molecular level. Recent works indicated rapid downregulation of P-gp activity (within minutes) via endothelin (ET) -1 stimulation of $ET_{B/A}$ receptors secondary to effects of TNF-α. Activation of $ET_{A/B}$ receptors led to NOS activation and PKC stimulation without any change in barrier permeability or distribution of TJ proteins (Hartz et al., 2006). Exposing brain capillaries to TNF-α or ET-1 for 6 hours resulted in an increase in P-gp transport activity and protein expression, and in addition to NOS/PKC activation NF-kB was implicated in these changes (Bauer et al., 2007). Interestingly, expression of BCRP protein was decreased. While being an interesting observation, these results are opposite to the decrease in P-gp function seen in vivo and in vitro under inflammatory conditions. Longer period of exposure or other mediators involved could be an explanation. Activation of PKC is of special interest since our previous work suggested that HIV-1 gp120 also induced activation of PKC and Ca^{2+} release in primary human BMVEC (Kanmogne et al., 2007), and inhibition of PKC isoforms prevented gp120-induced functional effects in BMVEC (increased permeability and leukocyte migration across monolayers). Experiments performed using primary BMVEC and autopsy brain tissues affected by HIVE clearly indicated a decrease in expression and function of P-gp and BCRP.

P-gp is known to localize in caveolae and inhibition of P-gp transport activity was associated with caveolin-1 phosphorylation (Barakat et al., 2007). Activation of tyrosine kinases, such as Src, was responsible for the tyrosine 14 phosphorylation of caveolin-1(Labrecque et al., 2004). Better understanding of the putative mechanisms underlying downregulation of transporters on the BBB during neuroinflammation is needed as ABC drug transporters transport a large array of drugs, the effects of inflammation may drastically affect drug bioavailability or tissue uptake, and subsequently, drug efficacy or toxicity (Ho & Piquette-Miller, 2006).

Recent data suggest that estradiol (E2) signaled through estrogen receptor beta to downregulate BCRP expression. Using rat brain capillaries, Hartz et al. (Hartz, Mahringer et al.) showed that E2 increased active PTEN, decreased active Akt, and increased phosphorylated, active GSK3β. Inhibition of PI3K or Akt decreased BCRP activity and protein expression, and inhibition of PTEN or GSK3β reversed the E2 effect on BCRP. Proteasome inhibitor abolished E2-mediated BCRP downregulation, suggesting internalization followed by transporter degradation. Treatment of mice with E2 reduced BCRP activity in brain capillaries within 1 hour; this reduction persisted for 24 hours. BCRP protein expression in brain capillaries was unchanged 1 hour after E2 application, and it was substantially diminished 6 and 24 hours after E2 treatment. Further studies will be necessary to demonstrate

how other ABC transporters are affected by inflammation and what are the mechanisms underlying such changes.

BLOOD-BRAIN BARRIER IMPAIRMENT IN NEUROPATHOLOGIC CONDITIONS

It is increasingly recognized that injury to the CNS, whether in the form of a neurodegenerative condition, traumatic brain injury, cerebral hemorrhage, or pathogen-mediated inflammation, features various degrees of BBB disruption and is associated with various degrees of inflammatory responses. The disruption can occur in the physical, enzymatic, transport, and immunological capacities of the BBB. Therefore, all of these regulatory barriers are at risk of dysfunction in CNS pathologies. However, before looking at specific examples of CNS pathology, consider that, aside from forming a barrier to blood components, the brain endothelium is also involved in clearing of CNS metabolic byproducts, inactivation of neurotransmitters, hemodynamic neurovascular coupling, neurotrophin support, and neurogenic coupling. In all, the BBB is a highly dynamic structure that allows for a neuronal environment, which is optimal for neuronal function and more importantly, synaptic communication. The following section will review various CNS pathologies with a focus on the BBB.

Blood-brain barrier dysfunction occurs in neurodegenerative diseases such as AD, Parkinson's disease (PD), and MS. It is not known whether disruption to the BBB in neurodegeneration occurs first or whether it is a consequence of the disease. Inflammation plays an important role in the pathogenesis of AD and anti-inflammatory drugs suppress glial activation and regulate amyloid precursor protein (APP) processing (Zhou et al., 2003). Microglia play critical roles in inciting inflammation and accumulation is seen at the site of senile plaques in AD brains. Microglia are activated by APP processing products, such as secreted APP and Aβ peptide, and induce neurotoxicity (Barger & Harmon, 1997; Ikezu et al., 2003) affecting Aβ deposition and neurodegenerative processes including synaptic and neuronal cell loss. Tg2576 transgenic APP mice reproduce many aspects of human disease including microglial-induced brain inflammation, Aβ plaque formation, dystrophic neurites, astrogliosis, microglial activation, and deficits in learning and memory (Hsiao et al., 1996; Frautschy et al., 1998). Tg2576 mice deficient for CD40 ligand, a signaling molecule participating in T-cell microglial immune responses, show a marked reduction in Aβ deposition, microglial reactions, astrogliosis, and APP processing (Tan et al., 2002).

There is experimental evidence that cerebral perfusion is decreased during aging and in AD (McGeer et al., 2005). It has been shown that widespread Aβ accumulation resulted in degeneration and endothelial cells leading to microvessel obliteration (Ferrer et al., 2004). Miao et al. (, 2005) investigated the temporal development of cerebral vascular amyloid and its associated pathology in Tg-SwDI mice. They demonstrated that with increasing age there is extensive accumulation of fibrillar vascular amyloid, particularly in cerebral microvessels, and accumulation of cerebral vascular amyloid was associated with reduced microvessel density, vascular cell apoptosis, and vascular cell loss. Notably, neuroinflammatory cells were associated with the cerebral microvascular amyloid. These animals exhibited elevated levels of the inflammatory cytokines IL-1β and IL-6. These findings support a role for cerebral microvascular amyloid in promoting localized neuroinflammation. As compared to control littermates, TgAPP and PS1/APPsw transgenic mice showed a significant increase in the following pro-inflammatory cytokines: TNF-α, IL-6, IL-12p40, IL-1α, IL-1β, and GM-CSF. Several cytokines (TNF-α, IL-6, IL-1α, and GM-CSF) showed an increase from control to Tg2576 to PS1/APPsw, suggesting that the amplitude of this cytokine response is dependent on brain Aβ levels, since PS1/APPsw mouse brains accumulate more Aβ than Tg2576 mouse brains (Patel et al., 2005).

Ujiie et al. demonstrated that BBB permeability is increased in the cerebral cortex of 10-month-old Tg2576 mice before development of AD pathology (Ujiie et al., 2003). Furthermore, when compared with their nontransgenic littermates, 4-month-old Tg2576 mice exhibit compromised BBB integrity in some areas of the cerebral cortex. Immunization with Aβ peptides or passive immunization with antibodies against Aβ has been reported to reduce plaque burden, neuritic dystrophy, early Tau pathology, microgliosis, as well as reversing learning and memory deficits. When Tg2576 mice were immunized with Aβ before and after the onset of AD-type neuropathology, BBB permeability, amyloid burden, and microgliosis were decreased (Dickstein et al., 2006). This suggested that the BBB is disrupted in AD mice, and once Aβ is removed, the integrity of the BBB is restored (Dickstein et al., 2006). Decrease in Aβ burden also resulted in diminished inflammation as evidenced by diminished microglial activation and decrease in reactive oxygen species (ROS) and cytokine production. Dickstein and colleagues assumed that TJ were affected in transgenic animals; however, TJ compromise was not investigated.

Accumulation of Aβ in the brain is determined by the rate of its generation versus clearance (Tanzi et al., 2004). Clearance can be accomplished via two major pathways: proteolytic degradation and receptor-mediated transport from the brain. Mounting evidence suggests that the low-density lipoprotein receptor-related protein (LRP) is involved in receptor-mediated efflux of Aβ across the BBB (reviewed in Zlokovic, 2005). In addition, it was shown in vitro that Aβ is transported by P-gp. Aβ deposition is significantly elevated in brain tissue of individuals with low expression of P-gp in brain endothelial cells. Vogelgesang et al. (Vogelgesang et al., 2004) investigated the association between cerebral amyloid angiopathy (CAA) and P-gp expression in brain tissue from 243 nondemented elderly cases (aged 50 to 91 years). Microvessels with high P-gp expression showed no Aβ deposition in their walls, and vice versa. At early stages, Aβ accumulation occurred in arterioles where P-gp expression was primarily low, and disappeared completely with the accumulation of Aβ. Initially, P-gp was upregulated in capillaries, suggesting a compensatory mechanism to increase Aβ clearance from the brain. Capillaries were usually affected at advanced stages of CAA, and P-gp was lost even in these vessels. Therefore, Aβ clearance may be altered in

individuals with diminished P-gp expression secondary to genetic or environmental effects (such as drug administration). These observations were strengthened by Cirrito et al. (2005), who demonstrated that Aβ microinjected into the CNS clear at half the rate in P-gp-null mice than in WT mice. When APP-transgenic mice were treated with P-gp inhibitor, Aβ levels within the brain interstitial fluid significantly increased within hours of treatment. APP-transgenic/P-gp-null mice had enhanced Aβ deposition compared with APP-transgenic, P-gp WT mice.

To assess association between Aβ deposition and signs of BBB impairment, we analyzed brain tissues from five patients with diagnosis of AD and five age-matched controls. Using double stain for BCRP and CD163 we demonstrated an association between diminished BCRP staining and increased CD163 (Fig. 3.3.1A,E) that correlated with intensity of Aβ deposition (Fig. 3.3.1D,H). These changes paralleled also diminished expression of claudin-5 (Fig. 3.3.1B,F). Microglial activation was detected in the same areas (Fig. 3.3.1C,G) as Aβ plaques (E,H) and infiltration of CD163⁺ macrophages (A,B,E,F). Similar alterations were found in animal models for AD. Analyses of APP, APP/CCL2, and WT mice indicated inverted association between signs of neuroinflammation, claudin-5, BCRP, and P-gp staining (Fig. 3.3.2); and neuroinflammation inversely correlated with P-gp, BCRP, and TJ protein expression. Diminished expression of TJ proteins was proportional to the level of microglial activation and formation of dense plaques (Fig. 3.3.2 A,B,C,D). Intensity of P-gp staining was attenuated in APP/CCL2 mice as compared to APP animals and associated with microglial reaction (Fig. 3.3.2 C,F). These data established a direct link between P-gp and metabolism in vivo and suggest that P-gp activity at the BBB could affect risk for developing AD as well as provide a novel diagnostic and therapeutic target.

Neurodegeneration resulting from inflammation and immune infiltration in the brain, as in the case of MS, exemplifies a breach in the immunological barrier that is provided by the BBB. Pathologically, MS features demyelination of nerve cells both in the brain and in the spinal cord, axonal damage, oligodendrocyte loss, and gliosis. The cause is a function of infiltrating subpopulations of immune cells into CNS that are activated and destroy neuronal cells. Although the brain undergoes very low-level immune surveillance, it is for the most part restrictive to immune cells at the BBB. Dysfunction of the BBB is a major hallmark of MS. McQuaid et al. (2009) showed that increased BBB permeability is associated with decreased expression of TJ proteins in brain capillary endothelial cells. TJ abnormalities were found in active lesions (42% of vessels affected), and they were also present in inactive lesions (23%) and in normal-appearing MS white matter (13%). TJ impairment was associated with leakage of the serum protein fibrinogen, which has recently been shown to be an activator of microglia. TJ abnormality and the resultant vascular permeability in both plaque-containing and normal-appearing white matter may impair tissue homeostasis having effects on MS progression, repair mechanisms, and drug delivery. The animal model for MS, experimental autoimmune encephalomyelitis (EAE), has been a great tool is discerning the

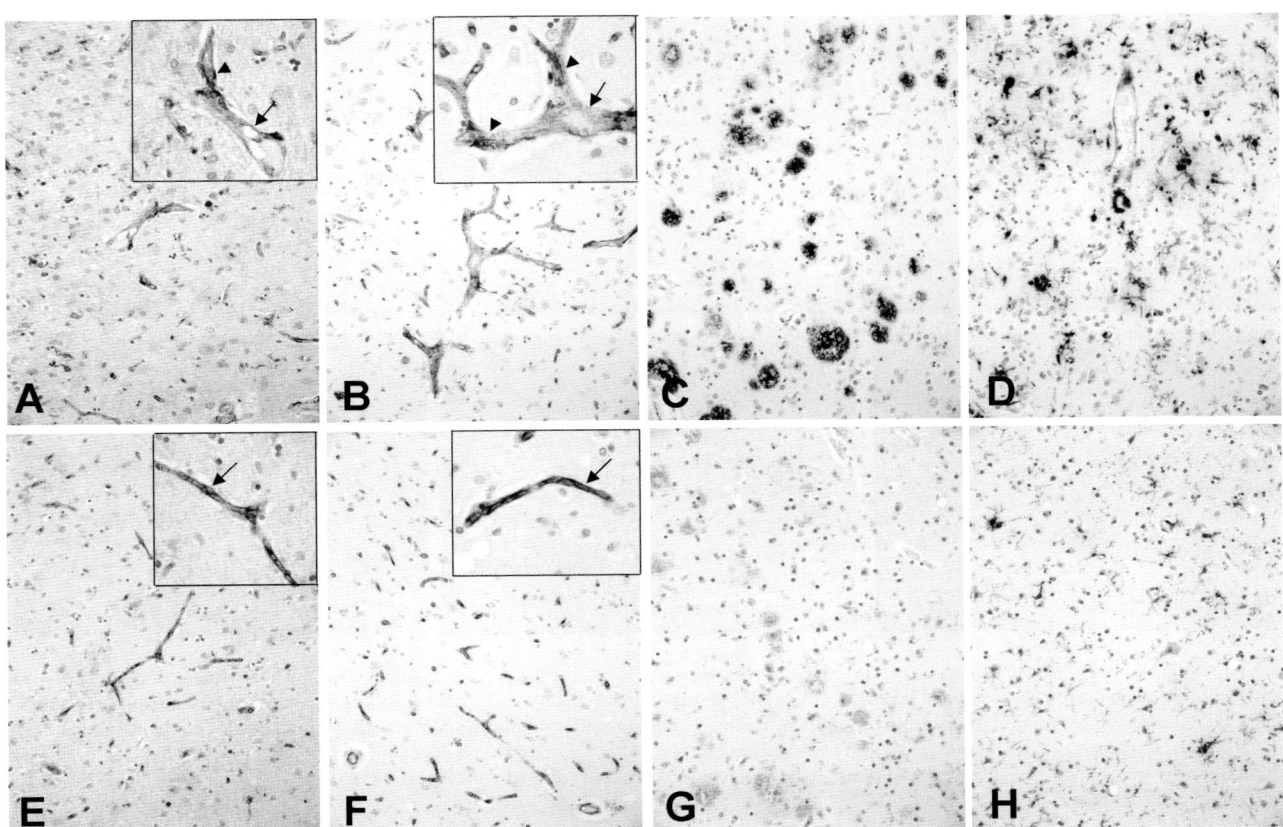

Figure 3.3.1 Microglial activation, TJ protein, and BCRP expression correlated with distribution of dense plaques in brain tissue with AD. (A, E) BCRP expression in AD brain tissues (brown, arrows) inversely correlated with accumulation of CD163+ perivascular macrophages (pink, arrowhead). (B,F) Claudin-5 immunostaining (brown, arrow) macrophages was diminished in AD brain showing prominent increase in CD163+ macrophages (pink, arrowhead) vs. preserved claudin-5 staining was associated with minimal presence of macrophages. These changes paralleled accumulation of Aβ within neuropil (C,G) and correlated with microglial activation (D,H). Serial brain section were stained with immunostained with Abs to BCRP/CD163 (A,E), claudin-5/CD163 (B,F), MHC class II (HLA-DR, C,G) and Aβ (D,H). Original magnification, panels A-H x 200, inserts panels A,B,E,F x 400.

mechanisms of aberrant immune-cell trafficking into the brain. Demyelinated white-matter focal plaques demonstrate an abundant infiltration of T cells and macrophages and damaged BBB. Suidan et al. (2008) showed that in vivo stimulation of CNS-infiltrating antigen-specific CD8 T cells initiates astrocyte activation, alteration of BBB TJ proteins, and increased CNS vascular permeability in a non-apoptotic manner. It was concluded that, despite having similar expansion of CD8 T cells in the brain as wild type and Fas ligand-deficient animals, perforin-deficient mice were resistant to TJ alterations and CNS vascular permeability. Therefore, CNS-infiltrating antigen-specific CD8 T cells have the capacity to initiate TJ disruption through a non-apoptotic perforin-dependent mechanism. Inflammation-driven leukocyte transendothelial migration in the brain is a multistep process, involving orchestrated immune-endothelial interactions that result in leukocyte rolling/adhesion, transmigration, accumulation in the perivascular space, and passage across the glial limitans. These transmigration events have been associated with deterioration of the BBB in 1) chronic inflammation of the endothelium that promotes leukocyte recruitment, and 2) regional breakdown of BBB TJ complexes. Indeed,

current antibody-based therapies to combat MS center on preventing the migration of T cell subpopulations into the CNS. This strategy shows promise in drastically restoring BBB function and limiting leukocyte transmigration into MS lesions. In addition to TJ (structural integrity), the transport function of BBB is also compromised in MS. Kooij et al. (2009) found that vascular P-gp expression and function were substantially diminished during MS and EAE. P-gp expression coincided with the presence of perivascular infiltrates consisting of lymphocytes. Lymphocyte interaction through ICAM-1 resulted in activation of NF-κB signaling pathway, which resulted in endothelial P-gp malfunction.

Our previous work indicated that there is a significant BBB impairment in HIVE. Major features include decrease in expression and post-translational modifications of TJ complexes mediated via activation of small GTPases (RhoA, Rac1) (Persidsky et al., 2006; Yamamoto et al., 2008) and CD40-CD40L signaling via cJUN-N-terminal kinase and mixed-lineage-kinase-3 leading to the subsequent activation of cJUN/AP-1 (activating-protein-1)(Ramirez et al., 2010). Furthermore, we found that both P-gp and BCRP expression

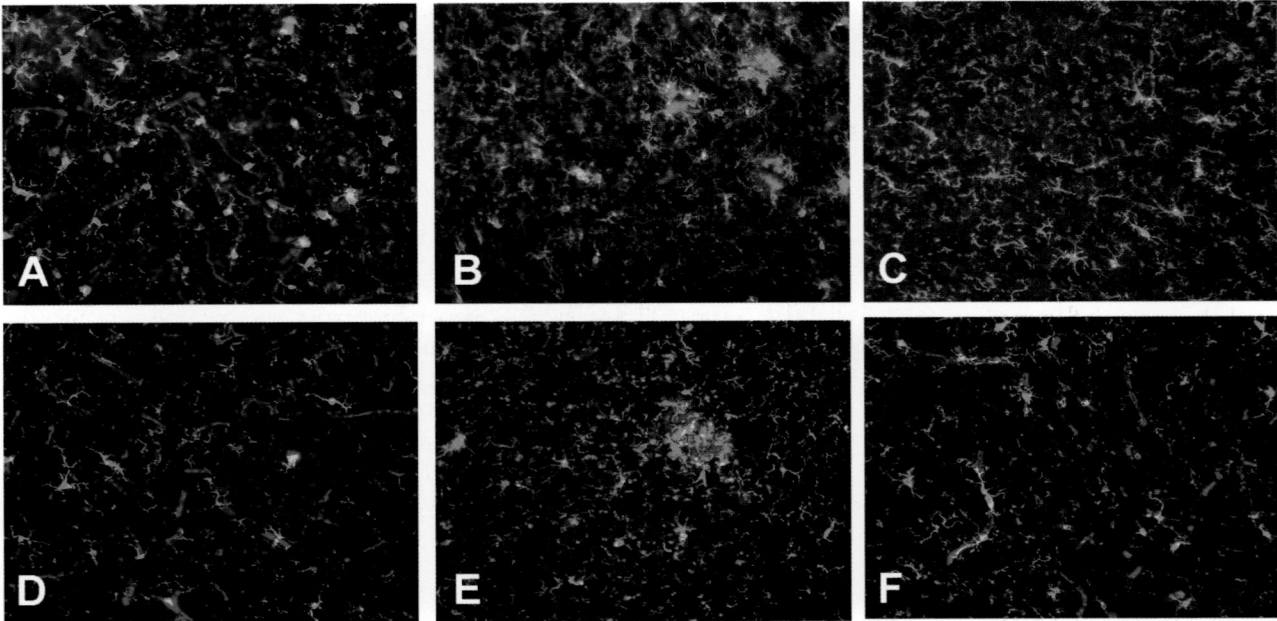

Figure 3.3.2 Expression of TJ and ABC transporter in the brain tissues of APP and APP/CCL2 transgenic mice. (A,D) Areas devoid of dense plaques demonstrated preserved claudin-5 staining in APP/CLL2 (red, A) and APP mice (B); however, microglial reaction (green, Iba1) was more prominent in APP/CCL2 mice when compared to APP animals. (B,E) Claudin-5 staining (red) was diminished in areas with plaque formation and prominent microglial activation (green). (C,F) P-gp expression (red) was attenuated in APP/CCL2 mice (C) as compared to APP animals (F). These changes paralleled intensity of microgliosis (green). Serial brain section were double immunostained with Abs to claudin-5/Iba1 (A,B,D,E), P-gp/Iba1 (C,F). Original magnification, panels A, B, C, D, E, F x 200.

were substantially decreased in human brain tissues affected by HIVE (Persidsky et al., 2006).

There is an accumulating body of evidence that the BBB is impaired in PD patients. Peripheral immunity contributes to the degenerative process of PD and may be responsible for the progressive nature of the disease (Monahan et al., 2008). Relatively recently it has been shown that in both PD patients and animal models of PD neuroinflammation appears to be a ubiquitous finding (Whitton, 2007). Usual features of inflammation were described including phagocyte activation, increased synthesis and release of proinflammatory cytokines, and complement activation. It is postulated that in the PD etiology the overactivation of microglia, the overproduction of cytokines and other proinflammatory mediators, as well as the release of destructive molecules such as reactive oxygen species, lead to neurodegeneration. This hypothesis is supported by diverse literature that is just beginning to come together to suggest that PD is, in part, an autoimmune disease. Recent findings point to the involvement of the BBB in PD, by disruptive changes to P-gp expression and function. Clinical studies using measurements of brain uptake of radiolabeled verapamil (a P-gp substrate) have shown high uptake of verapamil in PD patients as high as 18% above that of the control group. In PD, a breach to the TJ physical barrier can also be observed in animal models of PD. For example, significant leakage of fluorescently conjugated albumin from the vasculature to the brain parenchyma has been demonstrated the 6-hydroxydopamine PD animal model.

ANTI-INFLAMMATORY AND BLOOD-BRAIN BARRIER PROTECTIVE AGENTS

Understanding of the molecular mechanisms of BBB impairment as described above ultimately allows development of therapeutic approaches repairing BBB and preventing neurodegeration. Such strategies could be subdivided into ones restoring function of transporters, normalizing BBB tightness, and preventing leukocyte infiltration; however, as evidenced from a few examples given below, there is a significant overlap between them.

One of the potential and underappreciated targets is inhibition of GSK3β, a ubiquitous serine/threonine protein kinase. It is involved in numerous and diverse biological functions including: glycogen metabolism, regulation of cell division, differentiation, and apoptosis (Jope et al., 2007). Only recently, GSK3β has been recognized as a key regulator of the inflammatory response. The anti-inflammatory effects of GSK3β inhibition were documented in vitro and in several in vivo models of acute and chronic inflammation (Takada et al., 2004; Dugo et al., 2005; Jope et al., 2007). Anti-inflammatory effects of GSK3β inhibitors are mediated via suppression of the inflammatory response in the vascular endothelium. GSK3β inactivation prevented VCAM-1 upregulation by TNF-α in aortic endothelial cells (Eto et al,. 2005) and E-selectin expression in umbilical vein endothelium (Gong et al., 2006). GSK3β suppression enhanced endothelial barrier properties in pulmonary arterial endothelial cells (Liu et al., 2002). Anti-inflammatory and neuroprotective effects of GSK3β inhibition have been shown in models of stroke (Renet al., 2003) and spinal cord injury (Cuzzocreaet al., 2006). Interestingly, GSK3β activation was implicated in a "leakier" BBB in mice deficient of platelet endothelial cell adhesion molecule that developed more EAE (Graesser et al., 2002).

We have addressed the role of GSK3β in regulating inflammatory responses in the brain endothelium (Ramirez et al., 2010). We found high levels of active GSK3β by immunohistochemistry in brain endothelium in human brain tissue affected by neuroinflammation (HIVE). Using primary human BMVEC, we investigated the effects of GSK3β inhibition under neuroinflammatory conditions. Suppression of GSK3β activity in inflamed brain endothelium prevented the enhanced adhesion of leukocytes in vitro and in vivo, downregulated VCAM-1 expression, protected barrier function, and diminished migration of monocytes across BMVEC monolayers in response to relevant pro-inflammatory factors. Furthermore, GSK3β inhibition downregulated mRNA and secretion of numerous inflammatory factors (including IP-10/CXCL10, MCP-1/CCL2, IL-8/CXCL8, RANTES/CCL5, and Gro α/CXCL1) in TNFα-stimulated BMVEC. These results suggest that GSK3β is a potential target for the treatment of BBB injury associated with pro-inflammatory insult and leukocyte infiltration of the CNS, thus providing both an anti-inflammatory and neuroprotective effect. Accumulating evidence suggests that GSK3β inhibitors could be BBB protective under diverse inflammatory conditions.

Another potentially relevant target is peroxisome proliferator-activated receptors (PPARs), transcriptional regulators and members of a nuclear receptor family closely related to PPARα, PPARβ/δ, and PPARγ (Desvergne & Wahli, 1991). PPARs regulate adipocyte differentiation, insulin sensitivity, anti-inflammatory responses, and antiproliferative effects in certain tumors (Lehrke & Lazar, 2005). The lipid-lowering fibrates, which activate PPARα, and the insulin-sensitizing thiazolidinediones, which activate PPARγ, have proven useful as potent anti-inflammatory agents (Zingarelli & Cook, 2005). Activation of PPARs can lead to transrepression that negatively interferes with key transcription factors (e.g., NF-κB, AP-1, STAT1, and sp1) involved in inflammatory responses. Activation of PPARs downregulated the expression of pro-inflammatory genes such as IL-1β, IL-6, inducible nitric oxide synthase, cyclooxygenase-2, and various chemokines (Brown & Plutzky, 2007). PPARs were found to decrease endothelial-leukocyte interactions in models of atherosclerosis (Kurebayashi et al., 2005; Zandbergen & Plutzky, 2007). While such inhibitory effects on monocyte adhesion by PPAR activation were attributed to adhesion molecule suppression in the endothelial cells, the precise mechanism remains elusive.

The anti-inflammatory effects of PPARs in BMVEC have remained largely unexplored in the context of neuroinflammation. We tested whether PPARγ activation in cytokine-stimulated human BMVEC could control monocyte adhesion and migration (Ramirez et al., 2008). We found that PPARγ activation in BMVEC led to significant reduction of monocyte adhesion and migration in a BBB culture model.

Since Rho GTPases are key regulatory factors in endothelial cell-leukocyte interactions, we investigated effects of PPARγ activation on GTPase activity. Analysis of the Rho family of GTPases in cytokine-stimulated and PPAR agonist-treated BMVEC resulted in dose-dependent inhibition of Rac1 and RhoA that paralleled diminished monocyte adhesion and migration across BMVEC monolayer. PPARγ stimulation of inactivated BMVEC resulted in a significant decrease in the adhesion and transmigration of HIV-1-infected monocytes across brain endothelium. While PPARγ stimulation did not change barrier properties without inflammatory insult (including TJ expression, P-gp, or transendothelial electrical resistance as a measure of barrier function). Together, these observations provide a novel inhibitory mechanism of monocyte adhesion/migration by PPARγ ligands acting in endothelial cells forming the BBB. These findings are applicable to all neuroinflammatory conditions involving BBB injury secondary to endothelial engagement by leukocytes (ranging from stroke to encephalitis). Intriguingly, Rac1 inhibition in BMVEC recently has been discovered to increase neuronal viability due to broad upregulation of the genes relevant to neurovascular protection and endothelium-derived neurotrophic factors (like artemin) (Sawada et al., 2008).

Progesterone emerges as new compound that protects the BBB. Both preclinical and epidemiologic studies indicate that the hormone possesses neuroprotective capabilities (Stein et al., 2008). While research published to date has focused primarily on progesterone's effects on blunt traumatic brain injury, progesterone also appears to afford protection from several forms of acute CNS injury, including penetrating brain trauma, stroke, anoxic brain injury, and spinal cord injury. Progesterone provides its protective effects by protecting the BBB, decreasing development of cerebral edema, protecting TJ proteins, and downregulating inflammatory responses (expression of TNF-α and MMP-9) (Jiang et al., 2009). The exact mechanisms of progesterone action remain elusive and deserve further studies.

Another class of BBB protective compounds is cholesterol-lowering drugs, the statins (3-hydroxy-3-methylglutaryl coenzyme A reductase, HMG-CoA inhibitors). Several studies demonstrated the ability of statins to diminish leukocyte migration across BBB (MS, meningitis) and prevent glutamate-induced BBB disruption. Statins prevented BBB disruption via nitric-oxide (NO)-dependent pathways by decreasing release of intracellular Ca^{2+}, ROS generation by the NADPH-oxidase and activation of myosin light chain kinase (Kuhlmann et al., 2008).

Statins improved functional signs in the animal model of MS and reduced the number of gadolinium-enhancing lesions in MS. Ifergan et al. (2006) showed that statins reduced diffusion rates of bovine serum albumin and [$^{(14)}$C]-sucrose 50–60% across human brain endothelial cell monolayers through inhibition of isoprenylation. Statins had no effect on expression of TJ molecules (occludin, VE-cadherin, JAM-1, ZO-1 and -2). Statin treatment of endothelial cells significantly restricted the migration of MS patient-derived monocytes and lymphocytes across the human BBB in vitro, through a specific reduction in the secretion of the chemokines,

MCP-1/CCL2, and IP-10/CXCL10, by human brain endothelial cells.

In summary, BBB functions are clearly affected by neuroinflammation, and BBB impairment is a significant feature of diverse neuropathologic conditions as well as a contributing factor to pathogenesis. Better understanding of molecular mechanisms leading to BBB injury will result in new barrier-protective therapeutic strategies.

ACKNOWLEDGMENTS

We thank Brenda Morsey, Ryan Brodie, Nancy Reichenbach, Holly Dykstra, and Shongshan Fan for excellent technical support. This work was supported in part by research grants by the National Institutes of Health: MH65151, AA017398, AA015913, and DA025566.

REFERENCES

Barakat, S., Demeule, M., et al. (2007). Modulation of p-glycoprotein function by caveolin-1 phosphorylation. *J Neurochem, 101*(1), 1–8.

Barger, S. W. & Harmon, A. D. (1997). Microglial activation by Alzheimer amyloid precursor protein and modulation by apolipoprotein E. *Nature, 388*(6645), 878–81.

Bauer, B., Hartz, A. M., et al. (2007). Tumor necrosis factor alpha and endothelin-1 increase P-glycoprotein expression and transport activity at the blood-brain barrier. *Mol Pharmacol, 71*(3), 667–75.

Brown, J. D. & Plutzky, J. (2007). Peroxisome proliferator-activated receptors as transcriptional nodal points and therapeutic targets. *Circulation, 115*(4), 518–33.

Burridge, K. & Wennerberg, K. (2004). Rho and Rac take center stage. *Cell, 116*(2), 167–79.

Candelario-Jalil, E., Yang, Y., et al. (2009). Diverse roles of matrix metalloproteinases and tissue inhibitors of metalloproteinases in neuroinflammation and cerebral ischemia. *Neuroscience, 158*(3), 983–94.

Carvey, P. M., Hendey, B., et al. (2009). The blood-brain barrier in neurodegenerative disease: A rhetorical perspective. *J Neurochem, 111*(2), 291–314.

Chien, A. J. & Moon, R. T. (2007). WNTS and WNT receptors as therapeutic tools and targets in human disease processes. *Front Biosci, 12,* 448–57.

Cirrito, J. R., Deane, R., et al. (2005). P-glycoprotein deficiency at the blood-brain barrier increases amyloid-beta deposition in an Alzheimer disease mouse model. *J Clin Invest, 115*(11), 3285–90.

Cisternino, S., Mercier, C., et al. (2004). Expression, up-regulation, and transport activity of the multidrug-resistance protein Abcg2 at the mouse blood-brain barrier. *Cancer Res, 64*(9), 3296–301.

Cullere, X., Shaw, S. K., et al. (2005). Regulation of vascular endothelial barrier function by Epac, a cAMP-activated exchange factor for Rap GTPase. *Blood, 105*(5), 1950–5.

Cuzzocrea, S., Genovese, T., et al. (2006). Glycogen synthase kinase-3 beta inhibition reduces secondary damage in experimental spinal cord trauma. *J Pharmacol Exp Ther, 318*(1), 79–89.

Desvergne, B. & Wahli, W. (1991). Peroxisome proliferator-activated receptors: Nuclear control of metabolism. *Endocr Rev, 20*(5), 649–88.

Dickstein, D. L., Biron, K. E., et al. (2006). Abeta peptide immunization restores blood-brain barrier integrity in Alzheimer disease. *Faseb J, 20*(3), 426–33.

Dimitrijevic, O. B., Stamatovic, S. M., et al. (2005). Effects of the chemokine CCL2 on blood-brain barrier permeability during ischemia-reperfusion injury. *J Cereb Blood Flow Metab.*

Dugo, L., Collin, M., et al. (2005). GSK-3beta inhibitors attenuate the organ injury/dysfunction caused by endotoxemia in the rat. *Crit Care Med, 33*(9), 1903–12.

Etienne, S., Adamson, P., et al. (1998). ICAM-1 signaling pathways associated with Rho activation in microvascular brain endothelial cells. *J Immunol, 161*(10), 5755–61.

Eto, M., Kouroedov, A., et al. (2005). Glycogen synthase kinase-3 mediates endothelial cell activation by tumor necrosis factor-alpha. *Circulation, 112*(9), 1316–22.

Eugenin, E. A., Osiecki, K., et al. (2006). CCL2/monocyte chemoattractant protein-1 mediates enhanced transmigration of human immunodeficiency virus (HIV)-infected leukocytes across the blood-brain barrier: A potential mechanism of HIV-CNS invasion and NeuroAIDS. *J Neurosci, 26*(4), 1098–106.

Fernandez, C., Buyse, M., et al. (2004). Influence of the pro-inflammatory cytokines on P-glycoprotein expression and functionality. *J Pharm Pharm Sci, 7*(3), 359–71.

Ferrer, I., Boada Rovira, M., et al. (2004). Neuropathology and pathogenesis of encephalitis following amyloid-beta immunization in Alzheimer's disease. *Brain Pathol, 14*(1) 11–20.

Frautschy, S. A., Yang, F., et al. (1998). Microglial response to amyloid plaques in APPsw transgenic mice. *Am J Pathol, 152*(1), 307–17.

Fricker, G. & Miller, D. S. (2004). Modulation of drug transporters at the blood-brain barrier. *Pharmacology, 70*(4), 169–76.

Ge, S., Murugesan, N., et al. (2009). Astrocyte- and endothelial-targeted CCL2 conditional knockout mice: Critical tools for studying the pathogenesis of neuroinflammation. *J Mol Neurosci, 39*(1–2) 269–83.

Gong, R., Rifai, A., et al. (2006). Hepatocyte growth factor suppresses acute renal injury by inhibition of endothelial E-selectin. *Kidney Int, 69*(7), 1166–74.

Gonzalez, E., Rovin, B. H., et al. (2002). HIV-1 infection and AIDS dementia are influenced by a mutant MCP-1 allele linked to increased monocyte infiltration of tissues and MCP-1 levels. *Proc Natl Acad Sci USA, 99*(21), 13795–800.

Goralski, K. B., Hartmann, G., et al. (2003). Downregulation of mdr1a expression in the brain and liver during CNS inflammation alters the in vivo disposition of digoxin. *Br J Pharmacol, 139*(1), 35–48.

Graesser, D., Solowiej, A., et al. (2002). Altered vascular permeability and early onset of experimental autoimmune encephalomyelitis in PECAM-1-deficient mice. *J Clin Invest, 109*(3), 383–92.

Harkness, K. A., Adamson, P., et al. (2000). Dexamethasone regulation of matrix metalloproteinase expression in CNS vascular endothelium. *Brain, 123*(Pt 4), 698–709.

Hartz, A. M., Bauer, B., et al. (2006). Rapid modulation of P-glycoprotein-mediated transport at the blood-brain barrier by tumor necrosis factor-alpha and lipopolysaccharide. *Mol Pharmacol, 69*(2), 462–70.

Hartz, A. M., Mahringer, A., et al. 17-beta-Estradiol: A powerful modulator of blood-brain barrier BCRP activity. *J Cereb Blood Flow Metab.*

Hawkins, B. T. & Davis, T. P. (2005). The blood-brain barrier/neurovascular unit in health and disease. *Pharmacol Rev, 57*(2), 173–85.

Hirase, T., Kawashima, S., et al. (2001). Regulation of tight junction permeability and occludin phosphorylation byRhoA-p160ROCK-dependent and independent mechanism. *J Biol Chem, 276,* 10423–10431.

Ho, E. A. & Piquette-Miller, M. (2006). Regulation of multidrug resistance by pro-inflammatory cytokines. *Curr Cancer Drug Targets, 6*(4), 295–311.

Hsiao, K., Chapman, P., et al. (1996). Correlative memory deficits, A-beta elevation, and amyloid plaques in transgenic mice. *Science, 274*(5284) 99–102.

Hu, J., Van den Steen, P. E., et al. (2007). Matrix metalloproteinase inhibitors as therapy for inflammatory and vascular diseases. *Nat Rev Drug Discov, 6*(6), 480–98.

Ifergan, I., Wosik, K., et al. (2006). Statins reduce human blood-brain barrier permeability and restrict leukocyte migration: Relevance to multiple sclerosis. *Ann Neurol, 60*(1), 45–55.

Ikezu, T., Luo, X., et al. (2003). Amyloid precursor protein-processing products affect mononuclear phagocyte activation: Pathways for sAPP- and Abeta-mediated neurotoxicity. *J Neurochem, 85*(4), 925–34.

Jasmin, J. F., Malhotra, S., et al. (2007). Caveolin-1 deficiency increases cerebral ischemic injury. *Circ Res, 100*(5), 721–9.

Jiang, C., Wang, J., et al. (2009). Progesterone exerts neuroprotective effects by inhibiting inflammatory response after stroke. *Inflamm Res*, 58(9), 619–24.

Jope, R. S., Yuskaitis, C. J., et al. (2007). Glycogen synthase kinase-3 (GSK3): Inflammation, diseases, and therapeutics. *Neurochem Res*, 32(4–5), 577–95.

Kanmogne, G. D., Schall, K., et al. (2007). HIV-1 gp120 compromises blood-brain barrier integrity and enhance monocyte migration across blood-brain barrier: Implication for viral neuropathogenesis. *J Cereb Blood Flow Metab*, 27, 123–134.

Kooij, G., Backer, R., et al. (2009). P-glycoprotein acts as an immunomodulator during neuroinflammation. *PLoS One*, 4(12), e8212.

Kuhlmann, C. R., Gerigk, M., et al. (2008). Fluvastatin prevents glutamate-induced blood-brain-barrier disruption in vitro. *Life Sci*, 82(25–26), 1281–7.

Kurebayashi, S., Xu, X., et al. (2005). A novel thiazolidinedione MCC-555 down-regulates tumor necrosis factor-alpha-induced expression of vascular cell adhesion molecule-1 in vascular endothelial cells. *Atherosclerosis*, 182(1), 71–7.

Labrecque, L., Nyalendo, C., et al. (2004). Src-mediated tyrosine phosphorylation of caveolin-1 induces its association with membrane type 1 matrix metalloproteinase. *J Biol Chem*, 279(50), 52132–40.

Langford, D., Grigorian, A., et al. (2004). Altered P-glycoprotein expression in AIDS patients with HIV encephalitis. *J Neuropathol Exp Neurol*, 63(10), 1038–47.

Lehrke, M. & Lazar (2005). The many faces of PPARgamma. *Cell*, 123(6), 993–9.

Leslie, E. M., Deeley, R. G., et al. (2005). Multidrug resistance proteins: Role of P-glycoprotein, MRP1, MRP2, and BCRP (ABCG2) in tissue defense. *Toxicol Appl Pharmacol*, 204(3), 216–37.

Liebner, S., Corada, M., et al. (2008). Wnt/beta-catenin signaling controls development of the blood-brain barrier. *J Cell Biol*, 183(3), 409–17.

Lin, M. I., Yu, J., et al. (2007). Caveolin-1-deficient mice have increased tumor microvascular permeability, angiogenesis, and growth. *Cancer Res*, 67(6), 2849–56.

Liu, F., Schaphorst, K. L., et al. (2002). Hepatocyte growth factor enhances endothelial cell barrier function and cortical cytoskeletal rearrangement: Potential role of glycogen synthase kinase-3beta. *Faseb J*, 16(9), 950–62.

Mandi, Y., Ocsovszki, I., et al. (1998). Nitric oxide production and MDR expression by human brain endothelial cells. *Anticancer Res*, 18(4C), 3049–52.

Matter, K. & Balda, M. S. (2003). Signaling to and from tight junctions. *Nat Rev Mol Cell Biol*, 4(3), 225–36.

McGeer, E. G., Klegeris, A., et al. (2005). Inflammation, the complement system and the diseases of aging. *Neurobiol Aging*, 26 Suppl 1, 94–7.

McNeill, H. & Woodgett, J. R. (2010). When pathways collide: Collaboration and connivance among signalling proteins in development. *Nat Rev Mol Cell Biol*, 11(6), 404–13.

McQuaid, S., Cunnea, P., et al. (2009). The effects of blood-brain barrier disruption on glial cell function in multiple sclerosis. *Biochem Soc Trans*, 37(Pt 1), 329–31.

Miao, J., Vitek, M. P., et al. (2005). Reducing cerebral microvascular amyloid-beta protein deposition diminishes regional neuroinflammation in vasculotropic mutant amyloid precursor protein transgenic mice. *J Neurosci*, 25(27), 6271–7.

Monahan, A. J., Warren, M., et al. (2008). Neuroinflammation and peripheral immune infiltration in Parkinson's disease: An autoimmune hypothesis. *Cell Transplant*, 17(4), 363–72.

Neuwelt, E., Abbott, N. J., et al. (2008). Strategies to advance translational research into brain barriers. *Lancet Neurol*, 7(1), 84–96.

Patel, N. S., Paris, D., et al. (2005). Inflammatory cytokine levels correlate with amyloid load in transgenic mouse models of Alzheimer's disease. *J Neuroinflammation*, 2(1), 9.

Persidsky, G., Ghorpade, A., et al. (1999). Microglial and astrocyte chemokines regulate monocyte migration through blood-brain barrier in human immunodeficiency virus-1 encephalitis. *Am J Pathol*, 155, 1599–1611.

Persidsky, Y. & Gendelman, H. E. (2003). Mononuclear phagocyte immunity and the neuropathogenesis of HIV-1 infection. *J Leukoc Biol*, 74(5), 691–701.

Persidsky, Y., Heilman, D., et al. (2006). Rho-mediated regulation of tight junctions during monocyte migration across the blood-brain barrier in HIV-1 encephalitis (HIVE). *Blood*, 107(12), 4770–80.

Persidsky, Y., Ramirez, S. H., et al. (2006). Blood-brain barrier: Structural components and function under physiologic and pathologic conditions. *J Neuroimmune Pharmacology*, 1, 223–236.

Poller, B., Drewe, J., et al. Regulation of BCRP (ABCG2) and P-glycoprotein (ABCB1) by cytokines in a model of the human blood-brain barrier. *Cell Mol Neurobiol*, 30(1), 63–70.

Ramirez, S. H., Fan, S., et al. (2010a). Dyad of CD40/CD40 ligand fosters neuroinflammation at the blood brain barrier and is regulated via JNK signaling: Implications for HIV-1 encephalitis. *J Neurosci.30* (28): 9454–64.

Ramirez, S. H., Fan, S., et al. (2010b). Inhibition of glycogen synthase kinase 3beta (GSK3beta) decreases inflammatory responses in brain endothelial cells. *Am J Pathol*, 176(2), 881–92.

Ramirez, S. H., Heilman, D., et al. (2008). Activation of peroxisome proliferator-activated receptor gamma (PPARgamma) suppresses Rho GTPases in human brain microvascular endothelial cells and inhibits adhesion and transendothelial migration of HIV-1 infected monocytes. *J Immunol*, 180(3), 1854–65.

Reijerkerk, A., Kooij, G., et al. (2006). Diapedesis of monocytes is associated with MMP-mediated occludin disappearance in brain endothelial cells. *FASEB J*, 20(14), 2550–2.

Ren, M., Senatorov, V. V., et al. (2003). Postinsult treatment with lithium reduces brain damage and facilitates neurological recovery in a rat ischemia/reperfusion model. *Proc Natl Acad Sci USA*, 100(10), 6210–5.

Rosenberg, G. A. & Yang, Y. (2007). Vasogenic edema due to tight junction disruption by matrix metalloproteinases in cerebral ischemia. *Neurosurg Focus*, 22(5), E4.

Sawada, N., Salomone, S., et al. (2008). Regulation of endothelial nitric oxide synthase and postnatal angiogenesis by Rac1. *Circ Res*, 103(4), 360–8.

Schenkel, A. R., Mamdouh, Z., et al. (2004). Locomotion of monocytes on endothelium is a critical step during extravasation. *Nat Immunol*, 5(4), 393–400.

Schinkel, A. H. & Jonker, J. W. (2003). Mammalian drug efflux transporters of the ATP binding cassette (ABC) family: An overview. *Adv Drug Deliv Rev*, 55(1), 3–29.

Song, L., Ge, S., et al. (2007). Caveolin-1 regulates expression of junction-associated proteins in brain microvascular endothelial cells. *Blood*, 109(4), 1515–23.

Stamatovic, S. M., Dimitrijevic, O. B., et al. (2006). Protein kinase Calpha-RhoA cross-talk in CCL2-induced alterations in brain endothelial permeability. *J Biol Chem*, 281(13), 8379–88.

Stamatovic, S. M., Keep, R. F., et al. (2003). Potential role of MCP-1 in endothelial cell tight junction 'opening': Signaling via Rho and Rho kinase. *J Cell Sci*, 116(Pt 22), 4615–28.

Stamatovic, S. M., Keep, R. F., et al. (2009). Caveolae-mediated internalization of occludin and claudin-5 during CCL2-induced tight junction remodeling in brain endothelial cells. *J Biol Chem*, 284(28), 19053–66.

Stein, D. G., Wright, D. W., et al. (2008). Does progesterone have neuroprotective properties? *Ann Emerg Med*, 51(2), 164–72.

Suidan, G. L., McDole, J. R., et al. (2008). Induction of blood brain barrier tight junction protein alterations by CD8 T cells. *PLoS One*, 3(8), e3037.

Takada, Y., Singh, S., et al. (2004). Identification of a p65 peptide that selectively inhibits NF-kappa B activation induced by various inflammatory stimuli and its role in down-regulation of NF-kappaB-mediated gene expression and up-regulation of apoptosis. *J Biol Chem*, 279(15), 15096–104.

Tan, J., Town, T., et al. (2002). Role of CD40 ligand in amyloidosis in transgenic Alzheimer's mice. *Nat Neurosci*, 5(12), 1288–93.

Tanzi, R. E., Moir, R. D., et al. (2004). Clearance of Alzheimer's Abeta peptide: The many roads to perdition. *Neuron*, 43(5), 605–8.

Theron, D., Barraud de Lagerie, S., et al. (2003). Influence of tumor necrosis factor-alpha on the expression and function of P-glycoprotein in an immortalised rat brain capillary endothelial cell line, GPNT. *Biochem Pharmacol, 66*(4), 579–87.

Ujiie, M., Dickstein, D. L., et al. (2003). Blood-brain barrier permeability precedes senile plaque formation in an Alzheimer disease model. *Microcirculation, 10*(6), 463–70.

Vandenbroucke, E., Mehta, D., et al. (2008). Regulation of endothelial junctional permeability. *Ann N Y Acad Sci, 1123*, 134–45.

Vogelgesang, S., Warzok, R. W., et al. (2004). The role of P-glycoprotein in cerebral amyloid angiopathy; implications for the early pathogenesis of Alzheimer's disease. *Curr Alzheimer Res, 1*(2), 121–5.

Wettschureck, N. & Offermanns, S. (2002). Rho/Rho-kinase mediated signaling in physiology and pathophysiology. *J Mol Med, 80*(10), 629–38.

Whitton, P. S. (2007). Inflammation as a causative factor in the aetiology of Parkinson's disease. *Br J Pharmacol, 150*(8), 963–76.

Yamamoto, M., Ramirez, S. H., et al. (2008). Phosphorylation of claudin-5 and occludin by rho kinase in brain endothelial cells. *Am J Pathol, 172*(2), 521–33.

Yang, L., Froio, R. M., et al. (2005). ICAM-1 regulates neutrophil adhesion and transcellular migration of TNF-alpha-activated vascular endothelium under flow. *Blood, 106*(2), 584–92.

Zandbergen, F. & Plutzky, J. (2007). PPARalpha in atherosclerosis and inflammation. *Biochim Biophys Acta, 1771*(8), 972–82.

Zhang, W., Mojsilovic-Petrovic, J., et al. (2003). The expression and functional characterization of ABCG2 in brain endothelial cells and vessels. *Faseb J, 17*(14), 2085–7.

Zhao, Y. L., Du, J., et al. (2002). Shiga-like toxin II modifies brain distribution of a P-glycoprotein substrate, doxorubicin, and P-glycoprotein expression in mice. *Brain Res, 956*(2), 246–53.

Zhou, Y., Su, Y., et al. (2003). Nonsteroidal anti-inflammatory drugs can lower amyloidogenic Abeta42 by inhibiting Rho. *Science, 302*(5648), 1215–7.

Zingarelli, B. & Cook, J. A. (2005). Peroxisome proliferator-activated receptor-gamma is a new therapeutic target in sepsis and inflammation. *Shock, 23*(5), 393–9.

Zlokovic, B. V. (2005). Neurovascular mechanisms of Alzheimer's neurodegeneration. *Trends Neurosci, 28*(4), 202–8.

3.4

MECHANISMS OF VIRAL AND CELL ENTRY INTO THE CENTRAL NERVOUS SYSTEM

Eliseo A. Eugenin and Joan W. Berman

This chapter focuses on four mechanisms that have been proposed to explain how HIV crosses the blood-brain barrier (BBB) and gains access to the central nervous system (CNS). (1) Trojan horse model: Infected monocytes and perhaps CD4+ lymphocytes act as vehicles to transport the virus from the blood to the CNS and, subsequently, to recruit more inflammatory cells into the CNS. (2) Direct infection of BBB endothelial cells and astrocytes: These infected BBB cells either infect CNS parenchymal cells or release free virus into the CNS. (3) Transcytosis model: Internalization of HIV virus by endothelial cells or astrocytic foot processes, with subsequent transfer of the virus to CNS cells. (4) Viral entry due to BBB disruption: This theory is nonspecific and forms an element of the other three theories, in that entry of HIV into the brain ultimately depends on the loss of BBB integrity due to any cause, including causes associated with the other theories. Explanation of these theories is followed by a discussion of how current antiviral regimens influence the BBB in HIV-infected patients.

INTRODUCTION

HIV-1 infection of the central nervous system (CNS) has devastating consequences in a large number of individuals with AIDS. HIV-1 enters the brain early after infection, despite the success of combined antiretroviral treatment (cART), and approximately 50% of infected individuals develop some form of cognitive impairment, termed HIV-1-associated neurocognitive disorders (HAND). Infection and inflammation persist in the CNS, even in those individuals on effective therapy, as microglia/macrophages or other CNS cells such as astrocytes may serve as long-term reservoirs harboring HIV-1. The neuropathology of HIV-1 infection includes demyelination, reactive astrocytes, multinucleated giant cells, perivascular and parenchymal accumulation of macrophages, general inflammation, and neuronal injury and loss. There is also evidence of abnormal blood-brain barrier (BBB) permeability (see Persidsky, Zheng, Miller, & Gendelman, 2000; Strelow, Janigro, & Nelson, 2001; Diesing, Swindells, Gelbard, & Gendelman, 2002; Buckner, Luers, Calderon, Eugenin, & Berman, 2006; Eugenin et al., 2006a) and astrocyte dysfunction and apoptosis (Kleinschmidt, Neumann, Moller, Erfle, & Brack-Werner, 1994; Brack-Werner, 1999; Gonzalez-Scarano & Martin-Garcia, 2005; Eugenin & Berman, 2007; Borjabad,

Brooks, & Volsky, 2009; Churchill et al., 2009). This HIV-related CNS pathology has been attributed to both the presence of virus as well as to indirect effects of HIV-1 infection, including the elaboration of neurotoxic viral proteins, such as tat and gp120, and cytokines and chemokines, that may mediate alterations in CNS cells including apoptotic cell death and dysfunction (Corasaniti, Nistico, Costa, Rotiroti, & Bagetta, 2001a; Corasaniti et al., 2001b; Gonzalez-Scarano & Martin-Garcia, 2005; King, Eugenin, Buckner, & Berman, 2006; Eugenin & Berman, 2007; Eugenin et al., 2007).

HIV infection of the CNS ultimately causes cognitive and motor impairment in a large number of individuals (Spencer & Price, 1992; Robinson-Papp et al., 2008). The cellular basis and mechanisms by which HIV-1 crosses the BBB and then induces these neuropathologies are complex and incompletely understood. Based upon different findings and diverse approaches to examine how HIV gains access to the CNS, at least four different mechanisms have been proposed (see Figure. 3.4.1):

1. The "Trojan horse" model.
2. Direct HIV infection of BBB cells (endothelial cells and astrocytes).
3. Transcytosis model.
4. Nonspecific entry of HIV into the brain as a result of BBB disruption.

In all models, the integrity of the BBB is essential in regulating entry of HIV into the CNS. The BBB is a physical and metabolic barrier that separates the CNS from the periphery (see Chapter 3.1 by William A. Banks). The BBB is not rigid, and is comprised of dynamic vessels that are able to respond to rapid changes in the brain or in the blood (Huber, Egleton, & Davis, 2001; Buckner et al., 2006). The major functions of the BBB are to transmit signals from the blood to the brain and vice versa, exclude leukocytes and soluble factors present in the blood, and to select specific nutrients to transport into or out of the CNS (Pardridge, 1986; Rubin & Staddon, 1999). The BBB is composed mainly of endothelial cells (EC), induced to differentiate to CNS EC, in close contact with astrocytic end feet. EC differentiation to a BBB phenotype results in the expression of very specific systems of transport of metabolites to the brain, as well as high tight junction protein (TJP) expression to seal the intercellular gaps between EC-EC and EC-astrocytes,

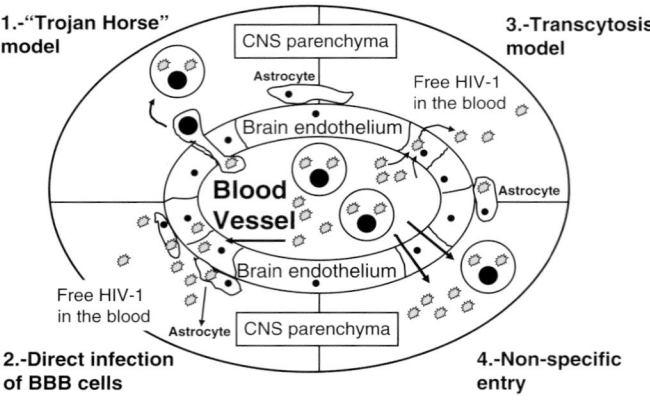

1.-"Trojan Horse" model

CNS parenchyma

Astrocyte

Brain endothelium

3.-Transcytosis model

Free HIV-1 in the blood

Blood Vessel

Astrocyte

Brain endothelium

Free HIV-1 in the blood

Astrocyte

CNS parenchyma

2.-Direct infection of BBB cells

4.-Non-specific entry

Figure 3.4.1 Schematic representation of the structure of the BBB and summary of different theories that explain HIV entry into the brain. We described four different complimentary theories: 1) Trojan horse model, 2) infection of BBB cells, 3) transcytosis model, and 4) nonspecific entry.

resulting in impermeability to most macromolecules and blood cells (Pardridge, 1986; Goldstein, 1988; Pardridge, Boado, & Farrell, 1990; Risau & Wolburg, 1990; Risau, 1991; Rubin & Staddon, 1999; Gloor et al., 2001; Strelow et al., 2001).

Tight junctions are comprised of continuous intercellular belts that produce multiple barriers and anchor the membranes of two adjacent cerebral EC or EC-astrocytes (see chapters 3.1 by William A. Banks; also, Tsukita & Furuse, 1999; Buckner et al., 2006; Roberts, Buckner, & Berman, 2010). Immunohistochemical and permeability data obtained from CNS vessels in diverse pathologies including HIV and SIV encephalitis, ischemia/reperfusion, and osmotic shock, showed significant tight junction disruption and an increase in BBB permeability (Dallasta et al., 1999; Tsukita & Furuse, 1999; Abbott, 2000; Boven, Middel, Verhoef, De Groot, & Nottet, 2000; Luabeya, Dallasta, Achim, Pauza, & Hamilton, 2000; Persidsky et al., 2000; Strelow et al., 2001; Mark & Davis, 2002; Gonzalez-Scarano & Martin-Garcia, 2005; Buckner et al., 2006; Eugenin et al., 2006a). In addition, in HIV infection, altered expression of chemoattractants by the BBB and associated cell types promotes enhanced leukocyte adhesion and transmigration into the brain across the CNS vessels (Gabuzda, He, Ohagen, & Vallat, 1998; Kelder, McArthur, Nance-Sproson, McClernon, & Griffin, 1998; Lavi, Kolson, Ulrich, Fu, & Gonzalez-Scarano, 1998; Sanders et al., 1998; Weiss, Downie, Lyman, & Berman, 1998; Weiss, Nath, Major, & Berman, 1999; Abbott, 2000; Wu et al., 2000; D'Aversa, Eugenin, & Berman, 2005; Gonzalez-Scarano & Martin-Garcia, 2005; Buckner et al., 2006; Eugenin et al., 2006a; Gendelman et al., 2009; Roberts et al., 2010), as well as increased permeability to small solutes that contribute to opening of the BBB and facilitate HIV invasion (Abbott, 2000; Stanimirovic & Satoh, 2000; Gloor et al., 2001). It is likely that, *in vivo*, the combination of BBB disruption, high expression of chemoattractants in the brain, and subsequent transmigration of uninfected, activated, or infected mononuclear cells is responsible for HIV's crossing of the BBB.

MECHANISM 1: THE "TROJAN HORSE" MODEL

This model is based on the concept that infected monocytes and perhaps CD4+ lymphocytes act as vehicles to transport the virus from the blood to the CNS. Although the specific events and factors involved in triggering leukocyte invasion are not completely understood, four observations support this model: 1) monocytes and T cells are the major target of HIV in the periphery, 2) immunohistological analysis of HIV-infected brains demonstrated accumulation of HIV-infected leukocytes, 3) HIV-infected leukocytes enhance the expression of adhesion molecules by brain EC, which facilitate interaction between HIV-infected leukocytes and CNS endothelium, the first step in the transmigration process (Wiley, Schrier, Nelson, Lampert, & Oldstone, 1986; Sasseville et al., 1992; Nottet & Gendelman, 1995; Sanders et al., 1998; Nottet, 1999; Persidsky et al., 1999; Gonzalez-Scarano & Martin-Garcia, 2005; Buckner et al., 2006; Eugenin et al., 2006b; Eugenin et al., 2006a), and 4) the expression of chemoattractants in the CNS of individuals with HIV encephalitis and/or dementia is high, most likely serving to recruit normal and HIV-infected leukocytes into the brain parenchyma (Nottet et al., 1995; Kelder et al., 1998; Weiss et al., 1998; Strelow et al., 2002; Gonzalez-Scarano & Martin-Garcia, 2005; Buckner et al., 2006; Eugenin et al., 2006a; Roberts et al., 2010). Many reports *in vivo* and *in vitro* support this theory and the molecular mechanisms of transmigration of leukocytes in other systems have been studied in detail. Some of the details are described in Section 3. Briefly, this model proposes that HIV-infected monocytes cross the BBB and infiltrate into the brain parenchyma in response to some factors, most likely chemokines, and then recruit more inflammatory cells into the CNS (Nottet, 1999; Wu et al., 2000; Strelow et al., 2001; Gonzalez-Scarano & Martin-Garcia, 2005; Buckner et al., 2006; Eugenin et al., 2006a; Roberts et al., 2010). The accumulation of uninfected and infected monocyte/macrophages after their transmigration across the BBB promotes the infection of CNS parenchymal cells (microglia, perivascular macrophages, and a small percentage of astrocytes) with HIV. Chemokine expression in the CNS is thus further enhanced, resulting in the recruitment of additional circulating leukocytes and resident immune cells to amplify the inflammatory/infection cascade and ultimately leading to neuronal impairment (Gonzalez-Scarano & Martin-Garcia, 2005; Buckner et al., 2006; King et al., 2006; Roberts et al., 2010).

Monocyte and T-cell transmigration across the BBB into the brain parenchyma requires cell- and tissue-specific mechanisms of leukocyte-endothelial interactions. This involves a variety of intracellular and extracellular cell-associated and soluble molecules (adhesion molecules, TJP, chemokine and cytokine receptors, and MMPs) and gradients of cytokines and chemokines secreted by both the transmigrating leukocytes as well as resident cells of the brain (Olson & Ley, 2002: Roberts et al., 2010; Buckner et al., 2006; Langer & Chavakis, 2009; Roberts et al., 2010). Leukocyte transmigration into the brain involves rolling of leukocytes along the endothelium, their firm adhesion, and subsequent diapedesis. The rolling and firm adhesion are well-characterized events during the transmigration process (Wu et al., 2000; Buckner et al., 2006; Weiss et al., 2009; Roberts et al., 2010). Oligosaccharides and proteins on the surface of monocytes (Lasky, 1992; Buckner et al., 2006; Langer & Chavakis, 2009; Weiss et al., 2009), and E-selectin or P-selectin on the surface of EC interact to reduce the velocity and establish a tethering between leukocyte-EC (Lasky, 1992; Buckner et al., 2006; Langer & Chavakis, 2009; Weiss et al., 2009; Roberts et al., 2010). This "tethering," as well as the elaboration of cytokines at the site of inflammation or injury, results in the expression or upregulation of another set of adhesion molecules, members of the immunoglobulin superfamily, I-CAM and V-CAM, on EC and also activate and/or increase the expression of integrin ligands for these Ig-superfamily proteins on the surface of leukocytes. This Ig-superfamily-integrin interaction ultimately facilitates diapedesis.

HIV infection *in vitro* and *in vivo* has been shown to increase adhesion molecule interactions involved in leukocyte transmigration. It was demonstrated that HIV-1 infection of human peripheral blood monocytes induces the increased expression of LFA-1, the β-integrin ligand for the EC adhesion molecule, I-CAM (Lafrenie et al., 1996a, b; Nottet, 1999; Buckner et al., 2006). Another study showed that soluble factors released by HIV-1-infected monocytes induce the expression of E-selectin and VCAM-1 by EC (Nottet et al., 1996). In addition, HIV-infected leukocytes expressed higher levels of specific chemokine receptors, such as CCR2, perhaps enabling these cells to sense lower amounts of CCL2 levels from the brain (Eugenin et al., 2006a). Both leukocytes infected with HIV (Dhawan, Vargo, & Meltzer, 1992; Dhawan et al., 1995), as well EC in close contact with HIV-infected leukocytes (Nottet, 1999; Borghi et al., 2000; Buckner et al., 2006), or treated with gp120 (Ren, Yao, & Chen, 2002) or with HIV-1 Tat protein (Lafrenie et al., 1996a, b; Nottet, 1999), have increased expression of adhesion molecules on their surfaces. In addition, E-selectin expression *in vivo*, as detected by immunohistochemical analysis of brain tissue of HIV-demented individuals, was dramatically increased as compared to nondemented people with AIDS (Nottet et al., 1996; Seilhean et al., 1997; Buckner et al., 2006). In macaques it was reported that VCAM-1 expression in vessels was increased in SIV-encephalitic brains (Sasseville et al., 1992).

Our data indicated that PECAM-1 expression within the CNS in HIV-infected individuals with HIV encephalitis is dysregulated, as compared to uninfected individuals (Eugenin et al., 2006b). We detected higher expression of PECAM-1 in encephalitic as compared to uninfected tissue. We also demonstrated a lack of colocalization between the intracellular and extracellular portion of this protein, suggesting a proteolytic process that affect this protein, such as shedding of the extracellular portion of PECAM-1 (Eugenin et al., 2006b). These changes in PECAM-1 were correlated with shedding of PECAM-1 into the sera in HIV-infected individuals as compared to uninfected individuals. We also detected that CCL2 treatment of HIV-infected peripheral blood mononuclear cells (PBMCs) causes shedding of PECAM-1. We did not find changes in serologic levels of soluble ICAM-1, suggesting

that shedding of PECAM-1 is not a nonspecific event of adhesion molecule cleavage by protease activation. All of the results were independent of cognitive and virological status. We suggest that this soluble PECAM-1 isoform binds to the extracellular portion of PECAM-1 on the surface of brain endothelial cells, helping to disrupt the BBB during the pathogenesis of HIV CNS infection by altering the PECAM-1-PECAM-1 homophilic interactions between two or more endothelial cells (Eugenin et al., 2006b).

Chemokines facilitate the directed migration of leukocytes to specific sites within the vasculature and activate leukocyte cell surface ligands for EC adhesion molecules, thus enhancing transmigration. Others and we demonstrated that chemokines and their receptors are more highly expressed in HIV-1 and SIV-encephalitic brain tissue as compared to normal brain, as well as by cultured microglia, astrocytes, and neurons (Sasseville et al., 1996; Conant et al., 1998; Gabuzda et al., 1998; Kelder et al., 1998; Lavi et al., 1998; Sanders et al., 1998; Albright et al., 1999; McManus et al., 2000b; McManus et al., 2000a). CCL2/MCP-1 is, to date, the most potent monocyte chemoattractant and is also chemotactic for activated T cells (Yla-Herttuala et al., 1991; Koch et al., 1992; Villiger, Terkeltaub, & Lotz, 1992; Brown, Covington, Newton, Ramage, & Welch, 1996) and microglia (Cross & Woodroofe, 1999; Eugenin, Dyer, Calderon, & Berman, 2005). Experiments in transgenic mice indicated that CCL2/MCP-1 is an essential chemokine for monocyte transmigration into the brain parenchyma (Fuentes et al., 1995; Gonzalez et al., 2002) and elevated levels of CCL2/MCP-1 have been detected in the CSF of individuals with AIDS dementia (Conant et al., 1998; Kelder et al., 1998). Thus, chemokines may play an important role in the recruitment of activated, infected monocytes and T cells into the CNS. Once infected leukocyte transmigration has occurred, CNS parenchymal cells, including macrophages and microglia, are susceptible to HIV infection. Chemokine-dependent microglial migration within the CNS could result in infection of microglia/ macrophages and astrocytes, fusion with other cells and amplification of the spread of HIV infection.

Our data indicated that CCL2/MCP-1 and HIV infection of PBMCs together disrupt the BBB, resulting in loss of impermeability and enhanced transmigration of HIV-infected leukocytes across the BBB (Eugenin et al., 2006a). This enhanced BBB permeability is characterized by loss of BBB integrity and reduction in TJP expression, such as ZO-1, occludin and claudin-1 (Eugenin et al., 2006a). HIV-infected monocytes and T cells transmigrated more exuberantly than uninfected cells in response to CCL2/MCP-1, in part due to their higher expression of CCR2, the receptor for CCL2/ MCP-1, as a result of HIV infection (Eugenin et al., 2006a). In addition, we demonstrated that CCL2/MCP-1 induces chemotaxis of human microglia, suggesting that uninfected cells can be induced to migrate to areas of active infection or BBB disruption where CCL2/MCP-1 is released in response to HIV products, such as tat (Eugenin et al., 2005).

Other factors that disrupt the BBB include leukotrienes, TNF-α, bradykinin, platelet-activating factor (PAF), glutamate, arachidonic acid, some chemokines, nitric oxide, substance P, and free radicals (Abbott, 2000, 2002; Gonzalez-Scarano & Martin-Garcia, 2005; Langer & Chavakis, 2009; Roberts et al., 2010). These factors are released during HIV infection and alter expression of matrix metalloproteinases (MMPs) in the BBB and the brain parenchyma. MMPs are expressed during development, healthy renewal of the brain, and during disease. Expression of MMP-2 and MMP-9 has been detected during the process of transmigration of leukocytes across the BBB in response to CCL2/MCP-1, suggesting the participation of these gelatinases during the transmigration of HIV-infected leukocytes into the brain (Eugenin et al., 2006a).

Recent data indicate that blocking MMP-9 using quantum-dot-siRNA nanoplex delivery maintains BBB integrity under basal and inflammatory conditions (Bonoiu et al., 2009). Also, high levels of MMP-1 and MMP-7 have been detected in human sera in correlation with brain injury induced by HIV infection of the CNS (Ragin et al., 2009). MMP-2, -7, and -9 are also elevated in the CSF of HIV-infected individuals with CNS compromise (Conant et al., 1999). These results indicate that at least MMP-1, -2, -7, and -9 are involved in the process of HIV-mediated invasion and enhanced transmigration into the brain.

However, the contribution of MMPs as well as other factors to leukocyte transmigration and changes in BBB permeability *in vivo* is difficult to evaluate. Thus, to understand the pathophysiological behavior of the BBB, it was necessary to develop experimental tissue culture models to examine the trafficking of cells, virus, bacteria, or drugs into the CNS. A variety of models have been used to study the BBB using EC and astrocytes from different species. We developed and characterized a model of the human BBB in which human fetal astrocytes and human umbilical vein EC (HUVEC) or human brain microvascular EC (BMVEC) are cultured on opposite sides of tissue culture inserts (Hurwitz, Berman, Rashbaum, & Lyman, 1993; Hurwitz, Berman, & Lyman, 1994; Eugenin & Berman, 2003; Eugenin et al., 2006a). Using this model we demonstrated that CCL2/MCP-1, as well as the HIV transactivator protein, Tat, induce monocyte transmigration across our co-culture model (Weiss et al., 1999). Tat-mediated transmigration was entirely due to tat-induced CCL2/MCP-1 expression by astrocytes, as neutralizing antibodies to CCL2/MCP-1 completely inhibited tat-induced transmigration (Weiss et al., 1999).

Recently it has been found that HIV clades in different areas of the world may result in different rates of HIV dementia, especially when comparing HIV clades B and C, including lower dementia rates in India as compared to the United States (Mishra, Vetrivel, Siddappa, Ranga, & Seth, 2008). Different groups examined the possibility that HIV-tat may contribute to the differences in the development of dementia. Tat C, obtained from an HIV isolated in India, was less potent in inducing CCL2 release from human astrocytes, induced less chemotaxis of leukocytes in response to Tat, and resulted in less neuropathology in a mouse model of cognitive compromise as compared to Tat B (Mishra et al., 2008; Rao et al., 2008; Rao, Eugenin, Berman, & Prasad, 2009b). In chemotaxis studies, Tat-induced migration of leukocytes was

CCL2/MCP-1 dependent, because blocking Tat or CCL2, using neutralizing antibodies, abolished migration of leukocytes (Rao et al., 2008; Rao et al., 2009b). Another group demonstrated that Tat C and Tat B have different effects in neuronal toxicity by a mechanism that involves binding to glutamate receptors (Li et al., 2008; Mishra et al., 2008). CCL2, shown to mediate CNS inflammation, and also can be neuroprotective against Tat-induced apoptosis (Eugenin, D'Aversa, Lopez, Calderon, & Berman, 2003b; Eugenin et al., 2007), suggesting that depending on the time course of release of CCL2/MCP-1, this key chemokine in neuroAIDS can play both roles, inflammatory as well as neuroprotective.

We demonstrated that HIV-infected monocytes and T cells transmigrate across our BBB model more than uninfected, activated, or unactivated leukocytes in response to CCL2/MCP-1 (Eugenin et al., 2006a). This increase in transmigration occurs only in the presence of CCL2 as a chemoattractant. The normal transmigration of leukocytes across BBB models does not result in disruption of barrier function (Burns et al., 1997; Burns et al., 2000). In our studies, the transmigration of HIV-infected PBMCs significantly enhanced the permeability of the BBB model at least ten-fold (Eugenin et al., 2006a; see also Fig. 3.4.2). Interestingly, this BBB disruption was CCL2/MCP-1 dependent, because the addition of HIV-infected cells alone to the top of the co-culture insert without chemokine in the bottom chamber did not disturb BBB permeability. This result suggests that CCL2/MCP-1 plus some other factor(s) released by HIV infected cells or expressed on their surface, serve to disrupt BBB permeability (Fig. 3.4.2). However, viral proteins other than Tat and gp120 must participate in this process, as we found that CCL2/MCP-1-mediated transmigration of leukocytes pretreated with HIV-1 Tat and/or gp120 proteins only increased the permeability of our BBB model by 2.5 fold, while the transmigration of HIV-infected leukocytes in response to CCL2/MCP-1 increased permeability tenfold (Fig. 3.4.2). Interestingly, CCL2/MCP-1 or HIV infection alone did not disrupt BBB integrity. Both together resulted in disruption. In addition, CCL3/MIP-1α, CCL4/MIP-1β, and CCL5/RANTES did not induce changes in BBB integrity after the transmigration of uninfected or HIV-infected leukocytes (Eugenin et al., 2006a).

In addition to CCL2, fractalkine has been associated with transmigration of HIV-infected leukocytes into the brain (Ancuta, Moses, & Gabuzda, 2004). Fractalkine (FKN, CX3CL1) exists as both membrane-anchored and soluble isoforms. Upon binding to its receptor, CX3CR1, FKN induces cell adhesion and chemoattraction to the sites of FKN release. Normally, like CCL2, FKN is constitutively expressed in the CNS, mainly by neurons and astrocytes (Harrison et al., 1998). However, upon activation, FKN expression and release is upregulated. In neuroAIDS, high expression of FKN has been detected in brains of individuals with HIV-associated dementia, with high expression mainly in astrocytes (Pereira, Middel, Jansen, Verhoef, & Nottet, 2001). Also, high levels of FKN have been detected in the CSF of HIV-infected people with cognitive compromise (Erichsen et al., 2003). Thus, FKN may be an important regulator of transmigration

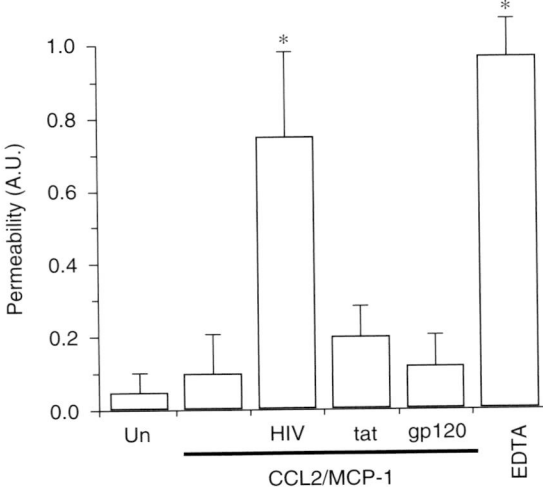

Figure 3.4.2 Alterations in BBB permeability by HIV-infected mononuclear cells in response to CCL2/MCP-1. After 24 h of transmigration of unactivated, activated, or HIV-infected cells, the permeability of the BBB model was determined. Albumin conjugated to Evans blue dye was added to the top of our co-culture model (EC side) for 30 min and the amount of albumin that crossed the BBB was quantified spectrophotometrically at 620 nm. Uninfected and activated peripheral mononuclear cells that transmigrated with or without CCL2/MCP-1 did not disrupt the BBB permeability, while HIV-infected cells (ADA virus) increased the permeability of BBB model only in the presence of CCL2/MCP-1 added to the bottom of the transwell. Leukocytes pretreated with HIV-soluble proteins, tat (10 ng/ml), or gp120 (50 ng/ml, CXCR4 strain) for 2.5 h did not increase the BBB permeability after transmigration in the presence of CCL2/MCP-1. EDTA (4 mM) was used as positive control. (n=4, *$p<0.05$ with respect to untreated conditions).

of leukocytes into the brain and of enhanced CNS inflammation during the neuropathogenesis of AIDS.

In the normal CNS, low levels of cytokine and chemokine expression may facilitate baseline trafficking of leukocytes into the brain for immune surveillance (Olson & Ley, 2002; Buckner et al., 2006; Roberts et al., 2010). Our data support the hypothesis that HIV-infected monocytes and T cells may be more sensitive to these baseline signals and therefore may transmigrate more exuberantly into the CNS, initiating a cascade of inflammatory events that ultimately results in BBB disruption. In contrast to our data, another group found that, while more activated monocytes migrate across their co-culture model than do unactivated cells, HIV infection did not increase further the number of monocytes that transmigrated. These differences may be due to culture conditions of the monocytes, extent of HIV infection, and differences in the time of transmigration assay, 24 as compared to 72 hours (Persidsky et al., 1999; Persidsky et al., 2000).

One reason that the transmigration of uninfected cells does not disrupt BBB permeability may be that they express TJP. Activated lymphocytes have been shown to express these proteins (Alexander et al., 1998). The potential formation of TJ between leukocytes-endothelium or leukocyte-astrocytes may help to maintain BBB integrity by sealing the membranes between different cell types (see Figure 3.4.1). Our preliminary

studies indicate that some TJP are increased on monocytes that transmigrate across our BBB model in response to CCL2. The finding that during the process of transmigration leukocytes express specific proteins in addition to TJ, not described previously in this kind of cell, such as potassium and chloride channels (Chung, Zelivyanskaya, & Gendelman, 2002; Gendelman et al., 2009), as well as gap junction channels (Eugenin, 2003), indicates new approaches to examine the transmigration process in normal and pathologic conditions. We demonstrated that monocytes/macrophage cells express the gap junction protein Cx43 and form functional gap junction channels after treatment with LPS plus IFN-gamma (Eugenin, Branes, Berman, & Saez, 2003a). This Cx43 expression facilitated the transmigration of these cells in response to CCL2/MCP-1 by establishing gap junction contacts with EC in our BBB model (Eugenin et al., 2003a). Interestingly, we recently found that HIV-1-infected leukocytes express Cx43. Gap junction channels may facilitate the transmigration or activation of HIV-infected leukocytes (Eugenin et al., 2003a). The continuation of these studies to address when, where, and how leukocytes express or alter their expression of TJ, GJ, or potassium and chloride channels may establish a correlation between BBB disruption and transmigration of HIV-infected cells into the brain.

In general, the Trojan horse model involves transmigration of HIV-infected monocytes into the CNS. This theory, however, does not discount the possibility that there are other sources of neuroinvasion, including infected CD4+ lymphocytes and/or cell free virions (see proposed mechanisms 3 and 4), present in high levels in the blood during the initial stages of HIV infection. It was demonstrated that lymphocytes from individuals with HIV migrate across endothelial barriers and that this is CD11a/CD18 (LFA-1) and CD49d/CD29 (VLA-4) dependent (Birdsall et al., 1997). The possible role of this migration is to spread HIV into CNS cells. In general, in brain sections of individuals with HIV, it is difficult to observe T-cell infiltration, probably because such infiltration may occur very early after HIV infection. The T cells may then egress to lymphoid organs, for example, to present viral and CNS antigens and for this reason are not detected in CNS tissue. Alternatively, HIV-infected T cells may not participate significantly in early CNS infection.

The development of more effective therapies resulted in a new syndrome in the HIV-infected population, mainly mediated by T cells, named immune reconstitution inflammatory syndrome (IRIS) (Miller et al., 2004; Riedel, Pardo, McArthur, & Nath, 2006). This syndrome is characterized by accumulation of CD8+ T cells within the brain. In addition, CD8+ T cells were detected in HIVE CNS tissue (Petito, Adkins, McCarthy, Roberts, Khamis, 2003) and in children with AIDS in association with vasculitis and endothelial damage (Katsetos et al., 1999). CD8+ T cell infiltration has also been detected during the late stages of SIV infection in perivascular regions (Lackner, Dandekar, & Gardner, 1991; Mankowski, Clements, & Zink, 2002; Kim et al., 2004). However, the mechanism of transmigration of these CD8+ T cells is unknown.

The phenotype of the cell population that transmigrates across the BBB in the context of HIV CNS infection has been examined in the past few years. Circulating CD16+ cells are expanded in different pathologies, including SIV and HIV infection (Thieblemont, Weiss, Sadeghi, Estcourt, & Haeffner-Cavaillon, 1995; Pulliam, Gascon, Stubblebine, McGuire, & McGrath, 1997; Otani et al., 1998; Fischer-Smith et al., 2001; Mavilio et al., 2005; Ancuta et al., 2006b; Ellery et al., 2007; Ziegler-Heitbrock, 2007; Ancuta et al., 2009) and maintain/support HIV infection even in the antiretroviral era. Accumulation of CD163/CD16 macrophages also has been described in HIV CNS infection (Fischer-Smith et al., 2008). CD169 has been identified on CD14+ cells as a marker of HIV disease progression (van der Kuyl et al., 2007). In macaques infected with SIV, a population of perivascular brain macrophages expressing CD163/CD68 is renewed by CD34 precursor cells, suggesting that CD163-positive cells cross the BBB during the time course of the disease (Soulas et al., 2009). We also found that the monocytes that transmigrate across our BBB model in response to CCL2 are CD14/CD16/CD166/CD11b/Mac387 and CD44v6 positive (Buckner et al., unpublished data). CD44v6 expression in monocytes also correlates with the development of SIV encephalitis, suggesting a role of this marker in disease progression (Marcondes, Lanigan, Burdo, Watry, & Fox, 2008). These populations, especially CD16 (+) monocytes, produce IL-6, CCL2, and MMP-9 by a mechanism that involves CX3CL1-expressing endothelial cells (Ancuta et al., 2006a), suggesting that this population may amplify BBB disruption and subsequent transmigration of leukocytes into the brain (Ancuta et al., 2006a).

MECHANISM 2: DIRECT HIV INFECTION OF BLOOD-BRAIN BARRIER CELLS (ENDOTHELIAL CELLS AND ASTROCYTES)

Another theory of CNS infection is the direct infection of BBB cells, primarily endothelial cells and/or astrocytes, by cell free HIV-1 that might then infect other parenchymal cells or release free virus into the CNS. The major targets of HIV in the brain are macrophages and microglia cells (Wiley et al., 1986; Budka, 1991). Some reports indicate that other CNS cells, such as endothelial cells, can be infected by HIV or SIV (Moses, Bloom, Pauza, & Nelson, 1993; Brack-Werner, 1999; Schweighardt & Atwood, 2001b, a; Schweighardt, Shieh, & Atwood, 2001; Strelow et al., 2001; Strelow, Janigro, & Nelson, 2002; Churchill et al., 2009).

The BBB is the major structural and functional barrier between the blood and the CNS parenchyma. Under physiological conditions, this barrier selectively regulates the trafficking of macromolecules and cells into the brain parenchyma. In HIV, alterations of the BMVEC have been observed in infected individuals with dementia (Petito & Cash, 1992; Power et al., 1993; Buttner, Mehraein, & Weis, 1996). Dysfunction of BMVEC has been associated with HIV entry into the brain by the different mechanisms discussed in this chapter. Another potential mechanism of BBB disruption is HIV-induced apoptosis of BMVEC. One study *in vivo* demonstrated that most

individuals with AIDS have brain endothelial apoptosis (Shi et al., 1996). Similar effects were also found in endothelial cells from macaques infected with SIV in the terminal stages of the disease (Adamson, Dawson, Zink, Clements, & Dawson, 1996). These data indicate that apoptosis of endothelial cells may contribute to the pathogenesis of neuroAIDS. However, the mechanisms and factors that contribute to brain endothelial cell apoptosis are still not identified.

Leukocyte infection by HIV, for the most part, is CD4 and CCR5 or CXCR4 receptor dependent (Dalgleish et al., 1984; Stantchev & Broder, 2001). Only a few reports have shown a potential HIV entry into endothelial cells by a CD4 and galactosylceramide-independent mechanism (Moses, Bloom, Pauza, & Nelson, 1993; Mankowski et al., 1994). Another hypothesis is that HIV can be transported by BMVEC from the blood to the CNS parenchyma by a mechanism that does not involve disruption of the barrier, with subsequent release of virus into the luminal surface. A small portion of the virus is degraded, and HIV proteins are also transported into the CNS parenchyma (Nakaoke, Ryerse, Niwa, & Banks, 2005).

Another key cell in the formation of the BBB is the astrocyte and its end-feet processes (see Fig. 3.4.3) that participates in many key functions of the brain, including maintenance of BBB integrity, neuron support (control of neurotransmitters and ion metabolism), protective functions (clearance and release of inflammatory and protective products), regulation of blood flow, and neuroimmune functions such as presentation of antigens or phagocytosis (Dong & Benveniste, 2001; Pender & Rist, 2001). HIV-1 infection in these cells is restricted to a very low percentage and is associated with minimal or no production of virus (Moses et al., 1993; Mankowski et al., 1994; Poland, Rice, & Dekaban, 1995; Schweighardt & Atwood, 2001b, a; Schweighardt et al., 2001; Eugenin & Berman, 2007).

HIV-1 infection of astrocytes is believed to be CD4 independent (Moses et al., 1993; Mankowski et al., 1994). Some reports concluded that this HIV infection is chemokine-receptor dependent, CCR5 and CXCR4 (Eugenin & Berman, 2007), or CD4 and CXCR4 independent when X4 isolates were used (Schweighardt & Atwood, 2001b, a; Schweighardt et al., 2001), while other groups indicated that astrocytes are not infected with HIV (Boutet et al., 2001). However, the basal expression of CCR5 and CXCR4 receptors on the surface of brain EC and astrocytes (Conant et al., 1994; Rottman et al., 1997; Sanders et al., 1998; Wu et al., 2000; Schweighardt & Atwood, 2001b, a; Schweighardt et al., 2001) is increased during pathological conditions such as in brains of children with AIDS (Vallat et al., 1998; McManus et al., 2000a), suggesting the possibility that in pathological conditions, chemokine receptor expression is increased and HIV entry is therefore facilitated during different stages of HIV CNS infection.

Our experiments with human astrocytes indicate that only a small population of astrocytes is infected with both CCR5 and CXCR4 dependent isolates of HIV-1 (Eugenin & Berman, 2007). The identification of a 260 kDa protein on the surface of fetal astrocytes that binds to gp120 (Ma, Geiger, & Nath, 1994) and that mediates HIV infection of some

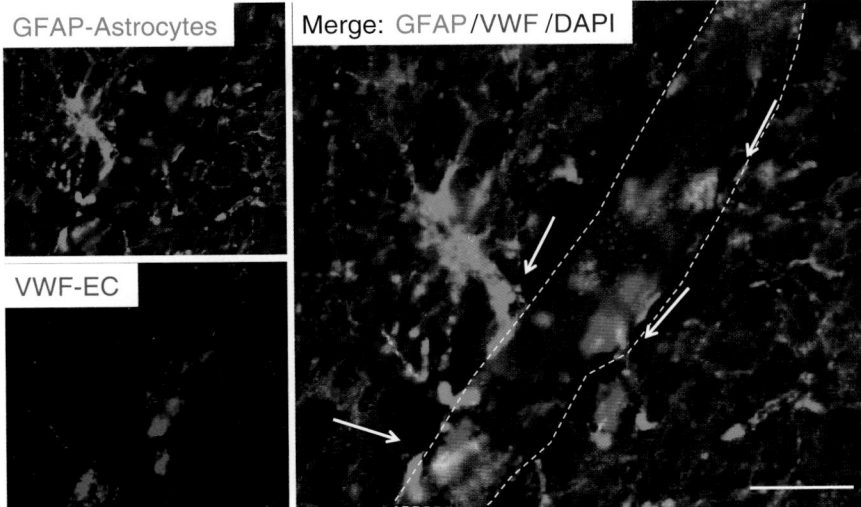

Figure 3.4.3 Astrocytes and astrocyte end-feet are important components of the BBB and participate in the pathology of neuroAIDS. CNS tissue obtained from an uninfected individual was examined by immunohistochemistry for GFAP (green staining), a marker for astrocytes, and von Willebrand factor (VWF, red staining), a marker for endothelium. Blue staining corresponds to DAPI labeling of nuclei. Arrows indicate the astrocyte end-feet in contact with the brain microvascular EC. The dotted lines indicate the shape of the blood vessel. Bar: 12.5 μm.

CD4-negative glial cell lines, indicates that these cells may have alternative pathways for HIV entry (Harouse et al., 1991b; Harouse, Laughlin, Pletcher, Friedman, & Gonzalez-Scarano, 1991a). Despite the low HIV infection of astrocytes, we found that these few infected cells amplify toxicity/inflammation to neighboring astrocytes and neurons through gap junction channels (Eugenin & Berman, 2007; unpublished data). These data suggest that gap junctions enable the exchange of toxic signals between connected cells. We showed that this new pathway, in the context of HIV, amplifies damage by dysregulating key factors in the neuropathogenesis of HIV, such as CCL2, that induces BBB disruption and transmigration of HIV-infected leukocytes into the CNS parenchyma as well as recruits additional monocytes into the CNS.

The improvement of the techniques to detect HIV DNA in single cells recently facilitated the quantification of the numbers of HIV-infected human astrocytes *in vivo*. These data indicated that up to 19% of the astrocytes isolated in dementia cases were positive for HIV DNA, without cross-contamination with other cell types (Churchill et al., 2009). *In vitro* experiments indicate that this infection can be transmitted to cells that support high viral replication by reactivation of the virus mediated by inflammatory factors (Brack-Werner, 1999). In agreement, *in vivo* studies demonstrated that areas of HIV-infected astrocytes correlated with high infiltration of monocytes/macrophages and macrophage-rich perivascular areas (Churchill et al., 2009). These data suggest that those HIV-infected astrocytes may release inflammatory factors, such as CCL2 (Eugenin & Berman, 2007), that enhance migration and recruitment of monocyte/macrophages to these areas, contributing to inflammation and to the subsequent cognitive impairment and dementia seen in many HIV-infected individuals.

The fact that HIV infection is low or nonproductive in EC and astrocytes does not mean that it does not contribute to

CNS pathology, as described above. This infection may have significant collateral effects independent of productive HIV infection, such as to 1) reduce TJP expression or other key proteins in the BBB to enhance the transmigration of infected cells (mechanism 1) or facilitate the crossing of cell free virus from the blood into the brain (mechanisms 2 and 3); 2) induce the production of soluble factors, such as chemokines, that recruit macrophage/microglia to the site of the infection and spread the virus by the infection of other cells that support productive HIV replication, such as monocyte/macrophage and microglia; and/or 3) induce apoptosis in brain EC and astrocytes that results in dysregulation of BBB integrity and neuronal metabolism, contributing to opening of the BBB as well as to neuronal impairment.

The major problem with this cell free virus theory is the low or nonproductive HIV infection of cells of the BBB. However, it is possible that specific combinations of factors within the CNS at the time of exposure to HIV enhance the replication and perhaps increase the production of HIV-1 in endothelial cells or astrocytes. The neuropeptide substance P, TNF-α, IL-1β, IFN-γ, IL-4, and glucocorticoids have been shown to enhance HIV-1 replication in latently infected astrocytes or leukocytes, and these activated astrocytes or leukocytes can then infect other cells (Tornatore, Nath, Amemiya, & Major, 1991; Janabi et al., 1998; Wang et al., 1998; Li, Douglas, Song, Sun, & Ho, 2001). Thus, astrocytes and endothelial cells may serve as important HIV reservoirs that, under certain conditions, can transfer the virus to other more replication-competent cells within the CNS.

MECHANISM 3: TRANSCYTOSIS MODEL

Another interesting hypothesis addressing how HIV-1 invades the CNS is by internalization of the HIV virion by endothelial cells or astrocytic foot processes by macropinocytosis or by endosomes, with subsequent transfer of the virus to CNS cells. Cell free virion transcytosis is dependent upon BBB integrity and uptake of HIV-1 by brain endothelial cells. The mechanism of HIV entry into these cells is controversial and it is not clear whether it is endosomal or by macropinocytosis (McClure, Marsh, & Weiss, 1988; Marechal, Clavel, Heard, & Schwartz, 1998; Marechal et al., 2001). Some studies indicated that HIV entry in nonsusceptible cells is pH independent, arguing against endosomal entry, while others found that it is pH dependent (McClure et al., 1988). In susceptible T cells, this entry is generally by pH-independent membrane fusion after interaction of the virus envelop with CD4 and a chemokine coreceptor (Berger, 1997). The differences in pH dependence may be due to cell type or to incubation times and differences in pharmacological approaches.

In vitro data indicate that HIV-1 DNA was found in human BMVEC (Poland et al., 1995). But in vivo the presence of HIV DNA or proteins in BMVEC or astrocytes does not exclude the possibility that HIV-infected T lymphocytes or monocytes (model of ¨Trojan horse¨) are the actual cells that are positive for HIV and are "trapped" during the transmigration process. This concern can be addressed in vitro, but in vivo it is very difficult to evaluate.

Despite these problems, compelling data in vitro supporting the hypothesis that HIV crosses the BBB by transcytosis are from studies with HIV-1 pseudovirions that express gp120 on their surface. The studies indicated that the internalization of the virions was pH dependent, and analysis by electron microscopy showed viral particles present in structures compatible with endosomes (Banks, Akerstrom, & Kastin, 1998; Banks et al., 2001). Unlike receptor-dependent uptake in productively infected cells, in abortive interactions the virus may be taken in by vesicular uptake mediated by macropinocytosis (Marechal et al., 2001). Macropinocytosis in BBB endothelial cells is dependent on intact lipid rafts and MAPK signaling (Liu et al., 2002). The macropinocytosis of HIV into CNS endothelial cells is supported by the presence of increased surface microvilli of CNS EC, abundance of cytoplasmic vesicles, and inhibition of HIV entry by dimethylamiloride (Liu et al., 2002). Interestingly, HIV virions in this study did not co-localize with caveolin-positive vesicles, as described during the transcytosis process in infection of BBB cells with SV40 in macaques (Pelkmans, Kartenbeck, & Helenius, 2001). Thus, it is possible that HIV may be different than SIV with regard to EC uptake. While the data obtained to support HIV-1 macropinocytosis and endocytosis are clear in the reports cited above, the question remains, how does the virus, after its internalization by CNS endothelium, transfer and replicate in CNS cells to expand HIV infection? The answer remains unknown.

MECHANISM 4: NONSPECIFIC ENTRY OF HIV INTO THE BRAIN AS A RESULT OF BLOOD-BRAIN BARRIER DISRUPTION

This theory combines the other three theories, because the nonspecific entry of HIV into the brain ultimately depends upon the loss of BBB integrity due to cytokines, chemokines, other inflammatory mediators, HIV infection of leukocytes, HIV soluble proteins, neurotransmitters, or direct infection or induction of apoptosis in EC or astrocytes. A common consequence of brain insult is an increase in the permeability of the BBB (Quagliarello, Long, & Scheld, 1986; Martiney, Berman, & Brosnan, 1992; Hurwitz et al., 1994; Soilu-Hanninen et al., 1994; Kim, Wass, & Cross, 1997; Dallasta et al., 1999; Rubin & Staddon, 1999; Gloor et al., 2001; Strelow et al., 2001; Mark & Davis, 2002). The reason for this increase is unknown, but there is a close correlation between the increase in blood and CSF cytokine levels induced by injury and the breakdown of the BBB. TNF-α often is a principal cause of permeability changes in the BBB, most likely by reduction in the TJP expression between EC-EC and EC-astrocyte that weakens the structure and function of the BBB. For example, systemic injection of TNF-α in animal models increased the permeability of the BBB (Abraham, Deli, Joo, Megyeri, & Torpier, 1996). During septic shock, TNF-α induces the expression of IL-1β and later IL-6. Both cytokines also increase the permeability of the BBB (Martiney et al., 1992; Cuff, Berman, & Brosnan, 1996; Kim et al., 1997; Farkas et al., 1998) and it has been shown that IL-1β reduced the expression of TJP in cultures of human fetal astrocytes (Duffy, John, Lee, Brosnan, & Spray, 2000).

Treatment of an in vitro model of BBB with HIV tat and gp120 (data not shown) or the addition of leukocytes treated with these proteins to the BBB model only minimally altered its integrity (Eugenin et al., 2006a; see also Fig. 3.4.3). One of the mechanisms that mediates this minimal disruption is degradation of the tight junction proteins zonula occludens-1 (ZO-1) and -2 (ZO-2) in BMVEC (Nakamuta et al., 2008). In addition, enhanced BBB disruption or HIV transport has been observed through activation of p38 pathways (Khan, Di Cello, Stins, & Kim, 2007; Dohgu & Banks, 2008), treatment with LPS (Wang, Sun, & Goldstein, 2008), oxidative stress (Price, Ercal Nakaoke, & Banks, 2005), and caveolin-1-dependent regulation of tat-induced alterations of TJP through ras modulation (Zhong et al., 2008). These mechanisms of alterations of BBB integrity may also contribute to both compromise of BBB integrity and enhanced transmigration. Additional research to establish the combination of events that results in enhanced transmigration of HIV-infected leukocytes into the brain is necessary.

Chemokine-mediated leukocyte transmigration may also contribute to BBB disruption. We demonstrated that CCL2/MCP-1-induced transmigration of HIV-infected leukocytes enhanced BBB permeability at least ten-fold with loss of TJP on the BBB (Eugenin et al., 2006a; see description of mechanism I). Additionally, elevated CCL2/MCP-1, CCL5/RANTES, and CXCL10/IP-10 levels have been found in the brain tissue and cerebrospinal fluid of infected individuals with HIV-1 encephalitis or AIDS dementia (Kelder et al., 1998; Kolb et al., 1999; McManus et al., 2000a). Therefore, it is possible to propose that high expression of specific chemokines in the brain parenchyma increases HIV leukocyte transmigration across the BBB, resulting in BBB disruption and enhanced entry of infected leukocytes, and perhaps free virion, into the CNS.

In addition, to their chemotactic properties, HIV-1 soluble proteins, such as Tat, gp120, Vpr, and Nef have been shown to induce cell death, either in solution, as secreted proteins, or when expressed on the surface of infected cells. Gp120 and gp160 are toxic to brain EC (Kanmogne, Kennedy, & Grammas, 2002) and this suggests that these HIV-1 proteins disrupt the BBB by the induction of EC apoptosis, perhaps by similar mechanisms to those described in T cells, neurons, CD8+ cells, and hematopoietic cells (Azad, 2000; Ullrich et al., 2000; Huang, Khan, Garcia-Barrio, Powell, & Bond, 2001) for which the cross linking of CD4-gp120 is essential to the induction of cell death. In addition, some reports demonstrated that tat induces apoptosis of EC (Jia et al., 2001; Park, Ullrich, Schoenberger, Ganju, & Groopman, 2001), although our laboratory has not detected this.

A different mechanism for BBB disruption has been described for the viral proteins, Vpr and Vpu. The addition of these proteins to cell cultures causes membrane permeability, an effect characteristic of viroporins. The formation of large membrane channels by viroporins impairs the ionic equilibrium of the cells that leads to apoptosis in many cell types (Gonzalez & Carrasco, 1998). The possible formation of these suicide channels in CNS endothelium during HIV infection could induce apoptosis and destabilize the BBB structure, resulting in nonspecific entry of HIV-infected cells and free virus into the CNS.

THE ROLE OF THE BLOOD-BRAIN BARRIER IN HIV INFECTION OF THE CENTRAL NERVOUS SYSTEM IN THE CURRENT ANTIRETROVIRAL ERA

Before the introduction of cART, HIV infection of the CNS was associated with the development of neurocognitive impairment and a large percentage of dementia in association with high mortality and morbidity. These cases were associated with major basal ganglia changes (Glass, Fedor, Wesselingh, & McArthur, 1995; Masliah et al., 1997; Boisse, Gill, & Power, 2008; Brew, Crowe, Landay, Cysique, & Guillemin, 2009). However, in the current cART era, the prevalence of dementia has decreased, but the prevalence of mild forms of cognitive impairment is increased. This is rapidly becoming a significant public health problem as individuals infected with HIV live longer (d'Arminio et al., 2004). In addition, the sites most affected by the virus shifted to the hippocampus and temporal cortex (Anthony & Bell, 2008).

Both dementia and mild and moderate cases of cognitive impairment are still occurring worldwide. However, in some countries where cART is not extensively available, in cases of drug toxicity, ineffective drug action, or in individuals that refuse treatment, these individuals show neurocognitive symptoms similar to those seen in the pre-ART era. In the current ART era, peripheral markers such as CD4 counts, blood viral copies, and certain inflammatory factors, are not good indicators of CNS dysfunction. In contrast, levels of viral replication and high levels of inflammatory factors within the CNS, such as CCL2, may be predictors of CNS cognitive impairment and correlate much better with CNS dysfunction than

peripheral markers (Ellis et al., 2002; Gonzalez-Scarano & Martin-Garcia, 2005; Anthony & Bell, 2008; Brew et al., 2009).

In addition to the BBB function as a physical barrier, specific BBB transporters of lipophilic drugs also control the final CNS concentration of therapeutics. These transporters include ABC transporters, soluble carrier super family members, multidrug-resistant protein, multidrug-resistance-associated protein, organic anion transporter, organic cation transporter, organic anion transporter, monocarboxylate transport system, and equilibriative nucleoside transporter (Tsuji, 2005). These transporters work in addition to other methods of BBB penetration, such as endocytosis or direct diffusion into the CNS parenchyma, and can alter the effective concentrations of the anti-HIV drugs into the CNS (Eilers, Roy, & Mondal, 2008; Varatharajan & Thomas, 2009).

The CNS penetration of these drugs into the CNS is divided into low, intermediate, and high (Letendre et al., 2008). Some example of these drugs are, low: saquinavir, ritonavir, and tenovir; intermediate: indiavir, efavirenz, and lamivudine; and high: abacavir, zidovudine, and nevirapine (see a complete list in Letendre et al., 2008).

The combination of the inefficiency of drugs in crossing the BBB and the activation of cellular systems that pump out some of the drugs resulted in the development of novel strategies to deliver therapies effectively into the CNS. Some of these novel approaches include the conjugation of drugs to molecules that render them more lipophilic, such as attachment of leucine-enkephalin to 1,4-dihydrotrigonellyl on its N-terminus (Prokai-Tatrai, Prokai, & Bodor, 1996).

More recently, the introduction of nanoparticles (Dou et al., 2007; Dou et al., 2009) and intranasal delivery of medications (Hanson & Frey, 2007) as effective ways to carry anti-HIV drugs have been used. Liposomes, dendrimers, micelles, and recently nanoparticles, are novel methods of CNS drug delivery that are currently under investigation (Rao, Ghorpade, & Labhasetwar, 2009a). These carriers are permeable to the BBB and are filled with specific combinations of drugs that are mostly impermeable to the BBB. Thus, these particles can then transport impermeable therapeutics across the BBB. Special characteristics of their surface, such as modifications of their polarity, conjugation to antibodies or proteins recognized by the BBB as necessary molecules within the CNS, facilitate their transport into the CNS parenchyma. In general these new delivery systems have been shown to have low toxicity and good levels of drug delivery (Rao et al., 2009a).

There are 22 clinical trials that target the neurocomplications of HIV infection (see (Kaul, 2009 or http://clinicaltrials.gov). One approach includes the use of antioxidants to reduce neuronal damage and loss. One of these therapies is selegiline, which inhibits monoamine oxidase B, resulting in decreased free radicals, increased superoxide dismutase and catalase, and increased synthesis of neurotrophic factors (Matsui & Kumagae, 1991; Tatton & Greenwood, 1991; Salo & Tatton, 1992; Ansari, Yu, Kruck, & Tatton, 1993). Another potential antioxidant therapy is a gene therapy system to deliver superoxide dismutase or glutathione peroxidase to neurons, which has been shown to decrease gp120-induced neuronal apoptosis in culture and in the caudate-putamen and substantia nigra of mice (Agrawal, Louboutin, Reyes, Van Bockstaele, & Strayer, 2006; Louboutin, Agrawal, Reyes, Van Bockstaele, & Strayer, 2009b, a). When both superoxide dismutase and glutathione peroxidase were delivered together, this also decreased tat-induced neuronal apoptosis (Agrawal, Louboutin, & Strayer, 2007).

Inflammation is one of the hallmarks of HAND and therapies to target this could potentially ameliorate some of the CNS consequences of HIV infection. Minocycline is a tetracycline derivative used in the treatment of bacterial infections. Minocycline can also be used for the treatment of inflammatory conditions and recent studies showed that it can cross the BBB and be neuroprotective (Stirling, Koochesfahani, Steeves, & Tetzlaff, 2005; Elewa, Hilali, Hess, Machado, & Fagan, 2006; Sapadin & Fleischmajer, 2006). Minocycline was shown to reduce HIV infection of microglia *in vitro* (Si et al., 2004) and another study demonstrated that it reduced the incidence and severity of encephalitis in SIV-infected macaques. A phase II clinical trial is underway in the United States (NIH, NIAID), as well as a clinical trial in Uganda to determine whether it reduces cognitive deficits in HIV-infected individuals (Zink et al., 2005; Follstaedt, Barber, & Zink, 2008).

Memantine, a noncompetitive NMDAR antagonist, is in use in Europe for the treatment of Alzheimer's disease and Parkinson's disease, and has recently been approved in the US for Alzheimer's disease treatment (Fleischhacker, Buchgeher, & Schubert, 1986; Rabey, Nissipeanu, & Korczyn, 1992; Winblad & Poritis, 1999; Reisberg et al., 2003; Tariot et al., 2004; Lipton, 2006). A recent phase II clinical trial of memantine in cognitively impaired HIV-infected adults found no significant improvement in cognitive dysfunction over a period of 16 weeks, but individuals treated with memantine did have an improvement in brain metabolism, as measured by N-acetyl aspartate to creatinine ratio using proton magnetic resonance spectroscopy (Schifitto et al., 2007). This study suggested that memantine may be an effective treatment for HAND, but that longer-term trials are necessary to determine its efficacy.

While there are some promising therapies currently in clinical trials using anti-HIV drugs as well as targeting inflammation and neuronal function, there is still no definitive treatment for the neurocognitive dysfunction that occurs in up to 50% of infected individuals. Thus, it is a high priority to continue and to expand research on the mechanisms of CNS infection and damage to identify new targets for interventional therapies.

FUTURE DIRECTIONS

We present four different mechanisms addressing how HIV invades the CNS. All of these models depend on BBB stability. The actual route by which HIV enters the brain most likely involves more than one mechanism, some of which may not yet be fully understood. The detailed examination of these mechanisms and their contribution to the pathogenesis of neuroAIDS should facilitate the design and implementation of novel strategies to inhibit HIV entry into the brain, and thus to limit some of the devastating consequences of HIV infection.

ACKNOWLEDGMENTS

This work was supported by the National Institute of Mental Health grant MH070297, MH075679, DA025567 and MH083497 to J. W. B. and E.A.E and by a KO1 grant from the National Institute of Mental Health (MH076679 to E.A.E.). We thank the NIH Centers for AIDS Research Grant (CFAR) AI-051519 and a CFAR pilot project (to E.A.E) at The Albert Einstein College of Medicine.

REFERENCES

Abbott, N. J. (2000). Inflammatory mediators and modulation of blood-brain barrier permeability. *Cell Mol Neurobiol, 20*, 131–147.

Abbott, N. J. (2002). Astrocyte-endothelial interactions and blood-brain barrier permeability. *J Anat, 200*, 629–638.

Abraham, C. S., Deli, M. A., Joo, F., Megyeri, P., & Torpier, G. (1996). Intracarotid tumor necrosis factor-alpha administration increases the blood-brain barrier permeability in cerebral cortex of the newborn pig: Quantitative aspects of double-labelling studies and confocal laser scanning analysis. *Neurosci Lett, 208*, 85–88.

Adamson, D. C., Dawson, T. M., Zink, M. C., Clements, J. E., & Dawson, V. L. (1996). Neurovirulent simian immunodeficiency virus infection induces neuronal, endothelial, and glial apoptosis. *Mol Med, 2*, 417–428.

Agrawal, L., Louboutin, J. P., & Strayer, D. S. (2007). Preventing HIV-1 Tat-induced neuronal apoptosis using antioxidant enzymes: Mechanistic and therapeutic implications. *Virology, 363*, 462–472.

Agrawal, L., Louboutin, J. P., Reyes, B. A., Van Bockstaele, E. J., & Strayer, D. S. (2006). Antioxidant enzyme gene delivery to protect from HIV-1 gp120-induced neuronal apoptosis. *Gene Ther, 13*, 1645–1656.

Albright, A. V., Shieh, J. T., Itoh, T., Lee, B., Pleasure, D., O'Connor, M. J., et al. (1999). Microglia express CCR5, CXCR4, and CCR3, but of these, CCR5 is the principal coreceptor for human immunodeficiency virus type 1 dementia isolates. *J Virol, 73*, 205–213.

Alexander, J. S., Dayton, T., Davis, C., Hill, S., Jackson, T. H., Blaschuk, O., et al. (1998). Activated T-lymphocytes express occludin, a component of tight junctions. *Inflammation, 22*, 573–582.

Ancuta, P., Moses, A., & Gabuzda, D. (2004). Transendothelial migration of CD16+ monocytes in response to fractalkine under constitutive and inflammatory conditions. *Immunobiology, 209*, 11–20.

Ancuta, P., Wang, J., & Gabuzda, D. (2006a). CD16+ monocytes produce IL-6, CCL2, and matrix metalloproteinase-9 upon interaction with CX3CL1-expressing endothelial cells. *J Leukoc Biol, 80*, 1156–1164.

Ancuta, P., Kunstman, K. J., Autissier, P., Zaman, T., Stone, D., Wolinsky, S. M., et al. (2006b). CD16+ monocytes exposed to HIV promote highly efficient viral replication upon differentiation into macrophages and interaction with T cells. *Virology, 344*, 267–276.

Ancuta, P., Liu, K. Y., Misra, V., Wacleche, V., Gosselin, A., Zhou, X/, et al. (2009). Transcriptional profiling reveals developmental relationship and distinct biological functions of CD16+ and CD16- monocyte subsets. *BMC Genomics, 10*, 403.

Ansari, K. S., Yu, P. H., Kruck, T. P., & Tatton, W. G. (1993). Rescue of axotomized immature rat facial motoneurons by R(-)-deprenyl: Stereospecificity and independence from monoamine oxidase inhibition. *J Neurosci, 13*, 4042–4053.

Anthony, I. C. & Bell, J. E. (2008). The neuropathology of HIV/AIDS. *Int Rev Psychiatry, 20*, 15–24.

Azad, A. A. (2000). Could Nef and Vpr proteins contribute to disease progression by promoting depletion of bystander cells and prolonged survival of HIV- infected cells? *Biochem Biophys Res Commun, 267*, 677–685.

Banks, W. A., Akerstrom, V., & Kastin, A. J. (1998). Adsorptive endocytosis mediates the passage of HIV-1 across the blood- brain barrier: Evidence for a post-internalization coreceptor. *J Cell Sci, 111*, 533–540.

Banks, W. A., Freed, E. O., Wolf, K. M., Robinson, S. M., Franko, M., & Kumar, V. B. (2001). Transport of human immunodeficiency virus type 1 pseudoviruses across the blood-brain barrier: Role of envelope proteins and adsorptive endocytosis. *J Virol, 75*, 4681–4691.

Berger, E. A. (1997). HIV entry and tropism: The chemokine receptor connection. *AIDS, 11*, S3–16.

Birdsall, H. H., Trial, J., Lin, H. J., Green, D. M., Sorrentino, G. W., Siwak, E. B., et al. (1997). Transendothelial migration of lymphocytes from HIV-1-infected donors: A mechanism for extravascular dissemination of HIV-1. *J Immunol, 158*, 5968–5977.

Boisse, L., Gill, M. J., & Power, C. (2008). HIV infection of the central nervous system: Clinical features and neuropathogenesis. *Neurol Clin, 26*, 799–819.

Bonoiu, A., Mahajan, S. D., Ye, L., Kumar, R., Ding, H., Yong, K. T., et al. (2009). MMP-9 gene silencing by a quantum dot-siRNA nanoplex delivery to maintain the integrity of the blood brain barrier. *Brain Res, 1282*, 142–155.

Borghi, M. O., Panzeri, P., Shattock, R., Sozzani, S., Dobrina, A., & Meroni, P. L. (2000). Interaction between chronically HIV-infected promonocytic cells and human umbilical vein endothelial cells: Role of proinflammatory cytokines and chemokines in viral expression modulation. *Clin Exp Immunol, 120*, 93–100.

Borjabad, A., Brooks, A. I., & Volsky, D. J. (2009). Gene expression profiles of HIV-1-infected glia and brain: Toward better understanding of the role of astrocytes in HIV-1-associated neurocognitive disorders. *J Neuroimmune Pharmacol.*

Boutet, A., Salim, H., Taoufik, Y., Lledo, P. M., Vincent, J. D., Delfraissy, J. F., et al. (2001). Isolated human astrocytes are not susceptible to infection by M- and T- tropic HIV-1 strains despite functional expression of the chemokine receptors CCR5 and CXCR4. *Glia, 34*, 165–177.

Boven, L. A., Middel, J., Verhoef, J., De Groot, C. J., & Nottet, H. S. (2000). Monocyte infiltration is highly associated with loss of the tight junction protein zonula occludens in HIV-1-associated dementia. *Neuropathol Appl Neurobiol, 26*, 356–360.

Brack-Werner, R. (1999). Astrocytes: HIV cellular reservoirs and important participants in neuropathogenesis. *AIDS, 13*, 1–22.

Brew, B. J., Crowe, S. M., Landay, A., Cysique, L. A., & Guillemin, G. (2009). Neurodegeneration and ageing in the HAART era. *J Neuroimmune Pharmacol, 4*, 163–174.

Brown, A. R., Covington, M., Newton, R. C., Ramage, R., & Welch, P. (1996). The total chemical synthesis of monocyte chemotactic protein-1 (MCP-1). *J Pept Sci, 2*, 40–46.

Buckner, C. M., Luers, A. J., Calderon, T. M., Eugenin, E. A., & Berman, J. W. (2006). Neuroimmunity and the blood-brain barrier: Molecular regulation of leukocyte transmigration and viral entry into the nervous system with a focus on neuroAIDS. *J Neuroimmune Pharmacol, 1*, 160–181.

Budka, H. (1991). Neuropathology of human immunodeficiency virus infection. *Brain Pathol, 1*, 163–175.

Burns, A. R., Walker, D. C., Brown, E. S., Thurmon, L. T., Bowden, R. A., Keese, C. R., et al. (1997). Neutrophil transendothelial migration is independent of tight junctions and occurs preferentially at tricellular corners. *J Immunol, 159*, 2893–2903.

Burns, A. R., Bowden, R. A., MacDonell, S. D., Walker, D. C., Odebunmi, T. O., Donnachie, E. M., et al. (2000) Analysis of tight junctions during neutrophil transendothelial migration. *J Cell Sci, 113*, 45–57.

Buttner, A., Mehraein, P., & Weis, S. (1996). Vascular changes in the cerebral cortex in HIV-1 infection. II. An immunohistochemical and lectinhistochemical investigation. *Acta Neuropathol, 92*, 35–41.

Chung, I., Zelivyanskaya, M., & Gendelman, H. E. (2002). Mononuclear phagocyte biophysiology influences brain transendothelial and tissue migration: Implication for HIV-1-associated dementia. *J Neuroimmunol, 122*, 40–54.

Churchill, M. J., Wesselingh, S. L., Cowley, D., Pardo, C. A., McArthur, J. C., Brew, B. J., et al. (2009). Extensive astrocyte infection is prominent in human immunodeficiency virus-associated dementia. *Ann Neurol, 66*, 253–258.

Conant, K., Tornatore, C., Atwood, W., Meyers, K., Traub, R., & Major, E. O. (1994). In vivo and in vitro infection of the astrocyte by HIV-1. *Adv Neuroimmunol, 4*, 287–289.

Conant, K., McArthur, J. C., Griffin, D. E., Sjulson, L., Wahl, L. M., & Irani, D. N. (1999). Cerebrospinal fluid levels of MMP-2, 7, and 9 are elevated in association with human immunodeficiency virus dementia. *Ann Neurol, 46*, 391–398.

Conant, K., Garzino-Demo, A., Nath, A., McArthur, J. C., Halliday, W., Power, C., et al. (1998). Induction of monocyte chemoattractant protein-1 in HIV-1 Tat-stimulated astrocytes and elevation in AIDS dementia. *Proc Natl Acad Sci USA, 95*, 3117–3121.

Corasaniti, M. T., Nistico, R., Costa, A., Rotiroti, D., & Bagetta, G. (2001a). The HIV-1 envelope protein, gp120, causes neuronal apoptosis in the neocortex of the adult rat: A useful experimental model to study neuroaids. *Funct Neurol, 16*(4), 31–38.

Corasaniti, M. T., Piccirilli, S., Paoletti, A., Nistico, R., Stringaro, A., Malorni, W., et al. (2001b). Evidence that the HIV-1 coat protein gp120 causes neuronal apoptosis in the neocortex of rat via a mechanism involving CXCR4 chemokine receptor. *Neurosci Lett, 312*, 67–70.

Cross, A. K. & Woodroofe, M. N. (1999). Chemokines induce migration and changes in actin polymerization in adult rat brain microglia and a human fetal microglial cell line in vitro. *J Neurosci Res, 55*, 17–23.

Cuff, C. A., Berman, J. W., & Brosnan, C. F. (1996). The ordered array of perivascular macrophages is disrupted by IL-1-induced inflammation in the rabbit retina. *Glia, 17*, 307–316.

d'Arminio, A., Sabin, C. A., Phillips, A. N., Reiss, P., Weber, R., Kirk, O., et al. (2004). Cardio- and cerebrovascular events in HIV-infected persons. *AIDS, 18*, 1811–1817.

D'Aversa, T. G., Eugenin, E. A., & Berman, J. W. (2005). NeuroAIDS: Contributions of the human immunodeficiency virus-1 proteins Tat and gp120 as well as CD40 to microglial activation. *J Neurosci Res, 81*, 436–446.

Dalgleish, A. G., Beverley, P. C., Clapham, P. R., Crawford, D. H., Greaves, M. F., & Weiss, R. A. (1984). The CD4 (T4) antigen is an essential component of the receptor for the AIDS retrovirus. *Nature, 312*, 763–767.

Dallasta, L. M., Pisarov, L. A., Esplen, J. E., Werley, J. V., Moses, A. V., et al. (1999). Blood-brain barrier tight junction disruption in human immunodeficiency virus-1 encephalitis. *Am J Pathol, 155*, 1915–1927.

Dhawan, S., Vargo, M., & Meltzer, M. S. (1992). Interactions between HIV-infected monocytes and the extracellular matrix: increased capacity of HIV-infected monocytes to adhere to and spread on extracellular matrix associated with changes in extent of virus replication and cytopathic effects in infected cells. *J Leukoc Biol, 52*, 62–69.

Dhawan, S., Weeks, B. S., Soderland, C., Schnaper, H. W., Toro, L. A., Asthana, S. P., et al. (1995). HIV-1 infection alters monocyte interactions with human microvascular endothelial cells. *J Immunol, 154*, 422–432.

Diesing, T. S., Swindells, S., Gelbard, H., & Gendelman, H. E. (2002). HIV-1-associated dementia: A basic science and clinical perspective. *AIDS Read, 12*, 358–368.

Dohgu, S. & Banks, W. A. (2008). Lipopolysaccharide-enhanced transcellular transport of HIV-1 across the blood-brain barrier is mediated by the p38 mitogen-activated protein kinase pathway. *Exp Neurol, 210*, 740–749.

Dong, Y. & Benveniste, E. N. (2001). Immune function of astrocytes. *Glia, 36*, 180–190.

Dou, H., Grotepas, C. B., McMillan, J. M., Destache, C. J., Chaubal, M., Werling, J., et al. (2009). Macrophage delivery of nanoformulated antiretroviral drug to the brain in a murine model of neuroAIDS. *J Immunol, 183*, 661–669.

Dou, H., Morehead, J., Destache, C. J., Kingsley, J. D., Shlyakhtenko, L., Zhou, Y., et al. (2007). Laboratory investigations for the morphologic, pharmacokinetic, and anti-retroviral properties of indinavir nanoparticles in human monocyte-derived macrophages. *Virology, 358*, 148–158.

Duffy, H. S., John, G. R., Lee, S. C., Brosnan, C. F., & Spray, D. C. (2000). Reciprocal regulation of the junctional proteins claudin-1 and connexin43 by interleukin-1beta in primary human fetal astrocytes. *J Neurosci, 20*, RC114.

Eilers, M., Roy, U., & Mondal, D. (2008). MRP (ABCC) transporters-mediated efflux of anti-HIV drugs, saquinavir and zidovudine, from human endothelial cells. *Exp Biol Med (Maywood), 233*, 1149–1160.

Elewa, H. F., Hilali, H., Hess, D. C., Machado, L. S., & Fagan, S. C. (2006). Minocycline for short-term neuroprotection. *Pharmacotherapy, 26*, 515–521.

Ellery, P. J., Tippett, E., Chiu, Y. L., Paukovics, G., Cameron, P. U., Solomon, A., et al. (2007). The CD16+ monocyte subset is more permissive to infection and preferentially harbors HIV-1 in vivo. *J Immunol, 178*, 6581–6589.

Ellis, R. J., Moore, D. J., Childers, M. E., Letendre, S., McCutchan, J. A., Wolfson, T., et al. (2002). Progression to neuropsychological impairment in human immunodeficiency virus infection predicted by elevated cerebrospinal fluid levels of human immunodeficiency virus RNA. *Arch Neurol, 59*, 923–928.

Erichsen, D., Lopez, A. L., Peng, H., Niemann, D., Williams, C., Bauer, M., et al. (2003). Neuronal injury regulates fractalkine: Relevance for HIV-1 associated dementia. *J Neuroimmunol, 138*, 144–155.

Eugenin, E. A. & Berman, J. W. (2003). Chemokine-dependent mechanisms of leukocyte trafficking across a model of the blood-brain barrier. *Methods, 29*, 351–361.

Eugenin, E. A. & Berman, J. W. (2007). Gap junctions mediate human immunodeficiency virus-bystander killing in astrocytes. *J Neurosci, 27*, 12844–12850.

Eugenin, E. A., Branes, M. C., Berman, J. W., & Saez, J. C. (2003a). TNF-alpha plus IFN-gamma induce connexin43 expression and formation of gap junctions between human monocytes/macrophages that enhance physiological responses. *J Immunol, 170*, 1320–1328.

Eugenin, E. A., Dyer, G., Calderon, T. M., & Berman, J. W. (2005). HIV-1 tat protein induces a migratory phenotype in human fetal microglia by a CCL2 (MCP-1)-dependent mechanism: Possible role in neuroAIDS. *Glia, 49*, 501–510.

Eugenin, E. A., D'Aversa, T. G., Lopez, L., Calderon, T. M., & Berman, J. W. (2003b). MCP-1 (CCL2) protects human neurons and astrocytes from NMDA or HIV-tat-induced apoptosis. *J Neurochem, 85*, 1299–1311.

Eugenin, E. A., Osiecki, K., Lopez, L., Goldstein, H., Calderon, T. M., & Berman, J. W. (2006a). CCL2/monocyte chemoattractant protein-1 mediates enhanced transmigration of human immunodeficiency virus (HIV)-infected leukocytes across the blood-brain barrier: A potential mechanism of HIV-CNS invasion and neuroAIDS. *J Neurosci, 26*, 1098–1106.

Eugenin, E. A., King, J. E., Nath, A., Calderon, T. M., Zukin, R. S., Bennett, M. V., et al. (2007). HIV-tat induces formation of an LRP-PSD-95-NMDAR-nNOS complex that promotes apoptosis in neurons and astrocytes. *Proc Natl Acad Sci USA, 104*, 3438–3443.

Eugenin, E. A., Gamss, R., Buckner, C., Buono, D., Klein, R. S., Schoenbaum, E. E., et al. (2006b). Shedding of PECAM-1 during HIV infection: A potential role for soluble PECAM-1 in the pathogenesis of neuroAIDS. *J Leukoc Biol, 79*, 444–452.

Eugenin, E. A., Branes, M. C., Berman, J. W., & Saez, J. C. (2003). TNF-a plus IFN-g induce connexin43 expression and formation of gap junctions between human monocytes/macrophages that enhance physiological responses. *J Immunol*, In press.

Farkas, G., Marton, J., Nagy, Z., Mandi, Y., Takacs, T., Deli, M. A., et al. (1998). Experimental acute pancreatitis results in increased blood-brain barrier permeability in the rat: A potential role for tumor necrosis factor and interleukin 6. *Neurosci Lett, 242*, 147–150.

Fischer-Smith, T., Tedaldi, E. M., & Rappaport, J. (2008). CD163/CD16 coexpression by circulating monocytes/macrophages in HIV: Potential biomarkers for HIV infection and AIDS progression. AIDS Res Hum Retroviruses, 24, 417–421.

Fischer-Smith, T., Croul, S., Sverstiuk, A. E., Capini, C., L'Heureux, D., Regulier, E. G., et al. (2001). CNS invasion by CD14+/CD16+ peripheral blood-derived monocytes in HIV dementia: Perivascular accumulation and reservoir of HIV infection. *J Neurovirol, 7*, 528–541.

Fleischhacker, W. W., Buchgeher, A., & Schubert, H. (1986). Memantine in the treatment of senile dementia of the Alzheimer type. *Prog Neuropsychopharmacol Biol Psychiatry, 10*, 87–93.

Follstaedt, S. C., Barber, S. A., & Zink, M. C. (2008). Mechanisms of minocycline-induced suppression of simian immunodeficiency virus encephalitis: Inhibition of apoptosis signal-regulating kinase 1. *J Neurovirol, 14*, 376–388.

Fuentes, M. E., Durham, S. K., Swerdel, M. R., Lewin, A. C., Barton, D. S., Megill, J. R., et al. (1995). Controlled recruitment of monocytes and macrophages to specific organs through transgenic expression of monocyte chemoattractant protein-1. *J Immunol, 155*, 5769–5776.

Gabuzda, D., He, J., Ohagen, A., & Vallat, A. V. (1998). Chemokine receptors in HIV-1 infection of the central nervous system. *Semin Immunol, 10*, 203–213.

Gendelman, H. E., Ding, S., Gong, N., Liu, J., Ramirez, S. H., Persidsky, Y., et al. (2009). Monocyte chemotactic protein-1 regulates voltage-gated K+ channels and macrophage transmigration. *J Neuroimmune Pharmacol, 4*, 47–59.

Glass, J. D., Fedor, H., Wesselingh, S. L., & McArthur, J. C. (1995). Immunocytochemical quantitation of human immunodeficiency virus in the brain: Correlations with dementia. *Ann Neurol, 38*, 755–762.

Gloor, S. M., Wachtel, M., Bolliger, M. F., Ishihara, H., Landmann, R., & Frei, K. (2001). Molecular and cellular permeability control at the blood-brain barrier. *Brain Res Brain Res Rev, 36*, 258–264.

Goldstein, G. W. (1988). Endothelial cell-astrocyte interactions. A cellular model of the blood- brain barrier. *Ann N Y Acad Sci, 529*, 31–39.

Gonzalez-Scarano, F. & Martin-Garcia, J. (2005). The neuropathogenesis of AIDS. *Nat Rev Immunol, 5*, 69–81.

Gonzalez, E., Rovin, B. H., Sen, L., Cooke, G., Dhanda, R., Mummidi, S., et al. (2002). HIV-1 infection and AIDS dementia are influenced by a mutant MCP-1 allele linked to increased monocyte infiltration of tissues and MCP-1 levels. *Proc Natl Acad Sci USA, 99*, 13795–13800.

Gonzalez, M. E. & Carrasco, L. (1998). The human immunodeficiency virus type 1 Vpu protein enhances membrane permeability. *Biochemistry, 37*, 13710–13719.

Hanson, L. R. & Frey, W. H., 2nd. (2007). Strategies for intranasal delivery of therapeutics for the prevention and treatment of neuroAIDS. *J Neuroimmune Pharmacol, 2*, 81–86.

Harouse, J. M., Laughlin, M. A., Pletcher, C., Friedman, H. M., & Gonzalez-Scarano, F. (1991a). Entry of human immunodeficiency virus-1 into glial cells proceeds via an alternate, efficient pathway. *J Leukoc Biol, 49*, 605–609.

Harouse, J. M., Bhat, S., Spitalnik, S. L., Laughlin, M., Stefano, K., Silberberg, D. H., et al. (1991b). Inhibition of entry of HIV-1 in neural cell lines by antibodies against galactosyl ceramide. *Science, 253*, 320–323.

Harrison, J. K., Jiang, Y., Chen, S., Xia, Y., Maciejewski, D., McNamara, R. K., et al. (1998). Role for neuronally derived fractalkine in mediating interactions between neurons and CX3CR1-expressing microglia. *Proc Natl Acad Sci USA, 95*, 10896–10901.

Huang, M. B., Khan, M., Garcia-Barrio, M., Powell, M., & Bond, V. C. (2001). Apoptotic effects in primary human umbilical vein endothelial cell cultures caused by exposure to virion-associated and cell membrane-associated HIV-1 gp120. *J Acquir Immune Defic Syndr, 27*, 213–221.

Huber, J. D., Egleton, R. D., & Davis, T. P. (2001). Molecular physiology and pathophysiology of tight junctions in the blood-brain barrier. *Trends Neurosci, 24*, 719–725.

Hurwitz, A. A., Berman, J. W., & Lyman, W. D. (1994). The role of the blood-brain barrier in HIV infection of the central nervous system. *Adv Neuroimmunol, 4*, 249–256.

Hurwitz, A. A., Berman, J. W., Rashbaum, W. K., & Lyman, W. D. (1993). Human fetal astrocytes induce the expression of blood-brain barrier specific proteins by autologous endothelial cells. *Brain Res, 625*, 238–243.

Janabi, N., Di Stefano, M., Wallon, C., Hery, C., Chiodi, F., & Tardieu, M. (1998). Induction of human immunodeficiency virus type 1 replication in human glial cells after proinflammatory cytokines stimulation: Effect of IFNgamma, IL1beta, and TNFalpha on differentiation and chemokine production in glial cells. *Glia, 23*, 304–315.

Jia, H., Lohr, M., Jezequel, S., Davis, D., Shaikh, S., Selwood, D., et al. (2001). Cysteine-rich and basic domain HIV-1 Tat peptides inhibit angiogenesis and induce endothelial cell apoptosis. *Biochem Biophys Res Commun, 283*, 469–479.

Kanmogne, G. D., Kennedy, R. C., & Grammas, P. (2002). HIV-1 gp120 proteins and gp160 peptides are toxic to brain endothelial cells and neurons: Possible pathway for HIV entry into the brain and HIV-associated dementia. *J Neuropathol Exp Neurol, 61*, 992–1000.

Katsetos, C. D., Fincke, J. E., Legido, A., Lischner, H. W., de Chadarevian, J. P., Kaye, E. M., et al. (1999). Angiocentric CD3(+) T-cell infiltrates in human immunodeficiency virus type 1-associated central nervous system disease in children. *Clin Diagn Lab Immunol, 6*, 105–114.

Kaul, M. (2009). HIV-1 associated dementia: Update on pathological mechanisms and therapeutic approaches. *Curr Opin Neurol, 22*, 315–320.

Kelder, W., McArthur, J. C., Nance-Sproson, T., McClernon, D., & Griffin, D. E. (1998). Beta-chemokines MCP-1 and RANTES are selectively increased in cerebrospinal fluid of patients with human immunodeficiency virus-associated dementia. *Ann Neurol, 44*, 831–835.

Khan, N. A., Di Cello, F., Stins, M., & Kim, K. S. (2007). Gp120-mediated cytotoxicity of human brain microvascular endothelial cells is dependent on p38 mitogen-activated protein kinase activation. *J Neurovirol, 13*, 242–251.

Kim, K. S., Wass, C. A., & Cross, A. S. (1997). Blood-brain barrier permeability during the development of experimental bacterial meningitis in the rat. *Exp Neurol, 145*, 253–257.

Kim, W. K., Corey, S., Chesney, G., Knight, H., Klumpp, S., Wuthrich, C., et al. (2004). Identification of T lymphocytes in simian immunodeficiency virus encephalitis: Distribution of CD8+ T cells in association with central nervous system vessels and virus. *J Neurovirol, 10*, 315–325.

King, J. E., Eugenin, E. A., Buckner, C. M., & Berman, J. W. (2006). HIV tat and neurotoxicity. *Microbes Infect, 8*, 1347–1357.

Kleinschmidt, A., Neumann, M., Moller, C., Erfle, V., & Brack-Werner, R. (1994). Restricted expression of HIV1 in human astrocytes: Molecular basis for viral persistence in the CNS. *Res Virol, 145*, 147–153.

Koch, A. E., Kunkel, S. L., Harlow, L. A., Johnson, B., Evanoff, H. L., Haines, G. K., et al. (1992). Enhanced production of monocyte chemoattractant protein-1 in rheumatoid arthritis. *J Clin Invest, 90*, 772–779.

Kolb, S. A., Sporer, B., Lahrtz, F., Koedel, U., Pfister, H. W., & Fontana, A. (1999). Identification of a T cell chemotactic factor in the cerebrospinal fluid of HIV-1-infected individuals as interferon-gamma inducible protein 10. *J Neuroimmunol, 93*, 172–181.

Lackner, A. A., Dandekar, S., & Gardner, M. B. (1991). Neurobiology of simian and feline immunodeficiency virus infections. *Brain Pathol, 1*, 201–212.

Lafrenie, R. M., Wahl, L. M., Epstein, J. S., Hewlett, I. K., Yamada, K. M., & Dhawan, S. (1996a). HIV-1-Tat protein promotes chemotaxis and invasive behavior by monocytes. *J Immunol, 157*, 974–977.

Lafrenie, R. M., Wahl, L. M., Epstein, J. S., Hewlett, I. K., Yamada, K. M., & Dhawan, S. (1996b). HIV-1-Tat modulates the function of monocytes and alters their interactions with microvessel endothelial cells. A mechanism of HIV pathogenesis. *J Immunol, 156*, 1638–1645.

Langer, H. F. & Chavakis, T. (2009). Leukocyte-endothelial interactions in inflammation. *J Cell Mol Med, 13*, 1211–1220.

Lasky, L. A. (1992). Selectins: Interpreters of cell-specific carbohydrate information during inflammation. *Science, 258*, 964–969.

Lavi, E., Kolson, D. L., Ulrich, A. M., Fu, L., & Gonzalez-Scarano, F. (1998). Chemokine receptors in the human brain and their relationship to HIV infection. *J Neurovirol, 4*, 301–311.

Letendre, S., Marquie-Beck, J., Capparelli, E., Best, B., Clifford, D., Collier, A. C., et al. (2008). Validation of the CNS Penetration-Effectiveness rank for quantifying antiretroviral penetration into the central nervous system. *Arch Neurol, 65*, 65–70.

Li W, Huang Y, Reid R, Steiner J, Malpica-Llanos T, Darden TA, et al. (2008). NMDA receptor activation by HIV-Tat protein is clade dependent. *J Neurosci, 28*, 12190–12198.

Li, Y., Douglas, S. D., Song, L., Sun, S., & Ho, W. Z. (2001). Substance P enhances HIV-1 replication in latently infected human immune cells. *J Neuroimmunol, 121*, 67–75.

Lipton, S. A. (2006). Paradigm shift in neuroprotection by NMDA receptor blockade: Memantine and beyond. *Nat Rev Drug Discov, 5*, 160–170.

Liu, N. Q., Lossinsky, A. S., Popik, W., Li, X., Gujuluva, C., Kriederman, B., et al. (2002). Human immunodeficiency virus type 1 enters brain microvascular endothelia by macropinocytosis dependent on lipid rafts and the mitogen-activated protein kinase signaling pathway. *J Virol, 76*, 6689–6700.

Louboutin, J. P., Agrawal, L., Reyes, B. A., Van Bockstaele, E. J., & Strayer, D. S. (2009a). HIV-1 gp120 neurotoxicity proximally and at a distance from the point of exposure: Protection by rSV40 delivery of antioxidant enzymes. *Neurobiol Dis, 34*, 462–476.

Louboutin, J. P., Agrawal, L., Reyes, B. A., Van Bockstaele, E. J., & Strayer, D. S. (2009b). A rat model of human immunodeficiency virus 1 encephalopathy using envelope glycoprotein gp120 expression delivered by SV40 vectors. *J Neuropathol Exp Neurol, 68*, 456–473.

Luabeya, M. K., Dallasta, L. M., Achim, C. L., Pauza, C. D., & Hamilton, R. L. (2000). Blood-brain barrier disruption in simian immunodeficiency virus encephalitis. *Neuropathol Appl Neurobiol, 26*, 454–462.

Ma, M., Geiger, J. D., & Nath, A. (1994). Characterization of a novel binding site for the human immunodeficiency virus type 1 envelope protein gp120 on human fetal astrocytes. *J Virol, 68*, 6824–6828.

Mankowski, J. L., Clements, J. E., & Zink, M. C. (2002). Searching for clues: Tracking the pathogenesis of human immunodeficiency virus central nervous system disease by use of an accelerated, consistent simian immunodeficiency virus macaque model. *J Infect Dis, 186* Suppl 2, S199–208.

Mankowski, J. L., Spelman, J. P., Ressetar, H. G., Strandberg, J. D., Laterra, J., Carter, D. L., et al. (1994). Neurovirulent simian immunodeficiency virus replicates productively in endothelial cells of the central nervous system in vivo and in vitro. *J Virol, 68*, 8202–8208.

Marcondes, M. C., Lanigan, C. M., Burdo, T. H., Watry, D. D., & Fox, H. S. (2008). Increased expression of monocyte CD44v6 correlates with the development of encephalitis in rhesus macaques infected with simian immunodeficiency virus. *J Infect Dis, 197*, 1567–1576.

Marechal, V., Clavel, F., Heard, J. M., & Schwartz, O. (1998). Cytosolic Gag p24 as an index of productive entry of human immunodeficiency virus type 1. *J Virol, 72*, 2208–2212.

Marechal, V., Prevost, M. C., Petit, C., Perret, E., Heard, J. M., & Schwartz, O. (2001). Human immunodeficiency virus type 1 entry into macrophages mediated by macropinocytosis. *J Virol, 75*, 11166–11177.

Mark, K. S. & Davis, T. P. (2002). Cerebral microvascular changes in permeability and tight junctions induced by hypoxia-reoxygenation. *Am J Physiol Heart Circ Physiol, 282*, H1485–1494.

Martiney, J. A., Berman, J. W., & Brosnan, C. F. (1992). Chronic inflammatory effects of interleukin-1 on the blood-retina barrier. *J Neuroimmunol, 41*, 167–176.

Masliah, E., Heaton, R. K., Marcotte, T. D., Ellis, R. J., Wiley, C. A., Mallory, M., et al (1997). Dendritic injury is a pathological substrate for human immunodeficiency virus-related cognitive disorders. HNRC Group. The HIV Neurobehavioral Research Center. *Ann Neurol, 42*, 963–972.

Matsui, Y. & Kumagae, Y. (1991). Monoamine oxidase inhibitors prevent striatal neuronal necrosis induced by transient forebrain ischemia. *Neurosci Lett, 126*, 175–178.

Mavilio, D., Lombardo, G., Benjamin, J., Kim, D., Follman, D., Marcenaro, E., et al. (2005). Characterization of CD56-/CD16+ natural killer (NK) cells: A highly dysfunctional NK subset expanded in HIV-infected viremic individuals. *Proc Natl Acad Sci USA, 102*, 2886–2891.

McClure, M. O., Marsh, M., & Weiss, R. A. (1988). Human immunodeficiency virus infection of CD4-bearing cells occurs by a pH-independent mechanism. *Embo J, 7*, 513–518.

McManus, C. M., Weidenheim, K., Woodman, S. E., Nunez, J., Hesselgesser, J., Nath, A., et al. (2000a). Chemokine and chemokine-receptor expression in human glial elements: Induction by the HIV protein, Tat, and chemokine autoregulation. *Am J Pathol, 156*, 1441–1453.

McManus, C. M., Liu, J. S., Hahn, M. T., Hua, L. L., Brosnan, C. F., Berman, J. W., et al. (2000b). Differential induction of chemokines in human microglia by type I and II interferons. *Glia, 29*, 273–280.

Miller, R. F., Isaacson, P. G., Hall-Craggs, M., Lucas, S., Gray, F., Scaravilli, F., et al. (2004). Cerebral CD8+ lymphocytosis in HIV-1 infected patients with immune restoration induced by HAART. *Acta Neuropathol, 108*, 17–23.

Mishra, M., Vetrivel, S., Siddappa, N. B., Ranga, U., & Seth, P. (2008). Clade-specific differences in neurotoxicity of human immunodeficiency virus-1 B and C Tat of human neurons: Significance of dicysteine C30C31 motif. *Ann Neurol, 63*, 366–376.

Moses, A. V., Bloom, F. E., Pauza, C. D., & Nelson, J. A. (1993). Human immunodeficiency virus infection of human brain capillary endothelial cells occurs via a CD4/galactosylceramide-independent mechanism. *Proc Natl Acad Sci USA, 90*, 10474–10478.

Nakamuta, S., Endo, H., Higashi, Y., Kousaka, A., Yamada, H., Yano, M., et al (2008). Human immunodeficiency virus type 1 gp120-mediated disruption of tight junction proteins by induction of proteasome-mediated degradation of zonula occludens-1 and -2 in human brain microvascular endothelial cells. *J Neurovirol, 14*, 186–195.

Nakaoke, R., Ryerse, J. S., Niwa, M., & Banks, W. A. (2005). Human immunodeficiency virus type 1 transport across the in vitro mouse brain endothelial cell monolayer. *Exp Neurol, 193*, 101–109.

Nottet, H. S. (1999). Interactions between macrophages and brain microvascular endothelial cells: Role in pathogenesis of HIV-1 infection and blood-brain barrier function. *J Neurovirol, 5*, 659–669.

Nottet, H. S. & Gendelman, H. E. (1995). Unraveling the neuroimmune mechanisms for the HIV-1-associated cognitive/motor complex. *Immunol Today, 16*, 441–448.

Nottet, H. S., Jett, M., Flanagan, C. R., Zhai, Q. H., Persidsky, Y., Rizzino, A., et al. (1995). A regulatory role for astrocytes in HIV-1 encephalitis. An overexpression of eicosanoids, platelet-activating factor, and tumor necrosis factor-alpha by activated HIV-1-infected monocytes is attenuated by primary human astrocytes. *J Immunol, 154*, 3567–3581.

Nottet, H. S., Persidsky, Y., Sasseville, V. G., Nukuna, A. N., Bock, P., Zhai, Q. H., et al (1996). Mechanisms for the transendothelial migration of HIV-1-infected monocytes into brain. *J Immunol, 156*, 1284–1295.

Olson, T. S. & Ley, K. (2002). Chemokines and chemokine receptors in leukocyte trafficking. *Am J Physiol Regul Integr Comp Physiol, 283*, R7–28.

Otani, I., Akari, H., Nam, K. H., Mori, K., Suzuki, E., Shibata, H., et al. (1998). Phenotypic changes in peripheral blood monocytes of cynomolgus monkeys acutely infected with simian immunodeficiency virus. *AIDS Res Hum Retroviruses, 14*, 1181–1186.

Pardridge, W. M. (1986). Blood-brain barrier transport of nutrients. *Nutr Rev, 44* Suppl, 15–25.

Pardridge, W. M., Boado, R. J., & Farrell, C. R. (1990). Brain-type glucose transporter (GLUT-1) is selectively localized to the blood-brain barrier. Studies with quantitative western blotting and in situ hybridization. *J Biol Chem, 265*, 18035–18040.

Park, I. W., Ullrich, C. K., Schoenberger, E., Ganju, R. K., & Groopman, J. E. (2001). HIV-1 Tat induces microvascular endothelial apoptosis through caspase activation. *J Immunol, 167*, 2766–2771.

Pelkmans, L., Kartenbeck, J., & Helenius, A. (2001). Caveolar endocytosis of simian virus 40 reveals a new two-step vesicular-transport pathway to the ER. *Nat Cell Biol, 3*, 473–483.

Pender, M. P. & Rist, M. J. (2001). Apoptosis of inflammatory cells in immune control of the nervous system: Role of glia. *Glia, 36*, 137–144.

Pereira, C. F., Middel, J., Jansen, G., Verhoef, J., & Nottet, H. S. (2001). Enhanced expression of fractalkine in HIV-1 associated dementia. *J Neuroimmunol, 115*, 168–175.

Persidsky, Y., Zheng, J., Miller, D., & Gendelman, H. E. (2000). Mononuclear phagocytes mediate blood-brain barrier compromise and neuronal injury during HIV-1-associated dementia. *J Leukoc Biol, 68*, 413–422.

Persidsky, Y., Ghorpade, A., Rasmussen, J., Limoges, J., Liu, X. J., Stins, M., et al. (1999). Microglial and astrocyte chemokines regulate monocyte migration through the blood-brain barrier in human immunodeficiency virus-1 encephalitis. *Am J Pathol, 155*, 1599–1611.

Petito, C. K. & Cash, K. S. (1992). Blood-brain barrier abnormalities in the acquired immunodeficiency syndrome: Immunohistochemical localization of serum proteins in postmortem brain. *Ann Neurol, 32*, 658–666.

Petito, C. K., Adkins, B., McCarthy, M., Roberts, B., Khamis, I. (2003). CD4+ and CD8+ cells accumulate in the brains of acquired immunodeficiency syndrome patients with human immunodeficiency virus encephalitis. *J Neurovirol, 9*, 36–44.

Poland, S. D., Rice, G. P., & Dekaban, G. A. (1995). HIV-1 infection of human brain-derived microvascular endothelial cells in vitro. *J Acquir Immune Defic Syndr Hum Retrovirol, 8*, 437–445.

Power, C., Kong, P. A., Crawford, T. O., Wesselingh, S., Glass, J. D., McArthur, J. C., et al. (1993). Cerebral white matter changes in acquired immunodeficiency syndrome dementia: Alterations of the blood-brain barrier. *Ann Neurol, 34*, 339–350.

Price, T. O., Ercal, N., Nakaoke, R., & Banks, W. A. (2005). HIV-1 viral proteins gp120 and Tat induce oxidative stress in brain endothelial cells. *Brain Res, 1045*, 57–63.

Prokai-Tatrai, K., Prokai, L., & Bodor, N. (1996). Brain-targeted delivery of a leucine-enkephalin analogue by retrometabolic design. *J Med Chem, 39*, 4775–4782.

Pulliam, L., Gascon, R., Stubblebine, M., McGuire, D., & McGrath, M. S. (1997). Unique monocyte subset in patients with AIDS dementia. *Lancet, 349*, 692–695.

Quagliarello, V. J., Long, W. J., & Scheld, W. M. (1986). Morphologic alterations of the blood-brain barrier with experimental meningitis in the rat. Temporal sequence and role of encapsulation. *J Clin Invest, 77*, 1084–1095.

Rabey, J. M., Nissipeanu, P., & Korczyn, A. D. (1992). Efficacy of memantine, an NMDA receptor antagonist, in the treatment of Parkinson's disease. *J Neural Transm Park Dis Dement Sect, 4*, 277–282.

Ragin, A. B., Wu, Y., Ochs, R., Scheidegger, R., Cohen, B. A., McArthur, J. C., et al. (2009). Serum matrix metalloproteinase levels correlate with brain injury in human immunodeficiency virus infection. *J Neurovirol, 1–7*.

Rao, K. S., Ghorpade, A., & Labhasetwar, V. (2009a). Targeting anti-HIV drugs to the CNS. *Expert Opin Drug Deliv, 6*, 771–784.

Rao, V. R., Eugenin, E. A., Berman, J. W., & Prasad, V. R. (2009b). Methods to study monocyte migration induced by HIV-infected cells. *Methods Mol Biol, 485*, 295–309.

Rao, V. R., Sas, A. R., Eugenin, E. A., Siddappa, N. B., Bimonte-Nelson, H., Berman, J. W., et al. (2008) HIV-1 clade-specific differences in the induction of neuropathogenesis. *J Neurosci, 28*, 10010–10016.

Reisberg, B., Doody, R., Stoffler, A., Schmitt, F., Ferris, S., & Mobius, H. J. (2003). Memantine in moderate-to-severe Alzheimer's disease. *N Engl J Med, 348*, 1333–1341.

Ren, Z., Yao, Q., & Chen, C. (2002). HIV-1 envelope glycoprotein 120 increases intercellular adhesion molecule-1 expression by human endothelial cells. *Lab Invest, 82*, 245–255.

Riedel, D. J., Pardo, C. A., McArthur, J., & Nath, A. (2006). Therapy insight: CNS manifestations of HIV-associated immune reconstitution inflammatory syndrome. *Nat Clin Pract Neurol, 2*, 557–565.

Risau, W. (1991). Induction of blood-brain barrier endothelial cell differentiation. *Ann N Y Acad Sci, 633*, 405–419.

Risau, W. & Wolburg, H. (1990). Development of the blood-brain barrier. *Trends Neurosci, 13*, 174–178.

Roberts, T. K., Buckner, C. M., & Berman, J. W. (2010). Leukocyte transmigration across the blood-brain barrier: Perspectives on neuroAIDS. *Front Biosci, 15*, 478–536.

Robinson-Papp, J., Byrd, D., Mindt, M. R., Oden, N. L., Simpson, D. M., & Morgello, S. (2008). Motor function and human immunodeficiency virus-associated cognitive impairment in a highly active antiretroviral therapy-era cohort. *Arch Neurol, 65*, 1096–1101.

Rottman, J. B., Ganley, K. P., Williams, K., Wu, L., Mackay, C. R., & Ringler, D. J. (1997). Cellular localization of the chemokine receptor CCR5. Correlation to cellular targets of HIV-1 infection. *Am J Pathol, 151*, 1341–1351.

Rubin, L. L. & Staddon, J. M. (1999). The cell biology of the blood-brain barrier. *Annu Rev Neurosci, 22*, 11–28.

Salo, P. T. & Tatton, W. G. (1992). Deprenyl reduces the death of motoneurons caused by axotomy. *J Neurosci Res, 31*, 394–400.

Sanders, V. J., Pittman, C. A., White, M. G., Wang, G., Wiley, C. A., & Achim, C. L. (1998). Chemokines and receptors in HIV encephalitis. *AIDS, 12*, 1021–1026.

Sapadin, A. N. & Fleischmajer, R. (2006). Tetracyclines: Nonantibiotic properties and their clinical implications. *J Am Acad Dermatol, 54*, 258–265.

Sasseville, V. G., Newman, W. A., Lackner, A. A., Smith, M. O., Lausen, N. C., Beall, D., et al. (1992). Elevated vascular cell adhesion molecule-1 in AIDS encephalitis induced by simian immunodeficiency virus. *Am J Pathol, 141*, 1021–1030.

Sasseville, V. G., Smith, M. M., Mackay, C. R., Pauley, D. R., Mansfield, K. G., Ringler, D. J., et al. (1996). Chemokine expression in simian immunodeficiency virus-induced AIDS encephalitis. *Am J Pathol, 149,* 1459–1467.

Schifitto, G., Navia, B. A., Yiannoutsos, C. T., Marra, C. M., Chang, L., Ernst, T., et al. (2007). Memantine and HIV-associated cognitive impairment: A neuropsychological and proton magnetic resonance spectroscopy study. *AIDS, 21,* 1877–1886.

Schweighardt, B. & Atwood, W. J. (2001a). HIV type 1 infection of human astrocytes is restricted by inefficient viral entry. *AIDS Res Hum Retroviruses, 17,* 1133–1142.

Schweighardt, B. & Atwood, W. J. (2001b). Glial cells as targets of viral infection in the human central nervous system. *Prog Brain Res, 132,* 721–735.

Schweighardt, B., Shieh, J. T., & Atwood, W. J. (2001). CD4/CXCR4-independent infection of human astrocytes by a T-tropic strain of HIV-1. *J Neurovirol, 7,* 155–162.

Seilhean, D., Dzia-Lepfoundzou, A., Sazdovitch, V., Cannella, B., Raine, C. S., Katlama, C., et al. (1997). Astrocytic adhesion molecules are increased in HIV-1-associated cognitive/motor complex. *Neuropathol Appl Neurobiol, 23,* 83–92.

Shi, B., De Girolami, U., He, J., Wang, S., Lorenzo, A., Busciglio, J., et al. (1996). Apoptosis induced by HIV-1 infection of the central nervous system. *J Clin Invest, 98,* 1979–1990.

Si, Q., Cosenza, M., Kim, M. O., Zhao, M. L., Brownlee, M., Goldstein, H., et al. (2004). A novel action of minocycline: Inhibition of human immunodeficiency virus type 1 infection in microglia. *J Neurovirol, 10,* 284–292.

Soilu-Hanninen, M., Eralinna, J. P., Hukkanen, V., Roytta, M., Salmi, A. A., & Salonen, R. (1994). Semliki Forest virus infects mouse brain endothelial cells and causes blood-brain barrier damage. *J Virol, 68,* 6291–6298.

Soulas, C., Donahue, R. E., Dunbar, C. E., Persons, D. A., Alvarez, X., & Williams, K. C. (2009). Genetically modified CD34+ hematopoietic stem cells contribute to turnover of brain perivascular macrophages in long-term repopulated primates. *Am J Pathol, 174,* 1808–1817.

Spencer, D. C. & Price, R. W. (1992). Human immunodeficiency virus and the central nervous system. *Annu Rev Microbiol, 46,* 655–693.

Stanimirovic, D. & Satoh, K. (2000). Inflammatory mediators of cerebral endothelium: A role in ischemic brain inflammation. *Brain Pathol, 10,* 113–126.

Stantchev, T. S. & Broder, C. C. (2001). Human immunodeficiency virus type-1 and chemokines: beyond competition for common cellular receptors. *Cytokine Growth Factor Rev, 12,* 219–243.

Stirling, D. P., Koochesfahani, K. M., Steeves, J. D., & Tetzlaff, W. (2005). Minocycline as a neuroprotective agent. *Neuroscientist, 11,* 308–322.

Strelow, L., Janigro, D., & Nelson, J. A. (2002). Persistent SIV infection of a blood-brain barrier model. *J Neurovirol, 8,* 270–280.

Strelow, L. I., Janigro, D., & Nelson, J. A. (2001). The blood-brain barrier and AIDS. *Adv Virus Res, 56,* 355–388.

Tariot, P. N., Farlow, M. R., Grossberg, G. T., Graham, S. M., McDonald, S., & Gergel, I. (2004). Memantine treatment in patients with moderate to severe Alzheimer disease already receiving donepezil: A randomized controlled trial. *JAMA, 291,* 317–324.

Tatton, W. G. & Greenwood, C. E. (1991). Rescue of dying neurons: A new action for deprenyl in MPTP parkinsonism. *J Neurosci Res, 30,* 666–672.

Thieblemont, N., Weiss, L., Sadeghi, H. M., Estcourt, C., & Haeffner-Cavaillon, N. (1995). CD14lowCD16high: A cytokine-producing monocyte subset which expands during human immunodeficiency virus infection. *Eur J Immunol, 25,* 3418–3424.

Tornatore, C., Nath, A., Amemiya, K., & Major, E. O. (1991). Persistent human immunodeficiency virus type 1 infection in human fetal glial cells reactivated by T-cell factor(s) or by the cytokines tumor necrosis factor alpha and interleukin-1 beta. *J Virol, 65,* 6094–6100.

Tsuji, A. (2005). Small molecular drug transfer across the blood-brain barrier via carrier-mediated transport systems. *NeuroRx, 2,* 54–62.

Tsukita, S. & Furuse, M. (1999). Occludin and claudins in tight-junction strands: Leading or supporting players? *Trends Cell Biol, 9,* 268–273.

Ullrich, C. K., Groopman, J. E., & Ganju, R. K. (2000). HIV-1 gp120- and gp160-induced apoptosis in cultured endothelial cells is mediated by caspases. *Blood, 96,* 1438–1442.

Vallat, A. V., De Girolami, U., He, J., Mhashilkar, A., Marasco, W., Shi, B., et al. (1998). Localization of HIV-1 co-receptors CCR5 and CXCR4 in the brain of children with AIDS. *Am J Pathol, 152,* 167–178.

van der Kuyl, A. C., van den Burg, R., Zorgdrager, F., Groot, F., Berkhout, B., & Cornelissen, M. (2007). Sialoadhesin (CD169) expression in CD14+ cells is upregulated early after HIV-1 infection and increases during disease progression. *PLoS One, 2,* e257.

Varatharajan, L. & Thomas, S. A. (2009). The transport of anti-HIV drugs across blood-CNS interfaces: Summary of current knowledge and recommendations for further research. *Antiviral Res, 82,* A99–109.

Villiger, P. M., Terkeltaub, R., & Lotz, M. (1992). Monocyte chemoattractant protein-1 (MCP-1) expression in human articular cartilage. Induction by peptide regulatory factors and differential effects of dexamethasone and retinoic acid. *J Clin Invest, 90,* 488–496.

Wang, H., Sun, J., & Goldstein, H. (2008). Human immunodeficiency virus type 1 infection increases the in vivo capacity of peripheral monocytes to cross the blood-brain barrier into the brain and the in vivo sensitivity of the blood-brain barrier to disruption by lipopolysaccharide. *J Virol, 82,* 7591–7600.

Wang, J., Harada, A., Matsushita, S., Matsumi, S., Zhang, Y., Shioda, T., et al. (1998). IL-4 and a glucocorticoid up-regulate CXCR4 expression on human CD4+ T lymphocytes and enhance HIV-1 replication. *J Leukoc Biol, 64,* 642–649.

Weiss, J. M., Downie, S. A., Lyman, W. D., & Berman, J. W. (1998). Astrocyte-derived monocyte-chemoattractant protein-1 directs the transmigration of leukocytes across a model of the human blood-brain barrier. *J Immunol, 161,* 6896–6903.

Weiss, J. M., Nath, A., Major, E. O., & Berman, J. W. (1999). HIV-1 Tat induces monocyte chemoattractant protein-1-mediated monocyte transmigration across a model of the human blood-brain barrier and upregulates CCR5 expression on human monocytes. *J Immunol, 163,* 2953–2959.

Weiss, N., Miller, F., Cazaubon, S., & Couraud, P. O. (2009). The blood-brain barrier in brain homeostasis and neurological diseases. *Biochim Biophys Acta, 1788,* 842–857.

Wiley, C. A., Schrier, R. D., Nelson, J. A., Lampert, P. W., & Oldstone, M. B. (1986). Cellular localization of human immunodeficiency virus infection within the brains of acquired immune deficiency syndrome patients. *Proc Natl Acad Sci USA, 83,* 7089–7093.

Winblad, B. & Poritis, N. (1999). Memantine in severe dementia: Results of the 9M-Best Study (Benefit and efficacy in severely demented patients during treatment with memantine). *Int J Geriatr Psychiatry, 14,* 135–146.

Wu, D. T., Woodman, S. E., Weiss, J. M., McManus, C. M., D'Aversa, T. G., Hesselgesser, J., et al. (2000). Mechanisms of leukocyte trafficking into the CNS. *J Neurovirol, 6* Suppl 1, S82–85.

Yla-Herttuala, S., Lipton, B. A., Rosenfeld, M. E., Sarkioja, T., Yoshimura, T., Leonard, E. J., et al. (1991). Expression of monocyte chemoattractant protein 1 in macrophage-rich areas of human and rabbit atherosclerotic lesions. *Proc Natl Acad Sci USA, 88,* 5252–5256.

Zhong, Y., Smart, E. J., Weksler, B., Couraud, P. O., Hennig, B., & Toborek, M. (2008). Caveolin-1 regulates human immunodeficiency virus-1 Tat-induced alterations of tight junction protein expression via modulation of the Ras signaling. *J Neurosci, 28,* 7788–7796.

Ziegler-Heitbrock, L. (2007). The CD14+ CD16+ blood monocytes: Their role in infection and inflammation. *J Leukoc Biol, 81,* 584–592.

Zink, M. C., Uhrlaub, J., DeWitt, J., Voelker, T., Bullock, B., Mankowski, J., et al. (2005). Neuroprotective and anti-human immunodeficiency virus activity of minocycline. *JAMA, 293,* 2003–2011.

3.5

MONOCYTE-MACROPHAGES AND VIRAL CENTRAL NERVOUS SYSTEM ENTRY

Georgette D. Kanmogne

Monocytes and macrophages play many roles in human immunodeficiency virus (HIV) infection. Importantly, monocytes and macrophages mediate viral persistence and dissemination of virus into organs and tissues, including organs and tissues of the central nervous system. This chapter provides an overview of interactions between monocytes and the blood-brain barrier (BBB) in HIV/AIDS, and describes proinflammatory factors and virotoxins that are known to alter BBB functions and properties. The chapter also explores molecular mechanisms involved in HIV-induced BBB dysfunction, and discusses potential strategies for preventing or reducing entry of HIV, and HIV-infected cells, into the brain.

INTRODUCTION

Monocytes and macrophages are productively infected by the human immunodeficiency virus (HIV) and are responsible for viral persistence and dissemination into organs and tissues of infected individuals (Wang, Rumbaugh, & Nath, 2006; Williams & Hickey, 2002; Zheng & Gendelman, 1997; Alexaki, Liu, & Wigdahl, 2008; Crowe, Zhu, & Muller, 2003; Ho, Cherukuri, & Douglas, 1994). It has been demonstrated that HIV-1 enters the brain in the early stages of infection, mostly through infected monocytes in a "Trojan horse" mechanism (for recent reviews, see Buckner, Luers, Calderon, Eugenin, & Berman, 2006; Gras & Kaul, 2010; Ivey, MacLean, & Lackner, 2009; Persidsky, Ramirez, Haorah, & Kanmogne, 2006b; Roberts, Buckner, & Berman, 2010; Yao, Bethel-Brown, Li, & Buch, 2010). The blood-brain barrier (BBB) is a semi-permeable capillary membrane that, under normal physiologic conditions, restricts the movements of cells, organic substances, ions, and proteins between the central nervous system (CNS) and peripheral circulation (Ballabh, Braun, & Nedergaard, 2004; Huber, Egleton, & Davis, 2001; Persidsky et al., 2006b). However, under diseases conditions such as HIV/AIDS its barrier function can breakdown. *In vitro* and *in vivo* studies show that HIV infection cause a breakdown in the barrier function of the brain endothelium, and this BBB breakdown causes infiltration of HIV and infected cells into the brain (, Berman, & Lyman, 1994; Ivey et al., 2009; Persidsky et al., 2006b; Persidsky, Zheng, Miller, & Gendelman, 2000; Trillo-Pazos & Everall, 1997). Once in the brain, HIV is disseminated to other CNS cells, including resident macrophages and microglia which become productively infected, release

virions, virotoxins, and inflammatory cytokines that cause neuronal injury (Dhillon et al., 2008; Eugenin et al., 2006a; Fantuzzi et al., 2000; Persidsky & Gendelman, 2003; Persidsky et al., 2000). Disease pathology ranges from mild brain atrophy and gliosis to robust viral replication, multinucleated giant cell formation, astrogliosis and microgliosis, myelin pallor, and neuronal loss (Everall, Hansen, & Masliah, 2005; Kaul, 2009; Kolson, 2002; Krebs, Ross, McAllister, & Wigdahl, 2000; Lawrence & Major, 2002; Yadav & Collman, 2009; Zheng & Gendelman, 1997). These pathological findings are collectively termed HIV-1 encephalitis (HIVE). HIVE is a common correlate to the later stages of behavioral, motor, neuropsychiatric, and neurologic consequences of disease termed HIV-associated neurocognitive disorders (HAND) (Ances & Ellis, 2007; Antinori et al., 2007; Boisse, Gill, & Power, 2008; Everall et al., 2005; Grant, Heaton, & Atkinson, 1995; McArthur, Steiner, Sacktor, & Nath, 2010; Woods, Moore, Weber, & Grant, 2009). Thus, BBB dysfunction is a critical feature of HIV neuropathogenesis, as it leads to infiltration of virus and infected mononuclear phagocytes (MP) into the brain, and neurodegeneration. This chapter will provide an overview of monocyte-BBB interactions in HIV/AIDS, the proinflammatory factors and virotoxins known to alter BBB functions and properties, and the molecular mechanisms involved in HIV-induced BBB dysfunction; the chapter also discusses potential strategies for preventing/reducing entry of HIV and infected cells into the brain.

MONOCYTES AND HIV INFECTION OF THE CENTRAL NERVOUS SYSTEM

HIV infection of mononuclear phagocytes (MP) has been demonstrated in the peripheral blood of infected individuals, as well as in several target organs and tissues, including the brain and lymphoid tissues (Wang et al., 2006; Williams & Hickey, 2002; Zheng & Gendelman, 1997). It has been demonstrated that BBB breakdown occurs in the early stages of HIV infection (Avison et al., 2004), and monocyte infection and trafficking plays a major role in viral dissemination, viral persistence, and maintenance of HIV reservoirs (Alexaki et al., 2008; Crowe et al., 2003; Ho et al., 1994). Furthermore, peripheral blood monocytes, monocytes-derived macrophages, and tissue macrophages from human donors are productively infected by HIV *in vivo* and *in vitro* (Crowe, Maslin, Ellery, & Kedzierska, 2004; Crowe et al., 2003; Crowe, 1995; Fischer-Smith et al., 2008). HIV-1 also alters the pathophysiology and function of MP and disrupts the innate immune response (Yao et al., 2010). In fact it has been demonstrated that following HIV-1 infection, monocytes and macrophages show impairment in phagocytosis of bacteria and opportunistic pathogens such as *Mycobacterium avium* complex, *Mycobacterium tuberculosis*, *Pneumocystis carinii*, *Toxoplasma gondii* and *Candida albicans* (reviewed in Kedzierska et al., 2003). HIV infection of monocytes/macrophages also impairs other effector functions such as cytokine and chemokine production, chemotaxis, accessory cell function, and microbicidal activities (Crowe et al., 2003; Crowe, 1995). This defective function of MP leads to impaired immune function and the reactivation and development of opportunistic infections and AIDS (Kedzierska & Crowe, 2002).

Monocytes and macrophages also play an important role in the dissemination of virus into tissues, HIV neuropathogenesis, and the development of neuroAIDS. It is well established that HIV enters the brain in the early stages of viral infection, mostly via infected and activated monocytes-macrophages (Hurwitz et al., 1994; Ivey et al., 2009; Persidsky et al., 2006b; Persidsky et al., 2000; Trillo-Pazos & Everall, 1997); this initiates viral spreading into the brain and development of neurological dysfunction in infected patients. There is also evidence of increased trafficking of CD14+/CD16+ peripheral blood monocytes into the CNS of HIVE patients, and macrophages derived from this monocyte subset constitute a major viral reservoir in the CNS (Fischer-Smith et al., 2001; Williams, Alvarez, & Lackner, 2001). Inflammatory cytokines and chemokines secreted by infected cells further increase infiltration of infected cells into the brain. MP in the brain serves as viral reservoirs and transmits HIV to resident microglia and macrophages; neurotoxins produced by these infected cells alter the function of other CNS cells, and induce neuronal injury and the development of HAND (Ances & Ellis, 2007; Boisse et al., 2008; Everall et al., 2005; Grant et al., 1995; McArthur et al., 2010; Woods et al., 2009).

MONOCYTE-BLOOD-BRAIN BARRIER INTERACTION AND VIRAL ENTRY INTO THE CENTRAL NERVOUS SYSTEM

HIV, VIRAL PROTEINS AND BBB DYSFUNCTION IN NEUROAIDS

The BBB is composed of endothelial cells, astrocytes foot processes, pericytes, and extracellular matrix, with endothelial cells forming the major component (Ballabh et al., 2004; Huber et al., 2001); and monocyte-BBB interactions are central to viral neuroinvasion and HIV neuropathogenesis (Banks, 1999; Banks, Ercal, & Price, 2006; Persidsky et al., 2006b; Toborek et al., 2005). Stins and colleagues showed that human brain microvascular endothelial cells (HBMEC) derived from children express the CD4 receptor (Stins et al., 2004; Stins et al., 2001) but other studies could not detect CD4 expression in primary, adult-derived HBMEC (Kanmogne, Grammas, &

Kennedy, 2000; Kanmogne, Kennedy, & Grammas, 2002). HBMEC express the HIV-1 co-receptors CCR5 and CXCR4 (Kanmogne et al., 2000; Kanmogne et al., 2007; Stins et al., 2004), and these co-receptors and proteoglycans facilitate HIV binding and uptake by brain endothelial cells, although no productive infection of HBMEC has been detected (Argyris et al., 2003; Kanmogne et al., 2002; Kanmogne et al., 2007). Exposure of the brain endothelium to HIV virions and infected MPs alters BBB function and properties. Exposure of HIV-1-infected monocytes to HBMEC decreased expression of JAM-A, occludin, and ZO-1, increased expression of adhesion molecules on the brain endothelium, and this was associated with increased BBB permeability and transendothelial migration of infected monocytes (Huang, Eum, Andras, Hennig, & Toborek, 2009; Nottet et al., 1996). It has been shown that Rho kinases and Rho GTPase mediate HIV-induced downregulation of occludin and claudin-5, claudin-5 phosphorylation, and increased monocyte migration in HIVE (Persidsky et al., 2006a; Ramirez et al., 2008; Yamamoto et al., 2008); and there is *in vitro* and *in vivo* evidence that HIV-1 virions and secreted viral proteins alter BBB integrity and function, and increase monocyte entry into the CNS (Hurwitz et al., 1994; Ivey et al., 2009; Persidsky et al., 2006b; Persidsky et al., 2000; Trillo-Pazos & Everall, 1997).

HIV gp120 Proteins

HIV enters and infects target cells by binding its envelope gp120 protein to cellular CD4 receptor or co-receptors such as CCR5 and CXCR4. Several studies, including ours, also showed that gp120 proteins derived from both macrophage-tropic and T-lymphocyte-tropic are toxic to HBMEC; disrupt tight junction (TJ) proteins; decrease expression of occludin, ZO-1, ZO-2, and claudin-5; increase release of lactate dehydrogenase; decrease transendothelial electrical resistance (TEER); and increase BBB permeability and monocyte transendothelial migration (Kanmogne et al., 2002; Kanmogne, Primeaux, & Grammas, 2005; Kanmogne et al., 2007; Stins et al., 2003; Stins et al., 2001). HIV-1 gp120 proteins upregulated expression of the adhesion molecules VCAM-1 and ICAM-1 in HBMEC (Stins et al., 2003; Stins et al., 2001), and studies further showed that the kinases and pathways mediating gp120 effects included PKCα/βII, PKC(pan)-βII, PCK-zeta/lambda, P38 MAPK, the signal transducers and activators of transcription (STAT)-1 pathways, and calcium signaling (Kanmogne et al., 2002; Kanmogne et al., 2005; Kanmogne et al., 2007; Khan, Di Cello, tins, & Kim, 2007; Persidsky et al., 2006b). HIV-1 gp120 protein also activates MP, causing secretions of TNF-α (D'Aversa, Eugenin, & Berman, 2005) and this can further exacerbate BBB dysfunction during monocytes-endothelial interaction and increase cellular infiltration into the CNS.

HIV Tat Proteins

Tat is release by HIV-infected cells, crosses the BBB, and is present in CNS tissues of infected individuals (Banks, Robinson, & Nath, 2005; Hudson et al., 2000). It has been demonstrated that Tat proteins alter the function of many cells including brain endothelial cells and other cells of the neurovascular unit (reviewed by Buckner et al., 2006; Li, Li, Steiner, & Nath, 2009; Wu et al., 2000). Tat induced MCP-1 secretion and migration of glial cells (Eugenin, Dyer, Calderon, & Berman, 2005; Weiss, Nath, Major, & Berman, 1999) and induced disruption of TJ proteins in brain endothelial cells (Andras et al., 2003). Tat also induced oxidative stress; upregulation of the adhesion molecules VCAM-1 and ICAM-1 in endothelial cells; and increased expression of IL-1β, TNF-α, MCP-1, and E-selectin in a human brain endothelial cell line via NFκB pathways (Huang et al., 2008; Mrowiec, Melchar, & Gorski, 1997). HIV-1 Tat also increased adhesion of monocytes and T cells to the endothelium *in vivo* and *in vitro*, and altered T-cell interaction with endothelial extracellular matrix proteins (Matzen et al., 2004; Mrowiec et al., 1997). These Tat-mediated effects have been shown to alter the BBB structure and function and promote MP trafficking into the CNS.

HIV Nef and Vpr Proteins

The accessory HIV proteins Nef and Vpr are expressed in infected CNS tissues and have been shown to be associated with BBB injury, HIV neuroinvasion, and HAD (Annunziata, 2003; Pomerantz, 2004; Ranki et al., 1995). Nef and Vpr from both T-lymphocyte-tropic and macrophage-tropic HIV-1 activated caspases and induced apoptosis in HBMEC (Acheampong et al., 2005; Choi et al., 2005). *In vivo* and *in vitro* studies showed that HIV-1 Nef-induced BBB disruption involved matrix metalloproteins (MMPs) activation, and MMPs inhibitors diminished Nef-induced BBB disruption (Bergonzini et al., 2009; Sporer et al., 2000). It has been shown that Vpr-derived peptides can reach endothelial mitochondria and induce cytochrome C release and apoptosis of brain endothelial cells (Borgne-Sanchez et al., 2007). This shows possible role of HIV-1 regulatory protein in HIV CNS invasion and neuropathogenesis.

PREVENTING HIV-VIRAL PROTEINS-INDUCED BLOOD-BRAIN BARRIER DYSFUNCTION

Targeting signaling pathways activated in the brain endothelium by HIV, viral proteins, and during monocyte-BBB interaction could provide strategies for preventing BBB injury in HIV/AIDS. *In vitro* and *ex-vivo* studies of microvessels isolated from infected humans showed that HAD is associated with increased disruption of TJ proteins and activation of STAT-1 on the brain endothelium (Chaudhuri et al., 2008a; Chaudhuri et al., 2008b). STAT-1 inhibitors decreased HIV-1- and gp120-induced cytokine secretion, and diminished HIV-1- and gp120-induced downregulation of TJ proteins (Chaudhuri, Duan, Morsey, Persidsky, & Kanmogne, 2008a; Chaudhuri, Yang, Gendelman, Persidsky, & Kanmogne, 2008b; Yang, Akhter, Chaudhuri, & Kanmogne, 2009; Yang, Singh, Bressani, & Kanmogne, 2010). HIV-1 gp120 BBB compromise also involved activation of PKC-α/β2 and PCK-zeta and inhibitors of PKC diminished HIV-induced

PKC activation (Kanmogne et al., 2007). Inhibitors of Rho kinases, Rho GTPase, and GSK3beta also diminished HIV-induced BBB compromise and TJ downregulation (Persidsky et al., 2006a; Ramirez et al., 2010; Ramirez et al., 2008).

Zhong and colleagues (Zhong et al., 2008) showed that HIV-1 Tat-induced downregulation of occludin, ZO-1, and ZO-2 in HBMEC involved caveolin-1 and activation of the Ras pathway (Zhong et al., 2008). Caveolin-1 silencing and pharmacological inhibition of Ras signaling attenuated Tat-induced downregulation of TJ proteins (Zhong et al., 2008). Injection of Tat proteins to mice decreased ZO-1 and occludin, upregulated COX-2 expression, and induced BBB disruption (Pu et al., 2007); these effects were attenuated by pretreatment of mice with the COX-2 inhibitor rofecoxib (Pu et al., 2007). Andras and colleagues (Andras et al., 2005) also showed that Tat-induced alterations of claudin-5 mRNA levels in brain EC could be partially reversed by inhibitors of MEK1/2 (U0126), VEGFR-2 (SU1498), PI3K (LY294002), the NFκB peptide SN50, and the calcium chelator BAPTA/AM (Andras et al., 2005). Overall, these studies showed that there are multiple pathways activated by HIV virions, viral proteins, and infected monocytes on the brain endothelium, and pharmacological inhibitors of these pathways diminished HIV-induced BBB compromise.

INFLAMMATION AND BLOOD-BRAIN BARRIER COMPROMISE IN NEUROAIDS

Inflammation plays a major role in BBB breakdown, drives monocyte recruitment into the CNS and HIV neuroinvasion, and CSF levels of MCP-1 correlate with BBB compromise in infected patients (Avison et al., 2004). HIV-1 infection of MPs induced cellular activation and increased expression and secretion of inflammatory cytokines and chemokines, including MCP-1, SDF-1α, and IL-6 (Dhillon et al., 2008; Eugenin et al., 2006a; Fantuzzi et al., 2000; Persidsky & Gendelman, 2003). These cytokines have been shown to enhance the expression of the adhesion molecules ICAM-1, VCAM-1, β-2 integrins, and PECAM on MPs and the vascular endothelium, activate voltage-gated ions channels, and increased transmigration of MPs across the BBB (Chaudhuri, Duan, Morsey, Persidsky, & Kanmogne, 2008a; Chaudhuri et al., 2008b; Eugenin et al., 2006b; Gendelman et al., 2009; Maslin et al., 2005; Mengozzi et al., 1999; Wu et al., 2000). Direct exposure of the brain endothelium to virions and secreted viral factors also induced expression of inflammatory cytokines and chemokines (Chaudhuri et al., 2008a; Chaudhuri et al., 2008b; Yang et al., 2009). This ongoing inflammation, activation of monocytes/macrophages, and opportunistic infections facilitates passages on infected MPs across the BBB and HIV neuroinvasion (Avison et al., 2004; Eugenin et al., 2006a).

Direct inflammation of the brain endothelium plays a major role in BBB dysfunction in neuroAIDS. Brain microvessels from HIV-infected humans and HAD patients showed increased cytokine expression (Chaudhuri et al., 2008b). Exposure of primary HBMEC to HIV-1 virions, gp120 proteins, or HIV-infected macrophages increased mRNA and protein levels of several proinflammatory cytokines and chemokines, including IL-6, IL-8, CCL2, CCL20, CX3CL1, CX3CL2, CX3CL3, CX3CL5, CX3CL6, CX3CL10, and TNF-α (Chaudhuri et al., 2008a Yang et al., 2009); interaction of HBMEC with infected macrophages further increased cytokine expression in both HBMEC and macrophages (Chaudhuri et al., 2008a; Chaudhuri et al., 2008b). HIV-1 gp120 transgenic mice showed increased expression of IP-10 and MCP-1 (Asensio et al., 2001). Exposure of brain endothelial cell cultures to Tat and injection of Tat to mice increased mRNA and protein levels of MCP-1 and TNF-α, as well as the adhesion molecules VCAM-1, ICAM-1, and E-selectin, leading to increased adherence of inflammatory cells to the endothelium and monocyte infiltration into the CNS (Lee, Eum, Nath, & Toborek, 2004; Pu et al., 2003).

PREVENTING INFLAMMATION-INDUCED BLOOD-BRAIN BARRIER DYSFUNCTION AND MONOCYTE CENTRAL NERVOUS SYSTEM MIGRATION IN NEUROAIDS

Several molecular pathways have been shown to be involved in HIV-1-, gp120-, and Tat-induced upregulation of inflammatory cytokines, inflammation-induced BBB compromise, and transendothelial migration of infected monocytes and infiltration of MP into the CNS. These molecular mechanisms include the NFκB, STAT1 (Chaudhuri et al., 2008a; Chaudhuri et al., 2008b), glycogen synthase kinase-3-beta (GSK-3β) (Ramirez et al., 2010), and peroxisome proliferator-activated receptor (PPAR) (Huang et al., 2009; Potula et al., 2008; Ramirez et al., 2008) pathways. Therefore, it is possible that pharmacological inhibitors of these pathways could reduce HIV-induced inflammation and monocyte migration across the BBB.

STAT1 is a member of the STAT family of transcription factors involved in upregulation of genes following signal by interferons and inflammatory cytokines such as IL-6. STAT1 inhibitors prevented HIV-1- and gp120-induced upregulation of IL-6, IL-8, and MCP-1 in HBMEC, and diminished HIV-1-, gp120-, and cytokine-induced transendothelial migration of monocytes (Chaudhuri et al., 2008a; Chaudhuri et al., 2008b; Yang et al., 2009). PPARs are nuclear receptors that have been shown to have anti-inflammatory properties. Activation and overexpression of PPAR-α and PPAR-γ diminished HIV-1 infection of MPs in animal models of neuroAIDS, diminished adhesion and transendothelial migration of infected monocytes (Potula et al., 2008; Ramirez et al., 2008), and attenuated HIV-induced dysregulation of junctional adhesion molecule A (JAM-A), occludin, and ZO-1 in HBMEC (Huang et al., 2009). Exposure of HIV-1 Tat proteins to HBMEC cell line decreased transactivation of PPAR-α and PPARγ, and increased IL-1β, TNF-α, CCL2, and E-selectin expression through NFκB pathways (Huang et al., 2008). Overexpression of PPARγ and PPAR-α significantly attenuated Tat-inducted upregulation of IL-1β, TNF-α, CCL2 and E-selectin, and prevented Tat-induced binding activity of NFκB (Huang et al., 2008). Inhibition of GSK-3β decreased inflammation in HBMEC (Ramirez et al., 2010).

Co-culture of HIV-infected macrophages with HBMEC induced expression of cyclooxygenase-2 (COX-2) in both cell types (Pereira, Boven, Middel, Verhoef, & Nottet, 2000); there is also evidence that overexpression of COX-2 modulates inflammatory reactions in Tat-injected mice, and COX inhibitors diminished Tat-induced inflammation (Flora, Pu, Hennig, & Toborek, 2006).

Overall, these data suggest that targeting STAT1, GSK-3β, PPARs, COX-2, and/or NFκB pathways could prevent HIV-induced inflammation in both MPs and brain endothelium. To control inflammation in HIV/AIDS, it is also critical to prevent opportunistic infections, which often induce release of bacterial endotoxins such as lipopolysaccharide (LPS); LPS induces monocyte activation and trafficking into the brain, potentiates HIV-induced monocyte entry into the brain, and HAD patients show elevated levels of LPS (Ancuta et al., 2008; Wang, Sun, & Goldstein, 2008).

OXIDATIVE STRESS, PROTEASES, AND BLOOD-BRAIN BARRIER COMPROMISE IN NEUROAIDS

Oxidative Stress

HIV-1 and viral proteins have been shown to induce oxidative stress in the brain endothelium, which contributes to BBB damage in infected patients and neuroAIDS (reviewed in Mollace et al., 2001). Exposure of brain endothelial cells to Tat proteins increased cellular oxidative stress, decreased levels of intracellular glutathione, and activated DNA binding of the transcription factors NFκB and activator protein 1 (AP1) (Toborek et al., 2003); injection of Tat to rats increased protein carbonylation (Aksenov et al., 2001). HIV-1 infection induces depletion of endogenous antioxidants and increased production of reactive oxygen species (ROS); and this is enhanced by chronic inflammation that is associated with activation of MPs (Elbim et al., 2001; Pace & Leaf, 1995). Free radicals are generated following HIV infection of macrophages, and IL-1β and TNF-α up-regulate inducible nitric oxide synthase (iNOS) in brain cells (Boven, Middel, Verhoef, De Groot, Nottet, 1999; Hori et al., 1999). This infection of macrophages results in increased production of superoxide anion and superoxide dismutase (SOD) (Boven et al., 1999; Boven et al., 2000), and brain tissues of HAD patients showed increased iNOS and SOD, compared to nondemented AIDS patients, with 70% of HIV-1p24+ MPs also expressing SOD (Boven et al., 1999). Co-culture of brain endothelial cells with infected MPs induced expression of endothelial NOS (Mollace et al., 2001), which suggest that close contact of infected MPs with the brain endothelium induce nitrotyrosine and peroxynitrite formation. In fact, brain tissues of HAD patients showed extensive nitrotyrosine immunoreactivity in perivascular areas, on MPs closed to the brain endothelium, and this was associated with decreased ZO-1 expression (Mollace et al., 2001). Thus, overproduction of free radicals can disrupt the BBB integrity and increase BBB permeability.

Glutathione (GSH) is an antioxidant that maintains the redox potential in cells, protects against ROS, and interacts directly with free radicals by acting as an electron donor in the reduction of peroxidase catalyzed by glutathione peroxidase (Forstermann, 2008; Mari, Morales, Colell, Garcia-Ruiz, & Fernandez-Checa, 2009; Oktyabrsky & Smirnova, 2007). Decreased levels of GSH in endothelial cells increased cell sensitivity to oxidative stress (Hurst, Heales, Dobbie, Barker, & Clark, 1998). GSH levels are decreased in the blood and CNS of HIV-infected patients (Pietarinen-Runtti, Lakari, Raivio, & Kinnula, 2000) and this is associated with poor survival (Herzenberg et al., 1997).

Altogether, these evidences suggests that oxidative stress and free radicals produced by infected cells play a role in monocytes-BBB interaction and transendothelial migration of monocytes, and further show that during interaction of infected MP with the brain endothelium, endothelial cells produce ROS which further contributes to BBB damage.

Proteases

Matrix metalloproteinases (MMPs) are zinc-dependent endopeptidases which are involved in the degradation of basement membranes, leading to BBB compromise and disruption of the neurovascular unit (Malemud, 2006; Milward, Fitzsimmons, Szklarczyk, & Conant, 2007). HIV-infected monocytes secrete MMPs that degrade basement membrane proteins (Dhawan, Toro, Jones, & Meltzer, 1992), and CSF of HAD patients showed increased levels of MMP-2, MMP-7, and MMP-9 (Conant et al., 1999). MMPs' transcription and expression are often controlled by redox reactions, growth factors, or cytokines, and MMPs are regulated by tissue inhibitor of metalloproteinases (TIMPs), which inhibits MMP activities (Malemud, 2006; Milward et al., 2007). Studies in TIMP-1 knock-out mice showed that TIMP-1 prevented BBB disruption in cerebral ischemia by inhibiting MMP9 activities (Fujimoto et al., 2008); In vivo studies showed that the antioxidant enzyme glutathione peroxidase protects the brain microvasculature against ischemia-reperfusion injury by inhibiting MMP-9 expression and reducing endothelial activation and inflammation (Wong, Bozinovski, Hertzog, Hickey, & Crack, 2008). These data suggest that destruction of the vascular extracellular matrix in neuroAIDS is associated with dysregulation of MMPs' and TIMPs' homeostasis.

PREVENTING OXIDATIVE STRESS AND MATRIX DEGRADATION IN NEUROAIDS

There is evidence that antioxidants and strategies aimed at reducing HIV-induced oxidative stress can prevent redox-induced BBB injury. Studies in mice models of HIV infection showed that HIV-1 Tat- induced alterations of ZO-1 and alteration of BBB integrity is mediated by redox reactions and ERK1/2 activation (Pu et al., 2005), and ERK inhibitor (U0126) and N-acetylcysteine, an antioxidant and glutathione precursor, attenuated Tat-induced ERK1/2 activation and infiltration of infected cells into the brain (Pu et al., 2005). Fluvastatin prevents glutamate-induced upregulation of ROS and BBB disruption (Kuhlmann et al., 2008), and targeting TIMP-1 could help abrogate HIV-induced increased MMPs activities and prevent degradation of endothelial matrix.

EFFECT OF ANTIRETROVIRAL THERAPY ON MONOCYTES, BLOOD-BRAIN BARRIER, AND VIRAL ENTRY INTO THE CENTRAL NERVOUS SYSTEM

Secreted viral factors and production of HIV proteins in vivo and vitro directly correlated with active viral replication and levels of viremia. Thus, it is likely that controlling viral infection, which leads to reduced viral load, decreased secretion of HIV proteins and other inflammatory factors, will diminish/abrogate BBB compromise in infected individuals, diminish monocyte trafficking into the CNS, and reduce viral neuroinvasion and the incidence or severity of neuroAIDS. Although there have been no studies examining the potential protective effects of antiretroviral therapy (ART) on the brain endothelium of HIV-infected individuals, human studies showed that ART significantly reduce both plasma and CSF viral load (Antinori et al., 2002; Robertson et al., 2004), decreased the prevalence of CNS opportunistic infections and HIVE (Langford, Letendre, Larrea, & Masliah, 2003), and improved neurocognitive and neurologic function in infected individuals (Robertson et al., 2004). Studies of SIV neuroAIDS models also showed that ART significantly reduced the number of infected/activated monocytes/macrophages in the brain of SIV-infected rhesus macaques, and reversed SIV-induced neuronal injury (Williams et al., 2005). It has also been suggested that ART benefits may be maximized by choosing ART drugs that reach therapeutic CNS levels (Webb, Mactutus, & Booze, 2009), but it is not known whether the effects of this class of ART on the brain endothelium and monocyte-endothelial interaction may be different from that of other available ART drugs.

Like the overall battle against HIV/AIDS, successfully reducing HIV-induced BBB compromise and entry of infected MP into the brain will depend on the continued success of ART. Langford and colleagues (Langford et al., 2003) showed that the emergence of HIV strains resistant to ART was associated with increased/resurgence in the frequency of HIVE and leukoencephalopathy; and further showed that HIV leukoencephalopathy in AIDS patients failing combination ART (cART) was characterized by massive infiltration of HIV-infected monocytes/macrophages into the brain and extensive white matter destruction. This suggest that ART failure may be associated with increased BBB compromise, increased monocyte-BBB interactions, and infiltration of infected/activated MPs into the CNS.

CONCLUSION

There are numerous evidences that HIV-1 infection and secreted viral toxins increase mRNA and proteins levels of inflammation-, oxidative stress-, and chemotaxis-inducing substances in monocytes, macrophages, and brain EC (Annunziata, 2003; Chaudhuri et al., 2008a; Elbim et al., 2001; Mollace et al., 2001; Pace & Leaf, 1995; Potula et al., 2008; Ramirez et al., 2008; Roberts et al., 2003; Toborek et al., 2003; Yang et al., 2009). HIV-1 infection increases expression of adhesion molecules and infected and activated

MPs are more likely to breach and cross the BBB. These inflammatory and redox reactions are further accentuated during monocyte-EC interactions, further increasing breach of the BBB integrity and infiltration of infected MPs into the brain (Banks, 1999; Banks et al., 2006; Nottet et al., 1996; Persidsky et al., 2006b; Toborek et al., 2005). Strategies aimed at reducing/preventing injury, inflammation, and oxidative stress in MPs and EC could reduce BBB injury and entry of HIV virions and infected monocytes into the CNS. To better design therapeutic approaches for preventing HIV-induced BBB compromise and CNS invasion by infected cells, it is critical to understand the molecular mechanisms involved. Current studies showed involvement of several molecular pathways in inflammation, oxidative stress, and BBB dysfunction induced by HIV-1 and viral proteins. These signaling pathways include the NFκB, STAT1 (Chaudhuri et al., 2008a; Chaudhuri et al., 2008b), GSK-3β (Ramirez et al., 2010), PPAR-α, PPAR-γ, rho kinases (Huang et al., 2009; Potula et al., 2008; Ramirez et al., 2008 Huang, 2008 #29), PCK, p38 MAPK, MEK1/2, Ras, and calcium signaling (Kanmogne et al., 2007; Pu et al., 2005). In most of these studies, pharmacological inhibitors of these pathways attenuate HIV-induced effects. It is important to determine whether there is crosstalk between these various signaling pathways or they act independently, and whether best protective strategies should be targeting these pathways individually or in combination. There is a need for *in vivo* and *in vitro* studies to determine both the beneficial and potential side effects of inhibiting these signaling pathways individually and/or simultaneously.

HIV virions and viral factors produced by infected cells directly cause BBB injury and entry of infected monocytes into the CNS; thus it is likely that by preventing/reducing infection of MPs, decreasing viral load and secretions of toxic viral factors, ART could reduce/abrogate HIV-induced BBB injury and viral invasion of the CNS. However, this will depend on the success of various ART regimens, as patients with ART failure show increased BBB injury and increased infiltration of infected MPs into the CNS (Langford et al., 2003). It is also not known whether ART can reverse HIV-induced BBB compromise, which occurs in the early stages of infection. Abdulle and colleagues (Abdulle, Hagberg, & Gisslen, 2005) studied a cohort of 38 HIV-infected patients before and during ART and showed that after 2 years of ART, CSF viral loads were significantly reduced, but the albumin ratio (CSF albumin/serum albumin) did not changed significantly, suggesting that ART did not significantly improve BBB integrity or function. In summary, to prevent monocyte and HIV entry into the brain, it is critical to prevent BBB compromise and monocyte activation, and this remains a major challenge.

ACKNOWLEDGMENTS

Dr Kanmogne is supported by grants from the National Institute of Mental Health (RO1 MH081780 and R21 MH80611).

REFERENCES

Abdulle, S., Hagberg, L., & Gisslen, M. (2005). Effects of antiretroviral treatment on blood-brain barrier integrity and intrathecal immunoglobulin production in neuroasymptomatic HIV-1-infected patients. *HIV Med, 6,* 164–169.

Acheampong, E. A., Parveen, Z., Muthoga, L. W., Kalayeh, M., Mukhtar, M., & Pomerantz, R. J. (2005). Human immunodeficiency virus type 1 Nef potently induces apoptosis in primary human brain microvascular endothelial cells via the activation of caspases. *J Virol, 79,* 4257–4269.

Aksenov, M. Y., Hasselrot, U., Bansal, A. K., Wu, G., Nath, A., Anderson, C., et al. (2001). Oxidative damage induced by the injection of HIV-1 Tat protein in the rat striatum. *Neurosci Lett, 305,* 5–8.

Alexaki, A., Liu, Y., & Wigdahl, B. (2008). Cellular reservoirs of HIV-1 and their role in viral persistence. *Curr HIV Res, 6,* 388–400.

Ances, B. M. & Ellis, R. J. (2007). Dementia and neurocognitive disorders due to HIV-1 infection. *Semin Neurol, 27,* 86–92.

Ancuta, P., Kamat, A., Kunstman, K. J., Kim, E. Y., Autissier, P., Wurcel, A., et al. (2008). Microbial translocation is associated with increased monocyte activation and dementia in AIDS patients. *PLoS One, 3,* e2516.

Andras, I. E., Pu, H., Deli, M. A., Nath, A., Hennig, B., & Toborek, M. (2003). HIV-1 Tat protein alters tight junction protein expression and distribution in cultured brain endothelial cells. *J Neurosci Res, 74,* 255–265.

Andras, I. E., Pu, H., Tian, J., Deli, M. A., Nath, A., Hennig, B., et al. (2005). Signaling mechanisms of HIV-1 Tat-induced alterations of claudin-5 expression in brain endothelial cells. *J Cereb Blood Flow Metab, 25,* 1159–1170.

Annunziata, P. (2003). Blood-brain barrier changes during invasion of the central nervous system by HIV-1. Old and new insights into the mechanism. *J Neurol, 250,* 901–906.

Antinori, A., Arendt, G., Becker, J. T., Brew, B. J., Byrd, D. A., Cherner, M., et al. (2007). Updated research nosology for HIV-associated neurocognitive disorders. *Neurology, 69,* 1789–1799.

Antinori, A., Giancola, M. L., Grisetti, S., Soldani, F., Alba, L., Liuzzi, G., et al. (2002). Factors influencing virological response to antiretroviral drugs in cerebrospinal fluid of advanced HIV-1-infected patients. *AIDS, 16,* 1867–1876.

Argyris, E. G., Acheampong, E., Nunnari, G., Mukhtar, M., Williams, K. J., & Pomerantz, R. J. (2003). Human immunodeficiency virus type 1 enters primary human brain microvascular endothelial cells by a mechanism involving cell surface proteoglycans independent of lipid rafts. *J Virol, 77,* 12140–12151.

Asensio, V. C., Maier, J., Milner, R., Boztug, K., Kincaid, C., Moulard, M., et al. (2001). Interferon-independent, human immunodeficiency virus type 1 gp120-mediated induction of CXCL10/IP-10 gene expression by astrocytes in vivo and in vitro. *J Virol, 75,* 7067–7077.

Avison, M. J., Nath, A., Greene-Avison, R., Schmitt, F. A., Bales, R. A., Ethisham, A., et al. (2004). Inflammatory changes and breakdown of microvascular integrity in early human immunodeficiency virus dementia. *J Neurovirol, 10,* 223–232.

Ballabh, P., Braun, A., & Nedergaard, M. (2004). The blood-brain barrier: An overview: structure, regulation, and clinical implications. *Neurobiol Dis, 16,* 1–13.

Banks, W. A. (1999). Physiology and pathology of the blood-brain barrier: Implications for microbial pathogenesis, drug delivery and neurodegenerative disorders. *J Neurovirol, 5,* 538–555.

Banks, W. A., Ercal, N., & Price, T. O. (2006). The blood-brain barrier in neuroAIDS. *Curr HIV Res, 4,* 259–266.

Banks, W. A., Robinson, S. M., & Nath, A. (2005). Permeability of the blood-brain barrier to HIV-1 Tat. *Exp Neurol, 193,* 218–227.

Bergonzini, V., Calistri, A., Salata, C., Del Vecchio, C., Sartori, E., Parolin, C., et al. (2009). Nef and cell signaling transduction: a possible involvement in the pathogenesis of human immunodeficiency virus-associated dementia. *J Neurovirol,* 1–11.

Boisse, L., Gill, M. J., & Power, C. (2008). HIV infection of the central nervous system: Clinical features and neuropathogenesis. *Neurol Clin, 26,* 799–819.

Borgne-Sanchez, A., Dupont, S., Langonne, A., Baux, L., Lecoeur, H., Chauvier, D., et al. (2007). Targeted Vpr-derived peptides reach mitochondria to induce apoptosis of alphaVbeta3-expressing endothelial cells. *Cell Death Differ, 14,* 422–435.

Boven, L. A., Gomes, L., Hery, C., Gray, F., Verhoef, J., Portegies, P., et al. (1999). Increased peroxynitrite activity in AIDS dementia complex: Implications for the neuropathogenesis of HIV-1 infection. *J Immunol, 162,* 4319–4327.

Boven, L. A., Middel, J., Verhoef, J., De Groot, C. J., Nottet, H. S. (2000). Monocyte infiltration is highly associated with loss of the tight junction protein zonula occludens in HIV-1-associated dementia. *Neuropathol Appl Neurobiol, 26,* 356–360.

Buckner, C. M., Luers, A. J., Calderon, T. M., Eugenin, E. A., & Berman, J. W. (2006). Neuroimmunity and the blood-brain barrier: Molecular regulation of leukocyte transmigration and viral entry into the nervous system with a focus on neuroAIDS. *J Neuroimmune Pharmacol, 1,* 160–181.

Chaudhuri, A., Duan, F., Morsey, B., Persidsky, Y., & Kanmogne, G. D. (2008a). HIV-1 activates proinflammatory and interferon-inducible genes in human brain microvascular endothelial cells: putative mechanisms of blood-brain barrier dysfunction. *J Cereb Blood Flow Metab, 28,* 697–711.

Chaudhuri, A., Yang, B., Gendelman, H. E., Persidsky, Y., & Kanmogne, G. D. (2008b). STAT1 signaling modulates HIV-1-induced inflammatory responses and leukocyte transmigration across the blood-brain barrier. *Blood, 111,* 2062–2072.

Choi, J., Walker, J., Boichuk, S., Kirkiles-Smith, N., Torpey, N., Pober, J. S., et al. (2005). Human endothelial cells enhance human immunodeficiency virus type 1 replication in CD4+ T cells in a Nef-dependent manner in vitro and in vivo. *J Virol, 79,* 264–276.

Conant, K., McArthur, J. C., Griffin, D. E., Sjulson, L., Wahl, L. M., & Irani, D. N. (1999). Cerebrospinal fluid levels of MMP-2, 7, and 9 are elevated in association with human immunodeficiency virus dementia. *Ann Neurol, 46,* 391–398.

Crowe, S., Maslin, C., Ellery, P., & Kedzierska, K. (2004). Culture of HIV in monocytes and macrophages. *Curr Protoc Immunol,* Chapter 12, Unit 12 14.

Crowe, S., Zhu, T., & Muller, W. A. (2003). The contribution of monocyte infection and trafficking to viral persistence, and maintenance of the viral reservoir in HIV infection. *J Leukoc Biol, 74,* 635–641.

Crowe, S. M. (1995). Role of macrophages in the pathogenesis of human immunodeficiency virus (HIV) infection. *Aust N Z J Med, 25,* 777–783.

D'Aversa, T. G., Eugenin, E. A., & Berman, J. W. (2005). NeuroAIDS: contributions of the human immunodeficiency virus-1 proteins Tat and gp120 as well as CD40 to microglial activation. *J Neurosci Res, 81,* 436–446.

Dhawan, S., Toro, L. A., Jones, B. E., & Meltzer, M. S. (1992). Interactions between HIV-infected monocytes and the extracellular matrix: HIV-infected monocytes secrete neutral metalloproteases that degrade basement membrane protein matrices. *J Leukoc Biol, 52,* 244–248.

Dhillon, N. K., Williams, R., Callen, S., Zien, C., Narayan, O., & Buch, S. (2008). Roles of MCP-1 in development of HIV-dementia. *Front Biosci, 13,* 3913–3918.

Elbim, C., Pillet, S., Prevost, M. H., Preira, A., Girard, P. M., Rogine, N., et al. (2001). The role of phagocytes in HIV-related oxidative stress. *J Clin Virol, 20,* 99–109.

Eugenin, E. A., Dyer, G., Calderon, T. M., & Berman, J. W. (2005). HIV-1 tat protein induces a migratory phenotype in human fetal microglia by a CCL2 (MCP-1)-dependent mechanism: Possible role in neuroAIDS. *Glia, 49,* 501–510.

Eugenin, E. A., Gamss, R., Buckner, C., Buono, D., Klein, R. S., Schoenbaum, E. E., et al. (2006a). Shedding of PECAM-1 during HIV infection: A potential role for soluble PECAM-1 in the pathogenesis of neuroAIDS. *J Leukoc Biol, 79,* 444–452.

Eugenin, E. A., Osiecki, K., Lopez, L., Goldstein, H., Calderon, T. M., & Berman, J. W. (2006b). CCL2/monocyte chemoattractant protein-1 mediates enhanced transmigration of human immunodeficiency virus (HIV)-infected leukocytes across the blood-brain barrier: A potential

mechanism of HIV-CNS invasion and neuroAIDS. *J Neurosci, 26,* 1098–1106.

Everall, I. P., Hansen, L. A., & Masliah, E. (2005). The shifting patterns of HIV encephalitis neuropathology. *Neurotox Res, 8,* 51–61.

Fantuzzi, L., Conti, L., Gauzzi, M. C., Eid, P., Del Corno, M., Varano, B., et al. (2000). Regulation of chemokine/cytokine network during in vitro differentiation and HIV-1 infection of human monocytes: Possible importance in the pathogenesis of AIDS. *J Leukoc Biol, 68,* 391–399.

Fischer-Smith, T., Bell, C., Croul, S., Lewis, M., & Rappaport, J. (2008). Monocyte/macrophage trafficking in acquired immunodeficiency syndrome encephalitis: Lessons from human and nonhuman primate studies. *J Neurovirol, 14,* 318–326.

Fischer-Smith, T., Croul, S., Sverstiuk, A. E., Capini, C., L'Heureux, D., Regulier, E. G., et al. (2001). CNS invasion by CD14+/CD16+ peripheral blood-derived monocytes in HIV dementia: Perivascular accumulation and reservoir of HIV infection. *J Neurovirol, 7,* 528–541.

Flora, G., Pu, H., Hennig, B., & Toborek, M. (2006). Cyclooxygenase-2 is involved in HIV-1 Tat-induced inflammatory responses in the brain. *Neuromolecular Med, 8,* 337–352.

Forstermann, U. (2008). Oxidative stress in vascular disease: Causes, defense mechanisms and potential therapies. *Nat Clin Pract Cardiovasc Med, 5,* 338–349.

Fujimoto, M., Takagi, Y., Aoki, T., Hayase, M., Marumo, T., Gomi, M., et al. (2008). Tissue inhibitor of metalloproteinases protect blood-brain barrier disruption in focal cerebral ischemia. *J Cereb Blood Flow Metab, 28,* 1674–1685.

Gendelman, H. E., Ding, S., Gong, N., Liu, J., Ramirez, S. H., Persidsky, Y., et al. (2009). Monocyte chemotactic protein-1 regulates voltage-gated K+ channels and macrophage transmigration. *J Neuroimmune Pharmacol, 4,* 47–59.

Grant, I., Heaton, R. K., & Atkinson, J. H. (1995). Neurocognitive disorders in HIV-1 infection. HNRC Group. HIV Neurobehavioral Research Center. *Curr Top Microbiol Immunol, 202,* 11–32.

Gras, G. & Kaul, M. (2010). Molecular mechanisms of neuroinvasion by monocytes-macrophages in HIV-1 infection. *Retrovirology, 7,* 30.

Herzenberg, L. A., De Rosa, S. C., Dubs, J. G., Roederer, M., Anderson, M. T., Ela, S. W., et al. (1997). Glutathione deficiency is associated with impaired survival in HIV disease. *Proc Natl Acad Sci USA, 94,* 1967–1972.

Ho, W. Z., Cherukuri, R., & Douglas, S. D. (1994). The macrophage and HIV-1. *Immunol Ser, 60,* 569–587.

Hori, K., Burd, P. R., Furuke, K., Kutza, J., Weih, K. A., & Clouse, K. A. (1999). Human immunodeficiency virus-1-infected macrophages induce inducible nitric oxide synthase and nitric oxide (NO) production in astrocytes: Astrocytic NO as a possible mediator of neural damage in acquired immunodeficiency syndrome. *Blood, 93,* 1843–1850.

Huang, W., Eum, S. Y., Andras, I. E., Hennig, B., & Toborek, M. (2009). PPARalpha and PPARgamma attenuate HIV-induced dysregulation of tight junction proteins by modulations of matrix metalloproteinase and proteasome activities. *FASEB J, 23,* 1596–1606.

Huang, W., Rha, G. B., Han, M. J., Eum, S. Y., Andras, I. E., Zhong, Y., et al. (2008). PPARalpha and PPARgamma effectively protect against HIV-induced inflammatory responses in brain endothelial cells. *J Neurochem, 107,* 497–509.

Huber, J. D., Egleton, R. D., & Davis, T. P. (2001). Molecular physiology and pathophysiology of tight junctions in the blood-brain barrier. *Trends Neurosci, 24,* 719–725.

Hudson, L., Liu, J., Nath, A., Jones, M., Raghavan, R., Narayan, O., et al. (2000). Detection of the human immunodeficiency virus regulatory protein tat in CNS tissues. *J Neurovirol, 6,* 145–155.

Hurst, R. D., Heales, S. J., Dobbie, M. S., Barker, J. E., & Clark, J. B. (1998). Decreased endothelial cell glutathione and increased sensitivity to oxidative stress in an in vitro blood-brain barrier model system. *Brain Res, 802,* 232–240.

Hurwitz, A. A., Berman, J. W., & Lyman, W. D. (1994). The role of the blood-brain barrier in HIV infection of the central nervous system. *Adv Neuroimmunol, 4,* 249–256.

Ivey, N. S., MacLean, A. G., & Lackner, A. A. (2009). Acquired immunodeficiency syndrome and the blood-brain barrier. *J Neurovirol, 15,* 111–122.

Kanmogne, G. D., Grammas, P., & Kennedy, R. C. (2000). Analysis of human endothelial cells and cortical neurons for susceptibility to HIV-1 infection and co-receptor expression. *J Neurovirol, 6,* 519–528.

Kanmogne, G. D., Kennedy, R. C., & Grammas, P. (2002). HIV-1 gp120 proteins and gp160 peptides are toxic to brain endothelial cells and neurons: possible pathway for HIV entry into the brain and HIV-associated dementia. *J Neuropathol Exp Neurol, 61,* 992–1000.

Kanmogne, G. D., Primeaux, C., & Grammas, P. (2005). HIV-1 gp120 proteins alter tight junction protein expression and brain endothelial cell permeability: Implications for the pathogenesis of HIV-associated dementia. *J Neuropathol Exp Neurol, 64,* 498–505.

Kanmogne, G. D., Schall, K., Leibhart, J., Knipe, B., Gendelman, H. E., & Persidsky, Y. (2007). HIV-1 gp120 compromises blood-brain barrier integrity and enhances monocyte migration across blood-brain barrier: Implication for viral neuropathogenesis. *J Cereb Blood Flow Metab, 27,* 123–134.

Kaul, M. (2009). HIV-1 associated dementia: Update on pathological mechanisms and therapeutic approaches. *Curr Opin Neurol, 22,* 315–320.

Kedzierska, K., Azzam, R., Ellery, P., Mak, J., Jaworowski, A., & Crowe, S. M. (2003). Defective phagocytosis by human monocyte/macrophages following HIV-1 infection: Underlying mechanisms and modulation by adjunctive cytokine therapy. *J Clin Virol, 26,* 247–263.

Kedzierska, K. & Crowe, S. M. (2002). The role of monocytes and macrophages in the pathogenesis of HIV-1 infection. *Curr Med Chem, 9,* 1893–1903.

Khan, N. A., Di Cello, F., Stins, M., & Kim, K. S. (2007). Gp120-mediated cytotoxicity of human brain microvascular endothelial cells is dependent on p38 mitogen-activated protein kinase activation. *J Neurovirol, 13,* 242–251.

Kolson, D. L. (2002). Neuropathogenesis of central nervous system HIV-1 infection. *Clin Lab Med, 22,* 703–717.

Krebs, F. C., Ross, H., McAllister, J., & Wigdahl, B. (2000). HIV-1-associated central nervous system dysfunction. *Adv Pharmacol, 49,* 315–385.

Kuhlmann, C. R., Gerigk, M., Bender, B., Closhen, D., Lessmann, V., & Luhmann, H. J. (2008). Fluvastatin prevents glutamate-induced blood-brain-barrier disruption in vitro. *Life Sci, 82,* 1281–1287.

Langford, T. D., Letendre, S. L., Larrea, G. J., & Masliah, E. (2003). Changing patterns in the neuropathogenesis of HIV during the HAART era. *Brain Pathol, 13,* 195–210.

Lawrence, D. M. & Major, E. O. (2002). HIV-1 and the brain: Connections between HIV-1-associated dementia, neuropathology and neuroimmunology. *Microbes Infect, 4,* 301–308.

Lee, Y. W., Eum, S. Y., Nath, A., & Toborek, M. (2004). Estrogen-mediated protection against HIV Tat protein-induced inflammatory pathways in human vascular endothelial cells. *Cardiovasc Res, 63,* 139–148.

Li, W., Li, G., Steiner, J., & Nath, A. (2009). Role of Tat protein in HIV neuropathogenesis. *Neurotox Res, 16,* 205–220.

Malemud, C. J. (2006). Matrix metalloproteinases (MMPs) in health and disease: An overview. *Front Biosci, 11,* 1696–1701.

Mari, M., Morales, A., Colell, A., Garcia-Ruiz, C., & Fernandez-Checa, J. C. (2009). Mitochondrial glutathione, a key survival antioxidant. *Antioxid Redox Signal, 11,* 2685–2700.

Maslin, C. L., Kedzierska, K., Webster, N. L., Muller, W. A., & Crowe, S. M. (2005). Transendothelial migration of monocytes: The underlying molecular mechanisms and consequences of HIV-1 infection. *Curr HIV Res, 3,* 303–317.

Matzen, K., Dirkx, A. E., oude Egbrink, M. G., Speth, C., Gotte, M., Ascherl, G., et al. (2004). HIV-1 Tat increases the adhesion of monocytes and T-cells to the endothelium in vitro and in vivo: Implications for AIDS-associated vasculopathy. *Virus Res, 104,* 145–155.

McArthur, J. C., Steiner, J., Sacktor, N., & Nath, A. (2010). Human immunodeficiency virus-associated neurocognitive disorders: Mind the gap. *Ann Neurol, 67,* 699–714.

Mengozzi, M., De Filippi, C., Transidico, P., Biswas, P., Cota, M., Ghezzi, S., et al. (1999). Human immunodeficiency virus replication induces monocyte chemotactic protein-1 in human macrophages and U937 promonocytic cells. *Blood, 93,* 1851–1857.

Milward, E. A., Fitzsimmons, C., Szklarczyk, A., & Conant, K. (2007). The matrix metalloproteinases and CNS plasticity: An overview. *J Neuroimmunol, 187,* 9–19.

Mollace, V., Nottet, H. S., Clayette, P., Turco, M. C., Muscoli, C., Salvemini, D., et al. (2001). Oxidative stress and neuroAIDS: Triggers, modulators and novel antioxidants. *Trends Neurosci, 24,* 411–416.

Mrowiec, T., Melchar, C., & Gorski, A. (1997). HIV-protein-mediated alterations in T cell interactions with the extracellular matrix proteins and endothelium. *Arch Immunol Ther Exp (Warsz), 45,* 255–259.

Nottet, H. S., Persidsky, Y., Sasseville, V. G., Nukuna, A. N., Bock, P., Zhai, Q. H., et al. (1996). Mechanisms for the transendothelial migration of HIV-1-infected monocytes into brain. *J Immunol, 156,* 1284–1295.

Oktyabrsky, O. N. & Smirnova, G. V. (2007). Redox regulation of cellular functions. *Biochemistry (Mosc), 72,* 132–145.

Pace, G. W. & Leaf, C. D. (1995). The role of oxidative stress in HIV disease. *Free Radic Biol Med, 19,* 523–528.

Pereira, C. F., Boven, L. A., Middel, J., Verhoef, J., & Nottet, H. S. (2000). Induction of cyclooxygenase-2 expression during HIV-1-infected monocyte-derived macrophage and human brain microvascular endothelial cell interactions. *J Leukoc Biol, 68,* 423–428.

Persidsky, Y. & Gendelman, H. E. (2003). Mononuclear phagocyte immunity and the neuropathogenesis of HIV-1 infection. *J Leukoc Biol, 74,* 691–701.

Persidsky, Y., Heilman, D., Haorah, J., Zelivyanskaya, M., Persidsky, R., Weber, G. A., et al. (2006a). Rho-mediated regulation of tight junctions during monocyte migration across the blood-brain barrier in HIV-1 encephalitis (HIVE). *Blood, 107,* 4770–4780.

Persidsky, Y., Ramirez, S. H., Haorah, J., & Kanmogne, G. D. (2006b). Blood-brain barrier: Structural components and function under physiologic and pathologic conditions. *J Neuroimmune Pharmacol, 1,* 223–236.

Persidsky, Y., Zheng, J., Miller, D., & Gendelman, H. E. (2000). Mononuclear phagocytes mediate blood-brain barrier compromise and neuronal injury during HIV-1-associated dementia. *J Leukoc Biol, 68,* 413–422.

Pietarinen-Runtti, P., Lakari, E., Raivio, K. O., & Kinnula, V. L. (2000). Expression of antioxidant enzymes in human inflammatory cells. *Am J Physiol Cell Physiol, 278,* C118–125.

Pomerantz, R. J. (2004). Effects of HIV-1 Vpr on neuroinvasion and neuropathogenesis. *DNA Cell Biol, 23,* 227–238.

Potula, R., Ramirez, S. H., Knipe, B., Leibhart, J., Schall, K., Heilman, D., et al. (2008). Peroxisome proliferator-activated receptor-gamma activation suppresses HIV-1 replication in an animal model of encephalitis. *AIDS, 22,* 1539–1549.

Pu, H., Hayashi, K., Andras, I. E., Eum, S. Y., Hennig, B., & Toborek, M. (2007). Limited role of COX-2 in HIV Tat-induced alterations of tight junction protein expression and disruption of the blood-brain barrier. *Brain Res, 1184,* 333–344.

Pu, H., Tian, J., Andras, I. E., Hayashi, K., Flora, G., Hennig, B., et al. (2005). HIV-1 Tat protein-induced alterations of ZO-1 expression are mediated by redox-regulated ERK 1/2 activation. *J Cereb Blood Flow Metab, 25,* 1325–1335.

Pu, H., Tian, J., Flora, G., Lee, Y. W., Nath, A., Hennig, B., et al. (2003). HIV-1 Tat protein upregulates inflammatory mediators and induces monocyte invasion into the brain. *Mol Cell Neurosci, 24,* 224–237.

Ramirez, S. H., Fan, S., Zhang, M., Papugani, A., Reichenbach, N., Dykstra, H., et al. (2010). Inhibition of glycogen synthase kinase 3beta (GSK3beta) decreases inflammatory responses in brain endothelial cells. *Am J Pathol, 176,* 881–892.

Ramirez, S. H., Heilman, D., Morsey, B., Potula, R., Haorah, J., & Persidsky, Y. (2008). Activation of peroxisome proliferator-activated receptor gamma (PPARgamma) suppresses Rho GTPases in human brain microvascular endothelial cells and inhibits adhesion and transendothelial migration of HIV-1 infected monocytes. *J Immunol, 180,* 1854–1865.

Ranki, A., Nyberg, M., Ovod, V., Haltia, M., Elovaara, I., Raininko, R., et al. (1995). Abundant expression of HIV Nef and Rev proteins in brain astrocytes in vivo is associated with dementia. *AIDS, 9,* 1001–1008.

Roberts, E. S., Zandonatti, M. A., Watry, D. D., Madden, L. J., Henriksen, S. J., Taffe, M. A., et al. (2003). Induction of pathogenic sets of genes in macrophages and neurons in neuroAIDS. *Am J Pathol, 162,* 2041–2057.

Roberts, T. K., Buckner, C. M., & Berman, J. W. (2010). Leukocyte transmigration across the blood-brain barrier: Perspectives on neuroAIDS. *Front Biosci, 15,* 478–536.

Robertson, K. R., Robertson, W. T., Ford, S., Watson, D., Fiscus, S., Harp, A. G., et al. (2004). Highly active antiretroviral therapy improves neurocognitive functioning. *J Acquir Immune Defic Syndr, 36,* 562–566.

Sporer, B., Koedel, U., Paul, R., Kohleisen, B., Erfle, V., Fontana, A., et al. (2000). Human immunodeficiency virus type-1 Nef protein induces blood-brain barrier disruption in the rat: Role of matrix metalloproteinase-9. *J Neuroimmunol, 102,* 125–130.

Stins, M. F., Pearce, D., Choi, H., Di Cello, F., Pardo, C. A., & Kim, K. S. (2004). CD4 and chemokine receptors on human brain microvascular endothelial cells, implications for human immunodeficiency virus type 1 pathogenesis. *Endothelium, 11,* 275–284.

Stins, M. F., Pearce, D., Di Cello, F., Erdreich-Epstein, A., Pardo, C. A., & Sik Kim, K. (2003). Induction of intercellular adhesion molecule-1 on human brain endothelial cells by HIV-1 gp120: role of CD4 and chemokine coreceptors. *Lab Invest, 83,* 1787–1798.

Stins, M. F., Shen, Y., Huang, S. H., Gilles, F., Kalra, V. K., & Kim, K. S. (2001). Gp120 activates children's brain endothelial cells via CD4. *J Neurovirol, 7,* 125–134.

Toborek, M., Lee, Y. W., Flora, G., Pu, H., Andras, I. E., Wylegala, E., et al. (2005). Mechanisms of the blood-brain barrier disruption in HIV-1 infection. *Cell Mol Neurobiol, 25,* 181–199.

Toborek, M., Lee, Y. W., Pu, H., Malecki, A., Flora, G., Garrido, R., et al. (2003). HIV-Tat protein induces oxidative and inflammatory pathways in brain endothelium. *J Neurochem, 84,* 169–179.

Trillo-Pazos, G. & Everall, I. P. (1997). From human immunodeficiency virus (HIV) infection of the brain to dementia. *Genitourin Med, 73,* 343–347.

Wang, H., Sun, J., & Goldstein, H. (2008). Human immunodeficiency virus type 1 infection increases the in vivo capacity of peripheral monocytes to cross the blood-brain barrier into the brain and the in vivo sensitivity of the blood-brain barrier to disruption by lipopolysaccharide. *J Virol, 82,* 7591–7600.

Wang, T., Rumbaugh, J. A., & Nath, A. (2006). Viruses and the brain: From inflammation to dementia. *Clin Sci (Lond), 110,* 393–407.

Webb, K. M., Mactutus, C. F., & Booze, R. M. (2009). The ART of HIV therapies: Dopaminergic deficits and future treatments for HIV pediatric encephalopathy. *Expert Rev Anti Infect Ther, 7,* 193–203.

Weiss, J. M., Nath, A., Major, E. O., & Berman, J. W. (1999). HIV-1 Tat induces monocyte chemoattractant protein-1-mediated monocyte transmigration across a model of the human blood-brain barrier and up-regulates CCR5 expression on human monocytes. *J Immunol, 163,* 2953–2959.

Williams, K., Alvarez, X., & Lackner, A. A. (2001). Central nervous system perivascular cells are immunoregulatory cells that connect the CNS with the peripheral immune system. *Glia, 36,* 156–164.

Williams, K., Westmoreland, S., Greco, J., Ratai, E., Lentz, M., Kim, W. K., et al. (2005). Magnetic resonance spectroscopy reveals that activated monocytes contribute to neuronal injury in SIV neuroAIDS. *J Clin Invest, 115,* 2534–2545.

Williams, K. C. & Hickey, W. F. (2002). Central nervous system damage, monocytes and macrophages, and neurological disorders in AIDS. *Annu Rev Neurosci, 25,* 537–562.

Wong, C. H., Bozinovski, S., Hertzog, P. J., Hickey, M. J., & Crack, P. J. (2008). Absence of glutathione peroxidase-1 exacerbates cerebral ischemia-reperfusion injury by reducing post-ischemic microvascular perfusion. *J Neurochem, 107,* 241–252.

Woods, S. P., Moore, D. J., Weber, E., & Grant, I. (2009). Cognitive neuropsychology of HIV-associated neurocognitive disorders. *Neuropsychol Rev, 19,* 152–168.

Wu, D. T., Woodman, S. E., Weiss, J. M., McManus, C. M., D'Aversa, T. G., Hesselgesser, J., et al. (2000). Mechanisms of leukocyte trafficking into the CNS. *J Neurovirol, 6* Suppl 1, S82–85.

Yadav, A. & Collman, R. G. (2009). CNS inflammation and macrophage/microglial biology associated with HIV-1 infection. *J Neuroimmune Pharmacol, 4,* 430–447.

Yamamoto, M., Ramirez, S. H., Sato, S., Kiyota, T., Cerny, R. L., Kaibuchi, K., et al. (2008). Phosphorylation of claudin-5 and occludin by rho kinase in brain endothelial cells. *Am J Pathol, 172,* 521–533.

Yang, B., Akhter, S., Chaudhuri, A., & Kanmogne, G. D. (2009). HIV-1 gp120 induces cytokine expression, leukocyte adhesion, and transmigration across the blood-brain barrier: Modulatory effects of STAT1 signaling. *Microvasc Res, 77,* 212–219.

Yang, B., Singh, S., Bressani, R., & Kanmogne, G. D. (2010). Cross-talk between STAT1 and PI3K/AKT signaling in HIV-1-induced blood-brain barrier dysfunction: Role of CCR5 and implications for viral neuropathogenesis. *J Neurosci Res.*

Yao, H., Bethel-Brown, C., Li, C. Z., & Buch, S. J. (2010). HIV neuropathogenesis: A tight rope walk of innate immunity. *J Neuroimmune Pharmacol.*

Zheng, J. & Gendelman, H. E. (1997). The HIV-1 associated dementia complex: A metabolic encephalopathy fueled by viral replication in mononuclear phagocytes. *Curr Opin Neurol, 10,* 319–325.

Zhong, Y., Smart, E. J., Weksler, B., Couraud, P. O., Hennig, B., & Toborek, M. (2008). Caveolin-1 regulates human immunodeficiency virus-1 Tat-induced alterations of tight junction protein expression via modulation of the Ras signaling. *J Neurosci, 28,* 7788–7796.

SECTION 4

CELLULAR AND VIRAL NEUROTOXICITY AND ABUSED DRUGS

Stuart A. Lipton

4.1

MONONUCLEAR PHAGOCYTE INFLAMMATION AND NEUROTOXICITY

Andrea Martinez-Skinner, Ari S. Nowacek, JoEllyn McMillan, and Howard E. Gendelman

Effective combination antiretroviral therapy has reduced the incidence and severity of HIV-associated neurocognitive impairments. Nonetheless, disease has continued and remains a serious source of disease morbidity associated with advanced viral infection and immune suppression. The disease conductors are mononuclear phagocytes (MP; blood-borne macrophages and microglia). A plethora of viral and cellular products secreted as a consequence of MP immune activation and viral infection incites an inflammatory cascade that elicits neurotoxicity, blood-brain barrier breakdown, and viral dissemination. The fundamental parts of the disease process can be readily understood by studies of MP biology and its particular unique functions during disease. Overall, an understanding of the molecular and biochemical bases of MP immunity has led to valuable insights into our understanding of disease processes. Such works will certainly lead to the development of new therapeutic strategies to prevent MP-associated neural insults.

OVERVIEW

Mononuclear phagocytes (MP; blood-borne macrophages, dendritic cells, tissue macrophages, and microglia) are primordial cells as reflected in both ontogeny and phylogeny. They function in broad ways through their abilities to act as scavengers, immune effectors, transport and antigen-presenting cells. Their phagocytic and immunomodulatory abilities enable them to work as sentinels to maintain tissue homeostasis during disease (Hickey, 2001; Hunter et al., 2009; Yoshioka et al., 2009; Suttles & Stout, 2009; Nestle, Di Meglio, Qin, & Nickoloff, 2009). MP find their origins from pluripotent stem cells (PSC) (van Furth, 1982). Early during embryonic development, PSC migrate from the mesoderm to the neuroectoderm where they reside as fetal macrophages (Chan, Kohsaka, & Rezaie, 2007; Monier et al., 2007; Streit, 2001). After development, in response to chemokines, monocytes emerge into the peripheral circulation then travel to tissue where they differentiate into macrophages (van Furth, 1982; Scheuerer et al., 2000).

Nervous system macrophages, commonly called microglial cells, are present throughout the central nervous system (CNS) (Lawson, Perry, Dri, & Gordon, 1990). They function in the removal of damaged tissue products including apoptotic cells and in immune sentry and surveillance (Bessis, Bechade, Bernard, & Roumier, 2007; Streit, 2001; Kreutzberg, 1996). Such surveillance functions include tissue remodeling that occurs during development as well as guiding axonal development within white matter tracts (Pollard, 2009; Milligan, Levitt, & Cunningham, 1991).

Parenchymal macrophages and microglia are differentiated embryonic and fetal progenitor cells (Streit & Xue, 2009). These form a dynamic network in tissue that continually survey and sample the microenvironment in which they inhabit; thus they have become known as the brain's immune system (Graeber & Streit, 1990; Tambuyzer, Ponsaerts, & Nouwen, 2009). Functions of brain MP include protection of the CNS from pathogens as well as from the consequences of neural trauma and disease. This is accomplished, in part, by engulfing and digesting cellular debris and pathogens. MP also stimulate a response to pathogens by activating lymphocytes and other immune cells. Thus, microglia function in both innate and adaptive immune responses.

MP BIOLOGY IN MAINTAINING HEALTH AND TISSUE HOMEOSTASIS

In maintaining tissue homeostasis, MP act as scavengers and immune effectors. MP immune activation is elicited in response to injury and microbial infections to clear debris, maintain tissue function, and eliminate microbial insults (Aderem & Underhill, 1999). Although their main functions are to phagocytize and eliminate pathogens and damaged neural tissue debris they also orchestrate adaptive immune responses (Town, Nikolic, & Tan, 2005; Herbein & Varin, 2010). To perform these functions, MP recruit other inflammatory cells by producing and secreting chemokines and cytokines such as monocyte chemotactic protein-1 (MCP-1), fractalkine, and stromal cell-derived factor-1α (SDF-1α) (Boven et al., 2000; Fantuzzi, Belardelli, & Gessani, 2003; Cotter et al., 2002; Peng et al., 2006). These recruited inflammatory cells include, but are not limited to, blood-borne macrophages and T effector cells (Persidsky et al., 1999). MP migrate from the bloodstream through the wall of microvessels in response to a stimulus, which can also potentially guide their migratory pathway (Butcher & Picker, 1996; Foxman, Campbell, & Butcher, 1997). The process of cell migration out of the bloodstream and movement within tissues begins with a stimulus signaling the cell to polarize, thus making a clear distinction between the front and the rear of the cell. Cell membrane extension can then occur by rearrangement of actin filaments, uprooting existing attachments to the surroundings, and forming what are termed lamellipodia and filopodia. Lamellipodia are characterized as broad, flat, sheet-like structures, whereas filopodia are characterized as thin, cylindrical, needle-like projections. Once frontal adhesion has occurred in the formation of the lamellipodia, the cell body will move forward through contractile forces of the actin filaments and formation of new attachments. The rear adhesion is then released and the cell contracts with the remaining portions forming attachments to the surroundings (Lauffenburger & Horwitz, 1996; Condeelis, 1993; Stossel, 1993; Howard & Oresajo, 1985; Wilkinson, 1986). Once at the site of infection or injury MP work to eliminate the pathogen and clear the tissue of injurious proteins and dead cells. The process of phagocytosis involves a portion of the macrophage membrane extending out into the environment to surround a protein or particle of interest followed by fully engulfing it into the cell and forming what is known as a phagosome. The phagosome then fuses with early endosomes and as it matures it is transported on microtubules, giving it the opportunity to interact with various components of the endosomal system (Swanson & Baer, 1995; Pizon, Desjardins, Bucci, Parton, & Zerial, 1994). There are a series of fusion and fission events that occur in which the vacuolar membrane and its contents mature and fuse with late endosomes and ultimately lysosomes to finally form the phagolysosome. The contents of the phagolysosome are then degraded. Macrophages contain toxic peroxides and enzymes that can result in their own death, but they are capable of digesting hundreds of bacteria or foreign particles before these components cause damage to the cells themselves.

In the course of digestion of the diseased environment, MP often present antigens of the pathogen to T cells. Once the pathogen has been ingested, lysosomal-associated enzymes digest pathogen-associated proteins into small peptides. These peptides are then attached to MHC class II molecules and are integrated into the cell membrane. The attached MHC class II molecule indicates to other white blood cells that despite having an antigen, it is not in itself a pathogen. CD4+ helper T-cells are then capable of recognizing and binding the peptide. Two signals are required for initial activation after the T-cell receptor binds the peptide. First, the CD4 receptor on the T-cell must interact appropriately with the MHC class II molecule on the macrophage. Second, the CD28 receptor on the T-cell must interact with the CD80 receptor on the macrophage. Once the T-cell is activated it can then produce an array of cytokines that provide signals to other immune cells. It can signal to other cells to proliferate or differentiate, as well as contribute to the establishment of an inflammatory environment. The production of antibodies by plasma cells enable better scavenging and clearing of bacteria by MP. Macrophages also possess toll-like receptors (TLR), which are cell-surface proteins that can detect broad patterns of pathogen-specific markers. Activation of these TLR is important in eliciting effector molecules that include antimicrobial peptides. Finally, macrophages can make use of the compliment pathway by the recognition of complement component 3-derived tags which signal the macrophage to recognize, ingest, and destroy the particle; this process is known as opsonization (Lodish, 2008). After the irritative stimulus has either subsided or been degraded, the activated macrophage will return to an inactive state and their numbers will decrease through either apoptosis or cell death.

MICROGLIA IMMUNITY AND CNS HOMEOSTASIS

A number of pathologic insults can affect the normal working of the nervous system, such as CNS injury, toxin exposure, infectious agents, and metabolic disturbances. Microglial cells tend to form the initial line of defense against most of these insults. They can function in parallel to the responses observed by peripheral monocytes, macrophages, and/or dendritic cells in attempts to clear the brain of the noxious insult and restore the homeostatic environment (Gehrmann, Matsumoto, & Kreutzberg, 1995; Kreutzberg, 1996; Graeber & Streit, 1990). When necessary, they can increase dramatically in number to combat disease and restore homeostasis. Activated microglia produce a variety of growth factors and cytokines that vary with the type and severity of the injury. Microglia also upregulate the expression of a variety of surface receptors; many of which are immunological in nature and are linked to mediating cell-cell interactions while others bind to serum components such as complement, thrombin, or immunoglobulins (Akiyama & McGeer, 1990; Fishman & Savitt, 1989; Graeber, Streit, & Kreutzberg, 1988; Moller et al., 2000).

Receptors that have been upregulated in microglial cells can function in a neuroprotective manner by binding serum proteins that could potentially leak into the CNS and damage neurons. These receptors are expressed during times of inactivation as well, suggesting that "mopping up" of serum proteins occurs continually to help maintain homeostasis (Akiyama & McGeer, 1990; Graeber et al., 1988). Receptors for lymphokines are also present on microglial cells that function in activating these cells into a single-minded pursuit of the pathogen.

LINKS BETWEEN INFLAMMATION, AUTOIMMUNITY, CANCER, AND DEGENERATIVE DISEASES

Macrophages can also be directly involved with disease mechanisms and work against the immune system in battles against both infectious and noninfectious diseases. This is thought to occur due to the functional nature of macrophages and their involvement in so many biological processes. It has been shown that macrophages can cause the formation of granulomas, sometimes even fusing to form multinucleated giant cells and inflammatory lesions. Events such as these occur after the macrophage ingests the pathogen, but instead of degradation and presentation the pathogen is able to replicate and induce apoptosis, subsequently bypassing the immune response and spreading the infection. In such instances macrophages function as reservoirs for disease.

One example is *L. pneumophila*, a facultative intracellular pathogen that uses the macrophage as a site to evade the immune system and replicate (Shuman & Horwitz, 1996; Vogel, Andrews, Wong, & Isberg, 1998). *L. pneumophila* are the bacteria that cause Legionnaires' disease, a severe infection resulting in pneumonia. Major outer membrane protein (MOMP) on the surface of the bacteria is fixed with complement component 3 that facilitates the binding of the macrophage through complement receptors found on the macrophage (Bellinger-Kawahara & Horwitz, 1990). Binding of the bacteria causes the host to form a "coiling phagosome," which is a pseudopod that spirals around the bacteria (Horwitz, 1984). Once the bacteria are internalized, the outer portion of the macrophage membrane coil will degrade and leave the bacteria in a single membrane phagosome (Horwitz, 1984; Marra, Horwitz, & Shuman, 1990). This phagosome does not acidify, nor does it fuse with the endosome or lysosome; instead it fuses with smooth vesicles forming a ribosome-studded vacuole composed of endoplasmic reticulum-derived membranes (Horwitz, 1983; Horwitz & Maxfield, 1984; Horwitz & Silverstein, 1980; Swanson & Isberg, 1995). The bacteria will then divide within the vacuole and rupture the macrophage, spreading further throughout the host.

Mycobacterium tuberculosis uses a similar mechanism to *L. pneumophila* to evade immune surveillance. *M. tuberculosis* can bind via compliment receptors, mannose receptors, or scavenger receptors found on the macrophage (Ernst, 1998; Schlesinger, Bellinger-Kawahara, Payne, & Horwitz, 1990; Schlesinger, 1993; Schorey, Carroll, & Brown, 1997). Once internalized it resides in a membrane-bound vacuole that resists lysosomal fusion and only mildly acidifies, thus preventing maturation into a phagolysosome (Sturgill-Koszycki et al., 1994; Hart, Armstrong, Brown, & Draper, 1972; Russell, 2001). The bacteria then multiply within the phagosome uninhibited and eventually rupture the macrophage (Flynn & Chan, 2001). The processed antigen is then recognized by infiltrating T cells, which activates the MP which then kill the bacteria (Chan, Xing, Magliozzo, & Bloom, 1992). An antibody-mediated immune response will not aid in the eradication of this particular bacteria due to its intracellular location; only a cell-mediated response via activation of macrophages will be of benefit. However, this activation causes the release of lytic enzymes and cytokines that can attract more monocytes, lymphocytes, and neutrophils, none of which are efficient at killing the bacteria and can aid in the progression of the disease (Fenton & Vermeulen, 1996; van Crevel, Ottenhoff, &

Van der Meer, 2002). Granulomatous focal lesions, consisting of macrophage-derived giant cells and lymphocytes, can form where the bacteria will cluster together in units, only multiplying in nearby inactive macrophages or spreading throughout the system causing lesions and further damage.

Macrophages can also cause disease through their activation and subsequent release of inflammatory factors that damage surrounding tissues. An increased number of activated macrophages and production of inflammatory mediators are a prominent feature of inflammatory lesions (Smeets et al., 2001). One such disease macrophages play a role in is rheumatoid arthritis (RA), a debilitating, chronic, systemic inflammatory disorder that affects many organs but primarily attacks synovial joints. It has been shown that the depletion of tumor necrosis factor (TNF), an inflammatory mediator produced by activated macrophages, is a successful treatment for RA, which gives credence to the macrophage's role in causing disease through their release of inflammatory factors (Kinne, Stuhlmuller, & Burmester, 2007; Tracey, Klareskog, Sasso, Salfeld, & Tak, 2008). Furthermore, the degree of joint erosion corresponds to the number of macrophages in the synovial tissue, suggesting that erosion may be in part due to the phagocytic function of macrophages (Mulherin, Fitzgerald, & Bresnihan, 1996; Tak & Bresnihan, 2000).

Systemic lupus erythematosus (SLE), a chronic inflammatory disease that can affect all organs, is another disease that is thought to be linked to macrophage dysfunction. SLE is characterized by high serum levels of autoantibodies to cytoplasmic and nuclear antigens (Harigai et al., 1992; Schnabel, Csernok, Isenberg, Mrowka, & Gross, 1995; Brito, Biamonti, Caporali, & Montecucco, 1994). Here the immune system of the host recognizes self-antigens and produces antibodies to rid the body of cells expressing the specific self-antigen and thus affects many organs. Some studies suggest that auto-antigens appear from impaired phagocytosis of apoptotic cells by macrophages. These apoptotic cells not efficiently cleared contain nuclear proteins that when present in high enough concentrations within the lymphatic system can trigger antinuclear immune responses (Herrmann et al., 1998).

Macrophages have also been shown to be involved in cancer. Many cancers arise from sites of chronic irritation and inflammation (Coussens & Werb, 2002). Angiogenesis facilitates tumor growth, invasion, and metastasis (Folkman, 1995; Folkman & Shing, 1992). Many studies suggest that cells adjacent to cancer cells such as fibroblasts, macrophages, neutrophils, and lymphocytes can interact with cancer cells and produce angiogenic factors (Kelly et al., 1994; Connolly, Stoddard, Harakas, & Feder, 1987; Fukumura et al., 1998). The macrophage is a primary inflammatory cell and activation of the macrophage can lead to the release of growth factors, proteolytic enzymes, cytokines, and inflammatory mediators, which are key angiogenic factors involved in facilitating growth and metastasis (Chen et al., 2005). Thus, via activation and release of inflammatory factors or through their inability to contain and degrade pathogens, macrophages can modulate disease processes.

MP IN THE PERSISTENCE AND PATHOGENESIS OF HIV-1 INFECTION

MP and CD4+ T lymphoyctes are natural targets of HIV-1. Despite their broad range of innate immune functions these cells are incapable of eradicating HIV-1. Indeed, MP are the main storage sites and machinery for HIV-1 in peripheral tissues and the nervous system. (Tardieu & Boutet, 2002) and can incite tissue damage.

In order for HIV to enter into the cell and replicate it must first attach to the host cell and allow its envelope to fuse with the host cell membrane to enter the cytoplasm. HIV attaches via the host cell receptor CD4 and a co-receptor, either CXCR4 or CCR5. Cells expressing the CD4 receptor include subsets of T cells, monocytes, macrophages, dendritic cells, and glial cells. It is the depletion of normally functioning CD4+ T cells that leads to immune deficiency and ultimately acquired immune deficiency syndrome (AIDS). The HIV-1 envelope glycoprotein 120 (gp120) found on the surface of the virus aids in this attachment step to form a complex between CD4 and the co-receptor, which functions as a key allowing the viral envelope to fuse with the host cell membrane.

Along with its RNA, HIV transports two important enzymes into the cell: reverse transcriptase and integrase. After the virus fuses with the cell, its RNA strand is reverse transcribed into double-stranded DNA via reverse transcription. Integrase then inserts the newly synthesized DNA into the host cells genome. Transcription of viral DNA can then occur. New viral proteins are synthesized from the translation of mRNA after the transcription of the integrated provirus; however, before they can become functional units these viral proteins must be cleaved by protease enzymes found in the viral core. The cleaved proteins are then assembled into new viral particles that can infect other cells after budding from the cell surface.

In the case of HIV infection and replication in the brain, studies have shown that only a small percentage of microglial cells are infected at any one time, suggesting they are not all equally able to be infected and replicate the virus (Tardieu & Boutet, 2002; Brack-Werner, 1999; Tornatore, Chandra, Berger, & Major, 1994; Saito et al., 1994). Macrophages/microglial cells that express CD4 and chemokine receptors such as CXCR4 and CCR5 are more susceptible to infection and are better able to replicate the virus than CD4- cells (He et al., 1997; Kozak et al., 1997; Gabuzda & Wang, 1999). Furthermore, activation of macrophage/microglial cells increases their ability to replicate the virus (Rich, Chen, Zack, Leonard, & O'Brien, 1992; Herbein & Varin, 2010; Yu et al., 2008). This is most likely due to metabolic modification and expression of new surface proteins as well as the production of soluble inflammatory mediators. Astrocytes, a subtype of glial cells, are less susceptible to HIV infection and do not effectively support viral replication. This could be due to the lack of CD4 expression causing limited penetration, transcriptional restriction, or other factors dependent on phenotypic expression that would reduce a cell's ability to host the virus (Brack-Werner,

1999). It is important to note that neurons are not directly infected with HIV but are damaged by the accumulation of activated macrophage/microglial cells that release neurotoxic mediators including cellular activation products and viral proteins. A summary of the processes of MP development, infection, migration, and neurotoxicity is provided in Figure 4.1.1.

MP INGRESS ACROSS THE BLOOD-BRAIN BARRIER (BBB)

Initial infection of HIV-1 in the CNS occurs by a process known as the "Trojan horse" mechanism (Meltzer et al. 1990). Perivascular macrophages within the CNS are replenished by monocytes that circulate in the blood, cross the BBB, and enter the CNS where they differentiate into macrophages. It is the trafficking of monocytes infected with HIV-1 across the BBB that establishes the initial infection and constitutes the "Trojan horse" mechanism. Furthermore, the differentiation of these infected monocytes in the CNS enhances their ability to replicate the virus. These infected macrophages then produce chemotactic and inflammatory mediators that work in concert to recruit monocytes and activate the resident CNS macrophages. This method of recruitment and activation is referred to as the "pull" mechanism.

There are many chemotactic and inflammatory mediators secreted by activated microglial cells. A list of these and the rest of the cytokines/chemokines discussed here are listed in Table 4.1.1. The cytokine MCP-1 is a major chemoattractant in the recruitment of monocytes across the BBB. It has been found that the levels of MCP-1 correlate to the levels of HIV-1 in the cerebral spinal fluid (CSF) (Kelder et al., 1998; Letendre et al., 1999). The main source of MCP-1 in the brain is microglial cells (Boven et al., 2000; Fantuzzi et al., 2003; Persidsky & Gendelman, 2003). MCP-1 is also produced by astrocytes in response to quinolinic acid (QA) as well as the HIV protein negative regulatory factor (Nef) (Guillemin, Croitoru-Lamoury, Dormont, D., Armati, & Brew, 2003; Lehmann, Masanetz, Kramer, & Erfle, 2006). MCP-1 disrupts the BBB and increases vascular permeability by affecting the arrangement of tight junction proteins and upregulating expression of matrix metalloproteinases MMP-2 and MMP-9 (Eugenin et al., 2006).

Fractalkine is a chemokine involved in the "pull" mechanism of cell attraction. It is produced by neurons and increases in response to inflammatory stimuli. It can be found in both membrane-bound and soluble forms (Fong et al., 2000; Harrison et al., 2001). Monocytes, brain microglia, T-cells, natural killer cells, dendritic cells, neurons, and astrocytes express the fractalkine receptor, CX3CR1. Fractalkine recruits CD16+ monocyte subsets to inflamed tissues (Ancuta et al., 2003). Also, fractalkine expressed by endothelial cells and induces CD16+ monocytes to produce IL-6, MCP-1, and MMP-9 (Ancuta, Wang, & Gabuzda, 2006c). Thus, the accumulation of this cytokine in inflamed endothelial beds and subsequent recruitment of CD16+ monocytes suggests a role

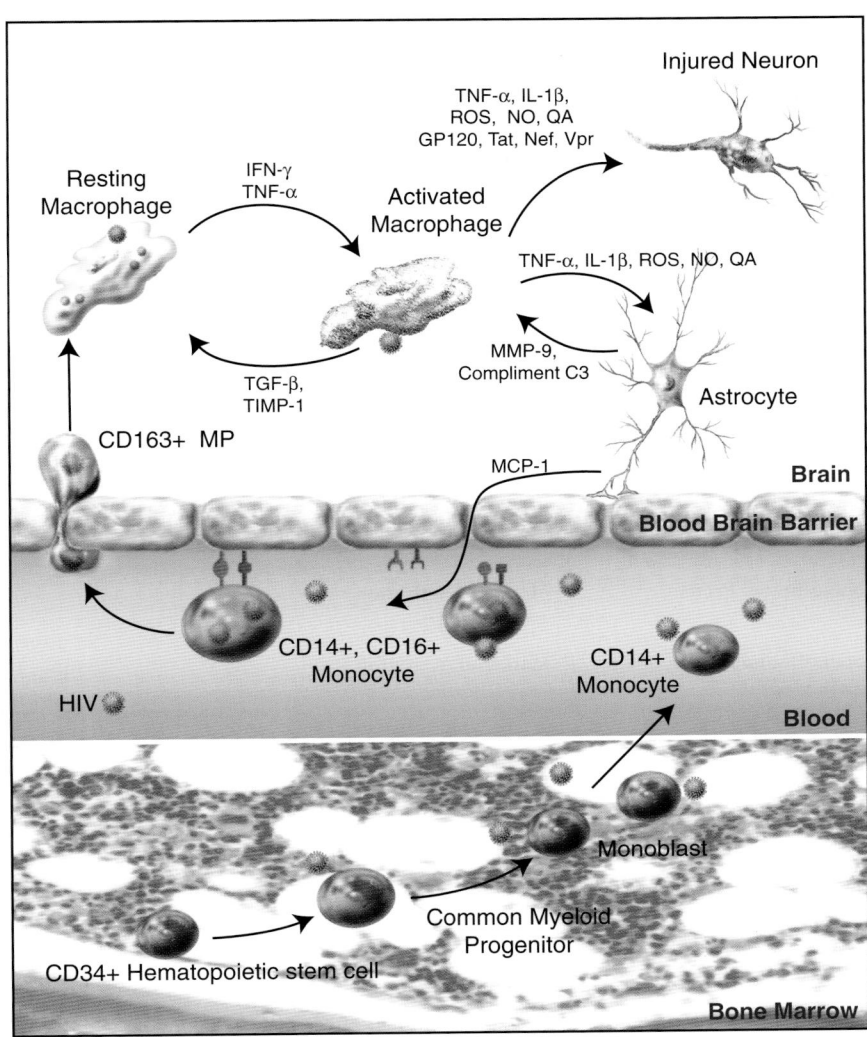

Figure 4.1.1 *MPs and the neuropathogenesis of HIV-1 infection.* Hematopoietic stem cells in the bone marrow differentiate into monocytes and enter the bloodstream. HIV-1-infected monocytes migrate into the brain in response to cytokines/chemokines and differentiate into macrophages where they can be infected at the blood brain barrier interface and; traffick HIV-1 into the brain. Within the CNS, infected macrophages activate surrounding cells such as astrocytes and resident microglia, inducing inflammation. Neurotoxic products, released from infected and immune activated macrophages/microglia directly and indirectly damage neurons. Furthermore, activation increases the release of cytokines/chemokines that further increases recruitment of neuroinflammatory cells to the site of inflammation.

in tissue injury. Activation of the fractalkine receptor may lead to a secondary wave of monocyte recruitment into the brain due to upregulation of MCP-1 followed by differentiation into macrophages triggered by IL-6.

Stromal cell-derived factor-1 alpha (SDF-1α) can contribute to the recruitment of inflammatory cells via activation of CXCR4 on monocytes enabling transmigration across the BBB (Rostasy et al., 2003; Peng et al., 2006). Lyn, a Src family kinase, is an important factor in this pathway. It acts by relaying the signal from CXCR4 activated by SDF-1α to two different regulatory events, both of which are necessary for transmigration. This signaling includes down regulation of an active epitope of monocyte β2 integrins which allows monocyte detachment from inflamed brain microvascular endothelial cells (BMVEC). This pathway is also responsible for chemotaxis as well as for decreasing monocyte attachment

to BMVECs and for their migration toward SDF-1α gradient (Malik et al., 2008).

Activated populations of blood monocytes were observed in HIV-1 infected patients with advanced disease. These cells are believed to have invasive properties that may allow them to cross the BBB and enter the CNS in response to chemokines like MCP-1, fractalkine, and others (Ancuta, Moses, & Gabuzda, 2004); this is referred to as the "push" mechanism. This invasive population of monocytes has been found in patients with HAD. Individuals with HIV-1 associated neurological defects were found to have an expanded population of CD14+ peripheral blood monocytes that co-expressed the marker CD16 (Pulliam, Gascon, Stubblebine, McGuire, & McGrath, 1997). Monocytes that express CD16, an Fc receptor (FCγ RIII) which is a receptor that binds to the Fc portion of an antibody, express higher levels of HLA-DR, CD86,

Table 4.1.1 CYTOKINES/CHEMOKINES AND MARKERS OF ACTIVATION

NAME	TYPE	ACTION	SOURCE
CCR5	Membrane-Bound Receptor	HIV Co-receptor	Monocytes Macrophages Microglial cells
CD4	Membrane-Bound Receptor	HIV Receptor Marker of Activation	Monocytes Macrophages Microglial cells T cells
CD14	Membrane-Bound Receptor Soluble receptor	Functions in Innate Immune System	Monocytes Macrophages Microglial cells
CD16	Membrane-Bound Receptor	Fc Receptor Functions in Innate Immune System	Monocytes Macrophages Microglial cells
CD23	Membrane-Bound Protein	Marker of Activation	Macrophages Microglial cells
CD40	Membrane-Bound Protein	Marker of Activation	Monocytes Macrophages Microglial cells
CD86	Membrane-Bound Protein	Marker of Activation	Monocytes Macrophages Microglial cells
CD163	Membrane-Bound Receptor	Prevents BBB from Breakdown and Leakage Marker of Activation Bacterial Sensor Haptoglobin-Hemoglobin Receptor	Monocytes Macrophages Microglial cells
CXCR4	Membrane-Bound Receptor	HIV Co-receptor SDF-1alpha Receptor	Monocytes Macrophages Microglial cellls
CX3CR1	Membrane-Bound Receptor	Fractalkine Receptor	Monocytes Macrophages Microglial cells T cells NK cells Dendritic cells Neurons Astrocytes
Eicosanoids	Intracellular Chemokine	Neurotoxic Affects Synaptic Transmission/Vascular Permeability	Macrophages Microglial cells
Fractalkine	Membrane-Bound Receptor Soluble Receptor	Marker of Activation Recruits CD16+ Monocytes Induces CD16+ Monocytes to Secrete IL-6, MCP-1, MMP-9 Adhesion, Chemoattraction Activates of Inflammatory cells Protects from GP120 Induced Apoptosis	Neurons Endothelial cells

Table 4.1.1 (CONTINUED)

NAME	TYPE	ACTION	SOURCE
Free Radicals	Intracellular Chemokine	Neurotoxic	Macrophages
			Microglial cells
Glutamate	Soluble Protein	Neurotransmitter	Glial cells
		Can be Neurotoxic in High Concentrations	Neurons
GP 120	Surface Protein	Aids in Attachment	HIV
		Increases Production of TNF-alpha	
		Inhibits Glutamate Recapture	
		Triggers Release of TNF-alpha, IL-1beta, IL-6, GM-CSF, Reactive Oxygen Species	
		Triggers Release of MCP-1, MIP-1alpha, MIP-1beta, RANTES	
		Induces Neuronal Apoptosis	
		Activates Macrophages and Microglial cells	
		Disrupts Ca2+ Homeostasis	
HLA-DR	Membrane-Bound Protein	Marker of Activation	Monocytes
			Macrophages
			Dendritic cells
			B cells
IFN-gamma	Intracellular Antigen	Potent Inducer of Soluble Inflammatory Mediators	T-helper Lymphocytes
		Induces Expression of QA	Monocytes
			Glial cells
IL-1beta	Membrane-Bound Protein	Marker of Activation	Monocytes
		Neurotoxic	Macrophages
		Induces Expression of ICAM-1, VCAM-1,	Microglial cells
		Induces Expression of E-selectin	
		Increases Expression of Ceramide	
MCP-1	Soluble Cytokine	Major Chemoattractant for Monocytes	Microglial cells
		Disrupts BBB	Astrocytes
		Increases Vascular Permeability	
		Affects Arrangement of Tight Junctions	
		Upregulates MMP-2 MMP-9	
M-CSF	Soluble Protein	Controls Survival	Monocytes
		Proliferation	Macrophages
		Differentiation	
		Increases CD14/CD16/CD163 Expression	
		Increases MIP-1alpha, MIP-1beta, RANTES	
MIP-1alpha	Soluble Protein	Involved in Recruitment at Low Concentrations	Macrophages
		Can Block HIV Entry by Blocking CCR5 at High Concentrations	Microglial cells
MIP-1beta	Intracellular Chemokine	Neurotoxic	Macrophages
		Involved in Recruitment at Low Concentrations	Microglial cells
		Can Block HIV Entry by Blocking CCR5 at High Concentrations	
Nef	Soluble Protein	Increases MCP-1	HIV

(Continues)

Table 4.1.1 CYTOKINES/CHEMOKINES AND MARKERS OF ACTIVATION (CONTINUED)

NAME	TYPE	ACTION	SOURCE
		Induces QA Production	
		Manipulates Host-cell Machinery	
NO	Free Radical	Neurotoxic	Macrophages
			Microglial cells
PAF		Excitotoxic	Endothelial cells
		Induces QA and TNF-alpha Production	Neutrophils
			Basophils
			Platelets
PGE-2	Intracellular Chemokine	Neurotoxic	Macrophages
			Microglial cells
Prostaglandin	Soluble Protein	Neurotoxic via Activation of NMDA Receptors	Macrophages
		Inhibits Glutamate Recapture	Microglial cells
QA	Soluble Protein	Increases MCP-1 Production	Macrophages
		Stimulates Release of MCP-1, RANTES, IL-8, SDF-1alpha, Fractalkine	Microglial cells
RANTES	Intracellular Antigen	Neurotoxicity	Macrophages
		Can Block HIV Entry by Blocking CCR5 at High Concentrations	Microglial cells
		Involved in Recruitment at Low Concentrations	
SDF-1alpha	Soluble protein	Activates CXCR4	Monocytes
		Recruits of Inflammatory cells	Macrophages
			Microglial cells
Tat	Soluble Protein	Induces QA Production	HIV
		Induces PAF Production	
		Inhibits Glutamate Recapture	
		Stimulates Production of IL-1beta, TNF-alpha, Il-6, TGF-beta	
		Activates Microglial cells	
		Stimulates Secretion of MCP-1, IL-8, IP-10, MIP-1a, MIP-1B, RANTES	
		Induces Apoptosis	
		Excitotoxic via Activation of NMDA Receptors	
		Alters Tight Junction Proteins	
TGF-beta	Intracellular Antigen	Neuroprotection from: Glutamate Toxicity, Hypoxia, gp120-mediate Injury	Macrophages
		Controls Astrocytosis	Microglial cells
TNF-alpha	Membrane-Bound Protein	Marker of Activation	Monocytes
		Pro-inflammatory	Macrophages
		Activates Macrophages and Astrocytes	Microglial cells
		Recruits Macrophages and Microglial cells	
		Potentiates Glutamate Neurotoxicity	
		Damages BBB	
		Increases Expression of ICAM-1	
		Increases Expression of VCAM-1	
		Increases MCP-1 Production	
		Directly Harms Neurons	

Table 4.1.1 (CONTINUED)

NAME	TYPE	ACTION	SOURCE
Vpr	Soluble Protein	Increases Ca2+ Mobilization Increases Expression of E-selectins Increases Fractalkine Production Induces Expression of QA Inhibits Gluatamate Recapture Induces PAF Production Induces Apoptosis Activates Glial cells Essential for Viral Replication Induces Secretion of Neurotoxins Changes Neuronal Membrane Proteins	HIV

CD40, tumor necrosis factor α (TNF-α), and interleukin 1β (IL-1β).

In HIV-1 encephalitis (HIVE), the majority of perivascular macrophages that accumulated in microglial nodules were CD14+/CD16+. Monocytes that are CD16+ are more susceptible to infection as well as harbor proviral DNA (Shiramizu et al., 2005; Ellery et al., 2007; Jaworowski et al., 2007). Furthermore, CD16-expressing monocytes differentiate into macrophages that are more efficient at promoting T-cell activation, virus transfer, and HIV-1 replication (Ancuta et al., 2006a; Ancuta et al., 2006b). Co-localization in the CNS between viral p24 antigen and both CD14 and CD16 within the CNS has been demonstrated, which suggests that these macrophages are the major reservoir for virus in the CNS (Fischer-Smith et al., 2001).

A scavenger receptor for haptoglobin-hemoglobin complex, CD163, is another surface marker which was found to be expressed by circulating monocytes in HIV-positive individuals and on CD16+ HIV-infected perivascular macrophages in HIVE brains (Fischer-Smith, Tedaldi, & Rappaport, 2008b; Fischer-Smith, Bell, Croul, Lewis, & Rappaport, 2008a). Parenchymal microglia are CD163-, which suggests that there is an increased influx of inflammatory monocytes across the BBB (Sulahian et al., 2000). CD163 may participate in macrophage activation as a monocyte/macrophage bacterial sensor in response to bacterial translocation from the gut into the systemic circulation (Fabriek et al., 2009). Furthermore, CD163 may protect the BBB from breakdown and leakage as a hemoglobin/haptoglobin scavenger molecule in perivascular macrophages (Borda et al., 2008).

There is evidence that early in infection there is damage to the gastrointestinal mucosa whereby there is a loss of mucosal lymphocytes that leads to translocation of bacterial endotoxin lipopolysaccharide (LPS) and causes a generalized systemic immune activation (Brenchley et al., 2006). LPS, along with other translocation products, can trigger monocyte activation through activation of CD14 and TLR. This results in release of soluble CD14 and pro-inflammatory cytokines contributing to a chronic systemic immune activation (Brenchley et al., 2006; Douek, 2007). Studies have shown that microbial translocation has been linked to increased monocyte activation in the development of dementia, suggesting a mechanism for the expansion of this invasive population (Ancuta et al., 2008). Also, in vivo studies of the BBB have shown that increased levels of LPS in circulation compromise the integrity of the BBB (Zhou, LaPointe, Clark, Zbytnuik, & Kubes, 2006). Compromise of the BBB via increased LPS and HIV-1 infection of monocytes may act synergistically to disrupt the BBB and increase transmigration of monocytes into the CNS (Wang, Sun, & Goldstein, 2008).

MP NEUROTOXICITY

Activation of microglia is responsible for combating disease in the CNS, but as discussed previously it can also lead to dysfunction. In the case of HIV-1 infection, macrophages actually aid in the trafficking and harboring of virus, thus allowing the virus to bypass the immune response. Microglia activation can also lead to neurotoxic consequences depending on their environment and intensity of cell marker expression.

Expression of cell markers resulting from activation is divided into membrane-bound proteins and intracellular antigens or mRNAs that are related to the production of soluble inflammatory mediators. Membrane-bound markers of activation in microglial cells include HLA-DR, CD4, CD23, and CD40. There are also membrane-bound cytokines/chemokines such as TNF-α and fractalkine (Nuovo & Alfieri, 1996; Tong et al., 2000; Dugas, Lacroix, Kilchherr, Delfraissy, & Tardieu, 2001; Peudenier, Hery, Montagnier, & Tardieu, 1991).

When macrophages/microglial cells are exposed to the viral proteins gp120 or transactivator of transcription (Tat) they increase their production of soluble inflammatory mediators such as TNF-α (Yeung et al., 1995; Nicolini, Ajmone-Cat,

Bernado, Levi, & Minghetti, 2001). TNF-α is pro-inflammatory and can further activate and recruit macrophages and microglial cells, activate astrocytes, and potentiate glutamate neurotoxicity as well as directly harm neurons. TNF-α is responsible for many events including damage to the BBB, increased expression of ICAM-1 adhesion molecule, vascular cell adhesion molecule 1 (VCAM-1), and MCP-1 (Strieter et al., 1989; Hurwitz, Lyman, & Berman, 1995). Furthermore, it causes increased expression of E-selectin on astrocytes and endothelial cells that result in infected macrophage transmigration across the BBB into the CNS (Collins et al., 1995; Fiala et al., 1996; Lee, Hou, & Benveniste, 1998). TNF-α can be toxic to neurons by indirectly overstimulating glutamate receptors (Gelbard et al., 1993), increasing the release of the excitotoxic neurotransmitter glutamate from astrocytes and microglia (Bezzi et al., 2001), as well as inhibiting the uptake of glutamate by astrocytes (Casado et al., 1993; Fine et al., 1996; Wang et al., 2003b). Overexpression of TNF-α can also lead to increased Ca^{2+} ion mobilization by overstimulating NMDA receptors by an indirect mechanism (Lipton, 1994), formation of NO, and superoxide toxicity (Bonfoco, Krainc, Ankarcrona, Nicotera, & Lipton, 1995).

Fractalkine expression by neurons and astrocytes also increases in response to stimulation by TNF-α. In addition to its role in the "pull" mechanism as discussed previously, fractalkine is responsible for adhesion, chemoattraction, and activation of inflammatory cells, including other macrophages and microglial cells (Tong et al., 2000; Erichsen et al., 2003), making it potentially neurotoxic. However, it is also able to protect neurons against gp120-induced apoptosis (Meucci & Miller, 1996). Thus, its ultimate effect on neuronal survival is still being explored.

Intracellular antigens or mRNAs that are markers of activation in macrophages/microglial cells include the cytokines: IL-1β, IFN-γ, TGF-β, and TGF-α as well as the chemokines: RANTES, MIP-1β, eicosanoids, free radicals, and PGE-2, many of which can be neurotoxic. IL-1β is neurotoxic and like TNF-α it also induces the expression of ICAM-1, VCAM-1, and E-selectin on endothelial cells and astrocytes which aid in the infiltration of monocytes into the CNS (Collins et al., 1995; Lee et al., 1998; Winkler & Beveniste, 1998). It has been found in higher concentrations in the cerebrospinal fluid (CSF) and brains of infected patients with HAD compared to infected patients without dementia (Gallo et al., 1989; Tyor et al., 1992; Zhao, Kim, Morgello, & Lee, 2001; Brabers & Nottet, 2006). IL-1β can also increase the expression of ceramide, which is thought to be involved in ROS formation and apoptosis in neurons (Haughey et al., 2004). IFN-γ, another intracellular antigen, is one of the most potent inducers of secretion of soluble inflammatory mediators by glial cells (Janabi, Chabrier, & Tardieu, 1996). It can be secreted by both activated CD4+ T-helper lymphocytes as well as activated monocytes that have crossed the BBB into the CNS. The intracellular antigen TGF-β is special in that it is neuroprotective. It protects neurons from glutamate toxicity, hypoxia, gp120-mediated injury (Vitkovic, Maeda, & Sternberg, 2001), and controls astrocytosis. Finally, the chemokines RANTES, MIP-1β, MIP-1α, eicosanoids, free radicals, and PGE-2 are normally expressed at low levels in macrophages/microglial cells; however, cytokine activation increases their concentration (Janabi et al., 1996; Janabi, Hau, & Tardieu, 1999).

Macrophage colony-stimulating factor (M-CSF) is a cytokine, specifically a hematopoietic growth factor that controls survival, proliferation, differentiation, and other functions in monocytes and macrophages. When macrophages are infected with HIV-1 they increase their production of M-CSF (Gruber, Weih, Boone, Smith, & Clouse, 1995). There are a number of factors that are then upregulated by the presence of M-CSF. These factors include the increased development of CD14+CD16+ and CD163+ monocytes that produce high levels of TNF-α and IL-1β, which, as discussed previously, lead to neurotoxicity (Li, Hangoc, & Broxmeyer, 2004; Buechler et al., 2000). Furthermore, M-CSF is also responsible for the increased levels of MIP-1α, MIP-1β, and RANTES. At higher concentrations these chemokines can block HIV-1 entry through the co-receptor CCR5, but in lower concentrations they may be involved in recruitment (Haine, Fischer-Smith, & Rappaport, 2006). Oddly, M-CSF can also block viral entry through upregulation of chemokines; however, it can also enhance viral entry by upregulating expression of CD4 receptors on monocytes and macrophages (Bergamini et al., 1994; Wang, Roderiquez, Oravecz, & Norcross, 1998). Due to the varying effects of M-CSF, it is thought to mediate activation of microglial cells which can result in the release of soluble inflammatory factors (Hao, Dheen, & Ling, 2002; Vincent, Selwood, & Murphy, 2002; Mitrasinovic et al., 2005).

Activated astrocytes and microglia release the chemokine NO, which is also a free radical and may contribute to neuronal death (Nuovo & Alfieri, 1996; Rostasy et al., 1999; Vincent et al., 1999; Zhao et al., 2001; Liu et al., 2002). Eicosanoids, a class of chemokines, can also lead to neurotoxicity. They are thought to influence the nervous system by affecting synaptic transmission and vascular permeability and flow (Sang & Chen, 2006; Chawengsub, Gautheir, & Campbell, 2009). The chemokine prostaglandin can lead to neurotoxicity directly by over activating NMDA receptors and indirectly by inhibiting glutamate recapture by astrocytes (Caruso, Durand, Watanobe, & Lasaga, 2006).

When macrophages are infected with HIV-1 they produce quinolinic acid (QA), a neurotoxin, in response to the viral proteins Tat and Nef. Nef manipulates the host's cellular machinery to aid in infection, survival, and replication (Brew et al., 1995; Nottet et al., 1996; Kerr et al., 1997; Heyes et al., 2001; Smith et al., 2001). Macrophages can also be stimulated to produce QA in response to TNF-α, IFN-γ, and IFN-α at concentrations that are neurotoxic (Pemberton, Kerr, Smythe, & Brew, 1997). QA is implicated in many inflammatory and neurodegenerative diseases including Alzheimer's disease, Huntington's disease, and amyotrophic lateral sclerosis (Heyes et al., 1991; Heyes et al., 2001; Sei et al., 1995; Guillemin et al., 2005). It can also stimulate astrocytes to release MCP-1, RANTES, and IL-8 as well as increase SDF-1α and fractalkine expression (Guillemin et al., 2003).

Glutamate is an excitotoxic neurotransmitter that can be released by activated or infected microglia (Jiang et al., 2001; Erdmann et al., 2007). HIV-1 proteins Tat and gp120 as well as microglia products such as TNF-α inhibit glutamate homeostasis by affecting the ability of astrocytes to re-uptake glutamate (Benos et al., 1994; Fine et al., 1996; Patton, Zhou, Bubien, Benveniste, & Benos, 2000). Platelet activating factor (PAF) can cause neuronal damage directly via excitotoxicity or through QA and TNF-α (Bito et al., 1992; Lipton, 1994; Smith et al., 2001; Bellizzi, Lu, Masliah, & Gelbard, 2005). PAF production is induced by HIV-1 Tat as well as by TNF-α (Del Sorbo et al., 1999; Arese, Ferrandi, Primo, Camussi, & Bussolino, 2001). Many cells produce PAF including neutrophils, basophils, platelets, and endothelial cells. Viral proteins, as noted above, can lead to neurotoxicity through direct and indirect means via activation of both macrophage and microglia. The HIV-1 envelope glycoprotein consists of two major subunits, the transmembrane domain gp41 and a non-covalently associated surface subunit gp120. HIV-1 envelope gp120 interacts with CD4, CCR5, and CXCR4 receptors to mediate infection of target cells by facilitating entry of the virus into the cell. It is also shed from virons and is released by infected cells (Dreyer, Kaiser, Offermann, & Lipton, 1990; Kaul & Lipton, 1999). Gp120 has been found to localize to microglia and multinucleated giant cells (Jones, Bell, & Nath, 2000). When gp120 interacts with receptors on macrophages and microglial cells it activates these cells and triggers the release of TNF-α, IL-1β, IL-6, granulocyte macrophage colony-stimulating factor (GM-CSF), and reactive oxygen species (Clouse et al., 1991; Corasaniti, Bagetta, Rotiroti, & Nistico, 1998; Viviani, Corsini, Binaglia, Galli, & Marinovich, 2001; Lee, Tomkowicz, Freedman, & Collman, 2005; Cheung, Ravyn, Wang, Ptasznik, & Collman, 2008). It also triggers macrophages/monocytes to release MCP-1, macrophage inflammatory protein-1α (MIP-1α), MIP-1β, and RANTES (Choe, Volsky, & Potash, 2001; Del Corno et al., 2001; Fantuzzi et al., 2001). Glycoprotein120 not only mediates infection but also activates macrophages and microglia. In rats, gp120 has also been shown to induce neuronal apoptosis via interaction with the CXCR4 receptor (Hesselgesser et al., 1997; Hesselgesser et al., 1998; Catani et al., 2000; Bachis & Mocchetti, 2004; Bachis, Biggio, Major, & Mocchetti, 2009). In humans, gp120 interaction with CCR5 can induce neuronal apoptosis (Xu et al., 2004). Glycoprotein120-induced apoptosis involves the disruption of calcium homeostasis, which subsequently leads to mitochondrial membrane disturbances and intrinsic activation of caspases and endonucleases (Dreyer et al., 1990; Lannuzel, Lledo, Lamghitnia, Vincent, & Tardieu, 1995; Mattson, Haughey, & Nath, 2005).

A virally encoded transactivator of transcription (Tat) is an HIV-1 protein that is released by infected cells (Chang, Samaniego, Nair, Buonaguro, & Ensoli, 1997). Tat can stimulate a pro-inflammatory response leading to the production of cytokines such as IL-1β, TNF-α, IL-6, and transforming growth factor-β (Zauli et al., 1992; Zauli et al., 1993; Lafrenie, Wahl, Epstein, Yamada, & Dhawan, 1997). When microglial cells are treated with Tat it causes activation and secretion of the chemokines MCP-1, IL-8, IP-10, MIP-1α, MIP-1β, and RANTES, all of which are chemotactic factors for monocytes. Studies have shown that Tat has toxic effects on CNS cells, especially neurons, and can induce apoptosis (Kruman, Nath, & Mattson, 1998; Bonavia et al., 2001; Bruce-Keller et al., 2003; Eugenin, D'Aversa, Lopez, Calderon, & Berman, 2003; Eugenin et al., 2007; Miagkov, Turchan, Nath, & Drachman, 2004; Singh et al., 2004; Pocernich, Sultana, Mohmmad-Abdul, Nath, & Butterfield, 2005; Aksenova et al., 2006). These toxic effects are mediated by cytokines, chemokines, and NO released by activated microglia (Polazzi, Levi, & Minghetti, 1999; Turchan-Cholewo et al., 2009). Tat can also lead to excitotoxicity and apoptosis via indirect activation of NMDA receptors (Haughey, Nath, Mattson, Slevin, & Geiger, 2001; Song, Nath, Geiger, Moore, & Hochman, 2003; Eugenin et al., 2007; Li et al., 2008). The inflammatory responses induced by Tat also affect astrocytes and endothelial cells which lead to further infiltration of monocytes into the brain (Pu et al., 2003). Tat may also contribute to the enhanced transmigration of monocytes and lymphocytes via disruption of the BBB by altering tight junction proteins (Andras et al., 2003; Toborek et al., 2003).

The HIV accessory protein Vpr may also play a role in neuronal injury directly by cytotoxic action and indirectly by the activation of glial cells with subsequent release of neurotoxic products (Jones et al., 2007). Vpr is an HIV-1-encoded virion-incorporated protein that is essential for viral replication in macrophages (Emerman, 1996; Subbramanian et al., 1998). When glial cells are treated with Vpr it induces the secretion of neurotoxins. When neurons are treated with soluble Vpr it leads to changes in neuronal membrane potentials and induces apoptosis (Patel, Mukhtar, & Pomerantz, 2000; Jones et al., 2007; Rom et al., 2009).

Neurotoxicity can alter CNS cell morphology and induce both cell proliferation and apoptosis. Chronic neurotoxicity can induce formation of lesions within white matter and cell loss within gray matter (Ketzler, Weis, Haug, & Budka, 1990; Everall et al., 1991). Programmed cell death is thought to be a major mechanism of neuronal damage (Adle-Biassette et al., 1995; Ohagen et al., 1999). Activated microglial cells, multinucleated giant cells, and p24-expressing cells have been found in areas of increased apoptotic neurons. Ultimately, chronic neurotoxicity can result in brain atrophy, which is commonly manifested as dementia.

ANTIRETROVIRAL AND ADJUNCTIVE THERAPIES LINK MP FUNCTION AND BIOLOGY

Antiretroviral therapy (ART) is the main treatment used to combat the neurotoxic effects of HIV-infected macrophages that have entered the brain. By suppressing viral replication within infected macrophages, many of the neurotoxic and inflammatory mediators released by these cells are eliminated. ART is effective at suppressing viral replication; however, these drugs have many pharmacokinetic, pharmacodynamic, and biodistribution limitations. These limitations make it difficult to maintain therapeutic drug levels and prevent these medications from effectively reaching all regions of the body. As a result, viral sanctuaries, regions where ART drugs cannot enter and virus can replicate unimpeded, are allowed to form. The CNS is a major viral sanctuary.

Since ART medications have a very limited ability to cross the BBB, much research has been done looking for adjunctive therapies that can either prevent the activation of macrophages/microglia or block the effects of their activation products. A few of these adjunctive therapies include minocycline, memantine, sodium valproate, PMS-601, lithium, and a variety of nanoformulated compounds. Minocycline is a tetracycline antimicrobial agent that mitigates microglial activation in vitro and in vivo. In vitro it reduces glutamate toxicity as well as caspase-independent and dependent mitochondrial-mediated cell death (Wang et al., 2003a). Work in an SIV model has shown that minocycline can decrease the expression of CNS inflammatory markers as well as inhibit viral replication (Si et al., 2004; Zink et al., 2005). Memantine, an uncompetitive NMDA receptor antagonist, is able to inhibit HIV-1 gp120-dependent calcium changes in neurons and astrocytes. It has also been shown to protect neurons from gp120-induced cell death (Lipton, 1992; Nath et al., 2000). In HIV-1-infected subjects, memantine can improve neuronal metabolism (Schifitto et al., 2007). Sodium valproate (VPA) has been shown to promote neurite outgrowth, which may serve as a mechanism to promote recovery in damaged neurons (Dou et al., 2003). VPA has been used in a pilot study of HIV-1-infected neurocognitively impaired subjects and showed evidence of improving both neuropsychological performance and the rate of metabolism within the brain (Schifitto et al., 2006). PMS-601, a PFA receptor antagonist, has also been proposed as adjunctive therapy. PAF has been found to reduce macrophage inflammatory mediator secretion, neuronal loss, and microgliosis (Eggert et al., 2009). Lithium, a drug traditionally used to treat bipolar disorder, has been found to protect neurons from neurotoxicity induced by HIV-infected macrophage secretion products (Dou et al., 2005) as well as from gp120-mediated toxicity (Everall et al., 2002).

An exciting new area of research has been the use of nanotechnology to increase circulation time, improve efficacy, and target delivery of drugs. By reformulating or repacking drugs, researchers have been able to overcome many of the limitations associated with traditionally manufactured medications. These methods have been applied to ART medications in an attempt to increase delivery of these drugs to HIV-infected organs. Of particular interest has been the use of macrophages and monocytes as vehicles to transport ART nanoparticles into the brain. We have been working with this very model in our own laboratories. We have been able to manufacture stable crystalline nanoparticles of atazanavir, indinavir, ritonavir, and efavirenz coated with a variety of surfactant coatings, collectively referred to as "nanoART." We have shown that macrophages are capable of both rapidly taking up ($\leq$ 30 min) and slowly releasing (> 15 days) nanoART in clinically significant amounts (Nowacek et al., 2009; Nowacek et al., 2010). In addition, we have demonstrated that nanoART loaded into macrophages have superior in vivo pharmacokinetics and efficacy over traditionally formulated drugs (Nowacek et al., 2009). Most importantly, we have also shown that nanoART-laden macrophages are able to cross the BBB and deliver drug specifically to HIV-infected regions of the brain (Dou et al., 2009). These results indicate that reformulating ART medications into nanoART and delivering them to the brain via monocytes and macrophages may be a promising new way to treat infective/inflammatory CNS disorders such as HIV encephalopathy.

SUMMARY AND CONCLUSIONS

Macrophages are complex cells that function in both innate and adaptive immunity as well as aid the body in multiple cellular processes. Their main function is to phagocytose pathogens and clear away debris in order to aid in remodeling after injury or disease. However, they also rid the body of damaged or dead cells, thereby aiding in the maintenance of homeostasis. In some diseases, such as HIV-1 infection, macrophages become dysfunctional and work against the body's immune system as well as directly cause harm through their activation and subsequent release of soluble factors. Thus, they are able to mediate neurotoxicity both directly and indirectly. By focusing on the pathways that lead to neurotoxicity, treatments can be developed to specifically target both the causes as well as the consequences of macrophage dysfunction.

ACKNOWLEDGMENTS

The work was supported by grants 2R01 NS034239, 2R37 NS36126, P01 NS31492, P20RR 15635, P01MH64570, and P01 NS43985 (to H.E.G.) from the National Institutes of Health.

The authors thank Ms. Robin Taylor for critical reading of the manuscript and outstanding graphic and literary support.

REFERENCES

Aderem, A. & Underhill, D. M. (1999). Mechanisms of phagocytosis in macrophages. *Annu Rev Immunol, 17,* 593–623.

Adle-Biassette, H., Levy, Y., Colombel, M., Poron, F., Natchev, S., Keohane, C., et al. (1995). Neuronal apoptosis in HIV infection in adults. *Neuropathol Appl Neurobiol, 21,* 218–27.

Akiyama, H. & McGeer, P. L. (1990). Brain microglia constitutively express beta-2 integrins. *J Neuroimmunol, 30,* 81–93.

Aksenova, M. V., Silvers, J. M., Aksenov, M. Y., Nath, A., Ray, P. D., Mactutus, C. F., et al. (2006). HIV-1 Tat neurotoxicity in primary cultures of rat midbrain fetal neurons: Changes in dopamine transporter binding and immunoreactivity. *Neurosci Lett, 395,* 235–9.

Ancuta, P., Autissier, P., Wurcel, A., Zaman, T., Stone, D., & Gabuzda, D. (2006a). CD16+ monocyte-derived macrophages activate resting T cells for HIV infection by producing CCR3 and CCR4 ligands. *J Immunol, 176,* 5760–71.

Ancuta, P., Kamat, A., Kunstman, K. J., Kim, E. Y., Autissier, P., Wurcel, A., et al. (2008). Microbial translocation is associated with increased monocyte activation and dementia in AIDS patients. *PLoS One, 3,* e2516.

Ancuta, P., Kunstman, K. J., Autissier, P., Zaman, T., Stone, D., Wolinsky, S. M., et al. (2006b). CD16+ monocytes exposed to HIV promote highly efficient viral replication upon differentiation into macrophages and interaction with T cells. *Virology, 344*, 267–76.

Ancuta, P., Moses, A., & Gabuzda, D. (2004). Transendothelial migration of CD16+ monocytes in response to fractalkine under constitutive and inflammatory conditions. *Immunobiology, 209*, 11–20.

Ancuta, P., Rao, R., Moses, A., Mehle, A., Shaw, S. K., Luscinskas, F. W., et al. (2003). Fractalkine preferentially mediates arrest and migration of CD16+ monocytes. *J Exp Med, 197*, 1701–7.

Ancuta, P., Wang, J., & Gabuzda, D. (2006c). CD16+ monocytes produce IL-6, CCL2, and matrix metalloproteinase-9 upon interaction with CX3CL1-expressing endothelial cells. *J Leukoc Biol, 80*, 1156–64.

Andras, I. E., Pu, H., Deli, M. A., Nath, A., Hennig, B., & Toborek, M. (2003). HIV-1 Tat protein alters tight junction protein expression and distribution in cultured brain endothelial cells. *J Neurosci Res, 74*, 255–65.

Areses, M., Ferrandi, C., Primo, L., Camussi, G., & Bussolino, F. (2001). HIV-1 Tat protein stimulates in vivo vascular permeability and lymphomononuclear cell recruitment. *J Immunol, 166*, 1380–8.

Bachis, A., Biggio, F., Major, E. O., & Mocchetti, I. (2009). M- and T-tropic HIVs promote apoptosis in rat neurons. *J Neuroimmune Pharmacol, 4*, 150–60.

Bachis, A. & Mocchetti, I. (2004). The chemokine receptor CXCR4 and not the N-methyl-D-aspartate receptor mediates gp120 neurotoxicity in cerebellar granule cells. *J Neurosci Res, 75*, 75–82.

Bellinger-Kawahara, C. & Horwitz, M. A. (1990). Complement component C3 fixes selectively to the major outer membrane protein (MOMP) of Legionella pneumophila and mediates phagocytosis of liposome-MOMP complexes by human monocytes. *J Exp Med, 172*, 1201–10.

Bellizzi, M. J., Lu, S. M., Masliah, E., & Gelbard, H. A. (2005). Synaptic activity becomes excitotoxic in neurons exposed to elevated levels of platelet-activating factor. *J Clin Invest, 115*, 3185–92.

Benos, D. J., Hahn, B. H., Bubien, J. K., Ghosh, S. K., Mashburn, N. A., Chaikin, M. A., et al. (1994). Envelope glycoprotein gp120 of human immunodeficiency virus type 1 alters ion transport in astrocytes: Implications for AIDS dementia complex. *Proc Natl Acad Sci U S A, 91*, 494–8.

Bergamini, A., Perno, C. F., Dini, L., Capozzi, M., Pesce, C. D., VENTURA, L., et al. (1994). Macrophage colony-stimulating factor enhances the susceptibility of macrophages to infection by human immunodeficiency virus and reduces the activity of compounds that inhibit virus binding. *Blood, 84*, 3405–12.

Bessis, A., Bechade, C., Bernard, D., & Roumier, A. (2007). Microglial control of neuronal death and synaptic properties. *Glia, 55*, 233–8.

Bezzi, P., Domercq, M., Brambilla, L., Galli, R., Schols, D., De Clercq, E., et al. (2001). CXCR4-activated astrocyte glutamate release via TNFalpha: Amplification by microglia triggers neurotoxicity. *Nat Neurosci, 4*, 702–10.

Bito, H., Nakamura, M., Honda, Z., Izumi, T., Iwatsubo, T., Seyama, Y., et al. (1992). Platelet-activating factor (PAF) receptor in rat brain: PAF mobilizes intracellular Ca2+ in hippocampal neurons. *Neuron, 9*, 285–94.

Bonavia, R., Bajetto, A., Barbero, S., Albini, A., Noonan, D. M., & Schettini, G. (2001). HIV-1 Tat causes apoptotic death and calcium homeostasis alterations in rat neurons. *Biochem Biophys Res Commun, 288*, 301–8.

Bonfoco, E., Krainc, D., Ankarcrona, M., Nicotera, P., & Lipton, S. A. (1995). Apoptosis and necrosis: Two distinct events induced, respectively, by mild and intense insults with N-methyl-D-aspartate or nitric oxide/superoxide in cortical cell cultures. *Proc Natl Acad Sci USA, 92*, 7162–6.

Borda, J. T., Alvarez, X., Mohan, M., Hasegawa, A., Bernardino, A., Jean, S., et al. (2008). CD163, a marker of perivascular macrophages, is up-regulated by microglia in simian immunodeficiency virus encephalitis after haptoglobin-hemoglobin complex stimulation and is suggestive of breakdown of the blood-brain barrier. *Am J Pathol, 172*, 725–37.

Boven, L. A., Middel, J., Breij, E. C., Schotte, D., Verhoef, J., Soderland, C., et al. (2000). Interactions between HIV-infected monocyte-derived macrophages and human brain microvascular endothelial cells result in increased expression of CC chemokines. *J Neurovirol, 6*, 382–9.

Brabers, N. A., & Nottet, H. S. (2006). Role of the pro-inflammatory cytokines TNF-alpha and IL-1beta in HIV-associated dementia. *Eur J Clin Invest, 36*, 447–58.

Brack-Werner, R. (1999). Astrocytes: HIV cellular reservoirs and important participants in neuropathogenesis. *AIDS, 13*, 1–22.

Brenchely, J. M., Price, D. A., Schacker, T. W., Asher, T. E., Silvestri, G., Rao, S., et al. (2006). Microbial translocation is a cause of systemic immune activation in chronic HIV infection. *Nat Med, 12*, 1365–71.

Brew, B. J., Corbeil, J., Pemberton, L., Evans, L., Saito, K., Penny, R., et al. (1995). Quinolinic acid production is related to macrophage tropic isolates of HIV-1. *J Neurovirol, 1*, 369–74.

Brito, J., Biamonti, G., Caporali, R., & Montecucco, C. (1994). Autoantibodies to human nuclear lamin B2 protein. Epitope specificity in different autoimmune diseases. *J Immunol, 153*, 2268–77.

Bruce-Keller, A. J., Chauhan, A., Dimayuga, F. O., Gee, J., Keller, J. N., & Nath, A. (2003). Synaptic transport of human immunodeficiency virus-Tat protein causes neurotoxicity and gliosis in rat brain. *J Neurosci, 23*, 8417–22.

Buechler, C., Ritter, M., Orso, E., Langmann, T., Klucken, J., & Schmitz, G. (2000). Regulation of scavenger receptor CD163 expression in human monocytes and macrophages by pro- and antiinflammatory stimuli. *J Leukoc Biol, 67*, 97–103.

Butcher, E. C. & Picker, L. J. (1996). Lymphocyte homing and homeostasis. *Science, 272*, 60–6.

Caruso, C., Durand, D., Watanobe, H., & Lasaga, M. (2006). NMDA and group I metabotropic glutamate receptors activation modulates substance P release from the arcuate nucleus and median eminence. *Neurosci Lett, 393*, 60–4.

Casado, M., Bendahan, A., Zafra, F., Danbolt, N. C., Aragon, C., Gimenez, C., et al. (1993). Phosphorylation and modulation of brain glutamate transporters by protein kinase C. *J Biol Chem, 268*, 27313–7.

Catani, M. V., Corasaniti, M. T., Navarra, M., Nistico, G., Finazzi-Agro, A., & Melino, G. 2000. gp120 induces cell death in human neuroblastoma cells through the CXCR4 and CCR5 chemokine receptors. *J Neurochem, 74*, 2373–9.

Chan, J., Xing, Y., Magliozzo, R. S., & Bloom, B. R. (1992). Killing of virulent Mycobacterium tuberculosis by reactive nitrogen intermediates produced by activated murine macrophages. *J Exp Med, 175*, 1111–22.

Chan, W. Y., Kohsaka, S., & Rezaie, P. (2007). The origin and cell lineage of microglia: New concepts. *Brain Res Rev, 53*, 344–54.

Chang, H. C., Samaniego, F., Nair, B. C., Buonaguro, L., & Ensoli, B. (1997). HIV-1 Tat protein exits from cells via a leaderless secretory pathway and binds to extracellular matrix-associated heparan sulfate proteoglycans through its basic region. *AIDS, 11*, 1421–31.

Chawengsub, Y., Gautheir, K. M., & Campbell, W. B. (2009). Role of arachidonic acid lipoxygenase metabolites in the regulation of vascular tone. *Am J Physiol Heart Circ Physiol, 297*, H495–507.

Chen, J. J., Lin, Y. C., Yao, P. L., Yuan, A., Chen, H. Y., Shun, C. T., et al. (2005). Tumor-associated macrophages: The double-edged sword in cancer progression. *J Clin Oncol, 23*, 953–64.

Cheung, R., Ravyn, V., Wang, L., Ptasznik, A., & Collman, R. G. (2008). Signaling mechanism of HIV-1 gp120 and virion-induced IL-1beta release in primary human macrophages. *J Immunol, 180*, 6675–84.

Choe, W., Volsky, D. J., & Potash, M. J. (2001). Induction of rapid and extensive beta-chemokine synthesis in macrophages by human immunodeficiency virus type 1 and gp120, independently of their coreceptor phenotype. *J Virol, 75*, 10738–45.

Clouse, K. A., Cosentino, L. M., Weih, K. A., Pyle, S. W., Robbins, P. B., Hochstein, H. D., et al. (1991). The HIV-1 gp120 envelope protein has the intrinsic capacity to stimulate monokine secretion. *J Immunol, 147*, 2892–901.

Collins, T., Read, M. A., Neish, A. S., Whitley, M. Z., Thanos, D., & Maniatis, T. (1995). Transcriptional regulation of endothelial cell adhesion molecules: NF-kappa B and cytokine-inducible enhancers. *FASEB J, 9,* 899–909.

Condeelis, J. (1993). Life at the leading edge: The formation of cell protrusions. *Annu Rev Cell Biol, 9,* 411–44.

Connolly, D. T., Stoddard, B. L., Harakas, N. K., & Feder, J. (1987). Human fibroblast-derived growth factor is a mitogen and chemoattractant for endothelial cells. *Biochem Biophys Res Commun, 144,* 705–12.

Corasaniti, M. T., Bagetta, G., Rotiroti, D., & Nistico, G. (1998). The HIV envelope protein gp120 in the nervous system: Interactions with nitric oxide, interleukin-1beta and nerve growth factor signalling, with pathological implications in vivo and in vitro. *Biochem Pharmacol, 56,* 153–6.

Cotter, R., Williams, C., Ryan, L., Erichsen, D., Lopez, A., Peng, H., et al. (2002). Fractalkine (CX3CL1) and brain inflammation: Implications for HIV-1-associated dementia. *J Neurovirol, 8,* 585–98.

Coussens, L. M. & Werb, Z. (2002). Inflammation and cancer. *Nature, 420,* 860–7.

Del Corno, M., Liu, Q. H., Schols, D., De Clercq, E., Gessani, S., Freedman, B. D., et al. (2001). HIV-1 gp120 and chemokine activation of Pyk2 and mitogen-activated protein kinases in primary macrophages mediated by calcium-dependent, pertussis toxin-insensitive chemokine receptor signaling. *Blood, 98,* 2909–16.

Del Sorbo, L., Demartino, A., Biancone, L., Bussolati, B., Conaldi, P. G., Toniolo, A., et al. 1999. The synthesis of platelet-activating factor modulates chemotaxis of monocytes induced by HIV-1 Tat. *Eur J Immunol, 29,* 1513–21.

Dou, H., Birunsingh, K., Faraci, J., Gorantla, S., Poluektova, L. Y., Maggirwar, S. B., et al. (2003). Neuroprotective activities of sodium valproate in a murine model of human immunodeficiency virus-1 encephalitis. *J Neurosci, 23,* 9162–70.

Dou, H., Ellison, B., Bradley, J., Kasiyanov, A., Poluektova, L. Y., Xiong, H., et al. (2005). Neuroprotective mechanisms of lithium in murine human immunodeficiency virus-1 encephalitis. *J Neurosci, 25,* 8375–85.

Dou, H., Grotepas, C. B., McMillan, J. M., Destache, C. J., Chaubal, M., Werling, J., et al. (2009). Macrophage delivery of nanoformulated antiretroviral drug to the brain in a murine model of neuroAIDS. *J Immunol, 183,* 661–9.

Douek, D. (2007). HIV disease progression: immune activation, microbes, and a leaky gut. *Top HIV Med, 15,* 114–7.

Dreyer, E. B., Kaiser, P. K., Offermann, J. T., & Lipton, S. A. 1990. HIV-1 coat protein neurotoxicity prevented by calcium channel antagonists. *Science, 248,* 364–7.

Dugas, N., Lacroix, C., Kilchherr, E., Delfraissy, J. F., & Tardieu, M. (2001). Role of CD23 in astrocytes inflammatory reaction during HIV-1 related encephalitis. *Cytokine, 15,* 96–107.

Eggert, D., Dash, P. K., Serradji, N., Dong, C. Z., Clayette, P., Heymans, F., et al. (2009). Development of a platelet-activating factor antagonist for HIV-1 associated neurocognitive disorders. *J Neuroimmunol, 213,* 47–59.

Ellery, P. J., Tippett, E., Chiu, Y. L., Paukovics, G., Cameron, P. U., Solomon, A., et al. (2007). The CD16+ monocyte subset is more permissive to infection and preferentially harbors HIV-1 in vivo. *J Immunol, 178,* 6581–9.

Emerman, M. (1996). HIV-1, Vpr and the cell cycle. *Curr Biol, 6,* 1096–103.

Erdmann, N., Zhao, J., Lopez, A. L., Herek, S., Curthoys, N., HEXUM, T. D., et al. 2007. Glutamate production by HIV-1 infected human macrophage is blocked by the inhibition of glutaminase. *J Neurochem, 102,* 539–49.

Erichsen, D., Lopez, A. L., Peng, H., Niemann, D., Williams, C., Bauer, M., et al. (2003). Neuronal injury regulates fractalkine: Relevance for HIV-1-associated dementia. *J Neuroimmunol, 138,* 144–55.

Ernst, J. D. (1998). Macrophage receptors for Mycobacterium tuberculosis. *Infect Immun, 66,* 1277–81.

Eugenin, E. A., D'Aversa, T. G., Lopez, L., Calderon, T. M., & Berman, J. W. (2003). MCP-1 (CCL2) protects human neurons and astrocytes from NMDA or HIV-tat-induced apoptosis. *J Neurochem, 85,* 1299–311.

Eugenin, E. A., King, J. E., Nath, A., Calderon, T. M., Zukin, R. S., Bennett, M. V., et al. (2007). HIV-tat induces formation of an LRP-PSD-95-NMDAR-nNOS complex that promotes apoptosis in neurons and astrocytes. *Proc Natl Acad Sci USA, 104,* 3438–43.

Eugenin, E. A., Osiecki, K., Lopez, L., Goldstein, H., Calderson, T. M., & Berman, J. W. (2006). CCL2/monocyte chemoattractant protein-1 mediates enhanced transmigration of human immunodeficiency virus (HIV)-infected leukocytes across the blood-brain barrier: A potential mechanism of HIV-CNS invasion and neuroAIDS. *J Neurosci, 26,* 1098–106.

Everall, I. P., Bell, C., Mallory, M., Langford, D., Adame, A., Rockestein, E., et al. (2002). Lithium ameliorates HIV-gp120-mediated neurotoxicity. *Mol Cell Neurosci, 21,* 493–501.

Everall, I. P., Luthert, P. J., & Lantos, P. L. (1991). Neuronal loss in the frontal cortex in HIV infection. *Lancet, 337,* 1119–21.

Fabriek, B. O., Van Bruggen, R., Deng, D. M., Ligtenberg, A. J., Nazmi, K., Schornagel, K., et al. (2009). The macrophage scavenger receptor CD163 functions as an innate immune sensor for bacteria. *Blood, 113,* 887–92.

Fantuzzi, L., Belardelli, F., & Gessani, S. (2003). Monocyte/macrophage-derived CC chemokines and their modulation by HIV-1 and cytokines: A complex network of interactions influencing viral replication and AIDS pathogenesis. *J Leukoc Biol, 74,* 719–25.

Fantuzzi, L., Canini, I., Belardelli, F., & Gessani, S. (2001). HIV-1 gp120 stimulates the production of beta-chemokines in human peripheral blood monocytes through a CD4-independent mechanism. *J Immunol, 166,* 5381–7.

Fenton, M. J. & Vermeulen, M. W. (1996). Immunopathology of tuberculosis: Roles of macrophages and monocytes. *Infect Immun, 64,* 683–90.

Fiala, M., Rhodes, R. H., Shapshak, P., Nagano, I., Martinez-Maza, O., Diagne, A., et al. (1996). Regulation of HIV-1 infection in astrocytes: expression of Nef, TNF-alpha and IL-6 is enhanced in coculture of astrocytes with macrophages. *J Neurovirol, 2,* 158–66.

Fine, S. M., Angel, R. A., Perry, S. W., Epstein, L. G., Rothstein, J. D., Dewhurst, S., et al. (1996). Tumor necrosis factor alpha inhibits glutamate uptake by primary human astrocytes. Implications for pathogenesis of HIV-1 dementia. *J Biol Chem, 271,* 15303–6.

Fischer-Smith, T., Bell, C., Croul, S., Lewis, M., & Rappaport, J. (2008a). Monocyte/macrophage trafficking in acquired immunodeficiency syndrome encephalitis: Lessons from human and nonhuman primate studies. *J Neurovirol, 14,* 318–26.

Fischer-Smith, T., Croul, S., Sverstiuk, A. E., Capini, C., L'Heureux, D., Regulier, E. G., et al. (2001). CNS invasion by CD14+/CD16+ peripheral blood-derived monocytes in HIV dementia: Perivascular accumulation and reservoir of HIV infection. *J Neurovirol, 7,* 528–41.

Fischer-Smith, T., Tedaldi, E. M., & Rappaport, J. (2008b). CD163/CD16 coexpression by circulating monocytes/macrophages in HIV: potential biomarkers for HIV infection and AIDS progression. *AIDS Res Hum Retroviruses, 24,* 417–21.

Fishman, P. S. & Savitt, J. M. (1989). Selective localization by neuroglia of immunoglobulin G in normal mice. *J Neuropathol Exp Neurol, 48,* 212–20.

Flynn, J. L. & Chan, J. (2001). Immunology of tuberculosis. *Annu Rev Immunol, 19,* 93–129.

Folkman, J. (1995). Seminars in Medicine of the Beth Israel Hospital, Boston. Clinical applications of research on angiogenesis. *N Engl J Med, 333,* 1757–63.

Folkman, J. & Shing, Y. 1992. Angiogenesis. *J Biol Chem, 267,* 10931–4.

Fong, A. M., Erickson, H. P., Zachariah, J. P., Poon, S., Schamberg, N. J., Imai, T., et al. (2000). Ultrastructure and function of the fractalkine mucin domain in CX(3)C chemokine domain presentation. *J Biol Chem, 275,* 3781–6.

Foxman, E. F., Campbell, J. J., & Butcher, E. C. (1997). Multistep navigation and the combinatorial control of leukocyte chemotaxis. *J Cell Biol, 139,* 1349–60.

Fukumura, D., Xavier, R., Sugiura, T., Chen, Y., Park, E. C., Lu, N., et al. (1998). Tumor induction of VEGF promoter activity in stromal cells. *Cell, 94,* 715–25.

Gabuzda, D. & Wang, J. (1999). Chemokine receptors and virus entry in the central nervous system. *J Neurovirol, 5,* 643–58.

Gallo, P., Frei, K., Rordorf, C., Lazdins, J., Tavolato, B., & Fontana, A. (1989). Human immunodeficiency virus type 1 (HIV-1) infection of the central nervous system: An evaluation of cytokines in cerebrospinal fluid. *J Neuroimmunol, 23,* 109–16.

Gehrmann, J., Matsumoto, Y., & Kreutzberg, G. W. (1995). Microglia: Intrinsic immuneffector cell of the brain. *Brain Res Brain Res Rev, 20,* 269–87.

Gelbard, H. A., Dzenko, K. A., Diloreto, D., Del Cerro, C., Del Cerro, M., & Epstein, L. G. (1993). Neurotoxic effects of tumor necrosis factor alpha in primary human neuronal cultures are mediated by activation of the glutamate AMPA receptor subtype: Implications for AIDS neuropathogenesis. *Dev Neurosci, 15,* 417–22.

Graeber, M. B. & Streit, W. J. (1990). Microglia: Immune network in the CNS. *Brain Pathol, 1,* 2–5.

Graeber, M. B., Streit, W. J., & Kreutzberg, G. W. (1988). Axotomy of the rat facial nerve leads to increased CR3 complement receptor expression by activated microglial cells. *J Neurosci Res, 21,* 18–24.

Gruber, M. F., Weih, K. A., Boone, E. J., Smith, P. D., & Clouse, K. A. (1995). Endogenous macrophage CSF production is associated with viral replication in HIV-1-infected human monocyte-derived macrophages. *J Immunol, 154,* 5528–35.

Guillemin, G. J., Croitoru-Lamoury, J., Dormont, D., Armati, P. J., & Brew, B. J. (2003). Quinolinic acid upregulates chemokine production and chemokine receptor expression in astrocytes. *Glia, 41,* 371–81.

Guillemin, G. J., Kerr, S. J., & Brew, B. J. (2005). Involvement of quinolinic acid in AIDS dementia complex. *Neurotox Res, 7,* 103–23.

Haine, V., Fischer-Smith, T., & Rappaport, J. (2006). Macrophage colony-stimulating factor in the pathogenesis of HIV infection: Potential target for therapeutic intervention. *J Neuroimmune Pharmacol, 1,* 32–40.

Hao, A. J., Dheen, S. T., & Ling, E. A. (2002). Expression of macrophage colony-stimulating factor and its receptor in microglia activation is linked to teratogen-induced neuronal damage. *Neuroscience, 112,* 889–900.

Harigai, M., Hara, M., Takahashi, N., Kitani, A., Hirose, T., Suzuki, K., et al. (1992). Presence of autoantibodies to peptidyl-prolyl cis-trans isomerase (cyclosporin A-binding protein) in systemic lupus erythematosus. *Clin Immunol Immunopathol, 63,* 58–65.

Harrison, J. K., Fong, A. M., Swain, P. A., Chen, S., Yu, Y. R., Salafranca, M. N., et al. (2001). Mutational analysis of the fractalkine chemokine domain. Basic amino acid residues differentially contribute to CX3CR1 binding, signaling, and cell adhesion. *J Biol Chem, 276,* 21632–41.

Hart, P. D., Armstrong, J. A., Brown, C. A., & Draper, P. (1972). Ultrastructural study of the behavior of macrophages toward parasitic mycobacteria. *Infect Immun, 5,* 803–7.

Haughey, N. J., Cutler, R. G., Tamara, A., McArthur, J. C., Vargas, D. L., Pardo, C. A., et al. (2004). Perturbation of sphingolipid metabolism and ceramide production in HIV-dementia. *Ann Neurol, 55,* 257–67.

Haughey, N. J., Nath, A., Mattson, M. P., Slevin, J. T., & Geiger, J. D. (2001). HIV-1 Tat through phosphorylation of NMDA receptors potentiates glutamate excitotoxicity. *J Neurochem, 78,* 457–67.

He, J., Chen, Y., Farzan, M., Choe, H., Ohagen, A., Gartner, S., et al. (1997). CCR3 and CCR5 are co-receptors for HIV-1 infection of microglia. *Nature, 385,* 645–9.

Herbein, G. & Varin, A. (2010). The macrophage in HIV-1 infection: From activation to deactivation? *Retrovirology, 7,* 33.

Herrmann, M., Voll, R. E., Zoller, O. M., Hagenhofer, M., Ponner, B. B., & Kalden, J. R. (1998). Impaired phagocytosis of apoptotic cell material by monocyte-derived macrophages from patients with systemic lupus erythematosus. *Arthritis Rheum, 41,* 1241–50.

Hesselgesser, J., Halks-Miller, M., Delvecchio, V., Peiper, S. C., Hoxie, J., Kolson, D. L., et al. (1997). CD4-independent association between HIV-1 gp120 and CXCR4: Functional chemokine receptors are expressed in human neurons. *Curr Biol, 7,* 112–21.

Hesselgesser, J., Taub, D., Baskar, P., Greenberg, M., Hoxie, J., Kolson, D. L. et al. (1998). Neuronal apoptosis induced by HIV-1 gp120 and the chemokine SDF-1 alpha is mediated by the chemokine receptor CXCR4. *Curr Biol, 8,* 595–8.

Heyes, M. P., Brew, B. J., Martin, A., Price, R. W., Salazar, A. M., Sidtis, J. J., et al. (1991). Quinolinic acid in cerebrospinal fluid and serum in HIV-1 infection: Relationship to clinical and neurological status. *Ann Neurol, 29,* 202–9.

Heyes, M. P., Ellis, R. J., Ryan, L., Childers, M. E., Grant, I., Wolfson, T., et al. (2001). Elevated cerebrospinal fluid quinolinic acid levels are associated with region-specific cerebral volume loss in HIV infection. *Brain, 124,* 1033–42.

Hickey, W. F. (2001). Basic principles of immunological surveillance of the normal central nervous system. *Glia, 36,* 118–24.

Horwitz, M. A. (1983). The Legionnaires' disease bacterium (Legionella pneumophila) inhibits phagosome-lysosome fusion in human monocytes. *J Exp Med, 158,* 2108–26.

Horwitz, M. A. (1984). Phagocytosis of the Legionnaires' disease bacterium (Legionella pneumophila) occurs by a novel mechanism: engulfment within a pseudopod coil. *Cell, 36,* 27–33.

Horwitz, M. A. & Maxfield, F. R. (1984). Legionella pneumophila inhibits acidification of its phagosome in human monocytes. *J Cell Biol, 99,* 1936–43.

Horwitz, M. A. & Silverstein, S. C. (1980). Legionnaires' disease bacterium (Legionella pneumophila) multiples intracellularly in human monocytes. *J Clin Invest, 66,* 441–50.

Howard, T. H. & Oresajo, C. O. (1985). The kinetics of chemotactic peptide-induced change in F-actin content, F-actin distribution, and the shape of neutrophils. *J Cell Biol, 101,* 1078–85.

Hunter, M., Wang, Y., Eubank, T., Baran, C., Nana-Sinkam, P., & Marsh, C. (2009). Survival of monocytes and macrophages and their role in health and disease. *Front Biosci, 14,* 4079–102.

Hurwitz, A. A., Lyman, W. D., & Berman, J. W. (1995). Tumor necrosis factor alpha and transforming growth factor beta upregulate astrocyte expression of monocyte chemoattractant protein-1. *J Neuroimmunol, 57,* 193–8.

Janabi, N., Chabrier, S., & Tardieu, M. (1996). Endogenous nitric oxide activates prostaglandin F2 alpha production in human microglial cells but not in astrocytes: A study of interactions between eicosanoids, nitric oxide, and superoxide anion (O2-) regulatory pathways. *J Immunol, 157,* 2129–35.

Janabi, N., Hau, I., & Tardieu, M. (1999). Negative feedback between prostaglandin and alpha- and beta-chemokine synthesis in human microglial cells and astrocytes. *J Immunol, 162,* 1701–6.

Jaworowski, A., Kamwendo, D. D., Ellery, P., Sonza, S., Mwapasa, V., Tadesse, E., et al. (2007). CD16+ monocyte subset preferentially harbors HIV-1 and is expanded in pregnant Malawian women with Plasmodium falciparum malaria and HIV-1 infection. *J Infect Dis, 196,* 38–42.

Jiang, Z. G., Piggee, C., Heyes, M. P., Murphy, C., Quearry, B., Bauer, M., et al. (2001). Glutamate is a mediator of neurotoxicity in secretions of activated HIV-1-infected macrophages. *J Neuroimmunol, 117,* 97–107.

Jones, G. J., Barsby, N. L., Cohen, E. A., Holden, J., Harris, K., Dickie, P., et al. (2007). HIV-1 Vpr causes neuronal apoptosis and in vivo neurodegeneration. *J Neurosci, 27,* 3703–11.

Jones, M. V., Bell, J. E., & Nath, A. (2000). Immunolocalization of HIV envelope gp120 in HIV encephalitis with dementia. *AIDS, 14,* 2709–13.

Kaul, M. & Lipton, S. A. (1999). Chemokines and activated macrophages in HIV gp120-induced neuronal apoptosis. *Proc Natl Acad Sci USA, 96,* 8212–6.

Kelder, W., McArthur, J. C., Nance-Sproson, T., McClernon, D., & Griffin, D. E. (1998). Beta-chemokines MCP-1 and RANTES are selectively increased in cerebrospinal fluid of patients with human immunodeficiency virus-associated dementia. *Ann Neurol, 44,* 831–5.

Kelly, C. P., Keates, S., Siegenberg, D., Linevsky, J. K., Pothoulakis, C., & Brady, H. R. (1994). IL-8 secretion and neutrophil activation by HT-29 colonic epithelial cells. *Am J Physiol, 267,* G991–7.

Kerr, S. J., Armati, P. J., Pemberton, L. A., Smythe, G., Tattam, B., & Brew, B. J. (1997). Kynurenine pathway inhibition reduces neurotoxicity of HIV-1-infected macrophages. *Neurology, 49,* 1671–81.

Ketzler, S., Weis, S., Haug, H., & Budka, H. (1990). Loss of neurons in the frontal cortex in AIDS brains. *Acta Neuropathol, 80,* 92–4.

Kinne, R. W., Stuhlmuller, B., & Burmester, G. R. (2007). Cells of the synovium in rheumatoid arthritis. Macrophages. *Arthritis Res Ther, 9,* 224.

Kozak, S. L., Platt, E. J., Madani, N., Ferro, F. E., Jr., Peden, K., & Kabat, D. (1997). CD4, CXCR-4, and CCR-5 dependencies for infections by primary patient and laboratory-adapted isolates of human immunodeficiency virus type 1. *J Virol, 71,* 873–82.

Kreutzberg, G. W. (1996). Microglia: A sensor for pathological events in the CNS. *Trends Neurosci, 19,* 312–8.

Kruman, II, Nath, A., & Mattson, M. P. (1998). HIV-1 protein Tat induces apoptosis of hippocampal neurons by a mechanism involving caspase activation, calcium overload, and oxidative stress. *Exp Neurol, 154,* 276–88.

Lafrenie, R. M., Wahl, L. M., Epstein, J. S., Yamada, K. M., & Dhawan, S. (1997). Activation of monocytes by HIV-Tat treatment is mediated by cytokine expression. *J Immunol, 159,* 4077–83.

Lannuzel, A., Lledo, P. M., Lamghitnia, H. O., Vincent, J. D., & Tardieu, M. (1995). HIV-1 envelope proteins gp120 and gp160 potentiate NMDA-induced [Ca2+]i increase, alter [Ca2+]i homeostasis and induce neurotoxicity in human embryonic neurons. *Eur J Neurosci, 7,* 2285–93.

Lauffenburger, D. A. & Horwitz, A. F. (1996). Cell migration: A physically integrated molecular process. *Cell, 84,* 359–69.

Lawson, L. J., Perry, V. H., Dri, P., & Gordon, S. (1990). Heterogeneity in the distribution and morphology of microglia in the normal adult mouse brain. *Neuroscience, 39,* 151–70.

Lee, C., Tomkowicz, B., Freedman, B. D., & Collman, R. G. (2005). HIV-1 gp120-induced TNF-{alpha} production by primary human macrophages is mediated by phosphatidylinositol-3 (PI-3) kinase and mitogen-activated protein (MAP) kinase pathways. *J Leukoc Biol, 78,* 1016–23.

Lee, S. J., Hou, J., & Benveniste, E. N. (1998). Transcriptional regulation of intercellular adhesion molecule-1 in astrocytes involves NF-kappaB and C/EBP isoforms. *J Neuroimmunol, 92,* 196–207.

Lehmann, M. H., Masanetz, S., Kramer, S., & Erfle, V. (2006). HIV-1 Nef upregulates CCL2/MCP-1 expression in astrocytes in a myristoylation- and calmodulin-dependent manner. *J Cell Sci, 119,* 4520–30.

Letendre, S. L., Lanier, E. R., & McCutchan, J. A. (1999). Cerebrospinal fluid beta chemokine concentrations in neurocognitively impaired individuals infected with human immunodeficiency virus type 1. *J Infect Dis, 180,* 310–9.

Li, G., Hangoc, G., & Broxmeyer, H. E. (2004). Interleukin-10 in combination with M-CSF and IL-4 contributes to development of the rare population of CD14+CD16++ cells derived from human monocytes. *Biochem Biophys Res Commun, 322,* 637–43.

Li, W., Huang, Y., Reid, R., Steiner, J., Malpica-Llanos, T., Darden, T. A., et al. 2008. NMDA receptor activation by HIV-Tat protein is clade dependent. *J Neurosci, 28,* 12190–8.

Lipton, S. A. (1992). Memantine prevents HIV coat protein-induced neuronal injury in vitro. *Neurology, 42,* 1403–1405.

Lipton, S. A. (1994). Neuronal injury associated with HIV-1 and potential treatment with calcium-channel and NMDA antagonists. *Dev Neurosci, 16,* 145–51.

Liu, X., Jana, M., Dasgupta, S., Koka, S., He, J., Wood, C., et al. (2002). Human immunodeficiency virus type 1 (HIV-1) tat induces nitric-oxide synthase in human astroglia. *J Biol Chem, 277,* 39312–9.

Lodish, H. F. (2008). *Molecular cell biology,* New York, W.H. Freeman.

Malik, M., Chen, Y. Y., Kienzle, M. F., Tomkowicz, B. E., Collman, R. G., & Ptasznik, A. (2008). Monocyte migration and LFA-1-mediated attachment to brain microvascular endothelia is regulated by SDF-1 alpha through Lyn kinase. *J Immunol, 181,* 4632–7.

Marra, A., Horwitz, M. A., & Shuman, H. A. (1990). The HL-60 model for the interaction of human macrophages with the Legionnaires' disease bacterium. *J Immunol, 144,* 2738–44.

Mattson, M. P., Haughey, N. J., & Nath, A. (2005). Cell death in HIV dementia. *Cell Death Differ,* 12 Suppl 1, 893–904.

Meucci, O. & Miller, R. J. (1996). gp120-induced neurotoxicity in hippocampal pyramidal neuron cultures: protective action of TGF-beta1. *J Neurosci, 16,* 4080–8.

Miagkov, A., Turchan, J., Nath, A., & Drachman, D. B. (2004). Gene transfer of baculoviral p35 by adenoviral vector protects human cerebral neurons from apoptosis. *DNA Cell Biol, 23,* 496–501.

Milligan, C. E., Levitt, P., & Cunningham, T. J. (1991). Brain macrophages and microglia respond differently to lesions of the developing and adult visual system. *J Comp Neurol, 314,* 136–46.

Mitrasinovic, O. M., Grattan, A., Robinson, C. C., LaPustea, N. B., Poon, C., Ryan, H., et al. (2005). Microglia overexpressing the macrophage colony-stimulating factor receptor are neuroprotective in a microglial-hippocampal organotypic coculture system. *J Neurosci, 25,* 4442–51.

Moller, T., Hanisch, U. K., & Ransom, B. R. (2000). Thrombin-induced activation of cultured rodent microglia. *J Neurochem, 75,* 1539–47.

Monier, A., Adle-Biassette, H., Delezoide, A. L., Evrad, P., Gressens, P., & Verney, C. (2007). Entry and distribution of microglial cells in human embryonic and fetal cerebral cortex. *J Neuropathol Exp Neurol, 66,* 372–82.

Mulherin, D., Fitzgerald, O., & Bresnihan, B. (1996). Synovial tissue macrophage populations and articular damage in rheumatoid arthritis. *Arthritis Rheum, 39,* 115–24.

Nath, A., Haughey, N. J., Jones, M., Anderson, C., Bell, J. E., & Geiger, J. D. (2000). Synergistic neurotoxicity by human immunodeficiency virus proteins Tat and gp120: Protection by memantine. *Ann Neurol, 47,* 186–94.

Nestle, F. O., Di Meglio, P., Qin, J. Z., & Nickoloff, B. J. (2009). Skin immune sentinels in health and disease. *Nat Rev Immunol, 9,* 679–91.

Nicolini, A., Ajmone-Cat, M. A., Bernado, A., Levi, G., & Minghetti, L. (2001). Human immunodeficiency virus type-1 Tat protein induces nuclear factor (NF)-kappaB activation and oxidative stress in microglial cultures by independent mechanisms. *J Neurochem, 79,* 713–6.

Nottet, H. S., Flanagan, E. M., Flanagan, C. R., Gelbard, H. A., Gendelman, H. E., & Reinhard, J. F., Jr. (1996). The regulation of quinolinic acid in human immunodeficiency virus-infected monocytes. *J Neurovirol, 2,* 111–7.

Nowacek, A. S., McMillan, J., Miller, R., Anderson, A., Rabinow, B., & Gendelman, H. E. (2010). Nanoformulated antiretroviral drug combinations extend drug release and antiretroviral responses in HIV-1-infected macrophages: Implications for neuroAIDS therapeutics. *J Neuroimmune Pharmacol.*

Nowacek, A. S., Miller, R. L., McMillan, J., Kanmogne, G., Kanmogne, M., Mosley, R. L., et al. (2009). NanoART synthesis, characterization, uptake, release and toxicology for human monocyte-macrophage drug delivery. *Nanomedicine (Lond), 4,* 903–17.

Nuovo, G. J. & Alfieri, M. L. (1996). AIDS dementia is associated with massive, activated HIV-1 infection and concomitant expression of several cytokines. *Mol Med, 2,* 358–66.

Ohagen, A., Ghosh, S., He, J., Huang, K., Chen, Y., Yuan, M., et al. (1999). Apoptosis induced by infection of primary brain cultures with diverse human immunodeficiency virus type 1 isolates: Evidence for a role of the envelope. *J Virol, 73,* 897–906.

Patel, C. A., Mukhtar, M., & Pomerantz, R. J. (2000). Human immunodeficiency virus type 1 Vpr induces apoptosis in human neuronal cells. *J Virol, 74,* 9717–26.

Patton, H. K., Zhou, Z. H., Bubien, J. K., Benveniste, E. N., & Benos, D. J. (2000). gp120-induced alterations of human astrocyte function: Na(+)/H(+) exchange, K(+) conductance, and glutamate flux. *Am J Physiol Cell Physiol, 279,* C700–8.

Pemberton, L. A., Kerr, S. J., Smythe, G., & Brew, B. J. (1997). Quinolinic acid production by macrophages stimulated with IFN-gamma, TNF-alpha, and IFN-alpha. *J Interferon Cytokine Res, 17*, 589–95.

Peng, H., Erdmann, N., Whitney, N., Dou, H., Gorantla, S., Gendelman, H. E., et al. (2006). HIV-1-infected and/or immune activated macrophages regulate astrocyte SDF-1 production through IL-1beta. *Glia, 54*, 619–29.

Persidsky, Y. & Gendelman, H. E. (2003). Mononuclear phagocyte immunity and the neuropathogenesis of HIV-1 infection. *J Leukoc Biol, 74*, 691–701.

Persidsky, Y., Ghorpade, A., Rasmussen, J., Limoges, J., Liu, X. J., Stins, M., et al. (1999). Microglial and astrocyte chemokines regulate monocyte migration through the blood-brain barrier in human immunodeficiency virus-1 encephalitis. *Am J Pathol, 155*, 1599–611.

Peudenier, S., Hery, C., Montagnier, L., & Tardieu, M. (1991). Human microglial cells: Characterization in cerebral tissue and in primary culture, and study of their susceptibility to HIV-1 infection. *Ann Neurol, 29*, 152–61.

Pizon, V., Desjardins, M., Bucci, C., Parton, R. G., & Zerial, M. (1994). Association of Rap1a and Rap1b proteins with late endocytic/phagocytic compartments and Rap2a with the Golgi complex. *J Cell Sci, 107* (Pt 6), 1661–70.

Pocernich, C. B., Sultana, R., Mohmmad-Abdul, H., Nath, A., & Butterfield, D. A. (2005). HIV-dementia, Tat-induced oxidative stress, and antioxidant therapeutic considerations. *Brain Res Brain Res Rev, 50*, 14–26.

Polazzi, E., Levi, G., & Minghetti, L. (1999). Human immunodeficiency virus type 1 Tat protein stimulates inducible nitric oxide synthase expression and nitric oxide production in microglial cultures. *J Neuropathol Exp Neurol, 58*, 825–31.

Pollard, J. W. (2009). Trophic macrophages in development and disease. *Nat Rev Immunol, 9*, 259–70.

Pu, H., Tian, J., Flora, G., Lee, Y. W., Nath, A., Hennig, B., et al. (2003). HIV-1 Tat protein upregulates inflammatory mediators and induces monocyte invasion into the brain. *Mol Cell Neurosci, 24*, 224–37.

Pulliam, L., Gascon, R., Stubblebine, M., McGuire, D., & McGrath, M. S. (1997). Unique monocyte subset in patients with AIDS dementia. *Lancet, 349*, 692–5.

Rich, E. A., Chen, I. S., Zack, J. A., Leonard, M. L., & O'Brien, W. A. (1992). Increased susceptibility of differentiated mononuclear phagocytes to productive infection with human immunodeficiency virus-1 (HIV-1). *J Clin Invest, 89*, 176–83.

Rom, I., Deshmane, S. L., Mukerjee, R., Khalili, K., Amini, S., & Sawaya, B. E. (2009). HIV-1 Vpr deregulates calcium secretion in neural cells. *Brain Res, 1275*, 81–6.

Rostasy, K., Egles, C., Chauhan, A., Kneissl, M., Bahrani, P., Yiannoutsos, C., et al. (2003). SDF-1alpha is expressed in astrocytes and neurons in the AIDS dementia complex: An in vivo and in vitro study. *J Neuropathol Exp Neurol, 62*, 617–26.

Rostasy, K., Monti, L., Yiannoutsos, C., Kneissl, M., Bell, J., Kemper, T. L., et al. (1999). Human immunodeficiency virus infection, inducible nitric oxide synthase expression, and microglial activation: Pathogenetic relationship to the acquired immunodeficiency syndrome dementia complex. *Ann Neurol, 46*, 207–16.

Russell, D. G. (2001). Mycobacterium tuberculosis: Here today, and here tomorrow. *Nat Rev Mol Cell Biol, 2*, 569–77.

Saito, Y., Sharer, L. R., Epstein, L. G., Michaels, J., Mintz, M., Louder, M., et al. (1994). Overexpression of nef as a marker for restricted HIV-1 infection of astrocytes in postmortem pediatric central nervous tissues. *Neurology, 44*, 474–81.

Sang, N. & Chen, C. (2006). Lipid signaling and synaptic plasticity. *Neuroscientist, 12*, 425–34.

Scheuerer, B., Ernst, M., Durrbaum-Landmann, I., Fleischer, J., Grage-Greibenow, E., Brandt, E., et al. (2000). The CXC-chemokine platelet factor 4 promotes monocyte survival and induces monocyte differentiation into macrophages. *Blood, 95*, 1158–66.

Schifitto, G., Navia, B. A., Yiannoutsos, C. T., Marra, C. M., Chang, L., Ernst, T., et al. (2007). Memantine and HIV-associated cognitive impairment: a neuropsychological and proton magnetic resonance spectroscopy study. *AIDS, 21*, 1877–86.

Schifitto, G., Peterson, D. R., Zhong, J., Ni, H., Cruttenden, K., Gaugh, M., Gendelman, H. E., et al. (2006). Valproic acid adjunctive therapy for HIV-associated cognitive impairment: A first report. *Neurology, 66*, 919–21.

Schlesinger, L. S. (1993). Macrophage phagocytosis of virulent but not attenuated strains of Mycobacterium tuberculosis is mediated by mannose receptors in addition to complement receptors. *J Immunol, 150*, 2920–30.

Schlesinger, L. S., Bellinger-Kawahara, C. G., Payne, N. R., & Horwitz, M. A. (1990). Phagocytosis of Mycobacterium tuberculosis is mediated by human monocyte complement receptors and complement component C3. *J Immunol, 144*, 2771–80.

Schnabel, A., Csernok, E., Isenberg, D. A., Mrowka, C., & Gross, W. L. (1995). Antineutrophil cytoplasmic antibodies in systemic lupus erythematosus. Prevalence, specificities, and clinical significance. *Arthritis Rheum, 38*, 633–7.

Schorey, J. S., Carroll, M. C., & Brown, E. J. (1997). A macrophage invasion mechanism of pathogenic mycobacteria. *Science, 277*, 1091–3.

Sei, S., Saito, K., Stewart, S. K., Crowley, J. S., Brouwers, P., KLEINER, D. E., et al. (1995). Increased human immunodeficiency virus (HIV) type 1 DNA content and quinolinic acid concentration in brain tissues from patients with HIV encephalopathy. *J Infect Dis, 172*, 638–47.

Shiramizu, B., Gartner, S., Williams, A., Shikuma, C., Ratto-Kim, S., Watters, M., et al. (2005). Circulating proviral HIV DNA and HIV-associated dementia. *AIDS, 19*, 45–52.

Shuman, H. A. & Horwitz, M. A. (1996). Legionella pneumophila invasion of mononuclear phagocytes. *Bacterial Invasiveness, 209*, 99–112.

Si, Q., Cosenza, M., Kim, M. O., Zhao, M. L., Brownlee, M., GOLDSTEIN, H., et al. (2004). A novel action of minocycline: Inhibition of human immunodeficiency virus type 1 infection in microglia. *J Neurovirol, 10*, 284–92.

Singh, I. N., Goody, R. J., Dean, C., Ahmad, N. M., Lutz, S. E., Knapp, P. E., et al. (2004). Apoptotic death of striatal neurons induced by human immunodeficiency virus-1 Tat and gp120: Differential involvement of caspase-3 and endonuclease G. *J Neurovirol, 10*, 141–51.

Smeets, T. J., Kraan, M. C., Galjaard, S., Youssef, P. P., Smith, M. D., & Tak, P. P. (2001). Analysis of the cell infiltrate and expression of matrix metalloproteinases and granzyme B in paired synovial biopsy specimens from the cartilage-pannus junction in patients with RA. *Ann Rheum Dis, 60*, 561–5.

Smith, D. G., Guillemin, G. J., Pemberton, L., Kerr, S., Nath, A., Smythe, G. A. et al. (2001). Quinolinic acid is produced by macrophages stimulated by platelet activating factor, Nef and Tat. *J Neurovirol, 7*, 56–60.

Song, L., Nath, A., Geiger, J. D., Moore, A., & Hochman, S. (2003). Human immunodeficiency virus type 1 Tat protein directly activates neuronal N-methyl-D-aspartate receptors at an allosteric zinc-sensitive site. *J Neurovirol, 9*, 399–403.

Stossel, T. P. (1993). On the crawling of animal cells. *Science, 260*, 1086–94.

Streit, W. J. (2001). Microglia and macrophages in the developing CNS. *Neurotoxicology, 22*, 619–24.

Streit, W. J. & Xue, Q. S. (2009). Life and death of microglia. *J Neuroimmune Pharmacol, 4*, 371–9.

Strieter, R. M., Wiggins, R., Phan, S. H., Wharram, B. L., Showell, H. J., Remick, D. G., et al. (1989). Monocyte chemotactic protein gene expression by cytokine-treated human fibroblasts and endothelial cells. *Biochem Biophys Res Commun, 162*, 694–700.

Sturgill-Koszycki, S., Schlesinger, P. H., Chakraborty, P., Haddix, P. L., Collins, H. L., Fok, A. K., et al. (1994). Lack of acidification in Mycobacterium phagosomes produced by exclusion of the vesicular proton-ATPase. *Science, 263*, 678–81.

Subbramanian, R. A., Kessous-Elbaz, A., Lodge, R., Forget, J., Yao, X. J., Bergeron, D., et al. (1998). Human immunodeficiency virus type 1 Vpr is a positive regulator of viral transcription and infectivity in primary human macrophages. *J Exp Med, 187*, 1103–11.

Sulahian, T. H., Hogger, P., Wahner, A. E., Wardwell, K., Goulding, N. J., Sorg, C., et al. (2000). Human monocytes express CD163, which is upregulated by IL-10 and identical to p155. *Cytokine, 12,* 1312–21.

Suttles, J. & Stout, R. D. (2009). Macrophage CD40 signaling: A pivotal regulator of disease protection and pathogenesis. *Semin Immunol, 21,* 257–64.

Swanson, J. A. & Baer, S. C. (1995). Phagocytosis by zippers and triggers. *Trends Cell Biol, 5,* 89–93.

Swanson, M. S. & Isberg, R. R. (1995). Association of Legionella pneumophila with the macrophage endoplasmic reticulum. *Infect Immun, 63,* 3609–20.

Tak, P. P. & Bresnihan, B. (2000). The pathogenesis and prevention of joint damage in rheumatoid arthritis: Advances from synovial biopsy and tissue analysis. *Arthritis Rheum, 43,* 2619–33.

Tambuyzer, B. R., Ponsaerts, P., & Nouwen, E. J. (2009). Microglia: Gatekeepers of central nervous system immunology. *J Leukoc Biol, 85,* 352–70.

Tardieu, M. & Boutet, A. (2002). HIV-1 and the central nervous system. *Curr Top Microbiol Immunol, 265,* 183–95.

Toborek, M., Lee, Y. W., Pu, H., Malecki, A., Flora, G., Garrido, R., et al. (2003). HIV-Tat protein induces oxidative and inflammatory pathways in brain endothelium. *J Neurochem, 84,* 169–79.

Tong, N., Perry, S. W., Zhang, Q., James, H. J., Guo, H., Brooks, A., et al. (2000). Neuronal fractalkine expression in HIV-1 encephalitis: Roles for macrophage recruitment and neuroprotection in the central nervous system. *J Immunol, 164,* 1333–9.

Tornatore, C., Chandra, R., Berger, J. R., & Major, E. O. (1994). HIV-1 infection of subcortical astrocytes in the pediatric central nervous system. *Neurology, 44,* 481–7.

Town, T., Nikolic, V., & Tan, J. (2005). The microglial "activation" continuum: from innate to adaptive responses. *J Neuroinflammation, 2,* 24.

Tracey, D., Klareskog, L., Sasso, E. H., Salfeld, J. G., & Tak, P. P. (2008). Tumor necrosis factor antagonist mechanisms of action: A comprehensive review. *Pharmacol Ther, 117,* 244–79.

Turchan-Cholewo, J., Dimayuga, V. M., Gupta, S., Gorospe, R. M., Keller, J. N., & Bruce-Keller, A. J. (2009). NADPH oxidase drives cytokine and neurotoxin release from microglia and macrophages in response to HIV-Tat. *Antioxid Redox Signal, 11,* 193–204.

Tyor, W. R., Glass, J. D., Griffin, J. W., Becker, P. S., McArthur, J. C., Bezman, L., et al. (1992). Cytokine expression in the brain during the acquired immunodeficiency syndrome. *Ann Neurol, 31,* 349–60.

Van Crevel, R., Ottenhoff, T. H., & Van der Meer, J. W. (2002). Innate immunity to Mycobacterium tuberculosis. *Clin Microbiol Rev, 15,* 294–309.

Van Furth, R. (1982). Current view on the mononuclear phagocyte system. *Immunobiology, 161,* 178–85.

Vincent, V. A., De Groot, C. J., Lucassen, P. J., Portegies, P., Troost, D., Tilders, F. J., et al. 1999. Nitric oxide synthase expression and apoptotic cell death in brains of AIDS and AIDS dementia patients. *AIDS, 13,* 317–26.

Vincent, V. A., Selwood, S. P., & Murphy, G. M., Jr. (2002). Proinflammatory effects of M-CSF and A beta in hippocampal organotypic cultures. *Neurobiol Aging, 23,* 349–62.

Vitkovic, L., Maeda, S., & Sternberg, E. (2001). Anti-inflammatory cytokines: Expression and action in the brain. *Neuroimmunomodulation, 9,* 295–312.

Viviani, B., Corsini, E., Binaglia, M., Galli, C. L., & Marinovich, M. (2001). Reactive oxygen species generated by glia are responsible for neuron death induced by human immunodeficiency virus-glycoprotein 120 in vitro. *Neuroscience, 107,* 51–8.

Vogel, J. P., Andrews, H. L., Wong, S. K., & Isberg, R. R. (1998). Conjugative transfer by the virulence system of Legionella pneumophila. *Science, 279,* 873–6.

Wang, H., Sun, J., & Goldstein, H. (2008). Human immunodeficiency virus type 1 infection increases the in vivo capacity of peripheral monocytes to cross the blood-brain barrier into the brain and the in vivo sensitivity of the blood-brain barrier to disruption by lipopolysaccharide. *J Virol, 82,* 7591–600.

Wang, J., Roderiquez, G., Oravecz, T., & Norcross, M. A. 1998. Cytokine regulation of human immunodeficiency virus type 1 entry and replication in human monocytes/macrophages through modulation of CCR5 expression. *J Virol, 72,* 7642–7.

Wang, X., Zhu, S., Drozda, M., Zhang, W., Stavrovskaya, I. G., Cattaneo, E., et al. (2003a). Minocycline inhibits caspase-independent and -dependent mitochondrial cell death pathways in models of Huntington's disease. *Proc Natl Acad Sci USA, 100,* 10483–7.

Wang, Z., Pekarskaya, O., Bencheikh, M., Chao, W., Gelbard, H. A., Ghorpade, A., et al. (2003b). Reduced expression of glutamate transporter EAAT2 and impaired glutamate transport in human primary astrocytes exposed to HIV-1 or gp120. *Virology, 312,* 60–73.

Wilkinson, P. C. (1986). The locomotor capacity of human lymphocytes and its enhancement by cell growth. *Immunology, 57,* 281–9.

Winkler, M. K. & Beveniste, E. N. (1998). Transforming growth factor-beta inhibition of cytokine-induced vascular cell adhesion molecule-1 expression in human astrocytes. *Glia, 22,* 171–9.

Xu, Y., Kulkosky, J., Acheampong, E., Nunnari, G., Sullivan, J., & Pomerantz, R. J. (2004). HIV-1-mediated apoptosis of neuronal cells: Proximal molecular mechanisms of HIV-1-induced encephalopathy. *Proc Natl Acad Sci U S A, 101,* 7070–5.

Yeung, M. C., Pulliam, L., & Lau, A. S. (1995). The HIV envelope protein gp120 is toxic to human brain-cell cultures through the induction of interleukin-6 and tumor necrosis factor-alpha. *AIDS, 9,* 137–43.

Yoshioka, N., Taniguchi, Y., Yoshida, A., Nakata, K., Nishizawa, T., Inagawa, H., et al. (2009). Intestinal macrophages involved in the homeostasis of the intestine have the potential for responding to LPS. *Anticancer Res, 29,* 4861–5.

Yu, W., Ramakrishnan, R., Wang, Y., Chiang, K., Sung, T. L., & Rice, A. P. (2008). Cyclin T1-dependent genes in activated CD4 T and macrophage cell lines appear enriched in HIV-1 co-factors. *PLoS One, 3,* e3146.

Zauli, G., Davis, B. R., Re, M. C., Visani, G., Furlini, G., & La Placa, M. (1992). tat protein stimulates production of transforming growth factor-beta 1 by marrow macrophages: A potential mechanism for human immunodeficiency virus-1-induced hematopoietic suppression. *Blood, 80,* 3036–43.

Zauli, G., Furlini, G., Re, M. C., Milani, D., Capitani, S., & La Placa, M. (1993). Human immunodeficiency virus type 1 (HIV-1) tat-protein stimulates the production of interleukin-6 (IL-6) by peripheral blood monocytes. *New Microbiol, 16,* 115–20.

Zhao, M. L., Kim, M. O., Morgello, S., & Lee, S. C. (2001). Expression of inducible nitric oxide synthase, interleukin-1 and caspase-1 in HIV-1 encephalitis. *J Neuroimmunol, 115,* 182–91.

Zhou, H., LaPointe, B. M., Clark, S. R., Zbytnuik, L., & Kubes, P. (2006). A requirement for microglial TLR4 in leukocyte recruitment into brain in response to lipopolysaccharide. *J Immunol, 177,* 8103–10.

Zink, M. C., Uhrlaub, J., DeWitt, J., Voelker, T., Bullock, B., Mankowski, J., et al. (2005). Neuroprotective and anti-human immunodeficiency virus activity of minocycline. *JAMA, 293,* 2003–11.

4.2

NEUROTOXICITY OF HIV-1 PROTEINS

Manja Meggendorfer, Ina Rothenaigner, Bianca Tigges,
Michelle Vincendeau, and Ruth Brack-Werner

Numerous experimental studies indicate that HIV proteins have the capacity to injure neurons and thus may contribute to neuronal demise in the brains of HIV-infected individuals. Potentially neurotoxic viral proteins include the envelope proteins (gp120 and gp41), Vpr, Tat, and Nef. In this section we will first give a brief general overview of the possible sources of neurotoxic HIV proteins in the brain, the experimental models used to study their neurotoxicity, and current concepts of the contributions of these viral proteins to neuronal injury. In the second section we will discuss the experimental evidence supporting neurotoxic activities of the individual HIV proteins indicated above in more detail and summarize recent developments.

POTENTIAL SOURCES OF HIV PROTEINS IN THE BRAIN

PRODUCTION OF NEUROTOXIC HIV PROTEINS BY INFECTED BRAIN CELLS

HIV can enter the brain early after systemic infection. Once in the brain, HIV can infect various cell types that permit HIV replication to different extents (reviewed in Kramer-Hammerle, Rothenaigner, Wolff, Bell, & Brack-Werner, 2005b). Production of infectious HIV particles is apparent mainly in brain macrophages and microglial cells. Thus, infected macrophages/microglial cells are potential sources of the neurotoxic HIV proteins Env and Vpr, which are contained in virus particles.

HIV can also enter and persist in astrocytes and recent studies indicate that *in vivo* infection of astrocytes may be more frequent than previously anticipated (Churchill et al., 2009). Productive HIV infection is only rarely detected in astrocytes, especially during long-term HIV infection, and astrocytes possess powerful mechanisms for restriction of HIV production (reviewed in Brack-Werner, 1999; Gorry et al., 2003; Kramer-Hammerle et al., 2005b). Nevertheless, astrocytes can express viral gene products normally generated in the early phase of HIV replication while blocking production of new virus particles. This infection phenotype has been referred to as "blocked early-stage latency" and can also occur in peripheral blood cells (Seshamma, Bagasra, Trono, Baltimore, & Pomerantz, 1992). The viral proteins produced during blocked early-stage latency include Tat and Nef, indicating that infected astrocytes can

contribute to the burden of these neurotoxic proteins in the brain.

Recently, evidence has accumulated that HIV-1 may also invade and persist in neural progenitor cell (NPC) populations (Lawrence et al., 2004; Rothenaigner et al., 2007; Schwartz et al., 2007; Schwartz & Major, 2006). HIV persistence was associated with long-term moderate production and release of HIV particles, followed by gradual virus shut down (Rothenaigner et al., 2007).

Finally, a few studies analyzing either brain tissue specimens from HIV-infected individuals or cultured cells exposed to HIV also reported detection of HIV markers in brain microvascular endothelial cells (BMVECs), mature neurons, and oligodendrocytes (reviewed in Kramer-Hammerle et al., 2005b). However, the majority of such studies did not observe evidence for HIV infection of these cells. Therefore, the current concept is that these cells are not infected by HIV and therefore do not produce neurotoxic HIV proteins. Still, it should be pointed out that the current data does not permit the definite exclusion of BMVECs, neurons, and oligodendrocytes as HIV targets in the brain.

ENTRY OF NEUROTOXIC HIV PROTEINS FROM PERIPHERAL SITES OF INFECTION INTO THE BRAIN

Infected cells can release the viral proteins gp120 (Cashion, Banks, Bost, & Kastin, 1999) and Tat (Banks, Robinson, & Nath, 2005). Both proteins can cross an intact blood-brain barrier. In addition, they may contribute to the breakdown of the blood-brain barrier (Kanmogne, Primeaux, & Grammas, 2005; Price, Uras, Banks, & Ercal, 2006), facilitating their access to the brain. This raises the possibility that these neurotoxic HIV proteins may enter the brain from peripheral sites of virus production and damage neurons.

GENERAL FEATURES OF HIV NEUROTOXICITY

PATHOLOGICAL MANIFESTATION OF HIV-ASSOCIATED NEURONAL DAMAGE

Visible signs of neuronal damage in the brains of HIV-infected individuals are selective neuronal loss (Everall,

Luthert, & Lantos, 1993) and decrease of dendritic and synaptic densities (Ellis, Langford, & Masliah, 2007). In addition, neuroinflammation is a prominent feature associated with HIV-1 infection and can occur in the absence of productive HIV infection (Anthony & Bell, 2008; Gartner, 2000). Neuroinflammation is apparent as activation of brain macrophages/microglia; infiltration of leukocytes, particularly monocytes; and reactive astrocytosis. Surprisingly, brain samples from individuals effectively treated with HAART (highly active antiretroviral therapy) also show ongoing neuroinflammation and increased presence of neurodegenerative proteins. Indeed, the level of neuroinflammation apparent as microglial activation in HAART-treated individuals is comparable to that detected in untreated AIDS patients (Anthony & Bell, 2008). This indicates that even efficient antiretroviral therapies are not able to prevent chronic neuroinflammation in HIV-infected individuals. Interestingly, neuroinflammation is also a hallmark of neurodegenerative diseases like Alzheimer's and there are overlaps in the host factors implicated in both HIV-associated neuronal injury and neurodegenerative diseases (Brew, Crowe, Landay, Cysique, & Guillemin, 2009; Jayadev & Garden, 2009; Ting, Brew, & Guillemin, 2009). This raises the possibility that detrimental effects of HIV infection may also promote neurodegenerative diseases and vice-versa.

caused by the exposure of neurons to toxic factors in their microenvironment rather than by direct HIV infection. Two nonexclusive general hypotheses have been proposed to explain HIV-1-induced neuronal injury (Kaul, 2008). The first hypothesis proposes neuronal demise to be a consequence of the direct exposure of neurons and neuronal progenitor cells to HIV proteins, mainly Env proteins, Vpr, Tat, and Nef. The second hypothesis proposes that neuronal damage is caused by the responses of non-neuronal cells (e.g., macrophages, glial cells, and astrocytes) to HIV. Thus HIV-infected macrophages, microglial cells, and astrocytes have been shown to secrete a plethora of factors that may contribute to neuronal damage (Gonzalez-Scarano & Martin-Garcia, 2005). In addition, exposure to HIV proteins can induce uninfected brain cells to produce factors that contribute to neuronal damage by various means (for examples, see Table 4.2.1). In general, the mechanisms of neuronal injury are complex, involving the interplay of numerous effector molecules (see Fig. 4.2.1). Furthermore, appearance of HIV-associated neurocognitive disturbances in only a subset of HIV-infected individuals suggests that the risk of neuronal injury is also influenced by factors associated with the age, metabolism, genetic predisposition, and co-morbid conditions of the infected individual as well as the characteristics of the viral genotypes (Jayadev & Garden, 2009).

CURRENT CONCEPTS FOR HIV-INDUCED NEURONAL DAMAGE

Since evidence for productive HIV infection of mature neurons is lacking (see above), neuronal injury is believed to be

EXPERIMENTAL SYSTEMS USED TO STUDY NEUROTOXICITY OF HIV PROTEINS

Various experimental systems have been used to study the neuropathogenic potential of HIV proteins. These include both

Table 4.2.1 EXAMPLES OF NEUROTOXIC CELLULAR FACTORS ACTIVATED BY EXPOSURE OF NON-NEURONAL CELLS TO HIV PROTEINS

CELLULAR FACTORS	ACTIVATED BY HIV-1 PROTEIN	EFFECTS
Arachidonic acids and their metabolites	gp120	Impairment of glutamate uptake by astrocytes
EAAs and related substances (glutamate, quinolinic acid, L-cystein, Ntox)	gp120, gp41	Excitotoxicity
Nitric oxide, peroxynitrite, superoxide anions	gp120, gp41, Tat, Nef	Oxidative injury
Metalloproteinase 2 (MMP-2)	gp120	Cleavage of SDF-1 to neurotoxic product
SDF-1	gp120	Ligand of CXCR4, apoptosis of neurons
IL-1β	gp120, gp41	Proinflammatory cytokine, stimulation of EAA release by macrophages and astrocytes, excitotoxicity via COX-2, release of SDF-1α by astrocytes
TNF-α	gp120, gp41, Tat, Nef	Proinflammatory cytokine, neurotoxic activities, impairment of glutamate uptake by astrocytes, induction of astrogenesis, inhibition of neurogenesis, stimulation of EAA release by macrophages and astrocytes
IL-6	gp41, Nef	stimulation of iNOS expression
β-chemokines (MIP-1β, RANTES)	gp41, Nef	Enhancement of neuronal survival
MCP-1	Tat, Nef	Chemoattraction of lymphocytes

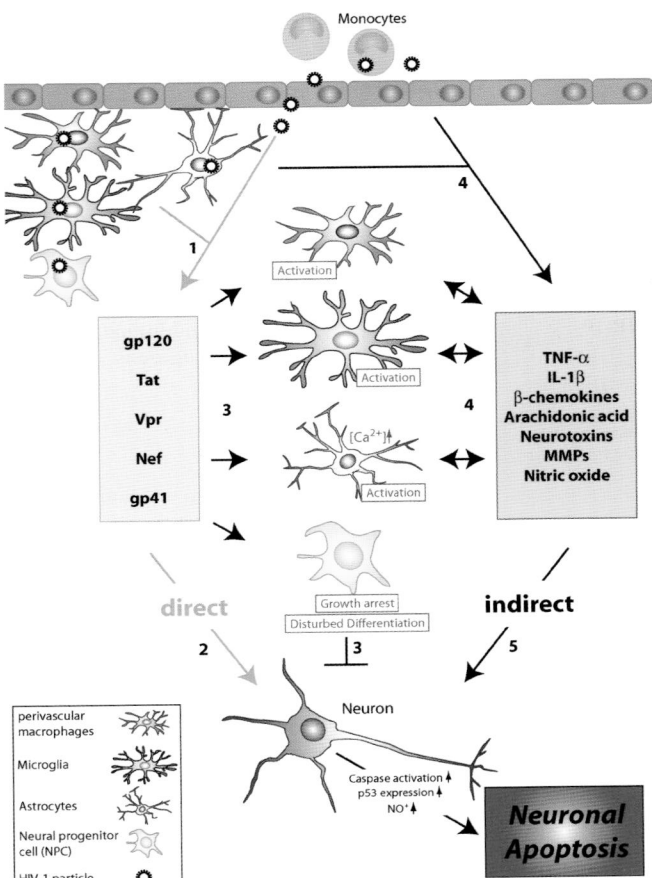

perivascular macrophages	
Microglia	
Astrocytes	
Neural progenitor cell (NPC)	
HIV-1 particle	●

Figure 4.2.1 *Potential neurotoxic effects of HIV-1 proteins.* HIV proteins, mainly gp120/gp41, Tat, Vpr, and Nef, can cause neuronal demise either directly (left) or indirectly (right) by responses elicited in non-neuronal cells. Thus, macrophages, microglial cells, and astrocytes have been shown to secrete a plethora of factors that may contribute to neuronal damage in response to HIV infection or exposure to HIV-1 proteins. (1) Potential sources of viral proteins in the brain are free virus particles and HIV-infected cells in the brain as well as virus particles and proteins that cross the blood-brain barrier. In the brain, productively infected cells may release HIV-1 structural proteins, like envelope proteins, whereas restrictedly infected cells, like astrocytes, are a preferential source of HIV-1 regulatory factors. (2) The HIV-envelope protein gp120 (glycoprotein 120), Vpr (viral protein R), Tat (transcriptional transactivator), and Nef (negative factor) have all been shown to be directly toxic to neurons. (3) Viral proteins can cause activation of macrophages, microglia, and astrocytes and impairment of neurogenesis and migration of NPCs, reducing neuronal regeneration. (4) Furthermore, HIV-1 proteins stimulate the production of neurotoxic and soluble factors, such as cytokines (including tumor-necrosis factor, TNF), quinolinic and arachidonic acid, and nitric oxide by glial cells. (5) Mechanisms leading to neuronal injury and/or death by soluble cellular factors involve excitotoxicity; for example, overstimulation of N-methyl-d-aspartate (NMDA) receptors with excessive influx of Ca^{2+}, formation of free radicals (nitric oxide and superoxide anion), and triggering of apoptotic pathways.

cell culture and animal models (Table 4.2.2). Cell-culture models consist of brain-derived fetal cells, tumor cell lines, and primary cells extracted from animal brains exposed to recombinant HIV proteins.

In addition, various animal models have been established. These include macaque models infected with specific isolates

Table 4.2.2 **EXAMPLES OF EXPERIMENTAL SYSTEMS USED TO STUDY NEUROTOXICITY OF HIV PROTEINS**

EXPERIMENTAL SYSTEMS	HIV-1 PROTEINS
Mixed primary cultures (human)	gp120, Nef
Primary neurons/ microglia/ macrophages (rodent)	gp120, gp41, Tat, Vpr, Nef
Primary fetal neurons/ astrocytes/ progenitor cells (human/mouse)	gp120, Nef
Cell-lines, tumor derived or transformed (human/mouse)	gp120, gp41, Tat, Vpr, Nef
SCID mouse	gp120, Nef
Sprague-Dawley rat	Tat
transgenic mice	Vpr
neonatal mice	Vpr
Wistar rat	Nef
Injection of HIV-1 protein in rodent brain	gp120

of the simian immunodeficiency virus as well as rodents (rat or mice) injected with recombinant HIV proteins or with transgenes for expression of various HIV proteins (Crews, Lentz, Gonzalez, Fox, & Masliah, 2008; Zink et al., 2006), or immunodeficient SCID mice with human-infected macrophages engrafted into the brain (Tyor, Power, Gendelman, & Markham, 1993).

MECHANISMS OF NEURONAL INJURY BY HIV PROTEINS

The mechanisms of neuronal injury by HIV proteins can involve direct interactions of these proteins with neurons as well as effects of these proteins on non-neuronal cells in the brain. The latter include astrocytes, macrophages/microglial cells, brain microvascular endothelial cells, and possibly also neural progenitor cells, which can all contribute to neuronal demise (see Table 4.2.3 and Fig. 4.2.1).

Neuronal injury and death involves apoptosis and damage by oxidative stress, excessive Ca^{2+} influx, and changes in lipid membrane composition (Mattson, Haughey, & Nath, 2005). Chemokine receptors and receptors for excitatory neurotransmitters, like the NMDA (N-methyl-D-aspartate-type glutamate) receptor are two types of cell surface receptors that are particularly important for the neurotoxic effects of HIV proteins. Chemokine receptors are widely expressed by various brain cells (Gonzalez-Scarano & Martin-Garcia, 2005). Binding of the HIV envelope protein gp120 to chemokine receptors like CXCR4 or CCR5 on neurons may activate intracellular signaling pathways and trigger apoptosis by elevation of intracellular Ca^{2+} levels (van de Bovenkamp et al., 2002). Interaction of gp120 and Tat with NMDA receptors on neurons can lead to the over-stimulation of these receptors and what is called excitotoxicity (Erdmann, Whitney, & Zheng, 2006), potentially leading to Ca^{2+} dysregulation and cell death. A natural

Table 4.2.3 SELECTED EFFECTS OF HIV-1 PROTEINS ON BRAIN CELLS WHICH MAY CONTRIBUTE TO CNS INJURY

NON-NEURONAL CELLS

HIV-1 PROTEINS	NEURONS	ASTROCYTES	MACROPHAGES/ MICROGLIA	BMVECS	NPCS
gpl20/gp41	Activation of chemokine and NMDA receptors; p53 activation; apoptosis	Changes in gene expression; diminished glutamate uptake; expression of iNOS; p53 activation	Upregulation of TNF-α, IL-lβ, EAAs, arachidonic acid, β-chemokines; p53 activation	Apoptosis	Inhibition of proliferation; interfering with migration via SDF-1
Tat	Activation of NMDA receptors; Ca-release; activation of NO; inhibition of tyrosine hydroxylase; decreased dopamine uptake; apoptosis	Upregulation of MCP-1; diminished glutamate uptake	Upregulation of TNF-α, IP-10	Apoptosis	Induction of astrogenesis and inhibition of neurogenesis
Vpr	Apoptosis; modulation of ion-channels; upregulation of H_2O_2; accumulation of HIF-1	Apoptosis; activation of caspase 6		Apoptosis	Impaired maturation of neurons; mitochondrial dysfunction
Nef	Apoptosis; modulation of [K⁺] channels	Apoptosis; upregulation of complement factor C3, MCP-1 and IP-10; changes in gene expression; induction of astrogenesis; increased MMP-9 activity	Recruitment of leukocytes; upregulation of proinflammatory factors MIP-1, IL-6, TNF-α; release of superoxide	Apoptosis	

ligand of NMDA receptors is the excitatory amino acid (EAA) glutamate, which is an important neurotransmitter. Prevention of excitotoxicity requires efficient clearance of glutamate by astrocytes in synaptic clefts. Both Tat and gp120 can downregulate glutamate uptake by astrocytes. Elevated production of glutamate by HIV-infected macrophages can also increase extracellular levels of glutamate (Erdmann et al., 2009). In addition, excitotoxicity can be exacerbated by various other cellular factors produced by activated astrocytes and macrophages/microglial cells like the pro-inflammatory cytokines TNF-α and IL-1ß (Kaul & Lipton, 2006).

Interestingly, HIV can also affect properties of neural progenitor cells. Thus, gp120 was shown to cause quiescence of neural progenitor cells (Krathwohl & Kaiser, 2004). Furthermore, chronically HIV-infected progenitor populations increase expression of glial cell markers and show morphological changes concomitant with glial progression (Rothenaigner et al., 2007), indicating that HIV infection can disturb the balance between *de novo* production of glial and neuronal cells.

Neuronal injury can also result from the damage or death of cells that fulfill important support functions for neurons (i.e., astrocytes), cells that contribute to the blood-brain barrier (i.e., BMVEC), and cells required for the *de novo* generation of neurons (i.e., neuronal progenitor cells). Thus, Vpr can induce apoptosis of astrocytes (Noorbakhsh et al., 2010) and Tat and gp120 can induce oxidative stress and apoptosis of BMVECs (Price et al., 2005).

NEUROPATHOGENIC POTENTIAL OF THE HIV ENVELOPE PROTEINS GP120 AND GP41

The HIV envelope proteins gp120 and gp41 are glycoproteins that associate with membranes and form heterotrimeric spikes on the envelope of virus particles (Roux & Taylor, 2007). Gp120 mediates the attachment of the virus to the host cell, whereas gp41 is required for the fusion of viral and target cell membranes. Both envelope proteins are derived from a highly glycosylated precursor protein with a molecular mass of 160 kDa, which is cleaved in the Golgi network by cellular proteases. Both proteins remain noncovalently associated and are initially expressed on the cell surface. A fraction of the gp120/gp41 molecules remains in complexed form and they are incorporated into budding virus particles. However, a large proportion of the gp120/gp41 complexes is dissolved, causing gp120 to be shed from both virus particles and infected cells (Cornblath & Hoke, 2006; Wyatt & Sodroski, 1998).

Gp120 binds to receptor molecules on the surface of human cells and the primary HIV receptor is CD4. In addition, gp120 interacts with cell-surface molecules like the chemokine receptors CXCR4 and CCR5, which play important roles as co-receptors in HIV infection. CXCR4 and CCR5 are both expressed on numerous cell types throughout the brain (Kaul, Zheng, Okamoto, Gendelman, & Lipton, 2005; Lavi, Kolson, Ulrich, Fu, & Gonzalez-Scarano, 1998; Martin-Garcia, Kolson, & Gonzalez-Scarano, 2002). The variable loops V1-V3 of gp120 determine the HIV-1 tropism, describing which co-receptor is predominately used for infection (Freed, 2001). Both coat proteins gp120 and gp41 have been identified as neurotoxins.

Effects of the glycoprotein gp120 on brain cell activity have been addressed in numerous studies, providing evidence for both direct mechanisms of neuronal damage or death and indirect or bystander effects (Tables 4.2.1 and 4.2.3) (reviewed in Cadet & Krasnova, 2007; Ghafouri, Amini, Khalili, & Sawaya, 2006; Gonzalez-Scarano & Martin-Garcia, 2005; Kaul et al., 2005; Kraft-Terry, Buch, Fox, & Gendelman, 2009; Mattson et al., 2005).

The transmembrane protein gp41 has been shown to be upregulated in tissues of the CNS (central nervous system) of HIV-infected patients with HIV-associated dementia (HAD) (Adamson, McArthur, Dawson, & Dawson, 1999b). In cell culture, gp41 is lethal to neurons, only in the presence of glia, suggesting an indirect mechanism on neuronal damage (reviewed in Cadet & Krasnova, 2007; Mattson et al., 2005).

DIRECT MECHANISMS OF GP120 NEUROTOXICITY

Cell culture experiments indicate that HIV gp120 can interact directly (i.e., independent of CD4) with chemokine receptors, like CXCR4 on neuronal cells of human and rodent origin. This interaction results in an increase of intracellular Ca^{2+} level, disrupting the cellular homeostasis and finally leading to neuronal cell death (Dreyer, Kaiser, Offermann, & Lipton, 1990; Meucci et al., 1998; Zheng et al., 1999). Experiments aiming at blocking the chemokine receptor signaling in some cases prevented this damaging process (Zheng et al., 1999). Gp120 initiated Ca^{2+} influx and apoptosis could be blocked by superoxide dismutase SOD1 (converts O_2^- to H_2O_2) and glutathione peroxidase GPx1 (converts H_2O_2 to H_2O). This suggests that O_2^- and H_2O_2 are required for gp120-induced apoptosis in neurons and that these molecules participate in pro-apoptotic pathways upstream of Ca^{2+} release in the pro-apoptotic signaling process (Agrawal et al., 2010). Gp120 can also induce neuronal cell death through direct interaction with the NMDA receptor. Neuronal apoptosis after excitotoxic insult could be attenuated by glutamate antagonists and blockade of calcium channels in human neurons (differentiated NT cells) (Wu, Price, Du, Hatch, & Terwilliger, 1996) and by antagonists that block the NMDA receptor in human neuroblastoma cells (Corasaniti et al., 1995).

Exposure of human NPCs to recombinant HIV coat protein promoted the quiescent state of these cells by CXCR4 signaling without producing apoptosis (Kaul et al., 2005; Krathwohl & Kaiser, 2004). The treated cells showed decreased incorporation of BrdU, decreased phosphorylation of ERK, and enhanced expression of the cyclin-dependent kinase inhibitors p21 and p27. The CXCR4 antagonist AMD3100 and a monoclonal antibody to CXCR4 could block these effects. The same effects were observed with CSF (cerebrospinal fluid) from HIV-positive demented patients. Furthermore, brain tissues from patients with dementia

contained fewer neural progenitor cells compared to healthy donors (Krathwohl & Kaiser, 2004). In a murine model for HAD and neurodegeneration, this decreased proliferation of adult neural progenitor cells was due to activation of the p38 MAPK/MAPKAPK2 cascade, resulting in a prolonged G1 phase (Okamoto et al., 2007). SDF-1/CXCR4 signaling regulates migration of NPCs in the cerebellum, dentate gyrus, and cortex, another important aspect of neurogenesis. It was shown that hCD4-primed gp120 can also alter the migration capacity of mouse neural progenitors by interfering with SDF-1-induced migration (Tran, Ren, & Miller, 2005).

Taken together, this direct toxicity of gp120 on neuronal cells can induce overactivation of chemokine receptors, oxidative stress, excitotoxicity, and impairment of neuronal regeneration.

INDIRECT MECHANISMS OF GP120 NEUROTOXICITY

Gp120 can interact with the chemokine receptors CXCR4 and CCR5 on macrophages, microglia, and astrocytes, leading to activation and release of neurotoxic factors that can trigger apoptosis in neurons by different ways (Tables 4.2.1 and 4.2.3).

HIV-1 gp120 is responsible for signaling the release of the pro-inflammatory factors IL-1ß and TNF-α from macrophages, in part through phosphatydilinositol-3 kinase and MAP kinase signaling (Cheung, Ravyn, Wang, Ptasznik, & Collman, 2008; Lee, Tomkowicz, Freedman, & Collman, 2005). By acting on microglia, gp120 also induces the production of TNF-α, IL-1ß, excitatory amino acids (EAAs), and related substances (like quinolinate, cystein, and Ntox), that produce excessive activation of NMDA receptor (reviewed in Garden, 2002; Kaul, Garden, & Lipton, 2001; Xiong et al., 2000). TNF-α and IL-1ß stimulate macrophages to release L-cystein and astrocytes to release glutamate, which both overstimulate the NMDA receptors on neurons and lead to apoptosis (Brabers & Nottet, 2006). Additionally, TNF-α may possibly directly activate caspase 8 in neurons via TNFR1, resulting in downstream activation of caspase 3 and neuronal death (Garden et al., 2002). TNF-α and arachidonic acid, released by activated microglia, lead to inhibition of glutamate uptake by astrocytes. Excitotoxicity is induced with increasing concentrations of extracellular glutamate (Fine et al., 1996; Genis et al., 1992; Kaul et al., 2001). The cell culture supernatant of human HIV-infected macrophages (monocyte derived) induced the proliferation and astrogenesis and inhibited neurogenesis of NPCs (Peng et al., 2008). This effect could be partially abrogated by a soluble TNFR1/2 antagonist, indicating that these effects are mediated in part by TNF-α. These observations were confirmed in SCID mice with HIV encephalitis, where injection of NPCs and monocyte-derived macrophages resulted in more astrocyte and less neuronal differentiation than after injection of NPCs alone (Peng et al., 2008). Upregulated levels of IL-1ß in microglia enhance the expression of COX-2, which converts arachidonic acid in prostaglandin E2 (PGE2). Elevated concentrations of PGE2 stimulate Ca^{2+}-dependent release of glutamate by astrocytes, giving excitotoxic insult on neurons, shown in the neocortex of rats (Corasaniti et al., 2001; Corasaniti, Rotiroti, Nappi, & Bagetta, 2003). IL-1ß additionally activates astrocytes to release SDF-1α, the natural ligand of CXCR4; this SDF-1α/CXCR4 signaling results in apoptosis in neurons (Brabers & Nottet, 2006; Peng et al., 2006; Zheng et al., 1999). HIV-infected macrophages or microglia also secrete SDF-1α, and also show gp120-induced expression of MMP-2, a metalloproteinase that cleaves SDF-1α, resulting in a neurotoxic variant of SDF-1α (Conant et al., 1999; Johnston et al., 2000; Zhang et al., 2003).

Recent studies reveal that microglia, astrocytes, and neurons all demonstrate p53 activation in response to HIV infection. The transcription factor p53 accumulates in nuclei of neurons, microglia, and astrocytes of HAD patients. Microglia from p53-deficient mice fail to induce neurotoxicity in response to the HIV coat protein gp120 in a co-culture system, supporting the hypothesis that p53 plays a pathogenic role in the chronic neuroinflammatory component of HIV-associated neurodegeneration, mediated by gp120. P53 activation altered gene expression in HAD, showing immunoreactivity for both Bax and p21 in neurons and glia from patients demonstrating elevated p53 immunoreactivity (Garden & Morrison, 2005; Jayadev et al., 2007).

Interaction of gp120 with astrocytes stimulates the expression of the inducible nitric oxide synthase (iNOS) (Mollace et al., 1993). The released nitric oxide (NO) may then react with superoxide anion (O_2^-) to form the neurotoxic peroxynitrite (ONOO⁻), a similar reaction that can occur within neurons after NMDA receptor stimulation or NO-dependent neurotoxicity induced by gp41 (Adamson et al., 1996; Lipton & Nicotera, 1998). Astrocytes normally protect neurons from excitotoxic damage by buffering the EAA glutamate. Gp120 induces intracellular alkalinization, leading to the inhibition of Na^+-dependent glutamate influx in human astrocytes (Patton, Zhou, Bubien, Benveniste, & Benos, 2000). Microarray analysis showed that HIV infection or exposure to gp120 altered significantly the overall program of gene expression in astrocytes. One impaired function of these cells was the downregulation of the EAAT2 glutamate transporter gene, losing their ability to transport L-glutamate (Wang et al., 2004).

Taken together, the indirect effects of gp120 on neuronal cells and the engagement of the chemokine receptors CXCR4, CCR5, and others by gp120 on macrophages, microglia, and astrocytes, lead to cell activation and release of neurotoxic factors or alterations of the extracellular glutamate levels, giving finally excitotoxic insult on neurons.

INDIRECT MECHANISMS OF GP41 NEUROTOXICITY

In brain tissues of HIV-infected patients, gp41 is detectable (Dickson, Lee, Mattiace, Yen, & Brosnan, 1993; Kure, Lyman, Weidenheim, & Dickson, 1990a; Kure, Weidenheim, Lyman, & Dickson, 1990b) and levels of gp41 correlate with the severity and progression of HAD (Adamson et al., 1999b; Adamson

et al., 1996). In both human and rodent cell cultures, recombinant gp41 can increase the expression of pro-inflammatory cytokines (like TNF-α, IL-1ß, and IL-6), chemokines (RANTES and MIP-1ß), and upregulates iNOS-mediated nitric oxide (NO) synthesis (Tables 4.2.1 and 4.2.3) (Koka et al., 1995a; Koka et al., 1995b; Merrill et al., 1992; Sheng, Hu, Hegg, Thayer, & Peterson, 2000). In these studies, NO was shown to be the major mediator of gp41-induced neurotoxicity. INOS–derived NO was also established as a major mediator of neurotoxic effects of gp41 in primary mixed cortical cultures derived from either neuronal NO synthase (nNOS) or inducible NO synthase (iNOS) knock-out mice (Adamson, Kopnisky, Dawson, & Dawson, 1999a). Neuroprotective effects of the NOS inhibitor L-nitroarginine methyl ester confirmed the role of NO in gp41 neurotoxicity.

NEUROPATHOGENIC POTENTIAL OF HIV TAT

The HIV-1 regulatory factor Tat is the transcriptional transactivator of HIV-1. It binds to a specific recognition element called TAR (transactivation response element) at the 5' end of HIV transcripts and promotes virus replication by activating HIV transcription (Romani et al., 2010). In addition, Tat is capable of modulating expression of numerous cellular genes (Pugliese, Vidotto, Beltramo, Petrini, & Torre, 2005). The presence of the Tat protein has been demonstrated in the brains of patients with HIV-1-associated brain pathology and in the brains of HIV-infected primates (Del Valle et al., 2000; Hudson et al., 2000). HIV-infected cells can secrete Tat and this extracellular Tat can be taken up by neighboring cells through binding to cell membrane receptors and internalization (Ferrari et al., 2003; Romani et al., 2010). Thus, Tat is able to affect both infected and uninfected cells. In the brain, Tat is actively secreted mainly from astrocytes, microglia, and macrophages. Neurons can internalize Tat primarily by the lipoprotein-related protein receptor (LRP) that is expressed on the cell surface. Unlike other LRP ligands, Tat escapes from the endosome degradation pathway and localizes to the cytoplasm and the nucleus. Tat may act in both cellular locations to affect signaling pathways, but exerts its main activity in the nucleus (Liu et al., 2000). Tat is the only ligand of LRP that induces substantial levels of apoptosis.

Multiple effects of extracellular and intracellular Tat on functions of brain cells have been shown, both in cell culture models and in animal models. Tat has proven to be a neurotoxin and can damage neurons by various means, involving direct and indirect mechanisms (King, Eugenin, Buckner, & Berman, 2006). As a consequence of secreted Tat, neuronal dysfunction can occur at sites distant from that of viral replication. In rat brains, Tat was shown to be transported along anatomical pathways to adjacent neuronal populations, for example, from the striatum to the *substantia nigra* (Bruce-Keller et al., 2003).

In addition, there are recent data suggesting an effect of Tat on the cellular composition of the developing brain, proposing maybe an influence of this HIV protein on neural progenitor cells. Anatomical results in adult rats after neonatal hippocampal injection of Tat demonstrated a decrease in the number of neurons and an increase in the numbers of astrocytes and oligodendrocytes. Furthermore it could be shown that the exposure to Tat negatively affected cognitive processes in neonatal and adult rats (Fitting, Booze, Hasselrot, & Mactutus, 2008a; Fitting, Booze, & Mactutus, 2008b). In cell culture, Tat interferes with the nerve growth factor-induced neuronal differentiation of PC12 cells and promotes a less differentiated, and therefore more immature, phenotype (Bergonzini et al., 2004).

The HIV-1 Tat protein is encoded by two exons of the HIV mRNA. The neurotoxicity of Tat was located within amino acids 1–72 encoded by the first *tat* exon (Nath et al., 1996). A recent study highlighted the specific role of the cysteine-rich domain of Tat in mediating neurotoxicity (Aksenov, Aksenova, Mactutus, & Booze, 2009). Neurotoxic activities of Tat proteins from different clades varied and these differences were attributed to differences in the sequences of the cysteine-rich regions (Mishra, Vetrivel, Siddappa, Ranga, & Seth, 2008). Interestingly, a different epitope of Tat was shown to contribute to indirect neurotoxic effects via a TNF-α-dependent mechanism (Buscemi, Ramonet, & Geiger, 2007).

HIV-positive substance abusers often develop more severe encephalitis and neuronal damage than patients who do not abuse. It has been shown for many drugs (e.g., cocaine, opiates, ethanol, methamphetamine) that they boost the Tat-induced neurotoxicity. Enhanced mitochondrial injury, oxidative stress, changes in control of dopamine homeostasis, and glial activation and glial death are likely mechanisms for the toxic synergy (Aksenov et al., 2006; Aksenov, Aksenova, Silvers, Mactutus, & Booze, 2008; Ferris, Frederick-Duus, Fadel, Mactutus, & Booze, 2009b; Hauser et al., 2009; Khurdayan et al., 2004; Self, Mulholland, Harris, Nath, & Prendergast, 2004; Theodore, Cass, & Maragos, 2006a; Theodore, Cass, & Maragos, 2006b).

DIRECT MECHANISMS OF TAT NEUROTOXICITY

There are several postulated mechanisms how Tat induces direct neuronal dysfunction and death (Table 4.2.1 and 4.2.3) (reviewed in King et al., 2006; Pocernich, Sultana, Mohmmad-Abdul, Nath, & Butterfield, 2005; Wallace, 2006). Tat neurotoxicity is thought to be mediated through excitotoxic mechanisms. Tat stimulates NMDA receptors and potentiates glutamate-induced excitotoxicity. The activation of NMDA receptors subsequently causes increase of intracellular calcium levels, promotes the generation of nitric oxide, and triggers pro-apoptotic signaling events. Recent data support the idea of a direct interplay between Tat and the NMDA receptor. Chandra et al. demonstrated that Tat releases Zn^{2+} from its binding site on the NMDA receptor on cultured rat hippocampal neurons (Chandra et al., 2005). When Zn^{2+} is bound to the NMDA receptor, the receptor has a reduced capacity to conduct Ca^{2+} through its channel. When Zn^{2+} is removed, the NMDA receptor is activated, increasing Ca^{2+} influx. Tat triggers the formation of a macromolecular complex involving the LRP-receptor, the postsynaptic density protein-95 (PSD-95), NMDA receptors, and nNOS at the neuronal plasma membrane. This complex leads to apoptosis in neurons negative as well as positive for NMDA receptors (Eugenin et al., 2007). Aksenova et al. showed that subpopulations of primary cultures of rat fetal neurons are resistant to Tat toxicity and that in these neurons the levels of the NR2A subunit of the NMDA receptor complex were significantly lower than in controls (Aksenova, Aksenov, Adams, Mactutus, & Booze, 2009). Another recent study demonstrated that the high level of Tat toxicity observed in human neurons involves specific developmental stages that correlate with expression of NMDA receptors, and that Tat toxicity is also dependent upon the species being analyzed (Eugenin et al., 2010). Another mechanism causing calcium dysregulation in neurons involves Tat-dependent release calcium from inositol 1,4,5-trisphosphate (IP3)-regulated intracellular stores, preceding extracellular calcium flux (Haughey, Holden, Nath, & Geiger, 1999). Tat-induced injury of neurons also causes increased oxidative stress (Pocernich et al., 2005). Tat triggers mitochondrial depolarization, the activation of nitric oxidase, generation of reactive oxygen species (ROS), and protein oxidation (Aksenov et al., 2006). Cellular damage and death following Tat administration have also been linked to activation of caspase and an increase in apoptosis. The induction of apoptosis is dependent on oxidative stress, on the binding of Tat to LRP receptor, as well as activation of the NMDA receptor. One neurological system that is involved in Tat-induced neurotoxicity is the dopaminergic system (Ferris et al., 2009a). Patients develop symptoms of dopamine deficiency and display increased sensitivity to dopaminergic-selective drugs as well as psychostimulants which act on dopaminergic neurons (Nath et al., 2000). Both *in vivo* and cell culture studies show that Tat inhibits tyrosine hydroxylase (TH) gene expression, the rate-limiting enzyme in the biosynthesis of dopamine (DA) (Bruce-Keller et al., 2003; Zauli et al., 2000). Consistently, decreased tyrosine hydroxylase immunoreactivity has been detected in the *substantia nigra* of HIV- positive humans (Silvers et al., 2006). In addition, Tat was shown to decrease dopamine uptake by the dopamine transporter (DAT) (Aksenova et al., 2006; Ferris, Frederick-Duus, Fadel, Mactutus, & Booze, 2009b; Wallace, Dodson, Nath, & Booze, 2006; Zhu, Mactutus, Wallace, & Booze, 2009). Another recent study found that in rat midbrain cell cultures the D1 dopamine receptor is also involved in the mechanism of Tat neurotoxicity. The authors suggest that Tat-mediated inhibition of DA re-uptake in "'presynaptic'" DA neurons may influence the activity of D1 dopamine receptors in "'postsynaptic'" neurons and trigger NMDA receptor-controlled apoptotic cascades through D1/NMDA receptor interactions (Silvers, Aksenova, Aksenov, Mactutus, & Booze, 2007).

INDIRECT MECHANISMS OF TAT NEUROTOXICITY

Tat induces indirect neurotoxicity through activating and increasing the production and release of various inflammatory mediators from activated glial cells and macrophages.

These released toxins damage neurons. Treatment with Tat led, for example, to increased secretion of cytokines (e.g., TNF-α), of interleukins (e.g., IL-6), and of chemokines (e.g., CCL2/MCP-1 and CXCL10/IP-10) (Buscemi et al., 2007; D'Aversa, Yu, & Berman, 2004; Pocernich et al., 2005). In addition, Tat increases infiltration of monocytes into the brain by upregulating production of chemotactic factors like monocyte chemoattractant protein-1 (MCP-1) by astrocytes. It was shown that the Tat-induced cytokine/chemokine and superoxide release from astrocytes, microglia, and macrophages is dependent in large part on the activation of the NADPH oxidase (Turchan-Cholewo et al., 2009; Williams et al., 2010). Another mechanism contributing to Tat-induced neurotoxicity is the fact that Tat restricts glutamate uptake by astrocytes which leads to extracellular glutamate accumulation and possibly neuronal toxicity (Zhou, Liu, Kim, Xiao, & He, 2004). Tat can also cause alterations in the blood-brain barrier, which also contributes to the toxicity on neurons (Price, Ercal, Nakaoke, & Banks, 2005).

NEUROPROTECTION AGAINST TAT-INDUCED NEUROTOXICITY

Several studies present factors that prevent Tat-induced neurotoxicity, at least in cell culture, often acting via prevention of Tat-induced oxidative stress; for example, steroids like estrogens or NMDA receptor blockers (King et al., 2006; Wallace, 2006).

One recent study showed for example the neuroprotective effect of the neurotrophic factor platelet-derived growth factor (PDGF) in cell culture and *in vivo*. PDGF could rescue dopaminergic neurons in the *substantia nigra* of rats (Yao et al., 2009). Another study showed a protective mechanism that occurs *in vivo*: Proteinase-activated receptor 2 (PAR-2) (a G-protein coupled receptor) is upregulated in conjunction with neuroinflammation in brain tissue from patients with HIV-1-associated dementia. This increased expression and subsequent activation of PAR-2 was shown to prevent neuronal cell death in cell culture and *in vivo* (Noorbakhsh et al., 2005).

To summarize, Tat is an important mediator of neurotoxicity in the HIV-infected brain and investigation of its role in HIV-associated neurodegeneration is important for understanding of the pathogenesis of HIV cognitive and motor dysfunction.

NEUROPATHOGENIC POTENTIAL OF HIV VPR

HIV-1 Vpr consists of 96 amino acids and has a predicted molecular weight of 14 kDa. It is packaged into virus particles via its interaction with the Gag precursor protein. Vpr has multiple activities and is important for the infection of nondividing cells, like macrophages (Romani & Engelbrecht, 2009). Vpr plays a role in various early events of the HIV-1 replication cycle, including transport of the viral DNA to the nucleus and its integration into the host genome. Vpr can also facilitate HIV expression by increasing the activity of the HIV LTR and inhibiting splicing, thus promoting production of HIV-1 mRNAs that encode viral structural proteins (Kilareski, Shah, Nonnemacher, & Wigdahl, 2009; Zhang & Aida, 2009).

Vpr has multiple effects on cells of the immune system, indicating that Vpr plays an important role for immunopathogenesis of AIDS (Majumder, Venkatachari, Srinivasan, & Ayyavoo, 2009). These include inhibition of cell proliferation, induction of apoptosis, and modulation of the production of various immune molecules.

DIRECT MECHANISMS OF VPR NEUROTOXICITY

Evidence has accumulated that Vpr may also affect the survival and function of cells of the central nervous system. Levels of Vpr are increased in the cerebrospinal fluids of HIV-1 dementia patients (Tungaturthi et al., 2003) and expression of Vpr was detected in brain tissue samples from individuals with HIV-1 encephalitis (Jones et al., 2007; Wheeler et al., 2006). Vpr has been shown to induce the apoptosis of cells in primary cultures of neurons from the hippocampus (Piller, Jans, Gage, & Jans, 1998), striatum, and cortex of rodents (Sabbah & Roques, 2005) and in cultures of a human cholinergic neuroblastoma cell line (Jones et al., 2007). Evidence for Vpr-induced apoptosis of neurons *in vivo* was obtained by examining Vpr-transgenic mice (Jones et al., 2007) and by ventricular injection of Vpr into neonatal mice (Cheng et al., 2007). Vpr was shown to form cation-selective ion channels in artificial membranes (Piller, Ewart, Premkumar, Cox, & Gage, 1996) and exposure of cultured neurons to Vpr led to changes in whole-cell currents (Jones et al., 2007; Piller et al., 1998). This suggests that Vpr may induce electrophysiological changes in neurons by forming channels in neuronal membranes.

Induction of apoptosis of neurons was associated with the activation or cleavage of caspases (Jones et al., 2007; Sabbah & Roques, 2005), and with oxidative stress apparent as increased production of H_2O_2 and accumulation of the HIF-1 transcription factor (Deshmane et al., 2009).

INDIRECT MECHANISMS OF VPR NEUROTOXICITY

Vpr may also cause neuronal damage by bystander effects. Thus apoptosis markers and activation of caspase 6 were detected in cultured human primary astrocytes exposed to Vpr and in transgenic mice expressing Vpr in microglia cells (Noorbakhsh et al., 2010). This suggests that the killing of astrocytes by Vpr may also contribute to Vpr-induced neuronal injury in the brain. Another potential bystander effect could be the impairment of the development of mature functional neurons. This is indicated by a study (Kitayama et al., 2008) showing that exposure of murine neural progenitor cells to Vpr impairs axonal outgrowth of developing neurons and causes mitochondrial dysfunction. Finally, Vpr has also been shown to affect the survival of BMVECs (Acheampong et al., 2002), indicating that Vpr may also interfere with blood-brain barrier functions.

NEUROPATHOGENIC POTENTIAL
OF HIV NEF

Nef is a small accessory protein of 27–35 kDa that increases viral persistence and pathogenicity by exerting multiple effects on host cells (Arhel & Kirchhoff, 2010). Nef can also affect the viability of brain cells, leading to the assumption that Nef might play a crucial role in HIV neuropathology (Kramer-Hammerle, Hahn, Brack-Werner, & Werner, 2005a; Mattson et al., 2005). Detection of Nef in supernatants of HIV-1-infected cultures and in sera of AIDS patients (Fujii, Otake, Tashiro, & Adachi, 1996) suggests the release of Nef by infected cells, and may facilitate access of peripheral Nef to the CNS. Extracellular Nef seems to activate various transcription factors and release of inflammatory factors in monocytes and macrophages (Tables 4.2.1 and 4.2.3) (Olivetta et al., 2003).

In the brain, Nef expression has been detected mainly in astrocytes of HIV-infected individuals (Ranki et al., 1995; Saito et al., 1994). Intracellular expression of Nef can have many different effects on astrocyte properties (see below and Table 4.2.3).

DIRECT MECHANISMS OF NEF
NEUROTOXICITY

Extracellular Nef may interfere directly with neuronal functions. Nef can cause cell death of neurons and apoptosis of astrocytes (Trillo-Pazos, McFarlane-Abdulla, Campbell, Pilkington, & Everall, 2000; Mattson et al., 2005). This was shown in human primary astrocytes and glioma cell lines as well as in mice brains (Acheampong et al., 2009; He, deCastro, Vandenbark, Busciglio, & Gabuzda, 1997; van Marle et al., 2004). Furthermore, Nef was also shown to influence the conductance of potassium channels (Kort & Jalonen, 1998), displaying similar activity as peptides of scorpion neurotoxins, with which it shares sequence similarities (Werner et al., 1991). This suggests that Nef is capable of altering electrophysiological properties of neurons.

INDIRECT MECHANISMS OF NEF
NEUROTOXICITY

Nef has been shown to compromise the blood-brain barrier (BBB) (Acheampong et al., 2005; Kohleisen et al., 1999). Sporer et al. observed increased permeability of the BBB in rats injected with Nef into the brain and ascribed this effect to increased activity of the matrix metalloprotease-9 (Sporer et al., 2000). In support, Nef was recently shown to activate matrix metalloproteinases produced by human cultured astrocytic glioma cells (Bergonzini et al., 2009).

In a rodent model, Nef promoted the recruitment of leukocytes (Koedel et al., 1999) to the brain. Furthermore, stable *nef* expression in astrocytes was shown to increase production of CCL2/MCP-1, which is a potent chemotactic protein for monocytes (Lehmann, Masanetz, Kramer, & Erfle, 2006). Stable *nef* expression also increased the expression of several activation markers in astrocytes (Kohleisen et al., 1999). Expression of *nef* in microglia led to priming of the

NADPH oxidase, enhancing the release of superoxide in response to various stimuli (Vilhardt et al., 2002). This suggests that *nef* expression in microglia may contribute to neuronal death by promoting oxidative stress in the brain.

The exposure of human monocyte/macrophages to Nef protein causes these cells to release various pro-inflammatory factors like MIP-1α and -ß, IL-6 and TNF-α (Olivetta et al., 2003).

It was also shown that recombinant Nef upregulates the production of the complement factor C3 by astrocytic and neuronal cell lines (Bruder et al., 2004; Speth et al., 2002).

Other studies also provide evidence that Nef can modulate cellular properties of astrocytes. Thus, Nef has been shown to increase activation and proliferation of astrocytes (Cosenza-Nashat, Si, Zhao, & Lee, 2006; Kohleisen et al., 1999; Richard et al., 1997; Robichaud & Poulin, 2000), alter their growth properties (Kramer-Hammerle et al., 2001) and change their gene expression profiles (Kramer-Hammerle et al., 2005a). Intracellular Nef interfered with cell signaling pathways in astrocytes, resulting in dysregulation of glutamate homeostasis (Kaul et al., 2001).

Taken together, the multiple effects of endogenously expressed *nef* and extracellular Nef on brain cells suggests a critical role for Nef in HIV-associated neuroinflammation and neurodegeneration.

CONCLUDING REMARKS

Numerous studies with cell culture and animal models demonstrate the potency of various HIV proteins to injure the brain. HIV proteins shown to have neurotoxic effects in these experimental systems include proteins in virus particles (e.g., the envelope proteins gp120 and gp41and Vpr), as well as viral proteins with regulatory functions in infected cells (e.g., Tat and Nef). Exposure of neurons to these HIV proteins can lead to neuronal cell death and cripple the functions of mature neurons. In addition, HIV proteins may interfere with self-renewal and differentiation capacities of neural progenitor cells, further reducing the already limited *de novo* production of neurons in adult human brains. Finally, HIV proteins can cause non-neuronal cells like microglia cells and astrocytes to produce a broad spectrum of cellular factors that can damage the brain. These include both factors that are directly toxic to neurons and other brain cells as well as factors that sustain and amplify neuroinflammation, and thus potentiate the effects of HIV infection of the brain.

It is clear that therapy and prevention of HIV-induced neuronal damage depends on the efficient suppression of HIV-protein production at both peripheral sites of infection and in the brain. The poor accession of many current antiretroviral drugs to the brain requires the development of novel antiretroviral drugs that target the brain. Furthermore, compounds are required to prevent expression of viral proteins from integrated HIV genomes in persistently HIV-infected cells in the brain, since elimination of infected cells is not a therapeutic option for the brain. Finally, like for other neurodegenerative diseases, compounds that prevent or at least control neuroinflammation can also be expected to be helpful in the treatment of HIV-associated neurodegeneration. The development of dedicated therapies to prevent damage of the brain by HIV is an important goal for future research efforts.

REFERENCES

Acheampong, E., Mukhtar, M., Parveen, Z., Ngoubilly, Ahmad, N., Patel, C., et al. (2002). Ethanol strongly potentiates apoptosis induced by HIV-1 proteins in primary human brain microvascular endothelial cells. *Virology, 304*, 222–34.

Acheampong, E. A., Parveen, Z., Muthoga, L. W., Kalayeh, M., Mukhtar, M., & Pomerantz. R/ J. (2005). Human Immunodeficiency virus type 1 Nef potently induces apoptosis in primary human brain microvascular endothelial cells via the activation of caspases. *J Virol, 79*, 4257–69.

Acheampong, E. A., Roschel, C., Mukhtar, M., Srinivasan, A., Rafi, M., Pomerantz, R. J., et al. (2009). Combined effects of hyperglycemic conditions and HIV-1 Nef: A potential model for induced HIV neuropathogenesis. *Virol J, 6*, 183.

Adamson, D. C., Kopnisky, K. L., Dawson, T. M., & Dawson, V. L. (1999a). Mechanisms and structural determinants of HIV-1 coat protein, gp41-induced neurotoxicity. *J Neurosci, 19*, 64–71.

Adamson, D. C., McArthur, J. C., Dawson, T. M., & Dawson, V. L. (1999b). Rate and severity of HIV-associated dementia (HAD): Correlations with Gp41 and iNOS. *Mol Med, 5*, 98–109.

Adamson, D. C., Wildemann, B., Sasaki, M., Glass, J. D., McArthur, J. C., Christov, V. I., et al. (1996). Immunologic NO synthase: Elevation in severe AIDS dementia and induction by HIV-1 gp41. *Science, 274*, 1917–21.

Agrawal, L., Louboutin, J. P., Marusich, E., Reyes, B. A., Van Bockstaele, E. J., & Strayer, D. S. (2010). Dopaminergic neurotoxicity of HIV-1 gp120: Reactive oxygen species as signaling intermediates. *Brain Res, 1306*, 116–30.

Aksenov, M. Y., Aksenova, M. V., Mactutus, C. F., & Booze, R. M. (2009). Attenuated neurotoxicity of the transactivation-defective HIV-1 Tat protein in hippocampal cell cultures. *Exp Neurol, 219*, 586–90.

Aksenov, M. Y., Aksenova, M. V., Nath, A., Ray, P. D., Mactutus, C. F., & Booze, R. M. (2006). Cocaine-mediated enhancement of Tat toxicity in rat hippocampal cell cultures: The role of oxidative stress and D1 dopamine receptor. *Neurotoxicology, 27*, 217–28.

Aksenov, M. Y., Aksenova, M. V., Silvers, J. M., Mactutus, C. F., & Booze, R. M. (2008). Different effects of selective dopamine uptake inhibitors, GBR 12909 and WIN 35428, on HIV-1 Tat toxicity in rat fetal midbrain neurons. *Neurotoxicology, 29*, 971–7.

Aksenova, M. V., Aksenov, M. Y., Adams, S. M., Mactutus, C. F., & Booze, R. M. (2009). Neuronal survival and resistance to HIV-1 Tat toxicity in the primary culture of rat fetal neurons. *Exp Neurol, 215*, 253–63.

Aksenova, M. V., Silvers, J. M., Aksenov, M. Y., Nath, A., Ray, P. D., Mactutus, C. F., et al. (2006). HIV-1 Tat neurotoxicity in primary cultures of rat midbrain fetal neurons: Changes in dopamine transporter binding and immunoreactivity. *Neurosci Lett, 395*, 235–9.

Anthony, I. C. & Bell, J. E. (2008). The neuropathology of HIV/AIDS. *Int Rev Psychiatry, 20*, 15–24.

Arhel, N. J. & Kirchhoff, F. (2010). Implications of nef: Host cell interactions in viral persistence and progression to AIDS. *Curr Top Microbiol Immunol, 339*, 147–75.

Banks, W. A., Robinson, S. M., & Nath, A. (2005). Permeability of the blood-brain barrier to HIV-1 Tat. *Exp Neurol, 193*, 218–227.

Bergonzini, V., Calistri, A., Salata, Del Vecchio, C., Sartori, E., Parolin, C., et al. (2009). Nef and cell signaling transduction: A possible involvement in the pathogenesis of human immunodeficiency virus-associated dementia. *J Neurovirol*, 1–11.

Bergonzini, V., Delbue, S., Wang, J. Y., Reiss, K., Prisco, M., Amini, S., et al. (2004). HIV-Tat promotes cellular proliferation and inhibits NGF-induced differentiation through mechanisms involving Id1 regulation. *Oncogene, 23*, 7701–11.

Brabers, N. A. & Nottet, H. S. (2006). Role of the pro-inflammatory cytokines TNF-alpha and IL-1beta in HIV-associated dementia. *Eur J Clin Invest, 36*, 447–58.

Brack-Werner, R. (1999). Astrocytes: HIV cellular reservoirs and important participants in neuropathogenesis. *AIDS, 13*, 1–22.

Brew, B. J., Crowe, S. M., Landay, A., Cysique, L. A., & Guillemin, G. (2009). Neurodegeneration and ageing in the HAART era. *J Neuroimmune Pharmacol, 4*, 163–74.

Bruce-Keller, A. J., Chauhan, A., Dimayuga, F. O., Gee, J., Keller, J. N., & Nath, A. (2003). Synaptic transport of human immunodeficiency virus-Tat protein causes neurotoxicity and gliosis in rat brain. *J Neurosci, 23*, 8417–22.

Bruder, C., Hagleitner, M., Darlington, G., Mohsenipour, I., Wurzner, R., Hollmuller, I., et al. (2004). HIV-1 induces complement factor C3 synthesis in astrocytes and neurons by modulation of promoter activity. *Mol Immunol, 40*, 949–61.

Buscemi, L., Ramonet, D., & Geiger, J. D. (2007). Human immunodeficiency virus type-1 protein Tat induces tumor necrosis factor-alpha-mediated neurotoxicity. *Neurobiol Dis, 26*, 661–70.

Cadet, J. L. & Krasnova, I. N. (2007). Interactions of HIV and methamphetamine: Cellular and molecular mechanisms of toxicity potentiation. *Neurotox Res, 12*, 181–204.

Cashion, M. F., Banks, W. A., Bost, K. L., & Kastin, A. J. (1999). Transmission routes of HIV-1 gp120 from brain to lymphoid tissues. *Brain Res, 822*, 26–33.

Chandra, T., Maier, W., Konig, H. G., Hirzel, K., Kogel, D., Schuler, T., et al. (2005). Molecular interactions of the type 1 human immunodeficiency virus transregulatory protein Tat with N-methyl-d-aspartate receptor subunits. *Neuroscience, 134*, 145–53.

Cheng, X., Mukhtar, M., Acheampong, E. A., Srinivasan, A., Rafi, M., Pomerantz, R. J., et al. (2007). HIV-1 Vpr potently induces programmed cell death in the CNS in vivo. *DNA Cell Biol, 26*, 116–31.

Cheung, R., Ravyn, V., Wang, L., Ptasznik, A., & Collman, R. G. (2008). Signaling mechanism of HIV-1 gp120 and virion-induced IL-1beta release in primary human macrophages. *J Immunol, 180*, 6675–84.

Churchill, M. J., Wesselingh, S. L., Cowley, D., Pardo, C. A., McArthur, J. C., Brew, B. J., et al. (2009). Extensive astrocyte infection is prominent in human immunodeficiency virus-associated dementia. *Ann Neurol, 66*, 253–8.

Conant, K., McArthur, J. C., Griffin, D. E., Sjulson, L., Wahl, L. M., & Irani, D. N. (1999). Cerebrospinal fluid levels of MMP-2, 7, and 9 are elevated in association with human immunodeficiency virus dementia. *Ann Neurol, 46*, 391–8.

Corasaniti, M. T., Maccarrone, M., Nistico, R., Malorni, W., Rotiroti, D., & Bagetta, G. (2001). Exploitation of the HIV-1 coat glycoprotein, gp120, in neurodegenerative studies in vivo. *J Neurochem, 79*, 1–8.

Corasaniti, M. T., Melino, G., Navarra, M., Garaci, E., Finazzi-Agro, A., Nistico, G. (1995). Death of cultured human neuroblastoma cells induced by HIV-1 gp120 is prevented by NMDA receptor antagonists and inhibitors of nitric oxide and cyclooxygenase. *Neurodegeneration, 4*, 315–21.

Corasaniti, M. T., Rotiroti, D., Nappi, G., & Bagetta, G. (2003). Neurobiological mediators of neuronal apoptosis in experimental neuroAIDS. *Toxicol Lett, 139*, 199–206.

Cornblath, D. R. & Hoke, A. (2006). Recent advances in HIV neuropathy. *Curr Opin Neurol, 19*, 446–50.

Cosenza-Nashat, M. A., Si, Q., Zhao, M. L., & Lee, S. C. (2006). Modulation of astrocyte proliferation by HIV-1: Differential effects in productively infected, uninfected, and Nef-expressing cells. *J Neuroimmunol, 178*, 87–99.

Crews, L., Lentz, M. R., Gonzalez, R. G., Fox, H. S., & Masliah, E. (2008). Neuronal injury in simian immunodeficiency virus and other animal models of neuroAIDS. *J Neurovirol, 14*, 327–39.

D'Aversa, T. G., Yu, K. O., & Berman, J. W. (2004). Expression of chemokines by human fetal microglia after treatment with the human immunodeficiency virus type 1 protein Tat. *J Neurovirol, 10*, 86–97.

Del Valle, L., Croul, S., Morgello, S., Amini, S., Rappaport, J., & Khalili, K. (2000). Detection of HIV-1 Tat and JCV capsid protein, VP1, in AIDS brain with progressive multifocal leukoencephalopathy. *J Neurovirol, 6*, 221–8.

Deshmane, S. L., Mukerjee, R., Fan, S., Del Valle, L., Michiels, C., Sweet, T., et al. (2009). Activation of the oxidative stress pathway by HIV-1 Vpr leads to induction of hypoxia-inducible factor 1alpha expression. *J Biol Chem, 284*, 11364–73.

Dickson, D. W., Lee, S. C., Mattiace, L. A., Yen, S. H., & Brosnan, C. (1993). Microglia and cytokines in neurological disease, with special reference to AIDS and Alzheimer's disease. *Glia, 7*, 75–83.

Dreyer, E. B., Kaiser, P. K., Offermann, J. T., & Lipton, S. A. (1990). HIV-1 coat protein neurotoxicity prevented by calcium channel antagonists. *Science, 248*, 364–7.

Ellis, R., Langford, D., & Masliah, E. (2007). HIV and antiretroviral therapy in the brain: Neuronal injury and repair. *Nat Rev Neurosci, 8*, 33–44.

Erdmann, N., Tian, C., Huang, Y., Zhao, J., Herek, S., Curthoys, N., et al. (2009). In vitro glutaminase regulation and mechanisms of glutamate generation in HIV-1-infected macrophage. *J Neurochem, 109*, 551–61.

Erdmann, N. B., Whitney, N. P., & Zheng, J. (2006). Potentiation of excitotoxicity in HIV-1-associated dementia and the significance of glutaminase. *Clin Neurosci Res, 6*, 315–328.

Eugenin, E. A., King, J. E., Hazleton, J. E., Major, E. O., Bennett, M. V., Zukin, R. S., et al. (2010). Differences in NMDA Receptor Expression During Human Development Determine the Response of Neurons to HIV-Tat-mediated Neurotoxicity. *Neurotox Res.*

Eugenin, E. A., King, J. E., Nath, A., Calderon, T. M., Zukin, R. S., Bennett, M. V., et al. (2007). HIV-tat induces formation of an LRP-PSD-95-NMDAR-nNOS complex that promotes apoptosis in neurons and astrocytes. *Proc Natl Acad Sci U S A, 104*, 3438–43.

Everall, I., Luthert, P., & Lantos, P. (1993). A review of neuronal damage in human immunodeficiency virus infection: Its assessment, possible mechanism and relationship to dementia. *J Neuropathol Exp Neurol, 52*, 561–6.

Ferrari, A., Pellegrini, V., Arcangeli, C., Fittipaldi, A., Giacca, M., & Beltram, F. (2003). Caveolae-mediated internalization of extracellular HIV-1 tat fusion proteins visualized in real time. *Mol Ther, 8*, 284–94.

Ferris, M. J., Frederick-Duus, D., Fadel, J., Mactutus, C. F., & Booze, R. M. (2009a). In vivo microdialysis in awake, freely moving rats demonstrates HIV-1 Tat-induced alterations in dopamine transmission. *Synapse, 63*, 181–5.

Ferris, M. J., Frederick-Duus, D., Fadel, J., Mactutus, C. F., & Booze, R. M. (2009b). The human immunodeficiency virus-1-associated protein, Tat1–86, impairs dopamine transporters and interacts with cocaine to reduce nerve terminal function: A no-net-flux microdialysis study. *Neuroscience, 159*, 1292–9.

Fine, S. M., Angel, R. A., Perry, S. W., Epstein, L. G., Rothstein, J. D., Dewhurst, S., et al. (1996). Tumor necrosis factor alpha inhibits glutamate uptake by primary human astrocytes. Implications for pathogenesis of HIV-1 dementia. *J Biol Chem, 271*, 15303–6.

Fitting, S., Booze, R. M., Hasselrot, U., & Mactutus, C. F. (2008a). Differential long-term neurotoxicity of HIV-1 proteins in the rat hippocampal formation: A design-based stereological study. *Hippocampus, 18*, 135–47.

Fitting, S., Booze, R. M., & Mactutus, C. F. (2008b). Neonatal intrahippocampal injection of the HIV-1 proteins gp120 and Tat: Differential effects on behavior and the relationship to stereological hippocampal measures. *Brain Res, 1232*, 139–54.

Freed, E. O. (2001). HIV-1 replication. *Somat Cell Mol Genet, 26*, 13–33.

Fujii, Y., Otake, K., Tashiro, M., & Adachi, A. (1996). Human immunodeficiency virus type 1 Nef protein on the cell surface is cytocidal for human CD4+ T cells. *FEBS Lett, 393*, 105–8.

Garden, G. A. (2002). Microglia in human immunodeficiency virus-associated neurodegeneration. *Glia, 40*, 240–51.

Garden, G. A., Budd, S. L., Tsai, E., Hanson, L., Kaul, M., D'Emilia, D. M., et al. (2002). Caspase cascades in human immunodeficiency virus-associated neurodegeneration. *J Neurosci, 22*, 4015–24.

Garden, G. A. & Morrison, R. S. (2005). The multiple roles of p53 in the pathogenesis of HIV associated dementia. *Biochem Biophys Res Commun, 331*, 799–809.

Gartner, S. 2000. HIV infection and dementia. *Science, 287*, 602–4.

Genis, P., Jett, M., Bernton, E. W., Boyle, T., Gelbard, H. A., Dzenko, K., et al. (1992). Cytokines and arachidonic metabolites produced during human immunodeficiency virus (HIV)-infected macrophage-astroglia interactions: Implications for the neuropathogenesis of HIV disease. *J Exp Med, 176*, 1703–18.

Ghafouri, M., Amini, S., Khalili, K., & Sawaya. B. E. (2006). HIV-1 associated dementia: Symptoms and causes. *Retrovirology, 3*, 28.

Gonzalez-Scarano, F. & Martin-Garcia, J. (2005). The neuropathogenesis of AIDS. *Nat Rev Immunol, 5*, 69–81.

Gorry, P. R., Ong, C., Thorpe, J., Bannwarth, S., Thompson, K. A., Gatignol, A., et al. (2003). Astrocyte infection by HIV-1: Mechanisms of restricted virus replication, and role in the pathogenesis of HIV-1-associated dementia. *Curr HIV Res, 1*, 463–73.

Haughey, N. J., Holden, C. P., Nath, A., & Geiger, J. D. (1999). Involvement of inositol 1,4,5-trisphosphate-regulated stores of intracellular calcium in calcium dysregulation and neuron cell death caused by HIV-1 protein tat. *J Neurochem, 73*, 1363–74.

Hauser, K. F., Hahn, Y. K., Adjan, V. V., Zou, S., Buch, S. K., Nath, A., et al. (2009). HIV-1 Tat and morphine have interactive effects on oligodendrocyte survival and morphology. *Glia, 57*, 194–206.

He, J., deCastro, C. M., Vandenbark, G. R., Busciglio, J., & Gabuzda, D. (1997). Astrocyte apoptosis induced by HIV-1 transactivation of the c-kit protooncogene. *Proc Natl Acad Sci USA, 94*, 3954–9.

Hudson, L., Liu, J., Nath, A., Jones, M., Raghavan, R., Narayan, O., et al. (2000). Detection of the human immunodeficiency virus regulatory protein tat in CNS tissues. *J Neurovirol, 6*, 145–55.

Jayadev, S. & Garden, G. A. (2009). Host and viral factors influencing the pathogenesis of HIV-associated neurocognitive disorders. *J Neuroimmune Pharmacol, 4*, 175–89.

Jayadev, S., Yun, B., Nguyen, H., Yokoo, H., Morrison, R. S., & Garden, G. A. (2007). The glial response to CNS HIV infection includes p53 activation and increased expression of p53 target genes. *J Neuroimmune Pharmacol, 2*, 359–70.

Johnston, J. B., Jiang, Y., van Marle, G., Mayne, M. B., Ni, W., Holden, J., et al. (2000). Lentivirus infection in the brain induces matrix metalloproteinase expression: Role of envelope diversity. *J Virol, 74*, 7211–20.

Jones, G. J., Barsby, N. L., Cohen, E. A., Holden, J., Harris, K., Dickie, P., et al. (2007). HIV-1 Vpr causes neuronal apoptosis and in vivo neurodegeneration. *J Neurosci, 27*, 3703–11.

Kanmogne, G. D., Primeaux, C., & Grammas, P. (2005). HIV-1 gp120 proteins alter tight junction protein expression and brain endothelial cell permeability: Implications for the pathogenesis of HIV-associated dementia. *J Neuropathol Exp Neurol, 64*, 498–505.

Kaul, M. (2008). HIV's double strike at the brain: Neuronal toxicity and compromised neurogenesis. *Front Biosci, 13*, 2484–94.

Kaul, M., Garden, G. A., & Lipton, S. A. (2001). Pathways to neuronal injury and apoptosis in HIV-associated dementia. *Nature, 410*, 988–94.

Kaul, M., & Lipton, S. A. (2006). Mechanisms of neuronal injury and death in HIV-1 associated dementia. *Curr HIV Res, 4*, 307–18.

Kaul, M., Zheng, J., Okamoto, S., Gendelman, H. E., & Lipton, S. A. (2005). HIV-1 infection and AIDS: Consequences for the central nervous system. *Cell Death Differ, 12* Suppl 1, 878–92.

Khurdayan, V. K., Buch, S., El-Hage, N., Lutz, S. E., Goebel, S. M., Singh, I. N., et al. (2004). Preferential vulnerability of astroglia and glial precursors to combined opioid and HIV-1 Tat exposure in vitro. *Eur J Neurosci, 19*, 3171–82.

Kilareski, E. M., Shah, S., Nonnemacher, M. R., & Wigdahl, B. (2009). Regulation of HIV-1 transcription in cells of the monocyte-macrophage lineage. *Retrovirology, 6*, 118.

King, J. E., Eugenin, E. A., Buckner, C. M., & Berman, J. W. (2006). HIV tat and neurotoxicity. *Microbes Infect, 8*, 1347–57.

Kitayama, H., Miura, Y., Ando, Y., Hoshino, S., Ishizaka, Y., & Koyanagi, Y. (2008). Human immunodeficiency virus type 1 Vpr inhibits axonal outgrowth through induction of mitochondrial dysfunction. *J Virol, 82*, 2528–42.

Koedel, U., Kohleisen, B., Sporer, B., Lahrtz, F., Ovod, V., Fontana, A., et al. (1999). HIV type 1 Nef protein is a viral factor for leukocyte recruitment into the central nervous system. *J Immunol, 163*, 1237–45.

Kohleisen, B., Shumay, E., Sutter, G., Foerster, R., Brack-Werner, R., Nuesse, M., et al. (1999). Stable expression of HIV-1 Nef induces changes in growth properties and activation state of human astrocytes. *AIDS, 13*, 2331–41.

Koka, P., K. He, K., Camerini, D., Tran, T., Yashar, S. S., & Merrill, J. E. (1995a). The mapping of HIV-1 gp160 epitopes required for interleukin-1 and tumor necrosis factor alpha production in glial cells. *J Neuroimmunol, 57*, 179–91.

Koka, P., He, K., Zack, J. A., Kitchen, S., Peacock, W., Fried, I., et al. (1995b). Human immunodeficiency virus 1 envelope proteins induce interleukin 1, tumor necrosis factor alpha, and nitric oxide in glial cultures derived from fetal, neonatal, and adult human brain. *J Exp Med, 182*, 941–51.

Kort, J. J. & Jalonen, T. O. (1998). The nef protein of the human immunodeficiency virus type 1 (HIV-1) inhibits a large-conductance potassium channel in human glial cells. *Neurosci Lett, 251*, 1–4.

Kraft-Terry, S. D., Buch, S. J., Fox, H. S., & Gendelman, H. E. (2009). A coat of many colors: Neuroimmune crosstalk in human immunodeficiency virus infection. *Neuron, 64*, 133–45.

Kramer-Hammerle, S., Hahn, A., Brack-Werner, R., & Werner, T. (2005a). Elucidating effects of long-term expression of HIV-1 Nef on astrocytes by microarray, promoter, and literature analyses. *Gene, 358*, 31–8.

Kramer-Hammerle, S., Kohleisen, B., Hohenadl, C., Shumay, E., Becker, I., Erfle, V., et al. (2001). HIV type 1 Nef promotes neoplastic transformation of immortalized neural cells. *AIDS Res Hum Retroviruses, 17*, 597–602.

Kramer-Hammerle, S., Rothenaigner, I., Wolff, H., Bell, J. E., & Brack-Werner, R. (2005b). Cells of the central nervous system as targets and reservoirs of the human immunodeficiency virus. *Virus Res, 111*, 194–213.

Krathwohl, M.D., & Kaiser, J. L. (2004). HIV-1 promotes quiescence in human neural progenitor cells. *J Infect Dis, 190*, 216–26.

Kure, K., Lyman, W. D., Weidenheim, K. M., & Dickson, D. W. (1990a). Cellular localization of an HIV-1 antigen in subacute AIDS encephalitis using an improved double-labeling immunohistochemical method. *Am J Pathol, 136*, 1085–92.

Kure, K., Weidenheim, K. M., Lyman, W. D., & Dickson, D. W. (1990b). Morphology and distribution of HIV-1 gp41-positive microglia in subacute AIDS encephalitis. Pattern of involvement resembling a multisystem degeneration. *Acta Neuropathol, 80*, 393–400.

Lavi, E., Kolson, D. L., Ulrich, A. M., Fu, L., & Gonzalez-Scarano, F. (1998). Chemokine receptors in the human brain and their relationship to HIV infection. *J Neurovirol, 4*, 301–11.

Lawrence, D. M., Durham, L. C., Schwartz, L., Seth, P., Maric, D., & Major, E. O. (2004). Human immunodeficiency virus type 1 infection of human brain-derived progenitor cells. *J Virol, 78*, 7319–28.

Lee, C., Tomkowicz, B., Freedman, B. D., & Collman, R. G. (2005). HIV-1 gp120-induced TNF-{alpha} production by primary human macrophages is mediated by phosphatidylinositol-3 (PI-3) kinase and mitogen-activated protein (MAP) kinase pathways. *J Leukoc Biol, 78*, 1016–23.

Lehmann, M. H., Masanetz, S., Kramer, S., & Erfle, V. (2006). HIV-1 Nef upregulates CCL2/MCP-1 expression in astrocytes in a myristoylation- and calmodulin-dependent manner. *J Cell Sci, 119*, 4520–30.

Lipton, S. A., & Nicotera, P. (1998). Calcium, free radicals and excitotoxins in neuronal apoptosis. *Cell Calcium, 23*, 165–71.

Liu, Y., Jones, M., Hingtgen, C. M., Bu, G., Laribee, N., Tanzi, R. E., et al. (2000). Uptake of HIV-1 tat protein mediated by low-density lipoprotein receptor-related protein disrupts the neuronal metabolic balance of the receptor ligands. *Nat Med, 6*, 1380–7.

Majumder, B., Venkatachari, N. J., Srinivasan, A., & Ayyavoo, V. (2009). HIV-1 mediated immune pathogenesis: Spotlight on the role of viral protein R (Vpr). *Curr HIV Res, 7*, 169–77.

Martin-Garcia, J., Kolson, D. L., & Gonzalez-Scarano, F. (2002). Chemokine receptors in the brain: Their role in HIV infection and pathogenesis. *AIDS, 16*, 1709–30.

Mattson, M. P., Haughey, N. J., & Nath, A. (2005). Cell death in HIV dementia. *Cell Death Differ, 12*, Suppl 1, 893–904.

Merrill, J. E., Koyanagi, Y., Zack, J., Thomas, L., Martin, F., & Chen, I. S. (1992). Induction of interleukin-1 and tumor necrosis factor alpha in brain cultures by human immunodeficiency virus type 1. *J Virol, 66*, 2217–25.

Meucci, O., Fatatis, A., Simen, A. A., Bushell, T. J., Gray, P. W., & Miller, R. J. (1998). Chemokines regulate hippocampal neuronal signaling and gp120 neurotoxicity. *Proc Natl Acad Sci U S A, 95*, 14500–5.

Mishra, M., Vetrivel, S., Siddappa, N. B., Ranga, U., & Seth, P. (2008). Clade-specific differences in neurotoxicity of human immunodeficiency virus-1 B and C Tat of human neurons: Significance of dicysteine C30C31 motif. *Ann Neurol, 63*, 366–76.

Mollace, V., Colasanti, M., Persichini, T., Bagetta, G., Lauro, G. M., & Nistico, G. (1993). HIV gp120 glycoprotein stimulates the inducible isoform of no synthase in human cultured astrocytoma cells. *Biochem Biophys Res Commun, 194*, 439–45.

Nath, A., Anderson, C., Jones, M., Maragos, W., Booze, R., Mactutus, C., et al. (2000). Neurotoxicity and dysfunction of dopaminergic systems associated with AIDS dementia. *J Psychopharmacol, 14*, 222–7.

Nath, A., Psooy, K., Martin, C., Knudsen, B., Magnuson, D. S., Haughey, N., et al. (1996). Identification of a human immunodeficiency virus type 1 Tat epitope that is neuroexcitatory and neurotoxic. *J Virol, 70*, 1475–80.

Noorbakhsh, F., Ramachandran, R., Barsby, N., Ellestad, K. K., Leblanc, A., Dickie, P., et al. (2010). MicroRNA profiling reveals new aspects of HIV neurodegeneration: Caspase-6 regulates astrocyte survival. *Faseb J.*

Noorbakhsh, F., Vergnolle, N., McArthur, J. C., Silva, C., Vodjgani, M., Andrade-Gordon, P., et al. (2005). Proteinase-activated receptor-2 induction by neuroinflammation prevents neuronal death during HIV infection. *J Immunol, 174*, 7320–9.

Okamoto, S., Kang, Y. J., Brechtel, C. W., Siviglia, E., Russo, R., & Clemente, A. (2007). HIV/gp120 decreases adult neural progenitor cell proliferation via checkpoint kinase-mediated cell-cycle withdrawal and G1 arrest. *Cell Stem Cell, 1*, 230–6.

Olivetta, E., Percario, Z., Fiorucci, G., Mattia, G., Schiavoni, I., Dennis, C., et al. (2003). HIV-1 Nef induces the release of inflammatory factors from human monocyte/macrophages: Involvement of Nef endocytotic signals and NF-kappa B activation. *J Immunol, 170*, 1716–27.

Patton, H. K., Zhou, Z. H., Bubien, J. K., Benveniste, E. N., & Benos, D. J. (2000). gp120-induced alterations of human astrocyte function: Na(+)/H(+) exchange, K(+) conductance, and glutamate flux. *Am J Physiol Cell Physiol, 279*, C700–8.

Peng, H., Erdmann, N., Whitney, N., Dou, H., Gorantla, S., Gendelman, H. E., et al. (2006). HIV-1-infected and/or immune activated macrophages regulate astrocyte SDF-1 production through IL-1beta. *Glia, 54*, 619–29.

Peng, H., Whitney, N., Wu, Y., Tian, C., Dou, H., Zhou, Y., et al. (2008). HIV-1-infected and/or immune-activated macrophage-secreted TNF-alpha affects human fetal cortical neural progenitor cell proliferation and differentiation. *Glia, 56*, 903–16.

Piller, S. C., Ewart, G. D., Premkumar, A., Cox, G. B., & Gage, P. W. (1996). Vpr protein of human immunodeficiency virus type 1 forms cation-selective channels in planar lipid bilayers. *Proc Natl Acad Sci USA, 93*, 111–5.

Piller, S. C., Jans, P., Gage, P. W., & Jans, D. A. (1998). Extracellular HIV-1 virus protein R causes a large inward current and cell death in cultured hippocampal neurons: implications for AIDS pathology. *Proc Natl Acad Sci USA, 95*, 4595–4600.

Pocernich, C. B., Sultana, R., Mohmmad-Abdul, H., Nath, A., & Butterfield, D. A. (2005). HIV-dementia, Tat-induced oxidative stress, and antioxidant therapeutic considerations. *Brain Res Brain Res Rev, 50,* 14–26.

Price, T. O., Ercal, N., Nakaoke, R., & Banks, W. A. (2005). HIV-1 viral proteins gp120 and Tat induce oxidative stress in brain endothelial cells. *Brain Res, 1045,* 57–63.

Price, T. O., Uras, F., Banks, W. A., & Ercal, N. (2006). A novel antioxidant N-acetylcysteine amide prevents gp120- and Tat-induced oxidative stress in brain endothelial cells. *Exp Neurol, 201,* 193–202.

Pugliese, A., Vidotto, V., Beltramo, T., Petrini, S., & Torre, D. (2005). A review of HIV-1 Tat protein biological effects. *Cell Biochem Funct, 23,* 223–7.

Ranki, A., Nyberg, M., Ovod, V., Haltia, M., Elovaara, I., Raininko, R., et al. (1995). Abundant expression of HIV Nef and Rev proteins in brain astrocytes in vivo is associated with dementia. *AIDS, 9,* 1001–8.

Richard, A., Robichaud, G., Lapointe, R., Bourgoin, S., Darveau, A., & Poulin, L. (1997). Interference of HIV-1 Nef in the sphingomyelin transduction pathway activated by tumour necrosis factor-alpha in human glial cells. *AIDS, 11,* F1–7.

Robichaud, G. A. & Poulin, L. (2000). HIV type 1 nef gene inhibits tumor necrosis factor alpha-induced apoptosis and promotes cell proliferation through the action of MAPK and JNK in human glial cells. *AIDS Res Hum Retroviruses, 16,* 1959–65.

Romani, B. & Engelbrecht, S. (2009). Human immunodeficiency virus type 1 Vpr: Functions and molecular interactions. *J Gen Virol, 90,* 1795–805.

Romani, B., Engelbrecht, S., & Glashoff, R. H. (2010). Functions of Tat: The versatile protein of human immunodeficiency virus type 1. *J Gen Virol, 91,* 1–12.

Rothenaigner, I., Kramer, S., Ziegler, M., Wolff, H., Kleinschmidt, A., & Brack-Werner, R. (2007). Long-term HIV-1 infection of neural progenitor populations. *AIDS, 21,* 2271–81.

Roux, K. H. & Taylor, K. A. (2007). AIDS virus envelope spike structure. *Curr Opin Struct Biol, 17,* 244–52.

Sabbah, E. N. & Roques, B. P. (2005). Critical implication of the (70–96) domain of human immunodeficiency virus type 1 Vpr protein in apoptosis of primary rat cortical and striatal neurons. *J Neurovirol, 11,* 489–502.

Saito, Y., Sharer, L. R., Epstein, L. G., Michaels, J., Mintz, M., Louder, M., et al. (1994). Overexpression of nef as a marker for restricted HIV-1 infection of astrocytes in postmortem pediatric central nervous tissues. *Neurology, 44,* 474–81.

Schwartz, L., Civitello, L., Dunn-Pirio, A., Ryschkewitsch, S., Berry, E., Cavert, W., et al. (2007). Evidence of human immunodeficiency virus type 1 infection of nestin-positive neural progenitors in archival pediatric brain tissue. *J Neurovirol, 13,* 274–83.

Schwartz, L. & Major, E. O. (2006). Neural progenitors and HIV-1-associated central nervous system disease in adults and children. *Curr HIV Res, 4,* 319–27.

Self, R. L., Mulholland, P. J., Harris, B. R., Nath, A., & Prendergast, M. A. (2004). Cytotoxic effects of exposure to the human immunodeficiency virus type 1 protein Tat in the hippocampus are enhanced by prior ethanol treatment. *Alcohol Clin Exp Res, 28,* 1916–1924.

Seshamma, T., Bagasra, O., Trono, D., Baltimore, D., & Pomerantz, R. J. (1992). Blocked early-stage latency in the peripheral blood cells of certain individuals infected with human immunodeficiency virus type 1. *Proc Natl Acad Sci USA, 89,* 10663–7.

Sheng, W. S., Hu, S., Hegg, C. C., Thayer, S. A., & Peterson, P. K. (2000). Activation of human microglial cells by HIV-1 gp41 and Tat proteins. *Clin Immunol, 96,* 243–51.

Silvers, J. M., Aksenov, M. Y., Aksenova, M. V., Beckley, J., Olton, P., Mactutus, C. F., et al. (2006). Dopaminergic marker proteins in the substantia nigra of human immunodeficiency virus type 1-infected brains. *J Neurovirol, 12,* 140–5.

Silvers, J. M., Aksenova, M. V., Aksenov, M. Y., Mactutus, C. F., & Booze, R. M. (2007). Neurotoxicity of HIV-1 Tat protein: Involvement of D1 dopamine receptor. *Neurotoxicology, 28,* 1184–90.

Speth, C., Schabetsberger, T., Mohsenipour, I., Stockl, G., Wurzner, R., Stoiber, H., et al. (2002). Mechanism of human immunodeficiency virus-induced complement expression in astrocytes and neurons. *J Virol, 76,* 3179–88.

Sporer, B., Koedel, U., Paul, R., Kohleisen, B., Erfle, V., Fontana, A., et al. (2000). Human immunodeficiency virus type-1 Nef protein induces blood-brain barrier disruption in the rat: Role of matrix metalloproteinase-9. *J Neuroimmunol, 102,* 125–30.

Theodore, S., Cass, W. A., & Maragos, W. F. (2006a). Involvement of cytokines in human immunodeficiency virus-1 protein Tat and methamphetamine interactions in the striatum. *Exp Neurol, 199,* 490–8.

Theodore, S., Cass, W. A., & Maragos, W. F. (2006b). Methamphetamine and human immunodeficiency virus protein Tat synergize to destroy dopaminergic terminals in the rat striatum. *Neuroscience, 137,* 925–35.

Ting, K. K., Brew, B. J., & Guillemin, G. J. (2009). Effect of quinolinic acid on human astrocytes morphology and functions: Implications in Alzheimer's disease. *J Neuroinflammation, 6,* 36.

Tran, P. B., Ren, D., & Miller, R. J. (2005). The HIV-1 coat protein gp120 regulates CXCR4-mediated signaling in neural progenitor cells. *J Neuroimmunol, 160,* 68–76.

Trillo-Pazos, G., McFarlane-Abdulla, E., Campbell, I. C., Pilkington, G. J., & Everall, I. P. (2000). Recombinant nef HIV-IIIB protein is toxic to human neurons in culture. *Brain Res, 864,* 315–26.

Tungaturthi, P. K., Sawaya, B. E., Singh, S. P., Tomkowicz, B., Ayyavoo, V., Khalili, K., et al. (2003). Role of HIV-1 Vpr in AIDS pathogenesis: Relevance and implications of intravirion, intracellular and free Vpr. *Biomed Pharmacother, 57,* 20–4.

Turchan-Cholewo, J., Dimayuga, V. M., Gupta, S., Gorospe, R. M., Keller, J. N., & Bruce-Keller, A. J. (2009). NADPH oxidase drives cytokine and neurotoxin release from microglia and macrophages in response to HIV-Tat. *Antioxid Redox Signal, 11,* 193–204.

Tyor, W. R., Power, C., Gendelman, H. E., & Markham, R. B. (1993). A model of human immunodeficiency virus encephalitis in scid mice. *Proc Natl Acad Sci USA, 90,* 8658–62.

van de Bovenkamp, M., Nottet, H. S., & Pereira, C. F. (2002). Interactions of human immunodeficiency virus-1 proteins with neurons: Possible role in the development of human immunodeficiency virus-1-associated dementia. *Eur J Clin Invest.* 32:619–27.

van Marle, G., Henry, S., Todoruk, T., Sullivan, A., Silva, C., Rourke, S. B., et al. 2004. Human immunodeficiency virus type 1 Nef protein mediates neural cell death: A neurotoxic role for IP-10. *Virology, 329,* 302–18.

Vilhardt, F., Plastre, O., Sawada, M., Suzuki, K., Wiznerowicz, M., Kiyokawa, E., et al. (2002). The HIV-1 Nef protein and phagocyte NADPH oxidase activation. *J Biol Chem, 277,* 42136–43.

Wallace, D. R. (2006). HIV neurotoxicity: Potential therapeutic interventions. *J Biomed Biotechnol, 2006,* 65741.

Wallace, D. R., Dodson, S., Nath, A., & Booze, R. M. (2006). Estrogen attenuates gp120- and tat1–72-induced oxidative stress and prevents loss of dopamine transporter function. *Synapse, 59,* 51–60.

Wang, Z., Trillo-Pazos, G., Kim, S. Y., Canki, M., Morgello, S., Sharer, L. R., et al. (2004). Effects of human immunodeficiency virus type 1 on astrocyte gene expression and function: potential role in neuropathogenesis. *J Neurovirol.* 10 Suppl 1:25–32.

Werner, T., Ferroni, S., Saermark, T., Brack-Werner, R., Banati, R. B., Mager, R., et al. 1991. HIV-1 Nef protein exhibits structural and functional similarity to scorpion peptides interacting with K+ channels. *AIDS 5,* 1301–8.

Wheeler, E. D., Achim, C. L., & Ayyavoo, V. (2006). Immunodetection of human immunodeficiency virus type 1 (HIV-1) Vpr in brain tissue of HIV-1 encephalitic patients. *J Neurovirol, 12,* 200–10.

Williams, R., Yao, H., Peng, F., Yang, Y., Bethel-Brown, C., & Buch, S. (2010). Cooperative induction of CXCL10 involves NADPH oxidase: Implications for HIV dementia. *Glia, 58,* 611–21.

Wu, P., Price, P., Du, B., Hatch, W. C., & Terwilliger, E. F. (1996). Direct cytotoxicity of HIV-1 envelope protein gp120 on human NT neurons. *Neuroreport, 7,* 1045–9.

Wyatt, R. & Sodroski, J. (1998). The HIV-1 envelope glycoproteins: Fusogens, antigens, and immunogens. *Science, 280*, 1884–8.

Xiong, H., Zeng, Y. C., Lewis, T., Zheng, J., Persidsky, Y., & Gendelman, H. E. (2000). HIV-1 infected mononuclear phagocyte secretory products affect neuronal physiology leading to cellular demise: relevance for HIV-1-associated dementia. *J Neurovirol, 6* Suppl 1, S14–23.

Yao, H., Peng, F., Fan, Y., Zhu, X., Hu, G., & Buch, S. J. (2009). TRPC channel-mediated neuroprotection by PDGF involves Pyk2/ERK/CREB pathway. *Cell Death Differ, 16*, 1681–93.

Zauli, G., Secchiero, P., Rodella, L., Gibellini, D., Mirandola, P., Mazzoni, M., et al. (2000). HIV-1 Tat-mediated inhibition of the tyrosine hydroxylase gene expression in dopaminergic neuronal cells. *J Biol Chem, 275*, 4159–65.

Zhang, K., McQuibban, G. A., Silva, C., Butler, G. S., Johnston, J. B., Holden, J., et al. (2003). HIV-induced metalloproteinase processing of the chemokine stromal cell derived factor-1 causes neurodegeneration. *Nat Neurosci, 6*, 1064–71.

Zhang, X., & Aida, Y. (2009). HIV-1 Vpr: A novel role in regulating RNA splicing. *Curr HIV Res, 7*, 163–8.

Zheng, J., Thylin, M. R., Ghorpade, A., Xiong, H., Persidsky, Y., et al. (1999). Intracellular CXCR4 signaling, neuronal apoptosis and neuropathogenic mechanisms of HIV-1-associated dementia. *J Neuroimmunol, 98*, 185–200.

Zhou, B. Y., Liu, Y., Kim, B., Xiao, Y., & He, J. J. (2004). Astrocyte activation and dysfunction and neuron death by HIV-1 Tat expression in astrocytes. *Mol Cell Neurosci, 27*, 296–305.

Zhu, J., Mactutus, C. F., Wallace, D. R., & Booze, R. M. (2009). HIV-1 Tat protein-induced rapid and reversible decrease in [3H]dopamine uptake: Dissociation of [3H]dopamine uptake and [3H]2beta-carbomethoxy-3-beta-(4-fluorophenyl)tropane (WIN 35,428) binding in rat striatal synaptosomes. *J Pharmacol Exp Ther, 329*, 1071–83.

Zink, M. C., Laast, V. A., Helke, K. L., Brice, A. K., Barber, S. A., Clements, J. E., et al. (2006). From mice to macaques—animal models of HIV nervous system disease. *Curr HIV Res, 4*, 293–305.

HIV-1 AND TAT

NEUROPATHOGENESIS AND THERAPEUTIC TARGETS

Wenxue Li, Guanhan Li, Joseph Steiner, and Avindra Nath

The Tat protein of the human immunodeficiency virus (HIV) has been implicated in the neuropathogenesis of HIV infection. This is the earliest protein to be produced by the proviral DNA in the infected cell. The protein not only drives the production and replication of the virus but is also actively released from the cell and then interacts with cell surface receptors of other uninfected cells in the brain, leading to cellular dysfunction. It may also be taken up by these cells and can then activate a number of host genes. The Tat protein is highly potent and has the unique ability to travel along neuronal pathways. It can also easily cross the blood-brain barrier. Importantly, its production is not impacted by the use of antiretroviral drugs once the proviral DNA has been formed. This chapter reviews the pleomorphic actions of Tat protein in relation to its effects on the nervous system.

INTRODUCTION

Human immunodeficiency virus (HIV) infection frequently results in neurological complications such as decreased cognition, depression, and motor dysfunction. Several terms have been used to describe the syndrome, including AIDS dementia complex and HIV-associated dementia. With the use of antiretroviral therapy, the severe forms of neurocognitive impairment are seldom seen, and more commonly milder forms persist. This has been termed HIV-associated neurocognitive disorders or HAND (Antinori et al., 2007). The pathophysiology of this disorder in the presence of antiretroviral drugs is clearly different than that in the pre-antiretroviral era and suggests a more important role for the Tat protein of HIV than previously anticipated. Tat is the first protein produced during viral replication. It plays a critical role in driving viral replication by transactivation of the promoter region of the virus, there is no effective treatment that blocks Tat activity, and it is produced by infected cells once the proviral DNA is formed even in the presence of available antiretroviral drugs. In this review, we discuss the pleomorphic actions of the Tat protein on the various cells types within the brain, the molecular basis of these interactions and the pharmacological approaches to date developed to try and block its activity.

TAT STRUCTURE

Tat is a transactivator of TAR (Tat associated region). It is a small protein of 101 amino acids but the length varies from strain to strain (Robert-Guroff et al., 1990). It is produced in the initial phase of viral transcription and localizes mainly to the nucleus and nucleolus (Stauber & Pavlakis, 1998). It is a highly basic protein, and therefore, has the potential for a nonspecific binding with different RNAs (Ruben et al., 1989). The primary role of Tat is to regulate (productive and processive) transcription from the HIV promoter region termed the long terminal repeat (LTR) (Rosen, Terwilliger, Dayton, Sodroski, & Haseltine, 1988). Residues 1–72 are encoded by the first exon and residues 73–101 or 104 are encoded by a second exon (Ruben et al., 1989). An 86 amino acid form of Tat, which exists in a few laboratory passaged virus strains (LAI, HXB2, and NL4–3), has been frequently used (Bilodeau, Domsic, & Stoltzfus, 1999). This version represents a truncated and not a naturally occurring full-length protein. Tat can be divided into six functional regions (Figure 4.3.1). Amino acids 1–48 represent a minimal activation domain of HIV-1 Tat required for LTR activation; the basic domain 49–72 contains a RKKRRQRRR motif, which confers TAR RNA binding and is important for nuclear localization signal (NLS) and uptake of Tat by cells (Jeang, Xiao, & Rich, 1999). Tat is believed to be functional as a monomer rather than a dimer. Mutations in the region 1–21 amino acids are tolerant to changes without loss of biologic activity; in contrast, changes in amino acids 25–40 are generally deleterious for transactivation. Sequences from 22–37, a cysteine-rich domain, binds with divalent cations like Zn^{2+} and Cd^{2+}. It has been shown that the Zn binding property is important for dimerization of Tat and subsequently affects its biological functions (Frankel, Bredt, & Pabo, 1988a). Moreover, it has been demonstrated that substitutions at cysteine residues 22, 25, 27, and 37 alter the transactivation of HIV LTR (Jeang et al., 1999). Acetylation of lysine at position 28 modulates the affinity and stability of Tat-cyclinT1-TAR complexes by enhancing an interaction with the cyclinT1 Tat-TAR recognition motif (D'Orso & Frankel, 2009). The cysteine residue at position 31 is critical for binding to the NMDA receptor on neurons and mediating neurotoxicity (Li et al., 2008). Chemotactic properties have also

I	II	III	IV	V	VI
1–20;	21–40;	41–48;	49–59;	60–72;	73–86/104;
Acidic/Pro rich	Cys rich/ZnF	Core	Basic	Glu rich	
First Exon					**Second Exon**

Figure 4.3.1 *Structural and functional domains of HIV-Tat protein.* The Tat protein is formed from two exons. The first exon is formed of 72 amino acids and the second exon varies in length and encodes amino acids 73 to 86 or 104. The protein is divided into six regions. The first five reside in the first exon. Of these, the cysteine-rich and the arginine-rich regions are important in mediating neurotoxicity through cell surface interactions. The nuclear localizing domain (amino acids 48–56) is important in the gene transactivation properties of Tat.

been attributed to this residue (Ranga et al., 2004). The second exon of Tat, 73–101 or 104 amino acids, is less studied. Findings from HIV and SIV (simian immunodeficiency virus) Tat are quite clear in demonstrating that this exon contributes towards optimal transactivation. There is also evidence that the second exon of HIV-1 Tat, in other assays, is important for transactivation, transrepression of transcription factors such as AP-1 and NF-kB, and virus replication. The RGD motif in the second exon that binds to integrin receptors is not found in HIV-2 and SIV Tat (Barillari, Gendelman, Gallo, & Ensoli, 1993). Moreover, the second exon has an ESKKKVE motif which is conserved in most HIV-1 Tat proteins and partially present in HIV-2 and SIV Tat (Kuppuswamy, Subramanian, Srinivasan, Chinnadurai, 1989). Nonetheless, it has been shown that cleavage of the C terminal of Tat between amino acids 68 and 69 by calpain-1 leads to increased neurotoxic properties (Passiatore, Rom, Eletto, & Peruzzi, 2009).

POST-TRANSLATIONAL MODIFICATIONS OF TAT AND THEIR ROLE IN ITS FUNCTION

Tat protein released from mammalian cells is 5,000-fold more neurotoxic than recombinant protein produced in *E. coli*. A major difference in the production of Tat in mammalian cells versus *E. coli* is the presence of unique post-translational modifications in the former. Tat has rather unique physical properties much unlike any other known protein. It has a pI of 9.4. It has a Cys-rich region that has the potential for forming dimers and polymers, binding to divalent cations (Frankel et al., 1988a; Frankel, Chen, Cotter, & Pabo, 1988b); a poly-Arg region that gives the molecule a highly positive change, to which several functions have been ascribed; several Lys residues that get acetylated (Kaehlcke et al., 2003; Kiernan et al., 1999) or methylated (Van Duyne et al., 2008); and several Ser and Thr residues that have the potential to get phosphorylated. Acetylation of the lysine residues has been shown to be critical for its ability to bind cyclin1 and thus mediate LTR transactivation (Desfosses et al., 2005). Tat has eight Lys residues in positions 12, 19, 28, 29, 41, 50 51, and 71. Interestingly the Lys residues in positions 28 and 29 are flanked by Cys residues in positions 27 and 30 and the Lys residues in positions 50 and 51 are flanked by Arg residues in positions 49 and 52. This suggests that the post-translational

modifcations are likely clustered and thus could have a major impact on its configuration and function (Table 4.3.1). The role of these physical properties and post-translational modifications in mediating Tat effects on brain cells have not been well studied, except that Cys31 to Ser mutation results in attenuation of Tat neurotoxicity. S-nitrosylation of the Cys in Tat can block its neurotoxic properties (Li et al., 2008). In an in vitro study, the Cys in Tat were also shown to be acetylated (Dormeyer, Dorr, Ott, & Schnolzer, 2003).

IMMUNE RESPONSES TO TAT

The immunological epitopes within Tat have not been studied in detail. Uninfected individuals have natural IgM antibodies directed against two portions of Tat (CTNCYCKKCCFH and GRKKRRQRRRPP), suggesting that this might be one basis for natural immunity against the virus (Rodman, Pruslin, To, & Winston, 1992). Interestingly, following a period of post-infection latency, the titers of natural antibodies decline and other Tat reactive antibodies do not rise (Zagury et al., 1998). This has made the use of Tat protein as an antigen for subunit vaccines extremely challenging. While, there is no information available regarding the antibody titers to Tat in patients with HIV-associated neurocognitive dysfunction, antibodies to the N or C terminal of Tat can form immune complexes that can bind to the NMDA receptor on neurons. These immune complexes can prevent activation of the receptor by Tat and even by other agonists of the receptor such as glutamate and quinolinic acid through stearic hinderance (Rumbaugh & Nath, unpublished observations).

TAT-MEDIATED HIV TRANSCRIPTION

HIV transcription is controlled primarily by Tat (Rosen et al., 1988). Transcription of the HIV provirus is characterized by an early, Tat-independent phase and a late, Tat-dependent phase. In the absence of Tat, a series of short transcripts are produced due to inefficient elongation by the recruited RNA pol II. However inefficient, this process results in the synthesis of a small fraction of full length viral transcripts leading to the synthesis of the Tat protein (Yedavalli, Benkirane, & Jeang, 2003). Tat, after binding to the hairpin loop (bulged RNA stem loop structure) TAR that is present at the 5'- terminus of all viral transcripts, rapidly leads to the synthesis of more Tat and the establishment of a positive regulatory loop. The optimal activity of Tat is further dictated by its association with two classes of cellular proteins, Tat-associated kinases (TAKs) (Deng et al., 2002) and Tat-associated histone acetyl transferases (HAT) (Marcello, Zoppe, & Giacca, 2001). Association of Tat and p-TEFb (TAK) with TAR leads to phosphorylation of the RNAPII CTD (Deng, Ammosova, Pumfery, Kashanchi, & Nekhai, 2002). Phosphorylation of RNAPII CTD renders otherwise nonprocessive RNAPII into productively elongating molecules. In addition to cellular kinases Tat also recruits cellular HATs. Two nuclear HATs, p300 and P/CAF, interact with and acetylate Tat on distinct lysine residues. The acetylation of the activator domain of Tat by P/CAF enhances the binding of Tat to the cellular factor CDK9/p-TEFb, whereas the acetylation of the TAR-binding domain by p300 promotes its dissociation from TAR element during early transcriptional elongation, and both events increase the activation of transcription from LTR (D'Orso & Frankel, 2009). Lysine methyl transferase Set7/9-KMT7 also methylates Tat, and this enhances Tat function (Pagans et al., 2010). The crystal structure of Tat bound to CDK9 and cyclin1 has recently been reported, which suggest that Tat binds through multiple interactions with these molecules (Tahirov et al., 2010). Tat-mediated LTR transactivation in astrocytes is unique and involves complex interactions with cellular transcription factors (Coyle-Rink et al., 2002) and may occur independent of TAR (Taylor et al., 1992).

ROLE OF TAT IN HIV REVERSE TRANSCRIPTION

It has been shown that Tat is able to stimulate efficient reverse transcription (Harrich, Ulich, Garcia-Martinez, & Gaynor, 1997). Tat binding to TAR RNA may alter TAR structure such that the initiation of reverse transcription is enhanced. Mutations of the Tat gene decrease the initiation of reverse transcription HIV-1 replication several thousand fold. Viruses lacking Tat are also defective in endogenous assays of reverse transcription, although these viruses contain similar levels of reverse transcriptase. These results indicate that the Tat protein, in addition to regulating the level of gene expression, is also important for efficient HIV-1 reverse transcription.

RELEASE AND UPTAKE OF TAT

Tat is released by infected lymphoid (Ensoli et al., 1993), monocytic cells (Turchan et al., 2001), and glial cells (Tardieu, Hery, Peudenier, Boespflug, & Montagnier, 1992) in vitro, by a leaderless but energy-dependent pathway (Chang, Samaniego, Nair, Buonaguro, & Ensoli, 1997) that does not involve any intracellular organelles (Rayne et al.). Monocytic (Johnston et al., 2001) and astrocytic cells (Chauhan et al., 2003) stably expressing Tat also release Tat extracellularly (Bruce-Keller et al., 2003). Both forms of Tat, that is, Tat formed by first exon only and that formed by first and second exon, are released

(Li et al., 2008; Malim & Cullen, 1991). Tat release occurs most optimally in low serum conditions (Ensoli et al., 1993) such as that present in the brain. Tat can be taken up readily by most cell types (Frankel & Pabo, 1988). This property of Tat has been exploited to deliver other proteins conjugated to Tat-derived peptides; a phenomenon called "protein transduction" (Ford, Darling, Souberbielle, & Farzaneh, 2000; Snyder & Dowdy, 2001). When full length Tat is taken up by cells it remains functionally active and can transactivate HIV expression. The basic domain that contains the arginine rich region is critical for the nuclear localization of Tat (Vives, Brodin, & Lebleu, 1997). The region derived from the second exon of Tat is important for the uptake of Tat (Ma & Nath, 1997). The mechanism of uptake involves interaction with the low-density lipoprotein receptor (Liu et al., 2000) and cell surface heparan sulfate proteoglycans (Tyagi et al., 2001). The transmembrane uptake of Tat is mediated through caveolar endocytosis (Fittipaldi et al., 2003) and clathrin-dependent endocytosis (Vendeville et al., 2004).

The cationic Tat peptide (amino acids 48–56), called the protein transduction domain (PTD) or cell penetrating peptide (CPP), is widely used as a vehicle for the intracellular delivery of macromolecules including oligonucleotides, peptides or proteins, low-molecular-mass drugs, nanoparticles, and liposomes (Schwarze, Ho, Vocero-Akbani, & Dowdy, 1999; Snyder & Dowdy, 2001). This approach has also been exploited for developing novel neuroprotective strategies (Spitere, Toulouse, O'Sullivan, & Sullivan, 2008; Wei, Miou, & Baudry, 2008). The mechanisms of the CPP-cargo translocation include macropinocytosis, clathrin-mediated endocytosis, and caveolae/lipid-raft-mediated endocytosis (Kaplan, Wadia, & Dowdy, 2005; Richard et al., 2005).

DETECTION OF TAT PROTEIN AND TRANSCRIPTS IN THE BRAIN

Several groups have demonstrated the presence of Tat protein in brains of patients with HIV encephalitis by immunostaining (Hofman et al., 1994; Hudson et al., 2000; Kruman, Nath, & Mattson, 1999; Liu et al., 2000; Valle et al., 2000a). Additionally, mRNA levels for *tat* are also elevated in brain tissue of patients with HIV dementia (Hudson et al., 2000; Wesselingh et al., 1993; Wiley, Baldwin, & Achim, 1996). In rhesus macaques with encephalitis due to a chimeric strain of HIV and the simian immunodeficiency virus, Tat has been demonstrated by immunostaining and by western blot analysis (Hudson et al., 2000). Immunostaining patterns suggest that Tat can be found in cytoplasm of perivascular macrophages, microglial nodules, and in glial cells which likely represent HIV-infected cells. However, interestingly, Tat can also be found in the nuclei of some neurons (Liu et al., 2000) and oligodendroglia (Valle et al., 2000b), which likely suggests that extracellular Tat was taken up by these cells. Tat can also be detected in the serum of patients with HIV infection in concentrations of about 1ng/ml (Westendorp et al., 1995) and concentrations of 4ng/ml have been reported in conditioned medium of HIV-infected cells (Albini et al., 1998a). While most studies using recombinant Tat protein use nM concentrations, the vast majority of the Tat protein in these preparations is polymerized or oxidized and hence, inactive. A recent study in which supernatants from Tat-transfected cells were directly used to cause neurotoxicity showed that low pM concentrations of Tat were sufficient to cause NMDA receptor activation and neurotoxicity (Li et al., 2008). In fact, cells stably transfected with Tat when injected into the brain cause significant alterations in histological markers of inflammation, synaptic density, and most importantly, in behavioral performance (Bruce-Keller et al., 2003; Chauhan et al., 2003).

EVOLUTION OF TAT MUTATIONS IN THE BRAIN

Tat sequences from the brain show distinct compartmentalization when compared to other tissues (Thomas et al., 2007). Non-synonymous/synonymous substitution (synonymous substitution is the substitution of one base for another in an exon of a gene coding for a protein, such that the amino acid sequence produced is not modified, while non-synonymous substitution leads to a change in the amino acid sequence) rates among the *tat* sequences derived from patients with HIV-associated neurocognitive impairment are significantly higher compared to the HIV-infected patient without neurocognitive impairment. The ratios of transversions (substitution of a purine for a pyrimidine or vice versa) to transitions (a mutation changing a purine to another purine nucleotide or a pyrimidine to another pyrimidine nucleotide) in the *tat* sequences are also significantly higher among the patients with HIV-associated neurocognitive impairment. Phylogenetic analyses show clustering of sequences from each clinical group among the brain-derived *tat* sequences (Bratanich et al., 1998). Comparison of matched brain- and spleen-derived *tat* sequences indicate that homology among brain-derived clones is greater than that between the brain- and spleen-derived clones. The brain-derived *tat* sequences are markedly heterogeneous in regions, which influence viral replication and intracellular transport (Mayne et al., 1998). Further, *tat* sequences from patients with HIV-associated neurocognitive impairment have different functional properties compared to those without associated neurocognitive impairment. For example, the former are not as efficient at transactivation of the LTR, but suppress the expression of proapoptotic genes and have a differential effect on several other host genes, features that promote it's neurotoxic potential (Boven et al., 2007). These studies indicate that differing selective forces act on the HIV *tat* gene in the brain, which may influence the development of neurocognitive impairment.

TRANSPORT OF TAT WITHIN THE BRAIN ALONG NEURONAL PATHWAYS

Tat can be transported in the brain along anatomical pathways both anterogradely and retrogradely. For example, when Tat-expressing cells were injected into the striatum, synaptic injury and gliosis was found in the substantia nigra and when the cells were injected into the hilus of the dentate gyrus, similar synaptic injury and gliosis was found in the CA3/4 region. Importantly, in both instances Tat could be detected at the sites of synaptic injury, clearly demonstrating the ability of Tat to be transported along these neurons (Bruce-Keller et al., 2003). Tat must have the ability to escape the proteolytic pathways within the cell and enter axonal transport systems. Consistent with the scenario, Tat can inhibit the proteolytic activity of the 20S proteasome (Huang et al., 2002; Seeger, Ferrell, Frank, & Dubiel, 1997), which may explain its ability to escape proteolysis in neurons. Further, these data suggest that Tat can be transported both retrogradely (from the striatum to the pars compacta region of the substantia nigra) and anterogradely (from the hilus to CA3/4). In another study, Tat was administered intranasally and then detected in the olfactory bulb, demonstrating its ability to travel along neuronal pathways; interestingly, dysregulation of several genes, including those involved in oxidative stress, were noted in other parts of the brain. These observations may have important implications for neuropathogenesis of retroviral infections, suggesting that Tat-induced neuronal damage and glial cell activation may occur at sites distant from the cells infected with the virus.

INTERACTIONS OF TAT WITH CELL SURFACE RECEPTORS

In the past years, Tat entry into cells was thought to be receptorless; however, recent studies have demonstrated that Tat transduction is receptor mediated. Heparan sulfate is the receptor for Tat, present on almost all types of cells and helps localize Tat to the cell membrane. Another receptor, the low-density lipoprotein receptor-related protein (LRP), helps internalize Tat by an endocytic process. However, both heparan sulfate and LRP are necessary for Tat entry in neuronal cells (Liu et al., 2000). In neurons, LRP, postsynaptic density protein-95 (PSD-95), and the N-methyl-d-aspartic acid (NMDA) receptors form a macromolecular complex which is stimulated by Tat, leading to neuronal injury (Eugenin et al., 2007). The core domain of Tat (aa 37–48) is directly involved in Tat interaction with LRP domains II, III, and IV. Tat can also bind directly to the NMDA receptor through cys-cys interactions with the extracellular domain of the NR-1 subunit (Li et al., 2008) and Tat-derived peptides can block NMDA receptor-mediated excitotoxicity (Vaslin, Rummel, & Clarke, 2009). Tat can also bind to the dopamine transporter in striatal neurons (Zhu, Mactutus, Wallace, & Booze, 2009). Tat shows conserved amino acids corresponding to critical sequences of some chemokines. Synthetic Tat and a peptide (CysL24–51) encompassing the "chemokine-like" region of Tat induces a rapid and transient Ca^{2+} influx in monocytes and macrophages, analogous to beta-chemokines. Cross-desensitization studies indicate that Tat shares receptors with MCP-1, MCP-3, and eotaxin and can displace beta-chemokines from chemokine receptors CCR2 and CCR3, but not CCR1, CCR4, and CCR5 (Albini et al., 1998b). Furthermore, Tat binds to chemokine receptor CXCR4; therefore it may act as an antagonist for virion binding to this receptor (Xiao et al., 2000). This directs pressure on HIV-1 CXCR4 strains to adapt to CCR5 tropic strains. However, neurons are not infected though they contain CXCR4 as well as CCR5. Thus Tat may disrupt neuronal function by interaction with CXCR4. Tat is also capable of inducing chemokine receptor expression. Tat can induce CXCR4 on both lymphocytes and monocytes/macrophages, whereas CCR5 and CCR3 are induced on monocytes/macrophages but not on lymphocytes (Huang et al., 1998; Secchiero, Zella, Capitani, Gallo, & Zauli, 1999; Weiss, Nath, Major, & Berman, 1999).

INTRACELLULAR TAT BINDING FACTORS

HIV Tat protein interacts intracellularly with host proteins which amplify or down modulate its effects on HIV transcription. A 110 kDa Tat-interacting protein (Tip) in the nucleus amplifies the Tat effect on LTR transactivation (Liu et al., 2002). Another Tip—60 kDa—also augments Tat-dependent HIV LTR transcription by interacting with various cellular transcription factors that belong to the nuclear histone acetyl transferase family. HIV Tat also interacts with a 26S proteosome, through Tat-binding protein-1 (Nelbock, Dillon, Perkins, & Rosen, 1990; Tanaka, Nakamura, Takagi, & Sato, 1997). Interestingly, another nuclear protein, pur alpha, also interacts directly with Tat. Residues 49–72 of Tat are critical for binding with pur alpha (Wortman et al., 2000). Pur alpha is a single-stranded DNA binding protein, which binds to RNA, with much lower affinity. Pur alpha and Tat also synergistically stimulate the JC virus promoter (Tada et al., 1990).

EFFECT OF TAT ON NEURONS

Intracerebral injection of Tat can be lethal to mice within hours of injection (Gourdou et al., 1990; Sabatier et al., 1991). In another animal model, Tat was shown to cause attenuation of spatial learning accompanied by suppression of long-term potentiation, the cellular basis of spatial learning in hippocampal slices (Li et al., 2004). In adult animals Tat affects preattentive processes and spatial memory (Fitting, Booze, & Mactutus, 2008). In a Tat transgenic model there is marked glial cell activation and neuronal loss (Kim et al., 2003a). Tat causes loss of selective populations of neurons in vitro and in vivo (Hayman et al., 1993; Jones, Olafson, Del Bigio, Peeling, & Nath, 1998; Magnuson, Knudsen, Geiger, Brownstone, & Nath, 1995; Maragos et al., 2003). Regions particularly susceptible to Tat neurotoxicity include the striatum (Hayman et al., 1993), dentate gyrus, and the CA3 region of the hippocampus (Maragos et al., 2003). These regions are rich in NMDA receptors (Malva, Carvalho, & Carvalho, 1998). Furthermore, neuropathological studies from patients with HIV infection show a preferential loss of neurons in the dentate gyrus (Maragos et al., 2003) and striatum (Everall, Barnes, Spargo, & Lantos, 1995). Consistent with these observations, there is a reduction in evoked dopamine in the striatum of the Tat-treated animals suggesting a dysfunction of nerve terminals (Ferris, Frederick-Duus, Fadel, Mactutus, & Booze, 2009). Specifically, in dopaminergic neurons, Tat-mediated neurotoxicity can be blocked by antagonists of the D1 dopaminergic receptor (Silvers, Aksenova, Aksenov, Mactutus, & Booze, 2007).

Tat produces dose-dependent depolarizations even in the presence of the sodium channel blocker tetrodotoxin, which suggests that Tat actions are independent of synaptic interactions (Magnuson et al., 1995; Perez, Probert, Wang, & Sharmeen, 2001). Tat also depolarizes the neuronal cell membrane when applied extracellularly to outside-out membrane patches providing strong evidence for direct excitation of neurons on the cell surface (Cheng et al., 1998). In contrast, neurotoxicity induced by gp120 is mediated primarily by indirect mechanisms. However, the polyamine site of the NMDA receptor (Prendergast et al., 2002) and Tat-induced phosphorylation of the NMDA receptor (Haughey, Nath, Mattson, Slevin, & Geiger, 2001) have also been implicated in Tat-mediated neurotoxicity. Tat treatment of neurons results in tyrosine (Y) phosphorylation of the NMDAR subunit 2A (NR2A) in a src kinase-dependent manner at Y1325. Phosphorylation of this site can also be found in the brain from patients with HIV encephalitis (King, Eugenin, Hazleton, Morgello, & Berman, 2010). Further, Tat binds to the extracellular domain of the NR1 subunit of the NMDA receptor via cysteine-cysteine interactions, which suggest a novel mechanism for excitation of this receptor (Li et al., 2008). Another unique feature of the electrophysiological property of Tat is that it does not show any evidence of desensitization upon repetitive applications (Cheng et al., 1998). The degree of desensitization of glutamate receptors may be inversely predictive of agonist toxicity (Brorson, Manzolillo, Gibbons, & Miller, 1995; Garthwaite, 1991; Jonas & Sakmann, 1992). The nondesensitizing actions of Tat would cause the potentially deleterious actions to persist during the prolonged periods in which neurons in HIV-1-infected brain would be exposed to Tat.

Tat induces dramatic increases in levels of intracellular calcium in neurons. There is an initial brief burst of intracellular calcium release through IP-3 sensitive pools followed by prolonged increases in cytoplasmic calcium resulting from an influx of extracellular calcium (Haughey et al., 1999). This is followed by mitochondrial calcium uptake, inhibition of complex IV of the electron transport chain, generation of reactive oxygen species, activation of caspases, and eventually results in apoptosis (Kruman et al., 1998; New, Ma, Epstein, Nath, & Gelbard, 1997; Norman, Perry, Kasischke, Volsky, & Gelbard, 2007). Tat-induced neuronal cell death can be prevented by excitatory amino acid receptor antagonists (Brailoiu, Brailoiu, Chang, & Dun, 2008; Magnuson et al., 1995), inhibitors of nitric oxide synthase and caspases, antioxidants and agents that stabilize mitochondrial membrane permeability, and IP-3 pools of intracellular calcium (Haughey et al., 1999; Kruman et al., 1998; Perry et al., 2005) and inhibition of glycogen synthase kinase-3beta by lithium (Maggirwar, Tong, Ramirez,

Gelbard, & Dewhurst, 1999; Sui et al., 2006). Downregulation of PTEN (phosphatase and tensin homolog deleted on chromosome 10), which is located upstream of glycogen synthase kinase-3beta, also protects against Tat neurotoxicity (Zhao et al., 2007). Tat also induces rapid loss of calcium from endoplasmic reticulum mediated by the ryanodine receptor, followed by the unfolded protein response and pathologic dilatation of the endoplasmic reticulum in cortical neurons. These morphological features can also be seen in the brain from patients with HIV encephalitis (Norman et al., 2008). Evidence of oxidative stress is also noted in vivo upon intrastriatal injections of Tat (Aksenov et al., 2001). Interestingly, Tat expression in glial cells has an antioxidative effect on the glial cells; however, upon release from these cells it causes oxidative stress and toxicity in neurons (Chauhan et al., 2003). Hence, these toxic effects are specific for neuronal cells. Other mechanisms have also been implicated in Tat-induced neurotoxicity. It has been shown that Tat can induce the expression of SDF-1 in neurons, which in turn upon release can cause neurotoxicity in other neurons (Langford, Sanders, Mallory, Kaul, & Masliah, 2002). Tat can synergize with other toxins such as gp120 (Bansal et al., 2000; Nath et al., 2000), glutamate (Wang, Barks, & Silverstein, 1999), and drugs of abuse to cause neurotoxicity (Nath et al., 2002). Following a brief exposure to Tat, subsequent application of physiological levels of glutamate can cause massive derangement in intracellular calcium, suggesting that the protein can sensitize the neurons to neurotoxic substances (Nath et al., 2000). In contrast, Tat may inhibit glutamate-mediated changes in intracellular calcium in astrocytes (Koller et al., 2001). The cysteine-rich region and the basic domain seem to be critical for causing neurotoxicity (Gourdou et al., 1990; Nath et al., 1996; Weeks et al., 1995). Neurotrophic factors can also protect against Tat-induced neurotoxicity through the induction of anti-apoptotic genes (Ramirez et al., 2001). Another mechanism by which Tat may affect synaptic function is by dysregulation of selected microRNAs, particularly neuronal mir-128, in primary cortical neurons, which further inhibits expression of the pre-synaptic protein SNAP25 (Eletto et al., 2008).

Tat also induces marked aggregation of neurons and astrocytes in developing cultures and causes the neuritic processes to coalesce into fascicles. These effects have been mapped to the RGD (arginine-glycine-aspartic acid) sequence within the second exon (Kolson et al., 1993). These observations may be important not only for the developing brain but also in adults as it may impair neurogenesis and gliogenesis.

EFFECT OF TAT ON GLIAL CELL FUNCTION

Besides direct neurotoxicity, Tat can also cause neurotoxicity by the release of neurotoxic substances from glial cells and macrophages. Tat can also alter glial cell function, which leads to loss of support function for neurons. For example, intraventricular injection of Tat showed prominent glial cell activation and infiltration of perivascular macrophages (Jones et al., 1998). Tat also has a number of effects on glial cell function. It stimulates the production of pro-inflammatory cytokines in the brain (Chen, Mayne, Power, & Nath, 1997; Pulliam et al., 2007) and neurotoxins in these cells. Tat induces a milieu of cytokines and chemokines in macrophages and astrocytes (D'Aversa, Yu, & Berman, 2004; Kutsch, Oh, Nath, & Benveniste, 2000; Weiss et al., 1999). Significant amongst these are tumor necrosis factor -α (TNF-α), monocyte chemoattractant factor-1 (MCP-1)/CCL-2, and CXCL-10 (Eugenin, Dyer, Calderon, & Berman, 2005; McManus et al., 2000). In fact, Tat is more potent than even lipopolysaccharide (LPS) in inducing TNF-α production (Chen et al., 1997) and may act on the TNF-α promoter (Darbinian et al., 2001). Cytokine induction in both cell types is NF-κB dependent (Conant et al., 1996). The epitope of Tat that induces TNF-α is different from the one that causes neurotoxicity (Buscemi, Ramonet, & Geiger, 2007). Tat-induced TNF-α can mediate neurotoxicity (New, Maggirwar, Epstein, Dewhurst, & Gelbard, 1998; Shi, Raina, Lorenzo, Busciglio, & Gabuzda, 1998; Sui et al., 2007). MCP-1/CCL-2 is a highly potent chemoattractant for monocytes. Levels of this chemokine are elevated in the CSF and brain of patients with HIV dementia (Conant, Ma, Nath, & Major, 1998). Interestingly, MCP-1/CCL-2 may protect neurons against Tat-induced neurotoxicity, suggesting that this chemokine may act as a double-edged sword (Eugenin, D'Aversa, Lopez, Calderon, & Berman, 2003). Tat-mediated MCP-1/CCL-2 production in astrocytes is mediated via kappa opiate receptors (Sheng, Hu, Lokensgard, & Peterson, 2003), is independent of the NF-kB pathway, but is mediated via cdk9 (Khiati et al.). Tat can synergize with gamma interferon to produce CXCL-10 (Dhillon et al., 2008) and can also induce endothelin-1 in astrocytes (Chauhan et al., 2007). Tat also induces matrix metalloproteinases (MMP) expression in astrocytes, which also facilitates monocyte transmigration by degradation of the extracellular matrix (Johnston et al., 2001; Ju et al., 2009). Quinolinic acid production, which is an excitotoxin, can also be induced by macrophages by Tat (Smith et al., 2001). Together, these studies suggest that Tat may be an important mediator of the inflammatory response in the brain. In a Tat transgenic model it was shown that ginkgo biloba extract could attenuate glial cell activation (Zou et al., 2007).

Differences in neurotoxic potential have been shown between Tat derived from patients with HIV dementia when compared to those without dementia. For example, macrophages expressing Tat from patients with HIV dementia exhibited elevated matrix metalloproteinase-2 and -7 release and caused neurotoxicity, but cells expressing Tat from non-demented patients did not exhibit enhanced MMP expression or cause neurotoxicity (Johnston et al., 2001). Tat can synergize with gamma interferon to induce iNOS expression in microglia (Polazzi et al., 1999). It can also induce iNOS in astrocytes (Liu et al., 2002). Independent of its effects on nitric oxide, Tat can also potently decrease cyclic AMP levels in microglia. This effect was not noted in astrocytes (Patrizio, Colucci, & Levi, 2001).

EFFECT OF TAT ON BLOOD-BRAIN BARRIER

The blood-brain barrier is formed of endothelial cells on the capillary luminal surface and astrocyte foot processes on the ablumenal surface. There is a basement membrane between the cells and the endothelial cells themselves are connected by tight junctions. Hence, any compromise in the endothelial or astrocytic cell function could impair the blood-brain barrier, leading to influx of serum proteins and leukocytes. Tat is capable of crossing the intact blood-brain barrier by a non-saturable mechanism with a unidirectional influx rate of about 0.490 microl/g/min. About 0.126% of an intravenous dose of Tat enters each gram of brain (Banks, Robinson, & Nath, 2005). Additionally, prolonged exposure of brain-derived endothelial cells to Tat may cause apoptosis (Kim et al., 2003b) or oxidative stress (Toborek et al., 2003). Tat can also induce IL-6 (Zidovetzki, Wang, Chen, Jeyaseelan, & Hofman, 1998) and IL-8 (Hofman, Chen, Incardona, Zidovetzki, & Hinton, 1999) expression on endothelial cells. Tat may also affect trafficking of leukocytes into the brain by inducing the expression of adhesion molecules, VCAM-1 and ICAM-1 in astrocytes (Woodman, Benveniste, Nath, & Berman, 1999). Tat-induced cytokine dysregulation in endothelial cells can be prevented by agonists of nuclear receptors, the peroxisome proliferator-activated receptors (Huang et al., 2008), or by simvastatin (Andras et al., 2008). Tat can also decrease the expression of several tight junction proteins; an effect that is mediated via calveolin-1 (Zhong et al., 2008). In contrast, cyclooxygenase-2 inhibitors attenuate Tat-induced alterations of occludin expression but have no effect on Tat-induced downregulation of zona occudens-1 expression or on increased blood-brain barrier permeability (Pu et al., 2007). Importantly, Tat induces the expression of P-glycoprotein and multidrug resistance-associated protein-1 on brain endothelial cells and astrocytes, which may have implications for delivery of antiretroviral drugs to the brain, since these efflux systems could prevent the CNS entry of these compounds (Hayashi et al., 2006; Hayashi et al., 2005; Zhong et al.). Further, as discussed above, some of the effects of Tat on chemokine expression, which may attract monocytes into the brain, matrix metalloproteinase production, which may degrade the extracellular matrix and alteration of astrocyte function, may also impair the blood-brain barrier. It remains unknown what the net effect might be of these seemingly opposite effects, that is, break down of the blood-brain barrier and the upregulation of multidrug resistance-associated protein on drug delivery to the CNS.

TAT AS A CHEMOATTRACTANT

Beside the ability of Tat to induce the production of chemokines and chemokine receptors, Tat may have some chemoattactant properties particularly for monocytes (Albini et al., 1998b). Significant sequence homology has been shown for Tat with several of the chemokines in key residues of functional importance in chemokines. These include a CCF motif,

an SYXR motif, which determines CXC/CC chemokine cell-type specificity (Lusti-Narasimhan et al., 1995), as well as a strongly conserved isoleucine. The greatest similarity is noted with the MCP/CCL family of chemokines (Albini et al., 1998b). Mutations in CC motif of Tat, particularly Cys in position 31 as is found naturally in clade C Tat, impairs its chemotactic properties (Ranga et al., 2004). Consistent with this observation, it is able to bind to CCR2 and CCR3 (Albini et al., 1998b).

EFFECT OF TAT ON AMYLOID DEPOSITION AND METABOLISM

Several in vitro and in vivo studies suggest that Tat increases deposition of amyloid in the brain and influences its metabolism (Giunta et al., 2009). This is important since both Tat and amyloid are neurotoxic and amyloid deposition increases with age, which may get accelerated by HIV infection. Tat can directly interact with the low density lipoprotein receptor and thus inhibit the uptake of its ligands including amyloid beta peptide (Liu et al., 2000). Further, the cysteine-rich domain of Tat interacts with neprilysin which is responsible for cleavage of secreted amyloid beta peptide and hence its clearance (Hersh, 2003).

INTERACTION OF TAT WITH DRUGS OF ABUSE IN MEDIATING NEURONAL INJURY

Methamphetamine and cocaine synergize with Tat to cause increased neurotoxicity (Turchan et al., 2001; Cai & Cadet, 2008). An in vivo study demonstrated the synergism between methamphetamine and Tat (Maragos et al., 2002). Animals treated with methamphetamine alone showed only a 7% reduction in striatal dopamine levels and Tat-treated animals showed only an 8% decline, but animals treated with both methamphetamine and Tat demonstrated a 65% reduction in striatal dopamine. This study might be particularly relevant, because the doses of methamphetamine and Tat used were equivalent to what might be seen in human disease. Subsequent microdialysis studies in this same animal model showed that the synergistic reduction in striatal dopamine is accompanied by significant decrease in dopamine release from the striatum (Cass, Harned, Peters, Nath, & Maragos, 2003) and a decrease in dopamine transporter due to loss of dopamine terminals (Theodore, Cass, Nath, & Maragos, 2007; Theodore, Stolberg, Cass, & Maragos, 2006b). Another possible mechanism for HIV-methamphetamine or cocaine interaction is via oxidative stress. Cocaine decreases mitochondrial respiration and increases the production of reactive oxygen species in animals (Boess, Ndikum-Moffor, Boelsterli, & Roberts, 2000). In one study (Flora et al., 2003), administration of either Tat or methamphetamine to mice increased markers of oxidative stress, including redox-regulated transcription factors in cortical, striatal, and hippocampal brain regions. Furthermore, the DNA-binding activities of these transcription factors were greater in mice injected with both Tat and methamphetamine, than with either Tat or methamphetamine alone. This same study also suggested Tat and methamphetamine may interact through changes in cell signaling and cytokine/chemokine expression. Mice treated with both agents had synergistic upregulation of intercellular adhesion molecule-1 (ICAM-1), tumor necrosis factor-alpha, and interleukin-1beta gene expression compared to mice treated with either agent alone. Interestingly, knock out animals lacking both receptors of tumor necrosis factor had no effect on dopamine levels when treated with Tat, suggesting that the Tat-mediated increase in tumor necrosis factor may contribute to the loss of dopaminergic terminals (Theodore et al., 2006a). Another study showed that Tat and methamphetamine interact to cause damage to calbindin-immunoreactive non-pyramidal neurons by dysregulating mitochondrial calcium metabolism, associated with increased levels of oxidative stress (Langford et al., 2004).

Morphine is the active metabolite of heroin and remarkable synergistic effects of Tat and morphine have been reported in glial cells. Sustained exposure to morphine and Tat causes dysfunction and death of both glial precursors and astrocytes, mediated by mu-opioid receptors through the activation of caspase-3 (Khurdayan et al., 2004). Similar changes have been reported in oligodendrocytes which also express the mu-opioid receptor (Hauser et al., 2009). Furthermore, recent studies have implicated astroglia as mediators for the proinflammatory effects of opiates in HIV-infected individuals. Combined opiate and Tat exposure synergistically destabilizes levels of intracellular calcium, increases reactive oxygen species, and causes massive release of proinflammatory chemokines in cultured striatal astroglia (El-Hage et al., 2005). The released chemokines include monocyte chemoattractant protein-1 (MCP-1) or CCL-2 and RANTES. MCP-1 triggers an influx of monocyte/macrophages and microglial activation.

INTERACTIONS BETWEEN HIV TAT AND OTHER VIRUSES

HERPES VIRUSES

Complex interactions occur with select herpes viruses such as cytomegalovirus (CMV), human herpesvirus-6 (HHV-6), and human herpesvirus-8 (HHV-8); however, no effect has been reported with other herpes viruses such as HSV-1 and HSV-2. In brain infections with HIV, co-infection with other viruses has been seen and synergistic association for severity or attenuation of the disease is reported. CMV and HHV-6 infection stimulate HIV replication and transactivate the HIV-1 promoter (the long terminal repeat or LTR) in astrocytes (McCarthy, Auger, He, & Wood, 1998). The level of this transactivation with immediate early genes, IE1/IE2, is similar to that following co-transfection with a Tat expression vector. Tat and CMV IE1/IE2 have a synergistic effect on HIV LTR transactivation; however, Tat effect or the synergistic effect is downregulated by another CMV product, UL44. Co-infection of HIV and HHV-6 and its

association with the severity of the disease has been seen in the brain. Tat upregulates HHV-6 replication by directly binding to the HHV-6 promoter or indirectly via activation of cellular factors (Garzino-Demo, Chen, Lusso, Berneman, & DiPaolo, 1996).

JC VIRUS

Another viral infection seen with HIV is JCV, where Tat plays a prominent role in activation of JCV in glial cells. HIV Tat can be detected in various JCV-infected cells as well as in uninfected oligodendrocytes from patients with PML and HIV infection, supporting the earlier in vitro findings that secreted Tat from the infected cells can be localized in the neighboring uninfected cells. The presence of Tat in oligodendrocytes is particularly interesting as this protein can up-modulate JCV gene transcription and several key cell cycle regulatory proteins including cyclin E, Cdk2, pRb, and SMAD (Stettner et al., 2009; Valle et al., 2000a). JCV contains sequences in the 5' end of the late RNA species with an extensive homology to HIV TAR. Site-directed mutagenesis studies show that critical G residues required for the function of HIV TAR that are conserved in the JCV TAR homolog play an important role in Tat activation of the JCV promoter. In addition, in vivo competition studies suggest that shared regulatory components mediate Tat activation of the JCV late and HIV-LTR promoters. These results suggest that the TAR homolog of the JCV late promoter is responsive to HIV Tat induction and thus may participate in the overall activation of the JCV late promoter mediated by this transactivation (Chowdhury, Traub, Durham, & Major, 1992; Chowdhury, Taylor, Chang, Rappaport, & Khalili, 1990). Further, JCV activation at transcriptional level is mediated by interaction of several inducible regulatory proteins such as NF-κB, C Jun/Ap-1 and NF-1 (Amemiya, Traub, Durham, & Major, 1989; Amemiya et al., 1992; Wortman et al., 2000). These regulatory proteins can be induced by HIV-Tat protein in glial cells or by cytokines that are induced by HIV proteins in glial cells (Atwood et al., 1995; Chen et al., 1997; Conant et al., 1996). The ability of Tat protein to enter into other cells as well as to induce production of cytokines, may thus make the latent JCV in oligodendrocytes or astrocytes target for activation and may thus be involved in the neuropathogenesis of PML in patients with HIV infection.

Conversely, infection of human astrocytes with HIV and JCV show a decrease in the level of HIV replication in cells that are co-infected with JCV. The agnoprotein of JCV through its N-terminal domain associates with Tat and the interaction causes the suppression of Tat-mediated HIV replication (Kaniowska et al., 2006). This could potentially promote the development of a latent reservoir of HIV in the brain.

NEUROTOXIC PROPERTIES OF TAT-LIKE PROTEINS FROM OTHER RETROVIRUSES

The Tat protein derived from maedi-visna virus that infects sheep has also been shown to be neurotoxic in a variety of in vitro and in vivo assays (Gourdou et al., 1990). Although this protein has not been studied as extensively as the HIV-Tat protein, similar mechanisms seem to be involved, such as the stimulation of excitatory amino acid receptors (Starling, Wright, Arbuthnott, & Harkiss, 1999), influx of extracellular calcium (Strijbos, Zamani, Rothwell, Arbuthnott, & Harkiss, 1995), and induction of nitric oxide synthase (Hayman et al., 1993). Similarly, the Tax protein of human T cell leukemia virus type-I can induce the production of cytokines and chemokines in glial cells (Arai et al., 1998; Szymocha et al., 2000) and brain endothelial cells (Rott, Tontsch, Fleischer, & Cash, 1993) and may result in neurotoxicity and destruction of myelin-producing cells (Ohya et al., 1997). Interestingly, monoclonal antibodies to Tax cross-react with a neuronal-specific protein, hnRNP A1, indicating molecular mimicry between the two proteins. These cross-reactive antibodies completely inhibit neuronal firing indicative of their pathogenic nature (Lee, Morcos, Jang, Stuart, & Levin, 2005b).

TAT AS A TARGET FOR DRUG DEVELOPMENT

Currently, available antiretroviral drugs have no effect on Tat production once the HIV proviral DNA is integrated.

Table 4.3.1 STRUCTURAL PROPERTIES OF TAT

TAT SEQUENCE: MEPVDPRLEP WKHPGSQPKT ACTNCYCKKC CFHCQVCFIT KALGISYGRK KRRPQRRRPQ GSQTHQVSLS KQ

AMINOACID	NUMBER OF RESIDUES IN TAT	PHYSICAL PROPERTIES/ POTENTIAL POST-TRANSLATIONAL MODIFICATION
Cys	7	Oxidation, acetylation, S-nitrosylation
Arg	7	positive charge
Lys	8	acetylation, methylation
Thr	4	phosphorylation, glycosylation
Ser	3 or 4	phosphorylation, glycosylation

Hence there is a critical need to develop compounds that may antagonize Tat function (see Table 4.3.1 and 4.3.2). Merck Pharmaceuticals screened a panel of natural compounds and discovered durhamycin (DurA) as a potent Tat inhibitor (IC 50 = 4.8 nM) (Jayasuriya et al., 2002). Methods for its synthesis have recently been developed (Pragani & Roush, 2008). Structural analogs of durhamycin were also isolated and evaluated for antagonism of Tat transactivation, with dur-

Table 4.3.2 PHARMACOLOGICAL COMPOUNDS THAT TARGET TAT-MEDIATED HIV REPLICATION

COMPOUND	INHIBITORY ACTIVITY (µM)	MECHANISM	PROS/CONS	REFERENCE
Durhamycin A	IC_{50}=0.0048 Tat-LTR; The IC_{50}=0.0116 for inhibition of HIV replication.	Tat-LTR	BBB penetration issues	(Jayasuriya et al., 2002)
keto/enol steroid 34a	IC_{50}=2.8 Tat-LTR transactivation and IC_{50}=2.1 HIV replication	Tat-LTR	Small therapeutic window	(Michne et al., 1995)
TDS 0, 1, 2	IC_{50}=0.5–1 HIV infect; TDS2 binds to Tat with 0.330 µM	Tat-TAR	Cons: cytotoxicity in PBMC 10 µM	(Montembault et al., 2004)
CGP74026	IC_{50}=0.020 for Tat-TAR complex inhibition. Blocks Tat-dependent LTR transactivation, IC_{50}=1.0	Tat-TAR	Primarily targets TAR	(Klimkait et al., 1998)
THP (A)	IC_{50}=0.05–0.1 for Tat binding to TAR	Tat-TAR	Primarily targets TAR	(Lapidot et al., 1995)
TR87	IC_{50}=0.147 HIV replication; Tat-TAR inhibition(FRET) K_i=1 µM; IC_{50}=1–5 µM Tat transactivation.	Tat-TAR	Primarily targets TAR; good therapeutic index in vitro and in vivo	(Hwang et al., 2003)
squaryldiamide	IC_{50}=7.7 for Tat-TAR binding inhibition. IC_{50}=12.4 for HIV replication	Tat-TAR	Primarily targets TAR; guanidine bioisostere to improve PK over TR87	(Lee et al., 2005a)
CGP 40336A	IC_{50}= 0.022 for Tat-TAR inhibition. IC_{50}=1.2 µM for Tat LTR transactivation.	Tat-TAR	Acridine derivative that competes with Tat for TAR binding.	(Hamy et al., 1998)
WP631	IC_{50}=0.1–1 for HIV replication; Blocked HIV infectivity at 0.1–0.2 µM.	TAR binding	DNA intercalator that blocks HIV replication; Toxicity and BBB issues.	(Kutsch et al., 2004)
CGA137053	IC_{50}=0.001–0.01 for Tat binding to TAR. IC_{50}=1–5 µM for LTR transactivation.	Tat-P-TEFb	TAR mimic that binds directly to Tat	(Hamy et al., 2000)
Ro24–7429	IC_{50}=0.1–1 HIV replication	Tat-cyclin T1	Primarily targets cyclin T1. Not effective at nontoxic doses in clinical trials.	(Hsu et al., 1993)
Prochlorperazine	IC_{50}<0.1 Cyclin T1:Tat-TAR	Tat:cyclin T1 -TAR interaction	Primarily targets TAR	(Lind et al., 2002)

hamycin B demonstrating one-tenth the potency as DurA and the DurA aglycone was inactive at 25 uM (Pragani & Roush, 2008). However, it has a molecular mass of 1307 daltons, and numerous saccharide moieties, which would likely make it too big and polar to cross the blood-brain barrier. Another group has used a structure-based drug design or computer-aided drug discovery approach to generate a 2D-NMR structure of Tat and synthesized a series of compounds called TDS that bind to Tat and inhibit HIV replication. This family of compounds consists of a triphenylene aromatic ring substituted with at least one carbon chain bearing a succinimide group which could occupy the hydrophobic pocket of Tat (Montembault et al., 2004). However, toxicity in leukocytes of the lead compound TDS2 may require additional modifications to these compounds (Montembault et al., 2004). Polyarginine-containing peptoid compounds mimicking the arginine-rich basic domain of Tat, such as CGP 74026 (Klimkait, Felder, Albrecht, & Hamy, 1998), bind potently to TAR with nano-molar potency and block Tat-dependent LTR transactivation around 1 micromolar. Other prior approaches had included the development of a benzodiazepine derivative (Ro5–3335 and Ro24–7429) as a potential Tat inhibitor (Hsu et al., 1991; Hsu et al., 1992), but it turned out that this compound was not binding to Tat but to cyclin T, a cellular cofactor essential for Tat (Hsu et al., 1993). Another study described a tetrahydro-pyrimidine derivative (THP A) able to bind to a polyarginine peptide (Lapidot, Ben-Asher, & Eisenstein, 1995). This polyarginine peptide binds to TAR but there was no evidence that tetrahydropyrimidine could bind to the basic region of Tat. Similarly, keto/enol epoxy steroids were found to act as Tat inhibitors, with potencies to block Tat-mediated LTR transactivation and HIV viral replication in the 2–3 μM range (Michne et al., 1995). Another group discovered that sulfonated stilbene derivatives (CGA137053) were capable of inhibiting Tat-TAR interactions in vitro at 3–10 nanomolar concentrations, by binding to Tat protein with nanomolar potency (Hamy et al., 2000). However, low micromolar concentrations of CGA137053 were required to block Tat-mediated LTR transactivation and HIV infection in leukocytes and macrophages. However, a number of studies describe molecules that bind to TAR and act as Tat competitors. One of these studies (Lind, Du, Fujinaga, Peterlin, & James, 2002) found compounds, such as prochlorperazine and acetylpromazine that bound to the TAR 5' bulge and could block Tat-TAR interactions and Tat transactivation at low micromolar ranges. Another compound, CGP40336A, is an acridine derivative that competes with Tat for TAR binding at 22 nM, but requires 1.2 μM to block Tat-mediated LTR transactivation (Hamy et al., 1998). The most interesting is a compound called TR87, which inhibits Tat-TAR interactions half maximally at 1 micromolar. It blocks Tat-mediated LTR transactivation at 1–5 μM; however, it inhibits HIV replication at high concentrations of 5 μM (Hwang et al., 2003). This same group synthesized a TR87 analog, squaryldiamide, with a guanidine bioisostere with improved pharmacokinetic properties, but required concentrations of 12 μM to block HIV replication (Lee, Cao, Ichiyama, & Rana, 2005a). These molecules can

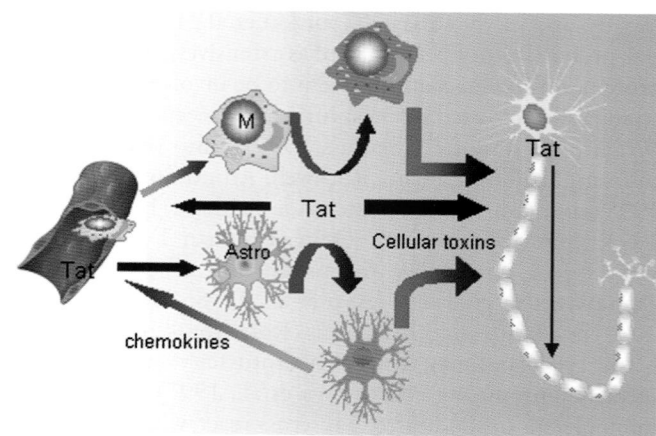

Figure 4.3.2 Tat-mediated cascades in HIV neuropathogenesis. Tat may cross the blood-brain barrier or be released extracellularly from HIV-infected macrophages/microglia and astrocytes in the brain. Tat may activate uninfected macrophages/microglia or astrocytes to release cytokines, chemokines, or other toxins which may adversely affect neuronal function. Tat itself has chemotactic properties for macrophages which may set up a positive feedback loop. Additionally, Tat may directly interact with neurons, causing neurodegeneration of axonal retraction. It may also be transported along neuronal pathways leading to synaptic injury and glial cell activation at distant sites.

inhibit only the Tat–TAR interaction but have no effect on the other Tat functions. Another molecule, bis-anthracycline WP631, which was developed as a DNA intercalator, can also prevent Tat-mediated transcription but these type of compounds would not be expected to have any effect on the extracellular effects of Tat (Kutsch et al., 2004). An ideal compound would be one that binds directly to Tat itself and can also cross the blood-brain barrier. A recent breakthrough has been the publication of the crystal structure of Tat bound to cyclin1 and CDK9. This shows that there is a major conformational change in these molecules upon interaction. This could potentially be exploited to develop a new class of antiviral compounds against Tat-mediated HIV replication (Tahirov et al., 2010).

CONCLUSIONS

In summary, the Tat protein of HIV is critical for viral replication and survival. The protein has evolved to where it escapes surveillance by the immune system. It can assume various shapes and forms, hence is capable of interacting with a large number of cell surface and intracellular molecules. In the brain it continues to evolve to develop potent glial and neuronal activating properties. While glial cell activation results in the induction of various detrimental cytokines and chemokines, neuronal activation results in impaired synaptic function, loss of neurites, and eventually in cell death. These complex cascades of events may be self-perpetuating (Figure 4.3.2), hence interruption of these cascades may be of therapeutic potential in patients at risk of developing HIV-associated neurocognitive impairment.

REFERENCES

Aksenov, M. Y., Hasselrot, U., Bansal, A. K., Wu, G., Nath, A., Anderson, C., et al. (2001). Oxidative damage induced by the injection of HIV-1 Tat protein in the rat striatum. *Neurosci Lett, 305*, 5–8.

Albini, A., Benelli, R., Giunciuglio, D., Cai, T., Mariani, G., Ferrini, S., et al. (1998a). Identification of a novel domain of HIV tat involved in monocyte chemotaxis. *J Biol Chem, 273*, 15895–900.

Albini, A., Ferrini, S., Benelli, R., Sforzini, S., Giunciuglio, D., Aluigi, M. G., et al. (1998b). HIV-1 Tat protein mimicry of chemokines. *Proc Natl Acad Sci U S A, 95*, 13153–8.

Amemiya, K., Traub, R., Durham, L., & Major, E. O. (1989). Interaction of a nuclear factor-1-like protein with the regulatory region of the human polyomavirus JC virus. *J Biol Chem, 264*, 7025–32.

Amemiya, K., Traub, R., Durham, L., & Major, E. O. (1992). Adjacent nuclear factor-1 and activator protein binding sites in the enhancer of the neurotropic JC virus. A common characteristic of many brain-specific genes. *J Biol Chem, 267*, 14204–11.

Andras, I. E., Rha, G., Huang, W., Eum, S., Couraud, P. O., Romero, I. A., et al. (2008). Simvastatin protects against amyloid beta and HIV-1 Tat-induced promoter activities of inflammatory genes in brain endothelial cells. *Mol Pharmacol, 73*, 1424–33.

Antinori, A., Arendt, G., Becker, J. T., Brew, B. J., Byrd, D. A., Cherner, M., et al. (2007). Updated research nosology for HIV-associated neurocognitive disorders. *Neurology, 69*, 1789–99.

Arai, M., Ohashi, T., Tsukahara, T., Murakami, T., Hori, T., Uchiyama, T., et al.(1998). Human T-cell leukemia virus type 1 Tax protein induces the expression of lymphocyte chemoattractant SDF-1/PBSF. *Virology, 241*, 298–303.

Atwood, W. J., Wang, L., Durham, L. C., Amemiya, K., Traub, R. G., & Major, E. O. (1995). Evaluation of the role of cytokine activation in the multiplication of JC virus (JCV) in human fetal glial cells. *J Neurovirol, 1*, 40–9.

Banks, W. A., Robinson, S. M., & Nath, A. (2005). Permeability of the blood-brain barrier to HIV-1 Tat. *Exp Neurol, 193*, 218–27.

Bansal, A. K., Mactutus, C. F., Nath, A., Maragos, W., Hauser, K. F., & Booze, R. M. (2000). Neurotoxicity of HIV-1 proteins gp120 and Tat in the rat striatum. *Brain Res, 879*, 42–9.

Barillari, G., Gendelman, R., Gallo, R. C., & Ensoli, B. (1993). The Tat protein of HIV, a growth factor for AIDS Kaposi sarcoma and cytokine activated vascular cells, induces adhesion of the same cell types by using integrin receptors recognizing the RGD amino acid sequence. *Proc Natl Acad Sci USA, 90*, 7941–7945.

Bilodeau, P. S., Domsic, J. K., & Stoltzfus, C. M. (1999). Splicing regulatory elements within Tat exon 2 of human immunodeficiency virus type 1 (HIV-1) are characteristic of group M but not group O HIV-1 strains. *J Virol, 73*, 9764–72.

Boess, F., Ndikum-Moffor, F. M., Boelsterli, U. A., & Roberts, S. M. (2000). Effects of cocaine and its oxidative metabolites on mitochondrial respiration and generation of reactive oxygen species. *Biochem Pharmacol, 60*, 615–23.

Boven, L. A., Noorbakhsh, F., Bouma, G., van der Zee, R., Vargas, D. L., Pardo, C., et al. (2007). Brain-derived human immunodeficiency virus-1 Tat exerts differential effects on LTR transactivation and neuroimmune activation. *J Neurovirol, 13*, 173–84.

Brailoiu, G. C., Brailoiu, E., Chang, J. K., & Dun, N. J. (2008). Excitatory effects of human immunodeficiency virus 1 Tat on cultured rat cerebral cortical neurons. *Neuroscience, 151*, 701–10.

Bratanich, A. C., Liu, C., McArthur, J. C., Fudyk, T., Glass, J. D., Mittoo, S., et al. (1998). Brain-derived HIV-1 tat sequences from AIDS patients with dementia show increased molecular heterogeneity. *J Neurovirol, 4*, 387–93.

Brorson, J. R., Manzolillo, P. A., Gibbons, S. J., & Miller, R. J. (1995). AMPA receptor desensitization predicts the selective vulnerability of cerebellar Purkinje cells to excitotoxicity. *J Neurosci, 15*, 4515–24.

Bruce-Keller, A. J., Chauhan, A., Dimayuga, F. O., Gee, J., Keller, J. N., & Nath, A. (2003). Synaptic transport of human immunodeficiency virus-Tat protein causes neurotoxicity and gliosis in rat brain. *J Neurosci, 23*, 8417–22.

Buscemi, L., Ramonet, D., & Geiger, J. D. (2007). Human immunodeficiency virus type-1 protein Tat induces tumor necrosis factor-alpha-mediated neurotoxicity. *Neurobiol Dis, 26*, 661–70.

Cai, N. S. & Cadet, J. L. (2008). The combination of methamphetamine and of the HIV protein, Tat, induces death of the human neuroblastoma cell line, SH-SY5Y. *Synapse, 62*, 551–2.

Cass, W. A., Harned, M. E., Peters, L. E., Nath, A., & Maragos, W. F. (2003). HIV-1 protein Tat potentiation of methamphetamine-induced decreases in evoked overflow of dopamine in the striatum of the rat. *Brain Res, 984*, 133–142.

Chang, H. C., Samaniego, F., Nair, B. C., Buonaguro, L., & Ensoli, B. (1997). HIV-1 tat protein exits from cells via a leaderless secretory pathway and binds to extracellelar matrix-associated heparan sulfate proteoglycan through its basic region. *AIDS, 11*, 1421–1431.

Chauhan, A., Hahn, S., Gartner, S., Pardo, C. A., Netesan, S. K., McArthur, J., et al. (2007). Molecular programming of endothelin-1 in HIV-infected brain: Role of Tat in up-regulation of ET-1 and its inhibition by statins. *Faseb J, 21*, 777–89.

Chauhan, A., Turchan, J., Pocernich, C., Bruce-Keller, A., Roth, S., Butterfield, D. A., et al. (2003). Intracellular human immunodeficiency virus Tat expression in astrocytes promotes astrocyte survival but induces potent neurotoxicity at distant sites via axonal transport. *J Biol Chem, 278*, 13512–9.

Chen, P., Mayne, M., Power, C., & Nath, A. (1997). The Tat protein of HIV-1 induces tumor necrosis factor-a production: Implications for HIV associated neurological diseases. *J Biol Chem, 272*, 22385–22388.

Cheng, J., Nath, A., Knudsen, B., Hochman, S., Geiger, J. D., Ma, M., et al. (1998). Neuronal excitatory properties of human immunodeficiency virus type 1 tat protein. *Neuroscience, 82*, 97–106.

Chowdhury, M., Taylor, J. P., Chang, C. F., Rappaport, J., & Khalili, K. (1992). Evidence that a sequence similar to TAR is important for induction of the JC virus late promoter by human immunodeficiency virus type 1 Tat. *J Virol, 66*, 7355–61.

Chowdhury, M., Taylor, J. P., Tada, H., Rappaport, J., Wong-Staal, F., Amini, S., et al. (1990). Regulation of the human neurotropic virus promoter by JCV-T antigen and HIV-1 tat protein. *Oncogene, 5*, 1737–42.

Conant, K., Garzino-Demo, A., Nath, A., McArthur, J. C., Halliday, W., Power, C., et al. (1998). Induction of monocyte chemotactic protein-1 in HIV-1 Tat-stimulated astrocytes and elevation in AIDS dementia. *Proceedings of the National Academy of Sciences, 95*, 3117–3121.

Conant, K., Ma, M., Nath, A., & Major, E. O. (1996). Extracellular HIV-1 Tat protein is associated with an increase in both NF-kappa B binding and protein kinase C activity in primary human astrocytes. *J Virol, 70*, 1384–1389.

Coyle-Rink, J., Sweet, T., Abraham, S., Sawaya, B., Batuman, O., Khalili, K., et al. (2002). Interaction between TGFbeta signaling proteins and C/EBP controls basal and Tat-mediated transcription of HIV-1 LTR in astrocytes. *Virology, 299*, 240–7.

D'Aversa, T. G., Yu, K. O., & Berman, J. W. (2004). Expression of chemokines by human fetal microglia after treatment with the human immunodeficiency virus type 1 protein Tat. *J Neurovirol, 10*, 86–97.

D'Orso, I. & Frankel, A. D. (2009). Tat acetylation modulates assembly of a viral-host RNA-protein transcription complex. *Proc Natl Acad Sci USA*.

Darbinian, N., Sawaya, B. E., Khalili, K., Jaffe, N., Wortman, B., Giordano, A., et al. (2001). Functional interaction between cyclin T1/cdk9 and Puralpha determines the level of TNFalpha promoter activation by Tat in glial cells. *J Neuroimmunol, 121*, 3–11.

Deng, L., Ammosova, T., Pumfery, A., Kashanchi, F., & Nekhai, S. (2002). HIV-1 Tat interaction with RNA polymerase II C-terminal domain (CTD) and a dynamic association with CDK2 induce CTD phosphorylation and transcription from HIV-1 promoter. *J Biol Chem, 277*, 33922–9.

Desfosses, Y., Solis, M., Sun, Q., Grandvaux, N., Van Lint, C., Burny, A., et al. (2005). Regulation of human immunodeficiency virus type 1 gene expression by clade-specific Tat proteins. *J Virol, 79*, 9180–91.

Dhillon, N., Zhu, X., Peng, F., Yao, H., Williams, R., Callen, S., et al. (2008). Molecular mechanism(s) involved in the synergistic induction of CXCL10 by human immunodeficiency virus type 1 Tat and interferon-gamma in macrophages. *J Neurovirol, 14*, 196–204.

Dormeyer, W., Dorr, A., Ott, M., & Schnolzer, M. (2003). Acetylation of the HIV-1 Tat protein: An in vitro study. *Anal Bioanal Chem, 376*, 994–1005.

El-Hage, N., Gurwell, J. A., Singh, I. N., Knapp, P. E., Nath, A., & Hauser, K. F. (2005). Synergistic increases in intracellular Ca2+, and the release of MCP-1, RANTES, and IL-6 by astrocytes treated with opiates and HIV-1 Tat. *Glia, 50*, 91–106.

Eletto, D., Russo, G., Passiatore, G., Del Valle, L., Giordano, A., Khalili, K., et al. (2008). Inhibition of SNAP25 expression by HIV-1 Tat involves the activity of mir-128a. *J Cell Physiol, 216*, 764–70.

Ensoli, B., Buonaguro, L., Barillari, G., Fiorelli, V., Gendelman, R., Morgan, R., et al. (1993). Release, uptake, and effects of extracellular human immunodeficiency virus type-1 Tat protein on cell growth and viral replication. *Journal of Virology, 67*, 277–287.

Eugenin, E. A., D'Aversa, T. G., Lopez, L., Calderon, T. M., & Berman, J. W. (2003). MCP-1 (CCL2) protects human neurons and astrocytes from NMDA or HIV-tat-induced apoptosis. *J Neurochem, 85*, 1299–311.

Eugenin, E. A., Dyer, G., Calderon, T. M., & Berman, J. W. (2005). HIV-1 tat protein induces a migratory phenotype in human fetal microglia by a CCL2 (MCP-1)-dependent mechanism: Possible role in NeuroAIDS. *Glia, 49*, 501–10.

Eugenin, E. A., King, J. E., Nath, A., Calderon, T. M., Zukin, R. S., Bennett, M. V., et al. (2007). HIV-tat induces formation of an LRP-PSD-95-NMDAR-nNOS complex that promotes apoptosis in neurons and astrocytes. *Proc Natl Acad Sci USA, 104*, 3438–43.

Everall, I., Barnes, H., Spargo, E., & Lantos, P. (1995). Assessment of neuronal density in the putamen in human immunodeficiency virus (HIV) infection. Application of stereology and spatial analysis of quadrats. *J Neurovirol, 1*, 126–9.

Ferris, M. J., Frederick-Duus, D., Fadel, J., Mactutus, C. F., & Booze, R. M. (2009). In vivo microdialysis in awake, freely moving rats demonstrates HIV-1 Tat-induced alterations in dopamine transmission. *Synapse, 63*, 181–5.

Fitting, S., Booze, R. M., & Mactutus, C. F. (2008). Neonatal intrahippocampal injection of the HIV-1 proteins gp120 and Tat: Differential effects on behavior and the relationship to stereological hippocampal measures. *Brain Res, 1232*, 139–54.

Fittipaldi, A., Ferrari, A., Zoppe, M., Arcangeli, C., Pellegrini, V., Beltram, F., et al. (2003). Cell membrane lipid rafts mediate caveolar endocytosis of HIV-1 Tat fusion proteins. *J Biol Chem, 278*, 34141–9.

Flora, G., Lee, Y. W., Nath, A., Hennig, B., Maragos, W., & Toborek, M. (2003). Methamphetamine potentiates HIV-1 Tat protein-mediated activation of redox-sensitive pathways in discrete regions of the brain. *Exp Neurol, 179*, 60–70.

Ford, K. G., Darling, D., Souberbielle, B., & Farzaneh, F. (2000). Protein transduction: A new tool for the study of cellular ageing and senescence. *Mech Ageing Dev, 121*, 113–21.

Frankel, A., Bredt, D., & Pabo, C. (1988a). Tat protein from immunodeficiency virus forms a metal-linked dimer. *Science, 240*, 70–73.

Frankel, A. D., Chen, L., Cotter, R. J., & Pabo, C. O. (1988b). Dimerization of the Tat protein from human immunodeficiency virus: A cysteine-rich peptide mimics the normal metal-linked dimer interface. *Proc Natl Acad Sci USA, 85*, 6297–300.

Frankel, A. D. & Pabo, C. O. (1988). Cellular uptake of the tat protein from human immunodeficiency virus. *Cell, 55*, 1189–93.

Garthwaite, J. (1991). Glutamate, nitric oxide and cell-cell signalling in the nervous system. *Trends Neurosci, 14*, 60–7.

Garzino-Demo, A., Chen, M., Lusso, P., Berneman, Z., & DiPaolo, J. A. (1996). Enhancement of TAT-induced transactivation of the HIV-1 LTR by two genomic fragments of HHV-6. *J Med Virol, 50*, 20–4.

Giunta, B., Hou, H., Zhu, Y., Rrapo, E., Tian, J., Takashi, M., et al. (2009). HIV-1 Tat contributes to Alzheimer's disease-like pathology in PSAPP mice. *Int J Clin Exp Pathol, 2*, 433–43.

Gourdou, I., Mabrouk, K., Harkiss, G., Marchot, P., Watt, N., Hery, F., et al. (1990). [Neurotoxicity in mice due to cysteine-rich parts of visna virus and HIV-1 Tat proteins]. *C R Acad Sci III, 311*, 149–55.

Hamy, F., Brondani, V., Florsheimer, A., Stark, W., Blommers, M. J., & Klimkait, T. (1998). A new class of HIV-1 Tat antagonist acting through Tat-TAR inhibition. *Biochemistry, 37*, 5086–95.

Hamy, F., Gelus, N., Zeller, M., Lazdins, J. L., Bailly, C., & Klimkait, T. (2000). Blocking HIV replication by targeting Tat protein. *Chem Biol, 7*, 669–76.

Harrich, D., Ulich, C., Garcia-Martinez, L. F., & Gaynor, R. B. (1997). Tat is required for efficient HIV-1 reverse transcription. *Embo J, 16*, 1224–35.

Haughey, N. J., Holden, C. P., Nath, A., & Geiger, J. D. (1999). Involvement of inositol 1,4,5-trisphosphate-regulated stores of intracellular calcium in calcium dysregulation and neuron cell death caused by HIV-1 protein tat. *J Neurochem, 73*, 1363–74.

Haughey, N. J., Nath, A., Mattson, M. P., Slevin, J. T., & Geiger, J. D. (2001). HIV-1 Tat through phosphorylation of NMDA receptors potentiates glutamate excitotoxicity. *J Neurochem, 78*, 457–467.

Hauser, K. F., Hahn, Y. K., Adjan, V. V., Zou, S., Buch, S. K., Nath, A., et al (2009). HIV-1 Tat and morphine have interactive effects on oligodendrocyte survival and morphology. *Glia, 57*, 194–206.

Hayashi, K., Pu, H., Andras, I. E., Eum, S. Y., Yamauchi, A., Hennig, B., et al (2006). HIV-TAT protein upregulates expression of multidrug resistance protein 1 in the blood-brain barrier. *J Cereb Blood Flow Metab, 26*, 1052–65.

Hayashi, K., Pu, H., Tian, J., Andras, I. E., Lee, Y. W., Hennig, B., et al. (2005). HIV-Tat protein induces P-glycoprotein expression in brain microvascular endothelial cells. *J Neurochem, 93*, 1231–41.

Hayman, M., Arbuthnott, G., Harkiss, G., Brace, H., Filippi, P., Philippon, V., et al. (1993). Neurotoxicity of peptide analogues of the transactivating protein tat from Maedi-Visna virus and human immunodeficiency virus. *Neuroscience, 53*, 1–6.

Hersh, L. B. (2003). Peptidases, proteases and amyloid beta-peptide catabolism. *Curr Pharm Des, 9*, 449–54.

Hofman, F. M., Chen, P., Incardona, F., Zidovetzki, R., & Hinton, D. R. (1999). HIV-1 tat protein induces the production of interleukin-8 by human brain-derived endothelial cells. *J Neuroimmunol, 94*, 28–39.

Hofman, F. M., Dohadwala, M. M., Wright, A. D., Hinton, D. R., & Walker, S. M. (1994). Exogenous tat protein activates central nervous system-derived endothelial cells. *J Neuroimmunol, 54*, 19–28.

Hsu, M. C., Dhingra, U., Earley, J. V., Holly, M., Keith, D., Nalin, C. M., et al. (1993). Inhibition of type 1 human immunodeficiency virus replication by a tat antagonist to which the virus remains sensitive after prolonged exposure in vitro. *Proc Natl Acad Sci USA, 90*, 6395–9.

Hsu, M. C., Schutt, A. D., Holly, M., Slice, L. W., Sherman, M. I., Richman, D. D., et al. (1991). Inhibition of HIV replication in acute and chronic infections in vitro by a Tat antagonist. *Science, 254*, 1799–802.

Hsu, M. C., Schutt, A. D., Holly, M., Slice, L. W., Sherman, M. I., Richman, D. D., et al. (1992). Discovery and characterization of an HIV-1 Tat antagonist. *Biochem Soc Trans, 20*, 525–31.

Huang, L., Bosch, I., Hofmann, W., Sodroski, J., & Pardee, A. B. (1998). Tat protein induces human immunodeficiency virus type 1 (HIV-1) coreceptors and promotes infection with both macrophage-tropic and T-lymphotropic HIV-1 strains. *J Virol, 72*, 8952–60.

Huang, W., Rha, G. B., Han, M. J., Eum, S. Y., Andras, I. E., Zhong, Y., et al. (2008). PPARalpha and PPARgamma effectively protect against HIV-induced inflammatory responses in brain endothelial cells. *J Neurochem, 107*, 497–509.

Huang, X., Seifert, U., Salzmann, U., Henklein, P., Preissner, R., Henke, W., et al. (2002). The RTP site shared by the HIV-1 Tat protein and the 11S regulator subunit alpha is crucial for their effects on proteasome function including antigen processing. *J Mol Biol, 323*, 771–82.

Hudson, L., Liu, J., Nath, A., Narayan, O., Male, D., Jones, M., et al. (2000). Detection of human immunodeficiency virus regulatory protein tat in CNS tissues. *J Neurovirol, 6*, 145–155.

Hwang, S., Tamilarasu, N., Kibler, K., Cao, H., Ali, A., Ping, Y. H., et al. (2003). Discovery of a small molecule Tat-trans-activation-responsive RNA antagonist that potently inhibits human immunodeficiency virus-1 replication. *J Biol Chem, 278*, 39092–103.

Jayasuriya, H., Lingham, R. B., Graham, P., Quamina, D., Herranz, L., Genilloud, O., et al (2002). Durhamycin A, a potent inhibitor of HIV Tat transactivation. *J Nat Prod*, 65, 1091–5.

Jeang, K. T., Xiao, H., & Rich, E. A. (1999). Multifaceted activities of the HIV-1 transactivator of transcription, Tat. *J Biol Chem*, 274, 28837–40.

Johnston, J. B., Zhang, K., Silva, C., Shalinsky, D. R., Conant, K., Ni, W., et al. (2001). HIV-1 Tat neurotoxicity is prevented by matrix metalloproteinase inhibitors. *Ann Neurol*, 49, 230–41.

Jonas, P. & Sakmann, B. (1992). Glutamate receptor channels in isolated patches from CA1 and CA3 pyramidal cells of rat hippocampal slices. *J Physiol (Lond)*, 455, 143–71.

Jones, M., Olafson, K., Del Bigio, M. R., Peeling, J., & Nath, A. (1998). Intraventricular injection of human immunodeficiency virus type 1 (HIV-1) Tat protein causes inflammation, gliosis, apoptosis, and ventricular enlargement. *J Neuropathol Exp Neurol*, 57, 563–570.

Ju, S. M., Song, H. Y., Lee, J. A., Lee, S. J., Choi, S. Y., & Park, J. (2009). Extracellular HIV-1 Tat up-regulates expression of matrix metalloproteinase-9 via a MAPK-NF-kappaB dependent pathway in human astrocytes. *Exp Mol Med*, 41, 86–93.

Kaehlcke, K., Dorr, A., Hetzer-Egger, C., Kiermer, V., Henklein, P., Schnoelzer, M., et al. (2003). Acetylation of Tat defines a cyclinT1-independent step in HIV transactivation. *Mol Cell*, 12, 167–76.

Kaniowska, D., Kaminski, R., Amini, S., Radhakrishnan, S., Rappaport, J., Johnson, E., et al. (2006). Cross-interaction between JC virus agnoprotein and human immunodeficiency virus type 1 (HIV-1) Tat modulates transcription of the HIV-1 long terminal repeat in glial cells. *J Virol*, 80, 9288–99.

Kaplan, I. M., Wadia, J. S., & Dowdy, S. F. (2005). Cationic TAT peptide transduction domain enters cells by macropinocytosis. *J Control Release*, 102, 247–53.

Khiati, A., Chaloin, O., Muller, S., Tardieu, M., & Horellou, P. (2010). Induction of monocyte chemoattractant protein-1 (MCP-1/CCL2) gene expression by human immunodeficiency virus-1 Tat in human astrocytes is CDK9 dependent. *J Neurovirol*, 16, 150–67.

Khurdayan, V. K., Buch, S., El-Hage, N., Lutz, S. E., Goebel, S. M., Singh, I. N., et al. (2004). Preferential vulnerability of astroglia and glial precursors to combined opioid and HIV-1 Tat exposure in vitro. *Eur J Neurosci*, 19, 3171–82.

Kiernan, R. E., Vanhulle, C., Schiltz, L., Adam, E., Xiao, H., Maudoux, F., et al (1999). HIV-1 tat transcriptional activity is regulated by acetylation. *Embo J*, 18, 6106–18.

Kim, B. O., Liu, Y., Ruan, Y., Xu, Z. C., Schantz, L., & He, J. J. (2003a). Neuropathologies in transgenic mice expressing human immunodeficiency virus type 1 Tat protein under the regulation of the astrocyte-specific glial fibrillary acidic protein promoter and doxycycline. *Am J Pathol*, 162, 1693–707.

Kim, T. A., Avraham, H. K., Koh, Y. H., Jiang, S., Park, I. W., & Avraham, S. (2003b). HIV-1 Tat-mediated apoptosis in human brain microvascular endothelial cells. *J Immunol*, 170, 2629–37.

King, J. E., Eugenin, E. A., Hazleton, J. E., Morgello, S., & Berman, J. W. (2010). Mechanisms of HIV-tat-induced phosphorylation of N-methyl-D-aspartate receptor subunit 2A in human primary neurons: implications for neuroAIDS pathogenesis. *Am J Pathol*, 176, 2819–30.

Klimkait, T., Felder, E. R., Albrecht, G., & Hamy, F. (1998). Rational optimization of a HIV-1 Tat inhibitor: Rapid progress on combinatorial lead structures. *Biotechnol Bioeng*, 61, 155–68.

Koller, H., Schaal, H., Freund, M., Garrido, S. R., von Giesen, H. J., Ott, M., et al. (2001). HIV-1 protein Tat reduces the glutamate-induced intracellular Ca2+ increase in cultured cortical astrocytes. *Eur J Neurosci*, 14, 1793–9.

Kolson, D. L., Buchhalter, J., Collman, R., Hellmig, B., Farrell, C. F., Debouck, C., et al. (1993). HIV-1 Tat alters normal organization of neurons and astrocytes in primary rodent brain cell cultures: RGD sequence dependence. *AIDS Res Hum Retroviruses*, 9, 677–85.

Kruman, I., Nath, A., & Mattson, M. P. (1998). HIV protein Tat induces apoptosis by a mechanism involving mitochondrial calcium overload and caspase activation. *Expt Neurol*, 154, 276–288.

Kruman, I. I., Nath, A., Maragos, W. F., Chan, S. L., Jones, M., Rangnekar, V. M., et al. (1999). Evidence that Par-4 participates in the pathogenesis of AIDS dementia. *Am J Pathol*, 155, 39–46.

Kuppuswamy, M., Subramanian, T., Srinivasan, A., Chinnadurai, G. (1989). Multiple functional domains of Tat, the trans-activator of HIV-1, defined by mutational analysis. *Nucleic Acids Res*, 17, 3551–61.

Kutsch, O., Levy, D. N., Bates, P. J., Decker, J., Kosloff, B. R., Shaw, G. M., et al. (2004). Bis-anthracycline antibiotics inhibit human immunodeficiency virus type 1 transcription. *Antimicrob Agents Chemother*, 48, 1652–63.

Kutsch, O., Oh, J., Nath, A., & Benveniste, E. N. (2000). Induction of the chemokines interleukin-8 and IP-10 by human immunodeficiency virus type 1 Tat in astrocytes. *J Virol*, 74, 9214–21.

Langford, D., Grigorian, A., Hurford, R., Adame, A., Crews, L., & Masliah, E. (2004). The role of mitochondrial alterations in the combined toxic effects of human immunodeficiency virus Tat protein and methamphetamine on calbindin positive-neurons. *J Neurovirol*, 10, 327–37.

Langford, D., Sanders, V. J., Mallory, M., Kaul, M., & Masliah, E. (2002). Expression of stromal cell-derived factor 1alpha protein in HIV encephalitis. *J Neuroimmunol*, 127, 115–26.

Lapidot, A., Ben-Asher, E., & Eisenstein, M. (1995). Tetrahydropyrimidine derivatives inhibit binding of a Tat-like, arginine-containing peptide, to HIV TAR RNA in vitro. *FEBS Lett*, 367, 33–8.

Lee, C. W., Cao, H., Ichiyama, K., & Rana, T. M. (2005a). Design and synthesis of a novel peptidomimetic inhibitor of HIV-1 Tat-TAR interactions: Squaryldiamide as a new potential bioisostere of unsubstituted guanidine. *Bioorg Med Chem Lett*, 15, 4243–6.

Lee, S. M., Morcos, Y., Jang, H., Stuart, J. M., & Levin, M. C. (2005b). HTLV-1 induced molecular mimicry in neurological disease. *Curr Top Microbiol Immunol*, 296, 125–36.

Li, S. T., Matsushita, M., Moriwaki, A., Saheki, Y., Lu, Y. F., Tomizawa, K., et al. (2004). HIV-1 inhibits long-term potentiation and attenuates spatial learning. *Ann Neurol*, 55, 362–71.

Li, W., Huang, Y., Reid, R., Steiner, J., Malpica-Llanos, T., Darden, T. A., et al. (2008). NMDA receptor activation by HIV-Tat protein is clade dependent. *J Neurosci*, 28, 12190–8.

Lind, K. E., Du, Z., Fujinaga, K., Peterlin, B. M., & James, T. L. (2002). Structure-based computational database screening, in vitro assay, and NMR assessment of compounds that target TAR RNA. *Chem Biol*, 9, 185–93.

Liu, X., Jana, M., Dasgupta, S., Koka, S., He, J., Wood, C., et al. (2002). Human immunodeficiency virus type-1 (HIV-1) Tat induces nitric oxide synthase in human astroglia. *J Biol Chem*, 277, 39312-9.

Liu, Y., Jones, M., Hingtgen, C. M., Bu, G., Laribee, N., Tanzi, R. E., et al. (2000). Uptake of HIV-1 tat protein mediated by low-density lipoprotein receptor-related protein disrupts the neuronal metabolic balance of the receptor ligands. *Nat Med*, 6, 1380–7.

Lusti-Narasimhan, M., Power, C. A., Allet, B., Alouani, S., Bacon, K. B., Mermod, J. J., et al. (1995). Mutation of Leu25 and Val27 introduces CC chemokine activity into interleukin-8. *J Biol Chem*, 270, 2716–21.

Ma, M. & Nath, A. (1997). Molecular determinants for cellular uptake of Tat protein of human immunodeficiency virus type 1 in brain cells. *J Virol*, 71, 2495–2499.

Maggirwar, S. B., Tong, N., Ramirez, S., Gelbard, H. A., & Dewhurst, S. (1999). HIV-1 Tat-mediated activation of glycogen synthase kinase-3-beta contributes to Tat-mediated neurotoxicity. *J Neurochem*, 73, 578–86.

Magnuson, D. S., Knudsen, B. E., Geiger, J. D., Brownstone, R. M., & Nath, A. (1995). Human immunodeficiency virus type 1 tat activates non-N-methyl-D-aspartate excitatory amino acid receptors and causes neurotoxicity. *Ann Neurol*, 37, 373–380.

Malim, M. H. & Cullen, B. R. (1991). HIV-1 structural gene expression requires the binding of multiple Rev monomers to the viral RRE: Implications for HIV-1 latency. *Cell*, 65, 241–8.

Malva, J. O., Carvalho, A. P., & Carvalho, C. M. (1998). Kainate receptors in hippocampal CA3 subregion: Evidence for a role in regulating neurotransmitter release. *Neurochem Int*, 32, 1–6.

Maragos, W. F., Tillman, P., Jones, M., Bruce-Keller, A. J., Roth, S., Bell, J. E., et al. (2003). Neuronal injury in hippocampus with human immunodeficiency virus transactivating protein, Tat. *Neuroscience, 117*, 43–53.

Maragos, W. F., Young, K. L., Turchan, J. T., Guseva, M., Pauly, J. R., Nath, A., et al. (2002). Human immunodeficiency virus-1 Tat protein and methamphetamine interact synergistically to impair striatal dopaminergic function. *J Neurochem, 83*, 955–63.

Marcello, A., Zoppe, M., & Giacca, M. (2001). Multiple modes of transcriptional regulation by the HIV-1 Tat transactivator. *IUBMB Life, 51*, 175–81.

Mayne, M., Bratanich, A. C., Chen, P., Rana, F., Nath, A., & Power, C. (1998). HIV-1 tat molecular diversity and induction of TNF-alpha: Implications for HIV-induced neurological disease. *Neuroimmunomodulation, 5*, 184–92.

McCarthy, M., Auger, D., He, J., & Wood, C. (1998). Cytomegalovirus and human herpesvirus-6 trans-activate the HIV-1 long terminal repeat via multiple response regions in human fetal astrocytes. *J Neurovirol, 4*, 495–511.

McManus, C. M., Weidenheim, K., Woodman, S. E., Nunez, J., Hesselgesser, J., Nath, A., et al. (2000). Chemokine and chemokine-receptor expression in human glial elements: induction by the HIV protein, Tat, and chemokine autoregulation. *Am J Pathol, 156*, 1441–53.

Michne, W. F., Schroeder, J. D., Bailey, T. R., Neumann, H. C., Cooke, D., Young, D. C., et al. (1995). Keto/enol epoxy steroids as HIV-1 Tat inhibitors: Structure-activity relationships and pharmacophore localization. *J Med Chem, 38*, 3197–206.

Montembault, M., Vo-Thanh, G., Deyine, A., Fargeas, V., Villieras, M., Adjou, A., et al. (2004). A possible improvement for structure-based drug design illustrated by the discovery of a Tat HIV-1 inhibitor. *Bioorg Med Chem Lett, 14*, 1543–6.

Nath, A., Haughey, N. J., Jones, M., Anderson, C., Bell, J. E., & Geiger, J. D. (2000). Synergistic neurotoxicity by human immunodeficiency virus proteins Tat and gp120: protection by memantine. *Ann Neurol, 47*, 186–94.

Nath, A., Hauser, K. F., Wojna, V., Booze, R. M., Maragos, W., Prendergast, M., et al. (2002). Molecular basis for interactions of HIV and drugs of abuse. *J Acquir Immune Defic Syndr, 31* Suppl 2, S62–9.

Nath, A., Psooy, K., Martin, C., Knudsen, B., Magnuson, D. S., Haughey, N., et al. (1996). Identification of a human immunodeficiency virus type 1 Tat epitope that is neuroexcitatory and neurotoxic. *J Virol, 70*, 1475–1480.

Nelbock, P., Dillon, P. J., Perkins, A., & Rosen, C. A. (1990). A cDNA for a protein that interacts with the human immunodeficiency virus Tat transactivator. *Science, 248*, 1650–1653.

New, D. R., Ma, M., Epstein, L. G., Nath, A., & Gelbard, H. A. (1997). Human immunodeficiency virus type 1 Tat protein induces death by apoptosis in primary human neuron cultures. *J Neurovirol, 3*, 168–73.

New, D. R., Maggirwar, S. B., Epstein, L. G., Dewhurst, S., & Gelbard, H. A. (1998). HIV-1 Tat induces neuronal death via tumor necrosis factor-alpha and activation of non-N-methyl-D-aspartate receptors by an NFkappaB- independent mechanism. *J Biol Chem, 273*, 17852–8.

Norman, J. P., Perry, S. W., Kasischke, K. A., Volsky, D. J., & Gelbard, H. A. (2007). HIV-1 transactivator of transcription protein elicits mitochondrial hyperpolarization and respiratory deficit, with dysregulation of complex IV and nicotinamide adenine dinucleotide homeostasis in cortical neurons. *J Immunol, 178*, 869–76.

Norman, J. P., Perry, S. W., Reynolds, H. M., Kiebala, M., De Mesy Bentley, K. L., Trejo, M., et al. (2008). HIV-1 Tat activates neuronal ryanodine receptors with rapid induction of the unfolded protein response and mitochondrial hyperpolarization. *PLoS ONE, 3*, e3731.

Ohya, O., Tomaru, U., Yamashita, I., Kasai, T., Morita, K., Ikeda, H., et al. (1997). HTLV-I induced myelomeneuropathy in WKAH rats: Apoptosis and local activation of the HTLV-I pX and TNF-alpha genes implicated in the pathogenesis. *Leukemia, 11* Suppl 3, 255–7.

Pagans, S., Kauder, S. E., Kaehlcke, K., Sakane, N., Schroeder, S., Dormeyer, W., et al. (2010). The cellular lysine methyltransferase Set7/9-KMT7 binds HIV-1 TAR RNA, monomethylates the viral transactivator Tat, and enhances HIV transcription. *Cell Host Microbe, 7*, 234–44.

Passiatore, G., Rom, S., Eletto, D., & Peruzzi, F. (2009). HIV-1 Tat C-terminus is cleaved by calpain 1: Implication for Tat-mediated neurotoxicity. *Biochim Biophys Acta, 1793*, 378–87.

Patrizio, M., Colucci, M., & Levi, G. (2001). Human immunodeficiency virus type 1 Tat protein decreases cyclic AMP synthesis in rat microglia cultures. *J Neurochem, 77*, 399–407.

Perez, A., Probert, A. W., Wang, K. K., & Sharmeen, L. (2001). Evaluation of HIV-1 Tat-induced neurotoxicity in rat cortical cell culture. *J Neurovirol, 7*, 1–10.

Perry, S. W., Norman, J. P., Litzburg, A., Zhang, D., Dewhurst, S., & Gelbard, H. A. (2005). HIV-1 transactivator of transcription protein induces mitochondrial hyperpolarization and synaptic stress leading to apoptosis. *J Immunol, 174*, 4333–44.

Polazzi, E., Levi, G., & Minghetti, L. (1999). Human immunodeficiency virus type 1 Tat protein stimulates inducible nitric oxide synthase expression and nitric oxide production in microglial cultures. *J Neuropathol Exp Neurol, 58*, 825–31.

Pragani, R. & Roush, W. R. (2008). Studies on the synthesis of durhamycin A: Stereoselective synthesis of a model aglycone. *Org Lett, 10*, 4613–6.

Prendergast, M. A., Rogers, D. T., Mulholland, P. J., Littleton, J. M., Wilkins, L. H., Jr., Self, R. L., et al. (2002). Neurotoxic effects of the human immunodeficiency virus type-1 transcription factor Tat require function of a polyamine sensitive-site on the N-methyl-D-aspartate receptor. *Brain Res, 954*, 300–7.

Pu, H., Hayashi, K., Andras, I. E., Eum, S. Y., Hennig, B., & Toborek, M. (2007). Limited role of COX-2 in HIV Tat-induced alterations of tight junction protein expression and disruption of the blood-brain barrier. *Brain Res, 1184*, 333–44.

Pulliam, L., Sun, B., Rempel, H., Martinez, P. M., Hoekman, J. D., Rao, R. J., et al. (2007). Intranasal tat alters gene expression in the mouse brain. *J Neuroimmune Pharmacol, 2*, 87–92.

Ramirez, S. H., Sanchez, J. F., Dimitri, C. A., Gelbard, H. A., Dewhurst, S., & Maggirwar, S. B. (2001). Neurotrophins prevent HIV Tat-induced neuronal apoptosis via a nuclear factor-kappaB (NF-kappaB)-dependent mechanism. *J Neurochem, 78*, 874–89.

Ranga, U., Shankarappa, R., Siddappa, N. B., Ramakrishna, L., Nagendran, R., Mahalingam, M., et al. (2004). Tat protein of human immunodeficiency virus type 1 subtype C strains is a defective chemokine. *J Virol, 78*, 2586–90.

Rayne, F., Debaisieux, S., Bonhoure, A., & Beaumelle, B. HIV-1 Tat is unconventionally secreted through the plasma membrane. *Cell Biol Int, 34*, 409–13.

Richard, J. P., Melikov, K., Brooks, H., Prevot, P., Lebleu, B., & Chernomordik, L. V. (2005). Cellular uptake of unconjugated TAT peptide involves clathrin-dependent endocytosis and heparan sulfate receptors. *J Biol Chem, 280*, 15300–6.

Robert-Guroff, M., Popovic, M., Gartner, S., Markham, P., Gallo, R. C., & Reitz, M. S. (1990). Structure and expression of tat-, rev-, and nef-specific transcripts of human immunodeficiency virus type 1 in infected lymphocytes and macrophages. *J Virol, 64*, 3391–8.

Rodman, T. C., Pruslin, F. H., To, S. E., & Winston, R. (1992). Human immunodeficiency virus (HIV) Tat-reactive antibodies present in normal HIV-negative sera and depleted in HIV-positive sera. Identification of the epitope. *J Exp Med, 175*, 1247–53.

Rosen, C. A., Terwilliger, E., Dayton, A., Sodroski, J. G., & Haseltine, W. A. (1988). Intragenic cis-acting art gene-responsive sequences of the human immunodeficiency virus. *Proc Natl Acad Sci USA, 85*, 2071–5.

Rott, O., Tontsch, U., Fleischer, B., & Cash, E. (1993). Interleukin-6 production in "normal" and HTLV-1 tax-expressing brain-specific endothelial cells. *Eur J Immunol, 23*, 1987–91.

Ruben, S., Perkins, A., Purcell, R., Joung, K., Sia, R., Burghoff, R., et al. (1989). Structural and functional characterization of human immunodeficiency virus tat protein. *J Virol, 63*, 1–8.

Sabatier, J. M., Vives, E., Marbrouk, K., et al. (1991). Evidence for neurotoxicity of tat from HIV. *Journal of Virology, 65*, 961–967.

Schwarze, S. R., Ho, A., Vocero-Akbani, A., & Dowdy, S. F. (1999). In vivo protein transduction: delivery of a biologically active protein into the mouse. *Science, 285*, 1569–1572.

Secchiero, P., Zella, D., Capitani, S., Gallo, R. C., & Zauli, G. (1999). Extracellular HIV-1 tat protein up-regulates the expression of surface CXC-chemokine receptor 4 in resting CD4+ T cells. *J Immunol, 162,* 2427–31.

Seeger, M., Ferrell, K., Frank, R., & Dubiel, W. (1997). HIV-1 tat inhibits the 20 S proteasome and its 11 S regulator-mediated activation. *J Biol Chem, 272,* 8145–8.

Sheng, W. S., Hu, S., Lokensgard, J. R., & Peterson, P. K. (2003). U50,488 inhibits HIV-1 Tat-induced monocyte chemoattractant protein-1 (CCL2) production by human astrocytes. *Biochem Pharmacol, 65,* 9–14.

Shi, B., Raina, J., Lorenzo, A., Busciglio, J., & Gabuzda, D. (1998). Neuronal apoptosis induced by HIV-1 Tat protein and TNF-alpha: Potentiation of neurotoxicity mediated by oxidative stress and implications for HIV-1 dementia. *J Neurovirol, 4,* 281–90.

Silvers, J. M., Aksenova, M. V., Aksenov, M. Y., Mactutus, C. F., & Booze, R. M. (2007). Neurotoxicity of HIV-1 Tat protein: involvement of D1 dopamine receptor. *Neurotoxicology, 28,* 1184–90.

Smith, D. G., Guillemin, G. J., Pemberton, L., Kerr, S., Nath, A., Smythe, G. A., et al. (2001). Quinolinic acid is produced by macrophages stimulated by platelet activating factor, Nef and Tat. *J Neurovirol, 7,* 56–60.

Snyder, E. L. & Dowdy, S. F. (2001). Protein/peptide transduction domains: Potential to deliver large DNA molecules into cells. *Curr Opin Mol Ther, 3,* 147–52.

Spitere, K., Toulouse, A., O'Sullivan, D. B., & Sullivan, A. M. (2008). TAT-PAX6 protein transduction in neural progenitor cells: A novel approach for generation of dopaminergic neurones in vitro. *Brain Res, 1208,* 25–34.

Starling, I., Wright, A., Arbuthnott, G., & Harkiss, G. (1999). Acute in vivo neurotoxicity of peptides from Maedi Visna virus transactivating protein Tat. *Brain Res, 830,* 285–91.

Stauber, R. H. & Pavlakis, G. N. (1998). Intracellular trafficking and interactions of the HIV-1 Tat protein. *Virology, 252,* 126–36.

Stettner, M. R., Nance, J. A., Wright, C. A., Kinoshita, Y., Kim, W. K., Morgello, S., et al. (2009). SMAD proteins of oligodendroglial cells regulate transcription of JC virus early and late genes coordinately with the Tat protein of human immunodeficiency virus type 1. *J Gen Virol, 90,* 2005–14.

Strijbos, P. J., Zamani, M. R., Rothwell, N. J., Arbuthnott, G., & Harkiss, G. (1995). Neurotoxic mechanisms of transactivating protein Tat of Maedi-Visna virus. *Neurosci Lett, 197,* 215–8.

Sui, Z., Sniderhan, L. F., Fan, S., Kazmierczak, K., Reisinger, E., Kovacs, A. D., et al. (2006). Human immunodeficiency virus-encoded Tat activates glycogen synthase kinase-3beta to antagonize nuclear factor-kappaB survival pathway in neurons. *Eur J Neurosci, 23,* 2623–34.

Sui, Z., Sniderhan, L. F., Schifitto, G., Phipps, R. P., Gelbard, H. A., Dewhurst, S., et al. (2007). Functional synergy between CD40 ligand and HIV-1 Tat contributes to inflammation: implications in HIV type 1 dementia. *J Immunol, 178,* 3226–36.

Szymocha, R., Brisson, C., Bernard, A., Akaoka, H., Belin, M. F., & Giraudon, P. (2000). Long-term effects of HTLV-1 on brain astrocytes: Sustained expression of Tax-1 associated with synthesis of inflammatory mediators. *J Neurovirol, 6,* 350–7.

Tada, H., Rappaport, J., Lashgari, M., Amini, S., Wong-Staal, F., & Khalili, K. (1990). Trans-activation of the JC virus late promoter by the tat protein of type 1 human immunodeficiency virus in glial cells. *Proc Natl Acad Sci USA, 87,* 3479–83.

Tahirov, T. H., Babayeva, N. D., Varzavand, K., Cooper, J. J., Sedore, S. C., & Price, D. H. (2010). Crystal structure of HIV-1 Tat complexed with human P-TEFb. *Nature, 465,* 747–51.

Tanaka, T., Nakamura, T., Takagi, H., & Sato, M. (1997). Molecular cloning and characterization of a novel TBP-1 interacting protein (TBPIP):enhancement of TBP-1 action on Tat by TBPIP. *Biochem Biophys Res Commun, 239,* 176–81.

Tardieu, M., Hery, C., Peudenier, S., Boespflug, O., & Montagnier, L. (1992). Human immunodeficiency virus type 1-infected monocytic cells can destroy human neural cells after cell-to-cell adhesion. *Annals of Neurology, 32,* 11–17.

Taylor, J. P., Pomerantz, R., Bagasra, O., Chowdhury, M., Rappaport, J., Khalili, K., et al. (1992). TAR-independent transactivation by Tat in cells derived from the CNS: A novel mechanism of HIV-1 gene regulation. *Embo J, 11,* 3395–403.

Theodore, S., Cass, W. A., Nath, A., & Maragos, W. F. (2007). Progress in understanding basal ganglia dysfunction as a common target for methamphetamine abuse and HIV-1 neurodegeneration. *Curr HIV Res, 5,* 301–13.

Theodore, S., Cass, W. A., Nath, A., Steiner, J., Young, K., & Maragos, W. F. (2006a). Inhibition of tumor necrosis factor-alpha signaling prevents human immunodeficiency virus-1 protein Tat and methamphetamine interaction. *Neurobiol Dis, 23,* 663–8.

Theodore, S., Stolberg, S., Cass, W. A., & Maragos, W. F. (2006b). Human immunodeficiency virus-1 protein tat and methamphetamine interactions. *Ann N Y Acad Sci, 1074,* 178–90.

Thomas, E. R., Dunfee, R. L., Stanton, J., Bogdan, D., Kunstman, K., Wolinsky, S. M., et al. (2007). High frequency of defective vpu compared with tat and rev genes in brain from patients with HIV type 1-associated dementia. *AIDS Res Hum Retroviruses, 23,* 575–80.

Toborek, M., Lee, Y. W., Pu, H., Malecki, A., Flora, G., Garrido, R., et al. (2003). HIV-Tat protein induces oxidative and inflammatory pathways in brain endothelium. *J Neurochem, 84,* 169–79.

Turchan, J., Anderson, C., Hauser, K. F., Sun, Q., Zhang, J., Liu, Y., et al. (2001). Estrogen protects against the synergistic toxicity by HIV proteins, methamphetamine and cocaine. *BMC Neurosci, 2,* 3.

Tyagi, M., Rusnati, M., Presta, M., & Giacca, M. (2001). Internalization of HIV-1 tat requires cell surface heparan sulfate proteoglycans. *J Biol Chem, 276,* 3254–61.

Valle, L. D., Croul, S., Morgello, S., Amini, S., Rappaport, J., & Khalili, K. (2000). Detection of HIV-1 Tat and JCV capsid protein, VP1, in AIDS brain with progressive multifocal leukoencephalopathy. *J Neurovirol, 6,* 221–8.

Van Duyne, R., Easley, R., Wu, W., Berro, R., Pedati, C., Klase, Z., et al. (2008). Lysine methylation of HIV-1 Tat regulates transcriptional activity of the viral LTR. *Retrovirology, 5,* 40.

Vaslin, A., Rummel, C., & Clarke, P. G. (2009). Unconjugated TAT carrier peptide protects against excitotoxicity. *Neurotox Res, 15,* 123–6.

Vendeville, A., Rayne, F., Bonhoure, A., Bettache, N., Montcourrier, P., & Beaumelle, B. (2004). HIV-1 Tat enters T cells using coated pits before translocating from acidified endosomes and eliciting biological responses. *Mol Biol Cell, 15,* 2347–60.

Vives, E., Brodin, P., & Lebleu, B. (1997). A truncated HIV-1 Tat protein basic domain rapidly translocates through the plasma membrane and accumulates in the cell nucleus. *J Biol Chem, 272,* 16010–7.

Wang, P., Barks, J. D., & Silverstein, F. S. (1999). Tat, a human immunodeficiency virus-1-derived protein, augments excitotoxic hippocampal injury in neonatal rats. *Neuroscience, 88,* 585–97.

Weeks, B. S., Lieberman, D. M., Johnson, B., Roque, E., Green, M., Lowenstein, P., et al. (1995). Neurotoxicity of the human immunodeficiency virus type 1 Tat transactivator to PC12 cells requires the Tat amino acid 49–58 basic domain. *Journal of Neuroscience Research, 42,* 34–40.

Wei, X., Miou, Z., & Baudry, M. (2008). Neuroprotection by cell permeable TAT-mGluR1 peptide in ischemia: Synergy between carrier and cargo sequences. *Neuroscientist, 14,* 409–14.

Weiss, J. M., Nath, A., Major, E. O., & Berman, J. W. (1999). HIV-Tat induces MCP-1-mediated monocyte transmigration and upregulates CCR5 expression on human monocytes. *J Immunol, 163,* 2953–2959.

Wesselingh, S. L., Power, C., Glass, J. D., Tyor, W. R., McArthur, J. C., Farber, J. M., et al. (1993). Intracerebral cytokine messenger RNA expression in acquired immunodeficiency syndrome dementia. *Ann Neurol, 33,* 576–582.

Westendorp, M. O., Frank, R., Ochsenbauer, C., Stricker, K., Dhein, J., Walczak, H., et al. (1995). Sensitization of T cells to CD95-mediated apoptosis by HIV-1 Tat and gp120. *Nature, 375,* 497–500.

Wiley, C. A., Baldwin, M., & Achim, C. L. (1996). Expression of regulatory and structural mRNA in the central nervous system. *AIDS, 10,* 943–947.

Woodman, S. E., Benveniste, E. N., Nath, A., & Berman, J. W. (1999). Human immunodeficiency virus type 1 TAT protein induces adhesion molecule expression in astrocytes. *J Neurovirol, 5,* 678–84.

Wortman, M. J., Krachmarov, C. P., Kim, J. H., Gordon, R. G., Chepenik, L. G., Brady, J. N., et al. (2000). Interaction of HIV-1 Tat with Puralpha in nuclei of human glial cells: Characterization of RNA-mediated protein-protein binding. *J Cell Biochem, 77,* 65–74.

Xiao, H., Neuveut, C., Tiffany, H. L., Benkirane, M., Rich, E. A., Murphy, P. M., et al. (2000). Selective CXCR4 antagonism by Tat: Implications for in vivo expansion of coreceptor use by HIV-1. *Proc Natl Acad Sci USA, 97,* 11466–71.

Yedavalli, V. S., Benkirane, M., & Jeang, K. T. (2003). Tat and trans-activation-responsive (TAR) RNA-independent induction of HIV-1 long terminal repeat by human and murine cyclin T1 requires Sp1. *J Biol Chem, 278,* 6404–10.

Zagury, J. F., Sill, A., Blattner, W., Lachgar, A., Le Buanec, H., Richardson, M., et al. (1998). Antibodies to the HIV-1 Tat protein correlated with nonprogression to AIDS: A rationale for the use of Tat toxoid as an HIV-1 vaccine [see comments]. *J Hum Virol, 1,* 282–92.

Zhao, T., Adams, M. H., Zou, S. P., El-Hage, N., Hauser, K. F., & Knapp, P. E. (2007). Silencing the PTEN gene is protective against neuronal death induced by human immunodeficiency virus type 1 Tat. *J Neurovirol, 13,* 97–106.

Zhong, Y., Hennig, B., & Toborek, M.(2010). Intact lipid rafts regulate HIV-1 Tat protein-induced activation of the Rho signaling and upregulation of P-glycoprotein in brain endothelial cells. *J Cereb Blood Flow Metab, 30,* 522–33.

Zhong, Y., Smart, E. J., Weksler, B., Couraud, P. O., Hennig, B., & Toborek, M. (2008). Caveolin-1 regulates human immunodeficiency virus-1 Tat-induced alterations of tight junction protein expression via modulation of the Ras signaling. *J Neurosci, 28,* 7788–96.

Zhu, J., Mactutus, C. F., Wallace, D. R., & Booze, R. M. (2009). HIV-1 Tat protein-induced rapid and reversible decrease in [3H]dopamine uptake: dissociation of [3H]dopamine uptake and [3H]2beta-carbomethoxy-3-beta-(4-fluorophenyl)tropane (WIN 35,428) binding in rat striatal synaptosomes. *J Pharmacol Exp Ther, 329,* 1071–83.

Zidovetzki, R., Wang, J. L., Chen, P., Jeyaseelan, R., & Hofman, F. (1998). Human immunodeficiency virus Tat protein induces interleukin 6 mRNA expression in human brain endothelial cells via protein kinase C- and cAMP-dependent protein kinase pathways. *AIDS Res Hum Retroviruses, 14,* 825–33.

Zou, W., Kim, B. O., Zhou, B. Y., Liu, Y., Messing, A., & He, J. J. (2007). Protection against human immunodeficiency virus type 1 Tat neurotoxicity by Ginkgo biloba extract EGb 761 involving glial fibrillary acidic protein. *Am J Pathol, 171,* 1923–35.

4.4

HIV-1 gp120

Shu-ichi Okamoto, Marcus Kaul, Ian Paul Everall,
Eliezer Masliah, and Stuart A. Lipton

This chapter reviews the neurotoxic effects of gp120, which has been implicated in the development of neurocognitive disorders. The toxic effects of Tat, which are discussed in detail in Chapter 4.3, are also briefly discussed. The major toxic action of gp120 is thought to be indirect, acting via NMDA receptors and other pathways, including GSK3β and the production of cytokines such as TNF-α, IL-1β, and IL-6. Therapeutic strategies designed to interfere with these neurotoxic pathways and prevent or reduce harm from gp120 are considered, as are other substances, such as Tat. Agents considered include NMDA receptor antagonists, antioxidants, chemokine and cytokine antagonists, neurotrophic factors, inhibitors of GSK3β, and of caspase, estrogen, and p38 MAPK antagonists.

INTRODUCTION

It is now clear that HIV infection of the brain is accompanied by a complex series of events that pathologically result in inflammatory changes, neuronal damage, and death. Clinically, those affected can develop a range of cognitive impairments, which can result in mild to profound dementia, now termed HIV-associated neurocognitive disorders (HAND), often with a poor prognosis if severe enough to be labelled HIV-associated dementia (HAD). The prevalence of HAND continues to increase despite highly active antiretroviral therapy (HAART) (McArthur, Steiner, Sacktor, & Nath, 2010). Understanding the pathogenic mechanisms which result in cellular damage may therefore identify pathways that can be targeted to ameliorate this process and thus prevent HAND. Two candidates implicated in pathogenesis are the envelope viral protein gp120 and the regulatory protein Tat. In this chapter a few of the salient features of the mechanisms of toxicity will be outlined which may be relevant to protective strategies against gp120. A more comprehensive review of neurotoxicity associated with Tat protein is covered in Chapter 4.3.

HIV infection of the brain results in a spectrum of neuropathological disorders, including a range of inflammatory changes, the best known being HIV encephalitis (HIVE), synaptic and dendritic damage, and neuronal loss (Budka et al., 1987; Budka et al., 1991; Everall, Luthert, & Lantos, 1991; Wiley et al., 1991; Everall, Luthert, & Lantos, 1993) HIVE is characterized by productive infection of cells of the monocytic/macrophage lineage accompanied by diffuse and nodular microgliosis, multinucleated giant cell formation, astrogliosis, and myelin pallor (Budka, 1991). While these remain the morphological hallmarks of the infection, fundamental questions still arise. The one most relevant to this chapter is what contribution do viral proteins make to this process and are there means by which this can be prevented.

Microglia, macrophages, and multinucleated giant cells are the main cellular targets within the brain for productive HIV infection (Kure, Lyman, Weidenheim, & Dickson, 1990a; Kure, Weidenheim, Lyman, & Dickson, 1990b; Kure, et al., 1991; Wiley, Schrier, Nelson, Lampert, & Oldstone, 1986). These infected cells then become cellular reservoirs of viral proteins and virus production. Similarly a small proportion of astrocytes are "restrictively" infected, whereby viral replication commences in a very small number of HIV-infected astrocytes (Brack-Werner, 1999). However, this does not go beyond the stage of production of regulatory proteins such as Tat. Thus, a milieu is established in the HIV-infected brain in which potentially toxic viral proteins are produced by at least two distinct cellular populations, which can then result in neuronal damage and death.

THE HIV-1 ENVELOPE PROTEIN gp120

The viral envelope protein gp120 is considered to play a significant role in the pathogenesis of neuronal damage. The impetus for this notion has arisen from animal and tissue culture studies. Systemic injection of gp120 into rats pathologically results in dystrophic changes in cortical pyramidal neurons, while behaviorally there is retardation in acquiring developmental milestones associated with complex motor behaviors (Hill, Mervis, Avidor, Moody, & Brenneman, 1993). Furthermore, direct intracerebral injection of gp120 resulted in memory impairment on water maze tasks in rats (Glowa et al., 1992) as well as other neurobehavioral disturbances (Barak et al., 2002). Toggas and colleagues (1994) inserted a truncated version of HIV-1$_{LAV}$ env gene encoding soluble gp120 into exon 1 of a modified murine glial fibrillary acidic protein (GFAP) gene. Astroglial cells expressed this construct at high levels in the neocortex, olfactory bulb, hippocampus, and tectum-selected white matter tracts. By quantitative neuropathological analysis they observed that there was extensive vacuolar degeneration of neuronal dendrites, a decrease in pre-synaptic terminals, loss of large cortical neurons, and widespread astrocytosis and microgliosis. These changes are similar to the inflammatory picture noted in individuals who died of AIDS (Budka et al. 1991) together with the neuronal damage and loss (Everall et al., 1991; Masliah, Ge, Achim, Hansen, & Wiley, 1992a; Masliah et al., 1992b; Weis, Haug, & Budka, 1993; Everall et al., 1999). It had also been noted that loss of large cortical neurons correlates with the onset and progression of HIV-associated dementia (HAD) (Asare et al., 1996). These observations in the murine model indicated a key role for gp120 in mediating HIV-related neuropathology. However, for a number of years a key stumbling block for promoting this hypothesis as a causative substrate of cognitive impairment was the failure to demonstrate gp120 in the brains of individuals who had died of AIDS. One explanation for this difficulty is that gp120 antibodies may only recognize the protein in particular conformations and that they did not detect the particular conformations present in the brain (Altmeyer, Mordelet, Girard, & Vidal, 1999). Recently, using a highly specific anti-gp120 antibody, immunopositive cells have been observed in multinucleated giant cells and those with microglial morphology (Jones, Bell, &Nath, 2000; Nath et al., 2000). These were primarily present perivascularly; they were often observed in clusters in the white matter but were more scattered in the grey matter. The staining occurred in many multinucleated giant cells. No staining was present in control brains and specificity was confirmed by Western blotting. However, while this observation provided an important piece of missing data, the confirmation of the role of gp120 in HIV-related neuropathology will be strengthened by replication of the observation by other groups.

Following from the concept that gp120 is a putative neurotoxin, investigators have begun assessing the potential mechanism(s) involved in this process. This has not proved a trivial task. Basically, it is postulated that there are two sequences of events. These are firstly that gp120 can have a direct neurotoxic effect, and secondly that the inflammatory process stimulated by gp120, and possibly other viral proteins, stimulates microglia and astrocytes to generate products, which are themselves inadvertently neurotoxic. These two processes are not mutually exclusive and it is probable that a combination of them both contribute to the overall scenario of HIV-related neurotoxicity. However, several lines of evidence suggest that the *predominant* pathway involves the secondary generation of macrophage/microglial toxins as well as effects on astrocytes after immune stimulation of these cells by gp120 or by viral infection itself that is initiated by gp120/ surface receptor interactions (Giulian, Vaca, & Noonan, 1990). Secretion of neurotoxins by mononuclear phagocytes infected with HIV-1 (Giulian et al., 1990; Lipton 1994a). HIV coat protein gp120 induces soluble neurotoxins in culture medium (Giulian, Wendt, Vaca, & Noonan, 1993; Bukrinsky et al., 1995; Lipton & Gendelman, 1995; Adamson et al., 1996; Giulian et al., 1996; Lipton, 1999; Kaul & Lipton, 1999; Yeh et al., 2000; Kaul & Lipton 2000; Kaul Garden, & Lipton, 2001; Garden et al., 2002). What is the evidence for either sequence of events?

The concept of potential direct gp120-mediated neurotoxicity was demonstrated by a number of groups. Work carried out in the late 1980s and early 1990s revealed the detrimental effects of gp120 on neurons (Table 4.4.1; Figure 4.4.1) (Brenneman et al., 1988; Kaiser, Offermann, & Lipton, 1990) Application of gp120 to rat striatal sections resulted in tissue loss and astrocytosis (Bansal et al., 2000). However, the predominant mechanism accounting for these findings is thought to involve interaction of gp120 with macrophages, which in turn are thought to release glutamate-like toxins onto neurons and to enhance excitotoxic insults, for example, by inhibiting glutamate reuptake or promoting glutamate release from astrocytes (Kaiser et al., 1990; Dreyer, Kaiser, Offermann, & Lipton, 1990) These effects of gp120 were shown to lead to excessive activation of glutamatergic NMDA receptors on neurons and consequent damage or apoptotic-like cell death (Lipton & Gendelman,1995; Kaul, 2000; Kaul, Garden, & Lipton, 2001; Lipton, Kaiser, Sucher, Dreyer, & Offerman, 1990; Lipton, Sucher, Kaiser, & Dreyer, 1991; Lipton,1992a; Lipton, 1992b; Lipton, 1993; Lipton & Rosenberg, 1994; Lipton, 1994; Gelbard et al., 1994; Kaul, 2002). Particular chemokines, such as SDF-1, were recently found to augment the release of glutamate from astrocytes triggered by gp120. Concerning in vivo results, at least five different laboratories have shown that gp120 injected into the brain can contribute to dendritic damage or apoptotic-like neuronal cell death (Lipton, Brenneman, Silverstein, Masliah, & Mucke, 1995). Nonetheless, not all workers have found this to be the case (Bagetta, Corasaniti, Finazzi-Agro, & Nistico, 1994). For example, a direct interaction of gp120 with neurons (Kaiser et al., 1990; Dreyer et al., 1990) was thought to involve interaction by gp120 with the glutamatergic NMDA receptors. Barks et al. (1997) injected gp120 into the CA1 region of perinatal rat hippocampus and failed to notice neuronal damage. However, when the rats were co-injected with gp120 and NMDA the hippocampal volume was reduced to a greater extent than when NMDA was injected on its own. Previously, synergistic neurotoxic effects between gp120 and glutamate

Table 4.4.1 **DIRECT AND INDIRECT NEUROTOXIC EFFECTS OF gp120**

Direct	CXCR4, CCR5
Indirect	NMDA receptors
	Ca (intracellular)
	NO
	TNFα
	IL-1
	IL-6
	β-chemokines
Chemokine-mediated	G protein coupled
	ERK 1/2
	p38 MAPK
	PI3K- PKB/AKT-GSK3β

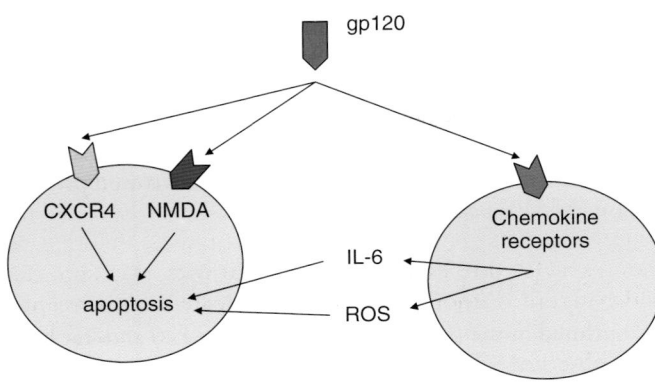

Figure 4.4.1 Neuronal death induced by direct and indirect effects of gp120.

had been reported in vitro (Lipton et al., 1991); again indicating involvement of the NMDA subtype of glutamate receptors in gp120-mediated neuronal damage. The V3 loop of gp120 has a relatively high affinity for the glycine coagonist site of the NMDA receptor (Pattarini, Pittaluga, & Raiteri, 1998) but it is not clear if this is relevant in HIV-associated dementia since the predominant effect of gp120 appears to be indirect via CD4 and chemokine receptors on macrophage and microglial cells and the subsequent release of glutamate-like toxins (Kaul et al., 2001). Moreover, direct effects of low (picomolar concentrations, the pathophysiologically relevant dose) of gp120 on NMDA receptor function have not been observed during patch-clamp recording of currents from either recombinant or native NMDA receptors (Lipton et al. 1991). Application of selective NMDA receptor antagonists, such as the channel blockers memantine and MK-801 (Lipton et al., 1991; Lipton, 1992c), prevented gp120-induced cell death (Lipton, 1992d; Corasaniti et al., 1995). Excessive activation of the NMDA receptor results in an increase in intracellular calcium concentration (Meucci et al., 1998) followed by nitric oxide generation, which may finally induce neuronal apoptosis (Corasaniti et al., 1995; Dawson, Dawson, Uhl, & Snyder, 1993). Further assessment of the cellular consequences of gp120 intracerebral injection revealed DNA fragmentation and electron microscopic features consistent with apoptosis, such as early compaction and marginalization of nuclear chromatin along the nuclear envelope followed by clumping of the nuclear envelope and enlargement of the endoplasmic reticulum (Bagetta et al., 1995; Bagetta et al., 1996a; Bagetta et al., 1996b). Corasaniti et al. (2001) recently extended this work demonstrating that gp120 neuronal apoptosis is mediated through binding to the CXCR4 chemokine receptor. Of course, this finding is predicted on the use of a gp120 from a CXCR4 (X4)-preferring HIV strain (Kaul & Lipton, 1999). Certain chemokines can block glutamatergic excitatory post-synaptic currents as well as gp120-induced neuronal apoptosis (Meucci et al., 1998). CXCR4 is expressed by a variety of macrophages, astrocytes as well as neurons, including hippocampal pyramidal neurons, suggesting the importance of binding to this receptor in mediating neurotoxicity (Lavi et al., 1997). Neuronal immunopositivity for CXCR4 was highest in regions such as the human hippocampus, superior temporal gyrus, amygdala, and thalamus. There were also a number of neurons immunopositive for CCR2 and CCR3 in similar anatomical regions to CXCR4 expression (van der Meer, Ulrich, Gonzalez-Scarano, & Lavi, 2000). Furthermore, the intensity of immunocytochemical CXCR4 staining was greater in HIV-infected cases (van der Meer et al., 2000). Finally, it would appear that the intracellular mechanism mediated by HIV-associated neuronal apoptosis involves overactivation of glycogen synthase kinase-3beta (GSK3β). GSK3β is a member of the canonical Wnt signaling pathway which plays a pivotal role in brain development (Dierick & Bejsovec, 1999; Joutel & Tournier-Lasserve, 1998) and in adult cytoskeletal maintenance (Hall, Lucas, & Salinas, 2000; Lucas, Goold, Gordon-Weeks, & Salinas, 1998; Lucas et al., 1997; Salinas, 1999). It is known that overactivation of this kinase results in apoptosis (Pap & Cooper, 1998; Pap & Cooper, 2002) and the role of Wnt signaling in neurodegeneration is currently being investigated (Joutel & Tournier-Lasserve, 1998; Mudher et al., 2001). Inhibition of this kinase has recently been shown to prevent gp120-associated neuronal death (Everall et al., 2002).

Additionally, gp120 appears to contribute to the development of HAND by interfering with neurogenesis in the adult hippocampus (Okamoto et al., 2007). Normally, neurogenesis occurs constitutively in the dentate gyrus throughout adulthood (Deng, Aimone, & Gage, 2010). Newly generated neurons functionally integrate into existing circuits and contribute to certain forms of learning and memory (Okamoto et al., 2007). Notably, neurogenesis in the dentate gyrus has recently been shown to be impaired in HIV patients with dementia (Krathwohl & Kaiser, 2004a; Krathwohl & Kaiser, 2004b). Mechanistically, one of our groups (Okamoto and colleagues) recently demonstrated that gp120 inhibits proliferation of adult neural progenitor cells in vitro and in vivo in the dentate gyrus of the hippocampus of gp120-transgenic mice via a p38 mitogen-activated protein kinase (MAPK) pathway (Okamoto et al., 2007). Specifically, HIV/gp120 arrests cell-cycle progression of adult neural progenitor cells at the G1 phase via activation of a cascade consisting of p38 MAPK—> MAPK-activated protein kinase 2 (a cell-cycle checkpoint kinase)—> Cdc25B/C. This eukaryotic Cdc25 phosphatase family was previously thought to be phosphorylated and hence inactivated in order to halt cell-cycle progression when DNA is damaged or incompletely replicated. Here, however, we showed for the first time that this cascade is also involved in arrest of neurogenesis from stem cells in neurodegenerative disorders. Our findings therefore define a molecular mechanism that compromises adult neurogenesis in HAND. Thus, gp120 may be involved in cognitive alterations in HIV patients by impairing neuronal differentiation in the hippocampal dentate gyrus.

INDIRECT MECHANISMS OF NEUROTOXICITY BY gp120

The HIV-1 envelope protein gp120 elicits the release of cytokines such as tumor necrosis factor-alpha (TNF-α), interleukin-1 (IL-1), and IL-6 as part of the immune response of the brain (Table 4.4.1) (Merrill et al., 1992; Yeung, Pulliam, & Lau, 1995; Ilyin & Plata-Salaman, 1997). However, within the brain this immune response can contribute to the neuronal damage and loss (Ensoli et al., 1999; Bjugstad, Flitter, Garland, Su, & Arendash, 1998)]. Behavioral experiments in rats have shown that some of the neurobehavioral abnormalities are linked to the cytokine production (Barak et al., 2002). Furthermore, gp120 can stimulate cysteine, quinolinate, and other potential excitotoxin release from human monocyte-derived macrophages in amounts which are neurotoxic (Yeh et al., 2000). In the previous section it was noted that gp120 in binding to neuronal CXCR4 receptors may mediate neuronal death (Meucci et al., 1998). However, the actions of gp120 are probably more complex as the neuronal apoptosis is probably mediated predominantly by activation of chemokine receptors on macrophages/microglia. Depletion of macrophages/microglia from mixed neuronal/glial cortical cultures or inhibition of macrophage/microglial activation by tuftsin-derived tripeptide (TKP) abrogates gp120-induced neuronal apoptosis (Kaul & Lipton, 1999). Gp120 from either CCR5 or CXCR4-tropic HIV-1 species stimulates the macrophage production of the β-chemokines such as macrophage inflammatory protein 1α (MIP-1α), MIP-1β, and RANTES, as well as TNF-α. This production may have complex effects as β-chemokines inhibit CCR5 HIV-1 infection in clinical studies (Cocchi et al., 1995; Cocchi et al., 2000; Zagury et al., 1998); however, chemokines have also been observed to increase viral replication (Kinter et al., 1998). These observations have been made mainly in CD4+ and CD8+ T cells and the activities of chemokines in macrophages/microglia may be more heterogeneous or manifest rapid desensitization as only 15% of adult microglia were found to be responsive to either α- or β-chemokines, while 27% were not responsive to either chemokine (Albright, Martin, O'Connor, & Gonzalez-Scarano, 2001). So, the functional effects of chemokines on resident brain macrophages and microglia require further investigation. Studies on primary rat mixed glial cell cultures co-cultured with primary rat hippocampal neurons have revealed that gp120 induces a significant increase in intracellular calcium which precedes neuronal death, while in the glial population there was a significant production of IL-1β which was then postulated to be responsible for the observed rise in reactive oxygen species which are involved in neurotoxicity (Viviani, Corsini, Binaglia, Galli, & Marinovich, 2001). In human primary cultures containing astrocytes and macrophages, exposure to gp120 caused upregulation of IL-6 and TNF-α, both putative neurotoxic agents (Yeung et al., 1995). Overall, gp120 appears to initiate neuronal damage and death through a complex cascade involving both direct and indirect neurotoxicity with the indirect route thought to be the predominant mechanism (Figure 4.4.1).

NEUROPROTECTION AGAINST gp120

The most rational avenue to investigate putative neuroprotective strategies is to intervene in demonstrated neurotoxic pathways. As the approaches are common to both viral proteins they will be considered together under particular strategies. The potential approaches that will be considered are antagonism of glutamate receptors, antagonism of cytokines/chemokines, neurotrophic support, inhibition of GSK3β, inhibition of caspase or mitogen–activated protein kinase (MAPK) cascades, and steroids.

NMDA RECEPTOR ANTAGONISTS

As outlined in the previous section, both gp120 and Tat have been observed to mediate neuronal damage by excitotoxicity (Lipton et al., 1991; Lipton, 1992a, Haughey et al., 2001; Nath & Geiger, 1998; Magnuson, 1995).However, the mechanisms of action of these proteins are not identical. Tat initially releases calcium from inositol 1,4,5-trisphosphate-regulated pools, followed by influx mediated by excitatory amino acid receptors (Haughey, Holden, Nath, & Geiger, 1999; Holden, Haughey, Nath, & Geiger, 1999). HIV gp120 may work via a variety of mechanisms to activate excitotoxicity and the NMDA receptor on neurons. The predominant pathways are thought to involve release of toxins from macrophages and/or astrocytes that result, either directly or indirectly, in excessive stimulation of NMDA receptors. For example, as mentioned earlier, gp120 leads to the release of macrophage TNF-α, which in turn acts via arachidonic acid to interfere with glutamate handling by astrocytes. Glutamate uptake by astrocytes is thus inhibited and, in fact, glutamate release ensues. Additionally, arachidonic acid is known to enhance NMDA receptor activation. Toxins released by gp120-stimulated macrophages, such as L-cysteine, also mimic the action of glutamate at the NMDA receptor. Overactivation of NMDA receptors leads to excessive influx of Ca^{2+} and subsequent overstimulation of enzymatic pathways and free radical generation, with consequent neuronal injury and apoptotic-like death (Kaul et al., 2002). Thus, investigators have assessed the potential of preventing the excessive rise in intraneuronal Ca^{2+} by use of either glutamate antagonists or calcium channel antagonists to prevent the rise in intracellular calcium that accompanies excitotoxic damage. Originally, Dreyer et al. (Dreyer et al., 1990), using rat ganglion cells, demonstrated that administration of picomolar concentrations of recombinant gp120 resulted in a significant increase in intracellular calcium concentration and significant neuronal loss, which could be prevented by either transiently lowering extracellular calcium or application of the dihydropyridine L-type voltage-dependent calcium antagonist nimodipine. NMDA receptor antagonists were also shown to be effective in combating gp120 neurotoxicity, including the clinically tolerated open-channel blocker memantine, with potential benefits in vivo for HAD as well in phase 1–2 human clinical trial (Lipton, 1992c; Schifitto et al., 2007). Transient release of inositol 1,4,5-triphosphate regulated intracellular calcium stores is essential for the subsequent delayed secondary increase in calcium via glutamate receptors (Haughey et al., 2001). It has been found that prevention of this release of intracellular calcium by inhibitors such as 8-(diethylamino)octyl-3,4,5-trimethoxybenzoate hydrochloride, xestospongin, or thapsigargin can interfere with tat-associated neuronal death (Haughey et al., 2001). Drugs such as riluzole, which among other actions inhibits glutamate releases, prevent gp120-mediated neurotoxicity and hence may have therapeutic potential in HIV dementia but this remains unclear (Sindou et al., 1994).

ANTIOXIDANTS

A phenomenon common to neurotoxicity mediated by HIV proteins is the induction of oxidative stress (Kruman, Nath, & Mattson, 1998; Foga, Nath, Hasinoff, & Geiger, 1997). Production of free radicals, mitochondrial injury, depletion of glutathione, and production of nitric oxide are some of the factors that contribute to viral protein-induced oxidative stress. Oxidized lipids and proteins can be detected in the brain and cerebrospinal fluid (CSF) of patients with HIV dementia and encephalitis (Turchan et al., 2003). Hence, antioxidants may play an important role in altering the progression of HIV dementia. Deprenyl has shown some efficacy in two previous studies on patients with HIV dementia (Sacktor et al., 2000; Roesler et al., 1998) and a much larger study using a transdermal form of the drug is currently underway. Other drugs such as didox, which has both antiretroviral and antioxidant effects, are also worthy of further consideration (Turchan et al., 2003).

TARGETING CYTOKINES AND CHEMOKINES

Chemokines and chemokine receptors play a critical role in inflammatory and neurodegenerative process HIV brain infection. They are expressed by neurons, astrocytes, and microglia. Chemokine receptors, which act as co-receptors, are crucial for the HIV-binding process. Following chemokine-receptor binding, conformational changes of the envelope region occur, allowing the fusion of cell membranes and the transport of the viral nucleocapsid into the host cell (Furuta, Wild, Weng, & Weiss, 1998). This is an important step to target viral entry inhibition. The macrophage-tropic strains, also known as nonsyncytium-inducing or R5 variants, predominantly use the chemokine receptor CCR5 and the T-cell-tropic strains, also known as syncytium-inducing or X4 variants, predominantly use CXCR4 receptors. It was first observed that in 1% of the global population, individuals who are homozygous for the 32-base-pair deletion in the CCR5 gene (CCR5Δ32) are prevented from HIV infection.

We found in previous studies that natural ligands for CCR5, such as MIP-1β/CCL4 and RANTES/CCL5, per se did not affect neuronal survival but abrogated gp120-induced neuronal death in mixed neuronal-glial cerebrocortical cell cultures. In contrast, the natural ligand of CXCR4, SDF-1/CXCL12, exerted a neurotoxic effect (Kaul & Lipton, 1999; Kaul, Ma, Medders, Desai, & Lipton, 2007). The somewhat surprising toxicity of SDF-1 was prevented in CXCR4-deficient cerebrocortical cultures confirming that, at least in our experimental system, this α-chemokine induced neuronal damage specifically via its physiological receptor. Another surprising observation in our studies was that physiological CCR5 ligands could also ameliorate or prevent the neurotoxic effects of CXCR4 stimulation by SDF-1, the receptor's exclusive natural ligand. Moreover, triple-immuno-fluorescence staining revealed almost 100% co-expression of both chemokine receptors in cerebrocortical neurons, and the selective CCR5 ligand MIP-1β/CCL4 suppressed CXCR4-mediated increases in neuronal intracellular free Ca^{2+}. Taken together, these findings strongly suggest that the neuroprotective effect of CCR5-binding MIP-1β/CCL4 and RANTES/CCL5 involves heterologous desensitization of CXCR4 receptors on neurons (Kaul et al., 2007). In the case of HIV-1/gp120, the neuroprotective effect of CCR5 ligands could be explained by interference with HIV co-receptors on microglia and macrophages, causing direct competition with gp120 for CCR5 binding. HIV co-receptors in the brain are also expressed on astrocytes and neurons (Rottman et al., 1997; Lavi et al., 1997; Hesselgesser & Horuk, 1999; Kaul et al., 2001). Moreover, the neurotoxicity of SDF-1 does not depend on microglial activation, and yet is blocked by CCR5 ligands (Kaul & Lipton, 1999; Bezzi et al., 2001). These results suggest that CCR5-dependent neuroprotection can also be mediated by cell types other than microglia, such as astrocytes and neurons themselves. Indeed, our studies suggested for the first time that neuroprotection by natural CCR5 ligands may be possible via heterologous desensitization of CXCR4 directly on neurons. Interestingly, we and others have observed that MIP-1β/CCL4 and RANTES/CCL5 also reduce neuronal death due to direct excitotoxic insult by NMDA, which is also consistent with a direct effect of these CCR5 ligands on neurons (Bruno, Copani, Besong, Scoto, & Nicoletti, 2000; Kaul & Lipton, 2001).

Finally, our neurotoxicity experiments in cerebrocortical cultures from CCR5 KO mice demonstrated a pivotal role for this receptor in both neuronal injury by gp120 and neuroprotection by β-chemokines (Kaul et al., 2007). Interestingly, the CCR5 ligands RANTES and MIP-1α/β have been found to be highly expressed in cerebrospinal fluid (CSF) of neurocognitively intact HIV-infected individuals, while the same chemokines were drastically diminished in the CSF of cognitively impaired AIDS patients (Letendre, Lanier, & McCutchan, 1999). These findings lend support to the hypothesis that endogenous CCR5 ligands may offer neuroprotection in the setting of neuroAIDS.

Investigations of the molecular mechanism of CCR5-dependent neuroprotection revealed that the pro-survival effect of CCR5 activation was abrogated by a dominant-interfering form of Akt, whereas wild-type (WT) Akt had no effect (Kaul et al., 2007). This observation was in line with findings in another study, which showed that neuronal Akt provided protection against excitotoxic insult (Digicaylioglu, Garden, Timberlake, Fletcher, & Lipton, 2004). In summary, it appears that CCR5 may be able to confer neuroprotection against HIV-induced neurotoxicity in case its natural ligands are present, whereas in situations where those neuroprotective β-chemokines are lacking, the receptor may primarily contribute to neuronal injury and demise such as after HIV/gp120 stimulation.

Concerning chemokines and possible neuroprotection, TAK-779 and PRO 140 are two CCR5 inhibitors that were reported to prevent gp120 binding to the CCR5 receptor (Baba et al., 1999; Olson, 2000). TAK-779 was reported to inhibit R5 variants at very low concentrations (Baba et al., 1999). Similar findings were also reported for PRO-140 (Trkola et al., 2007). However, there are no clinical trials available for these two inhibitors. Schering's SCH-C is another CCR5 antagonist and it was shown to interact at the V3 loop of gp120 and CCR5 (Reynes, Rouzier, & Kanouni, 2002). SCH-C was reported to have potent antiretroviral activity in SCID-hu Thy/Liv mice (Strizki et al., 2001). SCH-C was allowed to undergo clinical phase trials 1 and 2. However, due to a persistent level of HIV-1 RNA, it was discontinued (Eron, 2002). Similarly, the CXCR4 inhibitors ALX40–4C and T22 were observed to prevent the binding of gp120 and CXCR4 (Tamamura et al., 1998; O'Brien et al., 1996). Some in vitro studies have shown that CXCR4 ligands such as SDF-1α and β were found to be neurotoxic at low nanomolar concentrations (Kaul & Lipton, 1999) suggesting that their inhibition might be beneficial in HIV-associated dementia. Clinical trial of ALX40–4C was reported to have poor viral inhibitory response (Eron, 2002). However, the investigations into most of the chemokine entry inhibitors are still at their initial stages and awaiting clinical trials.

The elevated expression of pro-inflammatory cytokines such as TNFα, IL-1, and IL-6 following exposure to gp120 and Tat was mentioned previously. Activated microglial cells can be the main source of these cytokines. Homozygous HIV-1 transgenic mice (Tg26) express HIV-1 mRNA and gp120 along with large quantities of TNFα (De et al., 2002). Treatment of Tg26 mice with anti- TNFα antibody was demonstrated to reduce TNFα production as well as the accompanying HIV-1 pathology. However, cytokines such as IL-4, IL-10, and TGFβ-1 have anti-inflammatory properties (Turrin & Plata-Salaman, 2000). These cytokines were observed to inhibit the actions induced by pro-inflammatory cytokines (Ilyin & Plata-Salaman, 1997). Also, the CD200 receptor expressed by neurons was found to inhibit the neurotoxic effects of activated microglia (Hoek et al., 2000). The ligand for the CD200 receptor is produced by the microglial cells. Mice deficient in CD200 were observed to produce all the features accompanying microglial cell activation (Hoek et al., 2000). Furthermore, these microglial cells were less ramified, expressing increased levels of CD11b and CD45. Also, unlike in healthy brain tissue, these cells formed aggregates (Hoek et al., 2000).

NEUROTROPHIC FACTORS

The role of neurotrophic factors on neurogenesis during brain development is a well-established phenomenon (Cameron, Hazel, & McKay, 1998). Evidence indicates that fibroblast growth factor (FGF), nerve growth factor (NGF), and brain-derived growth factor (BDNF) all contribute towards neuronal functioning and survival. The gene expression of BDNF is enhanced during HIV infection of microglial cultures (Achim & Wiley, 1996). Additionally, in postmortem brains of HIVE patients, BDNF has been localized to neuronal perikarya and to the neuritic processes (Soontornniyomkij, Wang,

Pittman, Wiley, & Achim, 1998). In gp120-exposed neuronal cultures, BDNF was reported enhanced in a concentration-dependent manner (Barnea, Roberts, & Ho, 1999). Also, rats receiving cerebral injections of gp120 were observed to synergistically increase NGF levels in the hippocampus (Bagetta et al., 1996b). Either NGF or BDNF receptor binding initiates intracellular signaling pathways of PI3K and MAPK pathways (Yao & Cooper, 1995, Crowder & Freeman, 1998; Hetman, Kanning, Cavanaugh, & Xia, 1999). Both BDNF and NGF were reported to prevent Tat-induced neuronal apoptosis by activating the transcription factor NF-κB and promoting the expression of Bcl-2 (Ramirez et al., 2001).

FGFs function similarly to NGF and BDNF. Acidic FGF (FGF1) is primarily produced by neurons, whereas basic FGF (FGF2) by astrocytes. We have shown that fibroblast growth factor-1 (FGF1) inhibits GSK3β activity, as explained below (Hashimoto et al., 2002) and increased levels of FGF1 are expressed in surviving neurons in HIVE (Sagara et al., 2001; Everall et al., 2001). The increase in FGF1 correlates with improved cognitive performance and preservation of dendritic integrity (Everall et al., 2001). Furthermore, we have shown neuroprotection against gp120 by both lithium (Everall et al., 2002) and Wnt, both of which inhibit GSK3β. Lithium is a powerful inhibitor of GSK3β (Hedgepeth et al., 1997; Hedgepeth, 1999; Klein & Melton, 1996). This implies that inhibition of GSK3β is neuroprotective. Studies on FGF2 have indicated that this neurotrophic factor is expressed mainly by astrocytes as a response to brain injury to prevent neuronal damage and promote axonal sprouting (Abe, Aoyagi, & Saito, 2001; Fagan et al., 1997).

REGULATION OF GSK-3β BY WNT SIGNALING AND CYTOKINES

Alterations in Wnt signaling are currently being recognized as important in the pathogenesis of neurodegeneration (Joutel & Tournier-Lasserve, 1998; Mudher et al., 2001; Wodarz & Nusse, 1998; Axelrod, Matsuno, Artavanis-Tsakonas, & Perrimon, 1996). GSK-3β is regulated by the evolutionarily highly conserved Wnt signaling pathway (Figure 4.4.2). Specifically, in relation to HIV, it has been shown that HIV Tat protein increases GSK3β activity (Maggirwar, Tong, Ramirez, Gelbard, & Dewhurst, 1999). In the absence of a Wnt signal, GSK3β targets β-catenin for degradation; inhibition of GSK3β by a Wnt signal results in the stabilization of β-catenin, which can then translocate to the nucleus to activate transcription. Active GSK3β phosphorylates adenomatous polyposis coli (APC) and promotes the association of APC, axin, and β-catenin. Thus in the absence of a Wnt signal, β-catenin exists in the same complex and is phosphorylated by GSK-3β. This targets β-catenin for degradation. When Wnt signals via the frizzled receptor, the cytoplasmic protein dishevelled (dvl) binds to axin and acts to inhibit GSK3β phosphorylation of β-catenin and APC by an as yet poorly understood mechanism. It has been suggested that β-catenin is released from the complex via the action of Frat1 (Frequently arranged in advanced T-cell lymphomas-1), which interacts with dvl and axin. Thus as the result of a Wnt

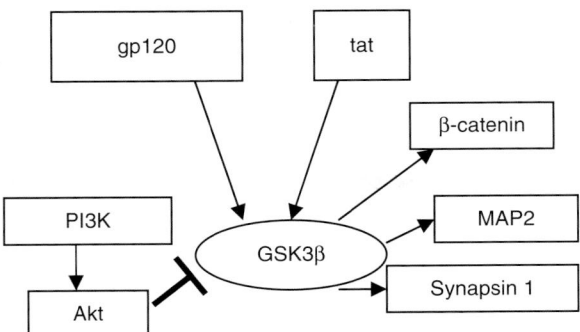

Figure 4.4.2 A schematic diagram of the interactions of (1) morphine, and TNF-α with PI3-kinase./Akt, and (2) PI3kinase/Akt with GSK3β. PI3kinase/Akt inhibits GSK3β.

signal a complex consisting of Frat1/DVl/GSK3β/axin is formed. This results in the dissociation of GSK3β from axin and the stabilization of β-catenin (Thomas et al., 1999; Dominguez & Green, 2000). The released β-catenin translocates to the nucleus where it forms a complex with TCF/Lef 1 to regulate transcription from Wnt target genes.

Wnt genes are expressed in postmitotic neurons during periods of axonal extension and synaptogenesis (Lucas & Salinas, 1997; Salinas, Fletcher, Copeland, Jenkins, & Nusse, 1994) and manipulation of Wnt signaling in cultured neurons results in perturbations of axonal modeling. The presence of Wnt7 reduces the amount of phosphorylated MAP1b in the growth cone and both Wnt7 and lithium result in increased spread area of the growth cone (Lucas et al., 1998). The importance of Wnt signaling in neurogenesis of developing brain and in plasticity in the developed brain is shown by the findings that overexpression of Wnt in Drosophila results in a massively increased CNS size (Richter, Hartmann, Reichert, 1998) and it has been reported that lithium treatment in humans increases grey matter in the cortex (Moore, Bebchuk, Wilds, Chen, & Manji, 2000a; 2000b). As explained above, both FGF1 and lithium were found to be neuroprotective against gp120 (Everall et al., 2002; Everall et al., 2001).

Additionally, a recent investigation has shown that the GSK3β-specific inhibitors AR-A014418 and B6B30 were able to ameliorate increases in the pro-apoptotic enzymes caspases-3 and -7 in primary human neurons in vitro following exposure to HIV$_{BaL}$ envelope (Nguyen et al., 2009). The neuroprotective effect of these specific inhibitors, at levels close to their IC$_{50}$ values for GSK3β, and having very little affinity for GSK3α, provide further support for GSK3β as a potential specific therapeutic target and may have important clinical implications for treatment of HAND. The neuroprotective effect of AR-A014418 observed for this investigation is in keeping with a previous study demonstrating the ability of AR-A014418 to protect N2A neuroblastoma cells against cell death mediated by inhibition of the phosphatidylinositol 3-kinase/protein kinase B survival pathway (Bhat et al., 2003). This work further suggests that inhibitors of GSK-3β may have clinical potential for the treatment of HAND.

Recently, one of our groups showed the therapeutic potential of the cytokines erythropoietin (EPO) and insulin-like

growth factor-I (IGF-I) in animal models of HAND. When administered transnasally, EPO plus IGF-I act in a synergistic fashion to activate the PI3K/Akt/GSK-3β pathway. The resulting phosphorylation of GSK-3β inhibits its activity. This acts to decrease hyperphosphorylation of tau protein and limit neuronal damage due to gp120 both in vitro and in vivo in HIV/gp120 transgenic mice (Kang et al., 2010). These results have been used to suggest that a human clinical trial of EPO plus IGF-I should be entertained for HAND.

STEROIDS

An emerging area of research is the association between HIV and steroid hormones. Glucocorticoids (GC) are steroid hormones secreted as a response to stressful situations by the adrenal glands. In hippocampal, cortical, and striatal cultures, GCs were demonstrated to exacerbate the neurotoxic effects of gp120 (Brooke & Sapolsky, 2000). On the contrary, estrogen was reported to have a neuroprotective effect against a range of insults. Estrogen was found to act by regulating calcium homeostasis (Mermelstein, Becker, & Surmeier, 1996), reducing free radical production (Behl et al., 1997), and influencing the growth of dendrites (Brinton, Tran, Proffitt, & Montoya, 1997). Howard et al. (2001) observed in gp120-treated primary hippocampal cultures reductions in lipid peroxidation and superoxide levels following estrogen treatment. Here, estrogen was found to prevent Tat-induced phosphorylation of MAP kinase, superoxide, and TNFα release. Estrogen has also been shown to modulate Bcl-2 and activate the AP-1 (Dubal, Wilson, & Wise, 1999; Uht, Anderson, Webb, & Kushner, 1997). The neuroprotective effects of estrogen have been extended to neurogenesis, whereby it's believed to actively stimulate neurogenesis in adult hippocampus (Behl, 2002).It has also been associated with the recovery of a range of neurodegenerative disorders in humans (Behl, 2002). The beneficial effects of estrogen may be brought about by its interactions with neurotrophic factors, including NGF and BDNF (Sohrabji, Miranda, & Toran-Allerand, 1995) and on apoptotic factors (Singer, Rogers, & Dorsa, 1998).

CASPASE INHIBITORS AND P38 MAPK ANTAGONISTS

Both gp120 and tat have been reported to activate, either directly or indirectly, neuronal caspases, serine proteases involved in apoptotic cell death (Kaul et al., 2001; Garden et al., 2002; Kruman et al., 1998). One example of an indirect pathway to caspase activation involves excessive NMDA receptor stimulation leading to mitochondrial Ca^{2+} overload, permeability pore transition, cytochrome c release, and activation of caspase-9 and -3 (the so-called intrinsic pathway to caspase activation and apoptotic cell death). Additionally, via a TNF-α-dependent pathway, gp120 can lead to caspase-8 activation in neurons, and presumably also lead to downstream activation of caspase-3 (the so-called extrinsic or non-mitochondrial pathway to caspase activation). Caspase inhibitors have been shown to ameliorate gp120-induced neuronal

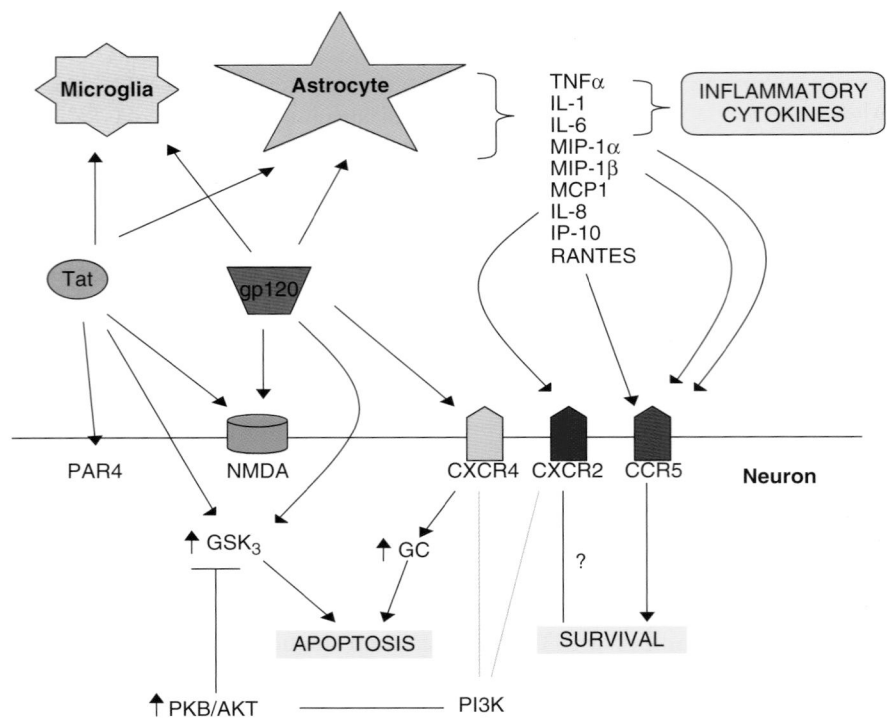

Figure 4.4.3 A schematic representation of the possible effects of gp120 on neuronal, microglial, and astrocyte cells that can lead to cellular death.

damage both in vitro and in the gp120-transgenic mouse, indicating that these drugs may hold therapeutic potential in HIV-associated dementia.

Additionally, gp120, possible via excessive NMDA receptor stimulation by macrophage toxins, leads to activation of the p38 MAPK pathway. Inhibition of this pathway, either by molecular interference or with relatively specific drugs, can be neuroprotective. As mentioned above, p38 MAPK is also involved in arrest of adult neural progenitor cells in HAND brains (Okamoto et al., 2007). These results suggest that p38 antagonists, currently being developed for other inflammatory diseases such as rheumatoid arthritis, might prove useful in combating HIV-related neuronal damage (Kaul et al., 2001).

CONCLUSION

In this chapter we have reviewed the neurotoxic effects of gp120, which have been implicated in neurocognitive disorders. This has highlighted the significant role played by gp120 and possibly other HIV proteins such as Tat and the various signaling pathways they interact with in order to produce these neurotoxic effects. The major toxic action of gp120 is thought to be indirect via NMDA receptors and other pathways, including GSK3β and production of cytokines such as TNF-α, IL-1β, and IL-6. These neurotoxic products are listed in Table 4.4.1. A schematic representation of these events is shown on Figure 4.4.3. To prevent gp120 and potential Tat neurotoxicity, we considered strategies to intervene in these

neurotoxic pathways. These include NMDA receptor antagonists, antioxidants, chemokine and cytokine antagonists, neurotrophic factors, inhibitors of GSK3β, estrogen, caspase inhibition, and p38 MAPK antagonists. NMDA receptor antagonists were reported to prevent the elevation of intracellular calcium concentrations associated with excitotoxic damage. NMDA receptor antagonists have been observed to prevent neuronal loss following administration of gp120 and Tat. The production of free radicals and NO, which are known to be downstream of excessive NMDA receptor activation, that follows HIV infection, is also thought to contribute to HAND. Antioxidants were reported to prevent progression towards dementia in HIV patients. Chemokine receptor antagonists were also reported to prevent binding of gp120. However, to date clinical studies have been less successful compared to in vitro studies. Although there are many reports of anti-inflammatory cytokine intervention for the prevention of neurotoxicity, this is less well reported in the area of HIV. IL-4, IL-10, and TGFβ have all been implicated in the inhibition pro-inflammatory cytokine production. Neurotrophic factors such as FGF, NGF, and BDNF have all been shown to be neuroprotective. FGF1 was reported to act by inhibiting the activity of GSK3β, thereby promoting neuronal survival, as do the synergistic combination of EPO plus IGF-I. Steroidal hormones, such as estrogen, and caspase and p38 MAPK inhibitors can also promote neuronal survival by regulating the levels of calcium and free radical production. It is evident that these various neurotoxic pathways are linked and the strategies we considered also interact with each other.

REFERENCES

Abe, K., Aoyagi, A., & Saito, H. (2001). Sustained phosphorylation of mitogen-activated protein kinase is required for basic fibroblast growth factor-mediated axonal branch formation in cultured rat hippocampal neurons. *Neurochemistry International*, 38(4), 309–15.

Achim, C. L. & Wiley, C. A. (1996). Inflammation in AIDS and the role of the macrophage in brain pathology. *Current Opinion in Neurology*, 9(3), 221–5.

Adamson, D. C., Wildemann, B., Sasaki, M., Glass, J. D., McArthur, J. C., Christov, V. I., et al. (1996). Immunologic NO synthase: Elevation in severe AIDS dementia and induction by HIV-1 gp41. *Science*, 274(5294), 1917–21.

Albright, A. V., Martin, J., O'Connor, M., & Gonzalez-Scarano, F. (2001). Interactions between HIV-1 gp120, chemokines, and cultured adult microglial cells. *Journal of Neurovirology*, 7(3), 196–207.

Altmeyer, R., Mordelet, E., Girard, M., & Vidal, C. (1999). Expression and detection of macrophage-tropic HIV-1 gp120 in the brain using conformation-dependent antibodies. *Virology*, 259(2), 314–23.

Asare, E., Dunn, G., Glass, McArthur, J., Luthert, P. Lantos, P., et al. (1996). Neuronal pattern correlates with the severity of human immunodeficiency virus-associated dementia complex. Usefulness of spatial pattern analysis in clinicopathological studies. *American Journal of Pathology*, 148(1), 31–8.

Axelrod, J. D., Matsuno, K., Artavanis-Tsakonas, S., & Perrimon, N. (1996). Interaction between Wingless and Notch signaling pathways mediated by dishevelled. *Science*, 271(5257), 1826–32.

Baba, M., Nishimura, O., Kanzaki, N., Okamoto, M., Sawada, H., Iizawa, Y., et al. (1999). A small-molecule, nonpeptide CCR5 antagonist with highly potent and selective anti-HIV-1 activity. *Proceedings of the National Academy of Sciences of the United States of America*, 96(10), 5698–703.

Bagetta, G., Corasaniti, T. M., Finazzi-Agro, A., & Nistico, G. (1994). Does the HIV-1 coat protein gp120 produce brain damage? *Trends in Pharmacological Sciences*, 15(10), 362–3.

Bagetta, G., Corasaniti, M. T., Berliocchi, L., Navarra, M., Finazzi-Agro, A., & Nistico, G. (1995). HIV-1 gp120 produces DNA fragmentation in the cerebral cortex of rat. *Biochemical & Biophysical Research Communications*, 211(1), 130–6.

Bagetta, G., Corasaniti, M. T., Malorni, W., Rainaldi, G., Berliocchi, L., Finazzi-Agro, A., et al. (1996a). The HIV-1 gp120 causes ultrastructural changes typical of apoptosis in the rat cerebral cortex. *Neuroreport*, 7(11), 1722–4.

Bagetta, G., Corasaniti, M. T., Aloe, L., Berliocchi, L., Costa, N., Finazzi-Agro, A., et al. (1996b). Intracerebral injection of human immunodeficiency virus type 1 coat protein gp120 differentially affects the expression of nerve growth factor and nitric oxide synthase in the hippocampus of rat. *Proceedings of the National Academy of Sciences of the United States of America*, 93(2), 928–33.

Bansal, A. K., Mactutus, C. F., Nath, A., Maragos, W., Hauser, K. F., & Booze, R. M. (2000). Neurotoxicity of HIV-1 proteins gp120 and Tat in the rat striatum. *Brain Research*, 879(1–2), 42–9.

Barak, O., Goshen, I., Ben-Hur, T., Weidenfeld, J., Taylor, A. N., & Yirmiya, R. (2002). Involvement of brain cytokines in the neurobehavioral disturbances induced by HIV-1 glycoprotein120. *Brain Research*, 933(2), 98–108.

Barks, J. D., Liu, X. H., Sun, R., & Silverstein, F. S. (1997). Gp120, a human immunodeficiency virus-1 coat protein, augments excitotoxic hippocampal injury in perinatal rats. *Neuroscience*, 76(2), 397–409.

Barnea, A., Roberts, J., & Ho, R. H. (1999). Evidence for a synergistic effect of the HIV-1 envelope protein gp120 and brain-derived neurotrophic factor (BDNF) leading to enhanced expression of somatostatin neurons in aggregate cultures derived from the human fetal cortex. *Brain Research*, 815(2), 349–57.

Behl, C., Skutella, T., Lezoualc'h, F., Post, A., Widmann, M., Newton, C. J., et al. (1997). Neuroprotection against oxidative stress by estrogens: structure-activity relationship. *Molecular Pharmacology*, 51(4), 535–41.

Behl, C. (2002). Sex hormones, neuroprotection and cognition. *Prog Brain Res*, 138, 135–42.

Bezzi, P., Domercq, M., Brambilla, L., Galli, R., Schols, D., De Clercq, E., et al. (2001). CXCR4-activated astrocyte glutamate release via TNFalpha: Amplification by microglia triggers neurotoxicity. *Nature Neurosci*, 4(7), 702–10.

Bhat, R., Xue, Y., Berg, S., Hellberg, S., Ormo, M., Nilsson, Y., et al. (2003). Structural insights and biological effects of glycogen synthase kinase 3-specific inhibitor AR-A014418. *J Biol Chem*, 278, 45937–45945.

Bjugstad, K. B., Flitter, W. D., Garland, W. A., Su, G. C., & Arendash, G. W. (1998). Preventive actions of a synthetic antioxidant in a novel animal model of AIDS dementia. *Brain Res*, 795(1–2), 349–57.

Brack-Werner, R. (1999). Astrocytes: HIV cellular reservoirs and important participants in neuropathogenesis. *AIDS*, 13(1), 1–22.

Brenneman, D. E., Westbrook, G. L., Fitzgerald, S. P., Ennist, D. L., Elkins, K. L., Ruff, M. R., et al. (1988). Neuronal cell killing by the envelope protein of HIV and its prevention by vasoactive intestinal peptide. *Nature*, 335(6191), 639–42.

Brinton, R. D., Tran, J., Proffitt, P., & Montoya, M. (1997). 17 beta-Estradiol enhances the outgrowth and survival of neocortical neurons in culture. *Neurochemical Research*, 22(11), 1339–51.

Brooke, S. M. & Sapolsky, R. M. (2000). The effects of steroid hormones in HIV-related neurotoxicity: A mini review. *Biological Psychiatry*, 48(9), 881–93.

Bruce-Keller, A. J., Barger, S. W., Moss, N. I., Pham, J. T., Keller, J. N., & Nath, A. (2001). Pro-inflammatory and pro-oxidant properties of the HIV protein Tat in a microglial cell line: attenuation by 17 beta-estradiol. *J Neurochemistry*, 78(6), 1315–24.

Bruno, V., Copani, A., Besong, G., Scoto, G., & Nicoletti, F. (2000). Neuroprotective activity of chemokines against N-methyl-D-aspartate or beta-amyloid-induced toxicity in culture. *Euro J Pharmacology*, 399(2–3), 117–21.

Budka, H., Costanzi, G., Cristina, S., Lechi, A., Parravicini, C., Trabattoni, R., et al. (1987). Brain pathology induced by infection with the human immunodeficiency virus (HIV). A histological, immunocytochemical, and electron microscopical study of 100 autopsy cases. *Acta Neuropathologica*, 75(2), 185–98.

Budka, H., Wiley, C. A., Kleihues, P., Artigas, J., Asbury, A. K., Cho, E. S., et al. (1991). HIV-associated disease of the nervous system: review of nomenclature and proposal for neuropathology-based terminology. *Brain Pathology*, 1(3), 143–52.

Bukrinsky, M. I., Nottet, H. S., Schmidtmayerova, H., Dubrovsky, L., Flanagan, C. R., Mullins, M. E., et al. (1995). Regulation of nitric oxide synthase activity in human immunodeficiency virus type 1 (HIV-1)-infected monocytes: implications for HIV-associated neurological disease. *J Exper Med*, 181(2), 735–45.

Cameron, H. A., Hazel, T. G., & McKay, R. D. (1998). Regulation of neurogenesis by growth factors and neurotransmitters. *J Neurobiology*, 36(2), 287–306.

Chang, H. C., Samaniego, C. F., Nair, B. C., Buonaguro, L., & Ensoli, B. (1997). HIV-1 Tat protein exits from cells via a leaderless secretory pathway and binds to extracellular matrix-associated heparan sulfate proteoglycans through its basic region. *AIDS*, 11(12), 1421–31.

Cheng, J., Nath, A., Knudsen, B., Hochman, S., Geiger, J. D., Ma, M., et al. (1998). Neuronal excitatory properties of human immunodeficiency virus type 1 Tat protein. *Neuroscience*, 82(1), 97–106.

Cocchi, F., DeVico, A. L., Garzino-Demo, A., Arya, S. K., Gallo, R. C., & Lusso, P. (1995). Identification of RANTES, MIP-1 alpha, and MIP-1 beta as the major HIV-suppressive factors produced by CD8+ T cells. *Science*, 270(5243), 1811–5.

Cocchi, F., DeVico, A. L., Yarchoan, R., Redfield, R., Cleghorn, F., Blattner, W. A., et al. (2000). Higher macrophage inflammatory protein (MIP)-1alpha and MIP-1beta levels from CD8+ T cells are associated with asymptomatic HIV-1 infection. *Proc Natl Acad Sci USA*, 97(25), 13812–7.

Conant, K., Garzino-Demo, A., Nath, A., McArthur, J. C., Halliday, W., Power, C., et al. (1998). Induction of monocyte chemoattractant protein-1 in HIV-1 Tat-stimulated astrocytes and elevation in AIDS dementia. *Proceedings of the National Academy of Sciences of the United States of America*, 95(6), 3117–21.

Corasaniti, M. T., Melino, G., Navarra, M., Garaci, E., Finazzi-Agro, A. & Nistico, G. (1995). Death of cultured human neuroblastoma cells induced by HIV-1 gp120 is prevented by NMDA receptor antagonists and inhibitors of nitric oxide and cyclooxygenase. *Neurodegeneration*, 4(3), 315–21.

Corasaniti, M. T., Piccirilli, S., Paoletti, A., Nistico, R., Stringaro, A., Malorni, W., et al. (2001). Evidence that the HIV-1 coat protein gp120 causes neuronal apoptosis in the neocortex of rat via a mechanism involving CXCR4 chemokine receptor. *Neurosci Letters*, 312(2), 67–70.

Crowder, R. J.& Freeman, R. S. (1998). Phosphatidylinositol 3-kinase and Akt protein kinase are necessary and sufficient for the survival of nerve growth factor-dependent sympathetic neurons. *J Neurosci*, 18(8), 2933–43.

Dawson, V. L., Dawson, T. M., Uhl, G. R., & Snyder. S. H. (1993). Human immunodeficiency virus type 1 coat protein neurotoxicity mediated by nitric oxide in primary cortical cultures. *Proceedings of the National Academy of Sciences of the United States of America*, 90(8), 3256–9.

De Swapan K., Devadas, K., & Notkins, A. L. (2002). Elevated levels of tumor necrosis factor alpha (TNF-alpha) in human immunodeficiency virus type 1-transgenic mice: Prevention of death by antibody to TNF-alpha. *Journal of Virology*, 76(22), 11710–4.

Deng, W., Aimone, J. B., & Gage, F. H. New neurons and new memories: How does adult hippocampal neurogenesis affect learning and memory? *Nature Reviews Neuroscience*, 11(5), 339–50.

Dierick, H. & Bejsovec, A. (1999). Cellular mechanisms of wingless/Wnt signal transduction. *Current Topics in Developmental Biology*, 43, 153–90.

Digicaylioglu, M., Garden, G., Timberlake, S., Fletcher, L., & Lipton, S. A. (2004). Acute neuroprotective synergy of erythropoietin and insulin-like growth factor I. *Proc Nat Acad Sci USA*, 101(26), 9855–60.

Dominguez, I., & Green, J. B. (2000). Dorsal downregulation of GSK3beta by a non-Wnt-like mechanism is an early molecular consequence of cortical rotation in early Xenopus embryos. *Development*, 127(4), 861–8.

Dreyer, E. B., Kaiser, P. K., Offermann, J. T., & Lipton, S. A. (1990). HIV-1 coat protein neurotoxicity prevented by calcium channel antagonists. *Science*, 248(4953), 364–7.

Dubal, D. B., Wilson, M. E., & Wise, P. M. (1999). Estradiol: A protective and trophic factor in the brain. *J Alzheimer's Disease*, 1, 265–274.

Ensoli, F., Fiorelli, V., Muratori, D. S., De Cristofaro, M., Vincenzi, L., Topino, S., et al. (1999). Immune-derived cytokines in the nervous system: Epigenetic instructive signals or neuropathogenic mediators? *Critical Reviews in Immunology*, 19(2), 97–116.

Eron, J. J., Jr. (2002) Expert offers help for PI-related heart disease. *AIDS Alert*, 17, 26–27, 14.

Everall, I. P., Luthert, P. J., & Lantos, P. L. (1991). Neuronal loss in the frontal cortex in HIV infection. *Lancet*, 337(8750), 1119–21.

Everall, I. P., Luthert, P. J., & Lantos, P. L. (1993). Neuronal number and volume alterations in the neocortex of HIV infected individuals. *Journal of Neurology, Neurosurgery & Psychiatry* 56(5):481–6.

Everall, I. P., Trillo-Pazos, G., Bell, C., Mallory, M., Sanders, V., & Masliah, E. (2001). Amelioration of neurotoxic effects of HIV envelope protein gp120 by fibroblast growth factor: A strategy for neuroprotection. *Journal of Neuropathology & Experimental Neurology*, 60(3), 293–301.

Everall, I. P., Bell, C., Mallory, M., Langford, D., Adame, A., Rockestein, E., et al. (2002). Lithium ameliorates HIV-gp120-mediated neurotoxicity. *Molecular & Cellular Neurosciences*, 21(3), 493–501.

Fagan, A. M., Suhr, S. T., Lucidi-Phillipi, C. A., Peterson, D. A., Holtzman, D. M., & Gage, F. H. (1997). Endogenous FGF-2 is important for cholinergic sprouting in the denervated hippocampus. *Journal of Neuroscience*, 17(7), 2499–511.

Foga, I. O., Nath, A., Hasinoff, B. B., & Geiger, J. D. (1997). Antioxidants and dipyridamole inhibit HIV-1 gp120-induced free radical-based oxidative damage to human monocytoid cells. *Journal of AIDS & Human Retrovirology*, 16(4), 223–9.

Furuta, R. A., Wild, C. T., Weng, Y., & Weiss, C. D. (1998). Capture of an early fusion-active conformation of HIV-1 gp41. [Erratum appears in Nat Struct Biol 1998 Jul;5(7):612]. *Nature Structural Biology*, 5(4), 276–9.

Garden, G. A., Budd, S. L., Tsai, E., Hanson, L., Kaul, M., D'Emilia, D. M., et al. (2002). Caspase cascades in human immunodeficiency virus-associated neurodegeneration. *J Neuroscience*, 22(10), 4015–24.

Gelbard, H. A., Nottet, H. S., Swindells, S., Jett, M., Dzenko, K. A., Genis, P., et al. (1994). Platelet-activating factor: A candidate human immunodeficiency virus type 1-induced neurotoxin. *J Virology*, 68(7), 4628–35.

Giulian, D., Vaca, K., & Noonan, C. A. (1990). Secretion of neurotoxins by mononuclear phagocytes infected with HIV-1. *Science*, 250(4987), 1593–6.

Giulian, D., E. Wendt, K. Vaca, & Noonan, C. A. (1993). The envelope glycoprotein of human immunodeficiency virus type 1 stimulates release of neurotoxins from monocytes. *Proc Natl Acad Sci USA*, 90 (7), 2769–73.

Giulian, D., Yu, J., Li, X., Tom, D., Li, J., Wendt, E., et al. (1996). Study of receptor-mediated neurotoxins released by HIV-1-infected mononuclear phagocytes found in human brain. *J Neuroscience*, 16(10), 3139–53.

Glowa, J. R., Panlilio, L. V., Brenneman, D. E., Gozes, I., Fridkin, M., & Hill, J. M. (1992). Learning impairment following intracerebral administration of the HIV envelope protein gp120 or a VIP antagonist. *Brain Res*, 570(1–2), 49–53.

Gonzalez, E., Rovin, B. H., Sen, L., Cooke, G., Dhanda, R., Mummidi, S., et al. (2002). HIV-1 infection and AIDS dementia are influenced by a mutant MCP-1 allele linked to increased monocyte infiltration of tissues and MCP-1 levels. *Proc Natl Acad Sci USA*, 99(21), 13795–800.

Guo, Q., Fu, W., Xie, J., Luo, H., Sells, S. F., Geddes, J. W., et al. (1998). Par-4 is a mediator of neuronal degeneration associated with the pathogenesis of Alzheimer disease. *Nature Medicine*, 4(8), 957–62.

Guo, Q., Xie, J., & Du, H. (2000). Par-4 induces cholinergic hypoactivity by suppressing ChAT protein synthesis and inhibiting NGF-inducibility of ChAT activity. *Brain Res*, 874(2), 221–32.

Hall, A. C., Lucas, F. R., & Salinas, P. C. (2000). Axonal remodeling and synaptic differentiation in the cerebellum is regulated by WNT-7a signaling. *Cell*, 100 (5), 525–35.

Hashimoto, M., Sagara, Y., Langford, D., Everall, I. P., Mallory, M., Everson, A., et al. (2002). Fibroblast growth factor 1 regulates signaling via the glycogen synthase kinase-3beta pathway. Implications for neuroprotection. *J Biol Chemistry*, 277(36), 32985–91.

Haughey, N. J., Holden, C. P., Nath, A., & Geiger, J. D. (1999). Involvement of inositol 1,4,5-trisphosphate-regulated stores of intracellular calcium in calcium dysregulation and neuron cell death caused by HIV-1 protein tat. *J Neurochemistry*, 73(4), 1363–74.

Haughey, N. J., Nath, A., Mattson, M. P., Slevin, J. T., & Geiger, J. D. (2001). HIV-1 Tat through phosphorylation of NMDA receptors potentiates glutamate excitotoxicity. *J Neurochemistry*, 78(3), 457–67.

Haughey, N. J. & Mattson, M. P. (2002). Calcium dysregulation and neuronal apoptosis by the HIV-1 proteins Tat and gp120. *JAIDS*, 31 Suppl 2, S55–61.

Hedgepeth, C. M., Conrad, L. J., Zhang, J., Huang, H. C., Lee, V. M., & Klein, P. S. (1997). Activation of the Wnt signaling pathway: A molecular mechanism for lithium action. *Developmental Biology*, 185(1), 82–91.

Hedgepeth, C. M., Deardorff, M. A., Rankin, K., & Klein, P. S. (1999). Regulation of glycogen synthase kinase 3beta and downstream Wnt signaling by axin. *Molecular & Cellular Biology*, 19(10), 7147–57.

Hesselgesser, J. & Horuk, R. (1999). Chemokine and chemokine receptor expression in the central nervous system. *J Neurovirology*, 5(1), 13–26.

Hetman, M., Kanning, K., Cavanaugh, J. E., & Xia, Z. (1999). Neuroprotection by brain-derived neurotrophic factor is mediated by extracellular signal-regulated kinase and phosphatidylinositol 3-kinase. *J Bio Chem*, 274(32), 22569–80.

Hill, J. M., Mervis, R. F., Avidor, R., Moody, T. W., & Brenneman, D. E. (1993). HIV envelope protein-induced neuronal damage and retardation of behavioral development in rat neonates. *Brain Res*, 603(2), 222–33.

Hoek, R. M., Ruuls, S. R., Murphy, C. A., Wright, G. J., Goddard, R., Zurawski, S. M., et al. (2000). Down-regulation of the macrophage lineage through interaction with OX2 (CD200). *Science*, 290 (5497), 1768–71.

Holden, C. P., Haughey, N. J., Nath, A., & Geiger, J. D. (1999). Role of Na+/H+ exchangers, excitatory amino acid receptors and voltage-operated Ca2+ channels in human immunodeficiency virus type 1 gp120-mediated increases in intracellular Ca2+ in human neurons and astrocytes. *Neuroscience*, 91(4), 1369–78.

Howard, S. A., Brooke, S. M., & Sapolsky, R. M. (2001). Mechanisms of estrogenic protection against gp120-induced neurotoxicity. *Experimental Neurology*, 168(2), 385–91.

Hudson, L., Liu, J., Nath, A., Jones, M., Raghavan, R., Narayan, O., et al. (2000). Detection of the human immunodeficiency virus regulatory protein tat in CNS tissues. *J Neurovirology*, 6(2), 145–55.

Ilyin, S. E. & Plata-Salaman, C. R. (1997). HIV-1 envelope glycoprotein 120 regulates brain IL-1beta system and TNF-alpha mRNAs in vivo. *Brain Res Bull*, 44(1), 67–73.

Jones, M., Olafson, K., Del Bigio, M. R., Peeling, J., & Nath, A. (1998). Intraventricular injection of human immunodeficiency virus type 1 (HIV-1) tat protein causes inflammation, gliosis, apoptosis, and ventricular enlargement. *J Neuropathology & Experimental Neurology*, 57 (6), 563–70.

Jones, M. V., Bell, J. E., &Nath, A. (2000). Immunolocalization of HIV envelope gp120 in HIV encephalitis with dementia. *AIDS*, 14(17), 2709–13.

Joutel, A. & Tournier-Lasserve, E. (1998). Notch signalling pathway and human diseases. *Seminars in Cell & Developmental Biology*, 9(6), 619–25.

Kaiser, P. K., Offermann, J. T., & Lipton, S. A. (1990). Neuronal injury due to HIV-1 envelope protein is blocked by anti-gp120 antibodies but not by anti-CD4 antibodies. *Neurology*, 40(11), 1757–61.

Kang, Y.-J., Digicaylioglu, M., Russo, R., Kaul, M., Achim, C. L., Fletcher, L., et al. (2010) (in press). Erythropoietin plus insulin-like growth factor-I protect against neuronal damage in a murine model of HIV-associated neurocognitive disorders. *Annals of Neurology*.

Kaul, M. & Lipton, S. A. (2000). The NMDA receptor - Its role in neuronal apoptosis and HIV-associated dementia. Science Online: NeuroAIDS. (www. sciencemag. org/NAIDS). 3, 1–12.

Kaul, M. & Lipton, S. A. (1999). Chemokines and activated macrophages in HIV gp120-induced neuronal apoptosis. *Proc Natl Acad Sci USA*, 96(14), 8212–6.

Kaul, M., Garden, G. A., & Lipton, S. A. (2001). Pathways to neuronal injury and apoptosis in HIV-associated dementia. *Nature*, 410(6831), 988–94.

Kaul, M., Ma, Q., Medders, K. E., Desai, M. K., & Lipton, S. A. (2007). HIV-1 coreceptors CCR5 and CXCR4 both mediate neuronal cell death but CCR5 paradoxically can also contribute to protection. *Cell Death & Differentiation*, 14(2), 296–305.

Kelder, W., McArthur, J. C., Nance-Sproson, T., McClernon, D., & Griffin, D. E. (1998). Beta-chemokines MCP-1 and RANTES are selectively increased in cerebrospinal fluid of patients with human immunodeficiency virus-associated dementia. *Annals of Neurology*, 44(5), 831–5.

Kinter, A., Catanzaro, A., Monaco, J., Ruiz, M., Justement, J., Moir, S., Arthos, J., et al. (1998). CC-chemokines enhance the replication of T-tropic strains of HIV-1 in CD4(+) T cells: Role of signal transduction. *Proc Natl Acad Sci USA*, 95(20), 11880–5.

Klein, P. S. & Melton, D. A. (1996). A molecular mechanism for the effect of lithium on development. *Proc Natl Acad Sci USA*, 93(16), 8455–9.

Krathwohl, M. D. & Kaiser, J. L. (2004). HIV-1 promotes quiescence in human neural progenitor cells. [Erratum appears in J Infect Dis. 2004 Dec 15;190(12):2198]. *J Infect Dis*, 190(2), 216–26.

Kruman, I. I., Nath, A., Maragos, W. F., Chan, S. L., Jones, M., Rangnekar, V. M., et al. (1999). Evidence that Par-4 participates in the pathogenesis of HIV encephalitis. *Amer J Path*, 155(1), 39–46.

Kruman, I. I., Nath, A., & Mattson, M. P. (1998). HIV-1 protein Tat induces apoptosis of hippocampal neurons by a mechanism involving caspase activation, calcium overload, and oxidative stress. *Experimental Neurology*, 154(2), 276–88.

Kure, K., Lyman, W. D., Weidenheim, K. M., & Dickson, D. W. (1990a). Cellular localization of an HIV-1 antigen in subacute AIDS encephalitis

using an improved double-labeling immunohistochemical method. *Amer J Path*, 136(5), 1085–92.

Kure, K., Weidenheim, K. M., Lyman, W. D., & Dickson, D. W. (1990b). Morphology and distribution of HIV-1 gp41-positive microglia in subacute AIDS encephalitis. Pattern of involvement resembling a multisystem degeneration. *Acta Neuropathologica*, 80 (4), 393–400.

Kure, K., Llena, J. F., Lyman, W. D., Soeiro, R., Weidenheim, K. M., Hirano, A., et al. (1991). Human immunodeficiency virus-1 infection of the nervous system: An autopsy study of 268 adult, pediatric, and fetal brains. *Human Pathology*, 22(7), 700–10.

Kutsch, O., Oh, J., Nath, A., & Benveniste, E. N. (2000). Induction of the chemokines interleukin-8 and IP-10 by human immunodeficiency virus type 1 tat in astrocytes. *J Virology*, 74(19), 9214–21.

Lavi, E., Strizki, J. M., Ulrich, A. M., Zhang, W., Fu, L., Wang, Q., et al. (1997). CXCR-4 (Fusin), a co-receptor for the type 1 human immunodeficiency virus (HIV-1), is expressed in the human brain in a variety of cell types, including microglia and neurons. *Amer J Path*, 151(4), 1035–42.

Letendre, S. L., Lanier, E. R., & McCutchan, J. A. (1999). Cerebrospinal fluid beta chemokine concentrations in neurocognitively impaired individuals infected with human immunodeficiency virus type 1. *J Infect Dis*, 180(2), 310–9.

Lipton, S. A., Kaiser, P. K., Sucher, N. J., Dreyer, E. B., & Offerman, J. T. (1990). AIDS virus coat protein sensitizes neurons to NMDA receptor-mediated toxicity. *Soc Neurosci Abstr*, 16, 28.

Lipton, S. A., Sucher, N. J., Kaiser, P. K., & Dreyer, E. B. (1991). Synergistic effects of HIV coat protein and NMDA receptor-mediated neurotoxicity. *Neuron*, 7(1), 111–8.

Lipton, S. A. (1992a). Models of neuronal injury in AIDS: Another role for the NMDA receptor? *Trends Neurosci*, 15(3), 75–9.

Lipton, S. A. (1992b). Requirement for macrophages in neuronal injury induced by HIV envelope protein gp120. *Neuroreport*, 3(10), 913–5.

Lipton, S. A. (1992c). Memantine prevents HIV coat protein-induced neuronal injury in vitro. *Neurology*, 42(7), 1403–5.

Lipton, S. A. (1992d). 7-Chlorokynurenate ameliorates neuronal injury mediated by HIV envelope protein gp120 in rodent retinal cultures. *Eur J Neurosci*, 4, 1411–15.

Lipton, S. A. (1993). Prospects for clinically tolerated NMDA antagonists: Open-channel blockers and alternative redox states of nitric oxide. *Trends in Neurosciences*, 16(12), 527–32.

Lipton, S. A. (1994a). HIV displays its coat of arms. [Erratum appears in Nature 1994 Jan 27;367(6461):320]. *Nature*, 367(6459), 113–4.

Lipton, S. A. (1994b). Ca2+, N-methyl-D-aspartate receptors, and AIDS-related neuronal injury. *Internatl Rev Neurobiology*, 36, 1–27.

Lipton, S. A. & Rosenberg, P. A. 1994. Excitatory amino acids as a final common pathway for neurologic disorders. *New Engl J Med*, 330(9), 613–22.

Lipton, S. A., Brenneman, D. E., Silverstein, F. S., Masliah, E., & Mucke, L. (1995). gp120 and neurotoxicity in vivo. *Trends in Pharmacological Sciences*, 16(4), 122.

Lipton, S. A. & Gendelman, H. E. (1995). Seminars in medicine of the Beth Israel Hospital, Boston. Dementia associated with the acquired immunodeficiency syndrome. *New Engl J Med*, 332(14), 934–40.

Lipton, S. A. (1999). *NO in AIDS-associated neurologic disease*. In F. Fang, (Ed.). *Nitric oxide and infection*. New York: Plenum.

Lucas, F. R. & Salinas, P. C. (1997). WNT-7a induces axonal remodeling and increases synapsin I levels in cerebellar neurons. *Developmental Biology*, 192(1), 31–44.

Lucas, F. R., Goold, R. G., Gordon-Weeks, P. R., &Salinas, P. C. (1998). Inhibition of GSK-3beta leading to the loss of phosphorylated MAP-1B is an early event in axonal remodelling induced by WNT-7a or lithium. *J Cell Science*, 111(Pt 10), 1351–61.

Maggirwar, S. B., Tong, N., Ramirez, S., Gelbard, H. A., & Dewhurst, S. (1999). HIV-1 Tat-mediated activation of glycogen synthase kinase-3-beta contributes to Tat-mediated neurotoxicity. *J Neurochemistry*, 73 (2), 578–86.

Magnuson, D. S., Knudsen, B. E., Geiger, J. D., Brownstone, R. M., & Nath, A. (1995). Human immunodeficiency virus type 1 tat activates non-N-methyl-D-aspartate excitatory amino acid receptors and causes neurotoxicity. *Annals of Neurology*, 37(3), 373–80.

Masliah, E., Ge, N., Achim, C. L., Hansen, L. A., & Wiley, C. A. (1992a). Selective neuronal vulnerability in HIV encephalitis. *Journal of Neuropathology & Experimental Neurology*, 51(6), 585–93.

Masliah, E., Achim, C. L., Ge, N., DeTeresa, R., Terry, R. D., & Wiley, C. A. (1992b). Spectrum of human immunodeficiency virus-associated neocortical damage. *Annals of Neurology*, 32(3), 321–9.

Mayne, M., Holden, C. P., Nath, A., & Geiger, J. D. (2000). Release of calcium from inositol 1,4,5-trisphosphate receptor-regulated stores by HIV-1 Tat regulates TNF-alpha production in human macrophages. *J Immunology*, 164(12), 6538–42.

McArthur, J. C., Steiner, J., Sacktor, N. & Nath, A. (2010). Human immunodeficiency virus-associated neurocognitive disorders mind the gap. *Annals of Neurology*, 67, 699–714.

McManus, C. M., Weidenheim, K., Woodman, S. E., Nunez, J., Hesselgesser, J., Nath, A., et al. (2000). Chemokine and chemokine-receptor expression in human glial elements: Induction by the HIV protein, Tat, and chemokine autoregulation. *American Journal of Pathology*, 156(4), 1441–53.

Medina, I., Ghose, S., & Ben-Ari, Y. (1999). Mobilization of intracellular calcium stores participates in the rise of [Ca2+]i and the toxic actions of the HIV coat protein GP120. *European Journal of Neuroscience*, 11(4), 1167–78.

Mermelstein, P. G., Becker, J. B., & Surmeier, D. J. (1996). Estradiol reduces calcium currents in rat neostriatal neurons via a membrane receptor. *J Neuroscience*, 16(2), 595–604.

Merrill, J. E., Koyanagi, Y., Zack, J., Thomas, L., Martin, F., & Chen, I. S. (1992). Induction of interleukin-1 and tumor necrosis factor alpha in brain cultures by human immunodeficiency virus type 1. *J Virology*, 66(4), 2217–25.

Meucci, O., Fatatis, A., Simen, A. A., Bushell, T. J., Gray, P. W., & Miller, R. J. (1998). Chemokines regulate hippocampal neuronal signaling and gp120 neurotoxicity. *Proc Natl Acad Sci USA*, 95(24), 14500–5.

Moore, G. J., Bebchuk, ·J. M., Wilds, I. B., Chen, G., & Manji, H. K. (2000a). Lithium-induced increase in human brain grey matter. [Erratum appears in Lancet 2000 Dec 16;356(9247):2104 Note: Menji HK [corrected to Manji HK]. *Lancet*, 356(9237), 1241–2.

Moore, G. J., Bebchuk, J. M., Hasanat, K., Chen, G., Seraji-Bozorgzad, N., Wilds, I. B., et al. (2000b). Lithium increases N-acetyl-aspartate in the human brain: in vivo evidence in support of bcl-2's neurotrophic effects? *Biological Psychiatry*, 48(1), 1–8.

Mudher, A., Chapman, S., Richardson, J., Asuni, A., Gibb, G., Pollard, C., et al. (2001). Dishevelled regulates the metabolism of amyloid precursor protein via protein kinase C/mitogen-activated protein kinase and c-Jun terminal kinase. *J Neuroscience*, 21(14), 4987–95.

Nath, A. & Geiger, J. (1998). Neurobiological aspects of human immunodeficiency virus infection: Neurotoxic mechanisms. *Progress in Neurobiology*, 54(1), 19–33.

Nath, A., Conant, K., Chen, P., Scott, C., & Major, E. O. (1999). Transient exposure to HIV-1 Tat protein results in cytokine production in macrophages and astrocytes. A hit and run phenomenon. *J Biological Chemistry*, 274(24), 17098–102.

Nath, A., Haughey, N. J., Jones, M., Anderson, C., Bell, J. E., & Geiger, J. D. (2000). Synergistic neurotoxicity by human immunodeficiency virus proteins Tat and gp120: Protection by memantine. *Annals of Neurology*, 47(2), 186–94.

New, D. R., Ma, M., Epstein, L. G., Nath, A., & Gelbard, H. A. (1997). Human immunodeficiency virus type 1 Tat protein induces death by apoptosis in primary human neuron cultures. *J Neurovirology*, 3(2), 168–73.

Nguyen, T. B., Lucero, G. R., Chana, G., Hult, B. J., Tatro, E. T., Masliah, E., et al. (2009) Glycogen synthase kinase-3beta (GSK-3beta) inhibitors AR-A014418 and B6B3O prevent human immunodeficiency virus-mediated neurotoxicity in primary human neurons. *J Neurovirol*, 15, 434–438.

O'Brien, W. A., Sumner-Smith, M., Mao, S. H., Sadeghi, S., Zhao, J. Q., & Chen I. S. (1996). Anti-human immunodeficiency virus type 1 activity of an oligocationic compound mediated via gp120 V3 interactions. *J Virology*, 70(5), 2825–31.

Oh, J. W., Schwiebert, L. M., & Benveniste, E. N. (1999). Cytokine regulation of CC and CXC chemokine expression by human astrocytes. *J Neurovirology*, 5(1), 82–94.

Okamoto, S., Kang, Y-J., Brechtel, C. W., Siviglia, E., Russo, R., Clemente, A., et al. (2007). HIV/gp120 decreases adult neural progenitor cell proliferation via checkpoint kinase-mediated cell-cycle withdrawal and G1 arrest. *Cell Stem Cell*, 1(2), 230–6.

Olson, W. (2000). Comparative and combinatorial analysis of the HIV-1 entry inhibitors 542, T-20 and PRO 140. Paper read at XIII International AIDS Conference, at Nagashima, Korea.

Pap, M., & Cooper, G. M. (1998). Role of glycogen synthase kinase-3 in the phosphatidylinositol 3-kinase/Akt cell survival pathway. *Journal of Biological Chemistry*, 273(32), 19929–32.

Pap, M. & Cooper, G. M. (2002). Role of translation initiation factor 2B in control of cell survival by the phosphatidylinositol 3-kinase/Akt/ glycogen synthase kinase 3beta signaling pathway. *Molecular & Cellular Biology*, 22(2), 578–86.

Pattarini, R., Pittaluga, A., & Raiteri, M. (1998). The human immunodeficiency virus-1 envelope protein gp120 binds through its V3 sequence to the glycine site of N-methyl-D-aspartate receptors mediating noradrenaline release in the hippocampus. *Neuroscience*, 87(1), 147–57.

Perez, A., Probert, A. W., Wang, K. K., & Sharmeen, L. (2001). Evaluation of HIV-1 Tat-induced neurotoxicity in rat cortical cell culture. *Journal of Neurovirology*, 7(1), 1–10.

Ramirez, S. H., Sanchez, J. F., Dimitri, C. A., Gelbard, H. A., Dewhurst, S., & Maggirwar, S. B. (2001). Neurotrophins prevent HIV Tat-induced neuronal apoptosis via a nuclear factor-kappaB (NF-kappaB)-dependent mechanism. *J Neurochemistry*, 78(4), 874–89.

Reynes, J., Rouzier, R., & Kanouni, T. (2002). Safety and antiviral effects of a CCR5 receptor antagonist in HIV-1. *9th Conference on Retroviruses and Opportunistic Infections*. Abstract 1.

Richter, S., Hartmann, B., Reichert, H. (1998). The wingless gene is required for embryonic brain development in Drosophila. *Development Genes & Evolution*, 208(1), 37–45.

Roesler, R., Quevedo, J., Walz, R., & Bianchin, M. (1998). A randomized, double-blind, placebo-controlled trial of deprenyl and thiotic acid in HIV-associated cognitive impairment. *Neurology*, 50(3), 645–51.

Rottman, J. B., Ganley, K. P., Williams, K., Wu, L., Mackay, C. R., & Ringler, D. J. (1997). Cellular localization of the chemokine receptor CCR5. Correlation to cellular targets of HIV-1 infection. *Amer J Path*, 151(5), 1341–51.

Sacktor, N., Schifitto, G., McDermott, M. P., Marder, K., McArthur, J. C., & Kieburtz, K. (2000). Transdermal selegiline in HIV-associated cognitive impairment: Pilot, placebo-controlled study. *Neurology*, 54(1), 233–5.

Salinas, P. C., Fletcher, C., Copeland, N. G., Jenkins, N. A., & Nusse, R. (1994). Maintenance of Wnt-3 expression in Purkinje cells of the mouse cerebellum depends on interactions with granule cells. *Development*, 120(5), 1277–86.

Salinas, P. C. (1999). Wnt factors in axonal remodelling and synaptogenesis. *Biochemical Society Symposia*, 65, 101–9.

Sanders, V. J., Pittman, C. A., White, M. G., Wang, G., Wiley, C. A., & Achim, C. L. (1998). Chemokines and receptors in HIV encephalitis. *AIDS*, 12(9), 1021–6.

Schifitto, G., Navia, B. A., Yiannoutsos, C. T., Marra, C. M., Chang, L., Ernst, T., et al. (2007). Memantine and HIV-associated cognitive impairment: A neuropsychological and proton magnetic resonance spectroscopy study. *AIDS*, 21(14), 1877–86.

Sindou, P., Couratier, P., Esclaire, F., Yardin, C., Bousseau, A., & Hugon, J. (1994). Prevention of HIV coat protein (gp120) toxicity in cortical cell cultures by riluzole. *J Neurological Sciences*, 126(2), 133–7.

Singer, C. A., Rogers, K. L., & Dorsa, D. M. (1998). Modulation of Bcl-2 expression: A potential component of estrogen protection in NT2 neurons. *Neuroreport*, 9(11), 2565–8.

Sohrabji, F., Miranda, R. C., & Toran-Allerand, C. D. (1995). Identification of a putative estrogen response element in the gene encoding brain-derived neurotrophic factor. *Proc Natl Acad Sci USA*, 92(24), 11110–4.

Soontornniyomkij, V., Wang, G., Pittman, C. A., Wiley, C. A., & Achim, C. L. (1998). Expression of brain-derived neurotrophic factor protein in activated microglia of human immunodeficiency virus type 1 encephalitis. *Neuropathology & Applied Neurobiology*, 24(6), 453–60.

Strizki, J. M., Xu, S., Wagner, N. E., Wojcik, L., Liu, J., Hou, Y., et al. (2001). SCH-C (SCH 351125), an orally bioavailable, small molecule antagonist of the chemokine receptor CCR5, is a potent inhibitor of HIV-1 infection in vitro and in vivo. *Proc Natl Acad Sci USA*, 98(22), 12718–23.

Tamamura, H., Imai, M., Ishihara, T., Masuda, M., Funakoshi, H., Oyake, H., et al. (1998). Pharmacophore identification of a chemokine receptor (CXCR4) antagonist, T22 ([Tyr(5,12),Lys7]-polyphemusin II), which specifically blocks T cell-line-tropic HIV-1 infection. *Bioorganic & Medicinal Chemistry*, 6(7), 1033–41.

Tardieu, M., Hery, C., Peudenier, S., Boespflug, O., & Montagnier, L. (1992). Human immunodeficiency virus type 1-infected monocytic cells can destroy human neural cells after cell-to-cell adhesion. *Annals of Neurology*, 32(1), 11–7.

Thomas, G. M., Frame, S., Goedert, M., Nathke, I., Polakis, P., & Cohen, P. (1999). A GSK3-binding peptide from FRAT1 selectively inhibits the GSK3-catalysed phosphorylation of axin and beta-catenin. *FEBS Letters*, 458(2), 247–51.

Toggas, S. M., Masliah, E., Rockenstein, E. M., Rall, G. F., Abraham, C. R., & Mucke, L. (1994). Central nervous system damage produced by expression of the HIV-1 coat protein gp120 in transgenic mice. *Nature*, 367(6459), 188–93.

Trkola, A., Ketas, T. J., Nagashima, K. A., Zhao, L., Cilliers, T., Morris, L., et al. (2001). Potent, broad-spectrum inhibition of human immunodeficiency virus type 1 by the CCR5 monoclonal antibody PRO 140. *J Virology*, 75(2), 579–88.

Turchan, J., Pocernich, C. B., Gairola, C., Chauhan, A., Schifitto, G., Butterfield, D. A., et al. (2003). Oxidative stress in HIV demented patients and protection ex vivo with novel antioxidants. *Neurology*, 60 (2), 307–14.

Turrin, N. P. & Plata-Salaman, C. R. (2000). Cytokine-cytokine interactions and the brain. *Brain Research Bulletin*, 51(1), 3–9.

Uht, R. M., Anderson, C. M., Webb, P., & Kushner, P. J. (1997). Transcriptional activities of estrogen and glucocorticoid receptors are functionally integrated at the AP-1 response element. *Endocrinology*, 138 (7), 2900–8.

van der Meer, P., Ulrich, A. M., Gonzalez-Scarano, F., & Lavi. E. (2000). Immunohistochemical analysis of CCR2, CCR3, CCR5, and CXCR4 in the human brain: Potential mechanisms for HIV dementia. *Experimental & Molecular Pathology*, 69(3), 192–201.

Viviani, B., Corsini, E., Binaglia, M., Galli, C. L., & Marinovich, M. (2001). Reactive oxygen species generated by glia are responsible for neuron death induced by human immunodeficiency virus-glycoprotein 120 in vitro. *Neuroscience*, 107(1), 51–8.

Weis, S., Haug, H., & Budka, H. (1993). Neuronal damage in the cerebral cortex of AIDS brains: A morphometric study. *Acta Neuropathologica*, 85(2), 185–9.

Wiley, C. A., Masliah, E., Morey, M., Lemere, C., DeTeresa, R., Grafe, M., et al. (1991). Neocortical damage during HIV infection. *Annals of Neurology*, 29(6), 651–7.

Wiley, C. A., Schrier, R. D., Nelson, J. A., Lampert, P. W., & Oldstone, M. B. (1986). Cellular localization of human immunodeficiency virus infection within the brains of acquired immune deficiency syndrome patients. *Proc Natl Acad Sci USA*, 83(18), 7089–93.

Wodarz, A. & Nusse, R. (1998). Mechanisms of Wnt signaling in development. *Annual Review of Cell & Developmental Biology*, 14, 59–88.

Xie, J., Chang, X., Zhang, X., & Guo, Q. (2001). Aberrant induction of Par-4 is involved in apoptosis of hippocampal neurons in presenilin-1 M146V mutant knock-in mice. *Brain Research*, 915(1), 1–10.

Yao, R. & Cooper, G. M. (1995). Requirement for phosphatidylinositol-3 kinase in the prevention of apoptosis by nerve growth factor. *Science*, 267(5206), 2003–6.

Yeh, M. W., Kaul, M., Zheng, J., Nottet, H. S., Thylin, M., Gendelman, H. E., et al. (2000). Cytokine-stimulated, but not HIV-infected, human monocyte-derived macrophages produce neurotoxic levels of l-cysteine. *J Immunology*, 164(8), 4265–70.

Yeung, M. C., Pulliam, L., & Lau, A. S. (1995). The HIV envelope protein gp120 is toxic to human brain-cell cultures through the induction of interleukin-6 and tumor necrosis factor-alpha. *AIDS*, 9(2), 137–43.

Zagury, D., Lachgar, A., Chams, V., Fall, L. S., Bernard, J., Zagury, J. F., et al. (1998). C-C chemokines, pivotal in protection against HIV type 1 infection. *Proc Natl Acad Sci USA*, 95(7), 3857–61.

HIV-1 AND CANNABINOIDS

Guy A. Cabral and Erinn S. Raborn

Marijuana, or Cannabis sativa, is a complex substance that contains a class of terpenoid-like compounds known as cannabinoids. These compounds can affect immune function directly by activating cannabinoid receptors on immune cells, and indirectly thorough their effect on neurons, which in turn alter the neuroendocrine axes. Tetrahydrocannabinol, or THC, the major psychoactive component of marijuana, acts primarily to suppress immune function. Since many individuals with HIV use multiple drugs, often including marijuana, the possibility of additional immunosuppression from cannabinoids, perhaps acting synergistically with immunosuppressive effects of other drugs, is particularly relevant. There are at this time no data that directly link marijuana use in humans either to greater susceptibility to HIV infection or to increased vulnerability to opportunistic infection or disease progression in HIV-infected individuals. Nonetheless, various in vivo and in vitro studies show a link between cannabinoids, immune suppression, and greater susceptibility to infection with bacteria, protozoa, and viruses. This chapter reviews many aspects of the complex interactions among cannabis, immune suppression, and HIV infection.

INTRODUCTION

Cannabinoids have been shown to alter the functional activities of a variety of cells in the immune system (reviewed in Cabral & Staab, 2005). These compounds can act indirectly on immune cells by targeting neurons in the central nervous system (CNS) and altering the activity of neuroendocrine axes or neurotransmission pathways (Tasker, 2004; Szabo & Schlicker, 2005; Cota, 2008). They also can act directly on such cells by activating cannabinoid receptors. This potential to modulate the functional activities of immune cells is especially poignant in view of the worldwide epidemic of infection with the human immunodeficiency virus (HIV), a virus that targets the immune system and renders individuals highly susceptible to opportunistic infections (Haverkos & Curran, 1982; Mansell, 1984; Friedman, Newton, & Klein, 2003). In addition, since many individuals with HIV infection use multiple drugs, there is a potential risk for synergistic or additive effects on immune function. Although there have been clinical reports of association between HIV infection and use of cannabinoids, data that directly link their use by humans as causative of greater susceptibility to infection or disease progression remain elusive. However, studies using various in vitro

and in vivo model systems have demonstrated a direct link between cannabinoid-induced immune dysfunction and greater susceptibility to infection with bacteria, protozoa, and viruses (Friedman et al., 2003; reviewed in Cabral & Staab, 2005). These collective observations suggest that greater susceptibility to infection in humans, including that to HIV, is not limited solely to illicit substances such as marijuana serving as vehicles for pathogens, but that these substances directly or indirectly affect the immune response.

CANNABINOIDS AND CANNABINOID RECEPTORS

Marijuana, or *Cannabis sativa*, is a highly complex substance that contains a class of terpenoid-like compounds known as cannabinoids. The term "phytocannabinoid" has been applied to these cannabinoids from the marijuana plant. These compounds, and those that are synthesized in the laboratory, are collectively referred to as "exogenous" cannabinoids. Delta-9-tetrahydrocannabinol (THC), cannabinol (CBN), and cannabidiol (CBD) have been the most prevalent and studied cannabinoids derived from *Cannabis sativa* (Fig. 4.5.1). THC is the major psychoactive component of marijuana. It also exerts immunomodulatory effects, primarily of an immunosuppressive nature. The purification and structural characterization of THC (Gaoni & Mechoulam, 1971) led to the chemical synthesis of various cannabinoid analogs. These synthetic compounds have been used extensively in structure-activity studies to characterize cannabinoid-mediated effects in vitro and in vivo and to define the mechanisms by which these effects are elicited. Some of the synthetic cannabinoids that have been studied extensively include CP55,940, HU-210, WIN55,212, JWH-015, ACEA, SR141716A, and SR144528 (Fig. 4.5.1). Studies in which naturally occurring cannabinoids such as THC, as well as synthetic cannabinoid compounds exemplified by CP55,940, were used have served as the basis for the identification of specific binding sites in mammalian brain and peripheral non-neuronal tissues which are now recognized as representing cannabinoid receptors (Matsuda, Lolait, Brownstein, Young, & Bonner, 1990; Munro, Thomas, & Abu-Shaar, 1993).

The initial evidence for the existence of a cannabinoid receptor was obtained through pharmacological assessment that indicated that THC treatment of neuroblastoma cells,

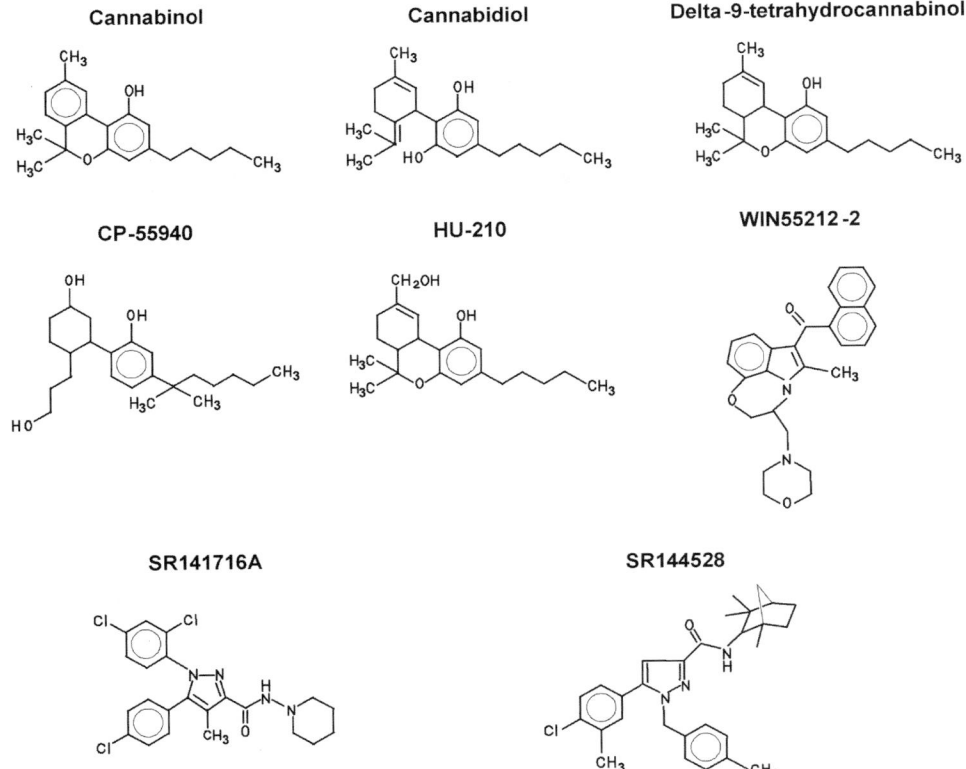

Figure 4.5.1 *Representative Exogenous and Synthetic Cannabinoids.* Cannabinol (CBN): 6,6,9-trimethyl-3-pentyl-benzo[c]chromen-1-ol; Cannabidiol (CBD): 2-[(1*R*,6*R*)-6-isopropenyl-3-methylcyclohex-2-en-1-yl]-5-pentylbenzene-1,3-diol; Delta-9-tetrahydrocannabinol (THC): (−)-(6a*R*,10a*R*)-6,6,9-trimethyl-3-pentyl-6a,7,8,10a-tetrahydro-6*H*-benzo[*c*]chromen-1-ol; CP55,940: 2-[(1R,2R,5R)-5-hydroxy-2-(3- hydroxypropyl)cyclo 2-en-1-yl]-5-pentylbenzene-1,3-diol; HU-210: (6a*R*,10a*R*)- 9-(Hydroxymethyl)- 6,6-dimethyl- 3-(2-methyloctan-2-yl)- 6a,7,10,10a-tetrahydrobenzo [c]chromen-1-ol; WIN 55,212–2: (R)-(+)-[2,3-Dihydro-5-methyl-3-(4-morpholinylmethyl)pyrrolo [1,2,3-de]-1,4-benzoxazin-6-yl]-1-napthalenylmethanone; SR141716A: 5-(4-chlorophenyl)-1-(2,4-dichlorophenyl)-4-methyl-N-piperidin-1-ylpyrazole-3-carboxamide; SR144528: (1S-endo)-5-(4-Chloro-3-methylphenyl)-1-((4-methylphenyl)methyl)-N-(1,3,3-trimethylbicyclo(2.2.1)hept-2-yl)-1H-pyrazole-3-carboxamide. THC is a partial agonist for CB₁ and CB₂. CP 55,940, HU-210 and WIN 55,212–2 are full agonists for CB₁ and CB₂. SR141716A is an antagonist for CB₁. SR144528 is an antagonist for CB₂. The International Union of Pure and Applied Chemistry (IUPAC) nomenclature is designated for each compound.

and that of other cannabinoids, resulted in inhibition of plasma membrane activity of adenylate cyclase, the enzyme that catalyzes the conversion of ATP to 3′, 5′-cyclic AMP (cAMP) and pyrophosphate (Howlett & Fleming, 1984; Howlett, 1985). This putative receptor subsequently was shown to require a guanine nucleotide binding complex, G_i, for activation since the inhibitory effect on adenylate cyclase was sensitive to treatment with pertussis toxin (PTX) (Howlett, Qualy, & Khachatrian, 1986), a protein-based AB5-type exotoxin produced by the bacterium *Bordetella pertussis* that catalyzes adenosine diphosphate (ADP) ribosylation. Follow-up studies using radiolabeled CP55,940 allowed for the identification of specific ligand binding sites in rat brains (Devane, Dysarz, Johnson, Melvin, & Howlett, 1988). This "neuronal" receptor, now referred to as CB₁, was subsequently cloned from a rat brain complementary DNA (cDNA) library (Matsuda et al., 1990). The cDNA encoded a 473 amino acid long, 7-transmembrane G protein-coupled receptor, which exhibited physiological properties consistent with those described previously (Howlett, 1985; Howlett et al., 1986), such as negative coupling to adenylate cyclase.

Radioligand binding and in situ mRNA hybridization studies demonstrated that the receptor was distributed throughout the brain and was localized predominantly in the cerebellum, cerebral cortex, hippocampus, basal ganglia, and spinal cord (Matsuda et al., 1990; Herkenham et al., 1990; Westlake, Howlett, Bonner, Matsuda, & Herkenham, 1994). The cloning of rat CB₁ was followed by that of human CB₁ (Fig. 4.5.2A), yielding a sequence that encoded a protein of 472 amino acids in length that was localized primarily to the brain but also was found in testis (Gerard, Mollereau, Vassart, & Parmentier, 1991). The psychotropic effects attributed to select cannabinoids are due to activation of the CB₁ (Agarwal et al., 2007; Kunos, Osei-Hyiaman, Batkai, Sharkey, & Makriyannis, 2008).

A second or "peripheral" cannabinoid receptor, the CB₂, was cloned from a human promyelocytic cell line (HL-60) cDNA library (Munro et al., 1993). The gene for this receptor encoded for a 360 amino acid long, 7-transmembrane G-protein coupled receptor. As in the case of CB₁, this receptor had an extracellular, glycosylated N-terminus and an intracellular C-terminus (Fig. 4.5.2B). A distinctive feature of the

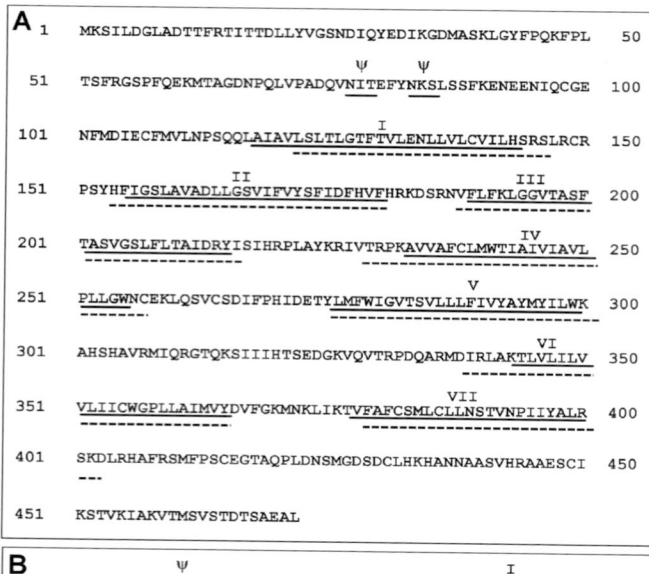

```
A 1    MKSILDGLADTTFRTITTDLLYVGSNDIQYEDIKGDMASKLGYFPQKFPL    50
                      ψ           ψ
   51   TSFRGSPFQEKMTAGDNPQLVPADQVNITEFYNKSLSSFKENEENIQCGE    100
                                        I
  101   NFMDIECFMVLNPSQQLAIAVLSLTLGTFTVLENLLVLCVILHSRSLRCR    150
                      II
  151   PSYHFIGSLAVADLLGSVIFVYSFIDFHVFHRKDSRNVLFKLGGVTASF    200
                 -----------------------
  201   TASVGSLFLTAIDRYISIHRPLAYKRIVTRPKAVVAFCLMWTIAIVIAVL    250
        -----------------                    ----------
                                         V
  251   PLLGWNCEKLQSVCSDIFPHIDETYLMFWIGVTSVLLLFIVYAYMYILWK    300
        --------                 ----------------------
  301   AHSHAVRMIQRGTQKSIIIHTSEDGKVQVTRPDQARMDIRLAKTLVLILV    350
                                                -----------
                                  VII
  351   VLIICWGPLLAIMVYDVFGKMNKLIKTVFAFCSMLCLLNSTVNPIIYALR    400
        ------------------      ----------------------
  401   SKDLRHAFRSMFPSCEGTAQPLDNSMGDSDCLHKHANNAASVHRAAESCI    450
        ---
  451   KSTVKIAKVTMSVSTDTSAEAL
```

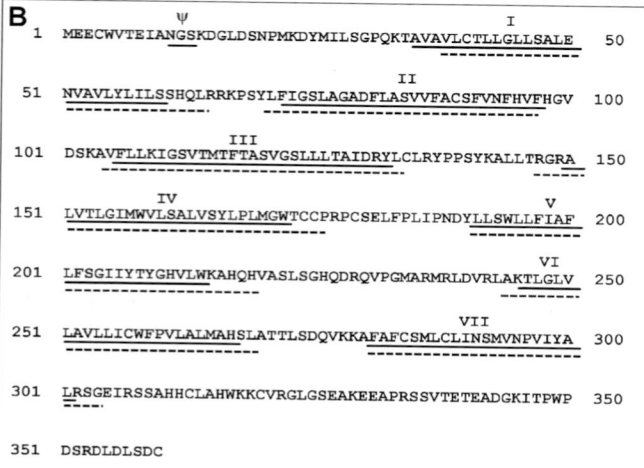

```
B 1    MEECWVTEIANGSKDGLDSNPMKDYMILSGPQKTAVAVLCTLLGLLSALE    50
                ψ                               I
                                               ----------
   51   NVAVLYLILSSHQLRRKPSYLFIGSLAGADFLASVVFACSFVNFHVFHGV    100
        ----------             ----------------------
                      III
  101   DSKAVFLLKIGSVTMTFTASVGSLLLTAIDRYLCLRYPPSYKALLTRGRA    150
               --------------------------
                  IV                               V
  151   LVTLGIMWVLSALVSYLPLMGWTCCPRPCSELFPLIPNDYLLSWLLFIAF    200
        -----------------                    -------------
  201   LFSGIIYTYGHVLWKAHQHVASLSGHQDRQVPGMARMRLDVRLAKTLGLV    250
        -------------------                       --------
                                  VII
  251   LAVLLICWFPVLALMAHSLATTLSDQVKKAFAFCSMLCLINSMVNPVIYA    300
        --------------         ----------------------
  301   LRSGEIRSSAHHCLAHWKKCVRGLGSEAKEEAPRSSVTETEADGKITPWP    350
        ----
  351   DSRDLDLSDC
```

Figure 4.5.2 *Human Cannabinoid Receptors.* (A) Amino acid sequence of the full-length human CB₁ receptor (CB₁). (B) Amino acid sequence of the full-length human CB₂ receptor. The putative asparagine-linked glycosylation sites are shown as Ψ. The solid underlines indicate the position of the seven transmembrane domains (I–VII) reported in the International Union of Pharmacology. XXVII. Classification of Cannabinoid Receptors (Howlett et al., 2002). The dashed lines indicate the position of the transmembrane regions reported in Cabral and Griffin-Thomas (2009).

Gomez del Pulgar, Guzman, & de Ceballos, 2005; Cabral & Marciano-Cabral, 2005; Fernandez-Ruiz et al., 2007). In addition, there is evidence for the existence of cannabinoid receptors other than CB_1 and CB_2, based primarily on in vivo studies in which CB_1 knockout or CB_1/CB_2 double-knockout mice have been used to investigate the pharmacology and pharmacokinetics of cannabinoids. However, a novel non-CB_1, non-CB_2 cannabinoid receptor that meets rigid pharmacological and functional criteria has yet to be cloned and characterized at the molecular level (Jarai et al., 1999; Di Marzo et al., 2000a; Breivogel, Griffin, Di Marzo, & Martin, 2001; Wiley & Martin, 2002).

The recognition that select exogenous and synthetic cannabinoids interacted with specific receptors in the CNS and immune systems led to the identification of endogenous cannabinoids or "endocannabinoids" (reviewed in Di Marzo, Bifulco, & De Petrocellis, 2004; Mechoulam, 2002). These lipid molecules are now recognized as constituents of a so-called endocannabinoid system in mammals that also includes cannabinoid receptors and the mediators responsible for endocannabinoid synthesis, metabolism and catabolism. Endocannabinoids (Fig. 4.5.3) are derivatives of integral components of the phospholipid bilayers of cellular membranes. Since these compounds are highly hydrophobic, it is postulated that they cannot translocate unassisted in aqueous cellular environments and, upon release through the mediation of transporters, activate cannabinoid receptors locally or on nearby cells. The first endocannabinoid to be identified was anandamide (arachidonoylethanolamide; AEA), which was isolated from porcine brain (Devane et al., 1992). A second endocannabinoid, 2-arachidonoylglycerol (2-AG), subsequently was isolated from canine gut (Mechoulam et al., 1995). It has been reported that 2-AG is the more bioactive and abundant endocannabinoid in the CNS, with concentrations reported to be considerably higher than those of anandamide (Stella, Schweitzer, & Piomelli, 1997; Di Marzo,

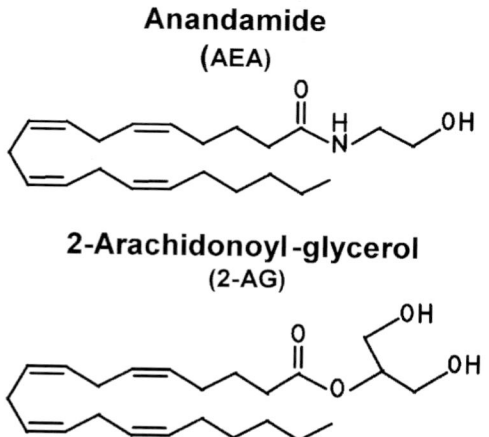

Figure 4.5.3 *Representative Endogenous Endocannabinoids.* Anandamide (*N*-arachidonoylethanolamine or AEA): (5*Z*,8*Z*,11*Z*,14*Z*)-*N*-(2-hydroxyethyl)icosa-5,8,11,14-tetraenamide; 2-Arachidonoylglycerol (2-AG): 1,3-Dihydroxy-2-propanyl (5*Z*,8*Z*,11*Z*,14*Z*)-5,8,11,14-eicosatetraenoate.

CB_2, however, was that its distribution was limited predominantly to cells and tissues of the immune system. Furthermore, the level of this receptor was found to vary among different immune cell populations, with B lymphocytes expressing the highest levels followed by macrophages, monocytes, natural killer (NK) cells, and polymorphonuclear cells, in that order (Galiegue et al., 1995; Schatz, Lee, Condie, Pulaski, & Kaminski, 1997). While initial studies suggested that the distribution of CB_2 was confined to peripheral non-neuronal sites, it is now recognized that this receptor can be expressed in vitro by macrophage-like cells purified from brain tissue as well as in the CNS during various states of inflammation (Carlisle, Marciano-Cabral, Staab, Ludwick, & Cabral, 2002; Carrier et al., 2004; Nunez et al., 2004; Ramirez, Blazquez,

Hill, Bisogno, Crossman, & Brotchie, 2000b). In addition, 2-AG appears to be the more robust endocannabinoid in terms of immunomodulatory activity (Lee, Yang, & Kaminski, 1995; Gonsiorek et al., 2000).

CANNABINOID EFFECTS ON IMMUNITY

There is a large body of data that indicates that cannabinoids alter immune responses in vitro and in vivo (reviewed in Cabral & Staab, 2005). Exogenous cannabinoids have been reported to suppress the antibody response of humans and animals (Friedman, Klein, & Specter, 1991; Klein, Friedman, & Specter, 1998) in a mode that implicates a cannabinoid receptor since inhibition of adenylate cyclase by a pertussis-toxin-sensitive G-protein-coupled mechanism has been observed (Kaminski, Koh, Yang, Lee, & Kessler, 1994). These compounds also have been reported to suppress a variety of activities of T lymphocytes (Kaminski, 1998; Klein et al., 2004). In vivo administration of THC to mice also has been shown to result in inhibition of natural killer (NK) cytolytic activity and to reduce significantly levels of interferon-gamma (IFNγ) (Massi, Fuzio, Vigano, Sacerdote, & Parolaro, 2000). Furthermore, administration of CB$_1$ and CB$_2$ receptor antagonists resulted in a complete reversal in the reduction of levels of IFNγ, suggesting that both cannabinoid receptors were involved in the network mediating NK cytolytic activity. In addition, exogenous cannabinoids have been reported to abolish the functional activities of macrophages and macrophage-like cells. THC, CP55,940, and HU-210 inhibited macrophage-like cell contact-dependent cytolysis of tumor cells and the processing of antigens (Klein, Kawakami, Newton, & Friedman, 1991; Burnette-Curley, & Cabral, 1995; McCoy, Matveyeva, Carlisle, & Cabral, 1999). Furthermore, treatment of macrophages from wild-type mice with THC prevented the activation of helper T cells, while treatment of macrophages from CB$_2$ knockout mice with this cannabinoid had little effect (Buckley et al., 2000), suggesting a functionally relevant role for the CB$_2$ in this process. Recently, it has been recognized that exogenous cannabinoids alter the expression of chemokines and cytokines, leading to perturbation in the homeostatic balance between pro-inflammatory (Th$_1$) and anti-inflammatory (Th$_2$) activities. For example, it has been shown that treatment of BALB/c mice with THC results in a decrease in levels of the pro-inflammatory Th$_1$ cytokines IFNγ and interleukin (IL)-12 in response to infection with *Legionella pneumophila* (Klein, Newton, Nakachi, & Friedman, 2000). This cannabinoid-mediated effect was found to be linked to both the CB$_1$ and CB$_2$ receptors. Conversely, cannabinoids have been implicated as increasing levels of Th$_2$-type cytokines. It was shown through the use of a mouse lung tumor model in which THC mediated a decrease in tumor immunogenicity (Zhu et al., 2000), that levels of the immune inhibitory Th$_2$ cytokines IL-10 and transforming growth factor (TGF) were augmented while the level of the immune stimulatory Th$_1$ cytokine IFNγ was downregulated. These collective results suggest that cannabinoid agonists alter the Th$_1$/Th$_2$

cytokine profile such that the balance of chemokine and cytokine functional activity shifts from that of Th$_1$ pro-inflammatory cytokines to that which favors Th$_2$-type anti-inflammatory cytokines. This shift may articulate a mode by which cannabinoid exposure may drive an anti-inflammatory response during early stages of pathogen invasiveness, rendering the host more susceptible to disease progression, including possibly that linked to HIV.

Endocannabinoids also have been reported to have effects on immune function, although these appear to be of shorter duration as compared to those exerted by exogenous cannabinoids. Anandamide at nanomolar concentrations has been shown to diminish the production of IL-6 and IL-8, while at higher concentrations (i.e., micromolar) to inhibit the production of tumor necrosis factor (TNF)-α, IFNγ, IL-4, and p75 TNF-α soluble receptors (Berdyshev et al., 1997). It has been suggested that this inhibition not only is a result of signaling through the CB$_2$, but that various endogenous fatty acid ethanolamides participate in the regulation of the immune response. In addition, anandamide has been shown to exert an inhibitory effect on the migration of CD8+ T lymphocytes in response to the chemokine stromal derived factor-1 (SDF-1) that was mediated through the CB$_2$ (Joseph, Niggermann, Zaenker, & Entschladen, 2004). However, there are reports that anandamide can act as a synergistic growth factor for primary murine marrow cells and hematopoietic growth factor (HGF)-dependent cell lines (Valk et al., 1997) and that it augments the production of IL-6 by astrocytes that have been infected with Theiler's murine encephalomyelitis virus (Molina-Holgado, Molina-Holgado, & Guaza, 1998). Nevertheless, the preponderance of the data that is available supports a role for anandamide in dampening immune responses.

On the other hand, 2-AG appears to act in an immune stimulatory role. This endocannabinoid has been reported to stimulate the release of nitric oxide (NO) from human immune and vascular tissues and invertebrate immunocytes by a mode linked to the CB$_1$ (Stefano, Bilfinger, Rialas, & Deutsch, 2000). In addition, hematopoietic cells expressing the CB$_2$ have been shown to migrate in response to 2-AG (Jorda et al., 2002) and it has been proposed that cell migration constitutes a major function of the CB$_2$ receptor upon stimulation with this endocannabinoid (Rayman et al., 2004). The migratory inducing capability of 2-AG has been extended to microglia (Walter et al., 2003) and to human peripheral blood monocytes and promyelocytic leukemia HL-60 cells that have been differentiated into macrophage-like cells (Kishimoto et al., 2003). The endocannabinoid also has been reported to accelerate production of chemokines by HL-60 cells (Kishimoto et al., 2004). Also, in studies in which receptor type-specific antibodies have been used, it has been demonstrated that the CB$_2$ is localized to lamellipodia of activated microglia (Walter et al., 2003), suggesting that this receptor plays a critical role in directed cellular migration. This observation, coupled with the report that rat microglia synthesize 2-AG in vitro and express CB$_2$ receptors (Carrier et al., 2004), suggests that microglia, and possibly other immune cells, harbor an endogenous cannabinoid system that may play an autocrine and/or paracrine role in cell migration and proliferation.

In summary, as immunomodulatory lipid molecules that have short half-lives, endocannabinoids appear to act locally to modulate immune functional activities. These effects most probably are of short duration and may be exerted in a mode in which overall homeostatic balance is maintained on the part of anandamide and 2-AG, respectively, acting as "cross-signaling" anti-inflammatory and inflammatory factors. In this context, exogenous cannabinoids introduced into the host may alter this endogenous homeostatic balance to which these endocannabinoids contribute. However, there is a paucity of data as to the extent to which such perturbation may impact HIV-associated neuropathogenesis.

CANNABINOID EFFECTS ON ANTI-MICROBIAL ACTIVITY

In view of the documentation that cannabinoids exert a multiplicity of effects on immune function in vitro and in animal models, it is not surprising that these compounds have been shown to dampen antimicrobial activities with these experimental systems. THC has been reported to inhibit macrophage extrinsic and intrinsic anti-herpesvirus activity (Morahan, Klykken, Smith, Harris, & Munson, 1979; Cabral & Vasquez, 1991; Cabral & Vasquez, 1992) and to suppress the growth restriction of the facultative intracellular bacterium *Legionella pneumophila*, the agent of Legionnaire's disease, in human and guinea pig macrophages and in A/J mouse peritoneal exudate macrophages (Arata, Klein, Newton, & Friedman, 1991; Arata, Newton, Klein, & Friedman, 1992). THC also has been reported to alter in vitro the capacity of macrophages to kill *Naegleria fowleri* (Burnette-Curley, Marciano-Cabral, Fischer-Stenger, & Cabral, 1993), a free-living amoeba that causes a fatal disease in humans known as primary amoebic meningoencephalitis (PAME) (Marciano-Cabral, 1988).

One of the earliest studies indicating that cannabinoids exacerbated resistance to microbes in vivo demonstrated enhanced susceptibility of mice to combinations of THC and live or killed gram-negative bacteria (Bradley, Munson, Dewey, & Harris, 1977). THC since has been shown to compromise the ability of BALB/c mice to resist experimental infection with herpes simplex virus (HSV) type 2 (HSV-2) or *Listeria monocytogenes* (Morahan et al., 1979). This observation has been extended to guinea pigs and mice in which it has been demonstrated that THC increases susceptibility to HSV-2 genital infection and elicits greater severity of herpes genitalis, higher mortalities, higher mean titers of virus shed from the vagina, suppression of antibody production to HSV-2, and a delay in the onset of the delayed hypersensitivity response (DHR) to HSV-2 (Mishkin & Cabral, 1985; Cabral, Lockmuller, & Mishkin, 1986a, b). THC also has been reported to augment murine retroviral-induced immunosuppression and infection (Specter, Lancz, Westrich, & Friedman, 1991). It was indicated that in vitro administration of THC to spleen cells from mice infected with Friend leukemia virus (FLV) resulted in a decrease in lymphocyte blastogenesis and NK cell activity beyond that seen with virus or THC alone. Moreover, when FLV and THC were co-administered to mice concurrently infected with HSV, mortality attributed to FLV infection occurred significantly more rapidly than in the absence of HSV or THC. In addition, in a hamster model, it has been indicated that THC enhances infection with *Treponema pallidum*, the causative agent of syphilis in humans (Paradise & Friedman, 1993). THC also has been reported to exacerbate brain infection in mice by the free-living opportunistic protozoan *Acanthamoeba*, an amoeba that causes granulomatous amoebic encephalitis (GAE) in humans (Marciano-Cabral, Ferguson, Bradley, & Cabral, 2001; Cabral & Marciano-Cabral, 2004). Furthermore, in murine models of GAE and atherosclerosis, macrophages and macrophage-like cells exposed to THC have been reported to display less migration to sites of infection (Cabral & Marciano-Cabral, 2004; Steffens et al., 2005). Thus, the collective data from in vitro and in vivo studies indicate that THC, as an immunosuppressive agent, decreases host resistance to a variety of microbial agents. This immunosuppressive property and attendant linkage to compromised host resistance may be extended to other cannabinoid agonists that signal through cannabinoid receptors. Furthermore, the recognition that cannabinoids compromise host resistance to a variety of infectious agents in animal models indicates a potential for these compounds to render the human host susceptible to opportunistic infections, including those individuals whose immune systems are already compromised as a result of HIV infection.

CANNABINOID EFFECTS ON HIV IN EXPERIMENTAL SYSTEMS

It has been indicated that enhanced syncytial formation, a phenomenon reported to serve as an indicator of HIV infection and cytopathicity (Dedera & Ratner, 1991; Nardacci et al., 2005), occurs in THC-treated MT-2 cells infected with cell-free HIV (Noe, Nyland, Ugen, Friedman, & Klein, 1998). In addition, the role of THC as a cofactor in the development and progression of HIV infection has been examined using the huPBL-SCID mouse, a hybrid in vivo model in which human peripheral blood leukocytes (PBLs) are implanted into severe combined immunodeficient mice and infected with an HIV reporter construct. In this in vivo paradigm, THC treatment was found to significantly increase the percentage of HIV-infected PBLs, increase the systemic viral load, and decrease the number of human IFN-γ-producing cells (Roth, Tashkin, Whittaker, Choi, & Baldwin, 2005). In addition, examination of brains of macaques with simian immunodeficiency virus (SIV)-induced encephalitis has led to the suggestion that the endocannabinoid system participates in the development of HIV-induced encephalitis (Benito et al., 2005). Expression of CB_2 was found to be induced in perivascular macrophages, microglial nodules, and T-lymphocytes. In addition, the endogenous cannabinoid-degrading enzyme FAAH was over-expressed in perivascular astrocytes as well as in astrocytic processes reaching cellular infiltrates. Based on these observations, it has been proposed that activation of the CB_2 that is expressed by immune cells results in reduction of their antiviral response and favors the entry of infected monocytes into the CNS. In contrast to these observations, the synthetic cannabinoid WIN 55,212–2 has been reported to inhibit HIV-1 expression in CD4+ lymphocytes and microglial cells in vitro (Peterson, Gekker, Hu, Cabral, & Lokensgard, 2004). This cannabinoid also has been reported to mediate inhibition of HIV-1 expression in microglia in a mode that involves cannabinoid receptors (Rock et al., 2007). Thus, the role of cannabinoids in modulating HIV infection using these experimental systems remains unresolved.

Recent studies indicate that cannabinoid agonists also can affect G protein-coupled receptors that serve as co-receptors for the HIV. It has been reported that activation of the CB_2 results in inhibition of the transendothelial migration of Jurkat T cells and primary human T lymphocytes by interfering with the CXCL12/CXCR4 chemokine receptor system (Ghosh, Preet, Groopman, & Ganju, 2006), suggesting that cannabinoids can indirectly target CXCR4 that functions as a co-receptor for T-lymphotropic strains of HIV. A similar observation in terms of a potential linkage to the CB_2 has been made for the chemokine receptor CCR5 that acts as the co-receptor for monotropic HIV (Raborn, Marciano-Cabral, Buckley, Martin, & Cabral, 2008). Activation of CB_2 with THC, CP55,940, or with the receptor-selective compound O-2137 resulted in inhibition of the chemotactic response of murine peritoneal macrophages to the chemokine ligand CCL5 (RANTES). In summary, our understanding of the role of exogenous and endogenous cannabinoids on the expression and functionality of receptors and co-receptors that are relevant in HIV infection is in its infancy. Nevertheless, the collective data to date suggest that $G_{i/o}$ protein-coupled receptors such as the CB_2 can "cross-talk" with other G protein-coupled receptors, especially chemokine receptors, to modulate HIV infection of T lymphocytes and monocytes.

CANNABINOIDS AND HIV-RELATED NEUROPATHOGENESIS IN EXPERIMENTAL SYSTEMS

The parenchyma of the brain is sequestered from the rest of the body by the blood-brain barrier (BBB), a selectively permeable barrier that consists of a continuous layer of microvascular endothelial cells that are interconnected by tight junctions. The BBB regulates the traffic of substances and cells that are present in the circulatory system. Perivascular macrophages are found in the region surrounding the endothelium of brain capillaries and are replenished through the migration of circulating monocytes. In addition, astrocytes are found in this region and play a critical homeostatic role in the BBB by maintaining contact with endothelial cells and regulating permeability of the endothelial layer through the release of soluble factors. It has been proposed that HIV enters the brain as a "Trojan horse" through its presence in infected monocytes that transmigrate the BBB to replenish the population of perivascular macrophages (reviewed in

Gonzalez-Scarano & Martin-Garcia, 2005). Once within the brain, infected monocytes acquire an activated phenotype and infect microglia. Infected perivascular macrophages and microglia not only produce HIV, but also release a plethora of factors such as the HIV-envelope glycoprotein gp120, the HIV transcriptional activator Tat, quinolinic acid, arachidonic acid, nitric oxide (NO), platelet-activating factor (PAF), and pro-inflammatory cytokines such as TNF-α. These factors, in combination or alone, promote further activation of perivascular macrophages, microglia, and astrocytes that leads to modification of BBB permeability, migration of additional monocytes from peripheral sites into the brain, and neurocytotoxicity.

Cannabinoids have been reported to inhibit HIV-1 gp120-mediated insults in brain microvascular endothelial cells (Lu et al., 2008). In experiments in which co-cultures of human brain microvascular endothelial cells (HBMEC) and human astrocytes were used as a model of the human blood-brain barrier, cannabinoid agonists inhibited HIV-1 gp120-induced calcium influx mediated by substance P, a neuropeptide that functions as a neurotransmitter and neuromodulator and is associated with inflammatory processes and pain; significantly inhibited permeability of HBMEC; and prevented tight junction protein downregulation of ZO-1, claudin-5, and JAM-1 in HBMEC. Furthermore, cannabinoid agonists were shown to inhibit the transmigration of human monocytes across the BBB. Since breakdown of the BBB is frequently observed in individuals with HIV-associated dementia (HAD), it was suggested that cannabinoid agonists have potential for ablating this effect. In addition, it has been reported that the exogenous cannabinoid WIN55,212–2 inhibits the expression of inducible NO synthase (iNOS) and NO release elicited from rat glioma C6 cells in response to Tat (Esposito et al., 2002). The inhibition in iNOS expression and NO release was found to be linked to the CB_1 receptor based on the use of cannabinoid receptor-selective antagonists. These results are consistent with those that demonstrated previously that cannabinoid-mediated inhibition of iNOS production and NO release by neonatal rat microglia produced in response to the bacterial immune modulator lipopolysaccharide (LPS) were linked to the CB_1 (Waksman, Olson, Carlisle, & Cabral, 1999). Furthermore, it was reported that treatment of C6 glioma cells with Tat plus IFN-γ also resulted in a significant inhibition of the uptake of the endocannabinoid anandamide while having no effect on anandamide hydrolysis, suggesting that the endocannabinoid system through the modulation of the L-arginine/NO pathway reduced Tat-induced cytotoxicity and was itself regulated by Tat. It was concluded that the endocannabinoid system protects rat glioma cells against HIV-1 Tat-induced cytotoxicity (Esposito et al., 2002).

Comparable to reports that cannabinoid agonists affect G protein-coupled receptors that function as co-receptors for the HIV at peripheral sites (Ghosh et al., 2006; Raborn et al., 2008), it has been reported that stromal cell-derived growth factor-1α (SDF-1α/CXCL120), a chemokine ligand for CXCR4 that also is a co-receptor involved in entry of

HIV-1, interacts with a physiological response to a cannabinoid (Benamar, Yondorf, Geller, Eisenstein, & Adler, 2009). Direct infusion of the exogenous cannabinoid agonist WIN55,212–2 into the preoptic anterior hypothalamus (POAH) of the rat, the primary brain area involved in thermoregulation, elicited a dose-related hypothermia. The hypothermic effect was attenuated by SDF-1α/CXCL12 microinjected directly into the POAH. Furthermore, the SDF-1α/CXCL12-induced attenuation of WIN55212–2-mediated hypothermia was reversed by an antagonist of SDF-1α/CXCL12 acting on its receptor CXCR4. The aminoalkylindole WIN55,212–2 also has been reported to inhibit the production of CX3CL1 (fractalkine) (Sheng, Hu, Ni, Rock, and Peterson, 2009), a chemokine shown to be neuroprotective and implicated as playing a role in HIV-1-associated neuropathogenesis. In these studies, the production of CX3CL1 by human astrocytes stimulated with IL-1β was inhibited by WIN55,212–2. The CB$_2$ receptor antagonist reversed the WIN55,212–2-induced suppression of CX3CL1, consistent with a linkage to a CB$_2$ receptor mode of action. It was indicated that the suppression of CX3CL1 production by the aminoalkylindole may involve the inhibition of the mitogen-activated protein (MAP) kinase signaling system. Thus, as in the case of studies which have implicated G protein-coupled heterologous signaling in immune cells at peripheral sites, there is emerging evidence that such action also is operative in the CNS and, as such, may be linked to modulation of HIV disease progression in that compartment.

CANNABINOIDS AND HUMAN HIV INFECTION AND AIDS

There have been a limited number of studies that have addressed the issue of effects of marijuana or cannabinoids on human HIV infection and AIDS. No conclusive data have been obtained as to potential risks and/or hazards associated with HIV infection and the use of marijuana or administration of cannabinoids in a therapeutic mode. A number of studies have indicated that marijuana or cannabinoid products have little deleterious effect on the immune system or on HIV infection (Kaslow et al., 1989; Coates et al., 1990; Struwe et al., 1993; Di Franco, Sheppard, Hunter, Tosteson, & Ascher, 1996; Wallace et al., 1998; Persaud, Klaskala, Tewari, Shultz, & Baum, 1999; Miller & Goodridge, 2000; Bredt et al., 2002). In a randomized, placebo-controlled 21-day clinical trial to examine the short-term effects of smoked marijuana on the viral load in 67 HIV-infected patients in an inpatient setting at the General Clinical Research Center at the San Francisco General Hospital, San Francisco, CA, smoked and oral cannabinoids did not appear to present a risk in individuals with HIV infection with respect to HIV RNA levels, CD4+ and CD8+ cell counts, or protease inhibitor levels (Abrams et al., 2003). In addition, the tolerability and efficacy of smoked marijuana and oral dronabinol, a schedule III controlled substance that contains THC approved for appetite stimulation in AIDS-related anorexia, maintenance in HIV-positive marijuana smokers was evaluated in a placebo-controlled within-subjects study (Haney et al., 2007). Both marijuana and dronabinol were reported to be well tolerated. Furthermore, as compared to placebo, marijuana and dronabinol increased daily caloric intake and body weight in HIV-positive marijuana smokers. Also, in a phase II, double-blind, placebo-controlled crossover clinical trial to assess the impact of smoked cannabis on HIV-associated distal sensory predominant polyneuropathy (DSPN), smoked cannabis was found generally to be well tolerated and effective when added concomitantly with analgesis therapy in patients with refractory pain due to HIV DSPN (Ellis et al., 2009). However, it has been suggested that, while the precise role of cannabinoids in pain management requires further evaluation, these compounds may be more effective in the management of chronic neuropathic pain as compared to acute pain in humans (Beaulieu & Ware, 2007).

In contrast, there are reports that marijuana use is associated with compromised health status among HIV-infected individuals. In an assessment of oral manifestations of tumor and opportunistic infections in AIDS-affected men with Kaposi's sarcoma (KS), past or present infections with CMV, hepatitis, venereal diseases, and gastrointestinal microorganisms were shown to occur in more than 70% of individuals and oral candidiasis was confirmed in 57% (Lozada, Silverman, Migliorati, Conant, & Volberding, 1983). Heavy marijuana smoking was identified as the most common habit among these individuals. Marijuana also has been identified as a risk factor among men referred for possible AIDS (Newell et al., 1985). Smoking illicit drugs such as marijuana was one of several factors that increased the risk of bacterial pneumonia in HIV-seropositive drug users (Caiaffa et al., 1994). In an examination of risk factors for HIV–AIDS among youth in Cape Town, South Africa, for young men one of the HIV risk factors identified was use of Dagga (marijuana) (Simbayi et al., 2005). In addition, immunoepidemiological studies using univariant and multivariant analyses have indicated an association between marijuana use and progression of HIV seropositivity to development of symptomatic AIDS (Tindall et al., 1988). An examination of the impact of ethanol and Marinol/marijuana on HIV+/AIDS patients undergoing azidothymidine (AZT), azidothymidine/dideoxycytidine (AZT/DDC), or dideoxyinosine (DDI) therapy indicated that Marinol/marijuana was associated with declining health status in both the AZT and AZT/DDC groups (Whitfield, Bechtel, & Starich, 1997). However, in HIV+/AIDS patients with the lowest CD4+ counts undergoing DDI monotherapy, utilization of Marinol/marijuana did not seem to have a deleterious impact.

In summary, definitive data that directly link the use of marijuana in a recreational or therapeutic mode, or exposure to cannabinoid compounds, to greater susceptibility to HIV infection or to disease progression in humans have yet to be obtained. Evaluation of multiple immunological parameters has revealed little or no major perturbation in humans. The preponderance of evidence that use or ingestion of these substances is detrimental in the context of HIV infection has been almost exclusively derivative of correlative epidemiological studies. Clearly, there is a need for the conduct of longitudinal epidemiological assessment of human populations to elucidate the risks in terms of immune status and health that may be associated with marijuana use or cannabinoid exposure, especially as related to HIV infection. This issue is particularly relevant as applied to HIV-associated neuropathies for which there are essentially no data available regarding the functional impact of marijuana or cannabinoids on immunologically active cells within the brain that harbor HIV or elicit inflammatory or neurocytotoxic factors.

SUMMARY AND FUTURE PERSPECTIVES

Cannabinoids have been shown to alter the functional activities of a variety of immune cells at peripheral sites and in the CNS. While there is a large body of data from animal models that these effects of cannabinoids on immunity are linked to decreased resistance to infectious agents, a comparable linkage in humans has yet to be obtained, at least as relates to long-terms effects. A major confound in resolving this issue is that individuals who use marijuana in a recreational mode also partake of other substances that have immune-suppressing potential. On the other hand, patients who use marijuana or select cannabinoid formulations for therapeutic purposes already have underlying health conditions that may render them immune compromised or susceptible to infection. Many of the activities of cannabinoids are mediated through activation of cannabinoid receptors. The CB_1 appears to be functionally relevant for the overall homeostatic balance and regulation of the CNS (Marsicano et al., 2003; Cota et al., 2007). In this context, it has been suggested that the CB_1 may have potential as a molecular target for therapeutic attenuation of cognitive impairment and degeneration in select CNS disorders (Shen & Thayer, 1998; Pryce et al., 2003; Pryce & Baker, 2007). However, while many neuropathogenic processes are characterized by progressive decline in cognitive functions, a major hallmark of CNS pathologies is inflammation. Since the CB_2 has been linked to the modulation of immune responses and its expression by cells such as macrophages and microglia appears to be upregulated in response to stimuli (Carlisle et al., 2002), this receptor may serve as a selective molecular target for ablating untoward inflammatory responses. That is, cannabinoid agonists that selectively bind the CB_2 could prove useful for adjunctive therapeutic management of various neuropathological processes that have a neuroinflammatory component, including that related to HIV-associated neuroinflammation in which perivascular macrophages and microglia play a prominent role, especially during the early stages of HIV invasion of the brain. Thus, in targeting the CB_2, the prospect exists for the rational design of cannabinoid compounds that have low toxicity, that readily penetrate the BBB since these compounds are highly lipophilic, that exert minimal psychotropic effects since they activate the CB_2 rather than the CB_1, and that selectively target perivascular macrophages and microglia that are productively competent for HIV.

ACKNOWLEDGMENTS

Supported, in part, by NIDA/NIH award R01 DA05832.

REFERENCES

Abrams, D. I., Hilton, J. F., Leiser, R. J., et al. (2003). Short-term effects of cannabinoids in patients with HIV-1 infection: a randomized, placebo-controlled clinical trial. *Ann Intern Med*, 139, 258–66.

Agarwal, N., Pacher, P., Tegeder, I., et al. (2007). Cannabinoids mediate analgesia largely via peripheral type 1 cannabinoid receptors in nociceptors. *Nat Neurosci*, 10, 870–9.

Arata, S., Klein, T. W., Newton, C., & Friedman, H. (1991). Tetrahydrocannabinol treatment suppresses growth restriction of *Legionella pneumophila* in murine macrophage cultures. *Life Sci*, 49, 473–9.

Arata, S., Newton, C., Klein, T., & Friedman, H. (1992). Enhanced growth of *Legionella pneumophila* in tetrahydrocannabinol-treated macrophages. *Proc Soc Exp Biol Med*, 199, 65–7.

Beaulieu, P. & Ware, M. (2007). Reassessment of the role of cannabinoids in the management of pain. *Curr Opin Anaesthesiol*, 20, 473–7.

Benamar, K., Yondorf, M., Geller, E. B., Eisenstein, T. K., & Adler, M. W. (2009). Physiological evidence for interaction between the HIV-1 co-receptor CXCR4 and the cannabinoid system in the brain. *Br J Pharmacol*, 157, 1225–31.

Benito, C., Kim, W. K., Chavarria, I., et al. (2005). A glial endogenous cannabinoid system is upregulated in the brains of macaques with simian immunodeficiency virus-induced encephalitis. *J Neurosci*, 25, 2530–6.

Berdyshev, E. V., Boichot, E., Germain, N., Allain, N., Anger, J., & Lagente, V. (1997). Influence of fatty acid ethanolamides and D9-tetrahydrocannabinol on cytokine and arachidonate release by mononuclear cells. *Eur J Pharmacol*, 330, 231–40.

Bradley, S. G., Munson, A. E., Dewey, W. L., & Harris, L. S. (1977). Enhanced susceptibility of mice to combinations of delta 9-tetrahydrocannabinol and live or killed gram-negative bacteria. *Infect Immun*, 17, 325–9.

Bredt, B. M., Higuera-Alhino, D., Shade, S. B., Hebert, S. J., McCune, J. M., & Abrams, D. I. (2002). Short-term effects of cannabinoids on immune phenotype and function in HIV-1-infected patients. *J Clin Pharmacol*, 42, 82S–89S.

Breivogel, C. S., Griffin, G., Di Marzo, V., & Martin, B. R. (2001). Evidence for a new G protein-coupled cannabinoid receptor in mouse brain. *Mol Pharmacol*. 60, 155–63.

Buckley, N. E., McCoy, K. L., Mezey, E., et al. (2000). Immunomodulation by cannabinoids is absent in mice deficient for the cannabinoid CB(2) receptor. *Eur J Pharmacol*. 396, 141–9.

Burnette-Curley, D. & Cabral, G. A. (1995). Differential inhibition of RAW264.7 macrophage tumoricidal activity by delta 9tetrahydrocannabinol. *Proc Soc Exp Biol Med*, 210, 64–76.

Burnette-Curley, D., Marciano-Cabral, F., Fischer-Stenger, K., & Cabral, G. A. (1993). Delta-9-Tetrahydrocannabinol inhibits cell contact-dependent cytotoxicity of Bacillus Calmette-Guerin-activated macrophages. *Int J Immunopharmacol*, 15, 371–82.

Cabral, G. A. & Griffin-Thomas, L. (2009). Emerging role of the cannabinoid receptor CB_2 in immune regulation: Therapeutic prospects for neuroinflammation. *Expert Rev Mol Med*, 11, e3.

Cabral, G. A., Lockmuller, J. C., & Mishkin, E. M. (1986a). Delta 9-tetrahydrocannabinol decreases alpha/beta interferon response to herpes simplex virus type 2 in the B6C3F1 mouse. *Proc Soc Exp Biol Med*, 181, 305–11.

Cabral, G. A. & Marciano-Cabral, F. (2004). Cannabinoid-mediated exacerbation of brain infection by opportunistic amebae. *J Neuroimmunol*, 147, 127–30.

Cabral, G. A. & Marciano-Cabral, F. (2005). Cannabinoid receptors in microglia of the central nervous system: Immune functional relevance. *J Leukoc Biol*, 78,1192–7.

Cabral, G. A., Mishkin, E. M., Marciano-Cabral, F., Coleman, P., Harris, L., & Munson, A. E. (1986b). Effect of delta 9-tetrahydrocannabinol on herpes simplex virus type 2 vaginal infection in the guinea pig. *Proc Soc Exp Biol Med*, 182, 181–6.

Cabral, G. A. & Staab, A. (2005). Effects on the immune system. *Hand Exp Pharmacol*, 168, 385–423.

Cabral, G. A. & Vasquez, R. (1991). Effects of marijuana on macrophage function. *Adv Exp Med Biol*, 288, 93–105.

Cabral, G. A. & Vasquez, R. (1992). Delta 9-Tetrahydrocannabinol suppresses macrophage extrinsic antiherpesvirus activity. *Proc Soc Exp Biol Med*, 199, 255–63.

Caiaffa, W. T., Vlahov, D., Graham, N. M., et al. (1994). Drug smoking, *Pneumocystis carinii* pneumonia, and immunosuppression increase risk of bacterial pneumonia in human immunodeficiency virus-seropositive injection drug users. *Am J Respir Crit Care Med*, 150, 1493–8.

Carlisle, S. J., Marciano-Cabral, F., Staab, A., Ludwick, C., & Cabral, G. A. (2002). Differential expression of the CB2 cannabinoid receptor by rodent macrophages and macrophage-like cells in relation to cell activation. *Int Immunopharmacol*, 2, 69–82.

Carrier, E. J., Kearn, C. S., Barkmeier, A. J., et al. (2004). Cultured rat microglial cells synthesize the endocannabinoid 2-arachidonylglycerol, which increases proliferation via a CB2 receptor-dependent mechanism. *Mol Pharmacol*, 65, 999–1007.

Coates, R. A., Farewell, V. T., Raboud, J., et al. (1990). Cofactors of progression to acquired immunodeficiency syndrome in a cohort of male sexual contacts of men with human immunodeficiency virus disease. *Am J Epidemiol*, 132, 717–22.

Cota, D. (2008). The role of the endocannabinoid system in the regulation of hypothalamic-pituitary-adrenal axis activity. *J Neuroendocrinol*, 20, 35–8.

Cota, D., Steiner, M. A., Marsicano, et al. (2007). Requirement of cannabinoid receptor type 1 for the basal modulation of hypothalamic-pituitary-adrenal axis function. *Endocrinology*, 148, 1574–81.

Dedera, D. & Ratner, L. (1991). Demonstration of two distinct cytopathic effects with syncytium formation-defective human immunodeficiency virus type 1 mutants. *J Virol*, 65, 6129–36.

Devane, W. A., Dysarz, F. A., III, Johnson, M. R., Melvin, L. S., & Howlett, A. C. (1988). Determination and characterization of a cannabinoid receptor in rat brain. *Mol Pharmacol*, 34, 605–13.

Devane, W. A., Hanus, L., Breuer, A., et al. (1992). Isolation and structure of a brain constituent that binds to the cannabinoid receptor. *Science*, 258, 1946–9.

Di Franco, M. J., Sheppard, H. W., Hunter, D. J., Tosteson, T. D., & Ascher, M. S. (1996). The lack of association of marijuana and other recreational drugs with progression to AIDS in the San Francisco Men's Health Study. *Ann Epidemiol*, 6, 283–9.

Di Marzo, V., Bifulco, M., & De Petrocellis L. (2004). The endocannabinoid system and its therapeutic exploitation. *Nature Rev Drug Dis*, 3, 771–84.

Di Marzo, V., Breivogel, C. S., Tao, Q., et al. (2000a). Levels, metabolism, and pharmacological activity of anandamide in CB(1) cannabinoid receptor knockout mice: Evidence for non-CB(1), non-CB(2) receptor-mediated actions of anandamide in mouse brain. *J Neurochem*, 75, 2434–44.

Di Marzo, V., Hill, M. P., Bisogno, T., Crossman, A. R., & Brotchie, J. M. (2000b). Enhanced levels of endogenous cannabinoids in the globus pallidus are associated with a reduction in movement in an animal model of Parkinson's disease. *FASEB J*, 14, 1432–8.

Ellis, R. J., Toperoff, W., Vaida, F., et al. (2009). Smoked medicinal cannabis for neuropathic pain in HIV: A randomized, crossover clinical trial. *Neuropsychopharmacology*, 34, 672–80.

Esposito, G., Ligresti, A., Izzo, A.A., et al. (2002). The endocannabinoid system protects glioma cells against HIV-1 Tat protein-induced cytotoxicity. *J Biol Chem*, 277, 50348–54.

Fernandez-Ruiz, J., Romero, J., Velasco, G., Tolon, R. M., Ramos, J. A., & Guzman, M. (2007). Cannabinoid CB2 receptor: A new target for controlling neural cell survival? *Trends Pharmacol Sci*, 28, 39–45.

Friedman, H., Klein, T. W., & Specter, S. (1991). Immunosuppression by marijuana components. In R. Ader, D. L. Felten, & N. Cohen (Eds.). *Psychoneuroimmunology*, 2nd ed, pp. 931–53, Academic Press.

Friedman, H., Newton, C., & Klein, T. W. (2003). Microbial infections, immunomodulation, and drugs of abuse. *Clin Microbiol Rev*, 16, 209–19.

Galiegue, S., Mary, S., Marchand, J., et al. (1995). Expression of central and peripheral cannabinoid receptors in human immune tissues and leukocyte subpopulations. *Eur J Biochem*, 232, 54–61.

Gaoni, Y. & Mechoulam, R. (1971). The isolation and structure of delta-1-tetrahydrocannabinol and other neutral cannabinoids from hashish. *J Am Chem Soc*, 93, 217–24.

Gerard, C. M., Mollereau, C., Vassart, G., & Parmentier, M. (1991). Molecular cloning of a human cannabinoid receptor which is also expressed in testis. *Biochem J*, 279, 129–34.

Ghosh, S., Preet, A., Groopman, J. E., & Ganju, R. K. (2006). Cannabinoid receptor CB2 modulates the CXCL12/CXCR4-mediated chemotaxis of T lymphocytes. *Mol Immunol*, 43, 2169–79.

Gonsiorek, W., Lunn, C., Fan, X., Narula, S., Lundell, D., & Hipkin, R. W. (2000). Endocannabinoid 2-arachidonyl glycerol is a full agonist through human type 2 cannabinoid receptor: Antagonism by anandamide. *Mol Pharmacol*, 57, 1045–50.

Gonzalez-Scarano, F. & Martin-Garcia, J. (2005). The neuropathogenesis of AIDS. *Nat Rev Immunol*, 5, 69–81.

Haney, M., Gunderson, E. W., Rabkin, J., et al. (2007). Dronabinol and marijuana in HIV-positive marijuana smokers. Caloric intake, mood, and sleep. (2007). *J Acquir Immune Defic Syndr*, 45, 545–54.

Haverkos, H. W. & Curran, J.W. (1982). The current outbreak of Kaposi's sarcoma and opportunistic infections. *CA Cancer J Clin*, 32, 330–9.

Herkenham, M., Lynn, A. B., Little, M. D., et al. (1990). Cannabinoid receptor localization in brain. *Proc Natl Acad Sci. USA*, 87, 1932–6.

Howlett, A. C. (1985). Cannabinoid inhibition of adenylate cyclase. Biochemistry of the response in neuroblastoma cell membranes. *Mol Pharmacol*, 27, 429–36.

Howlett, A. C., Barth, F., Bonner, T. I., et al. (2002). International Union of Pharmacology. XXVII. Classification of cannabinoid receptors. *Pharmacol Rev*, 54, 162–202.

Howlett, A. C. & Fleming, R. M. (1984). Cannabinoid inhibition of adenylate cyclase. Pharmacology of the response in neuroblastoma cell membranes. *Mol Pharmacol*, 26, 532–8.

Howlett, A. C., Qualy, J. M., & Khachatrian, L. L. (1986). Involvement of GI in the inhibition of adenylate cyclase by cannabimimetic drugs. *Mol Pharmacol*, 29, 307–13.

Jarai, Z., Wagner, J. A., Varga, K., et al. (1999). Cannabinoid-induced mesenteric vasodilation through an endothelial site distinct from CB1 or CB2 receptors. *Proc Natl Acad Sci. USA*, 96, 14136–41.

Jorda, M. A., Verbakel, S. E., Valk, P. J., et al. (2002). Hematopoietic cells expressing the peripheral cannabinoid receptor migrate in response to the endocannabinoid 2-arachidonoylglycerol. *Blood*, 99, 2786–93.

Joseph, J., Niggermann, B., Zaenker, K. S., & Entschladen F. (2004). Anandamide is an endogenous inhibitor for the migration of tumor cells and T lymphocytes. *Cancer Immunol Immunother*, 53, 723–8.

Kaminski, N. E. (1998). Inhibition of the cAMP signaling cascade via cannabinoid receptors: A putative mechanism of immune modulation by cannabinoid compounds. *Toxicol Lett*, 102–103, 59–63.

Kaminski, N. E., Koh, W. S., Yang, K. H., Lee, M., & Kessler, F. (1994). Suppression of the humoral immune response by cannabinoids is partially mediated through inhibition of adenylate cyclase by a pertussis toxin-sensitive G-protein coupled mechanism. *Biochem Pharmacol*, 48, 1899–908.

Kaslow, R. A., Blackwelder, W. C., Ostrow, D. G., et al. (1989). No evidence for a role of alcohol or other psychoactive drugs in accelerating immunodeficiency in HIV-1-positive individuals. A report from the Multicenter AIDS Cohort Study. *JAMA*, 261, 3424–9.

Kishimoto, S., Gokoh, M., Oka, S., et al. (2003). 2-arachidonoylglycerol induces the migration of HL-60 cells differentiated into macrophage-like cells and human peripheral blood monocytes through the cannabinoid CB2 receptor-dependent mechanism. *J Biol Chem*, 278, 24469–75.

Kishimoto, S., Kobayashi, Y., Oka, S., Gokoh, M., Waku, K., & Sugiura, T. (2004). 2-Arachidonoylglycerol, an endogenous cannabinoid receptor ligand, induces accelerated production of chemokines in HL-60 cells. *J Biochem*, 135, 517–24.

Klein, T. W., Friedman, H., & Specter, S. (1998). Marijuana, immunity and infection. *J Neuroimmunol*, *83*, 102–15.

Klein, T. W., Kawakami, Y., Newton, C., & Friedman, H. (1991). Marijuana components suppress induction and cytolytic function of murine cytotoxic T cells in vitro and in vivo. *J Toxicol Environ Health*, *32*, 465–77.

Klein, T. W., Newton, C., Larsen, K., et al. (2004). Cannabinoid receptors and T helper cells. *J Neuroimmunol*, *147*, 91–4.

Klein, T. W., Newton, C. A., Nakachi, N., & Friedman, H. (2000). Delta-9- tetrahydrocannabinol treatment suppresses immunity and early IFN-gamma, IL-12, and IL-12 receptor beta 2 responses to *Legionella pneumophila* infection. *J Immunol*, *164*, 6461–6.

Kunos, G., Osei-Hyiaman, D., Batkai, S., Sharkey, K. A., & Makriyannis, A. (2008). Should peripheral CB_1 cannabinoid receptors be selectively targeted for therapeutic pain? *Trends Pharmacol Sci*, *30*, 1–7.

Lee, M., Yang, K. H., & Kaminski, N. E. (1995). Effects of putative cannabinoid receptor ligands, anandamide and 2-arachidonyl-glycerol, on immune function in $B_6C_3F_1$ mouse splenocytes. *J Pharmcol Exp Ther*, *275*, 529–36.

Lozada, F., Silverman, S. Jr, Migliorati, C. A., Conant, M. A., & Volberding, P. A. (1983). Oral manifestations of tumor and opportunistic infections in the acquired immunodeficiency syndrome (AIDS): Findings in 53 homosexual men with Kaposi's sarcoma. *Oral Surg Oral Med Oral Pathol*, *56*, 491–4.

Lu, T. S., Avraham, H. K., Seng, S., et al. (2008). Cannabinoids inhibit HIV-1 Gp120-mediated insults in brain microvascular endothelial cells. *J Immunol*, *181*, 6406–16.

Mansell, P. W. (1984). Acquired immune deficiency syndrome, leading to opportunistic infections, Kaposi's sarcoma, and other malignancies. *Crit Rev Clin Lab Sci*, *20*, 191–204.

Marciano-Cabral, F. (1988). Biology of *Naegleria* spp. *Microbiol Rev*, *52*, 114–33.

Marciano-Cabral, F., Ferguson, T., Bradley, S. G., & Cabral, G. (2001). Delta-9-tetrahydrocannabinol (THC), the major psychoactive component of marijuana, exacerbates brain infection by *Acanthamoeba*. *J Eukaryot Microbiol*, *48*, 4S–5S.

Marsicano, G., Goodenough, S., Monory, K., et al. (2003). CB1 cannabinoid receptors and on-demand defense against excitotoxicity. *Science*, *302*, 84–8.

Massi, P., Fuzio, D., Vigano, D., Sacerdote, P., & Parolaro, D. (2000). Relative involvement of cannabinoid CB(1) and CB(2) receptors in the Delta(9)-tetrahydrocannabinol-induced inhibition of natural killer activity. *Eur J Pharmacol*, *387*, 343–7.

Matsuda, L. A., Lolait, S. J., Brownstein, M. J., Young, A. C., & Bonner, T. I. (1990). Structure of a cannabinoid receptor and functional expression of the cloned cDNA. *Nature*, *346*, 561–4.

McCoy, K. L., Matveyeva, M., Carlisle, S. J., & Cabral, G. A. (1999). Cannabinoid inhibition of the processing of intact lysozyme by macrophages: Evidence for CB2 receptor participation. *J Pharmacol Exp Ther*, *289*, 1620–5.

Mechoulam, R. (2002). Discovery of endocannabinoids and some random thoughts on their possible roles in neuroprotection and aggression. *Prostaglandins Leukot Essent Fatty Acids*, *66*, 93–9.

Mechoulam, R., Ben Shabat, S., Hanus, L., et al. (1995). Identification of an endogenous 2-monoglyceride, present in canine gut, that binds to cannabinoid receptors. *Biochem Pharmacol*, *50*, 83–90.

Miller, J. M. Jr. & Goodridge, C. (2000). Antenatal marijuana use is unrelated to sexually transmitted infections during pregnancy. *Infect Dis Obstet Gynecol*, *8*, 155–7.

Mishkin, E. M. & Cabral, G. A. (1985). Delta-9-Tetrahydrocannabinol decreases host resistance to herpes simplex virus type 2 vaginal infection in the B6C3F1 mouse. *J Gen Virol*, *66*, 2539–49.

Molina-Holgado, F., Molina-Holgado, E., & Guaza, C. (1998). The endogenous cannabinoid anandamide potentiates interleukin-6 production by astrocytes infected with Theiler's murine encephalomyelitis virus by a receptor-mediated pathway. *FEBS Lett*, *433*, 139–42.

Morahan, P. S., Klykken, P. C., Smith, S. H., Harris, L. S., & Munson, A. E. (1979). Effects of cannabinoids on host resistance to *Listeria monocytogenes* and herpes simplex virus. *Infect Immun*, *23*, 670–4.

Munro, S., Thomas, K. L., & Abu-Shaar, M. (1993). Molecular characterization of a peripheral receptor for cannabinoids. *Nature*, *365*, 61–5.

Nardacci, R., Antinori, A., Larocca, L. M., et al. (2005). Characterization of cell death pathways in human immunodeficiency virus-associated encephalitis. *Am J Pathol*, *167*, 695–704.

Newell, G. R., Mansell, P. W., Wilson, M. B., Lynch, H. K., Spitz, M. R., & Hersh, E. M. (1985). Risk factor analysis among men referred for possible acquired immune deficiency syndrome. *Prev Med*, *14*, 81–91.

Noe, S. N., Nyland, S. B., Ugen, K., Friedman, H., & Klein, T. W. (1998). Cannabinoid receptor agonists enhance syncytia formation in MT-2 cells infected with cell free HIV-1MN. *Adv Exp Med Biol*, *437*, 223–9.

Nunez, E., Benito, C., Pazos, M. R., et al. (2004). Cannabinoid CB2 receptors are expressed by perivascular microglial cells in the human brain: An immunohistochemical study. *Synapse*, *53*, 208–13.

Paradise, L. J. & Friedman, H. (1993). Syphilis and drugs of abuse. *Adv Exp Med Biol*, *335*, 81–7.

Persaud, N. E., Klaskala, W., Tewari, T., Shultz, J., & Baum, M. (1999). Drug use and syphilis. Co-factors for HIV transmission among commercial sex workers in Guyana. *West Indian Med J*, *48*, 52–6.

Peterson, P. K., Gekker, G., Hu, S., Cabral, G., & Lokensgard, J. R. (2004). Cannabinoids and morphine differentially affect HIV-1 expression in CD4(+) lymphocyte and microglial cell cultures. *J Neuroimmunol*, *147*, 123–6.

Pryce, G., Ahmed, Z., Hankey, D. J. R., et al. (2003). Cannabinoids inhibit neurodegeneration in models of multiple sclerosis. *Brain*, *126*, 2191–202.

Pryce, G. & Baker, D. (2007). Control of spasticity in multiple sclerosis model is mediated by CB_1, not CB_2, cannabinoid receptors. *Br J Pharmacol*, *150*, 519–25.

Raborn, E. S., Marciano-Cabral, F., Buckley, N. E., Martin, B. R., & Cabral, G. A. (2008). The cannabinoid delta-9-tetrahydrocannabinol mediates inhibition of macrophage chemotaxis to RANTES/CCL5: Linkage to the CB_2 receptor. *J Neuroimmune Pharmacol*, *3*, 117–29.

Ramirez, B. G., Blazquez, C., Gomez del Pulgar, T., Guzman, M., & de Ceballos, M. L. (2005). Prevention of Alzheimer's disease pathology by cannabinoids: Neuroprotection mediated by blockade of microglial activation. *J Neurosci*, *25*, 1904–13.

Rayman, N., Lam, K. H., Laman, J. D., et al. (2004). Distinct expression profiles of the peripheral cannabinoid receptor in lymphoid tissues depending on receptor activation status. *J Immunol*, *172*, 2111–7.

Rock, R. B., Gekker, G., Hu, S., et al. (2007). WIN55,212–2-mediated inhibition of HIV-1 expression in microglial cells: Involvement of cannabinoid receptors. *J Neuroimmune Pharmacol*, *2*, 178–83.

Roth, M. D., Tashkin, D. P., Whittaker, K. M., Choi, R., & Baldwin, G. C. (2005). Tetrahydrocannabinol suppresses immune function and enhances HIV replication in the huPBL-SCID mouse. *Life Sci*, *77*, 1711–22.

Schatz, A. R., Lee, M., Condie, R. B., Pulaski, J. T., & Kaminski, N. E. (1997). Cannabinoid receptors CB1 and CB2: A characterization of expression and adenylate cyclase modulation within the immune system. *Toxicol Appl Pharmacol*, *142*, 278–87.

Shen, M. & Thayer, S. A. (1998). Cannabinoid receptor agonists protect cultured rat hippocampal neurons from excitotoxicity. *Mol Pharmacol*, *54*, 459–62.

Sheng, W. S., Hu, S., Ni, H. T., Rock, R. B., & Peterson, P. K. (2009). WIN55,212–2 inhibits production of CX3CL1 by human astrocytes: Involvement of p38 MAP kinase. *J Neuroimmune Pharmacol*, *4*, 244–8.

Simbayi, L. C., Kalichman, S. C., Jooste, S., Cherry, C., Mfecane, S., & Cain, D. (2005). Risk factors for HIV–AIDS among youth in Cape Town, South Africa. *AIDS Behav*, *9*, 53–61.

Specter, S., Lancz, G., Westrich, G., & Friedman, H. (1991). Delta-9-tetrahydrocannabinol augments murine retroviral induced immunosuppression and infection. *Int J Immunopharmacol*, *13*, 411–7.

Stefano, G. B., Bilfinger, T. V., Rialas, C. M., & Deutsch, D. G. (2000). 2-Arachidonyl-glycerol stimulates nitric oxide release from human immune and vascular tissues and invertebrate immunocytes by cannabinoid receptor 1. *Pharmacol Res*, *42*, 317–22.

Steffens, S., Veillard, N. R., Arnaud, C., et al. (2005). Low dose oral cannabinoid therapy reduces progression of atherosclerosis in mice. *Nature, 434,* 782–6.

Stella, N., Schweitzer, P., & Piomelli, D. (1997). A second endogenous cannabinoid that modulates long-term potentiation. *Nature, 388,* 773–8.

Struwe, M., Kaempfer, S. H., Geiger, C. J., et al. (1993). Effect of dronabinol on nutritional status in HIV infection. *Ann Pharmacother, 27,* 827–31.

Szabo, B. & Schlicker, E. (2005). Effects of cannabinoids on neurotransmission. *Hanb Exp Pharmacol, 168,* 327–65.

Tasker, J. (2004). Endogenous cannabinoids take the edge off neuroendocrine responses to stress. *Endocrinology, 145,* 5429–30.

Tindall, B., Cooper, D. A., Donovan, B., et al. (1988). The Sydney AIDS Project: Development of acquired immunodeficiency syndrome in a group of HIV seropositive homosexual men. *Aust N Z J Med, 18,* 8–15.

Valk, P., Verbakel, S., Vankan, Y., et al. (1997). Anandamide, a natural ligand for the peripheral cannabinoid receptor is a novel synergistic growth factor for hematopoietic cells. *Blood, 90,* 1448–57.

Waksman, Y., Olson, J. M., Carlisle, S. J., & Cabral, G. A. (1999). The central cannabinoid receptor (CB1) mediates inhibition of nitric oxide production by rat microglial cells. *J Pharmacol Exp Ther, 288,* 1357–1366.

Wallace, J. M., Lim, R., Browdy, B. L., et al. (1998). Risk factors and outcomes associated with identification of *Aspergillus* in respiratory specimens from persons with HIV disease. Pulmonary Complications of HIV Infection Study Group. *Chest, 114,* 131–137.

Walter, L., Franklin, A., Witting, A., et al. (2003). Nonpsychotropic cannabinoid receptors regulate microglial cell migration. *J Neurosci, 23,* 1398–405.

Westlake, T. M., Howlett, A. C., Bonner, T. I., Matsuda, L. A., & Herkenham, M. (1994). Cannabinoid receptor binding and messenger RNA expression in human brain: An in vitro receptor autoradiography and in situ hybridization histochemistry study of normal aged and Alzheimer's brains. *Neurosci, 63,* 637–52.

Whitfield, R. M., Bechtel, L. M., & Starich, G. H. (1997). The impact of ethanol and marinol/marijuana usage on HIV+/AIDS patients undergoing azidothymidine, azidothymidine/dideoxycytidine, or dideoxyinosine therapy. *Alcohol Clin Exp Res, 21,* 122–7.

Wiley, J. L. & Martin, B. R. (2002). Cannabinoid pharmacology: Implications for additional cannabinoid receptor subtypes. *Chem Phys Lipids, 121,* 57–63.

Zhu, L. X., Sharma, S., Stolina, M., et al. (2000). Delta-9-tetrahydrocannabinol inhibits antitumor immunity by a CB2 receptor-mediated, cytokine-dependent pathway. *J Immunol, 165,* 373–80.

4.6

HIV-1 AND METH

Howard S. Fox

The stimulant dextro (D)-methamphetamine hydrochloride (methamphetamine, meth) is a member of the amphetamine family of abused drugs. Meth is chemically related to amphetamine (dextroamphetamine), with the additional methyl group giving it enhanced lipophilicity, which increases its ability to cross the blood-brain barrier. Significant demographic overlap exists between those who use meth and those at risk for HIV infection. Several research groups have studied the interaction of meth and HIV in humans. HIV and meth appear to have adverse, additive effects on frontal and striatal neuronal and glial markers; and rates of neurocognitive impairment appear to be higher in HIV-positive individuals who use meth versus those who do not. This chapter presents the result of clinical trials, nonhuman primate studies, and nonprimate animal studies relevant to interactions between meth use and HIV. The chapter also discusses meth toxicity; the effects of meth on central nervous system function; and interactions among aging, chronic HIV infection, and meth use.

INTRODUCTION

Drugs of abuse are taken for their effects on the brain. While desired by the user, use of these substances can lead to functional and structural damage. The untoward effects of HIV on the brain are well described in this book. While there is a large overlap between those that use drugs of abuse and those that are affected by HIV, it remains unclear whether such drugs affect the course of HIV in infected individuals. While one focus is on end-effects on the brain, it is obvious that if drugs of abuse have effects on the immune system and the virus-host interplay throughout the stages of infection, this too will impact the effects of the virus on the central nervous system (CNS). Methamphetamine is a drug with the potential to be a key cofactor in HIV's effects on the brain, given its actions on the brain as well as the immune system, and its significant use in the HIV-infected population. Here, evidence for the effects of meth on HIV-infected individuals will be presented first, followed by lessons learned from animal studies and other experimental systems. Salient issues related to the effects of meth itself are then considered. When combined with the effects of HIV, as explored throughout this book, additional areas of potential interaction emerge.

METHAMPHETAMINE AND THE LINK TO HIV

The stimulant dextro (D)-methamphetamine hydrochloride (methamphetamine, meth) is a member of the amphetamine family of abused drugs, which have structural similarities to the monoamine neurotransmitter dopamine (Figure 4.6.1), and exert their effects through dopaminergic as well as other monoaminergic systems. Meth is chemically related to amphetamine (dextroamphetamine), with the additional methyl group giving it enhanced lipophilicity which increases its ability to cross the blood-brain barrier, and decreasing its enzymatic breakdown by monoamine oxidase, thus leading to prolonged effects. While both the levo and dextro isomers of amphetamine are active in the CNS, only the dextro isomer of meth shows CNS activity, and levo (L)-methamphetamine is used as a sympathomimetic vasoconstrictor in nasal decongestants. Both amphetamine and methamphetamine are available as pharmaceuticals, approved for treatment of attention-deficit hyperactivity disorder (ADHD) as well as narcolepsy (amphetamine) and obesity (methamphetamine); both are Schedule II controlled substances in the United States. Another related substituted amphetamine, 3,4-methylenedioxymethamphetamine (MDMA, ecstasy) is currently a Schedule I controlled substance, but is undergoing clinical trials for assisting therapy in the treatment of chronic posttraumatic stress disorder (PTSD) (Mithoefer, Wagner, Mithoefer, Jerome, & Doblin, 2010).

Meth is used illicitly for a variety of reasons and several of these, including maintaining alertness and energy as well as increasing libido and sexual pleasure, are linked to risk for HIV infection. The intersection between those who use meth and those at risk for HIV infection is profound, and for men who have sex with other men, meth users are three times more likely to become HIV infected than those who do not use meth, and the resulting the prevalence of HIV infection is significantly higher in meth users (Molitor, Truax, Ruiz, & Sun, 1998; Rotheram-Borus, Luna, Marotta, & Kelly, 1994; Chesney, Barrett, & Stall, 1998; Molitor et al., 1999; Vongsheree et al., 2001). Studies have clearly shown the association of meth use and HIV risk behaviors (Koblin et al., 2006; Plankey et al., 2007) and links between meth use and HIV incidence (Hurt et al., 2010; Buchacz et al., 2005; Lambert, Normand, Stall, Aral, & Vlahov, 2005). The link between meth and HIV exists not only in the United States,

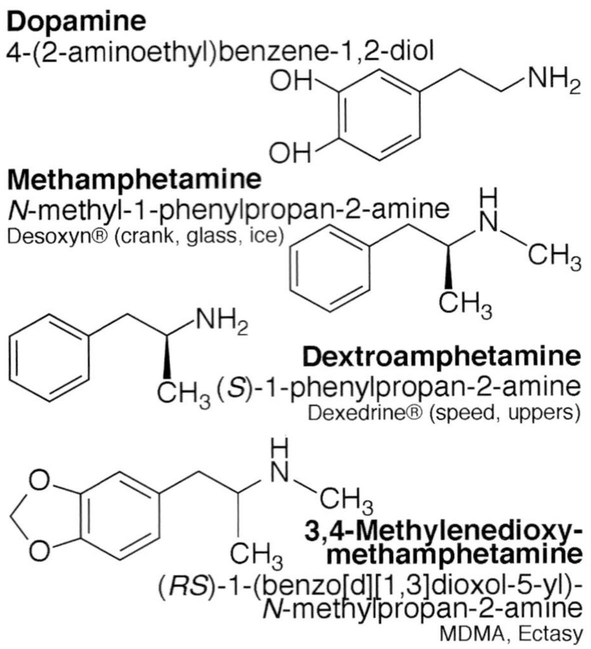

Dopamine
4-(2-aminoethyl)benzene-1,2-diol

Methamphetamine
N-methyl-1-phenylpropan-2-amine
Desoxyn® (crank, glass, ice)

Dextroamphetamine
(*S*)-1-phenylpropan-2-amine
Dexedrine® (speed, uppers)

3,4-Methylenedioxy-methamphetamine
(*RS*)-1-(benzo[d][1,3]dioxol-5-yl)-*N*-methylpropan-2-amine
MDMA, Ectasy

Figure 4.6.1 Dopamine and members of the amphetamine family. Note relatedness in their structures. The systematic (IUPAC) chemical names are given, as well as selected trade names, abbreviations, and slang (street) names of the drugs.

but in other countries as well (Vongsheree et al., 2001). Meth abuse has increased greatly in the United States, and worldwide meth abuse is a large and growing problem, with more users than those who take cocaine and heroin (Rawson et al., 2007; Roehr, 2005).

METHAMPHETAMINE AND HIV HUMAN STUDIES

The study of the effects of chronic use of drugs of abuse on people is complex for many reasons. Knowledge of the drug dose, extent of use, and purity and identity of contaminants is problematic. Users of illicit drugs also frequently use many different drugs and their drug use can be associated with a variety of social and medical conditions that themselves can affect diseases such as HIV infection. However, through careful selection of subjects and multivariate analysis of potential confounding factors, several investigative groups have performed excellent studies on the interaction of meth and HIV in people.

A link between meth use and HIV-associated neurocognitive disorder (HAND) in HIV infection was identified in a well-powered study of 200 individuals with and without HIV infection and with and without meth dependence. The group that was both HIV infected and meth dependent had a higher rate of neuropsychological impairment (58%) than those who were HIV infected but did not use meth (38%) or those who were not infected with HIV but did use meth (40%) (Rippeth et al., 2004). Proton magnetic resonance

spectroscopy (^{1}H-MRS) imaging studies have yielded a clue to these effects, revealing an additive effect of HIV and meth on abnormalities in frontal and striatal neuronal and glial markers (Chang, Ernst, Speck, & Grob, 2005). Magnetic resonance imaging (MRI) has revealed distinct changes due to HIV and meth, with decreased volume of cortical and subcortical regions in HIV, but increased cortical volumes with meth, with overlapping effects found in those who were HIV infected and used meth (Jernigan et al., 2005). The decrease in brain area volumes in HIV and increase in meth both correlated with neurocognitive impairment.

Other studies have pursued potential interactions related to plasma viral load, linked to progression of nearly all HIV-associated conditions. In a study of 230 subjects, levels of plasma virus are higher in HIV-infected meth users than non-meth users (Ellis et al., 2003). Interestingly, in this study this difference was limited to those on combination antiretroviral therapy (cART), and thus the effectiveness of cART may be compromised in meth users, due to compliance or metabolic factors. In another study of 193 subjects, analysis of factors linked to the presence of a detectable (greater than 400 copies per ml of plasma) viral load yielded two significant findings: homelessness and meth use (King et al., 2009). Additional work has shown a negative association between meth use and antiretroviral medication adherence (Halkitis, Kutnick, & Slater, 2005; Moss et al., 2004; Reback, Larkins, & Shoptaw, 2003), pointing to poor adherence to cART regimens as a cause of the increased viral load. However, plasma viral load and other plasma factors have not been correlated with HAND (Vitiello et al., 2007; Sun et al., 2010).

One clue to the brain changes was found in a gene-expression profiling study of brains from individuals with HIV infection (Masliah et al., 2004). Interestingly, 13 of these donors had been assessed for meth use, and comparison of three groups (all HIV infected; five without HIV encephalitis (HIVE) or meth use, four with HIVE but no meth use, and four with HIVE and meth use) revealed significant increased expression of a group of interferon-inducible genes in the brains of those with HIVE and meth use (Everall et al., 2005). While in the current era of treatment HIVE is not the neuropathological correlate of HAND (Everall et al., 2009), and the previous study was a post-mortem characterization of a limited number of samples, the concept that meth increases the host response/inflammatory aspect of HIV infection of the brain which leads to functional abnormalities is a strong candidate hypothesis in the mechanism of the CNS comorbidity of HIV and meth.

However, this is somewhat at odds with neuropathological examination of brains of meth users that manifested HIVE, in which less severe encephalitis was found than in those with HIVE who did not use meth, with lower levels of immunoreactive viral proteins, but a higher degree of loss of calbindin interneurons in the neocortex (Langford et al., 2003). Yet this points to an interesting correlation, in which loss of such interneurons (including parvalbumin interneurons), is linked to memory abnormalities in meth users with HIV (Chana et al., 2006).

METHAMPHETAMINE AND HIV–NONHUMAN PRIMATE STUDIES

Animal studies have numerous advantages in studies on both HIV and drugs of abuse, and have the distinct advantage of rigorous control of experimental conditions as opposed to studies on humans. However, studies in animals must take into account aspects that are often ignored. One of these is relevant physiological dosing of drugs of abuse. While much has been learned from acute high (neurotoxic) doses of meth, the relevance to the chronic administration found in most meth abusers is not clear. Numerous studies have been performed in rodents, yet there is an approximately tenfold shorter half-life of meth in rodents than in humans (Segal et al., 2006). Further complicating the dosing, human meth users do not start with the dose of meth that characterizes their chronic use; they begin with lower doses and gradually increase the dose and frequency of use as tolerance builds to both the positive and negative aspects of the drug's effects. Still, rodents have been indispensible in the assessment of potential mechanisms of meth neurotoxicity, including the role of monoamine metabolites, excitotoxicity, and oxidative and metabolic stress (Kita, Wagner, & Nakashima, 2003; Cadet, Jayanthi, & Deng, 2003).

The simian immunodeficiency virus (SIV) is closely related to HIV-1, and SIV infected monkeys are considered the best animal model for HIV infection and its sequelae, including CNS disorders (see Chapter 5.1: Simian Immunodeficiency Virus). Monkeys also show great similarities to humans in their response to drugs, metabolism, immune system, and CNS. Thus, in order to study the effects of meth on HIV infection, an escalating dosing administration protocol was designed for monkeys based on usage patterns in humans (Madden et al., 2005). This protocol involves a slow, steady ramp-up in dose, as well as frequent repeated doses (twice a day, five days a week, mimicking human chronic users where usage can occur in binges and users take meth 20 or more times a month, 1 to 3 times a day (Simon et al., 2002)). The initial work characterized both physiological changes in the body (Madden et al., 2005) as well as neurostructural and molecular changes in the brain (Coutinho, Flynn, Burdo, Mervis, & Fox, 2008) following this regimen. Intriguingly, interferons were found to be increased in the brains of meth-treated animals, perhaps foreshadowing the findings of interferon-induced genes in human meth users with HIVE described above (Everall et al., 2005).

This escalating-dose chronic treatment protocol has also been used by others studying the effects of meth on the monkey brain, revealing behavioral and neurochemical abnormalities (Melega et al., 2007). While this model has gained acceptance as mimicking the human condition, the dosing (approximately 7 mg/kg per week) could still be thought of as modest compared to human chronic meth users. For example, in an imaging study, revealing structural abnormalities in the brains of chronic meth users (described in more detail below), found that the subjects averaged 3.4 g of meth per week (Thompson et al., 2004). After normalizing for body weight and approximating drug purity, this corresponds to 25 mg/kg per week.

One potential issue with studies in the SIV/monkey system is that an unusual (relative to HIV/humans) rapid disease course occurs in approximately one-quarter of infected animals, related to a poor initial immune response and lack of control of the initial viremia to a steady state set point level, complicating the interpretation of group studies. Therefore, in order to assess potential effects of meth on SIV infection in monkeys, a group of animals were first infected with SIV and a group chosen matched for viral load in the stable phase of infection. Half of this group then received the escalating meth dose protocol, but now reaching 25 mg/kg per week, while the others received vehicle injections.

While not carried through to end-stage simian AIDS, interesting findings resulted from chronic meth administration in these SIV-infected animals (Marcondes, Flynn, Watry, Zandonatti, & Fox, 2010). No differences were found in plasma viral load or blood-lymphocyte subset numbers over the 23-week meth treatment period. However, a distinct activation of natural killer (NK) cells was present, as well as changes in CD8+ T cells. Moreover, there were increased numbers of activated macrophages/microglia and increased levels of virus in the brain. Since macrophages/microglia are the targets and repository for virus in the brain, and the products of infected and activated macrophages/microglia are prime candidates in the neuropathogenesis of HIV (as described in Chapter 4.1: Mononuclear Phagocyte Inflammation and Neurotoxicity), these latter two findings are likely linked to each other and potentially to the mechanism of meth's effects on HIV neuropathogenesis. In addition, increased activation of astrocytes was found in the meth-treated, HIV-infected monkeys, perhaps paralleling signs of glial activation found in imaging studies of chronic meth users (Thompson et al., 2004).

METHAMPHETAMINE AND HIV—OTHER MODELS

Another animal model for HIV is the feline immunodeficiency virus (FIV) model infection of cats (described in Chapter 5.2: Feline Immunodeficiency Virus). Meth has been found to increase the replication of FIV in cultured primary astrocytes (Gavrilin, Mathes, & Podell, 2002). In vivo, meth and FIV interact to alter brain metabolites (Cloak et al., 2004), and meth worsens the functional abnormalities induced in the CNS by FIV (Huitron-Resendiz et al., 2010).

Perhaps the best-studied interactions of meth and HIV have been investigated through in vivo studies in rodents and in vitro studies on a number of cell types, on the neurotoxic HIV accessory protein Tat. Such studies have consistently revealed that meth enhances the neuropathogenic effects of Tat (Turchan et al., 2001; Maragos et al., 2002; Flora et al., 2003; Cass, Harned, Peters, Nath, & Maragos, 2003; Conant et al., 2004; Langford et al., 2004; Theodore, Cass, & Maragos, 2006a; Theodore, Cass, & Maragos, 2006b; Theodore et al., 2006c; Cai et al., 2008). A more detailed description of Tat neurotoxicity can be found in Chapter 4.3: HIV-1 and Tat.

Three transgenic rodent models of HIV (see Chapter 5.4: Transgenics) have also been studied for the effects of meth on HIV. In one, the HIV-1 gp120 surface glycoprotein is expressed in astrocytes. Distinct differences are found between these mice and nontransgenic controls in stereotypic behaviors exhibited following meth treatment (Roberts, Maung, Sejbuk, Ake, & Kaul, 2010). In the second model, a Gag- and Pol-deficient HIV provirus is expressed fairly ubiquitously in transgenic rats. Studies of transgenic and control rats administered meth reveal increased behavioral sensitization and altered hyperthermic responses in the HIV-transgenic rats (Kass, Liu, Vigorito, Chang, & Chang, 2010; Liu et al., 2009). In the third, a transgenic mouse expressing a replication-competent HIV provirus in addition to human cyclin T1, meth administration increased viremia (Toussi et al., 2009). Thus, in spite of the caveat of dosing, these rodent studies have enabled a number of experimental paradigms to be performed. With the development of methods to simulate human meth dosing and drug levels in rodents (Segal et al., 2006), the use of these and other small animal models show great promise in helping uncover the neuropathogenic interactions of HIV and meth.

Other interesting findings have recently been identified through in vitro studies. Meth has been found to increase HIV replication in macrophages and the degree of infectivity of dendritic cells (Liang et al., 2008; Nair et al., 2009). Such studies can enable the identification of molecular mechanisms of how meth affects HIV infection and provide clues for effects to examine in vivo.

METH TOXICITY

Amphetamines are substrates for dopamine, norepinephrine, and serotonin transporters, leading to reverse transport and release of these neurotransmitters into the synapse. Reuptake of these molecules is also inhibited, leading to increased and prolonged effects at the synapse (Sulzer, Sonders, Poulsen, & Galli, 2005). While a possible receptor for some of meth's effects has been identified (Xie et al., 2009), its end effects of increasing the amounts of monoamine transmitters dominate its actions. Meth's effects on dopaminergic neuronal systems are profound and have been extensively studied. Stimulation of the dopaminergic mesolimbic reward pathway by meth is linked to meth use and addiction, whereas meth toxicity is largely documented within the nigrostriatal dopaminergic system.

A number of mechanisms have been investigated regarding meth's damaging effects, and oxidative stress is prominent among these. Excessive dopamine in the nerve terminals, released due to meth, is easily oxidized, leading to the production of dopamine quinones and superoxide radicals that can react with and modify and damage synaptic proteins (LaVoie et al., 1999). Nitric oxide, specifically its reactant product with superoxide radicals, peroxynitrite, also likely plays a role in meth neurotoxicity (Imam et al., 2001). In a number of experimental systems, treatment with antioxidants or other methods to reduce oxidative damage protected against meth's

neurotoxicity (Fukami et al., 2004; Kondo, Ito, & Sugita, 1994; De Vito et al., 1989; Cadet, Ali, & Epstein, 1994), pointing to a central role for these reactive chemical species.

Meth is metabolized by the mitochondrial cytochrome P450 (CYP) system, specifically the CYP2D6 isoenzyme. Genetic variability in this enzyme results in individuals who metabolize meth at different rates. Interestingly, chronic meth users who have an enzyme activity yielding heightened metabolism of meth have increased rates of cognitive impairment compared to those who have intermediate or lower levels of meth metabolism (Cherner et al., 2010). This implies that the oxidative metabolic products of meth are linked to the functional damage in meth users.

In addition to metabolizing meth, meth has damaging effects on mitochondria themselves. Not only are mitochondria susceptible to oxidative stress damage, but meth itself can inhibit the function of a number of the mitochondrial electron transport chain complexes (Brown, Quinton, & Yamamoto, 2005; Burrows, Gudelsky, & Yamamoto, 2000), leading to decreased energy production as well as signaling of pro-death apoptotic pathways in the neuron (Wu et al., 2007; Jimenez et al., 2004).

Further neurotoxic effects of meth have been ascribed to glutamate-mediated excitotoxicity (Battaglia et al., 2002; Sonsalla, Nicklas, & Heikkila, 1989; Stephans et al., 1994) and hyperthermia (Ali, Newport, Holson, Slikker, & Bowyer, 1994; Bowyer et al., 1994). The hyperthermia produced by meth has itself been linked to breakdown of the blood-brain barrier (BBB) (Kiyatkin, Brown, & Sharma, 2007); such damage to the BBB can induce numerous pathological changes in the CNS (see Chapter 3.1: Blood-Brain Barrier: Structure and Function, and Chapter 3.3: The blood-brain barrier in the setting of neuroinflammation). Other studies have similarly documented meth-induced damage to the BBB (Brandtzaeg, Dale, & Gabrielsen, 1992; Brandtzaeg, Jones, Flavell, & Fagerhol, 1988).

METH AND THE IMMUNE SYSTEM

Many of these toxic effects are not limited to neurons. All cells rely on mitochondria for energy production, and meth-induced damage to mitochondria has been identified in other cell types including astrocytes, endothelial cells, and cardiomyocytes (Yi et al., 2008; Lau, Senok, & Stadlin, 2000; He, 1995). Particularly germane to the HIV infection are the effects of meth on the immune system. A recent study detailed the effects of meth on mitochondria as well as cellular function in T lymphocytes (Potula et al., 2010). In this study, meth treatment had numerous effects on mitochondria, including increased superoxide production, decreased membrane potential, and lower levels of electron transport chain protein complexes. Functionally, meth-treated T cells showed lower levels of proliferation and IL-2 production. However, effects on antigen-specific immune responses were not determined in this in vitro study.

In contrast, in macrophages and dendritic cells (key immune cells in initiating immune responses), a different set of meth-induced changes was found (Talloczy et al., 2008). Meth is a weak base, and a number of cellular organelles, such as lysosomes and autophagolysosomes, maintain an acidic pH. Meth was found to collapse the physiological pH gradient in these organelles, leading to defective phagocytosis, antigen processing, and antigen presentation. Furthermore, meth impaired the ability of macrophages to control fungal infections such as those associated with HIV infection. These in vitro studies were then followed up in vivo in mice, revealing impairment of immunity to the fungal pathogen *Histoplasma capsulatum*, with inhibition of macrophage functions, antigen-specific T cell responses and antibody production, and altered cytokine production (Martinez, Mihu, Gacser, Santambrogio, & Nosanchuk, 2009).

A determination of the effects of meth on the immune system in vivo has been difficult to assess in chronic meth users. In keeping with the study on histoplasmosis above, other studies in experimental animals generally have found immunosuppressive effects (In, Son, Rhee, & Pyo, 2005; Yu et al., 2002), but others have given conflicting results, for example both stimulatory and inhibitory effects of meth on natural killer (NK) cells have been reported (Saito et al., 2006; Saito et al., 2008; In et al., 2005). Given the dosing issues with meth and rodents discussed above, and the paucity of studies in human meth users, the true nature of the effects of meth on the immune system in people remains unclear.

EFFECTS OF METH ON HUMAN CENTRAL NERVOUS SYSTEM FUNCTION

Meth is clearly associated with neuropsychological deficits, which are largely ascribed to its damage to frontostriatal systems (Scott et al., 2007). These deficits include problems in memory, executive functions, language, and motor skills. The effects of chronic meth use on monoamine neurons have been examined through positron emission tomography (PET) imaging studies, where persistent loss of the dopamine transporter (DAT) in the cortex and striatum, and serotonin transporters in the cortex, is found in chronic meth users (Sekine et al., 2003; Sekine et al., 2006; Volkow et al., 2001a; Volkow et al., 2001b). Other PET studies have revealed an activation of microglia (innate immune cells in the brain and targets for HIV infection) in regions rich in dopaminergic and serotonergic terminals, perhaps as a reaction to neuronal damage (Sekine et al., 2008). In addition to these PET studies, structural studies using high-resolution magnetic resonance imaging (MRI) have been performed on meth users. Loss of grey matter, including in the cortex and hippocampus, and increase in white matter was found, indicating neuronal damage and a potential reactive glial response (Thompson et al., 2004).

These studies have also shown linkage to functional abnormalities. PET revealed that striatal DAT deficits were correlated with motor slowing and memory impairment (Volkow et al., 2001b), whereas MRI studies showed that hippocampal deficits in meth users correlated with memory impairment on a word recall test (Thompson et al., 2004). While the exact links of neuropathologic changes to functional deficits are still being worked out, it is clear that meth abuse has broad and significant effects on the CNS and its functions.

AGING, CHRONIC HIV INFECTION, AND METH

Treatment with cART has fortunately improved both the quality of life as well as the lifespan of those infected with HIV. This now increases the time span in which meth may interact with HIV to lead to further immune impairment. However, the nature of such potential interaction remains speculative.

Perhaps more likely are effects on the CNS. As HIV-infected people age there may be an additional risk for neurocognitive disorders (see Chapter 7.8: Aging) and interactions with meth abuse such as those described above may be manifest in greater amount or severity. HIV-infected individuals are increasingly recognized as being at increased risk for a number of diseases that are typically associated with aging (Deeks et al., 2009); of note, the greatest risk factor for neurodegenerative diseases is age. While HIV used to be a disease of young adults, in the next three years it is estimated that more than half of HIV-infected individuals in the US will be greater than 50 years of age. These epidemiological trends suggest a risk of concomitant neurodegenerative disorders.

Speculations on interactions of meth and HIV in the CNS have focused largely on the striatum. Before the advent of combination antiretroviral therapy (cART), studies on HIV dementia and encephalitis often found symptoms and pathology linked to subcortical regions, specifically the striatum and other parts of the basal ganglia including the substantia nigra (SN) (Berger et al., 2000; Gray et al., 2001). While such a relationship no longer exists in the era of cART (Everall et al., 2009) decreased levels of dopamine and its metabolite homovanillic acid (HVA) are found in the basal ganglia of those with HIV compared to those without HIV infection, irrespective of cART or degree of neurocognitive impairment (Kumar et al., 2009). Others have found decreased HVA as well as another dopamine metabolite, 3,4-dihydroxy phenylacetic acid (DOPAC), in the cerebrospinal fluid (CSF) of HIV-infected people, which correlated with hyperechogenicity of the SN, as determined by transcranial ultrasound (Obermann et al., 2009). Studies in the SIV/monkey model have also revealed dopaminergic deficits (Scheller et al., 2005).

Meth clearly damages the dopaminergic nerve terminals in the nigrostriatal pathways, documented in the animal and human studies described above as well as post-mortem studies of the brains of chronic meth users (Wilson et al., 1996). This thus leads to the hypothesis of a synergistic damaging effect on dopaminergic systems of HIV and meth. While this interaction could take many forms, one possibility relates to parkinsonism.

Parkinson's disease (PD) is a primarily a disease of aging, affecting 0.8% of those over 65 years of age, and is the most common neurodegenerative movement disorder (Savitt, Dawson, & Dawson, 2006). Loss of dopaminergic neurons in

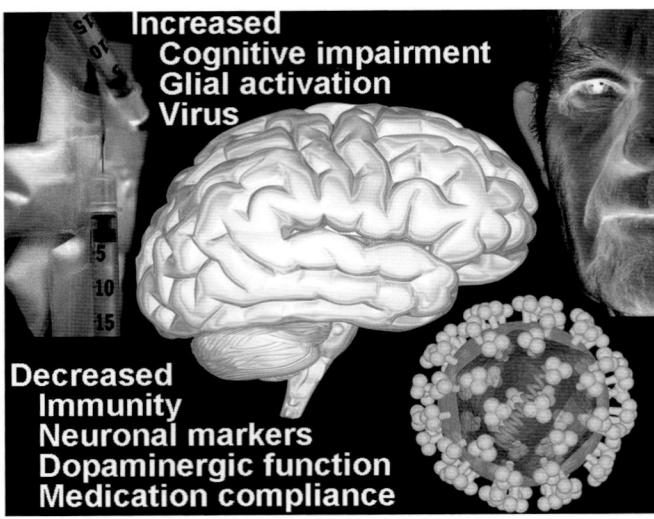

Figure 4.6.2 Meth, HIV, and aging can individually and collectively lead to neurodegenerative disorders.

the SN, and their terminals and dopamine itself in the striatum, underlies the pathology of PD and therein lays the potential link to HIV and meth. As described, damage to the striatum and dopaminergic dysregulation can be found in HIV, and motor dysfunction can be a prominent part of HIV-induced neurological disease (see Chapter 7.2: HIV-Associated Neurological Disorders); with frank HIV-related PD found predominantly late in the disease course (Tse et al., 2004). Similarly, meth produces damage to the nigrostriatal dopaminergic systems. PD-like dopaminergic damage and functional effects on the motor systems can be found in meth users (Volkow et al., 2001a). While the risk of PD in meth users is unclear, a retrospective study of PD patients (using spouses as controls) found that prolonged use of meth and/or amphetamine resulted in a significant eightfold increased risk of PD (Garwood, Bekele, McCulloch, & Christine, 2006). Aging, HIV, and meth may represent a triumvirate of damage leading to PD or neurodegenerative disorders (Figure 4.6.2).

SUMMARY

Due to the great overlap in the meth-using and HIV-infected (and at risk for infection) populations, meth is and will likely continue to be a relevant comorbid factor in HIV-induced disease, including HAND. Current findings indicate that effects on viral load in the blood may be due to lowered medication regimen compliance, whereas effects on the brain may be due to effects on immune cells or glia, whether primary or a secondary response to neuronal damage. Future efforts should focus of course on meth abstinence, as well as antiviral medications and regimens designed for enhanced compliance. Studies are needed on the effects of meth on the immune system in humans or systems relevant to people, and on the mechanisms by which meth results in increased HAND. Furthermore, as HIV-infected people age, the possibility of an increased risk for neurodegenerative disorders,

in particular PD, should be examined, especially in those who have used meth.

ACKNOWLEDGMENTS

The author's effort is supported by NIH grants DA032513, DA026146, MH073490, and MH062261. The author declares no conflict of interest.

REFERENCES

Ali, S. F., Newport, G. D., Holson, R. R., Slikker, W. Jr., & Bowyer, J. F. (1994). Low environmental temperatures or pharmacologic agents that produce hypothermia decrease methamphetamine neurotoxicity in mice. *Brain Res, 658*(1–2), 33–8.

Battaglia, G., Fornai, F., Busceti, C. L., Aloisi, G., Cerrito, F., De Blasi, A., et al. (2002). Selective blockade of mGlu5 metabotropic glutamate receptors is protective against methamphetamine neurotoxicity. *J Neurosci, 22*(6), 2135–41.

Berger, J. R. & Arendt, G. (2000). HIV dementia: The role of the basal ganglia and dopaminergic systems. *J Psychopharmacol, 14*(3), 214–21.

Bowyer, J. F., Davies, D. L., Schmued, L., Broening, H. W., Newport, G. D., Slikker, W. Jr., et al. 1994. Further studies of the role of hyperthermia in methamphetamine neurotoxicity. *J Pharmacol Exp Ther, 268*(3), 1571–80.

Brandtzaeg, P., Dale, I., & Gabrielsen, T. O. (1992). The leucocyte protein L1 (calprotectin): Usefulness as an immunohistochemical marker antigen and putative biological function. *Histopathology, 21*(2), 191–6.

Brandtzaeg, P., Jones, D. B., Flavell, D. J., & Fagerhol, M. K. (1988). Mac 387 antibody and detection of formalin resistant myelomonocytic L1 antigen. *J Clin Pathol, 41*(9), 963–70.

Brown, J. M., Quinton, M. S., & Yamamoto, B. K. (2005). Methamphetamine-induced inhibition of mitochondrial complex II: Roles of glutamate and peroxynitrite. *J Neurochem, 95*(2), 429–36.

Buchacz, K., McFarland, W., Kellogg, T. A., Loeb, L., Holmberg, S. D., Dilley, J., et al. (2005). Amphetamine use is associated with increased HIV incidence among men who have sex with men in San Francisco. *AIDS, 19*(13), 1423–4.

Burrows, K. B., Gudelsky, G., & Yamamoto, B. K. (2000). Rapid and transient inhibition of mitochondrial function following methamphetamine or 3,4-methylenedioxymethamphetamine administration. *Eur J Pharmacol, 398*(1), 11–8.

Cadet, J. L., Ali, S., & Epstein, C. (1994). Involvement of oxygen-based radicals in methamphetamine-induced neurotoxicity: Evidence from the use of CuZnSOD transgenic mice. *Ann N Y Acad Sci, 738*, 388–91.

Cadet, J. L., Jayanthi, S., & Deng, X. (2003). Speed kills: Cellular and molecular bases of methamphetamine-induced nerve terminal degeneration and neuronal apoptosis. *Faseb J, 17*(13), 1775–88.

Cai, N. S. & Cadet, J. L. (2008). The combination of methamphetamine and of the HIV protein, Tat, induces death of the human neuroblastoma cell line, SH-SY5Y. *Synapse, 62*(7), 551–2.

Cass, W. A., Harned, M. E., Peters, L. E., Nath, A., & Maragos, W. F. (2003). HIV-1 protein Tat potentiation of methamphetamine-induced decreases in evoked overflow of dopamine in the striatum of the rat. *Brain Res, 984*(1–2), 133–42.

Chana, G., Everall, I. P., Crews, L., Langford, D., Adame, A., Grant, I., et al. (2006). Cognitive deficits and degeneration of interneurons in HIV+ methamphetamine users. *Neurology, 67*(8), 1486–9.

Chang, L., Ernst, T., Speck, O., & Grob, C. S. (2005). Additive effects of HIV and chronic methamphetamine use on brain metabolite abnormalities. *Am J Psychiatry, 162*(2), 361–9.

Cherner, M., Bousman, C., Everall, I., Barron, D., Letendre, S., Vaida, F., et al. (2010). Cytochrome P450–2D6 extensive metabolizers are more vulnerable to methamphetamine-associated neurocognitive impairment: Preliminary findings. *J Int Neuropsychol Soc*, 1–12.

Chesney, M. A., Barrett, D. C., & Stall, R. (1998). Histories of substance use and risk behavior: Precursors to HIV seroconversion in homosexual men. *Am J Public Health*, 88(1), 113–6.

Cloak, C. C., Chang, L., Ernst, T., Barr, M. C., Huitron-Resendiz, S., Sanchez-Alavez, M., et al. (2004). Methamphetamine and AIDS: 1HMRS studies in a feline model of human disease. *J Neuroimmunol*, 147(1–2), 16–20.

Conant, K., St Hillaire, C., Anderson, C., Galey, D., Wang, J., & Nath, A. (2004). Human immunodeficiency virus type 1 Tat and methamphetamine affect the release and activation of matrix-degrading proteinases. *J Neurovirol*, 10(1), 21–8.

Coutinho, A., Flynn, C., Burdo, T. H., Mervis, R. F., & Fox, H. S. (2008). Chronic methamphetamine induces structural changes in frontal cortex neurons and upregulates type I interferons. *J Neuroimmune Pharmacol*, 3(4), 241–5.

De Vito, M. J. & Wagner, G. C. (1989). Methamphetamine-induced neuronal damage: A possible role for free radicals. *Neuropharmacology*, 28(10), 1145–50.

Deeks, S. G. & Phillips, A. N. (2009). HIV infection, antiretroviral treatment, ageing, and non-AIDS related morbidity. *BMJ*, 338, a 3172.

Ellis, R. J., Childers, M. E., Cherner, M., Lazzaretto, D., Letendre, S., & Grant, I. (2003). Increased human immunodeficiency virus loads in active methamphetamine users are explained by reduced effectiveness of antiretroviral therapy. *J Infect Dis*, 188(12), 1820–6.

Everall, I., Salaria, S., Roberts, E., Corbeil, J., Sasik, R., Fox, H., et al. (2005). Methamphetamine stimulates interferon inducible genes in HIV infected brain. *J Neuroimmunol*, 170(1–2), 158–71.

Everall, I., Vaida, F., Khanlou, N., Lazzaretto, D., Achim, C., Letendre, S., et al. (2009). Cliniconeuropathologic correlates of human immunodeficiency virus in the era of antiretroviral therapy. *Journal of Neurovirology*, 15(5–6), 360–70.

Flora, G., Lee, Y. W., Nath, A., Hennig, B., Maragos, W., & Toborek, M. (2003). Methamphetamine potentiates HIV-1 Tat protein-mediated activation of redox-sensitive pathways in discrete regions of the brain. *Exp Neurol*, 179(1), 60–70.

Fukami, G., Hashimoto, K., Koike, K., Okamura, N., Shimizu, E., & Iyo, M. (2004). Effect of antioxidant N-acetyl-L-cysteine on behavioral changes and neurotoxicity in rats after administration of methamphetamine. *Brain Res*, 1016(1), 90–5.

Garwood, E. R., Bekele, W., McCulloch, C. E., & Christine, C. W. (2006). Amphetamine exposure is elevated in Parkinson's disease. *Neurotoxicology*, 27(6), 1003–6.

Gavrilin, M. A., Mathes, L. E., & Podell, M. (2002). Methamphetamine enhances cell-associated feline immunodeficiency virus replication in astrocytes. *J Neurovirol*, 8(3), 240–9.

Gray, F., Adle-Biassette, H., Chretien, F., Lorin de la Grandmaison, G., Force, G., & Keohane. C. (2001). Neuropathology and neurodegeneration in human immunodeficiency virus infection. Pathogenesis of HIV-induced lesions of the brain, correlations with HIV-associated disorders and modifications according to treatments. *Clin Neuropathol*, 20(4), 146–55.

Halkitis, P. N., Kutnick, A. H., & Slater, S. (2005). The social realities of adherence to protease inhibitor regimens: Substance use, health care and psychological states. *J Health Psychol*, 10(4), 545–58.

He, S. Y. (1995). Methamphetamine-induced toxicity in cultured adult rat cardiomyocytes. *Nihon Hoigaku Zasshi*, 49(3), 175–86.

Huitron-Resendiz, S., Henriksen, S. J., Barr, M. C., Testa, M. P., Crawford, E., Parsons, L. H., et al. (2010). Methamphetamine and lentivirus interactions: Reciprocal enhancement of central nervous system disease. *Journal of Neurovirology*, 16(4), 268–78.

Hurt, C. B., Torrone, E., Green, K., Foust, E., Leone, P., & Hightow-Weidman, L. (2010). Methamphetamine use among newly diagnosed HIV-positive young men in North Carolina, United States, from 2000 to 2005. *PLoS ONE*, 5(6), e1 314.

Imam, S. Z., Newport, G. D., Itzhak, Y., Cadet, J. L., Islam, F., Slikker, W. Jr., et al. (2001). Peroxynitrite plays a role in methamphetamine-induced dopaminergic neurotoxicity: Evidence from mice lacking neuronal nitric oxide synthase gene or overexpressing copper-zinc superoxide dismutase. *J Neurochem*, 76(3), 745–9.

In, S. W., Son, E. W., Rhee, D. K., & Pyo, S. (2005). Methamphetamine administration produces immunomodulation in mice. *J Toxicol Environ Health A*, 68(23–24), 2133–45.

Jernigan, T. L., Gamst, A. C., Archibald, S. L., Fennema-Notestine, C., Mindt, M. R., Marcotte, T. D., et al. (2005). Effects of methamphetamine dependence and HIV infection on cerebral morphology. *Am J Psychiatry*, 162(8), 1461–72.

Jimenez, A., Jorda, E. G., Verdaguer, E., Pubill, D., Sureda, F. X., Canudas, A. M., et al. (2004). Neurotoxicity of amphetamine derivatives is mediated by caspase pathway activation in rat cerebellar granule cells. *Toxicol Appl Pharmacol*, 196(2), 223–34.

Kass, M. D., Liu, X., Vigorito, M., Chang, L., & Chang, S. L. (2010). Methamphetamine-Induced Behavioral and Physiological Effects in Adolescent and Adult HIV-1 Transgenic Rats. *J Neuroimmune Pharmacol*.

King, W. D., Larkins, S., Hucks-Ortiz, C., Wang, P. C., Gorbach, P. M., Veniegas, R., et al. (2009). Factors associated with HIV viral load in a respondent driven sample in Los Angeles. *AIDS Behav*, 13(1), 145–53.

Kita, T., Wagner, G. C., & Nakashima, T. (2003). Current research on methamphetamine-induced neurotoxicity: Animal models of monoamine disruption. *J Pharmacol Sci*, 92(3), 178–95.

Kiyatkin, E. A., Brown, P. L., & Sharma, H. S. (2007). Brain edema and breakdown of the blood-brain barrier during methamphetamine intoxication: Critical role of brain hyperthermia. *Eur J Neurosci*, 26(5), 1242–53.

Koblin, B. A., Husnik, M. J., Colfax, G., Huang, Y., Madison, M., Mayer, K., et al. (2006). Risk factors for HIV infection among men who have sex with men. *AIDS*, 20(5), 731–9.

Kondo, T., Ito, T., & Sugita, Y. (1994). Bromocriptine scavenges methamphetamine-induced hydroxyl radicals and attenuates dopamine depletion in mouse striatum. *Ann N Y Acad Sci*, 738, 222–9.

Kumar, A. M., Fernandez, J. B., Singer, E. J., Commins, D., Waldrop-Valverde, D., Ownby, R. L., et al. (2009). Human immunodeficiency virus type 1 in the central nervous system leads to decreased dopamine in different regions of postmortem human brains. *J Neurovirology*, 15(3), 257–74.

Lambert, E., Normand, J., Stall, R., Aral, S., & Vlahov, D. (2005). Introduction: New dynamics of HIV risk among drug-using men who have sex with men. *J Urban Health*, 82(1 Suppl 1), i1–8.

Langford, D., Adame, A., Grigorian, A., Grant, I., McCutchan, J. A., Ellis, R. J., et al. (2003). Patterns of selective neuronal damage in methamphetamine-user AIDS patients. *J Acquir Immune Defic Syndr*, 34(5), 467–74.

Langford, D., Grigorian, A., Hurford, R., Adame, A., Crews, L., & Masliah, E. (2004). The role of mitochondrial alterations in the combined toxic effects of human immunodeficiency virus Tat protein and methamphetamine on calbindin positive-neurons. *J Neurovirol*, 10(6), 327–37.

Lau, J. W., Senok, S., & Stadlin, A. (2000). Methamphetamine-induced oxidative stress in cultured mouse astrocytes. *Ann N Y Acad Sci*, 914, 146–56.

LaVoie, M. J. & Hastings, T. G. (1999). Dopamine quinone formation and protein modification associated with the striatal neurotoxicity of methamphetamine: Evidence against a role for extracellular dopamine. *J Neurosci*, 19(4), 1484–91.

Liang, H., Wang, X., Chen, H., Song, L., Ye, L., Wang, S. H., et al. (2008). Methamphetamine enhances HIV infection of macrophages. *Amer J Pathology*, 172(6), 1617–24.

Liu, X., Chang, L., Vigorito, M., Kass, M., Li, H., & Chang, S. L. (2009). Methamphetamine-induced behavioral sensitization is enhanced in the HIV-1 transgenic rat. *J Neuroimmune Pharmacol*, 4(3), 309–16.

Madden, L. J., Flynn, C. T., Zandonatti, M. A., May, M., Parsons, L. H., Katner, S. N., et al. (2005). Modeling human methamphetamine exposure in nonhuman primates: Chronic dosing in the rhesus macaque leads to behavioral and physiological abnormalities. *Neuropsychopharmacology*, 30(2), 350–9.

Maragos, W. F., Young, K. L., Turchan, J. T., Guseva, M., Pauly, J. R., Nath, A., et al. (2002). Human immunodeficiency virus-1 Tat protein and methamphetamine interact synergistically to impair striatal dopaminergic function. *J Neurochem*, 83(4), 955–63.

Marcondes, M. C., Flynn, C., Watry, D. D., Zandonatti, M., & Fox, H. S. (2010). Methamphetamine increases brain viral load and activates natural killer cells in simian immunodeficiency virus-infected monkeys. *Amer J Pathology, 177* (1), 355–61.

Martinez, L. R., Mihu, M. R., Gacser, A., Santambrogio, L., & Nosanchuk, J. D. (2009). Methamphetamine enhances histoplasmosis by immunosuppression of the host. *J Infectious Diseases, 200* (1), 131–41.

Masliah, E., Roberts, E. S., Langford, D., Everall, I., Crews, L, Adame, A., et al. (2004). Patterns of gene dysregulation in the frontal cortex of patients with HIV encephalitis. *J Neuroimmunol, 157* (1–2), 163–75.

Melega, W. P., Jorgensen, M. J., Lacan, G., Way, B. M., Pham, J., Morton, G., et al. (2007). Long-term methamphetamine administration in the Vervet monkey models aspects of a human exposure: Brain neurotoxicity and behavioral profiles. *Neuropsychopharmacology*.

Mithoefer, M. C., Wagner, M. T., Mithoefer, A. T., Jerome, I., & Doblin, R. (2010). The safety and efficacy of {+/-}3,4-methylenedioxymethamphetamine-assisted psychotherapy in subjects with chronic, treatment-resistant posttraumatic stress disorder: The first randomized controlled pilot study. *J Psychopharmacol*.

Molitor, F., Ruiz, J. D., Flynn, N., Mikanda, J. N., Sun, R. K., & Anderson, R. (1999). Methamphetamine use and sexual and injection risk behaviors among out-of-treatment injection drug users. *Am J Drug Alcohol Abuse, 25* (3), 475–93.

Molitor, F., Truax, S. R., Ruiz, J. D., & Sun, R. K. (1998). Association of methamphetamine use during sex with risky sexual behaviors and HIV infection among non-injection drug users. *West J Med, 168* (2), 93–7.

Moss, A. R., Hahn, J. A., Perry, S., Charlebois, E. D., Guzman, D., Clark, R. A., et al. (2004). Adherence to highly active antiretroviral therapy in the homeless population in San Francisco: A prospective study. *Clin Infect Dis, 39* (8), 1190–8.

Nair, M. P., Saiyed, Z. M., Nair, N., Gandhi, N. H., Rodriguez, J. W., Boukli, N., et al. (2009). Methamphetamine enhances HIV-1 infectivity in monocyte-derived dendritic cells. *J Neuroimmune Pharmacol, 4* (1), 129–39.

Obermann, M., Kuper, M., Kastrup, O., Yaldizli, O., Esser, S., Thiermann, J., et al. (2009). Substantia nigra hyperechogenicity and CSF dopamine depletion in HIV. *J Neurol, 256* (6), 948–53.

Plankey, M. W., Ostrow, D. G., Stall, R., Cox, C., Li, X., Peck, J. A., et al. (2007). The relationship between methamphetamine and popper use and risk of HIV seroconversion in the multicenter AIDS cohort study. *JAIDS, 45* (1), 85–92.

Potula, R., Hawkins, B. J., Cenna, J. M., Fan, S., Dykstra, H., Ramirez, S. H., et al. (2010). Methamphetamine causes mitochondrial oxidative damage in human T lymphocytes leading to functional impairment. *J Immunol*.

Rawson, R. A. & Condon, T. P. (2007). Why do we need an addiction supplement focused on methamphetamine? *Addiction, 102* Suppl 1, 1–4.

Reback, C. J., Larkins, S., & Shoptaw, S. (2003). Methamphetamine abuse as a barrier to HIV medication adherence among gay and bisexual men. *AIDS Care, 15* (6), 775–85.

Rippeth, J. D., Heaton, R. K., Carey, C. L., Marcotte, T. D., Moore, D. J., Gonzalez, R., et al. (2004). Methamphetamine dependence increases risk of neuropsychological impairment in HIV infected persons. *J Int Neuropsychol Soc, 10*(1), 1–14.

Roberts, A. J., Maung, R., Sejbuk, N. E., Ake, C., & Kaul, M. (2010). Alteration of Methamphetamine-induced stereotypic behaviour in transgenic mice expressing HIV-1 envelope protein gp120. *J Neurosci Methods, 186* (2), 222–5.

Roehr, B. (2005). Half a million Americans use methamphetamine every week. *BMJ, 331* (7515), 476.

Rotheram-Borus, M. J., Luna, G. C., Marotta, T., & Kelly, H. (1994). Going nowhere fast: Methamphetamine use and HIV infection. *NIDA Res Monogr, 143*:, 155–82.

Saito, M., Terada, M., Kawata, T., Ito, H., Shigematsu, N., Kromkhun, P., et al. (2008). Effects of single or repeated administrations of methamphetamine on immune response in mice. *Exp Anim, 57*(1), 35–43.

Saito, M., Yamaguchi, T., Kawata, T., Ito, H., Kanai, T., Terada, M., et al. (2006). Effects of methamphetamine on cortisone concentration, NK cell activity, and mitogen response of T-lymphocytes in female cynomolgus monkeys. *Exp Anim, 55* (5), 477–81.

Savitt, J. M., Dawson, V. L., & Dawson, T. M. (2006). Diagnosis and treatment of Parkinson disease: Molecules to medicine. *J Clin Invest, 116* (7), 1744–54.

Scheller, C., Sopper, S., Jenuwein, M., Neuen-Jacob, E., Tatschner, T., Grunblatt, E., et al. (2005). Early impairment in dopaminergic neurotransmission in brains of SIV-infected rhesus monkeys due to microglia activation. *J Neurochem*.

Scott, J. C., Woods, S. P., Matt, G. E., Meyer, R. A., Heaton, R. K., Atkinson, J. H., et al. (2007). Neurocognitive effects of methamphetamine: A critical review and meta-analysis. *Neuropsychol Rev, 17* (3), 275–97.

Segal, D. S. & Kuczenski, R. (2006). Human methamphetamine pharmacokinetics simulated in the rat: Single daily intravenous administration reveals elements of sensitization and tolerance. *Neuropsychopharmacology, 31* (5), 941–55.

Sekine, Y., Minabe, Y., Ouchi, Y., Takei, N., Iyo, M., Nakamura, K., et al. (2003). Association of dopamine transporter loss in the orbitofrontal and dorsolateral prefrontal cortices with methamphetamine-related psychiatric symptoms. *Am J Psychiatry, 160* (9), 1699–701.

Sekine, Y., Ouchi, Y., Sugihara, G., Takei, N., Yoshikawa, E., Nakamura, K., et al. (2008). Methamphetamine causes microglial activation in the brains of human abusers. *J Neurosci, 28* (22), 5756–61.

Sekine, Y., Ouchi, Y., Takei, N., Yoshikawa, E., Nakamura, K., Futatsubashi, M., et al. (2006). Brain serotonin transporter density and aggression in abstinent methamphetamine abusers. *Arch Gen Psychiatry, 63* (1), 90–100.

Simon, S. L., Richardson, K., Dacey, J., Glynn, S., Domier, C. P., Rawson, R. A. et al. (2002). A comparison of patterns of methamphetamine and cocaine use. *J Addict Dis, 21* (1), 35–44.

Sonsalla, P. K., Nicklas, W. J., & Heikkila, R. E. (1989). Role for excitatory amino acids in methamphetamine-induced nigrostriatal dopaminergic toxicity. *Science, 243* (4889), 398–400.

Stephans, S. E. & Yamamoto, B. K. (1994). Methamphetamine-induced neurotoxicity: roles for glutamate and dopamine efflux. *Synapse, 17* (3), 203–9.

Sulzer, D., Sonders, M. S., Poulsen, N. W., & Galli, A. (2005). Mechanisms of neurotransmitter release by amphetamines: A review. *Prog Neurobiol, 75* (6), 406–33.

Sun, B., Abadjian, L., Rempel, H., Calosing, C., Rothlind, J., & Pulliam, L. (2010). Peripheral biomarkers do not correlate with cognitive impairment in highly active antiretroviral therapy-treated subjects with human immunodeficiency virus type 1 infection. *Journal of Neurovirology, 16* (2), 115–24.

Talloczy, Z., Martinez, J., Joset, D., Ray, Y., Gacser, A., Toussi, S., et al. (2008). Methamphetamine inhibits antigen processing, presentation, and phagocytosis. *PLoS Pathog, 4* (2), e28.

Theodore, S., Cass, W. A., & Maragos, W. F. (2006a). Involvement of cytokines in human immunodeficiency virus-1 protein Tat and methamphetamine interactions in the striatum. *Exp Neurol, 199* (2), 490–8.

Theodore, S., Cass, W. A., & Maragos, W. F. (2006b). Methamphetamine and human immunodeficiency virus protein Tat synergize to destroy dopaminergic terminals in the rat striatum. *Neuroscience, 137* (3), 925–35.

Theodore, S., Cass, W. A., Nath, A., Steiner, J., Young, K., & Maragos, W. F. (2006c). Inhibition of tumor necrosis factor-alpha signaling prevents human immunodeficiency virus-1 protein Tat and methamphetamine interaction. *Neurobiol Dis, 23* (3), 663–8.

Thompson, P. M., Hayashi, K. M., Simon, S. L., Geaga, J. A., Hong, M. S., Sui, Y., et al. (2004). Structural abnormalities in the brains of human subjects who use methamphetamine. *J Neurosci, 24* (26), 6028–36.

Toussi, S. S., Joseph, A., Zheng, J. H., Dutta, M., Santambrogio, L., & Goldstein, H. (2009). Short communication: Methamphetamine treatment increases in vitro and in vivo HIV replication. *AIDS Res Hum Retroviruses*, 25 (11), 1117–21.

Tse, W., Cersosimo, M. G., Gracies, J. M., Morgello, S., Olanow, C. W., & Koller, W. (2004). Movement disorders and AIDS: A review. *Parkinsonism Relat Disord*, 10 (6), 323–34.

Turchan, J., Anderson, C., Hauser, K. F., Sun, Q., Zhang, J., Liu, Y., et al. (2001). Estrogen protects against the synergistic toxicity by HIV proteins, methamphetamine and cocaine. *BMC Neurosci*, 2 (1), 3.

Vitiello, B., Goodkin, K., Ashtana, D., Shapshak, P., Atkinson, J. H., Heseltine, P. N., et al. (2007). HIV-1 RNA concentration and cognitive performance in a cohort of HIV-positive people. *AIDS*, 21 (11), 1415–22.

Volkow, N. D., Chang, L., Wang, G. J., Fowler, J. S., Franceschi, D., Sedler, M., et al. (2001a). Loss of dopamine transporters in methamphetamine abusers recovers with protracted abstinence. *J Neurosci, 21* (23), 9414–8.

Volkow, N. D., Chang, L., Wang, G. J., Fowler, J. S., Leonido-Yee, M., Franceschi, D., et al. (2001b). Association of dopamine transporter reduction with psychomotor impairment in methamphetamine abusers. *Am J Psychiatry, 158* (3), 377–82.

Vongsheree, S., Sri-Ngam, P., Ruchusatsawat, N., Thaisri, H., Puangtabtim, W., Phutiprawan, T., et al. (2001). High HIV-1 prevalence among metamphetamine users in central Thailand, 1999–2000. *J Med Assoc Thai, 84* (9), 1263–7.

Wilson, J. M., Kalasinsky, K. S., Levey, A. I., Bergeron, C., Reiber, G., Anthony, R. M., et al. (1996). Striatal dopamine nerve terminal markers in human, chronic methamphetamine users. *Nat Med, 2* (6), 699–703.

Wu, C. W., Ping, Y. H., Yen, J. C., Chang, C. Y., Wang, S. F., Yeh, C. L., et al. (2007). Enhanced oxidative stress and aberrant mitochondrial biogenesis in human neuroblastoma SH-SY5Y cells during methamphetamine induced apoptosis. *Toxicol Appl Pharmacol, 220* (3), 243–51.

Xie, Z. & Miller, G. M. (2009). A receptor mechanism for methamphetamine action in dopamine transporter regulation in brain. *J Pharmacol Exp Ther, 330* (1), 316–25.

Yi, S. H., Ren, L., Yang, T. T., Liu, L., Wang, H., & Liu, Q. (2008). Myocardial lesions after long-term administration of methamphetamine in rats. *Chin Med Sci J, 23* (4), 239–43.

Yu, Q., D. Zhang, M. Walston, J. Zhang, Y. Liu, and R. R. Watson. (2002). Chronic methamphetamine exposure alters immune function in normal and retrovirus-infected mice. *Int Immunopharmacol, 2* (7), 951–62.

4.7

HIV-1 AND OPIOIDS

Toby K. Eisenstein, Jessica Breslow, Changcheng Song, Mathew J. Finley,
William D. Cornwell, Sumedha Chugh, Joseph J. Meissler, and Thomas J. Rogers

The opioid drugs of abuse have marked effects on many aspects of the immune system. As one example, μ-, κ-, and δ-opioid receptors are expressed on several hematopoietic cell populations, and opioid ligands selective for these receptors can influence HIV replication when added to human lymphoid, monocytic, or microglial cultures in vitro. Nonetheless, determining whether opioid abuse alters the progression of HIV infection has proven difficult. Epidemiological studies are complicated by the fact that drug abusers typically take combinations of drugs, which may include cocaine, marijuana, alcohol, and/or nicotine from cigarette smoke, and these drugs can have opposing effects on cells of the immune system. Even when groups of individuals use the same combination of drugs, the ratios among the drugs, the doses, and the frequency of dosing is far from uniform. In addition, although laboratory evidence points to many potential direct and indirect pathways by which opioids might influence viral replication, the absence of small animal models to test HIV infectivity has imposed significant challenges. It is hoped that new studies currently underway, using the SIV/macaque model, will address more directly the influence of opioids on the progression of AIDS and the development of HIV-associated neurodegeneration. This chapter reviews many lines of research bearing on the influence of exogenous opioids on HIV disease.

INTRODUCTION: DRUGS OF ABUSE AND HIV EPIDEMIOLOGIC INTERSECTIONS

During the earlier years of the AIDS epidemic (1996), one-third of HIV-infected individuals in the United States were identified as intravenous drug users (IVDUs) (CDC, 1996). As the epidemic became more controlled, the at-risk populations have shifted somewhat, so that in 2007, cases of HIV due to high-risk heterosexual contact increased, concomitantly lowering the percentage of IVDU-associated cases to 12.9% (Grigoryan et al., 2009). However, intravenous drug abuse is presently still the third most frequent risk factor for HIV infection in the United States (Grigoryan et al., 2009). This staggering intersection of these two afflictions raises the possibility of causality, although higher rates of HIV in IVDUs could simply be due to increased exposure to the virus. In fact, transmission of HIV by contaminated needles is, undoubtedly, a major mode of infection in the drug

abusing population, as strategies to reduce needle sharing and to encourage disinfection if sharing occurs, do reduce the risk of viral transmission (Chaisson et al., 1987; Des Jarlais et al., 1988; Friedland et al., 1985; McCoy et al., 1998). High-risk sexual behavior, which is associated with drug use, also correlates with HIV infection, probably due to greater risk of exposure to the virus. However, there are other hypotheses for how drugs of abuse might lead to increased rates of HIV infection. There is in vitro evidence that opioids and other drugs of abuse increase HIV replication (see below). Also, several abused drugs, in particular opioids, have been shown to induce significant immunosuppression. These observations have raised the question as to whether the drugs themselves may lead to increased sensitivity to infection with HIV or to faster progression of the disease (Donahoe & Falek, 1988). Epidemiologic studies have led to mixed conclusions on this point, with some studies showing a faster progression to AIDS in IVDUs (Selwyn et al., 1992; Rothenberg et al., 1986; Des Jarlais et al., 1987), and others not (Margolick et al., 1994; Margolick et al., 1992). Two studies have concluded that drug use slows progression to AIDS (Spijkerman et al., 1995; Spijkerman et al., 1996). It is important to take cognizance of the variables that can confound the epidemiologic studies and conclusions. First, most abusers use more than one drug, including cocaine, marijuana, nicotine, and alcohol, and few epidemiologic studies have tried to control for this very important variable (Crum et al., 1996). One interesting report found that intravenous cocaine lead to a higher risk of HIV infection than heroin abuse without cocaine (Anthony et al., 1991). A more recent study found that smoking crack cocaine was an independent risk factor for HIV seroconversion among IVDUs (DeBeck et al., 2009). In another study, crack cocaine itself was found to facilitate HIV progression (Baum et al., 2008), which shows the importance of identifying the spectrum of drugs being abused in HIV-infected populations used for epidemiologic studies, as different classes of drugs may have opposite, additive, or super-additive effects. A primary consideration is that in most epidemiologic studies investigators relied on either self-reports or drug screening at intervals of months as the basis for documentation of drug usage, both relatively unreliable criteria for assessment. Second, it is documented that severity of initial infection (Vanhems et al., 1998; Lindback et al., 1994; Veugelers et al., 1997), as well as HIV viral load, are predictors of clinical progression and survival (Lyles et al., 1999),

338

but there are no epidemiologic studies testing whether the threshold for HIV infection (i.e., the minimal infectious dose) is altered by drugs of abuse. Third, the metrics applied by several of the early epidemiologic studies to determine HIV progression were rather insensitive, such as decline in CD4 counts. The range of CD4 counts was quite large among the drug and non-drug-user cohorts, so that subtle changes may have been missed (Margolick et al., 1994). Fourth, in the era of highly active antiretroviral therapy (HAART), drug abuse may lead to reduced adherence to antiviral regimens (Baum et al., 2008). Fifth, drug abusers have increased incidence of other infections (Hussey & Katz, 1950; Louria et al., 1967; Haverkos & Lange, 1990) including hepatitis B and C (Garfein et al., 1996), right side endocarditis (Reiner et al., 1976; Levine, 1991), soft tissue abscesses (Haverkos & Lange, 1990), and pneumonia (Scheidegger & Zimmerli, 1989), all of which may alter immune function in ways that could impinge on the capacity to contain HIV replication or could lead to HIV activation through stimulation or suppression of the immune system. Finally, there may be differences in alteration of immune function and effects on HIV burden resulting from differences in frequency of drug use, drug dosage, and in frequency, severity, and duration of episodes of withdrawal. Chronic opioid abusers, compared with novice users, may keep themselves from withdrawal by maintaining their habit. Withdrawal from heroin in humans has been reported to be immunosuppressive, which could affect HIV progression (Govitrapong et al., 1998). Data from studies with monkeys suggest that chronic use of morphine is less detrimental to progression of SIV than withdrawal (Donahoe et al., 1993; Donahoe et al., 2009). The reader is referred to an excellent review by Donahoe and Vlahov that discusses the above points in depth (Donahoe & Vlahov, 1998). In summary, knowing the particular drug(s) used and the pattern of use are essential. The term "drug abuse" does not denote anything about the specifics of the drug and does not constitute a single entity.

The complexities of the epidemiologic reports make laboratory studies testing the effects of drugs of abuse on HIV progression very attractive. However, the lack of direct infectivity of HIV for any small animal has stymied a direct attack on the question. There are, however, two reports in the literature testing the effect of opioids on simian immunodeficiency virus (SIV) progression in monkeys, and one study testing the effect of cocaine on HIV load in severe-combined immunodeficiency (SCID) mice inoculated with human lymphoid cells harboring HIV. There are also studies on the effects of drugs of abuse on other infections, some of which are retroviral, and others are opportunistic infections in AIDS. In addition, there are a number of reports where abused drugs, in particular opioids, were added to human lymphocytes, macrophages, or microglia infected with HIV, and significant effects on viral replication were observed. Drugs of abuse have also been found to alter chemokines and chemokine receptor expression or signaling, with obvious implications for changing HIV infectivity. Together, these findings, which will be reviewed in this chapter, present robust evidence that drugs of abuse have the potential to alter the course of HIV infection in humans.

EFFECTS OF DRUGS OF ABUSE ON IN VITRO REPLICATION OF HIV

Peterson and colleagues (Peterson et al., 1990) reported in one of the earlier studies that morphine treatment promoted the growth of HIV in vitro. They showed that peripheral blood mononuclear cells (PBMCs) from normal humans, when co-cultured with morphine in the presence of HIV-infected lymphocytes, resulted in an increase in HIV-1 infectivity. This effect was reversible with a specific opioid receptor antagonist, suggesting that the morphine mediated its effects directly through classical opioid receptors. This group (Peterson et al., 1994) also showed that co-culture of a chronically infected promonocytic cell line, U1, with lipopolysaccharide (LPS)-stimulated human fetal brain cells, enhanced HIV replication. Moreover, pretreatment of the brain cells with morphine before the addition of LPS augmented the capacity of the brain cells to induce HIV replication. Neutralizing antibodies against tumor necrosis factor (TNF)-α and interleukin (IL)-6 blocked the effect of morphine in these cultures. These studies suggested that the mechanism by which morphine acted as a cofactor for enhanced HIV replication was dependent on increased production of these cytokines by the LPS-stimulated brain cells (Peterson et al., 1994). Additional studies have shown that morphine stimulates HIV replication in primary cultures of human Kupffer cells (Schweitzer et al., 1991). While the mechanism of the enhanced replication is not clear, there is evidence that morphine may act directly to stimulate HIV replication, based on data that morphine activates an HIV/long terminal repeat (LTR)-CAT fusion gene transfected into a human neuroblastoma cell line (Squinto et al., 1990).

Studies reported by the Ho laboratory (Li et al., 2002) showed that methadone and morphine induced an increase in HIV replication in fetal brain microglia and in human monocyte-derived macrophages (MDMs). Moreover, both morphine and methadone upregulated CCR5 expression by these MDMs. The increase in chemokine receptor expression may be responsible for the increase in HIV replication. Of particular note is the finding that both morphine and methadone upregulated HIV replication in "latently" infected PBMCs collected from asymptomatic patients. Additional studies showed that morphine blocked the ability of CD8+ T cells to inhibit HIV expression using the chronically infected cell lines U1 and J1.1 (Wang et al., 2005). Interferon-γ (IFN-γ), a potent antiviral cytokine produced in part by CD8+ T cells, was depressed as a result of morphine treatment in these studies (Wang et al., 2005).

It is important to mention that morphine is a relatively nonselective opioid agonist, and as such, is able to activate μ-, κ-, and δ-opioid receptors, although it has greater affinity for the μ receptor. Work carried out by several laboratories has shown that these receptors can mediate diverse effects on the immune system, and in some cases the effects can be opposing. Rogers and Peterson (2003) have suggested that μ- and κ-opioids can mediate pro- and anti-inflammatory activities, respectively, and these two types of opioids can exert opposing effects on HIV-1 replication in vitro. For example, Peterson and colleagues (Chao et al., 1996) showed that κ-opioid receptor ligands downregulated HIV-1 expression in acutely infected microglial cells. It is interesting that additional studies, reported by Sharp et al. (1998), have shown that activation of the δ-opioid receptor also inhibits HIV replication in the Jurkat CD4+ T cell line. These findings point out the dichotomy in the responses of cells of the immune system to μ-, κ-, and δ- opioid agonists.

Finally, the effects of opioids on HIV replication in peripheral blood leukocytes can be mediated through the modulation of co-receptor expression. For example, morphine upregulates the expression of both CCR5 and CXCR4, and these changes are associated with significantly increased susceptibility to infection with both R5 and X4 strains of HIV-1 (Steele et al., 2003). Evidence will be reviewed later in this chapter that also shows that opioids exert a significant influence on the expression of chemokines.

DRUGS OF ABUSE AND ANIMAL MODELS OF HIV OR SIV INFECTION

The SIV macaque model of human HIV infection is currently the best experimental animal model system for the study of the immune response to the viral infection in vivo. A number of practical advances have been made which have greatly enhanced the utility of this model, including the development of a significant number of nonhuman primate immunological and virological reagents. The macaque model allows for analysis of the activities of opioids administered over an extended period of time, and in this way, mirrors much more closely the human drug abuse condition. Further, this experimental infection removes the confounding factor of use of multiple drugs, as is the case for most human drug abusers. In addition, the macaque model also offers the opportunity to evaluate neurological consequences of the viral infection to a greater degree than alternative animal model systems.

- The results of studies carried out to evaluate the influence of morphine on SIV disease progression have been somewhat inconsistent. Donahoe and colleagues (Donahoe et al., 1993; Donahoe et al., 2009) reported that monkeys maintained on morphine exhibit slower SIV disease progression as measured by decline in CD4 counts and by time to death. This study utilized a virus that is only mildly virulent (SIV$_{SMM9}$), and as a consequence, the full range of pathological consequences of the SIV infection may not have been apparent in this experimental system. In contrast, the Chuang laboratory (Chuang et al., 1997) reported that monkeys given chronic morphine had more rapid progression of their infection, and the virus evolved more rapidly so that it escaped recognition by antisera raised to the infecting strain. The weakness in the latter studies is that they were based on relatively small numbers of animals. Interestingly, Carneiro et al. (1999) have reported that injection drug use in humans leads to a 62 % greater mutation rate of the HIV Env genes when compared to control subjects. In more recent work reported by Kumar and colleagues (Kumar et al., 2004), a mixture of three different viruses were used, including T cell and macrophage-tropic SIV/HIV

recombinants strains (SHIV$_{KU1B}$ and SHIV$_{89.6P}$) and a macrophage-tropic SIV strain (SIV-17E-Fr). The results showed that both morphine-treated and control animals showed rapid T cell depletion, but the morphine-treated animals exhibited a reduced tendency to recover normal levels of CD4+ T-cells. At least part of the variability in these model systems may be attributable to differences in major histocompatibility complex (MHC) haplotype, with Mamu A*01 animals generally having a slower rate of disease progression, while Mamu B01 animals typically are predisposed to the rapid progressor phenotype (Boyer et al., 2006). The MHC haplotypes are not reported in these studies, and consequently it is impossible to surmise their contribution to the results just reviewed. Clearly, the overall effect of morphine on HIV replication and disease development in vivo is complicated by several factors, including the influence of the opioids on the virus, and the immune competence of the subject.

DRUGS OF ABUSE AND ANIMAL MODELS OF INFECTION FOR NON-HIV RETROVIRUSES, OF OPPORTUNISTIC INFECTION SEEN IN AIDS, AND OF OTHER INFECTIONS

The lack of a convenient animal model for HIV has prompted experiments using other retroviruses that infect rodents as surrogate models with which to evaluate the effects of drugs of abuse on infection. Several laboratories have suggested using Friend leukemia virus (FLV) as a model for mouse AIDS or MAIDS (Watson et al., 1988). Morphine administered to mice infected with FLV resulted in acute mortality (Veyries et al., 1995). In contrast, like the monkeys given SIV, morphine-tolerant mice had no alteration in progression of FLV (Starec et al., 1991). In pigs that were tolerant to morphine, there was also no effect on progression of swine herpes virus (Risdahl et al., 1993). Interestingly, met-enkephalin, an opioid peptide with some selectivity for the delta opioid receptor, synergized with AZT in inhibiting FLV replication in vitro (Sin et al., 1996). Morphine has been reported to sensitize to systemic herpes simplex virus, type 1 (HSV-1) infection in mice (Panaslak et al., 1990). A single dose of morphine has also been found to potentiate the development of HSV-1 encephalitis in mice (Lioy et al., 2006), suggesting that the drug opened the blood-brain barrier. Evidence for this effect has been published using slow-release morphine pellets (Ni et al., 2000). Investigation of the mechanisms by which morphine might alter susceptibility to HSV-1 showed that a single injection of the drug suppressed Th1 cytokines, IFN-γ and IL-12, but upregulated anti-viral cytokines IFN-α and IFN-β. Glucocorticoid elevation was partially involved in some of these alterations (Sheridan & Moynihan, 2005). It is not clear how these results fit with observations from the other laboratories that morphine sensitizes to HSV-1 infection, as a rise in the α/β interferons would be expected to be protective.

Salmonella are opportunistic organisms in AIDS patients, with increased incidence and severity of gastrointestinal illness and systemic infection reported (Gruenewald et al., 1994;

Celum et al., 1987; Angulo & Swerdlow, 1995; Kao et al., 2005; MacLennan et al., 2010). An older literature found that treatment of guinea pigs with opium was a technique to increase their sensitivity to oral Salmonella (as well as Shigella) infection (Takeuchi, 1967; Takeuchi, 1971). More contemporary studies in Eisenstein's laboratory have shown that morphine given to mice by slow-release pellet, at the same time as *Salmonella typhimurium* given orally, resulted in orders of magnitude increases in susceptibility to the bacterium, as measured by survival and burden of organisms in Peyer's patches, mesenteric lymph nodes, spleen, and liver (MacFarlane et al., 2000). In contrast, morphine given by osmotic mini-pump over the same period of time was less effective (Feng et al., 2006a). Sensitization by morphine was mainly mediated by the μ opioid receptor as selective κ and δ opioid agonists had little effect in potentiating Salmonella infection (Feng et al., 2006a), and μ opioid receptor knockout mice were not sensitized (Breslow et al., 2010). Morphine's capacity to alter infection by the oral route correlated with its ability to inhibit gastric transit. Morphine pellet implantation also induced sepsis in mice, as opioid-treated animals had a spontaneous increase in the number of enteric organisms in liver and spleen (Hilburger et al., 1997). This effect may be due to changes in intestinal permeability. A related finding is that morphine sensitizes animals to endotoxic shock induced by injection of lipopolysaccharide (LPS) extracted from Gram-negative bacteria (Hilburger et al., 1997; Roy et al., 1999; Ocasio et al., 2004; Greeneltch et al., 2004). This effect is hypothesized to be related to the morphine-mediated release of pro-inflammatory cytokines induced by the organisms seeding into the bloodstream from the intestinal tract (Hilburger et al., 1997). Administration of morphine has complications, as continuous exposure to the drug can lead to tolerance to analgesic and almost all other effects of morphine, as well as leading to addiction (dependence). Cessation of morphine administration can lead to withdrawal characterized by signs of physical dependence, which in mice is best quantitated by jumping. Only a few studies have investigated the effect of chronic morphine administration on susceptibility to infection and only two have tested the effect of withdrawal. Eisenstein showed that animals exposed to morphine by extended release pellets for 96 hours became tolerant to the effects of the drug on Salmonella infection (MacFarlane et al., 2000). Abrupt withdrawal induced sepsis (Feng et al., 2006b) and sensitized to both systemic and oral Salmonella infection (Feng et al., 2005; Feng et al., 2006b). Sensitization to oral Salmonella infection by withdrawal from morphine was much weaker than the effect of morphine given simultaneously with the first exposure to Salmonella (Feng et al., 2006a). Thus, in regard to Salmonella infection, acute drug exposure sensitizes to infection, mice become tolerant to the sensitizing effect, and withdrawal of the drug again increases sensitization, but to a markedly lesser extent than acute exposure.

Morphine has also been shown to alter the pathogenesis of Gram-positive pathogens. Mice treated with morphine slow-release pellets were sensitized to infection with *Streptococcus pneumoniae* as assessed by bacterial burdens in the organs and increased mortality. Opioid treatment caused delayed neutrophil recruitment which correlated with lower levels of chemokines (Wang et al., 2005). In vitro morphine treatment also decreased *S. pneumoniae* phagocytosis and killing by alveolar macrophages (Wang et al., 2008), which was accompanied by suppression of phosphorylation of IRF-3, ATF2, and NF-κBp65 and inhibition of levels of the antimicrobial peptide S100A8/19 (Ma et al., 2010). Morphine has also been demonstrated to sensitize to *Listeria monocytogenes* in a murine model of infection (Asakura et al., 2006). When morphine was administered twice, at 12 hr intervals before Listeria inoculation, animals showed increased mortality as well as increased bacterial burdens in the spleen and liver, and increased frequency of dissemination to the central nervous system.

In contrast to the above studies, morphine was shown to inhibit multiplication of a mouse virulent strain of *Mycobacterium tuberculosis* given intravenously (Singh et al., 2008). The drug was given twice by subcutaneous injection, on days 0 and 15 over a large range of doses. Necropsy studies showed that morphine suppressed growth of the Mycobacteria in the lung and spleen at doses in the range of 5 mg/kg to 50 mg/kg in a naloxone-reversible fashion with a shallow U-shaped dose-response curve. Morphine also suppressed in vitro growth of the Mycobacteria in peritoneal macrophages. These effects seemed to be mediated by morphine-induced nitric oxide. The reason for the opposite effects of morphine in this infection model compared to other infections where the drug has been tested are unknown, particularly since opioid drug abusers are at increased risk for infection with *Mycobacterium tuberculosis* (Durante et al., 1998).

Candida albicans is a persistent opportunistic pathogen in AIDS. Morphine administration markedly sensitized mice to Candida infection and also to *Klebsiella pneumoniae*, an effect attributed to decreased function of phagocytic cells (Tubaro et al., 1983). In addition, morphine has been investigated for its effects on several parasitic infections. A seminal paper was the report that morphine sensitizes to murine infection with an avirulent strain of *Toxoplasma gondii* (Chao et al., 1990). Animals exposed to both parasite and drug succumbed acutely. Singh's laboratory found a dose-dependent, biphasic modulatory effect of morphine on *Plasmodium berghei* infection (Singh et al., 1993) and *Leishmania donovani* infection in mice and hamsters, respectively, in which a low dose suppressed and a high dose potentiated the infections (Singal et al., 2002; Singh & Singal, 2007) Part of the effect of morphine on Plasmodium was due to modulation of their ability to induce colony-stimulating factors by mouse peritoneal macrophages (Singh & Singh, 2000).

EFFECTS OF OPIOIDS ON IMMUNE RESPONSES

NATURAL KILLER CELL FUNCTION

Among the effects of morphine on the immune system, the suppression of Natural Killer (NK) cell activity is one of the first to be discovered and among the most well documented.

Morphine has been shown to suppress NK activity in rat spleens when given subcutaneously (Shavit et al., 1986; Shavit et al., 1987) or when given into the periaqueductal gray region of the brain (Weber & Pert, 1989). Human volunteers given morphine showed a similar reduction in NK activity in the peripheral blood over a 24-hr time period (Yeager et al., 1995). In rats, there is some evidence to suggest that the alterations in NK activity may not be by direct action on the immune cells, but may be mediated by adrenergic neurotransmitters (Carr et al., 1994) or by release of glucocorticoids (Freier & Fuchs, 1994), although contrary data is published (Band et al., 1992). Evidence for a neural mediated pathway of NK cell immunosuppression is supported by the observation that N-methyl-morphine, which does not pass the blood-brain barrier, is inactive (Shavit et al., 1986). The role of the μ opioid receptor in the action of morphine on NK cells is supported by reversal of its effects by naltrexone (Shavit et al., 1984; Shavit et al., 1987), and by the finding that mice with genetic deletion of the μ opioid receptor fail to demonstrate suppressed NK cell activity in response to morphine (Gavériaux-Ruff et al., 1998).

ANTIBODY RESPONSES

It is well established that morphine administration in vivo in mice leads to a reduced ability of murine B cells to respond to the mitogen, bacterial lipopolysaccharide (LPS) (Bryant et al., 1987; Bryant et al., 1991). In addition, morphine inhibits antibody production to sheep erythrocytes (Lefkowitz & Chiang, 1975; Bussiere et al., 1992) and tetanus toxoid (Eisenstein et al., 1990). The suppression of antibody formation is blocked by administration of naltrexone, and this demonstrates that the opioid receptors are required for the immunosuppression (Bussiere et al., 1992; Gavériaux-Ruff et al., 1998). Rahim et al. (2001) used minipumps to administer several different opioids continuously to mice for 48 hours, and found that the opioid agonist morphine sulfate, the κ-opioid selective agonist trans-3,4-dichloro-N-methyl-N-[7-(1-pyrroliidinyl) cyclohexyl] benzene-acetamide methanesulfonate (U50,488H), and deltorphin II (δ_2 selective agonist), each inhibited the capacity of spleen cells to make an ex vivo antibody response to sheep red blood cells. The effect of each opioid agonist was blocked by administration of opioid-receptor selective antagonists, namely H-D-phe-cys-tyr-D-trp-arg-thr-pen-thr-NH$_2$ (CTAP; μ-opioid selective), nor-binaltorphimine (κ-opioid selective), or naltriben (δ_2-opioid selective). These results suggest that immunosuppression may be induced via μ-, κ-, or δ_2-opioid receptors. An interesting aspect of this study was that each of the opioids tested yielded a U-shaped dose-response curve in which maximal inhibition of antibody formation was observed in the 0.5 to 2.0 mg/kg/day range. The reason that higher doses do not inhibit is unexplained. Few studies have investigated the effect of more chronic administration of opioids on antibody responses and these have been reviewed (Eisenstein et al., 2006). Continuous exposure to morphine via implantation of extended release morphine pellets leads to tolerance to the immunosuppressive effects by 96 hr after commencing drug delivery (Bussiere et al., 1993). Withdrawal from morphine has been shown to induce another round of immunosuppression in mice (Rahim et al., 2002; West et al., 1999). In addition to effects on systemic antibody responses, opioids have been shown to inhibit mucosal antibody responses. Carr found that β-endorphin suppressed production of non-specific IgM, IgG, and IgA production from Concanavalin A (ConA)-stimulated murine Peyer's patch cells (Carr et al., 1990). Morphine has also been shown to block mouse secretory IgA responses to cholera toxin using ex vivo ileal organ cultures or in gastrointestinal lavage fluids taken from opioid-treated mice (Peng et al., 2001; Dinari et al., 1989).

Studies carried out in vitro have also demonstrated that opioid administration is suppressive for antibody responses. Taub et al. (1991) treated mouse splenocytes with morphine, the μ-opioid-selective agonist [D-ala^2, N-Me-Phe^4, Gly-ol^5] enkephalin (DAMGO), or the κ selective agonist, U50,488H, and found that anti-erythrocyte antibody responses were significantly suppressed. These studies showed that the inhibitory effect was dose dependent, and the immunosuppressive effects could be blocked with either naloxone, a non-selective opioid receptor antagonist, or with receptor selective opioid antagonists (Taub et al., 1991). These studies were the first demonstration of immunosuppression by an exogenous kappa selective agonist. Finally, it also appears that δ-opioids induce significant immunosuppression in vitro in Peyer's patch lymphocytes (Carr et al., 1990). The δ-opioid receptor agonist oxymorphindole decreased total IgM, but not total IgA or IgG production. In vitro responses to morphine and to U50,488H were demonstrated to have activity on spleen cells of some mouse strains, but not others (Eisenstein et al., 1995). Morphine has also been reported to decrease IgM secretion by human peripheral blood B cells (Vassou et al., 2008). These results confirm the evidence from in vivo analysis that shows that μ-, κ-, and δ-opioids can participate in the regulation of immunoglobulin synthesis.

Attempts to determine the mechanism by which opioids inhibit antibody responses are complicated by the fact that this type of immune response is the result of interactions among several distinct cell populations. Experiments carried out with isolated populations of immune cells have demonstrated that the inhibitory activity of the κ-opioid agonist U50,488H is mediated directly through both accessory cell and T cell populations (Guan et al., 1994). This result is consistent with studies reported by Eisenstein's laboratory (Bussiere et al., 1993) which showed that the inhibition of antibody responses following morphine administration in vivo can be reversed by the addition of non-opioid-treated macrophages or the macrophage products IL-1, IL-6, or by interferon-γ.

OPIOIDS AND APOPTOSIS

One mechanism by which morphine might exert immunosuppressive effects, and also alter HIV infection, is via induction of apoptosis in cells of the immune system. There is definitive evidence showing that morphine added to human lymphocytes in vitro induces apoptosis (Nair et al., 1997). Similarly, morphine increases apoptosis in macrophages, apparently through induction of nitric oxide and Fas and Fas ligand (Singhal et al., 1998; Singhal et al., 2002). Morphine given to mice or rats systemically induces apoptosis in the thymus and spleen, which may be mediated by release of glucocorticoids or by upregulation of Fas (Fuchs & Pruett, 1993; Yin et al., 1999; Singhal et al., 1997). Thus, in vivo apoptosis may result from both direct and mediated effects on cells of the immune system.

PHAGOCYTIC CELL FUNCTION

Several studies have demonstrated that the in vivo administration of morphine inhibits the ability of peritoneal macrophages and neutrophils to phagocytize the pathogenic yeast *Candida albicans*. Tubaro et al. (1983) showed that morphine induced reduced phagocytosis by both mouse and rabbit polymorphonuclear leukocytes. Rojavin et al. (1993) administered morphine by implantation of a slow-release morphine pellet and showed a decrease in phagocytic activity of C. albicans by murine peritoneal macrophages. In contrast, Pacifici et al. (1994) found that mice injected with the synthetic opioid methadone exhibited no discernable change in phagocytic activity. It is not clear why methadone and morphine fail to exert similar immunomodulatory effects, but there are known differences in how the two opioids interact with opioid receptors.

Several laboratories have shown that in vitro treatment of mouse peritoneal macrophages with morphine suppresses phagocytic cell function. Casellas et al. (1991) reported that acute exposure of mouse peritoneal macrophages to morphine inhibited the phagocytosis of sheep erythrocytes; however, this effect in mouse and human cells was attenuated by chronic exposure of the phagocytes in vitro to the drug, suggesting that tolerance developed (Delgado-Velez et al., 2008). Other laboratories have also reported that morphine inhibits phagocytosis. Szabo et al. (1993) showed that administration of morphine or μ-, δ-, and κ-selective agonists inhibited the ability of macrophages to phagocytize C. albicans. These inhibitory effects were reversed by use of the respective selective antagonists. The results indicate that μ-, δ-, and κ-opioid receptors play a role in the regulation of macrophage function in response to opioid agonists. Using phagocytosis of red blood cells by mouse peritoneal macrophages, it was also found that μ and δ opioid receptors, but not κ receptors, mediated uptake of the cells (Tomassini et al., 2003). Morphine fails to inhibit phagocytosis in a μ-opioid receptor knockout mouse (Roy et al., 1998a). Morphine added to murine alveolar macrophages decreased phagocytosis and killing of *Streptococcus pneumoniae* (Wang et al., 2008). A contrasting study by Peterson et al. (1995), found that morphine treatment of microglial cells stimulated the phagocytosis of *M. tuberculosis* strain H37Rv. However, Sowa et al. (1997) demonstrated morphine treatment of swine microglia inhibited the phagocytosis of non-opsonized *Cryptococcus neoformans*. Treatment with pertussis toxin reversed the inhibitory effects of morphine. These findings indicate that

morphine stimulated the phagocytosis of *M. tuberculosis* and inhibited the microglial cell phagocytosis *of C. neoformans* via μ-opioid receptors coupled to a pertussis toxin-sensitive G_i/G_o protein. Singh demonstrated a dose effect of morphine on in vitro growth of *Leishmania donovani* in murine peritoneal macrophages, where low doses (10^{-9} to 10^{-11} M) inhibited replication of the parasite, but high doses (10^{-5} M) potentiated their growth (Singh & Singal, 2007). Thus, dosage may be an important variable in understanding conflicting results in the literature on effects of opioids on immune function.

Treatment with morphine has also been reported to inhibit microbicidal effector pathways of phagocytes. Superoxide production induced by opsonized zymosan or phorbol myristate acetate in human peripheral blood mononuclear cells was reduced by morphine in a naloxone blockable fashion (Peterson et al., 1987a).

Further, opioids have been shown to interfere with phagocyte mobilization. Roy's laboratory has shown that morphine given in vivo or in vitro suppressed macrophage colony formation from bone marrow cells in culture (Roy et al., 1991). Morphine administration is reported to inhibit granulocyte activation and aggregation by inhibiting the N-formyl-methionyl-leucyl-phenylalanine (fMLF)-induced upregulation of the β_2 integrin, CD11b-CD18, on human granulocytes (Mazzone et al., 1990). Results from several laboratories have shown that morphine and the endogenous opioid peptides β-endorphin, met-enkephalin, and dynorphin directly induce chemotaxis of human monocytes and neutrophils (Van Epps & Saland, 1984; Ruff et al., 1985; Makman et al., 1995; Grimm et al., 1998). On the other hand, pre-treatment with a number of opioids leads to an inhibition of the ability of neutrophils, monocytes, or microglial cells to exhibit chemotaxis to either complement-derived chemotactic factors (Perez-Castrillon et al., 1992; Liu et al., 1992; Chao et al., 1997) or to the chemokines MIP-1α, RANTES, MCP-1, or IL-8 (Grimm et al., 1998). The results of Grimm et al. (1998) suggest that the activation of the μ- and δ-opioid receptors leads to the desensitization of the chemokine receptors CCR1, CCR2, CXCR1, and CXCR2. This opioid-induced desensitization will be discussed in more detail below. These studies are in apparent conflict with the results of Simpkins et al. (1984), who found that pre-treatment with β-endorphin enhanced the chemotaxis directed to fMLF. The nature of the disparity in these results is not clear; however, the postulated capacity of β-endorphin to interact with a receptor distinct from the classical opioid receptors (Hazum et al., 1979) may be involved.

CYTOKINE EXPRESSION

One mechanism of immunomodulation induced by opioids may be related to alterations in the expression of various cytokines. Peterson et al. (1987b) reported naloxone-reversible suppression of IFN-γ production when human PBMCs were pretreated for 3 hours with morphine followed by ConA stimulation. Dose-dependent inhibition of both IL-2 and IL-4 production was observed when murine splenocytes were incubated for 24 hours with relatively high concentrations of morphine and then stimulated with ConA (Jessop & Taplits, 1991). Lysle et al. (1993) showed that morphine injected subcutaneously into rats induced a naltrexone-reversible, dose-dependent suppression of splenic lymphocyte IL-2 and IFN-γ production. Roy et al. (1997) showed that IL-2 production was decreased in a dose-dependent manner in thymocytes pretreated with relatively high doses of morphine and stimulated with phytohemagglutin and IL-1. More extensive analysis revealed that the decrease in IL-2 production was the result of a decrease in IL-2 mRNA transcription which appeared to be due to a reduction in the level of the transcriptional activator component *fos*, a necessary element controlling the synthesis of IL-2. In human PBMCs and in mouse splenocytes, Roy has presented evidence that morphine polarizes immune cells towards a Th2 response (Roy et al., 2001). Chao et al. (1992) demonstrated a naloxone-reversible increase in TGF-β production following morphine treatment of LPS- or PHA-stimulated PBMCs. The morphine-induced inhibition of IL-2 and IFN-γ production may be explained by the well-documented immunosuppressive activity of TGF-β. On the other hand, LPS-stimulated murine peritoneal macrophages pretreated with a low dose of morphine (50 nM) exhibited a naloxone-reversible increase in TNF-α and IL-6 (Roy et al., 1998b). Cells receiving a high concentration of morphine (50 μM) in vitro exhibited a decrease in IL-6 and TNF-α production that was not reversible with naloxone. It was determined that low doses of morphine augment LPS-induced NF-κB levels, whereas high doses of morphine reduced NF-κB levels, suggesting that opioids may be affecting cytokine production at the transcriptional level (Roy et al., 1998b). This result is consistent with studies on peritoneal macrophages taken 48 hours after in vivo treatment with morphine via extended release pellets, which show that opioid administration induced an increase in the expression of IL-12 in murine peritoneal macrophages (Peng et al., 2000). Opposite results were reported by the Sacerdote laboratory when peritoneal macrophages were harvested 1 hr after subcutaneous injection of morphine at a dose of 20 mg/kg. There was a reduction in baseline levels of IL-1β, TNF-α, and IL-12, and a more marked inhibition of elevation of these cytokines following LPS stimulation, which was dependent on RelB, a regulator of NF-κB (Martucci et al., 2007). Morphine has also been reported to inhibit the increase in TNF-α and IL-6 induced in human peripheral blood monocytes by bacterial peptidoglycan, but the effect was evident only at high concentrations of the opioid (10^{-5} and 10^{-4} M). Further, if morphine was applied to unfractionated peripheral blood cells, no inhibition of IL-6 was observed, suggesting that the lymphocytes produce something that counteracts the immunosuppression (Bonnet et al., 2008). Withdrawal from morphine has also been shown to result in a decrease in IL-12 production in animals receiving either bacterial LPS or live Salmonella (Feng et al., 2005a; Feng et al., 2005b; Kelschenbach et al., 2005). Exogenous IL-12 decreased the bacterial burdens in morphine withdrawn mice. The effect on IL-12 was selective, as TNF-α and nitric oxide levels increased (Feng et al., 2005a).

Both κ- and δ-selective agonists have also been found to alter cytokine expression. Studies carried out by Belkowski et al. (1995) showed that the κ-opioid receptor agonist U50,488H suppressed LPS-induced levels of IL-1 and TNF-α produced by the murine macrophage-like cell line P388D$_1$. Alicea et al. (1996) reported that resident peritoneal macrophages, stimulated with LPS and treated with U50,488H, exhibited decreased production of IL-1, TNF-α, and IL-6. Guan et al. (1997) determined that murine thymocytes stimulated with staphylococcal enterotoxin B (SEB) in the presence of activated macrophages exhibited significantly reduced IL-2 production following administration of U50,488H at concentrations as low as 1nM. Shahabi and Sharp (1995) observed that murine splenic CD4+ T-cells treated with the δ-opioid receptor agonist deltorphin and then stimulated with anti-CD3 exhibited an increase in IL-2 production when deltorphin was given at a low concentration (10^{-11}M). However, a decrease in IL-2 production was observed following deltorphin administration at a higher concentration (10^{-7} M), revealing an unexpected biphasic modulation of lymphokine production. House et al. (1996) found that the administration of either [D-Pen^2, D-Pen^5] enkephalin (DPDPE) or deltorphin, delta agonists, elevated anti-CD3-induced IL-2, IL-4 and IL-6 production. These results are consistent with studies carried out with Jurkat T cells transfected with the δ-opioid receptor which showed that δ-opioid agonist administration elevates the production of IL-2 (Hedin et al., 1997).

In summary, there are conflicting reports on the effects of morphine and other opioids on cytokine production depending on whether the drug is given in vivo or applied to cells in vitro. Variables that might affect the outcome of these studies include dose of the drugs, time of assay after exposure to the drug, and interactions between cells of the immune system.

EFFECTS OF DRUGS OF ABUSE ON CHEMOKINES AND CHEMOKINE RECEPTOR EXPRESSION

Chemokines and chemokine receptors are crucial for HIV infectivity (Bleul et al., 1996; Alkhatib et al., 1997; Dragic et al., 1996; Feng et al., 1996; Oberlin et al., 1996). Drugs of abuse have been shown to modulate both chemokine levels and chemokine receptor expression, with obvious implications for altering susceptibility to HIV infection. Morphine administration has been shown to alter the expression of both α- and β-chemokines. Morphine treatment of astrocyte cell lines in vitro results in a dose-dependent reduction in the mRNA transcription and protein secretion of the α-chemokine, IL-8, and the β-chemokines, MIP-1β and MCP-1 (Mahajan et al., 2002; Mahajan et al., 2005). Morphine treatment of microglial cell cultures also inhibited production of the β-chemokine RANTES, induced in response to LPS and IL-1β stimulation (Hu et al., 2000). More importantly, the morphine-induced immunomodulation of both astrocytes and microglial cells was reversed by the addition of the μ-opioid receptor antagonist β-funaltrexamine (β-FNA), implicating a role for a classic opioid receptor. The downregulation of IL-8 production by astrocytes has been associated with increased susceptibility to the induction of apoptosis (Saas et al., 1999). Additionally, it has been suggested that the reduced level of MIP-1β could potentially limit the ability of this chemokine to protect against HIV-1 (by competing for binding to CCR5, a co-receptor for HIV-1) in the CNS (Mahajan et al., 2002). Furthermore, these chemokines have been found to be expressed in the CNS during multiple stages of mouse hepatitis virus (MHV) infection, which supports the relevance of these immunological mediators in inflammatory disease states of the brain (Lane et al., 1998).

Recent studies have shown that treatment of unstimulated or PHA-stimulated PBMCs with the μ-opioid agonist DAMGO induced the expression of the pro-inflammatory chemokines MCP-1, RANTES, and interferon-inducible protein-10 (IP-10) (Wetzel et al., 2000). These studies also showed that μ-opioid activation results in significant induction of IP-10 and RANTES expression in HIV-infected PBMCs. Supporting these findings, IP-10 induction by the μ-opioid receptor can be blocked by pre-treatment with β-FNA (Davis et al., 2007). It has been suggested that the induction of these chemokines is likely to promote the replication of HIV, in part through the attraction of uninfected cells to the site of opioid expression and chemokine induction (Wetzel et al., 2000).

Chemokine receptor expression is an additional crucial component of the immune response that may be targeted in the intravenous drug abuser. Recent studies have shown that the expression of both CCR5 and CXCR4, the two major HIV-1 co-receptors, are induced by activation of the μ-opioid receptor (Steele et al., 2003). These studies demonstrated that either morphine, or the μ-selective agonist, DAMGO, induces co-receptor expression in both monocytes and activated T cells. This effect is reversible by treatment with either the non-selective opioid antagonist naloxone or the μ-opioid selective antagonist CTAP. More recent studies have determined that DAMGO can regulate chemokine (RANTES) and chemokine receptor (CXCR4) expression via a TGF-β-dependent pathway (Happel et al., 2008). Interestingly, DAMGO also induced expression of MCP-1, IP-10, and CCR5, but in a TGF-β-independent manner. Finally, the elevated level of co-receptor expression induces an increase in monocyte and T cell virus uptake, leading to an increase in HIV-1 replication (Steele et al., 2003). It is interesting that human astrocyte cell lines cultured with morphine exhibit a significant up-regulation of CCR5, CCR3, and CXCR4 expression (Mahajan et al., 2002). Morphine also significantly increased CCR5 expression in human blood monocyte-derived macrophages (Guo et al., 2002). Additionally, methadone, an opioid agonist commonly used in the treatment of opioid dependency, elevated mRNA and protein levels of CCR5 in a human lymphocytic cell line (Suzuki et al., 2002a).

Studies reported by Lokensgard et al. (2002) showed that, in contrast to the results reviewed above for the μ-opioid agonists DAMGO and morphine, CD4+ T cells exhibited a significant reduction in CXCR4 expression following treatment with κ-opioid agonists. The inhibition of CXCR4 expression was associated with reduced susceptibility to HIV-1 infection in this T-cell population. The opposing effects of μ- and κ-opioid agonists on co-receptor expression are most likely due to distinct signaling properties for these receptors. However, the nature of the differences in the effects between these two classes of opioid compounds remains undefined.

EFFECTS OF DRUGS OF ABUSE ON CHEMOKINE RECEPTOR FUNCTION

Studies have shown that pretreatment with either endogenous or exogenous opioids results in an inhibition of the chemotactic response to a number of chemokines. Grimm and his colleagues (Grimm et al., 1998) have reported that pre-treatment of primary monocytes with the endogenous opioid met-enkephalin significantly inhibited the chemotactic responses to either MCP-1 or MIP-1α. Similarly the chemotactic response of human neutrophils to IL-8 was inhibited by pre-incubation with met-enkephalin. Further analysis showed that more selective μ- and δ-opioid agonists also induced significant suppression of the chemotactic response to MIP-1α, RANTES, and MCP-1. Analysis of these results as well as additional data from the Rogers laboratory (Rogers et al., 2000; Szabo et al., 2003; Steele et al., 2002) showed that the μ- and δ-opioids inhibited the function of the chemokine receptors CCR1, CCR2, CCR5, CXCR1, and CXCR2, but not CXCR4, through heterologous desensitization. In contrast with these opioids, administration of κ-opioids was able to induce heterologous desensitization of CXCR4 in a bi-directional manner (Finley et al., 2008), suggesting that the κ-opioids exhibit stronger cross-desensitizing activity than the μ- or δ-opioids.

The heterologous desensitization of chemokine receptors by opioids has significant consequences for the functions of cells of the immune system. Each of these chemokine receptors has a well-established role in promoting inflammatory responses. This is particularly true for both CCR2 and CCR5 (Zhou et al., 1998; Boring et al., 1998; Kurihara et al., 1997; Kuziel et al., 1997). It has been shown that the capacity of μ-opioids to induce desensitization of CCR5 but not CXCR4, resulted in short-term inhibition of HIV-1 binding and uptake of R5, but not X4, strains (Szabo et al., 2003). These findings suggest that the μ- and δ-opioids may promote T-cell tropism during HIV-1 infection by inhibiting the capacity of CCR5 to serve as a viral co-receptor.

The biochemical mechanism of heterologous desensitization is typically due to target receptor phosphorylation. Activation of the μ-opioid receptor has been shown to alter G protein coupling of CCR5, and induce phosphorylation of CCR5 in Chinese hamster ovary (CHO) cells co-expressing μ-opioid and CCR5 (Chen et al., 2004). Opioid-mediated cross-desensitization of CCR5 could be blocked by the general PKC inhibitor calphostin C, but not by the calcium-dependent classic PKC inhibitor Go6976 (Zhang et al., 2003). Western blotting analysis and immunofluorescent staining experiments further showed that only calcium-independent PKCs were activated upon opioid stimulation, suggesting opioids achieve desensitization of this chemokine receptor via a pathway involving primarily calcium-independent PKC isotypes (Zhang et al., 2003).

Opioid receptors and chemokine receptors have been shown to form heterodimers. In both human CEMx174 lymphocytes and monkey lymphocytes, CCR5, but not CD4, forms heterodimers with all three subtypes of opioid receptors (μ, δ, and κ), based on data from co-immunoprecipitation and western blot analysis (Suzuki et al., 2002b). Chemical cross-linking experiments indicate that these receptors are closely situated on the cell membrane with an intermolecular distance less than 11.4A. The μ-opioid receptor and CCR5 also forms heterodimers in CHO cells, and the level of heterodimer is not affected by DAMGO or RANTES treatment (Chen et al., 2004). Additional studies using fluorescence resonance energy transfer (FRET) also show that CCR5 can form either homodimers or a heterodimer with CCR2 (Hernanz-Falcon et al., 2004; El-Asmar et al., 2005). Given the complexity of CCR5 oligomerization, the direct interaction of μ-opioid and CCR5 could contribute to the mutual regulation of their functions (Zhang et al., 2003).

EFFECTS OF OPIOIDS ON THE BLOOD-BRAIN BARRIER (BBB)

The increased incidence of the neurological complications of AIDS in opioid drug abusers suggests that opioids may promote elevated viral loads in the brain. In an R5-tropic SIV/macaque model, morphine-treated animals with subclinical disease had a clear tendency toward higher virus loads in the CNS (Marcario et al., 2008). In addition, while chronic morphine treatment alone does not significantly alter BBB integrity (based on BBB biomarker expression), treatment with morphine in combination with HIV-1 Tat protein modulates BBB permeability (Yousif et al., 2008). Following treatment, transendothelial electrical resistance is decreased and transendothelial migration is enhanced across the BBB in primary brain microvascular endothelial cells (Mahajan et al., 2008). In addition, opiates and HIV-1 Tat synergize to increase intracellular calcium, and the release of MCP-1, RANTES, and IL-6 by astrocytes (El-Hage et al., 2005). Without Tat, μ-opioid agonists inhibit enhanced intracellular calcium responses in activated astrocytes co-cultured with brain endothelial cells. Astrocytes appear to be key participants in the effects of opioids on the resistance to HIV in the brain. Astrocytes play a number of active roles in the brain, including the secretion or absorption of neural transmitters and maintenance of the blood-brain barrier. Immunohistochemical and calcium flux analysis indicates that μ-, δ-, and κ-opioid receptors are expressed by cultured murine astrocytes (Stiene-Martin et al., 1998). Disruptions of astrocyte function and inflammatory signaling may contribute to accelerated neuropathogenesis in HIV-infected opioid drug abusers.

In contrast to the studies just reviewed on astrocyte function, it should be pointed out that evidence suggests that opioids may attenuate vascular endothelial cell function. Studies using intravital microscopy in mice have suggested that morphine administration inhibits leukocyte rolling and adhesion to vascular endothelial cells by stimulation of nitric oxide (Ni et al., 2000). Similar decreases in leukocyte adhesion were observed in the rat mesentery following morphine treatment (House et al., 2001). Morphine has been shown to up-regulate NO production in human vascular endothelial cells (Stefano et al., 1995; Stefano et al., 1998). It appears that more work is necessary in order to more fully understand the mechanism(s) responsible for the influence of opioid drugs of abuse on the integrity of the blood-brain barrier, and its function during HIV infection.

DRUGS OF ABUSE AND NEUROINFLAMMATORY DISEASE STATES

Evidence in the pre-HAART era shows that frequent opiate use among HIV-infected individuals resulted in increased disease progression of HIV encephalitis (HIVE) and HIV-associated dementia (HAD) (Bell et al., 1996; Chiesi et al., 1996; Martinez et al., 1995); These observations suggest that frequent opioid abuse promotes increased neurologic disease progression in AIDS. The nature of the opioid effect on the progression of neuroAIDS remains unclear, but HIV does not appear to induce productive infection in neurons, in part because CD4 is absent and CCR5 expression is low, and HIV strains isolated from brain tissue of AIDS patients are almost exclusively R5-tropic (Strizki et al., 1996; Shieh et al., 1998; Albright et al., 1999; Gorry et al., 2001). As mentioned above, animal models suggest that the combination of Tat and morphine can mediate inflammatory effects on astrocytes and microglial cells. Tat has been shown to induce the expression of MCP-1 in murine brain tissue, as well as induce an influx of monocytes to the brain (Pu et al., 2003). It was later shown that astrocytes were responsible for the production of both MCP-1 and CCL5/RANTES (El-Hage et al., 2005). In addition, morphine enhanced this Tat-induced chemokine expression. It is widely assumed that HIV is transported to the brain via the "Trojan horse" concept where HIV-infected monocytes carry the virus into the brain.

Results from a number of studies suggest that MCP-1/CCL2 is a key mediator of inflammation within the brain during HIV infection. Tat and/or morphine show a reduced capacity to increase glial cell activation in the striatum of CCR2 knock-out mice, when compared to wild-type mice (El-Hage et al., 2006a). This work was confirmed, in part, by the observation that microglial cell activity increased in the striatum of Tat-inducible transgenic mice following induction of Tat expression, together with morphine delivery in the brain (Bruce-Keller et al., 2008). Finally, more recent studies show that the MCP-1 activity in this model is dependent on the expression of CCL5, since Tat and morphine were not able to induce MCP-1 expression in CCL5 knock-out mice (El-Hage et al., 2008).

It has been reported that Tat has other effects that contribute to neuroinflammation. For example, Tat can also modulate the inflammatory activity of morphine via regulation of the expression of the μ-opioid receptor. Treatment of microglial cells with morphine downregulates the expression of the μ-opioid receptor (Turchan-Cholewo et al., 2008). However, the addition of Tat prevents this reduction, and also increases the intracellular stores of the μ-opioid receptor. In addition, Tat can also damage neurons and oligodendrocytes by inducing caspase-3 activity, which can lead to apoptosis (Bruce-Keller et al., 2008; El-Hage et al., 2006b). The damage to oligodendrocytes can result in myelin pallor (Gray & Lescs, 1993), and these events collectively may contribute to HIV-associated dementia.

Murine animal model data suggest that direct addition of morphine to the striatum can induce a neuroinflammatory state characterized by MCP-1 expression and chemotaxis of monocytes to the brain. Presumably upon HIV infection of these individuals, the monocytes are already primed to be both readily infectable by HIV and traffic to the brain where virus can be released for microglia to become infected (Yadav & Collman, 2009; Steele et al., 2003). The release of Tat by infected macrophages and microglia, along with the chronic opioid use, may combine to create an opiate-driven, self-perpetuating feedback mechanism, resulting in chronic neuroinflammation, with bystander effects of neuronal destruction caused by the collective participation of astrocytes, microglia, macrophages, Tat, and the opioid.

SUMMARY

The opioid drugs of abuse have profound immunomodulatory effects on virtually all aspects of the immune system. There is substantial evidence that μ-, κ-, and δ-opioid receptors are expressed on several hematopoietic cell populations, although it is very likely that the expression of these receptors varies greatly among cell types, and activation typically induces upregulation of their expression. Unfortunately, reagents that would allow for the sensitive quantitation of these receptors are not available at this time. An equally important issue is the nature of the cell populations that are the source of relevant endogenous opioid ligands, and the precise conditions under which these natural opioids are produced. It should be appreciated that the administration of heroin, morphine, or other opioid drugs establishes an unusual source of elevated levels of opioid agonists, and the balance between endogenous and exogenous agonists is a component of the complex interplay between opioid drugs and the cells of the immune system. Little is known about the influence of chronic administration of opioid drugs on the bioavailability of endogenous opioid ligands, and even less is known about the bioavailability of μ-, κ-, and δ-opioid ligands for cells and tissues of the immune system in the drug-abusing subject. Finally, the chronic administration of opioids creates the significant additional issue of tolerance and withdrawal for the cells of the immune system.

Each of the three classes of opioid ligands selective for the different opioid receptors has been shown to alter levels of HIV replication when added to human lymphoid, monocytic, or microglial cultures in vitro. Further, opioids have been shown to have profound effects on chemokine receptor expression and chemokine levels, providing further opportunity for direct modulation of HIV infectivity at the level of co-receptor expression or competition for the co-receptor. Alteration of chemokine levels by these drugs may also affect cell trafficking to sites of HIV infection. The opioids alter cytokine levels, which could influence the state of activation of lymphocytes and macrophages, creating environments with varying degrees of permissiveness for HIV replication. Further, under the appropriate circumstances these drugs induce apoptosis, with the potential to decrease the available lymphocyte population targeted by HIV or to release HIV from infected cells.

It is extremely important to appreciate that in almost all cases, the drug abusing subject self-administers a combination of drugs in addition to the opioids, and this commonly includes cocaine, marijuana, alcohol, and cigarette smoke. In some cases these drugs have opposing effects on cells of the immune system, particularly cocaine, as compared to marijuana and opioids. As drug abusers usually use more than one drug, in varying doses, ratios, frequencies, and durations, attempts to ascertain the effects of drug abuse on HIV progression using epidemiological approaches have been hampered, yielding results that are not definitive and must be interpreted with caution. It has proven difficult to obtain direct in vivo laboratory evidence to support the hypothesis that drugs of abuse alter the progression of HIV infection because of the absence of small animal models to test HIV infectivity. There are new studies currently underway using the SIV/macaque model that will hopefully address in a direct way the influence of opioids on the progression of AIDS, and the development of neurodegeneration associated with the retrovirus infection. The current laboratory evidence all points to many potential direct and indirect pathways by which opioids may influence viral replication and also the intensity of the immune response to the virus. In a developing age of individualized medicine, it should be appreciated that no two HIV-infected opioid drug abusers have the same immune status. The influence of the opioid drugs of abuse are complex, and when this is combined with the diverse effects on immune function that occur with the virus infection, there is almost certainly a unique level of immune competence for each individual patient.

ACKNOWLEDGMENTS

We thank Dr. Martin Adler, Director Emeritus and Senior Advisor of CSAR, Temple University School of Medicine, for critical reading of the manuscript. This work was supported by NIDA grants T32DA-07237, DODW81XWH-06-1-0147, DA06650, DA25532, DA11130, DA11134, P30-DA13429, PO1-DA23860, DA14223, and DA14230.

REFERENCES

Albright, A. V., Shieh, J. Itoh, T., Lee, B., Pleasure, D., O'Connor, M. J., et al. (1999). Microglia express CCR5, CXCR4, and CCR3, but of these, CCR5 is the principal coreceptor for human immunodeficiency virus type 1 dementia isolates. *J Virol, 73*, 205–13.

Alicea, C., Belkowski, S., Eisenstein, T. K., Adler, M. W., & Rogers, T. J. (1996). Inhibition of primary murine macrophage cytokine production in vitro following treatment with the μ-opioid agonist U50,488H. *J Neuroimmunol, 64*, 83–90.

Alkhatib, G., Ahuja, S. S., Light, D., Mummidi, S., Berger, E. A., & Ahuja, S. K. (1997). CC chemokine receptor 5-mediated signaling and HIV-1 co-receptor activity share common structural determinants. *J Biol, Chem, 272*, 19771–76.

Angulo, F. J. & Swerdlow, D. L. (1995). Bacterial enteric infections in persons infected with human immunodeficiency virus. *Clin Infect Dis, 21*, S84–S93.

Anthony, J. C., Vlahov, D., Nelson, K. E., Cohn, S., Astemborski, J., & Solomon, L. (1991). New evidence on intravenous cocaine use and the risk of infection with human immunodeficiency virus type 1. *Am J Epidemiol, 134*, 1175–89.

Asakura, H., Kawamoto, K., Igimi, S., Yamamoto, S., & Makino, S. (2006). Enhancement of mice susceptibility to infection with *Listeria monocytogenes* by the treatment of morphine. *Microbiol Immunol, 50*, 543–47.

Band, L. C., Pert, A., Williams, W., de Costa, B. R., Rice, K. C., & Weber, R. J. (1992). Central μ-opioid receptors mediate suppression of natural killer cell activity *in vivo. Prog Neuroendocrinimmunol, 5*, 95–101.

Baum, M. K., Rafie, C., Lai, S., Sales, S., Page, B., & Campa, A. (2008). Crack-cocaine use accelerates HIV disease progression in a cohort of HIV-positive drug users. *J AIDS, 50*, 93–99.

Belkowski, S. M., Alicea, C., Eisenstein, T. K., Adler, M. W., & Rogers, T. J. (1995). Inhibition of IL-1 and TNF-α production following treatment of macrophages with the kappa opioid agonist U50,488H. *J Pharmacol Exp Ther, 273*, 1491–96.

Bell, J. E., Donaldson, Y. K., Lowrie, S., McKenzie, C. A., Elton, R. A., Chiswick, A., et al. (1996). Influence of risk group and zidovudine therapy on the development of HIV encephalitis and cognitive impairment in AIDS patients. *AIDS, 10*, 493–99.

Bleul, C. C., Farzan, M., Choe, H., Parolin, C., Clark-Lewis, I., Sodroski, J., et al. (1996). The lymphocyte chemoattractant SDF-1 is a ligand for LESTR/fusin and blocks HIV-1 entry. *Nature, 382*, 829–33.

Bonnet, M. P., Beloeil, H., Benhamou, D., Mazoit, J. X., & Asehnoune, K. (2008). The mu-opioid receptor mediates morphine-induced tumor necrosis factor and interleukin-6 inhibition in toll-like receptor 2-stimulated monocytes. *Anesth Analg, 106*, 1142–49.

Boring, L., Gosling, J., Cleary, M., & Charo, I. F. (1998). Decreased lesion formation in CCR2-/- mice reveals a role for chemokines in the initiation of atherosclerosis. *Nature, 394*, 894–97.

Boyer, J. D., Kumar, S., Robinson, T., Parkinson, R., Wu, L., Lewis, M., et al. (2006). Initiation of antiretroviral therapy during chronic SIV infection leads to rapid reduction in viral loads and the level of T-cell immune response. *J Med Primatol, 35*, 202–9.

Breslow, J. M., Feng, P., Meissler, J. J., Pintar, J. E., Gaughan, J., Adler, M. W., et al. (2010). Potentiating effect of morphine on oral *Salmonella enterica* serovar Typhimurium infection is mu-opioid receptor dependent. *Microbial Pathogenesis, 49*, 330–5.

Bruce-Keller, A. J., Turchan-Cholewo, J., Smart, E. J., Geurin, T., Chauhan, A., Reid, R., et al. (2008). Morphine causes rapid increases in glial activation and neuronal injury in the striatum of inducible HIV-1 Tat transgenic mice. *Glia, 56*, 1414–27.

Bryant, H. U., Bernton, E. W., & Holaday, J. W. (1987). Immunosuppressive effects of chronic morphine treatment in mice. *Life Sci, 41*, 1731–38.

Bryant, H. U., Bernton, E. W., Kenner, J. R., & Holaday, J. W. (1991). Role of adrenal cortical activation in the immunosuppressive effects of chronic morphine treatment. *Endocrinology, 128*, 3253–58.

Bussiere, J. L., Adler, M. W., Rogers, T. J., & Eisenstein, T. K. (1992). Differential effects of morphine and naltrexone on the antibody response in various mouse strains. *Immunopharmacol Immunotoxicol, 14*, 657–73.

Bussiere, J. L., Adler, M. W., Rogers, T. J., & Eisenstein, T. K. (1993). Cytokine reversal of morphine-induced suppression of the antibody response. *J Pharmacol Exp Ther, 264*, 591–97.

Carneiro, M., Yu, X-F., Lyles, C., Templeton, A., Weisstein, A. E., Safaeian, M., et al. (1999). The effect of drug-injection behavior on genetic evolution of HIV-1. *J Infect Dis, 180*, 1025–32.

Carr, D. J. J., Mayo, S., Gebhardt, B. M., & Porter, J. (1994). Central α-adrenergic involvement in morphine-mediated suppression of splenic natural killer cell activity. *J Neuroimmunol, 53*, 53–63.

Carr, D. J. J., Radulescu, R. T., de Costa, B. R., Rice, K. C., & Blalock, J. E. (1990). Differential effect of opioids on immunoglobulin production by lymphocytes isolated from Peyer's patches and spleen. *Life Sci, 47*, 1059–69.

Casellas, A. M., Guardiola, H., & Renaud, F. L. (1991). Inhibition of phagocytosis in peritoneal macrophages. *Neuropeptides, 18*, 35–40.

Centers for Disease Control. (1996). *HIV/AIDS surveillance report.* 7 ed. Atlanta: US Department of Health and Human Services.

Celum, C. L., Chaisson, R. E., Rutherford, G. W., Barnhart, J. L., & Echenberg, D. F. (1987). Incidence of Salmonellosis in patients with AIDS. *J Infect Dis, 156*, 998–1002.

Chaisson, R. E., Moss, A. R., Onishi, R., Osmond, D., & Carlson, J. R. (1987). Human immunodeficiency virus infection in heterosexual intravenous drug users in San Francisco. *Am J Pub Health, 77*, 169–72.

Chao, C. C., Gekker, G., Hu, S., Sheng, W. S., Shark, K. B., Bu, D-F., et al. (1996). κ-opioid receptors in human microglia downregulate human immunodeficiency virus-1 expression. *Proc Natl Acad Sci USA, 93*, 8051–56.

Chao, C. C., Hu, S., Molitor, T. W., Zhou, Y., Murtaugh, M. P., Tsang, M., et al. (1992). Morphine potentiates transforming growth factor-β release from human peripheral blood mononuclear cell cultures. *J Pharmacol Exp Ther, 262*, 19–24.

Chao, C. C., Hu, S., Shark, K. B., Sheng, W. S., Gekker, G., & Peterson, P. K. (1997). Activation of mu opioid receptors inhibits microglial cell chemotaxis. *J Pharmacol Exp Ther, 281*, 998–1003.

Chao, C. C., Sharp, B. M., Pomeroy, C., Filice, G. A., & Peterson, P. K. (1990). Lethality of morphine in mice infected with *Toxoplasma gondii. J Pharmacol Exp Ther, 252*, 605–9.

Chen, C., Li, J., Bot, G., Szabo, I., Rogers, T. J., & Liu-Chen, L-Y. (2004). Heterodimerization and cross-desensitization between the mu-opioid receptor and the chemokine CCR5 receptor. *Eur J Pharmacol, 483*, 175–86.

Chiesi, A., Seeber, A. C., Dally, L. G., Floridia, M., Rezza, G. & Vella, S. (1996). AIDS dementia complex in the Italian National AIDS Registry: temporal trends (1987–93) and differential incidence according to mode of transmission. *J Neurol Sci, 144*, 107–13.

Chuang, L. F., Killam, K. F. Jr., Chuang, R. Y. (1997). SIV infection of macaques: a model for studying AIDS and drug abuse. *Addiction Biol, 2*, 421–430.

Crum, R. M., Galai, N., Cohn, S., Celentano, D. D., & Vlahov, D. (1996). Alcohol use and T-lymphocyte subsets among injection drug users with HIV-1 infection: A prospective analysis. *Alcohol Clin Exp Res, 20*, 364–71.

Davis, R. L., Buck, D. J., Saffarian, N., & Stevens, C. W. (2007). The opioid antagonist, beta-funaltrexamine, inhibits chemokine expression in human astroglial cells. *J Neuroimmunol, 186*, 141–49.

DeBeck, K., Kerr, T., Li, K., Fischer, B., Buxton, J., Montaner, J., et al. (2009). Smoking of crack cocaine as a risk factor for HIV infection among people who use injection drugs. *Can Med Assoc J, 181*, 585–89.

Delgado-Velez, M., Lugo-Chinchilla, A., Lizardo, L., Morales, I., Robles, Y., Bruno, N., et al. (2008). Chronic exposure of human macrophages in vitro to morphine and methadone induces a putative tolerant/dependent state. *J Neuroimmunol, 196*, 94–100.

Des Jarlais, D. C., Friedman, S. R., & Stoneburner, R. L. (1988). HIV infection and intravenous drug use: Critical issues in transmission dynamics, infection outcomes, and prevention. *Rev Infect Dis, 10*, 151–58.

Des Jarlais, D. C., Friedman, S. R., Marmor, M., Cohen, H., Mildvan, D., Yancovitz, N., et al. (1987). Development of AIDS, HIV seroconversion and potential co-factors for T4 cell loss in a cohort of intravenous drug users. *AIDS, 1*, 105–111.

Dinari, G., Ashkenazi, S., Marcus, H., Rosenbach, Y., & Zahavi, I. (1989). The effect of opiates on the intestinal immune response to cholera toxin in mice. *Digestion, 44*, 14–19.

Donahoe, R. M., Byrd, L. D., McClure, H. M., Fultz, P., Brantley, M., Marsteller, F., et al. (1993). Consequences of opiate-dependency in a monkey model of AIDS. *Adv Exp Med Biol, 335*, 21–28.

Donahoe, R. M. & Falek, A. (1988). Neuroimmunomodulation by opiates and other drugs of abuse: Relationship to HIV infection and AIDS. In T.P. Bridge (Ed.). *Psychological, neuropsychiatric, and substance abuse aspects of AIDS* (pp. 145–58). New York: Raven Press.

Donahoe, R. M., O'Neil, S. P., Marsteller, F. A., Novembre, F. J., Anderson, D. C., Lankford-Turner, P., et al. (2009). Probable deceleration of progression of simian AIDS affected by opiate dependency: Studies with a rhesus macaque/SIVsmm9 model. *J AIDS, 50,* 241–49.

Donahoe, R. M. & Vlahov, D. (1998). Opiates as potential cofactors in progression of HIV-1 infections to AIDS. *J Neuroimmunol, 83,* 77–87.

Dragic, T., Litwin, V., Allaway, G. P., Martin, S. R., Huang, Y., Nagashima, K. A., et al. (1996). HIV-1 entry into CD4+ cells is mediated by the chemokine receptor CC-CKR-5. *Nature, 381,* 667–73.

Durante, A. J., Selwyn, P. A., & O'Connor, P. G. (1998). Risk factors for and knowledge of Mycobacterium tuberculosis infection among drug users in substance abuse treatment. *Addict, 93,* 1393–401.

Eisenstein, T. K., Meissler, J. J. Jr., Geller, E. B., & Adler, M. W. (1990). Immunosuppression to tetanus toxoid induced by implanted morphine pellets. *Ann NY Acad Sci, 594,* 377–79.

Eisenstein, T. K., Meissler, J. J. Jr., Rogers, T. J., Geller, E. B., & Adler, M. W. (1995). Mouse strain differences in immunosuppression by opioids *in vitro. J Pharmacol Exp Ther, 275,* 1484–89.

Eisenstein, T. K., Rahim, R. T., Feng, P., Thingalaya, N. K., & Meissler, J. J. (2006). Effects of opioid tolerance and withdrawal on the immune system. *J Neuroimm Pharmacol, 1,* 237–49.

El-Asmar, L., Springael, J. Y., Ballet, S., Andrieu, E. U., Vassart, G., & Parmentier, M. (2005). Evidence for negative binding cooperativity within CCR5-CCR2b heterodimers. *Mol Pharmacol, 67,* 460–469.

El-Hage, N., Bruce-Keller, A. J., Knapp, P. E., & Hauser, K. F. (2008). CCL5/RANTES gene deletion attenuates opioid-induced increases in glial CCL2/MCP-1 immunoreactivity and activation in HIV-1 Tat-exposed mice. *J Neuroimm Pharmacol, 3,* 275–85.

El-Hage, N., Gurwell, J. A., Singh, I. N., Knapp, P. E., Nath, A., & Hauser, K. F. (2005). Synergistic increases in intracellular Ca2+, and the release of MCP-1, RANTES, and IL-6 by astrocytes treated with opiates and HIV-1 Tat. *Glia, 50,* 91–106.

El-Hage, N., Wu, G., Ambati, J., Bruce-Keller, A. J., Knapp, P. E., & Hauser, K. F. . (2006a). CCR2 mediates increases in glial activation caused by exposure to HIV1 Tat and opiates. *J Neuroimmunol, 178,* 9–16.

El-Hage, N., Wu, G., Wang, J., Ambati, J., Knapp, P. E., Reed, J. L., et al. (2006b). HIV-1 Tat and opiate-induced changes in astrocytes promote chemotaxis of microglia through the expression of MCP-1 and alternative chemokines. *Glia, 53,* 132–46.

Feng, P., Meissler, J. J. Jr., Adler, M. W., & Eisenstein, T. K. (2005a). Morphine withdrawal sensitizes mice to lipopolysaccharide: Elevated TNF-alpha and nitric oxide with decreased IL-12. *J Neuroimmunol, 164,* 57–65.

Feng, P., Rahim, R. T., Cowan, A., Liu-Chen, L-Y., Peng, X., Gaughan, J., et al. (2006a). Effects of mu, kappa or delta opioids administered by pellet or pump on oral Salmonella infection and gastrointestinal transit. *Eur J Pharmacol, 534,* 250–257.

Feng, P., Truant, A. L., Meissler, J. J. Jr., Gaughan, J. P., Adler, M. W., & Eisenstein, T. K. (2006b). Morphine withdrawal lowers host defense to enteric bacteria: Spontaneous sepsis and increased sensitivity to oral *Salmonella enterica* serovar Typhimurium infection. *Infect Immun, 74,* 5221–26.

Feng, P., Wilson, Q. M., Meissler, J. J. Jr., Adler, M. W., & Eisenstein, T. K. (2005b). Increased sensitivity to *Salmonella enterica* serovar Typhimurium infection in mice undergoing withdrawal from morphine is associated with suppression of interleukin-12. *Infect Immun, 73,* 7953–59.

Feng, Y., Broder, C. C., Kennedy, P. E., & Berger, E. A. (1996). HIV-1 entry cofactor: Functional cDNA cloning of a seven-transmembrane, G protein-coupled receptor. *Science, 272,* 872–77.

Finley, M. J., Chen, X., Bardi, G., Davey, P., Geller, E. B., Zhang, L., et al. (2008). Bi-directional heterologous desensitization between the major HIV-1 co-receptor CXCR4 and the kappa-opioid receptor. *J Neuroimmunol, 197,* 114–23.

Freier, D. O. & Fuchs, B. A. (1994). A mechanism of action for morphine-induced immunosuppression: Corticosterone mediates morphine-induced suppression of natural killer cell activity. *J Pharmacol Exp Ther, 270,* 1127–33.

Friedland, G. H., Harris, C., Butkus-Small, C., Shine, D., Moll, B., Darrow, W., et al. (1985). Intravenous drug abusers and the acquired immunodeficiency syndrome (AIDS). Demographic, drug use, and needle-sharing patterns. *Arch Intern Med, 145,* 1413–17.

Fuchs, B. A. & Pruett, S. B. (1993). Morphine induces apoptosis in murine thymocytes *in vivo* but not *in vitro*: Involvement of both opiate and glucocorticoid receptors. *J Pharmacol Exp Ther, 266,* 417–23.

Garfein, R. S., Vlahov, D., Galai, N., Doherty, M. C., & Nelson, K. E. (1996). Viral infections in short-term injection drug users: The prevalence of the hepatitis C, hepatitis B, human immunodeficiency, and human T-lymphotropic viruses. *Am J Pub Health, 86,* 655–61.

Gavériaux-Ruff, C., Matthes, H. W. D., Peluso, J., & Kieffer, B. L. (1998). Abolition of morphine-immunosuppression in mice lacking the mu-opioid receptor gene. *Proc Natl Acad Sci USA, 95,* 6326–30.

Gorry, P. R., Bristol, G., Zack, J. A., Ritola, K., Swanstrom, R., Birch, C. J., et al. (2001). Macrophage tropism of human immunodeficiency virus type 1 isolates from brain and lymphoid tissues predicts neurotropism independent of coreceptor specificity. *J Virol, 75,* 10073–89.

Govitrapong, P., Suttitum, T., Kotchabhakdi, N., & Uneklabh, T. (1998). Alterations of immune functions in heroin addicts and heroin withdrawal subjects. *J Pharmacol Exp Ther, 286,* 883–89.

Gray, F. & Lescs, M. C. (1993). HIV-related demyelinating disease. *Eur J Med, 2,* 89–96.

Greeneltch, K. M., Haudenschild, C. C., Keegan, A. D., & Shi, Y. (2004). The opioid antagonist naltrexone blocks acute endotoxic shock by inhibiting tumor necrosis factor-α production. *Brain Behav.Immun, 18,* 476–84.

Grigoryan, A., Shouse, R. L., Durant, T., Mastro, T. D., Espinoza, L., Chen, M., et al. (2009). HIV infection among injection-drug users— 34 States, 2004–2007. *Morbidity and Mortality Weekly Report, 58,* 1291–95.

Grimm, M. C., Ben-Baruch, A., Taub, D. D., Howard, O. M. Z., Resau, J. H., Wang, J. M., et al. (1998). Opiates transdeactivate chemokine receptors: δ and μ opiate receptor-mediated heterologous desensitization. *J Exp Med, 188,* 317–25.

Gruenewald, R., Blum, S., & Chan, J. (1994). Relationship between human immunodeficiency virus infection and Salmonellosis in 20- to 59-year-old residents of New York City. *Clin Infect Dis, 18,* 358–63.

Guan, L., Eisenstein, T. K., Adler, M. W., & Rogers, T. J. (1997). Inhibition of T cell superantigen responses following treatment with the κ-opioid U50,488H. *J Neuroimmunol, 75,* 163–68.

Guan, L., Townsend, R., Eisenstein, T. K., Adler, M. W., & Rogers, T. J. (1994). Both T cells and macrophages are targets of κ-opioid-induced immunosuppression. *Brain Behav Immun, 8,* 229–40.

Guo, C. J., Li, Y., Tian, S., Wang, X., Douglas, S. D., & Ho, W. Z. (2002). Morphine enhances HIV infection of human blood mononuclear phagocytes through modulation of beta-chemokines and CCR5 receptor. *J Invest Med, 50,* 435–42.

Happel, C., Steele, A. D., Finley, M. J., Kutzler, M. A., & Rogers, T. J. (2008). DAMGO-induced expression of chemokines and chemokine receptors: The role of TGF-beta1. *J Leukoc Biol, 83,* 956–63.

Haverkos, H. W. & Lange, R. W. (1990). Serious infections other than human immunodeficiency virus among intravenous drug users. *J Infect Dis, 161,* 894–902.

Hazum, E., Chang, K-J., & Cuatrecasas, P. (1979). Specific nonopiate receptors for β-endorphin. *Science, 205,* 1033–35.

Hedin, K. E., Bell, M. P., Kalli, K. R., Huntoon, C. J., Sharp, B. M., & McKean, D. J. (1997). Mu-opioid receptors expressed by Jurkat T cells enhance IL-2 secretion by increasing AP-1 complexes and activity of the NF-AT/AP-1-binding promoter element. *J Immunol, 159,* 5431–40.

Hernanz-Falcon, P., Rodriguez-Frade, J. M., Serrano, A., Juan, D., del Sol, A., Soriano, S. F., et al. (2004). Identification of amino acid residues crucial for chemokine recptor dimerization. *Nature Immunol, 5,* 216–23.

Hilburger, M. E., Adler, M. W., Truant, A. L., Meissler, J. J. Jr., Satishchandran, V., Rogers, T. J., et al. (1997). Morphine induces sepsis in mice. *J Infect Dis, 176,* 183–88.

House, R. V., Thomas, P. T., & Bhargava, H. N. (1996). A comparative study of immunomodulation produced by in vitro exposure to delta opioid receptor agonist peptides. *Peptides, 17*, 75–81.

House, S. D., Mao, X., Wu, G. D., Espinelli, D., Li, W. X., & Chang, S. L. (2001). Chronic morphine potentiates the inflammatory response by disrupting interleukin-1β modulation of the hypothalamic-pituitary-adrenal axis. *J Neuroimmunol, 118*, 227–85.

Hu, S., Chao, C. C., Hegg, C. C., Thayer, S., & Peterson, P. K. (2000). Morphine inhibits human microglial cell production of, and migration towards, RANTES. *J Psychopharmacol, 14*, 238–43.

Hussey, H. H. & Katz, S. (1950). Infections resulting from narcotic addiction. *Am J Med, 9*, 186–93.

Jessop, J. J. & Taplits, M. S. (1991). Effect of high doses of morphine on Con-A induced lymphokine production in vitro. *Immunopharm, 22*, 175–84.

Kao, P. T., Liu, C. P., Lee, C. M., & Hung, Y. C. (2005). Non-typhi *Salmonella* adrenal abscess in an HIV-infected patient. *Scand J Infect Dis, 37*, 370–372.

Kelschenbach, J., Barke, R. A., & Roy, S. (2005). Morphine withdrawal contributes to Th cell differentiation by biasing cells toward the Th2 lineage. *J Immunol, 175*, 2655–65.

Kumar, R., Torres, C., Yamamura, Y., Rodriguez, I., Martinez, M., Staprans, S., et al. (2004). Modulation by morphine of viral set point in rhesus macaques infected with simian immunodeficiency virus and simian-human immunodeficiency virus. *J Virol, 78*, 11425–28.

Kurihara, T., Warr, G., Loy, J., & Bravo, R. (1997). Defects in macrophage recruitment and host defense in mice lacking the CCR2 chemokine receptor. *J Exp Med, 186*, 1757–62.

Kuziel, W. A., Morgan, S. J., Dawson, T. C., Griffin, S., Smithies, O., Ley, K., et al. (1997). Severe reduction in leukocyte adhesion and monocyte extravasation in mice deficient in CC chemokine receptor 2. *Proc Natl Acad Sci USA, 94*, 12053–58.

Lane, T. E., Asensio, N., Yu, N., Paoletti, A. D., Campbell, I. L., & Buchmeier, M. J. (1998). Dynamic regulation of α- and β-chemokine expression in the central nervous system during mouse hepatitis virus-induced demyelinating disease. *J Immunol, 160*, 970–978.

Lefkowitz, S. S. & C. Y. Chiang, C. Y. (1975). Effects of certain abused drugs on hemolysin forming cells. *Life Sci, 17*, 1763–68.

Levine, D. P. (1991). Infectious endocarditis in intravenous drug abusers. In D. P. Levine & J. D. Sobel (Eds.). *Infections in intravenous drug abusers* (pp. 251–85). New York: Oxford University Press.

Li, Y., X. Wang, Tian, S., Guo, C-J., Douglas, S. D., & Ho, W-Z. (2002). Methadone enhances human immunodeficiency virus infection of human immune cells. *J Infect Dis, 185*, 118–22.

Lindback, S., Brostrom, C., Karlsson, A., Gaines, H. (1994). Does symptomatic primary HIV-1 infection accelerate progression to CDC stage IV disease, CD4 count below 200 x (106)/l, AIDS, and death from AIDS? *Brit. Med.J, 309*, 1535–1537.

Lioy, D., Sheridan, P. A., Hurley, S. D., Walton, J. R., Martin, A. M., Olschowka, J. A., et al. (2006). Acute morphine exposure potentiates the development of HSV-1-induced encephalitis. *J Neuroimmunol, 172*, 9–17.

Liu, Y., Blackbourn, D. J., Chuang, L. F., Killam, K. F. Jr., & Chuang, R. Y. (1992). Effects of in vivo and in vitro administration of morphine sulfate upon Rhesus macaque polymorphonuclear cell phagocytosis and chemotaxis. *J Pharmacol Exp Ther, 263*, 533–39.

Lokensgard, J. R., Gekker, G., & Peterson, P. K. (2002). Mu-opioid receptor agonist inhibition of HIV-1 envelope glycoprotein-mediated membrane fusion and CXCR4 expression on CD4+ lymphocytes. *Biochem Pharmacol, 63*, 1037–41.

Louria, D. B, Hensle, T., & Rose, J. (1967). The major medical complications of heroin addiction. *Ann Int Med, 67*, 1–22.

Lyles, C. M., Graham, N. M. H., Astemborski, J., Vlahov, D., Margolick, J. B., Saah, A. J., et al. (1999). Cell-associated infectious HIV-1 viral load as a predictor of clinical progression and survival among HIV-1 infected injection drug users and homosexual men. *Eur J Epidemiol, 15*, 99–108.

Lysle, D. T., Coussons, M. E., Watts, V. J., Bennett, E. H., & Dykstra, L. A. (1993). Morphine-induced alterations of immune status: Dose dependency, compartment specificity and antagonism by naltrexone. *J Pharmacol Exp Ther, 265*, 1071–78.

Ma, J., Wang, J., Wan, J., Charboneau, R., Chang, Y., Barke, R. A., et al. (2010). Morphine disrupts interleukin-23 (IL-23)/IL-17-mediated pulmonary mucosal host defense against *Streptococcus pneumoniae* infection. *Infect Immun, 78*, 830–837.

MacFarlane, A. S., Peng, X., Meissler, J. J. Jr., Rogers, T. J., Geller, E. B., Adler, M. W., et al. (2000). Morphine increases susceptibility to oral *Salmonella typhimurium* infection. *J Infect Dis, 181*, 1350–1358.

MacLennan, C. A., Glichrist, J. J., Gordon, M. A., Cunningham, C. C., Cobbold, M., Goddall, M., et al . (2010). Dysregulated humoral immunity to nontyphoidal *Salmonella* in HIV-infected African adults. *Science, 328*, 508–12.

Mahajan, S. D., Aalinkeel, R., Sykes, D. E., Reynolds, J. L., Bindukumar, B., Fernandez, S. F., et al. (2008). Tight junction regulation by morphine and HIV-1 tat modulates blood-brain barrier permeability. *J Clin Immunol, 28*, 528–41.

Mahajan, S. D., Schwartz, S. A., Aalinkeel, R., Chawda, R. P., Sykes, D. E., Nair, M. P. N. (2005). Morphine modulates chemokine gene regulation in normal human astrocytes. *Clin Immunol, 115*, 323–32.

Mahajan, S. D., Schwartz, S. A., Shanahan, T. C., Chawda, R. P., & Nair, M. P. N. (2002). Morphine regulates gene expression of α- and β-chemokines and their receptors on astroglial cells via the opioid mu receptor. *J Immunol, 169*, 3589–99.

Makman, M. H., Bilfinger, T. V., & Stefano, G. B. (1995). Human granulocytes contain an opiate alkaloid-selective receptor mediating inhibition of cytokine-induced activation and chemotaxis. *J Immunol, 154*, 1323–30.

Marcario, J. K., Riazi, M., Adany, I., Kenjale, H., Fleming, K., Marquis, J., et al. (2008). Effect of morphine on the neuropathogenesis of SIVmac infection in Indian Rhesus macaques. *J Neuroimm Pharmacol, 3*, 12–25.

Margolick, J. B., Muñoz, A., Vlahov, D., Astemborski, J., Solomon, L., He, X-Y., et al. (1994). Direct comparison of the relationship between clinical outcome and change in CD4+ lymphocytes in human immunodeficiency virus-positive homosexual men and injecting drug users. *Arch Intern Med, 154*, 869–75.

Margolick, J. B., Muñoz, A., Vlahov, D., Solomon, L., Astemborski, J., Cohn, S., et al. (1992). Changes in T-lymphocyte subsets in intravenous drug users with HIV-1 infection. *JAMA, 267*, 1631–36.

Martinez, A. J., Sell, M., Mitrovics, T., Stoltenburg-Didinger, G., Iglesias-Rozas, J. R., Giraldo-Velasquez, M. A., et al. (1995). The neuropathology and epidemiology of AIDS. A Berlin experience. A review of 200 cases. *Pathol Res Pract, 191*, 427–43.

Martucci, C., Franchi, S., Lattauda, L., Panerai, A. E., & Sacerdote, P. (2007). Differential involvement of RelB in morphine-induced modulation of chemotaxis, NO, and cytokine production in murine macrophages and lymphocytes. *J Leukoc Biol, 81*, 344–54.

Mazzone, A., Ricevuti, G., Pasotti, D., Fioravanti, A., Marcoli, M., Lecchini, S., et al. (1990). Peptide opioids and morphine effects on inflammatory process. *Inflammation, 14*, 717–26.

McCoy, C. B., Metsch, L. R., Chitwood, D. D., Shapshak, P., & Comerford, S. T. (1998). Parenteral transmission of HIV among injection drug users: Assessing the frequency of multiperson use of needles, syringes, cookers, cotton, and water. *JAIDS, 18 Suppl 1* S25–S29.

Nair, M. P., Schwartz, S. A., Polasani, R., Hou, J., Sweet, A., & Chadha, K. C. (1997). Immunoregulatory effects of morphine on human lymphocytes. *Clin Diag Lab Immunol, 4*, 127–32.

Ni, X., Gritman, K. R., Eisenstein, T. K., Adler, M. W., Arfors, K. E., & Tuma, R. F. (2000). Morphine attenuates leukocyte/endothelial interactions. *Microvasc Res, 60*, 121–30.

Oberlin, E., Amara, A., Bachelerie, F., Bessia, C., Virelizier, J. L., Arenzana-Seisdedos, F., et al. (1996). The CXC chemokine SDF-1 is the ligand for LESTR/fusin and prevents infection by T-cell-line-adapted HIV-1. *Nature, 382*, 833–35.

Ocasio, F. M., Jiang, Y., House, S. D., & Chang. S. L. (2004). Chronic morphine accelerates the progression of lipopolysaccharide-induced sepsis to septic shock. *J Neuroimmunol, 149*, 90–100.

Pacifici, R., Patrini, G., Venier, I., Parolaro, D., Zuccaro, P., & Gori, E. (1994). Effect of morphine and methadone acute treatment on immunological activity in mice: pharmacokinetic and pharmacodynamic correlates. *J Pharmacol Exp Ther*, 269, 1112–16.

Panaslak, W., Gumulka, S., Kobus, M., & Luczak, M. (1990). The influence of morphine on development of HSV-1 and M-MSV virus infection in mice. *Acta Microbiol Pol*, 39, 215–18.

Peng, X., Cebra, J. J., Adler, M. W., Meissler, J. J., Jr., Cowan, A., Feng, P., et al. (2001). Morphine inhibits mucosal antibody responses and TGF-β mRNA in gut-associated lymphoid tissue following oral cholera toxin in mice. *J Immunol*, 167, 3677–81.

Peng, X., Mosser, D. M., Adler, M. W., Rogers, T. J., Meissler, J. J. Jr., & Eisenstein, T. K. (2000). Morphine enhances interleukin-12 and the production of other pro-inflammatory cytokines in mouse peritoneal macrophages. *J Leukoc Biol*, 68, 723–28.

Perez-Castrillon, J.-L., Perez-Arellanos, J-L., Carcia-Palomo, J-D., Jimeniz-Lopez, A., & de Castro, S. (1992). Opioids depress in vitro human monocyte chemotaxis. *Immunopharm*, 23, 57–61.

Peterson, P. K., Gekker, G., Hu, S., Anderson, W. R., Kravitz, F., Portoghese, P. S., et al. (1994). Morphine amplifies HIV-1 expression in chronically infected promonocytes cocultured with human brain cells. *J Neuroimmunol*, 50, 167–75.

Peterson, P. K., Gekker, G., Hu, S., Sheng, W. S., Molitor, T. W., & Chao, C. C. (1995). Morphine stimulates phagocytosis of *Mycobacterium tuberculosis* by human microglial cells: Involvement of a G protein-coupled opiate receptor. *Adv Neuroimmunol*, 5, 299–309.

Peterson, P. K., Sharp, B., Gekker, G., Brummitt, C., & Keane. W. F. (1987a). Opioid-mediated suppression of cultured peripheral blood mononuclear cell respiratory burst activity. *J Immunol*, 138, 3907–12.

Peterson, P. K., Sharp, B., Gekker, G., Brummitt, C., & Keane. W. F. (1987b). Opioid-mediated suppression of interferon-γ production by cultured peripheral blood mononuclear cells. *J Clin Invest*, 80, 824–31.

Peterson, P. K., Sharp, B. M., Gekker, G., Portoghese, P. S., Sannerud, K., & Balfour, H. H. Jr. (1990). Morphine promotes the growth of HIV-1 in human peripheral blood mononuclear cell cocultures. *AIDS*, 4, 869–73.

Pu, H., Tian, J., Flora, G., Lee, Y. W., Nath, A., Hennig, B., et al. (2003). HIV-1 Tat protein upregulates inflammatory mediators and induces monocyte invasion into the brain. *Mol Cell Neurosci*, 24, 224–37.

Rahim, R. T., Adler, M. W., Meissler, J. J. Jr., Cowan, A., Rogers, T. J., Geller, E. B., et al. (2002). Abrupt or precipitated withdrawal from morphine induces immunosuppression. *J Neuroimmunol*, 127, 88–95.

Rahim, R. T., Meissler, J. J., Jr., Cowan, A., Rogers, T. J., Geller, E. B., Gaughan, J., et al. (2001). Administration of mu-, kappa- or delta₂-receptor agonists via osmotic minipumps suppresses murine splenic antibody responses. *Int Immunopharm*, 1, 2001–9.

Reiner, N. E., Gopalakrishna, K. V., & Lerner, P. I. (1976). Enterococcal endocarditis in heroin addicts. *JAMA*, 235, 1861–63.

Risdahl, J. M., Peterson, P. K., Chao, C. C., Pijoan, C., & Molitor, T. W. (1993). Effects of morphine dependence on the pathogenesis of swine herpesvirus infection. *J Infec Dis*, 167, 1281–87.

Rogers, T. J. & Peterson, P. K. (2003). Opioid G protein-coupled receptors: Signals at the crossroads of inflammation. *Trends Immunol*, 24, 116–21.

Rogers, T. J., Steele, A. D., Howard, O. M. Z., & Oppenheim, J. J. (2000). Bidirectional heterologous desensitization of opioid and chemokine receptors. *Ann N Y Acad Sci*, 917, 19–28.

Rojavin, M., Szabo, I., Bussiere, J. L., Rogers, T. J., Adler, M. W., & Eisenstein, T. K. (1993). Morphine treatment in vitro or in vivo decreases phagocytic functions of murine macrophages. *Life Sci*, 53, 997–1006.

Rothenberg, R., Woelfel, M., Stoneburner, R., Milberg, J., Parker, R., & Truman, B. (1986). Survival with the acquired immunodeficiency syndrome. Experience with 5833 cases in New York City. *N Eng J Med*, 317, 1297–302.

Roy, S., Balasubramanian, S., Sumandeep, S., Charboneau, R., Wang, J., Melnyk, D., et al. (2001). Morphine directs T cells toward T$_{h2}$ differentiation. *Surgery*, 130, 304–9.

Roy, S., Barke, R. A., & Loh, H. H. (1998a). Mu-opioid receptor-knockout mice: Role of μ-opioid receptor in morphine-mediated immune functions. *Mol Brain Res*, 61, 190–194.

Roy, S., Cain, K. J., Chapin, R. B., Charboneau, R. G., Barke, R. A. (1998b). Morphine modulates NFκB activation in macrophages. *Biochem Biophys Res Comm*, 245, 392–96.

Roy, S., Chapin, R. B., Cain, K. J., Charboneau, R. G., Ramakrishnan, S., & Barke, R. A. (1997). Morphine inhibits transcriptional activation of IL-2 in mouse thymocytes. *Cell Immunol*, 179, 1–9.

Roy, S., Charboneau, R. G., & Barke, R. A. (1999). Morphine synergizes with lipopolysaccharide in a chronic endotoxemia model. *J Neuroimmunol*, 95, 107–14.

Roy, S., Ramakrishnan, S., Loh, H. H., & Lee, N. M. (1991). Chronic morphine treatment selectively suppresses macrophage colony formation in bone marrow. *Eur J Pharmacol*, 195, 359–63.

Ruff, M. R., Wahl, S. M., Mergenhagen, S., & Pert, C. B. (1985). Opiate receptor-mediated chemotaxis of human monocytes. *Neuropeptides*, 5, 363–66.

Saas, P. J., Boucraut, A. L., Quiquerez, V., Schnuriger, V., Perrin, G., Desplat-Jego, S., et al. (1999). CD95 (Fas/Apo-1) as a receptor governing astrocyte apoptotic or inflammatory responses: A key role in brain inflammation. *J Immunol*, 162, 2326–33.

Scheidegger, C. & Zimmerli, W. (1989). Infectious complications in drug addicts: Seven year review of 269 hospitalized narcotic abusers in Switzerland. *Rev Infect Dis*, 11, 486–93.

Schweitzer, C., Keller, F., Schmitt, M. P., Jaeck, D., Adloff, M., Schmitt, C. et al. (1991). Morphine stimulates HIV replication in primary cultures of human Kupffer cells. *Res Virol*, 142, 189–95.

Selwyn, P. A., Alcabes, P., Hartel, D., Buono, D., Schoenbau, E. E., Klein, R. S., et al. (1992). Clinical manifestations and predictors of disease progression in drug users with HIV infections. *N Eng J Med*, 327, 1697–703.

Shahabi, N. A. & Sharp, B. M. (1995). Antiproliferative effects of μ-opioids on highly purified CD4+ and CD8+ murine T cells. *J Pharmacol Exp Ther*, 273, 1105–13.

Sharp, B. M., Gekker, G., Li, M. D., Chao, C. C., & Peterson, P. K. (1998). Delta opioid suppression of human immunodeficiency virus-1 expression in T cells (Jurkat). *Biochem Pharmacol*, 56, 289–92.

Shavit, Y., Depaulis, A., Martin, F. C., Terman, G. W., Pechnick, R. N., Zane, C. J., et al. (1986). Involvement of brain opiate receptors in the immune-suppressive effect of morphine. *Proc Natl Acad Sci USA*, 83, 7114–17.

Shavit, Y., Lewis, J. W., Terman, G. W., Gale, R. P., & Liebeskind, J. C. (1984). Opioid peptides mediate the suppressive effect of stress on natural killer cell cytotoxicity. *Science*, 223, 188–90.

Shavit, Y., Martin, F. C., Yirmiya, R., Ben-Eliyahu, S., Terman, G. W., Weiner, H., et al. (1987). Effects of a single administration of morphine or footshock stress on natural killer cell cytotoxicity. *Brain Behav Immun*, 1, 318–28.

Sheridan, P. A. & Moynihan, J. A. (2005). Modulation of the innate immune response to HSV-1 following acute administration of morphine: Role of hypothalamo-pituitary-adrenal axis. *J Neuroimmunol*, 158, 145–52.

Shieh, J. T., Albright, A. V., Sharron, M., Gartner, S., Strizki, J., Doms, R. W., et al. (1998). Chemokine receptor utilization by human immunodeficiency virus type 1 isolates that replicate in microglia. *J Virol*, 72, 4243–49.

Simpkins, C. O., Dickey, C. A., & Fink, M. P. (1984). Human neutrophil migration is enhanced by beta-endorphin. *Life Sci*, 34, 2251–55.

Sin, J.-I., Plotnikoff, N., & Specter, S. (1996). Anti-retroviral activity of methionine enkephalin and AZT in a murine cell culture. *Int J Immunopharmacol*, 18, 305–9.

Singal, P., Kinhikar, A. G., Singh, S., & Singh, P. P. (2002). Neuroimmunomodulatory effects of morphine in *Leishmania donovani*-infected hamsters. *Neuroimmunomod*, 10, 261–69.

Singh, P. P. & Singal, P. (2007). Morphine-induced neuroimmunomodulation in murine visceral leishmaniasis: The role(s) of cytokines and nitric oxide. *J Neuroimm Pharmacol*, 2, 338–51.

Singh, P. P., Singh, S., Dutta, G. P., & Srimal, R. C. (1993). Immunomodulation by morphine in *Plasmodium berghei*-infected mice. *Life Sci, 54*, 331–39.

Singh, R. P., Jhamb, S. S., & Singh, P. P. (2008). Effects of morphine during Mycobacterium tuberculosis H37Rv infection in mice. *Life Sci, 82*, 301–14.

Singh, S. & Singh, P. P. (2000). Morphine modulation of plasmodial-antigens-induced colony-stimulating factors production by macrophages. *Life Sci, 67*, 1035–45.

Singhal, P. C., Bhaskaran, M., Patel, J., Patel, K., Kasinath, B. S., Duraisamy, S., et al. (2002). Role of P38 mitogen-activated protein kinase phosphorylation and Fas-Fas ligand interaction in morphine-induced macrophage apoptosis. *J Immunol, 168*, 4025–33.

Singhal, P. C., Reddy, K., Franki, N., Sanwal, & Gibbons, N. (1997). Morphine induces splenocyte apoptosis and enhanced mRNA expression of cathepsin-B. *Inflammation, 21*, 609–15.

Singhal, P. C., Sharma, P., Kapasi, A. A., Reddy, K., Franki, N., & Gibbons, N. (1998). Morphine enhances macrophage apoptosis. *J Immunol, 160*, 1886–93.

Sowa, G., Gekker, G., Lipovsky, M. M., Hu, S., Chao, C. C., Molitor, T. W., et al. (1997). Inhibition of swine microglial cell phagocytosis of *Cryptococcus neoformans* by femtomolar concentrations of morphine. *Biochem Pharmacol, 53*, 823–28.

Spijkerman, I. J., Koot, M., Keet, I. P., van den Hoek, A. J., Miedema, F., Coutinho, R. A. (1995). Lower prevalence and incidence of HIV-1 syncytium-inducing phenotype among injecting drug users compared with homosexual men. *AIDS, 9*, 1085–92.

Spijkerman, I. J., Langendam, M. W., Veugelers, P. J., van Ameijden, E. J., Keet, I. P., Geskus, R. B., et al. (1996). Differences in progression to AIDS between injection drug users and homosexual men with documented dates of seroconversion. *Epidemiology, 7*, 571–77.

Squinto, S. P., Mondal, D., Block, A. L., & Prakash, O. (1990). Morphine-induced transactivation of HIV-1 LTR in human neuroblastoma cells. *AIDS Res Human Retroviruses, 6*, 1163–68.

Starec, M., Rouveix, B., Sinet, M., Chau, F., Desforges, B., Pocidalo, J-J., et al. (1991). Immune status and survival of opiate- and cocaine-treated mice infected with Friend virus. *J Pharmacol Exp Ther, 259*, 745–50.

Steele, A. D., Henderson, E. E., & Rogers, T. J. (2003). µ-Opioid modulation of HIV-1 coreceptor expression and HIV-1 replication. *Virol, 309*, 99–107.

Steele, A. D., Szabo, I., Bednar, F., & Rogers, T. J. (2002). Interactions between opioid and chemokine receptors: Heterologous desensitization. *Cytok.Growth Factor Rev, 13*, 209–22.

Stefano, G. B., Hartman, A., Bilfinger, T. V., Magazine, H. I., Liu, Y., Casares, F., et al. (1995). Presence of the μ_3 opiate receptor in endothelial cells. *J Biol Chem, 270*, 30290–30293.

Stefano, G. B., Salzetl, M., & Bilfinger, T. V. (1998). Long-term exposure of human blood vessels to HIV gp120, morphine, and anandamide increases endothelial adhesion of monocytes: Uncoupling of nitric oxide release. *J Cardiovasc Pharmacol, 31*, 862–68.

Stiene-Martin, A., Zhou, R., Hauser, K. F. (1998). Regional, developmental, and cell cycle-dependent differences in mu, delta, and kappa-opioid receptor expression among cultured mouse astrocytes. *Glia, 22*, 249–59.

Strizki, J. M., Albright, A. V., Sheng, H., O'Connor, M., Perrin, L., & Gonzalez-Scarano, F. (1996). Infection of primary human microglia and monocyte-derived macrophages with human immunodeficiency virus type 1 isolates: Evidence of differential tropism. *J Virol, 70*, 7654–62.

Suzuki, S., Carlos, M. P., Chuang, L. F., Torres, J. V., Doi, R. H., & Chuang, R. Y. (2002a). Methadone induces CCR5 and promotes AIDS virus infection. *FEBS Lett, 519*, 173–77.

Suzuki, S., Chuang, L. F., Yau, P., Doi, R. H., & Chuang, R. Y. (2002b). Interactions of opioid and chemokine receptors: Oligomerization of *mu, kappa*, and *delta* with CCR5 on immune cells. *Exp Cell Res, 280*, 192–200.

Szabo, I., Rojavin, M., Bussiere, J. L., Eisenstein, T. K., Adler, M. W., & Rogers, T. J. (1993). Suppression of peritoneal macrophage phagocytosis of *Candida albicans* by opioids. *J Pharmacol Exp Ther, 267*, 703–6.

Szabo, I., M. Wetzel, A., Zhang, N., Steele, A. D., Kaminsky, D. E., Chen, C., et al. (2003). Selective inactivation of CCR5 and decreased infectivity of R5 HIV-1 strains mediated by opioid-induced heterologous desensitization. *J Leukoc Biol, 74*, 1074–82.

Takeuchi, A. (1967). Electron microscope studies of experimental Salmonella infection. I. Penetration into the intestinal epithelium by *Salmonella typhimurium. Amer J Path, 50*, 109–39.

Takeuchi, A. (1971). Penetration of the intestinal epithelium by various microorganisms. *Curr Top Pathol, 54*, 1–27.

Taub, D. D., Eisenstein, T. K., Geller, E. B., Adler, M. W., & Rogers, T. J. (1991). Immunomodulatory activity of µ- and κ-selective opioid agonists. *Proc Natl Acad Sci USA, 88*, 360–364.

Tomassini, N., Renaud, F. L., Roy, S., & Loh, H. H. (2003). Mu and delta receptors mediate morphine effects on phagocytosis by murine peritoneal macrophages. *J Neuroimmunol, 136*, 9–16.

Tubaro, E., Borelli, G., Croce, C., Cavallo, G., & Santiangeli, C. (1983). Effect of morphine on resistance to infection. *J Infec Dis, 148*, 656–66.

Turchan-Cholewo, J., Dimayuga, F. O., Ding, Q., Keller, J. N., Hauser, K. F., Knapp, P. E., et al. (2008). Cell-specific actions of HIV-Tat and morphine on opioid receptor expression in glia. *J Neurosci Res, 86*, 2100–2110.

Van Epps, D. E. & Saland, L. (1984). β-Endorphin and met-enkephalin stimulate human peripheral blood mononuclear cell chemotaxis. *J Immunol, 132*, 3046–53.

Vanhems, P., Lambert, J., Cooper, D. A., Perrin, L., Carr, A., Hirschel, B., et al. (1998). Severity and prognosis of acute human immunodeficiency virus type 1 illness: A dose-response relationship. *Clin Infect Dis, 26*, 323–29.

Vassou, D., Badogeorgou, E., Kampa, M., Dimitriou, H., Hatzoglou, A., & Castanas, E. (2008). Opioids modulate constitutive B-lymphocyte secretion. *Int Immunopharm, 8*, 634–44.

Veugelers, P. J., Kaldor, J. M., Strathdee, S. A., Page-Shafer, K. A., Schechter, M. T., Coutinho, R. A., et al. (1997). Incidence and prognositc significance of symptomatic primary human immunodeficiency virus type 1 infection in homosexual men. *J Infect Dis, 176*, 112–17.

Veyries, M.-L., Sinet, M., Desforges, B., & Rouveix, B. (1995). Effects of morphine on the pathogenesis of murine Friend retrovirus infection. *J Pharmacol Exp Ther, 272*, 498–504.

Wang, J., R. Barke, A., Charboneau, R., & Roy, S. (2005). Morphine impairs host innate immune response and increases susceptibility to *Streptococcus pneumoniae* lung infection. *J Immunol, 174*, 426–34.

Wang, J., Barke, R. A., Charboneau, R., Schwendener, R., & Roy, S. (2008). Morphine induces defects in early response of alveolar macrophages to *Streptococcus pneumoniae* by modulating TLR9-NFkB signaling. *J Immunol, 180*, 3594–600.

Wang, X., Tan, N., Douglas, D., Zhang, T., Wang, Y. J., & Ho, W. Z. (2005). Morphine inhibits CD8+ cell-mediated, noncytolytic, anti-HIV activity in latently infeted immue cells. *J Leukoc Biol, 78*, 772–76.

Watson, R. R., Prabhala, R. H., Darban, H. R., Yahya, M. D., & Smith, T. L. (1988). Changes in lymphocyte and macrophage subsets due to morphine and ethanol treatment during a retrovirus infection causing murine AIDS. *Life Sci, 43*, v–xi.

Weber, R. J. & Pert, A. (1989). The periaqueductal gray matter mediates opiate-induced immunosuppression. *Science, 245*, 188–90.

West, J. P., Dykstra, L. A., & Lysle, D. T. (1999). Immunomodulatory effects of morphine withdrawal in the rat are time dependent and reversible by clonidine. *Psychopharmacology, 146*, 320–327.

Wetzel, M. A., Steele, A. D., Eisenstein, T. K., Adler, M. W., Henderson, E. E., & Rogers, T. J. (2000). µ-opioid induction of monocyte chemoattractant protein-1, RANTES, and IFN-α-inducible protein-10 expression in human peripheral blood mononuclear cells. *J Immunol, 165*, 6519–24.

Yadav, A. & Collman, R. G. (2009). CNS inflammation and macrophage/microglial biology associated with HIV-1 infection. *J Neuroimm Pharmacol*, *4*, 430–447.

Yeager, M. P., Colacchio, T. A., Yu, C. T., Hildebrandt, L., Howell, A. L., Weiss, J., et al. (1995). Morphine inhibits spontaneous and cytokine-enhanced natural killer cell cytotoxicity in volunteers. *Anesthesiology*, *83*, 500–508.

Yin, D., Mufson, A., Wang, R., & Shi, Y. (1999). Fas-mediated cell death promoted by opioids. *Nature*, *397*, 218.

Yousif, S., Saubamea, B., Cisternino, S., Marie-Claire, C., Dauchy, S., Scherrmann, J. M., et al. (2008). Effect of chronic exposure to morphine on the rat blood-brain barrier: Focus on the P-glycoprotein. *J Neurochem*, *107*, 647–57.

Zhang, N., Hodge, D., Rogers, T. J., & Oppenheim, J. J. (2003). Ca²⁺-independent protein kinase Cs mediate heterologous desensitization of leukocyte chemokine receptors by opioid receptors. *J Biol Chem*, *278*, 12729–36.

Zhou, Y., Kurihara, T., Ryseck, R. P., Yang, Y., Ryan, C., Loy, J., et al. (1998). Impaired macrophage function and enhanced T cell-dependent immune response in mice lacking CCR5, the mouse homologue of the major HIV-1 coreceptor. *J Immunol*, *160*, 4018–25.

4.8

HIV-1 AND COCAINE

Shilpa Buch, Honghong Yao, and Sabita Roy

Cocaine has multiple and complex effects on cells infected with HIV-1. Many of these effects appear to promote HIV-1 infectivity and disease progression. Cocaine promotes virus replication in mononuclear phagocytes and, through its effects on IL-10, tends to promote a Th2 cellular phenotype, which benefits CXCR4-utilizing viruses. Cocaine can also upregulate the CCR5 receptor, and it acts synergistically with the toxic viral proteins Tat and gp120, exacerbating neuronal apoptosis. Additionally, cocaine exerts potent effects on microvascular permeability, thereby affecting the influx of virus-infected inflammatory cells into brain parenchyma. Epidemiological studies of drug abusers with AIDS link abuse of cocaine, even more than other drugs, to increased incidence of HIV seroprevalence and progression to AIDS. This chapter summarizes a wide range of cell culture and murine animal studies that have provided insight into the interactions of HIV-1 and cocaine in the pathogenesis of HAND.

INTRODUCTION

Drug users represent a significant proportion of the HIV-1-infected and at-risk population. The influences of concurrent drug abuse in HIV pathogenesis are also quite significant. In fact, intravenous drug use (IVDU) and HIV infections have become two linked global health crises. HIV-1 infection is one of the leading causes of death among Americans 25–44 years of age, and injection drug use accounts for one-third of all new cases of AIDS in the United States. According to the National Youth Risk Behavior Survey on Drug Abuse, it is estimated that in 2007 at least 3.3% Americans (aged 14 to 17) had tried some or the other form of cocaine during their lifetime. It has been demonstrated earlier that use of crack cocaine is a risk factor for acquisition of HIV infection and is also independently associated with progression to AIDS (Fiala et al., 1998; Larrat & Zierler, 1993; Webber, Schoenbaum, Gourevitch, Buono, & Klein, 1999). In recent years, emergence of a new cohort of HIV-infected individuals that are cocaine abusers has become evident. It is thus likely that interplay of HIV-1 and cocaine in HIV-infected cocaine abusers might be involved in progression of clinical AIDS.

The central nervous system (CNS) is a major target for HIV-1 infection. Within days following infection, HIV-1 enters the CNS where various brain resident cells can serve as reservoirs for HIV-1 (Clarke et al., 2006; Brack-Werner, 1999; Canki et al., 2001). In humans, HIV-1-associated neurocognitive disorders (HAND) occur in approximately one-third of infected patients. These symptoms can range from minor cognitive motor disorders that affect almost 50% of HIV+ individuals on antiretroviral therapy (ART), to severe encephalitis/dementia affecting almost 15 to 20% of those with AIDS but who do not receive treatment. Although ART has led to a decreased *incidence* of HAND, and has significantly increased longevity of HIV-infected individuals, there is a paradoxical accompaniment of increased *prevalence* of HAND in these people due to longer survival. Into this mix, and often elusive, is the interaction of HIV with other comorbid factor(s), such as abuse of illicit drugs, a condition that is prevalent both in HIV-infected cohorts, and in those with increased risk of contracting the virus. Adding another level of complexity to this mix is also the ability of the brain to function as a potential viral sanctuary due to the inability of most of the ARTs to effectively penetrate the blood-brain barrier (BBB).

The brain is also a target organ for cocaine. Cocaine impairs the functions of macrophages and CD4+ lymphocytes (Klein et al., 1993; Mao et al., 1996; Baldwin et al., 1997; Eisenstein & Hilburger, 1998; Friedman, Newton, & Klein, 2003) and enhances HIV-1 expression in these cells (Bagasra & Pomerantz, 1993; Peterson et al., 1990; Nair, Mahajan, Hou, Sweet, & Schwartz, 2000; Roth et al., 2002; Steele, Henderson, & Rogers, 2003). It has been postulated that cocaine may serve as a co-factor in the susceptibility and progression of HAND (Fiala et al., 1998; Larrat & Zierler, 1993; Webber et al., 1999). Epidemiological studies on drug abusers with AIDS link abuse of cocaine (by different routes), even more than other drugs, to increased incidence of HIV seroprevalence and progression to AIDS (Anthony et al., 1991; Baldwin, Roth, & Tashkin, 1998; Chaisson et al., 1989; Doherty, Garfein, Monterroso, Brown, & Vlahov, 2000; Chiasson et al., 1991). Cell culture and murine animal models have provided valuable tools to explore the synergistic interactions of HIV-1 and cocaine in the pathogenesis of HAND. This chapter summarizes these studies and the current understanding of the interplay of HIV infection and cocaine.

COCAINE-MEDIATED POTENTIATION OF HIV-1 REPLICATION IN VITRO AND IN VIVO

Despite the advent of antiretroviral therapy to combat AIDS, cocaine abusers with HIV-1 infection are becoming a newly emerging cohort of HIV-positive individuals. It is therefore critical to understand how the two agents interact to increase the disease severity. Various studies have focused on exploring how cocaine can enhance virus replication in the in vitro cell culture systems. Peterson et al. addressed this question very elegantly using the peripheral blood mononuclear cell (PBMC) co-culture system (Peterson et al., 1991; Peterson et al., 1992). Briefly, the system comprised of PBMCs from healthy donors incubated in the absence or presence of cocaine prior to activation with a plant lectin, phytohemagglutinin (PHA), and subsequently these cells were reconstituted with PBMCs that had been infected with a clinical isolate of HIV-1. The authors found that HIV replication, measured by the release of HIV p24 antigen in cell culture fluids was significantly enhanced in activated cells that had been exposed to cocaine (Peterson et al., 1991). It was further demonstrated that this effect of cocaine was mediated via the multifunctional cytokine, TGF-β. Since immune activation is considered critical for pathogenesis of HIV infection (Rosenberg & Fauci, 1989; Levy, 1989; Gallo, 1990), these in vitro studies by Peterson et al. suggest a clinical relevance of cocaine in disease pathogenesis.

Based on the premise that cocaine upregulated virus replication in activated PBMCs, the authors subsequently extended their earlier studies by asking the question whether cocaine could also enhance virus replication in PBMCs that had been activated with cytomegalovirus (CMV), a known enhancer of HIV replication in certain lymphocyte lines (Skolnik, Kosloff, & Hirsch, 1988; Clouse, Robbins, Fernie, Ostrove, & Fauci, 1989). Using the same co-culture system as described earlier, PBMCs from CMV-positive or CMV-negative donors were pre-treated with cocaine followed by culturing in the presence of HIV-infected PBMCs (Peterson et al., 1992). These studies demonstrated that while cocaine by itself was not able to trigger HIV-1 replication, in the presence of other activation signals of clinical relevance, such as CMV (Drew, 1988; Jacobson & Mills, 1988; Schooley, 1990; Skolnik, Kosloff, & Hirsch, 1988), cocaine was able to synergistically enhance virus replication. Furthermore, similar to the mitogen-stimulated PBMCs, the mechanism of cocaine-mediated upregulation of virus replication in CMV-stimulated PBMCs occurred via TGF-β with a possible involvement of another cytokine, TNF-α (Peterson et al., 1991; Peterson et al., 1992; Peterson et al., 1993).

Additional studies aimed at unraveling the role of cocaine have been carried out by Bagasra et al., wherein instead of using the co-culture system described earlier, which the authors argue may have inherent potential allogenic effects that could confound the data, PBMCs without any stimulation were used to assess the effects of cocaine on modulation of HIV-1 replication. It was found that cocaine-treated, unstimulated PBMCs, when infected with HIV-1, were also capable of responding with enhanced virus replication as evidenced by increased HIV-1p24 antigen levels, syncytium formation, and increased viral RNA compared to cells not treated with cocaine (Bagasra & Pomerantz, 1993).

The above findings were focused on mixed cell populations using the PBMC system. Further extension of these studies was carried out in a more relevant cell type, the microglia, which are the resident macrophages of the brain and are the target cells for virus replication in HAD (Reynolds et al., 2006). Microglia play a critical role in defense as well in the neuropathogenic effects of HIV-1. Similar to the effects of cocaine seen in HIV-infected PBMCs, cocaine also enhanced virus replication in microglial cells (Peterson et al., 1992; Bagasra & Pomerantz, 1993; Nair et al., 2000; Roth, Whittaker, Choi, Tashkin, & Baldwin, 2002). Assessment of p24 antigen levels in culture supernatants from the HIV-infected human microglial cells treated with cocaine showed a concentration-dependent increase in viral expression. Extension of these studies using κ-opioid receptor ligands further demonstrated suppression of cocaine-induced potentiation of HIV-1 replication in microglial cells. This effect was mediated by a down-modulation of CCR5, a co-receptor of HIV-1, involving the extracellular signal-regulated kinase1/2 (Gekker et al., 2004). More recently, it has been found that cocaine-induced HIV-1 expression in these cells also involved the sigma-1 (σ-1) receptors and the cytokine, TGF-β1 since the inhibitors specific for both σ-1 receptor and TGF-β1 effectively blocked cocaine-mediated enhancement of virus replication (Gekker et al., 2006). More recently, it has also been demonstrated that cocaine induces expression of the chemokine MCP-1 in brain microglia, resulting ultimately in increased transmigration of monocytes across the blood-brain barrier (Yao et al., 2010).

Although macrophages and microglial cells are the primary sources of HIV-1 replication in CNS (Minagar et al., 2002; Gonzalez-Scarano & Martin-Garcia, 2005), astrocytes are also susceptible to HIV-1 infection, albeit at lower levels (Brack-Werner, 1999; Canki et al., 2001; Conant et al., 1994). Astrocytes are integral components of the CNS since they maintain a homeostatic environment and actively participate in bi-directional communication with neurons (Brack-Werner, 1999; Dong & Benveniste, 2001; Hansson & Ronnback, 2003). Following initial infection with HIV-1, astrocytes exhibit a transient surge of viral replication that diminishes to low levels and often persists (Brack-Werner, 1999; Canki et al., 2001; Conant et al., 1994). It has been estimated that up to twenty percent of astrocytes can be infected with the virus in HIV-infected patients and remain as reservoirs for latent virus (Canki et al., 2001). Effect of cocaine on astrocytes in the context of HIV-1 infection has recently been reported by Reynolds et al (Reynolds et al., 2006). Since astrocytes constitute a major proportion of cells in the brain and, since significant numbers of astrocytes can be infected with HIV-1, and cocaine is known to act as a cofactor in HAND, these authors hypothesized that cocaine-induced increases in HIV-1 susceptibility and progression to HIV-encephalitis are mediated via the dysregulation of specific proteins critical for fostering neuroimmunopathogenesis of HIV-1 infection in these cells. The effect of cocaine on HIV-1 infectivity in normal human astrocytes was investigated and it was demonstrated that pre-treatment of astrocytes with cocaine prior to HIV-1 infection significantly upregulated the viral replication as monitored by a significant increase in LTR-R/U5 gene expression (Reynolds et al., 2006), representing early stages of reverse transcription of HIV-1. Using the p24 antigen assay, it was demonstrated that culture supernatants from astrocytes treated with cocaine exhibited increased virus replication at day 15 post-infection. Proteomic analysis by difference gel electrophoresis (DIGE) combined with protein identification through HPLC-MS/MS identified 22 proteins in normal human astrocytes that were differentially regulated by cocaine as compared to astrocytes that were not treated with cocaine. Specifically, these proteins comprised the intracellular signaling molecules, translation elongation factor, and molecular chaperones (Reynolds et al., 2006). These proteins were found to be critical in the neuropathogenesis of HIV-1 infection. These findings have clinical implications for HIV encephalitis (HIVE) since astrocytes make up a significant population of cells in the brain, and their responsiveness to cocaine and/or HIV-1 can lead to increased viral load and subsequent toxicity in the CNS. In addition to enhancing virus replication in astroglial cells in vitro, in vivo studies have suggested that cocaine administration in mice results in increased proliferation and expression of glial fibrillar acidic protein (GFAP) in the dentate gyrus (Fattore et al., 2002).

Interaction of cocaine and HIV-1 has also been evaluated in vivo under more physiologic conditions using a hybrid-mouse model (huPBL SCID mouse) infected with HIV-1 in the presence and absence of cocaine. In this model, systemic cocaine administration led to accelerated HIV-1 infection of human peripheral blood leukocytes (PBL), a decrease in CD4$^+$ cells, and a dramatic rise in circulating virus load (Roth et al., 2002). HIV infection is known to depress the hypothalamic-pituitary-adrenal axis (Kumar et al., 2002). Intriguingly, cocaine exposure to uninfected huPBL-SCID mice resulted in increased corticosterone production but, in concert with HIV-1 infection, resulted in depressed corticosterone production compared with the hu-PBL-SCID mice infected with HIV-1 alone (Roth et al., 2005). These authors also showed that cocaine induced an upregulation of CCR5 expression on peritoneal cells from HIV-infected, cocaine- treated huPBL-SCID mice, which preceded the increase in number of virally infected cells. Using the σ-1 receptor antagonist, Roth et al. demonstrated that cocaine acts via the σ-1 receptor since blocking this receptor abolished the effects of cocaine on HIV-1 replication (Roth et al., 2005).

IMMUNOMODULATORY EFFECTS OF COCAINE IN PERIPHERAL BLOOD LEUKOCYTES

Cocaine has multiple immunomodulatory effects including the ability to influence cytokine and chemokine release in immunoeffector cells (Baldwin, Roth, & Tashkin, 1998). In vitro studies using both mouse and human cells have consistently demonstrated that cocaine at physiological concentrations suppresses cytokine release from splenocytes, PBLs, and endothelial cells (Mao et al., 1997; Mao et al., 1996; Wang, Huang, & Watson, 1994; Watzl, Chen, Scuderi, Pirozhkov, & Watson, 1992). Cocaine has been found to inhibit the IL-2-induced production of IFN-γ and IL-8 by PBLs in a dose-responsive manner (Mao et al., 1997).

Cocaine was also shown to decrease IFN-γ mRNA expression in PBLs as determined by Northern and slot blot analyses, without affecting the stability of the mRNA. Nuclear run-on assays further demonstrated that cocaine downregulated the rate of IFN-γ transcription (Mao et al., 1996). Cocaine is also known to modulate the expression of IL-10, a Th2 cytokine that has been shown to promote HIV-1 replication (Stanulis, Jordan, Rosecrans, & Holsapple, 1997; Gardner et al., 2004).

The response of cocaine on mixed cultures such as PBMCs (Berkeley, Daussin, Hernandez, & Bayer, 1994; Delafuente & DeVane, 1991; Klein, Newton, & Friedman, 1988) is very different from its response in purified T cells (Klein et al., 1993). Using purified T cells, Klein et al. demonstrated that mitogen-stimulated proliferation of these cells was suppressed by cocaine via its down-modulation of calcium mobilization and IL-2 release (Klein et al., 1993). Interestingly, however, conflicting studies on cocaine-mediated release of IL-2 and calcium release were reported by Matsui et al (1992), when T cells were activated with anti-CD3 antibody. Cocaine can therefore have variable effects on lymphocyte responses depending upon the type of cells and the manner of activation of these cells.

Not only does cocaine have the ability to modulate cytokine expression, it has also been shown to affect the expression of chemokines, which are cytokines with chemoattractant properties. CCLs, or β-chemokines, play a significant role in resistance to HIV-1 infection and its clinical progression to AIDS. Cocaine has been reported to down-modulate expression of MIP-1β and the β-chemokine receptor, CCR5, a major HIV-1 co-receptor in normal PBMCs (Nair et al., 2000). Additionally, cocaine also selectively inhibited LPS-induced MIP-1β production by PBMCs isolated from HIV-infected patients (Nair et al., 2000). Cocaine-mediated decrease in the protective, anti-HIV chemokine may therefore be one the mechanisms by which cocaine can accelerate the progression of HIV-1 disease.

EFFECTS OF COCAINE ON HIV PROTEIN (TAT- AND GP120)-INDUCED NEUROTOXICITY

It is widely accepted that while neurodegeneration is one of the hallmark features of HAND, the virus does not infect neurons themselves. It has been implicated that the viral protein products, Tat and gp120, and not the virus per se, can exert neurotoxicity, both in vitro and in vivo (New, Ma, Epstein, Nath, & Gelbard, 1997; Bansal et al., 2000; Gurwell et al., 2001; Savio & Levi, 1993; Lipton, Sucher, Kaiser, & Dreyer, 1991; Kaul, Garden, & Lipton, 2001; Kaul & Lipton, 1999). Furthermore, emerging new in vitro data demonstrate that cocaine can amplify the neurotoxic responses of HIV-1 proteins, Tat and gp-120 (Turchan et al., 2001; Nath et al., 2002; Maragos et al., 2002; Gurwell et al., 2001). Evidence for the interactions of HIV-1 and cocaine in modulating neurotoxicity has been demonstrated in cell culture studies showing enhanced damage and oxidative stress in neurons exposed to Tat and gp120 in the presence of cocaine (Nath et al., 2000;

Koutsilieri et al., 1997). Detailed molecular mechanisms underlying the interaction between cocaine and gp120 have demonstrated that exposure of rat primary neurons to both cocaine and gp120 resulted in increased cell toxicity compared to cells treated with either factor alone. The combinatorial toxicity of cocaine and gp120 was accompanied by an increase in both caspase-3 activity and expression of the proapoptotic protein Bax. Furthermore, increased neurotoxicity in the presence of both the agents was associated with a concomitant increase in the production of intracellular reactive oxygen species and loss of mitochondrial membrane potential. Increased neurotoxicity mediated by cocaine and gp120 was ameliorated by NADPH oxidase inhibitor apocynin, thus underscoring the role of oxidative stress in this cooperation. Signaling pathways including c-jun N-terminal kinase (JNK), p38, extracellular signal-regulated kinase (ERK)/mitogen-activated protein kinases (MAPK), and nuclear factor (NF)-kB were also identified to be critical in the neurotoxicity induced by cocaine and gp120. These findings thus underscore the role of oxidative stress, and mitochondrial and MAPK signal pathways in combined cocaine and HIV gp120-mediated neurotoxicity as illustrated in Figure 4.8.1.

Similar potentiation of cocaine-mediated neurotoxicity has also been reported with yet another HIV protein—Tat. In this study using primary rat hippocampal cultures, it was shown that physiologically relevant doses of cocaine augmented Tat-mediated mitochondrial depolarization and

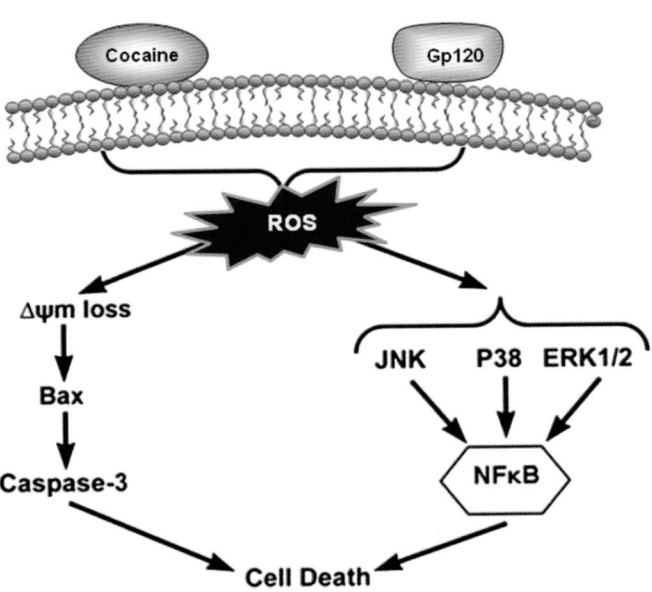

Figure 4.8.1 Schematic illustration of signaling pathways involved in the neurotoxicity mediated by cocaine and gp120 in rat primary neurons. Treatment of primary neurons with cocaine and gp120 results in increased intracellular ROS production, mitochondrial membrane potential loss, increased proapoptotic protein (Bax) expression, and increased caspase-3 activation. Other signaling pathways activated by both gp120 and cocaine involve the JNK, p38, and ERK/MAPK pathways converging in the activation of NF-kB and ultimately culminating in neuronal death.

intracellular production of reactive oxygen species (ROS), leading to enhanced oxidative stress and neurotoxicity (Aksenov et al., 2006). Additionally, treatment of hippocampal cells with a specific D1 dopamine receptor antagonist blocked the potentiation of Tat toxicity by cocaine (Aksenov et al., 2006). These findings led to the speculation that cocaine enhances Tat-mediated neurotoxicity via modulation of the D1 dopamine receptor-controlled signaling cascades (Aksenov et al., 2006). Neurologic impairment in patients with HAND is known to correlate with synaptodendritic injury. To investigate whether cocaine-mediated neurotoxicity could also involve a similar mechanism of injury, Yao et al. exposed hippocampal neurons to cocaine and observed increased neuronal beading in the presence of cocaine. Further investigation on the mechanisms underlying cocaine-mediated impairment of neuronal dendrites in primary hippocampal neurons involved downregulation of the neuronal plasticity gene Arc. Additionally, exposure of neurons to HIV-1 envelope protein gp120 resulted in enhanced loss of neuronal dendrites of neurons exposed to cocaine (Yao, Bethel-Brown, & Buch, 2009).

Corroboration of these in vitro findings was also done in vivo by Bagetta et al., demonstrating that subchronic intraperitoneal administration of cocaine to wild-type Wistar rats in combination with intracerebro-ventrical injection of recombinant HIV gp-120 resulted in the enhancement of iNOS expression and apoptosis in neurons in the neocortex region (Bagetta et al., 2004). Cocaine when administered alone, however, was not able to cause neuronal apoptosis. The addition of iNOS inhibitors minimized the neurotoxicity associated with gp120 and cocaine, thus suggesting that iNOS plays a critical role in gp120- and cocaine-induced neuronal apoptosis.

In addition to the neurotoxicity, decrease in neural stem cell proliferation engendered by gp120 also means that there are fewer progenitor cells present to differentiate in neurons, thus impairing neurogenesis (Kaul, Zheng, Okamoto, Gendelman, & Lipton, 2005). Recent observations indicate that drugs of abuse, including alcohol and opiates, impair adult neurogenesis in the hippocampus. Using 5'-bromo-2-deoxyuridine (BrdU) at the end of the drug treatments, it was reported that that long-term cocaine exposures significantly reduced cell proliferation in the dentate gyrus (DG) of the hippocampus. By labeling astrocytes using GFAP, we determined that long-term cocaine exposure caused increased activation of astrocytes. Further study was undertaken to dissect the mechanism underlying the activation of astrocytes; chronic exposures to cocaine increase the level of cytokines.

COCAINE AND THE BLOOD-BRAIN BARRIER (BBB)

The blood-brain barrier (BBB) normally functions as an interface between the blood and brain parenchyma, acting as a watch guard to inhibit the entry of ions, molecules, and infiltrating cells into the CNS. During progressive HIV-1 infection, however, there is a breach in this barrier (Burger et al., 1997; Nottet et al., 1996; Dallasta et al., 1999;

Avison et al., 2004), leading to influx of inflammatory cells into the brain, resulting in clinical and pathological abnormalities ranging from mild cognitive impairment to frank dementia. Cocaine, through its direct effect on brain microvascular endothelial cells (BMVECs) and its paracrine effects on the BBB via release of pro-inflammatory cytokines, augments HIV-1 neuroinvasion in HAD. Effects of cocaine on the enhancement of viral neuroinvasion through the BBB have been studied in great detail (Fiala et al., 2001; Fiala et al., 1998; Gan et al., 1999; Lee, Hennig, Fiala, Kim, & Toborek, 2001; Chang, Bersig, Felix, Fiala, & House, 2000). Exposure of brain endothelial cells to cocaine has been demonstrated to upregulate the expression of endothelial adhesion molecules like intracellular adhesion molecule-1 (ICAM-1), vascular cell adhesion molecule-1 (VCAM-1), and E-selectin and thus facilitating leukocyte migration across the endothelial monolayers (Gan et al., 1999). Our more recent findings using HBMECs have suggested cocaine-mediated induction of yet another novel adhesion molecule–activated leukocyte adhesion molecule (ALCAM) (Yao & Buch, unpublished observations). Additionally, cocaine has also been shown to upregulate dendritic cell-specific C type ICAM-3, grabbing nonintegrin (DC-SIGN) and matrix metalloproteinases (MMPs) in BMVECs, thereby suggesting that cocaine causes membrane permeability and endothelial transmigration of HIV-infected dendritic cells, which are the first line of defense against HIV infection (Nair et al., 2005). Chronic cocaine treatment has been reported to potentiate chemotactic

agent-induced leukocyte-endothelial cell adhesion (LEA) in rats (Chang et al., 2000). In addition, cocaine has been reported to decrease cellular glutathione levels, enhance DNA-binding activity of redox-regulated transcription factors (NF-kB and AP-1), and increase expression of TNF-α in human brain endothelial cells, thereby contributing to BBB dysfunction and enhanced leukocyte migration across the cerebral vessel (Lee et al., 2001). More recently, cocaine has also been shown to remodel BMVEC by upregulating transcription of genes critical in cytoskeleton organization, signal transduction, cell swelling, and vesicular trafficking (Fiala et al., 2005).

CONCLUSIONS

In summary, cocaine is a multifactorial agent that mediates its effects on several pathways in cells infected with HIV-1 (Figure 4.8.2). The drug not only promotes virus replication in PBMCs, macrophages, microglia, and astrocytes, but it can also shift the cytokine balance towards a Th2 response via its modulation of IL-10 (Stanulis et al., 1997; Gardner et al., 2004). Such a shift has been shown to promote enhancement of CXCR4-utilizing viruses (Buch et al., 2001; Dhillon et al., 2005; Buch et al., 2002). CNS infection with these X4 viruses is becoming increasingly more recognized (Hicks et al., 2002; Yi et al., 2003). Alternatively, cocaine can also upregulate the CCR5 co-receptor, and reciprocally inhibit its ligands, thereby

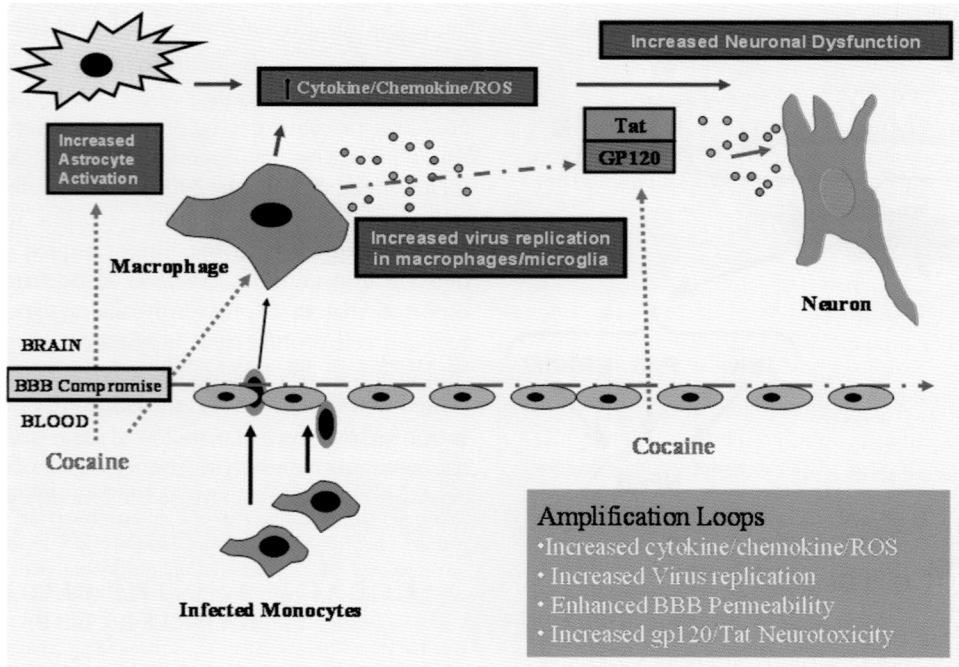

Figure 4.8.2 Overall interactive effects of cocaine and HIV-1 in the CNS. Cocaine exposure of macrophages, microglia, and astrocytes leads to enhanced virus replication and immunomodulation. Cocaine can also activate astrocyte function and proliferation. Cocaine by its interaction with viral proteins, Tat and gp120, augments neurotoxicity. Additionally, cocaine also exerts potent effects on microvascular permeability, thereby impacting the influx of virus-infected inflammatory cells in brain parenchyma. Thus, cocaine, by virtue of its multifactorial properties, aids in the progression and severity of HAND.

increasing virus infectivity. Cocaine can also modulate astroglial function and activation. Cocaine also causes interactive neurotoxicity with viral proteins Tat and gp120, thereby exacerbating neuronal apoptosis. Additionally, cocaine also exerts potent effects on microvascular permeability, thereby impacting the influx of virus-infected inflammatory cells in brain parenchyma. By amplifying the toxic responses that characterize HAND, cocaine skews the balance in favor of the virus leading to accelerated progression and severity of disease.

REFERENCES

Aksenov, M. Y., Aksenova, M. V., Nath, A., Ray, P. D., Mactutus, C. F., & Booze, R. M. (2006). Cocaine-mediated enhancement of Tat toxicity in rat hippocampal cell cultures: The role of oxidative stress and D1 dopamine receptor. *Neurotoxicology*, 27(2), 217–28.

Anthony, J. C., Vlahov, D., Nelson, K. E., Cohn, S., Astemborski, J., & Solomon, L. (1991). New evidence on intravenous cocaine use and the risk of infection with human immunodeficiency virus type 1. *Am J Epidemiol*, 134(10), 1175–1189.

Avison, M. J., Nath, A., Greene-Avison, R., Schmitt, F. A., Bales, R., A., Ethisham, A., et al. (2004). Inflammatory changes and breakdown of microvascular integrity in early human immunodeficiency virus dementia. *J Neurovirol*, 10 (4), 223–32.

Bagasra, O. & Pomerantz, R. J. (1993). Human immunodeficiency virus type 1 replication in peripheral blood mononuclear cells in the presence of cocaine. *J Infect Dis*, 168(5), 1157–1164.

Bagetta, G., Piccirilli, S., Del Duca, C., Morrone, L. A., Rombola, L., Nappi, G., et al. (2004). Inducible nitric oxide synthase is involved in the mechanisms of cocaine enhanced neuronal apoptosis induced by HIV-1 gp120 in the neocortex of rat. *Neurosci Lett*, 356 (3), 183–6.

Baldwin, G. C., Roth, M. D., & Tashkin, D. P. (1998). Acute and chronic effects of cocaine on the immune system and the possible link to AIDS. *J Neuroimmunol*, 83(1–2), 133–138.

Baldwin, G. C., Tashkin, D. P., Buckley, D. M., Park, A. N., Dubinett, S. M., & Roth, M. D. (1997). Marijuana and cocaine impair alveolar macrophage function and cytokine production. *Am J Respir Crit Care Med*, 156(5), 1606–1613.

Bansal, A. K., Mactutus, C. F., Nath, A., Maragos, W., Hauser, K. F., & Booze, R. M. (2000). Neurotoxicity of HIV-1 proteins gp120 and Tat in the rat striatum. *Brain Res*, 879(1–2), 42–49.

Berkeley, M. B., Daussin, S., Hernandez, M. C., & Bayer, B. M. (1994). In vitro effects of cocaine, lidocaine and monoamine uptake inhibitors on lymphocyte proliferative responses. *Immunopharmacol Immunotoxicol*, 16(2), 165–78.

Brack-Werner, R. (1999). Astrocytes: HIV cellular reservoirs and important participants in neuropathogenesis. *AIDS*, 13(1), 1–22.

Buch, S. J., Villinger, F., Pinson, D., Hou, Y., Adany, I., Li, Z., et al. (2002). Innate differences between simian-human immunodeficiency virus (SHIV)(KU-2)-infected rhesus and pig-tailed macaques in development of neurological disease. *Virology JID – 0110674*, 295(1), 54–62.

Buch, S., Pinson, D., King, C. L., Raghavan, R., Hou, Y., Li, Z., et al. (2001). Inhibitory and enhancing effects of IFN-gamma and IL-4 on SHIV(KU) replication in rhesus macaque macrophages: correlation between Th2 cytokines and productive infection in tissue macrophages during late-stage infection. *Cytokine JID – 9005353*, 13(5), 295–304.

Burger, D. M., Boucher, C. A., Meenhorst, P. L., Kraayeveld, C. L., Portegies, P., Mulder, J. W., et al. (1997). HIV-1 RNA levels in the cerebrospinal fluid may increase owing to damage to the blood-brain barrier. *Antivir Ther*, 2(2), 113–7.

Canki, M., Thai, J. N., Chao, W., Ghorpade, A., Potash, M. J., & Volsky, D. J. (2001). Highly productive infection with pseudotyped human immunodeficiency virus type 1 (HIV-1) indicates no intracellular restrictions to HIV-1 replication in primary human astrocytes. *J Virol*, 75(17), 7925–7933.

Chaisson, R. E., Bacchetti, P., Osmond, D., Brodie, B., Sande, M. A., & Moss, A. R. (1989). Cocaine use and HIV infection in intravenous drug users in San Francisco. *JAMA*, 261(4), 561–565.

Chang, S. L., Bersig, J., Felix, B., Fiala, M., & House, S. D. (2000). Chronic cocaine alters hemodynamics and leukocyte-endothelial interactions in rat mesenteric venules. *Life Sci*, 66(24), 2357–2369.

Chiasson, M. A., Stoneburner, R. L., Hildebrandt, D. S., Ewing, W. E., Telzak, E. E., & Jaffe, H. W. (1991). Heterosexual transmission of HIV-1 associated with the use of smokeable freebase cocaine (crack). *AIDS*, 5(9), 1121–1126.

Clarke, J. N., Lake, J. A., Burrell, C. J., Wesselingh, S. L., Gorry, P. R., & Li, P. (2006). Novel pathway of human immunodeficiency virus type 1 uptake and release in astrocytes. *Virology*, 348 (1), 141–55.

Clouse, K. A., Robbins, P. B., Fernie, B., Ostrove, J. M., & Fauci, A. S. (1989). Viral antigen stimulation of the production of human monokines capable of regulating HIV1 expression. *J Immunol*, 143(2), 470–5.

Conant, K., Tornatore, C., Atwood, W., Meyers, K., Traub, R., & Major, E. O. (1994). In vivo and in vitro infection of the astrocyte by HIV-1. *Adv Neuroimmunol*, 4 (3), 287–289.

Dallasta, L. M., Pisarov, L. A., Esplen, J. E., Werley, J. V., Moses, A. V., Nelson, J. A., et al. (1999). Blood-brain barrier tight junction disruption in human immunodeficiency virus-1 encephalitis. *Am J Pathol*, 155(6), 1915–27.

Delafuente, J. C. & DeVane, C. L. (1991). Immunologic effects of cocaine and related alkaloids. *Immunopharmacol Immunotoxicol*, 13(1–2), 11–23.

Dhillon, N., Sui, Y., Potula, R., Dhillon, S., Adany, I., Li, Z., et al. (2005). Inhibition of pathogenic SHIV replication in macaques treated with antisense DNA of Interleukin-4.

Doherty, M. C., Garfein, R. S., Monterroso, E., Brown, D., & Vlahov, D. (2000). Correlates of HIV infection among young adult short-term injection drug users. *AIDS*, 14(6), 717–726.

Dong, Y. & Benveniste, E. N. (2001). Immune function of astrocytes. *Glia*, 36(2), 180–90.

Drew, W. L. (1988). Cytomegalovirus infection in patients with AIDS. *J Infect Dis*, 158(2), 449–56.

Eisenstein, T. K. & Hilburger, M. E. (1998). Opioid modulation of immune responses: Effects on phagocyte and lymphoid cell populations. *J Neuroimmunol*, 83(1–2), 36–44.

Fattore, L., Puddu, M. C., Picciau, S., Cappai, A., Fratta, W., Serra, G. P., et al. (2002). Astroglial in vivo response to cocaine in mouse dentate gyrus: A quantitative and qualitative analysis by confocal microscopy. *Neuroscience*, 110(1), 1–6.

Fiala, M., Eshleman, A. J., Cashman, J., Lin, J., Lossinsky, A. S., Suarez, V., et al. (2005). Cocaine increases human immunodeficiency virus type 1 neuroinvasion through remodeling brain microvascular endothelial cells. *J Neurovirol*, 11(3), 281–291.

Fiala, M., Gan, X. H., Zhang, L., House, S. D., Newton, T., Graves, M. C., et al. (1998). Cocaine enhances monocyte migration across the blood-brain barrier. Cocaine's connection to AIDS dementia and vasculitis? *Adv Exp Med Biol*, 437, 199–205.

Fiala, M., Gujuluva, C., Berger, O., Bukrinsky, M., Kim, K. S., & Graves, M. C. (2001). Chemokine receptors on brain endothelia—keys to HIV-1 neuroinvasion? *Adv Exp Med Biol*, 493, 35–40.

Friedman, H., Newton, C., & Klein, T. W. (2003). Microbial infections, immunomodulation, and drugs of abuse. *Clin Microbiol Rev*, 16(2), 209–219.

Gallo, R. C. (1990). Mechanism of disease induction by HIV. *J Acquir Immune Defic Syndr*, 3(4), 380–9.

Gan, X., Zhang, L., Berger, O., Stins, M. F., Way, D., Taub, D. D., et al. (1999). Cocaine enhances brain endothelial adhesion molecules and leukocyte migration. *Clin Immunol*, 91(1), 68–76.

Gardner, B., Zhu, L. X., Roth, M. D., Tashkin, D. P., Dubinett, S. M., & Sharma, S. (2004). Cocaine modulates cytokine and enhances tumor growth through sigma receptors. *J Neuroimmunol*, 147(1–2), 95–98.

Gekker, G., Hu, S., Sheng, W. S., Rock, R. B., Lokensgard, J. R., & Peterson, P. K. (2006). Cocaine-induced HIV-1 expression in microglia involves sigma-1 receptors and transforming growth factor-beta1. *Int Immunopharmacol*, 6 (6), 1029–33.

Gekker, G., Hu, S., Wentland, M. P., Bidlack, J. M., Lokensgard, J. R., & Peterson, P. K. (2004). Kappa-opioid receptor ligands inhibit cocaine-induced HIV-1 expression in microglial cells. *J Pharmacol Exp Ther*, 309(2), 600–6.

Gonzalez-Scarano, F. & Martin-Garcia, J. (2005). The neuropathogenesis of AIDS. *Nat Rev Immunol*, 5(1), 69–81.

Gurwell, J. A., A. Nath, A., Sun, Q., Zhang, J., Martin, K. M., Chen, Y., et al. (2001). Synergistic neurotoxicity of opioids and human immuno-deficiency virus-1 Tat protein in striatal neurons in vitro. *Neuroscience*, 102(3), 555–63.

Hansson, E. & Ronnback, L. (2003). Glial neuronal signaling in the central nervous system. *FASEB J*, 17(3), 341–8.

Hicks, A., R. Potula, Y. J. Sui, F. Villinger, D. Pinson, I. Adany, I., et al. (2002). Neuropathogenesis of lentiviral infection in macaques: Roles of CXCR4 and CCR5 viruses and interleukin-4 in enhancing mono-cyte chemoattractant protein-1 production in macrophages. *Am J Pathol*, 161(3), 813–822.

Jacobson, M. A. & Mills, J. (1988). Serious cytomegalovirus disease in the acquired immunodeficiency syndrome (AIDS). Clinical findings, diagnosis, and treatment. *Ann Intern Med*, 108(4), 585–94.

Kaul, M., G. A. Garden, G. A., & Lipton. S. A. (2001). Pathways to neuronal injury and apoptosis in HIV-associated dementia. *Nature*, 410(6831), 988–994.

Kaul, M. & Lipton, S. A. (1999). Chemokines and activated macrophages in HIV gp120-induced neuronal apoptosis. *Proc Natl Acad Sci USA*, 96(14), 8212–8216.

Kaul, M., Zheng, J., Okamoto, S., Gendelman, H. E., & Lipton, S. A. (2005). HIV-1 infection and AIDS: Consequences for the central nervous system. *Cell Death Differ*, 12 Suppl 1, 878–92.

Klein, T. W., Matsui, K., Newton, C. A., Young, J., Widen, R. E., & Friedman, H. (1993). Cocaine suppresses proliferation of phytohe-magglutinin-activated human peripheral blood T-cells. *Int J Immunopharmacol*, 15(1), 77–86.

Klein, T. W., Newton, C. A., & Friedman, H. (1988). Suppression of human and mouse lymphocyte proliferation by cocaine. *Adv Biochem Psychopharmacol*, 44, 139–43.

Koutsilieri, E., Gotz, M. E., Sopper, S., Sauer, U., Demuth, M., ter Meulen, V., et al. (1997). Regulation of glutathione and cell toxicity following exposure to neurotropic substances and human immunodeficiency virus-1 in vitro. *J Neurovirol*, 3(5), 342–9.

Kumar, M., Kumar, A. M., Waldrop, D., Antoni, M. H., Schneiderman, N., & Eisdorfer, C. (2002). The HPA axis in HIV-1 infection. *J Acquir Immune Defic Syndr*, 31 Suppl 2, S89–93.

Larrat, E. P. & Zierler, S. (1993). Entangled epidemics: Cocaine use and HIV disease. *J Psychoactive Drugs*, 25(3), 207–221.

Lee, Y. W., Hennig, B., Fiala, M., Kim, K. S., & Toborek, M. (2001). Cocaine activates redox-regulated transcription factors and induces TNF-alpha expression in human brain endothelial cells. *Brain Res*, 920(1–2), 125–133.

Levy, J. A. (1989). Human immunodeficiency viruses and the pathogenesis of AIDS. *JAMA*, 261(20), 2997–3006.

Lipton, S. A., Sucher, N. J., Kaiser, P. K., & Dreyer, E. B. (1991). Synergistic effects of HIV coat protein and NMDA receptor-mediated neurotoxicity. *Neuron*, 7(1), 111–118.

Mao, J. T., Huang, M., Wang, J., Sharma, S., Tashkin, D. P., & Dubinett, S. M. (1996). Cocaine down-regulates IL-2-induced peripheral blood lymphocyte IL-8 and IFN-gamma production. *Cell Immunol*, 172(2), 217–223.

Mao, J. T., Zhu, L. X., Sharma, S., Chen, K., Huang, M., Santiago, S. J., et al. (1997). Cocaine inhibits human endothelial cell IL-8 production: The role of transforming growth factor-beta. *Cell Immunol*, 181(1), 38–43.

Maragos, W. F., Young, K. L., Turchan, J. T., Guseva, M., Pauly, J. R., Nath, A., et al. (2002). Human immunodeficiency virus-1 Tat protein and methamphetamine interact synergistically to impair striatal dopamin-ergic function. *J Neurochem*, 83(4), 955–63.

Matsui, K., Friedman, H., & Klein, T. W. (1992). Cocaine augments pro-liferation of human peripheral blood T-lymphocytes activated with anti-CD3 antibody. *Int J Immunopharmacol*, 14 (7), 1213–20.

Minagar, A., Shapshak, P., Fujimura, R., Ownby, R., Heyes, M., & Eisdorfer, C. (2002). The role of macrophage/microglia and astrocytes in the pathogenesis of three neurologic disorders: HIV-associated dementia, Alzheimer disease, and multiple sclerosis. *J Neurol Sci*, 202(1–2), 13–23.

Nair, M. P., Mahajan, S. D., Schwartz, S. A., Reynolds, J., Whitney, R., Bernstein, Z., et al. (2005). Cocaine modulates dendritic cell-specific C type intercellular adhesion molecule-3-grabbing nonintegrin expression by dendritic cells in HIV-1 patients. *J Immunol*, 174(11), 6617–26.

Nair, M. P. N., Mahajan, S., Hou, J., Sweet, A. M., & Schwartz, S. A. (2000). The stress hormone, cortisol, synergizes with HIV-1 gp-120 to induce apoptosis of normal human peripheral blood mononuclear cells. *Cell Mol Biol (Noisy.-le-grand)*, 46(7), 1227–1238.

Nath, A., Anderson, C., Jones, M., Maragos, W., Booze, R., Mactutus, C., et al. (2000). Neurotoxicity and dysfunction of dopaminergic systems associated with AIDS dementia. *J Psychopharmacol*, 14(3), 222–227.

Nath, A., Hauser, K. F., Wojna, V., Booze, R. M., Maragos, W., Prendergast, M., et al. (2002). Molecular basis for interactions of HIV and drugs of abuse. *J Acquir Immune Defic Syndr*, 31 Suppl 2, S62–S69.

New, D. R., Ma, M., Epstein, L. G., Nath, A., & Gelbard, H. A. (1997). Human immunodeficiency virus type 1 Tat protein induces death by apoptosis in primary human neuron cultures. *J Neurovirol*, 3 (2), 168–173.

Nottet, H. S., Persidsky, Y., Sasseville, V. G., Nukuna, A. N., Bock, P., Zhai, Q. H., et al. (1996). Mechanisms for the transendothelial migration of HIV-1-infected monocytes into brain. *J Immunol*, 156 (3), 1284–95.

Peterson, P. K., Gekker, G., Chao, C. C., Schut, R., Molitor, T. W., & Balfour, H. H. (1991). Cocaine potentiates HIV-1 replication in human peripheral blood mononuclear cell co-cultures. Involvement of transforming growth factor-beta. *J Immunol*, 146 (1), 81–84.

Peterson, P. K., Gekker, G., Chao, C. C., Schut, R., Verhoef, J., Edelman, C. K., et al. (1992). Cocaine amplifies HIV-1 replication in cytomega-lovirus-stimulated peripheral blood mononuclear cell co-cultures. *J Immunol*, 149(2), 676–680.

Peterson, P. K., Gekker, G., Schut, R., Hu, S., Balfour, Jr., H. H., & Chao, C. C. (1993). Enhancement of HIV-1 replication by opiates and cocaine: The cytokine connection. *Adv Exp Med Biol*, 335, 181–188.

Peterson, P. K., Sharp, B. M., Gekker, G., Portoghese, P. S., Sannerud, K., & Balfour, H. H. (1990). Morphine promotes the growth of HIV-1 in human peripheral blood mononuclear cell co-cultures. *AIDS*, 4(9), 869–873.

Reynolds, J. L., Mahajan, S. D., Bindukumar, B., Sykes, D., Schwartz, S. A., & Nair, M. P. (2006). Proteomic analysis of the effects of cocaine on the enhancement of HIV-1 replication in normal human astrocytes (NHA). *Brain Res*, 1123(1), 226–36.

Rosenberg, Z. F. & Fauci, A. S. (1989). Induction of expression of HIV in latently or chronically infected cells. *AIDS Res Hum Retroviruses*, 5(1), 1–4.

Roth, M. D., Tashkin, D. P., Choi, R., Jamieson, B. D., Zack, J. A., & Baldwin, G. C. (2002). Cocaine enhances human immunodeficiency virus replication in a model of severe combined immunodeficient mice implanted with human peripheral blood leukocytes. *J Infect Dis*, 185(5), 701–705.

Roth, M. D., Whittaker, K. M., Choi, R., Tashkin, D. P., & Baldwin, G. C. (2005). Cocaine and sigma-1 receptors modulate HIV infection, chemokine receptors, and the HPA axis in the huPBL-SCID model. *J Leukoc Biol*, 78(6), 1198–1203.

Savio, T. & Levi, G. (1993). Neurotoxicity of HIV coat protein gp120, NMDA receptors, and protein kinase C: A study with rat cerebellar granule cell cultures. *J Neurosci Res*, 34 (3), 265–272.

Schooley, R. T. (1990). Cytomegalovirus in the setting of infection with human immunodeficiency virus. *Rev Infect Dis*, 12 Suppl 7, S811–9.

Skolnik, P. R., Kosloff, B. R., & Hirsch, M. S. (1988). Bidirectional inter-actions between human immunodeficiency virus type 1 and cytomega-lovirus. *J Infect Dis*, 157 (3), 508–14.

Stanulis, E. D., Jordan, S. D., Rosecrans, J. A., & Holsapple, M. P. (1997). Disruption of Th1/Th2 cytokine balance by cocaine is mediated by corticosterone. *Immunopharmacology*, 37(1), 25–33.

Steele, A. D., Henderson, E. E., & Rogers, T. J. (2003). Mu-opioid modulation of HIV-1 co-receptor expression and HIV-1 replication. *Virology*, 309(1), 99–107.

Turchan, J., Anderson, C., Hauser, K. F., Sun, Q., Zhang, J., Liu, Y., et al. (2001). Estrogen protects against the synergistic toxicity by HIV proteins, methamphetamine, and cocaine. *BMC Neurosci*, 2(1), 3.

Wang, Y., Huang, D. S., & Watson, R. R. (1994). In vivo and in vitro cocaine modulation on production of cytokines in C57BL/6 mice. *Life Sci*, 54 (6), 401–411.

Watzl, B., Chen, G., Scuderi, P., Pirozhkov, S., & Watson, R. R. (1992). Cocaine-induced suppression of interferon-gamma secretion in leukocytes from young and old C57BL/6 mice. *Int J Immunopharmacol*, 14(6), 1125–31.

Webber, M. P., Schoenbaum, E. E., Gourevitch, M. N., Buono, D., & Klein, R. S. (1999). A prospective study of HIV disease progression in female and male drug users. *AIDS*, 13 (2), 257–262.

Yao, H., Bethel-Brown, C., & Buch, S. (2009). Cocaine exposure results in formation of dendritic varicosity in rat primary hippocampal neurons. *Am J Infect Dis*, 5(1), 26–30.

Yao, H., Yang, Y., Kim, K. J., Bethel-Brown, C., Gong, N., Funa, K., et al. (2010). Molecular mechanisms involving sigma receptor-mediated induction of MCP-1: Implication for increased monocyte transmigration. *Blood*.

Yi, Y., Chen, W., Frank, I., Cutilli, J., Singh, A., Starr-Spires, L., Sulcove, J., et al. (2003). An unusual syncytia-inducing human immunodeficiency virus type 1 primary isolate from the central nervous system that is restricted to CXCR4, replicates efficiently in macrophages, and induces neuronal apoptosis. *J Neurovirol*, 9(4), 432–441.

SECTION 5

ANIMAL MODELS

Howard S. Fox

5.1

SIMIAN IMMUNODEFICIENCY VIRUS

M. Christine Zink, Joseph L. Mankowski, David R. Graham,
Lucio Gama, and Janice E. Clements

An animal model using the pigtailed macaque co-infected with two SIV viruses recapitulates key clinical and pathological features of HIV infection of the peripheral and central nervous system (PNS, CNS). The pigtailed macaques in this model develop immunosuppression more rapidly than similarly co-infected rhesus macaques, and develop CNS lesions more frequently than either rhesus macaques or cynomologous monkeys when similarly co-infected. In this pigtail model, the majority of animals develop AIDS as well as CNS and PNS disease by 84 days post inoculation. Furthermore, this model recapitulates the acute, asymptomatic, and late stages of infection and disease in the CNS, making it possible to study stage-specific longitudinal viral and immunological changes and responses to therapies. This chapter discusses a range of important topics relevant to understanding SIV models of AIDS and neuroAIDS in general, as well as this pigtail model in particular. These topics include areas related to normal immune responses, genetic susceptibilities, pathogenesis of HIV disease, and preclinical testing of neuroprotective agents.

A simian immunodeficiency virus (SIV)/macaque model that recapitulates the key clinical and pathological features of HIV infection of the human central and peripheral nervous systems has been developed allowing for evaluation of neuroprotective therapeutics, longitudinal measures of immune and inflammatory parameters in the CNS, and the development of strategies that would purge latent reservoirs in the periphery, the CNS and PNS. SIV infection of macaques accurately replicates many features of HIV infection, including the development of encephalitis with characteristic histopathological changes and psychomotor impairment, making it an excellent model system to dissect the pathogenesis of HIV-associated neurological diseases (HAND) (Murray et al., 1992; Sharer et al., 1988; Witwer et al., 2009; Zink et al., 1997; Zink et al., 1999; Zink & Clements, 2002). Unlike most SIV models, which are confounded by variability in the incidence and time to onset of AIDS, CNS and PNS disease (Westmoreland et al., 1998), the pigtailed macaque model results in consistent and predictable onset of encephalitis by 84 days post infection (Zink et al., 1997).

The consistent accelerated SIV model of HIV encephalitis involves co-inoculation of pigtailed macaques with two viruses: a neurovirulent molecular clone (SIV/17E-Fr) and an immunosuppressive virus swarm (SIV/DeltaB670).

Inoculation with this combination of viruses results in rapid, acute virus replication in both the peripheral blood and the brain as measured by high plasma and CSF viral RNA levels that are detected as early as 3 days post inoculation and peak at 7 to 10 days post-inoculation (PI). Plasma levels peak at 10^8 to 10^9 copy eq/mL and CSF levels peak at 10^6 to 10^7 copy eq/mL (Fig. 5.1.1A). In the plasma there is a slight (approximately 1 log) but definite decline in plasma viral load that parallels the decline in viral load in HIV patients early after infection. However, plasma viral load rises again within weeks and remains high throughout infection. After acute infection, CSF viral loads decline by 2 to 3 logs at 14 to 21 days PI. Within 2 to 3 weeks, however, CSF viral loads again increase in macaques that develop moderate to severe neurological disease (Fig. 5.1.1A). After an initial decline there is recovery of peripheral blood CD4+ T cell numbers during acute infection; rapid, continued loss of CD4+ lymphocytes begins as early as 35 days PI, and the majority of animals have AIDS as well as CNS and PNS disease by 84 days post inoculation. (Zink et al., 1999) This model reproduces the acute, asymptomatic, and late stages of infection and disease in the CNS so that the viral and immunological changes that occur during these stages can be studied longitudinally.

A primary advantage of pigtailed macaques (*Macaca nemestrina*) in this model is that they develop immunosuppression more rapidly than rhesus macaques inoculated with the same viruses, and develop CNS lesions with a higher frequency than either rhesus macaques or cynomologous monkeys (Zink et al., 1997). During the last 10 years, this SIV pigtailed macaque model has proved invaluable in improving our understanding of the mechanisms of SIV/HIV-induced neurological disease, including the relationship between systemic and CNS viral replication, influence of the innate immune system on the development of CNS disease, and the identification of host genetic resistance to CNS disease (Barber et al., 2006; Dudaronek et al., 2007; Mankowski et al., 2008; Overholser et al., 2005; Ravimohan et al., 2009; Witwer et al., 2009). It also has been used to develop a robust simian model of highly-active antiretroviral drug therapy and has become the premier model for preclinical testing of drugs to ameliorate the CNS and PNS effects of HIV infection (Brice et al., 2010; Dinoso et al., 2009; Follstaedt et al., 2008; Szeto et al., 2010; Zink et al., 2005; Zink et al., 2010).

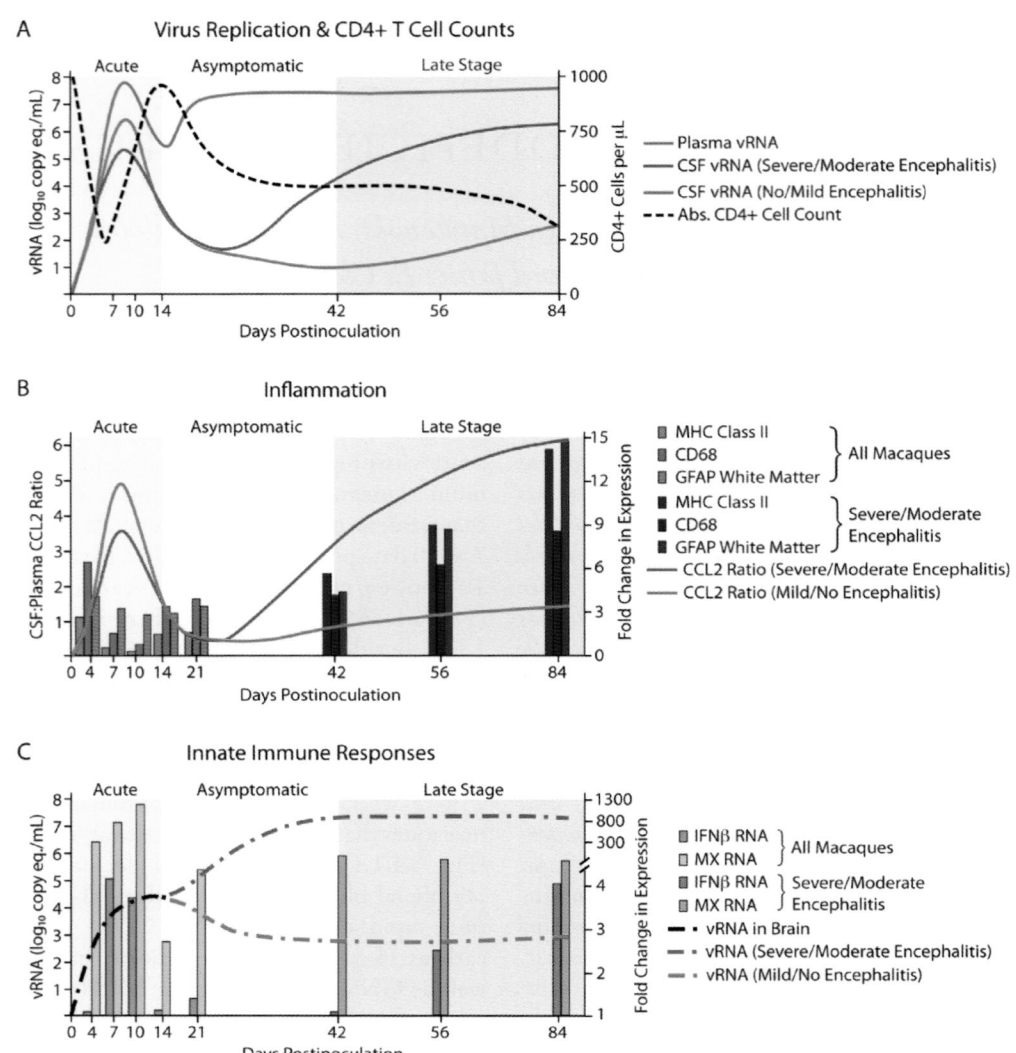

Figure 5.1.1 Viral, inflammatory, and immune parameters in the accelerated, consistent SIV/macaque model of HIV-associated neurological disease. (A) Viral RNA levels in plasma increase rapidly during the first 7 to 10 days after virus inoculation, decline by approximately 1 log, then increase again and remain at 10^7 to 10^8 for the remainder of the infection period. Viral RNA levels in CSF increase during acute infection, decline by several logs during the next 2 weeks, then increase again only in macaques that will develop moderate to severe encephalitis. CD4+ cell counts in peripheral blood decline during acute infection, recover briefly, then begin to decline again during the asymptomatic stage of infection. (B) CCL2 production in the CNS, expressed as the ratio of CCL2 in CSF:plasma rises during acute infection, declines by day 21 p.i., then increases again in macaques that will develop moderate to severe encephalitis. Markers of macrophage infiltration and activation (CD68 and MHC class II) are elevated in brain tissue during acute and terminal infection. In contrast, activation of astrocytes as measured by expression of GFAP in brain tissue increases gradually throughout infection. (C) During acute infection, when there is an increase in viral RNA in the brain, IFNβ and MX RNA are elevated in the brain. Viral RNA declines rapidly after expression of IFNβ and MX and rises again late in infection in conjunction with immunosuppression. IFNβ and MX RNA are again expressed at high levels during late-stage infection.

IDENTIFYING MECHANISMS OF VIRAL AND IMMUNE DAMAGE IN THE NERVOUS SYSTEM

The earliest stage of HIV infection in the CNS has been difficult to study in humans due to the inability to sample the brain during acute infection. Thus, it has been a challenge to evaluate acute immune and inflammatory responses in response to HIV. Using the accelerated, consistent SIV model as well as other SIV models, it has become clear that SIV infects the brain very early during infection and that innate immune responses are induced acutely in response (Fischer-Smith et al., 2008;

Roberts et al., 2004). In the accelerated SIV/macaque model, high levels of viral RNA are present in the CSF of all infected macaques during acute infection, regardless of whether those animals ultimately develop neurological lesions. By 4 days post-inoculation, SIV replication is detected in CD14+ macrophages in the brain and infection is accompanied by a widespread innate immune response (Witwer et al., 2009).

High levels of CSF viral RNA during acute infection could reflect several potential sources. They might indicate active virus replication in the meninges, since meningitis frequently is observed early in SIV infection (Zink et al., 1999). While it is possible that there is functional breakdown of the blood-brain barrier during acute infection, overt compromise of this barrier has not been shown and macaques do not show acute clinical signs of CNS disease. High CSF viral loads during acute infection could result from extensive trafficking of infected cells from the blood, through the brain parenchyma, and out into the CSF. Supporting this hypothesis is the observation that viral isolates from the brain of SIV-infected macaques at day 10 PI had sequences that were similar to those seen in the peripheral blood from the same animals (Babas et al., 2006). These data suggest that the brains of all infected individuals are exposed to virus during acute infection, but establishment of virus and long-term virus replication leading to neurological disease occurs only in a subset.

Trafficking of infected cells through the CNS clearly occurs during acute infection and the consequences of early exposure of the brain to virus and immune/inflammatory responses remains to be determined. In addition, the question remained as to whether the high levels of CSF virus during acute infection reflected virus solely from trafficking cells or also resulted from infected resident cells in the brain parenchyma, as the brain does not have the typical perivascular cuffs or microglial nodules containing virus-infected macrophages during acute infection. It therefore had been postulated that following acute infection, HIV was completely cleared from the brain. Under this hypothesis, the CNS deficits seen later in infection would occur because of reentry of virus into the CNS during late-stage disease when there is high viral load in peripheral blood and immune impairment (Alexaki et al., 2008; Gartner, 2000). However, in the accelerated SIV macaque model, while there is a substantial reduction in viral RNA levels in the brain after acute infection, SIV DNA levels remain constant in the brain from acute to late-stage disease, demonstrating that infected resident cells remain throughout infection (Clements, 2002). There also is a shift from transcriptionally active to inactive SIV DNA during the asymptomatic period (Barber et al., 2004a; Barber et al., 2006; Clements et al., 2005).

The SIV/macaque model also has been used to compare viral RNA in plasma, CSF, and different brain regions longitudinally throughout infection. There is no relationship between viral load in the plasma and the presence or severity of encephalitis. However, levels of CSF viral RNA after acute infection do correlate with the presence of CNS lesions. Additionally, the severity of CNS lesions directly correlates with levels of viral RNA and antigen in the brain (Zink et al., 1999). During terminal infection, CSF viral loads >10^4 copy eq/mg of brain RNA are seen only in macaques with CNS lesions or in animals in which CNS virus recently has developed escape mutations. At this stage of disease, there is a strong correlation between viral RNA levels in the brain and the severity of CNS lesions in this model (Clements et al., 2008; Witwer et al., 2009; Zink et al., 1999), which is consistent with what has been observed with HIV infection (Brew et al., 1997; Cinque et al., 1998; Di Stefano et al., 1998; Ellis et al., 1997; McArthur et al., 1997). Based on data derived from this model, CSF viral loads may be a good surrogate marker for encephalitis during post-acute stages of infection (Zink et al., 1999).

It long has been known that increased expression of macrophage markers such as CD68 and Ham56 in the brain of HIV-infected individuals correlates with the severity of neurological disease in HIV-infected individuals (Glass et al., 1995). In the SIV/macaque model there is a significant correlation in the CNS between viral load (viral RNA or gp41) and macrophage infiltration, the majority of which are not productively infected (Zink et al., 1999). The positive correlation between CNS viral load and macrophage infiltration suggests that virus infection of the CNS may signal the influx of additional macrophages into the brain, which could occur either via virus-induced expression of chemokines and/or indirectly through induction of chemokine-inducing cytokines. These chemokines signal the influx of macrophages from the peripheral blood, some of which are infected with or carrying virus, setting up a cycle of additional chemokine secretion and virus replication. Macrophage chemoattractant protein-1 or CCL2 likely plays a critical role in attracting macrophages to the brain as CCL2 levels are higher in the CSF than in the plasma during both acute and late-stage infection, suggesting the development of a concentration gradient (Fig. 5.1.1B) (Conant et al., 1998; Kelder et al., 1998; Zink et al., 2001). A strong correlation has been demonstrated in the SIV model between CSF levels of CCL2, as well as CCL2 mRNA expression in the brain and the number of macrophages in the brain as well as the severity of CNS disease (Mankowski et al., 2004; Witwer et al., 2009; Wright et al., 2006; Zink & Clements, 2002). These SIV studies suggest that levels of CCL2 in the CSF may be a biomarker for the severity of CNS disease in HIV-infected individuals.

OTHER SIV/MACAQUE MODELS OF HIV CNS DISEASE

An alternative consistent SIV model that results in rapid development of AIDS and CNS disease uses monoclonal antibody depletion of CD8+ T cells in rhesus macaques. This depletion causes accumulation of early monocytes/macrophages in the CNS, rapid disease progression, and a high incidence of encephalitis (Schmitz et al., 1999b; Schmitz et al., 1999a). This model was originally developed to examine the role of CD8+ T cells in control of SIV infection in the periphery. While CD8+ depletion results in monocyte/macrophage accumulation in the CNS, administration of anti-CD8+ monoclonal antibodies results in subject variability in the duration of CD8+ depletion (Schmitz et al., 1999b). Using this model, it has been proposed that perivascular macrophages and not parenchymal microglia are the primary monocyte/macrophage subpopulations infected with SIV in the brain (Williams et al., 2001). Because of the alterations to the immune system that are necessary to produce rapid disease progression in the CD8 depletion model, it may have limited usefulness for studying innate and adaptive immune responses to SIV and HIV and their role in the progression of CNS disease. However, this model and the accelerated CNS disease model in pigtailed macaques confirm the critical role of immune responses occurring in the periphery contributing to the progression and severity of CNS disease.

IMMUNE RESPONSES IN NATURAL AND NON-NATURAL HOSTS OF SIV INFECTION

Numerous species of old world monkeys, including sooty mangabeys (SM), African green monkeys (AG), and chimpanzees are naturally infected with SIV (Williams & Burdo, 2009). Much attention has been focused on these "natural" hosts of SIV infection since these animals have moderate to high viral loads in plasma, yet do not develop immunosuppression or CNS disease. Recent studies reveal that there are essential differences in the immune systems of these natural hosts of SIV as compared to non-natural hosts such as pig-tailed macaques (PM), rhesus macaques (RM), and humans. For example SM, unlike RM and PM, do not exhibit rapid depletion of CD4+ T cells in the circulation after infection (Gordon et al., 2007; Pandrea et al., 2007). Unlike humans and RM, natural hosts (SM and AG) also normally express low levels of activated CD4+/CCR5+ T cells in blood, lymph nodes, and gut-associated lymphoid tissues (GALT) (Pandrea et al., 2007). In human and RM GALT, more than 50% of CD4+ T cells are CCR5+, compared to less than 10% in SM and AG. Also a low frequency of CD4+CCR5+ T cells was seen in HIV-resistant chimpanzees (Pandrea et al., 2007). Surprisingly, there appear to be no appreciable differences in the number of CD8+CCR5+ T cells in HS, RM, SM, and AG in the peripheral blood and lymph nodes (Pandrea et al., 2007).

Bystander cell death also is limited in natural host species as compared to non-natural hosts (Chakrabarti et al., 2000; Silvestri et al., 2003; Silvestri et al., 2005; Villinger et al., 1996). One possible mechanism for resistance to bystander death in natural hosts may be a reduced susceptibility to cell cycle disruption, which has been seen in SM (Paiardini et al., 2004).

Recent studies have suggested that differences in innate immune system activation may be at the root of differences between NNH and NH. These studies suggest that in non-natural hosts innate immunity persists throughout infection, with ongoing production of high levels of IFNα (Mandl et al., 2008) secreted by plasmacytoid dendritic cells (pDCs) and macrophages resulting in upregulation of immunoregulatory molecules (PDL-1, PD-1, and TRAIL) on the increased numbers of CD4+ CCR5+ cells. This results in chronic immune activation eventually leading to immune exhaustion. At the same time, adaptive immune function is suppressed by pDC and macrophage production of indolamine 2,3, dioxygenase (IDO), which suppresses T cell function (Boasso & Shearer, 2007). IDO activation also has been shown to be elevated in the brains of SIV-infected macaques in our model (Zink et al., 2010). Besides having immunosuppressive functions, IDO activation also is the gatekeeper for kynurenine metabolism and results in the production of the NMDA receptor antagonist kynurenine and the NMDA receptor agonist quinolinic acid. Imbalances in kynurenine metabolism have been linked to several neurological diseases including Huntington's disease, schizophrenia, multiple sclerosis, and depressive disorders (Costantino, 2009; Kohl & Sperner-Unterweger, 2007; Kwidzinski & Bechmann, 2007).

The above studies emphasize the critical importance of understanding immune regulation of HIV. Control of SIV infection in the brain is a delicate balance between protective and hyperactivated innate and adaptive immune responses. In addition, there likely is a tight interplay between immune responses in the periphery and in the brain. The SIV/macaque accelerated model is ideal for these studies.

COORDINATED IMMUNE REGULATION OF SIV INFECTION IN THE CNS

SIV replication and accompanying innate immune responses in brain and in macrophages isolated from the brain are detectable as early as 4 days post-inoculation (Fig. 5.1.1C) (Witwer et al., 2009). At that time, there are increases in IFNβ, the IFNβ-induced gene MxA, and TNFα in the brain (Fig. 5.1.2). Induction of IFNβ, the first type I IFN to be produced in response to viral infection, reduces SIV replication in vitro in primary macaque macrophages, the major source of productive SIV replication in the brain, by a transcriptional mechanism. The early expression of IFNβ in the brain suggests that innate immune responses contribute significantly to suppression of acute SIV replication in the CNS (Barber et al., 2004a; Barber et al., 2006; Dudaronek et al., 2007; Ravimohan et al., 2009).

Acute infection is also accompanied by induction of the cytokines IL-6 and IL-10, and the chemokine CCL2, which is produced by both astrocytes and macrophages in the CNS during HIV and SIV infection (Conant et al., 1998; Kelder et al., 1998; McManus et al., 2000). CCL2 is believed to be a major factor in recruitment of peripheral blood monocytes and activated and infected lymphocytes into the brain during acute infection (Eugenin & Berman, 2003; Eugenin et al., 2006). Further, astrocyte CCL2 production has neuroprotective effects in astrocytes and neurons in vitro, inhibiting apoptosis (Eugenin et al., 2003). Cytokine/chemokine induction during acute infection is followed by control of the previously

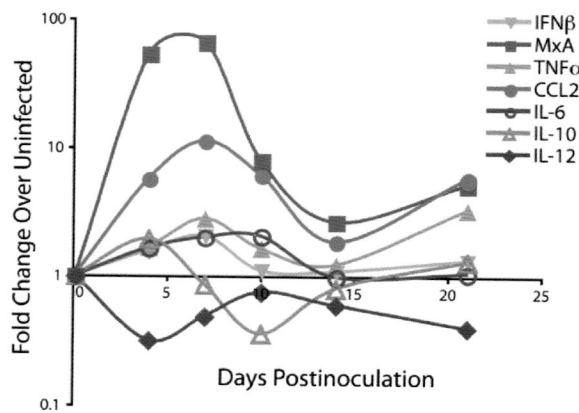

Figure 5.1.2 Coordinated expression of innate immune genes and cytokines in brain of SIV-infected macaques during acute infection in brain. A schematic of median values of mRNA levels for all cytokines measured by RT-PCR in brain tissue from uninfected and SIV-infected macaques euthanized at different time points (4, 7, 10, 14, and 21 days p.i.).

elevated inflammatory markers MHC Class II, CD68, and GFAP (Witwer et al., 2009).

Innate immune responses exemplified by expression of IFNβ, TNFα, and MxA decrease by day 14 following infection but begin to increase again as early as 21 days PI. In animals with moderate to severe encephalitis, CSF IL-6 and CCL2 levels were persistently elevated beginning at day 28 post-inoculation (Mankowski et al., 2004; Witwer et al., 2009). Median CSF CCL2 and Il-6 levels after days 28 and 42 PI, respectively, were significantly higher in animals with moderate to severe CNS lesions than in macaques with no or mild lesions, suggesting that these cytokines might be used as surrogate markers for neurological disease in HIV-infected patients.

These cytokine changes also are accompanied by induction of the dominant-negative isoform of the IFNβ downstream transcriptional regulatory pathway protein C/EBPβ, a member of the CCAAT/enhancer binding protein family of transcription factors. C/EBPβ is an important cytokine regulator and is involved in IFNβ anti-inflammatory control (Akira & Kishimoto, 1992, 1997; Ejarque-Ortiz et al., 2007; Li et al., 2007; Pope et al., 2000; Spooner et al., 2007). In addition to controlling virus infection, IFNβ-induced genes, particularly C/EBPβ, regulate inflammatory gene cascades, limiting inflammation and damage in tissues (Akira & Kishimoto, 1992; Kalvakolanu, 2003; Kim et al., 2002; Li et al., 2007; Poli, 1998; Pope et al., 2000). The ratio of the dominant-negative (C/EBPβ-3) isoform to the transcriptionally active (C/EBPβ-2) isoform is important in the regulation of transcription of cytokines, including the CCL2, IL-6, IL-10, and TNFα. C/EBPβ-3 levels in brain of SIV-infected macaques increase from 7–21 days correlating with the reduction of SIV mRNA in brain, as well as the level of acetylation of histone H4 downstream from the SIV transcriptional start site (Barber et al., 2006; Dudaronek et al., 2007). Thus, induction of the dominant-negative isoform of C/EBPβ and IFNβ leads to transcriptional repression of SIV, which may be important in the establishment of HIV and SIV latency. An inverse correlation between C/EBPβ-3:C/EBPβ-2 levels and SIV replication has been observed during late infection (Witwer et al., 2009).

These data suggest the following molecular model to describe the control of acute SIV/HIV replication in the CNS: CNS infection with SIV/HIV occurs during acute infection when full-length C/EBPβ predominates at the viral LTR. With chromatin remodeling events, LTR-dependent transcription occurs and full-length viral RNA is produced. The acute virus infection triggers IFNβ production in the brain, in turn inducing the alternative translation of dominant-negative C/EBPβ mRNA between 7 and 21 days post-inoculation. Chromatin remodeling events subside, and the production of full-length SIV RNA becomes undetectable (Cao et al., 1991; Vinson et al., 1989). The production of C/EBPβ-3 appears to occur through IFNβ-induced downstream activation of CUGBP1 and the formation of CUGP1-C/EBPβ complexes in macrophages (Dudaronek et al., 2007; Ravimohan et al., 2009).

Thus, there are mechanisms in the brain that induce coordinated control of both virus replication and the inflammatory cytokines produced in response to acute infection. It is likely that the inflammatory responses required to limit virus replication in the brain must also be tightly controlled so as to prevent the development of chronic inflammation that can trigger neuronal damage and cognitive impairment. These controlling responses provide an explanation for the lack of neurological deficits and CNS inflammation during acute HIV infection in the brain. Pathogenesis and encephalitis may result in part from a loss of this inflammation-limiting capacity. The coordinated control of virus replication and inflammation suggests that there are specific, possibly common, mechanisms in the brain that limit inflammatory processes produced in response to HIV and SIV infection.

GENETIC DETERMINANTS OF SUSCEPTIBILITY TO SIV CNS DISEASE

The SIV/macaque model has provided the first evidence for the existence of host genetic susceptibility to lentivirus-induced CNS disease. Previously, MHC Class I-restricted responses had been shown to be an important component of systemic immune responses to HIV and SIV infection (Borrow et al., 1994; Carrington & O'Brien, 2003). Multiple HLA alleles have been associated with altered HIV disease progression (Bailey et al., 2006; Fellay et al., 2007; Migueles et al., 2000). This also has been shown in pigtailed macaques and rhesus macaques, where the presence of the MHC Class I alleles Mane-A*10 and Mamu-A*01, respectively, have been linked to lower plasma viral loads and slower progression to AIDS (O'Connor et al., 2003; Sauermann, 2001; Smith et al., 2005a; Smith et al., 2005b).

The observed variability in the development of CNS disease in pigtailed macaques in the accelerated SIV macaque model, despite the fact that all animals develop high levels of persistent viremia and progression to AIDS, suggested that host genetic factors also may play a role in the development of CNS disease. A comparison of expression of the MHC Class I allele Mane-A*10 with the development of SIV CNS disease in pigtailed macaques revealed that animals expressing the Mane-A*10 allele had a 2.5 times reduced risk of developing SIV encephalitis compared to animals lacking this allele (Mankowski et al., 2008). Animals expressing Mane-A*10 also had lower levels of activated macrophages, SIV RNA, and neuronal dysfunction in the CNS. Notably, while animals expressing the allele showed decreased CSF and CNS SIV RNA, there was no difference in plasma viral load between Mane-A*10-positive and -negative macaques. A subset of macaques expressing the Mane-A*10 allele that did have high CNS viral loads developed escape mutations in SIV *gag*, while comparable Mane-A*10-negative animals had only wild-type virus (Mankowski et al., 2008). These data reveal that there are CNS-protective MHC Class I alleles that exert selective pressure on the virus and provide the first evidence of host genetic susceptibility to lentivirus-induced CNS disease. Based on these findings, it is imperative to understand the impact of MHC Class I alleles on disease outcomes in SIV/macaque models to assess treatment and prevention strategies.

THE ROLE OF MONOCYTES/ MACROPHAGES AND ASTROCYTES IN THE SIV/MACAQUE MODEL OF HIV

Monocytes originate in the bone marrow and circulate in the blood for a short period of time before migrating to tissues and organs. Some monocyte subpopulations express CCR5 and therefore are susceptible to HIV and SIV infection (Naif, 1998, Ellery 2007). Although the majority of productive viral replication during HIV infection is carried out by CD4+ T lymphocytes and tissue macrophages, new evidence shows that circulating monocytes also may represent an important reservoir for both latent and replicating virus, especially during combination antiretroviral therapy (cART) (Zhu, 2002, Crowe, 2003). Besides, because antiretroviral drugs do not block viral replication in monocytes as efficiently as they do in CD4+ cells, it is estimated that the mean half-life of HIV-1 DNA in the CD14+ monocyte population is longer than that in resting CD4+ lymphocytes (41.3 versus 23.5 months, respectively) in patients undergoing cART (Zhu, 2002).

Changes in the profile of monocyte subsets are clearly observed in both HIV and SIV infections, and may be associated with CNS disease. Of particular interest is the CD14+ CD16+ subpopulation, which seems to increase throughout infection, and correlates with the onset of HAD, probably due to its migratory capacity and ability to preferentially harbor the virus when compared to other subsets (Ellery, 2007). Other phenotypic alterations, such as reduction of some surface markers and general monocytosis, although not directly correlated to CNS disease, may reflect profound morphological changes in the bone marrow, and contribute to the overall state of immune activation observed in AIDS patients.

It is well known that cells of macrophage lineage are the main cells that productively replicate virus in the CNS during HIV or SIV infection (Chakrabarti et al., 1991; Dickson et al., 1991; Koenig et al., 1986; Kure et al., 1990; Lackner et al., 1991; Lackner et al., 1994; Lane et al., 1996; Price et al., 1988; Prospero-Garcia et al., 1996; Smith et al., 1995; Watry et al., 1995; Wiley et al., 1986). Inflammatory macrophages and activated microglial cells are major sources of neurotoxic proinflammatory molecules in the brains of infected individuals. Brain macrophages from patients with HAND express proinflammatory cytokines that can act synergistically with glutamate to induce neuronal apoptosis in vitro (Patton et al., 2000). Using the CD8 depletion SIV rhesus macaque model, Williams and colleagues reported that perivascular macrophages—and not resident parenchymal microglia—are the major cell population productively infected in the CNS during peak SIV viremia and among macaques with terminal disease and encephalitis (Williams et al., 2001). Studies of the SIV pigtailed macaque model during acute infection (4 days PI) concur with this finding. When cells of macrophage lineage were isolated from the brains of SIV-infected macaques, CD14+ perivascular macrophages had approximately 1 x 10^4 copy eq/μg RNA, whereas CD14-/CD11b+ microglia had a mean of only 60 copy eq/μg RNA (Witwer et al., 2009). This indicated that trafficking peripheral blood macrophages

transport virus into the brain during acute infection and very few microglia are replicating virus at that time.

Because of the essential functions of astrocytes in the CNS, their susceptibility to lentiviral infection may have important pathogenic consequences for HIV/SIV-associated CNS disease. Astrocytes expressing Nef protein are a prominent feature of pediatric HIV CNS disease (Blumberg et al., 1994), and in the SIV macaque model astrocytes also are nonproductively infected, expressing only Nef protein (Mori, 1992).

Productive infection of astrocytes can be achieved in vitro using the reproducibly neurovirulent SIV/17E-Fr molecular clone (Babas et al., 2003; Mankowski et al., 1997; Zink et al., 1999), but not the non-neurovirulent, lymphocyte-tropic molecular clone SIVmac239 (Overholser et al., 2003). However, macrophage tropism is not sufficient for replication of SIV in primary astrocytes—additional changes within the transmembrane portion of the *env* gene are necessary for the virus to enter and replicate in astrocytes, which it does via a CD4-independent mechanism (Overholser et al., 2005). With respect to the SIV/DeltaB670 viral swarm used in the accelerated SIV/macaque model, the macrophage-tropic, CD4-independent strains Cl-3 and Cl-12 are the only SIV genotypes that replicate efficiently in astrocyte cultures in vitro. These two strains also prominently replicate in the brain during early infection (10 and 21 days PI) (Babas et al., 2006). The early infection of astrocytes may contribute to the development of the innate immune response in the CNS (Barber et al., 2004a; Clements et al., 2002). Infected astrocytes also may contribute to the infiltration and activation of macrophages associated with SIV encephalitis, as astrocytes are the main CCL2 producers in the CNS (Conant et al., 1998; Dong & Benveniste, 2001; Eugenin & Berman, 2003; Zink et al., 2001).

SIV/MACAQUE MODELS FOR PRECLINICAL TESTING OF NEUROPROTECTIVE THERAPEUTICS

Despite the fact that many HIV-infected individuals in developed countries are treated with highly active (combination) antiretroviral drug regimens that target several stages of the viral replicative cycle, a substantial percentage still develop clinical signs of CNS and/or PNS disease (Kumar et al., 2007; Langford et al., 2006; Sacktor et al., 2001; Tozzi et al., 2001), perhaps because of the inability of many of these drugs to cross the blood-brain barrier. As a result, a number of clinical trials have been initiated to determine whether known neuroprotective agents such as amantidine and nerve growth factor-1 (NGF-1) have ameliorative effects on the CNS of HIV-infected individuals, but no single agent has emerged as the solution to both the inflammatory and neurodegenerative effects of HIV in the CNS (Clifford et al., 2002; McArthur et al., 2000; Sacktor et al., 2000; Schifitto et al., 2001).

The SIV macaque model provides a powerful tool for exploring the efficacy of novel neuroprotective drugs in the CNS. The antibiotic minocycline is one such potentially neuroprotective drug that was tested in the SIV/macaque model.

Minocycline has potent anti-inflammatory properties, effectively crosses the blood-brain barrier (Colovic & Caccia, 2008; Suk et al., 2001; Tikka et al., 2001), and is neuroprotective in animal models of multiple neurodegenerative diseases (Arvin et al., 2002; Chen et al., 2000; Du et al., 2001; Metz et al., 2004; Sanchez Mejia et al., 2001; Van Den Bosch et al., 2002; Wu et al., 2002). The anti-inflammatory and neuroprotective properties of minocycline might be linked to suppressed p38 mitogen-activated protein kinase activation, which is relevant to SIV as there is an increase in p38 activation in SIV encephalitis (Barber et al., 2004b). Furthermore, minocycline has the practical advantage of being readily available, inexpensive, relatively safe when administered long term, and approved by the US Food and Drug Administration for treatment of other medical conditions.

When SIV-infected macaques were treated with minocycline beginning during early asymptomatic infection, the incidence and severity of encephalitis was significantly reduced and viral RNA levels in the CSF and brain were significantly lower (Zink et al., 2005). In vitro, minocycline significantly inhibits replication of HIV and SIV in both primary macrophages and lymphocytes. Treatment with minocycline suppressed reactivation of HIV from a primary CD4+ T cell-derived model of HIV latency, and reduced reactivation of HIV from resting CD4+ T cell reservoirs from patients who have clinically undetectable viremia due to cART therapy. Minocycline alters T cell activation, blunting changes in expression of T cell activation/proliferation markers and cytokine secretion, many of which are critical for activation pathways that regulate HIV replication (Szeto et al., 2010). Minocycline also inhibits proliferation and activation of stimulated human CD4+ T cells and arrests cells in the G0/G1 phase of the cell cycle (unpublished data). Blocking of cells in the G0/G1 phase also may result in reduced SIV and HIV-1 viral production by decreasing the percentage of cells entering the G2/M phase. Our previous studies showed that minocycline reduced HIV and SIV replication in cultured peripheral blood lymphocytes, as measured by p24 and p27 production, respectively (Paiardini et al., 2004), and other labs have shown that inhibiting the cell cycle through G0/G1 caused a decrease in virus replication (Foli et al., 2007). HIV-1 can enter resting CD4+ T cells efficiently, but only short incomplete reverse transcripts are made. Complete reverse transcription requires transition of the infected cells through the cell cycle (Korin & Zack, 1998).

Partly as a result of the studies described above, clinical trials were initiated in the US and Africa to examine the potential efficacy of minocycline in improving neurocognitive deficits in HIV-infected individuals. In neither trial was neurocognitive improvement in minocycline-treated patients detected. However, it is important to critically examine the parameters that were used for these trials including the length of treatment, the selection of patients, and especially the timing at which minocycline treatment was initiated. The US trial recruited patients chronically infected with HIV, most of whom had been on cART therapy for years and now were experiencing unresolved neurological symptoms. Likewise, the clinical trial in Africa was not designed to address timing

of administration and likely selected for people who were in the middle to late stages of HIV infection. Recent studies on timing of cART therapy suggest that this may not be the patient population for whom therapy is most effective and that cART therapy that is initiated much earlier during infection is of greater benefit (Sterne et al., 2009; Zolopa et al., 2009). The same might be true of putative neuroprotective therapeutics such as minocycline. They might be most efficacious if administered before significant immune and/or CNS damage has occurred. Further, at the time of writing, biological samples obtained from patients in both trials have not yet been analyzed for the potential effect of minocycline treatment on viral or inflammatory markers known to impact CNS disease. In studies showing neuroprotective effects of minocycline in SIV-infected macaques, treatment was initiated very early in infection, right after the acute stage. It will be important to determine whether minocycline will prevent the development of neurocognitive changes when administered early during infection or whether it will prevent reactivation of virus replication in individuals for whom cART therapy has to be withdrawn. Regardless of the outcome of these clinical trials, the SIV/macaque model provides a rigorous platform for pre-clinical testing neuroprotective therapeutics. Additional drugs currently are being tested for their potential efficacy in suppressing neuroinflammation and for protecting neurons from the bystander effects of CNS inflammation.

SIV/MACAQUE MODEL OF cART

Since the CNS may represent a distinct viral reservoir in HIV, and most antiretroviral drugs do not cross the blood-brain barrier, it is critical to determine the extent to which non-CNS penetrant antiretrovirals nonetheless protect against CNS disease. Our SIV macaque model was therefore used to develop a model of cART in which SIV-infected macaques were treated with a combination of the nucleotide reverse transcriptase inhibitor tenofovir, the protease inhibitors saquinavir and atazanavir, and the investigational integrase inhibitor L-870812, most of which cross the blood-brain barrier to any significant extent (Letendre et al., 2008). Macaques were treated with this combination of antiretroviral drugs beginning at day 12 PI, right after acute infection. Plasma and CSF viral loads declined rapidly after initiating cART (Fig. 5.1.3A) with similar viral decay kinetics to HIV-infected individuals treated with cART (Fig. 5.1.3B) (Dinoso et al., 2009; Zink et al., 2010). The number of resting CD4+ T cells in blood and tissues that were latently infected with SIV was also similar to HIV-infected individuals on cART (Fig. 5.1.3B). These findings mirroring human results make this the first SIV macaque model using three or more classes of antiretroviral drugs. Brain viral RNA was undetectable in treated animals at necropsy but interestingly, viral DNA levels were not different from untreated SIV-infected macaques. CNS inflammation was significantly reduced, with decreased brain expression of MHC Class II and GFAP and reduced CSF CCL2 and IL-6 (Fig. 5.1.3C). Brains from treated macaques had significantly lower IFNβ, MxA, and IDO mRNA, suggesting suppressed immune hyperactivation

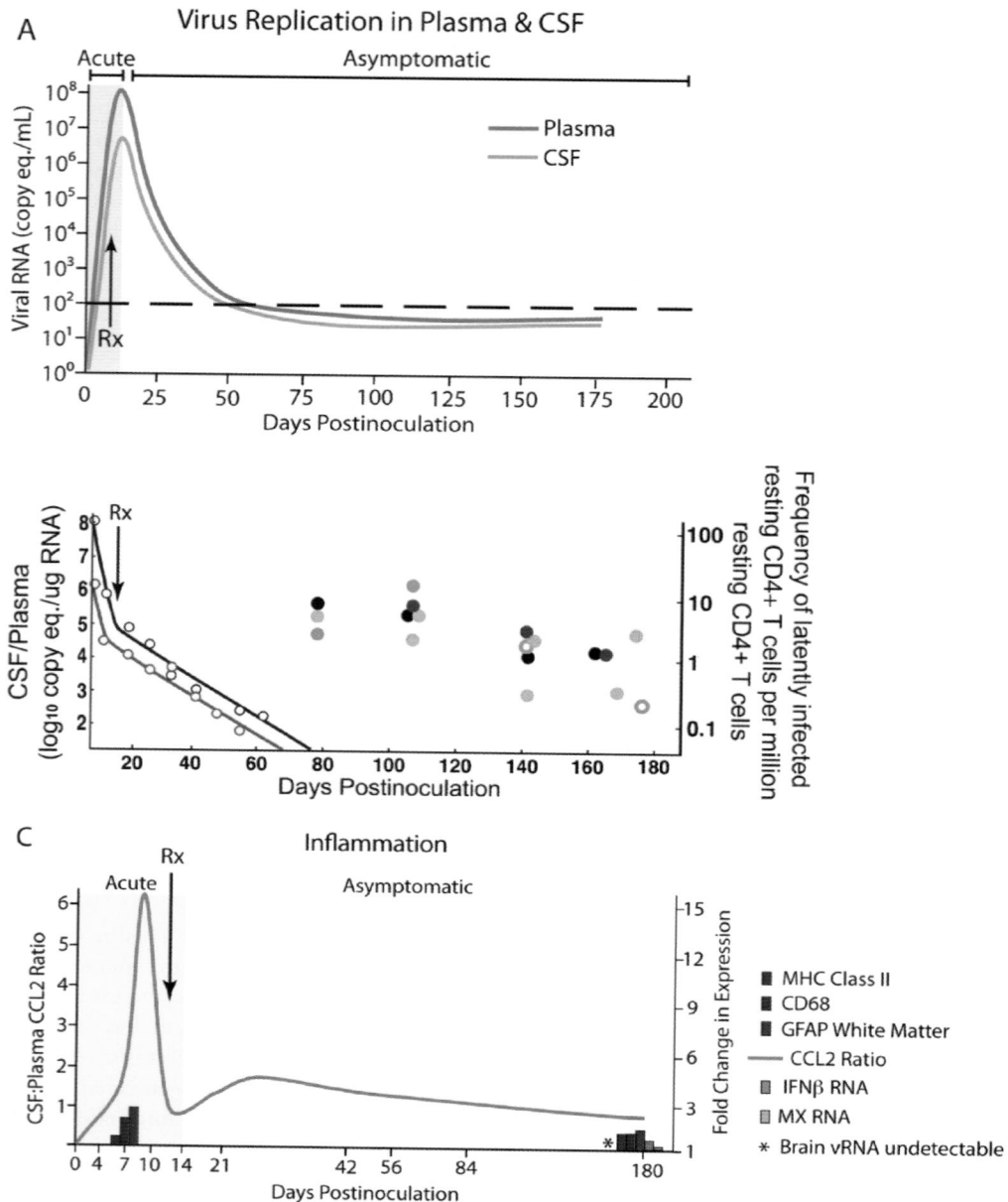

Figure 5.1.3 Virus replication and inflammation in SIV-infected macaques treated with cART. (A) Viral RNA levels in plasma and CSF increase rapidly during the first 7 to 10 days prior to cART treatment, which was initiated at 12 days p.i. Within a few days after initiation of cART, plasma and CSF viral load begin to decline. By approximately 60 days p.i., plasma and CSF viral load have declined to below the level of detection (approximately 100 copy eq./mL) and viral loads remained low throughout the remainder of the experiment. (B) The decline in plasma and CSF viral RNA occurred in two phases—an initial short-term rapid decline followed by a longer term slower decline similar to the two-phase decline seen in the plasma of HIV-infected individuals on cART. At 80 days p.i. there were 8 to 10 latently infected resting CD4+ T cells in the blood. These numbers declined gradually to approximately one latently infected resting CD4+ T cells per million by 175 days p.i. (C) CSF:Plasma CCL2 ratio, an estimate of the gradient of CCL2 in the brain as compared to the periphery, rose acutely, but declined significantly after initiation of cART therapy. Macrophage surface markers MHC Class II and CD68, astrocyte marker GFAP, and immune markers IFNα RNA and Mx RNA all were expressed at very low levels at necropsy as compared to untreated macaques (Figure 5.1.1). In addition, brain RNA was undetectable at necropsy.

and fewer CD4+ and CD8+ T cells, suggesting reduced trafficking of T cells from peripheral blood. Brain levels of CD68 protein and TNFα and IFNγ RNA, while reduced, were not significantly lower, indicating continued CNS inflammation, at least in some macaques, despite containment of CNS SIV replication. These data, generated in the rigorous, high viral load,

accelerated SIV/macaque model showed significant benefits of cART therapy on CNS virus replication and inflammation when treatment was initiated early in infection, even when the drugs did not cross the blood-brain barrier (Zink et al., 2010). This model is now established and will be used to determine the ideal stage of infection in which to initiate cART therapy, to determine whether it is possible to purge tissue reservoirs or virus, and to examine the ability of cART in combination with neuroprotective drugs to prevent neurological symptoms in HIV-infected individuals.

Similar results were observed in another SIV macaque model, in which rhesus macaques were inoculated with SIVmac251 that had been serially passaged in microgila (Marcondes et al., 2009). Rhesus macaques were treated with a regimen of tenofovir with or without the protease inhibitor nelfinavir, both of which are poorly CNS penetrant. Tenofovir monotherapy was shown to reverse neurophysiological abnormalities, which returned upon treatment cessation (Fox et al., 2000). Movement abnormalities were not affected by tenofovir treatment, however. In another study, early treatment with tenofovir and nelfinavir prevented development of characteristic neurophysiological and locomotor alterations following SIV infection, and significantly decreased brain viral load (Marcondes et al., 2009). Treatment also altered immune responses in the brain as indicated by decreased IFNα and the IFN-responsive gene G1P1 RNA and increased CCL5 RNA. Together, these studies showed decreased viral replication in the CNS following antiretroviral treatment in SIV-infected macaques, even when using a poorly CNS-penetrant cART regimen. However, there also appear to be residual immune responses that may contribute to inflammation and to CNS disease in HIV-infected individuals on cART.

CONCLUSIONS AND FUTURE DIRECTIONS

The development of CNS disease in SIV macaques depends on both host and viral factors. Based on the available evidence, it appears that SIV infection in the CNS induces an immediate, coordinated regulation of the innate immune system both in the periphery and the brain. Acute innate immune responses serve to control virus replication. However, these responses decrease following acute infection, likely in order to prevent the damaging effects of chronic inflammation. With late-stage disease, immune responses in the periphery and CNS become dysregulated coincident with development of encephalitis.

Host genes clearly can influence the risk of developing SIV CNS disease. These host factors have not been extensively studied, and there likely are multiple additional host factors influencing the development or severity of CNS disease.

SIV macaque models of HIV-associated CNS disease continue to be valuable not only in dissecting the immune and viral changes following SIV infection, but also in discovering therapeutic options for the prevention of CNS disorders in HIV. Questions about CNS penetrance and the timing of antiretroviral or neuroprotective therapy can be addressed in SIV macaque models. Additionally, the efficacy of novel neuroprotective and anti-inflammatory agents can be studied in the SIV/macaque model. The SIV/macaque model continues to provide unique advantages for studying the mechanisms of HIV-associated neurological disease that cannot solely be obtained from patient-based studies.

REFERENCES

Akira, S. & Kishimoto, T. (1992). IL-6 and NF-IL6 in acute-phase response and viral infection. *Immunol Rev, 127*, 25–50.

Akira, S. & Kishimoto, T. (1997). NF-IL6 and NF-kappa B in cytokine gene regulation. *Adv Immunol, 65*, 1–46.

Alexaki, A., Liu, Y., & Wigdahl, B. (2008). Cellular reservoirs of HIV-1 and their role in viral persistence. *Curr HIV Res, 6*(5), 388–400.

Arvin, K. L., et al. (2002). Minocycline markedly protects the neonatal brain against hypoxic-ischemic injury. *Ann Neurol, 52*(1), 54–61.

Babas, T., et al. (2003). Role of microglial cells in selective replication of simian immunodeficiency virus genotypes in the brain. *J Virol, 77*(1), 208–16.

Babas, T., et al. (2006). Progressive selection for neurovirulent genotypes in the brain of SIV-infected macaques. *AIDS, 20*(2), 197–205.

Bailey, J. R., et al. (2006). Maintenance of viral suppression in HIV-1-infected HLA-B*57+ elite suppressors despite CTL escape mutations. *J Exp Med, 203*(5), 1357–69.

Barber, S. A., et al. (2004a). Innate immune responses and control of acute simian immunodeficiency virus replication in the central nervous system. *J Neurovirol, 10* Suppl 1, 15–20.

Barber, S. A., et al. (2004b). Dysregulation of mitogen-activated protein kinase signaling pathways in simian immunodeficiency virus encephalitis. *Am J Pathol, 164*(2), 355–62.

Barber, S. A., et al. (2006). Mechanism for the establishment of transcriptional HIV latency in the brain in a simian immunodeficiency virus-macaque model. *J Infect Dis, 193*(7), 963–70.

Blumberg, B. M., Gelbard, H. A., & Epstein, L. G. (1994). HIV-1 infection of the developing nervous system: Central role of astrocytes in pathogenesis. *Virus Res, 32*(2), 253–67.

Boasso, A. & Shearer, G. M. (2007). How does indoleamine 2,3-dioxygenase contribute to HIV-mediated immune dysregulation. *Curr Drug Metab, 8*(3), 217–23.

Borrow, P., et al. (1994). Virus-specific CD8+ cytotoxic T-lymphocyte activity associated with control of viremia in primary human immunodeficiency virus type 1 infection. *J Virol, 68*(9), 6103–10.

Brew, B. J., et al. (1997). Levels of human immunodeficiency virus type 1 RNA in cerebrospinal fluid correlate with AIDS dementia stage. *J Infect Dis, 175*(4), 963–6.

Brice, A. K., et al. (2010). Minocycline blocks HIV- and mitogen-induced cell cycle progression by arresting CD4+ and CD8+ T cells in G0/G1. *Submitted.*

Cao, Z., Umek, R. M., & McKnight, S. L. (1991). Regulated expression of three C/EBP isoforms during adipose conversion of 3T3-L1 cells. *Genes Dev, 5*(9), 1538–52.

Carrington, M. & O'Brien, S. J. (2003). The influence of HLA genotype on AIDS. *Annu Rev Med, 54*, 535–51.

Chakrabarti, L., et al. (1991). Early viral replication in the brain of SIV-infected rhesus monkeys. *Am J Pathol, 139*(6), 1273–80.

Chakrabarti, L. A., et al. (2000). Normal T-cell turnover in sooty mangabeys harboring active simian immunodeficiency virus infection. *J Virol, 74*(3), 1209–23.

Chen, M., et al. (2000). Minocycline inhibits caspase-1 and caspase-3 expression and delays mortality in a transgenic mouse model of Huntington disease. *Nat Med, 6*(7), 797–801.

Cinque, P., et al. (1998). Cerebrospinal fluid HIV-1 RNA levels: Correlation with HIV encephalitis. *AIDS, 12*(4), 389–94.

Clements, J. E., et al. (2008). The accelerated simian immunodeficiency virus macaque model of human immunodeficiency virus-associated neurological disease: from mechanism to treatment. *J Neurovirol, 14*(4), 309–17.

Clements, J. E., et al. (2005). The central nervous system is a viral reservoir in simian immunodeficiency virus—infected macaques on combined antiretroviral therapy: A model for human immunodeficiency virus patients on highly active antiretroviral therapy. *J Neurovirol, 11*(2), 180–9.

Clements, J. E., et al. (2002). The central nervous system as a reservoir for simian immunodeficiency virus (SIV): Steady-state levels of SIV DNA in brain from acute through asymptomatic infection. *J Infect Dis, 186*(7), 905–13.

Clifford, D. B., et al. (2002). A randomized clinical trial of CPI-1189 for HIV-associated cognitive-motor impairment. *Neurology*, 59(10), 1568–73.

Colovic, M. & Caccia, S. (2008). Liquid chromatography-tandem mass spectrometry of I3,II8-biapigenin, the major biflavone in Hypericum perforatum extracts. *J Chromatogr B Analyt Technol Biomed Life Sci*, 863(1), 74–9.

Conant, K., et al. (1998). Induction of monocyte chemoattractant protein-1 in HIV-1 Tat-stimulated astrocytes and elevation in AIDS dementia. *Proc Natl Acad Sci USA*, 95(6), 3117–21.

Costantino, G. (2009). New promises for manipulation of kynurenine pathway in cancer and neurological diseases. *Expert Opin Ther Targets*, 13(2), 247–58.

Crowe, S., Zhu, T., Muller, W. A. (2003). The contribution of monocyte infection and trafficking to viral persistence, and maintenance of the viral reservoir in HIV infection. *J. Leukoc. Biol.* 74(5), 635-41.

Di Stefano, M., et al. (1998). Neurological disorders during HIV-1 infection correlate with viral load in cerebrospinal fluid but not with virus phenotype. *AIDS*, 12(7), 737–43.

Dickson, D. W., et al. (1991). Microglia in human disease, with an emphasis on acquired immune deficiency syndrome. *Lab Invest*, 64(2), 135–56.

Dinoso, J. B., et al. (2009). A simian immunodeficiency virus-infected macaque model to study viral reservoirs that persist during highly active antiretroviral therapy. *J Virol*, 83(18), 9247–57.

Dong, Y. & Benveniste, E. N. (2001). Immune function of astrocytes. *Glia*, 36(2), 180–90.

Du, Y., et al. (2001). Minocycline prevents nigrostriatal dopaminergic neurodegeneration in the MPTP model of Parkinson's disease. *Proc Natl Acad Sci USA*, 98(25), 14669–74.

Dudaronek, J. M., Barber, S. A., & Clements, J. E. (2007). CUGBP1 is required for IFNbeta-mediated induction of dominant-negative CEBPbeta and suppression of SIV replication in macrophages. *J Immunol*, 179(11), 7262–9.

Ejarque-Ortiz, A., et al. (2007). Upregulation of CCAAT/enhancer binding protein beta in activated astrocytes and microglia. *Glia*, 55(2), 178–88.

Ellery, P. J., Tippett, E., Chiu, Y. L., Paulkovics, G., Cameron, P. U., Solomon, A., Lewin, S. R., Gorry, P. R., Jaworowski, A., Greene, W. C., Sonza, S., Crowe, S. M. (2007). The CD16+ monocyte subset is more permissive to infection and preferentially harbors HIV-1 in vivo. *J. Immunol.* 178(10), 6581-9.

Ellis, R. J., et al. (1997). Cerebrospinal fluid human immunodeficiency virus type 1 RNA levels are elevated in neurocognitively impaired individuals with acquired immunodeficiency syndrome. HIV Neurobehavioral Research Center Group. *Ann Neurol*, 42(5), 679–88.

Eugenin, E. A. & Berman, J. W. (2003). Chemokine-dependent mechanisms of leukocyte trafficking across a model of the blood-brain barrier. *Methods*, 29(4), 351–61.

Eugenin, E. A., et al. (2003). MCP-1 (CCL2) protects human neurons and astrocytes from NMDA or HIV-tat-induced apoptosis. *J Neurochem*, 85(5), 1299–311.

Eugenin, E. A., et al. (2006). CCL2/monocyte chemoattractant protein-1 mediates enhanced transmigration of human immunodeficiency virus (HIV)-infected leukocytes across the blood-brain barrier: A potential mechanism of HIV-CNS invasion and neuroAIDS. *J Neurosci*, 26(4), 1098–106.

Fellay, J., et al. (2007). A whole-genome association study of major determinants for host control of HIV-1. *Science*, 317(5840), 944–7.

Fischer-Smith, T., Tedaldi, E. M., & Rappaport, J. (2008).CD163/CD16 coexpression by circulating monocytes/macrophages in HIV: Potential biomarkers for HIV infection and AIDS progression. *AIDS Res Hum Retroviruses*, 24(3), 417–21.

Foli, A., et al. (2007). A checkpoint in the cell cycle progression as a therapeutic target to inhibit HIV replication. *J Infect Dis*, 196(9), 1409–15.

Follstaedt, S. C., Barber, S. A., & Zink, M. C. (2008). Mechanisms of minocycline-induced suppression of simian immunodeficiency virus encephalitis: Inhibition of apoptosis signal-regulating kinase 1. *J Neurovirol*, 14(5), 376–88.

Fox, H. S., et al. (2000). Antiviral treatment normalizes neurophysiological but not movement abnormalities in simian immunodeficiency virus-infected monkeys. *J Clin Invest*, 106(1), 37–45.

Gartner, S. (2000). HIV infection and dementia. *Science*, 287(5453), 602–4.

Glass, J. D., Fedor, H., Wesselingh, S. L., McArthur, J. C. (1995). Immunocytochemical quantitation of human immunodeficiency virus in the brain: correlations with dementia, *Ann. Neurol.* 38(5), 755–762.

Gordon, S. N., et al. (2007). Severe depletion of mucosal CD4+ T cells in AIDS-free simian immunodeficiency virus-infected sooty mangabeys. *J Immunol*, 179(5), 3026–34.

Kalvakolanu, D. V. (2003). Alternate interferon signaling pathways. *Pharmacol Ther*, 100(1), 1–29.

Kelder, W., et al. (1998). Beta-chemokines MCP-1 and RANTES are selectively increased in cerebrospinal fluid of patients with human immunodeficiency virus-associated dementia. *Ann Neurol*, 44(5), 831–5.

Kim, M. O., et al. (2002) Interferon-beta activates multiple signaling cascades in primary human microglia. *J Neurochem*, 81(6), 1361–71.

Koenig, S., et al. (1986). Detection of AIDS virus in macrophages in brain tissue from AIDS patients with encephalopathy. *Science*, 233(4768), 1089–93.

Kohl, C. & Sperner-Unterweger, B. (2007). IDO and clinical conditions associated with depressive symptoms. *Curr Drug Metab*, 8(3), 283–7.

Korin, Y. D. & Zack, J. A. (1998). Progression to the G1b phase of the cell cycle is required for completion of human immunodeficiency virus type 1 reverse transcription in T cells. *J Virol*, 72(4), 3161–8.

Kumar, A. M., et al. (2007). Human immunodeficiency virus type 1 RNA Levels in different regions of human brain: quantification using real-time reverse transcriptase-polymerase chain reaction. *J Neurovirol*, 13(3), 210–24.

Kure, K., et al. (1990). Cellular localization of an HIV-1 antigen in subacute AIDS encephalitis using an improved double-labeling immunohistochemical method. *Am J Pathol*, 136(5), 1085–92.

Kwidzinski, E. & Bechmann, I. (2007). IDO expression in the brain: A double-edged sword. *J Mol Med*, 85(12), 1351–9.

Lackner, A. A., et al. (1994). Early events in tissues during infection with pathogenic (SIVmac239) and nonpathogenic (SIVmac1A11) molecular clones of simian immunodeficiency virus. *Am J Pathol*, 145(2), 428–39.

Lackner, A. A., et al. (1991). Localization of simian immunodeficiency virus in the central nervous system of rhesus monkeys. *Am J Pathol*, 139(3), 609–21.

Lane, J. H., et al. (1996). Neuroinvasion by simian immunodeficiency virus coincides with increased numbers of perivascular macrophages/microglia and intrathecal immune activation. *J Neurovirol*, 2(6), 423–32.

Langford, D., et al. (2006). Relationship of antiretroviral treatment to postmortem brain tissue viral load in human immunodeficiency virus-infected patients. *J Neurovirol*, 12(2), 100–7.

Letendre, S., et al. (2008). Validation of the CNS Penetration-Effectiveness rank for quantifying antiretroviral penetration into the central nervous system. *Arch Neurol*, 65(1), 65–70.

Li, H., et al. (2007). The interferon signaling network and transcription factor C/EBP-beta. *Cell Mol Immunol*, 4(6), 407–18.

Mandl, J. N., et al. (2008). Divergent TLR7 and TLR9 signaling and type I interferon production distinguish pathogenic and nonpathogenic AIDS virus infections. *Nat Med*, 14(10), 1077–87.

Mankowski, J. L., et al. (2004). Cerebrospinal fluid markers that predict SIV CNS disease. *J Neuroimmunol*, 157(1–2), 66–70.

Mankowski, J. L., et al. (2008). Natural host genetic resistance to lentiviral CNS disease: A neuroprotective MHC class I allele in SIV-infected macaques. *PLoS One*, 3(11), e3603.

Mankowski, J. L., et al. (1997). Pathogenesis of simian immunodeficiency virus encephalitis: Viral determinants of neurovirulence. *J Virol*, 71(8), 6055–60.

Marcondes, M. C., et al. (2009). Early antiretroviral treatment prevents the development of central nervous system abnormalities in simian immunodeficiency virus-infected rhesus monkeys. *AIDS, 23*(10), 1187–95.

McArthur, J. C., et al. (1997). Relationship between human immunodeficiency virus-associated dementia and viral load in cerebrospinal fluid and brain. *Ann Neurol, 42*(5), 689–98.

McArthur, J. C., et al. (2000). A phase II trial of nerve growth factor for sensory neuropathy associated with HIV infection. AIDS Clinical Trials Group Team 291. *Neurology, 54*(5), 1080–8.

McManus, C. M., et al. (2000). Chemokine and chemokine-receptor expression in human glial elements: Induction by the HIV protein, Tat, and chemokine autoregulation. *Am J Pathol, 156*(4), 1441–53.

Metz, L. M., et al. (2004). Minocycline reduces gadolinium-enhancing magnetic resonance imaging lesions in multiple sclerosis. *Ann Neurol, 55*(5), 756.

Migueles, S. A., et al. (2000). HLA B*5701 is highly associated with restriction of virus replication in a subgroup of HIV-infected long term nonprogressors. *Proc Natl Acad Sci U S A, 97*(6), 2709–14.

Mori, K., Ringler, D., & Desrosiers, R. (1992). Restricted replication of SIVmac239 in macrophages is determined by Env but is not due to restricted entry, *10th Annual Symposium of Nonhuman Primate Models for AIDS* (San Juan, Puerto Rico).

Murray, E. A., et al. (1992). Cognitive and motor impairments associated with SIV infection in rhesus monkeys. *Science, 255*(5049), 1246–9.

Naif, H. M., Li, S., Alali, M., Sloane, A., Wu, L., Kelly, M., Lynch, G., Lloyd, A., Cunningham, A. L. (1998) CCR5 expression correlates with susceptibility of maturing monocytes to human immunodeficiency virus type 1 infection. *J. Virol. 72*(1), 830-6.

O'Connor, D. H., et al. (2003). Major histocompatibility complex class I alleles associated with slow simian immunodeficiency virus disease progression bind epitopes recognized by dominant acute-phase cytotoxic-T-lymphocyte responses. *J Virol, 77*(16), 9029–40.

Overholser, E. D., et al. (2005). CD4-independent entry and replication of simian immunodeficiency virus in primary rhesus macaque astrocytes are regulated by the transmembrane protein. *J Virol, 79*(8), 4944–51.

Overholser, E. D., et al. (2003). Expression of simian immunodeficiency virus (SIV) nef in astrocytes during acute and terminal infection and requirement of nef for optimal replication of neurovirulent SIV in vitro. *J Virol, 77*(12), 6855–66.

Paiardini, M., et al. (2004). Cell-cycle dysregulation in the immunopathogenesis of AIDS. *Immunol Res, 29*(1–3), 253–68.

Pandrea, I., et al. (2007). Paucity of CD4+CCR5+ T cells is a typical feature of natural SIV hosts. *Blood, 109*(3), 1069–76.

Patton, H. K., et al. (2000). Gp120-induced alterations of human astrocyte function: Na(+)/H(+) exchange, K(+) conductance, and glutamate flux. *Am J Physiol Cell Physiol, 279*(3), C700–8.

Poli, V. (1998). The role of C/EBP isoforms in the control of inflammatory and native immunity functions. *J Biol Chem, 273*(45), 29279–82.

Pope, R., et al. (2000). Regulation of TNF-alpha expression in normal macrophages: The role of C/EBPbeta. *Cytokine, 12*(8), 1171–81.

Price, R. W., et al. (1988). The brain in AIDS: Central nervous system HIV-1 infection and AIDS dementia complex. *Science, 239*(4840), 586–92.

Prospero-Garcia, O., et al. (1996). Microglia-passaged simian immunodeficiency virus induces neurophysiological abnormalities in monkeys. *Proc Natl Acad Sci U S A, 93*(24), 14158–63.

Ravimohan, S., et al. (2009). Regulation of SIV mac 239 basal long terminal repeat activity and viral replication in macrophages: Functional roles of two CCAAT/enhancer-binding protein beta sites in activation and interferon beta-mediated suppression. *J Biol Chem, 285*(4), 2258–73.

Roberts, E. S., et al. (2004). Acute SIV infection of the brain leads to upregulation of IL6 and interferon-regulated genes: Expression patterns throughout disease progression and impact on neuroAIDS. *J Neuroimmunol, 157*(1–2), 81–92.

Sacktor, N., et al. (2000). Transdermal selegiline in HIV-associated cognitive impairment: Pilot, placebo-controlled study. *Neurology, 54*(1), 233–5.

Sacktor, N., et al. (2001). HIV-associated neurologic disease incidence changes: Multicenter AIDS Cohort Study, 1990–1998. *Neurology, 56* (2), 257–60.

Sanchez Mejia, R. O., et al. (2001). Minocycline reduces traumatic brain injury-mediated caspase-1 activation, tissue damage, and neurological dysfunction. *Neurosurgery, 48*(6), 1393–9; discussion 99–401.

Sauermann, U. (2001). Making the animal model for AIDS research more precise: The impact of major histocompatibility complex (MHC) genes on pathogenesis and disease progression in SIV-infected monkeys. *Curr Mol Med, 1*(4), 515–22.

Schifitto, G., et al. (2001). Long-term treatment with recombinant nerve growth factor for HIV-associated sensory neuropathy. *Neurology, 57*(7), 1313–6.

Schmitz, J. E., et al. (1999a). A nonhuman primate model for the selective elimination of CD8+ lymphocytes using a mouse-human chimeric monoclonal antibody. *Am J Pathol, 154*(6), 1923–32.

Schmitz, J. E., et al. (1999b). Control of viremia in simian immunodeficiency virus infection by CD8+ lymphocytes. *Science, 283*(5403), 857–60.

Sharer, L. R., et al. (1988). Comparison of simian immunodeficiency virus and human immunodeficiency virus encephalitides in the immature host. *Ann Neurol, 23* Suppl, S108–12.

Silvestri, G., et al. (2003). Nonpathogenic SIV infection of sooty mangabeys is characterized by limited bystander immunopathology despite chronic high-level viremia. *Immunity, 18*(3), 441–52.

Silvestri, G., et al. (2005). Divergent host responses during primary simian immunodeficiency virus SIVsm infection of natural sooty mangabey and nonnatural rhesus macaque hosts. *J Virol, 79*(7), 4043–54.

Smith, M. O., Heyes, M. P., & Lackner, A. A. (1995). Early intrathecal events in rhesus macaques (Macaca mulatta) infected with pathogenic or nonpathogenic molecular clones of simian immunodeficiency virus. *Lab Invest, 72*(5), 547–58.

Smith, M. Z., et al. (2005a). Analysis of pigtail macaque major histocompatibility complex class I molecules presenting immunodominant simian immunodeficiency virus epitopes. *J Virol, 79*(2), 684–95.

Smith, M. Z., et al. (2005b). The pigtail macaque MHC class I allele Mane-A*10 presents an immundominant SIV Gag epitope: identification, tetramer development and implications of immune escape and reversion. *J Med Primatol, 34*(5–6), 282–93.

Spooner, C. J., et al. (2007). Differential roles of C/EBP beta regulatory domains in specifying MCP-1 and IL-6 transcription. *Mol Immunol, 44*(6), 1384–92.

Sterne, J. A., et al. (2009). Timing of initiation of antiretroviral therapy in AIDS-free HIV-1-infected patients: A collaborative analysis of 18 HIV cohort studies. *Lancet, 373*(9672), 1352–63.

Suk, K., et al. (2001). Activation-induced cell death of rat astrocytes. *Brain Res, 900*(2), 342–7.

Szeto, G. L., et al. (2010) Minocycline Attenuates HIV Infection and Reactivation by Suppressing Cellular Activation in Human CD4(+) T Cells. *J Infect Dis.*

Tikka, T., et al. (2001). Minocycline, a tetracycline derivative, is neuroprotective against excitotoxicity by inhibiting activation and proliferation of microglia. *J Neurosci, 21*(8), 2580–8.

Tozzi, V., et al. (2001). Changes in neurocognitive performance in a cohort of patients treated with HAART for 3 years. *J Acquir Immune Defic Syndr, 28*(1), 19–27.

Van Den Bosch, L., et al. (2002). Minocycline delays disease onset and mortality in a transgenic model of ALS. *Neuroreport, 13*(8), 1067–70.

Villinger, F., et al. (1996). Immunological and virological studies of natural SIV infection of disease-resistant nonhuman primates. *Immunol Lett, 51*(1–2), 59–68.

Vinson, C. R., Sigler, P. B., & McKnight, S. L. (1989). Scissors-grip model for DNA recognition by a family of leucine zipper proteins. *Science, 246*(4932), 911–6.

Watry, D., et al. (1995). Transfer of neuropathogenic simian immunodeficiency virus with naturally infected microglia. *Am J Pathol, 146*(4), 914–23.

Westmoreland, S. V., Halpern, E., & Lackner, A. A. (1998). Simian immunodeficiency virus encephalitis in rhesus macaques is associated with rapid disease progression. *J Neurovirol, 4*(3), 260–8.

Wiley, C. A., et al. (1986). Cellular localization of human immunodeficiency virus infection within the brains of acquired immune deficiency syndrome patients. *Proc Natl Acad Sci U S A, 83*(18), 7089–93.

Williams, K. C. & Burdo, T. H. (2009). HIV and SIV infection: the role of cellular restriction and immune responses in viral replication and pathogenesis. *APMIS, 117*(5–6), 400–12.

Williams, K. C., et al. (2001). Perivascular macrophages are the primary cell type productively infected by simian immunodeficiency virus in the brains of macaques: Implications for the neuropathogenesis of AIDS. *J Exp Med, 193*(8), 905–15.

Witwer, K. W., et al. (2009). Coordinated regulation of SIV replication and immune responses in the CNS. *PLoS One, 4*(12), e8129.

Wright, E. K., Jr., Clements, J. E., & Barber, S. A. (2006). Sequence variation in the CC-chemokine ligand 2 promoter of pigtailed macaques is not associated with the incidence or severity of neuropathology in a simian immunodeficiency virus model of human immunodeficiency virus central nervous system disease. *J Neurovirol, 12*(6), 411–9.

Wu, D. C., et al. (2002). Blockade of microglial activation is neuroprotective in the 1-methyl-4-phenyl-1,2,3,6-tetrahydropyridine mouse model of Parkinson disease. *J Neurosci, 22*(5), 1763–71.

Zhu, T., Muthui, D., Holte, S., Nickle, D., Feng, F., Brodie, S., Hwangbo, Y., Mullins, J. I., Corey, L. (2002). Evidence for human immunodeficiency virus type 1 replication in vivo in CD14(+) monocytes and its potential role as a source of virus in patients on highly active antiretroviral therapy. *J. Virol. 76*(2), 707–16.

Zink, M. C. & Clements, J. E. (2002). A novel simian immunodeficiency virus model that provides insight into mechanisms of human immunodeficiency virus central nervous system disease. *J Neurovirol, 8* Suppl 2, 42–8.

Zink, M. C., et al. (2001), Increased macrophage chemoattractant protein-1 in cerebrospinal fluid precedes and predicts simian immunodeficiency virus encephalitis. *J Infect Dis, 184*(8), 1015–21.

Zink, M. C., et al. (1997). Pathogenesis of SIV encephalitis. Selection and replication of neurovirulent SIV. *Am J Pathol, 151*(3), 793–803.

Zink, M. C., et al. (2005), Neuroprotective and anti-human immunodeficiency virus activity of minocycline. *JAMA, 293*(16), 2003–11.

Zink, M. C., et al. (1999). High viral load in the cerebrospinal fluid and brain correlates with severity of simian immunodeficiency virus encephalitis. *J Virol, 73*(12), 10480–8.

Zink, M. C., et al. (2010). SIV-infected macaques treated with highly active antiretroviral therapy (HAART) have reduced CNS virus replication and inflammation but persistence of viral DNA. *Submitted.*

Zolopa, A., et al. (2009). Early antiretroviral therapy reduces AIDS progression/death in individuals with acute opportunistic infections: A multicenter randomized strategy trial. *PLoS One, 4*(5), e5575.

5.2

FELINE IMMUNODEFICIENCY VIRUS

Rick B. Meeker

Feline immunodeficiency virus (FIV) is a naturally occurring lentivirus that infects both domestic cats and free-ranging large cats. In domestic cats, FIV infection recapitulates most aspects of HIV-1 infection in humans, including the gradual development of immune deficiency and neurological symptoms. Both HIV and FIV viruses display a highly conserved tropism for the chemokine receptor, CXCR4, and rapidly penetrate the CNS, preferentially infecting microglia and macrophages. As with HIV-1, neuroinvasion by FIV produces a moderate and widespread inflammatory response that includes a small but progressive loss of neurons beginning in the asymptomatic stage of disease. These and other similarities have led to the use of FIV as a model to investigate HIV pathogenic mechanisms and potential therapies, with impressive results. This chapter summarizes advances in our understanding of FIV-associated CNS disease and efforts to develop new treatment strategies that prevent or reverse lentivirus-induced damage to the CNS.

INTRODUCTION

Animal models have provided essential data in our efforts to understand the processes that underlie the development of HIV-1-associated neurocognitive disorders (HAND), including HIV-associated dementia (HAD). Feline immunodeficiency virus (FIV) is a naturally occurring lentivirus that infects both domestic cats (Carpenter et al., 1998; Levy et al., 2006; Pedersen et al., 1987) and free-ranging large cats (Olmsted et al., 1992; Roelke et al., 2009). In domestic cats, FIV infection recapitulates most aspects of HIV-1 infection in humans, including the gradual development of immune deficiency and neurological symptoms. The similarities between FIV pathogenesis in domestic cats and HIV infection in humans has led to the use of the FIV model for the investigation of pathogenic mechanisms and potential therapeutics. Both in vitro and in vivo studies of neural tissue have provided important insights into the early penetration of virus into the central nervous system (CNS), infection and compartmentalization of virus within the nervous system, and the mechanisms of neuropathogenesis. In addition, several studies have begun to exploit this model for the development of therapeutics. This chapter summarizes advances in our understanding of FIV-associated CNS disease and efforts to develop new treatment strategies that prevent or reverse lentivirus-induced damage to the CNS.

THE STRUCTURE OF FIV AND ITS RELATIONSHIP TO HIV

FIV was first isolated by Pedersen et al. (1987) from a domestic cat with chronic AIDS-like symptoms. It has since been identified in both domestic and feral cat species worldwide at approximate seroprevalence rates ranging from 1% to 14% of the domestic feline population. Recent estimates of FIV infection in North America indicated that 2.5% of domestic cats entering clinics or shelters were seropositive for FIV (Levy, Scott, Lachtara, & Crawford, 2006). The genomic organization of FIV is similar to, although less complex than, the genome of HIV-1 (Figure 5.2.1). Like all mammalian lentiviruses, FIV contains three long open reading frames (ORFs) encoding the gag, pol, and env proteins, flanked on either side by long terminal repeats (LTRs) (Olmsted et al., 1989; Talbott et al., 1989). Three auxiliary ORFs contain the nonstructural regulatory genes, *tat* (de Parseval & Elder, 1999), *vif* (Shacklett & Luciw, 1994; Tomonaga et al., 1992), and *rev* (Kiyomasu et al., 1991; Phillips et al., 1992). Unlike the primate lentiviruses, the FIV genome includes dUTPase (Elder et al., 1992) and appears to lack functional equivalents of the HIV-1 accessory genes, *vpr*, *vpu*, and *nef*. Based on the genetic diversity of the *env* gene, FIV has been classified into five distinct subtypes which are distributed unequally among geographic regions (Bachmann et al., 1997). Phylogenetic analysis has further indicated that FIV may represent a more primitive lentivirus that has evolved independently of its primate counterparts (Elder & Phillips, 1993; Olmsted, Hirsch, Purcell, & Johnson, 1989).

FIV CELLULAR TROPISM AND PATHOGENESIS

In spite of differences in evolution and genomic organization, FIV and HIV-1 produce remarkably similar clinical syndromes within their respective hosts. Cats experimentally infected with FIV experience an acute flu-like illness, involving low-grade fever and transient lymphadenopathy, followed by an extended asymptomatic period that culminates in severe immunodeficiency with associated opportunistic infections (English et al., 1994). Like human AIDS, disease progression in FIV-infected cats is characterized by an inversion of the CD4/CD8 ratio that evolves due to a progressive decline in circulating CD4+ T cells (Ackley et al., 1990; Tompkins et al.,

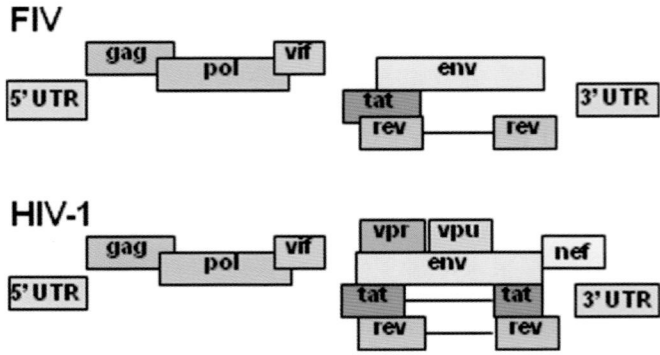

FIV

HIV-1

Figure 5.2.1 Comparison of the genomic structure of feline immunodeficiency virus (FIV) to that of human immunodeficiency virus-1 (HIV-1). Both viruses share common major structural (gag, env) and non-structural genes (pol), as well as several accessory genes (tat, rev, vif). However, FIV lacks sequences encoding vpr, vpu, and nef.

1991; Torten et al., 1991) accompanied by a sustained increase in activated CD8+ T cells (Bucci et al., 1998; Gebhard et al., 1999; Novotney et al., 1990; Willett et al., 1993). In addition to CD4+ and CD8+ T-lymphocytes (Brown et al., 1991; English et al., 1993), FIV also infects monocyte-derived cells (Beebe et al., 1994; Brunner & Pedersen, 1989; Dow et al., 1992; Willett & Hosie, 2008) and B-lymphocytes (English, Johnson, Gebhard, & Tompkins, 1993) in vivo, thereby exhibiting a slightly broader host cell range than the pattern of cell tropism displayed by HIV-1 (Levy, 1993). Although most primary isolates of FIV may target both T-lymphocytes and monocytes, productive infection in vivo is largely restricted to FIV-infected T-lymphocytes.

The molecular determinants of FIV cell tropism are incompletely understood, but some distinctions from HIV-1 are apparent. Unlike HIV-1, FIV does not appear to utilize CD4 as a high affinity, primary receptor (Brown et al., 1991; Dow et al., 1990; Hosie et al., 1993; Kawaguchi et al., 1992). Instead, CD134 is used as the primary receptor (Shimojima et al., 2004). However, CD134 appears to function similarly to CD4 by opening a CXCR4 binding site within the viral envelope (Willett et al., 1997; Willett et al., 2008). The use of the alpha chemokine receptor, CXCR4, as a co-receptor mimics HIV-1. Human and feline CXCR4 share significant homology, and both receptors are capable of mediating FIV- and HIV-1-related cell fusion (Willett et al., 1997). Infection of diverse cell types by both primary and cell-culture-adapted FIV isolates may be inhibited by antibodies to CXCR4 (Willett et al., 1997), the CXCR4-specific ligand, stromal-cell-derived factor-1α (SDF-1α) (Hosie et al., 1998; Richardson et al., 1999), and the selective CXCR4 antagonist, AMD3100 (Egberink et al., 1999; Richardson et al., 1999). To date, no alternative co-receptor has been identified for FIV. To explain the monocyte tropism, it has been suggested that the viral interaction with CD134 may become less stringent with disease progression and facilitate subsequent interactions with CXCR4. This would allow infection of cells expressing low levels of CXCR4 (Willett & Hosie, 2008). Transcripts of both CD134 and CXCR4 have been detected in dendritic

cells and macrophages in addition to lymphocytes, although detection of protein with available antibodies has been less reliable. Using an anti-feline CD134 monoclonal antibody, Willett et al. (2007) demonstrated a low level of CD134 expression on B cells and cultured macrophages which was enhanced by activation. In addition, activation of CD8+ T cells revealed weak CD134 expression, helping to explain the expansion of tropism to these cells during infection. However, the potential role of an unidentified co-receptor cannot be ruled out. Studies using soluble fusion proteins have demonstrated that some FIV surface glycoproteins fail to bind specifically to CXCR4, even though replication of the parent isolate may be inhibited by CXCR4 ligands (de Parseval & Elder, 2001). Studies by Troth et al. (2008) examining FIV infection of a variety of tissues in vivo showed that only approximately 50% of FIV-positive cells expressed detectable CXCR4. The role of specific co-receptors in infection of the CNS in particular remains unclear.

In HIV infection, virus is thought to penetrate into the brain via monocytes infected with CCR5-preferring strains of HIV. Usage of the beta chemokine receptor CCR5 affords tropism to macrophages and microglial cells within the brain (Albright et al., 1999; Albright et al., 2000; Alkhatib et al., 1996; He et al., 1997), thereby establishing a long-lived viral reservoir. Though FIV infection of mononuclear phagocytes is well documented (Beebe et al., 1994; Brunner & Pedersen, 1989; Dow, Dreitz, & Hoover, 1992; Dow et al., 1999), it is still unclear whether similar mechanisms govern FIV tropism for monocyte-derived cells. Feline PBMCs have been shown to express CCR5 receptor mRNA, which has 68% homology to human CCR5 (Kovacs et al., 1999). However, support for the use of beta chemokine receptors by FIV has been indirect. Infection of feline lymphocytes by some FIV isolates may be at least partially inhibited by the beta chemokine RANTES (Lerner & Elder, 2000) and FIV xenoinfection of primate cells may be partially attenuated by antibodies to human CCR3 and CCR5 (Johnston & Power, 2002). On the other hand, studies of FIV infection of cells engineered to express CCR5 have failed to demonstrate a role for CCR5 in infection (Willett et al., 2002). The authors suggested instead that CCR5 may enhance the expression and efficient use of CXCR4 by FIV. Additional studies are required to fully characterize the potential role of chemokine co-receptors in FIV infection of the CNS.

FIV INFECTION AND PATHOGENESIS

The similarities between FIV and HIV have led to the use of the FIV model not only for modeling neuropathogenesis but also for studies of the mechanisms of infection and immune suppression, the development of new therapeutic strategies and the development of vaccines. While a review of accomplishments in these areas is beyond the scope of the current review, it should be noted that significant advances in systemic pathogenesis have paralleled the CNS studies and highlight the broad utility of this model. Indeed, in 2002 the first vaccine for FIV was released. Subsequent work has followed this significant accomplishment to improve the vaccine strategies in ways that might facilitate vaccine development for HIV (Dunham, 2006; Lecollinet & Richardson, 2008; Uhl et al., 2008). Studies of infectious mechanisms have helped to clarify interactions of virus with host cell receptors that determine tropism (Willett, McMonagle, Logan, Samman, & Hosie, 2008; Willett & Hosie, 2008), the role of dendritic cells (Reggeti et al., 2008), and studies of viral latency (Assogba et al., 2007). Parallel immune studies have led to important insights into the mechanisms of immune suppression (Lehman et al., 2009; Mexas et al., 2008; Tompkins & Tompkins, 2008). As a result of this work, a variety of new therapeutic options to prevent infection and preserve immune function have been suggested (Dean et al., 2006; Heit et al., 2006; Maksaereekul et al., 2009; Mizukoshi et al., 2009; Willett et al., 2009). Together, these studies have not only advanced our understanding of viral pathogenesis but also provide a solid foundation for a better understanding of potential virus interactions with the CNS.

FIV NEUROTROPISM AND NEUROPATHOGENESIS

Like the primate lentiviruses, FIV rapidly penetrates the CNS of infected cats, producing a clinical syndrome that may include severe neurologic deficits. Studies of FIV neurotropism have demonstrated that 1) virus can be recovered from brain and CSF of cats infected by either peripheral or intrathecal inoculation with FIV (Dow, Poss, & Hoover, 1990; Johnston et al., 2002a; Macchi et al., 1998; Power et al., 1997) and, 2) FIV can infect a range of neural cells in vitro including microglia (Dow et al., 1990; Hein et al., 2000; Kawaguchi et al., 1992), choroid plexus macrophages (Bragg et al., 2002a), and, under certain conditions, feline astrocytes (Billaud et al., 2000; Danave et al., 1994; Dow et al., 1990; Kawaguchi et al., 1992; Yu et al., 1998).

As with HIV-1, the primary cellular targets of FIV within the CNS are microglia and macrophages, which appear capable of supporting a low-grade productive infection that accelerates dramatically in the presence of peripheral immune cells. Hein et al. (2000; 2001) have reported low levels of viral replication in microglia purified from FIV-infected cats that increased significantly following co-culture with peripheral blood mononuclear cells (PBMCs). Bragg et al. (2002a) observed a similar low level of FIV infection of choroid plexus macrophages. The choroid plexus macrophages, located just outside the blood-CSF barrier, have been considered an important potential target of circulating lentiviruses that could provide access to the CNS via the CSF/ventricular system. Although several studies had previously documented the presence of lentiviral transcripts within the choroid plexus of infected hosts (Beebe et al., 1994; Chen et al., 2000; Falangola et al., 1995; Petito et al., 1999), the function of the macrophages and the extent of trafficking is still unclear. Inoculation of cultures of feline choroid plexus macrophages with FIV$_{NCSU1}$ resulted in a small proviral burden similar to that detected in choroid plexus dissected from FIV-infected cats (Bragg, Childers, Tompkins, Tompkins, & Meeker, 2002a). Virus production was very weak or undetectable but increased dramatically in the presence of a permissive CD4+ feline T cell line. Thus, both microglia and macrophages have been shown to efficiently transfer FIV infection to PBMCs or a T-lymphocyte cell line, illustrating the potential of cell-cell interactions in the control of local viral replication.

Although most studies now indicate that wild-type strains of FIV do not directly infect astrocytes, some studies have indicated that astrocytes can be infected in vitro when exposed to infected PBMCs (Gavrilin et al., 2002). Cell-associated FIV$_{MD}$ was shown to give rise to a new astrocyte-tropic strain of FIV when co-cultured with primary feline astrocytes. This interaction has important implications for the development of reservoirs of viral quasispecies in the brain as well as their potential contribution to pathogenesis.

The above studies not only illustrate the cellular tropism of FIV but highlight the potential importance of cell-cell interactions in the transmission of infection. There is still much to learn about these interactions and the FIV model provides an opportunity to investigate the effects of cellular interactions at all stages of disease progression, including the early stages of infection and initiation of neurologic disease. In vivo studies in cats have clearly established the speed of FIV penetration into the CSF. High levels of FIV can be detected in the CSF within 1 week of infection often in parallel with the initial peak of systemic viremia (Liu et al., 2006a) and provirus is detected in brain parenchyma as early as 2–4 weeks after experimental inoculation (Poli et al., 1999; Ryan et al., 2003). An example of the close temporal relationship between plasma and CNS virus is illustrated in Figure 5.2.2A, for samples drawn from a single cat during the first 18 weeks after systemic inoculation with FIV. As with HIV, viral titers in CSF are typically lower than plasma, on average approximately 2%. However, the use of a neurovirulent strain, FIV$_{V1CSF}$, isolated from the CSF of an FIV-infected cat (Power, Moench, Peeling, Kong, & Langelier, 1997; Power et al., 1998) gave rise to CSF levels comparable to plasma. Intracerebral inoculation of the neurovirulent FIV$_{V1CSF}$, shown in Figure 5.2.2B, reverses the pattern with initial peak viral titers in CSF exceeding plasma, indicating that FIV can directly infect the CNS prior to the development of a robust systemic infection. CSF virus is maintained at higher levels and a significant proviral burden is seen in the brain (Liu et al., 2006a; Macchi et al., 1998). During the asymptomatic phase of disease progression it has been difficult to demonstrate virus production in the brain and in some cases there appears to be an early clearance of provirus (Ryan et al., 2003). As with HIV-1, significant questions remain regarding compartmentalization, viral evolution, and local control of viral replication in the CNS. The FIV model provides a versatile system for the investigation of these processes at all stages of pathogenesis.

Clinical evaluations of experimentally infected cats have further indicated that FIV rapidly penetrates the CNS and initiates a gradual and progressive neuropathogenesis. Neurologic deficits have been documented in cats experimentally inoculated with the primary isolate, FIV$_{MD}$ (Phillips et al., 1994; Podell et al., 1993; Podell et al., 1997; Podell et al.,

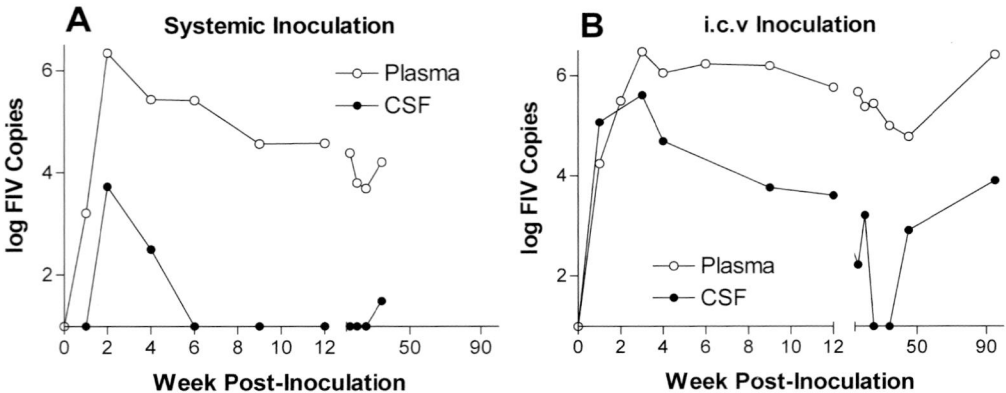

Figure 5.2.2 A. Example of FIV RNA titers in matched samples of plasma and CSF from a cat infected systemically (i.p.) with FIV_{NCSU1} at 0 weeks. Viral titers peak in both compartments at two weeks post-inoculation. By 6 weeks, CSF virus has been reduced to undetectable levels while plasma viral titers remain stable at 10^4–10^5 copies/ml. B. A cat inoculated with a similar titer of the neurotropic FIV_{V1CSF} showed an initial viral titer in CSF almost one log higher than plasma. CSF viral titers are sustained for at least 16 weeks, drop to undetectable levels and then reappear at high levels.

1999; Prospero-Garcia et al., 1994a), the infectious molecular clone, FIV_{PPR}(Phillips et al., 1996; Phipps et al., 2000), and the cerebrospinal fluid-derived isolate, FIV_{V1CSF} (Power et al., 1998). Estimates of the frequency of FIV-related CNS disease suggest that clinically relevant neurologic deficits appear in 20–40% of FIV-infected cats, which is similar to the incidence of HAD in untreated HIV-1-infected patients. Symptoms observed in these cats include abnormal, stereotypic motor behaviors, anisocoria, increased aggression, increased cortical slow wave activity in quantitative electroencephalograms, prolonged latencies in brainstem-evoked potentials, delayed righting and pupillary reflexes, decreased nerve conduction velocities, marked changes in sleep architecture, and deficits in cognitive-motor functions. Using proton magnetic resonance spectroscopy (MRS), Power et al. (1998) and Podell et al. (1999) have both demonstrated reductions in the concentrations of the neuronal marker, N-acetyl-aspartate (NAA) and the NAA/choline or NAA/creatine ratio within the brains of FIV-infected cats.

Thus, the neurologic deficits detected by clinical examination correlate with in vivo estimates of neuronal damage measured by noninvasive imaging techniques.

Most, if not all, FIV-infected cats at necropsy show a characteristic neuropathology that resembles the profile typically seen in brains of patients infected with HIV-1, albeit less severe. Diffuse damage, involving widespread gliosis, myelin pallor, and microglial nodules with rare, multinucleated giant cells, have been observed in brains of FIV-infected cats (Abramo et al., 1995; Boche et al., 1996; Gunn-Moore et al., 1996; Hurtrel et al., 1992; Poli et al., 1997; Silvotti et al., 1997). In addition, multiple investigators have documented a significant neuronal loss within the FIV-infected cat brain (Meeker et al., 1997; Power, Moench, Peeling, Kong, & Langelier, 1997). Neuropathological changes seen in cats with feline AIDS are illustrated in Figure 5.2.3. In the frontal/parietal cortex of asymptomatic cats infected experimentally with FIV_{NCSU1}, large pyramidal cells within layers two/three and five appeared to be most vulnerable (Meeker,

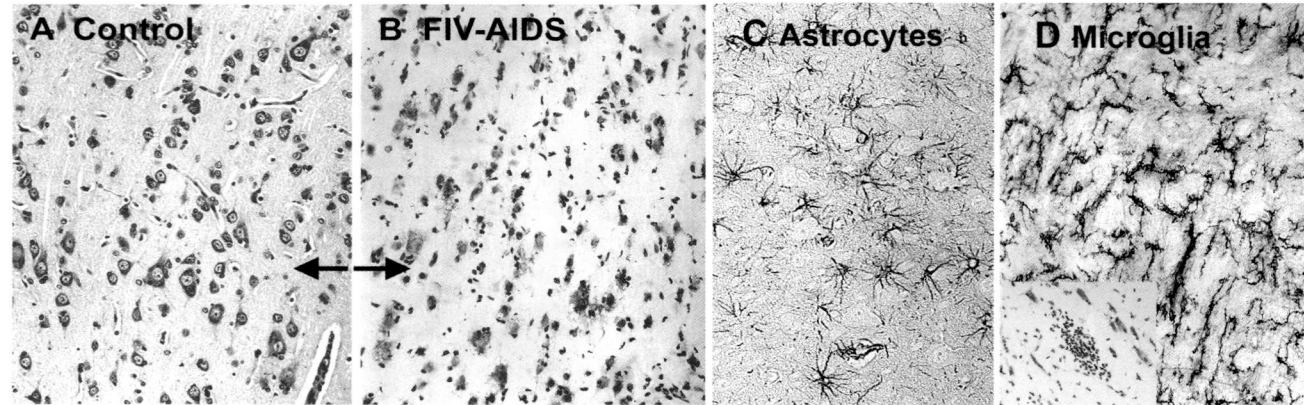

Figure 5.2.3 Neuropathological changes seen in the brains of FIV-infected cats. Cats with feline AIDS (FIV-AIDS) often show a significant loss of cortical pyramidal neurons (B, arrows) relative to uninfected cats (A). (C) A diffuse astrogliosis revealed by staining for glial fibrillary acidic protein (GFAP) is often seen. (D) Strong staining of CD18+ microglia in subcortical white matter. Glial nodules (inset) and scattered CD18+ monocytic cells (not shown) can also be seen scattered diffusely throughout the parenchyma.

Thiede, Hall, English, & Tompkins, 1997). Jacobson et al. (1997) found that large pyramidal neurons in cortical layers three and five also showed an increased immunoreactivity for neurofilament protein and Koirala et al. (2001) showed decreased immunoreactivity for MAP-2 and GAD following CNS infection by FIV. In the hippocampus of FIV-infected cats, a loss of somatostatin- or parvalbumin-immunoreactive neurons in the hippocampal hilus was correlated with increased Timms staining (sprouting) within the inner molecular layer (Mitchell et al., 1999).

The gradual appearance of neural damage in asymptomatic cats is consistent with the early appearance of altered sleep architecture at 10–12 months post-inoculation (p. i.) (Prospero-Garcia et al., 1994b), cortical atrophy by MRI at 12 months p. i. (Podell et al., 1993), decreased NAA and NAA/choline at 14 months (Podell et al., 1999), motor and spatial memory deficits at 12 months p. i. (Steigerwald et al., 1999), and the appearance of toxic activity in the CSF of FIV-infected cats as early as 4 months p. i. (Bragg et al., 2002b). These findings offer a clear indication that disease progresses steadily and that early therapeutic intervention is warranted to control the initiation and progression of neurodegenerative activity. This conclusion is supported by more recent studies that have used increasingly sophisticated behavioral measures to provide sensitive indices of cognitive function. Maingat et al. (2009) assessed the neurobehavioral performance of cats infected neonatally with a neurovirulent FIV chimera (FIV_{Ch}) in parallel with measures of infection and immune status. Behavioral measures included gait width for locomotor function and a modified T maze and object memory test for spatial memory. An increase in gait width was apparent by 15 weeks and deficits in memory and cognitive performance were seen at 12 and 15 weeks postinoculation. Infection also introduced greater variation in performance similar to the variations in host response to HIV infection. Poor performance on the behavioral tasks was associated with cortical viral burden and markers of T cell and monocyte/macrophage infiltration into the brain, based on feline CD3episilon and F4/80 mRNA expression, but not GFAP. It is noteworthy that parietal cortex viral burden was significantly correlated with the T cell marker CD3episilon but not the monocyte/macrophage marker F4/80, suggesting a potential role for T cells in the maintenance of viral burden. Markers of glutamate receptor signaling were suppressed in the FIV-infected cats and there was increased expression of the microglial activation marker Iba-1. Fewer Neu-N+ neurons were seen in the parietal cortex. These important studies established that cognitive deficits can emerge relatively quickly and provide valuable indices of neurocognitive performance that can potentially be used as sensitive measures of disease progression. Successful testing of cognitive function in cats using new tasks designed to be sensitive cognitive-motor deficits has also been reported (Meeker et al., 2010). These studies have begun to provide measures of cognitive function that parallel the measures used to define deficits in HIV-infected humans, providing useful endpoints for the valid translation of animal studies to human clinical trials.

FIV ENTRY INTO THE CENTRAL NERVOUS SYSTEM

Lentiviral neuropathogenesis begins with the entry of virus into the nervous system and control of this process and the associated inflammation is an important therapeutic goal. Evidence supports entry of virus within trafficking monocytes, T cells and perhaps penetration through a weak bloodbrain barrier, but the mechanisms that control this penetration in response to infection are still poorly understood. Studies with FIV have provided important new insights into these complex processes. Using an in vitro feline blood-brain barrier model composed of brain microvascular endothelial cells cultured on transwell membranes in combination with astrocytes and/or microglia, Hudson et al. (2005) evaluated the effects of FIV on the trafficking of PBMCs. By selectively exposing endothelium, astrocytes, or microglia to the FIV, the contribution of each virus-cell interaction to PBMC trafficking was assessed. Trafficking of PBMCs was enhanced by the presence of astrocytes independent of FIV. Addition of microglia inhibited this effect, indicating that astrocytes and microglia may play opposing roles in the control of immune cell trafficking. Exposure of astrocytes alone to FIV selectively increased the trafficking of CD8+ T cells, an effect that was again suppressed by the addition of microglia. Separate infection of the PBMCs mimicking the early stages of infection prior to penetration of FIV into the nervous system facilitated trafficking of CD4+ and CD8+ T cells (Hudson et al., 2008). Addition of FIV to other cell compartments in combination with the infected PBMCs resulted in different patterns of cell migration, including a general suppression of trafficking when the endothelial cells were exposed to FIV. Fletcher et al. (2006; 2009) used a similar system to explore the trafficking of cell-associated and cell-free FIV across the in vitro bloodbrain barrier. Cell-associated virus was found to cross much more efficiently. This trafficking was enhanced by the presence of tumor necrosis factor-α (TNF-α) or FIV on the brain side of the barrier. Together, these studies illustrate that cells and cytokines within the brain compartment can exert strong control over immune cell trafficking.

FIV may also enter the brain via the blood-CSF barrier at the choroid plexus epithelium. The choroid plexus stroma between the vasculature and the epithelium harbors a population of macrophages which can be infected with FIV (Bragg, Childers, Tompkins, Tompkins, & Meeker, 2002a). FIV is localized to the choroid plexus soon after infection and is associated with lymphocyte-rich perivascular infiltrates (Ryan et al., 2005). Trafficking of virus and immune cells through the choroid plexus could explain the rapid and efficient appearance of virus in the CSF. However, little is known about the potential function of trafficking macrophages and other immune cells into the cerebral ventricles. Inoculation of FIV directly into the ventricles has been shown to rapidly induce systemic infection with an efficiency that is greater than that seen with peripheral inoculation (Liu et al., 2006a). This highly efficient transfer of infectious virus via the CSF further established the importance of the protected brain reservoir as a general source of infectious virus.

MECHANISMS OF FIV NEUROPATHOGENESIS

Developing effective therapeutic strategies has been difficult, given that the mechanisms underlying lentivirus-induced neurotoxicity remain poorly understood. Efforts to unravel the molecular events that lead to neuronal dysfunction and cell death associated with FIV- and HIV-infection have been complicated by considerable evidence implicating a diverse range of putative neurotoxins, each of which might theoretically exert very different effects on neural cells. While the putative toxins are diverse, studies with both HIV-1 and FIV have identified several basic features of neuropathogenesis which can be summarized as follows: 1) CNS damage is thought to result from direct interactions between neurons and viral proteins as well as from the secretion of neurotoxins by macrophages/microglia in response to infectious or noninfectious interactions with the virus or viral proteins; 2) toxic accumulation of intracellular calcium is a common pathway by which the neurotoxins disable neurons, and 3) early pathological markers of neuronal dysfunction include neuritic beading and pruning of synapses and processes. Each of these effects can be studied in primary cultures of feline neural cells under well-controlled conditions.

The first studies to explore the mechanisms of FIV neurotoxicity in mixed neural cultures using the primary isolate, FIV$_{NCSU1}$, demonstrated rapid effects on neuronal function and survival (Meeker et al., 1996). Inoculation of primary feline neural cultures with infectious FIV in the presence of a small subtoxic concentration of glutamate (20 μM) resulted in swelling of neurons followed by death of a subset of neurons. The presence of FIV shifted the concentration-effect curve for glutamate toxicity approximately three-fold to the left, indicating an increase in the neuronal sensitivity to the glutamate. As with studies of the HIV-1 surface glycoprotein gp120 (Lipton et al., 1991), the effects of FIV were blocked by an NMDA receptor antagonist. Toxicity increased progressively over the first week post-inoculation, suggesting the gradual release of soluble toxic factors. Small amounts of FIV provirus were detected in these cultures at 18 days p. i., but no evidence of productive infection was observed during the period of toxin generation.

HIV-1 gp120 has been consistently implicated as a potent neurotoxin (Nath & Geiger, 1998), and there is evidence that the FIV surface glycoprotein possesses a comparable neurotoxic potential. Intracerebroventricular administration of the FIV envelope protein in rats (Prospero-Garcia et al., 1994c; Prospero-Garcia et al., 1999) reproduced the sleep disturbances and electrophysiologic abnormalities previously described in FIV-infected cats (Prospero-Garcia et al., 1994a) and HIV-1-infected patients (Darko et al., 1995). Similarly, inoculation of neuronal cultures with purified FIV$_{PPR}$ envelope protein(Bragg, 1999; Gruol et al., 1998) produced glutamate-dependent neuronal swelling and cell death similar to the pattern induced in vitro by infectious FIV (Gruol et al., 1998; Meeker, English, & Tompkins, 1996). Toxic effects were not induced by the envelope protein derived from FIV$_{34TF10}$, a less neurovirulent strain (Bragg, 1999).

Additional evidence that neurovirulence may be associated with specific FIV envelope sequences has been provided by Power et al. (1998), who characterized a unique, highly neurovirulent strain of FIV (FIV$_{V1CSF}$) isolated from the CSF of a cat with neurologic disease. FIV$_{V1CSF}$ stimulated greater secretion of neurotoxins from macrophages in vitro relative to FIV$_{Petaluma}$, a non-neurovirulent strain, even though both isolates replicated with equal efficiency in macrophages (Johnston et al., 2002b). Specific sequences within the envelope gene may be required for toxic interactions with the host cell. Evaluation of envelope variation in FIV-infected cats using heterodupex tracking assays have shown that variation can appear rapidly after infection, particularly in cats with neurological symptoms (Liu et al., 2006b). The dynamic nature of changes in the FIV envelope in CSF soon after infection is illustrated in Figure 5.2.4. The left lane of Figure 5.2.4 shows the inoculum with a single dense band at the bottom. As the envelope sequence changes the envelope DNA hybrids migrate slower, giving rise to additional bands. The changes in the band patterns over the first few weeks post-inoculation illustrate the rapid diversification of the envelope sequences. However, as with HIV, the relationship between specific envelope variants/co-receptor preference and CNS disease is not well understood. While CCR5-preferring variants of HIV-1 are predominant in the CNS, CXCR4-tropic strains induce neurotoxicity and can infect macrophages (Gorry et al., 2001; Ohagen et al., 1999). All FIV strains thus far have been shown to use CXCR4 as a co-receptor, but some strains can differ widely in their neurovirulence. For example, cats infected with FIV$_{Petaluma}$ fail to develop neurologic disease and macrophages infected in vitro with FIV$_{Petaluma}$ fail to release soluble neurotoxic factors (Power et al., 1998). Willett and Hosie (2008) have suggested that neurotropism may be due in part to differential stringency in the interaction of the virus with the primary receptor CD134. A more permissive interaction allows some viruses to take advantage of the lower expression of CXCR4 on cells of monocytic lineage.

The cellular location of envelope protein may also play a role in the pathogenic process. Noorbakhsh et al. (2006)

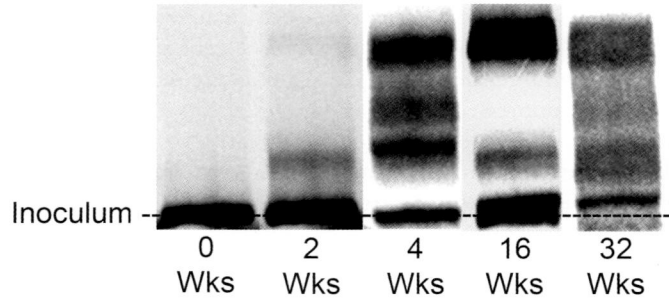

Inoculum -

| 0 Wks | 2 Wks | 4 Wks | 16 Wks | 32 Wks |

Figure 5.2.4 Rapid appearance of FIV envelope variants demonstrated by heteroduplex tracking assay (HTA). The left column shows a single dense band at the bottom corresponding to the inoculum. Mismatches of envelope sequences to the probe sequence (inoculum strain) delay the migration of DNA resulting in a pattern of bands that reflect different envelope variants. Increased diversity of envelope in the CSF of FIV-infected cats develops rapidly over time (weeks post-inoculation) and then decreases as the FIV titers decrease at 32 weeks.

assessed the toxic effects of FIV$_{V1CSF}$ envelope expressed extracellularly versus intracellularly. Extracellular exposure of feline macrophages to FIV$_{V1CSF}$ envelope protein generated the highest level of neurotoxic activity. Intracellular envelope expression using a Sindbis vector in macrophages and infection with FIV both resulted in supernatants with slightly less toxicity. However, a cellular stress response was induced by infection that was not seen with envelope alone. Induction of indolamine 2,3-dioxygenase (IDO), which has immunosuppressive properties, was seen with intracellular envelope expression in macrophages and infection of microglia. These results show that replication competence is not necessary for neurovirulence, but also indicate that cellular stress and potential immunosuppressive activity may contribute to the overall pathogenesis.

ASTROCYTES AND NEUROPATHOGENESIS

As noted above, neural cultures challenged in vitro with FIV experience a significant enhancement in glutamate-mediated neuronal responses (Gruol et al., 1998; Meeker, Thiede, Hall, English, & Tompkins, 1997). However, no differences in glutamate receptor binding were observed in cortical sections taken from FIV-infected and control cats (Meeker et al., 1997) and neonatally infected cats with well-characterized cognitive and behavioral deficits have shown no reductions in markers of glutamate receptor function (Maingat et al., 2009). One possible mechanism of facilitation is the failure to clear glutamate from the synaptic cleft because of dysfunctional amino acid transporters. Support for this argument has been provided by reports of suppressed uptake of glutamate by FIV-infected astrocytes in vitro (Yu, Billaud, & Phillips, 1998). Although astrocytes are a target for infection by some strains of FIV in vitro (Danave et al., 1994; Dow, Poss, & Hoover, 1990; Zenger et al., 1995), there is little evidence for direct infection by wild-type strains of FIV virus in vitro or in vivo. A potential exception is the infection of astrocytes via contact with infected T cells reviewed above. More work is needed to clarify the role of astrocytes in FIV infection and neuropathogenesis.

FIV AS A MODEL OF DISTAL SENSORY POLYNEUROPATHY

Distal sensory polyneuropathy (DSP) is a significant problem in HIV-infected individuals due to the debilitating effects and relatively high prevalence. The effects of HIV are compounded by the actions of antiretroviral drugs used to treat the infection which can themselves induce a DSP that is indistinguishable from that induced by HIV. Animal models that recapitulate the syndrome are badly needed to better understand both the pathogenesis and treatment. FIV-infected animals have been used to explore the mechanisms of DSP where infection of dorsal root ganglion (DRG) and treatment with didanosine (ddI) have been shown to synergize in their ability to damage DRG neurons as evidenced

by a decrease in neurite length and soma size in vitro and a loss of small diameter axons in sural nerve and footpad nerve endings in vivo (Zhu et al., 2007). Damage correlated with both a decrease in mitochondrial cytochrome C oxidase I and expression of brain-derived neurotrophic factor (BDNF) and its receptor, TrkB. The damage was significantly attenuated by BDNF treatment, suggesting that a loss of neurotrophin support may contribute to pathogenesis.

MACROPHAGE TOXINS AND NEURONAL INTRACELLULAR CALCIUM HOMEOSTASIS

In addition to harboring infection, microglia and macrophages can be activated by FIV or FIV-derived proteins to induce the release of neurotoxins. The interactions that trigger the release of neurotoxins by microglia and macrophages are poorly understood, and the FIV model is currently being exploited to examine these processes.

Macrophages and microglia inoculated with FIV release neurotoxins in much the same fashion as macrophages inoculated with HIV-1 (Giulian et al., 1990; Pulliam et al., 1991). Using feline neural cultures, the actions of FIV and macrophage-derived toxins have been examined in an effort to identify the intracellular processes that underlie neuropathogenesis. Since excessive intracellular calcium accumulation is widely considered a final common pathway leading to neuronal dysfunction and death, the role of various sources of calcium entry into the neuronal cytoplasm was investigated (Bragg et al., 2002c). In these early studies, approximately 64% of the neurons showed a very small acute calcium rise followed by a large delayed increase in intracellular calcium and swelling after approximately 30–60 min. Several key features of the responses of these neurons are illustrated in the responses of two representative neurons in Figure 5.2.5. Both neurons were from the same culture treated with a CSF-derived isolate of FIV$_{NCSU1}$. Neuron1 showed an acute calcium response followed by partial recovery and a delayed increase in intracellular calcium after approximately 40 min. Importantly, neuron 2 showed a negligible acute response but had a late destabilization of calcium similar to neuron 1 when corrected for the "resting" levels prior to the rise (115 fluorescence units, neuron 2 vs. 147, neuron 1). Thus, the destabilization of calcium in neurons is independent of the acute calcium response. However, the net accumulation of calcium is greater if the acute response is present. These responses were replicated in subsequent experiments with even greater calcium destabilization using conditioned medium from FIV-inoculated macrophages.

To identify the source of the calcium rise that led to toxicity, the neural cultures were treated with antagonists to block various routes of calcium entry into the cytosol. Xestospongin C, AP5, TTX, pertussis toxin, ω-conotoxin, and ruthenium red all partially attenuated toxin-induced cell death in response to a 24-hour exposure to conditioned medium from FIV-treated macrophages (Figure 5.2.6). This pharmacological profile indicated that all major sources of calcium may contribute to neuropathogenesis and toxicity was dependent on synaptic activity. Similar pharmacological profiles have been

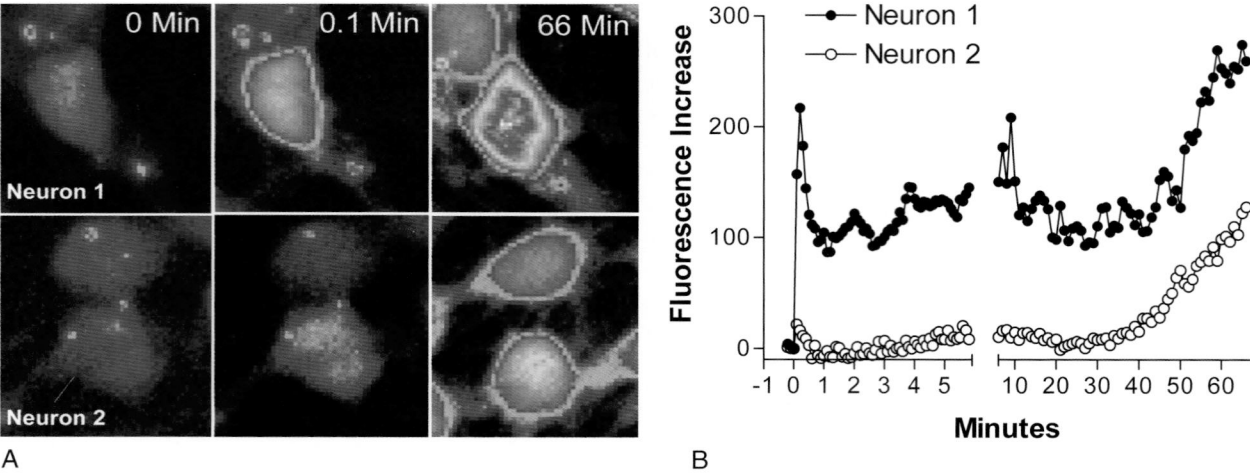

Figure 5.2.5 Calcium responses in two representative neurons from the same culture exposed to FIV collected from the CSF of an infected cat. **A.** Intracellular calcium was measured by the increase in fluorescence of the indicator dye Fluo-3 loaded at a concentration of 2 μM for 30 min at 37°. Neuron 1 shows a moderate acute response at 0.1 min followed by partial recovery and a steady delayed increase in calcium between 40 and 66 min. Neuron 2 failed to show an acute calcium response but showed a similar delayed increase illustrating the independence of the delayed response from the acute response. **B.** In neuron 1, the acute increase in calcium synergizes with the delayed increase resulting in a much higher net gain of intracellular calcium.

reported for the effects of the HIV envelope, gp120, tat proteins, and macrophage secretory products (Haughey et al., 1999; Holden et al., 1999; Lo et al., 1992; Zheng et al., 1999b; Zheng et al., 1999a). These observations are not consistent with a single source of excess calcium entry into the cytosol and did not support the involvement of direct excitotoxic processes. To explore the possibility that a downstream process responsible for the control of intracellular calcium homeostasis might contribute to the observed effects, the kinetics of intracellular calcium recovery were explored.

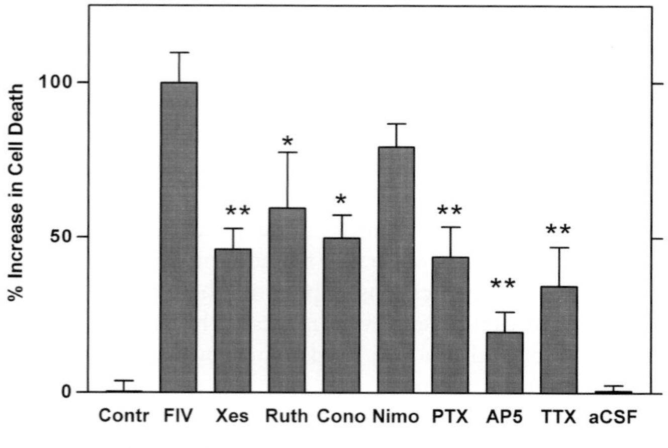

Figure 5.2.6 Pharmacological protection from cell death induced by supernatant from FIV-treated feline macrophages. Conditioned medium from choroid plexus macrophages exposed to FIV_{NCSU1} (FIV) was applied to primary feline cortical cultures in the presence of xestospongin C (Xes), ruthenium red (Ruth), ω-conotoxin (Cono), nimodipine (Nimo), pertussis toxin (PTX), 2-amino-5-phosphonopentanoic acid (AP5), tetrodotoxin (TTX) or artificial CSF (aCSF). The amount of cell death relative to conditioned medium (100%) was significantly reduced by most drugs, although each afforded only partial protection. (Reproduced from Bragg, et al., 2002c, with permission)

A brief (2 s) pulse of glutamate was used to stimulate a rapid calcium response in feline neurons followed by rapid washout. The glutamate pulse induced a much larger rise in intracellular calcium in treated neurons (Figure 5.2.7A). However, as illustrated by the recovery kinetics in Figure 5.2.7B, conditioned medium from FIV-treated macrophages decreased both the rate and extent of calcium recovery. Similar effects have been observed after incubation of rat cortical neurons in a 1:5 dilution of CSF from a subset of HIV-infected patients, suggesting the presence of similar toxin(s) in humans (Meeker et al., 2005).

A deficit in the ability of neurons to recover from increases in intracellular calcium would be expected to facilitate both acute and gradual intracellular calcium increases in response to many stimuli, including glutamate receptor activation. Moreover, the inability to recovery from a calcium load provides a consistent explanation for the diverse pharmacological effects described above and would predict the failure of therapeutic agents targeted to any one source of calcium mobilization. Although the targets of macrophage-derived targets remain unknown, likely candidates include calcium transporters or exchangers at the plasma membrane (Bragg, Boles, & Meeker, 2002c). Related studies employing various inhibitors of calcium transport or exchange suggested that damage to the sodium/calcium exchanger (NCX) may be partially responsible for the dysregulation of intracellular calcium homeostasis (Meeker, Boles, Robertson, & Hall, 2005).

A unique mechanism of neuronal damage has also been suggested by studies of FIV neuropathogenesis. These studies have shown that matrix metalloproteinase-2 (MMP-2) produced by inflammatory interactions in the nervous system cleaves the chemokine CXCL12 (also known as SDF-1), giving rise to a toxic fragment CXCL12(5–67) (Vergote et al., 2006; Zhang et al., 2003). This toxic fragment does not bind to the natural CXCL12 receptor CXCR4 but instead binds

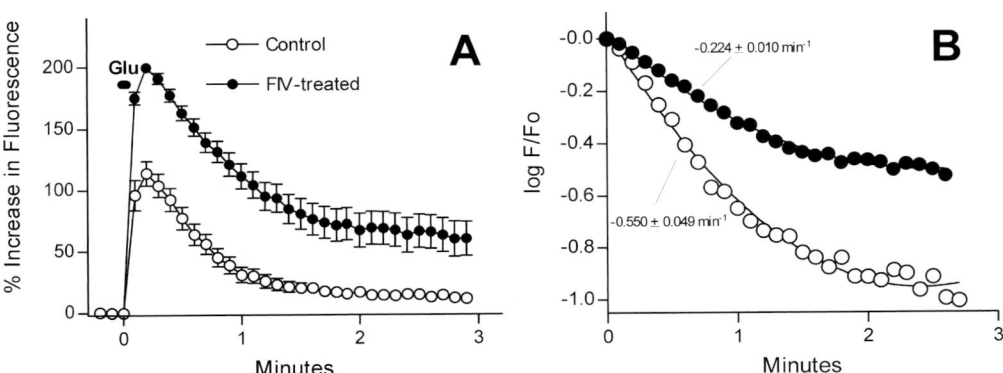

Figure 5.2.7 Effects of macrophage toxins on neuronal calcium homeostasis. A. Neurons exposed to conditioned medium from FIV-treated macrophages produced a greater increase in intracellular calcium in response to a brief pulse of glutamate and failed to recover completely. B. The rate of recovery from peak calcium fluorescence (Fo) following glutamate washout (slope of log F/Fo vs. time) was significantly slowed by the toxic medium. (Reproduced from Bragg, et al., 2002c, with permission).

to the chemokine receptor CXCR3. This interaction is toxic to neurons (Vergote et al., 2006). The toxicity may be due, in part, to the suppression of LC3 expression and associated neuronal autophagy (Zhu et al., 2009). Indeed, the improved neural function in response to antiretroviral therapy correlates with the restoration of these signaling pathways.

CALCIUM DYSREGULATION, NEUROPATHOGENESIS, AND THE DEVELOPMENT OF NEW THERAPEUTICS

Increases in intracellular calcium presumably give rise to changes that impair the function of neurons, but the

mechanisms responsible for neurological impairment are not known. Several potential pathological effects of excess calcium are illustrated in Figure 5.2.8. Calcium entering through NMDA receptors in the absence of adequate export may result in the activation of enzymes such as calpain, calcineurin, and glycogen synthase kinase-3β (GSK-3β). Overactivation of each of these enzymes may trigger a cascade leading to deleterious events such as damage to the sodium-calcium exchanger, uncoupling of Akt (protein kinase B) activity, depolymerization of actin, dephosphorylation of cyclic AMP response element binding protein (CREB), or hyper-phosphorylation of the microtubule binding protein, Tau. While we can only speculate on the possible pathways

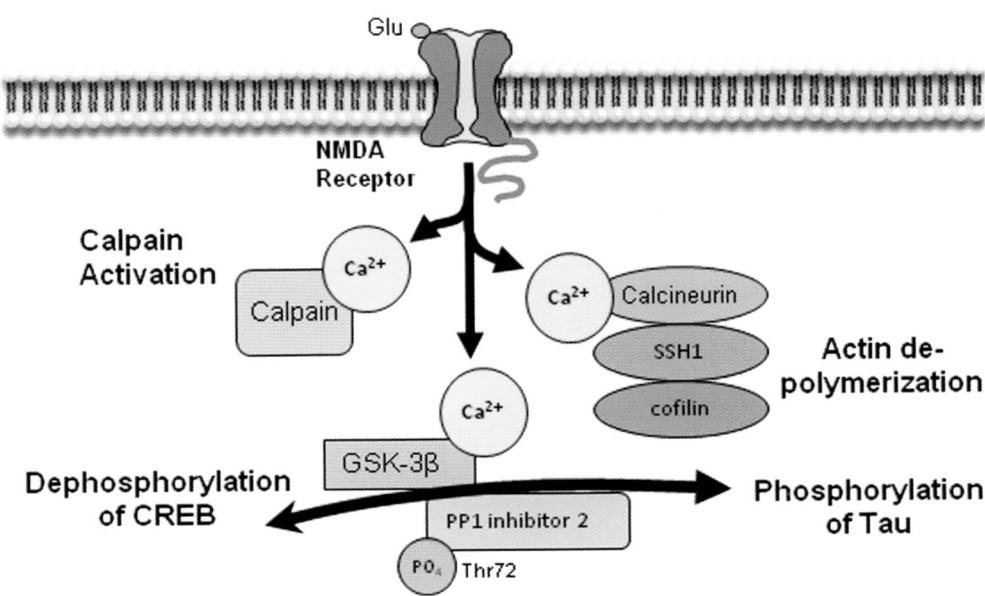

Figure 5.2.8 Calcium and neural dysfunction. Hypothetical pathogenic pathways activated by the accumulation of excess intracellular calcium. Overactivation of calpain may lead to GSK-3β activation, cleavage of the sodium-calcium exchanger, metabotropic glutamate receptor 1 truncation, or uncoupling of the neuroprotective, pro-survival signaling of Akt1/protein kinase B. Activation of calcium-calcineurin may activate the phosphatase, slingshot-1 (SSH1) which then activates cofilin by de-phosphorylation resulting in local actin breakdown. This may then lead to a loss of important scaffold domains. Indirect activation of GSK-3β phosphorylates and releases protein phosphatase-1 (PP1) inhibitor from PP1 thereby increasing PP1-mediated CREB dephosphorylation. The loss of phospho-CREB decreases many pro-survival functions of CREB. GSK-3β may also promote the hyperphosphorylation of the microtubule binding protein Tau leading to a destabilization of transport processes.

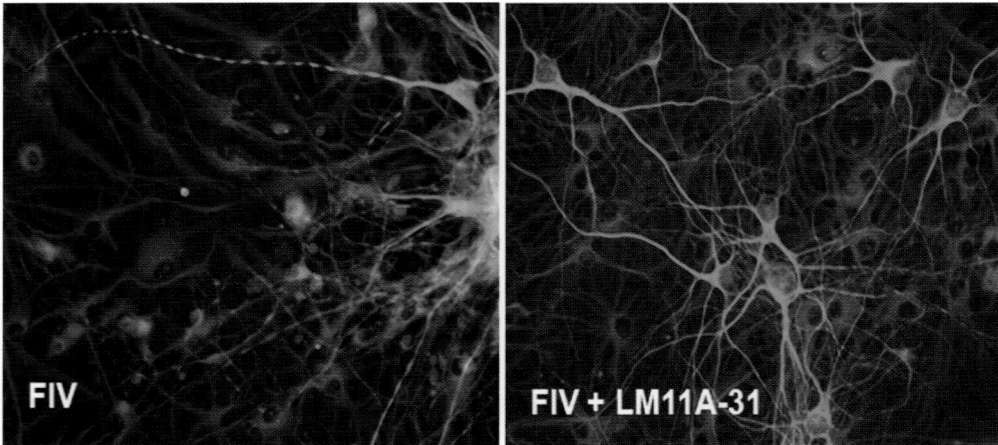

Figure 5.2.9 Neuroprotective efficacy of novel neurotrophin mimetics. Incubation of primary cortical feline neurons with FIV for 7 days resulted in areas of dendritic beading and a simplification of the network of neuronal processes, revealed by staining for MAP-2 (green). Many neurons also appear shrunken and have weak MAP-2 immunoreactivity. Co-incubation of cells with FIV plus 10 nM of the neurotrophin ligand, LM11A-31, almost completely reverses all signs of pathology in these cultures suggesting that this compound may be a potent new therapeutic option for the protection of neurons from damage caused by FIV or HIV. Astrocytes in the background are stained for GFAP (red) and nuclei are counterstained with bisbenzimide (blue).

leading to neural damage, the nature of the damage is well documented. The delayed destabilization of calcium in neurons in the above experiments correlates with the appearance of dendritic beading, neuronal swelling, and retraction of processes. In spite of often dramatic increases in calcium, dendritic beading, and neuronal swelling, very few neurons die, indicating that most of these early pathological changes are potentially reversible. Many of the deleterious effects of excess calcium noted above are offset by activity of Akt which acts to keep many of these pathways in check and promote pro-survival signaling. Recent work with cultured feline neurons has shown that non-peptide neurotrophin ligands that act through the p75 neurotrophin receptor to stimulate Akt are capable of reversing the damage seen in cultures infected with FIV. Figure 5.2.9 illustrates the reversal of dendritic beading and neuritic pruning seen seven days after inoculation of cultures with FIV. Cultures treated with 10 nM of the prototype neurotrophin mimetic, LM11A-31, with the FIV showed an almost normal morphology based on MAP-2 staining. Parallel studies showed a complete reversal of neuron death in these cultures. The feline model will serve as an excellent system for the future development of these and other therapeutic compounds.

SUMMARY

The FIV model has provided a comprehensive system for the analysis of both systemic and central nervous system pathologies. Although there are clear differences between the viral genome structures and cellular tropisms of FIV and HIV-1, the systemic and CNS diseases produced in their respective hosts are remarkably similar. Both viruses display a highly conserved tropism for the chemokine receptor, CXCR4, and rapidly penetrate the CNS with preferential infection of microglia and macrophages. As with HIV-1, neuroinvasion by FIV produces a moderate widespread inflammatory response that

includes a small but progressive loss of neurons beginning in the asymptomatic stage of disease. Once in the CNS, FIV envelope evolves rapidly although the link between specific envelope variants and CNS disease remains elusive. Studies using primary cell cultures from feline CNS have demonstrated that FIV, like HIV-1, is toxic to neural cells. These investigations have demonstrated 1) functional deficits in neurons and astrocytes that may promote neural dysfunction; 2) potential T-cell-astrocyte interactions that might support the emergence of astrocyte-tropic virus; 3) identification of the potential impact of choroid plexus-CSF virus trafficking; 4) the importance of virus interactions with CNS cells in the control of immune cell trafficking across the blood-brain barrier; 5) the identification of a novel mechanisms by which macrophage-derived toxins disrupt calcium homeostasis and by which MMP-2 generates toxic cleavage fragments of SDF-1; 6) development of behavioral paradigms that offer more sensitive tests of neural function; and 7) the identification of therapeutics that have the potential to reverse much of the damage induced by FIV.

These accomplishments demonstrate the important advantages this model offers for future investigations. Studies can be conducted at all stages of disease and can be complemented with parallel analyses of feline cell culture systems allowing a full range of translational studies. The FIV model should continue to be a valuable tool in the ongoing efforts to identify the mechanisms of HAND as well as for the design and evaluation of effective therapeutic strategies.

REFERENCES

Abramo, F., Bo, S., Canese, M. G., & Poli, A. (1995). Regional distribution of lesions in the central nervous system of cats infected with feline immunodeficiency virus. *AIDS Research & Human Retroviruses*, 11, 1247–1253.

Ackley, C. D., Yamamoto, J. K., Levy, N., Pedersen, N. C., & Cooper, M. D. (1990). Immunologic abnormalities in pathogen-free cats experimentally infected with feline immunodeficiency virus. *J Virol*, 64, 5652–5655.

Albright, A. V., Shieh, J. T., Itoh, T., Lee, B., Pleasure, D., O'Connor, M. J., et al. (1999). Microglia express CCR5, CXCR4, and CCR3, but of these, CCR5 is the principal coreceptor for human immunodeficiency virus type 1 dementia isolates. *J Virol*, 73, 205–213.

Albright, A. V., Shieh, J. T., O'Connor, M. J., & Gonzalez-Scarano, F. (2000). Characterization of cultured microglia that can be infected by HIV-1. *J Neurovirol*, 6 Suppl 1, S53–S60.

Alkhatib, G., Broder, C. C., & Berger, E. A. (1996). Cell type-specific fusion cofactors determine human immunodeficiency virus type 1 tropism for T-cell lines versus primary macrophages. *J Virol*, 70, 5487–5494.

Assogba, B. D., Leavell, S., Porter, K., & Burkhard, M. J. (2007). Mucosal administration of low-dose cell-associated feline immunodeficiency virus promotes viral latency. *J Infect Dis*, 195, 1184–1188.

Bachmann, M. H., Mathiason-Dubard, C., Learn, G. H., Rodrigo, A. G., Sodora, D. L., Mazzetti, P., et al. (1997). Genetic diversity of feline immunodeficiency virus: Dual infection, recombination, and distinct evolutionary rates among envelope sequence clades. *J Virol*, 71, 4241–4253.

Beebe, A. M., Dua, N., Faith, T. G., Moore, P. F., Pedersen, N. C., & Dandekar, S. (1994). Primary stage of feline immunodeficiency virus infection: Viral dissemination and cellular targets. *J Virol*, 68, 3080–3091.

Billaud, J. N., Selway, D., Yu, N., & Phillips, T. R. (2000). Replication rate of feline immunodeficiency virus in astrocytes is envelope dependent: Implications for glutamate uptake. *Virology*, 266, 180–188.

Boche, D., Hurtrel, M., Gray, F., Claessens-Maire, M. A., Ganiere, J. P., Montagnier, et al. (1996). Virus load and neuropathology in the FIV model. *Journal of Neurovirology* 2:377–387.

Bragg, D., Childers, T., Tompkins, M., Tompkins, W., & Meeker, R. (2002a). Infection of the choroid plexus by feline immunodeficiency virus. *J.Neurovirol*, 8, 211–224.

Bragg, D., Hudson, L., Liang, Y., Tompkins, M., Fernandes, A., & Meeker, R. (2002b). Choroid plexus macrophages proliferate and release toxic factors in response to feline immunodeficiency virus. *J Neurovirol*, 8, 225–239.

Bragg, D. C., Boles, J. C., & Meeker, R. B. (2002c). Destabilization of neuronal calcium homeostasis by factors secreted from choroid plexus macrophage cultures in response to feline immunodeficiency virus. *Neurobiol Dis*, 9, 173–186.

Bragg, D. C., Meeker R. B., Duff, B., English, R. V., & Tompkins, M. B. (1999). Neurotoxicity of FIV and FIV envelope protein in feline cortical cultures. *Brain Res*, 816, 431–437.

Brown, W. C., Bissey, L., Logan, K. S., Pedersen, N. C., Elder, J. H., & Collisson, E. W. (1991). Feline immunodeficiency virus infects both CD4+ and CD8+ T lymphocytes. *J Virol*, 65, 3359–3364.

Brunner, D. & Pedersen, N. C. (1989). Infection of peritoneal macrophages in vitro and in vivo with feline immunodeficiency virus. *J Virol*, 63, 5483–5488.

Bucci, J. G., English, R. V., Jordan, H. L., Childers, T. A., Tompkins, M. B., & Tompkins, W. A. (1998). Mucosally transmitted feline immunodeficiency virus induces a CD8+ antiviral response that correlates with reduction of cell-associated virus. *J Infect Dis*, 177, 18–25.

Carpenter, M. A., Brown, E. W., MacDonald, D. W., & O'Brien, S. J. (1998). Phylogeographic patterns of feline immunodeficiency virus genetic diversity in the domestic cat. *Virology*, 251, 234–243.

Chen, H., Wood, C., & Petito, C. K. (2000). Comparisons of HIV-1 viral sequences in brain, choroid plexus and spleen: Potential role of choroid plexus in the pathogenesis of HIV encephalitis. *J Neurovirol*, 6, 498–506.

Danave, I. R., Tiffany Castiglioni, E., Zenger, E., Barhoumi, R., Burghardt, R. C., & Collisson, E. W. (1994). Feline immunodeficiency virus decreases cell-cell communication and mitochondrial membrane potential. *J Virol*, 68, 6745–6750.

Darko, D. F., Mitler, M. M., & Henriksen, S. J. (1995). Lentiviral infection, immune response peptides, and sleep. *Adv Neuroimmunol*, 5, 57–77.

de Parseval, A. & Elder, J. H. (1999). Demonstration that orf2 encodes the feline immunodeficiency virus transactivating (tat) protein and characterization of a unique gene product with partial rev activity. *J Virol*, 73(1), 608–617.

de Parseval, A. & Elder, J. H. (2001). Binding of recombinant feline immunodeficiency virus surface glycoprotein to feline cells: Role of CXCR4, cell-surface heparans, and an unidentified non-CXCR4 receptor. *J Virol*, 75, 4528–4539.

Dean, G. A., LaVoy, A., Yearley, J., & Stanton, C. (2006). Cytokine modulation of the innate immune response in feline immunodeficiency virus-infected cats. *J Infect Dis*, 193, 1520–1527.

Dow, S., Poss, M., & Hoover, E. (1990). Feline immunodeficiency virus: A neurotropic lentivirus. *JAIDS*, 3, 658–668.

Dow, S. W., Dreitz, M. J., & Hoover, E. A. (1992). Feline immunodeficiency virus neurotropism: Evidence that astrocytes and microglia are the primary target cells. *Veterinary Immunology & Immunopathology*, 35, 23–35.

Dow, S. W., Mathiason, C. K., & Hoover, E. A. (1999). In vivo monocyte tropism of pathogenic feline immunodeficiency viruses. *J Virol*, 73, 6852–6861.

Dunham, S. P. (2006). Lessons from the cat: Development of vaccines against lentiviruses. *Vet Immunol Immunopathol*, 112, 67–77.

Egberink, H. F., De Clercq, E., van Vliet, A. L., Balzarini, J., Bridger, G. J., Henson, G., et al. (1999). Bicyclams, selective antagonists of the human chemokine receptor CXCR4, potently inhibit feline immunodeficiency virus replication. *J Virol*, 73, 6346–6352.

Elder, J. H., Lerner, D. L., Hasselkus-Light, C. S., Fontenot, D. J., Hunter, E., et al. (1992). Distinct subsets of retroviruses encode dUTPase. *J Virol*, 66, 1791–1794.

Elder, J. H. & Phillips, T. R. (1993). Molecular properties of feline immunodeficiency virus (FIV). *Infect Agents Dis*, 2, 361–374.

English, R., Johnson, C., Gebhard, D. H., & Tompkins, M. B. (1993). In vivo lymphocyte tropism of feline immunodeficiency virus. *J Virol*, 67, 5175–5186.

English, R. V., Nelson, P., Johnson, C. M., Nasisse, M., Tompkins, W. A., & Tompkins, M. B. (1994). Development of clinical disease in cats experimentally infected with feline immunodeficiency virus. *J Infect Dis*, 170, 543–552.

Falangola, M. F., Hanly, A., Galvao-Castro, B., & Petito, C. K. (1995). HIV infection of human choroid plexus: A possible mechanism of viral entry into the CNS. *J of Neuropathology and Experimental Science*, 54, 497–503.

Fletcher, N. F., Bexiga, M. G., Brayden, D. J., Brankin, B., Willett, B. J., Hosie, M. J., et al. (2009). Lymphocyte migration through the blood-brain barrier (BBB) in feline immunodeficiency virus infection is significantly influenced by the pre-existence of virus and tumour necrosis factor (TNF)-alpha within the central nervous system (CNS): Studies using an in vitro feline BBB model. *Neuropathol Appl Neurobiol*, 35, 592–602.

Fletcher, N. F., Brayden, D. J., Brankin, B., Worrall, S., & Callanan, J. J. (2006). Growth and characterisation of a cell culture model of the feline blood-brain barrier. *Veterinary Immunology and Immunopathology*, 109, 233–244.

Gavrilin, M. A., Mathes, L. E., & Podell, M. (2002). Methamphetamine enhances cell-associated feline immunodeficiency virus replication in astrocytes. *J Neurovirol*, 8, 240–249.

Gebhard, D. H., Dow, J. L., Childers, T. A., Alvelo, J. I., Tompkins, M. B., & Tompkins, W. A. (1999). Progressive expansion of an L-selectin-negative CD8 cell with anti-feline immunodeficiency virus (FIV) suppressor function in the circulation of FIV-infected cats. *J Infect Dis*, 180, 1503–1513.

Giulian, D., Vaca, K., & Noonan, C. A. (1990). Secretion of neurotoxins by mononuclear phagocytes infected with HIV-1. *Science*, 250, 1593–1596.

Gorry, P. R., Bristol, G., Zack, J. A., Ritola, K., Swanstrom, R., Birch, C. J., et al. (2001). Macrophage tropism of human immunodeficiency virus type 1 isolates from brain and lymphoid tissues predicts neurotropism independent of coreceptor specificity. *J Virol*, 75, 10073–10089.

Gruol, D. L., Yu, N., Parsons, K. L., Billaud, J. N., Elder, J. H., & Phillips, T. R. (1998). Neurotoxic effects of feline immunodeficiency virus, FIV-PPR. *J Neurovirol*, 4, 415–425.

Gunn-Moore, D. A., Pearson, G. R., Harbour, D. A., & Whiting, C. V. (1996). Encephalitis associated with giant cells in a cat with naturally occurring feline immunodeficiency virus infection demonstrated by in situ hybridization. *Vet Pathol*, 33, 699–703.

Haughey, N. J., Holden, C. P., Nath, A., & Geiger, J. D. (1999). Involvement of inositol 1,4,5-trisphosphate-regulated stores of intracellular calcium in calcium dysregulation and neuron cell death caused by HIV-1 protein tat. *J Neurochem*, 73, 1363–1374.

He, J., Chen, Y., Farzan, M., Choe, H., Ohagen, A., Gartner, S., et al. (1997). CCR3 and CCR5 are co-receptors for HIV-1 infection of microglia. *Nature*, 385, 645–649.

Hein, A., Martin, J. P., & Dorries, R. (2001). In vitro activation of feline immunodeficiency virus in ramified microglial cells from asymptomatically infected cats. *J Virol*, 75, 8090–8095.

Hein, A., Martin, J. P., Koehren, F., Bingen, A., & Dorries, R. (2000). In vivo infection of ramified microglia from adult cat central nervous system by feline immunodeficiency virus. *Virology*, 268, 420–429.

Heit, B., Jones, G., Knight, D., Antony, J. M., Gill, M. J., Brown, C., et al. (2006). HIV and other lentiviral infections cause defects in neutrophil chemotaxis, recruitment, and cell structure: Immunorestorative effects of granulocyte-macrophage colony-stimulating factor. *J Immunol*, 177, 6405–6414.

Holden, C. P., Haughey, N. J., Nath, A., & Geiger, J. D. (1999). Role of Na+/H+ exchangers, excitatory amino acid receptors and voltage-operated Ca2+ channels in human immunodeficiency virus type 1 gp120- mediated increases in intracellular Ca2+ in human neurons and astrocytes. *Neuroscience*, 91, 1369–1378.

Hosie, M. J., Broere, N., Hesselgesser, J., Turner, J. D., Hoxie, J. A., Neil, J. C., et al. (1998). Modulation of feline immunodeficiency virus infection by stromal cell-derived factor. *J Virol*, 72, 2097–2104.

Hosie, M. J., Willett, B. J., Dunsford, T. H., Jarrett, O., & Neil, J. C. (1993). A monoclonal antibody which blocks infection with feline immunodeficiency virus identifies a possible non-CD4 receptor. *J Virol*, 67,1667–1671.

Hudson, L. C., Bragg, D. C., Tompkins, M. B., & Meeker, R. B. (2005). Astrocytes and microglia differentially regulate trafficking of lymphocyte subsets across brain endothelial cells. *Brain Res*, 1058, 148–160.

Hudson, L. C., Tompkins, M. B., & Meeker, R. B. (2008). Endothelial cell suppression of peripheral blood mononuclear cell trafficking in vitro during acute exposure to feline immunodeficiency virus. *Cell Tissue Res*, 334, 55–65.

Hurtrel, M., Ganiere, J., Guelifi, J., Chakrabarti, L., Maire, M., Gray, F., et al. (1992). Comparison of early and late feline immunodeficiency virus encephalopathies. *AIDS*, 6, 399–406.

Jacobson, S., Henricksen, S. J., Prospero-Garcia, O., Phillips, T. R., Elder, J. H., Young, W. G., et al. (1997). Cortical neuronal cytoskeletal changes associated with FIV infection. *Journal of NeuroVirology*, 3, 283–289.

Johnston, J. B. & Power, C. (2002). Feline immunodeficiency virus xeno-infection: The role of chemokine receptors and envelope diversity. *J Virol*, 76, 3626–3636.

Johnston, J. B., Silva, C., & Power, C. (2002b). Envelope gene-mediated neurovirulence in feline immunodeficiency virus infection: Induction of matrix metalloproteinases and neuronal injury. *J Virol*. 76:2622–2633.

Johnston, J. B., Silva, C., & Power, C. (2002a). Envelope gene-mediated neurovirulence in feline immunodeficiency virus infection: Induction of matrix metalloproteinases and neuronal injury. *J Virol*, 76, 2622–2633.

Kawaguchi, Y., Maeda, K., Tohya, Y., Furuya, T., Miyazawa, T., Horimoto, T., et al. (1992). Replicative difference in early-passage feline brain cells among feline immunodeficiency virus isolates. *Archives of Virology*, 125, 347–354.

Kiyomasu, T., Miyazawa, T., Furuya, T., Shibata, R., Sakai, H., Sakuragi, J., et al. (1991). Identification of feline immunodeficiency virus rev gene activity. *J Virol*, 65, 4539–4542.

Koirala, T. R., Nakagaki, K., Ishida, T., Nonaka, S., Morikawa, S., & Tabira, T. (2001). Decreased expression of MAP-2 and GAD in the brain of cats infected with feline immunodeficiency virus. *Tohoku J Exp Med*, 195, 141–151.

Kovacs, E. M., Baxter, G. D., & Robinson, W. F. (1999). Feline peripheral blood mononuclear cells express message for both CXC and CC type chemokine receptors. *Arch Virol*, 144:273–285.

Lecollinet, S. & Richardson, J. (2008), Vaccination against the feline immunodeficiency virus: The road not taken. *Comp Immunol Microbiol Infect Dis*, 31, 167–190.

Lehman, T. L., O'Halloran, K. P., Fallon, S. A., Habermann, L. M., Campbell, J. A., Nordone, S., et al. (2009). Altered bone marrow dendritic cell cytokine production to toll-like receptor and CD40 ligation during chronic feline immunodeficiency virus infection. *Immunology*, 126, 405–412.

Lerner, D. L. & Elder, J. H. (2000). Expanded host cell tropism and cytopathic properties of feline immunodeficiency virus strain PPR subsequent to passage through interleukin-2-independent T cells. *J Virol*, 74:1854–1863.

Levy, J. A. (1993). Pathogenesis of human immunodeficiency virus infection. *Microbiol Rev*, 57:183–289.

Levy, J. K., Scott, H. M., Lachtara, J. L., & Crawford, P. C. (2006). Seroprevalence of feline leukemia virus and feline immunodeficiency virus infection among cats in North America and risk factors for seropositivity. *J Am Vet Med Assoc*, 228, 371–376.

Lipton, S., Sucher, N., Kaiser, P., & Dreyer, E. (1991). Synergistic effects of HIV coat protein and NMDA receptor-mediated neurotoxicity. *Neuron*, 7:111–118.

Liu, P., Hudson, L. C., Tompkins, M. B., Vahlenkamp, T. W., Colby, B., Rundle, C., et al. (2006a). Cerebrospinal fluid is an efficient route for establishing brain infection with feline immunodeficiency virus and transfering infectious virus to the periphery. *J Neurovirol*, 12:294–306.

Liu, P., Hudson, L. C., Tompkins, M. B., Vahlenkamp, T. W., & Meeker, R. B. (2006b). Compartmentalization and evolution of feline immunodeficiency virus between the central nervous system and periphery following intracerebroventricular or systemic inoculation. *J Neurovirol*, 12:307–321.

Lo, T. K., Fallert, C. J., Piser, T. M., & Thayer, S. A. (1992). HIV-1 envelope protein evokes intracellular calcium oscillations in rat hippocampal neurons. *Brain Res*, 594:189–196.

Macchi, S., Maggi, F., Di Iorio, C., Poli, A., Bendinelli, M., & Pistello, M. (1998). Detection of feline immunodeficiency proviral sequences in lymphoid tissues and the central nervous system by in situ gene amplification. *J Virol Methods*, 73, 109–119.

Maingat, F., Vivithanaporn, P., Zhu, Y., Taylor, A., Baker, G., Pearson, K., et al. (2009). Neurobehavioral performance in feline immunodeficiency virus infection: Integrated analysis of viral burden, neuroinflammation, and neuronal injury in cortex. *J Neurosci*, 29:8429–8437.

Maksaereekul, S., Dubie, R. A., Shen, X., Kieu, H., Dean, G. A., & Sparger, E. E. (2009). Vaccination with vif-deleted feline immunodeficiency virus provirus, GM-CSF, and TNF-alpha plasmids preserves global CD4 T lymphocyte function after challenge with FIV. *Vaccine*, 27:3754–3765.

Meeker, R., English, R., & Tompkins, M. (1996). Enhanced excitotoxicity in primary feline neural cultures exposed to feline immunodeficiency virus (FIV). *Journal of NeuroAIDS*, 1:1–27.

Meeker, R. B., Boles, J. C., Robertson, K. R., & Hall, C. D. (2005). Cerebrospinal fluid from human immunodeficiency virus—infected individuals facilitates neurotoxicity by suppressing intracellular calcium recovery. *J Neurovirol*, 11:144–156.

Meeker, R. B., Thiede, B. A., Hall, C., English, R., & Tompkins, M. (1997). Cortical cell loss in asymptomatic cats experimentally infected with feline immunodeficiency virus. *AIDS Res Hum Retroviruses*, 13, 1131–1140.

Mexas, A. M., Fogle, J. E., Tompkins, W. A., & Tompkins, M. B. (2008). CD4+CD25+ regulatory T cells are infected and activated during acute FIV infection. *Vet Immunol Immunopathol*, 126, 263–272.

Mitchell, T. W., Buckmaster, P. S., Hoover, E. A., Whalen, L. R., & Dudek, F. E. (1999). Neuron loss and axon reorganization in the dentate gyrus of cats infected with the feline immunodeficiency virus. *J Comp Neurol*, 411:563–577.

Mizukoshi, F., Baba, K., Goto, Y., Setoguchi, A., Fujino, Y., Ohno, K., et al. (2009). Antiviral activity of membrane fusion inhibitors that target gp40 of the feline immunodeficiency virus envelope protein. *Vet Microbiol*, 136:155–159.

Nath, A. & Geiger, J. (1998). Neurobiological aspects of human immunodeficiency virus infection: Neurotoxic mechanisms. *Prog Neurobiol*, 54:19–33.

Noorbakhsh, F., Tang, Q., Liu, S., Silva, C., van Marle, G., & Power, C. (2006). Lentivirus envelope protein exerts differential neuropathogenic effects depending on the site of expression and target cell. *Virology*, 348:260–276.

Novotney, C., English, R., Housman, J., Davidson, M., Nasisse, M., Jeng, C. R., et al. (1990). Lymphocyte population changes in cats naturally infected with feline immunodeficiency virus. *AIDS*, 4:1213–1218.

Ohagen, A., Ghosh, S. K., He, J., Huang, K., Chen, Y., Yuan, M., et al. (1999). Apoptosis induced by infection of primary brain cultures with diverse human immunodeficiency virus type 1 isolates: Evidence for a role of the envelope. *Journal of Virology*, 73, 897–906.

Olmsted, R., Hirsch, V., Purcell, R., & Johnson, P. (1989). Nucleotide sequence analysis of feline immunodeficiency virus: Genome organization and relationship to other lentiviruses. *Proc Natl Acad Sci*, 86, 8088–8092.

Olmsted, R. A., Langley, R., Roelke, M. E., Goeken, R. M., Adger-Johnson, D., Goff, J. P., et al. (1992). Worldwide prevalence of lentivirus infection in wild feline species: Epidemiologic and phylogenetic aspects. *J Virol*, 66, 6008–6018.

Pedersen, N. C., Ho, E. W., Brown, M. L., & Yamamoto J. K. (1987). Isolation of a T-lymphotropic virus from domestic cats with an immunodeficiency-like syndrome. *Science*, 235, 790–793.

Petito, C. K., Chen, H., Mastri, A. R., Torres-Munoz, J., Roberts, B., & Wood, C. (1999). HIV infection of choroid plexus in AIDS and asymptomatic HIV-infected patients suggests that the choroid plexus may be a reservoir of productive infection. *J Neurovirol*, 5, 670–677.

Phillips, T,. Prospero-Garcia, O., Puaoi, D., Lerner, D., Fox, H., Olmsted, R., et al. (1994). Neurological abnormalities associated with feline immunodeficiency virus infection. *J of General Virology*, 75, 979–987.

Phillips, T. R., Lamont, C., Konings, D. A., Shacklett, B. L., Hamson, C. A., Luciw, P. A., et al. (1992). Identification of the Rev transactivation and Rev-responsive elements of feline immunodeficiency virus. *J Virol*, 66, 5464–5471.

Phillips, T. R., Prospero-Garcia, O., Wheeler, D. W., Wagaman, P., Lerner, D. L., Fox, H. S., et al. (1996). Neurologic dysfunctions caused by a molecular clone of feline immunodeficiency virus, FIV-PPR. *J of Neurovirology*, 2, 388–396.

Phipps, A. J., Hayes, K. A., Buck, W. R., Podell, M., & Mathes, L. E. (2000). Neurophysiologic and immunologic abnormalities associated with feline immunodeficiency virus molecular clone FIV-PPR DNA inoculation. *J Acquir Immune Defic Syndr*, 23, 8–16.

Podell, M., Hayes, K., Oglesbee, M., & Mathes, L. (1997). Progressive encephalopathy associated with CD4/CD8 inversion in adult FIV-infected cats. *J Acquir Immune Defic Syndr Hum Retrovirol*, 15, 332–340.

Podell, M., Maruyama, K., Smith, M., Hayes, K. A., Buck, W. R., Ruehlmann, D. S., et al. (1999). Frontal lobe neuronal injury correlates to altered function in FIV-infected cats. *J Acquir Immune Defic Syndr*, 22, 10–18.

Podell, M., Oglesbee, M., Mathes, L., Krakowka, S., Olmstead, R., & Lafrado, L. (1993). AIDS-associated encephalopathy with experimental feline immunodeficiency virus infection. *Journal of AIDS*, 6, 758–771.

Poli, A., Abramo, F., Di Iorio, C., Cantile, C., Carli, M. A., Pollera, C., et al. (1997). Neuropathology in cats experimentally infected with feline immunodeficiency virus: A morphological, immunocytochemical, and morphometric study. *J Neurovirol*, 3, 361–368.

Poli, A., Pistello, M., Carli, M. A., Abramo, F., Mancuso, G., Nicoletti, E., et al. (1999). Tumor necrosis factor-alpha and virus expression in the central nervous system of cats infected with feline immunodeficiency virus. *J Neurovirol*, 5, 465–473.

Power, C., Buist, R., Johnston, J. B., Del Bigio, M. R., Ni, W., Dawood, M. R., et al. (1998). Neurovirulence in feline immunodeficiency virus-infected neonatal cats is viral strain specific and dependent on systemic immune suppression. *J Virol*, 72, 9109–9115.

Power, C., Moench, T., Peeling, J., Kong, P. A., & Langelier, T. (1997). Feline immunodeficiency virus causes increased glutamate levels and neuronal loss in brain. *Neuroscience*, 77, 1175–1185.

Prospero-Garcia, O., Herold, N., Phillips, T., Elder, J., Bloom, F., & Henriksen, S. (1994a). Sleep patterns are disturbed in cats infected with feline immunodeficiency virus. *Proc Natl Acad Sci*, 91, 12947–12951.

Prospero-Garcia, O., Herold, N., Phillips, T. R., Elder, J. H., Bloom, F. E., & Henriksen, S. J. (1994b). Sleep patterns are disturbed in cats infected with feline immunodeficiency virus. *Proc Natl Acad Sci USA*, 91, 12947–12951.

Prospero-Garcia, O., Herold, N., Waters, A., Phillips, T., Elder, J., & Henriksen, S. (1994c). Intraventricular administration of a FIV-envelope protein induces sleep architecture changes in rats. *Brain Research*, 659, 254–258.

Prospero-Garcia, O., Huitron-Resendiz, S., Casalman, S. C., Sanchez-Alavez, M., Diaz-Ruiz, O., Navarro, L., et al. (1999). Feline immunodeficiency virus envelope protein (FIVgp120) causes electrophysiological alterations in rats. *Brain Res*, 836, 203–209.

Pulliam, L., Herndier, B. G., Tang, N. M., & McGrath, M. S. (1991). Human immunodeficiency virus-infected macrophages produce soluble factors that cause histological and neurochemical alterations in cultured human brains. *J Clin Invest*, 87, 503–512.

Reggeti, F., Ackerley, C., & Bienzle, D. (2008). CD134 and CXCR4 expression corresponds to feline immunodeficiency virus infection of lymphocytes, macrophages and dendritic cells. *J Gen Virol*, 89:, 277–287.

Richardson, J., Pancino, G., Merat, R., Leste-Lasserre, T., Moraillon, A., Schneider-Mergener, J., et al. (1999). Shared usage of the chemokine receptor CXCR4 by primary and laboratory-adapted strains of feline immunodeficiency virus. *J Virol*, 73, 3661–3671.

Roelke, M. E., Brown, M. A., Troyer, J. L., Winterbach, H., Winterbach, C., Hemson, G., et al. (2009). Pathological manifestations of feline immunodeficiency virus (FIV) infection in wild African lions. *Virology*, 390, 1–12.

Ryan, G., Grimes, T., Brankin, B., Mabruk, M. J., Hosie, M. J., Jarrett, O., et al. (2005). Neuropathology associated with feline immunodeficiency virus infection highlights prominent lymphocyte trafficking through both the blood-brain and blood-choroid plexus barriers. *J Neurovirol*, 11, 337–345.

Ryan, G., Klein, D., Knapp, E., Hosie, M. J., Grimes, T., Mabruk, M. J., et al. (2003). Dynamics of viral and proviral loads of feline immunodeficiency virus within the feline central nervous system during the acute phase following intravenous infection. *J Virol*, 77, 7477–7485.

Shacklett, B. L. & Luciw, P. A. (1994). Analysis of the vif gene of feline immunodeficiency virus. *Virology*, 204, 860–867.

Shimojima, M., Miyazawa, T., Ikeda, Y., McMonagle, E. L., Haining, H., Akashi, H., et al. (2004). Use of CD134 as a primary receptor by the feline immunodeficiency virus. *Science*, 303, 1192–1195.

Silvotti, L., Corradi, A., Brandi, G., Cabassi, A., Bendinelli, M., Magnan, M., et al. (1997) FIV induced encephalopathy: Early brain lesions in the absence of viral replication in monocyte/macrophages. A pathogenetic model. *Vet Immunol Immunopathol*, 55, 263–271.

Steigerwald, E. S., Sarter, M., March, P., & Podell, M. (1999). Effects of feline immunodeficiency virus on cognition and behavioral function in cats. *J Acquir Immune Defic Syndr Hum Retrovirol*, 20, 411–419.

Talbott, R. L., Sparger, E. E., Lovelace, K. M., Fitch, W. M., Pedersen, N. C., Luciw, P. A., et al. (1989). Nucleotide sequence and genomic organization of feline immunodeficiency virus. *Proc Natl Acad Sci USA*, 86, 5743–5747.

Tomonaga, K., Norimine, J., Shin, Y. S., Fukasawa, M., Miyazawa, T., Adachi, A., et al. (1992). Identification of a feline immunodeficiency virus gene which is essential for cell-free virus infectivity. *J Virol*, 66, 6181–6185.

Tompkins, M. B., Nelson, P. D., English, R. V., & Novotney, C. (1991). Early events in the immunopathogenesis of feline retrovirus infections. *JAVMA*, 199, 1311–1315.

Tompkins, M. B. & Tompkins, W. A. (2008). Lentivirus-induced immune dysregulation. *Vet Immunol Immunopathol*, 123, 45–55.

Torten, M., Franchini, M., Barlough, J. E., George, J. W., Mozes, E., Lutz, H., et al. (1991). Progressive immune dysfunction in cats experimentally infected with feline immunodeficiency virus. *J Virol*, 65, 2225–2230.

Troth, S. P., Dean, A. D., & Hoover, E. A. (2008). In vivo CXCR4 expression, lymphoid cell phenotype, and feline immunodeficiency virus infection. *Vet Immunol Immunopathol*, 123, 97–105.

Uhl, E. W., Martin, M., Coleman, J. K., & Yamamoto, J. K. (2008). Advances in FIV vaccine technology. *Vet Immunol Immunopathol*, 123, 65–80.

Vergote, D., Butler, G. S., Ooms, M., Cox, J. H., Silva, C., Hollenberg, M. D., et al. (2006). Proteolytic processing of SDF-1alpha reveals a change in receptor specificity mediating HIV-associated neurodegeneration. *Proc Natl Acad Sci USA*, 103, 19182–19187.

Willett, B. J., Cannon, C. A., & Hosie, M. J. (2002). Upregulation of surface feline CXCR4 expression following ectopic expression of CCR5: Implications for studies of the cell tropism of feline immunodeficiency virus. *J Virol*, 76, 9242–9252.

Willett, B. J. & Hosie, M. J. (2008). Chemokine receptors and co-stimulatory molecules: Unravelling feline immunodeficiency virus infection. *Vet Immunol Immunopathol*, 123, 56–64.

Willett, B. J., Hosie, M. J., Callanan, J. J., Neil, J. C., & Jarrett, O. (1993). Infection with feline immunodeficiency virus is followed by the rapid expansion of a cd8+ lymphocyte subset. *Immunology*, 78, 1–6.

Willett, B. J., McMonagle, E. L., Logan, N., Samman, A., & Hosie, M. J. (2008). A single site for N-linked glycosylation in the envelope glycoprotein of feline immunodeficiency virus modulates the virus-receptor interaction. *Retrovirology*, 5, 77.

Willett, B. J., McMonagle, E. L., Logan, N., Schneider, P., & Hosie, M. J. (2009). Enforced covalent trimerisation of soluble feline CD134 (OX40)-ligand generates a functional antagonist of feline immunodeficiency virus. *Mol Immunol*, 46, 1020–1030.

Willett, B. J., McMonagle, E. L., Logan, N., Spiller, O. B., Schneider, P., & Hosie, M. J. (2007). Probing the interaction between feline immunodeficiency virus and CD134 by using the novel monoclonal antibody 7D6 and the CD134 (Ox40) ligand. *J Virol*, 81, 9665–9679.

Willett, B. J., Picard, L., Hosie, M. J., Turner, J. D., Adema, K., & Clapham, P. R. (1997). Shared usage of the chemokine receptor CXCR4 by the feline and human immunodeficiency viruses. *Journal of Virology*, 71, 6407–6415.

Yu, N., Billaud, J. N., & Phillips, T. R. (1998). Effects of feline immunodeficiency virus on astrocyte glutamate uptake: Implications for lentivirus-induced central nervous system diseases. *Proc Natl Acad Sci U S A*, 95, 2624–2629.

Zenger, E., Collisson, E. W., Barhoumi, R., Burghardt, R. C., Danave, I. R., & Tiffany-Castiglioni, E. (1995). Laser cytometric analysis of FIV-induced injury in astroglia. *Glia*, 13, 92–100.

Zhang, K., McQuibban, G. A., Silva, C., Butler, G. S., Johnston, J. B., Holden, J., et al. (2003). HIV-induced metalloproteinase processing of the chemokine stromal cell derived factor-1 causes neurodegeneration. *Nat Neurosci*, 6, 1064–1071.

Zheng, J., Ghorpade, A., Niemann, D., Cotter, R. L., Thylin, M. R., Epstein, L., et al. (1999a). Lymphotropic virions affect chemokine receptor-mediated neural signaling and apoptosis: Implications for human immunodeficiency virus type 1-associated dementia. *J Virol*, 73, 8256–8267.

Zheng, J., Thylin, M. R., Ghorpade, A., Xiong, H., Persidsky, Y., Cotter, R., et al. (1999b). Intracellular CXCR4 signaling, neuronal apoptosis and neuropathogenic mechanisms of HIV-1-associated dementia. *J Neuroimmunol*, 98, 185–200.

Zhu, Y., Antony, J. M., Martinez, J. A., Glerum, D. M., Brussee, V., Hoke, A., et al. (2007). Didanosine causes sensory neuropathy in an HIV/AIDS animal model: Impaired mitochondrial and neurotrophic factor gene expression. *Brain*, 130, 2011–2023.

Zhu, Y., Vergote, D., Pardo, C., Noorbakhsh, F., McArthur, J. C., Hollenberg, M. D., et al. (2009). CXCR3 activation by lentivirus infection suppresses neuronal autophagy: Neuroprotective effects of antiretroviral therapy. *FASEB J*, 23, 2928–2941.

5.3

CAPRINE ARTHRITIS ENCEPHALITIS VIRUS AND VISNA

Valgerdur Andrésdóttir, Sigurbjörg Torsteinsdóttir, and Gudmundur Georgsson[†]

Maedi-visna virus and caprine arthritis-encephalitis virus are lentiviruses that cause epizootics in, respectively, sheep and goats. These viruses do not cause overt immunosuppression, but the immune responses they engender are ineffective at eradicating the infections. Both viruses can cause encephalitis and both share important features with SIV and HIV infections, especially pertaining to the initial steps in the development of central nervous system (CNS) lesions. The main target cells for productive infection in the brain are cells of the monocyte/ macrophage lineage; and the mechanisms for virus entry into the CNS may be similar for all the lentiviruses. These viruses and their animal hosts are valuable models for aspects of HIV infection in humans, and are especially well suited for the study of AIDS neurology. This chapter describes these viruses and the pathogenic features they possess that are relevant to the modeling of human HIV infection.

INTRODUCTION

Maedi and visna are diseases that were brought to Iceland with the importation of apparently healthy sheep of the Karakul breed in 1933. Maedi (an Icelandic word for dyspnea) is an interstitial pneumonia, and visna (meaning wasting) is an encephalomyelitis. Epidemiological studies suggest that of the 20 sheep that were imported, two were healthy carriers, one giving rise to an epizootic of maedi in the northern part of the country, the other causing an epizootic of both maedi and visna in the southwest part of the country. Due to the long preclinical period and the insidious onset of maedi and visna, the diseases had spread unnoticed to many flocks when first recognized 6–7 years after the importation (Palsson, 1976). The diseases were described by Sigurdsson and coworkers (Sigurdsson, Grimsson, & Palsson, 1952; Sigurdsson & Palsson, 1958; Sigurdsson, Palsson, & Grimsson, 1957; Sigurdsson, Palsson, & Tryggvadottir, 1953). Virus was isolated from visna brains and maedi lungs (Sigurdardottir & Thormar, 1964; Sigurdsson, Thormar, & Palsson, 1960) and these were shown to be serologically related (Thormar & Helgadóttir, 1965). Transmission experiments indicated that visna and maedi were different organ manifestations of infection with the same virus, thus giving rise to the present name, maedi-visna virus (MVV) (Gudnadottir & Palsson, 1967;

Gudnadóttir & Pálsson, 1965). On the basis of these diseases, Sigurdsson formulated the concept of slow infections as different from acute and chronic infections (Sigurdsson, 1954b). The lentiviruses derive their name from Sigurdsson´s concept of slow infections (Lin & Thormar, 1970; Sigurdsson, 1954a; Haase, 1975). Additional manifestations of an MVV infection are mastitis (De Boer, Terpstra, Houwers, & Hendriks, 1979) and arthritis (Oliver et al., 1981). Lentiviruses of sheep have now been recognized worldwide and are variously called maedi-visna virus (MVV), ovine progressive pneumonia virus (OPPV), and ovine lentivirus (OvLV).

Caprine arthritis-encephalitis virus (CAEV) was originally isolated from an adult goat with arthritis (Crawford, Adams, Cheevers, & Cork, 1980). It was also shown to be the causative agent of a leukoencephalomyelitis of young goats that had been described by Cork and coworkers (Cork, Hadlow, Crawford, Gorham, & Piper, 1974a; Cork, Hadlow, Gorham, Piper, & Crawford, 1974b). An encephalomyelitis of goats described earlier in Germany may also have been caused by CAEV (Dahme, Stavrou, Deutschlander, Arnold, & Kaiser, 1973; Stavrou, Deutschlander, & Dahme, 1969). Further manifestations of infection of goats with CAEV are interstitial pneumonia (Cork et al., 1974a; Cork et al., 1974b) and mastitis (Kennedy-Stoskopf, Narayan, & Strandberg, 1985), that is, the target organs of CAEV are the same as of MVV.

The lentiviruses of sheep and goats do not cause immunodeficiency in the infected host. However, the virus establishes a lifelong infection, and persists and spreads in spite of an active immune response (Gudnadottir, 1974).

There is growing evidence for the occurrence of cross-species transmission of MVV and CAEV between sheep and goats. Thus, North American ovine lentiviruses have been characterized that are genetically more closely related to some CAEV strains than to MVV (Chebloune, Karr, Sheffer, Leung, & Narayan, 1996; Karr et al., 1996; Leroux, Chastang, Greenland, & Mornex, 1997; Rolland, Mooney, Valas, Perrin, & Mamoun, 2002; Valas, Benoit, Guionaud, Perrin, & Mamoun, 1997; Zanoni, 1998) and a number of studies have found evidence for natural transmission of the small ruminant lentiviruses from sheep to goats and vice versa (Gjerset, Jonassen, & Rimstad, 2007; Gjerset, Rimstad, Teige, Soetaert, & Jonassen, 2009; Shah et al., 2004). Infection of sheep by CAEV and goats by OPPV has also been shown experimentally (Banks, Adams, McGuire, & Carlson, 1983).

[†]Deceased

391

The differences in clinical and pathological manifestations may be both virus- and host- specific.

CLINICAL SIGNS AND PATHOLOGICAL LESIONS

In the majority of cases the CNS affection of MVV and CAEV infections is subclinical, although clinical visna was relatively common in some flocks during the epizootic in Iceland (Cork, 1976; Palsson, 1976; Phelps & Smith, 1993; Watt, Roy, McConnell, & King, 1990), and in recent years visna has been found in numerous sheep flocks in Spain (Benavides et al., 2006; Benavides et al., 2009).

The initial symptoms of visna often present with the sheep lagging behind when the flock is driven and the animal may fall for no evident reason. An ataxia and weakness of the hind legs may develop at an early stage, and the sheep lose weight. At this stage the sheep frequently rest on the distal ends of the metatarsals. The head is sometimes tilted to one side, and a fine trembling of the lips and facial muscles is sometimes observed as an early sign. The symptoms may progress slowly but steadily and lead to a paraplegia or total paralysis within a few months to one year. Sometimes the disease progresses in waves with short intervening remissions. There is a gradual loss of weight, but the sheep remain alert to the end and no difficulties are observed in feeding, defecation, or micturition (Palsson, 1976).

In sheep, the clinical signs are rarely observed before the age of 2 years, whereas the incubation period of the encephalitis in goats infected with CAEV can be much shorter. Thus, according to studies on goats in North America, neurological symptoms were mainly observed in 2–6 months old kids and only an occasional case was seen in adult goats (Cork, 1976; Norman & Smith, 1983). The dominant neurological signs were comparable with those observed in visna, that is, paresis and ataxia of the hindquarters, but the disease progression in goats, from initial signs to paralysis, is in general more rapid than in sheep, or as short as 2 weeks compared with several months (Cork, 1976; Norman & Smith, 1983; Palsson, 1976; Sundquist, Jonsson, Jacobsson, & Hammarberg, 1981). Other neurological signs occasionally found in goats are blindness, torticollis, nystagmus, and circling (Norman & Smith, 1983; Sundquist et al., 1981).

The localization and main features of the pathological lesions in the CNS are similar in sheep infected with MVV and goats infected with CAEV (Cork et al., 1974a; Georgsson, Nathanson, Palsson, & Petursson, 1976; Sundquist et al., 1981). A periventricular inflammation composed of mononuclear cells with preponderance of lymphocytes is conspicuous (Fig. 5.3.1). In visna it does sometimes border the entire ventricular system and may extend into the spinal cord around the central canal (Fig. 5.3.2). The inflammatory infiltrates are composed of lymphocytes and monocytes/macrophages. Immunophenotyping of the inflammatory infiltrates in visna has confirmed a preponderance of lymphocytes with a CD4/CD8 ratio of 1.3. Monocytes are approximately 10% of the inflammatory infiltrates (Torsteinsdottir et al., 1992). Glial nodules are also seen and in the most severe cases,

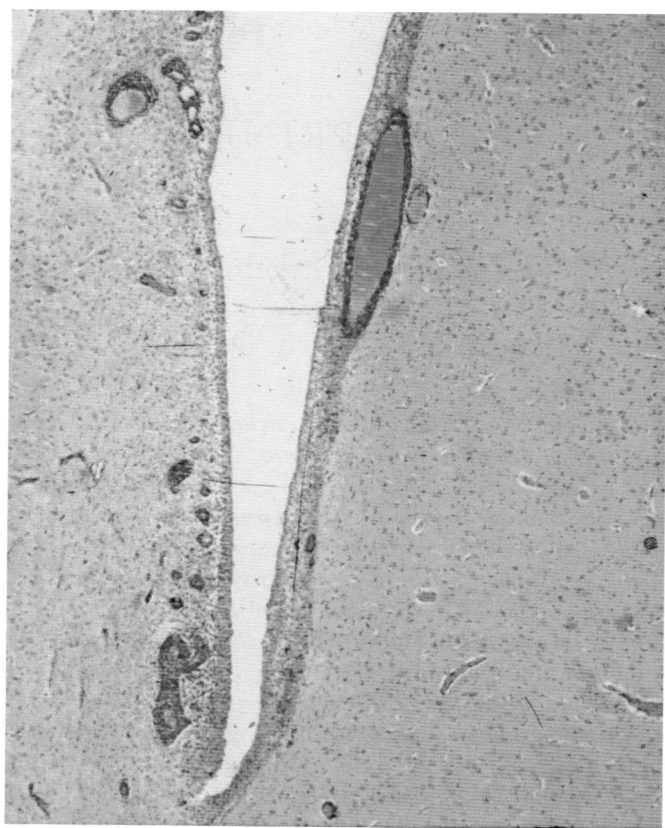

Figure 5.3.1 Visna of sheep. Lateral ventricle. Confluent periventricular inflammation. N. caudatus on the right and septum pellucidum on the left. Gallocyanin-eosin stain.

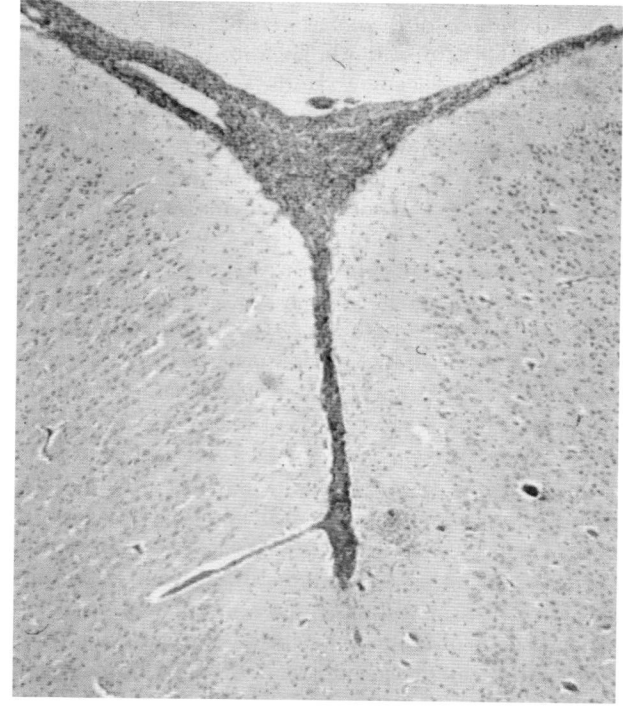

Figure 5.3.2 Visna of sheep. Spinal cord: conspicuous inflammation in commissura centralis around the central canal. Hematoxylin-eosin stain.

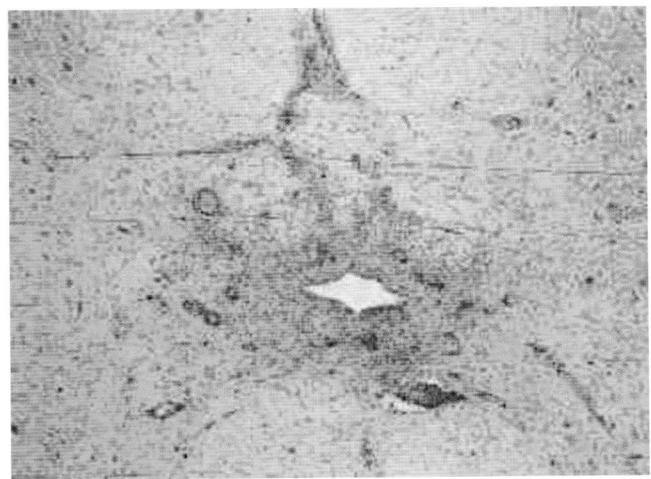

Figure 5.3.3 Visna of sheep. Intense infiltration of choroid plexus of lateral ventricle by lymphocytes forming regular lymph follicles. Hematoxylin-eosin stain.

necrotic changes. An additional early feature in both sheep and goats is meningitis (Cork et al., 1974a; Georgsson et al., 1976; Sundquist et al., 1981), usually present after 2 weeks in experimental visna (Petursson, Nathanson, Georgsson, Panitch, & Palsson, 1976). Inflammation of the choroid plexus in the lateral, third, and fourth ventricles is an early and common feature of the pathological lesions observed in visna. The inflammation varies in degree from discrete infiltration with lymphocytes, some macrophages, and plasma cells to very pronounced lymphoid proliferation with formation of lymphoid follicles with active germinal centers (Fig. 5.3.3).

The perivascular infiltrates, initially confined to the perivascular spaces, eventually invade the adjacent neuroparenchyma (Fig. 5.3.4A) and may lead to malacic foci with myelin breakdown of secondary type (Fig. 5.3.4B). In addition to foci of secondary demyelination, rather sharply demarcated foci of primary demyelination resembling chronic active or chronic silent plaques of multiple sclerosis (MS) occur in

goats (Cork & Davis, 1975) and have occasionally been observed in sheep that developed clinical signs several years after infection (Georgsson et al., 1982). The demyelinated plaques are mainly found in the spinal cord (Figs. 5.3.5; 5.3.6) and may show signs of remyelination, frequently with peripheral-type myelin.

Except for the plaques of primary demyelination, which are a late manifestation, the character of the pathological lesions does not change with time (Georgsson, 1990). Thus, the composition of the inflammatory infiltrates in sheep sacrificed 10 years after infection was similar to those observed 2 weeks after infection. The results of a long-term study indicate that lesion activity may be remitting, and inflammatory lesions that are not accompanied by breakdown of tissue may resolve and reappear later.

ROUTE OF ENTRY AND DETERMINANTS OF NEUROTROPISM

The sheep and goat lentiviruses can enter a wide variety of cell types both in vitro and in vivo. The identity of the cellular receptor(s) for these viruses has not been elucidated, but it appears that the receptor(s) is either a common molecule that is expressed on many cell types, or that the viruses have a choice of many receptors. Several lines of evidence suggest that there are strain differences in recognition of receptors. Thus, the Icelandic MVV strains K1772 and K1514 and the British strain EV1 can enter a variety of cell types from a wide range of species, while the North American MVV strains and CAEV are restricted to cells of ruminant species (Bruett & Clements, 2001; Gilden, Devlin, & Wroblewska, 1981; Hotzel & Cheevers, 2001, 2002; Jolly & Narayan, 1989; Lyall, Solanky, & Tiley, 2000; MacIntyre, Wintersgill, & Thormar, 1972; Mselli-Lakhal et al., 2000). MHC-II has been proposed as a possible receptor for visna virus (Dalziel et al., 1991). However, this can not be the only receptor since visna virus can infect a much wider range of cells than those

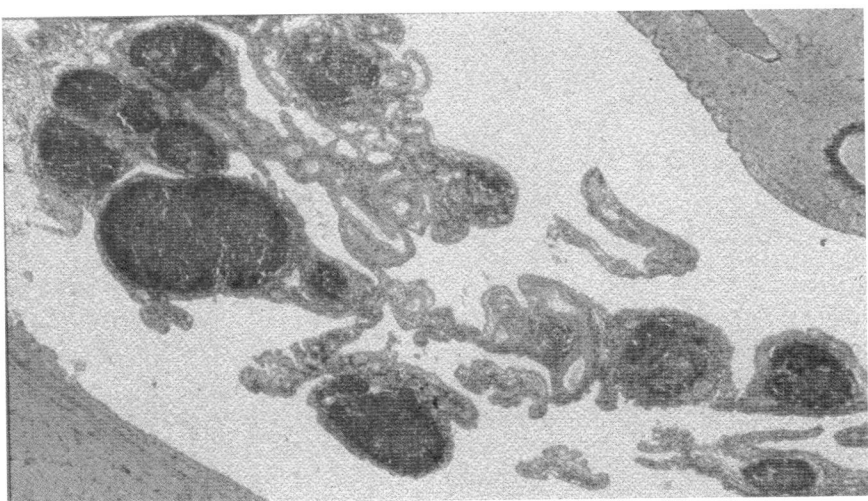

Figure 5.3.4 Visna of sheep. (a) Almost confluent inflammation of the white matter of centrum semiovale of cerebrum with some perivascular accentuation. Hematoxylin-eosin stain. (b) Same area at higher magnification shows breakdown of myelin (blue) and intense inflammation. Klüver-Barrera stain.

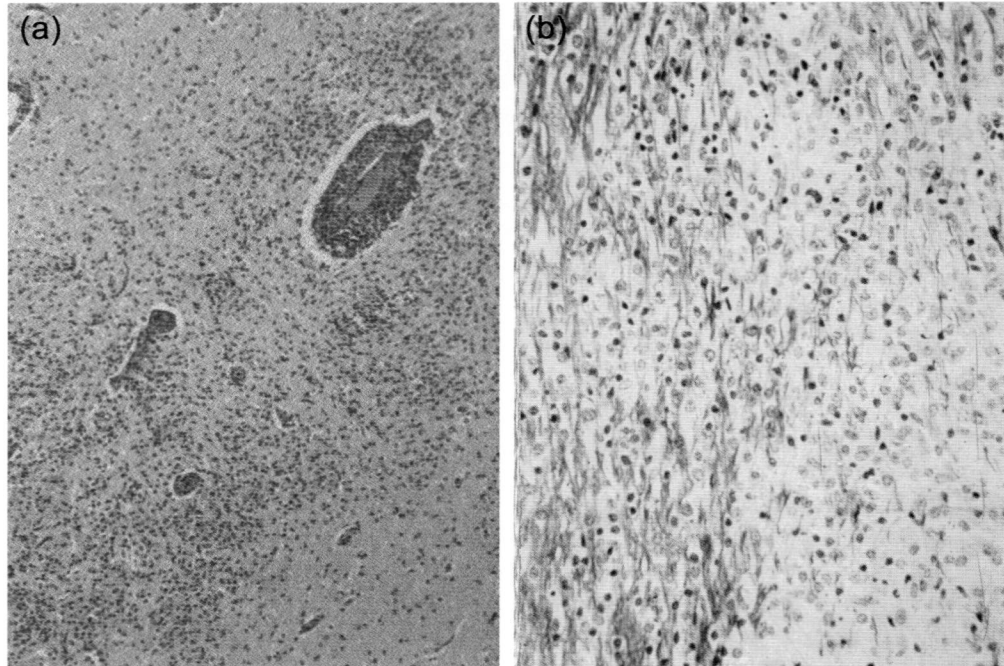

Figure 5.3.5 Leukoencephalomyelitis of goats. Spinal cord. Almost total demyelination of anterior and lateral columns on one side of the spinal cord. Weigert-Pal stain.

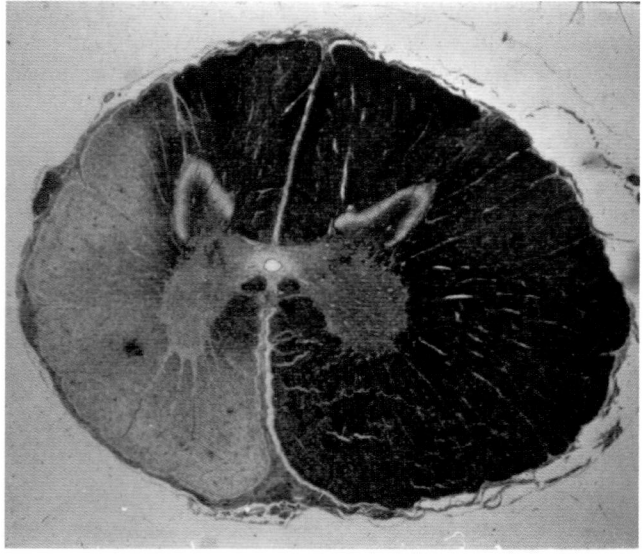

Figure 5.3.6 Visna of sheep. Spinal cord. Electron micrograph showing several demyelinated well-perserved axons. (Taken from Georgsson *et al.* (1982) with permission from Springer Verlag.)

that express class II antigen. Other candidates for the visna virus receptor are a 45 kDa protein that has serine/threonine kinase activity and a 30 kDa protein which is a chondroitin sulfate proteoglycan (Barber, Bruett, & Clements, 2000; Bruett, Barber, & Clements, 2000; Crane, Buzy, & Clements, 1991). In this connection it is interesting to note that heparan sulfate proteoglycans have been implicated as attachment receptors for HIV-1 (Mondor, Ugolini, & Sattentau, 1998;

Roderiquez et al., 1995; Saphire, Bobardt, Zhang, David, & Gallay, 2001).

Although MVV and CAEV can enter a variety of cells, the replication in vivo is highly restricted (Brahic, Stowring, Ventura, & Haase, 1981; Brodie et al., 1995; Haase, 1986; Haase, Stowring, Narayan, Griffin, & Price, 1977). Several studies have shown that the primary target cells of MVV and CAEV in vivo are cells of the monocyte lineage, and that viral replication is restricted until differentiation of the monocytes to macrophages (Adams et al., 1983; Clements et al., 1994; Gendelman et al., 1986; Gorrell, Brandon, Sheffer, Adams, & Narayan, 1992; Narayan, 1983). Replication has also been demonstrated in dendritic cells (Gorrell et al., 1992; Ryan, Tiley, McConnell, & Blacklaws, 2000). The restriction of virus replication in monocytes has been shown to be regulated at the transcriptional level. The virus infects monocytes and monocyte precursors in bone marrow and spleen, but infected monocytes do not express high levels of viral RNA and protein until they mature into macrophages. AP-1 and AP-4 binding sites in the LTR have been shown to be important in this regulation (Gabuzda, Hess, Small, & Clements, 1989; Gdovin & Clements, 1992; Hess, Small, & Clements, 1989; Saltarelli et al., 1990; Small et al., 1989).

Macrophages and microglia seem to be the main target cells of the virus in the brain (Adeyemo, Phadtare, & Williams, 1996; Ebrahimi, Allsopp, Fazakerley, & Harkiss, 2000; Zink, Gorrell, & Narayan, 1991) although a broad spectrum of cells in the CNS have been shown to be permissive for infection (Brodie et al., 1995 ; Ebrahimi et al., 2000 ; Georgsson et al., 1989 ; Sanna et al., 1999 ; Stowring et al., 1985 ; Zink et al., 1990). However, very few cells in the CNS are infected according to results of virus titrations, in situ hybridizations, and immuno-histochemical studies (Brodie et al., 1995; Georgsson et al., 1989; Petursson et al., 1976; Stowring et al., 1985).

The route of access to the CNS is most likely by the bloodstream, but the mechanism by which these viruses cross the blood-brain barrier has not been elucidated. The entrance into the CNS may be relatively nonspecific, depending mainly on the virus load. Activated monocytes may carry infection nonspecifically into the CNS in their capacity as immune surveillance cells of the CNS (Hickey, Hsu, & Kimura, 1991). Chebloune et al. reported that when MVV was inoculated intratracheally, virus could only be isolated from the brains of sheep that had at the same time been injected intramuscularly with brain white matter to induce experimental allergic encephalomyelitis. They proposed that activated T cells might migrate to the brain and provide chemotactic signals that promoted migration of latently infected monocytes and/or dendritic cells into the brain (Chebloune et al., 1998). However, this may not be the only route of brain entry, since we have found in experimental infections with the visna strains K1514 (Lutley et al., 1985) and the neurovirulent molecular visna clone KV1772 (Andresson et al., 1993) that these viruses enter the brain when inoculated intravenously or intratracheally in the absence of secondary infections (unpublished results). Other mechanisms that have been proposed for lentivirus entry are infection of endothelial cells of brain capillaries and subsequent release of virus into the brain, or infection of the choroid plexus (Chen, Wood, & Petito, 2000; Lackner et al., 1991; Patrick, Johnston, & Power, 2002; Zink, Spelman, Robinson, & Clements, 1998). There is some evidence to suggest that MVV may use both mechanisms of entry into the CNS, and that viral strains that can infect endothelial cells and cells of the choroid plexus are more neurovirulent than others. During the maedi-visna epizootic in Iceland, maedi, the pulmonary affection, was most prevalent. However, in some flocks, visna was the main cause of disease and death. Since there is only one sheep breed in the country, the epidemiology suggests that there were some virus strains that were more neurovirulent than others. The neurovirulent strains K1514 and K1772 are descendants of virus that was isolated from the brain of sheep from one of these flocks (Sigurdsson et al., 1960). Studies from our laboratory have shown that a repeat sequence present in the long terminal repeat (LTR) in these viruses determines the cell tropism of MVV. This duplication in the LTR broadens the cell tropism of the virus from being strictly macrophage tropic to being able to grow in a variety of cell types (Agnarsdottir et al., 2000). We have sequenced the LTR from the original paraffin-embedded, formalin-fixed brain sample of the visna-affected brain and found the duplication there as well. A field sample from another visna case had a different duplication in the LTR and there was an overlap between the two repeated sequences of 14 bp. The repeat sequence was not found in most lung-derived maedi strains. It therefore appears that the duplication in the LTR is associated with neurovirulent strains (Oskarsson et al., 2007).

A study of the distribution of viral antigens in the CNS in an experimental infection using the neurovirulent MVV strain K1772 revealed a variety of cell types productively infected. These included lymphocytes, plasma cells, macrophages, endothelial cells, pericytes, fibroblasts, and choroidal epithelial cells (Georgsson, Houwers, Palsson, & Petursson, 1989). Contrary to these findings, others have reported that although MVV can enter a variety of cell types, productive infection is strictly confined to macrophages (Brodie et al., 1995; Gendelman et al., 1985). In a study of 38 naturally infected sheep, it was found that 7 had lesions of the CNS. Viral proteins were only found in areas surrounding aggregates of mononuclear cells or lymphocytic nodules (Brodie et al., 1995). Together, these results suggest that the invasion of the brain by MVV in most cases probably is dependent on activated T cells or monocytes entering the brain and recruiting macrophages that may be infected. However, if the virus strain can infect the cells which comprise the blood-brain barrier, that is, endothelial cells or cells of the choroid plexus, it has easier access to the brain and, hence, is more neuroinvasive.

There are indications that neuroinvasiveness and neurovirulence are separate pathogenic determinants. Thus, a neuroadapted strain of MVV caused severe encephalitis typical of visna when inoculated intracerebrally. However, inoculation into the bone marrow resulted in persistent viremia but not encephalitis, indicating that the virus was not neuroinvasive (Craig et al., 1997). In a study from our laboratory, two MVV strains, one a lung isolate and the other a brain isolate, differed in inducing brain lesions when inoculated intracerebrally. However, the viral load of the two strains was similar judging from the frequency of virus isolations. These results indicate that there was a difference in neuropathogenesis of the two strains (Andresdottir et al., 1998).

The outcome of an infection by the small ruminant lentiviruses is to some extent host-specific. Thus, approximately tenfold greater concentration of Icelandic visna virus was required to cause a transient encephalitis in American Hampshire and Suffolk sheep than in Icelandic sheep (Griffin, Narayan, & Adams, 1978; Narayan, Griffin, & Silverstein, 1977; Petursson et al., 1976). The epidemic of maedi-visna in Iceland after the introduction of foreign sheep may be analogous to the situation with the simian viruses that appear relatively nonpathogenic in their natural hosts but become virulent on transmission to monkeys of other species (Hirsch & Johnson, 1994).

PATHOGENESIS

Replication of MVV and CAEV is highly restricted and unproductive in the infected animal. Very few cells are found to contain the viral DNA and many of those detected produce little or no viral RNA and even fewer detectable viral antigens (Haase, 1986). There is a great discrepancy between the frequency of productively infected cells and the extent and character of pathological lesions (Fig. 5.3.8A and B) (Georgsson et al., 1989). This indicates that a mechanism other than the direct lytic effect of the virus contributes to the evolution of CNS lesions. It has been reported that some peptides from the visna Tat protein are directly neurotoxic in rodents following

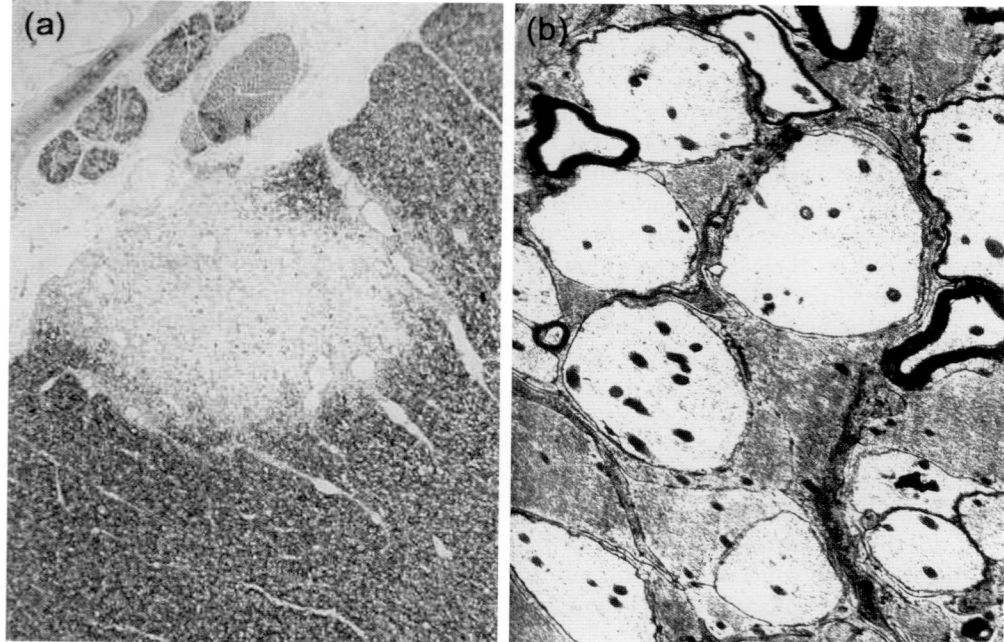

Figure 5.3.7 Visna of sheep. (a) *In situ* hybridization for viral DNA and RNA showing only two infected cells (black) in a big field of confluent inflammation in the white matter. Digoxigenin-tagged probe, substrate NBT/BCIP. Counterstaining with neutral red. (b) Higher magnification showing one ramified cell (microglia or macrophage) expressing p25 gag antigen detected by immunostaining with a monoclonal antibody. Peroxidase and DAB substrate. Counterstaining with hematoxylin-eosin.

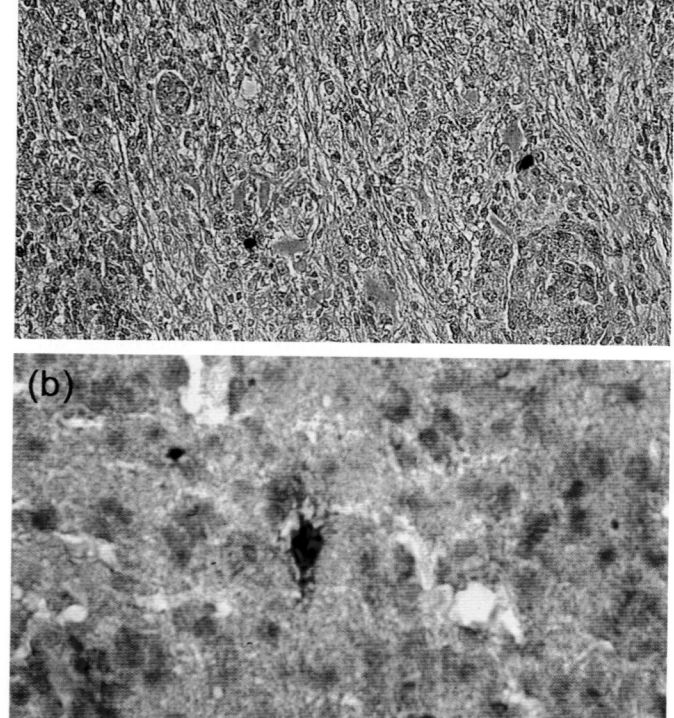

Figure 5.3.8 Visna of sheep. (a) Immunophenotyping of inflammatory cells in the white matter. CD4 black and CD8 lymphocytes yellow. Preponderance of CD4[+] lymphocytes perivascularly and CD8[+] lymphocytes in the diffusely infiltrated neuroparenchyma. (b) Immunostaining for MHC class II in the white matter adjacent to an intense inflammation shows an induction of class II expression on microglia.

injections into different areas of the central nervous system. The induced lesions, that is, microgliosis, astrocytosis, and neuronal loss were inhibited by nitric oxide (NO) synthase inhibitors and NMDA receptor antagonists, suggesting a complex mechanism for this pathological phenomenon (Hayman et al., 1993; Philippon et al., 1994; Starling, Wright, Arbuthnott, & Harkiss, 1999; Strijbos et al., 1995). It has also been reported that transgenic mice carrying the visna *tat* gene showed dramatic follicular lymphoproliferative disorders involving the lung, spleen, lymph nodes, and skin (Vellutini et al., 1994). It is unclear to what extent this effect of visna Tat may contribute to the production of the typical inflammatory and degenerative changes which characterize the lesions produced by infection with visna virus.

MVV- and CAEV-infected animals mount a fairly good virus-specific antibody response. Neutralizing antibodies depend on the virus strain. They are found in MVV infection (Petursson et al., 1976) but are very low or absent in infection with the American MVV strain (OvLV) and CAEV in goats (Craig et al., 1997; Klevjer-Anderson & Mcguire, 1982; Mcguire et al., 1990). The animals also develop cell-mediated immunity (Griffin et al., 1978; Larsen, Hyllseth, & Krogsrud, 1982; Sihvonen, 1981; Torsteinsdottir et al., 1992) and virus-specific cytotoxic T cells have been demonstrated both in MVV and CAEV infection (Blacklaws, Bird, Allen, & McConnell, 1994; Lee, McConnell, & Blacklaws, 1994; Lichtensteiger, Cheevers, & Davis, 1993). The immune response is considered to play a major role in the neuropathogenesis of MVV. Early lesions in experimental MVV infection of sheep were almost abolished by immunosuppressive treatment with antithymocyte serum and cyclophosphamide (Nathanson et al., 1976). Hyper-immunization with ovine

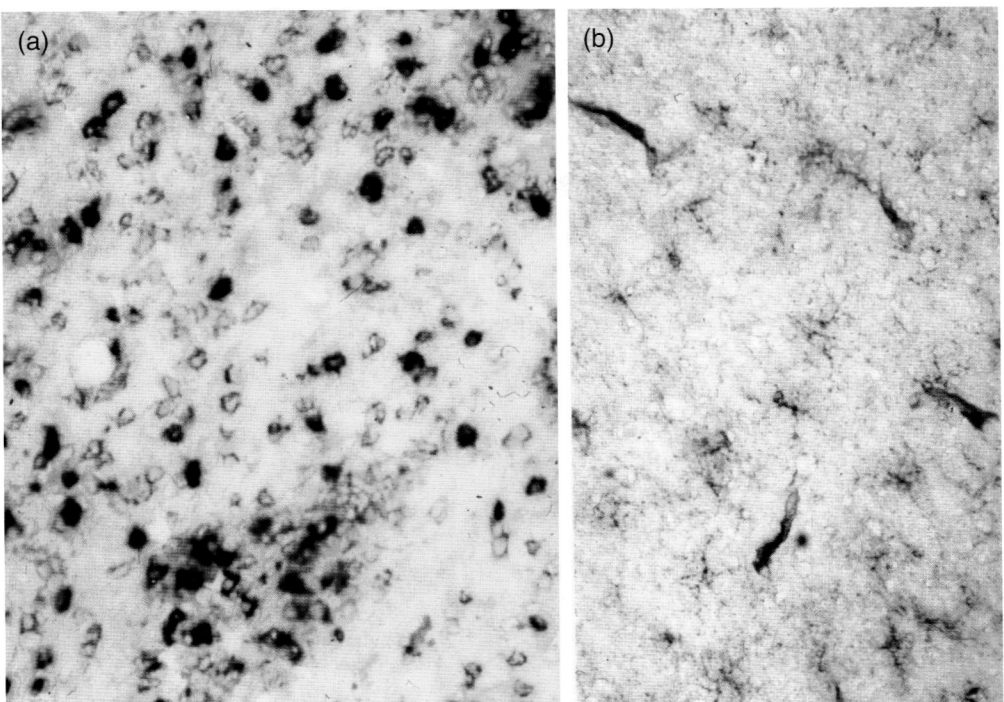

Figure 5.3.9 Visna of sheep. (a) Immunophenotyping of inflammatory cells in the white matter. CD4 black and CD8 lymphocytes yellow. Preponderance of CD4$^+$ lymphocytes perivascularly and CD8$^+$ lymphocytes in the diffusely infiltrated neuroparenchyma. (b) Immunostaining for MHC class II in the white matter adjacent to an intense inflammation shows an induction of class II expression on microglia.

and caprine lentiviruses has also been reported to increase the severity of the disease (Mcguire et al., 1986; Nathanson et al., 1981). It is likely that the damaging immune response is directed against virus-induced antigens rather than host antigens (Davies, Watt, Torsteinsdottir, & Carnegie, 1996; Panitch et al., 1976; Pétursson et al., 1979). Immune activation in the brain of visna-infected animals is well established. It appears that lesions may in large part be due to amplification of the immune response to viral antigens with a great influx of macrophages and lymphocytes and secretion of cytokines resulting in non-specific tissue damage (Pétursson et al., 1992). There is MVV-induced expression of class I and II MHC antigens in the brain of MVV-infected sheep (Bergsteinsdottir et al., 1998, Craig et al., 1997). The induction of MHC class II antigens was mainly found on microglia in or adjacent to inflammatory infiltrates of the white matter and correlated with severity of lesions (Fig. 5.3.9A and B) (Bergsteinsdottir et al., 1998). The induction of MHC molecules is probably due to cytokines secreted by inflammatory cells and activated microglia. Productive MVV infection of sheep microglia in vitro resulted in increased levels of mRNA of the proinflammatory cytokines TNF-α and interleukin-6 (Ebrahimi et al., 2000) and TNF-α expression was detected in perivascular macrophages in the brain of a sheep infected with neuroadapted virus (Craig et al., 1997). In vitro both MVV- and CAEV-infected macrophages have been reported to induce a unique interferon (LV-IFN) production of lymphocytes that induced MHC class II induction in a macrophage cell line. LV-IFN inoculated intracerebrally into visna-infected sheep enhanced MHC class II expression and

inflammation as compared to the animal which only received virus (Narayan & Cork, 1985; Zink et al., 1991). In MVV-infected sheep, mitogen-activated protein kinases (MAPK) are not only activated in the main target cells of MVV (macrophages/microglia) but also in nonsusceptible brain astrocytes. The MAPK activation was shown to correlate with virus-associated encephalitis (Barber et al., 2002).

In MVV infection there is infiltration of macrophages and both CD4- and CD8-positive T lymphocytes into the brain (Craig et al., 1997; Torsteinsdottir et al., 1992). The overall CD4/CD8 ratio in the CNS was shown to be within the normal range of blood but the distribution of these lymphocytes varied within the CNS lesions. CD4-positive lymphocytes were more numerous in perivascular sleeves, whereas CD8-positive lymphocytes predominated in the diffusely infiltrated neuroparenchyma, possibly as an indication of migration to their targets (Fig. 5.3.9A and B). Accordingly, the CD4/CD8 ratio was reversed in the CSF where the total number of CD8-positive lymphocytes correlated with the severity of lesions (Torsteinsdottir et al., 1992). It is not known if these CD8 cells are cytotoxic. Virus-specific CD8 cytotoxic T cells (CTL) have been isolated from the cerebrospinal fluid (CSF) of patients with AIDS dementia complex (Jassoy, Johnson, Navia, Worth, & Walker, 1992) and also from CSF and brains of SIV-infected rhesus macaques (Von Herrath, Oldstone, & Fox, 1995). The role played by CTL in the central nervous system in lentiviral infections is not clear. They may serve to inhibit viral replication but could also contribute to lesion development through cytokine production or cytotoxicity.

CONCLUSIONS

Although MVV and CAEV do not cause an overt immunodeficiency, they share several features pertinent for the establishment of neuropathological lesions with the primate lentiviruses. This holds especially true for the initial steps and early CNS lesions. The lesion pattern in the initial stages is similar; that is, it consists of meningitis, perivascular infiltrations especially of the deep white matter, and inflammation of the choroid plexus. Multinucleated giant cells which are prominent in HIV-1 and SIV infections are rare in MVV and practically nonexistent in infections with CAEV, possibly a reflection of differences in virus replication. The main target cells for productive infection in the brain are cells of the monocyte/macrophage lineage, and the mechanisms for virus entry into the CNS may be similar for all the lentiviruses. Differences in neuroinvasion and neurovirulence have been defined for MVV strains, and host susceptibility to neurological disease differs between sheep breeds. The availability of a neurotropic/neurovirulent infectious molecular clone of MVV provides a tool for determining the host and viral factors which play a role in MVV-induced development of neurological disease. The differences as well as the similarities of the neuropathogenesis in the various lentiviral systems may serve to enhance the understanding of the neurology of AIDS.

ACKNOWLEDGMENTS

We thank Gudmundur Pétursson for insightful comments and Gudrún Agnarsdóttir and Ólafur S. Andrésson for critically reading the manuscript.

REFERENCES

Adams, D. S., Klevjer-Anderson, P., Carlson, J. L., McGuire, T. C. & Gorham, J. R. (1983). Transmission and control of caprine arthritis-encephalitis virus. *Am J Vet Res*, 44, 1670–5.

Adeyemo, O., Phadtare, L. & Williams, C. (1996). The response of goat brain cells to infection by caprine arthritis-encephalitis virus. *Cell Mol Biol (Noisy-le-grand)*, 42, 1195–209.

Agnarsdottir, G., Thorsteinsdottir, H., Oskarsson, T., et al. (2000). The long terminal repeat is a determinant of cell tropism of maedi-visna virus. *J Gen Virol*, 81 Pt 8, 1901–5.

Andresdottir, V., Tang, X., Agnarsdottir, G., et al. (1998). Biological and genetic differences between lung- and brain-derived isolates of maedi-visna virus. *Virus Genes*, 16, 281–93.

Andresson, O. S., Elser, J. E., Tobin, G. J., et al. (1993). Nucleotide sequence and biological properties of a pathogenic proviral molecular clone of neurovirulent visna virus. *Virology*, 193, 89–105.

Banks, K. L., Adams, D. S., McGuire, T. C., & Carlson, J. (1983). Experimental infection of sheep by caprine arthritis-encephalitis virus and goats by progressive pneumonia virus. *Am J Vet Res*, 44, 2307–11.

Barber, S. A., Bruett, L., & Clements, J. E. (2000). Involvement of a membrane-associated serine/threonine kinase complex in cellular binding of visna virus. *Virology*, 274, 321–30.

Barber, S. A., Bruett, L., Douglass, B. R., Herbst, D. S., Zink, M. C., & Clements, J. E. (2002). Visna virus-induced activation of MAPK is required for virus replication and correlates with virus-induced neuropathology. *J Virol*, 76, 817–28.

Benavides, J., Gómez, N., Gelmetti, D., Ferreras, M. C., García-Pariente, C., Fuertes, M., et al. (2006). Diagnosis of the nervous form of maedi-visna infection with a high frequency in sheep in Castilla y Leon, Spain. *Vet Rec*, 158, 230–5.

Benavides, J., García-Pariente, C., Fuertes, M., Ferreras, M. C., García-Marín, J. F., Juste, R. A., et al. (2009). Maedi-visna: The meningoencephalitis in naturally occurring cases. *J Comp Pathol*, 140, 1–11.

Bergsteinsdottir, K., Arnadottir, S., Torsteinsdottir, S., et al. (1998). Constitutive and visna virus induced expression of class I and II major histocompatibility complex antigens in the central nervous system of sheep and their role in the pathogenesis of visna lesions. *Neuropathol Appl Neurobiol*, 24, 224–32.

Blacklaws, B. A., Bird, P., Allen, D., & McConnell, I. (1994). Circulating cytotoxic T lymphocyte precursors in maedi-visna virus-infected sheep. *J Gen Virol*, 75, 1589–96.

Brahic, M., Stowring, L., Ventura, P., & Haase, A. T. (1981). Gene expression in visna virus infection in sheep. *Nature*, 292, 240–2.

Brodie, S. J., Pearson, L. D., Zink, M. C., et al. (1995). Ovine lentivirus expression and disease. Virus replication, but not entry, is restricted to macrophages of specific tissues. *Am J Pathol*, 146, 250–63.

Bruett, L., Barber, S. A., & Clements, J. E. (2000). Characterization of a membrane-associated protein implicated in visna virus binding and infection. *Virology*, 271, 132–41.

Bruett, L. & Clements, J. E. (2001). Functional murine leukemia virus vectors pseudotyped with the visna virus envelope show expanded visna virus cell tropism. *J Virol*, 75, 11464–73.

Chebloune, Y., Karr, B., Sheffer, D., Leung, K., & Narayan, O. (1996). Variations in lentiviral gene expression in monocyte-derived macrophages from naturally infected sheep. *J Gen Virol*, 77, 2037–51.

Chebloune, Y., Karr, B. M., Raghavan, R., et al. (1998). Neuroinvasion by ovine lentivirus in infected sheep mediated by inflammatory cells associated with experimental allergic encephalomyelitis. *J Neurovirol*, 4, 38–48.

Chen, H., Wood, C., & Petito, C. K. (2000). Comparisons of HIV-1 viral sequences in brain, choroid plexus and spleen: Potential role of choroid plexus in the pathogenesis of HIV encephalitis. *J Neurovirol*, 6, 498–506.

Clements, J. E., Wall, R. J., Narayan, O., et al. (1994). Development of transgenic sheep that express the visna virus envelope gene. *Virology*, 200, 370–80.

Cork, L. C. (1976). Differential diagnosis of viral leukoencephalomyelitis of goats. *J Am Vet Med Assoc*, 169, 1303–6.

Cork, L. C. & Davis, W. C. (1975). Ultrastructural features of viral leukoencephalomyelitis of goats. *Lab Invest*, 32, 359–65.

Cork, L. C., Hadlow, W. J., Crawford, T. B., Gorham, J. R., & Piper, R. C. (1974a). Infectious leukoencephalomyelitis of young goats. *J Infect Dis*, 129, 134–41.

Cork, L. C., Hadlow, W. J., Gorham, J. R., Piper, R. C., & Crawford, T. B. (1974b). Pathology of viral leukoencephalomyelitis of goats. *Acta Neuropathol*, 29, 281–92.

Craig, L. E., Sheffer, D., Meyer, A. L., et al. (1997). Pathogenesis of ovine lentiviral encephalitis: Derivation of a neurovirulent strain by in vivo passage. *J Neurovirol*, 3, 417–27.

Crane, S. E., Buzy, J., & Clements, J. E. (1991). Identification of cell membrane proteins that bind visna virus. *J Virol*, 65, 6137–43.

Crawford, T. B., Adams, D. S., Cheevers, W. P., & Cork, L. C. (1980). Chronic arthritis in goats caused by a retrovirus. *Science*, 207, 997–9.

Dahme, E., Stavrou, D., Deutschlander, N., Arnold, W., & Kaiser, E. (1973). [Clinical and pathological findings in a transmissible granulomatous meningoencephalomyelitis (gMEM) in domestic goats]. *Acta Neuropathol*, 23, 59–76.

Dalziel, R. G., Hopkins, J., Watt, N. J., Dutia, B. M., Clarke, H. A., & McConnell, I. (1991). Identification of a putative cellular receptor for the lentivirus visna virus. *J Gen Virol*, 72, 1905–11.

Davies, J. M., Watt, N. J., Torsteinsdottir, S., & Carnegie, P. R. (1996). Mimicry of a 21.5 kDa myelin basic protein peptide by a maedi visna virus polymerase peptide does not contribute to the pathogenesis of encephalitis in sheep. *Vet Immunol Immunopathol*, 55, 127–39.

De Boer, G. F., Terpstra, C., Houwers, D. J., & Hendriks, J. (1979). Studies in epidemiology of maedi/visna in sheep. *Res Vet Sci*, 26, 202–8.

Ebrahimi, B., Allsopp, T. E., Fazakerley, J. K., & Harkiss, G. D. (2000). Phenotypic characterisation and infection of ovine microglial cells with Maedi-Visna virus. *J Neurovirol*, 6, 320–8.

Gabuzda, D. H., Hess, J. L., Small, J. A., & Clements, J. E. (1989). Regulation of the visna virus long terminal repeat in macrophages involves cellular factors that bind sequences containing AP-1 sites. *Mol Cell Biol*, 9, 2728–33.

Gdovin, S. L. & Clements, J. E. (1992). Molecular mechanisms of visna virus Tat: Identification of the targets for transcriptional activation and evidence for a post-transcriptional effect. *Virology*, 188, 438–50.

Gendelman, H. E., Narayan, O., Kennedy-Stoskopf, S., et al. (1986). Tropism of sheep lentiviruses for monocytes: susceptibility to infection and virus gene expression increase during maturation of monocytes to macrophages. *J Virol*, 58, 67–74.

Gendelman, H. E., Narayan, O., Molineaux, S., Clements, J. E., & Ghotbi, Z. (1985). Slow, persistent replication of lentiviruses: role of tissue macrophages and macrophage precursors in bone marrow. *Proc Natl Acad Sci USA*, 82, 7086–90.

Georgsson, G. (1990) Maedi-visna. Pathology and pathogenesis. In Pétursson and R. H., Hoff-Jörgensen (Eds.) *Maedi-visna and related diseases*. Boston: Kluwer Academic Publisher.

Georgsson, G., Houwers, D. J., Palsson, P. A., & Petursson, G. (1989). Expression of viral antigens in the central nervous system of visna-infected sheep: An immunohistochemical study on experimental visna induced by virus strains of increased neurovirulence. *Acta Neuropathol*, 77, 299–306.

Georgsson, G., Martin, J. R., Klein, J., Palsson, P. A., Nathanson, N., & Petursson, G. (1982). Primary demyelination in visna. An ultrastructural study of Icelandic sheep with clinical signs following experimental infection. *Acta Neuropathol*, 57, 171–8.

Georgsson, G., Nathanson, N., Palsson, P. A., & Petursson, G. (1976). The pathology of visna and maedi in sheep. *Front Biol*, 44, 61–96.

Gilden, D. H., Devlin, M., & Wroblewska, Z. (1981). The use of vesicular stomatitis (visna virus) pseudotypes to demonstrate visna virus receptors in cells from different species. *Arch Virol*, 67, 181–5.

Gjerset, B., Jonassen, C. M., & Rimstad, E. (2007). Natural transmission and comparative analysis of small ruminant lentiviruses in the Norwegian sheep and goat populations. *Virus Res*, 125, 153–61.

Gjerset, B., Rimstad, E., Teige, J., Soetaert, K., & Jonassen, C. M. (2009). Impact of natural sheep-goat transmission on detection and control of small ruminant lentivirus group C infections. *Vet Microbiol*, 135, 231–8.

Gorrell, M. D., Brandon, M. R., Sheffer, D., Adams, R. J., & Narayan, O. (1992). Ovine lentivirus is macrophagetropic and does not replicate productively in T lymphocytes. *J Virol*, 66, 2679–88.

Griffin, D. E., Narayan, O., & Adams, R. J. (1978). Early immune responses in visna, a slow viral disease of sheep. *J Infect Dis*, 138, 340–50.

Gudnadottir, M. (1974). Visna-maedi in sheep. *Prog Med Virol*, 18, 336–49.

Gudnadottir, M. & Palsson, P. A. (1967). Transmission of maedi by inoculation of a virus grown in tissue culture from maedi-affected lungs. *J Infect Dis*, 117, 1–6.

Gudnadóttir, M. & Pálsson, P. A. (1965). Successful transmission of visna by intrapulmonary inoculation. *Journal of Infectious Diseases*, 115, 217–225.

Haase, A. T. (1975). The slow infection caused by visna virus. *Curr Top Microbiol Immunol*. 72.101–56.

Haase, A. T. (1986). Pathogenesis of lentivirus infections. *Nature*, 322, 130–6.

Haase, A. T., Stowring, L., Narayan, P., Griffin, D., & Price, D. (1977). Slow persistent infection caused by visna virus: role of host restriction. *Science*, 195, 175–7.

Hayman, M., Arbuthnott, G., Harkiss, G., et al. (1993). Neurotoxicity of peptide analogues of the transactivating protein tat from Maedi-Visna virus and human immunodeficiency virus. *Neuroscience*, 53, 1–6.

Hess, J. L., Small, J. A., & Clements, J. E. (1989). Sequences in the visna virus long terminal repeat that control transcriptional activity and respond to viral trans-activation: Involvement of AP-1 sites in basal activity and trans-activation. *J Virol*, 63, 3001–15.

Hickey, W. F., Hsu, B. L., & Kimura, H. (1991). T-lymphocyte entry into the central nervous system. *J Neurosci Res*, 28, 254–60.

Hirsch, V. M. & Johnson, P. R. (1994). Pathogenic diversity of simian immunodeficiency viruses. *Virus Res*, 32, 183–203.

Hotzel, I. & Cheevers, W. P. (2001). Host range of small-ruminant lentivirus cytopathic variants determined with a selectable caprine arthritis-encephalitis virus pseudotype system. *J Virol*, 75, 7384–91.

Hotzel, I. & Cheevers, W. P. (2002). A maedi-visna virus strain K1514 receptor gene is located in sheep chromosome 3p and the syntenic region of human chromosome 2. *J Gen Virol*, 83, 1759–64.

Jassoy, C., Johnson, R. P., Navia, B. A., Worth, J., & Walker, B. D. (1992). Detection of a vigorous HIV-1-specific cytotoxic T lymphocyte response in cerebrospinal fluid from infected persons with AIDS dementia complex. *J Immunol*, 149, 3113–9.

Jolly, P. E. & Narayan, O. (1989). Evidence for interference, coinfections, and intertypic virus enhancement of infection by ovine-caprine lentiviruses. *J Virol*, 63, 4682–8.

Karr, B. M., Chebloune, Y., Leung, K., & Narayan, O. (1996). Genetic characterization of two phenotypically distinct North American ovine lentiviruses and their possible origin from caprine arthritis- encephalitis virus. *Virology*, 225, 1–10.

Kennedy-Stoskopf, S., Narayan, O., & Strandberg, J. D. (1985). The mammary gland as a target organ for infection with caprine arthritis-encephalitis virus. *J Comp Pathol*, 95, 609–17.

Klevjer-Anderson, P. & McGuire, T. C. (1982). Neutralizing antibody response of rabbits and goats to caprine arthritis-encephalitis virus. *Infect Immun*, 38, 455–61.

Lackner, A. A., Smith, M. O., Munn, R. J., et al. (1991). Localization of simian immunodeficiency virus in the central nervous system of rhesus monkeys. *Am J Pathol*, 139, 609–21.

Larsen, H. J., Hyllseth, B., & Krogsrud, J. (1982). Experimental maedi virus infection in sheep: early cellular and humoral immune response following parenteral inoculation. *Am J Vet Res*, 43, 379–83.

Lee, W. C., McConnell, I., & Blacklaws, B. A. (1994). Cytotoxic activity against maedi-visna virus-infected macrophages. *J Virol*, 68, 8331–8.

Leroux, C., Chastang, J., Greenland, T., & Mornex, J. F. (1997). Genomic heterogeneity of small ruminant lentiviruses: Existence of heterogeneous populations in sheep and of the same lentiviral genotypes in sheep and goats. *Arch Virol*, 142, 1125–37.

Lichtensteiger, C. A., Cheevers, W. P., & Davis, W. C. (1993). CD8+ cytotoxic T lymphocytes against antigenic variants of caprine arthritis-encephalitis virus. *J Gen Virol*, 74, 2111–6.

Lin, F. H. & Thormar, H. (1970). Ribonucleic acid-dependent deoxyribonucleic acid polymerase in visna virus. *J Virol*, 6, 702–4.

Lutley, R., Pétursson, G., Georgsson, G., Pálsson, P. A., & Nathanson, N. (Eds.) (1985) *Strains of visna virus with increased neurovirulence*. Luxembourg: Commision of the European Communities.

Lyall, J. W., Solanky, N., & Tiley, L. S. (2000). Restricted species tropism of maedi-visna virus strain EV-1 is not due to limited receptor distribution. *J Gen Virol*, 81, 2919–27.

MacIntyre, E. H., Wintersgill, C. J., & Thormar, H. (1972). Morphological transformation of human astrocytes by visna virus with complete virus production. *Nat New Biol*, 237, 111–3.

McGuire, T. C., Adams, D. S., Johnson, G. C., Klevjer-Anderson, P., Barbee, D. D., & Gorham, J. R. (1986). Acute arthritis in caprine arthritis-encephalitis virus challenge exposure of vaccinated or persistently infected goats. *Am J Vet Res*, 47, 537–40.

McGuire, T. C., O´Rourke, K. I., Knowles, D. P., & Cheevers, W. P. (1990). Caprine arthritis encephalitis lentivirus transmission and disease. *Current Topics in Microbiology and Immunology*, 160, 61–75.

Mondor, I., Ugolini, S., & Sattentau, Q. J. (1998). Human immunodeficiency virus type 1 attachment to HeLa CD4 cells is CD4 independent and gp120 dependent and requires cell surface heparans. *J Virol*, 72, 3623–34.

Mselli-Lakhal, L., Favier, C., Leung, K., et al. (2000). Lack of functional receptors is the only barrier that prevents caprine arthritis-encephalitis virus from infecting human cells. *J Virol*, 74, 8343–8.

Narayan, O. (1983). Role of macrophages in the immunopathogenesis of visna-maedi of sheep. *Prog Brain Res*, 59, 233–5.

Narayan, O. & Cork, L. C. (1985). Lentiviral diseases of sheep and goats: Chronic pneumonia leukoencephalomyelitis and arthritis. *Rev Infect Dis*, 7, 89–98.

Narayan, O., Griffin, D. E., & Silverstein, A. M. (1977). Slow virus infection: Replication and mechanisms of persistence of visna virus in sheep. *J Infect Dis*, 135, 800–6.

Nathanson, N., Martin, J. R., Georgsson, G., Palsson, P. A., Lutley, R. E., Petursson, G. (1981). The effect of post-infection immunization on the severity of experimental visna. *J Comp Pathol*, 91, 185–91.

Nathanson, N., Panitch, H., Palsson, P. A., Petursson, G., & Georgsson, G. (1976). Pathogenesis of visna. II. Effect of immunosuppression upon early central nervous system lesions. *Lab Invest*, 35, 444–51.

Norman, S. & Smith, M. C. (1983). Caprine arthritis-encephalitis: Review of the neurologic form in 30 cases. *J Am Vet Med Assoc*, 182, 1342–5.

Oliver, R. E., Gorham, J. R., Parish, S. F., Hadlow, W. J., & Narayan, O. (1981). Ovine progressive pneumonia: Pathologic and virologic studies on the naturally occurring disease. *Am J Vet Res*, 42, 1554–9.

Oskarsson, T., Hreggvidsdottir, H. S., Agnarsdottir, G., et al. (2007). Duplicated sequence motif in the long terminal repeat of maedi-visna virus extends cell tropism and is associated with neurovirulence. *J Virol*, 81, 4052–7.

Palsson, P. A. (Ed.) (1976) *Slow virus diseases of animals and man*, Amsterdam: North Holland Publishing Co.

Panitch, H., Petursson, G., Georgsson, G., Palsson, P. A., & Nathanson, N. (1976). Pathogenesis of visna. III. Immune responses to central nervous system antigens in experimental allergic encephalomyelitis and visna. *Lab Invest*, 35, 452–60.

Patrick, M. K., Johnston, J. B., & Power, C. (2002). Lentiviral neuropathogenesis: Comparative neuroinvasion, neurotropism, neurovirulence, and host neurosusceptibility. *J Virol*, 76, 7923–31.

Petursson, G., Nathanson, N., Georgsson, G., Panitch, H., & Palsson, P. A. (1976). Pathogenesis of visna. I. Sequential virologic, serologic, and pathologic studies. *Lab Invest*, 35, 402–12.

Pétursson, G., Andrésdóttir, V., Andrésson, Ó. S., et al. (Eds.) (1992). *Lentivirus diseases of sheep and goats: Maedi-visna and caprine arthritis-encephalitis*. Wallingford: C.A.B. International.

Pétursson, G., Martin, J. R., Georgsson, G., Nathanson, N., & Pálsson, P. A. (Eds.) (1979). *Visna. The biology of the agent and the disease*. The Hague - Boston – London: Martinus Nijhoff.

Phelps, S. L. & Smith, M. C. (1993). Caprine arthritis-encephalitis virus infection. *J Am Vet Med Assoc*, 203, 1663–6.

Philippon, V., Vellutini, C., Gambarelli, D., et al. (1994). The basic domain of the lentiviral Tat protein is responsible for damages in mouse brain: Involvement of cytokines. *Virology*, 205, 519–29.

Roderiquez, G., Oravecz, T., Yanagishita, M., Bou-Habib, D. C., Mostowski, H., & Norcross, M. A. (1995). Mediation of human immunodeficiency virus type 1 binding by interaction of cell surface heparan sulfate proteoglycans with the V3 region of envelope gp120-gp41. *J Virol*, 69, 2233–9.

Rolland, M., Mooney, J., Valas, S., Perrin, G., & Mamoun, R. Z. (2002). Characterisation of an Irish caprine lentivirus strain—SRLV phylogeny revisited. *Virus Res*, 85, 29–39.

Ryan, S., Tiley, L., McConnell, I., & Blacklaws, B. (2000). Infection of dendritic cells by the Maedi-visna lentivirus. *J Virol*, 74, 10096–103.

Saltarelli, M., Querat, G., Konings, D. A., Vigne, R., & Clements, J. E. (1990). Nucleotide sequence and transcriptional analysis of molecular clones of CAEV which generate infectious virus. *Virology*, 179, 347–64.

Sanna, E., Sanna, M. P., Vitali, C. G., et al. (1999). Proviral DNA in the brains of goats infected with caprine arthritis- encephalitis virus. *J Comp Pathol*, 121, 271–6.

Saphire, A. C., Bobardt, M. D., Zhang, Z., David, G., & Gallay, P. A. (2001). Syndecans serve as attachment receptors for human immunodeficiency virus type 1 on macrophages. *J Virol*, 75, 9187–200.

Shah, C., Huder, J. B., Boni, J., et al. (2004). Direct evidence for natural transmission of small-ruminant lentiviruses of subtype A4 from goats to sheep and vice versa. *J Virol*, 78, 7518–22.

Sigurdardottir, B. & Thormar, H. (1964). Isolation of viral agent from the lungs of sheep affected with maedi. *Journal of Infectious Diseases*, 114, 55–60.

Sigurdsson, B. (1954a). Observations on three slow infections of sheep (1). *British Veterinary Journal*, 110, 255–270.

Sigurdsson, B. (1954b). Observations on three slow infections of sheep (3). *British Veterinary Journal*, 110, 341–354.

Sigurdsson, B., Grimsson, H., & Palsson, P. A. (1952). Maedi, a chronic progressive infection of sheep's lungs. *Journal of Infectious Diseases*, 90, 233–241.

Sigurdsson, B. & Palsson, P. A. (1958). Visna of sheep. A slow demyelinating infection. *British Journal of Experimental Pathology*, 39, 519–528.

Sigurdsson, B., Palsson, P. A., & Grimsson, H (1957). Visna, a demyelinating transmissable disease of sheep. *Journal of Neuropathology and Experimental Neurology*, 14, 389–403.

Sigurdsson, B., Palsson, P. A., & Tryggvadottir, A. (1953). Transmission experiments with maedi. *Journal of Infectious Diseases*, 93, 166–175.

Sigurdsson, B., Thormar, H., & Palsson, P. A. (1960). Cultivation of visna virus in tissue culture. *Archiv fur die gesamte Virusforschung*, 10, 368–380.

Sihvonen, L. (1981). Early immune responses in experimental maedi. *Res Vet Sci*, 30, 217–22.

Small, J. A., Bieberich, C., Ghotbi, Z., Hess, J., Scangos, G. A., & Clements, J. E. (1989). The visna virus long terminal repeat directs expression of a reporter gene in activated macrophages, lymphocytes, and the central nervous systems of transgenic mice. *J Virol*, 63, 1891–6.

Starling, I., Wright, A., Arbuthnott, G., & Harkiss, G. (1999). Acute in vivo neurotoxicity of peptides from Maedi visna virus transactivating protein Tat. *Brain Res*, 830, 285–91.

Stavrou, D., Deutschlander, N., & Dahme, E. (1969). Granulomatous encephalomyelitis in goats. *J Comp Pathol*, 79, 393–6.

Stowring, L., Haase, A. T., Petursson, G., et al. (1985). Detection of visna virus antigens and RNA in glial cells in foci of demyelination. *Virology*, 141, 311–8.

Strijbos, P. J., Zamani, M. R., Rothwell, N. J., Arbuthnott, G., & Harkiss, G. (1995). Neurotoxic mechanisms of transactivating protein Tat of Maedi-Visna virus. *Neurosci Lett*, 197, 215–8.

Sundquist, B., Jonsson, L., Jacobsson, S. O., & Hammarberg, K. E. (1981). Visna virus meningoencephalomyelitis in goats. *Acta Vet Scand*, 22, 315–30.

Thormar, H. & Helgadóttir, H. (1965). A comparison of visna and maedi viruses II. Serological relationship. *Research in Veterinary Science*, 6, 456–465.

Torsteinsdottir, S., Georgsson, G., Gisladottir, E., Rafnar, B., Palsson, P. A., & Petursson, G. (1992). Pathogenesis of central nervous system lesions in visna: Cell-mediated immunity and lymphocyte subsets in blood, brain and cerebrospinal fluid. *J Neuroimmunol*, 41, 149–58.

Valas, S., Benoit, C., Guionaud, C., Perrin, G., & Mamoun, R. Z. (1997). North American and French caprine arthritis-encephalitis viruses emerge from ovine maedi-visna viruses. *Virology*, 237, 307–18.

Vellutini, C., Philippon, V., Gambarelli, D., et al. (1994). The maedi-visna virus Tat protein induces multiorgan lymphoid hyperplasia in transgenic mice. *J Virol*, 68, 4955–62.

von Herrath, M., Oldstone, M. B., & Fox, H. S. (1995). Simian immunodeficiency virus (SIV)-specific CTL in cerebrospinal fluid and brains of SIV-infected rhesus macaques. *Journal of Immunology*, 154, 5582–5589.

Watt, N. J., Roy, D. J., McConnell, I., & King, T. J. (1990). A case of visna in the United Kingdom. *Vet Rec*, 126, 600–1.

Zanoni, R. G. (1998). Phylogenetic analysis of small ruminant lentiviruses. *J Gen Virol*, 79, 1951–61.

Zink, M. C., Gorrell, M. D., & Narayan, O. (1991). The neuropathogenesis of visna virus infection in sheep. *Seminars in The Neurosciences*, 3, 125–130.

Zink, M. C., Spelman, J. P., Robinson, R. B., & Clements, J. E. (1998). SIV infection of macaques—modeling the progression to AIDS dementia. *J Neurovirol*, 4, 249–59.

Zink, M. C., Yager, J. A., & Myers, J. D. (1990). Pathogenesis of caprine arthritis encephalitis virus. Cellular localization of viral transcripts in tissues of infected goats. *Am J Pathol*, 136, 843–54.

5.4

TRANSGENICS

Sulie L. Chang and Marley D. Kass

The development and optimization of animal models for neuro-AIDS research is a challenging but necessary step toward delineating and effectively treating the central and peripheral neuropathologies that emerge with long-term HIV infection in humans. Because large-animal models, such as nonhuman primate models, are expensive and of limited availability, developing small-animal models of HIV disease, including with mice and rats, is important. Although certain aspects of HIV disease are modeled well by murine leukemia viruses and with the xenotransplantation of severe combined immunodeficient mice, there are situations where transgenic (Tg) models are uniquely valuable. Tg mice and rats expressing either the full HIV-1 genome or specific HIV-1 genes can mimic neuropathological abnormalities and cognitive, motor, and behavioral impairments observed in human HIV-1 disease. This chapter provides a detailed overview of transgenic murine models for HIV infection in humans.

INTRODUCTION

Combination antiretroviral therapy (cART) inhibits HIV-1 viral entry into cells and controls viral replication and helps restore immunity by impeding the actions of viral reverse transcriptase and viral protease. However, cART cannot eliminate the underlying infection (Sleasman & Goodenow, 2003; Barbaro et al. 2005; Gianotti & Lazzarin, 2005; Agbottah et al. 2006; Vigano et al. 2006). There is limited HIV-1 replication in HIV-1-infected patients receiving cART, but the persistent HIV-1 infection is associated with gradual neurodegeneration and may eventually progress to AIDS. The use of cART has dramatically increased survival rates over the past decade, but the incidence of HIV-associated neurocognitive disorders (HANDs) remains high (Woods et al. 2009). The pathogenesis of AIDS in the cART era is multifactorial. HIV-1 infection, adverse effects of long-term treatment with cART medication, and aging all contribute to the neuropathological and clinical outcomes. The mechanisms by which HIV-1 affects the central nervous system (CNS) are complex and can best be elucidated through the use of animal model systems.

The development and optimization of animal models for neuro-AIDS research is a challenging but necessary step toward delineating and effectively treating the central and peripheral neuropathologies that emerge with long-term HIV infection in humans. Because of the disadvantages of using large animal models, such as nonhuman primates, that

have high cost management and limited availability, establishing small animal models of HIV disease is of particular interest. Various rodent models, such as murine models of retrovirus encephalitis (e.g., murine leukemia viruses, MuLV), xenotransplant models in severe combined immunodeficient (SCID) mice, and transgenic (Tg) rodent models, have played an important role in elucidating HIV-1 pathogenesis and in advancing therapeutic interventions. Although certain aspects of HIV disease are modeled well by MuLV and SCID models, the use of Tg systems provides a unique opportunity to generate rodent models that mimic the pathology seen in HIV-infected individuals and to examine the pathological role of specific genes (Cazzin, et al. 2009). Despite several species-specific barriers that prevent rodents from supporting a robust and productive HIV-1 infection, genetic manipulations have been used to generate mice and rats transgenic for pro-inflammatory factors, the full HIV-1 genome, or specific HIV-1 genes. Tg mice and rats expressing either the full HIV-1 genome or specific HIV-1 genes mimic neuropathological abnormalities and cognitive, motor, and behavioral impairments that are observed in human HIV-1 disease.

TRANSGENIC MOUSE MODELS

In 1991, Dickie, et al. created a noninfectious proviral construct (pEVd1443) by deleting 3 kb of a sequence overlapping the *gag* and *pol* regions from an infectious clone of an integrated proviral plasmid (pNL4–3). A 7.4-kb *Eae* I/*Nae* I fragment containing the Env, Tat, Nef, Rev, Vif, Vpr, and Vpu genes, and the host's cell flanking sequences at the 5′ and 3′ regions was injected into fertilized FVB/N mouse eggs, and produced nine Tg founders. Tg progeny have the highest levels of HIV-1 gene expression in the skin, tail, and muscle. They also manifest renal disease associated with proteinuria, an AIDS-like cachexia syndrome, lymphoproliferation, thymic hypoplasia, dry, scaly hyperkeratotic skin, and early death (Dickie et al. 1991; Santoro et al. 1994; De et al. 1997). One Tg line of mice homozygous for the pNL4–3:d1443 mutant transgene, designated as Tg26, develops progressive renal dysfunction and glomerulosclerosis (Kopp et al. 1992). The Tg26 line has been used extensively as a model for HIV-associated nephropathy (HIVAN) (Nelson et al. 2003; Korgaonkar et al. 2008), and as a prototype to derive several Tg mutant lines that have been used to explore the role of HIV-1 Vpr in HIVAN (Dickie et al. 2004).

The *Tat* gene has been implicated as a key pathogenic factor in HIV-related neurological dysfunction (Zhong et al, 2008; Jayadev & Garden, 2009). HIV-1 Tg mice do not have a functional *Tat* gene, partly because mouse cyclin T is unable to facilitate interactions between *Tat* and the transactivation response element (TAR) (Wei et al. 1998; Fujinaga et al. 1999). The transactivational HIV-1 Tat protein has been identified as a possible pathogenetic mechanism of HIV-1 CNS dysfunction. In one Tat Tg mouse model, the integrity of the blood-brain barrier (BBB) is compromised by Tat, as indicated by increased permeability to albumin in brain microvascular endothelial cells (Avraham et al. 2004). This finding suggests that Tat may contribute to HIV-1 CNS disease during early stages of infection by altering BBB permeability, and, thereby, promoting viral entry.

Of the currently established Tat Tg mouse models, the neuropathology of a bigenic Tg line created by Kim et al. (2003) may be most relevant to neurological disorders in long-term HIV-1 patients. A doxycycline (Dox)-dependent and brain-targeted (astrocyte-specific glial fibrillary acid protein [GFAP] promoter) Tat Tg mouse line, designated as GT-Tg, was generated through cross-breeding two separate Tg mouse lines (Teton-GFAP [G-Tg] mice × TRE-Tat86 [T-Tg] mice). *Tat* expression, which is under regulatory control of a Dox-inducible GFAP promoter, is dependent on Dox administration and is found exclusively in astrocytes in GT-Tg bigenic mice. Neurobehavioral and developmental abnormalities, such as growth retardation, hunched posture, tremor, ataxia, hindlimb weakness, psychomotor slowing, seizure, or premature death, are induced by Dox in a dose-dependent manner in GT-Tg mice. Furthermore, apoptosis, astrocytosis, dendritic degeneration, and increased macrophage/monocyte and active T lymphocyte CNS infiltration are among the neuropathological features observed in GT-Tg mice. Studies have shown that the neuropathologies and behavioral phenotypes observed in GT-Tg mice can be reduced or slowed by food supplementation, specifically, green-tea-derived (−)-epigallocatechin-3-gallate (EGCG) (Rrapo et al. 2009) or ginkgo biloba extract (EGb) (Zhou et al. 2007), which attenuates Tat-induced astrocytosis and neuronal injury in GT-Tg mice. While cART is currently the most effective treatment for HIV-1 infection, it is not beneficial in ameliorating HIV-1-related neuroalterations and HANDs. The GT-Tg mice can be a useful animal model for exploring alternative approaches to treatment, such as the use of dietary supplements like EGCG and EGb in conjunction with cART.

With the advent of cART, the HIV-1-infected population is living longer, and aging HIV-1 patients may be at risk for developing age-related neurodegenerative disorders, such as Alzheimer's disease (AD). The adverse effects of cART itself may predispose aging HIV-1 patients to AD (Xu & Ikezu, 2009). AD-like pathologies, including elevated β-amyloid deposition and decreased CSF Aβ levels, have been observed in HIV-1-infected brains during autopsy (Brew et al., 2005; Green et al., 2005). This type of pathology likely impacts clinical HIV-1 disease outcomes, particularly those related to HAND. Guinta et al. (2009) characterized AD-like

pathology in GT-Tg mice, and found that HIV-1 Dox-dependent Tat induces neurodegeneration, tau phosphorylation, and decreased expression of the anti-apoptotic molecule Bcl-xL. To further characterize HIV-1 Tat-induced AD-like pathology, Guinta et al. (2009) crossed the Dox-inducible, brain-targeted Tat mouse with a doubly Tg mouse model of AD that carries presenilin 1 (PS) and amyloid precursor protein (APP) transgenes (Holcomb et al., 1998). To parallel the chronic condition in humans, for example, long-term CNS exposure to Tat in an aging organism, Dox was chronically administered to PSAPP/Tat Tg mice at 10 months of age. Compared to GT-Tg and PSAPP Tg mice, PSAPP/Tat Tg mice have a robust increase in Aβ deposition in the cingulate cortex (CC), hippocampus, and entorhinal cortex (EC), and also have a greater increase in tau phosphorylation in the cortex and a decreased Bcl-xL to Bax protein ratio.

Age-related neuroalterations are not the only the factors that can affect HIV-1 disease progression in the post-cART era. There is substantial comorbidity between HIV-1 infection and substance abuse disorders, and this comorbidity may increase the risk of neurological dysfunction in long-term HIV-1 patients. For example, in GT-Tg mice, morphine administration exacerbates astrocytosis, microglia/macrophage activation, and neuronal injury in the striatum (Bruce-Keller et al., 2008), suggesting that accelerated progression of HIV-1 disease in HIV-1-infected opiate users may be partially mediated by early changes in glial cells.

There are several other Tat Tg mouse models that recapitulate select features of chronic HIV-1 disease, such as tumorigenesis (Vogel et al., 1988; Corallini et al., 1993; Altavilla et al., 1999; De Benedictis et al., 2001; Altavilla et al., 2004), decreased antioxidant capacity via glutathione (GSH) depletion (Choi et al., 2000), immunologic abnormalities (Garza et al., 1996), and multiorgan disorders (Vellutini et al., 1995). Despite the relevance of these models to various health conditions that are associated with long-term HIV-1 infection, such as Kaposi's sarcoma and immunodeficiency, they are not ideal models for HIV-1-associated neurological dysfunction.

The viral envelope glycoprotein, gp120, has also been implicated in the pathogenesis of HIV-1 CNS disease, and gp120 Tg mice models can been used to address the role of gp120 in HIV-related neuropathology. Toggas et al. (1994) generated gp120 Tg mice that express secretable gp120 in astrocytes under the control of a GFAP promoter. Widespread dendritic degeneration, loss of presynaptic terminals, reactive astrocytosis, and microglial nodules are among the neuropathological abnormalities found in gp120 Tg mice. The BBB is also altered in gp120 Tg mice (Toneatto et al., 1999), and ex vivo analysis of both cultured brain endothelial cells and serum samples demonstrated that compromised functional endothelial integrity in gp120 Tg mice is dependent on circulating levels of gp120 (Cioni & Annunziata, 2002). Inhibition of gp120-induced caspase activation prevents dendritic degeneration in gp120 Tg mice (Garden et al., 2002). Neuronal injury in gp120 Tg mice may be caused partly by an overstimulation of caspase enzymes that is promoted directly by gp120, or indirectly through gp120-induced overstimulation of *N*-methyl-D-aspartate (NMDA) receptors which subsequently stimulate caspase enzymes. A gp120-induced elevation of matrix metalloproteinase (MMP)-2 protein and activity in gp120 Tg mouse brain may also contribute to the neurodegenerative environment produced by gp120 expression in gp120 Tg mice (Marshall et al., 1998).

The CNS of gp120 Tg mice was examined throughout development to determine the onset of structural damage (Toggas et al.,1996). Some minor CNS damage is detectable at one week of age, and by six weeks of age, the structural integrity of neuronal dendrites in gp120 Tg mice is severely compromised, with the neocortex, olfactory bulb, and hippocampus being the most prominently affected brain regions. Dendritic complexity and neuronal integrity is saved in gp120 Tg mice that are chronically treated with memantine from two days old. Hippocampal slice preparations from gp120 Tg mice have altered synaptic plasticity compared to slice preparations from control animals. Specifically, paired-pulse facilitation (PPF) and short term potentiation (STP) are enhanced and long-term potentiation (LTP) is reduced in gp120 Tg hippocampal slices (Krucker et al., 1998). Furthermore, gp120 Tg mice have aberrant hippocampal neurogenesis. There is a decreased number of adult neural progenitor cells (aNPCs) in the dentate gyrus of gp120 Tg mice. Gp120 inhibits aNPC proliferation in the hippocampus and slows cell-cycle kinetics both in vivo and in vitro (Okamoto et al., 2007). It is possible that HIV-1 gp120 leads to excitotoxic CNS damage in gp120 Tg mice through abnormal activation of NMDA receptor pathways. Support for a glutamatergic excitotoxic mechanism, that is, overstimulation of NMDA receptors, in gp120 Tg mice is twofold: (1) memantine, an NMDA receptor antagonist, inhibits neuronal injury in gp120 Tg mice (Toggas et al., 1996); and (2) gp120 Tg hippocampal mouse slices have augmented PPF and STP (Krucker et al., 1998), two facilitatory forms of plasticity that are mediated by NMDA receptors.

Expression of HIV-1 gp120 also causes neurobehavioral abnormalities in gp120 Tg mice that model those found in clinical observations in the HIV-1-infected population. Age-dependent differential effects of gp120 expression on performance are seen in gp120 Tg mice in the Morris water maze (MWM) and in open field activity. Specifically, open field behavior and performance in the MWM do not differ between young gp120 Tg mice (2–3 months old) and wild-type (WT) controls, whereas older gp120 Tg mice (12 months old) demonstrate decreased spontaneous behavior in an open field test as well as reduced swim velocity and impaired reference memory in the MWM compared to WT controls (D'Hooge et al., 1999). The age-dependent cognitive and neuromotor impairments observed in gp120 Tg mice parallel features of HAND that develop in patients with long-term HIV-1 infection, and are most likely caused by changes in synaptic plasticity and neurogenesis (Krucker et al., 1998; Okamoto et al., 2007), two cellular mechanisms that normally support learning and memory.

Behavioral responses to psychostimulant administration are also altered in gp120 Tg mice, and, more specifically, methamphetamine (meth)-induced stereotypic behavior is enhanced (Roberts, et al., 2010). Dopaminergic neurons in the substantia nigra and caudate putamen are hypersensitive to gp120-induced apoptosis (Agrawal et al., 2010), and it is, therefore, possible that the nigrostriatal and mesolimbic dopaminergic pathways are affected by gp120 and render gp120 Tg mice more sensitive to the stereotypic effects of meth. The interactive effects of meth and gp120 in the gp120 Tg mouse model are of particular interest given the high co-morbidity of meth abuse and HIV-1 infection in people.

Motor abnormalities are a prominent feature of chronic HIV-1 disease, and recent evidence suggests that extrapyramidal motor signs are increased in cART-treated patients as a result of the interactive effects of aging and HIV on motor function (Valcour, et al. 2009). Some motor impairment, however, can be attributed to changes in white matter, dorsal root ganglia, peripheral nerve fibers, or adverse effects of antiretroviral medications, and not HIV-related subcortical neuronal injury. As such, Tg systems can help to understand and treat HIV-1-associated peripheral neuropathies and spinal cord disease. Thomas et al. (1994) generated Tg mice that express the entire, infection-competent, HIV-1 genome in neurons. The transgene is under regulatory control of the human neurofilament subunit (NF-L) promoter, and is predominantly expressed in the anterior thalamic and spinal motor neurons. Pathologic evaluation revealed that there is reduced nerve fiber density, axonal degeneration, and impaired nerve conduction in sciatic nerves from NF-L-HIV Tg mice. A battery of neurobehavioral tests demonstrated that NF-L-HIV Tg mice have specific motor deficits, including decreased spontaneous activity and strength, and not generalized neurologic dysfunction.

The pathological and neurobehavioral characteristics of NF-L-HIV Tg mice are similar to aspects of distal sensory polyneuropathy (DSPN), a common neurological problem caused by HIV-1 infection and several antiretroviral therapies used during treatment (Ndir et al., 2002; Jose et al., 2007; Nicholas et al., 2007). DSPN, which is one of at least six HIV-1-associated peripheral neuropathies, is characterized by distal to proximal axonal degeneration, and presents as mild to moderate pain and/or weakness that begins in distal regions, such as the hands and feet, moves proximally up the extremities, and becomes more severe as the neuropathy advances. To mimic the concerted effects of HIV-1 and antiretroviral treatment on HIV-associated sensory neuropathy, Keswani et al. (2006) administered didanosine (DDI), a dideoxynucleoside reverse transcriptase inhibitor, to gp120 Tg mice. Gp120 Tg mice receiving chronic DDI treatment have an increased dying-back pattern in peripheral nerve fibers compared to untreated gp120 Tg mice. Accordingly, NF-L-HIV Tg and gp120 Tg mice can be used to model certain aspects of the peripheral neuropathies that develop and worsen with chronic HIV-1 infection and cART treatment.

In another Tg mouse model, HIV-1 gene expression is regulated by the myelin basic protein (MBP) gene, an oligodendrocyte-specific promoter. MBP/HIV-1 Tg mice develop a progressive white matter disorder in the spinal cord that is characterized as vacuolar myelopathy, and manifests clinically as late-onset paralysis (Goudreau et al., 1996). Subsequent studies using Tg mice expressing a MBP/HIV-1[Nef] mutant transgene demonstrated that expression of HIV-1 Nef in oligodendrocytes is sufficient to produce vacuolar myelopathy (Radja et al., 2003). Vacuolar myelopathy, a common pathogenic mechanism of spinal cord dysfunction, is associated with advanced HIV-1 infection, and is the most common pathological finding in spinal cord lesions of AIDS patients upon post mortem examination, regardless of clinical presentation (Eyer-Silva et al., 2001; Sartoretti-Schefer et al., 1997; Shimojima et al., 2005). The MBP/HIV and MBP/HIV[Nef.] Tg mice are among several Tg models that resemble characteristics of HIV-1-related spinal cord disease, and can, therefore, be of great utility in understanding spinal cord disorders in chronically infected HIV-1 patients.

TRANSGENIC RAT MODELS

In 2001, Reid et al. used the same proviral construct that was used to generate noninfectious HIV-1 Tg mice (Dickie et al., 1991) to create a noninfectious HIV-1 Tg rat model from Fisher/NHsd (F344) and Sprague-Dawley (SD) backgrounds. The HIV-1[gag -pol] clone pEVd1443 was microinjected into a fertilized egg and resulted in a female founder rat. The transgene founder was crossed with a WT F344 male, which resulted in normal offspring and two lines of HIV-1 Tg offspring. One HIV-1 Tg rat line contains a genotype with 20–25 copies of the plasmid and manifests a severe phenotype marked by very opaque cataracts, whereas the other HIV-1 Tg rat line contains only a few copies of the plasmid DNA and manifests a mild phenotype with very mild cataracts (Reid et al., 2001). HIV-1 Tg rats expressing the severe phenotype were produced through brother-sister mating, and are available through commercial breeders. Thus, research has focused on validating that HIV-1 Tg rat line as a small-animal model HIV-1 disease in the era of cART.

Similar to HIV-infected patients that, when given cART, have controlled viral replication but persistent HIV infection, there is no viral replication in the HIV-1 Tg rat, but viral proteins, including Env gp120, Nef, Tat, and Rev, are expressed in the blood and various tissues, including the lymph nodes, spleen, kidney, thymus, spinal cord, brain, and cutaneous epidermis (Reid et al., 2001; Mazzucchelli et al., 2004; Cedeno-Laurent et al., 2009; Peng et al., 2009). Thus, efficient HIV-1 gene expression occurs both peripherally and centrally in HIV-1 Tg rats, unlike in mice with the same transgene where gene expression is most pronounced in skin and muscle tissue. HIV-1 Tg rats develop clinical manifestations of AIDS that resemble those seen in humans, including dysregulated immune responses (Reid et al., 2001, 2004; Yadav et al., 2006, 2009; Chang et al., 2007; Royal et al., 2007), weight loss (Reid et al., 2004; Pruznak et al., 2008; Peng et al., 2009), cardiovascular (Kline et al., 2008; Otis et al., 2008; Pruznak et al., 2008; Hag et al., 2009) and respiratory dysfunction (Joshi et al., 2008; Lassiter et al., 2009), HIV-1-associated nephropathy (Reid et al., 2001; Ray et al., 2003), and dermatologic disorders (Reid et al., 2001; Cedeno-Laurent et al., 2009). There are, however, slight differences in the onset and severity of symptoms and overall disease progression in HIV-1 Tg rats that come from the commercially available strain sold through Harlan Laboratories and other populations bred by researchers. The inconsistent phenotypic transgene expression may be caused by one, or a combination, of three factors: (1) the presence of alternative alleles; (2) physiological-environmental interactions; and (3) modifier genes (Nadeau, 2001; Rao, 2001). These possibilities require a thorough investigation and further characterization of the HIV-1 Tg rat model. Nevertheless, the HIV-1 Tg rat is a promising model for neuroAIDS research.

HIV-1 viral protein expression appears to be age-dependent in this model. There is a higher peripheral expression in younger animals, and a higher central expression in older animals. Specifically, higher levels of Tat, gp120, Nef, and Vif are found in the spleen as well as higher Tat and Nef in the prefrontal cortex (PFC) of young (2–3 month old) HIV-1 Tg rats compared to older (10–11 month old) HIV-1 Tg rats. Higher levels of Tat, gp120, Nef, and Vif are seen in the spinal cord, cerebellum, and striatum of older HIV-1 Tg rats than in young HIV-1 Tg rats (Peng et al., 2009). The overall pattern of HIV-1 viral mRNA expression in the brain of HIV-1 Tg rats, for example, highest expression in the cerebellum, moderate expression in the striatum and cortex, and lowest expression in the PFC, hypothalamus, and hippocampus, is consistent with HIV-1 viral mRNA expression found in human brains during autopsy (Wiley et al., 1999; 1998). The decreased viral protein expression in the spleen of aged HIV-1 Tg rats may be related to increased apoptosis and loss of lymphocyte subsets (Reid et al., 2001). It is also important to consider that HIV-1-associated neurologic dysfunction may not correlate directly with the levels of protein expression, and may be related to chronic stress associated with the presence of HIV-1 viral proteins.

There is a variety of neuropsychological impairments that emerge in HIV-1-infected patients as the disease progresses. Cognitive and motor deficits, including behavioral inflexibility and decreased attention, working memory, and psychomotor speed, coincide with subcortical brain pathology. Using various behavioral assays, similar neurocognitive deficits have been found in HIV-1 Tg rats. The MWM is a task that is commonly used to evaluate learning and memory in rodents, and while not necessary, visual cues may be used during this task. HIV-1 Tg rats have congenital cataracts, and thus, performance in a traditional MWM could be confounded by their inability to use visual navigational cues as readily as control animals. To eliminate this disadvantage, Vigorito et al. (2007) developed a nonvisual MWM that contains intra-maze olfactory and tactile cues and an extra-maze auditory cue. This nonvisual apparatus was used to evaluate learning and memory in HIV-1 Tg rats (Fig. 5.4.1; Table 5.4.1). There was no difference in swim speed (meters/second) between HIV-1 Tg rats and control animals (unpublished data), indicating that HIV-1 Tg rats do not have motor deficits that affect performance in the water maze or affect the interpretation of learning and memory parameters. HIV-1 Tg rats were found to have longer escape latencies and longer swim paths than control animals during acquisition learning (a hippocampal-dependent task)

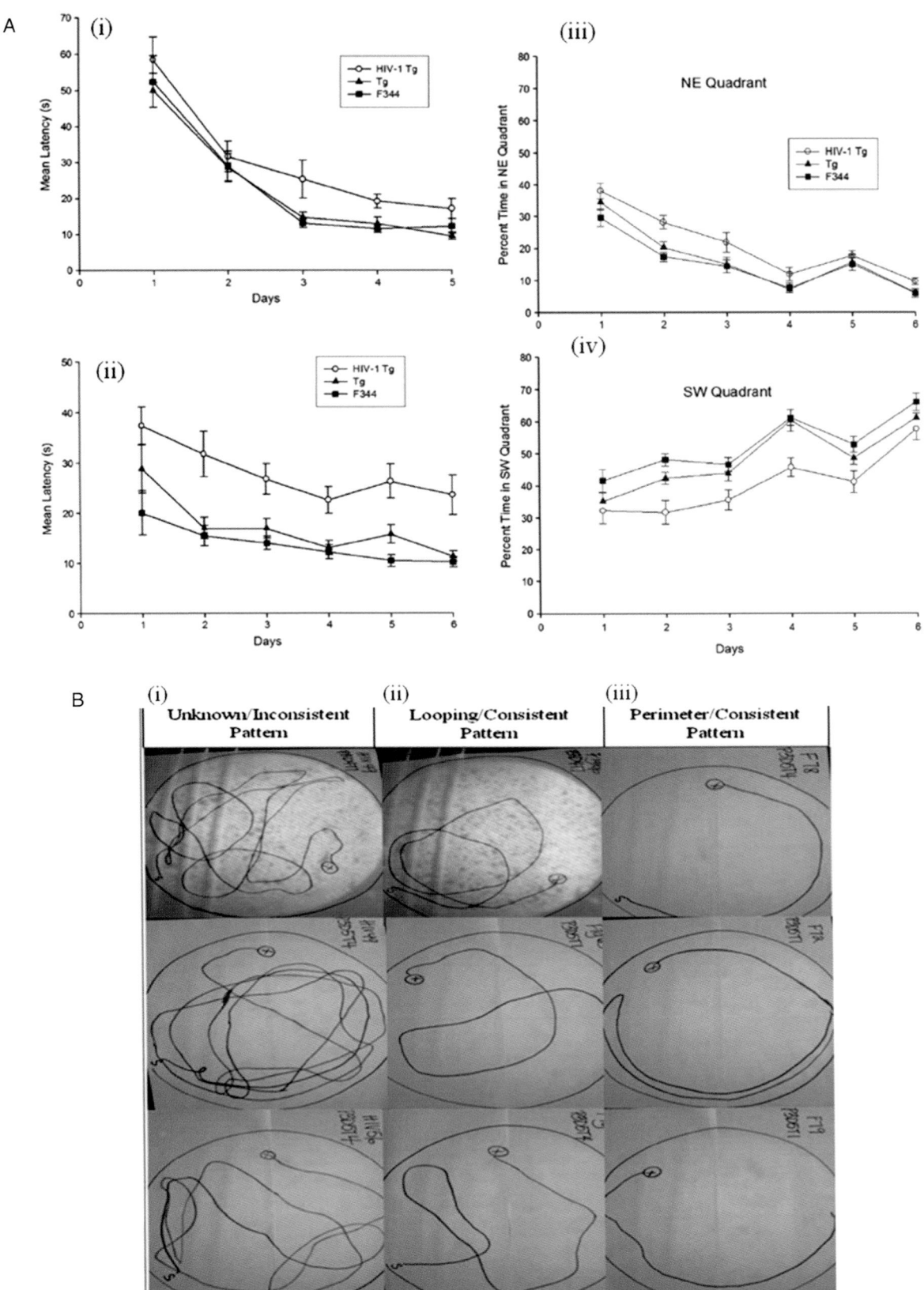

Figure 5.4.1 Performance of HIV-1 Tg rats in the non-visual MWM compared to non-Tg littermate (Tg) and WT (F344) controls during three testing phases. (A) Escape latencies during Phase 1, acquisition training. (i) The target quadrant (i.e., platform location) and the start location were fixed for all trials on all days. (ii) Escape latencies during Phase 2, reversal learning. The target quadrant was reversed from the NE quadrant to the SW quadrant, the platform location was randomized within the reversed target quadrant for each trial, and start locations were random. (iii) Percent of time spent searching in the NE quadrant (top right panel) and SW quadrant (bottom right panel) during six days of reversal learning in Phase 2. (B) Representative swim paths for three categories of swim patterns observed during Phase 3, five days of strategy reversal learning. (i) Unknown/Inconsistent; (ii) Looping/Consistent; and (iii) Perimeter/Consistent. (Reproduced from LaShomb, et al. 2009 with permission from Informa Healthcare.)

Table 5.4.1 NUMBER OF RATS BY GROUP SHOWING ONE OF THREE CATEGORIES OF SWIM PATTERNS IN PHASE 3

SWIM PATTERN	HIV-1TG	TG	F344
Perimeter	3 (23)	5 (38)	6 (46)
Mixed/loop	4 (31)	6 (46)	7 (54)
Inconsistent	6 (46)	2 (15)	0 (0)

Note: Numbers in parentheses are percentages.
$\chi 2 = 8.82$, $P = .03$.
(Reproduced from LaShomb et al., 2009 with permission from Informa Healthcare.)

in the nonvisual MWM (Vigorito et al., 2007). Severe impairment in reversal and new strategy learning, tasks that are dependent on subcortical and cortical structures, including the basal ganglia and the PFC, are also present in HIV-1 Tg rats (LaShomb et al., 2009).

Abnormal motor behavior is another complication that develops in HIV-infected patients, and, although HIV-1 Tg rats develop motor deficits similar to those seen in humans, the time of onset and severity of motor impairment varies. Reid et al. (2001) reported that circling behavior and hind limb paralysis emerge in HIV-1 Tg rats by five to nine months of age, and they also noted a brain pathology (i.e., changes in the caudate putamen and substantia nigra) that corresponds with the severity of the motor problems. However, this motor abnormality has not been reliably corroborated. Some laboratories report finding no evidence of motor dysfunction in HIV-1 Tg rats at seven months of age (Pruznak et al., 2008), whereas others report that disturbed gait and circling seldom develop in HIV-1 Tg rats at 18 to 22 months of age (Peng et al., 2010). Some studies have shown that HIV-1 Tg rats have less profound motor deficits than those initially reported by Reid et al. (2001), and such abnormalities recapitulate the psychomotor slowing seen in HIV-1 patients. Three-month old HIV-1 Tg rats spend less time rearing than WT controls (Liu et al., 2009), and six-month old HIV-1 Tg rats exhibit less vertical (that is, rearing) and horizontal (that is, travelling) activity than WT controls when tested in an open field (June et al., 2009). These findings demonstrate that the effects of transgene expression on spontaneous motor behavior are present in young, otherwise healthy, HIV-1 Tg rats. Furthermore, while clinical signs of psychomotor slowing remain present in HIV-1 Tg rats at six months of age, they are not accompanied by more extreme motor abnormalities, such as the circling and paralysis that Reid et al. (2001) observed in six-month old HIV-1 Tg rats. Motor function has also been assessed in HIV-1 Tg rats via an accelerating rotarod test, and HIV-1 Tg rats remained on the accelerating rotarod less time than WT controls (June et al., 2009). The rotarod test assesses motor skill learning and requires more than general locomotor ability and fitness because rodents must learn to continuously change their strategy as the velocity of the rotarod increases (Buitrago et al., 2004). The inability of HIV-1 Tg rats to remain on an accelerating rotarod may be due, in part, to a cognitive deficit and not poor motor coordination or balance given that HIV-1 Tg rats have (1) severe impairment in

strategy learning (LaShomb et al., 2009), and (2) good general locomotor ability and fitness, as indicated by performance in a running wheel (Chang & Vigorito, 2006).

HIV-1 transgene expression alters behavioral responses in HIV-1 Tg rats that are elicited by drugs with abuse potential. Chang and Vigorito (2006) administered increasing dosages of morphine to HIV-1 Tg and control rats and found that the morphine dose response curve is shifted to the left for HIV-1 Tg rats. More specifically, HIV-1 Tg rats have a greater sensitivity to the analgesic effects of morphine than WT controls, as indicated by longer tail flick latencies. HIV-1 Tg rats also have increased mu opioid receptor (MOR) mRNA expression in the hypothalamus and rostral brain, and this is probably a neural correlate of the morphine hypersensitivity. Similar to findings in gp120 Tg mice (Roberts et al., 2010), HIV-1 Tg rats have an altered behavioral response to meth treatment, which is characterized by an enhanced stereotypic response. Liu et al. (2009) showed that HIV-1 Tg rats develop behavioral sensitization of meth-induced stereotypic head movement at a faster rate than WT controls during six consecutive days of treatment. In HIV-1 Tg rats, meth treatment did not significantly change the expression of D1 or D2 dopamine receptors; however, it increased the D1/D2 ratio of dopamine receptor expression in the striatum and decreased the D1/D2 ratio in the PFC relative to saline controls (Fig. 5.4.2). Given that the PFC is integral to executive function, the elevated D1 expression and D1/D2 ratio in the PFC of saline-treated HIV-1 Tg rats compared to WT controls suggest that alterations in dopamine receptor subtypes may lead to damaged executive function in HIV-1-infected patients, whereby decision making is impaired and they are unable to inhibit drug-taking behaviors. The environment surrounding drug administration can modulate and, thereby, enhance or minimize the psychomotor-stimulating or behavior-sensitizing effects of psychostimulant drugs. The meth-potentiated behavioral response in HIV-1 Tg rats, however, has been dissociated from environmental modulation of meth-induced responses during the expression phase of a behavioral sensitization paradigm (Fig. 5.4.3; unpublished observation). Thus, the hypersensitivity to meth in HIV-1 Tg rats appears to be caused by transgene expression, and not by contextual modulation of drug-induced responses. It is possible that HIV-related neuronal injury in the nigrostriatal and mesolimbic dopaminergic neural networks leads to an increased sensitivity to the stimulating and reinforcing properties of meth in HIV-1 Tg rats.

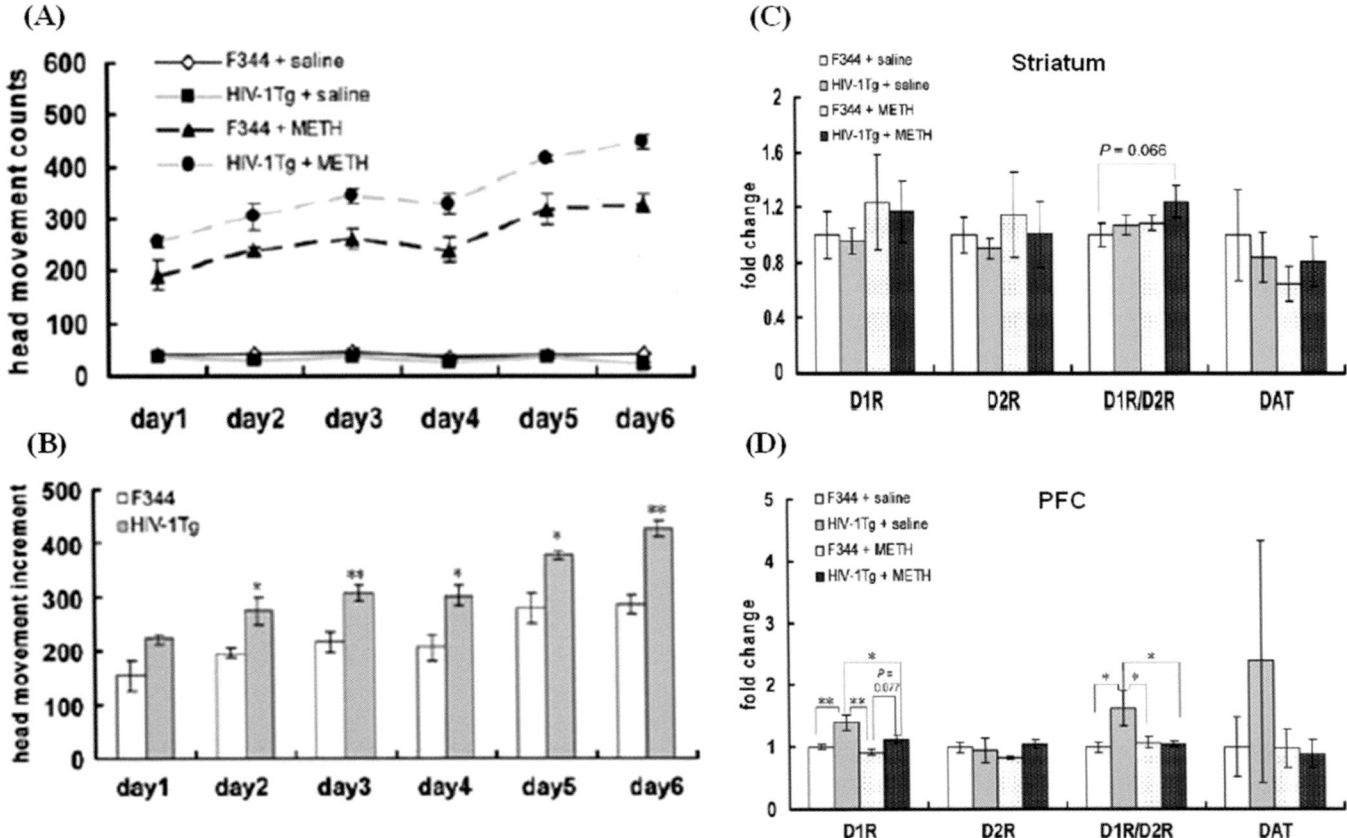

Figure 5.4.2 Behavioral and neuropathological analyses of HIV-1 Tg rats compared with WT (F344) controls. Half of each group received either 2.5 mg/kg meth or an equal volume of saline once per day on six consecutive days; the four treatment groups were: F344 + saline, HIV-1 Tg + saline, F344 + METH, and HIV-1 Tg + METH. (A) Head movement was quantified within three hours following injection on six consecutive treatment days. (B) Comparison of meth-induced head movement in HIV-1 Tg rats and in F344 control rats. (C) Dopamine receptors 1 (D1R) and 2 (D2R), dopamine transporter (DAT) expression, and the ratio of D1R to D2R in the striatum of HIV-1 Tg and F344 rats. (D) D1R, D2R, and DAT expression, and the ratio of D1R to D2R in the prefrontal cortex (PFC) of HIV-1 Tg and F344 rats. $^*p < 0.05$; $^{**}p < 0.01$. (Reproduced from Liu, et al. 2009 with permission from Springer.)

HIV-1 targets immune cells in the host, and T cells and macrophages, in particular, are recognized as sanctuaries for HIV. Ex vivo analysis of peripheral blood mononuclear cells (PBMCs) taken from HIV-1 Tg rats can help determine how immune cells interact with and spread the virus throughout various disease stages (Mazzucchelli et al., 2004). Before T-cell depletion occurs and full-blown AIDS develops, the immune system is altered by HIV infection, and immune abnormalities are present even in asymptomatic HIV-infected patients. In a like manner, immunologic dysfunction has been found in pre-symptomatic HIV-1 Tg rats. Converging evidence suggests that there is an imbalance between T helper-1 [Th1] (pro-inflammatory) and Th2 (anti-inflammatory) responses in HIV-1 Tg rats, and that the effects of the transgene on immune responses differ between early and advanced HIV disease. Thus, the HIV-1 Tg rat model provides an opportunity to elucidate the progression of dysregulated Th1 and Th2 responses and decreased immune function to HIV-1 CNS disease in vivo.

A delayed-type hypersensitivity (DTH) response to recall antigen (keyhole limphet hemocyanin, KLH) is attenuated in HIV-1 Tg rats. However, there is no difference between HIV-1 Tg and WT rats in anti-KLH-specific antibody (Ab) titers (Reid et al., 2001). This indicates that HIV-1 Tg rats have a defective Th1 response and a normal Th2 response. In another study (Chang et al., 2007), topical suffusion of N-formyl-methionyl-leucyl-phenylalanine (FMLP) demonstrated that five-month old HIV-1 Tg rats have a functional leukocyte endothelial adhesion (LEA) response. However, peripheral administration of lipopolysaccharide (LPS) failed to induce an LEA response, demonstrating that one of the first immune responses to infection is impaired in HIV-1 Tg rats (Fig. 5.4.4). Notably, LPS-induced increased serum levels of tumor necrosis factor-α (TNF-α), interleukin-β (IL-β), and IL-10 are higher in HIV-1 Tg rats than in WT controls and non-Tg littermates, despite the absence of an LPS-induced LEA response (Table 5.4.2). Royal et al. (2007) showed that mitogen-stimulated T cells in whole blood samples collected from three- to six-month old HIV-1 Tg rats have a greater number of cells expressing intracellular interferon-γ (IFN-γ), secrete higher levels of TNF-α, and have higher levels of surface MOR and MOR mRNA expression than WT rats. Additionally, HIV-1 gene expression in whole blood samples from HIV-1 Tg rats is increased by mitogen stimulation. HIV-1 gene

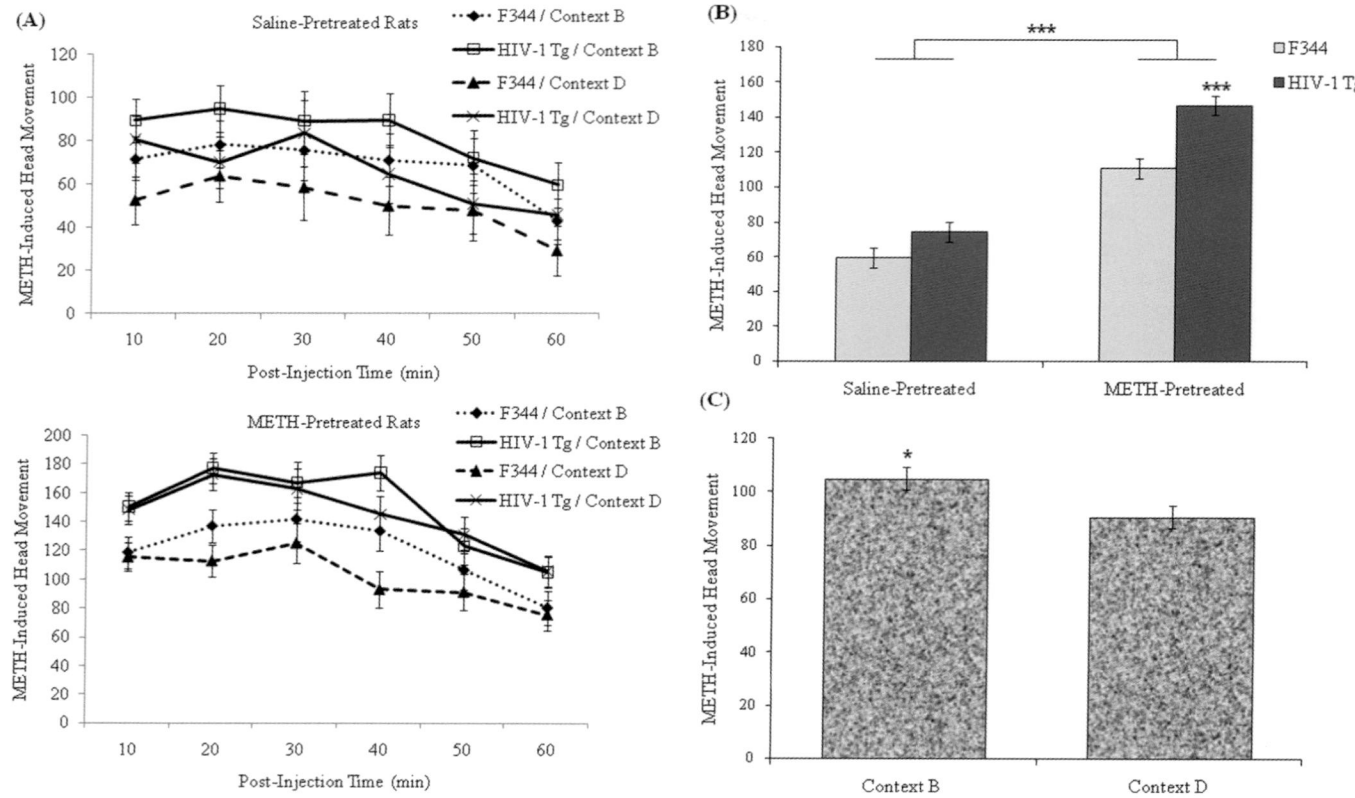

Figure 5.4.3 Behavioral data from the expression phase of a behavioral sensitization paradigm. (A) Summary of meth-induced head movement from all groups [drug pretreatment (2.5 mg/kg meth or saline) × context (Context B; bright surrounding, smooth surface, mint scent or Context D; dark surrounding, rough surface, vanilla scent) × strain (HIV-1 Tg rat or F344 WT controls)] up to 60 minutes post-injection during the expression phase. The response from all saline-pretreated rats to a low challenge dose of meth (0.5 mg/kg) is illustrated in the top panel, and the response from all meth-pretreated rats to a low challenge dose is illustrated in the bottom panel. (B) Expression of behavioral sensitization to meth-induced head movement in HIV-1 Tg rats compared to WT controls. meth-pretreated rats exhibited a larger stereotypic response after receiving a low challenge dose than saline-pretreated rats, demonstrating behavioral sensitization. This was enhanced in HIV-1 Tg rats compared to WT controls. (C) All animals that received a low challenge dose of meth in Context B exhibited a more robust acute stereotypic response than animals treated in Context D, regardless of HIV-1 status or drug pretreatment. * $p < 0.05$; *** $p < 0.001$.

expression and the resulting pro-inflammatory immune responses are also enhanced when HIV-1 Tg rats are fed a vitamin A-deficient diet, indicating that vitamin A deficiency may alter disease progression by increasing oxidative stress. However, this proposed mechanism for acceleration of HIV-1 disease requires further study. Nonetheless, malnutrition is associated with altered disease progression in chronically-infected HIV-1 patients, and these findings suggest that a vitamin A-enriched diet may have beneficial therapeutic effects and ameliorate HIV-1 disease progression.

Reid et al. (2004) demonstrated that mitogen-stimulated intracellular expression and production of IFN-γ in CD4$^+$ and CD8$^+$ cells is reduced in PBMCs in 12–15-month old HIV-1 Tg rats compared to age-matched WT controls; whereas, there is no difference in intracellular IL-10 expression between HIV-1 Tg and WT rats. The authors also found an opposite distribution of naïve and effector/memory cell phenotypic subsets of CD4$^+$ and CD8$^+$ T cells in peripheral blood T cells from HIV-1 Tg and WT rats, with the most abundant subpopulations of CD4$^+$ and CD8$^+$ cells being the CD45RC$^+$CD62L$^+$ naïve phenotype in HIV-1 Tg rats and the CD45RC$^-$CD62L$^-$ effector/memory phenotype in WT

controls. Furthermore, HIV-1 Tg rats have an increased susceptibility to activation-induced apoptosis of CD3$^+$ lymphocytes. Activation of naïve T cells and subsequent generation of effector/memory cells requires several signaling events, and the impaired Th1 responses in HIV-1 Tg rats may partly be a consequence of disrupted signaling events. Anti-CD3 stimulated CD4$^+$ T cells from PBMCs of 12–15-month old HIV-1 Tg rats have reduced expression of surface CD28 and an attenuated increase in IL-2, a cytokine dependent on CD28 signaling, compared to that of control animals. CD28-mediated signal transduction contributes to the expression of Bcl-xL, and Bcl-xL mRNA and protein expression in HIV-1 Tg rat CD4+ T cells is also reduced and accompanied by an increased activation-induced apoptosis that cannot be countered via co-stimulation with anti-CD3 plus anti-CD28 (Yadav et al., 2006). Pathogenetic mechanisms of neuronal apoptotic signaling and subsequent cortical and subcortical atrophy in HIV-1 Tg rats may be related to the peripheral reduction in Bcl-xL mRNA and protein expression. This is supported by converging evidence from Tg mouse models which demonstrated that GT-Tg and PSAPP/Tat Tg mice have decreased Bcl-xL to Bax protein ratios, accompanied by

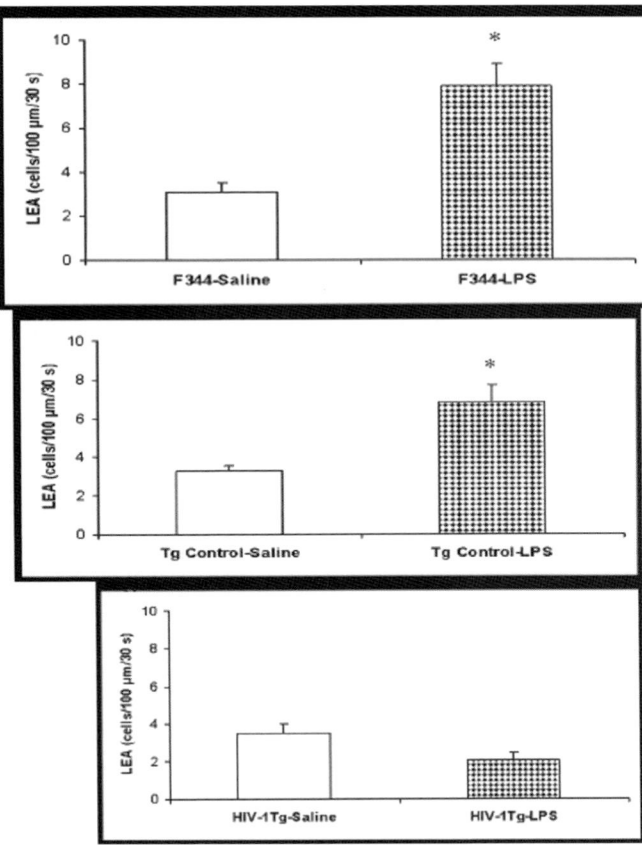

Figure 5.4.4 Intravital microscopy was used to examine leukocyte endothelial adhesion (LEA) in the mesentery of WT (F344) control rats (top panel), non-Tg littermate (Tg) control rats (middle panel), and HIV-1 Tg rats (bottom panel) two hours after injection (i.p.) with either 250 μg/kg LPS or saline. *$p < 0.05$. (Reproduced from Chang, et al. 2007 with permission from Science Publications.)

increased neurodegeneration in several brain regions (Giunta et al., 2009). Like GT-Tg and PSAPP/Tat Tg mice, HIV-1 Tg rats express Tat in the CNS and manifest neurocognitive and neuromotor deficits.

The health characteristics of HIV-1 Tg rats across their lifespan still require further elucidation, but, overall, HIV-1 Tg rats appear healthy and normal at younger ages despite

having immune irregularities. Although 2–3-month-old HIV-1 Tg rats have a slightly lower preference for a palatable sucrose solution than WT controls, they show no signs of anhedonia, indicating that subtle manifestations of sickness behavior are not present during early disease stages in HIV-1 Tg rats (Peng et al., 2009). Systemic disease begins to emerge between 7 and 10 months of age, and clinical wasting, followed by mortality, occurs at 19 months of age (Peng et al., 2009). At younger ages, HIV-1 Tg rats have lower body weight than control animals and, similar to the anorexia often reported in AIDS patients (Heckler & Kotler, 1990), also have lower spontaneous caloric intake (Peng et al., 2009). Notably, HIV-1 Tg rats are not anorexic, and the origin of the reduced body weight in HIV-1 Tg rats is multifactorial and not exclusively attributed to decreased food intake. Specifically, HIV-1 Tg rats gain less weight than pair-fed controls, and this is partly due to an elevated resting energy expenditure (Pruznak et al., 2008).

Long-term HIV-1 infection can lead to impaired alveolar macrophage immune function, and chronically infected patients are susceptible to infections of the lung, which are consequently a leading cause of death in HIV-1 patients (Thomas & Limper, 2007). Alveolar macrophage maturation and function is partly dependent on granulocyte-macrophage colony-stimulating factor (GM-CSF), a peptide secreted by alveolar epithelial cells (Trapnell, 2002). Immunosuppression of the pulmonary system in HIV-1 patients may be related to maladaptive changes in GM-CSF signaling and receptor expression. Antioxidant depletion and oxidant stress within the alveolar space have also been implicated in the lung diseases of chronically infected HIV-1 patients. The HIV-1 Tg rat model has been implemented to investigate possible mechanisms of compromised immune function in the pulmonary system. Joshi et al. (2008) found that HIV-1 Tg rats have decreased intracellular expression of the GM-CSF receptor β (GM-CSFRβ) subunit, and that zinc (Zn) levels in alveolar macrophages and fluid from the alveolar epithelial lining are decreased by gp120 expression. Interestingly, reduced GM-CSFRβ subunit expression is also seen in alveolar macrophages from WT controls when Zn depletion is induced in vitro, and conversely, GM-CSFRβ subunit expression in HIV-1 Tg rat alveolar macrophages

Table 5.4.2 SERUM LEVELS OF IL-1β, TNF-α, AND IL-10 IN WT (F344) CONTROL, NON-TG LITTERMATE (TG) CONTROL, AND HIV-1TG RATS AS DETERMINED BY ELISA

	F344 RATS		TG RATS		HIV-1TG RATS	
	SALINE	LPS	SALINE	LPS	SALINE	LPS
IL-1β (pg/mL)	80.5 ± 1.4	214.7 ± 2.6 *	98.3 ± 3.0	253.2 ± 5.7 *	204.8 ± 3.3	1392.0 ± 9.1 *#†
TNF-α (pg/mL)	129.7 ± 5.7	183.7 ± 3.5 *	129.5 ± 5.4	203.3 ± 5.6 *	112.7 ± 7.5	4557.1 ± 145.9 *#†
IL-10 (pg/mL)	127.4 ± 4.5	188.0 ± 2.1 *	125.6 ± 3.4	214.1 ± 2.7 *	136.4 ± 2.8	358.8 ± 9.8 *#†

N = 3 for each group.
*denotes $p < 0.05$ compared to animals without suffusion with FMLP; #denotes $p < 0.05$ compared to F344 control rats treated with LPS; †denotes $p < 0.05$ compared to Tg control rats treated with LPS.
(Reproduced from Chang et al., 2007 with permission from Science Publications.)

is increased when Zn supplementation is administered in vitro. The authors also identified an age-dependent modulation of reduced Zn levels in the bronchoalveolar lavage and alveolar macrophages, such that Zn depletion is enhanced with age in HIV-1 Tg rats. Another study (Lassiter et al., 2009) demonstrated that gp120 and Tat expression are associated with oxidative stress in the alveolar space. More specifically, HIV-1 Tg rats have decreased levels of GSH and increased levels of oxidized GSH (GSH disulfide, GSSG) in lung lavage fluid as well as increased levels of hydrogen peroxide (H_2O_2) in lung tissue compared to WT controls. HIV-1 transgene expression also impairs alveolar epithelial barrier function as indicated by a decreased ability to clear liquid from the lung after intra-tracheal saline challenge and reduced expression of two key tight junction proteins in the alveolar epithelium. Furthermore, when treated with gp120 or Tat in vitro, reduced expression of the tight junction proteins is also seen in alveolar epithelial cells from WT controls. Research has shown that the HIV-1 viral proteins, gp120 and Tat, compromise the blood-brain endothelial barrier and increase cell permeability through inducing oxidative stress (Price et al., 2005) and altering tight junction protein expression (Andras et al., 2003; Kanmogne et al., 2005). It appears that similar mechanisms increase susceptibility to lung disease in HIV-1-infected individuals.

Cardiac and skeletal myopathies, hypertension, and an increased risk for cardiovascular disease are among the myriad of health complications associated with HIV-1 infection in humans, and these aspects of chronic HIV-1 disease have also been identified in HIV-1 Tg rats. At seven months of age, HIV-1 Tg rats have enlarged relative heart masses and atrophied skeletal muscles, including the gastrocnemius, soleus, and plantaris muscles. Heart tissue taken from HIV-1 Tg rats has elevated GSSG:GSH ratios, lower levels of cysteine (Cys), and elevated levels of the oxidized form of Cys (cystine, Cyss) and Cyss:Cys ratios when compared to controls. Similar oxidative stress is present in HIV-1 Tg rat plantaris muscle tissue (Otis et al., 2008). Vascular oxidative stress and nitric oxide (NO) depletion are also observed in HIV-1 Tg rats at nine months of age, and GSH treatment restores aortic NO levels and improves endothelium-dependent relaxation (Kline et al., 2008). Ten- to 12-month old HIV-1 Tg rats have cardiovascular disease markers (Hag, et al., 2009). Aortic archs taken from HIV-1 Tg rats have a higher expression of genes that are implicated in endothelial dysfunction and accelerated atherogenesis than aortic archs taken from controls. While cardiovascular abnormalities and other peripheral myopathies have been partly attributed to anti-retroviral medications given to HIV-1 patients (Calza et al., 2008), the HIV-1 Tg rat model suggests that the presence of HIV-1 viral proteins can lead to these complications independent of the toxicity associated with antiretroviral treatment. More to the point, the expression of HIV-1 viral proteins may lead to altered cardiac and skeletal muscle morphologies by increasing oxidative stress, and dietary anti-oxidant supplementation may be an effective treatment in reducing such dysfunction.

SUMMARY

The prognosis for persons with AIDS has substantially changed in the era of cART, with a marked reduction in AIDS-related morbidity and mortality. However, cART medications do not eliminate the HIV-1 infection. The pathogenesis of HIV-1 CNS disease is a complex, multifactorial process that includes the interactive effects of chronic HIV-1-induced neuroinflammation, the adverse effects of cART medications, and age-related health complications. Transgenic (Tg) rodent models recapitulate many aspects of long-term HIV-1 infection, and can be used to explore the pathogenic mechanisms of neuro-AIDS as well as to validate novel therapeutic interventions in vivo. Tg mice expressing specific HIV-1 proteins can be utilized to evaluate the role of individual genes in chronic HIV-1 disease, and have, therefore, contributed substantially to neuro-AIDS research. However, in many aspects, the HIV-1 Tg rat model is superior to the Tg mouse models. HIV-1 Tg rats express seven of the nine HIV-1 genes in peripheral and central tissue, allowing researchers to examine the concerted effects of accessory and regulatory genes in a whole living organism. The HIV-1 Tg rat model is particularly well suited for studying both peripheral and central neuropathologies that develop with progressive immunologic dysfunction and systemic disease, whereas most Tg mouse models capture only select features of neurological dysfunction or systemic disease. Thus, while the HIV-1 Tg rat model cannot completely mimic natural HIV-1 infection, it parallels many characteristics that emerge in chronically infected HIV-1 patients, and will serve as a key experimental model in neuro-AIDS research.

REFERENCES

Agbottah, E., Zhang, N., Dadgar, S., Pumfrey, A., Wade, J. D., Zeng, C., et al. (2006). Inhibition of HIV-1 virus replication using small soluble Tat peptides. *Virology*, 345, 373–389.

Agrawal, L., Louboutin, J.-P., Marusich, E., Reyes, B. A. S., Van Bockstaele, E. J., & Strayer, D. S. (2010). Dopaminergic neurotoxicity of HIV-1 gp120: Reactive oxygen species as signaling intermediates. *Brain Res*, 1306, 116–130.

Altavilla, G., Caputo, A., Trabanelli, C., Cofana, B., Sabbioni, S., Menegatti, M. A., et al. (2004). Prevalence of liver tumours in HIV-1 *tat* -transgenic mice treated with urethane. *Eur J Cancer*, 40, 275–283.

Altavilla, G., Trabanelli, C., Merlin, M., Caputo, A., Lanfredi, M., Barbanti-Brodano, G., et al. (1999). Morphological, histological, immunohistological, and ultrastructural characterization of tumors, dysplastic and non-neoplastic lesions arising in BK virus/tat transgenic mice. *Am J Pathol*, 154, 1231–1244.

András, I. E., Pu, H., Deli, M. A., Nath, A., Henng, B., & Toborek, M. (2003). HIV-1 Tat protein alters tight junction protein expression and distribution in cultured brain endothelial cells. *J Neurosci Res*, 15, 255–265.

Avraham, H. K., Jiang, S., Lee, T.-H., Prakash, O., & Avraham, S. (2004). HIV-1 Tat- mediated effects on focal adhesion assembly and permeability in brain microvascular endothelial cells. *J Immunol*, 173, 6228–6233.

Barbaro, G., Scozzafava, A., Mastrolerenzo, A., & Supran, C. T. (2005). Highly active antiretroviral therapy: Current state of the art, new agents and their pharmacological interactions useful for improving therapeutic outcomes. *Curr Pharm Des*, 11, 1805–1843.

Brew, B. J., Pemberton, L., Blennow, K., Wallin, A., & Hagberg, L. (2005). CSF amyloid beta42 and tau levels correlate with AIDS dementia complex. *Neurology*, 65, 1490–1492.

Bruce-Keller, A. J., Turchan-Cholewo, J., Smart, E. J., Geurin, T., Cauhan, A., Reid, R., et al. (2008). Morphine causes rapid increases in glial activation and neuronal injury in the striatum of inducible HIV-1 Tat transgenic mice. *Glia*, 56, 1414–1427.

Buitrago, M. M., Schulz, J. B., Dichgans, J., & Luft, A. R. (2004). Short and long-term motor skill learning in an accelerated rotarod training paradigm. *Neurobiol Learn Mem*, 81, 211–216.

Calza, L., Manfredi, R., Pocaterra, D., & Chiodo, F. (2008). Risk of premature atherosclerosis and ischemic heart disease associated with HIV infection and antiretroviral therapy. *J Infect*, 57, 16–32.

Cazzin, C. & Ring, C. J. A. (2009). Recent advances in the manipulation of murine gene expression and its utility for the study of human neurological disease. *Biochim Biophys Acta*, doi:10.1016/j.bbadis.2009.11.005.

Cedeno-Laurent, F., Bryant, J., Fishelevich, R., Jones, O. D., Deng, A., Eng, M. L., et al. (2009). Inflammatory papillomatous hyperplasia and epidermal necrosis in a transgenic rat for HIV-1. *J Dermatol Sci*, 53, 112–119.

Chang, S. L., Ocasio, F., & Beltran, J. A. (2007). Immunodeficient parameters in the HIV-1 transgenic rat model. *Am J Infect Dis*, 3, 202–207.

Chang, S. L. & Vigorito, M. (2006). Role of HIV-1 infection in addictive behavior: A study of a HIV-1 transgenic rat model. *Am J Infect Dis* 2, 98–106.

Choi, J., Liu, R. M., Kundu, R. K., Sangiorgi, F., Wu, W., Maxson, R., et al. (2000). Molecular mechanism of decreased glutathione content in human immunodeficiency type 1 Tat-transgenic mice. *J Biol Chem* 275, 3693–3698.

Cioni, C. & Annunziata, P. (2002). Circulating gp120 alters the blood-brain barrier permeability in HIV-1 gp120 transgenic mice. *Neurosci Lett*, 330, 299–301.

Corallini, A., Altavilla., G., Pozzi, L., Bignozzi, F., Negrini, M., Rimessi, P., et al. (1993). Systemic expression of HIV-1 tat gene in transgenic mice induces endothelial proliferation and tumors of different histotypes. *Cancer Res*, 53, 5569–5575.

De, S. K., Wohlenberg, C. R., Marinos, N. J., Doodnauth, D., Bryant, J. L, & Notkins, A. L. (1997). Human chorionic gonadotropin hormone prevents wasting syndrome and death in HIV-1 transgenic mice. *J Clin Invest*, 99, 1484–1491.

De Benedictis, L., Mariotti, M., Dragoni, I., & Maier, J. A. M. (2001). Cloning and characterization of murine EDF-1. *Gene*, 275, 299–304.

D'Hooge, R., Franck, F., Mucke, L., & De Deyn, P. P. (1999). Age-related behavioural deficits in transgenic mice expressing the HIV-1 coat protein gp120. *Eur J Neurosci*, 11, 4398–4402.

Dickie, P., Felser, J., Eckhaus, M., Bryant, J., Silver, J., Marinos, N., et al. (1991). HIV-associated nephropathy in transgenic mice expressing HIV-1 genes. *Virology*, 185, 109–119.

Dickie, P., Roberts, A., Uwiera, R., Witmer, J., Sharma, K., & Kopp, J. B. (2004). Focal glomerulosclerosis in proviral and c-*fms* transgenic mice links expression to HIV-associated nephropathy. *Virology*, 322, 69–81.

Eyer-Silva, W. A., Auto, I., Pinto, J. F. C., & Morais-de-Sá, C. A. (2001). Myelopathy in a previously asymptomatic HIV-1-infected patient. *Infection*, 29, 99–102.

Fujinaga, K., Taube, R., Wimmer, J., Cujec, T. P., & Peterlin, B. M. (1999). Interactions between human cyclin T, Tat and the transactivation response element (TAR) are distributed by a cysteine to tyrosine substitution found in mouse cyclin T. *Proc Natl Acad Sci*, 96, 1285–1290.

Garden, G. A., Budd, S. L., Tsai, E., Hanson, L., Kaul, M., D'Emilia, D. M., et al. (2002). Caspase cascades in human immunodeficiency virus-associated neurodegeneration. *J Neurosci*, 22, 4015–4024.

Garza Jr, H. H., Prakash, O., & Carr, D. J. (1996). Aberrant regulation of cytokines in HIV-1 TAT72-transgenic mice. *J Immunol*, 156, 3631–3637.

Gianottia, N. & Lazzarin, A. (2005). Sequencing antiretroviral drugs for long-lasting suppression of HIV replication. *New Microbiol*, 28, 281–297.

Giunta, B., Hou, H., Zhu, Y., Rrapo, E., Tian, J., Takashi, M., et al. (2009). HIV-1 Tat contributes to Alzheimer's disease-like pathology in PSAPP mice. *Int J Exp Pathol*, 2, 433–443.

Goudreau, G., Carpenter, S., Beaulieu, N., & Jolicoeur, P. (1996). Vacuolar myelopathy in transgenic mice expressing human immunodeficiency virus type 1 proteins under the regulation of the myelin basic protein gene promoter. *Nat Med*, 2, 655–661.

Green, D. A., Masliah, E., Vinters, H. V., Beizai, P., Moore, D. J., & Achim, C. L. (2005). Brain deposition of beta-amyloid is a common pathogenic feature in HIV positive patients. *AIDS*, 19, 407–411.

Hag, A. M. F., Kristoffersen, U. S., Pedersen, S. F., Gutte, H., Lebech, A.-M., & Kjaer, A. (2009). Regional gene expression of LOX-1, VCAM-1, and ICAM-1 in aorta of HIV-1 transgenic rats. *PLoS ONE*, 4:e8170.

Heckler, L. M. & Kotler, D. P. (1990). Malnutrition in patients with AIDS. *Nutr. Rev*, 48, 393–401.

Holcomb, L., Gordon, M. N., McGowan, E., Yu, X., Benkovic, S. P., Jantzen, P., et al. (1998). Accelerated Alzheimer-type phenotype in transgenic mice carrying both mutant amyloid precursor protein and presenilin 1 transgenes. *Nat Med*, 4, 97–100.

Jayadev, S. & Garden, G. A. (2009). Host and viral factors influencing the pathogenesis of HIV-associated neurocognitive disorders. *J Neuroimmune Pharmacol*, 4, 175–189.

Jose, J., Saravu, K., Jimmy, B. & Shastry, B. A. (2007). Distal sensory polyneuropathy in human immunodeficiency virus patients and nucleoside analogue antiretroviral agents. *Ann Indian Acad Neurol*, 10, 81–87.

Joshi, P. C., Raynor, R., Fan, X., & Guidot, D. M. (2008). HIV-1 transgene expression in rats decreases alveolar macrophage zinc levels and phagocytosis. *Am J Respir Cell Mol Biol*, 39, 218–226.

June, H. L., Yang, A. R. S. T., Bryant, J. L., Jones, O., & Royall III, W. (2009). Vitamin A deficiency and behavioral and motor deficits in the human immunodeficiency virus type 1 transgenic rat. *J Neurovirol*, 15, 380–389.

Kanmogne, G., Primeaux, C., & Grammas, P. (2005). HIV-1 gp120 proteins alter tight junction protein expression and brain endothelial cell permeability: Implications for the pathogenesis of HIV-associated dementia. *J Neuropathol Exp Neurol*, 64, 498–505.

Keswani, S. C., Jack, C., Zhou, C., & Höke, A. (2006). Establishment of a rodent model of HIV-associated sensory neuropathy. *Neurobiol Dis*, 26, 10299–10304.

Kim, B. O., Liu, Y., Ruan, Y., Zao, C., Schantz, L., & He, J. J. (2003). Neuropathologies in trnasgenic mice expressing human immunodeficiency virus type 1 Tat protein under the regulation of the astrocyte-specific glial fibrillary acidic protein promoter and doxycycline. *Am J Pathol*, 162, 1693–1707.

Kline, E. R., Kleinhenz, D. J., Liang, B., Dikalov, S., Guidot, D. M., Hart, C. M., et al. (2008). Vascular oxidative stress and nitric oxide depletion in HIV-1 transgenic rats are reversed by glutathione restoration. *Am J Physiol Heart Circ Physiol*, 294, H2792–H2804.

Kopp, J. B., Klotman, M. E., Adler, S. H., Bruggeman, L. A., Dickie, P., Marinos, N. J., et al. (1992). Progressive glomerulosclerosis and enhanced renal accumulation of basement membrane components in mice transgenic for human immunodeficiency virus type 1 genes. *Proc Natl Acad Sci*, 89, 1577–1581.

Korgaonkar, S. N., Feng, X., Ross, M. D., Lu, T.-c., D'Agati, V. D., Iyengar, R., et al. (2008). HIV-1 upregulates VEGF in podocytes. *J Am Soc Nephrol*, 19, 877–883.

Krucker, T., Toggas, S. M., Mucke, L., & Siggins, G. R. (1998). Transgenic mice with cerebral expression of human immunodeficiency virus type-1 coat protein gp120 show divergent changes in short- and long-term potentiation in CA1 hippocampus. *Neuroscience*, 83, 691–700.

LaShomb, A. L., Vigorito, M., & Chang, S. L. (2009). Further characterization of the spatial learning deficit in the human immunodeficiency virus-1 transgenic rat. *J Neurovirol*, 15, 14–24.

Lassiter, C., Fan, X., Joshi, P. C., Jacob, B. A., Sutliff, R. L., Jones, D. P., et al. (2009). HIV-1 transgene expression in rats causes oxidant stress and alveolar epithelial barrier dysfunction. *AIDS Research and Therapy*, 6, doi:10.1186/1742–6405-6–1.

Liu, X., Chang, L., Vigorito, M., Kass, M., Li, H., & Chang, S. L. (2009). Methamphetamine-induced behavioral sensitization is enhanced in the HIV-1 transgenic rat. *J Neuroimmune Pharmacol*, 4, 309–316.

Marshall, D. C. L., Wyss-Coray, T., & Abraham, C. R. (1998). Induction of matrix metalloproteinase-2 in human immunodeficiency virus-1 glycoprotein 120 transgenic mouse brains. *Neurosci Lett*, 254, 97–100.

Mazzucchelli, R., Amadio, M., Curreli, S., Denaro, F., Bemis, K., Reid, W., et al. (2004). Establishment of an ex vivo model of monocytes-derived macrophages differentiated from peripheral blood mononuclear cells (PBMCs) from HIV-1 transgenic rats. *Mol Immunol*, 41, 979–984.

Nadeau, J. H. (2001). Modifier genes in mice and humans. *Nat Rev Genet*, 2, 165–174.

Ndir, A., Thiam, S., Canestri, A., Landman, R., Gueye, N. F., Diakhate, N., et al. (2002). Peripheral neuropathy in HIV-1 adult infected patients using Stavudine and Didanosine in a combination therapy with Efavirenz. *Int Conf AIDS*, 14, MoPeB3240.

Nelson, P. J., D'Agati, V. D., Gries, J.-M., Suarez, J.-R., and Gelman, I. H. (2003). Amelioration of nephropathy in mice expressing HIV-1 genes by the cyclin-dependent kinase inhibitor flavopiridol. *J Antimicrob Chemother*, 51, 921–929.

Nicholas, P. K, Mauceri, L., Ciampa, A. S., Corless, I. B., Raymond, N., Barry, D. J. et al. (2007). Distal sensory polyneuropathy in the context of HIV/AIDS. *J Assoc Nurses AIDS Care*, 18, 32–40.

Okamoto, S.-i., Kang, Y.-J., Brechtel, C. W., Siviglia, E., Russo, R., Clemente, A., Harrop, A., et al. (2007). HIV/gp120 decreases adult neural progenitor cell proliferation via checkpoint kinase-mediated cell-cycle withdrawal and G1 arrest. *Cell Stem Cell*, 1, 230–236.

Otis, J. S., Ashikhmin, Y. I., Brown, L. A. S., & Guidot, D. M. (2008). Effect of HIV-1-related protein expression on cardiac and skeletal muscles from transgenic rats. *AIDS Research and Therapy*, 5, doi:10.1186/1742–6405-5–8.

Peng, J., Vigorito, M., Liu, X., Zhou, D., Wu, X., & Chang, S. L. (2009). The HIV-1transgenic rat as a model for HIV-1-infected individuals on HAART. *J Neuroimmunol*, 218(1-2): 94–101.

Peng J, Michael Vigorito, Xiang Liu, Deng Zhou, X. Wu and Sulie L. Chang. (2010). The HIV-1 transgenic rat as a model for HIV-1 infected individuals on HAART. *Journal of Neuroimmunol*. 218(1–2): 94–101.

Price, T. O., Ercal, N., Nakaoke, R., & Banks, W. A. (2005). HIV-1 viral proteins gp120 and Tat induce oxidative stress in brain endothelial cells. *Brain Res*, 1045, 57–63.

Pruznak, A. M., Hong-Brown, L., Lantry, R., She, P., Frost, R. A., Vary, T. C., et al. (2008). Skeletal and cardiac myopathy in HIV-1 transgenic rats. *Am J Physiol Endocrinol Metab*, 295, E964–E973.

Radja, F., Kay, D. G., Albrecht, S., & Jolicoeur, P. (2003). Oligodendrocyte-specific expression of human immunodeficiency virus type 1 Nef in transgenic mice leads to vacuolar myelopathy and alters oligodendrocyte phenotype in vitro. *J Virol*, 77, 11745–11753.

Rao, B. J. (2001). New challenges in human genetics: Modifier genes. *J Biosci*, 26, 547.

Ray, P. E., Liu, X.-H., Robinson, L. R., Reid, W., Xu, L., Owens, J. W., et al. (2003). A novel HIV-1 transgenic model of childhood HIV-1-associated nephropathy. *Kidney Int*, 63, 2242–2253.

Reid, W., Abdelwahab, S., Sadowska, M., Huso, D., Neal, A., Ahearn, A., et al. (2004). HIV-1 transgenic rats develop T cell abnormalities. *Virology*, 321, 111–119.

Reid, W., Sadowska, M., Denaro, F., Rao, S., Foulke, J., Hayes, N., et al. (2001). An HIV-1 transgenic rat that develops HIV-related pathology and immunologic dysfunction. *Proc Natl Acad Sci USA*, 98, 9271–9276.

Roberts, A. J., Maung, R., Sejbuk, N. E., Ake, C., & Kaul, M. (2010). Alteration of methamphetamine-induced stereotypic behavior in transgenic mice expressing HIV-1 envelope protein gp120. *J Neurosci Methods*, 186, 222-225.

Royal III, W., Wang, H., Odell, J., Tran, H., & Bryant, J. L. (2007). A vitamin A-deficient diet enhances proinflammatory cytokine, Mu opioid receptor, and HIV-1 expression in the HIV-1 transgenic rat. *J Immunol*, 185, 29–36.

Rrapo, E., Zhu, Y., Tian, J., Hou, H., Smith, A., Fernandez, F., et al. (2009). Green tea-EGCG reduces GFAP associated neuronal loss in HIV-1 Tat transgenic mice. *Am J Transl Res*, 1, 72–79.

Santoretti-Schefer, S., Blättler, T, & Wichmann, W. (1997). Spinal MRI in vacuolar myelopathy, and correlation with histopathological findings. *Neuroradiology*, 39, 865–869.

Santoro, T. J., Bryant, J. L., Pellicoro, J., Klotman, M. E., Kopp, J. B., Bruggeman, L. A., et al. (1994). Growth failure and AIDS-like cachexia syndrome in HIV-1 transgenic mice. *Virology*, 201, 147–151.

Shimojima, Y., Yazaki, M., Kaneko, K., Fukushima, K., Morita, H., Hashimoto, T., et al. (2005). Characteristic spinal MDR findings of HIV-associated myelopathy in an AIDS patient. *Intern Med*, 44, 763–764.

Sleasman, J. W. & Goodenow, M. M. (2003). 13. HIV-1 infection. *J Allergy Clin Immunol*, 111, S582–S592.

Thomas, C. & Limper, A. (2007). Curent insights into the biology and pathogenesis of *Pneumocystis* pneumonia. *Nat Rev Microbiol*, 5, 298–308.

Thomas, F. P., Chalk, C., Lalonde, R., Robitaile, Y., & Jolicoeur, P. (1994). Expression of human immunodeficiency virus type 1 in the nervous system of transgenic mice leades to neurological disease. *J Virol*, 68, 7099–7107.

Toggas, S. M., Masliah, E., & Mucke, L. (1996). Prevention of HIV-1 gp120-induced neuronal damage in the central nervous system of transgenic mice by the NMDA receptor antagonist memantine. *Brain Res*, 706, 303–307.

Toggas, S. M., Masliah, E., Rockenstein, E. M., Rall, G. F., Abraham, C. R., & Mucke, L. (1994). Central nervous system damage produced by expression of the HIV-1 coat protein gp120 in transgenic mice. *Nature*, 367, 188–193.

Toneatto, S., Finco, O., van der Putten, H., Abrignani, S., & Annunziata, P. (1999). Evidence of blood-brain barrier alteration and activation in HIV-1 gp120 transgenic mice. *AIDS*, 13, 2343–2348.

Trapnell, B. (2002). Granulocyte macrophage-colony stimulating factor augmentation therapy in sepsis: is there a role? *Am J Respir Crit Care Med*, 166, 129–130.

Valcour, V., Watters, M. R., Williams, A. E., Sacktor, N., McMurtray, A., & Shikuma, C. (2008). Aging exacerbates extrapyramidal motor signs in the era of HAART. *J Neurovirol* 14, 362–367.

Van Rompay, K.K.A. 2009. Evaluation of antiretrovirals in animal models of HIV infection. *Antiviral Res*. doi:10.1016/j.antiviral.2009.07.008.

Vellunti, C., Horschowski, N., Philippon, V., Gambarelli, D., Nave, A., & Filippi, P. (1995). Development of lymphoid hyperplasia in transgenic mice expressing the HIV Tat gene. *AIDS Res Hum Retroviruses*, 11, 21–29.

Viganò, A., Trabattoni, D., Schneider, L., Ottaviani, F., Aliffi, A., Longhi, E., et al. (2006). Failure to eradicate HIV despite fully successful HAART initiated in the first days of life. *J Pediatr*, 148, 389–391.

Vigorito, M., LaShomb, A. L., & Chang, S. L. (2007). Spatial learning and memory in HIV-1 transgenic rats. *J Neuroimmune Pharmacol*, 2, 319–328.

Vogel, J., Hinrichs, S. H., Reynolds, R. K., Luciw, P. A., & Jay, G. (1988). The HIV Tat gene induces dermal lesions resembling Kaposi's sarcoma in transgenic mice. *Nature*, 335, 606–611.

Wei, P., Garber, M. E., Fang, S.-M., Fischer, W. H., & Jones, K. A. (1998). A novel CDK9-associated c-type cyclin interacts directly with HIV-1 Tat and mediates its high-affinity, loop-specific binding to TAR RNA. *Cell*, 92, 451–462.

Wiley, C. A., Achim, C. L., Christopherson, C., Kidnae, Y., Kwok, S., Masliah, E., et al. (1999). HIV mediates a productive infection of the brain. *AIDS*, 13:2055–2059.

Wiley, C. A., Soontornniyomkji, V., Radharkrishnan, L., Masliah, E., Mellors, J., Hermann, S. A., et al. (1998). Distribution of brain HIV load in AIDS. *Brain Pathol*, 8, 277–284.

Woods, S. P., Moore, D. J., Weber, E., & Grant, I. (2009). Cognitive and neuropsychology of HIV-associated neurocognitive disorders. *Neuropsychol Rev*, 19, 152–168.

Xu, J. & Ikezu, T. (2009). The comorbidity of HIV-associated neurocognitive neurocognitive disorders and alzheimer's disease: A foreseeable medical challenge in post-HAART era. *J Neuroimmune Pharmacol*, 4, 200–212.

Yadav, A., Fitzgerald, P., Sajadi, M. M., Gilliam, B., Lafferty, M. K., Redfield, R., et al. (2009). Increased expression of suppressor of cytokine signaling-1 (SOCS-1): A mechanism for dysregulated T helper-1 responses in HIV-1 disease. *Virology*, 385, 126–133.

Yadav, A., Pati, S., Nyugen, A., Barabitskaja, O., Mondal, P., Anderson, M., et al. (2006). HIV-1 transgenic rat CD4+ T cells develop decreased CD28 responsiveness and suboptimal Lck tyrosine dephosphorylation following activation. *Virology*, 353, 357–365.

Zhong, Y., Smart, E. J., Weksler, B., Couraud, P.-O., Hennig, B., & Toborek, M. (2008). Caveolin-1 regulates HIV-1 Tat-induced alterations of tight junction protein expression via modulation of the ras signaling. *J Neurosci*, 28, 7788–7796.

Zhou, W., Kim, B. O., Zhou, B. Y., Liu, Y., Messing, A., & He, J. J. (2007). Protection against human immunodeficiency virus type 1 Tat neurotoxicity by *Ginkgo biloba* extract EGb 761 involving glial fibrillary acidic protein. *Am J Pathol*, 171, 1923–1935.

5.5

MURINE MODELS FOR NEUROAIDS

Larisa Y. Poluektova

Among the animal models for HIV disease, nonhuman primates infected with SIV or chimeric SIV/HIV viruses best mimic human disease. However, limitations in cost and availability have limited the extent of research with these animals. For this and other reasons, mouse models, particularly those using immunodeficient and transgenic mice, have played an essential role. This chapter reviews these two important types of murine models.

INTRODUCTION

HIV-1-associated neurocognitive disorders (HAND) are a complex of neuropsychological impairments (Antinori et al., 2007). They represent a spectrum of disorders from very mild cognitive impairments to severe dementia. The pathogenesis and progression of brain damage despite nearly three decades of research remains incompletely understood. The toxicity mediated by viral proteins and host-specific immune responses are considered to be driving forces for the brain's glial cell activation and functional and structural neuronal damage. The nonhuman primates (for example, chimpanzees, rhesus, pigtail, and cynomologus macaques) infected with SIV provide the best model for human neuroAIDS. While lentiviral infections of primates have yielded insights into human disease, limitations in cost and availability have hampered sustained progress for investigations into disease pathogenesis and therapy.

What underlies nervous system disease is an interplay between viral replication in the periphery and that in the brain (Kraft-Terry et al., 2009). HIV-1 replication in lymphoid tissues induces activation of cellular and humoral immune responses, cytokines/chemokines secretion, development of immunologic impairments, and loss of CD4+ T lymphocytes and indirectly affects nervous system homeostasis. In turn, viral infection of the brain's resident microglia and blood-borne mononuclear phagocytes (MP; macrophages) with subsequent perivascular cuffing leads to the formation of multinucleated giant cells (MGC), microglial nodules, glial activation, and neuronal injury. These are characteristic histopathological features of advanced disease (Price et al., 1988; Johnson, McArthur, & Narayan, 1988; Gray et al., 1996) seen commonly before combination antiretroviral therapy (cART) became available. The progressive loss of the dendritic integrity of neurons, structural changes of axonal tracts, and neuronal loss resulted as a consequence

of persistent viral replication and immune compromise (Eden et al., 2007; Grovit-Ferbas & Harris-White, 2010). All these events represent the most severe pathological disease manifestation of neuroAIDS, called HIV-1-induced encephalitis (HIVE). This and more mild forms of disease, such as meningitis and more mild glial inflammatory responses ideally should be reproduced in neuroAIDS animal model systems.

The studies of HIV-1 infection of human cells in vivo was not possible before the discovery of the severe combined immunodeficiency (SCID) mice with a *scid* CB-17 mutation (Bosma, Custer, & Bosma, 1983). These mice contained an autosomal recessive mutation in the *prkdc* (DNA-dependent protein kinase, DNA-PK) gene resulting in losses in mature T and B lymphocytes. The mutation resulted in the ability of these mice to accept foreign tissues, allowing the engraftment of human cells. In September 1988, two landmark experiments sparked the development of humanized mice for human viral infections by transplanted human peripheral blood lymphocytes (hu-PBL) (Mosier et al., 1988) and fetal thymus/liver sandwich under the kidney capsule named SCID-hu Thy/Liv (McCune et al., 1988; Namikawa et al., 1988). The latter model allowed studies of human hematolymphoid differentiation and function.

When the *scid* mutation was transferred to a non-obese diabetic (NOD) mouse background, improved engraftment was realized (Shultz et al., 1995). Initially, the NOD background engraftment improvements were attributed to the low lytic activity of the C5 component of complement (due to 2 base-pair deletion in a 5' exon of the murine C5 gene; Baxter & Cooke 1993) with defects of macrophage function (defective regulation of colony-stimulating factor-1 and interferon-γ receptors, and reduced secretion of IL-1 in response to lipopolysaccharide, LPS) and natural killer (NK) cell activity. The animals can accept xenotransplantion of human hematopoietic stem cells (HSC), including those of liver, bone, thymus, and skin; made possible through defects in both adaptive and innate immunity. The murine polymorphism of signal regulatory protein-α (SIRP-α, CD172α)—the region in the insulin-dependent diabetes 13 (*Idd13*) locus on chromosome 2 containing a coding sequence polymorphism of *Sirpa*—is linked to the survival and subsequent development of human HSC in immune-compromised rodents. SIRP-α interacts with the widely expressed cell surface transmembrane glycoprotein CD47 (also called integrin-associated protein, IAP). The interaction of these ligands expressed on surface membranes of mouse macrophages and human HSC surfaces provides a negative "stop" signal for destruction of xenogeneic human cells (Takenaka et al., 2007; Takizawa & Manz, 2007).

Unfortunately, neither NOD/*scid* nor CB-17/*scid* mice were completely devoid of immune responses. Indeed, the mice continued to generate limited lymphocytes and immunoglobulin responses (Van Duyne et al., 2009). The significant restrictions derived from an incomplete blocking of DNA recombinations involved in T and B cell maturation lead to "leakiness" and production of limited functional mouse T and B cells. The lifespan of these animals was also limited to 7–8 months as a consequence of lymphoma and thymoma developments.

Description of X-chromosome-linked severe combined immunodeficiency in humans and its functional consequences, including the absence of NK activity and T cell reductions due to IL-2Rγ chain (IL-2Rγ$_c$) deficiency (Berry, 1970; Noguchi, Adelstein et al., 1993; Noguchi, Nakamura et al., 1993; Noguchi, Yi et al., 1993; Cao et al., 1993; Cao et al., 1995), enabled the creation of interleukin-2-receptor gamma-chain-deficient mice. Two types of mutations were generated—complete loss of the common cytokine receptor gamma chain (γ$_c$^{null}) (Cao et al., 1995; DiSanto et al., 1995) and deletion of its intracytoplasmic domain (γ$_c$-/-,(Ohbo et al., 1996; Ikebe et al., 1997; Sugamura et al., 1996). Further development of NOD/SCID animal models followed the addition of a (γ$_c$^{null}) mutation on NOD/ShiJic-*scid* background (NOG) (Ito et al., 2002) and by the realization of a NOD/LtSz-*scid* (NSG) (Shultz et al., 2005) rodent system at the Jackson Laboratories, Bar Harbor, Maine USA.

A genetic cross of γ$_c$^{null} or γ$_c$$^{-/-}$ with a (RAG2)-deficient strain has produced female mice doubly homozygous for the γc and RAG2 null alleles (γ$_c$$^{-/-}$/RAG2$^{-/-}$) (Goldman et al., 1998). These manipulations dramatically increased the utilities for "humanized mice" in a wide range of applications (Traggiai et al., 2004; Van Duyne et al., 2009; Gorantla, Sneller et al., 2007; Brehm et al., 2010). The rationale behind the creation of these doubly knockout mice reflects the fact that antigen recognition for B and T lymphocytes, respectively, is affected through the variable domains of immunoglobulin (Ig) or the T cell receptor (TCR) genes. Genes that encode the B and T cell receptors are assembled during the early stages of B and T lymphocyte differentiation from germline variable (V), diversity (D), and joining (J) regions that merge by a process referred to as V(D)J recombination. This recombination results in the expression of two lymphoid-specific recombination activating genes: RAG1 and RAG2. These genes are critical for cells to display V(D)J activity (Oettinger, 1996).

INTRACEREBRAL INJECTION OF HIV-1-INFECTED HUMAN MONOCYTE-DERIVED MACROPHAGES (MDM) AS A MODEL OF VIRAL ENCEPHALITIS (HIVE)

The discovery that HIV-1 persists in the resident brain macrophages and microglia (Gartner et al., 1986; Koenig et al., 1986) led to the idea that injecting human HIV-1-infected MDM into brains of CB-17/*scid* immunodeficient mice could reproduce the salient features of human neuropathology (Tyor et al., 1993). The reported histopathological findings in injected mice included a focal gliosis, MGC formation, and tumor necrosis factor alpha (TNF-α) expression. These findings were all sufficient to confirm that infected MDM are a primary driving force of HIV-1-mediated neuropathology. Nonetheless, the work failed to provide mechanisms for neuronal dysfunction.

The location of injected cells in the basal ganglia, the relevance of human macrophages as a primary cell type, the importance of viral infection and replication, neuronal damage due to traumatic injury, and xenoreactivity was subsequently developed (Persidsky et al., 1996). Due to significant similarities to human HIVE, the model allowed investigators to examine neuronal function with behavior testing. The multiple injection of HIV-infected macrophages (every month for 3 months to model a chronic state of infection) led to behavioral deficits and a decrease in motor abilities (by Morris water maze) when compared to controls and paralleled what has been seen in HIV-1 associated dementia (HAD) (Avgeropoulos et al., 1998). In a subsequent report, a single injection of HIV-1-infected MDM was found to impair spatial cognition and synaptic potentiation (Zink et al., 2002). Injection of infected MDM into the caudate and putamen of HIVE mice impaired synaptic function in the hippocampus and this impairment may be the underlying factor in cognitive dysfunction for HAD (Anderson et al., 2003). This model allowed investigation of the viral strain differences in viral neuropathogenesis (Nukuna et al., 2004). In these studies, and dependent on the viral strain, variable levels of neuroinflammatory reactions were elicited. The levels of neuropathologic changes, including microglial reactions, paralleled levels of viral infection and numbers of infected MDM. Later, the same model was used for direct comparison of neurotoxicity of two viral isolates—clade B and clade C—and confirmed the associations between neuroinflammation and HIV-1 strains (Rao et al., 2008). In the similar model (injection of human HIV-1-infected macrophages), were different strain of immunodeficient mice was used (C57bl/6-*scid*), the induction of type 1 interferon-α (IFN-α) expression in the brain was found. It is known that IFN-α can cause cognitive deficit. IFN-α levels in the brain correlated directly with working memory errors for diseased mice (Sas, Bimonte-Nelson, & Tyor, 2007).

Testing of adjunctive therapeutics has also received a boost with these murine disease models and has helped to guide clinical interventions. It was shown that dexamethasone therapy worsened HIV-1-associated neuropathology (Limoges et al., 1997) and as a result of these studies clinical investigations of dexamethasome were halted. The clinical observation that antiretroviral and anti-inflammatory therapy were able to reverse the most severe form of HAND, HAD (Gendelman et al. 1998) also greatly expanded potential therapeutic applications (Persidsky et al., 2001; Limoges et al., 2001; Limoges et al., 2000; Persidsky et al., 2001; Dou et al., 2003; Dou et al., 2005; Dou et al., 2006; Dou et al., 2007; Gorantla, Makarov, Roy et al.,

2010; Gorantla et al., 2008; Gorantla, Liu et al., 2007; Eggert et al., 2010; Eggert et al., 2009; Spitzenberger et al., 2007).

Translation of the rodent HIVE model from CB-17/*scid* to the newly developed backgrounds of NOD/*scid*, NOD/*scid*-γc*null* (NSG), or Balb/c-Rag2-/-γc-/- revealed that the absence of NK activity and the deficiency of macrophage functions [ability to secrete interleukin-1 (IL-1) and respond to interferon gamma (IFN-γ)] affected inflammatory reaction. Importantly, the levels of microglial and astrocyte activation as well as attraction of mouse peripheral macrophages were reduced in γc-deficient animals intracranially injected with human HIV-1-infected macrophages (unpublished observations). These animals compared to CB-17/*scid* mice revealed that transplantation of human PBL into the peritoneal cavity led to the spontaneous migration of human cells into the mouse brain as well as modest graft-versus-host disease (GVHD) (Gorantla, Makarov, Roy et al., 2010).

HIV-1-INFECTED HUMAN MDM INTRACRANIAL INJECTIONS AND PBL RECONSTITUTION (HU-PBL-HIVE)

Neuropathogenesis of HIV-1 infection-associated cognitive impairment has a strong correlation with efficacy of antiviral adaptive immune responses, the levels of activation of peripheral lymphoid system and CD4[+] cell decline (Munoz-Moreno et al., 2009), and the activation of brain microglia (Gendelman & Folks, 1999; Kraft-Terry et al., 2009). Activated CD8[+] cells and CD4[+] T cells are present in the CSF (Sadagopal et al., 2008) and perivascular cuffs of HIV-1 encephalitic brains (Katsetos et al., 1999; Coe et al., 1997; Singer et al., 1994), and are often found as scattering cells in white matter tracks (McCrossan et al., 2006). The neurological dysfunctions correlated with increased numbers of CD8[+] T cells in SIV-infected monkeys (McCrossan et al., 2006).

In order to find out the contribution of peripheral lymphocytes in HAND and assess adaptive immune responses for viral infection control in the brain, the next step was the combination of two procedures. First, reconstitution of NOD/*scid* mice with human PBL, second, transplantation of syngeneic HIV-1-infected macrophages into the brain (Poluektova et al., 2004; Poluektova et al., 2002). Such an hu-PBL-HIVE model showed that HIV-1-infected cells placed into the brain could induce cellular immune responses with an appearance of HIV-specific cytotoxic lymphocytes and low titer-specific antibodies in circulation (Gorantla et al., 2005). The presence of lymphocytes facilitates elimination of infected cells from the brain and the restoration of tissue integrity (Poluektova et al., 2004). The application of hu-PBL-HIVE mice allowed investigation of the effect of inhibition of indoleamine 2,3-dioxygenase (IDO). IDO activity is linked with immunosuppression by its ability to inhibit proliferation of cytotoxic T lymphocyte (CTL), and with neurotoxicity through the generation of quinolinic acid and other toxins. IDO is induced in macrophages by HIV-1 infection, and it is upregulated in macrophages in human brain tissue with HIVE. Using the hu-PBL-HIVE model, the ability of IDO inhibitor 1-methyl-d-tryptophan (1-MT) to stimulate the generation of CTL resulted in the clearance of virus-infected macrophages from the brain (Potula et al., 2005). In vivo findings obtained in this model underscored the ability of PPARγ agonists to reduce HIV-1 replication in lymphocytes and brain macrophages, thus offering a new therapeutic intervention in the brain and systemic infection (Potula et al., 2008).

An inherent problem was associated with the engraftment of hu-PBL into a mouse host. The GVHD was often observed when functional immune cells identified the host cells as foreign and subsequently initiated an immunologic response against the host. This response quickly spreads to become an established systemic attack, which results in the death of the host within 3–5 weeks. GVHD typically refers to the events associated with allogenic grafts and is not as well understood in xenogenic grafts. GVHD not only shortens the time window for experiments, it also can end up damaging brain tissue by in situ proliferating hu-PBL after injection of human macrophages as antigen-presenting cells (Poluektova, Gorantla, & Gendelman, 2004). The functionality of the surrogate "human immune system" is under scrutiny. The engrafted human T cells within the microenvironment of the mouse undergo significant phenotypic changes, such as losing naïve phenotype and ability to secrete IL-2 (Schneider & Gronvik, 1995), and upregulation of HLA-DR antigen expression and changes of the cell-surface markers is evident (Cao & Leroux-Roels, 2000). Moreover, the xenografted human T cells become anergic within the mouse, which suggests that *scid* mice, despite being able to support a human T cell system, may not always have a properly functional human immune system. Translation of this HIVE model from NOD/*scid* to the newly developed NSG backgrounds or Balb/c-Rag2-/-γ$_c$-/- revealed that in these more immune-deficient mice compared to CB-17/*scid* and NOD/*scid* mice, transplantation of human PBL into peritoneal cavity leads to their enhanced spontaneous migration into the mouse brain and results in GVH disease (Gorantla, Makarov, Roy et al., 2010).

TRUE "HUMANIZED" MICE

The long-term immune reconstitution of NSG mice by human HSC provides a new approach to study HAND. The major characteristics of these types of chimeric animals are: (1) the high rate of acceptance of human HSC; (2) stable population of mouse bone marrow; (3) occupancy of murine thymus with human thymocytes and their maturation in αβ, γδ, and regulatory T cells; (4) complete reconstitution of residual murine lymph nodes with human T, B, and dendritic cells; (5) formation of splenic white pulp (Figure 5.5.1); and (6) distribution of human cells of macrophage lineage throughout brain meninges and perivascular spaces (Figure 5.5.2). These "humanized" mice support chronic HIV-1 replication and recapitulate the course of human disease progression with loss of CD4[+] cells, development of HIV-1-specific CTL, and humoral antiviral immune

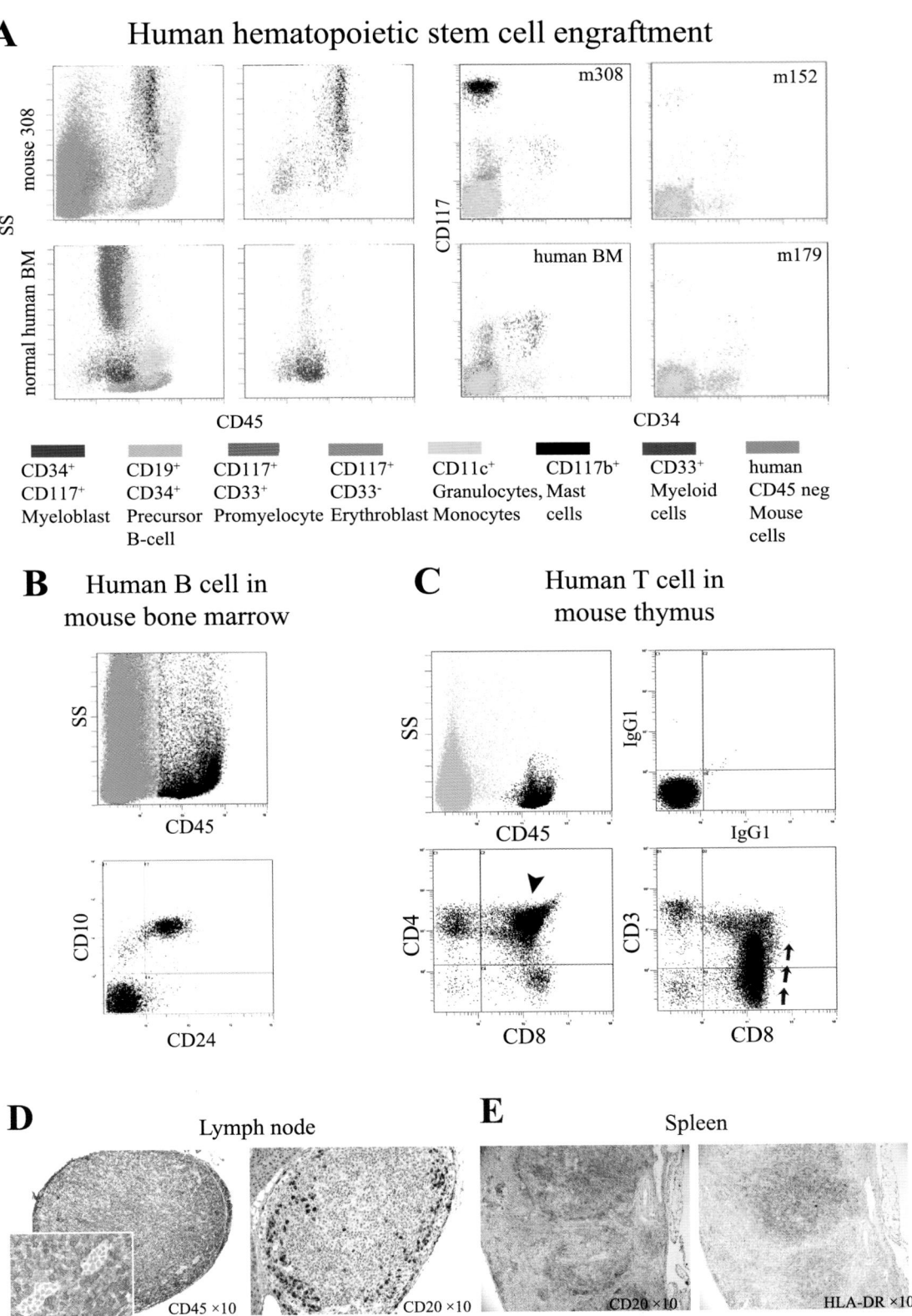

A Human hematopoietic stem cell engraftment

CD34+ CD117+ Myeloblast | CD19+ CD34+ Precursor B-cell | CD117+ CD33+ Promyelocyte | CD117+ CD33- Erythroblast | CD11c+ Granulocytes, Monocytes | CD117b+ Mast cells | CD33+ Myeloid cells | human CD45 neg Mouse cells

B Human B cell in mouse bone marrow

C Human T cell in mouse thymus

D Lymph node

CD45 ×10   ×40   CD20 ×10

E Spleen

CD20 ×10   HLA-DR ×10

Figure 5.5.1 Humanized mouse hematolymphoid tissues. Representative FACS panels of bone marrow (*A, B*), thymus (*C*), and immunohistological analysis of lymph node (*D*) and spleen (*E*). *A*, Human bone marrow (BM) cell subset distributions in engrafted mice compared to normal human BM. CD34+CD117+ myeloblasts, promyelocytes, erythroblasts, and B-cell precursors were detected. *B*, Plots demonstrate phenotypically normal appearing human B-cell precursors. These precursors are CD10, CD19, and CD24 positive and show differentiation (arrows) to mature B cells as evidenced by a loss of CD10 expression and a decrease in CD24 antigen density. *C*, Plots demonstrate that the majority of human cells isolated represent CD4 and CD8 dual positive common thymocytes (arrowhead) and there is generation of both CD4 and CD8 single positive, mature T cells with the characteristic increase in thymocyte CD3 density (arrows) that occurs during thymic maturation/selection. (Courtesy of Professor Samuel J. Pirruccelo, UNMC.) *D* and *E*, Representative sections from paraffin-embedded lymph nodes and spleen of "humanized" animal stained for human CD45, HLA-DR, and CD20 markers show fully populated nodule and splenic white pulp cells with lymphocyte, B cells and dendritic cell morphology (brown). Insert on CD45 lymph node panel shows high endothelial venules. Sections were counterstained with hematoxylin.

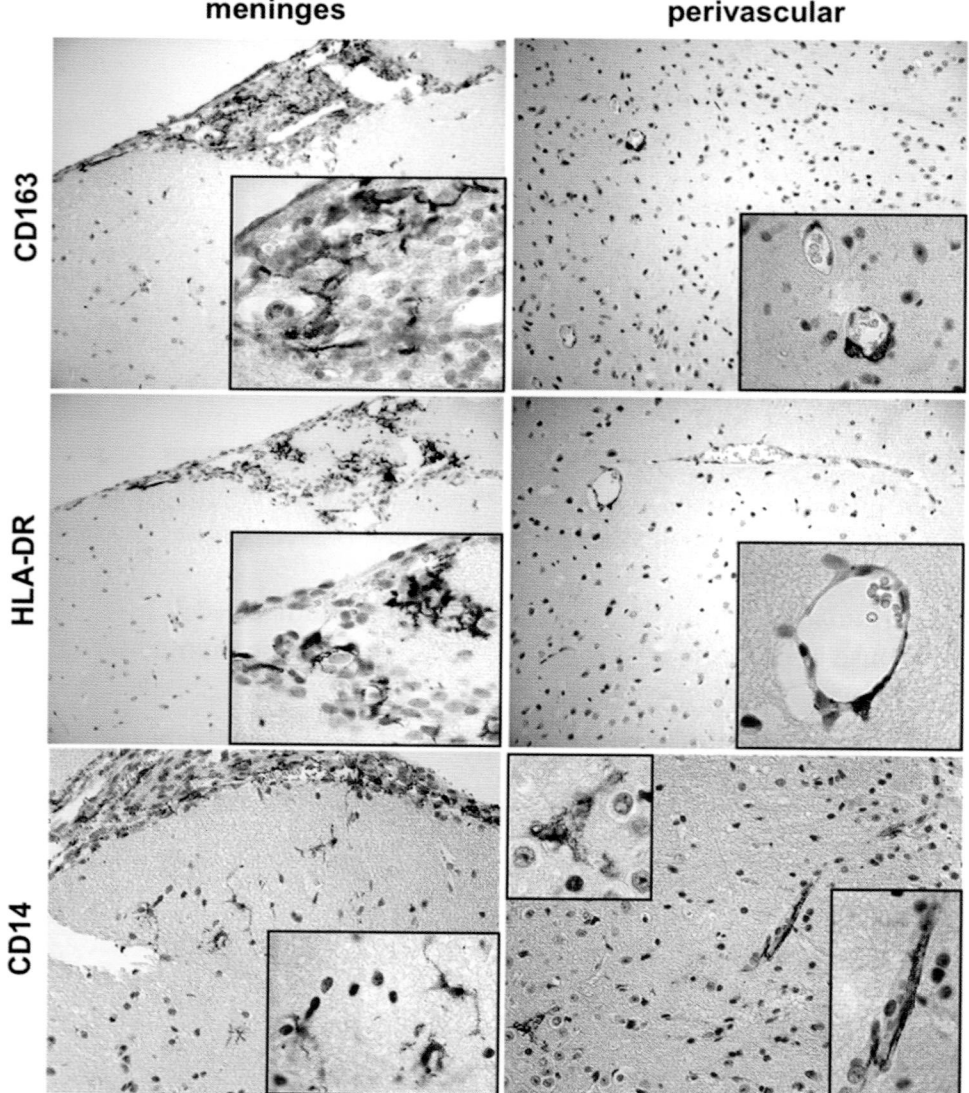

Figure 5.5.2 Human cells in meninges and brain perivascular spaces. Representative sections from paraffin-embedded brain of uninfected control animal stained for human CD163, HLA-DR, and CD14 markers show cells with macrophage, microglia, and dendritic cell morphology (brown). Sections were counterstained with hematoxylin. Original magnification × 200; Insets magnification × 1000.

responses (Watanabe, Terashima et al., 2007; Gorantla, Makarov, Finke-Dwyer et al., 2010; Brainard et al., 2009).

We investigated whether CNS pathologies could be seen in HIV-1-infected humanized mice. Several notable observations were made in regard to human cells infiltration, progressive HIV-1 infection, microglial activation and nodules formation, as well as the consequences of CD8+ cell depletion. The productive peripheral infection accelerated the entry of human cells (activated HLA-DR+ lymphocytes and macrophages) into the brain. This was seen by immunostaining for human CD163 and HLA-DR+ cells and by the expression of human HLA-DQ by real-time PCR. HIV-1 p24+ cells with macrophage and lymphocyte morphology in the meninges and perivascular spaces were observed. CD8+ T cell depletion initiated by cM-T807 antibodies two or five-seven weeks *post* infection accelerated the disease course, increased blood viral load, and resulted in increased HIV-1*gag* RNA and inducible nitric oxide syntase (iNOS) expression in the brain. The development of a meningitis and rarely meningoencephalitis was observed (Figure 5.5.3). These findings, taken together, demonstrated natural progression of virus-associated CNS disease in "humanized" rodents (Gorantla, Makarov, Finke-Dwyer et al., 2010).

FUTURE USE OF "HUMANIZED" MICE

The following need to be considered in further refinements of "humanized" mice for HAND: (1) the molecular pathways of HIV-1-related protein's toxicity. These may be different between human and mouse neurons, astrocytes, and microglia (Baumann et al., 2004). (2) Cross-reactivity between

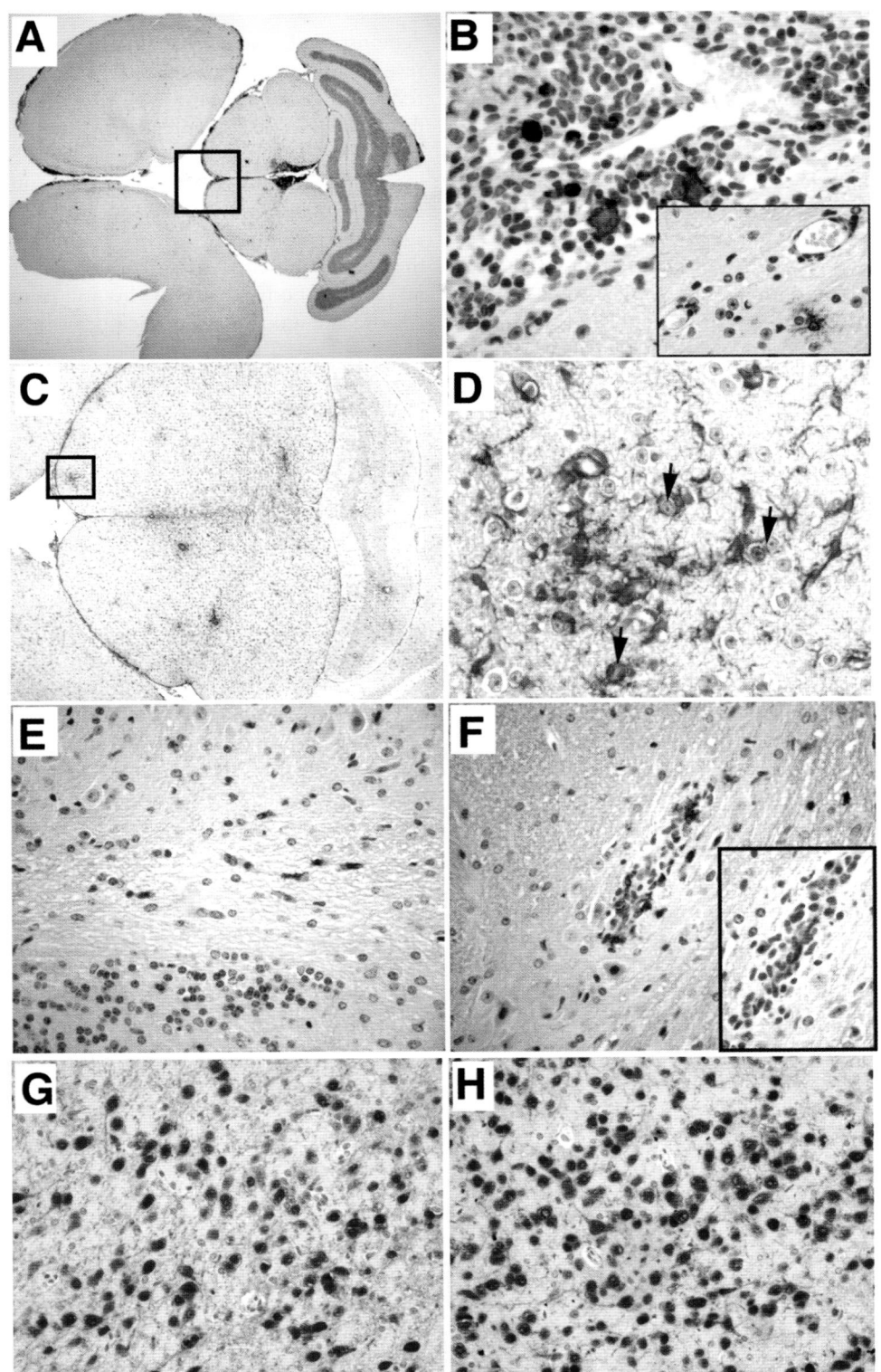

Figure 5.5. 3 Meningoencephalitis in HIV-1-infected and CD8$^+$ cell-depleted mice. Horizontal brain sections of a 29-week-old mouse #305 infected for 8 weeks and CD8$^+$ cell-depleted for 3 weeks is shown. Sections were stained for (*A*) human HLA-DR, (*B*) HIV-1p24 antigen and (*C* and *D*) mouse astrocytes (GFAP, Permanent Red) and microglia (Iba-1, DAB), (*E* and *F*) human CD8$^+$ cells, and the inset is the adjacent section stained for HIV-1p24, and (*G* and *H*) neuronal nuclear protein (NeuN, DAB) and MAP-2 (Permanent Red). Panel *A* shows accumulation of human cells in meninges and periaqueductal structures. Panel *B* represents magnified views of selected area on the adjacent section stained for viral protein showing viral cytopathic effects, perivascular-infected cells, and infected cells with microglial morphology. Panel *C* shows diffused activation of astrocytes and microglia, perivascular cuffs, and *D* is a magnified view of selected region showing activated phagocytizing microglial cells (arrows). Panels *E* and *F* show scattering CD8$^+$ cells in cerebellar white matter tracts (*E*) and perivascular infiltration of CD8$^+$ cells near HIV-1 p24 infected cell (*F* and inset). Panel *G* and *H* represent neuronal density in periaqueductal gray matter in the same mouse and in control reconstituted animal of the same age, respectively. Sections were counterstained with hematoxylin. Magnifications: *A* × 1, *B* × 20, inset × 400, *C* × 4, *D* × 400, *E, F* and inset × 400, *G* and *H* × 20.

human and mouse cytokine/chemokine receptor/ligand systems may preclude direct translation of "cytokine storm effects" generated by human HIV-1-infected cells in the murine cells (Mestas & Hughes 2004). (3) The molecular arrangements of human cell migration in the murine environment (Stefanidakis et al., 2008). (4) The maturation of the human immune system in a mouse requires ~6 months of time. The environmental pressure and T and B cell receptor repertoire development may be affected together with the profile and function of human lymphocytes. The nature of xenotransplantation makes it difficult to find a compromise between human versus mouse thymic environment for T and B cell repertoire development. In mice transplanted at birth with HSC, humoral and cellular immune responses are present but limited (Shultz et al., 2005; Watanabe, Terashima et al., 2007; Gorantla, Makarov, Finke-Dwyer et al., 2010). The use of NSG mice transplanted with fetal liver/thymus placed under the kidney capsule following intravenous infusion of HSC (BLT) shows promise (Brainard et al., 2009). These mice are arguably at an increased risk of GVH disease following maturation of *human* cells in *human* thymus. Selection of *human* cells in *mouse thymus* may be advantageous. A minor limitation is the requirement of low-dose irradiation for the HSC engraftments (Gamis & Nesbit, 1991; Devi, Hossain, & Bisht, 1999; Martin et al., 2001). The approach, however, reduces the ability of mice to develop a spatial memory (unpublished observations).

Recent observation showed that reconstitution can be achieved without irradiation (Watanabe, Ohta et al., 2007), or chemical myeloablation (Gorantla, Sneller et al., 2007). This provides a new opportunity to avoid functional memory deficits. Moreover, longer survival time of humanized animals will help to address issues of combining aging with chronic HIV-1 replication as two synergistic contributors in neurodegeneration. Lastly, the mechanisms for neuronal functional deficits and neurodegeneration require greater exploration. Nonetheless, and on balance, the recapitulation of brain inflammatory reactions and neuronal functional aberrations caused as a consequence of HIV-1 infection in humanized mice provides new opportunities for studies of disease pathobiology and for therapeutic testing and developments which will certainly see greater applications in the months and years ahead. This is a significant advance in the field, no doubt.

HIV PROVIRAL DNA AND SUBGENOMIC VIRAL FRAGMENT TRANSGENIC MICE

Mice have never been permissive for HIV-1 infection, so in order to study pathogenesis of disease, including neurologic complications, several approaches were used. One of them was the injection of viral genome into mouse germlines. A viral construct derived from the infectious molecular plasmids pNL4–3 was used to create transgenic mice (Leonard et al. 1988). During investigation, one of the seven founder mice (No. 13), which transmitted the HIV proviral DNA to its offspring, produced serum antibodies to virus as monitored by enzyme-linked immunosorbent assay. Immunoblotting demonstrated reactivity with the gpl20 envelope and p64 reverse transcriptase proteins of HIV. Southern blot analyses revealed that female mouse No. 13 contained two copies of proviral DNA at one integration site. Successive mating of mouse No. 13 with nontransgenic FVB/N males resulted in litters that developed a characteristic and fatal clinical syndrome in 45% of the pups. At approximately 10 to 14 days of age, affected F1 progeny were readily distinguishable from their unaffected littermates by their small size (approximately 50–80% of body weight of the non-transgenic littermates). All affected animals either died or were killed by siblings by 25 days of age. The major histologic abnormalities were found in the skin and lung. The introduction of the HIV provirus into the germline of mice bypasses the early events in the virus' life cycle including the binding of the particles to their receptor, the human CD4 molecule; a spreading infection in the newborn mice, unlikely in the absence of human CD4, cannot account for the abnormalities observed. Authors suggested that the synthesis of very small amounts of viral proteins or progeny particles may be sufficient to elicit the production of cellular proteins, which cause deleterious effects. Low-level HIV expression in macrophages might deregulate the synthesis or secretion of factors mediating chemotaxis, inflammation, or cell growth and result in the fatal disease observed. If the transgenic mice are not tolerant to HIV proteins, the observed splenomegaly and lymphadenopathy could be the result of a chronic immune response to the persistent production of viral proteins. Transgenic mice such as these are useful for studying the pathogensis of HIV-related diseases in man. Regrettably, these models were not useful for neuropathogenesis, because there was no detectable viral protein expression in the brain, nor were pathologic findings reported.

Transgenic mice bearing single or multiple HIV-1 genes have proven to be helpful in defining the tissue-specific pathological role of HIV-1 gene products, independent of immune deficiency or immunosuppression. Dickie and co-authors (Dickie et al. 1991) produced transgenic mice that bore copies of a defective HIV provirus. Five transgenic lines of mice were derived from four constructs: intact HIV-1 proviral DNA under the control of the HIV-1 long terminal repeat (LTR) or a chimeric HIV-1/MMTV LTR, a *gag-pol* deleted genome (a 3.1-kb deletion was made in the pNL4–3 HIV proviral genomic construct spanning HIV-1 gag and pol from bp 1443 to 4551), and the Nef gene. Transgenic mice variably expressed 6-, 4.3-, and 2-kb HIV-specific RNAs and HIV-related polypeptides in several tissues. The transgenic offspring from three independently derived mouse lines (Tg22c, Tg25, and Tg26) manifested renal disease associated with proteinuria, a high mortality rate, and HIV-specific gene expression in the kidney. Tg26 heterozygotes survived long enough to generate offspring and were sustained through heterozygous breeders. Despite the intrinsic limitations of HIV-1 Tat activity in rodent cells, the mRNA expression of HIV in the Tg26 model was readily detected in skin, skeletal muscle, and kidneys. Expression was also weakly detected in brain, eye, gastrointestinal tract, spleen, and thymus. Although transgene expression is one determinant of host cellular responses, it is the relative abundance of spliced or unspliced HIV mRNA that determines which gene products will be made in a particular cell type. In the Tg26 model, the unspliced message was readily detected in lymphoid tissue (thymus and spleen) and kidney while multiple spliced messages predominated in the other tissues (Bruggeman et al., 1994). Unfortunately, when tissue-specific factors that may be important in HIV-1 transcriptional and post-transcriptional regulation were explored in a mouse model containing a mutant provirus deleted in the *gag* and *pol* region, the brain analysis was not included (Bruggeman et al., 1994). In the similar model (*gag-pol* deletion mutant of the HIV-1 provirus pNL4–3), the brain expression was not detected (Santoro et al., 1994). When 2-, 4-, or 7-kb (full-length) mRNA species were calculated as a percentage of the total mRNA, two phenotypes of distribution were detected. Lymphoid tissue (thymus and spleen) and kidney had significantly greater amounts of unspliced Tat-coding RNA messages regardless of the level of expression. All other tissues expressed the multiple spliced messages encoding Tat, Rev, and Nef predominantly. The marked tissue-dependent patterns of HIV mRNA expression suggest a potential mechanism for the organ-specific manifestations of AIDS. These models made significant steps forward in understanding HIV-1-related nephrotoxicity (Lu, He, & Klotman, 2006; Rosenstiel et al., 2009), but not brain pathology. Mice that are transgenic for a full-length HIV-1 genome, with a deletion in *pol*, acquired the development of cataracts at 3–6 mo of age (Iwakura et al., 1992). Although accumulation of the Gag protein was also detected in the skin and brain, no apparent abnormality was observed in these tissues.

Transgenic mice expressing the full HIV genome under a CD4 promoter were designed to restrict expression solely to immune cells (Hanna et al., 1998). The human CD4 gene promoter sequences flanked by the enhancer of the mouse CD4 gene were used to express the whole HIV-1 coding sequences in Tg mice. A surrogate gene was expressed specifically in CD4$^+$ CD8$^+$ and CD4$^+$ CD8$^-$ thymic T cells, in peripheral CD4$^+$ CD8$^-$ T cells, and in macrophages. Expression of HIV-1 with this promoter mimic closely the expression of HIV-1 detected in HIV-1-infected individuals and indeed these Tg mice develop a severe AIDS-like disease, which was dependent on the levels of HIV-1 expression. Unfortunately, neither expression in the brain nor neuropathology was found.

The inability of murine cyclin T1 to associate with Tat during the formation of a complex with TAR RNA required for efficient transcription drive the generation of human cycline T1 transgenic mice. Hu-cycT1 transgenic mice were generated using a murine CD4 expression cassette encoding human cyclin T1 predicted to target transgene expression to CD4 T lymphocytes, macrophages, and dendritic cells. Expression of human cyclin T1 by the mouse cells rescued Tat function and permitted Tat-mediated transactivation of the HIV-1 LTR (Kwak et al., 1999). The effect of expression of the JR-CSF transgene combined with CD4-targeted expression of the human cyclin T1 gene in mouse lines transgenic for a full-length infectious proviral clone of a monocyte-tropic HIV-1 isolate, HIV-1$_{JR-C SF}$ (Paul et al., 2000) was studied (Sun et al., 2006; Sun et al., 2008). CD4 T lymphocytes and

myeloid lineage cells from these double-transgenic JR-CSF/hu-cycT1 mice displayed markedly increased HIV production compared to that of the JR-CSF mice. While mice did not have any sign of brain pathology, microglia and astrocytes in the brains of JR-CSF/hu-cycT1 mice displayed increased in vivo activation and CCL2/monocyte chemoattractant protein (MCP-1) production in response to lipopolysaccharide (LPS). The level of HIV production induced by granulocyte-macrophage colony-stimulating factor (GM-CSF) in the brains of JR-CSF/hu-cycT1 mice was almost twofold higher than the levels induced by GM-CSF in the brains of JR-CSF littermates. Despite inflammatory reaction induced by LPS and GM-CSF, neuronal abnormalities were not reported in these animals.

HIV transgenic mouse models can determine how different cell types and tissue compartments contribute to the overall disease process. In a natural infection, HIV-1 is highly productive at infecting lymphocytes, macrophages/dendritic cells, but does not efficiently and productively infect astrocytes (Trillo-Pazos et al., 2003; Wang et al., 2008), neurons (Pumarola-Sune et al., 1987; Nuovo et al., 1994; Ensoli, Ensoli, & Thiele, 1994; Torres-Munoz, Nunez, & Petito, 2008), endothelial cells (Bagasra et al., 1996), or oligodendrocytes (Gyorkey, Melnick, & Gyorkey, 1987) (reviewed in Bissel & Wiley, 2004). The nervous system can be affected by HIV-1 not only through the infected infiltrating lymphocytes and macrophages. Several tissue-specific expression models have been designed to study how expression of viral proteins in each cellular compartment (neurons, astrocytes, oligodendrocytes) individually will affect brain and peripheral nervous system.

A large proportion of patients with AIDS develop peripheral neuropathy, which has become the chief neurological syndrome in individuals infected with HIV-1 (reviewed in de Freitas, 2007). Transgenic mice that express the HIV genome in neurons under the transcriptional control of a neurofilament promoter were generated to elucidate the mechanisms of peripheral neuropathy (Thomas et al., 1994). The DNA construct used to generate the transgenic mice consisted of three fragments: the 5' upstream regulatory sequences of the gene for the human neurofilament subunit NF-L, which has been previously used to direct specific expression into cells of neuronal lineage; the entire open reading frame of the HIV genome, from which the 5' long terminal repeat, part of the 3' long terminal repeat, and part of the untranslated leader sequences were deleted; and the simian virus 40 polyadenylation signal. HIV RNA was detected in large motor neurons in the anterior horn of the spinal cord and brainstem motor neurons, in the anterior thalamic neurons, but not white matter tracks, when analyzed by in situ hybridization in combination with staining for neurophilaments. Viral RNA was not detected in dorsal root ganglia, peripheral nerve, thymus and spleen tissues, striated muscle, kidney, liver, and salivary gland tissues. HIV proteins were present in thalamic and spinal cord extract only. There was no evidence of inflammatory infiltrates, gliosis, vacuolation, or myelin abnormalities in brain or spinal cord tissue of any of the transgenic or control animals as assessed by semithin sections, the hematoxylin and eosin stain, and the Kluver-Barrera method. No differences between transgenic and control animals were detected in brain and spinal cord tissues by immunohistochemistry with antibodies to glial fibrillary acidic protein, neurofilaments, tyrosine-phosphorylated proteins, or ubiquitin. The neurobehavioral examination on the narrow suspension bar showed that transgenic mice fell more often and more quickly than controls and had less spontaneous activity in the T maze and the wooden box. However, the motor weakness and hypoactivity deficits were specific to the task and not indicative of a generalized neurological dysfunction. To explore the functional peripheral nerve deficit, the sciatic nerve was supramaximally stimulated at the sciatic notch, and the compound muscle action potential (CMAP) was recorded from the intrinsic foot muscles. Electrophysiological examination revealed a 30% reduction in the amplitude of the negative phase of the CMAP, consistent with a reduction in the number of functioning motor axons and indicating an impairment of nerve conduction.

Abnormalities were found in the nerves of 50% of all transgenic mice exhibiting a neurodegenerative phenotype at 7–12-months of age. In semithin sections, abnormal nerves showed a mild to moderate reduction in nerve fiber density and evidence of axonal degeneration. Fibers with thin myelin sheaths relative to axon caliber occurred in increased numbers. Due to the low frequency of pathologic findings, this model has not yet been used efficiently.

Vacuolar myelopathy (VM) in transgenic mice expressing complete HIV-1 genome under the regulation of the myelin basic protein gene promoter in oligodendrocytes (MBP/HIV^wt^) is similar to the expression of a single HIV-1 gene, *nef*, in oligodendrocytes (MBP/HIV^Nef^) (Goudreau et al., 1996; Radja et al., 2003). Histological examination of mouse spinal cords revealed a much higher incidence of pathology with vacuolar changes evident in the anterior and lateral, but rarely in the dorsal funiculi, in more than 70% of the Tg animals from four distinct Tg lines assessed. Despite robust Tg expression throughout the brain, vacuolation in brain white matter tracts was infrequently observed. None of these models have yet found their application in the neuroAIDS field.

TRANSGENIC MURINE MODELS BASED ON CELL-TYPE SPECIFIC SINGLE HIV-1 PROTEIN EXPRESSION

Tat Story

In 1988, Frankel and Pabo observed that the exogenous addition of a full-length 86-amino acid HIV-1 TAT protein to cells in culture resulted in cell membrane penetration and *trans*-activation of the HIV-1 promoter (Frankel & Pabo, 1988). Subsequent experimentation delineated the requirements for protein translocation and defined a small basic region spanning residues 49 to 58 of HIV-1 TAT responsible for cellular uptake (Vives, Brodin, & Lebleu, 1997). Tat is a transactivator of HIV-1 viral transcription, interacting with

the transactivation response element (TAR), located at the 5' end of all HIV-1 mRNAs. TAR-independent activity of Tat may be the result of cytokine activation. The direct involvement of Tat with damage to the CNS was suggested after the death of mice injected intracerebrally with a peptide representing the basic domain of Tat (reviewed in Rappaport et al., 1999; King et al., 2006).

Several models were made to study effects of systemic Tat protein expression. The introduction of the HIV *tat* gene under the control of the cellular proteolipoprotein promoter into the germline of mice demonstrated that, when expressed, the *tat* gene product induces lymphoid hyperplasia in spleen, lymph nodes, and lung, as is observed in AIDS patients, but was not expressed in the brain. During a long-term follow-up, all of the transgenic mice remained as healthy as their nontransgenic littermates housed in the same cages, as assessed by body weight, growth development, fertility, and life span. This observation suggested that despite the lymphoid disorders they developed, the transgenic animals were still able to resist a conventional antigen (Vellutini et al., 1994). It was completely different from the neurotoxicity (loss of ependymal cells and gray matter neurons) induced by direct infusion/injection of Tat protein in mouse brain (Philippon et al., 1994). When the TAT72 transgene (1–72 amino acids) was placed under the control of SV40 viral promoter to provide systemic expression (Garza, Prakash, & Carr, 1994), only T and NK cell functions were affected. The neurologic abnormalities were not reported (Garza, Prakash, & Carr, 1994). The transgenic mice in which HIV-1 Tat was expressed under the control of a chicken β-actin promoter; T cells, B cells, and monocytes contained Tat transcripts in readily detectable amounts, as well as in the brain (Kundu et al., 1999). Observation up to 15 months of age did not manifest any neurologic abnormalities to be reported (Choi et al., 2000).

Altogether, data drives the development of a Tat transgenic model targeting the brain specifically. A Tet-on system that uses a reverse tTA element (rtTA), which only becomes transcriptionally active when tetracycline or its derivatives such as doxycycline (Dox) were applied. The HIV-1 HXB2 Tat cDNA (86 amino acids in length) was used. Tet-on-GFAP transgene was crossbred with TRE-Tat86 transgene to obtain the Dox-regulated, brain-targeted Tat bigenic mice (Kim et al., 2003). After initiation of Dox treatment at 21 days of age for a 2-week period, growth failure, hunched posture, tremor, ataxia, hindlimb weakness, slow motor and cognitive movement, seizures, and finally death of all mice who survived the treatment period by 3 months of age were reported. Presumably dose-dependent accumulation of Tat protein induced complete collapse of the cerebellum, progressive loss of the cortex, significant vacuolation in the brain, and significant neuronal and dendritic changes in cerebellar, cortical, and hippocampal neurons. The apoptotic neurons appeared to be in a close proximity to Tat-positive regions including cerebellum, cortex, and hippocampus. Although inflammation (encephalitis or meningitis) was only occasionally observed, hydroencephalitis or edema was often present. The considerable increases in CD14-, CD4-, and CD8-positive cells, but fewer changes in CD68-positive cells, were found in the brain. The lymphocyte infiltration was associated with increased expression of interferon-γ. The damage observed after direct infusion/injection of Tat protein was reproduced in these mice. When Tat-transgenic mice were crossed with GFAP-null animals to determine the role of GFAP expression in Tat-induced pathologies, the significant increase in Tat accumulation in the brain and the attenuation of Tat-induced neurotoxicity was found (Zou et al., 2007). It was not associated with differences in astrocyte numbers. Such unpredicted findings raised the question about Tat toxicity associated with possible protein-protein interaction and functional role of secreted GFAP as intermediate filaments involved in gliosome formation and excretion (Bertelli et al., 2000); (Milanese et al., 2009).

Another brain-restricted, inducible transgenic mouse was created by crossing mice expressing the Tat gene (Tat1–86; HIV-1 IIIB) under the control of TRE with mice engineered to express a GFAP promoter-driven RTTA. Pure transgenic lines were derived by crossing homologous lines containing both the GFAP-RTTA and TRE-Tat genes (Bruce-Keller et al., 2008). To prevent fatal toxicity these animals were treated for only 2 days with Dox. Two days of Dox administration caused robust inductions of Tat mRNA expression in the cortex, striatum, and hippocampus of Tat(+) mice, without noticeable regional variation. It increased GFAP expression (astrogliosis), but not the proportion of F4/80- or Mac-1-positive cells of macrophage lineage. Moreover, the proportion of 3-nitrotyrosine [3-NT, a relatively specific marker of oxidative damage mediated by peroxynitrite, which is formed by the reaction of superoxide with nitric oxide (NO) on tyrosine residues in proteins or by reaction of nitrite and hydrogen peroxide-positive macrophages/microglia was not changed in Dox-treated animals. The direct neuronal toxicity of Tat was confirmed by finding an increased number of caspase-3-positive and, surprisingly, by the invariable number of TUNEL-positive (apoptotic) neurons in these mice (Bruce-Keller et al., 2008).

The significant differences in the range of neuropathology induced by systemic expression of Tat alone or in combination with other viral proteins (none) to strong toxicity mimicking direct injection of Tat protein (death) raised suspicions that such models reproduced free Tat protein toxicity, which might have different mechanisms such as cell-penetrating properties (Hervé, Ghinea, & Scherrmann, 2008), not directly related to HIV-1 induced neurologic complications.

Vpr Story

Vpr expression was also linked to the macrophage-specific murine exon 2 c-fms (M-CSF receptor) promoter in novel transgenic mouse lines (Jones et al., 2007). Vpr colocalized with F4/80 immunoreactivity, suggesting it was expressed principally in activated monocytoid cells in both perivascular and parenchymal regions. Vpr expression was highest in the cortex and basal ganglia, likely reflecting higher densities of microglia and perivascular macrophages in these regions (Lawson et al., 1990; Perry & Lawson, 1992). Three representative neuronal proteins, GAD65 (GABAergic neurons), VAChT (cholinergic

neurons), and synaptophysin (SYN, most synapses) in the brains of Tg and Wt animals were analyzed by Western blotting, revealing that all three neuronal proteins were reduced in the basal ganglia of Vpr Tg animals. However, the relative expression of GAD65 and VAChT was similar in the cerebral cortices of Vpr Tg animals when compared with wild type controls. Conversely, relative SYN levels were significantly higher in the Tg animal cortices. The following transcriptional changes were observed in the basal ganglia of transgenic animals: significantly lower transcript levels for the astrocyte-specific glutamate transporters EAAT1 and EAAT2 in the basal ganglia; and significantly reduced transcript levels for the neurotrophic molecules, IGF-1 and BDNF. Similarly, GFAP transcript levels were significantly reduced in both the cortex and basal ganglia of Vpr-transgenic animals compared to their wild-type littermate controls. The levels of the excitatory amino acid aspartate did not show a significant difference between transgenic animals and wild-type controls. Similarly, levels of glutamate were significantly higher in both cortex and basal ganglia of transgenic animals. A quantitative assay of motor activity revealed lower maximal levels of activity as well as reduced total levels of activity over the 45-min experimental period. Moreover, four-month-old Vpr transgenic animals appeared to be significantly more hyperexcitable compared to the wild type mice in three behavioral tests: the inverted screen test at 20 and 40 cm and the horizontal bar test. These observations highlighted the neurodegenerative changes mediated by Vpr at a molecular level in the absence of an inflammatory reaction in the brains of transgenic animals at one year of age (Noorbakhsh et al., 2010).

The in vivo expression of Vpr in the brains of mice failed to enhance both pro-inflammatory gene expression and macrophage activation, but highlighted the importance of astrocyte malfunction, independent of macrophage involvement, for neurodegeneration.

Env Story

As with the Tat protein story, the idea of an Env protein-based transgenic model came from the discovered in vivo neurotoxicity as a result of a subcutaneous (contrary to intracerebral Tat) injection of a small amount of gp-120 (Hill et al., 1993). In addition to the known in vitro toxicity of gp-120, authors observed developmental neurobehavior abnormalities. By day 3, gp120-treated rat pups took over 6 times longer to surface correctly in comparison to controls and had a delay in the first response of both forelimb placing and hindlimb placing. In the negative geotaxis test, gp120-treated pups responded significantly more slowly on day 6 than saline-treated pups. While simple behavior reflexes were preserved, more complex motor skills were retarded (Hill et al., 1993).

To achieve a brain-specific expression, the env gene of HIV-1$_{LAV}$ truncated to encode gp120 amino acids 1–509 was inserted into exon 1 of the modified murine GFAP gene. GFAP-gp-120 constructs were injected into fertilized murine (B6xSJL) oocytes (Toggas et al., 1994). The highest expression of gp-120 (in situ hybridization) was found in the neocortex, olfactory bulb, hippocampus, tectum, selected white matter tracts, and along the glia limitans. As in many other cases of transgenic expression of HIV-1 proteins (exception was Tat), Env protein well expressed in vitro in the C6 astrocytoma cell line was not found in vivo. The histologic evaluation performed on 1.5–2.5-month-old mice showed a dose-dependent (levels of RNA expression) reduction of neuropil-occupied areas in the cortex and hippocampus and expanded areas occupied by GFAP and F4/80 antigens. Vacuolizations of dendrites and a decrease in synapto-dendritic complexity along with a significant (40%) loss of large pyramidal neurons in the cortex was evident in the brains of 4-month-old animals. To explore potential functional alterations in neurons of gp120 tg mice and to determine if gp120 could alter synaptic plasticity, hippocampal slices from these animals were examined for changes in paired-pulse facilitation (PPF), short-term potentiation (STP), and long-term potentiation (LTP). They had reducedLTP in CA1, whereas both STP and PPF are enlarged, changes that may reflect physiological correlates of the histopathological alterations in this model. These animals with the highest levels of gp-120 transgene expression were analyzed at 1.5–2 mo of age (Krucker et al., 1998). It was the first model that successfully demonstrated neurotoxic effects of very low concentration (non-measurable) of HIV-1 envelope protein specifically expressed in the brain without any significant peripheral abnormalities and the absence of possible peripheral immune reaction (tolerance compared to other HIV-1 proteins constitutively expressed in transgenic mice?) to the brain-expressed foreign protein.

The transgenic mouse models carrying the HIV-1 *env* genes gp 120 and gp 41 (gp 160) under the control of the human light neurofilament (NFLgp160-Xba) and murine heavy neurofilament (NFHgp160) promoters were created later (Berrada et al., 1995; Michaud et al., 2001). To date, only in these murine models the expression of HIV-1 envelope protein was detected in neurons by immunohistochemistry performed with anti-gp41, anti-gp120, and human serum containing anti-HIV-1 antibodies. The Env products encoded by the transgenes were similar to the native moieties with respect to their processing (gp120 and gp41) and biological function (syncitia formation by transduced CD4+ HeLa cells). All mice maintained for 15 months have remained healthy regardless of copy number expression (1–30 full-length copies per haploid genome). Mice with a higher level of *env* mRNA expression in the cerebellum brainstem, lower in the forebrain, but not any other ectopic tissues, were analyzed for neuropathology. The most brain regions, which were shown in other studies to display perikaryal neurofilament immunoreactivity in normal adult mice, were also immunopositive for Env proteins in NFLgp160Xba and NFHgp160 transgenic mice, with the notable exception of the cerebral and cerebellar cortices. Morphologic evaluation and motor function of 3–4-month-old animals demonstrated no differences between the transgenic and the control. Numerous small abnormal dendritic swellings were found in and around the most intensely stained motor nuclei, such as the motor trigeminal and the facial nuclei. They were also present in the anterior gray horn of the spinal cord. Interestingly, these dendritic swellings were not stained with antibodies against

the phosphorylated neurofilament triplet or with the modified Bielschowsky method, which suggests that the neurofilaments were not involved in these changes. Minor axonal swellings were also observed in a region corresponding to the nucleus gracilis and to the gracilis and cuneate fascicles in the medulla and spinal cord, indicated that the Env proteins were axonally transported. Besides these neuritic changes, the GFAP reaction suggested early reactive astrocytosis in several areas of the CNS. This was particularly evident around or close to the immunoreactive structures in the brainstem and spinal cord (Berrada et al., 1995). Investigation of neuropathology in NFHgp160 transgenic mice at 3 and 12 months of age revealed accumulation of damaged neuronal structures, gliosis, and microglial reactivity with brain infiltration by immune cells. At 3 months of age, NFHgp160 transgenic mice had some evidence of a disturbance in distribution and/or size of the synapses. Synaptophysin immunostaining showed grain irregularities when compared to controls and occasional aggregates of larger grains were also present. The MAP-2 was also found slightly augmented for the transgenic animals in each sampled CNS area, but it reached statistical significance only in the cortex. By ultrastructure, at 3 months of age the initial lesion was a segmental watery degeneration of the neuronal dendritic tree. Its enhancement with some cytoskeletal markers (NF-a, NF-n, for example) without ultrastructural abnormalities of the cytoskeleton at that stage suggested a prefibrillogenesis derangement. At 12 months of age, the transgenic mice demonstrated chronic perivascular inflammation in the leptomeninges of the spinal cord and brainstem and also in the cerebellar white matter. The anterior gray horns of the spinal cord and the cranial nerve nuclei 5, 7, and 12 showed mild neuronal loss, with occasional degenerated or retracted acidophilic neurons. Beyond the watery dendritic and axonal changes, the morphometric analysis with the MAP-2 protein and the SYN immunostaining patterns suggested an increased density of the neuronal projections along with irregularities of synapses. Moreover, the neuronal loss became obvious at 12 months of age as degenerating neurons were observed by conventional histology. The gliosis that was already detected at 3 months by conventional histological and immunohistochemical techniques and confirmed by morphometric analysis is likely to be secondary to all these neuronal changes. However, the cellular reaction went beyond the reactive gliosis as chronic inflammation was found in the leptomeninges and white matter of the cerebellum at 12 months of age. The spleens of these animals also showed a reactive hyperplasia. Comparison of the findings in these two models (light or heavy NF promoters were used) suggests that association of gp160 with NF heavy chain is more detrimental. These two models (GFAP-gp120 and NFL+H-gp160) significantly contributed in understanding HIV-1 envelope protein-induced neurodegeneretion. There is a difference in effects of "nondetectable" in vivo expression of gp120 protein under GFAP promoter and strongly detectable gp120 and gp41 expression under NF promoters. In the first scenario we could suggest the delivery of gp120 in conjunction with GFAP protein-containing gliosomes directly to neuronal bodies or synaptic spaces at the sites of neuron-astrocyte cell-to-cell contacts (Quintanar, Franco, & Salinas, 2003). This interaction is more detrimental for neurons than in second scenario, when gp120+41 exist in association with nonsecreted neurofilaments (Petzold et al., 2010) and most probably contribute to the damage of synaptic structures as a result of axonal transportation of viral proteins. However, the question remains with how it could be used for the screening of new therapeutic strategies.

TRANSGENIC MURINE MODELS FOR SCREENING OF THERAPEUTICS

First attempt was done on GFAP-gp120 mice (Toggas et al., 1994). Line #2 with the highest trangene expression was treated with the NMDA receptor antagonist, memantine, starting on postnatal day 2 (because the minor degrees of damage were detectable in 1-week-old transgenic mice) with a loading dose of 20 mg/kg. Twenty-four hours later, mice were given a maintenance dose of 1 mg/kg, which was administered every 12 h for 6 weeks. Treatment reduced gp120–mediated toxicity as was shown by preservation of MAP-2 and SYN protein expression by the neurons (Toggas, Masliah, & Mucke, 1996). As an adjunctive therapy for HIV-1-associated neurologic application, memantine is being utilized in clinical studies where it has shown some preventive effects. During the initial 12-week open-label phase, participants randomized to memantine in the double-blind phase had a statistically significant improvement in NPZ-8 compared to those randomized to the placebo (Zhao et al., 2010).

Another therapeutic approach for HIV-1-associated neurodegeneration was tested on mice at 6 months of age (when damage already occurred). GFAP-gp120-transgenic mice were administered neuroprotective cytokines: 50U of erythropoietin (EPO) plus 2,000ng of insulin-like growth factor-I (IGF-I) intranasally for 4 months. Chronic treatment with transnasal EPO-IGF-I produced significant improvements (complete restoration up to wild type mice levels) in dendritic complexity (MAP-2+NeuN staining) and showed ~50% prevention of neuronal degeneration (assessed by the count of cells positive for phosphorylated PHF-1 tau) compared to untreated GFAP-gp120 transgenic mice. On the other hand, EPO-IGF-I manifested no significant effect on astrocytosis or microglial responses (Kang et al., 2010).

FUTURE STEPS IN TRANSGENICS FOR HAND PATHOGENESIS RESEARCH

An unlimited number of pathogenetic steps of HIV-1-mediated neuropathology can be studied in transgenic mice with a conditional expression of viral proteins under cell-specific host protein promoters. These are the fields for elucidation of the role of different type of cells and proteins in neurodegeneration. Combination of transgenic HIV-1-related protein expression with the Cre/lox system (site-specific recombinase technology), which is widely used in mice to achieve cell-type-specific "color" gene expression (Branda &

Dymecki, 2004; Livet et al., 2007; Madisen et al.), will open a new 90-color "brainbow" avenue.

CHIMERIC VIRUSES

HIV-1 pseudotyped with vesicular stomatitis virus (VSV) envelope glycoprotein (HIV/VSV) has been shown to productively infect murine astrocytes, lymphocytes, and macrophages. There are no intrinsic intracellular barriers for HIV-1 replication in primary mouse cells when virus entry is efficient (Nitkiewicz et al., 2004). Pseudotyped HIV was used to infect murine bone-marrow-derived macrophages (BMM) (Gorantla, Liu et al., 2007). Mouse bone-marrow macrophages may more adequately reflect cell trafficking compared to human monocyte-derived macrophages in the HIVE model (Nottet et al., 1996; Persidsky et al., 1996). The model is a conceptual advance because it allows bimodal study of both innate and adaptive immune responses that follow viral infection of macrophages in the brain. The problems seen in HIV/VSV HIVE mice are that infected mouse macrophages implanted in the brain were eliminated faster when compared with the HIVE-SCID mouse model. This may be due to an intact immune surveillance system resulting in a more limited neurodegeneration around the lesion observed. When HIV/VSV-infected BMM are injected into the mouse brain, HIV proteins are expressed by the infected BMM; however, the infection cannot spread to other mouse cells, including either uninfected remaining BMM or microglia, because the progeny virus from infected BMM is HIV, and not HIV/VSV. This model also lacks the formation of HIV-infected multinucleated giant cells in the brain, which is characteristic of the HIVE-SCID mouse model used in previous studies. Histopathological observations of brain tissues around the injection line showed lymphocyte infiltration representing the engagement of the adaptive immune system in this model. The loss of MAP-2 and NeuN staining markers, and degenerating neuronal cell bodies were found in the area of injection. By two weeks after injection of VSV-HIV-infected BMM the peripheral immune responses were detected to HIV-1gp120 protein by antigen-specific increased secretion of IFNγ in lymph nodes. By using this model of HIVE, the presence and neuromodulatory effects of T regulatory cells in HIV-1 associated neurodegeneration were demonstrated (Liu et al., 2009; Gong et al., 2010).

The host species range of HIV-1 from primate to rodent was expanded by replacing the coding region of its surface envelope glycoprotein, gp120, with the envelope-coding region from ecotropic MLV that restricts the replication of the virus to rodents (Potash et al., 2005). Two chimeric viruses, EcoHIV on a backbone of clade B NL4–3 and EcoNDK on a backbone of clade D were generated. EcoHIV and EcoNDK established systemic infection in mice after one inoculation. This experimental infection reproduced several major characteristics of HIV-1 infection of human beings, including viral targeting of lymphocytes and macrophages, induction of antiviral immune responses, neuroinvasiveness, and elevation of expression of inflammatory and antiviral factors in the brain.

Moreover, these models showed that mice are responsive to HIV-1 antigens, and that viral structural and regulatory proteins are produced in sufficient quantities during EcoHIV replication to elicit responses. The brains of EcoHIV-infected mice, most of which were killed 6 weeks after inoculation, had no overt signs of immune dysfunction or histological changes. However, the EcoHIV strain, which had the highest virus burden in the spleen and brain, showed significant increases in the expression of C3, IL-1β, MCP-1, and STAT-1. These models were not applied for neuropathogenesis studies, but were successfully used for the screening of antiviral drugs and vaccines (Hadas et al., 2007; Roshorm et al., 2009).

CONCLUSION

A model, by definition, is whatever can be utilized to reproduce a pattern of something existing. The use of human cells (macrophages, lymphocytes highly permissive for HIV-1) or "humanized" mice with lymphatics of human origin allows us to overcome issues of productive HIV-1 infection and generation of viral toxins. The incomplete overlap of human and mouse receptors and ligands, which are involved in HIV-1-mediated neuropathology, will remain a "dark" part of such models.

Transgenic mice that express single or multiple viral proteins are very instrumental, but have a lot of issues that are related to three questions: what to express, where to express, and what it means. Each time the transgenic model will require two important features/controls for clarification—conditional expression of viral proteins and, if it is a host protein-specific expression, the null-protein mice have to be used to understand the contribution of such cell-specific proteins (GFAP and NFs, as an example). Other dark components of transgenic models are the mysteries of how much the viral proteins themselves contribute to neurodegeneration and which part the host immune responses play. If in "humanized" mice and VSV-HIV chimeric virus models there are surrogates and normal immune responses are present, in transgenic models, immune responses may be completely absent or aberrant.

ACKNOWLEDGMENTS

I am very grateful to Edward Makarov, Jaclyn Knibbe, Santhi Gorantla, Tanuja Gutti, and Lana Reichardt for preparation of this review.

REFERENCES

Anderson, E. R., Boyle, J., Zink, W. E., Persidsky, Y., Gendelman, H. E., Xiong, H. (2003). Hippocampal synaptic dysfunction in a murine model of human immunodeficiency virus type 1 encephalitis. *Neuroscience*, 118(2), 359–69.

Antinori, A., Arendt, G., Becker, J. T., Brew, B. J., Byrd, D. A., Cherner, M., et al. (2007). Updated research nosology for HIV-associated neurocognitive disorders. *Neurology*, 69(18), 1789–99.

Avgeropoulos, N., Kelley, B., Middaugh, L., Arrigo, S., Persidsky, Y., Gendelman, H. E., et al. (1998). SCID mice with HIV encephalitis develop behavioral abnormalities. *J Acquir Immune Defic Syndr Hum Retrovirol*, 18(1), 13–20.

Bagasra, O., Lavi, E., Bobroski, L., Khalili, K., Pestaner, J. P., Tawadros, R., et al. (1996). Cellular reservoirs of HIV-1 in the central nervous system of infected individuals: Identification by the combination of in situ polymerase chain reaction and immunohistochemistry. *AIDS*, 10, 573–585.

Baumann, J. G., Unutmaz, D., Miller, M. D., Breun, S. K., Grill, S. M., Mirro, J., et al. (2004). Murine T cells potently restrict human immunodeficiency virus infection. *J Virol*, 78(22), 12537–47.

Baxter, A. G. & Cooke, A. (1993). Complement lytic activity has no role in the pathogenesis of autoimmune diabetes in NOD mice. *Diabetes*, 42(11), 1574–8.

Berrada, F., Ma, D., Michaud, J., Doucet, G., Giroux, L., & Kessous-Elbaz, A. (1995). Neuronal expression of human immunodeficiency virus type 1 env proteins in transgenic mice: Distribution in the central nervous system and pathological alterations. *J Virol*, 69(11), 6770–8.

Berry, C. L. (1970). Histopathological findings in the combined immunity-deficiency syndrome. *J Clin Pathol*, 23(3), 193–202.

Bertelli, E., Regoli, M., Gambelli, F., Lucattelli, M., Lungarella, G., & Bastianini, A. (2000). GFAP is expressed as a major soluble pool associated with glucagon secretory granules in A-cells of mouse pancreas. *J Histochem Cytochem*, 48(9), 1233–1242.

Bissel, S. J. & Wiley, C. A. (2004). Human immunodeficiency virus infection of the brain: Pitfalls in evaluating infected/affected cell populations. *Brain Pathol*, 14(1), 97–108.

Bosma, G. C., Custer, R. P., & Bosma, M. J. (1983). A severe combined immunodeficiency mutation in the mouse. *Nature*, 301, 527–30.

Brainard, D. M., Seung, E., Frahm, N., Cariappa, A., Bailey, C. C., Hart, W. K., et al. (2009). Induction of robust cellular and humoral virus-specific adaptive immune responses in HIV-infected humanized BLT mice. *J Virol*, 83(14), 7305–21.

Branda, C. S. & Dymecki, S. M. (2004). Talking about a revolution: The impact of site-specific recombinases on genetic analyses in mice. *Developmental Cell*, 6(1), 7–28.

Brehm, M. A., Cuthbert, A., Yang, C., Miller, D. M., DiIorio, P., Laning, J., et al. (2010). Parameters for establishing humanized mouse models to study human immunity: Analysis of human hematopoietic stem cell engraftment in three immunodeficient strains of mice bearing the IL2r[gamma]null mutation. *Clinical Immunology*, 135(1), 84–98.

Bruce-Keller, A. J., Turchan-Cholewo, J., Smart, E. J., Geurin, T., Chauhan, A., Reid, R., et al. (2008). Morphine causes rapid increases in glial activation and neuronal injury in the striatum of inducible HIV-1 Tat transgenic mice. *Glia*, 56(13), 1414–27.

Bruggeman, L. A., Thomson, M. M., Nelson, P. J., Kopp, J. B., Rappaport, J., Klotman, P. E., et al. (1994). Patterns of HIV-1 mRNA Expression in Transgenic Mice Are Tissue-Dependent. *Virology*, 202(2), 940–948.

Cao, T. & Leroux-Roels, G. (2000). Antigen-specific T cell responses in human peripheral blood leucocyte (hu-PBL)-mouse chimera conditioned with radiation and an antibody directed against the mouse IL-2 receptor beta-chain. *Clin Exp Immunol*, 122(1), 117–23.

Cao, X., Shores, E. W., Hu-Li, J., Anver, M. R., Kelsall, B. L., Russell, S. M., et al. (1995). Defective lymphoid development in mice lacking expression of the common cytokine receptor gamma chain. *Immunity*, 2(3), 223–238.

Cao, X., Kozak, C. A., Liu, Y. J., Noguchi, M., O'Connell, E., & Leonard, W. J. (1993). Characterization of cDNAs encoding the murine interleukin 2 receptor (IL-2R) gamma chain: chromosomal mapping and tissue specificity of IL-2R gamma chain expression. *Proc Natl Acad Sci U S A*, 90(18), 8464–8.

Choi, J., Liu, R-M., Kundu, R. K., Sangiorgi, F., Wu, W., Maxson, R., et al. (2000). Molecular mechanism of decreased glutathione content in human immunodeficiency virus type 1 Tat-transgenic mice. *Journal of Biological Chemistry*, 275(5), 3693–3698.

Coe, C. L., Reyes, T. M., Pauza, C. D., & Reinhard, J. F. Jr. (1997). Quinolinic acid and lymphocyte subsets in the intrathecal compartment as biomarkers of SIV infection and simian AIDS. *AIDS Res Hum Retroviruses*, 13(10), 891–7.

de Freitas, M. R. (2007). Infectious neuropathy. *Curr Opin Neurol*, 20(5), 548–52.

Devi, P. U., Hossain, M., & Bisht, K. S. (1999). Effect of late fetal irradiation on adult behavior of mouse: Dose-response relationship. *Neurotoxicol Teratol*, 21(2), 193–8.

Dickie, P., Felser, J., Eckhaus, M., Bryant, J., Silver, J., Marinos, N., et al. (1991). HIV-associated nephropathy in transgenic mice expressing HIV-1 genes. *Virology*, 185(1), 109–19.

DiSanto, J. P., Muller, W., Guy-Grand, D., Fischer, A., & Rajewsky, K. (1995). Lymphoid development in mice with a targeted deletion of the interleukin 2 receptor gamma chain. *Proc Natl Acad Sci U S A*, 92(2), 377–381.

Dou, H., Birusingh, K., Faraci, J., Gorantla, S., Poluektova, L. Y., Maggirwar, S. B., et al. (2003). Neuroprotective activities of sodium valproate in a murine model of human immunodeficiency virus-1 encephalitis. *J Neurosci*, 23(27), 9162–70.

Dou, H., Destache, C. J., Morehead, J. R., Mosley, R. L., Boska, M. D., Kingsley, J., et al. (2006). Development of a macrophage-based nanoparticle platform for antiretroviral drug delivery. *Blood*, 108(8), 2827–35.

Dou, H., Ellison, B., Bradley, J., Kasiyanov, A., Poluektova, L. Y., Xiong, H., et al. (2005). Neuroprotective mechanisms of lithium in murine human immunodeficiency virus-1 encephalitis. *J Neurosci*, 25(37), 8375–85.

Dou, H., Morehead, J., Destache, C. J., Kingsley, J. D., Shlyakhtenko, L., Zhou, Y., et al. (2007). Laboratory investigations for the morphologic, pharmacokinetic, and anti-retroviral properties of indinavir nanoparticles in human monocyte-derived macrophages. *Virology*, 358(1), 148–58.

Eden, A., Price, R. W., Spudich, S., Fuchs, D., Hagberg, L., & Gisslen, M. (2007). Immune activation of the central nervous system is still present after >4 years of effective highly active antiretroviral therapy. *The Journal of Infectious Diseases*, 196(12), 1779–1783.

Eggert, D., Dash, P. K., Gorantla, S., Dou, H., Schifitto, G., Maggirwar, S. B., et al. (2010). Neuroprotective activities of CEP-1347 in models of neuroAIDS. *J Immunol*, 184(2), 746–56.

Eggert, D., Dash, P. K., Serradji, N., Dong, C. Z., Clayette, P., Heymans, F., et al. (2009). Development of a platelet-activating factor antagonist for HIV-1 associated neurocognitive disorders. *J Neuroimmunol*, 213 (1–2), 47–59.

Ensoli, F., Ensoli, B., & Thiele, C. J. (1994). HIV-1 gene expression and replication in neuronal and glial cell lines with immature phenotype: Effects of nerve growth factor. *Virology*, 200(2), 668–76.

Frankel, A. D. & Pabo, C. O. (1988). Cellular uptake of the tat protein from human immunodeficiency virus. *Cell*, 55(6), 1189–1193.

Gamis, A. S. & Nesbit, M. E. (1991). Neuropsychologic (cognitive) disabilities in long-term survivors of childhood cancer. *Pediatrician*, 18 (1), 11–9.

Garza, H. H., Jr., Prakash, O., & Carr, D. J. (1994). Immunologic characterization of TAT72-transgenic mice: Effects of morphine on cell-mediated immunity. *Int J Immunopharmacol*, 16(12), 1061–70.

Gendelman, H. E. & Folks, D. G. (1999). Innate and acquired immunity in neurodegenerative disorders. *J Leukoc Biol*, 65(4), 407–8.

Gendelman, H. E., Zheng, J., Coulter, C. L., Ghorpade, A., Che, M., Thylin, M., et al. (1998). Suppression of inflammatory neurotoxins by highly active antiretroviral therapy in human immunodeficiency virus-associated dementia. *J Infect Dis*, 178(4), 1000–7.

Goldman, J. P., Blundell, M. P., Lopes, L., Kinnon, C., Di Santo, J. P., & Thrasher, A. J. (1998). Enhanced human cell engraftment in mice deficient in RAG2 and the common cytokine receptor gamma chain. *Br J Haematol*, 103, 335–42.

Gong, N., Liu, J., Reynolds, A. D., Gorantla, S., Mosley, R. L., & Gendelman, H. E. (2010). Brain ingress of regulatory T cells in a murine model of HIV-1 encephalitis. *J Neuroimmunol*, 230(1–2), 33–41.

Gorantla, S., Liu, J., Sneller, H., Dou, H., Holguin, A., Smith, L., et al. (2007). Copolymer-1 induces adaptive immune anti-inflammatory glial and neuroprotective responses in a murine model of HIV-1 encephalitis. *J Immunol*, 179(7), 4345–56.

Gorantla, S., Liu, J., Wang, T., Holguin, A., Sneller, H. M., Dou, H., et al. (2008). Modulation of innate immunity by copolymer-1 leads to neuroprotection in murine HIV-1 encephalitis. *Glia* 56(2), 223–32.

Gorantla, S., Makarov, E., Finke-Dwyer, J., Castanedo, A., Holguin, A., Gebhart, C. L., et al. (2010). Links between progressive HIV-1 infection of humanized mice and viral neuropathogenesis. *Am J Pathol*, 177(6), 2938–49.

Gorantla, S., Makarov, E., Finke-Dwyer, J., Gebhart, C. L., Domm, W., Dewhurst, S., et al. (2010). CD8+ cell depletion accelerates HIV-1 immunopathology in humanized mice. *J Immunol*, 184(12), 7082–91.

Gorantla, S., Makarov, E., Roy, D., Finke-Dwyer, J., Murrin, L. C., Gendelman, H. E., et al. (2010). Immunoregulation of a CB2 Receptor Agonist in a Murine Model of NeuroAIDS. *J Neuroimmune Pharmacol*, 5(3), 456–68.

Gorantla, S., Santos, K., Meyer, V., Dewhurst, S., Bowers, W. J., Federoff, H. J., et al. (2005). Human dendritic cells transduced with herpes simplex virus amplicons encoding human immunodeficiency virus type 1 (HIV-1) gp120 elicit adaptive immune responses from human cells engrafted into NOD/SCID mice and confer partial protection against HIV-1 challenge. *J Virol*, 79(4), 2124–32.

Gorantla, S., Sneller, H., Walters, L., Sharp, J. G., Pirruccello, S. J., West, J. T., et al. (2007). Human immunodeficiency virus type 1 pathobiology studied in humanized BALB/c-Rag2-/-gammac-/- mice. *J Virol*, 81 (6), 2700–12.

Goudreau, G., Carpenter, S., Beaulieu, N., & Jolicoeur, P. (1996). Vacuolar myelopathy in transgenic mice expressing human immunodeficiency virus type 1 proteins under the regulation of the myelin basic protein gene promoter. *Nat Med*, 2(6), 655–61.

Gray, F., Scaravilli, F., Everall, I., Chretien, F., An, S., Boche, D., et al. (1996). Neuropathology of early HIV-1 infection. *Brain Pathol*, 6 (1), 1–15.

Grovit-Ferbas, K. & Harris-White, M. (2010). Thinking about HIV: The intersection of virus, neuroinflammation and cognitive dysfunction. *Immunologic Research*, 1–19.

Gyorkey, F., Melnick, J. L., & Gyorkey, P. (1987). Human immunodeficiency virus in brain biopsies of patients with AIDS and progressive encephalopathy. *J Infect Dis*, 155(5), 870–6.

Hadas, E., Borjabad, A., Chao, W., Saini, M., Ichiyama, K., Potash, M. J., et al. (2007). Testing antiretroviral drug efficacy in conventional mice infected with chimeric HIV-1. *AIDS*, 21(8), 905–9

Hanna, Z., D. Kay, G., Cool, M., Jothy, S., Rebai, N., Jolicoeur, P. (1998). Transgenic mice expressing human immunodeficiency virus type 1 in immune cells develop a severe AIDS-like disease. *J Virol*, 72(1), 121–32.

Hervé, F., Ghinea, N., & Scherrmann, J-M. (2008). CNS delivery via adsorptive transcytosis. *The AAPS Journal*, 10(3), 455–472.

Hill, J. M., Mervis, R. F., Avidor, R., Moody, T. W., & Brenneman, D. E. (1993). HIV envelope protein-induced neuronal damage and retardation of behavioral development in rat neonates. *Brain Res*, 603 (2), 222–33.

Ikebe, M., Miyakawa, K., Takahashi, K., Ohbo, K., Nakamura, M., Sugamura, K., . (1997). Lymphohaematopoietic abnormalities and systemic lymphoproliferative disorder in interleukin-2 receptor gamma chain-deficient mice. *Int J Exp Pathol*, 78(3), 133–48.

Ito, M., Hiramatsu, H., Kobayashi, K., Suzue, K., Kawahata, M., Hioki, K., et al. (2002). NOD/SCID/gamma(c)(null) mouse: an excellent recipient mouse model for engraftment of human cells. *Blood*, 100(9), 3175–82.

Iwakura, Y., Shioda, T., Tosu, M., Yoshida, E., Hayashi, M., Nagata, T., et al. (1992). The induction of cataracts by HIV-1 in transgenic mice. *AIDS*, 6(10), 1069–75.

Johnson, R. T., McArthur, J. C., & Narayan, O. (1988). The neurobiology of human immunodeficiency virus infections. *FASEB J*, 2(14), 2970–2981.

Jones, G. J., Barsby, N. L., Cohen, E. A., Holden, J., Harris, K., Dickie, P., et al. (2007). HIV-1 Vpr causes neuronal apoptosis and in vivo neurodegeneration. *J Neurosci*, 27(14), 3703–3711.

Kang, Y. J., Digicaylioglu, M., Russo, R., Kaul, M., Achim, C. L., Fletcher, L., et al. (2010). Erythropoietin plus insulin-like growth factor-I protects against neuronal damage in a murine model of human immunodeficiency virus-associated neurocognitive disorders. *Ann Neurol*, 68(3), 342–52.

Katsetos, C. D., Fincke, J. E., Legido, A., Lischner, H. W., de Chadarevian, J. P., Kaye, E. M., et al. (1999). Angiocentric CD3(+) T-cell infiltrates in human immunodeficiency virus type 1-associated central nervous system disease in children. *Clin Diagn Lab Immunol*, 6(1), 105–14.

Kim, B. O., Liu, Y., Ruan, Y., Xu, Z. C., Schantz, L., & He, J. J. (2003). Neuropathologies in transgenic mice expressing human immunodeficiency virus type 1 Tat protein under the regulation of the astrocyte-specific glial fibrillary acidic protein promoter and doxycycline. *Am J Pathol*, 162(5), 1693–1707.

King, J. E., Eugenin, E. A., Buckner, C. M., & Berman, J. W. (2006). HIV tat and neurotoxicity. *Microbes and Infection*, 8(5), 1347–1357.

Kraft-Terry, S. D., Buch, S. J., Fox, H. S., & Gendelman, H. E. (2009). A coat of many colors: Neuroimmune crosstalk in human immunodeficiency virus infection. *Neuron*, 64(1), 133–45.

Krucker, T., Toggas, S. M., Mucke, L., & Siggins, G. R. (1998). Transgenic mice with cerebral expression of human immunodeficiency virus type-1 coat protein gp120 show divergent changes in short- and long-term potentiation in CA1 hippocampus. *Neuroscience*, 83(3), 691–700.

Kundu, R. K., Sangiorgi, F., Wu, L-Y., Pattengale, P. K., Hinton, D. R., Gill, P. S., et al. (1999). Expression of the human immunodeficiency virus-Tat gene in lymphoid tissues of transgenic mice is associated with B-cell lymphoma. *Blood*, 94(1), 275–282.

Kwak, Y. T., Ivanov, D., Guo, J., Nee, E., & Gaynor, R. B. (1999). Role of the human and murine cyclin T proteins in regulating HIV-1 tat-activation. *Journal of Molecular Biology*, 288(1), 57–69.

Lawson, L. J., Perry, V. H., Dri, P., & Gordon, S. (1990). Heterogeneity in the distribution and morphology of microglia in the normal adult mouse brain. *Neuroscience*, 39(1), 151–70.

Leonard, J. M., Abramczuk, J. W., Pezen, D. S., Rutledge, R., Belcher, J. H., Hakim, F., et al. (1988). Development of disease and virus recovery in transgenic mice containing HIV proviral DNA. *Science*, 242(4886), 1665–1670.

Limoges, J., Persidsky, Y., Poluektova, L., Rasmussen, J., Ratanasuwan, W., Zelivyanskaya, M., et al. (2000). Evaluation of antiretroviral drug efficacy for HIV-1 encephalitis in SCID mice. *Neurology*, 54(2), 379–89.

Limoges, J., Poluektova, L., Ratanasuwan, W., Rasmussen, J., Zelivyanskaya, M., McClernon, D. R., et al. (2001). The efficacy of potent anti-retroviral drug combinations tested in a murine model of HIV-1 encephalitis. *Virology*, 281(1), 21–34.

Liu, J., Gong, N., Huang, X., Reynolds, A. D., Mosley, R. L., & Gendelman, H. E. (2009). Neuromodulatory activities of CD4+CD25+ regulatory T cells in a murine model of HIV-1-associated neurodegeneration. *J Immunol*, 182(6), 3855–65.

Livet, J., Weissman, T. A., Kang, H., Draft, R. W., Lu, J., Bennis, R. A., et al. (2007). Transgenic strategies for combinatorial expression of fluorescent proteins in the nervous system. *Nature*, 450(7166), 56–62.

Lu, T-c., He, J. C., & Klotman, P. (2006). Animal models of HIV-associated nephropathy. *Current Opinion in Nephrology and Hypertension*, 15(3), 233–237.

Madisen, L., Zwingman, T. A., Sunkin, S. M., Oh, S. W., Zariwala, H. A., Gu, H., et al. A robust and high-throughput Cre reporting and characterization system for the whole mouse brain. *Nat Neurosci*, 13(1), 133–40.

Martin, C., Martin, S., Viret, R., Denis, J., Mirguet, F., Diserbo, M., et al. (2001). Low dose of the gamma acute radiation syndrome (1.5 Gy) does not significantly alter either cognitive behavior or dopaminergic and serotoninergic metabolism. *Cell Mol Biol (Noisy-le-grand)*, 47(3), 459–65.

McCrossan, M., Marsden, M., Carnie, F. W., Minnis, S., Hansoti, B., Anthony, I. C., et al. (2006). An immune control model for viral replication in the CNS during presymptomatic HIV infection. *Brain*, 129 (Pt 2), 503–16.

McCune, J. M., Namikawa, R., Kaneshima, H., Shultz, L. D., Lieberman, M., & Weissman, I. L. (1988). The SCID-hu mouse: Murine model for the analysis of human hematolymphoid differentiation and function. *Science*, 241(4873), 1632–1639.

Mestas, J. & Hughes, C. C. (2004). Of mice and not men: Differences between mouse and human immunology. *J Immunol*, 172(5), 2731–8.

Michaud, J., Fajardo, R., Charron, G., Sauvageau, A., Berrada, F., Ramla, D., et al. (2001). Neuropathology of NFHgp160 transgenic mice expressing HIV-1 env protein in neurons. *J Neuropathol Exp Neurol*, 60(6), 574–87.

Milanese, M., Bonifacino, T., Zappettini, S., Usai, C., Tacchetti, C., Nobile, M., et al. 2009. Chapter 21: Glutamate release from astrocytic gliosomes under physiological and pathological conditions. In *International review of neurobiology*: Academic Press. Vol. 85, pp. 295–318.

Mosier, D. E., Gulizia, R. J., Baird, S. M., & Wilson, D. B. (1988). Transfer of a functional human immune system to mice with severe combined immunodeficiency. *Nature*, 335(6187), 256–9.

Munoz-Moreno, J. A., Fumaz, C. R., Ferrer, M. J., Gonzalez-Garcia, M., Molto, J., Negredo, E., et al. (2009). Neuropsychiatric symptoms associated with efavirenz: Prevalence, correlates, and management. A neurobehavioral review. *AIDS Rev*, 11(2), 103–9.

Namikawa, R., Kaneshima, H., Lieberman, M., Weissman, I. L., & McCune, J. M. (1988). Infection of the SCID-hu mouse by HIV-1. *Science*, 242(4886), 1684–6.

Nitkiewicz, J., Chao, W., Bentsman, G., Li, J., Kim, S. Y., Choi, S. Y., et al. (2004). Productive infection of primary murine astrocytes, lymphocytes, and macrophages by human immunodeficiency virus type 1 in culture. *J Neurovirol*, 10(6), 400–8.

Noguchi, M., Nakamura, Y., Russell, S. M., Ziegler, S. F., Tsang, M., Cao, X., et al. (1993). Interleukin-2 receptor g chain: A functional component of the interleukin-7 receptor. *Science*, 272, 1877–1879.

Noguchi, M., Adelstein, S., Cao, X., & Leonard, W. J. (1993). Characterization of the human interleukin-2 receptor gamma chain gene. *J Biol Chem*, 268(18), 13601–8.

Noguchi, M., Yi, H., Rosenblatt, H. M., Filipovich, A. H., Adelstein, S., Modi, W. S., et al. (1993). Interleukin-2 receptor gamma chain mutation results in X-linked severe combined immunodeficiency in humans. *Cell*, 73(1), 147–57.

Noorbakhsh, F., Ramachandran, R., Barsby, N., Ellestad, K. K., LeBlanc, A., Dickie, P., et al. (2010). MicroRNA profiling reveals new aspects of HIV neurodegeneration: caspase-6 regulates astrocyte survival. *The FASEB Journal*, 24(6), 1799–1812.

Nottet, H. S., Persidsky, Y., Sasseville, V. G., Nukuna, A. N., Bock, P., Zhai, Q. H., et al. (1996). Mechanisms for the transendothelial migration of HIV-1-infected monocytes into brain. *J Immunol*, 156(3), 1284–95.

Nukuna, A., Gendelman, H. E., Limoges, J., Rasmussen, J., Poluektova, L., Ghorpade, A., et al. (2004). Levels of human immunodeficiency virus type 1 (HIV-1) replication in macrophages determines the severity of murine HIV-1 encephalitis. *J Neurovirol*, 10 Suppl 1, 82–90.

Nuovo, G. J., Gallery, F., MacConnell, P., & Braun, A. (1994). In situ detection of polymerase chain reaction-amplified HIV-1 nucleic acids and tumor necrosis factor-alpha RNA in the central nervous system. *Am J Pathol*, 144(4), 659–66.

Oettinger, M. A. (1996). Cutting apart V(D)J recombination. *Current Opinion in Genetics & Development*, 6(2), 141–145.

Ohbo, K., Suda, T., Hashiyama, M., Mantani, A., Ikebe, M., Miyakawa, K., et al. (1996). Modulation of hematopoiesis in mice with a truncated mutant of the interleukin-2 receptor gamma chain. *Blood*, 87(3), 956–967.

Paul, J. B., Wang, E-J., Pettoello-Mantovani, M., Raker, C., Yurasov, S., Goldstein, M. M., et al. (2000). Mice transgenic for monocyte-tropic HIV type 1 produce infectious virus and display plasma viremia: A new in vivo system for studying the postintegration phase of HIV replication. *AIDS Research and Human Retroviruses*, 16(5), 481–492.

Perry, V. H. & Lawson, L. J. (1992). Macrophages in the central nervous system. In C. Lewis & J. D. McGee (Eds.). *The macrophage*. Oxford, NY, Tokyo: Oxford University Press.

Persidsky, Y., Limoges, J., Rasmussen, J., Zheng, J., Gearing, A., & Gendelman, H. E. (2001). Reduction in glial immunity and neuropathology by a PAF antagonist and an MMP and TNF[alpha] inhibitor in SCID mice with HIV-1 encephalitis. *Journal of Neuroimmunology*, 114(1–2), 57–68.

Persidsky, Y., Limoges, J., McComb, R., Bock, P., Baldwin, T., Tyor, W., et al. (1996). Human immunodeficiency virus encephalitis in SCID mice. *Am J Pathol*, 149(3), 1027–1053.

Petzold, A., Groves, M., Leis, A., Scaravilli, F., & Stokic, D. (2010). Neuronal and glial cerebrospinal fluid protein biomarkers are elevated after West Nile virus infection. *Muscle & Nerve*, 41(1), 42–49.

Philippon, V., Vellutini, C., Gambarelli, D., Harkiss, G., Arbuthnott, G., Metzger, D., et al. (1994). The basic domain of the lentiviral Tat protein is responsible for damages in mouse brain: Involvement of cytokines. *Virology*, 205(2), 519–529.

Poluektova, L., Gorantla, S., Faraci, J., Birusingh, K., Dou, H., & Gendelman, H. E. (2004). Neuroregulatory events follow adaptive immune-mediated elimination of HIV-1-infected macrophages: Studies in a murine model of viral encephalitis. *J Immunol*, 172(12), 7610–7.

Poluektova, L. Y., Munn, D. H., Persidsky, Y., & Gendelman, H. E. (2002). Generation of cytotoxic T cells against virus-infected human brain macrophages in a murine model of HIV-1 encephalitis. *J Immunol*, 168(8), 3941–9.

Poluektova, L. Y., Gorantla, S., Gendelman, H. E. (2004). Studies of adaptive immunity in a murine model of HIV-1 encephalitis. In H. G. Gendelman, S. Lipton, & S. Swindells (Eds.). *Neurology of AIDS*. New York: Oxford University Press.

Potash, M. J., Chao, W., Bentsman, G., Paris, N., Saini, M., Nitkiewicz, J., et al. (2005). A mouse model for study of systemic HIV-1 infection, antiviral immune responses, and neuroinvasiveness. *Proceedings of the National Academy of Sciences of the United States of America*, 102(10), 3760–3765.

Potula, R., Poluektova, L., Knipe, B., Chrastil, J., Heilman, D., Dou, H., et al. (2005). Inhibition of indoleamine 2,3-dioxygenase (IDO) enhances elimination of virus-infected macrophages in an animal model of HIV-1 encephalitis. *Blood*, 106(7), 2382–90.

Potula, R., Ramirez, S. H., Knipe, B., Leibhart, J., Schall, K., Heilman, D., et al. (2008). Peroxisome proliferator-activated receptor-gamma activation suppresses HIV-1 replication in an animal model of encephalitis. *AIDS*, 22(13), 1539–49.

Price, R. W., Brew, B., Sidtis, J., Rosenblum, M., Scheck, A. C., & Cleary, P. (1988). The brain in AIDS: Central nervous system HIV-1 infection and AIDS dementia complex. *Science*, 239(4840), 586–592.

Pumarola-Sune, T., Navia, B. A., Cordon-Cardo, C., Cho, E. S., & Price, R. W. (1987). HIV antigen in the brains of patients with the AIDS dementia complex. *Ann Neurol*, 21(5), 490–6.

Quintanar, J. L., Franco, L. M., & Salinas, E. (2003). Detection of glial fibrillary acidic protein and neurofilaments in the cerebrospinal fluid of patients with neurocysticercosis. *Parasitology Research*, 90(4), 261–263.

Radja, F., Kay, D. G., & Albrecht, S., & Jolicoeur, P. (2003). Oligodendrocyte-specific expression of human immunodeficiency virus type 1 Nef in transgenic mice leads to vacuolar myelopathy and alters oligodendrocyte phenotype in vitro. *J Virol*, 77(21), 11745–11753.

Rao, V. R., A. R. Sas, E. A. Eugenin, N. B. Siddappa, H. Bimonte-Nelson, J. W. Berman, U. Ranga, W. R. Tyor, and V. R. Prasad. 2008. HIV-1 clade-specific differences in the induction of neuropathogenesis. *J Neurosci* 28(40), 10010–6.

Rappaport, J., Joseph, J., Croul, S., Alexander, G., Del Valle, L. Amini, S., et al. (1999). Molecular pathway involved in HIV-1-induced CNS pathology: Role of viral regulatory protein, Tat. *J Leukoc Biol*, 65(4), 458–65.

Rosenstiel, P., Gharavi, A., D'Agati, V., Klotman, P. (2009). Transgenic and infectious animal models of HIV-associated nephropathy. *J Am Soc Nephrol*, 20(11), 2296–304.

Roshorm, Y., Hong, J. P., Kobayashi, N., McMichael, A. J., Volsky, D. J., Potash, M. J., et al. (2009). Novel HIV-1 clade B candidate vaccines designed for HLA-B*5101(+) patients protected mice against chimaeric ecotropic HIV-1 challenge. *Eur J Immunol*, 39(7), 1831–40.

Sadagopal, S., Lorey, S. L., Barnett, L., Basham, R., Lebo, L., Erdem, H., et al. (2008). Enhancement of human immunodeficiency virus (HIV)-specific CD8+ T cells in cerebrospinal fluid compared to those in

blood among antiretroviral therapy-naive HIV-positive subjects. *J Virol*, 82(21), 10418–28.

Santoro, T. J., Bryant, J. L., Pellicoro, J., Klotman, M. E., Kopp, J. B., Bruggeman, L. A., et al. (1994). Growth failure and AIDS-like cachexia syndrome in HIV-1 transgenic mice. *Virology*, 201(1), 147–151.

Sas, A. R., Bimonte-Nelson, H. A., & Tyor, W. R. (2007). Cognitive dysfunction in HIV encephalitic SCID mice correlates with levels of Interferon-alpha in the brain. *AIDS*, 21(16), 2151–9.

Schneider, M. K. & Gronvik, K. O. (1995). Acute graft-versus-host reaction in SCID mice leads to an abnormal expansion of CD8+ V beta 14+ and a broad inactivation of donor T cells followed by a host-restricted tolerance and a normalization of the TCR V beta repertoire in the chronic phase. *Scand J Immunol*, 41(4), 373–83.

Shultz, L. D., Lyons, B. L., Burzenski, L. M., Gott, B., Chen, X., Chaleff, S., et al. (2005). Human lymphoid and myeloid cell development in NOD/LtSz-scid IL2R gamma null mice engrafted with mobilized human hemopoietic stem cells. *J Immunol*, 174(10), 6477–89.

Shultz, L. D., Schweitzer, P. A., Christianson, S. W., Gott, B., Schweitzer, I. B., Tennent, B., et al. (1995). Multiple defects in innate and adaptive immunologic function in NOD/LtSz-scid mice. *J Immunol*, 154(1), 180–91.

Singer, E. J., Syndulko, K., Fahy-Chandon, B., Schmid, P., Conrad, A., & Tourtellotte, W. W. (1994). Intrathecal IgG synthesis and albumin leakage are increased in subjects with HIV-1 neurologic disease. *J Acquir Immune Defic Syndr*, 7(3), 265–71.

Spitzenberger, T. J., Heilman, D., Diekmann, C., Batrakova, E. V., Kabanov, A. V., Gendelman, H. E., et al. (2007). Novel delivery system enhances efficacy of antiretroviral therapy in animal model for HIV-1 encephalitis. *J Cereb Blood Flow Metab*, 27(5), 1033–42.

Stefanidakis, M., Newton, G., Lee, W. Y., Parkos, C. A., & Luscinskas, F. W. (2008). Endothelial CD47 interaction with SIRPgamma is required for human T-cell transendothelial migration under shear flow conditions in vitro. *Blood*, 112(4), 1280–9.

Sugamura, K., Asao, H., Kondo, M., Tanaka, N., Ishii, N., Ohbo, K., et al. (1996). The interleukin-2 receptor gamma chain: Its role in the multiple cytokine receptor complexes and T cell development in XSCID. *Annu Rev Immunol*, 14, 179–205.

Sun, J., Zheng, J. H., Zhao, M., Lee, S., & Goldstein, H. (2008). Increased in vivo activation of microglia and astrocytes in the brains of mice transgenic for an infectious R5 human immunodeficiency virus type 1 provirus and for CD4-specific expression of human cyclin T1 in response to stimulation by lipopolysaccharides. *J Virol*, 82(11), 5562–72.

Sun, J., Soos, T., KewalRamani, V. N., Osiecki, K., Zheng, J. H., Falkin, L., et al. (2006). CD4-specific transgenic expression of human cyclin T1 markedly increases human immunodeficiency virus type 1 (HIV-1) production by CD4+ T lymphocytes and myeloid cells in mice transgenic for a provirus encoding a monocyte-tropic HIV-1 isolate. *J Virol*, 80(4), 1850–1862.

Takenaka, K., Prasolava, T. K., Wang, J. C., Mortin-Toth, S. M., Khalouei, S., Gan, O. I., et al. (2007). Polymorphism in Sirpa modulates engraftment of human hematopoietic stem cells. *Nat Immunol*, 8(12), 1313–23.

Takizawa, H., & Manz, M. G. (2007). Macrophage tolerance: CD47-SIRP-alpha-mediated signals matter. *Nat Immunol*, 8(12), 1287–9.

Thomas, F. P., Chalk, C., Lalonde, R., Robitaille, Y., & Jolicoeur, P. (1994). Expression of human immunodeficiency virus type 1 in the nervous system of transgenic mice leads to neurological disease. *J Virol*, 68(11), 7099–7107.

Toggas, S. M., Masliah, E., Rockenstein, E. M., Rall, G. F., Abraham, C. R., & Mucke, L. (1994). Central nervous system damage produced by expression of the HIV-1 coat protein gp120 in transgenic mice. *Nature*, 367(6459), 188–93.

Toggas, S. M., Masliah, E., & Mucke, L. (1996). Prevention of HIV-1 gp120-induced neuronal damage in the central nervous system of transgenic mice by the NMDA receptor antagonist memantine. *Brain Research*, 706(2), 303–307.

Torres-Munoz, J. E., Nunez, M., & Petito, C. K. (2008). Successful application of hyperbranched multidisplacement genomic amplification to detect HIV-1 sequences in single neurons removed from autopsy brain sections by laser capture microdissection. *J Mol Diagn*, 10(4), 317–324.

Traggiai, E., Chicha, L., Mazzucchelli, L., Bronz, L., Piffaretti, J. C., Lanzavecchia, A., et al. (2004). Development of a human adaptive immune system in cord blood cell-transplanted mice. *Science*, 304 (5667), 104–107.

Trillo-Pazos, G., Diamanturos, A., Rislove, L., Menza, T., Chao, W., Belem, P., et al. (2003). Detection of HIV-1 DNA in microglia/macrophages, astrocytes and neurons isolated from brain tissue with HIV-1 encephalitis by laser capture microdissection. *Brain Pathol*, 13 (2), 144–54.

Van Duyne, R., Pedati, C., Guendel, I., Carpio, L., Kehn-Hall, K., Saifuddin, M., et al. (2009). The utilization of humanized mouse models for the study of human retroviral infections. *Retrovirology*, 6 (1), 76.

Vellutini, C., Philippon, V., Gambarelli, D., Horschowski, N., Nave, K. A., Navarro, J. M., et al. (1994). The maedi-visna virus Tat protein induces multiorgan lymphoid hyperplasia in transgenic mice. *J Virol*, 68(8), 4955–4962.

Wang, T., Gong, N., Liu, J., Kadiu, I., Kraft-Terry, S., Schlautman, J., et al. (2008). HIV-1-infected astrocytes and the microglial proteome. *Journal of Neuroimmune Pharmacology*, 3(3), 173–186.

Watanabe, S., Terashima, K., Ohta, S., Horibata, S., Yajima, M., Shiozawa, Y., et al. (2007). Hematopoietic stem cell-engrafted NOD/SCID/IL2Rgamma null mice develop human lymphoid systems and induce long-lasting HIV-1 infection with specific humoral immune responses. *Blood*, 109(1), 212–8.

Watanabe, S, Ohta, S., Yajima, M., Terashima, K., Ito, M., Mugishima, H., et al. (2007). Humanized NOD/SCID/IL2R{gamma}null mice transplanted with hematopoietic stem cells under nonmyeloablative conditions show prolonged life spans and allow detailed analysis of human immunodeficiency virus type 1 pathogenesis. *J Virol*, 81(23), 13259–13264.

Zhao, Y., Navia, B., Marra, C., Singer, E., Chang, L., Berger, J., et al., and Aids Clinical Trial Group Team Adult. (2010). Memantine for AIDS dementia complex: Open-label report of ACTG 301. *HIV Clinical Trials*, 11(1),59–67.

Zink, W. E., Anderson, E., Boyle, J., Hock, L., Rodriguez-Sierra, J., Xiong, H., et al. (2002). Impaired spatial cognition and synaptic potentiation in a murine model of human immunodeficiency virus type 1 encephalitis. *J Neurosci*, 22(6), 2096–105.

Zou, W., Kim, B. O., Zhou, B. Y., Liu, Y., Messing, A., & He, J. J. (2007). Protection against human immunodeficiency virus type 1 Tat neurotoxicity by ginkgo biloba extract EGb 761 involving glial fibrillary acidic protein. *Am J Pathol*, 171(6), 1923–1935.

5.6

SIMIAN IMMUNODEFICIENCY VIRUS AND OPIATES

Shilpa Buch, Shannon Callen, Paul Cheney, and Anil Kumar

Substantial data support the notion that opioids negatively affect the immune system and potentiate HIV disease progression. In the central nervous system, morphine appears to exacerbate the neuropathogenesis of HIV through widespread disruption of astroglial and microglial function and potentiation of glial-derived cytokines and chemokines. Morphine exposure also reduces the threshold for neurotoxicity by potentiating the deleterious effects of marginally toxic inflammatory viral products. It is not surprising, therefore, that drug abusers are reported to have higher rates of both HIV encephalitis and HIV-associated neurological disorders compared to infected nondrug abusers. At the same time, and somewhat confusingly, there is evidence from epidemiological, clinical, and laboratory studies suggesting that opiates can actually have protective effects on the progression of HIV infections. One of the most promising models for clarifying this ambiguous situation is the nonhuman primate model, especially models using simian immunodeficiency virus (SIV) infection of macaque monkeys. This chapter describes research on HIV and opiates in general, with a particular focus on work involving the macaque monkey.

INTRODUCTION

AIDS is a cellular immune disorder that is an outcome of persistent HIV-1 infection. From the onset of the HIV/AIDS epidemic, the role of illicit drug use on HIV disease progression has been the focus of several investigations. Despite the recent advances in the development of potent antiretroviral therapies (ART) that are known to inhibit systemic HIV replication, concomitant use of drugs of abuse (e.g., cocaine, opiates, methamphetamine, and alcohol) is on the rise in patients as they continue to live longer. Drug abuse and its related consequences therefore constitute a major health problem in many parts of the world including the United States. In fact, the 2007 Centers for Disease Control (CDC) estimates indicated that one-third of total AIDS cases in the country were associated with injection drug users (IDU). The natural history and progression of HIV infection among IDU, however, remains ambiguous (Woody & Metzger, 1993; Alcabes & Friedland, 1995). The increase in number of HIV-infected individuals who are addicted to behavior-modifying drugs has resulted in a paradigm shift in AIDS-related research—raising the question whether such drugs of abuse

and/or host responses induced by these drugs can promote replication of the virus and, thus, enhance the pathogenesis of the infection and speed disease progression. One prospective study actually suggested that AIDS is the most frequent cause of death among IDUs (Brancato, Delvechio, & Simone, 1995). There are conflicting reports on the mortality rate among HIV-infected IDU, demonstrating on one hand, a survival advantage associated with IDU HIV-infected individuals, while other reports show lower survival rates among IDUs (Selwyn et al., 1992; Alcabes & Friedland, 1995). Among IDU, opiates are the most commonly injected drugs. Since intravenous drug use is a strong risk factor for HIV infection, it is plausible that opiate users do have a high risk of HIV infection.

In addition to epidemiological studies, various laboratory models have also been exploited to understand the mechanistic relationship between drug use and HIV disease progression. These laboratory studies have included in vitro and animal model experiments in which researchers have mimicked key drug-use and disease parameters to study specific influences of drugs of abuse on HIV infection and its progression. These laboratory models have proven extremely valuable since studying the ontogeny of HIV infection during the acute to the chronic stages in the drug-abusing human population remains an insurmountable challenge. Furthermore, the complexity as well as the heterogeneity of the human system, particularly the use of multiple drugs, presents an additional challenge for systematically characterizing the interplay of opioid abuse and HIV infection. This challenge has been met by performing such studies in a model for HIV infection that best recapitulates the disease—SIV infection of macaque monkeys. This chapter will cover the interplay of opiates and HIV infection in nonhuman primate models.

KINETICS OF HIV INFECTION

One of the peculiarities of the lentiviruses, specifically HIV, is their ability to infect cells of the host's immune system, causing persistent and lifelong infection (Narayan & Clements, 1989). It is now well established that the pathogenesis of HIV infection and the complex disease patterns caused by the virus revolve around the dystrophic effects of the infection first in the CD4+T cells and then later in cells of the macrophage lineage (Rosenberg & Fauci, 1991; Pantaleo, Graziosi, & Fauci, 1993). CCR5 and CD4 are critical co-receptors in the pathogenesis of HIV. In the early stages of infection, activated CD4+ T cells and resting memory cells, both expressing CCR5, are the primary substrates of viral replication (Alkhatib et al., 1996; Deng et al., 1996; Dragic et al., 1996). Initially, in contrast to the systemic immune system, most of the CD4+ T cells in the mucosal immune system are CCR5+/CD4+-activated memory T cells and thus over 60% of these cells are infected within days of virus exposure and are rapidly depleted (Mattapallil et al., 2005). Because activated cells are already transcribing DNA, infection of these cells would promote more robust viral replication (Lackner & Veazey, 2007). Naïve CD4+ T cells generally lack CCR5 receptors and therefore support little, if any, replication. Viremia becomes established early with virus located throughout the body including the thymus, spleen, peripheral lymphoid organs, and mucosal tissues (Douek et al., 2002; Lackner & Veazey, 2007; Mehandru et al., 2007). At this stage, mononuclear cells in the blood get activated and although large numbers of monocytes are also infected, macrophages derived from these cells show only minimal levels of viral replication. Shortly after viremia sets in and following the onset of seroconversion, virus can be found in the CNS where CD14+/CD45+ perivascular macrophages are the predominant cell types that become infected (Davis et al., 1992; Lackner, Vogel, Ramos, Kluge, & Marthas, 1994). While HIV appears in the CSF during this phase of infection (Gabuzda & Sobel, 1987), the nature of the infection in the CNS remains unknown. Early infection of the CNS is neither sustained nor productive but does result in monocyte and macrophage activation and enhanced entry of these cells into the CNS (Williams & Hickey, 2002). Increased levels of chemokines, activated monocytes, and adhesion molecules provide an important mix for potentiating entry of infected and uninfected cells into the CNS. Following the initial viremia, the increased viral replication is brought under control by CD8+ T cells. However, with the increased decline in CD4+ T cell numbers over time, the cell-mediated immune (CMI) responses become ineffective because CD4+ T lymphocytes are necessary for effective CD8+ T cell function (Fauci, 1988; Levy, 1993; Picker & Watkins, 2005). This, in turn, leads to the collapse of the cellular arm of the immune response and the loss of immunocompetence, thereby allowing opportunistic pathogens to proliferate.

Productive viral replication in the CNS coincides with severe loss of T-cell function. Although HIV or SIV (in the macaque model) enters the brain within days following primary infection, the late onset of neurological complications in HIV-infected individuals remains puzzling. It is still unclear whether: (a) neurological complications are due to virus reactivation during the late stage of infection; (b) there is a renewed phase of viral neuroinvasion in late stage disease; or (c) whether the virus is continuously replicating in the CNS at low levels.

In humans, HIV-1-associated neurocognitive disorders (HAND) occur in approximately one-third of infected patients. These symptoms can range from minor cognitive motor disorders that affect almost 50% of HIV+ individuals on ART, to severe encephalitis/dementia affecting almost 15% to 20% of those with AIDS but who do not receive treatment. Although ART has led to a decreased incidence of HAND, and has significantly increased longevity of HIV-infected individuals, there is a paradoxical accompaniment of increased prevalence of HAND in these people. Into this mix, and often elusive, is the interaction of HIV with other comorbid factor(s), such as abuse of illicit drugs, a condition that is prevalent both in HIV-infected cohorts and in those with increased risk of contracting the virus. As early events significantly affect the progression and likely specific outcomes in HIV infection, knowledge of the effects of drug abuse on the early events following infection is important. Adding another level of complexity to this story is the ability of the brain to function as a potential viral sanctuary due to the incapacity of most of the ARTs to effectively penetrate the blood-brain barrier (BBB).

Encephalitis is often characterized by extensive replication of the virus in macrophages in the brain (Koenig et al., 1986). This is accompanied by continuous recruitment of monocytes into the brain. Once in the brain, monocytes begin to differentiate into macrophages by expressing CD16 before crossing the BBB (Ancuta et al., 2006; Bissel, Wang, Trichel, Murphey-Corb, & Wiley, 2006). In the brain, the recruited macrophages become viral factories resulting in enhanced virus replication. Encephalitis, however, needs in addition to productive virus replication, activation of glia and increased expression of major histocompatibility complex class II (MHC II) (Dickson, Lee, Mattiace, Yen, & Brosnan, 1993; Dickson et al., 1994; Berman et al. 1999).

Although studies on humans with CNS disease have contributed significantly to our understanding of the pathogenesis of HAND, they only generate snapshots of the disease endpoint. This creates the need for an animal model system that will accurately reproduce the pathogenesis of HIV infection. However, since HIV does not cause disease in animals, the questions of disease pathogenesis have to be relegated to studies in macaques infected with SIV or chimeras of HIV and SIV (SHIVs) (Lackner et al., 1991; Lackner et al., 1994; Joag et al., 1997).

OPIATES AND THE IMMUNE SYSTEM

Opiates have been recognized to have an effect on immune function for over 100 years, when opium's influence on leukocyte phagocytosis was first described (Cantacuzene, 1898). Opiates belong to a family of CNS depressants and narcotic analgesics. The use of opiates typically creates physical as well as physiological dependence and tolerance. Belonging to this group of compounds are both natural and synthetic agents (e.g., heroin) that have analogous properties. In recent years, opioid abuse and withdrawal have become a major international public health concern. Opioid compounds such as morphine are known to produce powerful analgesia that is effective for pain management. Besides its therapeutic utility, morphine can also produce adverse events, and can interfere with various aspects of the immune system (Stefano et al., 1996; Friedman, Pross, & Klein, 2006).

It is well known that opioid receptors are present on many cell types located throughout the body, including monocytes and macrophages, T cells, B cells, PBMCs, neurons, and glial cells (Hauser et al., 2006; Roy, Wang, Kelschenbach, Koodie, & Martin, 2006). Opiates like morphine, as well as endogenous opioid peptides, exert their pharmacological and physiological effects by binding to their cognate endogenous receptors. As a consequence, opiates can modulate the immune system either directly via opioid receptors located on immune cells or indirectly via opioid receptors in the paraventricular nucleus (PVN) of the hypothalamus. Once activated by an appropriate ligand, opioid receptors in the PVN ultimately induce the release of cortisol and other glucocorticoids from the adrenal cortex. Opioid receptors are also located within the sympathetic nervous system, which when activated result in the release of epinephrine from the adrenal medulla and norepinephrine from sympathetic nerve terminals. The release of catecholamines and/or steroids may have a direct effect on immune cells (Roy et al., 2006).

Because heroin acts largely through its conversion to morphine in the brain, morphine is commonly used as a drug of choice to study the effects of opiates in vitro and in vivo. Morphine modulates both innate and adaptive immune responses and is known to have inhibitory effects on antibody and cellular immune responses, NK cell activity, cytokine expression, and phagocytic activity leading to increased susceptibility to a variety of infectious agents (Roy & Loh, 1996; Sharp, Roy, & Bidlack, 1998). This class of compounds acts as immunomodulators that modify the immune response to mitogens, antigens, and antibodies that cross-link the T-cell receptor (Sharp, 2003). In macrophages, activation of μ-opioid receptors leads to inhibition of phagocytosis (Szabo et al., 1993; Tomei & Renaud, 1997) and increased nitric oxide (NO) production which, in turn, can suppress lymphocyte proliferation (Fecho, Maslonek, Coussons-Read, Dykstra, & Lysle, 1994) or even induce macrophage apoptosis. Conversely, Chuang et al. have demonstrated that morphine was able to halt apoptosis leading to increased cell proliferation likely via the suppression of activated p53 and through activation of the MAPK signaling pathway. The authors contend this could provide a mechanism for infected cells to survive longer, allowing for greater viral replication (Chuang et al., 2005). Furthermore, morphine has also been shown to inhibit NF-κB DNA-binding in both neutrophils and monocytes (Welters et al., 2000). Since NF-κB DNA-binding is known to play a crucial role in the activation of inflammatory cytokines and adhesion molecules, immunosuppression mediated by morphine is likely attributable, at least partially, to morphine-induced inhibition of NF-κB activity (Ledebur & Parks, 1995). In addition to its impact on transcription factor activation, morphine has also been shown to polarize CD4+ T cells to a Th2 phenotype. Roy et al. have elegantly demonstrated that in CD4+ T cells, activation of μ-opioid receptors inhibits Th1 cytokines IL-2 and IFN-γ and potentiates Th2 cytokines IL-4 and IL-5,

ultimately biasing them towards a Th2 pathway (Roy et al., 2004; Roy, Wang, Charboneau, Loh, & Barke, 2005). Moreover, morphine modulates the entire immune system by its ability to favor expression of the TH2 cytokine, IL-4, while suppressing expression of the TH1 cytokine, IFN-γ, since the two are the cardinal cytokines regulating the development of cell-mediated immune responses.

Chronic morphine exposure has also been demonstrated to limit repair of damaged DNA in peripheral lymphocytes, leading to increased rate of host cell mutation and apoptosis (Madden, Wang, Lankford-Turner, & Donahoe, 2002). Morphine has been shown to induce expression of the HIV co-receptor CCR5 on neutrophils, monocytes, and macrophages (Miyagi et al., 2000; Suzuki, Chuang, Chuang, Doi, & Chuang, 2002). Upregulation of CCR5 receptor expression could be a major factor in increased viral replication. Importantly, morphine was found to increase production of the chemokine monocyte chemoattractant protein (MCP)-1 in neurons (Rock, Hu, Sheng, & Peterson, 2006). MCP-1 plays a significant role in neuroAIDS by activating macrophage function and attracting a variety of leukocytes to the areas of injury within the brain (McManus et al., 2000; Hauser et al., 2006).

OPIATES AND THE CENTRAL NERVOUS SYSTEM

In the brain, opiate receptors are located primarily in reward centers such as the ventral tegmental area (VTA), nucleus accumbens, caudate nucleus, and the thalamus, as well as the paraventricular nucleus of the hypothalamus. Activation of opiate receptors in reward pathways leads to increased release of dopamine from the VTA and a resulting euphoria that can lead to addiction. Chronic use may lead to psychological and physical dependence (De Vries & Shippenberg, 2002). Intracellular pathways modulated by morphine include upregulation of the cyclic AMP pathway that is observed in the locus ceruleus, a brain region critical for opiate addiction, in response to chronic opiate administration. This enhanced expression of the cyclic AMP pathway is known to contribute to opiate tolerance and dependence (De Vries & Shippenberg, 2002). Based on the pivotal role of IFN-γ in both glial activation and expression of MHC II in HAND, and since morphine inhibits expression of IFN-γ, it is not surprising to speculate that the drug has complex interactions with HIV and is also critical for preventing development of inflammatory lesions characteristic of HAND. In the CNS, morphine abuse exacerbates the neuropathogenesis of HIV through widespread disruption of astroglial and microglial function and potentiation of glial-derived cytokines and chemokines which may contribute to neuronal dysfunction, encephalitis, and neuronal death (Hauser et al., 2006). Morphine exposure also reduces the threshold for neurotoxicity by potentiating the deleterious effects of marginally toxic inflammatory viral products (Hu, Sheng, Lokensgard, & Peterson, 2005; Hauser et al., 2006).

OPIATES, HIV/AIDS, AND THE NONHUMAN PRIMATE MODEL

THE IMPACT OF OPIATES ON HIV AND AIDS HAS BEEN DIFFICULT TO DEFINE

The complex nature of drug addiction and its associated behavioral tendencies together with HIV infection have made understanding their interactions quite difficult. Although the effects of morphine on the immune system have been studied in great detail with many widely accepted conclusions, the interactions between virus, morphine, and the immune system have resulted in outcomes that are ambiguous at best. Many in vitro studies have been undertaken utilizing PBMCs, macrophages, and microglia, which clearly demonstrate enhanced viral replication in these cells in the presence of morphine (Peterson et al., 1990; Chuang, Killam, & Chuang, 1993; Peterson et al., 1993; Peterson et al., 1994). Morphine induces this effect through alterations in immune cell gene expression that results in significant upregulation of CCR5 co-receptor expression and inhibition of beta-chemokine production (Guo et al., 2002). This is further supported using a pharmacological approach and demonstrating that pretreatment with an opioid antagonist limits the morphine-mediated enhancement of viral replication primarily through abolishment of the upregulation of CCR5 receptor expression (Ho et al., 2003). A prospective study by Ronald et al. looking at an HIV-infected, drug-injecting cohort showed that concurrent heroin injection had an accelerating effect on the rate of disease progression, whereas no significant effects were found for use of other drugs (Ronald, Robertson, & Elton, 1994). The enigmatic nature of conclusions drawn from several epidemiological studies has driven the controversy surrounding the importance of morphine abuse in accelerating HIV infection and progression (Spijkerman et al., 1996; Bouwman et al., 1998; Thorpe et al., 2004).

The influence of concurrent drug abuse in AIDS is a burning issue, as drug abusers are reported to have higher rates of both HIV encephalitis (HIVE) and HIV-associated neurological disorders compared to infected nondrug abusers (Martinez et al., 1995; Bell et al., 1996; Chiesi et al., 1996; Goodkin et al. 1998; Nath, Maragos, Avison, Schmitt, & Berger, 2001). Neuropathologically, drug abusers tend to show greater levels of neuroinflammation as evidenced by microglial activation, astrocytosis, and CD8 lymphocytic infiltration (Tomlinson, Simmonds, Busuttil, Chiswick, & Bell, 1999; Anthony, Ramage, Carnie, Simmonds, & Bell, 2005). HIV infection and co-morbidities have been the subject of many reviews in recent years (Anthony & Bell, 2008; Hult, Chana, Masliah, & Everall, 2008; Nath et al., 2008).

MACAQUE MODELS OF MORPHINE AND SIV INFECTION HAVE STIMULATED CONTROVERSY SURROUNDING THE ROLE OF MORPHINE IN AIDS

SIV infection in macaques has proved to be an excellent model of HIV encephalopathy. Pathogenic chimeric SHIVs, which have the envelope of HIV-1 (HXB2) on a background of $SIV_{mac}239$, have also provided additional working models of HIV neurological disease. These chimeric viruses provide a unique opportunity to examine the effect of the HIV-1 envelope on the biology of the virus in the brain within the context of neurological disease. Both the SIV and SHIV macaque models of HIV infection have effectively recapitulated findings in HIV infection, demonstrating early virus neuroinvasion during systemic infection and CNS infection mediated by infected mononuclear cells and T cells that cross the BBB. The nonhuman primate models of neuroAIDS have shed light on a multitude of viral and host factor functions and interactions during both active and latent infection. However, despite the advantages of the macaque model systems, the prohibitive cost of macaques coupled with the development of HIV-related CNS pathologies in only a fraction of animals, a situation analogous to humans, have contributed to the fact that only a relatively meager number of research labs have adopted this model.

Further studies in macaque models of morphine and SIV infection have done little to resolve the controversy surrounding the role of morphine in AIDS. Some macaque studies have demonstrated that morphine may increase the severity and rate of HIV-1 disease progression. In one small pilot study using rhesus macaques, chronic morphine exposure resulted in a worsening of SIV infection (Chuang et al., 2005). Macaques were infected with SIVmac239 and chronically injected with either morphine or saline. The results showed increased plasma viremia in morphine-dependent animals compared to morphine-naïve animals. However, significantly higher plasma viral loads were detected only after 17 months of infection. Intriguingly, they found that morphine may induce mutations in the gag region of SIV genes in SIV-infected monkeys, which could contribute to a high frequency of genetic variability, allowing the virus to subvert host immune surveillance. Though this study had a small sample size, it suggested a trend toward better control of viral replication in animals not exposed to opioids (Suzuki et al., 2002; Chuang et al., 2005). In a larger study by Kumar et al., rhesus macaques were chronically injected with either morphine or saline. After morphine dependence was established, all animals were inoculated with a cocktail of three viruses including $SHIV_{KU-1B}$, $SHIV_{89.6P}$, and SIV 17E-Fr and followed for an additional 18 weeks. This viral cocktail is known to induce very rapid disease with precipitous loss of CD4+ T cells which fail to recover. This study concluded that morphine-treated animals have a greater loss of CD4+ T cells and a higher viral set point with greater CNS viral loads compared to untreated, infected controls (Kumar et al., 2004).

Notwithstanding the mounting data that opioids may negatively affect the immune system and potentiate HIV disease progression, there is evidence from epidemiological, clinical, and basic studies that opiate exposure may have protective effects on the progression of HIV infections (Donahoe & Vlahov, 1998; Kapadia, Vlahov, Donahoe, & Friedland, 2005; Donahoe et al., 2009). In a large, long-term study by Donahoe et al., rhesus macaques were chronically injected with either morphine or saline. After two weeks of injections, macaques were inoculated with the sooty mangabey strain of SIV (SIVmm9). These animals were then followed for over two years. This study found no evidence that opiates exacerbated the course of infection and the development of simian AIDS. In fact, of the 40% of animals that succumbed to AIDS and died prior to completion of the study, only one-quarter were exposed to morphine. Therefore, this study concluded that chronic morphine administration decelerates the progression of HIV with this effect most pronounced in animals with high viral set points which suggests that opiate dependency moderates disease distress associated with high viral virulence (Donahoe et al., 2009). It should be noted when evaluating these conclusions that SIVsmm9 is a slow progressing virus and does not cause a loss of circulating CD4+ T cells until late in the infection; unlike HIV infection which is characterized in the acute phase by a large decrease in the number of circulating CD4+ T cells, followed by a steady decline until a point is reached where the levels of viremia rises sharply and AIDS develops. Thus, the rhesus macaque/SIVsmm9 model may not be the most appropriate for studying the effects of chronic opiate exposure and HIV.

In another study by Marcario et al., rhesus macaques were divided into three groups (morphine only, morphine + virus, and virus only) to determine the effects of morphine on the pathogenesis of SIV. Morphine was chronically injected into two groups. After establishment of morphine dependence, animals were inoculated with SIVmacR71/17E and followed for 33 weeks. This virus causes the same type of disease in macaques that HIV causes in humans, but on a much faster timescale. This study concluded that morphine did not affect plasma or CSF viral titers, did not increase the incidence of neurological disease, nor did it affect disease progression compared to non-treated, virus-infected animals. However, there was a tendency for increased accumulation of virus in the brains of morphine-treated animals. Also, the morphine-treated animals developed a somewhat different type of CNS disease with lesions in the white matter of the brain, whereas untreated infected animals developed gray matter encephalitis (Marcario et al., 2008).

Differences in virus stocks and virulence of viruses used and different drug-dosing regimens may account for some or all of the incongruent conclusions of the preceding studies. These outcomes typify the complexities of opioids and HIV infection on the immune system.

CONCLUSION

Drug abuse is an important element in the HIV/AIDS epidemic. Even though our knowledge and understanding of the pathogenesis of HIV has dramatically increased since the initial discovery of the virus almost three decades ago, our ability to determine the role of drugs of abuse in altering immune function and viral-host interactions remains limited. The complexities of both HIV infection and drug abuse make it extremely difficult to draw conclusions from clinical and epidemiological data. However, nonhuman primate models have been shown to replicate key features of

HIV disease but on an accelerated timescale, and can be studied under more controlled environmental conditions compared to human studies and with much more invasive approaches. These models continue to show great promise for investigating the effects of drugs of abuse on lentivirus pathogenesis.

REFERENCES

Alcabes, P. & Friedland. G. (1995). Injection drug use and human immunodeficiency virus infection. *Clin Infect Dis*, 20(6), 1467–79.

Alkhatib, G., Combadiere, C., Broder, C. C., Feng, Y., Kennedy, P. E., Murphy, P. M., et al. (1996). CC CKR5: A RANTES, MIP-1alpha, MIP-1beta receptor as a fusion cofactor for macrophage-tropic HIV-1. *Science*, 272(5270), 1955–8.

Ancuta, P., Kunstman, K. J., Autissier, P., Zaman, T., Stone, D., Wolinsky, S. M., et al. (2006). CD16+ monocytes exposed to HIV promote highly efficient viral replication upon differentiation into macrophages and interaction with T cells. *Virology*, 344(2), 267–76.

Anthony, I. C. & Bell, J. E. (2008). The neuropathology of HIV/AIDS. *Int Rev Psychiatry*, 20(1), 15–24.

Anthony, I. C., Ramage, S. N., Carnie, F. W., Simmonds, P., & Bell, J. E. (2005). Influence of HAART on HIV-related CNS disease and neuroinflammation. *J Neuropathol Exp Neurol*, 64(6), 529–36.

Bell, J. E., Donaldson, Y. K., Lowrie, S., McKenzie, C. A., Elton, R. A., Chiswick, A., et al. (1996). Influence of risk group and zidovudine therapy on the development of HIV encephalitis and cognitive impairment in AIDS patients. *AIDS*, 10(5), 493–9.

Berman, N. E., Marcario, J. K., Yong, C., Raghavan, R., Raymond, L. A., Joag, S. V., et al. (1999). Microglial activation and neurological symptoms in the SIV model of neuroAIDS: Association of MHC-II and MMP-9 expression with behavioral deficits and evoked potential changes. *Neurobiol Dis*, 6(6), 486–98.

Bissel, S. J., Wang, G., Trichel, A. M., Murphey-Corb, M., & Wiley, C. A. (2006). Longitudinal analysis of activation markers on monocyte subsets during the development of simian immunodeficiency virus encephalitis. *J Neuroimmunol*, 177(1–2), 85–98.

Bouwman, F. H., Skolasky, R. L., Hes, D., Selnes, O. A., Glass, J. D., Nance-Sproson, T. E., et al. (1998). Variable progression of HIV-associated dementia. *Neurology*, 50(6), 1814–20.

Brancato, V., Delvechio, G., & Simone, P. (1995). Survival and mortality in a cohort of heroin addicts in 1985-1994. *Minerva Med*, 86(3), 97.

Cantacuzene, J. (1898). Nouvelles recherches sur le monde de destruction des vibrions dans l'organisme. *Ann Inst Pasteur*, 12, 273–300.

Chiesi, A., Vella, S., Dally, L. G., Pedersen, C., Danner, S., Johnson, A. M., et al. (1996). Epidemiology of AIDS dementia complex in Europe. AIDS in Europe Study Group. *J Acquir Immune Defic Syndr Hum Retrovirol*, 11(1), 39–44.

Chuang, L. F., Killam, Jr., K. F., & Chuang, R. Y. (1993). Increased replication of simian immunodeficiency virus in CEM x174 cells by morphine sulfate. *Biochem Biophys Res Commun*, 195(3), 1165–73.

Chuang, R. Y., Suzuki, S., Chuang, T. K., Miyagi, T., Chuang, L. F., & Doi, R. H. (2005). Opioids and the progression of simian AIDS. *Front Biosci*, 10, 1666–77.

Davis, L. E., Hjelle, B. L., Miller, V. E., Palmer, D. L., Llewellyn, A. L., Merlin, T. L., et al. (1992). Early viral brain invasion in iatrogenic human immunodeficiency virus infection. *Neurology*, 42(9), 1736–9.

De Vries, T. J. & Shippenberg, T. S. (2002). Neural systems underlying opiate addiction. *J Neurosci*, 22(9), 3321–5.

Deng, H., Liu, R., Ellmeier, W., Choe, S., Unutmaz, D., Burkhart, M., Di Marzio, P., et al. (1996). Identification of a major co-receptor for primary isolates of HIV-1. *Nature*, 381(6584), 661–6.

Dickson, D. W., Lee, S. C., Hatch, W., Mattiace, L. A., Brosnan, C. F., & Lyman, W. D. (1994). Macrophages and microglia in HIV-related CNS neuropathology. *Res Publ Assoc Res Nerv Ment Dis*, 72, 99–118.

Dickson, D. W., Lee, S. C., Mattiace, L. A., Yen, S. H., & Brosnan, C. (1993). Microglia and cytokines in neurological disease, with special reference to AIDS and Alzheimer's disease. *Glia*, 7(1), 75–83.

Donahoe, R. M., O'Neil S. P., Marsteller, F. A., Novembre, F. J., Anderson, D. C., Lankford-Turner, P., et al. (2009). Probable deceleration of progression of Simian AIDS affected by opiate dependency: Studies with a rhesus macaque/SIVsmm9 model. *J Acquir Immune Defic Syndr*, 50 (3), 241–9.

Donahoe, R. M. & Vlahov, D. (1998). Opiates as potential cofactors in progression of HIV-1 infections to AIDS. *J Neuroimmunol*, 83(1–2), 77–87.

Douek, D. C., Brenchley, J. M., Betts, M. R., Ambrozak, D. R., Hill, B. J., Okamoto, Y., et al. (2002). HIV preferentially infects HIV-specific CD4+ T cells. *Nature*, 417(6884), 95–8.

Dragic, T., Litwin, V., Allaway, G. P., Martin, S. R., Huang, Y., Nagashima, K. A., et al. (1996). HIV-1 entry into CD4+ cells is mediated by the chemokine receptor CC-CKR-5. *Nature*, 381(6584), 667–73.

Fauci, A. S. (1988). The human immunodeficiency virus: Infectivity and mechanisms of pathogenesis. *Science*, 239(4840), 617–22.

Fecho, K., Maslonek, K. A., Coussons-Read, M. E., Dykstra, L. A., & Lysle, D. T. (1994). Macrophage-derived nitric oxide is involved in the depressed concanavalin A responsiveness of splenic lymphocytes from rats administered morphine in vivo. *J Immunol*, 152(12), 5845–52.

Friedman, H., Pross, S., & Klein, T. W. (2006). Addictive drugs and their relationship with infectious diseases. *FEMS Immunol Med Microbiol*, 47(3), 330–42.

Gabuzda, D. H. & Sobel, R. A. (1987). HIV antigen in brains of patients with AIDS. *Ann Neurol*, 22(5), 668.

Goodkin, K., Shapshak, P., Metsch, L. R., McCoy, C. B., Crandall, K. A., Kumar, M., et al. (1998). Cocaine abuse and HIV-1 infection: Epidemiology and neuropathogenesis. *J Neuroimmunol*, 83(1–2), 88–101.

Guo, C. J., Li, Y., Tian, S., Wang, X., Douglas, S. D., & Ho, W. Z. (2002). Morphine enhances HIV infection of human blood mononuclear phagocytes through modulation of beta-chemokines and CCR5 receptor. *J Investig Med*, 50(6), 435–42.

Hauser, K. F., El-Hage, N., Buch, S., Nath, A., Tyor, W. R., Bruce-Keller, A. J., et al. (2006). Impact of opiate-HIV-1 interactions on neurotoxic signaling. *J Neuroimmune Pharmacol*, 1(1), 98–105.

Ho, W. Z., Guo, C. J., Yuan, C. S., Douglas, S. D., & Moss, J. (2003). Methylnaltrexone antagonizes opioid-mediated enhancement of HIV infection of human blood mononuclear phagocytes. *J Pharmacol Exp Ther*, 307(3), 1158–62.

Hu, S., Sheng, W. S., Lokensgard, J. R., & Peterson, P. K. (2005). Morphine potentiates HIV-1 gp120-induced neuronal apoptosis. *J Infect Dis*, 191(6), 886–9.

Hult, B., Chana, G., Masliah, E., & Everall, I. (2008). Neurobiology of HIV. *Int Rev Psychiatry*, 20(1), 3–13.

Joag, S. V., Adany, I., Li, Z., Foresman, L., Pinson, D. M., Wang, C., et al. (1997). Animal model of mucosally transmitted human immunodeficiency virus type 1 disease: Intravaginal and oral deposition of simian/human immunodeficiency virus in macaques results in systemic infection, elimination of CD4+ T cells, and AIDS. *J Virol*, 71(5), 4016–23.

Kapadia, F., Vlahov, D., Donahoe, R. M., & Friedland, G. (2005). The role of substance abuse in HIV disease progression: Reconciling differences from laboratory and epidemiologic investigations. *Clin Infect Dis*, 41(7), 1027–34.

Koenig, S., Gendelman, H. E., Orenstein, J. M., Dal Canto, M. C., Pezeshkpour, G. H., Yungbluth, M., et al. (1986). Detection of AIDS virus in macrophages in brain tissue from AIDS patients with encephalopathy. *Science*, 233(4768), 1089–93.

Kumar, R., Torres, C., Yamamura, Y., Rodriguez, I., Martinez, M., Staprans, S., et al. (2004). Modulation by morphine of viral set point in rhesus macaques infected with simian immunodeficiency virus and simian-human immunodeficiency virus. *J Virol*, 78(20), 11425–8.

Lackner, A. A., Smith, M. O., Munn, R. J., Martfeld, D. J., Gardner, M. B., Marx, P. A., et al. (1991). Localization of simian immunodeficiency virus in the central nervous system of rhesus monkeys. *Am J Pathol*, 139(3), 609–21.

Lackner, A. A. & Veazey, R. S. (2007). Current concepts in AIDS pathogenesis: Insights from the SIV/macaque model. *Annu Rev Med*, 58, 461–76.

Lackner, A. A., Vogel, P., Ramos, R. A., Kluge, J. D., & Marthas, M. (1994). Early events in tissues during infection with pathogenic (SIVmac239) and nonpathogenic (SIVmac1A11) molecular clones of simian immunodeficiency virus. *Am J Pathol*, 145(2), 428–39.

Ledebur, H. C. & Parks, T. P. (1995). Transcriptional regulation of the intercellular adhesion molecule-1 gene by inflammatory cytokines in human endothelial cells. Essential roles of a variant NF-kappa B site and p65 homodimers. *J Biol Chem*, 270(2), 933–43.

Levy, J. A. (1993). HIV pathogenesis and long-term survival. *AIDS*, 7(11), 1401–10.

Madden, J. J., Wang, Y., Lankford-Turner, P., & Donahoe, R. M. (2002). Does reduced DNA repair capacity play a role in HIV infection and progression in the lymphocytes of opiate addicts? *J Acquir Immune Defic Syndr*, 31 Suppl 2, S78–83.

Marcario, J. K., Riazi, M., Adany, I., Kenjale, H., Fleming, K., Marquis, J., et al. (2008). Effect of morphine on the neuropathogenesis of SIVmac infection in Indian Rhesus Macaques. *J Neuroimmune Pharmacol*, 3(1), 12–25.

Martinez, A. J., Sell, M., Mitrovics, T., Stoltenburg-Didinger, G., Iglesias-Rozas, J. R., Giraldo-Velasquez, M. A., et al. (1995). The neuropathology and epidemiology of AIDS. A Berlin experience. A review of 200 cases. *Pathol Res Pract*, 191(5), 427–43.

Mattapallil, J. J., Douek, D. C., Hill, B., Nishimura, Y., Martin, M., & Roederer, M. (2005). Massive infection and loss of memory CD4+ T cells in multiple tissues during acute SIV infection. *Nature*, 434(7037), 1093–7.

McManus, C. M., Weidenheim, K., Woodman, S. E., Nunez, J., Hesselgesser, J., Nath, A., et al. (2000). Chemokine and chemokine-receptor expression in human glial elements: Induction by the HIV protein, Tat, and chemokine autoregulation. *Am J Pathol*, 156(4), 1441–53.

Mehandru, S., Poles, M. A., Tenner-Racz, K., Manuelli, V., Jean-Pierre, P., Lopez, P., et al. (2007). Mechanisms of gastrointestinal CD4+ T-cell depletion during acute and early human immunodeficiency virus type 1 infection. *J Virol*, 81(2), 599–612.

Miyagi, T., Chuang, L. F., Doi, R. H., Carlos, M. P., Torres, J. V., & Chuang, R. Y. (2000). Morphine induces gene expression of CCR5 in human CEMx174 lymphocytes. *J Biol Chem*, 275(40), 31305–10.

Narayan, O. & Clements, J. E. (1989). Biology and pathogenesis of lentiviruses. *J Gen Virol*, 70(Pt 7), 1617–39.

Nath, A., Maragos, W. F., Avison, M. J., Schmitt, F. A., & Berger, J. R. (2001). Acceleration of HIV dementia with methamphetamine and cocaine. *J Neurovirol*, 7(1), 66–71.

Nath, A., Schiess, N., Venkatesan, A., Rumbaugh, J., Sacktor, N., & McArthur, J. (2008). Evolution of HIV dementia with HIV infection. *Int Rev Psychiatry*, 20(1), 25–31.

Pantaleo, G., Graziosi, C., & Fauci, A. S. (1993). The role of lymphoid organs in the pathogenesis of HIV infection. *Semin Immunol*, 5(3), 157–63.

Peterson, P. K., Gekker, G., Hu, S., Anderson, W. R., Kravitz, F., Portoghese, P. S., et al. (1994). Morphine amplifies HIV-1 expression in chronically infected promonocytes cocultured with human brain cells. *J Neuroimmunol*, 50(2), 167–75.

Peterson, P. K., Gekker, G., Schut, R., Hu, S., Balfour, H. H. Jr., & Chao, C. C. (1993). Enhancement of HIV-1 replication by opiates and cocaine: The cytokine connection. *Adv Exp Med Biol*, 335, 181–8.

Peterson, P. K., Sharp, B. M., Gekker, G., Portoghese, P. S., Sannerud, K., & Balfour, H. H. Jr. (1990). Morphine promotes the growth of HIV-1 in human peripheral blood mononuclear cell cocultures. *AIDS*, 4(9), 869–73.

Picker, L. J. & Watkins, D. I. (2005). HIV pathogenesis: The first cut is the deepest. *Nat Immunol*, 6(5), 430–2.

Rock, R. B., Hu, S., Sheng, W. S., & Peterson, P. K. (2006). Morphine stimulates CCL2 production by human neurons. *J Neuroinflammation*, 3, 32.

Ronald, P. J., Robertson, J. R., & Elton, R. A. (1994). Continued drug use and other cofactors for progression to AIDS among injecting drug users. *AIDS*, 8(3), 339–43.

Rosenberg, Z. F. & Fauci, A. S. (1991). Immunopathogenesis of HIV infection. *FASEB J*, 5(10), 2382–90.

Roy, S. & Loh, H. H. (1996). Effects of opioids on the immune system. *Neurochem Res*, 21(11), 1375–86.

Roy, S., Wang, J., Charboneau, R., Loh, H. H., & Barke, R. A. (2005). Morphine induces CD4+ T cell IL-4 expression through an adenylyl cyclase mechanism independent of the protein kinase A pathway. *J Immunol*, 175(10), 6361–7.

Roy, S., Wang, J., Gupta, S., Charboneau, R., Loh, H. H., & Barke, R. A. (2004). Chronic morphine treatment differentiates T helper cells to Th2 effector cells by modulating transcription factors GATA 3 and T-bet. *J Neuroimmunol*, 147(1-2), 78–81.

Roy, S., Wang, J., Kelschenbach, J., Koodie, L., & Martin, J. (2006). Modulation of immune function by morphine: Implications for susceptibility to infection. *J Neuroimmune Pharmacol*, 1(1), 77–89.

Selwyn, P. A., Alcabes, P., Hartel, D., Buono, D., Schoenbaum, E. E., Klein, R. S., et al. (1992). Clinical manifestations and predictors of disease progression in drug users with human immunodeficiency virus infection. *N Engl J Med*, 327(24), 1697–703.

Sharp, B. M. (2003). Opioid receptor expression and intracellular signaling by cells involved in host defense and immunity. *Adv Exp Med Biol*, 521, 98–105.

Sharp, B. M., Roy, S., & Bidlack, J. M. (1998). Evidence for opioid receptors on cells involved in host defense and the immune system. *J Neuroimmunol*, 83(1-2), 45–56.

Spijkerman, I. J., Langendam, M. W., Veugelers, P. J., van Ameijden, E. J., Keet, I. P., Geskus, R. B., et al. (1996). Differences in progression to AIDS between injection drug users and homosexual men with documented dates of seroconversion. *Epidemiology*, 7(6), 571–7.

Stefano, G. B., Scharrer, B., Smith, E. M., Hughes, T. K. Jr., Magazine, H. I., Bilfinger, T. V., et al. (1996). Opioid and opiate immunoregulatory processes. *Crit Rev Immunol*, 16(2), 109–44.

Suzuki, S., Chuang, A. J., Chuang, L. F., Doi, R. H., & Chuang, R. Y. (2002). Morphine promotes simian acquired immunodeficiency syndrome virus replication in monkey peripheral mononuclear cells: Induction of CC chemokine receptor 5 expression for virus entry. *J Infect Dis*, 185(12), 1826–9.

Szabo, I., Rojavin, M., Bussiere, J. L., Eisenstein, T. K., Adler, M. W., & Rogers, T. J. (1993). Suppression of peritoneal macrophage phagocytosis of Candida albicans by opioids. *J Pharmacol Exp Ther*, 267(2), 703–6.

Thorpe, L. E., Frederick, M., Pitt, J., Cheng, I., Watts, D. H., Buschur, S., et al. (2004). Effect of hard-drug use on CD4 cell percentage, HIV RNA level, and progression to AIDS-defining class C events among HIV-infected women. *J Acquir Immune Defic Syndr*, 37(3), 1423–30.

Tomei, E. Z. & Renaud, F. L. (1997). Effect of morphine on Fc-mediated phagocytosis by murine macrophages in vitro. *J Neuroimmunol*, 74(1-2), 111–6.

Tomlinson, G. S., Simmonds, P., Busuttil, A., Chiswick, A., & Bell, J. E. (1999). Upregulation of microglia in drug users with and without pre-symptomatic HIV infection. *Neuropathol Appl Neurobiol*, 25(5), 369–79.

Welters, I. D., Menzebach, A., Goumon, Y., Cadet, P., Menges, T., Hughes, T. K., et al. (2000). Morphine inhibits NF-kappaB nuclear binding in human neutrophils and monocytes by a nitric oxide-dependent mechanism. *Anesthesiology*, 92(6), 1677–84.

Williams, K. C. & Hickey, W. F. (2002). Central nervous system damage, monocytes and macrophages, and neurological disorders in AIDS. *Annu Rev Neurosci*, 25, 537–62.

Woody, G. E. & Metzger, D. S. (1993). Causes of death in injection-drug users. *N Engl J Med*, 329(22), 1661.

5.7

SIV AND FIV MODELS OF PERIPHERAL NEUROPATHY

Victoria A. Laast, Gigi Ebenezer, Justin C. McArthur, and Joseph L. Mankowski

Peripheral neuropathy frequently develops in HIV-infected patients. The most common clinical manifestation of HIV-induced peripheral nervous system (PNS) disease is distal sensory polyneuropathy. Many HIV-infected individuals receiving combination antiretroviral therapy develop HIV-induced PNS disease despite effective suppression of HIV replication in both plasma and the cerebrospinal fluid. Complicating the picture further, treatment of HIV infection with nucleoside reverse transcriptase inhibitors can itself produce a peripheral neuropathy, known as antiretroviral toxic neuropathy, that is clinically indistinguishable from HIV-mediated PNS damage. The fact that both HIV and antiretroviral treatment can damage the PNS complicates clinical studies of the pathogenesis of HIV-induced PNS disease. Animal models are essential to determine where and when initial neuronal injury occurs and to dissect out the effects of HIV infection from the effects of potentially neurotoxic antiretroviral drugs. This chapter provides a detailed overview of animal work in this area.

Peripheral neuropathy frequently develops in HIV-infected patients including those receiving antiretroviral therapy (Brinley et al., 2001; Kennedy et al., 2004; Keswani & Hoke, 2003; McArthur et al., 2005). The most common clinical manifestation of HIV-induced peripheral nervous system disease is distal sensory polyneuropathy (DSP), a debilitating syndrome with gradual onset of bilateral pain most pronounced in the soles of the feet (Cornblath & McArthur, 1988; Pardo et al., 2001). Although HIV-induced peripheral neuropathy is not life threatening, the relentless pain markedly impacts quality of life (McArthur et al., 2005; Simpson & Tagliati, 1994).

Many HIV-infected individuals receiving combination antiretroviral (cART) therapy develop HIV-induced PNS disease despite effective suppression of HIV replication in both plasma and CSF. Treatment of HIV infection with nucleoside reverse transcriptase inhibitors including zacitabine, stavudine, and didanosine, as well as protease inhibitors to control systemic viral replication, may induce unintended toxic neuropathy as a side effect (Cherry et al., 2003; Cherry et al., 2006; Cherry et al., 2008; Pettersen et al., 2006). The fact that both HIV and antiretroviral treatment can damage the PNS complicates clinically based studies of the pathogenesis of HIV-induced PNS disease. Antiretroviral toxic neuropathy (ATN) is clinically indistinguishable from HIV-mediated PNS damage. The reported incidence of HIV

neuropathy in cART-treated individuals varies from 13 to 52% depending on the cohort evaluated (Brinley et al., 2001; Cornblath & McArthur, 1988; Morgello et al., 2004; Schifitto et al., 2002).

HIV-induced PNS disease exhibits clinical features consistent with length-dependent nerve damage; however, the pathogenesis of HIV-induced damage to the sensory nociceptive pathway is poorly understood. The sites of primary damage in HIV-induced PNS disease remain to be established. Studies of the pathogenesis of HIV-induced PNS damage are severely limited by the inability to sample multiple components of the sensory pain pathway in HIV-infected individuals, highlighting the pressing need for a robust animal model. Animal models are essential to determine where and when initial neuronal injury occurs and to dissect out the effects of HIV infection separate from the effects of potentially neurotoxic antiretroviral drugs (Clements et al., 2008; Kennedy et al., 2004; Zhu et al., 2005). It is crucial to define the mechanisms underlying HIV PNS disease because this knowledge would direct appropriate therapeutic strategies.

AN SIV/MACAQUE MODEL OF HIV NEUROPATHY

An SIV/macaque model to study HIV peripheral nervous system (PNS) disease would be valuable for several reasons: 1) Macaque immune responses to SIV infection closely resemble immune responses in HIV-infected individuals, 2) SIV shares extensive homology with HIV including binding of SIV gp120 to the co-receptor CCR5 for viral entry, and 3) neurovirulent molecular SIV clones such as SIV/17E-Fr are available to advance studies of HIV-induced neurologic disease (Mankowski et al., 1997; Mankowski et al., 2002b; Mankowski et al., 2002a). Although the macaque model is used widely to study host and viral aspects of HIV CNS disease, the SIV-macaque model has only recently been examined in detail for the presence of lesions in somatosensory ganglia that parallel pathologic features of HIV-induced PNS disease (Clements et al., 2008; Laast et al., 2007).

Numerous studies have shown that SIV-infected macaques develop morphologic changes closely resembling HIV infection in the brain, including encephalitis with characteristic multifocal perivascular infiltrates of macrophages and formation of multinucleated giant cells (Fox et al., 1997; Lackner et al., 1991; Mankowski et al., 2002a; Williams et al., 2008; Zink et al., 2006). Because many SIV models vary widely with respect to incidence of encephalitis and progression to AIDS (Westmoreland et al., 1998), a refined pigtailed macaque model was developed at Johns Hopkins to study HIV encephalitis. This SIV model of HIV CNS disease, in which most macaques develop SIV encephalitis by 84 days post infection, entails inoculation of pigtailed macaques (*Macaca nemestrina*) with the neurovirulent molecular clone SIV/17E-Fr and an immunosuppressive virus swarm SIV/DeltaB670. The timing of disease progression from acute- to late-stage infection is highly reproducible in this model, with approximately 90% of SIV-infected macaques developing encephalitis within 3 months postinoculation (Zink et al., 1997).

To determine whether this SIV model developed to study HIV CNS disease also could serve as an SIV/macaque model of HIV–induced peripheral neuropathy, key components of the sensory pain pathway were evaluated, including samples of skin from distal leg, sural and sciatic nerves, and somatosensory ganglia, including dorsal root ganglia as well as trigeminal ganglia, collected from pigtailed macaques inoculated with SIV/17E-Fr and SIV/DeltaB670.

EPIDERMAL NERVE FIBER DENSITY DECLINES WITH SIV INFECTION

As skin biopsies are extremely useful to diagnose small sensory fiber neuropathies, they have supplanted sural nerve biopsies for diagnostic clinical purposes (Herrmann et al., 1999; Herrmann et al., 2004; Holland et al., 1997; McCarthy et al., 1995; Morgello et al., 2004; Polydefkis, 2002; Polydefkis et al., 2002). A correlation between epidermal nerve fiber (ENF) densities and neuropathic pain has been demonstrated by studies of HIV-infected patients (Polydefkis, 2002; Polydefkis et al., 2002). To determine whether epidermal nerve fiber loss also occurred with SIV infection, epidermal nerve fiber densities in footpad samples from SIV-infected macaques were measured following immunostaining for PGP9.5, and then were compared with ENF density in uninfected, age-matched animals. Immunostaining to detect PGP9.5, a pan-neuronal marker present in peripheral nerves, is widely used to identify epidermal nerve fibers in skin biopsy samples (Kennedy et al., 2000). Intra-epidermal nerve fiber density was significantly lower in SIV-infected macaques versus uninfected, age-matched animals. This striking loss of small sensory fibers in SIV-infected macaques parallels ENF decline in HIV-infected patients (Figure 5.7.1).

LESIONS IN SOMATOSENSORY GANGLIA OF SIV-INFECTED MACAQUES

Morphologic changes identified in the dorsal root ganglia (DRG) in HIV patients include infiltrates of macrophages,

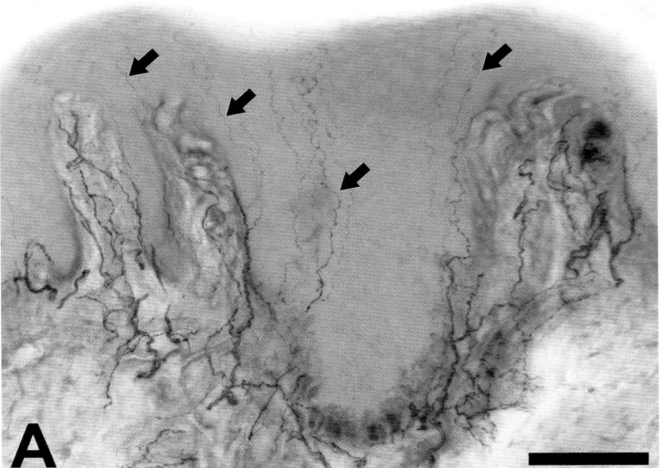

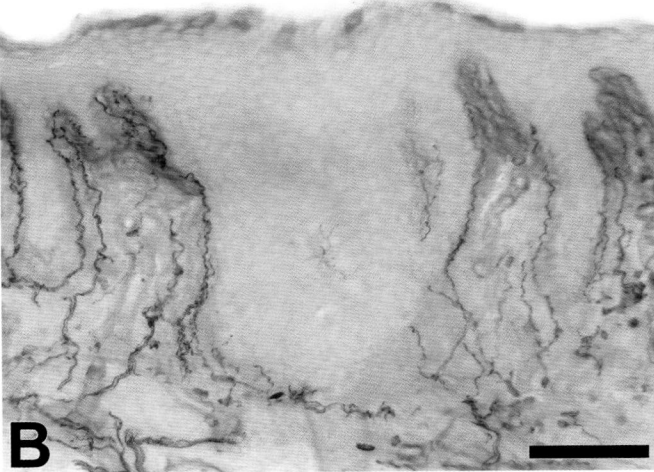

Figure 5.7.1 Representative sections of skin harvested from the plantar foot pad of control and SIV-infected animals at terminal stages of infection were immunostained for PGP 9.5 to evaluate epidermal nerve fiber alterations. Epidermal nerve fiber density (arrows denoting nerve fibers in epidermis) was much lower in SIV-infected animals (B) versus controls (A). Scale bars = 100 uM

loss of neurons, and the presence of Nageotte nodules (Esiri et al., 1993; Keswani & Hoke, 2003; Pardo et al., 2001). In our initial studies, we documented alterations in the trigeminal ganglia of SIV-infected macaques that closely resembled the alterations reported in the DRG from HIV-infected individuals (Laast et al., 2007). Somatosensory neurons in the trigeminal ganglia are structurally and functionally homologous to those of the DRG. Previous studies also have demonstrated that HIV-induced alterations in somatosensory ganglia are similar regardless of specific anatomic location of sensory ganglia (Scaravilli et al., 1992). Lesions in the trigeminal ganglia from SIV-infected macaques consisted of diffuse aggregates of infiltrating macrophages accompanied by scattered CD3+ lymphocytes. The presence of infiltrating macrophages adjacent to neurons, suggestive of neuronophagia, was frequent in animals with moderate to severe ganglionitis. In addition, Nageotte nodules, characterized by overt neuronal loss with replacement by both satellite cells and infiltrating mononuclear cells, were present in animals with severe ganglionitis (Laast et al., 2007). Follow-up studies have confirmed similar changes in the lumbar DRG in SIV-infected macaques. Taken together, these lesions in sensory ganglia from SIV-infected macaques demonstrate that SIV infection induces pathology in somatosensory ganglia that closely resembles the inflammatory lesions reported in dorsal root ganglia of HIV-infected individuals with distal sensory polyneuropathy (McArthur et al., 2005; Pardo et al., 2001).

In contrast with findings in ganglia, microscopic examination of toluidine blue-stained sections of sural and sciatic nerves did not reveal consistent development of overt neuritis or marked damage to myelinated fibers in SIV-infected macaques despite the presence of inflammatory changes in the DRG. Inflammatory lesions may still be present multifocally in peripheral nerves but may be difficult to detect given the extensive length of peripheral nerves. In humans, a similar paucity of lesions in sural nerves has also been reported (Gonzalez-Duarte et al., 2007; Gonzalez-Duarte et al., 2008).

INFLAMMATORY INFILTRATES IN SOMATOSENSORY GANGLIA

To measure infiltrating mononuclear cells identified in SIV-infected macaques, sections of ganglia were immunostained for the macrophage marker CD68. Total immunostaining for CD68-positive cells in ganglia was significantly higher in SIV-infected macaques examined at terminal stages of infection than in uninfected control animals. CD68 immunostaining also demonstrated a prominent resident population of CD68-positive macrophages located in the perineuronal compartment of ganglia in uninfected macaques. Although macrophage activation reflected by increased CD68 immunostaining of macrophages distributed diffusely throughout the perineuronal compartment appeared to be higher in SIV-infected macaques with ganglionitis than in control animals, the current lack of markers to differentiate between resident versus infiltrating macrophages limits our ability to resolve resident macrophage activation separate from infiltrating macrophages. It is likely that both macrophage populations contribute to inflammatory responses in sensory ganglia. In contrast with the increases in macrophages in SIV-infected macaques examined at terminal stages of disease, cytotoxic T cells (TIA-1+, CD3+) were present in variable numbers (Laast et al., 2007).

SIV REPLICATION IN SENSORY GANGLIA

To establish whether SIV was present in sensory ganglia of SIV-infected macaques at terminal stages of infection, trigeminal ganglia samples were immunostained for the SIV transmembrane protein gp41. Abundant SIV-infected cells were present amidst infiltrating mononuclear cells. In addition, SIV-positive cells were located diffusely in the perineuronal compartment, consistent with the distribution pattern of endogenous macrophages in ganglia. Most SIV-infected animals examined twelve weeks post-inoculation contained SIV in ganglia detected either by immunohistochemistry or in-situ hybridization. To identify the specific cell type/s in ganglia infected with SIV, sections were double immunostained for SIV gp41 and the macrophage marker Iba-1 and examined by laser confocal microscopy. Co-localization of SIV gp41 within Iba-1-positive macrophages demonstrated that macrophages were clearly the major cell type harboring SIV in sensory ganglia (Laast et al., 2007).

VIRUS DETECTION DURING ACUTE AND ASYMPTOMATIC INFECTION

To determine when macrophages in somatosensory ganglia were infected following SIV inoculation, we also examined ganglia from SIV-infected macaques euthanized during acute and asymptomatic infection. In two of six animals evaluated during acute infection, replicating SIV was detected by in situ hybridization; however, SIV RNA was not detected at 21 days post-inoculation. This trend, with low levels of SIV replication during acute infection in ganglia that is suppressed by 21 days post-inoculation, parallels the pattern of virus replication in the CNS of SIV-infected animals (Clements et al., 2005). During later stages of disease, as SIV-infected macaques transition into terminal disease when both AIDS and CNS disease develop, replicating SIV is abundant in ganglia. These findings demonstrate that sensory ganglia can be infected during acute infection but it remains to be determined whether gangliotropic viral strains actually do remain latent in sensory ganglia as proviral DNA throughout asymptomatic infection with re-emergence during later stages of disease. Although we identified SIV RNA by in situ hybridization in one-third of SIV-infected macaques during acute infection, it is probable that the use of more sensitive techniques including RT-PCR would uncover active infection in additional animals during acute infection. The SIV/macaque model offers the opportunity to address these critical questions.

NEURONAL LOSS IN TRIGEMINAL GANGLIA OF SIV-INFECTED MACAQUES

To determine whether neuronal loss developed in trigeminal ganglia of SIV-infected macaques, neuronal density in ganglia was measured using an unbiased stereological method, the area fraction fractionator technique. The area occupied by neurons in the trigeminal ganglia of SIV-infected macaques was significantly lower than control macaques, consistent with loss of neurons in the ganglia. The observed decline in neuronal density in ganglia was inversely correlated with the levels of macrophage infiltration. Given that the extent of macrophage infiltration in ganglia was co-linear with levels of SIVgp41, neurotoxic products generated by activated macrophages, including viral proteins, could mediate neuronal damage in sensory ganglia. Double-labeling studies showing SIV gp41 contained within macrophages in ganglia demonstrate the importance of macrophage-tropic SIV for inducing damage in somatosensory ganglia (Laast et al., 2007). It is possible that both resident and recruited macrophages develop an activated immunophenotype as well as support SIV replication within somatosensory ganglia. Local resident macrophages in particular are leading candidates for harboring latent SIV DNA in the peripheral nervous system.

SIV CNS disease is associated with replication of SIV in macrophages, resembling observations of SIV replication in trigeminal ganglia (Clements et al., 2002). To determine whether development of PNS disease closely paralleled SIV CNS disease within individual animals, we examined whether there was an association between host immune responses in SIV PNS disease versus SIV CNS disease. The presence of ganglionitis in trigeminal ganglia was not associated with concurrent encephalitis in the CNS in individual animals. This lack of concordance between development of SIV PNS and CNS disease in individual SIV-infected animals indicates that despite similarities such as replication of SIV in macrophages, there also are additional fundamental differences between the pathogenesis of lentiviral-induced CNS and PNS disease (Laast et al., 2007). Although resident populations of macrophages have been described in both PNS and the brain, important differences in barrier properties between the blood and these separate macrophage populations (such as the lack of a blood-ganglia barrier in the PNS versus the blood-brain barrier) influence regulation of macrophage activation and susceptibility to HIV infection (Esiri & Reading, 1989; Williams et al., 2001).

In summary, the presence of replicating SIV within macrophages in somatosensory ganglia coupled with neuronal loss demonstrates that this SIV/macaque model may be used to study the pathogenesis of HIV neuropathy. Initial studies that focused on the trigeminal ganglia to address these questions identified several parallels between SIV PNS disease and SIV CNS disease, including (1) replication of SIV predominantly within macrophages in ganglia; (2) the presence of SIV RNA in ganglia during acute infection, with reduction of SIV replication after acute infection; and (3) increases in CD68 immunostaining in the ganglia of SIV-infected animals, likely representing both recruitment of monocytes as well as activation of endogenous macrophage populations (Laast et al, 2007). Additional studies targeting pathologic and corresponding physiologic alterations in the PNS of SIV-infected pigtailed macaques will further our understanding of the pathogenesis of HIV PNS disease.

SIV IMPAIRS NERVE REGENERATION AFTER AXOTOMY

Given our findings that SIV induces damage to the peripheral nervous system, we extended our studies to determine whether SIV infection also influenced the capacity of peripheral nerves to regenerate. This is an important question with respect to development of therapeutics to treat HIV peripheral neuropathy. To define the normal features of nerve regeneration in macaques and study the impact of SIV-infection on nerve regeneration, we developed an excisional intracutaneous axotomy model in SIV-infected macaques specifically to study re-innervation in denervated skin. We examined the regenerative pattern of cutaneous nerves following nerve transection via intracutaneous axotomy in pigtailed macaques inoculated with SIV/17E-Fr and SIV/DeltaB670 as described for earlier PNS evaluation (Rajan et al., 2003; Ebenezer et al., 2007; Ebenezer et al., 2009).

Beginning two weeks after SIV inoculation, cutaneous axotomies were performed at two-week intervals on skin of the back using a circular skin punch to transect epidermis and dermis (Figure 5.7.2). These circular incisions served to uniformly transect epidermal axons to allow evaluation of subsequent epidermal nerve fiber regrowth into the healing region of skin post-axotomy. On the 70th day after the initial incision, we harvested all of the previous 3 mm punch incision sites to obtain skin samples containing excision sites from 14, 28, 42, 56, and 70 days post-axotomy. Samples were then examined after immunostaining for the pan-axonal marker PGP 9.5 and the Schwann cell marker p75 nerve growth factor receptor.

Epidermal nerve fiber length of regenerating sprouting collateral epidermal fibers that extended into the excisional site from the edge of the axotomy site and epidermal nerve fibers in the epidermis outside the axotomy site were both measured. The sprouting epidermal fibers (termed sprouts = S) reflected reinnervation into the excisional site previously denervated by the axotomy. The epidermal fibers outside the initial axotomy zone (termed normal = N) represented normal epidermal fiber length. By measuring both sprout and normal fiber lengths in each individual animal, we were able to calculate the ratio of sprout length to normal fiber length for each animal, thus controlling for any variation in normal fiber length between animals. In these studies, SIV-infection delayed epidermal nerve fiber regeneration and remodeling of new sprouts at every time point evaluated post-axotomy (Figure 5.7.3). Sprout length was shorter in SIV-infected animals than uninfected control macaques in the early time points after axotomy. These differences in epidermal nerve regeneration between control and SIV-infected animals demonstrate that SIV-infection impairs epidermal nerve fiber regeneration following nerve injury.

Because Schwann cell migration into the denervated epidermis may play a crucial role in guiding axonal regrowth, we also measured epidermal Schwann cell density in SIV-infected versus control animals to determine whether SIV infection altered Schwann cell migration patterns post-axotomy (Figure 5.7.3). In this study, we found slower migration of Schwann cells into the denervated epidermis following axotomy in SIV-infected animals, suggesting that SIV infection altered Schwann cell support of epidermal nerve fiber regeneration (Ebenezer et al., 2009).

These findings illustrate the value of the SIV/macaque model for investigating the mechanisms underlying HIV-induced alterations in cutaneous nerve regeneration.

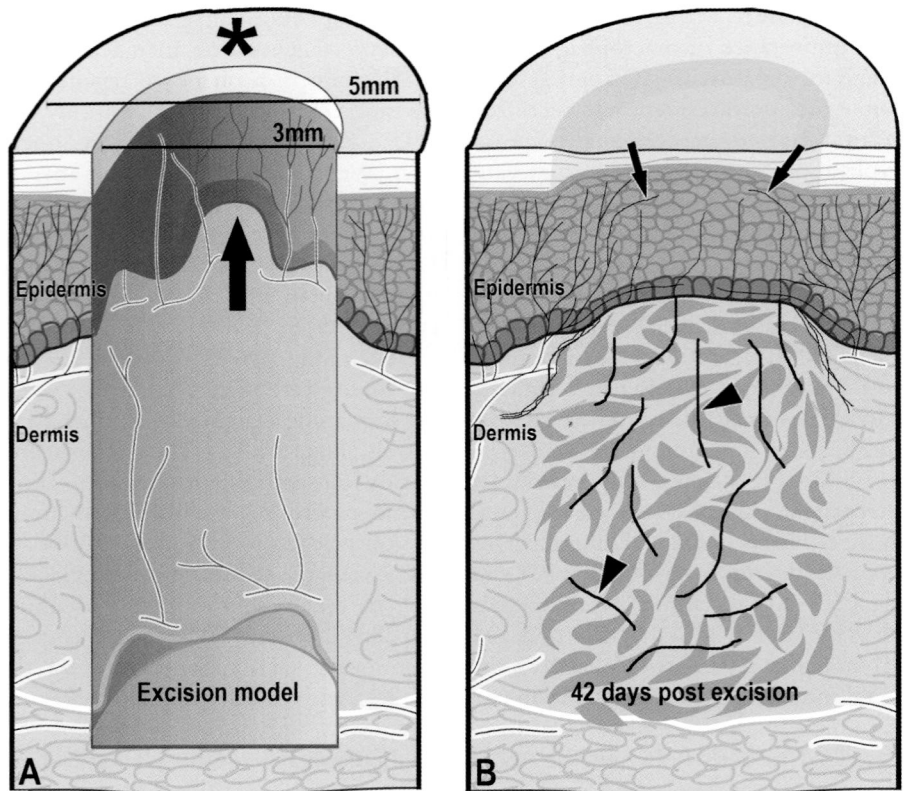

Figure 5.7.2 Circular cutaneous axotomies were performed at 2-week intervals on the dorsal interscapular skin using a 3 mm skin punch to transect epidermal axons (Fig. 5.7.2A). The central core containing epidermis and dermis was then removed (arrow), yielding an excisional axotomy. On the 70th day after the initial axotomy, a 5 mm circular biopsy punch (*) was used to harvest all of the previous 3 mm punch sites, providing samples containing axotomy sites that were 14, 28, 42, 56, and 70 days post-axotomy (Fig. 5.7.2A). By 42 days post-axotomy, collateral sprouts (arrows) and regenerating axons (arrowheads) had re-innervated the epidermis (Fig. 5.7.2B).

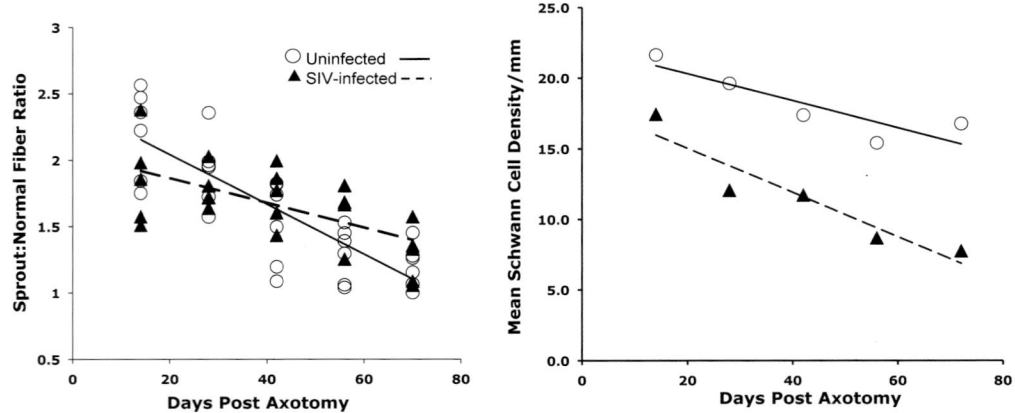

Figure 5.7.3 In contrast with uninfected macaques (circles, solid line), SIV-infected macaques (triangles, dashed line) had lower mean ratios of collateral sprout length (S) to normal nerve fiber length (N) at 14 day post-axotomy. Over time, the change in S: N ratio in SIV-infected macaques was significantly less than the S: N ratio in control macaques, indicating that SIV infection delayed epidermal fiber regeneration following axotomy (left panel). At every time point post-axotomy, the group of SIV-infected macaques (triangles, dashed line) consistently had lower mean Schwann cell density measurements than uninfected macaques (circles, solid line). In both infected and control animal groups, Schwann cell density was highest at the earliest time points post-axotomy and then declined at a similar rate for both groups over time (right panel).

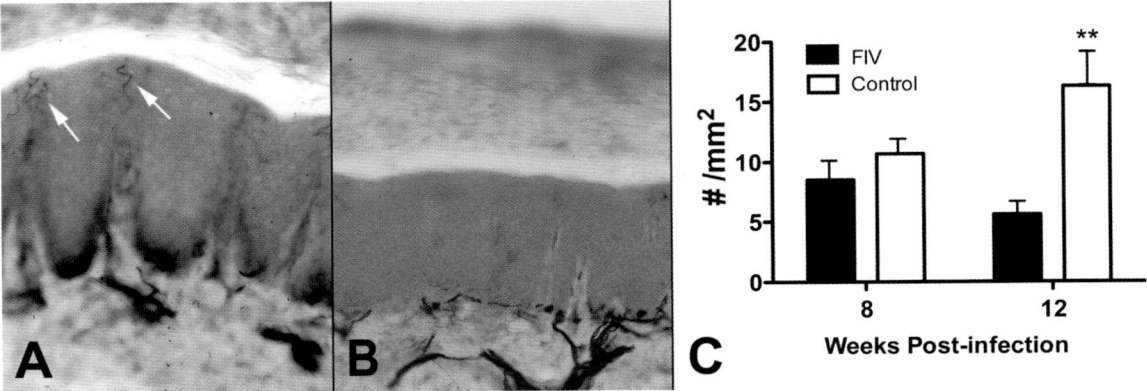

Figure 5.7.4 Abundant PGP 9.5-positive epidermal nerve fibers were present in skin from control cats (A), whereas FIV-infected cats had significant reduction in ENF 12 weeks post FIV-inoculation (B). Figure courtesy of Christopher Power.

Additional studies in SIV-infected macaques may help to define the specific Schwann cell-axon interactions relevant to the pathogenesis of HIV–associated sensory neuropathies. The relatively rapid regeneration time and the completeness of epidermal reinnervation in this macaque model provides a useful platform for assessing the efficacy of neurotrophic or regenerative drugs for sensory neuropathies including those caused by HIV. These findings also set the stage for examining neurotoxic damage caused by cART regimens including mitochondrial toxicity in the SIV/macaque model.

THE FIV MODEL OF HIV NEUROPATHY

Infection of domestic cats with feline immunodeficiency virus (FIV) is another valuable animal model for studying the pathogenesis of HIV neuropathy. Like HIV and SIV, FIV infection causes both immunosuppression and neurologic disease (Zink et al., 2006). The Power laboratory has established a model in which neurological and immune compromise develops in neonatally infected animals within 12 weeks of infection by using a chimeric infectious molecular clone, FIV-Ch, containing the full length V1CSF *env* on a Petaluma background (Kennedy et al., 2004). Similar to the SIV/macaque model for HIV PNS disease, FIV infection induces pathological events in the PNS like those seen in HIV sensory neuropathy, including alterations in the skin and dorsal root ganglia. Changes in nerves included reduced epidermal nerve fiber counts and myelinated fiber atrophy (reduced myelin sheath thickness) in sural nerves detected by morphometric analysis (Figure 5.7.4 and 5.7.5). Increased numbers of activated macrophages as well as elevated levels of TNF-α mRNA were also present in DRG and in the nerves. High levels of FIV RNA and DNA were detected in peripheral nerves in all FIV-infected cats. Of particular note with response to sensory perception, neurobehavioral studies demonstrated delayed

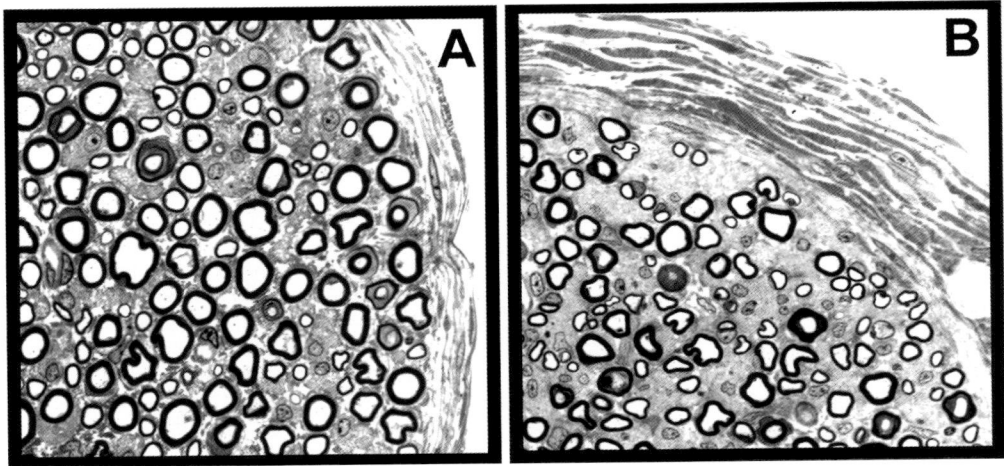

Figure 5.7.5 Control sural nerve from a cat demonstrates abundant myelinated fibers (A). In contrast, FIV-infected cats had a reduction in axonal density in sural nerve (B). Figure courtesy of Christopher Power.

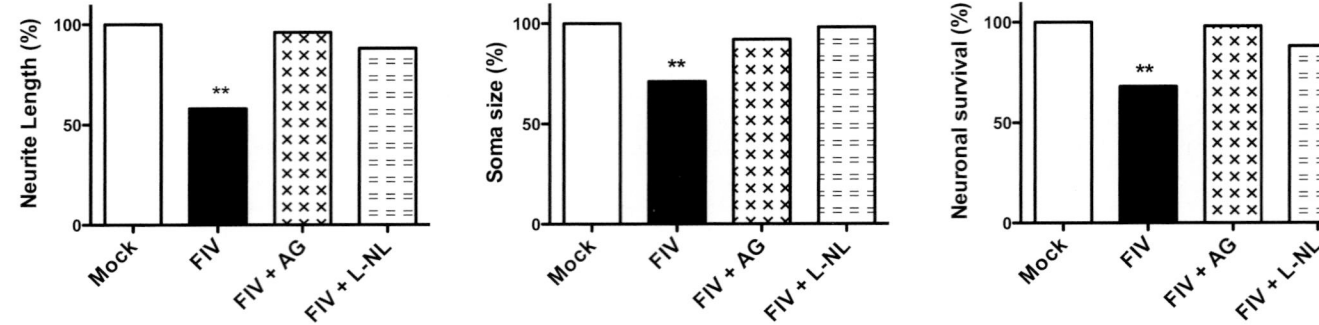

Figure 5.7.6 In ex vivo DRG cultures, treatment with the iNOS inhibitors aminoguanidine (AG) or (L-NIL) protected against FIV-induced neurite length reduction and soma size reduction. Treatment with these inhibitors also improved neuronal survival. Figure courtesy of Christopher Power.

withdrawal responses to a noxious thermal stimulus indicative of increased nociceptive thresholds in SIV-infected cats (Kennedy et al., 2004; Zhu et al., 2005)).

In this FIV model of HIV-induced peripheral neuropathy, high levels of CD3+ T cells were noted in DRG of infected cats. To study this observation using an ex vivo approach, FIV-infected lymphocytes were co-cultured with syngeneic DRG neurons, which induced neuronal damage and loss. This damage was found to be a consequence of CD40-CD154 mediated cell-to-cell interactions regulating contact between CD8+ T cells and neurons rather than a soluble factor (Zhu et al., 2006). This finding reinforces the premise that activated T cells may play crucial roles in neuronal damage.

In vivo findings in the FIV model were further extended by ex vivo studies using cultures consisting of primary feline sensory neurons, macrophages, and Schwann cells from DRG that were infected with the neurovirulent FIV strain V1-Ch. This approach demonstrated that FIV promoted damage and apoptosis of DRG neurons, which was mediated by STAT-1 activation as well as nitric oxide production by FIV-infected macrophages. Confirmatory studies demonstrated that the inducible nitric oxide synthase (iNOS) inhibitor aminoguanidine prevented neuronal injury in this model system (Figure 5.7.6). These experiments implicated STAT-1 and iNOS induction by activated macrophages in the DRG as a mechanism underlying neuronal damage and loss in the DRG with FIV infection (Zhu et al., 2005).

In addition to studying the pathogenesis of FIV-induced PNS damage, the FIV model has been used to study the mechanisms of antiretroviral toxic neuropathy induced by didanosine (ddI) superimposed upon FIV-induced damage using both in vivo and ex vivo approaches. In these studies, in DRG cultures, clinically relevant concentrations of ddI induced neuronal injury and corresponding reduced expression of both the neurotrophin BDNF and the mitochondrial cytochrome C oxidase subunit I gene (mtCOX I). Adding back BDNF to FIV-infected cultures reversed neuronal damage caused by FIV and ddI. In FIV-infected cats, treatment with ddI lowered plasma FIV loads; however, DRG FIV load was not reduced. Previously reported FIV-induced changes in withdrawal latency to a noxious stimulus and decline in epidermal nerve fibers were exacerbated by ddI treatment. These findings demonstrated that the additive damaging effects of FIV and ddI might be a consequence of impaired expression of both mitochondrial genes and neurotrophic factors (Zhu et al., 2007).

Further studies based in both the SIV and the FIV models of HIV-induced peripheral neuropathy will be crucial to advance our understanding of this insidious consequence of HIV infection. In particular, these animal models will be essential for defining mechanisms contributing to initial neuronal injury, to study the synergistic effects of HIV infection and neurotoxic antiretroviral drug regimens, and to develop new approaches to prevent and reverse damage to the peripheral nervous system in HIV-infected patients.

REFERENCES

Brinley, F. J., Jr., C. A. Pardo, and A. Verma. 2001. Human immunodeficiency virus and the peripheral nervous system workshop. *Arch Neurol* 58 (10):1561–6.

Cherry, C. L., J. C. McArthur, J. F. Hoy, and S. L. Wesselingh. 2003. Nucleoside analogues and neuropathy in the era of HAART. *J Clin Virol* 26 (2):195–207.

Cherry, C. L., A. Rosenow, J. S. Affandi, J. C. McArthur, S. L. Wesselingh, and P. Price. 2008. Cytokine genotype suggests a role for inflammation in nucleoside analog-associated sensory neuropathy (NRTI-SN) and predicts an individual's NRTI-SN risk. *AIDS Res Hum Retroviruses* 24 (2):117–23.

Cherry, C. L., R. L. Skolasky, L. Lal, J. Creighton, P. Hauer, S. P. Raman, R. Moore, K. Carter, D. Thomas, G. J. Ebenezer, S. L. Wesselingh, and J. C. McArthur. 2006. Antiretroviral use and other risks for HIV-associated neuropathies in an international cohort. *Neurology* 66 (6):867–73.

Clements, J. E., T. Babas, J. L. Mankowski, K. Suryanarayana, M. Piatak, Jr., P. M. Tarwater, J. D. Lifson, and M. C. Zink. 2002. The central nervous system as a reservoir for simian immunodeficiency virus (SIV): steady-state levels of SIV DNA in brain from acute through asymptomatic infection. *J Infect Dis* 186 (7):905–13.

Clements, J. E., M. Li, L. Gama, B. Bullock, L. M. Carruth, J. L. Mankowski, and M. C. Zink. 2005. The central nervous system is a viral reservoir in simian immunodeficiency virus–infected macaques on combined antiretroviral therapy: a model for human immunodeficiency virus patients on highly active antiretroviral therapy. *J Neurovirol* 11 (2):180–9.

Clements, J. E., J. L. Mankowski, L. Gama, and M. C. Zink. 2008. The accelerated simian immunodeficiency virus macaque model of human immunodeficiency virus-associated neurological disease: from mechanism to treatment. *J Neurovirol* 14 (4):309–17.

Cornblath, D. R., and J. C. McArthur. 1988. Predominantly sensory neuropathy in patients with AIDS and AIDS-related complex. *Neurology* 38 (5):794–6.

Ebenezer, G. J., P. Hauer, C. Gibbons, J. C. McArthur, and M. Polydefkis. 2007. Assessment of epidermal nerve fibers: a new diagnostic and predictive tool for peripheral neuropathies. *J Neuropathol Exp Neurol* 66 (12):1059–73.

Ebenezer, G. J., V. A. Laast, B. Dearman, P. Hauer, P. M. Tarwater, R. J. Adams, M. C. Zink, J. C. McArthur, and J. L. Mankowski. 2009. Altered cutaneous nerve regeneration in a simian immunodeficiency virus / macaque intracutaneous axotomy model. *J Comp Neurol* 514 (3):272–83.

Esiri, M. M., C. S. Morris, and P. R. Millard. 1993. Sensory and sympathetic ganglia in HIV-1 infection: immunocytochemical demonstration of HIV-1 viral antigens, increased MHC class II antigen expression and mild reactive inflammation. *J Neurol Sci* 114 (2):178–87.

Esiri, M. M., and M. C. Reading. 1989. Macrophages, lymphocytes and major histocompatibility complex (HLA) class II antigens in adult human sensory and sympathetic ganglia. *J Neuroimmunol* 23 (3):187–93.

Fox, H. S., L. H. Gold, S. J. Henriksen, and F. E. Bloom. 1997. Simian immunodeficiency virus: a model for neuroAIDS. *Neurobiol Dis* 4 (3–4):265–74.

Gonzalez-Duarte, A., K. Cikurel, and D. M. Simpson. 2007. Managing HIV peripheral neuropathy. *Curr HIV/AIDS Rep* 4 (3):114–8.

Gonzalez-Duarte, A., J. Robinson-Papp, and D. M. Simpson. 2008. Diagnosis and management of HIV-associated neuropathy. *Neurol Clin* 26 (3):821–32, x.

Herrmann, D. N., J. W. Griffin, P. Hauer, D. R. Cornblath, and J. C. McArthur. 1999. Epidermal nerve fiber density and sural nerve morphometry in peripheral neuropathies. *Neurology* 53 (8):1634–40.

Herrmann, D. N., M. P. McDermott, D. Henderson, L. Chen, K. Akowuah, and G. Schifitto. 2004. Epidermal nerve fiber density, axonal swellings and QST as predictors of HIV distal sensory neuropathy. *Muscle Nerve* 29 (3):420–7.

Holland, N. R., A. Stocks, P. Hauer, D. R. Cornblath, J. W. Griffin, and J. C. McArthur. 1997. Intraepidermal nerve fiber density in patients with painful sensory neuropathy. *Neurology* 48 (3):708–11.

Kennedy, J. M., A. Hoke, Y. Zhu, J. B. Johnston, G. van Marle, C. Silva, D. W. Zochodne, and C. Power. 2004. Peripheral neuropathy in lentivirus infection: evidence of inflammation and axonal injury. *Aids* 18 (9):1241–50.

Kennedy, W. R., G. Wendelschafer-Crabb, and D. Walk. 2000. Use of skin biopsy and skin blister in neurologic practice. *J Clin Neuromuscul Dis* 1 (4):196–204.

Keswani, S. C., and A. Hoke. 2003. Incidence of and risk factors for HIV-associated distal sensory polyneuropathy. *Neurology* 61 (2):279; author reply 279–80.

Laast, V. A., C. A. Pardo, P. M. Tarwater, S. E. Queen, T. A. Reinhart, M. Ghosh, R. J. Adams, M. C. Zink, and J. L. Mankowski. 2007. Pathogenesis of simian immunodeficiency virus-induced alterations in macaque trigeminal ganglia. *J Neuropathol Exp Neurol* 66 (1):26–34.

Lackner, A. A., S. Dandekar, and M. B. Gardner. 1991. Neurobiology of simian and feline immunodeficiency virus infections. *Brain Pathol* 1 (3):201–12.

Mankowski, J. L., J. E. Clements, and M. C. Zink. 2002a. Searching for clues: tracking the pathogenesis of human immunodeficiency virus central nervous system disease by use of an accelerated, consistent simian immunodeficiency virus macaque model. *J Infect Dis* 186 Suppl 2:S199–208.

Mankowski, J. L., M. T. Flaherty, J. P. Spelman, D. A. Hauer, P. J. Didier, A. M. Amedee, M. Murphey-Corb, L. M. Kirstein, A. Munoz, J. E. Clements, and M. C. Zink. 1997. Pathogenesis of simian immunodeficiency virus encephalitis: viral determinants of neurovirulence. *J Virol* 71 (8):6055–60.

Mankowski, J. L., S. E. Queen, P. M. Tarwater, K. J. Fox, and V. H. Perry. 2002b. Accumulation of beta-amyloid precursor protein in axons

correlates with CNS expression of SIV gp41. *J Neuropathol Exp Neurol* 61 (1):85–90.

McArthur, J. C., B. J. Brew, and A. Nath. 2005. Neurological complications of HIV infection. *Lancet Neurol* 4 (9):543–55.

McCarthy, B. G., S. T. Hsieh, A. Stocks, P. Hauer, C. Macko, D. R. Cornblath, J. W. Griffin, and J. C. McArthur. 1995. Cutaneous innervation in sensory neuropathies: evaluation by skin biopsy. *Neurology* 45 (10):1848–55.

Morgello, S., L. Estanislao, D. Simpson, A. Geraci, A. DiRocco, P. Gerits, E. Ryan, T. Yakoushina, S. Khan, R. Mahboob, M. Naseer, D. Dorfman, and V. Sharp. 2004. HIV-associated distal sensory polyneuropathy in the era of highly active antiretroviral therapy: the Manhattan HIV Brain Bank. *Arch Neurol* 61 (4):546–51.

Pardo, C. A., J. C. McArthur, and J. W. Griffin. 2001. HIV neuropathy: insights in the pathology of HIV peripheral nerve disease. *J Peripher Nerv Syst* 6 (1):21–7.

Pettersen, J. A., G. Jones, C. Worthington, H. B. Krentz, O. T. Keppler, A. Hoke, M. J. Gill, and C. Power. 2006. Sensory neuropathy in human immunodeficiency virus/acquired immunodeficiency syndrome patients: protease inhibitor-mediated neurotoxicity. *Ann Neurol* 59 (5):816–24.

Polydefkis, M. J. 2002. Peripheral neuropathy and HIV. *Hopkins HIV Rep* 14 (4):6–7.

Polydefkis, M., C. T. Yiannoutsos, B. A. Cohen, H. Hollander, G. Schifitto, D. B. Clifford, D. M. Simpson, D. Katzenstein, S. Shriver, P. Hauer, A. Brown, A. B. Haidich, L. Moo, and J. C. McArthur. 2002. Reduced intraepidermal nerve fiber density in HIV-associated sensory neuropathy. *Neurology* 58 (1):115–9.

Scaravilli, F., E. Sinclair, J. C. Arango, H. Manji, S. Lucas, and M. J. Harrison. 1992. The pathology of the posterior root ganglia in AIDS and its relationship to the pallor of the gracile tract. *Acta Neuropathol* 84 (2):163–70.

Schifitto, G., M. P. McDermott, J. C. McArthur, K. Marder, N. Sacktor, L. Epstein, and K. Kieburtz. 2002. Incidence of and risk factors for HIV-associated distal sensory polyneuropathy. *Neurology* 58 (12):1764–8.

Simpson, D. M., and M. Tagliati. 1994. Neurologic manifestations of HIV infection. *Ann Intern Med* 121 (10):769–85.

Westmoreland, S. V., J. B. Rottman, K. C. Williams, A. A. Lackner, and V. G. Sasseville. 1998. Chemokine receptor expression on resident and inflammatory cells in the brain of macaques with simian immunodeficiency virus encephalitis. *Am J Pathol* 152 (3):659–65.

Williams, K. C., S. Corey, S. V. Westmoreland, D. Pauley, H. Knight, C. deBakker, X. Alvarez, and A. A. Lackner. 2001. Perivascular macrophages are the primary cell type productively infected by simian immunodeficiency virus in the brains of macaques: implications for the neuropathogenesis of AIDS. *J Exp Med* 193 (8):905–15.

Williams, R., S. Bokhari, P. Silverstein, D. Pinson, A. Kumar, and S. Buch. 2008. Nonhuman primate models of NeuroAIDS. *J Neurovirol* 14 (4):292–300.

Zhu, Y., J. Antony, S. Liu, J. A. Martinez, F. Giuliani, D. Zochodne, and C. Power. 2006. CD8+ lymphocyte-mediated injury of dorsal root ganglion neurons during lentivirus infection: CD154-dependent cell contact neurotoxicity. *J Neurosci* 26 (13):3396–403.

Zhu, Y., J. M. Antony, J. A. Martinez, D. M. Glerum, V. Brussee, A. Hoke, D. Zochodne, and C. Power. 2007. Didanosine causes sensory neuropathy in an HIV/AIDS animal model: impaired mitochondrial and neurotrophic factor gene expression. *Brain* 130 (Pt 8):2011–23.

Zhu, Y., G. Jones, W. Tsutsui, S. Opii, S. Liu, C. Silva, D. A. Butterfield, and C. Power. 2005. Lentivirus Infection Causes Neuroinflammation and Neuronal Injury in Dorsal Root Ganglia: Pathogenic Effects of STAT-1 and Inducible Nitric Oxide Synthase. *J Immunol* 175 (2):1118–26.

Zink, M. C., A. M. Amedee, J. L. Mankowski, L. Craig, P. Didier, D. L. Carter, A. Munoz, M. Murphey-Corb, and J. E. Clements. 1997. Pathogenesis of SIV encephalitis. Selection and replication of neurovirulent SIV. *Am J Pathol* 151 (3):793–803.

Zink, M. C., V. A. Laast, K. L. Helke, A. K. Brice, S. A. Barber, J. E. Clements, and J. L. Mankowski. 2006. From mice to macaques–animal models of HIV nervous system disease. *Curr HIV Res* 4 (3):293–305.

5.8

ANIMAL MODELS AND BIOIMAGING

Eva-Maria Ratai, Margaret R. Lentz, and R. Gilberto González

Imaging has been used extensively to study the effect of HIV infection on the brain. However, because histological samples cannot typically be obtained and correlated with imaging results, human imaging results can be difficult to interpret. In contrast, imaging studies of animals can be performed in a controlled fashion, and the image results can be compared directly to histological findings. These points are important for the study of the neurological consequences of HIV infection. This chapter discusses the use of imaging modalities in the study of animal models for HIV infection.

INTRODUCTION

Imaging has been used extensively to study the effect of HIV infection on the brain. Due to its noninvasive nature, imaging is suitable for both cross-sectional and longitudinal studies where disease processes and effects of experimental therapies can be assessed. However, imaging in HIV+ individuals presents difficulties in interpretation. Imaging studies using animal models provide an excellent opportunity to understand the biological basis of the imaging changes produced by the AIDS virus. Studies may be performed in a controlled fashion and imaging results can be compared directly to histological results, which are typically difficult to obtain in patients. Extant animal models include simian immunodeficiency virus (SIV) infection of monkeys (Zink et al., 2002a; Williams et al., 2005), feline immunodeficiency virus (FIV) infection of cats (Podell et al., 1999), transgenic HIV mouse and rat models (Reid et al., 2001; Toggas et al., 1994), and a severe combined immunodeficient (SCID) mouse model where HIV-1-infected macrophages are injected into the brain (Persidsky et al., 1996). All of these models exhibit neuronal injury and inflammation that are comparable to that observed in HIV encephalitis (HIVE) (Persidsky et al., 1997; Persidsky et al., 2002; Zink et al., 2002b).

Neuroimaging has become a useful tool for the study of HIV-infected patients with neurological and/or cognitive symptoms. Structural neuroimaging methods such as magnetic resonance imaging (MRI) and computerized tomography (CT) are important for the diagnosis of cerebral opportunistic infections and determining atrophy due to later stages of HIV-associated dementia (HAD), but are limited in the evaluation of early cognitive changes (Aylward et al., 1993; Broderick et al., 1993; Dooneief et al., 1992; McArthur et al., 1990). Neuroimaging techniques that provide functional and biochemical information have proven to be more useful in the earlier stages of neuroAIDS. These techniques include magnetic resonance spectroscopy (MRS) (Chong et al., 1993), positron emission tomography (PET) (von Giesen et al., 2000), functional MRI (Chang et al., 2001), perfusion MRI (Tracey et al., 1998), and diffusion MRI (Filippi et al., 2001). Herein, we review studies of animal models using a variety of imaging modalities that have led to a better understanding of neuronal injury and neuroinflammation caused by HIV. We will first focus on the MRS findings in the simian, feline, and rodent models reflective of HIV-infection and subsequently discuss other imaging modalities in those animal models.

MAGNETIC RESONANCE SPECTROSCOPY

MRS offers the unique ability to measure metabolite levels in vivo in a noninvasive manner. Quantification of these metabolites can assist in the identification of disease, measuring the severity of injury, and/or monitoring a response to treatment. The brain is made up of many cell types—neurons, astrocystes, microglia, and oligodendrocytes—and studies using cell cultures and high field NMR spectroscopy have indicated each exhibits a distinct proton (^{1}H) MR spectrum (Urenjak et al., 1992; 1993). However, the in vivo MR spectrum of the brain (typically at 1.5 or 3T) represents a mixture of these cells resulting in many overlapping resonances. Figure 5.8.1 shows a typical in vivo ^{1}H MR spectrum from the white matter of the centrum semiovale of a human brain and a macaque brain, which are quite similar. ^{1}H MR spectra acquired with short echo times (as often used in HIV studies) are characterized by resonances arising primarily from N-acetylaspartate and N-acetylaspartylglutamate (collectively referred to as NAA), choline-containing compounds (Cho), *myo*-inositol (MI), and creatine-containing compounds (Cr). Resonance peaks from glutamate and glutamine overlap extensively at lower magnetic field strengths and are collectively referred to as Glx.

It is well documented that NAA is localized almost exclusively in neurons in the adult brain, and hence serves as an in vivo marker of neuronal health (Baslow, 2000). While its function is not completely understood, it plays multiple roles. NAA is the source of acetyl in myelin membrane biosynthesis (Chakraborty et al., 2001). It is also believed to act as an osmolyte (metabolic water pump) (Baslow, 2002),

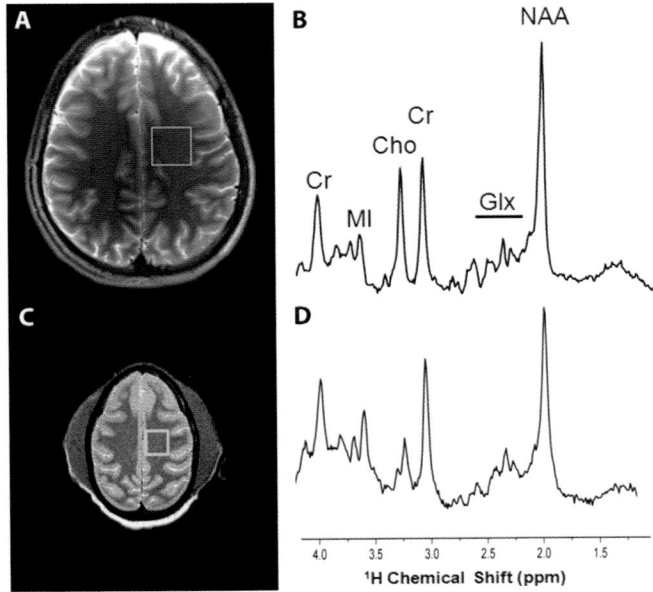

Figure 5.8.1 Representative proton MRS voxel locations from the white matter. The voxel size is 6 cm³ in the human [A] and 1.7 cm³ in the macaque [C]. MR spectroscopy acquired from the white matter of a healthy human brain [B] and healthy macaque brain [D] show highly similar spectra; the major difference is in the intensity of the Cho resonance. Spectra were acquired on a 3T MRI scanner (TE = 30 ms, TR = 2500 ms).

Much like HIV, the simian immunodeficiency virus productively infects CD4+ T lymphocytes, monocyte-derived cells, and microglia, the resident macrophage of the brain (Lackner et al., 1991; Zink et al., 1998). Analogous to patients with HIV encephalitis, rhesus macaques infected with pathogenic strains, such as SIVmac251, are prone to developing SIV encephalitis, the hallmarks of which include multinucleated giant cells, astrogliosis, microgliosis, and severe injury to the synaptodendritic apparatus of both excitatory and inhibitory neurons (Crews et al., 2008). Accordingly, SIV models are the premier model of AIDS neuropathogenesis (Schmitz et al., 1999; Zink et al., 2002a). While the standard SIV models using pathogenic strains typically result in progression to AIDS in 1 to 3 years after infection, they are due to the low percentage of animals which develop SIV encephalitis (~25%) (Westmoreland et al., 1998). However, this model allows for imaging as well as molecular and histopathologic examination of acute SIV infection, which is complex metabolically and occurs consistently in virtually all animals within the initial weeks of infection.

Imaging of Acute SIV and Early HIV Infection

Acute HIV infection is a time period when impairment/destruction of CD4+ T lymphocytes occurs and viral levels are uncontrolled due to a lack of the host's immune response (Altfeld et al., 2001a; Daar et al., 1991; Rosenberg et al., 1997). These events are similar to those that are manifest in chronic infection when HIV-related dementia is more likely to occur (McArthur et al., 1993). Rhesus macaques infected with SIVmac251 exhibit detectable viral levels in the blood within 4 days of infection, rapidly expanding to 10^7–10^9 copies/mL, 8–17 days after infection (Staprans et al., 1999). Much like observations in studies of acute HIV infection, a viral set point in the SIV model (~35–60 days post infection) helps to predict disease progression (Mellors et al., 1995; Staprans et al., 1999). Those maintaining high viral loads progress faster to AIDS, while those with lower viral loads during this time period became slow or intermediate progressors.

Perivascular monocytes, which transport virus into the brain at this time, have been observed in the brain at 12 and 14 days post infection, coinciding with the presence of virus in brain tissue and cerebrospinal fluid (Clay et al., 2007). Within the first 2 weeks of infection, presynaptic injury (20% reduction in synaptophysin), injury to GABAergic neurons, and a massive glial response (a two-fold increase in glial fibrillary-associated protein, GFAP) is observed in the presence of "subtle" perivascular infiltrates (Gonzalez et al., 2000). An ex vivo MRS analysis of neighboring brain tissues demonstrated abnormalities in neuronal metabolism reflected in a reduction in NAA/Cr from that of healthy control levels within the first weeks of infection, presumably in response to this insult. Subsequent studies indicated lower NAA/Cr levels observed during acute SIV infection correlated well with presynaptic injury (Figure 5.8.2), which would result in altered synaptic

a storage form of aspartate, and is coupled to lipid metabolism and energy generation (Moffett et al., 2007). Decreases in NAA or NAA/Cr are indicative of both neuronal injury and death (Cheng et al., 1997; Cheng et al., 2002; Lentz et al., 2005). The creatine resonance observed in vivo represents the sum of creatine and phosphocreatine, a high energy reservoir for ATP generation, and thus a marker for bioenergetics. Cr is frequently used as an internal standard, and is commonly considered to be relatively constant even in the presence of cellular pathology. However, elevated Cr levels have been reported in the frontal white matter of chronic HIV patients (Chang et al., 2002) and during acute SIV infection (Ratai et al., 2009). The choline-containing compounds detected by MRS include free choline, glycerophosphocholine, and phosphocholine. These compounds are primarily related to lipid membrane turnover (Hakumaki et al., 2000), and changes in Cho are typically interpreted as related to changes in the glial response in neuroAIDS. *Myo*-inositol is primarily located in microglia and believed to be essential for cell growth and a storage form for glucose (Ross, 1991). Alterations in MI levels within the context of this disease are poorly understood and commonly interpreted to be a reflection of microgliosis and inflammation (Brand et al., 1993). The Glx resonances represent the major excitatory neurotransmitter (glutamate) and its storage form (glutamine). Excess glutamate can be toxic to the neuronal environment and, in the healthy brain, is quickly absorbed by astrocytes and converted into glutamine for storage (Govindaraju et al., 2000; Kaul et al., 2001).

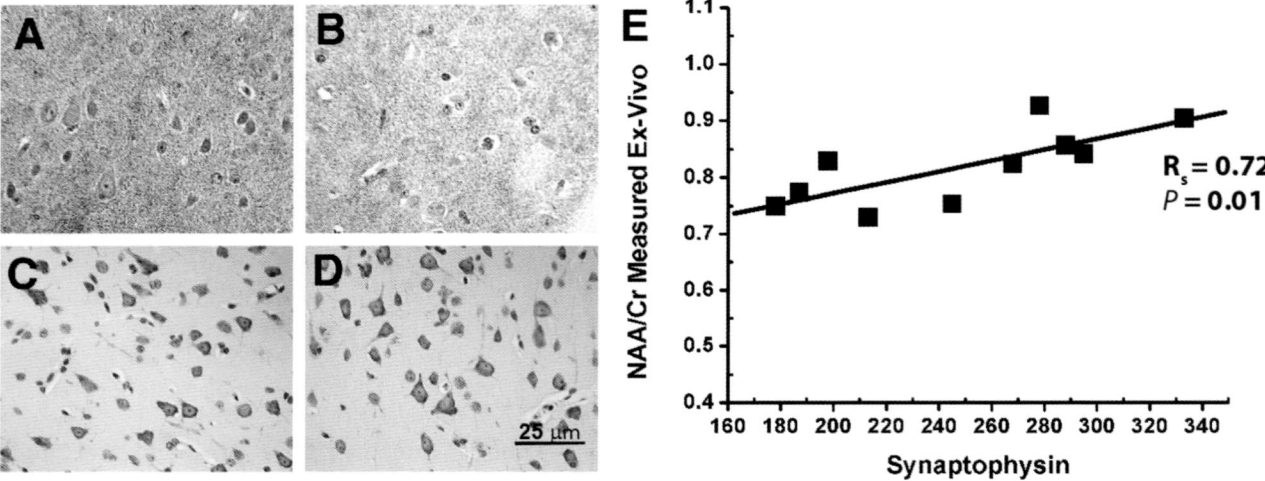

Figure 5.8.2 Photomicrographs of anti-synaptophysin [A and B] and cresyl violet [C and D] staining of an uninfected, healthy rhesus macaque [A and C] and a macaque 14 days after SIV-infection [B and D]. Acute SIV infection exhibits a decrease in synaptophysin expression [A and B], but no severe neuronal injury [C and D] or dendritic damage was observed. Synaptophysin levels were significantly correlated with NAA/Cr measured in frontal lobe tissue extracts [E]. Adapted with permission from Lentz et al., 2005.

transmission (Lentz et al., 2005) and may explain recent reports of neuropsychological impairment in HIV+ patients during the first year of infection (Moore et al., 2010; Peterson et al., 2010).

These ex vivo investigations led to the use of in vivo MRS as a means of monitoring lipid membrane turnover, neuronal and glial metabolism over the first months of SIV infection (Greco et al., 2004; Ratai et al., 2009). In these studies nearly all macaques ($N = 15$) had reductions in NAA/Cr (-8%) in the frontal cortex within the first two weeks of infection.

Myo-inositol levels were significantly elevated in both the frontal cortex and white matter regions, suggesting stimulation of glial metabolism within the first month of infection. Additionally, changes in lipid membrane turnover (Cho/Cr) in both the frontal cortex and white matter were pronounced and rapid in nature. These and more recent studies using the rapid progression, CD8-depletion SIV macaque model ($N = 28$, Figure 5.8.3) have shown that Cho/Cr levels increase greatly 11–12 days after infection (11–21%, depending on region), corresponding to the time of peak viremia.

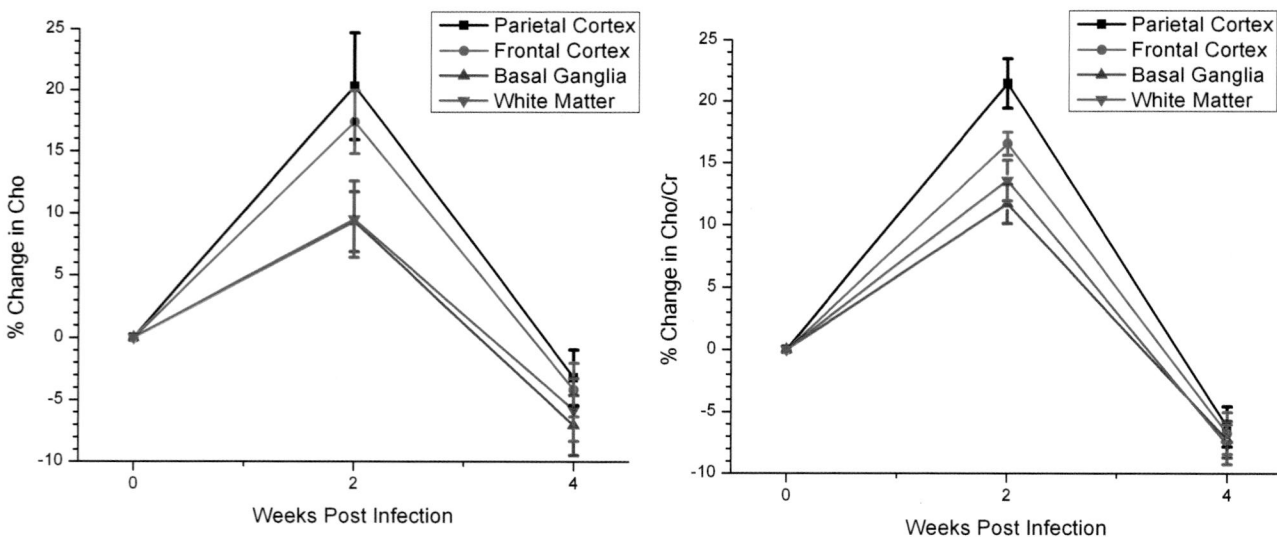

Figure 5.8.3 Average Cho (*left*) and Cho/Cr (*right*) levels in parietal cortex, frontal cortex, basal ganglia, and white matter regions of 23 rhesus macaques before SIV-infection, and 2 and 4 weeks post infection. Repeated-measures analysis of variance for all measures were highly significant ($P < 0.00001$). Subsequent matched-pair t-tests for both choline and Cho/Cr in all regions indicated large elevations from pre-infection levels at 2 weeks (all t-tests: $P < 0.006$) and large reductions between 2 weeks and 4 weeks (all t-tests: $P < 0.0003$). Reductions between pre-infection and 4 weeks were significant ($P \leq 0.03$) with the exception of Cho in the parietal and frontal cortices.

Between 12–18 days post infection, choline concentrations undergo a large reduction, resulting in Cho/Cr levels that are lower than pre-infection levels (Greco et al., 2004). Both GFAP and Cho/Cr levels were associated with changes in plasma viral RNA levels (Greco et al., 2004). While changes in Cho/Cr mirrored the changes in the astrocyte response (GFAP) in animals sacrificed over various time points during the first month of infection, they were not found to be correlated (Kim et al., 2005). These results indicate changes in choline are more complicated than a simple relationship with astrogliosis. Decreases in choline levels below baseline have rarely been reported in diseases not involving necrosis (Groeschel et al., 2006; Kreis et al., 1992; Taylor et al., 1996). Choline levels within the brain are typically believed to be elevated in a nearly global fashion in patients with AIDS, and these dynamic choline changes warrant further study (Meyerhoff et al., 1999; Mohamed et al., 2010).

The SIV macaque model demonstrates neuronal injury and gliosis in the central nervous system occurs early and that the relationship between these changes and events in the periphery are important (Clay et al., 2007; Greco et al., 2004). It has become evident that antiretroviral treatment for HIV may be most effective when initiated during acute/early infection (Altfeld et al., 2001b). Even if early SIV-induced brain injury is controlled (via therapy or host immune responses), it is plausible that the underlying neurotoxic mechanisms are similar for both early and late neuronal injury. Thus, the acute SIV model may be ideal for the study of the HIV-related neuropathogenesis, particularly in regards to examining the reversibility limits of neuronal injury related to HIV-associated neurologic disease.

Until recently, MRS studies in acute/early HIV infection patients remained relatively unexplored (Lentz et al., 2009). Eight subjects identified during acute HIV infection without gross neurologic symptoms were examined by MRS within 90 days of their evolving Western blot. As observed in the macaque model, lower NAA (-12%) and Glx (-14%) levels were observed in the frontal cortex of subjects compared to controls, suggesting the cortical gray matter may be more susceptible to early neuronal injury. Further longitudinal study of this cohort ($N = 9$, over six months) indicated lipid membrane turnover and glial metabolism in the frontal cortex and white matter are increasing over the first year of infection (Figure 5.8.4) (Lentz et al., 2010). Similar to that observed during acute SIV infection, changes in choline and glutamate+glutamine metabolism were related to changes in plasma viral loads. Using the MR/pathology studies from SIV models will allow for a better understanding of events occurring in the CNS during the initial year of infection and allow for the examination of questions such as the efficacy of early antiretroviral use on CNS disease in HIV+ individuals.

Imaging of Chronic SIV and HIV Infection

MRS studies of patients chronically infected with HIV have explored the relationships between cognitive impairment/

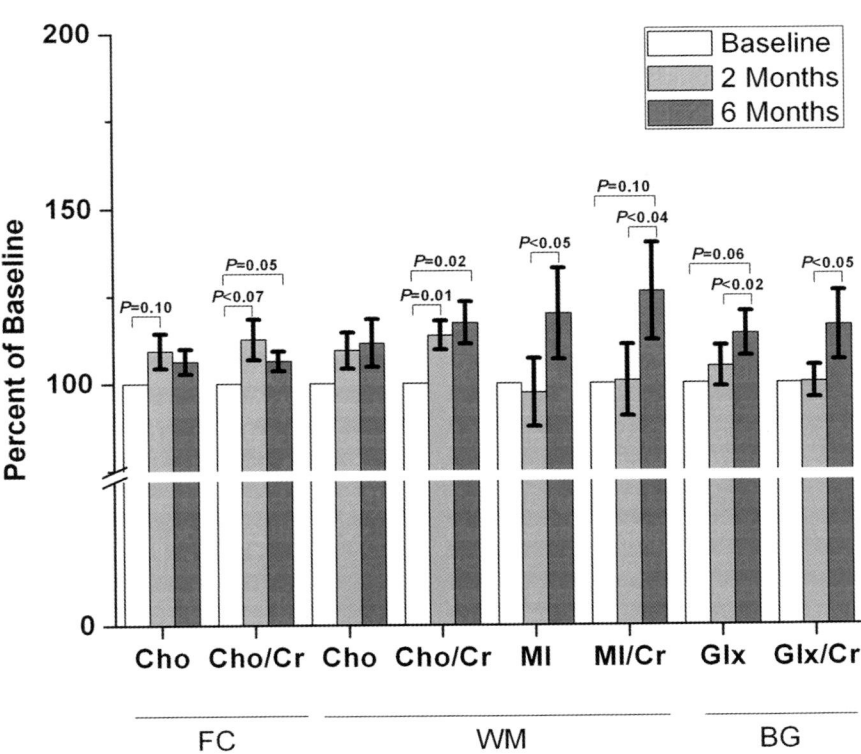

Figure 5.8.4 Metabolite changes occur within the first year of HIV infection. Specifically, elevations in the metabolites considered related to glial activation and lipid membrane turnover [Cho, Cho/Cr, MI, and MI/Cr] can be seen in the frontal cortex and white matter regions. All changes are significant ($P < 0.05$) or show strong trends towards significant changes ($P < 0.10$). Matched-pair t-test P values are shown.

dementia and neuronal metabolism (NAA). Decreases in NAA/Cr (-10%) are observed in those with minor cognitive motor dysfunction (Chang et al., 1999), while reductions of 15–28% from that observed in seronegative controls have been reported in those with severe cognitive impairment or AIDS dementia complex (Marcus et al., 1998; Meyerhoff et al., 1999; Moller et al., 1999; Salvan et al., 1997). While in vivo MRS is ideal for monitoring HIV-infected patients over time, the limited spectral resolution (Figure 5.8.5) and the inability to assess pathology make interpretation of MRS difficult.

The SIV macaque model provides the opportunity to better understand the biologic nature of these MRS observations in cognitively impaired patients chronically infected with HIV. For this purpose, extracted metabolites from frontal cortex tissue samples of 6 healthy control and 23 SIV-infected macaques moribund with AIDS were used to determine a metabolite profile of various stages of CNS pathology. In animals moribund with AIDS that had either mild or no encephalitis, lower levels of NAA/Cr (-13% from control levels) were observed, while reductions >20% corresponded to moderate and severe encephalitis (Lentz et al., 2008). Moreover, NAA/Cr levels were significantly related to the SIV inoculums used ($P < 0.0009$), and animals infected with SIVmac251 were found to have lower NAA/Cr levels (Lentz et al., 2008). Likewise, animals infected with

SIVmac251 have a greater incidence of SIVE and progress more rapidly to AIDS than those with SIVmac239 (Westmoreland et al., 1998) suggesting that further studies on the effects of specific viral clades and strains involved in HIV-associated neurologic disorders are necessary (Sacktor et al., 2009).

Additionally, metabolites not easily resolved using in vivo MRS can be examined at higher fields (14 Tesla) using either magic angle spinning MRS on whole tissue samples or liquid state MRS of extracted metabolites from these tissues (Gonzalez et al., 2000; Lentz et al., 2008). These include small molecules such as glutamate, γ-aminobutyric acid (GABA), taurine, and phosphocholine. Interestingly, in all macaques with AIDS, glutamate and GABA ratios were reduced from healthy control levels indicating that neuronal injury or death to both glutamateric and GABAergic neurons was occurring. Phosphocholine levels in all SIV-infected macaques were significantly elevated compared to controls (post-hoc Wilcoxon rank sum test: $P = 0.02$). The significance of this observation is not clear. It is possible that increases of phosphocholine are mechanistically related to the metabolism of sphingomyelin into ceramide, which has been shown to be a promoter of apoptosis in the context of neuroAIDS (Haughey et al., 2004).

MRS STUDIES IN AN ACCELERATED MACAQUE MODEL OF NEUROAIDS

The SIV macaque model is limited by the low rate of SIVE development and the length of time required for its evolution (Burudi et al., 2001; Westmoreland et al., 1998) making it inefficient for use in natural history and therapeutic studies (Fuller et al., 2004). Therefore, attention has turned to two rapidly progressing SIV macaque models. One model employs pigtailed macaques that are co-inoculated with two SIV strains (SIV/17E-Fr and SIVΔB670), which accelerates SIV CNS disease, producing SIVE in over 90% of these animals within 3 months (Zink et al., 2002a). The second model uses SIV-infected rhesus macaques which receive a monoclonal antibody to deplete the animal of CD8+ T lymphocytes soon after infection (Schmitz et al., 1999). In this model, over 85% of persistently CD8-depleted animals develop SIVE with a course of progression to terminal AIDS (Williams et al., 2005).

CD8+ T Lymphocyte Depletion Alone Does Not Produce MRS Changes or Neuropathological Abnormalities in the Macaque

Studies were undertaken to determine if CD8+ T lymphocyte depletion alone produced brain injury or altered its metabolism in the absence of SIV infection (Ratai et al., 2011b). Four rhesus macaques were examined before and after treatment with anti-CD8 antibody cM-T807 by in vivo MRS (TE/TR=30/3000, voxel size = 1.7 cm³) using a 7.0 T MRI scanner. No changes in metabolite concentrations or ratios were detected over time in the frontal cortex (FC), the subcortical white matter (WM), or basal ganglia (BG) (NAA/Cr shown in Figure 5.8.6A). Immunohistochemistry analysis on nondepleted control and CD8-depleted control (SIV-)

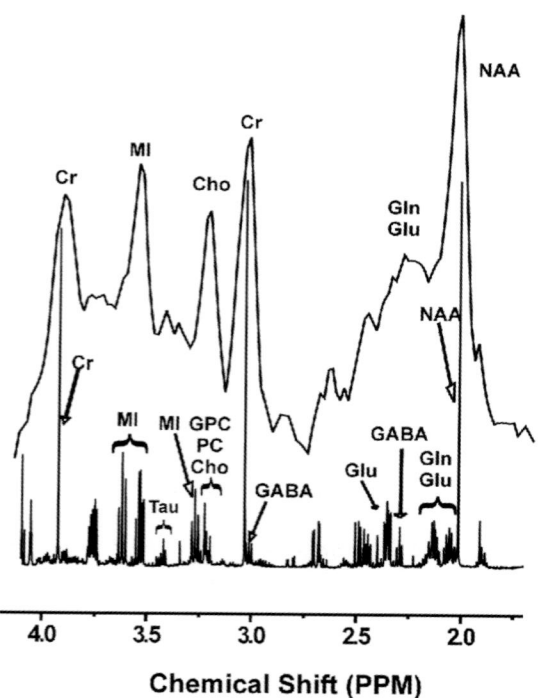

Figure 5.8.5 MR spectrum of the brain of a SIV-infected rhesus macaque obtained in vivo at 1.5 T overlaid on an *ex vivo* 14 T MR spectrum of metabolites extracted from the frontal cortex of the same animal. Note the higher resolution exhibited by the higher field spectrum of tissue extracts. Tau = taurine, GPC = glycerophosphocholine, PC = phosphocholine, GABA = γ-aminobutyric acid, Glu = glutamate, Gln = glutamine. Adapted with permission from Kim et al., 2005.

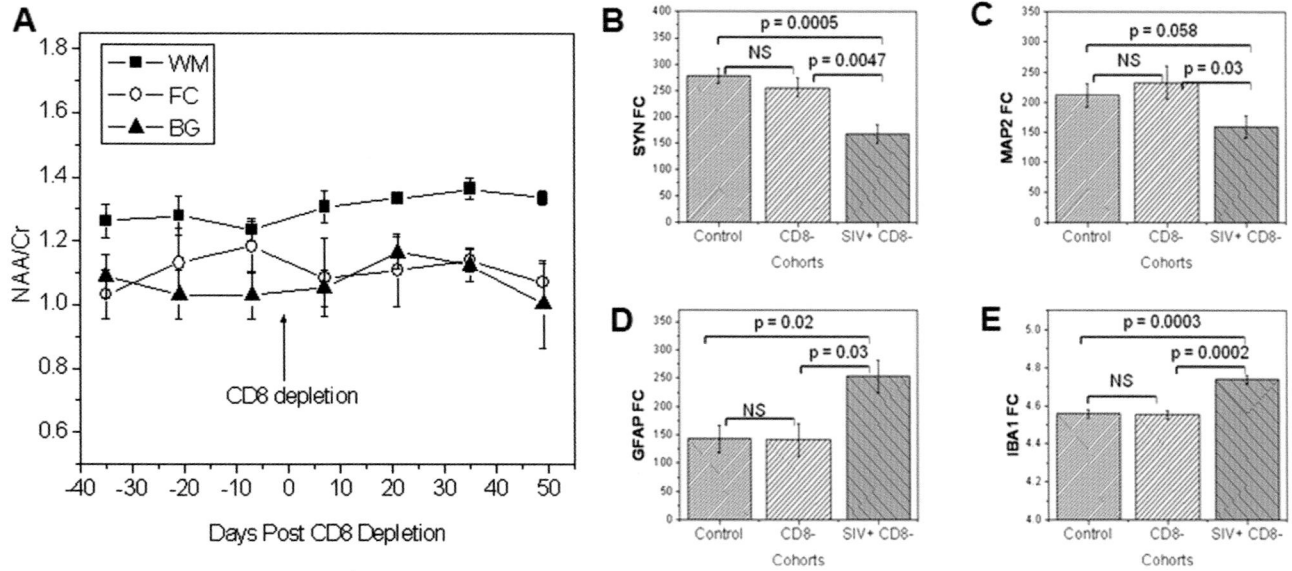

Figure 5.8.6 [A] Mean NAA/Cr levels of four uninfected CD8-depleted animals in the white matter, frontal cortex, and basal ganglia as a function of time post CD8-depletion. No significant changes were observed suggesting CD8-depletion alone has no significant effect on brain metabolism. Quantitative IHC reveals no difference between uninfected CD8-depleted and uninfected controls in [B] SYN, [C] MAP2, [D] GFAP and [E] IBA-1. These IHC measures in both control groups were significantly different from SIV-infected, CD8-depleted animals euthanized 8 weeks post infection.

animals indicate that pre-synaptic (synaptophysin) and dendritic (MAP2) integrity, as well as astrocyte (GFAP) and microglia (IBA-1) activation are similar in both control groups (Figure 5.8.6B). SIV-infected, CD8-depleted animals that were sacrificed 8 weeks after infection had elevated astrocyte and microglia activation, and reduced presynaptic and dendritic integrity compared to either control group. These results indicate alterations in brain metabolism and pathology observed in this accelerated model of neuroAIDS are a result of uncontrolled viral expansion and not CD8+ T lymphocyte depletion alone.

Severe Neuronal Injury Produced Shortly After SIV Infection in the CD8-Depleted Macaque Model

Data from both the rapid progression pigtail macaque and CD8-depletion rhesus macaque models support the critical role of the peripheral immune system in contributing to CNS disease progression and severity (Marcondes et al., 2001; Sopper et al., 1998). In vivo MRS studies performed at 1.5 Tesla of the SIV-infected, CD8-depleted macaque model identified profound neuronal injury that was detectable within weeks and was coincident with the expansion and infection of activated (CD16+) monocyte populations (Williams et al., 2005). Within 10 weeks of SIV infection, all untreated animals had postmortem evidence of SIVE characterized by multinucleated giant cells, perivascular infiltrates (CD16+), and SIVp27 protein in all brain sections examined. Postmortem analysis of NAA/Cr by ex vivo MRS and quantitative immunohistochemical measurements of synaptophysin (SYN) and MAP2 confirmed neuronal injury occurred in these animals. These observations suggest that activated monocyte and macrophage accumulation in the CNS are indicators of and

likely contributors to CNS neuronal injury (Williams et al., 2005).

Additional in vivo MRS studies performed at 3 Tesla found significant decreases in NAA/Cr in the frontal cortex, parietal cortex (PC), basal ganglia, and white matter (Figure 5.8.7A) (Ratai et al., 2011a). NAA and Cr concentrations were determined to assess whether changes in NAA and/or Cr were responsible for the observed changes in NAA/Cr in this model. Mean NAA concentrations declined relative to baseline measurements in the FC, BG, and WM, but were statistically significant only in the WM. The mean brain concentrations of Cr were elevated in all four regions, with statistical significance observed in the parietal cortex and white matter (Figure 5.8.7B). These observations are in accord with MRS studies of HIV-infected patients that found elevated creatine levels (Chang et al., 2002).

Changes in total creatine are associated with altered energy metabolism. It is believed that the virus enters the brain through infected monocytes that later differentiate into macrophages. A high metabolic demand in these brain regions due to monocyte infiltration, glial activation, and the brain's efforts towards neuronal repair may explain an increase in Cr. NAA decreases as a result of neuronal injury and is coupled to energy metabolism, and thus a decline in Cr would be expected in these cells. Our observations are explained if the expected decline in neuronal Cr is overcompensated by Cr elevations produced by the metabolic rates within activated astrocytes and microglia. Due to the large error involved in estimating metabolite concentrations in such small cohorts, the combinations of decreased NAA and increased Cr make the NAA/Cr ratio detected by MRS a sensitive, reliable marker for brain disease (Ratai et al., 2009, Ratai et al., 2011a).

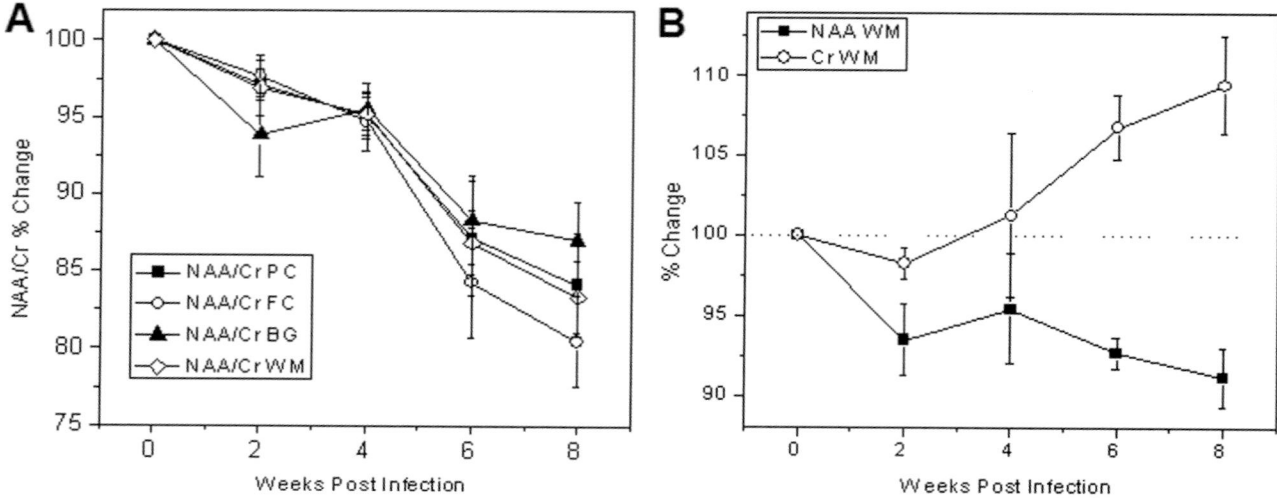

Figure 5.8.7 [A] NAA/Cr declines rapidly during disease progression in SIV-infected, CD8-depleted macaques, shown for four brain regions (PC: $P < 0.001$, FC: $P < 0.002$, BG: $P < 0.004$, WM: $P < 0.001$). In the 12 animals included in the analysis, declines in NAA/Cr had already reached significance by 2 weeks post infection (indicated by *). [B] Mean NAA concentrations in white matter of these animals declined relative to baseline measurements at all time points following infection ($P = 0.03$), while Cr concentrations were elevated ($P = 0.02$). Similar findings are observed in the other brain regions.

Alleviation of Neuronal Injury Using Antiretroviral Therapy and Minocycline

Accelerated macaque models, in combination with imaging studies, provide an exceptional opportunity to efficiently explore potential therapies that can control or reverse neuronal injury. Combined antiretroviral therapy (cART) with limited CNS penetration resulted in slightly decreased levels of plasma virus, a significant reduction in the number of activated and infected monocytes, and rapid, near-complete

reversal of neuronal injury (Williams et al., 2005). In the frontal cortex, declines in NAA/Cr from that of baseline were observed after 4 weeks of infection in all eight animals (paired T-test: $P < 0.001$, Figure 5.8.8A). After 4 weeks of treatment, results from in vivo MRS experiments demonstrated improved neuronal metabolism (NAA/Cr, +9%, $P < 0.03$). There was a significant difference in NAA/Cr levels between the cART-treated and untreated cohorts at their last scans before sacrifice in the frontal cortex and in the white

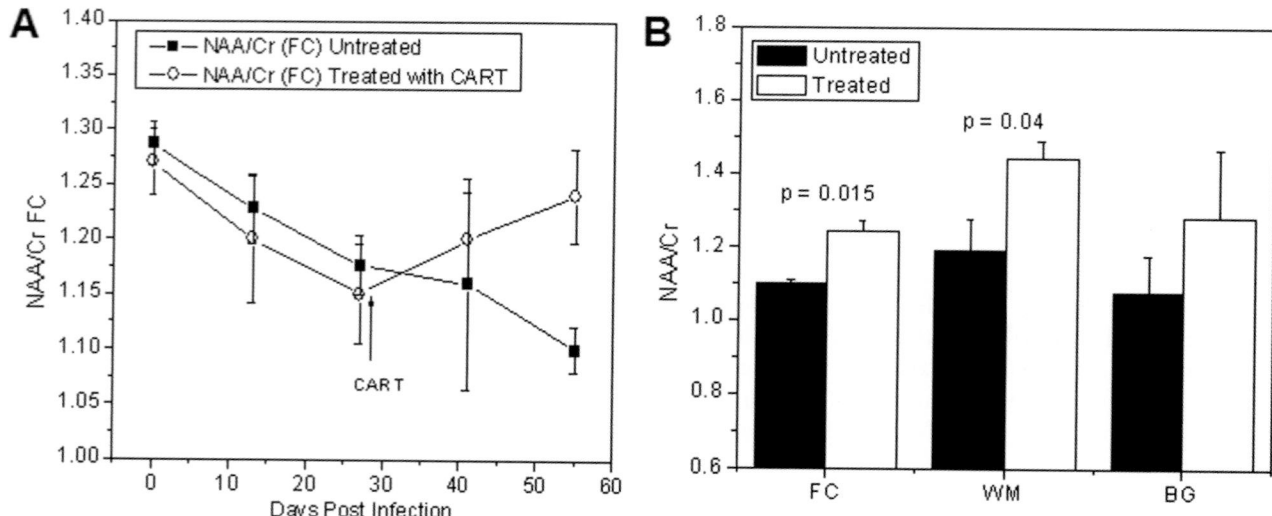

Figure 5.8.8 [A] Recovery of neuronal marker NAA/Cr with cART treatment in SIV infection. The arrow indicates the time point when daily cART was initiated. In the frontal cortex, a near-complete reversal of the NAA/Cr decline was seen in the four animals that underwent therapy. After 4 weeks of treatment, we observed an increase of 9% in NAA/Cr (Holm's t-test between 4 and 8 weeks, $P = 0.03$). [B] There was a significant difference in NAA/Cr between the treated and untreated cohorts at their last scans before sacrifice in the frontal cortex and in the white matter. Adapted with permission from González et al., 2006.

matter (Figure 5.8.8B) (González et al., 2006). Mean NAA/Cr levels in the BG were also improved in treated animals, although not significant, most likely because of greater measurement error. Immunohistochemistry revealed decreased synaptophysin, MAP2, and neuronal counts in animals scarified at 4 and 8 weeks post infection compared to uninfected controls. Animals that received antiretroviral therapy had higher levels of these neuronal markers. (Figure 5.8.9). Furthermore, astroglial activation by GFAP is decreased in animals receiving cART.

The persistence of minor neurological disease in HIV+ patients, despite antiretroviral therapy (Brodt et al., 1997; McArthur, 2004) and the increased prevalence of protracted forms of dementia, has led to a search for adjunctive therapies (Nath et al., 2008; Sacktor, 2002; Sacktor et al., 2002).

Zink et al. demonstrated minocycline possessed neuroprotective, anti-inflammatory, and possible anti-viral properties resulting in reduced severity of SIVE in studies using the pigtail SIV-macaque model (Follstaedt et al., 2008; Zink et al., 2005). Minocycline is a member of the tetracycline class of molecules with broad-spectrum antibiotic activity, which easily penetrates the blood-brain barrier and has a good clinical safety record (Domercq et al., 2004).

Ratai et al. have verified the neuroprotective properties of minocycline in the CD8-depleted, SIV-infected macaque model and demonstrated the utility of MRS in monitoring this neuronal protection (Ratai et al., 2010). MRS revealed that after 4 weeks of infection, daily MN treatment (orally administered) stabilized NAA/Cr indicating prevention of further neuronal injury (Figure 5.8.10A).

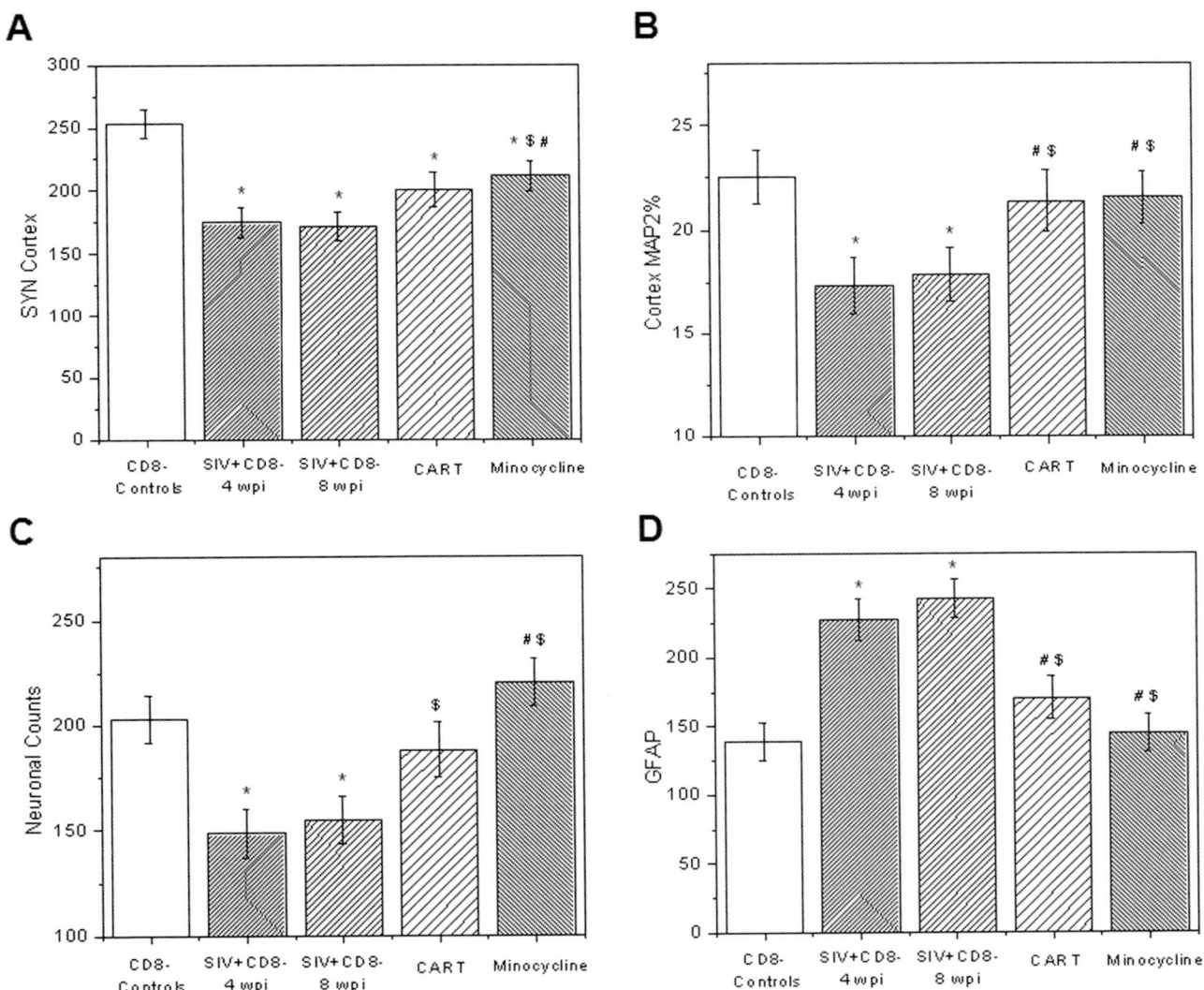

Figure 5.8.9 The use of either cART or minocycline helps preserve neuronal integrity [A, B, C] and decreases astrogliosis [D]. Synaptophysin (SYN), microtubule associated protein 2 (MAP2), neuronal counts, and glial fibrillary acetic protein (GFAP) levels were quantified in the cortices of 1) uninfected CD8-depleted control animals (CD8-controls), 2) SIV-infected, CD8-depleted untreated animals sacrificed at 4 weeks post infection (wpi) (SIV+/CD8–4 wpi), 3) SIV-infected, CD8-depleted untreated animals sacrificed at 8 wpi (SIV+/CD8–8 wpi), 4) cART-treated, SIV-infected, CD8-depleted animals (CART), and 5) MN-treated, SIV-infected, CD8-depleted animals. Symbols indicate a significant difference ($P \leq 0.05$) when a cohort is compared to either uninfected CD8-depleted controls (*), untreated SIV+/CD8-depleted macaques sacrificed at 4 wpi ($), or untreated SIV+/CD8-depleted animals sacrificed at 8 wpi (#).

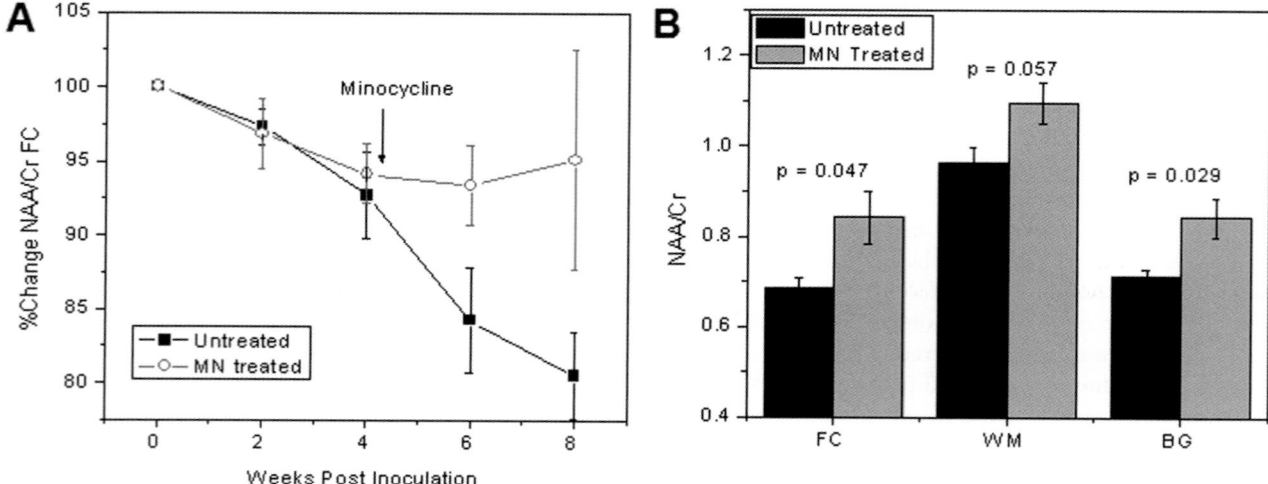

Figure 5.8.10 [A] NAA/Cr in the frontal cortex after SIV infection in untreated animals (solid squares) and animals treated daily with minocycline (circles). The arrow identifies the time point when minocycline (MN) treatment was initiated. [B] The SIV-infected, untreated animals exhibited lower levels of NAA/Cr at study endpoint (8 wpi) in all brain regions examined compared to animals that received MN (Ratai et al., 2010).

There was a significant difference in frontal cortex, white matter, and basal ganglia NAA/Cr between SIV-infected macaques that were MN treated and those that were untreated (Figure 5.8.10B). Neuroprotection by minocycline was supported by postmortem brain investigations on synaptophysin, MAP2, and neuronal counts. Additionally, microglial activation was reduced in the MN-treated animals, but not those animals treated with antiretrovirals. However, astrogliosis was decreased by either antiretroviral therapy or MN treatment.

MRS STUDIES OF FIV INFECTION

Several studies have examined neurologic disease induced by feline immunodeficiency virus in domestic cats as well as lions (Brennan et al., 2006; Maingat et al., 2009). Neurologic disease induced with FIV-infection typically is more profound during the developmental period of brain maturation, making this an ideal model for understanding neurologic complications observed in children infected with HIV (Belman, 1997; Podell et al., 1999). Like HIV, FIV is known to infect CD4+ T lymphocytes, causing immunosuppression, lentiviral encephalopathy, and neurobehavioral deficits (Phipps et al., 2000; Podell et al., 1997). A recent study demonstrated that motor and neurocognitive impairment in FIV-Ch-infected cats were closely coupled with increased viral burden in parietal cortex, increased microgliosis, and neuronal loss in the parietal cortex and hippocampus (Maingat et al., 2009). F4/80 and CD3ɛmRNA upregulation in FIV-infected brain tissues was observed, suggesting greater T cell and macrophage/microglial infiltration, both of which correlated with impaired performance on neurobehavioral testing. These observations emphasize the relationships between neurobehavioral deficits, neuroinflammation, viral abundance, and ensuing neurodegeneration.

In 1999, Podell and colleagues discovered cats infected with the FIV Maryland isolate had altered neuronal function (NAA and NAA/Cr reductions) between 8 and 14 months of infection (Podell et al., 1999). Oddly, lower NAA values were correlated with higher CD4+ lymphocyte function, but this may be due to the limited cohort size examined ($N = 6$). Longitudinal studies on cats infected at birth have indicated neurobehavioral deficits observed 12 weeks post infection coincide with neuronal injury (NAA/Cr, in vivo MRS) in the midfrontal sulci in animals inoculated with either V1CSF or with Petaluma virus and cyclosporine A (Power et al., 1998). Strong associations were observed between NAA/Cr and the ranking on the feline behavioral scale. In a similar study, animals infected with high viral titers of V1CSF had increased Cho/Cr and reduced NAA/Cr (in vivo MRS) in the frontal cortex compared to those that received low titers (Johnston et al., 2002). While all cats exhibited increased astrocytosis and activated macrophages in the brain tissue, cats receiving higher viral titers of V1CSF had reductions in neuronal processes (microtubule-associated protein-2), increased neuronal stress (c-fos), and dysmorphic neurons.

Glutamate-mediated neuronal injury is believed to contribute to lentiviral neuropathogenesis (Kaul et al., 2001). Power et al. discovered decreases in frontal lobe glutamate decarboxylase, the enzyme responsible for converting glutamate into GABA, consistent with increased glutamate of FIV–infected cats (Power et al., 1997). However, many FIV studies have reported reduction in glutamate, glutamate/creatine, or the glutamate/glutamine ratio in the cortex and white matter by MRS and high performance liquid chromatography (Johnston et al., 2002; Maingat et al., 2009). Analyses of ionotropic glutamate receptor transcript levels indicate GluR1, GluR5, and KA2 expression was suppressed in FIV+ animals (Maingat et al., 2009). These results suggest a disruption of the glutamate/glutamine balance could alter glutamate receptor expression and contribute to neuronal injury.

Most recently, the pediatric FIV model has been examined as a potential substance abuse model (Cloak et al., 2004). Methamphetamine abuse is rising among newly diagnosed HIV+ patients; however, little is known about the interactions between methamphetamines (MA) and HIV. In MRS studies of metabolites extracted from brain tissues, reductions in NAA, creatine, and glutamate in the frontal white matter due to FIV infection were observed, suggesting that neuronal injury was occurring, but it was not verified with pathology. In the same region, choline concentrations were increased in uninfected cats receiving methamphetamines. GABA levels of the frontal white matter were increased in animal cohorts that had repeated exposure to MA whether or not they were infected with FIV. GABA is an inhibitory neurotransmitter and is present in both glia and neurons, and its elevations may indicate ongoing disturbance to GABAergic neurons. In mouse and rat studies of other diseases, cell damage can lead to elevated GABA levels by several means (Saransaari et al., 1997), and increased GABA release may mediate neuroprotection (DeFazio et al., 2009).

MRS STUDIES OF MOUSE MODELS

Rodent models have been useful in elucidating pathogenic pathways associated with HIV neurologic disease, such as the migration and distribution of monocytes in brain tissue and the neurotoxic effects of specific viral proteins (Bruce-Keller et al., 2003; Okamoto et al., 2007; Zelivyanskaya et al., 2003). In a SCID mouse model, HIVE was induced focally into the striatum by the unilateral injection of HIV-1_{ADA}-infected human monocyte-derived macrophages (MDM) (Nelson et al., 2005). Metabolite concentrations were measured 7 days after injection in infected mice and were compared with sham-operated and unmanipulated controls using in vivo MRS imaging (MRSI at 7.0 Tesla). Spectroscopic examination revealed significant decreases in NAA and NAA/Cr levels both ipsilaterally and contralaterally to the site of injection in HIVE mice compared to sham-operated and unmanipulated cohorts. Additionally, histological sections were co-registered with MRSI voxels to allow comparison of the in vivo and postmortem data. It was shown that although significant decreases in NAA levels were observed in both the injected and contralateral hemispheres of HIVE mice compared to sham-operated controls, expression of synaptophysin and of glial markers (IBA-1 and GFAP) did not reveal significant differences in the contralateral hemispheres between the two cohorts. This finding suggests that decreasing NAA levels in general may be an early marker of neuronal dysfunction and may not indicate neuronal injury as detected by histology.

OTHER IMAGING MODALITIES

POSITRON EMISSION TOMOGRAPHY

PET is an imaging technique that detects signals generated by a positron-emitting radionuclide (tracer) which is part of a biologically relevant molecule. For example, ^{18}F-fluorodeoxyglucose (FDG), the most common PET tracer in use, is a fluorinated analogue of glucose, which is injected into a subject and allows physicians to determine the metabolic activity of a tumor in terms of glucose uptake. PET studies in HIV+ individuals have been used for imaging of glucose metabolism, abnormalities in the dopamine and serotonin systems, and microglia/macrophage activation (Andersen et al., 2010; Chang et al., 2008; Hammoud et al., 2005; Hammoud et al., 2010).

The majority of PET/autoradiography studies in SIV-infected macaques have focused on targeting the translocator protein (TSPO), previously referred to as peripheral benzodiazepine receptor, using (R)-1-(2-chlorphenyl)-N-methyl-N-(1-methylpropyl)-3-isoquinoline-carbox-amide, also known as (R)-PK11195. In the CNS, TSPO is expressed at low levels and is believed to be upregulated upon the activation of microglia and brain macrophages (Banati, 2002; Cagnin et al., 2002). Monocytes, which differentiate into macrophages in the brain, have an active role in the trafficking of virus into the brain, while microglia, the brain's resident immune cells, can also become infected (Kaul et al., 2001). Autoradiography studies using the tritium-labeled PK11195 tracer showed that pigtailed macaques with SIVE had higher binding in both gray and white matter regions compared to uninfected controls (Mankowski et al., 2003). Cell culture studies demonstrated that microglia and macrophages activated with lipopolysaccharide have increased PK11195 binding, and that this binding is reversed using an inhibitor of phosphatidylinositol-3 kinase (PI3-kinase). The PI3-kinase activation is important in promoting the survival of long-lived infected macrophages/microglia (Venneti et al., 2007). Studies on human postmortem brain tissues and cell cultures found that the tritium-labeled PK11195 tracer specifically binds to activated macrophages and microglia (Venneti et al., 2008a).

Two PET SIV-macaque studies, using both rapid progression models, have reported the uptake of [11C]-(R)-PK11195 in the frontal cortical gray matter, basal ganglia, frontal white matter, and hippocampus of animals with SIVE (Figure 5.8.11 A & B) (Venneti et al., 2004). [11C]-(R)-PK11195 levels in these regions were similar in uninfected controls and macaques lacking encephalitis. Postmortem examination using confocal microscopy and autoradiography (tritium PK11195) confirmed that the uptake was by abundant activated macrophages/microglia (CD68+) and not astrocytes (Figure 5.8.11 C & D). This suggested that PK11195 uptake was capable of predicting the development of SIVE and may be useful in treatment studies of neurologically impaired HIV+ patients. Longitudinal studies on six pigtailed macaques infected with SIVΔB670 revealed that retention of [11C]-(R)-PK11195 in the brain correlated with viral burden in the brain and cerebrospinal fluid as well as with brain regions containing both pre- and postsynaptic damage (decreases in SYN and MAP2) (Venneti et al., 2008a). Longitudinal changes in [11C]-(R)-PK11195 retention in the cortex, striatum, cerebellum, and brainstem correlated with changes in CD14+ monocyte and natural killer cell populations. Specifically, increased uptake of [11C]-(R)-PK11195 occurred when these monocyte populations in the

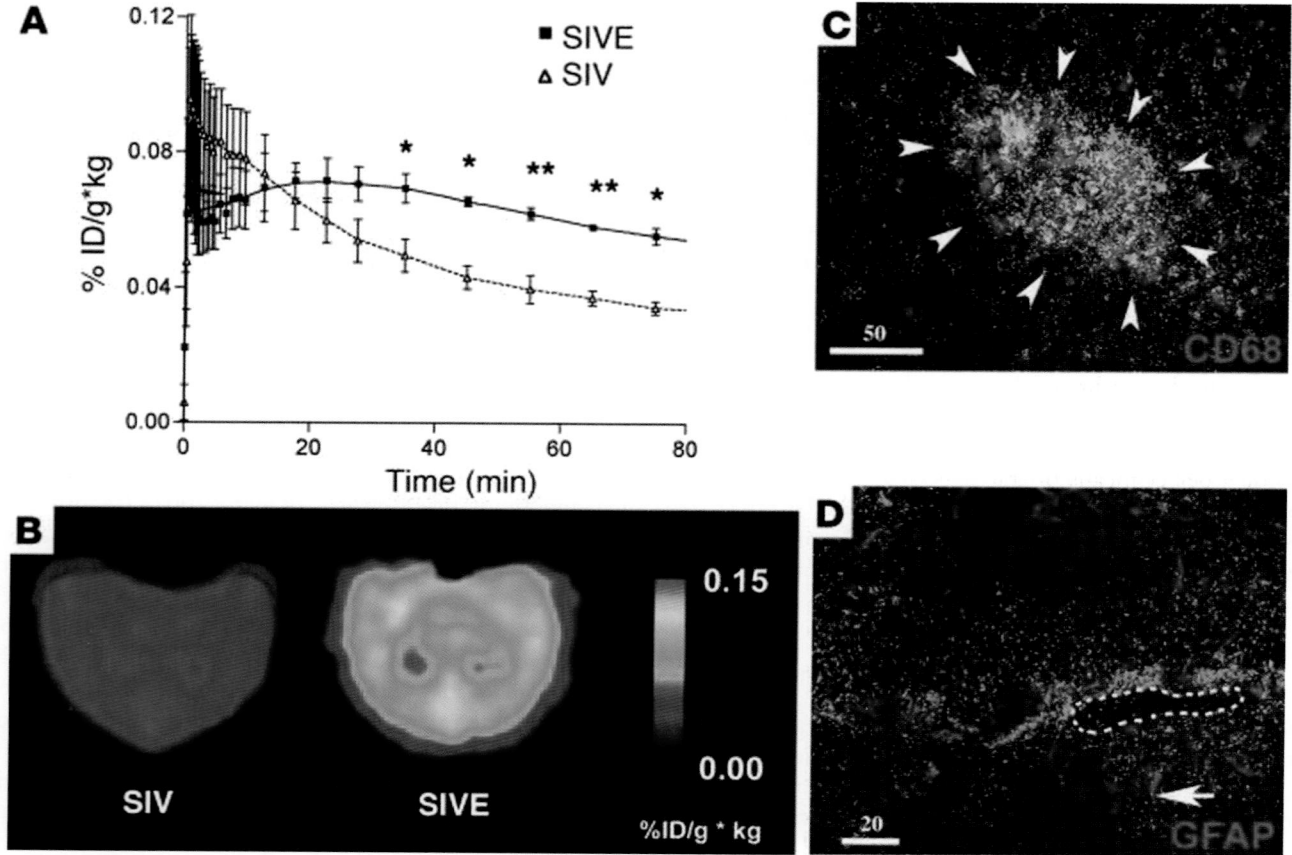

Figure 5.8.11 [A] SIVE macaques show increased [11C](R)-PK11195 retention and specific binding over time in the late scan frames (40–90 minutes) compared with SIV-infected, nonencephalitic macaques. [B] SIVE macaque brains show increased [11C](R)-PK11195–specific binding compared with SIV-infected, nonencephalitic macaques. [C & D] Combined [3H](R)-PK11195 autoradiography (green grains) and immunostaining for activated macrophages (C: CD68, red) or astrocytes (D: GFAP, red) in SIVE frontal cortex show that [3H](R)-PK11195–specific binding corresponds to macrophages, but not astrocytes. Scale bar in microns. Adapted with permission from Venneti et al., 2004.

blood were larger, suggesting that the development and progression of SIVE in vivo correlates with changes in immune cell populations in the periphery.

Despite the success of [11C]-(R)-PK11195 in models of SIVE, translational studies to HIV+ individuals have been less promising. While HIV+ subjects had retention of this PET microglia marker, it was incapable of distinguishing between patients with and without neurologic deficits (Hammoud et al., 2005; Wiley et al., 2006). One reason may be that this tracer can identify microglial activation, but not neuronal injury. Alternatively, it may be due to PK11195's low uptake. Therefore, ligands with greater binding affinity to TSPO are being explored for future use (Boutin et al., 2007; James et al., 2008; Venneti et al., 2008b).

CELL TRAFFICKING IN MACAQUE AND MOUSE MODELS

Monocytes and macrophages play a central role in the pathogenesis of neuroAIDS. It is generally agreed that key events in the initiation of neuronal injury are infection and activation of monocytes able to cross the blood-brain barrier (Kaul et al., 2001); however, many aspects regarding monocyte trafficking remain unexplored. Imaging studies of cell migration from peripheral blood into the CNS are possible using iron oxide labeled monocytes. Once accumulated in the brain tissue, properties such as the transverse relaxation time constant T_2 will be shorted, resulting in hypo-intensities on T_2^*-weighted images.

Using the SCID mouse model of HIVE, Zelivyanskaya et al. investigated the distribution of super-paramagnetic iron oxide (SPIO) labeled human monocytes in mouse brain tissue (Zelivyanskaya et al., 2003). After human monocytes labeled with SPIO particles were injected into the brain of SCID mice, high-field (7T) MRI and histological confirmation assays were used in parallel to monitor monocyte trafficking into and throughout the nervous system. Seven days post injection, monocytes were present in the ventricular system, corpus callosum, and throughout the brain, although they remained clustered in areas around the injection site. In a subsequent study, SPIO particles loaded into bone marrow-derived macrophages (BMM) were injected intravenously into HIVE mice, and BMM entry into the diseased brain regions was quantified (Liu et al., 2008). These data support the idea that cell migration can be monitored in vivo and provides an opportunity to assess monocyte mobility in the brain and its effects on neurodegenerative processes. It has been proposed that the same mononuclear phagocytes (MP) that serve as target cells and vehicles for dissemination of virus can be used to improve diagnostics and drug delivery (Beduneau et al., 2009).

The approach to monitor cell migration from peripheral blood into the central nervous system (CNS) in primates has been lacking. However, Clay et al. demonstrated acute monocyte brain infiltration using fluorescein dye-labeled monocytes into the choroid plexus stromata and perivascular spaces in the cerebra of rhesus macaques acutely infected with SIV between days 12 and 14 post infection (Clay et al., 2007). Future studies in SIV-macaques using SPIOs may provide a better means of tracking monocytes in vivo over the duration of infection.

SUMMARY AND FUTURE DIRECTIONS

The combination of imaging, virology, immunology, and molecular studies in animal models has led to a greater understanding of events inducing both inflammation and neuronal injury. Future imaging studies will revolve around the use of animal models such as the rapid progression macaque models for the efficient testing of novel therapies and for mechanistic studies of HIV-induced neuropathology. Enhancement of imaging techniques that currently suffer from low resolution such as microglia PET markers is likely to be important. Greater signal-to-noise and spatial resolution gained from higher field magnets may permit better quantification of those metabolites that overlap such as glutamate and glutamine and *myo*-inositol (Figure 5.8.12A). The use of MRI scanners with magnetic field strengths greater than 3T will allow for better image resolution and acquisition of metabolite maps with

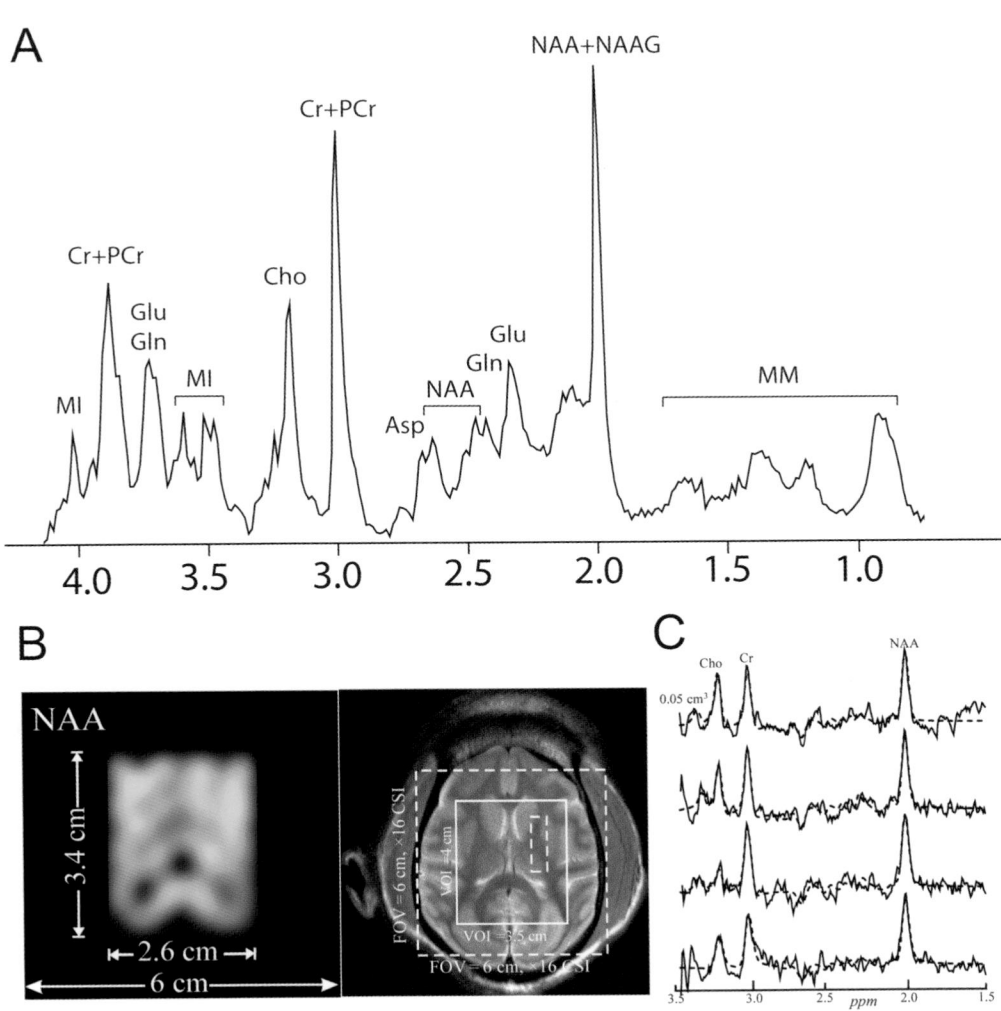

Figure 5.8.12 [A] Single voxel MR spectrum at 7 Tesla acquired from the parietal lobe of a primate (TE/TR = 30/3000 ms, voxel size 8 cm³). Higher field strength allow for better spectral resolution, allowing for better metabolite quantification. [B] Newly developed three-dimensional MRSI pulse sequence (TE/TR = 39/140 ms) resulting in 0.05 cm³ isotropic spatial resolution in macaques. Metabolic maps of NAA can be constructed (yellow) that correspond to the anatomy of that slice (note ventricles and midline). Adapted with permission from Gonen et al., 2008.

high spatial resolution. Recently, Gonen et al., have successfully implemented a 3D MR spectroscopy pulse sequence with a 0.05 cm^3 isotropic spatial resolution (Figure 5.8.12B) (Gonen et al., 2008). Novel imaging techniques using iron oxide particles or fluorescent agents should provide a means to directly monitor monocyte/macrophage trafficking into the brain (Bremer et al., 2003; Larson et al., 2003).

ACKNOWLEDGMENTS

Our own work was supported by NIH grants R01-NS050041, R21-NS059331, R01-NS040237 and K25-NS051129.

REFERENCES

Altfeld, M., Rosenberg, E. S., Shankarappa, R., et al. (2001). Cellular immune responses and viral diversity in individuals treated during acute and early HIV-1 infection. *J Exp Med*, 193, 169–80.

Altfeld, M. & Walker, B. D. (2001). Less is more? STI in acute and chronic HIV-1 infection. *Nat Med*, 7, 881–4.

Andersen, A. B., Law, I., Krabbe, K. S., et al. (2010). Cerebral FDG-PET scanning abnormalities in optimally treated HIV patients. *J Neuroinflammation*, 7.

Aylward, E. H., Henderer, J. D., McArthur, J. C., et al. (1993). Reduced basal ganglia volume in HIV-1-associated dementia: Results from quantitative neuroimaging. *Neurology*, 43, 2099–104.

Banati, R. B. (2002). Visualising microglial activation in vivo. *Glia*, 40, 206–17.

Baslow, M. H. (2000). Functions of N-acetyl-L-aspartate and N-acetyl-L-aspartylglutamate in the vertebrate brain: Role in glial cell-specific signaling. *J Neurochem*, 75, 453–9.

Baslow, M. H. (2002). Evidence supporting a role for N-acetyl-L-aspartate as a molecular water pump in myelinated neurons in the central nervous system. An analytical review. *Neurochem Int*, 40, 295–300.

Beduneau, A., Ma, Z., Grotepas, C. B., et al. (2009). Facilitated monocyte-macrophage uptake and tissue distribution of superparmagnetic iron-oxide nanoparticles. *PLoS One*, 4, e4343.

Belman, A. L. (1997). Pediatric neuro-AIDS. Update. *Neuroimaging Clin N Am*, 7, 593–613.

Boutin, H., Chauveau, F., Thominiaux, C., et al. (2007). 11C-DPA-713: A novel peripheral benzodiazepine receptor PET ligand for in vivo imaging of neuroinflammation. *J Nucl Med*, 48, 573–81.

Brand, A., Richter-Landsberg, C., & Leibfritz, D. (1993). Multinuclear NMR studies on the energy metabolism of glial and neuronal cells. *Dev Neurosci*, 15, 289–98.

Bremer, C., Mustafa, M., Bogdanov, A., Jr., et al. (2003). Steady-state blood volume measurements in experimental tumors with different angiogenic burdens a study in mice. *Radiology*, 226, 214–20.

Brennan, G., Podell, M. D., Wack, R., et al. (2006). Neurologic disease in captive lions (Panthera leo) with low-titer lion lentivirus infection. *J Clin Microbiol*, 44, 4345–52.

Broderick, D. F., Wippold, F. J., 2nd, Clifford, D. B., et al. (1993). White matter lesions and cerebral atrophy on MR images in patients with and without AIDS dementia complex. *AJR Am J Roentgenol*, 161, 177–81.

Brodt, H. R., Kamps, B. S., Gute, P., et al. (1997). Changing incidence of AIDS-defining illnesses in the era of antiretroviral combination therapy. *AIDS*, 11, 1731–8.

Bruce-Keller, A. J., Chauhan, A., Dimayuga, F. O., et al. (2003). Synaptic transport of human immunodeficiency virus-Tat protein causes neurotoxicity and gliosis in rat brain. *J Neurosci*, 23, 8417–22.

Burudi, E. M. E. & Fox, H. S. (2001). Simian immunodeficiency virus model of HIV-induced central nervous system dysfunction. *Adv Virus Research*, 56, 435–68.

Cagnin, A., Gerhard, A., & Banati, R. B. (2002). In vivo imaging of neuroinflammation. *Eur Neuropsychopharmacol*, 12, 581–6.

Chakraborty, G., Mekala, P., Yahya, D., et al (2001). Intraneuronal N-acetylaspartate supplies acetyl groups for myelin lipid synthesis: evidence for myelin-associated aspartoacylase. *J Neurochem*, 78, 736–45.

Chang, L., Ernst, T., Leonido-Yee, M., et al (1999). Cerebral metabolite abnormalities correlate with clinical severity of HIV-1 cognitive motor complex. *Neurology*, 52, 100–8.

Chang, L., Ernst, T., Witt, M. D., et al (2002). Relationships among brain metabolites, cognitive function, and viral loads in antiretroviral-naive HIV patients. *Neuroimage*, 17, 1638–48.

Chang, L., Speck, O., Miller, E. N., et al (2001). Neural correlates of attention and working memory deficits in HIV patients. *Neurology*, 57, 1001–7.

Chang, L., Wang, G. J., Volkow, N. D., et al (2008). Decreased brain dopamine transporters are related to cognitive deficits in HIV patients with or without cocaine abuse. *Neuroimage*, 42, 869–78.

Cheng, L. L., Ma, M. J., Becerra, L., et al (1997). Quantitative neuropathology by high resolution magic angle spinning proton magnetic resonance spectroscopy. *Proc Natl Acad USA*, 94, 6408–13.

Cheng, L. L., Newell, K., Mallory, A. E., et al (2002). Quantification of neurons in Alzheimer and control brains with ex vivo high resolution magic angle spinning proton magnetic resonance spectroscopy and stereology. *Magn Reson Imaging*, 20, 527–33.

Chong, W. K., Sweeney, B., Wilkinson, I. D., et al (1993). Proton spectroscopy of the brain in HIV infection: Correlation with clinical, immunologic, and MR imaging findings. *Radiology*, 188, 119–24.

Clay, C. C., Rodrigues, D. S., Ho, Y. S., et al (2007). Neuroinvasion of fluorescein-positive monocytes in acute simian immunodeficiency virus infection. *J Virol*, 81, 12040–8.

Cloak, C. C., Chang, L., Ernst, T., et al (2004). Methamphetamine and AIDS: 1HMRS studies in a feline model of human disease. *J Neuroimmunol*, 147, 16–20.

Crews, L., Lentz, M. R., Gonzalez, R. G., et al (2008). Neuronal injury in simian immunodeficiency virus and other animal models of neuroAIDS. *J Neurovirol*, 14, 327–39.

Daar, E. S., Moudgil, T., Meyer, R. D., et al (1991). Transient high levels of viremia in patients with primary human immunodeficiency virus type 1 infection. *N Engl J Med*, 324, 961–4.

DeFazio, R. A., Raval, A. P., Lin, H. W., et al (2009). GABA synapses mediate neuroprotection after ischemic and epsilonPKC preconditioning in rat hippocampal slice cultures. *J Cereb Blood Flow Metab*, 29, 375–84.

Domercq, M. & Matute, C. (2004). Neuroprotection by tetracyclines. *Trends Pharmacol Sci*, 25, 609–12.

Dooneief, G., Bello, J., Todak, G., et al (1992). A prospective controlled study of magnetic resonance imaging of the brain in gay men and parenteral drug users with human immunodeficiency virus infection. *Arch Neurol*, 49, 38–43.

Filippi, C. G., Ulug, A. M., Ryan, E., et al (2001). Diffusion tensor imaging of patients with HIV and normal-appearing white matter on MR images of the brain. *AJNR Am J Neuroradiol*, 22, 277–83.

Follstaedt, S. C., Barber, S. A., & Zink, M. C. (2008). Mechanisms of minocycline-induced suppression of simian immunodeficiency virus encephalitis: Inhibition of apoptosis signal-regulating kinase 1. *J Neurovirol*, 14, 376–88.

Fuller, R. A., Westmoreland, S. V., Ratai, E., et al (2004). A prospective longitudinal in vivo 1H MR spectroscopy study of the SIV/macaque model of neuroAIDS. *BMC Neurosci*, 5, 10.

Gonen, O., Liu, S., Goelman, G., et al (2008). Proton MR spectroscopic imaging of rhesus macaque brain in vivo at 7T. *Magn Reson Med*, 59, 692–9.

Gonzalez, R. G., Cheng, L. L., Westmoreland, S. V., et al (2000). Early brain injury in the SIV-macaque model of AIDS. *AIDS*, 14, 2841–9.

González, R.G., Greco, J.B., He, J., et al (2006). New insights into the neuroimmunity of SIV infection by magnetic resonance spectroscopy. *J Neuroimmune Pharmacol*, 1, 152–9.

Govindaraju, V., Young, K., & Maudsley, A. A. (2000). Proton NMR chemical shifts and coupling constants for brain metabolites. *NMR Biomed*, 13, 129–53.

Greco, J. B., Westmoreland, S. V., Ratai, E. M., et al (2004). In vivo 1H MRS of brain injury and repair during acute SIV infection in the macaque model of neuroAIDS. *Magn Reson Med*, 51, 1108–14.

Groeschel, S., Brockmann, K., Dechent, P., et al (2006). Magnetic resonance imaging and proton magnetic resonance spectroscopy of megalencephaly and dilated Virchow-Robin spaces. *Pediatr Neurol*, 34, 35–40.

Hakumaki, J. M. & Kauppinen, R. A. (2000). 1H NMR visible lipids in the life and death of cells. *Trends Biochem Sci*, 25, 357–62.

Hammoud, D. A., Endres, C. J., Chander, A. R., et al (2005). Imaging glial cell activation with [11C]-R-PK11195 in patients with AIDS. *J Neurovirol*, 11, 346–55.

Hammoud, D. A., Endres, C. J., Hammond, E., et al (2010). Imaging serotonergic transmission with [11C]DASB-PET in depressed and non-depressed patients infected with HIV. *Neuroimage*. 49, 2588–95.

Haughey, N. J., Cutler, R. G., Tamara, A., et al (2004). Perturbation of sphingolipid metabolism and ceramide production in HIV-dementia. *Ann Neurol*, 55, 257–67.

James, M. L., Fulton, R. R., Vercoullie, J., et al (2008). DPA-714, a new translocator protein-specific ligand: Synthesis, radiofluorination, and pharmacologic characterization. *J Nucl Med*, 49, 814–22.

Johnston, J. B., Silva, C., Hiebert, T., et al (2002). Neurovirulence depends on virus input titer in brain in feline immunodeficiency virus infection: Evidence for activation of innate immunity and neuronal injury. *J Neurovirol*, 8, 420–31.

Kaul, M., Garden, G. A., & Lipton, S. A. (2001). Pathways to neuronal injury and apoptosis in HIV-associated dementia. *Nature*, 410, 988–94.

Kim, J. P., Lentz, M. R., Westmoreland, S. V., et al (2005). Relationships between astrogliosis and 1H MR spectroscopic measures of brain choline/creatine and myo-inositol/creatine in a primate model. *AJNR Am J Neuroradiol*, 26, 752–9.

Kreis, R., Ross, B. D., Farrow, N. A., et al (1992). Metabolic disorders of the brain in chronic hepatic encephalopathy detected with H-1 MR spectroscopy. *Radiology*, 182, 19–27.

Lackner, A. A., Smith, M. O., Munn, R. J., et al (1991). Localization of simian immunodeficiency virus in the central nervous system of rhesus monkeys. *Am J Pathol*, 139, 609–21.

Larson, D. R., Zipfel, W. R., Williams, R. M., et al (2003). Water-soluble quantum dots for multiphoton fluorescence imaging in vivo. *Science*, 300, 1434–6.

Lentz, M. R., Burdo, T., Kim, H., et al (Submitted). Alterations in Brain Metabolism during the First Year of HIV-Infection. *Magn Reson Med*.

Lentz, M. R., Kim, J. P., Westmoreland, S. V., et al (2005). Quantitative neuropathologic correlates of changes in ratio of N-acetylaspartate to creatine in macaque brain. *Radiology*, 235, 461–8.

Lentz, M. R., Kim, W. K., Lee, V., et al (2009). Changes in MRS neuronal markers and T cell phenotypes observed during early HIV infection. *Neurology*, 72, 1465–72.

Lentz, M. R., Westmoreland, S. V., Lee, V., et al (2008). Metabolic markers of neuronal injury correlate with SIV CNS disease severity and inoculum in the macaque model of neuroAIDS. *Magn Reson Med*, 59, 475–84.

Lentz, M. R., Kim, W-K., Kim, H., Soulas, C., Lee, V., Venna, N., et al. (in press 2011). Alterations in Brain Metabolism during the First Year of Infection" *Journal of Neurovirology*.

Liu, Y., Uberti, M. G., Dou, H., et al (2008). Ingress of blood-borne macrophages across the blood-brain barrier in murine HIV-1 encephalitis. *J Neuroimmunol*, 200, 41–52.

Maingat, F., Vivithanaporn, P., Zhu, Y., et al (2009). Neurobehavioral performance in feline immunodeficiency virus infection: Integrated analysis of viral burden, neuroinflammation, and neuronal injury in cortex. *J Neurosci*, 29, 8429–37.

Mankowski, J. L., Queen, S. E., Tarwater, P. J., et al (2003). Elevated peripheral benzodiazepine receptor expression in simian immunodeficiency virus encephalitis. *J Neurovirol*, 9, 94–100.

Marcondes, M. C., Burudi, E. M., Huitron-Resendiz, S., et al (2001). Highly activated CD8(+) T cells in the brain correlate with early central nervous system dysfunction in simian immunodeficiency virus infection. *J Immunol*, 167, 5429–38.

Marcus, C. D., Taylor-Robinson, S. D., Sargentoni, J., et al (1998). 1H MR spectroscopy of the brain in HIV-1-seropositive subjects: Evidence for diffuse metabolic abnormalities. *Metab Brain Dis*, 13, 123–36.

McArthur, J. C. (2004). HIV dementia: An evolving disease. *J Neuroimmunol*, 157, 3–10.

McArthur, J. C., Hoover, D. R., Bacellar, H., et al (1993). Dementia in AIDS patients: Incidence and risk factors. Multicenter AIDS Cohort Study. *Neurology*, 43, 2245–52.

McArthur, J. C., Kumar, A. J., Johnson, D. W., et al (1990). Incidental white matter hyperintensities on magnetic resonance imaging in HIV-1 infection. Multicenter AIDS Cohort Study. *J Acquir Immune Defic Syndr*, 3, 252–9.

Mellors, J. W., Kingsley, L. A., Rinaldo, C. R., Jr., et al (1995). Quantitation of HIV-1 RNA in plasma predicts outcome after seroconversion. *Ann Intern Med*, 122, 573–9.

Meyerhoff, D. J., Bloomer, C., Cardenas, V., et al (1999). Elevated subcortical choline metabolites in cognitively and clinically asymptomatic HIV+ patients. *Neurology*, 52, 995–1003.

Moffett, J. R., Ross, B., Arun, P., et al (2007). N-Acetylaspartate in the CNS: From neurodiagnostics to neurobiology. *Prog Neurobiol*, 81, 89–131.

Mohamed, M. A., Lentz, M. R., Lee, V., et al (2010). Factor analysis of proton MR spectroscopic imaging data in HIV infection: Metabolite-derived factors help identify infection and dementia. *Radiology*, 254, 577–86.

Moller, H. E., Vermathen, P., Lentschig, M. G., et al (1999). Metabolic characterization of AIDS dementia complex by spectroscopic imaging. *J Magn Reson Imaging*, 9, 10–8.

Moore, D., Letendre, S., Deutsch, R., et al (2010). HIV-associated neurocognitive disorder in acute and early HIV infection. In: *17th Conference on Retroviruses and Opportunistic Infections*: San Francisco, CA.

Nath, A., Schiess, N., Venkatesan, A., et al (2008). Evolution of HIV dementia with HIV infection. *Int Rev Psychiatry*, 20, 25–31.

Nelson, J., Dou, H., Ellison, B., et al (2005). Coregistration of quantitative proton magnetic resonance spectroscopic imaging with neuropathological and neurophysiological analyses defines the extent of neuronal impairments in murine human immunodeficiency virus type-1 encephalitis. *J Neurosci Res*, 80, 562–75.

Okamoto, S., Kang, Y. J., Brechtel, C. W., et al (2007). HIV/gp120 decreases adult neural progenitor cell proliferation via checkpoint kinase-mediated cell-cycle withdrawal and G1 arrest. *Cell Stem Cell*, 1, 230–6.

Persidsky, Y., Buttini, M., Limoges, J., et al (1997). An analysis of HIV-1-associated inflammatory products in brain tissue of humans and SCID mice with HIV-1 encephalitis. *J Neurovirol*, 3, 401–16.

Persidsky, Y. & Gendelman, H. E. (2002). Murine models for human immunodeficiency virus type 1-associated dementia: The development of new treatment testing paradigms. *J Neurovirol*, 8 Suppl 2, 49–52.

Persidsky, Y., Limoges, J., McComb, R., et al (1996). Human immunodeficiency virus encephalitis in SCID mice. *Am J Pathol*, 149, 1027–53.

Peterson, J., Lee, E., Hecht, F., et al (2010). Neurocognitive performance during primary HIV-1 infection. In: *17th Conference on Retroviruses and Opportunistic Infections*: San Francisco, CA.

Phipps, A. J., Hayes, K. A., Buck, W. R., et al (2000). Neurophysiologic and immunologic abnormalities associated with feline immunodeficiency virus molecular clone FIV-PPR DNA inoculation. *J Acquir Immune Defic Syndr*, 23, 8–16.

Podell, M., Hayes, K., Oglesbee, M., et al (1997). Progressive encephalopathy associated with CD4/CD8 inversion in adult FIV-infected cats. *J Acquir Immune Defic Syndr Hum Retrovirol*, 15, 332–40.

Podell, M., Maruyama, K., Smith, M., et al (1999). Frontal lobe neuronal injury correlates to altered function in FIV-infected cats. *J Acquir Immune Defic Syndr*, 22, 10–8.

Power, C., Buist, R., Johnston, J. B., et al (1998). Neurovirulence in feline immunodeficiency virus-infected neonatal cats is viral strain specific and dependent on systemic immune suppression. *J Virol*, 72, 9109–15.

Power, C., Moench, T., Peeling, J., et al (1997). Feline immunodeficiency virus causes increased glutamate levels and neuronal loss in brain. *Neuroscience*, 77, 1175–85.

Ratai, E.M., Annamalai L., Burdo T., et al., (2011a). Brain creatine elevation and N-acetylaspartate reduction indicates neuronal dysfunction in the setting of enhanced glial energy metabolism in a macaque model of NeuroAIDS. *Magn Reson Med*. (in press)

Ratai, E. M., Pilkenton, S., He, J., et al (2011b). CD8+ lymphocyte depletion without SIV infection does not produce metabolic changes or pathological abnormalities in the rhesus macaque brain. *J Med Primatology* 2011 (in press).

Ratai, E. M., Bombardier, J. P., Joo, C. G., et al (2010). Proton magnetic resonance spectroscopy reveals neuroprotection by oral minocycline in a nonhuman primate model of accelerated neuroAIDS. *PLoS One*, 7, 5(5):e10523.

Ratai, E. M., Pilkenton, S. J., Greco, J. B., et al (2009). In vivo proton magnetic resonance spectroscopy reveals region specific metabolic responses to SIV infection in the macaque brain. *BMC Neurosci*, 10, 63.

Reid, W., Sadowska, M., Denaro, F., et al (2001). An HIV-1 transgenic rat that develops HIV-related pathology and immunologic dysfunction. *Proc Natl Acad Sci USA*, 98, 9271–6.

Rosenberg, E. S., Billingsley, J. M., Caliendo, A. M., et al (1997). Vigorous HIV-1-specific CD4+ T cell responses associated with control of viremia. *Science*, 278, 1447–50.

Ross, B. D. (1991). Biochemical considerations in 1H spectroscopy. Glutamate and glutamine; myo-inositol and related metabolites. *NMR Biomed*, 4, 59–63.

Sacktor, N. (2002). The epidemiology of human immunodeficiency virus-associated neurological disease in the era of highly active antiretroviral therapy. *J Neurovirol*, 8 Suppl 2, 115–21.

Sacktor, N., McDermott, M. P., Marder, K., et al (2002). HIV-associated cognitive impairment before and after the advent of combination therapy. *J Neurovirol*. 8, 136–42.

Sacktor, N., Nakasujja, N., Skolasky, R. L., et al (2009). HIV subtype D is associated with dementia, compared with subtype A, in immunosuppressed individuals at risk of cognitive impairment in Kampala, Uganda. *Clin Infect Dis*, 49, 780–6.

Salvan, A. M., Vion-Dury, J., Confort-Gouny, S., et al (1997). Brain proton magnetic resonance spectroscopy in HIV-related encephalopathy: Identification of evolving metabolic patterns in relation to dementia and therapy. *AIDS Res Hum Retroviruses*, 13, 1055–66.

Saransaari, P. & Oja, S. S. (1997). Enhanced taurine release in cell-damaging conditions in the developing and ageing mouse hippocampus. *Neuroscience* 79, 847–54.

Schmitz, J. E., Kuroda, M. J., Santra, S., et al (1999). Control of viremia in simian immunodeficiency virus infection by CD8+ lymphocytes. *Science*, 283, 857–60.

Sopper, S., Sauer, U., Hemm, S., et al (1998). Protective role of the virus-specific immune response for development of severe neurologic signs in simian immunodeficiency virus-infected macaques. *J Virol*, 72, 9940–7.

Staprans, S. I., Dailey, P. J., Rosenthal, A., et al (1999). Simian immunodeficiency virus disease course is predicted by the extent of virus replication during primary infection. *J Virol*, 73, 4829–39.

Taylor, J. S., Langston, J. W., Reddick, W. E., et al (1996). Clinical value of proton magnetic resonance spectroscopy for differentiating recurrent or residual brain tumor from delayed cerebral necrosis. *Int J Radiat Oncol Biol Phys*, 36, 1251–61.

Toggas, S. M., Masliah, E., Rockenstein, E. M., et al (1994). Central nervous system damage produced by expression of the HIV-1 coat protein gp120 in transgenic mice. *Nature*, 367, 188–93.

Tracey, I., Hamberg, L. M., Guimaraes, A. R., et al (1998). Increased cerebral blood volume in HIV-positive patients detected by functional MRI. *Neurology*, 50, 1821–6.

Urenjak, J., Williams, S. R., Gadian, D. G., et al (1992). Specific expression of N-acetylaspartate in neurons, oligodendrocyte-type-2 astrocyte progenitors, and immature oligodendrocytes in vitro. *J Neurochem*, 59, 55–61.

Urenjak, J., Williams, S. R., Gadian, D. G., et al (1993). Proton nuclear magnetic resonance spectroscopy unambiguously identifies different neural cell types. *J Neurosci*, 13, 981–9.

Venneti, S., Bonneh-Barkay, D., Lopresti, B. J., et al (2008a). Longitudinal in vivo positron emission tomography imaging of infected and activated brain macrophages in a macaque model of human immunodeficiency virus encephalitis correlates with central and peripheral markers of encephalitis and areas of synaptic degeneration. *Am J Pathol*, 172, 1603–16.

Venneti, S., Lopresti, B. J., Wang, G., et al (2004). PET imaging of brain macrophages using the peripheral benzodiazepine receptor in a macaque model of neuroAIDS. *J Clin Invest*, 113, 981–9.

Venneti, S., Wang, G., & Wiley, C. A. (2007). Activated macrophages in HIV encephalitis and a macaque model show increased [3H](R)-PK11195 binding in a PI3-kinase-dependent manner. *Neurosci Lett*, 426, 117–22.

Venneti, S., Wang, G., & Wiley, C. A. (2008b). The high affinity peripheral benzodiazepine receptor ligand DAA1106 binds to activated and infected brain macrophages in areas of synaptic degeneration: Implications for PET imaging of neuroinflammation in lentiviral encephalitis. *Neurobiol Dis*, 29, 232–41.

von Giesen, H. J., Antke, C., Hefter, H., *et al* (2000). Potential time course of human immunodeficiency virus type 1-associated minor motor deficits: Electrophysiologic and positron emission tomography findings. *Arch Neurol*, 57, 1601–7.

Westmoreland, S. V., Halpern, E., & Lackner, A. A. (1998). Simian immunodeficiency virus encephalitis in rhesus macaques is associated with rapid disease progression. *J Neurovirol*, 4, 260–8.

Wiley, C. A., Lopresti, B. J., Becker, J. T., et al (2006). Positron emission tomography imaging of peripheral benzodiazepine receptor binding in human immunodeficiency virus-infected subjects with and without cognitive impairment. *J Neurovirol*, 12, 262–71.

Williams, K., Westmoreland, S., Greco, J., et al (2005). Magnetic resonance spectroscopy reveals that activated monocytes contribute to neuronal injury in SIV neuroAIDS. *J Clin Invest*, 115, 2534–45.

Zelivyanskaya, M. L., Nelson, J. A., Poluektova, L., et al (2003). Tracking superparamagnetic iron oxide labeled monocytes in brain by high-field magnetic resonance imaging. *J Neurosci Res*, 73, 284–95.

Zink, M. C. & Clements, J. E. (2002a). A novel simian immunodeficiency virus model that provides insight into mechanisms of human immunodeficiency virus central nervous system disease. *J Neurovirol*, 8 Suppl 2, 42–8.

Zink, M. C., Spelman, J. P., Robinson, R. B., et al (1998). SIV infection of macaques—modeling the progression to AIDS dementia. *J Neurovirol*, 4, 249–59.

Zink, M. C., Uhrlaub, J., DeWitt, J., et al (2005). Neuroprotective and anti-human immunodeficiency virus activity of minocycline. *JAMA*, 293, 2003–11.

Zink, W. E., Anderson, E., Boyle, J., et al (2002b). Impaired spatial cognition and synaptic potentiation in a murine model of human immunodeficiency virus type 1 encephalitis. *J Neurosci*, 22, 2096–105.

SECTION 6

PERSONAL PERSPECTIVES IN LIVING WITH HIV/AIDS

Ian Paul Everall and Susan Swindells

6.1

HIV AND MY MENTAL HEALTH— A PERSONAL REFLECTION

Darren Kane

This chapter is a personal reflection, recalling the effect of contracting HIV as a young man. The author focuses on the mental impact of the diagnosis and the varying emotions that accompanied it, such as vulnerability, anxiety, denial, repression, confusion, and shame over his sexual identity as a gay male. The diagnosis and its conflicting emotions led to the author to experience depression and substance-abuse. Despite several difficult years, the author has been able to work through and process his HIV diagnosis and offers the reader a message of hope and self-realization.

At the age of nineteen, in my last year as a "teen," I was approaching a period in my life of increasing growth and exploration. The world was opening up to me and I was opening up to the world. While this was sometimes overwhelming for a boy as sheltered as I'd been, it was more often exciting. I was more enthusiastic than afraid. It was this spirit of enthusiasm that motivated me to engage with new ideas at university and to challenge many of my beliefs. It also took me to India, a part of the world I already felt drawn to when a good friend spontaneously invited me to come along with him.

My first trip to India was a rite of passage for me, coming at an age when the experience of independent travel in such a richly different culture could have a truly profound impact. And this it did. My late adolescent openness and willingness to trust allowed me to surrender to the experience of India, enough that it deeply shifted my perspective on the world and my place in it. But this process of change was as painful as it was wonderful. It was the beginning of my loss of innocence, which accelerated when I became unexplainably ill during a period of traveling alone. I'd never found it easy to be sick as it always confronted me with my fears. But I'd never been as afraid as I was this time—I was alone, I was sicker than I'd ever felt, and I had no idea why.

Returning to Australia several weeks later, I still hadn't fully recovered and was no wiser about what was going on inside my body. I was still in shock from the roughness of my experience in India. I felt vulnerable and weak compared with the strong, resilient state I'd originally left Australia in. Then began the process of medical investigation into what was wrong with me. I turned 20 in a state of transition, confusion, and fragility. The mystery of my neuropathic condition had not been fully solved. I was sent to a neurologist to have the diagnosis of Guillain-Barre syndrome confirmed.

He questioned me about the possibility that I'd contracted HIV, asking me coarsely and directly if I was gay. I'd only come out over the previous few years, so I was still very sensitive on the subject. His invasive questioning left me feeling embarrassed and deeply ashamed.

Certain of the possibility that I had HIV, the neurologist then pressured me into immediately having an HIV test. I feebly protested, saying that I was already planning to have one at the sexual health clinic where I'd been for previous tests. But, respecting his medical authority, I agreed to a test with the faith that it would turn out negative like the others had. When I returned to the neurologist the following week, it was for a consultation about my neuropathy. I wasn't expecting the test result for another week. He arrived late, pale-faced, and in a state of anxiety. He immediately sat me down and fired the result at me. I was HIV positive. Not expecting any result yet, let alone a positive one, I reeled with shock. Only a small part of me had seen this coming. It could never have prepared me for the reality of diagnosis.

An overwhelming wave of emotion overcame me in this moment, but I suppressed it. I didn't feel safe to express any of what I was feeling. I didn't really trust the man sitting opposite me. He wasn't experienced with HIV diagnosis, probably never having delivered one before. And he hadn't prepared me at all for the news he delivered. There had been no counseling, so there was no checking in that I grasped the gravity of the situation and that I anticipated the psychological reaction a positive diagnosis might provoke. Once the truth had come out, he then gave me a prognosis: 10 to 15 years. It was another assault on my senses. In that moment of deep vulnerability, I couldn't help but believe the death sentence I'd been given. I was staring the reality of HIV in the face and I'd be dead by 35. Although I didn't fully trust this neurologist, I wanted to. The words had been said and the traumatized state I was in allowed his prognosis to lodge itself in my psyche. I can now see that the lack of counseling and emotional support profoundly affected the impact the diagnosis had on me.

Through the experience of diagnosis, any afterglow that my waning innocence had left behind was crudely extinguished. Overall, it had been a traumatic loss of innocence. It felt as if my innocence was ripped away from me and that I had no chance to surrender it gracefully. I'd never felt so alone. My sense of invincibility was crushed. And at the same time I lost my sense of safety in the world. How could this have happened to me? Sure I'd taken risks. But so did many of my peers and they hadn't ended up with HIV. At the same time though, thanks to the wisdom I'd touched on in India, a part of me knew that it had happened for a reason. The painful reality was nonetheless overwhelming and I felt very ashamed about what had happened to me. Despite the support I had from family and friends, the loneliness of those first few months coming to terms with the diagnosis often made me want to die. All my pre-existing fears and insecurities came bubbling up to the surface. I became more anxious than ever. I'd always felt a bit different, but now I was on such a completely different page than most of my peers that I felt very isolated. This feeling continued for many years. Only more recently, in my late twenties, have I been able to reconcile with it.

In the diagnosis aftermath, I tried to go on with life as usual. I downplayed to myself the psychological and emotional impact of getting HIV, preferring to pretend it was no big deal and to try and just get over it. This would seem to work until I'd go into brief but intense periods of anxiety and depression. Initially, I used recreational drugs to numb the pain and get myself "out of it," but I could see that this was a downward spiral. So I followed my growing interest in leftist student politics and threw myself into political activism, opting to distract myself from the pain instead. I also started counseling because I could see I had issues to deal with and it seemed a normal step to take after diagnosis. But the counseling brought up such strong emotions in my 20-year-old self that I didn't want to go there and so I let it go fairly quickly.

My unconscious strategy was simple: deny, distract, and avoid. This I did in the context of constant emotional stress and anxiety. It was only recently, while studying to become a transpersonal counselor, that I discovered that these are telltale signs of post-traumatic stress. This response to the trauma of contracting HIV played itself out over the ensuing years. It's only in retrospect that I've been able to identify this undiagnosed condition in my history. My avoidance tendency both aided and concealed a deep-seated anger within me, which I channeled into my growing commitment to political activism. The radical circle I was mixing with shared the same distrust and lack of safety in the world. This was the period when George W. Bush came into power in the US and John Howard was reaching his zenith here, so there seemed plenty of reason to be distrustful! Our negative view and lack of trust was fuel for our anger and our activism was its outlet. But for me it became a vicious cycle that only led to depression and a sense of hopelessness. I felt judged, unsupported, and neglected by the world, despite the contradicting evidence in my personal life.

Eventually, I burnt out. Through the gentle observations of my close friends, I got an insight into the excessive expectations I had of myself, and the negativity it was fueling in me. My physical health was beginning to reflect my poor mental health. I was forced to accept my own limits and slow down. And thus, I allowed myself to the other extreme; spending a lazy summer on the dole, smoking pot. The lack of responsibility and the mind-expanding effects of the marijuana created a

space where I experienced a spiritual awakening. The faith I'd lost through political activism came flooding back stronger than ever.

At the same time, I was exploring using natural therapies to help restore my health and vitality. I decided that I needed to focus most of my energy on my health because if I didn't I thought it would deteriorate again. This possibility fueled my anxiety, motivating me to drop out of university and to quit my job. I was still only 21. I felt idle and useless in the urban environment that I now considered unhealthy. The prolonged marijuana use was also starting to make me depressed. So I left Melbourne to head for Byron Bay and be around people who were also trying to live their spiritual path through a pure lifestyle. I started practicing meditation daily. I stopped the marijuana and became a devout vegan, drifting around the Byron hinterland trying to find like-minded people.

I was obsessed with purifying myself, believing that this was the only way I might outlive my prognosis. I rejected the idea of HIV medication to the extent that I refused to have my blood tested, much to the dismay of my doctor. For the next 2 years I avoided seeing doctors altogether. I viewed pharmaceutical drugs as poisons that could do more damage than the virus. Of course, the effort to stick to these extremes meant that I did relapse into marijuana use sometimes. I always felt ashamed about this and disappointed with my frustrated efforts at self-purification. It reinforced my perception that I was imperfect, diseased, damaged, and therefore unworthy and inferior.

My extreme lifestyle began to disconnect me from mainstream society. Whenever I returned home to Melbourne, I sensed this more than ever. I was often withdrawn and had great difficulty expressing myself. I felt misunderstood by my family and society to the extent that I didn't feel I had a place here. So I took myself in self-imposed exile to Southeast Asia and eventually back to India, believing that these were cultures that better understood and supported a pure, spiritual lifestyle. But most of the time I was deeply lonely and unhappy. I maintained my obsessive habits around my diet, yoga practice, and meditation; hypervigilant in case I fell off the path and into a downward spiral. The irony is that I was already in a downward spiral mentally, emotionally, and physically. I desperately wanted to connect with people, which I did many times, only to have to say farewell to them so we could continue on our individual journeys. The constant anxiety continued and a pattern of depression initiated itself, worsening with each passing month. I was faced with all my self-hatred, my sense of taintedness, my shame. I'd tried to run away from it all, only to have it stand in my way at every step. My physical health and vitality started to deteriorate due to repeated parasitic infections, which I refused to treat with antibiotics. It was in Nepal that I finally cracked and threw in the towel, tired of searching and having to adjust to new places and people.

Coming home relieved my depression somewhat, thanks to the nurturing space my family provided. But my sense of failure in my attempts at self-purification still pervaded. I began counseling again, realizing again that I had major issues to deal with and needing support with my reintegration back into my own culture. Reluctantly, I finally treated the parasites and began the slow process of rebuilding my digestive system. But I still refused to have my blood tested. I believed that I could recover my health naturally and my rejection of medications remained. At this time, I even began to engage with AIDS dissident theories, which deny the connection between HIV and AIDS and sometimes even refute the existence of the virus altogether. This was painfully confusing as I became even less sure of who to trust. I therefore maintained my hypervigilance around my lifestyle, limiting my social life and avoiding work and study after attempts to do so proved too draining. It took two years of counseling for me to realize that it was my anxiety and lack of self-worth that was really draining me—that I was self-sabotaging out of fear that I wasn't good enough. The perfectionist inner critic within me was exposed and tamed, allowing me to begin to realize my own potential.

It was at this breakthrough point that I decided to have my blood tested again, for the first time in 4 years. Of course, my immune system was dangerously deficient. I realized that this was truly the cause of my pervasive health problems for the past 3 years. It finally felt real. There really was a virus in my body. As serious as this realization seems, it was actually a relief. I could let go of the confusion and the belief that I could only keep myself healthy through great effort and self-deprivation. I could stop blaming myself for being unwell. Most importantly, I could begin to fully trust in others' care again. This was profoundly healing. My anxiety eased up a bit and my general mental health immediately began to improve. It was like a weight had been lifted. Despite the challenges of adjusting to medication and finding a workable drug combination, I generally felt more secure and positive about the future.

A restored feeling of safety in the world allowed me to feel more confident in myself and with people and society. I felt a sense of place again. This encouraged me to take the important steps of finally finishing my bachelor's degree at 27, starting to work again, and exploring a career path that really resonates. My exploration led me last year to study transpersonal counseling. It was taught from an experiential learning approach, which gave me much new perspective on the past 10 years since I was infected. This vocation enables me to consciously bring in everything I've learned from my experience and use it to help others in their healing. This can only deeply assist my own continued healing.

Despite all the pain, doubt, shame, and confusion of those years of recovery from the trauma of contracting HIV at such a young age, a part of me was always conscious of the rich opportunity it created for my personal growth. This was the same part of me that knew way back at the time of diagnosis that it had happened for a reason. And this essential part of me was there with me all the time. It was gently reminding me that I wasn't worthless, that I needn't be ashamed, that I could trust in this experience, in other people, and in the universe. It was the part of me that I sometimes contacted in meditation or in random moments just when it all seemed to be getting too hard. I'd call this part of me my Higher Self. Although it was obscured and devalued so much of the time, it was what actually gave me back the faith that kept me from ending it all or continuing on self-destructive paths and downward spirals. It saved me. And it helped me see that having HIV could guide me towards what really matters in life—towards the meaning of life. So, as negative and heavy as this story may seem, there's hope in it too because the seed of self-realization was there from the beginning. And now that I'm 30 and I'm confidently outliving that prognosis, I trust that this growth will continue well into my thirties and beyond.

6.2

FEAR AND LOATHING
IN HIV MENTAL HEALTH CARE

Eric M. Glare

This is a personal reflection from someone in the medical community who has contracted HIV, allowing a unique perspective. He also received a diagnosis of Bipolar Type II after having contracted HIV, so he has experienced both the stigma of HIV, as well as the stigma of mental illness. The author details how both diagnoses impacted his life and his relationships, and talks about how he combats both stigmas by speaking publicly and openly about his experiences to others on behalf of people living with HIV (PLHIV) and poor mental health.

The moment I start to write it changes everything. The moment I stand up to advocate for people living with HIV (PLHIV) and poor mental health, I am no longer like the people I seek to represent. Silence is the essential attribute of PLHIV with mental health dysfunction. This silence, fear, and an overdose of self-loathing is the result of synergism between the stigma of HIV and the stigma of mental dysfunction.

I am very much a minority, of a minority, of a minority as a gay man living with HIV, bipolar type II, and cognitive dysfunction who speaks openly about the lived experience through the Positive Speakers Bureau, a program of People Living with HIV/AIDS Victoria based in Melbourne, Australia. I began publicly speaking on HIV to help out but very soon I realized that disclosing my story harnessed understanding and supported my health. Speaking out was the perfect tool to deflect and discard the burden of stigma I was continually exposed to.

I was not always open about living with HIV and ironically, fear of disclosing the need for an HIV test was the start of this whole mess. Irony seems to be a common thread. As a molecular biologist, I did HIV research before I contracted HIV. I was infecting brain astrocytes with HIV to see what would happen to their cytokine gene expression. Now my own brain is a walking experiment on the effect of HIV and this is my case study.

HIV INFECTION, DIAGNOSIS, AND GETTING ON WITH LIFE

I was cultivating HIV in the lab when I met my second long-term partner and it was very logical to talk about HIV testing. However, he was a serving member of the Australian Defence Force and in 1990 it was illegal for gays and lesbians to serve in the military. Asking for a HIV test would have meant an immediate dishonorable discharge because only gay men and injecting drug users were considered at risk. When the ban on gays was lifted in 1992, much noise was made in opposition to the HIV risk of gay soldiers. My partner could have sought testing outside the free "Rolls Royce" medical care provided on base, but was too afraid to do the necessary paperwork or to seek anonymous testing.

After 5 years of a cozy relationship, foreplay became sex without a condom. Four months later, I experienced what must have been my HIV seroconversion. At 29 years of age, I had contracted HIV. Fear gripped us both and it took another 3 years before the fear of not knowing led me to get tested behind my partner's back, and against his wishes. Devastating as that news was, I was confronted with another great disappointment that day. I was a rapid progressor with only 70 CD4 cells remaining. With such a low nadir, my gamble on the variance of HIV progression was to be my downfall. Ten days after my diagnosis, my partner received his positive test result. It was a story of fear and self-loathing, of love and tragedy of operatic proportions.

My partner and I stuck together and got on with our careers without telling anyone outside our medical care. We feared that if I disclosed my status I might inadvertently expose my partner and end his military career. In the end, he kept his secret and made his exit more than 5 years later on his own terms with 21 years of distinguished service with the option of another promotion if he wanted to stay.

In addition to my PhD studies on cytokines in asthma, I managed a project developing PCR-based assays of cytomegalovirus (CMV) viral load. We began the assay development in lung transplantation but when we wanted to extend the research to the HIV population in the late 1990s, many of my colleagues refused to allow the samples into the lab. It seemed important to them that two lab personnel were pregnant and others were planning to be in the near future. We were forced to transfer the project to the infectious diseases department of the hospital next door. Having seen the lack of principles of my seniors, it was not the time or place to acknowledge my own status.

BECOMING ILL

Eventually, my HIV status was assumed when I became ill with viral meningitis in 2002. One moment I was a post-doctoral researcher madly running after grants so that I still had a job in a year's time, and the next my career was over.

My brain had shut down whilst it fought a virus in my meninges, or at least that is the theory with such a default diagnosis.

Chronically ill with daily migraine-like headaches, I struggled to remember my phone number for the first 6 weeks. The lymphocytosis in my cerebrospinal fluid (CSF) from four lumbar punctures spaced over 3 months gradually resolved. The idea of a viral infection that was taking its time to be vanquished gave me some sympathy and somewhat counteracted the calls for me to "snap out of it." Nevertheless, I was continually told by everyone I came across that my ill health was entirely my fault and I was accused in equal measures of doing too much and not enough of the ordinary daily functions of life. This harassment and my severely depressed cognitive function made socializing an emotionally painful experience and a chore to be avoided. When I did socialize, I lagged behind or sat on the periphery trying to look included but avoiding conversation.

Unfortunately, although improved, the daily headaches continued, complete with immobilizing neck pain. I had become addicted to oxycodone and codeine in the painkillers I was cycling on a daily basis. Unable to significantly reduce the use of the painkillers myself, I had a 15-day dry-out procedure using an infusion of lidocaine. Not without risks, it worked.

When the fog of the past 6 months lifted, my brain took off. I was very happy to have my old friend the brain back, but my doctors were not so impressed with my psychosis. Looking back, I think it is a big discrepancy that I did not have formal counseling during this torrid time and that it took a drug-induced psychosis for me to start with my psychiatrist. I was more than ready and it was a big relief to begin to unpack the baggage of not only HIV infection and illness but my abusive childhood as well.

When I first came down with meningitis, my partner went cold, intimacy ended, and he did not want to touch me. He was afraid of contracting my mysterious virus. Even when that was no longer seemed a threat, I still reminded him every day when he came home from work that he too had HIV and one day he might be fighting for his life. He was very much against counseling for either of us but would not break off our relationship of more than 13 years. I was not fit for change, yet I needed resolution to get well.

With the help of my psychiatrist, I tried to put my life back together. Slowly, over a handful of months, I became stronger and eventually I broke off the relationship. Suddenly, I was free but very alone. I had lost my love, my friends, my career, and my health. I felt completely diminished, totally decimated.

Just one month later, two events happened that have had a profound effect on my life and health ever since. I joined the Positive Speakers Bureau and began a journey of self-discovery led by speaking out about my experiences. About the same time, I met my current partner who remains HIV negative. I told myself I was not having a relationship, but one day someone said to us that we looked like a nice couple and the bubble of denial burst.

One of the first things I did next was take him to meet my primary care doctor and then my psychiatrist. I realized he had to get acquainted with the issues and the support I had, fast, or

the relationship was not going to happen. Six and a half years on (he insisted on the half) as I write, it has been a tumultuous relationship, fraught to nonexistence many times, but we are still arguing together. We go to couple's counseling at an HIV service but we never see any other couples there. We rarely dare to mention the "L" word, love, but we have a connection that will not let go. We live for the moment and the short term, lest we be too afraid of the storm clouds over our future.

Moving in to his house should have been a historic moment to savor and celebrate but I was vomiting too much, too ill for that. I had never fully recovered from the meningitis, the gastrointestinal side effects of my ART regimen were increasingly debilitating, and I was chronically depressed. It was then that I noticed that increasing the dose of my antidepressant, citalopram, generally lifted my mood but did not change the fluctuations nor truly alleviate my depression.

BIPOLAR TYPE II DIAGNOSIS

A few weeks after changing to a new ART regime, my mood began to ultra-rapid cycle and I received a diagnosis of bipolar type II. I had become a collector of stigmatizing labels. For about 5 months, I had a cycle of about 3 to 5 days with a sharp drop from the peak of hypomania to the lowest level of depression, often within 24 hours. The quicker my mood dropped, the faster hope vanished, leaving me feeling breathlessly devastated.

Resolution was slow and tortuous as I took up lithium, gradually stepped down from citalopram, and then much later, the antipsychotic quetiapine was added. It was many months before I was confident enough to tell my story again or drive a car or ride my motorbike. I joked it was like watching grass grow in the desert of the Australian Outback during a drought. My vantage point, I dreamt, was a Luna Park roller coaster ride that ceased to be fun just moments after it started.

I have an understanding of my mood changes because my psychiatrist asked me to record mood scores three times a day. To be able to connect my mood with how I was feeling and the situations I found myself in was a tremendous benefit to both my partner and me. I wrote down "lead boots" several times before discovering others called it "lead coat depression." It was a cliché that fitted my experience perfectly. We came to understand my explosive anger was directly linked to my level of frustration and irritability. My mind had become my biggest traitor and I did not know what strife would happen next, but from my scores, I knew that tomorrow might be a different kind of agony. Knowing that was very important to me at the time.

I still experience labile moods and I need to be circumspect about when I go grocery shopping, when I drive my car, when to socialize or do public speaking. For the benefit of my audience, I have had to learn that there are times when I deserve a taxi or a lift from someone else.

I am not sure when I understood HIV-induced ongoing inflammation in the brain despite successful ART, but after receiving the diagnosis of bipolar II I knew that it applied to my brain. By the time I had left home as a teenager to go to university, my mother had complained that I was moody like my father and my grandfather. Now it seemed having HIV had tipped me over from being just moody to having bipolar. With the burden of HIV, bipolar, the meningitis event, and the medications and their side effects, it is anyone's guess how much each of these contribute to my cognitive dysfunction.

LIVING WITH COGNITIVE DYSFUNCTION

I have always had a brain that composed faster and with a greater vocabulary than my speech compartment delivered, but labile moods and cognitive dysfunction have changed it from the quirky end of diversity to an obvious defect that varies with my wellness. Sometimes every sentence of my story has to be squeezed from my brain as if it is someone else's story. I have difficulty with grammar, particularly composing around tense. Periodically, I have to rephrase what I was saying because I cannot pronounce an ordinary word. I may miss saying phrases and essential words like "not" in cannot, but my brain believes that my speech was complete which can be very confusing. I have learned to explain things in two or three different ways so that at least one makes sense.

Sometimes when I am speaking, it might be to 200 school kids 15-years old, and suddenly I will go to say a word and I have completely forgotten what it is. I might know what it feels like and that it starts with "r" but I cannot find it. Other times I run into what I call a hole, where I go from one word to where the next should be but inexplicably, I have completely lost where I was going, the phrase I just said and often the topic itself. It is as if in a split second my brain was reset to blank, but I am still acutely aware that I was supposed to be saying something.

How do I do public speaking like that? There is always someone who wants to tell me what I just said. Between them and my presentation guide, I move on. I think few people realize the extent of my memory loss or that my recovery is due more to being well versed in the topic rather than the return of my memory. Public speaking on HIV does require courage with my dysfunction but not as much as most people would think. What makes the difference is the lack of stigma. Because I stand up to say I made some mistakes and I contracted HIV, I get top marks every time. In fact, I have the opposite problem in that it is difficult to get constructive feedback about what worked and what did not. People are afraid of discouraging me.

If only mental health dysfunction were like that without all the stigma, without feeling blame or self-loathing, without being seen as a loose cannon not to be trusted.

LIVING WITH MENTAL ILLNESS STIGMA

Cognitive dysfunction is a concept rarely mentioned in the HIV sector unless it is the statistics showing it to be a common problem that is growing the longer we survive. It is almost never acknowledged at the individual level. I never mention HIV-associated neurocognitive disorder (HAND) because no one knows what I am talking about. Practitioners seem afraid of labeling PLHIV with a diagnosis that might lead to them being exposed to a cascade of stigma.

HIV mental health is only openly talked about in terms of situational depression. People say they are depressed because they lost their job when the reality of living with HIV might be that they were mentally unwell and therefore were unable to work and that made them feel more depressed. Fatigue is a much more acceptable symptom that I often hear used instead of disclosing depression. We fear being labeled a whiner, especially because we made mistakes that led to our HIV infection often many years ago. We fear the "slippery slope" of dementia and what the future might hold.

Describing poor mental health only through situational effects constantly suggests that there is some personal fault for being in that situation and a lack of control of one's response. I believe this denial is relief-seeking but never really relief-delivering. Knowing and understanding has been the start of healing for me. A lack of understanding prevents awareness and ability to explain our feelings and that impacts our uptake of health care. In contrast, a friend who talks to me openly about his mental health recently said to me, "I was getting a bit down, a bit too angry, so I talked to my doctor and now I have gone back on the antidepressants." It was as if he were talking about gastric reflux, not mental health.

Of course, mostly there is not a clear separation between situational and nonsituational depression. When I am down, situational issues get drawn into my mood like a monster vacuum cleaner out of control, sucking in the furnishings. Very soon my depression gets amplified and I feel terrible. When I try to let go of the issues, I feel just as bad and I feel my thinking latching back on or seeking other issues to despair about as if my brain requires an excuse for its agony. I know when a depressive episode is nearing its end when I am able to push these issues aside until circumstances allow some resolution of them. Even after it is over, for days or weeks if it has been severe, I still feel the drag of issues on my mood toward deeper depression.

If we cannot talk honestly and openly about depression, what happens to people when they learn that they have cognitive dysfunction? When I was trying to understand my cognitive dysfunction, I kept hearing people like me being called "a nutter" by others in the HIV sector. Such derogatory language is not only applied to those open about their diagnosis but to anyone who presents mentally unwell, perhaps with anxiety, or simply an unwell person who complains. My brain had "shattered" and was not always "together" but I was being told it had shrunk to the size of a walnut. No wonder there is fear and silence around mental ill-health.

Each of my diagnoses came with its own layer of stigma, in effect, doubling the burden on living. Knowing and understanding my mental health has helped me reject the stigma, push back fear and loathing, and break the silence. Drawing on my biological rationale and with a determination not to be on the scrap heap, I have taken every opportunity I can to improve my public speaking to prove the stigma wrong. Despite my denial, it does seem I have a focus on the future after all.

I will leave you with my motto: Talk about the negative things, find understanding, seek solutions, and do positive things known to help.

6.3

MEMORIES

James May

This is a personal account from a man who had been treating his HIV with natural therapies and his experience when he entered the hospital system not by his own choice. He discusses how jarring and terrifying the hospital experience was and how he felt like he had lost control over his treatment. Exacerbating his conflict is the mental impact of the disease, and the shame and denial that accompanied it. Eventually, the author is able to find a balance between alternative therapies, such as yoga and healthy eating, and the recommended medicinal treatments by HIV specialists, and he regains, control over his life and his diagnosis.

2006 is a year that haunts me in memories and dreams. I woke up in a hospital bed early one morning, held fast with restraints, a mental health guard watching over me. I had no idea where I was and little memory of what had happened. Slowly, it all trickled back.

I had felt terribly despondent for months. I'd dropped out of my university course after relentless bouts of insomnia and depression. A couple of intimate relationships had fallen by the wayside. The way I processed these circumstances was highly significant. I blamed myself for everything. I took sole responsibility for being unable to please the people in my life, meet their expectations, or make them happy.

It was winter in Melbourne and my health started to deteriorate. My energy was failing. It was a struggle to walk up the street to buy groceries. My legs felt like lead, I was short of breath. Pretty soon, I could hardly do the dishes, cook, or clean for myself. I was isolated from the outside world and spent most days wrapped in a blanket, huddled by the heater. Cold chills seared through my blood. It was impossible to warm up.

I was lost in my own mind, consumed with dark memories of the past, fears about the future. My world felt like it was falling apart. I couldn't understand what was going wrong with my mind and body. I thought it was just depression; I could work through it.

Unfortunately, things got worse. I was woken each night by drenching sweats that soaked the bed. Several weeks passed with barely any sleep at all. I was delirious and exhausted, trapped in the house, jumping at shadows. It felt like a chamber of horrors, but I was terrified of going out. Intense emotions were rising up: anger, fear, guilt, and shame. It felt like a diabolical force was taking me over.

I hated myself for being sick and useless, unable to get on with life. I refused to seek medical advice. I saw it as a failure, an admission of weakness, a loss of control. I'd been thriving with HIV for 6 years, relying on practices such as yoga and meditation as well as a rigorous regime of natural medicine and peak nutrition. My health had been stronger than it was prior to the diagnosis and I thought I could turn this around.

My behavior was quite erratic. A number of friends thought I was dealing with mental illness. My personality was changing; I was forgetful, distant, confused. I had wild mood swings; it felt like I was possessed. It was hard to explain or comprehend, but I knew it wasn't me.

A friend offered to take me in for awhile. I was grateful for the company but paranoid of everyone, struggling with all my might to hold onto sanity. I was still barely eating or sleeping. I had no appetite and shed several kilos in weight. Although I was quite malnourished and mentally unstable, I did my best to appear "normal." Calling upon psych services was the last thing I wanted, nor did my friend.

It was the only option in the end. One night we talked it over. We'd spent days grappling with the situation. What was going on in my head? What was the best course of action? I was terrified of being drugged and locked up in a hospital. This friend had stood by me the whole way but now she thought psychiatric help was a good idea.

We called the CATT (Community Assessment Treatment Team) and they came around to discuss the situation. I shut down when they arrived. I was too afraid to disclose anything. I did my best to appear calm and composed, make them believe I was in control. They stayed for half an hour and left, convinced that I was okay.

Shortly after, I experienced incredible fevers. It felt like I was suffocating, burning up. I stumbled around the house, delirious, losing track of where I was, what I was doing. The next thing I was on my hands and knees, chanting incoherent words, hallucinating wild flames and searing heat. I thought I was truly sick and evil (for being gay and HIV positive). I was plunging into the infernos of hell.

My friend called the CATT team again and within minutes, two men dragged me out of that house and into an ambulance. I didn't want to go but they used a measure of force. I recall lying on a trolley, a man with a stone-cold face watching over me. I don't recall being soothed or reassured. I felt nothing but fear and shame.

The next thing, I was dumped on the doorstep of a suburban hospital where nurses tied me down with restraints and left me on a trolley in the emergency room. It was painfully bright and chaotic and I was deep in psychosis, tossing and turning, trying to break free.

The nurses asked who I was and what was going on but I was too paranoid to speak, which fueled their contempt, perhaps thinking I was under the influence of drugs. The room was full of crying, wailing, injured people and the last thing I recall was being wheeled through starkly lit corridors by nurses whom I believed were aliens, carting me away for a cruel experiment. I recall them watching me, poking, and prodding me. Then they loaded me into a contraption for an MRI scan which I believed was some kind of torture chamber—the final descent into hell.

When I woke up, a mental health guard was stationed by the bed. The psychosis had lifted and I had no idea that HIV was involved. I was diagnosed with MAC (mycobacterium avium complex) and PCP (*Pneumocystis carinii* pneumonia). My T-cell count was 10 and viral load was off the scale. The doctors pumped me with Bactrim for the PCP, which was highly effective but caused debilitating nausea and headaches. The mental health guard was relieved a few days later and I was shifted to a private room as the hospital had no HIV/AIDS facility.

The hospitalization was traumatic. It was my first admission and I was completely overwhelmed by the procedures. I had no family present and felt too weak and vulnerable to assert myself. I was bombarded with regular injections, tests, and heavy doses of medication (around 25 tablets a day).

I found the attention from staff hard to cope with. Constant scrutiny from nurses, physicians, psychiatrists, dieticians, medical students, cleaners, and food staff. It was impossible to get any privacy or rest and I was given a variety of tranquillizers like Valium and temazepam. I became dependent on these drugs and they exacerbated my anxiety and delirium.

It felt like my health was being undermined. A system which was designed to provide healing was making me sicker each day. The procedures left me exhausted, I felt judged and scrutinized. The food was terrible; I could barely keep it down, let alone reap any nutritional benefit. Instead of healing, I was losing weight, feeling weaker, and becoming more depressed. I felt like I had to escape.

There was no room for me to question any of the treatments and little explanation was offered. Although many nurses were well meaning and compassionate, some were rude and insensitive. I was pressured by psychiatrists to take antidepressants and antipsychotics, even though the symptoms I presented with were HIV related. The doctors were particularly abrupt and patronizing, in light of the fact that I hadn't monitored the HIV regularly. They dismissed any beliefs I had about my health, especially regarding alternative medicine. They demanded I cease all this immediately, as it would undermine antiviral therapy.

There was so much going on in my personal life as well. Visits from friends who I had unresolved issues with. Calls from relatives I hadn't seen for years. I came from a dysfunctional home, fractured with alcohol and domestic violence. The community I grew up in was fiercely homophobic and I hadn't spoken to siblings for more than 10 years. I don't know if they even knew I was HIV positive.

The situation brought a lot of emotional baggage to the surface. I felt this had to be resolved to assist my recovery. My mother arrived and all the issues around my parents' alcoholism, violence, and homophobia were stirred up. They were directly involved in the destructive behavior that led to my HIV diagnosis. I had been living a high-risk lifestyle; a heavy user of drugs and alcohol since age fifteen. Having my mother present caused a great deal of tension and she was reluctant to engage with me. She was consumed with her own guilt about the past and anxiety about my condition. She left town before we had a chance to resolve anything.

I was discharged from hospital a month later, terrified of the outside world—55 kilos, extremely weak, and covered in cold sores. I looked vastly different and the world was vastly different. I had nowhere to live and was given accommodation at a residential support unit for people with HIV/AIDS and mental health issues.

I spent 6 months in that facility adjusting to antiviral drugs which boosted my immune system but made me feel extremely toxic, throw up everything I ate, and itch like crazy. I had neuropathy in my feet, a bout of shingles, and wild mood swings. The medication also caused anemia and had to be changed at one point to avert kidney failure.

The PCP resolved but the MAC caused complications with my lymphatic system and medication had to be adhered to for several months. For the next year, much of my time was taken up with hospital visits where I had fluid therapy, transfusions for low platelets, and pentamidine for PCP prophylaxis. There were ongoing tests and procedures such as x-rays, ultrasounds, MRIs, and regular checks for cytomegalovirus (CMV) retinitis.

I spent days in those clinics waiting for test results. A year later, the combination of antivirals was working well and the MAC was under control. My T cells were above 200 and I was virtually free of symptoms. I was around 65 kilos and living in private accommodations.

Those events are still with me. I have repeated bouts of insomnia and anxiety and a niggling fear of going through it again, although life has moved on and I monitor my immune system regularly. My T cells remain stable and my viral load is undetectable. I haven't had any bouts of illness since that time. I now use a combination of allopathic and complementary medicine which seems to be the most effective.

I had suspended contact with medical doctors prior to my hospitalization because I felt it was having a detrimental effect, emotionally and physically. Several general practitioners were judgmental about my lifestyle at the time I contracted the virus. They also made little effort to validate beliefs I had about the emotional/psychological aspects of the illness and the course of action I wanted to take regarding treatment.

They were determined to medicate in the first year of my diagnosis when it was clearly unnecessary. They tried to coerce me into doing things their way, which was heavy handed and disempowering. I also found the regimen of thrice monthly blood tests emotionally draining. Therefore, I chose to disconnect from the system.

I spent many years dealing with alternative practitioners such as naturopaths and Chinese herbalists. I found them far more comprehensive, supportive, and encouraging. They offered a great deal more time, personal empathy, and a holistic approach that was very effective and resonated with me.

I now have a healthy relationship with doctors in the HIV/AIDS sector who are equally supportive and encouraging. Although I only see them briefly, I always find them caring and helpful. I am sincerely grateful for the medication they prescribe and it's an essential part of my therapy. In hindsight, I would've been more discerning about whom I chose to consult after the diagnosis, although the clinics I attended were highly recommended for people with HIV/AIDS.

Although it was horrific, I am strangely grateful for the events of 2006. Although HIV was clearly involved in the psychological manifestations of the illness, many issues were confronting me at the time. The collapse of my immune system coincided with an emotional breakdown which, I believe, demonstrates a link between mental health and HIV disease progression.

I was deeply insecure for many years and had always carried a heavy burden of fear and shame associated with being gay. I had very low self-esteem and lived in emotional turmoil. I was dependent on drugs and alcohol as it was the only coping mechanism I knew at the time. Contracting HIV at 26 was devastating. The fear and shame was hugely magnified. I was living in chaos and didn't have the support networks or maturity to cope. It was also a big wake-up call,

a blessing in disguise. It gave me the motivation to deal with negative emotions that had consumed me for years. I stopped using drugs and alcohol and changed social networks. I adopted a lifestyle of spiritual practice and impeccable nutrition, paying close attention to my emotional health and self-development.

HIV/AIDS was the catalyst I needed to take control of my life and become the best person I could be. I couldn't have grown without it. My quality of life greatly surpassed the reality I endured prior to the diagnosis. Although, confronting being hospitalized with AIDS was the most life-affirming of all. It brought down barriers within me that seemed impossible to shift. It made me far more open, grateful, compassionate, and caring—for myself as well as others. I'd still carried a lot of shame and regret about contracting HIV and I was extremely hard on myself. I believe this contributed to the collapse of my immune system.

The last few years have been the most rewarding and productive. My spirituality and creativity have flourished; I'm more involved with the community, more emotionally centered. I feel far more at peace with being HIV positive and disclosing this to others. There's more intimacy in my life than ever before. As strange as it seems, I don't think I'd reverse the diagnosis if I could. It's brought too much faith, wisdom, and joy into my world. It's a gift that keeps me learning and growing, reaching out to others, and achieving things I never imagined. HIV/AIDS is the best thing that ever happened. I wouldn't be alive without it.

6.4

HIV DEMENTIA: A PATIENT'S PERSPECTIVE

LIVING WITH THE SUFFERING, THE DIAGNOSIS, AND THE UNCERTAINTIES

Karen

This chapter is the personal story of a young woman who experienced dementia caused by AIDS, most notably a four month period of memory loss. The chapter discusses the initial diagnosis, the treatment, and the eventual recovery, and the woman's reflections on what happened to her and her hopes for the future of becoming an advocate for people who have AIDS.

I am not supposed to be writing these words today. A few years ago, I might not have been able to understand them.

That I have memories to share—that I am alive at all—is a medical miracle. If you are reading this book, it is because you want to make miracles like mine possible. To conquer viruses, you will need to understand the other chapters in this book. To heal people—to connect with their hearts—you will need to read the next few pages.

You need, in short, to know my story.

My name is Karen, and I have AIDS.

Apparently, that was discovered on Friday, March 7, 1997. But I don't remember that day, or for that matter, much of the previous four months. I can only tell this story with the help of my family's memories.

The first time I thought something might be wrong was mid-December. I was trying to recover from a case of "strep" throat and thought all I needed was a few days bed rest, which my schedule as a teacher—Christmas break was approaching—would soon accommodate.

Those few days turned into my entire break. Normally, I am very active and spend my break shopping, baking, and getting caught up in the holiday bustle. But this year it was all I could do to get out of bed, move to a chair, and help my mom with a few "sit-down" jobs.

I was too tired to attend my brother's wedding reception 3 days after Christmas. That was when my family began to realize I had something more than a sore throat. So began the numerous doctor visits and the equally numerous diagnoses. My doctors thought I was suffering from depression, a viral infection, Lyme disease, and many other ailments.

First, we thought the throat infection was mononucleosis. No sooner was that ruled out then chronic fatigue syndrome was ruled in. My doctor eventually nixed that idea and thought it was lupus erythematosus. Soon lupus was eliminated as a possibility, and I was given a diagnosis of fibromyalgia syndrome.

In the meantime, I was still exhausted. But fatigue turned out to be only one symptom. One night, my father asked what I was eating for dinner. I told him I was eating a peanut butter and jelly sandwich—which would have been fine, except that I was eating soup. Another time my mother watched in disbelief as I mistook deodorant for lip gloss and brushed it across my lips.

On a Tuesday night in mid-February, my mother found me asleep in my car. I don't remember this, but I'm guessing I came home from work and was just too tired to make it to my bed. The next day at school would be my last. I was walking down the hall, and my principal asked me where I was going. I told him I was on my way to lunch. He said, "Karen, you just came from lunch." I couldn't teach, didn't recognize the children, or know what I was supposed to be doing.

Next, I went to see a neurologist. An MRI verified that there was some deterioration in my brain, so more tests followed to determine the cause. One week later we knew. The doctor called my parents and set up a meeting for the next morning. It was, to our family, Black Friday.

Although I was at that meeting, I do not remember it. A small part of me is almost glad. I cannot even begin to imagine how my parents must have felt upon learning the news that their oldest child had AIDS. I think everyone's initial reaction can be summed up in two words: pure shock.

Something this horrible is not supposed to happen to people like me. I come from a large Catholic family and went to Catholic schools my entire life. I don't smoke, rarely drink, do not sleep around, and have never used drugs.

Hours after we found out the news, my dad asked me if I knew what was wrong with me. I told him very matter-of-factly, "Yes, I have AIDS. I don't think they have a cure for that." They were the words everyone was thinking but no one wanted to say. Instead, they just brought a lump to everyone's throats.

TREATMENT

Three days after receiving a death sentence, from which there seemed to be no appeal, we met Dr. Gendelman at the

University of Nebraska Medical Center in Omaha. What he gave us was more precious than gemstones. In Dr. Gendelman, we found hope.

Dr. Gendelman told us the AIDS virus attacks different people in different ways but that having HIV affect the brain in such a devastating way with no other signs of the disease was rare. However, he said, there were new therapies available. He sounded cautiously optimistic. No one was expecting a miracle, but we certainly were praying for one. And with Dr. Gendelman and the new drugs on our side, we were a little more encouraged that our prayers were being heard.

Unfortunately, things would get much worse before they got better. One of the drugs I was taking caused sleeplessness. I went from sleeping 16 hours a day to hardly any sleep at all. The insomnia made the dementia that had now completely overtaken my brain all the worse.

Often I pretended I was teaching. I would get up several times during the middle of the night, go into the bathroom and conduct a class. Rubbing alcohol, shampoo bottles, and hairbrushes doubled as my students. My sister-in-law would often wake up, come in the bathroom and watch as I put Jessica, the rubbing alcohol, in a time out. Sometimes I walked around the house opening doors, looking for a room that wasn't there. Other times I stared at a towel and tried to read it like a book. One night my brother woke up because he heard the water running. He came upstairs and found me at the kitchen sink. I told him I was washing dishes and setting the table, but there were no dishes in sight.

Then other symptoms emerged. My hair started falling out. I lost a lot of weight. I had bags under my eyes, and I was getting very weak. I couldn't walk up the stairs without someone to lean on and my mother had to help me shower and get dressed.

I was also becoming feisty. One time at the hospital, I refused to get out of the car. My dad swung my legs out of the car, and I pulled them right back in. On our next visit, I had to go to the bathroom. I opened the door to get out while the car was still moving.

St. Patrick's Day in my very Irish family is normally a festive holiday. That was hardly the atmosphere this year. Dr. Gendelman called with devastating news. My viral count was over a million—one of the highest levels seen at the medical center. If the drugs did not kick in soon, I would be dead in 2 months.

RECOVERY

The sky started to clear a week later. The drugs were working! My behavior was still the same, but the tests showed otherwise. My viral count was down to 33,000—still dangerous, but compared to where it had been a week before, it was a cause for celebration.

My birthday was later that month. My entire family was in town and threw a big birthday party for me. My friends came over and brought me gifts. I argued with them, insisting that it was only November and my birthday wasn't until March. But they persisted. They showed me the date on the newspaper and pointed to the calendar. I got furious at everyone. I kept demanding, "How does everyone expect me to get better when you keep lying about what day it is?" When everyone woke up the next morning, I had turned all of the calendars in the house back to November.

My first big breakthrough was that Sunday. Two things happened. First, my niece—who is also my goddaughter—was crying. I decided to lay her down for a nap. I picked up all 25 pounds of her and carried her up the stairs. My entire family was there. Every single one of them stopped dead in their tracks and stared in amazement. A week earlier, I could hardly walk, let alone pick up a baby and carry her up the stairs.

The second event was even more special. It was the first day in 4 months that I remember. I was standing in the driveway saying goodbye to my brother and his family, who had apparently been with us for 2 weeks. I thought to myself, "They're leaving? I don't remember them being here." But just the awareness that they were with us even for that one day was a major breakthrough.

This wasn't just any Sunday. It was Easter Sunday. Later, my sister gave me a journal so I could start recording these amazing events. Inside of it she wrote:

I know you don't remember much of the last four months
    of your life, but try not to worry about that. Let your family
    and friends be your memory and we will help you fill in the gaps.
    In the meantime, I think a good day to begin on is Easter Sunday—
    the day Jesus rose from the dead and brought you back to us.

My recovery came in bits and pieces, most of which I didn't realize. One day I fed myself. The next day I took a shower. Soon after that I got dressed without any help.

And I suffered a few setbacks along the way. Right after Easter, I developed a horrible rash, then seizures. One night, after dinner, my arm began shaking. I thought it was because of all the drugs—I was taking 21 or 22 pills a day—but later that night when I was getting ready for bed, I felt a tingling sensation all the way from my brain down to my feet. I yelled for my parents, but they didn't hear me. They did, however, hear the bookcase crash, which I knocked down on my fall to the floor. My dad called 911 and my mom held me while the seizure ran its course. The scariest part of the seizure was that I was conscious of everything about it. The tingling, the numbness, the complete lack of control over my entire body, and, worst of all, the fact that it happened so fast without any sort of warning.

I stayed in the hospital for a few days. It was a horrible stay. There was a stranger in my room around the clock to monitor my condition, I had two spinal taps that left a constant pain in my head and back, and I got no sleep.

Having said that, something good did happen while I was in the hospital. I cried. Why is crying a good thing, you ask? The answer is simple. It was the first time that I had shed a tear since before this whole roller coaster ride began. Up to that point, I had showed no emotion. That first tear was a tear of amazement at the reality of the whole situation.

As my mother watched the tear roll down my cheek, she shed her own. Her tear was one of mixed emotions. There was heartache at the thought of watching me struggle with this disease and all the pains that go along with it. But mostly it was a tear of elation. Because finally, her daughter, who had been overpowered by this monster for so long, was not just fighting back, she was winning.

MY CONCLUDING THOUGHTS ON HAVING SURVIVED HIV DEMENTIA

The story you have just read is 13 years old. Today, my viral count is considered undetectable. Except for the occasional cold, I rarely get sick, and it never occurs to me that I might die from AIDS. I have been an assistant principal for the past 8 years. And I now take just three pills a day for AIDS. Dr. Gendelman tells me I am medical history in the making—the first case in which HIV had produced so much damage in the brain and then reversed itself.

One part of the story remains the same: AIDS survivors are still silenced by stigma. A curtain of ignorance still envelops this disease. People are afraid of it, and, to tell the truth, 5 years ago I might have been one of them. As a result, I feel that I cannot share an important part of my life with many people who are important to me.

Ignorance surrounds research into AIDS as well—a fact I have learned all too vividly. I am alive in large part because of groundbreaking research using "fetal cells" at the University of Nebraska Medical Center. When that research became public in the fall of 1999, a firestorm of controversy erupted. Elected officials condemned the research. Picketers marched outside the Medical Center, picketed at Dr. Gendelman's home—even harassed his family.

My family is very large, not to mention very Catholic. They, too, had a difficult time coming to terms with the research. But the moment we learned of its connection to my case, my family reached the obvious conclusion: In the most literal sense, this research *is* pro-life. I had a strong impulse to fight publicly for this research. I wrote an article for the local newspaper, but—because I was unwilling to confront, in such a public manner, the ignorance and bitterness that surround AIDS and fetal-cell research—I did so under a pseudonym.

Two trips to the emergency room a couple of years ago proved to be an eye opener for me that even some medical professionals do not know much about AIDS. The first trip revealed I had significant blood clotting in both lungs. The ER doctor in charge that day told me it was very common for AIDS patients to get blood clots. Let's ignore the fact that I have been on a birth control pill for over twenty years. Later that same year brought me back to the ER. This time I was told I had *Pneumocystis carinii* pneumonia (PCP), which only people with AIDS get. I did have pneumonia, but with a CD4 count in the 1300s, even I knew I didn't have PCP.

When I retire in a few years, I have decided I want to be an advocate for people who have AIDS. My goal would be to educate people about HIV/AIDS. My dream would be for the stigma and the ignorance to go away. The faces of AIDS come in all colors, sizes, and all over the world. No two AIDS patients look alike. Just because a person has lost some weight is not an indicator that they have AIDS. In fact, I have AIDS and I need to lose weight! Education is the key that unlocks ignorance.

I have learned many lessons on this journey. The foremost is this: I knew before—but especially appreciate now—both how fortunate I am to have such a loving family and what an indispensable role they played in my recovery.

For you, too, there is a moral to my story. It is this: The people you will treat are more than the sum of their diagnoses, viral counts, and brain scans. They are people. I know because Dr. Gendelman always treated me like one. Even when I was lost in the thickest fog of my dementia, he looked into my eyes and saw both a life worth saving and a heart worth knowing. I was, for him, always an individual with both feelings and fears.

Perhaps he could relate to my emotions so well because he seemed, so often, to share them. After seeing me at my worst and then improve just 2 weeks later, Dr. Gendelman could hardly contain his excitement. He was bursting with enthusiasm as he paraded his associates in to see me. I will never forget his words: "It's moments like these that make me proud to be a doctor." Turning to his colleagues, he shouted "It's time to find a cure." They hurried out of the room as if they couldn't wait to begin. As you join their search, may Dr. Gendelman's example be your guide.

6.5

MY VIRUS JUST TURNED TWENTY-ONE

A WOMAN'S PERSPECTIVE OF THE LONG-TERM PSYCHOLOGICAL IMPACT OF LIVING WITH HIV

Susan Paxton

This chapter discusses the long-term psychological impact of living with HIV, especially as a single mother raising a young child. The author highlights her constant worry of transmitting the virus to her son, as well as the loss of self-esteem that initially plagued her. The author discusses her journey to eventually becoming an openly HIV-positive person and the changing identity that came with the diagnosis.

My virus just turned twenty-one. The anniversary always follows 2 months after my son's birthday. His last birthday was a huge milestone in our lives—reaching twenty-one after finishing his undergraduate degree with honors in every subject—a cause for a great and joyous celebration. Now it's my virus' turn and I cannot say I am overwhelmed with joy about it. HIV has given my life an unwelcome and challenging edge and redefined my identity.

When I was told I had five to eight years to live, I was a single parent, the mother of a toddler whose father had walked out the year before because he could not cope with a partner who was constantly sick since giving birth—I contracted a never-ending flu, followed closely by meningitis, then pneumonia. Little did we know that 2 months after giving birth to my son, my body was responding savagely to HIV infection.

Being diagnosed with HIV was shattering. I had a life-threatening condition that was highly stigmatized. I was a modern-day leper. Over the next weeks and months, my self-esteem evaporated and the career I had built since returning to Australia slowly fizzled away. The nurse said to me, "You don't have to tell anybody about this if you don't want to." I am forever grateful for that advice. It made me understand that each person is responsible for protecting themselves from infection and I did not have to take on that responsibility for everybody. Health professionals would protect themselves by donning latex gloves if there was any risk of exposure to my blood—universal precautions were in place as protection from all infections, diagnosed or undiagnosed. I realized that I am one of the few who know whilst millions of people do not know they are HIV positive, just as I had not known for 2 years. Many people contract HIV from somebody who doesn't know they have the virus.

Although intellectually I knew nobody can catch HIV through casual contact, my irrational fear of infecting my son was enormous. I took him for three HIV tests to make sure he was negative. Then he fell over and cut his arm, and absent-mindedly I kissed his wound, so I waited 3 months then I took him for a fourth test, just in case; the terror of infecting him was always there. Little did I know until many years later, when research on the risks of HIV infection during breastfeeding was available, that the meningitis I got soon after I was HIV infected was in fact a blessing in disguise. I was told to stop breastfeeding the moment the doctor suspected my headache from hell might be meningitis, so until that point, my son was exclusively breastfed. Studies now indicate that mixed feeding increases the risk of HIV infection. Had I given him other food during the time I was breastfeeding him, it may have irritated and inflamed his delicate stomach lining, creating an opportunity for infection next time he ingested breast milk, particularly as my milk was highly laden with human immunodeficiency virus, being newly infected. With waves of relief I realized that my accidental "exclusive breastfeeding" may have been the best thing that happened in our mother-child relationship. My son is a lucky being.

Soon after I was diagnosed, I began to speak out about HIV to small groups of health care workers and, before long, to high school students. I knew that speaking out had a huge impact. People didn't talk much about HIV and AIDS. We'd had fear campaigns featuring the Grim Reaper striking death, and that was too scary to talk about and besides, the common perception was that HIV was a scourge of gay men and druggies. Most Australians believed that HIV would not affect them and meeting me allowed them to realize that no one is immune to HIV and that they also could be vulnerable to infection.

A year after my diagnosis, I woke up one morning feeling nauseous and lightheaded. I went to the bathroom, leaned over the basin and fell and smashed into the tap. When I regained consciousness I was lying in a pool of blood. A friend from overseas was staying with me at the time; she called the doctor who ran a surgery three doors away. When the doctor arrived, she bent down to look at my wound; no rubber gloves. I could barely speak but felt compelled to tell her, before she touched me, that I was HIV positive. As soon as my words drooled out, she recoiled, stood up and backed away. She said, "There is no way for me to attend to you here. You must come to the surgery in half an hour after I finish my home visits," and abruptly left. Ten minutes later my friend answered a telephone call: it was the doctor's secretary telling her they could not see me at the surgery because there was no way for them to dispose of the dressings. I asked my friend to drive me to Fairfield Hospital, the HIV-designated hospital at the time and a sanctuary for many of us living with HIV. It was on the other side of town and she did not have an international driver's license but she bundled me into the car and got me there. Five hours after the incident I received several stitches across the bridge of my nose and was left with a permanent scar, a reminder, every time I look in the mirror, of the unreasonable response certain people will have if I tell them I have HIV.

The first time I needed to see a dentist after this I was afraid, so I asked my HIV specialist to refer me to one at Fairfield Hospital. At the appointment, the dentist appeared as if ready to fight a toxic chemical spill. He had an enormous visor covering all of his face and I looked at him through layers of Perspex and could not stop tears from welling in my eyes. This is what I had become—a poisonous, untouchable creature from whom even those willing to treat me must shield themselves. I did not go for further dental care for many years.

After my diagnosis I had no sex for almost 7 years and believed nobody would ever want to touch me again. I could not contemplate telling a potential lover that I had HIV. I began to joke about a re-virginity party—I had heard that the vestal virgins of antiquity renewed their virginity by bathing in a sacred pool every seven years. Then I met somebody who was also positive and there was a mutual attraction. I was very shy after so long, but the experience did wonders for me and reconnected me to my being in a way I had forgotten. I am alone again now and I know many middle-aged women are alone, but I also know that HIV holds me back from initiating or exploring possibilities when many women would be more adventurous. I have constructed a cocoon that keeps me insulated from that type of dynamic social interaction.

Some years after my diagnosis, I unintentionally gained a PhD. I wanted to urge policy makers in the education system to engage speakers living with HIV in every school in Australia. I could see the difference my talks made. When I attempted, in the mid-90s, to convince people of influence that it's the most effective form of HIV preventive education, I was told there is no evidence. I asked, "What do you mean no evidence? I can see the changes in young people after my talks; and what about the evaluation sheets? There are hundreds of glowing reports of the impact of HIV-positive speakers in Melbourne alone." "It's not evidence." "So how does one get evidence?" "You have to do a study." A university research study? The idea seemed ludicrous. I was supposed to be dead or dying within a few years, and although I did not believe I would be, my slowly depleting immune system indicated otherwise. I decided to do a quick research study. Finding a supervisor who would take me on was perhaps the most challenging part of the exercise. Eventually, Wendy

Holmes at the Key Centre for Women's Health in Society offered to be my supervisor and I enrolled in a twelve-month Master of Science by research at the University of Melbourne. My study grew. I did a longitudinal matched control study involving over 1,200 high school students and conducted 15 focus-group discussions. Towards the end of my first year I was convinced of the need to upgrade to a PhD.

I found that the attitudes of young people do change after listening to a positive person; I was right. Still I asked more questions. What about the speakers? When I speak out, it is cathartic. Is it the same for other people? I decided to interview HIV-positive people who speak out in Africa, Asia, and Australia. At the time, I was the Australian representative on the Asia-Pacific Network of People Living with HIV and was privileged to attend many international HIV forums. Many of the people who were public about their HIV status were the very people attending these conferences. I spent much of my time at the International Congress on AIDS in Asia and the Pacific in Manila, Philippines in 1997, interviewing HIV-positive people who speak out, either to small closed groups or in the media. I immediately went on to the Global Network of People Living with HIV conference in Chiang Mai, Thailand, and spent days interviewing everybody I could find who did public speaking. Paradoxically, everybody said that speaking out was the most difficult, frightening thing they had ever done and it was also the most beneficial. It lifted the heavy burden of secrecy. People who were public in the media believed it was their best decision since their diagnosis. Many said their health had improved because they no longer had to lead a double life, constantly worrying about who knew and who did not know about their HIV status.

In 1999 I was preparing a presentation of my research findings for the next regional HIV Congress to be held in Kuala Lumpur. My son heard me practicing and later that evening said, "Mum, I think it would be a good idea if you went public about your HIV." "What makes you think that?" "I think it would be good for your health." For years, I had wanted to go be open in the media to educate more people about the realities of HIV, but my fear of subsequent discrimination against my son stopped me. I spoke out in schools, workplaces, hospitals, international meetings, but not in my local media. I replied, "I'll think about it."

In November 1999, two major incidents coincided in my life—my decision to go public and my decision to start taking triple combination antiretroviral drugs (ARVs). My immune system had gone up and down throughout the previous decade, like a rollercoaster built on a hillside—I had got on at the top and was now heading to the bottom trough before the engine cut out. I had only 50 CD-4 immune cells left, less than one-tenth of a "normal" healthy individual; there were millions of copies of HIV in every microliter of my blood. It was amazing that my body did not succumb to an AIDS-related infection. As my immune system plummeted, many friends urged me to start antiretroviral medication. It was 3 years since the discovery that triple combination ARV therapy was extremely effective in suppressing HIV. However, doctors were telling people to hit early and hit hard, and I saw young healthy men and women experiencing side effects of projectile vomiting and diarrhea and I was afraid. I believed I could manage my health without medical intervention. I brewed herbs foul and strong, and went to live in a cabin in the bush for 6 months, but my immune system would not bounce back. Eventually, I met a positive woman on a different regimen to that of most people I'd met. She was not using a protease inhibitor. In 1998, HIV researchers discovered that triple combination therapy did not need to include, in first-line treatment, the very toxic protease inhibitors. The combination of nucleoside and non-nucleoside reverse transcriptase inhibitors had few side effects.

Soon afterwards, I woke up one morning and realized the night sweats I had endured for almost a decade had stopped. I took this as a sign that my body had ceased its fight against the virus and I believed I was starting the process of dying. By then I could barely walk 200 meters without my coronary artery going into spasm; my hair was falling out; my face was constantly peeling off, leaving my skin red and raw. It was time to start treatment. I was terrified as I swallowed the first pill, and surprised I felt no effect. ARVs turned my life around. One afternoon, 2 weeks after I began medication, without forethought, I began running down the street; suddenly I became conscious that I was running, something I could not have done 2 weeks previously, and tears of joy welled inside me.

A few days after my decision to start ARVs, I received a letter saying I was nominated to carry the Olympic torch in the run-up to the Sydney 2000 Olympics. Did I want to accept? Of course I did. But if I was going to be part of the Olympic Torch Relay, I wanted to do so as an openly HIV-positive person to show that people with HIV can lead healthy, productive lives. I spoke to my mother and my son and they both gave their blessings so I said yes and I began my journey back to being a strong, energetic woman.

Six months later, I flew down Hoddle Street, Melbourne, and ever since my torch was set alight, I have felt free of the burden of secrecy. My personal experience of going public reflected my research findings. I am still on first-line therapy, I have an undetectable viral load and an immune system that is outrageously robust, and I am healthier than I was at any time during the 10 years between infection and starting ARV medication. My HIV specialist told me that it is possible that I might continue to take my medication every day and die of something unrelated to HIV. I am beginning to believe him. I am now in my 50s and it is likely that I may live into my 70s.

I have built a new career within the HIV sector: I have done further research studies including documenting AIDS discrimination, involvement of positive people in the HIV response, and access to HIV services; I have taught postgraduate students; I have assessed national HIV/AIDS programs in many countries in the Asia-Pacific region. What I enjoy doing most is training people living with HIV—women in particular—to speak out, advocate, develop their organizations, and become more involved in decision-making processes that affect their lives. I am proud of the work I have done and the impact I have had.

Because of my HIV, my relationship with my son has been intense. I brought him up alone and I always answered every question he asked because I was afraid that if I didn't, I might not be around to tell him when he needed the answers. I lived in fear that I may leave him an orphan before he finished school. Motherhood was also challenging because of my depleted energy and vitality. But he turned out well and I cannot flagellate myself about my shortcomings during that precious first decade of his childhood. My son is now a mature confident young man ready to go out into the world.

After two decades of being a parent living with, in, and around HIV, I now face an abyss alone, and I do not know what's on the other side. I have lost scores of peers, so I have a huge well of grief within me. It is deep and dark and thick and sometimes it's difficult to find my way through. For over a decade my survival as a parent and my income-earning capacity were precarious. I feel I lost so many parts of myself because of HIV. Perhaps my aloneness is no different to that of other single parents whose children are ready to leave the nest, but in my case, because I have no role models, no people who have gone before me, I lack clarity about where the next part of this rich tapestry that is my life can take me.

The pressure is lifted and I have greater freedom to live my life as I choose, free from the ties of parenthood, free from the worries of HIV illness. But, I am much older with fewer options so I find it hard to savor life alone. My identity for 20 years was shaped and coloured by being an HIV-positive single mother. I do not feel joy that my virus has just turned 21. I feel sad and I recognize the need to acknowledge this sadness so that I do not fall into depression now that perhaps the hardest part of the journey is over.

SECTION 7

CLINICAL AND PATHOLOGIC MANIFESTATIONS OF DISEASE

Igor Grant

7.1

PERSPECTIVE ON HIV CNS INFECTIONS

Richard W. Price

This chapter presents a retrospective view of the AIDS epidemic, focusing on the evolution of our understanding of the central nervous system complications of HIV infection. The presentation is structured in three main historical sections: First, the early years of disease recognition and symptomatic management, a period during which morbidity and mortality were little altered by medical intervention, culminating in the introduction of antiretroviral monotherapy. Second, the current era of combination antiretroviral therapy with its profound preventative and therapeutic effects. Third, the future, with its prospects for further refinements in prevention and therapy. The presentation provides a highly informed personal view, shaped by the author's experience, research, and clinical interests.

INTRODUCTION

With the appearance of this new and comprehensive 3rd edition of this book 30 years after the initial reports of the acquired immunodeficiency syndromes (AIDS) (Gottlieb, Schroff et al., 1981) and 25–30 years after initial recognition and characterization of the frequent neurological complications of human immunodeficiency virus (HIV) infection (Horowitz, Bentson et al., 1983; Snider, Simpson et al., 1983; Vieira, Frank et al., 1983; Navia, Cho et al., 1986; Navia, Jordan et al., 1986), it is an apt time to reflect on the what has happened over these years to our concepts of these conditions, to their prevention and treatment, and to the view of future needs. To this end, this chapter focuses on the interaction of HIV with the central nervous system (CNS), first defined clinically in its severe form in adults as the AIDS dementia complex (ADC) (Navia, Jordan et al., 1986), until present day spectrum of HIV-associated neurocognitive disorders (HAND) (Antinori et al., 2007). Thus, it is divided into three major historical sections: First, the early years of disease recognition and symptomatic management in which morbidity and mortality were little altered by medical intervention until the initial introduction of antiretroviral monotherapy; second, the current era of combination antiretroviral therapy (cART) with its profound prevention and treatment effects; and third, the coming years with their prospects for further refinements in prevention and therapy. This is largely a personal view based on the author's experience, research, and clinical interests.

THE EARLY YEARS: RECOGNITION AND EARLY TREATMENT OF ADC: 1981–1995

When AIDS was first recognized and the range of its clinical manifestations began to be categorized in the early 1980s, it was clear that the nervous system was among its common targets. Indeed, no level of the neuraxis was spared the effects of opportunistic infections (OIs) and other HIV-related conditions. As these complications were reported, it became evident that some of the most common ones were not simply related to OIs, but represented unique neurological disorders not previously found in the settings of other immunodeficiencies. Among these were aseptic meningitis, severe progressive encephalopathy, and myelopathy. Subsequently, these were found to relate to the AIDS retrovirus and not to an additional invading organism.

ASEPTIC MENINGITIS AND EARLY CNS INFECTION

Once HIV infection was identified, aseptic meningitis was reported as one of its common complications (Gabuzda & Hirsch, 1987). While at first described in association with headache and dementia, subsequent studies made it clear that mild cerebrospinal fluid (CSF) pleocytosis, usually with up to 20 cells per μL but at times higher, is common, characteristically asymptomatic, and occurs throughout the full spectrum of HIV infection from primary infection to ADC, though less frequently when blood CD4 counts fall below 50 cells per μL (Spudich, Nilsson et al., 2005).

In fact, this CSF cell response proved to be an indicator of the early and almost ubiquitous invasion of the nervous system, or at least the meninges, by HIV (Ellis, Hsia et al., 1997; McArthur, McClernon et al., 1997; Spudich, Nilsson et al., 2005), and appears to be largely clinically benign in the sense that it does not indicate clear neurological dysfunction at presentation and has not been shown to have prognostic significance. Indeed, it remains uncertain whether early asymptomatic HIV invasion is associated with subclinical, chronic brain injury (see below). However, it emphasizes one of the overall mysteries of HIV neuropathogenesis: How does a virus that invades the brain (or at least the meninges) early in the course of systemic infection without apparent sequelae subsequently cause a more invasive disease, HIV encephalitis (HIVE) manifesting as ADC with devastating clinical consequence? Is this switch from meningitis to encephalitis due to changes in the virus or alterations in the host?

AIDS DEMENTIA COMPLEX (ADC)

ADC was recognized early in the epidemic as a novel clinical-pathological entity in a number of centers, albeit using different names (Gopinathan, Laubenstein et al., 1983; Snider, Simpson et al., 1983). Although suspected by some to be a subacute encephalitis caused by CMV (Snider, Simpson et al., 1983), analysis of accumulating cases provided definition of a consistent constellation of symptoms and signs with distinct underlying pathology. The discovery of HIV was followed by its clinical and pathological association with ADC and HIVE (Shaw, Harper et al. 1985; Price, Brew et al. 1988).

Clinical Features

While variable from case to case, ADC was noted to have a cohesive pattern of disturbance in three components of neurological function—cognition, motor performance, and behavior. This pattern allowed definition of a core clinical phenotype (Navia, Jordan et al., 1986). Of these, cognitive and motor dysfunctions were most helpful in characterizing patients and defining diagnosis. In early and milder disease, patients presented with a variable pattern of inattention, reduced concentration, slowing of processing, and difficulty changing mental sets, along with slowed movements, clumsiness, and ataxia. Behaviorally, they manifested apathy, dulled personality, and in a subgroup, agitation, and mania. With progression, patients went on to show a more global dementia and paraplegia with urinary and fecal incontinence. The final stage was one of mutism and quadriparesis. On the basis of these clinical features, ADC was classified as a "subcortical dementia."

An empirical ADC staging system was also based on these features (Price & Brew 1988; Price & Sidtis 1990) in order to provide a vocabulary for describing the level of functional impairment (Table 7.1.1). This was modeled on other simple nervous system disease-staging schemes, and derived from a review of the cognitive, motor, and behavioral components of the patients encountered at Memorial Sloan-Kettering Cancer Center (MSKCC) in the pre-treatment era (Sidtis, Brew, & Price, unpublished) and has also been referred to as MSK staging.

Importantly, this staging was not intended as a basis for ADC diagnosis. Rather, it assumed an ADC diagnosis based on the clinical phenotype and setting, and then served to categorize the level of dysfunction in activities of daily living as obtained by the patient's history or as witnessed on direct examination. Thus, it relied on separate recognition of the clinical characteristics of the patient. Hence, at this early stage in disease recognition, there was no attempt to develop clear objective methods or criteria for diagnosis. In part, this was because the laboratory and neuroimaging characteristics of the condition were just emerging and also perhaps, in part, because the frequency and steady progression of the condition at that time in the absence of HIV therapy made recognition easier—the combination of the clinical phenotype and laboratory studies that ruled out other conditions was adequate, at least at MSKCC with an AIDS patient population comprised principally of middle-class, educated gay men. A research case-definition that followed a similar vocabulary was introduced by a task force of the American Academy of Neurology (1991). However, this case definition was, in fact, quite imprecise regarding specific clinical features, and also did not incorporate any more objective laboratory criteria in a more structured way.

While neuroimaging was an essential component of evaluation, it was used to rule out other conditions rather than

Table 7.1.1 ADC STAGING

ADC STAGE	CHARACTERISTICS
Stage 0 (Normal)	Normal mental and motor function
Stage 0.5 (Equivocal/subclinical)	Either minimal or equivocal symptoms of cognitive or motor dysfunction characteristic of ADC, or mild signs (snout response, slowed extremity movements), but *without impairment of work or capacity to perform activities of daily living* (ADL); gait and strength are normal
Stage 1 (Mild)	Unequivocal evidence (symptoms, signs, neuropsychological test performance) of functional intellectual or motor impairment characteristic of ADC, but able to perform *all but the more demanding aspects of work or ADL*; can walk without assistance
Stage 2 (Moderate)	Cannot work or maintain the more demanding aspects of daily life, but able to perform *basic activities of self-care*; ambulatory, but may require a single prop
Stage 3 (Severe)	*Major intellectual incapacity* (cannot follow news or personal events, cannot sustain complex conversation, considerable slowing of all output), *or motor disability* (cannot walk unassisted, requiring walker or personal support, usually with slowing and clumsiness of arms as well)
Stage 4 (End Stage)	Nearly vegetative; intellectual and social comprehension and responses are at a rudimentary level; nearly or absolutely mute; paraparetic or paraplegic with double incontinence

Adapted from Price & Sidtis, 1990.

provide a definitive ADC diagnosis. Characteristic cerebral atrophy and frequent diffuse, "fluffy" or "ground glass' white matter abnormalities were recognized as common and helpful in distinguishing ADC from progressive multifocal leukoencephalopathy (PML), but they were not considered sensitive or specific enough to be formally incorporated into diagnostic criteria. Likewise, routine CSF examination did not distinguish HIV encephalitis, since, as clearly documented later, elevations in cell count and protein are often seen in patients without this disorder (Spudich, Nilsson et al., 2005). Later, when CSF HIV RNA levels could be measured, it was noted that they could not be used for certain diagnosis because of the nearly universal presence of HIV in the CSF in asymptomatic patients. Likewise, while several inflammatory and neural biomarkers were noted to be characteristically altered in ADC, none were introduced into criteria for diagnosis (Cinque, Brew et al., 2006). Overall, the lack of diagnostic criteria related to either clinical phenotype or laboratory findings has continued as an important limitation in dealing with this disorder.

Neuropathology

Early descriptions noted that pathological changes were most prominent in subcortical structures and included: 1) Diffuse white matter pallor and associated gliosis; 2) multinucleated cell encephalitis; and 3) vacuolar myelopathy (Petito, Navia et al., 1985; Petito, Cho et al., 1986; Rosenblum, 1990; Budka, 1991; Wiley & Achim, 1994). Less common findings were diffuse or focal spongiform changes in the white matter and small areas of necrosis. The most common of these abnormalities was diffuse astrocytosis and white matter pallor that, in isolation, was associated with milder ADC. Inflammation was characteristically scant and consisted of a few perivascular lymphocytes and pigmented macrophages. Multinucleated cell encephalitis was a characteristic but not invariant finding. The term HIV encephalitis (HIVE) was supported by immunohistochemical and in situ hybridization studies showing that these multinucleated cells were infected by HIV (Pumarole-Sune, Navia et al., 1987; Vazeux, 1991; Wiley, Soontornniyomkij et al., 1998). However, infection of macrophages and microglia was not always accompanied by cell fusion and thus the term HIVE can be applied more broadly.

Productive HIV infection was confined to cells of the monocyte-macrophage lineage, including microglia, and these cells therefore play a pivotal role in pathogenesis. While astrocytes have also been reported to be infected, they characteristically do not produce progeny virus and their role is uncertain (Churchill, Wesselingh et al., 2009). More detailed pathological studies subsequently have elaborated on the cellular abnormalities, which include dendritic and synaptic changes (Moore, Masliah et al., 2006; Crews, Patrick et al., 2009) and increased amyloid precursor protein (APP) staining of neurons and axons, (Nebuloni, Pellegrinelli et al., 2001).

In the early description of ADC, it was recognized that some patients presented with a predominantly or exclusively myelopathic picture (Petito, Navia et al., 1985; Navia,

Cho et al., 1986; Di Rocco, 1999). Because of overlapping clinical features, this was included within the clinical definition of ADC. Pathologically, however, it is quite distinct and resembled subacute combined degeneration associated with vitamin B12 deficiency. Moreover, the vacuolar changes in the spinal cord did not correlate with the local presence of active HIV infection. Thus, while its epidemiological features and lack of alternative etiology suggested association with late HIV infection, it was less clearly related to an effect of local CNS infection. Indeed, vacuolar myelopathy remains a relatively neglected and still-puzzling aspect of HIV infection.

Pathogenesis

The correlation of HIVE with ADC has led to the generally accepted concept that CNS HIV infection is the cause of brain injury in this condition (Pumarole-Sune, Navia et al., 1987; Price, Brew et al., 1988; Wiley & Achim, 1994). However, because productive CNS HIV infection is supported in macrophages and related cells while the "functional elements" of the brain, particularly neurons, are not similarly infected, it seems that neuronal injury is the result of "indirect" processes, and that macrophages and related cells play a central role, not only in supporting HIV replication, but also serving as a key sources of virus- and cell-coded signals and toxins that lead to brain dysfunction. Ensuing years have elaborated upon these indirect injury pathways, and this is the focus of several segments of this book. At this point, it remains uncertain which particular neurotoxic pathways are most important in human disease, and it is likely that multiple overlapping and interacting processes are involved (Gonzalez-Scarano & Martin-Garcia, 2005).

Early Treatment

In the early years of antiretroviral therapy drug development, there was considerable interest in the treatment of ADC. In part, this was provoked by an early report of effective mitigation of neurological disease in three ADC cases (Yarchoan, Berg et al., 1987) by zidovudine monotherapy (then commonly referred to as AZT) and subsequent confirmation of this in a controlled clinical trial (Sidtis, Gatsonis et al., 1993). This was an important step. Not only did it show that treatment might be effective in treatment and prevention of ADC, it suggested that HIV infection was indeed its proximate cause and that its clinical deficits might be reversed, at least in part. Individual reports also documented reversal of CSF abnormalities (Hagberg, Andersson et al., 1991). As drug development accelerated, CNS disease became less and less an endpoint in clinical trials.

THE PRESENT: HAND IN THE ERA OF COMBINATION ANTIRETROVIRAL THERAPY: 1996–2010

While zidovudine monotherapy provided proof of ADC treatment concept, it required the development and broad implementation of effective cART for more widespread impact. Just as with systemic disease, cART has had a profound effect on all aspects of the neurological complications of HIV infection now referred to as HAND. In the developed world where cART is widely available, the severe neurological complications have markedly decreased (Sacktor, 2002; d'Arminio Monforte, Cinque et al., 2004). Indeed, these complications are now seen principally in population segments not being treated, either because of difficulty adhering to treatment or because they lie outside the umbrella of medical care. This includes individuals with severe psychiatric disease, drug abusers, the homeless, and those in socioeconomic settings isolated from therapeutic opportunity. Moreover, in celebrating this profound effect of antiretroviral therapy, it is important to remember that this is not yet the case in many resource-poor parts of the world that continue to bear the brunt of the expanding epidemic, including its effect on the nervous system (Robertson, Smurzynski et al., 2007).

The impact of cART has not been restricted to opportunistic CNS diseases, but equally and in parallel to ADC (d'Arminio Monforte, Cinque et al., 2004). Pharmacologically, this effect may appear remarkable. Despite the compartmentalized CNS infection underlying ADC/HIVE (Schnell, Spudich et al., 2009) and the blood-brain barriers that restrict full entry of many drugs (Letendre, Marquie-Beck et al., 2008), more severe ADC is largely prevented by standard cART regimens (Lescure, Omland et al., 2010). Additionally, CSF HIV infection generally appears to respond therapeutically to these regimens (Mellgren, Antinori et al., 2005; Price & Spudich, 2008), though with exceptions as discussed below.

On the other hand, there are a number of observations that suggest that treatment is imperfect in several respects. Since these are issues that need to be addressed in the future, they are considered in the next section.

THE FUTURE: EVOLVING TERMINOLOGY, TREATMENT REFINEMENT, AND PREVENTION OF NEUROLOGICAL MORBIDITY: 2011 -

Despite the extraordinary progress made in preventing and treating the more severe neurological complications of HIV, including ADC, there remain nagging issues suggesting that we still have more to do therapeutically. These include the observation that milder "neurocognitive impairment" may now have a high prevalence in treated patients (Antinori, Arendt et al., 2007; Robertson, Smurzynski et al., 2007; Simioni, Cavassini et al., 2010), the presence of continued, albeit low-level intrathecal immune activation in treated patients (Eden, Price et al., 2007; Yilmaz, Price et al., 2008; Hagberg, Cinque et al., 2010), and reported cases of discordant CSF responses or "CSF escape" in which the plasma HIV RNA level is suppressed below detection by conventional assays, but detected in the CSF at higher levels (Canestri, Lescure et al., 2010; Eden, Fuchs et al., 2010).

CONTINUING CNS MORBIDITY DESPITE TREATMENT

As the major CNS opportunistic diseases and ADC have disappeared in well-treated patient populations, attention of the community of neuro-HIV investigators has now turned to the less severe causes of neurological morbidity in HIV-infected patients—to the milder "neurocognitive impairments" embedded in two of the subcategories of HIV-associated neurocognitive disorders (HAND): asymptomatic neurocognitive impairment (ANI) and symptomatic minor neurocognitive disorder (MND) (Antinori, Arendt et al., 2007). As set out in the Frascati consensus definitions, these individuals are identified largely by performance on neuropsychological testing that is below established norms, with the two designations separated by the absence or presence of symptoms, though the MND group also displays minor difficulty in daily living. This is a useful step forward in that it takes into account the milder difficulties suffered by HIV-infected patients, particularly those on treatment. It also establishes criteria for diagnosis. On the other hand, these entities continue to suffer some of the same difficulties in definition and diagnosis as ADC. Thus, these milder disorders are defined by the presence of HIV infection and impaired performance on multidomain neuropsychological testing. However, they are not defined by a clear clinical phenotype, and both subcortical and cortical features have been reported (Brew, 2004). Hence, they are clinically amorphous without a clearly defined clinical presentation. They also are not defined by objective laboratory criteria. They thus share some of the uncertainties of ADC diagnosis, and may even extend them because of the mild nature of the deficits and the less clear association with active CNS HIV infection. Additionally, because they are lumped under the broad definition of HAND, the distinction from HAD is sometimes lost, leading to both lay and scientific misunderstanding. This misunderstanding may even, at times, obscure the profound effect of cART on more severe disease. Hence, as outlined in the original definition, ANI and MND should clearly be segregated from HAD. These milder entities are discussed in detail elsewhere in this volume.

PATHOGENESIS OF MILD NEUROCOGNITIVE IMPAIRMENT

Despite efforts to segregate them, inclusion of these milder disorders within the broad designation, HAND, carries an implicit association with HAD and perhaps with CNS HIV infection. However, in addition to an undefined clinical phenotype, they do not yet have a defined pathological or pathogenetic basis (Everall, Vaida et al., 2009). Indeed, even after eliminating the patients with non-HIV-related impaired performance, it is not yet clear that these diagnoses are a milder form of HAD/HIVE. Before considering the ways to ameliorate these milder disorders, it is thus reasonable to pose a number of fundamental questions, including:

1. What are the major causes of CNS injury in patients on treatment?

2. In that portion of patients in which CNS dysfunction is due to HIV, when did the injury occur?

3. If injury has continued on treatment, what are the mechanisms?

Causes of CNS Injury

There is likely to be a number of causes underlying the neuropsychological testing impairment in HIV-infected patients. Some of these will reflect the age susceptibilities of the normal population, while others may relate to the risk behaviors of HIV (particularly drug abuse). Importantly, some HIV-infected populations have a higher prevalence of smoking, hypertension, and other cardiovascular risk factors accounting for impairment in some patients as discussed above (Wright, Grund et al., 2010; Becker, Kingsley et al., 2009). Hepatitis C may also contribute to CNS injury or dysfunction, and clearly late-stage hepatic failure can have an impact, as noted at autopsy in some series (Everall, Vaida et al., 2009). However, in some, the higher incidence or prevalence of impairment may indeed relate more directly to HIV infection. In these, the critical questions relate to when and how this injury occurs.

Timing of Injury

For the clinician caring for the patient with neurological impairment, a critical question is: When did the underlying injury occur? And, importantly, is it continuing at the time of evaluation? Hence, it is imperative to know whether brain injury is *static* and due to past events, or *active* and will continue in the absence of effective intervention. At times, this can be discerned from the patient's history if there are complaints or evidence of progressive dysfunction. More often this evidence is absent, either because the injury is chronic and proceeds so slowly that recognition is difficult or because the injury is indeed static. Serial testing may be helpful in this regard if it shows continued deterioration. However, this practical and common difficulty underscores the need for more objective methods of discerning disease activity using biomarkers that discriminate active from static brain injury.

Even if dysfunction seems stable, the question can be asked whether the underlying disease process is still active, and whether, as in ADC/HIVE, there is a reversible component that might be therapeutically targeted. This is the premise of some clinical trials using neuropsychological testing as a main endpoint. While this may readily apply to untreated patients, it is less clear that it applies equally to patients on treatment with viral suppression, though this is an important issue requiring further study.

An alternative explanation for CNS dysfunction in patients on treatment is that they sustained brain injury during the period before they started cART. Even if such injury was subclinical, it may itself lead to impairment revealed by careful testing or reduce "brain reserve" and leave them vulnerable to other insults, including those associated with aging. If this is the main cause, the answer is implementation of earlier treatment to reduce this period of subclinical neuropathology.

Mechanisms of Injury in Patients on Therapy

Despite the assumption that CNS injury commonly continues in patients while on therapy, there is little known about the underlying mechanisms. Neuropathological studies do not show active CNS HIV infection, and CSF analysis, except for those patients with CSF viral escape discussed below, also failed to detect viral RNA using common methods. One possible clue may be the finding of continued low-level intrathecal immune activation in many patients on therapy. This is perhaps supported by the finding of mild elevations of CSF neopterin, although these levels are still below those commonly seen in untreated neuroasymptomatic patients (Eden, Price et al., 2007; Yilmaz, Price et al., 2008; Hagberg, Cinque et al., 2010). It is uncertain whether this persistent immunoactivation is a sign of indolent, yet undetectable HIV encephalitis, or a residual immunological abnormality independent of active CNS infection. These are obviously critical issues in planning therapy to prevent or treat this mild impairment.

Treatment Modalities

The only clearly effective tools for preventing and treating CNS HIV infection in those with systemic infection are antiviral drugs. One of the critical questions to be raised recently is whether it is important to tailor drug combinations on the basis of their CNS effects (Childers, Woods et al., 2008). Because many antiretroviral drugs achieved only poor CNS penetration (very often measured indirectly using the CSF concentration), there is worry that effective systemic therapy might not be adequate to suppress CNS infection and pathology. Arguing against the ubiquitous application of this is the prevention of overt ADC/HIVE by contemporary regimens, some of which achieve only poor CSF drug levels (Mellgren, Antinori et al., 2005; Price & Spudich, 2008). Additionally, although compartmentalized CSF drug resistance does occur, there is little evidence that the CNS serves as an important incubator for systemic resistance or as a major reservoir for persistent virus, despite suspicion that this may be the case. This is discussed in detail by Letendre elsewhere in this volume.

On the other hand, there may be settings where good drug penetration is important in addition to overt HIVE. A number of reports have documented patients with or without neurological symptoms in whom HIV RNA can be detected in CSF at a higher level than plasma and in those with plasma virus suppression (Canestri, Lescure et al., 2010), so called *CSF escape* or *discordance*. In some of these cases, CSF virus may be resistant to the systemic drug regimen. In our own series, we detected approximately 10% of patients showing this CSF viral escape, in the absence of symptoms (Eden, Fuchs et al., 2010). These cases raise the general question of whether and when CSF should be monitored in patients. This also is an area of controversy. Our own recommendation is to assess CSF, including its HIV RNA burden, in treated patients presenting with neurological symptoms not explained by other conditions. It then becomes part of the general evaluation that also includes neuroimaging.

DISSEMINATION OF TREATMENT

As with other aspects of HIV disease, one of the most important tasks is now to more broadly implement these successful measures to affected populations. This, of course, includes the enormous number of infected individuals in resource-poor areas of the world that now bear the brunt of the continuing epidemic. However, even in the developed world, there remain populations that need to be brought under the therapeutic umbrella. These include people with limited access to treatment or with difficulty in adhering to treatment related to socio-economic factors, substance abuse, psychiatric conditions, and the like. Since these are broad issues of health care delivery and not specific to neurological diseases, I will not discuss this further, but only emphasize the great need in this area. Clearly, broader treatment delivery measures can greatly reduce the overall neurological impact of HIV.

For those individuals out of reach of or who manage to slip through delivery systems and present with the late neurological complications of HIV, the diagnostic and therapeutic methods of earlier times still hold, though they may be made more difficult for a number of reasons. First, as time has passed, many clinicians are now less familiar with the clinical presentations of these disorders, and need to retrace the lessons of the past. Second, diagnosis may actually be more challenging now even for the experienced clinician because of the confounding background diseases and competing risks for neurological diseases in those patients most likely to progress to AIDS. The odds of AIDS-related neurological diagnoses may now be skewed away from the common disorders defined in the past. There is thus the continued need for education and improving the precision of these diagnoses using contemporary tools.

CONCLUSIONS

In looking toward the remaining problems in pathogenesis, diagnosis, and treatment of the CNS consequences of HIV infection, we should not lose track of the extraordinary progress that has been made, at least in the developed world. What was once termed a "dementia," implying a chronic and untreatable affliction of the CNS, affecting cognition, can now be largely prevented, and even in those cases missing preventative treatment and developing this disorder, we can now treat them with the hope of substantial reversal and restoration of function.

Lest those of us who are neurologists or neuroscientists become too proud of this, we might examine our own contribution to this progress. Perhaps we have added to the characterization of the disorder and its pathogenesis, and those of us treating these patients can be pleased with those that we have individually helped. On the other hand, we might also ask whether much of the extraordinary progress in treatment has been a result of focused efforts to target the nervous system or through advances in systemic therapy that fortunately apply to the CNS. This is an important consideration as we now look at whether earlier or broader targeting of CNS HIV infection is clinically important. We shall see. For myself, I suspect that future improvements in treatment will likely follow the same path of development—with advances in systemic therapy followed by neurological application. In the last few years, treatment effectiveness has been improved by the introduction of simplified and less toxic regimens resulting in better patient tolerance and adherence, and reduced treatment failure.

REFERENCES

(1991). Nomenclature and research case definitions for neurologic manifestations of human immunodeficiency virus-type 1 (HIV-1) infection. Report of a Working Group of the American Academy of Neurology AIDS Task Force. *Neurology*, *41*(6), 778–85.

Antinori, A., Arendt, G., et al. (2007). Updated research nosology for HIV-associated neurocognitive disorders. *Neurology*, *69*(18), 1789–99.

Becker, J. T., Kingsley, L., et al. (2009). Vascular risk factors, HIV serostatus, and cognitive dysfunction in gay and bisexual men. *Neurology*, *73*(16), 1292–9.

Brew, B. J. (2004). Evidence for a change in AIDS dementia complex in the era of highly active antiretroviral therapy and the possibility of new forms of AIDS dementia complex. *AIDS*, *18* Suppl 1, S75–8.

Budka, H. (1991). Neuropathology of human immunodeficiency virus infection. [Review]. *Brain Pathology*, *1*(3), 163–75.

Canestri, A., Lescure, F. X., et al. (2010). Discordance between cerebral spinal fluid and plasma HIV replication in patients with neurological symptoms who are receiving suppressive antiretroviral therapy. *Clin Infect Dis*, *50*(5), 773–8.

Childers, M. E., Woods, S. P., et al. (2008). Cognitive functioning during highly active antiretroviral therapy interruption in human immunodeficiency virus type 1 infection. *J Neurovirol*, *14*(6), 550–7.

Churchill, M. J., Wesselingh, S. L., et al. (2009). Extensive astrocyte infection is prominent in human immunodeficiency virus-associated dementia. *Ann Neurol*, *66*(2), 253–8.

Cinque, P., Brew, B. J., et al. (2006). Cerebrospinal fluid markers in central nervous system HIV infection and AIDS dementia complex. In *Handbook of clinical neurology: AIDS and HIV dementias*.

Crews, L., Patrick, C., et al. (2009). Molecular pathology of neuro-AIDS (CNS-HIV). *Int J Mol Sci*, *10*(3), 1045–63.

d'Arminio Monforte, A., Cinque, P., et al. (2004). Changing incidence of central nervous system diseases in the EuroSIDA cohort. *Ann Neurol*, *55*(3), 320–8.

Di Rocco, A. (1999). Diseases of the spinal cord in human immunodeficiency virus infection. *Semin Neurol*, *19*(2), 151–5.

Eden, A., Fuchs, D., et al. (2010). HIV-1 viral escape in cerebrospinal fluid of subjects on suppressive antiretroviral treatment. *Journal of Infectious Diseases*, In Press.

Eden, A., Price, R. W., et al. (2007). Immune activation of the central nervous system is still present after >4 years of effective highly active antiretroviral therapy. *J Infect Dis*, *196*(12), 1779–83.

Ellis, R. J., Hsia, K., et al. (1997). Cerebrospinal fluid human immunodeficiency virus type 1 RNA levels are elevated in neurocognitively impaired individuals with acquired immunodeficiency syndrome. HIV Neurobehavioral Research Center Group. *Ann Neurol*, *42*(5), 679–88.

Everall, I., Vaida, F., et al. (2009). Cliniconeuropathologic correlates of human immunodeficiency virus in the era of antiretroviral therapy. *J Neurovirol*, *15*(5–6), 360–70.

Gabuzda, D. H. & Hirsch, M. S. (1987). Neurologic manifestations of infection with human immunodeficiency virus. Clinical features and pathogenesis. [Review]. *Annals of Internal Medicine*, *107*(3), 383–91.

Gonzalez-Scarano, F. & Martin-Garcia, J. (2005). The neuropathogenesis of AIDS. *Nat Rev Immunol*, *5*(1), 69–81.

Gopinathan, G., Laubenstein, L., et al. (1983). Central nervous system manifestations of the acquired immunodeficiency syndrome (AIDS) in homosexual men. *Neurology, 33* [Suppl 2], 105.

Gottlieb, M. S., Schroff, R., et al. (1981). Pneumocystis carinii pneumonia and mucosal candidiasis in previously healthy homosexual men: Evidence of a new acquired cellular immunodeficiency. *N Engl J Med, 305*(24), 1425–31.

Hagberg, L., Andersson, M., et al. (1991). Effect of zidovudine on cerebrospinal fluid in patients with HIV infection and acute neurological disease. *Scandinavian Journal of Infectious Diseases, 23*(6), 681–5.

Hagberg, L., Cinque, P., et al. (2010). Cerebrospinal fluid neopterin: An informative biomarker of central nervous system immune activation in HIV-1 infection. *AIDS Res Ther, 7*, 15.

Horowitz, S. L., Bentson, J. R., et al. (1983). CNS toxoplasmosis in acquired immunodeficiency syndrome. *Arch Neurol, 40*(10), 649–52.

Lescure, F.-X., Omland, L. H., et al. (2010). Incidence and impact on mortality of severe neurocognitive disorders in persons with and without HIV: A Danish nationwide cohort study. *Clinical Infectious Diseases*, In press.

Letendre, S., Marquie-Beck, J., et al. (2008). Validation of the CNS Penetration-Effectiveness rank for quantifying antiretroviral penetration into the central nervous system. *Arch Neurol, 65*(1), 65–70.

McArthur, J. C., McClernon, D. R., et al. (1997). Relationship between human immunodeficiency virus-associated dementia and viral load in cerebrospinal fluid and brain. *Ann Neurol, 42*(5), 689–98.

Mellgren, A., Antinori, A., et al. (2005). Cerebrospinal fluid HIV-1 infection usually responds well to antiretroviral treatment. *Antivir Ther, 10*(6), 701–7.

Moore, D. J., Masliah, E., et al. (2006). Cortical and subcortical neurodegeneration is associated with HIV neurocognitive impairment. *AIDS, 20*(6), 879–87.

Navia, B., Cho, E. W., et al. (1986). The AIDS dementia complex: II. Neuropathology. *Ann Neurol, 19*, 525–535.

Navia, B., Jordan, B., et al. (1986). The AIDS dementia complex: I. Clinical Features. *Ann Neurol, 19*, 517–524.

Navia, B. A., Cho, E. S., et al. (1986). The AIDS dementia complex: II. Neuropathology. *Ann Neurol, 19*(6), 525–35.

Nebuloni, M., Pellegrinelli, A., et al. (2001). Beta amyloid precursor protein and patterns of HIV p24 immunohistochemistry in different brain areas of AIDS patients. *AIDS, 15*(5), 571–5.

Petito, C., Navia, B., et al. (1985). Vacuolar myelopathy pathologically resembling subacute combined degeneration in patients with acquired immunodeficiency syndrome (AIDS). *N Engl J Med, 312*, 874–879.

Petito, C. K., Cho, E. S., et al. (1986). Neuropathology of acquired immunodeficiency syndrome (AIDS): An autopsy review. *J Neuropathol Exp Neurol, 45*(6), 635–46.

Price, R. & Brew, B. (1988a). The AIDS dementia complex. *J of Infect Dis, 158*, 1079–1083.

Price, R. W., Brew, B., et al. (1988b). The brain in AIDS: Central nervous system HIV-1 infection and AIDS dementia complex. *Science, 239*(4840), 586–92.

Price, R. & Sidtis, J. (1990). Early HIV infection and the AIDS dementia complex. *Neurol, 40*, 323–326.

Price, R. W. & Spudich, S. (2008). Antiretroviral therapy and central nervous system HIV type 1 infection. *J Infect Dis, 197* Suppl 3, S294–306.

Pumarole-Sune, T., Navia, B., et al. (1987). HIV antigen in the brains of patients with the AIDS dementia complex. *Ann Neurol, 21*, 90–496.

Robertson, K. R., Smurzynski, M., et al. (2007). The prevalence and incidence of neurocognitive impairment in the HAART era. *AIDS, 21*(14), 1915–21.

Rosenblum, M. (1990). Infection of the central nervous system by the human immunodeficiency virus type 1: Morphology and relation to syndromes of progressive encephalopathy and myelopathy in patients with AIDS. *Pathol Ann, 25*, 117–169.

Sacktor, N. (2002). The epidemiology of human immunodeficiency virus-associated neurological disease in the era of highly active antiretroviral therapy. *J Neurovirol, 8* Suppl 2, 115–21.

Schnell, G., Spudich, S., et al. (2009). Compartmentalized human immunodeficiency virus type 1 originates from long-lived cells in some subjects with HIV-1-associated dementia. *PLoS Pathog, 5*(4), e1000395.

Shaw, G., Harper, M., et al. (1985). HTLV-III infection in brains of children and adults with AIDS encephalopathy. *Science, 227*, 177–182.

Sidtis, J. J., Gatsonis, C., et al. (1993). Zidovudine treatment of the AIDS dementia complex: results of a placebo-controlled trial. AIDS Clinical Trials Group. *Ann Neurol, 33*(4), 343–9.

Simioni, S., Cavassini, M., et al. (2010). Cognitive dysfunction in HIV patients despite long-standing suppression of viremia. *AIDS, 24*(9), 1243–50.

Snider, W. D., Simpson, D. M., et al. (1983). Neurological complications of acquired immune deficiency syndrome: Analysis of 50 patients. *Ann Neurol, 14*(4), 403–18.

Spudich, S. S., Nilsson, A. C., et al. (2005). Cerebrospinal fluid HIV infection and pleocytosis: Relation to systemic infection and antiretroviral treatment. *BMC Infect Dis, 5*, 98.

Vazeux, R. (1991). AIDS encephalopathy and tropism of HIV for brain monocytes/macrophages and microglial cells. [Review]. *Pathobiology, 59*(4), 214–8.

Vieira, J., Frank, E., et al. (1983). Acquired immune deficiency in Haitians: Opportunistic infections in previously healthy Haitian immigrants. *N Engl J Med, 308*(3), 125–9.

Wiley, C., Soontornniyomkij, V., et al. (1998). Distribution of brain HIV load in AIDS. *Brain Pathology, 8*, 277–284.

Wiley, C. A. & Achim, C. (1994). Human immunodeficiency virus encephalitis is the pathological correlate of dementia in acquired immunodeficiency syndrome [published erratum appears in Ann Neurol 1995 Jan;37(1):140]. *Annals of Neurology, 36*(4), 673–6.

Wright, E. J., Grund, B., et al.(2010). Cardiovascular risk factors associated with lower baseline cognitive performance in HIV-positive persons. *Neurology, 75*(10), 864–873.

Yarchoan, R., Berg, G., et al. (1987). Response of human-immunodeficiency-virus-associated neurological disease to 3'-azido-3'-deoxythymidine. *Lancet, 1*(8525), 132–5.

Yilmaz, A., Price, R. W., et al. (2008). Persistent intrathecal immune activation in HIV-1-infected individuals on antiretroviral therapy. *J Acquir Immune Defic Syndr, 47*(2), 168–73.

HIV-ASSOCIATED NEUROCOGNITIVE DISORDERS

Igor Grant and Ned Sacktor

A detailed overview of the neurocognitive disturbances associated with HIV infection is provided. The chapter discusses definitions, disease characteristics, and epidemiology. It includes a review of the neuropathological and disease-related correlates of cognitive disturbances, on risk factors that may contribute to cognitive complications, and on the impact of cognitive disturbances on social and occupational functioning, health, and early mortality. Therapeutic modalities are developed.

INTRODUCTION

In this chapter, we will define the various neurocognitive disturbances associated with HIV infection, describe their characteristics, and discuss our current understanding of their epidemiology. We shall also review the current state of the literature on neuropathological and disease-related correlates of cognitive disturbances, risk factors that may contribute to cognitive complications, and the significance of cognitive disturbances in terms of social-occupational functioning, health, and early mortality, as well as effects of treatment.

DEFINITIONS

Historically, terms were used to describe neurocognitive complications in ways that were often imprecise and sometimes contradictory. For example, neuropathological concepts such as encephalitis were applied to clinical phenomena; additionally, terms such as dementia were sometimes applied very broadly, so as to encompass even minor forms of cognitive disturbance. Such practices have created obvious difficulties in scientific and clinical communication; more importantly, lack of agreed-upon research definitions has hampered studies into the epidemiology, pathogenesis, prognosis, and treatment of these conditions. For these reasons, we have chosen in this chapter to provide definitions of the terms that we employ. Such definitions should increase the readability of our chapter; hopefully, they might also serve the broader purpose of sharpening our diagnostic terminology.

NEUROCOGNITIVE, NEUROBEHAVIORAL

If we view the brain as an apparatus for processing information, then it is useful to consider these information

management activities in terms of several processes. Examples of such neurocognitive processes or abilities include perceptual abilities, abstraction (conceptualization), executive functions, perceptual motor integration, learning, and remembering. Additionally, attention is usually regarded as a focusing and selecting process necessary for many of the other cognitive operations. Neurocognitive functioning can also be described in terms of its speed and efficiency, as well as its flexibility.

The term "neurobehavioral" more broadly encompasses the neurocognitive processes delineated above, plus other brain-mediated behaviors such as mood and affect, motivation, temperament, adaptive (coping) abilities, and personality. Generally speaking, significant changes in neurocognitive functioning are the most specific indicators of underlying pathologic changes in the brain. Other neurobehavioral changes can occur for many non-neuropathological reasons: For example, mood changes can be brought on by the realization of the seriousness of one's illness, and distortions in ability to cope secondary to the pain, discomfort, and disability associated with AIDS can produce apparent disturbance in personality. For these reasons, we shall focus our attention in this chapter specifically on neurocognitive complications.

NEUROCOGNITIVE ASSESSMENT

Information on cognitive functioning derives both from patient history (self-report) and direct examination. It goes without saying that a careful history should always be the starting point, and persons with HIV infection, particularly AIDS, ought to be questioned closely on possible changes in attention/concentration, mental efficiency, ability to learn and recall, or reduced psychomotor performance.

Unfortunately, the value of self-reported information depends heavily on subjective factors that are not always easy for the clinician to evaluate. For instance, some patients tend to deny problems, while others tend to amplify them. Also, terms such as "memory problems" or "difficulty in concentrating" can have very different meaning to different patients. For these reasons, as well as others, self-reported cognitive difficulties often do not correlate well with objective findings from neuropsychological testing or neurological examination.

Some data from the UC San Diego HIV Neurobehavioral Research Center (HNRC) illustrate this point (Figure 7.2.1). In this case, seropositive patients were asked about a number of subjective complaints that were then grouped into the

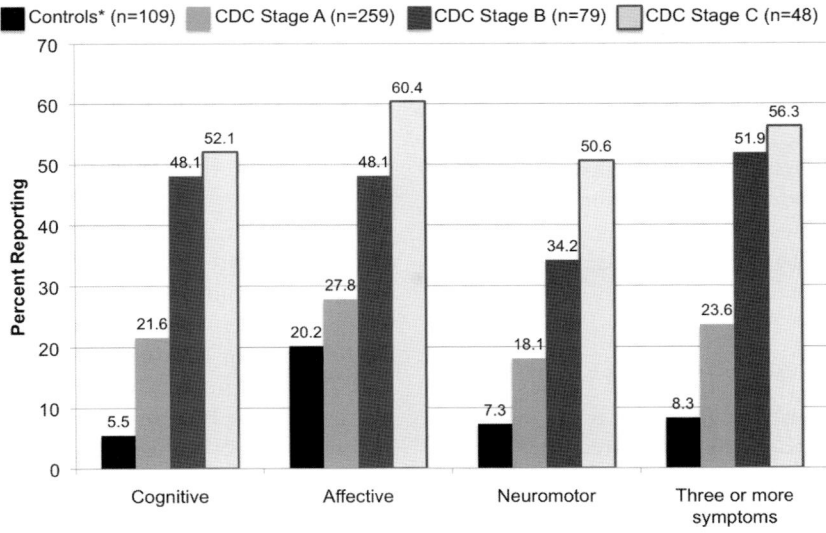

Figure. 7.2.1 Prevalence of cognitive, affective and neuromotor symptoms at different stages of HIV disease. Controls are HIV-negative "at risk" controls. For item content, see Figure 7.2.2. (Adapted from Mehta et al., 1996).

general categories of "cognitive" (example: complaint of memory loss), affective (example: feeling depressed or anxious), and neuromotor (example: gait disturbance). These clusters of self-reported complaints were then correlated with more objective indicators, including results of neuropsychological examination, mood measures, medical status, and neurological examination. As can be seen, "cognitive" self-reports were actually correlated better with mood measures than with neuropsychological and neurological measures (Figure 7.2.2).

For such reasons, it is essential that before a diagnosis of a neurocognitive disorder is made, the patient be examined by procedures that have documented validity and reliability. Ideally, neuropsychological testing should be accomplished,

but other approaches such as structured mental status examinations or cognitive screening procedures can also be used (for further discussion of this topic see Chapter 9.3 by Woods and colleagues).

NEUROPSYCHOLOGICAL TESTS

Neuropsychological tests can be viewed as probes of different cognitive abilities such as learning, recall, or perceptual motor skills. It is important to remember that there is no perfect test that corresponds exactly to a putative cognitive ability. Furthermore, tests vary in terms of their sensitivity and specificity, as well as the degree to which they are affected by

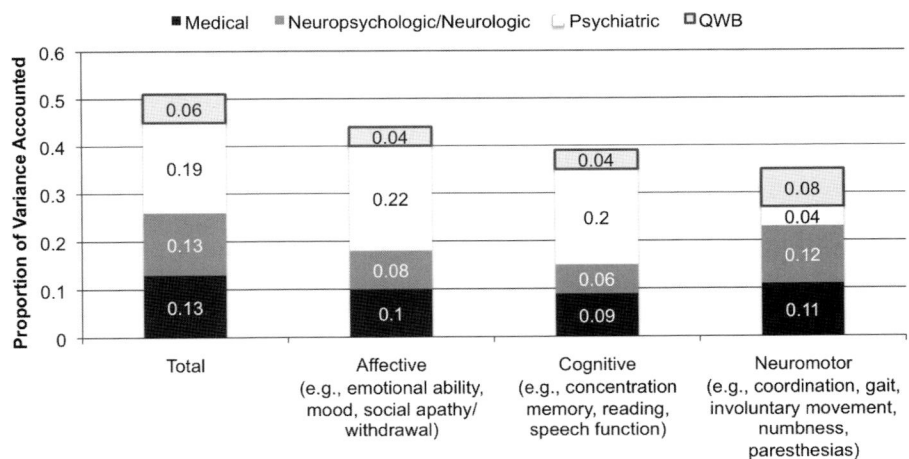

Figure. 7.2.2 Prediction of self-reported neurobehavioral symptoms. (From HNRC, unpublished data.) The predictor variables are as follows: Medical: CDC Classification, serum beta-2 microglobulin, absolute CD4 lymphocytes; Neuropsychological/Neurological: Global Neuropsychological Score, Overall Neurological Rating; Psychiatric: Depression/Dejection and Tension/Anxiety Profile of Mood States (POMS) Scores; QWB - Quality of Well-Being Score.

other general factors such as age, education, and cultural background. For this reason, it is important to assess cognitive ability domains utilizing more than one test of each domain.

It is also essential that a neuropsychological test abnormality not be equated to neurocognitive impairment. People can have difficulties with one or another neuropsychological test for many reasons, some of them non-neurological. Therefore, a clinical diagnosis cannot be based on a single test, or a very small grouping of tests that might not properly cover all relevant ability areas.

NEUROPSYCHOLOGICAL DEFICIT

We use the term neuropsychological deficit to refer to a clear-cut abnormality in a cognitive ability area. For example, a person might have been administered three tests of learning (e.g., a short story, a nonverbal test, and a list of words). Let us say such an individual scored below generally accepted norms on all of these tests. It would then be possible to conclude that such an individual has a learning deficit. However, to term an individual neurocognitively "impaired" requires that more than one ability area is deficient. In this example, if an individual had problems in learning only, and performed well in areas such as perceptual motor skills, executive functions, recall of information, and verbal skills, we would conclude that the person has a learning deficit and nothing more.

NEUROCOGNITIVE IMPAIRMENT

The term "neurocognitive (neuropsychological) impairment" is used when an individual has deficits in two or more cognitive areas, established by valid and reliable neuropsychological or mental status assessment.

DIAGNOSTIC CRITERIA FOR HIV NEUROCOGNITIVE COMPLICATIONS

Over the past 25 years, the diagnostic criteria for what are now termed HIV-associated neurocognitive disorders have been gradually refined. Some early examples include the Memorial Sloan Kettering (MSK) scheme, which contains gradations that range from minor cognitive disturbance to profound and incapacitating disorders (Price & Brew, 1988). It also integrates neurological deficits related to myelopathy, focusing on ambulatory function. While this scale has been useful in many contexts, it does not adequately separate the cognitive and behavioral impairments originating from brain disease specifically, from myelopathic impairments. A system developed by the World Health Organization (1988; Maj, 1990) also had some limitations, permitting dementia to be diagnosed even when relatively mild cognitive deficits of uncertain functional significance were present.

An advance was made in the publication by the American Academy of Neurology (AAN) (1991) of a diagnostic system that separated out the more severe forms of cognitive/motor disorder—termed HIV-associated dementia complex—from a new entity termed minor cognitive motor disorder (MCMD), which attempted to capture less profound forms of cognitive, motor, and other behavioral dysfunction (1991).

In 2006 the US National Institute of Mental Health convened a panel of international experts to consider possible updating of the AAN schema in light of emerging evidence. This resulted in the publication of a set of recommendations for diagnosing HIV-associated neurocognitive disorders (HAND) (Antinori et al., 2007). These "Frascati criteria" examined the presentation of neurocognitive disturbances in the post combination antiretroviral therapy (CART) era, which has been characterized by persistence of primarily milder forms of neurocognitive abnormality and decline in incidence and prevalence of the more profound disturbances (dementia). The Frascati criteria emphasized that the essential feature of HAND was cognitive disturbance; this revision eliminated the possibility of HIV neurocognitive disorders being diagnosed on the basis of neuromotor and noncognitive psychiatric changes such as changes in personality or mood. The Frascati criteria, which in good measure adopted criteria proposed earlier by the University of California San Diego, HIV Neurobehavioral Research Center (HNRC) Group (Grant & Atkinson, 1995), were found to correspond better than previous criteria to postmortem neuropathologic findings (Cherner et al., 2007).

The Frascati criteria proposed three levels of HAND: asymptomatic neurocognitive impairment (ANI) exists when an individual manifests decrements in at least two cognitive areas but these deficits are sufficiently subtle that they do not affect everyday functioning; mild neurocognitive disorder (MND) exists when a person has deficits in two or more cognitive areas that interfere at least mildly in day-to-day functioning; HIV-associated dementia (HAD) exists when neurocognitive impairment is so severe in nature that it interferes markedly in day-to-day functioning. Persons diagnosed with dementia are typically unable to work and some may not be able to care for themselves. Thus, the term dementia is reserved for those who have pervasive cognitive impairment that interferes markedly with day-to-day life. Figure 7.2.3 presents a schematic for the Frascati classification system. Table 7.2.1 (taken from Antinori et al., 2007) details these criteria.

It is hoped that general acceptance of the Frascati HAND criteria may replace less carefully defined concepts such as HIV encephalopathy and HIV dementia, thereby fostering better communication among scientists and clinicians, and affording improved cross study and international comparisons.

HAND PHENOMENOLOGY

In its milder forms, HAND presents as difficulties in learning new information, prospective memory (remembering to remember), some disturbance in attention, and slowing of information processing and output (reduced speed of cognitive processing and psychomotor slowing), and disturbance in executive functions (evaluating, planning, abstract reasoning). Typically, language skills are spared (aphasic difficulties

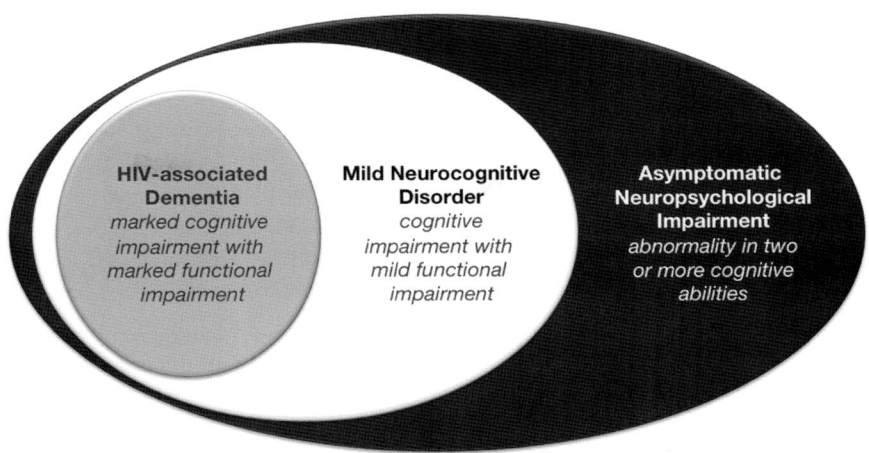

Figure 7.2.3 Schematic representation of the Frascati Criteria for HAND.

Table 7.2.1 REVISED RESEARCH CRITERIA FOR HIV-ASSOCIATED NEUROCOGNITIVE DISORDERS (HAND) (MODIFIED FROM HIV NEUROBEHAVIORAL RESEARCH CENTER CRITERIA)

*HIV-Associated Asymptomatic Neurocognitive Impairment (ANI)**

1. Acquired impairment in cognitive functioning, involving at least two ability domains, documented by performance of at least 1.0 SD below the mean for age-education-appropriate norms on standardized neuropsychological tests. The neuropsychological assessment must survey at least the following abilities: verbal/language; attention/working memory; abstraction/executive; memory (learning; recall); speed of information processing; sensory-perceptual, motor skills.

2. The cognitive impairment does not interfere with everyday functioning.

3. The cognitive impairment does not meet criteria for delirium or dementia.

4. There is no evidence of another preexisting cause for the ANI.[†]

* If there is a prior diagnosis of ANI, but currently the individual does not meet criteria, the diagnosis of ANI in remission can be made.
† If the individual with suspected ANI also satisfies criteria for a major depressive episode or substance dependence, the diagnosis of ANI should be deferred to a subsequent examination conducted at a time when the major depression has remitted or at least 1 month after cessation of substance use.

*HIV-1-Associated Mild Neurocognitive Disorder (MND)**

1. Acquired impairment in cognitive functioning, involving at least two ability domains, documented by performance of at least 1.0 SD below the mean for age-education-appropriate norms on standardized neuropsychological tests. The neuropsychological assessment must survey at least the following abilities: verbal/language; attention/working memory; abstraction/executive; memory (learning; recall); speed of information processing; sensory-perceptual, motor skills.
Typically, this would correspond to an MSK scale stage of 0.5 to 1.0.

2. The cognitive impairment produces at least mild interference in daily functioning (at least one of the following):
   a) Self-report of reduced mental acuity, inefficiency in work, homemaking, or social functioning.
   b) Observation by knowledgeable others that the individual has undergone at least mild decline in mental acuity with resultant inefficiency in work, homemaking, or social functioning.

3. The cognitive impairment does not meet criteria for delirium or dementia.

4. There is no evidence of another preexisting cause for the MND.[†]

* If there is a prior diagnosis of MND, but currently the individual does not meet criteria, the diagnosis of MND in remission can be made.
† If the individual with suspected MND also satisfies criteria for a severe episode of major depression with significant functional limitations or psychotic features, or substance dependence, the diagnosis of MND should be deferred to a subsequent examination conducted at a time when the major depression has remitted or at least 1 month after cessation of substance use.

*HIV-1-Associated Dementia (HAD)**

1. Marked acquired impairment in cognitive functioning, involving at least two ability domains; typically the impairment is in multiple domains, especially in learning of new information, slowed information processing, and defective attention/concentration. The cognitive impairment must be ascertained by neuropsychological testing with at least two domains 2 SD or greater than demographically corrected means. (Note that where neuropsychological testing is not available, standard neurological evaluation and simple bedside testing may be used, but this should be done as indicated in algorithm; see below).
Typically, this would correspond to an MSK scale stage of 2.0 or greater.

(Continued)

Table 7.2.1 (CONTINUED)

*HIV-1-Associated Dementia (HAD)**

2. The cognitive impairment produces marked interference with day-to-day functioning (work, home life, social activities).

3. The pattern of cognitive impairment does not meet criteria for delirium (e.g., clouding of consciousness is not a prominent feature); or, if delirium is present, criteria for dementia need to have been met on a prior examination when delirium was not present.

4. There is no evidence of another, preexisting cause for the dementia (e.g., other CNS infection, CNS neoplasm, cerebrovascular disease, preexisting neurologic disease, or severe substance abuse compatible with CNS disorder).[†]

* If there is a prior diagnosis of HAD, but currently the individual does not meet criteria, the diagnosis of HAD in remission can be made.
† If the individual with suspected HAD also satisfies criteria for a severe episode of major depression with significant functional limitations or psychotic features, or substance dependence, the diagnosis of HAD should be deferred to a subsequent examination conducted at a time when the major depression has remitted or at least 1 month has elapsed following cessation of substance use. Note that the consensus was that even when major depression and HAD occurred together, there is little evidence that pseudodementia exists and the cognitive deficits do not generally improve with treatment of depression.

such as naming problems and comprehension difficulties are rare), but there may be reduction in verbal fluency; for example, as indexed by number of words generated in a given period of time. This constellation of learning, attentional, executive, and cognitive slowing phenomena has sometimes been termed "subcortical" or "frontostriatal" in nature, reflecting some commonalities with conditions that involve damage to subcortical grey regions (e.g., Parkinson's disease, Huntington's disease) and white matter injury (e.g., multiple sclerosis). While it is true that the cognitive profile of HAND is not particularly similar to that seen in the "cortical" dementias (e.g., Alzheimer's disease, vascular dementias), it is also true to say that in different individuals the patterns of performance decrement may vary, reflecting the initially patchy nature of brain involvement. The likelihood that an impaired individual will have a deficit in a particular cognitive area is illustrated in Figure 7.2.4.

CHANGING EPIDEMIOLOGY OF HAND IN THE ART AND CART ERAS

The introduction of progressively more effective antiretroviral therapies (ART) has had a substantial impact on the epidemiology of HAND. (Note: in reviewing some of the studies below, particularly those from a decade ago or earlier, it is sometimes difficult to achieve precise equivalence of diagnostic terms. The Frascati criteria for HAND were only published in 2007, and although the AAN criteria were available from 2001 onward, these were not consistently applied in various studies. Therefore, the term "HIV dementia" as used in earlier studies may not be, strictly speaking, equivalent to the term HIV-associated dementia as proposed in Frascati. The ascertainment instruments utilized in various studies also did not necessarily include comprehensive neurocognitive testing; therefore, it is likely that milder cases of HAND were missed.

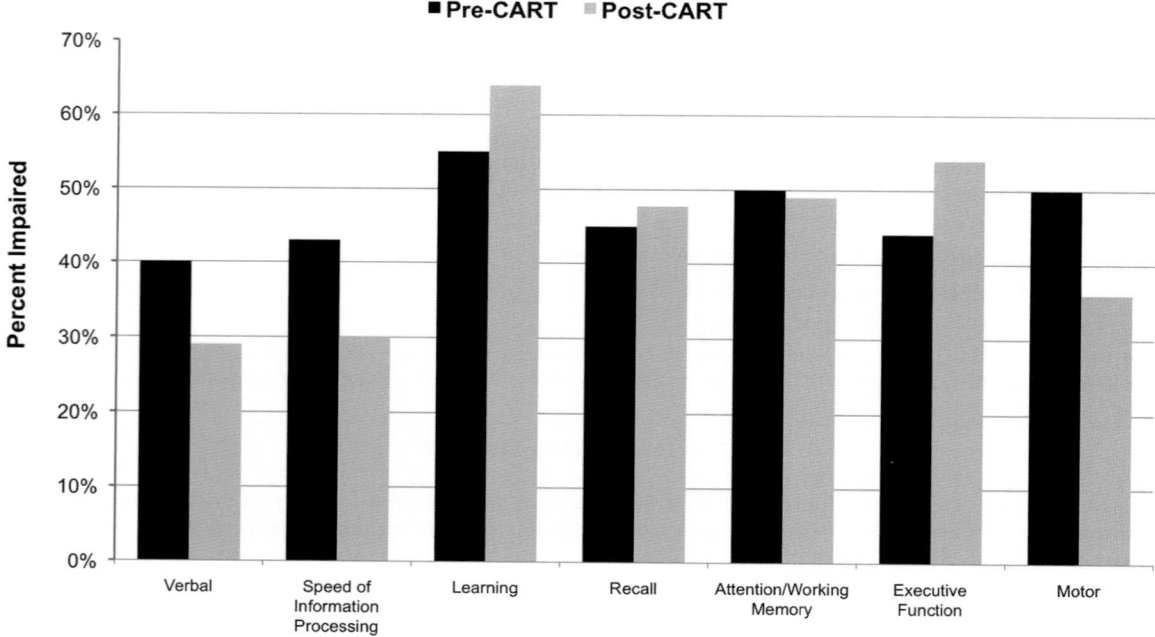

Figure 7.2.4 Neurocognitive impairment by domain in pre-CART versus CART eras. (Data from HNRC).

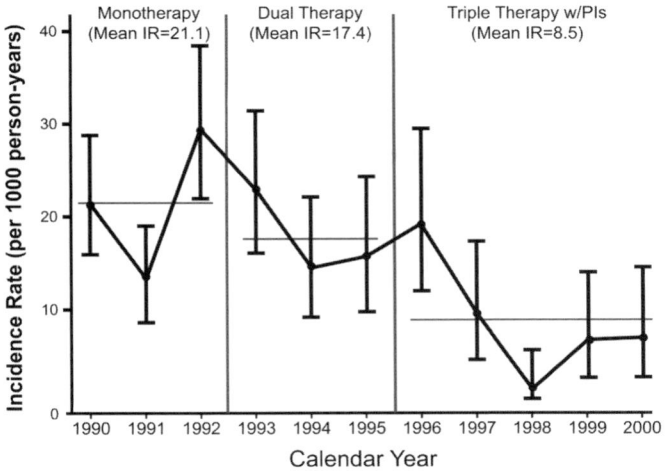

Figure 7.2.5 Incidence of dementia during three epochs of ARV treatment. IR, incidence rate; PIs, protease inhibitors.

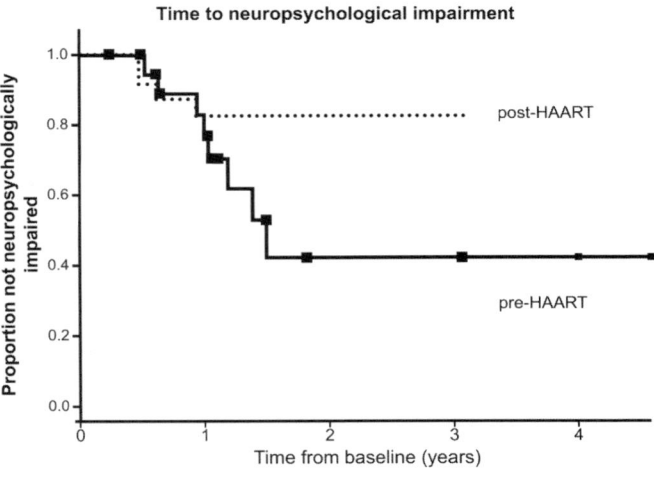

Figure 7.2.7 Kaplan-Meier survival estimate for distribution of time to neurocognitive impairment (in years) on or before December 31, 1995 (pre-HAART) versus on or after January 1, 1996 (post-HAART). Tic marks on curves represent censored observations. HAART, highly active antiretroviral therapy. (Deutsch et al., 2001).

It is probably reasonable to suggest that "HIV dementia" as used in some of these earlier studies would roughly equate to Frascati concepts of HIV associated dementia plus more severe presentations of mild neurocognitive disorder.)

With these cautions in mind, it is possible to generalize that more severe forms of HAND have declined since introduction of ART (i.e., mono therapy or dual therapy) and combined antiretroviral therapies (CART) (Brodt et al., 1997). For example, Sacktor and colleagues were able to analyze data from the Multicenter AIDS Cohort Study (MACS), a longitudinal cohort of gay/bisexual men from Baltimore, Pittsburgh, Chicago, and Los Angeles from 1990 to 1992, at which time mono therapy or no therapy were predominant forms of treatment (Sacktor et al., 2001). From 1993 to 1995, multidrug therapy without protease inhibitors

(i.e., dual therapy) and mono therapy were the predominant forms of treatment. From 1996 to the present CART has become the predominant approach. Characterizing treatment eras in this fashion, Sacktor et al. were able to demonstrate that frequency of the more severe forms of HIV-associated neurocognitive disorders has declined significantly (by about 50%) from the mono therapy/dual therapy eras to the CART era (Figure 7.2.5).

In the Johns Hopkins HIV clinic the incidence rate of HIV dementia has also decreased markedly in the years since the introduction of CART in 1996 (Figure 7.2.6).

The HNRC experience also bears out that the hazard of neurocognitive impairment has reduced significantly since the beginning of the era of CART (1996 and later) (Figure 7.2.7).

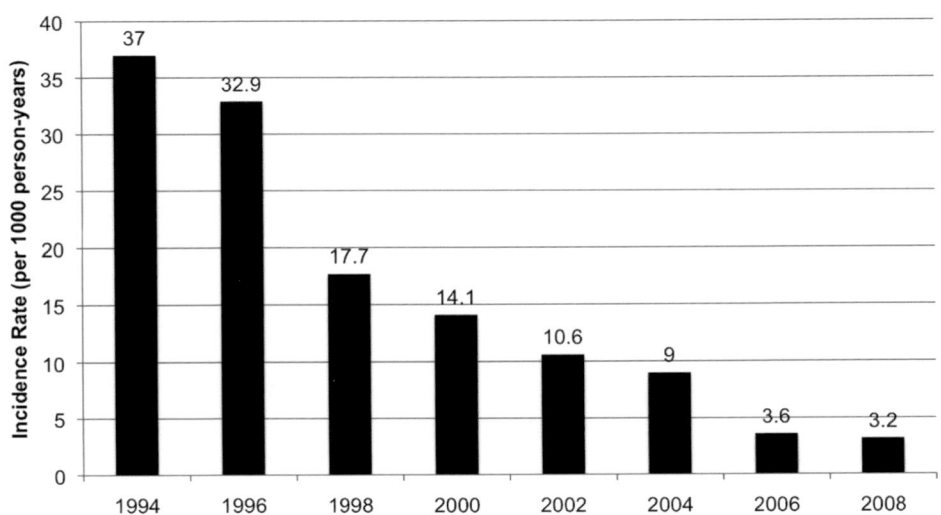

Figure 7.2.6 HIV dementia incidence rate in the years following introduction of CART. (Data from Johns Hopkins University).

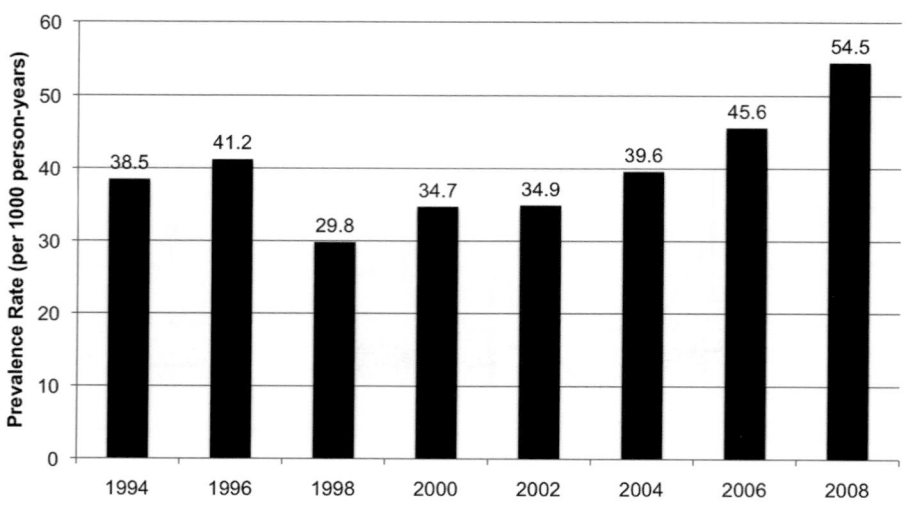

Figure 7.2.8 Neurocognitive disorders may be rising as those on CART survive longer. (Data from Johns Hopkins University).

Similarly, a European study of homosexual men (Raboud et al., 1997) found a decreased rate of HIV-associated CNS disease from 1992 to 1996. In the Multicenter Euro SIDA of 14 nations with 7,300 individuals, the incidence of HIV dementia also decreased by about 50% (Mocroft et al., 2000). The European CASCADE study tracked incidence of HIV dementia (i.e., severe neurocognitive impairment) among 15,380 seroconverters (Bhaskaran et al., 2008). The incidence pre CART era (pre 1997) was 6.49 per 1,000 person years, declining to 0.66 in the period 2003–2006. In addition to low current CD4, correlates of dementia risk post CART included older age at infection, chronicity of infection, and history of AIDS-defining events.

While the incidence of the more severe neurocognitive disorders has declined, overall prevalence of neurocognitive disorders may actually be increasing. In the Johns Hopkins HIV clinic, the prevalence rate has increased from approximately 30 per thousand patient years in 1998 to about 55 per thousand patient years by the year 2008 (Figure 7.2.8).

Data from the HNRC indicate that the overall proportion of people with neurocognitive impairment has not changed a great deal from 1997 through 2009. Because data from comparable comprehensive neuropsychological testings were available across the years, it was possible to compare more directly both frequencies and severities of impairments at different stages of disease. Figure 7.2.11 shows that overall frequency of HAND in HIV-infected people at all stages of disease declined somewhat from approximately 60% to 50%; this change was primarily due to reduction in HIV dementia (i.e., more disabling pervasive neurocognitive impairment).

The prevalence of moderate and mild forms of HAND has remained fairly stable (Cole et al., 2007; Tozzi et al., 2007). On more detailed analysis, it appears that, compared to the mono therapy/dual therapy eras, there is some increase in the proportion of persons with impairment at CDC Stages A (i.e., in the medically asymptomatic period of infection [Heaton, et al. 2011]). A recent analysis of the CNS HIV Anti-Retroviral Therapy Effects Research (CHARTER) and HNRC data

indicated that 36% of CART-era persons classified in CDC Stage A were cognitively impaired versus 29% of those in the pre-CART era. These increases occurred despite the fact that the proportion of persons with undetectable plasma viral load increased from 5% to 72% pre/post CART for those on ART (see Figure 7.2.9).

The reasons for persistence, and perhaps increased prevalence of milder forms of HAND in medically asymptomatic HIV-infected individuals is unclear. However, some clues come from the observation that the duration of infection in the CHARTER post-CART cases in CDC-A was significantly greater than among HNRC participants in the pre CART era (approximately 10 years versus 3 years). In addition, although in the main CD4 counts of post-CART individuals at time of evaluation were higher than those pre-CART, a larger proportion of post-CART CDC-A persons experienced nadir CD4s less than 200. Evidence that profound immunosuppression at some point in time may represent a "legacy event" predisposing to later neurocognitive impairment comes from further CHARTER data which indicate that cases least likely to be cognitively impaired were those who never experienced nadir CD4s under 200, and were currently virologically suppressed (Figure 7.2.10). These data are compatible with the idea that chronicity of infection, perhaps with attendant CD4 troughs, repeated viral load peaks, and bouts of neuroinflammation may contribute to HAND persistence.

RISK FACTORS FOR HAND

VIRAL FACTORS

Despite several years of intensive research, the host and viral factors which predispose to HAND remain poorly understood. From the virologic standpoint, some data suggest that some HIV clades might be less (e.g., clade C) or more (clade D) neuropathogenic. However, confirmation of these reports

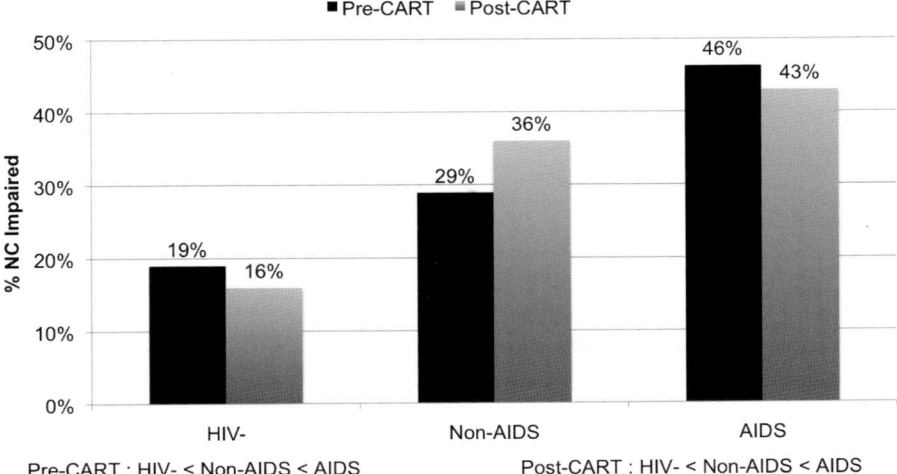

Figure 7.2.9 Increase in frequency of neurocognitive impairment is seen in non-AIDS cases in post CART era, possibly reflecting CART influenced longer survival of cases before experiencing an AIDS-defining condition. (Data from HNRC and CHARTER).

is required. In the case of clade C, some reports from studies in India indicate that neurocognitive impairment may be just as prevalent in those clade C-infected samples as in the clade B-infected western setting (Gupta et al., 2007; Sacktor et al., 2009). With respect to clades A and D, which are the predominant HIV subtypes in central and east Africa, one study suggests that in adults clade D is associated with an increased risk of dementia compared to clade A (Sacktor et al., 2009). The search for other genotypic and phenotypic variations has yielded few clues. It is possible that variations in the V3 loop may be associated with greater neuroadaptation, and possibly greater neuropathogenicity (Pillai et al., 2006). Another possible clue to a differential rate of neurovirulence by subtype comes from the observation that the *tat* gene in subtype C is associated with increased cell survival in rat hippocampal neuron cultures compared with subtype B (Li et al., 2008).

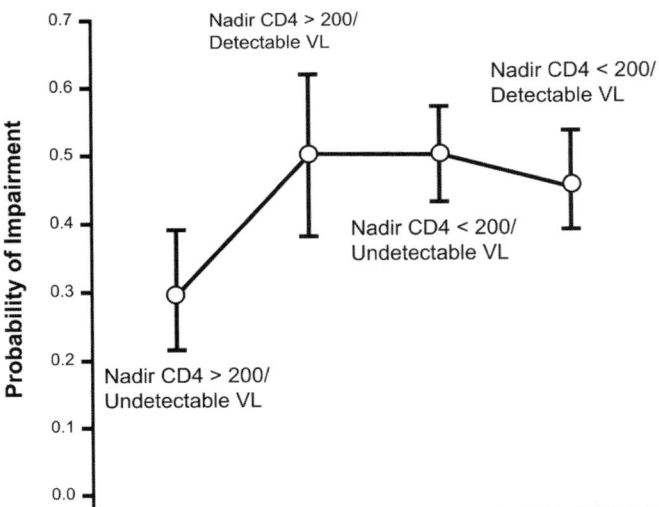

Figure 7.2.10 Reduced risk of HAND in those with absent history of severe immunosuppression and good virologic control.

Interestingly, development of ARV drug resistance appears to be associated with better neurocognitive performance (Hightower et al., 2009). This counterintuitive observation perhaps reflects lessened fitness of resistant strains.

HOST FACTORS

Since the initial descriptions of HIV dementia, it has been clear that some individuals are apparently spared, while others are severely affected, raising the potential that a genetic susceptibility exists, as it does for Alzheimer's disease. Polymorphisms in immune-response genes have been identified previously in published works. Specific polymorphisms in CCR2, the receptor for the potent chemoattractant MCP-1, and in the MCP-1 promoter, may affect the progression to neurocognitive impairment. In one study from UCSD, CSF levels of MCP-1 were influenced by polymorphisms in MCP-1 (-2578G/A) (Letendre et al., 2004a; Letendre et al., 2004b). The G allele appeared to be associated with higher expression of CSF MCP-1. Also, the E4 isoform for apolipoprotein E in some studies is associated with dementia specifically among older HIV+ individuals, possibly by making neurons more vulnerable to oxidative stress (Corder et al., 1998; Cutler et al., 2004; Valcour, Shikuma, Watters, & Sacktor, 2004a). Polymorphisms in the tumor necrosis factor-α (TNFα) promoter are also associated with HIV dementia, possibly by affecting neuronal vulnerability to TNFα-induced toxicity (Quasney et al., 2001). At this point, no genetic markers for HAND susceptibility have been conclusively identified and entered clinical practice.

HIV DISEASE FACTORS

Since neurological complications were first appreciated in the pretreatment era, it has been a consistent observation that as HIV disease progresses, the likelihood of neurocognitive disorder increases. In the CART era this relationship holds, as

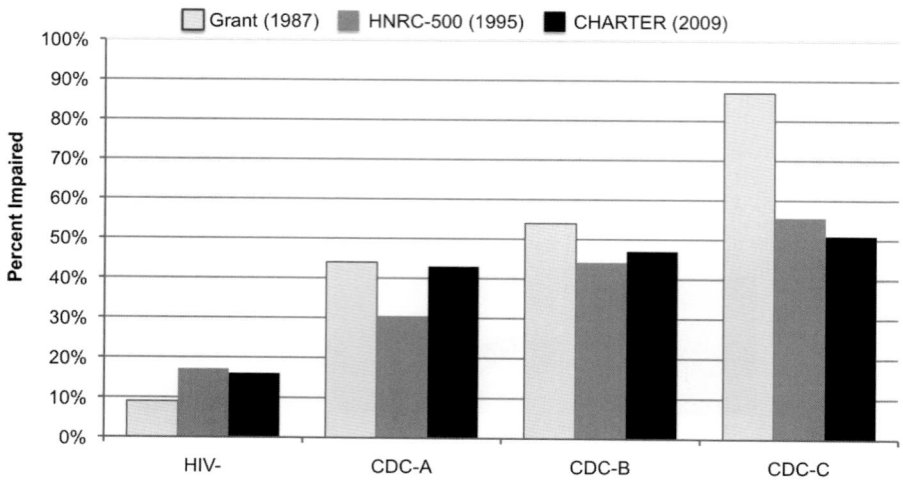

Figure 7.2.11 CHARTER data indicate that HAND persists despite modern ART. HIV- means HIV uninfected; CDC A, B, C means cases at Centers for Disease Control stages of HIV infection.

noted in recent CHARTER data (see Figure 7.2.11). In earlier studies high viral load and low current CD4 count were associated with HAND, but with combination treatment this association is less clear. The most consistent predictor of HAND is nadir CD4: those with lower nadirs (e.g., < 200) at any time are at higher risk of impairment (Heaton et al., 2010; Ellis et al., 2010; Munoz-Moreno et al., 2008; Robertson et al., 2007; Tozzi et al., 2005; Valcour et al., 2006).

AGING

Another characteristic that may increase risk of HAND is aging. With CART assuring longer survival, it is estimated that by 2015 as many as half of HIV-infected persons in developed countries may be over 50 years of age. Several studies have suggested that with increased age the likelihood of HAND increases. For example, in the Hawaii Aging Cohort, age greater than 50 was associated with about a twofold increased prevalence of dementia (25% versus 14%) and a threefold greater risk for dementia after adjusting for various demographic, comorbidity, and treatment variables (Valcour et al., 2004b). A similar increase was observed for minor cognitive motor disorder (45% versus 26%). The HNRC Group also found increased rate of impairment in older HIV-infected individuals (Cherner et al., 2004). It is possible that aging increases progression of HIV infection due to decreased ability to produce CD4, increased systemic inflammation, or less effective immunologic control of HIV replication. In addition, there may be interactions with other age-associated neurological diseases, including cerebral vascular disease and neurodegenerative conditions. Age-related changes in ARV neurotoxicity could also play a role.

DRUG ABUSE

Substance abuse may be another contributor to persistence of HAND. For example, methamphetamine increases likelihood of neurocognitive disturbance, both independently and may augment the neurological effects of HIV among dually affected persons (Rippeth et al., 2004; Chang, Ernst, Speck, & Grob, 2005). See Figure 7.2.12.

Similarly, alcoholism may potentiate HIV effects on the brain (Meyerhoff et al., 1995; Fein et al., 1998; Pfefferbaum et al., 2005; Pfefferbaum et al., 2006; Rosenbloom et al., 2007; Fama, Rosenbloom, Nichols, Pfefferbaum, & Sullivan, 2009). Substance abuse may also be associated with poorer medication adherence in some individuals, and/or enhanced viral replication or transmigration into the CNS due to stimulation of inflammatory cascades by stimulant drugs such as methamphetamine (Ellis et al., 2003; Hinkin et al., 2007; Toussi et al., 2009; Mellins et al., 2009; Applebaum et al., 2009; Baum et al., 2009).

HCV

HIV-infected persons may also be co-infected with hepatitis C virus (HCV), especially where injection drug use is a risk factor. In the CHARTER study 26% of 1,555 HIV+ persons attending HIV clinics tested positive for HCV antibody. In other series, HCV has been associated with neurocognitive impairment independently, and there may be an additive effect of HIV and HCV (Wu, Sullivan, Wang, Rotheram-Borus, & Detels, 2007; Ying, Robinson, & Fu-jie, 2009; Hilsabeck, Perry, & Hassanein, 2002; Forton et al., 2002; Ryan, Morgello, Isaacs, Naseer, & Gerits, 2004; Letendre et al., 2005; Cherner et al., 2005; Hilsabeck, Castellon, & Hinkin, 2005; Morgello et al., 2005; Perry et al., 2005). See Figure 7.2.13.

NEURORADIOLOGICAL CORRELATES OF HAND

The many changes found on structural and functional brain imaging are discussed in Chapters 9.1 and 9.2. In brief, HIV infection is associated with progressive atrophy within the gray and white matter in the brain, particularly in the later

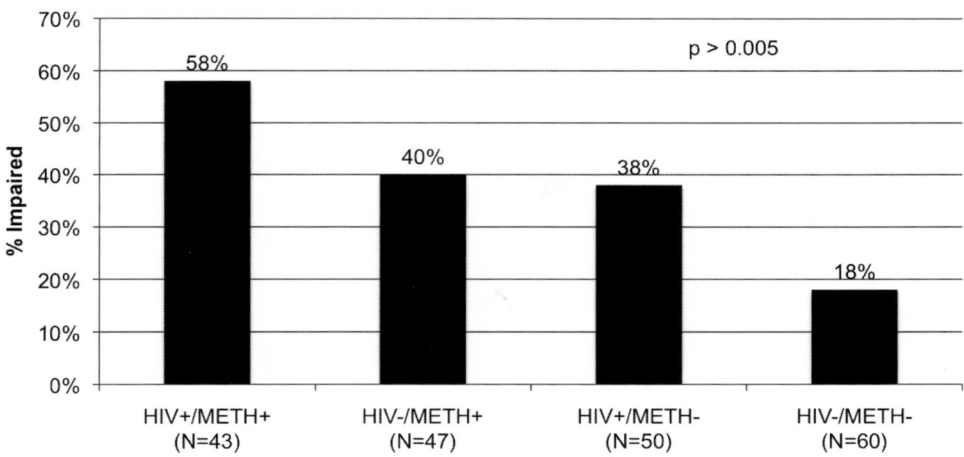

Figure 7.2.12 Global neuropsychological impairment in relation to HIV and methamphetamine risk status (Rippeth et al., 2004). HIV+ means HIV infected; METH+ means met diagnostic criteria for methamphetamine dependence.

stages of the disease (Hall et al., 1996; Dal Pan et al., 1992; Stout et al., 1998; Aylward et al., 1993; Tucker et al., 2004), and these findings persist despite CART (Cardenas et al., 2009). Structural MRI studies reveal that the degree of atrophy is correlated to the severity of neurocognitive dysfunction in both cross-sectional and longitudinal studies (Hall et al., 1996; Aylward et al., 1993; Tucker et al., 2004; Paul et al., 2008). Abnormal white matter signal, which may reflect areas of inflammation, is also observed (McMurtray, Nakamoto, Shikuma, & Valcour, 2008). Studies examining integrity of white matter tracts via diffusion tensor imaging (DTI) find increased mean diffusivity and reduced anisotropy (both thought to be indicators of fiber tract injury) in HIV+ persons (Chang, Yakupov, Nakama, Stokes, & Ernst, 2008), and such injury has been related to worse neurocognitive performance (Figure 7.2.14) (Gongvatana et al., 2009). However, DTI changes have also been reported in HIV+ persons in the absence of obvious neurocognitive impairment

(Pfefferbaum et al., 2009; Chen et al., 2009), suggesting that DTI might be picking up very early brain injury.

Various functional neuroimaging studies also reveal alterations in many HIV+ individuals, and these tend to be worse as the disease progresses. On MR spectroscopy, there tends to be reduced concentration of N-acetylaspartate, a putative marker of neuronal injury, and elevation in myo-inositol (perhaps reflecting gliosis or other inflammatory change) and choline (perhaps reflecting myelin damage) (Taylor et al., 2007; Chang et al., 2008; Pfefferbaum et al., 2009; Mohamed et al., 2010). Reduced glutamate has also been reported (Sailasuta, Shriner, & Ross, 2009). In several studies these metabolite changes were more common in the presence of neurocognitive impairment (Paul et al., 2008). Investigations utilizing various fMRI paradigms to probe function of circuitries subserving discrete cognitive operations tend to reveal patterns of reduced activation in certain regions (e.g., some frontal, basal ganglia, hippocampal), and

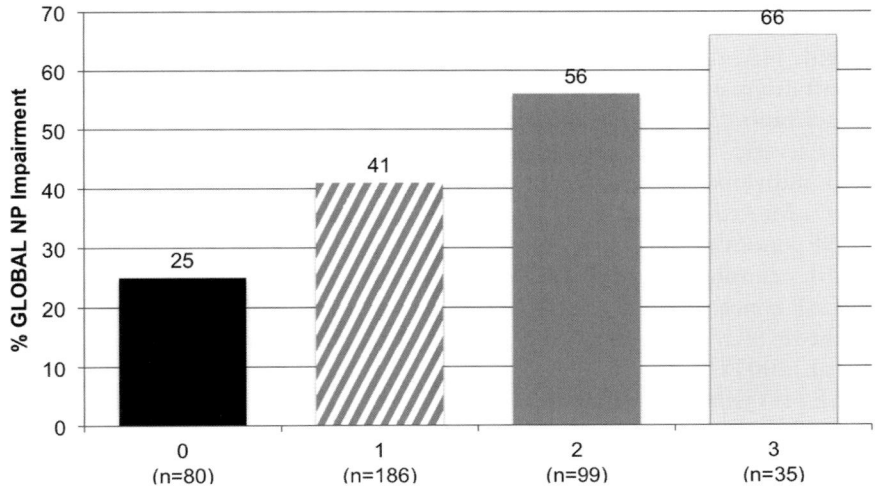

Figure 7.2.13 Rates of neurocognitive impairment by number of risk factors. The risk factors were HIV, HCV, and methamphetamine abuse.

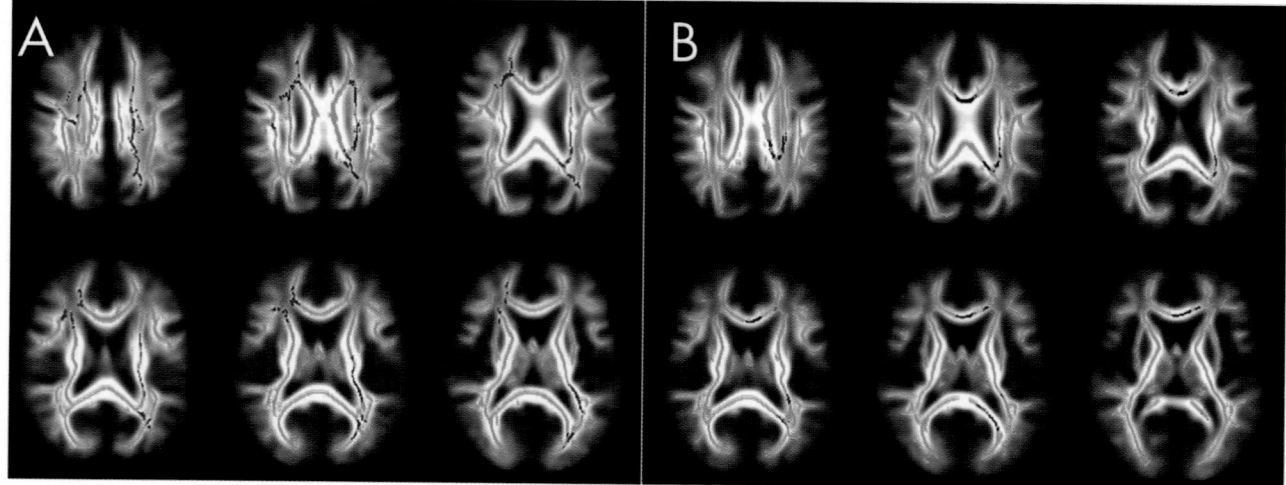

Figure 7.2.14 (A) Sample consecutive 5-mm slices showing voxels with significantly increased MD (in blue) in HIV+ participants with AIDS relative to seronegative participants, overlaid on white matter tract skeleton (green), and averaged FA image (grayscale). (B) Sample consecutive 5-mm slices showing voxels with significantly increased MD (in blue) in neurocognitively impaired relative to unimpaired HIV+ participants, overlaid on white matter tract skeleton (green), and averaged FA image (grayscale) MD = mean diffusivity; FA = fractional anisotropy.

increased activation in others (e.g., parietal, prefrontal and some frontal) in HIV+ individuals, suggesting hypofunction of some neural networks, accompanied by recruitment of others that might not usually come into play among unimpaired individuals (Maki et al., 2009; Chang et al., 2008; Melrose, Tinaz, Castelo, Courtney, & Stern, 2008). As with DTI, there have been some reports of fMRI changes in cognitively normal HIV+ individuals; for example, increased task-related activation of prefrontal and parietal areas (Ernst et al., 2009).

BIOMARKERS

No biomarker for HAND has yet entered clinical practice, although efforts are underway to develop a definitive biomarker. Those based on inflammatory byproducts are probably most likely to be promising, but further validation will be required before they can be used clinically (Price et al., 2007). In the absence of CART, CSF abnormalities are very common in individuals with HAND. These abnormalities include high CSF concentrations of HIV RNA, and elevated markers of immune activation. Concentrations of HIV RNA in CSF relate to the severity of neurological deficits only in CART-untreated individuals (Brew, Pemberton, Cunningham, & Law, 1997; McArthur et al., 1997), but in CART-treated patients CSF concentrations are not diagnostic and do not correlate with neurological status (McArthur et al., 2004). Decline in CSF concentrations of HIV RNA with CART relates with the reversal of neurological deficits (Ellis et al., 2000; Lee et al., 2003). Recent studies suggest that very low levels of CSF HIV RNA (less than 2 copies/ ml) may indicate persistent neurocognitive impairment (Best et al., 2009).

Various CSF markers of immune activation, or neuronal injury such as neopterin (Brew et al., 1990), β2 microglobulin (Brew et al., 1989), quinolinic acid (Heyes et al., 1991), and soluble Fas (Towfighi, Skolasky, St Hillaire, Conant, & McArthur, 2004), also relate with dementia severity but have not been validated adequately for clinical use. Other research markers including elevated sphingolipid products, indicative of oxidative stress, may indicate the continued activity of HIV-D (Haughey et al., 2004). Nitrosylated proteins, indicative of oxidative stress, also correlate with dementia severity (Li et al., 2008). Recently, the potentially harmful effects of gut-associated bacterial microbial products have been posited to play a role in CNS dysfunction. The translocation of these microbial products is indicated by elevated plasma levels of lipopolysaccharide (LPS), which in turn correlates with increased monocyte activation and HAND (Ancuta et al., 2008), and probably with impairment of the blood-brain barrier. Whether these products are directly injurious to the CNS is uncertain.

IMPLICATIONS OF HAND ON EVERYDAY FUNCTION

HIV, as any severe chronic illness, can be associated with reduced everyday functioning, including more unemployment, and in advanced disease, more need for help with activities of daily living. In regard to employment, multiple factors that include disease severity, psychological factors, socioeconomic status, and job discrimination can play into reduced workforce participation by persons with HIV (Braveman & Kielhofner, 2006). The introduction of CART has reduced disease-related unemployment, but this effect is most evident in better educated persons of higher social position (Dray-Spira, Gueguen, Ravaud, & Lert, 2007).

The contribution of HAND to disturbance in everyday functioning has received increasing attention (Gorman, Foley, Ettenhofer, Hinkin, & van Gorp, 2009). Although the degree of neurocognitive decrement found in persons with HIV tends to be mild, there is nevertheless significant impact on various measures of health related function. For example, Heaton et al. (1994) found that twice as many HIV+ people with HAND were unemployed compared to HIV+ non-HAND, and that neither mood changes nor several measures of severity of underlying disease accounted for this effect. Albert et al. (1995) reported that development of neurocognitive complications during a follow-up of HIV+ persons over an average of 4.5 years yielded a threefold increase in relative risk of reduced work hours, and confirmed that the neurocognitive effect could not be explained by other disease variables. The Dana Consortium (1996) also observed increased functional impairment in persons with minor cognitive motor disorder (MND in the Frascati classification). Neurocognitive impairments suggestive of frontal-subcortical dysfunction may contribute to employment difficulty (Twamley et al., 2006).

Increasingly, attempts are being made to apply various laboratory-based procedures to evaluate components of everyday function that may be disrupted by HAND. As an example, Heaton et al. (2004) deployed standardized functional evaluations that included laboratory measures of shopping, cooking, financial management, medication management, and vocational abilities. They observed that all of these indicators were affected in those with HAND, and that worse performance on measures of Abstraction/Executive Function, Learning, Attention/Working Memory and Verbal abilities most strongly and consistently predicted failures on the functional battery (Heaton et al., 2004). Similar results were reported in a pilot study of HIV+ Spanish-speaking persons (Mindt et al., 2003).

Automobile driving is another critical function in industrialized societies, and thus is receiving increased attention in relation to HAND. A series of studies by Marcotte and colleagues demonstrated that HIV+ persons with neurocognitive impairments were more likely to fail computer simulations of driving (Mindt et al., 2003; Marcotte et al., 1999) and that such failures were also related to on-road driving errors recorded by a driving instructor during actual driving (Marcotte et al., 2004). Disturbances in executive functioning were related to on-road driving impairments. Additionally, deficits in visual attention were associated with more accidents by history in the prior year (Marcotte et al., 2006).

Neurocognitive disorders associated with HIV can also reduce health-related quality of life; for example, as measured by the Quality of Well-Being (QWB) scale. As can be seen from Figure 7.2.15, there is a steady loss of quality-adjusted life-years in relation to increasing degree of neurocognitive impairment.

Additionally, neurocognitive impairment is associated with increased likelihood of mortality. This increased hazard of death applies not only to those who become frankly demented; for instance, Mayeux et al. (1993) reported earlier death in those who were neuropsychologically impaired but not demented. The HNRC group noted that diagnosis of mild neurocognitive disorder was associated with higher mortality risk. Also, when adjustments were made for disease indicators, those who were neurocognitively impaired, but did not meet criteria for MND, also had significantly reduced life expectancy (Ellis et al., 1996).

In summary, there are accumulating data to indicate that neurocognitive impairments are associated with reduced work efficiency, greater likelihood of unemployment, some reduction of health-related life quality, and earlier mortality.

NEUROCOGNITIVE STATUS OVER TIME

The temporal course of HAND is not clearly understood, with differing conclusions drawn from different studies. Data from large cohorts examined in the 1990s suggested that neurocognitive status remained relatively stable, with deteriorations seen primarily in those with advanced AIDS (Selnes et al., 1990; Selnes et al., 1992; Gastaut, Bolgert, & Brunet, 1990; Saykin et al., 1991; Helmstaedter, Hartmann, Niese, Brackmann, & Sass, 1992; Robertson et al., 1992; Whitt et al., 1993; Karlsen, Reinvang, & Froland, 1993). In contrast, observations from the HNRC cohorts suggested a more dynamic picture: Whereas about half of HIV+ individuals remained cognitively normal over a period of up to 8 years; of the remainder 11% were stably impaired; 18% improved from being initially impaired, and remained so; 19% had a course that fluctuated between impaired and unimpaired status; and only 4% underwent decline with no improvement on follow-up (see Figure 7.2.16). It remains to be seen if current CART, particularly with emphasis on long-term viral suppression, and perhaps use of more CNS-penetrating ARV, will modify this temporal pattern.

SUMMARY

Neurocognitive complications are common in HIV infection, manifesting most commonly as asymptomatic neurocognitive impairment or mild neurocognitive disorder, and less commonly as frank dementia. Current estimates are that

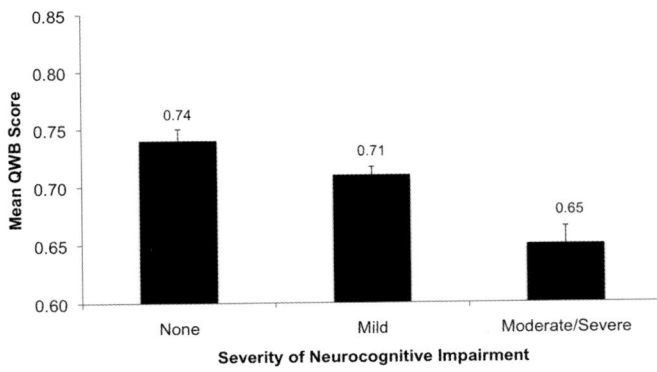

Figure 7.2.15 Quality of Well-Being (QWB) score by cognitive impairment severity. Note: Means (left to right) are based on baseline visits of 312, 186, and 75 HIV+ subjects respectively. The error bars shown are standard errors of the means. (From HNRC, unpublished data courtesy of Dr. Robert Kaplan).

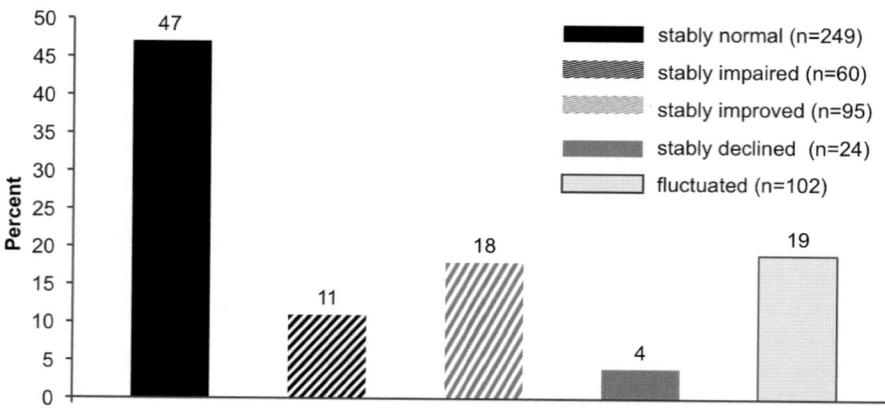

Figure 7.2.16 Neuropsychological course for neurocognitive states. In these data of HIV-infected persons followed up to 8 years by HNRC, 47% never manifested neurocognitive abnormality. Other patterns are as illustrated above.

in the context of CART fewer than 5% of individuals with AIDS will develop frank dementia and perhaps another 20–50% will develop lesser degrees of cognitive or motor dysfunction. Neurocognitive impairment is detected in perhaps a third of medically asymptomatic HIV-infected persons. Neurocognitive abnormalities in HIV reflect predominantly subcortical involvement, at least initially, with memory loss (i.e., learning difficulty), difficulties with speeded information processing, mental flexibility, and psychomotor slowing with disturbed motor control and incoordination in advanced cases. The development of sensitive and reliable neuropsychological test batteries now means that evolving neurocognitive impairment can be detected at a relatively early stage of HIV disease. Neurocognitive impairments detected in this manner predict presence of HIVE at autopsy, and may be related to injury of the synaptodendritic apparatus engendered by HIV products, host immune responses, or both. CART has reduced incidence of severe dementia, but milder forms of HAND persist, and, indeed, with long-term survival, its prevalence may be increasing in persons without traditional indicators of severe HIV disease such as severe immunosuppression or uncontrolled viremia. The factors contributing to HAND persistence in CART-treated persons are unclear, although experiencing more severe immunosuppression (e.g., CD4 < 200) at some point in time may be a risk. Subclinical immune reconstitution syndrome with systemic inflammatory response may be a factor in some cases where treatment has been associated with more, rather than less, neurocognitive impairment. As individuals with HIV survive into older age, there may be an acceleration of age-related neurological changes. Co-infection with HCV and drug abuse, particularly methamphetamine, may also contribute to impairment. Detection of HIV neurocognitive impairments may permit more timely initiation of neurologically directed therapies before irreversible neuronal damage and death have occurred. Such interventions may include use of ARV with better CNS penetration, or adjunctive neuroprotective treatments (e.g., lithium, SSRIs, statins, memantine, etc., have been speculated as possible agents). An important unanswered question is whether more aggressive ARV (e.g., beginning immediately when HIV infection is established, irrespective of CD4 or other criteria) may lessen likelihood of brain involvement that then persists as HAND.

ACKNOWLEDGMENTS

Support from the following awards assisted the authors in the preparation of this manuscript: MH62512 (HIV Neurobehavioral Research Center), DA26306 (Translational Methamphetamine AIDS Research Center), MH22005 (CNS HIV Anti-Retroviral Therapy Effects Research), and MH83506 (California NeuroAIDS Tissue Network), MH 71150 (Oxidative Stress Markers and HIV Dementia), MH 075673 (Center for Novel Therapeutics for HIV-associated Cognitive Disorders), NS 26643, RR00722, 73524, and the Charles A. Dana Foundation.

REFERENCES

Albert, S. M., Marder, K., Dooneief, G., Bell, K., Sano, M., Todak, G. et al. (1995). Neuropsychologic impairment in early HIV infection. A risk factor for work disability. *Arch Neurol*, 52, 525–30.

American Academy of Neurology AIDS Task Force. (1991). Nomenclature and research case definitions for neurologic manifestations of human immunodeficiency virus-type 1 (HIV-1) infection. Report of a Working Group of the American Academy of Neurology AIDS Task Force. *Neurology*, 41, 778–85.

Ancuta, P., Kamat, A., Kunstman, K. J., Kim, E. Y., Autissier, P., Wurcel, A., et al. (2008). Microbial translocation is associated with increased monocyte activation and dementia in AIDS patients. *Plos One*, 3, e2516.

Antinori, A., Arendt, G., Becker, J. T., Brew, B. J., Byrd, D. A., Cherner, M., et al. (2007). Updated research nosology for HIV-associated neurocognitive disorders. *Neurology*, 69, 1789–99.

Applebaum, A. J., Reilly, L. C., Gonzalez, J. S., Richardson, M. A., Leveroni, C. L. & Safren, S. A. (2009). The impact of neuropsychological functioning on adherence to HAART in HIV-infected substance abuse patients. *AIDS Patient Care STDS*, 23, 455–62.

Aylward, E. H., Henderer, J. D., McArthur, J. C., Brettschneider, P. D., Harris, G. J., Barta, P. E. et al. (1993). Reduced basal ganglia volume in

HIV-1-associated dementia: Results from quantitative neuroimaging. *Neurology*, 43, 2099–104.

Baum, M. K., Rafie, C., Lai, S., Sales, S., Page, B. & Campa, A. (2009). Crack-cocaine use accelerates HIV disease progression in a cohort of HIV-positive drug users. *J Acquir Immune Defic Syndr*, 50, 93–9.

Best, B. M., Letendre, S. L., Brigid, E., Clifford, D. B., Collier, A. C., Gelman, B. B., et al. (2009). Low atazanavir concentrations in cerebrospinal fluid. *AIDS*, 23, 83–87.

Bhaskaran, K., Mussini, C., Antinori, A., Walker, A. S., Dorrucci, M., Sabin, C., et al. (2008). Changes in the incidence and predictors of human immunodeficiency virus-associated dementia in the era of highly active antiretroviral therapy. *Ann Neurol*, 63, 213–21.

Braveman, B. & Kielhofner, G. (2006). HIV/AIDS and employment: the continuing challenge. *Work*, 27, 205–7.

Brew, B. J., Bhalla, R., Paul, M., Schwartz, M., & Price, R. W. (1989). CSF beta microglobulin as a marker of the presence and severity of AIDS dementia complex. *Conference on AIDS*. New York, NY.

Brew, B. J., Bhalla, R. B., Paul, M., Gallardo, H., Mcarthur, J. C., Schwartz, M. K., et al. (1990). Cerebrospinal-fluid neopterin in human-immunodeficiency-virus type-1 infection. *Annals of Neurology*, 28, 556–560.

Brew, B. J., Pemberton, L., Cunningham, P., & Law, M. G. (1997). Levels of human immunodeficiency virus type 1 RNA in cerebrospinal fluid correlate with AIDS dementia stage. *Journal of Infectious Diseases*, 175, 963–966.

Brodt, H. R., Kamps, B. S., Gute, P., Knupp, B., Staszewski, S. & Helm, E. B. (1997). Changing incidence of AIDS-defining illnesses in the era of antiretroviral combination therapy. *AIDS*, 11, 1731–8.

Cardenas, V., Meyerhoff, D., Studholme, C., Kornak, J., Rothlind, J., Lampiris, H., et al. (2009). Evidence for ongoing brain injury in human immunodeficiency virus-positive patients treated with antiretroviral therapy. *J Neurovirol*, 1–10.

Chang, L., Ernst, T., Speck, O., & Grob, C. S. (2005). Additive effects of HIV and chronic methamphetamine use on brain metabolite abnormalities. *Am J Psychiatry*, 162, 361–9.

Chang, L., Yakupov, R., Nakama, H., Stokes, B., & Ernst, T. (2008). Antiretroviral treatment is associated with increased attentional load-dependent brain activation in HIV patients. *J Neuroimmune Pharmacol*, 3, 95–104.

Chen, Y., An, H., Zhu, H., Stone, T., Smith, J. K., et al. (2009). White matter abnormalities revealed by diffusion tensor imaging in non-demented and demented HIV+ patients. *Neuroimage*, 47, 1154–62.

Cherner, M., Cysique, L., Heaton, R. K., Marcotte, T. D., Ellis, R. J., Masliah, E. et al. (2007). Neuropathologic confirmation of definitional criteria for human immunodeficiency virus-associated neurocognitive disorders. *J Neurovirol*, 13, 23–8.

Cherner, M., Ellis, R. J., Lazzaretto, D., Young, C., Mindt, M. R., Atkinson, J. H., et al. (2004). Effects of HIV-1 infection and aging on neurobehavioral functioning: preliminary findings. *AIDS*, 18 Suppl 1, S27–34.

Cherner, M., Letendre, S., Heaton, R. K., Durelle, J., Marquie-Beck, J., Gragg, B., et al. (2005). Hepatitis C augments cognitive deficits associated with HIV infection and methamphetamine. *Neurology*, 64, 1343–7.

Cole, M. A., Margolick, J. B., Cox, C., Li, X., Selnes, O. A., Martin, E. M., et al. (2007). Longitudinally preserved psychomotor performance in long-term asymptomatic HIV-infected individuals. *Neurology*, 69, 2213–20.

Corder, E. H., Robertson, K., Lannfelt, L., Bogdanovic, N., Eggertsen, G., Wilkins, J., et al. (1998). HIV-infected subjects with the E4 allele for APOE have excess dementia and peripheral neuropathy. *Nature Medicine*, 4, 1182–1184.

Cutler, R. G., Kelly, J., Storie, K., Pedersen, W. A., Tammara, A., Hatanpaa, K., et al. (2004). Involvement of oxidative stress-induced abnormalities in ceramide and cholesterol metabolism in brain aging and Alzheimer's disease. *Proceedings of the National Academy of Sciences of the United States of America*, 101, 2070–2075.

Dal Pan, G. J., McArthur, J. H., Aylward, E., Selnes, O. A., Nance-Sproson, T. E., Kumar, A. J., et al. (1992). Patterns of cerebral atrophy in HIV-1-infected individuals: results of a quantitative MRI analysis. *Neurology*, 42, 2125–30.

Dana Consortium on Therapy for HIV Dementia and Related Cognitive Disorders. (1996). Clinical confirmation of the American Academy of Neurology algorithm for HIV-1-associated cognitive/motor disorder. *Neurology*, 47, 1247–53.

Deutsch, R., Ellis, R. J., McCutchan, J. A., Marcotte, T. D., Letendre, S., Grant, I., et al. (2001). AIDS-associated mild neurocognitive impairment is delayed in the era of highly active antiretroviral therapy. *AIDS*, 15, 1898–9.

Dray-Spira, R., Gueguen, A., Ravaud, J. F., & Lert, F. (2007). Socioeconomic differences in the impact of HIV infection on workforce participation in France in the era of highly active antiretroviral therapy. *Am J Public Health*, 97, 552–8.

Ellis, R., Deutsch, R., Heaton, R. K., Marcotte, T., Nelson, J. A., Abramson, I., et al. (1996). Cognitive impairment is an independent risk factor for death in HIV infected individuals. *Neurology*, 46, A268.

Ellis, R. J., Childers, M. E., Cherner, M., Lazzaretto, D., Letendre, S., & Grant, I. (2003). Increased human immunodeficiency virus loads in active methamphetamine users are explained by reduced effectiveness of antiretroviral therapy. *J Infect Dis*, 188, 1820–6.

Ellis, R. J., Gamst, A. C., Capparelli, E., Spector, S. A., Hsia, K., Wolfson, T., et al. (2000). Cerebrospinal fluid HIV RNA originates from both local CNS and systemic sources. *Neurology*, 54, 927–936.

Ellis, R. J., Heaton, R. K., Letendre, S. L., Badiee, J., Munoz-Moreno, J., Vaida, F., et al. (2010). Higher CD4 nadir is associated with reduced rates of HIV-associated neurocognitive disorders in the CHARTER Study: Potential implications for early treatment initiation. *17th Conference on Retroviruses and Opportunistic Infections*. San Francisco, California.

Ernst, T., Yakupov, R., Nakama, H., Crocket, G., Cole, M., Watters, M., et al. (2009). Declined neural efficiency in cognitively stable human immunodeficiency virus patients. *Ann Neurol*, 65, 316–25.

Fama, R., Rosenbloom, M. J., Nichols, B. N., Pfefferbaum, A., & Sullivan, E. V. (2009). Working and episodic memory in HIV infection, alcoholism, and their comorbidity: baseline and 1-year follow-up examinations. *Alcohol Clin Exp Res*, 33, 1815–24.

Fein, G., Fletcher, D. J., & Di Sclafani, V. (1998). Effect of chronic alcohol abuse on the CNS morbidity of HIV disease. *Alcohol Clin Exp Res*, 22, 196S–200S.

Forton, D. M., Thomas, H. C., Murphy, C. A., Allsop, J. M., Foster, G. R., Main, J., et al. (2002). Hepatitis C and cognitive impairment in a cohort of patients with mild liver disease. *Hepatology*, 35, 433–9.

Gastaut, J. L., Bolgert, F., & Brunet, D. (1990). Early intellectual impairment in HIV seropositive patients. A longitudinal study (abstract). *Neurological and Neuropsychological Complications of HIV Infection*. Monterey, California.

Gongvatana, A., Schweinsburg, B. C., Taylor, M. J., Theilmann, R. J., Letendre, S. L., Alhassoon, O. M., et al. (2009). White matter tract injury and cognitive impairment in human immunodeficiency virus-infected individuals. *J Neurovirol*, 15, 187–95.

Gorman, A. A., Foley, J. M., Ettenhofer, M. L., Hinkin, C. H., & van Gorp, W. G. (2009). Functional consequences of HIV-associated neuropsychological impairment. *Neuropsychol Rev*, 19, 186–203.

Grant, I. & Atkinson, J. H. (1995). Psychiatric aspects of acquired immune deficiency syndrome. In: H. I. Kaplan & B. J. Sadock, (Eds.) *Comprehensive textbook of psychiatry*. 6th ed. Baltimore: Williams & Wilkins.

Gupta, J. D., Satishchandra, P., Gopukumar, K., Wilkie, F., Waldrop-Valverde, D., Ellis, R., et al. (2007). Neuropsychological deficits in human immunodeficiency virus type 1 clade C-seropositive adults from South India. *J Neurovirol*, 13, 195–202.

Hall, M., Whaley, R., Robertson, K., Hamby, S., Wilkins, J., & Hall, C. (1996). The correlation between neuropsychological and neuroanatomic changes over time in asymptomatic and symptomatic HIV-1-infected individuals. *Neurology*, 46, 1697–702.

Haughey, N. J., Cutler, R. G., Tamara, A., McArthur, J. C., Vargas, D. L., Pardo, C. A., et al. (2004). Perturbation of sphingolipid metabolism and ceramide production in HIV-dementia. *Annals of Neurology*, 55, 257–267.

Heaton, R. K., Clifford, D. B., Franklin, D. R., Woods, S. P., Ake, C., Vaida, F., et al. (2010). HIV-associated neurocognitive disorders

(HAND) persist in the era of potent antiretroviral therapy: The CHARTER Study. *Neurology*, 75, 2087–2096.

Heaton, R. K., Franklin, D. R., Ellis, R. J., McCutchan, J. A., Letendre, S. L., LeBlanc, S., et al. (2011). HIV-associated neurocognitive disorders before and during the era of combination antiretroviral therapy: Differences in rates, nature, and predictors. *Journal of Neurovirology*, 17, 3–16.

Heaton, R. K., Marcotte, T. D., Mindt, M. R., Sadek, J., Moore, D. J., Bentley, H., et al. (2004). The impact of HIV-associated neuropsychological impairment on everyday functioning. *J Int Neuropsychol Soc*, 10, 317–31.

Heaton, R. K., Velin, R. A., McCutchan, J. A., Gulevich, S. J., Atkinson, J. H., Wallace, M. R., et al. (1994). Neuropsychological impairment in human immunodeficiency virus-infection: Implications for employment. HNRC Group. HIV Neurobehavioral Research Center. *Psychosom Med*, 56, 8–17.

Helmstaedter, C., Hartmann, A., Niese, C., Brackmann, H. H., & Sass, R. (1992). Stage-independence and individual outcome of neuro-cognitive deficits in HIV. A follow-up study of 62 HIV-positive hemophilic patients. *Nervenarzt*, 63, 88–94.

Heyes, M. P., Brew, B. J., Martin, A., Price, R. W., Salazar, A. M., Sidtis, J. J., et al. (1991). Quinolinic acid in cerebrospinal-fluid and serum in HIV-1 infection: Relationship to clinical and neurological status. *Annals of Neurology*, 29, 202–209.

Hightower, G. K., Letendre, S. L., Cherner, M., Gibson, S. A., Ellis, R. J., Wolfson, T. J., et al. (2009). Select resistance-associated mutations in blood are associated with lower CSF viral loads and better neuropsychological performance. *Virology*, 394, 243–8.

Hilsabeck, R. C., Castellon, S. A., & Hinkin, C. H. (2005). Neuropsychological aspects of coinfection with HIV and hepatitis C virus. *Clin Infect Dis*, 41 Suppl 1, S38–44.

Hilsabeck, R. C., Perry, W., & Hassanein, T. I. (2002). Neuropsychological impairment in patients with chronic hepatitis C. *Hepatology*, 35, 440–6.

Hinkin, C. H., Barclay, T. R., Castellon, S. A., Levine, A. J., Durvasula, R. S., Marion, S. D., et al. (2007). Drug use and medication adherence among HIV-1 infected individuals. *AIDS Behav*, 11, 185–94.

Karlsen, N. R., Reinvang, I., & Froland, S. S. (1993). A follow-up study of neuropsychological function in asymptomatic HIV-infected patients. *Acta Neurol Scand*, 87, 83–7.

Lee, P. L., Yiannoutsos, C. T., Ernst, T., Chang, L., Marra, C. M., Jarvik, J. G., et al. (2003). A multi-center 1H MRS study of the AIDS dementia complex: validation and preliminary analysis. *J Magn Reson Imaging*, 17, 625–33.

Letendre, S., Marquie-Beck, J., Singh, K. K., de Almeida, S., Zimmerman, J., Spector, S. A., et al. (2004a). The monocyte chemotactic protein-1-2578G allele is associated with elevated MCP-1 concentrations in cerebrospinal fluid. *J Neuroimmunol*, 157, 193–6.

Letendre, S., Zheng, J., Yiannoutsos, C., Lopez, A., Ellis, R., Marquie-Beck, J., et al. (2004b). Chemokines correlate with cerebral metabolites on magnetic resonance spectroscopy: A substudy of ACTG 301 and 700. *11th Conference on Retroviruses and Opportunistic Infections*. San Francisco, CA.

Letendre, S. L., Cherner, M., Ellis, R. J., Marquie-Beck, J., Gragg, B., Marcotte, T., et al. (2005). The effects of hepatitis C, HIV, and methamphetamine dependence on neuropsychological performance: biological correlates of disease. *AIDS*, 19 Suppl 3, S72–8.

Li, W., Malpica-Llanos, T. M., Gundry, R., Cotter, R. J., Sacktor, N., McArthur, J., et al. (2008). Nitrosative stress with HIV dementia causes decreased L-prostaglandin D synthase activity. *Neurology*, 70, 1753–62.

Maj, M. (1990). Psychiatric aspects of HIV-1 infection and AIDS. *Psychol Med*, 20, 547–63.

Maki, P. M., Cohen, M. H., Weber, K., Little, D. M., Fornelli, D., Rubin, L. H., et al. (2009). Impairments in memory and hippocampal function in HIV-positive vs HIV-negative women: A preliminary study. *Neurology*, 72, 1661–8.

Marcotte, T. D., Heaton, R. K., Wolfson, T., Taylor, M. J., Alhassoon, O., Arfaa, K., et al. (1999). The impact of HIV-related neuropsychological

dysfunction on driving behavior. The HNRC Group. *J Int Neuropsychol Soc*, 5, 579–92.

Marcotte, T. D., Lazzaretto, D., Scott, J. C., Roberts, E., Woods, S. P., & Letendre, S. (2006). Visual attention deficits are associated with driving accidents in cognitively-impaired HIV-infected individuals. *J Clin Exp Neuropsychol*, 28, 13–28.

Marcotte, T. D., Wolfson, T., Rosenthal, T. J., Heaton, R. K., Gonzalez, R., Ellis, R. J., et al. (2004). A multimodal assessment of driving performance in HIV infection. *Neurology*, 63, 1417–22.

Mayeux, R., Stern, Y., Tang, M. X., Todak, G., Marder, K., Sano, M., et al. (1993). Mortality risks in gay men with human immunodeficiency virus infection and cognitive impairment. *Neurology*, 43, 176–82.

McArthur, J. C., McClernon, D. R., Cronin, M. F., NanceSproson, T. E., Saah, A. J., StClair, M., et al. (1997). Relationship between human immunodeficiency virus-associated dementia and viral load in cerebrospinal fluid and brain. *Annals of Neurology*, 42, 689–698.

McArthur, J. C., McDermott, M. P., McClernon, D., St Hillaire, C., Conant, K., Marder, K., et al. (2004). Attenuated central nervous system infection in advanced HIV/AIDS with combination antiretroviral therapy. *Archives of Neurology*, 61, 1687–1696.

McMurtray, A., Nakamoto, B., Shikuma, C., & Valcour, V. (2008). Cortical atrophy and white matter hyperintensities in HIV: The Hawaii Aging with HIV Cohort Study. *J Stroke Cerebrovasc Dis*, 17, 212–7.

Mehta, P., Gulevich, S. J., Thal, L. J., Jin, H., Olichney, J. M., McCutchan, J. A., et al. (1996). Neurological symptoms, not signs, are common in early HIV infection. *J NeuroAIDS*, 1(2), 67–85.

Mellins, C. A., Havens, J. F., McDonnell, C., Lichtenstein, C., Uldall, K., Chesney, M., et al. (2009). Adherence to antiretroviral medications and medical care in HIV-infected adults diagnosed with mental and substance abuse disorders. *AIDS Care*, 21, 168–77.

Melrose, R. J., Tinaz, S., Castelo, J. M., Courtney, M. G., & Stern, C. E. (2008). Compromised fronto-striatal functioning in HIV: An fMRI investigation of semantic event sequencing. *Behav Brain Res*, 188, 337–47.

Meyerhoff, D. J., MacKay, S., Sappey-Marinier, D., Deicken, R., Calabrese, G., Dillon, W. P., et al. (1995). Effects of chronic alcohol abuse and HIV infection on brain phosphorus metabolites. *Alcohol Clin Exp Res*, 19, 685–92.

Mindt, M. R., Cherner, M., Marcotte, T. D., Moore, D. J., Bentley, H., Esquivel, M. M., et al. (2003). The functional impact of HIV-associated neuropsychological impairment in Spanish-speaking adults: A pilot study. *J Clin Exp Neuropsychol*, 25, 122–32.

Mocroft, A., Katlama, C., Johnson, A. M., Pradier, C., Antunes, F., Mulcahy, F., et al. (2000). AIDS across Europe, 1994–98: The EuroSIDA study. *Lancet*, 356, 291–6.

Mohamed, M. A., Lentz, M. R., Lee, V., Halpern, E. F., Sacktor, N., Selnes, O., et al. (2010). Factor analysis of proton MR spectroscopic imaging data in HIV infection: Metabolite-derived factors help identify infection and dementia. *Radiology*, 254, 577–86.

Morgello, S., Estanislao, L., Ryan, E., Gerits, P., Simpson, D., Verma, S., et al. (2005). Effects of hepatic function and hepatitis C virus on the nervous system assessment of advanced-stage HIV-infected individuals. *AIDS*, 19 Suppl 3, S116–22.

Munoz-Moreno, J. A., Fumaz, C. R., Ferrer, M. J., Prats, A., Negredo, E., Garolera, M., et al. (2008). Nadir CD4 cell count predicts neurocognitive impairment in HIV-infected patients. *AIDS Res Hum Retroviruses*, 24, 1301–7.

Paul, R. H., Ernst, T., Brickman, A. M., Yiannoutsos, C. T., Tate, D. F., Cohen, R. A., et al. (2008). Relative sensitivity of magnetic resonance spectroscopy and quantitative magnetic resonance imaging to cognitive function among nondemented individuals infected with HIV. *J Int Neuropsychol Soc*, 14, 725–33.

Perry, W., Carlson, M. D., Barakat, F., Hilsabeck, R. C., Schiehser, D. M., Mathews, C., et al. (2005). Neuropsychological test performance in patients co-infected with hepatitis C virus and HIV. *AIDS*, 19 Suppl 3, S79–84.

Pfefferbaum, A., Adalsteinsson, E., & Sullivan, E. V. (2005). Cortical NAA deficits in HIV infection without dementia: Influence of alcoholism comorbidity. *Neuropsychopharmacology*, 30, 1392–9.

Pfefferbaum, A., Rosenbloom, M. J., Rohlfing, T., Adalsteinsson, E., Kemper, C. A., Deresinski, S., et al. (2006). Contribution of alcoholism to brain dysmorphology in HIV infection: effects on the ventricles and corpus callosum. *Neuroimage*, 33, 239–51.

Pfefferbaum, A., Rosenbloom, M. J., Rohlfing, T., Kemper, C. A., Deresinski, S., & Sullivan, E. V. (2009). Frontostriatal fiber bundle compromise in HIV infection without dementia. *AIDS*, 23, 1977–85.

Pillai, S. K., Pond, S. L., Liu, Y., Good, B. M., Strain, M. C., Ellis, R. J., et al. (2006). Genetic attributes of cerebrospinal fluid-derived HIV-1 env. *Brain*, 129, 1872–83.

Price, R. W. & Brew, B. J. (1988). The AIDS dementia complex. *J Infect Dis*, 158, 1079–83.

Price, R. W., Epstein, L. G., Becker, J. T., Cinque, P., Gisslen, M., Pulliam, L., et al. (2007). Biomarkers of HIV-1CNS infection and injury. *Neurology*, 69, 1781–1788.

Quasney, M. W., Zhang, Q., Sargent, S., Mynatt, M., Glass, J., & McArthur, J. (2001). Increased frequency of the tumor necrosis factor-alpha-308 A allele in adults with human immunodeficiency virus dementia. *Annals of Neurology*, 50, 157–162.

Raboud, J. M., Montaner, J. S., Rae, S., Kahn, J., Hammer, S. M., Katzenstein, D. A., et al. (1997). Meta-analysis of five randomized controlled trials comparing continuation of zidovudine versus switching to didanosine in HIV-infected individuals. *Antivir Ther*, 2, 237–47.

Rippeth, J. D., Heaton, R. K., Carey, C. L., Marcotte, T. D., Moore, D. J., Gonzalez, R., et al. (2004). Methamphetamine dependence increases risk of neuropsychological impairment in HIV-infected persons. *J Int Neuropsychol Soc*, 10, 1–14.

Robertson, K. R., Smurzynski, M., Parsons, T. D., Wu, K., Bosch, R. J., Wu, J., et al. (2007). The prevalence and incidence of neurocognitive impairment in the HAART era. *AIDS*, 21, 1915–21.

Robertson, K. R., Wilkins, J., Robertson, W., & Hall, C. (1992). Neuropsychological changes in HIV seropositive subjects over time: One and two year follow-up. (Abstract). *Neuroscience of HIV Infection: Basic and Clinical Frontiers*. Amsterdam.

Rosenbloom, M. J., Sullivan, E. V., Sassoon, S. A., O'Reilly, A., Fama, R., Kemper, C. A., et al. (2007). Alcoholism, HIV infection, and their comorbidity: Factors affecting self-rated health-related quality of life. *J Stud Alcohol Drugs*, 68, 115–25.

Ryan, E. L., Morgello, S., Isaacs, K., Naseer, M., & Gerits, P. (2004). Neuropsychiatric impact of hepatitis C on advanced HIV. *Neurology*, 62, 957–62.

Sacktor, N., Lyles, R. H., Skolasky, R., Kleeberger, C., Selnes, O. A., Miller, E. N., et al. (2001). HIV-associated neurologic disease incidence changes: Multicenter AIDS Cohort Study, 1990–1998. *Neurology*, 56, 257–60.

Sacktor, N., Nakasujja, N., Skolasky, R. L., Rezapour, M., Robertson, K., Musisi, S., et al. (2009). HIV subtype D is associated with dementia, compared with subtype A, in immunosuppressed individuals at risk of cognitive impairment in Kampala, Uganda. *Clin Infect Dis*, 49, 780–6.

Sailasuta, N., Shriner, K., & Ross, B. (2009). Evidence of reduced glutamate in the frontal lobe of HIV-seropositive patients. *NMR Biomed*, 22, 326–31.

Saykin, A. J., Janssen, R. S., Sprehn, G. C., Kaplan, J. E., Spira, T. J., & O'Connor, B. (1991). Longitudinal evaluation of neuropsychological function in homosexual men with HIV infection: 18-month follow-up. *J Neuropsychiatry Clin Neurosci*, 3, 286–98.

Selnes, O. A., McArthur, J. C., Royal, W., 3rd, Updike, M. L., Nance-Sproson, T., Concha, M., et al. (1992). HIV-1 infection and intravenous drug use: Longitudinal neuropsychological evaluation of asymptomatic subjects. *Neurology*, 42, 1924–30.

Selnes, O. A., Miller, E., McArthur, J., Gordon, B., Munoz, A., Sheridan, K., et al. (1990). HIV-1 infection: No evidence of cognitive decline during the asymptomatic stages. The Multicenter AIDS Cohort Study. *Neurology*, 40, 204–8.

Stout, J. C., Ellis, R. J., Jernigan, T. L., Archibald, S. L., Abramson, I., Wolfson, T., et al. (1998). Progressive cerebral volume loss in human immunodeficiency virus infection: A longitudinal volumetric magnetic resonance imaging study. HIV Neurobehavioral Research Center Group. *Arch Neurol*, 55, 161–8.

Taylor, M. J., Schweinsburg, B. C., Alhassoon, O. M., Gongvatana, A., Brown, G. G., Young-Casey, C., et al. (2007). Effects of human immunodeficiency virus and methamphetamine on cerebral metabolites measured with magnetic resonance spectroscopy. *J Neurovirol*, 13, 150–9.

Toussi, S. S., Joseph, A., Zheng, J. H., Dutta, M., Santambrogio, L., & Goldstein, H. (2009). Short communication: Methamphetamine treatment increases in vitro and in vivo HIV replication. *AIDS Res Hum Retroviruses*, 25, 1117–21.

Towfighi, A., Skolasky, R. L., St Hillaire, C., Conant, K., & McArthur, J. C. (2004). CSF soluble Fas correlates with the severity of HIV-associated dementia. *Neurology*, 62, 654–656.

Tozzi, V., Balestra, P., Bellagamba, R., Corpolongo, A., Salvatori, M. F., Visco-Comandini, U., et al. (2007). Persistence of neuropsychologic deficits despite long-term highly active antiretroviral therapy in patients with HIV-related neurocognitive impairment: Prevalence and risk factors. *J Acquir Immune Defic Syndr*, 45, 174–82.

Tozzi, V., Balestra, P., Lorenzini, P., Bellagamba, R., Galgani, S., Corpolongo, A., et al. (2005). Prevalence and risk factors for human immunodeficiency virus-associated neurocognitive impairment, 1996 to 2002: Results from an urban observational cohort. *J Neurovirol*, 11, 265–73.

Tucker, K. A., Robertson, K. R., Lin, W., Smith, J. K., An, H., Chen, Y., et al. (2004). Neuroimaging in human immunodeficiency virus infection. *J Neuroimmunol*, 157, 153–62.

Twamley, E. W., Narvaez, J. M., Sadek, J. R., Jeste, D. V., Grant, I., & Heaton, R. K. (2006). Work-related abilities in schizophrenia and HIV infection. *J Nerv Ment Dis*, 194, 268–74.

Valcour, V., Shikuma, C., Shiramizu, B., Watters, M., Poff, P., Selnes, O., et al. (2004a). Higher frequency of dementia in older HIV-1 individuals—The Hawaii Aging with HIV-1 Cohort. *Neurology*, 63, 822–827.

Valcour, V., Yee, P., Williams, A. E., Shiramizu, B., Watters, M., Selnes, O., et al. (2006). Lowest ever CD4 lymphocyte count (CD4 nadir) as a predictor of current cognitive and neurological status in human immunodeficiency virus type 1 infection—The Hawaii Aging with HIV Cohort. *J Neurovirol*, 12, 387–91.

Valcour, V. G., Shikuma, C. M., Watters, M. R., & Sacktor, N. C. (2004b). Cognitive impairment in older HIV-1-seropositive individuals: Prevalence and potential mechanisms. *AIDS*, 18 Suppl 1, S79–86.

Whitt, J. K., Hooper, S. R., Tennison, M. B., Robertson, W. T., Gold, S. H., Burchinal, M., et al. (1993). Neuropsychologic functioning of human immunodeficiency virus-infected children with hemophilia. *J Pediatr*, 122, 52–9.

World Health Organization. (1988). *Report on the consultation on the neuropsychiatric aspects of HIV infection*. Geneva: World Health Organization.

Wu, Z., Sullivan, S. G., Wang, Y., Rotheram-Borus, M. J., & Detels, R. (2007). Evolution of China's response to HIV/AIDS. *Lancet*, 369, 679–90.

Ying, L., Robinson, M., & Fu-jie, Z. (2009). Human immunodeficiency virus and hepatitis C virus co-infection: Epidemiology, natural history and the situation in China. *Chinese Medical Journal*, 122, 93–97.

7.3

THE CNS IN ACUTE AND EARLY INFECTION

Serena S. Spudich

The effect of HIV on the nervous system had been thought to become significant only years after systemic HIV infection occurs. However, around the time of HIV seroconversion, some individuals develop neurological signs and symptoms, and HIV has been documented in the cerebrospinal fluid and brain tissue early in the course of infection. The mechanisms involved in the central nervous system (CNS) response to initial infection, and the significance of early neuroinvasion for the natural history of CNS disease, establishment of a CNS reservoir of HIV, and the ultimate development of HIV-related neurological injury are only beginning to be understood. This chapter reviews what is known about the natural history and pathogenesis of systemic acute HIV and clinical neurological syndromes associated with seroconversion. The chapter also discusses more recent investigations into the relevance of early infection for the biological and neurocognitive aspects of HIV-related CNS disease.

INTRODUCTION

The effect of HIV in the nervous system has classically been thought to be significant only after many years of infection, paralleling the slow overt immunological decline which characterizes systemic disease (hence designation as a "lentivirus"). However, around the time of HIV seroconversion, a subgroup of individuals develop neurological signs and symptoms (Denning, 1988; Brew, 1989), and HIV has been documented in the cerebrospinal fluid and brain tissue in the first weeks to months after systemic HIV acquisition (Jones, 1988; Davis, 1992; Schacker, 1996; Pilcher, 2001). The mechanisms involved in the central nervous system response to initial infection, and the significance of this early neuroinvasion for the natural history of central nervous system infection, establishment of a central nervous system HIV reservoir, and the ultimate development of AIDS-related neurological injury are only beginning to be understood.

Following observations that acute simian immunodeficiency virus (SIV) infection causes very rapid massive infection and lysis of gut-associated lymphatic tissue, similar early loss of these lymphatics was recognized in human HIV infection (Schacker et al., 1996; Hecht, 2002; Veazey, 2004; Picker, 2006; Centlivre, 2007). In contrast to previously held assumptions that HIV was primarily latent in early infection and only led to immunodeficiency with the advent of CD4 T-cell decline in the blood, these recent findings have changed the focus to the first days and months of infection as crucial for viral pathogenesis. These studies have indicated that the rate of CD4 T cell decline is greatest during acute infection, critically impairing subsequent host immune control of HIV (Rosenberg, 2000; Walker, 2000; Davenport, 2006). The possibility that early treatment of patients during acute infection may preserve HIV-specific immune system responses has become a topic of intensive study (Kovacs, 2000; Rosenberg, et al. 2000; Khan, 2004; Guadalupe, 2006).

As a result, emphasis has recently been placed on evaluation of the virological and immunological events and effects of treatment during the early stages of infection, and on the consideration that the early entry of HIV into the nervous system may be a similarly seminal event, allowing for the establishment of autonomous infection which leads to the complications of HIV in the brain and spinal cord. A new focus on the effects of early HIV in the subsequent course of HIV infection has afforded insight and further opportunities for understanding the importance of acute and early infection for the central nervous system. This chapter reviews what is known about the natural history and pathogenesis of systemic acute HIV, clinical neurological syndromes associated with seroconversion, and more recent investigations into the relevance of early infection to the biological and neurocognitive aspects of HIV-related central nervous system disease.

BACKGROUND TO HIV IN THE CENTRAL NERVOUS SYSTEM

HIV-related nervous system injury has the potential to affect a significant portion of the 40 million infected individuals worldwide; long-term chronic exposure of the nervous system to HIV leads to overt HIV-associated dementia in 20–30% of untreated patients, both historically and in the current area where access to medications is limited (Navia, 1986; Wong, 2007). Though overall the incidence of opportunistic infections of the nervous system has greatly diminished in the current era, there is evidence that the central nervous system may be compromised in a large proportion of subjects chronically infected with HIV, even in the setting of antiretroviral therapy, which successfully suppresses systemic infection. A mild cognitive impairment is frequently detected in patients on successful antiretroviral therapy, which in some cases leads to impairment of quality of life and productive function (Sacktor, 2002; Heaton, 2004; Woods, 2009; Heaton, 2010). Central nervous system HIV infection is also associated with the establishment of a compartmentalized tissue reservoir that allows independent replication, mutation, and selection of viral quasispecies, with potential implications for systemic HIV disease progression and response to therapy. The early entry of HIV into the central nervous system may be a seminal event, allowing for the establishment of autonomous infection and coincident chronic inflammation which leads to HIV-related neurological complications.

OVERVIEW OF ACUTE AND EARLY INFECTION

Primary HIV infection is a term used to refer to the initial phase of infection, the first twelve months after exposure and inoculation. This period is further defined as either "acute infection" (before seroconversion and detection of antibodies to HIV), or "early/recent infection" (after seroconversion but within the first 12 months after infection) (Hecht et al., 2002; Stekler 2004; Zetola, 2007). Acute and early infection is characterized by a typical progression of initial exposure followed by a rapid and dramatic peak of HIV RNA in the plasma (Lindback, 2000a; Fiebig, 2003) which is associated with a clinical acute retroviral syndrome in a majority of individuals (Schacker et al. 1996; Hecht et al. 2002). This is accompanied by an increase in HIV antibody levels, detected by the fourth-generation enzyme immunosorbent assay (EIA) by day 21 after exposure, and a reduction of HIV RNA to a chronic stable level within months after exposure (Lindback et al., 2000a; Lindback, 2000b). The development of a less-sensitive EIA (LS-EIA) that requires higher levels of antibody to test fully reactive allows dating of HIV exposure which occurred within the previous 6 months in patients with positive standard serologies (Busch, 1995; Janssen, 1998; Kothe, 2003). Detection of a positive standard EIA and non-reactive LS-EIA is a well-established method of identifying recent infection (Hecht et al., 2002), which has been integrated into an overall framework for identification of recent infection, termed the Serologic Testing Algorithm for Recent HIV Seroconversion (STARHS) used in clinical studies worldwide (Murphy, 2008).

NATURAL HISTORY AND PATHOPHYSIOLOGY OF SYSTEMIC ACUTE AND EARLY HIV INFECTION

In the majority of cases of HIV transmission worldwide, systemic infection is initially established by HIV penetration through mucosal barriers. In the setting of mucosal invasion, initial infection involves only local target cells which display both the CD4 receptor and either CXC chemokine receptor 4 (CXCR4) or CC chemokine receptor 5 (CCR5), required for HIV entry (Royce, 1997). Replication within these cells leads to infection of local lymph nodes within three days and dissemination to widespread tissue compartments and blood within seven days (Zhang, 1999). In the ensuing three weeks, overwhelming infection of CD4+ memory T lymphocytes occurs throughout the body. CD4 memory T lymphocytes, predominantly housed in the gut-associated lymphoid tissue, undergo apoptosis or are the targets of killing by CD8+ cytotoxic T lymphocytes, reducing by over 80% the body's overall repository of this immune cell type during the first three to six weeks after HIV infection (Picker, 2006). Peripheral CD4+ T lymphocyte counts are reduced modestly during this period in most individuals, but not to a degree indicating the loss in overall body stores of CD4 T cells.

An abundance of CD4+ CCR5+ memory T lymphocytes available in the initial stages of infection and rapid unchecked viral replication leads to an immense increase in plasma viremia, peaking at 3–4 weeks after HIV exposure (Pilcher et al., 2001; Fiebig et al., 2003). While there is wide variability in plasma HIV RNA levels, systemic clinical syndromes, and immune responses during this period, many individuals manifest extremely high plasma viral loads, up to millions of viral particles per milliliter of blood. Besides the tremendous circulating blood viral burden at this point, dissemination of HIV into cellular components which serve as viral reservoirs is known to occur during this period (Finzi, 1997). An important target for infection are resting CD4+ memory T lymphocytes; a small proportion of these long-lived cells harbor HIV integrated within their chromosomes, serving as "long-lived" reservoirs for infection as they do not present surface viral particles and serve as targets for CD8+ cytotoxic T lymphocytes (Finzi, 1999).

Triggered in response to exponential viral replication, a cascade of host immune activation begins approximately two weeks after HIV exposure. This is characterized by migration of dendritic cells carrying viral particles to lymph nodes, recognition by naïve T lymphocytes, and subsequent differentiation of T lymphocytes into memory and effector cells, which are activated to perform functions ranging from cytotoxic killing, stimulation of other cells including macrophages, and secretion of cytokines that regulate further activation and expansion of cellular clones (Picker, 2006). In many pathological conditions, induction of such an immune cascade is an appropriate and effective adaptive immune response which fights and ultimately controls a microbe, but in HIV infection this process in most cases develops into a chronic, damaging response which is likely a critical determinant of systemic disease pathogenesis. In the acute and early period, the immune response is partially effective; induction of HIV-specific CD8+ T lymphocyte responses approximately four weeks after exposure contributes to the reduction in plasma HIV RNA levels observed at this point, though depletion of available target CD4+ T lymphocytes also slows the rate of viral replication (Koup, 1994; Letvin, 2003). A systemic plasma viral "set point" is commonly established by four to six months after exposure (Lindback et al., 2000a), though the level of this set-point varies greatly between individuals. The determinants of systemic viral set-point are not well understood, though there seem to be host genetic factors including variable responses based on specific HLA types (Kaslow, 1996).

Overall, by six months after infection, systemic features such as immune hyperactivation, viral load set-point, and to some extent CD4 trajectory, appear to be established, though immune responses may continue to evolve during this period. Peak systemic viral burden and dissemination to reservoirs, loss of CD4 memory T lymphocyte stores, and initiation of immune activation may all occur within the first six to eight weeks of infection, suggesting that many of the processes associated with long-term morbidity in HIV are established in the earliest stages of infection.

CLINICAL AND EPIDEMIOLOGICAL FEATURES OF ACUTE HIV INFECTION

SYSTEMIC ACUTE HIV INFECTION

To date, only a minority of individuals is diagnosed with HIV during the first year after initial infection. However, at least two-thirds of patients with HIV infection are estimated to experience a systemic acute retroviral syndrome, or overt clinical illness associated with the stages of viral invasion and immune activation/response to initial HIV infection (Schacker et al., 1996; Hecht et al., 2002). Typically occurring fourteen days after initial HIV exposure (Schacker et al., 1996; Lindback et al., 2000b), the syndrome is most often characterized by nonspecific signs and symptoms (see Table 7.3.1). Fever, fatigue, malaise, and anorexia occur in 70–90% of individuals with any clinical syndrome, and pharyngitis, diarrhea, nausea, and myalgias/arthralgias are experienced by approximately 50% of this group (Tindall, 1988; Schacker et al., 1996; Lindback et al., 2000b; Hecht et al., 2002). Mucous membrane apthous ulcers and a maculopapular rash on the torso and neck are typical dermatological manifestations. Focal and diffuse neurological symptoms may accompany, or more commonly follow, the onset of systemic illness in an estimated 10% of patients. Specific syndromes are discussed in detail below.

Table 7.3.1 CLINICAL FEATURES TYPICAL OF THE SYSTEMIC ACUTE HIV SEROCONVERSION SYNDROME

Fever

Fatigue

Pharyngitis

Lympadenopathy

Rash

Weight loss/loss of appetite

Diarrhea

Myalgias/arthralgias

Oral and genital ulcers

Nausea/vomiting

Headache

Night sweats

Many individuals experience multiple symptoms, though the constellation and severity of symptoms varies widely. Duration of illness usually ranges from 7 to 14 days, and in up to 90% of cases is severe enough to lead individuals to seek medical attention (Schacker et al., 1996; Kahn, 1998). In our experience, patients often describe the acute retroviral clinical syndrome as the most severe and prolonged illness they have experienced, associated often with pronounced fatigue and malaise. In one recent clinical study, only 17% of patients who sought medical attention for symptoms later identified as being those of the acute retroviral syndrome were diagnosed at presentation; more than half of this group had at least three visits before diagnosis was made. (Weintrob, 2003).

Unfortunately, standard methods of screening for HIV infection may miss the diagnosis during the earliest period of infection. Although the so-called "window-period" before antibody seroconversion has shortened considerably as the methods of detection have improved in sensitivity, there remains a period of four to six weeks in which current antibody tests, including rapid oral and blood tests, may be negative in a patient with early infection (Stekler, 2007; Stekler, 2009). Screening of all testing samples which are antibody negative with nucleic acid detection methods has been introduced in various clinical settings, using algorithms for broad screening, including pooled sample testing. These approaches have been associated with increased detection of acute infection (Zetola et al., 2007). However, these screening programs have not been widely instituted due to expense of the nucleic acid testing, delayed availability of results due to the pooling strategies and time for the polymerase chain reaction tests themselves, and limited patient and provider awareness of the value of detection of acute infection. Epidemiological data has suggested that the period of acute and early infection may be responsible for driving the HIV epidemic in areas of the Western and resource-limited world (Koopman, 1997; Wawer, 2005). This public health importance of identification of acute and early infection has led to a new focus on detection and perhaps treatment of acute infections in contexts where resources allow widespread screening.

CLINICAL NEUROLOGICAL SYNDROMES IN ACUTE HIV INFECTION

Clinical neurological manifestations in early infection have been well documented; a minority of patients with identified acute HIV infection manifests overt neurological signs and symptoms around the time of seroconversion (see Table 7.3.2). Many of these conditions have been described in clinical reports or case series, but the pathophysiology underlying these disorders has not been elucidated. "Aseptic" meningitis was one of the first neurological syndromes to be clearly linked to HIV (then HTLV-III) seroconversion, defined as either the presence of clinical signs of meningitis (Ho, 1985), or simply detection of a lymphocytic pleocytosis in the cerebrospinal fluid (De Caluwe, 1987). Mild to severe encephalopathy in the context of encephalitis or meningoencephalitis (Carne. 1985; Scarpini, 1991;

Table 7.3.2 REPORTED NEUROLOGICAL SYNDROMES
DURING ACUTE AND EARLY HIV INFECTION

Central Nervous System Disorders

- Aseptic meningitis (Ho, 1985; Caluwe, 1985)
- Encephalitis/Acute disseminated encephalomyelitis (Carne, 1985; Brew, 1989; Scarpini, 1991; Ben-Galim, 1996; Narciso, 2001; Newton, 2002; Meerseman, 2005; Douvoyiannis, 2009)
- Cerebellar ataxia (Scarpini, 1991)
- Myelopathy/Cauda equina syndrome (Denning, 1987; Zeman, 1991)
- Optic neuritis (Larsen, 1998)

Peripheral Nervous System Disorders

- Guillain-Barre syndrome/inflammatory polyneuropathy (Hagberg, 1986; Patton, 1990)
- Facial palsy (Piette, 1986; Krasner, 1993; Serrano, 2007)
- Peripheral neuritis (Calabrese, 1987; Brew,1989)
- Distal sensory polyneuropathy (Piette, 1986; Castellanos, 1994)

Ben-Galim, 1996; Douvoyiannis, 2009) as well as a clinical syndrome consistent with acute disseminated encephalomyelitis (Narciso, 2001; Mogensen, 2007) has been frequently described. Acute HIV infection should be sought in cases of acute unexplained neuropathies due to the frequency with which these develop in the context of seroconversion. Some individuals manifest cranial neuropathies including bilateral facial nerve paralysis (Calabrese, 1987; Hughes, 1992; Krasner, 1993; Serrano, 2007) or unilateral or bilateral optic neuritis (Larsen, 1998) in association with recent HIV infection. Acute inflammatory demyelinating peripheral neuropathies, brachial neuritis, meningoradiculitis, and ganglioneuronitis (Hagberg, 1986; Piette, 1986; Paton, 1990; Castellanos, 1994) may also occur. Acute myelopathy and cauda equina syndrome have been described in the literature and may be associated with lasting neurological sequelae (Denning, 1987; Zeman, 1991). Headaches or mood disorders occur in the majority of patients who have any systemic

symptoms of seroconversion (Tindall, 1989; Hecht et al., 2002; Taiwo, 2002; Aggarwal, 2003; Stekler, 2004).

Common features among these neurological syndromes are the typical time of onset of neurological symptoms (usually one to three weeks following initial development of fever/systemic symptoms and signs) (Denning, 1988), the typical self-limited nature of the clinical signs and symptoms, and their almost exclusive occurrence in the setting of a systemically symptomatic seroconversion. Figure 7.3.1 shows a timeline of the typical natural history of clinical and laboratory events during acute and early HIV infection. The spectrum of neurological conditions typically seen during this period is notably heterogeneous—the unifying link between the reported syndromes being that they are all neurological conditions which may occur as primarily autoimmune phenomena. The combination of the spectrum of clinical syndromes, their timing of onset, and their typical resolution without specific therapy suggests an abnormal host-mediated autoimmune etiology rather than a specific reaction to HIV-infection itself. The high level of systemic and central nervous system immune activation characterizing acute HIV infection plausibly serves as a substrate for immunologically mediated disorders of the nervous system in this context.

RHESUS MACAQUE MODELS OF HUMAN ACUTE HIV INFECTION IN THE NERVOUS SYSTEM

BACKGROUND TO SIV RHESUS MACAQUE MODELS OF NEUROAIDS

Human studies of individuals with acute infection have been historically difficult due to limited diagnosis and identification of patients during acute infection, and lack of confirmation of timing of infection in patients in the early but not acute stages. Use of a rhesus macaque model to investigate the early events in the nervous system after infection with simian

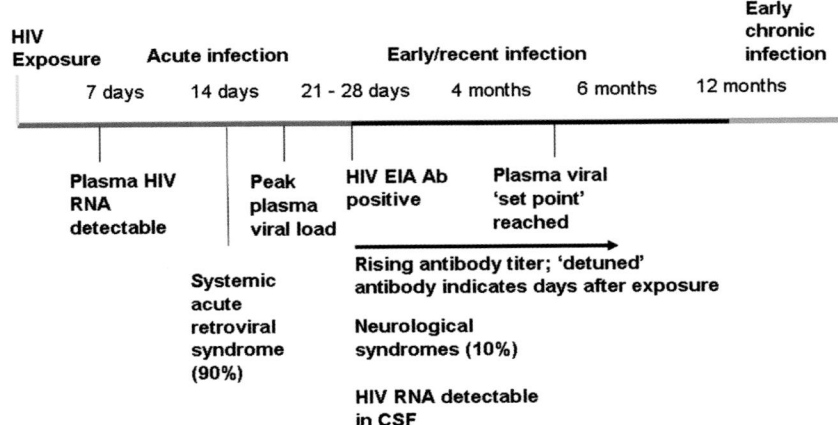

Figure 7.3.1 Timeline of Clinical and Laboratory Events in Acute and Early HIV Infection.

immunodeficiency virus (SIV) has contributed considerably to an understanding of the response of the primate nervous system to viral neuroinvasion. SIV shares significant homology with HIV and is associated in the macaque with similar clinical features both in terms of development of systemic immunosuppression and of encephalitis and cognitive and motor deficits in a proportion of chronically infected animals (Franchini, 1987; Lackner, 1991a; Murray, 1992). The macaque model allows for study of measures that parallel those used in human studies including cerebrospinal fluid markers and concentrations of cerebral metabolites as detected by magnetic resonance spectroscopy, as well as affords essentially unique studies of brain pathology in acute and early infection. Typical macaque SIV infection is similar to human HIV in that only 25% of infected animals develop overt dementia and associated encephalitis, the severity and time course of the disease is variable, and in most cases disease takes up to three years to develop (Westmoreland, 1998). Thus, investigators have used CD8+ lymphocyte depletion and neurovirulent strains to develop accelerated models of neuroAIDS that parallel human infection with HIV with a more rapid and inexorable course of encephalitis (Gold, 1998; Zink, 1999; Gonzalez, 2000; Williams, 2001; Clements, 2002; Mankowski, 2002; Nesbit, 2002; Barber, 2004).

PATHOPHYSIOLOGY OF ACUTE SIV IN THE CENTRAL NERVOUS SYSTEM IN THE RHESUS MACAQUE

The SIV macaque model has demonstrated that macrophages are a major target for SIV in the bone marrow and similarly in the central nervous system, and are a key means of viral entry across the blood-brain barrier (Kitagawa, 1991; Lackner, 1991b; Williams et al., 2001). Lymphocytes also appear to play a major role in trafficking into and persistently maintaining SIV infection within the primate nervous system (Stephens, 1995; Zhu, 1995). Viral invasion into the nervous system occurs within the first two weeks of infection, manifested by the presence of viral RNA in multiple areas of brain tissue as well as in cerebrospinal fluid (Smith, 1995; Lane, 1996). This neuroinvasion is associated with inflammatory T-cell reactions, cytokine production, microglial proliferation, and upregulation of genes involved in inflammatory pathways (Barber et al., 2004; Roberts, 2004; Witwer, 2009). Thus, neuroinflammation, which is directly associated with neurodegeneration in the primate brain, appears to be initiated by early entry of SIV (Bissel, 2002; Orandle, 2002). Clinically, the acute retroviral syndrome in macaques is associated not only with elevated body temperature but also with a profound decrease in motor activity; these behavioral changes last beyond the acute retroviral syndrome and are accompanied by abnormalities in sensory-evoked responses on electrophysiological testing (Horn, 1998).

The SIV macaque model has also allowed the identification of cerebrospinal fluid markers which have value when measured early in the disease course for prediction of development of later neurological disease. Levels of interleukin-6

(IL-6), monocyte chemoattractant protein-1 (MCP-1), and SIV RNA measured in the cerebrospinal fluid at day 28 after HIV inoculation have been significantly associated with the later development of severe SIV-associated central nervous system disease in a study of 18 macaques (Mankowski, 2004). These data support the concept that central nervous system immune responses are persistently active in some animals during the "asymptomatic" early period of infection and that such activation of the immune system is associated with later overt neurological injury. However, in this study, IL-6, MCP-1, and SIV RNA were elevated in all animals during acute infection, including four animals that did not eventually proceed to developing severe neurological disease. Such findings suggest that a prolonged abnormal neuroimmune activation which is sustained during the transition from acute to chronic infection may be a necessary substrate for development of neurological disease.

MAGNETIC RESONANCE SPECTROSCOPY DETECTION OF ACUTE SIV INFECTION-ASSOCIATED INFLAMMATION AND INJURY

In vivo magnetic resonance spectroscopy imaging techniques which noninvasively detect biochemical and physiological changes in the brain have been used to investigate early events in the macaque brain after infection with SIV. Typical findings in humans with the neuroasymptomatic chronic HIV infection include elevated choline and myoinositol (or elevated choline or myoinositol ratios relative to the standard, creatine) in subcortical white and gray matter (Cecil, 1998; Meyerhoff, 1999; Kivisakk, 2003; Boska, 2004), thought to reflect inflammatory processes or reactive gliosis. In the setting of late-stage disease, often accompanied by neurological signs and cognitive impairment, low cortical and subcortical n-acetylacetate (and n-acetylacetate ratios) are detected, reflective of neuronal injury (Meyerhoff, 1993; Meyerhoff, 1994; Kivisakk et al., 2003). In 15 macaques acutely infected through peripheral vein injection with SIV, by 11 days post inoculation, dramatic increases in choline and myoinositol ratios were detected in frontal gray matter, during the period of peak plasma viral load (Fuller 2004). By 13 days post infection, inflammatory metabolites were less prominent, but a mild decrease in n-acetylacetate ratios was observed, suggesting neuronal injury. At 27 days post infection, inflammation and neuronal markers had normalized except for a decrease in choline ratios, an unusual finding previously detected in human hepatic encephalopathy. These changes in cerebral metabolites suggesting initial inflammation followed by persistent abnormalities correlate with pathology findings in SIV macaques sacrificed early after SIV inoculation (Gonzalez et al., 2000; Clements et al., 2002). Though the SIV macaque model may be limited in generalizability to humans given the accelerated neuroAIDS disease model and the different primate species, these models suggest that initial infection with HIV might be associated with similar inflammatory changes and possibly associated neuronal damage in the brain during the early weeks or months after infection.

CENTRAL NERVOUS SYSTEM VIRAL COMPARTMENTALIZATION DURING EARLY SIV INFECTION

One of the central issues of HIV infection of the nervous system is the fact that it may be compartmentalized or isolated from that of systemic infection. Genetic comparisons of cerebrospinal fluid- and brain-derived viruses with those from plasma have shown sequence divergence in viral genes, including genes important to both chemokine coreceptor tropism and drug resistance, likely due to the presence of different selective pressures on HIV replication in the cerebrospinal fluid and periphery (Chiodi, 1989; Korber, 1994; O'Brien, 1994; Brew, 1996; Di Stefano, 1996a; Di Stefano, 1996b; Wong, 1997; Cunningham, 2000). However, what has been previously unknown is when central nervous system compartmentalization and presumably autonomous brain infection is established during the course of HIV. The heteroduplex tracking assay has been used to monitor evolution of HIV species in humans (Nelson, 1997; Ping, 1999) and has demonstrated compartmentalization of feline immunodeficiency (FIV) species in cerebrospinal fluid as compared to plasma within the first two months of infection (Liu, 2006). This approach has recently been utilized in an SIV macaque model to characterize viral genetic populations in plasma and cerebrospinal fluid in a longitudinal manner (Harrington, 2007). Using the heteroduplex tracking assay targeting the V1/V2 region of env, viral genetic populations in paired plasma and cerebrospinal fluid were characterized every two to four weeks throughout the course of infection in three macaques intravenously infected with SIVsm E660. In two macaques, genetic env populations in cerebrospinal fluid mirrored those in plasma at all sample time-points. In a third macaque, genetic env populations in cerebrospinal fluid permanently diverged from those in plasma by 31 days post infection, which preceded any detectable change in the plasma env population structure. This compartmentalized cerebrospinal fluid pattern was associated with elevated cerebrospinal fluid levels of the inflammatory marker MCP-1 and substantial brain macrophage infiltration on autopsy. Thus, variants that are unique to cerebrospinal fluid relative to plasma may emerge in primates during the first months of SIV infection, and such compartmentalization arises in the context of central nervous system inflammation (Harrington et al., 2007).

STUDIES OF THE HUMAN NERVOUS SYSTEM IN ACUTE AND EARLY HIV INFECTION

BRAIN PATHOLOGY DURING ACUTE AND EARLY HIV INFECTION

Pathological studies of the brain during the earliest stages after HIV exposure have been limited by availability of central nervous system tissues during acute and early infection (Gray, 1996). A few unique cases of acute HIV reveal brain pathology that may occur during an overwhelming, severe response to initial HIV infection. In one case, presumed acute infection (as indicated by multiple negative HTLV-III antibody tests in the context of HIV cultured from cerebrospinal fluid and brain tissue), was associated with cerebral angiitis resulting in narrowing of large and medium intracranial vessels with subsequent infarction in the basal ganglia and cerebral white matter led to severe encephalopathy and death (Yankner, 1986). The brain at autopsy showed widespread central nervous system angiitis with infiltration of mononuclear cells through all layers of large and medium-sized vessel walls. Few microglial nodules and multinucleated giant cells were identified, implying a distinct mechanism from the classic long-term changes of HIV encephalitis. In another case, an encephalopathy developed suddenly eight days after onset of a likely acute retroviral syndrome, resulting in coma within one day of neurological presentation and death within five days (Jones et al., 1988). Though a cerebrospinal fluid during life revealed a pleocytosis indicating inflammation, on autopsy, the brain parenchyma showed no vasculitis, macrophage or lymphocyte infiltration, nor multinucleated cells or microglial nodules. Instead, the tissue showed evidence of myelin pallor with some associated neuronal damage, suggesting acute demyelination. In another case, fatal widespread cortical necrosis of both cerebral hemispheres in the setting of confirmed HIV antibody seroconversion, occurring two weeks after a syndrome of fever, rash, and diarrhea, appeared to be mediated not by direct viral invasion of the brain, but instead by a widespread inflammatory response leading to perivenous infiltrates and cortical ischemia (Meersseman, 2005). Finally, a singular case of acute iatrogenic HIV infection by intravenous inoculation of infected white blood cells resulting in rapid overwhelming hepatorenal syndrome and death showed autopsy evidence of HIV nucleic acid and proviral DNA by day 15 after infection within the cerebral cortex (Davis, 1992). Rare cells infiltrating the perivascular and subpial spaces stained positive for gp41, and perivascular collections of mononuclear cells were present. This case may not be representative of typical mucous membrane transmission of HIV given the direct inoculation of an unusually high viral titer, but suggests that at least in some cases, HIV can populate the brain parenchyma itself within two weeks of systemic infection.

NEUROIMAGING DURING ACUTE AND EARLY HIV INFECTION

Imaging studies of patients during the earlier stages of HIV infection have been almost exclusively limited to asymptomatic HIV-infected individuals with chronic HIV infection. Various observational studies have detected global cerebral atrophy, cortical thinning, and evidence of cerebral inflammation on magnetic resonance spectroscopy in HIV-infected patients without symptoms evaluated before the advent of overt immunosuppression (Lopez-Villegas, 1997; Thompson, 2005). However, recent investigations have focused upon potential neuroimaging abnormalities in subjects around the time of seroconversion or shortly thereafter.

While little is known of the imaging characteristics of the central nervous system during acute and early infection, we hypothesized that in PHI subjects, abnormalities might be detected by high-field (4 Tesla) brain MRI and include T2 FLAIR abnormalities indicating inflammation or edema. We employed high-field (4 Tesla) brain MRI to examine brain MRI images in 28 individuals assessed at a median of three months after HIV infection (Ho, 2010). Only four of these subjects had discrete neurological symptoms during seroconversion (Guillain-Barré-like syndrome and facial palsy in one each and right arm pain/tingling in two). Neuroradiologists described and quantitated white matter abnormalities, atrophy, amd ventricular and sulcal enlargement. Only 54% of subjects had normal high-field brain imaging for age. Examples of representative abnormalities detected on neuroimaging are shown in Figure 7.3.2. White matter lesions were the predominant abnormality detected, and the prevalence of perivascular spaces was twice as high in patients as in controls.

Although nonspecific, punctuate white matter lesions could feasibly represent an acute inflammatory, ischemic, or demyelinating process related to early central nervous system exposure to HIV. Alternatively, these could reflect the presence of underlying comorbidities, including substance abuse.

In parallel with ongoing studies of the acute effects of SIV in the macaque model of neuroAIDS, Lentz and colleagues used 1.5 Tesla brain magnetic resonance imaging to identify cerebral metabolic abnormalities in eight individuals presenting within two months of seroconversion (Lentz, 2009). A comparison was made between absolute cerebral metabolite concentrations measured in two brain regions between subjects with recent infection (mean age of 39), those with chronic infection, and nine HIV-uninfected controls (mean age of 32). In the frontal cortex, lower concentrations of n-acetylacetate and combined glutamine and glutamate metabolites, putative neuronal markers, were measured in the early infection group as compared to the HIV-uninfected group.

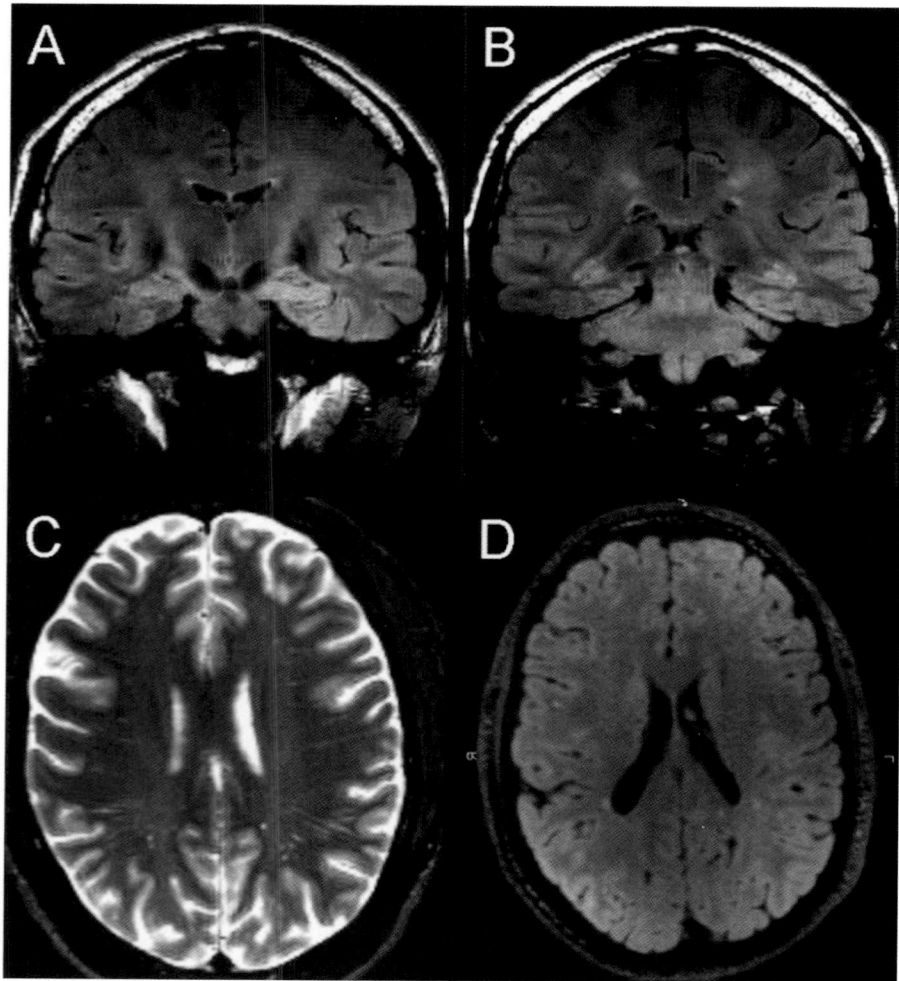

Figure 7.3.2 MRI images of cerebral abnormalities found in individuals with acute and early HIV infection. A & B) Diffuse white matter abnormalities in the basal ganglia and internal capsule on T2 FLAIR imaging in a 35-year-old man obtained 69 days after estimated HIV exposure. This subject had mononucleosis symptoms but no discrete neurological symptoms at the time of HIV seroconversion. C) Perivascular white matter hyperintensities identified on T2 imaging obtained 150 days after initial HIV infection in a 37-year-old man who presented with pharyngitis and rash at the time of HIV seroconversion. D) Initial scan in a 25-year-old man obtained 53 days after HIV infection who had cough and gastrointestinal symptoms at the time of seroconversion, showing multiple hyperintense foci in the deep WM of the frontal and parietal lobes on FLAIR imaging. Follow up scan one year after the initial imaging showed resolution of hyperintense lesions (Ho et al., 2010).

Chronically HIV-infected patients showed these differences as well as decreased n-acetylacetate in the centrum semiovale white matter. No changes in inflammatory or glial markers were noted. Since the finding of reduced n-acetylacetate may be influenced by the relatively older age of the primary infection subjects, larger studies are needed with age-matched subject groups and longitudinal follow-up to investigate the natural history of metabolite changes detected during early infection. However, detection of lower n-acetylacetate in the frontal white matter during early infection is suggestive of neuronal dysfunction or injury, which might be consistent with the high prevalence of aseptic meningitis and neurological symptoms in the subject group, or the effects of central nervous system dysfunction in the context of HIV seroconversion more generally.

CLINICAL LABORATORY STUDIES OF ACUTE AND EARLY HIV INFECTION IN THE CENTRAL NERVOUS SYSTEM

A small number of previous clinical laboratory studies have focused on the central nervous system effects of acute and early HIV infection in human subjects, mainly involving relatively small case series. One study comparing subjects with and without systemic symptoms of an acute retroviral syndrome around seroconversion demonstrated that neurocognitive impairment progressed more rapidly in those with any systemic symptoms (Wallace, 2001). No HIV viral load information was available to compare possible difference in viral burden between the two study groups, but potentially higher plasma HIV RNA levels, which directly correlate with the risk of an acute retroviral syndrome, were related to the more rapid development of neurological disease witnessed in the symptomatic group. Two studies have specifically investigated central nervous system involvement in the setting of acute and early HIV infection through neurological and cerebrospinal fluid examinations (Enting, 2001; Tambussi, 2002). In 22 subjects tested within two months after the onset of the acute retroviral syndrome, 11 subjects with neurological symptoms (including severe headache) had a higher cerebrospinal fluid HIV RNA level compared with a group with only fever or other systemic symptoms (Tambussi, 2002). A separate study longitudinally followed six individuals who initiated a five-drug antiretroviral regimen during the first six months after HIV infection (Enting, 2001). HIV RNA was detected in the cerebrospinal fluid in five of the six subjects at baseline. HIV RNA levels significantly declined after eight weeks of antiretroviral therapy, in parallel with initially elevated levels of cerebrospinal fluid beta-2-microglobulin, a marker of cellular immune activation. One subject with a quite elevated initial cerebrospinal fluid viral load still had not cleared HIV RNA from his cerebrospinal fluid when reevaluated at 48 weeks. In an observational study of HIV RNA levels in body fluids, five early infection subjects who underwent cerebrospinal fluid sampling had baseline cerebrospinal fluid HIV RNA levels significantly higher than historical controls with chronic infection (Pilcher et al. 2001). All five subjects had undetectable cerebrospinal fluid HIV

RNA levels six months after initiating antiretroviral therapy. Finally, in a study investigating neuroimmune activation during different stages of HIV infection, three subjects with acute infection (all within two weeks of onset of a clinical seroconversion syndrome) had elevated cerebrospinal fluid levels of beta-2-microglobulin and neopterin (a pteridine biomarker of macrophage activation) compared with historical controls, and also higher than those detected in blood (Sonnerborg 1989). One of these subjects had profound meningeal inflammation in the context of clinical aseptic meningitis, but the two others were neurologically asymptomatic. These findings, supported by our observations in a larger cohort (Spudich, 2011), demonstrate that central nervous system immune activation may be triggered in the very early stages of HIV infection, similar to the pattern seen in acute SIV in the rhesus macaque. Furthermore, such inflammatory processes are evident in subjects even in the absence of overt neurological symptoms or signs, suggesting that infection and immune dysregulation within the central nervous system are ubiquitous features of systemic HIV infection, even in individuals without clinical indicators of neurological disease.

To examine determinants of the HIV burden within the central nervous system during acute and early infection, we combined baseline data available from four study sites to identify the main predictors determining baseline HIV RNA levels in cerebrospinal fluid obtained from 96 subjects within the first six months after HIV exposure (Spudich, 2011). A multivariable model with cerebrospinal fluid HIV RNA level as the outcome included blood CD4 and CD8 count, plasma HIV RNA level, cerebrospinal fluid white blood cell count, and cerebrospinal fluid protein as possible predictors. In this simple model, levels of HIV RNA in the cerebrospinal fluid during acute and early infection were most strongly determined by plasma HIV in subjects with and without neurological symptoms. Both cerebrospinal fluid pleocytosis and cerebrospinal fluid protein were also independently associated with cerebrospinal fluid viral burden during this early period (Spudich et al., 2011).

Though a number of studies document the presence of HIV within the central nervous system very early during the course of infection, an essential remaining question is whether this presence of HIV and the neuroinflammation that may be associated with early and acute infection causes any damage to the nervous system during this early stage of disease. Measurement of cerebrospinal fluid neural markers, which, if elevated, provide an index of active neuronal breakdown, provides a window into potentially "subclinical" brain injury. Recently, Abdulle and colleages have shown that cerebrospinal fluid levels of the light subunit of neurofilament protein, while profoundly elevated (up to 10,000 nanograms per liter) in patients with HIV-associated dementia and also high in some untreated patients with neuroasymptomatic HIV infection, were slightly abnormal (ranging in value from 400–1900 nanograms/liter) in 4 of 16 subjects evaluated within three months of acquisition of HIV (Abdulle, 2007). Although the clinical significance of mild elevations in neurofilament protein levels is unknown, these findings suggest that a subset of individuals may sustain active injury to neurons during the period of early infection.

NEUROBEHAVIORAL EFFECTS OF ACUTE AND EARLY HIV INFECTION

Early in the HIV epidemic, a typical combination of cognitive, motor, and behavioral deficits was identified in infected subjects which was referred to as the AIDS dementia complex (now termed HIV-associated dementia) (Price, 1988; Price, 1990). Recently, a broader range of neurocognitive disorders has been identified as associated with HIV infection, including milder forms of disease. The use of neuropsychological testing in specific domains has been extensively validated for detection of cognitive impairment in HIV infection, indicating some degree of cognitive impairment in 35% of HIV-positive subjects in a meta-analysis of 57 studies (Dube, 2005). It is not presently understood whether the central nervous system effects of the earliest stages of HIV infection have a direct impact upon cognition and neurological function in subjects who have no overt neurological manifestations of disease. Subjects with very recent HIV infection have been shown to have a high prevalence of mood disorders, including depression, anxiety, and bipolar affective disorder (Atkinson, 2009). It is clear that in some cases these affective conditions were pre-morbid and directly influenced the risk of acquiring HIV. However, it is unclear whether the central nervous system effects of HIV itself may initiate or worsen mood disorders.

Recent investigations have suggested that patients with acute and early HIV infection have performance below age- and education-adjusted normative values on cognitive and motor aspects of neuropsychological testing (Moore, et al., 2011; Peterson, 2010) including both performance on comprehensive evaluations and on limited testing batteries with a strong emphasis on motor performance. A study involving a detailed neuropsychological assessment of seven cognitive domains in subjects assessed within one year of HIV infection, subjects with chronic HIV infection, and HIV-negative controls (Moore et al., 2011) demonstrated minimally worse global performance in subjects with recent infection as compared to HIV-negative controls. However, the recent infection group showed significantly worse performance than controls in the specific domain of learning. Though this effect was far less than that observed in the subjects with chronic infection, it indicates that there may be distinguishing features and circumscribed domains of cognitive impairment during the earliest stages of HIV infection. The presence of antiretroviral treatment (more common in the chronic infection group, but also characterizing some subjects in the early infection group) was a determinant of neuropsychological performance, suggesting that in the absence of treatment, additional abnormalities might be evident during the early stages of infection.

In an independent study, we performed neuromedical and laboratory assessments including neuropsychological testing in 37 antiretroviral-naïve individuals evaluated at a median of three and a half months after acquisition of HIV to assess for the presence and mediators of neurocognitive impairment

during this period (Peterson et al., 2010). Assessment of impairment was summarized as the NPZ4 (timed gait, grooved pegboard, nondominant finger tapping, and digit symbol). At baseline, 65% of subjects had evidence of impairment (greater than one standard deviation below the mean) on one or more NPZ4 tests. Proportions of subjects with impairment on one or more tests are shown in Figure 7.3.3. Whether this impairment reflects pre-morbid factors or an effect of HIV in the nervous system requires further study with well-matched uninfected control subjects. Additionally, elevated levels of cerebrospinal fluid cytokines mediating central nervous system migration of macrophages and T lymphocytes were associated with poorer performance on the baseline NPZ. Release of these chemokines may either initiate processes that result in neurocognitive deficits or serve as markers for immune processes that adversely affect neurocognitive function.

Importantly, patients included in each of these series had a high prevalence of comorbidities which could potentially confound neuropsychological testing results, including prominent drug and alcohol abuse as well as mood disorders, often directly related to their high risk for recent HIV acquisition. Further studies with comparison HIV-uninfected study subjects well matched for these demographics and comorbidities are needed to delineate the contribution of HIV versus these confounding factors in the early stages of infection.

ESTABLISHMENT OF CENTRAL NERVOUS SYSTEM COMPARTMENTALIZATION DURING EARLY HIV INFECTION

Despite a great interest in the genotypic and phenotypic characterization of HIV during early infection (Zhu, 1993; Simon, 2003), only limited studies have investigated early HIV compartmentalization in the central nervous system. Increased compartmentalization has been reported between blood and cerebrospinal fluid HIV populations in subjects with HIV-associated dementia, but the time that compartmentalization occurs during the course of HIV infection has been a subject of debate, and extensive compartmentalization has not been

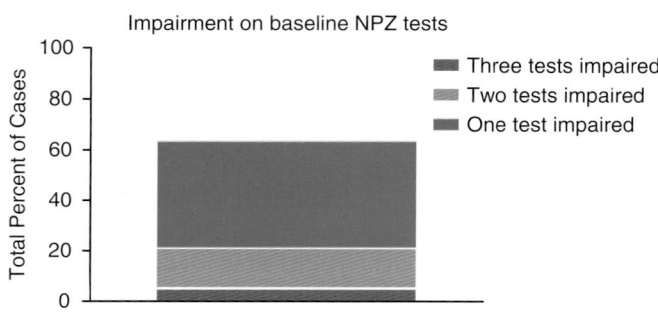

Figure 7.3.3 Percentages of early infection subjects with impairment on one, two, or three tests on baseline NPZ4 tests. At baseline, 24/37 (65%) of subjects with acute and early HIV infection had evidence of impairment on one or more NPZ4 tests (> 1 standard deviation below the mean). 43% (16) had one test impaired, 16% (6) had two tests impaired, and 5% (2) had three tests impaired (Peterson et al., 2010).

detected in primary infection subjects (Ritola, 2004; Harrington, 2009), suggesting that compartmentalization may occur later during chronic infection.

To assess HIV genetic compartmentalization early during infection, we have compared HIV populations between the peripheral blood and cerebrospinal fluid in 11 subjects enrolled within the first year of HIV acquisition, with analysis of longitudinal samples over 18 months in a subset of subjects (Schnell, 2009). We used the heteroduplex tracking assay targeting *env* and single genome amplification and sequence analysis of the full-length *env* gene to identify cerebrospinal fluid-compartmentalized variants and examine viral genotypes within the compartmentalized populations. Most early infection subjects had equilibrated HIV populations between the blood and cerebrospinal fluid compartments. However, compartmentalized HIV populations were detected in the cerebrospinal fluid of three primary infection subjects. In longitudinal follow-up, two subjects maintained unique or

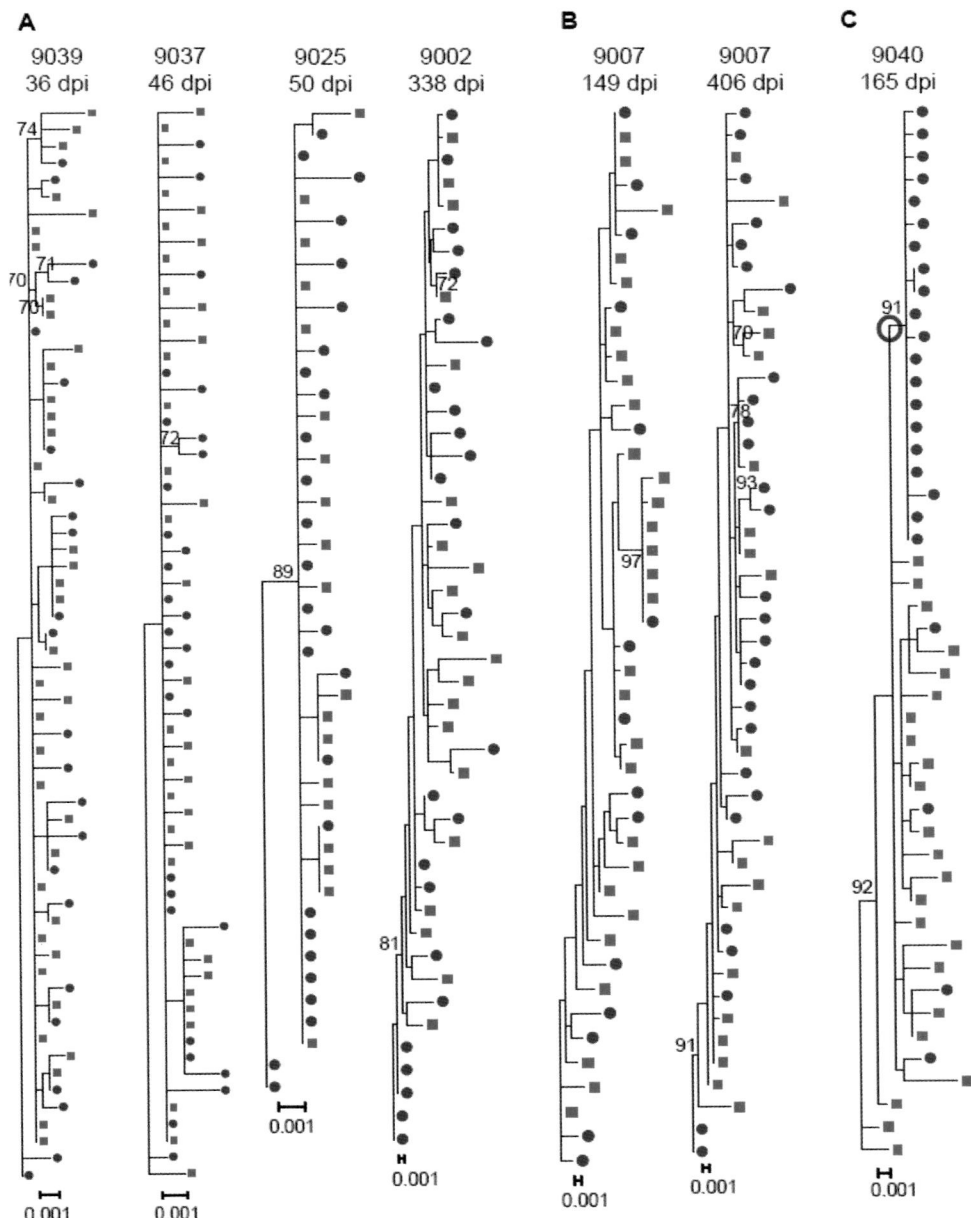

Figure 7.3.4 Phylogenetic analysis of plasma and cerebrospinal fluid HIV populations in early infection subjects. (A) Four examples of subjects whose HIV env sequences demonstrated equilibration between blood plasma and cerebrospinal fluid HIV-1 populations. (B) HIV-1 populations in subject 9007 showed equilibration at 149 days post infection (dpi), but became slightly discordant at 406 dpi. (C) Subject 9040 displayed significant compartmentalization of HIV species in the cerebrospinal fluid at 165 dpi. The blue circle illustrates the node of divergence for the compartmentalized cerebrospinal fluid sequences. Bootstrap numbers ≥70 are indicated at the appropriate nodes. Sequences obtained from the cerebrospinal fluid are labeled with solid circles, and plasma sequences are labeled with solid squares. Genetic distance between sequences is indicated by the distance scale bar at the bottom of the tree. Adapted from Schnell et al. (2009). Compartmentalization and Clonal Amplification of HIV-1 Variants in the Cerebrospinal Fluid during Primary Infection. Journal of Virology, with permission.

enriched populations in the central nervous system, while in one subject, initial compartmentalization later resolved. For examples of phylogenetic analyses demonstrating equilibrated and compartmentalized HIV-1 species, see Figure 7.3.4. The presence of distinct HIV populations in the cerebrospinal fluid indicates that independent HIV replication can occur in the central nervous system, even early after HIV transmission. Such early compartmentalization may have clinical significance in terms of guiding selection of central nervous system-targeted antiretroviral therapies, suggesting the need for independent central nervous system sampling for determination of antiretroviral sensitivities, and potentially as a biomarker of elevated risk of development of neurocognitive disease.

CONCLUSIONS

Clarification of the events in the in the central nervous system during the earliest stages of HIV infection is necessary to define the time course and pathophysiology of establishment of central nervous system infection and neurological injury associated with HIV. Clinically, characterization of central nervous system events in acute and early HIV infection has substantial implications for treatment strategies (Rausch, 2000). Identification of this primary stage of infection as a crucial period for establishment of central nervous system infection and injury may provide a new rationale of initiation of antiretroviral treatment in early HIV. Future studies focusing on the central nervous system in the setting of treatment initiated during the earliest stages of HIV infection are needed to assess the potential benefits of early intervention for neurocognitive outcomes. The determination of optimal timing for treatment initiation during the course of infection must be informed by knowledge of how such therapy influences the natural history of HIV in the central nervous system. Finally, correlation of abnormalities detected during the early stages of infection with the development of neurological morbidity in long-term follow-up may provide new insight into disease pathogenesis, yield valuable early biomarkers predictive of disease, and identify new targets for neuroprotective therapy.

REFERENCES

Abdulle, S., Mellgren, A., et al. (2007). CSF neurofilament protein (NFL)—a marker of active HIV-related neurodegeneration. *J Neurol*, 254(8), 1026–32.

Aggarwal, M. & Rein, J. (2003). Acute human immunodeficiency virus syndrome in an adolescent. *Pediatrics*, 112(4), e323.

Atkinson, J. H., Higgins, J. A., et al. (2009). Psychiatric context of acute/early HIV infection. The NIMH Multisite Acute HIV Infection Study: IV. *AIDS Behav*, 13(6), 1061–7.

Barber, S. A., Herbst, D. S., et al. (2004). Innate immune responses and control of acute simian immunodeficiency virus replication in the central nervous system. *J Neurovirol*, 10 Suppl 1, 15–20.

Ben-Galim, P., Shaked, Y., et al. (1996). Immediate immunosuppression caused by acute HIV-1 infection: A fulminant multisystemic disease 2 days post infection. *Infection*, 24(4), 332–5.

Betts, M. R., Price, D. A., et al. (2004). The functional profile of primary human antiviral CD8+ T cell effector activity is dictated by cognate peptide concentration. *J Immunol*, 172(10), 6407–17.

Bissel, S. J., Wang, G., et al. (2002). Macrophages relate presynaptic and postsynaptic damage in simian immunodeficiency virus encephalitis. *Am J Pathol*, 160(3), 927–41.

Boska, M. D., Mosley, R. L., et al. (2004). Advances in neuroimaging for HIV-1 associated neurological dysfunction: Clues to the diagnosis, pathogenesis and therapeutic monitoring. *Curr HIV Res*, 2(1), 61–78.

Brew, B. J., Dunbar, N., et al. (1996). Predictive markers of AIDS dementia complex: CD4 cell count and cerebrospinal fluid concentrations of beta 2-microglobulin and neopterin. *J Infect Dis*, 174(2), 294–8.

Brew, B. J., Perdices, M., et al. (1989). The neurological features of early and 'latent' human immunodeficiency virus infection. *Aust N Z J Med*, 19(6), 700–5.

Busch, M. P., Lee, L. L., et al. (1995). Time course of detection of viral and serologic markers preceding human immunodeficiency virus type 1 seroconversion: Implications for screening of blood and tissue donors. *Transfusion*, 35(2), 91–7.

Calabrese, L. H., Proffitt, M. R., et al. (1987). Acute infection with the human immunodeficiency virus (HIV) associated with acute brachial neuritis and exanthematous rash. *Ann Intern Med*, 107(6), 849–51.

Carne, C., Tedder, R, Smith, A, Sutherland, S, Elkington, S, Daly, H, et al. (1985). Acute encephalopathy coincident with seroconversion for anti-HTLV-III. *The Lancet*, 1206–1208.

Castellanos, F., Mallada, J., et al. (1994). Ataxic neuropathy associated with human immunodeficiency virus seroconversion. *Arch Neurol*, 51(3), 236.

Cecil, K. & Lenkinski, R. E. (1998). Proton MR spectroscopy in inflammatory and infectious brain disorders. *Neuroimaging Clinics of North America*, 8(4), 863–879.

Centlivre, M., Sala, M., et al. (2007). In HIV-1 pathogenesis the die is cast during primary infection. *AIDS*, 21(1), 1–11.

Chiodi, F., Valentin, A., et al. (1989). Biological characterizsation of paired human immunodeficiency virus type 1 isolates from blood and cerebrospinal fluid. *Virology*, 173, 178–187.

Clements, J. E., Babas, T., et al. (2002). The central nervous system as a reservoir for simian immunodeficiency virus (SIV): Steady-state levels of SIV DNA in brain from acute through asymptomatic infection. *J Infect Dis*, 186(7), 905–13.

Cunningham, P. H., Smith, D. G., et al. (2000). Evidence for independent development of resistance to HIV-1 reverse transcriptase inhibitors in the cerebrospinal fluid. *AIDS*, 14(13), 1949–54.

Davenport, M. P., Zhang, L., et al. (2006). Influence of peak viral load on the extent of CD4+ T-cell depletion in simian HIV infection. *J Acquir Immune Defic Syndr*, 41(3), 259–65.

Davis, L., Miller, V., Palmer, D., Llewellyn, A., Merlin, T., Young, S., et al. (1992). Early viral brain invasion in iatrogenic human immunodeficiency virus infection. *Neurology*, 42(9), 1736–1739.

De Caluwe, J. P., Dourov, N., et al. (1987). Mononucleosis-like illness and lymphocytic meningitis as the clinical presentation of an acute HIV infection. *Acta Clin Belg*, 42(5), 330–5.

Denning, D. W. (1988). The neurological features of acute HIV infection. *Biomed Pharmacother*, 42(1), 11–4.

Denning, D. W., Anderson, J., et al. (1987). Acute myelopathy associated with primary infection with human immunodeficiency virus. *Br Med J (Clin Res Ed)*, 294(6565), 143–4.

Di Stefano, M., Gray, F., et al. (1996a). Analysis of ENV V3 sequences from HIV-1-infected brain indicates restrained virus expression throughout the disease. *J Med Virol*, 49(1), 41–8.

Di Stefano, M., Wilt, S., et al. (1996b). HIV type 1 V3 sequences and the development of dementia during AIDS. *AIDS Res Hum Retroviruses*, 12(6), 471–6.

Douvoyiannis, M. & Litman, N. (2009). Acute encephalopathy and multi-organ involvement with rhabdomyolysis during primary HIV infection. *Int J Infect Dis*, 13(5), e299–304.

Dube, B., Benton, T., et al. (2005). Neuropsychiatric manifestations of HIV infection and AIDS. *J Psychiatry Neurosci, 30*(4), 237–46.

Enting, R., Prins, J., Jurriaans, S., Brinkman, K., Portegies, P., & Lange, J. (2001). Concentrations of human immunodeficiency virus type 1 (HIV-1) RNA in cerebrospinal fluid after antiretroviral treatment initiated during primary HIV-1 infection. *Clinical Infectious Diseases, 32*, 1095–1099.

Fiebig, E. W., Wright, D. J., et al. (2003). Dynamics of HIV viremia and antibody seroconversion in plasma donors: Implications for diagnosis and staging of primary HIV infection. *AIDS, 17*(13), 1871–9.

Finzi, D., Blankson, J., et al. (1999). Latent infection of CD4+ T cells provides a mechanism for lifelong persistence of HIV-1, even in patients on effective combination therapy [see comments]. *Nature Medicine, 5*(5), 512–7.

Finzi, D., Hermankova, M., et al. (1997). Identification of a reservoir for HIV-1 in patients on highly active antiretroviral therapy. *Science, 278*(5341), 1295–300.

Franchini, G., Gurgo, C., et al. (1987). Sequence of simian immunodeficiency virus and its relationship to the human immunodeficiency viruses. *Nature, 328*(6130), 539–43.

Fuller, R. A., Westmoreland, S. V., et al. (2004). A prospective longitudinal in vivo 1H MR spectroscopy study of the SIV/macaque model of neuroAIDS. *BMC Neurosci, 5*(1), 10.

Gold, L. H., Fox, H. S., et al. (1998). Longitudinal analysis of behavioral, neurophysiological, viral and immunological effects of SIV infection in rhesus monkeys. *J Med Primatol, 27*(2–3), 104–12.

Gonzalez, R. G., Cheng, L. L., et al. (2000). Early brain injury in the SIV-macaque model of AIDS. *AIDS, 14*(18), 2841–9.

Gray, F., Scaravilli, F., et al. (1996). Neuropathology of early HIV-1 infection. *Brain Pathol, 6*(1), 1–15.

Guadalupe, M., Sankaran, S., et al. (2006). Viral suppression and immune restoration in the gastrointestinal mucosa of human immunodeficiency virus type 1-infected patients initiating therapy during primary or chronic infection. *J Virol, 80*(16), 8236–47.

Hagberg, L., Malmvall, B. E., et al. (1986). Guillain-Barre syndrome as an early manifestation of HIV central nervous system infection. *Scand J Infect Dis, 18*(6), 591–2.

Harrington, P. R., Connell, M. J., et al. (2007). Dynamics of simian immunodeficiency virus populations in blood and cerebrospinal fluid over the full course of infection. *J Infect Dis, 196*(7), 1058–67.

Harrington, P. R., Schnell, G., et al. (2009). Cross-sectional characterization of HIV-1 env compartmentalization in cerebrospinal fluid over the full disease course. *AIDS, 23*(8), 907–15.

Heaton, R. K., Marcotte, T. D., et al. (2004). The impact of HIV-associated neuropsychological impairment on everyday functioning. *J Int Neuropsychol Soc, 10*(3), 317–31.

Heaton, R. K, Clifford, D. B., et al. (2010). HIV -associated neurocognitive disorders persist in the era of potent antiretroviral therapy. *Neurology*, in press.

Hecht, F. M., Busch, M. P., et al. (2002). Use of laboratory tests and clinical symptoms for identification of primary HIV infection. *AIDS, 16*(8), 1119–29.

Ho, D., Schooley, R., Kaplan, J., Allan, J., Groopman, J., Resnick, L., et al. (1985). Isolation of HTLV-III from cerebrospinal fluid and neural tissues of patients with neurologic syndromes related to the acquired immunodeficiency syndrome. *The New England Journal of Medicine, 313*(24), 1493–1497.

Ho, E., Lee, E., et al. (2010). Abnormalities in high-field brain MRI in primary HIV infection . 17th Conference on Retroviruses and Opportunistic Infections, San Francisco, CA.

Horn, T. F., Huitron-Resendiz, S., et al. (1998). Early physiological abnormalities after simian immunodeficiency virus infection. *Proc Natl Acad Sci USA, 95*(25), 15072–7.

Hughes, P. J., McLean, K. A., et al. (1992). Cranial polyneuropathy and brainstem disorder at the time of seroconversion in HIV infection. *Int J STD AIDS, 3*(1), 60–1.

Janssen, R. S., Satten, G. A., et al. (1998). New testing strategy to detect early HIV-1 infection for use in incidence estimates and for clinical and prevention purposes. *JAMA, 280*(1), 42–8.

Jones, H. R., Jr., Ho, D. D., et al. (1988). Acute fulminating fatal leukoencephalopathy as the only manifestation of human immunodeficiency virus infection. *Ann Neurol, 23*(5), 519–22.

Kahn, J. O. & Walker, B. D. (1998). Acute human immunodeficiency virus type 1 infection. *N Engl J Med, 339*(1), 33–9.

Kaslow, R. A., Carrington, M., et al. (1996). Influence of combinations of human major histocompatibility complex genes on the course of HIV-1 infection. *Nature Medicine, 2*(4), 405–11.

Khan, S. S., Smith, M. S., et al. (2004). Multiplex bead array assays for detection of soluble cytokines: Comparisons of sensitivity and quantitative values among kits from multiple manufacturers. *Cytometry B Clin Cytom, 61*(1), 35–9.

Kitagawa, M., Lackner, A. A., et al. (1991). Simian immunodeficiency virus infection of macaque bone marrow macrophages correlates with disease progression in vivo. *Am J Pathol, 138*(4), 921–30.

Kivisakk, P., Trebst, C., et al. (2003). Expression of CCR2, CCR5, and CXCR3 by CD4+ T cells is stable during a 2-year longitudinal study but varies widely between individuals. *J Neurovirol, 9*(3), 291–9.

Koopman, J. S., Jacquez, J. A., et al. (1997). The role of early HIV infection in the spread of HIV through populations. *J Acquir Immune Defic Syndr Hum Retrovirol, 14*(3), 249–58.

Korber, B. T., Kunstman, K. J., et al. (1994). Genetic differences between blood- and brain-derived viral sequences from human immunodeficiency virus type 1-infected patients: Evidence of conserved elements in the V3 region of the envelope protein of brain-derived sequences. *J Virol, 68*(11), 7467–7481.

Kothe, D., Byers, R. H., et al. (2003). Performance characteristics of a new less sensitive HIV-1 enzyme immunoassay for use in estimating HIV seroincidence. *J Acquir Immune Defic Syndr, 33*(5), 625–34.

Koup, R. A., Safrit, J. T., et al. (1994). Temporal association of cellular immune responses with the initial control of viremia in primary human immunodeficiency virus type 1 syndrome. *J Virol, 68*(7), 4650–5.

Kovacs, J. A., Lempicki, R. A., et al. (2000). In vivo labeling studies with bromodeoxyuridine (BrDU) and 2H-glucose demonstrate differential effects of HIV on lymphocyte and monocyte proliferation and substantially enhanced lymphocyte proliferation in HIV-infected pateints receiving IL-2 therapy . 7th Conference on Retroviruses and Opportunistic Infections, San Francisco.

Krasner, C. G. & Cohen, S. H. (1993). Bilateral Bell's palsy and aseptic meningitis in a patient with acute human immunodeficiency virus seroconversion. *West J Med, 159*(5), 604–5.

Lackner, A. A., Dandekar, S., et al. (1991a). Neurobiology of simian and feline immunodeficiency virus infections. *Brain Pathol, 1*(3), 201–12.

Lackner, A. A., Smith, M. O., et al. (1991b). Localization of simian immunodeficiency virus in the central nervous system of rhesus monkeys. *Am J Pathol, 139*(3), 609–21.

Lane, J. H., Sasseville, V. G., et al. (1996). Neuroinvasion by simian immunodeficiency virus coincides with increased numbers of perivascular macrophages/microglia and intrathecal immune activation. *J Neurovirol 2*(6), 423–32.

Larsen, M., Toft, P. B., et al. (1998). Bilateral optic neuritis in acute human immunodeficiency virus infection. *Acta Ophthalmol Scand, 76*(6), 737–8.

Lentz, M. R., Kim, W. K., et al. (2009). Changes in MRS neuronal markers and T cell phenotypes observed during early HIV infection. *Neurology, 72*(17), 1465–72.

Letvin, N. L. & Walker, B. D. (2003). Immunopathogenesis and immunotherapy in AIDS virus infections. *Nature Medicine, 9*(7), 861–6.

Lindback, S., Karlsson, A. C., et al. (2000a). Viral dynamics in primary HIV-1 infection. Karolinska Institutet Primary HIV Infection Study Group. *AIDS, 14*(15), 2283–91.

Lindback, S., Thorstensson, R., et al. (2000b). Diagnosis of primary HIV-1 infection and duration of follow-up after HIV exposure. Karolinska Institute Primary HIV Infection Study Group. *AIDS, 14*(15), 2333–9.

Liu, P., Hudson, L. C., et al. (2006). Compartmentalization and evolution of feline immunodeficiency virus between the central nervous system and periphery following intracerebroventricular or systemic inoculation. *J Neurovirol, 12*(4), 307–21.

Lopez-Villegas, D., Lenkinski, R. E., et al. (1997). Biochemical changes in the frontal lobe of HIV-infected individuals detected by magnetic resonance spectroscopy. *Proc Natl Acad Sci USA*, *94*(18), 9854–9.

Mankowski, J. L., Clements, J. E., et al. (2002). Searching for clues: Tracking the pathogenesis of human immunodeficiency virus central nervous system disease by use of an accelerated, consistent simian immunodeficiency virus macaque model. *J Infect Dis*, *186* Suppl 2, S199–208.

Mankowski, J. L., Queen, S. E., et al. (2004). Cerebrospinal fluid markers that predict SIV CNS disease. *J Neuroimmunol*, *157*(1–2), 66–70.

Meersseman, W., Van Laethem, K., et al. (2005). Fatal brain necrosis in primary HIV infection. *Lancet*, *366*(9488), 866.

Meyerhoff, D. J., Bloomer, C., et al. (1999). Elevated subcortical choline metabolites in cognitively and clinically asymptomatic HIV+ patients. *Neurology*, *52*(5), 995–1003.

Meyerhoff, D. J., MacKay, S., et al. (1993). Reduced brain N-acetylaspartate suggests neuronal loss in cognitively impaired human immunodeficiency virus-seropositive individuals: in vivo 1H magnetic resonance spectroscopic imaging. *Neurology*, *43*(3 Pt 1), 509–15.

Meyerhoff, D. J., MacKay, S., et al. (1994). N-acetylaspartate reductions measured by 1H MRSI in cognitively impaired HIV-seropositive individuals. *Magn Reson Imaging*, *12*(4), 653–9.

Mogensen, T. H., Marinovskij, E., et al. (2007). Acute demyelinizating encephalomyelitis (ADEM) as initial presentation of primary HIV infection. *Scand J Infect Dis*, *39*(6–7), 630–4.

Moore DJ, Letendre SL, Morris S, Umlauf A, Deutsch R, Smith DM, Little S, Rooney A, Franklin DR, Gouaux B, Leblanc S, Rosario D, Fennema-Notestine C, Heaton RK, Ellis RJ, Atkinson JH, Grant I, for the CHARTER Group. (2011). Neurocognitive functioning in acute or early HIV infection. *Journal of Neurovirology*, *17*(1), 50–57.

Murphy, G. & Parry. J. V. (2008). Assays for the detection of recent infections with human immunodeficiency virus type 1. *Euro Surveill*, *13*(36).

Murray, E. A., Rausch, D. M., et al. (1992). Cognitive and motor impairments associated with SIV infection in rhesus monkeys. *Science*, *255*(5049), 1246–9.

Narciso, P., Galgani, S., et al. (2001). Acute disseminated encephalomyelitis as manifestation of primary HIV infection. *Neurology*, *57*(8), 1493–6.

Navia, B. A., Jordan, B. D., et al. (1986). The AIDS dementia complex: I. Clinical features. *Ann Neurol*, *19*(6), 517–24.

Nelson, J. A., Fiscus, S. A., et al. (1997). Evolutionary variants of the human immunodeficiency virus type 1 V3 region characterized by using a heteroduplex tracking assay. *J Virol*, *71*(11), 8750–8.

Nesbit, C. E. & Schwartz, S. A. (2002). In vitro and animal models of human immunodeficiency virus infection of the central nervous system. *Clin Diagn Lab Immunol*, *9*(3), 515–24.

O'Brien, W. (1994). Genetic and biological basis of HIV-1 neurotropism. In R. Price & S. Perry (Eds.). *HIV, AIDS and the Brain*, pp. 47–70. New York: Raven Press, Ltd.

Orandle, M. S., MacLean, A. G., et al. (2002). Enhanced expression of proinflammatory cytokines in the central nervous system is associated with neuroinvasion by simian immunodeficiency virus and the development of encephalitis. *J Virol*, *76*(11), 5797–802.

Paton, P., Poly, H., et al. (1990). Acute meningoradiculitis concomitant with seroconversion to human immunodeficiency virus type 1. *Res Virol*, *141*(4), 427–33.

Peterson, J., Lee, E., et al. (2010). Neurocognitive performance during primary HIV-1 infection. 17th Conference on Retroviruses and Opportunistic Infections, San Francisco, CA.

Picker, L. J. (2006). Immunopathogenesis of acute AIDS virus infection. *Curr Opin Immunol*, *18*(4), 399–405.

Piette, A. M., Tusseau, F., et al. (1986). Acute neuropathy coincident with seroconversion for anti-LAV/HTLV-III. *Lancet*, *1*(8485), 852.

Pilcher, C. D., Shugars, D. C., et al. (2001). HIV in body fluids during primary HIV infection: Implications for pathogenesis, treatment and public health. *AIDS*, *15*(7), 837–45.

Ping, L. H., Nelson, J. A., et al. (1999). Characterization of V3 sequence heterogeneity in subtype C human immunodeficiency virus type 1 isolates from Malawi: Underrepresentation of X4 variants. *J Virol*, *73*(8), 6271–81.

Price, R. W. & Brew, B. J. (1988). The AIDS dementia complex. *J Infect Dis 158*(5): 1079–83.

Price, R. W. & Sidtis, J. J. (1990). Evaluation of the AIDS dementia complex in clinical trials. *J Acquir Immune Defic Syndr*, *3* Suppl 2, S51–60.

Rausch, D. M. (2000). Symposium HIV and the nervous system: Emerging issues. *Journal of Neurovirology*, *6*(Suppl 1), S1–S4.

Ritola, K., Pilcher, C. D., et al. (2004). Multiple V1/V2 env variants are frequently present during primary infection with human immunodeficiency virus type 1. *J Virol*, *78*(20), 11208–18.

Roberts, E. S., Burudi, E. M., et al. (2004). Acute SIV infection of the brain leads to upregulation of IL6 and interferon-regulated genes: Expression patterns throughout disease progression and impact on neuroAIDS. *J Neuroimmunol*, *157*(1–2), 81–92.

Rosenberg, E. S., Altfeld, M., et al. (2000). Immune control of HIV-1 after early treatment of acute infection. *Nature*, *407*(6803), 523–6.

Royce, R. A., Sena, A., et al. (1997). Sexual transmission of HIV. *N Engl J Med*, *336*(15), 1072–8.

Sacktor, N., McDermott, M. P., et al. (2002). HIV-associated cognitive impairment before and after the advent of combination therapy. *J Neurovirol*, *8*(2), 136–42.

Scarpini, E., Sacilotto, G., et al. (1991). Acute ataxia coincident with seroconversion for anti-HIV. *J Neurol*, *238*(6), 356–7.

Schacker, T., Collier, A. C., et al. (1996). Clinical and epidemiologic features of primary HIV infection. *Ann Intern Med*, *125*(4), 257–64.

Schnell, G., Price, R. W., et al. (2009). Compartmentalization and clonal amplification of HIV-1 variants in the cerebrospinal fluid during primary infection. *J Virol*.

Serrano, P., Hernandez, N., et al. (2007). Bilateral Bell palsy and acute HIV type 1 infection: Report of 2 cases and review. *Clin Infect Dis*, *44*(6), e57–61.

Simon, V., Padte, N., et al. (2003). Infectivity and replication capacity of drug-resistant human immunodeficiency virus type 1 variants isolated during primary infection. *J Virol*, *77*(14), 7736–45.

Smith, M. O., Heyes, M. P., et al. (1995). Early intrathecal events in rhesus macaques (Macaca mulatta) infected with pathogenic or nonpathogenic molecular clones of simian immunodeficiency virus. *Lab Invest*, *72*(5), 547–58.

Sonnerborg, A. B., von Stedingk, L. V., et al. (1989). Elevated neopterin and beta 2-microglobulin levels in blood and cerebrospinal fluid occur early in HIV-1 infection. *AIDS*, *3*(5), 277–83.

Spudich, S., Gisslen, M., et al. (2011). Central Nervous System Immune Activation Characterizes Primary HIV-1 Infection Even in Subjects with Minimal Cerebrospinal Fluid Viral Burden. *J Infect Dis*, in press.

Stekler, J. & Collier, A (2004). Primary HIV infection. *Current HIV/AIDS Reports*, *1*, 68–73.

Stekler, J., Maenza, J., et al. (2007). Screening for acute HIV infection: Lessons learned. *Clin Infect Dis*, *44*(3), 459–61.

Stekler, J. D., Swenson, P. D., et al. (2009). HIV testing in a high-incidence population: Is antibody testing alone good enough? *Clin Infect Dis*, *49*(3), 444–53.

Stephens, E. B., Liu, Z. Q., et al. (1995). Lymphocyte-tropic simian immunodeficiency virus causes persistent infection in the brains of rhesus monkeys. *Virology*, *213*(2), 600–14.

Taiwo, B. O. & Hicks, C. B. (2002). Primary human immunodeficiency virus. *South Med J*, *95*(11), 1312–7.

Tambussi, G., Gori, A., Capiluppi, B., Balotta, C., Papagno, L., Morandini, B., et al (2002). Neurological symptoms during primary human immunodeficiency virus (HIV) infection correlate with high levels of HIV RNA in cerebrospinal fluid. *Clinical Infectious Diseases*, *30*, 962–965.

Thompson, P. M., Dutton, R. A., et al. (2005). Thinning of the cerebral cortex visualized in HIV/AIDS reflects CD4+ T lymphocyte decline. *Proc Natl Acad Sci USA*, *102*(43), 15647–52.

Tindall, B., Barker, S., et al. (1988). Characterization of the acute clinical illness associated with human immunodeficiency virus infection. *Arch Intern Med*, *148*(4), 945–9.

Tindall, B., Hing, M., et al. (1989). Severe clinical manifestations of primary HIV infection. *AIDS*, *3*(11), 747–9.

Veazey, R. S. & Lackner, A. A. (2004). Getting to the guts of HIV pathogenesis. *J Exp Med*, *200*(6), 697–700.

Walker, B. D. & Rosenberg, E. S. (2000). Containing HIV after infection. *Nat Med*, *6*(10), 1094–5.

Wallace, M. R., Nelson, J. A., et al. (2001). Symptomatic HIV seroconverting illness is associated with more rapid neurological impairment. *Sex Transm Infect*, *77*(3), 199–201.

Wawer, M. J., Gray, R. H., et al. (2005). Rates of HIV-1 transmission per coital act, by stage of HIV-1 infection, in Rakai, Uganda. *J Infect Dis*, *191*(9), 1403–9.

Weintrob, A. C., Giner, J., et al. (2003). Infrequent diagnosis of primary human immunodeficiency virus infection: Missed opportunities in acute care settings. *Arch Intern Med*, *163*(17), 2097–100.

Westmoreland, S. V., Halpern, E., et al. (1998). Simian immunodeficiency virus encephalitis in rhesus macaques is associated with rapid disease progression. *J Neurovirol*, *4*(3), 260–8.

Williams, K. C., Corey, S., et al. (2001). Perivascular macrophages are the primary cell type productively infected by simian immunodeficiency virus in the brains of macaques: Implications for the neuropathogenesis of AIDS. *J Exp Med*, *193*(8), 905–15.

Witwer, K. W., Gama, L., et al. (2009). Coordinated regulation of SIV replication and immune responses in the CNS. *PLoS ONE*, *4*(12), e8129.

Wong, J. K., Ignacio, C. C., et al. (1997). In vivo compartmentalization of human immunodeficiency virus: Evidence from the examination of pol sequences from autopsy tissues. *J Virol*, *71*(3), 2059–2071.

Wong, M. H., Robertson, K., et al. (2007). Frequency of and risk factors for HIV dementia in an HIV clinic in sub-Saharan Africa. *Neurology*, *68*(5), 350–5.

Woods, S. P., Moore, D. J., et al. (2009). Cognitive neuropsychology of HIV-associated neurocognitive disorders. *Neuropsychol Rev*, *19*(2), 152–68.

Yankner, B. A., Skolnik, P. R., et al. (1986). Cerebral granulomatous angiitis associated with isolation of human T-lymphotropic virus type III from the central nervous system. *Ann Neurol*, *20*(3), 362–4.

Zeman, A. & Donaghy, M. (1991). Acute infection with human immunodeficiency virus presenting with neurogenic urinary retention. *Genitourin Med*, *67*(4), 345–7.

Zetola, N. M. & Pilcher, C. D. (2007). Diagnosis and management of acute HIV infection. *Infect Dis Clin North Am*, *21*(1), 19–48, vii.

Zhang, Z., Schuler, T., et al. (1999). Sexual transmission and propagation of SIV and HIV in resting and activated CD4+ T cells. *Science*, *286*(5443), 1353–7.

Zhu, G. W., Liu, Z. Q., et al. (1995). Pathogenesis of lymphocyte-tropic and macrophage-tropic SIVmac infection in the brain. *J Neurovirol*, *1*(1), 78–91.

Zhu, T., Mo, H., et al. (1993). Genotypic and phenotypic characterization of HIV-1 patients with primary infection. *Science*, *261*(5125), 1179–81.

Zink, M. C., Suryanarayana, K., et al. (1999). High viral load in the cerebrospinal fluid and brain correlates with severity of simian immunodeficiency virus encephalitis. *J Virol*, *73*(12), 10480–8.

7.4

HIV-1 NEUROPATHOLOGY

Benjamin B. Gelman and David J. Moore

After many years of extensive neuropathological examination several anomalies have been detected in the brains of HIV-infected people. These insights are highly valuable, yet can be quite difficult to prioritize with regard to their correlation with neurocognitive dysfunction, and their pathophysiological significance. That basic obstacle in the field was present prior to the discovery of highly active antiretroviral therapy (HAART), when infected populations were relatively young adults, and progression to end-stage acquired immunodeficiency syndrome (AIDS) was prevalent. In recent times it continues to be difficult to establish the cliniconeuropathological correlation, because HAART medicines dramatically modify the longitudinal progression of HIV/AIDS and the neuropathological outcomes. Added difficulties arise because HIV-1-infected populations often harbor multiple co-morbid conditions that can influence neurocognitive test performance and neuropathological outcome. Also, the population is much older than before and makes potential synergy with CNS aging an important influence. In this chapter the many neuropathological outcomes that have been described in subjects infected with HIV-1 are critically evaluated, and their potential relationship to the pathophysiology of HAND is discussed. Suggestions are made regarding principles that could channel the neuroAIDS "agenda" towards elucidating the pathophysiology and developing novel therapeutic approaches.

SCOPE OF COVERAGE

Neuropathological outcomes associated with HIV infection are of two broad types. In one, the changes are likely to be attributed directly to HIV-1 infection. The other category pertains to changes produced by a generalized immunological disturbance, which leads to increased vulnerability to opportunistic infection, neoplasms in the central nervous systems (CNS) and other changes that could impair neuropsychological function. The neuropathology of the opportunistic infections that are associated with HIV/AIDS has remained largely the same, although the prevalence of these CNS lesions has declined generally in the era of highly active antiretroviral therapy (HAART) (Masliah et al., 2000; Morgello et al., 2002). To avoid repetition, the reader is referred to outstanding contributions made by previous reviewers addressing opportunistic infection of the CNS (Budka, 1998; Petito, 1993). The main focus of this chapter is human (versus animal) neuropathological changes that are related to HIV-1 infection

itself, and their potential relationship to neurocognitive impairment in HIV-associated neurocognitive disorders (HAND). Key neurobiological changes found in human specimens may not be addressed in a comprehensive fashion herein because many worthwhile autopsy studies did not have neurocognitive data for comparison.

NOMENCLATURE OF HIV-ASSOCIATED NEUROCOGNITIVE DISORDERS

In order to understand the cliniconeuropathological relationship between HIV-associated neurocognitive impairment (NCI) and the associated neuropathological outcomes, a historical review of the nomenclature is essential. Definitions for the diagnosis of NCI have changed over time, and consequently, the association between a given neurocognitive diagnosis and the neuropathological outcome at autopsy strongly depends upon the criteria used to assign the clinical neurocognitive and neuropathological diagnoses. In the early days of the acquired immunodeficiency syndrome (AIDS) pandemic, clinicians noted the presence of abnormal neurological symptoms in many patients with advanced disease (Perry & Marotta, 1987; Snider et al., 1983). In some cases, a severe neurocognitive disturbance was observed and was termed AIDS dementia complex (ADC). The onset of ADC was usually insidious, but the diagnosis was confounded by rapidly progressing opportunistic infections in a high proportion of cases (Navia et al., 1986). In 1987, a comprehensive neuropsychological survey of HIV-associated neurocognitive deficits showed that objectively documented NCI could occur across all clinical stages of HIV/AIDS (i.e., asymptomatic, symptomatic, and AIDS) (Grant et al., 1987). Abnormal executive functions, episodic memory, and information processing speed were especially prevalent. In 1991, the AIDS Task Force of the American Academy of Neurology (AAN) published criteria that clinically classified two levels of neurocognitive impairment: 1) HIV-associated dementia (HAD) with motor, behavioral/psychosocial, or combined features; and 2) minor cognitive motor disorder (MCMD) (Janssen et al., 1991). The AAN system was later expanded to include added diagnostic refinement of less severely impaired people deemed as asymptomatic neuropsychological impairment (ANI) (Grant & Atkinson, 1999). "Subsyndromic neuropsychological impairment" was added to characterize patients with mild neurocognitive deficits that do not noticeably interfere with activities of daily living (ADLs). The latter category has become more prevalent than the more severe forms of impairment as the treatments to suppress HIV-1 replication have steadily improved. In 2007, the changing epidemiology of HIV/AIDS in HAART-treated populations led to further modifications known as the "Frascati criteria" (Antinori et al., 2007). The term HIV-associated neurocognitive disorders (HAND) was introduced in order to provide comprehensive guidelines to deal with comorbid conditions that can produce CNS effects, such as substance use and other neuropsychiatric disorders. The diagnosis of HAND is formally determined by assessment of at least five areas of neurocognitive functioning using a performance-based neuropsychological battery (e.g., executive functions, episodic memory, speed of information processing, motor skills, attention/working memory, language, and sensoriperception), which is evaluated using demographically appropriate normative data. These criteria may be adapted for resource-limited settings by using mental status exams such as the HIV Dementia Scale (Morgan et al., 2008; Power et al., 1995). A diagnosis of HAND can be assigned only when NCI cannot be attributed to a comorbid condition (e.g., psychosis) or delirium. Due to the high prevalence of CNS comorbidities in HIV populations, the updated criteria specify guidelines for dealing with "secondary" conditions (e.g., a remote history unlikely to have any residual cognitive effects), "contributing" conditions (e.g., a current condition in the setting of recent cognitive decline), and "confounding" conditions (e.g., an ongoing condition during test performance such as acute drug intoxication). A more structured approach to assigning declines in everyday functioning also is addressed using the Frascati criteria. All told, three diagnoses are possible in HAND: 1) asymptomatic neurocognitive impairment (ANI), 2) HIV-associated mild neurocognitive disorder (MND), and 3) HAD. The implicit assumption being made is that these are likely to be degrees, or clinical stages, of a single nosological entity known as HAND. Since there is but a single nosological entity pertaining to HIV-associated dementia that can be diagnosed at autopsy, underlying pathophysiologies and neuropathologies of the component diagnoses of HAND cannot be assumed to be identical to each other; neuropathological variation with each group is quite possible.

NOMENCLATURE OF HIV-ASSOCIATED NEUROPATHOLOGICAL CHANGES

The changing definitions of HAND over time exert substantial impact on attempts to define cliniconeuropathological correlations. Bedrock concepts regarding the neuropathology of HIV-associated brain dysfunction were developed in the first 15 years of the HIV pandemic, prior the era of HAART, and well before the Frascati criteria for HAND were developed (Budka, 1991). To understand how the neuropathology of HIV-1 infection relates to HAND, changing clinical patterns over time must be considered (McArthur,

2004; McArthur et al., 2010). In the early years of the pandemic, virus replication was relentless and progressed eventually to AIDS. Most AIDS patients were relatively young adults with profound immunodeficiency; few patients survived beyond one to three years or to older age. Under those conditions, pathological changes were very common in the CNS (Budka, 1991; Petito, 1993). The cause of death in people with AIDS was related to underlying CNS pathology in about 35% of the autopsies, second only to pulmonary failure (Klatt, 1988). At least 20% of patients had clinical impairment known as ADC (Navia et al., 1986). When the founding neuropathological principles of HIV/AIDS were established, these were the prevailing conditions (Budka 1991).

After HAART was introduced, the clinical scenario changed markedly (Sacktor et al., 1999a, 1999b, 2001). Effective medical suppression of HIV-1 replication produced a sharp decrease in AIDS morbidity and mortality in treated populations. In contrast to a relentless progression, HAART-era autopsy surveys reflect the end result of a more convoluted disease history that is intertwined with multiple kinds of responses to medical therapy, and is influenced by numerous associated comorbid conditions. Because HAART-treated patients can survive to older ages, a new spectrum of age-associated neuropathological changes became possible that were not germane to younger autopsy cohorts. Older decedents have longer biological "histories" of HIV-1 infection, can undergo widely varying exposures to HAART medicines, and can exhibit varying therapeutic responses. Attenuation of disease progress and prolonged survival in treated cohorts has produced a decrease in the severity of neurocognitive impairment, but not incidence (Tozzi et al., 2001), and a parallel decline in CNS-related mortality (Nuenburg et al., 2002; Morgello et al., 2002; Masliah et al., 2000). In subjects who had neurocognitive impairment prior to HAART, neurological status often showed substantial active improvement (reversal) with HAART (Sacktor et al., 1999a; Brew, 2004; McArthur et al., 2005). As patients live longer, a waxing and waning between normal neurocognitive performance and some form of neurocognitive impairment is perhaps the most commonly observed neurocognitive profile among HIV patients (McArthur, 2004; McArthur et al., 2010). Prolonged and less stereotypical battles between virus and human host with HAART is usually complicated further by other factors, including side effects of HAART drugs, longer cumulative exposure to CNS HIV infection, addiction to drugs of abuse, presence and treatment of psychiatric disturbances, and co-infection with other agents including hepatitis C virus (Bell, 2004). The neuropathology of HIV has probably evolved in parallel with shifting neurocognitive patterns, but unlike the clinical neurocognitive diagnoses, the neuropathological nomenclature is based upon cross-sectional samplings, has remained more constant over time, and strongly if not exclusively emphasizes HAD, which has become much less prevalent. Therefore, the neuropathological bases for a widely variable set of clinical patterns of HAND (cliniconeuropathological correlations) as observed in modern times remain to be elucidated.

NEUROPATHOLOGICAL OUTCOMES ASSOCIATED WITH HIV INFECTION

GROSS BRAIN ANATOMY

Gross brain anatomy remains clinically relevant due to the expanding technology of brain imaging. The gross brain in people with HIV-1 infection does not contain a highly characteristic or specific anomaly. Mild-to-moderate brain atrophy is a highly prevalent change in people with AIDS generally and is more prevalent in people with dementia (Gelman et al., 1996; McArthur et al., 2005). Brain ventricles are expanded the most in frontotemporal sectors, and there is mild sulcal widening. Cerebral atrophy is not, however, specific to infected people with HAND or HIV encephalitis (HIVE). When the atrophy was measured prior to the era of HAART, it was not linked solidly with any single histopathological change associated with the diagnosis of HIVE (Gelman & Guinto, 1992). An association of brain ventricular expansion at autopsy was evident in people with periventriculitis due to opportunistic CNS infection by cytomegalovirus (CMV) (Gelman et al., 1996). The increase in cerebrospinal fluid space volume can be observed prior to autopsy using either CT scanning or magnetic resonance imaging (MRI) (Gelman & Guinto, 1992; Archibald et al., 2004). MRI shows that the volume of white matter, caudate nucleus, hippocampus, and cerebral cortex all can be decreased (Archibald et al., 2004). Brain volume changes can occur with or without HIVE, although the HIVE cases are more likely to show increased white matter signal intensities. MRI also may reveal cortical thinning in primary sensorimotor, premotor, and visual areas of individuals with AIDS (Thompson et al., 2005). Gross brain morphology and spectroscopic changes are useful to follow clinical research cohorts longitudinally, but are not specific enough to screen for HIV-related neurocognitive impairments clinically. The neurohistological substrates behind these volume anomalies are not yet clear (Gelman, 1993).

HIV ENCEPHALITIS

A wide variety of abnormal CNS changes are possible in people with HIV/AIDS, with and without HAND, but there remains but a single nosologic entity identified thus far that addresses CNS HIV infection and CNS inflammatory reaction specifically. HIV encephalitis (HIVE) is the prime neuropathological candidate for causation of neurocognitive changes associated with HIV-1 infection (Budka, 1998; Cherner et al., 2002; McArthur et al., 2005). Before HAART, HIVE occurred in about 15 to 20% of decedents (Budka, 1998; Petito, 2003), a prevalence that was similar to the prevalence of HAD in clinical cohorts (McArthur et al., 2005). The incidence of HAD declined in the HAART era (Sacktor et al., 1999a,2001), but HIVE prevalence may not have undergone a parallel decrease in HAART-era autopsy cohorts (Jellinger et al., 2000; Masliah et al., 2000; Morgello et al., 2002; Vago et al., 2002; Neuenburg et al., 2002; Gray et al., 2003). The difference between autopsy and clinical surveys relates to the fact that autopsy cohorts are cross-sectional samplings enriched with people with end-stage AIDS, who are the most vulnerable to HIVE. Randomly selected populations of infected people probably have much less HIVE than before HAART.

HIVE is an inflammatory reaction of the brain in which HIV-infected macrophages and microglial cells infiltrate the CNS (Budka, 1991). It is usually a panencephalitis that affects gray and white matter both. The mononuclear inflammatory cells are most evident around blood vessels and within the perivascular spaces, but can be present in more diffuse patterns in brain parenchyma. The implicit assumption underlying the diagnosis of HIVE is that the inflammatory reaction is the putative response to replicating HIV-1 within the CNS compartment. The diagnosis is made based upon a constellation of descriptive changes that in most cases can be made using standard histological technique. HIVE is an accepted nosologic diagnosis that is essentially made in "all or none" fashion (Love & Wiley, 2008). The lack of an accepted histological grading system complicates the search for the cliniconeuropathological correlation because the clinical changes in HAND are subject to wide quantitative and qualitative variation. Individual morphological components of HIVE might contribute unique and different aspects to the spectrum of neuropsychological changes in HAND. A histological grading system for HIVE, which has not yet been incorporated into the nosology, might also segregate with the continuum of neurocognitive changes that is implied using the Frascati criteria for diagnosing HAND. The frequency and severity of the reaction in the brain is highly variable; each case may not contain every component as listed in Table 7.4.1. Evidence of replicating HIV-1 in the brain is the key component of the comprehensive picture, but often it is difficult to document histologically. Indeed, it was known early on that cases containing a mononuclear cell reaction often did not have evidence of strong HIV-1 antigenicity in macrophages as assessed using immunohistochemistry (Glass et al., 1995), or as implied by the presence of multinucleated cells (Love & Wiley, 2008). Recent biochemical measurements of HIV-1 mRNA in brain tissue also have shown that the burden of virus replication does not always correlate clearly with the severity of the inflammatory reaction. Evidence gathered in patients with HAD has indicated that the extent of macrophage infiltration may be linked more strongly to brain dysfunction than the burden of HIV-1 replication (Glass et al., 1995). Thus, each histological component of HIVE, and other related neurohistological anomalies present in HIV/AIDS, needs to be considered individually with regard to its potential role in brain dysfunction.

MACROPHAGES AND MULTINUCLEATED GIANT CELLS

The most distinctive individual histological change that occurs in HIVE is the formation of multinucleated giant cells (MNGC), which is considered a hallmark lesion (Budka, 1986; Budka et al., 1991). MNGCs are composed of fused mononuclear phagocytes actively infected with HIV-1

Table 7.4.1 CLINICONEUROPATHOLOGIC CORRELATION IN HAND

NEUROPATHOLOGICAL OR CLINICAL ABNORMALITY	DEMENTIA MEASURED ANTEMORTEM?	SIGNIFICANT CORRELATION SUGGESTED?	IN MORE THAN ONE COHORT?
Inflammation, Macrophages, and HIV			
HIV encephalitis	yes	yes	yes
HIV antigen, or RNA, or DNA	Yes	Possibly when HIV replication not suppressed	yes
Increased nitric oxide synthesis	Yes	Yes	yes
Increased brain density of macrophages	Yes	Yes	no
Increased tumor necrosis factor alpha synthesis	Yes	Yes	no
Increased matrix metalloproteinase activity	Yes	Yes	no
Increased monocyte chemoattractant protein-1	Yes	Yes	no
Interferon-induced immunoproteasome expression	Yes	Yes	no
Macrophage iron accumulation	No	unknown	no
White Matter Damage, Mixed Glial Cell Changes, Subcortical Damage			
Blood-brain barrier change	Yes	Yes	no
Apoptotic death of astrocytes	yes	Yes	yes
White matter lysosome expansion	yes	Yes	no
Increased fractalkine synthesis	yes	Yes	no
Increased chemokine receptor	No	unknown	no
Increased matrix metalloproteinase activity	No	unknown	no
Increased immunophilin synthesis	No	unknown	no
Neurodegeneration and Neuropil Damage			
Synaptodendritic damage	Yes	Yes	no
Dropout of neuron cell bodies	yes	inconclusive	yes
Loss of neuropil matrix components	no	unknown	yes
Active apoptotic death of neurons	yes	No	yes
Axon damage	yes	No	no
Neuronal channelopathies	yes	possibly	no
Brain Aging			
Fibrillary beta amyloid, diffuse	no	unknown	no
Fibrillary beta amyloid, argyrophilic	no	unknown	no
Ubiquitinylated aggresomes	no	unknown	no
Systemic Inflammation, Metabolic and/or Chronic and Acute Phase Responses			
Anemia of chronic inflammation	yes	Yes	yes
Increased plasma lipopolysaccharide	yes	Yes	yes
Blood-brain barrier changes	yes	Yes	yes

(Figure 7.4.1). In the setting of increased mononuclear inflammation, in a decedent known to have HIV-1 infection, the MNGC is a specific sign of HIVE when other diseases that form giant cells are excluded (such as tuberculosis, fungal infection, sarcoidosis, and other granulomatous reactions). HIV-1 glycoprotein 41 (gp41), a subunit of the virus envelope protein, is the putative fusion protein that leads to giant cell formation. As with the macrophage responses in HIVE, MNGCs most often appear in perivascular sectors of brain white matter, but can appear in any area. Doubt concerning the specificity for active HIV replication in a particular case can sometimes be resolved by demonstrating positive immunostaining for HIV-1 envelope protein within the inflammatory macrophages and microglia (i.e., HIV-1

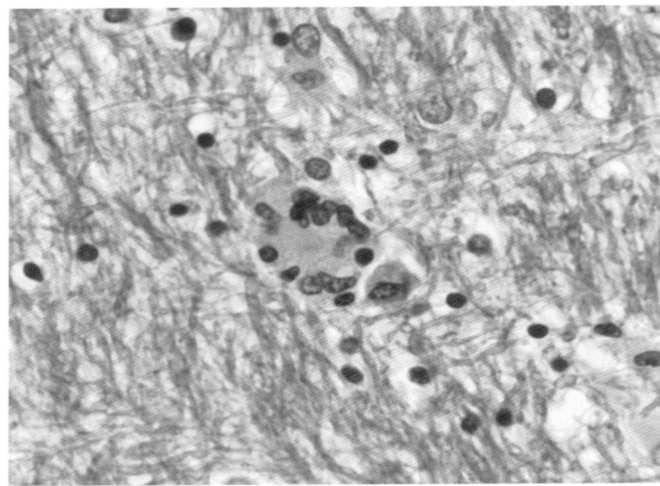

Figure 7.4.1 A typical multinucleated cell in white matter from a person with HIV encephalitis. Myelin is stained blue with Luxol Fast Blue.

gp41 and p24 antigens). In many cases of HIVE in routine pathology practice the specificity of the reaction for HIV-1 infection remains in doubt as discussed in more detail below.

MICROGLIAL NODULES, MICROGLIOSIS AND ENCEPHALITIS

A histological change that often is present in HIV-1-infected people, with and without HIVE, is multiple microglial nodules (MGN). Microglial cells (MGC) are the resident histiocytic macrophage population of the CNS, and MGNs are loosely aggregated clusters of activated MGCs (Figure 7.4.2). The proliferation and activation of microglia is considered to be highly important pathophysiologically because mononuclear phagocytes including MGCs are the main cell type to

host HIV-1 replication in the CNS. Nevertheless, MGNs are not specific to HIVE, nor are they required to diagnose it. MGNs can be produced by infection with other viruses and CNS pathogens, the most relevant examples being CMV encephalitis and CNS toxoplasmosis. Positive immunostaining for HIV-1 envelope antigens such as gp41 and p24 often helps to establish that inflammation is related to HIV-1 infection in the brain and is representative of HIVE. When there is residual doubt concerning the specificity of the microglial cell reaction for CNS HIV-1 infection, a diagnosis of microglial nodule encephalitis (MGNE) is made (Bell, 2004). When MGNE is diagnosed, specificity for CNS HIV-1 infection remains unclear even though no other infectious pathogen besides HIV-1 is known to be present. Whether MGNE is a subtype of HIVE that lacks the hallmark multinucleated giant cells is not clear (Love & Wiley, 2008). "Lumping" HIVE and MGNE together as one HIV-related brain pathology is sometimes reported in postmortem outcomes of HIV-1 infection (Everall et al., 2009). Nosologically, however, the rationale for lumping remains *sub judice*; HIVE and MGNE both can be diagnosed in the same material as two distinct entities (Bell, 2004).

In addition to nodular aggregates of activated microglial cells, a more diffusely distributed accumulation of activated microglial cells frequently occurs in people with HIV-1 infection, with and without HIVE. In routine hematoxylin- and eosin- (H and E) stained slides, they appear as abundant rod-shaped or dumbbell-shaped nuclei scatted in the neuropil and white matter ("rod cells"). The pattern is sometimes referred to as "diffuse microgliosis" (Figure 7.4.3). When immunostained for microglial cell markers such as HLAD, Iba1 or ferritin the cells exhibit the typical morphological characteristics of activated microglia, including an increase in the number and thickness of cell processes. The lesion was

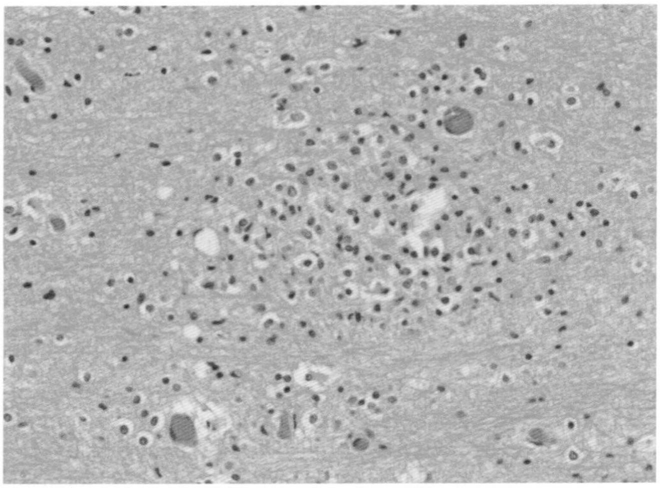

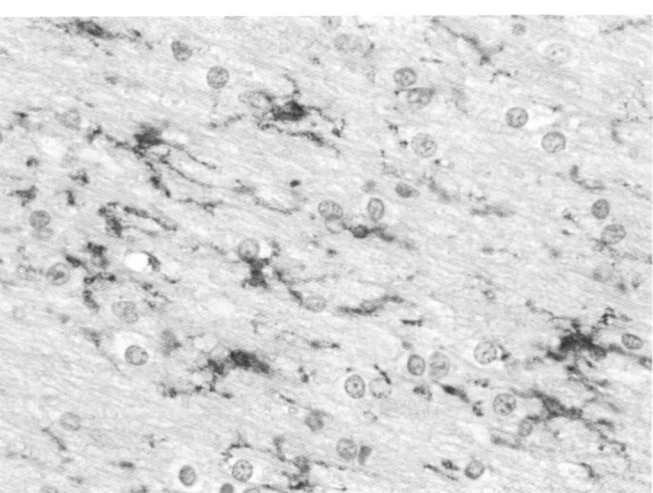

Figure 7.4.3 Diffuse microglial cell activation in brain cortex in a subject who did not have HIV encephalitis (HIVE). The branched cell processes of the activated microglial cells are stained brown (HLADR staining with CR3/43 antibody). Diffuse microglial cell activation can be observed with and without HIVE, and with or without microglial nodule encephalitis. Hematoxylin (blue) counterstaining.

Figure 7.4.2 A large, white matter microglial nodule in HIV encephalitis. The microglial cell nuclei are stained blue with hematoxylin and the neuropil is stained pink with eosin.

present in over 65% of decedents with end-stage AIDS prior to HAART (Gelman, 1993), with and without HIVE, and it showed some relationship to cerebral atrophy. In the HAART era the lesion still is still reported to occur with and without HIVE (Xing et al., 2009); it is not an explicit criterion for the nosological diagnosis however (Love & Wiley, 2008).

ASTROGLIAL HYPERTROPHY AND APOPTOSIS

Astroglial hypertrophy is present to some extent in the majority of HIVE cases, and often, is present in case material from HIV-infected people without the stigma of HIVE. It is most easily viewed in sections of white matter, but the intensity and regional pattern are highly variable (Figure 7.4.4). These astrocytic changes could represent a nonspecific neuropathological reaction to tissue injury or inflammation, which is often referred to as astroglial scarring, but also could participate in the multicellular inflammatory cascade that is believed to be neuropathogenic (Kaul et al., 2001). It also is possible that the astrocytes become hypertrophic and/or apoptotic in response to a relatively nonproductive and limited type of HIV-1 infection that occurs in these cells (Sabri et al., 2003; Thompson et al., 2004; Churchill et al., 2009). Using laser capture microdissection it was shown that a substantial proportion of the astrocytes in brain tissue from subjects with HAD contained HIV provirus DNA, with or without HIVE (Churchill et al., 2009). In addition to hypertrophy, apoptotic astrocytes have been observed in HIVE, and they were associated clinically with progressive worsening of HAND (Thompson et al., 2001). It remains to be determined whether or not programmed astrocyte death is a result of astrocyte HIV-1 infection, or alternatively, is the more general consequence of participating actively in antigen presentation and the inflammatory cascade that is postulated to occur (Kaul et al., 2001).

MYELIN CHANGES, LEUKOENCEPHALOPATHY AND THE BLOOD-BRAIN BARRIER

A characteristic pattern of change in HIVE is the appearance of rarefaction of myelin staining centered primarily about white matter blood vessels. The loss of white matter is usually angiocentric and is associated with increased numbers of macrophages, microglial cells, MNGCs, reactive astrocytes, or lymphocytes within the perivascular sectors (Figure 7.4.5). Macrophages in these numerous small sectors sometimes contain myelin debris, which demonstrates that degeneration of myelinated nerve fibers occurs to some extent. Sometimes, the microvasculature exhibits sclerotic changes, which suggests that microvascular damage and secondary ischemia play a role (Smith et al., 1990). A more diffuse decrease of myelin staining of white matter also occurs that is not restricted to the perivascular spaces. This loss of white matter is a common setting for the astroglial hypertrophy, as discussed above. It is possible that perivascular patterns of nerve fiber injury evolve into the more diffuse white matter lesions. Often the white matter exhibits a striking perivascular accumulation of macrophages that contain hemosiderin iron pigment (Gelman et al., 1992) (Figure 7.4.6).

HIVE is considered a panencephalitis, which means that it can affect gray and white matter both (Budka, 1991), but some examples reported recently had a strong predominance of white matter necrosis severe enough to be termed leukoencephalopathy (Langford et al., 2002). Most of the cases were linked to signs of HIVE and HIV-1 replication, and in some, increased perivascular mononuclear inflammation was present. The latter observation suggested that immune reconstitution produced by HAART might be a possible cause of leukoencephalopathy. This trend also was suggested to be present in a European autopsy cohort (Gray et al., 2003), although leukoencephalopathy was recognized generally as being fairly common in Europe prior to HAART (Budka, 1998). Another very unusual change that was recognized early in the HIV pandemic in patients with end-stage AIDS, and prior to

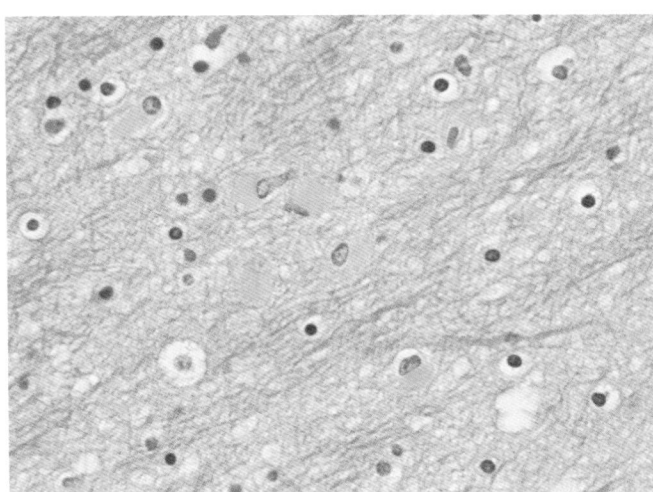

Figure 7.4.4 Astroglial hypertrophy in white matter in HIV encephalitis. Myelinated nerve fibers are stained blue with Luxol Fast Blue. Cytoplasm of the hypertrophic astrocyte is stained pink with eosin.

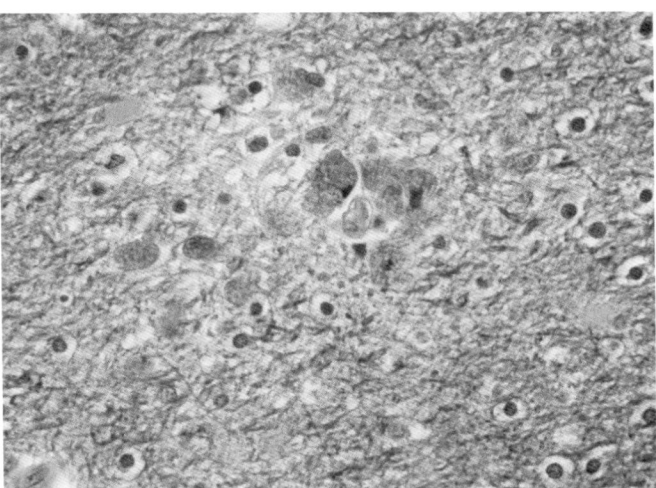

Figure 7.4.5 A white matter lesion with infiltrating macrophages that contain myelin debris stained with Luxol Fast Blue.

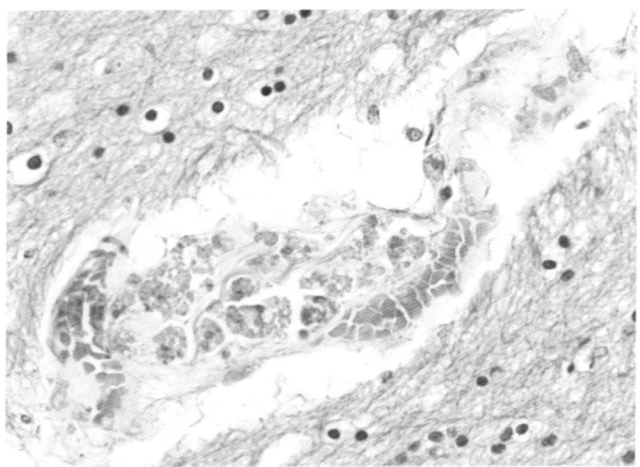

Figure 7.4.6 A blood vessel wall has perivascular accumulation of macrophages that contain abundant brown-stained iron pigment (hemosiderin). The change may be observed with and without HIVE and is associated with substantial white matter damage. Luxol Fast Blue and hematoxylin/eosin staining.

HAART, is a severe vacuolar degeneration of cerebral white matter, known as vacuolar leukoencephalopathy (Schmidbauer et al., 1990). The latter pattern is seldom if ever reported to occur in recent times.

"Myelin pallor" is yet another pattern of diffuse white matter change that may be present in HIVE. The white matter appears diffusely pale in response to myelin-specific histochemical stains such as luxol fast blue, without obvious localized inflammation. This abnormal tinctorial property of the white matter is not likely to reflect outright loss of myelinated nerve fibers because immunostaining for myelin protein is not abnormal. In this setting the lack of histochemical reaction for myelin reflects the leakage of plasma protein through the blood-brain barrier (BBB), which occurs preferentially in white matter and interferes with white matter staining technique (Power et al., 1993; Petito & Cash, 1992). This BBB leakage is reflected histologically by positive immunostaining of brain cells for plasma-derived protein. It was present in up to 50% of HIV-1-infected persons before HAART and may be an independent contributor to tissue damage above and beyond HIVE (Petito & Cash, 1992).

Magnetic resonance spectroscopy (MRS) in HIV-infected people suggests that there are biochemical anomalies in white matter that cannot be detected using routine histopathology. An increase in the ratio of choline to creatine (Cho/Cr) and a decrease in the N-acetylaspartate to Cr ratio (NAA/Cr) have been described in the white matter of people with HIV-1 infection. These chemical anomalies are taken to reflect, respectively, increased glial membrane lipid turnover, and decreased neuronal (axonal) integrity in HIV-infected people (Paul et al, 2008; Lentz et al, 2009, Ernst et al., 2003, Sacktor et al., 2005; Paul et al., 2007). Diffusion tensor imaging (DTI) of clinical cohorts has suggested that the microstructural organization of bundles of myelinated fiber tracts in white matter ("tractology") often is abnormal in HIV infected people (Wu et al., 2006; Müller-Oehring et al., 2010; Chen et al., 2009;

Gongvatana et al., 2009), although the conclusion of some reports is not in complete accord with that (Stebbins et al., 2007; Ragin et al., 2005). Histopathological causes of abnormal white matter "tractology" in AIDS are not clear as yet. Experimentally, infiltration of inflammatory cells in rodent brain produces a reversible disturbance in axon morphology that is correlated with abnormal white matter axial diffusivity (Xie et al., 2010). Axial diffusivity may not, therefore, be an effective marker for permanent changes in brain structure, which may explain why divergent results were obtained so far using DTI in different HIV-infected cohorts.

NEURODEGENERATION, POLIODYSTROPHY, AND SYNAPTODENDRITIC CHANGES

HIV-1 is not a neurotropic virus (i.e., it does not produce a latent or lytic infection of neurons). Nevertheless, it is widely believed that HIVE and HAND both are reflections of a neurodegenerative disease brought about as a secondary ("bystander") change associated with inflammatory cascades (Kaul et al., 2001). Neuropathological evidence supporting the presence of neurodegeneration rests on several observations made prior to the era of HAART, primarily in cases of HIVE in cross sectional observations: 1) There can be structural disorganization and vacuolization of the neuropil (poliodystrophy) as viewed in routine histological tissue sections (Budka et al., 1991); 2) Reports have described neurons and other brain cells undergoing apoptotic death (Petito & Roberts, 1995; Adle-Biassette, et al., 1999; Olano et al., 1996; Shi et al., 1996; Gray et al., 2000); 3) Cumulative dropout of neurons has been measured stereologically (Ketzler et al. 1990; Everall et al., 1991; Everall et al., 1993; Fischer et al., 1999); 4) The technique of Golgi impregnation shows that subtle disorganization of dendritic morphology of neurons can occur in HIVE (Masliah et al., 1992); 5) Immunohistology of synaptic and dendritic protein has revealed fine structural changes in the neuropil in HIVE that could represent subtle and/or early degeneration of neurons (Masliah et al., 1997; Everall et al., 1999); and 6) Axonal injury occurs in HIVE, as depicted in amyloid precursor protein (APP)-stained material (Giometto et al., 1997; Raja et al., 1997).

LYMPHOCYTE INFILTRATION AND IRIS

Immune reconstitution inflammatory syndrome (IRIS) is an adverse response that occurs in some people shortly after HIV-1 replication is suppressed by HAART (Shelburne et al., 2005; Venkataramana et al., 2006). Suppressing virus replication increases the number of circulating CD4 lymphocytes, which triggers an autoimmune-type of inflammatory reaction. IRIS is considered to be an over-response to a pre-existing infection, so the clinical picture can be one of an apparent paradoxical deterioration after HAART is started. It can produce serious and potentially fatal pathological effects in the CNS. In the CNS it can be a response to pre-existing infection with *Cryptococcus neoformans* (King et al., 2002; Wood et al, 1998), cytomegalovirus (Jacobson et al, 1997; Deayton et al., 2000), or papovavirus (the cause of progressive multifocal leukoencephalopathy [PML]) (Du Pasquier & Koralnik, 2003; Tantisiriwat et al., 1998; Corral et al, 2004), and possibly, HIVE (Langford et al., 2002; Miller et al., 2004). CNS inflammatory responses usually were blunted in people with immunodeficiency prior to HAART, whereas in IRIS, the inflammatory response is heightened pathologically. For example, a fatal inflammatory variant of PML was reported in which some white matter lesions contained abundant inflammatory cells with little-stained papovavirus (Corral et al., 2004; Miralles et al., 2001; Vendrely et al., 2005). These examples give the impression that "inflammatory PML" is more prevalent in the HAART era (Du Pasquier and Koralnik, 2003). IRIS-related relapsing meningitis due to *Cryptococcus neoformans* infection and CMV retinitis (King et al., 2002; Wood et al., 1998; Deayton et al., 2000) also are documented. Examples of heightened inflammation in white matter were suggested to be a form of IRIS in which HIVE was exacerbated (Langford et al., 2002). Two examples of panencephalitis with increased infiltration of T lymphocytes were associated with an IRIS-like worsening brain HIV infection (Miller et al., 2004). These reports imply that an unusual but dangerous inflammatory type of HIVE is possible after treatment with HAART is started.

Infiltration of CD4+ and CD8+ lymphocytes usually occurs in the brain of subjects with HIVE, with or without a history of HAART (Petito et al., 2003). These cells accumulate especially around neurons, in microglial nodules, and in perivascular areas. It is suggested that they could participate in the local inflammatory response of HIVE in end-stage AIDS patients. The perineuronal location of CD4+ cells provides the potential for lymphocyte-mediated neuronal injury or trans-receptor-mediated neuronal infection (Melzer et al., 2009). Another pattern of lymphocytic infiltration appears to be restricted to the leptomeninges, and is not clearly linked with HIVE. This pattern is recognized as "HIV-associated lymphocytic meningitis" (Budka, 1991) (Figure 7.4.7). Because it occurs at autopsy in late-stage AIDS, it is not equivalent to the clinically apparent aseptic meningitis that occurs during early-stage infection with HIV shortly after the virus is transmitted. It also is not likely to be equivalent to the lymphocytic infiltration associated with IRIS, because it was observed long before the era of HAART and IRIS. Its relationship to HIV-1 infection still remains unclear. The presence of a mild increase of perivascular and leptomeningeal lymphocytes in a brain without HIVE sometimes serves notice that there is underlying diffuse microglial cell activation in brain parenchyma.

BURNT OUT HIVE AND "NO NEUROPATHOLOGY"

When a person is treated with HAART successfully, one may observe at autopsy only nonspecific astrogliosis and damage to white or gray matter ("glial scars"), but no MNGCs, MGNE, inflammation, or other infectious agent. A diagnosis of "burnt out HIVE" is suggested to apply to these cases (Gray et al., 2003). There also are cases in which HIV-infected people are diagnosed with HAND clinically, but at autopsy, they do not

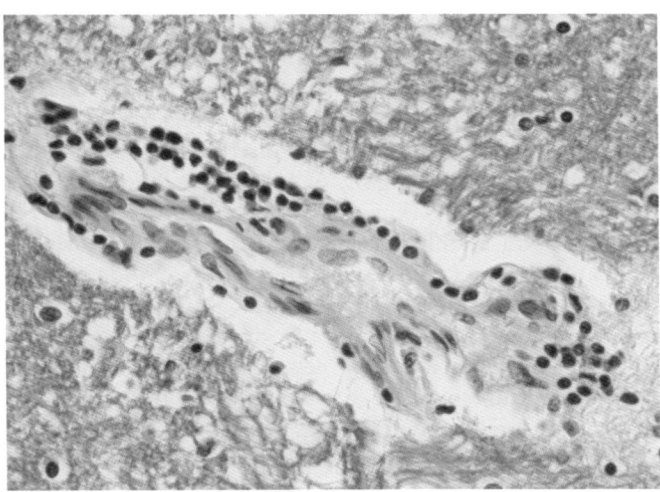

Figure 7.4.7 Round blue lymphocytes surround a blood vessel in a subject with HIV-associated lymphocytic meningitis (HLM). This lesion may be observed without HIV encephalitis. The appearance can resemble IRIS, but HLM was described years before the era of HAART and IRIS. Luxol Fast Blue and hematoxylin/eosin stains.

show active HIVE or other histopathological anomaly. This circumstance was observed prior to the HAART era (Wiley & Achim, 1994; Glass et al., 1993), and is not likely to reflect burnt out HIVE after HAART. This suggests that a predominantly functional, and possibly a metabolic, disturbance could occur in some cases that produces biochemical and physiological changes (versus anatomical) (Glass et al., 1993). In support of that suggestion, several acquired neuronal "channelopathies" have been observed in HIVE and HAD, in which ion channels that mediate membrane excitation are expressed atypically (Gelman et al., 2004). Another potential explanation is that some reported cases of HAD could possess substantial HIV-1 replication in the brain (but that was not specifically measured) yet do not exhibit a frank neuroinflammatory reaction due to generalized immunosuppression in end-stage AIDS. The highly critical issue that remains to be solved is whether or not the implied continuum for progressively severe impairment as diagnosed clinically using the Frascati criteria for HAND (Antinori et al., 2007), is paralleled by a unitary pathophysiology that is neuropathologically progressive in its severity. If the latter scenario should prove to be valid, the lack of neuropathological change might simply represent an early and mostly invisible stage on the continuum of a disease process that culminates with HAD and HIVE. Conversely, it is possible that the various degrees of HAND, and especially the highly prevalent mild forms, are produced by pathophysiological sequences that are neither continuous with HIVE, nor parallel to the progressively severe forms of HAND including HAD (Everall et al., 2009).

POTENTIAL EFFECTS OF BRAIN AGING AND SENILE DEMENTIA ON HAND

A qualitative change suggested to be of increased relevance in HAART-era brain specimens pertains to biological and pathological brain aging. Age was not considered to be highly germane in the early years of the HIV pandemic because patient cohorts were predominantly young adults. As patients survived to older ages, concern mounted regarding a potential clinical and neuropathological interaction with neurodegenerative diseases of aging such as the senile dementias (Brew et al., 2009). HIV-1 and aging could progress in parallel and produce additive effects on cognitive impairment, which was suggested in clinical surveys of older people (Valcour et al., 2004). Aging and HIV also could enter into mutual interaction and synergy. Both scenarios suggest that elderly HIV-infected people are at increased risk of age-associated neurocognitive impairment and disability. The neuropathological underpinnings of the potentially complex mix of persistent HIV-associated inflammation and the senile dementias remain to be elucidated. Morphological studies thus far have focused attention primarily on changes associated with senile dementia of the Alzheimer type (Nath & Hersh, 2005; Brew et al., 2009) such as the extracellular deposition of fibrillary aggregations of the beta fragment of amyloid precursor protein (Aβ plaque or diffuse plaque), and senile ("neuritic") plaques. Some reports have suggested that diffuse or senile plaques might be greater than expected in people with HIV/AIDS (Esiri et al., 1998; Rempel & Pulliam, 2005; Green et al., 2005). However, in studies of elderly subjects that controlled for the influence of chronological age, which is the most critical risk factor, there was no apparent association between HIV-1 infection and increased accumulation of diffuse Aβ plaque (Gelman et al., 2004; Anthony et al., 2006). Fibrillary Aβ accumulates in the brain in all human populations after the age of about 50 years (Yamaguchi et al., 2001; Caselli et al., 2009). The critical questions are whether the pathological signs of brain aging first appear at a younger age, and whether they accumulate at a more rapid pace relative to the person's chronological age. Even if changes associated with senile dementia are more prevalent in cross-sectional autopsy studies, the potential impact on HAND still would remain uncertain because senile plaque burden is not correlated strongly with the severity of senile dementia (Terry et al., 1991). Apparently, senile plaque burden is not a very good reflection of the cumulative loss of brain connectivity or brain cognitive function. In contrast, senile dementia and HAD both are correlated with measures of cumulative damage to the neuropil, such as with synaptophysin immunostaining (Masliah et al., 1997; Terry et al., 1991). Thus, cortical synaptodendritic changes could be a more relevant point of synergy between HAND and the senile dementias. Another potentially important focus of neurobiological synergy is the effect of microglial cell activation, which occurs in pathological brain aging and HIV infection both (Streit, 2005; Dipatre & Gelman, 1997; Gelman, 1993; Xing et al., 2009). The role played by the microglia in aging is unclear and could be neurodegenerative, neuroprotective, or both (Streit, 2005). If an "elderly variant" of HAD or HIVE is emerging that is qualitatively or quantitatively different from what has been observed in young adults, it has not been documented neuropathologically in a robust population of elderly and young subjects as yet.

CLINICONEUROPATHOLOGICAL CORRELATION

A great variety of brain abnormalities have been reported in HIV-infected people. Table 7.4.1 summarizes some key experimental findings made using brain specimens from people with HIV/AIDS generally. Most of these observations were made in selected decedents with HIVE. There are difficulties with this body of literature when trying to determine the cliniconeuropathological correlation with HAND: 1) Few neuropathological studies had the specimen resources necessary to compare outcomes to the severity of neurocognitive test performance prior to death; 2) Few significant clinical correlations have undergone independent replication in more than one cohort; 3) The literature tends to focus on the neuropathologic outcomes including HIVE (which is less prevalent in the post-HAART era) instead of the presence of a clinical neurocognitive diagnosis, which makes the clinical relevance of many neuropathological reports outdated; 4) Comorbid clinical conditions that can produce neurocognitive changes are very difficult to factor into or out of a retrospective autopsy study; 5) A standardized research paradigm to define dementia and comorbid conditions in HIV-1-infected people often was not used, and criteria for clinical diagnoses changed over time (see above); and 6) In vitro brain reconstitution systems can produce highly interesting results attributable to HIV-1 infection that are of unknown relevance to diseased brain tissue that is infected with HIV-1 (Kaul et al., 2001). It is difficult to compare all these kinds of studies to one another, which is the key to deriving the cliniconeuropathological correlation.

THE ROLE OF INFLAMMATION IN HAND

Abnormalities grouped according to macrophage dysfunction or HIV-1 infection of macrophages remain the best documented in terms of the cliniconeuropathological correlation (Williams & Hickey, 2002). HIVE remains a bellwether change in the diagnostic realm of autopsy neuropathology. It has been correlated with severe forms of HAND in multiple cohorts worldwide. HAART-era data continue to support that tenet, and indeed, the diagnosis of HIVE remains perhaps the only neuropathological category that has withstood the test of independent replication (Glass et al., 1993; Wiley & Achim, 1994; Bell et al., 1998; Cherner et al., 2002; Love & Wiley, 2008). Thus, the neuroAIDS field still emphasizes the connection between HAD and HIVE (and has avoided the disconnection), because it has provided useful insight into the pathophysiology (Williams & Hickey, 2002). One reason why the correlation between HAND and HIVE is frequently observed might be that there are several component changes that all can lead to the diagnosis of HIVE. Also, the diagnosis of HIVE does not discriminate according to its severity; the category is broadly inclusive and "all or none" (Love & Wiley, 2008). The lumping together of a constellation of changes instead of a single measurement stands a far better chance of including many different potential variants of HAND. Nevertheless, most evidence collected prior to and after the

HAART era shows that many people with HAND do not fall into the broad HIVE category, and conversely, people with HIVE may not have exhibited HAND. This was recently confirmed using 589 HAART-era brains in the largest cliniconeuropathological correlation study conducted thus far. In that study, 66 cases of HIVE were no more likely to have HAND than the cohort as a whole. As well, 29 cases of MGNE were not more likely to have HAND. This clearly suggests that etiologies other than HIVE and MGNE are more important in the pathophysiology of HAND in the era of HAART (Everall et al., 2009). We know little about what those factors might be, and the lack of clear-cut cliniconeuropathological correlation remains the premier paradox in the neuroAIDS field (Glass et al., 1993; Wiley & Achim, 1994; Everall et al., 2009). When the severity of neurocognitive change is compared specifically with the presence of MNGC, a correlation is not obvious, especially in people with mild impairment (Cherner et al., 2002). Professor Budka's impression that "we are not dealing with a uniform disease" still seems to hold true (Budka, 1998), even though the Frascati criteria for diagnosing HAND tend to imply otherwise. As yet, there is no specific hierarchical listing of pathological findings that has been linked incrementally to the great variation in CNS dysfunction that is observed clinically in HAND.

THE ROLE OF CNS HIV-1 REPLICATION IN HAND

Since the brain cells that are productively infected with HIV-1 are mononuclear phagocytes, and infection of those cells is a major criterion for the diagnosis of HIVE, one would expect that the presence of HIV-1 antigenicity, mRNA, and DNA in the brain to be strongly related to HAND. As already noted, these correlations are surprisingly weak (Glass et al., 1993; 1995). The most accessible compartment to assess HIV-1 replication in the CNS clinically is cerebrospinal fluid (CSF). The concentration of HIV RNA in CSF shows some degree of correlation with HAND when virus replication is not suppressed (Brew et al., 1997; Ellis et al., 2002), but after effective virus suppression with HAART, the correlation between CSF viral load and NP impairment may not persist (McArthur et al., 2004). Glass et al. (1995) undertook one of the only multiple comparisons in the field, so as to examine relative immunological and virological contributions to dementia. When brain HIV-1 antigenicity and the prevalence of brain macrophages were compared, NCI was correlated with macrophage staining very strongly and with HIV antigen staining much less strongly. This suggested that brain inflammation as detected histopathologically is the key driving force behind dementia, and not the burden of replicating HIV-1 in the brain (Williams & Hickey, 2002). Several other abnormal findings pertaining to macrophage activation have been observed in demented patients to support that suggestion. Examples include increased tumor necrosis factor alpha (TNFα) mRNA (Wesselingh et al., 1993; 1997), increased matrix metalloproteinase synthesis (Conant et al., 1999), increased monocyte chemoattractant protein-1 synthesis (Conant, et al., 1998), increased synthesis of inducible nitric oxide synthetase (Adamson et al., 1999; Vincent et al., 1999), and interferon-induced responses including immunoproteasome induction (Nguyen et al., 2010). Despite the substantial linkage of neurocognitive impairment with signs of macrophage activation, it is not obvious why macrophage activation would increase when the burden of replicating HIV-1 is not increased concomitantly. One explanation is that the mere contact of cells with neurotoxic components of HIV (such as HIV tat protein, HIV gp120 envelope protein or assembled virions) triggers lasting immune responses without substantial virus replication. In that proposed scenario, a "hit and run" type of macrophage activation could occur that is not produced by productive HIV-1 infection or virus accumulation (Nath et al., 1999). Another possible way that macrophages are activated is in response to HIV-1 infection of astrocytes (Thompson et al., 2004). Since astrocyte infection with HIV-1 produces only limited virus replication, astrocyte activation is not linked with the accumulation of virions or toxic proteins such as tat or gp120, but still could produce extensive changes in metabolic pathways (Kaul et al., 2001). It is interesting that Glass et al.'s now-classical brain macrophage correlation (Glass et al., 1995), which was derived prior to the HAART era, and other changes pertaining to macrophage activation were not replicated in multiple cohorts independently (Table 7.4.1). That fact tends to limit sharply cross-comparison between the various clinical correlations.

ROLE OF WHITE MATTER DAMAGE IN HAND

Since many of the defining changes of HIVE often affect white matter primarily, and HIVE is often correlated with HAND, white matter damage probably plays some role in producing HAND in some people. Indeed, subcortical structures are highly vulnerable in the setting of HIVE (Navia et al., 1986; Kure et al., 1991; Glass et al., 1995; Everall et al., 1995; Wiley & Achim, 1994; Bell, 2004), and the concentration of replicating HIV-1 is high in subcortical structures including white matter both (Achim et al., 1994). Animal models of HIVE also suggest that white matter damage seems to predominate in most cases (Xing et al., 2003; Raghavan et al., 1999). In addition to myelin loss, axon injury occurs in white matter myelinated nerve fibers (Giometto et al., 1997). Prior to HAART, it was shown that when the full spectrum of white matter injury was surveyed, there was a correlation with dementia in people with end-stage disease (Schmidbauer et al., 1992). However, when injured axons in white matter were examined specifically, a significant correlation with dementia was not apparent (Giometto et al., 1997). Sensitive neuroimaging techniques suggest that white matter changes and subcortical damage are clinically important (Jernigan et al., 1993). Brain spectroscopy (MRS) has shown that choline-containing compounds and myoinositol concentrations are increased, which suggests that membrane turnover is disturbed in white matter glial cells. These neuropathological indicators are harmonious with the fact that HAND is typical of a subcortical dementia (Lipton & Gendelman, 1995; Peavy et al., 1994).

Several other more specific changes pertaining to white matter that might lead to HAND are listed in Table 7.4.1.

In some of the cited work, correlation with dementia was pursued. For example, association between white matter "pallor" and clinical dementia was established in a single cohort (Glass et al., 1993; Power et al., 1993). Paleness of myelin staining was caused by leakage of plasma protein due to a blood-brain barrier (BBB) defect. Whether or not the BBB change in white matter actually causes dementia, or is an epiphenomenon is not clear. The mechanism for the change may be related to endothelial cell changes including a disruption of tight junction integrity (Smith et al., 1990; Dallasta et al., 1999). Another possible effect of a BBB disturbance would include increased access of plasma HIV-1 to the CNS compartment, which in turn could increase the amount of replicating HIV-1 in the brain. As well, an increase in the influx of HIV-1-infected mononuclear cells could occur and alter brain function. As already noted, the loss of myelinated fibers in subcortical white matter also is likely to be correlated with dementia, although very few studies have specifically addressed that correlation (Schmidbauer, 1992; Bell, 2004). Other evidence that abnormal cells of white matter may be related to neurocognitive impairment includes gene and protein expression in oligodendrocytes (Cosenza et al., 2002; Nguyen et al., 2010), increased fractalkine synthesis (Pereira et al., 2001), and expansion of the lysosome system. The lysosomal expansion might be related to abnormal membrane turnover in white matter as visualized by increased myoinositol concentrations using MRS (Gelman et al., 2005).

Similar to white matter pathology, white matter metabolic changes as detected using MRS show variable relationships to neuropsychological test performance, depending upon the population being studied (Ernst et al., 2003, Sactor et al., 2005; Paul et al., 2007). For example it was shown that nondemented subjects with HIV-1 infection have significantly higher Cho/Cr ratios in white matter relative to healthy uninfected controls (Paul et al. 2008). The abnormal MI/Cr in white matter was significantly correlated with measures of fine motor skill in nondemented subjects infected with HIV-1. In a statistically robust proton MRS study (Mahomed et al., 2010), the distribution of metabolites across different brain regions in 74 HIV-infected individuals was measured, including 34 with HIV-associated dementia. Compared to 20 HIV-seronegative controls a unitless "Cho factor" was elevated in the deep gray and white matter regions of HIV-positive subjects. An "NAA factor" was increased in subjects with dementia, and was correlated with impairment of psychomotor speed and executive function, which, in turn, are sometimes taken to reflect the function of frontal white matter (Filley, 2001). The NAA factor also was significantly related to metabolic anomalies in white matter. Since changes NAA signals are taken to represent anomalies in neuronal elements (versus glia), abnormal white matter axons may emit the abnormal NAA signals using MRS.

White matter tractology and altered nerve fiber microstructure using DTI have been compared to neuropsychological functioning in HIV infected people in a few studies, but the results thus far do not permit a clear conclusion. One study (Stebbins et al., 2007) found no association between fractional anisotropy (FA) or mean diffusivity of white matter and neuropsychological test performance. In contrast, another report suggested that reduced FA in the corpus callosum was indeed associated with dementia severity and motor speed (Wu et al., 2006). Similarly, abnormal mean diffusivity of white matter in several brain regions was related to a global index of neuropsychological impairment (Gongvatana et al., 2009). Experimentally, altered axial diffusivity detected using DTI is present when white matter undergoes inflammatory cell infiltration and reversible axonal disturbances (Xie et al., 2010). All these observations suggest that if HAND is reflected clinically by abnormal tractology using DTI, the underlying neuropathological substrate could turn out to be inflammatory cell infiltration (see above) with reversibly altered axonal morphology (see below), as opposed to the outright loss of myelinated nerve fibers (see Figure 7.4.5).

ROLE OF NEURONAL DAMAGE IN HAND

As noted already, neocortical damage also has been observed in HIVE (Wiley et al., 1991; Masliah et al., 1992). As well, subcortical structures that are vulnerable include the basal ganglia, which are composed of gray matter and neuronal cell bodies. HIV-1 does not infect neurons, but based upon early results in subjects with severe HIVE, it remains widely believed that HAND is a type of neurodegenerative disease. Neuropathological evidence supporting the presence of neurodegeneration rests on three main observations. 1) Reports have described neurons and other brain cells undergoing apoptotic death (Petito & Roberts, 1995; Adle-Biassette, et al., 1999; Olano et al., 1996; Shi et al., 1996); 2) Cumulative dropout of neurons has been measured stereologically (Ketzler et al. 1990; Everall et al., 1991); 3) Fine structural changes occur in the neuropil, which may represent subtle and/or early degeneration of neurons and has been related to antemortem HAND (Masliah et al., 1997; Everall et al., 1999, Moore et al., 2006). The meaning of the presence of apoptotic neurons remains unclear because correlation with dementia is not significant (Adle-Biassette et al., 1999; Gray et al., 2000). The lack of correlation does not mean that apoptosis does not play a role because the onset of functional changes may be delayed until a threshold amount of neuron death has accumulated (Terry et al., 1991; Jankovic, 2005). According to that principle, one would expect that the accumulated loss of neurons would be correlated strongly with HAD. But data comparing neuron density with HAD does not confirm that suggestion very consistently (Wiley et al., 1991;Everall et al., 1993; Everall et al., 1999; Weis et al., 1993; Everall et al., 1995; Asare et al., 1996; Seilhean et al., 1993; Korbo & West, 2000). For example, one study showed that loss of neurons occurred in one area of brain cortex, but not an adjacent sector of cortex. When neuron density was compared with dementia, linkage was not significant (Weis et al., 1993). In another study, the spatial arrangement of large and small neurons in brain cortex seemed to be related to dementia, but neuronal dropout itself was not correlated (Asare et al., 1996). Another study illustrated that neuronal subpopulations are affected quite selectively. Substantial loss of a subpopulation of small interneurons that immunostain for parvalbumin occurs in one sector of hippocampus (Masliah et al., 1992b). As for the mechanism of neurodegeneration, many scenarios have been verified experimentally that illustrate ways that HIV-1 and/or inflammation can produce neuronal injury (Kaul et al., 2001). Most of these exciting concepts were worked out in vitro; the challenge that remains is to verify that these postulated events take place in the brain cells of persons with HAND. These studies may be further limited because they focus on the most severe form of HAND (HAD) instead of considering the full spectrum of HAND, especially people with mild neurocognitive impairment.

A notable neuronal change that has withstood a test for correlation with neurocognitive dysfunction is synaptodendritic simplification (Masliah et al., 1997). A study that compared these synaptodendritic changes with neuronal dropout suggested that subtle synaptic changes relate to antemortem neurocognitive functioning, at least in the early stages of dysfunction. In contrast, full-blown neuronal loss was not an independent factor in people with mild impairment, which suggests that it is a late-stage event (Everall et al., 1999). An additional study showed that both subcortical and cortical synaptodendritic changes at autopsy were related to HAND (Moore et al., 2006). It is interesting that synaptodendritic simplification may be present without evidence of an inflammatory change, which contradicts the putative dogma that inflammation is the driving force behind dementia (Kaul et al., 2001; Williams & Hickey, 2002; Glass et al., 1995). Indeed, this lends support to the suggestion that multiple neuropathological pathways may exist that lead to HAND. The emphasis on neuronal elements in the neuropil such as synapses and dendrites is supported by studies showing that the extracellular proteoglycan matrix of neurons is degraded (Belichenko et al., 1997; Medina-Flores, 2004), possibly by macrophage proteases released into the extracellular compartment (Conant et al., 1999; Gelman et al., 1997).

Brain imaging studies have not resolved how cortical and subcortical gray matter anomalies are related to HAND. An MRI study showed severe cortical thinning in primary sensorimotor, premotor, and visual areas of individuals with AIDS generally. Cognitive deficits, specifically psychomotor deficits, were associated with pre-frontal and parietal volume loss (Thompson et al., 2005). Other clinical imaging results showed that caudate nucleus volume correlated significantly with measures of executive functions, and verbal learning, whereas putamen size correlated significantly with measures of processing speed and fine motor skills (Paul et al, 2008). MRS studies showed that decreased MI/Cr in the basal ganglia was correlated with neurocognitive performance. In contrast, no significant correlations were found between brain metabolites in parietal cortex and neuropsychological function (Paul et al., 2007). These clinical surveys lend some support to the suggestion that changes in regional brain volumes often are associated with HAND, but they do not identify the specific neuropathologies that produced abnormal neurocognitive test performance.

Although injured axons can be detected histologically in HIVE using ubiquitin and amyloid precursor protein (APP) staining, the apparent concentration of swollen and misshapen neuronal processes was not correlated significantly with the presence of severity of functional brain impairment (Giametto et al., 1997; Gelman et al., 2004). As noted previously in the discussion of neuronal death and senile plaques, the apparent lack of linkage could mean that axon damage is present transiently. The accumulated damage could eventually become inapparent due to "dropout" or repair of the damaged axons. If clinical symptoms and signs require a threshold amount of axon damage, an anomaly that is present transiently such as a swollen axon might not reflect accumulated damage over time as viewed cross-sectionally at autopsy. In contrast, clinical longitudinal studies using DTI might still be useful to detect transitory shifts in axon morphology, as reflected by abnormal white matter tractology (Xie et al., 2010). The changing white matter microstructural patterns may prove to be reflective of a waxing and waning pattern of neurocognitive anomalies that is often described.

SYSTEMIC AND FUNCTIONAL CHANGES IN HAND

A lack of neuropathological change, especially in gray matter, remains a numerically important category of neurocognitive impairment in HAND. As many as half of the demented patients with end-stage AIDS may fall into the category (Glass et al., 1993), and probably more than that in HAART-treated clinical cohorts with HAND. This ephemeral topic attracted very little attention formerly, but interest has increased because more subjects have mild neurocognitive impairment in the era of HAART (McArthur, 2004; McArthur et al., 2010; Heaton et al., 2010). One suggestion that addresses the lack of brain pathology is a systemic metabolic disturbance. Several systemic changes detected within the plasma compartment, but not within the CNS, have been correlated with severe neurological impairment (usually HAD). A prime example is that a type of anemia known as the "anemia of chronic inflammation" is correlated with HAD (McArthur et al., 1993). This implies that a persistent and possibly lower-grade systemic inflammatory reaction influences CNS function. In support of that, the concentration of lipopolysaccharide (LPS) in the plasma has been correlated significantly with HAD (Ancuta et al., 2008), which is linked to sepsis and/or systemic chronic inflammation of the enteric system. Another prevalent expression of systemic inflammation in end-stage AIDS is a profoundly catabolic wasting syndrome, which is produced by acute phase inflammatory reactants such as TNFα (Kotler, 2000). BBB disturbances in HAND also are likely to reflect a systemic process, because the brain vasculature is in direct and constant contact with blood plasma and circulating HIV-1. As with other systemic inflammatory correlates, BBB anomalies are correlated with HAND with and without HIVE (Power et al., 1993; Petito et al., 1993; Dallasta et al., 1999). The apparent linkage between HAND and systemic inflammation suggests that neurological anomalies could be a sensitive reflection of a broad spectrum of changes occurring systemwide in the whole organism. In that scenario, HIV-1 infection could produce an indolent metabolic encephalopathy, the pathophysiology of which is akin to what occurs in critically ill patients with the systemic inflammatory response syndrome (SIRS), which typically occurs due to a "cytokine storm" (Matsuda & Hattari, 2006). Thus, the lack of brain pathology in many patients with HAND might be explained by a catabolic type of metabolic encephalopathy (versus neurodegeneration or leukoencephalopathy) (Glass et al., 1993; Zheng & Gendelman, 1997). In support of that, results from a gene array showed that several genes involved in the excitation of neurons in brain cortex are expressed abnormally in people with HAD, with and without HIVE (Gelman et al., 2004a). The concept of acquired neuronal channelopathies agrees with results of cortical electroencephalographic (EEG) recordings in HAND, which show abnormal—and potentially reversible—postsynaptic potentials in demented people (Baldeweg & Gruzelier, 1997; Polich et al., 2000). The fact that HAND can improve after HAART (McArthur, 2004; Brew, 2004) also supports the concept of a reversible metabolic type of disturbance of neuronal function, in contrast to the irreversible dropout of neurons as occurs in a classical neurodegenerative disease, or with loss of myelin as in a leukoencephalopathy. These suggestions still must be weighed against the often-compelling evidence that certain neuronal populations are prone to drop out in people with end-stage AIDS and HIVE (Masliah et al., 1992a, Masliah et al., 1992b), and that leukoencephalopathy also can occur (Langford et al., 2002). Nevertheless, significant linkage between neuronal dropout or apoptosis, and the milder forms of HAND, has not been clearly documented. The suggested nosological classifications of HAND as being primarily a mild neurodegenerative disease and/or leukoencephalopathy are not generally substantiated neuropathologically, especially in people with the milder forms of HAND.

A CLINICONEUROPATHOLOGICAL NEUROAIDS AGENDA

The beneficial effect on CNS complications of suppressing HIV-1 replication with HAART is well established. Even though much progress has been made neurocognitive impairment still persists and great challenges lie ahead (McArthur, 2004; Heaton et al., 2010; McArthur et al., 2010). We need to elucidate the host factors that make specific people vulnerable and invulnerable to HAND and further understand how specific neuropathological observations are related to the pathophysiology of HAND (Masliah et al., 1997, Moore et al., 2006). Differences in virus strain and host factors both might produce CNS response variation (Dunfee et al., 2006; Diaz-Arrastia et al., 2004; Levine et al., 2009) and these need to be better understood. The cataloguing of human gene polymorphisms in the haplotype map (International HapMap Consortium, 2005) provides a prime opportunity to elucidate host genetic factors. Several host genetic determinant for systemic virus control have been identified already, but it remains to be seen if these, and other gene loci, exert any influence on host vulnerability to HAND, or immunological control of virus replication in the CNS (Levine et al., 2009).

The cliniconeuropathological correlation is only partly worked out because there are multiple disease categories and underlying pathophysiologies in play. In the future a more quantitative approach to the pathological characterization of these changes might bring added clarity to the cliniconeuropathological correlation. Specifically, a histological staging analogous to those established for research in the senile dementias (Braak et al., 1993) would be a worthwhile goal. Future studies need to pursue aggressively whether observed qualitative neuropathological changes are associated with the various degrees of impairment in HAND, and not just HAD. For example, the complex mixture of leukoencephalopathy-like and neurodegeneration-like changes that occur need to be linked individually with the results of specific neurocognitive task performance. In turn, the many possible neuropathological anomalies need to be mapped to particular brain circuits that can be linked to particular behavioral outcomes, analogous to what has been accomplished in the senile dementias (see Grober et al., 1999). Increased focus is needed to elucidate the effect of comorbid factors that can influence the clinical and pathological course of HIV diseases of the nervous system, such as drug addiction and mental illness. Ultimately, a hierarchical listing of pathological changes is needed that assigns relative importance, or lack of, to the development of HAND. This challenge appears daunting but is necessary to transform HAND from being a clinically described compendium of abnormal brain functions, into a neuropathologically defined disease process that can be mechanistically understood, therapeutically manipulated, and clinically controlled.

SUMMARY

Unlike the senile dementias, the cliniconeuropathological correlation for the full spectrum of HAND remains to be clearly elucidated. The main principles were worked out for HAD, the most severe form of HAND, prior to the HAART era. Those tenets are highly ripe for change given that HAART has decreased the prevalence of HAD sharply, and milder forms of HAND remain quite prevalent.

HIVE can exhibit varied faces and neuropathological features including elements of a neurodegenerative disease, a leukoencephalopathy, a polioencephalopathy, a panencephalopathy, and a metabolic encephalopathy. It is not yet clear how each of the various aspects leads to HAND.

HIVE remains an important neuropathological correlate of brain dysfunction in HIV-infected people in the HAART era. HIVE is the only outcome that has undergone substantial independent verification in multiple autopsy cohorts. HIVE also provides the field with a unifying concept to pursue pathophysiology. HIVE is nevertheless limited because: i) it represents a diverse constellation of anomalies that are not consistently correlated with milder forms of HAND, which are most prevalent in the post-HAART era; and ii) only a small proportion of people with HAND (as few as 5%) exhibit HIVE. The exact neuropathology for HAND in the remainder of cases remains unclear.

The criteria for a diagnosis of HIVE remain essentially intact but variants may have appeared in the HAART era. Examples include an increase in the number of cases with predominantly white matter necrosis (leukoencephalopathy), cases with only minimal or no pathological change (functional variant), cases that have scars without active apparent inflammation (burnt out), cases with age-associated degeneration (a potential senile variant), and cases in which IRIS has played a role (inflammatory variant). In the future it might be useful to establish a clinically validated "staging" of HIVE for comparison with the spectrum of clinical changes associated with HAND.

Very substantial disassociation between HAND and HIVE persists, and suggests that more than one underlying pathophysiology is present. Comorbid factors associated with HIV can produce neurocognitive dysfunction, and might combine with HIV to produce impairment without a recognized histomorphological change.

HAART has significantly decreased the prevalence of the most severe forms of HAND, but it did not decrease its overall prevalence and has introduced some new challenges. Initiation of therapy in an immunosuppressed patient with an ongoing pathological process can provoke immune reconstitution (IRIS), a pathological inflammatory response in the CNS that can be fatal. In addition, HAART drugs themselves might produce neurological side effects.

Because systemic inflammation and immunity are linked to HAND, more study is needed to understand how systemic immunity and CNS signaling via the neurovascular unit might drive abnormal neurocognitive test performance. More specifically, we need to address whether early treatment to prevent significant systemic immune compromise delays or prevents HAND.

HIV/AIDS might eventually prove to exacerbate diseases of brain aging, including the senile dementias, and vice versa. To address that issue the neurobiological interaction between persistent HIV-1 infection and brain aging needs to be elucidated with much greater precision using large cohorts of older HIV-infected people.

ACKNOWLEDGMENTS

The authors wish to acknowledge support of NIH awards to the Texas NeuroAIDS Research Center (U01MH083507, R24NS45491), and the California NeuroAIDS Tissue Network (U01MH083506, R24MH59745)

REFERENCES

Achim, C. L., Wang, R., Miners, D. K., & Wiley, C.A. (1994).Brain viral burden in HIV infection. *J Neuropathol Exp Neurol*, 53, 284–294.

Achim, C. L., Masliah, E., Schindelar, J., & Avramut, M. (2004). Immunophilin expression in the HIV-infected brain. *J Neuroimmunol*, 157, 126–132.

Adamson, D. C., McArthur, J. C., Dawson, T. M., & Dawson, V. L. (1999). Rate and severity of HIV-associated dementia (HAD): Correlations with Gp41 and iNOS. *Molecular Med*, 5, 98–109.

Adle-Biassette, H., Levy, Y., Colombel, M., Poron, F., Natchev, S., Keohane, C., et al. (1999). Neuronal apoptosis does not correlate with dementia in HIV infection but is related to microglial activation and axonal damage. *Neuropathol Appl Neurobiol*, 25, 125–133.

Ancuta, P., Kamat, A,. Kunstman, K. J., Kim, E-Y., Autissier, P., et al. (2008) Microbial translocation is associated with increased monocyte activation and dementia in AIDS patients. *PLoS ONE*, 3(6), e2516. doi:10.1371/journal.pone.0002516.

Anthony, I. C., Ramage, S. N., Carnie, F. W., Simmonds, P., & Bell, J. E. (2006). Accelerated tau deposition in the brains of individuals infected with human immunodeficiency virus-1 before and after the advent of highly active anti-retroviral therapy. *Acta Neuropathol*, 111(6), 529–538.

Antinori, A., Arendt, G., Becker, J. T., Brew, B. J., Byrd, D. A., Cherner, M., et al. (2007). Updated research nosology for HIV-associated neurocognitive disorders. *Neurology*, 69, 1789–1799.

Archibald, S. L., Masliah, E., Fennema-Notestine, C., Marcotte, T. D., Ellis, R. J., McCutchan, J. A., et al. (2004). Correlation of in vivo neuroimaging abnormalities with postmortem human immunodeficiency virus encephalitis and dendritic loss. *Arch Neurol*, 61, 369–376.

Asare, E., Dunn, G., Glass, J., et al. (1996). Neuronal pattern correlates with the severity of human immunodeficiency virus-associated dementia complex: Usefulness of spatial pattern analysis in clinicopathological studies. *Am J Pathol* 148, 31–38.

Baldeweg, T. & Gruzelier, J. H. (1997). Alpha EEG activity and subcortical pathology in HIV infection. *Int J Psychophysiol*, 26, 431–442.

Baue, A. E., Durham, R., & Faist, E. (1998). Systemic inflammatory response syndrome (Sirs), multiple organ dysfunction syndrome (Mods), multiple organ failure (Mof): Are we winning the battle? *Shock* 10(2), 79–89.

Belichenko, P. V., Miklossy, J., & Celio, M. R. (1997). HIV-I induced destruction of neocortical extracellular matrix components in AIDS victims. *Neurobiol Dis*, 4, 301–310.

Bell, J. E., Brettle, R. P., Chiswick, A., & Simmonds P. (1998). HIV encephalitis, proviral load and dementia in drug users and homosexuals with AIDS. Effect of neocortical involvement. *Brain*, 121 (Pt 11), 2043–2052.

Bell, J. E. (2004). An update on the neuropathology of HIV in the HAART era. *Histopathology*, 45, 549–559.

Braak, H., Braak, E., & Bohl, J. (1993). Staging of Alzheimer-related cortical destruction. *European Neurology, Basel, 33*, 403–408.

Brew, B. J., Pemberton, L., Cunningham, P., Law, & M. G. (1997). Levels of human immunodeficiency type 1 RNA in cerebrospinal fluid correlate with AIDS dementia stage. *J infect Dis*, 175, 963–966.

Brew, B. J. (2004). Evidence for a change in AIDS dementia complex in the era of highly active antiretroviral therapy and the possibility of new forms of AIDS dementia complex. *AIDS*, 18 (Suppl 1), S75–S78.

Brew, B. J., Crowe, S. M., Landay, A., Cysique, L. A., & Guillemin, G. (2009). Neurodegeneration and ageing in the HAART era. *J Neuroimmune Pharmacol*, 4,163–174.

Budka, H. (1998). HIV-associated neuropathology. In H. E. Gendelman, S. E. Lipton, L. Epstein, & S. Swindells (Eds.). *The Neurology of AIDS*. pp 241–260. New York: Chapman & Hall.

Budka, H. (1986). Multinucleated giant cells in brain: A hallmark of the acquired immune deficiency syndrome (AIDS). *Acta Neuropathol (Berl)*, 69, 253–258.

Budka, H. (1991). Neuropathology of human immunodeficiency virus infection. *Brain Pathology*, 1(3), 163–175.

Budka, H., Wiley, C. A., Kleihues, P., Artigas, J., Asbury, A. K., Cho, E. S., et al. (1991). HIV-associated disease of the nervous system: Review of nomenclature and proposal for neuropathology-based terminology. *Brain Pathology*, 1(3), 143–52.

Caselli, R. J., Dueck, A. C., Osborne, D., et al. (2009). Longitudinal modeling of age-related memory decline and the *APOE4* effect. *New Engl J Med* 361, 255–263.

Chen, Y., An, H., Zhu, H., Stone, T., Smith, J. K., Hall, C., et al. (2009). White matter abnormalities revealed by diffusion tensor imaging in non-demented and demented HIV+ patients. *Neuroimage, 47*(4), 1154–1162.

Cherner, M., Masliah, E., Ellis, R. J., Marcotte, T. D., Moore, D. J., Grant, I., et al. (2002). Neurocognitive dysfunction predicts postmortem findings of HIV encephalitis. *Neurology, 59*(10), 1563–1567.

Churchill, M. J., Wesselingh, S. L., Cowley, D., Pardo, C. A., McArthur, J. C., Brew, B. J., et al. (2009). Extensive astrocyte infection is prominent in human immunodeficiency virus-associated dementia. *Ann Neurol, 66*(2), 253–258.

Conant, K., McArthur, J. C., Griffin, D. E., Sjulson, L., Wahl, L. M., & Irani, D. N. (1999). Cerebrospinal fluid levels of MMP-2, 7, and 9 are elevated in association with human immunodeficiency virus dementia. *Ann Neurology, 46*, 391–398.

Conant, K., Garzino-Demo, A., Nath, A., McArthur, J. C., Halliday, W., Power, C., et al. (1998). Induction of monocyte chemoattractant protein-1 in HIV-1 Tat-stimulated astrocytes and elevation in AIDS dementia. *Proc Natl Acad Sci USA, 95*(6), 3117–3121.

Corral, I., Quereda, C., Garcia-Villanueva, M., Casado, J. L., Perez-Elias, M. J., Navas, E., et al. (2004). Focal monophasic demyelinating leukoencephalopathy in advanced HIV infection. *European Neurolog, 52*, 36–41.

Cosenza, M. A., Zhao, M-L., Shankar, S. L., Shafit-Zagardo, B., & Lee, S. C. (2002). Up-regulation of MAP2e-expressing oligodendrocytes in the white matter of patients with HIV-1 encephalitis. *Neuropathol Appl Neurobiol 28*, 480–488.

Deayton, J. R., Wilson, P., Sabin, C. A., Davey, C.C, Johnson, M. A., Emery, V. C., et al. (2000). Changes in the natural history of cytomegalovirus retinitis following the introduction of highly active antiretroviral therapy. *AIDS, 14*, 1163–1170.

Dallasta, L. M., Pisarov, L. A., Esplen, J. E., Werley, J. V., Moses, A. V., Nelson, J. A., et al. (1999). Blood-brain barrier tight junction disruption in human immunodeficiency virus-1 encephalitis. *Am J Pathol 155*(6), 1915–1927.

Diaz-Arrastia, R., Gong, Y., Kelly, C. J., & Gelman, B. B. (2004). Host genetic polymorphisms in HIV-related neurological disease. *J Neurovirol 10*, Suppl 1, 67–73.

DiPatre, P. L. & Gelman, B. B. (1997). Microglial cell activation in aging and Alzheimer's disease: Partial correlation with neurofibrillary tangle burden. *J Neuropathol Exp Neurol 56*, 137–143.

Dunfee, R. L, Thomas, E. R., Gorry, P. R., Taylor, J., Kunstman, K., Bell, J. M., et al. (2006). The HIV Env variant N283 enhances macrophage tropism and is associated with brain infection and dementia. *Proc. Natl. Acad. Sci. USA, 103*, 15160–15165.

Du Pasquier, R. A. & Koralnik, I. J. (2003). Inflammatory reaction in progressive multifocal leukoencephalopathy: Harmful or beneficial? *J Neurovirol, 9* Suppl 1, 25–31.

Ellis, R. J., Moore, D. J., Childers, M. E., Letendre, S., McCutchan, J. A., Wolfson, T., et al. (2002). Elevated cerebrospinal fluid HIV RNA levels predict progression to neuropsychological impairment in HIV infection. *Arch Neurol 59*(6), 923–928.

Ernst, T., Chang, L., & Arnold, S. (2003). Increased glial markers predict increased working memory network activation in HIV patients. *NeuroImage 19*(4), 1686–1693.

Esiri, M. M., Biddolph, S. C., & Morris, C. S. (1998). Prevalence of Alzheimer plaques in AIDS. *J Neurol Neurosurg Psych 65*, 29–33.

Everall, I. P., Luthert, P. J., & Lantos, P. L. (1991). Neuronal loss in the frontal cortex in HIV infection. *Lancet, 337*(8750), 1119–1121.

Everall, I., Luthert, P., & Lantos, P. (1993). A review of neuronal damage in human immunodeficiency virus infection: Its assessment, possible mechanism and relationship to dementia. *J Neuropathol Exp Neurol, 52*, 561–566.

Everall, I. P., Luthert, P. J., & Lantos, P. L. (1993). Neuronal number and volume alterations in the neocortex of HIV infected individuals. *J Neurol Neurosurg Psych, 56*, 481–486.

Everall, I. P., Glass, J. D., McArthur, J., Spargo, E., & Lantos, P. (1994). Neuronal density in the superior frontal and temporal gyri does not correlate with the degree of human immunodeficiency virus-associated dementia. *Acta Neuropathol (Berl), 88*, 538–544.

Everall, I., Barnes, H., Spargo, E., & Lantos, P. (1995). Assessment of neuronal density in the putamen in human immunodeficiency virus (HIV) infection. Application of stereology and spatial analysis of quadrats. *J Neurovirol, 1*, 126–129.

Everall, I. P., Heaton, R. K., Marcotte, T. D., Ellis, R. J., McCutchan, J. A., Atkinson, J. H., et al. (1999). Cortical synaptic density is reduced in mild to moderate human immunodeficiency virus neurocognitive disorder. HNRC Group. HIV Neurobehavioral Research Center. *Brain Pathology, 9*, 209–217.

Everall, I., Vaida, F., Khanlou, N., Lazzaretto, D., Achim, C., Letendre, S., et al. (2009). Cliniconeuropathologic correlates of human immunodeficiency virus in the era of antiretroviral therapy. *J Neurovirology, 15*, 360–370.

Filley, C. M. (2001). *The behavioral neurology of white matter*. New York: Oxford University Press. .

Fischer, C. P., Jorgen, G., Gundersen, H., & Pakkenberg, B. (1999). Preferential loss of large neocortical neurons during HIV infection: A study of the size distribution of neocortical neurons in the human brain. *Brain Researc, 828*(1–2), 119–126.

Gelman, B. B., Rodriguez, M. G., Wen, J., Campbell, G. A., & Herzog, N. (1992). Siderotic cerebral macrophages in the acquired immunodeficiency syndrome. *Arch Pathol Lab Med 116*, 509–516.

Gelman, B. B. & Guinto, F. C. Jr. (1992). Morphometry, histopathology, and tomography of cerebral atrophy in the acquired immunodeficiency syndrome. *Ann Neurol 32*, 32–40.

Gelman, B. B. (1993). Diffuse microgliosis associated with cerebral atrophy in the acquired immunodeficiency syndrome. *Ann Neurol, 34*, 65–70.

Gelman, B. B., Dholakia, S., Casper, K., Kent, T. A., Cloyd,M. W., Freeman, D. Jr. (1996). Expansion of the cerebral ventricles and correlation with acquired immunodeficiency syndrome: Neuropathology in 232 patients. *Arch Pathol Lab Med, 120*, 866–71.

Gelman, B. B., Wolf, D. A., Rodriguez-Wolf, M., West, B., Haque, A, & Cloyd, M. W. (1997). Mononuclear phagocyte hydrolytic enzyme activity associated with cerebral HIV infection. *Am J Pathol, 151*, 1437–1446.

Gelman, B. B., Soukup, V. M., Keherly, M. J., Schuenke, K. W., Holzer, C. E., Richey, J. L., et al. (2004a). Acquired neuronal channelopathies in HIV-associated dementia. *J Neuroimmunology, 157*, 111–119.

Gelman, B. B. & Schuenke, K. W. (2004b). Brain aging in AIDS: Increased ubiquitin-protein conjugate and correlation with decreased synaptic protein but not Aβ-stained diffuse plaque. *J Neurovirol, 10*:98–108.

Gelman, B. B., Soukup, V. M., Holzer, C. E. 3rd, Fabian, R. H., Schuenke, K. W., Keherly, M. J., et al. (2005). Potential role for white matter lysosome expansion in HIV-associated dementia. *J AIDS 39*, 422–425.

Giometto, B., An, S. F., Groves, M., Scaravilli, T., Geddes, J. F., Miller, R., et al. (1997). Accumulation of β-amyloid precursor protein in HIV encephalitis: Relationship with neuropsychological abnormalities. *Ann Neurol, 42*, 34–40.

Glass, J. D., Wesselingh, S. L., Selnes, O. A., & McArthur, J. C. (1993). Clinical-neuropathologic correlation in HIV-associated dementia. *Neurology, 43*:2230–2237.

Glass, J. D., Fedor, H., Wesselingh, S. L., & McArthur, J. C. (1995). Immunocytochemical quantitation of human immunodeficiency virus in the brain: Correlations with dementia. *Ann Neurol 38*, 755–762.

Glass, J. D. & Wesselingh, S. L. (1998). Viral load in HIV-associated dementia. *Ann Neurol 44*, 150–151.

Goebel, F. D. (2005). Immune reconstitution inflammatory syndrome (IRIS)—another new disease entity following treatment initiation of HIV infection. *Infection, 33*, 43–45.

Gongvatana, A., Schweinsburg, B. C., Taylor, M. J., Theilmann, R. J., Letendre, S. L., Alhassoon, O. M., et al. (2009). White matter tract injury and cognitive impairment in human immunodeficiency virus-infected individuals. *J Neurovirol, 15*(2), 187–195.

Grant, I., Atkinson, J. H., Hesselink, J. R., Kennedy, C. J., Richman, D. D., Spector, S. A., et al. (1987). Evidence for early central nervous system involvement in the acquired immunodeficiency syndrome (AIDS) and other human immunodeficiency virus (HIV) infections. Studies with neuropsychologic testing and magnetic resonance imaging. *Ann Intern Med.*, 107(6), 828–836.

Grant, I., Atkinson, J. H. (1999). Neuropsychiatric aspects of HIV infection and AIDS. In: B. J. Sadock & V. A. Sadock (eds.). *Kaplan and Sadock's comprehensive textbook of psychiatry/VII*, pp. 308–335. Baltimore: Williams & Wilkins.

Grassi, M. P., Clerici, F., Vago, L., Perin, C., Borella, M., Nebuloni, M., et al, (2002). Clinical aspects of the AIDS dementia complex in relation to histopathological and immunohistochemical variables. *European Neurology*, 47, 141–147.

Gray, F., Adle-Biassette, H., Brion, F., Ereau, T., le Maner, I., Levy, V., et al. (2000). Neuronal apoptosis in human immunodeficiency virus infection. *J Neurovirol*, 6 Suppl 1, S38–43.

Gray, F., Chretien, F., Vallat-Decouvelaere, A. V., & Scaravilli, F. (2003). The changing pattern of HIV neuropathology in the HAART era. *J Neuropathol Exp Neurol*, 62, 429–440.

Green, D. A., Masliah, E., Vinters, H. V., Beizai, P., Moore, D. J., & Achim, C. L. (2005). Brain deposition of beta-amyloid is a common pathologic feature in HIV positive patients. *AIDS*, 19, 407–411.

Grober, E., Dickson, D., Sliwinski, M. J., Buschke, H., Katz, M., Crystal, H., et al. (1999). Memory and mental status correlates of modified Braak staging. *Neurobiol Aging*, 20, 573–579.

Heaton, R. K., Grant, I., Butters, N., White, D. A., Kirson, D., Atkinson, J. H., et al. (1995). The HNRC 500—neuropsychology of HIV infection at different disease stages. HIV Neurobehavioral Research Center. *J Int Neuropsychol Soc*, 1, 231–251.

Heaton, R. K., Clifford, D. B., Franklin Jr., D. R., Woods, S. P., Ake, C., et al. (2010). HIV-associated neurocognitive disorders persist in the era of potent antiretroviral therapy. *Neurology*, 75(23), 2087–96.

The International HapMap Consortium. (2005). A haplotype map of the human genome. *Nature*, 437(7063), 1299–1320.

Jacobson, M. A., Zegans, M., Pavan, P. R., O'Donell, J. J., Settler, F., Rao, N., et al. (1997). Cytomegalovirus retinitis after initiation of highly active antiretroviral therapy. *Lancet*, 349:1143–1145.

Jankovic, J. (2005). Progression of Parkinson disease: Are we making progress in charting the course? *Arch Neurol*, 62(3), 351–352.

Janssen, R. S., Cornblath, D. R., Epstein, L. et al. (1991). Nomenclature and research case definitions for neurological manifestations of human immunodeficiency virus type-1 (HIV-1) infection. *Neurology*, 41, 778–785.

Jellinger, K. A., Setinek, U., Drlicek, M., Bohm, G., Steurer, A., & Lintner, F. (2000). Neuropathology and general autopsy findings in AIDS during the last 15 years. *Acta Neuropathol (Berl)*, 100, 213–220.

Jernigan, T. L., Archibald, S., Hesselink, J. R., Atkinson, H., Velin, R. A., McCutchan, J. A., et al. (1993). Magnetic resonance imaging morphometric analysis of cerebral volume loss in human immunodeficiency virus infection. *Arch Neurol*, 50(3), 250–255.

Kaul, M., Garden, G. A., & Lipton, S. A. (2001). Pathways to neuronal injury and apoptosis in HIV-associated dementia. *Nature*, 410, 988–994.

Ketzler, S, Weis, S., Haug, H., & Budka, H. (1990). Loss of neurons in the frontal cortex in AIDS brains. *Acta Neuropathol (Berl)*, 80, 92–94.

King, M. D., Perlino, C. A., Cinnamon, J., & Jernigan, J. A. (2002). Paradoxical recurrent meningitis following therapy of cryptococcal meningitis: An immune reconstitution syndrome after initiation of highly active antiretroviral therapy. *AIDS*, 13,724–726.

Klatt, E. C. (1988). Diagnostic findings in patients with acquired immune deficiency syndrome (AIDS). *J AIDS*, 1(5), 459–465.

Korbo, L. & West, M. (2000). No loss of hippocampal neurons in AIDS patients. *Acta Neuropathol*, 99, 529–533.

Kotler, D. P. (2000). Cachexia. *Ann Intern Med*, 133(8), 622–634.

Kure, K., Llena, J. F., Lyman, W. D., et al. (1991). Human immunodeficiency virus type 1 infection of the nervous system: An autopsy study of 268 adult, pediatric, and fetal brains. *Human Pathol*, 22, 700–710.

Langford, T. D., Letendre, S. L., Marcotte, T. D., Ellis, R. J., McCutchan, J. A., Grant, I., et al. (2002). Severe, demyelinating leukoencephalopathy in AIDS patients on antiretroviral therapy. *J AIDS*, 16, 1019–1029.

Lentz, M. R., Kim, W. K., Lee, V., Bazner, S., Halpern, E. F., Venna, N., et al. (2009). Changes in MRS neuronal markers and T cell phenotypes observed during early HIV infection. *Neurology*, 72(17), 1465–1472.

Levine, A. J., Singer, E. J., & Shapshak, P. (2009). The role of host genetics in the susceptibility for HIV-associated neurocognitive disorders. *AIDS Behav*, 13(1), 118–132.

Lipton, S. A. & Gendelman, H. L. (1995). Dementia associated with the acquired immunodeficiency syndrome. *N Engl J Med*, 332, 934–940.

Love, S. & Wiley, C. A. (2008). Viral infections. In S. Love, D. N. Louis, & D. W. Ellison, (Eds.). *Greenfield's neuropathology*, eighth edition. pp. 1343–1348. London: Edward Arnold Ltd.

Mohamed, M. A., Lentz, M. R., Lee, V., Halpern, E. F., Sacktor, N., Selnes, O., et al. (2010). Factor analysis of proton MR spectroscopic imaging data in HIV infection: Metabolite-derived factors help identify infection and dementia. *Radiology*, 254(2), 577–586.

Masliah, E., Achim, C. L., Ge, N., DeTeresa, R., Terry, R. D., & Wiley, C. A. (1992a). Spectrum of human immunodeficiency virus-associated neocortical damage. *Ann Neurol*, 32, 321–329.

Masliah, E., Ge, N., Achim, C. L., Hansen, L. A., & Wiley, C. A. (1992b). Selective neuronal vulnerability in HIV encephalitis. *J Neuropathol Exp Neurol*, 51, 585–593.

Masliah, E., DeTeresa, R. M., Mallory, M. E., & Hansen, L. A. (2000). Changes in pathological findings at autopsy in AIDS cases for the last 15 years. *AIDS*, 14, 69–74.

Masliah, E., Heaton, R. K., Marcotte, T. D., Ellis, R. J., Wiley, C. A., Mallory, M., et al. (1997). Dendritic injury is a pathological substrate for human immunodeficiency virus-related cognitive disorders. HNRC Group. The HIV Neurobehavioral Research Center. *Ann Neurol*, 42, 963–972.

Matsuda, N. & Hattori, Y. (2006). Systemic inflammatory response syndrome (SIRS): Molecular pathophysiology and gene therapy. *J Pharmacol Sci*, 101(3), 189–198.

McArthur, J. C., Hoover, D. R., Bacellar, H., Miller, E. N., Cohen, B. A., & Becker, J. T., et al. (1993). Dementia in AIDS patients: Incidence and risk factors. Multicenter AIDS Cohort Study. *Neurology*, 43(11), 2245–2252.

McArthur, J. C., McClernon, D. R., Cronin, M. F., Nance-Sproson, T. E., Saah, A. J., St Clair, M., et al. (1997). Relationship between human immunodeficiency virus-associated dementia and viral load in cerebrospinal fluid and brain. *Ann Neurol*, 42, 689–698.

McArthur, J. C. (2004). HIV dementia: An evolving disease. *J Neuroimmunology*, 157(1–2), 3–10.

McArthur, J. C., Brew, B., & Nath, A. (2005). Neurological complications of HIV infection. *Lancet Neurology 4*, 543–555.

McArthur, J. C., Steiner, J., Sacktor, N., & Nath, A. (2010). Human immunodeficiency virus-associated neurocognitive disorders: Mind the gap. *Ann Neurol*, 67, 699–714.

Medina-Flores, R., Wang, G., Bissel, S. J., Murphey-Corb, M., & Wiley, C. A. (2004). Destruction of extracellular matrix proteoglycans is pervasive in simian retroviral neuroinfection. *Neurobiol Disease*, 16, 604–616.

Melzer, N., Meuth, S. G., & Wiend, H. (2009). CD8+ T cells and neuronal damage: Direct and collateral mechanisms of cytotoxicity and impaired electrical excitability. *FASEB J*, 23, 3659–3673.

Miller, R. F., Isaacson, P. G., Hall-Craggs, M., Lucas, S., Gray, F., & Scaravilli, F., An, S. (2004). Cerebral CD8+ lymphocytosis in HIV-1 infected patients with immune restoration induced by HAART. *Acta Neuropathol*, 108, 17–23.

Miralles, P., Berenguer, J., Lacruz, C., Cosin, J., Lopez, J. C., Padilla, B., et al. (2001). Inflammatory reactions in progressive multifocal leukoencephalopathy after highly active antiretroviral therapy. *AIDS*, 15,1900–1902.

Moore, D. J., Masliah, E., Rippeth, J. D., Gonzalez, R., Carey, C. L., Cherner, M., et al. (2006). Cortical and subcortical neurodegeneration is associated with HIV neurocognitive impairment. *AIDS*, 20(6), 879–887.

Morgan, E. E., Woods, S. P., Scott, J. C., Childers, M., Beck, J. M., Ellis, R. J., et al. (2008). Predictive validity of demographically adjusted normative standards for the HIV Dementia Scale. *J Clin Exp Neuropsychol*, *30*(1), 83–90.

Morgello, S., Mahboob, R., Yakoushina, T., Khan, S., & Hague K. (2002). Autopsy findings in a human immunodeficiency virus-infected population over 2 decades: influences of gender, ethnicity, risk factors, and time. *Arch Pathol Lab Med*, *126*, 182–190.

Müller-Oehring, E. M., Schulte, T., Rosenbloom, M. J., Pfefferbaum, A., & Sullivan, E. V. (2010). Callosal degradation in HIV-1 infection predicts hierarchical perception: A DTI study. *Neuropsychologia*, *48*(4), 1133–1143.

Nath, A., Conant, K., Chen, P., Scott, C., & Major, E. O. (1999). Transient exposure to HIV-1 Tat protein results in cytokine production in macrophages and astrocytes. A hit and run phenomenon. *J Biol Chem*, *274*, 17098–17102.

Nath, A. & Hersh, L. B. (2005). Tat and amyloid: Multiple interactions. *AIDS*, *19*:203–204.

Navia, B. A., Cho, E. S., Petito, C. K., & Price, R. W. (1986). The AIDS dementia complex: II. Neuropathology. *Ann Neurol*, *19*, 525–535.

Neuenburg, J. K., Brodt, H. R., Herndier, B. G., Bickel, M., Bacchetti, P., Price, R. W., et al. (2002). HIV-related neuropathology, 1985 to 1999: Rising prevalence of HIV encephalopathy in the era of highly active antiretroviral therapy. *J AIDS*, *31*, 171–177.

Nguyen, T. N., Soukup, V. M, & Gelman, B. B. (2010). Persistent hijacking of brain proteasomes in HIV-associated dementia. *Am J Pathol*, *176*, 893–902.

Olano, J. P., Wolf, D. A., Keherly, M. J., Gelman, B. B. (1996). Quantifying apoptosis in banked human brains using flow cytometry. *J Neuropathol Exp Neurol*, *55*, 1164–1172.

Paul, R. H., Yiannoutsos, C. T., Miller, E. N., Chang, L., Marra, C. M., Schifitto, G., et al. (2007). Proton MRS and neuropsychological correlates in AIDS dementia complex: Evidence of subcortical specificity. *J Neuropsych Clin Neurosci*, *19*, 283–292.

Paul, R. H., Ernst, T., Brickman, A. M, Yiannoutsos, C. T., Tate, D. F., Cohen, R. A., et al. (2008). Relative sensitivity of magnetic resonance spectroscopy and quantitative magnetic resonance imaging to cognitive function among nondemented individuals infected with HIV. *J Int Neuropsychol Soc*, *14*, 725–733.

Peavy, G., Jacobs, D, Salmon, D. P, Butters, N., Delis, D. C., Taylor, M., et al. (1994). Verbal memory performance of patients with human immunodeficiency virus infection: Evidence of subcortical dysfunction. The HNRC Group. *J Clin Exp Neuropsychol*, *16*(4), 508–523.

Pereira, C. F., Middel, G., Jansen, J., Verhoef, H. S. L., & Nottet, M. (2001). Enhanced expression of fractalkine in HIV-1 associated dementia. *J Neuroimmunology*, *115*, 168–175.

Perry, S. & Marotta, R. F. (1987). AIDS dementia: A review of the literature. *Alzheimer Dis Assoc Disord*, *1*(4), 221–235.

Petito, C. K. (1993). Neuropathology of acquired immunodeficiency syndrome. In J. S. Nelson, J. E. Parisi, & S. S. Schochet Jr, (eds.). *Principles and practice of neuropathology*, pp. 88–108. Saint Louis: Mosby.

Petito, C. K. & Roberts, B. (1995). Evidence of apoptotic cell death in HIV encephalitis. *Amer J Pathol*, *146*, 1121–1130.

Petito, C. K. & Cash, K. S. (1992). Blood-brain barrier abnormalities in the acquired immunodeficiency syndrome: Immunohistochemical localization of serum proteins in postmortem brain. *Ann Neurol*, *32*(5), 658–666.

Petito, C. K., Adkins, B., McCarthy, M., Roberts, B., & Khamis, I. (2003). CD4+ and CD8+ cells accumulate in the brains of acquired immunodeficiency syndrome patients with human immunodeficiency virus encephalitis. *J Neurovirol*, *9*, 36–44.

Polich, J., Ilan, A., Poceta, J. S., Mitler, M. M., & Darko, D. F. (2000). Neuroelectric assessment of HIV: EEG, ERP, and viral load. *Int J Psychophysiology*, *38*, 97–108.

Power, C., Kong, P. A., Crawford, T. O., Wesselingh, S., Glass, J. D., McArthur, J. C., et al. (1993). Cerebral white matter changes in acquired immunodeficiency syndrome dementia: Alterations of the blood-brain barrier. *Ann Neurol*, *34*, 339–350.

Power, C., Selnes, O. A., Grim, J. A., & McArthur, J. C. (1995). HIV Dementia Scale: A rapid screening test. *Acquir Immune Defic Syndr Hum Retrovirol*. *8*(3), 273–278.

Raghavan, R., Cheney, P. D., Raymond, L. A., et al. (1999). Morphological correlates of neurobiological dysfunction in macaques infected with neurovirulent simian immunodeficiency virus. *Neuropathol Appl Neurobiol*, *25*, 285–294.

Raja, F., Sherriff, F. E., Morris, C. S., Bridges, L. R., & Esiri, M. M. (1997). Cerebral white matter damage in HIV infection demonstrated using beta-amyloid precursor protein immunoreactivity. *Acta Neuropathol (Berl)*, *93*, 184–189.

Rempel, H. C. & Pulliam, L. (2005). HIV-1 Tat inhibits neprilysin and elevates amyloid beta. *AIDS*, *19*, 127–135.

Sabri, F, Titanji, K, De Milito, A., & Chiodi, F. (2003). Astrocyte activation and apoptosis: Their roles in the neuropathology of HIV infection. *Brain Pathol*, *13*, 84–94.

Sacktor, N. C., Lyles, R. H., Skolasky, R. L., Anderson, D. E., McArthur, J. C., McFarlane, G., et al. (1999a). Combination antiretroviral therapy improves psychomotor speed performance in HIV-seropositive homosexual men. Multicenter AIDS Cohort Study (MACS). *Neurology*, *52*(8), 1640–1647.

Sacktor, N. C., Lyles, R. H., Skolasky, R., Anderson, D. E., McArthur, J. C., McFarlane, G. et al. (1999b). The multicenter AIDS Cohort Study. HIV-1 related neurological disease incidence changes in the era of highly active antiretroviral therapy. *Neurology*, *52*, A252–A253.

Sacktor, N., Lyles, R. H., Skolasky, R., Kleeberger, C., Selnes, O. A., Miller, E. N., et al. (2001). Multicenter AIDS Cohort Study. *Neurology*, *56*(2), 257–260.

Sacktor, N., Skolasky, R. L., Ernst, T., Mao, X, Selnes, O., Pomper, M. G., et al. (2005). A multicenter study of two magnetic resonance spectroscopy techniques in individuals with HIV dementia. *Jour Magn Res Imaging*, *21*(4), 325–333.

Schmidbauer, M., Huemer, M., Cristina, S, Trabattoni, G. R., & Budka, H. (1992). Morphological spectrum, distribution and clinical correlation of white matter lesions in AIDS brains. *Neuropathol Appl Neurobiol*, *18*, 489–501.

Schmidbauer, M., Budka, H., Okeda, R., Cristina, S., Lechi, A., & Trabattoni, G. R. (199). Multifocal vacuolar leucoencephalopathy: A distinct HIV-associated lesion of the brain. *Neuropathol Applied Neurobiol*, *16* 437–443.

Seilhean, D., Duyckaerts, C., Vazeux, R., Bolgert, F., Brunet, P., Katlama, C., et al. (1993). HIV-1-associated cognitive/motor complex: Absence of neuronal loss in the cerebral neocortex. *Neurology*, *43*(8), 1492–1499.

Sevigny, J. J., Albert, S. M., McDermott, M. P., McArthur, J. C., Sacktor, N., Conant, K., et al. (2004). Evaluation of HIV RNA and markers of immune activation as predictors of HIV-associated dementia. *Neurology*, *63*, 2084–2090.

Shelburne, S. A., Visnegarwala, F., Darcourt, J., Graviss, E. A., Giordano, T. P., White, A. C., et al. (2005). Incidence and risk factors for immune reconstitution inflammatory syndrome during highly active antiretroviral therapy. *AIDS*, *19*, 399–406.

Shi, B, De Girolami, U, He, J., Wang, S., Lorenzo, A., Busciglio, J., et al. (1996). Apoptosis induced by HIV-1 infection of the central nervous system. *J Clin Invest*, *98*, 1979–1990.

Smith, T. W., DeGirolami, U., Henin, D., Bolgert, F., & Hauw, J. J. (1990). Human immunodeficiency virus (HIV) leukoencephalopathy and the microcirculation. *J Neuropathol Exp Neurol*, *49*, 357–370.

Snider, D., Simpson, D. M., Nielsen, S., Gold, J., Metroka, C., & Posner, J. (1983). Neurological complications of AIDS: Analysis of 50 patients. *Ann Neurol*, *14*, 403–418.

Stebbins, G. T., Smith, C. A., Bartt, R. E., Kessler, H. A., Adeyemi, O. M., Martin, E., et al. (2007). HIV-associated alterations in normal-appearing white matter: A voxel-wise diffusion tensor imaging study. *J Acquir Immune Defic Syndr*, *46*(5), 564–573.

Streit, W. J. (2005). Microglia and neuroprotection: Implications for Alzheimer's disease. *Brain Research - Brain Research Reviews*, *48*, 234–239.

Tantisiriwat, W., Tebas, P., Clifford, D. B., Powderly, W. G., & Fichtenbaum, C. J. (1998). Progressive multifocal leukoencephalopathy in patients with AIDS receiving highly active antiretroviral therapy. *Clin Infect Dis*, 28, 1152–1154.

Terry, R. D., Masliah, E, Salmon, D. P., Butters, N., DeTeresa, R., Hill, R., et al. (1991). Physical basis of cognitive alterations in Alzheimer's disease: Synapse loss is the major correlate of cognitive impairment. *Ann Neurol*, 30, 572–580.

Thompson, K. A., McArthur, J. C., & Wesselingh, S. L. (2001). Correlation between neurological progression and astrocyte apoptosis in HIV-associated dementia. *Ann Neurol*, 49, 745–752.

Thompson, K. A., Churchill, M. J., Gorry, P. R., et al. (2004). Astrocyte-specific viral strains in HIV dementia. *Ann Neurol*, 56, 873–877.

Thompson, P. M., Dutton, R. A., Hayashi, K. M., Toga, A. W., Lopez, O. L., Aizenstein, H. J., et al. (2005). Thinning of the cerebral cortex visualized in HIV/AIDS reflects CD4+ T lymphocyte decline. *Proc Natl Acad Sci USA*, 102 (43), 15647–15652.

Tozzi, V., Balestra, P., Galgani, S., Narciso, P., Sampaolesi, A, Antinori, A., et al. (2001). Changes in neurocognitive performance in a cohort of patients treated with HAART for 3 years. *J Acquir Immune Defic Syndr*, 28(1), 19–27.

Tozzi, V., Balestra, P., Bellagamba, R., Corpolongo, A., Salvatori, M. F., et al. (2007). Persistence of neuropsychologic deficits despite long-term highly active antiretroviral therapy in patients with HIV-related neurocognitive impairment: Prevalence and risk factors. *J Acquir Immune Defic Syndr*, 45, 174–182.

Trillo-Pazos, G. & Everall, I. P. (1996). Neuronal damage and its relation to dementia in acquired immunodeficiency syndrome (AIDS). *Pathobiology*, 64(6), 295–307.

Valcour, V., Shikuma, C., Shiramizu, B., Watters, M, Poff, P., Selnes, O., et al. (2004). Higher frequency of dementia in older HIV-1 individuals. The Hawaii Aging with HIV-1 Cohort. *Neurology*, 63, 822–827.

Vago, L., Bonetto, S., Nebuloni, M., Duca, P., Carsana, L., Zerbi, P., et al. (2002). Pathological findings in the central nervous system of AIDS patients on assumed antiretroviral therapeutic regimens: Retrospective study of 1597 autopsies. *AIDS*, 16, 1925–1928.

Vendrely, A., Bienvenu, B., Gasnault, J., Thiebault, J. B., Salmon, D., & Gray, F. (2005). Fulminant inflammatory leukoencephalopathy associated with HAART-induced immune restoration in AIDS-related progressive multifocal leukoencephalopathy. *Acta Neuropathol (Berl)*, 109, 449–455.

Venkataramana, A., Pardo, C. A., McArthur, J. C., Kerr, D. A., Irani, D. N., Griffin, J. W., et al. (2006). Immune reconstitution inflammatory syndrome in the CNS of HIV-infected patients. *Neurology*, 67(3), 383–388.

Vincent, V. A., De Groot, C. J., Lucassen, P. J., Portegies, P., Troost, D., Tilders, F. J., et al. (1999). Nitric oxide synthase expression and apoptotic cell death in brains of AIDS and AIDS dementia patients. *AIDS*, 13, 317–326.

Weis, S., Haug, H., & Budka, H. (1993). Neuronal damage in the cerebral cortex of AIDS brains: A morphometric study. *Acta Neuropathol (Berl)*, 85, 185–189.

Wesselingh, S. L., Takahashi, K., Glass, J. D., McArthur, J. C., Griffin, J. W., & Griffin, D. E. (1997). Cellular localization of tumor necrosis factor mRNA in neurological tissue from HIV-infected patients by combined reverse transcriptase polymerase chain reaction in situ hybridization and immunohistochemistry. *J Neuroimmunol*, 74, 1–8.

Wesselingh, S. L., Power, C., Glass, J. D., Tyor, W. R., McArthur, J. C., Farber, J. M., et al. (1993). Intracerebral cytokine messenger RNA expression in acquired immunodeficiency syndrome dementia. *Ann Neurol*, 33, 576–582.

Wiley, C. A. & Achim, C. L. (1994). Human immunodeficiency virus encephalitis is the pathological correlate of dementia in acquired immunodeficiency syndrome. *Ann Neurol*, 36, 673–676.

Wiley, C. A., Masliah, E., Morey, M., Lemere, C., DeTeresa, R., Grafe, M., et al. (1991). Neocortical damage during HIV infection. *Ann Neurol*, 29(6), 651–657.

Williams, K. C. & Hickey, W. F. (2002). Central nervous system damage, monocytes and macrophages, and neurological disorders in AIDS. *Ann Rev Neurosci*, 25, 537–562.

Wood, M. L., MacGinley, R., Eisen, D .P, Allworth, A. M. (1998). HIV combination therapy: Partial immune reconstitution unmasking latent cryptococcal infection *AIDS*, 12, 1491–1494.

Wu, Y., Storey, P, Cohen, B. A., Epstein, L. G., Edelman, R. R., & Ragin, A. B. (2006). Diffusion alterations in corpus callosum of patients with HIV. *Am Jour Neuroradiology*, 27, 656–660.

Xing, H. Q., Moritoyo, T., Mori, K., Tadakuma, K., Sugimoto, C., Ono, F., et al. (2003). Simian immunodeficiency virus encephalitis in the white matter and degeneration of the cerebral cortex occur independently in simian immunodeficiency virus-infected monkey. *J Neurovirol*, 9, 508–18.

Xing, H. Q., Hayakawa, H., Gelpi, E., Kubota, R., Budka, H., & Izumo, S. (2009). Reduced expression of excitatory amino acid transporter 2 and diffuse microglial activation in the cerebral cortex in AIDS cases with or without HIV encephalitis. *J Neuropathol Exp Neurol*, 68, 199–209. doi: 10.1097/NEN.0b013e31819715df

Xie, M., Tobin, J. E., Budde, M. D., Chen, C-I., Trinkaus, K. C., Cross, A. H., et al. (2010). Rostrocaudal analysis of corpus callosum demyelination and axon damage across disease stages refines diffusion tensor imaging correlations with pathological features. *J Neuropathol Exptl Neurology*, 69(7), 704–716. doi: 10.1097/NEN.0b013e3181e3de90.

Yamaguchi, H., Sugihara, S., Ogawa, A., Oshima, N., & Ihara, Y. (2001). Alzheimer beta amyloid deposition enhanced by apoE epsilon4 gene precedes neurofibrillary pathology in the frontal association cortex of nondemented senior subjects. *J Neuropathol Exp Neurol*, 60, 731–739.

Zheng, J. & Gendelman, H. E. (1997). The HIV-1 associated dementia complex: A metabolic encephalopathy fueled by viral replication in mononuclear phagocytes. *Curr Opin Neurol*, 10, 319–325.

7.5

PERIPHERAL NEUROPATHY

Kathryn J. Elliott, Justin C. McArthur, and David M. Simpson

Peripheral neuropathies are the most common neurological complications associated with HIV infection. In the era since the introduction of highly active antiretroviral therapy (HAART), many patients on stable HIV therapy are free of opportunistic infections. However, at least one in two HIV-infected individuals will develop distal sensory polyneuropathy (DSP) (Morgello et al., 2004).

PATHOBIOLOGY

Preclinical models of HIV neuropathy and HIV neuropathic pain have been missing until very recently, which delayed research into the mechanisms of HIV neuropathic pain. Preclinical models include isolated cell cultures, in vitro nerve studies, and animal models. Given the complicated experience of neuropathic pain that requires not only sensory processing but an intact organism, the value of in vitro studies for shedding light on pain mechanisms is questionable. The recent development of animal models that approximate the human condition is a great advance to the field.

Initial studies of HIV neuropathy pathogenesis involved pathological examination from autopsies of patients who died with HIV infection. This neuropathological examination revealed distal degeneration of long axons (Pardo, McArthur, & Griffin, 2001). Additional pathological findings included infiltration of these involved nerves by macrophages (Pardo et al., 2001; Bradley et al., 1998). The dorsal root ganglia (DRG) shows evidence of both neuronal loss and a dying back of centrally projecting sensory neurons (Rance et al., 1988; Esiri, Morris, & Millard, 1993).

The focus on infected macrophages supports the concept that HIV enters the central nervous system (CNS) through HIV-infected monocytes that traverse the blood brain barrier (Nottet & Dhawan, 1998). It would not thus be surprising that infected monocytes/macrophages also play a putative role in the peripheral nervous system in HIV-related disorders. DRG macrophages express major histocompatibility (MHC) antigens as well as pro-inflammatory cytokines (Nagano et al., 1996). These data suggest that HIV neuropathic pain may in part be an inflammatory reaction to HIV infection.

Secretions from HIV-infected macrophages cause neurites in DRG culture to retract. This suggests that in this model, macrophages may be producing neurotoxins to peripheral nerve (Hahn et al., 2008). Blockade of chemokine receptors CXCR4 and CCR5 does not prevent the neurotoxic effects of the supernatants released by the activated macrophages, suggesting that these receptors do not mediate the neurotoxicity. HIV-infected macrophages release potentially neurotoxic substances such as the pro-inflammatory cytokines TNF-alpha, interferon-gamma, IL-6, nitric oxide, and glutamate (Jiang et al., 2001). Other substances released by HIV-infected macrophages that are potentially neurotoxic include the HIV protein Tat (Nath, 2002). In addition to the role of infected and activated macrophages in the pathogenesis of HIV neuropathic injury, there has been focus on the HIV envelope protein, glycoprotein (gp)120. This HIV protein binds to peripheral nerve and to DRG when studied with in vitro cell culture models, and gp120 may also contribute directly to neurotoxicity (Apostolski et al., 1993; Van den Berg et al., 1992). These findings implicating gp120 have led to the development of new animal models. In HIV infection, Schwann cells may play an important role in mediating HIV-1 gp120 nerve toxicity by producing the β-chemokine RANTES, which in turn causes TNF-α-mediated neuronal apoptosis and neuritic degeneration (Keswani et al., 2003). Thus, activated Schwann cells might actually induce nerve injury and degeneration. Figure 7.5.1 shows electron micrographs of Schwann cell abnormalities found in chronic neuropathy (see Figure 7.5.1). Two recent models of HIV neuropathy include the neonatal kitten model, and the rat model described below.

In one rodent model, HIV-gp120 was applied perineurally around the left sciatic nerve. HIV-gp120 was selected as the putative neurotoxic agent because HIV-related distal sensory neuropathy is considered to be an interaction between theglycoprotein (gp)120 and sensory neurons (Oh et al., 2001). This interaction produces a chemokine-driven, possibly inflammatory, secondary neuronal insult that produces HIV neuropathy and neuropathic pain syndrome (Melli et al., 2006).

Mechanical allodynia in this animal model was assessed with graded von Frey monofilaments (Wallace et al., 2007). The rodent equivalent of hyperalgesia was assessed with the Hargreaves plantar heat threshold assessment and time to hind paw withdrawal with a standardized heat stimulus was measured (Melli et al., 2006; Hargreaves et al., 1998). Cold allodynia was also determined with acetone application as has been described in an earlier model of sciatic nerve injury in the rat (Melli et al., 2006; Bridges, Ahmad, & Rice, 2001).

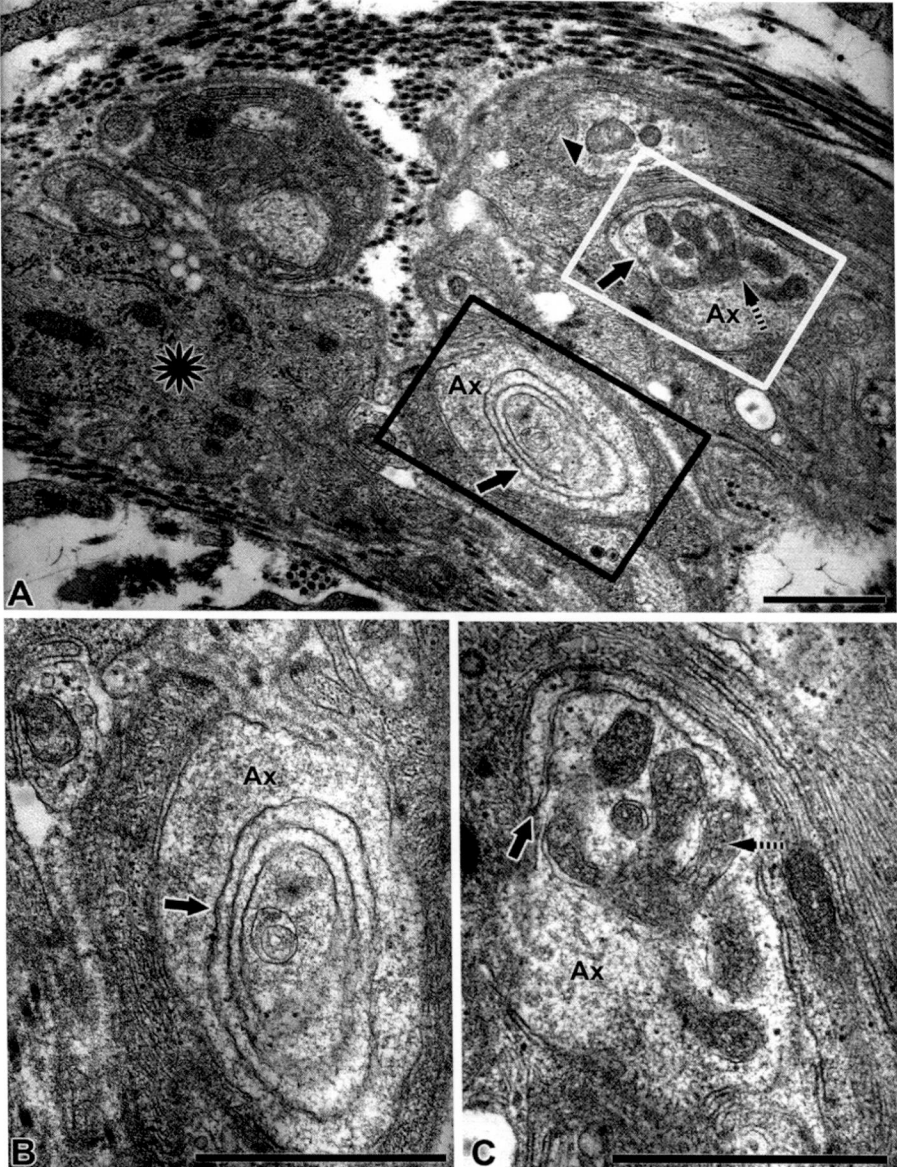

Figure 7.5.1 *Electron micrographs of Schwann cell abnormalities in chronic neuropathy patients.* A: A dermal nerve showing a denervated Schwann cell bands (asterisk). The black box identifies an axon (Ax) with Schwann cell ingrowths (arrow), seen at higher power in B. The white box identifies an axon with a Schwann cell ingrowth partially encircling a cluster of abnormally large mitochondria (broken arrow), seen at higher power in C. B: Schwann cell cytoplasmic ingrowths (arrow) spiraling and dividing axoplasm (ax). C: Long tongue of Schwann cell cytoplasmic ingrowths (arrow) curving around an enlarged mitochondrial cluster (broken arrow) and partitioning an area of axoplasm (ax). Scale bars = All 1 μm.

In this model, hypersensitivity to mechanical stimuli with von Frey hairs develops without any evidence of motor deficit (Melli et al., 2006). This is similar to the mechanical allodynia described in some patients with HIV neuropathy (Elliott, 1994). The behavioral response suggestive of neuropathic pain was accompanied by changes in the ipsilateral dorsal root ganglion.

In rats that received HIV-gp120, the chemokine CCL2 expression was increased in the ipsilateral dorsal root ganglion as compared to sham controls (Melli et al., 2006). Macrophages were also found in the peripheral nerve and the ipsilateral dorsal root ganglia as compared to controls (Melli et al., 2006). Gliosis in the spinal dorsal horn also occurred as well as a loss

of intraepidermal nerves (Melli et al., 2006). Figure 7.5.2 shows light and electron microscopic pictures of cutaneous nerves obtained from patients with chronic neuropathy (see Figure 7.5.2).

Intraepidermal nerve fibers, as assessed by nerve fiber density, are decreased in patients with HIV neuropathy, and their loss may be clinically associated with the extent of neuropathic pain experienced (Polydefkis et al., 2002).

Another approach to studying the role of gp120 in HIV neuropathy is the use of the transgenic gp120 mouse model. In this mouse model, the gp120 is under GFAP promoter control and Schwann cells in the peripheral nervous system (PNS) express it (Keswani et al., 2006). In a similar manner to

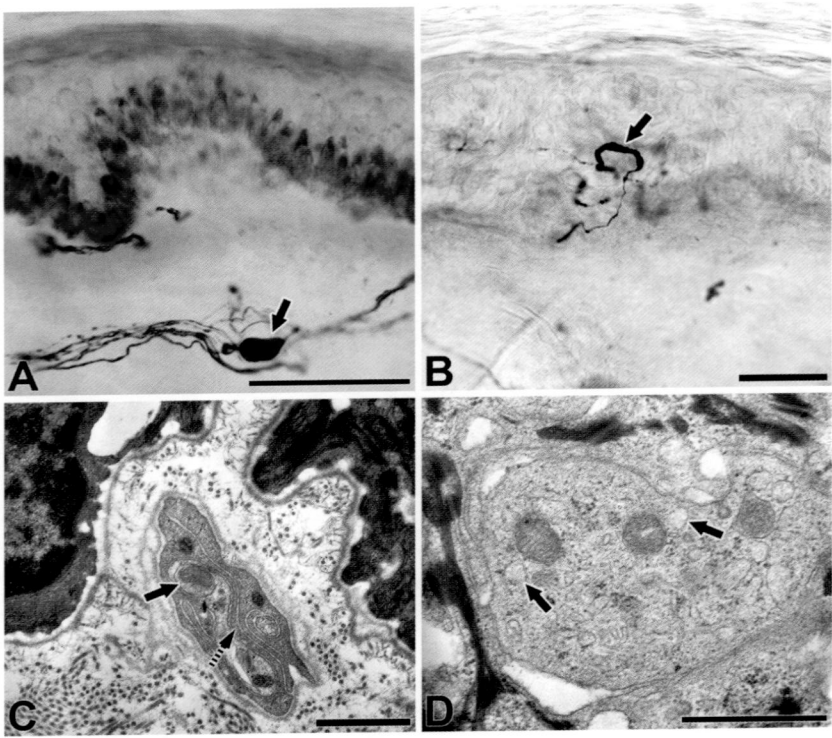

Figure 7.5.2 *Light and electron microscopic findings of cutaneous nerves in HIV neuropathy patients.* (A) Skin with loss of epidermal fibers and a fusiform axonal swelling in the dermis (arrows). Scale bar = 50 μm. (B) Skin showing a degenerating epidermal nerve fiber with attenuated segments (broken arrow). Scale bar = 50 μm. (C) Partially denervated Remak bundle with stacked lamellated Schwann cell processes (broken arrow) and an axon with enlarged mitochondria (arrow). Scale bar = 1 μm. (D) Globular axonal swelling (ax) containing accumulations of particulate organelles (arrows). Scale bar = 1 μm.

the neonatal kitten model with feline virus infection (FIV), administration of the antiretroviral agent didanosine reduced distal nerve fiber density, and in the kitten model, impaired mitochondrial function (Zhu et al., 2007). All of these models of HIV neuropathy have the potential to identify new agents that may lead to nerve regeneration or ameliorate neuropathic pain in patients with HIV neuropathy.

CLINICAL FEATURES

HIV DSP presents with slow onset and progression. Patients usually first describe either an unpleasant sensation under their toes bilaterally, or in the soles of their feet, often after they have been on their feet for a prolonged period of time. Neuropathic pain is a complex pathophysiological change that occurs from many insults to nerves such as trauma, compression, cancer, viral infections such as HIV, or metabolic derangements such as diabetes or renal failure (Elliott, 1994). It can be expected that specific symptoms of neuropathic pain vary greatly between patients (Max, 1990). It is important to consider alternative potentially treatable causes for the distal neuropathy and neuropathic pain before attributing the syndrome to HIV. Neuropathic symptoms often worsen with fatigue.

Symptoms of HIV DSP usually slowly ascend from the toes bilaterally to involve the feet and lower legs (Simpson & Olney, 1992). Neuropathic symptoms are often difficult for patients to describe. Patients may describe the sensations as akin to ants or worms under the skin. Along with the description of sensory loss, patients often experience abnormal sensations such as parasesthias and dysesthesias (Elliott, 1994). Paresthesias are abnormal tingling sensations that are not painful. Abnormal painful tingling sensations are labeled as dysesthetic. Other abnormal sensations include burning or shooting pains in the feet that can be spontaneous and are usually in the distribution of sensory impairment (Elliott, 1994).

Allodynia is a painful response to a normally nonpainful stimulus such as with the light touch of clothing (Elliott, 1994). Patients that experience allodynia sometimes cannot tolerate socks or shoes and wear sandals instead. Allodynia is often worse at night, and patients describe that bedclothes on the toes can become unbearable. Hyperpathia is another symptom of neuropathic injury and is an abnormally painful response to a normally painful stimulus such as light pin prick. Both allodynia and hyperpathia are considered manifestations of central sensitization (Elliott, 1994).

Central sensitization is the rubric under which the development of neuropathic pain is thought to develop following distal nerve injury. It is due to hyperactivity of peripheral sensory receptors that then leads to abnormal excitability in the pain pathways in the spinal cord dorsal horn and more rostral brain pathways controlling the experience and processing of pain (Elliott, 1994). There is abundant animal research to confirm the concept of central sensitization but little direct evidence in humans to confirm this.

After the patient describes abnormal sensory symptoms compatible with neuropathy, the clinician should examine the patient to confirm the diagnosis of DSP. One of the problems in comparing research studies of HIV DSP is that there is not a consensus definition of DSP. For example, most clinicians would probably consider a patient with the above described sensory symptoms as having DSP, possibly limited to small-fibers, even in the presence of a normal neurological examination. Research studies tend to be more stringent and it is common practice to require evidence of abnormal distal reflexes, most often reflected in decreased or absent ankle tendon reflexes bilaterally (as compared to knee reflexes) with some combination of distal sensory loss. The most commonly tested sensory modalities include impairment of distal vibration as assessed clinically with a tuning fork, and impairment of pin as assessed clinically with a disposable sharps. Sensory loss appears in a gradient such that the impairment will be most distal and as the clinician ascends up the foot and leg, normal sensation will return. This pattern of sensory loss is termed a stocking-glove distribution. Motor examination is usually normal in an uncomplicated HIV DSP and it is uncommon to have changes in reflexes aside from ankle reflexes.

NEUROTOXIC NEUROPATHY

Neurotoxic dideoxynucleoside ("d-drugs") antiretrovirals (ARV) have been implicated in causing a form of toxic neuropathy that is clinically indistinguishable from HIV DSP not associated with d-drug use (Elliott & Simpson, 2009). The history of d-drug exposure, including timing of onset and response to drug withdrawal, is a key feature in diagnosis.

D-drug ARVs are effective treatment for HIV and are commonly used in resource-limited settings where the cost of ARV is a significant consideration in drug access. D-drugs are no longer commonly used in the United States and other parts of the resource-rich world today because of their potential toxicity to peripheral nerve and other organ systems (Simpson & Olney, 1992). Didanosine (ddI), zalcitabine (ddC), and stavudine (d4T) not only cause peripheral nerve toxicity but also lipodystrophy and lactic acidosis (Pettersen et al., 2006; Simpson & Talgiati, 1995). The toxicity from d-drug use is additive (Moore et al., 2000). The mechanism by which d-drugs damage peripheral nerves is thought to be due to drug competition with thymidine triphosphate, which leads to acquired mitochondrial dysfunction and subsequent energy failure in peripheral nerve (Cui et al., 1997; Dalakas, 2001).

If an ARV drug is implicated in the development of HIV neuropathy then a first step is to consider withdrawal and consideration of an alternative ARV regimen that does not include a d-drug. This d-drug withdrawal is less of an option in some resource-limited settings where available antiretrovirals are limited and cost is an important consideration of access to treatment (Chien, 2007). HIV pharmacogenomic research on the individual patient risk of a genetic predisposition to toxic neuropathy may help predict at-risk patients in the future (Tozzi, Libertone, & Liuzzi, 2008).

Following d-drug withdrawal, neuropathic symptoms can take from 1 to 3 months to subside. A "coasting phenomenon" is occasionally observed, where symptom worsening occurs for several weeks to 2 months after d-drug discontinuation. Some patients have signs or symptoms of neuropathy after d-drug discontinuation. This may reflect nonreversible toxicity to the nerve from d-drug exposure, underlying HIV neuropathy, or the presence of another comorbidity implicated in DSP, such as diabetes mellitus or hepatitis C. Recently Cherry et al. showed that hepatitis C did not appear to be an important magnifying factor for HIV DSP (Cherry et al., 2010).

MONONEURITIS MULTIPLEX

The syndrome of mononeuritis multiplex (MM) refers to a condition in which two or more focal peripheral nerves are affected (Stewart, 1987). MM is less common in the post-HAART era in patients with uncomplicated HIV. Many patients with HIV develop other disorders of their CNS or PNS unrelated to their HIV infection, and this needs to be especially considered in a patient presenting with MM.

Vasculitis is an important cause of mononeuritis multiplex in patients without HIV (Davies et al., 1996). MM is often accompanied by moderate to severe neuropathic pain in the distribution of the affected peripheral nerves. Common nerves that are affected in MM include facial, ulnar, and common peroneal (Stewart, 1987).

An extensive search for infection, systemic vasculitis, or malignant infiltration (Stuebgen & Elliott, 1997; Turner et al., 2003) must be considered even in a patient with HIV disease. Cytomegalovirus (CMV) infection can cause MM in HIV patients that are severely immunosuppressed (i.e., CD4 < 50 cells/ml) (Said et al., 1991). HIV patients with MM are often co-infected with hepatitis C, a potential cause of MM.

Vasculitis confined to peripheral nerves presents as MM in approximately two-thirds of patients who develop MM without HIV infection (Davies et al., 1996; Dyck et al., 1987; Said et al., 1988). Ancillary tests, such as electromyography (EMG) and nerve conduction studies (NCS) are helpful in diagnosis, to establish the anatomy, physiology, and prognosis of the neuropathy (Tagliati et al., 1999). Biopsy of a clinically affected peripheral nerve may be necessary to establish an etiological diagnosis.

ACUTE INFLAMMATORY DEMYELINATING POLYNEUROPATHY

Acute inflammatory demyelinating polyneuropathy (AIDP), also known as Guillain-Barre syndrome (GBS), may occur in HIV infection (Griffin, Crawford, & McArthur, 1998). GBS usually appears early in the course of HIV infection and may be the presenting symptom of underlying HIV infection (Thorton, Latif, & Emmanuel, 1991). The clinical presentation of GBS associated with HIV is similar to GBS in HIV-uninfected patients. Patients develop rapidly ascending weakness, often preceded by tingling in the feet and back pain. There may be respiratory failure requiring ventilator support, and autonomic features.

Autonomic system involvement can lead to swings in blood pressure from hypotension requiring pressor support to severe hypertension, as well as cardiac tachyarrythmias or bradyarrythmias including heart block (Flachenecker, 2007). Autonomic involvement remains a cause of morbidity and mortality in patients with AIDP (Zollei et al., 2000; Alshekhlee et al., 2008). While the primary nerve pathology in AIDP is demyelination, axonal degeneration can also occur, which predicts a slower or incomplete recovery. GBS from HIV should be considered when the cerebrospinal fluid (CSF) evaluation, done as part of the routine evaluation of AIDP/GBS, shows pleocytosis in addition to an elevated protein level.

The treatment for AIDP associated with HIV is the same as with nonHIV AIDP. The clinician must provide supportive care, such as provision of adequate respiratory and circulatory support and should consider a trial of IVIG or plasmapheresis, especially if the patient is nonambulatory (Hughes et al., 2003). However controlled trials of these agents have not been performed in HIV-associated GBS. Clinicians should consider hospital admission on the first suspicion of this disorder as the course can be rapidly progressive, unpredictable, and life threatening.

CHRONIC INFLAMMATORY DEMYELINATING POLYNEUROPATHY

Chronic inflammatory demyelinating polyneuropathy (CIDP) is a rare complication of HIV. CIDP resembles AIDP, but the time course of the disease progression is slower (Griffin et al., 1998). Patients have weakness which can sometimes resemble the proximal weakness seen in myopathy, but there is loss of reflexes diffusely and a variable degree of sensory impairment. Electrodiagnostic studies reveal markedly slow distal latency and nerve conduction velocities, temporal dispersion, conduction block and prolonged late responses. While controlled studies have not been done, most provide similar treatment to HIV-negative CIDP, and includes IVIG, plasmapheresis or corticosteroids.

DIAGNOSIS

The initial step in diagnosis, management, and therapy of HIV-associated neuropathy and neuropathic pain involves acknowledgement that a diagnosis of HIV DSP is one of exclusion. In a patient with HIV and DSP, a search for treatable and potentially reversible causes is also a search for a diagnosis. Along with the general U.S. population, increasing weight and lifestyle choices are leading to many cases of subclinical metabolic syndrome and pre-diabetes, as well as frank type 2 diabetes that is predominantly lifestyle influenced.

There should be a comprehensive search for diabetes, and renal and liver disease, as well as micronutrient deficiency by assessing B12, folate, and vitamin D levels. Advancing age, substance and alcohol abuse also increase the risk of DSP. Psychiatric disorders should also be probed for as their presence makes the consideration of a future trial of opioids problematic. Electrophysiological studies can assist in the diagnosis of atypical neuropathy syndromes such as mononeuritis multiplex or demyelinating neuropathy.

TREATMENT

Correction of any underlying metabolic disorder such as diabetes mellitus (DM) may ameliorate both the neuropathy and the accompanying neuropathic pain syndrome. In general, controlled clinical trials for symptomatic treatment of neuropathic pain from HIV neuropathy have been disappointing. Gabapentin has shown some benefit in a small study (Hahn et al., 2004), as has smoked cannabis (Abrams et al., 2007). One large controlled study of a high-dose capsaicin patch (Simpson et al., 2008) has shown efficacy, although a second controlled study was negative. Trials with amitriptyline, pregabalin, lamotrigine, lidocaine patch, low-dose capsaicin (Paice et al., 2000), prosaptide, peptide T, acupuncture, and recombinant human nerve growth factor have been negative in HIV neuropathy (see Table 7.5.1 below). These data will be discussed in more detail below.

Animal studies have uncovered some of the pathophysiological changes that lead to neuropathic pain disorders that develop in a portion of patients who develop peripheral neuropathy (Bennett & Xie, 1988). These changes include peripheral nociceptor activation, neuroma formation, ectopic dorsal root ganglion discharges, reorganization of primary afferents such that tactile afferents begin to project to nociceptive regions of spinal cord, loss of inhibition in spinal cord, and central sensitization. These multiple mechanisms of neuropathic pain from HIV neuropathy support the clinical approach to use multiple analgesic therapies that target different pain mechanisms.

A common strategy for controlled clinical trials of symptomatic therapy of diverse neuropathic pain syndromes is to identify an animal model of neuropathic pain that identifies a new neuropathic pain agent and then to try it in a prototypical neuropathic pain syndrome disorder in patients (Fox et al., 2001; Jett et al., 1997).

Classes of adjuvant analgesics identified in this manner and found efficacious in such syndromes as postherpetic neuralgia and diabetic neuropathy pain have either not been found beneficial in patients with HIV neuropathic pain, or have not been studied in HIV neuropathic pain. For example, amitryptiline is an adjuvant analgesic with much data supporting its use in diverse neuropathic pain syndromes including postherpetic neuralgia, diabetic neuropathy, tension headache, migraine, fibromyalgia, and poststroke central neuropathic pain (Jett et al., 1997; Goldenberg, Felson, & Dinerman, 2005). Antidepressants, as a class of adjuvant analgesics, are frequently prescribed adjuvant analgesics for chronic pain (Loeser & Bonica, 2001). Amitryptiline is the most studied and oldest adjuvant antidepressant used in chronic neuropathic pain of diverse causes (French & Gronseth, 2008).

CLASSES OF EVIDENCE

Editors of numerous medical journals have recently decided to publish the level of evidence as a notation for each newly published therapeutic trial. For example, The Quality and Standards Subcommittee of the American Academy of Neurology has developed criteria for evaluating clinical trial evidence in an attempt to make the practice of neurology more "evidence based." Such criteria are clearly defined with proper attention to trial methodology and the accounting of study dropouts (French & Gronseth, 2008). The randomized and controlled trial must be in a representative sample and with relevant baseline characteristics presented and with equivalency across treatment groups as well as less then 20% dropout rate in order to have a Class I determination (Gross & Johnston, 2009). Table 7.5.1. lists the previously published clinical trials of analgesics in HIV neuropathy with a classification of the evidence.

Table 7.5.1 SYMPTOMATIC THERAPY FOR HIV NEUROPATHIC PAIN (FRENCH & GRONSETH, 2008; GROSS & JOHNSTON, 2009)

Class I	
Lidocaine patch. Estanislao 2004.	Class 1 Evidence: Negative Study (Estanislao et al., 2004).

Class II	
Pregabalin Simpson 2010.	No benefit in HIV neuropathic pain (Simpson et al., 2010).
Capsaicin Patch Simpson 2008.	Modest benefit from high dose patch (Simpson et al., 2008), earlier study with low dose capsaicin ineffective (Paice et al., 2000).

Class III	
Amitriptyline Kieburtz 1998	Class III evidence that amitriptyline is ineffective (Kieburtz et al., 1998).
Schaly 1998	Class III evidence that amitriptyline is ineffective (Shlay et al., 1998). (Dosages lower then in diabetic neuropathic pain studies that showed benefit.)
Lamotrigine Simpson 2000.	Class III evidence that lamotrigine is effective, smaller study size then Simpson 2003 (Simpson et al., 2000).
Simpson 2003.	Class III evidence that there is no benefit in HIV neuropathic pain and some benefit in d-drug neuropathic pain (Simpson, 2003).
Gabapentin Hahn 2004.	Class III evidence that there is benefit (Hahn et al., 2004).

Class IV	
Mexiletine Kemper 1998	No benefit
Cannabis Abrams 2007.	Modest benefit from smoked cannabis in HIV neuropathic pain (Abrams et al., 2007)
Opioids	No controlled trials in HIV neuropathic pain.

As compared with HIV neuropathic pain, abundant Class I evidence exists for the analgesic efficacy of the adjuvant analgesics in other peripheral neuropathic pain syndromes. Table 7.5.2 presents some of the Class 1 evidence for use of adjuvant analgesics in other peripheral non-HIV neuropathic pain disorders.

ANTIDEPRESSANTS

Multiple controlled trials in patients confirm the analgesic efficacy of tricyclic antidepressants in neuropathic pain. A Cochrane evidence-based review of the efficacy of antidepressants in the treatment of neuropathic pain identified 61 randomized controlled trials, and amitriptyline was by far the most-studied antidepressant (Saarto & Wiffen, 2009).

Amitriptyline's ability to relieve neuropathic pain is distinct from its efficacy in treating depression. Its analgesic efficacy can be observed even after the first or second dose, and usually in the first few days of treatment initiation if it is to be effective, in a dose range much smaller than its antidepressant dosage (i.e., 10 mg–25mg). In contrast, the antidepressant effect may take weeks or months. It is presumed that amitriptyline blocks the reuptake of serotonin and norepinephrine, in addtional to other neurotransmitters, throughout the central pathways including dorsal horn synapses that modulate the incoming neuropathic pain signals, as well as in the rostral

Table 7.5.2 THERAPIES FOR NEUROPATHIC PAIN WITH CLASS 1 EVIDENCE

AMITRIPTYLINE

Multiple Class 1 studies showing efficacy. See recent Cochrane review for descriptions of the many trials performed. Other antidepressants have less evidence to support their use(Saarto & Wiffen, 2009).

PREGABALIN

Multiple Class 1 studies showing efficacy in postherpetic neuralgia (Dworkin et al.; Sabatowski et al., 2004; Van Seventer et al., 2006). Multiple Class 1 studies showing efficacy in diabetic neuropathic pain (Lesser et al., 2004; Richter et al., 2005; Rosenstock et al., 2004).

GABAPENTIN

Multiple Class 1 studies showing efficacy in postherpetic neuralgia (Dworkin et al., 2007; Finnerup et al., 2005). Multiple Class 1 studies showing efficacy in diabetic neuropathic pain (Dworkin et al., 2007; Finnerup et al., 2005). Some evidence for efficacy in a study of mixed neuropathic pain conditons.

LIDOCAINE PATCH

Multiple Class 1 (as well as other classes) studies showing efficacy in PHN (Dworkin et al., 2007; Finnerup et al., 2005; Galer et al., 1999; Khaliq et al., 2007; Rowbotham et al., 1996; Argoff et al., 2004; Herrman et al., 2005; Barbano et al., 2004). 5% patch recommended as first line therapy for peripheral neuropathic pain (Finnerup et al., 2007). Similar efficacy to pregabalin in postherpetic neuralgia and diabetic neuropathy without pregabalin side effects (Baron et al., 2009).

signaling in the cerebrum and brainstem (Abdi, Lee & Chung, 1998; De Vry et al., 2004; Esser & Sawynok, 1999). In an earlier meta-analysis of controlled clinical trials of neuropathic pain of diverse causes and tricyclic antidepressants, one in three patients obtained more than 50% pain relief with a tricyclic antidepressant (McQuay & Moore, 1997).

However, the two published trials using the tricyclic antidepressant amitriptyline in HIV neuropathic pain found no additional efficacy of amitriptyline over placebo (Kieburtz et al., 1998; Shlay et al., 1998). It is not clear why a tricyclic antidepressant should show such benefit in post-herpetic neuralgia and diabetic neuropathy and not in HIV neuropathy. Patients with HIV neuropathic pain share many clinical characteristics with patients with post-herpetic neuralgia and diabetic distal neuropathy, so it is unlikely that the neuropathic pain symptom complex is significantly different. Despite the failure of these two early trials to show efficacy of amitriptyline in HIV neuropathic pain, the authors consider a trial of this inexpensive and readily available analgesic in some conditions where a patient with HIV has neuropathic pain. In a patient with a central pain syndrome from either cerebral infection, or from a severe deafferented zoster infection, amitriptyline may also be considered. Also, if an HIV patient has an element of diabetic neuropathy contributing to the neuropathic pain disorder, then amitriptyline may also be tried. Amitriptyline requires caution in the elderly as it can cause postural hypotension and increase the risk of falls. In the young HIV patient with neuropathic pain it will also be considered as there is an abundance of efficacy data from other neuropathic pain disorders.

This failure to demonstrate efficacy in HIV neuropathy with amitriptyline, the most studied adjuvant analgesic for neuropathic pain, has been unfortunately replicated in additional clinical trials with mexilitene, topical lidocaine, pregabalin, lamotrigine and low-dose capsaicin (Abrams et al., 2007; Kemper et al., 1998) (see Table 7.5.1). Duloxetine, an SNRI antidepressant with proven efficacy in painful diabetic neuropathy, is another option in the treatment of HIV neuropathy although it has not been examined in a controlled study.

ANTICONVULSANTS

Gabapentin is an off-patent anticonvulsant and adjuvant analgesic with demonstrated efficacy in several neuropathic pain states (see Table 7.5.2). Gabapentin blocks the alpha-2-delta subunit of the voltage gated calcium channel. Hahn and colleagues studied gabapentin for HIV neuropathic pain (Hahn et al., 2004). Each subject was randomized to receive either gabapentin at 400 mg/day to be titrated up to 2400 mg over two weeks, or matching placebo. The primary outcome measure of this study was the Visual Analogue Score (VAS) for pain (Hahn et al., 2004). The group that received gabapentin had a statistically decreased VAS for neuropathic pain than did the placebo-treated group (Hahn et al., 2004). Unfortunately, the study is flawed as the sample sizes were very small.

Pregabalin has a similar mechanism of action to gabapentin, with better bioavailability and linear pharmacokinetics.

There are multiple, large, and well-controlled studies showing pregabalin's analgesic efficacy in peripheral neuropathic pain (see Table 7.5.2). A recent, multicenter study evaluating the efficacy of pregabalin in HIV neuropathic pain revealed that both placebo and pregabalin showed substantial and similar reduction in pain (Simpson et al., 2010). Since methodological issues may have contributed to the failure of this study, a follow-up study is underway.

Lamotrigine is an anticonvulsant with mixed evidence supporting its use as an adjuvant analgesic (Simpson et al., 2000; Simpson et al., 2003.). There is some evidence that lamotrigine can act as an adjuvant analgesic in HIV neuropathic pain that is caused by neurotoxic HAART therapy (Simpson et al., 2003).

OTHER ADJUVANT ANALGESICS

Cannabis

Fifty subjects with painful HIV neuropathy were randomly assigned to smoke either cannabis cigarettes three times per day for five days or to smoke a placebo cigarette with the cannabinoids extracted (Abrams et al., 2007). While cannabis was superior to placebo in pain reduction, the study is limited as the numbers in each treatment arm are small, and there was a substantial rate of adverse events.

TOPICAL AGENTS

Lidocaine

In a small number of patients with a crossover design, randomized controlled trial of 5% lidocaine patch for 2 weeks as compared to placebo, there was no benefit seen in HIV neuropathic pain (Estanislao et al., 2004).

Capsaicin

A small, open-label study with high-dose capsaicin has shown efficacy (Simpson et al., 2007).More recent studies have evaluated a potent form of capsaicin in HIV neuropathic pain (Simpson et al., 2008). In a randomized controlled trial, 225 subjects received a single application of high-concentration capsaicin (8%) and 82 received a low-concentration capsaicin patch (0.04%) in a single 30, 60 or 90 minute treatment. The high-concentration patch group had a 23% reduction in pain scores at 12-week follow up and the control group hadan 11% reduction (p = 0.003) (Simpson et al., 2008). The high-dose capsaicin patch is now FDA approved in the US only for postherpetic neuralgia and is approved in Europe for all forms of peripheral neuropathic in non-diabetic patients.

As Table 7.5.1 reveals, HIV-neuropathy-specific analgesic clinical trials are of little help to guide clinicians, and the best evidence for adjuvant analgesics comes from Class I evidence from other peripheral neuropathic pain conditions described in Table 7.5.2. The problems with earlier HIV neuropathy research may in part reflect small sample sizes, and study designs that may not have optimally controlled for the placebo effect. In trying to determine which adjuvant analgesic to consider first in a patient with HIV neuropathic pain, it is helpful to consider the pain generator(s), as this may guide neuropathic pain therapy.

Controlled trials with single analgesic monotherapies do not adequately identify or treat many patients with neuropathic pain from HIV neuropathy or other neuropathic pain conditions. There is a small amount of clinical data and a large amount of clinical experience that supports the use of combination analgesic therapy that targets multiple pain generator(s) in patients with neuropathic pain (Gilron et al., 2005).

OPIOIDS FOR HIV NEUROPATHIC PAIN

Pain syndromes are common in patients with HIV and sometimes complicated with a disabling burden of neuropathic pain severity. Hewitt and colleagues recruited patients with HIV who were participating in a quality of life study to study pain syndromes in ambulatory patients with HIV (Hewitt et al., 1997). Ninety-five percent of the recruited subjects had AIDS and 61% reported frequent or persistent pain. Two to three different pain syndromes were described on average, in each subject. One-half described one or more neuropathic pain syndromes. Most of the neuropathic pain syndromes were due to polyneuropathy. The next most frequent neuropathic pain syndrome was radiculopathy, considered most often to be unrelated to HIV disease. Breitbart and colleagues additionally examined the pain burden experienced by these subjects. On a numerical scale of the Brief Pain Inventory (0–10), the mean pain intensity was 5.4 and the worst pain was 7.4, indicating that moderate to severe pain was common in this cohort (Brietbart et al., 1996). In the field of cancer pain (Elliott & Portenoy, 1997), the severity of the pain is used as a guide to determine if opioids are considered as part of treatment (Elliott & Pasternak, 1996; WHO, 1986). Given the burden of undertreated neuropathic pain from HIV, clinicians have borrowed from the approach to cancer pain by considering a trial of opioids in patients with severe to moderate HIV-associated neuropathic pain. Patients considered for an opioid analgesic trial would ideally have been considered for some of the adjuvant analgesics and topical agents discussed above.

Opioids are often considered after an insufficiently effective trial of a nonsteroidal anti-inflammatory drug (NSAID), topical agent, with an antidepressant such as amitriptyline or duloxetine, or anticonvulsant such as gabapentin or pregabalin. While there are ample data showing the efficacy of opioids in other neuropathic pain states, there are no controlled studies in HIV neuropathy to guide the clinician. Kalso and colleagues found short-term benefit using opioids for treatment of chronic pain disorders not related to HIV (Kalso et al., 2004). Eisenberg et al. reviewed 22 opioid trials for chronic neuropathic pain (Eisenberg, et al., 2005). Overall, opioids reduce pain intensity across studies by about 30%, a degree of efficacy at least matched by amitriptyline. Opioids are most often considered clinically as part of a combination analgesic therapy approach that includes consideration of a topical agent as well as an adjuvant analgesic to target multiple pain generators as well as to minimize the dose of opioids needed for adequate pain relief.

If opioids are considered to be a treatment option, the opioid should be preferably administered in an around-the-clock manner, and careful attention paid to side effects such as sedation, sleep apnea, and constipation. There are many opioid formulations available and there are no data in HIV neuropathic pain to guide selection of opioids such as codeine, oxycodone, morphine, or fentanyl patch, among many others. The degree of difficulty in treating an opioid addiction disorder increases with the more potent opioids, suggesting initial use of a less potent opioid in the lowest possible dosage.

Patients with HIV and neuropathic pain for which a trial of opioids may be considered should be carefully probed for a history of substance abuse. Passik et al. found that AIDS patients receiving opioids for pain, who had a history of substance abuse, were both more symptomatic and exhibited twice as many aberrant drug-taking behaviors as patients with cancer pain with no substance abuse history (Passik et al., 2006). Screening tools are available but rely heavily on patient honesty. Contracts may be another useful method to regulate the use of narcotics.

The analgesic use of methadone should be approached with special caution in patients with HIV, despite methadone's recent popularity as a potent analgesic for neuropathic pain. Methadone "respiratory" deaths may in fact be a result of methadone's newly recognized cardiac toxicity that can also cause sudden death via blockade of a cardiac potassium ion channel (Krantz et al.,2002 Krantz et al., 2009). The ability of methadone to induce torsade des pointes via QTc prolongation may be additive with HIV therapeutic drugs (HAART) (Anson et al., 2005).

ACKNOWLEDGMENTS

Figures are courtesy of Dr. G. Ebenezer, JHU Neurology.

REFERENCES

Abdi, S., Lee, D. H., & Chung, J. M. (1998). The anti-allodynic effects of amitriptyline, gabapentin, and lidocaine in a rat model of neuropathic pain. *Anesth Analg, 87,* 1360–1366.

Abrams, D. I., Jay, C. A., Shade, S. B., et al. (2007). Cannabis in painful HIV associated sensory neuropathy. *Neurology, 68,* 515–521.

Alshekhlee, A., Hussain, Z., Sultan, B. et al. (2008). Guillain Barre syndrome: Incidence and mortality rates in US hospitals. *Neurology, 70,* 1608–1613.

Anson, B. D., Weaver, J. G. R., Ackerman, M. J., et al. (2005). Blockade of HERG channels by HIV protease inhibitors. *Lancet, 365,* 682–686.

Apostolski, S., McAlarney, T., Quattrini, A., et al. (1993). The gp120 glycoprotein of human deficiency virus type 1 binds to sensory ganglion neurons. *Ann Neurol, 34,* 855–863.

Argoff, C. E., Galer, B. S., Jensen, M. P., et al. (2004). Effectiveness of the lidocaine patch 5% on pain qualities in three chronic pain states: Assessment with the Neuropathic Pain Scale. *Curr Med Res Opin, 20S,* 2, S21–S28.

Barbano, R. L., Herrmann, D. N., Hart-Gouleau, S., et al. (2004). Effectiveness, tolerability, and impact on quality of life of the 5% lidocaine patch in diabetic polyneuropathy. *Arch Neurol, 61,* 914–918.

Baron, R., Mayoral, V., Leijon, G., et al. (2009). Efficacy and safety of 5% lidocaine (Lignocaine) medicated plaster in comparison with pregabalin in patients with post-herpetic neuralgia and diabetic neuropathy. Interim analysis from an open-label, two-stage adaptive, randomized, controlled trial. *Clin Drug Invest, 29*, 231–241.

Bennett, G. J. & Xie, Y-K. (1988). A peripheral mononeuropathy in rat that produces disorders of pain sensation like those seen in man. *Pain, 33*, 87–107.

Bradley, W. G., Shapshak, P., Delgado, S., et al. (1998). Morphometric analysis of the peripheral neuropathy of AIDS. *Musch Nerve, 21*, 1188–1195.

Bridges, D., Ahmad, K., & Rice, A. S. (2001). The synthetic cannabinoid WIN55, 212–2 attenuates hyperalgesia and allodynia in a rat model of neuropathic pain. *Br J Pharmacol, 133*, 586–594.

Brietbart, W., McDonald, M. V., Rosenfeld, B., et al. (1996). Pain in ambulatory AIDS patients. I: Pain characteristics and medical correlates. *Pain, 68*, 315–321.

Cherry, C. L., Affandi, J. S., Brew, B. J., et al., (2010). Hepatitis C: Seropositivity is not a risk factor for sensory neuropathy among patients with HIV. *Neurology, 74*, 1538–1542.

Chien, C. V. (2007). HIV/AIDS drugs for sub-Saharan Africa: How do brand and generic supply compare? *PloS One, 2*, 2278.doi.10.1371/journal.pone.0000278 (2007). Accessed October 27, 2009.

Cui, L., Locatelli, L., Xie, M-Y., et al. (1997). Effect of nucleoside analogs on neurite regeneration and mitochondrial DN synthesis in PC-12 cells. *J Pharmacol Exp Ther, 280*, 1228–1234.

Dalakas, M. C. (2001). Peripheral neuropathy and antiretroviral drugs. *Journal of the Peripheral Nervous System (JPNS), 6*, 14–20.

Davies, L., Spies, J. M., Pollard, J. D., et al. (1996). Vasculitis confined to peripheral nerves. *Brain, 119*, 1441–1448.

De Vry, J., Kuhl, E., Franken-Kunkel, P., et al. (2004). Pharmacological characterization of the chronic constriction injury model of neuropathic pain. *Eur J Pharmacol, 491*, 137–148.

Dworkin, R. H., Corbin, A. E., Young, Jr J. P., et al. (2003)Pregabalin for the treatment of post-herpetic neuralgia: A randomized, placebo-controlled trial. *Neurology, 60*, 1274–1283.

Dworkin, R. H., O'Connor, A. B., Backonja, M., et al. (2007). Pharmacological management of neuropathic pain: Evidence-based recommendations. *Pain, 132*, 237–251.

Dyck, P. J., Benstead, T. J., Conn, D. L., et al. (1987). Nonsystemic vasculitic neuropathy. *Brain, 110*, 843–854.

Eisenberg, E., Lurie, Y., Braker, C., et al. Lamotrigine reduces painful diabetic neuropathy: A randomized controlled study.

Eisenberg, E., McNicol, E. D., & Carr, D. B. (2005). Efficacy and safety of Opioid agonists in the treatment of neuropathic pain of nonmalignant origin. *JAMA, 293*, 3043–3052.

Elliott, K. J 1994. (1994). Taxonomy and mechanisms of neuropathic pain. *Semin Neurol, 14*, 195–205.

Elliott, K. J. & Pasternak, G. (1996). Section 1: Symptomatic care pending diagnosis. *Conn's current therapy* Pp 1–4.

Elliott, K. J. & Portenoy, R. K. (1997). Cancer pain: Pathophysiology and syndromes. In T. L. Yaksh (ed.). *Anesthesia: Biologic foundations*, pp. 803–817. New York: Raven Press.

Elliott, K. J. & Simpson, D. M. (2009). Neurotoxic dideoxynucleoside antiretroviral therapy is not associated with progression of painful distal polyneuropathy. Priority Paper Evaluation, *HIV Ther, 3*.

Esiri, M. M., Morris, C. S., & Millard, P. R. (1993). Sensory ands sympathetic ganglia in HIV-1 infection: Immunocytochemical demonstration of HIV-1 viral antigens, increased MHC class II antigen expression and mild reactive inflammation. *J Neurol Sci, 1* 14, 178–187.

Esser, M. J. & Sawynok, J. (1999). Acute Amitriptyline in a rat model of neuropathic pain: Differential symptom and route effects. *Pain, 80*, 643–653.

Estanislao, L., Carter, K., McArthur, J., et al. (2004). A randomized controlled trial of 5% lidocaine gel for HIV associated Distal Sensory Neuropathy. *J AIDS, 37*, 1584–1586.

Finnerup, N. B., Otto, M., Jensen, T. S., et al. (2007). An evidence-based algorithm for the treatment of neuropathic pain. *Med Gen, M9*, 36.

Finnerup, N. B., Otto, M., McQuay, H. J., et al. (2005). Algorithm for neuropathic pain treatment: An evidence based proposal. *Pain, 118*, 289–305.

Flachenecker, P. (2007). Autonomic dysfunction in Guillain-Barre syndrome and multiple sclerosis. *J Neurol, 254*, S2 96–101.

Fox, A., et al. (2001). The role of central and peripheral Cannabinoid 1 receptors in the antihyperalgesic activity of cannabinoids in a model of neuropathic pain. *Pain, 92*, 91–100.

French, J. & Gronseth, G. (2008). Lost in the jungle of evidence: We need a compass. *Neurology, 71*, 1634–1638.

Galer, B. S., Rowbotham, M. C., Perander, J., et al. (1999). Topical lidocaine patch relieves postherpetic neuralgia more effectively than a vehicle topical patch: Results of an enriched enrollment study. *Pain, 80*, 533–538.

Gilron, I., et al. (2005). Morphine, gabapentin, or their combination for neuropathic pain. *N Engl J Med, 352*, 1324–1334.

Goldenberg, D. L., Felson, D. T., & Dinerman, H. (2005). A randomized controlled trial of amitryptiline and naproxen in the treatment of patients with fibromyalgia. *Arthritis and Rheumatism, 29*, 1371–1377.

Griffin, J. W., Crawford, T. O., & McArthur, J. C. (1998). Peripheral neuropathies associated with HIV infection. In H. E. Gendelman, S. A. Lipton, L. Epstein, & S. Swindells (eds.). *The neurology of AIDS*, Pp. 275–291. New York: Chapman & Hall, 1998.

Gross, R. A. & Johnston, K. C. (2009). Levels of evidence. Taking neurology to the next level. *Neurology, 72*, 8–10.

Hahn, K., Arendt, G., Braun, J. S., et al. (2004). A placebo-controlled trial of gabapentin for painful HIV-associated sensory neuropathies. *J Neurol, 251*, 1260–1266.

Hahn, K., Robinson, B., Anderson, C., et al. (2008). Differential effects of HIV infected macrophages on dorsal root ganglia neurons and axons. *Exp Neurol, 210*, 30–40.

Hargreaves, K., Dubner, R., Brown, F. F. C., et al. (1998). A new and sensitive method for measuring thermal nocioception in cutaneous hyperalgesia. *Pain, 32*, 77–88.

Hewitt, D. J., McDonald, M., Portenoy, R. K., et al. (1997). Pain syndromes and etiologies in ambulatory AIDS patients. *Pain, 70*, 117–123.

Herrman, D. N., Barbano, R. L., Hart-Gouleau, S., et al. (2005). An open label study of the lidocaine patch 5% in painful idiopathic sensory polyneuropathy. *Pain Med, 6*, 379–384.

Hughes, R. A. C., Wijdicks, E. F. M., Barohn, R., et al. (2003). Special Article. Practice parameter: Immunotherapy for Guillain-Barre syndrome. Report of the Quality Standards Subcommittee of the American Academy of Neurology. *Neurology, 61*, 736–740.

Jett, M. F., McGuirk, J., Waligora, D., et al. (1997). The effects of mexiletine, desipramine, and fluoxetine in rat models involving central sensitization. *Pain, 69*, 161–169.

Jiang, Z. G., Piggee, C., Heyes, M., et al. (2001). Glutamate is a mediator of neurotoxicity in secretions of activated HIV-1 infected macrophages. *J Neuroimmunol, 117*, 97–107.

Kalso, E., Edwards, J. E., Moore, R. A., & McQuay, H. J. (2004). Opioids in chronic noncancer pain: Systematic review of efficacy and safety. *Pain, 112*, 372–380.

Kemper, C. A., et al. (1998). Mexiletine for HIV-infected patients with painful peripheral neuropathy: A double-blind, placebo-controlled, crossover treatment trial. *J Acquir Immune Defic Syndr Hum Retrovirol, 19*, 367–372.

Keswani, S. C., Jack, C., Zhou, C., & Hoke, A. (2006). Establishment of a rodent model of HIV-associated sensory neuropathy. *The Journal of Neuroscience, 26*, 10299–10304.

Keswani, S. C., Polley, M., Pardo, C. A., et al. (2003). Schwann cell chemokine receptors mediate HIV-1 gp120 toxicity to sensory neurons. *Ann Neurol, 54*, 287–296.

Khaliq, W., Alam, S., & Puri, N. (2007). Topical lidocaine for the treatment of postherpetic neuralgia. *Cochrane Database Syst Rev, 2*, CD004846.

Kieburtz, K., et al. (1998). A randomized trial of amitriptyline and mexiletine for painful neuropathy in HIV infection. AIDS Clinical Trial Group 242 Protocol Team. *Neurology, 51*, 1682–1688.

Krantz, M. J., Lewkowiez, L., Hays, H., et al. (2002). Torsades de pointes associated with very high dose methadone. *Ann Intern Med, 137,* 501–504.

Krantz, M. J., Martin, J., Stimmel, B., et al. (2009). QTc interval screening in methadone treatment. Clinical guidelines. *Ann Intern Med, 150,* 387–395.

Lesser, H., Sharma, U., LaMoreaux, L., et al. (2004). Pregabalin relieves symptoms of painful diabetic neuropathy. *Neurology, 63,* 2104–2110.

Loeser, J. D. & Bonica, B. B. (2001). *Bonica's management of pain.*

Max, M. B. (1990). Towards a physiologically based treatment of patients with neuropathic pain. *Pain, 42,* 131–133.

McQuay, H. J. & Moore, R. A. (1997). Antidepressants and chronic pain. *BMJ, 314,* 763–764.

Melli, G., Keswani, S. C., Fishcer, A. et al. (2006). Spatially distinct and functionally independent mechanisms of axonal degeneration in a model of HIV-associated sensory neuropathy. *Brain, 129,* 1330–1338.

Moore, R. D., Wong, W. M., Keruly, J. C. et al. (2000). Incidence of neuropathy in HIV-infected patients on monotherapy versus those on combination therapy with didanosine, stavudine and hydroxyurea. *AIDS, 14,* 273–278.

Morgello, S., Estanislao, L., Simpson, D., et al. (2004). HIV-associated distal sensory polyneuropathy in the era of highly active antiretroviral therapy: The Manhattan HIV Brain Bank. *Arch Neurol, 61,* 546–551.

Nagano, I., Shapshak, .P, Yoshioka, M., et al. (1996). Parvalbumin and calbindin D-28k immunoreactivity in dorsal root ganglia in acquired immunodeficiency syndrome. *Neuropathol Appl Neurobiol, 22,* 293–301.

Nath, A. (2002). Human immunodeficiency virus (HIV) proteins in neuropathogenesis of HIV dementia. *J Infect Dis, 186*(Suppl 2), S193–S198.

Nottet, H. S. L. M. & Dhawan S. (1998). HIV-1 entry into brain: Mechanisms for the infiltration of HIV-1 infected macrophages across the blood-brain barrier. In H. E. Gendelman, S. A. Lipton, L. Epstein, & S. Swindells (Eds.). *The neurology of AIDS,* New York: Chapman & Hall.

Oh, S. B., Tran, P. B., Gillard, S. E., et al. (2001). Chemokines and glycoprotein 120 produce pain hypersensitivity by directly exciting primary nociceptive neurons. *J Neurosci, 21,* 5027–5035.

Paice, J. A., et al. (2000). Topical capsaicin in the management of HIV-associated peripheral neuropathy. *J Pain Symptom Management, 19,* 45–52.

Pardo, C. A., McArthur, J. C., & Griffin, J. W. (2001). HIV neuropathy: Insights in the pathology of HIV peripheral nerve disease. *J Periph Nerv Syst, 6,* 21–27.

Passik, S. D., Kirsh, K. L., Donaghy, K. B., et al. (2006). Pain and aberrant drug-related behaviors in medically ill patients with and without histories of substance abuse. *Clin J Pain, 22,* 173–181.

Pettersen, J. A., Jones, G., Worthington, C., et al. (2006). A sensory neuropathy in human immunodeficiency virus/acquired immunodeficiency syndrome patients: Protease-inhibitor mediated neurotoxicity. *Ann Neurol, 59,* 816–824.

Polydefkis, M., Yiannoutsos, C. T., Cohen, B. A., et al. (2002). Reduced intraepidermal nerve fiber density in HIV-associated sensory neuropathy. *Neurology, 58,* 115–119.

Rance, N. E., McArthur, J. C., Cornblath, D. R., et al. (1988). Gracile tract degeneration in patients with sensory neuropathy and AIDS. *Neurology, 38,* 265–271.

Richter, R. W., Portenoy, R., Sharma, U., et al. (2005). Relief of painful diabetic peripheral neuropathy with pregabalin: A randomized, placebo-controlled trial. *J Pain, 6,* 253, 260.

Rosenstock, J., Tuchman, M., La Moreaux, L., et al. (2004). Pregabalin for the treatment of painful diabetic peripheral neuropathy: A double-blind, placebo-controlled trial. *Pain, 110,* 628–638.

Rowbotham, M. C., Davies, P. S., Verkempinck, C., et al. (1996). Lidocaine patch: Double-blind controlled study of a new treatment method for post-herpetic neuralgia. *Pain, 65,* 39–44.

Sabatowski, R., Galvez, R., Cherry, D. A., et al. (2004). Pregabalin reduces pain and improves sleep and mood disturbances in patients with post-herpetic neuralgia: Results of a randomized, placebo-controlled clinical trial. *Pain, 109,* 26–35.

Saarto, T. & Wiffen, P. J. (2009). Antidepressants for neuropathic pain (Review). A Cochrane review, prepared and maintained by the Cochrane Collaboration, and published by the Cochrane Library, Issue 3, pp 1–77. John Wiley & Sons. http://www.thecochranelibrary.com

Said, G., Lacroix, C., Chemouilli, P. et al. (1991). Cytomegalovirus neuropathy in acquired immunodeficiency syndrome: A clinical and pathological study. *Ann Neurol, 29,* 139–146.

Said, G., Lacroix-Ciaudo, C., Fujimara, H., et al. (1988). The peripheral neuropathy of necrotizing arteritis: A clinicopathological study. *Ann Neurol, 23,* 461–465.

Shlay, J. C., et al. (1998). Acupuncture and amitriptyline for pain due to HIV-related peripheral neuropathy: A randomized controlled trial. Terry Beirn Community Programs for Clinical Research on AIDS. *JAMA, 280,* 1590–1595.

Simpson, D. M., et al. (2007). An open-label pilot study of high-concentration capsaicin patch in painful HIV neuropathy. *J Pain Symptom Management.*

Simpson, D. M. & Olney, R. K. (1992). Peripheral neuropathies associated with human immunodeficiency virus infection. *Neurol Clin, 10,* 685–711.

Simpson, D. M. & Talgiati, M. (1995). Nucleoside analogue-associated peripheral neuropathy in human immunodeficiency virus infection. *J Acquir Immune Defic Syndr Hum Retrovirol, 9,* 153–161.

Simpson, D. M., Brown, S., Tobias, J., et al. (2008). Controlled trial of high-concentration capsaicin patch for treatment of painful HIV neuropathy. *Neurology, 70,* 2305–2313.

Simpson, D. M., McArthur, J., Olney, R., et al. (2003). Lamotrigine for HIV-associated painful sensory neuropathies: A placebo-controlled trial. *Neurology, 60,* 1508–1514.

Simpson, D. M., Olney, R., McArthur, J. C., et al. (2000). A placebo-controlled trial of lamotrigine for painful HIV-associated neuropathy. *Neurology, 54,* 2115–2119.

Simpson, D. M., Schiffitto, G., Clifford, D. B., et al. (2010). Pregabalin for painful HIV neuropathy: A randomized, double-blind, placebo-controlled trial. *Neurology, 74,* 413–420

Stewart, J. D. (1987). *Focal peripheral neuropathies.* London: Elsevier.

Stuebgen, J. P. & Elliott, K. J. (1997). Malignant radiculopathy and plexopathy. *Handbook of clinical neurology,* pp. 71–82. Amsterdam: Elsevier.

Tagliati, M., Grinnell, J., Godbold, J., & Simpson, D. M. (1999). Peripheral nerve function in HIV infection: Clinical, electrophysiologic, and laboratory findings. *Arch Neurol, 56,* 84–89.

Thorton, C. A., Latif, A. S., & Emmanuel, J. C. (1991). Guillain-Barre syndrome associated with human immunodeficiency virus infection in Zimbabwe. *Neurology, 41,* 812–815.

Tozzi, V., Libertone, R., & Liuzzi, G. (2008). HIV Pharmacogenetics in clinical practice: Recent achievements and future challenges. *Curr HIV Res, 6,* 544–554.

Turner, M. R., Warren, J. D., Jacobs, J. M. et al. (2003). Microvasculitic paraproteinaemic polyneuropathy and B cell lymphoma. *J Peripher Nerv Syst, 8,* 100–107.

Van den Berg, L. H., Sadiq, S. A., Lederman, S., et al. (1992). The gp120 glycoprotein of HIV-1 binds to sulfatide and to the myelin associated glycoprotein. *J Neurosci Res, 33,* 513–518.

Van Seventer, R., Feister, H. A., Young, Jr J. P., et al. (2006). Efficacy and tolerability of twice-daily pregabalin for treating pain and related sleep interference in postherpetic neuralgia: A 13 week, randomized trial. *Curr Med Res Opin, 22,* 375–384.

Wallace, V. C., Blackbeard, J., Segerdahl, A., et al. (2007). Pharmacological, behavioral and mechanistic analysis of HIV-1 gp120 induced painful neuropathy. *Pain,* 2007 [Epub ahead of print].

World Health Organization. (1986). *Cancer pain relief.* Geneva, Switzerland: World Health Organization.

Zhu, Y., Antony, J. M., Martinez, J. A., et al. (2007). Didanosine causes sensory neuropathy in an HIV/AIDS animal model: Impaired mitochondrial and neurotrophic factor gene expression. *Brain, 130,* 2011–2023.

Zollei, E., Avramov, K., Gingl, Z. et al. (2000). Severe cardiovascular autonomic dysfunction in a patient with Guillain-Barre syndrome: A case report. *Autonomic Neuroscience: Basic and Clinical, 86,* 94–98.

7.6

SPINAL CORD DISEASE

Michael C. Previti and Christina M. Marra

HIV is associated with a relatively unique, noninflammatory, subacute myelopathy that has been referred to pathologically as vacuolar myelopathy (VM) and clinically as HIV-associated myelopathy. Most of what we know about VM or HIV-associated myelopathy comes from studies conducted before the advent of potent antiretroviral therapy. Vacuolar myelopathy may be less common in the current treatment era for reasons that have not been established. This chapter focuses on the pathological and clinical aspects of VM and HIV-associated myelopathy.

INTRODUCTION AND DIFFERENTIAL DIAGNOSIS

Myelopathy literally means "disease of the spinal cord." It can be due to an extrinsic process (outside the spinal cord), such as a tumor or abscess, or to an intrinsic process (within the spinal cord), such as tumor, demyelination, infection, or infarction. Myelitis refers to an inflammatory spinal cord process that is often attributed to infectious or parainfectious processes. Transverse myelitis is a clinical description that typically includes acute or subacute onset of ascending weakness, bowel and bladder dysfunction, and a discrete sensory level.

Spinal cord abnormalities that are of particular relevance to patients infected with human immunodeficiency virus (HIV) can be caused by metabolic, infectious, and neoplastic processes (Table 7.6.1). These include direct infection with cytomegalovirus (Mahieux et al., 1989), varicella zoster virus (Lionnet et al., 1996), herpes simplex viruses (Britton et al., 1985), *Mycobacterium tuberculosis* or other mycobacteria (Woolsey, Chambers, Chung, & Mcgarry, 1988; Bhigjee et al., 2001), and *Toxoplasma gondii* (Mehren, Burns, Mamani, Levy, & Laureno, 1988). Primary central nervous system lymphoma is considered in this infectious group because of its strong association with Epstein-Barr virus (Thurnher, Post, & Jinkins, 2000). *Treponema pallidum* spp. *pallidum*, the bacterium that causes syphilis, can cause a myelitis or a vasculitis leading to spinal cord infarction (Silber, 1989). Both Human T-cell leukemia virus I and II (HTLV I and II) can cause a chronic myelopathy in patients also infected with HIV (Beilke et al., 2004). Infectious causes of myelopathy in HIV-infected persons often affect other areas of the neuraxis (Henin, Smith, De Girolami, Sughayer, & Hauw, 1992), and they are discussed in detail in Chapters 8.4, 8.5, and 11.3 of this volume.

HIV is associated with a relatively unique, noninflammatory, subacute myelopathy that has been referred to pathologically as vacuolar myelopathy (VM) and clinically as HIV-associated myelopathy when pathological confirmation is not available. This entity is not due to direct infection of the cord. HIV-associated myelopathy should not be confused with HIV myelitis, which is an uncommon, rapidly progressive disease similar to transverse myelitis, and which is likely due to direct HIV infection of the spinal cord (Santosh, Bell, & Best, 1995; Henin et al., 1992).

Most of what we know about VM or HIV-associated myelopathy comes from studies conducted before the advent of potent antiretroviral therapy. Vacuolar myelopathy may be less common in the current treatment era, and the reason for this observation is not established. A simple explanation may be that VM is associated with advanced HIV disease, which is now less common than it was before potent antiretrovirals were available. Additionally, clinically defined HIV-associated

Table 7.6.1 DIFFERENTIAL DIAGNOSIS OF MYELOPATHY IN HIV-INFECTED INDIVIDUALS

METABOLIC ABNORMALITIES

Copper deficiency

Porto-systemic shunt

Vitamin B12 deficiency

Folate deficiency

INFECTIOUS CAUSES

Cytomegalovirus

Varicella zoster virus

Herpes simplex viruses types 1 and 2

Toxoplasma gondii

Mycobacterium tuberculosis

Treponema pallidum **spp.** *pallidum* **(syphilis)**

HTLV-I and HTLV-II

HIV myelitis

NONINFECTIOUS CAUSES

Vacuolar myelopathy/HIV-associated myelopathy

Lymphoma

myelopathy is likely underdiagnosed, particularly in patients with concomitant distal sensory peripheral neuropathy that may mask hyperreflexia and may overshadow sensory changes due to myelopathy itself. This chapter focuses on the pathological and clinical aspects of VM and HIV-associated myelopathy. We use the term VM in the context of studies that include pathological data and we use the term HIV-associated myelopathy when pathological confirmation is not available. It is important to emphasize that clinically, HIV-associated myelopathy is a diagnosis of exclusion. Thus, in synthesizing the literature, we have omitted case reports in which myelopathy could be reasonably attributed to a disorder other than HIV.

VACUOLAR MYELOPATHY AND HIV-ASSOCIATED MYELOPATHY

PATHOLOGY

Snider and colleagues first described the pathological findings of VM in 1983 (Snider et al., 1983). In one of nine autopsies in AIDS patients, a prominent vacuolar myelopathy with axonal swelling and astrocytosis was noted. Petito and coworkers reported a larger series of autopsy-defined VM in 1985. Thoracic and lumbar spinal cords were examined in 89 consecutive autopsies from patients with advanced AIDS; cervical cord from C2-C8 was not examined (Petito et al., 1985). Vacuolation of spinal white matter in association with lipid-filled macrophages was seen in 20 (22%) patients. Vacuoles were located primarily in the lateral spinal and posterior spinal cord at the middle to lower thoracic levels, and they did not follow specific anatomic tracts. The observed abnormalities were consistent with intramyelin formation of vacuoles, with lipid-laden macrophages within the vacuoles. Axons were disrupted in areas of severe abnormality. Histological severity was described as Grade I, mild (n = 8); Grade II, moderate (n = 7); and Grade III, marked (n = 5). Patients with Grade III changes had a progressive spastic ataxic myelopathy with urinary incontinence that developed over weeks to months. Similar but less frequent clinical findings were seen in patients with Grade II changes, and clinical findings consistent with myelopathy were infrequent in patients with Grade I changes. The pathological abnormalities resembled the changes seen in patients with subacute combined degeneration caused by vitamin B12 or folate deficiency. However, of 12 patients tested, serum B12 levels were normal in all and serum folate levels were normal in 11 of the 12. There was no evidence of opportunistic infection in any of the patients. A hematoxylin and eosin stain of a spinal cord with severe VM is shown in Figure 7.6.1.

ETIOLOGY

Three potential etiologies for VM have been put forth: abnormal B12 metabolism, direct HIV infection of the spinal cord,

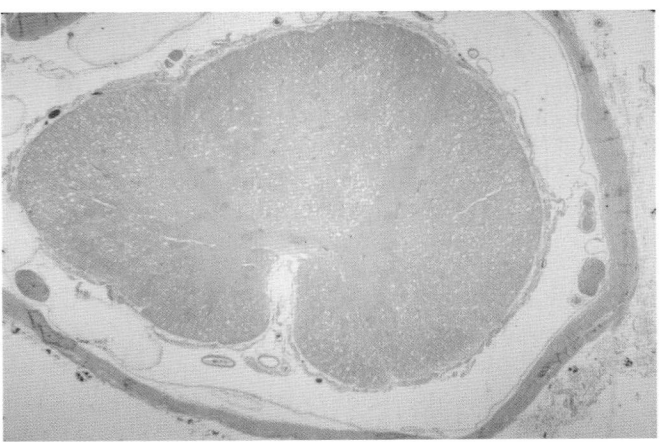

Figure 7.6.1 Hematoxylin and eosin stain of a thoracic spinal cord section from an HIV-infected patient showing extensive vacuolar change throughout the white matter that is not restricted to individual white matter tracts. Courtesy of Susan Morgello, MD.

or toxins. The fact that vacuolar myelopathy, as distinguished pathologically, is not exclusive to HIV suggests a metabolic or toxic cause. However, infection with an unidentified virus other than HIV remains a possibility.

Kamin and Petito reported 21 cases of VM in patients who were not infected with HIV (Kamin & Petito, 1991). Low- to mid-cervical specimens were not collected. Fourteen patients had been treated with prolonged courses of steroids before death, and only four were either immunocompetent or had no evidence of viral infection.

In the aforementioned studies, no patient with pathologically defined VM had evidence of vitamin B12 deficiency despite the pathological similarity between the two diagnoses. However, in a clinical study, Kieburtz and colleagues identified low serum B12 levels or abnormal Schilling test results or both in 10 (20%) of 49 patients referred for neurological evaluation in an HIV neurology clinic (Kieburtz, Giang, Schiffer, & Vakil, 1991). Abnormal B12 metabolism was significantly associated with a clinical diagnosis of neuropathy or myelopathy, and the strongest association was seen between abnormal B12 metabolism and combined neuropathy and myelopathy.

Di Rocco and colleagues postulated that HIV-associated myelopathy is a consequence not of B12 deficiency itself, but rather a deficiency of S-adenosyl methionine (SAM), which is the major methyl donor for myelin formation and repair. Vitamin B12 is an important cofactor for synthesis of SAM. In a study that included 18 HIV-infected patients with a clinical diagnosis of myelopathy, 13 HIV-infected patients without myelopathy, and 18 HIV-uninfected controls, cerebrospinal fluid (CSF) SAM concentration was lowest in the patients with HIV-associated myelopathy compared to the other two groups (Di Rocco et al., 2002). Of note, one HIV-infected patient without myelopathy but with low CSF SAM concentration went on to develop HIV-associated myelopathy six months later. Serum B12 and serum or red blood cell folate concentrations were normal in all patients.

Although there is uncertainty regarding the role of B12 metabolism in its pathogenesis, VM is likely not due to direct HIV infection of the spinal cord. Several authors have identified HIV within macrophages within or outside of vacuoles, including within the perivascular space, but not within neural tissue by in situ hybridization, immunohistochemistry, or electron microscopy (Maier, Budka, Lassmann, & Pohl, 1989; Eilbott et al., 1989; Rosenblum et al., 1989). Similarly, a study showed that severity of HIV-associated myelopathy, as measured by central conduction time, was not associated with CSF HIV RNA concentration (Geraci et al., 2000). Such findings have led to the speculation that macrophages themselves, or products of macrophages, damage myelin. This hypothesis is supported by the finding that the degree of myelin damage is proportional to the number of infiltrating macrophages (Eilbott et al., 1989). The deleterious effects of macrophages or macrophage products may be amplified when additional macrophages are recruited to phagocytose myelin debris.

Chief among the suggested macrophage-derived culprits is tumor necrosis factor-alpha (TNF-α). Several studies have investigated the potential role of this cytokine in VM. Tan and colleagues identified TNF-a in spinal cord macrophages and endothelial cells by immunocytochemistry in cases of VM and in controls (Tan, Guiloff, Henderson, Gazzard, & Miller, 1996). The amount of staining was greatest in spinal cords with VM compared to controls, but the intensity of staining was not related to the severity of VM, suggesting that cytokine damage may occur early or even trigger subsequent pathological changes. Tyor and colleagues, also using immunocytochemistry, showed that TNF-a staining was greater in spinal cord tissue from HIV-infected patients compared to controls and was seen in areas with the greatest macrophage infiltration, particularly in the posterior and lateral funiculi (Tyor et al., 1993). There was no correlation between degree of staining and pathological findings of VM or with severity of VM. These authors also suggested that production of a toxin such as TNF-a preceded and precipitated myelin injury.

A unifying hypothesis has been advanced to explain these divergent results. Specifically, HIV-infected macrophages release toxic cytokines, such as TNF-a, that injure myelin. Abnormalities in B12 metabolism, particularly decreased production of SAM, impair the host ability to repair damaged myelin (Tan & Guiloff, 1998).

CLINICAL ABNORMALITIES

The most comprehensive description of the clinical correlates of VM was provided by Dal Pan and colleagues based on a case control study of 215 autopsies that included examination of the spinal cord (Dal Pan, Glass, & Mcarthur, 1994). The 100 cases were patients with AIDS who had autopsy confirmation of VM. The 115 controls were individuals with AIDS but without pathological evidence of VM. Patients with VM had significantly more AIDS-defining illnesses than controls.

Neurological examination findings were available in 56 patients with VM and 15 of them had clinical findings consistent with myelopathy, including leg weakness, spasticity, and hyperreflexia. Onset of myelopathy symptoms was 3–16 weeks before examinations were performed. Eight of the 15 patients with evidence of myelopathy also had findings consistent with distal sensory peripheral neuropathy, and neuropathy was significantly more common in cases than controls. As in the series by Petito and colleagues (Petito et al., 1985), clinical severity of myelopathy was related to severity of pathological abnormalities. Specifically, clinical myelopathy was seen in none of the 17 patients with Grade I, 5 of 26 with Grade II, and 10 of 13 with Grade III pathology. These authors pointed out that a transverse myelitis-like picture with rapid onset of lower extremity weakness or spasticity, early bladder and bowel dysfunction, and a discrete sensory level argue against a diagnosis of HIV-associated myelopathy.

Di Rocco and colleagues developed a research clinical definition for HIV-associated myelopathy for use in clinical trials (Di Rocco et al., 2002). Although such rigor might not be necessary in clinical practice, the definition points out the salient clinical and diagnostic abnormalities of the disorder (Table 7.6.2). In addition to the clinical findings described above, abnormal tibial somatosensory-evoked potentials with prolonged conduction time (defined as interpeak latency between N21 and P27 greater than 2.5 standard deviations above normal) were considered diagnostic for HIV-associated myelopathy. A study from Denmark supports the importance of abnormal tibial somatosensory responses in the diagnosis of HIV-associated myelopathy (Helweg-Larsen et al., 1988). Among 23 unselected patients with AIDS, 16 had neurological abnormalities, most

Table 7.6.2 RESEARCH CRITERIA FOR DIAGNOSIS OF HIV-ASSOCIATED MYELOPATHY

CLINICAL CRITERIA

At least 4 of the following symptoms for at least 6 weeks:

1. **Lower extremity weakness**
2. **Unsteady, stiff or uncoordinated gait**
3. **Lower extremity stiffness or spasms**
4. **Lower extremity paresthesias or numbness**
5. **Urinary frequency, urgency, or incontinence**
6. **Erectile dysfunction in men**

At least 3 of the following signs:

1. **Lower extremity weakness**
2. **Spastic gait**
3. **Extensor plantar responses**
4. **Reduced vibration or position sense in the lower extremities**

Hyperactive reflexes or clonus in the lower extremities

No weakness or pyramidal signs in the upper extremities

ELECTROPHYSIOLOGICAL CRITERIA

1. **Abnormal tibial somatosensory-evoked potentials with prolonged central conduction time (CCT) and**
2. **Normal median nerve evoked potentials and CCT**

(Di Rocco et al., 2002)

commonly weakness, spasticity, and hyperreflexia of the legs. Central conduction time after tibial nerve stimulation was prolonged in all 16. In half of the 16, delay could not be attributed to peripheral neuropathy.

DIAGNOSIS

Screening Laboratory Tests

As noted above, there are many potential causes of myelopathy in HIV (Table 7.6.1), but the number that has a subacute onset and clinical features similar to HIV-associated myelopathy is limited. These include copper deficiency, porto-systemic shunt, syphilis, HTLV-I and HTLV-II infections and B12 or folate deficiency. These potential etiologies need to be excluded before a diagnosis of HIV-associated myelopathy can be made. Assessment of serum copper level; liver transaminases, ammonia, and coagulation factors; syphilis serological tests (for example, serum rapid plasma reagin test [RPR]; and serum fluorescent treponemal antibody-absorption [FTA-ABS] test or *T. pallidum* particle agglutingation [TPPA] test or *T. pallidum*-specific EIA or ELISA); HTLV serologic tests; and measurement of serum B12 and folate levels should be performed.

Cerebrospinal Fluid

Cerebrospinal fluid findings in patients with HIV-associated myelopathy are nonspecific. Generally, CSF white blood cells (WBCs) are within the normal range and CSF protein may be normal or mildly elevated (Dal Pan et al., 1994; Shimojima et al., 2005; Sartoretti-Schefer, Blattler, & Wichmann, 1997). One study showed that measurement of CSF HIV RNA levels was not diagnostically useful, although these results have not been replicated (Geraci et al., 2000). The value of CSF analysis is to exclude alternative infectious or neoplastic causes of myelopathy.

Neuroimaging

Magnetic resonance imaging of the spinal cord may be normal or abnormal in pathologically confirmed VM. In the study by Dal Pan and colleagues, 4 of 56 individuals with pathologically confirmed VM underwent magnetic resonance (MR) imaging of the thoracic spine; the study was normal in all (Dal Pan et al., 1994). A case report describes an HIV-infected patient who presented with clinical myelopathy who had high T2 signal abnormalities in the posterior columns of the cervical spinal cord with predominance in the gracile tract. Autopsy 10 weeks later showed vacuolar changes that corresponded to the abnormal areas on MR (Sartoretti-Schefer et al., 1997). In a study that included histopathological examination and postmortem MR in 30 HIV-infected patients, spinal cords from 9 showed vacuolar myelopathy; 6 of the 9 had MR abnormalities (Santosh et al., 1995). Of note, not all patients with clinical evidence of myelopathy had pathological abnormalities. This finding emphasizes the potential inaccuracy of a clinical diagnosis of VM.

In a study of 21 patients with clinically defined HIV-associated myelopathy, cord atrophy, primarily localized to the thoracic region, was present in 16 and increased intramedullary signal on T2-weighted images was evident in 6 individuals. Spinal cord MR was normal in 3 patients (Chong et al., 1999). The extent of the abnormality on MR was not related to clinical severity. Case reports similarly describe abnormal signal in the posterior columns affecting the gracile tracts in patients with clinically defined myelopathy (Shimojima et al., 2005).

The value of neuroimaging lies in its ability to identify alternative etiologies for HIV-associated myelopathy. Given that alternative etiologies often affect brain and cord, brain imaging should always accompany cord imaging in patients with suspected HIV-associated myelopathy.

TREATMENT

There is no proven treatment for HIV-associated myelopathy. Nonetheless, several case reports describe clinical, neuroimaging, and electrophysiological improvement after beginning antiretroviral therapy (Bizaare, Dawood, & Moodley, 2008; Staudinger & Henry, 2000; Fernandez-Fernandez, De La Fuente-Aguado, Ocampo-Hermida, & Iglesias-Castanon, 2004; Eyer-Silva et al., 2002). Because HIV-associated myelopathy occurs in advanced HIV, patients will likely meet current guidelines for antiretroviral therapy regardless of the neurological disorder. Even if they do not, antiretroviral therapy is likely the most reasonable treatment (see below).

Di Rocco and colleagues performed a controlled 12-week trial of L-methionine (3 gm by mouth twice a day) in HIV-associated myelopathy in 56 patients (Di Rocco et al., 2004). Stringent criteria were used to identify cases (Table 7.6.2), and the primary outcome was change in central conduction time. Secondary outcomes were measures of strength, spasticity, and urinary function. There was no benefit of L-methionine for any of the tested outcomes.

Cikurel and colleagues performed an open-label unblinded study of two infusions of intravenous immunoglobulin (IVIg) (2 gms given over 2 days at days 1 and 2 and days 29 and 30 after entry) for treatment of HIV-associated myelopathy in 17 patients (Cikurel, Schiff, & Simpson, 2009). The rationale for the study was that IVIg could mitigate a local inflammatory response that could contribute to myelin injury. Entry criteria were clinical and did not include central conduction time. Outcome was change in composite lower extremity strength scores at 28 (n = 17) and 56 (n = 10) weeks. Strength improved significantly at 28 weeks, but not at 56 weeks. A larger blinded study should be conducted to confirm these findings before IVIg can be recommended for treatment of HIV-associated myelopathy.

SUMMARY

Most of what we know about VM or HIV-associated myelopathy comes from studies conducted before the advent of potent antiretroviral therapy. The pathological abnormalities resemble the changes seen in subacute combined degeneration.

Clinically, HIV-associated myelopathy presents as subacute or chronic leg weakness, spasticity, and hyperreflexia. There is often concomitant peripheral neuropathy. Clinical severity is proportional to the severity of pathological abnormalities. The diagnosis of HIV-associated myelopathy is one of exclusion; there are no pathognomonic laboratory or imaging findings. There is no proven treatment for HIV-associated myelopathy, although some patients improve with potent antiretroviral therapy.

REFERENCES

Beilke, M. A., Theall, K. P., O'Brien, M., Clayton, J. L., Benjamin, S. M., Winsor, E. L., et al. (2004). Clinical outcomes and disease progression among patients coinfected with HIV and human T lymphotropic virus types 1 and 2. *Clin Infect Dis, 39*, 256–63.

Bhigjee, A. I., Madurai, S., Bill, P. L., Patel, V., Corr, P., Naidoo, M. N., et al. (2001). Spectrum of myelopathies in HIV seropositive South African patients. *Neurology, 57*, 348–51.

Bizaare, M., Dawood, H., & Moodley, A. (2008). Vacuolar myelopathy: A case report of functional, clinical, and radiological improvement after highly active antiretroviral therapy. *Int J Infect Dis, 12*, 442–4.

Britton, C. B., Mesa-Tejada, R., Fenoglio, C. M., Hays, A. P., Garvey, G. G., & Miller, J. R. (1985). A new complication of AIDS: Thoracic myelitis caused by herpes simplex virus. *Neurology, 35*, 1071–4.

Chong, J., Di Rocco, A., Tagliati, M., Danisi, F., Simpson, D. M., & Atlas, S. W. (1999). MR findings in AIDS-associated myelopathy. *AJNR Am J Neuroradiol, 20*, 1412–6.

Cikurel, K., Schiff, L., & Simpson, D. M. (2009). Pilot study of intravenous immunoglobulin in HIV-associated myelopathy. *AIDS Patient Care STDS, 23*, 75–8.

Dal Pan, G. J., Glass, J. D., & McArthur, J. C. (1994). Clinicopathologic correlations of HIV-1-associated vacuolar myelopathy: An autopsy-based case-control study. *Neurology, 44*, 2159–64.

Di Rocco, A., Bottiglieri, T., Werner, P., Geraci, A., Simpson, D., Godbold, J., et al. (2002). Abnormal cobalamin-dependent transmethylation in AIDS-associated myelopathy. *Neurology, 58*, 730–5.

Di Rocco, A., Werner, P., Bottiglieri, T., Godbold, J., Liu, M., Tagliati, M., et al. (2004). Treatment of AIDS-associated myelopathy with L-methionine: A placebo-controlled study. *Neurology, 63*, 1270–5.

Eilbott, D. J., Peress, N., Burger, H., Laneve, D., Orenstein, J., Gendelman, H. E., et al. (1989). Human immunodeficiency virus type 1 in spinal cords of acquired immunodeficiency syndrome patients with myelopathy: Expression and replication in macrophages. *Proc Natl Acad Sci USA, 86*, 3337–41.

Eyer-Silva, W. A., Couto-Fernandez, J. C., Caetano, M. R., Chequer-Fernandez, S. L., Pinto, J. F., Morais-De-Sa, C. A., et al. (2002). Remission of HIV-associated myelopathy after initiation of lopinavir in a patient with extensive previous exposure to highly active antiretroviral therapy. *AIDS, 16*, 2367–9.

Fernandez-Fernandez, F. J., De La Fuente-Aguado, J., Ocampo-Hermida, A., & Iglesias-Castanon, A. (2004). Remission of HIV-associated myelopathy after highly active antiretroviral therapy. *J Postgrad Med, 50*, 195–6.

Geraci, A., Di Rocco, A., Liu, M., Werner, P., Tagliati, M., Godbold, J., et al. (2000). AIDS myelopathy is not associated with elevated HIV viral load in cerebrospinal fluid. *Neurology, 55*, 440–2.

Helweg-Larsen, S., Jakobsen, J., Boesen, F., Arlien-Soborg, P., Brun, B., Smith, T., et al. (1988). Myelopathy in AIDS. A clinical and electrophysiological study of 23 Danish patients. *Acta Neurol Scand, 77*, 64–73.

Henin, D., Smith, T. W., De Girolami, U., Sughayer, M., & Hauw, J. J. (1992). Neuropathology of the spinal cord in the acquired immunodeficiency syndrome. *Hum Pathol, 23*, 1106–14.

Kamin, S. S. & Petito, C. K. (1991). Idiopathic myelopathies with white matter vacuolation in non-acquired immunodeficiency syndrome patients. *Hum Pathol, 22*, 816–24.

Kieburtz, K. D., Giang, D. W., Schiffer, R. B., & Vakil, N. (1991). Abnormal vitamin B12 metabolism in human immunodeficiency virus infection. Association with neurological dysfunction. *Arch Neurol, 48*, 312–4.

Lionnet, F., Pulik, M., Genet, P., Petitdidier, C., Davous, P., Lebon, P., et al. (1996) Myelitis due to varicella-zoster virus in two patients with AIDS: Successful treatment with acyclovir. *Clin Infect Dis, 22*, 138–40.

Mahieux, F., Gray, F., Fenelon, G., Gherardi, R., Adams, D., Guillard, A., et al. (1989). Acute myeloradiculitis due to cytomegalovirus as the initial manifestation of AIDS. *J Neurol Neurosurg Psychiatry, 52*, 270–4.

Maier, H., Budka, H., Lassmann, H., & Pohl, P. (1989). Vacuolar myelopathy with multinucleated giant cells in the acquired immune deficiency syndrome (AIDS). Light and electron microscopic distribution of human immunodeficiency virus (HIV) antigens. *Acta Neuropathol, 78*, 497–503.

Mehren, M., Burns, P. J., Mamani, F., Levy, C. S., & Laureno, R. (1988). Toxoplasmic myelitis mimicking intramedullary spinal cord tumor. *Neurology, 38*, 1648–50.

Petito, C. K., Navia, B. A., Cho, E. S., Jordan, B. D., George, D. C., & Price, R. W. (1985). Vacuolar myelopathy pathologically resembling subacute combined degeneration in patients with the acquired immunodeficiency syndrome. *N Engl J Med, 312*, 874–9.

Rosenblum, M., Scheck, A. C., Cronin, K., Brew, B. J., Khan, A., Paul, M., et al. (1989). Dissociation of AIDS-related vacuolar myelopathy and productive HIV-1 infection of the spinal cord. *Neurology, 39*, 892–6.

Santosh, C. G., Bell, J. E., & Best, J. J. (1995). Spinal tract pathology in AIDS: Postmortem MRI correlation with neuropathology. *Neuroradiology, 37*, 134–8.

Sartoretti-Schefer, S., Blattler, T., & Wichmann, W. (1997). Spinal MRI in vacuolar myelopathy, and correlation with histopathological findings. *Neuroradiology, 39*, 865–9.

Shimojima, Y., Yazaki, M., Kaneko, K., Fukushima, K., Morita, H., Hashimoto, T., et al. (2005). Characteristic spinal MRI findings of HIV-associated myelopathy in an AIDS patient. *Intern Med, 44*, 763–4.

Silber, M. H. (1989). Syphilitic myelopathy. *Genitourin Med, 65*, 338–41.

Snider, W. D., Simpson, D. M., Nielsen, S., Gold, J. W., Metroka, C. E., & Posner, J. B. (1983). Neurological complications of acquired immune deficiency syndrome: analysis of 50 patients. *Ann Neurol, 14*, 403–18.

Staudinger, R. & Henry, K. (2000). Remission of HIV myelopathy after highly active antiretroviral therapy. *Neurology, 54*, 267–8.

Tan, S. V. & Guiloff, R. J. (1998). Hypothesis on the pathogenesis of vacuolar myelopathy, dementia, and peripheral neuropathy in AIDS. *J Neurol Neurosurg Psychiatry, 65*, 23–8.

Tan, S. V., Guiloff, R. J., Henderson, D. C., Gazzard, B. G., & Miller, R. (1996). AIDS-associated vacuolar myelopathy and tumor necrosis factor-alpha (TNF alpha). *J Neurol Sci, 138*, 134–44.

Thurnher, M. M., Post, M. J., & Jinkins, J. R. (2000). MRI of infections and neoplasms of the spine and spinal cord in 55 patients with AIDS. *Neuroradiology, 42*, 551–63.

Tyor, W. R., Glass, J. D., Baumrind, N., Mcarthur, J. C., Griffin, J. W., Becker, P. S., et al. (1993). Cytokine expression of macrophages in HIV-1-associated vacuolar myelopathy. *Neurology, 43*, 1002–9.

Woolsey, R. M., Chambers, T. J., Chung, H. D., & Mcgarry, J. D. (1988). Mycobacterial meningomyelitis associated with human immunodeficiency virus infection. *Arch Neurol, 45*, 691–3.

7.7

MYOPATHY

Jessica Robinson-Papp, Kenneth A. Fox, David M. Simpson, and Susan Morgello

Skeletal muscle disorders associated with HIV infection are myriad. These disorders may present as initial symptoms of HIV disease or at any time during the course of infection. Diagnosis is not always straightforward, as multiple pathologies may coexist in the same patient and myopathies may be masked by concomitant central nervous system disorders. Neuromuscular disorders may be caused by HIV infection itself or arise secondarily as a result of a variety of processes that are associated with HIV infection, including as a treatment side effect. Furthermore, the insidious progression of most neuromuscular disorders may be overlooked in the advanced stages of AIDS, when other complications dominate the clinical picture. Prompt recognition of neuromuscular disease is important in HIV-infected patients, as therapy may dramatically improve the patient's quality of life. This chapter reviews the spectrum of myopathies that occurs in association with HIV infection and treatment. We describe the clinical, electrophysiological, and pathological features of these disorders, and discuss theories of pathogenesis and options for management.

INTRODUCTION

Skeletal muscle disorders associated with human immunodeficiency virus (HIV) infection are myriad, and may present as initial symptoms of HIV disease, or anywhere in the course of infection (Snider et al., 1983; Dalakas et al., 1986a, 1990; Lange et al., 1988; Simpson & Bender, 1988; Illa et al., 1991; Simpson et al., 1993a; Gherardi, 1994). They are not always straightforward to diagnose, as multiple pathologies may coexist in the same patient, and myopathies may be masked by concomitant central nervous system (CNS) disorders such as dementia, focal brain lesions, myelopathy, or peripheral neuropathy. Furthermore, the insidious progression of most neuromuscular complications may be overlooked in advanced stages of the acquired immunodeficiency syndrome (AIDS), when other complications dominate the clinical picture. Prompt recognition of neuromuscular disease is important in HIV-infected patients, as therapy may dramatically improve the patient's quality of life.

Muscle pathology may be primary (i.e., associated with HIV infection) or secondary to a variety of toxic, metabolic, infectious, neoplastic, and vasculitic processes (Table 7.7.1; Gherardi, 1994). Early series of neurologically affected AIDS patients reported cases of myopathy almost indistinguishable

from seronegative adults with idiopathic polymyositis (Snider et al., 1983; Dalakas et al., 1986a; Simpson & Bender, 1988). Additionally, HIV-wasting syndrome was described and recognized to be a form of myopathy in some individuals (Simpson et al., 1990). In 1987, the introduction of zidovudine (AZT) in the treatment of HIV disease opened a new chapter of myopathology, with the description of AZT-associated mitochondrial toxicity in skeletal muscle (Dalakas et al., 1990; Pezeshkpour et al., 1991; Mhiri et al., 1991; Arnaudo et al., 1991). As other antiretroviral medications became available, such as stavudine (d4T) and other nucleoside reverse transcriptase inhibitors (NRTIs), they too were implicated as causes of myopathy alone or in combination with AZT (Benbrik et al., 1997; Marcus et al., 2002; Rey et al., 1999; Falco et al., 2002; Miller et al., 2000; Mokrzycki et al., 2000; Simpson et al., 2003). The subsequent description of a neuromuscular weakness syndrome associated with antiretroviral therapy, and the recognition of the important role of muscle in the lipodystrophy syndrome, further supported mitochondrial toxicity as a common pathogenetic theme (Simpson et al., 2003; Gan et al., 2002; Kakuda, 2000). This chapter reviews the spectrum of myopathies that occur in association with HIV infection and in treatment. We describe the clinical,

Table 7.7.1 **HIV-ASSOCIATED MYOPATHIES**

Polymyositis
NRTI-associated myopathy
AZT
HIV-associated neuromuscular weakness syndrome
Nemaline rod myopathy
Inclusion body myositis
Cholesterol-lowering agent myopathy
Opportunistic Infections
Bacterial (*S. aureus*, others)
Fungal (*Pneumocystis carinii, Cryptococcus neoformans*)
Protozoal (*Toxoplasma gondii, Pleistophora (Microsporidia)*)
Neoplastic Infiltrates
Lymphoma
Kaposi's sarcoma

electrophysiological, and pathological features of these disorders, theories of pathogenesis, and management options.

DEFINITION

There are no clinical criteria specifically developed for the diagnosis of HIV myopathy. A similar situation was encountered in the early literature concerning seronegative polymyositis, where lack of a uniform definition for polymyositis ultimately led to the publication of more rigorous diagnostic criteria (Bohan & Peters, 1975; Mastaglia & Ojeda, 1985; Dalakas, 1991). Clinical and histopathological characteristics of HIV myopathy are similar to those of HIV-negative polymyositis. Thus, the diagnostic criteria of HIV-associated myopathy are analogous to those of polymyositis, as follows (Bohan & Peters, 1975; Mastaglia & Ojeda, 1985; Dalakas, 1991):

1) progressive, symmetrical weakness of limb-girdle muscles and neck flexors;

2) elevation of serum skeletal muscle enzymes, particularly creatine phosphokinase (CPK);

3) electromyographic abnormalities with short, brief, polyphasic motor unit action potentials that recruit with early and full interference patterns, with or without associated irritative activity;

4) muscle biopsy evidence of myofiber necrosis, phagocytosis, variation in fiber diameter, regeneration, and degeneration, with or without endomysial inflammatory infiltrates.

The diagnosis of polymyositis is considered definite when a patient fulfills all four criteria and probable when three criteria are positive. It is debated whether these diagnostic features have equal weight or whether muscle biopsy findings should be the diagnostic "gold standard" (Dalakas, 1991). In conventional clinical practice, it may be difficult to obtain muscle biopsy in all patients with suspected myopathy. We have adopted these four criteria in the evaluation of myopathic HIV-positive subjects and additionally consider a possible diagnosis of myopathy when two criteria are present and muscle biopsy results are not available.

HIV-infected patients present several challenges in the diagnosis of myopathy when using standard criteria. Central and peripheral nervous system diseases, classically considered to be an exclusion criteria in seronegative patients (Bohan & Peters, 1975), often coexist with myopathy in patients with AIDS. The symptoms of myalgia and fatigue are common and nonspecific in HIV-infected patients (Richman et al., 1987; Berman et al., 1988; Buskila & Gladman, 1990; Miller et al., 1991; Simpson et al., 1997) and should therefore be used with caution in the diagnosis of myopathy. Finally, the widespread use of AZT and other antiretroviral drugs complicates the diagnosis of HIV myopathy, as a toxic factor may be superimposed upon a primary inflammatory process (Lane et al., 1993; Morgello et al., 1995).

EPIDEMIOLOGY

Myopathy may occur at any time in the course of HIV disease and is not associated with any particular stage of immunosuppression (Simpson & Bender, 1988). Clinical experience suggests that HIV myopathy is rare in the highly active antiretroviral therapy (HAART) era, although the current prevalence and incidence is unknown. The majority of the epidemiological data available concerning HIV myopathy are from before the HAART era. In one series of 101 consecutive patients with HIV infection, 2 had polymyositis (Berman et al., 1988). A retrospective analysis of a large primary antiretroviral protocol (AIDS Clinical Trials Group (ACTG) 016), comparing the efficacy and safety of AZT ($n = 360$) to placebo ($n = 351$), found a 0.4% incidence of myopathy in the AZT-exposed group (Simpson et al., 1997). Pathological studies have reported a higher incidence of muscle disease in AIDS. Wrzolek et al. (1990) reported a series of 92 muscle specimens obtained at autopsy from HIV-infected subjects. Twenty-two (24%) revealed primary myopathic changes, including eight with inflammatory infiltrates and ten with necrotizing myopathy. Gabbai et al. (1990) reported 50 muscle biopsies in AZT-naive patients; 14 (28%) revealed muscle necrosis, phagocytosis, and inflammatory infiltrates. Fifty percent of primates infected with simian AIDS D retrovirus developed polymyositis with clinical, laboratory, and pathological features similar to those of the human disease (Dalakas et al., 1986b). There has been one HAART-era study that examined the prevalence of CPK elevations in HIV-infected patients. While transient elevations were relatively common (15%), sustained elevations in CPK, possibly reflecting muscle damage, were present in only 3.8% of evaluable patients (Manfredi et al., 2002). In a series of 379 advanced-stage HAART-era patients evaluated by a neurologist at the Manhattan HIV Brain Bank, only 4 (1%) displayed evidence of myopathy at baseline (Susan Morgello, personal communication).

CLINICAL FEATURES

The predominant presenting symptom of HIV myopathy is slowly progressive weakness of proximal limb muscles, with prominent involvement of neck and hip flexors (Dalakas et al., 1986a; Simpson & Bender, 1988; Manji et al., 1993). Patients typically complain of difficulty in rising from a chair, climbing stairs, or raising their arms above the shoulders. Other symptoms include fatigue, myalgia, muscle cramps, and dysphagia (Snider et al., 1983; Dalakas et al., 1986a; Simpson & Bender, 1988; Manji et al., 1993; Stern et al., 1987; Gonzales et al., 1988). Neurological examination typically reveals symmetric weakness of proximal muscle groups, with prominent involvement of neck flexors and limb-girdle groups and preserved deep tendon reflexes. Weak muscles may also be atrophic, although this finding is not specific to myopathy. Functional tests, including sustaining the arms above the head for 15 seconds and rising from both a seated position and squat, are helpful in the assessment of strength.

These functional tests are well suited for large-scale clinical studies, in which examinations are often performed by non-neurology personnel.

Several of the classic clinical features of polymyositis have poor specificity in HIV-infected subjects, due to the frequent occurrence of other neurological conditions, including peripheral neuropathy and myelopathy (Simpson & Tagliati, 1994). In particular, the slowly progressive AIDS-associated vacuolar myelopathy may initially present with symptoms of proximal weakness in the lower limbs (Dal Pan et al., 1994; see also Chapter 7.6 of this volume by Drs Previti and Marra). Fatigue, myalgia, and wasting are present in 25–50% of patients diagnosed with HIV myopathy (Simpson & Bender, 1988; Simpson et al., 1993a; Lange et al., 1988). Fatigue is a very common complaint of patients with AIDS, but there is little evidence that it results from altered muscle metabolism (Miller et al., 1991). Myalgia may be associated with polymyositis, usually early in the course of disease (Dalakas, 1994), but it is neither a sensitive nor specific symptom of myopathy in HIV-infected individuals (Tagliati et al., 1994). Myalgia occurs in as much as 44% of AZT-naive patients, and may have a slightly higher prevalence in patients taking AZT (Richman et al., 1987; Berman et al., 1988; Buskila & Gladman, 1990; Simpson et al., 1997). Like fatigue, there is no evidence that myalgia is associated with altered muscle metabolism (Miller et al., 1991).

The long term prognosis of HIV myopathy is not well established. Prior to the advent of HAART, follow-up was limited by the high mortality of HIV itself (Simpson & Bender, 1988). A more recent case series (n = 13) found that most patients improved over months to years with or without treatment (Johnson et al., 2003). Our experience has been more variable. While several of our patients with HIV-myopathy have responded to treatment, others have had stable or progressive weakness for many years.

LABORATORY STUDIES

The most sensitive serological test for HIV myopathy, as in other primary muscle disorders, is serum CPK level. CPK was elevated in 92% of patients with HIV myopathy in our retrospective series (Simpson et al., 1993a). CPK elevation parallels the degree of myonecrosis observed in coincident muscle biopsies, but does not correlate with weakness (Simpson & Wolfe, 1991). CPK is not a specific marker of myopathy in HIV-infected individuals. Our analysis of ACTG Protocol 016 (Simpson et al., 1997) indicated that the majority of patients with elevated CPK do not have limb weakness or other evidence of myopathy.

CPK levels are usually elevated to a moderate degree in HIV myopathy, with a median level of approximately 500 IU/l (Simpson et al., 1993a). Serum CPK levels greater than 1500 IU/l have been reported in association with acute rhabdomyolysis in HIV-infected patients (Chariot et al., 1994). Lactic acidosis is a well-recognized adverse effect of NRTI therapy, and a feature of HIV-associated neuromuscular weakness syndrome. Therefore, all patients with acute weakness in the setting of antiretroviral therapy should have both serum CPK and lactate measurements.

ELECTRODIAGNOSTIC FEATURES

Electromyography (EMG) is a useful tool in the diagnosis of myopathy. A myopathic EMG pattern is defined by short, brief motor-unit action potentials, recruiting with early and full interference pattern, with or without irritative activity. The diagnostic yield of needle EMG varies with the type of myopathy and may reach 90% in seronegative patients with adult idiopathic polymyositis (DeVere & Bradley, 1975). EMG is a sensitive and specific diagnostic test for HIV-associated myopathy. In our series of 50 patients with HIV-associated myopathy, 94% had myopathic EMG activity (Simpson et al., 1993a). The iliopsoas is the most sensitive muscle for diagnosis. Abnormal irritative activity (e.g., fibrillation potentials) is also present in many cases. In approximately 50% of our patients with HIV-associated myopathy, nerve conduction study abnormalities indicated concurrent distal symmetric polyneuropathy (Simpson & Bender, 1988).

HISTOPATHOLOGY AND PATHOGENESIS

Histological analysis of muscle biopsies from myopathic and nonmyopathic HIV-positive patients has provided diagnostic and pathogenetic insights. In evaluating the literature, it is important to distinguish cases of clinical myopathy from those with only myopathic findings on muscle biopsy, since there is not complete concordance between the two, and abnormalities on muscle biopsy may be found in asymptomatic patients (Grau et al., 1993). Descriptions of myopathology in symptomatic, AZT-naive patients are critical in distinguishing mechanisms of disease that are related or unrelated to drug toxicity.

Dalakas et al. (1986a) described two HIV-positive patients with clinical polymyositis. Muscle biopsies revealed myofiber necrosis and phagocytosis, and interstitial and interfascicular mononuclear cell inflammation, consistent with myositis (Fig. 7.7.1). HIV was detected immunohistochemically within CD4-positive cells in the inflammatory infiltrates (Dalakas et al., 1986a). Subsequent characterization of HIV-related myositis revealed that approximately 49% of the endomysial infiltrates were composed of CD8-positive cells, 38% of macrophages, and 13% of CD4-positive cells (Illa et al., 1991). In contrast to biopsies from seronegative individuals with polymyositis, biopsies from HIV-infected subjects showed a decreased percentage of CD4-positive cells, even in patients who were not lymphopenic. HIV was localized in interstitial inflammatory cells that were identified as macrophages (Illa et al., 1991; Chad et al., 1990).

In 1988, there were initial reports of AZT-naive patients with myopathy (Simpson & Bender, 1988; Gonzales et al., 1988). In these patients, structural myofiber abnormalities including rod and cytoplasmic bodies and basophilic granular

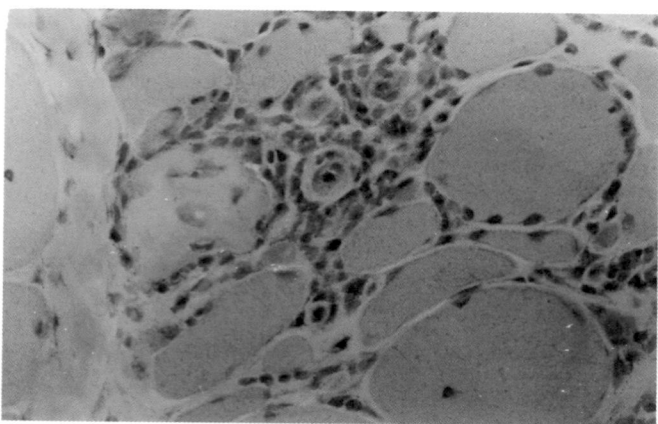

Figure 7.7.1 HIV-associated myositis. Displayed are prominent endomyseal inflammation, and myofiber necrosis and invasion. Modified trichrome stain; original magnification, 100 ×.

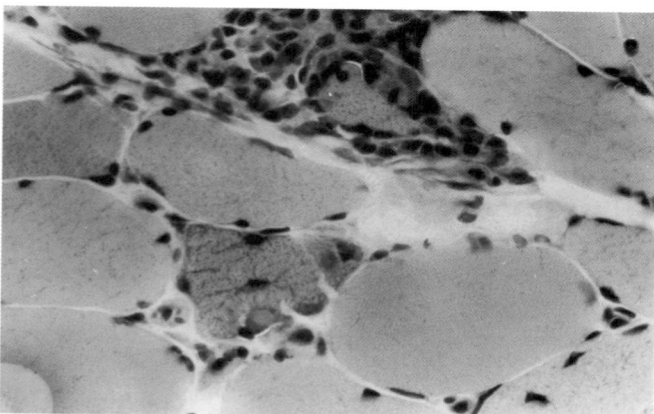

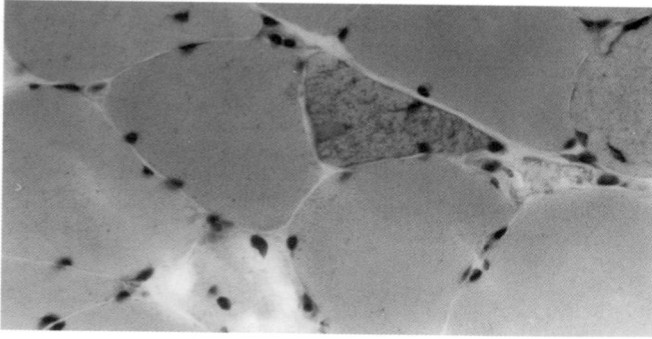

Figure 7.7.2 HIV myopathy in an AZT-naive patient. Degenerating basophilic myofibers with cytoplasmic bodies, (a) with and (b) without accompanying endomyseal inflammation. Hematoxylin and eosin stain; original magnification, 100 ×.

structural and inflammatory pathology. The pathogenesis of these entities was unknown, but was clearly unrelated to AZT. Attempts to identify virus within myofibers by immunohistochemistry, electron microscopy, and in situ hybridization were largely negative until 1994, when a study utilizing the technique of in situ reverse transcriptase polymerase chain reaction (RT-PCR) demonstrated HIV within endomyseal macrophages and myocyte nuclei (Seidman et al., 1994). While these results have not been replicated, they raise the possibility that myopathology in AZT-naive, HIV-positive individuals may be due in part to direct infection of myocytes.

Histological studies have advanced other theories of pathogenesis for HIV-associated myopathy. Several authors have suggested autoimmune mechanisms because of the inflammatory nature of some biopsies. The presence of CD8-positive lymphocytes together with diffuse expression of major histocompatibility complex (MHC) class I antigens on myofibers has led to speculation that HIV-myopathy is a T-cell-mediated and MHC class I-restricted cytotoxic process, similar to polymyositis in the absence of HIV infection (Dalakas et al., 1986a; Illa et al., 1991). Tubuloreticular inclusions have been identified by electron microscopy in capillary endothelia of HIV-positive myopathic patients (Lane et al., 1993). These inclusions are thought to be typical of autoimmune phenomena and, although not restricted to such processes, have been cited as evidence of primary immunological mechanisms in HIV-associated muscle disease. Recently, increased myocyte expression of toll-like receptor 3 has been described in HIV-associated myopathies, leading to speculation that this signaling pathway may be important in inflammatory cell recruitment to muscle in response to a viral stimulus (Schreiner et al., 2006).

Rarely, HIV-polymyositis has been reported to be part of a systemic CD8 lymphocytosis associated with a Sjögren-like syndrome, referred to as diffuse infiltrative lymphocytosis syndrome (Attarian et al., 2004). More recently, HIV-associated polymyositis has been noted during immune restoration with combination antiretroviral therapy (Sellier et al., 2000; Calza et al., 2004). In the patient described by Sellier and colleagues, myositis occurred in the context of a rapid increase in CD4+ T cell count and restored T-cell proliferative response to HIV-1 antigen. Clinical response to corticosteroids was evident, implicating an autoimmune etiology.

THE ROLE OF ANTIRETROVIRAL THERAPY

AZT

In 1987, AZT became widely used in HIV infection, following the results of several large clinical trials demonstrating clinical efficacy (Yarchoan et al., 1987; Volberding et al., 1990). Bessen et al. (1988) first reported a polymyositis-like syndrome in four AZT-treated patients, three of whom improved following AZT withdrawal (one with concomitant corticosteroid therapy). Several case reports confirmed this

material were identified (Simpson & Bender, 1988; Gonzales et al., 1988). Mononuclear cell inflammation was inconstant, ranging from severe to absent (Fig. 7.7.2). HIV could not be detected in these biopsies by either immunohistochemistry or in situ hybridization. Thus, by the late 1980s it became clear that symptomatic HIV-positive patients could display either HIV-related polymyositis, or a structural myopathy distinct from myositis, or possibly a disorder characterized by both observation, describing necrotizing myopathy in patients receiving high doses of AZT that improved with cessation of the drug (Helbert et al., 1988; Gorard et al., 1988; Gertner et al., 1989). Thus, it emerged that in some individuals, chronic, high-dose AZT could result in clinically significant muscle disease. However, one must bear in mind that this observation was made in an era when dosing schedules for AZT were much higher than current standards of administration. We are currently unaware of reports of AZT-induced myopathy with smaller dosing regimens typical of HAART-era therapeutics; while this does not preclude AZT-associated myotoxicity at a smaller dose range, it does raise a question about its clinical relevance in the HAART era.

There are no clinical features that differentiate myopathies due to HIV from those due to AZT (Simpson et al., 1993a; Gherardi, 1994; Manji et al., 1993). While some patients with HIV myopathy may improve with AZT withdrawal (Dalakas et al., 1990; Lane et al., 1993; Bessen et al., 1988; Gorard et al., 1988; Masahes et al., 1998), others do not (Simpson et al., 1993a; Gherardi, 1994; Manji et al., 1993; Espinoza et al., 1991; Till & MacDonnell, 1990). Some authors suggest that AZT may cause a myopathy only when underlying HIV-related polymyositis is present (Lane et al., 1993), thus exacerbating a pre-existing inflammatory myopathy (Berger et al., 1991; Walsh et al., 2002). When myopathic patients are rechallenged with AZT, some have not had recurrence of their myopathic symptoms (Helbert et al., 1988; Panegyres et al., 1988; Fischl et al., 1989). Cupler et al. (1994) reported that in patients with myopathy, AZT may be continued for at least 6 months without clinical or histological deterioration.

Epidemiological data to indicate the incidence of myopathy associated with high dose AZT therapy are sparse. None of the large antiretroviral therapy studies were originally designed to prospectively establish the diagnosis of myopathy. Our retrospective analysis of a large primary antiretroviral protocol (ACTG 016, discussed above), showed that the incidence of myopathy was 0.4% in the AZT-treated group (Simpson et al., 1997). In a prospective series of 118 patients, the incidence of myopathy in the AZT-treated group was 8% (7 of 88), although the small size of the control group and brief time of follow-up limited the significance of these data (Peters et al., 1993). We prospectively assessed the frequency of clinical and laboratory markers of myopathy in ACTG Protocol 175 (Simpson et al., 1998), a 2,467-patient study in which HIV-infected subjects were randomized to one of four antiretroviral treatment arms (AZT or ddI monotherapy, AZT/ddI, or AZT/ddC). There was no difference between treatment arms in the rate of myalgia or muscle weakness. The median CPK of subjects on AZT/ddC was significantly higher than that of those on other study treatments, although CPK levels did not correlate with symptoms of myopathy. Only six patients were diagnosed with myopathy during the study (AZT: 0; AZT/ddC: 1; AZT/ddI: 1; ddI:4).

Dalakas and colleagues (1990) described the histopathology of AZT-induced myopathy. Ragged red fibers (RRF) were present in all biopsies from AZT-treated patients, and the percentage of these RRF appeared to correlate with the severity

of clinical myopathy. Histological features of inflammatory myopathy, with varying degrees of inflammation, necrotic fibers, rod bodies, and cytoplasmic bodies were also present (Fig. 7.7.3). Electron microscopy confirmed mitochondrial abnormalities, with proliferation, enlargement, and paracrystalline inclusions (Fig. 7.7.4). Biopsies obtained from an AZT-naive control group contained no mitochondrial abnormalities (Dalakas et al., 1990). These authors published a more extensive pathological characterization of this myopathy in 1991, and these electron microscopic findings in 12 AZT-exposed patients were again described (Pezeshkpour et al., 1991). They concluded that AZT-treated patients displayed increased numbers of mitochondria with abnormal shape, size, and structure. They proposed the concept of an AZT-induced mitochondrial myopathy, due to inhibition of gamma polymerase and characterized by cytoplasmic bodies and mitochondrial abnormalities. To support this, investigators provided evidence of both in vitro mitochondrial abnormalities of human and animal muscle cells exposed to AZT (Lamperth et al., 1991) and in vivo impairment of muscle energy metabolism in AZT-treated patients (Sinnwell et al., 1995). Dalakas and co-workers (1994) reported depletion of carnitine and mitochondrial DNA (mtDNA) in muscle fibers of AZT-treated patients (Pezeshkpour et al., 1991; Arnaudo et al., 1991). Other groups described defects of mitochondrial enzymes, such as cytochrome c oxidase and reductase (Mhiri et al., 1991; Chariot et al., 1993), accumulation of cytokines in muscle fiber mitochondria (Gherardi et al., 1994), and mitochondrial oxidative dysfunction based on data obtained from ^{31}P magnetic resonance spectroscopy (MRS; Sinnwell et al., 1995; Weissman et al., 1992).

However, subsequent work suggested that the observed mitochondrial abnormalities were nonspecific. Chariot and colleagues (1996) reported cytochrome c oxidase deficiencies in the muscle of patients with HIV seronegative inflammatory myopathies. Cote et al. (2002) reported mitochondrial depletion in peripheral blood cells in HIV-infected subjects naïve to antiretroviral drugs. Our group reported 50 patients with

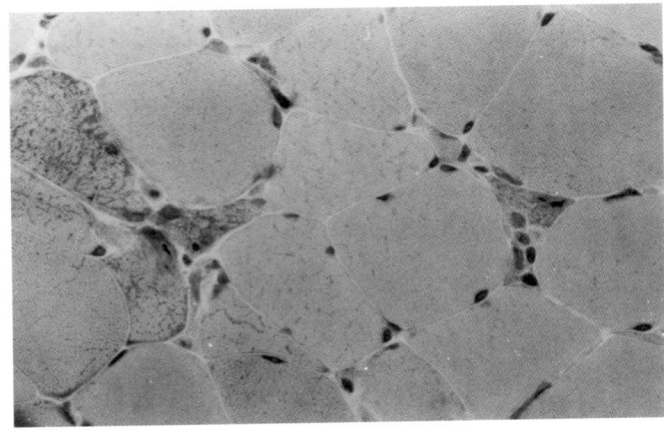

Figure 7.7.3 HIV myopathy in an AZT-treated patient. Degenerating myofibers with cytoplasmic bodies in the absence of inflammation. Modified trichrome stain; original magnification, 100 ×.

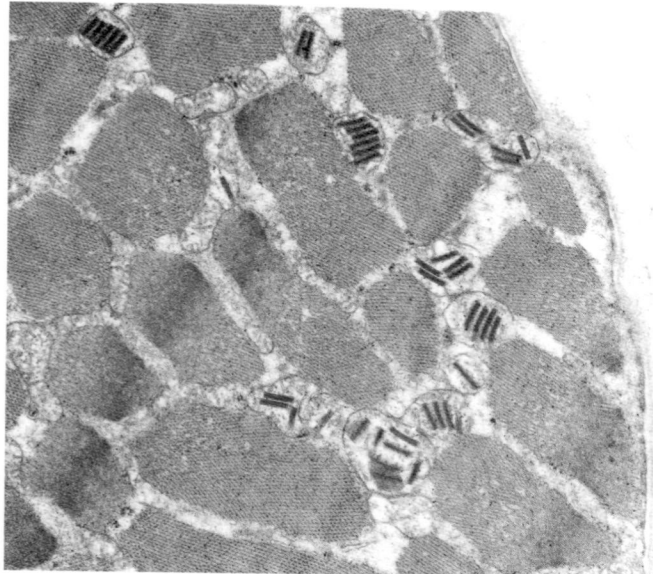

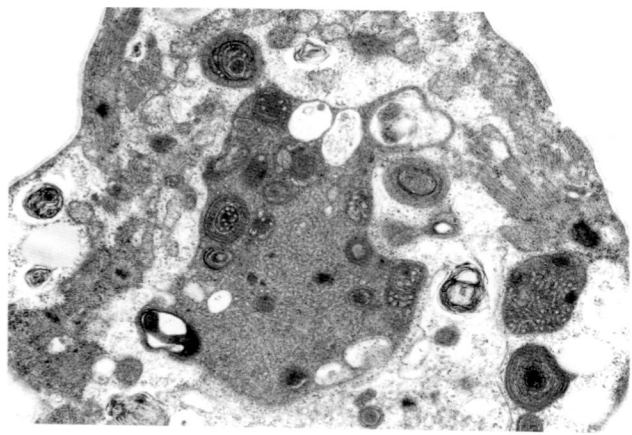

Figure 7.7.4 Electron micrographs of muscle biopsies from two patients with history of AZT exposure. (a) Paracrystalline intramitochondrial inclusions in a patient with a cumulative AZT dosage of 888 g and drug exposure at the time of biopsy. Original magnification, 5500 ×. (b) Abnormal mitochondria in a degenerating myofiber in a patient with cumulative dosage of 360 g and delay of 4.5 months between last AZT exposure and biopsy. Original magnification, 7500 ×.

argued that the degenerating myofibers seen in AZT-exposed patients exhibited a morphology distinct from the RRF originally described in mitochondrial myopathies by Olson et al. (1972). The AZT-exposed myofibers displayed extensive myofibrillar abnormalities, whereas, the RRF had aggregates of mitochondria with an intact myofibrillar apparatus. Furthermore, the percentage of RRF did not differ in symptomatic and asymptomatic AZT-treated patients.

Several studies showed atypical mitochondrial abnormalities or abnormalities outside of the mitochondria. Gherardi et al. (1994) demonstrated mitochondrial interleukin (IL)-1 expression, which led to the hypothesis that the myofibrillar disarray is cytokine mediated. Tubuloreticular inclusions, suggestive of autoimmune phenomena, were also demonstrated in symptomatic AZT-exposed patients (Lane et al., 1993). Schroder et al. (1992) reported a patient who developed necrotizing myopathy while on AZT, and displayed profound alterations in nuclear structure. These authors speculated that AZT might have effects on the myofiber nucleus to inhibit DNA synthesis, repair, and RNA transcription (Schroder et al., 1992). In yet another study of patients with AZT-related myopathy, segmental deficits in both mitochondrial and nuclear-encoded subunits of cytochrome c oxidase were seen in muscle biopsies, supporting drug effects at both the nuclear and cytoplasmic level (Yerroum et al., 2000).

Thus, the etiology of AZT-induced myopathy is currently unclear, with hypotheses including: mtDNA depletion, AZT-induced oxidative stress, direct inhibition of mitochondrial bioenergetic machinery, depletion of L-carnitine, and myofiber apoptosis (Scruggs & Naylor, 2008).

HIV-ASSOCIATED NEUROMUSCULAR WEAKNESS SYNDROME

In 2002, a rapidly ascending neuromuscular weakness syndrome, accompanied by lactic acidosis, was reported by the U. S. Food and Drug Administration (FDA) and Bristol Myers Squibb in over 30 HIV-infected patients (Marcus et al., 2002; Rey et al., 1999; Falco et al., 2002; Miller et al., 2000; Mokrzycki et al., 2000; Bristol Myers Squibb, data on file). We gathered additional cases of HIV-associated neuromuscular weakness syndrome (HANWS), totaling 69, and performed a retrospective analysis of clinical, laboratory, and metabolic features of this disorder (Simpson et al., 2003). Additional cases have since been reported (Vidal et al., 2007). Neurological manifestations ranged from a rapidly progressive sensorimotor neuropathy with areflexia, to subacutely progressive myopathy, with elevated CPK. Some cases progressed to respiratory failure and death. The cases were divided into possible, probable, and definite HANWS, depending on the ability to exclude confounding causes of weakness, and the availability of electrophysiological or pathological confirmation of neuromuscular pathology. All patients but one were on NRTI antiretroviral therapy at the time of clinical presentation. Forty-seven of 69 cases were taking d4T alone or in combination with another NRTI. In some cases, neuromuscular symptoms persisted with or even

either HIV- or AZT-associated myopathy, with analysis of 26 muscle biopsies. The biopsies from AZT-exposed and AZT-naive patients could not be distinguished by any individual histological finding. Abnormal mitochondria and few RRF were seen in both groups (Simpson et al., 1994). Other authors proposed that mitochondrial abnormalities reflected the degree of myofiber degeneration in HIV-positive individuals, regardless of AZT exposure (Kuncl & George, 1993; Lane et al., 1993; Morgello et al., 1995).

Adding to the controversy were studies that failed to find mitochondrial abnormalities in animal and in vitro models of AZT-induced myopathy. Herzberg and colleagues (1992) did not find abnormalities in cytochrome c oxidase and mitochondrial DNA in human muscle cells exposed to AZT. Reyes and colleagues (1992) did not observe weakness or RRF in hamsters treated with intraperitoneal AZT. Grau et al. (1993)

followed NRTI withdrawal. In cases where lactate levels were available, 81% were elevated. Electrophysiological studies, when available, mainly revealed axonal neuropathy; two patients had myopathic features. Of the 15 muscle biopsies performed, 3 revealed inflammation, and 4 had mitochondrial abnormalities, including mitochondrial DNA depletion and RRFs with decreased cytochrome oxidase staining and abnormalities in tissue oxidative phosphorylation complexes I, III, and IV. Nerve biopsies revealed a mixture of axonal and demyelinating neuropathies. In addition to NRTI withdrawal, patients received a variety of treatments for their neurologic deficits including intravenous immunoglobulin therapy (IVIg), corticosteroids, plasmapharesis, and dietary supplements, such as vitamins B_1 and B_{12}, carnitine, and coenzyme Q. Recovery was variable in the outcomes that were reported. Approximately one-quarter of these patients recovered completely, whereas 16% died. The remainder had persistent neurological deficits.

Until HANWS was described, the potential for adverse effects by nucleoside analogues other than AZT on human muscle cells had only been demonstrated in vitro. In 1997, Benbrik and colleagues compared, in vitro, the toxic effects of ddC, ddI, and AZT on human myocytes. In their study, cultured human muscle cells exposed to ddI, ddC, and AZT individually showed decreased proliferation and differentiation, significant lipid droplet accumulation, and increased lactate production, suggesting functional alterations in mitochondria. Similarly, Semino-Mora and colleagues (1997) observed that exposure of human myotubes in culture to fialuridine (FIAU), an experimental nucleoside analog used to treat patients with hepatitis B, leads to irreversible mitochondrial toxicity with histological changes similar to those caused by AZT. With the identification of HANWS, clinical muscle disease has been linked to antiretrovirals other than AZT. However, interpreting the muscle studies in isolation is inappropriate in these cases, given the degree of associated peripheral nerve and multisystem involvement. As with other forms of HIV-associated myopathy, the role of HIV infection itself and concomitant NRTI administration in disease pathogenesis remains speculative. The presence of lactic acidemia along with lipid accumulation, mitochondrial DNA depletion, and RRF in some muscle biopsies suggests mitochondrial toxicity as a pathogenetic mechanism, supporting in vitro study results. However, the variability in disease presentation and course implicates a multifactorial etiology for HANWS.

CHOLESTEROL-LOWERING AGENT MYOPATHY

Dyslipidemia is associated with the use of HAART (Henry, 1998; Fichtenbaum et al., 2002). Lipid-lowering agents are being utilized with increased frequency to reduce cardiovascular morbidity in HIV-positive patients (Dube et al., 2000; Hsyu et al., 2001). Myopathy in non-HIV patients resulting from the use of HMG-CoA reductase inhibitors (e.g., statins) is well described, although the precise pathogenetic mechanism remains undefined (Farmer, 2003).

Typical features include myalgia, proximal muscle weakness, and elevated serum CPK (Farmer, 2003). Occasionally, these cases progress to rhabdomyolysis (Farmer, 2003). Rhabdomyolysis is distinguished from other forms of myopathy by its rapid time course and higher CPK levels, which may result in complications such as renal failure. HIV-positive patients receiving HAART may be at particular risk for drug-induced rhabdomyolysis because of the potential for interaction between cholesterol-lowering agents and antiretrovirals, in particular protease inhibitors. ACTG Study A5047 (Fichtenbaum et al., 2002), which enrolled seronegative patients, found significant pharmacokinetic interactions between simvastatin or atorvastatin (although to a lesser extent) and the protease inhibitors, ritonavir and saquinavir. Protease inhibitors are thought to inhibit the hepatic metabolism of statin drugs through a common affinity for the cytochrome P450 system, increasing the potential for muscle toxicity by elevating statin concentrations in plasma (Fichtenbaum et al., 2002; Dube et al., 2000). Of the protease inhibitors, ritonavir has the most potent inhibitory effect on the cytochrome p450 in vitro (Von Moltke et al., 1998). Rhabdomyolysis has been reported in HIV patients on a variety of medication combinations, including: simvastatin and nelfinavir (Hsyu et al., 2001; Hare et al., 2002); simvastatin, indinavir, and ritonavir (Martin et al., 2000); atorvastatin and indinavir (Martin et al., 2000); atorvastatin and nelfinavir (Hsyu et al., 2001); simvastatin and a non-protease-inhibitor containing HAART regimen (delavirdine, lamivudine, d4T; Aboulafia & Johnston, 2000); clarithromycin, atorvastatin, and lopinavir/ritonavir (Mah Ming & Gill, 2003); abacavir and ciprofibrate (Fontaine et al., 2005); pravastatin, atazanavir, ritonavir, emtricitabine, and tenofovir (Mikhail et al., 2009); and simvastatin, amiodarone, and atazanavir (Schmidt et al., 2007). Weighing the potential side effects of combining protease inhibitors with statins and the cardiovascular morbidity of chronic hyperlipidemia has been identified as a significant dilemma in the care of HIV patients. Based on the available pharmacological and clinical data, the Adult AIDS Clinical Trial Group Cardiovascular Disease Focus Group recommends using either pravastatin or atorvastatin, along with regular monitoring of serum CPK level and viral load, when treating dyslipidemia in the setting of antiretroviral therapy (Dube et al., 2000). The use of other lipid-lowering agents, such as fibrates and niacin, in combination with protease inhibitors, has not been yet examined as closely as the statin drugs.

THE ROLE OF MUSCLE IN HIV-ASSOCIATED METABOLIC DISTURBANCES: WASTING AND THE LIPODYSTROPHY SYNDROME

HIV-associated wasting (HAW) is characterized by a reduction in lean body mass and has been defined as an involuntary weight loss of >10% (CDC, 1992). Additional clinical features include fever and chronic diarrhea. HAW is associated with increased morbidity and mortality and poorer functional status, and is considered an AIDS-defining illness (Wheeler et al., 1998; Grinspoon et al., 1999; CDC, 1992). Neurologic examination may reveal diffuse wasting and weakness, particularly in the lower extremities. The etiology of HAW is likely multifactorial. Although factors leading to inadequate nutrition, such as anorexia and malabsorption, play an important role, there is also evidence for altered muscle metabolism leading to an imbalance of protein synthesis and degradation (Dudgeon et al., 2006). The mechanisms by which HIV causes this is unclear, although it has been associated with higher viral loads and is partially reversed by HAART (Yarasheski et al., 2005). An indirect effect via abnormalities in cytokine production and endocrine function has been supported by the observation of derangement in these systems in patients with HAW (Roubenoff et al., 2002; Abad et al., 2002; Coodley et al., 1994). Cytokines alter protein metabolism within the muscle via several different mechanisms (Jackman & Kandarian, 2004). Elevated cytokine levels accelerate protein degradation via the ubiquitin-proteasome system. In addition, tumor necrosis factor-α (TNF-α) and interferon-γ (IFN-γ) inhibit muscle repair mechanisms. Hormones, including cortisol, testosterone, growth hormone, and other growth factors, may also play a role (Coodley et al., 1994). Grinspoon and colleagues (2001) reported relatively increased cortisol production in HAW, which may play a role in HAW via its catabolic effects. Testosterone exerts myotrophic effects via multiple mechanisms including protein synthesis (Kadi, 2008) and its deficiency has been associated with loss of muscle mass in HIV (Grinspoon et al., 1996). Perturbations in the growth hormone/insulin-like growth factor-I (GH/IGF-1) axis have also been associated with loss of muscle mass in HIV (Grinspoon et al., 1996), consistent with the known stimulatory effects of IGF-1 on protein metabolism and replication and differentiation of muscle precursor cells (Crown et al., 2000). Nutritional supplements, exercise regimens, hormonal therapies and cytokine modulation have been studied for the treatment of HAW. Nutritional strategies include increased caloric intake, amino acid supplementation with L-glutamine and L-arginine, antioxidants, and beta-hydroxy-beta-methylbutyrate, which is thought to limit proteolysis (Stack et al., 1996; Clark et al., 2000). Exercise therapy has focused on resistance training (Shevitz et al., 2005). Hormonal therapies include growth hormone, testosterone, and the testosterone analogue, nandrolone decanoate (Gelato et al., 2007; Kong & Edmonds, 2002; Gold et al., 2006). Cytokine-modulating treatments are aimed at suppressing TNF-α, and include thalidomide, pentoxifylline, and ketotifen (Kaplan et al., 2000; Combaret et al., 1999; Ockenga et al., 1996). Although treatment with HAART is typically indicated in patients with AIDS-defining illnesses including HAW, it probably does not increase lean body mass (McDermott et al., 2001).

The lipodystrophy syndrome is characterized by redistribution of fat from the limbs to the trunk and viscera, hyperlipidemia, and insulin resistance (Carr et al., 1998). ARVs, especially protease inhibitors, have been implicated in the pathogenesis of lipodystrophy (Mann et al., 1999). ARVs have multiple potential deleterious effects in adipose tissue.

ARVs may alter adipocyte gene expression leading to derangement in lipid metabolism within the adipocyte and secretion of proinflammatory cytokines (e.g., TNF-α and interleukin-6) which affect systemic glucose and lipid metabolism (Pacenti et al., 2006; Lihn et al., 2003). ARVs may also lead to mitochondrial toxicity in adipose tissue, causing compromise of metabolic pathways and increased cellular apoptosis (Buffet et al., 2005). Cellular apoptosis releases lipids into circulation and leads to reduced capacity for future peripheral lipid storage.

Recent data have supported an important role for skeletal muscle in the lipodystrophy syndrome. Several studies have shown increased intramyocellular lipid in HIV-positive patients with lipodystrophy (Luzi et al., 2003; Torriani et al., 2006; Gan et al., 2002). It is posited that lipid spill from injured peripheral adipocytes leads to increased lipid availability and subsequent storage within myocytes. The intramyocellular lipid may alter glucose entry and metabolism in the myocyte, contributing to insulin resistance. Other authors have suggested that alteration of glucose transport into the myocyte may be the cause rather than the effect of lipodystrophy (Stanley et al., 2009). ARVs may decrease the activity of glucose transporter 4 in the myocyte cell membrane, leading to decreased glucose uptake, insulin resistance, and hyperinsulinemia, which have been linked to obesity (Sathekge et al., 2010).

Treatment of lipodystrophy begins with alteration of the ARV regimen when possible (Stanley et al., 2009). Other therapeutics under study include leptin, diabetic medications (glitazones, metformin), growth hormone, statins, and uridine (Lee et al., 2006; Slama et al., 2008; Saint-Marc & Touraine, 1999; Luzi et al., 2005; Mallon et al., 2006; Sutinen et al., 2007).

THERAPY OF HIV-ASSOCIATED MYOPATHY

Corticosteroids are the mainstay of treatment in cases of non-HIV polymyositis. Numerous investigators have found corticosteroids to be effective in uncontrolled series of patients with HIV-associated myopathy (Dalakas et al., 1990; Mhiri et al., 1991; Manji et al., 1993; Chalmers et al., 1991; Johnson et al., 2003). Data from our randomized, placebo-controlled study of prednisone in HIV-associated myopathy support these observations (Simpson et al., 1993b). Corticosteroids are also beneficial in cases of wasting syndrome associated with myopathy (Simpson et al., 1990). Clinical trials indicate that the use of anabolic steroids such as oxandralone leads to improvement in muscle bulk and body weight in patients with AIDS wasting and myopathy (Berger et al., 1996). Although corticosteroids should be used cautiously in HIV-infected patients because of the risk of further immunosuppression, there is evidence that they provide benefit, with tolerable adverse effects regarding other HIV-associated diseases such as pneumocystis pneumonia (National Institutes of Health–University of California Expert Panel for Corticosteroids as Adjunctive Therapy for Pneumocystis Pneumonia, 1990).

Furthermore, in addition to other common side effects, such as hyperglycemia, gastrointestinal ulcers, and osteoporosis, one must remain aware that chronic steroid use may cause a distinct myopathy (Dalakas et al., 1987). Other treatments that have been used in non-HIV-associated myopathy, such as IVIg, plasma exchange, and chemotherapeutic agents, have not been studied in the HIV population specifically. Viard and colleagues (1992) report marked improvement with IVIg treatment in a patient with HIV-associated polymyositis that had been refractory to corticosteroids, plasma exchange, and chemotherapy; whereas, Johnson and colleagues (2003) report the treatment of three patients refractory to corticosteroids with IVIg, of whom two did not tolerate IVIg and one had no benefit.

Since it may be difficult to prospectively identify patients with NRTI myotoxicity, the initial management of patients with significant limb weakness and objective evidence of myopathy includes NRTI withdrawal when possible. The percentage of AZT-treated patients who show objective improvement in muscle strength following AZT withdrawal has varied from 18% to 100% in different series (Dalakas et al., 1990; Manji et al., 1993; Grau et al., 1993; Bessen et al., 1988; Chalmers et al., 1991). In our retrospective series, 4 of 15 (26%) patients with myopathy improved in strength after AZT was discontinued, suggesting that HIV itself or a related secondary mechanism is the major cause of myopathy. In the setting of HANWS, NRTI withdrawal showed similar variability with respect to clinical improvement. Additionally, given that mitochondrial toxicity may be contributing to the development of myopathy, dietary supplements such as riboflavin, vitamin C, antioxidants such as coenzyme Q10, and carnitine formulations may hasten recovery (Rosenfeldt et al., 2005). However, experience in using these compounds comes from cases of inherited mitochondrial myopathies and their efficacy is unproven in the setting of HIV myopathy.

OTHER MYOPATHIES IN THE SETTING OF HIV DISEASE

RHABDOMYOLYSIS

As described above, numerous HIV-positive patients with drug-induced rhabdomyolysis have been reported in the literature. These cases typically result from concommitant treatment with cholesterol-lowering agents and protease inhibitors, although a case has also been reported in association with raltegravir (Zembower et al., 2008). Additionally, rhabdomyolysis has been reported as an effect of HIV itself, either as part of an acute retroviral syndrome or later in the course of illness, or as a result of opportunistic infection of muscle (Chariot et al., 1994; Delo et al., 2006; McDonagh & Holman, 2003; Prabahar et al., 2008). Common clinical features include those seen in seronegative patients with rhabdomyolysis, such as muscle weakness and tenderness, myalgias, myoglobinuria, and renal impairment. When rhabdomyolysis occurs as part of the acute retroviral syndrome it may be associated with fever, maculopapular rash, and lymphadenopathy

(Delo et al., 2006; McDonagh & Holman, 2003). In addition, Douvoyiannis and Litman (2009) reported a case of rhabdomyolysis during primary HIV infection associated with encephalopathy and multiple organ involvement. Treatment of rhabdomyolysis is supportive with emphasis on adequate hydration, correction of any electrolyte abnormalities, and monitoring of renal function.

NEMALINE ROD MYOPATHY

Nemaline rod myopathy has been described in HIV-positive individuals (Simpson & Bender, 1988; Gherardi, 1994; Gonzales et al., 1988; Dalakas et al., 1987; Feinberg et al., 1998). In the general population, this form of myopathy is inherited as an autosomal dominant or recessive trait, and may manifest clinically in infancy through adulthood. Clinically, nemaline myopathy is characterized by indolent development of painless proximal muscle weakness, of which there is a considerable degree of variability, with or without CPK elevation (Gherardi, 1994; Cabello et al., 1990). EMG displays myopathic features (Simpson & Bender, 1988). Classically, the ultrastructural findings include aggregates of subsarcolemmal spindle-shaped myofibrillary components derived from Z-band thin filaments that occur predominantly in type 1 fibers (Ryan et al., 2003). In addition to the familial forms, nemaline rods occur in other muscle disorders, including polymyositis (Cape et al., 1970) and mitochondrial myopathy (Fukunaga et al., 1980). Unique histopathological and ultrastructural features in HIV-associated nemaline myopathy have been reported, consisting of intrasarcoplasmic changes, including granular degeneration and vacuoles, which were not seen in familial forms of the disorder (Feinberg et al., 1998). Coincidentally, the two patients with HIV-associated nemaline myopathy described by Feinberg's group developed myopathic symptoms prior to the diagnosis of HIV, suggesting that this form of myopathy may herald HIV infection. Still, the pathophysiological relationship of nemaline myopathy and HIV remains uncertain. As with HIV-associated polymyositis, it has been proposed that this unique form of rod body myopathy may be an epiphenomenon of systemic HIV infection, through autoimmune or other poorly defined mechanisms, rather than a distinct form of myopathy (Gherardi, 1994; Miro et al., 1999; Cabello et al., 1990). The treatment for HIV-associated nemaline myopathy has not been established. Some patients have mild symptoms that do not require treatment, or have symptoms that spontaneously regress (Miro et al., 1999). However, anecdotal improvement has been noted through administration of corticosteroids, IVIg, and plasma exchange (Feinberg et al., 1999; deSanctis et al., 2008).

INCLUSION BODY MYOSITIS

Inclusion body myositis (IBM) has also been described in the HIV population (Dalakas, 2002; Cupler et al., 1996; Freitas et al., 2008). In patients not infected with HIV, IBM is a sporadic inflammatory myopathy that typically occurs after the age of 50. In contrast to the other inflammatory myopathies,

IBM is characterized by early involvement of more distal musculature, most commonly in thigh extensors and forearm flexors (Tawil & Griggs, 2002). Serum CPK may be normal or elevated and EMG typically reveals a myopathic pattern (Tawil & Griggs, 2002). The diagnosis depends on characteristic findings on muscle biopsy, which include endomyseal inflammation (predominantly cytotoxic T-cells) and invasion of non-necrotic fibers, rimmed vacuoles, and intracellular amyloid deposits or 15–18 nm tubulofilamentous inclusions on electron microscroscopy (Tawil & Griggs, 2002). The pathophysiology of IBM remains unclear. However, it has been postulated that autoimmune mechanisms are involved, given its association with other autoimmune diseases (e.g., systemic lupus erythematosus) and other nonspecific markers of immune activation in serum (Tawil & Griggs, 2002). Cupler and colleagues (1996) reported two cases of biopsy-confirmed IBM occurring in HIV-positive patients. They found no difference between the histopathological and immunocytological features in the HIV-positive patients and those seen in non-HIV cases. HIV was undetectable in affected muscles. These authors proposed that systemic infection with HIV provokes superantigen stimulation of an endomyseal inflammatory response. Dalakas and colleagues (2007) described biopsies from four patients which revealed subsets of viral specific CD8(+) T cells surrounding muscle fibers. They proposed that these cells play an etiologic role in IBM by cross-reacting with antigens on the surface of muscle fibers. Loutfy and colleagues (2003) reported a patient with extensive antiretroviral exposure whose muscle biopsy revealed evidence of both IBM (rimmed vacuoles, intranuclear apple-green birefrigent inclusions with congo red staining) and RRF, suggesting that in some cases IBM may co-exist with antiretroviral-associated myopathology. At present, there is no effective treatment for IBM. Clinical trials using corticosteroids, IVIg, beta-interferon, and oxandrolone have yielded disappointing results.

OPPORTUNISTIC INFECTIONS

Infectious myositis is an increasingly recognized complication in the HIV-infected population (Hossain et al., 2000). The disease is typically characterized by fever, with pain and swelling localized to a single muscle or muscle group, usually of the lower limbs, potentially evolving into more diffuse muscle involvement and systemic toxicity (Al-Tawfiq et al., 2000; Biviji et al., 2002). As with other organ systems, advancing HIV infection and a decreasing CD4 count make skeletal muscle more susceptible to infection by both common and opportunistic pathogens. The pathogenesis of these infections in the HIV-infected patient is not well understood. It has been suggested that the predisposition to such infections is related to leukocyte dysfunction in the form of impaired chemotactic signaling, phagocytosis, and increased superoxide anion production (Widrow et al., 1991). Other coexisting factors that have been proposed to play a role in pathogenesis are overexertion of muscle, active parasitosis, malnutrition, local trauma, concomitant polymyositis, and NRTI-related mitochondrial toxicity (Al-Tawfiq et al., 2000). Initiation of antiretroviral

therapy may also unmask a previously mild or asymptomatic infectious myositis by causing an immune reconstitution inflammatory syndrome. This has been described in the setting of *Mycobacterium avium intracellulare* and *Mycobacterium tuberculosis* infection (Lawn et al., 2004; Chen et al., 2009).

Several bacteria have been isolated in cases of HIV-positive patients with symptomatic infectious myositis. *Staphylococcus aureus* remains the most prevalent pathogen in primary infection of muscle, in both HIV-infected patients and the general population (Gaut et al., 1988; Belec et al., 1991; Victor et al., 1989; Fox et al., 2004; Watts et al., 1987; Casado et al., 2001; Vassilopoulos et al., 1997; Hossain et al., 2000; Bureau & Cardinal, 2001; Medina et al., 1995; Husain & Singh, 2002; Blanche et al., 1998; Whitfeld et al., 1997). Bacillary angiomatosis, associated with *Bartonella henslae*, is well described in the HIV population. Although bacillary angiomatosis more typically involves organs other than muscle, myositis as the initial or most prominent feature of bacillary angiomatosis has occurred in several cases (Husain & Singh, 2002; Blanche et al., 1998; Whitfeld et al., 1997; Al-Tawfiq et al., 2000). Other bacterial pathogens isolated in symptomatic cases include *Salmonella* species (Vassilopoulos et al., 1997; Medina et al., 1995), *Streptococcus* species (Vassilopoulos et al., 1997; Chaterjee & Al-Hihi, 2007; Hull et al., 2008), *Escherichia coli* (Vilades et al., 1994), *Morganella morganii* (Arranz-Caso et al., 1996), *Citrobacter freundii* (Widrow et al., 1991), *Pseudomonas aeruginosa* (Lortholary et al., 1994), and *Mycobacterium avium intracellulare* (Wrzolek et al., 1989, 1990).

Disseminated fungal infections may also involve muscle. Pearl and Sieger (1996) reported a case of biopsy-confirmed *Pneumocystis carinii* in an HIV-positive patient with an intramuscular mass. *Cryptococcus neoformans* has been demonstrated in muscle in autopsy series, but has not been reported to be associated with clinical skeletal muscle disease (Wrzolek et al., 1990; O'Neill et al., 1998). A nodular myositis due to *Histoplasmosis* infection has also been reported (Goel et al., 2007).

Protozoal myositis has been described in several AIDS patients. Gherardi et al. (1992) described five patients with AIDS in whom *Toxoplasma gondii* caused multiorgan disease including an acute painful myopathy. Symptoms included fever, asthenia, and weight loss with muscle weakness, myalgias, and wasting. Laboratory tests revealed positive *Toxoplasma* serology and elevated serum CPK levels. Muscle biopsies demonstrated muscle fiber necrosis, inflammatory infiltrates, and *Toxoplasma* cysts in 0.5–4% of muscle fibers. Microsporidial myositis has also been described in HIV, including *Pleistophora* and *Trachipleistophora hominis* species (Ledford et al., 1985; Chupp et al., 1993; Curry et al., 2005).

Although these infections typically do not play a role in patients with HIV myopathy, it is important to consider them in the differential diagnosis of atypical cases, especially when the CD4 count drops below 200 (Casado et al., 2001; Vassilopoulos et al., 1997). Furthermore, the early stages of muscle infection may be difficult to differentiate from the more common HIV-related polymyositis or NRTI therapy toxicity (Bureau & Cardinal, 2001). Given that there exist specific and effective antibiotic treatments for most of these infections, early recognition is essential in order to avoid progression. Ultrasound, computed tomography (CT) and magnetic resonance imaging (MRI) are useful in helping to characterize the extent of the infectious process and provide direction for needle aspiration and surgical intervention (Bureau & Cardinal, 2001; Al-Tawfiq et al., 2000; Fox et al., 2004).

NEOPLASTIC INFILTRATES

Non-Hodgkin's lymphoma (NHL) is a frequent complication of AIDS, and affects muscle in about 9% of cases (Raphael et al., 1991). Chevalier and colleagues (1993) described two HIV-positive patients in whom muscle involvement was the first manifestation of an immunoblastic NHL. In both cases, the presenting finding was firm, warm, tender swelling adherent to the overlying skin. Immunoblastic lymphoma was identified by open muscle biopsy. Muscle lymphoma may be initially misdiagnosed for infection, myositis, or deep vein thrombosis, particularly when calf muscles are involved. CT or MRI of the lesion may show infiltration of the subcutaneous tissue by lymphoma (Chevalier et al., 1993), while in infectious myositis the process is usually limited to muscle (Heckenstein et al., 1991). In rare cases, Kaposi's sarcoma may develop in the muscles of patients with AIDS (Chevalier et al., 1993). Of note, the histopathological features of Kaposi's sarcoma are similar to those of bacillary angiomatosis, which may also involve muscle (see previous section) (Biviji et al., 2002). Treatment for these neoplasms is variable and beyond the scope of this chapter.

ACKNOWLEDGMENTS

J. R. P. was supported by K23NS066789. S. M. was supported by R24MH59724 and U01MH083501. We extend our gratitude to Lydia Estanislao, graduate of the NeuroAIDS fellowship at the Mount Sinai Medical Center, for her contributions.

REFERENCES

Abad, L. W., Schmitz, H. R., Parker, R., & Roubenoff, R. (2002). Cytokine responses differ by compartment and wasting status in patients with HIV infection and healthy controls. *Cytokine*, 18(5), 286–93.

Aboulafia, D. M. & Johnston, R. (2000). Simvastatin-induced rhabdomyolysis in an HIV-infected patient with coronary artery disease. *AIDS Patient Care STDS*, 14(1), 13–18.

Al-Tawfiq, J. A., Sarosi, G. A., & Cushing, H. E. (2000). Pyomyositis in the acquired immunodeficiency syndrome. *South Med J*, 93(3), 330–4.

Arnaudo, E., Dalakas, M., Shanske, S., et al. (1991). Depletion of muscle mitochondrial DNA in AIDS patients with zidovudine-induced myopathy. *Lancet*, 337, 508–10.

Arranz-Caso, J. A., Cuadrado-Gomez, L. M., Romanik-Cabrera, J., & Garcia-Tena, J. (1996). Pyomyositis caused by *Morganella morganii* in a patient with AIDS. *Clin Infect Dis*, 22(2), 372–3.

Attarian, S., Mallecourt, C., Donnet, A., Pouget, J., & Pellisier, J. F. (2004). Myositis in infiltrative lymphocytosis syndrome: Clinicopathological observations and treatment. *Neuromuscular Disorders*, 14(11), 740–3.

Belec, L., Di Costanzo, B., Georges, A. J., & Gherardi, R. (1991). HIV infection in African patients with tropical pyomyositis. *AIDS*, 5, 234.

Benbrik, E., Chariot, P., Bonavaud, S., et al. (1997). Cellular and mitochondrial toxicity of zidovudine (AZT), didanosine (ddI), and zalcitabine (ddC) on cultured human muscle cells. *J Neurol Sci*, 149, 19–25.

Berger, J. R., Shelbert, R., & Gregorius, J. B. (1991). Exacerbation of HIV-associated myopathy by zidovudine. *AIDS*, 4, 229–30.

Berger, J. R., Pall, L., Hall, C., Simpson, D. M., Berry, P., & Dudley, R. (1996). Oxandralone in AIDS wasting myopathy. *AIDS*, 10, 1657–62.

Berman, A., Espinoza, L. R., Diaz, J. D., et al. (1988). Rheumatic manifestations of human immunodeficiency virus infection. *Am J Med*, 85, 59–64.

Bessen, L. J., Greene, J. B., Louie, E., et al. (1988). Severe polymyositis-like syndrome associated with zidovudine therapy of AIDS and ARC. *New Engl J Med*, 318, 708.

Biviji, A. A., Paiement, G. D., & Steinbach, L. S. (2002). Musculoskeletal manifestations of human immunodeficiency virus infection. *J Am Acad Orthoped Surg*, 10, 312–20.

Blanche, P., Bachmeyer, C., Salmon-Ceron, D., & Sicard, D. (1998). Muscular bacillary angiomatosis in AIDS. *J Infect*, 37(2), 193.

Bohan, A. & Peters, J. B. (1975). Polymyositis and dermatomyositis. Part I. *New Engl J Med*, 292, 344–7.

Buffet, M., Schwarzinger, M., Amellal, B., Gourlain, K., Bui, P., Prevot, M., et al. (2005). Mitochondrial DNA depletion in adipose tissue of HIV-infected patients with peripheral lipoatrophy. *Journal of Clinical Virology*, 33(1), 60–4.

Bureau, N. J. & Cardinal, E. (2001). Imaging of musculoskeletal and spinal infections in AIDS. *Radiol Clin North Am*, 39(2), 343–55.

Buskila, D. & Gladman, D. (1990). Musculoskeletal manifestations of infection with human immunodeficiency virus. *Rev Infect Dis*, 12, 223–35.

Cabello, A., Martinez-Martin, P., Gutierrez-Rivas, E., & Madero, S. (1990). Myopathy with nemaline structures associated with HIV infection. *J Neurol*, 237, 64–5.

Calza, L., Manfredi, R., Colangeli, V., Freo, E., & Chiodo, F. (2004). Polymyositis associated with HIV infection during immune restoration induced by highly active anti-retroviral therapy. *Clinical and Experimental Rheumatology*, 22(5), 651–2.

Cape, C. A., Johnston, W. W., & Pitner, S. E. (1970). Nemaline structure in polymyositis. *Neurology*, 20, 494–502.

Carr, A., Samaras, K., Burton, S., Law, M., Freund, J., Chisholm, D. J., et al. (1998). A syndrome of peripheral lipodystrophy, hyperlipidaemia and insulin resistance in patients receiving HIV protease inhibitors. *AIDS*, 12(7), F51–8.

Casado, E., Olive, A., Holgado, S., Perez-Andres, R., Romeu, J., Lorenzo, J. C., et al. (2001). Musculoskeletal manifestations in patients positive for human immunodeficiency virus: correlation with CD4 count. *J Rheumatol*, 28, 802–4.

Centers for Disease Control and Prevention (1992). 1993 revised classification system for HIV infection and expanded surveillance case definition for AIDS among adolescents and adults. *MMWR Recomm Rep*, 41(RR-17), 1–19.

Chad, D., Smith, T., Blumenfeld, A., Fairchild, P., & DeGirolami, U. (1990). Human immunodeficiency virus (HIV)-associated myopathy: Immunocytochemical identification of an HIV antigen (gp41) in muscle macrophages. *Ann Neurol*, 28, 579–82.

Chalmers, A. C., Greco, C. M., & Miller, R. G. (1991). Prognosis in AZT myopathy. *Neurology*, 41, 1181–4.

Chariot, P., Monnet, I., & Gherardi, R. (1993). Cytochrome c reaction improves histopathological assessment of zidovudine myopathy. *Ann Neurol*, 34, 561–5.

Chariot, P., Ruet, E., Authier, F. J., Levy, Y., & Gherardi, R. (1994). Acute rhabdomyolysis in patients infected by human immunodeficiency virus. *Neurology*, 44, 1692–6.

Chariot, P., Ruet, E., Authier, F. J., Labes, D., Poron, F., & Gherardi, R. (1996). Cytochrome c oxidase deficiencies in the muscle of patients with inflammatory myopathies. *Acta Neuropathol (Berl)*, 91, 530–6.

Chatterjee, S. & Al-Hihi, M. (2007). Pneumococcal pyomyositis in a patient infected with human immunodeficiency virus. *The American Journal of Medicine, 120*, 5–6.

Chen, W. L., Lin, Y. F., Tsai, W. C., & Tsao, Y. T. (2009). Unveiling tuberculous pyomyositis: An emerging role of immune reconstitution inflammatory syndrome. *The American Journal of Emergency Medicine, 27*, 251.

Chevalier, X., Amoura, Z., Viard, I. P, Souissi, B., Sobel, A., & Gherardi, R. (1993). Skeletal muscle lymphoma in patients with the acquired immunodeficiency syndrome: A diagnostic challenge. *Arthritis Rheum, 36*, 426–7.

Chupp, G. L., Alroy, J., Adelman, I. S., Breen, J. C., & Skolnik, P. R. (1993). Myositis due to *Pleistophora* (*Microsporidia*) in a patient with AIDS. *Clin Infect Dis, 16*, 15–21.

Clark, R. H., Feleke, G., Din, M., Yasmin, T., Singh, G., Khan, F. A., et al. (2000). Nutritional treatment for acquired immunodeficiency virus-associated wasting using beta-hydroxy beta-methylbutyrate, glutamine, and arginine: A randomized, double-blind, placebo-controlled study. *JPEN, 24*(3), 133–9.

Combaret, L., Ralliere, C., Taillandier, D., Tanaka, K., & Attaix, D. (1999). Manipulation of the ubiquitin-proteasome pathway in cachexia: Pentoxifylline suppresses the activation of 20S and 26S proteasomes in muscles from tumor-bearing rats. *Molecular Biology Reports, 26*(1–2), 95–101.

Coodley, G. O., Loveless, M. O., Nelson, H. D., & Coodley, M. K. (1994). Endocrine function in the HIV wasting syndrome. *JAIDS, 7*(1), 46–51.

Cote, H. C., Brumme, Z. L., Craib, K. J., et al. (2002). Changes in mitochondrial DNA as a marker of nucleoside toxicity in HIV-infected patients. *New Engl J Med, 346*(11), 811–20.

Crown, A. L., He, X. L., Holly, J. M., Lightman, S. L., & Stewart, C. E. (2000). Characterisation of the IGF system in a primary adult human skeletal muscle cell model, and comparison of the effects of insulin and IGF-I on protein metabolism. *The Journal of Endocrinology, 167*(3), 403–15.

Cupler, E. J., Hench, K., Jay, C. A., et al. (1994). The natural history of zidovudine (AZT)-induced mitochondrial myopathy (ZIMM) [abstract]. *Neurology, 44*, AI32.

Cupler, E. J., Leon-Monzon, M., Miller, J., Semino-Mora, C., Anderson, T. L., & Dalakas, M. C. (1996). Inclusion body myositis in HIV-1 and HTLV-1 infected patients. *Brain, 119*(6), 1887–93.

Curry, A., Beeching, N. J., Gilbert, J. D., Scott, G., Rowland, P. L., & Currie, B. J. (2005). Trachipleistophora hominis infection in the myocardium and skeletal muscle of a patient with AIDS. *The Journal of Infection, 51*(3), e139–44.

Dal Pan, G. J., Glass, J. D., & McArthur, J. C. (1994). Clinicopathologic correlation of HIV-I associated vacuolar myelopathy: An autopsy based case-control study. *Neurology, 44*, 2159–64.

Dalakas, M. (1994). HIV or zidovudine myopathy [letter]? *Neurology, 44*, 360–1.

Dalakas, M. C. (1991). Polymyositis, dermatomyositis and inclusion body myositis. *New Engl J Med, 325*, 1497–8.

Dalakas, M. C. (2002). Understanding the immunopathogenesis of inclusion-body myositis: Present and future prospects [abstract]. *Rev Neurol (Paris), 158*(10, pt. 1), 948–58.

Dalakas, M. C., Pezeshkpour, G. H., Gravell, M., & Sever, J. L. (1986a). Polymyositis associated with AIDS retrovirus. *J Am Med Assoc, 256*, 2381–3.

Dalakas, M. C., London, W. T., Gravell, M., & Sever, J. L. (1986b). Polymyositis in an immunodeficiency disease in monkeys induced by a type D retrovirus. *Neurology, 36*, 569–72.

Dalakas, M. C., Pezeshkpour, G. H., & Flaherty, M. (1987). Progressive nemaline (rod) myopathy associated with HIV infection. *New Engl J Med, 317*, 1602–3.

Dalakas, M. C., Illa, I., Pezeshkpour, G. H., et al. (1990). Mitochondrial myopathy caused by long-term zidovudine therapy. *New Engl J Med, 322*, 1098–105.

Dalakas, M. C., Leon-Monzon, M. E., Bernardini, I., Gahl, W. A., & Jay, C. A. (1994). Zidovudine-induced mitochondrial myopathy is associated with muscle carnitine deficiency and lipid storage. *Ann Neurol, 35*, 482–7.

Dalakas, M. C., Rakocevic, G., Shatunov, A., Goldfarb, L., Raju, R., & Salajegheh, M. (2007). Inclusion body myositis with human immunodeficiency virus infection: Four cases with clonal expansion of viral-specific T cells. *Ann Neurol, 61*(5), 466–75.

Delo, D., Brett, A. S., & Postic, B. (2006). Primary HIV infection presenting with acute rhabdomyolysis. *The American Journal of the Medical Sciences, 332*(1), 46–7.

DeVere, R. & Bradley, W. G. (1975). Polymyositis: Presentation, morbidity and mortality. *Brain, 98*, 637–66.

de Sanctis, J. T., Cumbo-Nacheli, G., Dobbie, D., & Baumgartner, D. (2008). HIV-associated nemaline rod myopathy: Role of intravenous immunoglobulin therapy in two persons with HIV/AIDS. *The AIDS Reader, 18*, 90–4.

Douvoyiannis, M. & Litman, N. (2009). Acute encephalopathy and multiorgan involvement with rhabdomyolysis during primary HIV infection. *International Journal of Infectious Diseases: IJID: Official Publication of the International Society for Infectious Diseases, 13*(5), e299–304.

Dube, M. P., Sprecher, D., Henry, W. K., Aberg, J. A., Torriani, F. J., Hodis, H. N., et al.: Adult AIDS Clinical Trial Group Cardiovascular Disease Focus Group (2000). Preliminary guidelines for the evaluation and management of dyslipidemia in adults infected with human immunodeficiency virus and receiving antiretroviraltherapy: Recommendations of the Adult AIDS Clinical Trial Group Cardiovascular Disease Focus Group. *Clin Infect Dis, 31*(5), 1216–24.

Dudgeon, W. D., Phillips, K. D., Carson, J. A., Brewer, R. B., Durstine, J. L., & Hand, G. A. (2006). Counteracting muscle wasting in HIV-infected individuals. *HIV Medicine, 7*(5), 299–310.

Espinoza, L. R., Aguilar, J. L., Espinoza, C. G., et al. (1991). Characteristics and pathogenesis of myositis in human immunodeficiency virus infection. Distinction from azidothymidine-induced myopathy. *Rheum Dis Clin, 17*, 117–29.

Falco, V., Rodriguez, D., Ribera, E., et al. (2002). Severe nucleoside-associated lactic acidosis in HIV-infected patients: Report of 12 cases and review of the literature. *Cli Infect Dis, 34*, 838–46.

Farmer, J. A. (2003). Statins and myotoxicity. *Curr Atheroscler Rep, 5*(2), 96–100.

Feinberg, D. M., Spiro, A. J., & Weidenheim, K. M. (1998). Distinct light changes in human immunodeficiency virus-associated nemaline myopathy. *Neurology, 50*, 529–31.

Feinberg, D. M., Spiro, A. J., & Weidenheim, K. M. (1999). Response to: Comment on: *Neurology*, 1998, *50* (2), 529–31. Distinct light microscopic changes in HIV-associated nemaline myopathy. *Neurology, 53*(1), 241–2.

Fichtenbaum, C. J., Gerber, J. G., Rosenkranz, S. L., et al. (2002). Pharmacokinetic interactions between protease inhibitors and statins in HIV seronegative volunteers: ACTG Study A5047. *AIDS, 16*, 569–77.

Fischl, M., Gagnon, S., Uttamchandani, R., et al. (1989). Myopathy associated with long-term zidovudine therapy [abstract MBP 329]. Abstracts of the 5th International Conference on AIDS, Montreal, Canada.

Fontaine, C., Guiard-Schmid, J. B., Slama, L., Essid, A., Lukiana, T., Rondeau, E., et al. (2005). Severe rhabdomyolysis during a hypersensitivity reaction to abacavir in a patient treated with ciprofibrate. *AIDS (London, England), 19*(16), 1927–8.

Fox, L. P., Geyer, A. S., & Grossman, M. E. (2004). Pyomyositis: The Columbia Presbyterian Medical Center Experience—A case series. *J Am Acad Dermatol, 50*, 450–4.

Freitas, M. R., Neves, M. A., Nascimento, O. J., de Mello, M. P., Botelho, J. P., & Chimelli, L. (2008). Inclusion body myositis and HIV infection. *Arquivos De Neuro-Psiquiatria, 66*(2B), 428–30.

Fukunaga, H., Osame, M., & Igata, A. (1980). A case of nemaline myopathy with ophthalmoplegia and mitochondrial abnormalities. *J Neurol Sci, 46*, 169–77.

Gabbai, A. A., Schmidt, B., Castelo, A., Oliveira, A. S. B., & Lima, J. G. C. (1990). Muscle biopsy in AIDS and ARC: Analysis of 50 patients. *Muscle Nerve, 13*, 541–4.

Gan, S. K., Samaras, K., Thompson, C. H., Kraegen, E. W., Carr, A., Cooper, D. A., et al. (2002). Altered myocellular and abdominal fat partitioning predict disturbance in insulin action in HIV protease inhibitor-related lipodystrophy. *Diabetes, 51*, 3163–9.

Gaut, P., Wong, P. K., & Meyer, R. D. (1988). Pyomyositis in a patient with the acquired immunodeficiency syndrome. *Arch Intern Med, 148*, 1608–10.

Gelato, M., McNurlan, M., & Freedland, E. (2007). Role of recombinant human growth hormone in HIV-associated wasting and cachexia: Pathophysiology and rationale for treatment. *Clinical Therapeutics, 29*(11), 2269–88.

Gertner, E., Thum, J. R., Williams, D. N., et al. (1989). Zidovudine-associated myopathy. *Am J Med, 6*, 814–18.

Gherardi, R. K. (1994). Skeletal muscle involvement in HIV-infected patients. *Neuropathol Appl Neuropathol, 20*, 232–7.

Gherardi, R., Baudrimont, M., Lionnet, F., et al. (1992). Skeletal muscle toxoplasmosis in patients with acquired immunodeficiency syndrome: A clinical and pathological study. *Ann Neurol, 32*, 535–42.

Gherardi, R., Florea-Strat, A., Fromont, G., Poron, F., Sabourin, J.-C., & Authier, J. (1994). Cytokine expression in the muscle of HIV-infected patients: Evidence for interleukin-alpha accumulation in mitochondria of AZT fibers. *Ann Neurol, 36*, 752–8.

Goel, D., Prayaga, A. K., Rao, N., & Damodaram, P. (2007). Histoplasmosis as a cause of nodular myositis in an AIDS patient diagnosed on fine needle aspiration cytology. A case report. *Acta Cytologica, 51*(1), 89–91.

Gold, J., Batterham, M. J., Rekers, H., Harms, M. K., Geurts, T. B., Helmyr, P. M., et al. (2006). Effects of nandrolone decanoate compared with placebo or testosterone on HIV-associated wasting. *HIV Medicine, 7*(3), 146–55.

Gonzales, M. F., Olney, R. K., So, Y. T., et al. (1988). Subacute structural myopathy associated with human immunodeficiency virus infection. *Arch Neurol, 45*, 585–7.

Gorard, D. A., Henry, K., & Guiloff, R. J. (1988). Necrotizing myopathy and zidovudine. *Lancet, 1*, 1050–1.

Grau, J. M., Masanes, F., Pedro, E., et al. (1993). Human immunodeficiency virus type 1 infection and myopathy: Clinical relevance of zidovudine therapy. *Ann Neurol, 34*, 206–11.

Grinspoon, S., Corcoran, C., Lee, K., Burrows, B., Hubbard, J., Katznelson, L., et al. (1996). Loss of lean body and muscle mass correlates with androgen levels in hypogonadal men with acquired immunodeficiency syndrome and wasting. *The Journal of Clinical Endocrinology and Metabolism, 81*(11), 4051–8.

Grinspoon, S., Corcoran, C., Rosenthal, D., Stanley, T., Parlman, K., Costello, M., et al. (1999). Quantitative assessment of cross-sectional muscle area, functional status, and muscle strength in men with the acquired immunodeficiency syndrome wasting syndrome. *The Journal of Clinical Endocrinology and Metabolism, 84*(1), 201–6.

Grinspoon, S., Corcoran, C., Stanley, T., Rabe, J., & Wilkie, S. (2001). Mechanisms of androgen deficiency in human immunodeficiency virus-infected women with the wasting syndrome. *The Journal of Clinical Endocrinology and Metabolism, 86*(9), 4120–6.

Hare, C. B., Vu, M. P., Grunfeld, C., & Lampiris, H. W. (2002). Simvastatin–nelfinavir interaction implicated in rhabdomyolysis and death. *Clin Infect Dis, 35*, e111–12.

Heckenstein, J. L., Burns, D. K., Murphy, F. K., Jayson, H. T., & Bonte, F. J. (1991). Differential diagnosis of bacterial pyomyositis in AIDS: Evaluation with MR imaging. *Radiology, 179*, 653–8.

Helbert, M., Fletcher, T., Peddle, B., Harris, J. R. W., & Pinching, A. J. (1988). Zidovudine-associated myopathy. *Lancet, 1*, 689–90.

Henry, K. (1998). Lipid abnormalities associated with the use of protease inhibitors: Prevalence, clinical sequelae and treatment [abstract 12319]. 12th World AIDS Conference, Geneva, Switzerland.

Herzberg, N. H., Zorn, I., Zwart, R., Portegies, P., & Bolhuis, P. (1992). Major growth reduction and minor decrease in mitochondrial enzyme activity in cultured human muscle cells after exposure to zidovudine. *Muscle Nerve, 15*, 706–10.

Hossain, A., Reis, E. D., Soundararajan, K., Kerstein, M. D., & Hollier, L. H. (2000). Nontropical pyomyositis: Analysis of eight patients in an urban center. *Am Surg, 66*(11), 1064–6.

Hsyu, P., Shultz-Smith, M. D., Lillibridge, J. H., Lewis, R. H., & Kerr, B. M. (2001). Pharmacokinetic interactions between nelfinavir and 3-hydroxy-3-methylglutaryl coenzyme A reductase inhibitors atorvastatin and simvastatin. *Antimicrob Agents Chemother, 45*(12), 3445–50.

Hull, R., Gay, H., Giles, H., & Nowicki, M. (2008). *Streptococcus agalactiae* myositis in a child with perinatally acquired human immnodeficiency virus. *Southern Medical Journal, 101*(3), 317–9.

Husain, S. & Singh, N. (2002). Pyomyositis associated with bacillary angiomatosis in a patient with HIV infection. *Infection, 30*(1), 50–3.

Illa, I., Nath, A., & Dalakas, M. (1991). Immunocytochemical and virological characteristics of HIV-associated inflammatory myopathies: Similarities with seronegative patients. *Ann Neurol, 29*, 474–481.

Jackman, R. W. & Kandarian, S. C. (2004). The molecular basis of skeletal muscle atrophy. *American Journal of Physiology Cell Physiology, 287*(4), C834–43.

Johnson, R. W., Williams, F. M., Kazi, S., Dimachkie, M. M., & Reveille, J. D. (2003). Human immunodeficiency virus-associated polymyositis: A longitudinal study of outcome. *Arthritis and Rheumatism, 49*, 172–8.

Kadi, F. (2008). Cellular and molecular mechanisms responsible for the action of testosterone on human skeletal muscle. A basis for illegal performance enhancement. *British Journal of Pharmacology, 154*(3), 522–8.

Kakuda, T. N. (2000). Pharmacology of nucleoside and nucleotide reverse transcriptase inhibitor-induced mitochondrial toxicity. *Clin Ther, 22*, 685–708.

Kaplan, G., Thomas, S., Fierer, D. S., Mulligan, K., Haslett, P. A., Fessel, W. J., et al. (2000). Thalidomide for the treatment of AIDS-associated wasting. *AIDS Research and Human Retroviruses, 16*(14), 1345–55.

Kong, A. & Edmonds, P. (2002). Testosterone therapy in HIV wasting syndrome: Systematic review and meta-analysis. *The Lancet Infectious Diseases, 2*(11), 692–9.

Kuncl, R. W. & George, E. B. (1993). Toxic neuropathies and myopathies. *Curr Opin Neurol, 6*, 695–704.

Lamperth, L., Dalakas, M. C., Dagani, F., et al. (1991). Abnormal skeletal and cardiac muscle mitochondria induced by zidovudine (AZT) in human muscle *in vitro* and in an animal model. *Lab Invest, 65*, 742–51.

Lane, R. J. M., McLean, K. A., Moss, J., & Woodrow, D. F. (1993). Myopathy in HIV infection: The role of zidovudine and the significance of tubuloreticular inclusions. *Neuropathol Appl Neurobiol, 19*, 406–13.

Lange, D. J., Britton, C. B., Younger, D. S., et al. (1988). The neuromuscular manifestations of human immunodeficiency virus infections. *Arch Neurol, 45*, 1084–8.

Lawn, S. D., Bicanic, T. A., & Macallan, D. C. (2004). Pyomyositis and cutaneous abscesses due to mycobacterium avium: An immune reconstitution manifestation in a patient with AIDS. *Clinical Infectious Diseases: An Official Publication of the Infectious Diseases Society of America, 38*, 461–3.

Ledford, D. K., Overman, M. D., Gonzalvo, A., Cali A., Mester, S. W., & Lockey, R. F. (1985). Microsporidiosis myositis in a patient with acquired immunodeficiency syndrome. *Ann Intern Med, 102*, 628–630.

Lee, J. H., Chan, J. L., Sourlas, E., Raptopoulos, V., & Mantzoros, C. S. (2006). Recombinant methionyl human leptin therapy in replacement doses improves insulin resistance and metabolic profile in patients with lipoatrophy and metabolic syndrome induced by the highly active antiretroviral therapy. *The Journal of Clinical Endocrinology and Metabolism, 91*(7), 2605–11.

Lihn, A. S., Richelsen, B., Pedersen, S. B., Haugaard, S. B., Rathje, G. S., Madsbad, S., et al. (2003). Increased expression of TNF-alpha, IL-6, and IL-8 in HALS: Implications for reduced adiponectin expression and plasma levels. *American Journal of Physiology. Endocrinology and Metabolism, 285*(5), E1072–80.

Lortholary, O., Jehl, F., Petitjean, O., Cohen, P., Tarral, E., & Guillevin, L. (1994). Polymicrobial pyomyositis and bacteremia in a patient with AIDS. *Clin Infect Dis, 19*(3), 552–3.

Loutfy, M. R., Sheehan, N. L., Goodhew, J. E., & Walmsley, S. L. (2003). Inclusion body myositis: Another possible manifestation of antiretroviral-associated mitochondrial toxicity. *AIDS (London, England), 17*(8), 1266–7.

Luzi, L., Meneghini, E., Oggionni, S., Tambussi, G., Piceni-Sereni, L., & Lazzarin, A. (2005). GH treatment reduces trunkal adiposity in HIV-infected patients with lipodystrophy: A randomized placebo-controlled study. *European Journal of Endocrinology/European Federation of Endocrine Societies, 153*(6), 781–9.

Luzi, L., Perseghin, G., Tambussi, G., et al. (2003). Intramyocellular lipid accumulation and reduced whole body lipid oxidation in HIV lipodystrophy. *Am J Physiol Endocrinol Metab. 284*(2), E274-80.

Mah Ming, J. B. & Gill, M. J. (2003). Drug-induced rhabdomyolysis after concomitant use of clarithromycin, atorvastatin, and lopinavir/ritonavir in a patient with HIV. *AIDS Patient Care and STDs, 17*(5), 207–10.

Mallon, P. W., Miller, J., Kovacic, J. C., Kent-Hughes, J., Norris, R., Samaras, K., et al. (2006). Effect of pravastatin on body composition and markers of cardiovascular disease in HIV-infected men—a randomized, placebo-controlled study. *AIDS, 20*(7), 1003–10.

Manfredi, R., Motta, R., Patrono, D., Calza, L., Chiodo, F., & Boni, P. (2002). A prospective case-control survey of laboratory markers of skeletal muscle damage durring HIV disease and antiretroviral therapy. *AIDS, 16*(14), 1969–71.

Manji, H., Harrison, M. J. G., Round, J. M., et al. (1993). Muscle disease, HIV and zidovudine: The spectrum of muscle disease in HIV-infected individuals treated with zidovudine. *J Neurol, 240*, 479–88.

Mann, M., Piazza-Hepp, T., Koller, E., Struble, K., & Murray, J. (1999). Unusual distributions of body fat in AIDS patients: A review of adverse events reported to the food and drug administration. *AIDS Patient Care and STDs, 13*(5), 287–95.

Marcus, K., Truffa, M., Boxwell, D., & Toerner, J. (2002). Recently identified adverse events secondary to NRTI therapy in HIV-infected individuals: Cases from the FDA's adverse event reporting system (AERS). 9th Conference on Retroviruses and Opportunistic infections, Seattle.

Martin, C. M., Hoffman, V., & Berggren, R. E. (2000). Rhabdomyolysis in a patient receiving simvastain concurrently with highly active antiretroviral therapy [abstract 1297]. 40th Interscience Conference on Antimicrobial Agents and Chemotherapy, Toronto, September 2000.

Masahés, F., Barrientos, A., Cerebrian, M., Pediol, E., Miró, O., Casandemont, J., et al. (1998). Clinical, histological and molecular reversibility of Zidovudine myopathy. *J Neurol Sci, 169*, 226–8.

Mastaglia, F. L. & Ojeda, V. J. (1985). Inflammatory myopathies: Part2. *Ann Neurol, 17*, 317–23.

McDermott, A. Y., Shevitz, A., Knox, T., Roubenoff, R., Kehayias, J., & Gorbach, S. (2001). Effect of highly active antiretroviral therapy on fat, lean, and bone mass in HIV-seropositive men and women. *The American Journal of Clinical Nutrition, 74*(5), 679–86.

McDonagh, C. A. & Holman, R. P. (2003). Primary human immunodeficiency virus type 1 infection in a patient with acute rhabdomyolysis. *Southern Medical Journal, 96*(10), 1027–30.

Medina, F., Fuentes, M., Jara, L. J., Barile, L., Miranda, J. M., & Fraga, A. (1995). Salmonella pyomyositis in patients with the human immunodeficiency virus. *Br J Rheumatol, 34*(6), 568–71.

Mhiri, C., Baudrimont, M., Bonne, G., et al. (1991). Zidovudine myopathy: A distinctive disorder associated with mitochondrial dysfunction. *Ann Neurol, 29*, 606–14.

Mikhail, N., Iskander, E., & Cope, D. (2009). Rhabdomyolysis in an HIV-infected patient on anti-retroviral therapy precipitated by high-dose pravastatin. *Current Drug Safety, 4*(2), 121–2.

Miller, K. D., Cameron, M., Wood, L. V., Dalakas, M. C., & Kovacs, J. A. (2000). Lactic acidosis and hepatic steotosis associated with use of stavudine: Report of four cases. *Ann Intern Med, 133*, 192–6.

Miller, R. G., Carson, P. J., Moussavi, R. S., et al. (1991). Fatigue and myalgia in AIDS patients. *Neurology, 41*, 1603–7.

Miro, O., Grau, J. M., & Pedrol, E. (1999). Comment on: *Neurology*, 1998 Feb;50 (2), 529–31. Distinct light microscopic changes in HIV-associated nemaline myopathy. *Neurology 53*(1), 241–2.

Mokrzycki, M. H., Harris, C., May, H., Laut, J., & Palmisano, J. (2000). Lactic acidosis associated with stavudine administration: A report of 5 cases. *Clin Infect Dis, 30*, 198–200.

Morgello, S., Wolfe, D., Godfrey, E., Feinstein, R., Tagliati, M., & Simpson, D. (1995). Mitochondrial abnormalities in HIV-associated myopathy. *Acta Neuropathol, (Berl.) 90*, 366–74.

National Institutes of Health–University of California Expert Panel for Corticosteroids as Adjunctive Therapy for Pneumocystis Pneumonia (1990). Consensus statement on the use of corticosteroids as adjunctive therapy for pneumocystis pneumonia in the acquired immunodeficiency syndrome. *New Engl J Med, 323*, 1500–4.

Ockenga, J., Rohde, F., Suttmann, U., Herbarth, L., Ballmaier, M., & Schedel, I. (1996). Ketotifen in HIV-infected patients: Effects on body weight and release of TNF-alpha. *European Journal of Clinical Pharmacology, 50*(3), 167–70.

O'Neill, K. M., Ormsby, A. H., & Prayson, R. A. (1998). Cryptococcal myositis: A case report and review of the literature. *Pathology 30*, 316–17.

Olson, W., Engel, W., Walsh, G., & Einengler, R. (1972). Oculocraniosomatic neuromuscular disease with "ragged red" fibers. *Arch Neurol, 26*, 193–211.

Pacenti, M., Barzon, L., Favaretto, F., Fincati, K., Romano, S., Milan, G., et al. (2006). Microarray analysis during adipogenesis identifies new genes altered by antiretroviral drugs. *AIDS, 20*(13), 1691–705.

Panegyres, P. K., Tan, M., Kakulas, B. A., et al. (1988). Necrotising myopathy and zidovudine. *Lancet, 1*, 1050–1.

Pearl, G. S. & Sieger, B. (1996). Granulomatous *Pneumocystis carinii* myositis presenting as an intramuscular mass. *Clin Infect Dis, 22*(3), 577–8.

Peters, B. S., Winer, J., Landon, D. N., et al. (1993). Mitochondrial myopathy associated with chronic zidovudine therapy in AIDS. *Quart J Med, 86*, 5–15.

Pezeshkpour, G. H., Illa, I., & Dalakas, M. C. (1991). Ultrastructural characterics and DNA immunochemistry in HIV and AZT associated myopathies. *Hum Pathol, 22*, 1281–8.

Prabahar, M. R., Jain, M., Chandrasekaran, V., Indhumathi, E., & Soundararajan, P. (2008). Primary HIV infection presenting as nontraumatic rhabdomyolysis with acute renal failure. *Saudi Journal of Kidney Diseases and Transplantation, 19*(4), 636–42.

Raphael, M., Gentilhomme, O., Tulliez, M., Byron, P. A., Diebold, J., and the French Study Group of Pathology for Human Immunodeficiency Virus-Associated Tumors (1991). Histologic features of high grade non-Hodgkin's lymphomas in acquired immunodeficiency syndrome. *Arch Pathol Lab Med, 115*, 15–20.

Rey, P. M., Gouelp, J. P., Pennision-Besniere, I., & Chennebault, J. M. (1999). Severe lactic acidosis induced by nucleoside analogues in an HIV-infected man. *Ann Emerg Med, 34*, 282–4.

Reyes, M. G., Casanova, J., Varricchio, F., et al. (1992). Zidovudine myopathy [letter]. *Neurology 42*, 1252.

Richman, D. D., Fischl, M. A., Grieco, M. H., et al. (1987). The toxicity of azidothymidine (AZT) in the treatment of patients with AIDS and AIDS-related complex. A double-blind, placebo-controlled trial. *New Engl J Med, 317*, 192–7.

Rosenfeldt, F. L., Mijch, A., McCrystal, G., Sweeney, C., Pepe, S., Nicholls, M., et al. (2005). Skeletal myopathy associated with nucleoside reverse transcriptase inhibitor therapy: Potential benefit of coenzyme Q10 therapy. *International Journal of STD & AIDS, 16*(12), 827–9.

Roubenoff, R., Grinspoon, S., Skolnik, P. R., Tchetgen, E., Abad, L., Spiegelman, D., et al. (2002). Role of cytokines and testosterone in regulating lean body mass and resting energy expenditure in HIV-infected men. *American Journal of Physiology Endocrinology and Metabolism, 283*(1), E138–45.

Ryan, M. M., Ilkovski, B., Strickland, C. D., Schnell, C., Sanoudou, D., Midgett, C., et al. (2003). Clinical course correlates poorly with muscle pathology in nemaline myopathy. *Neurology, 60*(4), 665–73.

Saint-Marc, T. & Touraine, J. L. (1999). Effects of metformin on insulin resistance and central adiposity in patients receiving effective protease inhibitor therapy. *AIDS, 13*(8), 1000–2.

Sathekge, M., Maes, A., Kgomo, M., Stolz, A., Ankrah, A., & Van de Wiele, C. (2010). Evaluation of glucose uptake by skeletal muscle tissue and subcutaneous fat in HIV-infected patients with and without lipodystrophy using FDG-PET. *Nuclear Medicine Communications.* Epub ahead of print.

Schmidt, G. A., Hoehns, J. D., Purcell, J. L., Friedman, R. L., & Elhawi, Y. (2007). Severe rhabdomyolysis and acute renal failure secondary to concomitant use of simvastatin, amiodarone, and atazanavir. *JABFM, 20*(4), 411–6.

Schreiner, B., Voss, J., Wischhusen, J., Dombrowski, Y., Steinle, A., Lochmuller, H., et al. (2006). Expression of toll-like receptors by human muscle cells in vitro and in vivo: TLR3 is highly expressed in inflammatory and HIV myopathies, mediates IL-8 release and up-regulation of NKG2D-ligands. *The FASEB Journal, 20*(1), 118–20.

Schroder, J., Bertram, M., Schnabel, R., & Pfaff, U. (1992). Nuclear and mitochondrial changes of muscle fibers in AIDS after treatment with high doses of zidovudine. *Acta Neuropathol, (Berl.) 85*, 39–47.

Scruggs, E. R. & Naylor, A.J. (2008). Mechanisms of Zidovudine-induced mitochondrial toxicity and myopathy. *Pharmacology, 82*, 83–88.

Seidman, R., Peress, N., & Nuovo, G. (1994). In situ detection of polymerase chain reaction-amplified HIV-I nucleic acids in skeletal muscle in patients with myopathy. *Mod. Pathol. 7*, 369–75.

Sellier, P., Monsuez, J. J., Evans, J., et al. (2000). Human immunodeficiency virus-associated polymyositis during immune restoration with combination antiretroviral therapy. *Am J Med, 109*, 510–12.

Semino-Mora, C., Leon-Monzon, M., & Dalakas, M.C. (1997). Mitochondrial and cellular toxicity induced by fialuridine in human muscle *in vitro*. *Lab Invest, 76*, 487–95.

Shevitz, A.H., Wilson, I.B., McDermott, A.Y., et al. (2005). A comparison of the clinical and cost-effectiveness of 3 intervention strategies for AIDS wasting. *JAIDS, 38*(4), 399–406.

Simpson, D. M. & Bender, A. N. (1988). Human immunodeficiency virus-associated myopathy: analysis of 11 patients. *Ann Neurol 24*, 79–84.

Simpson, D. M. & Tagliati, M. (1994). Neurological manifestations of HIV infection. *Ann Intern Med, 121*, 769–85.

Simpson, D. M. & Wolfe, D. E. (1991). Neuromuscular complications of HIV infection and its treatment. *AIDS, 5*, 917–26.

Simpson, D. M., Bender, A. N., Farraye, J., et al. (1990). Human immunodeficiency virus wasting syndrome may represent a treatable myopathy. *Neurology, 40*, 535–8.

Simpson, D. M., Citak, K. A., Godfrey, E., Godbold, J., & Wolfe, D. (1993a). Myopathies associated with human immunodeficiency virus and zidovudine: Can their effects be distinguished? *Neurology, 43*, 971–6.

Simpson, D. M., Godbold, J., Hassett, J., et al. (1993b). HIV associated myopathy, and the effects of zidovudine and prednisone: Preliminary results of placebo-controlled trials [abstract]. *Clin Neuropathol, 12* (suppl. 1), S20.

Simpson, D. M., Citak, K. A. Godfrey, E., Godbold, L., & Wolfe, D. (1994). HIV or zidovudine myopathy [letter]? *Neurology, 44*, 362–3.

Simpson, D. M., Slasor, P., Dafni, U., et al. (1997). Analysis of myopathy in a placebo-controlled zidovudine trial. *Muscle Nerve, 20*, 382–5.

Simpson, D. M., Katzenstein, D. A., Hughes, M. D., Hammer, S. M., Williamson, D. L., Jiang, Q., et al. (1998). Neuromuscular function in HIV infection: Analysis of a placebo-controlled combination antiretroviral trial. AIDS Clinical Group 175/801 Study Team. *AIDS, 12*(18), 2425–32.

Simpson, D., Estanislao, L., Marcus, K., Truffa, M., McArthur, J., Lucey, B., et al. (2003). HIV-associated neuromuscular weakness syndrome [abstract]. 10th Conference on Retroviruses and Opportunistic Infections, Boston, Massachusetts, Feb. 12.

Sinnwell, T. M., Sivakumar, K., Soueidan, S., et al. (1995). Metabolic abnormalities in skeletal muscle of patients receiving zidovudine therapy observed by 31P in vivo magnetic resonance spectroscopy. *J Clin Invest, 96*, 126–31.

Slama, L., Lanoy, E., Valantin, M. A., Bastard, J. P., Chermak, A., Boutekatjirt, A., et al. (2008). Effect of pioglitazone on HIV-1-related lipodystrophy: A randomized double-blind placebo-controlled trial (ANRS 113). *Antiviral Therapy, 13*(1), 67–76.

Snider, W. D., Simpson, D. M., Nielsen, S., et al. (1983). Neurological complications of acquired immune deficiency syndrome: Analysis of 50 patients. *Ann Neurol, 14*, 403–18.

Stack, J. A., Bell, S. J., Burke, P. A., & Forse, R.A. (1996). High-energy, high-protein, oral, liquid, nutrition supplementation in patients with HIV infection: Effect on weight status in relation to incidence of secondary infection. *Journal of the American Dietetic Association, 96*(4), 337–41.

Stanley, T. L., Joy, T., Hadigan, C. M., Liebau, J. G., Makimura, H., Chen, C. Y., et al. (2009). Effects of switching from lopinavir/ritonavir to atazanavir/ritonovir on muscle glucose uptake and visceral fat in HIV-infected patients. *AIDS, 23*, 1349–57.

Stern, R., Gold, J., & DiCarlo, E. F. (1987). Myopathy complicating the acquired immunodeficiency syndrome. *Muscle Nerve, 10*, 318–22.

Sutinen, J., Walker, U. A., Sevastianova, K., Klinker, H., Hakkinen, A. M., Ristola, M., et al. (2007). Uridine supplementation for the treatment of antiretroviral therapy-associated lipoatrophy: A randomized, double-blind, placebo-controlled trial. *Antiviral Therapy 12*(1), 97–105.

Tagliati, M., Godbold, J., Hassett, J., Godfrey, E., Grinnell, J., & Simpson, D. (1994). Neuromuscular disorders in HIV infection: Cross-sectional cohort analysis of 250 patients [abstract]. *Neurology 44* (suppl. 2), A367.

Tawil, R. & Griggs, R. C. (2002). Inclusion body myositis. *Curr Opin Rheumatol, 14*(6), 653–7.

Till, M. & MacDonnell, K.B. (1990). Myopathy with human immunodeficiency virus type 1 (HIV-1) infection: HIV-1 or zidovudine. *Ann Intern Med, 113*, 492–4.

Torriani, M., Thomas, B. J., Barlow, R. B., Librizzi, J., Dolan, S., & Grinspoon, S. (2006). Increased intramyocellular lipid accumulation in HIV-infected women with fat redistribution. *J Appl Physiol, 100*(2), 609–14.

Vassilopoulos, D., Chalasani, P., Jurado, R. L., Workowski, K., & Agudelo, C. A. (1997). Musculoskeletal infections in patients with human immunodeficiency virus infection. *Medicine (Baltimore), 76*(4), 284–94.

Viard, J. P., Vittecoq, D., Lacroix, C., & Bach, J. F. (1992). Response of HIV-1-associated polymyositis to intravenous immunoglobulin. *Am J Med, 92*(5), 580–1.

Victor, G., Branley, L., Opal, S. M., & Mayer, K. H. (1989). Pyomyositis in a patient with the acquired immunodeficiency syndrome. *Arch Intern Med, 149*, 705–6.

Vidal, J. E., Clifford, D., Ferreira, C. M., & Oliveira A. C. (2007). HIV-associated neuromuscular weakness syndrome in Brazil: Report of the two first cases. *Arquivos De Neuro-Psiquiatria, 65*, 848–51.

Vilades, C., Garcia-Queralt, R., Rivas, I., Vidal, F., & Richart, C. (1994). Pyomyositis due to *Escherichia coli* in a patient infected by HIV. *Br. J. Rheumatol. 33*, 1728–32.

Volberding, P. A., Lagakos, S. W., Koch, M. A., et al. (1990). Zidovudine in asymptomatic human immunodeficiency virus infection: a controlled trial in persons with fewer than 500 CD4 positive cells per cubic millimeter. *New Engl J Med, 322*, 941–9.

Von Moltke, L. L., Greenblatt, D. J., Grassi, J. M., et al. (1998). Protease inhibitors of human cytochromes p450: High risk associated with ritonavir. *J Clin Pharmacol, 38*, 106–11.

Walsh, K., Kaye, K., Demaershalk, B., et al. (2002). AZT myopathy and HIV-1 polymyositis: One disease or two? *Can J Neurol Sci, 29*, 390–3.

Watts, R. A., Hoffbrand, B. I., Paton, D. F., & Davis, J. C. (1987). Pyomyositis associated with human immunodeficiency virus infection. *Br Med J (Clin Res Ed) 294*, 1524–5.

Weissman, J. D., Constantinitis, I., Hudgins, P., & Wallace, D. C. (1992). 31P magnetic resonance spectroscopy suggests impaired mitochondrial function in AZT-treated HIV-infected patients. *Neurology, 42*, 619–23.

Wheeler, D. A., Gibert, C. L., Launer, C. A., Muurahainen, N., Elion, R. A., Abrams, D. I., et al. (1998). Weight loss as a predictor of survival and disease progression in HIV infection. Terry Beirn community programs for clinical research on AIDS. *Journal of Acquired Immune Deficiency Syndromes and Human Retrovirology: Official Publication of the International Retrovirology Association, 18*(1), 80–5.

Whitfeld, M. J., Kaveh, S., Koehler, J. E., Mead, P., & Berger, T.G. (1997). Bacillary angiomatosis associated with myositis in a patient infected with human immunodeficiency virus. *Clin Infect Dis, 24*(4), 562–4.

Widrow, C. A., Kellie, S. M., Saltzman, B. R., & Mathur-Wagh, U. (1991). Pyomyositis in patients with the human immunodeficiency virus: An unusual form of disseminated bacterial infection. *Am J Med, 91*(2), 129–36.

Wrzolek, M. A., Rao, C., Kozlowski, P. B., & Sher, J. H. (1989). Muscle and nerve involvement in AIDS patients with disseminated *Mycobacterium avium intracellulare* infection [letter]. *Muscle Nerve, 12,* 247–9.

Wrzolek, M. A., Sher, J. H., Kozlowski, P. B., & Rao, C. (1990). Skeletal muscle pathology in AIDS: an autopsy study. *Muscle Nerve, 13,* 508–15.

Yarasheski, K. E., Smith, S. R., & Powderly, W. G. (2005). Reducing plasma HIV RNA improves muscle amino acid metabolism. *American Journal of Physiology Endocrinology and Metabolism, 288,* E278–84.

Yarchoan, R., Berg, G., Brouwers, P., et al. (1987). Response of human immunodeficicncy virus-associated neurological disease to 2'-azido-3'-deoxythymidine. *Lancet, 1,* 132–5.

Yerroum, M., Pham-Dang, C., Authier, F. J., Monnet, I., Gherardi, R., & Chariot, P. (2000). Cytochrome c oxidase deficiency in the msucle of pathients with zidovudine myopathy is segmental and affects both mitochondrial DNA- and nuclear DNA-encoded subunits *Acta Neuropathol, (Berl.) 100,* 82–6.

Zembower, T. R., Gerzenshtein, L., Coleman, K., & Palella, F. J. Jr. (2008). Severe rhabdomyolysis associated with raltegravir use. *AIDS (London, England) 22*(11), 1382–4.

7.8

AGING

Virawudh Soontornniyomkij and Cristian L. Achim

Dramatically improved survival due to highly active anti-retroviral therapy (HAART) and increases in newly diagnosed HIV infection in older adults have led to a growing number of older HIV-1 infected (HIV+) patients. In the United States, it has been estimated that 50% of individuals living with HIV will be 50 years old or older by 2015. Chronic comorbid conditions that are not specifically related to HIV are more common in older HIV+ adults than in their younger counterparts and chronic medication use for these conditions raises the risk of drug-drug interactions with HAART regimens. HIV-associated neurocognitive disorders (HAND) continue to affect the clinical outcome of HIV infection, even in the context of systemic viral suppression. Increasing evidence has suggested that HAND in older adults in the HAART era represent "deficits of multiple etiologies," including brain HIV variants, aging-related cerebro-vascular and neurodegenerative changes, chronic adverse effects of antiretroviral drugs, and other comorbid factors. This chapter surveys the complex interactions of HIV infection and aging as it affects the development of HAND.

INTRODUCTION

HIV+ adults who benefit from HAART have plasma viral loads below detectable levels, maintain immune function without significant opportunistic diseases, and live to old age. The dramatically improved survival due to HAART and increase in newly diagnosed HIV infection in older adults lead to the growing number of older HIV+ patients. In the United States, it has been estimated that 50% of individuals living with HIV will be 50 years and older by 2015 (Luther & Wilkin, 2007). Compared to HIV+ younger adults, older patients usually show better adherence to HAART and achieve systemic viral suppression, but may exhibit a slower immunologic recovery (as measured by CD4 cell count increases) (Luther & Wilkin, 2007). Chronic comorbid conditions unrelated to HIV are more common in older HIV+ adults than their younger counterparts (Tumbarello et al., 2003), which may affect the clinical outcome of HIV infection. A substantial proportion of older HIV+ patients are on chronic medications for comorbid conditions, such as hypertension, chronic airway disease, diabetes mellitus, arthritis, hepatitic C virus (HCV) infection, coronary artery disease, depression, renal disease, visual defects, and lipid disorders (Shah et al., 2002), resulting in increases of the long-term pill burden and risk of drug-drug interactions when they

concurrently receive HAART (Luther & Wilkin, 2007). Data from the Hawaii Aging with HIV Cohort showed that the odds of having HIV-1-associated dementia (HAD) among older adults were 3.26 times those in younger adults after adjusting for differences in education, race, current substance dependence, HAART status, viral load, CD4 cell count, and Beck Depression Inventory score (Valcour et al., 2004b).

In the current era of HAART, HAND continue to impact the clinical outcome of HIV infection, even in the context of systemic viral suppression (Brew et al., 2009; Nath et al., 2008). The incidence of severe cognitive impairment (i.e., HAD) has decreased; still, the overall prevalence of HAND has not declined (Heaton, et al., 2011), possibly because many patients with milder forms of HAND are living longer with persistent impairment (Cysique & Brew, 2009; Valcour et al., 2004c). Asymptomatic neurocognitive impairment affects 21–30% of asymptomatic HIV+ individuals and mild neurocognitive disorder comprises 5–20% of the HIV+ population overall (Woods et al., 2009). Among 1,316 HIV+ subjects who did not have severe comorbid risks for central nervous system (CNS) dysfunction, 33% had asymptomatic neurocognitive impairment, 12% mild neurocognitive disorder, and 2% HAD in a recent report from the CNS HIV Antiretroviral Therapy Effects Research (CHARTER) study of 1,555 HIV+ participants (Heaton et al., 2010). More variability in the clinical course has been observed, that is, cognitive deficits may progress, improve, fluctuate, or remain static over time (Grant, 2008; Nath et al., 2008). HAND in the pre-HAART era occurred primarily in the setting of high plasma viral loads and low CD4 cell counts (< 200/μl); in contrast, in the HAART era it may affect patients with lower plasma viral loads and higher CD4 cell counts (Brew, 2004; Nath et al., 2008). Among 843 CHARTER participants with minimal comorbidities, 30% of HAART-treated patients with undetectable plasma viral load (< 50 copies/ml) and nadir CD4 cell counts above two hundred developed HAND, compared to 47% of combined other minimal-comorbidities subgroups (Heaton et al., 2010). The nadir CD4 cell count and duration of HIV disease may be new risk factors for HAND (Antinori et al., 2007; Heaton et al., 2010; Nath et al., 2008). These findings suggest that successful control of systemic infection may not protect against HAND. This phenomenon may partly be explained by the use of different antiretroviral drug regimens with variable effectiveness on CNS penetration as measured by viral suppression in the cerebrospinal fluid (CSF) (Cysique & Brew, 2009; Letendre et al., 2008). It is largely unknown how well CSF viral loads reflect those in the brain parenchyma. Elevated CSF HIV RNA levels (> 200 copies/ml) were found to predict progression to neuropsychological deterioration in the areas of learning, attention and working memory, and motor function (i.e., deficits characteristic of HAND) after a median follow-up of 1.2 years (Ellis et al., 2002). Overall neuropsychological improvement was shown to correlate with being naïve to antiretroviral treatment, CNS-penetrating HAART regimen, and CSF viral suppression (Cysique & Brew, 2009; Letendre et al., 2004b). Taken together, these studies suggest that HIV burden in the CNS is prerequisite for the development of HAND, although other comorbid conditions are likely involved. Nonetheless, other studies have suggested that high CSF levels of HIV RNA and beta-2 microglobulin no longer predict the presence or severity of HAND in the HAART era, and this subset of affected patients may not respond to further CSF viral suppression, raising the possibility of a fixed or burnt-out form of HIV-associated neural injury (Brew, 2004).

Increasing evidence has suggested that HAND in older adults in the HAART era represents "deficits of multiple etiologies" (Antinori et al., 2007; Cysique & Brew, 2009), including brain HIV variants and viral loads, aging-related cerebrovascular and neurodegenerative changes, chronic adverse effects of antiretroviral agents, and other comorbid factors. The prevalence of HCV co-infection is particularly high among HIV+ intravenous drug users (Martin-Thormeyer & Paul, 2009). HCV seropositivity was shown to independently associate with worse neuropsychological performance after controlling for HIV seropositivity and methamphetamine dependence (Letendre et al., 2005). However, not all clinical studies have reported greater cognitive impairment in HCV/HIV co-infected patients (Martin-Thormeyer & Paul, 2009). Among intravenous drug users, more rapid HIV disease progression, higher prevalence of HAD, and more common postmortem HIV encephalitis have been observed, compared with other risk groups (Martin-Thormeyer & Paul, 2009). Also, methamphetamine dependence was shown to increase the risk of neuropsychological impairment in HIV+ patients (Rippeth et al., 2004). Among middle-aged and older subjects, insulin resistance was found to correlate with neurocognitive impairment (Valcour et al., 2006). Due to individual differences in viral, host, and comorbid factors (Jayadev & Garden, 2009), we can reasonably predict that there will be differential susceptibility among older HIV+ adults to the development and severity of HIV-associated neurocognitive impairment.

In summary, it will be important to: 1) understand the interactions among potential factors contributing to HIV-associated neural injury in old age; 2) identify a subset of HIV+ patients who are more susceptible to the development of HAND; and 3) identify accurate and practical biomarkers for detecting HIV-associated neural injury at stages earlier than the onset of clinical manifestation or poor neuropsychological performance, in order to allow disease-modifying therapeutic interventions, as well as evaluation of the response to treatment.

NEUROPATHOLOGIC CORRELATES OF HAND IN THE HAART ERA

In the pre-HAART era HAND was found to correlate with high levels of HIV burden in CSF (Brew, 2004) and brain parenchyma (i.e., HIV encephalitis) (Cherner et al., 2002; Wiley & Achim, 1994), as well as high levels of microglial activation (Glass et al., 1995) with aberrant cytokine expression (Anderson et al., 2002). HIV encephalitis was more common in injecting drug users than in other HIV risk categories (Bell et al., 1996). However, among HAART-treated patients, HAND can occur even in the setting of undetectable plasma and CSF viral loads (Brew, 2004). By definition, a diagnosis of HAND is made only after excluding pre-existing causes of neurocognitive impairment (e.g., other CNS infections, CNS neoplasms, cerebrovascular disease, pre-existing neurologic diseases, and severe substance abuse compatible with CNS disorder) (Antinori et al., 2007). Furthermore, there are comorbid conditions common in HIV+ patients in the HAART era (e.g., chronic adverse effects of specific antiretroviral agents, HCV infection, substance abuse, and brain aging; Cherner et al., 2005; Effros et al., 2008) that may interact with the effect of HIV in contributing to a compound of neural injury and neurocognitive impairment. In addition to the aging-related cerebrovascular and neurodegenerative changes, their presumptive underlying mechanisms may also take part in the development of HAND, including mitochondrial dysfunction and associated oxidative stress (Yankner et al., 2008), and disturbances in neuroglial regulation of cytokines and neurotrophic factors enhancing the pro-inflammatory response and neurotoxicity over neuroprotective and reparative measures (Valcour et al., 2004c). Therefore, the neuropathologic substrates of HAND in the HAART era may be more variable in association with lower levels of productive HIV replication, different from a classical form of HIV encephalitis.

Due to a substantial increase in life expectancy of HIV+ patients on HAART, the availability of autopsy brain studies is limited and (at least in the United Kingdom) confined to the patients who died of drug overdose or liver failure associated with HCV or hepatitis B virus (HBV) infection (Anthony & Bell, 2008). In our experience (California NeuroAIDS Tissue Network), the majority of the deaths are still associated with end-stage immunocompromise, systemic infection, and respiratory failure. In the HAART era, even with variable success in controlling systemic and CSF viral loads, autopsy brain studies have demonstrated dramatic reductions in the prevalence of HIV encephalitis, cytomegalovirus infection, and toxoplasmosis, but the frequency of malignant lymphoma and progressive multifocal leukoencephalopathy has remained stable (Anthony et al., 2005; Gray et al., 2003). Changes of the neuropathologic patterns in the HAART era reported in the literature appear to reflect a mixture of findings in HIV+ patients with differential success in controlling plasma and CSF viral burden, and with different combinations of comorbid conditions (Anthony et al., 2005; Everall et al., 2005; Everall et al., 2009; Gray et al., 2003; Jellinger et al., 2000; Langford et al., 2003b; Vago et al., 2002). There are only a few available neuropathologic studies that have included significant numbers of HIV+ patients with neuropsychological testing data (Cherner et al., 2002; Moore et al., 2006). Merely a history of receiving HAART does not guarantee success in plasma and CSF viral suppression. As HAND in patients with elevated CSF viral loads are potentially treatable with highly CNS-penetrating HAART regimens (Cysique & Brew, 2009), the focus has shifted on understanding the complex interactions between HIV and a variety of potential comorbid factors contributing to neural injury. To study the neuropathogenesis of HAND in patients who benefit from HAART, we need large prospective cohorts to study clinico-pathological correlates, beyond the levels of productive HIV replication in the brain, that may represent substrates for HAND, to verify antemortem neuroimaging findings, and finally to correlate with changes in CSF biomarkers. In-depth analyses should be attempted to explore potential associations between postmortem brain findings and other relevant parameters, such as HIV genetic variants, host genetic predisposition, antiretroviral regimens, HCV co-infection, and substance abuse. It will be also critical to recruit older HIV-seronegative individuals as controls in prospective cohorts conducting neuropsychological assessment, especially when milder forms of HAND have become more prevalent than HAD in old age.

Brain aging is perhaps the most important comorbid factor in the extended survival of HIV+ patients on HAART. During aging there is a progressive deficiency in the handling and clearance of misfolded proteins such as β-amyloid (Aβ), tau, and α-synuclein. The premature appearance of cerebral Aβ plaque deposition (Figure 7.8.1–A and B) and tau pathology (Figure 7.8.1–C) has been observed in subsets of HIV+ patients (Anthony et al., 2006; Esiri et al., 1998), and both of these lesions showed a tendency to be more common in HAART-treated patients (Anthony et al., 2006; Green et al., 2005) (see below). In addition, neuritic α-synuclein pathology was found in the substantia nigra in 16% of 73 brains of older HIV+ patients (aged 50–76 years, median 55) in the HAART era, but in none of 18 age-matched HIV-seronegative controls (Khanlou et al., 2009). In a magnetic resonance imaging (MRI) study in the HAART era, the severity of periventricular leukoaraiosis and volume of white matter lesions were found to correlate with age and systolic blood pressure, but not with HIV infection-related parameters, suggesting the

co-existence of aging-related cerebral small-vessel ischemic vascular disease (McMurtray et al., 2007).

NEUROINFLAMMATION AND NEURODEGENERATION

Consistent patterns of neural injury seen in the brains of cognitively impaired HIV+ patients include synaptodendritic degeneration, microglial activation, reactive astrocytosis, and in advanced stages, loss of selective neuronal populations. Some of the most vulnerable regions in the CNS include the frontal cortex, striatrum, and hippocampus, as well as the cerebral white matter. The extent of synaptodendritic injury, particularly in the striatum and hippocampus, correlates with the degree of neuropsychological impairment (Ellis et al., 2007; Moore et al., 2006). Postmortem brain studies of the combined effects of HIV and methamphetamine showed selective damage to frontal cortex calbindin-immunoreactive interneurons, particularly in the brains of HIV+ methamphetamine users with evidence of HIV encephalitis (Langford et al., 2003a), which was correlated with memory impairment (Chana et al., 2006).

In the brains of HAART-treated patients without detectable plasma viral loads, Anthony et al. (2005) observed increased microglial activation in the hippocampus and basal ganglia comparable to that seen in HIV encephalitis in the pre-HAART era. These patients did not have cognitive impairment, specific CNS pathology at autopsy, or HIV-1 p24 immunoreactivity in the brain. In this study, the possibility of confounding effects due to HCV infection could not be excluded, as 8 of 10 patients died of HCV-related pathology. However, it implies that in patients on HAART, the increased microglial activation without productive HIV replication may be insufficient to cause cognitive impairment.

In addition to autopsy studies, in vivo examination using proton magnetic resonance spectroscopy (MRS) plays a role in detecting neuronal damage and glial activation. An MRS study of 46 HIV+ patients naïve to antiretroviral therapy showed that glial activation in the frontal white matter was increased with age beyond that observed in HIV-seronegative controls, and neuronal damage in the basal ganglia was increased with age in the HIV+ group (Ernst & Chang, 2004). Another MRS study in HIV+ patients reported that glial

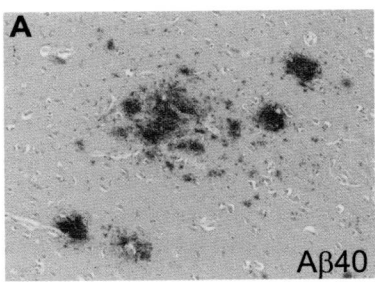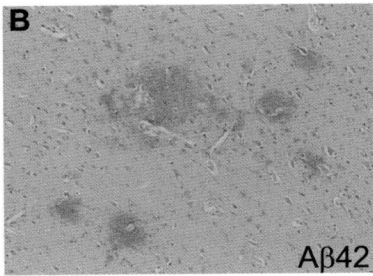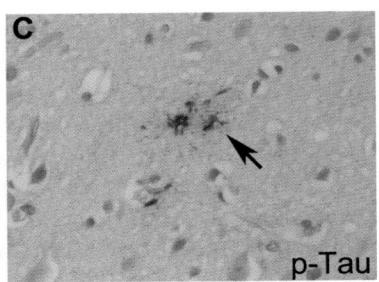

Aβ40

Aβ42

p-Tau

Figure 7.8.1 Diaminobenzidine immunoperoxidase staining on paraffin-embedded tissue sections from the mid-frontal cortex of a 56-year-old HIV+ male patient with mild neurocognitive disorder. Diffuse Aβ40 (A) and Aβ42 (B) parenchymal plaques are shown on the adjacent tissue sections. A neuritic plaque (C) contains dystrophic neurites immunoreactive for phosphorylated Ser202 Tau (p-Tau).

activation occurred during the neuro-asymptomatic stage, and further inflammatory activity and neuronal injury were associated with the development of cognitive impairment (Chang et al., 2004). By using MRS and contrast-enhanced MRI, Avison et al. (2004) found that the degree of blood-brain barrier (BBB) disruption in the basal ganglia correlated with the severity of cognitive impairment and glial cell activation, and that HAART might have a protective effect. One of the adverse effects of nucleoside reverse-transcriptase inhibitors (e.g., didanosine, stavudine, and zalcitabine) involving mitochondrial dysfunction and resultant oxidative stress (Valcour & Shiramizu, 2004) was evidenced on MRS by the presence of neuronal damage in the frontal region of HIV+ patients receiving didanosine and/or stavudine (Schweinsburg et al., 2005).

CEREBRAL Aβ DEPOSITION

Previous autopsy studies showed cerebral Aβ plaque deposition in the neocortex (Achim et al., 2009; Esiri et al., 1998; Green et al., 2005; Izycka-Swieszewska et al., 2000; Rempel & Pulliam, 2005) and hippocampus (Anthony et al., 2006) of HIV+ subjects. When compared to age-matched HIV-seronegative controls, this lesion was found to appear prematurely in some reports (Esiri et al., 1998; Rempel & Pulliam, 2005). In a study using brain specimens in the pre-HAART era, Esiri et al. (1998) found that the proportion of brains with Aβ plaques rose from 18% in the fourth decade to 50% in the seventh decade in the HIV+ group, compared to that in the HIV-seronegative control group from none to 36%. This study also showed that HIV-related pathologies (i.e., HIV encephalitis, HIV p24 immunoreactivity, opportunistic infections, and malignant lymphoma) did not predict the presence of cerebral Aβ plaque deposition (Esiri et al., 1998). Cerebral Aβ plaque deposition appeared more prevalent in HAART-treated patients, as Green et al. (2005) found it in 4% of 99 pre-HAART brains and 13% of 46 HAART brains. However, trivial or no correlative analysis among the Aβ accumulation, apolipoprotein E (ApoE) genotyping, and neurocognitive performance was available in these studies (Anthony et al., 2006; Esiri et al., 1998; Green et al., 2005). Interestingly, Khanlou et al. (2009) studied 36 brains of older HIV+ patients (50 years and older) in the HAART era and found none of them containing Aβ plaques in the neocortex or hippocampus. Aβ deposition in the walls of cerebral blood vessels (Figure 7.8.2) has been observed in subsets of HIV+ brains (Green et al., 2005; Khanlou et al., 2009).

Although comprehensive clinico-pathological correlative studies are not yet available to elucidate the mechanistic significance of cerebral Aβ deposition in the development of HAND, clinical studies applying quantitative assays of CSF proteins and molecular neuroimaging techniques have shed some light on this important issue. In a study by Clifford et al. (2009), in agreement with a report by Brew et al. (2005), Aβ42 levels in CSF (but not CSF Aβ40 levels) were decreased in patients with HAND similar to those in patients with mild dementia of the Alzheimer type (clinical dementia rating score of 0.5), when compared to

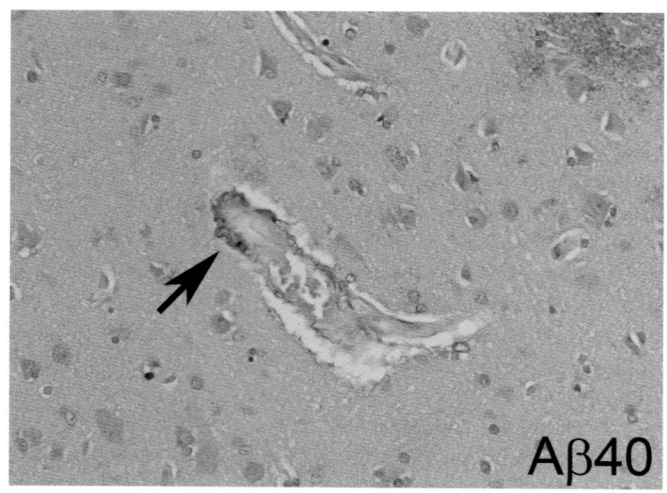

Figure 7.8.2 The wall of an intracortical artery is focally deposited by Aβ40 ("cerebral amyloid angiopathy") in the mid-frontal cortex of a 59-year-old HIV+ male patient with normal cognition, shown on diaminobenzidine immunoperoxidase staining.

the levels in subjects with normal cognition. Reductions in CSF Aβ42 levels were shown earlier to correlate with the presence of cerebral Aβ deposits taking up Pittsburgh Compound B (PiB) measured by positron-emission tomography (PET) in Alzheimer's disease (AD) patients, as well as elderly individuals with normal cognition (Fagan et al., 2006). Accordingly, the findings in CSF studies suggest the presence of cerebral Aβ accumulation in patients affected by HAND. In another report by Gisslen et al. (2009), Aβ42 levels in CSF were decreased in HIV+ patients with opportunistic CNS infections but not in those affected by HAD, as compared to the levels in those without neurological symptoms and signs. The mean age in the HAND group in the study by Clifford et al. (i.e., 48 years) was much higher than that in the HAD or opportunistic-infection group in the study by Gisslen et al. (i.e., 38 years). Moreover, most HIV+ patients in the former study were receiving antiretroviral therapy, while those in the latter study were untreated. Taken together, these studies support the notion that both brain aging and antiretroviral treatment may play a role in cerebral Aβ accumulation. The finding in the study by Brew et al. (2005) of decreased CSF Aβ42 levels in HIV+ subjects with normal cognition, compared to age-matched HIV-seronegative controls, suggests that the lone presence of cerebral Aβ deposition is not necessarily associated with cognitive impairment. Nonetheless, this finding was not confirmed in the study by Clifford et al. (2009), despite no apparent difference in age between the two study groups. In the study by Brew et al. (2005), CSF Aβ42 levels seemed to correlate inversely with the severity of AIDS dementia complex (ADC), and in the moderate ADC group the levels were lower in patients more than 40 years old.

As cerebral Aβ deposition is increasing with age in the brains of older adults in a predictable pattern of regional expansion (Thal et al., 2008), the premature appearance of Aβ plaques in a subset of HIV+ patients suggests that some

HIV-related factors play a role in disturbing cerebral Aβ metabolism in susceptible individuals. Brains of HIV+ patients involved by cerebral Aβ deposition contain Aβ plaques mostly of diffuse type (and rarely of neuritic type) (Esiri et al., 1998; Izycka-Swieszewska et al., 2000; Rempel & Pulliam, 2005), similar to those seen in HIV-seronegative elderly individuals with normal cognition (Thal et al., 2008). These findings suggest that the overall Aβ plaque burden is unlikely to predict neurocognitive impairment. In AD, where neuritic Aβ plaques and tau pathology are the histological hallmarks, increases of soluble Aβ40 in brain tissue (Näslund et al., 2000) and neocortical phosphorylated-tau (p-tau)+ neurofibrillary pathology (Thal et al., 2008) have been shown to correlate with the degree of cognitive impairment. Recent studies implicated soluble Aβ oligomers in amyloid neurotoxicity in AD (Cleary et al., 2005; Walsh et al., 2002). In addition to the extracellular deposition of Aβ, a smaller but significant fraction might accumulate intraneuronally (Gouras et al., 2005; LaFerla et al., 2007). In this context it would be of interest to assess tissue levels of different soluble Aβ isoforms, including intraneuronal Aβ42 oligomers (LaFerla et al., 2007), in brains of HIV+ patients in relation to other histological parameters and premortem data.

Intraneuronal Aβ accumulation has been reported in HIV+ brains (Achim et al., 2009; Green et al., 2005; Khanlou et al., 2009). Green et al. (2005) found cerebral intraneuronal Aβ accumulation in 39% of 99 pre-HAART brains and 54% of 46 HAART brains; no HIV-seronegative controls included in this study. Achim et al. (2009) reported increases of both the prevalence and level of intraneuronal Aβ accumulation associated with lysosomal structures in the mid-frontal cortex in HIV encephalitis brains (72% of 25), compared to HIV+ brains without significant CNS pathology (38% of 18), and the levels in the HIV encephalitis group increased with age. No significant intraneuronal Aβ accumulation was observed in 5 age-matched HIV-seronegative controls in this study. Khanlou et al. (2009) found intraneuronal Aβ accumulation in the neocortex or hippocampus in 35 of 36 brains from older HIV+ patients (50 years and older) in the HAART era, but no results on age-matched HIV-seronegative controls were available. It is of note that all these studies used the anti-Aβ(17–24) antibody (clone 4G8), which might cross-react with amyloid precursor protein (APP) or its other derivatives (LaFerla et al., 2007). Further studies using C-terminal specific antibodies against Aβ(1–40) and Aβ(1–42) are needed to characterize the intraneuronal Aβ accumulation in the brains of HIV+ patients in comparison with age-matched HIV-seronegative controls. In AD brains, it was Aβ42 immunoreactivity that was especially apparent within neurons (Gouras et al., 2005; LaFerla et al., 2007). The pathogenetic significance of intraneuronal Aβ accumulation is emphasized in AD but remains to be determined in HAND.

TAU PATHOLOGY

In an autopsy study by Anthony et al. (2006), the severity of tau pathology in the hippocampal formation was increased in HAART-treated patients without detectable plasma viral loads, when compared to that in the age-matched HIV-seronegative controls. These HAART-treated patients did not have cognitive impairment, HIV encephalitis, HIV p24 immunoreactivity, or opportunistic CNS infections. Although the tau pathology appeared more widespread, extending beyond the entorhinal cortex in the HIV+ groups when compared to that in the age-matched HIV-seronegative controls, only occasionally did it involve the temporal neocortex. The severity of tau pathology showed a tendency to increase with age in HIV+ patients, similar to that seen in the HIV-seronegative controls, but did not appear to correlate with the duration of HIV infection. Pre-HAART HIV+ cases with cognitive impairment did not show elevated levels of hippocampal tau pathology. Taken together, these findings suggest that HAART plays a role in the accelerated progression of tau pathology. Moreover, this accelerated tau pathology that is still confined to the hippocampal formation is not associated with frank cognitive impairment, in agreement with the observation in elderly individuals with intact cognition (Thal et al., 2008). However, more subtle cognitive impairment in hippocampus-related domains might have been detected upon comprehensive neuropsychological testing in this group of HAART-treated patients. The HIV replication in the brain does not appear to correlate with tau pathology. In this study, it is of note that all of nine HAART-treated patients ranged in age from 33 to 46 years, eight of whom died of HCV-related liver disease. Maybe if these patients had survived longer, they would have developed tau pathology extending to involve the neocortex enough to cause cognitive impairment (Thal et al., 2008).

A recent study by Clifford et al. (2009) showed that the elevation of total tau (t-tau) and p-tau181 levels in CSF, characteristic of AD, was absent in HAND patients, in agreement with earlier reports by Ellis et al. (1998) and Green et al. (2000). In contrast, Andersson et al. (1999) found increased CSF tau levels in patients with ADC, as well as those with other neurological complications. Gisslen et al. (2009) reported elevated CSF levels of t-tau but not p-tau181 in HAND patients without antiretroviral treatment. In another report by Brew et al. (2005), no increase in CSF p-tau181 levels was observed in AD patients, and the results on ADC patients appeared inconclusive. Overall, the relationship between HAND and CSF levels of t-tau and p-tau remains controversial. Nonetheless, it is possible that only in patients with severe HAND can elevation of p-tau levels in CSF be confirmed, where the severity of tau pathology in the brains of these patients approaches that found in AD brains. It is also reasonable to anticipate that decreases in CSF Aβ42 levels precede increases in p-tau levels in the natural course of HAND progression in old age, as it has been proposed in the development of AD in the general elderly population (Fagan et al., 2009). However, this temporal course of events may have an exception in opiate abusers, as Ramage et al. (2005) reported that p-tau+ pathology was more prevalent in HIV-seronegative opiate abusers (age < 40 years) than in age-matched non-drug controls and in the former had expanded beyond the entorhinal cortex to involve the subiculum, temporal neocortex, nucleus basalis of Meynert, and the locus ceruleus, without Aβ plaque deposition. Postmortem brain studies are needed to assess the severity of tau pathology in relation to the degree of neurocognitive impairment in the setting of HIV infection.

POTENTIAL MECHANISMS OF NEURAL INJURY IN OLDER HIV+ ADULTS ON HAART

To explore the potential mechanisms of neural injury in older HIV+ adults, it would be important to first consider the current understanding of changes in the aging brain that are relevant to pathologic features seen in HIV+ brains.

BRAIN AGING

A large proportion of elderly people is affected with a variable degree of cognitive decline in specific domains that is not attributable to a defined clinical entity of dementia (Lupien et al., 2005; Yankner et al., 2008). The differential susceptibility to the development of aging-related cognitive impairment may be driven by genetic polymorphisms, epigenetic phenomena, and dissimilar life-long environmental exposure to stressors (Goosens & Sapolsky, 2007). Mechanisms of brain aging have been proposed to involve cerebrovascular regulation, neuronal calcium homeostasis and synaptic plasticity, oxidative stress, neuroinflammation, and hypothalamic-pituitary-adrenal axis activity (Yankner et al., 2008).

In the cerebral vasculature, aging-related modifications in elastin and collagen compositions lead to thickening of vascular basement membranes and reduction in distensibility of blood vessels (Farkas & Luiten, 2001). Neocortical volume loss with increasing age is likely associated with a decrease in neuronal architectural complexity, rather than significant loss of neurons (Freeman et al., 2008; Yankner et al., 2008). Aging-related reductions in white matter density have been observed, particularly in the prefrontal cortex and anterior corpus callosum (Yankner et al., 2008).

According to cross-sectional studies of postmortem aging brains, the proportion of human brains involved by cerebral Aβ deposition and p-tau+ neurofibrillary pathology in various stages increases with age. Only a small minority of individuals older than 90 years remains free of these lesions (Thal et al., 2008). Diffuse Aβ plaques and vascular Aβ deposits first appear in the neocortex, while the p-tau+ neurofibrillary pathology occurs initially in the transentorhinal region, nucleus basalis of Meynert, and dorsal raphe nucleus (Geula et al., 2008; Sassin et al., 2000; Thal et al., 2008). These lesions then expand to involve additional brain regions in a predictable spatial pattern (Thal et al., 2008). In the neocortex, the temporal progression of Aβ and tau pathologies has been suggested to follow a stereotyped sequence: diffuse non-fibrillar Aβ plaques, Congo-red-stained (i.e., fibrillar Aβ) plaques associated with microglial activation, p-tau+ neuritic plaques and neuropil threads, and finally p-tau+ neurofibrillary tangles (Duyckaerts, 2004). It is the presence of p-tau+ lesions in the neocortex that is associated with neurocognitive impairment

(Morris & Price, 2001; Price, 1997). Although cerebral Aβ deposition and tau pathology appear to be independent processes (Duyckaerts, 2004), transgenic animal studies have suggested that Aβ triggers the progression of tau pathology and neuronal degeneration (Thal et al., 2008).

Progressive Aβ accumulation in the brain may be associated with decreased enzymatic degradation of Aβ, deficient efflux of soluble Aβ from the interstitial fluid (ISF), or increased influx of Aβ from the blood circulation (Zlokovic et al., 2005). In addition to receptor-mediated transcytosis of Aβ across BBB, Aβ elimination may be mediated by perivascular macrophages (Hawkes & McLaurin, 2009), via bulk flow of ISF into the ventricles (Abbott 2004), and through perivascular ISF drainage of soluble Aβ along the basement membranes of capillaries and arteries (Bell & Zlokovic, 2009; Carare et al., 2008). The cerebral cortical microvessels are innervated by the ipsilateral cholinergic nucleus basalis of Meynert, mediating vasodilatory response via activation of both muscarinic and nicotinic receptors, and by the noradrenergic locus ceruleus and serotonergic dorsal raphe nucleus, directing vasoconstriction (Sato & Sato, 1992). Neuronal tau pathology in the cholinergic nucleus basalis of Meynert in advancing age (Geula et al., 2008; Mesulam et al., 2004; Sassin et al., 2000) may contribute to deficiencies in dilatory regulation of cerebral microvessels and arteriolar pulsation, resulting in a decrease in perivascular drainage of ISF. In a rabbit cholinergic model of Aβ deposition reported by Roher et al. (2000), selective ablation of the cholinergic neurons of the nucleus basalis magnocellularis with consequent loss of their neocortical afferents, which was induced by unilateral intracerebroventricular injection of the ribosomal toxin saporin conjugated to an antibody raised against the p75 neurotrophin receptor, caused non-fibrillar Aβ deposits in cortical blood vessels and as perivascular diffuse plaques, as well as increased levels of Aβ40 and Aβ42 in the cerebral cortex measured by enzyme-linked immunosorbent assay (ELISA). A cross-sectional study of postmortem human brains has suggested that neuronal tau pathology in the nucleus basalis of Meynert precedes neocortical Aβ deposition, and that the gradual development of the former parallels the progression of the "Braak & Braak" neurofibrillary stages in the cerebral cortex (Sassin et al., 2000). Degenerative vascular changes (Farkas and Luiten 2001) may also compromise cerebral perivascular ISF drainage. The aging-related functional and structural alterations of intracortical blood vessels (Farkas & Luiten, 2001) may promote soluble Aβ to accumulate and be transformed into Aβ oligomers, insoluble Aβ intermediates, and Aβ fibrils within vascular basement membranes and parenchymal plaques (Nicoll et al., 2004; Roher et al., 2000).

Aβ is produced by neurons and can accumulate within neurons (LaFerla et al., 2007). Cellular oxidative/nitrosative stress promotes post-translational misfolding of proteins. Molecular chaperones (e.g., heat shock proteins) can facilitate proper folding of proteins and repair misfolded proteins, preventing protein oligomerization and aggregation. The ubiquitin-proteosome system can remove misfolded proteins, and the autophagy/lysosomal degradation is involved in clearance of toxic oligomers and aggregates (Hol & Scheper, 2008;

Nakamura & Lipton, 2009). In aging and neurodegenerative conditions, oxidative/nitrosative stress triggered by excessive NMDA receptor activation and/or mitochondrial dysfunction may lead to increasing protein misfolding and deficiencies in molecular chaperone or proteosome activities, resulting in intra- or extracellular accumulation of protein aggregates (e.g., p-tau and Aβ) (Balch et al., 2008; Nakamura & Lipton, 2009). Decreased expression of autophagy-inducing protein beclin 1 was observed in the frontal cortex of patients affected with early or advanced AD (Pickford et al., 2008). Several lines of evidence have suggested that soluble oligomers of misfolded proteins are neurotoxic, affecting neuronal connectivity and plasticity and triggering cell death signaling pathways, while protein aggregates may be an attempt by the cell to wall-off toxic material (Nakamura & Lipton, 2009).

Dysregulation of glucocorticoid signaling in the brain may also be involved in aging-related cognitive impairment. In an animal study, neuronal expression of the glucocorticoid receptor (GR) and FK506-binding protein (FKBP)52 proteins in the forebrain was increased in aged mice irrespective of their short-term memory performance compared to young mice in the single-trial object recognition test, while FKBP51 expression was decreased only in aged mice with memory impairment. Furthermore, the FKBP51/FKBP52 ratio correlated directly with the memory performance score in aged mice (Soontornniyomkij et al., 2010). In mammalian cells, the activity of GR is dependent on the relative levels of FKBP51 and FKBP52 in the cytoplasm where FKBP51 acts as an inhibitor and FKBP52 as a facilitator for nuclear translocation of GR upon hormone binding (Grad & Picard, 2007; Wochnik et al., 2005). These findings suggest that the combination of decreased FKBP51 expression and increased expression of GR and FKBP52 in forebrain may represent the molecular substrate for exaggerated genomic glucocorticoid signaling that adversely affects the functional condition of mice prior to the learning task and consequently predisposes them to develop short-term recognition memory impairment. It would be of interest to delineate the glucocorticoid signaling pathway in the brains of HIV+ patients with neurocognitive impairment.

INTERACTIONS AMONG CHRONIC HIV INFECTION, HAART, AND BRAIN AGING

There are several potential factors that may contribute to neural injury associated with chronic HIV infection in old age; including, but not limited to, HIV factors, antiretroviral agents, host factors, substance abuse, and HCV infection. Some of these factors may prematurely trigger or promote a cascade of metabolic disturbances that would otherwise occur only in the aging brain. For instance, postmortem studies showed cerebral Aβ accumulation (Esiri et al., 1998; Rempel & Pulliam, 2005) and tau pathology (Anthony et al., 2006) in the brains of HIV+ patients earlier than expected by age. When HIV+ patients live to their old age, it is anticipated that brain aging-related factors may interact with concurrent HIV-related factors in a direction that accelerates these metabolic disturbances to the point that leads to neural injury and

neurocognitive impairment. In addition to age, the duration of HIV disease may also play an important role in this regard. Cysique et al. (2004) reported the higher prevalence of HAND in older patients, especially in those who had low nadir CD4 cell counts and prolonged disease duration, compared to that in younger patients. However, clinical reports on the effects of aging and HIV-disease duration on the development of HAND remain inconsistent across different cohorts (Brew et al., 2009; Valcour et al., 2004c).

HIV-associated Factors

HIV enters the CNS via infected peripheral mononuclear cells early in the course of infection (An et al., 1999). The impact of different HIV clades on the risk of HAND remains controversial (Jayadev & Garden, 2009; Liner et al., 2007). Evidence of independent genetic evolution and development of antiretroviral drug resistance of HIV strains infecting blood and brain has supported the concept of viral compartmentalization, probably due to limited viral exchanges between brain and blood, as well as limited drug bioavailability in the CNS leading to a lower selection pressure on HIV replicating within the CNS (Lambotte et al., 2003). Likely, HIV replication in the CNS is an early trigger phenomenon, rather than a late proximate cause of neural injury, which is mediated primarily by the chronic inflammatory response, neuroglial activation, and dysregulation of cytokines and neurotrophic factors favoring neurotoxicity over neuroprotection.

Studies using transgenic mice and neural cell cultures have indicated that HIV-1 proteins, especially Tat and gp120, can induce glial cell activation, cytokine dysregulation, neurotoxicity, and BBB disruption (Ellis et al., 2007; Ivey et al., 2009). Current antiretroviral agents are primarily targeting either HIV-1 protease or reverse transcriptase. These modes of action may have no impact on HIV-1 Tat production once proviral DNA has been integrated in infected neuroglial cells, as in the nonproductive infection of astrocytes (Nath & Hersh, 2005). HIV-1 Tat peptides can inhibit neprilysin activity, an Aβ-degrading enzyme (Daily et al., 2006; Rempel & Pulliam, 2005), as well as interfere with microglial phagocytosis of Aβ42 (Giunta et al., 2008). Neuronal uptake of HIV-1 Tat through binding to the heparan sulfate proteoglycan and via low-density lipoprotein receptor-related protein (LRP)-mediated endocytosis inhibits neuronal clearance of physiological ligands for LRP, including ApoE4, APP, and Aβ (Liu et al., 2000). HIV-1 Tat also disturbs the ubiquitin-proteosome system, as well as the autophagy (Brew et al., 2009). Even in the absence of productive HIV replication in the brain, HIV-1 Tat may be able to disturb cerebral Aβ metabolism as long as the virus is sequestered in perivascular microglia/macrophages (Nath & Hersh, 2005). That HIV-1 Tat may disturb axonal transport is evidenced by the increased number of APP-immunoreactive neurons in close proximity to Tat expression in the basal ganglia of macaques with simian-human immunodeficiency virus encephalitis (Liu et al., 2000). In an HIV-1 gp120 transgenic mouse model of HIV neurodegeneration, expression of human APP751 reduced the extent of neuronal loss, synaptic degeneration, and gliosis, suggesting that APP expression has a neuroprotective effect (Mucke et al. 1995). Cytokines interleukin1β, tumor necrosis factor (TNF)-α, and interferon-γ, all of which are increased in HIV+ brains, are shown in vitro to stimulate γ-secretase-mediated cleavage of APP (Liao et al., 2004).

Antiretroviral Therapy

Major adverse effects of long-term HAART, especially protease inhibitors, include insulin resistance, hyperlipidemia, and fat redistribution (lipodystrophy), which may accelerate the development of atherosclerotic vascular disease (Grunfeld, 2008; Mallewa et al., 2008). In addition, the use of nelfinavir may promote cerebral Aβ accumulation, as this drug can inhibit insulin-degrading enzyme, an Aβ degrading enzyme in the CNS (Hamel et al., 2006). Nelfinavir and saquinavir at therapeutic dosages can inhibit proteasome peptidase activity and cause intracellular accumulation of polyubiquitinated proteins (Piccinini et al., 2005). Although cerebral Aβ deposition can be observed in the brains of HIV+ patients regardless of HAART status, it seems to be more prevalent in the HAART-treated group (Green et al., 2005). Nucleoside reverse transcriptase inhibitors (e.g., didanosine, stavudine, and zalcitabine) can induce mitochondrial dysfunction, resulting in oxidative stress and neuronal injury (Schweinsburg et al., 2005; Valcour & Shiramizu, 2004).

Leptin gene expression in adipose tissue was shown to be downregulated in HIV+ patients regardless of HAART status (Giralt et al., 2006). Leptin, an adipocyte-derived hormone, influences brain development and function, particularly in learning and memory domains by facilitating hippocampal synaptic plasticity and long-term potentiation via enhancing NMDA receptor-mediated calcium influx (Shanley et al., 2001), in addition to its impact on regulating food intake and body weight. It is possible that a leptin deficiency may affect neurocognitive function in HIV+ patients (see below).

Host Factors

Differential susceptibility to HIV-associated neural injury among HIV+ patients may be dependent on host genetic variations in the cytokine regulatory response to HIV replication or viral proteins (Ellis et al., 2007). For example, G/G homozygosity for the monocyte chemoattractant protein (MCP-1) promoter at position -2578 was associated with the increased risk of HAD (Gonzalez et al., 2002) and the elevated levels of MCP-1 in CSF (Letendre et al., 2004a). The TNF-α-308 allele 2 was also shown to associate with ADC (Pemberton et al,. 2008). Other than cytokines, neural cells can produce trophic factors, such as brain-derived neurotrophic factors (Soontornniyomkij et al., 1998), insulin-like growth factor 1, fibroblast growth factor 1, macrophage inflammatory protein 2, and stromal-derived factor 1α in response to injury or challenge (Ellis et al., 2007), which may be influenced by host genetic variations.

The ApoE ε4 allele was shown to correlate in non-demented elderly subjects with cerebral Aβ burden measured by PiB PET (Reiman et al., 2009; Rowe et al., 2007) and in AD brains with Aβ40 accumulation in senile plaques (Gearing et al., 1996; Mann et al., 1997) and vessel walls (Alonzo et al., 1998) previously seeded with Aβ42. Whether the ApoE ε4 allele predicts the presence and degree of cerebral Aβ deposition in HIV+ patients is currently unknown. Valcour et al. (2004a) reported that the ApoE ε4 allele conveyed the risk of HAD within the older group but not in the younger group. On the other hand, Pomara et al. (2008) found that the ApoE ε4 allele was associated with better baseline memory performance in HIV+ patients free from HAD. The relationship between the ApoE ε4 genotype and a clinical diagnosis of HAD remains controversial (Burt et al., 2008; Corder et al., 2008; Diaz-Arrastia et al., 2004; Dunlop et al., 1997; Pemberton et al., 2008; Pomara et al., 2008). However, it is possible that the ApoE ε4 allele increases the susceptibility for HAND, especially in older patients, by promoting cerebral Aβ accumulation.

Other Comorbid Factors

A range of substances of abuse, including opiates, cocaine, methamphetamine, and alcohol, are all known to increase immune suppression and enhance viral replication (Martin-Thormeyer & Paul, 2009). Increased microglial activation in the brain has been shown to correlate with intravenous drug use alone or with pre-symptomatic HIV infection (Tomlinson et al., 1999). More severe microglial reaction was associated with a history of methamphetamine abuse in HIV encephalitis brains (Langford et al., 2003a). In a postmortem brain study of HIV-seronegative opiate abusers died of drug overdose at age less than 40 years, p-tau+ pathology was more prevalent in the drug abusers than in age-matched non-drug controls (44% vs. 19%) and in the former had expanded beyond the entorhiral cortex to involve the subiculum, temporal neocortex, nucleus basalis of Meynert, and locus ceruleus (Ramage et al., 2005). Interactions between HIV-1 gp120 and Tat proteins and substances of abuse facilitate BBB disruption, release of TNF-α and other neurotoxic cytokines, up-regulate CCR5 expression, and increase oxidative stress (Martin-Thormeyer & Paul, 2009).

HCV crosses BBB and is present both in CSF and brain parenchyma (Martin-Thormeyer & Paul, 2009). In HIV+ subjects with HCV seropositivity, HCV RNA and proteins were found in brain tissue, with HCV immunoreactivity localized to astrocytes and perivascular macrophages, suggesting that HCV might undergo productive replication and cause neural injury in conjunction with HIV (Letendre et al., 2007). HCV seropositivity was also found to associate with elevated CSF levels of MCP-1, TNF-α, and soluble TNF receptor II (Letendre et al., 2005).

CLINICAL IMPLICATIONS

When HIV+ patients develop neurocognitive decline in their old age, it is important to distinguish between HAND (potentially with a brain-aging component) and neurodegenerative diseases, such as AD, vascular dementia, and diffuse Lewy body disease, although the concurrence of HAND and neurodegenerative diseases is possible (Brousseau et al., 2009). In addition to measurements of CSF HIV load, quantitative assays of selective proteins in CSF, PET neuroimaging scans, and selective host genotyping studies are considered to be potential candidate biomarkers for HAND. Nonetheless, a multimodal approach, rather than a single test, may be needed for screening and confirming the early development of HIV-associated neural injury, as it has been attempted in AD (Perrin et al., 2009).

As discussed above, Heaton et al. (2010) have reported that HAND, mostly in milder forms, persist in the HAART era and may correlate with the stage of systemic disease and detectable viral replication. Cherner et al. (2004) reported that older individuals with detectable virus in CSF had twice the prevalence of neuropsychological impairment of those with undetectable levels. In a study in Western Pennsylvania, the prevalence of cognitive disorders among HIV+ patients over 50 years of age was higher than in younger individuals (Becker et al., 2004). Nonetheless, the combined effects of aging and HIV infection on cognition are not uniform, probably due to large individual differences in a variety of co-factors of susceptibility among older HIV+ adults (Hardy & Vance, 2009).

There are still only a few and inconsistent reports about the neurocognitive profile in HIV+ aging subjects although it seems that some may be at greater risk to develop deficits in attention functioning (Hardy & Vance, 2009).

CSF BIOMARKERS

High CSF tau/Aβ42 or p-tau181/Aβ42 ratios have predicted cognitive decline in nondemented older individuals (Fagan et al., 2007), progression to AD in patients with mild cognitive impairment (Hansson et al., 2006), and more rapid progression of cognitive decline in mild AD patients (Snider et al., 2009). In the setting of HIV infection, clinical studies have shown a trend that Aβ42 levels in CSF are decreased in older HAND patients who have been receiving antiretroviral therapy (Brew et al., 2005; Clifford et al., 2009; Gisslen et al., 2009), as well as in some HIV+ subjects with normal cognition (Brew et al., 2005). Regarding the relationship between HAND and CSF levels of t-tau and p-tau, data from different clinical studies are conflicting (Brew et al., 2005; Clifford et al., 2009; Gisslen et al., 2009). It seems that clinical usefulness of CSF levels of Aβ42, t-tau, and p-tau as biomarkers for HAND awaits further investigations.

Among HIV+ men, lower CSF leptin levels and reduced CNS leptin uptake were shown to correlate with worse neuropsychological performance in learning and memory, after controlling for nadir CD4 cell counts, HAART exposure, and CSF HIV RNA levels; however, lipodystrophy was not assessed in this study (Huang et al., 2007). Byproducts of lipid peroxidation (isoprostanes) and RNA oxidation (8-hydroxyguanosine) may also be worthy of further investigation as candidate CSF biomarkers for HIV-associated neural injury. Furthermore, the ongoing advancement of mass spectrometry

can make unbiased proteomic analyses to discover novel predictive or surrogate biomarkers in CSF. The discovery of new candidate biomarkers without known relevance to the disease may provide clues into pathogenetic mechanisms that are currently underappreciated or not yet recognized (Perrin et al., 2009).

PET NEUROIMAGING

PET imaging studies of amyloid burden in the brain with the use of amyloid-binding radiotracers, like PiB (Bacskai et al., 2007; Fagan et al., 2006; Klunk et al., 2004) and FDDNP (Shoghi-Jadid et al., 2002; Small et al., 2006), have been conducted in elderly patients with or without cognitive impairment. PiB, a thioflavin-T derivative (Mathis et al., 2003), appears to bind fibrillar Aβ in cored plaques and vessel walls, but not neurofibrillary tangles or Lewy bodies at the tracer dosage used for PET scanning (Bacskai et al., 2007), whereas FDDNP labels both Aβ plaques and neurofibrillary tangles (Agdeppa et al., 2001). PiB does not label non-fibrillar Aβ (Bacskai et al., 2007; Cairns et al., 2009; Ikonomovic et al., 2008), which comprises the vast majority of Aβ deposits as diffuse plaques in early stages of cerebral amyloidosis. Nonetheless, as discussed above, the lone presence of diffuse plaques of non-fibrillar Aβ is not associated with neurocognitive impairment (Price, 1997; Thal et al., 2008). Only when Aβ plaques in the neocortex acquire increasing amounts of fibrillar Aβ and p-tau+ dystrophic neurites to become "neuritic plaques" and are accompanied by p-tau+ neuropil threads and neurofibrillary tangles, does neurocognitive decline emerge (Fagan et al., 2009; Price, 1997; Thal et al., 2008). As PiB uptake appears sensitive to the presence of fibrillar Aβ, PiB retention is a feature not only of AD, but also of cerebral amyloid angiopathy, non-demented elderly individuals with cerebral Aβ deposition at risk of AD (presumably "preclinical AD"), mild cognitive impairment, and other brain diseases with co-existent Aβ deposition (Aizenstein et al., 2008; Bacskai et al., 2007; Fagan et al., 2006; Johnson et al., 2007). In a subset of elderly individuals with normal cognition, decreased CSF Aβ42 levels were not accompanied by an increase in PiB uptake, suggesting that these subjects may have non-fibrillar Aβ42 deposits that do not retain PiB (Cairns et al., 2009; Fagan et al., 2006; Perrin et al., 2009). It remains to be seen whether these subjects are at risk of progression to neurocognitive impairment. In conjunction with PiB PET, PK11195 PET has been employed to detect increased expression of the peripheral benzodiazepine receptor by activated microglia (Perrin et al., 2009). An inverse correlation between neocortical PK11195 signal and cognitive performance was observed in AD patients (Edison et al., 2008).

As HIV+ patients treated with HAART in old age appear to be at risk of cerebral Aβ and tau pathologies and presumably resultant neurocognitive impairment, PET with ligands for relevant molecular markers may be applied as surrogate measures for identifying at-risk individuals to allow further investigations and early therapeutic interventions. It would be of interest to pursue longitudinal PET studies with the use of PiB, FDDNP, and PK11195 in HIV+ subjects.

THERAPEUTIC INTERVENTIONS

Recent studies have supported the benefit of CNS-penetrating HAART regimen in achieving CSF viral suppression and favorable neuropsychological outcome (Cysique & Brew, 2009; Letendre et al., 2008; Letendre et al., 2004b). However, despite this drug regimen there may be the persistence of low levels of chronic HIV replication in perivascular macrophages/microglia, as well as nonproductive HIV infection of astrocytes, which is sufficient to trigger a complex cascade of neural injury in the co-existence of a variety of comorbid factors, leading to neurocognitive impairment. Therefore, it may be important to also treat or control the modifiable comorbid conditions, such as lipid disorders, hypertension, insulin resistance, substance abuse, and HCV infection (Brew et al., 2009).

Furthermore, adjunctive therapies with agents that promote neural repair or prevent further neural injury have been in clinical trials. Inhibition of NMDA receptor activity is a mechanism that can reduce excessive Ca^{2+} influx, resultant overstimulation of neuronal nitric oxide synthase activity, and nitrosative/oxidative stress. Memantine acts as an open-channel inhibitor of NMDA receptor-coupled channel pore to preferentially block excessive NMDA receptor activity, while relatively sparing physiological activity (Nakamura & Lipton, 2009). Previous clinical trials of memantine failed to show a favorable effect on neuropsychological performance in HIV+ individuals with mild to moderate HAND, as did those of selegeline (a selective monoamine oxidase B inhibitor) (Cysique & Brew, 2009; Schifitto et al., 2009).

Cerebral Aβ deposition appears to prematurely involve a subset of HIV+ patients; however, to what extent it contributes to neurocognitive impairment remains to be seen. Nonsteriodal anti-inflammatory drugs like ibuprofen and indomethacin modulate the γ-secretase cleavage of APP, but their alleviating impact on cognitive decline in the elderly remains controversial (Thal et al., 2008). The benefits of β- and γ-secretase inhibitors have not been clinically proven in AD patients. Clinical trials of selective cyclo-oxygenase-2 inhibitors have failed to demonstrate any beneficial effect in AD patients (Firuzi & Praticò, 2006). Whether these groups of drugs would benefit patients with HAND is currently unknown.

CONCLUSIONS

HAND is a common complication of HIV infection even in patients who have achieved systemic viral suppression with HAART, and profoundly affects the clinical outcome, particularly in old age. Ongoing clinical and experimental research studies have made progress in understanding the complex interactions among HIV, host, and comorbid factors that lead to neural injury. Differences in these factors among HIV+ individuals may account for differential susceptibility to the development and severity of HIV-associated neurocognitive impairment. The neuropathologic correlates of HAND in the HAART era may be variable from one case to another, representing additive or synergistic effects of several contributing factors. The mechanistic significance of brain aging changes, especially cerebral Aβ and tau pathologies, in the development of HAND remains to be determined in large prospective cohort studies that allow systematic analysis to assess potential associations between the histological findings and clinical parameters like neuropsychological performance. A paramount goal is to identify accurate and practical biomarkers for detecting HIV-associated neural injury at stages earlier than the onset of clinical manifestation or abnormal neuropsychological testing, in order to allow disease-modifying therapeutic interventions, as well as objective evaluation of the response to treatment.

ACKNOWLEDGMENTS

The authors acknowledge support from NIH awards U01 MH83506 (California NeuroAIDS Tissue Network) and P30 MH62512 (HIV Neurobehavioral Research Center).

REFERENCES

Abbott, N. (2004). Evidence for bulk flow of brain interstitial fluid: Significance for physiology and pathology. *Neurochem Int, 45*(4), 545–552.

Achim, C., Adame, A., Dumaop, W., Everall, I., & Masliah, E. (2009). Increased accumulation of intraneuronal amyloid beta in HIV-infected patients. *J Neuroimmune Pharmacol, 4*(2), 190–199.

Agdeppa, E., Kepe, V., Liu, J., Flores-Torres, S., Satyamurthy, N., Petric, A., et al. (2001). Binding characteristics of radiofluorinated 6-dialkylamino-2-naphthylethylidene derivatives as positron emission tomography imaging probes for beta-amyloid plaques in Alzheimer's disease. *J Neurosci, 21*(24), RC189.

Aizenstein, H., Nebes, R., Saxton, J., Price, J., Mathis, C., Tsopelas, N., et al. (2008). Frequent amyloid deposition without significant cognitive impairment among the elderly. *Arch Neurol, 65*(11), 1509–1517.

Alonzo, N., Hyman, B., Rebeck, G., & Greenberg, S. (1998). Progression of cerebral amyloid angiopathy: Accumulation of amyloid-beta40 in affected vessels. *J Neuropathol Exp Neurol, 57*(4), 353–359.

An, S., Groves, M., Gray, F., & Scaravilli, F. (1999). Early entry and widespread cellular involvement of HIV-1 DNA in brains of HIV-1 positive asymptomatic individuals. *J Neuropathol Exp Neurol, 58*(11), 1156–1162.

Anderson, E., Zink, W., Xiong, H., & Gendelman, H. (2002). HIV-1-associated dementia: A metabolic encephalopathy perpetrated by virus-infected and immune-competent mononuclear phagocytes. *J Acquir Immune Defic Syndr, 31* Suppl 2, S43–54.

Andersson, L., Blennow, K., Fuchs, D., Svennerholm, B., & Gisslén, M. (1999). Increased cerebrospinal fluid protein tau concentration in neuro-AIDS. *J Neurol Sci, 171*(2), 92–96.

Anthony, I. & Bell, J. (2008). The Neuropathology of HIV/AIDS. *Int Rev Psychiatry, 20*(1), 15–24.

Anthony, I., Ramage, S., Carnie, F., Simmonds, P., & Bell, J. (2005). Influence of HAART on HIV-related CNS disease and neuroinflammation. *J Neuropathol Exp Neurol, 64*(6), 529–536.

Anthony, I., Ramage, S., Carnie, F., Simmonds, P., & Bell, J. (2006). Accelerated Tau deposition in the brains of individuals infected with human immunodeficiency virus-1 before and after the advent of highly active anti-retroviral therapy. *Acta Neuropathol, 111*(6), 529–538.

Antinori, A., Arendt, G., Becker, J., Brew, B., Byrd, D., Cherner, M., et al. (2007). Updated research nosology for HIV-associated neurocognitive disorders. *Neurology, 69*(18), 1789–1799.

Avison, M., Nath, A., Greene-Avison, R., Schmitt, F., Greenberg, R., & Berger, J. (2004). Neuroimaging correlates of HIV-associated BBB compromise. *J Neuroimmunol, 157*(1–2), 140–146.

Bacskai, B., Frosch, M., Freeman, S., Raymond, S., Augustinack, J., Johnson, K., et al. (2007). Molecular imaging with Pittsburgh Compound B confirmed at autopsy: A case report. *Arch Neurol, 64*(3), 431–434.

Balch, W., Morimoto, R., Dillin, A., & Kelly, J. (2008). Adapting proteostasis for disease intervention. *Science, 319*(5865), 916–919.

Becker, J., Lopez, O., Dew, M., & Aizenstein, H. (2004). Prevalence of cognitive disorders differs as a function of age in HIV virus infection. *AIDS, 18* Suppl 1, S11–18.

Bell, J., Donaldson, Y., Lowrie, S., McKenzie, C., Elton, R., Chiswick, A., et al. (1996). Influence of risk group and zidovudine therapy on the development of HIV encephalitis and cognitive impairment in AIDS patients. *AIDS, 10*(5), 493–499.

Bell, R. & Zlokovic, B. (2009). Neurovascular mechanisms and blood-brain barrier disorder in Alzheimer's disease. *Acta Neuropathol, 118*(1), 103–113.

Brew, B. (2004). Evidence for a change in AIDS dementia complex in the era of highly active antiretroviral therapy and the possibility of new forms of AIDS dementia complex. *AIDS, 18* Suppl 1, S75–78.

Brew, B., Crowe, S., Landay, A., Cysique, L., & Guillemin, G. (2009). Neurodegeneration and ageing in the HAART era. *J Neuroimmune Pharmacol, 4*(2), 163–174.

Brew, B., Pemberton, L., Blennow, K., Wallin, A., & Hagberg, L. (2005). CSF amyloid beta42 and tau levels correlate with AIDS dementia complex. *Neurology, 65*(9), 1490–1492.

Brousseau, K., Filley, C., Kaye, K., Kiser, J., Adler, L., & Connick, E. (2009). Dementia with features of Alzheimer's disease and HIV-associated dementia in an elderly man with AIDS. *AIDS, 23*(8), 1029–1031.

Burt, T., Agan, B., Marconi, V., He, W., Kulkarni, H., Mold, J., et al. (2008). Apolipoprotein (apo) E4 enhances HIV-1 cell entry in vitro, and the APOE epsilon4/epsilon4 genotype accelerates HIV disease progression. *Proc Natl Acad Sci U S A, 105*(25), 8718–8723.

Cairns, N., Ikonomovic, M., Benzinger, T., Storandt, M., Fagan, A., Shah, A., et al. (2009). Absence of Pittsburgh Compound B detection of cerebral amyloid beta in a patient with clinical, cognitive, and cerebrospinal fluid markers of Alzheimer disease: A case report. *Arch Neurol, 66*(12), 1557–1562.

Carare, R., Bernardes-Silva, M., Newman, T., Page, A., Nicoll, J., Perry, V., et al. (2008). Solutes, but not cells, drain from the brain parenchyma along basement membranes of capillaries and arteries: Significance for cerebral amyloid angiopathy and neuroimmunology. *Neuropathol Appl Neurobiol, 34*(2), 131–144.

Chana, G., Everall, I., Crews, L., Langford, D., Adame, A., Grant, I., et al. (2006). Cognitive deficits and degeneration of interneurons in HIV+ methamphetamine users. *Neurology, 67*(8), 1486–1489.

Chang, L., Lee, P., Yiannoutsos, C., Ernst, T., Marra, C., Richards, T., et al. (2004). A multicenter in vivo proton-MRS study of HIV-associated dementia and its relationship to age. *Neuroimage, 23*(4), 1336–1347.

Cherner, M., Ellis, R., Lazzaretto, D., Young, C., Mindt, M., Atkinson, J., et al. (2004). Effects of HIV-1 infection and aging on neurobehavioral functioning: Preliminary findings. *AIDS, 18* Suppl 1, S27–34.

Cherner, M., Letendre, S., Heaton, R., Durelle, J., Marquie-Beck, J., Gragg, B., et al. (2005). Hepatitis C augments cognitive deficits associated with HIV infection and methamphetamine. *Neurology, 64*(8), 1343–1347.

Cherner, M., Masliah, E., Ellis, R., Marcotte, T., Moore, D., Grant, I., et al. (2002). Neurocognitive dysfunction predicts postmortem findings of HIV encephalitis. *Neurology, 59*(10), 1563–1567.

Cleary, J., Walsh, D., Hofmeister, J., Shankar, G., Kuskowski, M., Selkoe, D., et al. (2005). Natural oligomers of the amyloid-beta protein specifically disrupt cognitive function. *Nat Neurosci, 8*(1), 79–84.

Clifford, D., Fagan, A., Holtzman, D., Morris, J., Teshome, M., Shah, A., et al. (2009). CSF biomarkers of Alzheimer disease in HIV-associated neurologic disease. *Neurology, 73*(23), 1982–1987.

Corder, E., Paganelli, R., Giunta, S., & Franceschi, C. (2008). Differential course of HIV-1 infection and APOE polymorphism. *Proc Natl Acad Sci U S A, 105*(46), E87.

Cysique, L. & Brew, B. (2009). Neuropsychological functioning and antiretroviral treatment in HIV/AIDS: A review. *Neuropsychol Rev, 19*(2), 169–185.

Cysique, L., Maruff, P., & Brew, B. (2004). Prevalence and pattern of neuropsychological impairment in human immunodeficiency virus-infected/acquired immunodeficiency syndrome (HIV/AIDS) patients across pre- and post-highly active antiretroviral therapy eras: A combined study of two cohorts. *J Neurovirol, 10*(6), 350–357.

Daily, A., Nath, A., & Hersh, L. (2006). Tat peptides inhibit neprilysin. *J Neurovirol, 12*(3), 153–160.

Diaz-Arrastia, R., Gong, Y., Kelly, C., & Gelman, B. (2004). Host genetic polymorphisms in human immunodeficiency virus-related neurologic disease. *J Neurovirol, 10* Suppl 1, 67–73.

Dunlop, O., Goplen, A., Liestøl, K., Myrvang, B., Rootwelt, H., Christophersen, B., et al. (1997). HIV dementia and apolipoprotein E. *Acta Neurol Scand, 95*(5), 315–318.

Duyckaerts, C. (2004). Looking for the link between plaques and tangles. *Neurobiol Aging, 25*(6), 735–739; discussion 743–746.

Edison, P., Archer, H., Gerhard, A., Hinz, R., Pavese, N., Turkheimer, F., et al. (2008). Microglia, amyloid, and cognition in Alzheimer's disease: An [11C](R)PK11195-PET and [11C]PIB-PET study. *Neurobiol Dis, 32*(3), 412–419.

Effros, R., Fletcher, C., Gebo, K., Halter, J., Hazzard, W., Horne, F., et al. (2008). Aging and infectious diseases: Workshop on HIV infection and aging: What is known and future research directions. *Clin Infect Dis, 47*(4), 542–553.

Ellis, R., Langford, D., & Masliah, E. (2007). HIV and antiretroviral therapy in the brain: Neuronal injury and repair. *Nat Rev Neurosci, 8*(1), 33–44.

Ellis, R., Moore, D., Childers, M., Letendre, S., McCutchan, J., Wolfson, T., et al. (2002). Progression to neuropsychological impairment in human immunodeficiency virus infection predicted by elevated cerebrospinal fluid levels of human immunodeficiency virus RNA. *Arch Neurol, 59*(6), 923–928.

Ellis, R., Seubert, P., Motter, R., Galasko, D., Deutsch, R., Heaton, R., et al. (1998). Cerebrospinal fluid tau protein is not elevated in HIV-associated neurologic disease in humans. HIV Neurobehavioral Research Center Group (HNRC). *Neurosci Lett, 254*(1), 1–4.

Ernst, T. & Chang, L. (2004). Effect of aging on brain metabolism in antiretroviral-naive HIV patients. *AIDS, 18* Suppl 1, S61–67.

Esiri, M., Biddolph, S., & Morris, C. (1998). Prevalence of Alzheimer plaques in AIDS. *J Neurol Neurosurg Psychiatry, 65*(1), 29–33.

Everall, I., Hansen, L., & Masliah, E. (2005). The shifting patterns of HIV encephalitis neuropathology. *Neurotox Res, 8*(1–2), 51–61.

Everall, I., Vaida, F., Khanlou, N., Lazzaretto, D., Achim, C., Letendre, S., et al. (2009). Cliniconeuropathologic correlates of human immunodeficiency virus in the era of antiretroviral therapy. *J Neurovirol, 15*(5–6), 360–370.

Fagan, A., Head, D., Shah, A., Marcus, D., Mintun, M., Morris, J., et al. (2009). Decreased cerebrospinal fluid Abeta(42) correlates with brain atrophy in cognitively normal elderly. *Ann Neurol, 65*(2), 176–183.

Fagan, A., Mintun, M., Mach, R., Lee, S., Dence, C., Shah, A., et al. (2006). Inverse relation between in vivo amyloid imaging load and cerebrospinal fluid Abeta42 in humans. *Ann Neurol, 59*(3), 512–519.

Fagan, A., Roe, C., Xiong, C., Mintun, M., Morris, J., & Holtzman, D. (2007). Cerebrospinal fluid tau/beta-amyloid(42) ratio as a prediction of cognitive decline in nondemented older adults. *Arch Neurol, 64*(3), 343–349.

Farkas, E. & Luiten, P. (2001). Cerebral microvascular pathology in aging and Alzheimer's disease. *Prog Neurobiol, 64*(6), 575–611.

Firuzi, O. & Praticò, D. (2006). Coxibs and Alzheimer's disease: Should they stay or should they go? *Ann Neurol, 59*(2), 219–228.

Freeman, S., Kandel, R., Cruz, L., Rozkalne, A., Newell, K., Frosch, M., et al. (2008). Preservation of neuronal number despite age-related cortical brain atrophy in elderly subjects without Alzheimer disease. *J Neuropathol Exp Neurol, 67*(12), 1205–1212.

Gearing, M., Mori, H., & Mirra, S. (1996). Abeta-peptide length and apolipoprotein E genotype in Alzheimer's disease. *Ann Neurol, 39*(3), 395–399.

Geula, C., Nagykery, N., Nicholas, A., & Wu, C. (2008). Cholinergic neuronal and axonal abnormalities are present early in aging and in Alzheimer disease. *J Neuropathol Exp Neurol, 67*(4), 309–318.

Giralt, M., Domingo, P., Guallar, J., Rodriguez de la Concepción, M., Alegre, M., Domingo, J., et al. (2006). HIV-1 infection alters gene expression in adipose tissue, which contributes to HIV- 1/HAART-associated lipodystrophy. *Antivir Ther, 11*(6), 729–740.

Gisslen, M., Krut, J., Andreasson, U., Blennow, K., Cinque, P., Brew, B., et al. (2009). Amyloid and tau cerebrospinal fluid biomarkers in HIV infection. *BMC Neurol, 9*(1), 63.

Giunta, B., Zhou, Y., Hou, H., Rrapo, E., Fernandez, F., & Tan, J. (2008). HIV-1 TAT inhibits microglial phagocytosis of Abeta peptide. *Int J Clin Exp Pathol, 1*(3), 260–275.

Glass, J., Fedor, H., Wesselingh, S., & McArthur, J. (1995). Immunocytochemical quantitation of human immunodeficiency virus in the brain: Correlations with dementia. *Ann Neurol, 38*(5), 755–762.

Gonzalez, E., Rovin, B., Sen, L., Cooke, G., Dhanda, R., Mummidi, S., et al. (2002). HIV-1 infection and AIDS dementia are influenced by a mutant MCP-1 allele linked to increased monocyte infiltration of tissues and MCP-1 levels. *Proc Natl Acad Sci U S A, 99*(21), 13795–13800.

Goosens, K. & Sapolsky, R. (2007). Stress and glucocorticoid contributions to normal and pathological aging. In D. Riddle (ed.). *Brain aging: Models, methods, and mechanisms*, pp. 305–314. New York: CRC Press.

Gouras, G., Almeida, C., & Takahashi, R. (2005). Intraneuronal Abeta accumulation and origin of plaques in Alzheimer's disease. *Neurobiol Aging, 26*(9), 1235–1244.

Grad, I. & Picard, D. (2007). The glucocorticoid responses are shaped by molecular chaperones. *Mol Cell Endocrinol, 275*(1–2), 2–12.

Grant, I. (2008). Neurocognitive disturbances in HIV. *Int Rev Psychiatry, 20*(1), 33–47.

Gray, F., Chrétien, F., Vallat-Decouvelaere, A., & Scaravilli, F. (2003). The changing pattern of HIV neuropathology in the HAART era. *J Neuropathol Exp Neurol, 62*(5), 429–440.

Green, A., Giovannoni, G., Hall-Craggs, M., Thompson, E., & Miller, R. (2000). Cerebrospinal fluid tau concentrations in HIV infected patients with suspected neurological disease. *Sex Transm Infect, 76*(6), 443–446.

Green, D., Masliah, E., Vinters, H., Beizai, P., Moore, D., & Achim, C. (2005). Brain deposition of beta-amyloid is a common pathologic feature in HIV positive patients. *AIDS, 19*(4), 407–411.

Grunfeld, C. (2008). Insulin resistance in HIV infection: Drugs, host responses, or restoration to health? *Top HIV Med, 16*(2), 89–93.

Hamel, F., Fawcett, J., Tsui, B., Bennett, R., & Duckworth, W. (2006). Effect of nelfinavir on insulin metabolism, proteasome activity and protein degradation in HepG2 cells. *Diabetes Obes Metab, 8*(6), 661–668.

Hansson, O., Zetterberg, H., Buchhave, P., Londos, E., Blennow, K., & Minthon, L. (2006). Association between CSF biomarkers and incipient Alzheimer's disease in patients with mild cognitive impairment: A follow-up study. *Lancet Neurol, 5*(3), 228–234.

Hardy, D. & Vance, D. 2009. The neuropsychology of HIV/AIDS in older adults. *Neuropsychol Rev, 19*(2), 263–272.

Hawkes, C. & McLaurin, J. (2009). Selective targeting of perivascular macrophages for clearance of beta-amyloid in cerebral amyloid angiopathy. *Proc Natl Acad Sci U S A, 106*(4), 1261–1266.

Heaton, R., Clifford, D., Franklin, Jr D., Woods, S., Ake, C., Vaida, F., et al. (2010). HIV-associated neurocognitive disorders persist in the era of potent antiretroviral therapy. *Neurology, 75*(23), 2087–2096.

Heaton, R. K., Franklin, D. R., Ellis, R. J., McCutchan, J. A., Letendre, S. L., Leblanc, S., . . . Grant, I. (2011). HIV-associated neurocognitive disorders before and during the era of combination antiretroviral therapy: Differences in rates, nature, and predictors. *J Neurovirol, 17*(1), 3–16.

Hol, E. & Scheper, W. (2008). Protein quality control in neurodegeneration: Walking the tight rope between health and disease. *J Mol Neurosci, 34*(1), 23–33.

Huang, J., Letendre, S., Marquie-Beck, J., Cherner, M., McCutchan, J., Grant, I., et al. (2007). Low CSF leptin levels are associated with worse learning and memory performance in HIV-infected men. *J Neuroimmune Pharmacol, 2*(4), 352–358.

Ikonomovic, M., Klunk, W., Abrahamson, E., Mathis, C., Price, J., Tsopelas, N., et al. (2008). Post-mortem correlates of in vivo PiB-PET amyloid imaging in a typical case of Alzheimer's disease. *Brain, 131*(Pt 6), 1630–1645.

Ivey, N., MacLean, A., & Lackner, A. (2009). Acquired immunodeficiency syndrome and the blood-brain barrier. *J Neurovirol, 15*(2), 111–122.

Izycka-Swieszewska, E., Zóltowska, A., Rzepko, R., Gross, M., & Borowska-Lehman, J. (2000). Vasculopathy and amyloid beta reactivity in brains of patients with acquired immune deficiency (AIDS). *Folia Neuropathol, 38*(4), 175–182.

Jayadev, S. & Garden, G. (2009). Host and viral factors influencing the pathogenesis of HIV-associated neurocognitive disorders. *J Neuroimmune Pharmacol, 4*(2), 175–189.

Jellinger, K., Setinek, U., Drlicek, M., Böhm, G., Steurer, A., & Lintner, F. (2000). Neuropathology and general autopsy findings in AIDS during the last 15 years. *Acta Neuropathol, 100*(2), 213–220.

Johnson, K., Gregas, M., Becker, J., Kinnecom, C., Salat, D., Moran, E., et al. (2007). Imaging of amyloid burden and distribution in cerebral amyloid angiopathy. *Ann Neurol, 62*(3), 229–234.

Khanlou, N., Moore, D., Chana, G., Cherner, M., Lazzaretto, D., Dawes, S., et al. (2009). Increased frequency of alpha-synuclein in the substantia nigra in human immunodeficiency virus infection. *J Neurovirol, 15*(2), 131–138.

Klunk, W., Engler, H., Nordberg, A., Wang, Y., Blomqvist, G., Holt, D., et al. (2004). Imaging brain amyloid in Alzheimer's disease with Pittsburgh Compound-B. *Ann Neurol, 55*(3), 306–319.

LaFerla, F., Green, K., & Oddo, S. (2007). Intracellular amyloid-beta in Alzheimer's disease. *Nat Rev Neurosci, 8*(7), 499–509.

Lambotte, O., Deiva, K., & Tardieu, M. (2003). HIV-1 persistence, viral reservoir, and the central nervous system in the HAART era. *Brain Pathol, 13*(1), 95–103.

Langford, D., Adame, A., Grigorian, A., Grant, I., McCutchan, J., Ellis, R., et al. (2003a). Patterns of selective neuronal damage in methamphetamine-user AIDS patients. *J Acquir Immune Defic Syndr, 34*(5), 467–474.

Langford, T., Letendre, S., Larrea, G., & Masliah,E. (2003b). Changing patterns in the neuropathogenesis of HIV during the HAART era. *Brain Pathol, 13*(2), 195–210.

Letendre, S., Cherner, M., Ellis, R., Marquie-Beck, J., Gragg, B., Marcotte, T., et al. (2005). The effects of hepatitis C, HIV, and methamphetamine dependence on neuropsychological performance: Biological correlates of disease. *AIDS, 19* Suppl 3, S72–78.

Letendre, S., Marquie-Beck,J., Capparelli, E., Best, B., Clifford, D., Collier, A., et al. (2008). Validation of the CNS Penetration-Effectiveness rank for quantifying antiretroviral penetration into the central nervous system. *Arch Neurol, 65*(1), 65–70.

Letendre, S., Marquie-Beck, J., Singh, K., de Almeida, S., Zimmerman, J., Spector, S., et al. (2004a). The monocyte chemotactic protein-1–2578G allele is associated with elevated MCP-1 concentrations in cerebrospinal fluid. *J Neuroimmunol, 157*(1–2), 193–196.

Letendre, S., McCutchan, J., Childers, M., Woods, S., Lazzaretto, D., Heaton, R., et al. (2004b). Enhancing antiretroviral therapy for human immunodeficiency virus cognitive disorders. *Ann Neurol, 56*(3),416–423.

Letendre, S., Paulino, A., Rockenstein, E., Adame, A., Crews, L., Cherner, M., et al. (2007). Pathogenesis of hepatitis C virus coinfection in the brains of patients infected with HIV. *J Infect Dis*, *196*(3), 361–370.

Liao, Y., Wang, B., Cheng, H., Kuo, L., & Wolfe, M. (2004). Tumor necrosis factor-alpha, interleukin-1beta, and interferon-gamma stimulate gamma-secretase-mediated cleavage of amyloid precursor protein through a JNK-dependent MAPK pathway. *J Biol Chem*, *279*(47), 49523–49532.

Liner, K., Hall, C., & Robertson, K. (2007). Impact of human immunodeficiency virus (HIV) subtypes on HIV-associated neurological disease. *J Neurovirol*, *13*(4), 291–304.

Liu, Y., Jones, M., Hingtgen, C., Bu, G., Laribee, N., Tanzi, R., et al. (2000). Uptake of HIV-1 tat protein mediated by low-density lipoprotein receptor-related protein disrupts the neuronal metabolic balance of the receptor ligands. *Nat Med*, *6*(12), 1380–1387.

Lupien, S., Schwartz, G., Ng, Y., Fiocco, A., Wan, N., Pruessner, J., et al. (2005). The Douglas Hospital Longitudinal Study of Normal and Pathological Aging: Summary of findings. *J Psychiatry Neurosci*, *30*(5), 328–334.

Luther, V. & Wilkin, A. (2007). HIV infection in older adults. *Clin Geriatr Med*, *23*(3), 567–583, vii.

Mallewa, J., Wilkins, E., Vilar, J., Mallewa, M., Doran, D., Back, D., et al. (2008). HIV-associated lipodystrophy: A review of underlying mechanisms and therapeutic options. *J Antimicrob Chemother*, *62*(4), 648–660.

Mann, D., Iwatsubo, T., Pickering-Brown, S., Owen, F., Saido, T., & Perry, R. (1997). Preferential deposition of amyloid beta protein (Abeta) in the form Abeta40 in Alzheimer's disease is associated with a gene dosage effect of the apolipoprotein E E4 allele. *Neurosci Lett*, *221*(2–3), 81–84.

Martin-Thormeyer, E. & Paul, R. (2009). Drug abuse and hepatitis C infection as comorbid features of HIV associated neurocognitive disorder: Neurocognitive and neuroimaging features. *Neuropsychol Rev*, *19*(2), 215–231.

Mathis, C., Wang, Y., Holt, D., Huang, G., Debnath, M., & Klunk, W. (2003). Synthesis and evaluation of 11C-labeled 6-substituted 2-arylbenzothiazoles as amyloid imaging agents. *J Med Chem*, *46*(13), 2740–2754.

McMurtray, A., Nakamoto, B., Shikuma, C., & Valcour, V. (2007). Small-vessel vascular disease in human immunodeficiency virus infection: The Hawaii aging with HIV cohort study. *Cerebrovasc Dis*, *24*(2–3), 236–241.

Mesulam, M., Shaw, P., Mash, D., & Weintraub, S. (2004). Cholinergic nucleus basalis tauopathy emerges early in the aging-MCI-AD continuum. *Ann Neurol*, *55*(6), 815–828.

Moore, D., Masliah, E., Rippeth, J., Gonzalez, R., Carey, C., Cherner, M., et al. (2006). Cortical and subcortical neurodegeneration is associated with HIV neurocognitive impairment. *AIDS*, *20*(6), 879–887.

Morris, J. & Price, A. (2001). Pathologic correlates of nondemented aging, mild cognitive impairment, and early-stage Alzheimer's disease. *J Mol Neurosci*, *17*(2), 101–118.

Mucke, L., Abraham, C., Ruppe, M., Rockenstein, E., Toggas, S., Mallory, M., et al. (1995). Protection against HIV-1 gp120-induced brain damage by neuronal expression of human amyloid precursor protein. *J Exp Med*, *181*(4), 1551–1556.

Nakamura, T. & Lipton, S. (2009). Cell death: Protein misfolding and neurodegenerative diseases. *Apoptosis*, *14*(4), 455–468.

Näslund, J., Haroutunian, V., Mohs, R., Davis, K., Davies, P., Greengard, P., et al. (2000). Correlation between elevated levels of amyloid beta-peptide in the brain and cognitive decline. *JAMA*, *283*(12), 1571–1577.

Nath, A. & Hersh, L. (2005). Tat and amyloid: Multiple interactions. *AIDS*, *19*(2), 203–204.

Nath, A., Schiess, N., Venkatesan, A., Rumbaugh, J., Sacktor, N., & McArthur, J. (2008). Evolution of HIV dementia with HIV infection. *Int Rev Psychiatry*, *20*(1), 25–31.

Nicoll, J., Yamada, M., Frackowiak, J., Mazur-Kolecka, B., & Weller, R. (2004). Cerebral amyloid angiopathy plays a direct role in the pathogenesis of Alzheimer's disease. Pro-CAA position statement. *Neurobiol Aging*, *25*(5), 589–597; discussion 603–604.

Pemberton, L., Stone, E., Price, P., van Bockxmeer, F., & Brew, B. (2008). The relationship between ApoE, TNFA, IL1a, IL1b and IL12b genes and HIV-1-associated dementia. *HIV Med*, *9*(8), 677–680.

Perrin, R., Fagan A., & Holtzman, D. (2009). Multimodal techniques for diagnosis and prognosis of Alzheimer's disease. *Nature*, *461*(7266), 916–922.

Piccinini, M., Rinaudo, M., Anselmino, A., Buccinnà, B., Ramondetti, C., Dematteis, A., et al. (2005). The HIV protease inhibitors nelfinavir and saquinavir, but not a variety of HIV reverse transcriptase inhibitors, adversely affect human proteasome function. *Antivir Ther*, *10*(2), 215–223.

Pickford, F., Masliah, E., Britschgi, M., Lucin, K., Narasimhan, R., Jaeger, P., et al. (2008). The autophagy-related protein beclin 1 shows reduced expression in early Alzheimer disease and regulates amyloid beta accumulation in mice. *J Clin Invest*, *118*(6), 2190–2199.

Pomara, N., Belzer, K., Silva, R., Cooper, T., & Sidtis, J. (2008). The apolipoprotein E epsilon4 allele and memory performance in HIV-1 seropositive subjects: Differences at baseline but not after acute oral lorazepam challenge. *Psychopharmacology (Berl)*, *201*(1), 125–135.

Price, J. (1997). Diagnostic criteria for Alzheimer's disease. *Neurobiol Aging*, *18*(4 Suppl), S67–70.

Ramage, S., Anthony, I., Carnie, F., Busuttil, A., Robertson, R., & Bell, J. (2005). Hyperphosphorylated tau and amyloid precursor protein deposition is increased in the brains of young drug abusers. *Neuropathol Appl Neurobiol*, *31*(4), 439–448.

Reiman, E., Chen, K., Liu, X., Bandy, D., Yu, M., Lee, W., et al. (2009). Fibrillar amyloid-beta burden in cognitively normal people at 3 levels of genetic risk for Alzheimer's disease. *Proc Natl Acad Sci U S A*, *106*(16), 6820–6825.

Rempel, H. & Pulliam, L. (2005). HIV-1 Tat inhibits neprilysin and elevates amyloid beta. *AIDS*, *19*(2), 127–135.

Rippeth, J., Heaton, R., Carey, C., Marcotte, T., Moore, D., Gonzalez, R., et al. (2004). Methamphetamine dependence increases risk of neuropsychological impairment in HIV infected persons. *J Int Neuropsychol Soc*, *10*(1), 1–14.

Roher, A., Kuo, Y., Potter, P., Emmerling, M., Durham, R., Walker, D., et al. (2000). Cortical cholinergic denervation elicits vascular A beta deposition. *Ann N Y Acad Sci*, *903*, 366–373.

Rowe, C., Ng, S., Ackermann, U., Gong, S., Pike, K., Savage, G., et al. (2007). Imaging beta-amyloid burden in aging and dementia. *Neurology*, *68*(20), 1718–1725.

Sassin, I., Schultz, C., Thal, D., Rüb, U., Arai, K., Braak, E., et al. (2000). Evolution of Alzheimer's disease-related cytoskeletal changes in the basal nucleus of Meynert. *Acta Neuropathol*, *100*(3), 259–269.

Sato, A. & Sato, Y. (1992). Regulation of regional cerebral blood flow by cholinergic fibers originating in the basal forebrain. *Neurosci Res*, *14*(4), 242–274.

Schifitto, G., Yiannoutsos, C., Ernst, T., Navia, B., Nath, A., Sacktor, N., et al. (2009). Selegiline and oxidative stress in HIV-associated cognitive impairment. *Neurology*, *73*(23), 1975–1981.

Schweinsburg, B., Taylor, M., Alhassoon, O., Gonzalez, R., Brown, G., Ellis, R., et al. (2005). Brain mitochondrial injury in human immunodeficiency virus-seropositive (HIV+) individuals taking nucleoside reverse transcriptase inhibitors. *J Neurovirol*, *11*(4), 356–364.

Shah, S., McGowan, J., Smith, C., Blum, S., & Klein, R. (2002). Comorbid conditions, treatment, and health maintenance in older persons with human immunodeficiency virus infection in New York City. *Clin Infect Dis*, *35*(10), 1238–1243.

Shanley, L., Irving, A., & Harvey, J. (2001). Leptin enhances NMDA receptor function and modulates hippocampal synaptic plasticity. *J Neurosci*, *21*(24), RC186.

Shoghi-Jadid, K., Small, G., Agdeppa, E, Kepe, V., Ercoli, L., Siddarth, P., et al. (2002). Localization of neurofibrillary tangles and beta-amyloid plaques in the brains of living patients with Alzheimer disease. *Am J Geriatr Psychiatry*, *10*(1), 24–35.

Small, G., Kepe, V., Ercoli, L., Siddarth, P., Bookheimer, S., Miller, K., et al. (2006). PET of brain amyloid and tau in mild cognitive impairment. *N Engl J Med*, *355*(25), 2652–2663.

Snider, B., Fagan, A., Roe, C., Shah, A., Grant, E., Xiong, C., et al. (2009). Cerebrospinal fluid biomarkers and rate of cognitive decline in very mild dementia of the Alzheimer type. *Arch Neurol, 66*(5), 638–645.

Soontornniyomkij, V., Risbrough, V., Young, J., Wallace, C., Soontornniyomkij, B., Jeste, D., et al. (2010). Short-term recognition memory impairment is associated with decreased expression of FK506 binding protein 51 in the aged mouse brain. *Age, 32*(3), 309–322.

Soontornniyomkij, V., Wang, G., Pittman, C., Wiley, C., & Achim, C. (1998). Expression of brain-derived neurotrophic factor protein in activated microglia of human immunodeficiency virus type 1 encephalitis. *Neuropathol Appl Neurobiol, 24*(6), 453–460.

Thal, D., Griffin, W., & Braak, H. (2008). Parenchymal and vascular Abeta-deposition and its effects on the degeneration of neurons and cognition in Alzheimer's disease. *J Cell Mol Med, 12*(5B), 1848–1862.

Tomlinson, G., Simmonds, P., Busuttil, A., Chiswick, A., & Bell, J. (1999). Upregulation of microglia in drug users with and without pre-symptomatic HIV infection. *Neuropathol Appl Neurobiol, 25*(5), 369–379.

Tumbarello, M., Rabagliati, R., De Gaetano Donati, K., Bertagnolio, S., Tamburrini, E., Tacconelli, E., et al. (2003). Older HIV-positive patients in the era of highly active antiretroviral therapy: Changing of a scenario. *AIDS, 17*(1), 128–131.

Vago, L., Bonetto, S., Nebuloni, M., Duca, P., Carsana, L., Zerbi, P., et al. (2002). Pathological findings in the central nervous system of AIDS patients on assumed antiretroviral therapeutic regimens: Retrospective study of 1597 autopsies. *AIDS, 16*(14), 1925–1928.

Valcour, V., Sacktor, N., Paul, R., Watters, M., Selnes, O., Shiramizu, B., et al. (2006). Insulin resistance is associated with cognition among HIV-1-infected patients: The Hawaii Aging with HIV Cohort. *J Acquir Immune Defic Syndr, 43*(4), 405–410.

Valcour, V., Shikuma, C., Shiramizu, B., Watters, M., Poff, P., Selnes, O., et al. (2004a). Age, apolipoprotein E4, and the risk of HIV dementia: The Hawaii Aging with HIV Cohort. *J Neuroimmunol, 157*(1–2), 197–202.

Valcour, V., Shikuma, C., Shiramizu, B., Watters, M., Poff, P., Selnes, O., et al. (2004b). Higher frequency of dementia in older HIV-1 individuals: The Hawaii Aging with HIV-1 Cohort. *Neurology, 63*(5), 822–827.

Valcour, V., Shikuma, C., Watters, M., & Sacktor, N. (2004c). Cognitive impairment in older HIV-1-seropositive individuals: Prevalence and potential mechanisms. *AIDS, 18* Suppl 1, S79–86.

Valcour, V. & Shiramizu, B. (2004). HIV-associated dementia, mitochondrial dysfunction, and oxidative stress. *Mitochondrion, 4*(2–3), 119–129.

Walsh, D., Klyubin, I., Fadeeva, J., Cullen, W., Anwyl, R., Wolfe, M., et al. (2002). Naturally secreted oligomers of amyloid beta protein potently inhibit hippocampal long-term potentiation in vivo. *Nature, 416*(6880), 535–539.

Wiley, C. & Achim, C. (1994). Human immunodeficiency virus encephalitis is the pathological correlate of dementia in acquired immunodeficiency syndrome. *Ann Neurol, 36*(4), 673–676.

Wochnik, G., Rüegg, J., Abel, G., Schmidt, U., Holsboer, F., & Rein, T. (2005). FK506-binding proteins 51 and 52 differentially regulate dynein interaction and nuclear translocation of the glucocorticoid receptor in mammalian cells. *J Biol Chem, 280*(6), 4609–4616.

Woods, S., Moore, D., Weber, E., & Grant, I. (2009). Cognitive neuropsychology of HIV-associated neurocognitive disorders. *Neuropsychol Rev, 19*(2), 152–168.

Yankner, B., Lu, T., & Loerch, P. (2008). The aging brain. *Annu Rev Pathol, 3*, 41–66.

Zlokovic, B., Deane, R., Sallstrom, J., Chow, N., & Miano, J. (2005). Neurovascular pathways and Alzheimer amyloid beta-peptide. *Brain Pathol, 15*(1), 78–83.

7.9

ADDICTION

R. Douglas Bruce

Substance use disorders can increase the risk of HIV infection directly, through the sharing of needles among injection drug users, and indirectly, through facilitation of high-risk sexual contacts. It is therefore not surprising that many HIV-infected patients have one or more substance use disorders. Substance use can impede adherence to HIV treatment regimens, resulting in significant morbidity and mortality, including the development of HIV resistance. Evidence-based treatments for substance use disorders, consisting of psychosocial support, mental health counseling, and pharmacotherapy for addiction, are necessary to improve health outcomes in this population. This chapter focuses on pharmacotherapy for substance use disorders.

INTRODUCTION

Substance use disorders include a range of behaviors from the abuse of a substance such as a drug or alcohol to dependence upon that substance. The diagnosis is based on the behavioral, cognitive, and physiological symptoms as well as the maladaptive patterns of drug use and varied consequences related to use. Substance use disorders have many well-known adverse consequences for the individual and for society, including, but not limited to, the promotion of risk-related behaviors leading to the acquisition of HIV and hepatitis B or C. Alcohol consumption, for example, is associated with risky sexual behaviors that increase the risk of HIV acquisition (Hendershot, Stoner, George, & Norris, 2007). Alcohol consumption is common in HIV clinical settings. Chander and colleagues reported on a cross-sectional study of 951 HIV-infected patients at 14 primary care sites in the US and found that 40% of the sample reported some alcohol use in the 4 weeks prior to the interview, with 11% meeting criteria for hazardous drinking (Chander et al., 2008). Illicit drug use is well known to enhance HIV risk behaviors, either through the direct means of needle or syringe sharing or the indirect means of facilitating sexual risk (Metzger et al., 1993). These problems remain large, multinational issues as seen by the approximately 15.9 million individuals in 148 countries that inject drugs of abuse, and where it is estimated that 3 million of these are HIV infected (Mathers et al., 2008). It is therefore not surprising that many HIV-infected patients have one or more substance use disorders involved in the etiology of their HIV infection that further complicates their ongoing treatment of HIV and other acquired diseases such as hepatitis B or C (Bruce & Altice, 2007). Ongoing substance use can impede adherence to HIV therapy, resulting in significant morbidity and mortality, including the development of HIV resistance (Maru et al., 2007; Kozal, 2009).Evidence-based treatments for substance use disorders, consisting of psychosocial support, mental health counseling, and pharmacotherapy for addiction (also termed medication-assisted treatment [MAT]), are necessary to improve health outcomes in this population. This chapter focuses on the pharmacotherapy involved in the treatment of substance use disorders.

NEUROBIOLOGY OF ADDICTION

Despite the possibility of negative health consequences from substance use disorders, individuals continue to engage in use for a variety of reasons. Some individuals consume drugs and/or alcohol *to feel good*—that is, to have novel feelings, sensations, and experiences—while others take them *to feel better*—that is, to lessen the symptoms of anxiety, fears, depression, and hopelessness (Stefanis & Kokkevi, 1986; Castenada, Galanter, & Franco, 1989). In support of the self-medication hypothesis is the finding that prevalence of major depressive disorder is upwards of 50% among opioid-dependent patients in some cross-sectional studies (Blatt, Rounsaville, Eyre, & Wilber, 1984). Not all substance use disorders constitute addiction, however. Addiction is a severe manifestation of a substance use disorder and is characterized by a compulsive behavior that is reinforcing—pleasurable or rewarding—where there is loss of control in limiting the intake of that substance (Kresina, Bruce, & McCance-Katz, 2009). Extensive research over the past fifty years has mapped the neurobiology of the brain related to substance dependence and the wide-ranging and complex neurobiological adaptations resulting from the chronic use of these substances (Chao & Nestler, 2004; Stimmel & Kreek, 2000; DiChiara & North, 1992; Nestler & Aghajanian, 1997). These adaptations can be long lasting in their effects. Some data have suggested, for example, that at least two years of opioid-agonist therapy may be required to stabilize neuronal changes acquired while using short-acting opioids such as heroin (Kaufman et al., 1999). In the case of methamphetamine use and HIV, some changes are correlated with actual neuronal damage that may or may not be completely reversible (Letendre et al., 2005; Jernigan et al., 2005; Chang, Ernst, Speck, & Grob, 2005; Rippeth et al., 2004).

Understanding why some people become addicted to substances and others do not will help clarify strategies for prevention and treatment. Vulnerability to addiction is on a spectrum between genetics (biology) and environmental factors (Figure 7.9.1). Specifically, some individuals are more genetically susceptible, and some more resistant, to specific addictions (Volkow et al., 2009; Nestler, 2001).Volkow and colleagues demonstrated this idea of genetic susceptibility elegantly in a study examining nonaddicted individuals' experience of methylphenidate (a stimulant) and found that the experience associated with the substance was related to the concentration of dopamine 2 receptors (Figure 7.9.2) (Volkow et al., 1999). The concentration of dopamine 2 receptors, therefore, correlated with the experience—the genetic predetermination of the number of receptors increased the probability of a pleasure response associated with use and thereby increased the risk of ongoing self-administration of the substance to maintain that pleasurable feeling. Some individuals may not be genetically predisposed to find a particular substance as reinforcing; however, these individuals may reside in environments that promote or make easily available particular substances. Tobacco is an example. Although many African Americans may be genetically predisposed to having slower metabolism of nicotine at CYP 2A6 with resultant greater side-effects from use and theoretically less use, African Americans smoke in abundance (Benowitz, 2008; Johnstone et al., 2006).There may be many environmental reasons for African Americans to smoke related to socioeconomics, but one interesting common factor is the abundance of menthol cigarettes that are smoked by African Americans (Richter, Beistle, Pederson, & O'Hegarty, 2008). Possibly, the environmental addition of menthol has moderated some of the theoretical genetic protective effects of slower nicotine metabolism (Allen & Unger, 2007).

The specific neurobiological mechanisms of addiction are related to several different pathways associated with dopamine and serotonin, chief of which is dopamine release in the nucleus accumbens (Di Chiara & Imperato, 1988a, 1988b; Nestler, Hope, & Widnell, 1993; Neslter, Alreja, & Aghajanian, 1994; Nestler, Berhow, & Brodkin, 1996). The nucleus accumbens (NA) is one of the neurobiological regions involved in reward and salience. Studies in rats have clearly demonstrated that the natural rewards of food and sex are associated with increases of dopamine in the NA of approximately 150% and 200%, respectively (Bassareo & Di Chiara, 1997). In contrast, dopamine increased in the NA over 1000% above basal levels with amphetamine, 300% with cocaine, 200% with nicotine,

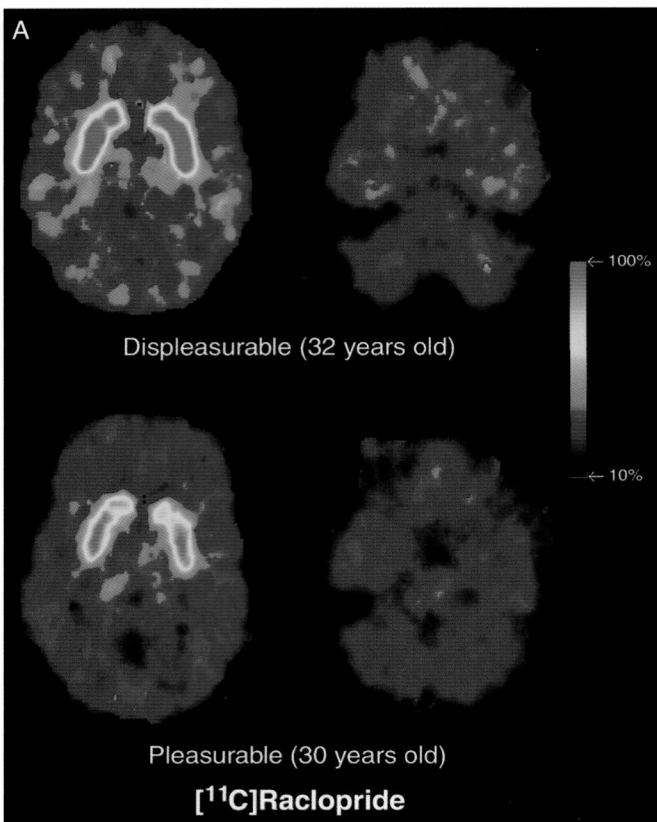

Displeasurable (32 years old)

← 100%

← 10%

Pleasurable (30 years old)

[^{11}C]Raclopride

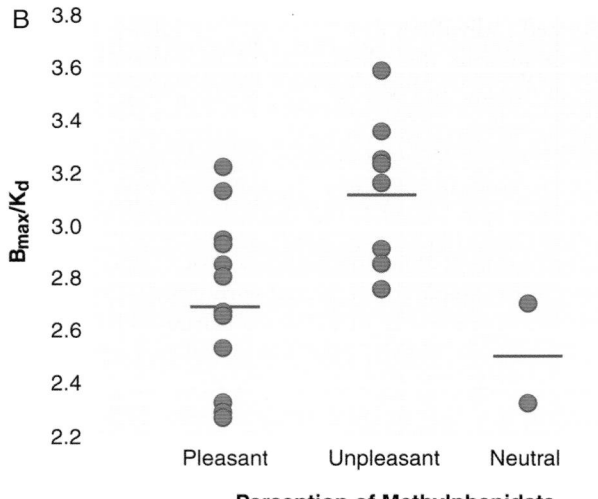

Figure 7.9.2 *Dopamine Receptors and the Response to Methylphenidate.* As a group, subjects with higher dopamine receptor levels (top panel) found methylphenidate (MP) unpleasant, while subjects with lower receptor levels (lower panel) found MP pleasant. Adapted with permission from Volkow and colleagues (Volkow et al., 1999).

and from approximately 150% to 200% above basal levels at different doses of morphine (Di Chiara & Imperato, 1988a). Such results help explain the common finding that substance dependent patients will engage in significant risk to obtain drugs because the end goal of drug use is more rewarding neurobiologically. In essence, the overwhelming physical and psychological reward that comes from the use of a substance

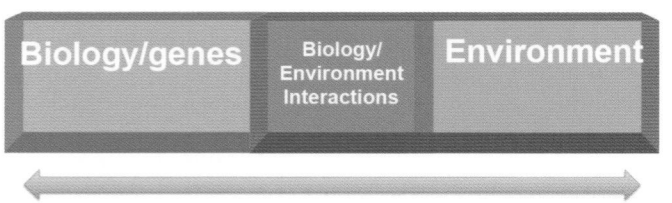

Figure 7.9.1 The Continuum between Biology and Environment.

stimulates a neurobiological system designed to preserve the individual. Opioids, for example, are a better neurobiological reward than food and so opioid-dependent patients will "ingest" heroin to "feed" this neurobiological pathway rather than eating actual food to preserve the body. Hence, opioid-dependent individuals are often underweight and malnourished. This neurobiology assists in framing why individuals will place themselves at risk for infectious diseases, physical and psychological trauma, and incarceration. The individual's brain has been primed to expect an exogenous opioid such as heroin and the brain will do all it can to move the individual to obtaining and using the opioid (Nestler, 2004). This neurobiology, which explains some of the individual's behavior, is in tension with the very real possibility of the individual making informed choices that go against this neurobiological programming (otherwise sobriety could never occur). These choices, however, become more difficult because of the neurobiological effect of addiction upon mechanisms of reward and salience, memory and learning, motivation and drive, and inhibitory control as illustrated in Figure 7.9.3 (Volkow, Fowler, & Wang, 2004). This emphasizes the challenge of treating the substance user: If, for example, medical providers are unable to have patients cease a lesser neurobiological reward such as being sexually abstinent, by counseling the patient on the risks of sexually transmitted diseases, providers must look beyond simple advice and consider the appropriate use of pharmacotherapy which may assist the patient in achieving sobriety.

Addicted individuals often suffer a host of maladies that further complicate the physical and psychological consequences of dependency and withdrawal and, in turn, craving and relapse to drug and alcohol use. These include social factors (e.g., the effects of homelessness), psychological stress (e.g., fear of domestic violence), and comorbid mental illness (e.g., post-traumatic stress disorder), which can interact with each other in varying ways and to varying degrees to negatively affect cognitive function (Drake, Wallach, & McGovern, 2005; Kresina et al., 2005; Rollins et al., 2005). In addition, both HIV and hepatitis C can independently cause neurocognitive dysfunction, making therapies based on neurocognitive ability more difficult (e.g., Alcoholics Anonymous and cognitive behavioral therapy) (Forton et al., 2005; Shaham, Erb, & Stewart, 2000; Soogoor et al., 2006; Parsons et al., 2006; Cysique, Maruff, & Brew, 2006; Waldrop-Valverde et al., 2006; Laskus et al., 2005). Individuals with the stressors and neurocognitive impairment as detailed above are all the more in need of medication-assisted treatment to reduce risk-taking behavior and assist in the stabilization of their other medical and psychiatric diseases.

PHARMACOLOGICAL THERAPIES FOR ADDICTION

Treatment for addiction includes pharmacologic treatment, behavioral therapies, medical treatment for complications of addiction (e.g., HIV and hepatitis C), and social services. In some sense, treating addiction with pharmacological therapies is less complicated than managing HIV infection with antiretroviral therapy, in that resistance does not develop to treatments for addiction. If a practitioner can manage the pharmacotherapy of HIV infection, that medical provider is already well equipped to incorporate pharmacological therapies for addiction. The following sections provide an overview of medication treatment strategies for addictions commonly seen in HIV clinical practice and are summarized in Table 7.9.1.

Table 7.9.1 SUMMARY TABLE OF PHARAMCOTHERAPIES

MEDICATION	DOSAGE AND RECOMMENDATIONS	STRENGTH OF EVIDENCE
Alcohol Dependence		
Acamprosate	666 mg TID	CI
Disulfiram	250 mg qD	CI
Naltrexone	100 mg qD	AI
Topiramate	Start at 25 mg qD and titrate to maximum of 300 mg qD	AI
Cocaine Dependence		
Disulfiram	250 mg qD	AI
Modafinil	200 or 400 mg qD	BI
Methamphetamine Dependence		
Bupropion	150 mg BID	BI
Modafinil	200 mg qD	BI
Opioid Dependence		
Buprenorphine	Individualize dosing based upon use: Range 8 to 32 mg sublingually qD	AI

(Continued)

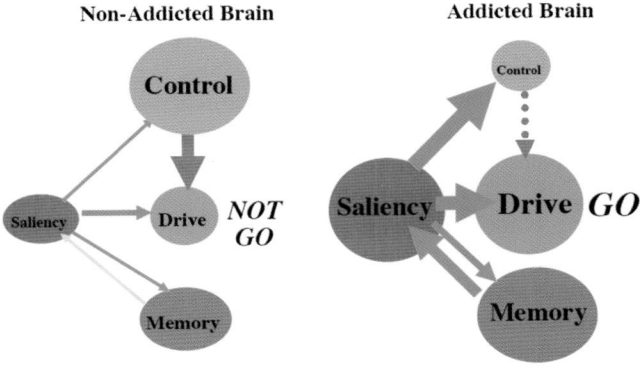

Figure 7.9.3 An addiction model proposed by Volkow and colleagues, taking into consideration imaging findings documenting abnormalities in brain circuits involving various pathways related to inhibitory control, saliency (or reward), memories, and motivation/drive. Adapted with permission from Volkow et al., 2004.

Table 7.9.1 (CONTINUED)

MEDICATION	DOSAGE AND RECOMMENDATIONS	STRENGTH OF EVIDENCE
Methadone	Individualize dose with higher doses (> 100 mg) showing improved retention	AI
Naltrexone	Various dosing with 50 mg to 100 mg either daily or three times weekly. Inferior to buprenorphine and methadone.	CI
Nicotine Dependence		
Nicotine Replacement	All forms work. Key is to find the form the patient will use	AI
Bupropion	Either 150 mg BID or 300 mg qD (SR only)	AI
Varenicline	Individualize dose with titration to effect with a goal of 1 mg BID	AI

A: Strong recommendation for the statement
B: Moderate recommendation for the statement
C: Optional recommendation for the statement
I: One or more randomized trials with clinical outcomes and/or validated laboratory endpoints.
II: One or more well-designed, nonrandomized trials or observational cohort studies with long-term clinical outcomes.
III: Expert Opinion

ALCOHOL

Alcohol use ranges from hazardous drinking to dependence and the effective treatment of these alcohol use disorders (AUDs) is critically important for the patient with HIV infection because alcohol dependence can result in ongoing risky sexual behaviors and compromise antiretroviral therapy (ARV) by influencing both access and adherence to ARVs (Samet, Walley, & Bridden, 2007). Bing and colleagues reported on a large nationally representative probability sample of 2,864 HIV-infected individuals receiving care in the US in 1996. This study reported on use within the prior 12 months and found that at least 53% of HIV-infected individuals attending clinic reported some alcohol use, with 18% reporting heavy or frequent heavy alcohol use (Bing et al., 2001). This high prevalence of alcohol use among HIV-infected patients was recently confirmed in a study of 1,555 people attending HIV clinics at six cities in the US. In this cross-sectional study, 55% met criteria for alcohol abuse or dependence at some point in their lives (Heaton et al., 2010). In addition to HIV, alcohol has well-known negative effects upon the course of hepatitis C (HCV) treatment and HIV/HCV co-infected patients with hazardous drinking are of special concern. Of particular concern is the interaction between alcohol and abacavir. Abacavir is the only ARV that shares alcohol's metabolic pathway. McDowell and colleagues examined the pharmacokinetic interaction between abacavir and ethanol in 24 HIV-infected men and found the AUC of abacavir increased 41%. It is not known if this increase in AUC correlates to increased toxicity (McDowell et al., 2000).

As in all chemical dependencies, a comprehensive approach to the treatment of alcohol dependence integrates psychosocial treatment with pharmacologic treatments (Weiss & Kueppenbender, 2006). In the physiologically dependent patient, a structured withdrawal utilizing benzodiazepines or barbiturates is also necessary and typically occurs on an inpatient unit. Afterwards, a combination of pharmacological and psychosocial treatments should be utilized to maintain abstinence and can be prescribed by a primary care provider (Bruce, Kresina, & McCance-Katz, 2010). The specific pharmacological treatments for alcohol dependence are described in detail below in alphabetical order.

ACAMPROSATE

Acamprosate is a structural analogue of the GABA neurotransmitter and is U. S. Food and Drug Administration (FDA) approved for the treatment of alcohol dependence (Thomson, 2006). Studies have suggested that acamprosate facilitates the function of GABA receptors and/or may attenuate the effect of glutamate at NMDA-type receptors. The cumulative effect results in restoration of a balance between neuronal excitation and inhibition in the central nervous system that is hypothesized to be altered in chronic alcoholics and plays a role in relapse (Thomson, 2006; Littleton, 1995; Mason et al., 2002). Sixteen trials with a total of more than 4,500 patients have demonstrated a modest advantage over placebo in maintaining abstinence from alcohol (Mason, 2001). A large, randomized controlled trial comparing naltrexone, acamprosate, or a combined behavioral intervention, however, did not demonstrate a benefit of acamprosate over placebo and was inferior to naltrexone (Anton et al., 2006). Acamprosate dosing of two capsules, three times a day, raises an obvious concern regarding medication adherence and may account for some of the lack of benefit in these trials (Mason, 2001). This greater pill burden, compared to naltrexone and disulfiram, may be of particular importance in patients with HIV who may have competing priorities for adherence with large numbers of medications to be taken daily.

DISULFIRAM

Disulfiram was first discovered as a possible treatment for alcoholism in 1937 by E.E. Williams and became the first FDA-approved treatment for alcohol dependence in 1951 (Suh et al., 2006). Disulfiram works by blocking the oxidation of alcohol, resulting in 5 to 10 times increased levels of acetaldehyde, which produces flushing, headache, nausea, vomiting, sweating, chest pain, palpitations, and tachycardia. The psychopharmacological principle of disulfiram was aversive conditioning. The goal was for the patient to experience the aversive effect of disulfiram in the presence of alcohol; that is, precipitate a disulfiram reaction with the hope that the patient would avoid future alcohol use. This was achieved by titrating the exact dose of disulfiram to the minimum dose required to experience aversion when administered alcohol. Over time, physicians stopped having patients purposefully experience the disulfiram-alcohol interaction. Instead, physicians described the interaction, hoping the fear of an adverse effect rather than aversive conditioning itself would be sufficient to reduce alcohol consumption. The description of the interaction rather than the actual aversive experience is materially different and may be one reason that Fuller and colleagues found disulfiram to be no different than placebo in a randomized controlled trial of 605 veterans (Fuller et al., 1986). Adherence is an obvious additional and likely more important issue, as a failure to ingest disulfiram means alcohol can be consumed without concern for a disulfiram reaction. Typically adherence support is necessary to achieve an improved rate of abstinence and occurs when a treatment provider and/or significant other monitors ingestion. The interactions of disulfiram with HIV medications are unknown, but are presently being studied. Disulfiram is bioactivated by cytochrome P450 3A4 to metabolites that inhibit the metabolism of alcohol (Madan, Parkinson, & Faiman, 1998). Thus, the co-administration of medications that alter hepatic metabolizing enzyme function, such as some antiretroviral medications, could alter the effectiveness of disulfiram.

NALTREXONE

Naltrexone, an opioid receptor antagonist, is the most studied and consistently most effective pharmacotherapy for alcohol dependence (Anton et al., 2006). Opioid receptor antagonists bind to but do not activate the receptor, and they prevent activation by full and partial agonists. Alcohol appears to stimulate receptor-mediated dopamine release through a complex mechanism involving gamma-aminobutyric acid and the endogenous opioid system. The involvement of the opioid receptor system appears to constitute the reinforcing effects of alcohol; therefore, by blocking the μ-opioid receptor, naltrexone acts to decrease the reinforcement associated with that behavior; likely tied, ultimately, to the dopamine reward (O'Malley & Froehlich, 2003; O'Malley, 1996; O'Brien, 2005; Gianoulakis, Krishnan, & Thavundayil, 1996). Patients on naltrexone-based pharmacotherapy while drinking alcohol have a decrease in heavy drinking days while those who are abstinent tend to have prolonged abstinence and relapses of reduced severity (Balldin et al., 2003; Petrakis et al., 2005; Monterosso et al., 2001). The currently recommended dosage is 100 mg/d, and vigilance for hepatotoxicity must be maintained (Anton et al., 2006). Expert opinion suggests that even lower doses of naltrexone may be effective in the treatment of alcohol dependence; therefore, medical providers should be encouraged to prescribe naltrexone, as even low doses of 25 mg may have clinical benefit.

As with all pharmacotherapies for addiction, treatment effectiveness is a function of medication adherence. An injectable formulation is available which provides therapeutic plasma concentrations of naltrexone over a 30-day period in an attempt to provide adherence support. Importantly, some patients with HIV disease may require opioids for chronic pain or for the treatment of opioid dependence (e.g., methadone and buprenorphine as described below) and naltrexone, as an opioid antagonist, will antagonize opioid activity, making it ineffective. HIV medical providers should carefully consider the possible need of opioid pain therapy before prescribing naltrexone to alcohol-dependent patients with HIV.

TOPIRAMATE

The anticonvulsant topiramate, which appears to act at gamma-aminobutyric acid receptors, has been shown to be effective for alcohol dependence in several studies, but is not approved by the Food and Drug Administration (FDA) for the treatment of alcohol dependence (Johnson et al., 2003; Johnson et al., 2008; Kenna et al., 2009). Doses vary by study, but generally treatment is started at low doses (e.g., 25 mg/d) with titration to a maximum dose of 300 mg/d over 6 weeks. Topiramate has proved useful in decreasing alcohol consumption and reducing symptoms of withdrawal. Naltrexone, an opioid antagonist, cannot be prescribed to patients on opioids (e.g., methadone or buprenorphine); therefore, topirimate is a possibility for alcohol-dependent patients receiving treatment with opioids. Studies evaluating its efficacy and safety among HIV-infected patients on ARVs have not been conducted.

BENZODIAZEPINES

Although benzodiazepines may be prescribed for therapeutic purposes, they can also be abused and result in physiological dependence (Denis, Fatseas, Lavie, & Auriacombe, 2006). Benzodiazepines vary greatly in pharmacokinetic parameters such as absorption, half-life, and metabolic pathway (Wynn et al., 2005). The benzodiazepines most prone to abuse are those with a rapid onset of action and short-half life (e.g., alprazolam and midazolam). In one convenient sample of buprenorphine injectors in Malaysia, those seeking to obtain euphoria not present in the injected buprenorphine also injected midazolam. The midazolam use resulted in amnesia regarding the events after use (Bruce et al., 2008). This anterograde amnesia is characteristic of all benzodiazepine use and is an effect to which the individual never develops tolerance (Roth & Roehrs, 1992). Additionally, these users may participate in riskier sexual behaviors and/or may be assaulted due to the increased impairment of the benzodiazepine with little recollection of the events (Djezzar, Questel, Burin, & Dally, 2009). Additionally, sex workers may gravitate towards benzodiazepines as their amnesia-inducing quality may be a welcome relief from the trauma related to some sex work (Roxburgh, Degenhardt, & Breen, 2005). This inability to remember events, conversations, and lessons learned impedes progress during psychosocial treatments for drug and alcohol dependence.

Substance users often consider benzodiazepines to be less dangerous than heroin or cocaine because benzodiazepines are tablets made by pharmaceutical companies while heroin is illicit. Benzodiazepine users may not be aware of the withdrawal risks of benzodiazepines and may incorrectly believe they have panic attacks when in reality the increasing anxiety they are experiencing is the result of benzodiazepine withdrawal (Bruce et al., 2008). As with alcohol withdrawal, abrupt withdrawal of benzodiazepines can result in seizures and death. Structured withdrawal from alcohol and benzodiazepines is necessary to safely withdraw from these substances and benzodiazepines or barbiturates can be employed to structurally withdraw patients (Hayner & Inaba, 1983; Ravi et al., 1990; Hayner, Galloway, & Wiehl, 1993).

Pharmacological therapies for benzodiazepine abuse are lacking and typically patients are transferred from benzodiazepines with a shorter half-life and higher abuse potential (e.g., alprazolam) to ones with a longer half-life and theoretically a lower abuse potential (e.g., clonazepam). In other instances, alternatives to a benzodiazepine may be sought to treat the symptoms of protracted withdrawal or underlying anxiety that may have promoted the benzodiazepine abuse.

Several pharmacological interactions of particular concern among individuals taking ARVs and benzodiazepines have been described (Bruce, Altice, & Friedland, 2008). In summary, patients should be cautioned about combining delavirdine (Tran, Gerber, & Kerr, 2001), ritonavir (Hsu, Granneman, & Bertz, 1998), ketoconazole (Albengres, Le Louet, & Tillement, 1998), clarithromycin (Dresser, Spence, & Bailey, 2000), and atazanavir (Le Tiec, Barrail, Goujard, & Taburet, 2005) with midazolam, triazolam, flunitrazepam, or alprazolam to avoid the potential for toxicity. Such combinations could lead to elevated plasma concentrations of these benzodiazepines with increased sedation and respiratory depression.

CANNABIS

In a study by Heaton and colleagues, 1,555 HIV-infected patients at several sites in the US were surveyed as part of a study to assess the prevalence of neurocognitive deficits in this population. This study found a lifetime cannabis use of approximately 30% in this population, with a much lower percentage (1–2%) currently using.

Among the substances described in this chapter, cannabis may seem to be the least hazardous. This misunderstanding often leads clinical providers to refrain from discussions with patients regarding the use of cannabis. As a general rule in pulmonology, the inhaling of smoke from any burning substance remains hazardous for alveolar tissue. The long-term effects of cannabis smoking are difficult to assess as many cannabis users also smoke tobacco.

Published data demonstrate a benefit to short-term cannabis use during hepatitis C (HCV) treatment likely because the cannabis ameliorates the anorexia and anxiety induced by the interferon (Fischer et al., 2006; Sylvestre, Clements, & Malibu, 2006).Chronic use, however, appears to promote hepatic fibrosis, possibly through a cannabinoid-mediated mechanism (Hezode et al., 2005).

Cannabis does not result in physiological dependence like alcohol or benzodiazepines. The main stay of treatment, therefore, remains psychosocial support rather than pharmacological treatments. Cannabis users with underlying mental illness, such as an anxiety disorder,who are using cannabis as a means to treat that disorder, will require other pharmacological treatments if they are going to cease cannabis use.

COCAINE

Cocaine hydrochloride is a water-soluble salt that can be injected or taken by nasal insufflation ("snorted"). Although cocaine hydrochloride cannot effectively be smoked because it is heat labile, it can be chemically converted to a base ("crack") that can be smoked. The onset of action from pulmonary absorption of "crack" and injection of cocaine are comparable and occur in seconds. Cocaine's half-life is short, resulting in the need for frequent administration and active cocaine users may use cocaine as many as 20 times a day.

Cocaine accelerates HIV replication (Roth et al., 2002) and may act as a cofactor in the pathogenesis of HIV and may increase susceptibility to HIV through the suppression of HIV-protective chemokines and/or the upregulation of the HIV co-receptor, CCR5 (Nair et al., 2001; Nair et al., 2000).

Cocaine inhibits the reuptake of dopamine from the synaptic cleft, thereby increasing levels of dopamine in the nucleus accumbens and VTA (Huang, Gu, & Zhan, 2009). This rapid increase in dopamine produces the reinforcing effects of cocaine. Extensive work has gone into studying various behavioral and pharmacological treatments for cocaine dependence (Vocci & Ling, 2005). Several medications have been investigated for cocaine dependence, including tiagabine (Sofuoglu et al., 2005; Winhusen et al., 2005; Gorelick, Gardner, & Xi, 2004; Gonzalez et al., 2003), topiramate (Johnson, 2005; Kampman et al., 2004), and several other agents including modafinil. Modafinil has shown some promise in the treatment of cocaine dependence (Umanoff, 2005; Donovan et al., 2005; Dackis et al., 2005; Dackis et al., 2003; Hart et al., 2008; Martinez-Raga, Knecht, & Cepeda, 2008). The most recent and largest randomized controlled trial, however, did not demonstrate a statistical benefit of modafinil over placebo in the primary outcome of weekly percent of cocaine non-use. This study was a double-blind randomized control trial of modafinil 200 mg, 400 mg, or placebo in a total of 210 treatment-seeking cocaine-dependent patients over a 12-week period (Anderson et al., 2009). Although this study did not show a benefit in the primary outcome measure, interest in modafinil continues due to reports of decreased cocaine craving among patients and possible benefits with sleep normalization (Anderson et al.,2009). Specifically, in a small randomized trial of modafinil 400 mg or placebo (total of 20 patients), morning-dosed modafinil was found to promote nocturnal sleep, normalize sleep architecture, and decrease daytime sleepiness in abstinent cocaine users (Morgan, et al., 2010).

The most promising agent to date remains disulfiram. After an effect of decreasing cocaine use was observed in patients with joint alcohol-cocaine dependence, disulfiram was found to reduce cocaine use in cocaine-dependent patients receiving methadone. Six randomized controlled trials have now shown the efficacy of disulfiram in treating cocaine dependence (Carroll et al., 1998; Carroll et al., 2000; George et al., 2000; Petrakis et al., 2000; Carroll et al., 2004). Disulfiram acts by inhibiting dopamine beta-hydroxylase activity, thus increasing dopamine levels in the synaptic cleft via a mechanism somewhat similar to that of cocaine. Compared with cocaine, which has a rapid onset of action and rapid attenuation of effect, disulfiram is slow acting. The goal of pharmacological therapy for cocaine is to relieve the craving for dopamine by maintaining stable, elevated levels. Taking cocaine in addition to disulfiram frequently results in a less rewarding, dysphoric response caused by excessive amounts of dopamine.

Although the dose of disulfiram that has been studied most extensively is 250 mg/d, the exact dosing in HIV and HCV co-infected patients has not been evaluated and treatment should likely be started at around 125 mg/d (half a tablet) because of the lack of data in this patient group, the concern about potential effects of disulfiram on aspartate aminotransferase and alanine aminotransferase levels, and possible pharmacological interactions with HIV therapies as disulfiram is bioactivated by CYP 3A4 (Madan et al., 1998). As discussed with alcohol dependence, adherence remains a problem with disulfiram. Treatment works well for motivated patients and for patients receiving disulfiram along with methadone maintenance.

Primary care physicians can help increase the beneficial use of this valuable resource in their cocaine-dependent patients. Because pharmacotherapies for cocaine dependence are an ongoing area of development, it is important for medical providers to have available the assistance of addiction medicine experts to provide consultation for patients who continue to struggle with cocaine use despite ongoing pharmacotherapy and counseling. Not all patients will want to use pharmacotherapy and it is critical that encounters with medical providers remain nonjudgmental if patients are going to be engaged in care rather than risk losing them to follow-up and diminish the likelihood of risk reduction interventions.

METHAMPHETAMINE

Methamphetamine is a stimulant that is similar in chemical structure to amphetamine but has more profound neurobiological effects on the central nervous system. It can be smoked, snorted, injected, ingested orally, or administered rectally. Like cocaine, methamphetamine ingestion produces stimulation and similar feelings of euphoria; however, methamphetamine has a much longer duration of action (6 to 8 hours after a single dose). Tolerance develops rapidly and escalation of dose and frequency is required. As is the case with other substances of abuse and dependence, methamphetamine use is associated with high-risk sexual behaviors (Halkitis, Mukherjee, & Palamar, 2009; Rawson et al., 2008).

Methamphetamine can have profound effects on the central nervous system, such as a loss of dopamine transporters in the brain and slowing of motor reactions and memory loss (Kalechstein, Newton, & Green, 2003; Rendell, Mazur, & Henry, 2009; Volkow et al., 2001a, 2001b). The neurocognitive effects associated with methamphetamine use are exacerbated in HIV-infected patients and the combination of methamphetamine use and HIV may result in permanent neurobiological changes as seen in Figure 7.9.4 (Volkow et al., 2001a; Chana et al., 2006; Everall et al., 2005). Methamphetamine increases HIV replication and also increases the expression of CCR5 on macrophages and these

events may contribute to the immunopathogenesis of HIV-infected methamphetamine users and may contribute to the greater neurocognitive effects seen in these individuals (Toussi et al., 2009; Liang et al., 2008; Cadet & Krasnova, 2007). Reduced neurocognitive performance in the HIV-infected methamphetamine user can severely compromise HIV clinical care and is associated with HIV nonadherence and the development of HIV resistance. Trials of selegeline, ondansetron, paroxetine, and sertraline have not demonstrated efficacy with high attrition rates (Piasecki et al., 2002; Shoptaw et al., 2006). The two most promising pharmacotherapies to date are buproprion and modafinil, as described below.

In a study by Shoptaw and colleagues, bupropion 150 mg twice daily was no more effective than placebo in reducing methamphetamine use through the planned analyses; however, in secondary analyses it did produce some reduction in methamphetamine use among *mild* users of methamphetamine (Shoptaw et al., 2008). There was a reduction in tobacco use among those assigned to the bupropion arm as is consistent with known effects of bupropion (Hurt et al., 1997). Given the tolerability of this medication and the known reduction in tobacco use, it should be considered as a first-line pharmacotherapy agent for methamphetamine use until further studies demonstrated a more beneficial agent.

One promising study by McElhiney and colleagues reported on the use of modafinil in combination with cognitive behavioral therapy among HIV-infected men who have sex with men (MSM). The study was a small, single-blinded pilot of 13 patients on modafinil for 12 weeks followed by a 4-week placebo phase with 18 sessions of cognitive behavioral therapy (CBT) over the 16-week study. The starting dose of modafinil was 50 mg/day for those on HIV therapy and 100 mg/day for those not taking HIV therapy. Doses were titrated up to 200 mg/day in the absence of clinical response and significant side effects. At the conclusion of the study, ten subjects completed, with six of the ten reducing methamphetamine use by over 50% (McElhiney et al., 2009). This pilot, however, was small and the absence of a control arm to control for the effect of CBT confounds the result. Shearer and colleagues conducted a double-blind placebo-controlled trial among 80 methamphetamine users for 10 weeks with an additional 12 weeks of follow-up. Eighty subjects were randomly assigned to modafinil 200 mg/day or placebo and no specific counseling method was utilized in this study. Reductions in systolic blood pressure and weight gain were statistically better in the modafinil group compared to placebo; however, there was no difference in methamphetamine abstinence or craving (Shearer et al., 2009). In both studies, subjects who accessed counseling had improved outcomes and so clinicians may consider its use in the motivated patient who is currently engaged in treatment and did not experience a benefit with bupropion.

As with disulfiram for cocaine dependence, bupropion and modafinil are not panaceas for methamphetamine use. Pharmacological therapy may tip the balance for some patients in favor of greater stability of behaviors and better participation in HIV disease care; however, ongoing counseling will be required to assist patients in reducing their ongoing use of methamphetamines.

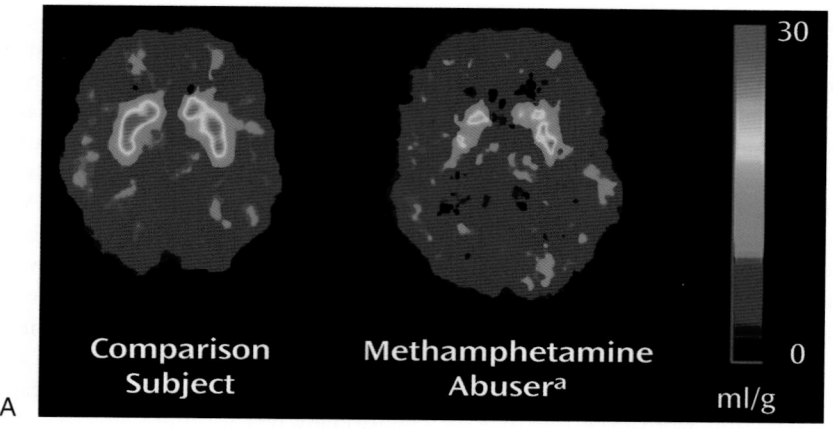

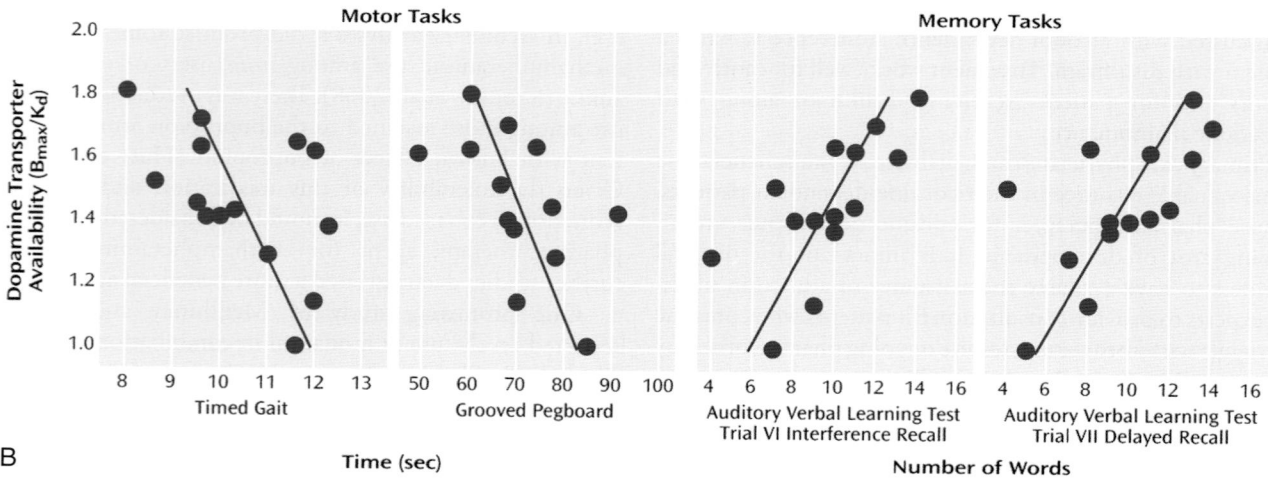

Figure 7.9.4 *Dopamine Transporters in Methamphetamine Users.* Adapted with permission from Volkow et al., 2001.

OPIOIDS

There are a number of opioids with abuse potential. Heroin is a short-acting, semisynthetic opioid produced from opium. Heroin is heat stable and may be smoked, sniffed, or injected (Bruce & Altice, 2007). Onset is seconds after injection and euphoria lasts approximately 1 hour, followed by 1–4 hours of sedation. As a consequence, most heroin injectors will inject 2–4 times per day. Some heroin users will mediate the sedating effects of heroin by ingesting a stimulant such as combining a small amount of cocaine with the heroin (aka, a "speedball") or will smoke "crack" shortly after injection. The unsterile method of use, unpredictable concentrations in street samples, adulterants in the injection mixture and the lifestyle necessary to procure heroin, are responsible for most heroin-associated medical complications. In addition to heroin, other opioids, typically short acting ones, such as Vicodin®, Percocet®, and Oxycontin® have a history of being crushed and either sniffed or injected. All opioids act through the same neurobiochemical system, whereby the μ-opioid receptor is activated, resulting in increases in dopamine in the nucleus accumbens and ventral tegmental area (Johnson & Glick, 1993; Self et al., 1995). This increase in dopamine constitutes the rewarding effect of opioid use and plays a strong role in ongoing dependence upon opioids.

The rationale for treating heroin dependence with a long-acting opioid such as buprenorphine or methadone is to satisfy the brain's craving for an opioid in a safe and controlled manner. The aim of providing medication-assisted treatment (MAT), therefore, is to provide cross-tolerance through activation of the μ-opioid receptor, preventing withdrawal and relieving craving for opioids. Additionally, MAT provides a blockade that attenuates the euphoric effect of exogenous opioids. In contrast to heroin, the use of which is characterized by rapidly alternating states of craving and satiety, MAT permits a steady release of dopamine, bringing some stability to the patient's neurobiology and some organization to what is essentially a chaotic neurocognitive environment. This, in turn, allows patients and providers to concentrate on deriving and maximizing the benefits of HIV therapy. In addition to MAT, naltrexone, an opioid antagonist, has been used for the treatment of opioid dependence but is inferior to MAT (Schottenfeld, Chawarski, & Mazlan, 2008).

BUPRENORPHINE

Buprenorphine has been studied since 1978 as a synthetic partial opioid agonist for the treatment of pain (Jasinski, Pevnick, & Griffith, 1978). Unlike full agonists (e.g., heroin, methadone, and morphine) which increase receptor-specific effects in a dose-dependent manner, dose increases of buprenorphine increase receptor specific effects up to a plateau of effects, such as respiratory depression (Walsh et al., 1994; Liguori, Morse, & Bergman, 1996), as graphically represented in Figure 7.9.5 (Ling & Smith, 2002; Fiellin & O'Connor, 2002). As with all opioids, a potential for abuse exists (Tzschentke, 2002; seet & Lim, 2006). To combat this potential for abuse, buprenorphine was combined with naloxone (Suboxone®), though buprenorphine alone (Subutex®) is also available. In Suboxone®, the naloxone (NTX) has limited bioavailability when administered sublingually. However, when crushed and injected, NTX has increased bioavailability and the potential to precipitate opioid withdrawal in buprenorphine maintained subjects (Robinson et al., 1993; Comer & Collins, 2002).The exact ability of this to decrease abuse, however, is unclear as various reports have demonstrated ongoing injection in the setting of Suboxone® use (Bruce et al., 2008; Bruce et al., 2009). More importantly in preventing diversion, buprenorphine can precipitate opioid withdrawal in opioid-maintained (e.g., heroin or methadone) subjects because it binds to the μ-receptor with greater affinity than heroin, thereby rapidly dislodging the heroin and slowly stimulating the receptor (Clark, Lintzeris, & Muhleisen, 2002; Geenwald et al., 2002). Finally, buprenorphine dissociates slowly from the μ-receptor; therefore, its effects at the receptor site are long acting and can allow for alternate day dosing (Johnson et al., 1995; Fudala, Jaffe, Dax, & Johnson, 1990).

Several randomized, controlled trials have demonstrated buprenorphine's efficacy in managing opioid withdrawal (Gowling, Ali, & White, 2002; Mattick et al., 2002)and opioid dependence (Johnson et al., 2000; Doran et al., 2003). In one study by Johnson and colleagues, the mean percentage in opioid-negative urine toxicology was comparable between "high dose" methadone and buprenorphine over the 17 weeks of the study. However, buprenorphine was inferior to methadone in retaining patients in the study. Specifically, the percentage of patients retained in treatment over 17 weeks was 58% with buprenorphine, compared with 73% with high-dose methadone (Johnson et al., 2000).

The FDA approved both Suboxone® and Subutex® in October of 2002 and buprenorphine was classified as a Class III controlled substance, thereby allowing its prescription in primary care clinics by properly trained physicians under the Drug Addiction Treatment Act (DATA) of 2000. The goal was to expand access to pharmacological treatments by avoiding the highly regulated methadone clinics. In the primary care setting where methadone cannot currently be prescribed for opioid dependence, buprenorphine remains the best option for the treatment of opioid dependence, as it has been shown to be superior to naltrexone (Schottenfeld, Chawarski, & Mazlan, 2008).

METHADONE

Methadone is a full opioid agonist that can be administered once daily because of its relatively constant plasma levels over a 24-hour period. Daily dosing regimens are variable and patient-specific. Higher doses, over 100 mg, are typically more effective than lower doses (e.g., 40–50 mg) in reducing illicit opioid use (Strain et al., 1999). While lower doses suppress heroin withdrawal symptoms, higher doses may be required to block the μ-opioid receptor, thereby limiting both craving and blocking the effects of exogenous opioids (Donny et al., 2002). Since methadone takes 2 to 6 hours to attain peak levels, it does not provide a euphoric sensation when properly dosed in stabilized patients. Dependency develops rapidly, and missed doses result in severe opioid withdrawal symptoms, which translate into greater retention in treatment when compared to buprenorphine or naltrexone (Johnson et al., 2000; Liu & Wang, 1984).

Over the past forty years, methadone has demonstrated an ability to improve health outcomes in heroin-dependent patients (Mattick, Breen, Kimber, & Davoli, 2002; Marsch, 1998; Yoast et al., 2001; Barnett, Zaric, & Brandeau, 2001). Methadone has been shown to decrease injection of heroin and therefore to moderate this HIV risk-taking behavior (Dolan, Hall, & Wodak, 1996; Donny et al., 2002; Qian et al., 2008). Metzger and colleagues demonstrated this with their report of the dramatic reduction in HIV incidence among those who entered methadone compared to those who continued to inject heroin (Metzger et al., 1993). Chronic maintenance with methadone prevents relapse to injection-related behavior and maintains patients in treatment (Murray, 1998). Methadone maintenance has been shown to be effective in decreasing psychosocial and medical morbidity associated with opioid dependence, including increasing access to and retention on HIV therapy (Lucas et al., 2006). Furthermore, in addition to its benefit in decreasing the spread of HIV among injection drug users, it improves overall health status and is associated with decreased criminal activity and improved social functioning (Marsch, 1998; Stenbacka, Leifman, & Romelsjo, 2003; Gossop, Marsden, Stewart, & Rolfe, 2000; Davstad et al., 2009). The use of methadone as

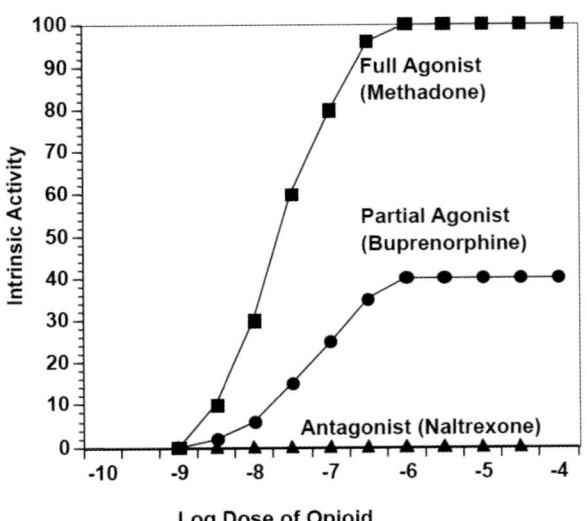

Figure 7.9.5 *Intrinsic activity of Various Opioids upon the Opioid Receptor.*

pharmacotherapy for opioid dependence has repeatedly demonstrated that methadone is effective in primary and secondary HIV prevention (Kerr et al., 2004) and is cost-effective to society (Doran et al., 2003).

In the US, methadone maintenance must be provided within the context of specialized programs specifically registered with federal and state authorities to dispense methadone for the treatment of opioid dependence. Medical providers who treat HIV-infected heroin users should be familiar with the local methadone program and be aware of the referral process necessary to help patients access treatment. Unfortunately, in many places access to treatment is more difficult than obtaining illicit substances. Medical providers must therefore be able to provide effective support to the patient, including motivational enhancement, if the patient is to access treatment effectively.

Important pharmacological interactions between methadone/buprenorphine and HIV therapies have been reviewed extensively in the literature (Bruce et al., 2010; Bruce et al., 2006; Bruce, Altice, Gourevitch, & Friedland, 2006). Table 7.9.2 provides a summary of these pharmacological interactions.

Table 7.9.2 INTERACTIONS BETWEEN ANTIRETROVIRALS AND METHADONE AND BUPRENORPHINE

MEDICATION	METHADONE	BUPRENORPHINE	ANTI-RETROVIRAL THERAPY	COMMENTS
Nucleoside Reverse Transcriptase Inhibitors (NRTI)				
Abacavir (ABC)[a]	↑ clearance	Not studied	↓ C_{max}	No dose change required for METH. Alcohol increases AUC of ABC by 41% with unknown clinical significance
Didanosine (ddI)	No clinical effect	No clinical effect	METH ↓ ddI AUC by 57% for buffered tablet, partially corrected by EC capsule No BUP effect on ddI	No dose adjustments necessary when EC capsule used with METH patients.
Emtriva (FTC)	Not studied	Not studied	Not studied	
Festinavir	Not studied	Not studied	Not studied	
Lamivudine (3TC)	No clinical effect	No clinical effect	No effect of BUP on 3TC	AZT/3TC co-formulation studied only with METH. No dose adjustments necessary
Stavudine (d4T)	No clinical effect	Not studied	↓ d4T AUC_{12h} by 23% and C_{max} by 44%	No dose adjustments necessary
Tenofovir (TDF)	No clinical effect	No clinical effect	No significant effect on TDF by BUP	No dose adjustments necessary
Zalcitabine (ddC)	Not studied	Not studied	Not studied	
Zidovudine (AZT)	No clinical effect	No clinical effect	↑ AZT AUC by 40%	Watch for AZT related toxicity (symptoms and laboratory). Dose reductions of zidovudine may be required.
Non-Nucleoside Reverse Transcriptase Inhibitors (NNRTI)				
Delavirdine (DLV)	↑ AUC by 19%; ↑ C_{max} by 10%	↑ AUC by 400%, without clinical effect	No clinical effect	No dose adjustments necessary; however, should be used with caution as long-term effects (>7 days) unknown.
Efavirenz (EFV)	↓ AUC by 57%	No clinical effect	No clinical effect	Opioid withdrawal form METH common. METH dose increase likely necessary.
Etravirine (ETV)	No clinical effect (only 100 BID of etravirine studied)	Not studied	No clinical effect	No dose adjustments necessary
Lersivirine	No clinical effect	Not studied	Not studied	No dose adjustments necessary
Nevirapine (NVP)	↓ AUC by 46%	No clinical effect	No clinical effect	Opioid withdrawal form METH common. METH dose increase likely necessary.

(Continued)

Table 7.9.2 (CONTINUED)

MEDICATION	METHADONE	BUPRENORPHINE	ANTI-RETROVIRAL THERAPY	COMMENTS
Rilpivirine (TMC278)	↓ AUC by 22%	Not studied	No clinical effect	Monitoring for symptoms of METH withdrawal is recommended.
Protease Inhibitors (PI)				
Amprenavir (AMP)	↓ AUC of R-METH by 13%	Not studied	↓ AUC by 30%	No dose adjustments necessary.
Atazanavir (ATV)	No effect	↑ AUC by 167%	No effect	Some individuals may experience oversedation. Slower titration upwards of BUP may be advisable.
Darunavir	↓ S-METH AUC by 36% and ↓ R-METH AUC by 15%	↑ nor BUP AUC by 46%	No clinical effect	No ARV dose change when combined with METH or BUP. Four subjects out of 16 in METH study reported mild opioid withdrawal, but no dose adjustments were needed.
Fosamprenavir (fAMP)	↓ AUC R-METH by 18%	Not studied	No clinical effect	No dose adjustments necessary
Indinavir (IND)	No clinical effect	Not studied	↓ C_{max} between 16% and 28% and ↑ C_{min} between 50% and 100%	Differences do not appear to be clinically significant
Lopinavir/ ritonavir (LPV/r)	↓ AUC by 26–36%	No clinical effect	Not studied	↓ AUC of METH caused by lopinavir. One study reported opioid withdrawal symptoms in 27% of patients. METH dose increase may be necessary in some patients.
Nelfinavir	↓ AUC by 40%	No clinical effect	↓ AUC of active M8 metabolite by 48%	Despite ↓ METH AUC, clinical withdrawal is usually absent and *a priori* dosage adjustments are not needed. Decrease in AUC of M8 unlikely to be clinically significant.
Ritonavir (RTV)	↓ AUC by 37% in one study and no effect in another (see text)	↑ AUC by 157%	Not studied	No dosage adjustments necessary
Saquinavir (SQV)	↓ AUC by 20–32%	Not studied	Not studied	Saquinavir boosted with ritonavir studied. Despite ↓ METH AUC, clinical withdrawal was not reported.
Tipranavir (TPV)	↓ AUC by 50%[a]	↓ norBUP by 80%	No ARV dose change when combined with METH. TPV/r AUC and C_{max} decreased 19% and 25% respectively compared to historical controls in the presence of BUP	METH dose may need to be increased. TPV may be less effective with BUP, but no dosage adjustments necessary in BUP.
Integrase				
Elvitegravir	Not studied	Not studied	Not studied	
Raltegravir	No clinical effect	No clinical effect	No clinical effect.	No dosage adjustments necessary.
Entry Inhibitors				
Maraviroc	Not studied	Not studied	Not studied	
Enfurvitide	Not studied	Not studied	Not studied	

[a] Decrease in methadone not specified as AUC or C_{max}. NRTI, nucleoside reverse transcriptase inhibitors; NNRTI, non-nucleoside reverse transcriptase inhibitors; PI, protease inhibitor; AUC, area under curve; METH, methadone; BUP, buprenorphine; norBUP, norbuprenorphine. (Adapted with permission from Bruce et al., 2006)

NALTREXONE

Naltrexone is a long-acting, pure opioid antagonist that competitively inhibits the euphoric effects of opioids at the μ-opioid receptor and has been in use for the treatment of opioid dependence for decades (Farren, O'Malley, & Rounsaville, 1997). The major strength of naltrexone is the absence of opioid-related side effects and therefore no risk of overdose, no negative consequences upon cessation (e.g., withdrawal), and no possibility for diversion. Additionally, as discussed earlier, naltrexone has some beneficial effects in the treatment of moderate alcoholism, a common comorbid condition among opioid users (Marmot et al., 1999; Aditya et al., 2004).Unlike methadone, there is no positive reinforcement for taking the medication (e.g., relieving craving or withdrawal symptoms) and no negative reinforcement upon abrupt discontinuation (e.g., opioid withdrawal). The effectiveness of naltrexone treatment, therefore, depends greatly upon the motivation of the patient and the patient's social support system (Baros et al., 2007; Greenstein et al., 1983). Indeed, the drug is most effective among "white collar" opioid users, such as health care professionals, and has achieved its best results when treatment was contingent upon continued employment (Roth, Hogan, & Farren, 1997; Washton, Gold, & Pottash, 1984).

The dosing of naltrexone is variable, and 50 mg daily, 100/150 mg twice weekly, and 100/100/150 three times weekly have all been studied (Kirchmayer, Davoli, & Verster, 2002). In clinical practice, the patients are told to take the medication daily, given the increased risk of nonadherence with this medication. Treatment initiation generally requires an effective, supervised medical withdrawal from opioids for at least 5–7 days prior to treatment initiation to prevent the precipitation of severe opioid withdrawal. The efficacy and safety of naltrexone for the treatment of opioid dependence has been demonstrated in several randomized, controlled clinical trials (Gonzalez & Brogden, 1988). Systematic meta-analysis, however, indicates that naltrexone is no better than placebo except when used in combination with behavioral therapy, and this effect was explained primarily by subject motivation (Kirchmayer et al., 2002). Schottenfeld and colleagues reported on the first double-blind placebo controlled study of naltrexone and buprenorphine in 126 patients in Malaysia. Buprenorphine with standardized counseling was associated with a longer duration of abstinence compared with drug counseling alone or drug counseling with naltrexone, suggesting that, where feasible, μ-opioid agonists such as buprenorphine or methadone should be preferred over antagonists such as naltrexone (Schottenfeld et al., 2008; Mazlan, Schottenfeld, & Chawarski, 2006).Because of a lack of positive reinforcing effects with naltrexone, low patient motivation, and poor clinician acceptability, naltrexone is not widely prescribed for the treatment of opioid dependence.

A one-month injectable depo-naltrexone formulationhas renewed interest in naltrexone as a treatment for opioid dependence. The injectable formulation has the potential to improve adherence. Studies comparing opioid agonists such as buprenorphine and methadone to the depot formulation of naltrexone, however, have yet to be conducted. Current evidence to date weighs in favor of the opioid agonists buprenorphine and methadone. Naltrexone should only be used in the highly motivated patient with a strong social support who can assist in adherence.

TOBACCO

Cigarette smoking is prevalent among HIV-infected patients at rates above the national average, and HIV-infected substance users almost universally smoke cigarettes (Tesoriero et al., 2008; Burkhalter et al., 2005).Nicotine is a potent stimulant and one of the most difficult substances for patients to quit. Advising patients to stop smoking does help, and encouragement to quit should be offered repeatedly to all smokers, regardless of underlying motivation (Stead, Bergson, & Lancaster, 2008). With regard to pharmacotherapy, nicotine replacement is efficacious (Amodei & Lamb, 2010). Bupropion, however, doubles quit rates, with doses of 150 mg to 300 mg effective (Hurt et al., 1997). Because bupropion is metabolized by cytochrome P450 2D6, pharmacokinetic interactions with nelfinavir, ritonavir, and efavirenz need to be considered, and in the case of ritonavir, dose reductions may be necessary, although no studies have formally evaluated these interactions.

Varenicline, a partial nicotine receptor agonist, is FDA approved for the treatment of nicotine dependence and, in comparative studies, was superior to bupropion (Gonzales et al., 2006; West, Baker, Cappelleri, & Bushmakin, 2008). There is a concern that varenicline may exacerbate some serious neuropsychiatric symptoms (including the extremes of suicidality and homicidality); however, individuals with mental illness have a high prevalence of smoking and it is unclear if varenicline has a direct effect on promoting such symptoms or if the effect is unrelated and due to bias or confounding (Hughes, 2008). Because HIV-infected substance users have a higher proportion of mental illness than the general population, such concerns should be taken seriously and medical providers should follow patients closely. A slow upward titration of varenicline is necessary to minimize side effects in this patient population.

REDUCING HIV RISK BEHAVIORS AND RETAINING PATIENTS IN TREATMENT

Those who work in HIV medicine are familiar with the concept of reducing HIV risk behaviors as a goal of treatment. Sometimes the "success" of treating substance dependence will have to be not the cessation of use, but the return of a patient to the next medical appointment. Decreasing the frequency of adverse events related to a behavior is also a success, as is changing substance use behavior. A patient, for example, might transition from injecting to smoking a substance and thereby avoid endocarditis. Of course, practitioners want to remove risk-taking behaviors altogether; however, small changes can still improve health-related outcomes through a reduction in some

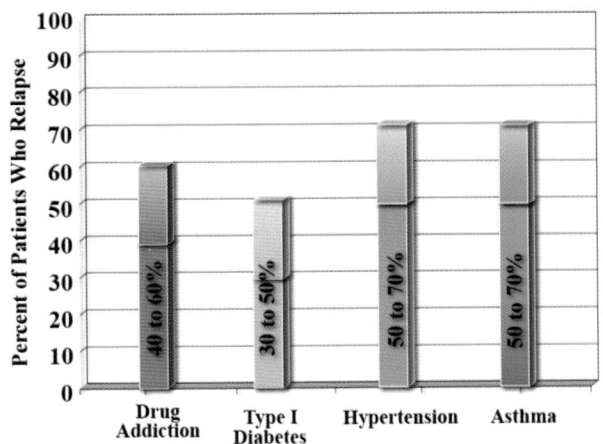

Figure 7.9.6 *Relapse Rates Are Similar Between Addiction and Other Chronic Diseases.*

of the medical consequences of addiction and increased participation in HIV medical care. This patient-centered treatment that sees even small changes as a success is classically termed "harm reduction."

The concept of reducing risk-taking as it relates to health outcomes is not unique to the treatment of addiction. Like other chronic illnesses, relapse rates in addiction are similar to those in diabetes, hypertension, and asthma (Figure 7.9.6) (McLellan et al., 2000). Unfortunately, primary care providers and society as a whole tend to moralize addiction, with relapse often confirming in the mind of the medical provider the categorical failure of the substance user. Instead, relapses should be seen and responded to in the same way as relapses in patients with hypertension. Patients should be reminded of how much better they were feeling when they were taking their medications and of the health benefits that accrued during treatment, with encouragement to resume treatment as those health benefits can be obtained once again.

Medical providers cannot know in advance when the use of pharmacotherapy might tip the balance in favor of an improved health outcome, such as assisting a patient in the reduction or cessation of a substance, thereby reducing the adverse consequences of that substance use, and improving patient participation and benefit in HIV therapy. Medical providers, therefore, should offer pharmacotherapy to all patients in need and work with those patients to overcome barriers both to accepting the medications and ongoing counseling.

ACKNOWLEDGMENTS

R. D. Bruce received funding for this research from the National Institute on Drug Abuse (K23 DA 022143).

REFERENCES

Aditya, G. S., Mahadevan, A., Santosh, V., Chickabasaviah, Y. T., Ashwathnarayanarao, C. B., & Krishna, S. S. (2004). Cysticercal chronic basal arachnoiditis with infarcts, mimicking tuberculous pathology in endemic areas. *Neuropathology, 24*, 320–5.

Albengres, E., Le Louet, H., & Tillement, J. P. (1998). Systemic antifungal agents. Drug interactions of clinical significance. *Drug Saf, 18*, 83–97.

Allen, B., Jr. & Unger, J. B. (2007). Sociocultural correlates of menthol cigarette smoking among adult African Americans in Los Angeles. *Nicotine Tob Res, 9*, 447–51.

Amodei, N. & Lamb, R. J. (2010). The role of nicotine replacement therapy in early quitting success. *Nicotine Tob Res, 12*, 1–10.

Anderson, A. L., Reid, M. S., Li, S. H., et al. (2009). Modafinil for the treatment of cocaine dependence. *Drug Alcohol Depend, 104*, 133–9.

Anton, R. F., O'Malley, S. S., Ciraulo, D. A., et al. (2006). Combined pharmacotherapies and behavioral interventions for alcohol dependence: the COMBINE study: A randomized controlled trial. *JAMA, 295*, 2003–17.

Balldin, J., Berglund, M., Borg, S., et al. (2003). A 6-month controlled naltrexone study: Combined effect with cognitive behavioral therapy in outpatient treatment of alcohol dependence. *Alcoholism: Clinical & Experimental Research, 27*, 1142–9.

Barnett, P. G., Zaric, G. S., & Brandeau, M. L. (2001). The cost-effectiveness of buprenorphine maintenance therapy for opiate addiction in the United States. *Addiction, 96*, 1267–78.

Baros, A. M., Latham, P. K., Moak, D. H., Voronin, K., & Anton, R. F. (2007). What role does measuring medication compliance play in evaluating the efficacy of naltrexone? *Alcohol Clin Exp Res, 31*, 596–603.

Bassareo, V. & Di Chiara, G. (1997). Differential influence of associative and nonassociative learning mechanisms on the responsiveness of prefrontal and accumbal dopamine transmission to food stimuli in rats fed ad libitum. *J Neurosci, 17*, 851–61.

Benowitz, N. L. (2008). Clinical pharmacology of nicotine: Implications for understanding, preventing, and treating tobacco addiction. *Clin Pharmacol Ther, 83*, 531–41.

Bing, E. G., Burnam, M. A., Longshore, D., et al. (2001). Psychiatric disorders and drug use among human immunodeficiency virus-infected adults in the United States. *Arch Gen Psychiatry, 58*, 721–8.

Blatt, S. J., Rounsaville, B., Eyre, S. L., & Wilber, C. (1984). The psychodynamics of opiate addiction. *J Nerv Ment Dis, 172*, 342–52.

Bruce, R. D. & Altice, F. L. (2007). Clinical care of the HIV-infected drug user. *Infect Dis Clin North Am, 21*, 149–79, ix.

Bruce, R., Altice, F. L., & Friedland, G. H. (2008). A review of pharmacokinetic drug interactions between drugs of abuse and antiretroviral medications: Implications and management for clinical practice. *Expert Review of Clinical Pharmacology, 1*, 115–27.

Bruce, R. D., Altice, F. L., Gourevitch, M. N., & Friedland, G. H. (2006). Pharmacokinetic drug interactions between opioid agonist therapy and antiretroviral medications: Implications and management for clinical practice. *J Acquir Immune Defic Syndr, 41*, 563–72.

Bruce, R. D., Govindasamy, S., Sylla, L., Kamarulzaman, A., & Altice, F. L. (2009). Lack of reduction in buprenorphine injection after introduction of co-formulated buprenorphine/naloxone to the Malaysian market. *Am J Drug Alcohol Abuse, 35*, 68–72.

Bruce, R. D., Govindasamy, S., Sylla, L., Haddad, M. S., Kamarulzaman, A., & Altice, F. L. (2008). Case series of buprenorphine injectors in Kuala Lumpur, Malaysia. *Am J Drug Alcohol Abuse, 34*, 511–7.

Bruce, R. D., Kresina, T. F., & McCance-Katz, E. F. (2010). Medication-assisted treatment and HIV/AIDS: Aspects in treating HIV-infected drug users. *AIDS, 24*, 331–40.

Bruce, R. D., McCance-Katz, E., Kharasch, E. D., Moody, D. E., & Morse, G. D. (2006). Pharmacokinetic interactions between buprenorphine and antiretroviral medications. *Clin Infect Dis, 43* Suppl 4, S216–23.

Burkhalter, J. E., Springer, C. M., Chhabra, R., Ostroff, J. S., & Rapkin, B. D. (2005). Tobacco use and readiness to quit smoking in low-income HIV-infected persons. *Nicotine Tob Res, 7*, 511–22.

Cadet, J. L. & Krasnova, I. N. (2007). Interactions of HIV and methamphetamine: Cellular and molecular mechanisms of toxicity potentiation. *Neurotox Res, 12*, 181–204.

Carroll, K. M., Fenton, L. R., Ball, S. A., et al. (2004). Efficacy of disulfiram and cognitive behavior therapy in cocaine-dependent outpatients: A randomized placebo-controlled trial. *Archives of General Psychiatry*, 61, 264–72.

Carroll, K. M., Nich, C., Ball, S. A., McCance, E., & Rounsavile, B. J. (1998). Treatment of cocaine and alcohol dependence with psychotherapy and disulfiram. *Addiction*, 93, 713–27.

Carroll, K. M., Nich, C., Ball, S. A., McCance, E., Frankforter, T. L., & Rounsaville, B. J. (2000). One-year follow-up of disulfiram and psychotherapy for cocaine-alcohol users: Sustained effects of treatment. *Addiction*, 95, 1335–49.

Casteneda, R., Galanter, M., & Franco, H. (1989). Self-medication among addicts with primary psychiatric disorders. *Compr Psychiatry*, 30, 80–3.

Chana, G., Everall, I. P., Crews, L., et al. (2006). Cognitive deficits and degeneration of interneurons in HIV+ methamphetamine users. *Neurology*, 67, 1486–9.

Chander, G., Josephs, J., Fleishman, J. A., et al. (2008). Alcohol use among HIV-infected persons in care: Results of a multisite survey. *HIV Med*, 9, 196–202.

Chang, L., Ernst, T., Speck, O., & Grob, C. S. (2005). Additive effects of HIV and chronic methamphetamine use on brain metabolite abnormalities. *Am J Psychiatry*, 162, 361–9.

Chao, J. & Nestler, E. J. (2004). Molecular neurobiology of drug addiction. *Annual Review of Medicine*, 55, 113–32.

Clark, N. C., Lintzeris, N., & Muhleisen, P. J. (2002). Severe opiate withdrawal in a heroin user precipitated by a massive buprenorphine dose. *Med J Aust*, 176, 166–7.

Comer, S. D. & Collins, E. D. (2002). Self-administration of intravenous buprenorphine and the buprenorphine/naloxone combination by recently detoxified heroin abusers. *Journal of Pharmacology & Experimental Therapeutics*, 303, 695–703.

Cysique, L. A., Maruff, P., & Brew, B. J. (2006). The neuropsychological profile of symptomatic AIDS and ADC patients in the pre-HAART era: A meta-analysis. *Journal of the International Neuropsychological Society*, 12, 368–82.

Dackis, C. A., Kampman, K. M., Lynch, K. G., Pettinati, H. M., & O'Brien, C. P. (2005). A double-blind, placebo-controlled trial of modafinil for cocaine dependence.[see comment]. *Neuropsychopharmacology*, 30, 205–11.

Dackis, C. A., Lynch, K. G., Yu, E., et al. (2003). Modafinil and cocaine: A double-blind, placebo-controlled drug interaction study. *Drug & Alcohol Dependence*, 70, 29–37.

Davstad, I., Stenbacka, M., Leifman, A., & Romelsjo, A. (2009). An 18-year follow-up of patients admitted to methadone treatment for the first time. *J Addict Dis*, 28, 39–52.

Denis, C., Fatseas, M., Lavie, E., & Auriacombe, M. (2006). Pharmacological interventions for benzodiazepine mono-dependence management in outpatient settings. *Cochrane Database Syst Rev*, 3, CD005194.

Di Chiara, G. & Imperato, A. (1988a). Drugs abused by humans preferentially increase synaptic dopamine concentrations in the mesolimbic system of freely moving rats. *Proc Natl Acad Sci U S A*, 85, 5274–8.

Di Chiara, G. & Imperato, A. (1988b). Opposite effects of mu and kappa opiate agonists on dopamine release in the nucleus accumbens and in the dorsal caudate of freely moving rats. *J Pharmacol Exp Ther*, 244, 1067–80.

Di Chiara, G. & North, R. A. (1992). Neurobiology of opiate abuse. *Trends in Pharmacological Sciences*, 13, 185–93.

Djezzar, S., Questel, F., Burin, E., & Dally, S. (2009). Chemical submission: Results of 4-year French inquiry. *Int J Legal Med*, 123, 213–9.

Dolan, K., Hall, W., & Wodak, A. (1996). Methadone maintenance reduces injecting in prison.[see comment]. *BMJ*, 312, 1162.

Donny, E. C., Walsh, S. L., Bigelow, G. E., Eissenberg, T., & Stitzer, M. L. (2002). High-dose methadone produces superior opioid blockade and comparable withdrawal suppression to lower doses in opioid-dependent humans. *Psychopharmacology (Berl)*, 161, 202–12.

Donovan, J. L., DeVane, C. L., Malcolm, R. J., et al. (2005). Modafinil influences the pharmacokinetics of intravenous cocaine in healthy cocaine-dependent volunteers. *Clinical Pharmacokinetics*, 44, 753–65.

Doran, C. M., Shanahan, M., Mattick, R. P., Ali, R., White, J., & Bell, J. (2003). Buprenorphine versus methadone maintenance: A cost-effectiveness analysis. *Drug Alcohol Depend*, 71, 295–302.

Drake, R. E., Wallach, M. A., & McGovern, M. P. (2005). Future directions in preventing relapse to substance abuse among clients with severe mental illnesses. *Psychiatric Services*, 56, 1297–302.

Dresser, G. K., Spence, J. D., & Bailey, D. G. (2000). Pharmacokinetic-pharmacodynamic consequences and clinical relevance of cytochrome P450 3A4 inhibition. *Clin Pharmacokinet*, 38, 41–57.

Everall, I., Salaria, S., Roberts, E., et al. (2005). Methamphetamine stimulates interferon inducible genes in HIV infected brain. *J Neuroimmunol*, 170, 158–71.

Farren, C. K., O'Malley, S., & Rounsaville, B. (1997). Naltrexone and opiate abuse. In S. M. Stine & T. R. Kosten (Eds.). *New treatments for opiate dependence, The Guilford substance abuse series* (pp 104–123). Guilford, CT: Guilford Press.

Fiellin, D. A. & O'Connor, P. G. (2002). Clinical practice. Office-based treatment of opioid-dependent patients. *N Engl J Med*, 347, 817–23.

Fischer, B., Reimer, J., Firestone, M., Kalousek, K., Rehm, J., & Heathcote, J. (2006). Treatment for hepatitis C virus and cannabis use in illicit drug user patients: Implications and questions. *Eur J Gastroenterol Hepatol*, 18, 1039–42.

Forton, D. M., Allsop, J. M., Cox, I. J., et al. (2005). A review of cognitive impairment and cerebral metabolite abnormalities in patients with hepatitis C infection. *AIDS*, 19 Suppl 3, S53–63.

Fudala, P. J., Jaffe, J. H., Dax, E. M., & Johnson, R. E. (1990). Use of buprenorphine in the treatment of opioid addiction. II. Physiologic and behavioral effects of daily and alternate-day administration and abrupt withdrawal. *Clin Pharmacol Ther*, 47, 525–34.

Fuller, R. K., Branchey, L., Brightwell, D. R., et al. (1986). Disulfiram treatment of alcoholism. A Veterans Administration cooperative study. *JAMA*, 256, 1449–55.

George, T. P., Chawarski, M. C., Pakes, J., Carroll, K. M., Kosten, T. R., & Schottenfeld, R. S. (2000). Disulfiram versus placebo for cocaine dependence in buprenorphine-maintained subjects: A preliminary trial. *Biological Psychiatry*, 47, 1080–6.

Gianoulakis, C., Krishnan, B., & Thavundayil, J. (1996). Enhanced sensitivity of pituitary beta-endorphin to ethanol in subjects at high risk of alcoholism.[erratum appears in Arch Gen Psychiatry 1996 Jun;53(6):555]. *Archives of General Psychiatry*, 53, 250–7.

Gonzalez, J. P. & Brogden, R. N. (1988). Naltrexone. A review of its pharmacodynamic and pharmacokinetic properties and therapeutic efficacy in the management of opioid dependence. *Drugs*, 35, 192–213.

Gonzales, D., Rennard, S. I., Nides, M., et al. (2006). Varenicline, an alpha4beta2 nicotinic acetylcholine receptor partial agonist, versus sustained-release bupropion and placebo for smoking cessation: A randomized controlled trial. *JAMA*, 296, 47–55.

Gonzalez, G., Sevarino, K., Sofuoglu, M., et al. (2003). Tiagabine increases cocaine-free urines in cocaine-dependent methadone-treated patients: Results of a randomized pilot study. *Addiction*, 98, 1625–32.

Gorelick, D. A., Gardner, E. L., & Xi, Z. X. (2004). Agents in development for the management of cocaine abuse. *Drugs*, 64, 1547–73.

Gossop, M., Marsden, J., Stewart, D., & Rolfe, A. (2000). Patterns of improvement after methadone treatment: 1 year follow-up results from the National Treatment Outcome Research Study. *Drug Alcohol Depend*, 60, 275–86.

Gowing, L., Ali, R., & White, J. (2002). Buprenorphine for the management of opioid withdrawal. *Cochrane Database SystRev*, CD002025.

Greenstein, R. A., Evans, B. D., McLellan, A. T., & O'Brien, C. P. (1983). Predictors of favorable outcome following naltrexone treatment. *Drug & Alcohol Dependence*, 12, 173–80.

Greenwald, M. K., Schuh, K. J., Hopper, J. A., Schuster, C. R., & Johanson, C. E. (2002). Effects of buprenorphine sublingual tablet maintenance on opioid drug-seeking behavior by humans. *Psychopharmacology (Berl)*, 160, 344–52.

Halkitis, P. N., Mukherjee, P. P., & Palamar, J. J. (2009). Longitudinal modeling of methamphetamine use and sexual risk behaviors in gay and bisexual men. *AIDS Behav*, 13, 783–91.

Hart, C. L., Haney, M., Vosburg, S. K., Rubin, E., & Foltin, R. W. (2008). Smoked cocaine self-administration is decreased by modafinil. *Neuropsychopharmacology, 33*, 761–8.

Hayner, G. N. & Inaba, D. S. (1983). A pharmacological approach to outpatient benzodiazepine detoxification. *J Psychoactive Drugs, 15*, 99–104.

Hayner, G., Galloway, G., & Wiehl, W. O. (1993). Haight Ashbury free clinics' drug detoxification protocols—Part 3: Benzodiazepines and other sedative-hypnotics. *J Psychoactive Drugs, 25*, 331–5.

Heaton, R., Clifford, D. B., Franklin, D. R., Woods, S. P., Ake, C,. Vaida, F., et al. (2010). HIV-associated neurocognitive disorders persist in the era of potent antiretroviral therapy. *Neurology*, in press.

Hendershot, C. S., Stoner, S. A., George, W. H., & Norris, J. (2007). Alcohol use, expectancies, and sexual sensation seeking as correlates of HIV risk behavior in heterosexual young adults. *Psychol Addict Behav, 21*, 365–72.

Hezode, C., Roudot-Thoraval, F., Nguyen, S., et al. (2005). Daily cannabis smoking as a risk factor for progression of fibrosis in chronic hepatitis C. [see comment][erratum appears in Hepatology. 2005 Aug;42(2):506 Note: Pawlostky, Jean-Michel [corrected to Pawlotsky, Jean-Michel]]. *Hepatology, 42*, 63–71.

Huang, X., Gu, H. H., & Zhan, C. G. (2009). Mechanism for cocaine blocking the transport of dopamine: Insights from molecular modeling and dynamics simulations. *J Phys Chem B, 113*, 15057–66.

Hughes, J. R. (2008). Smoking and suicide: A brief overview. *Drug Alcohol Depend, 98* 169–78.

Hurt, R. D., Sachs, D. P., Glover, E. D., et al. (1997). A comparison of sustained-release bupropion and placebo for smoking cessation. *N Engl J Med, 337*, 1195–202.

Hsu, A., Granneman, G. R., & Bertz, R. J. (1998). Ritonavir. Clinical pharmacokinetics and interactions with other anti-HIV agents. [erratum appears in Clin Pharmacokinet 1998 Dec;35(6):473]. *Clinical Pharmacokinetics, 35*, 275–91.

Jasinski, D. R., Pevnick, J. S., & Griffith, J. D. (1978). Human pharmacology and abuse potential of the analgesic buprenorphine: A potential agent for treating narcotic addiction. *Arch Gen Psychiatry, 35*, 501–16.

Jernigan, T. L., Gamst, A. C., Archibald, S. L., et al. (2005). Effects of methamphetamine dependence and HIV infection on cerebral morphology. *Am J Psychiatry, 162*, 1461–72.

Johnson, B. A. (2005). Recent advances in the development of treatments for alcohol and cocaine dependence: Focus on topiramate and other modulators of GABA or glutamate function. *CNS Drugs, 19*, 873–96.

Johnson, D. W. & Glick, S. D. (1993). Dopamine release and metabolism in nucleus accumbens and striatum of morphine-tolerant and nontolerant rats. *Pharmacol Biochem Behav, 46*, 341–7.

Johnson, B. A., Ait-Daoud, N., Bowden, C. L., et al. (2003). Oral topiramate for treatment of alcohol dependence: A randomised controlled trial. *Lancet, 361*, 1677–85.

Johnson, R. E., Chutuape, M. A., Strain, E. C., Walsh, S. L., Stitzer, M. L., & Bigelow, G. E. (2000). A comparison of levomethadyl acetate, buprenorphine, and methadone for opioid dependence. *N Engl J Med, 343*, 1290–7.

Johnson, R. E., Eissenberg, T., Stitzer, M. L., Strain, E. C., Liebson, I. A., & Bigelow, G. E. (1995). Buprenorphine treatment of opioid dependence: Clinical trial of daily versus alternate-day dosing. *Drug Alcohol Depend, 40*, 27–35.

Johnson, B. A., Rosenthal, N., Capece, J. A., et al. (2008). Improvement of physical health and quality of life of alcohol-dependent individuals with topiramate treatment: US multisite randomized controlled trial. *Arch Intern Med, 168*, 1188–99.

Johnstone, E., Benowitz, N., Cargill, A., et al. (2006). Determinants of the rate of nicotine metabolism and effects on smoking behavior. *Clin Pharmacol Ther, 80*, 319–30.

Kalechstein, A. D., Newton, T. F., & Green, M. (2003). Methamphetamine dependence is associated with neurocognitive impairment in the initial phases of abstinence. *J Neuropsychiatry Clin Neurosci, 15*, 215–20.

Kampman, K. M., Pettinati, H., Lynch, K. G., et al. (2004). A pilot trial of topiramate for the treatment of cocaine dependence. *Drug & Alcohol Dependence, 75*, 233–40.

Kaufman, M. J., Pollack, M. H., Villafuerte, R. A., et al. (1999). Cerebral phosphorus metabolite abnormalities in opiate-dependent polydrug abusers in methadone maintenance. *Psychiatry Research, 90*, 143–52.

Kenna, G. A., Lomastro, T. L., Schiesl, A., Leggio, L., & Swift, R. M. (2009). Review of topiramate: An antiepileptic for the treatment of alcohol dependence. *Curr Drug Abuse Rev, 2*, 135–42.

Kerr, T., Wodak, A., Elliott, R., Montaner, J. S., & Wood, E. (2004). Opioid substitution and HIV/AIDS treatment and prevention. *Lancet, 364*, 1918–9.

Kirchmayer, U., Davoli, M., & Verster, A. (2002). Naltrexone maintenance treatment for opioid dependence. *Cochrane Database Syst Rev*, CD001333.

Kirchmayer, U., Davoli, M., Verster, A. D., Amato, L., Ferri, A., & Perucci, C. A. (2002). A systematic review on the efficacy of naltrexone maintenance treatment in opioid dependence. *Addiction, 97*, 1241–9.

Kozal, M. J. (2009). Drug-resistant human immunodefiency virus. *Clin Microbiol Infect, 15* Suppl 1, 69–73.

Kresina, T. F., Bruce, R. D., & McCance-Katz, E. F. (2009). Medication-assisted treatment in the treatment of drug abuse and dependence in HIV/AIDS infected drug users. *Curr HIV Res, 7*, 354–64.

Kresina, T. F., Bruce, R. D., Cargill, V. A., & Cheever, L. W. (2005). Integrating care for hepatitis C virus (HCV) and primary care for HIV for injection drug users coinfected with HIV and HCV. *Clinical Infectious Diseases, 41*, S83–S8.

Laskus, T., Radkowski, M., Adair, D. M., Wilkinson, J., Scheck, A. C., & Rakela, J. (2005). Emerging evidence of hepatitis C virus neuroinvasion. *AIDS, 19* Suppl 3, S140–4.

Letendre, S. L., Cherner, M., Ellis, R. J., et al. (2005). The effects of hepatitis C, HIV, and methamphetamine dependence on neuropsychological performance: Biological correlates of disease. *AIDS, 19* Suppl 3, S72–8.

Le Tiec, C., Barrail, A., Goujard, C., & Taburet, A. M. (2005). Clinical pharmacokinetics and summary of efficacy and tolerability of atazanavir. *Clinical Pharmacokinetics, 44*, 1035–50.

Ling, W. & Smith, D. (2002). Buprenorphine: Blending practice and research. *J Subst Abuse Treat, 23*, 87–92.

Liang, H., Wang, X., Chen, H., et al. (2008). Methamphetamine enhances HIV infection of macrophages. *Am J Pathol, 172*, 1617–24.

Liguori, A., Morse, W. H., & Bergman, J. (1996). Respiratory effects of opioid full and partial agonists in rhesus monkeys. *J Pharmacol Exp Ther, 277*, 462–72.

Littleton, J. (1995). Acamprosate in alcohol dependence: How does it work? *Addiction, 90*, 1179–88.

Liu, S. J. & Wang, R. I. (1984). Relationship of plasma level and pharmacological activity of methadone. *NIDA Res Monogr, 49*, 128–35.

Lucas, G. M., Mullen, B. A., Weidle, P. J., Hader, S., McCaul, M. E., & Moore, R. D. (2006). Directly administered antiretroviral therapy in methadone clinics is associated with improved HIV treatment outcomes, compared with outcomes among concurrent comparison groups. *Clin Infect Dis, 42*, 1628–35.

Madan, A., Parkinson, A., & Faiman, M. D. (1998). Identification of the human P-450 enzymes responsible for the sulfoxidation and thiono-oxidation of diethyldithiocarbamate methyl ester: Role of P-450 enzymes in disulfiram bioactivation. *Alcohol Clin Exp Res, 22*, 1212–9.

Marmot, M. G., Siegrist, J., Theorell, T., & Feeney, A. (1999). Health and the psychosocial environment of work. In M. G. Marmot & R. Wilkinson, (Eds.). *Social determinants of health*. Oxford: Oxford University Press.

Marsch, L. A. (1998). The efficacy of methadone maintenance interventions in reducing illicit opiate use, HIV risk behavior and criminality: A meta-analysis. *Addiction, 93*, 515–32.

Martinez-Raga, J., Knecht, C., & Cepeda, S. (2008). Modafinil: A useful medication for cocaine addiction? Review of the evidence from neuropharmacological, experimental and clinical studies. *Curr Drug Abuse Rev, 1*, 213–21.

Maru, D. S., Kozal, M. J., Bruce, R. D., Springer, S. A., & Altice, F. L. (2007). Directly administered antiretroviral therapy for HIV-infected drug users does not have an impact on antiretroviral resistance: Results from a randomized controlled trial. *J Acquir Immune Defic Syndr, 46,* 555–63.

Mason, B. J. (2001). Treatment of alcohol-dependent outpatients with acamprosate: A clinical review. *Journal of Clinical Psychiatry, 62* Suppl 20, 42–8.

Mason, B. J., Goodman, A. M., Dixon, R. M., et al. (2002). A pharmacokinetic and pharmacodynamic drug interaction study of acamprosate and naltrexone. *Neuropsychopharmacology, 27,* 596–606.

Mathers, B. M., Degenhardt, L., Phillips, B., et al. (2008). Global epidemiology of injecting drug use and HIV among people who inject drugs: A systematic review. *Lancet, 372,* 1733–45.

Mattick, R. P., Breen, C., Kimber, J., & Davoli, M. (2002). Methadone maintenance therapy versus no opioid replacement therapy for opioid dependence (Cochrane Review). *Cochrane Database Syst Rev,* CD002209.

Mattick, R. P., Kimber, J., Breen, C., & Davoli, M. (2002). Buprenorphine maintenance versus placebo or methadone maintenance for opioid dependence (Cochrane Review). *Cochrane Database Syst Rev,* CD002207.

Mazlan, M., Schottenfeld, R. S., & Chawarski, M. C. (2006). New challenges and opportunities in managing substance abuse in Malaysia. *Drug Alcohol Rev, 25,* 473–8.

McDowell JA, Chittick GE, Stevens CP, Edwards KD, Stein DS (2000). Pharmacokinetic interaction of abacavir (1592U89) and ethanol in human immunodeficiency virus-infected adults. Antimicrobial Agents & Chemotherapy, *44:*1686-1690.

McElhiney, M. C., Rabkin, J. G., Rabkin, R., & Nunes, E. V. (2009). Provigil (modafinil) plus cognitive behavioral therapy for methamphetamine use in HIV+ gay men: A pilot study. *Am J Drug Alcohol Abuse, 35,* 34–7.

McLellan, A. T., Lewis, D. C., O'Brien, C. P., & Kleber, H. D. (2000). Drug dependence, a chronic medical illness: Implications for treatment, insurance, and outcomes evaluation. *JAMA, 284,* 1689–95.

Metzger, D. S., Woody, G. E., McLellan, A. T., et al. (1993). Human immunodeficiency virus seroconversion among intravenous drug users in- and out-of-treatment: An 18-month prospective follow-up. *Journal of Acquired Immune Deficiency Syndromes, 6,* 1049–56.

Monterosso, J. R., Flannery, B. A., & Pettinati, H. M., et al. (2001). Predicting treatment response to naltrexone: The influence of craving and family history. American Journal on *Addictions, 10,* 258–68.

Morgan, P. T., Pace-Schott, E., Pittman, B., Stickgold, R., & Malison, R. T. (2010). Normalizing effects of modafinil on sleep in chronic cocaine users. *Am J Psychiatry.*

Murray, J. B. (1998). Effectiveness of methadone maintenance for heroin addiction. *Psychological Reports, 83,* 295–302.

Nair, M. P., Chadha, K. C., Hewitt, R. G., Mahajan, S., Sweet, A., & Schwartz, S. A. (2000). Cocaine differentially modulates chemokine production by mononuclear cells from normal donors and human immunodeficiency virus type 1-infected patients. *Clinical & Diagnostic Laboratory Immunology, 7,* 96–100.

Nair, M. P., Mahajan, S., Chadha, K. C., et al. (2001). Effect of cocaine on chemokine and CCR-5 gene expression by mononuclear cells from normal donors and HIV-1 infected patients. *Adv Exp Med Biol, 493,* 235–40.

Nestler, E. J. (2001). Psychogenomics: Opportunities for understanding addiction. [see comment]. *Journal of Neuroscience, 21,* 8324–7.

Nestler, E. J. (2004). Molecular mechanisms of drug addiction. *Neuropharmacology, 47* Suppl 1, 24–32.

Nestler, E. J. & Aghajanian, G. K. (1997). Molecular and cellular basis of addiction. *Science 278,* 58–63.

Nestler, E. J., Alreja, M., & Aghajanian, G. K. (1994). Molecular and cellular mechanisms of opiate action: Studies in the rat locus coeruleus. *Brain Research Bulletin, 35,* 521–8.

Nestler, E. J., Berhow, M. T., & Brodkin, E. S. (1996). Molecular mechanisms of drug addiction: Adaptations in signal transduction pathways. *Molecular Psychiatry, 1,* 190–9.

Nestler, E. J., Hope, B. T., & Widnell, K. L. (1993). Drug addiction: A model for the molecular basis of neural plasticity. *Neuron, 11,* 995–1006.

O'Brien, C. P. (2005). Anticraving medications for relapse prevention: A possible new class of psychoactive medications. *American Journal of Psychiatry, 162,* 1423–31.

O'Malley, S. S. (1996). Opioid antagonists in the treatment of alcohol dependence: Clinical efficacy and prevention of relapse. *Alcohol & Alcoholism, 31* Suppl 1, 77–81.

O'Malley, S. S & Froehlich, J. C. (2003). Advances in the use of naltrexone: An integration of preclinical and clinical findings. *Recent Dev Alcohol, 16,* 217–45.

Parsons, T. D., Tucker, K. A., Hall, C. D., et al. (2006). Neurocognitive functioning and HAART in HIV and hepatitis C virus co-infection. *AIDS, 20,* 1591–5.

Petrakis, I. L., Carroll, K. M., Nich, C., et al. (2000). Disulfiram treatment for cocaine dependence in methadone-maintained opioid addicts. *Addiction, 95,* 219–28.

Petrakis, I. L., Poling, J., Levinson, C., et al. (2005). Naltrexone and disulfiram in patients with alcohol dependence and comorbid psychiatric disorders. *Biological Psychiatry, 57,* 1128–37.

Piasecki, M. P., Steinagel, G. M., Thienhaus, O. J., & Kohlenberg, B. S. (2002). An exploratory study: The use of paroxetine for methamphetamine craving. *J Psychoactive Drugs, 34,* 301–4.

Qian, H. Z., Hao, C., Ruan, Y., et al. (2008). Impact of methadone on drug use and risky sex in China. *J Subst Abuse Treat, 34,* 391–7.

Ravi, N. V., Maany, I., Burke, W. M., Dhopesh, V., & Woody, G. E. (1990). Detoxification with phenobarbital of alprazolam-dependent polysubstance abusers. *J Subst Abuse Treat, 7,* 55–8.

Rawson, R. A., Gonzales, R., Pearce, V., Ang, A., Marinelli-Casey, P., & Brummer, J. (2008). Methamphetamine dependence and human immunodeficiency virus risk behavior. *J Subst Abuse Treat, 35,* 279–84.

Rendell, P. G., Mazur, M., & Henry, J. D. (2009). Prospective memory impairment in former users of methamphetamine. *Psychopharmacology (Berl), 203,* 609–16.

Rippeth, J. D., Heaton, R. K., Carey, C. L., et al. (2004). Methamphetamine dependence increases risk of neuropsychological impairment in HIV infected persons. *J Int Neuropsychol Soc, 10,* 1–14.

Richter, P., Beistle, D., Pederson, L., & O'Hegarty, M. (2008). Small-group discussions on menthol cigarettes: Listening to adult African American smokers in Atlanta, Georgia. *Ethn Health, 13,* 171–82.

Robinson, G. M., Dukes, P. D., Robinson, B. J., Cooke, R. R., & Mahoney, G. N. (1993). The misuse of buprenorphine and a buprenorphine-naloxone combination in Wellington, New Zealand. *Drug & Alcohol Dependence, 33,* 81–6.

Rollins, A. L., O'Neill, S. J., Davis, K. E., & Devitt, T. S. (2005). Substance abuse relapse and factors associated with relapse in an inner-city sample of patients with dual diagnoses. *Psychiatric Services, 56,* 1274–81.

Roth, T. & Roehrs, T. A. (1992). Issues in the use of benzodiazepine therapy. *J Clin Psychiatry, 53 Suppl,* 14–8.

Roth, A., Hogan, I., & Farren, C. (1997). Naltrexone plus group therapy for the treatment of opiate-abusing health care professionals. *J Subst Abuse Treat, 14,* 19–22.

Roth, M. D., Tashkin, D. P., Choi, R., Jamieson, B. D., Zack, J. A., & Baldwin, G. C. (2002). Cocaine enhances human immunodeficiency virus replication in a model of severe combined immunodeficient mice implanted with human peripheral blood leukocytes. *Journal of Infectious Diseases, 185,* 701–5.

Roxburgh, A., Degenhardt, L., & Breen, C. (2005). Drug use and risk behaviours among injecting drug users: A comparison between sex workers and non-sex workers in Sydney, Australia. *Harm Reduct J, 2,* 7.

Samet, J. H., Walley, A. Y., & Bridden, C. (2007). Illicit drugs, alcohol, and addiction in human immunodeficiency virus. *Panminerva Med, 49,* 67–77.

Schottenfeld, R. S., Chawarski, M. C., & Mazlan, M. (2008). Maintenance treatment with buprenorphine and naltrexone for heroin dependence in Malaysia: A randomised, double-blind, placebo-controlled trial. *Lancet, 371,* 2192–200.

Seet, R. C. & Lim, E. C. (2006). Intravenous use of buprenorphine tablets associated with rhabdomyolysis and compressive sciatic neuropathy. *Annals of Emergency Medicine, 47,* 396–7.

Self, D. W., McClenahan, A. W., Beitner-Johnson, D., Terwilliger, R. Z., & Nestler, E. J. (1995). Biochemical adaptations in the mesolimbic dopamine system in response to heroin self-administration. *Synapse, 21,* 312–8.

Shaham, Y., Erb, S., & Stewart, J. (2000). Stress-induced relapse to heroin and cocaine seeking in rats: A review. *Brain Research—Brain Research Reviews, 33,* 13–33.

Shearer, J., Darke, S., Rodgers, C., et al. (2009). A double-blind, placebo-controlled trial of modafinil (200 mg/day) for methamphetamine dependence. *Addiction, 104,* 224–33.

Shoptaw, S., Heinzerling, K. G., Rotheram-Fuller, E., et al. (2008). Randomized, placebo-controlled trial of bupropion for the treatment of methamphetamine dependence. *Drug Alcohol Depend, 96,* 222–32.

Shoptaw, S., Huber, A., Peck, J., et al. (2006). Randomized, placebo-controlled trial of sertraline and contingency management for the treatment of methamphetamine dependence. *Drug Alcohol Depend, 85,* 12–8.

Sofuoglu, M., Poling, J., Mitchell, E., & Kosten, T. R. (2005). Tiagabine affects the subjective responses to cocaine in humans. *Pharmacology, Biochemistry & Behavior, 82,* 569–73.

Soogoor, M., Lynn, H. S., Donfield, S. M., et al. (2006). Hepatitis C virus infection and neurocognitive function. *Neurology, 67,* 1482–5.

Stead, L. F., Bergson, G., & Lancaster, T. (2008). Physician advice for smoking cessation. *Cochrane Database Syst Rev,* CD000165.

Stenbacka, M., Leifman, A., & Romelsjo, A. (2003). The impact of methadone treatment on registered convictions and arrests in HIV-positive and HIV-negative men and women with one or more treatment periods. *Drug and Alcohol Review, 22,* 27–34.

Stefanis, C. N. & Kokkevi, A. (1986). Depression and drug use. *Psychopathology, 19* Suppl 2, 124–31.

Stimmel, B. & Kreek, M. J. (2000). Neurobiology of addictive behaviors and its relationship to methadone maintenance. *Mt Sinai J Med, 67,* 375–80.

Strain, E. C., Bigelow, G. E., Liebson, I. A., & Stitzer, M. L. (1999). Moderate- vs high-dose methadone in the treatment of opioid dependence: A randomized trial. *JAMA, 281,* 1000–5.

Suh, J. J., Pettinati, H. M., Kampman, K. M., & O'Brien, C. P. (2006). The status of disulfiram: A half of a century later. *Journal of Clinical Psychopharmacology, 26,* 290–302.

Sylvestre, D. L., Clements, B. J., & Malibu, Y. (2006). Cannabis use improves retention and virological outcomes in patients treated for hepatitis C. *Eur J Gastroenterol Hepatol, 18,* 1057–63.

Tesoriero, J. M., Gieryic, S. M., Carrascal, A., & Lavigne, H. E. (2008). Smoking among HIV positive New Yorkers: Prevalence, frequency, and opportunities for cessation. *AIDS Behav.*

Thomson (2006). Acamprosate. MICROMEDEX.

Toussi, S. S., Joseph, A., Zheng, J. H., Dutta, M., Santambrogio, L., & Goldstein, H. (2009). Short communication: Methamphetamine treatment increases in vitro and in vivo HIV replication. *AIDS Res Hum Retroviruses, 25,* 1117–21.

Tran, J. Q., Gerber, J. G., & Kerr, B. M. (2001). Delavirdine: Clinical pharmacokinetics and drug interactions. *Clin Pharmacokinet, 40,* 207–26.

Tzschentke, T. M. (2002). Behavioral pharmacology of buprenorphine, with a focus on preclinical models of reward and addiction. *Psychopharmacology (Berl), 161,* 1–16.

Umanoff, D. F. (2005). Trial of modafinil for cocaine dependence. [comment]. *Neuropsychopharmacology, 30,* 2298; author reply 9–300.

Vocci, F. & Ling, W. (2005). Medications development: Successes and challenges. *Pharmacology & Therapeutics, 108,* 94–108.

Volkow, N. D., Chang, L., Wang, G. J., et al. (2001a). Association of dopamine transporter reduction with psychomotor impairment in methamphetamine abusers. *Am J Psychiatry, 158,* 377–82.

Volkow, N. D., Chang, L., Wang, G. J., et al. (2001b). Low level of brain dopamine D2 receptors in methamphetamine abusers: Association with metabolism in the orbitofrontal cortex. *Am J Psychiatry, 158,* 2015–21.

Volkow, N. D., Fowler, J. S., & Wang, G. J. (2004). The addicted human brain viewed in the light of imaging studies: Brain circuits and treatment strategies. *Neuropharmacology, 47* Suppl 1, 3–13.

Volkow, N. D., Fowler, J. S., Wang, G. J., Baler, R., & Telang, F. (2009). Imaging dopamine's role in drug abuse and addiction. *Neuropharmacology, 56* Suppl 1, 3–8.

Volkow, N. D., Wang, G. J., Fowler, J. S., et al. (1999). Prediction of reinforcing responses to psychostimulants in humans by brain dopamine D2 receptor levels. *Am J Psychiatry, 156,* 1440–3.

Waldrop-Valverde, D., Ownby, R. L., Wilkie, F. L., Mack, A., Kumar, M., & Metsch, L. (2006). Neurocognitive aspects of medication adherence in HIV-positive injecting drug users. *AIDS & Behavior, 10,* 287–97.

Walsh, S. L., Preston, K. L., Stitzer, M. L., Cone, E. J., & Bigelow, G. E. (1994). Clinical pharmacology of buprenorphine: Ceiling effects at high doses. *Clin Pharmacol Ther, 55,* 569–80.

Washton, A. M., Gold, M. S., & Pottash, A. (1984). Successful use of naltrexone in addicted physicians and business executives. *Advances in Alcohol & Substance Abuse, 4,* 89–96.

Weiss, R. D. & Kueppenbender, K. D. (2006). Combining psychosocial treatment with pharmacotherapy for alcohol dependence. *J Clin Psychopharmacol, 26* Suppl 1, S37–42.

West, R., Baker, C. L., Cappelleri, J. C., & Bushmakin, A. G. (2008). Effect of varenicline and bupropion SR on craving, nicotine withdrawal symptoms, and rewarding effects of smoking during a quit attempt. *Psychopharmacology (Berl), 197,* 371–7.

Winhusen, T. M., Somoza, E. C., Harrer, J. M., et al. (2005). A placebo-controlled screening trial of tiagabine, sertraline, and donepezil as cocaine dependence treatments. *Addiction, 100* Suppl 1, 68–77.

Yoast, R., Williams, M. A., Deitchman, S. D., & Champion, H. C. (2001). Report of the Council on Scientific Affairs: Methadone maintenance and needle-exchange programs to reduce the medical and public health consequences of drug abuse. *J Addict Dis, 20,* 15–40.

Wynn, G. H., Cozza, K. L., Zapor, M. J., Wortmann, G. W., & Armstrong, S. C. (2005). Med-psych drug-drug interactions update. Antiretrovirals, part III: Antiretrovirals and drugs of abuse. *Psychosomatics, 46,* 79–87.

SECTION 8

PATHOGENESIS OF COMORBID CONDITIONS

Igor Grant

8.1

NEUROAIDS AS AN INFLAMMATORY DISORDER

Denise R. Cook*, Stephanie A. Cross*, Samantha S. Soldan, and Dennis L. Kolson

The pathological basis for the neurological complications of AIDS involves complex interactions between multiple cell types within both the brain and the periphery. This review focuses on the role for inflammation in the development of HIV-associated neurocognitive disorders (HAND). Specifically, evidence for inflammation in HAND pathogenesis in the pre-antiretroviral therapy (ART) and post-ART eras is discussed. The biology of HIV infection and subsequent CNS invasion is emphasized, with particular focus on chemokines and chemokine receptors. Because chronic neuroinflamation has also been implicated in other infectious and non-infectious CNS disorders, such as multiple sclerosis (MS), Alzheimer's disease (AD), Parkinson's disease (PD) and HTLV-1-associated myelopathy/tropical spastic paraparesis (HAM/TSP), these are also reviewed. The status of current adjunctive therapies for HAND and their relationship to such neuroinflammatory disorders is also included. Understanding common pathways of neuroinflammation will lead to the identification of biomarkers for classification, diagnosis, and clinical prognosis, as well as to the development of novel treatment modalities for HAND and other neuroinflammatory disorders of the CNS.

INTRODUCTION

Advances in antiretroviral therapies for HIV infection have improved virological control and greatly increased the life expectancy of infected individuals. However, despite the availability of these potent antiviral drugs, the prevalence of HIV-associated neurocognitive disorders (HAND) has persisted and even increased (McArthur et al., 2003; Robertson et al., 2007; Sacktor et al., 2002), emphasizing the need for effective adjunctive neuroprotective therapies. Inflammation in the brain and in the periphery is a driving force in the neuropathogenesis of HAND, MS, HAM/TSP, and probably also AD and PD. As these conditions share common features in their pathogenic processes, identifying common mechanisms and developing targeted treatment modalities will not only benefit HAND patients, but likely also be effective in other neuroinflammatory disorders.

PATHOLOGICAL CHARACTERISTICS OF NEUROAIDS

CLINICAL CHARACTERISTICS OF HIV-ASSOCIATED NEUROCOGNITIVE DISORDERS (HAND)

According to recent estimates, over 33 million people are currently living with HIV-1 worldwide (WHO, 2009). HIV-1 infection has devastating consequences for the immune system, resulting in immunodeficiency marked by profound CD4$^+$ T-cell depletion. In addition, neurologic disorders involving the CNS and the peripheral nervous system (PNS) affect between 40–70% of HIV-positive individuals at some point during the course of infection (McArthur et al., 2005). Although opportunistic infections of the CNS and PNS associated with HIV-induced immunodeficiency have become far less common because of the availability of antiretroviral therapy (ART) (Mamidi et al., 2002; Habata et al., 1999; Roullet, 1999), the prevalence of primary HIV-induced neurological disorders has increased (Antinori et al., 2007). Conditions directly induced by HIV-1 include peripheral neuropathies, vacuolar myelopathies, and HIV-associated neurocognitive disorders (HAND) (Childs et al., 1999; McArthur et al., 2003; McArthur et al., 2005; Antinori et al., 2007).

HAND are comprised of three conditions of increasingly severe cognitive impairment and interference with activities of daily living: (1) HIV-associated asymptomatic neurocognitive impairment (ANI), (2) HIV-associated mild neurocognitive disorder (MND), and (3) HIV-associated dementia (HAD) (Antinori et al., 2007; Grant, 2008). The diagnosis of ANI, the least severe of the HAND conditions, describes individuals who have mild cognitive impairment, revealed by formal neuropsychological testing, that does not affect day-to-day functioning and does not meet criteria for delirium or dementia. In the more severe MND, increased cognitive impairment interferes with daily functioning as determined by self-reporting or by observation of others. Again, individuals with MND do not meet the criteria for delirium or dementia. HAD, the most severe form of HAND, is typically diagnosed

---

* DRC and SAC contributed equally to this work.

during end-stage HIV infection, primarily in patients with low CD4+ T-cell counts. In HAD, cognitive impairment is associated with marked interference with day-to-day functioning and HAD is considered a significant independent risk factor for death due to AIDS (Liner et al., 2008). Since the inception of ART, the incidence of HAD, defined as the percentage of new HAD cases diagnosed in a given year, has decreased (Sacktor et al., 2002; McArthur et al., 2004; Nath et al., 2008). However, the prevalence of HAD, defined as the overall number of HAD cases, is rising owing to the increased life span of HIV patients (McArthur et al., 2003; Robertson et al., 2007; Sacktor et al., 2002). There is also evidence of ongoing neurodegeneration that may manifest as ANI or MND in patients without evidence of active HIV disease, contributing to the continued prevalence of HAND in the ART era. Moreover, the onset of HAND during ART-controlled clinical latency underscores the need for adjunctive neuroprotective therapies, because no current therapies would be expected to improve neurologic outcomes in the absence of viral replication (Sacktor et al., 2002; Antinori et al., 2007; Brew, 2004).

PATHOLOGY OF HAND: EVIDENCE FOR NEUROINFLAMMATION

HIV-1 enters the brain early in the course of infection via infected macrophages and lymphocytes (Petito et al., 1986; Ho et al., 1985; Koenig et al., 1986). Subsequently, the virus persists in the CNS primarily in perivascular macrophages and microglia and increased numbers of macrophages and microglia have been found to correlate with the severity of HAND (Glass et al., 1995). In general, intrathecal replication of HIV-1 is controlled by CD8+ T cells (Sadagopal et al., 2008; McCrossan et al., 2006), and cerebral spinal fluid (CSF) viral load has been found to correlate with both viral load in the brain and the degree of cognitive dysfunction in HAND (Brew et al., 1997; Ellis et al., 2002; Ellis et al., 1997; Ellis et al., 2000; McArthur et al., 1997). Importantly, in addition to the initial neuroinvasion and infection of macrophages and microglia, it is believed that HIV infection and immune activation in the periphery and ongoing neuroinvasion of activated monocytes play a role in the development of HAND (Gartner, 2000; Banks et al., 2006).

The pathological hallmarks of HIV infection in the brain in the pre-ART era, collectively termed HIV encephalitis (HIVE), include monocyte infiltration and accumulation of perivascular monocyte-derived macrophages (MDM), formation of microglial nodules and multinucleated giant cells (syncytia) due to HIV-driven fusion of MDM/microglia, and widespread reactive microgliosis and astrogliosis. (Wiley & Achim, 1994; Gendelman et al., 1994; Lawrence & Major, 2002; Adle-Biassette et al., 1999; Masliah et al., 1997; Petito et al., 1986). Since the initiation of widespread ART (1996/7), however, at least one study suggests the presence of "burnt out" HIVE in some individuals dying with AIDS (see below) (Gray et al., 2003). MDM and microglia are the primary CD4+ cells in the CNS and the major sources of productive HIV infection in the brain (McArthur et al., 2003;

Gonzalez-Scarano & Martin-Garcia, 2005; Kolson & Gonzalez-Scarano, 2000; Kaul et al., 2001) and clinical disease severity correlates more strongly with the amount of monocyte infiltration and MDM/microglia activation than with the quantity of infected cells or viral load (Glass et al., 1995; Adle-Biassette et al., 1999), suggesting that MDM/microglia play a predominant role in the neuroinflammation and neurotoxicity seen in HAND. Immune activation of MDM/microglia is demonstrated by expression of CD14 (lipopolysaccharide receptor), CD16, CD68, and MHC class II *in vivo* (Swindells et al., 1999; Anderson et al., 2002; Fischer-Smith et al., 2004; Bell, 2004). Furthermore, CSF markers of immune activation and inflammation are commonly detected in individuals with HAND. These markers include CCL2 (monocyte chemoattractant protein-1, MCP-1) (Conant et al., 1998; Chang et al., 2004), β2 microglobulin (Brew et al., 1992; Brew et al., 1996; Enting et al., 2000; McArthur et al., 1992), quinolinic acid (Heyes et al., 1991; Heyes et al., 2001; Brew et al., 1995; Achim et al., 1993), arachidonic acid metabolites (Griffin et al., 1994; Genis et al., 1992), oxidative stress markers (Haughey et al., 2004; Schifitto et al., 2009a), and platelet activating factor (PAF) (Gelbard et al., 1994).

Although most studies demonstrate that neurons are not infected by HIV, neuronal loss is common in HAND and post-mortem studies of HAND patients have revealed morphological changes in neurons including loss of synaptic density, dendritic simplification, and vacuolization (Petito et al., 1986; Masliah et al., 1997). This neuronal damage induced by HIV infection affects multiple regions of the brain and several neuronal subtypes. HIV antigen is commonly detected in the thalamus, basal ganglia, and central white matter and neuronal damage and loss has been reported in the frontal cortex, cerebellum, putamen, and substantia nigra, although the distribution of HIV antigen might be altered in individuals receiving ART (Everall et al., 1991; Ketzler et al., 1990).

CHANGES IN NEUROPATHOLOGY OF HAND IN THE ERA OF ART

The most effective current therapy for HAND is treatment of the underlying HIV infection with ART. Neuropsychological performance is improved in AIDS patients treated with ART and the CNS penetration of antiretroviral drugs directly correlates with decreased CSF viral loads and improved neurocognitive performance (Letendre et al., 2008). However, some recent studies suggest that ART drugs might demonstrate CNS neurotoxicity in treated patients, with associated poorer neurocognitive performance (Schweinsburg et al., 2005; Marra et al., 2009). Unfortunately, although ART can improve cognition, it does not fully eradicate impairments. In addition, patients who have had ART exposure before developing HAND do not appear to respond as well to a change in their ART regimen, indicating the presence of drug-resistant viruses in the CNS or the emergence of a burnout phase of the disease (Brew et al., 2007).

The era of ART has changed the neuropathology of HIV-1 infection (Table 8.1.1) (Boisse et al., 2008; Brew, 2004;

Anthony et al., 2005). Before the introduction of ART, neuroinflammation was frequently observed in HIV-infected patients and usually increased throughout the progression of disease from the asymptomatic stage to AIDS and HAD. Inflammation is less severe during ART, but it appears to be persistent within the macrophage/microglial populations (Gray et al., 2003). Furthermore, ART seems to have limited the severity of pathological changes characteristic of HIVE. As described by Gray and colleagues (Gray et al., 2003), the persistent pathological findings in ART-experienced individuals include neuronal loss with apoptosis, astrocytosis, myelin pallor, and at least a few activated microglia and perivascular macrophages. Distinctly absent are multinucleated giant cells and microglial nodules.

Although for the most part ART has limited the persistent infiltration of HIV-infected lymphocytes into the CNS (Anthony & Bell, 2008), it should be noted that an exception to this occurs during neurologic immune reconstitution inflammatory syndrome (neuroIRIS). NeuroIRIS is a relatively rare (less than 1% of those who initiate ART) consequence of the introduction of ART in highly immuno-suppressed patients and is marked by a severe deterioration in neurologic status that is characterized by massive lymphocytosis, extensive demyelination, and white matter damage (Boisse et al., 2008; Anthony et al., 2005). In neuroIRIS there is a paradoxical clinical deterioration in spite of improved CD4$^+$ T-cell counts and decreased viral loads (McCombe et al., 2009). Despite the overall effectiveness of ART in limiting the infiltration of infected cells into the CNS, neuroinflammation still persists. However, the primary sites of neuroinflammation are different (Table 8.1.1); a strong

involvement of the basal ganglia was observed pre-ART, whereas post-ART specimens display prominent signs of inflammation in the hippocampus and adjacent parts of the entorhinal and temporal cortex (Anthony et al., 2005; Ho et al., 1985). Notably, these autopsy studies have demonstrated microglial activation in brains of individuals treated with ART comparable to those of patients with fully developed, pre-ART AIDS, although HIVE (when defined as the presence of HIV-infected multinucleated giant cells) is much less common now. Overall, these studies confirm the notion that neuroinflammation continues to be associated with HIV CNS infection in ART-experienced individuals, albeit without HIVE.

BIOLOGY OF HIV INFECTION AND INVASION OF THE BRAIN

As mentioned above, HIV-1 traffics into the brain early in the course of infection via infected monocytes and lymphocytes (Dunfee et al., 2006). Despite retroviral therapy, HIV-1 persists in the CNS throughout the duration of infection in parenchymal microglia and perivascular macrophages (Petito et al., 1986; Ho et al., 1985; Koenig et al., 1986). Because increased numbers of microglia and macrophages correlate with the severity of pre-mortem HAND, these cell types probably mediate neurological impairment (Petito et al., 1986; Glass et al., 1995; Anthony et al., 2005). Multiple pro-inflammatory cytokines, including interleukin (IL)-1β, tumor necrosis factor-alpha (TNF-α), and IL-6 are elevated in the CNS and/or CSF of patients with HAND (Oster et al., 1987;

Table 8.1.1 CHANGES IN THE NEUROPATHOLOGY OF HAND IN THE ERA OF ART

	PRE ART	POST ART
CSF viral load	viral load correlates with cognitive dysfunction (Brew et al., 1997, Ellis et al., 2002, Ellis et al., 1997, Ellis et al., 2000, McArthur et al., 1997)	CSF viral load is decreased with treatment and higher CSF ART drug penetrance is associated with lower viral load (Letendre et al., 2008)
Cognitive dysfunction	severe in HAD and improved when patients begin ART (Letendre et al., 2008)	variable and less severe (McArthur et al., 2004, Antinori et al., 2007, Heaton et al., 2010)
Associative biomarkers of dementia	CSF viral load, decreased CD4$^+$ T-cells, increased levels of CCL2 (von Giesen et al., 2005, Bandaru et al., 2007)	increased levels of CCL2, β2 microglobulin, quinolinic acid, arachidonic acid metabolites, oxidative stress markers, platelet activating factor (Bandaru et al., 2007)
Major pathological findings	multinucleated giant cells, microglial nodules, neuronal loss, astrocytosis, myelin pallor, activated microglia and perivascular macrophages	neuronal loss, astrocytosis, myelin pallor, activated microglia and perivascular macrophages.
Multinucleated giant cells and microglial nodules	present	absent
Neuroinflammation	severe and progressive	less severe, but chronic
Site of neuroinflammation	basal ganglia (Ho et al., 1985)	hippocampus and entorhinal and temporal cortex (Anthony et al., 2005)
Microglial activation	present	present
CNS Complications from Tx	N/A	neuroIRIS (rare <1%) (Boisse et al., 2008)

Perrella et al., 1992; Achim et al., 1993; Foli et al., 1997). The pro-inflammatory environment within the CNS is a result of cytokine release from monocytes/macrophages stimulated by either direct viral infection or by shed viral proteins (Rappaport et al., 1999; Sundar et al., 1991) and astrocyte activation without productive infection but with immune activation (Sabri et al., 2003; Kramer-Hammerle et al., 2005). Inflammatory mediators modulate the permeability of the blood-brain barrier, the entry of infected monocytes into the CNS, and peripheral processes that contribute to the neurological complications of HIV. Thus, understanding the mechanisms responsible for HIV entry into the CNS and the modulation of replication within the monocyte/macrophage reservoir are important for developing targeted therapeutics for HAND.

INTEGRITY OF THE BLOOD-BRAIN BARRIER (BBB): ROLE FOR NEUROINFLAMMATION

The blood-brain barrier (BBB) separates the CNS from the periphery and modulates the traffic of low-molecular-weight nutrients, peptides, proteins, and cells in and out of the brain. The integrity and traffic across the BBB can be impacted by many factors, including HIV-dependent cytotoxicity towards cellular BBB components, chemotactic gradients, and the regulation of adhesion molecules and tight junction proteins (Figure 8.1.1). Progressive HIV infection and immune compromise result in the breakdown of the BBB (Dallasta et al., 1999; Kanmogne et al., 2002; Persidsky et al., 2000), which permits the entry of free virus, lymphocytes, and infected and/or activated monocytes into the CNS.

The BBB is composed of brain microvascular endothelial cells (BMECs) that are connected by intercellular junctions to form a semipermeable monolayer. HIV infection increases the permeability of the BBB by compromising the integrity of the tight junctions. Brain regions with HIVE demonstrate an accumulation of activated/infected perivascular macrophages and a decrease in the tight junction membrane proteins zonula occludens (ZO-1) and occludin (Dallasta et al., 1999; Persidsky et al., 2006). TNF-α production by activated/infected macrophages can directly increase the permeability

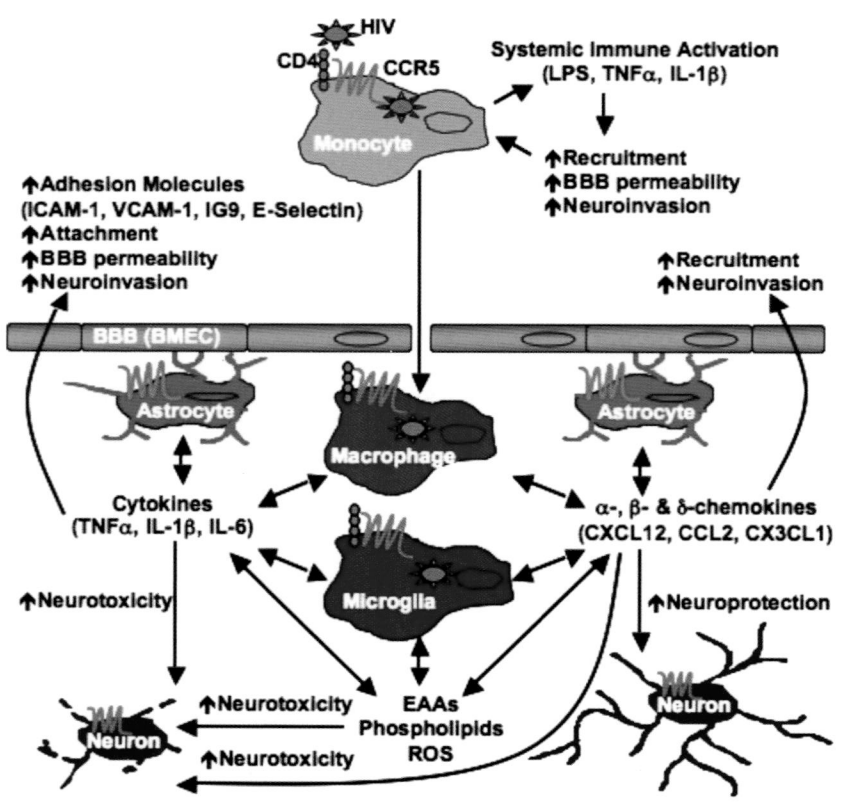

Figure 8.1.1 Role for inflammation via cytokines and chemokines in HIV neuroinvasion and neurodegeneration. HIV-infected monocytes cross the BBB, differentiate into macrophages, and productively infect microglia and other macrophages. Infected and/or activated macrophages/microglia and immune activated astrocytes release pro-inflammatory cytokines which promote monocyte neuroinvasion by increasing expression of adhesion molecules required for monocyte attachment and increasing BBB permeability. This pro-inflammatory environment is enhanced by LPS- and cytokine-induced systemic immune activation, which promotes monocyte recruitment and further BBB permeability. Together, the resulting neuroinflammation can directly and indirectly cause neuronal loss. Infected and/or activated macrophages/microglia and astrocytes also release chemokines, which can serve as both neurotoxic pro-inflammatory factors and neuroprotectants against HIV-induced neurotoxicity. Cytokines and chemokines can undergo reciprocal modulation by additional neurotoxic factors released from infected and/or activated macrophages/microglia, including excitatory amino acids (EAAs), phospholipids and reactive oxygen species (ROS).

of the BBB to free virus (Fiala et al., 1997). However, these profound structural changes of the BBB are late events associated with encephalitis and HIV neuroinvasion is an early and continuing process.

HIV enters the CNS compartment through infected monocytes that cross the BBB via trans-endothelial migration, and this process is particularly enhanced by monocyte immune activation (Figure 8.1.1). Infected and immune-activated monocytes induce adhesion molecules on BMECs, thereby increasing transmigration during HIV infection. In HIVE brain tissue, viral load and pro-inflammatory cytokines correlate with levels of the adhesion molecules E-selectin and VCAM-1 (Nottet et al., 1996; Persidsky et al., 1997; Hurwitz et al., 1994; Sasseville et al., 1994). Exposure to TNF-α stimulates astrocytes to produce ICAM-1, VCAM-1, IG9, and E-selectin, all of which promote monocyte attachment and transmigration (Hurwitz et al., 1994). Following HIV infection, inflammatory cytokines promote the expression of adhesion molecules on BMECs and thereby promote the transmigration of activated/infected monocytes into the brain. Whether compromise to the BBB is as common now in the ART era as in the pre-ART (HIVE) era remains to be determined.

INFLAMMATION IN THE PERIPHERY

Pathology in the periphery may also be involved in the development of HAND (Figure 8.1.1) (Gartner, 2000). Neurological complications following HIV infection have been associated with an expanded population of circulating blood monocytes expressing markers of activation (Pulliam et al., 1997). These activated CD14+/CD16+ monocytes produce TNF-α and IL-1β, which contribute to inflammation in the periphery and further activation of other immune cells (Thieblemont et al., 1995). CD16+ monocytes are particularly susceptible to HIV infection, are capable of tissue invasion, and they compose the majority of the accumulated perivascular macrophages in patients with HIVE (Shiramizu et al., 2005; Ellery et al., 2007; Jaworowski et al., 2007). Peripheral activation of monocytes leads to an enhancement of infected and invasive monocytes that can be recruited into the CNS by chemokines (chemotactic cytokines), as discussed in detail below.

In the gastrointestinal tract, HIV infection also causes microbial translocation, in which HIV-driven depletion of gut-associated lymphoid tissue (GALT) results in leakage of bacteria into the bloodstream and subsequently increases systemic bacterial lipopolysaccharide (LPS) (Brenchley et al., 2006; Douek, 2007). LPS increases monocyte transmigration into the CNS by contributing to the systemic immune activation of chronic HIV infection. In addition to priming peripheral monocytes for neuroinvasion, bacterial LPS can also compromise the integrity of the BBB. In vitro studies demonstrate that LPS-stimulated macrophages create gaps between endothelial cells of an artificial BBB, resulting in enhanced monocyte transmigration (Zhou et al., 2006; Persidsky et al., 1997; Wang et al., 2008). Notably, studies in SIV-infected rhesus macaques and HIV-infected humans

correlate higher levels of plasma LPS, LPS-binding protein, and soluble CD14 with increased HAND severity (Ancuta et al., 2008) and more rapid progression towards AIDS (Brenchley et al., 2006). Thus, the neurological complications of HIV are not exclusively mediated by pathological processes within the CNS, and components of systemic immune activation also play a significant role in the development of HAND.

In summary, inflammatory mediators contribute to HIV infection of the brain by affecting components of both the CNS and the peripheral compartments. Pro-inflammatory cytokines activate a neuroinvasive subset of monocytes in the periphery, compromise the integrity of the BBB, and promote the transmigration of infected monocytes into the CNS. In addition to mediating HIV neuroinvasion, inflammatory mediators also promote the accumulation of macrophages in the brain. These cells serve as a primary reservoir for HIV in the CNS and contribute to the pathogenesis of HAND via the release of neurotoxic and inflammatory cellular products, which can activate noninfected cells (macrophages/microglia, astrocytes). Understanding the role of inflammation in mediating HIV infection of the CNS could provide new therapeutic targets for HAND and other neuroinflammatory diseases.

MECHANISMS OF HIV-INDUCED NEURODEGENERATION: ROLES FOR CHEMOKINES, CHEMOKINE RECEPTORS, AND INFLAMMATION

Monocyte infiltration and macrophage/microglia activation are thought to initiate HAND pathogenesis through both systemic and CNS inflammatory signaling (Kaul et al., 2001; Yadav & Collman, 2009; Kraft-Terry et al., 2009). Following systemic inflammation and monocyte infiltration, activated and/or infected macrophages/microglia within the CNS can release a variety of neurotoxic factors, including viral proteins (gp120, Tat), pro-inflammatory cytokines (TNF-α, IL-1β, IL-6), interferons (IFN-α, IFN-β, IFN-γ), excitatory amino acids (glutamate, quinolinic acid), phospholipids (platelet activating factor, arachidonic acid), and reactive oxygen species (Scorziello et al., 1998; Song et al., 2003; Maragos et al., 2003; Jiang et al., 2001; Brenneman et al., 1988; Gelbard et al., 1993; Wesselingh et al., 1993; Brew et al., 1995; Gelbard et al., 1994; Genis et al., 1992; Gendelman et al., 1998; Boven et al., 1999). Many of these factors can undergo reciprocal modulation by chemokines. Indeed, chemokines and chemokine receptors expressed within the CNS have central roles in HIV neuropathogenesis, from the function of chemokine receptors in mediating infection of the macrophage/microglia reservoir, to the seemingly dichotomous roles of chemokines as neurotoxic pro-inflammatory factors and neuroprotectants against HIV-induced neurotoxicity (Collman & Yi, 1999; Gonzalez-Scarano & Martin-Garcia, 2005; Martin-Garcia et al., 2002; Doms, 2000). Here, we focus on the α-, β-, and δ-chemokine subfamilies in relation to HAND pathogenesis.

α-CHEMOKINES

The α-chemokines, which bind CXCR chemokine receptors, affect HAND neuropathogenesis by enhancing neuroinvasion, promoting astrocyte activation, and directly acting as neurotoxic or neuroprotective factors (Figure 8.1.1). Increased expression of several α-chemokines has been documented in the CSF and brain tissue of HAD patients, including CXCL10 (γ-interferon-inducible protein 10, IP-10) and CXCL12 (stromal cell-derived factor-1, SDF-1) (Kolb et al., 1999; Rostasy et al., 2003; Cinque et al., 2005; Zhang et al., 1998). *In vitro* studies demonstrate that CXCL10 is expressed in microglia and astrocytes, and that gp120, Tat, TNF-α and IFN-γ can act independently or synergistically to increase CXCL10 release (Asensio et al., 2001; Kutsch et al., 2000; D'Aversa et al., 2004; Dhillon et al., 2008a; Williams et al., 2009a; Williams et al., 2009b). In turn, soluble CXCL10 can directly induce apoptosis in neurons (van Marle et al., 2004; Sui et al., 2004; Sui et al., 2006a) and increase neuroinflammation through leukocyte recruitment into the CNS (Kolb et al., 1999; Asensio et al., 2001; Dhillon et al., 2008a).

Like CXCL10, CXCL12 is a potent chemoattractant that can increase recruitment, adhesion, and transendothelial migration of monocytes into the CNS (Malik et al., 2008; Peled et al., 1999; Malik et al., 2008; Wu et al., 2000; Rostasy et al., 2003; Peng et al., 2006). CXCL12 is expressed in astrocytes, microglia, and neurons, and exposure to LPS or IL-1β from HIV-infected and/or activated macrophages can increase CXCL12 release (Peng et al., 2006; Bajetto et al., 1999; Ohtani et al., 1998). Conversely, CXCL12 can trigger astrocytic release of TNF-α and glutamate, causing neuronal damage and apoptosis (Bezzi et al., 2001). Like CXCL10, CXCL12 can also act as a direct neurotoxin. It can undergo proteolytic cleavage by matrix metallic proteinase-2, which changes its co-receptor specificity from CXCR4 to CXCR3, the receptor for CXCL10, and enhances its neurotoxicity (Zhang et al., 2003; Vergote et al., 2006). The neurotoxic properties of native, non-cleaved CXCL12 are controversial as CXCL12 exposure produces either neuroprotective or neurodegenerative responses depending on the experimental conditions (Hesselgesser et al., 1998; Kaul & Lipton, 1999; Zheng et al., 1999a; Zheng et al., 1999b; Khan et al., 2004; Lazarini et al., 2000).

β-CHEMOKINES

Like α-chemokines, β-chemokines, which bind CCR receptors, can mediate neurotoxic and neuroprotective effects against HIV-induced neurotoxicity (Figure 8.1.1). Several ligands in the β-chemokine subfamily are expressed at increased levels during HIV infection, including CCL2, CCL3 (macrophage inflammatory protein-1α, MIP-1α), CCL4 (MIP-1β), and CCL5 (regulated on activation, normal T cell expressed and secreted, RANTES; Kelder et al., 1998). Interestingly, CCL2 CSF levels increase in SIV-infected macaques and HIV-infected individuals prior to neurocognitive impairments and correlate with severity of dementia, suggesting that CCL2 can be a predictive marker for clinical HAND (Kelder et al., 1998; Dhillon et al., 2008b; Zink et al., 2001; Cinque et al., 1998; Zink et al., 1998; Sevigny et al., 2004; Sevigny et al., 2007; Ragin et al., 2006). *In vitro* studies demonstrate that CCL2 is expressed and released from endothelial cells, macrophages, microglia, and astrocytes during HIV infection and in response to gp120, Tat, TNF-α, IL-1β, IFN-β, and IFN-γ (Conant et al., 1998; D'Aversa et al., 2004; Mengozzi et al., 1999; Choe et al., 2001; McManus et al., 2000; Gu et al., 1997; Guillemin et al., 2003; Lehmann et al., 2006). HIV infection of macrophages increases their expression of the CCL2 receptor, CCR2, and concomitantly increases CCL2-mediated recruitment and transmigration of HIV-infected monocytes into the CNS (Eugenin et al., 2006; Park et al., 2001). Thus, inflammation following HIV infection establishes a cycle of monocyte/macrophage activation and neuroinvasion mediated by CCL2. However, CCL2 also provides neuroprotection against Tat-induced neurotoxicity (Eugenin et al., 2003; Yao et al., 2009), suggesting that increased expression of CCL2 during HIV infection may play a destructive and/or protective role. Additionally, the potential CNS destructive role for CCL2 in HIV infection thus appears to be driven through its enhancement of monocyte transendothelial migration and not direct effects on neurons.

While elevated CCL2 CSF levels are associated with an increased risk of HAND, the association of CCL3, CCL4, and CCL5 with HAND is unclear (Letendre et al., 1999). CCL3, CCL4, and CCL5 can all serve as ligands for the CCR5 receptor and can suppress CCR5-mediated HIV infection (Cocchi et al., 1995). Studies also demonstrate that CCL3, CCL4, and CCL5 are expressed and released from microglia and astrocytes during HIV infection and in response to Tat (D'Aversa et al., 2004; El-Hage et al., 2005; Cota et al., 2000; Si et al., 2002), and can ameliorate excitatory amino acid- and gp120-induced neurotoxicity *in vitro* (Kaul & Lipton, 1999; Bruno et al., 2000; D'Aversa et al., 2004; Meucci et al., 1998; Meucci et al., 2000). The neuroprotective effects of CCL5 could be mediated by CCL2 induction (Eugenin et al., 2003). Together, these studies suggest that β-chemokines play important roles in modulating neuroinflammation and neurotoxicity during HIV infection and that they could express either protective or destructive effects within the CNS inflammatory microenvironment.

δ-CHEMOKINES

CX3CR1 and its unique ligand, CX3CL1 (fractalkine), are the only known receptor-ligand pair in the δ-chemokine subfamily. Furthermore, CX3CL1 is the only chemokine expressed in higher amounts in the CNS than in peripheral tissues, suggesting a potentially critical role in modulating HAND pathogenesis (Figure 8.1.1) (Bajetto et al., 2001; Cotter et al., 2002; Re & Przedborski, 2006). It is expressed as a membrane-anchored form on the cell surface or as a soluble form, which can be proteolytically released from the cell. CX3CL1 expression is elevated in serum, CSF, and brain tissue of HAD patients (Pereira et al., 2001; Erichsen et al., 2003; Sporer et al., 2003) and *in vitro* studies suggest that exposure to purified HIV virus, gp120, TNF-α, IL-1β, IFN-γ, or glutamate increases expression of soluble and membrane-bound forms of CX3CL1 in neurons and astrocytes (Erichsen et al., 2003; Chapman et al., 2000a; Maciejewski-Lenoir et al., 1999). Both forms of CX3CL1 can serve as potent CNS leukocyte chemoattractants and can mediate monocyte adhesion and transendothelial migration across the BBB (Ancuta et al., 2003; Harrison et al., 1998; Chapman et al., 2000b; Imai et al., 1997; Tong et al., 2000). In addition to recruiting activated peripheral blood monocytes, fractalkine can trigger the production of IL-6 and CCL2 by CD16+ monocytes (Ancuta et al., 2003). Elevated CCL2 levels can lead to further recruitment of monocytes to the brain while IL-6 can activate and promote the differentiation of monocytes into macrophages, which could promote neurodegeneration. CX3CL1 differentially modulates other neuroinflammatory factors as well, increasing secretion of TNF-α and IL-8, from monocytes and macrophages (Ancuta et al., 2003; Ancuta et al., 2006; Cotter et al., 2002), while inhibiting TNF-α, IL-1β, and IL-6 release from LPS-activated microglia and attenuating cytokine-mediated neuronal loss *in vivo* and *in vitro* (Mizuno et al., 2003; Cardona et al., 2006).

Like β-chemokines, CX3CL1 can also promote neuronal survival, as it can protect against gp120- and Tat-induced neurotoxicity *in vitro* (Meucci et al., 1998; Meucci et al., 2000; Deiva et al., 2004; Limatola et al., 2005). While it is unclear what factors maintain the *in vivo* balance between these neurotoxic and neuroprotective functions of CX3CL1 and other chemokines, the dysregulation of chemokine signaling likely significantly contributes to HAND pathogenesis. These processes are central to neurodegenerative diseases such as HIV infection and multiple sclerosis, and have implications for other neuroinflammatory diseases (Savarin-Vuaillat & Ransohoff, 2007; Li & Ransohoff, 2008; Kaul & Lipton, 2006; Ransohoff, 1999; Ransohoff & Zamvil, 2007).

INFLAMMATORY MARKERS IN NEUROAIDS AND OTHER NEUROINFLAMMATORY DISEASES

Chronic neuroinflammation and elevated levels of pro-inflammatory cytokines and chemokines are associated with several neurodegenerative disorders of the CNS including HAND, MS, AD, PD, and HAM/TSP (Block & Hong, 2005; Mrak & Griffin, 2005; Sawada et al., 2006; Grant et al., 2002). In the CNS, macrophages/microglia are the principal mediators of inflammation and, when activated, secrete pro-inflammatory cytokines (including TNF-α, IL-1β, and IL-6), chemokines (including CCL2 and CCL3), and adhesion molecules (ICAM-1, VCAM-1) that promote inflammation. Regardless of the factor initiating microglia activation, a chronic inflammatory response in the brain can contribute to the death of vulnerable neuronal populations and understanding common mechanisms in these neuroinflammatory disorders could identify common targets for

broadly-protective drugs. Additionally, more reliable biomarkers for neuroinflammatory diseases are needed in order to make early and accurate diagnoses, monitor the course of disease progression, and predict a patient's response to therapy.

INFLAMMATION IN NEURODEGENERATIVE DISEASES ASSOCIATED WITH AGING

HAND shares clinical features with normal aging including the deterioration of cognitive abilities and working memory (Alirezaei et al., 2008; Kaul, 2009). Of interest, diffusion tensor imaging studies, where diffusion is an indicator of neuroinflammation, have shown altered water diffusion within specific brain regions in HIV-infected patients in comparison to normally aging control patients (Chang et al., 2008). These data suggest that even a well-controlled HIV infection may accelerate aging and promote neurodegeneration. In addition, there are several pathological features shared between HAND and neurodegenerative diseases associated with aging, including AD and PD (Brew et al., 2009; Esiri et al., 1998; Khanlou et al., 2009; Chang et al., 2008). These include neuroinflammation, oxidative stress, and cellular degradation pathways (Brew et al., 2009; Nath et al., 2008; Lovell & Markesbery, 2007).

The neuropathology of HAND is clearly distinguishable from AD at autopsy, although there are some shared features. HAND demonstrates less atrophy and fewer neurofibrillary tangles in plaques, which are the hallmarks of AD. Amyloid beta (Aβ) deposition, which precedes symptoms in AD, has also been described in the brains of HIV-infected individuals, although its potential role in HAND symptoms is controversial (Brew et al., 2009; Esiri et al., 1998). Aβ deposition has pro-inflammatory effects that accelerate neurodegeneration *in vitro* (Craft et al., 2006). In AD brains, microglia localize to amyloid plaques (McGeer et al., 1987) and upregulate human leukocyte antigen-DR (HLA-DR) and complement in addition to several pro-inflammatory cytokines that are also implicated in HAND pathogenesis (IL-1β, IL-6, and TNFα) (Eikelenboom et al., 2002; McGeer et al., 1987; McGeer & McGeer, 2010, Sheng et al., 1998). Notably, a transgenic mouse model for a familial AD mutation of amyloid precursor protein recapitulates this proinflammatory effect of Aβ deposition and astrocytes and microglia expressing IL-1β, IL-6, TGF-β, and TNF-α surround plaques (Qiao et al., 2001). In addition to common expression of cytokines that are believed to be involved in the pathogenesis of AD and HAND, LPS concentrations are elevated in both disorders (Ancuta et al., 2008; Herber et al., 2006).

As with AD, HAND also shares some similar neuropathological features with PD. The presence of α-synuclein-positive inclusions in the cell bodies (Lewy bodies) and processes (Lewy neuritis) in the substantia nigra is the neuropathological hallmark of PD. Lewy bodies have also been observed in autopsied brains of HIV-infected individuals (Brew et al., 2009; Esiri et al., 1998; Khanlou et al., 2009; Kaul, 2009) and dopamine deficiency is found in both disorders. However, whether neuroinflammation in PD is a consequence or a cause of the selective loss of dopaminergic neurons in the substantia nigra is unknown. Evidence for neuroinflammation in PD includes increased CSF levels of proinflammatory cytokines, including TNF-α, IL-1β, IL-6, TGF-β, and IFN-γ (Hunot et al., 1999; Vawter et al., 1996). Moreover, single nucleotide polymorphisms associated with increased production of cytokines and chemokines are overrepresented in PD cohorts and may confer increased susceptibility to PD (Hakansson et al., 2005b; Hakansson et al., 2005a; Kruger et al., 2000).

Although the role for neuroinflammation in AD and PD is not completely understood, inflammatory mediators may be used as both biomarkers and targets for drug development for these disorders. For example, platelet inflammatory biomarkers, like cyclooxygenase 2 (COX-2) and phospholipase A_2 could be exploited as peripheral inflammatory biomarkers (Casoli et al., 2010). COX-2 and its homolog COX-1 are pro-inflammatory proteins that are used by activated microglia to synthesize a variety of inflammatory mediators and are elevated in AD brains. Both COX-1 and COX-2 are targets of non-steroidal anti-inflammatory drugs (NSAIDS), and there is a link between chronic use of NSAIDS and a reduced risk for AD and PD (Breitner et al., 1995; Chen et al., 2003). Moreover, biomarkers identified in AD, PD, and other diseases related to aging may also be relevant in HAND. In a recent study, β-Amyloid$_{(1-42)}$(Aβ42) measurements in the CSF of HAND patients were found to be similar to those found in patients with AD and significantly decreased compared to those in normal controls and HIV-infected individuals with normal cognitive function (Clifford et al., 2009). However, HAND patients had normal or slightly depressed levels of CSF tau and tau phosphorylated at threonine 181 (p-Tau181), which distinguished them from patients with AD (Clifford et al., 2009). The detection of pro-inflammatory proteins in the periphery may, in the future, be exploited as useful biomarkers in a wide spectrum of neurodegenerative disorders.

OTHER CHRONIC PROGRESSIVE, INFLAMMATORY DISORDERS OF THE CNS WITH KNOWN OR SUSPECTED VIRAL ETIOLOGY

Neuroinflammation is a major component of other disorders of the CNS with known or suspected viral etiology including HAM/TSP and MS. The human retrovirus HTLV-1 (human T-lymphotropic virus type I) causes HAM/TSP in a small percentage (<5%) of infected individuals. The incubation period between infection with HTLV-I and the development of HAM/TSP is typically long (20–30 years) and the clinical hallmark of this chronic progressive neurologic disorder is a gradual onset of lower extremity weakness (Osame et al., 1990; McFarlin & Blattner, 1991). HTLV-I is predominantly CD4⁺T-cell-tropic. However, CD8⁺ T cells, astrocytes, monocytes/macrophages, and microglia may also become infected and serve as viral reservoirs (Nagai et al., 2001b; Nagai et al., 2001a; Hoffman et al., 1992; Watabe et al., 1989). As in HAND, monocytes/macrophages are believed to

contribute to the pathogenesis of HAM/TSP. However, in contrast to the pathogenesis of HAND/HIV-1 infection of the CNS, much of the neurodegeneration resulting from HTLV-I infection is caused directly by HTLV-I Tax-specific cytotoxic T cells (CTLs) restricted to immunodominant epitopes of HTLV-I gene products (predominantly Tax) (Elovaara et al., 1993; Jacobson et al., 1990b). These HTLV-I-specific CTLs are readily detected in the peripheral blood lymphocytes (PBLs), CSF, and active inflammatory lesions of HAM/TSP patients (Levin et al., 1997; Greten et al., 1998). HTLV-I Tax-specific CTLs secrete many proinflammatory cytokines and chemokines including IFN-γ, TNF-α, CCL3, CCL4, and IL-16 (Biddison et al., 1997). In addition, HTLV-I Tax *trans*-activates many host genes and HTLV-I-infected astrocytes secrete high levels of IL-1α, IL-6, TNF-α, and matrix metalloproteinases (MMPs) (Szymocha et al., 2000a; Szymocha et al., 2000b). Increased levels of HTLV-I tax mRNA, an increased frequency of HTLV-I Tax-specific CD8+ T cells, and high proviral loads correlate with disease severity in HAM/TSP and provide good biomarkers of disease progression (Yamano et al., 2002). Other candidate HAM/TSP biomarkers, CD244 (a signaling lymphocyte activation molecule [SLAM] family receptor) and SLAM-associated protein (SAP), were found to be significantly higher in HAM/TSP compared to asymptomatic carriers and uninfected individuals and both may be used as biomarkers for neurodegeneration in HTLV-I-infected individuals (Enose-Akahata et al., 2009).

Another prototypic neuroinflammatory disease with some neuropathological similarities to HAND is MS. MS is the most common inflammatory disease of the CNS, with a prevalence that ranges between 2 and 150 per 100,000 (Rosati, 2001). The etiology of MS is unknown. In part, this is attributable to the variability of this disease, suggesting that many factors may be involved in the development of MS (reviewed in Soldan et al., 2008). However, it is generally believed that genetic, immunological, and environmental factors contribute to MS pathogenesis. Infectious agents have been implicated in the pathogenesis of MS for over 100 years but no single causative agent has been identified. Again, unlike HAND, MS is chiefly a T-cell-mediated neuroinflammatory disorder. However, in both MS and HAND an inflammatory cascade contributes to disease pathogenesis. Although the neuroinflammatory nature of MS has been confirmed at all stages, inflammation tends to decrease after decades of disease, as irreversible neuronal degeneration accumulates. Such neuroinflammation is detectable through brain magnetic resonance imaging (MRI) as the presence of gadolinium-enhancing lesions, which represent areas of inflammation associated with leakiness of capillary endothelial cells and infiltration of serum components into the brain parenchyma. Analysis of CSF often reveals markers of neuroinflammation, as does examination of autopsied brain specimens (see below).

The overexpression of several proinflammatory cytokines, including TNF-α, IFN-γ, IL-12, IL-6 and CXCL10 have been demonstrated in MS brain specimens (Bartosik-Psujek & Stelmasiak, 2005; Ubogu et al., 2006; Frohman et al., 2006;

Miljkovic et al., 2002; Drulovic et al., 1998; Drulovic et al., 1997). Importantly, an increase in TNF-α expression in peripheral blood mononuclear cells has been found to precede MS relapses and inflammatory activity (Rieckmann et al., 1995). In contrast, anti-inflammatory cytokines (IL-4, IL-10, and TGF-β) and other chemokines (CCL2 and CCL5) are downregulated during MS disease exacerbations (Rieckmann et al., 1995; Mahad et al., 2002a; Mahad et al., 2002b; Malmestrom et al., 2006). The altered expression of these cytokines promotes disease pathogenesis by upregulating MHC and adhesion molecule expression on endothelial and glial cells, activating macrophages, recruiting TH-1 cells, and/or by directly damaging oligodendrocytes and myelin sheaths. In addition, soluble adhesion molecules such as ICAM-1 and E-selectin are elevated in the sera of MS patients while soluble vascular cell adhesion molecules VCAM-1 and E-selectin are increased in the CSF of MS patients, thereby promoting the trafficking of activated T cells into the CNS (Dore-Duffy et al., 1995).

Another long-standing diagnostic biomarker for MS is the presence of oligoclonal bands, which represent intrathecally expressed immunoglobin. While the presence of oligoclonal bands clearly suggests neuroinflammation in the CSF, the MS-relevant reactive antigens have not yet been identified. CSF oligoclonal bands are also present in HAM/TSP and in these individuals they have been found to be chiefly directed against HTLV-I (Jacobson et al., 1990a). More reliable biomarkers that can be assayed in the peripheral blood and CSF of MS patients are still being sought due to the high cost of frequent MRI and its poor reliability to detect neuronal degeneration, axonal loss, and to some extent, spinal cord lesions.

There are many molecules with the potential for more specific clinical diagnostic and prognostic application in MS including auto-antibodies, virus antibodies, transcription factors, molecules in the nitric oxide pathway, neuronal breakdown products, apolipoprotein E (a marker for cognitive dysfunction in AD), molecules in the amyloid precursor protein pathway, cytokines, and chemokines among others (reviewed in Harris & Sadiq, 2009). Several biomarkers of MS inflammatory disease activity are also of interest in HAND, including IL-6 and osteopontin, which are both upregulated in HAND and in MS lesions (Cannella & Raine, 1995; Burdo et al., 2008; Frei et al., 1991) and CCL2, which is downregulated during MS exacerbations and increased in HAND (Kelder et al., 1998). Further assessment of these biomarkers and the use of proteomics and microarray technologies to discover new and specific biomarkers for neuroinflammatory diseases will ultimately improve diagnosis and treatment of these disabling neuroinflammatory disorders.

THERAPEUTIC CONSIDERATIONS

Given the complexity of the pathogenesis of HIV-associated neurodegeneration, multiple cell types and cellular processes are under investigation as therapeutic targets. Ongoing clinical trials are examining drugs that target overall neuronal survival in addition to reducing neuroinflammation. It is likely that a combination of classes of drugs will be necessary to ameliorate the neurocognitive decline in HIV patients receiving ART.

ART is increasingly effective in reducing morbidities and mortality in HIV-1-infected patients. While ART has significantly decreased the incidence of HAD, presumably by lowering systemic viral loads, current efforts are focused on improving the penetration of ART past the BBB. Improved penetration or retention of bioavailable ART drugs in the CNS may slow HAND progression by decreasing CNS viral replication and reducing concomitant release of neurotoxins from infected and activated macrophages/microglia (Letendre et al., 2008; Ellis et al., 2007; Spitzenberger et al., 2007). However, a recent study demonstrated that ART regimens with strong CNS penetration and reduced CSF viral loads were associated with poorer neurocognitive outcomes (Marra et al., 2009). While further clinical studies are needed, this study highlights the importance of considering drug toxicity when promoting ART in the CNS. Furthermore, effective therapies for HAND will likely require combination therapy that not only targets viral load, but also addresses the indirect pathways known to contribute to HIV-associated neurodegeneration.

Clinical similarities between HIV-associated neurodegeneration and other neurodegenerative diseases have prompted investigation into currently approved neuroprotective therapies in HAND (Table 8.1.2). Memantine (Namenda), approved in the treatment for Alzheimer's disease, is a non-competitive NMDA receptor antagonist that also increases levels of brain-derived neurotrophic factor (BDNF) and conserves dopamine function in SIV-infected macaques (Meisner et al., 2008). Both *in vitro* and *in vivo* animal studies have shown that memantine inhibits gp120 and Tat-induced neurotoxicity (Nath et al., 2000; Toggas et al., 1996; Anderson et al., 2004). A short-term clinical trial in HAND patients demonstrated that memantine improved neuronal metabolism (as judged by magnetic resonance spectroscopy/MRS), indicative of neuroprotection, but did not cause significant neurocognitive improvement (Schifitto et al., 2007a). Nevertheless, this study suggests a potential beneficial effect of memantine, even following short-term administration, although a longer-term follow-up study in this patient cohort failed to reveal a clinically demonstrable neurological benefit (Zhao et al., 2010).

Selegiline (Deprenyl), a monoamine oxidase B (MAO-B) inhibitor used in the treatment of early-stage Parkinson's disease, has shown some promise in clinical trials for HAND. Selegiline is proposed to act as a neuroprotectant by reducing the antioxidant burden of the cell (Magyar & Szende, 2004). Early trials with orally or transdermally administered selegiline demonstrated some improvement in psychomotor speed (The Dana Consortium, 1998; Sacktor et al., 2000). However, recent studies have shown neither a reduction in biomarkers of oxidative stress nor evidence of cognitive improvement with short-term (24 weeks) transdermal selegiline (Schifitto, Yiannoutsos, et al., 2009a; Schifitto, Zhang, et al., 2007). While memantine and selegiline have shown

Table 8.1.2 THERAPEUTICS UNDER CONSIDERATION FOR HAND

GENERIC (BRAND) NAME	MOLECULAR TARGET	EFFECTS/ROLE	REFERENCES
Memantine (Namenda)	NMDA receptor antagonist	Increases BDNF levels, conserves dopamine function, inhibits gp120 and Tat-induced neurotoxicity, improves neuronal metabolism, short-term treatment provided no neurocognitive impairment	(Meisner et al., 2008, Nath et al., 2000, Toggas et al., 1996, Anderson et al., 2004, Schifitto et al., 2007a, Zhao et al., 2010)
Selegiline (Deprenyl)	MAO-B Inhibitor	Proposed to reduce antioxidant burden of cell, may improve psychomotor speed, no clinical evidence of cognitive improvement over 24-week treatment	(Sacktor et al., 2000, Magyar and Szende, 2004, The Dana Consortium, 1998, Schifitto et al., 2009a, Schifitto et al., 2007b)
Sodium valproate and lithium	GSK-3β inhibitor	Reduces neurotoxicity, improved neuropsychological performance	(Ances et al., 2008, Tong et al., 2001, Dou et al., 2003, Everall et al., 2002, Schifitto et al., 2006, Letendre et al., 2006, Schifitto et al., 2009b)
SSRIs— citalopram, paroxetine	Serotonin transporter	May decrease HIV viral levels in CSF, improved adherence to ART	(Ances et al., 2008, Letendre et al., 2007)
Minocycline	5-lipoxygenase and others	Decreases CCL2 levels in CSF, improves SIV encephalitis, suppresses HIV replication, and inhibits secretion of TNF-α, IFN-γ, and IL-2 by lymphocytes	(Copeland and Brooks, 2010, Colovic and Caccia, 2003, Si et al., 2004, Zink et al., 2005, Szeto et al., 2010)
PMS-601	Platelet-activating factor (PAF) receptor antagonist	Reduces neurotoxicity, microgliosis and TNF-α, CCL3, CCL4 and CCL5 secretion by macrophages	(Martin et al., 2000, Eggert et al., 2009b)
Copolymer-1 (Copaxone)	Myelin basic protein analog, shifts T cell responses from Th1 → Th2	Decreases microgliosis, astrogliosis, neurotoxicity, and TNF-α and IL-12 levels	(Gorantla et al., 2007, Gorantla et al., 2008)
CEP-1347	Semisynthetic inhibitor of mixed lineage kinases	Anti-apoptotic, decreases monocyte secretion of TNF-α, reduces microgliosis and neurotoxicity	(Sui et al., 2006b, Eggert et al., 2009a, Bodner et al., 2002)

some effectiveness, they are clearly not potential monotherapies for HAND. In addition to using such drugs prior to neurocognitive decline, effective neuroprotective therapies will likely have to be used in combination and over the duration of viral infection in order to have maximal clinical benefit.

In addition to therapies for neurodegenerative diseases, compounds in clinical use for neuropsychiatric disorders are also under investigation in HAND (Ances et al., 2008). Sodium valproate (VPA) and lithium are approved for treatment of bipolar disorder and related mood disorders, and both inhibit glycogen synthase kinase-3β and provide neuroprotection against HIV-induced toxicity *in vitro* and in mouse models of HIVE (Tong et al., 2001; Dou et al., 2003; Everall et al., 2002). Several small pilot studies have demonstrated improved neuropsychological performance in HAND patients following short-term VPA or lithium therapy (Schifitto et al., 2006; Letendre et al., 2006; Schifitto, Yiannoutsos, et al., 2009). Additional studies using selective serotonin reuptake inhibitors (SSRIs), including citalopram and paroxetine, are also under consideration as adjunctive therapies for HAND (Ances et al., 2008; Letendre et al., 2007).

Other adjunctive therapies for HAND are focused on targeting inflammation cascades that contribute to neurotoxicity.

Minocycline is a broad-spectrum tetracycline antimicrobial that is currently in phase I clinical trials for HAND (Copeland & Brooks, 2010). Minocycline is capable of efficiently crossing the BBB and can suppress HIV replication in microglia, macrophages, and lymphocytes (Colovic & Caccia, 2003; Si et al., 2004; Zink et al., 2005; Szeto et al., 2010). In addition, minocycline has anti-inflammatory properties and can inhibit the secretion of the inflammatory cytokines TNF-α, IFN-γ, and IL-2 by lymphocytes (Szeto et al., 2010). Experimental studies using SIV-infected macaques demonstrated that minocycline decreased CSF levels of CCL2, a marker of CNS inflammation, and decreased the severity of encephalitis (Zink et al., 2005).

In addition to minocycline, several other therapies that have anti-HIV and anti-inflammatory effects are also being considered as adjunctive therapy for HAND. PMS-601, a platelet-activating factor (PAF) receptor antagonist, reduces neurotoxicity, microgliosis, and macrophage secretion of the inflammatory mediators TNF-α, CCL3, CCL4, and CCL5 *in vitro* and in a mouse model of HIVE (Martin et al., 2000; Eggert et al., 2009b). Copolymer-1 (COP-1 or Copaxone) is a clinically approved immune modulator used in the treatment of MS. In addition to decreasing levels of TNF-α and IL-12, COP-1 decreases microgliosis, astrogliosis, and neurotoxicity in a mouse model of HIVE (Gorantla et al., 2007;

Gorantla et al., 2008). CEP-1347 is an anti-apoptotic immune modulator that decreases monocyte secretion of TNF-α and macrophage secretion of chemokines, including CCL4 and CXCL10 (Sui et al., 2006b; Eggert et al., 2009a). CEP-1347 reduces microgliosis and HIV-mediated neurotoxicity *in vitro* and reduces signs of HIVE in a mouse model (Bodner et al., 2002; Sui et al., 2006b; Eggert et al., 2009a). As our understanding of the complex nature of HAND pathogenesis evolves, it is becoming clear that adjunctive therapies that address not only viral burden in the CSF but also the contribution of processes such as inflammation are critical for successful clinical management of HAND. In addition, the development of adjunctive therapies for HAND will contribute to and likely improve the clinical management of other neuroinflammatory disorders, including AD, PD, and MS.

ACKNOWLEDGMENTS

DRC and SAC contributed equally to this work and are listed alphabetically. This manuscript was was supported by NIH grants NS043994 (DLK), NS27405 (DLK), T32 AI07632 (DRC), F31 NS066791 (DRC), T32 AG000255 (SAC), and NS074626 (SSS). The authors declare that there are no conflicts of interest.

REFERENCES

Achim, C. L., Heyes, M. P., & Wiley, C. A. (1993). Quantitation of human immunodeficiency virus, immune activation factors, and quinolinic acid in AIDS brains. *J Clin Invest, 91,* 2769–2775.

Adle-Biassette, H., Chretien, F., Wingertsmann, L., Hery, C., Ereau, T., Scaravilli, F., et al. (1999). Neuronal apoptosis does not correlate with dementia in HIV infection but is related to microglial activation and axonal damage. *Neuropathol Appl Neurobiol, 25,* 123–133.

Alirezaei, M., Kiosses, W. B., Flynn, C. T., Brady, N. R., & Fox, H. S. (2008). Disruption of neuronal autophagy by infected microglia results in neurodegeneration. *PLoS One, 3,* e2906.

Ances, B. M., Letendre, S. L., Alexander, T., & Ellis, R. J. (2008). Role of psychiatric medications as adjunct therapy in the treatment of HIV associated neurocognitive disorders. *Int Rev Psychiatry, 20,* 89–93.

Ancuta, P., Kamat, A., Kunstman, K. J., Kim, E. Y., Autissier, P., Wurcel, A., et al. (2008). Microbial translocation is associated with increased monocyte activation and dementia in AIDS patients. *PLoS One, 3,* e2516.

Ancuta, P., Rao, R., Moses, A., Mehle, A., Shaw, S. K., Luscinskas, F. W., et al. (2003). Fractalkine preferentially mediates arrest and migration of CD16+ monocytes. *J Exp Med, 197,* 1701–1707.

Ancuta, P., Wang, J., & Gabuzda, D. (2006). CD16+ monocytes produce IL-6, CCL2, and matrix metalloproteinase-9 upon interaction with CX3CL1-expressing endothelial cells. *J Leukoc Biol, 80,* 1156–1164.

Anderson, E., Zink, W., Xiong, H., & Gendelman, H. E. (2002). HIV-1-associated dementia: A metabolic encephalopathy perpetrated by virus-infected and immune-competent mononuclear phagocytes. *J Acquir Immune Defic Syndr, 31* Suppl 2, S43–54.

Anderson, E. R., Gendelman, H. E., & Xiong, H. (2004). Memantine protects hippocampal neuronal function in murine human immunodeficiency virus type 1 encephalitis. *J Neurosci, 24,* 7194–7198.

Anthony, I. C. & Bell, J. E. (2008). The Neuropathology of HIV/AIDS. *Int Rev Psychiatry, 20,* 15–24.

Anthony, I. C., Ramage, S. N., Carnie, F. W., Simmonds, P., & Bell, J. E. (2005). Influence of HAART on HIV-related CNS disease and neuroinflammation. *J Neuropathol Exp Neurol, 64,* 529–536.

Antinori, A., Arendt, G., Becker, J. T., Brew, B. J., Byrd, D. A., Cherner, M., et al. (2007). Updated research nosology for HIV-associated neurocognitive disorders. *Neurology, 69,* 1789–1799.

Asensio, V. C., Maier, J., Milner, R., Boztug, K., Kincaid, C., Moulard, M., et al. (2001). Interferon-independent, human immunodeficiency virus type 1 gp120-mediated induction of CXCL10/IP-10 gene expression by astrocytes in vivo and in vitro. *J Virol, 75,* 7067–7077.

Bajetto, A., Bonavia, R., Barbero, S., Florio, T., & Schettini, G. (2001). Chemokines and their receptors in the central nervous system. *Front Neuroendocrinol, 22,* 147–184.

Bajetto, A., Bonavia, R., Barbero, S., Piccioli, P., Costa, A., Florio, T., et al. (1999). Glial and neuronal cells express functional chemokine receptor CXCR4 and its natural ligand stromal cell-derived factor 1. *J Neurochem, 73,* 2348–2357.

Bandaru, V. V., Mcarthur, J. C., Sacktor, N., Cutler, R. G., Knapp, E. L., Mattson, M. P., et al. (2007). Associative and predictive biomarkers of dementia in HIV-1-infected patients. *Neurology, 68,* 1481–1487.

Banks, W. A., Ercal, N., & Price, T. O. (2006). The blood-brain barrier in neuroAIDS. *Curr HIV Res, 4,* 259–266.

Bartosik-Psujek, H. & Stelmasiak, Z. (2005). Correlations between IL-4, IL-12 levels and CCL2, CCL5 levels in serum and cerebrospinal fluid of multiple sclerosis patients. *J Neural Transm, 112,* 797–803.

Bell, J. E. (2004). An update on the neuropathology of HIV in the HAART era. *Histopathology, 45,* 549–559.

Bezzi, P., Domercq, M., Brambilla, L., Galli, R., Schols, D., De Clercq, E., et al. (2001). CXCR4-activated astrocyte glutamate release via TNFalpha: Amplification by microglia triggers neurotoxicity. *Nat Neurosci, 4,* 702–710.

Biddison, W. E., Kubota, R., Kawanishi, T., Taub, D. D., Cruikshank, W. W., Center, D. M., et al. (1997). Human T cell leukemia virus type I (HTLV-I)-specific CD8+ CTL clones from patients with HTLV-I-associated neurologic disease secrete proinflammatory cytokines, chemokines, and matrix metalloproteinase. *J Immunol, 159,* 2018–2025.

Block, M. L. & Hong, J. S. (2005). Microglia and inflammation-mediated neurodegeneration: Multiple triggers with a common mechanism. *Prog Neurobiol, 76,* 77–98.

Bodner, A., Maroney, A. C., Finn, J. P., Ghadge, G., Roos, R., & Miller, R. J. (2002). Mixed lineage kinase 3 mediates gp120IIIB-induced neurotoxicity. *J Neurochem, 82,* 1424–1434.

Boisse, L., Gill, M. J., & Power, C. (2008). HIV infection of the central nervous system: Clinical features and neuropathogenesis. *Neurol Clin, 26,* 799–819.

Boven, L. A., Gomes, L., Hery, C., Gray, F., Verhoef, J., Portegies, P., et al. (1999). Increased peroxynitrite activity in AIDS dementia complex: Implications for the neuropathogenesis of HIV-1 infection. *J Immunol, 162,* 4319–4327.

Breitner, J. C., Welsh, K. A., Helms, M. J., Gaskell, P. C., Gau, B. A., Roses, A. D., et al. (1995). Delayed onset of Alzheimer's disease with non-steroidal anti-inflammatory and histamine H2 blocking drugs. *Neurobiol Aging, 16,* 523–530.

Brenchley, J. M., Price, D. A., Schacker, T. W., Asher, T. E., Silvestri, G., Rao, S., et al. (2006). Microbial translocation is a cause of systemic immune activation in chronic HIV infection. *Nat Med, 12,* 1365–1371.

Brenneman, D. E., Westbrook, G. L., Fitzgerald, S. P., Ennist, D. L., Elkins, K. L., Ruff, M. R., et al. (1988). Neuronal cell killing by the envelope protein of HIV and its prevention by vasoactive intestinal peptide. *Nature, 335,* 639–642.

Brew, B. J. (2004). Evidence for a change in AIDS dementia complex in the era of highly active antiretroviral therapy and the possibility of new forms of AIDS dementia complex. *AIDS, 18* Suppl 1, S75–78.

Brew, B. J., Bhalla, R. B., Paul, M., Sidtis, J. J., Keilp, J. J., Sadler, A. E., et al. (1992). Cerebrospinal fluid beta 2-microglobulin in patients with AIDS dementia complex: An expanded series including response to zidovudine treatment. *AIDS, 6,* 461–465.

Brew, B. J., Corbeil, J., Pemberton, L., Evans, L., Saito, K., Penny, R., et al. (1995). Quinolinic acid production is related to macrophage tropic isolates of HIV-1. *Journal of Neurovirology, 1*, 369–374.

Brew, B. J., Crowe, S. M., Landay, A., Cysique, L. A., & Guillemin, G. (2009). Neurodegeneration and ageing in the HAART era. *J Neuroimmune Pharmacol, 4*, 163–174.

Brew, B. J., Dunbar, N., Pemberton, L., & Kaldor, J. (1996). Predictive markers of AIDS dementia complex: CD4 cell count and cerebrospinal fluid concentrations of beta 2-microglobulin and neopterin. *J Infect Dis, 174*, 294–298.

Brew, B. J., Halman, M., Catalan, J., Sacktor, N., Price, R. W., Brown, S., et al. (2007). Factors in AIDS dementia complex trial design: Results and lessons from the abacavir trial. *PLoS Clin Trials, 2*, e13.

Brew, B. J., Pemberton, L., Cunningham, P., & Law, M. G. (1997). Levels of human immunodeficiency virus type 1 RNA in cerebrospinal fluid correlate with AIDS dementia stage. *J Infect Dis, 175*, 963–966.

Bruno, V., Copani, A., Besong, G., Scoto, G., & Nicoletti, F. (2000). Neuroprotective activity of chemokines against N-methyl-D-aspartate or beta-amyloid-induced toxicity in culture. *Eur J Pharmacol, 399*, 117–121.

Burdo, T. H., Ellis, R. J., & Fox, H. S. (2008). Osteopontin is increased in HIV-associated dementia. *J Infect Dis,198*, 715–722.

Cannella, B. & Raine, C. S. (1995). The adhesion molecule and cytokine profile of multiple sclerosis lesions. *Ann Neurol, 37*, 424–435.

Cardona, A. E., Pioro, E. P., Sasse, M. E., Kostenko, V., Cardona, S. M., Dijkstra, I. M., et al. (2006). Control of microglial neurotoxicity by the fractalkine receptor. *Nat Neurosci, 9*, 917–924.

Casoli, T., Di Stefano, G., Balietti, M., Solazzi, M., Giorgetti, B., & Fattoretti, P. (2010). Peripheral inflammatory biomarkers of Alzheimer's disease: The role of platelets. *Biogerontology*.

Chang, L., Ernst, T., St Hillaire, C., & Conant, K. (2004). Antiretroviral treatment alters relationship between MCP-1 and neurometabolites in HIV patients. *Antivir Ther, 9*, 431–440.

Chang, L., Wong, V., Nakama, H., Watters, M., Ramones, D., Miller, E. N., et al. (2008). Greater than age-related changes in brain diffusion of HIV patients after 1 year. *J Neuroimmune Pharmacol, 3*, 265–274.

Chapman, G. A., Moores, K., Harrison, D., Campbell, C. A., Stewart, B. R., & Strijbos, P. J. (2000a). Fractalkine cleavage from neuronal membranes represents an acute event in the inflammatory response to excitotoxic brain damage. *J Neurosci, 20*, RC87.

Chapman, G. A., Moores, K. E., Gohil, J., Berkhout, T. A., Patel, L., Green, P., et al. (2000b). The role of fractalkine in the recruitment of monocytes to the endothelium. *Eur J Pharmacol, 392*, 189–195.

Chen, H., Zhang, S. M., Hernan, M. A., Schwarzschild, M. A., Willett, W. C., Colditz, G. A., et al. (2003). Nonsteroidal anti-inflammatory drugs and the risk of Parkinson disease. *Arch Neurol, 60*, 1059–1064.

Childs, E. A., Lyles, R. H., Selnes, O. A., Chen, B., Miller, E. N., Cohen, B. A., et al. (1999). Plasma viral load and CD4 lymphocytes predict HIV-associated dementia and sensory neuropathy. *Neurology, 52*, 607–613.

Choe, W., Volsky, D. J., & Potash, M. J. (2001). Induction of rapid and extensive beta-chemokine synthesis in macrophages by human immunodeficiency virus type 1 and gp120, independently of their coreceptor phenotype. *J Virol, 75*, 10738–10745.

Cinque, P., Bestetti, A., Marenzi, R., Sala, S., Gisslen, M., Hagberg, L., et al. (2005). Cerebrospinal fluid interferon-gamma-inducible protein 10 (IP-10, CXCL10) in HIV-1 infection. *J Neuroimmunol, 168*, 154–63.

Cinque, P., Vago, L., Mengozzi, M., Torri, V., Ceresa, D., Vicenzi, E., et al. (1998). Elevated cerebrospinal fluid levels of monocyte chemotactic protein-1 correlate with HIV-1 encephalitis and local viral replication. *AIDS, 12*, 1327–1332.

Clifford, D. B., Fagan, A. M., Holtzman, D. M., Morris, J. C., Teshome, M., Shah, A. R., et al. (2009). CSF biomarkers of Alzheimer disease in HIV-associated neurologic disease. *Neurology, 73*, 1982–1987.

Cocchi, F., Devico, A. L., Garzino-Demo, A., Arya, S. K., Gallo, R. C., & Lusso, P. (1995). Identification of RANTES, MIP-1 alpha, and MIP-1 beta as the major HIV-suppressive factors produced by CD8+ T cells. *Science, 270*, 1811–1815.

Collman, R. G. & Yi, Y. (1999). Cofactors for human immunodeficiency virus entry into primary macrophages. *J Infect Dis, 179* Suppl 3, S422–426.

Colovic, M. & Caccia, S. (2003). Liquid chromatographic determination of minocycline in brain-to-plasma distribution studies in the rat. *J Chromatogr B Analyt Technol Biomed Life Sci, 791*, 337–343.

Conant, K., Garzino-Demo, A., Nath, A., Mcarthur, J. C., Halliday, W., Power, C., et al. (1998). Induction of monocyte chemoattractant protein-1 in HIV-1 Tat-stimulated astrocytes and elevation in AIDS dementia. *Proc Natl Acad Sci U S A, 95*, 3117–3121.

Copeland, K. F. & Brooks, J. I. (2010). A novel use for an old drug: The potential for minocycline as anti-HIV adjuvant therapy. *J Infect Dis, 201*, 1115–1117.

Cota, M., Kleinschmidt, A., Ceccherini-Silberstein, F., Aloisi, F., Mengozzi, M., Mantovani, A., et al. (2000). Upregulated expression of interleukin-8, RANTES and chemokine receptors in human astrocytic cells infected with HIV-1. *J Neurovirol, 6*, 75–83.

Cotter, R., Williams, C., Ryan, L., Erichsen, D., Lopez, A., Peng, H., et al. (2002). Fractalkine (CX3CL1) and brain inflammation: Implications for HIV-1-associated dementia. *J Neurovirol, 8*, 585–598.

Craft, J. M., Watterson, D. M., & Van Eldik, L. J. (2006). Human amyloid beta-induced neuroinflammation is an early event in neurodegeneration. *Glia, 53*, 484–490.

D'aversa, T. G., Yu, K. O., & Berman, J. W. (2004). Expression of chemokines by human fetal microglia after treatment with the human immunodeficiency virus type 1 protein Tat. *J Neurovirol, 10*, 86–97.

Dallasta, L. M., Pisarov, L. A., Esplen, J. E., Werley, J. V., Moses, A. V., Nelson, J. A., et al. (1999). Blood-brain barrier tight junction disruption in human immunodeficiency virus-1 encephalitis. *Am J Pathol, 155*, 1915–1927.

Deiva, K., Geeraerts, T., Salim, H., Leclerc, P., Hery, C., Hugel, B., et al. (2004). Fractalkine reduces N-methyl-d-aspartate-induced calcium flux and apoptosis in human neurons through extracellular signal-regulated kinase activation. *Eur J Neurosci, 20*, 3222–3232.

Dhillon, N., Zhu, X., Peng, F., Yao, H., Williams, R., Qiu, J., et al. (2008a). Molecular mechanism(s) involved in the synergistic induction of CXCL10 by human immunodeficiency virus type 1 Tat and interferon-gamma in macrophages. *J Neurovirol, 14*, 196–204.

Dhillon, N. K., Williams, R., Callen, S., Zien, C., Narayan, O. & Buch, S. (2008b). Roles of MCP-1 in development of HIV-dementia. *Front Biosci, 13*, 3913–3918.

Doms, R. W. (2000). Beyond receptor expression: The influence of receptor conformation, density, and affinity in HIV-1 infection. *Virology, 276*, 229–237.

Dore-Duffy, P., Newman, W., Balabanov, R., Lisak, R. P., Mainolfi, E., Rothlein, R., et al. (1995). Circulating, soluble adhesion proteins in cerebrospinal fluid and serum of patients with multiple sclerosis: Correlation with clinical activity. *Ann Neurol, 37*, 55–62.

Dou, H., Birusingh, K., Faraci, J., Gorantla, S., Poluektova, L. Y., Maggirwar, S. B., et al. (2003). Neuroprotective activities of sodium valproate in a murine model of human immunodeficiency virus-1 encephalitis. *J Neurosci, 23*, 9162–9170.

Douek, D. (2007). HIV disease progression: Immune activation, microbes, and a leaky gut. *Top HIV Med, 15*, 114–117.

Drulovic, J., Mostarica-Stojkovic, M., Levic, Z., Mesaros, S., Stojsavljevic, N., Popadic, D., et al. (1998). Serum interleukin-12 levels in patients with multiple sclerosis. *Neurosci Lett, 251*, 129–132.

Drulovic, J., Mostarica-Stojkovic, M., Levic, Z., Stojsavljevic, N., Pravica, V., & Mesaros, S. (1997). Interleukin-12 and tumor necrosis factor-alpha levels in cerebrospinal fluid of multiple sclerosis patients. *J Neurol Sci, 147*, 145–150.

Dunfee, R., Thomas, E. R., Gorry, P. R., Wang, J., Ancuta, P., & Gabuzda, D. (2006). Mechanisms of HIV-1 neurotropism. *Curr HIV Res, 4*, 267–278.

Eggert, D., Dash, P. K., Gorantla, S., Dou, H., Schifitto, G., Maggirwar, S. B., et al. (2009a). Neuroprotective Activities of CEP-1347 in Models of NeuroAIDS. *J Immunol*.

Eggert, D., Dash, P. K., Serradji, N., Dong, C. Z., Clayette, P., Heymans, F., et al. (2009b). Development of a platelet-activating factor antagonist for HIV-1 associated neurocognitive disorders. *J Neuroimmunol, 213,* 47–59.

Eikelenboom, P., Bate, C., Van Gool, W. A., Hoozemans, J. J., Rozemuller, J. M., Veerhuis, R., et al. (2002). Neuroinflammation in Alzheimer's disease and prion disease. *Glia, 40,* 232–239.

El-Hage, N., Gurwell, J. A., Singh, I. N., Knapp, P. E., Nath, A., & Hauser, K. F. (2005). Synergistic increases in intracellular Ca2+, and the release of MCP-1, RANTES, and IL-6 by astrocytes treated with opiates and HIV-1 Tat. *Glia, 50,* 91–106.

Ellery, P. J., Tippett, E., Chiu, Y. L., Paukovics, G., Cameron, P. U., Solomon, A., et al. (2007). The CD16+ monocyte subset is more permissive to infection and preferentially harbors HIV-1 in vivo. *J Immunol, 178,* 6581–6589.

Ellis, R., Langford, D., & Masliah, E. (2007). HIV and antiretroviral therapy in the brain: Neuronal injury and repair. *Nat Rev Neurosci, 8,* 33–44.

Ellis, R. J., Gamst, A. C., Capparelli, E., Spector, S. A., Hsia, K., Wolfson, T., et al. (2000). Cerebrospinal fluid HIV RNA originates from both local CNS and systemic sources. *Neurology, 54,* 927–936.

Ellis, R. J., Hsia, K., Spector, S. A., Nelson, J. A., Heaton, R. K., Wallace, M. R., et al. (1997). Cerebrospinal fluid human immunodeficiency virus type 1 RNA levels are elevated in neurocognitively impaired individuals with acquired immunodeficiency syndrome. HIV Neurobehavioral Research Center Group. *Ann Neurol, 42,* 679–688.

Ellis, R. J., Moore, D. J., Childers, M. E., Letendre, S., Mccutchan, J. A., Wolfson, T., et al. (2002). Progression to neuropsychological impairment in human immunodeficiency virus infection predicted by elevated cerebrospinal fluid levels of human immunodeficiency virus RNA. *Arch Neurol, 59,* 923–928.

Elovaara, I., Koenig, S., Brewah, A. Y., Woods, R. M., Lehky, T., & Jacobson, S. (1993). High human T cell lymphotropic virus type 1 (HTLV-1)-specific precursor cytotoxic T lymphocyte frequencies in patients with HTLV-1-associated neurological disease. *J Exp Med, 177,* 1567–1573.

Enose-Akahata, Y., Matsuura, E., Oh, U., & Jacobson, S. (2009). High expression of CD244 and SAP regulated CD8 T cell responses of patients with HTLV-I associated neurologic disease. *PLoS Pathog, 5,* e1000682.

Enting, R. H., Foudraine, N. A., Lange, J. M., Jurriaans, S., Van Der Poll, T., Weverling, G. J., et al. (2000). Cerebrospinal fluid beta2-microglobulin, monocyte chemotactic protein-1, and soluble tumour necrosis factor alpha receptors before and after treatment with lamivudine plus zidovudine or stavudine. *J Neuroimmunol, 102,* 216–221.

Erichsen, D., Lopez, A. L., Peng, H., Niemann, D., Williams, C., Bauer, M., et al. (2003). Neuronal injury regulates fractalkine: Relevance for HIV-1 associated dementia. *J Neuroimmunol, 138,* 144–155.

Esiri, M. M., Biddolph, S. C., & Morris, C. S. (1998). Prevalence of Alzheimer plaques in AIDS. *J Neurol Neurosurg Psychiatry, 65,* 29–33.

Eugenin, E. A., D'Aversa, T. G., Lopez, L., Calderon, T. M., & Berman, J. W. (2003). MCP-1 (CCL2) protects human neurons and astrocytes from NMDA or HIV-tat-induced apoptosis. *J Neurochem, 85,* 1299–1311.

Eugenin, E. A., Osiecki, K., Lopez, L., Goldstein, H., Calderon, T. M., & Berman, J. W. (2006). CCL2/monocyte chemoattractant protein-1 mediates enhanced transmigration of human immunodeficiency virus (HIV)-infected leukocytes across the blood-brain barrier: A potential mechanism of HIV-CNS invasion and NeuroAIDS. *J Neurosci, 26,* 1098–1106.

Everall, I. P., Bell, C., Mallory, M., Langford, D., Adame, A., Rockestein, E., et al. (2002). Lithium ameliorates HIV-gp120-mediated neurotoxicity. *Mol Cell Neurosci, 21,* 493–501.

Everall, I. P., Luthert, P. J., & Lantos, P. L. (1991). Neuronal loss in the frontal cortex in HIV infection. *Lancet, 337,* 1119–1121.

Fiala, M., Looney, D. J., Stins, M., Way, D. D., Zhang, L., Gan, X., et al. (1997). TNF-alpha opens a paracellular route for HIV-1 invasion across the blood-brain barrier. *Mol Med, 3,* 553–564.

Fischer-Smith, T., Croul, S., Adeniyi, A., Rybicka, K., Morgello, S., Khalili, K., et al. (2004). Macrophage/microglial accumulation and proliferating cell nuclear antigen expression in the central nervous system in human immunodeficiency virus encephalopathy. *Am J Pathol, 164,* 2089–2099.

Foli, A., Saville, M. W., May, L. T., Webb, D. S., & Yarchoan, R. (1997). Effects of human immunodeficiency virus and colony-stimulating factors on the production of interleukin 6 and tumor necrosis factor alpha by monocyte/macrophages. *AIDS Res Hum Retroviruses, 13,* 829–839.

Frei, K., Fredrikson, S., Fontana, A., & Link, H. (1991). Interleukin-6 is elevated in plasma in multiple sclerosis. *J Neuroimmunol, 31,* 147–153.

Frohman, E. M., Racke, M. K., & Raine, C. S. (2006). Multiple sclerosis—the plaque and its pathogenesis. *N Engl J Med, 354,* 942–955.

Gartner, S. (2000). HIV infection and dementia. *Science, 287,* 602–604.

Gelbard, H. A., Dzenko, K. A., Diloreto, D., Del Cerro, C., Del Cerro, M., & Epstein, L. G. (1993). Neurotoxic effects of tumor necrosis factor alpha in primary human neuronal cultures are mediated by activation of the glutamate AMPA receptor subtype: Implications for AIDS neuropathogenesis. *Dev Neurosci, 15,* 417–422.

Gelbard, H. A., Nottet, H. S., Swindells, S., Jett, M., Dzenko, K. A., Genis, P., et al. (1994). Platelet-activating factor: A candidate human immunodeficiency virus type 1-induced neurotoxin. *J Virol, 68,* 4628–4635.

Gendelman, H. E., Lipton, S. A., Tardieu, M., Bukrinsky, M. I., & Nottet, H. S. (1994). The neuropathogenesis of HIV-1 infection. *J Leukoc Biol, 56,* 389–398.

Gendelman, H. E., Zheng, J., Coulter, C. L., Ghorpade, A., Che, M., Thylin, M., et al. (1998). Suppression of inflammatory neurotoxins by highly active antiretroviral therapy in human immunodeficiency virus-associated dementia. *J Infect Dis, 178,* 1000–1007.

Genis, P., Jett, M., Bernton, E. W., Boyle, T., Gelbard, H. A., Dzenko, K., et al. (1992). Cytokines and arachidonic metabolites produced during human immunodeficiency virus (HIV)-infected macrophage-astroglia interactions: Implications for the neuropathogenesis of HIV disease. *J Exp Med, 176,* 1703–1718.

Glass, J. D., Fedor, H., Wesselingh, S. L., & McArthur, J. C. (1995). Immunocytochemical quantitation of human immunodeficiency virus in the brain: Correlations with dementia. *Ann Neurol, 38,* 755–762.

Gonzalez-Scarano, F. & Martin-Garcia, J. (2005). The neuropathogenesis of AIDS. *Nat Rev Immunol, 5,* 69–81.

Gorantla, S., Liu, J., Sneller, H., Dou, H., Holguin, A., Smith, L., et al. (2007). Copolymer-1 induces adaptive immune anti-inflammatory glial and neuroprotective responses in a murine model of HIV-1 encephalitis. *J Immunol, 179,* 4345–4356.

Gorantla, S., Liu, J., Wang, T., Holguin, A., Sneller, H. M., Dou, H., et al. (2008). Modulation of innate immunity by copolymer-1 leads to neuroprotection in murine HIV-1 encephalitis. *Glia, 56,* 223–232.

Grant, C., Barmak, K., Alefantis, T., Yao, J., Jacobson, S., & Wigdahl, B. (2002). Human T cell leukemia virus type I and neurologic disease: Events in bone marrow, peripheral blood, and central nervous system during normal immune surveillance and neuroinflammation. *J Cell Physiol, 190,* 133–159.

Grant, I. 2008. Neurocognitive disturbances in HIV. *Int Rev Psychiatry, 20,* 33–47.

Gray, F., Chretien, F., Vallat-DeCouvelaere, A. V., & Scaravilli, F. (2003). The changing pattern of HIV neuropathology in the HAART era. *J Neuropathol Exp Neurol, 62,* 429–440.

Greten, T. F., Slansky, J. E., Kubota, R., Soldan, S. S., Jaffee, E. M., Leist, T. P., et al. (1998). Direct visualization of antigen-specific T cells: HTLV-1 Tax11–19- specific CD8(+) T cells are activated in peripheral blood and accumulate in cerebrospinal fluid from HAM/TSP patients. *Proc Natl Acad Sci U S A, 95,* 7568–7573.

Griffin, D. E., Wesselingh, S. L., & McArthur, J. C. (1994). Elevated central nervous system prostaglandins in human immunodeficiency virus-associated dementia. *Ann Neurol, 35,* 592–597.

Gu, L., Rutledge, B., Fiorillo, J., Ernst, C., Grewal, I., Flavell, R., et al. (1997). In vivo properties of monocyte chemoattractant protein-1. *J Leukoc Biol, 62,* 577–580.

Guillemin, G. J., Croitoru-Lamoury, J., Dormont, D., Armati, P. J., & Brew, B. J. (2003). Quinolinic acid upregulates chemokine production and chemokine receptor expression in astrocytes. *Glia, 41,* 371–381.

Habata, Y., Fujii, R., Hosoya, M., Fukusumi, S., Kawamata, Y., Hinuma, S., et al. (1999). Apelin, the natural ligand of the orphan receptor APJ, is abundantly secreted in the colostrum. *Biochim Biophys Acta, 1452*, 25–35.

Hakansson, A., Westberg, L., Nilsson, S., Buervenich, S., Carmine, A., Holmberg, B., et al. (2005a). Interaction of polymorphisms in the genes encoding interleukin-6 and estrogen receptor beta on the susceptibility to Parkinson's disease. *Am J Med Genet B Neuropsychiatr Genet, 133B*, 88–92.

Hakansson, A., Westberg, L., Nilsson, S., Buervenich, S., Carmine, A., Holmberg, B., et al. (2005b). Investigation of genes coding for inflammatory components in Parkinson's disease. *Mov Disord, 20*, 569–573.

Harris, V. K. & Sadiq, S. A. (2009). Disease biomarkers in multiple sclerosis: Potential for use in therapeutic decision making. *Mol Diagn Ther, 13*, 225–244.

Harrison, J. K., Jiang, Y., Chen, S., Xia, Y., Maciejewski, D., McNamara, R. K., et al. (1998). Role for neuronally derived fractalkine in mediating interactions between neurons and CX3CR1-expressing microglia. *Proc Natl Acad Sci U S A, 95*, 10896–10901.

Haughey, N. J., Cutler, R. G., Tamara, A., McArthur, J. C., Vargas, D. L., Pardo, C. A., et al. (2004). Perturbation of sphingolipid metabolism and ceramide production in HIV-dementia. *Ann Neurol, 55*, 257–267.

Heaton, R. K., Clifford, D. B., Franklin D. R. Jr, Woods, S. P., Ake C., Vaida F., Ellis, R. J., Letendre, S. L., Marcotte, T. D., Atkinson, J. H., Rivera-Mindt, M., Virgil, O. R., Taylor, M. J., Collier, A. C., Marra, C. M., Gelman, B. B., McArthur, J. C., Morgello, S., Simpson, D. M., McCutchan, J. A., Abramson, I., Gamst, A., Fennema-Notestine, C., Jernigan, T. L., Wong, J., Grant, I.; CHARTER Group. (2010). HIV-associated neurocognitive disorders persist in the era of potent antiretroviral therapy: CHARTER Study. *Neurol, 75*, 2087–2096.

Herber, D. L., Maloney, J. L., Rot, L. M., Freeman, M. J., Morgan, D., & Gordon, M. N. (2006). Diverse microglial responses after intrahippocampal administration of lipopolysaccharide. *Glia, 53*, 382–391.

Hesselgesser, J., Taub, D., Baskar, P., Greenberg, M., Hoxie, J., Kolson, D. L., et al. (1998). Neuronal apoptosis induced by HIV-1 gp120 and the chemokine SDF-1 alpha is mediated by the chemokine receptor CXCR4. *Curr Biol, 8*, 595–598.

Heyes, M. P., Brew, B. J., Martin, A., Price, R. W., Salazar, A. M., Sidtis, J. J., et al. (1991). Quinolinic acid in cerebrospinal fluid and serum in HIV-1 infection: Relationship to clinical and neurological status. *Ann Neurol, 29*, 202–209.

Heyes, M. P., Ellis, R. J., Ryan, L., Childers, M. E., Grant, I., WolfsonO, T., et al. (2001). Elevated cerebrospinal fluid quinolinic acid levels are associated with region-specific cerebral volume loss in HIV infection. *Brain, 124*, 1033–1042.

Ho, D. D., Rota, T. R., Schooley, R. T., Kaplan, J. C., Allan, J. D., Groopman, J. E., et al. (1985). Isolation of HTLV-III from cerebrospinal fluid and neural tissues of patients with neurologic syndromes related to the acquired immunodeficiency syndrome. *N Engl J Med, 313*, 1493–1497.

Hoffman, P. M., Dhib-Jalbut, S., Mikovits, J. A., Robbins, D. S., Wolf, A. L., Bergey, G. K., et al. (1992). Human T-cell leukemia virus type I infection of monocytes and microglial cells in primary human cultures. *Proc Natl Acad Sci U S A, 89*, 11784–11788.

Hunot, S., Dugas, N., Faucheux, B., Hartmann, A., Tardieu, M., Debre, P., et al. (1999). FcepsilonRII/CD23 is expressed in Parkinson's disease and induces, in vitro, production of nitric oxide and tumor necrosis factor-alpha in glial cells. *J Neurosci, 19*, 3440–3447.

Hurwitz, A. A., Berman, J. W., & Lyman, W. D. (1994). The role of the blood-brain barrier in HIV infection of the central nervous system. *Adv Neuroimmunol, 4*, 249–256.

Imai, T., Hieshima, K., Haskell, C., Baba, M., Nagira, M., Nishimura, M., et al. (1997). Identification and molecular characterization of fractalkine receptor CX3CR1, which mediates both leukocyte migration and adhesion. *Cell, 91*, 521–530.

Jacobson, S., Gupta, A., Mattson, D., Mingioli E., & McFarlin, D. E. (1990a). Immunological studies in tropical spastic paraparesis. *Ann Neurol, 27*, 149–156.

Jacobson, S., Shida, H., McFarlin, D. E., Fauci, A. S., & Koenig, S. (1990b). Circulating CD8+ cytotoxic T lymphocytes specific for HTLV-I pX in patients with HTLV-I associated neurological disease. *Nature, 348*, 245–248.

Jaworowski, A., Kamwendo, D. D., Ellery, P., Sonza, S., Mwapasa, V., Tadesse, E., et al. (2007). CD16+ monocyte subset preferentially harbors HIV-1 and is expanded in pregnant Malawian women with Plasmodium falciparum malaria and HIV-1 infection. *J Infect Dis, 196*, 38–42.

Jiang, Z. G., Piggee, C., Heyes, M. P., Murphy, C., Quearry, B., Bauer, M., et al. (2001). Glutamate is a mediator of neurotoxicity in secretions of activated HIV-1-infected macrophages. *J Neuroimmunol, 117*, 97–107.

Kanmogne, G. D., Kennedy, R. C., & Grammas, P. (2002). HIV-1 gp120 proteins and gp160 peptides are toxic to brain endothelial cells and neurons: Possible pathway for HIV entry into the brain and HIV-associated dementia. *J Neuropathol Exp Neurol, 61*, 992–1000.

Kaul, M. (2009). HIV-1 associated dementia: Update on pathological mechanisms and therapeutic approaches. *Curr Opin Neurol, 22*, 315–320.

Kaul, M., Garden, G. A., & Lipton, S. A. (2001). Pathways to neuronal injury and apoptosis in HIV-associated dementia. *Nature, 410*, 988–994.

Kaul, M. & Lipton, S. A. (1999). Chemokines and activated macrophages in HIV gp120-induced neuronal apoptosis. *Proc Natl Acad Sci U S A, 96*, 8212–8216.

Kaul, M. & Lipton, S. A. (2006). Mechanisms of neuroimmunity and neurodegeneration associated with HIV-1 infection and AIDS. *J Neuroimmune Pharmacol, 1*, 138–151.

Kelder, W., McArthur, J. C., Nance-Sproson, T., McClernon, D., & Griffin, D. E. (1998). Beta-chemokines MCP-1 and RANTES are selectively increased in cerebrospinal fluid of patients with human immunodeficiency virus-associated dementia. *Ann Neurol, 44*, 831–835.

Ketzler, S., Weis, S., Haug, H., & Budka, H. (1990). Loss of neurons in the frontal cortex in AIDS brains. *Acta Neuropathol, 80*, 92–94.

Khan, M. Z., Brandimarti, R., Patel, J. P., Huynh, N., Wang, J., Huang, Z., et al. (2004). Apoptotic and antiapoptotic effects of CXCR4: Is it a matter of intrinsic efficacy? Implications for HIV neuropathogenesis. *AIDS Res Hum Retroviruses, 20*, 1063–1071.

Khanlou, N., Moore, D. J., Chana, G., Cherner, M., Lazzaretto, D., Dawes, S., et al. (2009). Increased frequency of alpha-synuclein in the substantia nigra in human immunodeficiency virus infection. *J Neurovirol, 15*, 131–138.

Koenig, S., Gendelman, H. E., Orenstein, J. M., Dal Canto, M. C., Pezeshkpour, G. H., Yungbluth, M., et al. (1986). Detection of AIDS virus in macrophages in brain tissue from AIDS patients with encephalopathy. *Science, 233*, 1089–1093.

Kolb, S. A., Sporer, B., Lahrtz, F., Koedel, U., Pfister, H. W., & Fontana, A. (1999). Identification of a T cell chemotactic factor in the cerebrospinal fluid of HIV-1-infected individuals as interferon-gamma inducible protein 10. *J Neuroimmunol, 93*, 172–181.

Kolson, D. L. & Gonzalez-Scarano, F. (2000). HIV-1 and dementia. *Journal of Clinical Investigation, 106*, 11–13.

Kraft-Terry, S. D., Buch, S. J., Fox, H. S., & Gendelman, H. E. (2009). A coat of many colors: Neuroimmune crosstalk in human immunodeficiency virus infection. *Neuron, 64*, 133–145.

Kramer-Hammerle, S., Rothenaigner, I., Wolff, H., Bell, J. E., & Brack-Werner, R. (2005). Cells of the central nervous system as targets and reservoirs of the human immunodeficiency virus. *Virus Res, 111*, 194–213.

Kruger, R., Hardt, C., Tschentscher, F., Jackel, S., Kuhn, W., Muller, T., et al. (2000). Genetic analysis of immunomodulating factors in sporadic Parkinson's disease. *J Neural Transm, 107*, 553–562.

Kutsch, O., Oh, J., Nath, A., & Benveniste, E. N. (2000). Induction of the chemokines interleukin-8 and IP-10 by human immunodeficiency virus type 1 tat in astrocytes. *J Virol, 74*, 9214–9221.

Lawrence, D. M. & Major, E. O. (2002). HIV-1 and the brain: Connections between HIV-1-associated dementia, neuropathology and neuroimmunology. *Microbes Infect, 4*, 301–308.

Lazarini, F., Casanova, P., Tham, T. N., De Clercq, E., Arenzana-Seisdedos, F., Baleux, F., et al. (2000). Differential signalling of the chemokine receptor CXCR4 by stromal cell-derived factor 1 and the HIV glycoprotein in rat neurons and astrocytes. *Eur J Neurosci, 12*, 117–125.

Lehmann, M. H., Masanetz, S., Kramer, S., & Erfle, V. (2006). HIV-1 Nef upregulates CCL2/MCP-1 expression in astrocytes in a myristoylation- and calmodulin-dependent manner. *J Cell Sci, 119*, 4520–4530.

Letendre, S., Marquie-Beck, J., Capparelli, E., Best, B., Clifford, D., Collier, A. C., et al. (2008). Validation of the CNS Penetration-Effectiveness rank for quantifying antiretroviral penetration into the central nervous system. *Arch Neurol, 65*, 65–70.

Letendre, S. L., Lanier, E. R., & McCutchan, J. A. (1999). Cerebrospinal fluid beta chemokine concentrations in neurocognitively impaired individuals infected with human immunodeficiency virus type 1. *J Infect Dis, 180*, 310–319.

Letendre, S. L., Marquie-Beck, J., Ellis, R. J., Woods, S. P., Best, B., Clifford, D. B., et al. (2007). The role of cohort studies in drug development: Clinical evidence of antiviral activity of serotonin reuptake inhibitors and HMG-CoA reductase inhibitors in the central nervous system. *J Neuroimmune Pharmacol, 2*, 120–127.

Letendre, S. L., Woods, S. P., Ellis, R. J., Atkinson, J. H., Masliah, E., Van Den Brande, G., et al. (2006). Lithium improves HIV-associated neurocognitive impairment. *AIDS, 20*, 1885–1888.

Levin, M. C., Lehky, T. J., Flerlage, A. N., Katz, D., Kingma, D. W., Jaffe, E. S., et al. (1997). Immunologic analysis of a spinal cord-biopsy specimen from a patient with human T-cell lymphotropic virus type I-associated neurologic disease. *N Engl J Med, 336*, 839–845.

Li, M. & Ransohoff, R. M. (2008). Multiple roles of chemokine CXCL12 in the central nervous system: A migration from immunology to neurobiology. *Prog Neurobiol, 84*, 116–131.

Limatola, C., Lauro, C., Catalano, M., Ciotti, M. T., Bertollini, C., Di Angelantonio, S., et al. (2005). Chemokine CX3CL1 protects rat hippocampal neurons against glutamate-mediated excitotoxicity. *J Neuroimmunol, 166*, 19–28.

Liner, K. J., 2nd, Hall, C. D., & Robertson, K. R. (2008). Effects of antiretroviral therapy on cognitive impairment. *Curr HIV/AIDS Rep, 5*, 64–71.

Lovell, M. A. & Markesbery, W. R. (2007). Oxidative damage in mild cognitive impairment and early Alzheimer's disease. *J Neurosci Res, 85*, 3036–3040.

Maciejewski-Lenoir, D., Chen, S., Feng, L., Maki, R., & Bacon, K. B. (1999). Characterization of fractalkine in rat brain cells: Migratory and activation signals for CX3CR-1-expressing microglia. *J Immunol, 163*, 1628–1635.

Magyar, K. & Szende, B. (2004). (-)-Deprenyl, a selective MAO-B inhibitor, with apoptotic and anti-apoptotic properties. *Neurotoxicology, 25*, 233–242.

Mahad, D. J., Howell, S. J., & Woodroofe, M. N. (2002a). Expression of chemokines in cerebrospinal fluid and serum of patients with chronic inflammatory demyelinating polyneuropathy. *J Neurol Neurosurg Psychiatry, 73*, 320–323.

Mahad, D. J., Howell, S. J., & Woodroofe, M. N. (2002b). Expression of chemokines in the CSF and correlation with clinical disease activity in patients with multiple sclerosis. *J Neurol Neurosurg Psychiatry, 72*, 498–502.

Malik, M., Chen, Y. Y., Kienzle, M. F., Tomkowicz, B. E., Collman, R. G., & Ptasznik, A. (2008). Monocyte migration and LFA-1-mediated attachment to brain microvascular endothelia is regulated by SDF-1 alpha through Lyn kinase. *J Immunol, 181*, 4632–4637.

Malmestrom, C., Andersson, B. A., Haghighi, S., & Lycke, J. (2006). IL-6 and CCL2 levels in CSF are associated with the clinical course of MS: Implications for their possible immunopathogenic roles. *J Neuroimmunol, 175*, 176–182.

Mamidi, A., Desimone, J. A., & Pomerantz, R. J. (2002). Central nervous system infections in individuals with HIV-1 infection. *J Neurovirol, 8*, 158–167.

Maragos, W. F., Tillman, P., Jones, M., Bruce-Keller, A. J., Roth, S., Bell, J. E., et al. (2003). Neuronal injury in hippocampus with human immunodeficiency virus transactivating protein, Tat. *Neuroscience, 117*, 43–53.

Marra, C. M., Zhao, Y., Clifford, D. B., Letendre, S., Evans, S., Henry, K., et al. (2009). Impact of combination antiretroviral therapy on cerebrospinal fluid HIV RNA and neurocognitive performance. *AIDS, 23*, 1359–1366.

Martin-Garcia, J., Kolson, D. L., & Gonzalez-Scarano, F. (2002). Chemokine receptors in the brain: Their role in HIV infection and pathogenesis. *AIDS, 16*, 1709–1730.

Martin, M., Serradji, N., Dereuddre-Bosquet, N., Le Pavec, G., Fichet, G., Lamouri, A., et al. (2000). PMS-601, a new platelet-activating factor receptor antagonist that inhibits human immunodeficiency virus replication and potentiates zidovudine activity in macrophages. *Antimicrob Agents Chemother, 44*, 3150–3154.

Masliah, E., Heaton, R. K., Marcotte, T. D., Ellis, R. J., Wiley, C. A., Mallory, M., et al. (1997). Dendritic injury is a pathological substrate for human immunodeficiency virus-related cognitive disorders. HNRC Group. The HIV Neurobehavioral Research Center. *Ann Neurol, 42*, 963–972.

McArthur, J. C., Brew, B. J., & Nath, A. (2005). Neurological complications of HIV infection. *Lancet Neurol, 4*, 543–555.

McArthur, J. C., Haughey, N., Gartner, S., Conant, K., Pardo, C., Nath, A., et al. (2003). Human immunodeficiency virus-associated dementia: An evolving disease. *Journal of Neurovirology, 9*, 205–221.

McArthur, J. C., McClernon, D. R., Cronin, M. F., Nance-Sproson, T. E., Saah, A. J., St Clair, M., et al. (1997). Relationship between human immunodeficiency virus-associated dementia and viral load in cerebrospinal fluid and brain. *Ann Neurol, 42*, 689–698.

McArthur, J. C., McDermott, M. P., McClernon, D., St Hillaire, C., Conant, K., Marder, K., et al. (2004). Attenuated central nervous system infection in advanced HIV/AIDS with combination antiretroviral therapy. *Arch Neurol, 61*, 1687–1696.

McArthur, J. C., Nance-Sproson, T. E., Griffin, D. E., Hoover, D., Selnes, O. A., Miller, E. N., et al. (1992). The diagnostic utility of elevation in cerebrospinal fluid beta 2-microglobulin in HIV-1 dementia. Multicenter AIDS Cohort Study. *Neurology, 42*, 1707–1712.

McCombe, J. A., Auer, R. N., Maingat, F. G., Houston, S., Gill, M. J., & Powe, C. (2009). Neurologic immune reconstitution inflammatory syndrome in HIV/AIDS: Outcome and epidemiology. *Neurology, 72*, 835–841.

McCrossan, M., Marsden, M., Carnie, F. W., Minnis, S., Hansotti, B., Anthony, I. C., et al. (2006). An immune control model for viral replication in the CNS during presymptomatic HIV infection. *Brain, 129*, 503–516.

McFarlin, D. E. & Blattner, W. A. (1991). Non-AIDS retroviral infections in humans. *Annu Rev Med, 42*, 97–105.

McGeer, E. G. & McGeer, P. L. (2010). Neuroinflammation in Alzheimer's disease and mild cognitive impairment: A field in its infancy. *J Alzheimers Dis, 19*, 355–361.

McGeer, P. L., Itagaki, S., Tago, H., & McGeer, E. G. (1987). Reactive microglia in patients with senile dementia of the Alzheimer type are positive for the histocompatibility glycoprotein HLA-DR. *Neurosci Lett, 79*, 195–200.

McManus, C. M., Liu, J. S., Hahn, M. T., Hua, L. L., Brosnan, C. F., Berman, J. W., et al. (2000). Differential induction of chemokines in human microglia by type I and II interferons. *Glia, 29*, 273–280.

Meisner, F., Scheller, C., Kneitz, S., Sopper, S., Neuen-Jacob, E., Riederer, P., et al. (2008). Memantine upregulates BDNF and prevents dopamine deficits in SIV-infected macaques: A novel pharmacological action of memantine. *Neuropsychopharmacology, 33*, 2228–2236.

Mengozzi, M., De Filippi, C., Transidico, P., Biswas, P., Cota, M., Ghezzi, S., et al. (1999). Human immunodeficiency virus replication induces monocyte chemotactic protein-1 in human macrophages and U937 promonocytic cells. *Blood, 93*, 1851–1857.

Meucci, O., Fatatis, A., Simen, A. A., Bushell, T. J., Gray, P. W., & Miller, R. J. (1998). Chemokines regulate hippocampal neuronal signaling and gp120 neurotoxicity. *Proc Natl Acad Sci U S A, 95*, 14500–14505.

Meucci, O., Fatatis, A., Simen, A. A., & Miller, R. J. (2000). Expression of CX3CR1 chemokine receptors on neurons and their role in neuronal survival. *Proc Natl Acad Sci U S A, 97,* 8075–8080.

Miljkovic, D., Drulovic, J., Trajkovic, V., Mesaros, S., Dujmovic, I., Maksimovic, D., et al. (2002). Nitric oxide metabolites and interleukin-6 in cerebrospinal fluid from multiple sclerosis patients. *Eur J Neurol, 9,* 413–418.

Mizuno, T., Kawanokuchi, J., Numata, K., & Suzumura, A. (2003). Production and neuroprotective functions of fractalkine in the central nervous system. *Brain Res, 979,* 65–70.

Mrak, R. E. & Griffin, W. S. (2005). Glia and their cytokines in progression of neurodegeneration. *Neurobiol Aging, 26,* 349–354.

Nagai, M., Brennan, M. B., Sakai, J. A., Mora, C. A., & Jacobson, S. (2001a). CD8(+) T cells are an in vivo reservoir for human T-cell lymphotropic virus type I. *Blood, 98,* 1858–1861.

Nagai, M., Yamano, Y., Brennan, M. B., Mora, C. A., & Jacobson, S. (2001b). Increased HTLV-I proviral load and preferential expansion of HTLV-I Tax-specific CD8+ T cells in cerebrospinal fluid from patients with HAM/TSP. *Ann Neurol, 50,* 807–812.

Nath, A., Haughey, N. J., Jones, M., Anderson, C., Bell, J. E., & Geiger, J. D. (2000). Synergistic neurotoxicity by human immunodeficiency virus proteins Tat and gp120: Protection by memantine. *Ann Neurol, 47,* 186–194.

Nath, A., Schiess, N., Venkatesan, A., Rumbaugh, J., Sacktor, N., & McArthur, J. (2008). Evolution of HIV dementia with HIV infection. *Int Rev Psychiatry, 20,* 25–31.

Nottet, H. S., Persidsky, Y., Sasseville, V. G., Nukuna, A. N., Bock, P., Zhai, Q. H., et al. (1996). Mechanisms for the transendothelial migration of HIV-1-infected monocytes into brain. *J Immunol, 156,* 1284–1295.

Ohtani, Y., Minami, M., Kawaguchi, N., Nishiyori, A., Yamamoto, J., Takami, S., et al. (1998). Expression of stromal cell-derived factor-1 and CXCR4 chemokine receptor mRNAs in cultured rat glial and neuronal cells. *Neurosci Lett, 249,* 163–166.

Osame, M., Janssen, R., Kubota, H., Nishitani, H., Igata, A., Nagataki, S., et al. (1990). Nationwide survey of HTLV-I-associated myelopathy in Japan: Association with blood transfusion. *Ann Neurol, 28,* 50–56.

Oster, W., Lindemann, A., Horn, S., Mertelsmann, R., & Herrmann, F. (1987). Tumor necrosis factor (TNF)-alpha but not TNF-beta induces secretion of colony stimulating factor for macrophages (CSF-1) by human monocytes. *Blood, 70,* 1700–1703.

Park, I. W., Wang, J. F., & Groopman, J. E. (2001). HIV-1 Tat promotes monocyte chemoattractant protein-1 secretion followed by transmigration of monocytes. *Blood, 97,* 352–358.

Peled, A., Grabovsky, V., Habler, L., Sandbank, J., Arenzana-Seisdedos, F., Petit, I., et al. (1999). The chemokine SDF-1 stimulates integrin-mediated arrest of CD34(+) cells on vascular endothelium under shear flow. *J Clin Invest, 104,* 1199–211.

Peng, H., Erdmann, N., Whitney, N., Dou, H., Gorantla, S., Gendelman, H. E., et al. (2006). HIV-1-infected and/or immune activated macrophages regulate astrocyte SDF-1 production through IL-1beta. *Glia, 54,* 619–629.

Pereira, C. F., Middel, J., Jansen, G., Verhoef, J., & Nottet, H. S. (2001). Enhanced expression of fractalkine in HIV-1 associated dementia. *J Neuroimmunol, 115,* 168–175.

Perrella, O., Guerriero, M., Izzo, E., Soscia, M., & Carrieri, P. B. (1992). Interleukin-6 and granulocyte macrophage-CSF in the cerebrospinal fluid from HIV infected subjects with involvement of the central nervous system. *Arq Neuropsiquiatr, 50,* 180–182.

Persidsky, Y., Heilman, D., Haorah, J., Zelivyanskaya, M., Persidsky, R., Weber, G. A., et al. (2006). Rho-mediated regulation of tight junctions during monocyte migration across the blood-brain barrier in HIV-1 encephalitis (HIVE). *Blood, 107,* 4770–4780.

Persidsky, Y., Stins, M., Way, D., Witte, M. H., Weinand, M., Kim, K. S., et al. (1997). A model for monocyte migration through the blood-brain barrier during HIV-1 encephalitis. *J Immunol, 158,* 3499–3510.

Persidsky, Y., Zheng, J., Miller, D., & Gendelman, H. E. (2000). Mononuclear phagocytes mediate blood-brain barrier compromise and neuronal injury during HIV-1-associated dementia. *J Leukoc Biol, 68,* 413–422.

Petito, C. K., Cho, E. S., Lemann, W., Navia, B. A., & Price, R. W. (1986). Neuropathology of acquired immunodeficiency syndrome (AIDS): An autopsy review. *J Neuropathol Exp Neurol, 45,* 635–646.

Pulliam, L., Gascon, R., Stubblebine, M., McGuire, D., & McGrath, M. S. (1997). Unique monocyte subset in patients with AIDS dementia. *Lancet, 349,* 692–695.

Qiao, X., Cummins, D. J., & Paul, S. M. (2001). Neuroinflammation-induced acceleration of amyloid deposition in the APPV717F transgenic mouse. *Eur J Neurosci, 14,* 474–482.

Ragin, A. B., Wu, Y., Storey, P., Cohen, B. A., Edelman, R. R., & Epstein, L. G. (2006). Monocyte chemoattractant protein-1 correlates with subcortical brain injury in HIV infection. *Neurology, 66,* 1255–1257.

Ransohoff, R. M. (1999). Mechanisms of inflammation in MS tissue: Adhesion molecules and chemokines. *J Neuroimmunol, 98,* 57–68.

Ransohoff, R. M. & Zamvil, S. S. (2007). Neuroimmunotherapeutics comes of age. *Neurotherapeutics, 4,* 569–570.

Rappaport, J., Joseph, J., Croul, S., Alexander, G., Del Valle, L., Amini, S., et al. (1999). Molecular pathway involved in HIV-1-induced CNS pathology: Role of viral regulatory protein, Tat. *J Leukoc Biol, 65,* 458–465.

Re, D. B. & Przedborski, S. (2006). Fractalkine: Moving from chemotaxis to neuroprotection. *Nat Neurosci, 9,* 859–861.

Rieckmann, P., Albrecht, M., Kitze, B., Weber, T., Tumani, H., Broocks, A., et al. (1995). Tumor necrosis factor-alpha messenger RNA expression in patients with relapsing-remitting multiple sclerosis is associated with disease activity. *Ann Neurol, 37,* 82–88.

Robertson, K. R., Smurzynski, M., Parsons, T. D., Wu, K., Bosch, R. J., Wu, J., et al. (2007). The prevalence and incidence of neurocognitive impairment in the HAART era. *AIDS, 21,* 1915–1921.

Rosati, G. (2001). The prevalence of multiple sclerosis in the world: An update. *Neurol Sci, 22,* 117–139.

Rostasy, K., Egles, C., Chauhan, A., Kneissl, M., Bahrani, P., Yiannoutsos, C., et al. (2003). SDF-1alpha is expressed in astrocytes and neurons in the AIDS dementia complex: An in vivo and in vitro study. *J Neuropathol Exp Neurol, 62,* 617–626.

Roullet, E. (1999). Opportunistic infections of the central nervous system during HIV-1 infection (emphasis on cytomegalovirus disease). *J Neurol, 246,* 237–243.

Sabri, F., Titanji, K., De Milito, A., & Chiodi, F. (2003). Astrocyte activation and apoptosis: Their roles in the neuropathology of HIV infection. *Brain Pathol, 13,* 84–94.

Sacktor, N., McDermott, M. P., Marder, K., Schifitto, G., Selnes, O. A., McArthur, J. C., et al. (2002). HIV-associated cognitive impairment before and after the advent of combination therapy. *Journal of Neurovirology, 8,* 136–142.

Sacktor, N., Schifitto, G., McDermott, M. P., Marder, K., McArthur, J. C., & Kieburtz, K. (2000). Transdermal selegiline in HIV-associated cognitive impairment: Pilot, placebo-controlled study. *Neurology, 54,* 233–235.

Sadagopal, S., Lorey, S. L., Barnett, L., Basham, R., Lebo, L., Erdem, H., et al. (2008). Enhancement of human immunodeficiency virus (HIV)-specific CD8+ T cells in cerebrospinal fluid compared to those in blood among antiretroviral therapy-naive HIV-positive subjects. *J Virol, 82,* 10418–10428.

Sasseville, V. G., Newman, W., Brodie, S. J., Hesterberg, P., Pauley, D., & Ringler, D. J. (1994). Monocyte adhesion to endothelium in simian immunodeficiency virus-induced AIDS encephalitis is mediated by vascular cell adhesion molecule-1/alpha 4 beta 1 integrin interactions. *Am J Pathol, 144,* 27–40.

Savarin-Vuaillat, C. & Ransohoff, R. M. (2007). Chemokines and chemokine receptors in neurological disease: Raise, retain, or reduce? *Neurotherapeutics, 4,* 590–601.

Sawada, M., Imamura, K., & Nagatsu, T. (2006). Role of cytokines in inflammatory process in Parkinson's disease. *J Neural Transm* Suppl, 373–381.

Schifitto, G., Navia, B. A., Yiannoutsos, C. T., Marra, C. M., Chang, L., Ernst, T., et al. (2007). Memantine and HIV-associated cognitive impairment: A neuropsychological and proton magnetic resonance spectroscopy study. *AIDS, 21,* 1877–1886.

Schifitto, G., Peterson, D. R., Zhong, J., Ni, H., Cruttenden, K., Gaugh, M., et al. (2006). Valproic acid adjunctive therapy for HIV-associated cognitive impairment: A first report. *Neurology, 66*, 919–921.

Schifitto, G., Yiannoutsos, C. T., Ernst, T., Navia, B. A., Nath, A., Sacktor, N., et al. (2009). Selegiline and oxidative stress in HIV-associated cognitive impairment. *Neurology, 73*, 1975–1981.

Schifitto, G., Zhang, J., Evans, S. R., Sacktor, N., Simpson, D., Millar, L. L., et al. (2007). A multicenter trial of selegiline transdermal system for HIV-associated cognitive impairment. *Neurology, 69*, 1314–1321.

Schifitto, G., Zhong, J., Gill, D., Peterson, D. R., Gaugh, M. D., Zhu, T., et al. (2009). Lithium therapy for human immunodeficiency virus type 1-associated neurocognitive impairment. *J Neurovirol, 15*, 176–186.

Schweinsburg, B. C., Taylor, M. J., Alhassoon, O. M., Gonzalez, R., Brown, G. G., Ellis, R. J., et al. (2005). Brain mitochondrial injury in human immunodeficiency virus-seropositive (HIV+) individuals taking nucleoside reverse transcriptase inhibitors. *J Neurovirol, 11*, 356–364.

Scorziello, A., Florio, T., Bajetto, A., & Schettini, G. (1998). Intracellular signalling mediating HIV-1 gp120 neurotoxicity. *Cell Signal, 10*, 75–84.

Sevigny, J. J., Albert, S. M., McDermott, M. P., McArthur, J. C., Sacktor, N., Conant, K., et al. (2004). Evaluation of HIV RNA and markers of immune activation as predictors of HIV-associated dementia. *Neurology, 63*, 2084–2090.

Sevigny, J. J., Albert, S. M., McDermott, M. P., Schifitto, G., McArthur, J. C., Sacktor, N., et al. (2007). An evaluation of neurocognitive status and markers of immune activation as predictors of time to death in advanced HIV infection. *Arch Neurol, 64*, 97–102.

Sheng, J. G., Griffin, W. S., Royston, M. C., & Mrak, R. E. (1998). Distribution of interleukin-1-immunoreactive microglia in cerebral cortical layers: implications for neuritic plaque formation in Alzheimer's disease. *Neuropathol Appl Neurobiol, 24*, 278–283.

Shiramizu, B., Gartner, S., Williams, A., Shikuma, C., Ratto-Kim, S., Watters, M., et al. (2005). Circulating proviral HIV DNA and HIV-associated dementia. *AIDS, 19*, 45–52.

Si, Q., Cosenza, M., Kim, M. O., Zhao, M. L., Brownlee, M., Goldstein, H. et al. (2004). A novel action of minocycline: Inhibition of human immunodeficiency virus type 1 infection in microglia. *J Neurovirol, 10*, 284–292.

Si, Q., Kim, M. O., Zhao, M. L., Landau, N. R., Goldstein, H., & Lee, S. (2002). Vpr- and Nef-dependent induction of RANTES/CCL5 in microglial cells. *Virology, 301*, 342–353.

Soldan, S. S., Wu, G., Markowitz, C., & Kolson, D. L. (2008). Multiple Sclerosis and other demyelinating diseases. In: T. Ikezu & H. E. Gendelman (eds.). *Neuroimmune pharmacology*, Springer.

Song, L., Nath, A., Geiger, J. D., Moore, A., & Hochman, S. (2003). Human immunodeficiency virus type 1 Tat protein directly activates neuronal N-methyl-D-aspartate receptors at an allosteric zinc-sensitive site. *J Neurovirol, 9*, 399–403.

Spitzenberger, T. J., Heilman, D., Diekmann, C., Batrakova, E. V., Kabanov, A. V., Gendelman, H. E., et al. (2007). Novel delivery system enhances efficacy of antiretroviral therapy in animal model for HIV-1 encephalitis. *J Cereb Blood Flow Metab, 27*, 1033–1042.

Sporer, B., Kastenbauer, S., Koedel, U., Arendt, G., & Pfister, H. W. (2003). Increased intrathecal release of soluble fractalkine in HIV-infected patients. *AIDS Res Hum Retroviruses, 19*, 111–116.

Sui, Y., Potula, R., Dhillon, N., Pinson, D., Li, S., Nath, A., et al. (2004). Neuronal apoptosis is mediated by CXCL10 overexpression in simian human immunodeficiency virus encephalitis. *Am J Pathol, 164*, 1557–1566.

Sui, Y., Stehno-Bittel, L., Li, S., Loganathan, R., Dhillon, N. K., Pinson, D., et al. (2006a). CXCL10-induced cell death in neurons: Role of calcium dysregulation. *Eur J Neurosci, 23*, 957–964.

Sui, Z., Fan, S., Sniderhan, L., Reisinger, E., Litzburg, A., Schifitto, G., et al. (2006b). Inhibition of mixed lineage kinase 3 prevents HIV-1 Tat-mediated neurotoxicity and monocyte activation. *J Immunol, 177*, 702–711.

Sundar, S. K., Cierpial, M. A., Kamaraju, L. S., Long, S., Hsieh, S., Lorenz, C., et al. (1991). Human immunodeficiency virus glycoprotein (gp120) infused into rat brain induces interleukin 1 to elevate pituitary-adrenal activity and decrease peripheral cellular immune responses. *Proc Natl Acad Sci U S A, 88*, 11246–11250.

Swindells, S., Zheng, J., & Gendelman, H. E. (1999). HIV-associated dementia: New insights into disease pathogenesis and therapeutic interventions. *AIDS Patient Care STDS, 13*, 153–163.

Szeto, G. L., Brice, A. K., Yang, H. C., Barber, S. A., Siliciano, R. F., & Clements, J. E. (2010). Minocycline attenuates HIV infection and reactivation by suppressing cellular activation in human CD4+ T cells. *J Infect Dis, 201*, 1132–1140.

Szymocha, R., Akaoka, H., Brisson, C., Beurton-Marduel, P., Chalon, A., Bernard, A., et al. (2000a). Astrocytic alterations induced by HTLV type 1-infected T lymphocytes: A role for Tax-1 and tumor necrosis factor alpha. *AIDS Res Hum Retroviruses, 16*, 1723–1729.

Szymocha, R., Brisson, C., Bernard, A., Akaoka, H., Belin, M. F., & Giraudon, P. (2000b). Long-term effects of HTLV-1 on brain astrocytes: Sustained expression of Tax-1 associated with synthesis of inflammatory mediators. *J Neurovirol, 6*, 350–357.

The Dana Consortium. (1998). A randomized, double-blind, placebo-controlled trial of deprenyl and thioctic acid in human immunodeficiency virus-associated cognitive impairment. The Dana Consortium on the Therapy of HIV Dementia and Related Cognitive Disorders *Neurology, 50*, 645–651.

Thieblemont, N., Weiss, L., Sadeghi, H. M., Estcourt, C., & Haeffner-Cavaillon, N. (1995). CD14lowCD16high: A cytokine-producing monocyte subset which expands during human immunodeficiency virus infection. *Eur J Immunol, 25*, 3418–3424.

Toggas, S. M., Masliah, E., & Mucke, L. (1996). Prevention of HIV-1 gp120-induced neuronal damage in the central nervous system of transgenic mice by the NMDA receptor antagonist memantine. *Brain Res, 706*, 303–307.

Tong, N., Perry, S. W., Zhang, Q., James, H. J., Guo, H., Brooks, A., et al. (2000). Neuronal fractalkine expression in HIV-1 encephalitis: roles for macrophage recruitment and neuroprotection in the central nervous system. *J Immunol, 164*, 1333–1339.

Tong, N., Sanchez, J. F., Maggirwar, S. B., Ramirez, S. H., Guo, H., Dewhurst, S., et al. (2001). Activation of glycogen synthase kinase 3 beta (GSK-3beta) by platelet activating factor mediates migration and cell death in cerebellar granule neurons. *Eur J Neurosci, 13*, 1913–1922.

Ubogu, E. E., Cossoy, M. B., & Ransohoff, R. M. (2006). The expression and function of chemokines involved in CNS inflammation. *Trends Pharmacol Sci, 27*, 48–55.

Van Marle, G., Henry, S., Toduruk, T., Sullivan, A., Silva, C., Rourke, S. B., et al. (2004). Human immunodeficiency virus type 1 Nef protein mediates neural cell death: A neurotoxic role for IP-10. *Virology, 329*, 302–318.

Vawter, M. P., Dillon-Carter, O., Tourtellotte, W. W., Carvey, P., & Freed, W. J. (1996). TGFbeta1 and TGFbeta2 concentrations are elevated in Parkinson's disease in ventricular cerebrospinal fluid. *Exp Neurol, 142*, 313–322.

Vergote, D., Butler, G. S., Ooms, M., Cox, J. H., Silva, C., Hollenberg, M. D., et al. (2006). Proteolytic processing of SDF-1alpha reveals a change in receptor specificity mediating HIV-associated neurodegeneration. *Proc Natl Acad Sci U S A, 103*, 19182–19187.

Von Giesen, H. J., Adams, O., Koller, H., & Arend, G. (2005). Cerebrospinal fluid HIV viral load in different phases of HIV-associated brain disease. *J Neurol, 252*, 801–807.

Wang, H., Sun, J., & Goldstein, H. (2008). Human immunodeficiency virus type 1 infection increases the in vivo capacity of peripheral monocytes to cross the blood-brain barrier into the brain and the in vivo sensitivity of the blood-brain barrier to disruption by lipopolysaccharide. *J Virol, 82*, 7591–7600.

Watabe, K., Saida, T., & Kim, S. U. (1989). Human and simian glial cells infected by human T-lymphotropic virus type I in culture. *J Neuropathol Exp Neurol, 48*, 610–619.

Wesselingh, S. L., Power, C., Glass, J. D., Tyor, W. R., McArthur, J. C., Farber, J. M., et al. (1993). Intracerebral cytokine messenger RNA expression in acquired immunodeficiency syndrome dementia. *Ann Neurol, 33*, 576–582.

WHO. (2009). AIDS Epidemic update 2009. Available: http://www.unaids.org/en/KnowledgeCentre/HIVData/EpiUpdate/EpiUpdArchive/2009/default.asp.

WILEY, C. A. & ACHIM, C. (1994). Human immunodeficiency virus encephalitis is the pathological correlate of dementia in acquired immunodeficiency syndrome. *Ann Neurol*, *36*, 673–676.

Williams, R., Dhillon, N. K., Hegde, S. T., Yao, H., Peng, F., Callen, S., et al. (2009a). Proinflammatory cytokines and HIV-1 synergistically enhance CXCL10 expression in human astrocytes. *Glia*, *57*, 734–743.

Williams, R., Yao, H., Dhillon, N. K., & Buch, S. J. (2009b). HIV-1 Tat co-operates with IFN-gamma and TNF-alpha to increase CXCL10 in human astrocytes. *PLoS One*, *4*, e5709.

Wu, D. T., Woodman, S. E., Weiss, J. M., McManus, C. M., D'Aversa, T. G., Hesselgesser, J., et al. (2000). Mechanisms of leukocyte trafficking into the CNS. *J Neurovirol*, *6* Suppl 1, S82–85.

Yadav, A. & Collman, R. G. (2009). CNS inflammation and macrophage/microglial biology associated with HIV-1 infection. *J Neuroimmune Pharmacol*.

Yamano, Y., Nagai, M., Brennan, M., Mora, C. A., Soldan, S. S., Tomaru, U., et al. (2002). Correlation of human T-cell lymphotropic virus type 1 (HTLV-1) mRNA with proviral DNA load, virus-specific CD8(+) T cells, and disease severity in HTLV-1-associated myelopathy (HAM/TSP). *Blood*, *99*, 88–94.

Yao, H., Peng, F., Dhillon, N., Callen, S., Bokhari, S., Stehno-Bittel, L., et al. (2009). Involvement of TRPC channels in CCL2-mediated neuroprotection against tat toxicity. *J Neurosci*, *29*, 1657–1669.

Zhang, K., Rana, F., Silva, C., Ethier, J., Wehrly, K., Chesebro, B., et al. (2003). Human immunodeficiency virus type 1 envelope-mediated neuronal death: Uncoupling of viral replication and neurotoxicity. *J Virol*, *77*, 6899–6912.

Zhang, L., He, T., Talal, A., Wang, G., Franke, S. S., & Ho, D. D. (1998). In vivo distribution of the human immunodeficiency virus/simian immunodeficiency virus coreceptors: CXCR4, CCR3, and CCR5. *J Virol*, *72*, 5035–5045.

Zhao, Y., Navia, B. A., Marra, C. M., Singer, E. J., Chang, L., Berger, J., et al. (2010). Memantine for AIDS dementia complex: open-label report of ACTG 301. *HIV Clin Trials*, *11*, 59–67.

Zheng, J., Ghorpade, A., Niemann, D., Cotter, R. L., Thylin, M. R., Epstein, L., et al. (1999a). Lymphotropic virions affect chemokine receptor-mediated neural signaling and apoptosis: Implications for human immunodeficiency virus type 1-associated dementia. *J Virol*, *73*, 8256–8267.

Zheng, J., Thylin, M. R., Ghorpade, A., Xiong, H., Persidsky, Y., Cotter, R., et al. (1999b). Intracellular CXCR4 signaling, neuronal apoptosis and neuropathogenic mechanisms of HIV-1-associated dementia. *J Neuroimmunol*, *98*, 185–200.

Zhou, H., Lapointe, B. M., Clark, S. R., Zbytnuik, L., & Kubes, P. (2006). A requirement for microglial TLR4 in leukocyte recruitment into brain in response to lipopolysaccharide. *J Immunol*, *177*, 8103–8110.

Zink, M. C., Coleman, G. D., Mankowski, J. L., Adams, R. J., Tarwater, P. M., Fox, K., et al. (2001). Increased macrophage chemoattractant protein-1 in cerebrospinal fluid precedes and predicts simian immunodeficiency virus encephalitis. *J Infect Dis*, *184*, 1015–1021.

Zink, M. C., Spelman, J. P., Robinson, R. B., & Clements, J. E. (1998). SIV infection of macaques—modeling the progression to AIDS dementia. *J Neurovirol*, *4*, 249–59.

Zink, M. C., Uhrlaub, J., Dewitt, J., Voelker, T., Bullock, B., Mankowski, J., Tarwater, P., Clements, J. & Barber, S. (2005). Neuroprotective and anti-human immunodeficiency virus activity of minocycline. *JAMA*, *293*, 2003–11.

8.2

NEURONAL INJURY, WHITE MATTER DISEASE, AND NEUROTROPHIC FACTORS

T. Dianne Langford, Ian Paul Everall, and Eliezer Masliah

The patterns of neurodegeneration in acquired immune deficiency syndrome (AIDS) patients, with special attention to neuronal injury, white matter disease, and the potential role of neurotrophic factors, are reviewed. On the cellular level, there is evidence that neuronal damage in AIDS might start in synapses and dendrites and then spread to the rest of the neuron, leading to cell death by apoptosis. Anatomically, neurodegeneration affects primarily the striato-cortical, cortico-cortical, and limbic intrinsic/inhibitory circuitries. Whether these circuitries are affected simultaneously or as part of an anatomical progression is unknown. Differences in the relative levels of specific receptors across neuronal populations may influence their vulnerability to distinct HIV-related neurotoxins. The emergence of combination anti-retroviral therapy (cART)-resistant HIV strains may have contributed to more aggressive forms of HIV encephalitis (HIVE). However, since not all patients with HIVE display neurodegeneration and motor-cognitive impairment, it is possible that, in some cases, the host is capable of producing trophic factors that protect neuronal, glial, and endothelial cell populations from HIV-associated toxicity. Identification of new trophic factors and improved understanding of neuro-protective mechanisms may lead to new treatments for HIVE in the cART era.

INTRODUCTION

With the advent of more effective combination antiretroviral therapy (cART) and the longer survival of acquired immune deficiency syndrome (AIDS) patients, the pathogenesis of HIV encephalitis (HIVE) has been transformed from a sub-acute, neuroinflammatory disorder with florid neurological alterations, to a chronic and protracted condition (Langford et al., 2003). In agreement with these changes in the natural history of AIDS, recent studies show that although the frequency of HIV-related central nervous system (CNS) lesions and dementia among HIV-infected patients has decreased, the prevalence of HIVE and more subtle forms of motor-cognitive impairment has increased (Deutsch et al., 2001; Neuenburg et al., 2002; Vago et al., 2002). In the pre-cART era, prevalence rates for HIV-associated dementia (HAD) ranged from 5–20% among patients with AIDS, while rates for those suffering from minor cognitive and motor deficits reached 30% (Power et al., 2002). Without antiretrovirals,

the mean survival of patients with HAD was only three to six months (Power et al., 2002). Despite cART, neurocognitive alterations in patients with HIV infection continue to pose a significant problem with HIV-associated neurocognitive disorders (HAND) reported in approximately 40% of treated patients, especially in those with advanced immunosuppression (McArthur et al., 1993; Grant et al., 1995; Dore et al., 1999; Letendre et al., 2010; Heaton et al., 2010). However, there is still no therapeutic strategy targeted toward protecting the CNS from HIV-mediated neuronal damage and cell death, although regimens with increased CNS-penetrating efficiencies may improve cognitive functioning (Letendre et al., 2010; Liner et al., 2010). The combination of cART with adjuvant therapies that target neurotoxic processes may represent a means to diminish, prevent, or reverse HIV-mediated neuronal damage (Dreyer et al., 1990; Thorns & Masliah, 1999; Everall et al., 2001). For example, in some animal models of HIVE, and in *in vitro* systems, blocking the action of platelet-activating factor (PAF) lessened reactive gliosis, the formation of multinucleated giant cells (MNGC) and microglial nodules (MGN), and decreased neurodegeneration (Eggert et al., 2009). In studies using the SIV-infected macaque model of HIVE, treatment with memantine, a drug that blocks the NMDA receptor, was shown to increase production of brain-derived neurotrophic factor (BDNF), thereby lessening dopamine deficits in this model (Meisner et al., 2008). Studies such as these with PAF support the possibility that adjuvant therapies to cART may be able to protect or lessen the severity of HIV-associated CNS damage. Therefore, identifying the neuronal populations selectively vulnerable to HIV and a better understanding of the mechanisms of HIV-associated neurodegeneration involved in AIDS might contribute to the development of new and improved treatments for HIVE.

The relationship among HIVE, cognitive impairment, and neurodegeneration is complex. Pathologically, the brain is affected by dendritic and synaptic damage, neuronal loss (Figure 8.2.1) and by a spectrum of inflammatory changes (Figure 8.2.2) (Everall et al., 1997; Cherner et al., 2002). Further complicating this picture, patients with AIDS also show varying degrees of damage to the cerebral microvasculature and white matter (Figures 8.2.2a, d, f and 8.2.3b-d). Increased viral load is associated with worsening neuronal damage, and this damage correlates with the onset of early cognitive impairment (Masliah et al., 1992a; Masliah et al.,

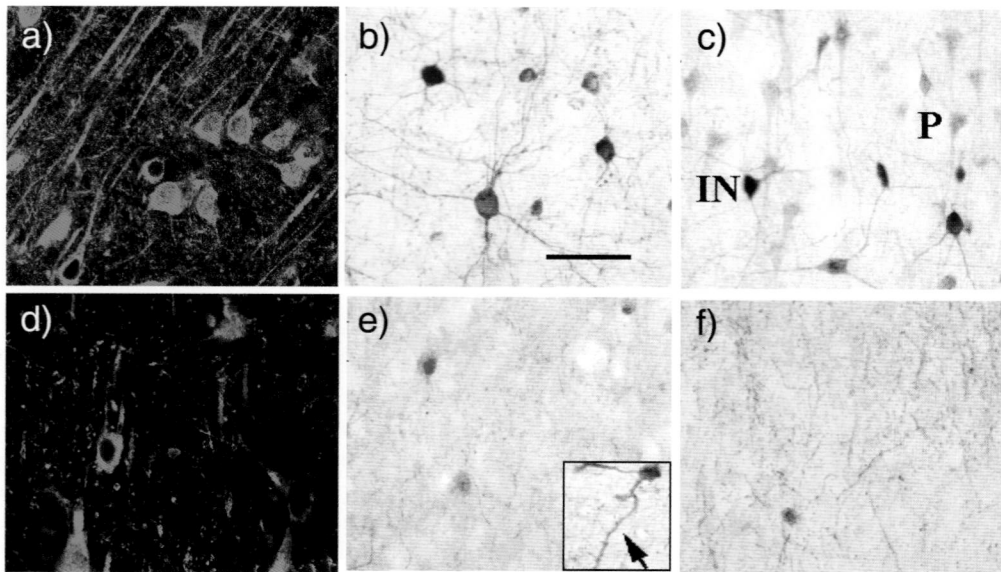

Figure 8.2.1 *Patterns of Neurodegeneration in HIV Encephalitis* Panels (a-c) are sections from the frontal cortex of an age-matched HIV-negative patient. Panels (d-f) are sections from the frontal cortex of an HIVE patient. (a, d) Immunofluorescence labeling of pyramidal neurons and dendrites with anti-microtubule-associated protein-2 (MAP-2) antibody (green). (d) Note the neuronal damage in the HIVE patient's brain as evidenced by the loss of dendritic complexity indicated by loss of green fluorescence. (b, e) Immunohistochemical labeling of calbindin-positive neurons in an HIV-negative (b) and an HIVE patient (e). The inset in (e) shows aberrant sprouting (arrow) of a damaged neuron in an HIVE patient. (c, f) Immunohistochemical labeling of parvalbumin (PV)-positive pyramidal (P) and interneurons (IN) in an HIV-negative (c) and an HIVE patient (f). Scale bar = 50 microns.

1997; Everall et al., 1999). Nonetheless, while approximately 70% of HIVE patients show cognitive impairment and neurodegeneration, the remaining 30% are cognitively unimpaired and their neuronal populations are well preserved (Table 8.2.1) (Masliah et al., 1996b; Everall et al., 2001). Such observations suggest that among the factors responsible for relative sparing of neurons and cognition, these individuals may have the capacity to produce neurotrophic factors capable of protecting neurons against the deleterious effects of HIV. In this context, the patterns of neurodegeneration in AIDS patients with special

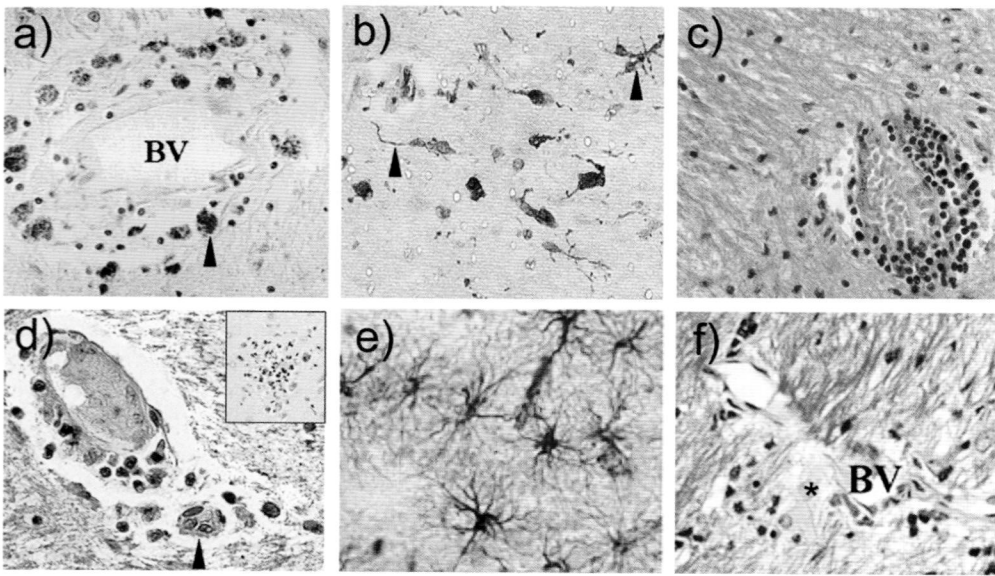

Figure 8.2.2 *Neuropathological Hallmarks Observed in HIV Encephalitis.* All sections are from the frontal cortex. (a) HIV-infected macrophages surrounding a damaged blood vessel (BV) with expansion of the perivascular space. Macrophages are immunolabeled with anti-HIV p24 antibody (arrowhead, brown) and the section is counterstained with hematoxylin. (b) Microglia labeled with anti-CD45 antibody (arrowheads, brown). (c) Hematoxylin and eosin-stained section showing perivascular cuffing of a damaged blood vessel by inflammatory cells. (d) Hematoxylin and eosin-stained section showing a multinucleated giant cell (arrowhead) adjacent to a damaged blood vessel. Inset is a microglial nodule. (e) Astroglial activation detected by anti-glial fibroblast acidic protein (GFAP) antibody immunolabeling (brown). (f) Myelin stained with Luxol fast blue showing loss of myelin (asterisk) around a damaged blood vessel (BV).

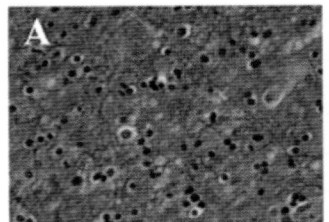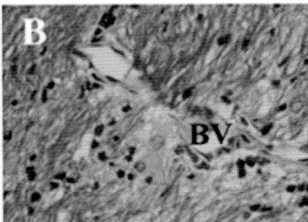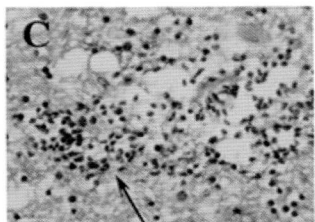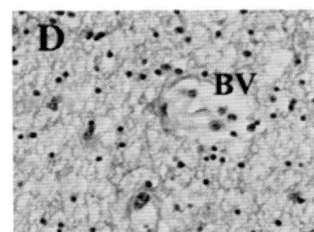

Figure 8.2.3 *Patterns of demyelination in the white matter of patients with HIV-associated leukoencephalopathy.* All images are from the frontal cortex. Sections are stained with Luxol fast blue and counter-stained with hematoxylin. (A) Normal brain with intact myelin (blue). (B-C) Cases with mild-to-moderate demyelination, most apparent around blood vessels (BV) with infiltrating inflammatory cells (arrow). (D) Severe case of leukoencephalopathy with extensive myelin loss and loss of blood vessel (BV) architecture. (Reprinted from Langford et al., 2002, with permission).

emphasis on neuronal injury, white matter disease, and the potential role of neurotrophic factors in HIV CNS disease progression are reviewed in this chapter.

PATTERNS OF NEURONAL INJURY IN AIDS PATIENTS

Neuronal damage includes dendritic simplification of pyramidal neurons (compare Figure 8.2.1a with d), and selective loss of interneuronal populations (compare 8.2.1b with e, and c with f). In addition to neuronal loss, aberrant sprouting (Figure 8.2.1e, inset) and dystrophic synaptodendritic connections are features of HIVE in AIDS patients (Ellis et al., 2007).

Other hallmarks of HIVE include extensive damage to microvessels of the blood-brain barrier (BBB) caused by infiltration of HIV-infected cells and inflammatory cells into the brain (8.2.2a, c, d (Dallasta et al., 1999; Langford & Masliah, 2001). Likewise, microgliosis (Figure 8.2.2d), the formation of MGN (8.2.2d, inset), MNGC (8.2.2d, arrowhead) and astrogliosis (8.2.2e) are common in HIVE, as well (Budka, 1991; Masliah et al., 1994a; Masliah et al., 1996a).

The neurodegenerative process affects primarily the stria-to-cortical, cortico-cortical, and limbic intrinsic/inhibitory circuitries (Table 8.2.2) (Masliah et al., 1996b). It is not known if these circuitries are affected simultaneously or if there is a temporal progression of the neurodegenerative process from one site to another. The neuronal populations most severely affected in these regions include large pyramidal neurons in the neocortex (Budka et al., 1987; Everall et al., 1991; Wiley et al., 1991; Masliah et al., 1992a; Weis et al., 1993; Masliah et al., 1997), spiny neurons in the putamen (Masliah et al., 1996a; Masliah et al., 1992b), medium-sized neurons in the globus pallidus, and interneurons in the hippocampus (Table 8.2.2) (Masliah et al., 1992b; Fox et al., 1997). Using image analysis techniques, a statistically significant 30–50% decrease in the number of large neurons (200 to 500 μm^2) was identified in the frontal, parietal and temporal cortices of HIVE cases. This damage was accompanied by a reduction in neocortical width (up to 20%) and astrogliosis (Budka, 1991; Gray et al., 1991; Wiley et al., 1991; Everall et al., 1992; Weis et al., 1993; Everall et al., 1994; Asare et al., 1996; Everall et al., 1997). Budka et al. label this condition as diffuse poliodystrophy (Budka, 1991). Consistent with these neuropathological studies, analyses of the brains of AIDS patients and observations in animal models show similar alterations in neuronal markers such as decreased *N*-acetyl-aspartate evidenced by nuclear magnetic resonance spectroscopy (Wilkinson et al., 1997; Marcus et al., 1998; Gonzalez et al., 2000).

Studies in experimental animal models, as well as observations in the brains of AIDS patients, indicate that neuronal damage might begin in synapses and dendrites and then spread to the rest of the neuron, thereby activating pathways leading to cell death via apoptosis (Masliah et al., 1997; Everall et al., 1999). In fact, recent proteomic analyses report that concentrations of pre- and post-synaptic proteins are inversely

Table 8.2.1 PERCENTAGE OF AIDS PATIENTS WITH HIV ENCEPHALITIS (HIVE) AND/OR NEURODEGENERATION (ND) INDICATING COGNITIVE STATUS AND LEVELS OF FIBROBLAST GROWTH FACTOR-1 (FGF1) OBSERVED IN THE BRAINS OF THE FOUR GROUPS

GROUP (N)	HIVE	ND	COGNITIVE STATUS	FGF1 LEVELS	% CASES
1	–	–	Normal	Unchanged	29
2	–	+	Impaired	⇓ 70%	17
3	+	–	Normal	⇑ 50%	23
4	+	+	Impaired	⇓ 30%	31

HIVE, HIV encephalitis; ND, neurodegeneration; FGF1, fibroblast growth factor-1.
+, present; –, absent. (Data from HNRC neuropathologic series, E. Masliah, personal communication)

Table 8.2.2 CIRCUITIES IN BRAIN REGIONS AFFECTED BY HIV NEURODEGENERATION

CELL TYPE†	CORTICAL LAYER	CB	PV	SOM	NT[*]	AIDS STATUS[f]
Neocortex						
Retzuis-Cajal	1	-	-	-	Glu	?
MS Spiny Pyramidal	2/3	+/-	-	-	Glu	+
Double-bouquet	2/3	+	+	+	GABA	+
Axo-axonal (chandelier)	2/3	+	-	-	GABA	?
Basket	2/3	+	+	+/-	GABA	+
MS spiny stellate	4	+/-	-	-	?	?
Basket (clutch)	4	+	+	+/-	GABA	?
Large pyramidal	5	+/-	-	-	Glu	+
Martinotti	6	-	-	+	NPY, GABA	-
Hippocampus						
Granular	Dentate	+/-	-	-	Glu	-
Pyramidal	CA1–4	+/-	-	-	Glu	-
Basket	CA1–4	-	+	-	GABA	+
O/A interneurons	Oriens	+/-	-	+	GABA	+
L/M interneurons	Lacunosum	+/-	-	-	GABA	?
Basket	Hilus	+/-	-	?	GABA	?
Mossy	Hilus	?	?	?	GABA	?
Basal Ganglia						
Giant Spiny	NA	+	+	-	GABA, peptides	-
Other Spiny	NA	+	+	-	GABA, peptides	-
Giant Spiny	NA	-	-	-	Ach	+
MS (few spines)	NA	-	+/-	-	GABA	+
MS (smooth)	NA	-	+/-	-	GABA	?

(For review of brain anatomy, physiology and neuronal cell types, see (Peters & Jones, 1984a; Peters & Jones, 1984b).
† MS, mid-sized; O/A, oreins/alveus; L/M, lacunosum/molecular.
CB, Calbindin; **PV**, parvalbumin; **SOM**, somatostatinergic; **NT**, neurotransmitter; +, present; -, absent; +/-, occasionally present; ?, unknown.
‡ Glu, glutamate; GABA, γ-aminobutyric acid; NPY, neuropeptide
Y; Ach, acetylcholine.
f +, affected; -, not affected; ?, unknown.

related to viral replication in the brain (Gelman & Nguyen, 2010; Nguyen et al. 2010). Moreover, in HIVE there is caspase-3 activation, as well as pro-apoptotic gene expression (James et al., 1999; Garden et al., 2002). Studies in the brains of HIVE patients show evidence of DNA fragmentation as determined by the TUNEL assay in neurons, glia and endothelial cells (Adle-Biassette et al., 1995; Everall et al., 1997; Wiley et al., 2000; Gray et al., 2001). New data demonstrate that microRNAs, which are small noncoding RNA molecules that regulate gene expression in physiological and pathological conditions, are differentially expressed in the brains of HIVE patients. Gene families and biological processes targeted by upregulated microRNA species include caspase-6 activation, suggesting that differentially regulated microRNAs affect cell death programs in HIVE brains (Noorbakhsh et al., 2010). The mechanisms involved in neuronal and synaptic degeneration in AIDS patients are complex, but most evidence supports the contention that infected and/or activated microglia/macrophages release toxic factors (such as viral proteins, excitotoxins and/or inflammatory cytokines and chemokines) that, in turn, damage neurons by multiple mechanisms (Gendelman et al., 1994; Bezzi et al., 2001; Kaul et al., 2001). These factors may also activate astrocytes to produce chemokines and cytokines that affect neuronal functioning (Pulliam et al., 1991; Benveniste, 1994; Minagar et al., 2002). As HIVE progresses, different neurotoxic factors are released and it is likely that during this time, diverse neuronal populations are affected in the areas of the CNS most vulnerable, including the frontal cortex, basal ganglia, hippocampus, and white matter.

In the neocortex, at least two sets of neuronal populations are differentially susceptible to damage mediated by HIV-1 (Table 8.2.2) (Masliah et al., 1992b; Masliah et al., 1996a). These populations include: 1) pyramidal neurons that express microtubule-associated protein 2 (MAP2) (Figure 8.2.1a, d), neurofilament (NF), glutamate and cytokine/chemokine receptors, and low levels of calcium-binding proteins; and 2) interneurons with high expression levels of both cytokine/chemokine receptors and the calcium-binding proteins, calbindin (CB) (Figure 8.2.1b, e) and parvalbumin (PV) (Figure 8.2.1c, f) (Masliah et al., 1994b). Furthermore, neurons vulnerable to HIV toxicity also express high levels of chemokine receptors, such as CXCR4, and low levels of trophic factor receptors, such as fibroblast growth factor receptor (FGFR), neurotrophin factor receptors (NTFR) for nerve growth factor (NGF), or BDNF (Figures 8.2.4, 8.2.5) (Sanders et al., 2000; Ahmed et al., 2008; Crews et al., 2009). Therefore, differences in the relative levels of glutamate receptors, growth factor receptors, chemokine/cytokine receptors, and calcium-binding

proteins in different neuronal populations may determine their selective vulnerability to distinct HIV-induced neuro-toxins during the course of HIVE (Table 8.2.3) (Masliah, 1996; Hesselgesser & Horuk, 1999). In the hippocampus of HIVE patients, pyramidal neurons are relatively spared; however, there is a significant loss of PV-immunoreactive interneurons in the CA3 region (Masliah et al., 1992b; Masliah et al., 1994a; Masliah et al., 1996a), which contains neurons that express cytokine receptors such as interleukin 1β (IL-1β), IL-6, and tumor necrosis factor α (TNFα). Dysfunction of the dopaminergic system is also implicated to play a critical role in the clinical manifestation of HAD (Lopez et al., 1999; Nath et al., 2000; Zauli et al., 2000). Moreover, in the basal ganglia of HIVE patients, there is significant loss of large spiny neurons that express MAP2 and glutamate receptors; however, neurons that express CB are somewhat spared (Table 8.2.3) (Mucke et al., 1995; Masliah et al., 1996a). Likewise, somatostatin-immunoreactive neurons express glutamate receptors

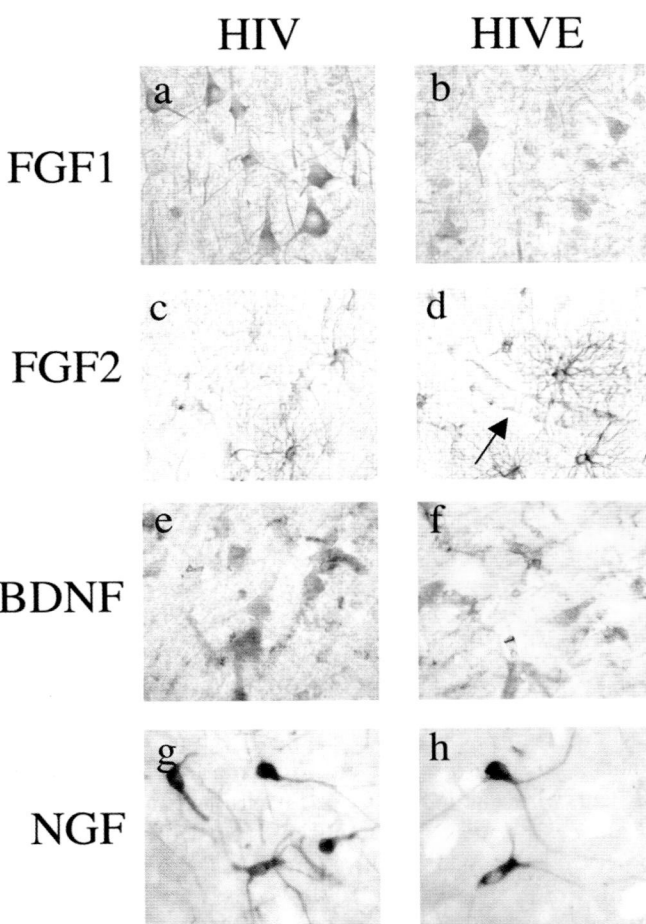

Figure 8.2.4 *Trophic factor expression in the brains of HIVE patients is reduced compared to that in HIV patients without encephalitis.* (a, b) FGF1 in the frontal cortex of HIV versus HIVE. FGF1 is mainly expressed in neurons. In HIVE, FGF1 expression in pyramidal neurons is reduced in cases with neurodegeneration. (c, d) FGF2 in the frontal cortex of HIV versus HIVE. FGF2 is localized to astroglia and around vessels. In HIVE, FGF2 expression is increased around blood vessels (arrow). (e, f) BDNF in the hippocampus of HIV versus HIVE. BDNF is expressed by pyramidal neurons. In HIVE, neuronal BDNF is reduced and microglial cells express BDNF, as well. (g, h) NGF in the hippocampus of HIV versus HIVE. NGF is expressed in small neurons in CA3–4 and dentate. In HIVE, NGF immunoreactive neurons are fewer. Trophic factors are immunolabeled with specific antibodies and detected with DAB staining. FGF, fibroblast growth factor; BDNF, brain-derived growth factor; NGF, neuron growth factor.

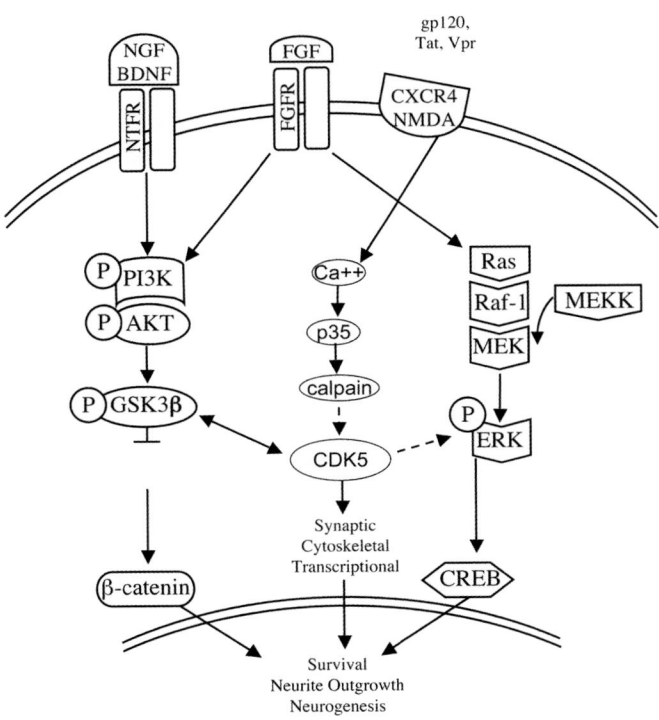

Figure 8.2.5 *Schematic representation of neurotrophic factor signaling in neurons in the presence of HIV.* HIV-mediated alterations may affect GSK3β, ERK, and/or cytoskeletal, synaptic, or transcriptional activities. FGF receptor (FGFR)-mediated signaling may stabilize normal signaling or block HIV-mediated disruptions in these pathways through PI3K/AKT/GSK3β phosphorylation, leading to β-catenin translocation into the nucleus, or increased ERK1/2 phosphorylation and cell survival. Neurotrophic factor receptor (NTFR) signaling is mediated through binding of neuronal growth factor (NGF) or brain-derived growth factor (BDNF) to maintain neuron fitness and survival. Disruption of these signaling pathways by HIV proteins (gp120, Tat, Vpr) through NMDA or CXCR4 can lead to cell death. Viral proteins (gp120, Tat, Vpr) and other neurotoxins may signal through the NMDA or CXCR4 to alter intracellular calcium (Ca++), thereby inducing downstream signaling through calpain and CDK5. FGF, BDNF, and NGF have been shown to regulate CXCR4 expression, thereby preventing apoptosis.

TROPHIC FACTOR*	CELL TARGET	HIV PROTEIN	REFERENCE
FGF1	Pyramidal neurons	gp120	Everall, 2001; Hashimoto, 2002
NGF	Glutaminergic, cholinergic, cerebellar neurons and neuroblastoma cells	gp120, Tat	Bezzi, 2001; Hesselgesser, 1999; Ramirez, 2001
BDNF	Somatostatinergic, dopaminergic, nigrostriatal and cerebellar neurons, and neuroblastoma cells	gp120, Tat	Ramirez, 2001; Mocchetti, 2007; Barnea, 1999; Nosheny, 2007
PDGF	Dopaminergic and neuroblastoma cells	gp120, Tat	Zhu, 2009; Peng, 2008a; Peng, 2008b; Yao, 2009
GDNF	Dopaminergic neurons	gp120, Tat	Lopez, 1999; Nath, 2000; Zauli, 2000
SDF	Cortical neurons and neuroblastoma cells	gp120, Tat	Bagetta, 1996; Corasaniti, 2001; Peruzzi, 2002; Langford, 2002
IGF	Glutaminergic and GABA neurons	HIV proteins	Wang, 2006
Estrogen	Cortical neurons and neuroblastoma cells	gp120	Corasaniti, 2005; Russo, 2005

* FGF, fibroblast growth factor; NGF, neuronal growth factor; BDNF, brain-derived neurotrophic factor; PDGF, platelet-derived growth factor; GDNF, glial-derived growth factor; SDF-stromal-derived growth factor; IGF, insulin-like growth factor; GABA, gamma aminobutyric acid

and may therefore be susceptible to HIV-mediated damage (Fox et al., 1997; Ramirez et al., 2001). Somatostatin immunoreactivity in interneurons in the frontal cortex, hippocampal pyramidal and non-pyramidal neurons, and neurons in the globus pallidus is significantly reduced in HIVE (Table 8.2.2). These findings in human autopsy cases are consistent with studies in transgenic mice showing that overexpression of HIV gp120 results in significant damage to MAP2-immunoreactive pyramidal neurons in the neocortex, while PV-immunoreactive interneurons are spared (Toggas et al., 1994; Masliah et al., 1996b; Campbell et al., 1993; Campbell et al., 1997). In contrast, transgenic mice that express high levels of IL-6 display widespread loss of PV-immunoreactive interneurons in the hippocampus (Campbell et al., 1997). Regional differences in the patterns of selective damage to neurons in patients with HIVE, as well as in transgenic mice, suggest that neurons in the neocortex are more vulnerable to direct damage mediated by HIV-derived proteins, while cytokines and chemokines might play a more significant role in neuropathogenesis in the hippocampus and basal ganglia (Table 8.2.2).

It is anticipated that in the cART era, the shift of HIVE from a subacute neuroinflammatory condition to a chronic, more subtle process (Langford et al., 2003) with neurodegeneration, particularly involving synapses and dendrites will become a more prominent feature. Due to the chronic state of HIVE, degeneration of neuronal populations that usually are unaffected by acute HIVE may also occur. Other factors such as toxicity triggered by cART and the emergence of more aggressive and drug resistant HIV strains may also play roles in the increased susceptibility of distinct neuronal populations to HIV-mediated toxic events.

In conclusion, HIV does not directly injure neurons by productive infection, but rather by inducing the production of inflammatory factors from infected or activated macrophages, microglia and astrocytes. Likewise, HIV perturbs the expression of proteins in synaptic compartments, thereby disrupting neuronal communication (Gelman & Nguyen, 2010). These indirect mechanisms of toxicity lead to damage of select neuronal populations and white matter tracts, and in many cases result in neurocognitive impairment.

WHITE MATTER DISEASE IN HIV ENCEPHALITIS

In addition to the classical neuropathological features associated with HIVE, such as the formation of MNGC, MGN, and reactive gliosis (Figure 8.2.2) (Budka et al., 1991), initial studies also show that the degenerative process in HIVE includes white matter alterations (Figure 8.2.3). Diffuse damage to the white matter is detected more frequently in patients with cognitive impairment and is characterized in life by diffuse or focal hyperintensities by MRI, and at autopsy is observed as mild to moderate myelin loss and astrogliosis (Smith et al., 1990; Budka, 1991; Aylward et al., 1995). Although cART may improve cognitive impairment (Sacktor et al., 2002), HIV-infected patients treated with potent cART more frequently display extensive focal white matter lesions on neuroimaging studies compared to those not taking antiretrovirals (Ammassari et al., 1998; Ammassari et al., 2000). After the mid-1990s when combination therapy was widely used, a shift in CNS HIV-associated pathology was observed (Gray et al., 2001; Langford et al., 2003). In the later 1990s, the percentage of HIV patients with HIVE increased, whereas the percentage with non-Hodgkin's lymphoma and toxoplasmosis decreased, and cytomegalovirusencephalitis, cryptococcosis, and HIV patients with no CNS alterations remained unchanged (Jellinger et al., 2000; Masliah et al., 2000). Recent diffuser tensor imaging studies in HIV patients taking cART indicated that cognitive impairment was related to white matter damage, but white matter injury was not associated with viral loads or estimated CNS penetration of antiretroviral drug regimens (Gongvatana et al., 2009). HIV patients with AIDS exhibited more widespread white matter damage than the non-AIDS HIV patients.

Furthermore, and probably due to the emergence of resistance, a surge in the frequency of HIVE (Neuenburg et al., 2002), and in particular of a highly destructive form of HIV-associated leukoencephalopathy (HAL), has been observed. In this regard, we reported seven autopsy cases of leukoencephalopathy in antiretroviral-experienced patients with AIDS (Langford et al., 2002). Clinically, all seven patients were severely immunosuppressed, had poorly controlled HIV replication despite cART, and had HIV-associated cognitive impairment. Neuropathologically, all seven patients had intense perivascular infiltration of virus as detected by HIV-gp41 immunoreactive monocytes/macrophages and lymphocytes, widespread myelin loss, axonal injury, microgliosis, and astrogliosis (see Figure 8.2.3 for case examples). The extent of damage observed in these cases exceeds that described prior to the use of cART. Furthermore, brain tissue demonstrated high levels of HIV RNA, but no evidence of other viral pathogens. In this model, white matter damage begins with perivascular infiltration by HIV-infected monocytes, which may occur as a consequence of antiretroviral-associated immune restoration. Massive infiltration by immune cells injures brain endothelial cells and is followed by myelin loss, axonal damage, and astrogliosis (Figures 8.2.2, 8.2.3).

In addition to these more severe forms of white matter damage, during the cART era focal white matter lesions without mass effect or contrast enhancement have become a more frequent observation (Ammassari et al., 2000). Compared with the white matter injury that occurred prior to the use of cART, the leukoencephalopathy we describe differs primarily in its severity. In the past, perivascular infiltration by mononuclear cells and myelin loss was less extensive, white matter atrophy was milder, and HIV levels in the brain were lower (Smith et al., 1990). In comparison, our cases are characterized by massive perivascular macrophage infiltration, extensive demyelination, and evidence of very high levels of HIV replication in the brain. These observations are consistent with recent reports of an increased incidence of focal white matter lesions in cART-treated patients (Ammassari et al., 2000) and of an unexpectedly high incidence of "not determined" leukoencephalopathy in AIDS patients (Antinori et al., 2000). Taken together, our findings provide evidence for the emergence of a severe form of HAL.

Leukoencephalopathy in HIV-infected individuals may result from HIV-, immune-, opportunistic-, or drug-based mechanisms. HIV itself could injure white matter by damaging oligodendrocytes or brain endothelial cells or by injuring myelin via myelinotoxic viral proteins, such as gp120 or Tat (Arese et al., 2001). Although the brain is normally immune-privileged, the immune system can injure white matter by several mechanisms, including the release of pro-inflammatory cytokines such as TNF-α (Wesselingh et al., 1993; Sato-Matsumura et al., 1998). The phagocytosis of myelin by macrophages as observed in immune-mediated demyelinating diseases such as acute disseminated encephalomyelitis may occur in HIV infection, as well. Reactivated infection with opportunistic viruses, such as human herpes virus-6 or JC-virus (Monno et al., 1998), can also damage the white matter in the brains of AIDS patients. Prescribed (e.g., HIV protease inhibitors) or illicit (e.g., CNS stimulants, such as methamphetamine) drugs may penetrate the BBB and injure myelin, as well (Bell et al., 1998; Chana et al., 2006). Finally, immune reconstitution inflammatory syndrome (IRIS) may contribute to extensive white matter damage as evidenced by changing patterns on imaging. IRIS usually develops weeks or months after cART initiation in response to an underlying opportunistic infection (OI), when the immune system recovers. In some cases, IRIS can occur in the absence of detection of an OI and presents as T-cell mediated encephalitis (Johnson & Nath, 2009; McCombe et al., 2009). These conditions warrant further study and increased vigilance among those who provide healthcare for HIV-infected individuals.

HIV ENCEPHALITIS, NEURODEGENERATION, AND COGNITIVE IMPAIRMENT

Characterization of the neuronal populations affected in AIDS patients has provided a better understanding of the mechanisms contributing to cognitive impairment. However, the relationships among HIVE, neurodegeneration, and HAD are more complex than neuronal loss because death of neurons might be a later event preceded by synaptodendritic damage and white matter loss. Further complicating the analyses of the neuropathological correlates of HAD are the heterogeneous medical and neuropsychological characteristics of patients with HIV-associated cognitive impairments (Masliah et al., 1997; Gray et al., 2001; Heaton et al.,2010). Recent cohort studies in cART-experienced patients indicate that although many individuals have good virologic responses to antiretroviral drugs, they continue to suffer from mild to moderate cognitive impairments (Letendre et al., 2009; Heaton et al.,2010). Likewise, not all patients with HIVE develop dementia and not all demented AIDS patients have HIVE (Table 8.2.1). In comparison, most patients with cognitive impairment do have neurodegeneration, and those with a normal neuropsychological profile show preservation of their synaptodendritic architecture (Everall et al., 1999; Cherner et al., 2002). Four diagnostic categories based on impaired performance on neuropsychological testing are recognized: 1) neuropsychological impairment, likely due to causes other than HIV (NPI-O); 2) asymptomatic neuropsychological impairment, likely due to HIV (NPI); 3) minor cognitive motor disorder (MCMD); and 4) HAD. Assignment of one of the three sub-dementia diagnoses does not necessarily portend progression to dementia, although co-existing depression may be an early manifestation of HAD (Stern et al., 2001). In one study, 18 of 19 subjects with antemortem neurocognitive impairment had evidence of HIV-related brain disease at autopsy (positive predictive value = 95%). The sensitivity and specificity of neurocognitive impairment in detecting the occurrence of HIVE were 67% and 92%, respectively (Cherner et al., 2002). These findings support the use of neuropsychological assessment to predict HIV-related brain disease and thereby help identify HIV patients who may benefit from treatments targeting HIV CNS disease.

Virus specific factors may also contribute to the development of HAND and/or HAD. Studies of differences in viral sequence compartmentalization in the blood versus cerebrospinal fluid (CSF) showed that in patients with no neurocognitive alterations, HIV *env* gene sequences were more similar in CSF and blood; whereas, during development of severe HAND, *env* sequence partitioning between CSF and blood became much more distinct (Ritola et al., 2005; Strain et al., 2005; Pillai et al., 2006). Taken together, data from several studies suggests that "signature sequences" predictive of HAND may be detectable in the blood or CSF prior to HAND onset (Harrington et al., 2009).

Based on these data, viral and host molecular alterations observed in AIDS patients during the progression of HAND or HIVE might be better understood by recognizing four groups of AIDS patients based on the presence or absence of HIVE and neurodegeneration (Table 8.2.1): 1) without HIVE or neurodegeneration (-/-); 2) without HIVE, but with neurodegeneration (-/+); 3) HIVE, without neurodegeneration (+/-); and 4) HIVE and neurodegeneration (+/+). While the pathogenesis of the degenerative process in the last group can be explained in part by the known neurotoxic effects of HIV proteins and the neuroinflammatory response, the mechanisms responsible for the paradoxical findings in groups 2 and 3 are more complex. Neurodegeneration in AIDS patients with no evidence of HIVE (or other CNS OI pathology) might be associated with systemic inflammatory or infectious processes. For example, bacterial lipopolysaccharide (LPS) may directly or indirectly activate macrophages that in turn cross the BBB and promote neuronal injury when CD4 is expressed by cells in the brain (Buttini et al., 1998). Supporting this possibility, previous animal studies have shown that systemic LPS injection triggers microgliosis with increased expression of TNF-α and other cytokines. Furthermore, in the transgenic mouse model, expression of human CD4 in the CNS results in neurodegeneration (Buttini et al., 1998; Maingat et al.). Neurodegeneration in the absence of HIV and/or an inflammatory process in the brain might also be observed in cases where cART reduced viral burden to undetectable levels, but the antiretroviral agents are also triggering neuronal toxicity. Regarding those patients with HIVE but without evidence of neurodegeneration (group 3), it has been proposed that enhanced production of neurotrophic factors might contribute to the protection of the CNS from HIV toxicity (Everall et al., 2001; Langford & Masliah, 2002). Among such factors, increased expression of fibroblast growth factor 1 (FGF1) ameliorates the neurotoxic effects of HIV proteins. In cases with neither HIVE nor neurodegeneration, mild to moderate levels of FGF1 immunoreactivity were observed in pyramidal neurons, while in cases with HIVE without neurodegeneration, FGF1 levels were significantly elevated (Figure 8.2.4 a, b). In contrast, individuals with both HIVE and neurodegeneration showed low levels of neuronal FGF1 immunoreactivity (Everall et al., 2001). Furthermore, studies in primary human neuronal cultures treated with the HIV envelope protein gp120 showed that FGF1 was protective against gp120 neurotoxicity in a dose-dependent manner (Everall et al., 2001). Taken together, these results support the notion that increased levels of certain neurotrophic factors, such as FGF1, might protect the CNS from the neurotoxic effects of HIV. Molecular mechanisms involved in FGF and other neurotrophic factor-mediated protection are discussed below.

NEUROTROPHIC FACTORS AND HIV INFECTION OF THE CENTRAL NERVOUS SYSTEM

Neurotrophins such as NGF, BDNF, platelet-derived growth factor (PDGF), and neurotrophin 3 (NT3) are produced by neurons and glial cells to promote neuronal survival and growth (Table 8.2.3) (Encinas et al., 2000). These factors may regulate or be regulated by the neuroinflammatory response (NIR) and will be discussed in more detail in the following sections. Interactions among neurotrophic factors, NIR components, and viral proteins work in concert to influence cell fitness.

Through molecular mimicry, the virus or viral proteins can exploit the host cell's machinery by binding to host cell receptors to disrupt normal cell signaling (Asensio & Campbell, 1999; Langford & Masliah, 2002). For example, the HIV-encoded angiogenic Tat peptide mimics signaling properties of vascular endothelial cell growth factor (VEGF) to induce cerebral endothelial cell functioning (Scheidegger et al., 2001). Studies also indicate that Tat mimicry of VEGF correlates with increased microvessel density in AIDS-related diffuse large B-cell and Burkitt lymphomas (Nyagol et al., 2008). Molecular mimicry by HIV proteins also includes exploitation of chemokine receptors by both Tat and gp120 to promote the NIR and viral infection of host cells (Berger et al., 1999; Murphy, 2001). Numerous examples of viral mimicry exist and include homologues of cytokines, chemokines, and neurotrophic growth factors or their receptors (Lalani & McFadden, 1999; Alcami & Koszinowski, 2000; Murphy et al., 2001), leading to the dysregulation of host-mediated immune responses.

Neurotrophic factors play diverse roles during the progression of CNS infection by promoting increased viral replication or cooperating with viral and/or NIR molecules to alter neurotransmission. Trophic factors may also provide neuronal protection against toxic inflammatory factors produced in response to macrophage/microglial HIV infection, such as cytokines, chemokines or harmful viral products released by infected cells (Tables 8.2.1, 8.2.3). For example, in some patients with HIVE, levels of FGF1, FGF2, BDNF, and

NGF are elevated (Figure 8.2.4) (Boven et al., 1999; Saarelainen et al., 2001). Studies in a small group (n = 18) of HIV patients with HIV-associated cognitive disorder indicated that levels of FGF2 and BDNF were significantly lower than levels in control patients, whereas levels of NGF were elevated in HIV patients compared to control (Albrecht et al., 2006). Interestingly, recent studies have also shown that gp120 cooperation with BDNF enhances somatostatin neurotransmission in HIVE, which otherwise is severely impaired in disease (Barnea et al., 1999; Ramirez et al., 2001). In addition, NGF and BDNF play important roles in neuronal survival in HIV infection by activating the NF-κB, thereby inducing expression of the anti-apoptotic Bcl-2 gene that protects neurons from the pro-apoptotic effects of HIV-Tat (Table 8.2.3) (Ramirez et al., 2001). On the other hand, gp120 has been shown to affect the expression of both NGF and nitric oxide synthase in rodent models of disease (Bagetta et al., 1996; Corasaniti et al., 1998). Also, Tat has been shown to cooperate with p35 signaling in neurons to dysregulate the NGF pathway, thereby decreasing neuronal survival and disrupting differentiation (Peruzzi et al., 2002; Darbinian et al., 2008).

Platelet-derived growth factor-mediated neuroprotection against both gp120 and Tat is reported in studies with SHSY-5Y neuroblastoma cells (Peng et al., 2008a; Peng et al., 2008b; Zhu et al., 2009). Pathways through which PDGF protects differentiated neurons from gp120 and Tat both involve blocking apoptosis; however, the signaling cascades differ. For example, PDGF protects neurons from gp120-mediated toxicity via the phosphatidylinositol 3' kinase (PI3K)/AKT/GSK3β pathway (Peng et al., 2008a; Peng et al., 2008b). On the other hand, neurons are protected from Tat by PDGF regulation of extracellular glutamate and intracellular calcium levels (Zhu et al., 2009). Further studies show that intrastriatal delivery of PDGF in mice protects dopaminergic neurons in the substantia nigra from Tat toxicity via transient receptor potential canonical channel signaling (Yao et al., 2009).

FIBROBLAST GROWTH FACTORS IN HIV ENCEPHALITIS

As described in the previous section, trophic factors play important roles in the pathogenesis of HIVE by regulating the NIR, protecting neurons against toxins, and modulating viral replication. In addition, trophic factors may interact with viral proteins and chemokines in regulating the permeability of the BBB and in the process of angiogenesis in response to CNS damage (Salcedo et al., 1999; Arese et al., 2001; Persidsky et al., 2001; Toschi et al., 2001). Among the trophic factors involved in viral encephalitis, special attention has been placed on the role of FGF in the progression of these disorders. The FGF family includes at least 13 trophic factors that are important in neurogenesis and angiogenesis (Klint & Claesson-Welsh, 1999; Reuss & von Bohlen und Halbach, 2003). Of interest in the brain are FGF1 (acidic, aFGF) that is produced by neurons and is primarily neurotrophic, and FGF2 (basic, bFGF) that is produced by glial cells and is angiotrophic (Walicke & Baird, 1988; Eckenstein, 1994; Klint & Claesson-Welsh, 1999).

Fibroblast growth factors maintain a broad range of neurons, including those selectively vulnerable to virus-derived factors (Thorns & Masliah, 1999; Abe & Saito, 2001; Everall et al., 2001). Furthermore, FGFs sustain the integrity of the BBB and levels are altered in patients with HIVE (Figure 8.2.4a-d) (Boven et al., 1999; Everall et al., 2001). Consequently, their potential value in the treatment of neurological disorders is under investigation. This is important for patients with AIDS because neurocognitive alterations in this population continue to be a significant problem (McArthur et al., 1993; Grant et al., 1995; Starace et al., 1998; Dore et al., 1999; Heaton et al., 2010). However, to date there are no therapeutic strategies targeted toward protecting the CNS and/or preventing neuronal damage and death due to HIV infection.

Since not all patients with HIVE show cognitive impairment and neurodegeneration (Wiley & Achim, 1994), some individuals may have the capacity to produce neurotrophic factors that protect neurons against the deleterious effects of HIV. Supporting this possibility, studies have shown that levels of FGF1 are increased in HIVE patients with preserved neuronal architecture and that FGF1 protects primary cultured neurons from the neurotoxic effects of gp120 (Everall et al., 2001). Moreover, in HIV patients with Kaposi's sarcoma, high levels of FGF2 (Faris et al., 1998) produced by the tumor are associated with a decreased risk for neuronal degeneration and neurological impairment (Liestael et al., 1998). In contrast, neurodegeneration in patients with HIV is associated with low levels of FGF1 expression (Everall et al., 2001). While mechanisms by which FGF1 might be neuroprotective against HIV are not completely clear, several possibilities include antagonism of excitatory amino acid toxicity that blocks gp120 interaction with NMDA/glutamate receptors (Dreyer et al., 1990; Inklestein et al., 1993). In addition, FGF downregulates CXCR4 receptors, which are co-receptors for HIV cellular entry (Sanders et al., 2000) and important mediators of gp120 neurotoxicity (Kaul & Lipton, 1999). Alternatively, the signaling pathway downstream of the FGF-receptor 1 may mediate neuroprotective effects of FGF1 by activating tyrosine kinase pathways (Klint et al., 1999; Hashimoto et al., 2002). An array of signal transduction molecules are activated by growth factor binding and FGF receptor dimerization (Figure 8.2.5). Through PI3K signaling (Klint & Claesson-Welsh, 1999; Williams & Doherty, 1999), FGF induces sustained activation of the mitogen-activated protein (MAP) kinases ERK1 and 2, which are downstream of Ras in the pathway (Klint et al., 1999). MAP kinase activation is important in mediating a number of neurotrophic effects, although independent pathways may also be activated (Renaud et al., 1996). Furthermore, FGF binding activates Ras and the PI3K/AKT pathways, which in turn stabilize cAMP response element-binding protein (CREB) and membrane-associated β-catenin (Maggirwar et al., 1999). Degradation of β-catenin is promoted by GSK3β and FGF inhibits endogenous GSK3β, possibly through p90

(Torres et al., 1999) or the PI3K/AKT signaling cascade (Hashimoto et al., 2002). While activation of GSK3ß might lead to cell death, inhibition is associated with cell survival (Pap & Cooper, 1998). In fact, FGF1 has been shown to be neuroprotective via regulation of the GSK3ß pathway both *in vivo* and *in vitro* (Hashimoto et al., 2002; Crews et al., 2009). Further supporting a role of this pathway in HIVE, studies show that FGF1 alters GSK3ß activity and that in HIV-infected cells Tat is capable of inducing GSK3ß (Maggirwar et al., 1999). In summary, FGF1 might be neuroprotective against HIV via regulation of intracellular signaling pathways important for cell survival (Figure 8.2.5).

Although beyond the scope of this chapter, a brief mention of potential protective properties of FGF2 in maintaining BBB integrity is warranted. Brain levels of FGF2 have been shown to correlate positively with an intact BBB in HIV patients (Persidsky et al., 2000; Ullrich et al., 2000; Huang et al., 2001; Toborek et al., 2003). Likewise, in vitro studies indicate that FGF2 protects cerebral endothelial cells of the BBB against gp120-mediated toxicity via PI3K-MEK-ERK signaling (Langford et al., 2005). Brain levels of FGF2 are decreased in HIVE patients compared to HIV patients without encephalitis (Figure 8.2.4c, d). Thus, FGFs play important roles in protecting CNS cells, regulating the NIR and influencing HIV replication and infection by mediating co-receptor expression.

BRAIN-DERIVED NEUROTROPHIC FACTOR IN HIV ENCEPHALITIS

Brain-derived neurotrophic factor is a member of the neurotrophin family that includes NGF and the neurotrophins 3 and 4/5. Recent evidence has shown that BDNF is neuroprotective against gp120 both *in vivo* and *in vitro* (Bachis & Mocchetti, 2005; Nosheny et al., 2007). Studies suggest that BDNF exerts its protective effects by regulating neuronal expression of CXCR4 (Bachis et al., 2003; Ahmed et al., 2008). BDNF binds to the tyrosine kinase receptor, TrkB, and induces its dimerization. In turn, phosphorylation of ERK downregulates the expression of the HIV co-receptor, CXCR4, by inhibiting caspase-3 (Nosheny et al., 2007). Following the binding of HIV-gp120 to the CD4 receptor, secondary interactions with CXCR4 facilitate viral entry into permissive cells. In neurons expressing CXCR4, binding of gp120 induces the caspase cascade resulting in neuronal apoptosis. *In vitro* and *in vivo* studies indicate that BDNF induces CXCR4 internalization and blocks caspase-3 (Bachis et al., 2003; Mocchetti & Bachis, 2004; Mocchetti et al., 2007). Interestingly, CXCR4 internalization is also induced by FGF (Sanders et al., 2000), suggesting that neuroprotective properties of some neurotrophic factors may share common mechanisms.

In conclusion, a common theme begins to emerge in which cytokines, chemokines, trophic factors, and viral proteins converge to modulate host response to neurodegenerative infectious diseases. There is increasing evidence supporting a role for neuro-regulatory interactions of trophic factors and the NIR during viral infection, providing potential targets for the development of new therapeutic approaches.

SUMMARY

Dendritic simplification and axonal damage of pyramidal neurons, selective loss of interneurons, BBB damage, white matter pallor, astrogliosis, and microgliosis characterize the degenerative process in HIV infection of the CNS. Neuronal populations susceptible to HIV neurotoxins include pyramidal cells with glutamate and cytokine/chemokine receptors and low levels of calcium-binding proteins, as well as interneurons with cytokine/chemokine receptors and high levels of calcium-binding proteins. Therefore, differences in the relative levels of receptors across different neuronal populations may influence their selective vulnerability to distinct HIV-related neurotoxins during the course of HIVE. While damage to pyramidal neurons in the neocortex and limbic system might result in cognitive deficits, damage to interneurons in the neocortex and basal ganglia may be associated with motor deficits. Demyelination and vascular damage may also contribute to the neurological dysfunction in AIDS patients by interfering with axonal transmission. In particular, the emergence of cART-resistant HIV strains may contribute to more aggressive forms of HIVE with extensive white matter destruction. However, since not all patients with HIVE display neurodegeneration and motor-cognitive impairment, it is possible that in some cases the host is capable of producing trophic factors that protect neuronal, glial, and endothelial cell populations from HIV-mediated toxicity. Among these factors, FGF and BDNF have been shown to play prominent roles in neuronal protection. Both operate by receptor-mediated regulation of signaling molecules in the PI3K/AKT pathways that transduce cell survival signals and oppose the pro-apoptotic cascades triggered by HIV proteins (Figure 8.2.5). Neurotrophic factors modulate the NIR, which plays a central role in the pathogenesis of the neurodegenerative process. Identification of new trophic factors and a better understanding of their potential neuroprotective properties is important in the development of new treatments for HIVE in the cART era.

ACKNOWLEDGMENTS

This work was supported by NIH grants MH62962, MH59745, MH45294, DA12065.

REFERENCES

Abe, K. & Saito, H. (2001). Effects of basic fibroblast growth factor on central nervous system functions. *Pharmacol Res, 43,* 307–312.

Adle-Biassette, H., Levy, Y., Colombel, M., Poron, F., Natchev, S., Keohane, C. et al. (1995). Neuronal apoptosis in HIV infection in adults. *Neuropathol Appl Neurobiol, 21,* 218–227.

Ahmed, F., Tessarollo, L., Thiele, C. & Mocchetti, I. (2008). Brain-derived neurotrophic factor modulates expression of chemokine receptors in the brain. *Brain Res, 1227,* 1–11.

Albrecht, D., Garcia, L., Cartier, L., Kettlun, A. M., Vergara, C., Collados, L., et al. (2006). Trophic factors in cerebrospinal fluid and spinal cord of patients with tropical spastic paraparesis, HIV, and Creutzfeldt-Jakob disease. *AIDS Res Hum Retroviruses, 22,* 248–254.

Alcami, A. & Koszinowski, U. H. (2000). Viral mechanisms of immune evasion. *Immunol Today, 21,* 447–455.

Ammassari, A., Cingolani, A., Pezzotti, P., De Luca, D. A., Murri, R., Giancola, M. L., et al. (2000). AIDS-related focal brain lesions in the era of highly active antiretroviral therapy. *Neurology, 55,* 1194–1200.

Ammassari, A., Scoppettuolo, G., Murri, R., Pezzotti, P., Cingolani, A., Del Borgo, C., et al. (1998). Changing disease patterns in focal brain lesion-causing disorders in AIDS. *J Acquir Immune Defic Syndr Hum Retrovirol, 18,* 365–371.

Antinori, A., Ammassari, A., Luzzati, R., Castagna, A., Maserati, R., Rizzardini, G., et al. (2000). Role of brain biopsy in the management of focal brain lesions in HIV-infected patients. Gruppo Italiano Cooperativo AIDS & Tumori. *Neurology, 54,* 993–997.

Arese, M., Ferrandi, C., Primo, L., Camussi, G., & Bussolino, F. (2001). HIV-1 Tat protein stimulates in vivo vascular permeability and lymphomononuclear cell recruitment. *J Immunol, 166,* 1380–1388.

Asare, E., Dunn, G., Glass, J., McArthur, J., Luthert, P., Lantos, P. et al. (1996). Neuronal pattern correlates with the severity of human immunodeficiency virus-associated dementia complex. Usefulness of spatial pattern analysis in clinicopathological studies. *Am J Pathol, 148,* 31–38.

Asensio, V. C. & Campbell, I. L. (1999). Chemokines in the CNS: Plurifunctional mediators in diverse states. *Trends Neurosci, 22,* 504–512.

Aylward, E. H., Brettschneider, P. D., McArthur, J. C., Harris, G. J., Schlaepfer, T. E., Henderer, J. D., et al. (1995). Magnetic resonance imaging measurement of gray matter volume reductions in HIV dementia. *Am J Psychiatry, 152,* 987–994.

Bachis, A., Major, E. O., & Mocchetti, I. (2003). Brain-derived neurotrophic factor inhibits human immunodeficiency virus-1/gp120-mediated cerebellar granule cell death by preventing gp120 internalization. *J Neurosci, 23,* 5715–5722.

Bachis, A. & Mocchetti, I. (2005). Brain-derived neurotrophic factor is neuroprotective against human immunodeficiency virus-1 envelope proteins. *Ann N Y Acad Sci, 1053,* 247–257.

Bagetta, G., Corasaniti, M. T., Aloe, L., Berliocchi, L., Costa, N., Finazzi-Agro, A., & Nistico, G. (1996). Intracerebral injection of human immunodeficiency virus type 1 coat protein gp120 differentially affects the expression of nerve growth factor and nitric oxide synthase in the hippocampus of rat. *Proc Natl Acad Sci U S A, 93,* 928–933.

Barnea, A., Roberts, J., & Ho, R. H. (1999). Evidence for a synergistic effect of the HIV-1 envelope protein gp120 and brain-derived neurotrophic factor (BDNF) leading to enhanced expression of somatostatin neurons in aggregate cultures derived from the human fetal cortex. *Brain Res, 815,* 349–357.

Bell, J. E., Brettle, R. P., Chiswick, A., & Simmonds, P. (1998). HIV encephalitis, proviral load and dementia in drug users and homosexuals with AIDS. Effect of neocortical involvement. *Brain, 121,* 2043–2052.

Benveniste, E. N. (1994). Cytokine circuits in brain. Implications for AIDS dementia complex. *Res Publ Assoc Res Nerv Ment Dis, 72,* 71–88.

Berger, E. A., Murphy, P. M., & Farber, J. M. (1999). Chemokine receptors as HIV-1 coreceptors: Roles in viral entry, tropism, and disease. *Annu Rev Immunol, 17,* 657–700.

Bezzi, P., Domercq, M., Brambilla, L., Galli, R., Schols, D., De Clercq, E., et al. (2001). CXCR4-activated astrocyte glutamate release via TNFalpha: Amplification by microglia triggers neurotoxicity. *Nat Neurosci, 4,* 702–710.

Boven, L. A., Middel, J., Portegies, P., Verhoef, J., Jansen, G. H., & Nottet, H. S. (1999). Overexpression of nerve growth factor and basic fibroblast growth factor in AIDS dementia complex. *J Neuroimmunol, 97,* 154–162.

Budka, H. (1991). Neuropathology of human immunodeficiency virus infection. *Brain Pathol, 1,* 163–175.

Budka, H., Costanzi, G., Cristina, S., Lechi, A., Parravicini, C., Trabattoni, R. et al. (1987). Brain pathology induced by infection with the human immunodeficiency virus (HIV). A histological, immunocytochemical, and electron microscopical study of 100 autopsy cases. *Acta Neuropathol, 75,* 185–198.

Budka, H., Wiley, C. A., Kleihues, P., Artigas, J., Asbury, A. K., Cho, E. S., et al. (1991). HIV-associated disease of the nervous system: Review of nomenclature and proposal for neuropathology-based terminology. *Brain Pathol, 1,* 143–152.

Buttini, M., Westland, C. E., Masliah, E., Yafeh, A. M., Wyss-Coray, T., & Mucke, L. (1998). Novel role of human CD4 molecule identified in neurodegeneration. *Nat Med, 4,* 441–446.

Campbell, I. L., Abraham, C. R., Masliah, E., Kemper, P., Inglis, J. D., Oldstone, M. B., et al. (1993). Neurologic disease induced in transgenic mice by cerebral overexpression of interleukin 6. *Proc Natl Acad Sci USA, 90,* 10061–10065.

Campbell, I. L., Stalder, A. K., Chiang, C. S., Bellinger, R., Heyser, C. J., Steffensen, S., et al. (1997). Transgenic models to assess the pathogenic actions of cytokines in the central nervous system. *Mol Psychiatry, 2,* 125–129.

Chana, G., Everall, I. P., Crews, L., Langford, D., Adame, A., Grant, I., et al. (2006). Cognitive deficits and degeneration of interneurons in HIV+ methamphetamine users. *Neurology, 67,* 1486–1489.

Cherner, M., Masliah, E., Ellis, R. J., Marcotte, T. D., Moore, D. J., Grant, I., et al. (2002). Neurocognitive dysfunction predicts postmortem findings of HIV encephalitis. *Neurology, 59,* 1563–1567.

Corasaniti, M. T., Bagetta, G., Rotiroti, D., & Nistico, G. (1998). The HIV envelope protein gp120 in the nervous system: Interactions with nitric oxide, interleukin-1beta and nerve growth factor signalling, with pathological implications in vivo and in vitro. *Biochem Pharmacol, 56,* 153–156.

Crews, L., Patrick, C., Achim, C. L., Everall, I. P., & Masliah, E. (2009). Molecular pathology of neuro-AIDS (CNS-HIV). *Int J Mol Sci, 10,* 1045–1063.

Dallasta, L. M., Pisarov, L. A., Esplen, J. E., Werley, J. V., Moses, A. V., Nelson, J. A., et al. Blood-brain barrier tight junction disruption in human immunodeficiency virus-1 encephalitis. *Am J Pathol, 155,* 1915–1927.

Darbinian, N., Darbinyan, A., Czernik, M., Peruzzi, F., Khalili, K., Reiss, K., et al. (2008). HIV-1 Tat inhibits NGF-induced Egr-1 transcriptional activity and consequent p35 expression in neural cells. *J Cell Physiol, 216,* 128–134.

Deutsch, R., Ellis, R. J., McCutchan, J. A., Marcotte, T. D., Letendre, S., & Grant, I. (2001). AIDS-associated mild neurocognitive impairment is delayed in the era of highly active antiretroviral therapy. *AIDS, 15,* 1898–1899.

Dore, G. J., Correll, P. K., Li, Y., Kaldor, J. M., Cooper, D. A., & Brew, B. J. (1999). Changes to AIDS dementia complex in the era of highly active antiretroviral therapy. *AIDS, 13,* 1249–1253.

Dreyer, E. B., Kaiser, P. K., Offermann, J. T., & Lipton, S. A. (1990). HIV-1 coat protein neurotoxicity prevented by calcium channel antagonists. *Science, 248,* 364–367.

Eckenstein, F. P. (1994). Fibroblast growth factors in the nervous system. *J Neurobiol, 25,* 1467–1480.

Eggert, D., Dash, P. K., Serradji, N., Dong, C. Z., Clayette, P., Heymans, F., et al. (2009). Development of a platelet-activating factor antagonist for HIV-1 associated neurocognitive disorders. *J Neuroimmunol, 213,* 47–59.

Ellis, R., Langford, D., & Masliah, E. (2007). HIV and antiretroviral therapy in the brain: Neuronal injury and repair. *Nat Rev Neurosci, 8,* 33–44.

Encinas, M., Iglesias, M., Liu, Y., Wang, H., Muhaisen, A., Cena, V., et al. (2000). Sequential treatment of SH-SY5Y cells with retinoic acid and brain-derived neurotrophic factor gives rise to fully differentiated, neurotrophic factor-dependent, human neuron-like cells. *J Neurochem, 75,* 991–1003.

Everall, I., Gray, F., Barnes, H., Durigon, M., Luthert, P., & Lantos, P. (1992). Neuronal loss in symptom-free HIV infection. *Lancet, 340,* 1413.

Everall, I., Gray, F., & Masliah, E. (1997). Neurological and neuropsychiatric manifestations of HIV-1 infection, 1st ed. New York: Chapman and Hall.

Everall, I. P., Glass, J. D., McArthur, J., Spargo, E., & Lantos, P. (1994). Neuronal density in the superior frontal and temporal gyri does not correlate with the degree of human immunodeficiency virus-associated dementia. *Acta Neuropathol, 88,* 538–544.

Everall, I. P., Heaton, R. K., Marcotte, T. D., Ellis, R. J., McCutchan, J. A., Atkinson, J. H., et al. (1999). Cortical synaptic density is reduced in mild to moderate human immunodeficiency virus neurocognitive disorder. HNRC Group. HIV *Neurobehavioral Research Center. Brain Pathol, 9,* 209–217.

Everall, I. P., Luthert, P. J., & Lantos, P. L. (1991). Neuronal loss in the frontal cortex in HIV infection. *Lancet, 337,* 1119–1121.

Everall, I. P., Trillo-Pazos, G., Bell, C., Mallory, M., Sanders, V., & Masliah, E. (2001). Amelioration of neurotoxic effects of HIV envelope protein gp120 by fibroblast growth factor: A strategy for neuroprotection. *J Neuropathol Exp Neurol, 60,* 293–301.

Faris, M., Ensoli, B., Kokot, N., & Nel, A. E. (1998). Inflammatory cytokines induce the expression of basic fibroblast growth factor (bFGF) isoforms required for the growth of Kaposi's sarcoma and endothelial cells through the activation of AP-1 response elements in the bFGF promoter. *AIDS, 12,* 19–27.

Fox, L., Alford, M., Achim, C., Mallory, M., & Masliah, E. (1997). Neurodegeneration of somatostatin-immunoreactive neurons in HIV encephalitis. *J Neuropathol Exp Neurol, 56,* 360–368.

Garden, G. A., Budd, S. L., Tsai, E., Hanson, L., Kaul, M., D'Emilia, D. M., et al. (2002). Caspase cascades in human immunodeficiency virus-associated neurodegeneration. *J Neurosci, 22,* 4015–4024.

Gelman, B. B. & Nguyen, T. P. (2010). Synaptic Proteins Linked to HIV-1 Infection and Immunoproteasome Induction: Proteomic Analysis of Human Synaptosomes. *J Neuroimmune Pharmacol, 5,* 92–102.

Gendelman, H. E., Lipton, S. A., Tardieu, M., Bukrinsky, M. I., & Nottet, H. S. (1994). The neuropathogenesis of HIV-1 infection. *J Leukoc Biol, 56,* 389–398.

Gongvatana, A., Schweinsburg, B. C., Taylor, M. J., Theilmann, R. J., Letendre, S. L., Alhassoon, O. M., et al. (2009). White matter tract injury and cognitive impairment in human immunodeficiency virus-infected individuals. *J Neurovirol, 15,* 187–195.

Gonzalez, R. G., Cheng, L. L., Westmoreland, S. V., Sakaie, K. E., Becerra, L. R., Lee, P. L., et al. (2000). Early brain injury in the SIV-macaque model of AIDS. *AIDS, 14,* 2841–2849.

Grant, I., Heaton, R. K., Atkinson, J. H., and H. G. (1995). Current topics in microbiology and immunology. In M. B. Oldstone, & L. Vitovic, (Eds.). *HIV and dementia,* pp. 9–30. Heidelberg: Springer-Verlag.

Gray, F., Adle-Biassette, H., Chretien, F., Lorin de la Grandmaison, G., Force, G., & Keohane, C. (2001). Neuropathology and neurodegeneration in human immunodeficiency virus infection. Pathogenesis of HIV-induced lesions of the brain, correlations with HIV-associated disorders and modifications according to treatments. *Clin Neuropathol, 20,* 146–155.

Gray, F., Haug, H., Chimelli, L., Geny, C., Gaston, A., Scaravilli, F., et al. (1991). Prominent cortical atrophy with neuronal loss as correlate of human immunodeficiency virus encephalopathy. *Acta Neuropathol, 82,* 229–233.

Harrington, P. R., Schnell, G., Letendre, S. L., Ritola, K., Robertson, K., Hall, C., et al. (2009). Cross-sectional characterization of HIV-1 env compartmentalization in cerebrospinal fluid over the full disease course. *AIDS, 23,* 907–915.

Hashimoto, M., Sagara, Y., Langford, D., Everall, I. P., Mallory, M., Everson, A., et al. (2002). Fibroblast growth factor 1 regulates signaling via the glycogen synthase kinase-3beta pathway. Implications for neuroprotection. *J Biol Chem, 277,* 32985–32991.

Heaton RK, Clifford DB, Franklin Jr DR, Woods SP, Ake C, Vaida F, Ellis RJ, Letendre SL, Marcotte TD, Atkinson JH, Rivera-Mindt M, Vigil OR, Taylor MJ, Collier AC, Marra CM, Gelman BB, McArthur JC, Morgello S, Simpson DM, McCutchan JA, Abramson I, Gamst A, Fennema-Notestine C, Jernigan TL, Wong J, Grant I, the CHARTER Group. (2010). HIV-associated neurocognitive disorders persist in the era of potent antiretroviral therapy. *Neurology, 75,* 2087–2096.

Hesselgesser, J. & Horuk, R. (1999). Chemokine and chemokine receptor expression in the central nervous system. *J Neurovirol, 5,* 13–26.

Huang, M. B., Khan, M., Garcia-Barrio, M., Powell, M., & Bond, V. C. (2001). Apoptotic effects in primary human umbilical vein endothelial cell cultures caused by exposure to virion-associated and cell membrane-associated HIV-1 gp120. *J Acquir Immune Defic Syndr, 27,* 213–221.

Inklestein, S. P., Kemmou, A., Caday, C. G., & Berlove, D. J. (1993). Basic fibroblast growth factor protects cerebrocortical neurons against excitatory amino acid toxicity in vitro. *Stroke, 24,* 141–143.

James, H. J., Sharer, L. R., Zhang, Q., Wang, H. G., Epstein, L. G., Reed, J. C., et al. (1999). Expression of caspase-3 in brains from paediatric patients with HIV-1 encephalitis. *Neuropathol Appl Neurobiol, 25,* 380–386.

Jellinger, K. A., Setinek, U., Drlicek, M., Bohm, G., Steurer, A., & Lintner, F. (2000). Neuropathology and general autopsy findings in AIDS during the last 15 years. *Acta Neuropathol, 100,* 213–220.

Johnson, T. & Nath, A. (2009). Neurological complications of immune reconstitution in HIV-infected populations. *Ann N Y Acad Sci, 1184,* 106–120.

Kaul, M., Garden, G. A., & Lipton, S. A. (2001). Pathways to neuronal injury and apoptosis in HIV-associated dementia. *Nature, 410,* 988–994.

Kaul, M. & Lipton, S. A. (1999). Chemokines and activated macrophages in HIV gp120-induced neuronal apoptosis. *Proc Natl Acad Sci U S A, 96,* (1999) 8212–8216.

Klint, P. & Claesson-Welsh, L. (1999). Signal transduction by fibroblast growth factor receptors. *Front Biosci, 4,* D165–177.

Klint, P., Kanda, S., Kloog, Y., & Claesson-Welsh, L. (1999). Contribution of Src and Ras pathways in FGF-2 induced endothelial cell differentiation. *Oncogene, 18,* 3354–3364.

Lalani, A. S. & McFadden, G. (1999). Evasion and exploitation of chemokines by viruses. *Cytokine Growth Factor Rev, 10,* 219–233.

Langford, D., Hurford, R., Hashimoto, M., Digicaylioglu, M., & Masliah, E. (2005). Signalling mediated protection of endothelial cells from HIV-gp120. *BMC Neurosci, 6,* 8.

Langford, D. & Masliah, E. (2001). Crosstalk between components of the blood brain barrier and cells of the CNS in microglial activation in AIDS. *Brain Pathol, 11,* 306–312.

Langford, D. & Masliah, E. (2002). Role of trophic factors on neuroimmunity in neurodegenerative infectious diseases. *J Neurovirol, 8,* 625–638.

Langford, T. D., Letendre, S. L., Larrea, G. J., & Masliah, E. (2003). Changing patterns in the neuropathogenesis of HIV during the CART era. *Brain Pathol, 13,* 195–210.

Langford, T. D., Letendre, S. L., Marcotte, T. D., Ellis, R. J., McCutchan, J. A., Grant, I., et al. (2002). Severe, demyelinating leukoencephalopathy in AIDS patients on antiretroviral therapy. *AIDS, 16,* 1019–1029.

Letendre, S. L., Ellis, R. J., Ances, B. M., & McCutchan, J. A. (2010). Neurologic complications of HIV disease and their treatment. *Top HIV Med, 18,* 45–55.

Letendre, S. L., Ellis, R. J., Everall, I., Ances, B., Bharti, A., & McCutchan, J. A. (2009). Neurologic complications of HIV disease and their treatment. *Top HIV Med, 17,* 46–56.

Liestael, K., Goplen, A. K., Dunlop, O., Bruun, J. N., & Maehlen, J. (1998). Kaposi's sarcoma and protection from HIV dementia. *Science, 280,* 361–362.

Liner, K. J., 2nd, Ro, M. J., & Robertson, K. R. (2010). HIV, antiretroviral therapies, and the brain. *Curr HIV/AIDS Rep, 7,* 85–91.

Lopez, O. L., Smith, G., Meltzer, C. C., & Becker, J. T. (1999). Dopamine systems in human immunodeficiency virus-associated dementia. *Neuropsychiatry Neuropsychol Behav Neurol, 12,* 184–192.

Maggirwar, S. B., Tong, N., Ramirez, S., Gelbard, H. A., & Dewhurst, S. (1999). HIV-1 Tat-mediated activation of glycogen synthase kinase-3-beta contributes to Tat-mediated neurotoxicity. *J Neurochem, 73,* 578–586.

Maingat, F., Viappiani, S., Zhu, Y., Vivithanaporn, P., Ellestad, K. K., Holden, J., et al. (2010). Regulation of lentivirus neurovirulence by lipopolysaccharide conditioning: Suppression of CXCL10 in the brain by IL-10. *J Immunol, 184*, 1566–1574.

Marcus, C. D., Taylor-Robinson, S. D., Sargentoni, J., Ainsworth, J. G., Frize, G., Easterbrook, P. et al. (1998). 1H MR spectroscopy of the brain in HIV-1-seropositive subjects: Evidence for diffuse metabolic abnormalities. *Metab Brain Dis, 13*, 123–136.

Masliah, E. (1996). In vivo modeling of HIV-1-mediated neurodegeneration. *Am J Pathol, 149*, 745–750.

Masliah, E., Achim, C. L., Ge, N., De Teresa, R., & Wiley, C. A. (1994a). Cellular neuropathology in HIV encephalitis. *Res Publ Assoc Res Nerv Ment Dis, 72*, 119–131.

Masliah, E., Achim, C. L., Ge, N., DeTeresa, R., Terry, R. D., & Wiley, C.A. (1992a). Spectrum of human immunodeficiency virus-associated neocortical damage. *Ann Neurol, 32*, 321–329.

Masliah, E., DeTeresa, R. M., Mallory, M. E., & Hansen, L. A. (2000). Changes in pathological findings at autopsy in AIDS cases for the last 15 years. *AIDS, 14*, 69–74.

Masliah, E., Ge, N., Achim, C. L., DeTeresa, R., & Wiley, C. A. (1996a). Patterns of neurodegeneration in HIV encephalitis. *J Neuro AIDS, 1*, 161–173.

Masliah, E., Ge, N., Achim, C. L., Hansen, L. A., & Wiley, C. A. (1992b). Selective neuronal vulnerability in HIV encephalitis. *J Neuropathol Exp Neurol, 51*, 585–593.

Masliah, E., Ge, N., Achim, C. L., & Wiley, C. A. (1994b). Cytokine receptor alterations during HIV infection in the human central nervous system. *Brain Res, 663*, 1–6.

Masliah, E., Ge, N., & Mucke, L. (1996b). Pathogenesis of HIV-1 associated neurodegeneration. *Crit Rev Neurobiol, 10*, 57–67.

Masliah, E., Heaton, R. K., Marcotte, T. D., Ellis, R. J., Wiley, C. A., Mallory, M., et al. (1997). Dendritic injury is a pathological substrate for human immunodeficiency virus-related cognitive disorders. HNRC Group. The HIV Neurobehavioral Research Center. *Ann Neurol, 42*, 963–972.

McArthur, J. C., Hoover, D. R., Bacellar, H., Miller, E. N., Cohen, B. A., Becker, J. T., et al. (1993). Dementia in AIDS patients: Incidence and risk factors. Multicenter AIDS Cohort Study. *Neurology, 43*, 2245–2252.

McCombe, J. A., Auer, R. N., Maingat, F. G., Houston, S., Gill, M. J., & Power, C. (2009). Neurologic immune reconstitution inflammatory syndrome in HIV/AIDS: Outcome and epidemiology. *Neurology, 72*, 835–841.

Meisner, F., Scheller, C., Kneitz, S., Sopper, S., Neuen-Jacob, E., Riederer, P., et al. (2008). Memantine upregulates BDNF and prevents dopamine deficits in SIV-infected macaques: A novel pharmacological action of memantine. *Neuropsychopharmacology, 33*, 2228–2236.

Minagar, A., Shapshak, P., Fujimura, R., Ownby, R., Heyes, M., & Eisdorfer, C. (2002). The role of macrophage/microglia and astrocytes in the pathogenesis of three neurologic disorders: HIV-associated dementia, Alzheimer disease, and multiple sclerosis. *J Neurol Sci, 202*, 13–23.

Mocchetti, I. & Bachis, A. (2004). Brain-derived neurotrophic factor activation of TrkB protects neurons from HIV-1/gp120-induced cell death. *Crit Rev Neurobiol, 16*, 51–57.

Mocchetti, I., Nosheny, R. L., Tanda, G., Ren, K., Meyer, E. M. (2007) Brain-derived neurotrophic factor prevents human immunodeficiency virus type 1 protein gp120 neurotoxicity in the rat nigrostriatal system. Ann *N Y Acad Sci, 1122*, 144–154.

Monno, L., Di Stefano, M., Zimatore, G. B., Andreula, C. F., Appice, A., Perulli, L. M., et al. (1998). Measurement of viral sequences in cerebrospinal fluid of AIDS patients with cerebral white-matter lesions using polymerase chain reaction. *AIDS, 12*, 581–590.

Mucke, L., Masliah, E., & Campbell, I. L. (1995). Transgenic models to assess the neuropathogenic potential of HIV-1 proteins and cytokines. *Curr Top Microbiol Immunol, 202*, 187–205.

Murphy, C. L., Eulitz, M., Hrncic, R., Sletten, K., Westermark, P., Williams, T., et al. (2001). Chemical typing of amyloid protein contained in formalin-fixed paraffin-embedded biopsy specimens. *Am J Clin Pathol, 116*, 135–142.

Murphy, P. M. (2001). Viral exploitation and subversion of the immune system through chemokine mimicry. *Nat Immunol, 2*, 116–122.

Nath, A., Anderson, C., Jones, M., Maragos, W., Booze, R., Mactutus, C., et al. (2000). Neurotoxicity and dysfunction of dopaminergic systems associated with AIDS dementia. *J Psychopharmacol, 14*, 222–227.

Neuenburg, J. K., Brodt, H. R., Herndier, B. G., Bickel, M., Bacchetti, P., Price, R. W., et al. (2002). HIV-related neuropathology, 1985 to 1999: Rising prevalence of HIV encephalopathy in the era of highly active antiretroviral therapy. *J Acquir Immune Defic Syndr, 31*, 171–177.

Nguyen, T. P., Soukup, V. M., & Gelman, B. B. (2010). Persistent hijacking of brain proteasomes in HIV-associated dementia. *Am J Pathol, 176*, 893–902.

Noorbakhsh, F., Ramachandran, R., Barsby, N., Ellestad, K. K., Leblanc, A., Dickie, P., et al. (2010). MicroRNA profiling reveals new aspects of HIV neurodegeneration: Caspase-6 regulates astrocyte survival. *FASEB J.*

Nosheny, R. L., Ahmed, F., Yakovlev, A., Meyer, E. M., Ren, K., Tessarollo, L., et al. (2007). Brain-derived neurotrophic factor prevents the nigrostriatal degeneration induced by human immunodeficiency virus-1 glycoprotein 120 in vivo. *Eur J Neurosci, 25*, 2275–2284.

Nyagol, J., De Falco, G., Lazzi, S., Luzzi, A., Cerino, G., Shaheen, S., et al. (2008). HIV-1 Tat mimetic of VEGF correlates with increased microvessels density in AIDS-related diffuse large B-cell and Burkitt lymphomas. *J Hematop, 1*, 3–10.

Pap, M. & Cooper, G. M. (1998). Role of glycogen synthase kinase-3 in the phosphatidylinositol 3-Kinase/Akt cell survival pathway. *J Biol Chem, 273*, 19929–19932.

Peng, F., Dhillon, N., Callen, S., Yao, H., Bokhari, S., Zhu, X., et al. (2008a). Platelet-derived growth factor protects neurons against gp120-mediated toxicity. *J Neurovirol, 14*, 62–72.

Peng, F., Dhillon, N. K., Yao, H., Zhu, X., Williams, R., & Buch, S. (2008b). Mechanisms of platelet-derived growth factor-mediated neuroprotection—implications in HIV dementia. *Eur J Neurosci, 28*, 1255–1264.

Persidsky, Y., Limoges, J., Rasmussen, J., Zheng, J., Gearing, A., & Gendelman, H. E. (2001). Reduction in glial immunity and neuropathology by a PAF antagonist and an MMP and TNFalpha inhibitor in SCID mice with HIV-1 encephalitis. *J Neuroimmunol, 114*, 57–68.

Persidsky, Y., Zheng, J., Miller, D., & Gendelman, H. E. (2000). Mononuclear phagocytes mediate blood-brain barrier compromise and neuronal injury during HIV-1-associated dementia. *J Leukoc Biol, 68*, 413–422.

Peruzzi, F., Gordon, J., Darbinian, N., & Amini, S. (2002). Tat-induced deregulation of neuronal differentiation and survival by nerve growth factor pathway. *J Neurovirol, 8*, Suppl 2 91–96.

Peters, A. & Jones, E. (1984a). Cellular components of the cerebral cortex. In: A. Peters (Ed.). *Cerebral cortex*. New York: Plenum Press.

Peters, A. & Jones, E. (1984b). Functional properties of cortical cells. In: E. Peters E. (Ed.). *Cerebral cortex*. New York: Plenum Press.

Pillai, S. K., Pond, S. L., Liu, Y., Good, B. M., Strain, M. C., Ellis, R. J., et al. (2006). Genetic attributes of cerebrospinal fluid-derived HIV-1 env. *Brain, 129*, 1872–1883.

Power, C., Gill, M. J., & Johnson, R. T. (2002). Progress in clinical neurosciences: The neuropathogenesis of HIV infection: Host-virus interaction and the impact of therapy. *Can J Neurol Sci, 29*, 19–32.

Pulliam, L., Herndier, B. G., Tang, N.M., & McGrath, M. S. (1991). Human immunodeficiency virus-infected macrophages produce soluble factors that cause histological and neurochemical alterations in cultured human brains. *J Clin Invest, 87*, 503–512.

Ramirez, S. H., Sanchez, J. F., Dimitri, C. A., Gelbard, H.A., Dewhurst, S., & Maggirwar, S. B. (2001). Neurotrophins prevent HIV Tat-induced neuronal apoptosis via a nuclear factor-kappaB (NF-kappaB)-dependent mechanism. *J Neurochem, 78*, 874–889.

Renaud, F., Desset, S., Oliver, L., Gimenez-Gallego, G., Van Obberghen, E., Courtois, Y., et al. (1996). The neurotrophic activity of fibroblast growth factor 1 (FGF1) depends on endogenous FGF1 expression and is independent of the mitogen-activated protein kinase cascade pathway. *J Biol Chem, 271*, 2801–2811.

Reuss, B. & von Bohlen und Halbach, O. (2003). Fibroblast growth factors and their receptors in the central nervous system. *Cell Tissue Res, 313,* 139–157.

Ritola, K., Robertson, K., Fiscus, S. A., Hall, C., & Swanstrom, R. (2005). Increased human immunodeficiency virus type 1 (HIV-1) env compartmentalization in the presence of HIV-1-associated dementia. *J Virol, 79,* 10830–10834.

Saarelainen, T., Vaittinen, S., & Castren, E. (2001). trkB-receptor activation contributes to the kainate-induced increase in BDNF mRNA synthesis. *Cell Mol Neurobiol, 21,* 429–435.

Sacktor, N., McDermott, M. P., Marder, K., Schifitto, G., Selnes, O. A., McArthur, J. C., et al. (2002). HIV-associated cognitive impairment before and after the advent of combination therapy. *J Neurovirol, 8,* 136–142.

Salcedo, R., Wasserman, K., Young, H. A., Grimm, M. C., Howard, O. M., Anver, M. R., et al. (1999). Vascular endothelial growth factor and basic fibroblast growth factor induce expression of CXCR4 on human endothelial cells: In vivo neovascularization induced by stromal-derived factor-1alpha. *Am J Pathol, 154,* 1125–1135.

Sanders, V. J., Everall, I. P., Johnson, R. W., & Masliah, E. (2000). Fibroblast growth factor modulates HIV coreceptor CXCR4 expression by neural cells. HNRC Group. *J Neurosci Res, 59,* 671–679.

Sato-Matsumura, K. C., Berger, J., Hainfellner, J. A., Mazal, P., & Budka, H. (1998). Development of HIV encephalitis in AIDS and TNF-alpha regulatory elements. *J Neuroimmunol, 91,* 89–92.

Scheidegger, P., Weiglhofer, W., Suarez, S., Console, S., Waltenberger, J., Pepper, M. S., et al. (2001). Signalling properties of an HIV-encoded angiogenic peptide mimicking vascular endothelial growth factor activity. *Biochem J, 353,* 569–578.

Smith, T. W., DeGirolami, U., Henin, D., Bolgert, F., & Hauw, J. J. (1990). Human immunodeficiency virus (HIV) leukoencephalopathy and the microcirculation. *J Neuropathol Exp Neurol, 49,* 357–370.

Starace, F., Dijkgraaf, M., Houweling, H., Postma, M., & Tramarin, A. (1998). HIV-associated dementia: Clinical, epidemiological and resource utilization issues. *AIDS Care, 10,* Suppl 2 S113–21.

Stern, Y., McDermott, M. P., Albert, S., Palumbo, D., Selnes, O. A., McArthur, J., et al. (2001). Factors associated with incident human immunodeficiency virus-dementia. *Arch Neurol, 58,* 473–479.

Strain, M. C., Letendre, S., Pillai, S. K., Russell, T., Ignacio, C. C., Gunthard, H. F., et al. (2005). Genetic composition of human immunodeficiency virus type 1 in cerebrospinal fluid and blood without treatment and during failing antiretroviral therapy. *J Virol, 79,* 1772–1788.

Thorns, V. & Masliah, E. (1999). Evidence for neuroprotective effects of acidic fibroblast growth factor in Alzheimer disease. *J Neuropathol Exp Neurol, 58,* 296–306.

Toborek, M., Lee, Y. W., Pu, H., Malecki, A., Flora, G., Garrido, R., et al. (2003). HIV-Tat protein induces oxidative and inflammatory pathways in brain endothelium. *J Neurochem, 84,* 169–179.

Toggas, S. M., Masliah, E., Rockenstein, E. M., Rall, G. F., Abraham, C. R., & Mucke, L. (1994). Central nervous system damage produced by expression of the HIV-1 coat protein gp120 in transgenic mice. *Nature, 367,* 188–193.

Torres, M. A., Eldar-Finkelman, H., Krebs, E.G., & Moon, R. T. (1999). Regulation of ribosomal S6 protein kinase-p90(rsk), glycogen synthase kinase 3, and beta-catenin in early Xenopus development. *Mol Cell Biol, 19,* 1427–1437.

Toschi, E., Barillari, G., Sgadari, C., Bacigalupo, I., Cereseto, A., Carlei, D., et al. (2001). Activation of matrix-metalloproteinase-2 and membrane-type-1-matrix-metalloproteinase in endothelial cells and induction of vascular permeability in vivo by human immunodeficiency virus-1 Tat protein and basic fibroblast growth factor. *Mol Biol Cell, 12,* 2934–2946.

Ullrich, C. K., Groopman, J. E., & Ganju, R. K. (2000). HIV-1 gp120- and gp160-induced apoptosis in cultured endothelial cells is mediated by caspases. *Blood, 96,* 1438–1442.

Vago, L., Bonetto, S., Nebuloni, M., Duca, P., Carsana, L., Zerbi, P., et al. (2002). Pathological findings in the central nervous system of AIDS patients on assumed antiretroviral therapeutic regimens: Retrospective study of 1597 autopsies. *AIDS, 16,* 1925–1928.

Walicke, P. A. & Baird, A. (1988). Neurotrophic effects of basic and acidic fibroblast growth factors are not mediated through glial cells. *Brain Res, 468,* 71–79.

Weis, S., Haug, H., & Budka, H. (1993). Neuronal damage in the cerebral cortex of AIDS brains: A morphometric study. *Acta Neuropathol, 85,* 185–189.

Wesselingh, S. L., Power, C., Glass, J. D., Tyor, W. R., McArthur, J. C., Farber, J. M., et al. (1993). Intracerebral cytokine messenger RNA expression in acquired immunodeficiency syndrome dementia. *Ann Neurol, 33,* 576–582.

Wiley, C.A. & Achim, C. (1994) Human immunodeficiency virus encephalitis is the pathological correlate of dementia in acquired immunodeficiency syndrome. *Ann Neurol, 36,* 673–676.

Wiley, C. A., Achim, C. L., Hammond, R., Love, S., Masliah, E., Radhakrishnan, L., et al. (2000). Damage and repair of DNA in HIV encephalitis. *J Neuropathol Exp Neurol, 59,* 955–965.

Wiley, C. A., Masliah, E., Morey, M., Lemere, C., DeTeresa, R., Grafe, M., et al. (1991). Neocortical damage during HIV infection. *Ann Neurol, 29,* 651–657.

Wilkinson, I. D., Lunn, S., Miszkiel, K. A., Miller, R. F., Paley, M. N., Williams, I., et al. (1997). Proton MRS and quantitative MRI assessment of the short term neurological response to antiretroviral therapy in AIDS. *J Neurol Neurosurg Psychiatry, 63,* 477–482.

Williams, E. J. & Doherty, P. (1999). Evidence for and against a pivotal role of PI 3-kinase in a neuronal cell survival pathway. *Mol Cell Neurosci, 13,* 272–280.

Yao, H., Peng, F., Fan, Y., Zhu, X., Hu, G., & Buch, S. J. (2009). TRPC channel-mediated neuroprotection by PDGF involves Pyk2/ERK/CREB pathway. *Cell Death Differ, 16,* 1681–1693.

Zauli, G., Secchiero, P., Rodella, L., Gibellini, D., Mirandola, P., Mazzoni, M., et al. (2000). HIV-1 Tat-mediated inhibition of the tyrosine hydroxylase gene expression in dopaminergic neuronal cells. *J Biol Chem, 275,* 4159–4165.

Zhu, X., Yao, H., Peng, F., Callen, S., & Buch, S. (2009). PDGF-mediated protection of SH-SY5Y cells against Tat toxin involves regulation of extracellular glutamate and intracellular calcium. *Toxicol Appl Pharmacol, 240,* 286–291.

8.3

PATHOBIOLOGY OF HIV-RELATED NEUROPATHIES

Nicholas W. S. Davies and Bruce J. Brew

HIV-associated neuropathies remain the cause of considerable morbidity. The pathobiology of these neuropathies is complex, resulting from many mechanisms through which HIV interacts with the immune and nervous systems. Additional complexity arises because antiretroviral medications can themselves cause or contribute to neuropathy, both directly and through the metabolic complications of long-term treatment. This chapter presents a general conceptual framework for understanding the neuropathies and then discusses specific neuropathies. The concepts discussed are time locking, layering, and nonspecific pathology. The specific neuropathies discussed are distal symmetrical sensory polyneuropathy, antiretroviral toxic neuropathies, inflammatory demyelinating neuropathies, mononeuritic multiplex, diffuse infiltrative lymphocytosis syndrome, cytomegalovirus polyradiculopathy, syphilitic polyradiculopathy, human T-lymphotropic virus neuropathy, and statin neuropathy.

INTRODUCTION

The pathobiology of HIV-related neuropathies is complex, in part, due to the diversity of etiologies. This review will first discuss a general conceptual framework for understanding the neuropathies and then delineate each using an etiologic classification. The previous chapters have discussed the possible etiologic agents for each of the limited patterns of clinical presentation, so this approach should be "user friendly."

The general conceptual framework that should be applied to this topic is discussed in detail elsewhere (Brew, 2001). With the exception of the final principle, it consists of a set of principles that apply to all the neurologic complications of HIV disease. These include time locking, layering, and non-specific pathology. Here, their specific relevance to the pathobiology of the neuropathies will be emphasized.

TIME LOCKING

The first principle, time locking, refers to the observation that the neurologic complications are time locked to the degree of advancement of HIV disease as assessed by the CD4 cell count. The inflammatory demyelinating neuropathies, for example, are seen in patients with normal or mildly depressed CD4 cell counts. Distal symmetrical sensory polyneuropathy (DSPN) on the other hand most often occurs in advanced HIV

disease—usually CD4 cell counts below 200/μL. However, with the advent of combined antiretroviral therapy (cART) leading to significant rises in CD4 cell counts, patients may present with complications, such as DSPN, at a CD4 cell count that is much higher than previously expected. This different presentation may influence the pathobiology in ways that at present are only speculative. For example, DSPN could be characterized by a more prominent inflammatory infiltrate in patients who commence cART and have a significant improvement in immune function.

LAYERING

The next principle pertinent to the pathobiology of the neuropathies is that of layering. As HIV-infected patients are living longer, they are increasingly likely to develop complications of the disease, its treatment, or other illnesses. This may alter the more classic neuropathologic appearance of certain complications. For example, patients may develop a neuropathy related to diabetes, which in turn is related to protease inhibitor therapy, on a background of a mild toxic neuropathy from stavudine. In such a case, the neuropathology will be characterized by involvement of all sizes of axons, which would be atypical for diabetic neuropathy. Not only may the neuropathology be different but there may also be a more marked discordance between the "dose" of the inducing agent and the neuropathologic severity: patients are "exposed" to more potentially neuropathic agents such as antiretroviral drugs, diabetes, as well as lipid lowering agents. In the resource-poor world, particularly in children, malnutrition may also be an important cofactor for neuropathy in HIV (Esteban et al., 2009). Worldwide, the median age of cART-treated patients is rising and the independent effects of aging require consideration in relation to the nervous system. Lastly, peripheral nervous system repair is impaired in HIV-infected persons compared to controls (Hahn et al., 2007). Hence, as these factors accumulate they result in layering and less "reserve."

NONSPECIFIC PATHOLOGY

The final principle is that the pathology of HIV-related neuropathies is by and large not complication-specific: most lead to axonal changes with reactive infiltrates. This is different from the other neurologic complications of HIV of the neuraxis, especially those involving the brain, where for the most part there are complication-specific neuropathologic findings. Therefore, biopsy alone usually does not assist differentiation between HIV-related neuropathies, an important principle when it comes to diagnosis. Indeed, it indicates that the pathobiologies of HIV-related neuropathies are likely to share at least some common mechanistic pathways.

Thus, the pathobiology of HIV-related neuropathies is rarely pure. More often the findings are the result of a number of disease processes. The clinician should be cognizant of this when translating the neuropathological features of the conditions below into the management of individual patients.

HIV-RELATED DISTAL SYMMETRICAL SENSORY POLYNEUROPATHY

The most common neurologic complication of HIV is the development of a distal symmetrical sensory polyneuropathy (DSPN) that is directly related to HIV. As discussed in the previous chapter, in the pre-cART era it occurred more frequently in patients with CD4 cell counts below $200/\mu L$. Since cART, rather than markers of HIV disease severity, demographic features such as older age appear increasingly important DSPN risk factors (Robinson-Papp & Simpson, 2009; Schifitto et al., 2005); and in contrast to HIV-associated neurocognitive syndrome (HAND), nadir CD4 count does not appear to be an independent risk factor for DSPN (Smyth et al., 2007). The concurrence of type 2 diabetes mellitus and hypertriglyceridemia are associated with increased risk of

DSPN (Ances et al., 2009), although others have failed to show an association of glucose dysmetabolism and neuropathy in HIV (Sheth et al., 2007). However, the latter study, a retrospective analysis of a public HIV dataset, has serious methodological flaws. First, a low proportion of patients were reported as suffering from a peripheral neuropathy (5%); second, fasting sugars were available for only 20% of patients with neuropathy and 12% without. Third, the proportion of patients with glucose dysmetabolism was highest in patients without neuropathy, suggesting considerable bias in selection of individuals who had fasting sugar measured. Interestingly, raised triglycerides in particular are associated with painful idiopathic chronic axonal neuropathy in the HIV seronegative (Hughes et al., 2004). In diabetic neuropathy, raised triglycerides are a better predictor for disease progression than glycosylated hemoglobin and appear independent of other known risk factors (Wiggin et al., 2009). Measurement of serum triglycerides is a surrogate marker for activity of the endogenous lipid transport pathway. Whether the association between elevated triglycerides and neuropathy serves solely as a marker of deranged metabolism or in addition it plays a key role in pathobiology of neuronal damage has yet to be established. Figure 8.3.1 summarizes the key pathogenetic factors relating neuropathy caused by HIV or its treatment.

Neuropathologically, DSPN is characterized by a length-dependent sensory axonal neuropathy; however, it is important to note that the histopathological description is based upon studies prior to cART. The loss of intradermal fibers is an early phenomenon (Brinley et al., 2001) (see Figures 8.3.2 and 8.3.3). All sizes of axon can be involved in contrast to diabetic

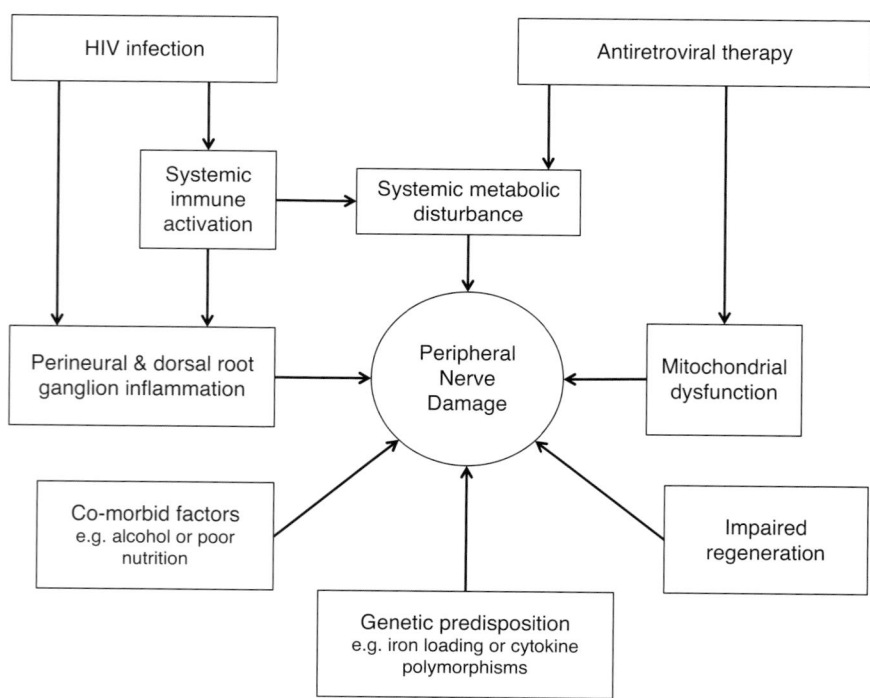

Figure 8.3.1 Overview of the pathiobiological factors associated with HIV-related distal symmetrical sensory polyneuropathy and antiretroviral toxic neuropathy.

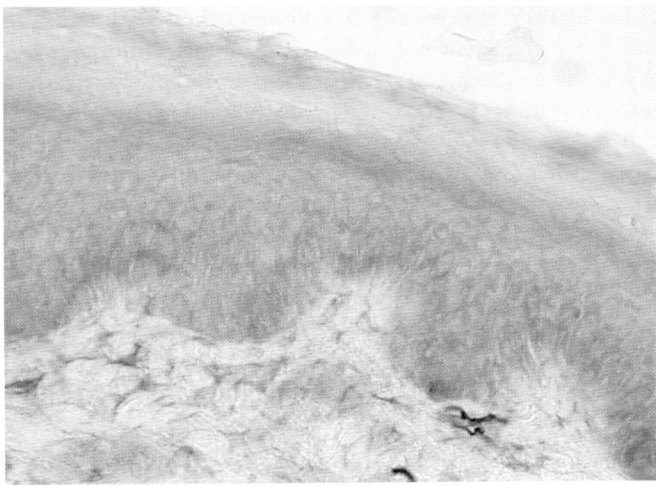

Figure 8.3.2 Skin biopsy showing no nerve fibers in the epidermis of a patient with severe sensory neuropathy secondary to HIV (50μm section stained with PGP x 400) (Courtesy Dr. C. Cherry).

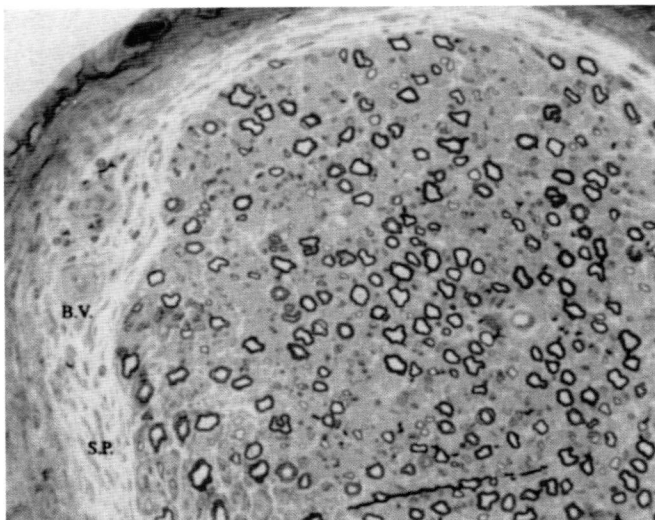

Figure 8.3.4 Sural nerve biopsy of a patient with distal symmetrical sensory neuropathy. There is edema and a mild mononuclear infiltrate in the subepineural space (SP) adjacent to the blood vessel (BV) (toluidine blue x 10).

and uremic neuropathies where smaller fibers are preferentially affected (Brinley et al., 2001). Small and large myelinated fibers are affected (Griffin et al., 1998) but especially unmyelinated fibers, at least in children (Araujo et al., 2000) (see Figures 8.3.4 and 8.3.5). Demyelination can be seen, but where this occurs it is not segmental and results from axonal damage. Interestingly, there is a gradient of damage with loss of intradermal fibers being greater than axonal loss in peripheral nerves, which in turn is more marked than loss of neurons in DRG (Brinley et al., 2001). These findings suggest an axonal "dying-back" in a length-dependent manner; which is further supported by the observed loss of DRG neurons' centrally directed extensions and degeneration of the gracile tracts within the spinal cord (Brinley et al., 2001; Rance et al., 1988).

Importantly, many of these findings, including decreased epidermal nerve fiber density, can occur in patients without DSPN (McCarthy et al., 1995). However, a fall in density below threshold levels of epidermal nerve fibers or Meissner's corpuscles, is associated with symptomatic DSPN (Herrmann et al., 2007; Herrmann et al., 2006). Curiously, prominent inflammatory infiltrates of mononuclear cells in the epineurium occur infrequently in contrast to the greater prominence of these cells in the brain in HAND. There is no evidence to indicate immune-complex deposition as a mechanism for neuronal damage (Dalakas & Pezeshkpour, 1988; de la Monte et al., 1988).

Neurovirologically, HIV viral transcripts and antigens are absent from the axons. However, perivascular macrophages

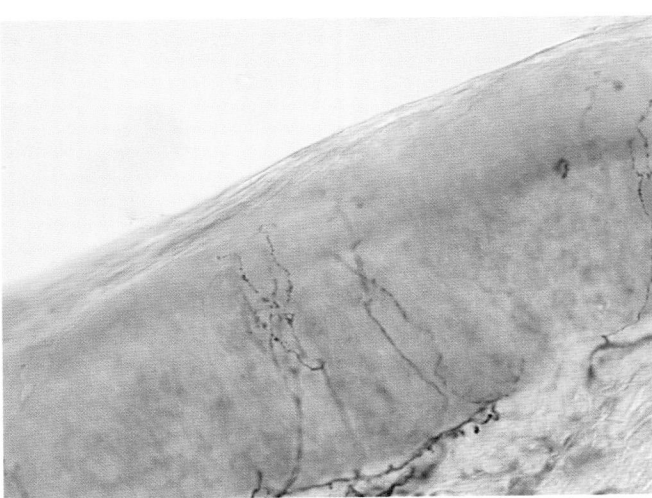

Figure 8.3.3 Skin biopsy showing normal nerve fiber density in the epidermis of a patient without neuropathy (50μm section stained with PGP x 400).

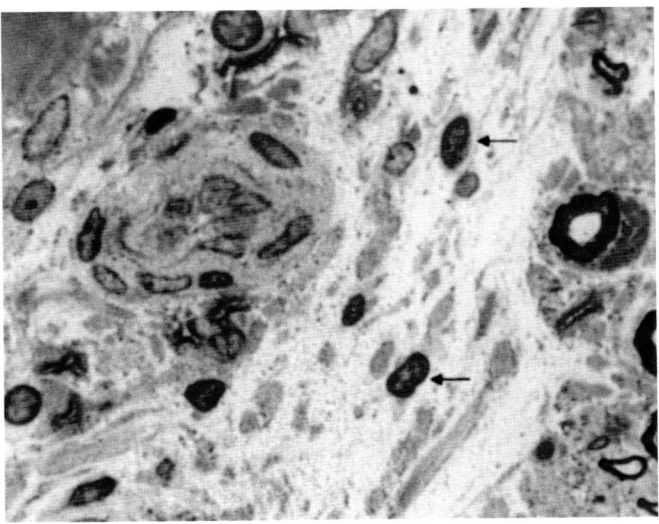

Figure 8.3.5 High power view of the same sural nerve biopsy showing edema and a mild mononuclear infiltrate in the subepineural space (toluidine blue x 40).

and Langerhans cells in the skin adjacent to the terminal axons do harbor HIV, which is predominantly CCR5 tropic (Brinley et al., 2001; Jones et al., 2005). In tissue from patients with DSPN perineural macrophages, unlike Schwann cells, show productive HIV infection (Hahn et al., 2008). Similarly, satellite cells that are close to DRG also support HIV infection (Brinley et al., 2001). However, it would be wrong to think that these cells contain abundant HIV; at least in one study, p24 mRNA in perivascular macrophages was found in 6 of 13 specimens and only 2 of 5 DRG cells (Rizzuto et al., 1995). Similar results have been obtained by other investigators (Shapshak et al., 1995). Importantly, HIV can be recovered from such cells even in patients who do not have DSPN (Esiri et al., 1993; Yoshioka et al., 1994). This appears to be related to the degree of advancement of HIV disease as determined by the CD4 cell count but this relationship may not hold true in cART-treated patients who have been living with HIV for many years. In addition, it is unusual for DSPN to worsen upon immune reconstitution following initiation of cART, perhaps suggesting that load of virus in peripheral nerve or DRG is not the critical determinant in neuropathy pathobiology. To date, no peripheral nerve-tropic HIV species has been reported. However, the possibility of such a strain is not inconceivable as it might be difficult to identify in blood, being "lost" amongst more dominant species (Brew & Tomlinson, 2004).

More consistent than the finding of recoverable HIV are the following neuroimunological observations. Firstly, there is an abundance of activated macrophages in both the peripheral nerves and DRG; and secondly, DSPN correlates with degree of macrophage activation (Jones et al., 2005). These macrophages express tumor necrosis factor alpha (TNF-α), nitric oxide (NO), interleukin-1, and interleukin-6 (Shapshak et al., 1995; Esiri et al., 1993; Yoshioka et al., 1994; Tyor et al., 1993). Furthermore, the inflammation persists, raising speculation that perhaps patients with DSPN might have a local deficit in immune regulation; or that in those patients receiving cART, HIV within macrophages is inadequately treated (Brew & Tomlinson, 2004).

The pathogenesis of DSPN is still not resolved. Nonetheless, it is related in some way to HIV infection: The neuropathological, neurovirological, and neuroimmunological findings in patients without DSPN almost certainly reflect subclinical disease (see Figure 8.3.7). Currently, there are three schools of thought. One holds that the disorder is primarily a consequence of disturbed function and loss of DRG leading to the dying back neuropathy and spinal cord changes characterized by degeneration of the gracile tracts (Rance et al., 1988; Scaravilli et al., 1992). Certainly, DRG do not have a blood-brain or blood-nerve barrier and are therefore susceptible to the products of systemic HIV disease. However, the clinical phenotype of DSPN is markedly different to other neurological conditions where the DRG is the principle target of immunopathogenesis. The second states that the axon is the primary site and that the DRG changes are secondary to axonal damage. Injury would be a consequence of immune activation of the perivascular macrophages, satellite cells, and the Langerhans cells, driven

either by HIV infection of the cells per se or more likely as an indirect consequence of a product of adjacent infected cells. A few infected cells, by virtue of release of a "product," could lead to widespread immune activation of adjacent cells, a so-called "cascade" effect. The third school of thought holds that neither DRG nor the axon is primary and that in fact both are equally important, with infected and activated cells of mononuclear/macrophage lineage that are "turned over" from the bone marrow mediating damage. At least in chimeric rats, up to 80% of these cells are replaced every three months (Brinley et al., 2001).

A candidate toxic product could be the HIV protein gp120, which in the early 1990s was shown to bind to neural glycolipids and glycoproteins as well as DRG (van den Berg et al., 1992; Apostolski et al., 1993). Following exposure to rat sciatic nerve, gp120 causes axonal swelling, increased TNF-α expression and intense activation of astrocytes and microglia in the spinal cord as well as allodynia (Herzberg & Sagen, 2001). Others have shown behavioral changes in rats compared to controls following sciatic nerve injection of gp120, including persistent mechanical hypersensitivity, thigomatic (anxiety-like) behavior but no alteration in sensitivity to hot or cold (Wallace, Blackbeard, Pheby et al., 2007). Histologically, the latter model revealed reduced intraepidermal nerve fiber density with expression of the cell stress marker ATF-3 in small diameter sensory neurons. Furthermore, increased caspase-3 expression was found in the DRG as well as upregulation of CCL2 (monocyte chemotactic protein-1), although in HIV patients with DSPN CCL2 is not elevated in blood or CSF (Schifitto et al., 2005). In a third model, injection of gp120 into rat paws caused localized allodynia and at the DRG neuronal stimulation with substance P release, a neurotransmitter known to be important in the pathophysiology of pain (Oh et al., 2001).

In vitro gp120, at picomolar concentrations, induces DRG sensory neuron neuritic pruning and apoptosis in a caspase-3

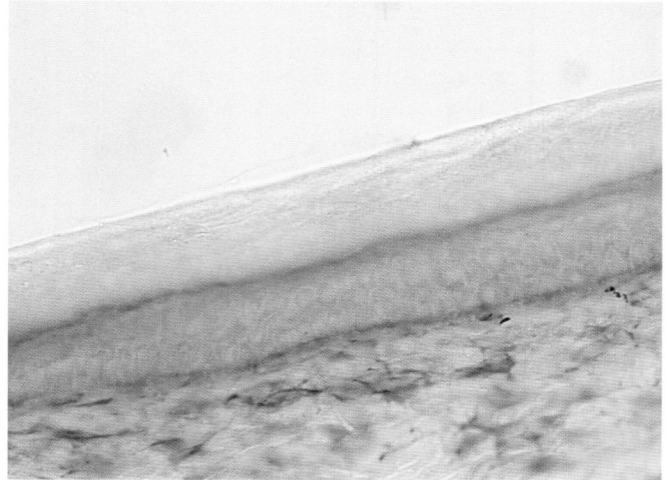

Figure 8.3.6 Skin biopsy showing no nerve fibers in the epidermis of a patient with severe antiretroviral toxic neuropathy (50μm section stained with PGP x 400) (Courtesy Dr. C. Cherry).

dependent manner (Keswani, Polley et al., 2003). The mechanism for this observation involves both paracrine and autocrine processes. CXCR4 receptors on Schwann cells can be stimulated by gp120 as well as their ligand stromal cell-derived factor-1 alpha (SDF-1α), resulting in RANTES (regulated-on-activation normal T-cell expressed and secreted) secretion. RANTES exerts a direct toxic effect on sensory neurons by its agonist effect on neuronal CCR5 receptors and indirectly through TNF-α production, which independently leads to neuronal apoptosis in this model. Interestingly, in addition to its action at the DRG, gp120 can cause axonal injury in a Schwann cell-independent manner through its ligand action at axonal CCR5 and CXCR4 receptors (Melli et al., 2006). There is no evidence to indicate axonal transport of gp120 in the peripheral nervous system, reinforcing the likelihood of local production of this toxin at the site of neural damage (Ahmed et al., 2009). Unfortunately, peptide T, an in vitro inhibitor of gp120 binding, was not clinically efficacious in the treatment of DSPN (Simpson et al., 1996).

Others have identified CCR5- and CXCR4-independent mechanisms through which supernatants of cultured HIV-infected macrophages (either CCR5 or CXCR4-tropic strains) cause cell body and axonal injury independently (Hahn et al., 2008). Whilst the mediator(s) of these observations in the model remain to be elucidated at the level of the cell body, mechanistically there is evidence for production of reactive oxygen species and mitochondrial dysfunction. However, the mechanism in the model accounting for axonal injury appears to differ and, in contrast to the cell body damage, it is not ameliorated by antioxidants.

Other macrophage-produced potentially toxic products include NO, neurotoxic amine (Ntox), and HIV tat, nef, and vpr proteins. Whilst in DSPN, increased macrophage NO is found in DRG (Nagano et al., 1996), lower levels of nitrosylated proteins were found in the sciatic nerves of patients with DSPN compared to HIV patients and negative controls without neuropathy (Hahn et al., 2008). However, this counterintuitive finding might relate to timing during the disease process as tissue was obtained postmortem and could represent "burnt out disease." The roles of other factors in sensory neuron damage remains to be established. However, the growing body of evidence supports pathogenetic mechanisms through which independent damage to the axon and cell body occur. Importantly, these findings are in keeping the pathological observations at the DRG as well as the clinical phenotype of a length dependent axonal neuropathy. A recently reported macaque SIV model of DSPN, which appears closely to mimic that in humans, could considerably advance understanding in this area (Mankowski et al., 2010). Importantly, it will allow study of the complete sensory pathway from epidermis to dorsal columns during the development of neuropathy.

ANTIRETROVIRAL TOXIC NEUROPATHY

Another common sensory neuropathy found in HIV patients is that related to the toxicity of certain antiretroviral drugs, in particular the dideoxynucleoside reverse transcriptase inhibitors stavudine (d4T), didanosine (ddI), and dideoxycytidine (ddC), especially when combined with hydroxyurea (Cherry et al., 2003). These have been termed nucleoside neuropathies, or antiretroviral toxic neuropathies (ATN). Initial reports suggested that the protease inhibitors indinavir, saquinavir, nelfinavir, and ritonavir might also cause ATN (Lichtenstein et al., 2005; Pettersen et al., 2006). Furthermore, Pettersen et al. showed in vitro that indinavir was toxic to DRG and more recently in a cross-sectional study others have reported indinavir to be an independent risk factor for ATN (Cherry et al., 2009). Multivariate analysis of a different large cohort of HIV patients indicated that the association between protease inhibitors grouped together and ATN was not independent of other known neuropathy risk factors (Ellis et al., 2008). However, in contrast to the agents identified in the initial reports, secondary analysis by individual protease inhibitor showed a small increased ATN risk for amprenavir and lopinavir. When the criteria for diagnosis of neuropathy were adjusted to increase its specificity, thereby identifying patients with greater severity of symptoms, lopinavir, nelfinavir, and saquinavir were associated with DSPN (odds ratios ranging between 1.25–1.86) after adjustment for concomitant risk factors. Hence, the independent risk of protease inhibitors in ATN appears possible, but small, and has yet fully to be confirmed.

As discussed in the previous chapter, ATN usually develops within weeks of commencement of the drug and is reversible once the drug is ceased. Certain patients appear constitutively susceptible to ATN as there does not appear to be a cumulative effect of prolonged exposure to dideoxynucleosides (Arenas-Pinto et al., 2008). Increased height and age are key risk factors for manifesting ATN (Cherry et al., 2009). Apart from the temporal relationship to the drug and elevated serum lactate concentrations in those with pain (Brew et al., 2003), there is no established way of distinguishing the neuropathy from DSPN. This appears to be true of the neuropathologic findings as well (Brinley et al., 2001). However, it should be remembered that few patients with this disorder have been studied, as in clinical practice the drug is stopped and most of the time the patient improves, obviating the need for further assessment. Similarly, it is extremely rare for a patient to die in the context of ATN, thereby making full autopsy study of the condition uncommon. Be that as it may, there are several skin biopsy studies, which have shown significant decrease in epidermal nerve fiber density (Griffin et al., 2001) (see Figure 8.3.6).

Studies to elucidate the pathogenetic mechanisms of ATN were initially hampered by a lack of animal models. The majority of authors report that animals exposed to prolonged high doses of dideoxynucleoside analogues do not develop a sensory neuropathy, including noninfected primates exposed to up to 600 mg/kg d4T per day for 12 months (Cherry et al., 2003). One group has described a dose-dependent increase in persistent mechanical hypersensitivity and anxiety-like behavior with ddC showing a reduction in C-fiber axon terminals in the rats' hind paws and modest microgliosis in the cord (Wallace, Blackbeard, Segerdahl et al., 2007). However, the addition of perineural gp120 to systemic ddC not only

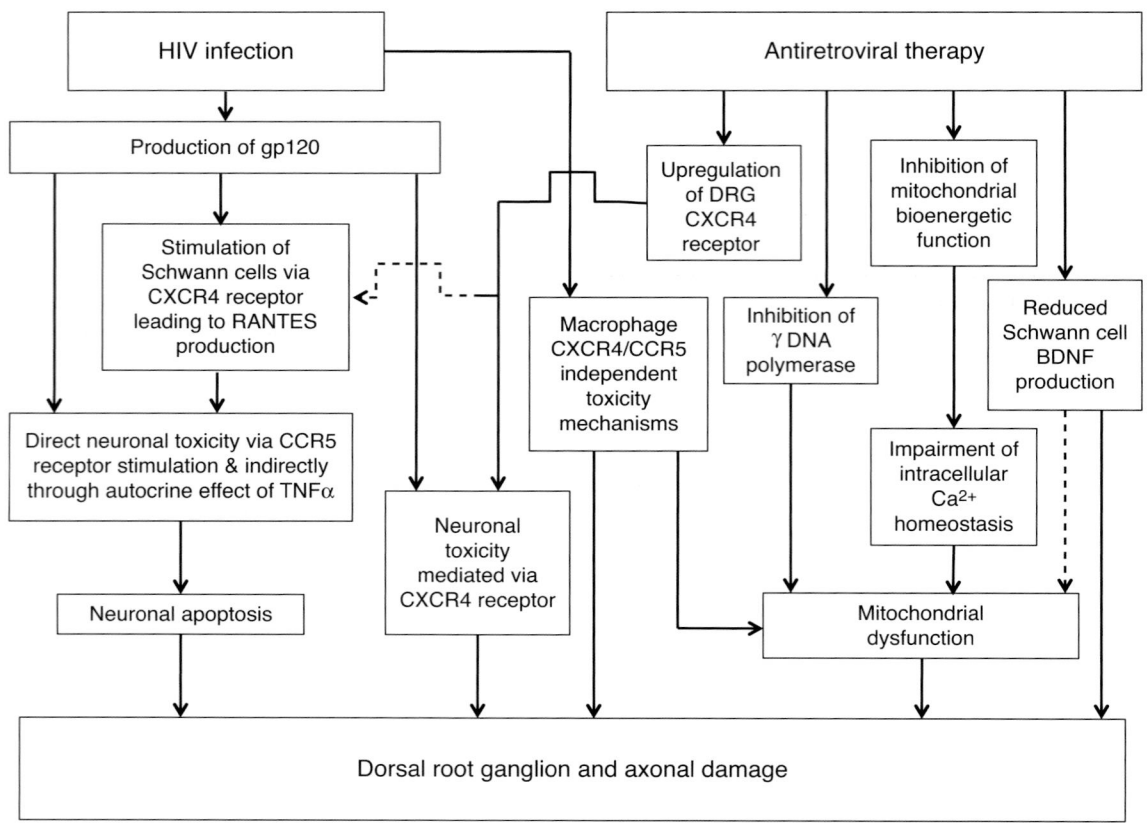

Figure 8.3.7 The cellular mechanisms proposed to underlie the pathobiology of HIV-related distal symmetrical sensory polyneuropathy and antiretroviral toxic neuropathy. The dashed lines indicate hypothetical routes of damage for which validation from further experimental study is required. BDNF, brain-derived neurotrophin factor; RANTES, regulated-on-activation normal T-cell expressed and secreted; TNFα, transforming growth factor alpha.

exacerbated the behavioral changes but also caused DRG histological change more typical of that found in humans. Similarly, another recent in vivo model of ATN required not only drug exposure but also retroviral infection (Zhu et al., 2007). Therefore, for ATN to manifest it appears that a synergy is required between drug and retrovirus; and for disease modeling, use of a susceptible animal is essential. Recent work has identified one possible substrate for this synergy. CXCR4 and its agonist SDF-1α, but not CCR5, were upregulated in DRG neurons and glia of Sprague-Dawley rats exposed to a single dose of ddC (Bhangoo et al., 2007). As explained earlier, the CXCR4 receptor is likely to have a key role in mediating the neurotoxicity of gp120. Interestingly in this model, an antagonist of CXCR4 inhibited ddC-induced pain hypersensitivity.

Mitochondrial dysfunction appears key to ATN pathogenesis with evidence stemming from laboratory studies as well as clinical observations. Dideoxynucleoside analogs were noted to be cytotoxic in vitro and to cause reversible inhibition of mitochondrial reproduction prior to their widespread clinical use. Variability in toxicity between tissues is explained through differences in expression of thymidine kinase isoforms, which are necessary for phosphorylation of nucleoside analogs to their active compounds (Dalakas, 2001). The substrate for their toxicity is thought to be inhibition of

gamma DNA polymerase, a nuclear-encoded mitochondrial enzyme essential for mitochondrial DNA replication (Lewis & Dalakas, 1995). The dideoxynucleoside analogs are more potent inhibitors of this enzyme than other nucleoside reverse transcriptase inhibitors (Cherry et al., 2003). However, an in vitro model of ATN showed impairment of mitochondrial bioenergetic function and necrotic neuronal cell death shortly after drug exposure. This would suggest mechanisms of mitochondrial toxicity other than DNA depletion for which slower rates of impairment would be anticipated (Keswani, Chander et al., 2003). Other ATN models have yet to confirm whether neuronal death is predominantly through necrosis as opposed to apoptosis.

Clinical evidence supporting the role of mitochondrial dysfunction includes the following observations. Firstly, ATN is a length-dependent sensory axonal neuropathy sharing similarities with neuropathies found in primary mitochondrial disorders. Secondly, in some patients with painful neuropathy, an elevation of lactic acid is found (Brew et al., 2003); and thirdly, cases of antiretroviral therapy precipitating manifestation of inherited mitochondrial disorders, such as Leber's hereditary optic neuropathy, are reported. Genetic studies in HIV-infected patients reveal that European mitochondrial haplogroup T and the Leber's hereditary optic neuropathy 4917G polymorphism are associated with increased odds ratios of developing ATN of 5.4 and 5.5, respectively (Hulgan et al., 2005; Canter et al., 2008). Histological studies of peripheral nerves from HIV patients treated with ddC show reduced numbers of mitochondria and reduced cellular mitochondrial DNA levels (Dalakas et al., 2001). Furthermore, in sural nerves from HIV patients with neuropathy there is a greater frequency of mitochondrial deletion mutations compared to controls and an increased deletion mutation frequency distally compared to mitochondria in matched DRG (Lehman et al., 2010). However, evidence of systemically raised levels of oxidative stress has not been found in ATN (Hulgan et al., 2006).

An informative animal model of ATN is that of feline immunodeficiency virus-infected cats treated with ddI (Zhu et al., 2007). It demonstrated that therapeutic amounts of ddI caused DRG neuronal injury with evidence of mitochondrial dysfunction in neurons and reduced brain-derived neurotrophin factor (BDNF) expression by Schwann cells. Not only is BDNF a trophic factor for growth and maturation of neurites as well as its roles in neuronal and synaptic function, it also improves mitochondrial respiratory coupling and has been shown to protect neurons from gp120-induced neuronal degeneration (Nosheny et al., 2005; Zhu et al., 2007). Intriguingly, BDNF receptors (TrkB) are found on mitochondrial membranes, but further characterization of this neurotrophic factor's influence on mitochondria in ATN is required. Others have demonstrated in a rat model that ddC, ddI, and d4T cause dose-dependent mechanical hypersensitivity and allodynia (Joseph et al., 2004). In contrast to models of painful diabetic neuropathy or cancer chemotherapy-induced neuropathy, these findings were not attenuated by inhibition of second messengers in primary afferent nociceptor peripheral terminals. Instead, intracellular calcium modulators reduced the mechanical hypersensitivity induced by ddC. Interestingly, this observation was also seen with the antiparasitic drug suranim, which is known to cause a neuropathy mediated by mitochondrial toxicity. Furthermore, C-fibers in ddC-treated rats showed electrophysiological changes. Sustained suprathreshold stimuli led to a greater proportion of interspike intervals falling between 0.1–0.3 s than in controls (Joseph et al., 2004). The authors hypothesized that the reported electrophysiological abnormalities might arise from a failure of mitochondrial calcium buffering. Recently, in ATN but not DSPN patients, we have observed in vivo electrophysiological disturbances of motor neurons (Ng et al., 2010). These include depolarization of the internodal membrane (fanned-in threshold electrotonus, increased resting IV slope, reduced superexcitability) with sparing of nodal properties (absolute threshold, strength-duration time constant, refractoriness), which could also reflect mitochondrial dysfunction. Whilst the number of patients studied was small and the observations require validation in other cohorts, this neurophysiological technique might offer a diagnostic adjunct to distinguish ATN from "pure" DSPN.

Other studies have indicated roles for non-mitochondrial-related genetic polymorphisms in the pathobiology of ATN. These including iron-loading C282Y heterozygotes being associated with decreased risk of ATN (Kallianpur et al., 2006);

as well as several cytokine polymorphisms either carrying increased risk of ATN or being protective respectively (Cherry et al., 2008).

The spectrum of adverse metabolic side effects associated with antiretrovirals continues to expand. For example tenofovir, a nucleotide reverse transcriptase inhibitor, is increasingly recognized to be nephrotoxic in some patients. Whether such newly recognized metabolic adverse effect might contribute to the layering of insults noted in HIV patients remains conjecture at present. However, given the likelihood that antiretroviral therapy will remain a lifelong necessity for HIV patients, it is possible that further HIV medications will be associated with peripheral nerve toxicity; particularly when combined with the additional effects of aging.

INFLAMMATORY DEMYELINATING NEUROPATHIES

Both acute and chronic inflammatory demyelinating neuropathies occur in HIV disease. As discussed in the previous chapter, they mimic their non-HIV counterparts both clinically and neuropathologically. There is segmental demyelination and remyelination with predominant perivenular infiltrates, but most investigators consider that the lymphocytic and macrophage infiltrates are more prominent and that there is greater axonal loss (Brinley et al., 2001). Indeed, the infiltrates are mostly composed of CD8 lymphocytes in the demyelinating form of the acute disorder while studies of the "axonal" variety of the acute form have been extremely limited and in one case showed minimal inflammation, no demyelination, and the changes of Wallerian degeneration (Griffin et al., 1998).

MONONEURITIS MULTIPLEX

This form of neuropathy occurs uncommonly either at a time when the immune system is relatively preserved or in advanced disease. Neuropathologically, it is characterized by lymphocytic infiltrates with destruction of the vessel wall, often with marked inflammatory infiltrates affecting the endoneurium and capillaries (Said & Lacroix, 2005). At the early phase of HIV disease, it may be related to the deposition of immune complexes directed against either hepatitis B or C. In some, no clear etiology apart from HIV can be found. In advanced HIV disease there is evidence of productive cytomegalovirus (CMV) infection of endothelial cells with typical inclusions, evidence of focal demyelination, and Wallerian degeneration (Libman et al., 1995; Younger et al., 1996).

DIFFUSE INFILTRATIVE LYMPHOCYTOSIS SYNDROME

This is also a rare complication exclusive to HIV disease, affecting patients with moderately depressed CD4 cell counts. As discussed elsewhere, patients present with subacute onset of a painful distal symmetrical sensorimotor neuropathy associated with parotidomegaly and a sicca syndome (Moulignier et al., 1997; Gherardi et al., 1998), although an isolated lumbosacral plexopathy with neuropathy has recently been described (Chahin et al., 2009). Diffuse infiltrative lymphocytosis syndrome results from a CD8 T-cell expansion, which is thought to be a hyperimmune reaction to HIV. Neuropathologically the disorder is strikingly characterized by the presence of CD8 lymphocytic angiocentric infiltrates in the epineurium and endoneurium usually without disruption of the vessel wall (Moulignier et al., 1997). There is frequently no evidence of monoclonality of the infiltrating cells (Gherardi et al., 1998). In contrast to DSPN, there is evidence of significant productive infection by HIV with 10^5 times greater HIV proviral DNA load in homogenized nerve compared to that in other HIV-associated neuropathies (Gherardi et al., 1998).

CYTOMEGALOVIRUS POLYRADICULOPATHY

CMV infection in a small number of patients with advanced HIV disease may lead to a polyradiculopathy, as discussed in the previous chapter (de Gans et al., 1990; Kim & Hollander, 1993). Neuropathologically, there are predominantly polymorphonuclear inflammatory infiltrates in the nerve roots with areas of necrosis and, on occasion, mild myelitis (Miller et al., 1990). Productive CMV infection can be found in inflammatory cells, endothelial, Schwann, and ependymal cells (Miller et al., 1990).

SYPHILITIC POLYRADICULOPATHY

A rare complication is a polyradiculopathy related to syphilis (Lanska et al., 1988; Winston et al., 2005). The neuropathological features have not been described, but it is presumably a consequence of meningovascular syphilis.

HUMAN T-LYMPHOTROPIC VIRUS TYPES 1 AND 2 NEUROPATHY

Occasionally, HIV-infected patients are co-infected with human T-lymphotropic virus type-I (HTLV-I) or 2 (HTLV-2) (Said et al., 1988). Symptomatic HTLV-1 patients usually have a myelopathy, which can be associated with a distal symmetric sensory neuropathy. However, amongst the HTLV-1-infected without myelopathy, multivariate analysis shows HTLV-1 infection per se not to be an independent neuropathy risk factor (Biswas et al., 2009). The neuropathology is that of a mixed axonal and demyelinating neuropathy with perineural and perivascular inflammatory infiltrates very similar to those occurring in the spinal cord. Infection with both HIV and HTLV-1 increases the risk of DSPN (Harrison et al., 1997). Similarly, HIV co-infection with HTLV-2 also increases the risk of DSPN compared to those only infected with HIV; however, this difference is mitigated by treatment with cART (Zehender et al., 1995; Zehender et al., 2002).

STATIN NEUROPATHY

Rarely, drugs of the lipid-lowering class, the statins, may lead to a distal symmetrical sensory neuropathy (Phan et al., 1995). The neuropathologic features have not been well defined but it appears to be an axonal neuropathy. Due to the increasing age of HIV patients and greater prevalence of the lipid-raising side effects of antiretroviral drugs, there is greater statin use in this cohort. How this will interact with DSPN or ATN is yet to be determined. However, two observations are noteworthy. Firstly, some side effects of statins are thought to result from mitochondria-related mechanisms (Beltowski et al., 2009). Secondly, in diabetes mellitus concomitant use of statins may actually reduce the risk of sensory neuropathy (Davis et al., 2008). Thus there is reason to think that a neuropathy dominantly related to statin therapy will become increasingly common in HIV infected patients.

CONCLUSIONS

The pathobiology of HIV-associated neuropathies is complex, resulting from the myriad of mechanisms through which HIV interacts with the immune and nervous systems. An added layering of complexity results from the adverse effects of antiretroviral medications and the metabolic complications of long-term HIV treatment. HIV-associated neuropathies remain the cause of considerable morbidity. Understanding the pathobiology of HIV-associated neuropathies, particularly in the context of the marked increase in longevity and rising age of HIV-infected patients, remains a major goal to achieve improvement in patients' quality-of-life.

REFERENCES

Ahmed, F., MacArthur, L., De Bernardi, M. A., & Mocchetti, I. (2009). Retrograde and anterograde transport of HIV protein gp120 in the nervous system. *Brain Behav Immun*, 23(3), 355–64.

Ances, B. M., Vaida, F., Rosario, D., Marquie-Beck, J., Ellis, R. J., Simpson, D. M., et al. (2009). Role of metabolic syndrome components in HIV-associated sensory neuropathy. *AIDS*, 23(17), 2317–22.

Apostolski, S., McAlarney, T., Quattrini, A., Levison, S. W., Rosoklija, G., Lugaressi, A., et al. (1993). The gp120 glycoprotein of human immunodeficiency virus type 1 binds to sensory ganglion neurons. *Ann Neurol*, 34(6), 855–63.

Araujo, A. P., Nascimento, O. J., & Garcia, O. S. (2000). Distal sensory polyneuropathy in a cohort of HIV-infected children over five years of age. *Pediatrics*, 106(3), E35.

Arenas-Pinto, A., Bhaskaran, K., Dunn, D., & Weller, I. V. (2008). The risk of developing peripheral neuropathy induced by nucleoside reverse transcriptase inhibitors decreases over time: Evidence from the Delta trial. *Antivir Ther*, 13(2), 289–95.

Beltowski, J., Wojcicka, G., & Jamroz-Wisniewska, A. (2009). Adverse effects of statins—mechanisms and consequences. *Curr Drug Saf*, 4(3), 209–28.

Bhangoo, S. K., Ren, D., Miller, R. J., Chan, D. M., Ripsch, M. S., Weiss, C., et al. (2007). CXCR4 chemokine receptor signaling mediates pain hypersensitivity in association with antiretroviral toxic neuropathy. *Brain Behav Immun*, 21(5), 581–91.

Biswas, H. H., Engstrom, J. W., Kaidarova, Z., Garratty, G., Gibble, J. W., Newman, B. H., et al. (2009). Neurologic abnormalities in

HTLV-I- and HTLV-II-infected individuals without overt myelopathy. *Neurology*, 73(10), 781–9.

Brew, B. (2001). Principles of HIV neurology. In *HIV neurology*. New York: Oxford University Press.

Brew, B. J., Tisch, S., & Law, M. (2003). Lactate concentrations distinguish between nucleoside neuropathy and HIV neuropathy. *AIDS*, 17(7), 1094–1096.

Brew, B. J. & Tomlinson, S. E. (2004). HIV neuropathy: Time for new therapies. *Drug Discovery Today: Disease Models*, 1(2), 171–176.

Brinley, F. J., Jr., Pardo, C. A., & Verma, A. (2001). Human immunodeficiency virus and the peripheral nervous system workshop. *Arch Neurol*, 58(10), 1561–6.

Canter, J. A., Haas, D. W., Kallianpur, A. R., Ritchie, M. D., Robbins, G. K., Shafer, R. W., et al. (2008). The mitochondrial pharmacogenomics of haplogroup T: MTND2*LHON4917G and antiretroviral therapy-associated peripheral neuropathy. *Pharmacogenomics*, 8(1), 71–77.

Chahin, N., Temesgen, Z., Kurtin, P. J., Spinner, R. J., & Dyck, P. J. (2009). HIV lumbosacral radiculoplexus neuropathy mimicking lymphoma: Diffuse infiltrative lymphocytosis syndrome (DILS) restricted to nerve? *Muscle Nerve*, 41(2), 276–82.

Cherry, C. L., Affandi, J. S., Imran, D., Yunihastuti, E., Smyth, K., Vanar, S., et al. (2009). Age and height predict neuropathy risk in patients with HIV prescribed stavudine. *Neurology*, 73(4), 315–20.

Cherry, C. L., McArthur, J. C., Hoy, J. F., & Wesselingh, S. L. (2003). Nucleoside analogues and neuropathy in the era of HAART. *J Clin Virol*, 26(2), 195–207.

Cherry, C. L., Rosenow, A., Affandi, J. S., McArthur, J. C., Wesselingh, S. L., & Price, P. (2008). Cytokine genotype suggests a role for inflammation in nucleoside analog-associated sensory neuropathy (NRTI-SN) and predicts an individual's NRTI-SN risk. *AIDS Res Hum Retroviruses*, 24(2), 117–23.

Dalakas, M. C. (2001). Peripheral neuropathy and antiretroviral drugs. *J Peripher Nerv Syst*, 6(1), 14–20.

Dalakas, M. C. & Pezeshkpour, G. H. (1988). Neuromuscular diseases associated with human immunodeficiency virus infection. *Ann Neurol*, 23 Suppl, S38–S48.

Dalakas, M. C., Semino-Mora, C., & Leon-Monzon, M. (2001). Mitochondrial alterations with mitochondrial DNA depletion in the nerves of AIDS patients with peripheral neuropathy induced by 2'3'-dideoxycytidine (ddC). *Lab Invest*, 81(11), 1537–44.

Davis, T. M., Yeap, B. B., Davis, W. A., & Bruce, D. G. (2008). Lipid-lowering therapy and peripheral sensory neuropathy in type 2 diabetes: The Fremantle Diabetes Study. *Diabetologia*, 51(4), 562–6.

de Gans, J., Portegies, P., Tiessens, G., Troost, D., Danner, S. A., & Lange, J. M. (1990). Therapy for cytomegalovirus polyradiculomyelitis in patients with AIDS: Treatment with ganciclovir. *AIDS*, 4(5), 421–425.

de la Monte, S. M., Gabuzda, D. H., Ho, D. D., Brown, Jr. R. H., Hedley-Whyte, E. T., Schooley, R. T., et al. (1988). Peripheral neuropathy in the acquired immunodeficiency syndrome. *Ann Neurol*, 23(5), 485–92.

Ellis, R. J., Marquie-Beck, J., Delaney, P., Alexander, T., Clifford, D. B., McArthur, J. C., et al. (2008). Human immunodeficiency virus protease inhibitors and risk for peripheral neuropathy. *Ann Neurol*, 64(5), 566–72.

Esiri, M. M., Morris, C. S., & Millard, P. R. (1993). Sensory and sympathetic ganglia in HIV-1 infection: Immunocytochemical demonstration of HIV-1 viral antigens, increased MHC class II antigen expression and mild reactive inflammation. *J Neurol Sci*, 114(2), 178–87.

Esteban, P. M., Thahn, T. G., Bravo, J. F., Roca, L. K., Quispe, N. M., Montano, S. M., et al. (2009). Malnutrition associated with increased risk of peripheral neuropathy in Peruvian children with HIV infection. *J Acquir Immune Defic Syndr*, 52(5), 656–8.

Gherardi, R. K., Chretien, F., Delfau-Larue, M. H., Authier, F. J., Moulignier, A., Roulland-Dussoix, D., et al. (1998). Neuropathy in diffuse infiltrative lymphocytosis syndrome: An HIV neuropathy, not a lymphoma. *Neurology*, 50(4), 1041–1044.

Griffin, J. W., Crawford, T. O., & McArthur, J. C. (1998). Peripheral neuropathies associated with HIV infection. In H. E. Gendelman, H. L. Lipton, L. Epstein & S. Swindells (Eds.). *The neurology of AIDS*. New York: Chapman and Hall.

Griffin, J. W., McArthur, J. C., & Polydefkis, M. (2001). Assessment of cutaneous innervation by skin biopsies. *Curr Opin Neurol*, 14(5), 655–9.

Hahn, K., Robinson, B., Anderson, C., Li, W., Pardo, C. A., Morgello, S., et al. (2008). Differential effects of HIV infected macrophages on dorsal root ganglia neurons and axons. *Exp Neurol*, 210(1), 30–40.

Hahn, K., Triolo, A., Hauer, P., McArthur, J. C., & Polydefkis, M. (2007). Impaired reinnervation in HIV infection following experimental denervation. *Neurology*, 68(16), 1251–6.

Harrison, L. H., Vaz, B., Taveira, D. M., Quinn, T. C., Gibbs, C. J., de Souza, S. H., et al. (1997). Myelopathy among Brazilians coinfected with human T-cell lymphotropic virus type I and HIV. *Neurology*, 48(1), 13–18.

Herrmann, D. N., Boger, J. N., Jansen, C., & Alessi-Fox, C. (2007). In vivo confocal microscopy of Meissner corpuscles as a measure of sensory neuropathy. *Neurology*, 69(23), 2121–7.

Herrmann, D. N., McDermott, M. P., Sowden, J. E., Henderson, D., Messing, S., Cruttenden, K., et al. (2006). Is skin biopsy a predictor of transition to symptomatic HIV neuropathy? A longitudinal study. *Neurology*, 66(6), 857–861.

Herzberg, U. & Sagen, J. (2001). Peripheral nerve exposure to HIV viral envelope protein gp120 induces neuropathic pain and spinal gliosis. *J Neuroimmunol*, 116(1), 29–39.

Hughes, R. A., Umapathi, T., Gray, I. A., Gregson, N. A., Noori, M., Pannala, A. S., et al. (2004). A controlled investigation of the cause of chronic idiopathic axonal polyneuropathy. *Brain*, 127(Pt 8), 1723–30.

Hulgan, T., Haas, D. W., Haines, J. L., Ritchie, M. D., Robbins, G. K., Shafer, R. W., et al. (2005). Mitochondrial haplogroups and peripheral neuropathy during antiretroviral therapy: An adult AIDS clinical trials group study. *AIDS*, 19(13), 1341–9.

Hulgan, T., Hughes, M., Sun, X., Smeaton, L. M., Terry, E., Robbins, G. K., et al. (2006). Oxidant stress and peripheral neuropathy during antiretroviral therapy: An AIDS clinical trials group study. *J Acquir Immune Defic Syndr*, 42(4), 450–4.

Jones, G., Zhu, Y., Silva, C., Tsutsui, S., Pardo, C. A., Keppler, O. T., et al. (2005). Peripheral nerve-derived HIV-1 is predominantly CCR5-dependent and causes neuronal degeneration and neuroinflammation. *Virology*, 334(2), 178–193.

Joseph, E. K., Chen, X., Khasar, S. G., & Levine, J. D. (2004). Novel mechanism of enhanced nociception in a model of AIDS therapy-induced painful peripheral neuropathy in the rat. *Pain*, 107 (1–2), 147–58.

Kallianpur, A. R., Hulgan, T., Canter, J. A., Ritchie, M. D., Haines, J. L., Robbins, G. K., et al. (2006). Hemochromatosis (HFE) gene mutations and peripheral neuropathy during antiretroviral therapy. *AIDS*, 20(11), 1503–13.

Keswani, S. C., Chander, B., Hasan, C., Griffin, J. W., McArthur, J. C., & Hoke, A. (2003). FK506 is neuroprotective in a model of antiretroviral toxic neuropathy. *Ann Neurol*, 53(1), 57–64.

Keswani, S. C., Polley, M., Pardo, C. A., Griffin, J. W., McArthur, J. C., & Hoke, A. (2003). Schwann cell chemokine receptors mediate HIV-1 gp120 toxicity to sensory neurons. *Ann Neurol*, 54(3), 287–296.

Kim, Y. S. & Hollander, H. (1993). Polyradiculopathy due to cytomegalovirus: Report of two cases in which improvement occurred after prolonged therapy and review of the literature. *Clin Infect Dis*, 17(1), 32–37.

Lanska, M. J., Lanska, D. J., & Schmidley, J. W. (1988). Syphilitic polyradiculopathy in an HIV-positive man. *Neurology*, 38(8), 1297–301.

Lehman, H., Mankowski, J. L., & Hoke, A. (2010). Mitochondrial dysfunction in HIV and SIV-associated sensory neuropathy. In *17th Conference on Retroviruses and Opportunistic Infections*. San Francisco.

Lewis, W. & Dalakas, M. C. (1995). Mitochondrial toxicity of antiviral drugs. *Nat Med*, 1(5), 417–22.

Libman, B. S., Quismorio, Jr., F. P., & Stimmler, M. M. (1995). Polyarteritis nodosa-like vasculitis in human immunodeficiency virus infection. *J Rheumatol*, 22(2), 351–5.

Lichtenstein, K. A., Armon, C., Baron, A., Moorman, A. C., Wood, K. C., et al. (2005). Modification of the incidence of drug-associated symmetrical peripheral neuropathy by host and disease factors in the HIV outpatient study cohort. *Clin Infect Dis*, 40(1), 148–157.

Mankowski, J. L., Laast, V., Dorsey, J., Pardo, C., Hauer, P., Adams, R. D., et al. (2010). A SIV macaque model of HIV-induced peripheral neuropathy. In *17th Conference on Retroviruses and Opportunistic Infections*. San Francisco.

McCarthy, B. G., Hsieh, S. T., Stocks, A., Hauer, P., Macko, C., Cornblath, D. R., et al. (1995). Cutaneous innervation in sensory neuropathies: Evaluation by skin biopsy. *Neurology*, 45(10), 1848–55.

Melli, G., Keswani, S. C., Fischer, A., Chen, W., Hoke, A. (2006). Spatially distinct and functionally independent mechanisms of axonal degeneration in a model of HIV-associated sensory neuropathy. *Brain*, 129 (Pt 5), 1330–8.

Miller, R. G., Storey, J. R., Greco, C. M. (1990). Ganciclovir in the treatment of progressive AIDS-related polyradiculopathy. *Neurology*, 40(4), 569–74.

Moulignier, A., Authier, F. J., Baudrimont, M., Pialoux, G., Belec, L., Polivka, M., et al. (1997). Peripheral neuropathy in human immunodeficiency virus-infected patients with the diffuse infiltrative lymphocytosis syndrome. *Ann Neurol*, 41 (4), 438–445.

Nagano, I., Shapshak, P., Yoshioka, M., Xin, K. Q., Nakamura, S., & Bradley, W. G. (1996). Parvalbumin and calbindin D-28 k immunoreactivity in dorsal root ganglia in acquired immunodeficiency syndrome. *Neuropathol Appl Neurobiol*, 22(4), 293–301.

Ng, K., Kishore, K., Brew, B. J., & Burke, D. (2010). Axonal excitability in viral distal sensory polyneuropathy and nucleoside neuropathy in HIV patients. *J Neurol Neurosurg Psychiatry*, Accepted for publication.

Nosheny, R. L., Mocchetti, I., Bachis, A. (2005). Brain-derived neurotrophic factor as a prototype neuroprotective factor against HIV-1-associated neuronal degeneration. *Neurotox Res*, 8(1–2), 187–98.

Oh, S. B., Tran, P. B., Gillard, S. E., Hurley, R. W., Hammond, D. L., & Miller, R. J. (2001). Chemokines and glycoprotein120 produce pain hypersensitivity by directly exciting primary nociceptive neurons. *J Neurosci*, 21(14), 5027–35.

Pettersen, J. A., Jones, G., Worthington, C., Krentz, H. B., Keppler, O. T., Hoke, A., et al. (2006). Sensory neuropathy in human immunodeficiency virus/acquired immunodeficiency syndrome patients: Protease inhibitor-mediated neurotoxicity. *Ann Neurol*, 59(5), 816–824.

Phan, T., McLeod, J. G., Pollard, J. D., Peiris, O., Rohan, A., & Halpern, J. P. (1995). Peripheral neuropathy associated with simvastatin. *J Neurol Neurosurg Psychiatry*, 58(5), 625–8.

Rance, N. E., McArthur, J. C., Cornblath, D. R., Landstrom, D. L., Griffin, J. W., & Price, D. L. (1988). Gracile tract degeneration in patients with sensory neuropathy and AIDS. *Neurology*, 38(2), 265–71.

Rizzuto, N., Cavallaro, T., Monaco, S., Morbin, M., Bonetti, B., Ferrari, S., et al. (1995). Role of HIV in the pathogenesis of distal symmetrical peripheral neuropathy. *Acta Neuropathol*, 90(3), 244–50.

Robinson-Papp, J. & Simpson, D. M. (2009). Neuromuscular diseases associated with HIV-1 infection. *Muscle Nerve*, 40(6), 1043–53.

Said, G., Goulon-Goeau, C., Lacroix, C., Feve, A., Descamps, H., & Fouchard, M. (1988). Inflammatory lesions of peripheral nerve in a patient with human T-lymphotropic virus type I-associated myelopathy. *Ann Neurol*, 24(2), 275–7.

Said, G. & Lacroix, C. (2005). Primary and secondary vasculitic neuropathy. *J Neurol*, 252(6), 633–41.

Scaravilli, F., Sinclair, E., Arango, J. C., Manji, H., Lucas, S., & Harrison, M. J. (1992). The pathology of the posterior root ganglia in AIDS and

its relationship to the pallor of the gracile tract. *Acta Neuropathol*, 84(2), 163–70.

Schifitto, G., McDermott, M. P., McArthur, J. C., Marder, K., Sacktor, N., McClernon, D. R., et al. (2005). Markers of immune activation and viral load in HIV-associated sensory neuropathy. *Neurology*, 64(5), 842–848.

Shapshak, P., Nagano, I., Xin, K., Bradley, W., McCoy, C. B., Sun, N. C., et al et al. (1995). HIV-1 heterogeneity and cytokines. Neuropathogenesis. *Adv Exp Med Biol*, 373, 225–38.

Sheth, S. G., Rao, C. V., Tselis, A., & Lewis, R. A. (2007). HIV-related peripheral neuropathy and glucose dysmetabolism: Study of a public dataset. *Neuroepidemiology*, 29(1–2), 121–124.

Simpson, D. M., Dorfman, D., Olney, R. K., McKinley, G., Dobkin, J., So, Y., et al. (1996). Peptide T in the treatment of painful distal neuropathy associated with AIDS: Results of a placebo-controlled trial. The Peptide T Neuropathy Study Group. *Neurology*, 47(5), 1254–9.

Smyth, K., Affandi, J. S., McArthur, J. C., Bowtell-Harris, C., Mijch, A. M., Watson, K., et al. (2007). Prevalence of and risk factors for HIV-associated neuropathy in Melbourne, Australia 1993–2006. *HIV Med*, 8(6), 367–73.

Tyor, W. R., Glass, J. D., Baumrind, N., McArthur, J. C., Griffin, J. W., Becker, P. S., et al. (1993). Cytokine expression of macrophages in HIV-1-associated vacuolar myelopathy. *Neurology*, 43(5), 1002–9.

van den Berg, L. H., Sadiq, S. A., Lederman, S., & Latov, N. (1992). The gp120 glycoprotein of HIV-1 binds to sulfatide and to the myelin associated glycoprotein. *J Neurosci Res*, 33(4), 513–8.

Wallace, V. C., Blackbeard, J., Pheby, T., Segerdahl, A. R., Davies, M., Hasnie, F., et al. (2007). Pharmacological, behavioural and mechanistic analysis of HIV-1 gp120-induced painful neuropathy. *Pain*, 133(1–3), 47–63.

Wallace, V. C., Blackbeard, J., Segerdahl, A. R., Hasnie, F., Pheby, T., McMahon, S. B., et al. (2007). Characterization of rodent models of HIV-gp120 and antiretroviral-associated neuropathic pain. *Brain*, 130(Pt 10), 2688–2702.

Wiggin, T. D., Sullivan, K. A., Pop-Busui, R., Amato, A., Sima, A. A., & Feldman, E. L. (2009). Elevated triglycerides correlate with progression of diabetic neuropathy. *Diabetes*, 58(7), 1634–40.

Winston, A., Marriott, D., & Brew, B. (2005). Early syphilis presenting as a painful polyradiculopathy in an HIV-positive individual. *Sex Transm Infect*, 81(2), 133–4.

Yoshioka, M., Shapshak, P., Srivastava, A. K., Stewart, R. V., Nelson, S. J., Bradley, W. G., . (1994). Expression of HIV-1 and interleukin-6 in lumbosacral dorsal root ganglia of patients with AIDS. *Neurology*, 44(6), 1120–30.

Younger, D. S., Rosoklija, G., Neinstedt, L. J., Latov, N., Jaffe, I. A., & Hays, A. P. (1996). HIV-1 associated sensory neuropathy: A patient with peripheral nerve vasculitis. *Muscle Nerve*, 19(10), 1364–6.

Zehender, G., Colasante, C., Santambrogio, S., De Maddalena, C., Massetto, B., Cavalli, B., et al. (2002). Increased risk of developing peripheral neuropathy in patients coinfected with HIV-1 and HTLV-2. *J Acquir Immune Defic Syndr*, 31(4), 440–7.

Zehender, G., De Maddalena, C., Osio, M., Cavalli, B., Parravicini, C., Moroni, M., et al. (1995). High prevalence of human T cell lymphotropic virus type II infection in patients affected by human immunodeficiency virus type 1-associated predominantly sensory polyneuropathy. *J Infect Dis*, 172(6), 1595–8.

Zhu, Y., Antony, J. M., Martinez, J. A., Glerum, D. M., Brussee, V., Hoke, A., et al. (2007). Didanosine causes sensory neuropathy in an HIV/AIDS animal model: Impaired mitochondrial and neurotrophic factor gene expression. *Brain*, 130(Pt 8), 2011–23.

8.4

CNS COMORBIDITIES

Georgette D. Kanmogne and David B. Clifford

This chapter gives a structured overview of the major HIV-related opportunistic and non-opportunistic infections of the CNS, including discussion of their interactions with immune reconstitution inflammatory syndrome (IRIS), stressing their pathogenesis, how they are affected by combination antiretroviral therapy, and the influence of geographic setting on prevalence, morbidity, and mortality. Part I discusses opportunistic infections (OIs). Considered are cytomegalovirus, cryptococcus, toxoplasmosis, and progressive multifocal leukoencephalopathy. Part II discusses IRIS and its interactions with specific OIs. Part III considers non-opportunistic infectious CNS complications, especially primary CNS lymphoma (closely associated with Epstein-Barr virus) and HIV encephalopathy.

INTRODUCTION

The human immunodeficiency virus (HIV) enters the brain in the early stages of infection and this infection of the central nervous system (CNS) commonly results in behavioral, motor, and cognitive impairments that range from mild to severe (Ghafouri et al., 2006; Grant, 2005; McArthur, 2004). Despite advances with antiretroviral therapy, the brain continues to be a common site of HIV-related infectious and noninfectious complications; in fact, neurological dysfunction has been reported as a clinical manifestation of AIDS in 39–70% of patients (Bacellar et al., 1994; Levy et al., 1985; Snider et al., 1983) and 76–83% of brain autopsies continue to show observable neuropathological abnormalities (Jellinger et al., 2000; Masliah et al., 2000; Vago et al., 2002). This chapter will provide an overview on the current/major HIV-related opportunistic and non-opportunistic infections of the CNS, their pathogenesis, effects of combination antiretroviral therapy (cART) on these complications, and the influence of geographic settings on their prevalence, morbidity, and mortality.

OPPORTUNISTIC INFECTIONS OF THE CENTRAL NERVOUS SYSTEM

It is estimated that up to 80% of patients with AIDS die from infections other than HIV (Chimelli et al., 1992; Kasper & Buzoni-Gatel, 1998; Moreno et al., 2010; Zelman & Mossakowski, 1998). These infections are caused by organisms that do not normally afflict healthy individuals and usually occur late in the course of disease, in patients with low CD4 T-cell count (below 200 cells/μl) (Kasper & Buzoni-Gatel, 1998; Moreno et al., 2010; Roullet, 1999). Cytomegalovirus encephalitis, cryptococcal meningitis (CM), cerebral toxoplasmosis, and progressive multifocal leukoencephalopathy (PML) are the most common opportunistic infections (OI) of the CNS in HIV-infected patients.

CYTOMEGALOVIRUS (CMV) INFECTION

Human cytomegalovirus (HCMV), or beta-herpes virus 5, is a herpes virus that is prevalent throughout the world (for a recent review, see Cannon et al., 2010). Following initial infection, HCMV resides in T cells and can remain latent and asymptomatic in the infected host throughout life. However, infection can reactivate in individuals with weakened immune system such as HIV/AIDS patients, causing life-threatening illness that contributes to increased morbidity and mortality. In fact, HCMV infection is one of the most important OI in the late stages of AIDS and can affect multiple organs, including the CNS (Anders & Goebel, 1999; Roullet, 1999). CMV infection constitutes an AIDS case definition and CMV-induced encephalitis is found in about 25% of CNS lesions in AIDS patients (Gray et al., 1988; Petito et al., 1986; Snider et al., 1983).

Pathology and Pathogenesis

Common CMV infection sites include the retina, gastrointestinal tract, liver, lung, and nervous system (Drew, 1992; McCutchan, 1995). Following immune suppression, reactivation and dissemination of HCMV leads to infection of the brain, meninges, nerve roots, and spinal cord (Drew, 1992; McCutchan, 1995; Roullet, 1999). In fact, HCMV has been detected in multiple CNS cell types, including endothelial cells, glia, neurons, and monocytes-macrophages (Morgello et al., 1987; Wiley et al., 1986); and dual infection of cells with HIV-1 and CMV has been documented in the brain and retina of HIV-infected humans (Belec et al., 1990; Nelson et al., 1988; Skolnik et al., 1989). In the CNS, HCMV cause necrotic and inflammatory lesions in the roots of the cauda equina, conus terminalis, and lumbar segments of the spinal cord (Drew, 1992; McCutchan, 1995; Roullet, 1999). About 30% of patients show focal signs indicative of brainstem or cerebellar involvement (Roullet, 1999), and brain tissues from patients with CMV encephalitis showed extensive necrosis, a high number of activated microglia, hemorrhage, and diffuse inflammatory infiltrates consisting predominantly of macrophages (Morgello et al., 1987; Wiley et al., 1986). The ability of HCMV to infect and replicate in these brain cells was also confirmed by *in vitro* studies. Primary brain endothelial cells and cell lines of astrocytoma, glioblastoma, and neuroblastoma origin have been shown to yield measurable titers of progeny CMV virus (Jault et al., 1994; Poland et al., 1990), and studies of human brain cell aggregates showed that HCMV preferentially infect monocyte-derived macrophages and microglial cells (Pulliam, 1991). This suggests that in the human host, CMV and HIV-1 co-infect the same cells; the effect of this dual infection on disease pathology is not known but it is likely that it does worsen patients' condition and increase morbidity and mortality.

CMV infection is associated with inflammation, increased levels of serum nitrate and nitric oxide synthase, urokinase plasminogen activator receptor (uPAR), and increased expression of TGF-β (Dighiero et al., 1994; Kossmann et al., 2003; Nebuloni et al., 2009; Torre et al., 1996). TGF-β has been identified in the brain of HIV-infected individuals, as well as brains of HIV-CMV co-infected individuals (Wahl et al., 1991), which suggests an association between TGF-β and HIV- and/or CMV-mediated brain pathology in AIDS patients with CMV encephalitis. Kossmann and colleagues showed increased expression of TGF-β in brain tissues of HIV+ individuals with CMV encephalitis, compared to HIV+ individuals without CMV infection and HIV- controls (Kossmann et al., 2003). These studies also showed co-localization of CMV and TGF-β in human and murine astrocytes, and showed that CMV infection of astrocytes induced the production of TGF-β, which in turn enhanced productive CMV expression. Increased CMV titers correlated with increased TGF-β mRNA and proteins and the levels of CMV released by astrocytes decreased significantly in the presence of TGF-β antibodies, and increased in the presence of exogenous TGF-β (Kossmann et al., 2003). Studies by Lokensgard and colleagues (Lokensgard et al., 1999) also showed that CMV replicates in primary human astrocytes and induced cytopathic effects.

cART, Morbidity, and Mortality

Before the cART era, CMV was a major cause of morbidity and mortality in Western countries and up to 50% of HIV-infected individuals developed CMV end-organ diseases, including CMV diseases of the central and peripheral nervous system (Chimelli et al., 1992; Gray et al., 1991; Matthiessen et al., 1992). However, occurrence of CMV disease in developed countries has declined dramatically with cART, with most cases observed only in late AIDS cases (Torre et al., 2005). In the cART era, a progressive reduction in the incidence of cerebral toxoplasmosis was observed in developed countries (Anders & Goebel, 1999; Maschke et al., 2000; Neuenburg et al., 2002; Torre et al., 2005) and cART-induced immune reconstitution is often associated with significant decrease in blood CMV titers (O'Sullivan et al., 1999).

However, CMV encephalitis and other CNS OI still occur in patients with advanced immunosuppression, especially in those who failed cART, and their incidence and prevalence is much higher in developing countries where access to cART is limited.

CRYPTOCOCCOSIS

Cryptococcosis is a fungal disease caused by fungus of the genus *Cryptococcus*. *Cryptococcus* is endemic in many parts of the world and *Cryptococcus gattii* causes infections in immunocompetent individuals, while *Cryptococcus* (C) *neoformans*, the most prominent and medically important species, infects immunocompromised individuals such as HIV/AIDS patients (Chayakulkeeree & Perfect, 2006; Morgan et al., 2006). This fungus generally enters the human body through inhalation into the lung and can remain dormant and asymptomatic for long periods. However, following immune suppression, infection can reactivate and spread to several organs including the brain and spinal cord, where it causes meningitis. Thus, it is believed that in HIV-seropositive patients, most episodes of cryptococcal meningitis represent reactivation of latent infection, which may have been acquired many years earlier. Cryptococcosis is the first opportunistic infection that occurs in over a quarter of patients who develop AIDS (Kovacs et al., 1985), and CM is one of the most important HIV-related OI. In countries with a high HIV/AIDS prevalence, *Cryptococcus* is one of the most common cause of meningitis (Bekondi et al., 2006; Bogaerts et al., 1999; Heyderman et al., 1998; Hovette et al., 1999; Schutte et al., 2000) and is considered as a leading causes of opportunistic neuro-infection and infectious morbidity and mortality in AIDS patients (for reviews, see Jarvis & Harrison, 2007; Satishchandra et al., 2007).

Pathology and Pathogenesis

Cryptococcus generally enters the human body through inhalation and depending on the host immune system, the clinical manifestations can range from asymptomatic colonization of the respiratory tract to widespread dissemination, including into the CNS. HIV-associated CM usually presents as a chronic or subacute meningo-encephalitis in profoundly immunosuppressed patients (CD4 cell counts <200 cells/μl), with severe acute or subacute headache and fever; in later stages of the disease patients may experience visual disturbance and altered mental status (Jarvis & Harrison, 2007; Satishchandra et al., 2007; Subramanian & Mathai, 2005). It is believed that cryptococcal-induced visual impairment either results from direct fungal invasion of the optic nerve or from increased intracranial pressure (Rex et al., 1993). Clinical signs may also include meningism, papilloedema, cranial nerve, and reduced conscious level (Jarvis & Harrison, 2007; Satishchandra et al., 2007; Subramanian & Mathai, 2005). Diagnosis is usually confirmed by positive India ink staining, presence of cryptococcal antigen in the serum or cerebrospinal fluids (CSF), and/or increased CSF opening pressures (Feldmesser et al., 1996; Morgan et al., 2006). CSF analysis usually reveals lymphocytic pleocytosis with increased protein levels (Satishchandra et al., 2007; Subramanian & Mathai, 2005).

It has been suggested that the increased virulence and infectivity of *C. neoformans* is partly due to melanin, phenoloxidase, and proteases (Brueske, 1986; Casadevall et al., 2000; Kwon-Chung & Rhodes, 1986; Satishchandra et al., 2007). In fact, there is evidence that phenoloxidase, an enzyme present in *C. neoformans*, induces melanin production and this melanin acts as a virulence factor by making *Cryptococcus* resistant to leukocyte attack and by decreasing lymphocyte proliferation (Satishchandra et al., 2007). The anti-phagocytic properties of the fungal carbohydrate capsule were also demonstrated in studies showing that noncapsular mutant forms of *Cryptococcus* lack pathogenicity (Kwon-Chung & Rhodes, 1986). It has also been suggested that the affinity of phenoloxidase to L-dopamine play a role in the CNS predisposition to *C. neoformans* infection (Jarvis & Harrison, 2007; Satishchandra et al., 2007; Subramanian & Mathai, 2005). Other studies showed evidence of increased levels of vascular endothelial growth factor (VEGF), a mediator of vascular permeability, in the CSF of patients with cryptococcal diseases but these studies did not show any correlation between VEGF levels and CSF opening pressure (Coenjaerts et al., 2004). Over half of HIV+ patients with CM have CSF pressures > 25 cm H_2O and a third of these patients have pressures >35 cm H_2O (reviewed in Jarvis & Harrison, 2007; Satishchandra et al., 2007; Subramanian & Mathai, 2005). This raised CSF pressure manifests as severe headache, papilloedema, and progressive loss of vision, hearing impairment, and decreased level of consciousness (Denning et al., 1991), and is associated with cognitive impairment and cranial nerve lesions (Satishchandra et al., 2007). The exact mechanism for such severe headache is not known, but there have been suggestions that it may due to meningeal involvement, raised intracranial tension, or thrombosis (Satishchandra et al., 2007). A significant proportion of patients who survive can develop neurological sequelae, including visual loss, decreased mental capacity, hearing loss, permanent cranial nerve palsies, and hydrocephalus (Satishchandra et al., 2007).

cART, Morbidity, and Mortality

A defective production of interferon (IFN)-γ and tumor necrosis factor (TNF)-α has been observed in HIV+ patients with CM and a recent study showed improved treatment when standard antifungal therapy was supplemented with IFN-γ (Pappas et al., 2004). There is also direct *in vivo* evidence that IFN-γ is important for the clearance of cryptococcal infection in HIV-infected patients (Siddiqui et al., 2005). Cryptococcocal diseases have increased significantly in the era of HIV/AIDS epidemic and cryptococcosis is an AIDS-defining opportunistic infection. However, with widespread use of cART and the resulting increase in CD4+ cell counts and immune reconstitution, its incidence has decreased significantly in developed countries (Dromer et al., 2004; Kaplan et al., 2000; Mirza et al., 2003; van Elden et al., 2000); in these settings, CM is now seen mostly in patients with limited access to health care who present with late-stage HIV infection (Kaplan et al., 2000; Mirza et al., 2003). Studies of HIV+ patients with CM in Botswana and South Africa showed that cART at the time of first admission with CM was associated with a lower risk of death during antifungal therapy (Letendre et al., 2008b).

Cryptococcosis remains a major opportunistic infection in resource-limited countries and is the leading cause of meningitis in sub-Saharan Africa (SSA). Park and colleagues recently estimated the global burden of CM and found a high number of cases and associated death, with the highest in SSA (Park et al., 2009). In case series studies of HIV-infected patients, *C. neorfomans* was responsible for 26.5%, 31%, and 45% of cerebral meningitis in Malawi (Gordon et al., 2000), Central African Republic (Bekondi et al., 2006), and Zimbabwe (Hakim et al., 2000), respectively. Studies of cohorts of HIV-infected individuals in these settings also showed that CM was responsible for 13 to 44% of all deaths (Corbett et al., 2002; French et al., 2002; Okongo et al., 1998). Cryptococcosis is also the leading cause of meningitis in Rwanda (Bogaerts et al., 1999) and Zimbabwe (Heyderman et al., 1998), and studies in two different cities in South Africa showed 64% (Moosa & Coovadia, 1997) and 43% (Bergemann & Karstaedt, 1996) in-hospital mortality for HIV+ patients with CM. These studies also showed a high proportion of cases with coma (24%) and advanced systemic illnesses (29%) (McCarthy et al., 2006). Thus, these high in-hospital mortalities may be due to late diagnosis/delay in seeking medical care, or inadequacy of initial medical care. In fact, in many SSA countries, some individuals rely primarily on traditional medicine and only seek hospital care when traditional medicine doesn't work and disease condition has worsened.

In another prospective population- and laboratory-based surveillance of a cART-naïve population in South Africa, 97% of the 2,753 incident cases of cryptococcosis identified had meningitis, in-hospital mortality was 27%, and death risk factors included altered mental status, coma, or wasting syndrome (McCarthy et al., 2006). Cryptococcosis is also a major opportunistic infection in Asia and South America, including India (Kumarasamy et al., 2003; Satishchandra et al., 2007; Subramanian & Mathai, 2005) and Brazil (Pappalardo and Melhem, 2003), and accounts for up to 20% of AIDS-defining illnesses in Thailand (Chariyalertsak et al., 2001). A study of 411 HIV/AIDS patients in India found that meningitis was the most common CNS infection in patients, accounting for 39.4% of cases (Teja et al., 2005).

CM is generally fatal if untreated. Mortality risk factors in patients with HIV-associated CM include: 1) a high organism burden at baseline (high CSF levels of *Cryptococcus* or cryptococcal antigen) (Diamond & Bennett, 1974; Letendre et al., 2008b); 2) an abnormal mental status (Brouwer et al., 2004; Saag et al., 1992); 3) high CSF opening pressures (≥ 250 mm H_2O) (Graybill et al., 2000); 4) a poor inflammatory response in the CSF (Graybill et al., 2000; Saag et al., 1992; van der Horst et al., 1997); and 5) low CSF cell counts and glucose levels (Subramanian & Mathai, 2005). Even with optimal antifungal and cART treatment, the 10-week mortality in developed countries remains at 10–25% (Lortholary et al., 2006). A recent retrospective study of 202 patients with cryptococcosis in the United States, 85% of whom had CNS involvement, showed a 30-day mortality of 14% (Sajadi et al., 2009). Mortality is much higher is developing countries, with a 10-week mortality of 37% in South Africa despite antifungal and cART treatment (Bicanic et al., 2007), and only 19 days median survival in Zambia (Mwaba et al., 2001); which was less or equal to median survival in the absence of antifungal therapy (Heyderman et al., 1998; Maher & Mwandumba, 1994; Mwaba et al., 2001).

TOXOPLASMOSIS

Toxoplasmosis is an infectious disease caused by *Toxoplasma* (T.) *gondii*, a parasitic protozoa of the genus toxoplasma. *T. gondii* is a food- and water-borne pathogen that infects animals and humans, it is a frequent cause of opportunistic infection in AIDS patients where it affects mostly the CNS, but may also affect the eyes, lungs, heart, and gastrointestinal tract (Holliman, 1988; New & Holliman, 1994; Pavesio & Lightman, 1996). CNS toxoplasmosis is the most common cause of intracerebral lesions in AIDS patients and symptoms include headache, fever, seizure, hemiplegia, and hemiparesis; symptoms can range from lethargy to coma, and loss of memory to dementia (Cohen, 1999; Del Valle & Pina-Oviedo, 2006; Kumar et al., 2010; Smith et al., 2008).

Pathology and Pathogenesis

Animals and humans are infected by ingesting contaminated food and vertical in-utero transmission also occurs (for recent reviews, see Dubey, 2008; Hide et al., 2009; Smith, 2009)). *T. gondii* infection is mostly asymptomatic and latent in immunocompetent individuals. Initial infection is characterized by nonspecific symptoms and subsequent formation of cysts that often remain in latent form in many organs (Dunlop et al., 1996). There is evidence that once *T. gondii* enters the tissues, it rapidly induces a potent IFN-γ-dependent cell-mediated immunity that controls its replication and facilitates the formation of dormant cysts, which ensure its survival (Dunlop et al., 1996). It has also been shown that this cell-mediated immunity is associated with increased expression of interleukin (IL)-12, TNF-α, and IL-1β in macrophages and T cells, which promote HIV replication (Filisetti & Candolfi, 2004; Sarciron & Gherardi, 2000).

In individuals with weakened immune system, such as HIV/AIDS patients, reactivation of toxoplasma cysts and reactivation of latent infection and dissemination of toxoplasmosis occurs, causing life-threatening disease, especially CNS disease involving encephalitis (Dubey, 2008; Hill & Dubey, 2002; Pereira-Chioccola et al., 2009). In fact, it is estimated that over 95% of toxoplasmic encephalitis cases are due to reactivation of latent infection following progressive immune suppression, and this often occur in individuals with CD4 T-lymphocyte counts below 100 cells/μl (Dannemann et al., 1992; Renold et al., 1992). Toxoplasmosis is one of the most common opportunistic infection in AIDS patients and it is estimated that 30 to 50% of HIV+ patients latently infected with *T. gondii* subsequently develop toxoplasmic

encephalitis (Luft & Remington, 1992; New & Holliman, 1994). Ocular infections by *T. gondii* cause lesions in the optic nerves, which can result in impaired vision and spread of the parasite to other CNS cells (Pavesio & Lightman, 1996). Once in the CNS, the parasite undergoes a rapid multiplication and destroys neuronal and glial cells (Carruthers & Suzuki, 2007; Kasper & Buzoni-Gatel, 1998; Wilson & Hunter, 2004).

There is evidence that in *T. gondii* infection, cytokines such as IL-4, IL-6, IL-7, and IL-15 are involved in the host immune response and dendritic cells and granulocytes are important modulators for establishing long-term CD8+ T-cell immunity to *T. gondii* (Beaman et al., 1994; Kasper et al., 1995; Khan & Kasper, 1996; Suzuki et al., 1996). Because *T. gondii* can infect a wide range of tissues and cells, it has been suggested that attachment of the parasite to host cell is a receptor-mediated interaction involving either a highly conserved cellular receptor or different receptors recognized by *T. gondii* (Grimwood et al., 1996; Kasper & Buzoni-Gatel, 1998). This hypothesis of a receptor-mediated interaction is supported by studies showing that attachment of *T. gondii* to the hosts' cells can be inhibited by antibodies to *T. gondii* surface antigen (Mineo & Kasper, 1994); extracellular matrix protein laminin enhance the attachment of *T. gondii* to macrophages and laminin-derived peptides inhibited parasite binding (Furtado et al., 1992).

cART, Morbidity, and Mortality

Toxoplasmic encephalitis is fatal in the absence of treatment. With widespread use of cART and improved immune status, the incidence of toxoplasmosis and other HIV-induced OI have significantly decreased in developed countries; however, these OI are still occurring in large numbers of individuals in developing countries, especially in SSA countries where access to cART is limited and HIV infection is often diagnosed in the late stages when patients have progressed to AIDS. Even when cART is available, these OI may still occur in cases of cART failure, decreased immune function and reactivation of latent toxoplasma cysts in tissues. Recent studies showed that despite cART, toxoplasmic encephalitis was the most common opportunistic infection in HIV-infected individuals in Cuba (Alfonso et al., 2009). Toxoplasmic encephalitis still represents the most common cerebral mass lesion in HIV-infected individuals, and in the US, it affects 18–25% of AIDS patients during the course of their disease (reviewed in Kasper & Buzoni-Gatel, 1998), with 16% mortality (Skolasky et al., 1999). Pre-cART studies showed a very high incidence and prevalence of cerebral toxoplasmosis in many countries, including 21 to 34% in Brazil (Chimelli et al., 1992; Wainstein et al., 1992), and 37% in France (Matthiessen et al., 1992); and post-cART studies showed a prevalence of 16.3% in Poland (Zelman & Mossakowski, 1998). Mortality due to HIV-induced toxoplasmic encephalitis remains high in resource-limited countries, including 25.5% mortality in Brazil despite increased cART use (Passos et al., 2000). Mortality is likely much higher in other resource-limited countries where diagnostic facilities are scarce, availability of treatment is limited and patients are often diagnosed at very late stages of infection (Paul et al., 2007).

PROGRESSIVE MULTIFOCAL LEUKOENCEPHALOPATHY

Progressive multifocal leukoencephalopathy (PML) is a disorder caused by a polyomavirus called JC virus (JCV). JCV is ubiquitous throughout the world and studies showed that 39 to 58% of the general population has JCV antibodies (Egli et al., 2009; Gordon & Khalili, 1998; Kean et al., 2009). Thus, JCV is found in many individuals and infection is usually asymptomatic. However, viral reactivation can occur following immunosuppression or use of immunosuppressive drugs (Gheuens et al., 2010; Major, 2010; Tan & Koralnik, 2010). Reactivated virus enters the brain and causes lytic infection of CNS cells, especially oligodendrocytes, astrocytes, and neurons (Cinque et al., 2009; Koralnik, 2006; Sweet et al., 2002; Tan & Koralnik, 2010). This cytolytic destruction of CNS myelin-producing cells results in widespread damage of myelin sheets in the nerves brain white matter, with sometime additional damages in the gray matter (Drake et al., 2007; Sweeney et al., 1994; Tan & Koralnik, 2010). Symptoms and clinical signs include severe headaches, seizures, neck stiffness, and behavioral, motor, cognitive, and visual impairments, which often lead to life-threatening disability and death within weeks to few months (Cinque et al., 2009; Drake et al., 2007; Koralnik, 2006; Tan & Koralnik, 2010).

Unlike other HIV- associated OI, PML incidence and prevalence has not changed with cART, and remain at about 4–5% (Antinori et al., 2001; Drake et al., 2007). Other studies showed that among HIV/AIDS patients with CNS complications, the proportion of those with PML was 25% in the US (Skolasky et al., 1999), 9.3% in Poland (Zelman & Mossakowski, 1998), and 10.7% in Brazil (Chimelli et al., 1992). Study of 50 HIV+ individuals with seizure showed that 6% of seizure cases were due to PML (Dore et al., 1996). Another study of 281 HIV+ individuals in Italy with neurological abnormalities and focal brain lesions showed that PML was the major diagnosis in 18.2% (Ammassari et al., 2000). PML prevalence and incidence have been reported to be very low in Africa and India (Shankar et al., 2003); this is likely due to technical challenges with PML diagnosis, underreporting and/or under-diagnosis. In fact, many clinical settings in these resource-limited areas may not routinely perform biopsy, JCV PCR, or imaging procedures required for accurate PML diagnosis.

A number of factors has been shown to be predictors of improved survival in HIV+ PML patients. These include a higher CD4+ T cells count (above 100 cells/μl) at PML diagnosis (Berger et al., 1998; Drake et al., 2007), use of cART post PML diagnosis (Clifford et al., 1999; Drake et al., 2007; Geschwind et al., 2001; Miralles et al., 1998), a rise in CD4+ T cells count following initiation of cART (Gasnault et al., 1999), the presence of JCV-specific cytotoxic T-lymphocytes (Marzocchetti et al., 2009), a low baseline level of JCV-DNA in the CSF at diagnosis, and clearance of JCV from the CSF following cART treatment (Yiannoutsos et al., 1999).

Treatment, Morbidity, and Mortality

There is currently no effective treatment for PML, and in the pre-cART era mortality for HIV/AIDS individuals with PML was very high, with death often occurring within months following the first clinical manifestation of disease (Berger et al., 1998; Cinque et al., 2009). However, cohort studies showed a significant increase in survival in cART-treated PML patients (Clifford et al., 1999; De Luca et al., 2000; Dworkin et al., 1999; Tassie et al., 1999). Antinori and colleagues showed that survival of patients with HIV-associated PML had increased from 10% in the pre-cART era to 50% in cART era (Antinori et al., 2003). A review of 87 cases of HIV-associated PML in Australia and Hong Kong showed that median survival increased from 14 weeks in the pre-cART to 64 weeks in the cART era (Drake et al., 2007). A retrospective study of 97 patients with HIV-associated PML showed that cART increased median survival by 6 weeks (Geschwind et al., 2001), while a prospective study of 12 cases by Miralles and colleagues (Miralles et al., 1998) showed that cART increased the cumulative probability of survival in HIV+ PML patients, with a median survival of 78 weeks in patients who received cART, compared to 9 weeks in historical cohorts who had not received cART. Another prospective study by Clifford and colleagues (Clifford et al., 1999) also showed significant increase in survival, with 46.4 weeks median survival in HIV+ PML patients on cART, compared to 11 weeks in historical control cohorts. A recent Swiss HIV cohort study showed that cART significantly reduced PML incidence and attributable 1-year mortality (Khanna et al., 2009). However, PML can occur in patients receiving cART (Cinque et al., 2003; Tantisiriwat et al., 1999).

The mechanisms through which cART reduces PML morbidity and mortality are not known. It is possible that HIV directly stimulates JCV gene expression and by reducing HIV load, cART suppresses JCV replication, reducing JCV load and JCV-induced damage to CNS cells and tissues. This possibility of HIV-JCV interaction is supported by studies showing that the HIV-1 tat protein transactivates the JCV late promoter in glial cells (Tada et al., 1990) and cART decreases JCV load in the CSF (Taoufik et al., 1998).

IMMUNE RECONSTITUTION INFLAMMATORY SYNDROME

One of the important clinical developments related to HIV disease and therapy has been the recognition of the phenomenon of immune reconstitution disease (IRD) or immune reconstitution inflammatory syndrome (IRIS) (French, 2009). With the development of cART, initiation of therapy routinely results in marked decline in the HIV viral loads followed by gradual increases in CD4-lymphocyte counts accompanied by the return of effective immune responses. The beneficial aspects of this, including prompt reduction in mortality, clearing of some chronic opportunistic problems, and marked reduction of new opportunistic complications, has been dramatic. However, the period of immune reconstitution has also been marked by sometimes clinically important paradoxical worsening due to inflammatory conditions. In general, the possibility of IRIS should be considered whenever new or worsening inflammatory clinical conditions occur in the setting of declining HIV viral load and increasing CD4 counts (see website of the International Network for the Study of HIV-associated IRIS (INSHI), http://www.inshi.umn.edu/home.html). While strict criteria for IRIS may be required in the research setting, it is likely that the spectrum of such conditions is quite wide, and when looked for will be found to be very common in the treatment initiation period. The duration of risk varies somewhat but is most common in the first 3–6 months following initiation of effective cART. However, later complications may still occur. In general, the risk for IRIS is greater for patients in whom immune deficiency is advanced at the time of initiation or change in therapy (very low CD4 counts), and in whom opportunistic conditions are present (French et al., 2004).

The most common and clear forms of IRIS complicate opportunistic pathogens in the CNS, most often CM or PML. Perhaps the most typical presentation is a patient presenting untreated for HIV with one of these opportunistic diseases. With the initiation of therapy for the OI and initiation of cART, the anticipated improvement in meningitis may be punctuated by increasing evidence of inflammatory complications even while primary cultures show response to the therapy. In the case of PML, the typically noninflammatory lesions of PML in the setting of advanced HIV with lesions that are without mass effect or MR enhancement, may transform to include both of these features as a result of inflammatory response. Simplistically, it is easy to understand this by considering the newly competent immune system identifying and responding to the opportunistic pathogen antigens present in the nervous system. At times, the inflammatory response may be so severe that it becomes life threatening, and requires direct therapy to modulate the inflammation.

One of the major questions in therapeutics in this setting has been whether it is important to treat the opportunistic disease first, before starting HIV therapy. The rationale for this approach would be that control of the OI and reduction of the antigen load might protect the patient from detrimental IRIS reactions. However, since this problem occurs in the face of very advanced HIV, the risks associated with longer duration of immune deficiency due to delay of HIV therapy are also substantial. An important randomized trial comparing early versus delayed initiation of HIV therapy suggested that early initiation of HIV therapy is probably preferred (Zolopa et al., 2009).

Perhaps more interesting, at times the opportunistic diseases appear to present in an inflammatory form only after the initiation of the cART therapy. Simplistically, one can think of this as "unmasking" the opportunistic disease, which may have been present in an early preclinical form, causing no recognizable symptoms until the irritation of an inflammatory response brought it to light. This is actually not a rare phenomenon, making it possible that it is more complicated than a simple unmasking phenomenon, and may additionally reflect the propensity of an activated immune system spreading pathogens to the vulnerable brain. In any case, the clinical appearance of OI presenting during the first months of HIV therapy may differ and reflect a greater inflammatory component than has been traditionally associated with the conditions.

While the simplistic view of IRIS as an appropriate response to an antigenic stimulus may be appropriate in some cases, it is also likely that in other cases the pathophysiological story is more complicated with dysregulation of the immune response as it is recovering, resulting in imbalance between mechanisms of effector and regulatory immune mechanisms, making it possible to have a poorly regulated and deleterious immune response in this setting.

CRYPTOCOCCAL IRIS

IRIS has been recognized in the setting of CM, causing paradoxical increasing symptoms and signs of inflammatory disease in the setting of treatment for the OI (Lortholary et al., 2005). Signs and symptoms include increasing headache, photophobia, vomiting, meningismus, papilledema, and seizures, developing in the face of improving immune status and treatment for CM (Boulware et al., 2010). Careful evaluation of a series of patients presenting with CM demonstrated that the patients presenting with less initial CSF inflammation at the diagnosis of CM were more likely to develop IRIS than those with better immune reaction at baseline. Over time, the critical and sometimes difficult distinction between disease driven by IRIS versus failing CM therapy appeared to be reflected by inflammatory CSF cytokine profiles. Elevations in IFN-γ, TNF-α, granulocyte colony-stimulating factor, vascular-endothelial growth factor, and eotaxin (CCL11) were found with IRIS, distinguish it from failing CM therapy (Boulware et al., 2010). The complications of the inflammatory meningitis may be lethal and active therapy, including CSF drainage and corticosteroid therapy, is sometimes required to address this complication.

PROGRESSIVE MULTIFOCAL LEUKOENCEPHALOPATHY IRIS

The clinical appearance and behavior of PML associated with IRIS is critical to recognize. In this setting, IRIS is probably required for the survival of the patient, and thus historically development of inflammatory responses, often detected by new slight contrast enhancement on MR scans of the brain in lesions of PML, was considered a good prognostic indicator in this notoriously lethal disease. With improved rates of survival typically in the range of 50% in the cART era (Antinori et al., 2001; Clifford et al., 1999; Miralles et al., 1998), it is almost certain that beneficial cART is occurring in at least half of PML patients (De Luca et al., 2008). However, IRIS may also be causing some of the deaths associated with PML in the cART era, since IRIS may transform the normally non-mass-producing and contrast media-unenhanced lesions typical of PML into tumor-like lesions with dangerous mass effect and contrast enhancement (see Figure 8.4.1). In lethal cases, or those in whom brain biopsy was undertaken, it is typical to find marked inflammatory responses, often with predominance of CD8 lymphocytes that may form perivascular cuffing that would be highly atypical of PML (Gray et al., 2005; Vendrely et al., 2005). It is also potentially of importance that the presentation of PML in the setting of variably reconstituting immune system has likely compromised the sensitivity of JC virus detection in the CSF, since over time with immune reconstitution, the already relatively low JC viral loads sometimes found in PML further decline. Recent reports emphasize the decline of viral loads and sensitivity of PCR testing of CSF in the era of cART therapy (Marzocchetti et al., 2005). The decreased viral load typically seen in the setting of PML associated with cART emphasizes the need for highly sensitive and reliable JC PCR assays. Even with the optimal assays, negative CSF may be encountered in this setting, making brain biopsy the only practical way to determine with certainty the etiology of the brain lesion.

Because of the considerable mortality of IRIS in PML, active treatment with corticosteroids has been undertaken. It is certainly true that often the IRIS is mild enough that it can be managed prospectively without direct intervention. It is unfortunate when those unaware of this complication fail to recognize it, attributing progression and clinical deterioration to PML alone, doom their patient to die without intervention. While concerns about the risk of corticosteroid use while attempting to treat an OI are reasonable, a recent review of a retrospective case series supports aggressive corticosteroid use with evidence that earlier and more aggressive steroid use was applied in those that survived this complication (Tan et al., 2009). Many experts recommend high-dose treatment,

typically infusions of 1 gram IV methylprednisolone daily for five days. In some cases, this may need to be repeated after 4–6 weeks, as the IRIS reaction may last several months before gradually resolving.

HIV-ASSOCIATED IRIS

A potentially very important form of IRIS may occur much more rarely in cART-treated patients, and draws attention to the possibility that dysregulated inflammatory responses to HIV during HIV therapy could be an important explanation for acute or perhaps more subtle brain damage. Sometimes in the period following change or initiation of cART, inflammatory CNS disease develops without any evidence of other opportunistic pathogens, with the exception of the HIV virus, which is known to invade the brain early in infection and to remain present in the central nervous system throughout the course. While the dramatic examples of this problem are relatively few and reported along with more typical IRIS from OI (Gray et al., 2005; McCombe et al., 2009; Miller et al., 2004; Venkataramana et al., 2006), and consist of patients developing inflammatory encephalopathy during successful cART therapy, often with marked white matter changes and on biopsy the presence of inflammatory changes with CD8 cellular infiltration. The described cases have tended to be quite a serious clinical problem with substantial mortality. Other reports of inflammatory white matter syndromes continue to be emphasized in patients during cART and may well have pathophysiology related to cART. The earlier report of Langford (Langford et al., 2002) described inflammatory encephalitis in failing cART patients, which

PML IRIS after two months of cART

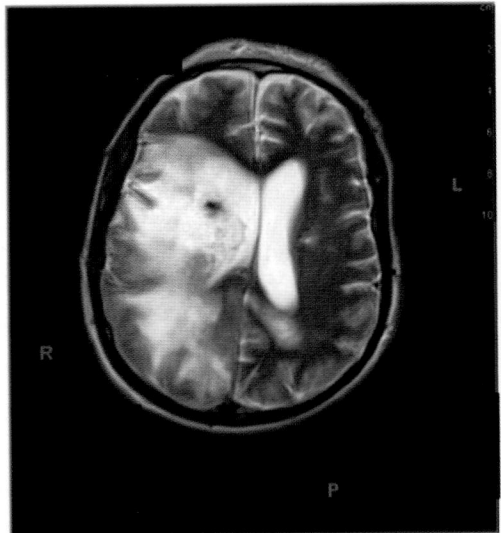 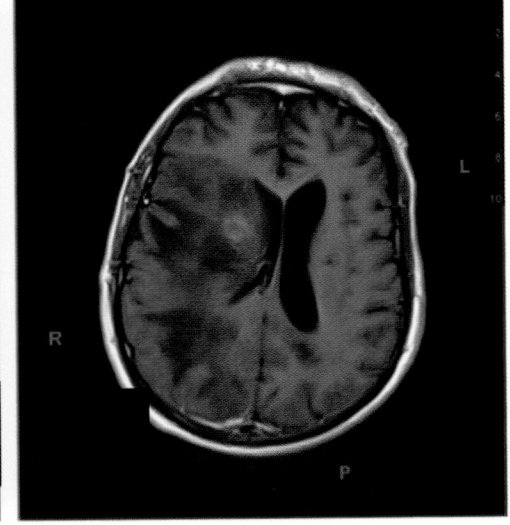

T2 weighted MRI   T1 with gadolinium

Figure 8.4.1 *PML in HAART era may violate previous rules of MR diagnosis.* This scan shows a PML lesion two months after effective HIV therapy initiated during an immune reconstitution inflammatory syndrome (IRIS) phase. Unlike classic PML where the lesion has no mass effect and no contrast enhancement with gadolinium, this figure demonstrates massive swelling of the brain accompanied by contrast enhancement during gadolinium infusion. Such a reaction could easily be confused with primary central nervous system lymphoma. Because of varying degrees of IRIS, lesions of PML have more diverse presentation on imaging than in the past.

was pathologically consistent with HIV IRIS. More recently, a series of cases of inflammatory encephalopathy was similarly reported in cART-treated patients and might be more examples of HIV-associated IRIS (Lescure, 2010). Further study of the biology of these cases is required, while the therapeutic approach used combines optimizing the CNS HIV therapy, while use of corticosteroids or even more potent anti-inflammatory therapy.

OTHER OPPORTUNISTIC INFECTIONS AND IRIS

IRIS is a clinically much less important entity for other CNS pathogens, although virtually any CNS infection may be associated with enhanced inflammatory components. While toxoplasma encephalitis is one of the most common CNS OI in HIV, it has surprisingly rarely been associated with clinically meaningful IRIS responses (Pfeffer et al., 2009). Herpes viruses certainly do involve the CNS and are sometimes exacerbated by IRIS, so the possibility that either varicella CNS manifestations or herpes simplex 2 may be enhanced by immune reconstitution remains a consideration (Clark et al., 2004; French, 2009). It is also likely that neurosyphilis may occasionally be triggered during immune reconstitution, and careful consideration of inflammatory responses in the CNS should always include evaluation for syphilis. Finally, tuberculosis is commonly complicated by IRIS in systemic disease, and it is likely that this is the case also for CNS manifestations of tuberculosis that may be especially encountered in the developing world.

NON-OPPORTUNISTIC INFECTIONS OF THE CNS

PRIMARY CNS LYMPHOMA

Primary CNS lymphoma (PCNSL) is the most common brain neoplasm in AIDS patients and both toxoplasma encephalitis and PCNSL are the most common causes of mass lesions in HIV+ patients (for recent reviews, see Bayraktar et al., 2010; Gerstner & Batchelor, 2010). Organs affected include the CNS, eyes, leptomeninges, or spinal cord (reviewed in Gerstner & Batchelor, 2010; Grimm et al., 2008), and the most frequent clinical findings include focal neurological deficits and seizures (Bayraktar et al., 2010). PCNSL occurs in both immunocompetent and immunocompromised individuals and accounts for about 4% of all primary brain tumors (Bayraktar et al., 2010). Other studies showed a PCNSL prevalence of 3 to 10%, with a higher-than-normal prevalence in patients with AIDS (Beral et al., 1991; Levy et al., 1985; Navarro et al., 1998; Schulz et al., 1996). However, studies in India showed a very low prevalence and incidence of HIV-associated PCNSL (0.01 to 0.07%) (Agarwal et al., 2009; Kumari et al., 2009; Paul et al., 2008). In a study of 281 HIV+ individuals with neurological abnormalities and focal brain lesions in Italy, PCNSL was the major diagnosis in 26.7% (Ammassari et al., 2000).

Pathology and Pathogenesis

AIDS-associated PCNSL is almost always associated with the presence of Epstein-Barr virus (EBV). Various studies demonstrated that the EBV genome and/or proteins are present in PCNSL tumor cells of over 90% in immunocompromised patients, with other studies showing EBV genome in almost 100% of HIV-associated non-Hodgkin lymphoma (NLH) cases (Auperin et al., 1994; Brink et al., 1998; Cinque et al., 1993; De Luca et al., 1995; Hamilton-Dutoit et al., 1993; Morgello, 1992). Thus, the presence of EBV DNA in the CSF is a marker of PCNSL. EBV DNA has also been detected in brain tissues and plasma of patients with PCNSL (Cinque et al., 1993; Hamilton-Dutoit et al., 1993; Morgello, 1992). Possible factors that contribute to lymphoma development include HIV-induced immunosuppression, impaired immune surveillance, cytokine release and deregulation, and chronic antigenic stimulation (Bayraktar et al., 2010; Gerstner & Batchelor, 2010; Grimm et al., 2008). In fact, it has been shown that these alterations are associated with the development of oligoclonal B-cell expansion (Knowles, 1996). It is believed that in immunosuppressed individuals, the impaired immune surveillance and resulting disregulation of cytokine expression cause chronic antigenic stimulation, and this antigenic stimulation induce polyclonal B-cell proliferation (De Luca et al., 1995; Knowles, 1996; Morgello, 1992; Wong et al., 2010). This is supported by studies demonstrating that IL-10 dysregulation play a role in EBV-associated PCNSL (Wong et al., 2010), and patients with AIDS-related lymphomas showed increased IL-10 production associated with the presence of EBV in lymphoma cells (De Luca et al., 1995). In fact the presence of single nucleotide polymorphism rs1800871_T or rs1800872_A in the IL-10 gene promoter is associated with lower IL-10 production and release (Breen et al., 2003; Shin et al., 2000), and a recent multicenter cohort study showed that HIV+ individuals with at least one copy of either rs1800871_T or rs1800872_A allele were at decreased risk of PCNSL (Wong et al., 2010). Increased levels of serum and CSF lactate dehydrogenase (LDH) (Bayraktar et al., 2010) and soluble CD23 (Bossolasco et al., 2001) were also associated with increased risk of developing PCNSL in HIV+ individuals. It has also been shown that irrespective of absolute CD4+ T cell counts, HIV-positive patients who subsequently developed PCNS lymphoma lacked EBV-specific CD4+ T cell function (Gasser et al., 2007). Thus EBV and dysregulation of cytokine expression and T-cell function play a major role in PCNSL pathogenesis.

Treatment, Morbidity, and Mortality

PCNSL is generally associated with a poor prognosis and short survival, with a median survival of just few weeks to few months following diagnosis (Bayraktar et al., 2010; Corti et al., 2004; Rubio et al., 1995). It has been shown that even with anticancer therapy, only about 10% of patients survive beyond 1 year (Sparano, 2001) and increased levels of LDH (> or = 300 U/L) and alkaline phosphatase (> or = 500 U/L) have also been associated with poor prognosis (Navarro et al., 1998; Rubio et al., 1995).

Evidence suggests that cART has decreased the incidence of PCNSL, improved its prognosis, and prolonged survival (Chow et al., 2001; Gerstner & Batchelor, 2007; Sparano, 2001). In a study of 41 HIV+ and 45 HIV- individuals with PCNSL, Bayraktar and colleagues (Bayraktar et al., 2010) showed that survival was significantly better in the HIV- group compared to the HIV+ group. cART was associated with improved survival, but survival for HIV+ individuals on cART was still lower than survival in the HIV- group. A prospective study of 281 HIV+ patients with neurological abnormalities showed a strong decline of AIDS-related PCNSL during the cART era (Ammassari et al., 2000). A study by Sparano and colleagues (Sparano et al., 1999) in New York, showed that compared to the pre-cART period, the annual number of first admission for non-Hodgkin's lymphoma (NHL), including PCNSL, decreased by 63%. Another study of 25 patients in the US showed that receipt of cART resulted in marked increase in the survival of patients with AIDS-associated PCNSL (Skiest & Crosby, 2003). Survival of these patients ranged from 7.5 to over 70 months, while for patients who received radiation alone without cART, the median survival was 5.6 months (Skiest & Crosby, 2003). In this study, other factors that were associated with improved survival included increase in CD4+ T-cell counts and decreased viral load following cART (Skiest & Crosby, 2003). cART use by patients with AIDS-related lymphomas is also associated with decreased frequency of meningeal involvement (Navarro et al., 2008).

HIV ENCEPHALOPATHY

Pathology and Pathogenesis

HIV encephalopathy is caused primarily by HIV infection and fueled by immune activation of CNS cells and virotoxins, including viral proteins, cytokines, and chemokines, secreted by infected brain macrophages and microglia (for recent reviews, see Dhillon et al., 2008; Gras & Kaul, 2010; Kraft-Terry et al., 2009; Kraft-Terry et al., 2010; Yadav & Collman, 2009). Current evidence demonstrates that following HIV infection, the resulting inflammation as well as the virus and secreted viral proteins induces a breach in the BBB integrity, allowing HIV and infected mononuclear phagocytes to invade the CNS (Gras & Kaul, 2010; Kanmogne et al., 2007; Persidsky et al., 2006; Roberts et al., 2010). Virus and toxic products secreted by infected brain mononuclear phagocytes and glial cells induce neuroinflammation, neurodegeneration, and encephalopathy (Gras & Kaul, 2010; Kraft-Terry et al., 2009). Disease pathology ranges from mild brain atrophy and gliosis to robust viral replication, multinucleated giant cell formation, astro- and micro-gliosis, myelin pallor, and neuronal loss (Boisse et al., 2008; Everall et al., 1993; Everall et al., 1991; Ketzler et al., 1990; Price et al., 1988). HIV encephalitis is a common correlate to later stages of behavioral, motor, neuropsychiatric, and neurological syndromes termed AIDS dementia complex or HIV-associated neurocognitive disorder (HAND) (Antinori et al., 2007; Boisse et al., 2008; Ghafouri et al., 2006; McArthur et al., 1993). Detailed descriptions of the clinical, pathological, and neurobehavioral effects of HAND are provided in Chapter 7.3.

The mechanism by which HIV infection leads to neuroinvasion and encephalopathy is multifactorial and has been shown to involve direct viral infection of brain mononuclear phagocytes, dysfunction, and injury of brain endothelial cells, astrocytes, oligodendrocytes, and neurons induced directly by HIV and secreted viral factors (Boisse et al., 2008; Everall et al., 1993; Everall et al., 1991; Gras & Kaul, 2010; Ketzler et al., 1990; Kraft-Terry et al., 2009; Price et al., 1988). HIV proteins that have been shown to induce injury of CNS cells include gp120, gp41, Tat, Nef, Vpr, and Rev (Bergonzini et al., 2009; Gras & Kaul, 2010; Kanmogne et al., 2007; Li et al., 2009; Persidsky et al., 2006; Roberts et al., 2010; Toborek et al., 2003). Encephalopathy generally occurs in the late stages of HIV infection and is associated with low levels of CD4+ T cells (below 200 cells/µl) and high plasma viral loads. Encephalopathy is also sometimes seen as the first sign of the onset of AIDS (Rigardetto et al., 1999).

Progressive HIV encephalopathy (PHE) is also common among perinatally HIV-infected children; it is an important cause of morbidity and mortality and is characterized by delayed neurological development, acquired microcephaly, brain atrophy, and neuromotor deficits (Mitchell, 2006; Scarmato et al., 1996). Similar to adult HIV encephalopathy, PHE neuropathogenesis involves HIV itself and secreted viral proteins, as well as viral-induced cytokines and chemokines that promote ongoing CNS inflammation and injury of CNS cells, including neurons and astrocytes (Hamid et al., 2008; McCoig et al., 2004; Mitchell, 2006). Pediatric HIV+ patients with PHE also showed low blood CD8+ T-lymphocytes (Sanchez-Ramon et al., 2003), increased expression of caspase-3 in CNS tissues and neuronal apoptosis (Gelbard et al., 1995; James et al., 1999), and increased expression and activation of NFκB (Dollard et al., 1995).

cART, Morbidity, and Mortality in HIV-induced Encephalopathy and PHE

Before the era of cART, encephalopathy developed in 20 to 30% of untreated AIDS patients. Widespread use of cART in developed countries has led to a decrease in the incidence of HIV-associated encephalopathy, although there is increase in the prevalence of HAND as patients live longer with the disease and are more likely to develop cognitive impairments (Brew et al., 2009; Price & Spudich, 2008; Wright, 2009). A prospective multicenter cohort study in the US showed a decrease in HIV-associated dementia (HAD) incidence from 21 cases per 1000 person-years in the pre-cART era to 10.5 cases per 1000 person-years in the cART era (Sacktor et al., 2001). Studies in Australia also showed a decreased HAD incidence in the cART era compared to the pre-cART era, with simultaneous increase in prevalence and increased patients survival from 5 to 19.6 months in the pre-cART to over 39 months in the cART era (Dore et al., 1999; Dore et al., 2002). The EuroSIDA cohort study showed a 10-fold decrease in HIV-induced CNS diseases with cART (d'Arminio Monforte et al., 2004).

Similar trends have been observed for PHE. Before cART became widely available, PHE was reported in 13–35% of children with HIV-1 infection and in 35–50% of children with AIDS (reviewed in Cooper et al., 1998; Lobato et al., 1995; Van Rie et al., 2007); current evidence shows that cART has dramatically reduced the incidence and prevalence of PHE and data suggest that cART can prevent or reverse PHE in children (Shanbhag et al., 2005). A retrospective study by Shanbhag and colleagues showed a decrease of PHE prevalence from 29.6% in children born before 1996, to 12% in children born after 1996 (Shanbhag et al., 2005). Another study showed a current PHE incidence of 1.6% and a prevalence of 10% in the US (Chiriboga et al., 2005). A recent prospective study of 2,575 children perinatally infected with HIV-1 between 2000–2006 in over 80 sites in the U.S.A. showed a PHE prevalence of 8.93% and a decrease in incidence from 1.16 person-years in 2001 to 0.38 person-years in 2006 (Nachman et al., 2009). cART use and improved immune function in HIV+ children in South America and Asia was also associated with improved neurological, neuropsychological, and immunological conditions, and decreased risk of HPE (Hamid et al., 2008; Saavedra-Lozano et al., 2006).

Some antiretroviral drugs have better CNS penetration than others (Letendre et al., 2008a; Patel et al., 2009) and it is possible that cART regimens including these high CNS-penetrating drugs may be more effective at preventing or reducing the risk of encephalopathy and other CNS complications in infected individuals. In a large U.S.A. prospective cohort study of 2,398 perinatally HIV-infected children enrolled over a 14-year period (1993–2006), Patel and colleagues (Patel et al., 2009) evaluated the impact of cART and CNS- penetrating antiretroviral regimens on the incidence of HIV encephalopathy and survival after diagnosis of HIV encephalopathy. Over a median 6.4 years follow-up, they observed a 10-fold decline in incidence of HIV-associated encephalopathy, beginning in 1996. cART regimens were associated with a 50% decrease in the incidence of HIV encephalopathy compared with non-cART group. Of the 77 HIV encephalopathy cases observed in this study, 60% were children who never took cART and the majority of deaths (62%) occurred in this group. On the contrary, by the end of the follow-up period, only 2% of the 1,741 children who received high CNS-penetrating cART regimens had a diagnosis of HIV encephalopathy, while of the 267 children who received a medium CNS-penetrating regimen and the 264 children on a low CNS-penetrating regimen, 9% and 7% respectively had a diagnosis of HIV encephalopathy by the end of the follow-up period (Patel et al., 2009). cART use is also associated with improved overall survival (Gortmaker et al., 2001; Patel et al., 2008; Patel et al., 2009) and use of high CNS-penetrating antiretroviral regimens after diagnosis of HIV encephalopathy reduced the risk of death by 74% compared with low CNS-penetrating regimens (Patel et al., 2009).

However, cART does not eliminate HIV from the CNS and does not prevent encephalopathy in all patients.

For example, in the CHARTER study of 1555 HIV infected cases, the majority of whom were receiving cART, about half had some degree of neurocognitive impairment (Heaton, et al., 2010); the rates of impairment were not substantially different from a pre cART cohort (Heaton et al., 2011). Langford and colleagues showed severe and demyelinating leukoencephalopathy in AIDS patients on cART (Langford et al., 2002) and other studies have shown mixed benefits of CNS-penetrating cART drugs (Cysique et al., 2004; Cysique et al., 2006). In a study of 97 AIDS patients on a stable cART regimen, Cysique and colleagues (Cysique et al., 2004) found no direct benefit of CNS-penetrating cART drugs. Both patients receiving CNS-penetrating and non-CNS-penetrating drugs performed similarly on neuropsychological tests and showed cognitive impairment compared to controls. In another study, these authors followed up 101 AIDS patients over 27 months and found a significant cognitive decline (8% to 34%) over the study period, despite undetectable plasma viral load, and low nadir CD4 was significantly associated with cognitive decline (Cysique et al., 2006). This is corroborated by other clinical observations showing occurrence of HAD, despite cART (Brew et al., 2009; Gras & Kaul, 2010; Liner et al., 2008; Nath & Sacktor, 2006). In a prospective cohort study of 1,160 subjects participating in the ACTG antiretroviral trial, Robertson and colleagues showed that cognitive impairment was sustained in 22% of participants and an additional 21% further developed impairment during the study period (Robertson et al., 2007). Sevigny and colleagues followed up 203 nondemented AIDS patients with low CD4 (<200/µl) or with a CD4<300/µl with cognitive impairment over a median 20.7 months; during this period, 36% developed HAD despite an undetectable plasma viral load in 21% and an undetectable CSF viral load in 43% (Sevigny et al., 2004). In this study, the cumulative incidence of HAD was 20% at 1 year and 33% at 2 years, and neither plasma nor CSF HIV RNA levels were associated with time of development of HAD (Sevigny et al., 2004).

It is possible that for individuals with advanced disease, extensive CNS damage may have already occurred and cART may not reverse the damages. In fact, for some of these studies showing little or no cART effect on HIV-induced neurocognitive impairment, including CNS-penetrating drugs, participants were at the advanced stages of infection and had developed AIDS (Cysique et al., 2004; Cysique et al., 2006; Sevigny et al., 2004). It is well known that antiretroviral drugs do not completely cross the BBB and their concentrations in the CNS and CSF are often several folds lower than their blood concentrations. Optimal levels of antiretroviral drugs in the CNS are likely necessary to stop active HIV replication within the brain and prevent further neuropathological damage and cognitive decline. Nevertheless, there is increasing evidence that cART, especially regimens containing high CNS-penetrating drugs such as abacavir, delavirdine, lamivudine, stavudine, zidovudine, efavirenz, nevirapine, amprenavir, atazanavir, ritonavir, and indinavir (Letendre et al., 2008a; Patel et al., 2009), reduces viral burden, improves cognitive function, and decreases the risk of HIV-associated CNS diseases in infected individuals. However, this is not true for resource-limited countries where the majority of HIV-infected adults and children do not have access to antiretroviral drugs and the incidence and prevalence of encephalopathy likely resembles or exceeds that observed in developed countries before widespread use of cART (Ellis, 2010; Kanmogne et al., 2010; Njamnshi et al., 2009; Robertson et al., 2010; Sacktor et al., 2007).

DISCUSSION

Current evidence suggests that with widespread cART usage, the incidence of several HIV-associated opportunistic and nonopportunistic complications has dramatically declined in developed countries (Brew et al., 2009; d'Arminio Monforte et al., 2004; Dore et al., 2002; Neuenburg et al., 2002; Price & Spudich, 2008; Sacktor, 2002; Sacktor et al., 2001; Torre et al., 2005; Wright, 2009). However, CNS complications still occur (Nath & Sacktor, 2006; Heaton, et al., 2010) and brain involvement continues to be a frequent finding at autopsy (Jellinger et al., 2000). This suggest that although combination cART decreases overall mortality and prevalence of many HIV-associated CNS OI, these therapies may be less effective in preventing direct HIV-1 effects on the brain, especially in cases with advanced disease (Cysique et al., 2004; Cysique et al., 2006; Sevigny et al., 2004). Paradoxically, adequate therapies against opportunistic pathogens, as well as adequate cART and immune reconstitution, have been associated with IRIS and worsening clinical conditions.

Available data underscore the heavy burden of infectious CNS OI in resource-limited areas, including CM, CMV encephalitis, and toxoplasmosis (Bekondi et al., 2006; Bergemann and Karstaedt, 1996; Bicanic et al., 2007; Bogaerts et al., 1999; Hakim et al., 2000; Heyderman et al., 1998; McCarthy et al., 2006; Moosa & Coovadia, 1997; Mwaba et al., 2001; Pappalardo & Melhem, 2003; Park et al., 2009; Passos et al., 2000; Satishchandra et al., 2007; Subramanian & Mathai, 2005). There is also evidence of high occurrence of noninfectious CNS complications in these settings (Clifford et al., 2007; Kanmogne et al., 2010; Njamnshi et al., 2009; Robertson et al., 2010; Sacktor et al., 2007). Considering the continuous high incidence and prevalence of these diseases in resource-limited countries and associated high mortality, there is a critical need for a better understanding of the epidemiology, pathology, and pathogenesis of these diseases in these developing countries that are home to over two-thirds of persons living with HIV/AIDS. There is also a need for a better understanding of the effect of co-infection of HIV and opportunistic pathogens on disease pathogenesis. A recent African study of HIV/AIDS patients showed that the presence of pulmonary tuberculosis in HIV-infected individuals was a risk factor for the development of CM (Jarvis et al., 2009). As these pathogens primarily invades the lungs before disseminating into the brain, it is not known what molecular, biological, or physiological interactions occurs between them in the context of HIV infection and likely accelerate disease progression, morbidity, and mortality. In addition to tuberculosis, malaria is also endemic in many regions with high HIV/AIDS prevalence and affects the CNS. It is not known what effect plasmodium-HIV coinfection may have on the CNS. It is also likely that inflammation and damages induced by opportunistic pathogens in the human host further increase/accentuate direct HIV-induced CNS injury. In fact, high levels of matrix metalloproteinase (MMP)-9 are found in the CSF of HIV-infected patients with cryptococcosis, cytomegalovirus encephalitis, and tuberculous meningitis (Liuzzi et al., 2000). MMPs degrade components of the extracellular matrix and increased MMP-9 in these patients can induce/increase degradation of the blood-brain barrier, inducing/increasing transendothelial migration of HIV-infected cells into the brain and development of HIV-associated CNS damages.

In addition to current efforts to provide cART to a larger number of HIV-infected individuals, improved monitoring, adequate treatment, and control of OI in this population are critically important (McCutchan, 2009). More routine screening, early detection, and treatment of HIV-associated opportunistic diseases should be encouraged, as late diagnosis is often associated with increased morbidity and high mortality (Moreno et al., 2010). For example, using serum cryptococcal antigen test in at risk patients to screen for early cryptococcal diseases could be beneficial, as non-meningeal cryptococcal infection often precedes meningitis but is often under-recognized or misdiagnosed (Driver et al., 1995; French et al., 2002; Tassie et al., 2003). Resource-limited countries also have major deficiencies in diagnostic technology, especially modern molecular and neuroimaging modalities that are used for diagnosis and management of CNS diseases in the developed world. It is likely that diagnostic imprecision will impede accurate epidemiological studies and clinical management of HIV-associated neurological diseases in these settings. Thus, for a better and global control of HIV-induced opportunistic and nonopportunistic complications, improvements in diagnostic capabilities, availability of treatment, and effective prevention measures are urgently needed in resource-limited settings. Improved and standardized diagnostic tools, equivalent to Western standards, will enable more accurate comparisons of research data across countries and cultures, a better understanding of disease epidemiology in developing countries, and determine the effects of other factors such as HIV clades diversity on disease pathology and pathogenesis.

ACKNOWLEDGMENTS

Dr. Kanmogne is supported by NIMH grants RO1 MH081780 and R21 MH80611. Dr. Clifford is supported by NINDS grant U01 NS32228, NIAID grant U01 A169495, and NIMH grants 2R01 MH058076, 1R21 MH083489, and 22005.

REFERENCES

Agarwal, P. A., Menon, S., Smruti, B. K., & Singhal, B. S. (2009). Primary central nervous system lymphoma: A profile of 26 cases from Western India. *Neurol India, 57,* 756–763.

Alfonso, Y., Fraga, J., Fonseca, C., Jimenez, N., Pinillos, T., Dorta-Contreras, A. J., et al. (2009). Molecular diagnosis of *Toxoplasma gondii* infection in cerebrospinal fluid from AIDS patients. *Cerebrospinal Fluid Res, 6,* 2.

Ammassari, A., Cingolani, A., Pezzotti, P., De Luca, D. A., Murri, R., Giancola, M. L., et al. (2000). AIDS-related focal brain lesions in the era of highly active antiretroviral therapy. *Neurology, 55,* 1194–1200.

Anders, H. J. & Goebel, F. D. (1999). Neurological manifestations of cytomegalovirus infection in the acquired immunodeficiency syndrome. *Int J STD AIDS, 10,* 151–159; quiz 160–151.

Antinori, A., Ammassari, A., Giancola, M. L., Cingolani, A., Grisetti, S., Murri, R., et al. (2001). Epidemiology and prognosis of AIDS-associated progressive multifocal leukoencephalopathy in the HAART era. *J Neurovirol, 7,* 323–328.

Antinori, A., Arendt, G., Becker, J. T., Brew, B. J., Byrd, D. A., Cherner, M., et al. (2007). Updated research nosology for HIV-associated neurocognitive disorders. *Neurology, 69,* 1789–1799.

Antinori, A., Cingolani, A., Lorenzini, P., Giancola, M. L., Uccella, I., Bossolasco, S., et al. (2003). Clinical epidemiology and survival of progressive multifocal leukoencephalopathy in the era of highly active antiretroviral therapy: Data from the Italian Registry Investigative Neuro AIDS (IRINA). *J Neurovirol, 9* Suppl 1, 47–53.

Auperin, I., Mikolt, J., Oksenhendler, E., Thiebaut, J. B., Brunet, M., Dupont, B., et al. (1994). Primary central nervous system malignant non-Hodgkin's lymphomas from HIV-infected and non-infected patients: Expression of cellular surface proteins and Epstein-Barr viral markers. *Neuropathol Appl Neurobiol, 20,* 243–252.

Bacellar, H., Munoz, A., Miller, E. N., Cohen, B. A., Besley, D., Selnes, O. A., et al. (1994). Temporal trends in the incidence of HIV-1-related neurologic diseases: Multicenter AIDS Cohort Study, 1985–1992. *Neurology, 44,* 1892–1900.

Bayraktar, S., Bayraktar, U. D., Ramos, J. C., Stefanovic, A., & Lossos, I. S. (2010). Primary CNS lymphoma in HIV positive and negative patients: Comparison of clinical characteristics, outcome and prognostic factors. *J Neurooncol.*

Beaman, M. H., Hunter, C. A., & Remington, J. S. (1994). Enhancement of intracellular replication of *Toxoplasma gondii* by IL-6. Interactions with IFN-gamma and TNF-alpha. *J Immunol, 153,* 4583–4587.

Bekondi, C., Bernede, C., Passone, N., Minssart, P., Kamalo, C., Mbolidi, D., et al. (2006). Primary and opportunistic pathogens associated with meningitis in adults in Bangui, Central African Republic, in relation to human immunodeficiency virus serostatus. *Int J Infect Dis, 10,* 387–395.

Belec, L., Gray, F., Mikol, J., Scaravilli, F., Mhiri, C., Sobel, A., et al. (1990). Cytomegalovirus (CMV) encephalomyeloradiculitis and human immunodeficiency virus (HIV) encephalitis: Presence of HIV and CMV co-infected multinucleated giant cells. *Acta Neuropathol, 81,* 99–104.

Beral, V., Peterman, T., Berkelman, R., & Jaffe, H. (1991). AIDS-associated non-Hodgkin lymphoma. *Lancet, 337,* 805–809.

Bergemann, A. & Karstaedt, A. S. (1996). The spectrum of meningitis in a population with high prevalence of HIV disease. *QJM, 89,* 499–504.

Berger, J. R., Pall, L., Lanska, D., & Whiteman, M. (1998). Progressive multifocal leukoencephalopathy in patients with HIV infection. *J Neurovirol, 4,* 59–68.

Bergonzini, V., Calistri, A., Salata, C., Del Vecchio, C., Sartori, E., Parolin, C., et al. (2009). Nef and cell signaling transduction: a possible involvement in the pathogenesis of human immunodeficiency virus-associated dementia. *J Neurovirol,* 1–11.

Bicanic, T., Meintjes, G., Wood, R., Hayes, M., Rebe, K., Bekker, L. G., et al. (2007). Fungal burden, early fungicidal activity, and outcome in cryptococcal meningitis in antiretroviral-naive or antiretroviral-experienced patients treated with amphotericin B or fluconazole. *Clin Infect Dis, 45,* 76–80.

Bogaerts, J., Rouvroy, D., Taelman, H., Kagame, A., Aziz, M. A., Swinne, D., et al. (1999). AIDS-associated cryptococcal meningitis in Rwanda (1983–1992): Epidemiologic and diagnostic features. *J Infect, 39,* 32–37.

Boisse, L., Gill, M. J., & Power, C. (2008). HIV infection of the central nervous system: Clinical features and neuropathogenesis. *Neurol Clin, 26,* 799–819.

Bossolasco, S., Nilsson, A., de Milito, A., Lazzarin, A., Linde, A., Cinque, P., et al. (2001). Soluble CD23 in cerebrospinal fluid: A marker of AIDS-related non-Hodgkin's lymphoma in the brain. *AIDS, 15,* 1109–1113.

Boulware, D. R., Bonham, S. C., Meya, D. B., Wiesner, D. L., Park, G. S., Kambugu, A., et al. (2010). Paucity of initial cerebrospinal fluid inflammation in cryptococcal meningitis is associated with subsequent immune reconstitution inflammatory syndrome. *J Infect Dis, 202,* 962–970.

Breen, E. C., Boscardin, W. J., Detels, R., Jacobson, L. P., Smith, M. W., O'Brien, S. J., et al. (2003). Non-Hodgkin's B cell lymphoma in persons with acquired immunodeficiency syndrome is associated with increased serum levels of IL10, or the IL10 promoter -592 C/C genotype. *Clin Immunol, 109,* 119–129.

Brew, B. J., Crowe, S. M., Landay, A., Cysique, L. A., & Guillemin, G. (2009). Neurodegeneration and ageing in the HAART era. *J Neuroimmune Pharmacol, 4,* 163–174.

Brink, N. S., Sharvell, Y., Howard, M. R., Fox, J. D., Harrison, M. J., & Miller, R. F. (1998). Detection of Epstein-Barr virus and Kaposi's sarcoma-associated herpesvirus DNA in CSF from persons infected with HIV who had neurological disease. *J Neurol Neurosurg Psychiatry, 65,* 191–195.

Brouwer, A. E., Rajanuwong, A., Chierakul, W., Griffin, G. E., Larsen, R. A., White, N. J., et al. (2004). Combination antifungal therapies for HIV-associated cryptococcal meningitis: A randomised trial. *Lancet, 363,* 1764–1767.

Brueske, C. H. (1986). Proteolytic activity of a clinical isolate of Cryptococcus neoformans. *J Clin Microbiol, 23,* 631–633.

Cannon, M. J., Schmid, D. S., & Hyde, T. B. (2010). Review of cytomegalovirus seroprevalence and demographic characteristics associated with infection. *Rev Med Virol, 20,* 202–213.

Carruthers, V. B. & Suzuki, Y. (2007). Effects of Toxoplasma gondii infection on the brain. *Schizophr Bull, 33,* 745–751.

Casadevall, A., Rosas, A. L., & Nosanchuk, J.D. (2000). Melanin and virulence in Cryptococcus neoformans. *Curr Opin Microbiol, 3,* 354–358.

Chariyalertsak, S., Sirisanthana, T., Saengwonloey, O., & Nelson, K. E. (2001). Clinical presentation and risk behaviors of patients with acquired immunodeficiency syndrome in Thailand, 1994–1998: Regional variation and temporal trends. *Clin Infect Dis, 32,* 955–962.

Chayakulkeeree, M. & Perfect, J. R. (2006). Cryptococcosis. *Infect Dis Clin North Am, 20,* 507–544, v–vi.

Chimelli, L., Rosemberg, S., Hahn, M. D., Lopes, M. B., & Netto, M. B. (1992). Pathology of the central nervous system in patients infected with the human immunodeficiency virus (HIV): A report of 252 autopsy cases from Brazil. *Neuropathol Appl Neurobiol, 18,* 478–488.

Chiriboga, C. A., Fleishman, S., Champion, S., Gaye-Robinson, L., & Abrams, E. J. (2005). Incidence and prevalence of HIV encephalopathy in children with HIV infection receiving highly active anti-retroviral therapy (HAART). *J Pediatr, 146,* 402–407.

Chow, K. U., Mitrou, P. S., Geduldig, K., Helm, E. B., Hoelzer, D., & Brodt, H. R. (2001). Changing incidence and survival in patients with aids-related non-Hodgkin's lymphomas in the era of highly active anti-retroviral therapy (HAART). *Leuk Lymphoma, 41,* 105–116.

Cinque, P., Bossolasco, S., Brambilla, A. M., Boschini, A., Mussini, C., Pierotti, C., et al. (2003). The effect of highly active antiretroviral therapy-induced immune reconstitution on development and outcome of progressive multifocal leukoencephalopathy: Study of 43 cases with review of the literature. *J Neurovirol 9 Suppl, 1,* 73–80.

Cinque, P., Brytting, M., Vago, L., Castagna, A., Parravicini, C., Zanchetta, N., et al. (1993). Epstein-Barr virus DNA in cerebrospinal fluid from patients with AIDS-related primary lymphoma of the central nervous system. *Lancet, 342,* 398–401.

Cinque, P., Koralnik, I. J., Gerevini, S., Miro, J. M., & Price, R. W. (2009). Progressive multifocal leukoencephalopathy in HIV-1 infection. *Lancet Infect Dis, 9,* 625–636.

Clark, B. M., Krueger, R. G., Price, P., & French, M. A. (2004). Compartmentalization of the immune response in varicella zoster virus immune restoration disease causing transverse myelitis. *AIDS, 18,* 1218–1221.

Clifford, D. B., Mitike, M. T., Mekonnen, Y., Zhang, J., Zenebe, G., Melaku, Z., et al. (2007). Neurological evaluation of untreated human immunodeficiency virus infected adults in Ethiopia. *J Neurovirol, 13,* 67–72.

Clifford, D. B., Yiannoutsos, C., Glicksman, M., Simpson, D. M., Singer, E. J., Piliero, P. J., et al. (1999). HAART improves prognosis in HIV-associated progressive multifocal leukoencephalopathy. *Neurology, 52,* 623–625.

Coenjaerts, F. E., van der Flier, M., Mwinzi, P. N., Brouwer, A. E., Scharringa, J., Chaka, W. S., et al. (2004). Intrathecal production and secretion of vascular endothelial growth factor during Cryptococcal Meningitis. *J Infect Dis, 190,* 1310–1317.

Cohen, B. A. (1999). Neurologic manifestations of toxoplasmosis in AIDS. *Semin Neurol, 19,* 201–211.

Cooper, E. R., Hanson, C., Diaz, C., Mendez, H., Abboud, R., Nugent, R., et al. (1998). Encephalopathy and progression of human immunodeficiency virus disease in a cohort of children with perinatally acquired human immunodeficiency virus infection. Women and Infants Transmission Study Group. *J Pediatr, 132,* 808–812.

Corbett, E. L., Churchyard, G. J., Charalambos, S., Samb, B., Moloi, V., Clayton, T. C., et al. (2002). Morbidity and mortality in South African gold miners: Impact of untreated disease due to human immunodeficiency virus. *Clin Infect Dis, 34,* 1251–1258.

Corti, M., Villafane, F., Trione, N., Schtirbu, R., Yampolsky, C., & Narbaitz, M. (2004). [Primary central nervous system lymphomas in AIDS patients]. *Enferm Infecc Microbiol Clin, 22,* 332–336.

Cysique, L. A., Maruff, P., & Brew, B. J. (2004). Antiretroviral therapy in HIV infection: Are neurologically active drugs important? *Arch Neurol, 61,* 1699–1704.

Cysique, L. A., Maruff, P., & Brew, B. J. (2006). Variable benefit in neuropsychological function in HIV-infected HAART-treated patients. *Neurology, 66,* 1447–1450.

d'Arminio Monforte, A., Cinque, P., Mocroft, A., Goebel, F. D., Antunes, F., Katlama, C., et al. (2004). Changing incidence of central nervous system diseases in the EuroSIDA cohort. *Ann Neurol, 55,* 320–328.

Dannemann, B., McCutchan, J. A., Israelski, D., Antoniskis, D., Leport, C., Luft, B., et al. (1992). Treatment of toxoplasmic encephalitis in patients with AIDS. A randomized trial comparing pyrimethamine plus clindamycin to pyrimethamine plus sulfadiazine. The California Collaborative Treatment Group. *Ann Intern Med, 116,* 33–43.

De Luca, A., Ammassari, A., Pezzotti, P., Cinque, P., Gasnault, J., Berenguer, J., et al. (2008). Cidofovir in addition to antiretroviral treatment is not effective for AIDS-associated progressive multifocal leukoencephalopathy: A multicohort analysis. *AIDS, 22,* 1759–1767.

De Luca, A., Antinori, A., Cingolani, A., Larocca, L. M., Linzalone, A., Ammassari, A., et al. (1995). Evaluation of cerebrospinal fluid EBV-DNA and IL-10 as markers for in vivo diagnosis of AIDS-related primary central nervous system lymphoma. *Br J Haematol, 90,* 844–849.

De Luca, A., Giancola, M. L., Ammassari, A., Grisetti, S., Paglia, M. G., Gentile, M., et al. (2000). The effect of potent antiretroviral therapy and JC virus load in cerebrospinal fluid on clinical outcome of patients with AIDS-associated progressive multifocal leukoencephalopathy. *J Infect Dis, 182,* 1077–1083.

Del Valle, L. & Pina-Oviedo, S. (2006). HIV disorders of the brain: Pathology and pathogenesis. *Front Biosci, 11,* 718–732.

Denning, D. W., Armstrong, R. W., Lewis, B. H., & Stevens, D. A. (1991). Elevated cerebrospinal fluid pressures in patients with cryptococcal meningitis and acquired immunodeficiency syndrome. *Am J Med, 91,* 267–272.

Dhillon, N. K., Williams, R., Callen, S., Zien, C., Narayan, O., & Buch, S. (2008). Roles of MCP-1 in development of HIV-dementia. *Front Biosci, 13,* 3913–3918.

Diamond, R. D. & Bennett, J. E. (1974). Prognostic factors in cryptococcal meningitis. A study in 111 cases. *Ann Intern Med, 80,* 176–181.

Dighiero, P., Reux, I., Hauw, J. J., Fillet, A. M., Courtois, Y., & Goureau, O. (1994). Expression of inducible nitric oxide synthase in cytomegalovirus-infected glial cells of retinas from AIDS patients. *Neurosci Lett, 166,* 31–34.

Dollard, S. C., James, H. J., Sharer, L. R., Epstein, L. G., Gelbard, H. A., & Dewhurst, S. (1995). Activation of nuclear factor kappa B in brains from children with HIV-1 encephalitis. *Neuropathol Appl Neurobiol, 21,* 518–528.

Dore, G. J., Correll, P. K., Li, Y., Kaldor, J. M., Cooper, D. A., & Brew, B. J. (1999). Changes to AIDS dementia complex in the era of highly active antiretroviral therapy. *AIDS, 13,* 1249–1253.

Dore, G. J., Law, M. G., & Brew, B. J. (1996). Prospective analysis of seizures occurring in human immunodeficiency virus type-1 infection. *J NeuroAIDS, 1,* 59–69.

Dore, G. J., Li, Y., McDonald, A., Ree, H., & Kaldor, J. M. (2002). Impact of highly active antiretroviral therapy on individual AIDS-defining illness incidence and survival in Australia. *J Acquir Immune Defic Syndr, 29,* 388–395.

Drake, A. K., Loy, C. T., Brew, B. J., Chen, T. C., Petoumenos, K., Li, P. C., et al. (2007). Human immunodeficiency virus-associated progressive multifocal leucoencephalopathy: Epidemiology and predictive factors for prolonged survival. *Eur J Neurol, 14,* 418–423.

Drew, W. L. (1992). Cytomegalovirus infection in patients with AIDS. *Clin Infect Dis, 14,* 608–615.

Driver, J. A., Saunders, C. A., Heinze-Lacey, B., & Sugar, A. M. (1995). Cryptococcal pneumonia in AIDS: Is cryptococcal meningitis preceded by clinically recognizable pneumonia? *J Acquir Immune Defic Syndr Hum Retrovirol, 9,* 168–171.

Dromer, F., Mathoulin-Pelissier, S., Fontanet, A., Ronin, O., Dupont, B., & Lortholary, O. (2004). Epidemiology of HIV-associated cryptococcosis in France (1985–2001): Comparison of the pre- and post-HAART eras. *AIDS, 18,* 555–562.

Dubey, J.P. (2008). The history of Toxoplasma gondii—the first 100 years. *J Eukaryot Microbiol, 55,* 467–475.

Dunlop, O., Rootwelt, V., Sannes, M., Goplen, A. K., Abdelnoor, M., Skaug, K., et al. (1996). Risk of toxoplasmic encephalitis in AIDS patients: Indications for prophylaxis. *Scand J Infect Dis, 28,* 71–73.

Dworkin, M. S., Wan, P. C., Hanson, D. L., & Jones, J. L. (1999). Progressive multifocal leukoencephalopathy: Improved survival of human immunodeficiency virus-infected patients in the protease inhibitor era. *J Infect Dis, 180,* 621–625.

Egli, A., Infanti, L., Dumoulin, A., Buser, A., Samaridis, J., Stebler, C., et al. (2009). Prevalence of polyomavirus BK and JC infection and replication in 400 healthy blood donors. *J Infect Dis, 199,* 837–846.

Ellis, R. (2010). HIV and antiretroviral therapy: Impact on the central nervous system. *Prog Neurobiol, 91,* 185–187.

Everall, I., Luthert, P., & Lantos, P. (1993). A review of neuronal damage in human immunodeficiency virus infection: Its assessment, possible mechanism and relationship to dementia. *J Neuropathol Exp Neurol, 52,* 561–566.

Everall, I. P., Luthert, P. J., & Lantos, P.L. (1991). Neuronal loss in the frontal cortex in HIV infection. *Lancet, 337,* 1119–1121.

Feldmesser, M., Harris, C., Reichberg, S., Khan, S., & Casadevall, A. (1996). Serum cryptococcal antigen in patients with AIDS. *Clin Infect Dis, 23,* 827–830.

Filisetti, D. & Candolfi, E. (2004). Immune response to Toxoplasma gondii. *Ann Ist Super Sanita, 40,* 71–80.

French, M. A. (2009). HIV/AIDS: Immune reconstitution inflammatory syndrome: A reappraisal. *Clin Infect Dis, 48,* 101–107.

French, M. A., Price, P., & Stone, S. F. (2004). Immune restoration disease after antiretroviral therapy. *AIDS, 18,* 1615–1627.

French, N., Gray, K., Watera, C., Nakiyingi, J., Lugada, E., Moore, M., et al. (2002). Cryptococcal infection in a cohort of HIV-1-infected Ugandan adults. *AIDS, 16,* 1031–1038.

Furtado, G. C., Slowik, M., Kleinman, H. K., & Joiner, K. A. (1992). Laminin enhances binding of Toxoplasma gondii tachyzoites to J774 murine macrophage cells. Infect *Immun, 60,* 2337–2342.

Gasnault, J., Taoufik, Y., Goujard, C., Kousignian, P., Abbed, K., Boue, F., et al. (1999). Prolonged survival without neurological improvement in patients with AIDS-related progressive multifocal leukoencephalopathy on potent combined antiretroviral therapy. *J Neurovirol, 5,* 421–429.

Gasser, O., Bihl, F. K., Wolbers, M., Loggi, E., Steffen, I., Hirsch, H. H., et al. (2007). HIV patients developing primary CNS lymphoma lack EBV-specific CD4+ T cell function irrespective of absolute CD4+ T cell counts. *PLoS Med, 4,* e96.

Gelbard, H. A., James, H. J., Sharer, L. R., Perry, S. W., Saito, Y., Kazee, A. M., et al. (1995). Apoptotic neurons in brains from paediatric patients with HIV-1 encephalitis and progressive encephalopathy. *Neuropathol Appl Neurobiol, 21,* 208–217.

Gerstner, E. & Batchelor, T. (2007). Primary CNS lymphoma. *Expert Rev Anticancer Ther, 7,* 689–700.

Gerstner, E. R. & Batchelor, T. T. (2010). Primary central nervous system lymphoma. *Arch Neurol, 67,* 291–297.

Geschwind, M. D., Skolasky, R. I., Royal, W. S., & McArthur, J.C. (2001). The relative contributions of HAART and alpha-interferon for therapy of progressive multifocal leukoencephalopathy in AIDS. *J Neurovirol, 7,* 353–357.

Ghafouri, M., Amini, S., Khalili, K., & Sawaya, B. E. (2006). HIV-1 associated dementia: Symptoms and causes. *Retrovirology, 3,* 28.

Gheuens, S., Pierone, G., Peeters, P., & Koralnik, I. J. (2010). Progressive multifocal leukoencephalopathy in individuals with minimal or occult immunosuppression. *J Neurol Neurosurg Psychiatry, 81,* 247–254.

Gordon, J. & Khalili, K. (1998). The human polyomavirus, JCV, and neurological diseases (review). *Int J Mol Med, 1,* 647–655.

Gordon, S. B., Walsh, A. L., Chaponda, M., Gordon, M. A., Soko, D., Mbwvinji, M., et al. (2000). Bacterial meningitis in Malawian adults: Pneumococcal disease is common, severe, and seasonal. *Clin Infect Dis, 31,* 53–57.

Gortmaker, S. L., Hughes, M., Cervia, J., Brady, M., Johnson, G. M., Seage, G. R., 3rd, et al. (2001). Effect of combination therapy including protease inhibitors on mortality among children and adolescents infected with HIV-1. *N Engl J Med, 345,* 1522–1528.

Grant, I., Sacktor, N., & McArthur, J. (2005). HIV neurocognitive disorders. In H. E. Gendelman, I. Grant, I. P. Everall, S. A. Lipton, & S. Swindells (Eds.). The neurology of AIDS, pp. 357–373. New York: Oxford University Press.

Gras, G. & Kaul, M. (2010). Molecular mechanisms of neuroinvasion by monocytes-macrophages in HIV-1 infection. *Retrovirology, 7,* 30.

Gray, F., Bazille, C., Adle-Biassette, H., Mikol, J., Moulignier, A., & Scaravilli, F. (2005). Central nervous system immune reconstitution disease in acquired immunodeficiency syndrome patients receiving highly active antiretroviral treatment. *J Neurovirol, 11* Suppl 3, 16–22.

Gray, F., Geny, C., Lionnet, F., Dournon, E., Fenelon, G., Gherardi, R., et al. (1991). [Neuropathologic study of 135 adult cases of acquired immunodeficiency syndrome (AIDS)]. *Ann Pathol, 11,* 236–247.

Gray, F., Gherardi, R., Keohane, C., Favolini, M., Sobel, A., & Poirier, J. (1988). Pathology of the central nervous system in 40 cases of acquired immune deficiency syndrome (AIDS). *Neuropathol Appl Neurobiol, 14,* 365–380.

Graybill, J. R., Sobel, J., Saag, M., van Der Horst, C., Powderly, W., Cloud, G., et al. (2000). Diagnosis and management of increased intracranial pressure in patients with AIDS and cryptococcal meningitis. The NIAID Mycoses Study Group and AIDS Cooperative Treatment Groups. *Clin Infect Dis, 30,* 47–54.

Grimm, S. A., McCannel, C. A., Omuro, A. M., Ferreri, A. J., Blay, J. Y., Neuwelt, E. A., et al. (2008). Primary CNS lymphoma with intraocular involvement: International PCNSL Collaborative Group Report. *Neurology, 71,* 1355–1360.

Grimwood, J., Mineo, J. R., & Kasper, L.H. (1996). Attachment of Toxoplasma gondii to host cells is host cell cycle dependent. *Infect Immun, 64,* 4099–4104.

Hakim, J. G., Gangaidzo, I. T., Heyderman, R. S., Mielke, J., Mushangi, E., Taziwa, A., et al. (2000). Impact of HIV infection on meningitis in Harare, Zimbabwe: A prospective study of 406 predominantly adult patients. *AIDS, 14,* 1401–1407.

Hamid, M. Z., Aziz, N. A., Zulkifli, Z. S., Norlijah, O., & Azhar, R. K. (2008). Clinical features and risk factors for HIV encephalopathy in children. *Southeast Asian J Trop Med Public Health, 39,* 266–272.

Hamilton-Dutoit, S. J., Raphael, M., Audouin, J., Diebold, J., Lisse, I., Pedersen, C., et al. (1993). In situ demonstration of Epstein-Barr virus small RNAs (EBER 1) in acquired immunodeficiency syndrome-related lymphomas: Correlation with tumor morphology and primary site. *Blood, 82,* 619–624.

Heaton, R.K., Clifford, D.B., Franklin, Jr D.R., Woods, S.P., Ake, C., Vaida, F., et al. (2010). HIV-associated neurocognitive disorders persist in the era of potent antiretroviral therapy. *Neurology, 75,* 2087–2096.

Heaton, R. K., Franklin, D. R., Ellis, R. J., McCutchan, J. A., Letendre, S. L., Leblanc, S., et al. (2011). HIV-associated neurocognitive disorders before and during the era of combination antiretroviral therapy: Differences in rates, nature, and predictors. *Journal of Neurovirology, 17(1),* 3–16.

Heyderman, R. S., Gangaidzo, I. T., Hakim, J. G., Mielke, J., Taziwa, A., Musvaire, P., et al. (1998). Cryptococcal meningitis in human immunodeficiency virus-infected patients in Harare, Zimbabwe. *Clin Infect Dis, 26,* 284–289.

Hide, G., Morley, E. K., Hughes, J. M., Gerwash, O., Elmahaishi, M. S., Elmahaishi, K. H., et al. (2009). Evidence for high levels of vertical transmission in Toxoplasma gondii. *Parasitology, 136,* 1877–1885.

Hill, D. & Dubey, J. P. (2002). Toxoplasma gondii: Transmission, diagnosis and prevention. *Clin Microbiol Infect, 8,* 634–640.

Holliman, R. E. (1988). Toxoplasmosis and the acquired immune deficiency syndrome. *J Infect, 16,* 121–128.

Hovette, P., Soko, T. O., Raphenon, G., Camara, P., Burgel, P. R., & Garraud, O. (1999). Cryptococcal meningitis in AIDS patients: An emerging opportunistic infection in Senegal. *Trans R Soc Trop Med Hyg, 93,* 368.

James, H. J., Sharer, L. R., Zhang, Q., Wang, H. G., Epstein, L. G., Reed, J. C., et al. (1999). Expression of caspase-3 in brains from paediatric patients with HIV-1 encephalitis. *Neuropathol Appl Neurobiol, 25,* 380–386.

Jarvis, J. N., Boulle, A., Loyse, A., Bicanic, T., Rebe, K., Williams, A., et al. (2009). High ongoing burden of cryptococcal disease in Africa despite antiretroviral roll out. *AIDS, 23,* 1182–1183.

Jarvis, J. N. & Harrison, T. S. (2007). HIV-associated cryptococcal meningitis. *AIDS, 21,* 2119–2129.

Jault, F. M., Spector, S. A., & Spector, D. H. (1994). The effects of cytomegalovirus on human immunodeficiency virus replication in brain-derived cells correlate with permissiveness of the cells for each virus. *J Virol, 68,* 959–973.

Jellinger, K. A., Setinek, U., Drlicek, M., Bohm, G., Steurer, A., & Lintner, F. (2000). Neuropathology and general autopsy findings in AIDS during the last 15 years. *Acta Neuropathol, 100,* 213–220.

Kanmogne, G. D., Kuate, C. T., Cysique, L. A., Fonsah, J. Y., Eta, S., Doh, R., et al. (2010). HIV-associated neurocognitive disorders in sub-Saharan Africa: A pilot study in Cameroon. *BMC Neurol, 10,* 60.

Kanmogne, G. D., Schall, K., Leibhart, J., Knipe, B., Gendelman, H. E., & Persidsky, Y. (2007). HIV-1 gp120 compromises blood-brain barrier integrity and enhances monocyte migration across blood-brain barrier: Implication for viral neuropathogenesis. *J Cereb Blood Flow Metab, 27,* 123–134.

Kaplan, J. E., Hanson, D., Dworkin, M. S., Frederick, T., Bertolli, J., Lindegren, M. L., et al. (2000). Epidemiology of human immunodeficiency virus-associated opportunistic infections in the United States in the era of highly active antiretroviral therapy. *Clin Infect Dis, 30* Suppl 1, S5–14.

Kasper, L. H. & Buzoni-Gatel, D. (1998). Some opportunistic parasitic infections in AIDS: Candidiasis, pneumocystosis, cryptosporidiosis, toxoplasmosis. *Parasitol Today, 14,* 150–156.

Kasper, L. H., Matsuura, T., & Khan, I. A. (1995). IL-7 stimulates protective immunity in mice against the intracellular pathogen, Toxoplasma gondii. *J Immunol, 155,* 4798–4804.

Kean, J. M., Rao, S., Wang, M., & Garcea, R.,L. (2009). Seroepidemiology of human polyomaviruses. *PLoS Pathog, 5,* e1000363.

Ketzler, S., Weis, S., Haug, H., & Budka, H. (1990). Loss of neurons in the frontal cortex in AIDS brains. *Acta Neuropathol, 80,* 92–94.

Khan, I. A. & Kasper, L. H. (1996). IL-15 augments CD8+ T cell-mediated immunity against Toxoplasma gondii infection in mice. *J Immunol, 157,* 2103–2108.

Khanna, N., Elzi, L., Mueller, N. J., Garzoni, C., Cavassini, M., Fux, C. A., et al. (2009). Incidence and outcome of progressive multifocal leukoencephalopathy over 20 years of the Swiss HIV Cohort Study. *Clin Infect Dis, 48,* 1459–1466.

Knowles, D. M. (1996). Etiology and pathogenesis of AIDS-related non—Hodgkin's lymphoma. *Hematol Oncol Clin North Am, 10,* 1081–1109.

Koralnik, I. J. (2006). Progressive multifocal leukoencephalopathy revisited: Has the disease outgrown its name? *Ann Neurol, 60,* 162–173.

Kossmann, T., Morganti-Kossmann, M. C., Orenstein, J. M., Britt, W. J., Wahl, S. M., & Smith, P. D. (2003). Cytomegalovirus production by infected astrocytes correlates with transforming growth factor-beta release. *J Infect Dis, 187,* 534–541.

Kovacs, J. A., Kovacs, A. A., Polis, M., Wright, W. C., Gill, V. J., Tuazon, C. U., et al. (1985). Cryptococcosis in the acquired immunodeficiency syndrome. *Ann Intern Med, 103,* 533–538.

Kraft-Terry, S. D., Buch, S. J., Fox, H. S., & Gendelman, H. E. (2009). A coat of many colors: Neuroimmune crosstalk in human immunodeficiency virus infection. *Neuron, 64,* 133–145.

Kraft-Terry, S. D., Stothert, A. R., Buch, S., & Gendelman, H. E. (2010). HIV-1 neuroimmunity in the era of antiretroviral therapy. *Neurobiol Dis, 37,* 542–548.

Kumar, G. G., Mahadevan, A., Guruprasad, A. S., Kovoor, J. M., Satishchandra, P., Nath, A., et al. (2010). Eccentric target sign in cerebral toxoplasmosis: neuropathological correlate to the imaging feature. *J Magn Reson Imaging, 31,* 1469–1472.

Kumarasamy, N., Solomon, S., Flanigan, T. P., Hemalatha, R., Thyagarajan, S. P., & Mayer, K. H. (2003). Natural history of human immunodeficiency virus disease in southern India. *Clin Infect Dis, 36,* 79–85.

Kumari, N., Krishnani, N., Rawat, A., Agarwal, V., & Lal, P. (2009). Primary central nervous system lymphoma: Prognostication as per international extranodal lymphoma study group score and reactive CD3 collar. *J Postgrad Med, 55,* 247–251.

Kwon-Chung, K. J. & Rhodes, J. C. (1986). Encapsulation and melanin formation as indicators of virulence in Cryptococcus neoformans. *Infect Immun, 51,* 218–223.

Langford, T. D., Letendre, S. L., Marcotte, T. D., Ellis, R. J., McCutchan, J. A., Grant, I., et al. (2002). Severe, demyelinating leukoencephalopathy in AIDS patients on antiretroviral therapy. *AIDS, 16,* 1019–1029.

Lescure, F. X., Gray, F., Savatovsky, J., et. al.(2010). Lymphocytes T8 infiltrative encephalitis: A new form of neurological complication in HIV infection. XVIII International AIDS Conference

Letendre, S., Marquie-Beck, J., Capparelli, E., Best, B., Clifford, D., Collier, A. C., et al. (2008a). Validation of the CNS Penetration-Effectiveness rank for quantifying antiretroviral penetration into the central nervous system. *Arch Neurol, 65,* 65–70.

Letendre, S., McCutchan, J. A., & Ellis, R. J. (2008b). Highlights of the 15th conference on retroviruses and opportunistic infections. Neurologic complications of HIV disease and their treatment. *Top HIV Med, 16,* 15–22.

Levy, R. M., Bredesen, D. E., & Rosenblum, M. L. (1985). Neurological manifestations of the acquired immunodeficiency syndrome (AIDS): Experience at UCSF and review of the literature. *J Neurosurg, 62,* 475–495.

Li, W., Li, G., Steiner, J., & Nath, A. (2009). Role of Tat protein in HIV neuropathogenesis. *Neurotox Res, 16,* 205–220.

Liner, K. J., 2nd, Hall, C. D., & Robertson, K. R. (2008). Effects of antiretroviral therapy on cognitive impairment. *Curr HIV/AIDS Rep, 5,* 64–71.

Liuzzi, G. M., Mastroianni, C. M., Santacroce, M. P., Fanelli, M., D'Agostino, C., Vullo, V., et al. (2000). Increased activity of matrix metalloproteinases in the cerebrospinal fluid of patients with HIV-associated neurological diseases. *J Neurovirol, 6,* 156–163.

Lobato, M. N., Caldwell, M. B., Ng, P., & Oxtoby, M. J. (1995). Encephalopathy in children with perinatally acquired human immunodeficiency virus infection. Pediatric Spectrum of Disease Clinical Consortium. *J Pediatr, 126,* 710–715.

Lokensgard, J. R., Cheeran, M. C., Gekker, G., Hu, S., Chao, C. C., & Peterson, P. K. (1999). Human cytomegalovirus replication and modulation of apoptosis in astrocytes. *J Hum Virol, 2,* 91–101.

Lortholary, O., Fontanet, A., Memain, N., Martin, A., Sitbon, K., & Dromer, F. (2005). Incidence and risk factors of immune reconstitution inflammatory syndrome complicating HIV-associated cryptococcosis in France. *AIDS, 19,* 1043–1049.

Lortholary, O., Poizat, G., Zeller, V., Neuville, S., Boibieux, A., Alvarez, M., et al. (2006). Long-term outcome of AIDS-associated cryptococcosis in the era of combination antiretroviral therapy. *AIDS, 20,* 2183–2191.

Luft, B. J. & Remington, J. S. (1992). Toxoplasmic encephalitis in AIDS. *Clin Infect Dis, 15,* 211–222.

Maher, D. & Mwandumba, H. (1994). Cryptococcal meningitis in Lilongwe and Blantyre, Malawi. *J Infect, 28,* 59–64.

Major, E. O. (2010). Progressive multifocal leukoencephalopathy in patients on immunomodulatory therapies. *Annu Rev Med, 61,* 35–47.

Marzocchetti, A., Di Giambenedetto, S., Cingolani, A., Ammassari, A., Cauda, R., & De Luca, A. (2005). Reduced rate of diagnostic positive detection of JC virus DNA in cerebrospinal fluid in cases of suspected progressive multifocal leukoencephalopathy in the era of potent antiretroviral therapy. *J Clin Microbiol, 43,* 4175–4177.

Marzocchetti, A., Tompkins, T., Clifford, D. B., Gandhi, R. T., Kesari, S., Berger, J. R., et al. (2009). Determinants of survival in progressive multifocal leukoencephalopathy. *Neurology, 73,* 1551–1558.

Maschke, M., Kastrup, O., Esser, S., Ross, B., Hengge, U., & Hufnagel, A. (2000). Incidence and prevalence of neurological disorders associated with HIV since the introduction of highly active antiretroviral therapy (HAART). *J Neurol Neurosurg Psychiatry, 69,* 376–380.

Masliah, E., DeTeresa, R. M., Mallory, M. E., & Hansen, L. A. (2000). Changes in pathological findings at autopsy in AIDS cases for the last 15 years. *AIDS, 14,* 69–74.

Matthiessen, L., Marche, C., Labrousse, F., Trophilme, D., Fontaine, C., & Vedrenne, C. (1992). [Neuropathology of the brain in 174 patients who died of AIDS in a Paris hospital 1982–1988]. *Ann Med Interne (Paris), 143,* 43–49.

McArthur, J. C. (2004). HIV dementia: An evolving disease. *J Neuroimmunol, 157,* 3–10.

McArthur, J. C., Hoover, D. R., Bacellar, H., Miller, E. N., Cohen, B. A., Becker, J. T., et al. (1993). Dementia in AIDS patients: Incidence and risk factors. Multicenter AIDS Cohort Study. *Neurology, 43,* 2245–2252.

McCarthy, K. M., Morgan, J., Wannemuehler, K. A., Mirza, S. A., Gould, S. M., Mhlongo, N., et al. (2006). Population-based surveillance for cryptococcosis in an antiretroviral-naive South African province with a high HIV seroprevalence. *AIDS, 20,* 2199–2206.

McCoig, C., Castrejon, M. M., Saavedra-Lozano, J., Castano, E., Baez, C., Lanier, E. R., et al. (2004). Cerebrospinal fluid and plasma concentrations of proinflammatory mediators in human immunodeficiency virus-infected children. *Pediatr Infect Dis J, 23,* 114–118.

McCombe, J. A., Auer, R. N., Maingat, F. G., Houston, S., Gill, M. J., & Power, C. (2009). Neurologic immune reconstitution inflammatory syndrome in HIV/AIDS: Outcome and epidemiology. *Neurology, 72,* 835–841.

McCutchan, J. A. (1995). Cytomegalovirus infections of the nervous system in patients with AIDS. *Clin Infect Dis, 20,* 747–754.

McCutchan, J. A. (2009). Management of HIV in resource limited settings. *Curr Opin Infect Dis, 22,* 464–470.

Miller, R. F., Isaacson, P. G., Hall-Craggs, M., Lucas, S., Gray, F., Scaravilli, F., et al. (2004). Cerebral CD8+ lymphocytosis in HIV-1 infected patients with immune restoration induced by HAART. *Acta Neuropathol, 108,* 17–23.

Mineo, J. R. & Kasper, L. H. (1994). Attachment of Toxoplasma gondii to host cells involves major surface protein, SAG-1 (P30). *Exp Parasitol, 79,* 11–20.

Miralles, P., Berenguer, J., Garcia de Viedma, D., Padilla, B., Cosin, J., Lopez-Bernaldo de Quiros, J. C., et al. (1998). Treatment of AIDS-associated progressive multifocal leukoencephalopathy with highly active antiretroviral therapy. *AIDS, 12,* 2467–2472.

Mirza, S. A., Phelan, M., Rimland, D., Graviss, E., Hamill, R., Brandt, M. E., et al. (2003). The changing epidemiology of cryptococcosis: An update from population-based active surveillance in 2 large metropolitan areas, 1992–2000. *Clin Infect Dis, 36,* 789–794.

Mitchell, C. D. (2006). HIV-1 encephalopathy among perinatally infected children: Neuropathogenesis and response to highly active antiretroviral therapy. *Ment Retard Dev Disabil Res Rev, 12,* 216–222.

Moosa, M. Y., & Coovadia, Y. M. (1997). Cryptococcal meningitis in Durban, South Africa: A comparison of clinical features, laboratory findings, and outcome for human immunodeficiency virus (HIV)-positive and HIV-negative patients. *Clin Infect Dis, 24,* 131–134.

Moreno, S., Mocroft, A., & Monforte, A. (2010). Medical and societal consequences of late presentation. *Antivir Ther, 15* Suppl 1, 9–15.

Morgan, J., McCarthy, K. M., Gould, S., Fan, K., Arthington-Skaggs, B., Iqbal, N., et al. (2006). Cryptococcus gattii infection: Characteristics and epidemiology of cases identified in a South African province with high HIV seroprevalence, 2002–2004. *Clin Infect Dis, 43,* 1077–1080.

Morgello, S. (1992). Epstein-Barr and human immunodeficiency viruses in acquired immunodeficiency syndrome-related primary central nervous system lymphoma. *Am J Pathol, 141,* 441–450.

Morgello, S., Cho, E. S., Nielsen, S., Devinsky, O., & Petito, C. K. (1987). Cytomegalovirus encephalitis in patients with acquired immunodeficiency syndrome: An autopsy study of 30 cases and a review of the literature. *Hum Pathol, 18,* 289–297.

Mwaba, P., Mwansa, J., Chintu, C., Pobee, J., Scarborough, M., Portsmouth, S., et al. (2001). Clinical presentation, natural history, and cumulative death rates of 230 adults with primary cryptococcal meningitis in Zambian AIDS patients treated under local conditions. *Postgrad Med J, 77,* 769–773.

Nachman, S. A., Chernoff, M., Gona, P., Van Dyke, R. B., Dankner, W. M., Seage, G. R., et al. (2009). Incidence of noninfectious conditions in perinatally HIV-infected children and adolescents in the HAART era. *Arch Pediatr Adolesc Med, 163,* 164–171.

Nath, A. & Sacktor, N. (2006). Influence of highly active antiretroviral therapy on persistence of HIV in the central nervous system. *Curr Opin Neurol, 19,* 358–361.

Navarro, J. T., Ribera, J. M., Oriol, A., Vaquero, M., Romeu, J., Batlle, M., et al. (1998). International prognostic index is the best prognostic factor for survival in patients with AIDS-related non-Hodgkin's lymphoma treated with CHOP. A multivariate study of 46 patients. *Haematologica, 83,* 508–513.

Navarro, J. T., Vall-Llovera, F., Mate, J. L., Morgades, M., Feliu, E., & Ribera, J. M. (2008). Decrease in the frequency of meningeal involvement in AIDS-related systemic lymphoma in patients receiving HAART. *Haematologica, 93,* 149–150.

Nebuloni, M., Cinque, P., Sidenius, N., Ferri, A., Lauri, E., Omodeo-Zorini, E., et al. (2009). Expression of the urokinase plasminogen activator receptor (uPAR) and its ligand (uPA) in brain tissues of human immunodeficiency virus patients with opportunistic cerebral diseases. *J Neurovirol, 15,* 99–107.

Nelson, J. A., Reynolds-Kohler, C., Oldstone, M. B., & Wiley, C. A. (1988). HIV and HCMV coinfect brain cells in patients with AIDS. *Virology, 165,* 286–290.

Neuenburg, J. K., Brodt, H. R., Herndier, B. G., Bickel, M., Bacchetti, P., Price, R. W., et al. (2002). HIV-related neuropathology, 1985 to 1999: Rising prevalence of HIV encephalopathy in the era of highly active antiretroviral therapy. *J Acquir Immune Defic Syndr, 31,* 171–177.

New, L. C. & Holliman, R. E. (1994). Toxoplasmosis and human immunodeficiency virus (HIV) disease. *J Antimicrob Chemother, 33,* 1079–1082.

Njamnshi, A. K., Bissek, A. C., Ongolo-Zogo, P., Tabah, E. N., Lekoubou, A. Z., Yepnjio, F. N., et al. (2009). Risk factors for HIV-associated neurocognitive disorders (HAND) in sub-Saharan Africa: The case of Yaounde-Cameroon. *J Neurol Sci, 285,* 149–153.

O'Sullivan, C. E., Drew, W. L., McMullen, D. J., Miner, R., Lee, J. Y., Kaslow, R. A., et al. (1999). Decrease of cytomegalovirus replication in human immunodeficiency virus infected-patients after treatment with highly active antiretroviral therapy. *J Infect Dis, 180,* 847–849.

Okongo, M., Morgan, D., Mayanja, B., Ross, A., & Whitworth, J. (1998). Causes of death in a rural, population-based human immunodeficiency virus type 1 (HIV-1) natural history cohort in Uganda. *Int J Epidemiol, 27,* 698–702.

Pappalardo, M. C. & Melhem, M. S. (2003). Cryptococcosis: A review of the Brazilian experience for the disease. *Rev Inst Med Trop Sao Paulo, 45,* 299–305.

Pappas, P. G., Bustamante, B., Ticona, E., Hamill, R. J., Johnson, P. C., Reboli, A., et al. (2004). Recombinant interferon-gamma 1b as adjunctive therapy for AIDS-related acute cryptococcal meningitis. *J Infect Dis, 189,* 2185–2191.

Park, B. J., Wannemuehler, K. A., Marston, B. J., Govender, N., Pappas, P. G., & Chiller, T. M. (2009). Estimation of the current global burden of cryptococcal meningitis among persons living with HIV/AIDS. *AIDS, 23,* 525–530.

Passos, L. N., Araujo Filho, O. F., & Andrade Junior, H. F. (2000). Toxoplasma encephalitis in AIDS patients in Sao Paulo during 1988 and 1991. A comparative retrospective analysis. *Rev Inst Med Trop Sao Paulo, 42,* 141–145.

Patel, K., Hernan, M. A., Williams, P. L., Seeger, J. D., McIntosh, K., Van Dyke, R. B., et al. 92008). Long-term effectiveness of highly active antiretroviral therapy on the survival of children and adolescents with HIV infection: A 10-year follow-up study. *Clin Infect Dis, 46,* 507–515.

Patel, K., Ming, X., Williams, P. L., Robertson, K. R., Oleske, J. M., & Seage, G. R., 3rd. (2009). Impact of HAART and CNS-penetrating antiretroviral regimens on HIV encephalopathy among perinatally infected children and adolescents. *AIDS, 23,* 1893–1901.

Paul, R. H., Laidlaw, D. H., Tate, D. F., Lee, S., Hoth, K. F., Gunstad, J., et al. (2007). Neuropsychological and neuroimaging outcome of HIV-associated progressive multifocal leukoencephalopathy in the era of antiretroviral therapy. *J Integr Neurosci, 6,* 191–203.

Paul, T., Challa, S., Tandon, A., Panigrahi, M., & Purohit, A. (2008). Primary central nervous system lymphomas: Indian experience, and review of literature. *Indian J Cancer, 45,* 112–118.

Pavesio, C. E. & Lightman, S. (1996). Toxoplasma gondii and ocular toxoplasmosis: Pathogenesis. *Br J Ophthalmol, 80,* 1099–1107.

Pereira-Chioccola, V. L., Vidal, J. E., & Su, C. (2009). Toxoplasma gondii infection and cerebral toxoplasmosis in HIV-infected patients. *Future Microbiol, 4,* 1363–1379.

Persidsky, Y., Ramirez, S. H., Haorah, J., & Kanmogne, G. D. (2006). Blood-brain barrier: Structural components and function under physiologic and pathologic conditions. *J Neuroimmune Pharmacol, 1,* 223–236.

Petito, C. K., Cho, E. S., Lemann, W., Navia, B. A., & Price, R. W. (1986). Neuropathology of acquired immunodeficiency syndrome (AIDS): An autopsy review. *J Neuropathol Exp Neurol, 45,* 635–646.

Pfeffer, G., Prout, A., Hooge, J., & Maguire, J. (2009). Biopsy-proven immune reconstitution syndrome in a patient with AIDS and cerebral toxoplasmosis. *Neurology, 73,* 321–322.

Poland, S. D., Costello, P., Dekaban, G. A., & Rice, G. P. (1990). Cytomegalovirus in the brain: In vitro infection of human brain-derived cells. *J Infect Dis, 162,* 1252–1262.

Price, R. W., Brew, B., Sidtis, J., Rosenblum, M., Scheck, A. C., & Cleary, P. (1988). The brain in AIDS: Central nervous system HIV-1 infection and AIDS dementia complex. *Science, 239,* 586–592.

Price, R. W. & Spudich, S. (2008). Antiretroviral therapy and central nervous system HIV type 1 infection. *J Infect Dis, 197* Suppl 3, S294–306.

Pulliam, L. (1991). Cytomegalovirus preferentially infects a monocyte derived macrophage/microglial cell in human brain cultures: Neuropathology differs between strains. *J Neuropathol Exp Neurol, 50,* 432–440.

Renold, C., Sugar, A., Chave, J. P., Perrin, L., Delavelle, J., Pizzolato, G., et al. (1992). Toxoplasma encephalitis in patients with the acquired immunodeficiency syndrome. *Medicine (Baltimore), 71,* 224–239.

Rex, J. H., Larsen, R. A., Dismukes, W. E., Cloud, G. A., & Bennett, J. E. (1993). Catastrophic visual loss due to Cryptococcus neoformans meningitis. *Medicine (Baltimore), 72*, 207–224.

Rigardetto, R., Vigliano, P., Boffi, P., Marotta, C., Raino, E., Arfelli, P., et al. (1999). Evolution of HIV-1 encephalopathy in children. *Panminerva Med, 41*, 221–226.

Roberts, T. K., Buckner, C. M., & Berman, J. W. (2010). Leukocyte transmigration across the blood-brain barrier: Perspectives on neuroAIDS. *Front Biosci, 15*, 478–536.

Robertson, K., Liner, J., Hakim, J., Sankale, J. L., Grant, I., Letendre, S., et al. (2010). NeuroAIDS in Africa. *J Neurovirol, 16*, 189–202.

Robertson, K. R., Smurzynski, M., Parsons, T.D., Wu, K., Bosch, R. J., Wu, J., et al. (2007). The prevalence and incidence of neurocognitive impairment in the HAART era. *AIDS, 21*, 1915–1921.

Roullet, E. (1999). Opportunistic infections of the central nervous system during HIV-1 infection (emphasis on cytomegalovirus disease). *J Neurol, 246*, 237–243.

Rubio, R., Pulido, F., Pintado, V., Diaz-Mediavilla, J., Flores, E., Serrano, M., et al. (1995). [Non-Hodgkin's lymphomas associated with the acquired immunodeficiency syndrome. A multicenter clinical study of 77 cases]. *Med Clin (Barc), 104*, 481–486.

Saag, M. S., Powderly, W. G., Cloud, G. A., Robinson, P., Grieco, M. H., Sharkey, P. K., et al. (1992). Comparison of amphotericin B with fluconazole in the treatment of acute AIDS-associated cryptococcal meningitis. The NIAID Mycoses Study Group and the AIDS Clinical Trials Group. *N Engl J Med, 326*, 83–89.

Saavedra-Lozano, J., Ramos, J. T., Sanz, F., Navarro, M. L., de Jose, M. I., Martin-Fontelos, P., et al. (2006). Salvage therapy with abacavir and other reverse transcriptase inhibitors for human immunodeficiency-associated encephalopathy. *Pediatr Infect Dis J, 25*, 1142–1152.

Sacktor, N. (2002). The epidemiology of human immunodeficiency virus-associated neurological disease in the era of highly active antiretroviral therapy. *J Neurovirol, 8* Suppl 2, 115–121.

Sacktor, N., Lyles, R. H., Skolasky, R., Kleeberger, C., Selnes, O. A., Miller, E. N., et al. (2001). HIV-associated neurologic disease incidence changes: Multicenter AIDS Cohort Study, 1990–1998. *Neurology, 56*, 257–260.

Sacktor, N., Nakasujja, N., Robertson, K., & Clifford, D. B. (2007). HIV-associated cognitive impairment in sub-Saharan Africa—the potential effect of clade diversity. *Nat Clin Pract Neurol, 3*, 436–443.

Sajadi, M. M., Roddy, K. M., Chan-Tack, K. M., & Forrest, G. N. (2009). Risk factors for mortality from primary cryptococcosis in patients with HIV. *Postgrad Med, 121*, 107–113.

Sanchez-Ramon, S., Bellon, J. M., Resino, S., Canto-Nogues, C., Gurbindo, D., Ramos, J. T., et al. (2003). Low blood CD8+ T-lymphocytes and high circulating monocytes are predictors of HIV-1-associated progressive encephalopathy in children. *Pediatrics, 111*, E168–175.

Sarciron, M. E. & Gherardi, A. (2000). Cytokines involved in Toxoplasmic encephalitis. *Scand J Immunol, 52*, 534–543.

Satishchandra, P., Mathew, T., Gadre, G., Nagarathna, S., Chandramukhi, A., Mahadevan, A., et al. (2007). Cryptococcal meningitis: Clinical, diagnostic and therapeutic overviews. *Neurol India, 55*, 226–232.

Scarmato, V., Frank, Y., Rozenstein, A., Lu, D., Hyman, R., Bakshi, S., et al. (1996). Central brain atrophy in childhood AIDS encephalopathy. *AIDS, 10*, 1227–1231.

Schulz, T. F., Boshoff, C. H., & Weiss, R. A. (1996). HIV infection and neoplasia. *Lancet, 348*, 587–591.

Schutte, C. M., Van der Meyden, C. H., & Magazi, D. S. (2000). The impact of HIV on meningitis as seen at a South African Academic Hospital (1994 to 1998). *Infection, 28*, 3–7.

Sevigny, J. J., Albert, S. M., McDermott, M. P., McArthur, J. C., Sacktor, N., Conant, K., et al. (2004). Evaluation of HIV RNA and markers of immune activation as predictors of HIV-associated dementia. *Neurology, 63*, 2084–2090.

Shanbhag, M. C., Rutstein, R. M., Zaoutis, T., Zhao, H., Chao, D., & Radcliffe, J. (2005). Neurocognitive functioning in pediatric human immunodeficiency virus infection: Effects of combined therapy. *Arch Pediatr Adolesc Med, 159*, 651–656.

Shankar, S. K., Satishchandra, P., Mahadevan, A., Yasha, T. C., Nagaraja, D., Taly, A. B., et al. (2003). Low prevalence of progressive multifocal leukoencephalopathy in India and Africa: Is there a biological explanation? *J Neurovirol, 9* Suppl 1, 59–67.

Shin, H. D., Winkler, C., Stephens, J. C., Bream, J., Young, H., Goedert, J. J., et al. (2000). Genetic restriction of HIV-1 pathogenesis to AIDS by promoter alleles of IL10. *Proc Natl Acad Sci U S A, 97*, 14467–14472.

Siddiqui, A. A., Brouwer, A. E., Wuthiekanun, V., Jaffar, S., Shattock, R., Irving, D., et al. (2005). IFN-gamma at the site of infection determines rate of clearance of infection in cryptococcal meningitis. *J Immunol, 174*, 1746–1750.

Skiest, D. J. & Crosby, C. (2003). Survival is prolonged by highly active antiretroviral therapy in AIDS patients with primary central nervous system lymphoma. *AIDS, 17*, 1787–1793.

Skolasky, R. L., Dal Pan, G. J., Olivi, A., Lenz, F. A., Abrams, R. A., & McArthur, J. C. (1999). HIV-associated primary CNS lymorbidity and utility of brain biopsy. *J Neurol Sci, 163*, 32–38.

Skolnik, P. R., Pomerantz, R. J., de la Monte, S. M., Lee, S. F., Hsiung, G. D., Foos, R. Y., et al. (1989). Dual infection of retina with human immunodeficiency virus type 1 and cytomegalovirus. *Am J Ophthalmol, 107*, 361–372.

Smith, A. B., Smirniotopoulos, J. G., & Rushing, E. J. (2008). From the archives of the AFIP: Central nervous system infections associated with human immunodeficiency virus infection: Radiologic-pathologic correlation. *Radiographics, 28*, 2033–2058.

Smith, J. E. (2009). Tracking transmission of the zoonosis Toxoplasma gondii. *Adv Parasitol, 68*, 139–159.

Snider, W. D., Simpson, D. M., Nielsen, S., Gold, J. W., Metroka, C. E., & Posner, J. B. (1983). Neurological complications of acquired immune deficiency syndrome: Analysis of 50 patients. *Ann Neurol, 14*, 403–418.

Sparano, J. A. (2001). Clinical aspects and management of AIDS-related lymphoma. *Eur J Cancer, 37*, 1296–1305.

Sparano, J. A., Anand, K., Desai, J., Mitnick, R. J., Kalkut, G. E., & Hanau, L. H. (1999). Effect of highly active antiretroviral therapy on the incidence of HIV-associated malignancies at an urban medical center. *J Acquir Immune Defic Syndr, 21* Suppl 1, S18–22.

Subramanian, S. & Mathai, D. (2005). Clinical manifestations and management of cryptococcal infection. *J Postgrad Med, 51* Suppl 1, S21–26.

Suzuki, Y., Yang, Q., Yang, S., Nguyen, N., Lim, S., Liesenfeld, O., et al. (1996). IL-4 is protective against development of toxoplasmic encephalitis. *J Immunol, 157*, 2564–2569.

Sweeney, B. J., Manji, H., Miller, R. F., Harrison, M. J., Gray, F., & Scaravilli, F. (1994). Cortical and subcortical JC virus infection: Two unusual cases of AIDS associated progressive multifocal leukoencephalopathy. *J Neurol Neurosurg Psychiatry, 57*, 994–997.

Sweet, T. M., Del Valle, L., & Khalili, K. (2002). Molecular biology and immunoregulation of human neurotropic JC virus in CNS. *J Cell Physiol, 191*, 249–256.

Tada, H., Rappaport, J., Lashgari, M., Amini, S., Wong-Staal, F., & Khalili, K. (1990). Trans-activation of the JC virus late promoter by the tat protein of type 1 human immunodeficiency virus in glial cells. *Proc Natl Acad Sci U S A, 87*, 3479–3483.

Tan, C. S. & Koralnik, I. J. (2010). Progressive multifocal leukoencephalopathy and other disorders caused by JC virus: Clinical features and pathogenesis. *Lancet Neurol, 9*, 425–437.

Tan, K., Roda, R., Ostrow, L., McArthur, J., & Nath, A. (2009). PML-IRIS in patients with HIV infection: Clinical manifestations and treatment with steroids. *Neurology, 72*, 1458–1464.

Tantisiriwat, W., Tebas, P., Clifford, D. B., Powderly, W. G., & Fichtenbaum, C. J. (1999). Progressive multifocal leukoencephalopathy in patients with AIDS receiving highly active antiretroviral therapy. *Clin Infect Dis, 28*, 1152–1154.

Taoufik, Y., Gasnault, J., Karaterki, A., Pierre Ferey, M., Marchadier, E., Goujard, C., et al. (1998). Prognostic value of JC virus load in cerebrospinal fluid of patients with progressive multifocal leukoencephalopathy. *J Infect Dis, 178*, 1816–1820.

Tassie, J. M., Gasnault, J., Bentata, M., Deloumeaux, J., Boue, F., Billaud, E., et al. (1999). Survival improvement of AIDS-related progressive multifocal leukoencephalopathy in the era of protease inhibitors. Clinical Epidemiology Group. French Hospital Database on HIV. *AIDS, 13*, 1881–1887.

Tassie, J. M., Pepper, L., Fogg, C., Biraro, S., Mayanja, B., Andia, I., et al. (2003). Systematic screening of cryptococcal antigenemia in HIV-positive adults in Uganda. *J Acquir Immune Defic Syndr, 33*, 411–412.

Teja, V. D., Talasila, S. R., & Vemu, L. (2005). Neurologic manifestations of HIV infection: An Indian hospital-based study. *AIDS Read, 15*, 139–143, C133.

Toborek, M., Lee, Y. W., Pu, H., Malecki, A., Flora, G., Garrido, R., et al. (2003). HIV-Tat protein induces oxidative and inflammatory pathways in brain endothelium. *J Neurochem, 84*, 169–179.

Torre, D., Ferrario, G., Speranza, F., Orani, A., Fiori, G. P., & Zeroli, C. (1996). Serum concentrations of nitrite in patients with HIV-1 infection. *J Clin Pathol, 49*, 574–576.

Torre, D., Speranza, F., & Martegani, R. (2005). Impact of highly active antiretroviral therapy on organ-specific manifestations of HIV-1 infection. *HIV Med, 6*, 66–78.

Vago, L., Bonetto, S., Nebuloni, M., Duca, P., Carsana, L., Zerbi, P., et al. (2002). Pathological findings in the central nervous system of AIDS patients on assumed antiretroviral therapeutic regimens: Retrospective study of 1597 autopsies. *AIDS, 16*, 1925–1928.

van der Horst, C. M., Saag, M. S., Cloud, G. A., Hamill, R. J., Graybill, J. R., Sobel, J. D., et al. (1997). Treatment of cryptococcal meningitis associated with the acquired immunodeficiency syndrome. National Institute of Allergy and Infectious Diseases Mycoses Study Group and AIDS Clinical Trials Group. *N Engl J Med, 337*, 15–21.

van Elden, L. J., Walenkamp, A. M., Lipovsky, M. M., Reiss, P., Meis, J. F., de Marie, S., et al. (2000). Declining number of patients with cryptococcosis in the Netherlands in the era of highly active antiretroviral therapy. *AIDS, 14*, 2787–2788.

Van Rie, A., Harrington, P. R., Dow, A., & Robertson, K. (2007.) Neurologic and neurodevelopmental manifestations of pediatric HIV/AIDS: A global perspective. *Eur J Paediatr Neurol, 11*, 1–9.

Vendrely, A., Bienvenu, B., Gasnault, J., Thiebault, J. B., Salmon, D., & Gray, F. (2005). Fulminant inflammatory leukoencephalopathy associated with HAART-induced immune restoration in AIDS-related progressive multifocal leukoencephalopathy. *Acta Neuropathol, 109*, 449–455.

Venkataramana, A., Pardo, C. A., McArthur, J. C., Kerr, D. A., Irani, D. N., Griffin, J. W., et al. (2006). Immune reconstitution inflammatory syndrome in the CNS of HIV-infected patients. *Neurology, 67*, 383–388.

Wahl, S. M., Allen, J. B., McCartney-Francis, N., Morganti-Kossmann, M. C., Kossmann, T., Ellingsworth, L., et al. (1991). Macrophage- and astrocyte-derived transforming growth factor beta as a mediator of central nervous system dysfunction in acquired immune deficiency syndrome. *J Exp Med, 173*, 981–991.

Wainstein, M. V., Ferreira, L., Wolfenbuttel, L., Golbspan, L., Sprinz, E., Kronfeld, M., et al. (1992). [The neuropathological findings in the acquired immunodeficiency syndrome (AIDS): A review of 138 cases]. *Rev Soc Bras Med Trop, 25*, 95–99.

Wiley, C. A., Schrier, R. D., Denaro, F. J., Nelson, J. A., Lampert, P. W., & Oldstone, M. B. (1986). Localization of cytomegalovirus proteins and genome during fulminant central nervous system infection in an AIDS patient. *J Neuropathol Exp Neurol, 45*, 127–139.

Wilson, E. H. & Hunter, C. A. (2004). The role of astrocytes in the immunopathogenesis of toxoplasmic encephalitis. *Int J Parasitol, 34*, 543–548.

Wong, H. L., Breen, E. C., Pfeiffer, R. M., Aissani, B., Martinson, J. J., Margolick, J. B., et al. (2010). Cytokine signaling pathway polymorphisms and AIDS-related non-Hodgkin lymphoma risk in the multicenter AIDS cohort study. *AIDS, 24*, 1025–1033.

Wright, E. J. (2009). Neurological disease: The effects of HIV and antiretroviral therapy and the implications for early antiretroviral therapy initiation. *Curr Opin HIV AIDS, 4*, 447–452.

Yadav, A. & Collman, R. G. (2009). CNS inflammation and macrophage/microglial biology associated with HIV-1 infection. *J Neuroimmune Pharmacol, 4*, 430–447.

Yiannoutsos, C. T., Major, E. O., Curfman, B., Jensen, P. N., Gravell, M., Hou, J., et al. (1999). Relation of JC virus DNA in the cerebrospinal fluid to survival in acquired immunodeficiency syndrome patients with biopsy-proven progressive multifocal leukoencephalopathy. *Ann Neurol, 45*, 816–821.

Zelman, I. B. & Mossakowski, M. J. (1998). Opportunistic infections of the central nervous system in the course of acquired immune deficiency syndrome (AIDS). Morphological analysis of 172 cases. *Folia Neuropathol, 36*, 129–144.

Zolopa, A., Andersen, J., Powderly, W., Sanchez, A., Sanne, I., Suckow, C., et al. (2009). Early antiretroviral therapy reduces AIDS progression/death in individuals with acute opportunistic infections: A multicenter randomized strategy trial. *PLoS One, 4*, e5575.

8.5

OPPORTUNISTIC INFECTIONS

Joseph R. Berger and Bruce A. Cohen

"As it takes two to mask a quarrel,
so it takes two to make a disease,
the microbe and its host." CHARLES V. CHAPIN [1856–1941], Papers, "The Principles of Epidemiology"

The focus of this chapter is on common and not-so-common infections of both the central and peripheral nervous systems seen in AIDS patients. It is organized by the nature of the infecting organism. Part I discusses viral opportunists—herpes viruses (cytomegalovirus, herpes simplex, varicella-zoster) and JC virus. Part II discusses bacteria—including mycobacteria tuberculosis, atypical mycobacteria, leprosy, syphilis, bartonella, listeria, and nocardia. Part III discusses fungus—cryptococcus, coccidiomycosis, histoplasmosis, blastomycosis, aspergillus, mucormycosis, candida albicans, sporotrichosis, and cladosporiosis. Part IV discusses parasites—toxoplasmosis, acanthamoeba, trypanosoma cruzi (Chagas disease), strongyloides stercoralis, cysticercosis. Part V discusses algae.

INTRODUCTION

Remarkable achievements in the treatment of HIV infection over the past 15 years have resulted in significant change in the epidemiology of the neurological opportunistic infections associated with HIV/AIDS. The availability of combination highly active antiretroviral therapy (HAART) has led not only to prolonged suppression of HIV replication, but also reconstitution of the immune system. Not unexpectedly, the frequency of most of these neurological opportunistic infections has declined in successfully treated individuals (Jellinger et al., 2000; Sacktor et al., 2001; Vago et al., 2002). Nonetheless, there still remains a reservoir of individuals whose first presentation of HIV is with a neurologic opportunistic infection, and a group of patients in whom even HAART therapy fails to maintain control of evolving species of resistant HIV, resulting in recurrent or persistent immune suppression and the potential for neurological opportunistic infection. The brain remains the second most common organ affected by HIV-related pathology (Masliah et al., 2000; Jellinger et al., 2000). When analyzed by the occurrence of AIDS-defining illness, some studies have shown little or no reduction in the proportion of common neurological opportunistic infections (Manfredi, Calza et al., 2001). While effective antiretroviral therapy has led to reduction in morbidity

and mortality, recovery of immune function attending their use has also been associated with the immune reconstitution inflammatory syndrome (IRIS) which not infrequently complicates the treatment of CNS opportunistic infection. The spectrum of HIV-associated neurological opportunistic infections in the era of HAART remains broad, including representatives of viruses, bacteria, fungi, and unicellular and multicellular parasites. Table 8.5.1 lists the CNS infections detected in a composite autopsy series of 926 patients with AIDS from seven separate studies (Kure, Llena et al., 1991). This chapter is devoted to the common and not so common infections of the central and peripheral nervous system seen in patients with the acquired immunodeficiency syndrome (AIDS). It has been organized by the nature of the opportunistic infection, namely, viruses, bacteria, fungi, and parasites.

VIRUSES

HERPES VIRUSES

Cytomegalovirus

Human cytomegalovirus (CMV) is a ubiquitous herpes virus acquired throughout life. In the United States, 60–80% of adults have serologic evidence of infection and 90% or more of HIV-infected patients acquire CMV (Drew, Mintz et al., 1981; Bale, 1984; Drew, 1988). Primary infection is usually asymptomatic in young healthy adults but may be associated with a transient mononucleosis-like syndrome (Klemola et al., 1969).

In the early years of the AIDS pandemic, CMV was a common and initially devastating opportunistic infection. With the introduction of HAART, however, the incidence of opportunistic CMV infections has dramatically declined. In the large Multicenter AIDS Cohort Study, the risk of opportunistic CMV infection was found to be reduced by 90% during the years of HAART therapy in comparison to rates observed in the era of monotherapy (Detels et al., 2001).

Cytomegalovirus	15.8%
Toxoplasmosis	13.6%
Cryptococcus	7.6%
Progressive multifocal leukoencephalopathy.	4.0%
HSV encephalitis.	1.6%
Candidiasis	1.1%
HZV encephalitis	0.6%
Histoplasmosis	0.4%
Tuberculosis	0.3%
Aspergillosis	0.3%

Neuropathologic series have described a range of pathology, from isolated cytomegalic cells to severe necrotizing hemorrhagic encephalitis, myelitis, or neuritis. In the brain, cytomegalocytes may be found in isolation or in association with microglial nodules. The most common neuropathologic pattern is a diffuse microglial nodular encephalitis disseminated in deep gray and to a lesser degree in white matter locations (Morgello et al., 1987; Vinters et al., 1989). Molecular diagnostic techniques increase the sensitivity of CMV detection and have identified CMV antigens or DNA in one-third or more of AIDS brains in the pre-HAART era. CMV is localized in microglial nodules, macrophages, astrocytes, oligodendrocytes, neurons, ependymal cells, endothelia, and meninges (Wiley & Nelson, 1988; Schmidbauer et al., 1989; Belec et al., 1990).

A necrotizing ventriculitis is seen in about 10% of cases with acute and chronic inflammatory infiltrates, cytomegalic cells, associated vasculitis, and meningitis with involvement of choroid plexus and cranial nerve roots and centrifugal extension of inflammation. Dystrophic calcification occurs in some instances (Morgello et al., 1987; Vinters et al., 1988; Kalayjian et al., 1993).

Focal necrotizing encephalitis and myelitis due to CMV results in discrete areas of parenchymal injury with variable degrees of associated inflammatory cell infiltration, cytomegalic cells, and hemorrhages. Multiple foci in both deep gray and white matter regions are present, often beyond what is apparent by imaging studies obtained in life. Macrophage infiltration may be prominant and vascular involvement leads to infarction and hemorrhage (Morgello et al., 1987; Vinters et al., 1988; Gungor et al., 1993).

CMV polyradiculomyelitis is usually characterized by a necrotizing radiculitis with associated vasculitis and segmental thrombosis, and a polymorphonuclear or mixed meningitis which may extend into the spinal cord (Eidelberg et al., 1986; Mahieux et al., 1989; Miller et al., 1990). Necrotizing myelitis may be associated (Jacobsen et al., 1988; Miller et al., 1990). Demyelination of nerve or spinal cord may be seen in conjunction with necrotizing radiculitis (Moskowitz et al., 1984; Bishopric et al., 1985).

Peripheral nerves may be affected by a multifocal necrotizing neuritis and arteritis with polymorphonuclear infiltration resulting in endoneurial necrosis. Cytomegalic cells may or may not be present. Involvement is characteristically asymmetric (Said et al., 1991; Roullet et al., 1994). CMV multifocal neuritis may affect cranial nerves (Small et al., 1989). Necrotizing optic neuritis may result from extension of CMV retinitis (Grossnik-Laus et al., 1987). Dorsal root ganglionitis has been found in association with necrotizing myelitis due to CMV (Tucker et al., 1985). Cytomegalocytes containing CMV-specific antigens have been found in Schwann cells (Bishopric et al., 1985; Grafe & Wiley, 1989), and demyelinating neuropathy has been attributed to CMV (Robert et al., 1989; Cornford et al., 1992; Morgello & Simpson, 1994).

In studies done prior to the HAART era, the frequency with which CMV could be found in neuromuscular tissue appeared to increase with survival following diagnosis of AIDS. In a series of 115 adult autopsies, 27% had light microscopic evidence of CMV in perineurial, epineurial, perimysial, or epimysial sites, usually in endothelia. The frequency increased from 19% in those having AIDS for three months or less to 46% in those having AIDS for two years or longer (Cornford et al., 1992).

The neuropathologic features are most suggestive of hematogenous dissemination to the CNS and peripheral nerve. Subsequent extension of infection may involve seeding by virus entering CSF as well as by contiguous extension (Morgello et al., 1987; Wiley & Nelson, 1988).

Clinical Features of CMV Neurologic Disease in AIDS

Several recognizable clinical syndromes in AIDS patients are associated with CMV opportunistic infection. These may occur in isolation or in concurrent or sequential combination (Cinque, Cleator et al., 1998; Anders & Goebel, 1999). Disseminated CMV infection is virtually always present, although it may not be recognized prior to neurologic presentation.

CMV ENCEPHALITIS Small case series and case reports have identified a number of clinical presentations of CMV encephalitis in AIDS (Arribas et al., 1996). A subacute diffuse encephalopathy evolving over weeks is characterized by impairments of cognition and sensorium, apathy, and withdrawal from normal activities. Confusion and disorientation contrast with HIV encephalopathy, in which sensorium tends to be preserved, and the course evolves more rapidly. Neurologic examination reveals slowing of cognition, impairment of memory and attention, and variable motor features, including hyperreflexia, ataxia, and weakness (Holland, Power et al., 1994). When ventriculitis is present, cranial neuropathies, nystagmus, and progressive ventricular enlargement may be seen (Kalayjian, Cohen et al., 1993). Progressive CMV encephalitis has been reported in an HIV-infected infant acquiring CMV infection in utero (Curless, Scott et al., 1987). A patient presenting with acute CMV encephalitis at the time of HIV seroconversion has been described (Berger, Bucher et al., 1996).

Patients with multifocal necrotizing encephalitis may complain of headache and localized symptoms. Fever and focal neurologic findings may be present on examination (Edwards et al., 1985; Laskin et al., 1987; Masdeu et al., 1988). A patient with hypopituitarism due to focal CMV infection of the hypothalamus has been described (Sullivan, Kelley et al., 1992). Brainstem encephalitis, with ataxia, oculomotor disturbances, quadraparesis, and bulbar dysfunction, has been described in occasional cases. Progressive confusion and obtundation may evolve. Autopsy studies revealed multifocal necrotizing encephalitis, with ventriculitis in one case and microglial nodular encephalitis with ventriculitis in another. A third case revealed widespread CMV infection with prevalent involvement of posterior fossa structures (Fuller et al., 1989; Pierelli et al., 1997).

Uncommonly, CMV may present as a mass lesion affecting brain or spinal cord. Pain and focal neurological findings including weakness, sensory loss, and aphasia have been described. Imaging studies reveal ring-enhancing mass lesions with or without mass effect and surrounding edema (Dyer et al., 1995; Moulignier et al., 1996; Huang et al., 1997). In one case, thallium-201 radionucleide scanning revealed increased uptake suggestive of tumor (Gorniak, Kramer et al., 1997). Diagnosis has required stereotactic brain biopsy.

Acute onset of neurologic deficit may occur in patients with cerebral infarctions resulting from CMV vasculitis and may progress in a stepwise fashion (Kieburtz, Eskin et al., 1993). Acute subarachnoid hemorrhage (Hawley, Schaefer et al., 1983) and intracerebral hemorrhage (Hawley, Schaefer et al., 1983; Dyer et al., 1995) have also been described.

Virtually all patients with CMV encephalitis will have systemic infection, which may occur despite maintenance antiviral therapy for CMV (Schwarz, Loeschke et al., 1990; Berman & Kim, 1994) as a result of emergent viral resistance. Autopsy studies of patients with CMV encephalitis commonly disclose involvement of other organs (Kalayjian, Cohen et al., 1993; Holland, Power et al., 1994).

Cerebral imaging studies are of limited sensitivity and even less specificity in patients with CMV encephalitis. Often they are negative or show nonspecific atrophy in patients with diffuse encephalitis (Clifford, Arribas et al., 1996). Ependymal or meningeal enhancement may be suggestive of CMV ventriculitis when present (Grafe, Press et al., 1990; Kalayjian, Cohen et al., 1993; Holland, Power et al., 1994), and areas of focal infarction or necrosis may be visualized (Masdeu, Small et al., 1988; Grafe, Press et al., 1990). Patchy or diffuse leukoencephalopathy can be seen in patients with CMV encephalitis (Miller, Lucas et al., 1997). Patients with ring-enhancing mass lesions due to CMV and one with a hemorrhagic mass have been described (Dyer, French et al., 1995; Moulignier, Mikol et al., 1996; Huang, McMeeking et al., 1997). Progressive ventricular enlargement may suggest ventriculitis (Kalayjian, Cohen et al., 1993).

Cerebrospinal fluid findings also vary. Most patients have nonspecific protein elevation. Glucose may be normal or decreased. Leukocytes may be absent or a modest lymphocytesis may be present (Holland, Power et al., 1994). A prominent pleocytosis with polymorphonuclear leukocytes may occur in patients with ventriculitis (Kalayjian, Cohen et al., 1993). CMV can rarely be cultured from CSF of patients with subacute encephalitis (Dix, Waitzman et al., 1985) or meningoencephalitis (Edwards, Messing et al., 1985). Specific oligoclonal bands directed at CMV antigens have been reported (Franciotta, Zardini et al., 1996). Identification of CMV DNA in the CSF using polymerase chain reaction amplification techniques is sensitive and specific (see below).

NECROTIZING MYELITIS Necrotizing myelitis due to CMV in HIV-infected patients is most commonly seen in association with polyradiculitis (Moskowitz et al., 1984; Tucker, Dix et al., 1985; Jacobsen, Mills et al., 1988), which is discussed below. Occasional cases of necrotizing myelitis in the absence of a typical polyradiculitis syndrome have been described, presenting with acute or progressive paraplegia and disturbances of urinary and rectal sphincter functions. Reflexes are preserved or enhanced in the legs unless concurrent neuropathy is present, and a sensory level may be demonstrable (Said et al., 1991; Gungor, Funk et al., 1993). Pathologic studies may reveal necrosis of both gray and white matter structures (Vinters, Kwok et al., 1989).

A patient with a demyelinating myelopathy involving the posterior columns associated with astrocytic gliosis, spongy changes with foamy macrophages, and numerous cytomegalic cells has been described. Necrosis or perivascular inflammation was not seen. Clinical features were compatible with a myelopathy (Moskowitz, Gregorios et al., 1984).

POLYRADICULOMYELITIS CMV polyradiculomyelitis in HIV-infected patients presents subacutely over days to a few weeks. Initial symptoms of paresthesias or dysesthetic pain localized to perineal and lower extremity regions are followed by a rapidly progressive paraparesis with hypotonia and diminished or absent lower extremity reflexes. Urinary retention is characteristic and rectal sphincter incontinence is common. Variable sensory findings are overshadowed by the motor features. Babinski reflexes and a sensory level may indicate an associated myelitis. With time, symptoms progress by ascending to involve the upper limbs and sometimes the cranial nerves (Tucker, Dix et al., 1985; Eidelberg, Sotrel et al., 1986; Behar, Wiley et al., 1987; Miller, Storey et al., 1990; Cohen, McArthur et al., 1993; So & Olney, 1994; Anders & Goebel, 1998).

Cerebrospinal fluid is usually characterized by a polymorphonuclear pleocytosis and a prominent elevation of protein. Hypoglycorrhachia is often present. Cases without these abnormalities have been reported, however (Miller, Fox et al., 1996). CMV may be cultured from CSF; however, successful demonstration of growth may take weeks (Tucker, Dix et al., 1985; Cohen, McArthur et al., 1993; So & Olney, 1994). Fortunately, current polymerase amplification techniques for identifying CMV DNA provide more sensitive and rapid diagnostic measures (see below).

MRI may be normal or reveal enhancement of the conus medullaris, cauda equina, meninges, and nerve roots in about one-third of cases (Bazan, Jackson et al., 1991; Talpos, Tien et al., 1991; Whiteman, Dandapani et al., 1994; Anders, Weiss et al., 1998). Electrophysiologic studies reveal features of an axonal neuropathy with acute denervation changes. Variable slowing of nerve conduction may also be present (Behar, Wiley et al., 1987; Miller, Storey et al., 1990).

The appearance of acute cauda equina syndrome in a patient with AIDS is suggestive of CMV when polymorphonuclear pleocytosis is present in CSF; however, the syndrome is not pathognomonic. Other conditions which may produce a cauda equina syndrome in AIDS patients include lymphomatous meningitis, syphilis, toxoplasmosis, other herpes viruses, cryptococcus, or bacterial meningitis.

MULTIFOCAL NEURITIS A progressive multifocal motor and sensory neuropathy which evolves over weeks to months has been demonstrated to result from CMV infection in AIDS. Initial paresthesiae and dysesthesiae are quickly followed by prominent motor weakness which involves both upper and lower limbs asymmetrically. Neurogenic atrophy may be prominent. Electrophysiologic studies reveal features of an axonal neuropathy with diminished sensory and motor nerve amplitudes and denervation changes. CMV viremia is often present. CSF may be normal or show nonspecific protein elevation. Nerve biopsy reveals a necrotizing neuritis with mononuclear and polymorphonuclear infiltrates and cytomegalocytes localized around endoneurial capillaries in nerve trunks and roots. Necrotizing arteritis may be present (Robert, Geraghty et al., 1989; Said, Lacroix et al., 1991; Roullet, Assuerus et al., 1994). Cranial nerves may be similarly affected (Small, McPhaul et al., 1989). A patient with a multifocal neuropathy revealing both necrotizing and demyelinating pathology has been described (Morgello & Simpson, 1994). Neuromuscular pathology due to CMV was found in 27% of a series of 115 AIDS autopsies, predominantly localized to perineurial and epineurial regions (Cornford, Ho et al., 1992).

Diagnosis of CMV Neurologic Disease in AIDS

Diagnosis of neurologic CMV infections during life in AIDS patients has been hindered until recently by the rarity of positive cultures from cerebrospinal fluid and the limited sensitivity and specificity of other diagnostic studies. Treatment was often empiric, when histopathologic confirmation of the diagnosis could not be obtained. The recent development of molecular diagnostic techniques and their application to cerebrospinal fluid analysis now provides the opportunity to diagnose and treat patients with CMV infection of the nervous system with increased sensitivity and potentially efficacy.

Detection of CMV DNA in CSF following polymerase chain reaction amplification (PCR) has been found to be highly sensitive and specific for CMV infection of the nervous system in retrospective studies (Cinque, Vago et al., 1992; Wolf & Spector, 1992; Gozlan, Salord et al., 1992; Clifford, Buller et al., 1993). A prospective study found sensitivity and specificity of CSF PCR to be over 90%, with positive and negative predictive values of 86 and 97%, respectively (Gozlan, el Amrani et al., 1995). Quantification of CMV DNA levels

has been correlated with histopathologic evidence of CNS infection in brain or spinal cord with the highest levels found in patients with ventriculoencephalitis (Arribas, Clifford et al., 1995). In contrast, a retrospective autopsy series found low specificity of CSF detection of CMV DNA for CMV encephalitis, though limited spinal cord and radicular tissue could be assessed (Achim, Nagra et al., 1994). It is now possible to quantify the CMV genomes in a sample of CSF and higher values can be used to discriminate productive from latent CMV infection (Wildemann, Haas et al., 1998).

In patients with polymorphonuclear CSF pleocytosis, detection of the CMV lower matrix phosphoprotein pp65 within neutrophil nuclei provided a rapid diagnostic test for CMV (Revello, Percivalle et al., 1994). Large atypical cells believed to be macrophages revealed positive immunoperoxidase staining with antisera directed at CMV in a patient determined to have CMV encephalitis and polyradiculitis (Marmaduke, Brandt et al., 1991). In situ hybridization with digoxigenin-labeled CMV probes detected CMV DNA in CSF cells of six patients with suspected CMV encephalitis, one of whom was confirmed at autopsy . Similar detection of CMV DNA in peripheral blood neutrophils was present in all six cases (Musiani, Zerbini et al., 1994).

Therapy of CMV Neurologic Disease in AIDS

At the time of this writing, three antiviral agents with efficacy against CMV patients are available for use. All three are virustatic and in the setting of persistent immune suppression require continued suppressive maintenance therapy during which viral resistance may emerge. Optimal regimens for treatment of CMV neurologic disease in AIDS are yet to be devised.

Ganciclovir (9-(1,3, -dihydroxy -2-propoxymethyl)-guanine) is an acyclic nucleoside which requires intracellular phosphorylation for efficacy. The first phosphorylation step is dependent on a viral phosphotransferase and the accumulation within infected cells imparts some selectivity to the agent (Matthews & Boehme, 1988). Clinical studies have established efficacy against CMV DNA polymerase in patients with CMV retinitis and gastroenteritis. Hematologic toxicity, particularly neutropenia and thrombocytopenia, is a common problem in the use of ganciclovir (1986; Laskin, Cederberg et al., 1987; Dieterich, Chachoua et al., 1988). Resistance related to deficient production of the viral phosphotransferase mediating the first intracellular phosphorylation has been shown to emerge during continued suppressive therapy (Erice, Chou et al., 1989).

Foscarnet (trisodium phosphonoformate) is also virustatic, exerting its effect against CMV DNA polymerase without requiring phosphorylation. It has some efficacy against the reverse transcriptase of HIV, as well (Palestine et al., 1991), and showed a benefit on survival compared to ganciclovir in patients treated for CMV retinitis (1996). Renal toxicity is the most significant adverse effect, though seizures and paresthesias may also be seen. Anemia and electrolyte disturbances and mild myelosuppression, which is aggravated by concomitant antiretroviral therapy, may also occur (Palestine et al., 1991). While foscarnet is active against ganciclovir-resistant strains of CMV, resistance to this agent may also emerge. Concurrent use of both agents may provide additional efficacy in patients with CMV retinitis or gastrointestinal disease despite failure of monotherapy with each (Dieterich, Poles et al., 1993; 1996).

Cidofovir is a nucleotide analogue of cytosine which selectively inhibits CMV DNA synthesis. In contrast to ganciclovir, cidofovir is phosphorylated to the active diphosphate form by intracellular host enzymes rather than those of the infecting virus. In vitro, it has broad activity against a broad spectrum of herpes viruses. Two major dose-limiting side effects are nephrotoxicity and ocular hypotony, which can lead to blindness if therapy is continued. Cidofovir is given intravenously with hydration and probenecid to limit uptake of the drug by renal tubules. In a prospective multicenter trial of individuals with AIDS and CMV retinitis progressing despite ganciclovir or foscarnet therapy, cidofovir was effective in delaying further progression of retinitis (Lalezari, Holland et al., 1998).

No prospective studies on treatment of neurologic CMV infections have been carried out to date. Case reports have been mixed, though some indications of potential efficacy can be found. In CMV encephalitis, response to ganciclovir in a patient with biopsy proven focal CMV encephalitis has been documented (Sullivan, Kelley et al., 1992). Encephalitis has occurred, however, despite maintenance ganciclovir therapy for CMV retinitis, suggesting the emergence of viral resistance (Schwarz, Loeschke et al., 1990; Berman & Kim, 1994). The addition of foscarnet reversed obtundation and improved CSF inflammation in a similar patient transiently, but recrudescence followed reduction in dosage several weeks later (Enting, de Gans et al., 1992). In patients with ventriculoencephalitis, response has been poor. Many of these patients were already exposed to ganciclovir because of prior CMV retinal or gastrointestinal disease (Kalayjian, Cohen et al., 1993), although one patient failed to respond to primary initiation of therapy (Price, Digioia et al., 1992). A patient who developed encephalitis one week following initiation of ganciclovir therapy for CMV retinitis responded to the addition of foscarnet at split doses of 180 mg/kg/day and was maintained on an alternating regimen of ganciclovir and foscarnet until cardiopulmonary death seven months later (Peters, Timm et al., 1992). Another patient who presented with CMV meningoencephalitis as his first opportunistic infection responded to ganciclovir with survival exceeding a year (Cohen, 1996). In an open observational series, 23 of 31 patients with CMV encephalitis or myelitis responded to a combined regimen of ganciclovir and foscarnet induction; however, 10 of the 22 patients subsequently relapsed in a median time of 126 days (Anduze-Faris, Fillet et al. 2000). Cases of successful treatment of ganciclovir-refractory CMV encephalitis with cidofovir have been reported (Blick, Garton et al., 1997; Sadler, Morris-Jones et al., 1997).

In patients with polyradiculomyelitis, a number of reports have noted response to prompt initiation of ganciclovir therapy. Response could be slow, requiring several months before neurologic improvement was seen. (Graveleau, Perol et al., 1989; Miller, Storey et al., 1990; Cohen, McArthur et al., 1993;

Kim & Hollander, 1993; Anders, Weiss et al., 1998). Other patients have failed to respond despite initiation of therapy (Jacobsen, Mills et al., 1988; de Gans, Portegies et al. 1990). Progression of polyradiculomyelitis in spite of ganciclovir has been shown to be associated with CMV resistance (Cohen, McArthur et al., 1993). Addition of foscarnet resulted in gradual improvement has resulted (Decker, Tarver et al., 1994). Improvement in two patients followed combined therapy with both agents after ganciclovir in one and foscarnet in the other failed as monotherapy (Karmochkine, Molina et al., 1994).

Multifocal neuropathy responds initially to therapy with ganciclovir; however, relapse of neuropathy or development of CMV polyradiculitis or encephalitis appears common. As much as 75% of patients with multifocal neuropathy may die of disseminated CMV infection (Said, Lacroix et al., 1991; Roullet, Assuerus et al., 1994).

Some authorities have recommended initial therapy with ganciclovir and foscarnet in combination for AIDS-associated CMV neurologic disease, recognizing that potential adverse effects are more likely (Kaplan, Benson et al., 2009).

Limited sensitivity of imaging studies and slow recovery in responsive patients has hindered decision making on modification of therapy. The best guidance for therapeutic efficacy may come from serial CSF studies. In patients with polyradiculomyelitis, resolution of polymorphonuclear leukocytosis and hypoglycorrhachia occurs quickly. Persistence appears indicative of viral resistance (Cohen, McArthur et al., 1993). The availability of PCR analysis for CMV DNA in CSF offers a means of serial monitoring, and small series suggest that this may be a useful marker of therapeutic response or failure (Cinque, Baldanti et al., 1995; Cohen, 1996).

Recent literature suggests that it may be possible to discontinue maintenance therapy against prior CMV opportunistic infection when immune reconstitution results in prolonged elevation of CD4 lymphocyte counts (Kirk, Reiss et al., 2002). It is currently recommended that secondary prophylaxis be discontinued when CD4+ counts > 100 cells/ul are sustained for 3–6 months, but that prophylaxis be reinstituted if CD4+ counts subsequently drop below this level (Kaplan, Benson et al., 2009). CMV opportunistic disease may recur in spite of robust increases in total CD4 counts, however, when deficits in CMV-specific CD4 T-cell responses persist (Komanduri, Feinberg et al., 2001).

Immune Reconstitution Disease

A case of CMV ventriculitis emerging 10 days following the institution of HAART, associated with a documented increase in CD4+ count from 42 to 159 cells/ul, and responding to therapy with ganciclovir and foscarnet has been reported (Janowicz, Johnson et al., 2005). A patient developing CMV polyradiculitis a month following HAART initiation, who recovered with ganciclovir treatment, has also been described (Majumder, Mandal et al., 2007). Both of these cases likely represent unmasking of latent CMV infection following immune reconstitution.

Herpes Simplex Virus (HSV)

Herpes simplex virus type 1 is commonly acquired early in life, while serologic evidence of HSV-2 infection increases with age and numbers of sexual partners. As much as 70% and 90% of sexually active heterosexual and homosexual men respectively, residing in some parts of the United States, may have serologic evidence of HSV-2 infection (Nahmias, Lee et al., 1990). HSV-2 is acquired through contact with infected mucosa where virus may be shed. Transport by retrograde axonal flow may lead to colonization of sacral ganglia and latency (Baringer, 1974). HSV-1 can also establish latency in the nervous system and has been recovered from trigeminal, superior cervical, and vagus ganglia (Baringer & Swoveland, 1973; Warren, Brown et al., 1978).

HSV-1 produces sporadic necrotizing encephalitis in apparently normal adults with a predilection to involve the temporal and inferior frontal regions of the brain. HSV-2 produces aseptic meningitis which may be recurrent (Craig & Nahmias, 1973). Despite the widespread prevalence and neurotropism of HSV, clinical reports of neurologic infections in HIV-infected patients are sparse, and may be confounded by concurrent opportunistic processes, particularly CMV. It has been suggested that a vigorous immune response may be an important element in the typical presentation of neurologic HSV infection and that the absence of normal immune responses may modify the neuropathology. An anergic patient with Hodgkin's disease and HSV encephalitis was noted to have limited neuronal loss and myelin damage (Price, Chernik et al., 1973). Another individual developed chronic encephalopathy while on steroid therapy. Biopsied brain tissue grew HSV but revealed no necrotizing features and only modest inflammation (Sage, Weinstein et al., 1985). It has been suggested that the paucity of inflammatory changes in some immunosuppressed individuals with fatal herpetic encephalitis indicates that an intact immune response is not required for severe neurological injury and that the incidence of HSV encephalitis may be underestimated in immune-suppressed populations as a result of alterations in the neuropathology (Schiff & Rosenblum, 1998).

Necrotizing temporal encephalitis has been reported occasionally in HIV-infected patients. Some atypical features may be present, such as the lack of a diffuse meningeal reaction and abundant viral inclusions several weeks after onset (Tan, Guiloff et al., 1993). Concurrent CMV ventriculoencephalitis and HSV-1 necrotizing temporal encephalitis has been described. Immunohistochemical and situ hybridization studies revealed two discrete processes (Vital, Monlun et al., 1995; Chretien, Belec et al., 1996). Two patients with lymphadenopathy and HIV-infection had temporal encephalitis with necrosis and intense inflammatory responses. HSV-2 grew from cultures of biopsied brain (Chretien, Belec et al., 1996).

The clinical presentations in these patients were acute, with fever, headache, confusion and lethargy, seizures, and in one case, hemiparesis. EEG revealed focal slowing or periodic discharges over the involved temporal and frontal regions. CT scans were normal in two and abnormal in one, revealing a localized hypodensity in the involved temporal lobe.

Cerebrospinal fluid was acellular in two and showed 11 mononuclear cells/mm^3 and 19 erythrocytes/mm^3 in another. Protein was elevated in two cases, normal in one, and glucose was normal in two. Cultures were unrevealing and PCR analysis failed to reveal HSV DNA in CSF of one patient obtained after 11 days of therapy. In each case diagnosis was established histopathologically, from biopsy tissue in three instances and at autopsy in one (Dix, Waitzman et al., 1985; Tan, Weldon-Linne et al,. 1993; Vital, Monlun et al., 1995). PCR amplification techniques now allow rapid detection of HSV-1 DNA in CSF of patients with herpetic encephalitis (Rowley, Whitley et al., 1990; Kessler, Muhlbauer et al., 2000) and are useful in monitoring successful antiviral therapy (Domingues, Fink et al., 1998).

Several patients with ventriculoencephalitis have been found to have both CMV and HSV in areas of ependymal and subependymal necrosis. In one patient, necrotizing retinitis due to both CMV and HSV was present in association with a necrotizing ventriculitis. Immunohistochemistry identified extensive CMV staining in necrotic regions while HSV staining in the brain occurred mainly in the endothelia of small arterioles and large venules (Pepose, 1984). In another, productive CMV ventriculitis occurred in association with anatomically separated HSV-1 temporal encephalitis (Chretien, Belec et al., 1996). In three other cases, immunostaining also revealed evidence of both viruses in necrotic regions but evidence of CMV appears to have been more extensive (Laskin, Stahl-Bayliss et al., 1987). In a large autopsy series of 82 cases of AIDS-associated CMV encephalitis, concomitant HSV infection was found in 16% of cases. Double label immunostaining revealed cytomegalic cells containing both CMV and HSV antigens usually within or at the borders of necrotic lesions. Although the high frequency of HSV-positive cells in some cases suggested that both viruses contributed to the necrotizing encephalitis, the relatively low percentage of cases with concomitant prominent HSV infection suggested to the authors that CMV was the predominant pathogen in the majority of the cases (Vago, Nebuloni et al., 1996).

Clinical presentations in these patients were acute delirium and seizures in one; subacute progressive ataxia, weakness, seizures and lethargy over six weeks in another; fever and headache in a third; and gradual deterioration over several months in a fourth, who also had treated CNS toxoplasmosis. The fifth patient was not noted to have a neurologic illness in life (Pepose, Hilborne et al., 1984; Laskin, Stahl-Bayliss et al., 1987; Chretien, Belec et al., 1996). While it would seem on the basis of current understanding that HSV may have been incidental to the CMV encephalitis in these patients, it is intriguing to speculate on possible synergies between the two herpes viruses.

Two patients with HIV infection and HSV brainstem encephalitis have been described, presenting with acute ataxia, fever, and disorientation. Magnetic resonance imaging (MRI) revealed several foci of increased signal on T2-weighted images without mass effect. Fatal progression ensued despite therapy with acyclovir. Autopsy revealed diffuse HSV infection of oligodendroglia, most intensely in the brainstem and cerebellum, though other regions also showed staining.

Demyelination with relative preservation of axons and minimal inflammation was observed. The HSV isolate recovered was found to be fivefold more virulent than a laboratory strain when inoculated into mice (Hamilton, Achim et al., 1995; Moulignier, Mikol et al., 1996). HSV DNA has also been identified in neuronal nuclei of an HIV-infected patient with microglial nodular brainstem encephalitis by in situ hybridization (Schmidbauer, Budka et al., 1989).

A diffuse meningoencephalitis in HIV-infected patients has been associated with HSV-2. The clinical presentation is nonspecific, with fever, headache, lethargy or delirium, tremors, or seizures in variable combinations. Imaging studies may be normal or, as in one case, reveal subdural fluid collections. A patient with central diabetes insipidus and HSV-2 meningoencephalitis has been described. Cerebrospinal fluid may yield a lymphocytic pleocytosis with reported cell counts as high as 720/mm³. Erythrocytosis may be present. Protein is usually elevated and may be markedly increased. In one patient, IgM antibodies to HSV were found in CSF and the CSF/serum index was elevated, indicating local production. HSV can be cultured from CSF, though cultures are often unrevealing. Brain biopsy in one patient yielded HSV-2 on culture. Concurrent herpetic lesions may be present in patients with meningitis (Dahan, Haettich et al., 1988; Gateley, Gander et al., 1990; Madhoun, DuBois et al., 1991). HSV-1 (Yamamoto, Tedder et al., 1991), and HSV-2 (Picard, Dekaban et al., 1993; Cohen, Rowley et al., 1994; Tedder, Ashley et al., 1994) DNA has been identified through PCR amplification in CSF of patients with recurrent meningitis.

HSV MYELITIS AND RADICULITIS Herpes genitalis has been shown to cause a lumbosacral radiculitis, producing paresthesiae and neuralgia in the perineum and lower extremities and urinary retention (Caplan, Kleeman et al., 1977). Meningitis and ascending myelitis may occur in association with (Craig & Nahmias, 1973; Wiley, Sofrin et al., 1987) or in the absence of vesicular eruptions (Klastersky, Cappel et al., 1972; Bergstrom, Vahlne et al., 1990). HSV-2 has been identified by immunohistochemical staining in spinal cord, chronically inflamed peripheral nerves, and dorsal root ganglia (Wiley, VanPatten et al. 1987). HIV-infected patients with apparent HSV-2 lumbosacral radiculitis (Madhoun, DuBois et al., 1991) and ascending myelitis have been described (Britton, Mesa-Tejada et al., 1985). Concurrent CMV infection was present in a patient presenting with a subacute polyradiculomyelitis. CSF revealed a polymorphonuclear pleocytosis with depressed glucose and elevated protein. At autopsy, CMV infection involved the brain, spinal cord, and some cranial nerves. HSV-2 staining was present by immunohistochemistry to a lesser degree. HSV-2 was cultured from cervical spinal cord, suggesting dual infection. The strain was identical to that cultured from a perirectal ulcer (Tucker, Dix et al., 1985).

A patient with necrotizing anterior spinal arteritis and associated myelomalacia had Cowdry type A intranuclear inclusions which stained positively for HSV-2 by immunohistochemistry. A small focus of CMV positive cells was seen and thought to be a superinfection. The clinical presentation

evolved over three months and consisted of low back pain, paresthesias and neuralgia in the perineum and lower extremities, followed by asymmetric leg weakness and urinary retention. Reflexes were lost in the involved limbs and a thoracic sensory level was present. Cerebrospinal fluid was acellular with elevated protein and normal glucose. CSF cultures were unrevealing (Britton, Mesa-Tejada et al., 1985).

Treatment of Neurologic HSV Infections in AIDS

Acyclovir [9-(2-hydroxyethoxymethyl)guanine], is the initial antiviral agent of choice for patients with HSV neurologic infection. Acyclovir is phosphorylated intracellularly to its active triphosphate form with the first phosphorylation dependent on a virus specified thymidine kinase. The triphosphate form binds HSV DNA polymerase and acts as a chain terminator (Whitley & Gnann, 1993).

The efficacy of acyclovir therapy of HSV neurologic infection has been variable in HIV-infected patients. Progression of HSV encephalitis has occurred in some cases in spite of therapy (Tan, Guiloff et al., 1993; Hamilton, Achim et al., 1995). Acyclovir treatment of cutaneous lesions failed to prevent progressive myelitis in a patient with HSV-2 infection (Britton, Mesa-Tejada et al., 1985). Improvement of encephalopathy but not an associated radiculomyelitis occurred in a patient with perianal HSV-2 (Madhoun, DuBois et al., 1991). In contrast, stabilization of HSV-2 encephalitis occurred in two patients given acyclovir following progression on vidarabine therapy (Dix, Waitzman et al., 1985).

Treatment of HSV infections is complicated by the emergence of acyclovir-resistant strains which have altered or absented thymidine-kinase activity (Erlich, Mills et al., 1989; Englund, Zimmerman et al., 1990). Acyclovir-resistant isolates have been thought to lack neurovirulence; however, a recent case of relapsing and ultimately fatal meningoencephalitis due to HSV-2 has been reported in which serial viral isolates demonstrated the emergence of acyclovir resistance during therapy. The addition of vidarabine was associated with transient improvement; however, rapid deterioration ensued a week later and repeat CSF yielded HSV-lacking thymidine kinase activity (Gateley, Gander et al., 1990). Persistence of HSV DNA in CSF of acyclovir-treated cases may suggest a resistant strain (Najioullah, Bosshard et al., 2000). An alternative therapy is foscarnet, which has been successfully used to treat acyclovir-resistant mucocutaneous lesions in HIV-infected individuals (Chatis, Miller et al., 1989; Safrin, Crumpacker et al., 1991; Safrin, 1992). The clinical setting is an important factor in choice of therapy as a case of HSV encephalitis in a patient on chronic therapy with foscarnet was found to be caused by a resistant strain (Read, Vilar et al., 1998).

VARICELLA-ZOSTER VIRUS (VZV)

Varicella-zoster virus produces distinct clinical syndromes in humans: chicken-pox and a variety of neurological syndromes resulting from reactivation of the virus. Restriction enzyme analysis has shown no detectable difference between matched viral isolates obtained during distinct episodes of chicken pox and subsequent zoster, indicating that both syndromes are caused by the same virus (Ilyid, Oakes et al., 1977), usually acquired in childhood. Decline in immune competence is associated with recurrent VZV, which presents as segmental radiculitis most commonly. The age adjusted risk of VZV radiculitis in HIV-infected individuals has been reported to be 17 times that of a noninfected homosexual control population, although occurrence did not predict faster progression to AIDS (Buchbinder, Katz et al., 1992). A community-based study in New York City reported that VZV radiculitis in a group of homosexual men was associated with the development of AIDS in almost 73% (Melbye, Grossman et al., 1987). The frequency of CNS zoster in autopsy series of AIDS patients has ranged from 2–4.4% (Petito, Cho et al., 1986; Gray, Belec et al., 1994).

The manifestations of segmental VZV radiculitis are similar in HIV and noninfected individuals, with a cutaneous eruption characterized by pain and vesicles on an erythematous base in a dermatomal distribution. The trunk is most commonly affected, followed by the face and extremities. Pain may occur without cutaneous lesions, or cutaneous dissemination may occur, suggesting viremia (Gelb, 1993). VZV DNA has been detected in circulating mononuclear cells during clinical VZV eruptions (Gilden, Devlin et al., 1989). Dermatomal zoster may be recurrent and multi-segmental in AIDS patients.

VZV may cause Ramsey-Hunt syndrome or herpes zoster oticus with a vesicular eruption in the auricle and external auditory canal and facial weakness (Mishell & Applebaum, 1990). Segmental myoclonus may precede or occur in association with VZV radiculitis (Koppel & Daras, 1992).

VZV Infection of the CNS in AIDS

VZV infection of the CNS in AIDS patients may produce a variety of neuropathology. A recent classification identified five clinicopathologic patterns: multifocal encephalitis, ventriculitis, acute meningomyeloradiculitis with necrotizing vasculitis, focal necrotizing myelitis, and vasculopathy resulting in cerebral infarction. Multiple patterns were found to occur in individual patients, all of whom were immunosuppressed with CD4 counts below 300/mm³ (Gray, Belec et al., 1994). Of clinical significance, a history of cutaneous VZV was absent in up to one-third of cases (Morgello, Block et al., 1988; Chretien, Gray et al., 1993; Gray, Belec et al., 1994; Moulignier, Pialoux et al., 1995).

VZV ENCEPHALITIS A leukoencephalitis with pathologic, radiologic, and clinical features resembling progressive multifocal leukoencephalitis has been demonstrated in several HIV-infected patients. Discrete ovoid or round lesions suggestive of PML are found in white matter with a predilection for gray-white junctions and periventicular regions. Zoster lesions also may be confluent and may occur in brain stem and cerebellar sites in addition to the cerebral hemispheres. Central cavitation necrosis with peripheral edema, reactive astrocytosis, and microglial proliferation comprise the architecture of the lesions and relative sparing of axons may or may not be seen in demyelinated regions. A necrotizing ventriculitis with associated vasculitis, similar to that caused by CMV, may be present. Cowdry type A inclusion bodies are found in astrocytes, oligodendroglia, macrophages, endothelial cells, ependyma, and neurons. When cutaneous zoster is associated, it may be recent or remote in occurrence and is often recurrent (Ryder, Croen et al., 1986; Morgello, Block et al., 1988; Gilden, Murray et al., 1988; Gray, Mohr et al., 1992; Gray, Belec et al., 1994; Amlie-Lefond, Kleinschmidt-DeMasters et al., 1995). The location of lesions in the periventricular regions and gray-white junctions suggests hematogenous dissemination to the CNS (Morgello, Block et al., 1988; Gray, Belec et al., 1994). Other cases where VZV is present in restricted distribution along discrete pathways indicate that trans-synaptic spread of VZV also occurs (Rosenblum, 1989; Rostad, Oson et al., 1989).

The most frequent clinical presentation in HIV-infected patients with VZV encephalitis is a diffuse subacute encephalopathy with headache, fever, cognitive deficits, lethargy or delirium, seizures, and variable focal deficits, evolving over weeks (Ryder, Croen et al., 1986; Morgello, Block et al., 1988). Acute encephalitis may be seen (Gray, Mohr et al., 1992; Aygun, Finelli et al., 1998) and a case of chronic progressive encephalitis evolving over months has been reported (Gilden, Murray et al., 1988; Weaver, Rosenblum et al., 1999). Isolated brainstem encephalitis has been described (Rosenblum, 1989; Moulignier, Pialoux et al., 1995) and a case of ophthalmic zoster followed by chronic progressive dissemination through the visual system (with some involvement of adjacent structures) over an 11-month period has been documented (Rostad, Oson et al., 1989).

Both CT and MRI scans may be normal (Ryder, Croen et al., 1986; Morgello, Block et al., 1988; Poscher, 1994), or show nonspecific lesions with or without peripheral contrast enhancement (Gilden, Murray et al., 1988; Rostad, Oson et al., 1989; Gray, Mohr et al., 1992; Moulignier, Pialoux et al., 1995). Recently, it has been suggested that MRI features characteristic of VZV include multiple well-defined discrete spherical or "target-like" lesions, often occurring in a regional distribution within the white matter. These evolve into confluent lesions with cavitation and both homogenous and ring-enhancing patterns following contrast infusion. Both infarctions and hemorrhages may be seen (deAngelis, Weaver et al., 1994; Aygun, Finelli et al., 1998; Weaver, Rosenblum et al., 1999).

Cerebrospinal fluid may be normal (Moulignier, Pialoux et al., 1995) but more often reveals features of a viral meningitis. Moderate lymphocytic pleocytosis, marked pleocytosis or acellular CSF may be seen. Protein elevation may be moderate or substantial. Glucose concentrations are usually normal (Dix, Bredesen et al., 1985; Ryder, Croen et al., 1986; Morgello, Block et al., 1988; Gilden, Murray et al., 1988; Gray, Mohr et al., 1992; Poscher, 1994). On occasion, VZV can be cultured from CSF, though this is infrequent (Dix, Bredesen et al., 1985) VZV-specific IgG antibodies may be detected by immunofluorescent assay in CSF of patients with meningo-encephalitis or meningomyelitis (Poscher, 1994; de Silva, Mark et al., 1996). Polymerase chain reaction amplification of

VZV DNA in CSF offers a sensitive and specific means of diagnosis (Rosemberg & Lebon, 1991; Shoji, Honda et al., 1992).

VZV Myelitis in HIV-infected Patients

Myelopathy is an uncommon complication of cutaneous VZV, occurring in less than 1% of cases. Symptoms and signs of spinal cord involvement usually begin within three weeks of the rash and progress to maximal deficit within another three weeks. Occasional cases where myelopathy preceded or followed the rash by up to ten weeks have been reported (Devinsky, Cho et al., 1991). In HIV-infected patients, the interval between cutaneous eruptions and the onset of myelopathy may be measured in months. Recurrent cutaneous lesions at multiple dermatomal levels may precede CNS disease (Devinsky, Cho et al., 1991; Gilden, Beinlich et al., 1994; Snoeck, Gerard et al., 1994). Myelopathy may appear prior to the cutaneous eruption (Gomez-Tortosa, Gadea et al., 1994; de Silva, Mark et al., 1996) or as an acute or subacute meningomyeloradiculitis in the absence of a cutaneous eruption (Vinters, Guerra et al., 1988; Chretien, Gray et al., 1993; Gray, Belec et al., 1994\).

A neuropathologic series including both HIV-infected and non-HIV-infected cases with VZV myelitis revealed extensive hemorrhagic necrotizing myelitis with vasculitis and thrombosis in dorsal root ganglia, and abnormalities of posterior nerve roots varying from lymphocytic infiltration to hemorrhagic necrosis. The most extensive pathologic changes were in the dorsal horns, ranging from focal necrosis with mild capillary proliferation and wedge-shaped demyelination to extensive necrotizing vasculitis and myelitis (Devinsky, Cho et al., 1991). Similar necrotizing myeloradiculitis and vasculitis has been found in HIV-infected patients presenting with rapidly progressive radiculomyelopathy. Cowdry type A inclusion bodies may not be seen even in the fulminant cases, or may occur so rarely as to hinder neuropathologic diagnosis. Immunohistochemistry and in situ hybridization techniques are more sensitive. Myelitis may be diffuse or restricted to segments associated with cutaneous eruptions (Vinters, Guerra et al., 1988; Chretien, Gray et al., 1993; Gray, Belec et al., 1994; de Silva, Mark et al., 1996). A case of spinal cord infarction in association with VZV ventriculitis and vasculitis involving surrounding leptomeningeal vessels has been described (Kenyon, Dulaney et al., 1996).

Clinical presentations of VZV myelitis in HIV-infected patients may be acute or subacute with progressive weakness, sensory impairment, and urinary sphincter dysfunction, often preceded by localized back pain. Evolution of symptoms may occur over days to weeks and may then accelerate rapidly to paraplegia (Vinters, Guerra et al., 1988; Gilden, Beinlich et al., 1994; Gomez-Tortosa, Gadea et al., 1994; Snoeck, Gerard et al., 1994). An acute rapidly progressive course may occur in some cases, culminating in paraplegia and urinary retention. Polyradicular involvement may produce loss of lower extremity reflexes, resulting in a picture similar to CMV polyradiculomyelitis (Vinters, Guerra et al., 1988; Chretien, Gray et al., 1993; Gray, Belec et al., 1994; Kenyon, Dulaney et al., 1996).

MRI may reveal non-enhancing focal intramedullary abnormalities (Gilden, Beinlich et al., 1994; de Silva, Mark et al., 1996), or prominant enlargement of the spinal cord with more extensive transverse abnormalities (Chretien, Gray et al., 1993; de Silva, Mark et al., 1996). Enhancing margins suggestive of meningitis or vasculitis may be seen (Snoeck, Gerard et al., 1994; Kenyon, Dulaney et al., 1996). On occasion, imaging may be normal (Gomez-Tortosa, Gadea et al., 1994). Cerebrospinal fluid may be normal or reveal nonspecific protein elevation and lymphocytic pleocytosis in more gradually evolving cases (Devinsky, Cho et al., 1991; Gilden, Beinlich et al., 1994; Gomez-Tortosa, Gadea et al., 1994; de Silva, Mark et al., 1996). In patients with more rapidly progressive necrotizing myelitis, CSF may contain a mixed lymphocytic and polymorphonuclear pleocytosis with predominance of either cell type (20–200 cells/mm^3), erythrocytosis (400–7300 cells/mm^3), and marked protein elevations (to 780 mg/dl) (Vinters, Guerra et al., 1988; Chretien, Gray et al., 1993; Snoeck, Gerard et al., 1994); Gray, Belec et al., 1994; Kenyon, Dulaney et al., 1996). VZV may be recovered from CSF (Snoeck, Gerard et al., 1994), but more commonly cultures are unrevealing.

VZV Vasculopathy in HIV-Infected Patients

Vascular lesions associated with VZV may involve large or small vessels and may be inflammatory or bland. They often occur in conjunction with other manifestations of CNS VZV in HIV-infected patients (Gray, Belec et al., 1994). Herpes zoster ophthalmicus may be complicated by contralateral hemiparesis resulting from infarction of arteries of the circle of Willis ipsilateral to the involved trigeminal nerve in both HIV-infected and uninfected patients. The interval between acute ophthalmic zoster and the infarction may be as long as a year in HIV-infected individuals (Zaraspe-Yoo, Miletich et al., 1984; Eidelberg, Sotrel et al., 1986; Pillai, Mahmood et al., 1989; Carneiro, Ferro et al., 1991, Rousseau, Perronne et al., 1993), and may be associated with VZV encephalitis (Gray, Belec et al., 1994; Amlie-Lefond, Kleinschmidt-DeMasters et al., 1995) or meningomyeloradiculitis (Gray, Belec et al., 1994). Recurrent cerebral infarctions may be the presenting manifestation of VZV encephalitis in HIV-infected individuals in the absence of cutaneous zoster (Amlie-Lefond, Kleinschmidt-DeMasters et al., 1995; Aygun et al., 1998).

Neuropathologic studies reveal noninflammatory vascular lesions of large leptomeningeal or small, deep penetrating arteries, with intimal or fibromuscular proliferation and focal thrombosis (Eidelberg, Sotrel et al., 1986; Morgello, Block et al., 1988; Gray, Belec et al., 1994; Amlie-Lefond, Kleinschmidt-DeMasters et al., 1995). In other individuals, necrotizing arteritis with transmural inflammation may involve large and small vessels (Gilden, Murray et al., 1988; Gray, Belec et al., 1994; Amlie-Lefond, Kleinschmidt-DeMasters et al., 1995; Kenyon, Dulaney et al., 1996). Immunohistochemical staining may reveal VZV in sites of vascular necrosis (Gray, Belec et al., 1994).

Magnetic resonance imaging studies reveal infarction patterns in small or large vessel territories (Eidelberg, Sotrel et al., 1986; Rousseau, Perronne et al., 1993). The combination of multifocal ischemic and hemorrhagic infarctions with deep white matter lesions may be suggestive of VZV in the context of AIDS (Amlie-Lefond, Kleinschmidt-DeMasters et al., 1995). Cerebral arteriography may show features of vasculitis (Carneiro, Ferro et al., 1991; Rousseau, 1994). Cerebrospinal fluid may be normal in VZV-related cerebral infarction, though more commonly nonspecific protein elevation is present. Modest pleocytosis may be present and glucose levels are normal or mildly decreased (Eidelberg, Sotrel et al., 1986; Carneiro, Ferro et al., 1991). Polymerase chain reaction amplification techniques allow identification of zoster DNA in CSF samples from patients with VZV vasculopathy (Amlie-Lefond, Kleinschmidt-DeMasters et al., 1995). A recent study suggests that the detection of anti-VZV IgG antibody in CSF by enzyme immunoassay is more sensitive than PCR in patients with Zoster vasculopathy (Nagel, Forghani et al., 2007).

Therapy of VZV in HIV-Infected Patients

In patients with cutaneous zoster, treatment with acyclovir may accelerate healing and alleviate acute pain (Wood, Ogan et al., 1988; Huff, Bean et al., 1988; Harding & Porter, 1991). The benefit of acyclovir for post herpetic neuralgia is less clear, with some reports noting a decreased incidence following seven or ten days of oral acyclovir (Huff, Bean et al., 1988; Harding & Porter, 1991), while others report no impact (Wood, Ogan et al., 1988; Wood, Johnson et al., 1994). Currently, valacyclovir or famciclovir are preferred because of improved pharmacokinetic properties and dosing regimen (Kaplan, Benson et al., 2009).

Treatment of CNS zoster in HIV-infected patients has been variable in cases reported to date. Progression of disease has occurred despite acyclovir or ganciclovir in patients with myelopathy (Chretien, Gray et al., 1993; Gilden, Beinlich et al., 1994). One patient survived without improvement of his paraplegia (Gomez-Tortosa, Gadea et al., 1994). The availability of PCR amplification has allowed detection of VZV DNA in CSF with subsequent institution of successful antiviral therapy (de Silva, Mark et al., 1996). Patients with acute encephalitis have also failed to respond to ganciclovir or acyclovir (Gray, Mohr et al., 1992; Amlie-Lefond, Kleinschmidt-DeMasters et al., 1995). One patient presenting with multiple cerebral infarctions was diagnosed by identification of VZV DNA in CSF after PCR amplification and appears to have stabilized on acyclovir therapy continued in maintenance dosages of 2400mg/day, though reported follow-up is limited to five months (Amlie-Lefond et al., 1995). Another, diagnosed by brain biopsy, improved with combined therapy using ganciclovir and foscarnet (Aygun, Finelli et al., 1998). Two patients with zoster retinitis and vasculopathy appear to have stabilized on high doses of oral acyclovir (3000 and 3200 mg/day) for as long as two years; however, one appeared to develop VZV encephalitis when the dose was reduced to 2000 mg/day (Rousseau, 1994). Four patients with meningitis due to VZV responded to intravenous acyclovir or ganciclovir. In each case, MRI scans of the brain revealed no parenchymal lesions (Poscher, 1994).

One therapeutic problem which may arise is resistance to acyclovir; however, relying on a lack of clinical improvement following 10 days of acyclovir therapy may overestimate the frequency of acyclovir resistance in HIV-infected persons and a 21-day course of therapy without response has been recommended in these patients before suspecting acyclovir resistance (Saint-Leger, Caumes et al., 2001). Acyclovir resistance is the consequence of absent or low production of viral thymidine kinase (TK), altered TK substrate specificity, or altered viral DNA polymerase. Infections with TK-negative variants are cross-resistant to other agents activated by viral TK, for example, ganciclovir, but are usually less virulent (Hayden, 2005). A patient with VZV meningoradiculitis who was found to develop resistance to acyclovir during therapy was treated with foscarnet, resulting in stabilization of his neurologic symptoms, though no improvement was seen. Subsequent dosage reduction of foscarnet from 180mg/kg/day to 90 mg/kg/day was followed by the occurrence of necrotizing retinitis and isolation of VZV from CSF. Despite increase in foscarnet dosage, gradual clinical deterioration ensued (Snoeck, Gerard et al., 1994). Vidarabine has activity against VZV, but has failed to prevent encephalitis in HIV-infected patients with ophthalmic zoster (Cole, Meisler et al., 1984). Foscarnet has been recommended for patients suspected to have acyclovir-resistant cutaneous zoster (Balfour, Benson et al., 1994); however, VZV resistance to foscarnet has also been described (Visse, Dumont et al., 1998). Assessment of drug sensitivity should be performed if the opportunity arises, but response may best be assessed by serial clinical and CSF monitoring. Combination therapy may provide more effective treatment. Earlier diagnosis and institution of effective antiviral therapy using PCR analysis of CSF specimens may prevent development of irreversible necrotizing encephalitis or myeloradiculitis. More recently, cidofovir has been suggested as another alternative (Kaplan, Benson et al., 2009).

IMMUNE RECONSTITUTION-RELATED ZOSTER INFECTIONS

Dermatomal zoster has been reported to increase in frequency following initiation of HAART, and related to increased numbers of CD8+ lymphocytes (Domingo, Torres et al., 2001). A case of transverse myelitis associated with increased numbers of CD8+ lymphocytes and NK cells in CSF but not blood, successfully treated with valacyclovir has been reported (Clark, Krueger et al., 2004), as have two cases of zoster encephalitis (Torok, Kambugu et al., 2008).

JC VIRUS

Progressive Multifocal Leukoencephalopathy

Progressive multifocal leukoencephalopathy (PML) is a demyelinating disease of the central nervous system that results from infection of oligodendrocytes with JC virus, a papovavirus (Richardson, 1988). This disorder was crystallized as a distinct entity in 1958 when Aström, Mancall, and Richardson identified the disorder on the basis of its unique pathological features (Astrom, Mancall et al., 1958). In 1965, viral particles morphologically typical of the papovaviruses were detected by electron microscopic studies in the brains of patients dying of PML (Zurhein & Chou, 1965) and, in 1971, JCV (named after the initials of the patient from whom it was first isolated) was cultivated and identified (Padgett, Walker et al., 1971).

Until the acquired immunodeficiency syndrome (AIDS) epidemic, experience with this disease was limited. A comprehensive review of PML published in 1984 found only 230 reported cases (Brooks & Walker, 1984). Within one year of the initial description of AIDS in 1981, PML was recognized as an associated disorder (Gottlieb, Schroff et al., 1981; Masur, Michelis et al., 1981; Siegal, Lopez et al., 1981; Miller, Barrett et al., 1982; Bedri, Weinstein et al., 1983). Until the time that HAART was introduced, approximately 4% to 5% of all HIV-infected individuals developed PML (Berger, Kaszovitz et al., 1987). Following the use of HAART, the incidence of PML in most populations studied has appeared to decline (Subsai, Kanoksri et al., 2006; Engsig, Hansen et al., 2009; Khanna, Elzi et al., 2009). In the intervals 1995–96, 1997–99, and 2000–2006, incidence rates declined from 3.3 per 1000 person-years to 1.8 and 1.3, respectively, in one Danish study (Engsig, Hansen et al., 2009). However, some studies have failed to reveal a reduction in the incidence of PML when the pre-HAART era was compared to the post-HAART era (Antinori, Ammassari et al., 2001; Yoritaka, Ohta et al., 2007). A study from Brazil reveals that among opportunistic infections of the brain, PML is only exceeded only by cerebral toxoplasmosis, cryptococcal meningoencephalitis, and CNS tuberculosis (Vidal et al., 2008). Despite HAART, HIV infection continues to be the greatest risk factor for PML. A study of national U.S. inpatient diagnosis codes from 1995 to 2005 identified 9,675 cases of PML in which HIV accounted for 7,934 (82%) (Molloy & Calabrese, 2009) and an autopsy study of 589 brains collected since 1999 by the National NeuroAIDS Tissue Consortium found PML in 28 (5%) (Everall, Vaida et al., 2009).

Earlier studies have suggested that by middle adulthood, as much as 80 to 90% of the population has IgG antibodies against JC virus and seroconversion rates have exceeded 90% in some urban areas (Walker & Padgett, 1983). More recent studies of JCV seroepidemiology using enzyme immunoassay studies suggests that seroprevalence rates may be considerably lower (Antonsson, Green et al., 2010; Knowles, Pipkin et al., 2003; Kean, Rao et al., 2009). No disease has been convincingly associated with acute infection, although Blake and colleagues reported meningoencephalitis identified by a rise of IgM titers to JCV in a 13-year-old girl (Blake, Pillay et al., 1992). Although the overwhelming majority of people have antibodies to JCV by adulthood, indicating prior exposure to the virus, the occurrence of PML in the absence of an underlying disorder, generally one associated with impaired cellular immunity, is quite unusual. Indeed, it is but a small minority of persons with a predisposing disorder who ultimately develop disease, suggesting that the presence of JCV and immunodeficiency are not by themselves sufficient conditions for the development of the disorder. In this respect, the development of PML in patients treated with natalizumab for multiple sclerosis and Crohn's disease has been very instructive for understanding the pathogenesis of PML (Berger, Houff et al., 2009). Natalizumab is an $\alpha 4\beta 1$ integrin inhibitor that mobilizes premature B cells, potential repositories of latent JC virus, from the marrow and also prevents inflammatory cells, including JC virus-specific cytotoxic T lymphocytes, from entering the brain (Berger, 2010). Neither MS or Crohn's disease had not been previously reported to occur in association with PML and the observation strongly implicates not only failed CNS immunosurveillance, but also the potential contribution of JCV-infected B cell release and activation in the genesis and expression of neurotropic forms of JCV.

Prior to the AIDS epidemic, the male to female ratio of PML approximated 1:1. The AIDS epidemic transformed this ratio from 5:1 (Holman, Janssen et al., 1991) to 8:1 (Berger, Pall et al., 1998). However, a changing pattern of infection with increasing numbers of women affected by AIDS as opposed to homosexual men has brought this ratio closer to parity. Furthermore, instead of affecting chiefly elderly individuals (Brooks & Walker, 1984), as was observed in studies prior to AIDS, PML has been a disease of the young and middle-age populations affected by AIDS. The greatest incidence is in individuals between the ages of 20 and 50 years (Brooks & Walker, 1984; Berger, Bucher et al., 1996). PML is rarely observed in immunosuppressed children, perhaps chiefly the result of the lower percentages of children who have been exposed to JCV. However, despite its rarity in this age group, it has been described in both HIV-infected children (Henson, Roseblum et al., 1991; Berger, Scott et al., 1992; Berger, Pall et al., 1998) and those with other underlying causes of immunodeficiency (Katz, Berger et al., 1994).

Despite the ubiquity of JCV infection, the mechanism of its spread remains uncertain. The demonstration of JCV DNA in tonsillar tissue (Monaco, Atwood et al., 1996) suggests that dissemination via an oropharyngeal route is likely, though remains unproven. The high prevalence of antibodies in the adult population and the rarity of PML in children supports the contention that PML is the consequence of reactivation of JCV in individuals who have become immunosuppressed. Additionally, high titers of IgM antibody specific for JCV, anticipated if PML were the result of acute infection, are not observed (Padgett & Walker 1983). Other support is forthcoming in those rare instances when recovery of JCV from blood or tissues obtained months to years before the development of PML and were essentially genetically identical to virus recovered from the brain or CSF at the time of diagnosis (Fedele, Ciardi et al., 2003; Major, 2010).

Until the mid 1980s, the overwhelming majority of patients with PML had lymphoproliferative disorders as the underlying cause of their immunosuppression (Brooks & Walker, 1984). Lymphoproliferative diseases remained the most common underlying illness for the development of PML until the AIDS pandemic. In a review of 69 pathologically confirmed cases and 40 virologically and pathologically confirmed cases of PML performed in 1984, Brooks and Walker found lymphoproliferative diseases accounted for 62.2% of the cases. In that series (Brooks & Walker, 1984), immune deficiency states were seen in 16.1%, but AIDS represented only 3% of the total number of cases. Since the AIDS pandemic, the frequency with which this formerly rare disorder was seen has increased substantially.

PML occurring in association with AIDS was reported within one year of the initial recognition of AIDS in 1981 (Gottlieb, Schroff et al., 1981; Masur, Michelis et al., 1981; Siegal, Lopez et al., 1981; Miller, Barrett et al., 1982). Since then, this formerly rare disease has become remarkably common. AIDS has been estimated to be the underlying disease for PML in 55% to more than 85% of all current cases (Major, Amemiya et al., 1992). Based on reporting of AIDS to the Centers for Disease Control (CDC) between 1981 and June 1990, 971 of 135,644 (0.72%) individuals with AIDS were reported to have PML (Holman, Janssen et al., 1991). This likely is an underestimate, since to be included in the CDC AIDS reporting system, PML cases must have pathologic confirmation. A study of PML among patients with AIDS in the San Francisco Bay area estimated a prevalence of PML of 0.3% (Gillespie, Chang et al., 1991). The findings of these investigators suggested that PML in HIV-infected patients was underestimated by as much as 50% (Gillespie, Chang et al., 1991). The intrinsic nature of mortality data, inaccurate diagnosis, and incomplete reporting may affect these estimates. Other types of studies suggest that the incidence of PML in AIDS cases is substantially higher than that reported by the CDC, with estimates of 1–5% in clinical studies and as a high as 10% in pathological series (Krupp, Lipton et al., 1985; Stoner, Ryschkewitsch et al., 1986; Berger, Kaszovitz et al., 1987; Kure, Llena et al., 1991; Kuchelmeister, Gullotta et al., 1993; Whiteman, Post et al., 1993). In one large, retrospective, hospital-based, clinical study (Berger, Kaszovitz et al., 1987), PML occurred in approximately 4% of patients hospitalized with AIDS. In a combined series of seven neuropathological studies comprising a total of 926 patients with AIDS (Kure, Llena et al., 1991), 4.0% had PML. Similarly, a neuropathology series from Switzerland detected PML in more than 7% of their patients dying with AIDS (Lang, Miklossy et al., 1989). A pathological study based on 548 consecutive, unselected autopsies between 1983 and 1991 performed on patients with AIDS by the Broward County (Florida) Medical Examiner revealed that 29 (5.3%) had PML confirmed at autopsy (Whiteman, Post et al., 1993). Yet another recent neuropathologic review, based on autopsies between 1985 and 1992, found 21 (9.8%) cases of PML in 215 individuals dying with AIDS (Kuchelmeister, Gullotta et al., 1993), but may have been influenced by the numerous referral cases from outside that study center (Kuchelmeister, Gullotta et al., 1993). The increasing frequency with which PML has been observed since the inception of the AIDS epidemic is attested to by a twelvefold increase in the disorder when the four year intervals 1981–1984 and 1991–1994 were compared in a series from south Florida (Berger, Bucher et al., 1996). Of 156 cases of PML in this series, only two were associated with immunodeficient states other than AIDS (Berger, Bucher et al., 1996). Bacellar and colleagues, studying the temporal trends in incidence of HIV-related neurologic disease in the Multicenter AIDS Cohort, noted that the average annual incidence rate of PML was 0.15/100 person-years, with a yearly rate of increase of 24% between 1985 and 1992 (Bacellar, Munoz et al., 1994). After adjusting for the CD4 lymphocyte count, there appeared to be no residual calendar trends in the incidence rate of PML (Bacellar, Munoz et al., 1994).

Macroscopically, the cardinal feature of PML is demyelination. Demyelination may, on rare occasion, be unifocal, but typically occurs as a multifocal process. These lesions may occur in any location in the white matter; however, they have a predilection for the parieto-occipital regions. Not infrequently, lesions involve gray matter (von Einsiedel, Fife et al., 1993) and are also found involving cerebellum, brainstem and, exceptionally, the spinal cord (Bauer, 1969; Kuchelmeister, Gullotta et al., 1993; von Einsiedel, Fife et al., 1993). In an autopsy series of 21 cases, 17 cases showed PML foci in infratentorial structure, 13 cases in cerebellum, 13 cases in brainstem, and 10 cases in both regions (Kuchelmeister, Gullotta et al., 1993). The lesions ranged in size from 1 mm to several centimeters (Astrom, Mancall et al., 1958; Richardson, 1970); larger lesions are not infrequently the result of coalescence of multiple smaller lesions.

The histopathological hallmarks of PML are a triad (Astrom, Mancall et al., 1958; Richardson, 1970) of multifocal demyelination; hyperchromatic, enlarged oligodendroglial nuclei; and enlarged bizarre astrocytes with lobulated hyperchromatic nuclei. The latter may be seen to undergo mitosis and appear to be quite malignant. In situ hybridization for JCV antigen allows for detection of the virion in the infected cells. Electron microscopic examination will reveal the JC virus in the nucleus of the oligodendroglial cells. These virions measure 28 to 45 nm in diameter and appear singly or in dense crystalline arrays (Zurhein & Chou, 1965; Zurhein, 1967). Less frequently, the virions are detected in reactive astrocytes and they are uncommonly observed in macrophages that are engaged in removing the affected oligodendrocytes (Mazlo & Herndon, 1977; Mazlo & Tariska, 1982).

Even though neuropathologic findings of PML do not reveal fundamental differences between cases with AIDS and non-AIDS PML, according to some investigators the former group more frequently tends to present with extensive lesions having particularly destructive, necrotizing character (Schmidbauer, Budka et al., 1990; Kuchelmeister, Gullotta et al., 1993). Whether these pathological changes has been tempered by HAART is unknown. Some investigators (Kuchelmeister, Gullotta et al., 1993; Berger & Concha, 1995) have suggested that AIDS-associated PML may present infratentorial lesions more frequently than non-AIDS PML cases, although others have not found a substantial difference (von Einsiedel, Fife et al., 1993).

CLINICAL FEATURES The clinical hallmark of PML is the presence of focal neurological disease associated with radiographic evidence of white matter disease generally occurring in the absence of mass effect. Emphasis needs to be placed on the focal features of this disease, particularly those that are apparent on clinical examination. The presence of focal findings on neurological examination is quite helpful in distinguishing this disorder from HIV dementia, which may be radiographically very similar. The most common presentations include weakness, gait abnormalities, speech disorders, visual deficits, and cognitive abnormalities. Table 8.5.1 summarizes the initial neurologic manifestations in four separate clinical series of patients with PML unrelated to AIDS (Brooks & Walker, 1984) and AIDS-associated PML (Berger, Kaszovitz et al., 1987; von Einsiedel, Fife et al., 1993; Berger & Concha, 1995).

Weakness is typically a hemiparesis, but monoparesis, hemiplegia, and quadriparesis may be observed with progression of disease. On occasion, the patient may present with a rapidly progressive flaccid hemiparesis that over time evolves into a spastic weakness. In older series, weakness is present in more than 80% of patients at the time of diagnosis (Arthur, Dagostin et al., 1989), but the improvement in the diagnostic modalities (in particular, MRI) and better familiarity with the disorder allows for earlier diagnosis. Other motor disturbances, including impaired dexterity, may also be observed. Limb and trunk ataxia resulting most often from cerebellar involvement is detected in 10%. A high proportion of patients with AIDS-associated PML will ultimately develop cerebellar lesions. Nearly one-third of patients have cerebellar signs at the time of diagnosis (Brooks & Walker, 1984; von Einsiedel, Fife et al., 1993). Extrapyramidal disease, at least at onset, is rare, but bradykinesia and rigidity may be detected in a substantial minority of patients with advanced disease (Richardson, 1970, Richardson, 1974). Dystonia and severe dysarthria have also been observed as a consequence of lesions in the basal ganglia (Singer, Berger et al., 1993; Singer, Stoner et al., 1994). Not unexpectedly, lesions due to PML in the basal ganglia are chiefly a reflection of involvement of medullated fibers coursing through this region rather than involvement of the deep gray matter (Whiteman, Post et al., 1993). For the most part, the presentation of the AIDS patient with PML does not appear to be substantially different from that of patients with PML complicating other immunosuppressive conditions except perhaps for a higher frequency of focal motor deficits, dysarthria, and limb incoordination (Krupp, Lipton et al., 1985; Berger, Kaszovitz et al., 1987; Berger, Bucher et al., 1996). The latter two may be a reflection of a greater frequency of infratentorial lesions in AIDS-related PML.

Neuro-ophthalmic symptoms occur in up to 50% of patients with PML and are the presenting manifestation in 30%–45% (Brooks & Walker, 1984). The most common visual deficits are homonymous hemianopsia or quadrantanopsia due to lesions of the optic radiations. Prior to AIDS and the introduction of MRI, cortical blindness was present at the time of diagnosis in up to 8% and occurred more commonly as the disease progressed (Brooks & Walker, 1984). Cortical blindness does not appear to be as frequent in the AIDS population as reported in previous series (Berger, Bucher et al., 1996). Other ophthalmic manifestations include optic aphasia, alexia without agraphia, and ocular motor abnormalities (Berger, Bucher et al., 1996). Optic atrophy is not seen.

The spectrum of cognitive changes observed is quite broad. Unlike the HIV-associated neurocognitive disorders (HAND), which may present as fluctuating, static, or slowly progressive neurocognitive deficits, the mental impairments of PML are often more rapidly advancing and typically occur in conjunction with focal neurological deficits. Among the abnormalities seen are personality and behavioral changes, poor attention, motor impersistence, memory impairment, dyslexia, dyscalculia, and the alien hand syndrome. A global dementia occurring in the absence of focal neurological disease is rarely the presenting manifestation of PML (Brooks & Walker, 1984; von Einsiedel, Fife et al., 1993). Weakness, cognitive disturbance, speech abnormalities, headache, gait problems, and visual disorders are the most common symptoms reported by patients with HIV-associated PML, whereas, in descending order of frequency, hemiparesis, abnormal gait, cognitive impairment, dysarthria, aphasia, and hemisensory loss were the most frequent signs (Berger, Pall et al., 1998). Other clinical manifestations that are observed less frequently, including sensory disturbances, vertigo, and seizures (Brooks & Walker, 1984; Berger, Kaszovitz et al., 1987; von Einsiedel, Fife et al., 1993; Berger, Bucher et al., 1996). Seizures may be seen and have been attributed to lesions that affect cortical gray matter (von Einsiedel, Fife et al., 1993). There appears to be a difference in the frequencies of the clinical manifestations occurring with HIV-associated PML in comparison to PML consequent to other immunosuppressive conditions.

In AIDS patients, as in those with other underlying diseases, PML usually progresses inexorably to death within a mean of four months (Brooks & Walker, 1984; Berger, Kaszovitz et al., 1987). Small clinical studies suggested that approximately 80% of patients with PML succumb within one year from the time of diagnosis (Kuchelmeister, Gullotta et al., 1993; Brooks & Walker, 1984; Berger, Kaszovitz et al., 1987; von Einsiedel, Fife et al., 1993; Moore & Chaisson, 1996); however, the largest series to date (Berger, Bucher et al., 1996) indicates that 80% die within 6 months of the diagnosis and the median survival is 3.5 months.

On occasion, individuals with PML experience clinical, radiographic, and pathological recovery, which, in some instances, may be complete. Often this includes full neurological recovery in the absence of specific therapeutic intervention (Berger & Mucke, 1988; Whiteman, Post et al., 1993). In our own experience, five pathologically confirmed AIDS patients with PML have exhibited both neurological recovery and survival in excess of one year (Berger, 1996). In one patient, survival from time of diagnosis was 92 months. Another patient had total remyelination in the previously affected areas at the time of autopsy more than 2 years after the diagnosis was first established (Berger, 1996). Survival exceeding 1 year was observed in 9% of pathologically proven cases in our experience (Berger, 1996). There was no correlation with treatment regimens, including the use of cytosine arabinoside. However, there appeared to be an association with PML as the heralding manifestation of AIDS, higher CD4 counts (often >200 cells/mm^3), inflammatory infiltration on biopsy, and contrast enhancement on CT scan or MRI (Berger, 1996). Others have described an improvement in AIDS-associated PML in association with the use of aggressive antiretroviral therapy (Fiala, Cone et al., 1988; Conway, Halliday et al., 1990; Singer, Stoner et al., 1994).

PML-IRIS has been seen regularly since the introduction of HAART. One study found that 26% of newly diagnosed HIV-associated PML was complicated by IRIS. In the largest study of PML-IRIS to date, Tan and colleagues identified 54 patients, of whom 36 had their PML unmasked at the time of IRIS and 18 had worsening of their PML (Tan, Roda et al., 2009). PML-IRIS is characterized by worsening clinical and radiographic features and typically, but not invariably, contrast-enhancing lesions on magnetic resonance imaging developing at a time that the HIV viral load has declined and CD4 count is normalizing. It has been reported to develop from 1 week to 26 months after the introduction of combined ART. While no controlled trials have been performed regarding the management strategies, corticosteroids seem to improve survival, particularly when administered early (Tan, Roda et al., 2009). However, some studies have failed to reveal an altered mortality with PML-IRIS (Falco, Olmo et al., 2008) and corticosteroid administration in this population is not without risk (Berger, 2009).

DIAGNOSIS The diagnosis of PML is strongly supported by radiographic imaging, but currently confirmation requires brain biopsy. Computed tomography (CT) of the brain reveals hypodense lesions of the affected white matter that generally do not enhance with contrast and almost always exhibit no mass effect. These lesions may have a "scalloped" appearance as a result of the subcortical arcuate fibers lying directly beneath the cortex (Whiteman, Post et al., 1993). With a higher sensitivity, magnetic resonance imaging (MRI) shows patchy or confluent hyperintense lesions on T2-weighted images in the affected regions. As with CT scan, contrast enhancement is an exception; however, contrast enhancement has been observed with both brain imaging techniques in approximately 5% to 10% of pathologically confirmed cases of PML (Whiteman, Post et al., 1993; Berger, Bucher et al., 1996). The enhancement observed is typically faint and peripheral. Mass effect in association with PML may be seen on rare occasions (Berger, Bucher et al., 1996). When present, it is usually quite subtle (Berger, Bucher et al., 1996).

The lesions of PML have a predilection for the frontal and parieto-occipital lobes (Whiteman, Post et al., 1993), but may occur virtually anywhere (Figure 8.5.1). Lesions may be unifocal, but in general are multiple and bihemispheric. Involvement of the basal ganglia, external capsule, and posterior fossa structures (cerebellum and brainstem) is not uncommon (Whiteman, Post et al., 1993). One-third to one-half of all patients will eventually have involvement of the posterior fossa and in 5–10% of patients the disease activity was isolated to these structures (Berger, Bucher et al., 1996).

Other diseases may cause white matter disease, especially in association with HIV infection. The demyelination observed with HIV dementia may be radiographically indistinguishable from that of PML. Clinically, however, PML is associated with focal neurological disease and is more rapidly progressive. Radiographic distinctions include a greater propensity of PML lesions to involve the subcortical white matter, its hypointensity on T1WI images, its rare enhancement, and more frequent occurrence of infratentorial lesions

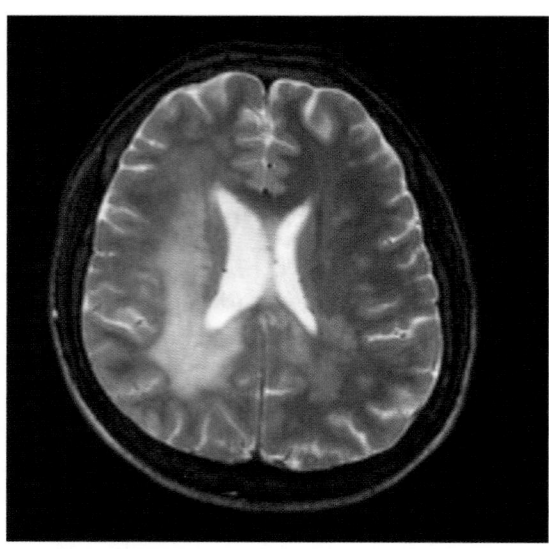

Figure 8.5.1 PML. This T2-weighted axial MRI shows a large hyperintense signal abnormality of the white matter of the right cerebral hemisphere from PML and several small lesions on the left side.

(Whiteman, Post et al., 1993). Cytomegalovirus (CMV) may also cause demyelinating lesions. Typically these lesions are located in the periventricular white matter and centrum semiovale, and subependymal enhancement is observed (Sze & Zimmerman, 1988; Bowen & Post, 1991). MRI images similar to those seen in PML have been recently described in a patient with dementia and extrapyramidal symptoms secondary to systemic lupus erythematosus (Kaye, Neuwelt et al., 1992).

Cerebrospinal Fluid and Other Studies

With the exception of polymerase chain reaction performed on cerebrospinal fluid (CSF) for the presence of JCV, other studies applied to CSF are nondiagnostic. The routine studies performed on CSF are usually normal (Brooks & Walker, 1984; Berger, 1987; von Einsiedel, Fife et al., 1993). In patients with PML-complicating HIV infection, the CSF abnormalities typically reflect those observed as a consequence of the HIV infection. These abnormalities may include a mononuclear pleocytosis ($\leq$20 cells/cu mm), elevated protein ($\leq$65 mg/dl), and borderline low glucose (Marshall, Brey et al., 1988; Navia, Jordan et al., 1986). PML in the absence of AIDS may be associated with a slight elevation in the CSF protein, a mild lymphocytic pleocytosis, and the presence of myelin basic protein (Brooks & Walker, 1984; Berger, 1987).

Until the early 1990s, the diagnosis of PML relied exclusively on typical histopathologic changes and detection of JC virus in brain samples from biopsies or at autopsy. JCV can be detected by electron microscopy or isolated in cell cultures, viral antigens can be detected by immunocytochemistry, and viral DNA can be detected by in situ hybridization or PCR (Zurhein & Chou, 1965; Padgett, Walker et al., 1971; Tornatore, Berger et al., 1992; Moret, Guichard et al., 1993). By electron microscopy using negative staining technique, papova-like particles were observed in two of three CSF samples from patients with clinical and neuroradiologic evidence of PML but not in 12 controls with AIDS (Orefice, Campanella et al., 1993).

The application of PCR for the detection of JCV DNA in CSF samples has been enormously helpful in establishing the diagnosis premortem with procedures that are less invasive than brain biopsy (Weber, Turner et al., 1990). Based on a series of 110 CSF samples, 28 PML cases, and 82 controls, Weber et al. reported 82% sensitivity and 100% specificity for diagnosis of PML with PCR (Weber, Bodemer et al., 1994). Yet another large cohort, 156 individual CSF samples, revealed a 92% sensitivity and specificity (McGuire, Barhite et al., 1994). With an overall sensitivity of 61%, Aksamit and Kost reported a specificity above 99% in a large sample size, 470 CSF samples (Aksamit & Kost, 1994). False positive samples might depend on the stage of the disease or on technical variation, such as set of primers and amount of CSF analyzed (Gibson, Field et al., 1981; Moret, Guichard et al., 1993; Weber, Bodemer et al., 1994). The range of sensitivity of JCV PCR in proficient laboratories is between 10 and 1 copy equivalents per 10 microl of CSF (Weber, Bodemer et al., 1994). Supersensitive quantitative real time PCR (Elfaitouri, Hammarin et al., 2006) and other techniques (Glass & Venter, 2009) have substantially improved the sensitivity of CSF PCR for JCV, but have not completely eliminated falsely negative studies.

Serum antibodies are not helpful in establishing the diagnosis, since 80% or more of the population show seropositivity to antibodies against JC virus by adulthood (Taguchi, Kajioka et al., 1982). JCV DNA was detected in the peripheral blood lymphocytes by PCR in nearly 30% of HIV-infected patients without PML (Dubois, Lafon et al., 1996). Intrathecal antibody synthesis of JCV-specific antibody can be performed (Weber, Trebst et al., 1997), but has not been used as a diagnostic method. Therefore, this test is not particularly useful in diagnosing the disorder. The electroencephalogram may show focal slowing, but, like other studies, is also nondiagnostic.

Currently, the diagnosis is established by the appropriate clinical manifestations and radiological findings coupled with the presence of a positive CSF PCR for JCV DNA. Other diagnostic possibilities need be excluded. If the CSF PCR remains negative and the clinical suspicion high for the disorder, a brain biopsy, still considered the gold standard for diagnosis, is required for confirmation.

Differential Diagnosis

The large increase in the incidence of PML in the last decades of the 20th Century has been due to the AIDS epidemic, and therefore, the majority of PML cases will present in AIDS patients. With increasing frequency, clinicians find themselves confronted by HIV-infected patients with cognitive impairment and a cranial MRI showing "hyperintense signal abnormalities on T2-weighted image (T2WI) characteristic of PML" due to the HIV dementia (AIDS dementia complex). It is the presence of these white matter lesions detected on MRI that frequently leads to the incorrect diagnosis of PML. HIV dementia may be the initial manifestation of AIDS in up to 3.0% of adult AIDS patients (Janssen,

Nwanyanwu et al., 1992; McArthur, Hoover et al., 1993), and has an estimated annual incidence of close to 7% following the diagnosis of AIDS. As many as one-third or more of AIDS patients will develop the disorder prior to death (McArthur, Hoover et al., 1993), although the frequency and severity of the disorder appears to have been positively impacted by the widespread use of highly active antiretroviral therapy (Sacktor, 2002).

Cardinal features include an insidiously progressive psychomotor slowing, impaired memory, and apathy (McArthur, Hoover et al., 1993; Price & Brew, 1988). Early complaints of forgetfulness, difficulty concentrating and manipulating complex tasks, problems reading, general slowness, headache, and fatigue are classic. Because of the advanced degree of immunosuppression, AIDS patients with HIV dementia or PML generally exhibit similar constitutional features, including, wasting, global alopecia, oral thrush and hairy leukoplakia, seborrheic dermatitis, and generalized lymphadenopathy. The patient with HIV dementia commonly has slow mental processing (bradyphrenia), abnormalities of saccadic and pursuit eye movements, diminished facial expression, low-volume, poorly articulated speech, impaired coordination and balance, postural tremor, poor dexterity, and a slow clumsy gait. Unlike PML, focal neurological findings are uncharacteristic and suggest an alternative diagnosis. CSF examination is most valuable in eliminating the possibility of other disorders. Pathological examination reveals brain atrophy and meningeal fibrosis. The most common histopathological feature of this illness is white matter pallor, associated with an astrocytic reaction chiefly distributed perivascularly in periventricular and central white matter (Navia, Cho et al., 1986). There is no evidence of myelin breakdown or loss of myelin basic protein. Multinucleate giant cells secondary to virus-induced macrophage fusion is the pathologic hallmark of the disease (Sharer, 1992). Other pathological features include microglial nodules, diffuse astrocytosis, and perivascular mononuclear inflammation (Navia, Cho et al., 1986).

In HIV dementia, the most commonly reported abnormality on CT of the brain is cerebral atrophy; however, low density white matter abnormalities are also frequently observed. CT scan is quite helpful in ruling out focal mass lesions as a cause of a patient's altered mental status (Katz, Berger et al., 1994). On MRI, large areas of white matter lesions are observed diffused over a large area, typically in the centrum semiovale and periventricular white matter (Olsen, Longo et al., 1988; Post, Tate et al., 1988). Less commonly, localized involvement with ill-defined margins (patchy) or small foci less than 1 cm in diameter (punctate) are observed (Olsen, Longo et al., 1988). These white matter abnormalities are frequently mistaken for PML and the history, clinical findings, and, to a lesser extent, CSF parameters are quite helpful in distinguishing between the two disorders (Griffin, McArthur et al., 1991; Royal, Selnes et al., 1994). The clinician needs to be mindful that these conditions are not mutually exclusive and that both conditions may coexist in the same patient.

HIV dementia and PML are not the only disorders of white matter occurring in AIDS in the absence of mass-producing lesions. Incidental white matter abnormalities are not uncommonly observed in HIV-infected individuals and do not appear to have any clinical significance (McArthur, Kumar et al., 1990). The appearance of white matter abnormalities in the absence of mass lesions can be seen with other HIV-related neurological disorders, including: i) a rare acute, diffuse,rapidly fatal leukoencephalopathy due to HIV; ii) an HIV-associated granulomatous angiitis; iii) a multifocal necrotizing leukoencephalopathy with a predilection for the pons; iv) a relapsing and remitting illness clinically indistinguishable from multiple sclerosis; v) CMV ventriculoencephalitis; vi) VZV encephalitis; and vii) other viral opportunistic infections (Olsen, Longo et al., 1988; Post, Tate et al., 1988).

TREATMENT Unequivocally, effective therapy of PML has remained elusive, whether specific antiviral therapy directed at the JC virus or attempts to enhance cellular immunity. A variety of treatment regimens has been proposed on the basis of anecdotal reports and small series. No randomized, double-blind therapeutic regimen has yet been completed, and the observation that PML may remain stable for long periods of time or even remit in the rare patient highlights the inadequacies of anecdotal reports suggesting the value of a specific therapy. The rarity of PML prior to the AIDS epidemic precluded practical therapeutic trials.

The nucleoside analogue, cytosine arabinoside, which is effective in suppressing JCV replication in vitro (Hou & Major, 1998) proved to be of no benefit in a clinical trial of HIV-associated PML when administered either intravenously or intrathecally and compared to antiretroviral therapy alone (Hall, Dafni et al., 1998). Similarly, topotecan has also been demonstrated to suppress JCV replication (Kerr, Chang et al., 1993), but is very difficult to administer in an immunosuppressed population and is without demonstrated efficacy clinically. An improved understanding of the mechanisms of JCV attachment and cellular entry has suggested that drugs that block the 5HT-2a serotonin receptor (e.g., mirtazapine) necessary for the former or that block clathirin-dependent cell entry (e.g., chlorpromazine) may prove useful in treating PML, but other than anecdotal reports, there has been no substantive confirmation supporting these therapies (Verma, Cikurel et al., 2007; Cettomai & McArthur, 2009; Lanzafame, Ferrari et al., 2009). An analysis of 2,000 off-the-shelf drugs and biological agents for effects on JCV revealed that the antimalarial drug, mefloquine, had anti-JCV activity (Brickelmaier, Lugovskoy et al. 2009). An ongoing clinical study is addressing whether it is capable of suppressing CSF JCV titers, but its use in natalizumab-associated PML appears not to be particularly promising (Clifford, DeLuca et al., 2010).

Additional study will be required to determine whether mefloquine or other antiviral agents will be successful in treating PML. Other proposed therapeutic strategies include the use of synthetic oligonucleotides designed to inhibit JCV genes or immunotherapies, such as, dendritic cell vaccines (Marzocchetti, Lima et al., 2009). Short of a successful antiviral agent for JCV, the most important therapeutic strategy is to restore normal adaptive immune function.

For HIV-associated PML that requires the use of effective combined ART to suppress HIV replication.

OTHER JCV-ASSOCIATED DISEASES

PML remains the most common of JCV-related neurological disorders; however, others have been described. JC virus granule cell neuronopathy has been observed both in association with PML and in isolation. This disorder results in a progressive cerebellar ataxia that advances over the course of weeks to months before plateauing. The disorder eventuates in dysarthria, limb and truncal ataxia, and gait ataxia that precludes independent ambulation. The first description in the AIDS population (Tagliati, Simpson et al., 1998) identified JCV in the granule cells of one patient, but an understanding of the true pathogenesis awaited more detailed analysis (Koralnik, Wuthrich et al., 2005). Isolated cases of JCV encephalopathy (Wuthrich, Dang et al., 2009) and JCV meningitis (Behzad-Behbahani, Klapper et al., 2003) have also been observed in immunosuppressed hosts, but have yet to be described with HIV infection.

BACTERIA

MYCOBACTERIA TUBERCULOSIS

HIV/AIDS predisposes to infection with tuberculosis. In some populations, one-third or more of the cases of tuberculosis occur in association with HIV infection (Pitchenik, Burr et al., 1987). These patients are more often Mycobacteria tuberculosis culture-negative and the majority are not known to be seropositive at the time of diagnosis of tuberculosis (Pitchenik, Burr et al., 1987). The incidence of tuberculosis occurring in association with AIDS is related to risk group. Pitchenik and colleagues observed that AIDS patients with tuberculosis in south Florida were more often younger (ages 25 to 44 years) and were more often of African American or of Haitian ancestry (Pitchenik, Burr et al., 1987). Intravenous drug abusers also appear to be at greater risk (Sunderam, McDonald et al., 1986). The percentage of AIDS patients with tuberculosis varies with locale (Nunn & McAdam, 1988), with the highest incidence in the United States among HIV-infected Haitians in south Florida, 60% of whom have tuberculosis (Pitchenik, Cole et al., 1984). High rates of tuberculosis among HIV-infected persons have been found worldwide (Nunn & McAdam, 1988). The highest rates of HIV-TB are in sub-Saharan Africa (Lawn & Churchyard, 2009), which has been estimated to account for 79% of the disease burden. There are approximately 1.37 million new cases of HIV-TB worldwide in 2007 (Lawn &Churchyard, 2009).

TUBERCULOUS MENINGITIS The clinical spectrum of CNS tuberculosis with HIV infection includes meningitis, cerebral abscesses, and tuberculomas (Bishburg, Sunderam et al., 1986); meningitis is the most common of these neurological complications and is typically characterized by seizures, altered mental status, and fever with meningismus (Bishburg, Sunderam et al., 1986). Although HIV infection appears to increase the risk for meningitis with *M. tuberculosis*, it does not appear to alter the clinical manifestations, response to therapy, or prognosis of the disease (Berenguer, Moreno et al., 1992). Tuberculous meningitis presents in a subacute fashion, preceded by a period of two to eight weeks of nonspecific symptoms which include malaise, anorexia, fatigue, fever, myalgias, and headache. In one large series, headache was reported by 86% of patients (Kent, Crowe et al., 1993). Neck stiffness is reported by about one-quarter of patients, but meningismus is detected in higher numbers at the time of examination (Kent, Crowe et al., 1993). Bulging fontanelles develop in infants. Patients become increasingly irritable. Nausea, vomiting, confusion, and seizures ensue. Behavioral disturbances including psychosis may also be observed (Daif, Obeid et al., 1992). A history of tuberculosis is obtained in approximately one-half of cases of childhood tuberculous meningitis (Lincoln, 1947) and in up to 12% of adult cases (Barrett-Connor, 1967; Traub, Colchester et al., 1984; Ogawa, Smith et al., 1987).

Although some series report that fever is absent in up to 20% of patients with tuberculous meningitis, a low-grade fever is typically present except in the elderly and immunosuppressed. Teoh and Humphries (1991) state that in their experience the fever is rarely in excess of 39° C. when the tuberculous involvement is limited to the meninges alone. Indeed, in the HIV-infected population, the cardinal features of tuberculous meningitis are often absent. In a Brazilian study of 108 co-infected persons, only 15% had concomitant fever, headache, and meningeal signs (Croda, Vidal et al., 2009).

Meningismus is noted in the adult patients, but is not invariable (Barrett-Connor, 1967; Traub, Colchester et al., 1984; Ogawa, Smith et al., 1987). Cranial nerve palsies are common. In descending order of frequency, the sixth cranial nerve is most commonly affected, followed by the third, fourth, seventh, second, eighth, tenth, eleventh, and twelfth (Lincoln, Sordillo et al., 1960; Traub, Colchester et al., 1984). Papilledema is frequently observed and, on occasion, fundoscopic examination may reveal choroid tubercles, which are yellow lesions with indistinct borders present either singly or in clusters. Their presence is convincing evidence of the disease, but they appear in only about 10% of cases of tuberculous meningitis not associated with miliary tuberculosis (Illingworth & Lorber, 1956; Lincoln, Sordillo et al., 1960). Visual impairment should be not immediately be ascribed solely to tuberculous meningitis. Optochiasmatic arachnoiditis, tuberculomas compressing the optic nerves and ethambutol toxicity in treated patients need to be considered (Teoh & Humphries, 1991). Ophthalmoplegia may result from involvement of the third, fourth, or sixth cranial nerves. Alternatively, ophthalmoplegia due to parenchymal lesions resulting in gaze palsies and internuclear ophthalmoplegia may be observed, the consequence of vasculitic lesions or tuberculoses. Facial palsy and hearing loss attend the less frequent involvement of the seventh and eight cranial nerves, respectively. Among the neurological signs observed are hemiparesis and hemiplegia and a wide variety of movement disorders, including chorea, hemiballismus, athetosis, cerebellar ataxia, and myoclonus (Alarcon, Duenas et al., 2000). These abnormalities are usually the consequence of infarction due to tuberculous vasculitis, but may occur as the result of mass lesions from tuberculoma or tuberculous abscesses. Involuntary movements may be observed in as many as 13%, occur more commonly in children and, in rare instances, may persist after treatment (Udani, Parekh et al., 1971). Seizures, either focal or generalized, may occur during the acute illness or months after treatment.

A higher incidence of intracranial tuberculomas (Bishburg, Sunderam et al., 1986; Dube, Holtom et al., 1992) and tuberculous brain abscesses (Velasco-Martinez, Guerrero-Espejo et al., 1995) is noted with HIV infection, although this observation has been questioned (Pagnoux, Genereau et al., 2000). Typically, these lesions are characterized by ring-enhancing masses on radiographic imaging. These lesions may occur as the heralding manifestation of HIV infection and may also be seen in the absence of positive tuberculin skin tests and abnormal chest radiographs (Velasco-Martinez, Guerrero-Espejo et al., 1995). Tuberculomas and tuberculous abscesses may result in seizures as well, but most often present as focal neurological disturbances resulting from mass lesions that may lead to brain herniation. In rare instances, paraparesis may attend an associated myelopathy due to proliferative granulomatous meningitis secondary to M. tuberculosis (Vlcek, Burchiel et al., 1984) or may occur as a consequence of spinal abscess (Doll, Yarbro et al., 1987).

Diagnosis in HIV-Infected Patients

RADIOGRAPHIC STUDIES Computed tomography (CT) or magnetic resonance imaging (MRI) of the head often reveals thickening and enhancement of the meninges, particularly the basilar meninges, with hydrocephalus, infarction (Bullock & Welchman, 1982; Witrack & Ellis, 1985), edema (often located periventricularly) (Bullock & Welchman, 1982), and mass lesion due to associated tuberculoma or tuberculous abscess. In all patients, whether HIV infected (Villoria, de la Torre et al., 1992) or not, hydrocephalus appears to be the single most common abnormality seen in tuberculous meningitis on CT or MRI. It has been reported in 80% of patients (Offenbacher, Fazekas et al., 1991) and was detected in 100% of 30 children with CNS tuberculosis in another (Waecker & Connor, 1990). Ventricular dilatation is seen in about 50% of HIV-infected persons with tuberculous meningitis (Davis, Rastogi et al., 1993; Villoria, de la Torre et al., 1992). The degree of hydrocephalus correlates with the duration of the disease (Bhargava, Gupta et al., 1982). Enhancement of the meninges is observed in approximately 50–60%, and infarctions, the third most common CT finding, are seen in about one fourth of patients (Offenbacher, Fazekas et al., 1991; Villoria, de la Torre et al., 1992)). The latter is a consequence of reactive endarteritis obliterans occurring as a consequence of the bathing of arteries that course though the thick, gelatinous exudate located at the base of the brain. Arteritis occurs in approximately 30 to 40% of cases with basilar meningitis (Leiguarda, Berthier et al., 1988) and the middle cerebral artery and small perforating branches to the basal ganglia are the vessels most often affected (Sheller & Des Prez, 1986). Radiographic imaging of the diffuse infiltration of the brain parenchyma by small granulomas (<5 mm) in the course of miliary tuberculosis may reveal multiple, small, contrast-enhancing intraparenchymal lesions (Gee, Bazan et al., 1992; Kchouk, Zouiten et al., 1992; Eide, Gean et al., 1993). In a series of AIDS patients studied by Villoria (Villoria, de la Torre et al., 1992), 37% exhibited parenchymal enhancement.

Distinguishing infarction from inflammation due to tuberculosis may be difficult on cranial MR (Offenbacher, Fazekas et al., 1991). Angiography is characterized by a hydrocephalic pattern of the vessels, narrowing of the vessels at the base of the brain, and narrowed or occluded small and medium-sized vessels with few collaterals (Lehrer, 1966). Radiographic clues to the presence of intracranial tuberculosis include multiloculated abscesses, cisternal enhancement, basal ganglia infarction, and communicating hydrocephalus, which are not findings associated with primary central nervous system lymphoma (PCNSL) or toxoplasma encephalitis (Whiteman, Espinoza et al., 1995). SPECT scans are negative and, therefore, helpful in distinguishing these lesions from PCNSL.

LABORATORY DIAGNOSIS Routine laboratory studies provide few clues to the diagnosis of tuberculosis. Erythrocyte sedimentation rate and the peripheral white cell count are often elevated, but not invariably so. In fact, leukopenia may also be observed and the differential white blood cell count is not particularly helpful. Hyponatremia may indicate the syndrome of inappropriate antidiuretic hormone (Smith & Godwin-Austen, 1980). In the presence of miliary dissemination, cultures of extraneural sites, such as the bone marrow and lung, may be positive.

In the non-HIV-infected population, the chest X-ray in adult patients reveals abnormalities consistent with pulmonary tuberculosis in 25 to 50% of patients (Stockstill & Kauffman, 1983; Traub, Colchester et al., 1984; Clark, Metcalf et al., 1986). Radiographic findings include miliary disease, apical scarring, hilar adenopathy and the Ghon complex. Skin testing for delayed hypersensitivity to tuberculosis with purified protein derivative (PPD) is not invariably positive either. PPD-positivity has been reported in 40–65% of adults with tuberculosis meningitis (Haas, Madhavan et al., 1977; Ogawa, Smith et al., 1987; Clark, Metcalf et al., 1986) and in 85–90% of children (Steiner & Portugaleza, 1973; Sumaya, Simek et al., 1975; Idriss, Sinno et al., 1976). A negative PPD is even more common with HIV infection. Therefore, both the chest X-ray and the PPD may be negative in the face of tuberculous meningitis, so a high index of suspicion for the diagnosis must be held for the prompt initiation of therapy. The presence of tuberculosis can be highly suspected on the basis of newer serological studies that can rapidly detect TB antigens or using immunologic assays which measure the production of interferon-γ by TB-specific T lymphocytes exposed to M. tuberculosis antigens (QuantiFERON and T-SPOT TB tests) (Al-Zamel, 2009). However, these tests are not diagnostic of tuberculous meningitis and may lack sensitivity.

Cerebrospinal fluid (CSF) analysis is pivotal in diagnosing tuberculous meningitis. As with other forms of bacterial meningitis, the opening pressure should be elevated. However, approximately half of both adult and pediatric patients have normal opening pressures at the time of study (Singhal, Bhagwati et al., 1975; Ogawa, Smith et al., 1987; Leiguarda, Berthier et al., 1988). The CSF may appear xanthochromic due to elevated protein concentrations, and spinal block may result in the Froin's syndrome, clot formation of CSF after removal of any red blood cells due to the presence of high concentration of serum proteins, including fibrinogen. Reported median CSF white blood cell count range from 63 (Traub, Colchester et al., 1984) to 283 cells/cu mm (Barrett-Connor, 1967). On occasion, the CSF white cell count may be normal (Klein, Damsker et al., 1985; Ogawa, Smith et al., 1987) or, at the other extreme, exceed 4000 cell/cu mm (Karadanis & Shulman, 1976). In the early stages of infection, a significant number of polymorphonuclear cells may be observed, but over the course of several days to weeks are typically replaced by lymphocytes. The persistent predominance of polymorphonuclear cells may result in mistaken diagnosis (Mizutani, Kurosawa et al., 1993; Pardiwalla, Yeolekar et al., 1992). A higher frequency of normocellular CSF is seen with HIV-associated tuberculous meningitis than otherwise (Cecchini, Ambrosioni et al., 2009). Rarely, cells other than lymphocytes are observed, such as plasma cells and eosinophils; however, their presence should suggest some other underlying process. In general, an elevated CSF protein is the rule, with values usually in the 100 to 200 mg/dl range (Kent, Crowe et al., 1993); values may occasionally exceed 1 to 2 gm/dl, but may be normal in more than a third of patients (Berenguer, Moreno et al., 1992). The CSF glucose is low, with values usually less than 50% of serum glucose and a median values of CSF glucose reported between 18 mg/dl (Barrett-Connor, 1967) and 45 mg/dl (Haas, Madhavan et al., 1977). In culture-proven cases, the CSF glucose tends to be lower than in presumptive tuberculous meningitis (Traub, Colchester et al., 1984; Ogawa, Smith et al., 1987). Low CSF chloride and elevated CSF C-reactive protein (Vaishnavi, Dhand et al., 1992) are nonspecific markers of tuberculous meningitis with limited application.

The hallmark of diagnosis of tuberculous meningitis is the demonstration of M. tuberculosis in the CSF. Typically, no more than 25% of cases have identifiable M. tuberculosis when acid-fast stains are performed on spun specimens of the CSF (Hinman, 1967; Sumaya, Simek et al., 1975; Klein, Damsker et al., 1985) and in one study (Davis, Rastogi et al., 1993), acid-fast stains of CSF sediment were positive in only 4%. The percentages of positive smears may improve with increased numbers of specimens (Kennedy & Fallon, 1979). Cultures of the CSF for M. tuberculosis are not invariably positive either. Rates of positivity for clinically diagnosed cases range from 25% (Traub, Colchester et al., 1984) to 70% (Alvarez & McCabe, 1984) in patients without AIDS, but are considerably lower in the presence of HIV infection. Rates of positive CSF cultures have varied between 3% and 10% in this population (Small, Schecter et al. 1991; Berenguer, Moreno et al., 1992). Mycobacterial cultures require several weeks before they are positive.

The frequency of false negative CSF stains and cultures for M. tuberculosis and the long duration for positive cultures to become available have served as an impetus to the development of alternative diagnostic tests on the CSF that are based on the detection of the organism immunologically or by PCR, detection of antibody to M. tuberculosis, or the detection of substances in the CSF that are believed to be unique to M. tuberculosis (Daniel, 1987). With respect to the latter, measurement of the radiolabeled bromide partition ratio following the administration of oral or intravenous([84]Br) ammonium bromide was one of the earliest tests employed (Smith, Taylor et al., 1955). It has been reported to have both a sensitivity and specificity on the order of 90% (Mann, Macfarlane et al., 1982; Coovadia, Dawood et al., 1986)). Gas-liquid chromatography has been used to identify a basic indole in the CSF believed to be relatively specific for tuberculosis meningitis (Brooks, Choudhary et al., 1977). Tests of the CSF for the presence of tuberculostearic acid, a component of the mycobacteria cell wall, has been reported to have sensitivity and specificity in excess of 90% (French, Teoh et al., 1987), and those of CSF adenosine deaminase (ADA) have been reported between 73% to 100% and 71% to 99%, respectively (Mann, Macfarlane et al., 1982; Coovadia, Dawood et al., 1986; Ribera, Martinez-Vazquez et al., 1987). In a study of 180 adults with meningitis of various etiologies, CSF ADA levels ≥ 10 IU/L had a sensitivity of 48% and a specificity of 100% in patients with tuberculous meningitis (Lopez-Cortes, Cruz-Ruiz et al. 1995). Antibodies directed to M. tuberculosis can be detected immunologically with enzyme linked immunosorbent assay (ELISA) with varying success (Kalish, Radin et al., 1983; Watt, Zaraspe et al., 1988). Similarly, a variety of immunological techniques have been employed to detect M. tuberculosis antigen in the CSF with high levels of sensitivity and specificity reported (Sada, Ruiz-Palacios et al., 1983; Krambovitis, McIllmurray et al., 1984; Kadival, Samuel et al., 1987; Radhakrishnan & Mathai, 1990).

Since the early 1990s, PCR has been applied to CSF specimens to detect M. tuberculosis DNA (Kaneko, Onodera et al., 1990; Narita, Matsuzono et al., 1992; Donald, Victor et al. 1993). This test may remain positive four or more weeks after the initiation of treatment (Donald, Victor et al., 1993). A recent study suggests that the PCR assay has a sensitivity of 70.5% and specificity of 87.5%. (Bhigjee, Padayachee et al., 2007) Targeting multiple sites of the TB genome with conventional PCR did not improve the yield and real-time PCR was more sensitive (Bhigjee, Padayachee et al. 2007). With the exception of the radiolabeled bromide partition ratio, the results of all these tests are available within hours, a distinct advantage over the long wait for mycobacterial cultures.

Therapy in HIV-Infected Patients

Tuberculous meningitis should be considered a medical emergency. When the disease is strongly suspected, treatment should be started empirically even before confirmation by microbiological or molecular diagnostic techniques. The antimicrobials used in the treatment of tuberculous meningitis can be divided into first and second-line agents. The former include isoniazid, rifampin, pyrazinamide, ethambutol, and streptomycin. Peak levels of isoniazid (INH) following oral administration exceed levels needed to inhibit most strains of M. tuberculosis in vitro (0.025–0.05 ug/ml) by one hundred-fold (Mandel & Sande, 1985). Penetration through inflamed meninges is excellent, with CSF concentrations 90% that of serum; however, in the absence of inflammation, the penetration is about 20% of serum levels (Forgan-Smith, Ellard et al., 1973). Drug toxicity reactions with INH include hepatotoxicity, peripheral neuropathy when pyridoxine is not co-administered, and alterations in mental state. The usual daily dose is 5–10 mg/kg/day. Rifampin achieves high serum levels after oral administration, and CSF levels are approximately 20% of serum levels in the presence of meningeal inflammation (D'Oliveira, 1972). Adverse reactions include renal, hematologic, and hepatic disorders. The latter seem to be particularly frequent in individuals receiving INH concomitantly. The usual dose is 10–20 mg/kg/day in children and 10 mg/kg/day in adults, up to 600 mg daily. Pyrazinamide has its effect on intracellular rather than extracellular organisms and penetrates the CSF extremely well. Hepatotoxicity is the chief toxicity, and the usual dose is 20–35 mg/kg/day. Ethambutol achieves CSF concentrations of 10% to 50% of serum levels in the presence of meningeal inflammation (Bobrowitz, 1972). The chief toxicity of this tuberculostatic drug is optic neuritis, which develops in as many as 1% of persons on the currently recommended dose of 15 to 25 mg/kg/day. Careful attention to visual acuity and color perception is required of patients on this drug. Streptomycin was the initial drug demonstrated to be efficacious in the treatment of tuberculous meningitis. It must be given parenterally and requires meningeal inflammation for penetration, with CSF levels approximately one-quarter of that of the serum (Zintel, Flippin et al., 1945). Vestibular disorders due to ototoxicity are its chief adverse effect. Currently recommended doses are 20–40 mg/kg/day in children and 1 g daily in adults. The second-line agents for the treatment of tuberculous include para-aminosalicylic acid (PAS), cycloserine, and the aminoglycosides: amikacin and kanamycin. There are a number of recommended regimens for the treatment of tuberculous meningitis (Table 8.5.2) that depend on whether the M. tuberculosis is likely to be drug resistant or not. While three-drug regimens have been employed successfully, the high morbidity and mortality of the disorder coupled with the increasing frequency of multidrug resistant organisms may warrant more aggressive regimens. The British Infection Society recommends that treatment of all forms of CNS tuberculosis should consist of four drugs (isoniazid, rifampicin, pyrazinimide, ethambutol) for 2 months followed by two drugs (isoniazid and rifampicin) for at least 10 months (Thwaites, Fisher et al., 2009).

In the absence of diagnostic uncertainty regarding the nature of a mass lesion or life threatening mass effect from tuberculoma or tuberculous abscess, surgical evacuation need not be necessary as good response to antituberculous therapy often leads to favorable results (Thonell, Pendle et al., 2000).

IRIS is not infrequently observed in HIV-infected persons with tuberculous meningitis. In one South African study, 41% of patients developing IRIS had TB-IRIS (Murdoch,

Table 8.5.2 MEDICAL RESEARCH COUNCIL CLASSIFICATION OF TUBERCULOUS MENINGITIS

STAGE I (EARLY):

nonspecific symptoms and signs

consciousness undisturbed

no focal neurological signs

STAGE II (INTERMEDIATE):

consciousness disturbed but not comatose nor delirious

signs of meningeal irritation

minor focal neurological signs, e.g., cranial nerve palsies

STAGE III (ADVANCED):

seizures

abnormal movements

stupor or coma

severe neurological deficits, e.g., paresis

Table 8.5.3 THE NEUROLOGICAL COMPLICATIONS OF TUBERCULOSIS (AFTER WOOD 1988)

Meningeal

Purulent tuberculous meningitis

1. disseminated miliary tuberculosis
2. focal caseating plaques
3. inflammatory caseous meningitis
4. proliferative meningitis

Serous tuberculous meningitis

Cerebral

Tuberculous encephalopathy

Tuberculoma

Tuberculous brain abscess

Cerebral infarction

Tuberculous of the skull

Spinal

Spinal tuberculoma

Tuberculous spinal abscess

Tuberculous spinal osteomyelitis

Necrotizing myelopathy

Tuberculous radiculomyelitis

Venter et al., 2008). Paradoxical neurological TB-IRIS accounts for 12% of all TB-IRIS cases and exhibits a significant short-term morbidity (Pepper, Marais et al. 2009). Despite the risk of IRIS, the prognosis of HIV-infected individuals with tuberculosis who are naïve to ART is better when HAART is started concomitant with antituberculosis medication than when it is introduced after the completion of such therapy (Abdool Karim, Naidoo et al.).

Prognosis in HIV-Infected Patients

A method for staging the severity of the tuberculous meningitis was developed by the British Medical Research Council in 1948 (1948) for purposes of classification in the initial trials of streptomycin in tuberculous meningitis Table 8.5.3. This schema has proven useful for grading the initial severity of the illness and for purposes of prognosis.

In the absence of treatment, tuberculous meningitis is invariably fatal in AIDS, although rare spontaneous recoveries had been reported prior to the AIDS epidemic. Following the introduction of isoniazid in 1952, the survival rates of tuberculous meningitis approached their present rates of 70% to 80% (Lepper & Spies, 1963). In the non-HIV infected population, poor prognosis has been correlated with advanced stages by the classification of the British Medical Research Council; extremes of age (Smith & Vollum, 1956; Lincoln, Sordillo et al., 1960; Hinman, 1967; Lepper & Spies, 1963; Weiss & Flippin, 1965), coexistent miliary disease (Lorber, 1954; Wasz-Hockert & Donner, 1962; Lepper & Spies, 1963), extraordinarily high CSF protein levels with spinal block (Weiss & Flippin, 1965), and markedly reduced CSF glucose (Wasz-Hockert & Donner, 1962).

In AIDS patients, a CD4 lymphocyte count of less than 22 cells/cu mm and illness lasting more than 14 days before hospital admission were poor prognostic signs (Berenguer, Moreno et al., 1992). The association of mortality with a profoundly low CD4+ lymphocyte count (<50 cells/μL) has

been a consistent observation (Cecchini, Ambrosioni et al., 2009). The severity of tuberculous meningitis as characterized by clinical neurological features (Torok, Chau et al., 2008; Cecchini, Ambrosioni et al., 2009), a low serum sodium (Torok, Chau et al., 2008), decreased CSF lymphocyte count (Torok, Chau et al. 2008), and multidrug resistant organisms (Cecchini, Ambrosioni et al., 2009), are independent variables for mortality. The overall mortality in one large series was 33% in the HIV-infected population with tuberculous meningitis, but mortality directly attributable to the meningitis was 21%, equal to that of a non-HIV infected control group (Berenguer, Moreno et al., 1992). This has not been universally observed as in one retrospective study, mortality rates were 63.3% in HIV-infected persons compared to 17.5% for non-HIV-infected (Cecchini, Ambrosioni et al., 2009) and were 41% at one month in another (Ganiem, Parwati et al., 2009). Dube and colleagues (Dube, Holtom et al., 1992) when comparing tuberculous meningitis in patients with and without HIV infection found that the only significant difference between the two groups was the increased incidence of intracerebral mass lesions in the HIV-infected group. The mortality does not appear to have changed significantly by HAART. In one study, mortality of tuberculous meningitis was 41% at 9 months and was actually higher in those who had been on HAART (Croda, Vidal et al. 2009); however, in those just initiating HAART in tandem with tuberculous meningitis, prognosis is better (Siika, Ayuo et al. 2008).

Within two weeks of the initiation of effective treatment, clinical improvement is noted. However, it is not unusual to observe transient worsening in clinical and CSF parameters following the initiation of therapy, probably occurring as an immunological phenomenon akin to the Jarisch-Herxheimer reaction in syphilis. Resolution of the fever may require weeks. CSF glucose levels return to normal within 2 months in 50% of patients and within 6 months in almost all, whereas the CSF pleocytosis requires more than 6 months to resolve in 25% and the CSF protein remains elevated in 40% at this time (Lepper & Spies, 1963; Barrett-Connor, 1967).

Continued alteration in level of consciousness in the early stages of the disease may be the result of concomitant hydrocephalus or hyponatremia. Later, 2 to 18 months after the initiation of adequate antituberculous therapy, enlarging intracranial tuberculomata may result in clinical deterioration. In the non-HIV infected population (Teoh, Humphries et al. 1987), organisms isolated from these enlarging tuberculomata are sensitive to the antibiotic employed and their appearance appears to be an immunological phenomenon. Surgery can usually be avoided with the administration of corticosteroids and continued antituberculous therapy.

Data derived in the pre-AIDS era indicate that the rate of sequelae among survivors is quite variable. These sequelae include cognitive disturbances, seizures, hemiparesis, ataxia, and persistent cranial nerve palsies (Ogawa, Smith et al., 1987; Smith & Vollum, 1956; Donner & Wasz-Hockert, 1962).

Visual impairment often accompanies optic atrophy (Mooney, 1956). The neurological sequelae are likely to be similar in the AIDS population.

ATYPICAL MYCOBACTERIA

Atypical (non-tuberculous) mycobacteria were recognized as pathogens in the 1950s and, until the AIDS epidemic, chiefly resulted in localized pulmonary disease in middle-aged persons with pre-existing lung disease (Wolinsky, 1979). Mycobacterium avium-intracellulare (MAI) and other atypical mycobacteria infections occur frequently in AIDS and are often extrapulmonary in nature (Pumarola-Sune, Navia et al., 1987). As these organisms are frequently isolated from soil, the route of infection is believed to be environmental. In the AIDS patient, symptomatic disease may be the result of reactivation of latent infection. The most common atypical mycobacterium observed in the AIDS patient is MAI; however, other atypical mycobacteria are also seen (Nunn & McAdam, 1988), including brain abscess and meningitis in association with *Mycobacterium kansasii* (Haas, Madhavan et al., 1977; Bergen, Yangco et al., 1993; Gordon & Blumberg, 1992) and at least one case of leprosy in association with AIDS (Lamfers, Bastiaans et al., 1987). In reality, these are two distinct organisms, but they are bacteriologically very similar and difficult

Table 8.5.4 CHEMOTHERAPEUTIC REGIMENS FOR TUBERCULOUS MENINGITIS [ZUGER 1991]

LOW PROBABILITY OF DRUG RESISTANCE

Drug	Usual Daily Dose	Maximum Dose	Duration
Isoniazid	5 to10 mg/kg	300 mg	6 months
Rifampin	10 to 20 mg/kg	600 mg	6 months
Pyrazinamide or	15 to 30 mg/kg	2500 mg	2 months
Isoniazid	5 to 10 mg/kg	300 mg	9 months
Rifampin	10 to 20 mg/kg	600 mg	9 months
Ethambutol or	15 to 25 mg/kg		2 months
Streptomycin	15 mg/kg	1000 mg	2 months
Isoniazid	5 to 10 mg/kg	300 mg	2 months
	15 mg/kg*	900 mg	8 months
Rifampin	10 to 20 mg/kg	600 mg	1 month
	10 to 20 mg/kg*	600 mg	8 months

HIGH PROBABILITY OF DRUG RESISTANCE

	Drug	Maximum Dose	Duration
(A)	Isoniazid	5 to 10 mg/kg	1 year
	Rifampin	25 mg/kg	1 year
	Pyrazinamide	15 to 30 mg/kg	2 months
	Ethambutol or	25 mg/kg	2 months
	Streptomycin	15 mg/kg	2 months
(B)	In cases of documented drug resistance, chemotherapy must be tailored to the demonstrated sensitivities.		

* Twice weekly

to distinguish. MAI is diagnosed pre-mortem in 15 to 20% of AIDS patients and in as many as 50% post-mortem (Hawkins, Gold et al. 1986). In the latter, recovery of the organism is chiefly from the spleen and lymph node, but dissemination elsewhere is not uncommon. Symptoms of MAI typically include fever, malaise, night sweats, generalized weakness, and weight loss (Young, Inderlied et al., 1986; Hawkins, Gold et al., 1986). In one study, MAI was the most common bacteremia observed in patients with AIDS (Whimbey, Gold et al., 1986). Despite the frequency of mycobacterial infection, involvement of the CNS is not as common as may be expected and is most frequently due to *Mycobacteria tuberculosis*.

In contrast to *M. tuberculosis*, patients with MAI have single or multiple mass lesions twice as commonly as meningitis. In a study from New York, MAI was cultured from the CSF in 15 of 16 cases with atypical mycobacterial meningitis complicating AIDS (Jacob, Henein et al., 1993). The other case was the due to *M. fortuitum* (Jacob, Henein et al., 1993). CT characteristics are diverse, and, in general, mirror those seen in tuberculous meningitis in the absence of HIV infection. Hydrocephalus and meningeal enhancement were observed on CT in approximately one-half of all patients in one study in which intravenous drug abusers constituted more than 90% of the population (Villoria, de la Torre et al., 1992). Radiographic studies are often helpful in suggesting the presence of CNS tuberculosis.

Optimal regimens in the treatment of CNS disease due to atypical mycobacteria, such as MAI, have not been precisely defined. A four-drug regimen is required for treating MAI (Kemper, Meng et al., 1992). Current recommendations include using azithromycin (500–1000 mg daily) and clarithromycin (500–1000 mg/day) in combination with ethambutol (15 mg/kg/day) or clofazimine (100 mg/day). Alternative regimens include the use of ciprofloxacin and rifampicin. Further study will be required to determine the best regimen. There are insufficient data to determine the duration of therapy in patients with CNS atypical tuberculosis, and, in general, treatment of this disorder is disappointing.

LEPROSY

Hansen's disease is characterized by three cardinal features, namely, hypoesthetic skin lesions, thickened peripheral nerves, and positive skin smears for the bacilli. The expression of Hansen's disease is chiefly dependent on the host response to the causative organism, *M. leprae*. Numerous, small, diffusely though symmetrically distributed skin lesions typify lepromatous leprosy. When advanced, the skin of the face and earlobes is diffusely thickened giving the distinctive "onine facies" appearance. Peripheral nerve involvement results in widespread symmetric loss of sensation. In tuberculoid leprosy, the skin lesions are single or few and asymmetrically distributed. These lesions are typically depigmented, raised, hypoesthetic and have well-defined borders. The peripheral nerve involvement is confined to smaller dermal nerves in cooler parts of the body. The most commonly observed form is borderline leprosy, which has features of both lepromatous and tuberculoid leprosy.

While HIV has been demonstrated to significantly worsen other mycobacterial disorders, in particular, tuberculosis and atypical tuberculosis, with an increase in proliferation of the micro-organism, there have been, paradoxically, no reports suggesting a similar phenomenon in individuals co-infected with HIV and *M. leprae*. Indeed, there has been no evidence that the expression of the disease as assessed by the ratio of lepromatous to tuberculoid disease when HIV-infected individuals are compared to uninfected controls is altered. This paradox remains poorly understood, but is likely the consequence of preserved cell-mediated immunity at the site of infection despite its abrogation systemically (Ustianowski, Lawn et al., 2006).

However, more than ten persons with IRIS in leprosy have been reported (Chow, Okinaka et al., 2009). In about 80%, leprosy was unmasked by the institution of HAART (Ustianowski, Lawn et al., 2006). Forty percent developed a neuritis (Ustianowski, Lawn et al., 2006). Management of leprosy-IRIS with corticosteroids was generally successful, but could require a prolonged course and, in one instance, azathioprine was instituted as a corticosteroid-sparing measure (Ustianowski, Lawn et al., 2006).

SYPHILIS

The incidence of neurosyphilis is difficult to evaluate because of underreporting, difficulty in establishing the diagnosis, diverse clinical presentations, and arrest of the illness by treatment with antibiotics for other infections (Koffman, 1956; Hooshmand, Escobar et al., 1972; Joyce-Clark & Molteno, 1978; Luxon, Lees et al., 1979; Norbeno & Sorenson, 1981; Burke & Schaberg, 1985). There had been a threefold increase in the nationwide incidence of primary and secondary syphilis in the United States from its nadir in 1957 to 1983 (1984), and the incidence continued to increase thereafter (1988). Between 1955 and 1958, the annual rate of infectious (primary and secondary) syphilis fell to approximately 4/100,000 (Fleming, 1964), the lowest recorded in the US, and it changed very little between 1960 to 1985 (Aral & Holmes, 1990). However, rates among white men showed sharp increases during this time period and were largely attributed to homosexual practices (Aral & Holmes, 1990). Since 1982, the rate of syphilis among homosexual white men had decreased, presumably in response to altered sexual behavior in response to AIDS (Aral & Holmes, 1990). However, the decline in incidence of infectious syphilis was not observed in other segments of the population in the United States at that time. In 2001, the Centers for Disease Control and Prevention regarded syphilis as a re-emerging public health threat (CDC, 2009). Thereafter, the rate of all cases of syphilis began to decline in the United States through 2005, when a consistent increase was observed through at least 2008 when 13,500 cases of primary and secondary syphilis were reported, the highest number since 1995 (CDC, 2009). The majority of reported cases of syphilis in the US has been in men who have sex with men (CDC, 2009). The risk groups for the acquired immunodeficiency syndrome (AIDS) encompass these same groups (Guinan, Thomas et al., 1984; Friedland & Klein, 1987); thus, it is not surprising to find syphilis and infection with the human immunodeficiency virus (HIV) occurring together. Furthermore, epidemiological studies have suggested that syphilis, like other genital ulcerative diseases, serves as a cofactor for the acquisition of HIV infection (Guinan, Thomas et al., 1984; Greenblatt, Lukehart et al., 1988; Holmberg, Stewart et al., 1988; Pepin, Plummer et al., 1989; Simonsen, Cameron et al., 1988; Stamm, Handsfield et al., 1988).

Despite the fact that general reviews of the neurological complications of HIV infection have reported low rates of neurosyphilis (Snider, Simpson et al., 1983; Levy, Bredesen et al., 1985; McArthur, 1987; Berger, 1987), neurosyphilis is surprisingly common in HIV infection. In a retrospective chart review study from south Florida Katz and Berger (1989) estimated that neurosyphilis, strictly defined by the presence of reactive CSF VDRL, was diagnosed in approximately 1.5% of HIV-infected patients hospitalized at a large public health hospital in South Florida. An expansion of this study confirmed this estimate (Katz, Berger et al., 1993), which concorded remarkably well with the estimates from a prospective longitudinal study from the same institution (Berger, 1991). In that study, a history of syphilis and/or a reactive serum FTA-ABS was observed in 43.3% of 180 asymptomatic HIV-seropositive subjects and 50.6% of 77 neurologically symptomatic HIV-seropositive subjects in comparison to 26.1% of HIV-seronegative controls with similar risk factors for HIV infection (Berger, 1991). Three (1.8%) neurologically asymptomatic subjects and 3.3% of the neurologically symptomatic subjects had neurosyphilis (Berger, 1991). The former is virtually identical to the 2.0% incidence of a reactive CSF VDRL found by Appleman et al. (Appleman, Marshall et al., 1988) in asymptomatic, HIV-infected U.S. servicemen undergoing lumbar puncture. Similarly, in a Brazilian study, Livramento et al. (Livramento, Machado et al., 1989) found 10 (5.9%) cases of neurosyphilis among 170 patients with AIDS and neurological syndromes. In another study, 9.1% of HIV-infected patients undergoing lumbar puncture because of a reactive serology with no history of recent treatment for syphilis had a reactive CSF VDRL (Holtom, Larsen et al., 1992).

CLINICAL FEATURES Anecdotal reports suggest that the clinical manifestations of syphilis may be altered when occurring in association with HIV infection. Among the unusual manifestations reported are peculiar ocular manifestations and rashes, lues maligna, gummas, osteitis, and pneumonitis (Marra, 1996). False negative serological responses (Hicks, Benson et al., 1987; Strobel, Beauclair et al., 1989), an unusually aggressive neurosyphilis (Johns, Tierney et al., 1987), and poor therapeutic responses of neurosyphilis to penicillin (Musher, Hamill et al., 1990) have also been described.

Concomitant human immunodeficiency virus (HIV) infection may significantly alter the natural history of neurosyphilis (Johns, Tierney et al., 1987; Katz & Berger, 1989; Katz, Berger et al., 1993). Syphilis appears to be not only more aggressive, but also more difficult to treat when it occurs in association with HIV infection (Berry, Hooton et al., 1987; Katz, Berger et al., 1993; Musher, Hamill et al., 1990). These observations suggest that the host's immune response is critical in controlling this infection. The inability of the HIV-infected patient to establish delayed hypersensitivity to

T. pallidum may prevent secondary syphilis from evolving to latency or may cause a spontaneous relapse from a latent state. This impairment of delayed hypersensitivity may account for a more rapid progression of neurosyphilis in HIV-infected individuals than would otherwise be expected. *T. pallidum* can be isolated from the CSF of HIV-seropositive patients with primary, secondary, and latent syphilis following currently recommended CDC penicillin therapy (Lukehart, Hook et al., 1988). Neurosyphilis has been reported following CDC-recommended therapy for early syphilis of the HIV-infected individual (Berry, Hooton et al., 1987), and it has also been reported that erythromycin has failed to cure secondary syphilis in a patient infected with HIV (Duncan, 1989).

In HIV infection, an acute, symptomatic, syphilitic meningitis during the course of secondary syphilis is not uncommon. A decrease in the latent period prior to the development of some neurosyphilitic manifestations, such as meningovascular syphilis and general paresis, has been suggested. The development of meningovascular syphilis within four months of primary infection despite the administration of accepted penicillin regimens (Johns, Tierney et al., 1987) and the neurologic relapse of syphilis in HIV-infected individuals after appropriate doses of benzathine penicillin for secondary syphilis (Berry, Hooton et al., 1987) have been reported. In one large study (Katz, Berger et al., 1993), the most common forms of neurosyphilis observed with HIV infection were syphilitic meningitis (64% of cases) and meningovascular syphilis (27%). Syphilitic meningitis is characterized by headaches, meningismus, photophobia, impaired vision, and cranial nerve palsies (chiefly—in descending order of frequency—VII, VIII, VI, and II), while hearing loss, tinnitus, and vertigo may be observed in isolation or in combination. Encephalopathic features resulting from vascular compromise or increased intracranial pressure may be observed. These include confusion, lethargy, seizures, aphasia, and hemiplegia. Acute sensorineural hearing loss and acute optic neuritis may occur in association with syphilitic meningitis or independently. Meningovascular syphilis may affect the brain or spinal cord and, although it typically occurs 6 to 7 years after the initial infection, the latency for this and other forms of neurosyphilis may be considerably shorter in the presence of concomitant HIV infection. The nature of the neurological features are dependent on the area of the brain or spinal cord affected. Many of the stroke eponyms described at the turn of the 19th century, such as, Weber's, Claude's, and Benedikt's syndromes, were the consequence of meningovascular syphilis producing discrete lesions of the brainstem. The neurological manifestations include aphasia, hemiparesis, hemianesthesia, diplopia, vertigo, dysarthria, and a variety of brainstem syndromes. Computed tomography and magnetic resonance imaging are invaluable diagnostic aids.

Other unusual manifestations of syphilis that have been reported in association with HIV infection include unexplained fever (Chung, Pien et al., 1983), bilateral optic neuritis with blindness (Zambrano, Perez et al., 1987), Bell's palsy and severe bilateral sensorineural hearing loss (Fernandez-Guerrero, Miranda et al., 1988), syphilitic polyradiculopathy (Lanska, Lanska et al., 1988), and syphilitic cerebral gumma presenting as a mass lesion (Berger, Waskin et al., 1992; Regal, Demaerel et al., 2005; Morshed, Lee et al., 2008; Weinert, Scheffel et al., 2008). Syphilitic meningomyelitis (Berger, Scott et al., 1992) has also been reported and is characterized by slowly progressive weakness and paresthesia of the lower extremities. Eventually, bowel and bladder incontinence and paraplegia supervene. Examination reveals a spastic paraparesis or paraplegia with brisk lower extremity reflexes, loss of the superficial abdominal reflexes and impaired sensory perception with vibratory and position sense being disproportionately affected.

Ocular syphilis was seen in 36% of one large cohort with neurosyphilis (Katz, Berger et al., 1993). Syphilitic eye disease in AIDS patients has only recently been documented (Zaidman, Weinberg et al., 1983; Zaidman, 1986; Carter, Hamill et al., 1987; Zambrano, Perez et al., 1987; Stoumbos & Klein, 1987; Passo & Rosenbaum, 1988; Becerra, Ksiazek et al., 1989; Levy, Liss et al., 1989; Joyce, Haye et al., 1989). Several comprehensive reviews (Palestine, Rodrigues et al., 1984; Freeman, Lerner et al., 1984; Gal, Pollack et al., 1984) fail to mention syphilis as an etiology of ocular complaints in AIDS patients. Eye disease may occur in all stages of syphilis infection. Uveitis and perineuritis are more common in early (primary and secondary) syphilis, whereas chorioretinitis, optic atrophy, and pupillary abnormalities are found more often in late infection (Spoor, Wynn et al., 1983). These later manifestations may be signs of progressive disease and require treatment equally as aggressive as that used in the management of neurosyphilis. Conjunctivitis may result from chancre or gummas of the conjunctiva or occur in association with papular syphilides (Spoor, Wynn et al., 1983). Papilledema may result from the sustained increased intracranial pressure of syphilitic meningitis. Optic perineuritis or optic neuritis may mimic papilledema. Syphilitic retinitis may be difficult to differentiate from that of cytomegalovirus (Stoumbos & Klein, 1987).

As noted, HIV infection may alter the natural history of syphilis as well as the response to treatment. Norris states that "immunosuppression of T-cell responses can lead to poor clearance of *T. pallidum* and more severe infection" (Norris, 1988). Animal experimentation performed over several decades has revealed that immunosuppression from corticosteroid therapy modifies the expression of *T. pallidum* infection. For instance, Turner and Hollander (1957) demonstrated that the administration of cortisone to rabbits infected intradermally with *T. pallidum* (Nichols strain) resulted in quickly enlarging dermal lesions that did not ulcerate and with organisms "literally swarming over the entire preparation" quite unlike that observed in untreated animals. Corticosteroid therapy has been used to enhance the speed with which *T. pallidum* can be recovered from rabbits who have undergone intratesticular inoculation of potentially infectious material for diagnostic purposes.

The role of immunosuppression on the course of syphilis in humans is uncertain. Two individuals with an unusual presentation of syphilis in the face of immunosuppression for organ transplantation have been described (Petersen, Mead et al., 1983; Johnson, Norris et al., 1988). Syphilitic meningitis, presumably resulting from a recrudescence of previously treated syphilis, has also been described in a 30-year-old homosexual man who was immunosuppressed following a kidney transplant, but also was HIV infected (Clark & Carlisle, 1988). Among the evidence for a significant role of cell-mediated immunity in syphilis is: 1) passive transfer of syphilis-immune serum is only partially protective; 2) untreated, syphilis may progress despite the presence of immobilizing antibodies; 3) delayed hypersensitivity to treponemal antigens develops in late secondary, latent, and tertiary syphilis; 4) granulomatous lesions characterize tertiary syphilis; and 5) immunization with killed organisms is usually unsuccessful, whereas immunization with live, attenuated organisms has produced immunity (Musher & Schell, 1975). Conceivably, the inability of HIV patients to establish delayed hypersensitivity may prevent secondary syphilis from evolving to latency or may cause a spontaneous relapse from the latent state. The impairment of delayed hypersensitivity probably accounts for the acute development and rapid progression of neurologic disease in AIDS patients, mirroring the nature of other CNS infections in AIDS, such as toxoplasmosis and progressive multifocal leukoencephalopathy. The pathogen in each of these instances exists in a latent state, becoming evident only after the onset of immunosuppression.

DIAGNOSING NEUROSYPHILIS Diagnosing neurosyphilis can be quite problematic. Several different diagnostic schemata have been used to establish the diagnosis; however, all have relied on indirect evidence of the presence of *T. pallidum*, as the organism is fastidious and requires the rather cumbersome use of animal inoculation for culture verification. Examples of the diagnostic schemata for neurosyphilis proffered in the literature include:

1. Reactive serum FTA or microhemagglutination *T. pallidum* (MHA-TP) in association with one of the following:

   a. reactive CSF VDRL,

   b. CSF pleocytosis (≥ 5 cells/cu mm), or

   c. increased CSF protein (greater than 46 mg%).

   (Burke & Schaberg, 1985)

2. Reactive serum FTA in association with one of the following:

   a. neurological or ophthalmological disease unexplained by other illnesses,

   b. reactive CSF FTA and increased CSF cell count (>5 cells/cu mm), or

   c. reactive CSF FTA with progressive neurological symptoms without other explanation.

   (Hooshmand, Escobar et al., 1972)

3. Reactive CSF VDRL in the absence of gross blood contamination of the CSF

   (Katz & Berger, 1989).

In the setting of HIV, the diagnosis of neurosyphilis can be particularly difficult due to the CSF abnormalities observed with the former. Table 8.5.5 provides a diagnostic schema for neurosyphilis occurring with HIV.

The Centers for Disease Control and Prevention (CDC) requires 1) any syphilis stage and 2) a reactive CSF VDRL for the diagnosis of "confirmed" neurosyphilis. "Presumptive" syphilis is any stage syphilis with an abnormal CSF protein or white blood cell count, but negative CSF VDRL.

Though it is the most specific test for neurosyphilis, the CSF VDRL, as well as other nontreponemal tests, may be insensitive to the diagnosis of neurosyphilis. In their classic monograph on neurosyphilis, Merritt and colleagues (Merritt, Adams et al., 1946) state that the Wasserman and the Davis-Hinton, earlier nontreponemal tests, were negative in a high percentage of patients with neurosyphilis. For instance, the CSF Wasserman or Davis-Hinton were negative in 28% of patients with tabes dorsalis. Other investigators have demonstrated the presence of pathologically confirmed neurosyphilis in the face of a negative CSF VDRL (Burke, 1972). Recently, HIV-infected patients have been described with an initially nonreactive CSF VDRL that reverted to reactive following treatment for neurosyphilis (Feraru, Aronow et al., 1990). Similarly, the absence of a reactive serum nontreponemal study, like the VDRL, is not a reliable means of excluding the diagnosis of neurosyphilis (Jaffe, Larsen et al., 1978; Wolters, 1987) as these studies are often negative in patients with latent or tertiary syphilis. In untreated neurosyphilis, cardiovascular and congenital syphilis, the serum VDRL was nonreactive in 30% (Deacon, Lucas et al., 1966). Likewise, in a study of neurosyphilis, the serum VDRL was reactive in only 61% (Harner, Smith et al., 1968). Specific serum treponemal tests, for example, FTA-ABS and MHA-TP, are expected to be positive in the presence neurosyphilis (Jaffe, Larsen et al., 1978), although Mapelli (Mapelli, Pavoni et al., 1981) reported a rate of only 70% for reactive serum FTA and 65% for *T. pallidum* immobilization tests (TPI) in the association with neurosyphilis.

Conversely, the CSF VDRL is believed to be extremely specific with few falsely reactive studies (Thomas, 1964), though patients with falsely reactive CSF VDRL have been reported in association with a spinal ependymoma (Delaney, 1976) and meningeal carcinomatosis (Madiedo, Ho et al., 1980). A falsely positive CSF VDRL can also be produced by blood contamination of the CSF; however, even at serum VDRL titers of 1:256, gross blood contamination is required to result in a false positive study (Izzat, Bartruff et al., 1971). Parenthetically, as many as 4% of patients with neurosyphilis have a reactive CSF nontreponemal test, but a nonreactive serum test (Dewhurst, 1969).

The value of specific treponemal antibody studies on the CSF for diagnosing neurosyphilis remains controversial. Some investigators (Escobar, Dalton et al., 1970; Davis & Schmitt, 1989) have proposed using the CSF FTA-ABS as a sensitive screening modality. The correlation of serum FTA titers to CSF titers suggests the presence of blood diffusion into the CSF (Traviesa, Prystowsky et al., 1978; Jaffe, Larsen et al., 1978), a finding which had previously been demonstrated (Ribault & Colombani, 1964). This diffusion may seriously detract from the specificity of the test for diagnosing neurosyphilis. Small amounts of blood contamination of the CSF may also invalidate a reactive CSF FTA-ABS (Davis & Sperry, 1979). Other studies have been touted for diagnosing neurosyphilis, such as the MHA-TP (Kinnunen & Hillbom, 1986), a 19S IgM to a treponemal antigen (Luger, Schmidt et al., 1972), determination of intrathecal synthesis of anti-treponemal antibody (Van Eijk, Wolters et al., 1987), and polymerase chain reaction using synthetic DNA probes for *T. pallidum* (Noordhoek, Wieles et al., 1990).

Relying on nonspecific CSF abnormalities in order to diagnose neurosyphilis in the face of HIV infection is fraught with difficulty, as the CSF in HIV-infected patients is frequently abnormal. Marshall and colleagues (Marshall, Brey et al., 1988) found that 63% of over 400 CSF analyses performed in HIV-infected U.S. servicemen were abnormal. These abnormalities included a CSF pleocytosis, increased CSF protein, and increased CSF IgG levels and IgG synthesis (Marshall, Brey et al., 1988), abnormalities that are also observed with neurosyphilis. Importantly, a CSF pleocytosis is less common in HIV infection when the peripheral blood CD4+ T cell counts are less than 200/μL, when plasma HIV viremia is controlled, and when the patient is taking antiretroviral therapy (Marra, Maxwell et al., 2007). Muller, Moskophidis et al., (1988) proposed measuring intrathecal synthesis of specific IgG in these patients to distinguish between the two disorders; however, a satisfactory means of distinguishing between the two disorders remains to be established.

Peripheral blood analysis is helpful in establishing the diagnosis of neurosyphilis. Titers of serum rapid plasma reagin (RPR) greater than 1:32 increase the odds for the presence of neurosyphilis (Libois, De Wit et al., 2007). Interestingly, a retrospective analysis suggests that neurosyphilis is more common when the serum RPR titer is greater than 1:128 compared to less than 1:32 or when the peripheral blood CD4+ T cells counts were less than 350/μL (Ghanem, Moore et al., 2008). Using CD4 cell count and RPR titers in individuals with concurrent HIV infection and syphilis improves the ability to identify asymptomatic neurosyphilis (Ghanem, Moore et al., 2009).

An approach to diagnosing neurosyphilis in the HIV-infected individual is outlined in Table 8.5.5. Marra (Marra, Gary et al., 1996) has incorporated the CDSF FTA-ABS or MHA-TP into an algorithm for the diagnoses of neurosyphilis. If reactive, treatment for neurosyphilis is recommended. PCR for *T. pallidum* DNA may be of value in some instances of neurosyphilis (Michelow, Wendel et al., 2002), but did not appear to offer more sensitivity than routine laboratory measures in a study of HIV-infected persons with neurosyphilis (Marra, Gary et al., 1996).

Treatment of Neurosyphilis in HIV-Infected Patients

Perhaps no other disease has been as dramatically affected by the discovery of penicillin as syphilis. However, the adequacy of currently recommended treatment regimens remains a question. In fact, there have been no controlled, randomized, prospective studies as to the optimal dose or duration of therapy in neurosyphilis. The treponemicidal level of penicillin is 0.03 mcg/ml. Though the organism has

Table 8.5.5 DIAGNOSING NEUROSYPHILIS IN THE FACE OF HIV INFECTION

DEFINITE NEUROSYPHILIS

1. + blood treponemal serology e.g. FTA- ABS, MHA-TP, etc
2. + CSF VDRL

PROBABLE NEUROSYPHILIS

1. + blood treponemal serology
2. - CSF VDRL
3. CSF mononuclear pleocytosis (>20 cells/cu mm)

or

< CSF protein (>60mg/dl)

4. neurological complications compatible with neurosyphilis, such as, cranial nerve palsies, stroke, etc. or evidence of ophthalmological syphilis

POSSIBLE NEUROSYPHILIS

1. + blood treponemal serology
2. - CSF VDRL
3. CSF mononuclear pleocytosis (>20 cells/cu mm)

or

< CSF protein (>60mg/dl)

4. no neurological or ophthalmological complications compatible with syphilis

been demonstrated to be capable of acquiring plasmids that produce penicillinase, there is no evidence that penicillin has lost its efficacy in the treatment of *T. pallidum*. If penicillin levels become subtherapeutic, the spirochetes begin regenerating within 18 to 24 hours. The Centers for Disease Control (CDC) recommends using 2.4 million units of benzathine penicillin intramuscularly at weekly intervals for three weeks in the treatment of neurosyphilis, but the recordable penicillin levels in the CSF during treatment fail to reach treponemicidal levels. The concentration of penicillin in the CSF is typically unmeasurable, probably not exceeding 0.0005 mcg/ml, which is 1% to 2% of the serum levels. Furthermore, viable treponemes have been recovered from the CSF of individuals at the completion of therapy. Another "recommended" regimen is procaine penicillin 600,000 units intramuscularly daily for 15 days. This regimen, too, may fail to achieve treponemicidal levels of penicillin in the CSF. Ideally, treatment of neurosyphilis should be 12 to 24 million units of crystalline aqueous penicillin administered intravenously daily (2 to 4 million units every four hours) for a period of 10 to 14 days. This regimen generally requires hospitalization. Because of the expense of treatment, we have occasionally resorted to the placement of an indwelling catheter and self-administered infusions at home in reliable, well-motivated patients. The penicillin should be administered at no less than four hour intervals to maintain the penicillin levels consistently at or above treponemicidal values, avoiding subtherapeutic troughs that occur when

administered at less frequent intervals. An alternative approach to the use of parenteral penicillin is the daily oral administration of amoxicillin 3.0 grams and probenicid 1.0 gram for 14 days. This regimen achieves treponemicidal levels of amoxicillin in the CSF.

In patients who are penicillin allergic, erythromycin 500 mg four times daily or tetracycline 500 mg four times daily for a period of 30 days has been recommended. Erythromycin does not diffuse readily into the brain and CSF, nor has its efficacy been demonstrated in the treatment of neurosyphilis. Similarly, oral therapy with tetracycline yields very low CSF tetracycline concentrations and it, too, has unproven efficacy in the treatment of neurosyphilis. Ideally, in the penicillin-allergic patient with unequivocally established, clinically manifest neurosyphilis, the prudent course is hospitalization, desensitization to penicillin, and subsequent high-dose aqueous penicillin treatment.

Recommendations altering the standard follow-up regimens and treatment of HIV-infected patients with syphilis have been suggested (Kinloch-de Loes, Radeff et al., 1988; Berger, 1990). At the present time, it is unknown whether secondary prophylaxis, that is, continuous administration of penicillin following the initial treatment, is necessary for syphilis. However, careful follow-up is certainly indicated. In general, serum RPR or VDRL titers should decline fourfold at 6 months and eightfold by 12 months after treatment of primary and secondary syphilis, and fourfold at 12 months following treatment for latent syphilis (Romanowski, Sutherland et al., 1991). The decline in serum titers in HIV-infected persons with infectious syphilis (Telzak, Greenberg et al., 1991) or HIV-uninfected persons with neurosyphilis (Nitrini & Spina-Franca, 1987) may not be as brisk. Furthermore, serum titers may not reflect the activity of the CNS disease in HIV-infected persons (Bayne, Schmidley et al., 1986; Berry, Hooton et al., 1987). With respect to CSF parameters, the cell counts typically normalize within 3 to 6 months, although CSF protein may remain elevated in approximately 50% at this time (Nitrini & Spina-Franca, 1987). CSF Wasserman tests remained abnormal in 90% of patients at 19 to 24 months (Nitrini & Spina-Franca, 1987). Other investigators have noted a normalization of CSF cell count and protein within 8 months and reversion to nonreactivity of the CSF VDRL by 10 months in 95% of patients with HIV (Marra, Longstreth Jr. et al., 1992). Marra (Marra, Gary et al., 1996) recommends that after treatment for neurosyphilis in HIV-infected persons, serum non-treponemal tests should be obtained monthly for the first 3 months and then every 3 to 6 months until nonreactive or repeatedly reactive at a titer of <1:8. The CSF should be re-examined at 3 months after therapy and every 6 months thereafter until normal.

BARTONELLA

Two members of the genus Bartonella, *Bartonella quintana* (formerly, *Rochalimaea quintana*) and *Bartonella henselae* (formerly, *Rochalimaea henselae*) are agents of severe and potentially fatal disease in HIV-infected persons (Regnery,

Childs et al., 1995). Infection with *B. henselae* has been associated with traumatic contact with cats (scratches or bites) and domestic cats appear to be a reservoir for this infection (Regnery, Childs et al., 1995). *B. henselae* causes several disorders, including bacillary angiomatosis, peliosis hepatis, lymphadenitis, aseptic meningitis with bacteremia, and cat-scratch disease (Wong, Dolan et al., 1995). Bacillary angiomatosis resulting from *B. henselae* in HIV-infected persons often presents with vascular skin lesions resembling Kaposi's sarcoma, frequently accompanied by fever and anemia (Moore, Russell et al., 1995). Other manifestations may include lung nodules with mediastinal adenopathy, peripheral adenopathy, pleural effusions, ascites, and lesions of the liver and spleen (Moore, Russell et al., 1995). In some communities, such as the San Francisco Bay area, infection with *B. quintana* appears to be more common than that due to *B. henselae*. Bartonellosis in the HIV-infected person can last for years and result in both cutaneous lesions and bacteremia.

Neurological disorders associated with *B. henselae* include cerebral and retinal bacillary angiomatosis, cat-scratch-related encephalitis, myelitis, cerebral arteritis, and retinitis (Schwartzman, Marchevsky et al., 1990). Contrast-enhancing intracerebral mass lesions due to bacillary angiomatosis in which *B. henselae* can be demonstrated pathologically by silver staining has been described in an HIV-infected individual (Sprach, Panther et al., 1992). When paired sera and CSF from 50 HIV-infected patients with neurologic disease were screened for the presence of reactive antibodies, Schwartzman and colleagues (Schwartzman, Marchevsky et al., 1990) detected *B. henselae*-specific IgG antibody in 32% of serum samples and 26% of CSF specimens. In comparison, only 4 to 5.5% of HIV-infected persons without neurologic disease had serological evidence of *B. henselae* infection (Schwartzman, Marchevsky et al., 1990). These investigators describe three patients in detail. One patient presented with Bell's palsy and later developed uveitis, other cranial nerve palsies, ataxia, and limb incoordination. Cranial MRI showed extensive white matter disease of both hemispheres evidenced by hyperintense signal abnormalities on T2-weighted image. CSF PCR was also positive for *B. henselae*. In the absence of specific therapy, slow clearing of clinical and radiographic findings was noted (Schwartzman, Marchevsky et al., 1990). Two other patients presented with sudden onset of disorientation and hallucinations followed by progressive dementia and death. In both, CSF PCR was also positive for *B. henselae* (Schwartzman, Marchevsky et al., 1990). The frequency with which *B. henselae* results in neurological disease in the HIV-infected population requires further study, but the disorder may be more common than its current level of clinical recognition.

Diagnosing the neurological manifestations of *Bartonella* is important, as it is a treatable disorder. There have been no randomized controlled clinical trials to evaluate antimicrobial treatment of bartonellosis in the HIV-infected population; a variety of antimicrobials, including erythromycin, doxycycline, rifampin, clarithromycin, and azithromycin have resulted in complete or partial clearing (Knobler, Silvers et al., 1988; Berger, McCarthy et al., 1989; Schlossberg, Morad et al., 1989;

Kemper, Lombard et al., 1990; Schwartzman, Marchevsky et al., 1990 ; Kaplan, Benson et al., 2009). Therapy should be continued for at least 3 months (Kaplan, Benson et al., 2009).

LISTERIA

Despite the frequent association of *Listeria monocytogenes* infection in individuals with other causes of impaired cell-mediated immunity, such as malignancy and post-organ transplantation, this infection is surprisingly rare in patients with AIDS. This relative infrequency has led to speculation (Jacobs & Murray, 1986; Mullin & Sheppell, 1987), but no explanation has been forthcoming. Occasionally, *L. monocytogenes* has been reported as a cause of sepsis or meningitis in this population (Decker, Simon et al., 1991; Kales & Holzman, 1990). In a study encompassing the years 1981 to 1988, an increased incidence of listeriosis in three medical centers in New York City was attributed to an increased incidence of concomitant, predisposing HIV infection (Kales & Holzman, 1990). The clinical manifestations of *L. monocytogenes* in the HIV-infected population did not appear to be different than that in those individuals without risk factors for HIV (Kales & Holzman, 1990). In addition to acute meningitis (Kales & Holzman, 1990; Gould, Belok et al., 1986; Koziol, Rielly et al., 1986; Decker, Simon et al., 1991; Levy, Bredesen et al., 1988), *L. monocytogenes* may also result in a chronic meningitis (Gould, Belok et al., 1986) and in brain abscesses (Patey, Nedelec et al., 1989; Harris, Marquez et al., 1980) in patients with AIDS. Penicillin or ampicillin with or without gentamycin is the preferred regimen for *L. monocytogenes* infection (Decker, Simon et al., 1991). Penicillin and ampicillin appear to be equally efficacious. Trimethoprim-sulfamethoxazole also has been successfully used to treat listerosis in the immunocompromised host (Spitzer, Hammer et al., 1986).

NOCARDIA

Like *L. monocytogenes*, *Nocardia asteroides* is an intracellular bacterium that is observed with increased frequency in immunocompromised individuals; however, it has been reported relatively infrequently in AIDS (Kim, Minamoto et al., 1991). Underreporting may be the consequence of the growth properties of Nocardia, the presence of other organisms, the common use of sulfonamides for treatment of patients with AIDS, and a low index of suspicion among physicians (Kim, Minamoto et al., 1991). The lung appears to be the most common site of infection with *N. asteroides*. In a study of 30 AIDS patients with nocardiosis, pulmonary disease was observed in 21, extrapulmonary disease in 8, and pulmonary and extra-pulmonary disease in one (Uttamchandani, Daikos et al., 1994). Brain abscess is the neurological manifestation most often observed (Sharer & Kapila, 1985; Holtz, Lavery et al., 1985; Adair, Beck et al., 1987; Idemyor & Cherubin, 1992; Bishburg, Eng et al., 1989; Uttamchandani, Daikos et al., 1994; Off, Lynn et al., 1997; Minamoto & Sordillo, 1998). Nocardia may also result in meningitis (Perez Perez, Garcia-Martos et al., 1990), and the organism has been isolated from the CSF in the absence of brain abscess (Alamo & Garcia Herruzo, 1991). Nocardia may respond to sulfonamides, but limited penetration into abscess cavities may necessitate surgical evacuation. Norden and colleagues (Norden, Ruben et al., 1983) recommend employing nonsurgical measures only when the number or distribution of lesions makes surgery technically unfeasible or when the patient's initial response to antimicrobial therapy is excellent (Norden, Ruben et al., 1983). Off and colleagues documented a clinical and imaging response, using both contrast MRI and indium 111 radionucleide scanning, to amikacin, imipenem, and ceftriaxone in combination (Off, Lynn et al., 1997). Delayed diagnosis, extensive disease, and early discontinuation of treatment have been associated with poor outcome (Uttamchandani, Daikos et al., 1994).

OTHER BACTERIAL INFECTIONS OF THE CNS

The spectrum of bacteria that can lead to meningitis and brain abscess in AIDS is extensive. Isolated case reports and small series indicate that meningitis may occur with non-typhoidal *Salmonella* (Fraimow, Wormser et al., 1990), *Klebsiella pneumoniae* (Holder & Halkias, 1988), and *Haemophilus influenzae* (Steinhart, Reingold et al., 1992). Brain abscess in the absence of meningitis may also occur with *Salmonella* (Glaser, Morton-Kute et al., 1985; Holtz, Lavery et al., 1985).

FUNGI

CRYPTOCOCCUS

Cryptococcus neoformans is recognized as the second most common opportunistic infection affecting the CNS, and the most common cause of opportunistic meningitis in AIDS patients. The frequency of cryptococcal infections in HIV-infected patients has been estimated at 5–10%, prior to widespread use of triazole antibiotics (Dismukes, 1988; Powderly, 1993). Cryptococcus is the first opportunistic infection in 45–75% of patients in whom it occurs (Kovacs, Kovacs et al., 1985; Chuck & Sande, 1989; Clark, Greer et al., 1990). While the majority of AIDS patients with cryptococcal disease have meningitis, pneumonitis, dermatitis, osteomyelitis, myocarditis, pericarditis, gastroenteritis, and arthritis also occur. Cryptococcal prostatitis is of special concern because it may serve as a reservoir for recurrence following therapy (Larsen, Bozzette et al. 1989). Most cryptococcal infections in HIV-infected patients occur when CD4 lymphocyte counts fall below 100/mm³ (Nightingale, Cal et al., 1992; Powderly, 1993). Although the incidence of AIDS-associated cryptococcal meningitis has declined in the United States coincident with widespread use of combination anti-retroviral therapy (Sacktor, Lyles et al., 2001), this has not been universally observed despite the introduction of HAART in less developed areas of the world (Oliveira, Greco et al., 2006; Jarvis, Boulle et al., 2009). Cryptococcosis is now the most common cause of adult meningitis in Southern and East Africa, where it is a major cause of HIV-related mortality (Park, Wannemuehler et al., 2009).

Cryptococcus neoformans is a common soil fungus found throughout the world. Areas contaminated by pigeon droppings are particularly likely to contain this organism. Antigenic variations in the polysaccharide capsule are used to define four serotypes, of which A and D most commonly cause human infections. Human infection is usually acquired by inhalation of spores. The initial pulmonary infection is generally asymptomatic. Hematogenous dissemination results in seeding of other organs.

Cryptococcus is cleared by neutrophils and macrophages in a process which is mediated by complement, interferon, and T lymphocyte-derived lymphokines. The polysaccharide capsule is a virulence factor which may inhibit phagocytosis and leukocyte migration, but may also activate the alternative complement pathway. Cryptococcus has a particular affinity for the CNS, perhaps due to the absence of complement and soluble anticryptococcal factors present in serum, and a diminished inflammatory response to the agent in brain tissue. Clinical infection occurs in both apparently normal and immunocompromised individuals (Dismukes, 1992).

Neuropathology

Cryptococcus neoformans proliferates in the subarachnoid space, resulting in leptomeningeal opacification with a gelatinous appearance. In HIV-infected individuals, the initial inflammatory response may be sparse and discrete, resulting in focal collections of macrophages and formation of giant cells. Focal granulomas composed of macrophages, lymphocytes, giant cells, and fungi may be seen. The organisms extend along Virchow-Robin spaces where clusters of fungi may distend the perivascular space into adjacent parenchyma. Intracerebral abscesses and cryptococcomas may be found in some cases. Mucicarmine staining demonstrates the capsule of the organism (Vinters & Anders, 1990; Lang, Miklossy et al., 1990). A recent postmortem study demonstrated direct evidence of cryptococcal cells in the arachnoid granulations in greater proportion to the rest of the brain parenchyma, and demonstrated a relationship between the mean number of organisms and CSF opening pressures during treatment, a common and significant cause of morbidity and mortality in this disease. In one of the patients who died on the second day of antifungal therapy, invasion of pontine and midbrain parenchyma without an associated inflammatory response was seen, indicating the potential for encephalitis as well as meningitis in this setting (Loyse, Wainwright et al.).

Clinical Features

HIV-infected patients with cryptococcal meningitis most commonly complain of headache and fever, though these symptoms occur in only 67–82% of some large series. Nausea or emesis occurs in about 45% of cases, while photophobia and meningismus are remarkably uncommon, occurring in less than a third of cases. Seizures occur in 4–18%, and cognitive impairment or alterations in sensorium occur in 17–24%. Cranial neuropathies are seen in up to 15%. Focal neurologic deficits are uncommon, occurring in 5–15% of cases. Dizziness, cerebellar ataxia, and syncope have also been noted as presenting features (Kovacs, Kovacs et al., 1985; Zuger, Louie et al., 1986; Chuck & Sande, 1989; Clark, Greer et al., 1990; Rozenbaum & Goncalves, 1994).

Visual symptoms may occur in up to 21% of cases and neuro-ophthalmic findings in up to 33% (Jabs, Green et al., 1989; Rozenbaum & Goncalves, 1994). Visual symptoms may include transient, abrupt, or progressive loss of visual acuity in one or both eyes due to increased intracranial pressure (Denning, Armstrong et al., 1991), necrotizing optic neuropathy from cryptococcal infiltration (Ofner & Baker, 1987; Cohen & Glasgow, 1993), or compression of the optic nerve with vascular compromise (Lipson, Freeman et al., 1989). Diplopia may occur intermittently or persistently due to cranial neuropathy, and skew deviation or nystagmus may also be seen (Keane, 1991; Friedman, 1991; Keane, 1993). Papilledema may occur in 1.5–12% of cases (Jabs, Green et al., 1989; Rozenbaum & Goncalves, 1994). Visual field deficits may be homonomous, bitemporal, or altitudinal (Golnik, Newman et al., 1991; Friedman, 1991; Garrity, Herman et al., 1993). Visual symptoms may be the first indication of recurrent cryptococcal meningitis in patients on maintenance antibiotic therapy (Golnik, Newman et al., 1991).

Psychiatric symptoms may also be presenting features of cryptococcal meningitis. Psychosis (Clark, Greer et al., 1990) and behavioral changes (Saag, Powderly et al., 1992) have been noted. Mania as an isolated presenting symptom has been described in two patients, one of whom responded to successful therapy of his meningitis with complete resolution of the manic syndrome (Johannessen & Wilson, 1988).

In some cases, no signs of neurologic disease are present and diagnosis results from evaluation of systemic symptoms (Zuger, Louie et al., 1986; Rozenbaum & Goncalves, 1994).

Diagnosis

Radiology
CT imaging is insensitive to cryptococcal meningitis, revealing nonspecific atrophy or no abnormalities in most instances (Post, Kursunoglu et al., 1985; Popovich, Arthur et al., 1990; Tien, Chu et al., 1991). MRI is more sensitive than CT, but still substantially underestimates the lesion burden found on pathologic examination (Mathews, Alo et al., 1992).

Contrast-enhanced imaging with MRI may reveal meningeal enhancement, but appears to do so less frequently than in non-HIV-infected patients with cryptococcal meningitis. Parenchymal cryptococcomas may appear as enhancing mass lesions within the parenchyma (Zuger, Louie et al., 1986; Tien, Chu et al., 1991; Andreula, Burdi et al., 1993). Miliary nodular-enhancing leptomeningeal lesions have been noted uncommonly (Tien, Chu et al., 1991). In the abseynce of pathological confirmation, it is difficult to exclude the possibility of concurrent opportunistic pathology accounting for enhancing mass lesions (Mathews, Alo et al., 1992).

Nonenhancing foci (which may be numerous in the basal ganglia and midbrain, displaying signal intensities similar to CSF) represent dilated Virchow-Robin spaces. On pathologic examination these may be filled with clusters of cryptococci and mucinous secretions. These collections have been referred to as gelatinous pseudocysts by some authors (Popovich, Arthur et al., 1990; Tien, Chu et al., 1991; Mathews, Alo et al., 1992; Andreula, Burdi et al., 1993).

Cerebrospinal Fluid
In contrast to non-HIV-infected individuals with cryptococcal meningitis, CSF abnormalities may be subtle in AIDS patients. Opening pressure is elevated in about two-thirds and may exceed 500 mm of water. Pleocytosis is lacking or modest in most instances, though occasionally vigorous mixed inflammatory responses are seen. Hypoglycorrhachia and elevated protein levels are found in up to three-fourths of cases.

India ink stains will disclose cryptococci in 70–94% of patients with positive CSF cultures. However, in over 90% of patients with meningitis, cryptococcal antigen titers in CSF are positive (Kovacs, Kovacs et al., 1985; Zuger, Louie et al., 1986; Chuck & Sande, 1989; Clark, Greer et al., 1990; Saag, Powderly et al., 1992; Rozenbaum & Goncalves, 1994). This means that cryptococci are cultured from CSF in virtually all patients with meningitis; however, occasional individuals with parenchymal cryptococcomas and no meningitis have had sterile CSF (Zuger, Louie et al., 1986).

Serologic Studies
Cryptococcal antigen titers in serum are usually elevated in patients with cryptococcal meningitis, in some cases even when antigen titers in CSF are negative (Chuck & Sande, 1989). The level of serum cryptococcal antigen and changes in response to therapy do not appear to reliably reflect CSF responses (Eng, Bishburg et al., 1986; Clark, Greer et al., 1990; Powderly, 1993).

Serum cryptococcal antigen titers may reflect disease disseminated to other organs, which occurs in conjunction with meningitis in up to one-half of cases. Most common sites for extrameningeal infection are the lungs, blood, urine, and bone marrow, but virtually any organ may be involved (Kovacs, Kovacs et al., 1985; Larsen, Bozzette et al., 1989; Clark, Greer et al., 1990; Rozenbaum & Goncalves, 1994).

Therapy in HIV-infected Patients

The optimal antibiotic regimen for cryptococal meningitis in HIV-infected patients has yet to be devised. Early series reported acute mortalities within six weeks of the completion of therapy of 18 to 37%. Much of this early mortality occured in the first two weeks (Kovacs, Kovacs et al., 1985; Chuck & Sande, 1989; Clark, Greer et al., 1990; Saag, Powderly et al., 1992). A variety of treatment regimens were used both within and between studies. Even with current regimens, 10-week mortalities from 10–25% are seen in the developed world and up to 43% in resource-poor environments (Jarvis & Harrison, 2007).

The drug of choice for cryptococcal meningitis has been amphotericin B, a polyene antibiotic which binds to ergosterol in the cryptococcal membrane, altering its permeability. Renal toxicity, which is related to the cumulative dose administered, is the major limiting adverse effect. During infusion, acute reactions commonly occur with fevers, chills, rigors, headache, and nausea, which may be mitigated by pretreatment with hydrocortisone, nonsteroidal anti-inflammatory agents, antiemetics, and antihistamines. Other potential adverse reactions include seizures, phlebitis, anemia, and edema (Sugar, Stern et al., 1990). Dosages used have ranged from 0.3 to 1.0 mg/kg/day, with higher doses given for shorter periods before reduction to a maintenance regimen (Kovacs, Kovacs et al., 1985; Zuger, Louie et al., 1986; Chuck & Sande, 1989; Clark, Greer et al., 1990; Larsen, Leal et al., 1990; Saag, Powderly et al., 1992; White, Cirrincione et al., 1992; de Lalla, Pellizzer et al., 1995). A large randomized trial in 1997 established the current recommendation of amphotericin B deoxycholate 0.7mg/kg/day (van der Horst, Saag et al., 1997).

Attempts to mitigate toxicity from amphotericin B therapy have included incorporation into liposomes (Coker, Murphy et al., 1991; Coker, Murphy et al., 1991) and infusion of amphotericin in a fat emulsion (Leake, Appleyard et al., 1994). At least three preparations of amphotericin B in lipid emulsion are available. They are as effective as amphotericin B in the treatment of cryptococcal meningitis and have less nephrotoxicity; however, they are far more expensive. Therefore, they are recommended only in the setting of pre-existing renal failure

In studies prior to AIDS, amphotericin B was found to be more effective in treating cryptococcal meningitis when administered with flucytosine, an oral antimycotic metabolized to 5-fluorouracil within fungal cells, which inhibits fungal DNA and RNA synthesis. Flucytosine may also inhibit purine and pyramidine uptake by fungi. Myelosuppression from the usual doses of 100–150 mg/kg/day may be problematic in AIDS patients, however, limiting its use, as can gastrointestinal reactions and hepatotoxicity (Sugar, Stern et al., 1990; Powderly, 1993).

The development of triazole agents, which inhibit cytochrome P450 enzyme activity by limiting fungal ergosterol synthesis (Sugar, Stern et al., 1990), has had a major impact on control of cryptococcal infections in AIDS. Fluconazole has a higher CSF penetration than itraconazole, though both have shown efficacy in AIDS patients with cryptococcal meningitis (Stern, Hartman et al., 1988; Sugar & Saunders, 1988; Denning, Tucker et al., 1989; Nightengale, 1995). Fluconazole has been used as an induction therapy in doses of 400–1200 mg daily in resource-poor environments lacking access to or the capability to adequately monitor amphotericin therapy. Higher doses of fluconazole have greater fungicidal activity and appear to be well tolerated (Longley, Muzoora et al., 2008).

Currently, the recommended initial treatment for AIDS-associated cryptococcal meningitis is amphotericin B deoxycholate 0.7mg/kg/day with flucytosine 100mg/kg/day in four divided doses for two weeks in those with normal renal function. For individuals with impaired renal function, lipid formulations of amphotericin can be substituted in doses of 4–6 mg/kg/day. After two weeks, if clinical improvement and sterilization on repeat CSF cultures is demonstrated, induction therapy can be discontinued and fluconaxole 400 mg/kg/day can be substituted for eight weeks. Fluconazole in doses of 400–800mg daily combined with flucytosine is considered an alternative to amphotericin B but is recommended only for those unable to tolerate or unresponsive to standard treatment. (Kaplan, Benson et al., 2009).

Elevated CSF opening pressure is seen in over half of patients with HIV-associated cryptococcal meningitis and has been related to short-term mortality in some studies. (Graybill, Sobel et al., 2000). Repeated lumbar punctures and the placement of an intraventricular drain is warranted in those individuals with high intracranial pressure associated with cryptococcal meningitis. When the elevated intracranial pressure is refractory, lumbar drains or lumbar peritoneal shunts have been utilized (Fessler, Sobel et al., 1998). A more recent series in which repeated lumbar punctures were routinely used, found a relationship between initial fungal burden measured by count of crytpococcal colony-forming units to increased CSF pressure, but no relationship of the intracranial pressure to mortality, which was 12% at two weeks and 26% at 10 weeks. An interesting finding in this study was that the initial opening pressure was not significantly related to the CSF pressure at day 14; however, the number of colony-forming units and the initial CSF cryptococcal antigen titer were, suggesting not only that the fungal burden was related to CSF pressure but that CSF pressure elevations could be biphasic and occur after the initial presentation (Bicanic, Brouwer et al., 2009). Randomized controlled trials regarding treatment of IRIS have not yet been done; however, use of corticosteroids is commonly considered and one case report suggests a beneficial response in a patient with cryptococcal meningoradiculitis (Brunel, Makinson et al., 2009).

Studies have not consistently identified patient factors predicting outcome. Among the factors associated with higher mortality have been neurologic impairment on initiation of therapy (Clark, Greer et al., 1990; Saag, Powderly et al., 1992), hyponatremia, positive cultures of extrameningeal specimens (Chuck & Sande, 1989), abnormal CT scan (Clark, Greer et al., 1990), cryptococcal antigen titer in CSF (Zuger, Louie et al., 1986; Saag, Powderly et al., 1992), and CSF white blood cells less than 20/mm^3 (Zuger, Louie et al., 1986; Chuck & Sande, 1989). As noted above, initial CSF pressure has been inconsistently associated with mortality.

Prevention of Relapse
Early series of AIDS patients with cryptococcal meningitis treated only with acute therapy were associated with relapse rates of 50–60% (Kovacs, Kovacs et al., 1985; Zuger, Louie et al., 1986; Clark, Greer et al., 1990). Open label trials of fluconazole (Sugar & Saunders, 1988) and itraconazole (deGans, Eeftinck Schattenkerk et al., 1988; Denning, Tucker et al., 1989) and a retrospective series in which some patients were given amphotericin B or ketoconazole (Chuck & Sande, 1989), suggested survival benefit for maintenance therapy.

A large placebo controlled trial documented a 19% persistence of positive CSF cultures following six weeks of primary therapy with amphotericin alone or in combination with flucytosine, and a significant benefit for fluconazole 100–200 mg/day in preventing relapse in patients with sterile CSF (Bozzette, Larsen et al., 1991). Subsequently, a study comparing fluconazole 200 mg/day to amphotericin B 1.0 mg/kg/week found the former agent to be more effective with less toxicity (Powderly, Saag et al., 1992) and the current recommendation is to use fluconazole for secondary prophylaxis until immune reconstitution occurs (Kaplan, Benson et al., 2009).

Despite maintenance therapy, recurrent cryptococcal meningitis occurs in up to 2–16% of AIDS patients (Chuck & Sande, 1989; Clark, Greer et al., 1990; Bozzette, Larsen et al., 1991; Powderly, Saag et al., 1992). Serum cryptococcal antigen is not a reliable marker for CNS infection (Eng, Bishburg et al., 1986; Bozzette, Larsen et al., 1991). CSF cryptococcal antigen titers decline with successful therapy, but subsequent rises with recurrence are apparently acute and not predicted by routine monitoring of CSF (Bozzette, Larsen et al., 1991). Persistence of cryptococcus in the prostate despite sterilization of CSF has been shown (Larsen, Bozzette et al., 1989). Molecular genetic studies have revealed clonal identity of serial isolates obtained from three AIDS patients with recurrent meningitis (Spitzer, Spitzer et al., 1993). Though prospective studies are yet to be done on the natural history of persistently positive cultures in patients with suppression of clinical disease, it seems likely that recurrence results from sequestered organisms in CSF or elsewhere.

Failures of primary or secondary prophylactic therapy might potentially be due to resistant fungi. A case in which resistance to fluconazole appeared to evolve during therapy has been reported (Paugam, Dupouy-Camet et al., 1994) and another in which resistance of a *Cryptococcus neoformans* var. *gattii* species to fluconazole was noted (Peetermans, Bobbaers et al., 1993). The latter species is uncommonly reported as a cause of cryptococcal meningitis in HIV-infected patients.

Another small series noted no change in sensitivity of serial isolates to either fluconazole or amphotericin, but noted wide variation in the dose sensitivity to fluconazole among different isolates (Casadevall, Spitzer et al., 1993). Higher doses of fluconazole to 800 mg/day have been reported to be effective salvage therapy in patients failing conventional therapy with either fluconazole or amphotericin (Berry, Rinaldi et al., 1992). At least one well-characterized isolate with resistance to amphotericin B has been described in a patient who responded to high dose fluconazole (Powderly, Saag et al., 1992).

Immune Reconstitution Syndrome

Immune reconstitution syndrome has been reported in 8.3–30% of patients with cryptococcal meningitis associated with AIDS and the initiation of combination anti-retroviral therapy in retrospective studies (Shelburne, Darcourt et al., 2005; Lortholary, Fontanet et al., 2005). Two recent prospective studies reported frequencies of 13 and 17%. The mortality rate among patients developing IRIS was 7.7% and 36.3% respectively in these prospective studies, but in neither of them was the mortality significantly different for IRIS patients than for similar patients not developing IRIS (Sungkanuparph, Filler et al., 2009; Bicanic, Meintjes et al., 2009).

The occurrence of IRIS in patients with cryptococcal meningitis following the initiation of combined antiretroviral therapy is most commonly about 30 days, but ranged from about 2 weeks to 2 months in the prospective series and as long as a year in the retrospective reports. Recurrent presenting symptoms do not reliably discriminate IRIS from recrudescent cryptococcal meningitis, but negative CSF cultures are required and CSF pleocytosis may be higher than in patients with recrudescent meningitis. Prediction of which patients will develop IRIS based on presenting disease features is unreliable. A higher initial serum cryptococcal antigen titer was predictive in one prospective study, but no features were predictive in the other. Higher CSF pressures, lower CD4+ lymphocyte counts with a more vigorous response to HAART, early initiation of HAART within 2 months of diagnosis of cryptococcosis, and fungemia or disseminated cryptococcosis were related to the occurrence of IRIS in the retrospective studies, but were not confirmed as risk factors in the prospective studies (Shelburne, Darcourt et al., 2005; Lortholary, Fontanet et al., 2005; Sungkanuparph, Filler et al., 2009; Bicanic, Meintjes et al., 2009).

Primary Prophylaxis

The safety and efficacy of triazole antibiotics has raised the possibility of primary prevention in susceptible immunosuppressed HIV-infected individuals. An open label trial showed a reduced rate of cryptococcal meningitis in patients with CD4 levels $\leq$ 68/mm^3 given 100 mg/day fluconazole compared to controls from the previous two years seen in the same site (Nightengale, 1995). A prospective clinical study demonstrated benefit of primary prophylaxis with fluconazole to prevent opportunistic cryptococcal infection in patients with CD4 counts <50/ul (Powderly, Finkelstein et al., 1995); however, current guidelines for the United States do not recommend routine prophylaxis for cryptococcosis because of the low incidence of the disease and the potential risks, drug interactions, and cost of the antifungal agents. Recommendations for primary prophylaxis in areas of higher prevalence are likely to differ.

Therapy-Supportive Measures

Elevated intracranial pressure is common in patients with cryptococcal meningitis and may result in hydrocephalus. It has been postulated that sustained elevations in intracranial pressure may contribute to early mortality by impairing cerebral circulation (Denning, Armstrong et al., 1991). Therapeutic modalities include drainage by serial lumbar punctures, ventricular drainage, and acetazolamide.

Acute visual loss in patients with HIV-associated cryptococcal meningitis may be transient, abrupt, or progressive and may result from increased intracranial pressure (Denning, Armstrong et al., 1991), necrotizing optic neuropathy due to cryptococcal invasion (Cohen & Glasgow, 1993), or constrictive arachnoiditis (Lipson, Freeman et al., 1989). Patients with papilledema and severely impaired vision may respond to antibiotic therapy alone (Golnik, Newman et al., 1991), ventricular shunting of CSF (Tan, 1988), or lysis of arachnoid adhesions (Maruk, Nakano et al., 1988). Optic nerve sheath fenestration resulted in visual recovery of two patients with cryptococcal meningitis who had persistent associated papilledema and visual loss despite antibiotic therapy (Garrity, Herman et al., 1993).

COCCIDIOMYCOSIS

Coccidioides immitis grows as a mold with septate hyphae in soil of hot semiarid regions of the Southwestern United States, Northern Mexico, and Central and South America. Bat and rodent droppings enhance growth. Infection of humans usually results from inhalation of aerosolized arthroconidia, which is optimized when dry conditions exist. Inhaled arthroconidia form spherules at body temperature which then rupture, releasing endospores. With intact cellular immunity, granulomatous tissue reactions limit but do not eradicate infection, and reactivation may occur with immunosuppression. It is uncertain whether disseminated infection in AIDS patients results from acute infection or reactivation (Bronnimann, Adam et al., 1987; Fish, Ampel et al., 1990; Ampel, Dols et al., 1993; Wheat, 1995)).

HIV-infected patients with CNS coccidioidomycosis present with meningitis (Fish, Ampel et al., 1990; Galgiani, Catanzaro et al., 1993), meningoencephalitis, myelitis or radiculitis (Mischel & Vinters, 1995), or cerebral abscesses which may be single or multiple (Jarvik, Hesselink et al., 1988; Levy, Bredesen et al., 1988). The occurrence of CNS disease appears to be uncommon despite immunosuppression, with only nine cases in a large retrospective review of 77 HIV-infected patients (Fish, Ampel et al., 1990), and none in a prospective series of 170 patients over a median follow up of almost a year (Ampel, Dols et al., 1993).

Neuropathologic reports of CNS coccidioidomycosis in HIV-infected patients describe a necrotizing granulomatous meningitis with abundant fungi, extending along Virchow-Robin spaces to involve underlying brain. Adjacent vessels are affected by extension of inflammation and an endarteritis obliterans may result. Organisms may be found in the adventitia of involved vessels. Cavitary necrosis results in abscess formation. Both granulomatous and suppurative meningitis are described (Jarvik, Hesselink et al., 1988; Mischel & Vinters, 1995).

HIV-infected patients with coccidioidal meningitis may have a prominant CSF pleocytosis with elevated protein and hypoglycorrhachia. In five of nine cases in a large review, organisms were cultured from CSF and complement fixation antibodies to coccidiodes were found in the other four. Immunosuppression as measured by CD4 lymphocytes varied, with four of eight patients tested having levels above 200/mm³ (Fish, Ampel et al., 1990). Another case was proven at autopsy after CSF studies proved unrevealing (Mischel & Vinters, 1995).

Patients with cerebral abscesses will present with headaches and fever, and may lack focal neurologic findings. Imaging studies are nonspecific and may show small enhancing lesions without mass effect. CSF in patients with abscesses may be normal (Jarvik, Hesselink et al., 1988; Levy, Bredesen et al., 1988).

Limited reports of treatment for CNS coccidioidomycosis in HIV-infected patients reveal some success. Of nine patients reviewed in a large retrospective series, three survived 5–21 months following therapy with amphotericin B, ketoconazole, or fluconazole. Mortality for the entire series of 77 patients with HIV infection and coccidioidomycosis was significantly related to CD4 levels (Fish, Ampel et al., 1990). In a series of 50 patients with coccidioidal meningitis, 9 of whom also had HIV-infection, fluconazole in doses of 400 mg/day produced responses in 6 of the 9 with survivals of 9–26 months. In two, recrudescent coccidioidomycosis appeared to contribute to their mortality (Galgiani, Catanzaro et al., 1993).

Current recommendations call for initial treatment of coccidioidal meningitis with fluconazole 400–800 mg daily. Itraconazole has also been used. If unsuccessful, amphotericin B may be required. Even with successful antifungal therapy, hydrocephalus may develop and require shunting (Kaplan, Benson et al., 2009).

HISTOPLASMOSIS

Histoplasma capsulatum is an ascomycete which grows in soil particularly where enriched by guano from birds or bats. The hyphae contain tuberculate microconidia and infectious macroconidia, which are usually acquired by inhalation. Disruption of soil by natural phenomena or construction activities enhances aerosolized spread. Distribution of the fungus is worldwide, with the highest prevalence in temperate and tropical environments. In the United States, endemic areas include the North Central and South Central regions (Dismukes, 1992; Wheat, 1995).

Histoplasmosis may occur in 2–5% of AIDS patients from endemic areas compared to less than 1% of those from other regions. In cities with particularly high prevalence, such as Indianapolis, Indiana; Kansas City, Kansas; and Nashville and Memphis, Tennessee, up to 25% of AIDS patients may be affected. Histoplasmosis may represent the first AIDS-related illness in up to 75% of such individuals, occurring alone or as a co-infection with another pathogen (Johnson, Khardori et al., 1988; Wheat, Batteiger et al., 1990).

Following inhalation, histoplasma transforms into a yeast at body temperature. With intact immune function, the host contains infection by mononuclear phagocytosis and granuloma formation.

The organism parasitizes macrophages, which provide a means of dissemination in immune-compromised individuals. In HIV-infected individuals with histoplasmosis, dissemination appears to occur in 95% of cases, usually when CD4 counts fall below 200/mm³. HIV-infected patients may acquire primary infection with subsequent dissemination or experience reactivation of previously contained infection as immune compromise occurs (Johnson, Khardori et al., 1988; Wheat, Batteiger et al., 1990).

The CNS is affected in up to 20% of cases with a mononuclear meningitis extending to adjacent vessels, resulting in endothelial proliferation, granulomatous vasculitis, and fibrinoid necrosis. A granulomatous necrotizing encephalitis may be seen with single or multiple abscesses (Anaissie, Fainstein et al., 1988; Wheat, Connolly-Stringfield et al., 1990; Wheat, Batteiger et al., 1990; Weidenheim, Nelson et al., 1992). In addition to affecting CNS, dissemination from the lungs may produce septicemia with high mortality or involve the skin or almost any organ system (Wheat, 1995).

CNS histoplasmosis typically presents with headache and fever, confusion or mental status changes, lethargy, or obtundation and cranial neuropathies. Focal neurologic findings may be seen in about 10% and seizures occur in about 10–30% of cases. Meningismus is uncommon, occurring in about 10%. Stroke syndromes may be the presenting features resulting from meningovasculitis, with thrombosis of basal or meningeal vessels, or septic embolization from infected heart valves (Wheat, Connolly-Stringfield et al., 1990; Wheat, 1995).

Cerebrospinal fluid may reveal a lymphocytic pleocytosis with protein elevation and hypoglycorrachia in patients with meningitis; however, some patients have normal CSF or nonspecific protein elevation. Isolation of histoplasma takes weeks, when it is recovered. Histoplasma antigen levels are detected in about 40% and antibodies to histoplasma in 60% or more of patients though cross reactions limit antibody specificity for acute infection (Wheat, Connolly-Stringfield et al., 1990; Wheat, Batteiger et al., 1990). Cerebral imaging studies may be normal, or show contrast-enhancing mass lesions, infarction patterns without enhancement, or meningeal enhancement (Anaissie, Fainstein et al., 1988; Wheat, Connolly-Stringfield et al., 1990; Weidenheim, Nelson et al., 1992).

Histoplasma capsulatum may be recovered from blood, bone marrow, respiratory secretions, or bronchoalveolar lavage fluid in about 85% of HIV-infected patients with disseminated histoplasmosis (Wheat, Batteiger et al., 1990; Wheat, 1995). In a mixed series of HIV and non-HIV-infected individuals with histoplasmosis, histoplasma antigen was detected by radioimmuno- or enzyme immunoassays in CSF or serum in about 40%, or in urine in 60% of cases. Cross reactions may occur with coccidioides. Antigen elevations may herald recurrent disease (Wheat, Kohler et al., 1989; Wheat, Connolly-Stringfield et al., 1991). Serologic tests are of limited value in patients from endemic regions, though high levels occur in about 60% of patients with CNS histoplasmosis with or without associated HIV infection (Wheat, Connolly-Stringfield et al., 1990; Wheat, Batteiger et al., 1990). Neuropathologic specimens obtained at biopsy or autopsy yield organisms on culture or by demonstration with methenamine silver stains in about 80% of cases of antemortem histoplasmosis (Wheat, Connolly-Stringfield et al., 1990; Wheat, Batteiger et al., 1990; Weidenheim, Nelson et al., 1992).

Prognosis for AIDS patients with CNS histoplasmosis has been poor, with mortality exceeding 60% in spite of therapy (Wheat, Batteiger et al., 1990). Amphotericin B in doses up to 1.0 mg/kg/day for initial therapy may be used, but CNS relapse has occurred despite cumulative dosages of two grams

(Weidenheim, Nelson et al., 1992). The optimal regimen is unestablished but current recommendations are initiation with amphotericin B followed by maintenance therapy with itraconazole (Kaplan, Benson et al., 2009).

Triazole agents may be of value. Itraconazole in doses of 200–400 mg/day has appeared to prevent relapse in HIV-infected patients with histoplasmosis, though data on CNS involvement were limited. Fluconazole offers better CNS penetration and may be preferable for maintenance therapy in patients with CNS histoplasmosis, though resistance to fluconazole has been seen (Wheat, 1995).

For patients with mass lesions, resection and antifungal therapy may be superior to antibiotic therapy alone, though little data exist for AIDS patients with histoplasmomas (Wheat, Connolly-Stringfield et al., 1990).

No evidence exists at present to support primary prophylaxis for histoplasmosis in HIV-infected patients. One small study failed to show benefit from fluconazole (Nightengale, 1995).

BLASTOMYCOSIS

Blastomyces dermatitides is an ascomycete with pear-shaped conidia found in the Northeast, Southeast, North Central, and South Central regions of the United States and Southern Canada. Cases have also been reported from Africa, India, the Middle East, Europe (Witzig, Hoadley et al. 1994), and South America. (Cury, Pulido et al., 2003) The organism is found in moist acidic soil containing organic matter and usually is acquired by inhalation. At body temperature, it transforms to a broad-based budding yeast. Neutrophilis and lymphocytes respond to infection with pyogranuloma formation in normal hosts. With immune suppression, disseminated infection may occur (Pappas, Pottage et al., 1992; Wheat, 1995).

Blastomycosis has not been commonly reported in AIDS patients to date, with only 24 documented cases as of 1994. CNS disease occurred in 46%, which is five to ten times the rate expected from non-HIV associated case series. The mortality rate of 54% is five times the expected rate. Most cases in HIV-infected patients occurred with CD4 counts less than 200/mm³ (Witzig, Hoadley et al., 1994).

Neuropathologic findings in autopsied cases reveal basilar meningitis or necrotizing arteritis and encephalitis with abscess formation. Organisms may be seen clustered around vessel walls and in meninges. Granuloma formation is often lacking (Harding, 1991; Fraser, Keath et al., 1991; Pappas, Pottage et al., 1992; Tan, Weldon-Linne et al., 1993).

Clinical neurologic features are nonspecific and include fever and headache, lethargy, progressive obtundation, seizures, and variable focal signs. Single or multiple enhancing mass lesions may be present (Figure 8.5.2), or a lymphocytic meningitis which may occasionally yield the organism on culture (Harding 1991; Pappas, Pottage et al., 1992; Witzig, Hoadley et al., 1994). Isolated CNS disease without apparent pulmonary involvement may occur as a presenting manifestation (Pappas, Pottage et al., 1992) or as a site of recurrence following treatment (Witzig, Hoadley et al., 1994). Most patients are diagnosed from pulmonary specimens obtained at

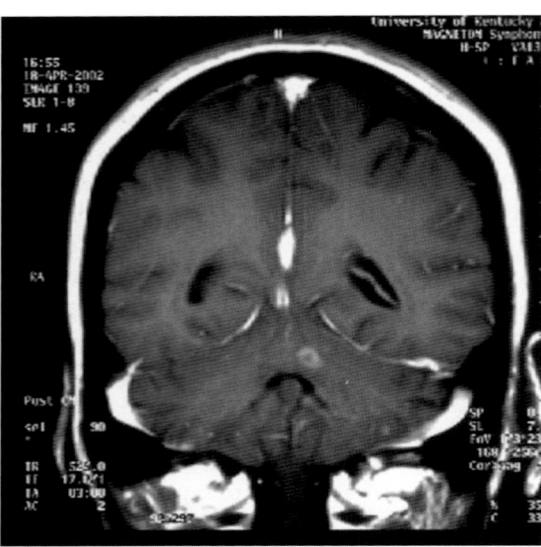

Figure 8.5.2 Blastomycosis. This contrast-enhanced coronal T1 MRI shows enhancing lesions diffusely affecting the cerebellum in an HIV-infected person with CNS blastomycosis.

bronchoscopy; however, culture of cutaneous ulcerating lesions, blood, CSF, or cerebral abscess fluid may also yield blastomyces. Histopathologic diagnosis on biopsy or autopsy material may yield organisms before cultures, which may require weeks to grow. Serologic studies have not been positive in most reported patients (Pappas, Pottage et al., 1992; Witzig, Hoadley et al., 1994).

Diagnosed cases of blastomycosis in AIDS patients have been treated initially with amphotericin B followed by maintenance therapy with ketoconazole or fluconazole. One patient was treated initially with ketoconazole. Most patients failed to respond (Fraser, Keath et al., 1991; Pappas, Pottage et al., 1992; Tan, Weldon-Linne et al., 1993; Witzig, Hoadley et al., 1994); however, one individual initially given 800 mg of amphotericin followed by 400 mg/day of ketoconazole maintenance therapy appeared to respond to treatment (Pappas, Pottage et al., 1992). Itraconazole in doses of 200–400 mg/day has been effective in non-HIV infected patients with blastomycosis and may prove useful in future AIDS patients (Wheat, 1995).

ASPERGILLUS

Aspergillus species are ubiquitous in most soils, especially on dead leaves, compost piles, decaying vegetation, and grain stockpiles, and are generally acquired by inhalation. Colonization of the respiratory tract without tissue invasion commonly occurs. Polymorphonuclear granulocytes respond to the mycelial form, while macrophages kill the conidia (Minamoto, Barlam et al., 1992). Invasive aspergillosis occurs in individuals with impaired neutrophil and macrophage function related to neutropenia, steroid therapy, or both. Some authors consider broad-spectrum antibiotic therapy, intravenous drug use, hyperglycemia or diabetes, alcoholism, and chronic pulmonary disease, particularly if cavitary, to be additional risk factors (Singh, Yu et al., 1991; Pursell, Telzak et al., 1992;

Minamoto, Barlam et al., 1992; Lortholary, Meyohas et al., 1993). When invasion occurs, contiguous extension may lead to infection of cranial sinuses, dural sinuses, or spinal structures (Woods & Goldsmith, 1990; Strauss & Fine, 1991; Hall & Farrior, 1993). An affinity for vascular invasion leads to hematogenous dissemination and necrotizing vasculitis. CNS involvement occurs in one-third to one-half of cases reported in HIV-infected individuals, compared to 10–25% in series of other immunosuppressed patients. *Aspergillus fumigatus* and *Aspergillus flavus* account for most cases of CNS aspergillosis in HIV-infected patients (Singh, Yu et al., 1991; Minamoto, Barlam et al., 1992; Pursell, Telzak et al., 1992). Spread to the CNS may also occur by septic embolization from colonized heart valves resulting in infarction and formation of mycotic aneurysms or abscesses (Henochowicz, Mustafa et al., 1985; Cox, DiDio et al., 1990).

Neuropathologic examination reveals a necrotizing vasculitis with hemorrhagic infarctions, and microscopic or macroscopic abscess formation. Meningitis may be present with neutrophilic inflammation. Fungi with regular acute or right angle branching septate hyphae may be demonstrated (Asnis, Chitkara et al., 1988; Vinters & Anders, 1990; Woods & Goldsmith, 1990; Carrazana, Rossitch et al., 1991). Dural thrombosis may be the result of extension from infected cranial sinuses (Strauss & Fine, 1991; Hall & Farrior, 1993). Extension from the lungs may result in vertebral osteomyelitis and meningomyelitis (Woods & Goldsmith, 1990) or myelopathy may result from epidural abscess formation (Go, Ziring et al., 1993).

CNS aspergillosis is difficult to diagnose in life. Patients may present with fever and headache, and changes in sensorium or mentation. Patients with abscesses or infarctions may have focal findings on examination (Woods & Goldsmith, 1990; Singh, Yu et al., 1991; Carrazana, Rossitch et al., 1991; Pursell, Telzak et al., 1992). Acute embolic infarction in an AIDS patient with fever and headache may be the presenting feature (Henochowicz, Mustafa et al., 1985). Fever, back pain, and features of myelopathy developing over months have been reported in patients with necrotizing meningomyelitis (Woods & Goldsmith, 1990) and compressive myelopathy from epidural abscess (Go, Ziring et al., 1993). Facial neuropathy occurs with otomastoiditis and is often preceded by otalgia and otorhea. Subsequent headache and lethargy are associated with CNS extension (Strauss & Fine, 1991; Hall & Farrior, 1993; Lyos, Malpica et al., 1993).

Cerebrospinal fluid may show a lymphocytic or neutrophilic pleocytosis (Woods & Goldsmith, 1990; Carrazana, Rossitch et al., 1991) or be unremarkable despite basal meningitis (Asnis, Chitkara et al., 1988; Woods & Goldsmith, 1990). Cultures often fail to yield the organism.

Cerebral imaging studies may demonstrate enhancing mass lesions typical of abscesses or non-enhancing abnormalities characteristic for infarctions (Hofflin & Remington, 1985; Singh, Yu et al., 1991; Pursell, Telzak et al., 1992). White matter lesions may resemble progressive multifocal leukoencephalopathy (Woods & Goldsmith, 1990). CT scans may be normal or show nonspecific atrophy in patients with meningitis

(Asnis, Chitkara et al., 1988). MRI is more sensitive than CT, but failed to reveal a necrotizing myelitis in one reported case (Woods & Goldsmith, 1990).

Diagnosis of invasive aspergillosis is difficult in life. Sputum cultures are insufficient because of the frequency of colonization. Histopathologic demonstration or culture from a sterile space is required (Minamoto, Barlam et al., 1992). Bronchoalveolar lavage fluid may have a high yield (Lortholary, Meyohas et al., 1993).

Therapy of CNS aspergillosis in diagnosed patients with HIV infection has been discouraging in most instances. Amphotericin B in doses of 0.5–1.0 mg/kg/day has been used without convincing success. One patient with mastoiditis extending to the cerebellum and lateral sinus survived hospitalization and abscess resection but was immediately lost to follow-up (Hall & Farrior, 1993). Itraconazole has in vitro activity against aspergillus and has been used successfully in patients with bronchopulmonary disease (Minamoto, Barlam et al., 1992; Jennings & Hardin, 1993). Amphotericin B and itraconazole in combination have resulted in sterilization of cultures from HIV-infected patients with invasive aspergillosis but not documented CNS disease (Lortholary, Meyohas et al., 1993).

MUCORMYCOSIS

Infection by Mucorales species: rhizopus, mucor, and absidia, are uncommonly reported in HIV-infected patients. Rhinocerebral mucormycosis is most often associated with uncontrolled diabetes. A case has been described in an AIDS patient in association with maxillary and ethmoid sinusitis, who progressed to develop cerebral infarction. Diagnosis was obtained at biopsy of the sinus lesion and therapy with amphotericin B produced clinical stabilization until death six months later from cytomegalovirus infection (Blatt, Lucey et al., 1991).

Isolated CNS mucormycosis is most often reported in conjunction with intravenous drug use where concurrent HIV infection may be present. Presentation with fever and lethargy with progressive development of focal deficits occurred in reported cases. Imaging studies revealed infarctions or were normal, and CSF, where available, revealed a lymphocytic pleocytosis and elevated protein with no organisms on fungal cultures. Relatively high CD4 lymphocyte counts in some cases suggest that intravenous drug use might have been a more important factor than immunosuppression (Cuadrado, Guerrero et al., 1988; Skolnik & De La Monte, 1990)). The course of other cases associated with lymphopenia may have been influenced by immunosuppression, though HIV infection can only be presumed (Wetli, Weiss et al., 1984; Micozzi & Wetli, 1985). Therapy with amphotericin has been successful when biopsy established the diagnosis in life (Skolnik & De La Monte, 1990).

CANDIDA ALBICANS

Candida albicans is a common mucocutaneous infection in the oropharynx and esophagus of HIV-infected individuals.

Candidal fungemia may disseminate infection to other organs, including the CNS, where it may result in meningitis or cerebral abscess formation. Intravenous drug use is an independent risk factor.

Despite the frequency of candidiasis in HIV-infected patients, reports of CNS involvement are sparse; some represent only neuropathologic findings at autopsy, apparently unrecognized in life (Snider, Simpson et al., 1983; Levy, Bredesen et al., 1985; Petito, Cho et al., 1986; Kure, Llena et al., 1991). Symptoms may be subtle and unappreciated in life (Koppel, Wormser et al., 1985).

In cases providing clinical information, features may be nonspecific with ring-enhancing mass lesions and focal findings (Pitlik, Fainstein et al., 1983) or meningitis with either neurotrophilic (Ehni & Ellison, 1987) or mononuclear (Bruinsma-Adams, 1991) predominance. In the latter case, candidal meningitis was the presenting manifestation of AIDS. In candidal meningitis the fungus may be recovered from CSF.

A case of disseminated candidemia resulting in colonization of cerebral arteries resulting in acute cerebral infarction has been reported. CSF was benign, but blood cultures revealed the organism. Treatment with amphotericin B was unsuccessful (Kieburtz, Eskin et al., 1993).

Treatment of patients with candidal meningitis or abscess with amphotericin has had mixed success. Two patients appeared to respond to surgical drainage and amphotericin (Pitlik, Fainstein et al., 1983) alone or with five flucytosine (Levy, Pons et al., 1984). One patient with meningitis responded to amphotericin and five flucytosine with resolution of symptoms and sterilization of CSF, which was maintained for several months by weekly maintenance amphotericin (Ehni & Ellison, 1987).

The role of azole therapy for CNS candidiasis is presently unestablished. Reports of responses can be found (Sanches-Portocarrero, Perez-Cecilia et al., 1993), although resistance may emerge in patients on continuing therapy (Heinic, Stevens et al., 1993).

SPOROTRICHOSIS

Sporothrix schenkii is a ubiquitous soil fungus which is found in association with both living and decaying vegetation. It may infect dogs and cats as well as humans, and percutaneous introduction may occur in florists, nursery or forestry workers, landscapers, gardeners, and others with similar exposures.

Clinical infection usually results in a nodular or ulcerating cutaneous lesion which may spread locally through lymphatic channels. Pulmonary disease is less common. Hematogenous dissemination may occur in immune compromised hosts, most commonly producing arthritis, but occasionally a lymphocytic meningitis (Dismukes, 1992).

Two cases of *Sporothrix schenkii* meningitis in HIV-infected patients with cutaneous sporotrichosis have been reported. One patient developed lymphocytic meningitis with hypoglycorrhachia two months following apparently successful therapy of cutaneous disease with amphotericin B and while on maintenance therapy with fluconazole. Serum and CSF antibodies with an elevated IgG index were present, and the organism was subsequently isolated from CSF. Reinstitution of amphotericin B at 1mg/kg/day failed to prevent progression, and meningitis due to *S. schenkii* was confirmed at autopsy (Penn, Goldstein et al., 1992).

A second case occurred in an agricultural worker with a CD4 court of 17/mm³. Progressive cutaneous lesions developed despite fluconazole therapy. An MRI done because of hyponatremia revealed nonenhancing lesions in the brainstem, basal ganglia, and centrum semiovale. After he developed seizures, despite therapy with amphotericin B, a lumbar puncture revealed a neutrophilic pleocytosis with hypoglycorrhachia and elevated protein. Yeasts were identified on a spun CSF specimen and culture of CSF yielded sporothrix. Addition of high-dose fluconazole, itraconazole, and potassium iodide failed to prevent progression. At autopsy, a diffuse meningitis and ventriculitis with thrombotic endarteritis producing infarctions corresponding to the MRI lesions was demonstrated. Yeasts were present in the meninges and infiltrating adjacent vessels. Postmortem sensitivity testing revealed resistance to the agents employed, but sensitivity to ketoconazole, miconazole, and flucytosine (Donabedian, O'Donnell et al., 1994).

CLADOSPORIOSIS

Cladosporiosis (*Xylohypha bantiana*) is a fungal plant pathogen that on rare occasions may cause fungal brain abscess. It has been reported in both immunologically normal individuals (Banerjee, Mohapatra et al., 1989) as well as the immunosuppressed, including patients with AIDS. An example of the latter is the report of an intravenous drug user presenting with fever, headache, and focal neurologic deficits, who was found to have multiple contrast-enhancing lesions on CT scan. Empiric therapy for toxoplasmosis failed to prevent progressive deterioration over seven weeks. Autopsy disclosed cladosporiosis (Colon, 1988).

PARASITES

CNS TOXOPLASMOSIS

Toxoplasma gondii is the most common cause of cerebral mass lesions in AIDS patients. Estimates of its prevalence vary geographically and among populations in accordance with serologic evidence of exposure, which ranges from 3–45% in the United States to as high as 80% in parts of Europe (Clumeck, 1991; Hunter & Remington, 1994). Estimates of the frequency of symptomatic toxoplasmosis in the United States range from 6% (Achim, Nagra et al., 1994) to a third of seropositive individuals (Luft & Remington, 1992). In a series from New York City, 2.5% of AIDS patients had CNS toxoplasmosis (Achim, Nagra et al., 1994). In a treatment study of dideoxyinosine, toxoplasmic encephalitis occurred in 11% of all patients and 25% of those with positive serology and immunosuppression as reflected by CD4 lymphocyte counts less than 100/mm³ (Oksenhendler, Charreau et al., 1994).

More recently, with the common use of HAART and primary prophylaxis, the frequency of toxoplasmic encephalitis has declined even in populations with high rates of infestation. In a review of the French Hospital Database on HIV comparing periods prior to and following the onset of HAART therapy, the incidence rate of toxoplasmic encephalitis declined from 3.9 to 1.0 cases per hundred person years (Abgrall, Rabaud et al., 2001). However, in some parts of the world, toxoplasmic encephalitis remains a major opportunistic infection even in the HAART era. In an Italian registry of patients with neurologic complications of AIDS compiled between 2000 and 2002, new onset toxoplasmic encephalitis was the most frequent neurologic disorder occurring in 26% of the cohort. Among these individuals were 11% with CD4+ counts > 200 cells/ul and 12% with undetectable HIV viral loads (Antinori, Larussa et al., 2004).

T. gondii is usually acquired by ingestion of raw or poorly cooked red meat which contains tissue cysts. Cats are the definitive hosts of this obligate intracellular protozoan and excrete oocysts in their feces. Contact with contaminated material provides another source of transmission of infection. The infection has been transmitted by transfusion of infected blood and transplantation of infected organs. Transplacental transmission occurs.

Excreted oocysts may survive more than a year. *T. gondii* organisms released from ingested oocysts enter intestinal mucosal cells, where replication results in trophozoites which disseminate via the bloodstream or lymphatics, infect nucleated host cells and multiply within vacuoles. With continued division, rupture of the cell leads to contiguous spread of infection with progressive necrosis. Both humoral and cellular immune responses are important in containment of the infection, but even with effective responses, eradication of the parasite does not occur. Consequently, *T. gondii* cysts may persist in any organ, though they are particularly common in brain, myocardium, skeletal muscle, and lymph nodes. Dormant organisms remain viable (Masur, 1992).

Immune competent individuals who acquire toxoplasmosis may have a transient flu-like illness with fever, malaise, and lymphadenopathy or, more commonly, suffer no clinical symptoms. With loss of immune competence, reactivation of latent infection leads to the emergence of clinical disease. Because not all AIDS patients with serologic evidence of toxoplasma infection develop clinical disease, it has been suggested that host factors, including genetic susceptibility or variation in strain virulence, may be important pathogenetic elements (Luft & Remington, 1992). Evidence derived largely from studies of murine toxoplasmosis suggests that interferon gamma is critical for resistance to both acute infection with *T. gondii* and subsequent reactivation of latent infestation. Upregulation of interferon gamma by dendritic cell secretion of interleukin 12 appears to be an important inducer of interferon gamma in both T cells and non-T cells. CD8 T- lymphocytes are considered to be the major efferent limb in resistance against acute infection and are important regulators of the numbers of cysts, although it is thought that humoral immunity may also play a role. Activation of macrophages, microglia, and astrocytes by interferon gamma appear to be important in suppression of *T. gondii* by a number of mechanisms, which may include generation of NO by iNOS, depletion of tryptophan pools by indolamine dioxygenase, genetic control of resistance factors, limitation of sources of intracellular iron, and generation of reactive oxygen intermediates (Hunter & Remington, 1994; Suzuki, 2002).

In most AIDS patients, low levels of IgG antibodies and lack of IgM antibodies to *T. gondii* suggest reactivation of latent infection; however, occasional reported cases are more typical of acute infection (Leport, Raffi et al., 1988; Renold, Sugar et al., 1992). Pathologically proven or clinically responsive cases of presumed toxoplasmic encephalitis may occur in 15–20% of AIDS patients (Porter & Sande, 1992). Studies on stored sera indicate that some cases of seronegative toxoplasmosis may result from loss of previous antibody responses (Renold, Sugar et al., 1992). Immune competence as indicated by CD4 lymphocyte levels is significantly compromised in the majority of AIDS patients with toxoplasmic encephalitis, with CD4 counts less than 200/mm^3 in about 90% and less than 100/mm^3 in about two-thirds of cases (Porter & Sande, 1992).

Neuropathology

Toxoplasmic encephalitis is characterized pathologically by hemorrhagic or coagulative necrosis with a mixed inflammatory reaction. Granulomas may be present and microglial nodules containing encysted organisms or free tachyzoites may be found. Organisms are best demonstrated with immunoperoxidase stains. Hematoxylin-eosin staining may fail to reveal organisms in up to half of cases with positive immunoperoxidase stains (Luft, Brooks et al., 1984). Vascular involvement is prominent and results in infarction and vasculitis. Less often, small hemorrhages may be found (Israelski & Remington, 1988; Cornford, Holden et al., 1992). A granular ependymitis may be seen in the ventricular walls (Gray, Gherardi et al., 1988).

Less active lesions may consist of small microglial aggregates with encysted or free organisms. Necrotizing lesions may be circumscribed or poorly demarcated with organisms evident peripherally. As organized abscesses develop, a rim of macrophages surrounds the area of necrosis and rare encysted bradyzoites are found around chronic abscesses (Luft, Brooks et al., 1984; Navia, Cho et al., 1986; Petito, Cho et al., 1986; Farkesh, MacCabee et al., 1986; Gray, Gherardi et al., 1988; Lang, Miklossy et al., 1990; Burns, Risser et al., 1991; Cornford, Holden et al., 1992). Histologic features may vary with the degree of immune suppression. More intense lymphocytic and plasmocytic responses with fibrous capsular formation may be seen in those with more competent immune systems, while more modest inflammation without capsules may be seen in those with more advanced immune suppression (Falangola, Reichler et al., 1994).

Clinical Features

The most common clinical presentation is a subacute illness evolving over days to weeks, characterized by fever, headache, often confusion or cognitive disturbances, and focal neurologic findings on examination, including hemiparesis, ataxia, cranial neuropathies, aphasias, visual field defects, and sensory impairments (Navia, Jordan et al., 1986; Israelski & Remington, 1988; Luft & Remington, 1992; Porter & Sande, 1992; Renold, Sugar et al., 1992). A patient presenting with panhypopituitarism has been reported (Milligan, Katz et al., 1984). Seizures are presenting features in up to 24–29% of patients (Porter & Sande, 1992; Renold, Sugar et al., 1992) and a patient presenting with a diffuse subacute encephalopathy and continuous focal discharges on electroencephalography resembling herpetic encephalitis has been described (Carrazana, Rossitch et al., 1989).

Meningoencephalitis presenting with diffuse encephalopathy and cerebrospinal fluid inflammation in the absence of parenchymal lesions detectable by computerized tomography has been reported (Caramello, Forno et al., 1993; Artigas, Grosse et al., 1994). Subacutely progressive fatal encephalopathy in patients lacking focal findings or radiographic evidence of parenchymal lesions has been found to be due to diffuse toxoplasmic encephalitis with or without positive toxoplasmic serology (Gray, Gherardi et al., 1989). Two cases of diffuse toxoplasmic encephalitis following a more prolonged course more typical of HIV encephalopathy have been reported (Arendt, Hefter et al., 1991).

The tendency of toxoplasmic encephalitis to occur in the basal ganglia has resulted in a number of descriptions of patients with movement disorders, including chorea, ballistic movements (Nath, Jankovic et al., 1987; Deway & Jankovic, 1989)), focal dystonia (Tolge & Factor, 1991), choreoathetosis (Maggi, de Mari et al., 1996), and akathisia (Carrazana, Rossitch et al., 1989). The movements are often unilateral, reflecting localization of the underlying lesions and may persist despite resolution of the abscesses following antibiotic therapy. The movements may respond to symptomatic treatment (Nath, Hobson et al., 1993). Two patients with thalamic pain syndrome due to toxoplasmic abscesses which persisted despite effective antibiotic therapy responded to amitryptilene (Gonzales, Herskovitz et al., 1992).

Occasional patients with a brainstem encephalitis due to *T. gondii* have been reported with oculomotor weakness and contralateral ataxia (Kure, Harris et al., 1989) or hemiplegia, ipsilateral rubral tremor, or complete external ophthalmoplegia (Daras, Koppel et al., 1994). Parinaud's syndrome and pineal region abscess have also been reported (Daras, Koppel et al., 1994; Poon, Behbahani et al., 1994).

Microscopic hemorrhage in necrotic regions is a neuropathologic finding in toxoplasmic encephalitis. Clinically apparent intracerebral hemorrhage has occasionally been noted, perhaps due to toxoplasmic arteritis or endothelial parasitism (Levy, Bredesen et al., 1985; Chaudhari, Singh et al., 1989; Trenkwalder, Trenkwalder et al., 1992).

A patient with progressive obstructive hydrocephalus in the absence of other abnormalities on CT scan was found to have multifocal necrotic lesions in the periaqueductal region and in the basal ganglia and cerebellum (Nolla-Salas, Ricart et al., 1987). Patients with progressive obstructive hydrocephalus in the absence of parenchymal lesions on MRI have been found to have a necrotizing ependymitis due to *T. gondii* (Eggers, Vortmeyer et al., 1995; de Silva, Raychaudhuri et al., 2005; Sell, Sander et al., 2005).

Psychiatric symptoms as an isolated presenting feature of toxoplasmic encephalitis were described in 12 of 53 hospitalized French AIDS patients. Depression, psychomotor slowing, bipolar disease, dementia, and schizophrenic syndromes were seen (Linard, Beau et al., 1992).

A few patients with toxoplasmic myelitis have been reported. Necrotizing myelitis presenting with rapidly progressive upper limb weakness and paresthesias (Mehren, Burns et al., 1988), thoracic pain followed after two months by progressive leg weakness, and urinary and fecal incontinence (Herskovitz, Siegel et al., 1989), and an acute conus medullaris syndrome (Overhage, Greist et al., 1990; Harris, Smith et al., 1990) have been described.

T. gondii may also produce a myositis concurrent with or in the absence of CNS infection. Fever and myalgias with weakness, wasting, and elevated creatine kinase levels comprise the clinical features (Gherardi, Baudrimont et al., 1992).

Diagnosing Toxoplasmosis

Radiology

Most AIDS patients with toxoplasmic encephalitis will have multiple discrete mass lesions revealed by imaging procedures. Lesions are most commonly located at the cortical gray-white matter junctions and in the basal ganglia, but also may be found in the brainstem and cerebellum. Following contrast infusion, homogenous or ring enhancement is typical, though some lesions exhibit marginal enhancement or fail to enhance at all (Post, Kursunoglu et al., 1985; Levy, Bredesen et al., 1985; Navia, Jordan et al., 1986; Farkesh, MacCabee et al., 1986; Rovira, Post et al., 1991; Porter & Sande, 1992; Renold, Sugar et al., 1992). Double doses of contrast with delayed imaging sequences increase the sensitivity of cranial computed tomography (Post, Kursunoglu et al., 1985).

Magnetic resonance imaging (MRI) is more sensitive than CT and may reveal additional lesions (Ciricillo & Rosenblum, 1990; Porter & Sande, 1992) (Figure 8.5.3). Isolated toxoplasmic abscesses may occur in up to 14% of cases (Renold, Sugar et al,. 1992; Porter & Sande, 1992) and false negative MRI scans in patients with toxoplasmic encephalitis have been noted; however, solitary enhancing lesions on MRI were four times more likely to be lymphomas than toxoplasmic abscesses in a large series from San Francisco (Ciricillo & Rosenblum, 1990).

A number of studies have explored the value of metabolic imaging in diagnosis of CNS mass lesions in AIDS patients. Most of these have used single photon emission computed tomography (SPECT) in the differentiation of CNS lymphoma from CNS infection. In the majority of these cases, the CNS infections proved to be toxoplasmic encephalitis; however, the technique is not useful in distinguishing among different infectious etiologies for cerebral abscesses. Initial studies found the majority of lymphomas to demonstrate

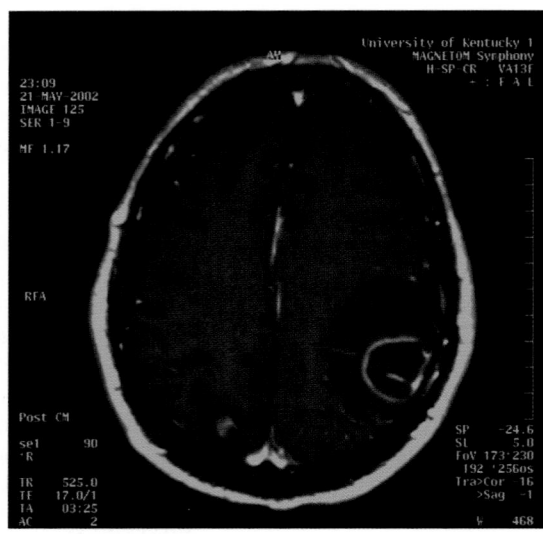

Figure 8.5.3 Cerebral toxoplasmosis. Figure 8.5.3a (left) is a fluid-attenuated inversion recovery (FLAIR) axial MRI showing a large area of edema surrounding an oval toxoplasmosis abscess in the right basal ganglia. Figure 8.5.3b (right) shows the underlying lesion enhanced by gadolinium on contrast-enhanced T1-weighted MRI.

increased uptake with thallium 201-SPECT while abscesses were characterized by hypometabolism (O'Malley, Ziessman et al., 1994; Ruiz, Ganz et al., 1994); however, more recent studies have found more modest accuracy (D'Amico, Messa et al., 1997; Lorberboym, Wallach et al., 1998; Licho, Litofsky et al., 2002). It has been suggested that sensitivity and specificity may be increased with the use of three-hour delayed imaging to assess radionucleide retention (Lorberboym, Wallach et al., 1998), and in combination with serum titers for *T. gondii* IgG > 1:256 (Skiest, Erdman et al., 2000).

Effective antibiotic therapy results in parallel clinical and radiologic responses in most patients, with up to 95% showing improvement within two weeks (Porter & Sande, 1992). Some radiologic lesions may persist for six weeks and resolution may take as long as six months (Levy, Rosenbloom et al., 1986). Radiologic worsening despite clinical improvement may occur in the first three weeks of therapy (Luft & Remington, 1992).

Cerebrospinal Fluid

CSF in patients with cerebral toxoplasmosis is usually unremarkable or nonspecific, with modest protein elevation being the most common abnormality. Occasionally, a lymphocytic pleocytosis is seen (Navia, Petito et al., 1986; Porter and Sande, 1992). Patients with meningoencephalitis or meningomyelitis may show a mixed pleocytosis with prominent protein elevations and normal or depressed glucose levels (Mehren, Burns et al., 1988; Herskovitz, Siegel et al., 1989; Overhage, Greist et al., 1990; Caramello, Forno et al., 1993). *T. gondii* has occasionally been cultured from CSF of patients with meningoencephalitis (Caramello, Forno et al., 1993; Eggers, Gross et al., 1995).

IgG antibodies to *T. gondii* may be detected in CSF and may occasionally show fourfold elevations on serial specimens in the absence of similar changes in serum (Navia, Petito et al., 1986;

Porter & Sande, 1992). Toxoplasma-specific IgG antibody indices may be elevated in about two-thirds of patients with toxoplasmic encephalitis. CSF antibodies are not usually found in patients with serum antibodies but no CNS disease (Potasman, Resnick et al., 1988; Orefice, Carrieri et al., 1992). IgA antibodies to the P30 surface protein of *T. gondii* were found in two-thirds of CSF samples from patients with acute toxoplasmic encephalitis, but only 15% of paired serum samples, and none of a small control group with other opportunistic infections in a recent study (Mastroianni, Mengoni et al., 1994). An ELISA containing pooled *Toxoplasma gondii*-secreted antigens was able to distinguish sera from symptomatic cerebral toxoplasmosis from those with chronic asymptomatic toxoplasmosis (Meira, Costa-Silva et al., 2008).

Polymerase chain reaction amplification techniques have been used to detect *T. gondii* DNA in CSF and serum. Unfortunately, sensitivity varies from 11.5% to 65% using probes directed at the B1 gene (Parmley, Goebel et al., 1992; Novati, Castagna et al., 1994; Eggers, Vortmeyer et al., 1995; Cingolani, De Luca et al., 1996). In one study, PCR in CSF demonstrated *T. gondii*-specific DNA in two-thirds of patients with toxoplasmic encephalitis but no control patients without CNS disease whether seropositive or not (Schoondermark-van de Ven, Galama et al., 1993). Serial PCR amplification studies to detect the P30 surface protein of *T. gondii* in serum correlated with parasitemia in another recent study but were negative in some patients with toxoplasmic encephalitis (Dupouy-Camet, de Souza et al., 1993).

A study using reverse transcriptase-PCR (RT-PCR) retrospectively identified tachyzoite - specific surface antigen 1 (SAG-1) in CSF of 63.6% of subjects with a first attack of toxoplasmic encephalitis in comparison to 36.4% detected by nested PCR (n-PCR). Bradyzoite-specific surface antigen 4 (SAG-4) was detected in 75% of relapsing toxoplasmic encephalitis using RT-PCR compared to 62.5% by n-PCR and matric-associated antigen -1 (MAG-1), which is localized in cyst walls, was detected in 100% of relapsing patients by RT-PCR compared to 62.5% by n-PCR. This small study found additionally that RT-PCR detected SAG-1 only in patients with a first episode of toxoplasmic encephalitis while SAG-4 and MAG-1 were found exclusively in relapsing disease. (Cultrera, Seraceni et al., 2002). Recently, a study comparing real-time PCR for detecting the B1 gene of *T. gondii* in blood and CSF of patients with cerebral toxoplasmosis compared to AIDS patients with other neurological diseases found a sensitivity of 35.3%, specificity and positive predictive values of 100%, and a negative predictive value of 44.7% in CSF while sensitivity in blood was only 1.5% with a negative predictive value of 365%. The authors concluded that CSF PCR offered low sensitivity but high specificity while PCR on blood was not useful for diagnosis (Correia, Melo et al., 2010). PCR techniques can also be used to detect *T. gondii* DNA in brain-biopsy specimens (Johnson, Butcher et al., 1993).

Treatment

The treatment of choice for AIDS patients with CNS toxoplasmosis is a combined regimen of sulfadiazine and pyrimethamine given initially in induction doses of 4–8 gm/day and 50–75 mg/day, respectively. A 100–200 mg initial dose of pyrimethamine is given the first day. To counteract myelosuppression from the pyrimethamine, leukovorin in doses of 10–15 mg/day is given concurrently (Kovacs, 1995). Acute treatment should be continued for at least six weeks if there is clinical and radiological response and may be required for longer periods if the response is incomplete. Cotrimoxazole is considered an alternative option which is well tolerated and less expensive than pyrimethamine–sulfadiazine and can be used parenterally (Kaplan, Benson et al., 2009). In a recent observational report of 83 patients followed for a mean of about 3 years, 10–50 mg/kg/day (15–75mg/kg/day for obtunded patients) cotrimoxazole was given initially for 3–5 days followed by 7.5–37.5 mg/kg/day once clinical improvement was seen for another 4–6 weeks, after which 160/800mg qd was given orally. Efficacy was reported as 85.5%, with relapses over the follow-up period in 30% (Beraud, Pierre-Francois et al., 2009). Response in most patients with CNS toxoplasmosis is rapid, typically beginning within days, and radiologic improvements are evident within two to three weeks, though occasional patients respond over six weeks or longer (Navia, Petito et al., 1986; Porter and Sande, 1992).

Patients intolerant to sulfa can be given clindamycin in split doses of 2400–4800 mg/day initially in combination with the pyrimethamine and leukovorin. Efficacy in acute treatment appears to be similar (Dannemann, McCutchan et al., 1992; Luft, Hafner et al., 1993); however, relapse rates in patients on maintenance regimens may be higher in those taking clindamycin compared to those on sulfadiazine (Porter & Sande, 1992). Some patients will be intolerant to both sulfa and clindamycin. Alternative options include atovaquone (Kovacs, 1992; Iribarren, Goenaga et al., 1994), pyrimethamine and azithromycin (Saba, Morlat et al., 1993), pyrimethamine and dapsone (Ward, 1992), pyrimethamine and doxycycline (Hagberg, Palmertz et al., 1993), or pyrimethamine and clarithromycin (Fernandez-Martin, Leport et al., 1991). These alternative options have not been shown to have equivalent efficacy to date (Cinque, Baldanti et al., 1995). A phase II trial using an atovaquone suspension in combination with either pyrimethamine or sulfadiazine demonstrated a 75% acute response rate after six weeks with the former regimen and an 82% response with the latter; however, 34 of 39 subjects discontinued maintenance treatment during the 48-week follow-up phase (Chirgwin, Hafner et al., 2002).

The speed with which clinical and radiographic response occurs permits presumptive diagnosis and empiric initiation of therapy in AIDS patients with typical clinical and radiographic features and positive serology for *T. gondii* (Cohn, McMeeking et al., 1989). Opinions vary for patients lacking toxoplasmic serology or with single lesions by MRI, and we tend to favor early biopsy to establish a firm diagnosis in single lesions in patients with negative serology and in those who fail to respond rapidly to antibiotic therapy directed at *T. gondii*. Induction antibiotic regimens are continued for six weeks with repeat imaging studies at two to three weeks. Progressive disease at any site should prompt consideration of biopsy to exclude a concurrent or alternate pathology. Occasionally, mixed pathologies may occur within the same lesion (Cohen, 1999). In vitro secretion of antitoxoplasmic antibodies by peripheral blood mononuclear cells may be useful as a surrogate marker of response of toxoplasmic encephalitis to therapy (Lacascade, Conge et al., 2000).

Following successful acute therapy, relapse rates of 30–60% were previously reported in patients who discontinued antibiotics (Porter & Sande, 1992; Richards, Kovacs et al., 1995), and were noted to occur despite maintenance antibiotics in up to 20% (Renold, Sugar et al., 1992; Porter & Sande, 1992). Patients with persistent enhancement of lesions on neuroimaging studies following initial antibiotic therapy were found to be at increased risk of recurrence in one series (Laissy, Soyer et al., 1994). Maintenance regimens continue acute therapy at reduced dosages of 2 gm/day sulfadiazine or 1200–1800 mg/day clindamycin with pyrimethamine 50–75 mg/day and leukovorin. Daily maintenance therapy with sulfadiazine and pyrimethamine has been shown to be superior to intermittent regimens in preventing recurrence of toxoplasmic encephalitis (Podzamczer, Miro et al., 1995). Pyrimethamine alone is less effective than in combination maintenance regimens with clindamycin or sulfadiazine (de Gans, Portegies et al., 1992). Proposed alternative regimens for secondary prophylaxis include dapsone, dapsone with pyrimethamine, atovaquone, or aerosolized pentamidine (Kaplan, Benson et al., 2009).

More recently, with the availability of HAART and resulting immune reconstitution, studies have demonstrated the safety of discontinuing secondary prophylaxis when sustained elevation of CD4 lymphocyte levels are achieved and HAART is continued (Soriano, Dona et al., 2000; Kirk, Reiss et al., 2002). However, continued monitoring is required as recurrent toxoplasmic encephalitis has been seen even with prolonged and sustained elevations of CD4 (Kirk, Reiss et al., 2002; Antinori, Larussa et al., 2004). Current guidelines on prophylaxis for opportunistic infections in HIV-infected individuals do consider discontinuation of secondary prophylaxis following sustained increases in CD4 counts >200 cells/mm^3 on HAART to be reasonable. Resumption of prophylaxis is recommended if CD4 counts drop below this level (Masur, Kaplan et al., 2002; Kaplan, Benson et al., 2009).

Primary prophylaxis for toxoplasmic encephalitis is now common practice among physicians treating HIV-infected patients with immune suppression (CD4+ count < 100 cell/ml) and serologic evidence of infection. Trimethoprim-sulfamethoxazole 160mg/800mg taken twice daily two times weekly was found to prevent toxoplasmic encephalitis in a small uncontrolled series (Carr, Tindall et al., 1992). Dapsone 50 mg/day plus pyrimethamine 50 mg/week has also been shown to have efficacy in primary prevention (Girard, Landman et al., 1993). In contrast, trials of primary prophylaxis for pneumocystis pneumonia have yielded mixed results, with one study finding neither trimethoprim-sulfamethoxazole three times weekly with or without pyrimethamine 25 mg weekly, nor dapsone 100 mg and pyrimethamine 25 mg weekly effective in preventing initial episodes of toxoplasmosis in HIV-infected patients seropositive for *T. gondii*

(Mallolas, Zamora et al., 1993). Another open label trial found a fixed combination of 500 mg sufadoxine and 25 mg pyridoxine, supplemented with 15 mg of leukovorin, twice weekly safe and effective in preventing toxoplasma encephalitis in AIDS patients with CD4 levels < 100 cells/mm3 (Schurmann, Bergmann et al., 2002). At present, primary prophylaxis with daily trimethoprim-sulfamethoxazole or dapsone and pyrimethamine is recommended for HIV-infected patients with CD4 counts less than 100/mm^3 and seropositivity to *T. gondii* (Masur, Kaplan et al., 2002; Kaplan, Benson et al., 2009). Recent studies have demonstrated that primary prophylaxis can be safely discontinued when CD4 counts rise to sustained levels >200/mm3 (Mussini, Pezzotti et al., 2000), and current guidelines now recommend such discontinuation (Masur, Kaplan et al., 2002; Kaplan, Benson et al., 2009).

Immune Reconstitution Syndrome with Toxoplasmic Encephalitis

Only a few cases of immune reconstitution syndrome associated with cerebral toxoplasmosis have been reported to date. In one recent report, Cerebral toxoplasmosis was seen 3 months following initiation of HAART with a documented increase in CD4+ cells from 130 to 290/mm3. The patient presented with focal onset secondary generalized seizures and was found to have a large right frontal T2 signal abnormality with associated enhancement and lesser involvement of the left frontal white matter. Empiric treatment for cerebral toxoplasmosis was initiated but discontinued a week later when a serum toxoplasmic IgG antibody serology was negative. The patient worsened and brain biopsy revealed both an intense CD8+ lymphocytic immune response typical of IRIS and the presence of *T. gondii* tachyzoites and bradyzoites. Resumption of treatment of cerebral toxoplasmosis led to almost complete resolution. In this case, the restoration of immune function led to the unmasking of cerebral toxoplasmosis (Pfeffer, Prout et al., 2009).

ACANTHAMOEBA

Acanthamoeba are commonly found in moist soil in warm climactic regions and can produce human infection when acquired by inhalation or cutaneous contact. Hematogenous spread from pulmonary or cutaneous foci may provide entry to the CNS resulting in a subacute or chronic encephalitis, in contrast to the more fulminant encephalitis produced by *Naegleria*, which is contracted from swimming in infested water and invades the CNS by way of the olfactory tract (Bottone 1993). The normal immune response is both humoral and granulomatous (Sison, Kemper et al. 1995).

Meningoencephalitis resulting from *Acanthamoeba* or leptomyxid amebic infestation has been reported in HIV-infected patients. Clinical features are nonspecific, with fever and headache with or without focal neurologic findings on examination. Meningismus or signs of increased intracranial pressure may be present. Seizures may be a presenting feature (Wiley, Sofrin et al., 1987; Anzil, Rao et al., 1991; Gardner,

Martinez et al., 1991; Di Gregorio, Rivasi et al., 1992; Gordon, Steinberg et al. 1992; Tan, Guiloff et al., 1993). Nodular papular or pustular cutaneous lesions precede amebic encephalitis in half the cases (Tan, Guiloff et al., 1993; Sison, Kemper et al., 1995).

Cerebral imaging studies may show hypodensities or mass lesions with enhancement (Wiley, Sofrin et al., 1987 ; Gardner, Martinez et al., 1991 ; Martinez, Gonzalez-Mediero et al., 2000) or without (Gordon, Steinberg et al., 1992), following contrast infusion. Lesions vary in size. Mass effect may (Gardner, Martinez et al., 1991; Gordon & Blumberg, 1992; Martinez, Gonzalez-Mediero et al., 2000) or may not be present (Gardner, Martinez et al., 1991).

Cerebrospinal fluid may show a neutrophilic pleocytosis with protein elevation (Wiley, Sofrin et al., 1987) or be acellular (Gardner, Martinez et al., 1991; Gordon, Steinberg et al., 1992). Organisms have not been recovered from CSF in HIV-infected patients to date, and diagnosis has been made histopathologically by brain biopsy (Gordon & Blumberg, 1992) or at autopsy. Cutaneous lesions when present may yield a diagnosis on histopathologic examination (Tan, Guiloff et al., 1993; Sison, Kemper et al., 1995).

Neuropathologic examination reveals necrotizing arteritis and fibrinoid necrosis (Wiley, Sofrin et al., 1987; Di Gregorio, Rivasi et al., 1992). A thrombo-occlusive angiitis involving thin-walled vessels may be seen (Gardner, Martinez et al., 1991). A suppurative meningitis may be extensive (Wiley, Sofrin et al., 1987). Amoebic trophozoites can be demonstrated with periodic acid-Schiff and methenamine silver stains. Encysted organisms may also be seen (Wiley, Sofrin et al., 1987; Gardner, Martinez et al., 1991; Gordon, Steinberg et al., 1992; Di Gregorio, Rivasi et al., 1992).

It has been suggested that the rapidly progressive course seen in most AIDS patients with acanthamoeba encephalitis may be due to diminished ability to mount an effective granulomatous response. While no specific therapy has been identified for acanthamoeba encephalitis, a non-HIV-infected patient has been reported to respond to sulfamethazine (Cleland, Lawande et al., 1982). An AIDS patient with *Acanthamoeba castellanii* producing a localized mass lesion was successfully treated with surgical excision followed by fluconazole and sulfadiazine antibiotic therapy (Martinez, Gonzalez-Mediero et al., 2000).

TRYPANOSOMA CRUZI (CHAGAS DISEASE)

Trypanosoma cruzi is a flagellated parasite, endemic in rural Mexico and Central and South America, has been estimated to infect 16–18 million people in the Western Hemisphere, often without overt clinical symptoms. Acute meningoencephalitis may occur at the onset of infection, typically in childhood. The disease is acquired from fecal material in soil with inoculation through skin breaks or mucous membranes. Transmission via contaminated needles or blood transfusion is known, as is transplacental infection of newborn infants. Ingestion of contaminated food has been implicated. Meningoencephalitis may occur in the acute phase, but in most individuals, chronic latency ensues. Chronic infection most commonly affects the heart, producing cardiomyopathy with congestive heart failure or arrhythmia, or the autonomic cells of the gut, resulting in megaesophagus or megacolon. CNS disease in chronic *T. cruzi* infection in HIV-infected patients is the most common manifestation, with myocarditis the second (Diazgranados, Saavedra-Trujillo et al., 2009; (Rosemberg, Chaves et al., 1992; Rocha, de Meneses et al., 1994; Ferreira, Nishioka Sde et al., 1997).

Despite the widespread prevalence of *T. cruzi* infestation, a limited number of patients with HIV infection and Chagas' disease has been reported to date. However, of the 23 cases reviewed in 1994 by Rocha and colleagues, 20 were found to have multifocal CNS disease. Where noted, most had diminished CD4 lymphocyte counts (Rocha, de Meneses et al., 1994). The most common clinical presentation of CNS involvement were features of a meningoencephalitis with headache and fever, often with focal findings on neurologic examination and sometimes with seizures (Del Castillo, Mendoza et al., 1990; Ferreira, Nishioka Sde et al., 1991; Gluckstein, Ciferri et al., 1992; Solari, Saavedra et al., 1993; Metze & Maciel, 1993; Ferreira, Nishioka Sde et al., 1997). One patient presented with progressive ataxia and emesis due to progressive hydrocephalus resulting from meningoencephalitis (Rosemberg, Chaves et al., 1992).

Cerebral imaging studies in 16 patients revealed focal or multifocal lesions in 15. Following contrast infusion, ring-enhancement patterns were common, though some nonenhancing or irregular enhancing lesions were also seen. Mass effect was common but not always seen (Rocha, de Meneses et al., 1994). The principal differential considerations are toxoplasmosis or lymphoma.

Cerebrospinal fluid studies reported in nine cases revealed lymphocytic pleocytosis in seven. Moderate to marked protein elevation occurred in all eight cases noted, and hypoglycorrhachia was reported in five of eight (Rocha, de Meneses et al., 1994). Cell counts are typically less than 100/μL. *T. cruzi* trypomastigotes can be identified in Giemsa-stained CSF. Motile parasites can sometimes be seen in fresh unstained CSF specimens (Ferreira, Nishioka Sde et al., 1997). Antibodies to *T. cruzi* are not usually found in CSF (Gluckstein, Ciferri et al., 1992; Metze & Maciel, 1993). In a recent case report, Lages-Silva and colleagues used PCR techniques to document *T. cruzi* in CSF and to monitor the course of Chagasic meningoencephalitis during therapy (Lagues-Silva, Ramirez et al., 2002). The parasite can be demonstrated in blood smears; however, positive blood cultures are found in the setting of chronic disease (Ferreira, Nishioka Sde et al., 1997).

Empiric therapy for toxoplasmosis was initiated on presentation in a number of reported cases. Correct diagnosis was subsequently made from pathological analysis of biopsy or autopsy tissue. Histopathological features include multifocal hemorrhagic necrosis with amastigotes of *T. cruzi* demonstrable intracellularly in glia, macrophages, endothelial cells, and less commonly, neurons by methenamine silver stains. Free amastigotes may be seen in perivascular and intercellular spaces (Del Castillo, Mendoza et al., 1990; Gluckstein, Ciferri et al., 1992; Solari, Saavedra et al., 1993; Rocha, de Meneses et al., 1994). Purulent meningitis and vasculitis has been noted in some instances (Rosemberg, Chaves et al., 1992; Solari, Saavedra et al., 1993).

Therapy in two cases following biopsy diagnosis appeared to be beneficial. One patient stabilized neurologically with residual deficits and radiologic lesions following four weeks of nifurtimox before dying of pneumocystis pneumonia several months later (Del Castillo, Mendoza et al., 1990). Another was treated initially with benznidazole 400mg/day followed by itraconazole and fluconazole 400 mg/day, resulting in resolution of fever and stabilization of neurologic symptoms. Maintenance therapy with benznidazole 200 mg/day was associated with clinical stabilization, though with persistent lesions radiographically over a nine-month period (Solari, Saavedra et al., 1993). A recent review recommends benznidazole 5 mg/kg daily split into two doses for 60–90 days, or nifurtimox 8–10 mg/kg daily split into three doses, with induction therapy continuing for 60–120 days (Diazgranados, Saavedra-Trujillo et al., 2009). Others have suggested benznidazole 5–8 mg/kg daily for 30–60 days or nifurtimox 8–10 mg/kg for 90–120 days (Kaplan, Benson et al., 2009). Although no standard regimen for secondary prophylaxis currently is established, authors suggest benznidazole 3–5 mg/kg or nifurtimox 5 mg/kg three times weekly (Diazgranados, Saavedra-Trujillo et al., 2009; Ferreira, Nishioka Sde et al., 1997).

Despite the frequency of infestation in endemic areas where HIV infection is increasingly being found, CNS opportunistic infection with *T. cruzi* appears uncommon to date. Only one instance was found in a neuropathologic series of 252 HIV autopsy cases from Brazil (Chimelli, Rosemberg et al., 1992). Nonetheless, awareness of this parasite, which mimics toxoplasmosis in its clinical and imaging features, should prompt aggressive diagnostic evaluation in HIV-infected patients from endemic areas with compatible clinical presentations and risk factors for inoculation (Diazgranados, Saavedra-Trujillo et al., 2009).

STRONGYLOIDES STERCORALIS

Strongyloides stercoralis are an intestinal nematode found in moist soil in tropical and semi tropical areas including the Southeastern United States. Ingestion results in colonization of the intestine, which is usually asymptomatic. Sexual transmission may occur. Both humoral and cellular immunity appear important in control of the infestation and disseminated disease occurs in individuals with immune compromise due to steroids, cytotoxic drugs, or systemic disease. A hyperinfection syndrome in which the infective filariform larvae may carry intestinal bacteria to distant sites including the meninges may result (Maayan, Wormser et al., 1987; Dutcher, Marcus et al., 1990).

Only a few cases of HIV-infected patients with meningitis associated with the *Strongyloides* hyperinfection syndrome have been reported. In some instances, other risk factors such as steroid and cytotoxic therapy for an AIDS patient with systemic lymphoma were present. The organism was recovered from CSF and stool samples (Dutcher, Marcus et al., 1990).

Gastrointestinal symptoms may precede neurologic features with anorexia, weight loss, and diarrhea (Armignacco, Capecchi et al., 1989; Harcourt-Webster, Scaravilli et al., 1991 ; Morgello, Soifer et al., 1993). Subsequent purulent meningitis has been reported due to *E. coli* (Maayan, Wormser et al., 1987; Armignacco, Capecchi et al., 1989) or *Streptococcus bovis* (Jain, Agarwal et al., 1994).

Thiabendozole therapy has been tried but proved unsuccessful in two instances (Dutcher, Marcus et al., 1990; Jain, Agarwal et al., 1994), and failed to prevent hyperinfection syndrome in another patient with AIDS (Harcourt-Webster, Scaravilli et al., 1991).

Cerebral infestation by *Strongyloides* in two patients produced a granulomatous ependymitis and subependymitis with viable larvae in cortex and white matter in one and white matter and cerebral vessels resulting in infarctions in another. Neither had meningitis nor any inflammatory response to the larvae (Morgello, Soifer et al., 1993).

CYSTICERCOSIS (TAENIA SOLIUM)

Neurocysticercosis are a common infestation in Mexico and parts of Central and South America, Africa, and Asia. Often acquired by ingestion, they may be asymptomatic or cause seizures, meningitis, hydrocephalus, cerebral abscess, or infarction. Thornton, Houston et al. (1992) reported four cases from a series of 107 HIV-infected patients from Zimbabwe, 13 of whom had intracranial mass lesions. All four presented with headaches and seizures or focal deficits on examination. Multiple cystic lesions were present on CT scans. The frequency of cysticercosis producing 30% of cerebral mass lesions in an HIV-infected population was compared to a non-HIV-infected series of 51 intracranial mass lesions in which only 6% were due to neurocysticercosis. The authors suggest the increased frequency may be due to reactivation in a setting of immune suppression (Thornton, Houston et al., 1992).

In contrast, a case of asymptomatic neurocysticercosis and cryptococcal meningitis was reported in an AIDS patient with the speculation that immune suppression might prevent the emergence of neurocysticercosis symptoms, resulting from the host inflammatory response to the parasite (White, Dakik et al., 1995). An autopsy series from Mexico noted only one case of neurocysticercosis in 97 AIDS patients compared to three cases in 197 controls, suggesting that the association between HIV-infection and neurocysticercosis might be coincidental (Barron-Rodriguez, Jessurun et al., 1990).

ALGAE

A case of meningitis due to *Prototheca wickerhamii* in an HIV-infected intravenous drug user co-infected with cryptococcal meningitis has been reported. Treatment with amphotericin B and five fluorocytosine appeared to suppress the fungal infection; however, *P. wickerhamii* was isolated from a subsequent CSF sample. Autopsy disclosed both cryptococcal and prothecal meningitis (Kaminski, Kapila et al., 1992).

IRIS WITH OPPORTUNISTIC INFECTIONS

The immune reconstitution inflammatory syndrome (IRIS) follows the institution of HAART and is defined as a paradoxical deterioration of the clinical status attributable to the recovery of the immune system (Shelburne, Hamill et al., 2002). While IRIS has been described with a wide variety of opportunistic infections, it may also result from an inflammatory immune response mounted to noninfectious antigens. The noninfectious forms of IRIS include autoimmune disorders, such as Graves' disease; malignancies, such as worsening of Kaposi's sarcoma; and other inflammatory conditions including sarcoidosis and inflammation at tattoo sites (Dhasmana, Dheda et al., 2008). Conversely, IRIS need not always be associated with HIV infection. It has been observed after the removal of natalizumab therapy in multiple sclerosis patients with PML (Clifford, DeLuca et al., 2010). Individuals may develop IRIS before the underlying opportunistic infection has been recognized. In fact, patients may be asymptomatic with respect to the infection, only for it to blossom into an aggressive illness at the time it is unmasked by the immune reconstitution. Alternatively, and more commonly, the opportunistic infection had been recognized but worsens dramatically at the time of immune recovery. Diagnosis requires that there is an increase of CD4+ T-lymphocytes and a decrease in HIV viral load subsequent to treatment with antiretroviral therapies (usually, but not necessarily, including a protease inhibitor), symptoms consistent with an infectious/inflammatory disorder while on ART, and symptoms that cannot be explained by other disorders, such as a newly acquired infection (Tan, Roda et al., 2009). No radiographic criteria have been incorporated into the diagnosis, but contrast enhancement is often observed on CT or MRI, reflective of the inflammatory process. Similarly, there are no specific cerebrospinal fluid abnormalities. IRIS has been associated with numerical increases in CD4+ T-lymphocytes which typically starts 1 to 2 weeks after initiation of HAART and continues for 2 to 3 months (Autran, Carcelain et al., 1997), but it is likely that other components of the immune system are as important to its pathogenesis (Shelburne, Hamill et al., 2002). Some investigators have proposed that an inappropriate or delayed restoration of impaired regulatory immune mechanisms predisposes to an uncontrolled antigen-specific response (Ruhwald & Ravn, 2007). Pathological examination of IRIS affected tissue reveals a brisk perivascular infiltration of CD8+ - T lymphocytes (Miller, Isaacson et al., 2004; Dhasmana, Dheda et al., 2008). Nonetheless, its pathogenesis remains poorly understood (Dhasmana, Dheda et al., 2008).

The form of IRIS that is characterized by the unmasking of an opportunistic infection may be prevented by thoroughly screening the patient in advance of the initiation of ART. IRIS can be life threatening and therefore, aggressive management may be necessitated. Typically, high-dose corticosteroid therapy has been employed to reduce the inflammatory response; however, in circumstances in which the illness is unresponsive to corticosteroids, interrupting ART may be required (Dhasmana, Dheda et al., 2008). Other therapies are dependent on the underlying disorder. The best therapy will require additional study.

REFERENCES

(1948). Streptomycin treatment of tuberculous meningitis. Report of the committee on streptomycin in tuberculosis trials. *Lancet, 1*, 582–597.

(1984). Syphilis-United States, 1983. *Morbidity and Mortality Weekly Report*, CDDC. Atlanta. 33, 433–441.

(1986). Treatment of serious cytomegalovirus infections with 9-(1,3-dihydroxy-2-propoxymethyl)guanine in patients with AIDS and other immunodeficiencies. Collaborative DHPG Treatment Study Group. *N Engl J Med, 314*(13), 801–805.

(1988). Continuing increase in infectious syphilis—United States. *Morbidity and Mortality Weekly Report*. CDC. Atlanta 3735–3738.

(1988). Recommendations for diagnosing and treating syphilis in HIV-infected patients. *Morbidity and Mortality Weekly Report*. CDC. Atlanta. 37, 600–608.

(1996). Combination foscarnet and ganciclovir therapy vs monotherapy for the treatment of relapsed cytomegalovirus retinitis in patients with AIDS. The Cytomegalovirus Retreatment Trial. The Studies of Ocular Complications of AIDS Research Group in Collaboration with the AIDS Clinical Trials Group. *Arch Ophthalmol, 114*(1), 23–33.

Abdool K., Naidoo, K., et al. Timing of initiation of antiretroviral drugs during tuberculosis therapy. *N Engl J Med, 362*(8), 697–706.

Abgrall, S., Rabaud, C., et al. (2001). Incidence and risk factors for toxoplasmic encephalitis in human immunodeficiency virus-infected patients before and during the highly active antiretroviral therapy era. *Clin Infect Dis, 33*(10), 1747–1755.

Achim, C. L., Nagra, R. M., et al. (1994). Detection of cytomegalovirus in cerebrospinal fluid autopsy specimens from AIDS patients. *J Infect Dis, 169*(3), 623–627.

Adair, J. C., Beck, A. C., et al. (1987). Nocardial cerebral abscess in the acquired immunodeficiency syndrome. *Arch Neurol, 44*(5), 548–550.

Aksamit, A. J. & Kost, S. (1994). PCR detection of JC virus in PMS and control CSF. *Neuroscience of HIV infection. Basis and clinical frontiers.*

Al-Zamel, F. A. (2009). Detection and diagnosis of Mycobacterium tuberculosis. *Expert Rev Anti Infect Ther, 7*(9), 1099–1108.

Alamo, C. & Garcia Herruzo, J. G. (1991). Nocardiosis in a patient with AIDS. *Revista Clinica Espanola, 188*, 83–84.

Alarcon, F., Duenas, G., et al. (2000). Movement disorders in 30 patients with tuberculous meningitis. *Mov Disord, 15*(3), 561–569.

Alvarez, S. & McCabe, W. R. (1984). Extrapulmonary tuberculosis revisited: A review of experience at Boston City and other hospitals. *Medicine (Baltimore), 63*(1), 25–55.

Amlie-Lefond, C., Kleinschmidt-DeMasters, B. K. et al. (1995). The vasculopathy of varicella-zoster virus encephalitis." *Ann Neuro, l 37*(6), 784–790.

Ampel, N. M., Dols, C. L., et al. (1993). Coccidioidomycosis during human immunodeficiency virus infection: Results of a prospective study in a coccidioidal endemic area. *Am J Med, 94*(3), 235–240.

Anaissie, E., Fainstein, V., et al. (1988). Central nervous system histoplasmosis. An unappreciated complication of the acquired immunodeficiency syndrome. *Am J Med, 84*(2), 215–217.

Anders, H. J. & Goebel, F. D. (1998). Cytomegalovirus polyradiculopathy in patients with AIDS. *Clin Infect Dis, 27*(2), 345–352.

Anders, H. J. & Goebel, F. D. (1999). Neurological manifestations of cytomegalovirus infection in the acquired immunodeficiency syndrome. *Int J STD AIDS, 10*(3), 151–159; quiz 160–151.

Anders, H. J., Weiss, N., et al. (1998). Ganciclovir and foscarnet efficacy in AIDS-related CMV polyradiculopathy. *J Infect. 36*(1), 29–33.

Andreula, C. F., Burdi, N., et al. (1993). CNS cryptococcosis in AIDS: Spectrum of MR findings. *J Comput Assist Tomogr. 17*(3), 438–441.

Anduze-Faris, B. M., Fillet, A. M., et al. (2000). Induction and mainte-nance therapy of cytomegalovirus central nervous system infection in HIV-infected patients. *AIDS, 14*(5), 517–524.

Antinori, A., Ammassari, A., et al. (2001). Epidemiology and prognosis of AIDS-associated progressive multifocal leukoencephalopathy in the HAART era. *J Neurovirol, 7*(4), 323–328.

Antinori, A., Larussa, D., et al. (2004). Prevalence, associated factors, and prognostic determinants of AIDS-related toxoplasmic encephalitis in the era of advanced highly active antiretroviral therapy. *Clin Infect Dis,39*(11), 1681–1691.

Antonsson, A., Green, A. C., et al. Prevalence and stability of antibodies to the BK and JC polyomaviruses—a long-term longitudinal study of Australians. J Gen Virol,.

Anzil, A. P., Rao, C. et al. (1991). Amebic meningoencephalitis in a patient with AIDS caused by a newly recognized opportunistic patho-gen. Leptomyxid ameba. *Arch Pathol Lab Med, 115*(1), 21–25.

Appleman, M. E., Marshall, D. W., et al. (1988). Cerebrospinal fluid abnormalities in patients without AIDS who are seropositive for the human immunodeficiency virus. *J Infect Dis, 158*(1), 193–199.

Aral, S. O. & Holmes, K. K. (1990). Epidemiology of sexual behaviour and sexually transmitted diseases. *Sexually transmitted diseases*, pp. 19–36. New York: McGraw-Hill.

Arendt, G., Hefter, H., et al. (1991). Two cases of cerebral toxoplasmosis in AIDS patients mimicking HIV-related dementia. *J Neurol, 238*(8), 439–442.

Armignacco, O., Capecchi, A., et al. (1989). Strongyloides stercoralis hyperinfection and the acquired immunodeficiency syndrome. *Am J Med, 86*(2), 258.

Arribas, J. R., Clifford, D. B., et al. (1995). Level of cytomegalovirus (CMV) DNA in cerebrospinal fluid of subjects with AIDS and CMV infection of the central nervous system. *J Infect Dis, 172*(2), 527–531.

Arribas, J. R., Storch, G. A., et al. (1996). Cytomegalovirus encephalitis. *Ann Intern Med, 125*(7), 577–587.

Arthur, R. R., Dagostin, S., et al. (1989). Detection of BK virus and JC virus in urine and brain tissue by the polymerase chain reaction. *J Clin Microbiol, 27*(6), 1174–1179.

Artigas, J., Grosse, G., et al. (1994). Severe toxoplasmic ventriculom-eningoencephalomyelitis in two AIDS patients following treatment of cerebral toxoplasmic granuloma. *Clinical Neuropathology, 13*, 120–126.

Asnis, D. S., Chitkara, R. K., et al. (1988). Invasive aspergillosis: An unusual manifestation of AIDS. *N Y State J Med, 88*(12), 653–655.

Astrom, K. E., Mancall, E. L., et al. (1958). Progressive multifocal leuko-encephalopathy; a hitherto unrecognized complication of chronic lymphatic leukaemia and Hodgkin's disease. *Brain, 81*(1), 93–111.

Autran, B., Carcelain, G., et al. (1997). Positive effects of combined anti-retroviral therapy on CD4+ T cell homeostasis and function in advanced HIV disease. *Science, 277*(5322), 112–116.

Aygun, N., Finelli, D. A., et al. (1998). Multifocal varicella-zoster virus leukoencephalitis in a patient with AIDS: MR findings. *AJNR Am J Neuroradiol, 19*(10), 1897–1899.

Bacellar, H., Munoz, A., et al. (1994). Temporal trends in the incidence of HIV-1-related neurologic diseases: Multicenter AIDS Cohort Study. *Neurology, 44*, 1892–1900.

Bale, J. F., Jr. (1984). Human cytomegalovirus infection and disorders of the nervous system. *Arch Neurol, 41*(3), 310–320.

Balfour, H. H., Jr., Benson, C., et al. (1994). Management of acyclovir-resistant herpes simplex and varicella-zoster virus infections. *J Acquir Immune Defic Syndr, 7*(3), 254–260.

Banerjee, U., Mohapatra, A. K., et al. (1989). Cladosporiosis (cerebral phaeohyphomycosis) of brain—a case report. *Mycopathologia, 105*(3), 163–166.

Baringer, J. R. (1974). Recovery of herpes simplex virus from human sacral ganglions. *N Engl J Med, 291*(16), 828–830.

Baringer, J. R. & Swoveland, P. (1973). Recovery of herpes-simplex virus from human trigeminal ganglions. *N Engl J Med, 288*(13), 648–650.

Barrett-Connor, E. (1967). Tuberculous meningitis in adults. *South Med J, 60*(10), 1061–1067.

Barron-Rodriguez, L. P., Jessurun, J., et al. (1990). The prevalence of inva-sive amebiasis and cysticercosis is not increased in Mexican patients dying of AIDS. International Conference on AIDS. San Francisco: 253.

Bauer, W., Chamberlin W., & Horenstein, S. (1969). Spinal demyelina-tion in progressive multifocal leukoencephalopathy. *Neurology, 19*.

Bayne, L. L., Schmidley, J. W., et al. (1986). Acute syphilitic meningitis. Its occurrence after clinical and serologic cure of secondary syphilis with penicillin G. *Arch Neurol, 43*(2), 137–138.

Bazan, C., 3rd, Jackson, C., et al. (1991). Gadolinium-enhanced MRI in a case of cytomegalovirus polyradiculopathy. *Neurology, 41*(9), 1522–1523.

Becerra, L. I., Ksiazek, S. M., et al. (1989). Syphilitic uveitis in human immunodeficiency virus-infected and noninfected patients. *Ophthalmology, 96*(12), 1727–1730.

Bedri, J., Weinstein, W., et al. (1983). Progressive multifocal leukoenceph-alopathy in acquired immunodeficiency syndrome. *N Engl J Med, 309*(8), 492–493.

Behar, R., Wiley, C., et al. (1987). Cytomegalovirus polyradiculoneuropa-thy in acquired immune deficiency syndrome. *Neurology, 37*(4), 557–561.

Behzad-Behbahani, A., Klapper, P. E., et al. (2003). BKV-DNA and JCV-DNA in CSF of patients with suspected meningitis or encephalitis. *Infection, 31*(6), 374–378.

Belec, L., Tayot, J., et al. (1990). Cytomegalovirus encephalopathy in an infant with congenital acquired immunodeficiency syndrome. *Neuropediatrics, 21*(3), 124–129.

Beraud, G., Pierre-Francois, S., et al. (2009). Cotrimoxazole for treatment of cerebral toxoplasmosis: An observational cohort study during 1994–2006. *Am J Trop Med Hyg, 80*(4), 583–587.

Berenguer, J., Moreno, S., et al. (1992). Tuberculous meningitis in patients infected with the human immunodeficiency virus. *N Engl J Med, 326*(10), 668–672.

Bergen, G. A., B. G. Yangco, et al. (1993). Central nervous system infec-tion with *Mycobacterium kansasii*. *Ann Intern Med, 118*(5), 396.

Berger, D. S., Bucher, G., et al. (1996). Acute primary human immunode-ficiency virus type 1 infection in a patient with concomitant cytomeg-alovirus encephalitis. *Clin Infect Dis, 23*(1), 66–70.

Berger, J. R. (1987). Syphilis of the spinal cord. In R. A. Davidoff *Handbook of the spinal cord*, pp. 491–538. New York: Marcel Dekker.

Berger, J. R. (1990). Neurosyphilis. In *Current therapy in neurologic dis-ease,*. pp. 143–147. Philadelphia, PA: Dekker.

Berger, J. R. (1991). Neurosyphilis in human immunodeficiency virus type 1-seropositive individuals. A prospective study. *Arch Neurol, 48*(7), 700–702.

Berger, J. R. (1996). Prolonged survival in pathologically-proven AIDS-associated PML. (Abstract). *J Neurvirology, 2*: 31.

Berger, J. R. (2009). Steroids for PML-IRIS: a double-edged sword? *Neurology, 72*(17), 1454–1455.

Berger, J.R. (2010). Progressive multifocal leukoencephalopathy and newer biological agents. Drug Saf. 1;33(11):969-83.

Berger, J. R. & Concha, M. (1995). Progressive multifocal leukoenceph-opathy: The evolution of a disease once considered rare. *J Neurovirol, 1*(1), 5–18.

Berger, J. R., Houff, S. A., et al. (2009). Monoclonal antibodies and progressive multifocal leukoencephalopathy. *Mabs, 1*(6), 583–589.

Berger, J. R., Kaszovitz, B., et al. (1987). Progressive multifocal leukoen-cephalopathy associated with human immunodeficiency virus infection. A review of the literature with a report of sixteen cases. *Ann Intern Med, 107*(1), 78–87.

Berger, J. R., McCarthy, M., et al. (1989). Serological and cerebrospinal fluid parameters related to syphilis in HIV asymptomatic seroposi-tives. Fifth International Conference on AIDS . Montreal, CA: 361.

Berger, J. R. & Mucke, L. (1988). Prolonged survival and partial recovery in AIDS-associated progressive multifocal leukoencephalopathy. *Neurology, 38*(7), 1060–1065.

Berger, J. R., Pall, L., et al. (1998). Progressive multifocal leukoencephal-opathy in patients with HIV infection. *J Neurovirol, 4*(1), 59–68.

Berger, J. R., Scott, G., et al. (1992). Progressive multifocal leukoencephal-opathy in HIV-1-infected children. *AIDS, 6*(8), 837–841.

Berger, J. R., Waskin, H., et al. (1992). Syphilitic cerebral gumma with HIV infection. *Neurology, 42*(7), 1282–1287.

Bergstrom, J., Vahlne, A., et al. (1990). Primary and recurrent herpes simplex virus type 2 induced meningitis. *Journal of Infectious Diseases, 162,* 322–330.

Berman, S. M. & Kim, R. C. (1994). The development of cytomegalovirus encephalitis in AIDS patients receiving ganciclovir. *Am J Med, 96*(5), 415–419.

Berry, A. J., Rinaldi, M., et al. (1992). Use of high dose fluconazole as salvage therapy for cryptococcal meningitis in patients with AIDS. *Antimicrobial Agents and Chemotherapy, 36,* 690–692.

Berry, C. D., Hooton, T. M., et al. (1987). Neurologic relapse after benzathine penicillin therapy for secondary syphilis in a patient with HIV infection. *N Engl J Med,316*(25), 1587–1589.

Bhargava, B. S., Gupta, A. K., et al. (1982). Tuberculous meningitis, a CT study. *British Journal of Radiology, 55,* 189–196.

Bhigjee, A. I., Padayachee, R., et al. (2007). Diagnosis of tuberculous meningitis: Clinical and laboratory parameters. *Int J Infect Dis, 11*(4), 348–354.

Bicanic, T., Brouwer, A. E., et al. (2009). Relationship of cerebrospinal fluid pressure, fungal burden and outcome in patients with cryptococcal meningitis undergoing serial lumbar punctures. *AIDS, 23*(6), 701–706.

Bicanic, T., Meintjes, G., et al. (2009). Immune reconstitution inflammatory syndrome in HIV-associated cryptococcal meningitis: A prospective study. *J Acquir Immune Defic Syndr, 51*(2), 130–134.

Bishburg, E., Eng, R. H., et al. (1989). Brain lesions in patients with acquired immunodeficiency syndrome. *Arch Intern Med, 149*(4), 941–943.

Bishburg, E., Sunderam, G., et al. (1986). Central nervous system tuberculosis with the acquired immunodeficiency syndrome and its related complex. *Ann Intern Med, 105*(2), 210–213.

Bishopric, G., Bruner, J., et al. (1985). Guillain-Barre syndrome with cytomegalovirus infection of peripheral nerves. *Arch Pathol Lab Med, 109*(12), 1106–1108.

Blake, K., Pillay, D., et al. (1992). JC virus associated meningoencephalitis in an immunocompetent girl. *Arch Dis Child, 67*(7), 956–957.

Blatt, S. P., Lucey, D. R., et al. (1991). Rhinocerebral zygomycosis in a patient with AIDS. *J Infect Dis, 164*(1), 215–216.

Blick, G., Garton, T., et al. (1997). Successful use of cidofovir in treating AIDS-related cytomegalovirus retinitis, encephalitis, and esophagitis. *J Acquir Immune Defic Syndr Hum Retrovirol, 15*(1), 84–85.

Bobrowitz, E. D. (1972). Ethambutol in tuberculous meningitis. *Chest, 61,* 629–632.

Bottone, E. J. (1993). Free-living amebas of the genera Acanthamoeba and Naegleria: An overview and basic microbiologic correlates. *Mt Sinai J Med, 60*(4), 260–270.

Bowen, B. C. & Post, M. J. (1991). Intracranial infections. In S. W. Atlas (ed.). *Magnetic resonance imaging of the brain and spine.* New York: Raven Press.

Bozzette, S. A., Larsen, R. A., et al. (1991). A placebo-controlled trial of maintenance therapy with fluconazole after treatment of cryptococcal meningitis in the acquired immunodeficiency syndrome. California Collaborative Treatment Group. *N Engl J Med, 324*(9), 580–584.

Brickelmaier, M., Lugovskoy, A., et al. (2009). Identification and characterization of mefloquine efficacy against JC virus in vitro. *Antimicrob Agents Chemother, 53*(5), 1840–1849.

Britton, C. B., Mesa-Tejada, R., et al. (1985). A new complication of AIDS: Thoracic myelitis caused by herpes simplex virus. *Neurology, 35,* 1071–1074.

Bronnimann, D. A., Adam, R. D., et al. (1987). Coccidioidomycosis in the acquired immunodeficiency syndrome. *Ann Intern Med, 106*(3), 372–379.

Brooks, B. R. & Walker, D. L. (1984). Progressive multifocal leukoencephalopathy. *Neurol Clin, 2*(2), 299–313.

Brooks, J. B., Choudhary, G., et al. (1977). Electron capture gas chromatography detection and mass spectrum identification of 3-(2'-keto-hexyl)indoline in spinal fluids of patients with tuberculous meningitis. *J Clin Microbiol, 5*(6), 625–628.

Bruinsma-Adams, I. K. (1991). AIDS presenting as Candida albicans meningitis: A case report. *AIDS, 5*(10), 1268–1269.

Brunel, A. S., Makinson, A., et al. (2009). HIV-related immune reconstitution cryptococcal meningoradiculitis: orticosteroid response. *Neurology, 73*(20), 1705–1707.

Buchbinder, S. P., Katz, M. H., et al. (1992). Herpes zoster and human immunodeficiency virus infection. *J Infect Dis, 166*(5), 1153–1156.

Bullock, M. R. & Welchman, J. M. (1982). Diagnostic and prognostic features of tuberculous meningitis on CT scanning. *J Neurol Neurosurg Psychiatry, 45*(12), 1098–1101.

Burke, A. W. (1972). Syphilis in a Jamaican psychiatric hospital. A review of 52 cases including 17 of neurosyphilis. *Br J Vener Dis, 48*(4), 249–253.

Burke, J. M. & Schaberg, D. R. (1985). Neurosyphilis in the antibiotic era. *Neurology, 35*(9), 1368–1371.

Burns, D. K., Risser, R. C., et al. (1991). The neuropathology of human immunodeficiency virus infection. The Dallas, Texas, experience. *Arch Pathol Lab Med, 115*(11), 1112–1124.

Caplan, L. R., Kleeman, F. J., et al. (1977). Urinary retention probably secondary to herpes genitalis. *N Engl J Med, 297*(17), 920–921.

Caramello, P., Forno, B., et al. (1993). Meningoencephalitis caused by Toxoplasma gondii diagnosed by isolation from cerebrospinal fluid in an HIV-positive patient. *Scand J Infect Dis, 25*(5), 663–666.

Carneiro, A. V., Ferro, J., et al. (1991). Herpes zoster and controlateral hemiplegia in an African patient infected with HIV-1. *Acta Med Port, 4*(2), 91–92.

Carr, A., Tindall, B., et al. (1992). Low-dose trimethoprim-sulfamethoxazole prophylaxis for toxoplasmic encephalitis in patients with AIDS. *Ann Intern Med, 117*(2), 106–111.

Carrazana, E. J., Rossitch, E., Jr., et al. (1991). Isolated central nervous system aspergillosis in the acquired immunodeficiency syndrome. *Clin Neurol Neurosurg, 93*(3), 227–230.

Carrazana, E. J., Rossitch, Jr., E., et al. (1989). Parkinsonian symptoms in a patient with AIDS and cerebral toxoplasmosis. *J Neurol Neurosurg Psychiatry, 52*(12), 1445–1447.

Carrazana, E. J., Rossitch, Jr., E., et al. (1989). Cerebral toxoplasmosis masquerading as herpes encephalitis in a patient with the acquired immunodeficiency syndrome. *Am J Med, 86*(6 Pt 1), 730–732.

Carter, J. B., Hamill, R. J., et al. (1987). Bilateral syphilitic optic neuritis in a patient with a positive test for HIV. Case report. *Arch Ophthalmol, 105*(11), 1485–1486.

Casadevall, A., Spitzer, E. D., et al. (1993). Susceptibilities of serial Cryptococcus neoformans isolates from patients with recurrent cryptococcal meningitis to amphotericin B and fluconazole. *Antimicrob Agents Chemother, 37*(6), 1383–1386.

CDC. (2009). Sexually Transmitted Disease Surveillance, 2008: National Surveillance Data for Chlamydia, Gonorrhea, and Syphilis. http://www.cdc.gov/std/stats08/2008survFactSheet.PDF.

Cecchini, D., Ambrosioni, J., et al. (2009). Tuberculous meningitis in HIV-infected and non-infected patients: Comparison of cerebrospinal fluid findings. *Int J Tuberc Lung Dis, 13*(2), 269–271.

Cettomai, D. & McArthur, J. C. (2009). Mirtazapine use in human immunodeficiency virus-infected patients with progressive multifocal leukoencephalopathy. *Arch Neurol, 66*(2), 255–258.

Chatis, P. A., Miller, C. H., et al. (1989). Successful treatment with foscarnet of an acyclovir-resistant mucocutaneous infection with herpes simplex virus in a patient with acquired immunodeficiency syndrome. *N Engl J Med, 320*(5), 297–300.

Chaudhari, A. B., Singh, A., et al. (1989). Haemorrahe in cerebral toxoplasmosis. *S Afr Med J, 76,* 272–274.

Chimelli, L., Rosemberg, S., et al. (1992). Pathology of the central nervous system in patients infected with the human immunodeficiency virus (HIV): A report of 252 autopsy cases from Brazil. *Neuropathol Appl Neurobiol, 18*(5), 478–488.

Chirgwin, K., Hafner, R., et al. (2002). Randomized phase II trial of atovaquone with pyrimethamine or sulfadiazine for treatment of toxoplasmic encephalitis in patients with acquired immunodeficiency syndrome: ACTG 237/ANRS 039 Study. AIDS Clinical Trials Group 237/Agence Nationale de Recherche sur le SIDA, Essai 039. *Clin Infect Dis, 34*(9), 1243–1250.

Chow, D., Okinaka, L., et al. (2009). Hansen's disease with HIV: A case of immune reconstitution disease. *Hawaii Med J, 68*(2), 27–29.

Chretien, F., Belec, L., et al. (1996). Herpes simplex virus type 1 encephalitis in acquired immunodeficiency syndrome. *Neuropathol Appl Neurobiol*, 22(5), 394–404.

Chretien, F., Gray, F., et al. (1993). Acute varicella-zoster virus ventriculitis and meningo-myelo-radiculitis in acquired immunodeficiency syndrome. *Acta Neuropathol*, 86(6), 659–665.

Chuck, S. L. & Sande, M. A. (1989). Infections with Cryptococcus neoformans in the acquired immunodeficiency syndrome. *N Engl J Med*, 321(12), 794–799.

Chung, W. M., Pien, F. D., et al. (1983). Syphilis: A cause of fever of unknown origin. *Cutis*, 31(5), 537–540.

Cingolani, A., De Luca, A., et al. (1996). PCR detection of Toxoplasma gondii DNA in CSF for the differential diagnosis of AIDS-related focal brain lesions. *J Med Microbiol*, 45(6), 472–476.

Cinque, P., Baldanti, F., et al. (1995). Ganciclovir therapy for cytomegalovirus (CMV) infection of the central nervous system in AIDS patients: Monitoring by CMV DNA detection in cerebrospinal fluid. *J Infect Dis*, 171(6), 1603–1606.

Cinque, P., Cleator, G. M., et al. (1998). Diagnosis and clinical management of neurological disorders caused by cytomegalovirus in AIDS patients. European Union Concerted Action on Virus Meningitis and Encephalitis. *J Neurovirol*, 4(1), 120–132.

Cinque, P., Vago, L., et al. (1992). Cytomegalovirus infection of the central nervous system in patients with AIDS: Diagnosis by DNA amplification from cerebrospinal fluid. *J Infect Dis*, 166(6), 1408–1411.Ciricillo, S. F. & Rosenblum, M. L. (1990). Use of CT and MR imaging to distinguish intracranial lesions and to define the need for biopsy in AIDS patients. *J Neurosurg*, 73(5), 720–724.

Clark, B. M., Krueger, R. G., et al. (2004). Compartmentalization of the immune response in varicella zoster virus immune restoration disease causing transverse myelitis. *AIDS*, 18(8), 1218–1221.

Clark, R. & Carlisle, J. T. (1988). Neurosyphilis and HIV infection. *South Med J*, 81(9), 1204–1205.

Clark, R. A., Greer, D., et al. (1990). Spectrum of Cryptococcus neoformans infection in 68 patients infected with human immunodeficiency virus. *Rev Infect Dis*, 12(5), 768–777.

Clark, W. C., Metcalf, Jr., J. C., et al. (1986). Mycobacterium tuberculosis meningitis: A report of twelve cases and a literature review. *Neurosurgery*, 18(5), 604–610.

Cleland, P. G., Lawande, R. V., et al. (1982). Chronic amebic meningoencephalitis. *Arch Neurol*, 39(1), 56–57.

Clifford, D., Buller, R. S., et al. (1993). Use of polymerase chain reaction to domonstrate cytomegalovirus DNA in CSF of patients with human immunodeficiency virus infection. *Neurology*, 43, 75–79.

Clifford, D. B., Arribas, J. R., et al. (1996). Magnetic resonance brain imaging lacks sensitivity for AIDS associated cytomegalovirus encephalitis. *J Neurovirol* 2(6), 397–403.

Clifford, D. B., DeLuca, A., et al. (2010). Natalizumab-associated progressive multifocial leukoencephalopathy in patients with multiple sclerosis: Lessons from 28 cases. *Lancet Neurol*.

Clumeck, N. (1991). "Some aspects of the epdiemiology of toxoplasmosis and pneumocystosis in AIDS in Europe. *Eur J Clin Microbiol Infect Dis*, 10, 177–178.

Cohen, B. A. (1996). Prognosis and response to therapy of cytomegalovirus encephalitis and meningomyelitis in AIDS. *Neurology*, 46(2), 444–450.

Cohen, B. A. (1999). Neurologic manifestations of toxoplasmosis in AIDS. *Semin Neurol*, 19(2): 201–211.

Cohen, B. A., McArthur, J. C., et al. (1993). Neurologic prognosis of cytomegalovirus polyradiculomyelopathy in AIDS. *Neurology*, 43(3 Pt 1), 493–499.

Cohen, B. A., Rowley, A. H., et al. (1994). Herpes simplex type 2 in a patient with Mollaret's meningitis: Demonstration by polymerase chain reaction. *Ann Neurol*, 35(1), 112–116.

Cohen, D. B. & Glasgow, B. J. (1993). Bilateral optic nerve cryptococcosis in sudden blindness in patients with acquired immune deficiency syndrome. *Ophthalmology*, 100(11), 1689–1694.

Cohn, J. A., McMeeking, A. et al. (1989). "Evaluation of the policy of empiric treatment of suspected Toxoplasma encephalitis in patients with the acquired immunodeficiency syndrome." *Am J Med*, 86(5), 521–527.

Coker, R. J., Murphy, S. M., et al. (1991). Experience with liposomal amphotericin B (AmBisome) in cryptococcal meningitis in AIDS. *J Antimicrob Chemother*, 28 Suppl B, 105–109.

Cole, E. L., Meisler, D. M., et al. (1984). Herpes zoster ophthalmicus and acquired immune deficiency syndrome. *Arch Ophthalmol*, 102(7), 1027–1029.

Colon, L. G. (1988). Cerebral cladosporiosis in AIDS. (Abstract). *Journal of Neuropathology and Experimental Neurology*, 47, 387.

Conway, B., Halliday, W. C., et al. (1990). Human immunodeficiency virus-associated progressive multifocal leukoencephalopathy: Apparent response to 3'-azido-3'-deoxythymidine. *Rev Infect Dis*, 12(3), 479–482.

Coovadia, Y. M., Dawood, A., et al. (1986). Evaluation of adenosine deaminase activity and antibody to Mycobacterium tuberculosis antigen 5 in cerebrospinal fluid and the radioactive bromide partition test for the early diagnosis of tuberculosis meningitis. *Arch Dis Child*, 61(5), 428–435.

Cornford, M. E., Ho, H. W., et al. (1992). Correlation of neuromuscular pathology in acquired immune deficiency syndrome patients with cytomegalovirus infection and zidovudine treatment. *Acta Neuropathol*, 84(5), 516–529.

Cornford, M. E., Holden, J. K., et al. (1992). Neuropathology of the acquired immune deficiency syndrome (AIDS): Report of 39 autopsies from Vancouver, British Columbia. *Can J Neurol Sci*, 19(4), 442–452.

Correia, C. C., Melo, H. R., et al. (2010). Influence of neurotoxoplasmosis characteristics on real-time PCR sensitivity among AIDS patients in Brazil." *Trans R Soc Trop Med Hyg*, 104(1), 24–28.

Cox, J. N., DiDio, F., et al. (1990). Aspergillus endocarditit and myocarditis in a patient with the acquired immunodeficiency syndrome (AIDS). *Virchows Archives [A]*, 417, 255–259.

Craig, C. P. & Nahmias, A. J. (1973). Different patterns of neurologic involvement with herpes simplex virus types 1 and 2: Isolation of herpes simplex virus type 2 from the buffy coat of two adults with meningitis. *J Infect Dis*, 127(4), 365–372.

Croda, M. G., Vidal, J. E., et al. (2009). Tuberculous meningitis in HIV-infected patients in Brazil: Clinical and laboratory characteristics and factors associated with mortality. *Int J Infect Dis*.

Cuadrado, L. M., Guerrero, A., et al. (1988). Cerebral mucormycosis in two cases of acquired immunodeficiency syndrome. *Arch Neurol*, 45(1), 109–111.

Cultrera, R., Seraceni, S., et al. (2002). Efficacy of a novel reverse transcriptase-polymerase chain reaction (RT-PCR) for detecting Toxoplasma gondii bradyzoite gene expression in human clinical specimens. *Mol Cell Probes*, 16(1), 31–39.

Curless, R. G., Scott, G. B., et al. (1987). Progressive cytomegalovirus encephalopathy following congenital infection in an infant with acquired immunodeficiency syndrome. *Childs Nerv Syst*, 3(4), 255–257.

Cury, P. M., Pulido, C. F., et al. (2003). Autopsy findings in AIDS patients from a reference hospital in Brazil: Analysis of 92 cases. *Pathol Res Pract*, 199(12), 811–814.

D'Amico, A., Messa, C., et al. (1997). Diagnostic accuracy and predictive value of 201T1 SPET for the differential diagnosis of cerebral lesions in AIDS patients. *Nucl Med Commun*, 18(8), 741–750.

D'Oliveira, J. J. (1972). Cerebrospinal fluid concentrations of rifampin in meningeal tuberculosis. *Am Rev Respir Dis*, 106(3), 432–437.

Dahan, P., Haettich, B., et al. (1988). Meningoradiculitis due to herpes simplex virus disclosing HIV infection. *Ann Rheum Dis*, 47 (5), 440.

Daif, A., Obeid, T., et al. (1992). Unusual presentation of tuberculous meningitis. *Clin Neurol Neurosurg*, 94(1), 1–5.

Daniel, T. M. (1987). New approaches to the rapid diagnosis of tuberculous meningitis. *J Infect Dis*, 155(4), 599–602.

Dannemann, B., McCutchan, J. A., et al. (1992). "Treatment of toxoplasmic encephalitis in patients with AIDS. A randomized trial comparing pyrimethamine plus clindamycin to pyrimethamine plus sulfadiazine.

The California Collaborative Treatment Group. *Ann Intern Med*, *116*(1), 33–43.

Daras, M., Koppel, B. S., et al. (1994). Brainstem toxoplasmosis in patients with acquired immunodeficiency syndrome. *J Neuroimaging*, *4*(2), 85–90.

Davis, L. E., Rastogi, K. R., et al. (1993). Tuberculous meningitis in the southwest United States: A community-based study. *Neurology*, *43*(9), 1775–1778.

Davis, L. E. & Schmitt, J. W. (1989). Clinical significance of cerebrospinal fluid tests for neurosyphilis. *Ann Neurol*, *25*(1), 50–55.

Davis, L. E. & Sperry, S. (1979). The CSF-FTA test and the significance of blood contamination. *Ann Neurol*, *6*(1), 68–69.

de Gans, J., Portegies, P., et al. (1992). Pyrimethamine alone as maintenance therapy for central nervous system toxoplasmosis in 38 patients with AIDS. *J Acquir Immune Defic Syndr*, *5*(2), 137–142.

de Gans, J., Portegies, P., et al. (1990). Therapy for cytomegalovirus polyradiculomyelitis in patients with AIDS: Treatment with ganciclovir. *AIDS*, *4*(5), 421–425.

de Lalla, F., Pellizzer, G., et al. (1995). Amphotericin B as primary therapy for cryptococcosis in patients with AIDS: Reliability of relatively high doses administered over a relatively short period. *Clin Infect Dis*, *20*(2), 263–266.

de Silva, S. M., Mark, A. S., et al. (1996). Zoster myelitis: Improvement with antiviral therapy in two cases. *Neurology*, *47*(4), 929–931.

de Silva, T., Raychaudhuri, M., et al. (2005). Ventriculitis and hydrocephalus: An unusual presentation of toxoplasmosis in an adult with human immunodeficiency virus. *J Neurol Neurosurg Psychiatry*, *76*(8), 1074.

Deacon, W. E., Lucas, J. B., et al. (1966). Fluorescent treponemal pallikum antibody absorption (FTA-ABS) test for syphilis. *JAMA*, *198*, 624–628.

deAngelis, L. M., Weaver, S., et al. (1994). Herpes zoster (HVA) encephalitis in immunocompromised patients. (Abstract). *Neurology*, *44*(Suppl 2), A332.

Decker, C. F., Simon, G. L., et al. (1991). Listeria monocytogenes infections in patients with AIDS: report of five cases and review. *Rev Infect Dis*, *13*(3), 413–417.

Decker, C. F., Tarver, 3rd, J. H., et al. (1994). Prolonged concurrent use of ganciclovir and foscarnet in the treatment of polyradiculopathy due to cytomegalovirus in a patient with AIDS. *Clin Infect Dis*, *19*(3), 548–549.

deGans, J., Eeftinck Schattenkerk, J. K., et al. (1988). Itraconazole as maintenance treatment for cryptococcal meningitis inthe acquired immune deficiency syndrome. *British Medical Journal*, *296*, 339.

Del Castillo, M., Mendoza, G., et al. (1990). AIDS and Chagas' disease with central nervous system tumor-like lesion. *Am J Med*, *88*(6), 693–694.

Delaney, P. (1976). False positive serology in cerebrospinal fluid associated with a spinal cord tumor. *Neurology*, *26*(6 PT 1), 591–593.

Denning, D. W., Armstrong, R. W., et al. (1991). Elevated cerebrospinal fluid pressures in patients with cryptococcal meningitis and acquired immunodeficiency syndrome. *Am J Med*, *91*(3), 267–272.

Denning, D. W., Tucker, R. M., et al. (1989). Itraconazole therapy for cryptococcal meningitis and cryptococcosis. *Arch Intern Med*, *149*(10), 2301–2308.

Detels, R., Tarwater, P., et al. (2001). Effectiveness of potent antiretroviral therapies on the incidence of opportunistic infections before and after AIDS diagnosis. *AIDS*, *15*(3), 347–355.

Devinsky, O., Cho, E. S., et al. (1991). Herpes zoster myelitis. *Brain*, *114* (Pt 3), 1181–1196.

Deway, R. B. & Jankovic, J. (1989). Hemiballism-hemichorea: clinical and pharmacologic finding in 21 patients. *Arch Neurol*, *46*, 862–867.

Dewhurst, K. (1969). The composition of the cerebro-spinal fluid in the neurosyphilitic psychoses. *Acta Neurol Scand*, *45*(1), 119–123.

Dhasmana, D. J., Dheda, K., et al. (2008). "mmune reconstitution inflammatory syndrome in HIV-infected patients receiving antiretroviral therapy : Pathogenesis, clinical manifestations and management. *Drugs*, *68*(2), 191–208.

Di Gregorio, C., Rivasi, F., et al. (1992). Acanthamoeba meningoencephalitis in a patient with acquired immunodeficiency syndrome. *Arch Pathol Lab Med*, *116*(12), 1363–1365.

Diazgranados, C. A., Saavedra-Trujillo, C. H., et al. (2009). Chagasic encephalitis in HIV patients: Common presentation of an evolving epidemiological and clinical association. *Lancet Infect Dis*, *9*(5), 324–330.

Dieterich, D. T., Chachoua, A., et al. (1988). Ganciclovir treatment of gastrointestinal infections caused by cytomegalovirus in patients with AIDS. *Rev Infect Dis*, *10* Suppl 3, S532–537.

Dieterich, D. T., Poles, M. A., et al. (1993). Concurrent use of ganciclovir and foscarnet to treat cytomegalovirus infection in AIDS patients. *J Infect Dis*, *167*(5), 1184–1188.

Dismukes, W. E. (1988). Cryptococcal meningitis in patients with AIDS. *J Infect Dis*, *157*(4), 624–628.

Dismukes, W. E. (1992). Sporotrichosis. In J. B. Wyngaarden, L. H. Smith Jr., & J. C. Bennett *Cecil's textbook of medicine*, pp. 1897–1898. Philadelphia: W. B. Saunders.

Dix, R. D., Bredesen, D. E., et al. (1985). Recovery of herpesviruses from cerebrospinal fluid of immunodeficient homosexual men. *Ann Neurol*, *18*(5), 611–614.

Dix, R. D., Waitzman, D. M., et al. (1985). Herpes simplex virus type 2 encephalitis in two homosexual men with persistent lymphadenopathy. *Ann Neurol*, *17*(2), 203–206.

Doll, D. C., Yarbro, J. W., et al. (1987). Mycobacterial spinal cord abscess with an ascending polyneuropathy. *Ann Intern Med*, *106*(2), 333–334.

Domingo, P., Torres, O. H., et al. (2001). Herpes zoster as an immune reconstitution disease after initiation of combination antiretroviral therapy in patients with human immunodeficiency virus type-1 infection. *Am J Med*, *110*(8), 605–609.

Domingues, R. B., Fink, M. C., et al. (1998). Diagnosis of herpes simplex encephalitis by magnetic resonance imaging and polymerase chain reaction assay of cerebrospinal fluid. *J Neurol Sci*, *157*(2), 148–153.

Donabedian, H., O'Donnell, E., et al. (1994). Disseminated cutaneous and meningeal sporotrichosis in an AIDS patient. *Diagn Microbiol Infect Dis*, *18*(2), 111–115.

Donald, P. R., Victor, T. C., et al. (1993). Polymerase chain reaction in the diagnosis of tuberculous meningitis. *Scand J Infect Dis*, *25*(5), 613–617.

Donner, M. & Wasz-Hockert, O. (1962). Late neurologic sequelae of tuberculous meningitis. *Acta Paediatr 51*(Suppl 141), 34–42.

Drew, W. L. (1988). Cytomegalovirus infection in patients with AIDS. *J Infect Dis*, *158*, 449–456.

Drew, W. L., Mintz, L., et al. (1981). Prevalence of cytomegalovirus infection in homosexual men. *J Infect Dis*, *143*(2), 188–192.

Dube, M. P., Holtom, P. D., et al. (1992). Tuberculous meningitis in patients with and without human immunodeficiency virus infection. *Am J Med*, *93*(5), 520–524.

Dubois, V., Lafon, M. E., et al. (1996). Detection of JC virus DNA in the peripheral blood leukocytes of HIV-infected patients. *AIDS*, *10*(4), 353–358.

Duncan, W. C. (1989). Failure of erythromycin to cure secondary syphilis in a patient infected with the human immunodeficiency virus. *Arch Dermatol*, *125*(1), 82–84.

Dupouy-Camet, J., de Souza, S. L., et al. (1993). Detection of Toxoplasma gondii in venous blood from AIDS patients by polymerase chain reaction. *J Clin Microbiol*, *31*(7), 1866–1869.

Dutcher, J. P., Marcus, S. L., et al. (1990). Disseminated strongyloidiasis with central nervous system involvement diagnosed antemortem in a patient with acquired immunodeficiency syndrome and Burkitts lymphoma. *Cancer*, *66*(11), 2417–2420.

Dyer, J. R., French, M. A., et al. (1995). Cerebral mass lesions due to cytomegalovirus in patients with AIDS: Report of two cases. *J Infect*, *30*(2), 147–151.

Edwards, R. H., Messing, R., et al. (1985). Cytomegalovirus meningoencephalitis in a homosexual man with Kaposi's sarcoma: Isolation of CMV from CSF cells. *Neurology*, *35*(4), 560–562.

Eggers, C., Gross, U., et al. (1995). Limited value of cerebrospinal fluid for direct detection of Toxoplasma gondii in toxoplasmic encephalitis associated with AIDS. *J Neurol*, *242*(10), 644–649.

Eggers, C., Vortmeyer, A., et al. (1995). Cerebral toxoplasmosis in a patient with the acquired immunodeficiency syndrome presenting as obstructive hydrocephalus. *Clin Neuropathol*, *14*(1), 51–54.

Ehni, W. F. & Ellison, 3rd, R. T. (1987). Spontaneous Candida albicans meningitis in a patient with the acquired immune deficiency syndrome. *Am J Med*, *83*(4), 806–807.

Eide, F. F., Gean, A. D., et al. (1993). Clinical and radiographic findings in disseminated tuberculosis of the brain. *Neurology*, *43*(7), 1427–1429.

Eidelberg, D., Sotrel, A., et al. (1986). Thrombotic cerebral vasculopathy associated with herpes zoster. *Ann Neurol*, *19*(1), 7–14.

Eidelberg, D., Sotrel, A., et al. (1986). Progressive polyradiculopathy in acquired immune deficiency syndrome. *Neurology*, *36*(7), 912–916.

Elfaitouri, A., Hammarin, A. L., et al. (2006). Quantitative real-time PCR assay for detection of human polyomavirus infection. *J Virol Methods*, *135*(2), 207–213.

Eng, R. H., Bishburg, E., et al. (1986). Cryptococcal infections in patients with acquired immune deficiency syndrome. *Am J Med*, *81*(1), 19–23.

Englund, J. A., Zimmerman, M. E., et al. (1990). Herpes simplex virus resistant to acyclovir. A study in a tertiary care center. *Ann Intern Med*, *112*(6), 416–422.

Engsig, F. N., Hansen, A. B., et al. (2009). Incidence, clinical presentation, and outcome of progressive multifocal leukoencephalopathy in HIV-infected patients during the highly active antiretroviral therapy era: A nationwide cohort study. *J Infect Dis*, *199*(1), 77–83.

Enting, R., de Gans, J., et al. (1992). Ganciclovir/foscarnet for cytomegalovirus meningoencephalitis in AIDS. *Lancet*, *340*(8818), 559–560.

Erice, A., Chou, S., et al. (1989). Progressive disease due to ganciclovir-resistant cytomegalovirus in immunocompromised patients. *N Engl J Med*, *320*(5), 289–293.

Erlich, K. S., Mills, J., et al. (1989). Acyclovir-resistant herpes simplex virus infections in patients with the acquired immunodeficiency syndrome. *N Engl J Med*, *320*(5), 293–296.

Escobar, M. R., Dalton, H. P., et al. (1970). Fluorescent antibody tests for syphilis using cerebrospinal fluid; clinical correlation in 150 cases. *Am J Clin Pathol*, *53*, 886–890.

Everall, I., Vaida, F., et al. (2009). Cliniconeuropathologic correlates of human immunodeficiency virus in the era of antiretroviral therapy. *J Neurovirol*, *15*(5–6), 360–370.

Falangola, M. F., Reichler, B. S., et al. (1994). Histopathology of cerebral toxoplasmosis in human immunodeficiency virus infection: A comparison between patients with early-onset and late-onset acquired immunodeficiency syndrome. *Hum Pathol*, *25*(10), 1091–1097.

Falco, V., Olmo, M., et al. (2008). Influence of HAART on the clinical course of HIV-1-infected patients with progressive multifocal leukoencephalopathy: Results of an observational multicenter study. *J Acquir Immune Defic Syndr*, *49*(1), 26–31.

Farkesh, A. E., MacCabee, P. J., et al. (1986). CNS toxoplasmosis in acquired immune deficiency syndrome. *J Neurol Neurosurg Psychiatry*, *49*, 744–748.

Fedele, C. G., Ciardi, M. R., et al. (2003). Identical rearranged forms of JC polyomavirus transcriptional control region in plasma and cerebrospinal fluid of acquired immunodeficiency syndrome patients with progressive multifocal leukoencephalopathy. *J Neurovirol*, *9*(5), 551–558.

Feraru, E. R., Aronow, H. A., et al. (1990). Neurosyphilis in AIDS patients: initial CSF VDRL may be negative. *Neurology*, *40*(3 Pt 1), 541–543.

Fernandez-Guerrero, M. L., Miranda, C., et al. (1988). The treatment of neurosyphilis in patients with HIV infection. *JAMA*, *259*(10), 1495–1496.

Fernandez-Martin, J., Leport, C., et al. (1991). Pyrimethamine-clarithromycin combination for therapy of acute Toxoplasma encephalitis in patients with AIDS. *Antimicrob Agents Chemother*, *35*(10), 2049–2052.

Ferreira, M. S., Nishioka Sde, A., et al. (1991). Acute fatal Trypanosoma cruzi meningoencephalitis in a human immunodeficiency virus-positive hemophiliac patient. *Am J Trop Med Hyg*, *45*(6), 723–727.

Ferreira, M. S., Nishioka Sde, A., et al. (1997). Reactivation of Chagas' disease in patients with AIDS: Report of three new cases and review of the literature. *Clin Infect Dis*, *25*(6), 1397–1400.

Fessler, R. D., Sobel, J., et al. (1998). Management of elevated intracranial pressure in patients with Cryptococcal meningitis. *J Acquir Immune Defic Syndr Hum Retrovirol*, *17*(2), 137–142.

Fiala, M., Cone, L. A., et al. (1988). Responses of neurologic complications of AIDS to 3'-azido-3'-deoxythymidine and 9-(1,3-dihydroxy-2-propoxymethyl) guanine. I. Clinical features. *Rev Infect Dis*, *10*(2), 250–256.

Fish, D. G., Ampel, N. M., et al. (1990). Coccidioidomycosis during human immunodeficiency virus infection, a review of 77 patients. *Medicine*, *69*, 384–391.

Fleming, W. L. (1964). Syphilis through the ages. *Medical Clinics of North America*, *48*, 587–612.

Forgan-Smith, R., Ellard, G. A., et al. (1973). Pyrazinamide and other drugs in tuberculous meningitis. *Lancet*, *2*(7825), 374.

Fraimow, H. S., Wormser, G. P., et al. (1990). Salmonella meningitis and infection with HIV. *AIDS*, *4*(12), 1271–1273.

Franciotta, D., Zardini, E. et al. (1996). Antigen-specific oligoclonal IgG in AIDS-related cytomegalovirus and toxoplasma encephalitis. *Acta Neurol Scand*, *94*(3), 215–218.

Fraser, V. J., Keath, E. J., et al. (1991). Two cases of blastomycosis from a common source: Use of DNA restriction analysis to identify strains. *J Infect Dis*, *163*(6), 1378–1381.

Freeman, W. R., Lerner, C. W., et al. (1984). A prospective study of the ophthalmologic findings in the acquired immune deficiency syndrome. *Am J Ophthalmol*, *97*(2), 133–142.

French, G. L., Teoh, R., et al. (1987). Diagnosis of tuberculous meningitis by detection of tuberculostearic acid in cerebrospinal fluid. *Lancet*, *2*(8551), 117–119.

Friedland, G. H. & Klein, R. S. (1987). Transmission of the human immunodeficiency virus. *N Engl J Med*, *317*(18), 1125–1135.

Friedman, D. I. (1991). Neuro-ophthalmic manifestations of human immunodeficiency virus infection. *Neurol Clin*, *9*(1), 55–72.

Fuller, G. N., Guiloff, R. J., et al. (1989). Combined HIV-CMV encephalitis presenting with brainstem signs. *J Neurol Neurosurg Psychiatry*, *52*(8), 975–979.

Gal, A., Pollack, A., et al. (1984). Ocular findings in the acquired immunodeficiency syndrome. *Br J Ophthalmol*, *68*(4), 238–241.

Galgiani, J. N., Catanzaro, A., et al. (1993). Fluconazole therapy for coccidioidal meningitis. The NIAID-Mycoses Study Group. *Ann Intern Med*, *119*(1), 28–35.

Ganiem, A. R., Parwati, I., et al. (2009). The effect of HIV infection on adult meningitis in Indonesia: A prospective cohort study. *AIDS*, *23*(17), 2309–2316.

Gardner, H. A., Martinez, A. J., et al. (1991). Granulomatous amebic encephalitis in an AIDS patient. *Neurology*, *41*(12), 1993–1995.

Garrity, J. A., Herman, D. C., et al. (1993). Optic nerve sheath decompression for visual loss in patients with acquired immunodeficiency syndrome and cryptococcal meningitis with papilledema. *Am J Ophthalmol*, *116*(4), 472–478.

Gateley, A., Gander, R. M., et al. (1990). Herpes simplex virus type 2 meningoencephalitis resistant to acyclovir in a patient with AIDS. *J Infect Dis*, *161*(4), 711–715.

Gee, G. T., Bazan, 3rd, C., et al. (1992). Miliary tuberculosis involving the brain: MR findings. AJR *Am J Roentgenol*, *159*(5), 1075–1076.

Gelb, L. D. (1993). Varicella zoster virus: Clinical aslpects. In B. Roizman, R. J. Whitley & C. Lopez, *The human herpesviruses*, pp. 281–308. New York: Raven Press.

Ghanem, K. G., Moore, R. D., et al. (2008). Neurosyphilis in a clinical cohort of HIV-1-infected patients. *AIDS*, *22*(10), 1145–1151.

Ghanem, K. G., Moore, R. D., et al. (2009). Lumbar puncture in HIV-infected patients with syphilis and no neurologic symptoms. *Clin Infect Dis*, *48*(6), 816–821.

Gherardi, R., Baudrimont, M., et al. (1992). Skeletal muscle toxoplasmosis in patients with acquired immunodeficiency syndrome: A clinical and pathological study. *Ann Neurol*, *32*(4), 535–542.

Gibson, P. E., Field, A. M., et al. (1981). Occurrence of IgM antibodies against BK and JC polyomaviruses during pregnancy. *J Clin Pathol*, *34*(6), 674–679.

Gilden, D. H., Beinlich, B. R., et al. (1994). Varicella-zoster virus myelitis: An expanding spectrum. *Neurology*, *44*(10), 1818–1823.

Gilden, D. H., Devlin, M., et al. (1989). Persistence of varicella-zoster virus DNA in blood mononuclear cells of patients with varicella or zoster. *Virus Genes*, *2*(4), 299–305.

Gilden, D. H., Murray, R. S., et al. (1988). Chronic progressive varicella-zoster virus encephalitis in an AIDS patient. *Neurology*, *38*(7), 1150–1153.

Gillespie, S. M., Chang, Y., et al. (1991). Progressive multifocal leukoencephalopathy in persons infected with human immunodeficiency virus, San Francisco, 1981–1989. *Ann Neurol*, *30*(4), 597–604.

Girard, P. M., Landman, R., et al. (1993). Dapsone-pyrimethamine compared with aerosolized pentamidine as primary prophylaxis against Pneumocystis carinii pneumonia and toxoplasmosis in HIV infection. The PRIO Study Group. *N Engl J Med*, *328*(21), 1514–1520.

Glaser, J. B., Morton-Kute, L., et al. (1985). Recurrent Salmonella typhimurium bacteremia associated with the acquired immunodeficiency syndrome. *Ann Intern Med*, *102*(2), 189–193.

Glass, A. J. & Venter, M. (2009). Improved detection of JC virus in AIDS patients with progressive multifocal leukoencephalopathy by T-antigen specific fluorescence resonance energy transfer hybridization probe real-time PCR: Evidence of diverse JC virus genotypes associated with progressive multifocal leukoencephalopathy in Southern Africa. *J Med Virol*, *81*(11), 1929–1937.

Gluckstein, D., Ciferri, F., et al. (1992). Chagas' disease: Another cause of cerebral mass in the acquired immunodeficiency syndrome. *Am J Med*, *92*(4), 429–432.

Go, B. M., Ziring, D. J., et al. (1993). Spinal epidural abscess due to Aspergillus sp in a patient with acquired immunodeficiency syndrome. *South Med J*, *86*(8), 957–960.

Golnik, K. C., Newman, S. A., et al. (1991). Cryptococcal optic neuropathy in the acquired immune deficiency syndrome. *J Clin Neuroophthalmol*, *11*(2), 96–103.

Gomez-Tortosa, E., Gadea, I., et al. (1994). Development of myelopathy before herpes zoster rash in a patient with AIDS. *Clin Infect Dis*, *18*(5), 810–812.

Gonzales, G. R., Herskovitz, S., et al. (1992). Central pain from cerebral abscess: Thalamic syndrome in AIDS patients with toxoplasmosis. *Neurology*, *42*(5), 1107–1109.

Gordon, S. M. & Blumberg, H. M. (1992). Mycobacterium kansasii brain abscess in a patient with AIDS. *Clin Infect Dis*, *14*(3), 789–790.

Gordon, S. M., Steinberg, J. P., et al. (1992). Culture isolation of Acanthamoeba species and leptomyxid amebas from patients with amebic meningoencephalitis, including two patients with AIDS. *Clin Infect Dis*, *15*(6), 1024–1030.

Gorniak, R. J., Kramer, E. L., et al. (1997). Thallium-201 uptake in cytomegalovirus encephalitis. *J Nucl Med*, *38*(9), 1386–1388.

Gottlieb, M. S., Schroff, R., et al. (1981). Pneumocystis carinii pneumonia and mucosal candidiasis in previously healthy homosexual men: Evidence of a new acquired cellular immunodeficiency. *N Engl J Med*, *305*(24), 1425–1431.

Gould, I. A., Belok, L. C., et al. (1986). Listeria monocytogenes: A rare cause of opportunistic infection in the acquired immunodeficiency syndrome (AIDS) and a new cause of meningitis in AIDS. A case report. *AIDS Res*, *2*(3), 231–234.

Gozlan, J., el Amrani, M., et al. (1995). A prospective evaluation of clinical criteria and polymerase chain reaction assay of cerebrospinal fluid for the diagnosis of cytomegalovirus-related neurological diseases during AIDS. *AIDS*, *9*(3), 253–260.

Gozlan, J., Salord, J. M., et al. (1992). Rapid detection of cytomegalovirus DNA in cerebrospinal fluid of AIDS patients with neurologic disorders. *J Infect Dis*, *166*(6), 1416–1421.

Grafe, M. R., Press, G. A., et al. (1990). Abnormalities of the brain in AIDS patients: Correlation of postmortem MR findings with neuropathology. *AJNR Am J Neuroradiol*, *11*(5), 905–911; discussion 912–903.

Grafe, M. R. & Wiley, C. A. (1989). Spinal cord and peripheral nerve pathology in AIDS: The roles of cytomegalovirus and human immunodeficiency virus. *Ann Neurol*, *25*(6), 561–566.

Graveleau, P., Perol, R., et al. (1989). Regression of cauda equina syndrome in AIDS patient being treated with ganciclovir. *Lancet*, *2*(8661), 511–512.

Gray, F., Belec, L., et al. (1994). Varicella-zoster virus infection of the central nervous system in the acquired immune deficiency syndrome. *Brain*, *117* (Pt 5), 987–999.

Gray, F., Gherardi, R., et al. (1988). Pathology of the central nervous system in 40 cases of acquired immune deficiency syndrome (AIDS). *Neuropathol Appl Neurobiol*, *14*(5), 365–380.

Gray, F., Gherardi, R., et al. (1989). Diffuse 'encephalitic' cerebral toxoplasmosis in AIDS. Report of four cases. *J Neurol*, *236*(5), 273–277.

Gray, F., Mohr, M., et al. (1992). Varicella-zoster virus encephalitis in acquired immunodeficiency syndrome: Report of four cases. *Neuropathol Appl Neurobiol*, *18*(5), 502–514.

Graybill, J. R., Sobel, J., et al. (2000). Diagnosis and management of increased intracranial pressure in patients with AIDS and cryptococcal meningitis. The NIAID Mycoses Study Group and AIDS Cooperative Treatment Groups. *Clin Infect Dis*, *30*(1), 47–54.

Greenblatt, R. M., Lukehart, S. A., et al. (1988). Genital ulceration as a risk factor for human immunodeficiency virus infection. *AIDS*, *2*(1), 47–50.

Griffin, D. E., McArthur, J. C., et al. (1991). Neopterin and interferon-gamma in serum and cerebrospinal fluid of patients with HIV-associated neurologic disease. *Neurology*, *41*(1), 69–74.

Grossnik-Laus, H. E., Frank, K. E., et al. (1987). Cytomegalovirus retinitis and optic neuritis in acquired immune deficiency syndrome. Report of a case. *Ophthalmology*, *94*(12), 1601–1604.

Guinan, M. E., Thomas, P. A., et al. (1984). Heterosexual and homosexual patients with the acquired immunodeficiency syndrome. A comparison of surveillance, interview, and laboratory data. *Ann Intern Med*, *100*(2), 213–218.

Gungor, T., Funk, M., et al. (1993). Cytomegalovirus myelitis in perinatally acquired HIV. *Arch Dis Child*, *68*(3), 399–401.

Haas, E. J., Madhavan, T., et al. (1977). Tuberculous meningitis in an urban general hospital. *Arch Intern Med*, *137*(11), 1518–1521.

Hagberg, L., Palmertz, B., et al. (1993). Doxycycline and pyrimethamine for toxoplasmic encephalitis. *Scand J Infect Dis*, *25*(1), 157–160.

Hall, C. D., Dafni, U., et al. (1998). Failure of cytarabine in progressive multifocal leukoencephalopathy associated with human immunodeficiency virus infection. AIDS Clinical Trials Group 243 Team [see comments]." *N Engl J Med*, *338*(19), 1345–1351.

Hall, P. J. & Farrior, J. B. (1993). Aspergillus mastoiditis. *Otolaryngol Head Neck Surg*, *108*(2), 167–170.

Hamilton, R. L., Achim, C., et al. (1995). Herpes simplex virus brainstem encephalitis in an AIDS patient. *Clin Neuropathol*, *14*(1), 45–50.

Harcourt-Webster, J. N., Scaravilli, F., et al. (1991). Strongyloides stercoralis hyperinfection in an HIV positive patient. *J Clin Pathol*, *44*(4), 346–348.

Harding, C. V. (1991). Blastomycosis and opportunistic infections in patients with acquired immunodeficiency syndrome. An autopsy study. *Arch Pathol Lab Med*, *115*(11), 1133–1136.

Harding, S. P. & Porter, S. M. (1991). Oral acyclovir in herpes zoster ophthalmicus. *Curr Eye Res*, *10* Suppl, 177–182.

Harner, R. E., Smith, J. L., et al. (1968). The FTA-ABS test in late syphilis. A serological study in 1,985 cases. *JAMA*, *203*(8), 545–548.

Harris, J. O., Marquez, J., et al. (1980). Listeria brain abscess in the acquired immunodeficiency syndrome. (Letter). *Arch Neurol*, *46*, 250.

Harris, T. M., Smith, R. R., et al. (1990). Toxoplasmic myelitis in AIDS: Gadolinium-enhanced MR. *J Comput Assist Tomogr*, *14*(5), 809–811.

Hawkins, C. C., Gold, J. W., et al. (1986). Mycobacterium avium complex infections in patients with the acquired immunodeficiency syndrome. *Ann Intern Med*, *105*(2), 184–188.

Hawley, D. A., Schaefer, J. F., et al. (1983). Cytomegalovirus encephalitis in acquired immunodeficiency syndrome. *Am J Clin Pathol*, *80*(6), 874–877.

Hayden, F. G. (2005). Antiviral Drugs (Other than Antiretrovirals). In G. L. Mandell, J. E. Bennett, & R. Dolin *Mandell, Douglas, and Bennett's principles and practice of infectious diseases*, pp. 514–551. Philadelphia: Elsevier Churchill Livingstone.

Heinic, G. S., Stevens, D. A., et al. (1993). Fluconazole-resistant Candida in AIDS patients. Report of two cases. *Oral Surg Oral Med Oral Pathol*, 76(6), 711–715.

Henochowicz, S., Mustafa, M., et al. (1985). Cardiac aspergillosis in acquired immune deficiency syndrome. *Am J Cardiol*, 55(9), 1239–1240.

Henson, J., Roseblum, M., et al. (1991). Amplication of JC nirus DNA from brain and cerebrospinal fluid of patients with progressive multifocal leukoencephalopahty. *Neurology*, 41, 11967–11971.

Herskovitz, S., Siegel, S. E., et al. (1989). Spinal cord toxoplasmosis in AIDS. *Neurology*, 39(11), 1552–1553.

Hicks, C. B., Benson, P. M., et al. (1987). Seronegative secondary syphilis in a patient infected with the human immunodeficiency virus (HIV) with Kaposi sarcoma. A diagnostic dilemma. *Ann Intern Med*, 107(4), 492–495.

Hinman, A. R. (1967). Tuberculous meningitis at Cleveland Metropolitan General Hospital 1959 to 1963. *Am Rev Respir Dis*, 95(4), 670–673.

Hofflin, M. & Remington, J. (1985). Tissue culture isolationof toxoplasma fromblood of a patient with AIDS. *Arch Intern Med*, 145, 925–926.

Holder, C. K. & Halkias, D. (1988). Case report: Relapsing, bacteremic Klebsiella pneumoniae miningityis in an AIDS patient. *Am J Med Sci*, 295, 55–59.

Holland, N. R., Power, C., et al. (1994). Cytomegalovirus encephalitis in acquired immunodeficiency syndrome (AIDS). *Neurology*, 44(3 Pt 1), 507–514.

Holman, R. C., Janssen, R. S., et al. (1991). Epidemiology of progressive multifocal leukoencephalopathy in the United States: Analysis of national mortality and AIDS surveillance data. *Neurology*, 41(11), 1733–1736.

Holmberg, S. D., Stewart, J. A., et al. (1988). Prior herpes simplex virus type 2 infection as a risk factor for HIV infection. *JAMA*, 259(7), 1048–1050.

Holtom, P. D., Larsen, R. A., et al. (1992). Prevalence of neurosyphilis in human immunodeficiency virus-infected patients with latent syphilis. *Am J Med*, 93(1), 9–12.

Holtz, H. A., Lavery, D. P., et al. (1985). Actinomycetales infection in the acquired immunodeficiency syndrome. *Ann Intern Med*, 102(2), 203–205.

Hooshmand, H., Escobar, M. R., et al. (1972). Neurosyphilis. A study of 241 patients. *JAMA*, 219(6), 726–729.

Hou, J. & Major, E. O. (1998). The efficacy of nucleoside analogs against JC virus multiplication in a persistently infected human fetal brain cell line. *J Neurovirol*, 4(4), 451–456.

Huang, P. P., McMeeking, A. A., et al. (1997). Cytomegalovirus disease presenting as a focal brain mass: Report of two cases. *Neurosurgery*, 40(5), 1074–1078; discussion 1078–1079.

Huff, J. C., Bean, B., et al. (1988). Therapy of herpes zoster with oral acyclovir. *Am J Med*, 85(2A), 84–89.

Hunter, C. A. & Remington, J. S. (1994). Immunopathogenesis of toxoplasmic encephalitis. *J Infect Dis*, 170(5), 1057–1067.

Idemyor, V. & Cherubin, C. E. (1992). Pleurocerebral Nocardia in a patient with human immunodeficiency virus. *Ann Pharmacother*, 26(2), 188–189.

Idriss, Z. H., Sinno, A. A., et al. (1976). Tuberculous meningitis in childhood. Forty-three cases. *Am J Dis Child*, 130(4), 364–367.

Illingworth, R. S. & Lorber, J. (1956). Tubercles of the choroid. *Arch Dis Child*, 31(160), 467–469.

Ilyid, J. P., Oakes, J. E., et al. (1977). Compairson of the DNAs of varicella-zoster viruses isolated from clinical cases of varicella and herpes zoster. *Virology*, 82, 345–352.

Iribarren, J. A., Goenaga, J., et al. (1994). Atovaquone in cerebral toxoplasmosis: Preliminary experience. (Abstract PB0626). International Conference on AIDS. 10: 153.

Israelski, D. M. & Remington, J. S. (1988). Toxoplasmic encephalitis in patients with AIDS. *Infect Dis Clin North Am*, 2(2), 429–445.

Izzat, N. N., Bartruff, J. K., et al. (1971). Validity of the VDRL test on cerebrospinal fluid contaminated by blood. *Br J Vener Dis*, 47(3), 162–164.

Jabs, D. A., Green, W. R., et al. (1989). Ocular manifestations of acquired immune deficiency syndrome. *Ophthalmology*, 96(7), 1092–1099.

Jacob, C. N., Henein, S. S., et al. (1993). Nontuberculous mycobacterial infection of the central nervous system in patients with AIDS. *South Med J*, 86(6), 638–640.

Jacobs, J. L. & Murray, H. W. (1986). Why is Listeria monocytogenes not a pathogen in the acquired immunodeficiency syndrome? *Arch Intern Med*, 146(7), 1299–1300.

Jacobsen, M. A., Mills, J., et al. (1988). Failure of antiviral therapy for acquired immunodeficiency syndrome related cytomegalovirus myelitis. *Arch Neurol*, 45, 1090–1092.

Jaffe, H. W., Larsen, S. A., et al. (1978). Tests for treponemal antibody in CSF. *Arch Intern Med*, 138(2), 252–255.

Jain, A. K., Agarwal, S. K., et al. (1994). Streptococcus bovis bacteremia and meningitis associated with Strongyloides stercoralis colitis in a patient infected with human immunodeficiency virus. *Clin Infect Dis*, 18(2), 253–254.

Janowicz, D. M., Johnson, R. M., et al. (2005). Successful treatment of CMV ventriculitis immune reconstitution syndrome. *J Neurol Neurosurg Psychiatry*, 76(6), 891–892.

Janssen, R. S., Nwanyanwu, O. C., et al. (1992). Epidemiology of human immunodeficiency virus encephalopathy in the United States. *Neurology*, 42(8), 1472–1476.

Jarvik, J. G., Hesselink, J. R., et al. (1988). Coccidioidomycotic brain abscess in an HIV-infected man. *West J Med*, 149(1), 83–86.

Jarvis, J. N., Boulle, A., et al. (2009). High ongoing burden of cryptococcal disease in Africa despite antiretroviral roll out. *AIDS*, 23(9), 1182–1183.

Jarvis, J. N. & Harrison, T. S. (2007). HIV-associated cryptococcal meningitis. *AIDS*, 21(16), 2119–2129.

Jellinger, K. A., Setinek, U., et al. (2000). Neuropathology and general autopsy findings in AIDS during the last 15 years. *Acta Neuropathol*, 100(2), 213–220.

Jennings, T. S. & Hardin, T. C. (1993). Treatment of aspergillosis with itraconazole. *Ann Pharmacother*, 27(10), 1206–1211.

Johannessen, D. J. & Wilson, L. G. (1988). Mania with cryptococcal meningitis in two AIDS patients. *J Clin Psychiatry*, 49(5), 200–201.

Johns, D. R., Tierney, M., et al. (1987). Alteration in the natural history of neurosyphilis by concurrent infection with the human immunodeficiency virus. *N Engl J Med*, 316(25), 1569–1572.

Johnson, J. D., Butcher, P. D., et al. (1993). Application of the polymerase chain reaction to the diagnosis of human toxoplasmosis. *J Infect*, 26(2), 147–158.

Johnson, P. C., Khardori, N., et al. (1988). Progressive disseminated histoplasmosis in patients with acquired immunodeficiency syndrome. *Am J Med*, 85(2), 152–158.

Johnson, P. C., Norris, S. J., et al. (1988). Early syphilitic hepatitis after renal transplantation. *J Infect Dis*, 158(1), 236–238.

Joyce-Clark, N. & Molteno, A. C. B. (1978). Modified neurosyphilis in the Cape Peninsula. *S Afr Med J*, 53, 10–14.

Joyce, P. W., Haye, K. R., et al. (1989). Syphilitic retinitis in a homosexual man with concurrent HIV infection: Case report. *Genitourin Med*, 65(4), 244–247.

Kadival, G. V., Samuel, A. M., et al. (1987). Radioimmunoassay for detecting Mycobacterium tuberculosis antigen in cerebrospinal fluids of patients with tuberculous meningitis. *J Infect Dis*, 155(4), 608–611.

Kalayjian, R. C., Cohen, M. L., et al. (1993). Cytomegalovirus ventriculoencephalitis in AIDS. A syndrome with distinct clinical and pathologic features. *Medicine (Baltimore)*, 72(2), 67–77.

Kales, C. P. & Holzman, R. S. (1990). Listeriosis in patients with HIV infection: Clinical manifestations and response to therapy. *J Acquir Immune Defic Syndr*, 3(2), 139–143.

Kalish, S. B., Radin, R. C., et al. (1983). The enzyme-linked immunosorbent assay method for IgG antibody to purified protein derivative in cerebrospinal fluid of patients with tuberculous meningitis. *Ann Intern Med*, 99(5), 630–633.

Kaminski, Z. C., Kapila, R., et al. (1992). Meningitis due to Prototheca wickerhamii in a patient with AIDS. *Clin Infect Dis*, 15(4), 704–706.

Kaneko, K., Onodera, O., et al. (1990). Rapid diagnosis of tuberculous meningitis by polymerase chain reaction (PCR). *Neurology, 40*(10), 1617–1618.

Kaplan, J. E., Benson, C., et al. (2009). Guidelines for prevention and treatment of opportunistic infections in HIV-infected adults and adolescents: Recommendations from CDC, the National Institutes of Health, and the HIV Medicine Association of the Infectious Diseases Society of America. *MMWR Recomm Rep, 58*(RR-4), 1–207; quiz CE201–204.

Karadanis, D. & Shulman, J. A. (1976). Recent survey of infectious meningitis in adults: Review of laboratory findings in bacterial, tuberculous and aseptic meningitis. *S Med J, 69*, 449–457.

Karmochkine, M., Molina, J. M., et al. (1994). Combined therapy with ganciclovir and foscarnet for cytomegalovirus polyradiculomyelitis in patients with AIDS. *Am J Med, 97*(2), 196–197.

Katz, D. A. & Berger, J. R. (1989). Neurosyphilis in acquired immunodeficiency syndrome. *Arch Neurol, 46*(8), 895–898.

Katz, D. A., Berger, J. R., et al. (1993). Neurosyphilis. A comparative study of the effects of infection with human immunodeficiency virus. *Arch Neurol, 50*(3), 243–249.

Katz, D. A., Berger, J. R., et al. (1994). Progressive multifocal leukoencephalopathy complicating Wiskott-Aldrich syndrome. Report of a case and review of the literature of progressive multifocal leukoencephalopathy with other inherited immunodeficiency states. *Arch Neurol, 51*(4), 422–426.

Kaye, B. R., Neuwelt, C. M., et al. (1992). Central nervous system systemic lupus erythematosus mimicking progressive multifocal leucoencephalopathy. *Ann Rheum Dis, 51*(10), 1152–1156.

Kchouk, M., Zouiten, F., et al. (1992). [Cerebral miliary tuberculosis. Apropos of 5 cases and review of the literature]. *J Radiol, 73*(11), 589–593.

Kean, J. M., Rao, S., et al. (2009). Seroepidemiology of human polyomaviruses. *PLoS Pathog, 5*(3), e1000363.

Keane, J. R. (1991). Neuro-ophthalmologic signs of AIDS: 50 patients. *Neurology, 41*(6), 841–845.

Keane, J. R. (1993). Intermittent third nerve palsy with cryptococcal meningitis. *J Clin Neuroophthalmol, 13*(2), 124–126.

Kemper, C. A., Lombard, C. M., et al. (1990). Visceral bacillary epithelioid angiomatosis: Possible manifestations of disseminated cat scratch disease in the immunocompromised host: A report of two cases. *Am J Med, 89*(2), 216–222.

Kemper, C. A., Meng, T. C., et al. (1992). Treatment of Mycobacterium avium complex bacteremia in AIDS with a four-drug oral regimen. Rifampin, ethambutol, clofazimine, and ciprofloxacin. The California Collaborative Treatment Group. *Ann Intern Med, 116*(6), 466–472.

Kennedy, D. H. & Fallon, R. J. (1979). Tuberculous meningitis. *JAMA, 241*(3), 264–268.

Kent, S. J., Crowe, S. M., et al. (1993). Tuberculous meningitis: A 30-year review. *Clin Infect Dis, 17*(6), 987–994.

Kenyon, L. C., Dulaney, E., et al. (1996). Varicella-zoster ventriculo-encephalitis and spinal cord infarction in a patient with AIDS. *Acta Neuropathol, 92*(2), 202–205.

Kerr, D. A., Chang, C. F., et al. (1993). Inhibition of human neurotropic virus (JCV) DNA replication in glial cells by camptothecin. *Virology, 196*(2), 612–618.

Kessler, H. H., Muhlbauer, G., et al. (2000). Detection of Herpes simplex virus DNA by real-time PCR. *J Clin Microbiol, 38*(7), 2638–2642.

Khanna, N., Elzi, L., et al. (2009). Incidence and outcome of progressive multifocal leukoencephalopathy over 20 years of the Swiss HIV Cohort Study. *Clin Infect Dis, 48*(10), 1459–1466.

Kieburtz, K. D., Eskin, T. A., et al. (1993). Opportunistic cerebral vasculopathy and stroke in patients with the acquired immunodeficiency syndrome. *Arch Neurol, 50*(4), 430–432.

Kim, J., Minamoto, G. Y., et al. (1991). Nocardial infection as a complication of AIDS: Report of six cases and review. *Rev Infect Dis, 13*(4), 624–629.

Kim, Y. S. & Hollander, H. (1993). Polyradiculopathy due to cytomegalovirus: Report of two cases in which improvement occurred after prolonged therapy and review of the literature. *Clin Infect Dis, 17*(1), 32–37.

Kinloch-de Loes, S., Radeff, B., et al. (1988). AIDS meets syphilis: Changing patterns of the syphilitic infection and its treatment. *Dermatologica, 177*(5), 261–264.

Kinnunen, E. & Hillbom, M. (1986). The significance of cerebrospinal fluid routine screening for neurosyphilis. *J Neurol Sci, 75*(2), 205–211.

Kirk, O., Reiss, P., et al. (2002). Safe interruption of maintenance therapy against previous infection with four common HIV-associated opportunistic pathogens during potent antiretroviral therapy. *Ann Intern Med, 137*(4), 239–250.

Klastersky, J., Cappel, R., et al. (1972). Ascending myelitis in association with herpes-simplex virus. *N Engl J Med, 287*(4), 182–184.

Klein, N. C., Damsker, B., et al. (1985). Mycobacterial meningitis. Retrospective analysis from 1970 to 1983. *Am J Med, 79*(1), 29–34.

Klemola, E., von Essen, R., et al. (1969). Cytomegalovirus mononucleosis in previously healthy individuals. Five new cases and follow-up of 13 previously published cases. *Ann Intern Med, 71*(1), 11–19.

Knobler, E. H., Silvers, D. N., et al. (1988). Unique vascular skin lesions associated with human immunodeficiency virus. *JAMA, 260*(4), 524–527.

Knowles, W. A., Pipkin, P., et al. (2003). Population-based study of antibody to the human polyomaviruses BKV and JCV and the simian polyomavirus SV40. *J Med Virol, 71*(1), 115–123.

Koffman, O. (1956). The changing pattern of neurosyphilis. *Can Med Assoc J, 74*, 807–812.

Komanduri, K. V., Feinberg, J., et al. (2001). Loss of cytomegalovirus-specific CD4+ T cell responses in human immunodeficiency virus type 1-infected patients with high CD4+ T cell counts and recurrent retinitis. *J Infect Dis, 183*(8), 1285–1289.

Koppel, B. S. & Daras, M. (1992). Segmental myoclonus preceding herpes zoster radiculitis. *Eur Neurol, 32*(5), 264–266.

Koppel, B. S., Wormser, G. P., et al. (1985). Central nervous system involvement in patients with acquired immune deficiency syndrome (AIDS). *Acta Neurol Scand, 71*(5), 337–353.

Koralnik, I. J., Wuthrich, C., et al. (2005). JC virus granule cell neuronopathy: A novel clinical syndrome distinct from progressive multifocal leukoencephalopathy. *Ann Neurol, 57*(4), 576–580.

Kovacs, J. A. (1992). Efficacy of atovaquone in treatment of toxoplasmosis in patients with AIDS. The NIAID-Clinical Center Intramural AIDS Program. *Lancet, 340*(8820), 637–638.

Kovacs, J. A. (1995). Toxoplasmosis in AIDS: Keeping the lid on. *Ann Intern Med, 123*(3), 230–231.

Kovacs, J. A., Kovacs, A. A., et al. (1985). Cryptococcosis in the acquired immunodeficiency syndrome. *Ann Intern Med, 103*(4), 533–538.

Koziol, K., Rielly, K. S., et al. (1986). Listeria monocytogenes meningitis in AIDS. *Cmaj, 135*(1), 43–44.

Krambovitis, E., McIllmurray, M. B., et al. (1984). Rapid diagnosis of tuberculous meningitis by latex particle agglutination. *Lancet, 2*(8414), 1229–1231.

Krupp, L. B., Lipton, R. B., et al. (1985). Progressive multifocal leukoencephalopathy: Clinical and radiographic features. *Ann Neurol, 17*(4), 344–349.

Kuchelmeister, K., Gullotta, F., et al. (1993). Progressive multifocal leukoencephalopathy (PML) in the acquired immunodeficiency syndrome (AIDS). A neuropathological autopsy study of 21 cases. *Pathol Res Pract, 189*(2), 163–173.

Kure, K., Harris, C., et al. (1989). Solitary midbrain toxoplasmosis and olivary hypertrophy in a patient with acquired immunodeficiency syndrome. *Clin Neuropathol, 8*(1), 35–40.

Kure, K., Llena, J. F., et al. (1991). Human immunodeficiency virus-1 infection of the nervous system: An autopsy study of 268 adult, pediatric, and fetal brains. *Hum Pathol, 22*(7), 700–710.

Lacascade, C., Conge, A. M., et al. (2000). In vitro anti-Toxoplasma gondii antibody production by peripheral blood mononuclear cells in the diagnosis and the monitoring of toxoplasmic encephalitis in AIDS-related brain lesions. *J Acquir Immune Defic Syndr, 25*(3), 256–260.

Lagues-Silva, E., Ramirez, L. E., et al. (2002). Chagasic meningoencephalitis in a patient with acquired immunodeficiency syndrome: Diagnosis, follow-up and genetic characterization of Trypanosoma cruzi. *Clin Infect Dis, 34*, 118–123.

Laissy, J. P., Soyer, P., et al. (1994). Persistent enhancement after treatment for cerebral toxoplasmosis in patients with AIDS: Predictive value for subsequent recurrence. *AJNR Am J Neuroradiol, 15*(9), 1773–1778.

Lalezari, J. P., Holland, G. N., et al. (1998). Randomized, controlled study of the safety and efficacy of intravenous cidofovir for the treatment of relapsing cytomegalovirus retinitis in patients with AIDS. *J Acquir Immune Defic Syndr Hum Retrovirol, 17*(4), 339–344.

Lamfers, E. J., Bastiaans, A. H., et al. (1987). Leprosy in the acquired immunodeficiency syndrome. *Ann Intern Med, 107*(1), 111–112.

Lang, W., Miklossy, J., et al. (1990). Definition and incidence of AIDS-associated CNS lesions. *Prog AIDS Pathol, 2*, 89–101.

Lang, W., Miklossy, J., et al. (1989). Neuropathology of the acquired immune deficiency syndrome (AIDS): A report of 135 consecutive autopsy cases from Switzerland. *Acta Neuropathol, 77*(4), 379–390.

Lanska, M. J., Lanska, D. J., et al. (1988). Syphilitic polyradiculopathy in an HIV-positive man. *Neurology, 38*(8), 1297–1301.

Lanzafame, M., Ferrari, S., et al. (2009). Mirtazapine in an HIV-1 infected patient with progressive multifocal leukoencephalopathy. *Infez Med, 17*(1), 35–37.

Larsen, R. A., Bozzette, S. A., et al. (1989). Persistant cryptococcus neoformans infection of the prostate after successful treatment of meningitis. *Ann Intern Med, 111*, 125–128.

Larsen, R. A., Leal, M. A., et al. (1990). Fluconazole compared with amphotericin B plus flucytosine for cryptococcal meningitis in AIDS. A randomized trial. *Ann Intern Med, 113*(3), 183–187.

Laskin, O. L., Cederberg, D. M., et al. (1987). Ganciclovir for the treatment and suppression of serious infections caused by cytomegalovirus. *Am J Med, 83*(2), 201–207.

Laskin, O. L., C. M. Stahl-Bayliss, et al. (1987). Concomitant herpes simplex virus type 1 and cytomegalovirus ventriculoencephalitis in acquired immunodeficiency syndrome. *Arch Neurol, 44*(8), 843–847.

Lawn, S. D. & Churchyard, G. (2009). Epidemiology of HIV-associated tuberculosis. *Curr Opin HIV AIDS, 4*(4), 325–333.

Leake, H. A., Appleyard, M. N., et al. (1994). Successful treatment of resistant cryptococcal meningitis with amphotericin B lipid emulsion after nephrotoxicity with conventional intravenous amphotericin B. *J Infect, 28*(3), 319–322.

Lehrer, H. (1966). The angiographic triad in tuberculous meningitis. A radiographic and clinicopathologic correlation. *Radiology, 87*(5), 829–835.

Leiguarda, R., Berthier, M., et al. (1988). Ischemic infarction in 25 children with tuberculous meningitis. *Stroke, 19*(2), 200–204.

Leport, C., Raffi, F., et al. (1988). Treatment of central nervous system toxoplasmosis with pyrimethamine/sulfadiazine combination in 35 patients with the acquired immunodeficiency syndrome. Efficacy of long-term continuous therapy. *Am J Med, 84*(1), 94–100.

Lepper, M. H. & Spies, H. W. (1963). The present status of the treatment of tuberculosis of the central nervous system. *Ann N Y Acad Sci, 106*, 106–123.

Levy, J. H., Liss, R. A., et al. (1989). Neurosyphilis and ocular syphilis in patients with concurrent human immunodeficiency virus infection. *Retina, 9*(3), 175–180.

Levy, R. M., Bredesen, D. E., et al. (1985). Neurological manifestations of the acquired immunodeficiency syndrome (AIDS): Experience at UCSF and review of the literature. *J Neurosurg, 62*, 475–495.

Levy, R. M., Bredesen, D. E., et al. (1988). Opportunistic central nervous system pathology in patients with AIDS. *Ann Neurol, 23* Suppl, S7–12.

Levy, R. M., Pons, V. G., et al. (1984). Central nervous system mass lesions in the acquired immunodeficiency syndrome (AIDS). *J Neurosurg, 61*(1), 9–16.

Levy, R. M., Rosenbloom, S., et al. (1986). Neuroradiologic findings in AIDS: A review of 200 cases. *AJR Am J Roentgenol, 147*(5), 977–983.

Libois, A., De Wit, S., et al. (2007). HIV and syphilis: When to perform a lumbar puncture. *Sex Transm Dis, 34*(3), 141–144.

Licho, R., Litofsky, N. S., et al. (2002). Inaccuracy of Tl-201 brain SPECT in distinguishing cerebral infections from lymphoma in patients with AIDS. *Clin Nucl Med, 27*(2), 81–86.

Linard, F., Beau, P., et al. (1992). Toxoplasmosis with an onset of isolated psychiatric disturbance (12 cases). (Abstract PUB 7316). International Conference on AIDS . 8: 101.

Lincoln, E. M. (1947). Tuberculous meningitis in children; with special reference to serous meningitis; tuberculous meningitis. *Am Rev Tuberc, 56*(2), 75–94.

Lincoln, E. M., Sordillo, V. R., et al. (1960). Tuberculous meningitis in children. A review of 167 untreated and 74 treated patients with special reference to early diagnosis. *J Pediatr, 57*, 807–823.

Lipson, B. K., Freeman, W. R., et al. (1989). Optic neuropathy associated with cryptococcal arachnoiditis in AIDS patients. *Am J Ophthalmol, 107*(5), 523–527.

Livramento, J. A., Machado, L. R., et al. (1989). [Cerebrospinal fluid abnormalities in 170 cases of AIDS]. *Arq Neuropsiquiatr, 47*(3), 326–331.

Longley, N., Muzoora, C., et al. (2008). Dose response effect of high-dose fluconazole for HIV-associated cryptococcal meningitis in southwestern Uganda. *Clin Infect Dis, 47*(12), 1556–1561.

Lopez-Cortes, L. F., Cruz-Ruiz, M., et al. (1995). Adenosine deaminase activity in the CSF of patients with aseptic meningitis: Utility in the diagnosis of tuberculous meningitis or neurobrucellosis. *Clin Infect Dis, 20*(3), 525–530.

Lorber, J. (1954). The results of treatment of 549 cases of tuberculous meningitis. *Am Rev Tuberc, 69*(1), 13–25.

Lorberboym, M., Wallach, F., et al. (1998). Thallium-201 retention in focal intracranial lesions for differential diagnosis of primary lymphoma and nonmalignant lesions in AIDS patients. *J Nucl Med, 39*(8), 1366–1369.

Lortholary, O., Fontanet, A., et al. (2005). Incidence and risk factors of immune reconstitution inflammatory syndrome complicating HIV-associated cryptococcosis in France. *AIDS, 19*(10), 1043–1049.

Lortholary, O., Meyohas, M. C., et al. (1993). Invasive aspergillosis in patients with acquired immunodeficiency syndrome: Report of 33 cases. French Cooperative Study Group on Aspergillosis in AIDS. *Am J Med, 95*(2), 177–187.

Loyse, A., Wainwright, H., et al. Histopathology of the arachnoid granulations and brain in HIV-associated cryptococcal meningitis: Correlation with cerebrospinal fluid pressure. *AIDS, 24*(3), 405–410.

Luft, B. J., Brooks, R. G., et al. (1984). Toxoplasmic encephalitis in patients with acquired immune deficiency syndrome. *JAMA, 252*(7), 913–917.

Luft, B. J., Hafner, R., et al. (1993). Toxoplasmic encephalitis in patients with the acquired immunodeficiency syndrome. Members of the ACTG 077p/ANRS 009 Study Team. *N Engl J Med, 329*(14), 995–1000.

Luft, B. J. & Remington, J. S. (1992). Toxoplasmic encephalitis in AIDS. *Clin Infect Dis, 15*(2), 211–222.

Luger, A., Schmidt, B. L., et al. (1972). Diagnosis of neurosyphilis by examination of cerebrospinal fluid. *Br J Vener Dis, 48*, 1–10.

Lukehart, S. A., Hook, 3rd, E. W., et al. (1988). Invasion of the central nervous system by Treponema pallidum: Implications for diagnosis and treatment. *Ann Intern Med, 109*(11), 855–862.

Luxon, L., Lees, A. J., et al. (1979). Neurosyphilis today. *Lancet, 1*(8107), 90–93.

Lyos, A. T., Malpica, A., et al. (1993). Invasive aspergillosis of the temporal bone: An unusual manifestation of acquired immunodeficiency syndrome. *Am J Otolaryngol, 14*(6), 444–448.

Maayan, S., Wormser, G. P., et al. (1987). Strongyloides stercoralis hyperinfection in a patient with the acquired immune deficiency syndrome. *Am J Med, 83*(5), 945–948.

Madhoun, Z. T., DuBois, D. B., et al. (1991). Central diabetes insipidus: A complication of herpes simplex type 2 encephalitis in a patient with AIDS. *Am J Med, 90*(5), 658–659.

Madiedo, G., Ho, K. C., et al. (1980). False-positive VDRL and FTA in cerebrospinal fluid. *JAMA, 244*(7), 688–689.

Maggi, P., de Mari, M., et al. (1996). Choreoathetosis in acquired immune deficiency syndrome patients with cerebral toxoplasmosis. *Mov Disord, 11*(4), 434–436.

Mahieux, F., Gray, F., et al. (1989). Acute myeloradiculitis due to cytomegalovirus as the initial manifestation of AIDS. *J Neurol Neurosurg Psychiatry*, 52(2), 270–274.

Major, E. O. (2010). Lexington, Kentucky.

Major, E. O., Amemiya, K., et al. (1992). Pathogenesis and molecular biology of progressive multifocal leukoencephalopathy, the JC virus-induced demyelinating disease of the human brain. *Clin Microbiol Rev* 5(1), 49–73.

Majumder, S., S. K. Mandal, et al. (2007). "Multiorgan involvement due to cytomegalovirus infection in AIDS. *Braz J Infect Dis*, 11(1), 176–178.

Mallolas, J., Zamora, L., et al. (1993). Primary prophylaxis for Pneumocystis carinii pneumonia: A randomized trial comparing cotrimoxazole, aerosolized pentamidine and dapsone plus pyrimethamine. *AIDS*, 7(1), 59–64.

Mandel, G. L. & Sande, M. A. (1985). Drugs used in the chemotherapy of tuberculosis and leprosy. In A. G. Gilman, L. Goodman, T. W. Rall, & F. Murad (eds.). *The pharmacological basis of therapeutics*, pp. 1199–1218. New York: Macmillan.

Manfredi, R., Calza, L., et al. (2001). Lack of change in the distribution of AIDS-defining opportunistic diseases and the related degree of immunodeficiency during the periods before and after the introduction of highly active antiretroviral therapy. *Eur J Clin Microbiol Infect Dis*, 20(6), 410–413.

Mann, M. D., Macfarlane, C. M., et al. (1982). The bromide partition test and CSF adenosine deaminase activity in the diagnosis of tuberculosis meningitis in children. *S Afr Med J*, 62(13), 431–433.

Mapelli, G., Pavoni, M., et al. (1981). Neurosyphilis today. *Eur Neurol*, 20(4), 334–343.

Marmaduke, D. P., Brandt, J. T., et al. (1991). Rapid diagnosis of cytomegalovirus in the cerebrospinal fluid of a patient with AIDS-associated polyradiculopathy. *Arch Pathol Lab Med*, 115(11), 1154–1157.

Marra, C. M. (1996). Syphilis, human immunodeficiency virus, and the nervous system. In J. R. Berger & R. M. Levy *AIDS and the nervous system*, pp. 677–691. New York: Lippincott-Raven.

Marra, C. M., Gary, D. W., et al. (1996). Diagnosis of neurosyphilis in patients infected with human immunodeficiency virus type 1. *J Infect Dis*, 174(1), 219–221.

Marra, C. M., Longstreth Jr., W. T., et al. (1992). Resolution of SCF abnormalities in neursyplilis: Influence of stage and HIV infection. Abstract. *Neurology*, 42(Suppl 3), 212.

Marra, C. M., Maxwell, C. L., et al. (2007). Interpreting cerebrospinal fluid pleocytosis in HIV in the era of potent antiretroviral therapy. *BMC Infect Dis*, 7, 37.

Marshall, D. W., Brey, R. L., et al. (1988). Spectrum of cerebrospinal fluid findings in various stages of human immunodeficiency virus infection. *Arch Neurol*, 45(9), 954–958.

Martinez, M. S., Gonzalez-Mediero, G., et al. (2000). Granulomatous amebic encephalitis in a patient with AIDS: Isolation of Acanthamoeba sp. dgroup II from brain tissue and successful treatment with sulfadiazine and fluconazole. *J Clin Microbiol*, 38, 3892–3895.

Maruk, C. H., Nakano, T., et al. (1988). Loss of vision due to cryptococcal optochiasmatic arachnoiditis and optocurative surgical exploration. *Neurol Medica Chirurgica (Toydyo)*, 28, 695–697.

Marzocchetti, A., Lima, M., et al. (2009). Efficient in vitro expansion of JC virus-specific CD8(+) T-cell responses by JCV peptide-stimulated dendritic cells from patients with progressive multifocal leukoencephalopathy. *Virology*, 383(2), 173–177.

Masdeu, J. C., Small, C. B., et al. (1988). Multifocal cytomegalovirus encephalitis in AIDS. *Ann Neurol*, 23(1), 97–99.

Masliah, E., DeTeresa, R. M., et al. (2000). Changes in pathological findings at autopsy in AIDS cases for the last 15 years. *AIDS*, 14(1), 69–74.

Mastroianni, C. M., Mengoni, C., et al. (1994). Ig A antibodies to P30 of toxoplasma gondii in AIDS patients with cerebral toxoplasmosis. (Abstract PBO 634). International Conference on AIDS . 10: 155.

Masur, H. (1992). Toxoplasmosis. In J. B. Wyngaarden, L. H. Smith Jr., & J. C. Bennett *Cecil's textbook of medicine*, pp.1987–1991. Philadelphia: W. B. Saunders.

Masur, H., Kaplan, J. E., et al. (2002). Guidelines for preventing opportunistic infections among HIV-infected persons—2002. Recommendations of the U.S. Public Health Service and the Infectious Diseases Society of America. *Ann Intern Med*, 137(5 Pt 2), 435–478.

Masur, H., Michelis, M. A., et al. (1981). An outbreak of community-acquired Pneumocystis carinii pneumonia: Initial manifestation of cellular immune dysfunction. *N Engl J Med*, 305(24). 1431–1438.

Mathews, V. P., Alo, P. L., et al. (1992). AIDS-related CNS cryptococcosis: Radiologic-pathologic correlation. *AJNR Am J Neuroradiol*, 13(5), 1477–1486.

Matthews, T. & Boehme, R. (1988). Antiviral activity and mechanism of action of ganciclovir. *Rev Infect Dis*, 10 Suppl 3, S490–494.

Mazlo, M. & Herndon, R. M. (1977). Progressive multifocal leukoencepahlopathy: Ultrastructural findings in two brain biopsies. *Neuropathol Appl Neurobiol*, 3, 323–339.

Mazlo, M. & Tariska, I. (1982). Are astrocytes infected in progressive multifocal leukoencephalopathy (PML)? *Acta Neuropathol*, 56(1), 45–51.

McArthur, J. C. (1987). Neurologic manifestations of AIDS. *Medicine (Baltimore)*, 66(6), 407–437.

McArthur, J. C., Hoover, D. R., et al. (1993). Dementia in AIDS patients: Incidence and risk factors. Multicenter AIDS Cohort Study. *Neurology*, 43(11), 2245–2252.

McArthur, J. C., Kumar, A. J., et al. (1990). Incidental white matter hyperintensities on magnetic resonance imaging in HIV-1 infection. Multicenter AIDS Cohort Study. *J Acquir Immune Defic Syndr*, 3(3), 252–259.

McGuire, D., Barhite, D., et al. (1994). PCR-based assay of JC virus DNA in spinal fluid of HIV-1 infected patients: High sensistvity and specificity for PML. *Neuroscience of HIV Infection. Basic and Clinical Frontiers*.

Mehren, M., Burns, P. J., et al. (1988). Toxoplasmic myelitis mimicking intramedullary spinal cord tumor. *Neurology*, 38(10), 1648–1650.

Meira, C. S., Costa-Silva, T. A., et al. (2008). Use of the serum reactivity against Toxoplasma gondii excreted-secreted antigens in cerebral toxoplasmosis diagnosis in human immunodeficiency virus-infected patients. *J Med Microbiol*, 57(Pt 7), 845–850.

Melbye, M., Grossman, R. J., et al. (1987). Risk of AIDS after herpes zoster. *Lancet*, 1(8535), 728–731.

Merritt, H. H., Adams, R. D., et al. (1946). *Neurosyphilis*. New York: Oxford University Press.

Metze, K. & Maciel, Jr., J. A. (1993). AIDS and Chagas' disease. *Neurology*, 43(2), 447–448.

Michelow, I. C., Wendel, Jr., G. D., et al. (2002). Central nervous system infection in congenital syphilis. *N Engl J Med*, 346(23), 1792–1798.

Micozzi, M. S. & Wetli, C. V. (1985). Intravenous amphetamine abuse, primary cerebral mucormycosis, and acquired immunodeficiency. *J Forensic Sci*, 30(2), 504–510.

Miller, J. R., Barrett, R. E., et al. (1982). Progressive multifocal leukoencephalopathy in a male homosexual with T-cell immune deficiency. *N Engl J Med*, 307(23), 1436–1438.

Miller, R. F., Fox, J. D., et al. (1996). Acute lumbosacral polyradiculopathy due to cytomegalovirus in advanced HIV disease: CSF findings in 17 patients. *J Neurol Neurosurg Psychiatry*, 61(5), 456–460.

Miller, R. F., Isaacson, P. G., et al. (2004). Cerebral CD8+ lymphocytosis in HIV-1 infected patients with immune restoration induced by HAART. *Acta Neuropathol*, 108(1), 17–23.

Miller, R. F., Lucas, S. B., et al. (1997). Comparison of magnetic resonance imaging with neuropathological findings in the diagnosis of HIV and CMV associated CNS disease in AIDS. *J Neurol Neurosurg Psychiatry*, 62(4), 346–351.

Miller, R. G., Storey, J. R., et al. (1990). Ganciclovir in the treatment of progressive AIDS-related polyradiculopathy. *Neurology*, 40(4), 569–574.

Milligan, S. A., Katz, M. S., et al. (1984). Toxoplasmosis presenting as panhypopituitarism in a patient with the acquired immune deficiency syndrome. *Am J Med*, 77(4), 760–764.

Minamoto, G. Y., Barlam, T. F., et al. (1992). Invasive aspergillosis in patients with AIDS. *Clin Infect Dis*, 14(1), 66–74.

Minamoto, G. Y. & Sordillo, E. M. (1998). Disseminated nocardiosis in a patient with AIDS: Diagnosis by blood and cerebrospinal fluid cultures. *Clin Infect Dis*, *26*(1), 242–243.

Mischel, P. S. & Vinters, H. V. (1995). Coccidioidomycosis of the central nervous system: Neuropathological and vasculopathic manifestations and clinical correlates. *Clin Infect Dis*, *20*(2), 400–405.

Mishell, J. H. & Applebaum, E. L. (1990). Ramsay-Hunt syndrome in a patient with HIV infection. *Otolaryngol Head Neck Surg*, *102*(2), 177–179.

Mizutani, T., Kurosawa, N., et al. (1993). Atypical manifestations of tuberculous meningitis. *Eur Neurol*, *33*(2), 159–162.

Molloy, E. S. & Calabrese, L. H. (2009). Progressive multifocal leukoencephalopathy: A national estimate of frequency in systemic lupus erythematosus and other rheumatic diseases. *Arthritis Rheum*, *60*(12), 3761–3765.

Monaco, M. C., Atwood, W. J., et al. (1996). JC virus infection of hematopoietic progenitor cells, primary B lymphocytes, and tonsillar stromal cells: Implications for viral latency. *J Virol*, *70*(10), 7004–7012.

Mooney, A. J. (1956). Some ocular sequelae of tuberculous meningitis. *Am J Ophthalmol*, *41*, 753–768.

Moore, E. H., Russell, L. A., et al. (1995). Bacillary angiomatosis in patients with AIDS: Multiorgan imaging findings. *Radiology*, *197*(1), 67–72.

Moore, R. D. & Chaisson, R. E. (1996). Natural history of opportunistic disease in an HIV-infected urban clinical cohort. *Ann Intern Med*, *124*(7), 633–642.

Moret, H., Guichard, M., et al. (1993). Virological diagnosis of progressive multifocal leukoencephalopathy: Detection of JC virus DNA in cerebrospinal fluid and brain tissue of AIDS patients. *J Clin Microbiol*, *31*(12), 3310–3313.

Morgello, S., Block, G. A., et al. (1988). Varicella-zoster virus leukoencephalitis and cerebral vasculopathy. *Arch Pathol Lab Med*, *112*(2), 173–177.

Morgello, S., Cho, E. S., et al. (1987). Cytomegalovirus encephalitis in patients with acquired immunodeficiency syndrome: An autopsy study of 30 cases and a review of the literature. *Hum Pathol*, *18*(3), 289–297.

Morgello, S. & Simpson, D. M. (1994). Multifocal cytomegalovirus demyelinative polyneuropathy associated with AIDS. *Muscle Nerve*, *17*(2), 176–182.

Morgello, S., Soifer, F. M., et al. (1993). Central nervous system Strongyloides stercoralis in acquired immunodeficiency syndrome: A report of two cases and review of the literature. *Acta Neuropathol*, *86*(3), 285–288.

Morshed, M. G., Lee, M. K., et al. (2008). Neurosyphilitic gumma in a homosexual man with HIV infection confirmed by polymerase chain reaction. *Int J STD AIDS*, *19*(8), 568–569.

Moskowitz, L. B., Gregorios, J. B., et al. (1984). Cytomegalovirus. Induced demyelination associated with acquired immune deficiency syndrome. *Arch Pathol Lab Med*, *108*(11), 873–877.

Moulignier, A., Mikol, J., et al. (1996). AIDS-associated cytomegalovirus infection mimicking central nervous system tumors: A diagnostic challenge. *Clin Infect Dis*, *22*(4), 626–631.

Moulignier, A., Pialoux, G., et al. (1995). Brain stem encephalitis due to varicella-zoster virus in a patient with AIDS. *Clin Infect Dis*, *20*(5), 1378–1380.

Muller, F., Moskophidis, M., et al. (1988). Intrathecal synthesis of specific IgG in syphilitic patients with human immunodeficiency virus 1 infection. *J Neurol*, *235*(4), 252–253.

Mullin, G. E. & Sheppell, A. L. (1987). Listeria monocytogenes and the acquired immunodeficiency syndrome. *Arch Intern Med*, *147*(1), 176.

Murdoch, D. M., Venter, W. D., et al. (2008). Incidence and risk factors for the immune reconstitution inflammatory syndrome in HIV patients in South Africa: A prospective study. *AIDS*, *22*(5), 601–610.

Musher, D. M., Hamill, R. J., et al. (1990). Effect of human immunodeficiency virus (HIV) infection on the course of syphilis and on the response to treatment. *Ann Intern Med*, *113*(11), 872–881.

Musher, D. M. & Schell, R. F. (1975). The immunology of syphilis. *Hosp Pract (Off Ed)*, *10*, 45–50.

Musiani, M., Zerbini, M., et al. (1994). Rapid diagnosis of cytomegalovirus encephalitis in patients with AIDS using in situ hybridisation. *J Clin Pathol*, *47*(10), 886–891.

Mussini, C., Pezzotti, P., et al. (2000). Discontinuation of primary prophylaxis for Pneumocystis carinii pneumonia and toxoplasmic encephalitis in human immunodeficiency virus type I-infected patients: the changes in opportunistic prophylaxis study. *J Infect Dis*, *181*(5), 1635–1642.

Nagel, M. A., Forghani, B., et al. (2007). The value of detecting anti-VZV IgG antibody in CSF to diagnose VZV vasculopathy. *Neurology*, *68*(13), 1069–1073.

Nahmias, A. J., Lee, F. K., et al. (1990). Seroepidemiologic and sociological patterns of herpes simplex virus infection in the world. *Scand J Infect Dis*, *69*, 19–36.

Najioullah, F., Bosshard, S., et al. (2000). Diagnosis and surveillance of herpes simplex virus infection of the central nervous system. *J Med Virol*, *61*(4), 468–473.

Narita, M., Matsuzono, Y., et al. (1992). Nested amplification protocol for the detection of Mycobacterium tuberculosis. *Acta Paediatr*, *81*(12), 997–1001.

Nath, A., Hobson, D. E., et al. (1993). Movement disorders with cerebral toxoplasmosis and AIDS. *Mov Disord*, *8*(1), 107–112.

Nath, A., Jankovic, J., et al. (1987). Movement disorders and AIDS. *Neurology*, *37*(1), 37–41.

Navia, B. A., Cho, E. S., et al. (1986). The AIDS dementia complex: II. *Neuropathology Ann Neurol*, *19*(6), 525–535.

Navia, B. A., Jordan, B. D., et al. (1986). "The AIDS dementia complex: I. Clinical features. *Ann Neurol*, *19*(6), 517–524.

Navia, B. A., Petito, C. K., et al. (1986). Cerebral toxoplasmosis complicating the acquired immune deficiency syndrome: Clinical and neuropathological findings in 27 patients. *Ann Neurol*, *19*(3), 224–238.

Nightengale, S. D. (1995). Initial therapy for acquired immunodeficiency syndrome-associated cryptococcus with fluconazole. *Arch Intern Med*, *155*, 538–540.

Nightingale, S. D., Cal, S. X., et al. (1992). Primary prophylaxis with fluconazole against systemic fungal infections in HIV-positive patients. *AIDS*, *6*(2), 191–194.

Nitrini, R. & Spina-Franca, A. (1987). Penicilinoterapia intravenosa em altas doses na neurossifillis. Estudo de 62 casos. II. Avalic o do liquido cefalorraqueano. *Arquivos de Neuropsiququiatria*, *45*, 231–241.

Nolla-Salas, J., Ricart, C., et al. (1987). Hydrocephalus: An unusual CT presentation of cerebral toxoplasmosis in a patient with acquired immunodeficiency syndrome. *Eur Neurol*, *27*(2), 130–132.

Noordhoek, G. T., Wieles, B., et al. (1990). Polymerase chain reaction and synthetic DNA probes: A means of distinguishing the causative agents of syphilis and yaws? *Infect Immun*, *58*(6), 2011–2013.

Norbeno, O. & Sorenson, P. (1981). The incidence and cllinical presentation of neurosyphilis in Greater Copenhagen 1974 through 1978. *Acta Neurol Scand*, *63*, 237–246.

Norden, C. W., Ruben, F. L., et al. (1983). Nonsurgical treatment of cerebral nocardiosis. *Arch Neurol*, *40*(9), 594–595.

Norris, S. J. (1988). The immunology of sexually transmitted diseases . Boston: Kluwer Academic Publishers.

Novati, R., Castagna, A., et al. (1994). Polynerase chain reaction for toxoplasma gondii DNA in the cerebrospinal fluid of AIDS patients with focal brain lesions. *AIDS*, *8*, 1691–1694.

Nunn, P. P. & McAdam, K. P. (1988). Mycobacterial infections and AIDS. *Br Med Bull*, *44*(3), 801–813.

O'Malley, J. P., Ziessman, H. A., et al. (1994). Diagnosis of intracranial lymphoma in patients with AIDS: Value of 201TI single-photon emission computed tomography. *AJR Am J Roentgenol*, *163*(2), 417–421.

Off, G., Lynn, W. A., et al. (1997). Cerebral nocardia abscesses in a patient with AIDS: Correlation of magnetic resonance and white cell scanning images with neuropathological findings. *J Infect*, *35*, 311–313.

Offenbacher, H., Fazekas, F., et al. (1991). MRI in tuberculous meningoencephalitis: Report of four cases and review of the neuroimaging literature. *J Neurol*, *238*(6), 340–344.

Ofner, S. & Baker, R. S. (1987). Visual loss in cryptococcal meningitis. *J Clin Neuroophthalmol*, 7(1), 45–48.

Ogawa, S. K., Smith, M. A., et al. (1987). Tuberculous meningitis in an urban medical center. *Medicine (Baltimore)*, 66(4), 317–326.

Oksenhendler, E., Charreau, I., et al. (1994). Toxoplasma gondii infection in advanced HIV infection. *AIDS*, 8(4), 483–487.

Oliveira, J. F., Greco, D. B., et al. (2006). Neurological disease in HIV-infected patients in the era of highly active antiretroviral treatment: A Brazilian experience. *Rev Soc Bras Med Trop*, 39(2), 146–151.

Olsen, W. L., Longo, F. M., et al. (1988). White matter disease in AIDS: Findings at MR imaging. *Radiology*, 169(2), 445–448.

Orefice, G., Campanella, G., et al. (1993). Presence of papova-like viral particles in cerebrospinal fluid of AIDS patients with progressive multifocal leukoencephalopathy. An additional test for 'in vivo' diagnosis. *Acta Neurol, (Napoli)* 15(5), 328–332.

Orefice, G., Carrieri, P. B., et al. (1992). Cerebral toxoplasmosis and AIDS. Clinical, neuroradiological and immunological findings in 15 patients. *Acta Neurol (Napoli)*, 14(4–6), 493–502.

Overhage, J. M., Greist, A., et al. (1990). Conus medullaris syndrome resulting from *Toxoplasma gondii* infection in a patient with the acquired immunodeficiency syndrome. *Am J Med*, 89(6), 814–815.

Padgett, B. & Walker, D. (1983). Virologic and serologic studies of progressive multifocal leukoencephalopathy. In J. Sever & D. L. Madden (Eds.). *Polyomaviruses and human neurological disease*. New York: Alan R. Liss, Inc.

Padgett, B. L., Walker, D. L., et al. (1971). Cultivation of papova-like virus from human brain with progressive multifocal leucoencephalopathy. *Lancet*, 1(7712), 1257–1260.

Pagnoux, C., Genereau, T., et al. (2000). Brain tuberculomas. *Ann Med Interne* (Paris), 151(6), 448–455.

Palestine, A. G., Polis, M. A., et al. (1991). A randomized, controlled trial of foscarnet in the treatment of cytomegalovirus retinitis in patients with AIDS. *Ann Intern Med*, 115(9), 665–673.

Palestine, A. G., Rodrigues, M. M., et al. (1984). Ophthalmic involvement in acquired immunodeficiency syndrome. *Ophthalmology*, 91(9), 1092–1099.

Pappas, P. G., Pottage, J. C., et al. (1992). Blastomycosis in patients with the acquired immunodeficiency syndrome. *Ann Intern Med*, 116(10), 847–853.

Pardiwalla, F. K., Yeolekar, M. E., et al. (1992). Persistent neutrophilic meningitis. An unusual presentation of tuberculous meningitis. *J Assoc Physicians India*, 40(9), 632–633.

Park, B. J., Wannemuehler, K. A., et al. (2009). Estimation of the current global burden of cryptococcal meningitis among persons living with HIV/AIDS. *AIDS*, 23(4), 525–530.

Parmley, S. F., Goebel, F. D., et al. (1992). Detection of *Toxoplasma gondii* in cerebrospinal fluid from AIDS patients by polymerase chain reaction. *J Clin Microbiol*, 30(11), 3000–3002.

Passo, M. S. & Rosenbaum, J. T (1988). Ocular syphilis in patients with human immunodeficiency virus infection. *Am J Ophthalmol*, 106(1), 1–6.

Patey, O., Nedelec, C., et al. (1989). Listeria monocytogenes septicemia in an AIDS patient with a brain abscess. *Eur J Clin Microbiol Infect Dis*, 8(8), 746–748.

Paugam, A., Dupouy-Camet, J., et al. (1994). Increased fluconazole resistance of *Cryptococcus neoformans* isolated from a patient with AIDS and recurrent meningitis. *Clin Infect Dis*, 19(5), 975–976.

Peetermans, W., Bobbaers, H., et al. (1993). Fluconazole-resistant *Cryptococcus neoformans* var gattii in an AIDS patient. *Acta Clin Belg*, 48(6), 405–409.

Penn, C. C., Goldstein, E., et al. (1992). Sporothrix schenckii meningitis in a patient with AIDS. *Clin Infect Dis*, 15(4), 741–743.

Pepin, J., Plummer, F. A., et al. (1989). The interaction of HIV infection and other sexually transmitted diseases: An opportunity for intervention. *AIDS*, 3(1), 3–9.

Pepose, J. S. (1984). Skin test with varicella-zoster virus antigen for ophthalmic herpes zoster. *Am J Ophthalmol*, 98(6), 825–827.

Pepose, J. S., Hilborne, L. H., et al. (1984). Concurrent herpes simplex and cytomegalovirus retinitis and encephalitis in the acquired immune deficiency syndrome (AIDS). *Ophthalmology*, 91(12), 1669–1677.

Pepper, D. J., Marais, S., et al. (2009). Neurologic manifestations of paradoxical tuberculosis-associated immune reconstitution inflammatory syndrome: A case series. *Clin Infect Dis*, 48(11), e96–107.

Perez Perez, M., Garcia-Martos, P., et al. (1990). [Nocardia caviae meningitis in a patient with HIV infection]. *Rev Clin Esp*, 187(7), 374–375.

Peters, M., Timm, U., et al. (1992). Combined and alternating ganciclovir and foscarnet in acute and maintenance therapy of human immunodeficiency virus-related cytomegalovirus encephalitis refractory to ganciclovir alone. A case report and review of the literature. *Clin Investig*, 70(5), 456–458.

Petersen, L. R., Mead, R. H., et al. (1983). Unusual manifestations of secondary syphilis occurring after orthotopic liver transplantation. *Am J Med*, 75(1), 166–170.

Petito, C. K., Cho, E. S., et al. (1986). Neuropathology of acquired immunodeficiency syndrome (AIDS): An autopsy review. *J Neuropathol Exp Neurol*, 45(6), 635–646.

Pfeffer, G., Prout, A., et al. (2009). Biopsy-proven immune reconstitution syndrome in a patient with AIDS and cerebral toxoplasmosis. *Neurology*, 73(4), 321–322.

Picard, F. J., Dekaban, G. A., et al. (1993). Mollaret's meningitis associated with herpes simplex type 2 infection. *Neurology*, 43(9), 1722–1727.

Pierelli, F., Tilia, G., et al. (1997). Brainstem CMV encephalitis in AIDS: Clinical case and MRI features. *Neurology*, 48(2), 529–530.

Pillai, S., Mahmood, M. A., et al. (1989). Herpes zoster ophthalmicus, contralateral hemiplegia, and recurrent ocular toxoplasmosis in a patient with acquired immune deficiency syndrome-related complex. *J Clin Neuroophthalmol*, 9(4), 229–233; discussion 234–225.

Pitchenik, A. E., Burr, J., et al. (1987). Human T-cell lymphotropic virus-III (HTLV-III) seropositivity and related disease among 71 consecutive patients in whom tuberculosis was diagnosed. A prospective study. *Am Rev Respir Dis*, 135(4), 875–879.

Pitchenik, A. E., Cole, C., et al. (1984). Tuberculosis, atypical mycobacteriosis, and the acquired immunodeficiency syndrome among Haitian and non-Haitian patients in south Florida. *Ann Intern Med*, 101(5), 641–645.

Pitlik, S. D., Fainstein, V., et al. (1983). Spectrum of central nervous system complications in homosexual men with acquired immune deficiency syndrome. *J Infect Dis*, 148(4), 771–772.

Podzamczer, D., Miro, J. M., et al. (1995). Twice-weekly maintenance therapy with sulfadiazine-pyrimethamine to prevent recurrent toxoplasmic encephalitis in patients with AIDS. Spanish Toxoplasmosis Study Group. *Ann Intern Med*, 123(3), 175–180.

Poon, T. P., Behbahani, M., et al. (1994). Pineal toxoplasmosis mimicking pineal tumor in an AIDS patient. *J Natl Med Assoc*, 86(7), 550–552.

Popovich, M. J., Arthur, R. H., et al. (1990). CT of intracranial cryptococcosis. *AJNR Am J Neuroradiol*, 11(1), 139–142.

Porter, S. B. & Sande, M. A (1992). Toxoplasmosis of the central nervous system in the acquired immunodeficiency syndrome. *N Engl J Med*, 327(23), 1643–1648.

Poscher, M. E. (1994). Successful treatment of varicella zoster virus meningoencephalitis in patients with AIDS: Report of four cases and review. *AIDS*, 8(8), 1115–1117.

Post, M. J., Kursunoglu, S. J., et al. (1985). Cranial CT in acquired immunodeficiency syndrome: spectrum of diseases and optimal contrast enhancement technique. *AJR Am J Roentgenol*, 145(5), 929–940.

Post, M. J., Tate, L. G., et al. (1988). CT, MR, and pathology in HIV encephalitis and meningitis. *AJR Am J Roentgenol*, 151(2), 373–380.

Potasman, I., Resnick, L., et al. (1988). Intrathecal production of antibodies against *Toxoplasma gondii* in patients with toxoplasmic encephalitis and the acquired immunodeficiency syndrome (AIDS). *Ann Intern Med*, 108(1), 49–51.

Powderly, W. G. (1993). Cryptococcal meningitis and AIDS. *Clin Infect Dis*, 17(5), 837–842.

Powderly, W. G., Finkelstein, D., et al. (1995). A randomized trial comparing fluconazole with clotrimazole troches for the prevention of fungal infections in patients with advanced human immunodeficiency virus infection. NIAID AIDS Clinical Trials Group. *N Engl J Med*, *332*(11)700–705.

Powderly, W. G., Saag, M. S., et al. (1992). A controlled trial of fluconazole or amphotericin B to prevent relapse of cryptococcal meningitis in patients with the acquired immunodeficiency syndrome. The NIAID AIDS Clinical Trials Group and Mycoses Study Group. *N Engl J Med*, *326*(12), 793–798.

Price, R., Chernik, N. L., et al. (1973). Herpes simplex encephalitis in an anergic patient. *Am J Med*, *54*(2), 222–228.

Price, R. W. & Brew, B. J (1988). The AIDS dementia complex. *J Infect Dis*, *158*(5), 1079–1083.

Price, T. A., Digioia, R. A., et al. (1992). Ganciclovir treatment of cytomegalovirus ventriculitis in a patient infected with human immunodeficiency virus. *Clin Infect Dis*, *15*(4), 606–608.

Pumarola-Sune, T., Navia, B. A., et al. (1987). HIV antigen in the brains of patients with the AIDS dementia complex. *Ann Neurol*, *21*(5), 490–496.

Pursell, K. J., Telzak, E. E., et al. (1992). Aspergillus species colonization and invasive disease in patients with AIDS. *Clin Infect Dis*, *14*(1), 141–148.

Radhakrishnan, V. V. & Mathai, A (1990). Detection of mycobacterial antigen in cerebrospinal fluid: Diagnostic and prognostic significance. *J Neurol Sci*, *99*(1), 93–99.

Read, R. C., Vilar, F. J., et al. (1998). AIDS-related herpes simplex virus encephalitis during maintenance foscarnet therapy. *Clin Infect Dis*, *26*(2), 513–514.

Regal, L., Demaerel, P., et al. (2005). Cerebral syphilitic gumma in a human immunodeficiency virus-positive patient. *Arch Neurol*, *62*(8), 1310–1311.

Regnery, R. L., Childs, J. E., et al. (1995). Infections associated with Bartonella species in persons infected with human immunodeficiency virus. *Clin Infect Dis*, *21* Suppl 1, S94–98.

Renold, C., Sugar, A., et al. (1992). Toxoplasma encephalitis in patients with the acquired immunodeficiency syndrome. *Medicine (Baltimore)*, *71*(4), 224–239.

Revello, M. G., Percivalle, E., et al. (1994). Diagnosis of human cytomegalovirus infection of the nervous system by pp65 detection in polymorphonuclear leukocytes of cerebrospinal fluid from AIDS patients. *J Infect Dis*, *170*(5), 1275–1279.

Ribault, J. & Colombani, J (1964). Le test d'immuno-fluorescence applique au diagnostic de las syphilis. Comparison avec le test de Nelson et la serologic classique. Il Etude de 411 liquides cephalorachidiens. *Pathologie et Biologie (Paris)*, *12*, 276–285.

Ribera, E., Martinez-Vazquez, J. M., et al. (1987). Activity of adenosine deaminase in cerebrospinal fluid for the diagnosis and follow-up of tuberculous meningitis in adults. *J Infect Dis*, *155*(4), 603–607.

Richards, F. O., Jr., Kovacs, J. A., et al. (1995). Preventing toxoplasmic encephalitis in persons infected with human immunodeficiency virus. *Clin Infect Dis*, *21* Suppl 1, S49–56.

Richardson, E. P., Jr. (1970). Progressive jultifocal leukoencephalopahty. In G. W.,Vinken (Ed.). *Handbook of Clinical Neurology* (pp. 486–499). North Holland, NY: Elsevier.

Richardson, E. P., Jr. (1974). Our evolving understanding of progressive jultifocal leukoencepahlopathy. *Ann N Y Acad Sci*, *230*, 258–264.

Richardson, E. P., Jr. (1988). Progressive multifocal leukoencephalopathy 30 years later. *N Engl J Med*, *318*(5), 315–317.

Robert, M. E., Geraghty, J. J., 3rd, et al. (1989). Severe neuropathy in a patient with acquired immune deficiency syndrome (AIDS). Evidence for widespread cytomegalovirus infection of peripheral nerve and human immunodeficiency virus-like immunoreactivity of anterior horn cells." *Acta Neuropathol*, *79*(3), 255–261.

Rocha, A., de Meneses, A. C., et al. (1994). Pathology of patients with Chagas' disease and acquired immunodeficiency syndrome. *Am J Trop Med Hyg*, *50*(3), 261–268.

Romanowski, B., Sutherland, R., et al. (1991). Serological response to treatment of infectious syphilis. *Ann Intern Med*, *114*, 1005–1009.

Rosemberg, F. & Lebon, P. (1991). Amplification and characterization of herpes virus DNA in cerebrospinal fluid from patients with acute encephalitis. *J Clin Microbiol*, *29*, 2412–2417.

Rosemberg, S., Chaves, C. J., et al. (1992). Fatal meningoencephalitis caused by reactivation of Trypanosoma cruzi infection in a patient with AIDS. *Neurology*, *42*(3 Pt 1), 640–642.

Rosenblum, M. K. (1989). Bulbar encephalitis complicating trigeminal zoster in the acquired immune deficiency syndrome. *Hum Pathol*, *20*(3), 292–295.

Rostad, S. W., Oson, K., et al. (1989). Trans-sympatic spread of varicella-zoster virus through the visual system: A mechanism of viral dissemination in the central nervous system. *Hum Pathol*, *20*, 174–179.

Roullet, E., Assuerus, V., et al. (1994). Cytomegalovirus multifocal neuropathy in AIDS: analysis of 15 consecutive cases. *Neurology*, *44*(11), 2174–2182.

Rousseau, F., Perronne, C., et al. (1993). Necrotizing retinitis and cerebral vasculitis due to varicella-zoster virus in patients infected with the human immunodeficiency virus. *Clin Infect Dis*, *17*(5), 943–944.

Rousseau, P. (1994). Giant cell arteritis. *Arch Fam Med*, *3*(7), 628–632.

Rovira, M. J., Post, M. J., et al. (1991). Central nervous system infections in HIV-positive persons. *Neuroimaging Clinics of North America*, *1*, 179–200.

Rowley, A. H., Whitley, R. J., et al. (1990). Rapid detection of herpes-simplex-virus DNA in cerebrospinal fluid of patients with herpes simplex encephalitis. *Lancet*, *335*(8687), 440–441.

Royal, W., 3rd, Selnes, O. A., et al. (1994). Cerebrospinal fluid human immunodeficiency virus type 1 (HIV-1) p24 antigen levels in HIV-1-related dementia. *Ann Neurol*, *36*(1), 32–39.

Rozenbaum, R. & Goncalves, A. J. (1994). Clinical epidemiological study of 171 cases of cryptococcosis. *Clin Infect Dis*, *18*(3), 369–380.

Ruhwald, M. & Ravn, P. (2007). Immune reconstitution syndrome in tuberculosis and HIV-co-infected patients: Th1 explosion or cytokine storm? *AIDS*, *21*(7), 882–884.

Ruiz, A., Ganz, W. I., et al. (1994). Use of thalllium-201 SPECT to differentiate cerebral lymphoma from toxoplasma encephalitis in AIDS patients. *Am J Neuroradiology*, *15*, 1885–1894.

Ryder, J. W., Croen, K., et al. (1986). Progressive encephalitis three months after resolution of cutaneous zoster in a patient with AIDS. *Ann Neurol*, *19*(2), 182–188.

Saag, M. S., Powderly, W. G., et al. (1992). Comparison of amphotericin B with fluconazole in the treatment of acute AIDS-associated cryptococcal meningitis. The NIAID Mycoses Study Group and the AIDS Clinical Trials Group. *N Engl J Med*, *326*(2), 83–89.

Saba, J., Morlat, P., et al. (1993). Pyrimethamine plus azithromycin for treatment of acute toxoplasmic encephalitis in patients with AIDS. *Eur J Clin Microbiol Infect Dis*, *12*(11), 853–856.

Sacktor, N. (2002). The epidemiology of human immunodeficiency virus-associated neurological disease in the era of highly active antiretroviral therapy. *J Neurovirol*, 8 Suppl 2, 115–121.

Sacktor, N., Lyles, R. H., et al. (2001). HIV-associated neurologic disease incidence changes: Multicenter AIDS Cohort Study, 1990–1998. *Neurology*, *56*(2), 257–260.

Sada, E., Ruiz-Palacios, G. M., et al. (1983). Detection of mycobacterial antigens in cerebrospinal fluid of patients with tuberculousmeningitis by enzyme-linked immunosorbent assay. *Lancet*, *2*(8351), 651–652.

Sadler, M., Morris-Jones, S., et al. (1997). Successful treatment of cytomegalovirus encephalitis in an AIDS patient using cidofovir. *AIDS*, *11*(10), 1293–1294.

Safrin, S. (1992). Treatment of acyclovir-resistant herpes simplex virus infections in patients with AIDS. *J Acquir Immune Defic Syndr*, 5 Suppl 1, S29–32.

Safrin, S., Crumpacker, C., et al. (1991). A controlled trial comparing foscarnet with vidarabine for acyclovir-resistant mucocutaneous herpes simplex in the acquired immunodeficiency syndrome. The AIDS Clinical Trials Group. *N Engl J Med*, *325*(8), 551–555.

Sage, J. I., Weinstein, M. P., et al. (1985). Chronic encephalitis possibly due to herpes simplex virus: two cases. *Neurology*, *35*(10), 1470–1472.

Said, G., Lacroix, C., et al. (1991). Cytomegalovirus neuropathy in acquired immunodeficiency syndrome: A clinical and pathological study. *Ann Neurol*, *29*(2), 139–146.

Saint-Leger, E., Caumes, E., et al. (2001). Clinical and virologic characterization of acyclovir-resistant varicella-zoster viruses isolated from 11 patients with acquired immunodeficiency syndrome. *Clin Infect Dis, 33*(12), 2061–2067.

Sanches-Portocarrero, J., Perez-Cecilia, E., et al. (1993). Meningitis pro candida alvicans en 2 adictos a drogas pro via parenteral, revision de la literatura. *Enfermedades Infecciosas y Microbiologia Clinica, 11,* 244–249.

Schiff, D. & Rosenblum, M. K. (1998). Herpes simplex encephalitis (HSE) and the immunocompromised: A clinical and autopsy study of HSE in the settings of cancer and human immunodeficiency virus-type 1 infection. *Hum Pathol, 29*(3), 215–222.

Schlossberg, D., Morad, Y., et al. (1989). Culture-proved disseminated cat-scratch disease in acquired immunodeficiency syndrome. *Arch Intern Med, 149*(6), 1437–1439.

Schmidbauer, M., Budka, H., et al. (1989). Herpes simplex virus (HSV) DNA in microglial nodular brainstem encephalitis. *J Neuropathol Exp Neurol, 48*(6), 645–652.

Schmidbauer, M., Budka, H., et al. (1990). Progressive multifocal leukoencephalopathy (PML) in AIDS and in the pre-AIDS era. A neuropathological comparison using immunocytochemistry and in situ DNA hybridization for virus detection. *Acta Neuropathol, 80*(4), 375–380.

Schoondermark-van de Ven, E., Galama, J., et al. (1993). Value of the polymerase chain reaction for the detection of *Toxoplasma gondii* in cerebrospinal fluid from patients with AIDS. *Clin Infect Dis, 16*(5), 661–666.

Schurmann, D., Bergmann, F., et al. (2002). Effectiveness of twice-weekly pyrimethamine-sulfadoxine as primary prophylaxis of *Pneumocystis carinii* pneumonia and toxoplasmic encephalitis in patients with advanced HIV infection. *Eur J Clin Microbiol Infect Dis, 21*(5), 353–361.

Schwartzman, W. A., Marchevsky, A., et al. (1990). Epithelioid angiomatosis or cat scratch disease with splenic and hepatic abnormalities in AIDS: Case report and review of the literature. *Scand J Infect Dis, 22*(2), 121–133.

Schwarz, T. F., Loeschke, K., et al. (1990). CMV encephalitis during ganciclovir therapy of CMV retinitis. *Infection, 18*(5), 289–290.

Sell, M., Sander, B., et al. (2005). Ventriculitis and hydrocephalus as the primary manifestation of cerebral toxoplasmosis associated with AIDS. *J Neurol, 252*(2), 234–236.

Sharer, L. R. (1992). Pathology of HIV-1 infection of the central nervous system. A review. *J Neuropathol Exp Neurol, 51*(1), 3–11.

Sharer, L. R. & Kapila, R. (1985). Neuropathologic observations in acquired immunodeficiency syndrome (AIDS). *Acta Neuropathol, 66*(3), 188–198.

Shelburne, S. A., 3rd, Darcourt, J., et al. (2005). The role of immune reconstitution inflammatory syndrome in AIDS-related *Cryptococcus neoformans* disease in the era of highly active antiretroviral therapy. *Clin Infect Dis, 40*(7), 1049–1052.

Shelburne, S. A., 3rd, Hamill, R. J., et al. (2002). Immune reconstitution inflammatory syndrome: Emergence of a unique syndrome during highly active antiretroviral therapy. *Medicine (Baltimore), 81*(3), 213–227.

Sheller, J. R. & Des Prez, R. M. (1986). CNS tuberculosis. *Neurol Clin, 4*(1), 143–158.

Shoji, H., Honda, Y., et al. (1992). Detection of varicella-zoster virus DNA by polymerase chain reaction in cerebrospinal fluid of patients with herpes zoster meningitis. *J Neurol, 239*(2), 69–70.

Siegal, F. P., Lopez, C., et al. (1981). Severe acquired immunodeficiency in male homosexuals, manifested by chronic perianal ulcerative herpes simplex lesions. *N Engl J Med, 305*(24), 1439–1444.

Siika, A. M., Ayuo, P. O., et al. (2008). Admission characteristics, diagnoses and outcomes of HIV-infected patients registered in an ambulatory HIV-care programme in western Kenya. *East Afr Med J, 85*(11), 523–528.

Simonsen, J. N., Cameron, D. W., et al. (1988). Human immunodeficiency virus infection among men with sexually transmitted diseases. Experience from a center in Africa. *N Engl J Med, 319*(5), 274–278.

Singer, C., Berger, J. R., et al. (1993). Akinetic-rigid syndrome in a 13-year-old girl with HIV-related progressive multifocal leukoencephalopathy. *Mov Disord, 8*(1), 113–116.

Singer, E. J., Stoner, G. L., et al. (1994). AIDS presenting as progressive multifocal leukoencephalopathy with clinical response to zidovudine. *Acta Neurol Scand, 90*(6), 443–447.

Singh, N., Yu, V. L., et al. (1991). Invasive aspergillosis in AIDS. *South Med J 84*(7), 822–827.

Singhal, B. S., Bhagwati, S. N., et al. (1975). Raised intracranial pressure in tuberculous meningitis. *Neurol India, 23*(1), 32–39.

Sison, J. P., Kemper, C. A., et al. (1995). Disseminated acanthamoeba infection in patients with AIDS: Case reports and review. *Clin Infect Dis, 20*(5), 1207–1216.

Skiest, D. J., Erdman, W., et al. (2000). SPECT thallium-201 combined with Toxoplasma serology for the presumptive diagnosis of focal central nervous system mass lesions in patients with AIDS. *J Infect, 40*(3), 274–281.

Skolnik, P. R. & De La Monte, S. M. (1990). Case records of the Massachusetts General Hospital, Case52–1990. *N Engl J Med, 26,* 1823–1833.

Small, P. M., McPhaul, L. W., et al. (1989). Cytomegalovirus infection of the laryngeal nerve presenting as hoarseness in patients with acquired immunodeficiency syndrome. *Am J Med, 86*(1), 108–110.

Small, P. M., Schecter, G. F., et al. (1991). Treatment of tuberculosis in patients with advanced human immunodeficiency virus infection. *N Engl J Med, 324*(5), 289–294.

Smith, H. V., Taylor, L. M., et al. (1955). The blood-cerebrospinal fluid barrier in tuberculous meningitis and allied conditions. *J Neurol Neurosurg Psychiatry, 18*(4), 237–249.

Smith, H. V. & Vollum, R. L. (1956). The treatment of tuberculous meningitis. *Tubercle, 37*(5), 301–320.

Smith, J. & Godwin-Austen, R. (1980). Hypersecretion of anti-diuretic hormone due to tuberculous meningitis. *Postgrad Med J, 56*(651), 41–44.

Snider, W. D., Simpson, D. M., et al. (1983). Neurological complications of acquired immune deficiency syndrome: Analysis of 50 patients. *Ann Neurol, 14*(4), 403–418.

Snoeck, R., Gerard, M., et al. (1994). Meningoradiculoneuritis due to acyclovir-resistant varicella zoster virus in an acquired immune deficiency syndrome patient. *J Med Virol, 42*(4), 338–347.

So, Y. T. & Olney, R. K. (1994). Acute lumbosacral polyradiculopathy in acquired immunodeficiency syndrome: Experience in 23 patients. *Ann Neurol, 35*(1), 53–58.

Solari, A., Saavedra, H., et al. (1993). Successful treatment of *Trypanosoma cruzi* encephalitis in a patient with hemophilia and AIDS. *Clin Infect Dis, 16*(2), 255–259.

Soriano, V., Dona, C., et al. (2000). Discontinuation of secondary prophylaxis for opportunistic infections in HIV-infected patients receiving highly active antiretroviral therapy. *AIDS, 14*(4), 383–386.

Spitzer, E. D., Spitzer, S. G., et al. (1993). Persistence of initial infection in recurrent *Cryptococcus neoformans* meningitis. *Lancet, 341*(8845), 595–596.

Spitzer, P. G., Hammer, S. M., et al. (1986). Treatment of Listeria monocytogenes infection with trimethoprim-sulfamethoxazole: Case report and review of the literature. *Rev Infect Dis, 8*(3), 427–430.

Spoor, T. C., Wynn, P., et al. (1983). Ocular syphilis. Acute and chronic. *J Clin Neuroophthalmol, 3*(3), 197–203.

Sprach, D. H., Panther, L. A., et al. (1992). Intrracerebral bacillary angiomatosis in a patient with human immunodeficiency virus. *Ann Intern Med, 116,* 740–742.

Stamm, W. E., Handsfield, H. H., et al. (1988). The association between genital ulcer disease and acquisition of HIV infection in homosexual men. *JAMA, 260*(10), 1429–1433.

Steiner, P. & Portugaleza, C. (1973). Tuberculous meningitis in children. A review of 25 cases observed between the years 1965 and 1970 at the Kings County Medical Center of Brooklyn with special reference to the problem of infection with primary drug-resistant strains of M. tuberculosis. *Am Rev Respir Dis, 107*(1), 22–29.

Steinhart, R., Reingold, A. L., et al. (1992). Invasive Haemophilus influenzae infections in men with HIV infection. *JAMA, 268*(23), 3350–3352.

Stern, J. J., Hartman, B. J., et al. (1988). Oral fluconazole therapy for patients with acquired immunodeficiency syndrome and cryptococcosis: Experience with 22 patients. *Am J Med, 85*(4), 477–480.

Stockstill, M. T. & Kauffman, C. A. (1983). Comparison of cryptococcal and tuberculous meningitis. *Arch Neurol, 40*(2), 81–85.

Stoner, G. L., Ryschkewitsch, C. F., et al. (1986). JC papovavirus large tumor (T)-antigen expression in brain tissue of acquired immune deficiency syndrome (AIDS) and non-AIDS patients with progressive multifocal leukoencephalopathy. *Proc Natl Acad Sci U S A, 83*(7), 2271–2275.

Stoumbos, V. D. & Klein, M. L. (1987). Syphilitic retinitis in a patient with acquired immunodeficiency syndrome-related complex. *Am J Ophthalmol, 103*(1), 103–104.

Strauss, M. & Fine, E. (1991). Aspergillus otomastoiditis in acquired immunodeficiency syndrome. *Am J Otol, 12*(1), 49–53.

Strobel, M., Beauclair, P., et al. (1989). [Seronegative syphilis in AIDS]. *Presse Med, 18*(29), 1440.

Subsai, K., Kanoksri, S., et al. (2006). Neurological complications in AIDS patients receiving HAART: A 2-year retrospective study. *Eur J Neurol, 13*(3), 233–239.

Sugar, A. M. & Saunders, C. (1988). Oral fluconazole as suppressive therapy of disseminated cryptococcosis in patients with acquired immunodeficiency syndrome. *Am J Med, 85*(4), 481–489.

Sugar, A. M., Stern, J. J., et al. (1990). Overview: Treatment of cryptococcal meningitis. *Rev Infect Dis, 12* Suppl 3, S338–348.

Sullivan, W. M., Kelley, G. G., et al. (1992). Hypopituitarism associated with a hypothalamic CMV infection in a patient with AIDS. *Am J Med, 92*(2), 221–223.

Sumaya, C. V., Simek, M., et al. (1975). Tuberculous meningitis in children during the isoniazid era. *J Pediatr, 87*(1), 43–49.

Sunderam, G., McDonald, R. J., et al. (1986). Tuberculosis as a manifestation of the acquired immunodeficiency syndrome (AIDS). *JAMA, 256*(3), 362–366.

Sungkanuparph, S., Filler, S. G., et al. (2009). Cryptococcal immune reconstitution inflammatory syndrome after antiretroviral therapy in AIDS patients with cryptococcal meningitis: A prospective multicenter study. *Clin Infect Dis, 49*(6), 931–934.

Suzuki, Y. (2002). Immunopathogenesis of cerebral toxoplasmosis. *J Infect Dis, 186* Suppl 2, S234–240.

Sze, G. & Zimmerman, R. D. (1988). The magnetic resonance imaging of infections and inflammatory diseases. *Radiol Clin North Am, 26*(4), 839–859.

Tagliati, M., Simpson, D., et al. (1998). Cerebellar degeneration associated with human immunodeficiency virus infection. *Neurology, 50*(1), 244–251.

Taguchi, F., Kajioka, J., et al. (1982). Prevalence rate and age of acquisition of antibodies against JC virus and BK virus in human sera. *Microbiol Immunol, 26*(11), 1057–1064.

Talpos, D., Tien, R. D., et al. (1991). Magnetic resonance imaging of AIDS-related polyradiculopathy. *Neurology, 41*(12), 1995–1997.

Tan, B., Weldon-Linne, C. M., et al. (1993). Acanthamoeba infection presenting as skin lesions in patients with the acquired immunodeficiency syndrome. *Arch Pathol Lab Med, 117*(10), 1043–1046.

Tan, C. T. (1988). Intracranial hypertension causing visual failure in cryptococcus meningitis. *J Neurol Neurosurg Psychiatry, 51*(7), 944–946.

Tan, K., Roda, R., et al. (2009). PML-IRIS in patients with HIV infection: Clinical manifestations and treatment with steroids. *Neurology, 72*(17), 1458–1464.

Tan, S. V., Guiloff, R. J., et al. (1993). Herpes simplex type 1 encephalitis in acquired immunodeficiency syndrome. *Ann Neurol, 34*(4), 619–622.

Tedder, D. G., Ashley, R., et al. (1994). Herpes simplex virus infection as a cause of benign recurrent lymphocytic meningitis. *Ann Intern Med, 121*(5), 334–338.

Telzak, E. E., Greenberg, M. S., et al. (1991). Syphilis treatment response in HIV-infected individuals. *AIDS, 5*(5), 591–595.

Teoh, R. & Humphries, M. J. (1991). Tuberculous meningitis. In H. P. Lambert (Ed.). *Infections of the central nervous system* (pp. 189–206). Philadelphia: B. C. Decker.

Teoh, R., Humphries, M. J., et al. (1987). Symptomatic intracranial tuberculoma developing during treatment of tuberculosis: A report of 10 patients and review of the literature. *Q J Med, 63*(241), 449–460.

Thomas, E. W. (1964). Some aspects of neurosyphilis. *Med Clin N America, 48*, 699–705.

Thonell, L., Pendle, S., et al. (2000). Clinical and radiological features of South African patients with tuberculomas of the brain. *Clin Infect Dis, 31*(2), 619–620.

Thornton, C. A., Houston, S., et al. (1992). Neurocysticercosis and human immunodeficiency virus infection. A possible association. *Arch Neurol, 49*(9), 963–965.

Thwaites, G., Fisher, M., et al. (2009). British Infection Society guidelines for the diagnosis and treatment of tuberculosis of the central nervous system in adults and children. *J Infect, 59*(3), 167–187.

Tien, R. D., Chu, P. K., et al. (1991). Intracranial cryptococcosis in immunocompromised patients: CT and MR findings in 29 cases. *AJNR Am J Neuroradiol, 12*(2), 283–289.

Tolge, C. F. & Factor, S. A. (1991). Focal dystonia secondary to cerebral toxoplasmosis in a patient with acquired immune deficiency syndrome. *Mov Disord, 6*(1), 69–72.

Tornatore, C., Berger, J. R., et al. (1992). Detection of JC virus DNA in peripheral lymphocytes from patients with and without progressive multifocal leukoencephalopathy. *Ann Neurol, 31*(4), 454–462.

Torok, M. E., Chau, T. T., et al. (2008). Clinical and microbiological features of HIV-associated tuberculous meningitis in Vietnamese adults. *PLoS One, 3*(3), e1772.

Torok, M. E., Kambugu, A., et al. (2008). Immune reconstitution disease of the central nervous system. *Curr Opin HIV AIDS, 3*(4), 438–445.

Traub, M., Colchester, A. C., et al. (1984). Tuberculosis of the central nervous system. *Q J Med, 53*(209), 81–100.

Traviesa, D. C., Prystowsky, S. D., et al. (1978). Cerebrospinal fluid findings in asymptomatic patients with reactive serum fluorescent treponemal antibody absorption tests. *Ann Neurol, 4*(6), 524–530.

Trenkwalder, P., Trenkwalder, C., et al. (1992). Toxoplasmosis with early intracerebral hemorrhage in a patient with the acquired immunodeficiency syndrome. *Neurology, 42*(2), 436–438.

Tucker, T., Dix, R. D., et al. (1985). Cytomegalovirus and herpes simplex virus ascending myelitis in a patient with acquired immune deficiency syndrome. *Ann Neurol, 18*(1), 74–79.

Turner, T. B. & Hollander, D. H. (1957). Biology of the treponematoses based on studies carried out at the International Treponematosis Laboratory Center of the Johns Hopkins University under the auspices of the World Health Organization. *Monogr Ser World Health Organ*, (35), 3–266.

Udani, P. M., Parekh, U. C., et al. (1971). Neurological and related syndromes in CNS tuberculosis. Clinical features and pathogenesis. *J Neurol Sci, 14*(3), 341–357.

Ustianowski, A. P., Lawn, S. D., et al. (2006). Interactions between HIV infection and leprosy: A paradox. *Lancet Infect Dis, 6*(6), 350–360.

Uttamchandani, R. B., Daikos, G. L., et al. (1994). Nocardiosis in 30 patients with advanced human immunodeficiency virus infection: Clinical features and outcome. *Clin Infect Dis, 18*(3), 348–353.

Vago, L., Bonetto, S., et al. (2002). Pathological findings in the central nervous system of AIDS patients on assumed antiretroviral therapeutic regimens: Retrospective study of 1597 autopsies. *AIDS, 16*(14), 1925–1928.

Vago, L., Nebuloni, M., et al. (1996). Coinfection of the central nervous system by cytomegalovirus and herpes simplex virus type 1 or 2 in AIDS patients: Autopsy study on 82 cases by immunohistochemistry and polymerase chain reaction. *Acta Neuropathol, 92*(4), 404–408.

Vaishnavi, C., Dhand, U. K., et al. (1992). C-reactive proteins, immunoglobulin profile and mycobacterial antigens in cerebrospinal fluid of patients with pyogenic and tuberculous meningitis. *J Hyg Epidemiol Microbiol Immunol, 36*(3), 317–325.

van der Horst, C. M., Saag, M. S., et al. (1997). Treatment of cryptococcal meningitis associated with the acquired immunodeficiency syndrome. National Institute of Allergy and Infectious Diseases Mycoses Study Group and AIDS Clinical Trials Group. *N Engl J Med, 337*(1), 15–21.

Van Eijk, V. F. W., Wolters, E. C., et al. (1987). Effect of early and late syphilis on central nervous: cerebrospinal fluid changes and neurological deficit. *Genitourin Med, 63*, 77–82.

Velasco-Martinez, J. J., Guerrero-Espejo, A., et al. (1995). Tuberculous brain abscess should be considered in HIV/AIDS patients. *AIDS 9*(10), 1197–1199.

Verma, S., Cikurel, K., et al. (2007). Mirtazapine in progressive multifocal leukoencephalopathy associated with polycythemia vera. *J Infect Dis, 196*(5), 709–711.

Vidal, J. E., Penalva de Oliveira, A. C., et al. (2008). AIDS-related progressive multifocal leukoencephalopathy: A retrospective study in a referral center in Sao Paulo, Brazil. *Rev Inst Med Trop Sao Paulo, 50*(4), 209–212.

Villoria, M. F., de la Torre, J., et al. (1992). Intracranial tuberculosis in AIDS: CT and MRI findings. *Neuroradiology, 34*(1), 11–14.

Vinters, H. V. & Anders, K. H. (1990). *Neuropathology of AIDS*. Boca Raton, FL: CRC Press.

Vinters, H. V., Guerra, W. F., et al. (1988). Necrotizing vasculitis of the nervous system in a patient with AIDS-related complex. *Neuropathol Appl Neurobiol, 14*(5), 417–424.

Vinters, H. V., Kwok, M. K., et al. (1989). Cytomegalovirus in the nervous system of patients with the acquired immune deficiency syndrome. *Brain, 112* (Pt 1), 245–268.

Visse, B., Dumont, B., et al. (1998). Single amino acid change in DNA polymerase is associated with foscarnet resistance in a varicella-zoster virus strain recovered from a patient with AIDS. *J Infect Dis, 178* Suppl 1, S55–57.

Vital, C., Monlun, E., et al. (1995). Concurrent herpes simplex type 1 necrotizing encephalitis, cytomegalovirus ventriculoencephalitis and cerebral lymphoma in an AIDS patient. *Acta Neuropathol, 89*(1), 105–108.

Vlcek, B., Burchiel, K. J., et al. (1984). Tuberculous meningitis presenting as an obstructive myelopathy. Case report. *J Neurosurg, 60*(1), 196–199.

von Einsiedel, R. W., Fife, T. D., et al. (1993). Progressive multifocal leukoencephalopathy in AIDS: A clinicopathologic study and review of the literature. *J Neurol, 240*(7), 391–406.

Waecker, N. J., Jr. & Connor, J. D. (1990). Central nervous system tuberculosis in children: A review of 30 cases. *Pediatr Infect Dis, J 9*(8), 539–543.

Walker, D. & Padgett, B. (1983). The epidimiology of human polyomaviruses. In J. Sever & D. L. Madden (Eds.). *Polyomaviruses and human neurological disease* (pp. 99–106. New York: Alan R. Liss, Inc.

Ward, D. (1992). Dapsone/pyrinethamine for the treatment of toxoplasmic encephalitis (Abstract POP3277). *International Conference on AIDS, 8*, 133.

Warren, K. G., Brown, S. M., et al. (1978). Isolation of latent herpes simplex virus from the superior cervical and vagus ganglions of human beings. *N Engl J Med, 298*(19), 1068–1069.

Wasz-Hockert, O. & Donner, M. (1962). Results of the treatment of 191 children with tuberculous miningitis in the years 1949-1954. *Acta Paediatr, 51*(Suppl 141), 7–25.

Watt, G., Zaraspe, G., et al. (1988). Rapid diagnosis of tuberculous meningitis by using an enzyme-linked immunosorbent assay to detect mycobacterial antigen and antibody in cerebrospinal fluid. *J Infect Dis, 158*(4), 681–686.

Weaver, S., Rosenblum, M. K., et al. (1999). Herpes varicella zoster encephalitis in immunocompromised patients. *Neurology, 52*(1), 193–195.

Weber, T., Bodemer, M., et al. (1994). Enhanced sensitivity of JC Virus DNA detection in CSF by nested primer PCR (Abstract). *Neuroscience of HIV infection. Basis and Clinical Frontiers.*

Weber, T., Trebst, C., et al. (1997). Analysis of the systemic and intrathecal humoral immune response in progressive multifocal leukoencephalopathy. *J Infect Dis, 176*(1), 250–254.

Weber, T., Turner, R. W., et al. (1990). JC virus detected by polymerase chain reaction in cerebrospinal fluid of AIDS patients with progressive multifocal leukoencephalopathy. *Proceedings from the Satellite Meeting of the International Conference on AIDS.* 100.

Weidenheim, K. M., Nelson, S. J., et al. (1992). Unusual patterns of histoplasma capsulatuum in a patient with the acquired immunodeficiency virus. *Hum Pathol, 23*, 581–586.

Weinert, L. S., Scheffel, R. S., et al. (2008). Cerebral syphilitic gumma in HIV-infected patients: Case report and review. *Int J STD AIDS, 19*(1), 62–64.

Weiss, W. & Flippin, H. F. (1965). The changing incidence and prognosis of tuberculous meningitis. *Am J Med Sci, 250*, 46–59.

Wetli, C. V., Weiss, S. D., et al. (1984). Fungal cerebritis from intravenous drug abuse. *J Forensic Sci, 29*(1), 260–268.

Wheat, J. (1995). Endemic mycoses in AIDS: A clinical review. *Clin Microbiol Rev, 8*(1), 146–159.

Wheat, L. J., Batteiger, B. E., et al. (1990). Histoplasma capsulatum infections of the central nervous system. A clinical review. *Medicine (Baltimore), 69*(4), 244–260.

Wheat, L. J., Connolly-Stringfield, P., et al. (1991). Histoplasmosis relapse in patients with AIDS: detection using Histoplasma capsulatum variety capsulatum antigen levels. *Ann Intern Med, 115*(12), 936–941.

Wheat, L. J., Connolly-Stringfield, P. A., et al. (1990). Disseminated histoplasmosis in the acquired immune deficiency syndrome: Clinical findings, diagnosis and treatment, and review of the literature. *Medicine (Baltimore), 69*(6), 361–374.

Wheat, L. J., Kohler, R. B., et al. (1989). Significance of Histoplasma antigen in the cerebrospinal fluid of patients with meningitis. *Arch Intern Med, 149*(2), 302–304.

Whimbey, E., Gold, J. W., et al. (1986). Bacteremia and fungemia in patients with the acquired immunodeficiency syndrome. *Ann Intern Med, 104*(4), 511–514.

White, A. C., Jr., Dakik, H., et al. (1995). Asymptomatic neurocysticercosis in a patient with AIDS and cryptococcal meningitis. *Am J Med, 99*(1), 101–102.

White, M., Cirrincione, C., et al. (1992). Cryptococcal meningitis: Outcome in patients with AIDS and patients with neoplastic disease. *J Infect Dis, 165*(5), 960–963.

Whiteman, M., Espinoza, L., et al. (1995). Central nervous system tuberculosis in HIV-infected patients: Clinical and radiographic findings. *AJNR Am J Neuroradiol, 16*(6), 1319–1327.

Whiteman, M. L., Dandapani, B. K., et al. (1994). MRI of AIDS-related polyradiculomyelitis. *J Comput Assist Tomogr, 18*(1), 7–11.

Whiteman, M. L., Post, M. J., et al. (1993). Progressive multifocal leukoencephalopathy in 47 HIV-seropositive patients: Neuroimaging with clinical and pathologic correlation. *Radiology, 187*(1), 233–240.

Whitley, R. J. & Gnann, J. W., Jr. (1993). Antiviral therapy. In B. Rosiman, R. J. Whitley & C. Lopez (Eds.). *The human herpesviruses* (pp. 329–348). New York: Raven Press.

Wildemann, B., Haas, J., et al. (1998). Diagnosis of cytomegalovirus encephalitis in patients with AIDS by quantitation of cytomegalovirus genomes in cells of cerebrospinal fluid. *Neurology, 50*(3), 693–697.

Wiley, C., Sofrin, R. E., et al. (1987). Acanthomoeba meningoencephalitis in an AIDS patient. *J Infect Dis, 155*, 130–133.

Wiley, C. A. & Nelson, J. A. (1988). Role of human immunodeficiency virus and cytomegalovirus in AIDS encephalitis. *Am J Pathol, 133*(1), 73–81.

Wiley, C. A., VanPatten, P. D., et al. (1987). Acute ascending necrotizing myelopathy caused by herpes simplex virus type 2. *Neurology, 37*(11), 1791–1794.

Witrack, B. J. & Ellis, G. T. (1985). Intracranial tuberculosis: Manifestations on computerized tomography. *S Med, J 78*, 386–392.

Witzig, R. S., Hoadley, D. J., et al. (1994). Blastomycosis and human immunodeficiency virus: Three new cases and review. *South Med J, 87*(7), 715–719.

Wolf, D. G. & Spector, S. A. (1992). Diagnosis of human cytomegalovirus central nervous system disease in AIDS patients by DNA amplification from cerebrospinal fluid. *J Infect Dis, 166*(6), 1412–1415.

Wolinsky, E. (1979). Nontuberculous mycobacteria and associated diseases. *Am Rev Respir Dis, 119*(1), 107–159.

Wolters, E. C. (1987). Neurosyphilis: A changing diagnostic problem? *Eur Neurol, 26*(1), 23–28.

Wong, M. T., Dolan, M. J., et al. (1995). Neuroretinitis, aseptic meningitis, and lymphadenitis associated with *Bartonella (Rochalimaea) henselae* infection in immunocompetent patients and patients infected with human immunodeficiency virus type 1. *Clin Infect Dis, 21*(2), 352–360.

Wood, M. J., Johnson, R. W., et al. (1994). A randomized trial of acyclovir for 7 days or 21 days with and without prednisolone for treatment of acute herpes zoster. *N Engl J Med, 330*(13), 896–900.

Wood, M. J., Ogan, P. H., et al. (1988). Efficacy of oral acyclovir treatment of acute herpes zoster. *Am J Med, 85*(2A), 79–83.

Woods, G. L. & Goldsmith, J. C. (1990). Aspergillus infection of the central nervous system in patients with acquired immunodeficiency syndrome. *Arch Neurol, 47*(2), 181–184.

Wuthrich, C., Dang, X., et al. (2009). Fulminant JC virus encephalopathy with productive infection of cortical pyramidal neurons. *Ann Neurol, 65*(6), 742–748.

Yamamoto, L. J., Tedder, D. G., et al. (1991). Herpes simplex virus type 1 DNA in cerebrospinal fluid of a patient with Mollaret's meningitis. *N Engl J Med, 325*(15), 1082–1085.

Yoritaka, A., Ohta, K., et al. (2007). Prevalence of neurological complications in Japanese patients with AIDS after the introduction of HAART. *Rinsho Shinkeigaku, 47*(8) 491–496.

Young, L. S., Inderlied, C. B., et al. (1986). Mycobacterial infections in AIDS patients, with an emphasis on the Mycobacterium avium complex. *Rev Infect Dis, 8*(6), 1024–1033.

Zaidman, G. W. (1986). Neurosyphilis and retrobulbar neuritis in a patient with AIDS. *Ann Ophthalmol, 18*(9), 260–261.

Zaidman, G. W., Weinberg, R. S., et al. (1983). Acquired syphilitic uveitis in homosexuals. *Ophthalmology, 90*(Aug. Suppl), 106–107.

Zambrano, W., Perez, G. M., et al. (1987). Acute syphilitic blindness in AIDS. *J Clin Neuroophthalmol, 7*(1), 1–5.

Zaraspe-Yoo, E., Miletich, R., et al. (1984). Herpes zoster ophthalmicus with contralateral hemiplegia in a patient with autoimmune deficiency syndrome (AIDS) (Abstract). *Neurology, 34*(Suppl 1), 229.

Zintel, H. A., Flippin, H. F., et al. (1945). Studies on streptomycin in man. I. Absorption, distribution, excretion and toxicity. *Am J Med Sci, 210*, 421–430.

Zuger, A., Louie, E., et al. (1986). Cryptococcal disease in patients with the acquired immunodeficiency syndrome. Diagnostic features and outcome of treatment. *Ann Intern Med, 104*(2), 234–240.

Zurhein, G. (1967). Polyoma-like virions in a human demyelinating disease. *Acta Neurolpathologica, 8*, 57–68.

Zurhein, G. & Chou, S. M. (1965). Particles resembling papova viruses in human cerebral demyelinating disease. *Science, 148*, 1477–1479.

8.6

PROGRESSIVE MULTIFOCAL LEUKOENCEPHALOPATHY

Maria G. Chiara and Eugene O. Major

Progressive multifocal leukoencephalopathy (PML), caused by the JC Virus (JCV), is a demyelinating disease of the white matter of the human brain. It is one of the principal opportunistic infections afflicting HIV-1-positive individuals and is an AIDS-defining illness. The role of the immune system in the pathogenesis of PML is complex. Interactions between the JC and HIV viruses further complicate the picture. Normally held in check by the immune system, JCV can become lethally active in AIDS patients either early in the progression of AIDS or in the months immediately following initiation of highly active antiretroviral treatment (HAART) in the form of immune reconstitution inflammatory syndrome (IRIS). This chapter provides an overview of many aspects of PML in AIDS, including reviews of the pathology, diagnosis, and incidence of PML, and of the association of PML with IRIS; a comparison of PML in AIDS versus in other immunosuppressive disorders; a discussion of PML pathogenesis from viral latency through demyelination; and a discussion of PML in patients undergoing pharmacologic immunosuppression.

INTRODUCTION

JC virus infection is the cause of progressive multifocal leukoencephalopathy (PML), a demyelinating disease of the white matter of the human brain that is one of the principal opportunistic infections (OIs) in HIV-1-seropositive individuals. PML occurs in approximately 1-3% of HIV-1-infected persons and is an AIDS-defining illness. The role of the immune system in the pathogenesis of PML, however, is complex, as well as the interactions between both of the viruses (Figure 8.6.1). Under normal circumstances, the host's immune response holds JCV infection in check from acute infection or the subsequent reactivation from sites of latency before the virus can enter the brain. However, PML can occur in AIDS patients early on, or in the months immediately following HAART therapy as the immune system begins reconstitution. The relationship between JCV infection in cells of the nervous system and cells of the immune system has led to investigations of viral pathogenesis both in AIDS and other immune-system-modifying diseases, as well as their therapies. The number of AIDS patients dying from PML in AIDS has declined since the introduction of HAART therapy, but the incidence of PML in HIV-1

infection remains high compared with other neurological complications.

PROGRESSIVE MULTIFOCAL LEUKOENCEPHALOPATHY IS A VIRAL-INDUCED DEMYELINATING DISEASE OF THE HUMAN BRAIN

There is the classic "triad" of clinical signs that raises suspicion of PML:1) Cognitive impairments, (including subcortical aspects of dementia with mental slowness), disorientation, and behavioral changes could all be among the first indication of PML; 2) Motor dysfunctions such as lack of coordination, gait disturbances, ataxia, and more severely, hemiparesis, are as common as cognitive problems which raise suspicion of PML; and 3) visual deficits like hemianopsia (Weber, 2008). Other clinical signs, though not as common, are seizures, language problems, and headaches. The clinical course of PML has been described as progressive and is almost always fatal, with death occurring within anywhere from weeks to months from the time of diagnosis. More recently, AIDS patients with PML undergoing HAART therapy have been able to restore their immune system functions and as many as 10–20% are surviving much longer with some resolution of PML lesions. The reason for this is related to CD4 and CD8 T cell rebound, which enters the brain to clear infection. However, this immune reconstitution has some negative effect, in that inflammation occurs due to the inflammatory nature of the immune response, identified as IRIS or immune reconstitution inflammatory syndrome (Berger, 2009b; Clifford et al., 2010). Patients with higher levels of CD8$^+$ cytotoxic T cells to the viral capsid protein showed a better prognosis that correlated with a less progressive course of disease (Du Pasquier et al., 2006; Wuthrich et al., 2006; Chen et al., 2008). No such correlation exists with humoral immunity since PML patients have substantial antibody titers to the same viral capsid protein before and during disease (Ryschkewitsch et al., 2010). The majority of the world's population has antibodies to JCV that remain throughout life. However, the role of antiviral antibody as neutralizing/protective is not understood.

In PML, typical demyelinated plaque areas show irregular borders, surrounding macrophages, and bizarre astrocytes.

Neurotropic viruses

JCV/PML   HIV-1/AIDS

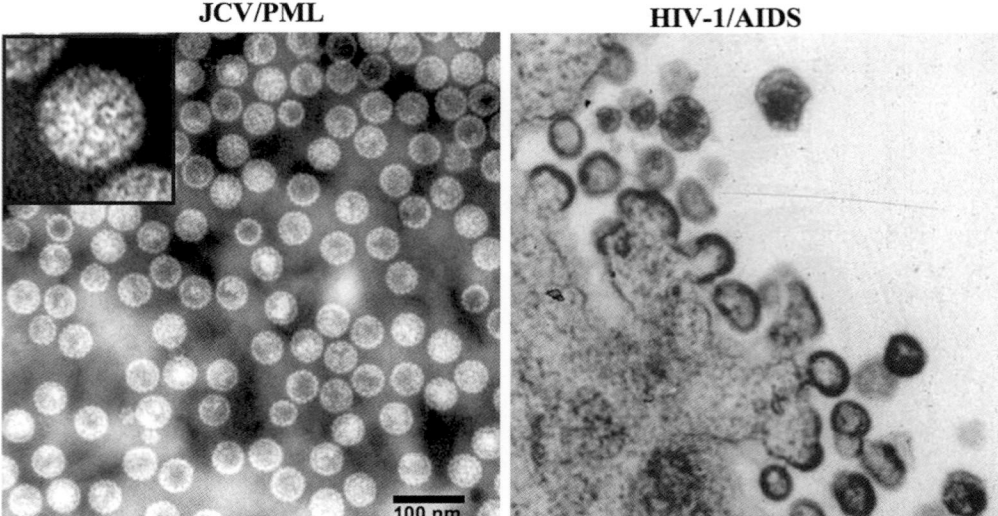

Figure 8.6.1 Electron microscopy of assembled virion particles. A) JCV mature virion particles 40 nm diameter; and B) HIV-1 virion particles budding from infected astrocytes in cultures (Imperiale et al., 2007).

The nuclei of infected oligodendrocytes are substantially enlarged due to the assembly of mature virion particles that tend to remain intranuclear. Infectious virus is disseminated to neighboring oligodendrocytes gradually as cell death occurs through a necrotic, lytic process (Seth et al., 2004), although apoptosis leading to cell degeneration may also occur (Richardson-Burns et al., 2002). Due to this process, lesions progressively enlarge in time ranging from weeks to months, and may become confluent. Consequently, plaque lesions are usually asymmetrical, and diffuse with ill-defined borders as

seen in subcortical white matter bilateral in the cerebral hemispheres and in some cases in the cerebellum. On magnetic resonance imaging (MRI), the lesions can be hyperintense on T2-weighted and FLAIR sequences and hypointense on T1-weighted sequences. The lesions can be located up against the cerebral cortex with damage to the U fibers (Figure 8.6.2A). PML lesions usually do not show edema, mass effect, or gadolinium enhancement—characteristics that help differentiate these lesions from those of multiple sclerosis (Yousry et al., 2006).

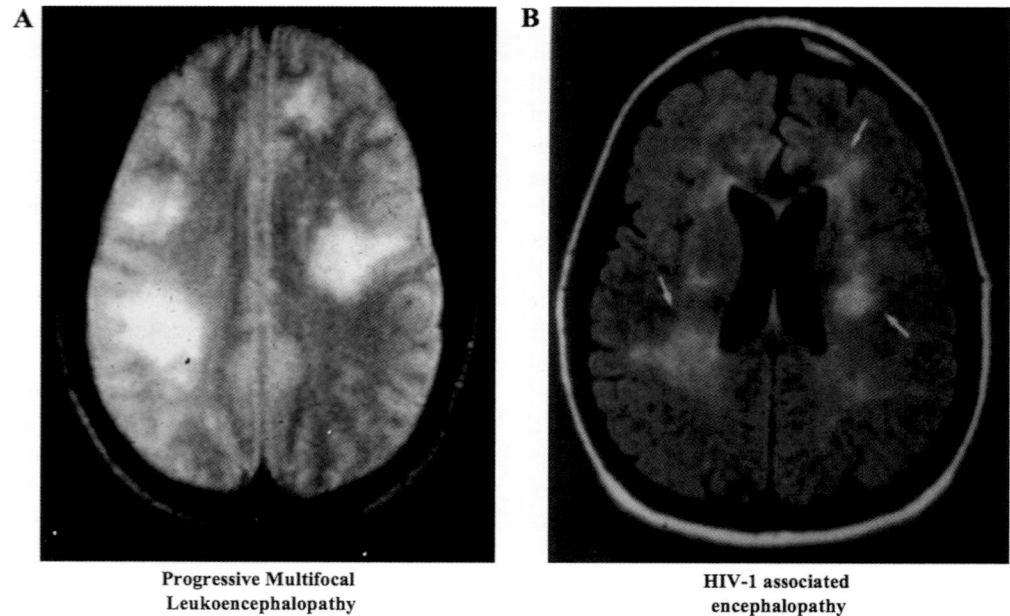

Figure 8.6.2 Brain magnetic resonance imaging (MRI) of white matter lesions. A) subcortical white matter demyelination in brain of progressive multifocal leukoencephalopathy (PML)-associated encephalopathy; and B) human immunodeficiency virus 1 (HIV-1)-associated encephalopathy with diffuse periventricular lesions.

Evidence of such symptoms, along with the characteristic lesions shown by MRI, can be sufficient for a diagnosis of PML. However, other encephalopathies, like HIV-1-associated brain infection or CNS tumors, can complicate the diagnosis (Figure 8.6.2B). Evidence of the presence of JCV DNA or protein is considered the defining criterion for the confirmation of a PML diagnosis. In the past, immuno-cytochemistry using antibodies that detect viral proteins in brain tissue has been used. But since these antibodies are cross reactive to other viruses; their specificity is not reliable. In situ DNA hybridization, using probes that are highly specific to JCV DNA, has replaced enzyme-linked immunosorbent assays (ELISA) based on antibodies measurement and is readily used in biopsy and autopsy tissues (Houff et al., 1989). However, this method requires biopsy samples that are not always available. With the rapid development of the quantization of polymerase chain reaction technology, qPCR, primers and probes for the detection of JCV DNA represent the most state-of-the-art method (Ryschkewitsch et al., 2004). The sensitivity and specificity of qPCR for JCV DNA allows detection of 100 to 10 copies per ml of the viral DNA in tissues including the cerebral spinal fluid (CSF), the most widely used clinical sample available for the confirmatory diagnosis of PML. Therefore, CSF testing using qPCR has become the current standard showing 98% specificity and over 90% sensitivity depending on the laboratory and its performance using this assay.

INCIDENCE OF PML IN AIDS AND ESTIMATES OF PROLONGED SURVIVAL WITH HAART

Prior to the mid 1980s, before the pandemic of HIV-1 infection, PML was a very rare disease occurring only in patients with underlying neoplastic diseases, organ transplants, or other immune system dysfunctions. While the overall incidence in various patient populations is estimated at 1 per million, the exact incidence is not accurately known, since PML is not a Centers for Disease Control (CDC) reportable disease, and may therefore be under diagnosed, or in some cases, not reported in patients with severe acute, underlying neoplastic diseases (Carson et al., 2009b; Yorita Christensen et al., 2010).

PML rarely occurs in young patients, it more frequently occurs in males within the third to fifth decade as compared with females. PML continues as an AIDS-defining illness with a modest reduction, even with the beginning of HAART therapy. There has been a steeper decline, several folds, in deaths of AIDS patients due to PML since the introduction of HAART therapy. More PML patients are surviving longer, although with continued neurological disability. Recently, PML has been described in another, more unexpected population: in patients with autoimmune diseases treated with biological therapies that do not directly suppress immunity but rather alter normal immune functions by selectively blocking adhesion of VLA 4 on T and B cells to the cell adhesion molecules, MAdCAM-1 and VCAM-1. This prevents entry

Table 8.6.1 INCIDENCE OF PML IN VARIOUS UNDERLYING CONDITIONS

HIV/AIDS	$1:10^2$
Natalizumab MS treated patients	$1:10^3$
Rituximab patients with lymphoproliferative diseases	$1:5^4–10^5$
Chemotherapy treatment in organ transplant patients	$1:10^6–10^7$

into tissues such as the gut or brain. These observations provide a strong link between JCV infection in cells of the immune and nervous systems that point to the importance of the tissue origin of JCV latency. However, the mechanisms that give rise to PML in HIV-1-infected individuals probably differ from individuals with other immune suppressive conditions. This is exemplified in the incidence of PML in AIDS patients at approximately 1–3% as compared with immune suppressive chemotherapy for transplants patients at approximately 0.07% or patients treated with immune modulatory therapies such as natalizumab, an adhesion molecule inhibitor used in multiple sclerosis and Crohn's disease patients at 0.1% or rituximab that ablates circulating B cells used for hematologic malignancies estimated at 0.05%. (Table 8.6.1) (Carson et al., 2009b). Between the period of 2002–2005, 85% of all PML cases regardless of underlying disease occurred in HIV-1-infected individuals (Yorita Christensen et al., 2010).

Several studies have evaluated the effect of HAART therapy on the incidence and survival of PML in HIV-1-infected individuals. In a Danish cohort of AIDS patients, Engsig et al. (2009) reported 47 cases of PML among 4639 HIV-1-infected persons, both before the introduction of HAART, and early and late into the HAART therapy. Survival was higher in the HAART-treated group with a median of 1.8 years more compared with 0.4 years in the untreated group. Higher CD4 counts were predictive of longer survival. In this study, however, 53% of the cases of PML were diagnosed without any virological data for JCV. In a Swiss cohort of HIV-1 patients from 1988 to 2007, 159 PML patient records were evaluated for treatment and outcome; 89 before and 70 after HAART therapy. There was a twofold increased survival rate of 1 year in the treated group, although CD4 counts were similar in both groups (Khanna et al., 2009). Factors that explained the differences between these groups were PML as the primary indication of AIDS, low HIV RNA levels, JCV-specific cytotoxic T cells, and low JCV DNA load in the CSF at time of PML diagnosis. In a more recent report, Lima et al. (2010) reported an increase in 1 year survival from 10% to 50% in HAART-treated PML patients with partial or stable improvement. Most of the patients had detectable CD8+ cytotoxic T cells that were JCV specific. In this review of case reports, 25% of cases did not have virologic data to confirm the diagnosis.

PML IN AIDS PATIENTS EXPERIENCING IMMUNE RECONSTITUTION INFLAMMATORY SYNDROME—IRIS

The use of combination antiretroviral drugs or HAART therapy dramatically reduces the HIV load in the peripheral circulation and restores or "reconstitutes" the number and physiology of CD4 and other T cells. One of the unintended consequences of this action is the infiltration of inflammatory cells into the brain, causing a substantial inflammatory process (Berger, 2003). The inflammation can be damaging to the brain so AIDS patients, with or without PML, are treated with steroids to lessen the inflammation (Cinque et al., 2001). The positive aspects of IRIS in PML patients are its potential attenuation of infection and the clearance of JCV from lesion areas as evidenced by a drop in the viral load in the CSF over time. In a review of PML patient records from the literature produced between 1998 and 2007, as well as at the Johns Hopkins Hospital between 2004 and 2007, there were 54 cases identified. PML and IRIS occurred simultaneously in 36 cases, while in 18 cases the pre-existing PML developed IRIS over a broad time range of 1 week to 26 months. The extended time from initiation of HAART therapy and IRIS might suggest that JCV infection may establish a persistence in the brain with pathological impact until a more active infection takes place, stimulating IRIS. Those patients with earlier IRIS demonstrated more lesions on MRI scans, a shorter survival time, and higher death rate. Generally, however, MRI images of the lesions in PML-IRIS patients show contrast enhancement with pronounced inflammation (Tan et al., 2009a). Brain tissues were also characterized by the presence of macrophages and CD8+ T lymphocytes, which may be JCV specific. Steroid therapy was initiated in patients for a period ranging from weeks to months in order to limit the intensity of the inflammatory response.

In another study of 20 PML patients from 1997–2006 at the U.C. San Diego HIV clinic, eight PML cases were diagnosed with PML within 6 months of beginning HAART therapy, with a mean of 6 weeks, described as "unmasked" PML (Sidhu et al., 2010). This patient group differed from the Hopkins group since they survived longer and also had lesions predominantly in the cerebellum. Three of these cases did not have evidence of IRIS, indicating that HAART therapy may have been the unique factor that promotes JCV infection leading to PML or "unmasks" the infection's process. There is evidence of JCV infection in the internal granule layer in the cerebellum which may show a more delayed immune reaction (Du Pasquier et al., 2003; Wuthrich et al., 2009a). PML cases diagnosed prior to HAART, or more than 6 months after initiation of HAART, showed similarities in clinical progression and diagnostic features with high HIV loads in the peripheral circulation and poor survival.

THE ASSOCIATION OF HIV-1 AND JCV INFECTION IN AIDS-PML PATIENTS

The incidence of PML is greater in HIV-1+ patients when compared with other immune-compromising underlying diseases and remains a substantial neurological complication in AIDS. Even in the widespread use of cART, or in some cases because of it, HIV-1 infection accounts for approximately 85% of all PML cases, at least in those reported. There may be several distinct features of HIV-1 infection that account for this high proportion of PML in AIDS patients. One factor may be the extent and duration of immune suppression that HIV-1 causes, damaging T cell responses to JCV infection following reactivation from latency. Another factor could be the trafficking of JCV-infected cells, such as B lymphocytes, into the brain across a damaged blood-brain barrier, and finally, a molecular mechanism of interaction between these two viruses is probably the most relevant factor to explain the high incidence of PML in AIDS (White et al., 2009).

The most likely active HIV-1 candidate factor that augments JCV infection is the transactivating nonstructural protein, Tat, which is essential for successful HIV infection and acts both directly and indirectly on the JCV genome. Using reporter genes transduced into glial type cells, Tat increases expression from the late promoter of JCV effecting RNA synthesis, the stability of the mRNA, and translation (Tada et al., 1990). While it is known that HIV-1 rarely, if at all, infects oligodendrocytes, Tat has been identified in some infected and noninfected oligodendrocytes in PML brain tissue. Tat can be secreted from infected monocytes and macrophages and taken up by neighboring cells (Del Valle et al., 2000). This observation was also confirmed when exogenous Tat was added in cultures of JCV-infected oligodendroglioma cells. In these cells, Tat associated with a cellular DNA binding transcription factor, purα, and increased JCV replication (Daniel et al., 2004). Purα can bind to the JCV multifunctional T protein as well as Tat, suggesting the probable role in interactions between these two viruses. The transcriptional stimulation by Purα occurs from both the JCV early and late promoters as well as the HIV-1 LTR (White et al., 2009). There is a high affinity binding of the Tat-Purα complex to the HIV TAR element activating JCV late gene expression. Independently, Tat also binds the TAR RNA element to augment HIV-1 transcription.

Tat also increases expression from the JCV "archetype" structure of its promoter always found in JCV secreted in the urine. In experiments in which COS 7 cells expressed Tat and the SV40 T protein, the levels of expression of reporter genes from the JCV late promoter increased (Nukuzuma et al., 2009). This observation was expanded in recent experiments that showed Tat increased the JCV archetype variant in HeLa cells, not normally permissive to infection, tenfold more than non-Tat-expressing cells (Gosert et al., 2010). Perhaps these observations could be relevant to in vivo infection because persistent JC viruria and increasing JCV DNA in AIDS patients may be predictive for PML (Grabowski et al., 2009).

The observations of molecular interactions between HIV and JCV provide mechanistic pathways that account for the high incidence of PML in AIDS patients even with HAART therapy that separates HIV-1 infection from other immune suppressive conditions like chemotherapy, neoplastic diseases, or biological therapies for autoimmune diseases in which PML is seen, but at much lower frequencies (Berger, 2003).

THE PATHOGENESIS OF PML FROM VIRAL LATENCY TO DEMYELINATION

The biology of JCV is summarized in a chapter on the family of polyomaviruses (Imperiale et al., 2007). Although the JC viral receptor, alpha 2–6-linked sialic acid, is found in many cell types, (Neu et al., 2009), JCV displays a very narrow cellular host range; it productively infects oligodendrocytes and astrocytes of the human brain, stromal cells in tonsillar tissues, and at low levels B cells and CD34[+] hematopoietic stem cells. While JCV infection has not been found in cerebral neurons or in human neuronal cultures, there are reports of infection in cerebellar granule cell neurons in patients with motor dysfunctions and nontypical PML (Du Pasquier et al., 2003; Wuthrich et al., 2009a). This observation is intriguing and suggests the potential for other CNS diseases associated with JCV infection beyond PML (Wuthrich et al., 2009b). Consequently, the host range for JCV may be controlled at the intracellular level, in the nuclei, dependent on host cell transcription factors that recognize the viral promoter DNA sequences for viral RNA and protein synthesis. Since viral DNA is infectious, the cell receptor can be bypassed by directly placing JCV DNA into cells. Even following viral DNA "transfection" into a wide range of cell types in culture experiments, infection takes place only in those cells in which evidence of infection comes from clinical tissues. Such cells share common DNA-binding proteins that promote infection (Marshall et al., 2010a). Investigations of the molecular nature of JCV in susceptible cells have turned attention to sites that might support viral persistence or latency.

There are three organs that are currently thought to harbor latent infection from various supporting studies: the kidney/urine, the brain, and bone marrow/lymphoid tissues. Several studies have shown that 10 to 30% of the population shed JCV in the urine, indicating kidney latency, mostly with no pathological significance (Kitamura et al., 1990; Markowitz et al., 1993). The arrangement of the non-coding viral regulatory region sequences found in urine-derived virus, however, are substantially different from those found in pathological tissues like the brain and lymphoid cells. There are studies showing that these kidney derived regulatory sequences can undergo a "rearrangement" during extensive DNA replication that might ultimately resemble those found in pathological tissues. When the virus is isolated from the urine it is not infectious for human glial cells and does not infect epithelial cells in culture, a paradox that remains unsolved since large amounts of virus can be shed in the urine. There is also the intriguing report of the possibility of a more neurovirulent phenotype of JCV following analysis of gene sequences of its capsid protein used for cell attachment. There were also amino acids in viral sequences found in PML brain tissues that differed from those in kidney isolates from non-PML patients (Sunyaev et al., 2009).

Because of the close association of PML with the immune system, lymphoid tissues from PML patients were probed for evidence of JCV infection. Spleen and bone marrow were shown to have JCV DNA sequences in AIDS patients (Houff et al., 1988), as well as B cells in the peripheral circulation using in situ DNA hybridization (Tornatore et al., 1992).

Tonsil tissue as well as lymphocytes from tonsils taken from juvenile non-PML patients also had JCV DNA (Monaco et al., 1998). Stromal cells from tonsillar tissue were also shown to be highly susceptible to JCV infection in culture as were CD34[+] cells and B lymphocytes (Monaco et al., 1996). In non-AIDS PML patients, bone marrow biopsy tissues that were taken anywhere from months to years prior to the development of PML also showed JCV DNA sequences that were similar if not identical to those sequences from the patients' brain tissues at the time of diagnosis of PML (Berger et al., 1995; Carson et al., 2009). A recent study of bone marrow from both HIV positive and negative patients with or without PML showed a high prevalence of bone marrow tissues with JCV DNA as well as expression of the viral T protein (Tan et al., 2009b), confirming these earlier observations. JCV DNA can also be found in plasma or serum from PML and non-PML patients, indicating that viremia occurs as would be expected for dissemination of the virus to lymphoid organs and kidneys that can be monitored using qPCR assays. In a number of surveys of the normal population, it seems that approximately 1–2% demonstrates viremia at some time, again not surprising for a virus that is so widely spread and can reactivate from latency. This observation is consistent with other DNA-containing viruses that are ubiquitous like CMV and HHV 6 in which viremia in the normal population may exceed 5% (Berger et al., 2009a). CMV also latently infects CD34[+] cells in the bone marrow. Without an animal model for PML (none exists at this point), evidence for the tissue origins of viral latency, reactivation, and trafficking to the brain depends on patients' tissues and their disease progression. The cumulative evidence for the pathogenesis of JCV from the initial site of infection to the brain best fits a critical intermediate role for the immune system, with initial infection in lymphoid cells that may amplify infection, disseminating the virus through infected lymphocytes or through viremia to other organs like the kidney and bone marrow and then reactivation at times of immune dysfunction that allows virus to enter the brain and pass infection to its final target cell, the oligodendrocyte. The molecular biology of JCV also fits this model of pathogenesis in which tonsillar stromal cells, B lymphocytes, and CD34[+] hematopoietic cells all share increased expression of specific DNA binding, transcriptional proteins that are essential for JCV multiplication, unlike cells that are not susceptible to productive infection (Gallia et al., 1997).

PML IN PATIENTS RECEIVING BIOLOGICAL THERAPIES FOR AUTOIMMUNE AND OTHER DISEASES

Non-AIDS patients who are at risk for PML usually either fall into the category of immunosuppression for allograft protection or neoplastic diseases of the immune system. However, PML has now been recognized in patients treated with monoclonal antibodies that are immune modulatory; natalizumab that is a selective adhesion molecule inhibitor blocking T and B cell binding to VLA 4 and rituximab that ablates CD20 cells from the peripheral circulation (Major, 2010). Understanding the links of these biological therapeutics, humanized monoclonal antibodies, with PML mush, begin with their effect on the functions of the immune system. Natalizumab binds the α4 integrin, β1, and β7 epitopes on T and B cells blocking those cells from attaching to the VCAM, and MadCAM respectively blocking their extravasation into the brain or gut (von Andrian et al., 2003). Since both multiple sclerosis (MS) and Crohns' disease show inflammatory T cells as a significant part of their pathology, preventing access of these cells to target organs has shown substantial clinical effects (Kappos et al., 2007; Verbeeck et al., 2008; Hutchinson et al., 2009). Rituximab binds the CD20 receptor on B cells, initiating complement-dependent cytolysis with clearance from the peripheral circulation. Natalizumab induces a leukocytosis for a time period of weeks to months. CD4 and CD8 ratios in the CSF of natalizumab patients have inverted for at least six months (Stuve et al., 2007; Stuve, 2008a; Stuve et al., 2008b). The binding of natalizumab on integrin molecules is not limited to T and B cells. Blocking cellular adhesion molecules also prevents homing of CD34+ hematopoietic progenitor cells in the bone marrow and of pre B cells in the marginal zones of lymph nodes (Lu et al., 2002). The consequences of this mode of action is migration of CD34+ and pre B cells into the peripheral circulation either from the bone marrow, certainly for CD34+ cells, and lymph nodes. This has been shown in natalizumab-treated patients within days to weeks from the start of therapy (Bonig et al., 2008; Zohren et al., 2008). Gene expression analysis using genome microarray methods of peripheral lymphocytes in these patients showed a pattern of upregulation of several genes active in B cell differentiation (Lindberg et al., 2008).

JCV DNA has been found in bone marrow and lymph nodes of patients anywhere from months to years prior to PML. It is found in the peripheral circulation in B cells or as a free virus, and can infect B cells in culture and uses host cell factors for its genome expression. Some of the critical host factors that promote JCV synthesis are shared with genes involved in B cell differentiation that are upregulated in natalizumab patients, members of the POU family domain (Lindberg et al., 2008). A particular DNA-binding site on the JCV promoter sequences is the Spi B binding site. It is essential for progression of pre B to mature B cell development and is highly represented in the JCV regulatory genome (Marshall et al., 2010b). A likely set of circumstances that links PML with natalizumab would then be the latency of JCV DNA in the bone marrow in CD34+ and/or pre B cells that migrate into the peripheral circulation due to the blocking of their integrins to VCAM, initiation of B cell differentiation due to upregulation of appropriate genes in that pathway, and activation of JCV synthesis using the same host molecular machinery as cells which are differentiated into CD19/CD20 B cells (Houff et al., 1988; Major et al., 1992; Ransohoff, 2005). Virus multiplication, measured as viremia, can take place in the peripheral circulation and enter into the brain either cell-free or in B cells. Once in the brain, since immune surveillance is hampered, JCV can pass infection to the oligodendrocyte. This scenario ties together many of the data from laboratory investigations to clinical observations. It also would suggest that JCV latency

may be rare in the bone marrow and would require factors that not only promote migration of the rare latently infected cells but also stimulation or reactivation of JCV DNA. The action of rituximab, however, is different. By depleting the peripheral circulation of B cells, the B precursors or pre B cells in lymph nodes, spleen, and bone marrow will continually function to replace the population. It may be that under rare circumstances rituximab fails to eliminate some of those B cells that if latently infected could traffic to the brain and initiate infection in the oligodendrocyte. This would happen only rarely and would require a combination of events, including a rare latent infection in pre B cells, the failure of treatment to eliminate these cells, perhaps not yet expressing the CD20 marker, and the subsequent entry of virus into the brain.

The loss of immune surveillance may be another factor for PML, but perhaps more relevant for other viral, bacterial, and fungal infections in the use of these therapies (Berger et al., 2009a). In natalizumab-treated MS patients, the observation that CD4+/CD8+ ratios in the CSF 6 months after cessation of drug were inverted and at lower levels than nontreated MS patients indicated that immune reactivity can be impaired in the CNS as expected (Stuve, 2008a). It is generally assumed that HIV-1 infection results in loss of immune surveillance that contributes to the risk of PML in addition to the specific viral interactions between HIV-1 and JCV.

CONCLUSION

PML is no longer as rare a disease as Creutzfeldt-Jakob (CJD) or subacute sclerosing panencephalitis (SSPE), infectious encephalopathies that frequently are described together with extremely low incidence. The incidence of PML remains relatively stable in HIV-1-infected individuals at approximately 1-3% and in natalizumab-treated MS patients at 0.1%. Other patient populations with underlying immune compromised conditions, such as lymphoproliferative diseases treated with rituximab, show an approximate incidence of 0.05% to 0.001% and organ transplants treated with chemotherapy show an even lower incidence of 0.0001% (Table 8.6.1). These incidence rates, with orders of magnitude differences, suggest specific mechanisms responsible for JCV reactivation that leads to infection of oligodendrocytes. PML in the context of AIDS presents a different mechanism than other immune-compromised conditions because JCV and HIV-1 do interact at the cellular and molecular levels. PML in patients treated with natalizumab points to drug release of latently infected cells from the bone marrow or other immune compartments perhaps with a greater efficiency than rituximab. Both of these monoclonal antibody therapies are immune modulatory with effects on immune surveillance as well. The very low incidence of PML in immune-suppressed patients on small molecule drugs like mycophenylate, perhaps does not affect reservoirs of viral latency but only the inability to control infection once initiated. The link between these underlying conditions and their treatment needs further, focused investigation since there are currently no effective antiviral drugs to prevent or modify JCV infection.

One new drug, CMX001, a lipid-ester derivative of cidofo-vir, has shown effectiveness against JCV in cultures (see Jiang et al., 2010; Marshall et al., 2010a for a thorough review of therapies for PML), and has been used as compassionate treatment in six PML patients. Clinical trials of this drug are being planned in various patient populations. The outcome of such trials will be informative and perhaps guide to a better understanding of JCV pathogenesis leading to PML.

REFERENCES

Berger, J. R. (2003). Progressive multifocal leukoencephalopathy in acquired immunodeficiency syndrome: explaining the high incidence and disproportionate frequency of the illness relative to other immunosuppressive conditions. *J Neurovirol, 9* Suppl 1, 38–41.

Berger, J. R. (2009b). Steroids for PML-IRIS: A double-edged sword? *Neurology, 72*(17), 1454–1455.

Berger, J. R. & Concha, M. (1995). Progressive multifocal leukoencephalopathy: The evolution of a disease once considered rare. *J Neurovirol, 1*(1), 5–18.

Berger, J. R. & Houff, S. (2009a). Opportunistic infections and other risks with newer multiple sclerosis therapies. *Ann Neurol, 65*(4), 367–377.

Bonig, H., Wundes, A., Chang, K. H., Lucas S., & Papayannopoulou, T. (2008). Increased numbers of circulating hematopoietic stem/progenitor cells are chronically maintained in patients treated with the CD49d blocking antibody natalizumab. *Blood, 111*(7), 3439–3441.

Carson, K. R., Evens A. M., Richey, E. A., Habermann, T. M., Focosi, D., Seymour, J. F., et al. (2009). Progressive multifocal leukoencephalopathy after rituximab therapy in HIV-negative patients: A report of 57 cases from the Research on Adverse Drug Events and Reports project. *Blood, 113*(20), 4834–4840.

Carson, K. R., Focosi, D., Major, E. O., Petrini, M., Richey, E. A., West, D. P., et al. (2009). Monoclonal antibody-associated progressive multifocal leucoencephalopathy in patients treated with rituximab, natalizumab, and efalizumab: A review from the Research on Adverse Drug Events and Reports (RADAR) project. *Lancet Oncol, 10*(8), 816–824.

Chen, Y., Trofe, J., Gordon, J., Autissier, P., Woodle, E. S., & Koralnik, I. J. (2008). BKV and JCV large T antigen-specific CD8+ T cell response in HLA A*0201+ kidney transplant recipients with polyomavirus nephropathy and patients with progressive multifocal leukoencephalopathy. *J Clin Virol 42*(2), 198–202.

Cinque, P., Pierotti, C., Vigano, M. G., Bestetti, A., Fausti, C., Bertelli, D., et al. (2001). The good and evil of HAART in HIV-related progressive multifocal leukoencephalopathy. *J Neurovirol, 7*(4), 358–363.

Clifford, D. B., De Luca, A., Simpson, D. M., Arendt, G., Giovannoni, G., & Nath, A. (2010). Natalizumab-associated progressive multifocal leukoencephalopathy in patients with multiple sclerosis: Lessons from 28 cases. *Lancet Neurol, 9*(4), 438–446.

Daniel, D. C., Kinoshita, Y., Khan, M. A., Del Valle, L., Khalili, K., Rappaport, J., et al. (2004). Internalization of exogenous human immunodeficiency virus-1 protein, Tat, by KG-1 oligodendroglioma cells followed by stimulation of DNA replication initiated at the JC virus origin. *DNA Cell Biol, 23*(12), 858–867.

Del Valle, L., Croul, S., Morgello, S., Amini, S., Rappaport, J., & Khalili, K. (2000). Detection of HIV-1 Tat and JCV capsid protein, VP1, in AIDS brain with progressive multifocal leukoencephalopathy. *J Neurovirol, 6*(3), 221–228.

Du Pasquier, R. A., Corey, S., Margolin, D. H., Williams, K., Pfister, L. A., De Girolami, U., et al. (2003). Productive infection of cerebellar granule cell neurons by JC virus in an HIV+ individual. *Neurology, 61*(6), 775–782.

Du Pasquier, R. A., Stein, M. C., Lima, M. A., Dang, X., Jean-Jacques, J., Zheng, Y., et al. (2006). JC virus induces a vigorous CD8+ cytotoxic T cell response in multiple sclerosis patients. *J Neuroimmunol, 176*(1–2), 181–186.

Engsig, F. N., Hansen, A. B., Omland, L. H., Kronborg, G., Gerstoft, J., Laursen, A. L., et al. (2009). Incidence, clinical presentation, and outcome of progressive multifocal leukoencephalopathy in HIV-infected patients during the highly active antiretroviral therapy era: A nationwide cohort study. *J Infect Dis,199*(1), 77–83.

Gallia, G. L., Houff, S. A., Major, E. O., & Khalili, K. (1997). Review: JC virus infection of lymphocytes—revisited. *J Infect Dis, 176*(6), 1603–1609.

Gosert, R., Kardas, P., Major, E. O., & Hirsch, H. H. (2010). Rearranged JC virus non-coding control regions found in progressive multifocal leukoencephalopathy increase virus early gene expression and replication rate. *J Virol*.

Grabowski, M. K., Viscidi, R. P., Margolick, J. B., Jacobson, L. P., & Shah, K. V. (2009). Investigation of pre-diagnostic virological markers for progressive multifocal leukoencephalopathy in human immunodeficiency virus-infected patients. *J Med Virol, 81*(7), 1140–1150.

Houff, S. A., Katz, D., Kufta, C. V., & Major, E. O. (1989). A rapid method for in situ hybridization for viral DNA in brain biopsies from patients with AIDS. *AIDS, 3*(12), 843–845.

Houff, S. A., Major, E. O., Katz, D. A., Kufta, C. V., Sever, J. L., Pittaluga, S., et al. (1988). Involvement of JC virus-infected mononuclear cells from the bone marrow and spleen in the pathogenesis of progressive multifocal leukoencephalopathy. *N Engl J Med, 318*(5), 301–305.

Hutchinson, M., Kappos, L., Calabresi, P. A., Confavreux, C., Giovannoni, G., Galetta, S. L., et al. (2009). The efficacy of natalizumab in patients with relapsing multiple sclerosis: Subgroup analyses of AFFIRM and SENTINEL. *J Neurol 256*(3), 405–415.

Imperiale, M. J., Major, E. O. Polyomaviruses. (2007). In: D.M. Knipe, P.M. Howley, D.E. Griffin, R.A. Lamb, M.A. Martin, B. Roizman, and S.E. Straus (eds.): *Fields Virology*, 5th Edition, Lippincott Williams & Wilkins, Philadelphia.

Jiang, Z. G., Cohen, J., Marshall, L. J., & Major, E. O. (2010). Hexadecyloxypropyl-cidofovir, CMX001, suppresses JC virus replication in human fetal brain SVG cell cultures. *Antimicrob Agents Chemother*.

Kappos, L., Bates, D., Hartung, H. P., Havrdova, E., Miller, D., Polman, C. H., et al. (2007). Natalizumab treatment for multiple sclerosis: Recommendations for patient selection and monitoring. *Lancet Neurol 6*(5), 431–441.

Khanna, N., Elzi, L., Mueller, N. J., Garzoni, C., Cavassini, M., Fux, C. A., et al. (2009). Incidence and outcome of progressive multifocal leukoencephalopathy over 20 years of the Swiss HIV Cohort Study. *Clin Infect Dis, 48*(10),1459–1466.

Kitamura, T., Aso, Y., Kuniyoshi, N., Hara, K., & Yogo, Y. (1990). High incidence of urinary JC virus excretion in nonimmunosuppressed older patients. *J Infect Dis, 161*(6), 1128–1133.

Lima, M. A., Bernal-Cano, F., Clifford, D. B., Gandhi, R. T., & Koralnik, I. J. (2010). Clinical outcome of long-term survivors of progressive multifocal leukoencephalopathy. *J Neurol Neurosurg Psychiatry*.

Lindberg, R. L., Achtnichts, L., Hoffmann, F., Kuhle, J., & Kappos, L. (2008). Natalizumab alters transcriptional expression profiles of blood cell subpopulations of multiple sclerosis patients. *J Neuroimmunol, 194*(1–2), 153–164.

Lu, T. T. & Cyster, J. G. (2002). Integrin-mediated long-term B cell retention in the splenic marginal zone. *Science, 297*(5580), 409–412.

Major, E. O. (2010). Progressive multifocal leukoencephalopathy in patients on immunomodulatory therapies. *Annu Rev Med, 61*, 35–47.

Major, E. O., Amemiya, K., Tornatore, C. S., Houff, S. A., & Berger, J. R. (1992). Pathogenesis and molecular biology of progressive multifocal leukoencephalopathy, the JC virus-induced demyelinating disease of the human brain. *Clin Microbiol Rev, 5*(1), 49–73.

Markowitz, R. B., Thompson, H. C., Mueller, J. F., Cohen, J. A., & Dynan, W. S. (1993). Incidence of BK virus and JC virus viruria in human immunodeficiency virus-infected and -uninfected subjects. *J Infect Dis, 167*(1), 13–20.

Marshall, L. J., Dunham, L. D., & Major, E. O. (2010b). The transcription factor spi-B binds unique sequences present in the tandem repeat promoter/enhancer of JC virus and supports viral activity. *J Gen Virol*.

Marshall, L. J. & Major, E. O. (2010a). Molecular regulation of JC virus tropism: Insights into potential therapeutic targets for progressive multifocal leukoencephalopathy. *J Neuroimmune Pharmacol*, 5(3), 404–417.

Monaco, M. C., Atwood, W. J., Gravell, M., Tornatore, C. S., & Major, E. O. (1996). JC virus infection of hematopoietic progenitor cells, primary B lymphocytes, and tonsillar stromal cells: Implications for viral latency. *J Virol*, 70(10), 7004–7012.

Monaco, M. C., Jensen, P. N., Hou, J., Durham, L. C., & Major, E. O. (1998). Detection of JC virus DNA in human tonsil tissue: Evidence for site of initial viral infection. *J Virol*, 72(12), 9918–9923.

Neu, U., Stehle, T., & Atwood, W. J. (2009). The Polyomaviridae: Contributions of virus structure to our understanding of virus receptors and infectious entry. *Virology*, 384(2), 389–399.

Nukuzuma, S., Kameoka, M., Sugiura, S., Nakamichi, K., Nukuzuma, C., Miyoshi, I., et al. (2009). Archetype JC virus efficiently propagates in kidney-derived cells stably expressing HIV-1 Tat. *Microbiol Immunol*, 53(11), 621–628.

Ransohoff, R. M. (2005). Natalizumab and PML. *Nat Neurosci*, 8(10), 1275.

Richardson-Burns, S. M., Kleinschmidt-DeMasters, B. K., DeBiasi, R. L., & Tyler, K. L. (2002). Progressive multifocal leukoencephalopathy and apoptosis of infected oligodendrocytes in the central nervous system of patients with and without AIDS. *Arch Neurol*, 59(12), 1930–1936.

Ryschkewitsch, C., Jensen, P., Hou, J., Fahle, G., Fischer, S., & Major, E. O. (2004). Comparison of PCR-southern hybridization and quantitative real-time PCR for the detection of JC and BK viral nucleotide sequences in urine and cerebrospinal fluid. *J Virol Methods*, 121(2), 217–221.

Ryschkewitsch, C. F., Jensen, P. N., Monaco, M. C., & Major, E. O. (2010). JC virus persistence following progressive multifocal leukoencephalopathy in multiple sclerosis patients treated with natalizumab. *Ann Neurol*, 68(3), 384–391.

Seth, P., Diaz, F., Tao-Cheng, J. H., & Major, E. O. (2004). JC virus induces nonapoptotic cell death of human central nervous system progenitor cell-derived astrocytes. *J Virol*, 78(9), 4884–4891.

Sidhu, N. & McCutchan, J. A. (2010). Unmasking of PML by HAART: Unusual clinical features and the role of IRIS. *J Neuroimmunol*, 219(1–2), 100–104.

Stuve, O. (2008a). The effects of natalizumab on the innate and adaptive immune system in the central nervous system. *J Neurol Sci*, 274(1–2), 39–41.

Stuve, O., Cravens, P. D., Singh, M. P., Frohman, E. M., Phillips, J. T., Remington, G.,et al. (2007). High incidence of post-lumbar puncture headaches in patients with multiple sclerosis treated with natalizumab: Role of intrathecal leukocytes. *Arch Neurol*, 64(7), 1055–1056.

Stuve, O., Gold, R., Chan, A., Mix, E., Zettl, U., & Kieseier, B. C. (2008b). Alpha4-Integrin antagonism with natalizumab: Effects and adverse effects. *J Neurol*, 255 Suppl 6, 58–65.

Sunyaev, S. R., Lugovskoy, A., Simon, K., & Gorelik, L. (2009). Adaptive mutations in the JC virus protein capsid are associated with

progressive multifocal leukoencephalopathy (PML). *PLoS Genet*, 5(2), e1000368.

Tada, H., Rappaport, J., Lashgari, M., Amini, S., Wong-Staal, F., & Khalili, K. (1990). Trans-activation of the JC virus late promoter by the tat protein of type 1 human immunodeficiency virus in glial cells. *Proc Natl Acad Sci U S A*, 87(9), 3479–3483.

Tan, C. S., Dezube, B. J., Bhargava, P., Autissier, P., Wuthrich, C., Miller, J., et al. (2009b). Detection of JC virus DNA and proteins in the bone marrow of HIV-positive and HIV-negative patients: Implications for viral latency and neurotropic transformation. *J Infect Dis*, 199(6), 881–888.

Tan, K., Roda, R., Ostrow, L., McArthur, J., & Nath, A. (2009a). PML-IRIS in patients with HIV infection: Clinical manifestations and treatment with steroids. *Neurology*, 72(17), 1458–1464.

Tornatore, C., Berger, J. R., Houff, S. A., Curfman, B., Meyers, K., Winfield, D., et al. (1992). Detection of JC virus DNA in peripheral lymphocytes from patients with and without progressive multifocal leukoencephalopathy. *Ann Neurol*, 31(4), 454–462.

Verbeeck, J., Van Assche, G., Ryding, J., Wollants, E., Rans, K., Vermeire, S., et al. (2008). JC viral loads in patients with Crohn's disease treated with immunosuppression: Can we screen for elevated risk of progressive multifocal leukoencephalopathy? *Gut*, 57(10), 1393–1397.

von Andrian, U. H. & Engelhardt, B. (2003). Alpha4 integrins as therapeutic targets in autoimmune disease. *N Engl J Med*, 348(1), 68–72.

Weber, T. (2008). Progressive multifocal leukoencephalopathy. *Neurol Clin*, 26(3), 833–854, x-xi.

White, M. K., Johnson, E. M., & Khalili, K. (2009). Multiple roles for Puralpha in cellular and viral regulation. *Cell Cycle*, 8(3), 1–7.

Wuthrich, C., Cheng, Y. M., Joseph, J. T., Kesari, S., Beckwith, C., Stopa, E., et al. (2009a). Frequent infection of cerebellar granule cell neurons by polyomavirus JC in progressive multifocal leukoencephalopathy. *J Neuropathol Exp Neurol*, 68(1), 15–25.

Wuthrich, C., Dang, X., Westmoreland, S., McKay, J., Maheshwari, A., Anderson, M. P., et al. (2009b). Fulminant JC virus encephalopathy with productive infection of cortical pyramidal neurons. *Ann Neurol*, 65(6), 742–748.

Wuthrich, C., Kesari, S., Kim, W. K., Williams, K., Gelman, R., Elmeric, D., et al. (2006). Characterization of lymphocytic infiltrates in progressive multifocal leukoencephalopathy: Co-localization of CD8(+) T cells with JCV-infected glial cells. *J Neurovirol*, 12(2), 116–128.

Yorita Christensen, K. L., Holman, R. C., Hammett, T. A., Belay, E. D., & Schonberger, L. B. (2010). Progressive multifocal leukoencephalopathy deaths in the USA, 1979–2005. *Neuroepidemiology*, 35(3), 178–184.

Yousry, T. A., Major, E. O., Ryschkewitsch, C., Fahle, G., Fischer, S., Hou, J., et al. (2006). Evaluation of patients treated with natalizumab for progressive multifocal leukoencephalopathy. *N Engl J Med*, 354(9), 924–933.

Zohren, F., Toutzaris, D., Klarner, V., Hartung, H. P., Kieseier, B., & Haas, R. (2008). The monoclonal anti-VLA-4 antibody natalizumab mobilizes CD34+ hematopoietic progenitor cells in humans. *Blood*, 111(7), 3893–3895.

8.7

NEOPLASMS

Alexis Demopoulos and Lauren Abrey

Intracranial mass lesions are common in HIV-infected individuals, especially those with the AIDS. These mass lesions may have infectious or neoplastic etiologies. This chapter focuses on neoplastic lesions, though in some cases the distinction between neoplasms and other lesions is blurred because neoplasia can be closely associated with infectious agents (e.g., Epstein-Barr virus). Primary central nervous system lymphomas (PCNSL), gliomas, and leiomyosarcomas all occur with increased frequency in the HIV-positive population and are discussed. Of these conditions, primary central nervous system lymphomas, an AIDS-defining illness, is the most common and developed in greatest detail.

INTRODUCTION

Intracranial mass lesions are common in human immunodeficiency virus (HIV)-infected individuals, especially those with the acquired immune deficiency syndrome (AIDS). Imaging is often atypical in these patients and distinguishing infectious etiologies from neoplasia on the basis of routine imaging studies alone is difficult. Infectious etiologies include toxoplasmosis, progressive multifocal leukoencephalopathy (PML), HIV encephalopathy, cytomegalovirus (CMV) encephalitis, bacterial or fungal brain abscess, tuberculoma, and syphilitic gumma. Primary central nervous system lymphomas (PCNSL), gliomas, and leiomyosarcomas all occur with increased frequency in the HIV positive population. Of these, the majority are PCNSL, an AIDS-defining illness by criteria established by the Centers for Disease Control. When CD4+ lymphocyte counts are robust, HIV-infected individuals may present with the same intracranial tumors that afflict the general population, including meningiomas, brain metastases, and cerebrovascular disorders. Intracranial mass lesions do not always represent a single process. Up to 6% of biopsy-proven AIDS-related PCNSL demonstrate concurrent opportunistic infections (Chang, 1995; Gildenberg, 2000; Stenzel, 2004).

While infection is a straightforward complication of impaired immunity, the mechanisms behind the development of cancer in the setting of immunosuppression are complex. Viruses play a role in oncogenesis. Virtually all immunodeficiency-associated non-Hodgkin's lymphoma (nHL), including PCNSL, contain Epstein-Barr virus (EBV) (MacMahon, 1991). EBV is not found in non-AIDS-related PCNSL (Cingolani, 1998). EBV is a viral oncogenic factor that probably promotes neoplastic growth through several mechanisms in the unique setting of inadequate immune function (Hsu & Glaser, 2000). Chronic antigenic stimulation and cytokine overproduction are associated with oligoclonal B-cell expansion. The presence of a monoclonal B-cell population displaying a variety of genetic lesions, including EBV infection, c-myc gene rearrangement, bcl-6 gene rearrangement, ras gene mutations, and p53 mutations/deletions suggests more than one pathogenic mechanism is operational in the development and progression of AIDS-associated lymphomas (Carbone & Gloghini, 2005; Epeldegui, 2010).

In a process known as "latency," EBV transforms adult primary B cells into continually growing lymphoblastoid cell lines expressing viral nuclear proteins (EBNA-1, EBNA-2, EBNA-3A, EBNA-3B, EBNA-3C, and EBNA-LP) and integral membrane proteins (LMP-1, LMP-2A, and LMP-2B) (Kieff, 1998) . LMP-1 expression induces upregulation of adhesion molecules (LFA-1, ICAM-1, LFA-3), B-cell activation markers (CD23, CD30, CD40, CD71), transcriptional factors (STAT-1), and anti-apoptotic genes (Bcl-2, BclxL, Mcl1, A20). Thus, EBV appears to be a central effector of altered cell growth, survival, adhesion, invasion, and even antiviral potential in EBV-infected cells (Fries, 1996; Miller, 1995; Wang, 1985, 1990; Yoshizaki et al., 1998). A majority of AIDS PCNSL expresses EBNA-2, LMPs, and EBERs, a pattern referred to as type III latency, which is associated with a variety of cellular effects, including upregulation of transforming gene products Bcl-2 and IRF-7 with concurrent inactivation of tumor suppressor gene products p53 and Rb (Cingolani, 2005; Ivers, 2004).

In normal individuals, a small number of circulating B cells enters the CNS (Paludan, 2003). During the course of HIV infection, EBV-specific T cells progressively lose the capacity to produce interferon-gamma in response to EBV peptides (van Baarle, 2001). In addition, EBV-positive B lymphocytes occur more frequently in the CNS of HIV-infected individuals than in normal brains. As HIV infection progresses, the number of EBV-specific T cells also decreases (Anthony, 2003). This combination of increased B-cell infection, upregulation of oncogenes, impaired T-cell immunity, and escape of EBV-infected cells to the relatively immunoprivileged CNS may set the stage for EBV-driven lymphoma development.

While the HIV virus itself is not generally considered oncogenic (Kieff, 1998), some studies suggest a direct role since components of the viral genome are incorporated into HIV-associated non-B-cell lymphomas (Shiramizu, 1994) and HIV gene products may stimulate growth of Kaposi's sarcoma (Albini, 1995).

A healthy immune system may be important in tumor surveillance and prevention in certain malignancies. Lymphomas, especially PCNSL, were described in solid-organ transplant recipients and other conditions of congenital or acquired immune dysfunction before the AIDS epidemic (Grulich et al., 2007). Effective immune surveillance is felt to play an important role in malignant melanoma genesis (Balsamo, 2009). Malignant melanoma is a well-known, non-AIDS-defining malignancy seen in both HIV/AIDS patients and transplant recipients (Laing et al., 2006). When it occurs in transplant recipients, it can develop de novo many years after receiving the transplant or a preexistent melanocytic lesion can become activated and have accelerated growth after the patient starts receiving immunosuppressive medications to facilitate organ retention. Malignant melanoma has also very recently been reported as a complication in three patients treated for multiple sclerosis with the immunosuppressive drug, natalizumab (Mullen, Vartanian, & Atkins, 2008; Polman et al., 2006). Interestingly, patients with malignant gliomas rarely experience spread of their disease to other organs. When kidneys, livers, or lungs are transplanted from a brain tumor patient into immunosuppressed transplant recipients, gliomas have arisen in those organs. Whether this represents iatrogenic inhibition of immune surveillance for cancer cells or growth of micrometastases in the setting of prolonged survivals is unknown (Collignon, 2004).

The interaction between infection, immunity, and cancer development provides a unique opportunity to further our knowledge of microbiology, immunology, and oncology. Recent advances in these fields provide fascinating insight into the development of successful treatment and prevention strategies.

PRIMARY CENTRAL NERVOUS SYSTEM LYMPHOMAS

EPIDEMIOLOGY

With the onset of the AIDS epidemic, the annual incidence of PCNSL increased steadily in the general population from a low of 0.15/100,000 population before AIDS (1973–84), to a high of 0.48 after AIDS (1985–97) (Olson et al., 2002, Eby et al., 1988). In the HIV positive population, the incidence of PCNSL ranges from 2 to 13%, with an autopsy incidence of about 10% (Loureiro et al., 1988). Prior to the introduction of HAART, the lifetime actuarial risk of developing PCNSL in HIV-positive patients approached 40%. One in nine patients with any non-Hodgkin's lymphoma has AIDS. About 1% of non-Hodgkin's lymphoma in the general population will be a PCNSL, while 15% of HIV-related lymphomas are PCNSL (Cote et al., 1997).

The introduction of highly active antiretroviral therapy (HAART) reduced the incidence of AIDS PCNSL in multiple large cohort studies (Besson, 2001; Ammassari, 2000). One European multicenter study—the EuroSIDA group—performed a prospective, observational cohort study consisting of 8,556 HIV-infected patients enrolled from 1994–1999. With 26,764 person-years of prospective follow-up (PYF), they reported significant differences in the incidence of lymphoma pre- and post-HAART (Kirk, Pedersen, & Cozzi-Lepri, 2001). All lymphomas decreased from 1.99 events/100 PYF to 0.83 events/100 PYF (p<0.001). AIDS PCNSL reduction decreased impressively from 1.29 events/100 PYF to 0.57 events/100 PYF (p<0.001). A retrospective analysis of 214 cases of AIDS lymphoma demonstrated a steady increase in incidence of all AIDS lymphomas from 1983 to 1994 to a high of 14.8 cases per 1000 patient years, followed by a steady decline from 1994 to 2002 to a low of 3.7 cases per 1000 patient years. There was a more pronounced decline in AIDS PCNSL over the same period, from a high of 5.3 per 1000 patient years, to a low of 0.32 per 1000 patient years. Meningeal involvement from systemic lymphoma also decreased, from 14% to 7% in the pre- and post-HAART eras, respectively (Wolf et al., 2005).

RISK FACTORS

In the pre-HAART era, approximately two-thirds of patients had AIDS-defining conditions prior to the development of PCNSL, underscoring how immune function must be significantly impaired before PCNSL arises (Gill et al., 1985; Goldstein et al., 1991). Peripheral CD4 lymphocyte count and viral load (pVL) remain the most significant risk factors for the development of PCNSL. The incidence of nHL in patients with CD4 <50 cells/uL is 20-fold higher than those with counts >350 cells/uL. No significant association with the nadir CD4 count has been established (Bower et al., 1999). Other investigators report CD4 counts generally less than 50/uL (Raez et al., 1998; DeMario et al., 1998; Forsyth, 1996). In a study of 111 AIDS PCNSL patients, median CD4 counts were 37, as opposed to 189 in a comparable population of AIDS-related systemic lymphoma. At diagnosis, 34% were not taking anti-retrovirals, PCNSL followed an AIDS diagnosis by a median of 487 days, and the median number of prior AIDS-defining illness was 1.8 (Newell, 2004).

As discussed earlier, AIDS PCNSL almost always occurs in the setting of EBV infection. MacMahon found EBV transcripts and viral protein expression in all 21 cases of AIDS PCNSL studied (MacMahon, Glass, & Hayward, 1991). The route of HIV transmission does not appear to be an independent risk factor for PCNSL (Kirk et al., 2001; Holly & Lele, 1997). As with the HIV negative population, no established occupational, chemical, or environmental PCNSL causes exist (Holly et al., 1997).

CLINICAL PRESENTATION

AIDS PCNSL patients have a younger median age of onset than non-AIDS PCNSL (37 years vs. 60 years). Presentation in AIDS patients appears to differ from the general population in three important ways: the symptoms arise more rapidly (over days to weeks, as opposed to weeks or months); seizures are more frequent, comprising the presenting complaint about 20% of the time; and constitutional, or "B symptoms," (including fever, night sweats, and weight loss) are reported in up to 80% of AIDS-related PCNSL, but are essentially unknown in the non-HIV PCNSL population (Baumgartner et al., 1990). Clinical presentations are otherwise similar to that of the general PCNSL population, with confusion the most common complaint; nonfocal neurologic complaints (headache, nausea or vomiting), weakness, and ataxia or cerebellar finding each seen about one-third of the time; and cranial nerve dysfunction or seizures are less common (Table 8.7.1).

AIDS PCNSL is an aggressive disease that may spread to leptomeninges, the spinal cord, or eye. Systemic AIDS lymphomas (which make up 80% of AIDS lymphomas) have a demonstrated propensity to spread extranodally into the CNS and the leptomeninges more frequently than non-AIDS systemic lymphomas (Mazhar et al., 2006). Leptomeningeal dissemination is probably underreported. Whether from systemic or primary central nervous system lymphoma, leptomeningeal disease (LMD) can present with increased intracranial pressure or multifocal neurological deficits. Cranial nerve dysfunction and absent deep tendon reflexes are highly suspicious for LMD. Patients rarely present with spinal cord involvement, but spinal cord signs can herald relapsing disease. Ocular lymphoma is present in up to one-quarter of all PCNSL patients. Worsening visual acuity, including floaters, suggests ocular lymphoma, with involvement of the vitreous, uvea, or retina. Since asymptomatic ocular lymphoma is common, slit-lamp examination should be performed in all newly diagnosed PCNSL patients. It may disclose corneal precipitate, anterior cell and flare, vitreitis, or subretinal infiltrate. Findings may mimic uveitis. When present, ocular disease is often bilateral. Neuro-ophthalmologic evaluation is often helpful. Vitrectomy confirms the diagnosis, although prior corticosteroid treatment may cause false-negative results. In PCNSL patients, a computed tomography (CT) scan of the chest, abdomen, and pelvis or positron emission tomography (PET) scan can exclude systemic disease. Bone marrow aspirates are rarely helpful.

PATHOLOGY

By definition, PCNSL is confined to the nervous system. Although imaging studies typically show a solitary, ring-enhancing lesion, AIDS PCNSL is often found to be diffuse, with multifocal tumors at autopsy. Cerebral lesions are most common, but tumors may occur in the cerebellum, basal ganglia, and brainstem (Loureiro et al., 1988; Zacharia, 2008). Lymphoma cells tend to be distributed along vascular channels as perivascular cuffs. They are of B-cell origin, display large cell and immunoblastic histologies, and uniformly exhibit EBV-associated DNA. Necrosis and atypical features are not uncommon. Small noncleaved cell lymphomas or mixed large and small cell lymphomas are infrequent. Unlike immunocompetent patients, both systemic AIDS lymphoma and AIDS PCNSL patients demonstrate high percentage of high-grade subtypes, frequent extranodal sites of disease, increased percentage of advanced disease, low response rate to combined modality therapy, and elevated mortality rates. T-cell lymphomas are rare, although a reactive perivascular T-cell infiltrate is typical and may create confusion, especially in the setting of corticosteroid administration.

WORK-UP AND DIFFERENTIAL DIAGNOSIS

Because PCNSL patients often present with lower CD4 counts, higher pVL, and overall greater degrees of immunodeficiency, this population is at risk for opportunistic infections that mimic PCNSL. In a study of focal brain lesions in HIV-infected individuals from 1991 through 1999, the major diagnoses in 281 patients were toxoplasmic encephalitis (36.4%), primary CNS lymphoma (26.7%), progressive multifocal leukoencephalopathy (18.2%), and focal HIV encephalopathy (5.0%). In a subset analysis, the authors identified a lower incidence of both toxoplasmosis and lymphoma in the post-HAART years (1996–99). The proportion of PML cases remained stable, while the "other" category increased. Additional diseases presenting with focal brain lesions included herpes simplex encephalitis, Kaposi's sarcoma, tuberculosis, aspergillosis, cryptococcus, and gliomas (Ammassari et al., 2000).

Corticosteroids are best avoided until a diagnosis is secure or tissue is obtained. They may induce resolution of all sites of disease or convert enhancing disease to nonenhancing disease. This strong lymphocytic effect is transient and noncurative. When given even 24 hours before a brain biopsy or CSF analysis, steroids can render tissue nondiagnostic. While many PCNSL lesions shrink radiographically after corticosteroid

Table 8.7.1 **PRESENTING COMPLAINTS IN PATIENTS WITH PCNSL**

	N = 20	N = 26	N = 54	N = 66
Behavioral changes	70 %	73 %	69 %	24 %
Nausea/vomiting/headache	45	38	37	15
Ataxia/Cerebellar findings	40	42	15	21
Weakness	20	42	52	11
Cranial Nerve dysfunction	15	19	31	no data
Seizures	5	23	15	13
Reference	Grote 1989	Herrlinger 1998	Braus 1992	Hochberg 1988

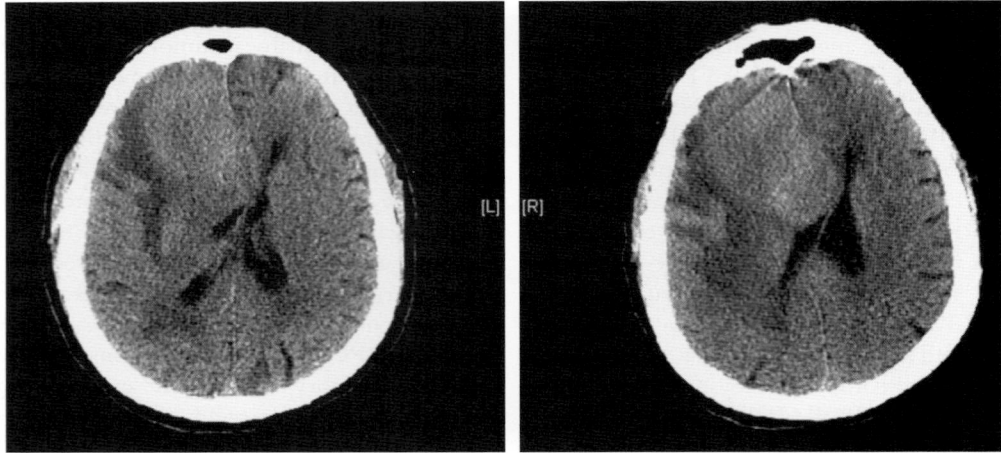

Figure 8.7.1 Two CT imaging studies of a PCNSL patient before (left) and one week after (right) administration of high dose steroids (40mg of dexamethasone daily). While steroid responsiveness occurs in a majority of PCNSL lesions, some do not change and may even—as in this example—continue to grow. Avoiding corticosteroids improves diagnostic accuracy.

administration, some do not (Figure 8.7.1). Moreover, other etiologies may also appear to improve, including malignant gliomas. Conversely, underlying opportunistic infections may worsen with further immunosuppression. Indeed, in the absence of a pressing medical need such as impending herniation, corticosteroids are best avoided.

LABORATORY STUDIES

Magnetic resonance imaging of AIDS PCNSL lesions have characteristics distinct from non-AIDS PCNSL. The lesions of non-AIDS PCNSL are usually periventricular, may involve the corpus callosum, and are often unifocal. They are bright on T2, dark on T1, homogeneously enhance, and typically bright on DWI sequences (Figure 8.7.2). AIDS PCNSL lesions are heterogenous, often peripheral or cortically based, rarely involve the corpus callosum and are usually multifocal (Baumgartner et al., 1990; Hochberg & Miller, 1988; So, Beckstead, & Davis, 1986). Gradient echo planar sequences may reveal subacute hemorrhage in AIDS PCNSL, but this is rarely clinically significant (Epstein, Goudsmit, & Sharer, 1988; Forsyth, Yahalom, & DeAngelis,

1994; McArthur, 1987). The dense uniform contrast enhancement typical of non-AIDS PCNSL tumors is less common in AIDS PCNSL lesions (Cellerier, Chiras, Gray, Metzger, & Bories, 1984; DeAngelis et al., 1990; O'Neill & Illig, 1989; Schwaighofer et al., 1989), which generally show ring enhancement (Ciricillo & Rosenblum, 1990; Forsyth et al., 1994; Goldstein et al., 1991; Levy, Bredesen, & Rosenblum, 1985; Remick et al., 1990; So et al., 1986). Central tumor necrosis produces the ring enhancement found in AIDS PCNSL and is occasionally found in non-AIDS patients (Remick et al., 1990). Ring enhancement is also typical for cerebral toxoplasmosis and may be seen in abscesses and even PML. Progressive multifocal leukoencephalopathy (PML) is usually not associated with significant mass effect (Giancola et al., 2008). Diffusion weighted imaging is usually positive in non-AIDS PCNSL, but may be negative in AIDS PCNSL (Zacharia, Law, Naidich, & Leeds, 2008). A ring of DWI positivity may indicate a cerebral abscess.

Newer imaging technologies may be useful to distinguish PCNSL from opportunistic infections. Perfusion and permeability MRI may be helpful. In one study, lymphomas were readily distinguished from high grade gliomas and

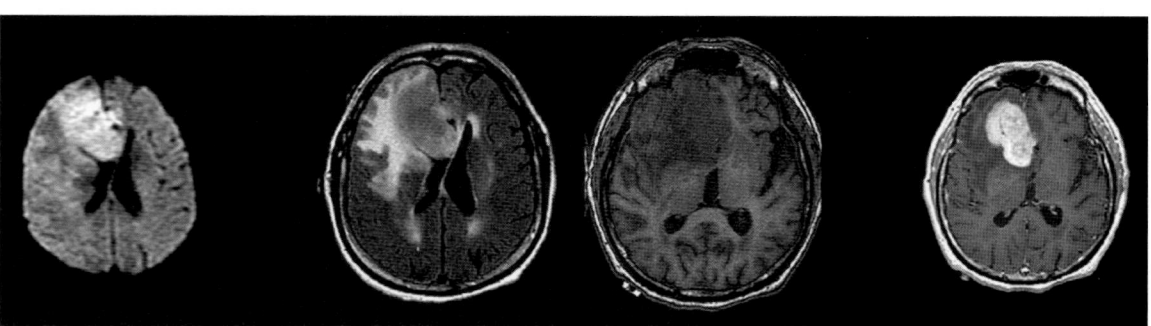

Figure 8.7.2 Magnetic resonance imaging characteristics of PCNSL. From left to right: DWI, T2-FLAIR, T1-precontrast, and T1 postcontrast sequences. Same patient.

brain metastases as the former demonstrate slower rates of contrast uptake (Weber et al., 2006). FDG-PET studies can guide stereotactic biopsy to the most metabolically active portion of the tumor. Relatively high uptake signal on thallium-201 SPECT studies suggests neoplasia, while low uptake is consistent with infection. When compared with brain biopsy and/or autopsy data, SPECT accuracy remains controversial. Even PML may demonstrate high thallium-201 uptake on SPECT (Port et al., 1999). Given the variety of diseases indistinguishable by imaging, SPECT data alone is probably inadequate to establish a diagnosis or to determine treatment (Licho, Litofsky, Senitko, & George, 2002).

Lumbar puncture with cerebrospinal fluid (CSF) sampling may establish the diagnosis and obviate the need for brain biopsy. However, CSF analysis can be entirely normal, especially if the disease lies in a deep parenchymal location or corticosteroids have been administered. Reasons to avoid a lumbar puncture include evidence of intracranial herniation, large posterior fossa lesions with mass effect, concurrent coagulopathy, strong suspicion for intracranial abscess, or an infection overlaying the skin at the procedure site. Once performed, the opening pressure should be recorded and CSF sent for laboratory analysis. In general, the first and last tubes are sent with about 1 cc of CSF for cell count with differential. The second tube is sent to chemistry and immunology for protein, glucose, and immunologic studies, including PCR for immunoglobulin heavy chain (IgH) rearrangement (about 4cc), and tube three for microbiology studies, including gram stain, bacterial and fungal cultures, viral studies, including JC virus, EBV DNA PCR, and CMV (5cc). Flow cytometry specimens are sent without fixative and if CSF white blood cell counts are known to be low, more fluid will be required for informative testing. Cytology should be mixed in a 1:1 solution with fixative immediately after the procedure, with as much fluid as possible sent for staining. Occasionally, immunostains for CD19+ lymphocytes are helpful.

Falsely negative CSF cytology is common. Flow cytometry has a higher yield than cytology and should be prioritized. The diagnostic utility of flow cytometry for detecting lymphoma cells in the CSF was evaluated in 51 newly diagnosed and 9 previously treated lymphoma patients at risk for leptomeningeal disease. Flow cytometry using multiple antibody panels for light chains and B- and T-cell antigens demonstrated a much higher sensitivity over conventional CSF cytology. Cytology was positive in 1 (2%) patient, while flow cytometry markers were positive in 11 (22%) of the same patients (P ≤ .002). The single patient in whom involvement was detected by both methods had the highest percentage of tumor cells in the CSF (99%) (Hegde et al., 2005). The accuracy of CSF analysis is increased by multiple lumbar punctures, large volumes of CSF, and obtaining fluid prior to corticosteroid administration.

PCR for immunoglobulin heavy chain (IgH) gene rearrangement has emerged as a valuable adjunct to cytological evaluation of CSF. In a study of 282 patients with nHL, dissemination of lymphoma into the CSF was detected in 33/205 (16%) by cytology, 8/217 (4%) by MRI, and 19/171

(11%) by PCR. The relative frequency was 17.4% (49 of 282 patients). PCR was positive in 6/19 (32%) with positive cytology, 1/13 (8%) with suspicious cytology, and 10/105 (10%) with negative cytology (Fischer et al., 2008). In a smaller study of 73 patients, PCR was positive in 4/8 (50%) with positive cytology, 1/5 (20%) with nonconclusive cytology, and 10/59 (18%) with negative cytology (Ekstein et al., 2006).

In AIDS PCNSL, but not other PCNSL, EBV DNA sequences can be detected by polymerase chain reaction (PCR) in the cerebrospinal fluid (CSF). The presence of EBV in CSF is diagnostic for AIDS PCNSL. EBV DNA PCR has an established sensitivity of 80–100% and specificity of 93–100%. The test has been positive in a patient before they developed symptomatic or radiographic PCNSL (Al-Shahi et al., 2000). EBV DNA in the CSF is not seen in non-AIDS PCNSL. In one series of HIV-infected patients with focal brain lesions, EBV DNA sequences were detected in the CSF in 24 of 30 patients (80%) with PCNSL compared none of 61 patients without PCNSL (Cingolani, 2000). As the incidence of AIDSL PCNSL declines in the post-HAART era and PCR techniques become increasing sensitive, the positive predictive value of CSF EBV DNA detection has been challenged. There may be an increased risk for false positive results in unselected patient populations (Corcoran, 2008; Cinque, 2004; Ivers, 2004). Bossolasco and colleagues performed PCR to quantify CSF EBV DNA in 42 patients with AIDS-related lymphoma. Twenty patients had PCNSL and 22 systemic NHL, including 12 with central nervous system involvement (CNS-NHL). EBV DNA was detected in the CSF from 16/20 (80%) patients with PCNSL, 7/22 (32%) with systemic NHL, 8/12 (67%) with CNS-NHL, and 2/16 (13%) of HIV-infected patients with other CNS disorders. Importantly, the viral EBV DNA titers were significantly higher in the CSF from patients with AIDS PCNSL or CNS-NHL compared to patients with systemic NHL or other CNS disease (Bossolasco, Cinque, & Ponzoni, 2002). In the appropriate clinical context, CSF EBV DNA remains a valuable aid in the diagnosis of AIDS PCNSL.

Combining EBV PCR data with thallium-201 SPECT, one study reported a sensitivity of 76.9%, a specificity of 100%, a negative predictive value of 85.7%, and a positive predictive value of 100%. Unfortunately, 12 of their 31 patients (39%) lacked a histological diagnosis either through biopsy or autopsy (Antinori, De Rossi, & Ammassari, 1999). Moreover, using EBV PCR data alone, they had a sensitivity of 84.5%, a specificity of 100%, a negative predictive value of 90%, and a positive predictive value of 100%, results comparable to earlier PCR studies (Cingolani et al., 1998).

Stereotactic brain biopsy establishes diagnosis in 88% of cases. Complication rates in one study of 435 AIDS patients undergoing brain biopsy were 8% morbidity and 3% mortality. The authors concluded that the rates were not significantly different from the non-HIV population (Luzzati et al., 1996; Skloasky et al., 1999). The relative merit of brain biopsy versus empiric toxoplasmosis therapy remains a matter of longstanding debate and beyond the scope of this discussion. However, in situations where toxoplasmosis appears unlikely (e.g., progression of rapid neurologic decline despite appropriate anti-toxoplasmosis therapies) or in the setting of rapid patient deterioration, brain biopsy is probably required (Skolasky et al., 1999; Mathews, Barba, & Fullerton, 1995; Antinori et al., 2000). Other risk factors for biopsy-related complications include poor functional status, thrombocytopenia, and multiple lesions at presentation. Surgical resection is rarely of therapeutic benefit in PCNSL.

THERAPEUTIC STRATEGIES

Standard therapeutic strategies for non-AIDS PCNSL include methotrexate-based chemotherapy regimen, followed by 45 Gy whole brain radiation therapy without a boost (Abrey, DeAngelis, & Yahalom, 1998; Nelson et al., 1992; Pollack, Lunsford, Flickinger, & Dameshek, 1989). While the combination of MTX-based chemotherapy and cranial radiation therapy (RT) is effective, significant neurological morbidity may occur, especially in adults >60 years of age. If radiation therapy is omitted in this population, survival may not be compromised and neurological morbidity is greatly reduced (Gerstner, 2008). Adjuvant high-dose cytarabine should be given after RT or the methotrexate regimen. Although at least half of patients who achieve a complete remission will eventually relapse, survival with this approach ranges between 30 and 60 months in immunocompetent patients (Abrey, 2000; Batchelor, 2008; DeAngelis, 2002).

Because the profoundly immunocompromised are at greatest risk of AIDS PCNSL, these patients have a much worse prognosis than non-AIDS patients. They tolerate cytotoxic chemotherapies poorly and develop more infectious complications. Bone marrow toxicity and a high rate of opportunistic infections frequently complicate treatment regimens. Before antiretroviral therapy, mean survival was 42 days without treatment. Whole brain RT in isolation resulted in a survival between three to four months (Baumgartner et al., 1990; Donahue, Sullivan, & Cooper, 1995).

NCCN guidelines for AIDS PCNSL include methotrexate-based chemotherapy regimens, whole brain radiation therapy, and the initiation of HAART therapy. However, a survey of treatment patterns and prognosis in 184 patients with AIDS and PCNSL by Kreisl and colleagues showed 46% patients received RT alone, 10% received chemotherapy and RT, 4% had chemotherapy alone and a substantial number (40%) received no tumor-directed treatment at all (Kreisl, 2008). Without treatment, patients can be expected to live weeks. Radiation increases survival to a median of 3.5 months. Long-term survivors remain a small minority. In one study, less than 20% of patients who completed radiation therapy lived one year or more (Newell, 2004). Receiving any radiation, completing radiation, and the delivery of at least 30cGy (or more) of radiation therapy have all been associated with improved prognosis (Newell, 2004; Skolasky, 1999; Raez, 1998). About 10% of patients will experience disease progression during radiotherapy (Baumgartner, 1990; Donahue et al., 1995). Opportunistic infections remain the principal cause of death following therapy (Jacomet, 1997; Forsyth, 1994).

Initiation of HAART has been reported to improve survival even without chemotherapy, suggesting improved outcome due to immune system recovery (Hoffman et al., 2001). McGowan and Shah were the first to describe an AIDS PCNSL patient who achieved CR after receiving dexamethasone for 8 weeks and a switch from a two-drug to a three-drug HAART regimen (McGowan & Shah, 1998). Another case report describes a 40-year-old antiretroviral-naïve man whose AIDS PCNSL resolved with HAART initiation, without chemotherapy or RT (Aboulafia & Puswella, 2007). Unfortunately, the majority of AIDS PCNSL patients will have already been on HAART for many years, and robust immune reconstitution responses are unlikely in that population.

The ability to deliver adequate chemotherapy and RT has improved following the introduction of HAART. Small institutional series published median survivals approaching a year, in contrast to an expected 10% of patients surviving that long following RT alone. In one study, 15 individuals with a mean CD4 count of 30 cells/mL and a median Karnofsky performance status (KPS) of 50 received high-dose methotrexate (3 g/m^2 every 14 days for 6 cycles) (Jacomet et al., 1997). The complete response rate was 50% with a median survival of 10 months. Tosi evaluated oral zidovudine (2, 4, and 6 mg/m^2) and IV MTX at 1gm/m^2 (moderate-dose) plus leucovorin rescue weekly for three to six cycles. In 29 patients with a median CD4 count of 133/uL, 46% had a complete response and the median survival was 12 months (Tosi et al., 1997). Antiviral therapy and biologic modifiers produced responses in four of five patients treated with parenteral zidovudine (1.6 g twice daily), ganciclovir (5 mg/kg twice daily), and interleukin 2 (2 million units twice daily). Among six patients, one remained in complete remission with > 4 years' follow-up, three patients died from complications of progressive PCNSL, and two patients exhibited favorable responses and remained in complete remission at 28 months and 52 months. Grade 3/4 myelosuppression was uniformly noted, but there were no clinically significant hemorrhagic or infectious complications (Aboulafia, 2006). As gancyclovir is active against EBV and can render CSF EBV DNA PCR negative (Bossolasco, 2006), further studies applying a regimen of induction intravenous zidovudine, ganciclovir, and IL-2 followed by maintenance subcutaneous IL-2 and oral ganciclovir were planned (Aboulafia, 2006).

SYSTEMIC NON-HODGKIN'S LYMPHOMA

HIV-positive patients with systemic nHL are at high risk of leptomeningeal dissemination of their disease. Therefore, performing a staging lumbar puncture for CSF cytology is suggested, with consideration of CNS prophylaxis. Levine published a review of 11 different chemotherapy regimens for systemic nHL prior to HAART therapy. He found median survivals ranging from 2.6 months to 15 months (median of 6 months) (Levine, 1992). Vaccher and colleagues began a trial of cyclophosphamide, doxorubicin, vincristine, and prednisone (CHOP) chemotherapy in the pre-HAART era and continued the study into the post-HAART period. Their treatment groups had similar demographics, lymphoma characteristics, HIV status, and treatment, that is, the number of cycles and chemotherapy dose. The response rates were similar between the two groups. Severe anemia and autonomic neurotoxicity were significantly greater in the patients who received CHOP-HAART compared with the patients who received CHOP alone (33% vs. 7% and 17% vs. none, respectively). Opportunistic infection rates and mortality were lower in the CHOP-HAART patients than in the CHOP patients (18% vs. 52% and 38% vs. 85%, respectively). The median survival for CHOP-HAART patients was not reached, whereas the median survival of CHOP patients was 7 months (P = 0.03) (Vaccher et al., 2001). A recent study of Rituximab plus concurrent infusional EPOCH (etoposide, doxorubicin, vincrisitne, and prednisone) chemotherapy demonstrated tolerability of this regimen, although patients with CD4 counts less than 50/uL had higher death rates (Sparano, 2010).

CONCLUSION

In summary, survival remains significantly lower for patients with AIDS PCNSL than for AIDS systemic lymphoma or non-AIDS PCNSL, reflecting both the highly aggressive nature of the disease and the complications inherent to chemotherapy administration in this population. HAART administration improves outcomes, especially in HAART naïve patients. Radiation therapy prolongs survival. Clinical trials incorporating chemo- and antiviral therapies promise improved outcomes. Favorable prognostic indicators include higher Karnofsky score and an absence of prior or concomitant opportunistic infections.

LEIOMYOSARCOMAS AND LEIOMYOMAS

In immunocompetent individuals, leiomyomas (LM) and leiomyosarcomas (LMS) are uterine smooth-muscle tumors found mainly in women. Alternative sites of disease, particularly involvement of the central nervous system, are exceedingly rare, estimated to occur in 2/1,000,000 persons per year. These tumors are thought to arise from the mesenchyma of the blood vessels in bone, dura, or subarachnoid space (Varela-Duran, Oliva, & Rosai, 1979). LM and LMS have been increasingly recognized as a complication of immunodeficiency and intercurrent EBV infection (Choi et al., 1997). These tumors typically involve the liver, lung, and gastrointestinal tract, but have been described in adrenal tissue, kidney, brain, and spine. While intraocular LM involving the ciliary body have been described, LM of the iris are probably melanocyte-derived neoplasms (Foss et al., 1994). McClain found the EBV receptor, CD21, in 6 of 7 HIV-positive patients with leiomyosarcoma and in none of 7 HIV-negative patients with leiomyosarcoma (McClain et al., 1995).

Children are affected more often than adults, making LM and LMS the second most frequently found solid tumors in the HIV-positive pediatric population. Children with congenital immune deficiencies are also at risk, including subacute combined immunodeficiency and ataxia-telangiectasia (Jensen et al., 1997; Mierau, Greffe, & Weeks, 1997; Reyes, Abuzaitoun, De Jong, Hanson, & Langston, 2002). Although rare in HIV positive adults and adult solid organ transplant recipients, LM and LMS are increasingly recognized complications of immunodeficiency. Currently, a dozen case reports now describe HIV-related brain and spine LM and LMS presenting as painful dural-based lesions (Table 8.7.2).

In the 13 HIV-positive adult cases reported to date, the median age was 35 there was no sex preference. The average CD4 count was low, with a range from 2 to 81 cells/uL although not all reports included this data. Most patients had longstanding HIV infection, with an AIDS-defining infection such as PCP pneumonia prior to diagnosis. One patient tested negative for HIV infection one month prior to resection and seroconverted two months after surgery

Table 8.7.2 LEIOMYOMA AND LEIOMYOSARCOMA CASE REPORT SUMMARY

AUTHOR	AGE	CD4 COUNT (/uL)	PRIOR AIDS DEFINING ILLNESS	TYPE	TUMOR LOCATION	PRESENTING COMPLAINT	EBV	OUTCOME
Bargiela 1999	32/F	*	yes	LM	occipital lobe	headache	*	died before intervention, fungal pneumonia
Bejjani 1999	38/M	*	no	LMS	sphenoid wing	facial pain	*	stable (12 months)
Blumenthal 1998	44/M	23	yes	LMS	cavernous sinus	headache, facial pain, CN VI palsy	yes	stable (5 years)
Brown 1999	34/F	34	yes	LMS	pontine cistern	headache, facial pain, facial weakness, slurred speech, gait difficulty, and ataxia	yes	clinical improvement, progressive disease

(Continued)

Table 8.7.2 (CONTINUED)

AUTHOR	AGE	CD4 COUNT (/uL)	PRIOR AIDS DEFINING ILLNESS	TYPE	TUMOR LOCATION	PRESENTING COMPLAINT	EBV	OUTCOME
Choi 1997	9/M	0	yes	LM	two: cervical spine - C7 & thoracic spine - T3/4	paraparesis, urinary incontinence	*	clinical improvement
Citow 2000	31/F	3	yes	LM	pontine cistern and lung	headache, CN IV palsy, and fevers with eye pain	no	stable disease
Karpinski 1999	26/M	20	yes	LM	two: sphenoid wing & cervical spine - C2/3	intermittent headaches and progressive neck pain	yes	*
Kleinschmidt 1998	35/F	81	yes	LM	cavernous sinus	facial pain, right CN VI palsy	yes	no clinical improvement, progressive disease
Litofsky 1998	50/M	27	no	LMS	occipital lobe	hemiparesis	yes	stable (8 months)
Mierau 1999	14/F	-	SCID	LMS	two: transverse sinus & sigmoid sinus	incidental finding (work-up for chronic sinusitis)	yes	clinical improvement (21 months)
Morgello 1997	35/M	16	yes	LMS	cervical spine - C6	painful radiculopathy with weakness	yes	died 4 weeks post-op, urosepsis
Ritter 2000	5/F	*	yes	LMS	cavernous sinus	incidental finding (surveillance imaging)	yes	minimal progression
Ritter 2000	35/F	*	yes	LMS	thoracic spine - T3/T4	paraparesis	yes	*
Savici 1995	28/M	*	yes	LM	cervical spine - C6/7	quadraparesis	*	*
Steel 1993	52/M	2	yes	LM	thoracic spine - T3	painful radiculopathy without weakness	*	clinical improvement

NB: - patient with SCID, not HIV positive.
* indicates data was not reported; not all data available from all case reports.

(Bejjani et al., 1999). Among adults and children with immunodeficiency, pain was the most distinctive presenting complaint, occurring in all but three adult patients. Facial pain was frequent and resembled trigeminal neuralgia. Lesions were dural-based, whether occurring in the spinal canal or in the intracranial compartment. Most were associated with vascular structures such as venous sinuses or adjacent arteries, including the vertebral artery in two patients. On imaging studies, all tumors enhanced with gadolinium and resembled meningiomas or schwannomas (Figure 8.7.3). All brain and spine tumors were EBV positive, a finding consistent with the pediatric literature on systemic HIV-related leiomyomas.

Resection was the mainstay of therapy and most did not receive additional therapy. A few patients received post-surgery radiotherapy and the outcomes, when reported, were favorable. One patient could not undergo complete resection, but had stable disease after receiving liposomal doxorubicin with concomitant HAART. There were three reported deaths. One occurred prior to surgery and was attributed to sepsis secondary to pneumonia (Bargiela, Rey, Diaz, & Martinez, 1999). Another died seven months after presentation of "other intracranial disease," presumably an unrelated opportunistic infection (Kleinschmidt-DeMaster et al., 1998). The last died of urosepsis four days after resection of a spinal lesion (Morgello, Kotsianti, Gumprecht, & Moore, 1997). Due to the small sample size and the variability of both methods and length of follow-up, few conclusions may be drawn from this data; however, overall survival appears excellent in most patients.

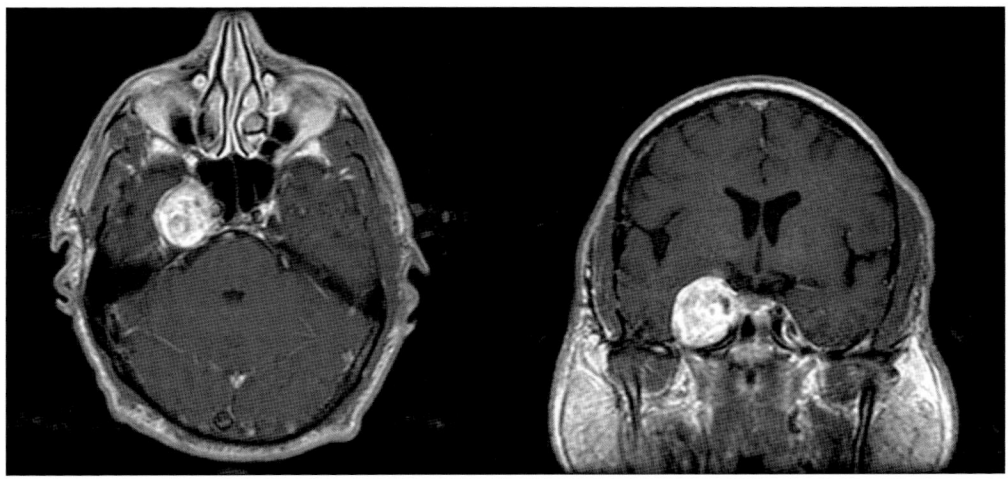

Figure 8.7.3 Leiomyosarcoma of the cavernous sinus. MRI: Axial T1 and coronal T1 images after gadolinium administration; note the homogeneous enhancement, dural base, and involvement of the right carotid artery at the level of the cavernous sinus.

GLIOMAS

Gliomas are a heterogenous group of brain tumors arising from glial components of the CNS. These neoplasms are rare, affecting about 16,500 people in the US each year. The overall incidence is 6/100,000 people/year, but there is a bimodal distribution, with increased risk in children and seniors. The incidence is 19.2/100,000 in those over 65 years old (Davis et al., 1998). Risk factors include cranial RT, hereditary syndromes, and male sex, with men predominating over women at a ratio of 7:5. A minority of patients has identifiable risk factors and the etiology of these neoplasms is unknown. Although associated with ataxia telangiectasia, immunodeficiency has only recently been recognized as a risk factor for glioma development. HIV-positive individuals and, to a lesser degree, solid organ transplant recipients have an increased risk for developing gliomas. Buttner and Weis published a review of 48 brain tumors occurring in the HIV population. They estimated that the incidence of gliomas was about 0.05% in this population, or 50/100,000. [Buttner and Weis, 1999] A National Cancer Institute study found a similar significantly increased relative risk of 3.5 for the development of gliomas in the AIDS population (Goedert, Cote, & Virgo, 1998).

The mechanism by which immune dysfunction predisposes to glioma development is unknown. In those tumors that have been studied, there is no evidence of EBV or other viral infection. Unfortunately, how these neoplasms develop in immunocompetent persons is also unknown, confounding any potential explanation. No viral factor has been identified and while many environmental influences have been proposed, only cranial irradiation has an established cause-effect relationship. Current hypotheses for non-AIDS glioma development emphasize the impact of genetic mutations acquired over the lifetime of the individual. Glioblastoma multiforme (GBM) formation is thought to be either de novo (primary GBMs) or due to the progression of a lower grade glioma to a higher grade one through the acquisition of additional mutations (secondary GBMs). How immunosuppression or an infectious pathogen induces these genetic abnormalities is unknown.

There are now sixty published case reports of non-lymphomatous brain tumors arising in AIDS patients (Table 8.7.3). They include 56 gliomas, 2 peripheral neuroectodermal tumors, 1 meningioma and 1 choroid plexus papilloma. Among the gliomas, there were 18 low grade astrocytomas (including 2 fibrillary and 1 pilocytic), 9 anaplastic astrocytomas (1 of the spinal cord), and 15 glioblastoma multiforme (2 of the spinal cord). WHO grading was unavailable in 6. In addition, 4 ependymomas,

Table 8.7.3 AIDS-ASSOCIATED GLIOMAS AND OTHER PRIMARY BRAIN TUMORS

LESION PATHOLOGY AT DIAGNOSIS	N=
Low grade astrocytoma	18
- 15 intracranial	
- 2 fibrillary	
- 1 pilocytic	
Anaplastic astrocytoma	9
- 8 intracranial	
- 1 spinal	
Glioblastoma Multiforme	15
- 13 intracranial	
- 2 spinal	
Astrocytoma - unknown grade	6
- 1 brainstem	
- 1 thalamic	
Oligodendroglioma	1
Ependymoma	4
Subependymoma	3
Meningioma	1
PNET	1
Medulloblastoma	1
Choroid plexus papilloma	1

3 subependymomas, and 1 oligodendroglioma have been reported. Although data is incomplete, most patients were younger men, typically in the fourth decade of life. They presented with headaches, seizures, and focal neurological deficits typical for intracranial mass lesions. Many patients were treated empirically with antitoxoplasmosis therapy before diagnosis via brain biopsy.

The prognosis of patients with AIDS-related gliomas is not necessarily worse than the non-AIDS population. Most patients do poorly, but selected patients can do well with aggressive treatment. Moreover, standard therapies, including resection, radiation and chemotherapy, do not usually exacerbate immune dysfunction related to HIV infection. Patients typically die from complications of their brain tumors and not because of an AIDS-related opportunistic infection.

Recently, two large retrospective studies suggested that solid organ transplant recipients are also at significantly increased risk of developing gliomas (Schiff et al., 2001; Detry et al., 2000). While cyclosporine and other immunosuppressant drugs may be mutagenic, a clear cause-and-effect relationship remains to be established. Whether an infectious agent or an impaired immune system was responsible is unknown (Frank et al., 1998). Several authors have suggested that cyclosporine itself is not mutagenic, but that the level of immunosuppression necessary for organ transplantation leads to impaired immunosurveillance for mutated cells and the subsequent development of cancer.

Interestingly, because primary brain tumors rarely metastasize outside the CNS, patients with gliomas are acceptable solid organ donors. There are now a dozen case reports describing gliomas in recipients of organs from patients with gliomas. The gliomas are identical by molecular analysis, indicating that these brain tumors were transmitted. More unusual, these tumors had widespread dissemination outside the CNS. On the one hand, the tumor may have developed the capacity to spread extra-neurally before donation and the organ donor died of brain disease before clinically evident disease arose. On the other hand, an effective immune response may have been able to control the malignancy systemically, while the immunoprivileged nature of the CNS prevented an adequate immune response from crossing the blood-brain barrier and controlling central disease. Whether aggressive tumor characteristics or impaired immunity led to the widespread dissemination of an otherwise locally invasive disease remains unknown.

While the development of gliomas in AIDS, ataxia telangiectasia, and solid organ transplant recipients appears related to impaired immunosurveillance, no oncogenic virus has been established. One candidate is another herpes virus, human cytomegalovirus (HCMV). One recently published study in immunocompetent patients reported HCMV DNA and mRNA in 27/27 gliomas and 0/5 non-neoplastic controls (Cobb et al., 2002). On the other hand, while HCMV may have oncogenic potential, HCMV ventriculitis, encephalitis, and TORCH infections are well-known entities, none of which are known to result in glioma formation. No investigator has looked for HCMV in gliomas affecting immunocompromised patients, a task made difficult by the rarity of these patients.

In conclusion, immunosuppressed patients are at greater risk for developing gliomas and do poorly once these tumors arise. The etiology of these tumors in healthy population is unknown. Why immune system dysfunction should result in a predisposition to this tumor is similarly unestablished. Further advances in glioma biology may help to explain etiology and provide insight into new therapies.

REFERENCES

[No authors listed] (2000). Highly active antiretroviral therapy and incidence of cancer in human immunodeficiency virus-infected adults. *Journal of the National Cancer Institute, 92*, 1823–30.

Abati, A., Dunleavy, K., Filie, A., et al. (2005). High incidence of occult leptomeningeal disease detected by flow cytometry in newly diagnosed aggressive B-cell lymphomas at risk for central nervous system involvement: the role of flow cytometry versus cytology. *Blood, 105*(2), 496–502.

Abdel-Wahab, M., Berson, A., Brandon, A. H., et al. (1997). Palliation of AIDS-related primary lymphoma of the brain: Observations from a multi-institutional database. *International Journal of Radiation Oncology Biology Physics, 38*(3), 601–5.

Aboulafia, D., Ambinder, R. F., Dezube, B. J., et al. (2009). Rituximab plus concurrent infusional EPOCH chemotherapy is highly effective in HIV-associated, B-cell non-Hodgkin's lymphoma. *Blood.*

Aboulafia, D. M, Puswella, A. L. (2007). Highly active antiretroviral therapy as the sole treatment for AIDS-related primary central nervous system lymphoma: a case report with implications for treatment. *AIDS Patient Care STDS, 21*, 900–7.

Aboulafia, D. M., Miles, S. A., Ratner, L., et al. (2006). AIDS Associated Malignancies Clinical Trials Consortium. Antiviral and immunomodulatory treatment for AIDS-related primary central nervous system lymphoma: AIDS Malignancies Consortium pilot study 019. *Clinical Lymphoma Myeloma, 6*(5), 399–402.

Abrams, R. A., Dal Pan, G. J., Lenz, F. A., et al. (1999). HIV-associated primary CNS lymorbidity and utility of brain biopsy. *Journal of Neurological Science, 163*, 32–8.

Abrey, L. E., DeAngelis, L. M., Elkin, E. B., et al. (2008). Treatment patterns and prognosis in patients with human immunodeficiency virus and primary central system lymphoma. *Leukemia and Lymphoma, 49*(9), 1710–6.

Abrey, L. E., DeAngelis, L. M., & Yahalom, J. (1998). Long-term survival in primary CNS lymphoma. *Journal of Clinical Oncology, 16*, 859–63.

Abrey, L. E., Yahalom, J., & DeAngelis, L. M. (2000). Treatment for primary CNS lymphoma: The next step. *Journal of Clinical Oncology, 18*, 3144–50.

Abuzaitoun, O., De Jong, A., Hanson, C., et al. (2002). Epstein-Barr virus-associated smooth muscle tumors in ataxia-telangiectasia: A case report and review. *Human Pathology, 33*, 133–6.

Agan, B. K., Armstrong, A., Blazes, D. L., et al. (2005). Incidence and risk factors for the occurrence of non-AIDS-defining cancers among human immunodeficiency virus-infected individuals. *Cancer, 104*(7), 1505–11.

Ajisawa, A., Hagiwara, S., Kanbe, T., et al. (2010). Whole brain radiation alone produces favorable outcomes for AIDS-related primary central nervous system lymphoma in the HAART era. *European Journal of Hematology.*

Albini, A., Barillari, G., Benelli, et al. (1995). Angiogenic properties of human immunodeficiency virus type 1 Tat protein. *Proceedings of the National Academy of Sciences U S A, 92*(11), 4838–42.

Alexander, R. A., Foss, A. J., Garner, A., et al. (1994). Are most intraocular "leiomyomas" really melanocytic lesions? *Ophthalmology, 101*, 919–24.

Al-Shahi, R., Bower, M., Gazzard, B. G., et al. (2000). Cerebrospinal fluid Epstein-Barr virus detection preceding HIV-associated primary central nervous system lymphoma by 17 months. *Journal of Neurology, 247*(6), 471–2.

Amaker, B. H., Broaddus, W. C., Graham, R. S., et al. (2000). Central nervous system leiomyosarcoma in patients with acquired immunodeficiency syndrome. Report of two cases. *Journal of Neurosurgery, 92,* 688–92.

Ambinder, R. F. & Flinn, I. W. (1996). AIDS primary central nervous system lymphoma. *Current Opinion in Oncology, 8*(5), 373–6. 9026061

Ammassari, A., Antinori, A., Cingolani, A., et al. (1997). Diagnosis of AIDS-related focal brain lesions: a decision-making analysis based on clinical and neuroradiologic characteristics combined with polymerase chain reaction assays in CSF. *Neurology, 48*(3), 687–94.

Ammassari, A., Antinori, A., & De Rossi, G. (1999). Value of combined approach with thallium-201 single-photon emission computed tomography and Epstein-Barr virus DNA polymerase chain reaction in CSF for the diagnosis of AIDS-related primary CNS lymphoma. *Journal of Clinical Oncology, 2,* 554–60.

Ammassari, A., Antinori, A., Luzzati, R., et al. (2000). Role of brain biopsy in the management of focal brain lesions in HIV-infected patients. Gruppo Italiano Cooperativo AIDS & Tumori. *Neurology, 54,* 993–7.

Ammassari, A., Cingolani, A., Pezzotti, P., et al. (2000). AIDS-related focal brain lesions in the era of highly active antiretroviral therapy. *Neurology, 55,* 1194–200.

Anthony, I. C., Crawford, D. H., & Bell, J. E. B. (2003). Lymphocytes in the normal brain: Contrasts with HIV-associated lymphoid infiltrates and lymphomas. *Brain, 126*(Pt 5), 1058–67.

Antin, J. H., O'Neill, B., Schiff, D., et al. (2001). Gliomas arising in organ transplant recipients: An unrecognized complication of transplantation? *Neurology, 57,* 1486–8.

Antinori, A., Ammassari, A., Luzzati, R., et al. (2000). Role of brain biopsy in the management of focal brain lesions in HIV-infected patients. Gruppo Italiano Cooperativo AIDS & Tumori. *Neurology, 54,* 993–7.

Antinori, A., Bossolasco, S., Cingolani, A., et al. (2004). Positive predictive value of Epstein-Barr virus DNA detection in HIV-related primary central nervous system lymphoma. *Clinical Infectious Diseases, 39*(9), 1396–7; author reply 1397–8.

Antinori, A., De Rossi, G., & Ammassari, A. (1999). Value of combined approach with thallium-201 single-photon emission computed tomography and Epstein-Barr virus DNA polymerase chain reaction in CSF for the diagnosis of AIDS-related primary CNS lymphoma. *Journal of Clinical Oncology, 2,* 554–60.

Antinori, A., Ammassari, A., De Luca, A., et al. (1997). Diagnosis of AIDS-related focal brain lesions: A decision-making analysis based on clinical and neuroradiologic characteristics combined with polymerase chain reaction assays in CSF. *Neurology 48,* 687–94.

Balsamo, M., Boitano, M., Cantoni, C., et al. (2009). Vitale M. Melanoma-associated fibroblasts modulate NK cell phenotype and antitumor cytotoxicity. *Proceedings of the National Academy of Sciences U S A.*

Barba, D., Fullerton, S. C., & Mathews, C. (1995). Early biopsy versus empiric treatment with delayed biopsy of non-responders in suspected HIV-associated cerebral toxoplasmosis: A decision analysis. *AIDS, 9,* 1243–50.

Barba, D., Hansen, L. A., Karpinski, N. C., et al. (1999). Case of the month: March- A 26 year old HIV positive male with dura-based masses. *Brain Pathology, 9,* 609–10.

Barditch-Crovo, P. A., Brown, H. G., Burger, P. C., et al. (1999). Intracranial leiomyosarcoma in a patient with AIDS. *Neuroradiology, 41,* 35–9.

Bargiela, A., Rey, J. L., Diaz, J. L., & Martinez, A. (1999). Meningeal leiomyoma in an adult with AIDS: CT and MRI with pathological correlation. *Neuroradiology, 41,* 696–8.

Barlas, S., Brem, S., Davis, F. G., et al. (1998). Survival rates in patients with primary malignant brain tumors stratified by patient age and tumor histological type: An analysis based on Surveillance, Epidemiology, and End Results (SEER) data, 1973–91. *Journal of Neurosurgery, 88,* 1–10.

Batchelor, T. T., Carson, K. A., Gerstner, E. R., et al. (2008). Long-term outcome in PCNSL patients treated with high-dose methotrexate and deferred radiation. *Neurology, 70*(5), 401–2

Baumgartner, J. E., Rachlin, J. R., Beckstead, J. H., et al. (1990). Primary central nervous system lymphomas: Natural history and response to radiation therapy in 55 patients with acquired immunodeficiency syndrome. *Journal of Neurosurgery, 73,* 206–11.

Beckstead, J. H., Davis, R. L., So, Y. T. (1986). Primary central nervous system lymphoma in acquired immune deficiency syndrome: A clinical and pathological study. *Annals of Neurology, 20,* 566–72.

Bejjani, G. K., Santi, R., Schwartz, A., et al. (1999). Primary dural leiomyosarcoma in a patient infected with human immunodeficiency virus: Case report. *Neurosurgery, 44,* 199–202.

Besson, C., Goubar, A., Gabarre, J., et al. (2001). Changes in AIDS-related lymphoma since the era of highly active antiretroviral therapy. *Blood, 98,* 2339–44.

Biggar, R. J., Blattner, W. A., Cote, T. R., et al. (1997). Non-Hodgkin's lymphoma among people with AIDS: Incidence, presentation and public health burden. AIDS/Cancer Study Group. *International Journal of Cancer, 73*(5), 645–50

Bonk, C., Frank, S., Haroske, G., et al. (1998). Transmission of glioblastoma multiforme through liver transplantation. *Lancet, 352,* 31.

Bonner, H., Martz, K. L., Nelson, D. F., et al. (1992). Non-Hodgkin's lymphoma of the brain: Can high dose, large volume radiation therapy improve survival? Report on a prospective trial by the Radiation Therapy Oncology Group (RTOG): RTOG 8315. *International Journal of Radiation Oncology Biology Physics, 23,* 9–17.

Bories, J., Cellerier, P., Chiras, J., et al. (1984). Computed tomography in primary lymphoma of the brain. *Neuroradiology, 26,* 485–92.

Boshoff, C. & Weiss, R. (2002). AIDS-related malignancies. *National Review of Cancer, 2,* 373–82.

Bossolasco, S., Cinque, P., & Ponzoni, M. (2002). Epstein-Barr virus DNA load in cerebrospinal fluid and plasma of patients with AIDS-related lymphoma. *Journal of Neurovirology, 8,* 432–8.

Bossolasco S, Falk KI, Ponzoni M, et al. (2006). Ganciclovir is associated with low or undetectable Epstein-Barr virus DNA load in cerebrospinal fluid of patients with HIV-related primary central nervous system lymphoma. *Clinical Infectious Diseases. 42,* e21-5.

Bower, M., Fife, K., Kirk, S., et al. (1999). Treatment outcome in presumed and confirmed AIDS-related primary cerebral lymphoma. *European Journal of Cancer, 35*(4), 601–4.

Bracci, P., Holly, E. A., & Lele, C. (1997). Non-Hodgkin's lymphoma in homosexual men in the San Francisco Bay Area: Occupational, chemical, and environmental exposures. *Journal of Acquired Immune Deficiency Syndrome and Human Retrovirology, 15,* 223–31.

Braus, D. F., Muller-Hermelink, H. K., Mundinger, F., et al. (1992). Primary cerebral malignant non-Hodgkin's lymphomas: A retrospective clinical study. *Journal of Neurology, 239,* 117–24.

Bredesen, D. E., Levy, R. M., & Rosenblum, M. L. (1985). Neurologic manifestations of the acquired immunodeficiency syndrome (AIDS): Experience at UCSF and review of the literature. *Journal of Neurosurgery, 62,* 475–95.

Brew, B. J., Bryant, M., Cooper, S. G., et al. (2004). Human immunodeficiency virus-related primary central nervous system lymphoma: Factors influencing survival in 111 patients. *Cancer, 100*(12), 2627–36.

Broder, S., Feuerstein, I. M., Jaffe, E. S., et al. (1990). Development of non-Hodgkin lymphoma in a cohort of patients with severe human immunodeficiency virus (HIV) infection on long-term antiretroviral therapy. *Annals of Internal Medicine, 113*(4), 276–82.

Brodt, H. R., Fichtlscherer, S., Wolf, T., et al. (2005). Changing incidence and prognostic factors of survival in AIDS-related non-Hodgkin's lymphoma in the era of highly active antiretroviral therapy (HAART). *Leukemia and Lymphoma, 46,* 207–15.

Brown, H. G., Burger, P. C., Olivi, A., Sills, A. K., Barditch-Crovo, P. A., & Lee, R. R. (1999). Intracranial leiomyosarcoma in a patient with AIDS. *Neuroradiology, 41,* 35–9.

Burger, P. C., Eby, N. L., Flannelly, C. M., et al. (1998). Increasing incidence of primary brain lymphoma in the US. *Cancer, 62,* 2461–5.

Burgi, A., Brodine, S., & Wegner, S. (2005). Incidence and risk factors for the occurrence of non-AIDS-defining cancers among human immunodeficiency virus-infected individuals. *Cancer, 104,* 1505–11.

Büttner A, Weis S. (1999) Non-lymphomatous brain tumors in HIV-1 infection: a review. *Journal of Neurooncology*, 41, 81–8.

Cabral, L., Cai, J. P., Raez, L., et al. (1999). Treatment of AIDS-related primary central nervous system lymphoma with zidovudine, ganciclovir, and interleukin 2. *AIDS Research and Human Retroviruses*, 15, 713–9.

Callan, M. F., Hovenkamp, E., Kostense, S., et al. (2001). Dysfunctional Epstein-Barr virus (EBV)-specific CD8(+) T lymphocytes and increased EBV load in HIV-1 infected individuals progressing to AIDS-related non-Hodgkin lymphoma. *Blood*, 98(1), 146–155.

Carbone A., Gloghini A.(2005) AIDS-related lymphomas: from pathogenesis to pathology. *British Journal of Haematology*, 130, 662-670.

Cassileth, P. A., Feun, L., Patel, P., et al. (1998). Natural history and prognostic factors for survival in patients with acquired immune deficiency syndrome (AIDS)-related primary central nervous system lymphoma (PCNSL).*Critical Reviews in Oncology/Hematology*, 9(3–4), 199–208. 10201628

Cellerier, P., Chiras, J., Gray, F., Metzger, J., & Bories, J. (1984). Computed tomography in primary lymphoma of the brain. *Neuroradiology*, 26, 485–92.

Chamberlain, M. C. & Kormanik, P. A. (1999). AIDS-related central nervous system lymphomas. *Journal of Neuro-oncology*, 43, 269–76.

Chang, L., Chiang, F. L., Cornford, M. E., et al. (1995). Radiologic-pathologic correlation. Cerebral toxoplasmosis and lymphoma in AIDS. *American Journal of Neuroradiology*, 16, 1653–63.

Choi, S., Krieger, M. D., Levy, M. L., et al. (1997). Spinal extradural leiomyoma in a pediatric patient with acquired immunodeficiency syndrome: Case report. *Neurosurgery*, 40, 1080–2.

Ciacci, J. D., Levy, R. M., Tellez, C., et al. (1999).Lymphoma of the central nervous system in AIDS. *Seminars in Neurology*, 19(2), 213–21.

Cingolani, A., De Luca, A., Larocca, L. M., et al. (1998). Minimally invasive diagnosis of acquired immunodeficiency syndrome-related primary central nervous system lymphoma. *Journal of the National Cancer Institute*, 90, 364–9.

Cingolani, A., Fassone, L., Gastaldi, R., et al. (2000). Epstein-Barr virus infection is predictive of CNS involvement in systemic AIDS-related non-Hodgkin's lymphomas. *Journal of Clinical Oncology*, 18, 3325–30.

Cingolani A, Fratino L, Scoppettuolo G, Antinori A. (2005). Changing pattern of primary cerebral lymphoma in the highly active antiretroviral therapy era. *Journal of Neurovirology.*11*(Suppl)*, 38-44.

Cinque, P., Cingolani, A., Bossolasco, S., & Antinori, A. Positive predictive value of Epstein-Barr virus DNA detection in HIV-related primary central nervous system lymphoma. *Clin Infect Dis*, 39(9), 1396–7; author reply 1397–8.

Ciricillo, S. F. & Rosenblum, M. L. (1990). Use of CT and MR imaging to distinguish intracranial lesions and to define the need for biopsy in AIDS patients. *Journal of Neurosurgery*, 73, 720–24.

Citow, J. S. & Kranzler, L. (2002). Multicentric intracranial smooth-muscle tumor in a woman with human immunodeficiency virus. *Journal of Neurosurgery*, 93, 701–3.

Clemens, M., Herrlinger, U., Schabet, M., et al. (1998). Clinical presentation and therapeutic outcome in 26 patients with primary CNS lymphoma. *Acta Neurologica Scandinavica*, 97, 257–64.

Cobbs, C. S., Harkins, L., Samanta, M., et al. (2002). Human cytomegalovirus infection and expression in human malignant glioma. *Cancer Research*, 62, 3347–50.

Cohen, J. I., Meier, J., Straus, S. E., et al. (1993). NIH conference. Epstein-Barr virus infections: Biology, pathogenesis, and management. *Annals of Internal Medicine*, 118, 45–58.

Collignon FP, Holland EC, Feng S. (2004). Organ donors with malignant gliomas: an update. *American Journal of Transplantation 4*, 15–21.

Cooper, J. S., Donahue, B. R., & Sullivan, J. W. (1995). Additional experience with empiric radiotherapy for presumed human immunodeficiency virus-associated primary central nervous system lymphoma. *Cancer*, 76, 328–32.

Corcoran, C., Hardie, D. R., Myer, L., et al. (2008). The predictive value of cerebrospinal fluid Epstein-Barr viral load as a marker of primary central nervous system lymphoma in HIV-infected persons. *Journal of Clinical Virology*, 42(4), 433–6.

Corn, B. W., Donahue, B. R., Rosenstock, J. G., Cooper, J. S., Xie, Y., Brandon, A. H., et al. Palliation of AIDS-related primary lymphoma of the brain: Observations from a multi-institutional database. *Int J Radiat Oncol Biol Phys*, 38(3), 601–5.

Corvi, F., Litofsky, N. S., Pihan, G., et al. (1998). Intracranial leiomyosarcoma: A neuro-oncological consequence of acquired immunodeficiency syndrome. *Journal of Neurooncology*, 40, 179–83.

Cote, T. R., Goedert, J. J., & Virgo, P. (1998). Spectrum of AIDS-associated malignant disorders. *Lancet*, 351, 1833–9.

Cote, T. R., Biggar, R. J., Rosenberg, P. S., et al. (1997) Non-Hodgkin's lymphoma among people with AIDS: Incidence, presentation and public health burden. AIDS/Cancer Study Group. *International Journal of Cancer*, 73, 645–50

Cozzi-Lepri, A., Kirk, O., & Pedersen, C. (2001). Non-Hodgkin lymphoma in HIV-infected patients in the era of highly active antiretroviral therapy. *Blood*, 98, 3406–12.

Dameshek, H. L., Flickinger, J. C., Lunsford, L. D., et al. (1989). Prognostic factors in the diagnosis and treatment of primary central nervous system lymphoma. *Cancer*, 63, 939–47.

Davis, F. G., Freels, S., Grutsch, J., Barlas, S., & Brem, S (1998). Survival rates in patients with primary malignant brain tumors stratified by patient age and tumor histological type: An analysis based on Surveillance, Epidemiology, and End Results (SEER) data, 1973–91. *Journal of Neurosurgery*, 88, 1–10.

DeAngelis, L. M., Seiferheld, W., Schold, S. C., et al. (2002) Combination chemotherapy and radiotherapy for primary central nervous system lymphoma: Radiation Therapy Oncology Group Study 93–10. *Journal of Clinical Oncology*, 20, 4643–8.

DeAngelis, L. M., Cirrincione, C., Heinemann, M. H., et al. (1990). Primary CNS lymphoma: Combined treatment with chemotherapy and radiotherapy. *Neurology*, 40, 80–6.

DeAngelis, L. M. & Forsyth, P. A. (1996). Biology and management of AIDS-associated primary CNS lymphomas. *Hematology/Oncology Clinics of North America*, 10(5), 1125–34. 8880200

DeAngelis, L. M., Yahalom, J., Heinemann, M. H., Cirrincione, C., Thaler, H. T., & Krol, G. (1990). Primary CNS lymphoma: Combined treatment with chemotherapy and radiotherapy. *Neurology*, 40, 80–6.

Delbouille, M. H., Detry, O., Hans, M. F., et al. (2000). Organ donors with primary central nervous system tumor. *Transplantation*, 70, 244–8; Discussion 251–2.

DeMario, M. D. & Liebowitz, D. N. (1998). Lymphomas in the immunocompromised patient. *Seminars in Oncology*, 25(4), 492–502.

Detry, O., Honore, P., Hans, M. F., Delbouille, M. H., Jacquet, N., & Meurisse, M. (2000). Organ donors with primary central nervous system tumor. *Transplantation*, 70, 244–8; Discussion 251–2.

Di Gennaro, G., Spina, M., Vaccher, E., et al. (2001). Concomitant cyclophosphamide, doxorubicin, vincristine, and prednisone chemotherapy plus highly active antiretroviral therapy in patients with human immunodeficiency virus-related, non-Hodgkin lymphoma. *Cancer*, 91, 155–63.

Diamond, C., Migliozzi, J. A., Remick, S. C., et al. (1990). Primary central nervous system lymphoma in patients with and without the acquired immune deficiency syndrome: A retrospective analysis and review of the literature. *Medicine*, 69, 345–60.

Dickson, D. W., Goldstein, J. D., Moser, F. G., et al. (1991). Primary central nervous system lymphoma in acquired immune deficiency syndrome. A clinical and pathologic study with results of treatment with radiation. *Cancer*, 67, 2756–65.

Dickson, D. W., Goldstein, J. D., Rubenstein, A., et al. (1990). Primary central nervous system lymphoma in a pediatric patient with acquired immune deficiency syndrome. *Cancer*, 66, 2503–08.

Donahue, B. R., Sullivan, J. W., & Cooper, J. S. (1995). Additional experience with empiric radiotherapy for presumed human immunodeficiency virus-associated primary central nervous system lymphoma. *Cancer, 76*, 328–32.

Eby, N. L., Grufferman, S., Flannelly, C. M., Schold, S. C. Jr., Vogel, F. S., & Burger, P. C. (1988). Increasing incidence of primary brain lymphoma in the US. *Cancer, 62*, 2461–5.

Egger, M., Ledergerber, B., & Telenti, A. (1999). Risk of HIV related Kaposi's sarcoma and non-Hodgkin's lymphoma with potent antiretroviral therapy: Prospective cohort study. Swiss HIV Cohort Study. *British Medical Journal, 319*, 23–4.

Ekstein, D., Ben-Yehuda, D., Slyusarevsky, E., Lossos, A., et al. (2006). CSF analysis of IgH gene rearrangement in CNS lymphoma: Relationship to the disease course. *Journal of Neurological Sciences, 247*(1), 39–46.

Epeldegui M, Vendrame E, Martínez-Maza O. (2010). HIV-associated immune dysfunction and viral infection: role in the pathogenesis of AIDS-related lymphoma. *Immunology Research, 48*, 72-83.

Epstein, L. G., Goudsmit, J., & Sharer, L. R. (1988). Neurological and neuropathological features of human immunodeficiency virus infection in children. *Annals of Neurology, 23*, Suppl:S19–23

Epstein, L. G., Sharer, L. R., & Goudsmit, J. (1988). Neurological and neuropathological features of human immunodeficiency virus infection in children. *Annals of Neurology, 23*, Suppl:S19–23

Farese, V. L., Girard, P. M., Jacomet, C., Lebrette, M. G., et al. (1997). Intravenous methotrexate for primary central nervous system non-Hodgkin's lymphoma in AIDS. *AIDS, 11*, 1725–30.

Fine, H. A. & Maher, E. A. (1999). Primary CNS lymphoma. *Seminars in Oncology, 26*(3), 346–56.

Fine, H. A. & Mayer, R. J. (1993). Primary central nervous system lymphoma. *Annals of Internal Medicine, 119*(11), 1093–104.

Fischer, L., Martus, P., Weller, M., Klasen, H. A., et al. (2008) Meningeal dissemination in primary CNS lymphoma: Prospective evaluation of 282 patients. *Neurology, 71*(14), 1102–8.

Flinn, I. W. & Ambinder, R. F. (1996). AIDS primary central nervous system lymphoma. *Opin Oncol, 8*(5), 373–6. 9026061

Forsyth, P. A. & DeAngelis, L. M. (1996) Biology and management of AIDS-associated primary CNS lymphomas. *Hematology Oncology Clinics of North America, 10*, 1125–34.

Forsyth, P. A., Yahalom, J., & DeAngelis, L. M. (1994). Combined-modality therapy in the treatment of primary central nervous system lymphoma in AIDS. *Neurology, 44*, 1473–78.

Foss, A. J., Pecorella, I., Alexander, R. A., Hungerford, J. L., & Garner, A. (1994). Are most intraocular "leiomyomas" really melanocytic lesions? *Ophthalmology, 101*, 919–24.

Fram, E. K., Jacobowitz, R., Johnson, B. A., et al. (1997). The variable MR appearance of primary lymphoma of the central nervous system: Comparison with histopathologic features. *American Journal of Neuroradiology, 18*(3), 563–72. 9090424

Frank, S., Muller, J., Bonk, C., Haroske, G., Schackert, H. K., & Schackert, G. (1998). Transmission of glioblastoma multiforme through liver transplantation. *Lancet, 352*, 31.

Fries KL, Miller WE, Raab-Traub N. (1996). Epstein-Barr virus latent membrane protein 1 blocks p53-mediated apoptosis through the induction of the A20 gene. *Journal of Virology. 70*, 8653–9.

Gathe, Jr. J. C., Gildenberg, P. L., & Kim, J. H. (2000). Stereotactic biopsy of cerebral lesions in AIDS. *Clinical Infectious Diseases, 30*, 491–9.

George, M., Licho, R., Litofsky, N. S., et al. (2002). Inaccuracy of Tl-201 brain SPECT in distinguishing cerebral infections from lymphoma in patients with AIDS. *Clinical Nuclear Medicine, 27*, 81–6.

Gerstner, E. R., Carson, K. A., Grossman, S. A., et al. (2008). Long-term outcome in PCNSL patients treated with high-dose methotrexate and deferred radiation. *Neurology, 70*, 401–2

Gherlinzoni, F., Mazza, P., Tosi, P., et al. (1997). 3'-Azido 3'-deoxythymidine + methotrexate as a novel antineoplastic combination in the treatment of human immunodeficiency virus-related non-Hodgkin's lymphomas. *Blood, 89*, 419–25.

Giancola, M. L., Rizzi, E. B., Lorenzini, P., et al. (2008). Progressive multifocal leukoencephalopathy in HIV-infected patients in the era of

HAART: Radiological features at diagnosis and follow-up and correlation with clinical variables. *AIDS Research in Human Retroviruses, 24*, 155–62.

Gildenberg, P. L., Gathe, J. C. Jr., & Kim, J. H. (2000). Stereotactic biopsy of cerebral lesions in AIDS. *Clin Infect Dis, 30*(3), 491–9.

Gill, P. S., Levine, A. M., Loureiro, C., et al. (1988). Autopsy findings in AIDS-related lymphoma. *Cancer, 62*, 735–9.

Gill, P. S., Levine, A. M., Meyer, P. R., et al. (1985). Primary central nervous system lymphoma in homosexual men. Clinical, immunologic, and pathologic features. *American Journal of Medicine, 78*, 742–8.

Glaser, S. L. & Hsu, J. L. (2000). Epstein-Barr virus-associated malignancies: Epidemiologic patterns and etiologic implications. *Critical Reviews in Oncology/Hematology, 34*, 27–53.

Glass, J. D., Hayward, S. D., & MacMahon, E. M. (1991). Epstein-Barr virus in AIDS-related primary central nervous system lymphoma. *Lancet, 338*, 969–73.

Goedert, J. J., Cote, T. R., & Virgo, P. (1998). Spectrum of AIDS-associated malignant disorders. *Lancet, 351*, 1833–9.

Goldstein, J. D., Dickson, D. W., Moser, F. G., et al. (1991). Primary central nervous system lymphoma in acquired immune deficiency syndrome. A clinical and pathologic study with results of treatment with radiation. *Cancer, 67*, 2756–65.

Goldstein, J. D., Dickson, D. W., Rubenstein, A., et al. (1990). Primary central nervous system lymphoma in a pediatric patient with acquired immune deficiency syndrome. *Cancer, 66*, 2503–08.

Gordon, K. B., Heinemann, M., Peterson, K., et al. (1993). The clinical spectrum of ocular lymphoma. *Cancer, 72*, 843–49.

Granzmann, M. B., Hamilton-Dutoit, S. J., Pallesen, G., et al. (1991). AIDS-related lymphoma: Histopathology, immunophenotype, and association with Epstein-Barr virus as demonstrated by in situ nucleic acid hybridization. *American Journal of Pathology, 138*, 149–63.

Greffe, B. S., Mierau, G. W., & Weeks, D. A. (1997). Primary leiomyosarcoma of brain in an adolescent with common variable immunodeficiency syndrome. *Ultrastructural Pathology, 21*, 301–5.

Grulich, A. E., vanLeeuwen, M. T., Falster, M. O., et al. (2007) Incidence of cancers in people with HIV/AIDS compared with immunosuppressed transplant recipients: A meta-analysis. *Lancet, 370*, 59–67.

Gumprecht, J. P., Kotsianti, A., Morgello, S., et al. (1997). Epstein-Barr virus-associated dural leiomyosarcoma in a man infected with human immunodeficiency virus. *Journal of Neurosurgery, 86*, 883–7.

Guterman, K. S., Hair, L. S., & Morgello, S. (1996). Epstein-Barr virus and AIDS-related primary central nervous system lymphoma. Viral detection by immunohistochemistry, RNA in situ hybridization, and polymerase chain reaction. *Clinical Neuropathology, 15*(2), 79–86.

Hamilton-Dutoit, S. J., Pallesen, G., Granzmann, M. B., et al. (1991). AIDS-related lymphoma: Histopathology, immunophenotype, and association with Epstein-Barr virus as demonstrated by in situ nucleic acid hybridization. *American Journal of Pathology, 138*, 149–63.

Hegde U, Filie A, Little RF, et al. (2005). High incidence of occult leptomeningeal disease detected by flow cytometry in newly diagnosed aggressive B-cell lymphomas at risk for central nervous system involvement: the role of flow cytometry versus cytology. *Blood, 105*, 496–502.

Herndier, B. G., McGrath, M. S., & Shiramizu, B. (1994). Identification of a common clonal human immunodeficiency virus integration site in human immunodeficiency virus-associated lymphomas. *Cancer Research, 54*(8), 2069–72.

Herrlinger, U., Schabet, M., Clemens, M., et al. (1998). Clinical presentation and therapeutic outcome in 26 patients with primary CNS lymphoma. *Acta Neurologica Scandinavica, 97*, 257–64.

Hesselink, J. R., Press, G. A., Schwaighofer, B. W., et al. (1989). Primary intracranial CNS lymphoma: MR manifestations. *American Journal of Neuroradiology, 10*, 725–29.

Hochberg, F. H. & Miller, D. C. (1988). Primary central nervous system lymphoma. *Journal of Neurosurgery, 68*, 835–53.

Hoffmann, C., Tabrizian, S., Wolf, E., et al. (2001). Survival of AIDS patients with primary central nervous system lymphoma is dramatically improved by HAART-induced immune recovery. *AIDS*, *15*, 2119–27.

Holly, E. A. & Lele, C. (1997). Non-Hodgkin's lymphoma in HIV-positive and HIV-negative homosexual men in the San Francisco Bay Area: Allergies, prior medication use, and sexual practices. *Journal of Acquired Immune Deficiency Syndrome and Human Retrovirology*, *152*, 11–22.

Hsu, J. L. & Glaser, S. L. (2000). Epstein-Barr virus-associated malignancies: Epidemiologic patterns and etiologic implications. *Critical Reviews in Oncology/Hematology*, *34*, 27–53.

Hurd, D., Manivel, J. C., Nakhleh, R. E., et al. (1989). Central nervous system lymphomas. Immunohistochemical and clinicopathologic study of 26 autopsy cases. *Archives of Pathology and Laboratory Medicine*, *113*, 1050–56.

Illig, J. J. & O'Neill, B. P. (1989). Primary central nervous system lymphoma. *Mayo Clinic Proceedings*, *64*, 1005–20.

Ivers LC, Kim AY, Sax PE. (2004). Predictive value of polymerase chain reaction of cerebrospinal fluid for detection of Epstein-Barr virus to establish the diagnosis of HIV-related primary central nervous system lymphoma. *Clinical Infectious Diseases*, *38*, 1629–32.

Jacomet, C., Girard, P. M., Lebrette, M. G., et al. (1997). Intravenous methotrexate for primary central nervous system non-Hodgkin's lymphoma in AIDS. *AIDS*, *11*, 1725–30.

Janney, C. A., Olson, J. E., Rao, R. D., et al. (2002). The continuing increase in the incidence of primary central nervous system non-Hodgkin lymphoma: A surveillance, epidemiology, and end results analysis. *Cancer*, *95*, 1504–10.

Jenson, H. B., Leach, C. T., McClain, K. L., et al. (1995). Association of Epstein-Barr virus with leiomyosarcomas in children with AIDS. *New England Journal of Medicine*, *332*, 12–8.

Jenson, H. B., Leach, C. T., McClain, K. L., et al. (1997). Benign and malignant smooth muscle tumors containing Epstein-Barr virus in children with AIDS. *Leukemia Lymphoma*, *27*, 303–14.

Johnson, B. A., Fram, E. K., Johnson, P. C., & Jacobowitz, R. (1977). The variable MR appearance of primary lymphoma of the central nervous system: Comparison with histopathologic features. *AJNR Am J Neuroradiol*, *18*(3), 563–72. 9090424

Jorgensen, J. L., Kroll, M. H., & Vilchez, R. A. (2002). Systemic non-Hodgkin lymphoma in HIV-infected patients in the era of highly active antiretroviral therapy. *Blood*, *99*, 4250–1.

Kaplan, L. D. & Sandler, A. S. (1996). Diagnosis and management of systemic non-Hodgkin's lymphoma in HIV disease. *Hematology Oncology Clinics of North America*, *10*(5), 1111–24. 8880199

Karpinski, N. C., Yaghmai, R., Barba, D., & Hansen, L. A. Case of the month: March 1999—A 26 year old HIV positive male with dura-based masses. *Brain Pathology*, *9*, 609–10.

Kieff, E. (1998). Current perspectives on the molecular pathogenesis of virus-induced cancers in human immunodeficiency virus infection and acquired immunodeficiency syndrome. *Journal of National Cancer Institute Monographs*, *23*, 7–14.

Kinjo, N., Miyagi, K., Mukawa, J., et al. (1995). Astrocytoma linked to familial ataxia-telangiectasia. *Acta Neurochirurgica* (Wien), *135*, 87–92.

Kirk, O., Pedersen, C., & Cozzi-Lepri, A. (2001). Non-Hodgkin lymphoma in HIV-infected patients in the era of highly active antiretroviral therapy. *Blood*, *98*, 3406–12.

Klein, G. (1994). Epstein-Barr virus strategy in normal and neoplastic B cells. *Cell*, *77*, 791–3.

Liebowitz, D. (1995). Epstein-Barr virus—an old dog with new tricks. *New England Journal of Medicine*, *332*, 55–7.

Kleinschmidt-DeMasters, B. K., Mierau, G. W., Sze, C. I., et al (1998). Unusual dural and skull-based mesenchymal neoplasms: A report of four cases. *Human Pathology*, *29*, 240–5.

Kreisl, T. N., Panageas, K. S., Elkin, E. B., Deangelis, L. M., & Abrey, L. E. (2008). Treatment patterns and prognosis in patients with human immunodeficiency virus and primary central system lymphoma. *Leuk Lymphoma*, *49*(9), 1710–6.

Laing, M. E., Moloney, F. J., Kay, E. W., et al. (2006) Malignant melanoma in transplant patients: A review of five cases. *Clinical Experimental Dermatology*, *31*, 662–64

Ledergerber, B., Telenti, A., & Egger, M. (1999). Risk of HIV related Kaposi's sarcoma and non-Hodgkin's lymphoma with potent antiretroviral therapy: Prospective cohort study. Swiss HIV Cohort Study. *British Medical Journal*, *319*, 23–4.

Lee, R. R., Miseljic, S., Port, J. D., et al. (1999) Progressive multifocal leukoencephalopathy demonstrating contrast enhancement on MRI and uptake of thallium-201: A case report. *Neuroradiology*, *41*, 895–8.

Levine, A. M. (1992). Acquired immunodeficiency syndrome-related lymphoma. *Blood*, *80*, 8–20.

Levy, R. M., Bredesen, D. E., & Rosenblum, M. L. (1985). Neurologic manifestations of the acquired immunodeficiency syndrome (AIDS): Experience at UCSF and review of the literature. *Journal of Neurosurgery*, *62*, 475–95.

Li, S., Palmer, M., Tyler, K. L., et al. (2002). Quantitative CSF PCR in Epstein-Barr virus infections of the central nervous system. *Annals of Neurology*, *52*, 543–8.

Licho, R., Litofsky, N. S., Senitko, M., & George, M. (2002). Inaccuracy of Tl-201 brain SPECT in distinguishing cerebral infections from lymphoma in patients with AIDS. *Clinical Nuclear Medicine*, *27*, 81–6.

Lim, G. H., Pell, M. F., Steel, T. R., et al. (1993). Spinal epidural leiomyoma occurring in an HIV-infected man. *Journal of Neurosurgery*, *79*, 442–5.

Litofsky, N. S., Pihan, G., Corvi, F., & Smith, T. W. (1998). Intracranial leiomyosarcoma: a neuro-oncological consequence of acquired immunodeficiency syndrome. *Journal of Neurooncology*, *40*, 179–83.

Loureiro, C., Gill, P. S., Meyer, P. R., Rhodes, R., Rarick, M. U., & Levine, A. M. (1988). Autopsy findings in AIDS-related lymphoma. *Cancer*, *62*, 735–9.

Luzzati, R., Ferrari, S., Nicolato, A., et al. (1996). Stereotactic brain biopsy in human immunodeficiency virus-infected patients. *Archives of Internal Medicine*, *156*, 565–8.

MacMahon, E. M., Glass, J. D., & Hayward, S. D. (1991). Epstein-Barr virus in AIDS-related primary central nervous system lymphoma. *Lancet*, *338*, 969–73.

Maher, E. A. & Fine, H. A. (1999). Primary CNS lymphoma. *Seminars in Oncology*, *26*(3), 346–56.

Mathews, C., Barba, D., & Fullerton, S. C. (1995). Early biopsy versus empiric treatment with delayed biopsy of non-responders in suspected HIV-associated cerebral toxoplasmosis: A decision analysis. *AIDS*, *9*, 1243–50.

Mazhar, D., Stebbing, J., Lewis, R., Nelson, M., Gazzard, B. G., & Bower, M. (2006). The management of meningeal lymphoma in patients with HIV in the era of HAART: Intrathecal depot cytarabine is effective and safe. *Blood*, *107*(8), 3412–4.

McArthur, J. C. (1987). Neurologic manifestations of AIDS. *Medicine*, *66*, 407–37.

McClain, K. L., Leach, C. T., Jenson, H. B., et al. (1995). Association of Epstein-Barr virus with leiomyosarcomas in children with AIDS. *New England Journal of Medicine*, *332*, 12–8.

McGowan, J. P. & Shah, S. (1998). Long-term remission of AIDS-related primary central nervous system lymphoma associated with highly active antiretroviral therapy. *AIDS*, *12*(8), 952–4.

Mierau, G. W., Greffe, B. S., & Weeks, D. A. (1997). Primary leiomyosarcoma of brain in an adolescent with common variable immunodeficiency syndrome. *Ultrastructural Pathology*, *21*, 301–5.

Miller CL, Burkhardt AL, Lee JH, et al. (1995). Integral membrane protein 2 of Epstein-Barr virus regulates reactivation from latency through dominant negative effects on protein-tyrosine kinases. *Immunity*, *2*, 155–66.

Miyagi, K., Mukawa, J., Kinjo, N., et al. (1995). Astrocytoma linked to familial ataxia-telangiectasia. *Acta Neurochirurgica (Wien)*, *135*, 87–92.

Morgello, S., Kotsianti, A., Gumprecht, J. P., & Moore, F. (1997). Epstein-Barr virus-associated dural leiomyosarcoma in a man infected with human immunodeficiency virus. *Journal of Neurosurgery*, *86*, 883–7.

Mullen, J. T., Vartanian, T. K., & Atkins, M. B. (2008). Melanoma complicating treatment with natalizumab for multiple sclerosis. *New England Journal of Medicine, 358*, 647–48.

Munz, C. & Paludan, C (2003). CD4+ T cell responses in the immune control against latent infection by Epstein-Barr virus. *Current Molecular Medicine, 3*(4), 341–7.

Nagai, H., Odawara, T., Ajisawa, A., Hagiwara, S., Watanabe, T., Uehira, T., et al. (2010). Whole brain radiation alone produces favourable outcomes for AIDS-related primary central nervous system lymphoma in the HAART era. *Eur J Haematol*, 2013–2301.

Nakhleh, R. E., Manivel, J. C., Hurd, D., et al. (1989). Central nervous system lymphomas. Immunohistochemical and clinicopathologic study of 26 autopsy cases. *Archives of Pathology and Laboratory Medicine, 113*, 1050–56.

Nelson, D. F., Martz, K. L., Bonner, H., et al. (1992). Non-Hodgkin's lymphoma of the brain: Can high dose, large volume radiation therapy improve survival? Report on a prospective trial by the Radiation Therapy Oncology Group (RTOG): RTOG 8315. *International Journal of Radiation Oncology Biology Physics, 23*, 9–17.

Newell ME, Hoy JF, Cooper SG, et al. (2004). Human immunodeficiency virus-related primary central nervous system lymphoma: factors influencing survival in 111 patients. *Cancer, 100*, 2627–36.

Oliva, H., Rosai, J., & Varela-Duran, J. (1979). Vascular leiomyosarcoma: The malignant counterpart of vascular leiomyoma. *Cancer, 44*, 1684–91.

Olson, J. E., Janney, C. A., Rao, R. D., et al. (2002). The continuing increase in the incidence of primary central nervous system non-Hodgkin lymphoma: A surveillance, epidemiology, and end results analysis. *Cancer, 95*, 1504–10.

O'Neill, B. P. & Illig, J. J. (1989). Primary central nervous system lymphoma. *Mayo Clinic Proceedings, 64*, 1005–20.

Paludan, C. & Munz, C. (2003). CD4+ T cell responses in the immune control against latent infection by Epstein-Barr virus. *Curr Mol Med, 3*(4), 341–7. 12776989

Pels, H., Staib, P., Stenzel, W., et al. (2004). Concomitant manifestation of primary CNS lymphoma and toxoplasma encephalitis in a patient with AIDS. *Journal of Neurology, 251*:764–6.

Peterson, K., Gordon, K. B., Heinemann, M., et al. (1993). The clinical spectrum of ocular lymphoma. *Cancer 72*, 843–49.

Pluda, J. M., Yarchoan, R., Jaffe, E. S., Feuerstein, I. M., Solomon, D., Steinberg, S. M., et al. (1990). Development of non-Hodgkin lymphoma in a cohort of patients with severe human immunodeficiency virus (HIV) infection on long-term antiretroviral therapy. *Ann Intern Med, 113*(4), 276–82. 1973886

Pollack, I. F., Lunsford, L. D., Flickinger, J. C., & Dameshek, H. L. (1989). Prognostic factors in the diagnosis and treatment of primary central nervous system lymphoma. *Cancer, 63*, 939–47.

Polman, C. H., O'Connor, P. W., Havrdova, E., et al. (2006) A randomized, placebo-controlled trial of natalizumab for relapsing multiple sclerosis. *New England Journal of Medicine, 354*, 899–910.

Port, J. D., Miseljic, S., Lee, R. R., et al. (1999). Progressive multifocal leukoencephalopathy demonstrating contrast enhancement on MRI and uptake of thallium-201: A case report. *Neuroradiology, 41*, 895–8.

Porter, S. B. & Sande, M. A. (1992). Toxoplasmosis of the central nervous system in the acquired immunodeficiency syndrome. *New England Journal of Medicine, 327*, 1643–8.

Raez, L., Cabral, L., Cai, J. P., et al. (1999). Treatment of AIDS-related primary central nervous system lymphoma with zidovudine, ganciclovir, and interleukin 2. *AIDS Research and Human Retroviruses, 15*, 713–9.

Raez, L. E., Patel, P., Feun, L., et al. (1998). Natural history and prognostic factors for survival in patients with acquired immune deficiency syndrome (AIDS)-related primary central nervous system lymphoma (PCNSL). *Critical Reviews in Oncology, 9*(3–4), 199–208.

Remick, S. C., Diamond, C., Migliozzi, J. A., et al. (1990). Primary central nervous system lymphoma in patients with and without the acquired immune deficiency syndrome: A retrospective analysis and review of the literature. *Medicine, 69*, 345–60.

Reyes, C., Abuzaitoun, O., De Jong, A., Hanson, C., & Langston, C. (2002). Epstein-Barr virus-associated smooth muscle tumors in ataxia-telangiectasia: A case report and review. *Human Pathology, 33*, 133–6.

Ritter, A. M., Amaker, B. H., Graham, R. S., Broaddus, W. C., & Ward, J. D. (2000). Central nervous system leiomyosarcoma in patients with acquired immunodeficiency syndrome. Report of two cases. *Journal of Neurosurgery, 92*, 688–92.

Sandler, A. S. & Kaplan, L. D. (1996). Diagnosis and management of systemic non-Hodgkin's lymphoma in HIV disease. *Hematol Oncol Clin North Am, 10*(5), 1111–24. 8880199

Schiff, D., O'Neill, B., Wijdicks, E., Antin, J. H., & Wen, P. Y. (2001). Gliomas arising in organ transplant recipients: An unrecognized complication of transplantation? *Neurology, 57*, 1486–8.

Schindler, E., Thurnher, M. M., & Thurnher, S. A. (1997).CNS involvement in AIDS: Spectrum of CT and MR findings. *European Radiology, 7*(7), 1091–7

Schwaighofer, B. W., Hesselink, J. R., Press, G. A., et al. (1989). Primary intracranial CNS lymphoma: MR manifestations. *American Journal of Neuroradiology, 10*, 725–29.

Shiramizu, B., Herndier, B. G., & McGrath, M. S. (1994). Identification of a common clonal human immunodeficiency virus integration site in human immunodeficiency virus-associated lymphomas. *Cancer Res, 54*(8), 2069–72.

Skolasky, R. L., Dal Pan, G. J., Olivi, A., Lenz, F. A., Abrams, R. A., & McArthur, J. C. (1999). HIV-associated primary CNS lymorbidity and utility of brain biopsy. *Journal of Neurological Science, 163*, 32–8.

Sloan, D. B., Slusher, M. M., Stanton, C. A., et al. (1992). Acquired immunodeficiency syndrome-related primary intraocular lymphoma. *Archives of Ophthalmology, 110*, 1614–17.

So, Y. T., Beckstead, J. H., & Davis, R. L. (1986). Primary central nervous system lymphoma in acquired immune deficiency syndrome: A clinical and pathological study. *Annals of Neurology, 20*, 566–72.

Sparano, J. A. (2001). Clinical aspects and management of AIDS-related lymphoma. *European Journal of Cancer, 37*, 1296–305.

Sparano, J. A., Lee, J. Y., Kaplan, L. D., et al. (2010) Rituximab plus concurrent infusional EPOCH chemotherapy is highly effective in HIV-associated, B-cell non-Hodgkin's lymphoma. *Blood, 115*, 3008–16.

Stanton, C. A., Sloan, D. B., Slusher, M. M., et al. (1992). Acquired immunodeficiency syndrome-related primary intraocular lymphoma. *Archives of Ophthalmology, 110*, 1614–17.

Steel, T. R., Pell, M. F., Turner, J. J., & Lim, G. H. (1993). Spinal epidural leiomyoma occurring in an HIV-infected man. *Journal of Neurosurgery, 79*, 442–5.

Stenzel, W., Pels, H., Staib, P., et al. (2004). Concomitant manifestation of primary CNS lymphoma and Toxoplasma encephalitis in a patient with AIDS. *J Neurol, 251*, 764.

Straus, S. E., Cohen, J. I., Tosato, G., & Meier, J. (1993). NIH conference. Epstein-Barr virus infections: Biology, pathogenesis, and management. *Annals of Internal Medicine, 118*, 45–58.

Thurnher, M. M., Thurnher, S. A., & Schindler, E. (1997). CNS involvement in AIDS: Spectrum of CT and MR findings. *Eur Radiol, 7*(7), 1091–7.

Tosi, P., Gherlinzoni, F., Mazza, P., et al. (1997). 3'-Azido 3'-deoxythymidine + methotrexate as a novel antineoplastic combination in the treatment of human immunodeficiency virus-related non-Hodgkin's lymphomas. *Blood, 89*, 419–25.

Vaccher, E., Spina, M., di Gennaro, G., et al. (2001). Concomitant cyclophosphamide, doxorubicin, vincristine, and prednisone chemotherapy plus highly active antiretroviral therapy in patients with human immunodeficiency virus-related, non-Hodgkin lymphoma. *Cancer, 91*, 155–63.

van Baarle, D., Hovenkamp, E., Callan, M. F., Wolthers, K. C., Kostense, S., Tan, L. C., et al. (2001). Dysfunctional Epstein-Barr virus (EBV)-specific CD8(+) T lymphocytes and increased EBV load in HIV-1 infected individuals progressing to AIDS-related non-Hodgkin lymphoma. *Blood*, 98(1), 146–155. 11418474

Varela-Duran, J., Oliva, H., & Rosai, J. (1979). Vascular leiomyosarcoma: The malignant counterpart of vascular leiomyoma. *Cancer*, 44, 1684–91.

Vilchez, R. A., Jorgensen, J. L., & Kroll, M. H. (2002). Systemic non-Hodgkin lymphoma in HIV-infected patients in the era of highly active antiretroviral therapy. *Blood*, 99, 4250–1.

Vilchez, R. A., Kozinetz, C. A., Jorgensen, J. L., Kroll, M. H., & Butel, J. S. (2002). AIDS-related systemic non-Hodgkin's lymphoma at a large community program. *AIDS Research and Human Retroviruses*, 18, 237–42.

Wang D, Liebowitz D, Kieff E. (1985) An EBV membrane protein expressed in immortalized lymphocytes transforms established rodent cells. *Cell*, 43, 831–40.

Wang F, Tsang SF, Kurilla MG, Cohen JI, Kieff E. (1990) Epstein-Barr virus nuclear antigen 2 transactivates latent membrane protein LMP1. *Journal of Virology*, 64, 3407–16.

Weber, M. A., Zoubaa, S., Schlieter, M., et al. (2006). Diagnostic performance of spectroscopic and perfusion MRI for distinction of brain tumors. *Neurology*, 66(12), 1899–906.

Weinberg, A., Li, S., Palmer, M., & Tyler, K. L. (2002). Quantitative CSF PCR in Epstein-Barr virus infections of the central nervous system. *Annals of Neurology*, 52, 543–8.

Wolf T, Brodt HR, Fichtlscherer S, et al. (2005) Changing incidence and prognostic factors of survival in AIDS-related non-Hodgkin's lymphoma in the era of highly active antiretroviral therapy (HAART). *Leukemia and Lymphoma*, 46, 207–15.

Yoshizaki T, Sato H, Furukawa M, Pagano JS. (1998). The expression of matrix metalloproteinase 9 is enhanced by Epstein-Barr virus latent membrane protein 1. *Proceedings of the National Academy of Sciences (USA)*, 31, 3621–6.

Zacharia, T. T., Law, M., Naidich, T. P., & Leeds, N. E. (2008). Central nervous system lymphoma characterization by diffusion-weighted imaging and MR spectroscopy. *Journal of Neuroimaging*, 18(4), 411–7.

8.8

HEPATITIS C

Li Ye and Wenzhe Ho

Hepatitis C virus (HCV) affects over 170 million people world wide and 4 million people in the United States. It is a major cause of chronic hepatitis, liver cirrhosis, and hepatocellular carcinoma. It also causes a variety of extrahepatic syndromes, including cryoglobulinemia, glomerulonephritis, porphyria cutanea tarda, and neurological dysfunctions. Co-infection of HIV and HCV is very common among injection drug users. In patients with HIV infection, HCV co-infection accelerates HIV disease progression and is an important source of increased HIV-associated morbidity and mortality. The combination of interferon-alpha (IFN-α) and ribavirin is currently the only available treatment for HCV infection. This treatment has a success rate of only about 50% and is often associated with serious side-effects. This chapter focuses on the role of HCV infection in neurological dysfunction. Topics covered include: HCV infection in the central nervous system (CNS), HCV and neurological dysfunction, HCV and depression, mechanisms of HCV-associated cognitive impairment, effects of anti-HCV therapy on cognitive functioning, and the impact of HIV-HCV co-infection on cognitive functioning.

INTRODUCTION

Hepatitis C virus (HCV) infection has emerged as the second major viral epidemic after HIV, affecting over 170 million people in the world and 4 million Americans (Alter, 1999; Shepard et al., 2005; Armstrong et al., 2006). HCV infection is a major cause of chronic hepatitis, liver cirrhosis and hepatocellular carcinoma worldwide (Alter, 2002). HIV-HCV co-infection is very common among injection drug users (IDUs), as rates of HCV infection among IDUs are extremely high ranging from 70%–90% (Crofts et al., 1994; Goldberg et al., 1998; Samuel et al., 2001). In patients with HIV infection, HCV displays increased persistence and accelerated progression, and thus co-infection with HCV has become an important source of morbidity and mortality among people infected with HIV (Thomas, 2002; Murray et al., 2008). The combination of interferon-alpha (IFN-α) and ribavirin is currently the only available treatment for HCV infection. This treatment, however, not only has a low success rate (about 50%) but is often associated with serious side effects (Hayashi & Takehara, 2006). HCV infection is also associated with a variety of extrahepatic syndromes, including cryoglobulinemia, glomerulonephritis, porphyria

cutanea tarda and neurological dysfunctions (Hoofnagle, 2002). This chapter focuses on the role of HCV infection in neurological dysfunction.

HCV INFECTION IN THE CNS

HCV can cross the blood-brain-barrier (BBB) and present in both the cerebrospinal fluid (CSF) and brain tissue (Maggi et al., 1999; Laskus et al., 2002; Murray et al., 2008). HCV has been identified in a variety of nervous system tissues and fluids, both in HCV mono-infected patients and those co-infected with HIV (Forton et al. 2004; Morgello et al., 2005; Forton et al., 2006). Some of the HCV sequences identified in the peripheral systems (mononuclear cells and lymph nodes) and the brain are very similar, suggesting that the virus can cross the BBB, perhaps through infected leukocytes (Forton et al., 2004; Laskus et al., 2004). However, diversification of the virus was also recently reported (Murray et al., 2008; Martin-Thormeyer & Paul, 2009). It has been suggested that HCV may replicate within the central nervous system (CNS), although the specific brain targets infected by HCV remain to be determined. Several studies demonstrated negative-strand replication intermediates and brain-specific quasispecies in HCV-infected subjects (Laskus et al., 2002; Radkowski et al., 2002; Vargas et al., 2002; Forton et al., 2004). It was also reported that HCV proteins (Core and NS5A) exist in brain astrocytes from people co-infected with HCV and HIV (Letendre et al., 2007). Wilkinson et al. found HCV presence in CD68[+] cells (macrophages and microglia) of frontal cortex and subcortex white matter (Wilkinson et al., 2009). The presence of HCV antigens in the brain along with evidence of HCV diversification in the brain (Bagaglio et al., 2005; Murray et al., 2008; Martin-Thormeyer & Paul, 2009) suggests that the brain may represent a site of persistent HCV viral replication among co-infected patients.

HCV AND NEUROLOGICAL DYSFUNCTION

There are large amounts of data indicated that there is association between impairment of brain function and HCV infection. Patients with HCV infection manifested impairments in the quality of life, fatigue, and depression, which are more common than patients with liver disease of other etiology (Barkhuizen et al., 1999; Foster, 1999; Kenny-Walsh, 1999; Singh et al., 1999). HCV infection was associated with cognitive dysfunction (Forton et al., 2002; Hilsabeck et al., 2002). Using proton magnetic resonance spectroscopy (1H MRS), investigators have demonstrated that there were elevated choline/creatine ratios in basal ganglia and white matter in patients with mild HCV disease, which were not present in healthy volunteers or patients with hepatitis (Forton et al., 2001; Forton et al., 2002). The similar abnormalities in choline/active rations in people infected with HCV were also reported by other researchers (Weissenborn et al., 2004; McAndrews et al., 2005). Such 1H MRS changes related to HCV infection differ from those seen in hepatic encephalopathy, where the choline ratios are depressed (Taylor-Robinson, 2001), but are similar to those found in patients with HIV infection (Marcus et al. 1998; Meyerhoff et al., 1999). Additional evidence for the biological basis of HCV-related cognitive dysfunction is recently reported, showing differences in gene expression patterns between brain tissue from HCV-positive and HCV-negative patients (Laskus et al., 2005; Wilkinson et al., 2009). However, despite these findings, it remains to be determined whether HCV infection itself and/or its associated factors contribute to neuropsychological and neuropsychiatric symptomatology. Apparently, more accurate and objective measures of cerebral function are required in order to determine the nature and degree of cerebral dysfunction related to HCV infection.

There is growing evidence showing that many people infected with HCV have fundamental cognitive deficits, which are unrelated to indices of liver dysfunction, viral load, or genotype of the virus (Forton et al., 2001; Forton et al., 2002; Hilsabeck et al., 2002; Kramer et al., 2002; Hilsabeck et al., 2003; Taylor et al., 2004; Weissenborn et al., 2004; Fontana et al., 2005; Kramer et al., 2005; McAndrews et al., 2005). A number of studies have been carried out to evaluate neuropsychological parameters in HCV-infected subjects (Forton et al., 2002; Cordoba et al., 2003; Martin et al., 2004; von Giesen et al., 2004; Weissenborn et al., 2004; Cherner et al., 2005; Letendre et al., 2005; McAndrews et al., 2005; Karaivazoglou et al., 2007). These studies vary markedly in their inclusion criteria, type of control group, statistical design, and choice and breadth of neuropsychological tests. However, these studies reported that HCV-infected individuals with mild liver disease performed worse than uninfected control subjects in at least one cognitive parameter. These studies also demonstrated that HCV infection is indeed associated with increased risk for cognitive impairments, particularly those related to ability of attention, concentration, and verbal learning. These cognitive impairments are not related to the extent of fatigue, depression, or the reduction of health-related quality of life (Weissenborn et al., 2009). In addition, there is no association between HCV-related cognitive impairment and history of intravenous drug users (IVDUs), history of psychiatric disorder and depressive symptoms. To establish a clear profile of HCV-associated cognitive impairment, however, still requires more extensive studies with well-characterized study subjects. Future research is also needed in order to address predictors of cognitive dysfunction in HCV-infected subjects, as well as the effect of antiviral treatment on cognitive function.

HCV AND DEPRESSION

Depression is a common finding in HCV-infected individuals (Foster et al., 1998; Dwight et al., 2000; Kraus et al., 2000; Goulding et al., 2001; Fontana et al., 2002). However, the relationship between HCV and depression is extremely complex. Currently, there is little biological evidence that HCV infection itself can cause depression. HCV infection is highly prevalent among IDUs, many of whom have depression (Kraus et al., 2001). Clinically, IFN-α-based treatment may precipitate in or exacerbate depression (Zdilar et al., 2000). HCV-positive IDUs had significantly lower positive affect scores than HCV-negative drug users (Kraus et al., 2001). However, it has also been reported there was no difference in psychological morbidity between HCV-positive and HCV-negative drug users, although in both of the studies, the effect of HCV may have been masked by the high background prevalence of depression in active drug users (Grassi et al., 2001). It is possible that patients with depression may have a higher incidence of HCV infection. Conversely, depression may exist as a secondary phenomenon to HCV infection. This reactive depression may be related to the diagnosis and concerns over long-term health, or may be secondary to symptoms such as fatigue and cognitive impairment (McDonald et al., 2002).

MECHANISM(S) OF HCV-ASSOCIATED COGNITIVE IMPAIRMENT

DIRECT EFFECTS OF HCV

The etiology of cognitive dysfunction exhibited by people infected with HCV is unknown. Several mechanisms have been proposed to explain HCV-associated cognitive impairment (Fig. 8.8.1). One mechanism proposed is that cognitive dysfunction associated with HCV infection is due to the virus itself infecting the brain (Fig. 8.8.1) (Forton et al., 2005; Laskus et al., 2005). This speculation is based on the reports showing that HCV replicates in peripheral blood mononuclear cells (PBMCs) and bone marrow (Cribier et al., 1995; Sansonno et al., 1996; Okuda et al., 1999; Roque Afonso et al., 1999), which serve as precursors for microglial cells and perivascular macrophages within the brain (Morsica et al., 1997; Maggi et al., 1999; Flugel et al., 2001; Laskus et al., 2002; Radkowski et al., 2002; Forton et al., 2004). Thus, it is proposed that HCV is introduced into CNS via a "Trojan horse" mechanism, which is similar to what is proposed for HIV-mediated neuronal injury in the CNS (Meyerhoff et al., 1999). The Trojan horse hypothesis suggests that cerebral dysfunction occurs secondary to infection of monocytes, which are believed to migrate into the CNS, as HCV-infected monocytes can release neurotoxic cytokines

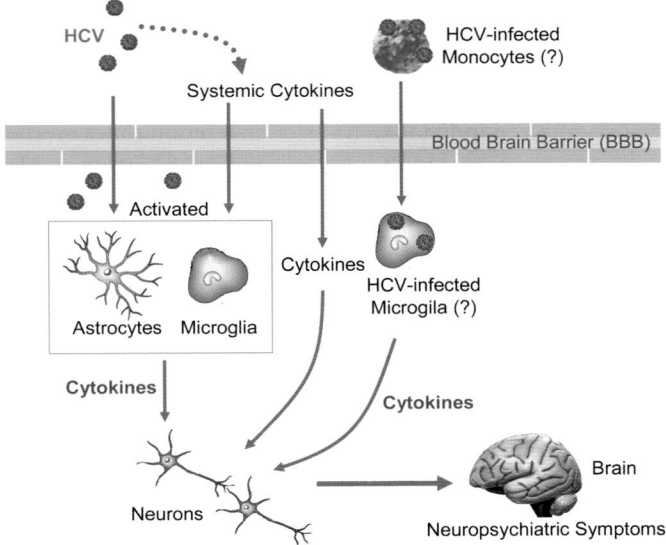

Figure 8.8.1 The schematic diagram of possible mechanisms of HCV-associated neurological dysfunction.

that impair neurons. This hypothesis is supported by evidence that HCV can replicate in human macrophages (Caussin-Schwemling et al., 2001; Laskus et al., 2004). There have been no reports showing that HCV can replicate in neuronal cells. Thus, any effect of HCV itself on neuronal injury, if any, is likely to be minimal. In vivo studies have shown that the replication of HCV quasispecies is very low and sometimes undetectable in the brain (Radkowski et al., 2002; Forton et al., 2004). Despite of high titer of HCV in serum, HCV RNA is not always detectable in the cerebrospinal fluid of HCV-infected patients (Morsica et al., 1997; Laskus et al., 2002), and when detectable, CSF viral loads have been found to be much lower than those in serum (Maggi et al., 1999). Several studies demonstrated there was no relationship between viral load in serum and cognitive dysfunction (Hilsabeck et al., 2002; Hilsabeck et al., 2003; Weissenborn et al., 2004; Fontana et al., 2005; McAndrews et al., 2005). Thus, these findings do not support direct effect of HCV on neuronal injury.

EFFECTS OF THE INFLAMMATORY PROCESS

Chronic activation of the immune system has also been considered as a mechanism responsible for cognitive dysfunction in patients with chronic HCV, as HCV in the CNS could produce an inflammatory cascade, which is similar to HIV infection in the brain (Morgello et al., 2005; Paul et al., 2007; Forton et al., 2008; Martin-Thormeyer & Paul, 2009). There is increasing evidence of cytokine-mediated cognitive dysfunction (Wilson et al., 2002; Lee et al., 2004; Meyers et al., 2005). It is well known that cytokines involve in positive and negative feedback loops within the brain. It is likely that people infected with HCV have increased levels of cytokines such as interleukin (IL)-2, IL-4, IL-10, and interferons (IFNs) (Cacciarelli et al,. 1996). Some of these cytok-

ines including IFN-α and tumor necrosis factor-alpha (TNF-α) may cross the BBB, especially at the site of the organum vasculosum laminae terminalis, to affect brain functioning (Farkkila et al., 1984; Shibata & Blatteis, 1991; Pan & Kastin, 1999). It is also possible that HCV and/or its proteins in the brain induce the local production of inflammatory cytokines, resulting in neuronal injury. Radkowski et al. demonstrated that macrophages infected with HCV in vitro could produce TNF-α and IL-8 (Radkowski et al., 2004).

In addition to the involvement of local inflammation in the CNS, cytokines have been reported to affect brain functioning indirectly by transmitting signals via the vagus nerve or other visceral afferent neuronal pathways and by binding to the cerebral vascular endothelium and inducing secondary messengers such as prostaglandins and nitric oxide (Licinio et al., 1998; Kronfol & Remick, 2000). Moreover, some cytokines have been shown to have neuromodulatory effects on the CNS through activation of neuroendocrine pathways and various neurotransmitter systems (Wilson et al, 2002; Wrona, 2006). Microglia are known to release excitatory amino acids that can induce neuronal cell death via excitotoxicity, and they can exert a neuromodulary role through the release of neurotoxins and other neurochemicals (Peterson et al., 1997). It has also been proposed that brain infection with HCV could potentially lead to free radical damage. Adair et al. demonstrated downregulation of oxidative phosphorylation genes in the brains of HCV-infected patients (Adair et al., 2005). This finding is of significance as oxidative phosphorylation is a critical source of cell energy and neurons are susceptible to reduced energy sources due to high metabolic rates. High levels of free radicals in the brain may be produced as a consequence of disruption in energy-dependent calcium homeostasis.

Although both virological and immunological hypotheses have been proposed to explain HCV-infected associated cognitive impairment, more specific mechanisms have yet to be investigated. Virological theories of HCV-associated cognitive impairment generally support in part the involvement of immunologic response in neuronal cognitive dysfunctioning. This concern is based on the report that the subjective cognitive complaints do not always correlate with objective performance on cognitive tests (Hilsabeck et al., 2003). In order to prove the direct role of HCV in neurological damage, it is of importance to establish an objective method to measure neuropsychological deficits for HCV-infected patients. Thus, a critical step toward validating a virological model is to confirm that HCV-infected patients have measurable neuropsychological deficits upon testing.

EFFECTS OF ANTI-HCV THERAPY ON COGNITIVE FUNCTIONING

Unfortunately, IFN-α, the primary antiviral cytokine for treatment of HCV infection, has been reported to impair cognitive functioning in both healthy volunteers (Smith et al., 1988) and clinical populations (Adams et al., 1984; Pavol et al., 1995; Valentine et al., 1998; Capuron et al., 2001). Although information about the effects of IFN-α on cognitive functioning in HCV patients is still limited, a few studies reported a negative impact of IFN-α on the CNS. Kamei et al. found diffuse slowing on quantitative electro-encephalogram and reduced performances on a cognitive screening measure after IFN-α therapy, which could be reversed after the end of treatment (Kamei et al., 1999; Kamei et al., 2002). One other study reported hypometabolism in the bilateral prefrontal and right parietal cortex, hypermetabolism in the bilateral putamen, right thalamus, left occipital cortex, and reduced verbal learning after 3 months of IFN-α therapy (Juengling et al., 2000). It has also been revealed that although there were no significant differences on simple attentional measures, the IFN-α-treated group performed significantly worse than the untreated patients on a measure of complex attention and working memory (Hilsabeck et al., 2005). In addition, several studies indicate that IFN-α treatment adversely affects frontal-subcortical systems in HCV patients and the prefrontal lobe functions of working memory may be the most vulnerable (Amodio et al., 2005; Capuron et al., 2005; Kraus et al., 2005; Lieb et al., 2006).

IMPACT OF HIV-HCV CO-INFECTION ON COGNITIVE FUNCTIONING

The interest in the effect of HIV-HCV co-infection on cognitive functioning is partially based on the observations that the prevalence of co-infection is very high in some populations of HIV-infected patients and co-infected subjects exhibit more severe cognitive dysfunction than individuals with mono-infection (Martin-Thormeyer & Paul, 2009). Given the high rate of transmission through percutaneous exposure, it is not surprising that individuals infected with HIV through injection drug use are at a high risk of being co-infected with HCV compared to individuals infected with HIV through sexual activity, although HCV can be transmitted by sexual contact. The prevalence of co-infection is estimated to range from 44% to as high as 95% among IDUs (Sulkowski et al., 2002; Verucchi et al., 2004; Matthews & Dore, 2008). These numbers translate to approximately 300,000 co-infected individuals in the US. HCV has now been recognized as an important "cognitive" comorbidity to HIV infection. However, the mechanisms that drive these cognitive symptoms largely remain unknown.

A number of studies have shown the impact of interactions between HCV and HIV on the CNS and neuropsychological function (Martin et al., 2004; Ryan et al., 2004; von Giesen et al., 2004; Cherner et al., 2005; Clifford et al., 2005; Letendre et al., 2005; Perry et al., 2005; Richardson et al., 2005). However, these studies could not prove that HCV has an additive effect on HIV-associated cognitive impairment. Several studies reported more severe neuropsychological impairment among co-infected patients than mono-infected individuals (Cherner et al., 2005; Clifford et al., 2005; Letendre et al., 2005; Richardson et al., 2005), as co-infected subjects had decreased processing speed and psychomotor speed. One study observed significantly slower reaction times among co-infected patients compared to individuals with either HIV or HCV mono-infection (von Giesen et al., 2004). This finding is supported by the report showing that co-infected individuals had slower reaction times on the task compared to mono-infected subjects (Martin et al., 2004). It was reported that 80% of a co-infected group met criteria for cognitive impairment compared to 69% of an HIV mono-infected group that met criteria for impairment (Hilsabeck et al., 2005). Further, it has also been reported that the primary cognitive domain affected among the co-infected subjects was psychomotor slowing, with 84% of the co-infected individuals impaired in this domain compared to 56% of the mono-infected individuals (Clifford et al., 2005). However, the findings that there is greater cognitive impairment among co-infected subjects could not be confirmed in other studies. One study indicated that there were no significant differences between co-infected patients and a comparison group of HCV mono-infected patients (Perry et al., 2005). Several other studies also failed to find significant differences between co-infected and mono-infected persons on individual neuropsychological measures, although trends for greater impairment in co-infected persons were suggested (Ryan et al., 2004; von Giesen et al., 2004). Interestingly, although there was no difference in neuropsychological measures, one report demonstrated a differential pattern of impairment on a cognitive task of reaction time and response inhibition, with HCV-infected patients exhibiting overall slowed processing speed and HIV-infected patients showing impaired executive ability (Martin et al., 2004).

SUMMARY

It is evident from laboratory and epidemiologic studies that HCV infection is associated with neurological dysfunction. However, because many confounding factors (HIV co-infection, drugs of abuse, liver damage, IFN-α treatment, etc.) are involved in HCV infection, the etiology of neurological dysfunctions exhibited by HCV-infected people remains to be determined. Apparently, more studies are needed in order to determine how HCV infection itself and/or its associated factors contribute to neuropsychological and neuropsychiatric symptomatology. With development of more sensitive/accurate measures of HCV in the brain and newly developed neuroimaging/neurometabolic technology, it is feasible to elucidate the mechanism(s) responsible for HCV-mediated neurological dysfunction in the future.

REFERENCES

Adair, D. M., Radkowski, M., Jablonska, J., et al. (2005). Differential display analysis of gene expression in brains from hepatitis C-infected patients. *AIDS, 19* Suppl 3, S145–150.

Adams, F., Quesada, J. R., & Gutterman, J. U. (1984). Neuropsychiatric manifestations of human leukocyte interferon therapy in patients with cancer. *JAMA, 252*(7), 938–941.

Alter, M. J. (1999). Hepatitis C virus infection in the United States. *J Hepatol, 31* Suppl 1, 88–91.

Alter, M. J. (2002). Prevention of spread of hepatitis C. *Hepatology, 36* 5 Suppl 1, S93–98.

Amodio, P., De Toni, E. N., Cavalletto, L., et al. (2005). Mood, cognition and EEG changes during interferon alpha (alpha-IFN) treatment for chronic hepatitis C. *J Affect Disord, 84*(1), 93–98.

Armstrong, G. L., Wasley, A., Simard, E. P., McQuillan, G. M., Kuhnert, W. L., & Alter, M. J. (2006). The prevalence of hepatitis C virus infection in the United States, 1999 through 2002. *Ann Intern Med, 144*(10), 705–714.

Bagaglio, S., Cinque, P., Racca, S., et al. (2005). Hepatitis C virus populations in the plasma, peripheral blood mononuclear cells and cerebrospinal fluid of HIV/hepatitis C virus-co-infected patients. *AIDS, 19* Suppl 3, S151–65.

Barkhuizen, A., Rosen, H. R., Wolf, S., Flora, K., Benner, K. & Bennett, R. M. (1999). Musculoskeletal pain and fatigue are associated with chronic hepatitis C: A report of 239 hepatology clinic patients. *Am J Gastroenterol, 94*(5), 1355–1360.

Cacciarelli, T. V., Martinez, O. M., Gish, R. G., Villanueva, J. C. & Krams, S. M. (1996). Immunoregulatory cytokines in chronic hepatitis C virus infection: Pre- and posttreatment with interferon alfa. *Hepatology, 24*(1), 6–9.

Capuron, L., Pagnoni, G., Demetrashvili, M., et al. (2005). Anterior cingulate activation and error processing during interferon-alpha treatment. *Biol Psychiatry, 58*(3), 190–196.

Capuron, L., Ravaud, A., & Dantzer, R. (2001). Timing and specificity of the cognitive changes induced by interleukin-2 and interferon-alpha treatments in cancer patients. *Psychosom Med, 63*(3), 376–386.

Caussin-Schwemling, C., Schmitt, C., & Stoll-Keller, F. (2001). Study of the infection of human blood derived monocyte/macrophages with hepatitis C virus in vitro. *J Med Virol, 65*(1), 14–22.

Cherner, M., Letendre, S., Heaton, R. K., et al. (2005). Hepatitis C augments cognitive deficits associated with HIV infection and methamphetamine. *Neurology, 64*(8), 1343–1347.

Clifford, D. B., Evans, S. R., Yang, Y., & Gulick, R. M. (2005). The neuropsychological and neurological impact of hepatitis C virus co-infection in HIV-infected subjects. *AIDS, 19* Suppl 3, S64–71.

Cordoba, J., Flavia, M., Jacas, C., et al. (2003). Quality of life and cognitive function in hepatitis C at different stages of liver disease. *J Hepatol, 39*(2), 231–238.

Cribier, B., Schmitt, C., Bingen, A., Kirn, A., & Keller, F. (1995). In vitro infection of peripheral blood mononuclear cells by hepatitis C virus. *J Gen Virol, 76* (Pt 10), 2485–2491.

Crofts, N., Hopper, J. L., Milner, R., Breschkin, A. M., Bowden, D. S., & Locarnini, S. A. (1994). Blood-borne virus infections among Australian injecting drug users: Implications for spread of HIV. *Eur J Epidemiol, 10*(6), 687–694.

Dwight, M. M., Kowdley, K. V., Russo, J. E., Ciechanowski, P. S., Larson, A. M., & Katon, W. J. (2000). Depression, fatigue, and functional disability in patients with chronic hepatitis C. *J Psychosom Res, 49*(5), 311–317.

Farkkila, M., Iivanainen, M., Roine, R., et al. (1984). Neurotoxic and other side effects of high-dose interferon in amyotrophic lateral sclerosis. *Acta Neurol Scand, 70*(1), 42–46.

Flugel, A., Bradl, M., Kreutzberg, G. W., & Graeber, M. B. (2001). Transformation of donor-derived bone marrow precursors into host microglia during autoimmune CNS inflammation and during the retrograde response to axotomy. *J Neurosci Res, 66*(1), 74–82.

Fontana, R. J., Bieliauskas, L. A., Back-Madruga, C., et al. (2005). Cognitive function in hepatitis C patients with advanced fibrosis enrolled in the HALT-C trial. *J Hepatol, 43*(4), 614–622.

Fontana, R. J., Walsh, J., Moyer, C. A., Lok, A. S., Webster, S., & Klein, S. (2002). High-dose interferon alfa-2b and ribavirin in patients previously treated with interferon: Results of a prospective, randomized, controlled trial. *J Clin Gastroenterol, 34*(2), 177–182.

Forton, D. M., Allsop, J. M., Cox, I. J., et al. (2005). A review of cognitive impairment and cerebral metabolite abnormalities in patients with hepatitis C infection. *AIDS, 19* Suppl 3, S53–63.

Forton, D. M., Allsop, J. M., Main, J., Foster, G. R., Thomas, H. C., & Taylor-Robinson, S. D. (2001). Evidence for a cerebral effect of the hepatitis C virus. *Lancet, 358*(9275), 38–39.

Forton, D. M., Hamilton, G., Allsop, J. M., et al. (2008). Cerebral immune activation in chronic hepatitis C infection: A magnetic resonance spectroscopy study. *J Hepatol, 49*(3), 316–322.

Forton, D. M., Karayiannis, P., Mahmud, N., Taylor-Robinson, S. D., & Thomas, H. C. (2004). Identification of unique hepatitis C virus quasispecies in the central nervous system and comparative analysis of internal translational efficiency of brain, liver, and serum variants. *J Virol, 78*(10), 5170–5183.

Forton, D. M., Taylor-Robinson, S. D., & Thomas, H. C. (2006). Central nervous system changes in hepatitis C virus infection. *Eur J Gastroenterol Hepatol, 18*(4), 333–338.

Forton, D. M., Thomas, H. C., Murphy, C. A., et al. (2002). Hepatitis C and cognitive impairment in a cohort of patients with mild liver disease. *Hepatology, 35*(2), 433–439.

Forton, D. M., Thomas, H. C., & Taylor-Robinson, S. D. (2004). Central nervous system involvement in hepatitis C virus infection. *Metab Brain Dis, 19*(3–4), 383–391.

Foster, G. R. (1999). Hepatitis C virus infection: Quality of life and side effects of treatment. *J Hepatol, 31* Suppl 1, 250–254.

Foster, G. R., Goldin, R. D., & Thomas, H. C. (1998). Chronic hepatitis C virus infection causes a significant reduction in quality of life in the absence of cirrhosis. *Hepatology, 27*(1), 209–212.

Goldberg, D., Cameron, S., & McMenamin, J. (1998). Hepatitis C virus antibody prevalence among injecting drug users in Glasgow has fallen but remains high. *Commun Dis Public Health, 1*(2), 95–97.

Goulding, C., O'Connell, P., & Murray, F. E. (2001). Prevalence of fibromyalgia, anxiety and depression in chronic hepatitis C virus infection: Relationship to RT-PCR status and mode of acquisition. *Eur J Gastroenterol Hepatol, 13*(5), 507–511.

Grassi, L., Mondardini, D., Pavanati, M., Sighinolfi, L., Serra, A., & Ghinelli, F. (2001). Suicide probability and psychological morbidity secondary to HIV infection: A control study of HIV-seropositive, hepatitis C virus (HCV)-seropositive and HIV/HCV-seronegative injecting drug users. *J Affect Disord, 64*(2–3), 195–202.

Hayashi, N. & Takehara, T. (2006). Antiviral therapy for chronic hepatitis C: Past, present, and future. *J Gastroenterol, 41*(1), 17–27.

Hilsabeck, R. C., Hassanein, T. I., Carlson, M. D., Ziegler, E. A., & Perry, W. (2003). Cognitive functioning and psychiatric symptomatology in patients with chronic hepatitis C. *J Int Neuropsychol Soc, 9*(6), 847–854.

Hilsabeck, R. C., Hassanein, T. I., Ziegler, E. A., Carlson, M. D., & Perry, W. (2005). Effect of interferon-alpha on cognitive functioning in patients with chronic hepatitis C. *J Int Neuropsychol Soc, 11*(1), 16–22.

Hilsabeck, R. C., Perry, W., & Hassanein, T. I. (2002). Neuropsychological impairment in patients with chronic hepatitis C. *Hepatology, 35*(2), 440–446.

Hoofnagle, J. H. (2002). Course and outcome of hepatitis C. *Hepatology, 36*(5 Suppl 1), S21–29.

Juengling, F. D., Ebert, D., Gut, O., et al. (2000). Prefrontal cortical hypometabolism during low-dose interferon alpha treatment. *Psychopharmacology (Berl), 152*(4), 383–389.

Kamei, S., Sakai, T., Matsuura, M., et al. (2002). Alterations of quantitative EEG and mini-mental state examination in interferon-alpha-treated hepatitis C. *Eur Neurol, 48*(2), 102–107.

Kamei, S., Tanaka, N., Mastuura, M., et al. (1999). Blinded, prospective, and serial evaluation by quantitative-EEG in interferon-alpha-treated hepatitis-C. *Acta Neurol Scand, 100*(1), 25–33.

Karaivazoglou, K., Assimakopoulos, K., Thomopoulos, K., et al. (2007). Neuropsychological function in Greek patients with chronic hepatitis C. *Liver Int, 27*(6), 798–805.

Kenny-Walsh, E. (1999). Clinical outcomes after hepatitis C infection from contaminated anti-D immune globulin. Irish Hepatology Research Group. *N Engl J Med, 340*(16), 1228–1233.

Kramer, L., Bauer, E., Funk, G., et al. (2002). Subclinical impairment of brain function in chronic hepatitis C infection. *J Hepatol, 37*(3), 349–354.

Kramer, L., Hofer, H., Bauer, E., et al. (2005). Relative impact of fatigue and subclinical cognitive brain dysfunction on health-related quality of life in chronic hepatitis C infection. *AIDS, 19* Suppl 3, S85–92.

Kraus, M. R., Schafer, A., Csef, H., Faller, H., Mork, H., & Scheurlen, M. (2001). Compliance with therapy in patients with chronic hepatitis C: Associations with psychiatric symptoms, interpersonal problems, and mode of acquisition. *Dig Dis Sci, 46*(10), 2060–2065.

Kraus, M. R., Schafer, A., Csef, H., Scheurlen, M., & Faller, H. (2000). Emotional state, coping styles, and somatic variables in patients with chronic hepatitis C. *Psychosomatics, 41*(5), 377–384.

Kraus, M. R., Schafer, A., Wissmann, S., Reimer, P., & Scheurlen, M. (2005). Neurocognitive changes in patients with hepatitis C receiving interferon alfa-2b and ribavirin. *Clin Pharmacol Ther, 77*(1), 90–100.

Kronfol, Z. & Remick, D. G. (2000). Cytokines and the brain: Implications for clinical psychiatry. *Am J Psychiatry, 157*(5), 683–694.

Laskus, T., Radkowski, M., Adair, D. M., Wilkinson, J., Scheck, A. C., & Rakela, J. (2005). Emerging evidence of hepatitis C virus neuroinvasion. *AIDS, 19* Suppl 3, S140–144.

Laskus, T., Radkowski, M., Bednarska, A., et al. (2002). Detection and analysis of hepatitis C virus sequences in cerebrospinal fluid. *J Virol, 76*(19), 10064–10068.

Laskus, T., Radkowski, M., Jablonska, J., et al. (2004). Human immunodeficiency virus facilitates infection/replication of hepatitis C virus in native human macrophages. *Blood, 103*(10), 3854–3859.

Laskus, T., Wilkinson, J., Gallegos-Orozco, J. F., et al. (2004). Analysis of hepatitis C virus quasispecies transmission and evolution in patients infected through blood transfusion. *Gastroenterology, 127*(3), 764–776.

Lee, B. N., Dantzer, R., Langley, K. E., et al. (2004). A cytokine-based neuroimmunologic mechanism of cancer-related symptoms. *Neuroimmunomodulation, 11*(5), 279–292.

Letendre, S., Paulino, A. D., Rockenstein, E., et al. (2007). Pathogenesis of hepatitis C virus coinfection in the brains of patients infected with HIV. *J Infect Dis, 196*(3), 361–370.

Letendre, S. L., Cherner, M., Ellis, R. J., et al. (2005). The effects of hepatitis C, HIV, and methamphetamine dependence on neuropsychological performance: Biological correlates of disease. *AIDS, 19* Suppl 3, S72–78.

Licinio, J., Kling, M. A., & Hauser, P. (1998). Cytokines and brain function: Relevance to interferon-alpha-induced mood and cognitive changes. *Semin Oncol, 25*(1 Suppl 1), 30–38.

Lieb, K., Engelbrecht, M. A., Gut, O., et al. (2006). Cognitive impairment in patients with chronic hepatitis treated with interferon alpha (IFNalpha): Results from a prospective study. *Eur Psychiatry, 21*(3), 204–10.

Maggi, F., Giorgi, M., Fornai, C., et al. (1999). Detection and quasispecies analysis of hepatitis C virus in the cerebrospinal fluid of infected patients. *J Neurovirol, 5*(3), 319–323.

Marcus, C. D., Taylor-Robinson, S. D., Sargentoni, J., et al. (1998). 1H MR spectroscopy of the brain in HIV-1-seropositive subjects: Evidence for diffuse metabolic abnormalities. *Metab Brain Dis, 13*(2), 123–136.

Martin-Thormeyer, E. M. & Paul, R. H. (2009). Drug abuse and hepatitis C infection as comorbid features of HIV associated neurocognitive disorder: Neurocognitive and neuroimaging features. *Neuropsychol Rev, 19*(2), 215–231.

Martin, E. M., Novak, R. M., Fendrich, M., et al. (2004). Stroop performance in drug users classified by HIV and hepatitis C virus serostatus. *J Int Neuropsychol Soc, 10*(2), 298–300.

Matthews, G. V. & Dore, G. J. (2008). HIV and hepatitis C coinfection. *J Gastroenterol Hepatol, 23*(7 Pt 1), 1000–1008.

McAndrews, M. P., Farcnik, K., Carlen, P., et al. (2005). Prevalence and significance of neurocognitive dysfunction in hepatitis C in the absence of correlated risk factors. *Hepatology, 41*(4), 801–808.

McDonald, J., Jayasuriya, J., Bindley, P., Gonsalvez, C., & Gluseska, S. (2002). Fatigue and psychological disorders in chronic hepatitis C. *J Gastroenterol Hepatol, 17*(2), 171–176.

Meyerhoff, D. J., Bloomer, C., Cardenas, V., Norman, D., Weiner, M. W., & Fein, G. (1999). Elevated subcortical choline metabolites in cognitively and clinically asymptomatic HIV+ patients. *Neurology, 52*(5), 995–1003.

Meyers, C. A., Albitar, M., & Estey, E. (2005). Cognitive impairment, fatigue, and cytokine levels in patients with acute myelogenous leukemia or myelodysplastic syndrome. *Cancer, 104*(4), 788–793.

Morgello, S., Estanislao, L., Ryan, E., et al. (2005). Effects of hepatic function and hepatitis C virus on the nervous system assessment of advanced-stage HIV-infected individuals. *AIDS, 19* Suppl 3, S116–122.

Morsica, G., Bernardi, M. T., Novati, R., Uberti Foppa, C., Castagna, A., & Lazzarin, A. (1997). Detection of hepatitis C virus genomic sequences in the cerebrospinal fluid of HIV-infected patients. *J Med Virol, 53*(3), 252–254.

Murray, J., Fishman, S. L., Ryan, E., et al. (2008). Clinicopathologic correlates of hepatitis C virus in brain: A pilot study. *J Neurovirol, 14*(1), 17–27.

Okuda, M., Hino, K., Korenaga, M., Yamaguchi, Y., Katoh, Y., & Okita, K. (1999). Differences in hypervariable region 1 quasispecies of hepatitis C virus in human serum, peripheral blood mononuclear cells, and liver. *Hepatology, 29*(1), 217–222.

Pan, W. & Kastin, A. J. (1999). Penetration of neurotrophins and cytokines across the blood-brain/blood-spinal cord barrier. *Adv Drug Deliv Rev, 36*(2–3), 291–298.

Paul, S., Javed, U., Tevendale, R., Lanford, J., & Liu, R. (2007). Acquired factor VIII inhibitor in an HIV-infected patient after treatment with pegylated interferon-alpha 2a and ribavirin. *AIDS, 21*(6), 784–785.

Pavol, M. A., Meyers, C. A., Rexer, J. L., Valentine, A. D., Mattis, P. J., & Talpaz, M. (1995). Pattern of neurobehavioral deficits associated with interferon alfa therapy for leukemia. *Neurology, 45*(5), 947–950.

Perry, W., Carlson, M. D., Barakat, F., et al. (2005). Neuropsychological test performance in patients co-infected with hepatitis C virus and HIV. *AIDS, 19* Suppl 3, S79–84.

Peterson, P. K., Hu, S., Salak-Johnson, J., Molitor, T. W., & Chao, C. C. (1997). Differential production of and migratory response to beta chemokines by human microglia and astrocytes. *J Infect Dis, 175*(2), 478–481.

Radkowski, M., Bednarska, A., Horban, A., et al. (2004). Infection of primary human macrophages with hepatitis C virus in vitro: Induction of tumour necrosis factor-alpha and interleukin 8. *J Gen Virol, 85*(Pt 1), 47–59.

Radkowski, M., Wilkinson, J., Nowicki, M., et al. (2002). Search for hepatitis C virus negative-strand RNA sequences and analysis of viral sequences in the central nervous system: Evidence of replication. *J Virol, 76*(2), 600–608.

Richardson, J. L., Nowicki, M., Danley, K., et al. (2005). Neuropsychological functioning in a cohort of HIV- and hepatitis C virus-infected women. *AIDS, 19*(15), 1659–1667.

Roque Afonso, A. M., Jiang, J., Penin, F., et al. (1999). Nonrandom distribution of hepatitis C virus quasispecies in plasma and peripheral blood mononuclear cell subsets. *J Virol, 73*(11), 9213–9221.

Ryan, E. L., Morgello, S., Isaacs, K., Naseer, M., & Gerits, P. (2004). Neuropsychiatric impact of hepatitis C on advanced HIV. *Neurology, 62*(6), 957–962.

Samuel, M. C., Doherty, P. M., Bulterys, M., & Jenison, S. A. (2001). Association between heroin use, needle sharing and tattoos received in prison with hepatitis B and C positivity among street-recruited injecting drug users in New Mexico, USA. *Epidemiol Infect, 127*(3), 475–484.

Sansonno, D., De Vita, S., Cornacchiulo, V., Carbone, A., Boiocchi, M., & Dammacco, F. (1996). Detection and distribution of hepatitis C virus-related proteins in lymph nodes of patients with type II mixed cryoglobulinemia and neoplastic or non-neoplastic lymphoproliferation. *Blood, 88*(12), 4638–4645.

Shepard, C. W., Finelli, L., & Alter, M. J. (2005). Global epidemiology of hepatitis C virus infection. *Lancet Infect Dis, 5*(9), 558–567.

Shibata, M. & Blatteis, C.M. (1991). Human recombinant tumor necrosis factor and interferon affect the activity of neurons in the organum vasculosum laminae terminalis. *Brain Res, 562*(2), 323–326.

Singh, N., Gayowski, T., Wagener, M. M., & Marino, I. R. (1999). Quality of life, functional status, and depression in male liver transplant recipients with recurrent viral hepatitis C. *Transplantation, 67*(1), 69–72.

Smith, A., Tyrrell, D., Coyle, K., & Higgins, P. (1988). Effects of interferon alpha on performance in man: a preliminary report. *Psychopharmacology (Berl), 96*(3), 414–416.

Sulkowski, M. S., Moore, R. D., Mehta, S. H., Chaisson, R. E., & Thomas, D. L. (2002). Hepatitis C and progression of HIV disease. *JAMA, 288*(2), 199–206.

Taylor-Robinson, S. D. (2001). Applications of magnetic resonance spectroscopy to chronic liver disease. *Clin Med, 1*(1), 54–60.

Taylor, M. J., Letendre, S. L., Schweinsburg, B. C., et al. (2004). Hepatitis C virus infection is associated with reduced white matter N-acetylaspartate in abstinent methamphetamine users. *J Int Neuropsychol Soc, 10*(1), 110–113.

Thomas, D. L. (2002). Hepatitis C and human immunodeficiency virus infection. *Hepatology, 36*(5 Suppl 1), S201–209.

Valentine, A. D., Meyers, C. A., Kling, M. A., Richelson, E., & Hauser, P. (1998). Mood and cognitive side effects of interferon-alpha therapy. *Semin Oncol, 25*(1 Suppl 1), 39–47.

Vargas, H. E., Laskus, T., Radkowski, M., et al. (2002). Detection of hepatitis C virus sequences in brain tissue obtained in recurrent hepatitis C after liver transplantation. *Liver Transpl, 8*(11), 1014–1019.

Verucchi, G., Calza, L., Manfredi, R., & Chiodo, F. (2004). Human immunodeficiency virus and hepatitis C virus coinfection: Epidemiology, natural history, therapeutic options and clinical management. *Infection, 32*(1), 33–46.

von Giesen, H. J., Heintges, T., Abbasi-Boroudjeni, N., et al. (2004). Psychomotor slowing in hepatitis C and HIV infection. *J Acquir Immune Defic Syndr, 35*(2), 131–137.

Weissenborn, K., Krause, J., Bokemeyer, M., et al. (2004). Hepatitis C virus infection affects the brain-evidence from psychometric studies and magnetic resonance spectroscopy. *J Hepatol, 41*(5), 845–851.

Weissenborn, K., Tryc, A. B., Heeren, M., et al. (2009). Hepatitis C virus infection and the brain. *Metab Brain Dis, 24*(1), 197–210.

Wilkinson, J., Radkowski, M., & Laskus, T. (2009). Hepatitis C virus neuroinvasion: Identification of infected cells. *J Virol, 83*(3), 1312–1319.

Wilson, C. J., Finch, C. E., & Cohen, H. J. (2002). Cytokines and cognition—the case for a head-to-toe inflammatory paradigm. *J Am Geriatr Soc, 50*(12), 2041–2056.

Wrona, D. (2006). Neural-immune interactions: An integrative view of the bidirectional relationship between the brain and immune systems. *J Neuroimmunol, 172*(1–2), 38–58.

Zdilar, D., Franco-Bronson, K., Buchler, N., Locala, J. A., & Younossi, Z. M. (2000). Hepatitis C, interferon alfa, and depression. *Hepatology, 31*(6), 1207–1211.

8.9

HIV AND PSYCHIATRIC COMORBIDITIES

Timothy B. Nguyen and Ian Paul Everall

HIV-positive individuals experience higher rates of all categories of mental illness compared to the general population. A wide range of factors may help explain this finding, including factors specific to the sexual minority status of gay men, factors associated with injection drug use, the stress of serious physical illness, and the likelihood that persons with severe mental illness may engage in high-risk sexual or drug-related behavior more frequently than those without mental illness. This chapter discusses the impact of psychiatric disorders and substance abuse on the course of HIV infection and disease. Specific psychiatric disorders covered include major depressive disorder, anxiety disorders, psychotic disorders, mania, and substance abuse, including the abuse of alcohol. The impact of aging is also considered.

INTRODUCTION

By definition, HIV infection is characterized by its comorbid disorders or diseases. Historically, the comorbidities were recognized long before the discovery of HIV. In the early 1980s, the first reported comorbidities were of rare opportunistic infections such as *Pneumocystis carinii* pneumonia and the tumor Kaposi's sarcoma in previously healthy young gay men (Centers for Disease Control, 1981a, 1981b). As the number of unusual infections increased, the collection of these morbidities gained the status of a syndrome called gay-related immune deficiency syndrome (GRID), which was later renamed acquired immune deficiency syndrome (AIDS). The syndrome was identified as affecting the four "H's: homosexuals, hemophiliacs, heroin users, and Haitians (Centers for Disease Control, 1982). In 1983, a retrovirus termed HTLV-III was discovered to be the cause of these unusual and life-threatening opportunistic infections and was renamed HIV.

Beginning in 1996, the advent of highly active antiretroviral therapy (HAART) significantly lowered the morbidity and mortality rate of AIDS and, today, HIV-infected individuals are living far more extended and normalized lives. However, these individuals often suffer from a new set of comorbidities that can drastically reduce the quality of life and efficacy of HIV therapy, and have been described in depth in many chapters of this book. In this chapter, we will concentrate on psychiatric disorders and substance abuse in relation to their impact on the course of HIV infection and disease.

PREVALENCE OF PSYCHIATRIC COMORBIDITIES

Prior to the advent of HAART, individuals living with HIV faced mental health problems related to stigma and the stress of living with falling CD4 counts, the emergence of AIDS-related illnesses, and the prospect of dying. In addition, the bereavement of partners, friends, health, and career/life expectations added to the hardship of living with HIV.

Today, stigmatic issues persist and the HIV community continues to experience high levels of mental illness compared to the general population. Cross-sectional data from two longitudinal and nationally representative samples compare the prevalence of psychiatric disorders of the general U.S. population to the HIV-infected population in Table 8.9.1. Using the fully structured World Mental Health Composite International Diagnostic Interview (CIDI; Kessler & Ustun, 2004), the U.S. National Comorbidity Survey Replication (NCS-R; Kessler, Chiu, Demler, Merikangas, & Walters, 2005) screened 9,282 individuals for DSM-IV disorders between 2001 and 2003 and showed that 26.2% of the general U.S. population suffered from a psychiatric disorder prevalent over 12 months. Screening for the same psychiatric disorders, the HIV Cost and Services Utilization Study (HCSUS; Bing et al., 2001) screened 2,864 HIV+ individuals using the University of Michigan Composite International Diagnostic Interview (UM-CIDI) based on DSM-III and found that 47.9% of their participants suffered from a psychiatric disorder, confirming estimates from earlier smaller scale studies (Atkinson et al., 1988). Although the surveys are separated by four years and are based on slightly different diagnostic criteria, it is clear that the frequency of psychiatric morbidity in the HIV+ population is significantly elevated in all categories.

While the NCS-R and HCSUS are currently the two largest and nationally representative psychiatric surveys to date, a meta-analysis of several smaller studies in multiple settings between 1988 and 1998 reported that the frequency of major depressive disorder (N = 2,596) was twofold higher in HIV+ subjects than in HIV- subjects regardless of symptomatic or state of disease progression (Ciesla & Roberts, 2001). To examine the relationship between HIV and comorbid psychiatric disorders, researchers have investigated several psychosocial, behavioral, and biological domains associated with HIV risk behaviors and disease progression and have identified a growing list of predicting risk factors for HIV and psychiatric illness.

Table 8.9.1 PREVALENCE OF MAJOR PSYCHIATRIC DISORDERS IN THE U.S. GENERAL POPULATION COMPARED TO THE HIV COMMUNITY

PSYCHIATRIC DISORDER	PREVALENCE IN SURVEY POPULATION (%)	
	NCS-R *(N = 9,282)*	*HCSUS* *(N = 2,864)*
Major depressive disorder	6.7	36.0
Dysthymic disorder	1.5	26.5
General anxiety disorder	3.1	15.8
Panic disorder	2.7	10.5
Any drug or alcohol use disorder	10.3	50.1
Any psychiatric disorder	26.2	47.9

Figures of the general US population from Kessler et al., 2005 and those for the HIV+ population from Bing et al., 2001. Abbreviations: NCS-R - US National Comorbidity Survey Replication; HCSUS - HIV Cost and Services Utilization Study

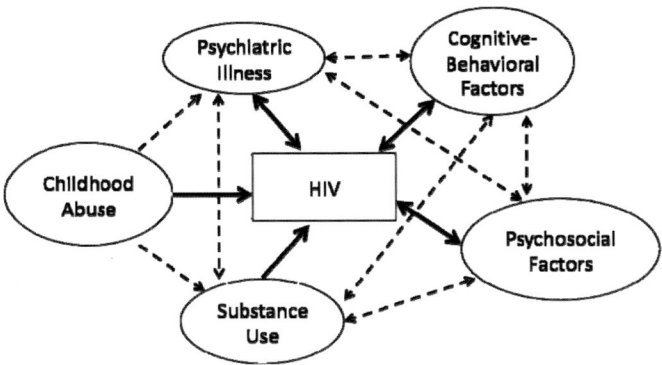

Figure 8.9.1 *Theoretical Model of Various Factors Related to HIV Risk Behavior.* Solid lines represent associations to HIV. Dashed lines represent interrelated associations across different domains. Adapted from Mead and Sikkema, 2005.

RISK FACTORS OF HIV AND PSYCHIATRIC ILLNESS

Men who have sex with men (MSM), substance users, individuals with sexual abuse history, and individuals with preexisting mental illness are populations disproportionately affected by HIV and several correlative factors have been proposed to influence high-risk behaviors among these groups. High-risk behavior such as having unprotected sexual intercourse, multiple/casual sex partners, and injection drug use are the predominant modes of HIV transmission. Figure 8.9.1 illustrates an adapted theoretical model from Meade and Sikkema (2005), linking several interrelated domains to HIV.

Sexual minorities, particularly MSM and self-identified gay and bisexual individuals, represent a population with a unique psychosocial background that continues to have the highest rates of HIV infection despite community-wide safe sex and needle-exchange intervention campaigns (Sullivan et al., 2009). A recent study by Cochran and Mays (2009) surveyed 2,272 adult Californians, including 652 self-identified sexual minorities selected from the California Quality of Life Survey to investigate the associations between sexual orientation, mental health/substance abuse, and HIV infection. The interview consisted of a fully structured computer-assisted telephone interview of several modules of the CIDI-short form, which identifies individuals with a high probability of receiving a 1-year diagnosis of a psychiatric disorder (Kessler, Andrews, Mroczek, Ustun, & Wittchen, 1998). The authors reported that minority sexual orientation was associated with elevated probable rates of affective, anxiety, and substance use disorders (Table 8.9.2).

The survey also showed that HIV+ sexual minorities reported higher rates of probable psychiatric morbidity than

Table 8.9.2 1-YEAR PREVALENCE OF PROBABLE MAJOR PSYCHIATRIC DISORDERS BY SEXUAL ORIENTATION

1-YEAR PROBABLE PSYCHIATRIC DISORDER	EXCLUSIVELY HETEROSEXUAL (N = 2,004) % (SE)	LESBIAN/GAY (N = 150) % (SE)	BISEXUAL (N = 67) % (SE)	HOMOSEXUALLY EXPERIENCED HETEROSEXUAL (N = 51) % (SE)
Major depressive disorder				
Men	8.7 (1.1)	21.5 (3.2)	15.7 (6.0)	30.7 (10.8)
Women	14.4 (1.3)	24.7 (4.6)	35.8 (5.8)	17.9 (6.8)
Generalized anxiety disorder				
Men	5.9 (0.9)	15.4 (2.9)	15.6 (5.9)	15.8 (7.9)
Women	7.6 (0.9)	9.2 (2.9)	20.3 (4.8)	13.3 (6.7)
Panic disorder				
Men	3.0 (0.6)	8.2 (2.2)	4.6 (3.0)	5.5 (4.0)
Women	7.1 (0.9)	8.1 (3.1)	21.2 (5.1)	14.4 (7.0)

(Continued)

Table 8.9.2 (CONTINUED)

1-YEAR PROBABLE PSYCHIATRIC DISORDER	EXCLUSIVELY HETEROSEXUAL (N = 2,004) % (SE)	LESBIAN/GAY (N = 150) % (SE)	BISEXUAL (N = 67) % (SE)	HOMOSEXUALLY EXPERIENCED HETEROSEXUAL (N = 51) % (SE)
Alcohol dependency				
Men	6.3 (0.9)	8.9 (2.2)	13.0 (6.0)	29.2 (11.2)
Women	2.8 (0.6)	4.7 (2.2)	12.8 (4.0)	15.0 (6.3)
Drug dependency				
Men	2.8 (0.6)	4.1 (1.7)	5.6 (3.8)	14.8 (10.6)
Women	1.9 (0.5)	0.3 (0.3)	7.5 (3.0)	6.6 (4.6)
Meets criteria for at least one disorder				
Men	18.2 (1.5)	26.9 (3.7)	36.3 (7.6)	61.8 (12.0)
Women	22.9 (1.5)	27.8 (4.7)	56.2 (6.0)	38.7 (9.8)

From Cochran and Mays, 2009.

those who were HIV- or exclusively heterosexual (Table 8.9.3). This association was especially noticeable for panic disorder, which rose from a frequency of approximately 3% in individuals not known to have HIV infection to 25% in those who reported to have HIV. Similar associations were also found for generalized anxiety and drug dependency disorders. However, it should be noted that HIV status was obtained by self-disclosure and it cannot be excluded that the findings of the HIV+ group are predominantly due to the knowledge of one's status.

Proposed psychosocial factors of sexual minorities that influence psychiatric morbidity and high-risk behavior include theories of harmful anti-gay stigma, discrimination, and victimization (Austin, Roberts, Corliss, & Molnar,

2008; Corliss, Cochran, & Mays, 2002; Mays & Cochran, 2001; Meyer, 2003). Anti-gay discrimination still remains as one of the few socially accepted and institutionally sanctioned forms of prejudice (Viad, 1995). Knowledge of one's sexual orientation develops during early childhood years and, unlike ethnic discrimination, childhood development as a gay or lesbian individual is a unique experience where the formative years developing parental buffers against the stigma is rarely shared by a family that has experienced the same discrimination. As a result, gay youth often develop internalized homophobia by turning the negative beliefs and stereotypes about homosexuality towards themselves and grow up in fear of rejection and alienation. Internalized homophobia has been linked to low self-esteem and

Table 8.9.3 1-YEAR PREVALENCE OF PROBABLE MAJOR PSYCHIATRIC DISORDERS BY SEXUAL ORIENTATION AND DISCLOSED HIV STATUS

Morbidity Indicator		SEXUAL ORIENTATION MINORITY	
	Exclusively Heterosexual (n = 948) % (SE)	*No HIV Infection Reported (n = 127) % (SE)*	*HIV Infection Reported (n = 27) % (SE)*
Major depressive disorder	8.7 (1.1)	18.0 (3.0)	40.2 (7.7)
Generalized anxiety disorder	5.9 (0.9)	13.2 (2.6)	26.4 (7.1)
Panic attack	3.0 (0.6)	3.5 (1.2)	24.8 (6.9)
Alcohol dependency	6.3 (0.9)	13.5 (2.9)	9.5 (5.0)
Drug dependency	2.8 (0.6)	4.9 (2.4)	11.4 (5.3)

From Cochran and Mays, 2009.

depression, maladaptive coping styles, and low social support (Nicholson & Long, 1990; Shidlo, 1994; Turner, Hays, & Coates, 1993). Furthermore, studies of young gay, bisexual, and African-American MSM found that internalized homophobia is associated with risky sexual behavior (Folch, Munoz, Zaragoza, & Casabona, 2009; Herek, 1995; Meyer & Dean, 1998; Stokes & Peterson, 1998). Internalized homophobia has also been found to negatively affect public HIV-prevention interventions, as affected individuals are less likely to respond to campaigns that aim to reduce HIV-related sexual risk behavior (Huebner, Davis, Nemeroff, & Aiken, 2002).

Substance abusers, particularly injecting drug users (IDUs), account substantially to the HIV epidemic. It is estimated that 15.9 million people inject drugs worldwide, 20–40% of them might be HIV+, and that injection drug use is responsible for 30% of HIV infections outside of Africa (Mathers et al., 2008). Cocaine, heroin, and crystal methamphetamine (meth) are common injection drugs that can transmit HIV by needle transmission. Additionally, meth and cocaine use has been shown to indirectly promote HIV transmission by decreasing inhibitions and engaging in impulsive risky sexual behavior (Kjome et al., 2010; Semple, Zians, Grant, & Patterson, 2006). Meth users are more likely to be HIV+, have multiple sex partners, and engage in unprotected sex (Rawson et al., 2008; Semple et al., 2006). Meth is commonly used to enhance sexual desire and its use is increasing among gay men, sex workers, and the HIV+ population (Colfax & Shoptaw, 2005; Shoptaw, 2006; Shoptaw & Reback, 2007). Additionally, there is a strong association with injection drug use and psychological distress, particularly with depression (Bousman et al., 2009).

Persons with severe mental illness have also been reported to be more likely to engage in high-risk sexual behavior, substance abuse, and often report a history of childhood sexual abuse (Meade & Sikkema, 2007). HIV prevalence rates of individuals with mental illness have been estimated to be eight times the U.S. population rate (Rosenberg et al., 2001). Independent of mental illness, individuals with a history of childhood abuse are at direct risk for HIV, as this group has been purported to have sex at an earlier age, have multiple sex partners, and have higher rates of sexually transmitted infections (Arriola, Louden, Doldren, & Fortenberry, 2005).

It is clear that HIV and psychiatric illness involve a complicated heterogeneous relationship between several psychosocial, behavioral, and biological domains and persons who suffer from a combination of risk factors may be at increased risk for HIV compared to those with a single risk factor.

PSYCHIATRIC DISORDERS AND HIV DISEASE

HIV infection crosses the blood-brain barrier early after primary systemic exposure and exhibits deleterious effects on the central nervous system (CNS). While the exact mechanisms continue to be under active investigation, studies investigating the comorbidity of psychiatric disorders have highlighted important aspects of the neuropathology of HIV and of common psychiatric disorders within the HIV+ population.

MAJOR DEPRESSIVE DISORDER

As previously noted, the rate of major depressive disorder (MDD) in the HIV-infected community is significantly elevated compared to the general population. The high rates of MDD may be indicative of either pre-existing MDD, maladaptive coping, the side effects of HAART, a biological mechanism underlying MDD caused by HIV, or a combination of these factors. Atkinson et al. (2008) noted that, of many HIV+ individuals who have MDD, many depressive episodes represent recurrences where the first episode preceded diagnosis of HIV. Maladaptive coping styles, particularly avoidant behavior, have been significantly associated with severity of depression and quality of life (Gore-Felton et al., 2006).

Biological evidence suggests that HIV may exacerbate physiological correlates of MDD related to chronic stress. Compared to controls, individuals with HIV have elevated levels of systemic cortisol, detectable changes in the immune system, and suffer significant cellular changes in the brain. Elevated cortisol is a consistent correlate found in both HIV and MDD patients and clinical studies of patients with MDD have demonstrated reduced metabolic cortisol deactivation (Romer et al., 2009) and higher levels of cortisol in the saliva, plasma, and urine compared to matched healthy controls (Gold, Goodwin, & Chrousos, 1988; Nemeroff & Evans, 1984). Elevated cortisol levels have also been measured in HIV patients (Kumar, Kumar, Waldrop, Antoni, & Eisdorfer, 2003; Kumar et al., 2002) and have been associated with increased viral load and depressed mood (Antoni et al., 2005; Barroso, Burrage, Carlson, & Carlson, 2006).

The consequences of elevated cortisol have been coupled with volumetric brain reductions in the hippocampus (Lupien et al., 1998; McEwen, 1997; Sapolsky, 1996), dysregulation of glucocorticoid signaling and the hypothalamus-pituitary-adrenal axis negative feedback loop (Kumar et al., 2003; Tatro, Everall, Kaul, & Achim, 2009; Webster, Knable, O'Grady, Orthmann, & Weickert, 2002), and a reduction in dendritic length and synaptic number (Tata & Anderson, 2010). Gene expression studies have highlighted alterations of gene pathways involved in stress, neurogenesis, and neurodegeneration related to elevated cortisol and shared by both HIV and MDD. In particular, a gene expression study of autopsy brains have implicated neurotrophic fibroblast growth factors (FGFs), important promoters of neuronal and glial survival and plasticity, to play a role in cellular changes associated with MDD, schizophrenia, and bipolar disorder (Gaughran, Payne, Sedgwick, Cotter, & Berry, 2006). Downregulation of *FGF1* and *FGF2* has been shown in autopsied MDD brains (Evans et al., 2004; Otsuki et al., 2008) and in primary human brain aggregates after chronic cortisol exposure (Salaria et al., 2006). FGF dysregulation has also been detected in autopsied brains of HIV+ patients (Boven et al., 1999) and exogenous addition of *FGF1* has been found to neuroprotect against the HIV envelope protein gp120 in primary human brain cultures

(Everall et al., 2001). In addition to gene expression changes, Tatro et al. (2009) reported that the immunophilin proteins FKBP51 and FKBP52, which regulate cortisol signaling from the cell cytoplasm into the nucleus, are also dysregulated in HIV+ individuals with MDD and that this is accompanied by significant downregulation in the brain of regulatory micro-RNAs, which in turn affect mRNA and subsequent gene protein product production (Tatro, Everall, Masliah, et al., 2009; Tatro et al., 2010). While the exact mechanisms are incompletely understood, these studies suggest that HIV infection in the CNS may alter a host of hormonal, genetic, and cellular regulatory mechanisms that may underlie the etiology and pathogenesis of comorbid MDD.

ANXIETY DISORDERS

While some studies, including the HCSUS, have shown that symptoms of anxiety are elevated among individuals with HIV compared to the general population, there is little evidence to suggest that anxiety is caused by HIV itself. A controlled 2-year longitudinal study using the Structured Clinical Interview for DSM-IV for anxiety disorder of 173 HIV+ homosexual men and 84 HIV- homosexual controls reported that anxiety disorder was related to the symptoms of fatigue and physical dysfunction associated with HIV but found no significant differences in prevalence rates between the groups (Sewell et al., 2000). This suggests that specific persistent anxiety over six months, as outlined by DSM-IV, is not a normative response to HIV but may be a response to a persistent focus on death and mortality when experiencing disease symptoms. Adjustment disorder and posttraumatic stress disorder (PTSD) have also been reported to be elevated among HIV patients as a response to HIV diagnosis (Kelly et al., 1998; Olley, Zeier, Seedat, & Stein, 2005). However, the relationship between acute anxiety and HIV may merely be due to adaptive coping post-diagnosis (Atkinson et al., 2009). Further studies of PTSD in HIV patients stipulate that it is heavily influenced by intense psychosocial stigma (Adewuya et al., 2009) and is more likely to occur in patients with pre-existing psychiatric illness or history of traumatic events (Koopman et al., 2002).

PSYCHOTIC DISORDERS

Psychosis within the HIV population may be due to pre-existing psychotic disorders or HIV itself, with prevalence rates ranging between 0.5%–15% (de Ronchi et al., 2000; Sewell et al., 1994). Individuals with pre-existing mental illness, such as schizophrenia or schizoaffective disorder, are at elevated risk for HIV infection because individuals with these disorders often exhibit poor judgment, high-risk sexual behavior, and engage in substance use (Cournos, McKinnon, & Sullivan, 2005; Dolder, Patterson, & Jeste, 2004). Schizophrenic HIV+ patients exhibit greater morbidity and mortality and have more difficulty engaging and maintaining contact with HIV health care services due to complications related to schizophrenic symptoms (paranoia, delusions, negative symptoms, etc.) which may cause difficulty

complying with medical care, including medication, and explaining their symptoms accurately to physicians (Sewell, 1996).

It has been suggested that the deleterious effects of HIV in the CNS may cause psychotic symptoms, particularly in the later stages of illness with the development of HIV-associated dementia (de Ronchi et al., 2000; Navia & Price, 1987). The development of new-onset psychotic symptoms includes grandiose delusions that may also be accompanied by auditory, visual, and olfactory hallucinations that were not present prior to HIV infection (Sewell et al., 1994). While still unclear, evidence suggests that the pathogenesis of new-onset psychosis may be due to subcortical neurodegeneration, HIV encephalitis, or opportunistic infections (Alciati et al., 2001; Harris, Jeste, Gleghorn, & Sewell, 1991). Unfortunately, the effects of substance abuse, aging, cognitive impairment, and dementia are often confounding variables difficult to control in HIV+ patients presenting with psychosis. Additionally, the antiretroviral drugs such as efavirenz have reported to cause acute psychotic side effects and highlight the need to further investigate the side effects of HAART in relation to neuropsychiatry (Arendt, de Nocker, von Giesen, & Nolting, 2007; de la Garza, Paoletti-Duarte, Garcia-Martin, & Gutierrez-Casares, 2001).

MANIA

Mania, marked by euphoric, impulsive, hypersexual, and irritable/violent behavior, is a risk factor for contracting and transmitting HIV. Mania may present in HIV+ patients as primary pre-existing mania/bipolar disorder or can develop secondarily from the neurotoxic effects of HIV in the CNS. Studies suggest that secondary mania due to HIV may be pathogenically distinct from pre-existing primary mania (Lyketsos et al., 1993; Lyketsos, Schwartz, Fishman, & Treisman, 1997). Table 8.9.4 summarizes the manic symptoms from a recent study comparing 64 HIV- patients with primary mania to 61 HAART-naïve HIV+ patients with secondary mania from Uganda (Nakimuli-Mpungu, Musisi, Mpungu, & Katabira, 2006). The study showed that HIV-related secondary mania presented with more irritable, aggressive, and talkative manic symptoms; higher rates of hallucinations and delusions; and a depressed mean CD4 count of 392 cells/mm^3 compared to 823 cells/mm^3 in controls. Thus, compared to primary mania, secondary mania from HIV may be clinically and immunologically distinct.

AGING

Since 1996, the number of HIV+ patients aged 50 or older has greatly increased with the success of HAART and it is expected that 50% of HIV+ individuals will be in this age group by 2015 (Collaboration, 2008; Kirk & Goetz, 2009). While still under investigation, it seems possible that aging and psychopathology may increase HIV-related morbidity and mortality. Untreated HIV may progress more rapidly in older HIV+ patients due to lower rates of immune reconstitution (Mussini et al., 2008). Elderly HIV+ patients tend to

Table 8.9.4 MANIC SYMPTOMS REPORTED BY 125 PATIENTS PRESENTING WITH PRIMARY MANIA OR HIV-RELATED SECONDARY MANIA IN UGANDA

SYMPTOM	PRIMARY MANIA, HIV- (N = 64) %	SECONDARY MANIA, HIV+ (N = 61) %	P VALUE
Excessive happiness	89.1	36.1	<0.001
Undressing in public	65.6	68.9	0.701
Violent and aggressive behavior	92.2	98.4	0.107
Possessed by spirits	54.7	59	0.625
Paranoid delusions	79.7	91.8	0.05
Visual hallucinations	15.6	93.4	<0.001
Auditory hallucinations	15.6	67.2	<0.001

Adapted from Nakimuli-Mpungu, Musisi, Mpungu, & Katabira, 2006.

have greater numbers of age-related comorbidities and may experience significant side effects of multiple-drug interactions and chronic HAART toxicity from long-term use (Gebo, 2008; Gebo & Justice, 2009; Simone & Appelbaum, 2008). Additionally, older HIV+ patients are more likely to have neurocognitive and psychiatric problems and age may be a significant predictor of HIV-associated neurocognitive disorder (HAND) and the development of HIV-associated dementia (HAD; Becker, Lopez, Dew, & Aizenstein, 2004; Valcour et al., 2004). Recently, Achim et al. (2009) showed that chronic HIV-mediated inflammation in the brain may increase the risk of early brain aging by interfering with the clearance of abnormal protein aggregate amyloid β, which is also found in Alzheimer's and other neurodegenerative diseases, in pyramidal neurons in the frontal cortex of HIV+ patients. HIV+ patients with encephalitis had greater amounts of amyloid β accumulation than HIV+ patients without encephalitis and this suggests that plaques of amyloid β may be biologically linked to worsened cognitive impairment in older HIV+ patients and may share common pathogenic mechanisms with Alzheimer's disease.

ALCOHOL AND SUBSTANCE ABUSE

Alcohol abuse is common among the HIV+ population, with prevalence of up to 50% (Samet, Phillips, Horton, Traphagen, & Freedberg, 2004). While also a predominant risk factor, alcohol is an immunosuppressant and its abuse has been shown to accelerate HIV disease progression. Alcoholics tend to have lower CD4+ cell counts, higher viral loads, and poorer adherence to HAART (Baum et al., 2010; Samet, Horton, Meli, Freedberg, & Palepu, 2004). While alcohol abuse is known to affect the systemic response to HIV infection, the effect of alcohol and HIV in the brain remains unclear. One study of 40 HIV+, 38 alcoholics, and 47 individuals with comorbid HIV and alcoholism showed that the comorbid group exhibited greater episodic memory impairment (Fama, Rosenbloom, Nichols, Pfefferbaum, & Sullivan, 2009). A molecular study of mice co-exposed to the HIV viral protein Tat and ethanol exhibited greater oxidative stress and induction of inflammatory cytokines in the hippocampus and corpus striatum

(Flora et al., 2005). Enhanced neuroinflammation and impaired immune response has also been shown in mice co-exposed to HIV-1 infected monocyte-derived macrophages and ethanol (Potula et al., 2006). These studies demonstrate that alcohol may be a significant synergistic cofactor in the progression of HIV infection in the CNS.

In addition to increasing the risk of transmitting HIV, meth and cocaine abuse contribute to neurocognitive decline in HIV+ individuals. Compared to the general public and HIV+/non-meth users, HIV+/meth users have significantly higher rates of cognitive impairment (Rippeth et al., 2004) and biological evidence supports an exacerbating neurotoxic effect of meth and HIV in the CNS. Proton magnetic resonance spectroscopy has shown significantly diminished levels of the neuronal integrity marker N-acetylaspartate in HIV+/meth users compared to HIV+/non-meth users (Chang, Ernst, Speck, & Grob, 2005) and patients with HAND who used meth suffer greater loss of calbindin-binding inhibitory GABAergic interneurons in the frontal cortex compared to non-meth users, which can exacerbate the neurotoxicity of pyramidal cells in the brain (Chana et al., 2006). Furthermore, gene expression studies from autopsy brain tissue have shown that the interferon-stimulated neuroinflammatory genes STAT-1, IFP35, and ISG15 are further dysregulated by as much as fivefold in HIV+/meth users as compared to HIV+/non-meth users (Everall et al., 2005). Active meth users have higher plasma viral loads when receiving HAART (Ellis et al., 2003), and reduced virologic suppression has been linked to magnetic resonance spectroscopic evidence of compromised neuronal integrity (Taylor et al., 2007). Similarly, longitudinal studies following HIV+ individuals using crack cocaine have shown that cocaine may independently enhance HIV disease progression and predict AIDS-related mortality (Baum et al., 2009; Cook et al., 2008).

CONCLUSION

As presented in this chapter, the comorbidities associated with HIV infection have changed over the decades. The initial life-threatening opportunistic infection are far less common and have been replaced by complex and interconnected comorbidities around challenging behaviors, impulsivity, and personality issues together with mental health problems. Additionally, the prevalence of mental health disorders, drugs, and alcohol use in the HIV+ population pose significant obstacles that are far more challenging for clinicians and health care services to manage and add significantly to the difficulty of treating HIV infection. HIV and psychiatric disorders have a bidirectional relationship and are influenced by significant psychosocial, behavioural, and biological risk factors. It is becoming clear that assessing and addressing these comorbidities is beyond the expertise of traditional HIV physicians and nurses and will probably require a re-engineering of HIV treatment teams that embrace mental health/addiction specialists. The ability to assess and manage behaviors, personality issues, and mental illness will maximize the opportunity of HIV+ patients to engage with health services and adhere to treatment plans. In addition, current research programs are still elucidating the correlation of psychiatric risk factors and biological mechanisms underlying these comorbid pathologies in a manner that will hopefully improve mental health interventions.

REFERENCES

Achim, C. L., Adame, A., Dumaop, W., Everall, I. P., & Masliah, E. (2009). Increased accumulation of intraneuronal amyloid beta in HIV-infected patients. *J Neuroimmune Pharmacol, 4*(2), 190–199.

Adewuya, A. O., Afolabi, M. O., Ola, B. A., Ogundele, O. A., Ajibare, A. O., Oladipo, B. F., et al. (2009). Post-traumatic stress disorder (PTSD) after stigma related events in HIV infected individuals in Nigeria. *Soc Psychiatry Psychiatr Epidemiol, 44*(9), 761–766.

Alciati, A., Fusi, A., D'Arminio Monforte, A., Coen, M., Ferri, A., & Mellado, C. (2001). New-onset delusions and hallucinations in patients infected with HIV. *J Psychiatry Neurosci, 26*(3), 229–234.

Antoni, M. H., Cruess, D. G., Klimas, N., Carrico, A. W., Maher, K., Cruess, S., et al. (2005). Increases in a marker of immune system reconstitution are predated by decreases in 24-h urinary cortisol output and depressed mood during a 10-week stress management intervention in symptomatic HIV-infected men. *J Psychosom Res, 58*(1), 3–13.

Arendt, G., de Nocker, D., von Giesen, H. J., & Nolting, T. (2007). Neuropsychiatric side effects of efavirenz therapy. *Expert Opin Drug Saf, 6*(2), 147–154.

Arriola, K. R., Louden, T., Doldren, M. A., & Fortenberry, R. M. (2005). A meta-analysis of the relationship of child sexual abuse to HIV risk behavior among women. *Child Abuse Negl, 29*(6), 725–746.

Atkinson, J. H., Heaton, R. K., Patterson, T. L., Wolfson, T., Deutsch, R., Brown, S. J., et al. (2008). Two-year prospective study of major depressive disorder in HIV-infected men. *J Affect Disord, 108*(3), 225–234.

Atkinson, J. H., Higgins, J. A., Vigil, O., Dubrow, R., Remien, R. H., Steward, W. T., et al. (2009). Psychiatric context of acute/early HIV infection. The NIMH Multisite Acute HIV Infection Study: IV. *AIDS Behav, 13*(6), 1061–1067.

Atkinson, J. H., Jr., Grant, I., Kennedy, C. J., Richman, D. D., Spector, S. A., & McCutchan, J. A. (1988). Prevalence of psychiatric disorders among men infected with human immunodeficiency virus. A controlled study. *Arch Gen Psychiatry, 45*(9), 859–864.

Austin, S. B., Roberts, A. L., Corliss, H. L., & Molnar, B. E. (2008). Sexual violence victimization history and sexual risk indicators in a community-based urban cohort of "mostly heterosexual" and heterosexual young women. *Am J Public Health, 98*(6), 1015–1020.

Barroso, J., Burrage, J., Carlson, J., & Carlson, B. W. (2006). Salivary cortisol values in HIV-positive people. *J Assoc Nurses AIDS Care, 17*(3), 29–36.

Baum, M. K., Rafie, C., Lai, S., Sales, S., Page, B., & Campa, A. (2009). Crack-cocaine use accelerates HIV disease progression in a cohort of HIV-positive drug users. *J Acquir Immune Defic Syndr, 50*(1), 93–99.

Baum, M. K., Rafie, C., Lai, S., Sales, S., Page, J. B., & Campa, A. (2010). Alcohol use accelerates HIV disease progression. *AIDS Res Hum Retroviruses, 26*(5), 511–518.

Becker, J. T., Lopez, O. L., Dew, M. A., & Aizenstein, H. J. (2004). Prevalence of cognitive disorders differs as a function of age in HIV virus infection. *AIDS, 18 Suppl 1,* S11–18.

Bing, E. G., Burnam, M. A., Longshore, D., Fleishman, J. A., Sherbourne, C. D., London, A. S., et al. (2001). Psychiatric disorders and drug use among human immunodeficiency virus-infected adults in the United States. *Arch Gen Psychiatry, 58*(8), 721–728.

Bousman, C. A., Cherner, M., Ake, C., Letendre, S., Atkinson, J. H., Patterson, T. L., et al. (2009). Negative mood and sexual behavior among non-monogamous men who have sex with men in the context of methamphetamine and HIV. *J Affect Disord, 119*(1–3), 84–91.

Boven, L. A., Middel, J., Portegies, P., Verhoef, J., Jansen, G. H., & Nottet, H. S. (1999). Overexpression of nerve growth factor and basic fibroblast growth factor in AIDS dementia complex. *J Neuroimmunol, 97*(1–2), 154–162.

Centers for Disease Control. (1981a). Kaposi's sarcoma and pneumocystis pneumonia—New York City and California. *Morbidity and Mortality Weekly Report, 30,* 305–308.

Centers for Disease Control. (1981b). Pneumocystis pneumonia—Los Angeles. *Morbidity and Mortality Weekly Report, 30,* 250–252.

Centers for Disease Control. (1982). Current Trends Update on acquired immune deficiency syndrome (AIDS) - United States. *MMWR, 31*(37), 507–508,513–514.

Chana, G., Everall, I. P., Crews, L., Langford, D., Adame, A., Grant, I., et al. (2006). Cognitive deficits and degeneration of interneurons in HIV+ methamphetamine users. *Neurology, 67*(8), 1486–1489.

Chang, L., Ernst, T., Speck, O., & Grob, C. S. (2005). Additive effects of HIV and chronic methamphetamine use on brain metabolite abnormalities. *Am J Psychiatry, 162*(2), 361–369.

Ciesla, J. A. & Roberts, J. E. (2001). Meta-analysis of the relationship between HIV infection and risk for depressive disorders. *Am J Psychiatry, 158*(5), 725–730.

Cochran, S. D. & Mays, V. M. (2009). Burden of psychiatric morbidity among lesbian, gay, and bisexual individuals in the California Quality of Life Survey. *J Abnorm Psychol, 118*(3), 647–658.

Colfax, G. & Shoptaw, S. (2005). The methamphetamine epidemic: Implications for HIV prevention and treatment. *Curr HIV/AIDS Rep, 2*(4), 194–199.

Collaboration, T. A. T. C. (2008). Life expectancy of individuals on combination antiretroviral therapy in high-income countries: A collaborative analysis of 14 cohort studies. *Lancet, 372*(9635), 293–299.

Cook, J. A., Burke-Miller, J. K., Cohen, M. H., Cook, R. L., Vlahov, D., Wilson, T. E., et al. (2008). Crack cocaine, disease progression, and mortality in a multicenter cohort of HIV-1 positive women. *AIDS, 22*(11), 1355–1363.

Corliss, H. L., Cochran, S. D., & Mays, V. M. (2002). Reports of parental maltreatment during childhood in a United States population-based survey of homosexual, bisexual, and heterosexual adults. *Child Abuse Negl, 26*(11), 1165–1178.

Cournos, F., McKinnon, K., & Sullivan, G. (2005). Schizophrenia and comorbid human immunodeficiency virus or hepatitis C virus. *J Clin Psychiatry, 66 Suppl 6,* 27–33.

de la Garza, C. L., Paoletti-Duarte, S., Garcia-Martin, C., & Gutierrez-Casares, J. R. (2001). Efavirenz-induced psychosis. *AIDS, 15*(14), 1911–1912.

de Ronchi, D., Faranca, I., Forti, P., Ravaglia, G., Borderi, M., Manfredi, R., et al. (2000). Development of acute psychotic disorders and HIV-1 infection. *Int J Psychiatry Med, 30*(2), 173–183.

Dolder, C. R., Patterson, T. L., & Jeste, D. V. (2004). HIV, psychosis and aging: past, present and future. *AIDS, 18 Suppl 1*, S35–42.

Ellis, R. J., Childers, M. E., Cherner, M., Lazzaretto, D., Letendre, S., & Grant, I. (2003). Increased human immunodeficiency virus loads in active methamphetamine users are explained by reduced effectiveness of antiretroviral therapy. *J Infect Dis, 188*(12), 1820–1826.

Evans, S. J., Choudary, P. V., Neal, C. R., Li, J. Z., Vawter, M. P., Tomita, H., et al. (2004). Dysregulation of the fibroblast growth factor system in major depression. *Proc Natl Acad Sci U S A, 101*(43), 15506–15511.

Everall, I. P., Salaria, S., Roberts, E., Corbeil, J., Sasik, R., Fox, H., et al. (2005). Methamphetamine stimulates interferon inducible genes in HIV infected brain. *J Neuroimmunol, 170*(1–2), 158–171.

Everall, I. P., Trillo-Pazos, G., Bell, C., Mallory, M., Sanders, V., & Masliah, E. (2001). Amelioration of neurotoxic effects of HIV envelope protein gp120 by fibroblast growth factor: A strategy for neuroprotection. *J Neuropathol Exp Neurol, 60*(3), 293–301.

Fama, R., Rosenbloom, M. J., Nichols, B. N., Pfefferbaum, A., & Sullivan, E. V. (2009). Working and episodic memory in HIV infection, alcoholism, and their comorbidity: baseline and 1-year follow-up examinations. *Alcohol Clin Exp Res, 33*(10), 1815–1824.

Flora, G., Pu, H., Lee, Y. W., Ravikumar, R., Nath, A., Hennig, B., et al. (2005). Proinflammatory synergism of ethanol and HIV-1 Tat protein in brain tissue. *Exp Neurol, 191*(1), 2–12.

Folch, C., Munoz, R., Zaragoza, K., & Casabona, J. (2009). Sexual risk behaviour and its determinants among men who have sex with men in Catalonia, Spain. *Euro Surveill, 14*(47).

Gaughran, F., Payne, J., Sedgwick, P. M., Cotter, D., & Berry, M. (2006). Hippocampal FGF-2 and FGFR1 mRNA expression in major depression, schizophrenia and bipolar disorder. *Brain Res Bull, 70*(3), 221–227.

Gebo, K. A. (2008). Epidemiology of HIV and response to antiretroviral therapy in the middle aged and elderly. *Aging health, 4*(6), 615–627.

Gebo, K. A. & Justice, A. (2009). HIV infection in the elderly. *Curr Infect Dis Rep, 11*(3), 246–254.

Gold, P. W., Goodwin, F. K., & Chrousos, G. P. (1988). Clinical and biochemical manifestations of depression. Relation to the neurobiology of stress (2). *N Engl J Med, 319*(7), 413–420.

Gore-Felton, C., Koopman, C., Spiegel, D., Vosvick, M., Brondino, M., & Winningham, A. (2006). Effects of quality of life and coping on depression among adults living with HIV/AIDS. *J Health Psychol, 11*(5), 711–729.

Harris, M. J., Jeste, D. V., Gleghorn, A., & Sewell, D. D. (1991). New-onset psychosis in HIV-infected patients. *J Clin Psychiatry, 52*(9), 369–376.

Herek, G. G. & Glunt, E.K. (1995). Identity and community among gay and bisexual men in the AIDS era: Preliminary findings from the Sacramento Men's Health Study. In G. M. Herek, Greene, B. (Ed.), *Psychological perspectives on lesbian and gay Issues: AIDS, identity and community: The HIV epidemic and lesbian and gay men*. Thousand Oaks, CA: Sage.

Huebner, D. M., Davis, M. C., Nemeroff, C. J., & Aiken, L. S. (2002). The impact of internalized homophobia on HIV preventive interventions. *Am J Community Psychol, 30*(3), 327–348.

Kelly, B., Raphael, B., Judd, F., Perdices, M., Kernutt, G., Burnett, P., et al. (1998). Posttraumatic stress disorder in response to HIV infection. *Gen Hosp Psychiatry, 20*(6), 345–352.

Kessler, R. C., Andrews, G., Mroczek, D., Ustun, B., & Wittchen, H. (1998). The World Health Organization Composite International Diagnostic Interview Short-Form (CIDI-SF). *Int J Methods Psychiatr Res, 7*, 171–185.

Kessler, R. C., Chiu, W. T., Demler, O., Merikangas, K. R., & Walters, E. E. (2005). Prevalence, severity, and comorbidity of 12-month DSM-IV disorders in the National Comorbidity Survey Replication. *Arch Gen Psychiatry, 62*(6), 617–627.

Kessler, R. C., & Ustun, T. B. (2004). The World Mental Health (WMH) Survey Initiative Version of the World Health Organization (WHO) Composite International Diagnostic Interview (CIDI). *Int J Methods Psychiatr Res, 13*(2), 93–121.

Kirk, J. B. & Goetz, M. B. (2009). Human immunodeficiency virus in an aging population, A complication of success. *J Am Geriatr Soc, 57*(11), 2129–2138.

Kjome, K. L., Lane, S. D., Schmitz, J. M., Green, C., Ma, L., Prasla, I., et al. (2010). Relationship between impulsivity and decision making in cocaine dependence. *Psychiatry Res, 178*(2), 299–304.

Koopman, C., Gore-Felton, C., Azimi, N., O'Shea, K., Ashton, E., Power, R., et al. (2002). Acute stress reactions to recent life events among women and men living with HIV/AIDS. *Int J Psychiatry Med, 32*(4), 361–378.

Kumar, M., Kumar, A. M., Waldrop, D., Antoni, M. H., & Eisdorfer, C. (2003). HIV-1 infection and its impact on the HPA axis, cytokines, and cognition. *Stress, 6*(3), 167–172.

Kumar, M., Kumar, A. M., Waldrop, D., Antoni, M. H., Schneiderman, N., & Eisdorfer, C. (2002). The HPA axis in HIV-1 infection. *J Acquir Immune Defic Syndr, 31 Suppl 2*, S89–93.

Lupien, S. J., de Leon, M., de Santi, S., Convit, A., Tarshish, C., Nair, N. P., et al. (1998). Cortisol levels during human aging predict hippocampal atrophy and memory deficits. *Nat Neurosci, 1*(1), 69–73.

Lyketsos, C. G., Hanson, A. L., Fishman, M., Rosenblatt, A., McHugh, P. R., & Treisman, G. J. (1993). Manic syndrome early and late in the course of HIV. *Am J Psychiatry, 150*(2), 326–327.

Lyketsos, C. G., Schwartz, J., Fishman, M., & Treisman, G. (1997). AIDS mania. *J Neuropsychiatry Clin Neurosci, 9*(2), 277–279.

Mathers, B. M., Degenhardt, L., Phillips, B., Wiessing, L., Hickman, M., Strathdee, S. A., et al. (2008). Global epidemiology of injecting drug use and HIV among people who inject drugs: A systematic review. *Lancet, 372*(9651), 1733–1745.

Mays, V. M. & Cochran, S. D. (2001). Mental health correlates of perceived discrimination among lesbian, gay, and bisexual adults in the United States. *Am J Public Health, 91*(11), 1869–1876.

McEwen, B. S. (1997). Possible mechanisms for atrophy of the human hippocampus. *Mol Psychiatry, 2*(3), 255–262.

Meade, C. S. & Sikkema, K. J. (2005). HIV risk behavior among adults with severe mental illness: A systematic review. *Clin Psychol Rev, 25*(4), 433–457.

Meade, C. S., & Sikkema, K. J. (2007). Psychiatric and psychosocial correlates of sexual risk behavior among adults with severe mental illness. *Community Ment Health J, 43*(2), 153–169.

Meyer, I. H. (2003). Prejudice, social stress, and mental health in lesbian, gay, and bisexual populations: Conceptual issues and research evidence. *Psychol Bull, 129*(5), 674–697.

Meyer, I. H. & Dean, L. (1998). Internalized homophobia, intimacy, and sexual behavior among gay and bisexual men. In G. M. Herek (Ed.), *Stigma and sexual orientation: Understanding prejudice against lesbians, gay men and bisexuals*. Thousand oaks, CA: Sage.

Mussini, C., Manzardo, C., Johnson, M., Monforte, A., Uberti-Foppa, C., Antinori, A., et al. (2008). Patients presenting with AIDS in the HAART era: A collaborative cohort analysis. *AIDS, 22*(18), 2461–2469.

Nakimuli-Mpungu, E., Musisi, S., Mpungu, S. K., & Katabira, E. (2006). Primary mania versus HIV-related secondary mania in Uganda. *Am J Psychiatry, 163*(8), 1349–1354; quiz 1480.

Navia, B. A. & Price, R. W. (1987). The acquired immunodeficiency syndrome dementia complex as the presenting or sole manifestation of human immunodeficiency virus infection. *Arch Neurol, 44*(1), 65–69.

Nemeroff, C. B. & Evans, D. L. (1984). Correlation between the dexamethasone suppression test in depressed patients and clinical response. *Am J Psychiatry, 141*(2), 247–249.

Nicholson, W. D. & Long, B. C. (1990). Self-esteem, social support, internalized homophobia, and coping strategies of HIV+ gay men. *J Consult Clin Psychol, 58*(6), 873–876.

Olley, B. O., Zeier, M. D., Seedat, S., & Stein, D. J. (2005). Post-traumatic stress disorder among recently diagnosed patients with HIV/AIDS in South Africa. *AIDS Care, 17*(5), 550–557.

Otsuki, K., Uchida, S., Watanuki, T., Wakabayashi, Y., Fujimoto, M., Matsubara, T., et al. (2008). Altered expression of neurotrophic factors in patients with major depression. *J Psychiatr Res, 42*(14), 1145–1153.

Potula, R., Haorah, J., Knipe, B., Leibhart, J., Chrastil, J., Heilman, D., et al. (2006). Alcohol abuse enhances neuroinflammation and impairs immune responses in an animal model of human immunodeficiency virus-1 encephalitis. *Am J Pathol, 168*(4), 1335–1344.

Rawson, R. A., Gonzales, R., Pearce, V., Ang, A., Marinelli-Casey, P., & Brummer, J. (2008). Methamphetamine dependence and human immunodeficiency virus risk behavior. *J Subst Abuse Treat, 35*(3), 279–284.

Rippeth, J. D., Heaton, R. K., Carey, C. L., Marcotte, T. D., Moore, D. J., Gonzalez, R., et al. (2004). Methamphetamine dependence increases risk of neuropsychological impairment in HIV-infected persons. *J Int Neuropsychol Soc, 10*(1), 1–14.

Romer, B., Lewicka, S., Kopf, D., Lederbogen, F., Hamann, B., Gilles, M., et al. (2009). Cortisol metabolism in depressed patients and healthy controls. *Neuroendocrinology, 90*(3), 301–306.

Rosenberg, S. D., Goodman, L. A., Osher, F. C., Swartz, M. S., Essock, S. M., Butterfield, M. I., et al. (2001). Prevalence of HIV, hepatitis B, and hepatitis C in people with severe mental illness. *Am J Public Health, 91*(1), 31–37.

Salaria, S., Chana, G., Caldara, F., Feltrin, E., Altieri, M., Faggioni, F., et al. (2006). Microarray analysis of cultured human brain aggregates following cortisol exposure: Implications for cellular functions relevant to mood disorders. *Neurobiol Dis, 23*(3), 630–636.

Samet, J. H., Horton, N. J., Meli, S., Freedberg, K. A., & Palepu, A. (2004). Alcohol consumption and antiretroviral adherence among HIV-infected persons with alcohol problems. *Alcohol Clin Exp Res, 28*(4), 572–577.

Samet, J. H., Phillips, S. J., Horton, N. J., Traphagen, E. T., & Freedberg, K. A. (2004). Detecting alcohol problems in HIV-infected patients: use of the CAGE questionnaire. *AIDS Res Hum Retroviruses, 20*(2), 151–155.

Sapolsky, R. M. (1996). Why stress is bad for your brain. *Science, 273*(5276), 749–750.

Semple, S. J., Zians, J., Grant, I., & Patterson, T. L. (2006). Methamphetamine use, impulsivity, and sexual risk behavior among HIV-positive men who have sex with men. *J Addict Dis, 25*(4), 105–114.

Sewell, D. D. (1996). Schizophrenia and HIV. *Schizophr Bull, 22*(3), 465–473.

Sewell, D. D., Jeste, D. V., Atkinson, J. H., Heaton, R. K., Hesselink, J. R., Wiley, C., et al. (1994). HIV-associated psychosis: A study of 20 cases. San Diego HIV Neurobehavioral Research Center Group. *Am J Psychiatry, 151*(2), 237–242.

Sewell, M. C., Goggin, K. J., Rabkin, J. G., Ferrando, S. J., McElhiney, M. C., & Evans, S. (2000). Anxiety syndromes and symptoms among men with AIDS: A longitudinal controlled study. *Psychosomatics, 41*(4), 294–300.

Shidlo, A. (1994). Internalized homophobia: Conceptual and empirical issues in measurement. In B. Greene & G. M. Herek, (Eds.). *Lesbian and gay psychology: Theory, research and clinical applications.* Thousand Oaks, CA: Sage.

Shoptaw, S. (2006). Methamphetamine use in urban gay and bisexual populations. *Top HIV Med, 14*(2), 84–87.

Shoptaw, S. & Reback, C. J. (2007). Methamphetamine use and infectious disease-related behaviors in men who have sex with men: Implications for interventions. *Addiction, 102 Suppl 1*, 130–135.

Simone, M. J. & Appelbaum, J. (2008). HIV in older adults. *Geriatrics, 63*(12), 6–12.

Stokes, J. P., & Peterson, J. L. (1998). Homophobia, self-esteem, and risk for HIV among African American men who have sex with men. *AIDS Educ Prev, 10*(3), 278–292.

Sullivan, P. S., Hamouda, O., Delpech, V., Geduld, J. E., Prejean, J., Semaille, C., et al. (2009). Reemergence of the HIV epidemic among men who have sex with men in North America, Western Europe, and Australia, 1996–2005. *Ann Epidemiol, 19*(6), 423–431.

Tata, D. A. & Anderson, B. J. (2010). The effects of chronic glucocorticoid exposure on dendritic length, synapse numbers and glial volume in animal models: Implications for hippocampal volume reductions in depression. *Physiol Behav, 99*(2), 186–193.

Tatro, E. T., Everall, I. P., Kaul, M., & Achim, C. L. (2009). Modulation of glucocorticoid receptor nuclear translocation in neurons by immunophilins FKBP51 and FKBP52: Implications for major depressive disorder. *Brain Res, 1286*, 1–12.

Tatro, E. T., Everall, I. P., Masliah, E., Hult, B. J., Lucero, G., Chana, G., et al. (2009). Differential expression of immunophilins FKBP51 and FKBP52 in the frontal cortex of HIV-infected patients with major depressive disorder. *J Neuroimmune Pharmacol, 4*(2), 218–226.

Tatro, E. T., Scott, E. R., Nguyen, T. B., Salaria, S., Banerjee, S., Moore, D. J., et al. (2010). Evidence for Alteration of Gene Regulatory Networks through MicroRNAs of the HIV-infected brain: Novel analysis of retrospective cases. *PLoS One, 5*(4), e10337.

Taylor, M. J., Schweinsburg, B. C., Alhassoon, O. M., Gongvatana, A., Brown, G. G., Young-Casey, C., et al. (2007). Effects of human immunodeficiency virus and methamphetamine on cerebral metabolites measured with magnetic resonance spectroscopy. *J Neurovirol, 13*(2), 150–159.

Turner, H. A., Hays, R. B., & Coates, T. J. (1993). Determinants of social support among gay men: The context of AIDS. *J Health Soc Behav, 34*(1), 37–53.

Valcour, V., Shikuma, C., Shiramizu, B., Watters, M., Poff, P., Selnes, O., et al. (2004). Higher frequency of dementia in older HIV-1 individuals: the Hawaii Aging with HIV-1 Cohort. *Neurology, 63*(5), 822–827.

Viad, U. (1995). *Virtual equality: The mainstreaming of gay & lesbian liberation.* New York: Doubleday.

Webster, M. J., Knable, M. B., O'Grady, J., Orthmann, J., & Weickert, C. S. (2002). Regional specificity of brain glucocorticoid receptor mRNA alterations in subjects with schizophrenia and mood disorders. *Mol Psychiatry, 7*(9), 985–994, 924.

SECTION 9

DIAGNOSTICS AND BIOMARKERS

Igor Grant

9.1

BIOIMAGING

Linda Chang, Ute Feger, and Thomas M. Ernst

Many neuroimaging studies have evaluated changes in brain structure and function in patients with HIV-associated brain disorders. Most of these were conducted to assess the neuroanatomical or neurophysiological substrates underlying the HIV-associated neurocognitive disorder (HAND). The ultimate goal of these neuroimaging studies was to improve the understanding of common cognitive deficits in HIV patients, such as deficits in sustained attention, mental flexibility, motor function, speed of information processing, short-term and working memory, executive function, and verbal fluency. In this chapter, we review and discuss early neuroimaging studies using computed tomography (CT) and other techniques that involve ionizing radiation, such as single-photon emission computed tomography (SPECT) and positron emission tomography (PET). We also review functional magnetic resonance imaging (MRI) studies, specifically perfusion MRI and BOLD-fMRI (blood oxygenation level dependent-functional MRI), and magnetic resonance spectroscopy (MRS) studies, in both HAND- and HIV-neuroasymptomatic individuals. We also propose future directions for the application of these techniques to improve our understanding of the pathophysiology of HIV-associated brain injury and for use in the monitoring of treatment.

Numerous neuroimaging studies have evaluated changes in the brain structure and function in HIV-associated brain disorders. The majority of these studies were conducted to assess the neuroanatomical or neurophysiological substrate underlying the HIV-associated neurocognitive disorder (HAND). The ultimate goal of these neuroimaging studies was to improve the understanding of common cognitive deficits in HIV patients such as decreased sustained attention, mental flexibility, motor function, speed of information processing, short-term and working memory, executive function, and verbal fluency. Earlier in the AIDS epidemic, many structural and functional neuroimaging studies also evaluated opportunistic brain lesions, which have become much less common in the United States and the developed countries since the introduction of highly active antiretroviral therapy (HAART).

Structural imaging studies such as CT and MRI are widely used clinically to evaluate HIV patients who develop neurological symptoms. CT, in particular, was applied to early studies of children infected with HIV when MRI was considered higher risk due to the need for sedation. However, structural MRI is generally much more sensitive and specific than CT in assessing brain abnormalities. Furthermore, functional or physiological neuroimaging techniques may be even more sensitive and can provide objective and noninvasive surrogate markers to monitor the severity of brain injury, as well as the effects of treatments, even when structural imaging scans are read as normal by clinicians.

Various nuclear medicine techniques, such as SPECT and PET also have been applied to evaluate HIV dementia. SPECT studies evaluated changes in cerebral blood flow (Shielke et al., 1990; Holman et al., 1992; Sacktor et al., 1995; Christensson et al., 1999), while PET studies evaluated cerebral glucose metabolism (Rottenberg et al., 1987; Rottenberg et al., 1996; Villemagne et al., 1996) or specific receptors, such as those that bind to dopamine transporters, microglia and fibrillary amyloid in the brain. Both blood flow and metabolism are thought to reflect underlying brain function. Nuclear medicine techniques, however, involve radiation and therefore have limited use for monitoring progression of disease or treatment effects when repeat measurements are necessary.

Several magnetic resonance (MR) techniques, including perfusion MRI (pMRI) and blood oxygenation level dependent-functional MR imaging (BOLD-fMRI), and MR spectroscopy (MRS) do not involve ionizing radiation and are widely available commercially. Therefore, they are particularly useful for clinical applications and for monitoring treatment effects. Phosphorous (^{31}P) and proton (^{1}H) MRS have also been applied to study brain chemical changes associated with HIV. While ^{1}H MRS has been used in over 40 clinical studies of HIV-associated brain injury as well as opportunistic infections or neoplasms in patients with AIDS, only a few studies have applied ^{31}P MRS to evaluate the high-energy phosphate metabolism in HIV-associated dementia. Since most functional MRI techniques were developed over the past 10–15 years, many technical issues are still being improved and evaluated, and fewer studies have used functional MRI to evaluate HIV brain injury.

We will review and discuss the early neuroimaging studies using CT and other neuroimaging techniques that involve ionizing radiation, such as SPECT and PET. In addition, we will review functional MRI studies, specifically perfusion MRI and BOLD-fMRI, and MRS studies, in both HAND- and HIV-neuroasymptomatic individuals. We also propose future directions for the application of these studies to improve our understanding of the pathophysiology of HIV-associated brain injury and for treatment monitoring.

COMPUTER TOMOGRAPHY STUDIES IN HIV-INFECTED CHILDREN AND ADULTS

Computer tomography (CT), also known as computed axial tomography (CAT) is an imaging method widely used in the clinical and emergency room settings. CT uses x-ray images and digital geometry to produce 2-dimensional cross-sectional or 3-D reconstructed images of body parts, such as the head. When compared to other imaging modalities, CT is usually more readily available, faster, less expensive, and less likely to require a person to be sedated or anesthetized. In children, sedation or anesthesia is typically needed for MRI scans, which are more susceptible to motion artifacts; therefore, CT has been used to study the effects of HIV in the brains of children infected with the virus.

The majority of children infected with HIV acquired the virus through vertical transmission from their mothers, primarily from exposure at the time of birth. The incidence for vertical transmission of HIV has declined by two-thirds after the introduction of zidovudine (ZDV) prophylaxis during the perinatal period (Fiscus et al., 1996), and is extremely rare now in the United States due to the prophylactic treatments of the infected mothers during pregnancy and at birth. However, the incidence of HIV encephalopathy in infants born to HIV-positive mothers in developing countries remains high. Worldwide, there is a large cohort of perinatally HIV-infected children, with 2.1 million infected children currently under 15 years of age and 430,000 newly infected infants each year. Most of the CT studies evaluated HIV-infected children between ages 1 month to 13 years at

Table 9.1.1 HEAD CT STUDIES OF HIV-INFECTED INDIVIDUALS

REFERENCE	SUBJECTS	MEDICATION	FINDINGS
CT Studies in HIV-Infected Children			
Tahan et al., *Brazil J Infect Dis* 2007	88 HIV-infected children 84 HIV-exposed but seronegative (ages 1-36 months)	Not specified	82% of HIV-infected children had neurological alterations, but only 45 (55%) had head CT, and 10% with abnormal scans (calcification of basal ganglia in one, others had cerebral atrophy)
Martin et al., *Dev Neuropsychol* 2006	41 HIV-infected children (ages 6-16 years)	≥1yr of HAART	20 (50%) with minimal to moderately abnormal scans on a 100 mm VAS (DeCarli, 1993: white matter abnormalities, intra cerebral calcifications, ventricular enlargement, subarachnoid dilatation). Children with abnormal CTs had low averaged FSIQ and poorer executive function, but those with normal CT had normal IQs and cognitive function
Rotta et al., *J Tropical Pediatrics* 2003	24 HIV+children (live) 13 had CT 25 HIV+children (dead) 18 had CT (live children ages > 9 years)	All live HIV+ children were on ART	2 (15%) of the live children and 12 (66%) of the dead children had altered cranial CT scans (78% had cortical atrophy; 22% calcification in basal ganglia)
Blanchette et al., *Dev Neuropsychol* 2002	14 HIV children with vertical transmission (2 asymptomatic, 8 mildly symptomatic, and 4 AIDS) 11 controls (6.3–14.2 years)	12 HIV subjects were on ART (3 on NRTI+PI, 9 on NRTI combinations)	50% of patients showed brain abnormalities, including brain atrophy (n = 1), calcification (n = 1), ventricular enlargement (n = 4), white matter abnormalities (n = 5). HIV-infected children had normal cognitive performance, but slower on finger tapping and less strong on hand dynamometer. Those with CT abnormalities tended to show worse performance on visual spatial skills.
Brouwers et al., *J NeuroVirol* 2000	39 HIV symptomatic children age 0.5 and 13yr (34 with vertical transmission)	Not specified (children were enrolled in clinical trials)	Severity of cortical atrophy correlated with CSF but not plasma HIV RNA copies.
Wolters et al., *Pedeatrics* 1995	36 HIV-infected children (ages 5.5, 1-10 years) with (n = 15) and without encephalopathy (n = 21); 34 had CT 20 uninfected siblings	Before treatment	All children with encephalopathy had at least one CT abnormality (mild to severe atrophy; White Matter hypodensity, calcification of basal ganglia); 73% of non-encephalopathic children had some CT abnormalities (minimal cortical atrophy); HIV children with encephalopathy had lower language scores than non-encephalitic children; abnormality score on CT correlated with poorer performance on language scores.
DeCarli et al., *Ann Neurol* 1993	83 HIV-infected children (ages 4.8 +/-4 years, 54 with and 29 without encephalopathy)	Not specified (children were enrolled in clinical trials)	86% had abnormal ratings (ventricular enlargement, cortical atrophy, leukoariosis, cerebral calcification). Those with encephalopathy had 2–3 times higher severity scores for each of these abnormalities than non-encephalopathic patients. All patients with calcifications had encephalopathy.

(Continued)

Table 9.1.1 (CONTINUED)

REFERENCE	SUBJECTS	MEDICATION	FINDINGS
	CT Studies in HIV-Infected Adults		
Davis et al., *AJNR 2007*	82 AIDS Patients with systemic non-Hodgkin lymphoma (ages: mean 43, 23–77 years)	31 no ART 52 on ART	The presence of malignant cells in CSF (n = 17) had worse survival, but menningeal enhancements (n = 3) or brain lesions (n = 7) on CT did not show difference in survival (or improved diagnosis).
Graham et al., *AJNR* 2007	178 HIV patients with uncomplicated headaches had 204 CT scans with and without contrast	Not specified	76 of 204 scans (37.3%) were positive; of these, 58 (76.3%) had atrophy, and 18 (23.8%) had mass lesions and white matter lesions. All cases with mass lesions and white matter lesions had CD4 <200 cells/uL.
Korbo et al., *Neuroradiol* 2002	13 HIV+IC (CD4 >400 cells/uL) 19 HIV+ID (CD4<400 cells/uL) 44 seronegative controls	28 treated with AZT	Ventricle size: HIV+ID (27, 8-80 mL) > HIV+IC (23, 10-72 mL) > SN controls (15, 6-54 mL). On follow-up CT scans (2-6 scans), time dependent increase of ventricle size seen in HIV+IC but not in HIV+ID group.
Brightbill et al., *AJNR* 1995	35 Patients with documented neurosyphillis (32 HIV+ and 3 HIV-)	Not specified	11 of 35 (31%) had normal CT, 8(23%) had cerebral infarction, 7(20%) had non-specific white matter lesions, 2(6%) had cerebral gummas & meningitis
Whiteman et al., *Radiology* 1993	47 HIV patients with pathologically documented progressive multileukoencephalopathy (PML)	Not mentioned but primarily pre-ART	36 CT and 29 MR scans were performed in these 47 patients. Lesions were hypoattenuated on CT but hyperintense on T2-weighted MR scans, and were located in the periventricular and subcortical white matter. MRI demonstrated greater sensitivity than CT for detecting the extent and number of lesions.

time of study. However, more recent neuroimaging studies of children with HIV infection rely on MR techniques (see MRS studies below).

Studies in the pre-HAART area showed CNS abnormalities in 70–80% of HIV-infected children, reaching up to 100% when diagnosed with encephalopathy (Wolters et al., 1995) (Table 9.1.1). Typical findings on cranial CT include the most commonly seen ventricular dilatation and cortical atrophy, followed by hypodensities and calcifications in the basal ganglia (Wolters et al., 1995; DeCarli et al., 1993). Children with HIV encephalopathy also had poorer language scores when compared to those without encephalopathy (Wolters et al., 1995). In the pre-HAART era, the extent of cortical atrophy, but not calcification of the basal ganglia, correlated with the amount of viral RNA present in the cerebrospinal fluid, indicating that different neuropathic processes might be responsible for basal ganglia lesions (Brouwers et al., 2000). More recent studies in children treated with antiretroviral medications did not find correlations between cranial CT abnormalities and HIV viral load (Lazareff et al., 1996). Furthermore, a higher percentage of HIV-infected children, age 1–3 years, exhibited alterations in neurodevelopment, especially in psychomotor functioning when compared to age-matched HIV-seronegative children, but CT abnormalities did not always coincide with the cognitive findings (Tahan et al., 2006). Therefore, the sensitivity and specificity of CT for detecting brain injury associated with HIV is limited.

In a more recent study of HIV-infected children treated with antiretroviral medication (ages 6–12), only half of the children exhibited CNS abnormalities similar to those typically observed in untreated children, including brain atrophy, ventricle enlargement, and basal ganglia calcification. ART-treated HIV-positive children with CNS abnormalities suffered from poorer neurodevelopment and cognitive deficits, especially in executive functioning (Martin et al., 2006). These findings confirmed earlier results by Blanchette et al. who also found 50% abnormal brain CT scans and poorer performance on tasks involving visual–motor and visual–spatial processing in a group of HIV-infected ART-treated children in the same age range (Blanchette et al., 2002). HIV-infected children in a Brazilian cohort, age 9 years and older, with ART treatment for about 5 years, also showed a higher frequency of CT abnormalities (78%), and similar findings of cortical atrophy and basal ganglia calcification were observed. Neurological symptoms such as delayed psychomotor development and acute encephalitis were also reported. The higher incidence of CNS alterations in the CT scans might be due to lack of ART in the early years of the infection (Rotta et al., 2003).

Only few studies used CT to study HIV-infected adults, and many of these studies were conducted retrospectively in individuals who had CT as a screening tool for neurological symptoms (Table 9.1.1). Whiteman et al. evaluated patients with progressive multifocal leukoencephalopathy (PML) using both CT and MRI, and found MRI to be more sensitive in detecting the extent and number of PML lesions (Whiteman et al., 1993). Wolter et al. evaluated CT abnormalities in 35 patients (32 with HIV infection) who had documented neurosyphilis (by CSF or biopsy) and found that 31% had normal CT, 23% had cerebral infarction, 20% had non specific white matter lesions, and 6% had cerebral gumma. Another large retrospective analyses of 204 head CTs from 178 HIV patients who had uncomplicated headaches found that 37.3% had positive scans; of these, the majority (76%) had atrophy and 23% had mass lesions or white matter lesions (all of these had CD4 <200 cells/μL) (Graham et al., 2000). Davis et al. also reviewed head CT scans in 82 HIV patients who presented with AIDS-related systemic non-Hodgkin lymphoma (ARL), and found that head CT only detected meningeal enhancement in 3 patients and brain lesions in 7 patients. The presence of malignant cells in the CSF (found in 17 patients) predicted worse survival; therefore, head CT did not offer additional prognostic information following a lumbar puncture in patients with ARL (Davies et al., 2007).

Korbo et al. performed a quantitative analyses of ventricular volumes of HIV patients and found that those with immunodeficiency (CD4<400 cells/μL) had greater ventricular dilatation (n = 27, 8–80 mL) than seronegative controls (n = 15, 6–54 mL), while HIV patients who were immunocompetent (CD4>400 cells/μL) only had mild ventricular dilatations (n = 23, 10–72 mL) (Korbo, Praestholm, & Skot, 2002). Surprisingly, time-dependent increases in the ventricle size were observed only in the HIV immunocompetent group at follow-up scans, suggesting ongoing brain injury in these HIV patients (up to six time points; three subjects were followed up to 100 months and most were followed up to 40 months).

Overall, CT has limited value in the research setting for the evaluation of brain changes in patients with HIV. Even in the clinical setting, a recent study of HIV patients who presented with neurological symptoms found that MRI detected cranial abnormalities in more than twice as many patients as did CT (74% compared to 32%, n = 54 and 38, respectively) (Wilson et al., 2010). Hence, MRI appears to be more cost effective and provides more expedient diagnoses for the optimal management of HIV patients presenting with neurological symptoms.

NUCLEAR MEDICINE TECHNIQUES: SPECT AND PET

SINGLE-PHOTON EMISSION COMPUTED TOMOGRAPHY (SPECT)

SPECT is a nuclear medicine technique that uses a SPECT camera with gamma detectors to detect radiation from a radioactive gamma-emitting isotope (radionuclide) that may be bound to a drug (radiopharmaceutical). The gamma camera rotates around the patient (typically 360 degree coverage is required) and acquires raw data from which a computer can reconstruct projection images, which are 2-dimensional views of the distribution of the radionuclide or radiopharmapharmaceutical in the brain. Typical scan time is 20–30 minutes. The radioactive drug may be inhaled (e.g., Xenon-133) or injected intravenously [e.g., ^{99m}Technitium-hexa-methyl-propylene amine oxime (^{99m}Tc-HMPAO) or ^{123}Iodine (^{123}I)-amphetamine] into the patient or subject prior to the scan.

The most common radiopharmaceutical to study the effects of HIV was ^{99m}Tc-HMPAO; other radioligands used include ^{123}I-amphetamine, ^{99m}Tc-exametazime, and ^{133}Xenon (Table 9.1.2). All of these compounds evaluate relative cerebral perfusion, since they are typically carried by blood flow and are perfused into various organs throughout the body. Some of the ligands undergo metabolism by the tissues and may become trapped in the tissue until the drugs are further metabolized. In the meantime, the radionuclide also

Table 9.1.2 BRAIN SPECT STUDIES IN HIV-INFECTED INDIVIDUALS

REFERENCE	NUMBER OF SUBJECTS	RADIOTRACER USED	BRAIN REGIONS EVALUATED	FINDINGS
Samuelsson et al., Eur J Neurol 2006	28 HIV patients stable on ARVs and followed 7 years	^{99m}Tc-HMPAO	All cortical regions reviewed visually	No major neurological, neuropsychological, or SPECT abnormalities were note over 7 years (3 scans); the proportion of HIV patients with focal or patchy hypoperfusion increased. The abnormalities were most often seen in the parietal regions.
Modi et al., J Neurol Sci 2002	15 HIV patients with new onset seizures	^{99m}Tc-HMPAO	Whole brain reviewed visually	All had perfusion defects in the left or right temporal lobes. 13 patients had generalized seizures and 2 had status epilepticus; all had normal structural scans (CT and MRI) and normal neurological examinations.
Ernst et al., J Magn Reson Imaging 2000	24 HIV+CMC 34 SN controls	^{133}Xeon (used to calibrate for absolute blood flow) ^{99m}Tc-HMPAO	Whole brain SPECT co-registered to four MRS voxel locations	On SPECT, only decreased rCBF in temporoparietal white matter. On MRS, HIV subjects had lower total creatine in basal ganglia and increased myoinositol in both basal ganglia and temporoparietal white matter. MRS is more sensitive and detects abnormalities in region that showed normal SPECT perfusion.
Christensson et al., Scan J Inf 1999	25 HIV (non-demented) 25 controls (no SPECT)	^{99m}Tc-HMPAO	Whole brain, cortical regions	Both the 99mTc-HMPAO uptake and functional level slowly decrease over time, but the regional cerebral blood flow decrease could be masked by a direct HIV-induced inflammation in the brain, which would lead to increased tracer uptake instead (found unexpected correlation with increased uptake and poorer cognitive performance)

(Continued)

Table 9.1.2 (CONTINUED)

REFERENCE	NUMBER OF SUBJECTS	RADIOTRACER USED	BRAIN REGIONS EVALUATED	FINDINGS
Schwartz et al: AJR 1994	27 AIDS 45 CFS 14 depressed 38 controls	^{99m}Tc-HMPAO	8 cortical and subcortical regions in each hemisphere	Visually counted perfusion defects in the 8 ROIs. AIDS patients (9.15/patient), chronic fatigue syndrome patients (CFS, 6.53), depressed patients (6.43), and healthy controls (1.66). SPECT detects similar abnormalities in these pathologies.
Sacktor et al., Arch Neurol 1995b	10 HIV+ 5 HIV+	^{99m}Tc-HMPAO	Qualitative and quantitative analyses for asymmetry of tracer uptakes	No increased frequency of focal defects in HIV subjects with cognitive impairment compared to those without cognitive deficits. Global tracer uptake (reflecting CBF) correlated inversely with motor speed in HIV subjects.
Sacktor et al., Arch Neurol 1995a	12 HIV+ 8 HIV+MCMD 10 SN controls	^{99m}Tc-exametazime	Compared left and right side tracer uptakes	15/20 of HIV-positive subjects (8/12 HIV and 7/8 of HIV+MCMD), and 2/10 of HIV-negative subjects had abnormal SPECT scans ($\geq$ 2 "focal defects" - >20% asymmetry - in cortical and subcortical regions).
Rosci et al 1992, AIDS	82 HIV (39 had SPECT)	^{99m}Tc-HMPAO	Visual analyses for asymmetry of tracer uptakes	Cerebral perfusion abnormalities were detected in 31 out of 39 (79%) subjects who underwent SPECT. There were high incidence of abnormal SPECT and of poor cognitive performance in asymptomatic HIV-1-infected patients, and the lack of correlation between immunological status and degree of cognitive deficits.
Holman et al., 1992 J Nucl Med 1992	20 HIV (all men) 20 cocaine users (all men) 20 controls (13 women)	^{99m}Tc-HMPAO	Visual rating of "focal defects" in 7 brain regions on each side	Compared to controls, HIV subjects and cocaine users had more focal perfusion defects in frontal, temporal or parietal cortices, but no difference between HIV and cocaine users. No abnormal defects were observed in any subject group in the primary visual cortex and cerebellum.
Masdeu et al., J Nucl Med 1991	32 HIV (29 M / 3 F) 15 non-HIV psychosis (13 M/ 2F) 6 controls (5 M / 1 F)	^{123}Iodo-amphetamine.	Visual rating (4 points) in cortex and white matter	Multifocal cortical and subcortical areas of hypoperfusion in HIV. In 4 cases, cognitive improvement after 6-8 weeks of zidovudine (AZT) therapy was reflected in amelioration of SPECT findings. 7 of 9 HIV subjects with normal cognition were still identified to have the HIV pattern (with multiple focal defects).
Pohl et al., J Nucl Med 1988	12 HIV encephalopathy	^{123}I-amphetamine or ^{99m}Tc-HMPAO	Visual rating of focal defects	Multiple focal tracer uptake defects in the cerebral cortex, similar regions for both tracers in majority of patients; pattern of defects similar to other brain diseases and hence is not specific but very sensitive for detecting pathology.

undergoes decay and has a limited half-life (typically less than 120 minutes) for the imaging. Cerebral perfusion represents the health of the brain tissue, and all of the SPECT studies were performed with the subjects at rest.

HIV-infected individuals without focal opportunistic brain lesions, and even those with relatively normal appearing structural imaging, tended to show multiple "focal defects" by visual inspection on SPECT with one of the radioligands. These focal perfusion defects may represent dysfunctional brain tissue, especially in those with minimal-to-no apparent brain atrophy on structural imaging. However, since brain atrophy is common amongst HIV-infected individuals, partial volume effects of these low resolution SPECT images may lead to apparent perfusion defects. The earlier studies aimed to "diagnose" HIV encephalopathy by demonstrating characteristic focal perfusion defects on SPECT images (Holman et al., 1992; Pohl et al., 1998; Masdeu et al., 1991). Therefore, several SPECT studies compared the patterns of focal perfusion defects between HIV-infected individuals without focal brain lesions, to those with other non-structural brain disorders (e.g., cocaine or heroin dependence (Holman et al., 1992), chronic fatigue syndrome or depression (Schwartz et al., 1994), or non-HIV psychosis (Brass et al., 1994). These earlier studies concluded that SPECT is sensitive for detecting abnormal focal perfusion defects but were not specific for diagnosing HIV encephalopathy since various other brain disorders had similar patterns and number of focal defects. Furthermore, perhaps due to the heterogeneous populations studied in these retrospective studies and the lack of detailed clinical correlations, the earlier brain SPECT studies did not find clear relationships between abnormalities on SPECT and neurocognitive function or immunological parameters (Rosci et al., 1996).

Later prospective SPECT studies confirmed the higher prevalence of focal perfusion defects in HIV-infected individuals (Sacktor et al., 1995), but no difference was seen between HIV subjects with or without cognitive impairments, perhaps due to the small sample size in lower global perfusion in these individuals was associated with slower motor function (Sacktor et al., 1995). Another brain SPECT study in a larger sample of participants, however, found unexpectedly that higher perfusion was associated with poorer cognitive performance (Christensson et al., 1999). Another SPECT study evaluated HIV-infected individuals with new onset seizures and found focal perfusion defects primarily in the temporal lobes (Modi et al., 2002).

Furthermore, some SPECT studies aimed to evaluate longitudinal brain changes in HIV-individuals and found that focal defects tend to increase over time (Christensson et al., 1999), especially in the parietal brain regions (Samuelsson et al., 2006); however, such changes could be due to normal aging or age-associated brain atrophy as well. One study also documented improvement of focal perfusion defects in four HIV-patients after they were treated with AZT (Masdeu et al., 1991). In contrast, HIV patients who were treated with HAART showed increased perfusion which was thought to be due to ongoing neuroinflammation (Christensson et al., 1999).

Lastly, one study evaluated co-registered and partial volume-corrected and [133]Xenon-calibrated 99TcHMPAO SPECT and ^{1}H MRS in the same HIV-infected individuals, in order to determine whether absolute regional cerebral blood flow or absolute concentration (after correction for partial volume effect due to atrophy) measured on MRS would be more sensitive for detecting brain injury (Figure 9.1.1). This study found that MRS abnormalities, with elevated myo-inositol indicating glial activation, could be detected in brain regions that showed normal perfusion (Ernst et al., 2000). Therefore, given the radiation involved and the low specificity of SPECT, its utility for the evaluation and monitoring of HIV-associated brain injury or treatment effects is limited.

POSITRON EMISSION TOMOGRAPHY (PET)

Imaging by positron emission tomography (PET) measures the distribution of positron emitting nuclides using detectors that are tuned specifically to 511keV. High image sensitivity is achieved by using a ring of detectors to ensure capturing of cross sections and by filtering out background noise due to the phenomena of coincidence counting. As the radioisotope undergoes positron emission decay, the positron emitted encounters its antiparticle, an electron. The two forms of matter annihilate each other, producing a pair of gamma rays of 511 keV moving in opposite directions of each other from the point of the annihilation reaction. A scintillator in the scanning device detects these gamma photons that transformed into a burst of light and the signal is enhanced by photomultiplier. Photons that do not arrive in the same timing window of a few nanoseconds will be ignored. This unique mechanism allows for the usage of radionuclide in the picomolar range and therefore significantly reduces the radiation when compared to other imaging techniques that involve radiation, such as SPECT. However, the radionuclides used in PET require a cyclotron and have a short half-life ranging from 20 to 110 min; therefore, radioisotope production

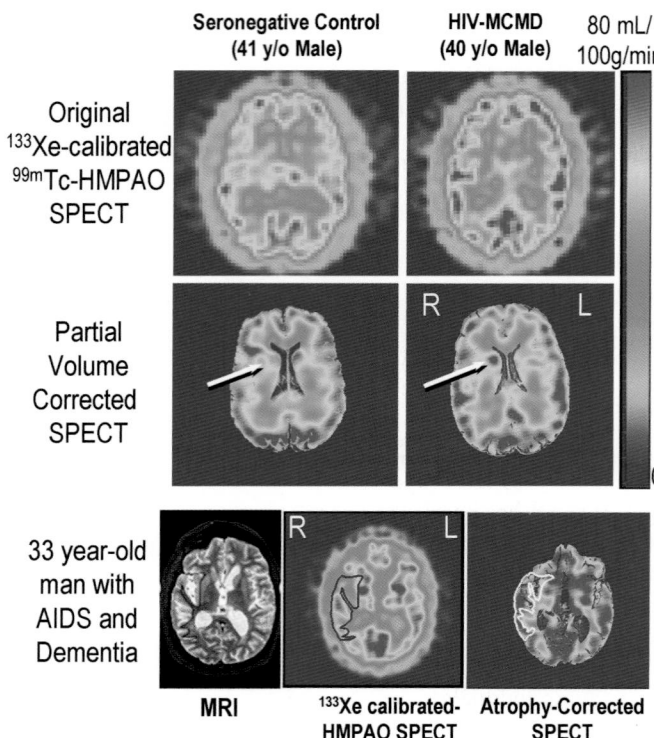

Figure 9.1.1 Top 4 Panels: SPECT images showing the improved delineation of regional cerebral blood flow (rCBF) in specific anatomical regions, after co-registration with the subjects' structural MRI, and correction for partial volume effects from the CSF (lower images). Arrows point to the higher rCBF in the right caudate of the HIV-MCMD subject compared to that in the seronegative control subject. Bottom row: SPECT images of an AIDS patient with dementia showing right temporal lobe atrophy, with enlarged right Sylvian fissure on MRI, and the apparent hypoperfusion or a focal defect in the right temporal lobe before partial volume (or atrophy) correction on the SPECT.

and the PET imaging must be an expeditious and well-coordinated process and in the close vicinity of the imaging facility. Another advantage of PET is its higher resolution of (~3-5 mm) compared to SPECT (~10mm), due to the coincidence detection of the gamma radiation from annihilations of the photons and electrons. However, SPECT is more readily available in hospitals and substantially less costly.

RADIOISOTOPES AND TRACERS USED TO EVALUATE HIV-ASSOCIATED BRAIN DISEASES

Characteristic nuclides used for PET scanning are isotopes with short half-lives such as carbon-11 (~20 min), nitrogen-13 (~10 min), oxygen-15 (~2 min), and fluorine-18 (~110 min). These radioisotopes are chemically integrated into compounds utilized in normal cell metabolism such as glucose, or molecules that bind to receptors or interact with other drugs. These so-called radiotracers create a wide range of application for PET as any compound from biological pathways can be used as long as they can be radio-labeled. Depending on the molecule used, a high tissue as well as metabolic specificity can be achieved. The most commonly used radiotracer, especially for the earlier PET studies of HIV patients, is fluorine-18 (^{18}F) fluorodeoxyglucose

(FDG). This tracer is taken up by any cells that utilize glucose and is subsequently phosphorylated by hexokinase. Oxygen needed for glycolyis is replaced by the radioactive-labeled ^{18}flourine, and the FDG is then trapped in the cell until it decays.

[^{11}C]cocaine and [^{11}C]raclopride are examples of ligand-receptor specific PET tracers. [^{11}C]cocaine binds to the pre-synaptic dopamine receptor (DAT), whereas [^{11}C]raclopride interacts with the postsynaptic dopamine 2 receptor (D2R). These tracers when combined together depict the dopamine metabolism in CNS, which is particularly vulnerable to drugs of abuse or HIV infection.

Another tracer for a neurotransmitter receptor is 3-^{11}C-amino-4-(2dimethylaminomethylphenylsulfanyl) benzonitrile ([^{11}C]DASB), which binds to the serotonin transporter (5-hydroxytryptamine transporter or 5-HTT). [^{11}C]DASB has been proven to be superior to other radiopharmaceuticals such as [^{11}C]McN5652 and [^{123}I]β-CIT for evaluating the serotonergic system. Its higher selectivity and greater specific binding makes it an ideal candidate for studying disease pathologies with imbalances in serotonin cycling such as depression, which is prevalent amongst HIV-infected individuals.

Recently PET studies in HIV patients have also evaluated the extent of glial activation by means of the new radioligand [^{11}C]1-[2-chlorphenyl]-N-methyl-N-[1-methyl-propyl-]-3-isoquinoline carboxamide ([^{11}C]-R-PK11195), which is selective for the peripheral benzodiazepine receptor (PBR). PBR itself is widely expressed throughout the body, especially in steroid-producing tissues, but only ependymal and glial cells express this receptor in the CNS (Casellas, Galiegue, & Basile, 2002). Lastly, the Pittsburg compound B ([^{11}C]PiB), or N-methyl-[11C]2-(4-methylaminophenyl)-6-hydroxybenzothiazole, has been applied to assess HIV-infected individuals for its specific binding to fibrillary amyloid in the brain, which is involved in the formation of amyloid plaques, a pathological hallmark of Alzheimer disease.

PET STUDIES IN NEURO-HIV/AIDS

HIV-RELATED NEUROLOGICAL COMPLICATIONS IN THE PRE- AND EARLY HAART ERA

More than 20 studies have employed PET to evaluate the effects of HIV infection or AIDS in the brain (Table 9.1.3).

Table 9.1.3 PET STUDIES OF BRAIN CHANGES ASSOCIATED WITH HIV-INFECTION

REFERENCE	NUMBER OF SUBJECTS	TRACER(S) USED	RECEPTORS OR BRAIN REGIONS EVALUATED,	ANTIRETROVIRAL TREATMENT	FINDINGS
Ances et al., Neurology 2010	10 HIV+ unimpaired 20 community unimpaired controls	^{11}C-PiB	Fibrillary amyloid plaque binding in prefrontal, temporal, precuneus, gyrus rectus	All on HAART (from CHARTER)	Cognitively unimpaired HIV+ participants, even those with low CSF Aβ42 (<500 pg/mL, n = 4), do not have increased PiB binding, which suggesting different Aβ or plaque formation in unimpaired HIV subjects compared to preclinical Alzheimer's disease.
Andersen et al., J Neuro-inflammation 2010	21 HIV with abnormal PET 17 HIV with normal PET	^{18}F-FDG	Glucose metabolism; Whole brain (using Neurostat and normalized z-scores)	ARVs for ≥3 years with no virological failure.	Lower glucose metabolism in frontal (anterior cingulate) cortex; 55% HIV patients studied had abnormal scans (lower z-scores) and they tended to have higher circulating levels of TNF-α and IL-6.
Hammoud et al., Neuroimage 2010	9 HIV+ Depressed 9 HIV+Not depressed 7 controls	^{11}C -DASB	serotonin transporter (5-HTT)-specific 11 brain structures	All HIV were on ARVs except for two in each group (who had past HAART)	HIV+ND subjects had lower mean regional 5-HTT BP to HC. HIV+D had higher 5- HTT-BP values than HIV-ND in most regions. After correction for the false discovery rate, only the insula showed significantly lower binding in HIV subjects compared to controls.
Chang et al., Neuroimage 2008	24 HIV 11 HIV+Coc 14 SN controls	^{11}C-cocaine ^{11}C-raclopride	DAT and D2R Striatum/ putamen and caudate	34 of 35 HIV patients were on stable ARVs (averaged 2 yrs)	Both HIV subject groups had lower DAT in putamen, HIV+COC also had lower DAT in caudate. Lower D2R in HIV subjects was due to nicotine use. Lower DAT was associated with poorer cognitive scores.
Georgiou et al., J NucI Med 2008	17 HIV+IDU 13 IDU 29 SN controls	^{18}F-FDG	Glucose metabolism; (Whole brain voxel-based analyses using SPM)	Information not available	HIV+IDU subjects had more extensive lower relative metabolism in cortical regions and higher relative metabolism in subcortical regions than those seen in IDU only compared to SN controls.

(Continued)

Table 9.1.3 (CONTINUED)

REFERENCE	NUMBER OF SUBJECTS	TRACER(S) USED	RECEPTORS OR BRAIN REGIONS EVALUATED,	ANTIRETROVIRAL TREATMENT	FINDINGS
Wiley et al., J NeuroVirol 2006	6 HIV+ cognitively impaired 6 HIV+non-impaired 5 SN controls	^{11}C (R)-PK11195	Peripheral benzodiazepine receptors (PBR) 10 brain regions	All on ARVs	No higher retention of the tracer in the in brain parenchyma of the 12 HIV subjects compared to 5 controls
Hammoud et al., J NeuroVirol 2005	5 HIV+ cognitively impaired 5 HIV+non-impaired 5 controls	^{11}C (R)-PK11195	PBR 8 cortical regions and one white matter	7 were on ARVs, 3 were not on ARV	Higher retention or tracer in 5 of 8 brain regions in HIV HAD, and in 5 regions in HIV overall when compared to controls
Wang et al., Brain 2004	10 HIV subjects with HAD 5 HIV non-impaired 13 SN controls	^{11}C-cocaine ^{11}C-raclopride	Dopamine transporter (DAT) and D2 Receptor (DR2) binding in Putamen, caudate, ventral striatum	14 were on ARVs, one was ARV-naïve	HIV subjects with HAD had lower [C-11] cocaine binding (reflecting lower DAT) than SN controls in putamen and ventral striatum. DAD2 receptor binding showed a trend to be lower. HIV subjects with higher viral load had lower DAT.
Von Giessen et al., Arch Neurol 2000	19 HIV (normal motor function to minor motor disorder) 15 SN controls	^{18}F-FDG	Glucose metabolism In 5 regions in each hemisphere	16 on ARVs (9 on HAART)	7 HIV subjects showed hypermetabolism in the basal ganglia, but 9 showed hypometabolism in the frontomesial cortical (anterior cingulate). Metabolic activities did not correlate with motor slowing
Wiseman et al., J Neuropsychiatry and Clin Neurosci 1999	10 HIV 9 HIV+MCMD 10 SN Controls	^{15}O-H$_2$0	Relative cerebral blood flow, SPM, during rest and short-term memory	All HIV-MCMD took ARVs (pre-protease inhibitors)	Brain activation during rest and low level automatic processing is normal in MCMD but abnormal during effortful retrieval of memory and organizational processes
Rottenberg et al., J Nuc Med 1996	21 HIV (4 ADC stage 0, 12 stage 0.5, 4 stage 1, one stage 2) 43 controls	^{18}F-FDG	Glucose metabolism Whole brain - 40 Volumes of Interests (VOIs)–scaled subprofiled model / PCA	15 with ARV treatment, 6 without ARVs	Higher metabolism in caudate & putamen and lower metabolism in remaining 36 VOIs in HIV than controls. SSM/PCA showed components that correlated with older age, cerebral atrophy and ADC stage; Follow-up PET at 6 months (n = 12) and 12 months (n = 4)
Depas et al., J Nucl Med 1995	HIV children (3 with & 5 without encephalopathy; ages 2.2-5.5 ears)	^{18}F-FDG	Glucose metabolism 5 ROIs each hemisphere on MRI co-registered to PET images	All on AZT	The 3 children with encephalopathy (P-2B/D1) had subcortical hypermetabolism and diffuse hypometaboism in the cortex; those without encephalopathy (P-2/A) only had right temporo-occipital hypometabolism.
Hinkin et al., J Neuropsychiatry Clin Neurosci 1995	10 with AIDS (Each had PET scans at baseline and 6 months later)	^{18}F-FDG	Glucose metabolism Whole brain	6 of 10 were on AZT	Increased metabolism in basal ganglia and parietal lobe, but no change in neuropsychological test (NPT) performance. PET may be more sensitive than NPT.
Van Gorp et al., J Neuropsychiatry Clin Neurosci 1992	17 AIDS 14 SN controls	^{18}F-FDG	Glucose metabolism Whole brain	14 were on AZT	Relative regional hypermetabolism in the basal ganglia and thalamus; temporal lobe metabolism correlated with ADC stage.
Brunetti et al., J Nucl Med 1989	4 HIV patients with ADC (before and after AZT)	^{18}F-FDG	Glucose metabolism Cortical ROIs (on 5 slices)	Treatment with AZT	3 adults and one 11-year old child all showed improved metabolism in cortical regions after AZT treatment.

In the late 1980s and early to mid-1990s, PET imaging studies focused on opportunistic CNS lesions and AIDS dementia complex, and evaluated the effect of the first antiretroviral medication, zidovudine (AZT). With the development of highly active antiretroviral therapy (HAART), PET has also been applied to evaluate the effects of comorbid conditions, such as drug of abuse, depression, and neuroinflammation associated with HIV CNS infection.

The major opportunistic brain lesions in HIV patients include CNS toxoplasmosis and CNS lymphomas. Computed tomography (CT) and magnetic resonance imaging (MRI) can demonstrate these focal or multifocal contrast-enhancing lesions, but definitive diagnosis without histopathological confirmation is difficult (Navia et al., 1986; Pitlik et al. 1983). PET imaging with (^{18}F) fluorodeoxyglucose (FDG) showed that CNS lymphoma lesions had significantly higher glucose utilization and uptake of the tracer than nonmalignant lesions, such as toxoplasmosis, regardless of the evaluation method (e.g., semiquantitative analysis, standardized uptake ratio or visual evaluation) (Hoffman, Waskin, & Schiffer, 1993; Villringer et al., 1995; Heald et al., 1996). However, due to its high costs, PET is rarely performed in the clinical setting for the differential diagnosis of focal brain lesions in AIDS. PET may also be useful for monitoring treatment effects, such as the evaluation of tumor hypoxia and the efficacy of gene therapy which have not yet been performed for CNS lymphoma. A detailed discussion regarding the use of PET for differential diagnosis and treatment monitoring of focal brain lesions in AIDS is beyond the scope of this chapter; for further reading, please see Review (Roelcke & Leenders, 1999).

AIDS dementia complex (ADC), the old terminology to describe HAND, occurs in 20–40% in HIV-positive subjects without HAART and 5–10% with HAART, although milder forms of cognitive deficits may occur in 30–50% of those infected with HIV. ADC is characterized clinically by severe cognitive, behavioral, and motor abnormalities in the absence of opportunistic infection. In earlier PET studies that evaluated ADC, subcortical brain regions (thalamus and basal ganglia) show relative hypermetabolism, while cortical and subcortical gray matter show relative hypometabolism with disease progression (Rottenberg et al., 1987). These findings were corroborated by later PET studies (Rottenberg et al., 1996; Bridge et al., 1989; Bridge et al., 1991; van Gorp et al., 1992; Hinkin et al., 1995; O'Doherty et al., 1997), which specified the striatum as the basal ganglia substructure showing relative hypermetabolism (Rottenberg et al., 1996). Additionally, generalized reduced cortical uptake of glucose was observed in HIV subjects with older age, greater brain atrophy, and greater severity of ADC (Rottenberg et al., 1996). This pattern of hypermetabolism in the basal ganglia and hypometabolism in the cortex of the brains of HIV-infected adults was also seen in a small FDG PET study of HIV-infected children with (n = 3) and without (n = 5) neurological involvement (Depas et al., 1995). These children showed hypometabolism primarily in posterior brains regions, which contrasts to the generalized or more anterior cortical hypometabolism seen in the adult HIV patients (Depas et al., 1995). These different patterns of hypometabolism could reflect the unique pattern of injury in the developing brain. These studies also demonstrate that metabolic changes can be detected in the brains of neurologically or neuropsychologically normal individuals.

When the first HIV antiretroviral medication, azidothymidine (AZT, a nucleoside analog reverse transcriptase inhibitor (NRTI) also known as Zidovudine or Retrovir) became available, PET was used to evaluate the effect of AZT in four HIV patients in 1989. Three adults and one 11-year-old child with ADC were studied before and after AZT. The study found reversal of cortical abnormalities, or overall increase in glucose metabolism, which accompanied immunological and neurological improvement in these patients (Brunetti et al., 1989). Another study of 10 AIDS patients who were evaluated at baseline and 6 months later reported increased basal ganglia and parietal lobe glucose metabolism at follow-up, with no change in their neuropsychological performance; hence, the authors concluded that PET may be more sensitive than neuropsychological evaluations for ADC (Hinkin et al., 1995). A case report of an HIV patient who was studied with PET before and 12 weeks after intranasal Peptide T, however, found "improved" (decreased) glucose metabolism in many brain regions after treatment (Villemagne et al., 1996). Although PET may be useful for assessing or elucidating the neuropathophysiology associated with HAD, the radiation exposure and the high cost of the technique limit its use as a biomarker to monitor the effects of treatment.

OTHER PET STUDIES TO EVALUATE HIV-ASSOCIATED NEUROCOGNITIVE DISORDER

The basal ganglia are key brain regions affected by HIV infection (Petito, 1993; Berger & Nath, 1997), and likely mediate the motor and cognitive disorders seen in patients with HAND (Arendt et al., 1990). Von Giesen et al. found that HIV-infected individuals with normal motor performance had hypermetabolism in the basal ganglia, those with moderate slowing (MCMD) showed striatal hypometabolism, while only those with more severe motor and cognitive deficits had wide spread hypometabolism in the basal ganglia (von Giesen et al., 2000). Another FDG PET study that evaluated HIV patients who were stable on medication for a minimum of 3 years without virological failures, found that 55% showed "abnormal PET" images, with lower glucose metabolism primarily in the anterior cingulate cortex (Andersen et al., 2010), using a software that generated normalized z-scores for the regional glucose uptake. Although these patients were all "neurologically intact," no information regarding their cognitive functioning were available, and those with "abnormal PET" scans tended to have higher levels of circulating TNF-α and interleukin-6 (Andersen et al., 2010).

Since the basal ganglia has the highest density of dopaminergic synapses, Wang et al. and Chang et al. used [^{11}C]cocaine and [^{11}C]raclopride to assess the dopamine transporters (DAT) and dopamine D2 receptors (D2R) in HIV patients with and without cognitive deficits (Figure 9.1.2). The initial study found that DAT was lower in the putamen and ventral striatum of 10 HIV-infected individuals with dementia, but

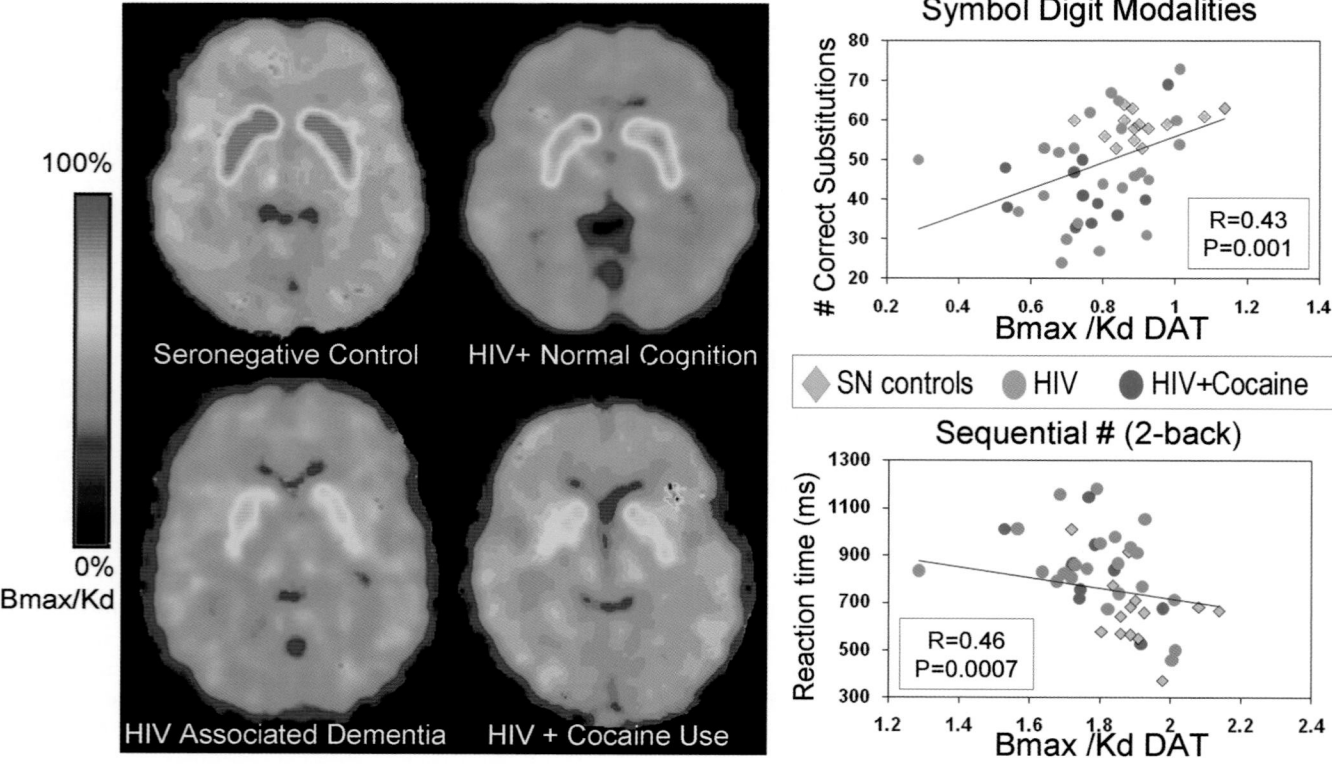

Figure 9.1.2 Left Panel: Representative PET images showing decreasing level of ^{11}C-cocaine binding (Bmax/Kd) in a seronegative control subject, an HIV+ subject with normal cognition, an HIV subject with HAND and an HIV subject with a history of cocaine-dependence. Right scatter plots: Subjects with lower dopamine transporter density (lower ^{11}[C]-cocaine Bmax/Kd) had poorer performance on Symbol Digit Modalities and a working memory task (2-back). Similar correlations were observed with the Auditory Verbal Learning Test and other working memory tests (data not shown, see Chang et al., 2008). Figures are modified from those presented in Chang et al., 2008; Wang et al., 2004.

not in five HIV subjects without dementia, compared to the 13 SN controls. In addition, higher viral load in these HIV subjects was associated with lower DAT. With a larger sample size (35 HIV subjects and 14 SN controls), lower DAT in both putamen and caudate were associated with poorer performance on several neurocognitive tests that evaluated psychomotor function (Chang et al., 2008). However, the dopamine D2 receptor density was only slightly reduced (Wang et al., 2004), which was found in the follow-up study to be reduced only in those who were active nicotine smokers (Chang et al., 2008). These studies clearly demonstrate that HIV infection has a deleterious effect on the dopaminergic system. Since the dopaminergic system mediates attention and working memory, dopaminergic deficits could in turn lead to the psychomotor and motor deficits seen in patients with HAND. These findings suggest that HIV patients may benefit from treatments that enhance the dopaminergic function or protect them from dopaminergic cell injury.

Neuroinflammation associated with HIV infection also plays a major role in the development of HAND. Peripheral immune cells, but more likely residential glial cells such as astrocytes and microglia, are involved in the inflammatory process (McArthur et al., 2003). PET Imaging with [^{11}C]-R-PK11195, a tracer specifically binding to the peripheral benzodiazepine receptor (PBR) on glial cells helps to identify

areas of immune activation in the brain. Assessment of encephalitic SIV-infected macaque brains with the PBR specific tracer showed increased binding in the frontal white and grey matter. Postmortem analyses showed that cells with [^{11}C]-R-PK11195 binding were of macrophage/microglial origin in the frontal white matter. No clear association in the grey matter with [^{11}C]-R-PK11195 signals was observed, suggesting a different subpopulation of microglia or infiltrating macrophages that predominate in the white matter in SIV/HIV encephalitis (Mankowski et al., 2003). Similarly Venneti et al. showed significantly higher binding of [^{11}C]-R-PK11195 in SIV-infected macaques with encephalitis in the frontal white and gray matter, basal ganglia, and hippocampal areas. Again, cells of [^{11}C]-R-PK11195 binding were found to be macrophages (Venneti, Wang, & Wiley, 2007).

The [^{11}C]-R-PK11195 tracer was subsequently applied by Hammoud et al. to study ten HIV–infected individuals (five had HAD and seven were stable on antiretroviral medications) and five SN controls. They found greater binding of the tracer in the thalamus, putamen, frontal, temporal and occipital cortex of patients with HAD, but no difference in HIV patients without cognitive deficits, compared to SN controls (Hammoud et al., 2005). In contrast, Wiley et al. found no difference in the retention of the PRB tracer between 12 HIV-infected individuals (6 with and 6 without cognitive impairment) and 5 SN control subjects (Wiley et al., 2006). These disparate findings might be due to the different levels of cognitive impairment in the HIV groups investigated, HIV HAD (Hammoud et al., 2005) versus HIV with minor cognitive impairment (Wiley et al., 2006) or to other methodological differences, since the tracers were synthesized at different institutions. Although these studies involved small sample sizes, this tracer may not be sensitive enough to detect the neuroinflammation. However, if future studies could validate higher PBR binding in HIV patients with cognitive impairment, it would further demonstrate that microglia and macrophages are involved in the cognitive impairment and that neuroinflammation is an ongoing process despite antiretroviral treatment.

PET AND DRUG ABUSE IN HIV PATIENTS

Illicit drug use is a major risk factor for acquiring HIV, for example, by sharing needles or increasing risky sexual behaviors. Drugs of abuse could also accelerate HIV-associated brain injury and drug users also may be more nonadherent to HIV therapy. Cocaine, a psychostimulant that binds to the presynaptic dopamine re-uptake transporter, is often abused by HIV-infected individuals. Chang et al. used [11C]cocaine and [11C]raclopride to assess DATs and the post synaptic dopamine D2 receptors (D2R) in HIV-infected individuals with and without a history of cocaine dependence, and found that HIV-infected abstinent cocaine users had further decreases of DAT in the putamen and caudate, but no decrease in D2R (except in individuals who were nicotine smokers), compared to seronegative controls (Chang et al., 2008). Those with the lowest DAT, primarily the HIV+ cocaine users, had the poorest cognitive performance and psychomotor speed, even after correcting for age, education, intelligence, mood, and nicotine use. This study demonstrates that despite prolonged abstinence from cocaine abuse (average 2 years) and stable treatment with antiretroviral medications, the density of DAT remained abnormally low, which likely contributed to the cognitive deficits in these individuals. Therefore, cocaine abuse likely exacerbates the neurotoxicity associated with HIV, possibly via enhanced viral replication, in agreement with in vivo and in vitro preclinical studies (Roth et al., 2002; Scheller et al., 2000; Czub et al., 2004).

Injection drug use (IDU) is common in HIV-infected subjects, may increase the risk for HIV transmission, and some of these drugs are also neurotoxic. An FDG PET study of HIV patients with IDU (primarily heroin and cocaine) found more extensive relative hypermetabolism in various subcortical regions, but lower relative metabolism in the medial frontal lobes and right inferior frontal and temporal cortices compared to IDU or to seronegative non-drug users (Georgiou et al., 2008). The authors concluded that IDU and HIV infection might have a synergistic effect in terms of neurotoxicity. However, these data are difficult to interpret due to the limited clinical information regarding the subjects' antiretroviral treatment status or other drugs of abuse, which could be potential confounds for the data presented.

PET TO EVALUATE DEPRESSION IN HIV PATIENTS

Major depression is prevalent in HIV-infected persons, with rates of current depression being at least twice that of the general population (Ferrando & Freyberg, 2008). Depression has direct negative effects on the brain, but may also lead to poorer treatment adherence (Catz et al., 2000), greater prevalence of substance abuse (Kalichman, Kelly, & Rompa, 1997), poorer HIV viral control (Horberg et al., 2007), and, if left untreated, can promote risk-taking behaviors (Kopnisky, Stoff, & Rausch, 2004). Alteration in the serotonergic system is generally thought to be involved in the neuropathophysiology of depression, which might be enhanced in HIV-infected patients. PET imaging with [11C]DASB, a serotonin transporter (5-HTT)-specific radiopharmaceutical showed lower levels of 5-HTT in HIV-infected subjects compared to controls, suggesting HIV-induced loss or alteration of serotonergic neurons (Hammoud et al., 2010)[65]. However, within the HIV group, patients with depression showed higher binding of [11C]DASB; this was interpreted by the investigators to indicate a higher density of 5-HTT that might have led to increased clearance of extracellular serotonin which in turn could contribute to the greater depressive symptoms in these individuals (Hammoud et al., 2010). However, since the HIV subjects as a group have lower 5-HTT than controls, other mechanisms likely contribute to the depressive symptoms. Given the small sample size of HIV patients with depression (n = 9) in this study, future larger studies are needed to further evaluate the effects of HIV on the serotonergic system.

PET AND BRAIN FIBRILLAR AMYLOID IN HIV PATIENTS

Since neuropathology studies of brains with HIV encephalitis (HIVE) showed higher levels of intraneuronal amyloid beta (Ab) immunoreactivity compared to HIV+ cases with no HIVE (Achim et al., 2009), there has been recent interest to evaluate amyloid deposition in the HIV-infected brain. A new study used the Pittsburgh compound B (11C-PiB) to evaluate for possible fibrillar beta-amyloid deposition in the brains of cognitive unimpaired HIV patients (Ances et al., 2010). The study evaluated 10 unimpaired HIV patients and 20 community nondemented control subjects, and found no increased 11C-PiB binding in the unimpaired HIV patients, even in those with low CSF levels of Ab42 <500pg/mL. In contrast, the community controls with low CSF Ab42 levels did have elevated 11C-PiB binding. The findings from this study suggest that the processes involved in the formation of amyloid plaques may be different in HIV compared to Alzheimer's disease. However, the sample size is rather small in the HIV subjects with the low CSF Ab42 levels (n = 4). Therefore, future studies with a larger sample size, evaluating the effects of APOE genotype, and longitudinal follow-up are needed.

In summary, nuclear medicine techniques are highly sensitive and many tracers are specific for assessing certain receptors or neurochemical targets, but they expose the subjects to radiation and therefore have limited use for monitoring progression of disease or treatment effects when repeat measurements are needed.

MR TECHNIQUES: MR SPECTROSCOPY AND FUNCTIONAL MRI

Magnetic resonance (MR) techniques, including high resolution structural MRI, ^{1}H MRS, pMRI, and BOLD-fMRI, do not involve ionizing radiation and are widely available commercially. Therefore, they are particularly useful for clinical applications and for monitoring treatment effects. Quantitative analyses of structural MRI has been shown to be sensitive for assessing brain injury in HIV (see Chapter 8.1, this volume). MRS has been used to identify chemical structures in vitro since the 1950s, however, since the late 1980s, it has been applied in vivo to study human metabolism. Proton MRS has been applied in more than 30 clinical studies of HIV associated brain injury, as well as opportunistic infections or neoplasms in patients with AIDS, while phosphorus (^{31}P) MRS has been applied to only few studies to evaluate the high-energy phosphate metabolites in HIV-associated dementia. In contrast, functional MRI techniques were developed just 15–20 years ago; many technical issues are still being improved and evaluated; hence, only a dozen clinical reports are available.

METHODOLOGICAL ASPECTS OF BRAIN MRS STUDIES

Proton (^{1}H) and Phosphorus (^{31}P) MRS

MR spectroscopy can detect metabolite resonances from several nuclei, most commonly ^{1}H and ^{31}P. A typical ^{1}H MR in vivo spectrum from the human brain has 4-6 major metabolite peaks (Figure 9.1.3). The N-acetyl (NA) peak is located at 2.02 ppm, and predominantly reflects the neuronal marker N-acetylaspartate (NAA) (Birken & Oldendorf, 1989). The total creatine (tCR) resonance at 3.0 ppm consists of the sum of the creatine and phosphocreatine signals (total creatine). Choline-containing compounds (CHO) resonate at 3.2 ppm and include water-soluble choline compounds, primarily free choline, phosphocholine, and glycero-phospho-choline (Miller et al., 1996). The signals from myo-inositol (MI), a glial marker that is only present in glial cells, resonate at 3.56 ppm (Brand, Richter-Landsberg, & Leibfritz, 1993). Glutamate plus glutamine (GLX, 2.1-2.7 ppm, with overlapping peaks) and gamma (γ)-amino butyric acid (GABA), which resonates at 2.0 ppm and 3.0 ppm, can be separated and assessed accurately only with customized MR sequences and/or editing techniques. Since ^{1}H MRS can measure metabolites that represent a neuronal marker (NA) and a glial marker (MI), it is particularly valuable for the in vivo

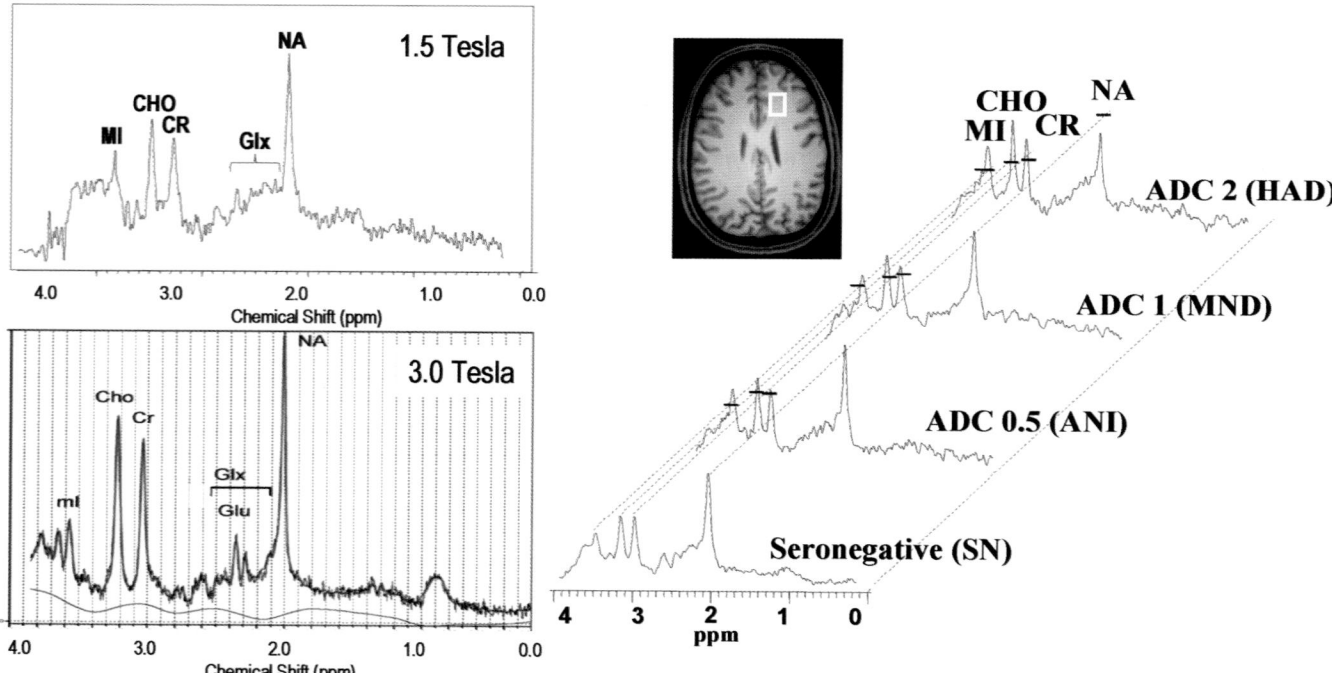

Figure 9.1.3 Left: Typical ^{1}H MR spectra acquired from the frontal white matter of a healthy volunteer on a 1.5 Tesla MR scanner (top) and 3.0 Tesla (bottom); both acquisitions used a short echo-time (TE) PRESS sequence (TR/TE = 3000/30ms). Note improved signal-to-noise and better separation of metabolite peaks in the MR spectrum acquired at the higher magnetic field. The major metabolite peaks include N-acetyl peak (NA, 2.02 ppm), glutamate and glutamine (Glx, 2.1–2.5 ppm), total creatine (CR, 3.0 ppm), choline-containing compounds (CHO, 3.2 ppm), and myo-inositol (MI). MI typically would collapse into a "pseudo-singlet" on 1.5 Tesla while Glutamate is difficult to delineate on the 1.5 Tesla spectrum. Right: Typical MR spectra from HIV-infected individuals compared to a SN control. CHO and MI are elevated even with asymptomatic neurocognitive impairment (ANI), whereas lower NA is found only in the individual with frank dementia.

non-invasive evaluation of neuronal integrity and glial responses in HIV associated brain injury.

^{31}P MRS allows the measurement of several compounds that are involved in high-energy phosphate metabolism, including adenosine triphosphate (ATP), phosphocreatine (PCr), and inorganic phosphate (Pi). ^{31}P MRS can also measure tissue pH by evaluating the relative shift between the Pi and PCr resonances (Figure 9.1.4). While the earliest in vivo MRS study of HIV brain disease used ^{31}P MRS, most of the studies used ^{1}H MRS because ^{31}P MRS has relatively lower signal-to-noise ratio and is limited to assessing predominantly high-energy phosphate metabolism.

METABOLITE CONCENTRATIONS VERSUS METABOLITE RATIOS

The result of MRS studies can be reported as ratios between metabolites, such as NA/CR, or as metabolite concentrations. The majority of published MRS studies in HIV patients report "metabolite ratios," and commonly used tCR or CHO as a reference. Total creatine and CHO, however, have been shown to vary with HIV disease stage (Suhy et al., 2000; Chang et al., 2002) as well as with subject age (Suhy et al., 2000; Chang et al., 1996; Zhong et al., 2002). Furthermore, a change in metabolite ratio can be caused by a change in the numerator or denominator metabolite, or both, and hence cannot be interpreted easily. Therefore, metabolite concentrations are preferable but typically require additional measurements and more complicated data analyses. The water signal from the brain is commonly used as a concentration reference for these measurements (Barker et al., 1993). To obtain accurate metabolite concentrations, it is also important to correct for the partial volume of cerebrospinal fluid (CSF) and the variable proportion of gray and white matter in MRS voxels, since CSF does not contain significant amounts of the major brain metabolites and could dilute the true metabolite

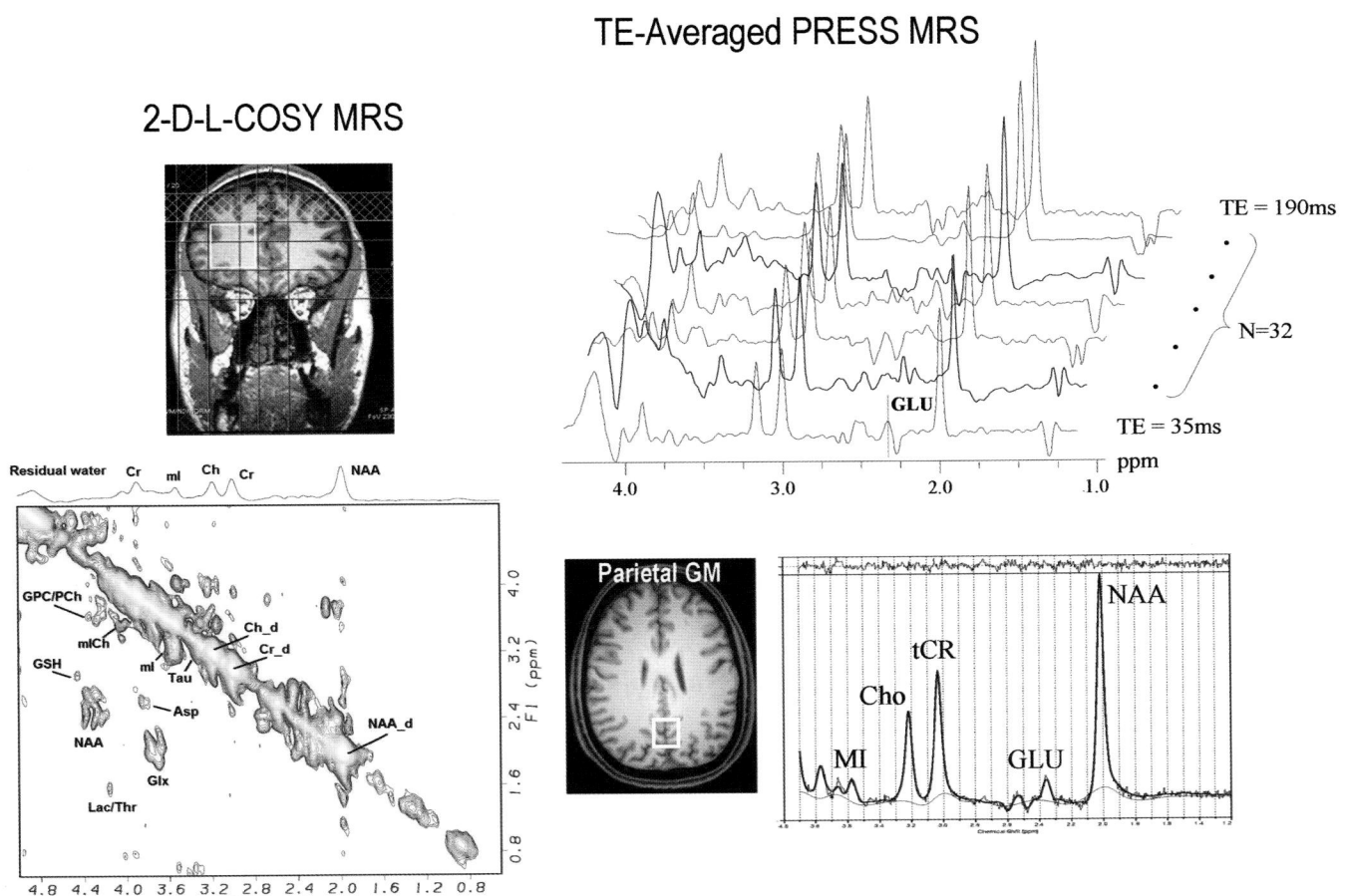

Figure 9.1.4 Left: Typical 2-D-L-COSY MRS from the dorsolateral prefrontal white matter of a 14 year old HIV-infected boy showing additional chemicals that can be delineated, such as GABA, Threonine/ Lactate, and Aspartate, compared to the 1-D MRS shown on top of the 2-D-MRS. The Spectrum was acquired with a 3T Trio-TIM MRI scanner (TR/TE = 2s/30ms), 2048 complex t2 points for the 1st spectral and 100 t1 increments for the 2nd spectral dimensions; 8 NEX per t1 increment (Courtesy of Dr. Albert Thomas from UCLA). Right: Representative MR spectrum from the parietal gray matter using the TE (echo time) averaged PRESS technique. Top image shows the multiple (n = 32 in this case) echo-times required to acquire the spectra, and the bottom image shows the averaged spectrum with well defined glutamate and myoinositol peaks, with markedly attenuated glutamine and macromolecule signals. The spectrum was also acquired from a 3 Tesla Trio-TIM scanner (Figure modified from Ernst et al., 2010).

concentrations (Ernst, Kreis, & Ross, 1993), and the variable proportion of gray-to-white matter may increase the inter-subject variability (Hetherington et al., 1994; Schuff et al., 2001).

MAJOR TECHNICAL CONSIDERATIONS IN MRS STUDIES

A strong static magnetic field is very important for MRI and MRS, since a higher magnetic field generally increases the signal strength and the spectral resolution between metabolite peaks (Figure 9.1.3). Therefore, more recent MRS studies in HIV infected individuals are performed at 3 or 4 Tesla field strength, as compared to the earlier studies that were conducted on 1.5 Tesla scanners (Table 9.1.4). The technical advantages of higher magnetic fields may also result in better reproducibility; for example, studies in our laboratory showed that the intra-subject variability for NAA, CR, CHO was 4-5% at 4 Tesla, but 6-7% at 1.5 Tesla. The smaller variability at higher fields may ultimately allow smaller sample sizes for clinical studies.

Another important MRS acquisition parameter for localized ^{1}H MRS is the "echo time" (TE). Short echo times (typically < 40ms) make it possible to detect all major metabolites, including NA, CR, CHO, MI, glutamate (Glu) plus glutamine (Gln), lactate, as well as some macromolecules. However, short-TE spectra may be crowded and exhibit a poorly defined baseline due to the presence of macromolecules. Hence, early ^{1}H MRS studies commonly used long echo times (typically >100ms), at which only NA, CR, and CHO

Table 9.1.4 PROTON MRS STUDIES OF HIV PATIENTS TREATED WITH ANTIRETROVIRAL MEDICATIONS

REFERENCES	NUMBER OF SUBJECTS	MRS METHOD	BRAIN REGIONS EVALUATED	ANTIRETROVIRAL MEDICATIONS	FINDINGS
Ernst et al., JMRI 2010	45 HIV (18 HAND; 27 unimpaired) 46 SN controls	3 Tesla MRI TE-averaged PRESS	4 brain regions Frontal cortex Frontal WM Basal Ganglia Parietal cortex	All on HAART (39 on nucleoside reverse transcriptase inhibitors)	Compared to controls, HIV subjects with cognitive deficits had lower Glu in the parietal gray matter, while those without cognitive deficits tended to show higher basal ganglia Glu. Lower parietal and frontal gray matter Glu were associated with greater number of NRTIs, and were predictive of poorer cognitive performance.
Mohamed et al., Magn Reson Imaging 2010	86 HIV+ (21 with HAD, 31 HIV+ MCI 34 HIV+NC)	3 Tesla MRI PRESS TR/TE = 2000/45 ms	2 voxels: Frontal white matter Basal Ganglia	All on HAART	Compared to both the MCI and NC groups, HAD subjects had lower glutamate+glutamine (Glx) and higher myo-inositol in the frontal white matter, but lower NAA in the basal ganglia. Lower Glx and NAA were associated with poor cognitive performance (Trail B, Digit Symbol, and Pegboard)
Banakar et al., JMRI 2008	10 HIV youths 11 SN controls (all 9-21 yrs)	1.5 Tesla MRI 2D-L-COSY	Left Frontal region	All on HAART	HIV-infected youths (infected since neonate) had elevated ratios of myo-inositol, GABA, and threonine-lactate (all relative to creatine or choline), as well as NAA/CR.
Schifitto et al., AIDS 2008	145 HIV ARV-stable subjects (51 had both baseline and wk 16 MRS)	1.5 Tesla MRI Multicenter MRS PROBE-p TR/TE = 3000/35 ms	3 voxels: Frontal gray matter, frontal white matter and parietal cortex	Stable on ARVs, studied before and after Memantine 40 mg qd x16 wks (ACTG 301/700)	61% of Memantine group and 85% of Placebo group reached the 40 mg dose at 16 weeks. No improvement on NPZ-8 but significant improvement on MRS (NA/Cr in frontal white matter and parietal cortex) after memantine
Chang et al., JNIP 2006	42 HIV (21 with chronic marijuana use) 54 SN controls (24 with chronic marijuana use)	4 Tesla MRI PRESS TR/TE = 3000/30 ms	6 brain regions: Frontal WM Basal ganglia Thalamus Parietal WM Occipital Cortex Cerebellar Vermis	38 of 42 HIV were on HAART	HIV infection (independent of MJ) was associated with trends for reduced NA in the parietal white matter and increased CHO in the basal ganglia. In contrast, MJ (independent of HIV) was associated with decreased basal ganglia NA, CHO, and glutamate, with increased thalamic creatine. HIV + MJ had normalization of the reduced glutamate in frontal white matter. HIV subjects had slower reaction times.

(Continues)

Table 9.1.4 (CONTINUED)

REFERENCES	NUMBER OF SUBJECTS	MRS METHOD	BRAIN REGIONS EVALUATED	ANTIRETROVIRAL MEDICATIONS	FINDINGS
Keller et al., Neurology 2006	12 HIV children studied with MRS at 24 weeks and 42 weeks (10 months) later	1.5 Tesla PRESS TR/TE = 3000/30 ms T2 decay for CSF correction and concentrations	5 voxels: Frontal GM R & L frontal WM R basal ganglia R hippocampus	11 stable on HAART, and one on 2 ARVs, during this 10 months period	Brain metabolites and metabolite ratios were all stable across the 3 time points during this 10 month follow-up period. Similarly, CD4, CD4%, viral load and clinical signs were all stable. Cognitive test showed improvement on spatial memory (practice effect vs. development).
Schweinsburg et al., J NeuroVirol 2005	18 HIV ddI+/- d4T 14 HIV AZT+3TC 16 HIV (no ARV) 17 SN controls	1.5 Tesla PRESS TR/TE = 3000/35 ms Ref to unsuppressed water	2 voxels: Frontal GM Frontal WM	18 on NRTIs (ddI and/or d4T); 14 on AZT + 3TC	HIV patients who were on didanosine (ddI) and/or stavudine (d4T) had 11.4% lower NAA in frontal WM compared to SN controls, and NAA levels of the other HIV+ groups were intermediate. NRTIs may lead to neuronal injury.
Chang et al., Antivir Ther 2004	39 HIV ARV naïve subjects before and 3 months after HAART	1.5 Tesla PRESS TR/TE = 3000/30 ms T2 decay for CSF correction and concentrations	3 voxels: Frontal GM Frontal WM Basal ganglia	HAART x 3 months	After HAART, MRS showed no change despite improvement on systemic variables (CD4, viral load, MCP-1) and CSF variables (viral load, MCP-1). CSF MCP-1, but not serum MCP-1, correlated inversely with the neuronal component before HAART and positively with the glial component after HAART.
Chang et al., Antivir Ther 2003	33 HIV ARV-naïve subjects had MRS before and 3 months after HAART	1.5 Tesla PRESS TR/TE = 3000/30 ms T2 decay for CSF correction and concentrations	3 voxels: Frontal GM Frontal WM Basal ganglia	HAART x 3 months	Despite improvements on CD4 and suppression of systemic and CSF viral load, elevated brain metabolites (choline compounds and myoinositol levels), as well as abnormalities on neuropsychological tests (including CalCAP) persisted after 3 months of HAART
Stankoff et al., Neurology 2001	HIV = 11 completed 9 month follow-up during HAART (from 22 at baseline);	1.5 Tesla STEAM TR/TE = 1500/136/18ms Studies performed at baseline, 3, 6 & 9 mo	3 voxels: Centrum semi-ovale Frontal WM; Medial parieto-occipital GM	At baseline: 19 were on HAART; one on two nucleosides; two were on no meds	Five were cognitively unimpaired and had normal NA/CR that remained normal. Six were cognitively impaired and showed improvement on NA/CR and MI/CR.
Chang et al., Neurology 1999	HIV = 16; Controls = 15	1.5 Tesla PRESS TR/TE = 3000/30 ms	3 voxels: Frontal GM Frontal WM Basal ganglia	Baseline: ≤ 2 ARVs (3 were on no meds); After HAART: 3-4 ARVs	14 of 16 who tolerated HAART showed reversal of initially elevated [MI] in frontal white matter and basal ganglia, and initially elevated CHO/CR in frontal cortex.
Wilkinson et al., JNNP 1997	HIV = 5 (ADC subjects before and after AZT)	1.5 Tesla PRESS TR/TE = 1600/135 ms	Single voxel, 8 cm³; parieto-occipital region	Before and after Zidovudine (ZDV)	Before AZT, NA/(NA+CHO+CR) was >2SD below the mean in 4/5 subjects. All 5 subjects showed increased NA/(NA+CHO+CR) ratio after AZT. Two subjects who deteriorated subsequently had concomitant decrease in NA/(NA+CHO+CR).
Salvan et al., AIDS Res Hum Retroviruses 1997	HIV = 11 (from a larger study of 112);	1.5 Tesla PRESS TR/TE = 1600/135 ms	Single voxel parietal	11 patients were followed up after ZDV	14% with normal MRI had abnormal MRS regardless of neurological status; neuroasymptomatic patients and ADC subjects both had elevated CHO/CR while ADC subjects also had decreased NA/CR
McConnell et al., AIDS Res Hum Retroviruses 1994	HIV = 6 (from total of 10 patients studied)	1.5 Tesla PRESS TR = 2000 ms; TE = 40/270 ms	Single voxel, 27mL temporoparietal region (including GM + WM)	4 were on ddI only; 2 were on ZDV, ddI ± NVP	NA/CR decreased in all HIV subjects on follow-up studies, most severe in those with progressive neurological impairment

ARV = antiretrovirals; ZDV = zidovudine; ddI = didanosine; NVP = neverapine; NRTI = nucleoside reverse transcriptase inhibitors; HAART = highly active antiretroviral therapy
PRESS = point resolved spectroscopy; L-COSY = localized chemical shift correlated spectroscopy; WM = white matter; GM = gray matter

could be detected. Longer TE also attenuates MR signals, requiring longer acquisition time or larger volumes of interest, and is rarely used in recent MRS studies. To address the issue of crowded or overlapping MR signals in the short TE spectrum, several novel MRS techniques have been developed and applied to the study of HIV-infected brain recently.

One of these novel MRS techniques is two-dimensional (2D) localized chemical shift correlated spectroscopy (L-COSY), which converts a crowded, overlapping 1D MR spectrum to a better resolved 2D spectrum through the addition of a second spectral dimension (Figure 9.1.4, left panel). In 2D-L-COSY MRS, there are two frequency axes (F1 & F2); F2 detects the "conventional" chemical shift of metabolites, while F1 detects J-coupling (indirect spin-spin coupling) between protons connected through covalent bonds through chemically shifted peaks indirectly along the F1 frequency axis. In addition to the metabolite ratios that are commonly reported using 1D ^{1}H-MRS metabolites, metabolites at physiological concentrations around 1mM, such as phosphocholine (PCh), phosphoethanolamine (PE), free aspartate (Asp), γ-aminobutyrate (GABA), threonine+lactate (Thr+Lac), and Glu+Gln (Glx) may also be detected using 2DL-COSY (Thomas et al., 2001; Banakar et al., 2008).

Other new MRS techniques utilize an editing approach to detect metabolites that are hidden underneath the major singlet-resonances. For instance, γ-amino-butyric acid (GABA, an important inhibitory neurotransmitter) and glutathione (GSH, a major antioxidant) are water soluble compounds at millimolar concentrations in the brain, which is sufficient for in vivo detection with ^{1}H MRS. In humans, detection of these metabolites typically requires the use of spectral editing techniques, since their resonances are obscured by the much larger total creatine (tCR) signal at 3.0 ppm. This is possible because the GABA and GSH resonances show J-coupling, whereas the tCR signal is a singlet.

There are two main techniques for spectral editing in vivo. First, editing in the human brain can be achieved by means of a double quantum coherence (DQC) filter, for instance for GSH (Trabesinger et al., 1999; Trabesinger & Boesiger, 2001). The DQC filter provides "single-shot" editing and entirely eliminates the signals from uncoupled spins, such as tCR, but leads to a significant attenuation of the GSH signal compared to other methods. The second method uses a difference editing technique in combination with LCModel analysis (Terpstra, Henry, & Gruetter, 2003). This technique, which has been labeled "MEGA-PRESS" or "BASING," yields a higher signal-to-noise ratio (SNR) than the DQC filtering method, but is not single-shot and involves an add-subtract cycle. Specifically, selective inversion of coupled methyl or methylene groups (with chemical shifts different from that of the resonance of interest) will invert the resonance of interest, but not the overlying singlet. Therefore, subtraction of spectra with selective inversion from those without will enhance the coupled resonance of interest, while eliminating the uncoupled singlets (Figure 9.1.4, right panel). The MEGA-PRESS method is used more commonly in vivo, due to its higher SNR compared to DQC filtering. The situation is very similar for GABA, since the C2-GABA resonance of interest

(at 3.05ppm) is obscured by the 3.0ppm tCR peak. Again, a variety of editing methods have been proposed (Henry et al., 2001; Hetherington, Newcomer, & Pan, 1998; Keltner et al., 1997; Mescher et al., Shen & Rothman, 2001; Wilman & Allen, 1995), including MEGA-PRESS (Terpstra, Ugurbil, & Gruetter, 2001).

SINGLE VOXEL MRS VERSUS MRS IMAGING (MRSI)

MRS can be performed in a single volume of interest (i.e., voxel) at a time (which is termed "single voxel" or "localized" MRS) or in rectangular array of voxels that cover a larger brain region or a few slices (MRS imaging, or "MRSI"). Localized MRS studies allow robust acquisitions at short echo time; however, the long cumulative scan time limits spectral acquisition to only a few voxels. In contrast, MRSI studies make it possible to cover large brain areas, but commonly suffer from poorer spectral resolution, variable magnetic field homogeneity throughout the brain, and are commonly performed at long echo times in order to suppress strong unwanted lipid signals from the scalp. Therefore, essentially all but one published MRSI studies in HIV patients reported only results of NA, CR and CHO.

MRS STUDIES IN HIV PATIENTS

^{31}P MRS in HIV Dementia

Only four ^{31}P MRS studies evaluated HIV associated brain injury. The first study was performed using a 3-cm thick axial slice and found reduced PCr and adenosine triphosphate (Bottomley et al., 1990). Another study also found that HIV patients had lower ATP/Pi and PCr/Pi ratios compared with the control group; furthermore, the ATP/Pi as well as the PCr/Pi ratios correlated negatively with overall severity of neuropsychiatric impairment (Deicken et al., 1991). These findings suggest that HIV brain infection might impair cellular oxidative metabolism. Alcohol and HIV were shown to cumulatively reduce PCr and phosphodiester; successive decreases in phosphodiester and PCr were observed in seronegative (SN) nonalcoholics, followed by SN alcoholics, then HIV nonalcoholics, and HIV alcoholics (Meyerhoff et al., 1995). Another ^{31}P MRS study additionally found more alkaline pH in the cerebellum of patients with HIV (Figure 9.1.5); the investigators proposed that HIV infection might have activated the astrocytic Na+/H+ exchanger (Patton et al., 2001). These four studies demonstrate that ^{31}P MRS may be useful for assessing in vivo high-energy metabolism and the pH in the brain. This knowledge should ultimately improve our understanding of the pathophysiology of HIV brain injury.

^{1}H MRS in HIV Patients

More than 30 ^{1}H MRS studies have been performed in both adult and pediatric patients with HIV infection, using localized MRS and MRSI techniques, long or short echo times,

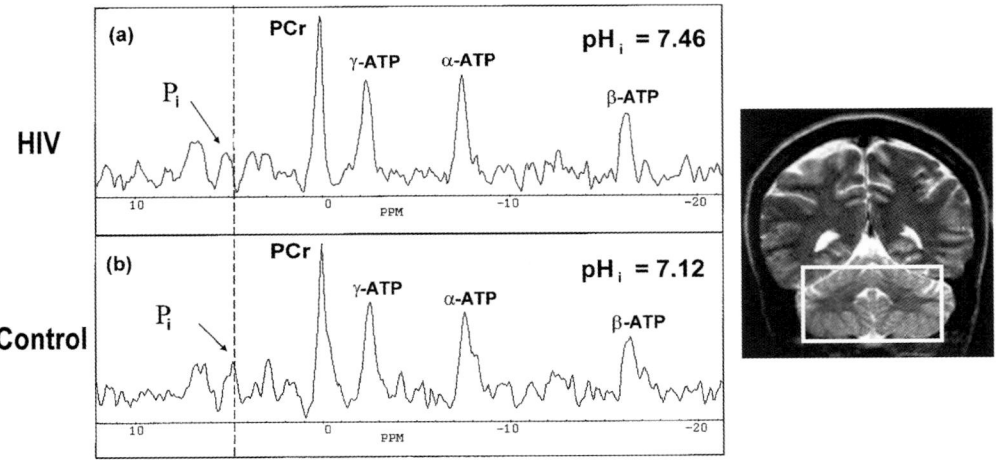

Figure 9.1.5 Selected ³¹P-MR spectra from the cerebellum in an HIV-infected patient (a) and a healthy volunteer (b); both acquired at 4.1 Tesla field strength. Each spectrum was acquired from an 11.5 ml voxel. Phosphocreatine (PCr) was used as an internal reference and was assigned a chemical shift of 0.0 ppm. The chemical shift of inorganic phosphate (Pi) vs. PCr was used for pH$_i$ determination. The spectra are shown with baseline correction. (Courtesy from Patton et al., modified from Patton et al., 2001).

1-D, 2-D or editing approaches, at different field strengths (1.5, 3, or 4 Tesla), and before or after antiretroviral treatment. More recent studies also evaluated HIV patients who had no neuropsychiatric symptoms or were asymptomatic for cognitive deficits. The majority of the studies used localized spectroscopy techniques that evaluated one to six brain regions; only six studies used MRSI. In order to maximize the signal-to-noise ratio, earlier studies used larger voxels, 8-64 mL (Menon, Ainsworth, & Cox, 1992; Chong et al., 1993; McConnell et al., 1994); metabolite concentrations from these larger volumes typically contained combined signals from white matter, gray matter and/or CSF. More recent MRS studies used smaller voxel sizes (0.8 to 3 mL), which allowed better separation of white and gray matter regions. Earlier localized MRS studies employed long echo times which only allowed measurements of NA, CR, and CHO, but the subsequent studies that used short-echo times (19-35ms) confirmed earlier studies that HIV dementia is associated with decreased NA (or NA/CR) and elevated CHO (or CHO/CR), and additionally found elevated glial marker MI (or MI/CR), especially in those with more severe dementia. The newest MRS studies, especially those with higher field strength or the newer 2-D or editing techniques, also found alterations in brain Glu levels (Ernst et al., 2010) or Glx (Mohamed et al., 2010), and possible alterations in GABA and Asp, in patients with or without HAND(Banaker et al., 2008).

LONG-ECHO TIME LOCALIZED ¹H MRS STUDIES IN HIV PATIENTS

The earliest MRS studies were performed at long echo times (TE > 100 ms). The first case report appeared in 1990 (Menon et al., 1990) and the first small study by the same group in 1992 (Menon et al., 1992). A year later, the first large series of MRS in HIV patients (n = 103) confirmed the early observations that decreased NA/Cr and elevated CHO/CR were present in HIV patients, especially in those with diffuse MRI

abnormalities (Chong et al., 1993). A multicenter study, across three sites, used long echo-time MRS and further confirmed that patients with CDC IV had the lowest NA/CR and NA/CHO (Paley et al., 1996). Another large study found elevation of CHO/CR in both neuroasymptomatic patients and those with AIDS dementia complex (ADC), while the ADC patients additionally had lower NA/CR (Salvan et al., 1997). These studies demonstrate that metabolite abnormalities can be detected with proton MRS, and that the pattern evolves with disease severity.

SHORT ECHO TIME MRS STUDIES IN HIV PATIENTS

The first short echo time MRS study in HIV patients appeared in 1993 (Jarvik et al., 1993). The short echo time studies confirmed findings from earlier long echo time studies, and primarily used the single voxel approach (Jarvik et al., 1993; Paley et al., 1995; Laubenberger et al., 1996; Tracey et al., 1996; English et al., 1997; Chang et al., 1999), except for one that used MRSI (Lopez-Villegas, Lenkinski, & Frank, 1997). Most studies concurred that decreased NA/Cr or NA/Cho were more commonly observed in HIV patients with cognitive impairment, but not in those who were neurologically asymptomatic (Menon et al., 1992; Paley et al., 1996; Salvan et al., 1997; Laubenberger et al., 1996; Tracey et al., 1996; Chang et al., 1999; Chong et al., 1994). The decreased ratios were commonly interpreted as decreases in NAA, which is a neuronal marker, and hence were thought to reflect neuronal loss in the HIV patients. However, prior to HAART, studies that measured metabolite concentrations generally found decreased NA only at later stages of the disease, but relatively normal NA levels during early stages of cognitive impairment (Chang et al., 1999; Barker, Lee, & McArthur, 1995) or in those with no cognitive deficits (Meyerhoff et al., 1999) (see also Figures 9.1.3 & 9.1.6). Recent studies in subjects chronically infected with HIV for more than a decade are beginning

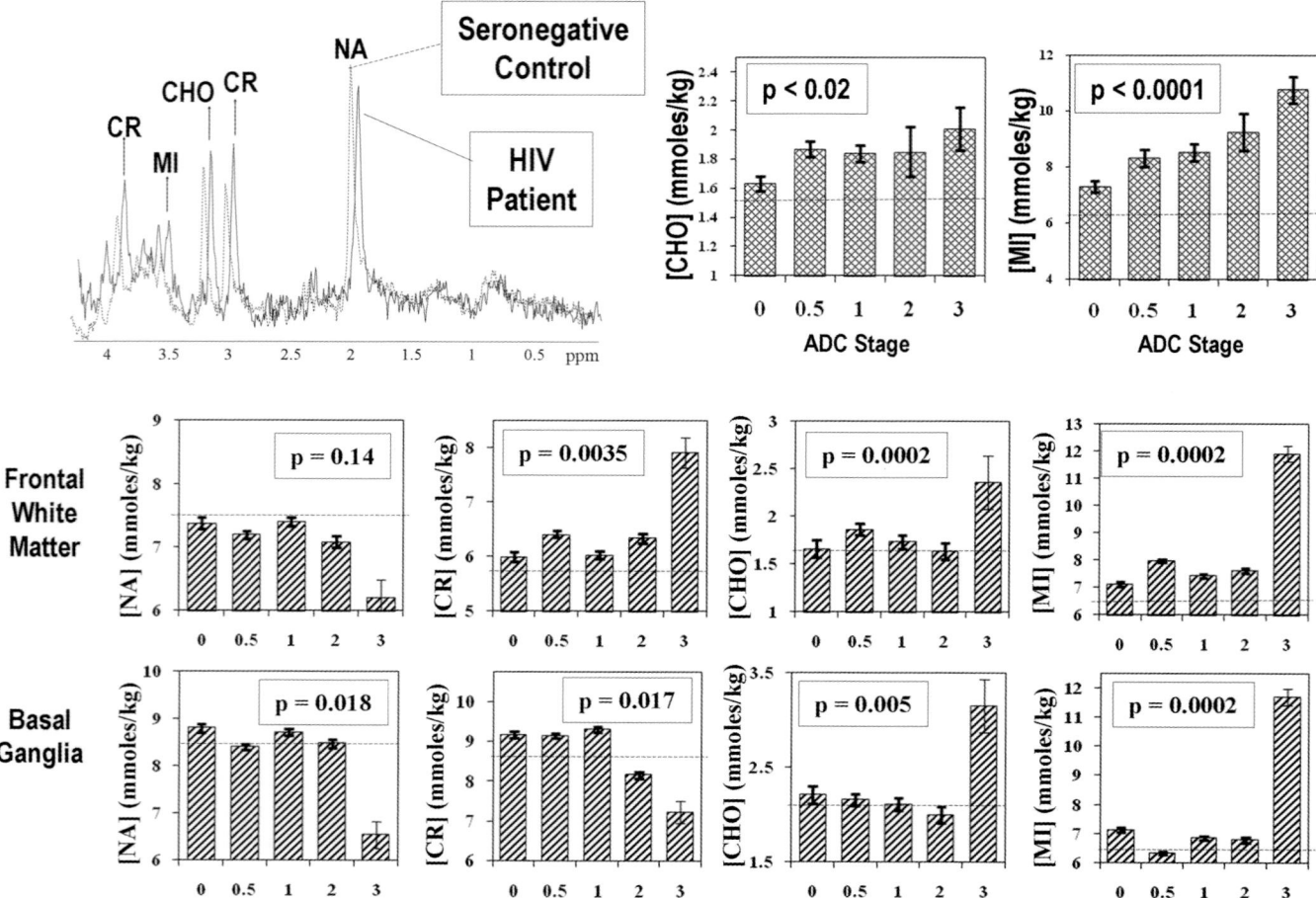

Figure 9.1.6 Top left: Compared to a seronegative control subject, an HIV patient (ADC stage 2) has decreased NA and increases in CR, CHO and MI in the frontal white matter. Both MR spectra were acquired on a 4 Tesla MR scanner (PRESS sequence, TR/TE = 3000/30ms, 64 averages). Metabolite changes are dependent on AIDS dementia complex (ADC) stages: Top right: Note gradual increases in choline and myoinositol in frontal white matter of HIV patients with increasing disease stage (data presented in Chang et al., 1999). The bottom two rows show that metabolite changes vary regionally and with disease stage. For instance, total creatine increases in the frontal white matter but decreases with the severity of dementia in the basal ganglia (data presented in Chang et al., 2002). The horizontal dashed lines in each graph indicate the mean value in the SN controls.

to show decreased NAA, more commonly decreased NA/CR, even in those with mild cognitive deficits (see below).

The CR peak is frequently used as an internal reference for MRS; however, it may change depending on disease stage and brain region in HIV patients (Figure 9.1.6). Concentration measurements illustrated that decreased NA/CR may be due to either a normal [NA], or mildly decreased [NA] along with elevated [CR], especially in the basal ganglia, during the cognitively asymptomatic stage (Chang et al., 1999; Chang et al., 1999b). Therefore, the prior finding of decreased NA/CR in HIV patients (Menon et al., 1990; Jarvik et al., 1993; Paley et al., 1995; Meyerhoff et al., 1993), even in those who were neurologically asymptomatic (Suwanwelaa et al., 2000), may reflect elevated CR rather than decreased NA. In the later stages of ADC, [CR] is significantly elevated in the frontal lobe, but decreased in the basal ganglia, along with decreased [NA] (Chang et al., 2002) (Figure 9.1.3). The elevation in [CR] may also obscure concomitant increases in CHO and MI. This emphasizes the

importance of metabolite concentration measurements and the ambiguity caused by using CR as an internal reference.

Short TE studies also demonstrated increased CHO/CR ratio in HIV patients (Jarvik et al., 1993; Tracey et al., 1996; English et al., 1997; Chang et al., 1999). Elevated CHO might be due to increased cellularity since neuropathological studies have shown increased number of macrophages and microglia cells in the brains of AIDS patients. Alternatively, higher choline compounds might be related to increased cell membrane break down and release of soluble choline compounds due to direct or indirect effects of HIV infection. Studies that evaluated metabolite concentrations indeed found elevated CHO both in patients with minor cognitive motor disorder (MCMD) and, even more so, in those with ADC (Figures 9.1.3 & 9.1.6) (Chang et al., 1999; Barker, Lee, & McArthur, 1995; Meyerhoff et al., 1999).

Elevated MI/CR or MI, which is observable only at short-echo times, has been reported at various stages of HIV dementia (Laubenberger et al., 1996; Chang et al., 1999;

Lopez-Villegas, Lenkinski, & Frank, 1997; von Giesen et al., 2001). Since MI is present primarily in glial cells (Brand et al., 1993) and has the putative function of regulating the cellular osmotic environment and maintaining the cell volume (Graf, Guggino, & Turnheim, 1993), glial activation or hypertrophy would be associated with elevated cytoplasmic MI. Measurement of MI concentrations in HIV patients further support this hypothesis since MI levels increase with dementia severity (Figures 9.1.3 & 9.1.6), especially in the frontal white matter where glial activation has been observed in neuropathological studies (Power et al., 1993).

REGIONAL VARIATIONS IN METABOLITE ABNORMALITIES

The frontal brain regions had been difficult to evaluate due to magnetic susceptibility problems in many of the earlier localized MRS studies; therefore, parietal or occipital brain regions were typically evaluated. However, technical advances such as adjustments of the slice order (Ernst & Chang, 1996), have made it possible to evaluate the frontal lobe and subcortical brain regions, including the basal ganglia and the thalamus. Elevated CHO/CR or MI/CR ratios, as well as CHO and MI concentrations, have been observed in the frontal white matter of neuroasymptomatic HIV patients or those with mild dementia (English et al., 1997), whereas similar changes in the frontal gray matter and basal ganglia are more often observed in those with more severe dementia (Chang et al., 1999; von Giesen et al., 2001) (also see Figure 9.1.6).

Regional variations can be more efficiently evaluated with spectroscopic imaging techniques (Lopez-Villegas et al., 1997;

Barker et al., 1995; Meyerhoff et al., 1999; Meyerhoff et al., 1993; Meyerhoff et al., 1994; Meyerhoff et al., 1996; Marcus et al., 1998; Moller et al., 1999). All but one (Barker et al., 1995) of these studies found no significant regional variations, and confirmed the findings of localized MRS with respect to HIV brain injury. Therefore, the general consensus from single-slice MRSI studies was that metabolite abnormalities occur diffusely throughout the brain. However, spectroscopic imaging using a multi-slice technique found higher CHO and lower NA in the frontal white matter of patients with AIDS dementia complex and lower CD4 count, but primarily higher CHO without decreased NA in the frontal white matter in patients with only MCMD and higher CD4 count (Figure 9.1.7). Since these regional changes are not always evident on all the slices, multi-slice MRSI may ensure a more comprehensive assessment of regional brain metabolite abnormalities. One study used a grid of small voxels (6x6x10mm) at short echo-time, and found elevated MI/CR in the frontal white matter of neuroasymptomatic HIV patients but only decreased NA/CR and normal MI/CR in the gray matter of patients with ADC (Lopez-Villages et al., 1997). These findings are consistent with a localized MRS study that found elevated MI levels in the frontal lobe of patients without dementia, and further elevation of both CR and MI in those with dementia (Chang et al., 2002).

MRS STUDIES OF HIV PATIENTS AFTER ANTIRETROVIRAL (ARV) TREATMENTS

Several longitudinal MRS studies evaluated the effects of ARV treatment in HIV patients. One of these followed seven HIV

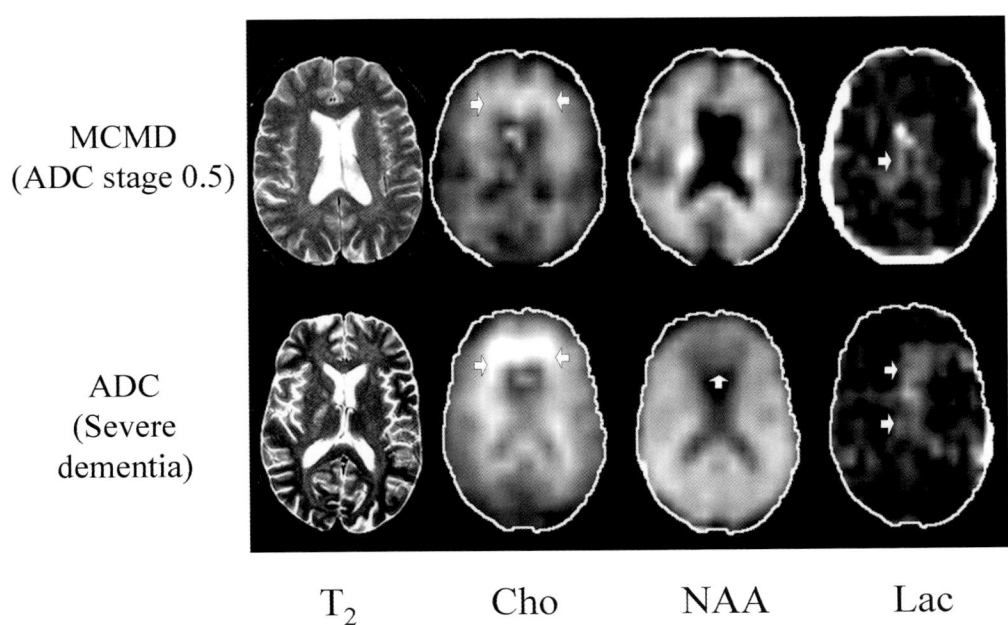

Figure 9.1.7 Spectroscopic imaging in two patients with HIV. Top row: 58-year-old HIV patient with mild cognitive motor disorder and CD4 count of 300 cells/μL; note mildly elevated choline compounds in the frontal white matter region with relatively normal NAA. Bottom row: 35-year-old HIV patient with AIDS dementia complex and CD4 count of 143 cells/μl shows further elevation of choline compounds and decreased NAA in the frontal brain region. Spectroscopic images were acquired on a 1.5 Tesla MR scanner (PRESS, TR/TE=2300/272ms); (Courtesy of Dr. Peter Barker, modified from Barker, Lee, & McArthur, 1995).

patients over one year, and found that NA/CR further decreased in all subjects despite treatment with one to three ARVs in six of these patients (McConnell et al., 1994). In contrast, other studies found primarily improvements in metabolite ratios or concentrations in HIV patients after antiretroviral treatment. One study evaluated five patients before and after zidovudine (ZDV) treatment, and found that NA/(CR+CHO+CR) improved (increased) 4 to 13 weeks after treatment along with clinical improvement in all patients, but the ratio decreased later in two patients who deteriorated (Wilkinson et al., 1997). Another study also followed 11 patients after 1000mg/day of ZDV, and found metabolite improvements only in those with decreased NA/CR at baseline but not in those with initially elevated CHO/CR (Salvan et al., 1997). A study of two pediatric patients similarly found normalization of the initially decreased NA/CR and disappearance of the lactate peaks 4 to 8 months after antiretrovirals (Pavlakis et al., 1998). Since these studies relied on metabolite ratios, changes in NA/CR or NA/(CR+CHO+CR) may in fact be due to decreases in the initially elevated CR and CHO after treatment.

The possible normalization of CR or CHO after ARV treatment was demonstrated in several MRS studies that evaluated the effects of highly active antiretroviral therapy (HAART) on brain metabolites. One study found that HIV patients had normalization of the initially increased MI and CHO levels (prior to HAART) in the frontal white matter and basal ganglia, after a mean follow-up period of 9 months on HAART (Chang et al., 1999). Another study followed a group of HIV patients who were already started on HAART over a period of 9 months and found that only those with cognitive impairment and lower NA/CR and higher MI/CR at baseline showed improvement on the metabolite abnormalities (Stankoff et al., 2001). A more systematic study of ARV-naïve HIV patients found that although viral loads and CD4 counts may rebound dramatically and rapidly (within one to three months) after HAART, the metabolite abnormalities (elevated CHO and MI) may persist or increased further after 3 months of HAART (Chang et al., 2000), and improve only after 6–9 months (Chang et al., 2001a). This study also further demonstrated that the relationship between macrophage chemotatic protein (MCP-1) and brain metabolites of HIV patients was altered after HAART. Specifically, despite the normalization of plasma and CSF MCP-1 after 3 months of HAART, the NAA was associated with CSF MCP-1 only at baseline while MI was associated with MCP-1 after HAART (Chang et al., 2004). Therefore, future medication trials using MRS metabolite measurements as surrogate markers should have follow-up evaluations longer than 6 months after treatment.

Although HIV patients may show significant improvements in psychomotor speed after 6 months of HAART (Sacktor et al., 1999), cognitive testing may be affected by practice effects, mood disorders, education, or cultural influences. Since regional metabolites on MRS correlated well with selected measures of neuropsychological tests (Chang et al., 2002; Lopez-Villages et al., 1997; Meyerhoff et al., 1999), the combination of cognitive testing and MRS might provide confirmatory and complementary information regarding treatment effects. The ACTG 301/700 trial that assessed changes in NPZ-8 and MRS markers after 16 weeks of memantine in HAART stable HIV patients found that frontal white matter NA/CR, but not NPZ-8, normalized (improved) after memantine, which suggests that MRS may be a more sensitive tool for monitoring treatment effects (Schifitto et al., 2007).

Since HIV is a chronic disease that required long-term ARV treatment, it is possible that some of the ARVs might have deleterious effects on the brain. One study that evaluated HIV-infected individuals who were taking non-nucleoside reverse transcriptase inhibitors (NRTIs), such as didanosine (ddI) and/or stavudine (d4T) had 11.4% lower NAA in frontal WM compared to SN controls, and NAA levels of the other HIV+ groups were intermediate. These findings suggest that ARVs, NRTIs in particular, might lead to neuronal injury since they could be neurotoxic to the mitochondria (Schweinsburg et al., 2005).

DETECTION OF METABOLITE ABNORMALITIES IN NONDEMENTED HIV PATIENTS

As described earlier, HIV patients tend to have elevated CHO/CR and MI/CR during the early stages and additional decreased NA/CR in later stages of ADC. However, some studies found no decreased NA/CR (Salvan et al., 1997; Marcus et al., 1998) but elevated CHO/CR (Salvan et al., 1997) or CHO (Meyerhoff et al., 1999), while others reported decreased NA/CR (Suwanwelaa et al., 2000; Wilkinson et al., 1997), in those who were systemically asymptomatic (Wilkinson et al., 1997), CDC groups A & B (Moller et al., 1999) or neurologically asymptomatic (Suwanwelaa et al., 2000; Marcus et al., 1998). In several studies, neuropsychological tests were also performed to ensure the neuroasymptomatic status of the subjects (Chang et al., 2002; Meyerhoff et al., 1999; Jarvik et al., 1996). These discrepant findings might be due to differing medication status of the subjects, since the two studies that found no change in CHO/CR or CHO levels during the asymptomatic stage were performed in subjects who were antiretroviral medication-naïve (Chang et al., 2002; Suwanwelaa et al., 2000). Alternatively, the changing disease pattern of HIV dementia also might contribute to these differing observations, since the more recent studies tend to observe little or no change in CHO during the early stages of HIV dementia (Chang et al., 2002; Suwanwelaa et al., 2000; von Giesen et al., 2001; Marcus et al., 1998).

Since elevated cytokines and chemokines associated with systemic inflammation might lead to glial activation (Conant et al., 1998), the putative glial marker MI might be elevated during the neuroasymptomatic stage of the disease. Although two MRS studies found normal MI/CR ratios (Suwanwelaa et al., 2000; von Giesen et al., 2001), MRS studies that measured concentrations typically found elevation of both MI and CR in the frontal white matter (Chang et al., 2002), which would tend to attenuate abnormalities in MI/CR. These findings again stress the importance of metabolite concentration measurements, especially while assessing small changes in the brain metabolites.

Lastly, an early study of asymptomatic HIV patients found a higher "marker peak"/CR ratio (Jarvik et al., 1996), while other studies found no change in Glx/CR in the same frequency range (2.1–2.5 ppm) on the MR spectrum (Chang et al., 1999; Marcus et al., 1998). However, since the metabolites in this spectral region are particularly difficult to quantify, due to the presence of macromolecules and overlapping peaks from Glu, Gln and GABA, these metabolites may be more accurately assessed and better separated at higher magnetic fields. More recent studies of HIV-infected individuals treated with HAART found lower Glx and/or glutamate (Glu) in the frontal white matter, more so in those with greater cognitive deficits, using higher magnetic field, specifically 4 Tesla (Chang et al., 2006) or 3 Tesla (Mohamed et al., 2010). Novel techniques such as TE-averaged PRESS or 2-D-LCOSY may be better suited to assess brain glutamate levels (see below).

MRS ABNORMALITIES IN PEDIATRIC HIV PATIENTS

Fewer MRS studies evaluated brain metabolites in pediatric HIV patients due to the small population of vertically infected children in the developed countries. Perinatally infected youths, however, may have the longest possible exposure to ongoing infection in their brains and may present a unique population to evaluate how the infection alters brain development. Several MRS studies demonstrated that its usefulness for monitoring of HIV infected children, due to its sensitivity for assessing brain pathology and its safety for repeat measurements.

Neonates born to HIV positive mothers were found to have lower NA/CR, higher CHO/CR, and higher "marker-region peak"/CR compared to neonate controls with HIV negative mothers (Cortey et al., 1994). Since the majority of these babies were not infected, these abnormalities were thought to be related to the indirect effects of HIV, such as intrauterine growth retardation. Another study further observed increased lipid signals in the centrum semiovale of 20 HIV-infected children; 5 with encephalopathy additionally showed decreased NA and increased MI relative to all the other metabolites (Salvan et al., 1998). The largest series included 45 children with AIDS and found lower NA/CR in those with encephalopathy; however, those who were neuroasymptomatic showed normal NA/CR but lower CHO/CR in the basal ganglia region (Lu et al., 1996). Furthermore, two children with AIDS encephalopathy showed normalization of NA/CR and disappearance of lactate in the basal ganglia after treatment with ZDV (Pavlakis et al., 1998).

A study that evaluated metabolite concentrations in five brain regions found that compared to 13 seronegative controls, 20 HIV-infected children had lower CHO in the left frontal white matter, and those with higher viral load (>5000 copies/mL) also had lower CHO, CR and MI in the basal ganglia but higher CHO in the anterior cingulate cortex (Keller et al., 2004). In addition, the HIV subjects did not show the normal (as seen in the controls) age-dependent increase in [NAA] in the frontal white matter and right hippocampus, but had age-dependent increases in myo-inositol levels in the frontal white matter instead. In the HIV subjects, the elevated MI in the frontal white matter and elevated CHO (which suggested a greater inflammatory response) in the anterior cingulate were associated with higher plasma viral load. These HIV children also had poorer spatial memory, and delayed memory performance correlated with elevated CHO in the hippocampus. These data suggest ongoing neuroinflammation in selected brain regions, which again demonstrate the importance of assessing multiple brain regions, and that normal brain development may be delayed in these HIV-infected children. These findings provide a strong argument for early aggressive treatment of infants with HIV before the development of encephalopathy. Twelve of these 20 children were followed over 10 months, and were re-assessed at 6 months and 10 months; no further deterioration of their brain metabolites were found along with their stable clinical course and cognitive assessments (Keller et al., 2006).

A recent study demonstrated the feasibility of using the novel 2D-L-COSY MRS to detect brain metabolite abnormalities associated with brain development in 10 HIV-infected youths and 11 controls (Banaker et al., 2008) (also see Figure 9.1.4). The HIV-infected children had elevated ratios of myo-inositol, GABA, and threonine-lactate (all relative to creatine or choline), as well as NAA/CR. These elevated metabolite ratios may be due to lower levels of CHO and CR, which had been reported in HIV-infected children, especially in the neuroasymptomatic children (Keller et al., 2004). However, assuming the levels of CR and CHO were not altered in these subjects, the elevated GABA ratio would suggest higher density of inhibitory interneurons in the frontal cortex, which is contrary to findings in adult HIV patients at autopsy (Chana et al., 2006). On the other hand, the HIV-infected developing brain may show compensatory responses that are different than HIV-infected adults and may lead to elevated GABA instead.

GLUTAMATE AND OTHER BRAIN METABOLITE ABNORMALITIES IN HIV PATIENTS

In addition to 2D-L-COSY, other novel MRS techniques can remove or separate the Glu peak from the overlapping peaks, such as Gln, tCR and macromolecules. A study that used the TE-averaged PRESS technique found that compared to 46 SN controls, 21 adult HIV subjects with cognitive deficits had lower Glu in the parietal gray matter, while 21 adult HIV subjects without cognitive deficits show trends for higher basal ganglia Glu (Ernst et al., 2010). Lower parietal and frontal gray matter Glu were associated with greater number of NRTIs, and were predictive of poorer cognitive performance. The lower Glu in the parietal cortex might have resulted from reduced astrocytic reuptake of Glu, secondary excitotoxicity, and mitochondrial toxicity from antiretroviral treatments. The lower parietal Glu in patients with HAND is consistent with another 3-Tesla study that found lower Glx (which contains primarily Glu signals) in the frontal white matter of HIV patients with HAD and treated with HAART (Mohamed et al., 2010). Therefore, the glutamatergic system may play an important role in the pathophysiology of HAND or possible deleterious effects of NRTIs. Brain Glu accurately assessed by ^{1}H MRS may be a useful early surrogate marker for monitoring disease severity and treatment effects.

PERFUSION AND FUNCTIONAL MRI TO EVALUATE HIV PATIENTS

Perfusion MRI can measure regional cerebral blood volume (rCBV) and blood flow (rCBF); the latter can also be obtained by nuclear medicine techniques (see above). One of the disadvantages of past nuclear medicine and perfusion MRI studies is that brain "function" was evaluated at rest. In contrast, blood-oxygenation-level-dependent (BOLD) functional MRI (fMRI) allows the direct observation of brain activation while subjects are performing cognitive tasks. This approach is analogous to performing a "stress test" for the brain. However, despite the large number of studies demonstrating cognitive deficits in HIV brain infection, there are only a few perfusion MRI studies that evaluated cerebral perfusion (Table 9.1.4) and several BOLD-fMRI studies that assessed the neural substrate of cognitive abnormalities in HIV patients (Table 9.1.5). We will review some of the technical aspects of perfusion MRI and BOLD fMRI, and discuss the findings of these published studies.

METHODOLOGICAL AND TECHNICAL ASPECTS OF PERFUSION MRI

The advent of ultrafast MRI techniques, such as echo planar imaging (EPI), has made it possible to scan the entire brain in a few seconds, with very little motion artifacts. By repeatedly scanning the brain at this high temporal resolution, it is possible to assess the functional and physiological state of the brain, including cerebral perfusion. The earliest perfusion MRI technique used an intravenous bolus injection of an MR contrast agent, and is called "dynamic susceptibility contrast" (DSC) pMRI (Rosen, Belliveau, & Chien, 1989). Following the bolus injection, the slightly magnetic contrast agent travels

Table 9.1.5 CEREBRAL BLOOD FLOW OR VOLUME MEASURED WITH MRI IN HIV SUBJECTS

REFERENCE	SUBJECTS	METHOD	BRAIN REGIONS EVALUATED	ARV MEDICATION	FINDINGS
Ances et al., J Infect DIs 2010	26 HIV 25 SN controls	Arterial Spin Labeling	Visual cortex (studied at rest and with visual stimulation)	15 (~60%) were on HAART	HIV subjects had lower baseline resting blood flow than SN controls. HIV serostatus and age independently affected fMRI measures, but no interaction occurred.
Ances et al., Neurology 2009	22 HIV (GDS < 0.5) 11 HIV (GDS ≥ 0.5) 26 SN controls	Arterial Spin Labeling	ROIs planed in lenticular nuclei (LN) and visual cortex (VC)	27 (82%) were on HAART	HIV subjects including neuropsychologically unimpaired, had reduced rCBF within the LN and VC compared to SN controls. Reduced LN rCBF was found in HIV subjects with early stages of the infection (<1 year of seroconversion) and in those infected chronically, whereas rCBF in the VC was diminished only in subjects with longer duration of HIV infection.
Ances et al., Neurology 2006	23 HIV (GDS<1) 19 HIV (GDS≥1) 17 SN controls	Arterial Spin Labeling	Bilateral Caudate (manually segmented)	15 (65%) of HIV GDS<1 and 17 (89%) of HIV GDS≥1 on HAART	HIV neuroasymptomatic subjects (global deficit score or GDS ≥1) had significantly lower caudate blood flow and volume compared to seronegative controls, and those who were "subsyndromic" (GDS <1) had a trend for lower rCBF in the caudate.
Chang et al., Neurology 2000	19 HIV+CMC 15 SN Controls	Dynamic Susceptibility Contrast	Whole brain with voxel-based analyses	18 were on ARVs (13 were on HAART)	Compared to controls, HIV subjects had lower rCBF in bilateral inferior lateral frontal cortices and medial parietal cortex, but higher rCBF in the posterior inferior parietal white matter. The rCBF abnormalities correlated with most clinical variables (CD4, plasma viral load, Karnofsky score and HIV dementia scale).
Tracey et al., Neurology 1998	13 HIV 11 controls	Dynamic Susceptibility Contrast	ROIs places in deep and cortical gray matter	10 were on ARVs (8 with AZT)	Significant increases in dynamic CBV were found in the deep and cortical gray matter of HIV-positive (HIV+) patients, especially those with definite cognitive impairment. One patient with cognitive impairment showed reversal of the increased rCBV that paralleled clinical improvement after initiation of zidovudine monotherapy.

to the brain via the heart, and causes a transient change in the MR signal in the brain (Axel, 1980). The signal change in each voxel is related to the intra-vascular concentration of contrast agent. High speed imaging is used to scan the entire brain every few seconds, immediately before, during, and after the bolus injection. The rCBV and rCBF can then be calculated from the signal-versus-time curves. The clinical advantages of DSC pMRI are its robustness and short scan time (approximately 2 minutes). However, DSC pMRI has a tendency to overestimate blood flow in larger vessels, so that accurate determination of absolute blood flow and volume are difficult, and the gadolinium contrast-agent used may have severe side effects in some individuals, especially those with poor renal function.

A more recent perfusion MRI technique, continuous arterial spin labeling (CASL), utilizes the subject's own blood as an internal contrast agent (Detre et al., 1992; Sliva et al., 1995; Wong, Buxton, & Frank, 1997; Buxton et al., 1998). Rather than tracking the time course of a bolus of contrast agent as in DSC pMRI, the scanner tracks the time course of a magnetically labeled "bolus" of arterial blood. Short time periods (seconds) of labeling are alternated with periods without labeling, and the difference in resulting MR images can be converted into maps representing rCBF throughout the brain. One of the difficulties of ASL is that the signal changes between the labeled and unlabeled conditions are relatively small, on the order of 1% or less, compared to 10% or more for the DSC technique. Therefore, ASL techniques tend to be very sensitive to subject motion, and may require relatively long scan times (on the order of 10 minutes) to attenuate the noise.

PERFUSION MRI STUDIES IN HIV BRAIN INJURY

The first perfusion MRI study used the DSC technique and evaluated rCBV in 13 HIV-positive patients and 7 healthy control subjects. HIV patients were found to have increased relative rCBV in the deep gray matter and cortical gray matter compared to control subjects (Tracey et al., 1998). The deep gray matter abnormalities were more severe in patients with mild to moderate dementia (ADC stages 1 or 2; n=9) compared to those with ADC stages 0 or 0.5. These findings were thought to reflect subcortical inflammatory changes, and were in general agreement with prior PET findings of increased subcortical glucose metabolism during the early stages of HIV dementia (Rottenberg et al., 1987; Arendt, 1995). However, the increased rCBV on perfusion MRI was inconsistent with the findings of several previous nuclear medicine studies that found decreased cortical perfusion in patients with HIV brain injury (see above). This difference might be due to a discordant relationship between rCBV (from pMRI) and rCBF (from SPECT) especially in a disease state, or due to differences in ARV treatment since one SPECT study noted that patients who were taking HAART had higher perfusion (Christensson et al., 1999). Furthermore, regional CBF is related to regional neuronal activity (Raichele, 1987), while the relationship between rCBV and neuronal activity is less clear.

Another DSC-pMRI study evaluated rCBF in the whole brains (voxel-by-voxel comparisons) of 19 HIV patients with mild dementia and 15 seronegative control subjects (Chang et al., 2000), and found that HIV patients had lower rCBF bilaterally in the inferior lateral frontal cortices and in an inferior medial parietal region, but higher rCBF bilaterally in the posterior inferior parietal white matter (Figure 9.1.8). The rCBF abnormalities were associated with CD4 count, plasma viral load, Karnofsky score and HIV dementia scale. The finding of decreased rCBF in the frontal cortex was consistent with previous findings from PET and SPECT studies, which also observed frontal hypoperfusion. It was speculated that increased perfusion in the parietal white matter might be related to reactive inflammatory processes or glial proliferation, which may be associated with higher blood flow.

Ances et al are the only investigators to use ASL-MRI to evaluate resting cerebral blood flow (CBF) in HIV infected individuals (Ances et al., 2006; Ances et al., 2009; Ances et al., 2010). In the first study, HIV neuroasymptomatic subjects (global deficit score ≥1) had significantly lower caudate blood flow and volume compared to seronegative controls, and those who were "subsyndromic" (GDS <1) had a trend for lower rCBF in the caudate (Ances et al., 2006) (Figure 9.1.9). A follow-up study found that HIV subjects who were neuropsychologically unimpaired (GDS<0.5) had reduced rCBF within the lenticular nuclei (LN) and visual cortex compared to SN controls. Reduced LN rCBF was found in HIV subjects with early stages of the infection (<1 year of seroconversion) as well as in those infected chronically, whereas more extensive reduced rCBF was seen in the visual cortex of subjects with longer duration of HIV infection (Ances et al., 2009). These studies demonstrated that resting rCBF using ASL-MRI, similar to those seen in HMPAO SPECT, could be sensitive for presymptomatic detection of brain perfusion abnormalities and may be a useful noninvasive neuroimaging biomarker for assessing HIV in the brain.

Perfusion MRI techniques typically have higher resolution than SPECT or PET, and can assess brain perfusion at rest or during activated states (i.e., during a cognitive task). However, BOLD-fMRI is typically used to assess cognitive function in HIV patients, since it affords approximately 5 times greater signal changes during brain activation than ASL as well as much higher temporal resolution (seconds compared minutes).

METHODOLOGICAL AND TECHNICAL ASPECTS OF BOLD-fMRI

BOLD-fMRI relies on the detection of MRI signal changes in brain regions that are activated while subjects perform a task during scanning. fMRI is based on a cascade of events during brain activation that begins with increased neuronal firing and increased glycolysis. These cellular events eventually lead to increased blood flow and blood oxygenation in activated brain regions. Because deoxyhemoglobin, but not oxyhemoglobin, is paramagnetic, changes in blood oxygenation alter the magnetic properties of the brain tissue, which ultimately can be

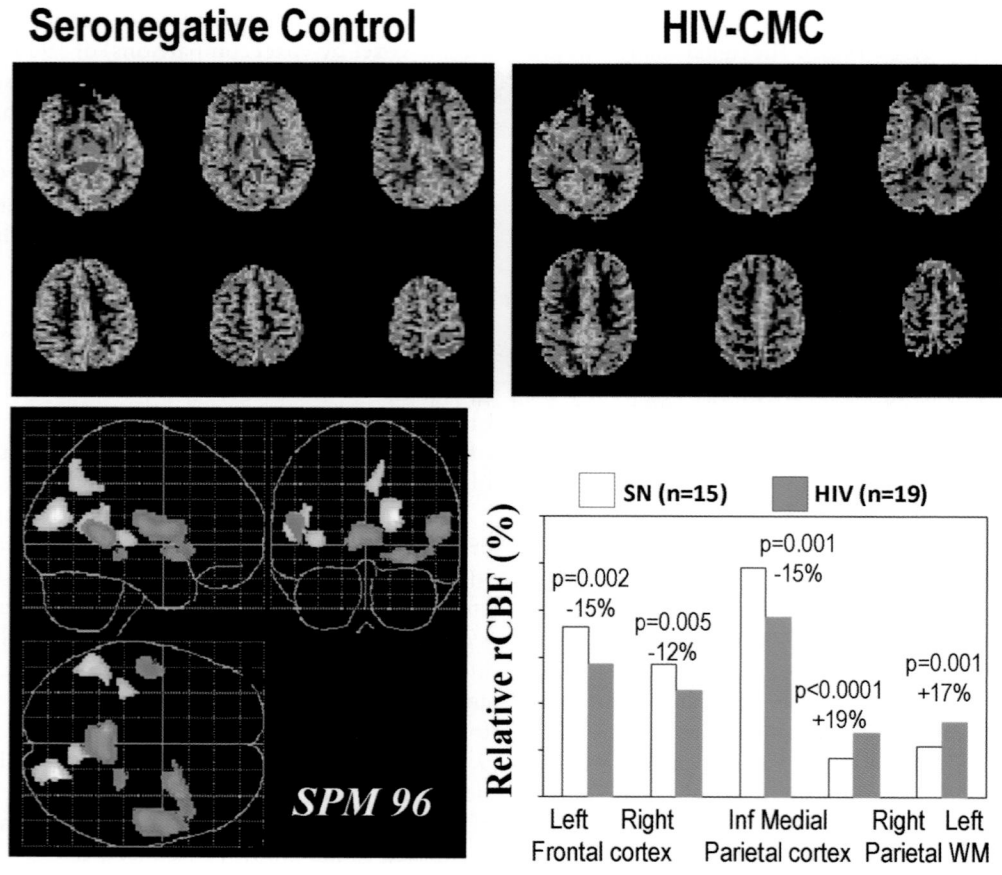

Figure 9.1.8 Top row: Perfusion MRI in a seronegative control (left) and in an HIV patient (ADC stage 2, right). Bottom row: Group comparison (voxel-by-voxel basis using statistical parametric mapping, SPM) between seronegative controls and HIV patients (modified from Chang et al., 2000).

detected with appropriate MRI sequences. The signal changes occurring during such "blood-oxygenation level dependent" (BOLD) fMRI scans are small (typically a few percent), but scale with the magnetic field strength. Therefore, higher magnetic field strengths generally yield better contrast to noise and hence may require a smaller sample size for the BOLD-fMRI studies. Earlier fMRI studies were performed at field strength of 1.5 Tesla while the more recent studies were performed at 3 or 4 Tesla MR scanners (Table 9.1.5). Several excellent reviews of the technical issues involved in fMRI studies have been published (Ogawa et al., 1993; Turner et al., 1993; Jezzard & Turner, 1996; Howseman & Bowtell, 1999). Importantly, since fMRI is very sensitive to motion, which might yield "false activation," subjects with at most mild dementia and who can follow instructions have been studied to date. The HIV patients at the earliest stages of the brain injury, however, might benefit most from treatments and evaluations with neuroimaging.

NEURAL CORRELATES OF WORKING MEMORY DEFICITS IN HIV PATIENTS

Several BOLD-fMRI studies evaluated working memory in HIV-patients (Chang et al., 2001; Ernst et al., 2002; Tomasi et al., 2006). In the first study, HIV patients and seronegative controls were scanned while performing several working memory tasks (0-back, 1-back, and 2-back) that required different levels of working memory load, and two tasks that additionally involved arithmetic skills (1-increment and 2-increment task). All tasks activated the lateral prefrontal cortices (LPFC), the posterior parietal cortices (PPC), the supplementary motor area (SMA), and less consistently the caudate nuclei bilaterally (Figure 9.1.10). In seronegative subjects, brain activation (% BOLD signal change) and total activated brain volume increased with task difficulty (e.g., from 0-back, 1-back, to 2-back), probably due to modulation of the attention network (Chang et al., 2001). It is well known that attention influences information processing in the brain by altering the firing rate of neurons that are sensitive to a specific attribute. For example, modulatory effects of attention on neural activity have been demonstrated by single-cell recordings (Moran & Desimone, 1985), by event-related potentials (Mangun, Hillyard, & Luck, 1993), by PET (Kawashima, O'Sullivan, & Roland, 1995), and by fMRI (Courtney et al., 1997; Speck et al., 2000; Tomasi et al., 2005; Tomasit et al., 2003).

Compared to control subjects, HIV patients showed similar increases in brain activation and total activated volume for

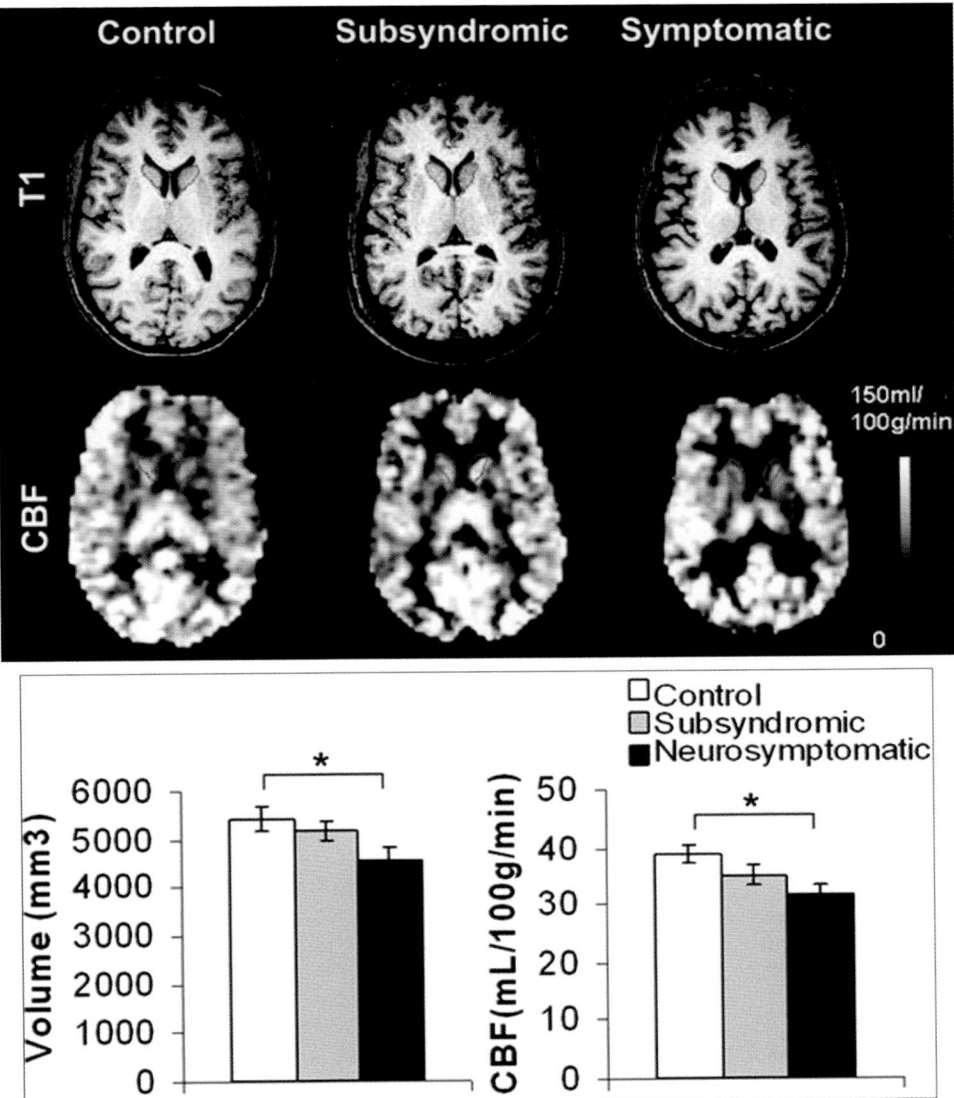

Figure 9.1.9 Top panel: MR images showing structural MRI (top row) and arterial spin labeling perfusion MRI images (bottom row) in a control, a subsyndromic, and a neurosymptomatic HIV subjects. Bottom panel: Caudate volumes and cerebral blood flow from the caudate were both lower in the neurosymptomatic subjects and show a trend to be lower in the subsyndromic subjects compared to controls. (Courtesy of Dr. Beau Ances; modified from Ances et al., 2006).

the simpler tasks (0-back and 1-back) but not for the more difficult tasks (2-back and 2-increment). These results suggest that HIV patients require greater activation of neural circuits (i.e., increased attentional modulation) to perform the simpler tasks, and to compensate for reduced efficiency of neural processing associated with the brain injury. However, with more difficult tasks, available network resources may be exhausted, and performance may suffer. Thus, increased brain activation (and exhausting the usage of brain reserve) is probably the direct neural correlate of the working memory deficits in some HIV patients.

To further test this hypothesis, HIV patients with completely normal cognitive performance on a battery of neuropsychological tests were studied and found to have increased brain activation despite normal performance during fMRI (Ernst et al., 2002). Therefore, BOLD-fMRI can detect pre-symptomatic abnormalities on brain activation. However,

compared to control subjects, asymptomatic HIV-patients had higher activation only in the lateral prefrontal cortex. These results suggest that mild brain injury, such as that caused by neuroinflammation, is present even in cognitively unimpaired HIV patients, and that they had to use their neural reserve networks to compensate for the impairments in neural processing.

A follow-up study to further "stress" the cognitive reserve network was performed by modulating the acoustic noise level of the MR scan (which can be substantial) while the subjects performed a series of N-back tasks. Compared with SN subjects, HIV patients showed lower activation with louder noise and lower neuronal marker *N*-acetylaspartate in prefrontal and parietal cortices. This study also evaluated the competing use of the working memory network between acoustic noise level and cognitive load, and found

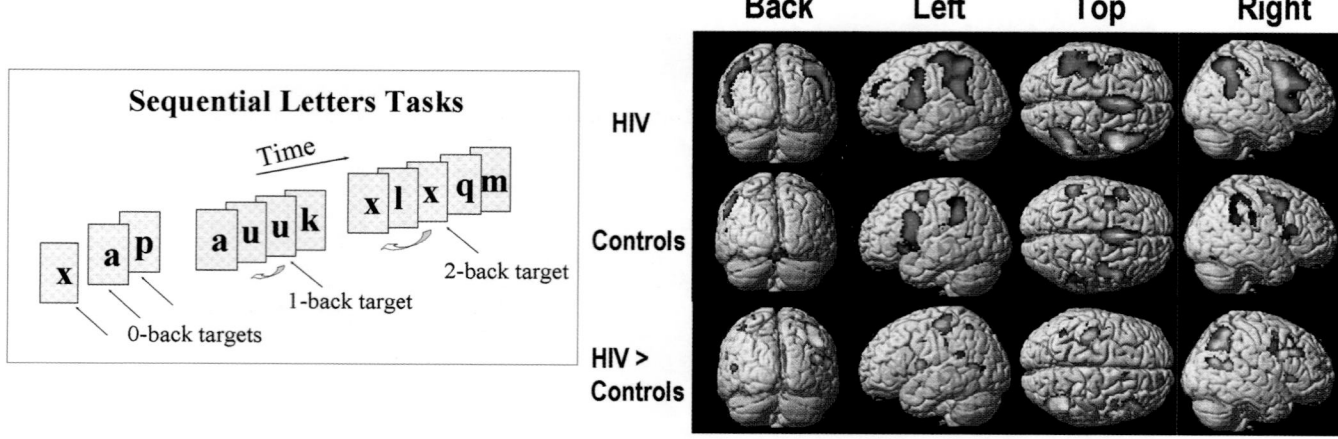

Figure 9.1.10 Left: Activation paradigm for the sequential letter (N-back) tasks used during the BOLD fMRI evaluation of working memory in the subjects. Right: SPM maps showing regions of significant brain activation on the brain surfaces in 11 seronegative control men (top row) and 11 HIV-infected men (middle row) and the group differences at T ≥ 3.1, p≤0.001 (Data presented in Chang et al., 2001).

Table 9.1.6 BOLD-FMRI STUDIES IN HIV PATIENTS

REFERENCE	SUBJECTS	COGNITION EVALUATED	METHOD &TASKS	MEDICATION	FINDINGS
Ernst et al., Ann Neurol 2009	32 HIV+ men (cognitively normal over one-year) 31 SN men	Visual attention (with increasing load)	3 Tesla MRI Tracking of 2, 3, or 4 balls	Stable on ARVs	Longitudinal study at baseline and one year later; each subject at two fMRI scans. HIV: increase in signal: prefrontal and posterior parietal cortices for the more difficult tasks. Controls: decreases in brain activation in these regions.
Maki et al., Neurology 2009	7 HIV+ women 4 SN women	Delayed verbal episodic memory	3 Tesla MRI Encoding and recognition task	3 on ARVs 4 without ARVs	Compared to SN subjects, HIV subjects had decreased activation during encoding but increased activation in hippocampi and parahippocampal gyrus (L>R) during delayed recognition. These alterations correlated with worse episodic verbal memory.
Melrose et al., Behav Brain Res 2008	11 HIV+ 11 Controls	Semantic event sequencing task	3 Tesla MRI Picture sequencing and object discrimination task	10 HIV on ARVs; 4 on antidepressants	HIV showed hypoactivation of the left caudate, left dorsolateral prefrontal cortex, and bilateral ventral prefrontal cortex less functional connectivity between the caudate and prefrontal cortex and basal ganglia regions increased activation of right postcentral/ supramarginal gyrus, and greater connectivity between the caudate and this same anterior parietal region.
Chang et al., J Neuro-Immune Pharmacol 2008	12 HIV+ARV 12 HIV+ no ARV 18 SN controls	Visual attention (with increasing load)	3 Tesla MRI Tracking of 2, 3, or 4 balls	12 on ARVs 12 no ARVs	HIV subjects showed greater load-dependent increases in brain activation in the right frontal regions compared to SN. HIV+ARV additionally showed greater load-dependent increases in activation compared to SN in bilateral superior frontal regions and a lower %accuracy on the performance of the most difficult task (tracking 4 balls). ROI analyses further demonstrated that SN showed load-dependent decreases (with repeated trials despite increasing difficulty), while HIV subjects showed load-dependent increases in activation with the more difficult tasks, especially those on ARVs.
Ances et al., J NeuroVirol 2008	12 HIV+high-CPE 12 HIV+ low CPE 10 controls	Primary visual activation	black-and-white flickering checker-board (8 Hz) and at rest	all stable on HAART	BOLD in motor hand area–evaluated effects of HAART (MHA) of the parietal cortex: HIV+ low-CPE had greater BOLD fMRI response amplitude than HIV+ high-CPE or seronegative controls

(Continued)

Table 9.1.6 (CONTINUED)

REFERENCE	SUBJECTS	COGNITION EVALUATED	METHOD &TASKS	MEDICATION	FINDINGS
Juengst et al., J Neurosci Methods 2007	19 HIV ANI 11 HIV MCMD/ HAD 16 controls	Simple sensory-motor function	Simple reaction time, press when word appears	Not specified	The HRF of MNCD/HAD subjects did not return to baseline after 16 s, suggesting subtle alterations in neuronal function.
Tomasi et al., Ann Neurol 2006	10 HIV men (cognitively unimpaired) 15 SN men	Working Memory and Acoustic Noise Interference	4 Tesla MRI, N-back tasks with letters (0-back, 1-back & 2-back) & MRS	7 on ARVs 3 on no ARVs	Compared with SN subjects, HIV patients showed reduced activation with louder noise and had lower *N*-acetylaspartate in prefrontal and parietal cortices. Competing use of the working memory network between louder noise and cognitive load showed lower dynamic range of the hemodynamic responses these regions in HIV patients. These findings suggest reduced reserve capacity of the working memory network in HIV patients and additional stress (e.g., loud noise) might exhaust the impaired network for more demanding tasks.
Castelo et al., Neurology 2006	14 HIV men (cognitively unimpaired) 14 SN controls	Episodic memory encoding (novel vs. repeated stimuli)	3 Tesla MRI, Encoding task (during fMRI), recognition task (outside scanner)	10 on ARVs; 4 were on no ARVs	Both HIV and SN controls recruited bilateral medial temporal lobes and inferior prefrontal gyri, the HIV group demonstrated significantly reduced signal intensity changes in the right posterior hippocampus, right inferior frontal gyrus, and left lingual gyrus. Additionally, the HIV group exhibited more activity within lateral frontal and posterior parietal regions. Pattern similar to aging subjects.
Chang et al., Ann Neurol 2004	18 HIV (2 cognitively normal, 10 ANI, 6 MND) 18 controls; 14M/4F in each group	Visual attention (with increasing load)	4 Tesla MRI, Tracking of 2, 3, or 4 balls	15 were stable on ARVs; 3 were on no ARVs	HIV subjects had less activation in the normal visual attention network (dorsal parietal, bilateral prefrontal, and cerebellar regions) but greater activation in adjacent or contralateral brain regions (reserve networks); HIV also had load-dependent increases in the reserve network regions (right prefrontal and parietal regions) but less in regions that showed a saturation effect with increasing load (which had none or little reserve).
Ernst et al., NeuroImage 2003	14 HIV (7 with HAND; 7 unimpaired)	Working memory (with increasing load)	1.5 Tesla MRI, N-back tasks with letters (0-back, 1-back & 2-back)	13 stable on ARVs; one ARV-naïve	BOLD signals in the working memory network (posterior parietal cortex and lateral prefrontal cortex) correlated with concentrations of glial metabolites in the frontal white matter and basal ganglia.
Ernst et al., Neurology 2002	10 HIV (cognitively unimpaired) 10 SN controls	Working memory (with increasing load)	1.5 Tesla MRI N-back tasks with letters (0-back, 1-back & 2-back)	9 stable on ARVs; one ARV-naïve	HIV subjects showed greater amplitude and extent of activation in the lateral prefrontal cortex compared to SN controls matched for age, sex, education, handedness, and cognitive performance.
Chang et al., Neurology 2001	11 HIV men 11 SN men	Working memory (with increasing load)	1.5 Tesla MRI N-back tasks with letters (0-back, 1-back & 2-back, 1-up, 2-up)	All stable on ART expect for one	Compared to SN controls, HIV subjects showed greater activation in the parietal regions for the simpler task, and additionally had greater activation the frontal lobes for the more difficult tasks.

that HIV subjects had lower dynamic range of the hemodynamic responses in their prefrontal and parietal cortices. These findings again suggest reduced reserve capacity of the working memory network in HIV patients and that additional stress (e.g., loud noise) might exhaust the impaired network for more demanding tasks (Tomasi et al., 2006).

The abnormalities found in the frontal lobe (LPFC) is consistent with the notion that the frontostriatal system is often most severely affected in patients with HIV dementia

(Rottenberg et al., 1987; Barker et al., 1995; Power et al., 1993; Kure et al., 1990). In particular, the dopaminergic system, which has a major role in regulating working memory function in the prefrontal cortices (Goldman-Rakic, 1996), has been shown to be affected in patients with HAND, both clinically (Berger et al., 1994; Lopez et al., 1999) and on PET studies that measured the dopamine transporters (Chang et al., 2008; Wang et al., 2004).

NEURAL CORRELATES OF EPISODIC MEMORY DEFICITS IN HIV PATIENTS

An event-related fMRI study by Castelo et al. evaluated episodic memory in cognitively unimpaired HIV and SN subjects, using a paradigm that assessed encoding of novel versus repeated stimuli. Both HIV and SN controls recruited brain regions involved in encoding (bilateral medial temporal lobes and inferior prefrontal gyri), but the HIV group demonstrated significantly reduced BOLD signals in the right posterior hippocampus, right inferior frontal gyrus, and left lingual gyrus. Additionally, the HIV group exhibited more activity within lateral frontal and posterior parietal regions. These findings suggest that the hippocampal function may be altered by HIV infection (Castelo et al., 2006). This pattern of abnormality is similar to that found in episodic memory and working memory fMRI studies in aging subjects (Daselaar et al., 2003; Gutchess et al., 2005), as well as in fMRI studies that evaluated working memory and attention in HIV subjects with and without cognitive impairments (Table 9.1.5). Therefore, these changes are also consistent with abnormalities seen in the attentional network (see below).

Another fMRI study reported findings of episodic memory during both encoding and retrieval (20 minutes later) in 7 HIV-infected and 4 seronegative women. This preliminary study essentially validated the findings by Castelo of decreased temporal lobe activation during encoding; however, subjects also showed increased activation in the hippocampi and parahippocampal regions during the retrieval phase of the episodic memory task (Maki et al., 2009).

NEURAL CORRELATES OF ATTENTION DEFICITS IN HIV PATIENTS

Attention is another cognitive domain that is mediated by the dopaminergic system and is often affected in HIV patients. Of note, attention is also needed for working memory and for the majority of cognitive tasks. Therefore, several studies evaluated attention with BOLD-fMRI (Table 9.1.5). One study was performed on a 4 Tesla MR scanner, using a well-validated parametrically designed visual attention task that required tracking of an increasing number of moving balls (Chang et al., 2004) amongst a set of ten balls. Compared with SN controls, HIV subjects showed similar task performance (accuracies and reaction times) but decreased activation in the normal visual attention network (dorsal parietal, bilateral

prefrontal, and cerebellar regions) and increased activation in adjacent or contralateral brain regions. Cognitive performance (assessed with NPZ-8), CD4, and viral load all correlated with activated BOLD signals in brain regions that activated more in HIV subjects. Furthermore, HIV subjects activated more than SN controls in brain regions that showed load-dependent increase in activation (right prefrontal and right parietal regions) but less in regions that showed a saturation effect with increasing load (Chang et al., 2004). These findings again suggest that HIV-associated brain injury reduces the efficiency of the normal attention network, thus requiring reorganization and increased usage of neural reserves to maintain performance during attention-requiring tasks. Exceeding the brain reserve capacity may eventually lead to attention deficits and cognitive impairment in HIV patients (Figure 9.1.11).

EFFECTS OF ANTIRETROVIRAL MEDICATIONS ON BRAIN FUNCTION ASSESSED WITH BOLD-fMRI

Using a visual attention task, Chang et al. evaluated the effects of antiretroviral medications (primarily HAART) in HIV patients (Chang et al., 2008). Consistent with earlier studies, HIV subjects, both with or without ARV treatment, showed greater load-dependent increases in brain activation in the right frontal regions (involved in visual attention) compared to SN. Compared to SN controls, HIV+ individuals taking ARVs additionally showed greater load-dependent increases in activation in bilateral superior frontal regions and lower performance accuracy for the most difficult task (tracking four balls). Region of interest analyses further demonstrated that SN controls showed load-dependent decreases (probably due to practice effects despite increasing difficulty), while HIV subjects showed load-dependent increases in activation with more difficult tasks, especially those on ARVs (Figure 9.1.12). These findings suggest that chronic ARV treatment may lead to greater requirement of the attentional network reserve and hence less efficient usage of the network and less practice effects (not able to adapt) in these HIV patients. As the brain has a limited reserve capacity, exhausting the reserve capacity in HIV+ARV would lead to declined performance with more difficult tasks that require more attention.

In contrast to this study, Ances et al. evaluated the effects of high versus low CSF penetrating effectiveness (CPE) combined antiretroviral treatment (cART) in HIV-infected individuals during a visual stimulation task with flickering checkerboards and found that the 12 HIV+ patients who were taking low-CPE cART had greater BOLD-fMRI response amplitude than the 12 HIV+ patients who were taking high-CPE cART or the 10 seronegative controls. The authors concluded that more efficient suppression of CNS HIV replication by high-CPE cART most likely reduces the metabolic demand in brain microenvironments where HIV is replicating, thereby leading to a greater normalization of the BOLD fMRI response.

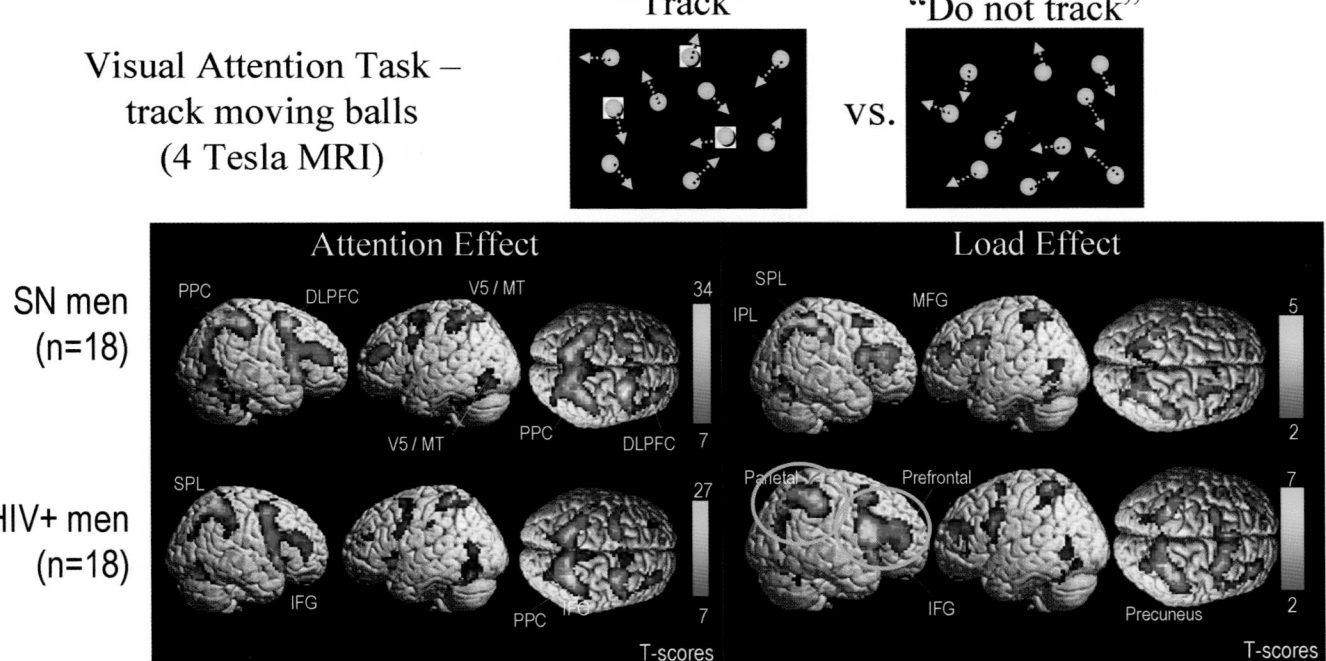

Figure 9.1.11 Left panel: Statistical maps of group brain activation (surface renderings) showing less activation, or decreased usage of the normal visual attention network, in 18 HIV subjects (bottom row) compared to 18 seronegative control men (top row) during the ball-tracking (visual attention) task (shown above brain maps). Right panel: Group analyses of load-dependent brain activation showing greater load-dependent activation in the HIV subjects (right bottom) compared to seronegative control men (right top), especially in the right prefrontal and parietal regions (in blue circles, further analyses showed these brain regions to be adjacent to the visual attention network). These findings demonstrated HIV subjects had greater usage of these load-dependent regions (reserve brain network). Figure modified from data presented in Chang et al., 2004.

DECLINE NEURAL EFFICIENCY IN HIV PATIENTS AFTER ONE-YEAR

Finally, an fMRI study compared brain activation changes at baseline and one-year later, using a visual attention task of increasing difficulty (tracking 2, 3, or 4 balls) between 32 neurocognitively normal HIV-subjects (all on stable ARV treatment) and 31 seronegative control subjects (Ernst et al., 2009). Both subject groups showed no changes in neurocognitive or fMRI task performance over 1 year. The most important finding was that on the more difficult tasks, brain activation increased in the HIV subjects, but decreased in the SN controls, in the prefrontal and posterior parietal cortices over this one-year follow up period. This suggests that SN controls had improved neural efficiency, that is, a practice effect, over this 1 year follow-up; conversely, the HIV subjects appeared to have declined neural efficiency after 1 year and therefore required more attentional resources to maintain the task performance on fMRI. As discussed above, both ARV treatment and neuroinflammation (as assessed by elevated glial markers on MRS) are associated with increased BOLD signals on fMRI. Therefore, increased brain activation or declined neural efficiency in these cognitively and clinically stable HIV-infected individuals may be related to their ARV treatment status, ongoing CNS infection, neuroinflammation, or a combination of these factors.

SUMMARY, CONCLUSIONS, AND FUTURE DIRECTIONS

Numerous neuroimaging studies have evaluated the direct or indirect effects of HIV infection on the brain, in addition to those that evaluated opportunistic brain lesions (not covered in this Chapter). These studies included HIV patients who were neurologically asymptomatic, subjects at various stages of HIV dementia (or HAND), and pediatric HIV populations. Structural imaging techniques, such as CT and MRI, are useful for screening for brain pathology or for the presence of opportunistic infections. Quantitative morphometric MRI additionally may be useful for assessing the severity of HIV-associated brain injury (see Chapter 8.1). Nuclear medicine techniques, including SPECT and PET, are highly sensitive to changes in cerebral perfusion or metabolism, but may be non-specific and can be subjected to confounding effects of brain atrophy in HIV. However, radionuclides that bind to specific receptors may provide better understanding of the pathophysiology associated with HAND and the common co-morbid conditions (e.g., drug abuse, depression, and others).

MRS is the most widely used neuroimaging technique to evaluate HAND. The majority of the MRS studies concurred that early brain injury (ANI or MND) is associated with subtle increases in MI and/or CHO in the white

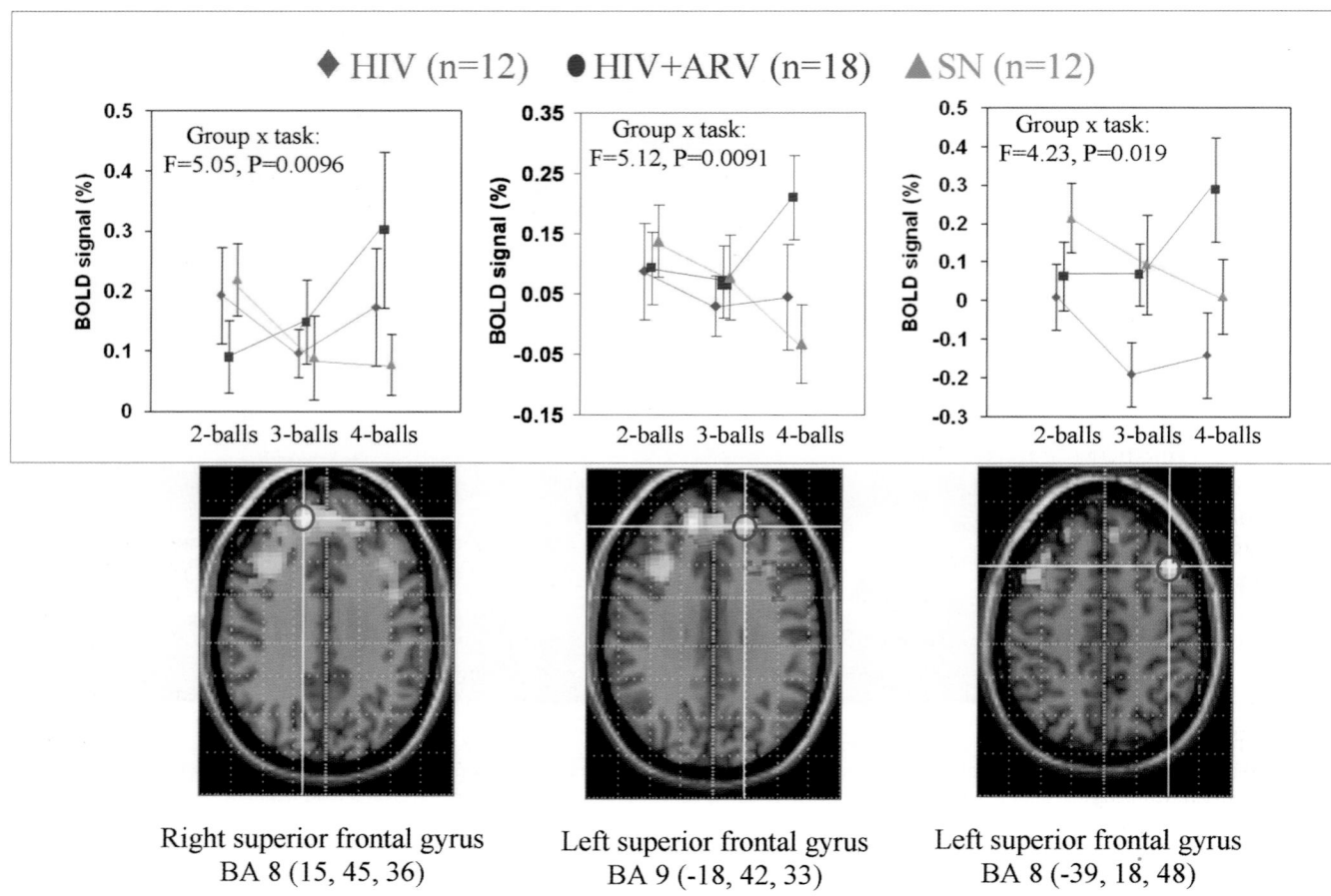

♦ HIV (n=12) ● HIV+ARV (n=18) ▲ SN (n=12)

Right superior frontal gyrus
BA 8 (15, 45, 36)

Left superior frontal gyrus
BA 9 (-18, 42, 33)

Left superior frontal gyrus
BA 8 (-39, 18, 48)

Figure 9.1.12 Top row: Region of interest (ROI) analyses at local maxima of significant clusters (see red circles in maps below), showing interaction effects between attentional load and group status. Load-dependent increases in BOLD signals were observed in the HIV+ subjects taking ARVs (HIV+ARV, blue squares) while BOLD signals decreased with increased attentional load in the SN subjects (green triangles), and the HIV+subjects not taking ARV (NARV) had decreased BOLD signals from tracking 2-balls to 3-balls, but increased BOLD with tracking 4-balls (red dots). These findings indicate greater usage of the brain network with more difficult tasks (tracking 3 or 4 balls) in the HIV+ARV group, but less usage or greater efficiency with repeating the task despite increasing difficulty (practice effects) in the SN subjects. Bottom row: Parametric maps showing brain regions with significantly greater attentional load effect in HIV+ARV subjects than SN subjects (cluster size > 100 voxels; *t*-scores >2.38); (permission obtained from Springer, Chang et al., 2008).

matter, indicating subclinical glial activation. Conversely, more severe injury (HAD) is associated with marked decreases in NA along with further increases in CHO and MI, suggesting neuronal damage or loss and further glial activation. More recent MRS studies that evaluated brain glutamate levels, using more advanced MRS technique (e.g., TE-averaged PRESS) also found decreased brain glutamate in those with more severe cognitive deficits. These progressive metabolite changes, with early glial activation and subsequent neuronal loss, are consistent with those observed in neuropathology studies. Several MRS studies also evaluated the effects of antiretroviral or neuroprotective treatments in HIV patients and found "improvement" of brain metabolites in HIV patients after treatment. Since MRS may provide additional objective surrogate markers to monitor treatment effects, future clinical trials may benefit from the use of MRS, and other quantitative MR techniques, in addition to the current approach of neuropsychological assessments.

Although MRS and some of the psychometrics appear to be well-correlated (Chang et al., 2002; Meyerhoff et al., 1999), the sensitivity and specificity for treatment efficacy between these two techniques remain to be determined. Likewise, the relationship or relative sensitivity and specificity of MRS to other neuroimaging techniques, including CT, structural MRI, SPECT, PET, and functional MRI, have not been evaluated extensively. Most studies found MRS to be more sensitive than structural MRI in the determination of brain injury, but they did not use sophisticated, state of the art image processing software that could quantify cortical and subcortical volumes, cortical thickness or surface areas. One study evaluated co-registered quantitative ^{1}H MRS and quantitative ^{133}Xenon-calibrated ^{99m}TcHMPAO SPECT; despite a lack of correlation between rCBF (on SPECT) and metabolite concentrations (from MRS) in any of the brain regions evaluated, MRS was found to be more sensitive than SPECT for detecting early brain injury in HIV dementia (Ernst et al., 2000). Another recent study also found good correlation between total creatine measured with MRS and brain activation on BOLD-fMRI, suggesting an up-regulated oxidative metabolic state may contribute to the increased prefrontal activation in patients with mild HIV dementia (Ernst, Chang, & Arnold, 2003). The study that evaluated both caudate volume and perfusion with CASL found lower perfusion and volumes in the caudate of HIV patients, but the study was not powered to determine the sensitivity of the two techniques (Ances et al., 2006). Future studies using more than one neuroimaging modality in the same subjects are needed to determine the optimal method, and whether the various techniques can provide complementary information to further elucidate the pathogenesis of HIV brain injury.

With continued technical and methodological advances, future nuclear medicine studies will most likely include pharmacologically more specific tracers, MRS studies will likely involve spectroscopic imaging, two-dimensional MRS, and other editing techniques to further assess regional changes and additional metabolites of interest (e.g. glutamate, GABA, glutathione, etc.), while BOLD-fMRI will provide complementary information regarding brain activation, as well as functional connectivity between activated regions, both during cognitive tasks and at rest. More research is needed to determine the sensitivity of these techniques for detecting early brain injury so that neuroprotective treatments might be implemented at the earliest stages. With further methodological improvements, these techniques may ultimately become more "user-friendly" and can be applied in routine clinical settings for assessments of the severity of brain injury and to monitor treatment effects.

Lastly, several comorbid factors might exacerbate HIV-associated brain injury. First, whether chronic ARVs may exacerbate neuroinflammation and neuronal injury remains somewhat controversial. The majority of the neuroimaging studies of HIV patients who are maintained on HAART or ARVs, especially with regimens that contain NRTIs, have shown possible increased neuroinflammation or neuronal injury, such as the increased perfusion seen on SPECT (Christensson et al., 1999), further elevation of choline and myo-inositol (Chang et al., 2000; Chang et al., 2004) or decreased NAA seen on MRS (Schweinsburg et al., 2005), and increased brain activation on BOLD-fMRI compared to HIV patients without ARVs (Chang et al., 2008). Second, both licit and illicit drugs of abuse are more commonly abused or used by HIV-infected individuals. Several neuroimaging studies have already shown additive or interactive effects of alcohol (Pfefferbaum, Adalsteinsson, & Sullivan, 2005), methamphetamine (Taylor et al., 2000; Chang et al., 2005), cocaine (Chang et al., 2008), heroin (Georgiou et al., 2008) and marijuana (Chang et al., 2006), on HIV-associated brain injury. Third, as the HIV-infected population is aging, many more age-related neurological disorders (e.g., Alzheimer's disease or Parkinson's disease) will likely further impact their brains, and more research using non-invasive neuroimaging techniques will be needed to evaluate for these possible cumulative or interactive effects of aging or age-related disorders and HIV.

ACKNOWLEDGMENTS

This work was partially supported by the National Institute on Drug Abuse (K24-DA16170 to L.C.), the National Institute of Mental Health (2R01-MH61427) and Core resources from the National Center for Research Resources (G12-RR003061, P20-RR011091), and the National Institute on Neurological Disorders and Strokes (U54-NS56883).

REFERENCES

Achim, C. L., et al. (2009). Increased accumulation of intraneuronal amyloid beta in HIV-infected patients. *J Neuroimmune Pharmacol*, 4(2), 190–199.

Ances, B. M., et al. (2006). Caudate blood flow and volume are reduced in HIV+ neurocognitively impaired patients. *Neurology*, 66(6), 862–866.

Ances, B. M., et al. (2009). Resting cerebral blood flow: A potential biomarker of the effects of HIV in the brain. *Neurology*, 73(9), 702–708.

Ances, B. M., et al. (2010a). Cognitively unimpaired HIV-positive subjects do not have increased 11C-PiB: A case-control study. *Neurology*, 75(2), 111–115.

Ances, B. M., et al. (2010b). HIV infection and aging independently affect brain function as measured by functional magnetic resonance imaging. *The Journal of Infectious Diseases*, 201, 336–340.

Andersen, A. B., et al. (2010). Cerebral FDG-PET scanning abnormalities in optimally treated HIV patients. *J Neuroinflammation*, 7(1), 13.

Arendt, G., et al. (1990). Motor dysfunction in HIV-infected patients without clinically detectable central-nervous deficit. *J Neurol*, 237(6), 362–368.

Arendt, G. (1995). Imaging methods as a diagnostic tool in neuro-AIDS. A review. *Bildgebung*, 62(4), 310–319.

Axel, L. (1980). Cerebral blood flow determination by rapid-sequence computed tomography. *Radiology*, 137, 679–686.

Banakar, S., et al. (2008). Two-dimensional 1H MR spectroscopy of the brain in human immunodeficiency virus (HIV)-infected children. *J Magn Reson Imaging*, 27(4), 710–717.

Barker, P., et al. (1993). Quantitation of proton NMR spectra of the human brain using tissue water as an internal concentration reference. *NMR in Biomedicine*, 6(1), 89–94.

Barker, P. B., Lee, R. R., & McArthur, J. C. (1995). AIDS dementia complex: Evaluation with proton MR spectroscopic imaging. *Radiology*, 195, 58–64.

Berger, J. R., et al. (1994). Cerebrospinal fluid dopamine in HIV-1 infection. *Acquired Immunodeficiency Syndrome*, 8(1), 67–71.

Berger, J. & Nath, A. (1997). HIV dementia and the basal ganglia. *Intervirology*, 40(2-3), 122–131.

Birken, D. L. & Oldendorf, W. H. (1989). N-acetyl-L-aspartic acid: A literature review of a compound prominent in 1H-NMR spectroscopic studies of brain. *Neuroscience and Biobehaviour Reviews*, 13, 23–31.

Blanchette, N., et al. (2002). Cognitive development in school-age children with vertically transmitted HIV infection. *Dev Neuropsychol*, 21(3), 223–241.

Bottomley, P. A., et al. (1990). AIDS dementia complex: Brain high-energy phosphate metabolite deficits. *Radiology*, 176, 407–411.

Brand, A., Richter-Landsberg, C., & Leibfritz, D. (1993). Multinuclear NMR studies on the energy metabolism of glial and neuronal cells. *Developmental Neurosciences*, 15, 289–298.

Brass, L. M., et al. (1994). The role of single photon emission computed tomography brain imaging with 99mTc-Bicisate in the localization and definition of mechanism of ischemic stroke. *Journal of Cerebral Blood Flow and Metabolism*, 14(Suppl. 1), S91–S98.

Bridge, T. P., et al. (1989). Improvement in AIDS patients on peptide T. *Lancet*, 2(8656), 226–227.

Bridge, T. P., et al. (1991). Results of extended peptide T administration in AIDS and ARC patients. *Psychopharmacol Bull*, 27(3), 237–245.

Brouwers, P., et al. (2000). Cerebrospinal fluid viral load is related to cortical atrophy and not to intracerebral calcifications in children with symptomatic HIV disease. *J Neurovirol, 6*(5), 390–397.

Brunetti, A., et al. (1989). Reversal of brain metabolic abnormalities following treatment of AIDS dementia complex with 3'-azido-2,'3'-dideoxythymidine (AZT, zidovudine): A PET-FDG study. *Journal of Nuclear Medicine, 30*(5), 581–590.

Buxton, R., et al. (1998). A general kinetic model for quantitative perfusion imaging with arterial spin labeling. *Magnetic Resonance in Medicine, 40*(3), 383–396.

Casellas, P., Galiegue, S., & Basile, A. S. (2002). Peripheral benzodiazepine receptors and mitochondrial function. *Neurochem Int, 40*(6), 475–486.

Castelo, J. M., et al. (2006). Altered hippocampal-prefrontal activation in HIV patients during episodic memory encoding. *Neurology, 66*(11), 1688–1695.

Catz, S. L., et al. (2000). Patterns, correlates, and barriers to medication adherence among persons prescribed new treatments for HIV disease. *Health Psychol, 19*(2), 124–133.

Chana, G., et al. (2006). Cognitive deficits and degeneration of interneurons in HIV+ methamphetamine users. *Neurology, 67*(8), 1486–1489.

Chang, L., et al. (1996). In vivo proton magnetic resonance spectroscopy of the normal human aging brain. *Life Sciences, 58*(22), 2049–2056.

Chang, L., et al. (1999a). Cerebral metabolite abnormalities correlate with clinical severity of HIV-cognitive motor complex. *Neurology, 52*(1), 100–108.

Chang, L., et al. (1999b). Highly active antiretroviral therapy reverses brain metabolite abnormalities in mild HIV dementia. *Neurology, 53,* 782–789.

Chang, L., et al. (2000a). Perfusion MRI detects rCBF abnormalities in early stages of HIV-cognitive motor complex. *Neurology, 54,* 389–396.

Chang, L., et al. (2000b). Cerebral metabolite abnormalities in antiretroviral-naïve HIV patients before and after HAART. *Neurology, 54,* S47.002.

Chang, L., et al. (2001a). Cerebral metabolite changes during the first nine months of HAART. *Neurology, 56,* S63.001.

Chang, L., et al. (2001b). Neural correlates of attention and working memory deficits in HIV patients. *Neurology, 57,* 1001–1007.

Chang, L., et al. (2002). Relationships among cerebral metabolites, cognitive function and viral loads in antiretroviral-naïve HIV patients. *NeuroImage, 17*(3), 1638–1648.

Chang, L., et al. (2004a). Adaptation of the attention network in human immunodeficiency virus brain injury. *Annals of Neurology, 56*(2), 259–272.

Chang, L., et al. (2004b). Antiretroviral treatment alters relationship between MCP-1 and neurometabolites in HIV patients. *Antiviral Therapy, 9*(3), 431–440.

Chang, L., et al. (2005). Additive effects of HIV and chronic methamphetamine use on brain metabolite abnormalities. *American Journal of Psychiatry, 162*(2), 361–369.

Chang, L., et al. (2006). Combined and independent effects of chronic marijuana use and HIV on brain metabolites. *Journal of NeuroImmune Pharmacology, 1,* 65–76.

Chang, L., et al. (2008). Antiretroviral treatment is associated with increased attentional load-dependent brain activation in HIV patients. *J Neuroimmune Pharmacol, 3*(2), 95–104.

Chong, W. K., et al. (1993). Proton spectroscopy of the brain in HIV infection: Correlation with clinical, immunologic and MR imaging findings. *Radiology, 188,* 119–124.

Chong, W. K., et al. (1994). Localized cerebral proton MR spectroscopy in HIV infection and AIDS. *American Journal of Neuroradiology, 15,* 21–25.

Christensson, B., et al. (1999). SPECT and 99mTc-HMPAO in subjects with HIV infection: Cognitive dysfunction correlates with high uptake. *Scandinavian Journal of Infectious Diseases, 31*(4), 349–354.

Conant, K., et al. (1998). Induction of monocyte chemoattractant protein-1 in HIV-1 tat-stimulated astrocytes and elevation in AIDS dementia. *Proceedings of the National Academy of Sciences, USA, 95,* 3117–3121.

Cortey, A., et al. (1994). Proton MR spectroscopy of brain abnormalities in neonates born to HIV-positive mothers. *American Journal of Neuroradiology, 15,* 1853–1859.

Courtney, S. M., et al. (1997). Transient and sustained activity in a distributed neural system for human working memory. *Nature, 386,* 608–611.

Czub, S., et al. (2004). Modulation of simian immunodeficiency virus neuropathology by dopaminergic drugs. *Acta Neuropathol (Berl), 107*(3), 216–226.

Daselaar, S., et al. (2003). Neuroanatomical correlates of episodic encoding and retrieval in young and elderly subjects. *Brain, 126*(Pt 1), 43–56.

Davies, C. L., et al. (2007). Outcome in AIDS-related systemic non-Hodgkin lymphoma and leptomeningeal disease is not predicted by a CT brain scan. *AJNR Am J Neuroradiol, 28*(10), 1988–1990.

DeCarli, C., et al. (1993). The prevalence of computed tomographic abnormalities of the cerebrum in 100 consecutive children symptomatic with the human immune deficiency virus. *Ann Neurol, 34*(2), 198–205.

Deicken, R. F., et al. (1991). Alterations in brain phosphate metabolite concentrations in patients with Human Immunodeficiency Virus infection. *Archives of Neurology, 48,* 203–209.

Depas, G., et al. (1995). Functional brain imaging in HIV-1-infected children born to seropositive mothers. *J Nucl Med, 36*(12), 2169–2174.

Detre, J. A., et al. (1992). Perfusion imaging. *Magnetic Resonance in Medicine, 23,* 37–45.

English, C., et al. (1997). Elevated frontal lobe cytosolic choline levels in minimal or mild AIDS dementia complex patients: A proton magnetic resonance spectroscopy study. *Biological Psychiatry, 41*(41), 500–502.

Ernst, T., Kreis, R. & Ross, B. D. (1993). Absolute quantitation of water and metabolites in the human brain. I: Compartments and water. *Journal of Magnetic Resonance,* B102, 1–8.

Ernst, T., et al. (2000). Changes in cerebral metabolism are detected prior to perfusion changes in early HIV-CMC: A coregistered (1)H MRS and SPECT study. *Journal of Magnetic Resonance Imaging, 12*(6), 859–865.

Ernst, T., et al. (2002). Abnormal brain activation on functional MRI in cognitively asymptomatic HIV patients. *Neurology, 59*(9), 1343–1349.

Ernst, T., et al. (2009). Declined neural efficiency in cognitively stable human immunodeficiency virus patients. *Annals of Neurology, 65*(3), 316–325.

Ernst, T., et al. (2010). Lower brain glutamate is associated with cognitive deficits in HIV patients: A new mechanism for HIV-associated neurocognitive disorder. *J Magn Reson Imaging,* (in press).

Ernst, T. & Chang, L. (1996). Elimination of artifacts in short echo time 1H MR spectroscopy of the frontal lobe. *Magnetic Resonance in Medicine, 36,* 462–468.

Ernst, T., Chang, L., & Arnold, S. (2003). Increased glial markers predict increased working memory network activation in HIV patients. *Neuroimage, 19*(4), 1686–1693.

Ferrando, S. J. & Freyberg, Z. (2008). Treatment of depression in HIV positive individuals: A critical review. *Int Rev Psychiatry, 20*(1), 61–71.

Fiscus, S., et al. (1996). Perinatal HIV infection and the effect of zidovudine therapy on transmission in rural and urban counties. *JAMA, 275*(19), 1483–1488.

Georgiou, M. F., et al. (2008). Analysis of the effects of injecting drug use and HIV-1 infection on 18F-FDG PET brain metabolism. *J Nucl Med, 49*(12), 1999–2005.

Goldman-Rakic, P. (1996). Regional and cellular fractionation of working memory. *Proceedings of the National Academy of Sciences USA, 93*(24), 13473–13480.

Graf, J., Guggino, W., & Turnheim, K. (1993). Volume regulation in transporting epithelia, in interactions in cell volume and cell function. In F. Lang & D. Häussinger (Eds.). pp. 67–1117. Springer-Verlag: Heidelberg.

Graham, C. R., et al. (2000). Screening CT of the brain determined by CD4 count in HIV-positive patients presenting with headache. *American Journal of Neuroradiology*, 21(3), 451–454.

Gutchess, A. H., et al. (2005). Aging and the neural correlates of successful picture encoding: Frontal activations compensate for decreased medial-temporal activity. *J Cogn Neurosci*, 17(1), 84–96.

Hammoud, D. A., et al. (2005). Imaging glial cell activation with [11C]-R-PK11195 in patients with AIDS. *J Neurovirol*, 11(4), 346–355.

Hammoud, D. A., et al. (2010). Imaging serotonergic transmission with [11C]DASB-PET in depressed and non-depressed patients infected with HIV. *Neuroimage*, 49(3), 2588–2595.

Heald, A. E., et al. (1996). Differentiation of central nervous system lesions in AIDS patients using positron emission tomography (PET). *Int J STD AIDS*, 7(5), 337–346.

Henry, P. G., et al. (2001). Brain GABA editing without macromolecule contamination. *Magnetic Resonance in Medicine*, 45(3), 517–520.

Hetherington, H., et al. (1994). Evaluation of cerebral gray and white matter metabolites differences by spectroscopic imaging at 4.1T. *Magnetic Resonance in Medicine*, 32(5), 565–571.

Hetherington, H., Newcomer, B., & Pan, J. (1998). Measurements of human cerebral GABA at 4.1 T using numerically optimized editing pulses. *Magnetic Resonance in Medicine*, 39(1), 6–10.

Hinkin, C., et al. (1995). Cerebral metabolic change in patients with AIDS: Report of a six-month follow-up using positron-emission tomography. *Journal of Neuropsychiatry and Clinical Neurosciences*, 7, 180–187.

Hoffman, J. M., Waskin, H. A., & Schiffer, T. (1993). FDG-PET in differentiating lymphoma from nonmalignant central nervous system lesions in patients with AIDS. *Journal of Nuclear Medicine*, 34, 567–575.

Holman, B.L., et al. (1992). A comparison of brain perfusion SPECT in cocaine abuse and AIDS dementia complex. *Journal of Nuclear Medicine*, 33, 1312–1315.

Horberg, M. A., et al. (2007). Effect of clinical pharmacists on utilization of and clinical response to antiretroviral therapy. *J Acquir Immune Defic Syndr*, 44(5), 531–539.

Howseman, A. & Bowtell, R. (1999). Functional magnetic resonance imaging: Imaging techniques and contrast mechanisms. *Philos Trans R Soc Lond B Biol Sci*, 354(1387), 1179–1194.

Jarvik, J. G., et al. (1993). Proton MR spectroscopy of HIV-infected patients: Characterization of abnormalities with imaging and clinical correlation. *Radiology*, 186, 739–744.

Jarvik, J. G., et al. (1996). Proton spectroscopy in asymptomatic HIV-infected adults: Initial results in a prospective cohort study. *Journal of Acquired Immune Deficiency Syndromes and Human Retrovirology*, 13(3), 247–253.

Jezzard, P. & Turner, R. (1996). Magnetic resonance imaging methods for study of human brain function and their application at high magnetic field. *Computerized Medical Imaging and Graphics*, 20(6), 467–481.

Kalichman, S. C., Kelly, J. A., & Rompa, D. (1997). Continued high-risk sex among HIV seropositive gay and bisexual men seeking HIV prevention services. *Health Psychol*, 16(4), 369–373.

Kawashima, R., O'Sullivan, B. T., & Roland, P. E. (1995). Positron-emission tomography studies of cross-modality inhibition in selective attentional tasks: Closing the "mind's eye." *Proceedings of the National Academy of Sciences*, 92, 5969–5972.

Keller, M., et al. (2004). Altered neurometabolite development in HIV-infected children: Correlation with neuropsychological tests. *Neurology*, 62(10), 1810–1817.

Keller, M. A., et al. (2006). Cerebral metabolites in HIV-infected children followed for 10 months with 1H-MRS. *Neurology*, 66(6), 874–879.

Keltner, J., et al. (1997). In vivo detection of GABA in human brain using a localized double-quantum filter technique. *Magnetic Resonance in Medicine*, 137, 366–371.

Kopnisky, K. L., Stoff, D. M., & Rausch, D. M. (2004). Workshop report: The effects of psychological variables on the progression of HIV-1 disease. *Brain Behav Immun*, 18(3), 246–261.

Korbo, L., Praestholm, J., & Skot, J. (2002). Early brain atrophy in HIV infection: A radiological-stereological study. *Neuroradiology*, 44(4), 308–313.

Kure, K., et al. (1990). Morphology and distribution of HIV-1 gp41-positive microglia in subacute AIDS encephalitis. *ACTA Neuropathologica (Berlin)*, 80, 393–400.

Laubenberger, J., et al. (1996). HIV-related metabolic abnormalities in the brain: Depiction with proton MR spectroscopy with short echo times. *Radiology*, 199, 805–810.

Lazareff, J. A., et al. (1996). Proton magnetic resonance spectroscopic imaging of pediatric low-grade astrocytomas. *Child's Nervous System*, 12(3), 130–135.

Lu, D., et al. (1996). Proton MR spectroscopy of the basal ganglia in healthy children and children with AIDS. *Radiology*, 199(2), 423–428.

Lopez, O., et al. (1999). Dopamine systems in human immunodeficiency virus-associated dementia. *Neuropsychiatry Neuropsychology Behavior and Neurology*, 12(3), 184–192.

Maki, P. M., et al. (2009). Impairments in memory and hippocampal function in HIV-positive versus HIV-negative women: A preliminary study. *Neurology*, 72(19), 1661–1668.

Mangun, G. R., Hillyard, S.A., & Luck, S. J. (1993). Electro-cortical substrates of visual selective attention, in attention and performance XIV. In D. E. Meyer & S. Kornblum, (Eds.). Cambridge, MA: MIT Press.

Mankowski, J. L., et al. (2003). Elevated peripheral benzodiazepine receptor expression in simian immunodeficiency virus encephalitis. *J Neurovirol*, 9(1), 94–100.

Marcus, C., et al. (1998). 1H MR spectroscopy of the brain in HIV-1 seropositive subjects: Evidence for diffuse metabolic abnormalities. *Metabolic Brain Disorders*, 13(2), 123–136.

Martin, S. C., et al. (2006). Cognitive functioning in school-aged children with vertically acquired HIV infection being treated with highly active antiretroviral therapy (HAART). *Dev Neuropsychol*, 30(2), 633–657.

Masdeu, J. C., et al. (1991). Single photon emission computed tomography in human immunodeficiency virus encephalopathy: A preliminary report. *Journal of Nuclear Medicine*, 32, 1471–1475.

McArthur, J. C., et al. (2003). Human immunodeficiency virus-associated dementia: An evolving disease. *J Neurovirol*, 9(2), 205–221.

McConnell, J. R., et al. (1994). Prospective utility of cerebral proton magnetic resonance spectroscopy in monitoring HIV infection and its associated neurological impairment. *AIDS Research and Human Retroviruses*, 10, 977–982.

Menon, D. K., et al. (1990). Proton MR spectroscopy and imaging of the brain in AIDS: Evidence for neuronal loss in regions that appear normal with imaging. *Journal of Computer Assisted Tomography*, 16, 882–885.

Menon, D. K., Ainsworth, J. G., & Cox, I. J. (1992). Proton MR spectroscopy of the brain in AIDS dementia complex. *Journal of Computer Assisted Tomography*, 16, 538–542.

Mescher, M., et al. Simultaneous in vivo spectral editing and water suppression. *NMR Biomed*, 11(6), 266–272.

Meyerhoff, D., et al. (1994). N-acetylaspartate reductions measured by 1H MRSI in cognitively impaired HIV-seropositive individuals. *Magnetic Resonance Imaging*, 12, 653–659.

Meyerhoff, D., et al. (1999). Elevated subcortical choline metabolites in cognitively and clinically asymptomatic HIV+ patients. *Neurology*, 52(5), 995–1003.

Meyerhoff, D. J., et al. (1993). Reduced brain N-acetylaspartate suggests neuronal loss in cognitively impaired immunodeficiency virus-seropositive individuals: In vivo 1H magnetic resonance spectroscopic imaging. *Neurology*, 43, 509–515.

Meyerhoff, D. J., et al. (1995). Effects of chronic alcohol abuse and HIV infection on brain phosphorus metabolites. *Alcoholism, Clinical and Experimental Research*, 19(3), 685–692.

Meyerhoff, D., Weiner, M., & Fein, G. (1996). Deep gray matter structures in HIV infection: A proton MR spectroscopic study. *American Journal of Neuroradiology*, 17, 973–978.

Miller, B. L., et al. (1996). In vivo ^{1}H MRS choline: Correlation with in vitro chemistry/histology. *Life Sciences, 58*(22), 1929–1935.

Modi, G., et al. (2002). New onset seizures in HIV-infected patients without intracranial mass lesions or meningitis—a clinical, radiological and SPECT scan study. *Journal of Neurological Sciences, 202*(1-2), 29–34.

Mohamed, M. A., et al. (2010). Brain metabolism and cognitive impairment in HIV infection: A 3-T magnetic resonance spectroscopy study. *Magn Reson Imaging.*

Moller, H., et al. (1999). Metabolic characterization of AIDS dementia complex by spectroscopic imaging. *Journal of Magnetic Resonance Imaging, 9*(1), 10–18.

Moran, J. & Desimone, R. (1985). Selective attention gates visual processing in the extrastriate cortex. *Science, 229,* 782–784.

Navia, B. A., et al. (1986). Cerebral toxoplasmosis complicating the acquired immune deficiency syndrome: Clinical and neuropathological findings in 27 patients. *Annals of Neurology, 19,* 224–238.

O'Doherty, M. J., et al. (1997). PET scanning and the human immunodeficiency virus-positive patient. *J Nucl Med, 38*(10), 1575–1583.

Ogawa, S., et al. (1993). Functional brain mapping by blood oxygenation level-dependent contrast magnetic resonance imaging. A comparison of signal characteristics with a biophysical model. *Biophysical Journal, 64,* 803–812.

Paley, M., et al. (1995). Short echo time proton spectroscopy of the brain in HIV infection/AIDS. *Magnetic Resonance Imaging, 13*(6), 871–875.

Paley, M., et al. (1996). A multicenter proton magnetic spectroscopy study of neurological complications of AIDS. *AIDS Research in Human Retroviruses, 12*(3), 213–222.

Patton, H., et al. (2001). Alkaline pH changes in the cerebellum of asymptomatic HIV-infected individuals. *NMR in Biomedicine, 14*(1), 12–18.

Pavlakis, S. G., et al. (1998). Brain lactate and N-acetylaspartate in pediatric AIDS encephalopathy. *American Journal of Neuroradiology, 19*(2), 383–385.

Petito, C. K. (1993). What causes brain atrophy in human immunodeficiency virus infection? *Ann Neurol, 34*(2), 128–129.

Pfefferbaum, A., Adalsteinsson, E., & Sullivan, E. V. (2005). Cortical NAA deficits in HIV infection without dementia: Influence of alcoholism comorbidity. *Neuropsychopharmacology, 30*(7), 1392–1399.

Pitlik, S. D., et al. (1983). Spectrum of central nervous system complications in homosexual men with acquired immune deficiency syndrome. *J Infect Dis, 148*(4), 771–772.

Pohl, P., et al. (1998). Single photon emission computed tomography in AIDS dementia complex. *J Nucl Med, 29,* 1382–1386.

Power, C., et al. (1993). Cerebral white matter changes in acquired immunodeficiency syndrome dementia: Alterations of the blood-brain barrier. *Annals of Neurology, 34,* 339–350.

Raichle, M. (1987). Circulatory and metabolic correlates of brain function in normal humans. In V. Mountcastle, F. Plum, & S. Geiger (Eds.). Handbook of physiology—The nervous system (pp. 643–674). American Physiological Society.

Roelcke, U. & Leenders, K. L. (1999). Positron emission tomography in patients with primary CNS lymphomas. *J Neurooncol, 43*(3), 231–236.

Rosci, M. A., et al. (1996). Methods for detecting early signs of AIDS dementia complex in asymptomatic subjects: A quantitative tomography study of 18 cases. *AIDS, 6*(11), 1309–1316.

Rosen, B. R., Belliveau, J. W., & Chien, D. (1989). Perfusion imaging by nuclear magnetic resonance. *Magnetic Resonance Quarterly, 5,* 263–281.

Roth, M. D., et al. (2002). Cocaine enhances human immunodeficiency virus replication in a model of severe combined immunodeficient mice implanted with human peripheral blood leukocytes. *Journal of Infectious Diseases, 185*(5), 701–705.

Rotta, N. T., et al. (2003). Follow-up of patients with vertically-acquired HIV infection who are more than 9 years old. *J Trop Pediatr, 49*(4), 253–255.

Rottenberg, D. A., et al. (1987). The metabolic pathology of the AIDS dementia complex. *Annals of Neurology, 22,* 700–706.

Rottenberg, D. A., et al. (1996). Abnormal cerebral glucose metabolism in HIV-1 seropositive subjects with and without dementia. *Journal of Nuclear Medicine, 37*(7), 1133–1141.

Sacktor, N., et al. (1995). A comparison of cerebral SPECT abnormalities in HIV-positive homosexual men with and without cognitive impairment. *Archives of Neurology, 52,* 1170–1173.

Sacktor, N., et al. (1999). Combination antiretroviral therapy improves psychomotor speed performance in HIV-seropositive homosexual men. Multicenter AIDS Cohort Study (MACS). *Neurology, 52*(8), 1640–1647.

Salvan, A., et al. (1997a). Brain proton magnetic resonance spectroscopy in HIV-related encephalopathy: Identification of evolving metabolic patterns in relation to dementia and therapy. *AIDS Research in Human Retroviruses, 13,* 1055–1066.

Salvan, A., et al. (1997b). Cerebral metabolic alterations in human immunodeficiency virus related encephalopathy detected by proton magnetic resonance spectroscopy. Comparison using short and long echo times. *Investigational Radiology, 32*(8), 485–495.

Salvan, A.-M., et al. (1998). Localized proton magnetic resonance spectroscopy of the brain in children infected with human immunodeficiency virus with and without encephalopathy. *Pediatric Research, 44*(5), 755–762.

Samuelsson, K., et al. (2006). The nervous system in early HIV infection: A prospective study through 7 years. *Eur J Neurol, 13*(3), 283–291.

Scheller, C., et al. (2000). Dopamine activates HIV in chronically infected T lymphoblasts. *Journal of Neural Transmission, 107*(12) 1483–1489.

Schifitto, G., et al. (2007). Memantine and HIV-associated cognitive impairment: A neuropsychological and proton magnetic resonance spectroscopy study. *AIDS, 21*(14), 1877–1886.

Schwartz, R. B., et al. (1994). SPECT imaging of the brain: Comparison of findings in patients with chronic fatigue syndrome, AIDS dementia complex, and major unipolar depression. *American Journal of Roentgenology, 162,* 943–951.

Schweinsburg, B. C., et al. (2005). Brain mitochondrial injury in human immunodeficiency virus-seropositive (HIV+) individuals taking nucleoside reverse transcriptase inhibitors. *J Neurovirology, 11*(4), 356–364.

Schuff, N., et al. (2001). Region and tissue differences of metabolites in normally aged brain using multislice 1H magnetic resonance spectroscopic imaging. *Magnetic Resonance in Medicine, 45*(5), 899–907.

Shen, J. & Rothman, D. L. (2001). In vivo GABA editing with complete metabolite suppression and reduced macromolecule contamination at low Bo field strengths. In *International society for magnetic resonance in medicine.* Glasgow, Scotland, UK.

Shielke, E., et al. (1990). Reduced cerebral blood flow in early stages of human immunodeficiency virus infection. *Archives of Neurology, 47,* 1342–1345.

Silva, A. D., et al. (1995). Multislice MRI of rat brain during amphetamine stimulation using arterial spin labeling. *Magnetic Resonance in Medicine, 33,* 209–214.

Speck, O., et al. (2000). Gender differences in the functional organization of the brain for working memory. *NeuroReport, 11*(11), 1–5.

Stankoff, B., et al. (2001). Clinical and spectroscopic improvement in HIV-associated cognitive impairment. *Neurology, 56*(1), 112–115.

Suhy, J., et al. (2000). ^{1}H MRSI comparison of white matter and lesions in primary progressive and relapsing-remitting MS. *Multiple Sclerosis, 6*(3), 148–155.

Suwanwelaa, N., et al. (2000). Magnetic resonance spectroscopy of the brain in neurologically asymptomatic HIV-infected patients. *Magnetic Resonance Imaging, 18*(7), 859–865.

Tahan, T. T., et al. (2006). Neurological profile and neurodevelopment of 88 children infected with HIV and 84 seroreverter children followed from (1995) to (2002). *Braz J Infect Dis, 10*(5), 322–326.

Taylor, M., et al. (2000). MR spectroscopy in HIV and stimulant dependence HNRC Group. HIV Neurobehavioral Research Center. *Journal of International Neuropsychological Society, 2000. 6*(1), 83–85.

Terpstra, M., Henry, P. G., & Gruetter, R. (2003). Measurement of reduced glutathione (GSH) in human brain using LCModel analysis of difference-edited spectra. *Magnetic Resonance in Medicine, 50*(1), 19–23.

Terpstra, M., Ugurbil, K., & Gruetter, R. (2001). Direct in vivo measurement of cerebral GABA in humans using MEGA-editing at 7 Tesla. In *International society for magnetic resonance in medicine.* Glasgow, Scotland, UK.

Thomas, M. A., et al. (2001). Localized two-dimensional shift correlated MR spectroscopy of human brain. *Magnetic Resonance in Medicine, 46*(1), 58–67.

Tomasi, D., et al., (2005). fMRI-acoustic noise alters brain activation during working memory tasks. *NeuroImage, 27*(2), 377–386.

Tomasi, D., et al. (2003). *The Effect of Practice in Visual Attention Processing: A functional MRI study at 4 Tesla.* In International Society of Magnetic Resonance in Medicine, Eleventh Annual Meeting. Toronto, Canada.

Tomasi, D., et al. (2006). The human immunodeficiency virus reduces network capacity: Acoustic noise effect. *Ann Neurol, 59*(2), 419–423.

Trabesinger, A. H., et al. (1999). Detection of glutathione in the human brain in vivo by means of double quantum coherence filtering. *Magnetic Resonance in Medicine, 42*(2) 283–289.

Trabesinger, A. H. & Boesiger, P. (2001). Improved selectivity of double quantum coherence filtering for the detection of glutathione in the human brain in vivo. *Magnetic Resonance Medicine, 45*(4), 708–710.

Tracey, I., et al. (1996). Brain choline-containing compounds are elevated in HIV-positive patients before the onset of AIDS dementia complex: A proton magnetic resonance spectroscopic study. *Neurology, 46,* 783–788.

Tracey, I., et al. (1998). Increased cerebral blood volume in HIV-positive patients detected by functional MRI. *Neurology, 50*(6), 1821–1826.

Turner, R., et al. (1993). Functional mapping of the human visual cortex at 4 and 1.5 Tesla using deoxygenation contrast EPI. *Magnetic Resonance Medicine, 29,* 277–279.

van Gorp, W.G., et al. (1992). Cerebral metabolic dysfunction in AIDS: Findings in a sample with and without dementia. *J Neuropsychiatry Clin Neurosci, 4*(3), 280–287.

Venneti, S., Wang, G., & Wiley, C. A. (2007). Activated macrophages in HIV encephalitis and a macaque model show increased [3H] (R)-PK11195 binding in a PI3-kinase-dependent manner. *Neurosci Lett, 426*(2), 117–122.

Villemagne, V., et al. (1996). Peptide T and glucose metabolism in AIDS dementia complex. *Journal of Nuclear Medicine, 37*(7), 1177–1180.

Villringer, K., et al. (1995). Differential diagnosis of CNS lesions in AIDS patients by FDG-PET. *J Comput Assist Tomogr, 19*(4), 532–536.

von Giesen, H., et al. (2000). Potential time course of human immunodeficiency virus type 1-associated minor motor deficits: Electrophysiologic and positron emission tomography findings. *Archives of Neurology, 57*(11), 1601–1607.

von Giesen, H., et al. (2001). Basal ganglia metabolite abnormalities in minor motor disorder associated with human immunodeficiency virus type 1. *Archives of Neurology, 58*(8), 1281–1286.

Wang, G. J., et al. (2004). Decreased brain dopaminergic transporters in HIV-associated dementia patients. *Brain, 127*(Pt 11), 2452–2458.

Whiteman, M. L. H., et al. (1993). Progressive multifocal leukoencephalopathy in 47 HIV-seropositive patients: Neuroimaging with clinical and pathologic correlation. *Radiology, 187,* 233–240.

Wiley, C. A. (2006). Positron emission tomography imaging of peripheral benzodiazepine receptor binding in human immunodeficiency virus-infected subjects with and without cognitive impairment. *J Neurovirol, 12*(4), 262–271.

Wilkinson, I., et al. (1997). Cerebral proton magnetic resonance spectroscopy in asymptomatic HIV infection. *Acquired Immunodeficiency Syndrome, 11*(3), 289–295.

Wilkinson, I. D., et al. (1997). Proton MRS and quantitative MRI assessment of the short term neurological response to antiretroviral therapy in AIDS. *Journal of Neurology, Neurosurgery and Psychiatry, 63*(4), 477–482.

Wilman, A. & Allen, P. (1995). Yield enhancement of a double-quantum filter sequence designed for the edited detection of GABA. *Journal of Magnetic Resonance, 109*(Series B), 169–174.

Wilson, A. J., et al. (2010). A comparison of computed tomography and magnetic resonance brain imaging in HIV-positive patients with neurological symptoms. *Int J STD AIDS, 21*(3), 198–201.

Wolters, P. L., et al. (1995). Differential receptive and expressive language functioning of children with symptomatic HIV disease and relation to CT scan brain abnormalities. *Pediatrics, 95*(1), 112–119.

Wong, E. C., Buxton, R. B., & Frank, L. R. (1997). Implementation of quantitative perfusion imaging techniques for functional brain mapping using pulsed arterial spin labeling. *NMR Biomed, 10*(4-5), 237–249.

Zhong, K., et al. (2002). Gender and age effects in human white matter on MR spectroscopy at 4 Tesla. In Tenth Annual Meeting of the International Society of Magnetic Resonance in Medicine. Honolulu, HI.

MAGNETIC RESONANCE IMAGING

Terry L. Jernigan, Sarah L. Archibald, and Christine Fennema-Notestine

This chapter reviews reports of structural and biological changes in the brains of individuals living with HIV infection. This information has come almost exclusively from magnetic resonance imaging, which is the most sensitive method available for characterizing structural damage to brain tissue in vivo. Because the incidence of focal opportunistic infections of the central nervous system has declined with the introduction of antiretroviral therapies (ART), this chapter focuses on individuals with no evidence of such infections. Thus, this is a review of imaging findings associated with chronic HIV-infection per se. This information has become increasingly important as more potent ARTs reduce viral replication, improve immune function, and increase longevity in HIV+ individuals.

INTRODUCTION

In this chapter, reports of structural and biological changes in the brains of individuals living with HIV-infection (HIV+) will be reviewed. Almost exclusively, this information has come from magnetic resonance imaging (MRI), the most sensitive available method for characterizing structural damage to brain tissue in vivo. Although the increased risks in HIV+ individuals for focal opportunistic infections of the central nervous system (CNS) are well known (see Sibtain & Chinn, 2002, for a review of the radiologic correlates), the incidence has declined with the introduction of antiretroviral therapies (ART) (Clements et al., 2005; d'Arminio Monforte et al., 2004; Ferrando, Rabkin, van Gorp, Lin, & McElhiney, 2003; Letendre et al., 2008; Maschke et al., 2000; Sacktor et al., 2001; Strazielle & Ghersi-Egea, 2005) and this chapter will focus on the findings in those individuals with no evidence of such infections. That is, the review will focus on the findings associated with chronic HIV-infection per se. This information has become increasingly important as more potent ARTs yield reduced viral replication, improved immune function, and increased longevity in HIV+ individuals.

As the following review explains, a series of early cross-sectional studies described the range and approximate incidence of radiologic abnormalities in patients at different stages of disease progression. Morphometric studies revealed more subtle aspects of the pattern of neurodegeneration present in AIDS patients. However, concerns about cohort effects (e.g., associated with use of clinical samples, variable substance use histories in controls and patients, choice of risk-group for

controls, etc.) have complicated the interpretation of cross-sectional studies. For this reason, longitudinal studies are particularly valuable, and the importance of pursuing comprehensive longitudinal studies is discussed. Also of particular interest are studies with neuropathological correlation and those of treatment effects on brain structural abnormalities.

CROSS-SECTIONAL STUDIES

Early studies of HIV+ adults focused on the prevalence of focal radiologic abnormalities, usually manifest as areas of increased signal on T2-weighted images, associated with lymphoma, toxoplasmosis, and progressive multifocal leuko-encephalopathy (Levy, Bredesen, & Rosenblum, 1988; Levy, Rosenbloom, & Perrett, 1986; Post et al., 1986; Sibtain, Butt, & Connor, 2007); however, most authors noted that even in the absence of such focal findings, evidence of cerebral atrophy (in the form of enlarged ventricles and subarachnoid spaces) and diffuse white matter hyperintensity were often present. These studies summarized the findings in clinical samples, and most individuals examined were patients with AIDS. In one of the larger clinic-based studies, for example, Olsen et al. (1988) reviewed MR findings in 365 AIDS cases and noted that 31% had white matter signal abnormalities. These authors distinguished between focal high-signal lesions, which were most often associated with CNS opportunistic infections, and the more common pattern of diffuse white matter hyperintensity, which they attributed to direct viral infection of the brain. In another retrospective study, 47 patients with AIDS and AIDS-related complex (ARC) were examined (Flowers et al., 1990). In this study, there was evidence of white matter signal abnormalities and cerebral and cerebellar atrophy, although 62% of these individuals had pathologically confirmed CNS opportunistic infections. Another clinical study focused on visual evidence of cerebral atrophy in HIV+ patients (Elovaara et al., 1990). These authors compared findings in 72 patients with those in 34 controls. Visual evidence of cerebral, cerebellar, and brainstem atrophy were all reported to be more frequent in patients. Patients with more advanced disease had more severe atrophy. Those with cognitive deficits had somewhat more central atrophy, but there was poor correlation between cognitive impairment and other radiologic abnormalities.

Several later MR studies attempted to determine prospectively the range of abnormalities present in the population of

HIV+ individuals at large. Post et al. (1991) examined 119 HIV+ subjects, 95 of whom were asymptomatic. MR images were evaluated clinically and cerebral atrophy and white matter hyperintensities, as well as focal lesions, were considered positive findings. Such findings were present in 23 cases; however, only 13% of asymptomatic patients had abnormal scans, while 46% of symptomatic patients did. In another large study of matched HIV+ and HIV- individuals, clinical assessments of the presence of focal white matter hyperintensities yielded very low rates in both groups, but modest increases in the rate among individuals with AIDS (Bornstein et al., 1992). Thus, although the rate of nonfocal findings, such as enlarged CSF spaces and diffuse white matter hyperintensity, can be quite high in clinical samples drawn retrospectively (especially of AIDS cases), most prospective studies (particularly those that include asymptomatic seropositive subjects) yielded quite low rates of abnormality.

In all of the studies reviewed above, MR images were evaluated clinically for evidence of visually apparent abnormalities. Because the criteria used to define and classify such abnormalities varied from study to study, it is difficult to compare results across studies. However, studies applying quantitative methods for assessing brain morphology have revealed abnormalities that may not be apparent on clinical inspection of the images and provide more objective criteria

for defining the abnormalities. In early quantitative work, 25 HIV+ individuals at different CDC stages were studied with a quantitative measure of ventricular size (Levin et al., 1990). These authors found that ventricular size was related to CDC stage (the five CDC-IV cases had larger ventricles than did asymptomatic cases), as well as to speed of information processing. A similar study of ventricular size (Moeller & Backmund, 1990), using x-ray computed tomography (CT) rather than MRI, also found evidence of ventricular enlargement only in the patients with AIDS.

In studies conducted within the authors' laboratory, MR morphometric analyses have been applied to data from HIV+ subjects and matched HIV- controls. In these studies, it has been possible to estimate the volumes of gray and white matter structures as well as fluid spaces within the brain. Thus, when evidence of atrophy in the form of increased CSF is present, the pattern of tissue volume loss can be examined to attempt to identify the most vulnerable anatomical targets of HIV infection. Quantitative measurements of the amount of signal hyperintensity in the cerebral white matter have also been applied in these studies. Figure 9.2.1 illustrates graphically the outcome of such a morphometric analysis.

The first study conducted using these methods was a cross-sectional analysis of the initial baseline examinations from a prospective, longitudinal study (Jernigan et al., 1993).

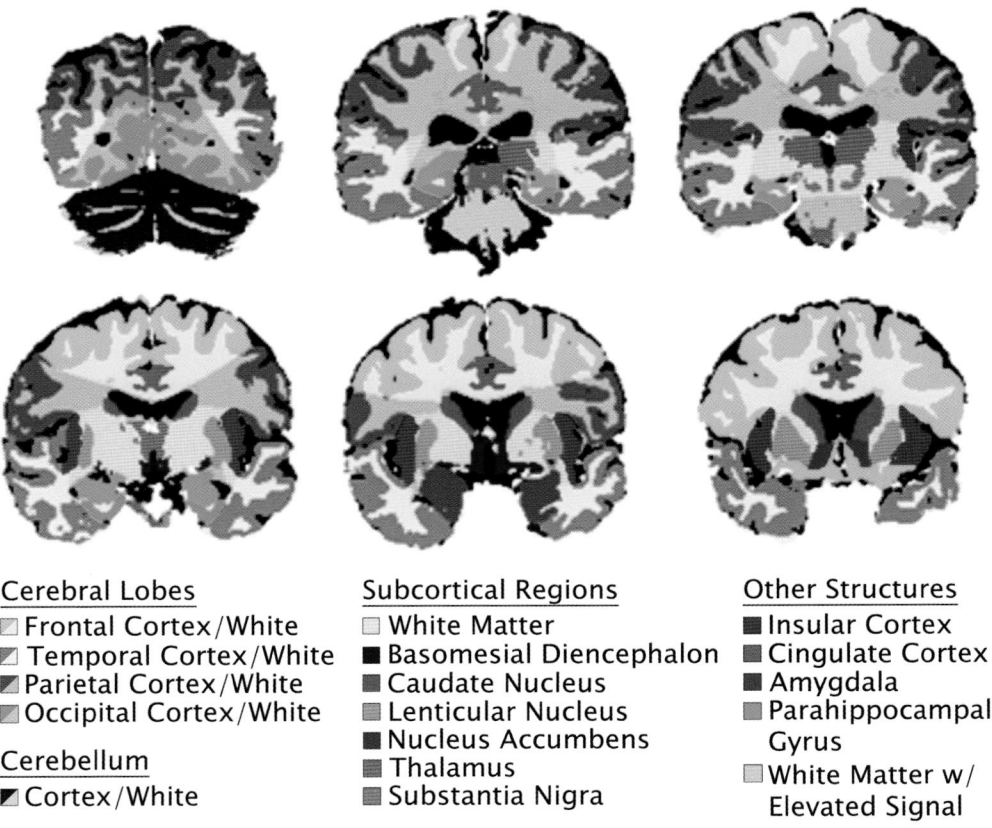

Cerebral Lobes
- Frontal Cortex/White
- Temporal Cortex/White
- Parietal Cortex/White
- Occipital Cortex/White

Cerebellum
- Cortex/White

Subcortical Regions
- White Matter
- Basomesial Diencephalon
- Caudate Nucleus
- Lenticular Nucleus
- Nucleus Accumbens
- Thalamus
- Substantia Nigra

Other Structures
- Insular Cortex
- Cingulate Cortex
- Amygdala
- Parahippocampal Gyrus
- White Matter w/ Elevated Signal

Figure 9.2.1 Coronal sections from an image volume that has been subjected to morphometric analysis. Skull and extracranial regions have been discarded and tissues have been segmented. Trained anatomists have designated the boundaries of different brain structures and regions, so that the volume of each can be estimated. These structures have been color-coded in the image to illustrate the placement of the boundaries. Regions within white matter with abnormally high signal values on T2-weighted images are also identified and color-coded in yellow.

We compared HIV+ men, with and without medical symptoms, to a matched group of men from the same risk group who were seronegative (HIV-). In addition, we examined a second age- and education-matched group of men not known to be members of any group "at high risk" for exposure to HIV. All of the subjects studied were neurologically normal. Briefly, the results confirmed and extended earlier imaging reports of brain volume loss, in the form of CSF increases, in HIV+ subjects. Like in previous studies, evidence for volume loss was strongest in the medically symptomatic subjects. While the results of secondary analyses suggested that this volume loss in the symptomatic subjects was largely attributable to substantial loss of white matter volume, there was also evidence for cerebral gray matter loss. Comparisons of HIV+ symptomatic with HIV+ asymptomatic subjects suggested that the caudate nuclei and the limbic structures in the temporal lobe might be the gray matter structures most severely affected as HIV-infection progressed. This pattern of volume loss in the HIV+ symptomatic subjects was also present when they were compared to HIV- "low-risk" controls of similar age and education. However, the presence of similar (lower) volumes of these structures in the HIV- high-risk controls complicated the interpretation of the gray matter losses in the symptomatic subjects. This study was informative, but the results underscored the limitations of cross-sectional studies, and the difficulty in defining the appropriate "controls" for studies of HIV+ individuals.

Another early MR study employing quantitative methods was conducted by Hestad et al. (1993). In this study, planimetric indices of regional atrophy were acquired and correlated with neuropsychological measures in a group of HIV+ individuals at different stages of the illness. Ventricular size and two linear ratios (a bifrontal ratio intended to measure frontal lobe atrophy, and a bi-caudate ratio intended to measure caudate atrophy) were measured. Correlation analyses suggested that atrophy, particularly as assessed by the bi-caudate ratio, was associated with significant performance decrements on behavioral measures of visuo-motor speed and verbal fluency. Subsequent studies by this group of investigators (Aylward et al., 1995; Aylward et al., 1993) employed MR volumetrics of basal ganglia and cerebral cortex. The focus of these studies was the presence of the dementia complex in HIV+ individuals. Groups of demented and nondemented HIV+ individuals were compared to HIV- controls. The results suggested that some generalized brain volume loss appeared to be present in HIV+ individuals regardless of the presence of dementia, but the demented patients had further losses in cerebral white matter and gray matter, particularly in basal ganglia and posterior cortex.

More recent cross-sectional MR morphometry studies have provided additional information about the extent and pattern of HIV-related brain abnormalities in individuals who are treated with more potent antiretroviral therapies than were the individuals studied in earlier reports. Using methods similar to those applied in our earlier studies, we reported (Jernigan et al., 2005) that HIV-related cerebral gray matter alterations were, as noted previously, very prominent in the caudate nucleus and the hippocampus; but in this group of HIV+ individuals, cortical volume loss was more significant, and the pattern suggested more loss in frontal and temporal lobe areas.

In another study, computational morphometry was applied to map the cortical structural abnormalities associated with HIV infection. Thompson et al. (2005) compared cortical thickness maps in 26 AIDS patients, of whom 13 were on ART therapies, and 14 controls. They reported thinning of 15% in primary sensory, motor, and premotor regions in AIDS patients relative to controls. Degree of immune suppression was related to cortical thinning in frontopolar and peri-sylvian regions, and cognitive deficits were associated with a fronto-parietal pattern of thinning. Viral load showed no association with degree of cortical thinning.

An unexpected result was reported by Castelo et al. (2007), who used computational morphometry to measure the volumes of subcortical structures in 22 HIV+ individuals and 22 matched seronegative controls. Most of the seropositive participants were on stable antiviral medication and the HIV+ group exhibited only mild functional impairments in motor and psychomotor speed. The HIV+ participants had significantly increased volume of the putamen, and this apparent hypertrophy of the putamen was associated with degree of psychomotor slowing and increased CD4 count. The authors speculated that hypertrophy of striatal structures in these relatively intact HIV+ participants might parallel the earlier findings of basal ganglia hypermetabolism on positron emission tomography (Rottenberg et al., 1996). In the latter study it was observed that asymptomatic patients exhibited hypermetabolism, but patients at more advanced stages of disease progression exhibited hypometabolism. Castelo et al. suggest that hypertrophy may reflect inflammatory tissue responses to the presence of viral proteins or other pathogens, an explanation we also considered to be a plausible explanation for striatal hypertrophy in methamphetamine abusers (Jernigan et al., 2005). As the authors point out, this explanation is consistent with the findings in other studies of reduced striatal volumes, usually most pronounced in participants at more advanced stages of disease progression, when chronic, or sporadic, exposure to pathogens results in cumulative tissue damage.

The cerebellum also has been studied in HIV in vivo (Klunder et al., 2008). In a comparison of 19 HIV+ with 15 HIV- participants, evidence for cerebellar atrophy, particularly in posterior vermis, was present in the HIV+ group. There was little association between the degree of atrophy and disease-related variables in this small sample of HIV+ individuals; however, surprisingly, severity of depressive symptoms was correlated with severity of cerebellar atrophy. A postmortem morphometric study from our group, described in more detail below, also reported significant cerebellar atrophy associated with white matter volume loss and increased CSF spaces (Archibald et al., 2004).

Recently, Cohen et al. (2010) reported the results of a large study of 82 HIV+ individuals, 69 of whom were described as neuroasymptomatic and 13 of whom were diagnosed with some degree of the AIDS dementia complex (ADC). MR images were processed with voxel-based morphometry and an atlas labeling scheme to estimate volumes of gray and white matter structures and ventricles. The demented subgroup had less cerebral gray matter and larger ventricles than the asymptomatic group. Models were constructed to examine the relationships between disease-related variables and brain volumes. History of advanced immune suppression, as indexed by nadir CD4, was associated with volume loss in white matter and in several cortical and subcortical gray matter structures. Longer duration of infection was also a factor that predicted more brain volume loss in several models. Presence of detectable HIV-RNA in plasma showed an inconsistent relationship with brain volumes in this study, but this factor was more often related to volume variability in the subcortical structures.

Finally, we recently reported initial cross-sectional neuroimaging findings from the CNS HIV Antiretroviral Therapy Effects Research (CHARTER) initiative, a large longitudinal study examining a diverse group of HIV+ individuals at several sites in the United States (Jernigan et al., 2011). Multispectral image analysis produced volumes of ventricular and sulcal CSF; cortical and subcortical gray matter; total cerebral white matter; and white matter with abnormal signal values in 251 HIV+ individuals. Using simultaneous multiple regression, and controlling for demographic and MRI instrument variables, we observed that severity of prior immunosuppression (as indexed by lower CD4 nadir) was related to white matter and subcortical gray matter volume loss as well as evidence for damage in the remaining white matter (indexed by T2 signal hyperintensity). Relatively higher current CD4 than nadir CD4, unexpectedly, was related to lower white and subcortical gray volumes and increased CSF. Detectable CSF viral load was also related to lower white matter volume. There was preliminary evidence that increased cumulative exposure to ART was associated with lower white matter and higher sulcal CSF volumes and this effect did not appear to be mediated by estimated duration of infection.

Unfortunately, the number of neuroimaging studies of HIV infection in children is small, and these are retrospective studies of children imaged for clinical indications. An early x-ray CT study (Price et al., 1988), revealed a low rate of focal mass lesions (relative to that reported in adults), but a high rate of enlargement of the CSF spaces (57%) in clinical cases. The authors also noted occasional calcifications in basal ganglia and white matter. A second retrospective CT study of 100 pediatric cases (DeCarli, Civitello, Brouwers, & Pizzo, 1993) revealed abnormalities in 86% of cases. The findings included, in order of prevalence: ventricular enlargement, cortical atrophy, leukoaraiosis and cerebral calcifications. These authors noted that cerebral calcifications were strongly associated with vertical transmission and the presence of encephalopathy; however, there was no relationship to measures of viral load. Interestingly, a more recent MR and CT study (Johann-Liang, Lin, Cervia, Stavola, & Noel, 1998), also of patients imaged for clinical purposes, revealed very similar radiologic findings. Of 33 children studied, 45% were assessed as showing cerebral atrophy and 27% had basal ganglia calcifications. Only one child had a mass lesion, and three had "white matter disease." Both ventricular enlargement and the presence of basal

ganglia calcifications were strongly associated with more advanced CDC stage and, unlike in the earlier study, increased plasma HIV RNA.

In summary, the cross-sectional studies of HIV-infected individuals have shown that HIV-1 infection in adults is associated with an increased prevalence of radiologically detectable focal lesions associated with lymphoma, toxoplasmosis, and progressive multifocal leukoencephalopathy. Even in the absence of these focal findings, however, many HIV+ individuals, particularly those with AIDS, appear on neuroimaging evaluation to have cerebral, cerebellar, or brainstem atrophy and signal abnormality in cerebral white matter. MR morphometry studies confirm, with quantitative methods, that the CSF spaces are larger in medically symptomatic patients; and these studies suggest that tissue loss may be most severe in the white matter and basal ganglia, but there is definite evidence for limbic and cortical damage as well. Studies of children are less definitive, but it appears that cerebral atrophy is also a very common finding in pediatric cases. Focal lesions due to opportunistic CNS infections may be less common in pediatric cases, but cerebral calcification is frequently observed, particularly in the basal ganglia. These calcifications, as well as cerebral atrophy, are most common in children with very advanced illness (i.e., high viral load and severe immunosuppression).

The cross-sectional studies confirm that, while the damage to brain tissues associated with chronic infection may be less severe, it continues to be measurable with imaging in a large number of individuals on modern therapies, even when viral levels are reasonably well controlled. There is growing evidence implicating a role for inflammatory processes in the tissue, perhaps triggered by low-level viral exposure, and possibly in some instances exacerbated by immune reconstitution. Effects on MRI volumetric measures may differ depending on whether inflammatory processes or neurodegenerative processes predominate. More evidence from longitudinal studies is needed to elucidate the dynamic processes that give rise to changes in brain morphology in infected individuals.

LONGITUDINAL STUDIES

Although imaging has sometimes been obtained in follow-up studies of individual cases with CNS complications of AIDS, prospective longitudinal studies of neuroimaging results in HIV-infection are rare. In an early study by Post et al. (1992), 31 HIV+ patients with abnormal findings on an initial MR examination (20 asymptomatic and 11 symptomatic) were followed with repeat MR one to two years later. Abnormal findings on initial images were cerebral atrophy and white matter lesions. All 31 patients continued to have abnormal findings on repeated examination. Twenty-seven cases exhibited no significant change. In one case, MR abnormalities, as well as clinical symptoms, improved. In the remaining three cases there was worsening both of MR abnormalities and clinical symptoms, consistent with HIV encephalopathy.

As described previously, an initial cross-sectional morphometric study from our group (Jernigan, et al., 1993) provided clear evidence for brain volume loss, particularly in cerebral white matter, in symptomatic HIV+ individuals. However, the presence of lower volumes of some brain structures in the seronegative "high-risk" controls made it difficult to conclude from this study how gray matter structures were affected. The pattern of losses we observed in the symptomatic patients may to some extent have been associated with factors other than HIV that were present in the risk group as a whole. A longitudinal study of the HIV+ and HIV- "high-risk" subjects, however, confirmed progressive loss of volume in specific structures in the HIV+ group.

A total of 109 (86 HIV+ and 23 HIV-) subjects with MRI morphometric data from two or more examinations (separated by at least 6 months) were included in our longitudinal study (Stout et al., 1998). Medically asymptomatic (CDC-A) and medically symptomatic (CDC-C) patients had significantly higher slopes for cortical CSF than seronegative controls, suggesting that volume loss progresses over the course of HIV disease, even within the medically asymptomatic phase. Increases in ventricular CSF were significantly greater only in the CDC-C subjects, though the values in the CDC-A subjects appeared to be intermediate between controls and CDC-C subjects. White matter volume declined more steeply in CDC-C than in CDC-A subjects. Among the gray matter measures, the caudate nucleus volume showed steeper decline in the CDC-C subjects than in other groups. In additional analyses, subjects who progressed over the follow-up period from one CDC stage to the next were compared to nonprogressing subjects in CDC-A&B. The progressors had significantly higher slopes for the ventricular measure and significantly steeper decreases in caudate volumes.

Furthermore, within the HIV+ group as a whole, rate of decline in CD4 lymphocytes was significantly related to decreasing caudate and cerebral white matter volumes. In summary, these results confirmed that HIV-infection was associated with progressive cerebral volume loss that began in the medically asymptomatic stage and was accelerated in the more advanced stages of the illness. The regional analysis showed that striatum and cerebral white matter were affected, beginning relatively early in the course of the disease, and that volume losses in these structures lead to secondary increases in CSF volume (Figure 9.2.2).

Our study was conducted relatively early in the epidemic and thus best represents the course of CNS involvement when available treatments had only limited effectiveness. A more recent longitudinal study of 39 treated HIV+ individuals and 30 HIV- controls (Cardenas et al., 2009) provides a better picture of the course of infection since more potent therapies became available. A comparison of baseline MRI to repeated imaging after a 24-month follow-up revealed that, as in our earlier study, loss of white matter volume was significantly greater in the HIV+ participants. Though the rate of gray matter loss did not differ between the groups overall, individuals with lower CD4 counts exhibited greater loss of thalamic and caudate loss, as well as white matter loss, over time. This study also provided some evidence that lack of viral suppression accelerated brain tissue loss.

The longitudinal studies reviewed here suggest that even in the era of potent therapies modest progressive damage to white matter, and some gray matter structures, occurs over time, at least in a subset of patients. Taken together with the cross-sectional studies, these results raise questions about the

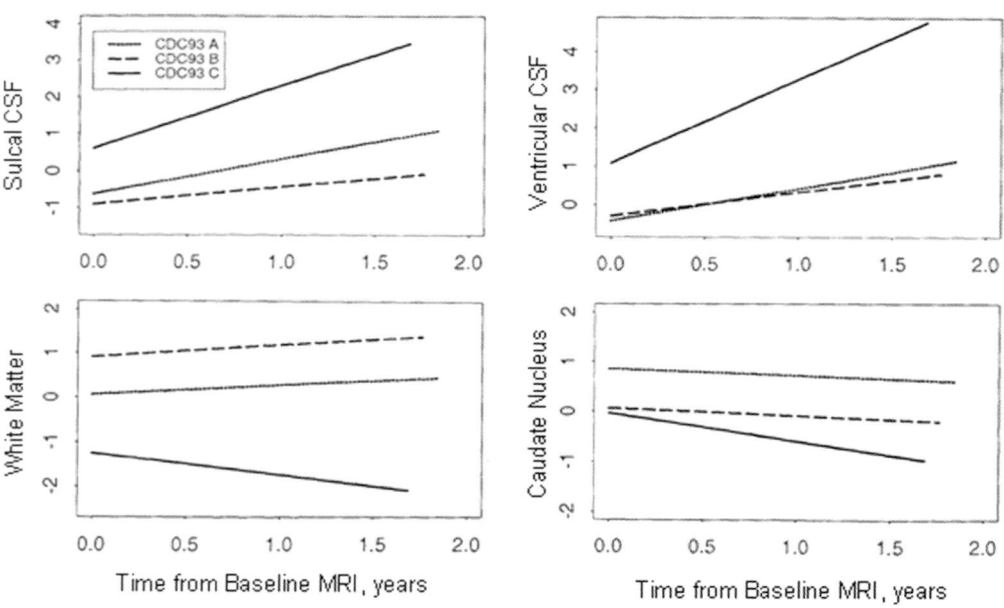

Figure 9.2.2 Mean baseline values and slopes for volumes of brain structures computed from serial MR images for three subgroups of HIV+ participants in a longitudinal study. Slopes shown for the brain volumes are standardized to the slopes for the HIV-control participants (these are not shown because, by definition, this group had a mean value of 0 with standard deviation of 1). CDC93 A, B, C refers to persons in stages A, B, or C of disease per the Centers for Disease Control Schema (1992). Figure from Stout et al., 1998.

factors contributing to ongoing brain injury in HIV+ individuals, for example, whether they are entirely due to continuing viral replication, whether inflammation plays a significant role, and whether chronic medication exposure contributes. A few longitudinal studies have examined the relationship of in vivo structural MRI to later autopsy findings, or have compared in vivo structural MRI findings before and after treatment.

STUDIES WITH POSTMORTEM CORRELATION

An early neuropathology study (Gelman & Guinto, 1992) examined the relationship between ventricular enlargement, measured at autopsy, and evidence of HIV-related histopathological abnormalities. The patients with ventricular enlargement had significantly more AIDS-related pathology. In vivo CT was available for a subset of these cases. In these, the correlation between the magnitude of ventricular enlargement observed in vivo and postmortem was good, suggesting that patients with radiologic evidence of atrophy are likely to have AIDS-related neuropathology.

In vivo MRI obtained shortly before death was available in 35 patients studied by Miller et al. (1997). Nineteen of these cases had diffuse signal hyperintensity in the white matter on MRI. The focus of the report was on the relationship between this finding and postmortem evidence of HIV leukoencephalopathy, HIV encephalitis, and CMV encephalitis. Ten cases with diffuse white matter hyperintensity had HIV encephalitis (and associated leukoencephalopathy) on subsequent autopsy examination, however three had CMV encephalitis, one had both HIV and CMV encephalitis, three had lymphoma, and two had "nonspecific inflammation." Among the eight cases without diffuse white matter hyperintensity, a few also had HIV encephalitis, one of these with associated leukoencephalopathy; however, many of them had CMV encephalitis (6). The authors concluded that diffuse white matter hyperintensity on MR could be caused by HIV-related or CMV-related pathology, or by nonspecific causes. It would appear from this study that diffuse white matter hyperintensity may be considerably more strongly associated with HIV encephalitis than with CMV encephalitis.

We correlated neuroanatomical changes measured in vivo shortly before death with the autopsy results in 22 deceased participants (Archibald et al., 2004). No subjects with CNS opportunistic infections other than CMV were included in the study. All MRI data were obtained within approximately 1 year of death. This study revealed that, irrespective of the autopsy diagnosis, patients dying with AIDS had suffered degenerative changes in the cerebrum as indexed by reduced white matter and caudate nucleus volumes. Patients meeting neuropathological criteria for HIV-encephalitis also had increased high-signal abnormalities in the remaining white matter relative to those with CMV-encephalitis or those without evidence of CMV- or HIV-encephalitis (Figure 9.2.3). Importantly, these high-signal abnormalities were associated with a decrease in dendritic complexity in the

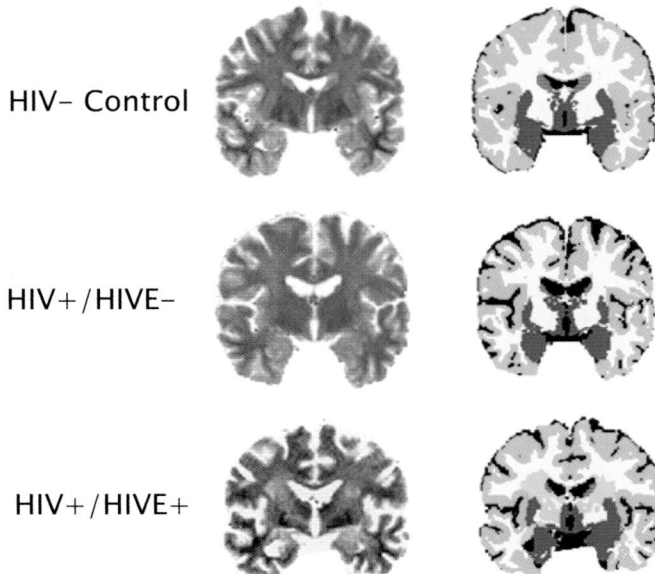

HIV− Control

HIV+/HIVE−

HIV+/HIVE+

Figure 9.2.3 Antemortem MRI morphometric results for HIV+ cases who died with postmortem diagnoses of HIV encephalitis (bottom row) or no encephalitis (middle row). The top row provides comparisons to uninfected controls. The cerebral cortex is shown in green, underlying white matter is shaded a lighter green and subcortical gray matter structures of the basal ganglia and diencephalon are shown in a darker green. However, for emphasis, the caudate nucleus is shown in magenta and areas within white matter with abnormally elevated signal are shown in yellow. Cerebrospinal fluid (CSF) is shown in black. Smaller caudate and white matter volumes (accompanied by increased CSF) are strongly associated with HIV. Increased volume of signal elevation in white matter has been associated with HIV and pathologically verified HIV encephalitis.

cortex, suggesting a link between the white matter damage and cortical degeneration.

STUDIES OF TREATMENT EFFECTS IN ADULTS

Soon after the advent of antiretroviral therapy (ART), anecdotal evidence emerged regarding treatment effects on the MRI appearance of CNS abnormalities. Case studies revealed mixed results and focused on the effects on focal lesions, often associated with opportunistic CNS infections. An early study by Tozzi et al. (1993) followed 30 patients with the AIDS dementia complex who were treated with zidovudine (ZDV). Thirteen of the patients showed clinical improvement, and six of these had some detectable regression of the severity of their white matter abnormalities on MRI. The authors of this study concluded that some regression of brain structural changes (and clinical status) occurred as a result of ZDV treatment of demented AIDS patients, however the gains were often transient and relapse occurred commonly over 6 months of treatment in their patients.

Later, Filippi et al. (1998) examined the effects of introducing protease inhibitors into the treatment regime for AIDS patients with HIV encephalopathy. Of the 16 patients studied, 9 received protease inhibitors and 7 did not. On initial MR examinations, all of the patients had signal hyperintensities in white matter and/or basal ganglia. The results were very encouraging. Of the nine treated patients, 89% showed clinical improvement and regression of white matter changes on MRI at a follow-up that was on average 5 months after the initiation of treatment. By contrast, 86% of the patients who were not treated with protease inhibitors deteriorated clinically. Two of the patients treated with protease inhibitors had complete, or near complete, resolution of their high signal abnormalities on MRI.

The results of a study of highly active antiretroviral therapy (HAART) by Thurnher et al. (2000) also provided encouraging results, but the observations differed somewhat from those of the earlier study. Four patients with the AIDS dementia complex were studied. On initial imaging, all had bilateral periventricular white matter hyperintensity, some had additional high signal abnormalities in basal ganglia and thalamus, and three had cerebral atrophy. All patients had two or three follow-up MR examinations after initiation of HAART, and on average patients were followed over 20 months. At the earliest follow-up examinations, performed an average of 6 months after treatment was modified, patients showed clinical improvement but worsening of white matter abnormalities or degree of atrophy. Interestingly, however, abnormalities within deep gray matter structures tended to normalize by this time. Later follow-up examinations showed regression of white matter abnormalities relative to those observed at the earlier follow-up. This study suggests that treatment-related regression of structural abnormalities may lag behind clinical improvement, and continued progression of abnormalities may occur during the early stage of treatment.

Tozzi et al. (2009) examined the change in neurocognitive performance before HAART initiation and at follow-up in 185 participants, about half of whom had neuropsychological impairment. They examined the relationship to the CNS penetration-effectiveness (CPE) of the HAART medications to cognitive change. Higher CPE was associated with greater improvements in several domains and this correlation was stronger in the impaired participants. This study suggests the type of HAART drugs with respect to their ability to penetrate the CNS is important for neurocognitive outcome. The neuroimaging correlates of the effects of different treatment regimens are being examined in our group and others.

STUDIES OF TREATMENT EFFECTS IN CHILDREN

Unfortunately, few systematic studies of treatment effects in children have included neuroimaging assessments. An initial study of ZDV infusion treatments of a small group of children (DeCarli et al., 1991) showed reduction of the ventricular brain ratio on CT after six months of treatment. These changes occurred concurrently with evidence of cognitive improvement. No group studies of neuroimaging findings in HAART treated children are available; however, a case study (Tepper et al., 1998) yielded promising results. The eight-year-old

child had undergone several courses of monotherapy but had developed a moderately severe encephalopathy accompanied by evidence of cerebral atrophy on MRI. Six months after initiation of HAART, clinical symptoms had substantially improved and significant regression of cerebral atrophy was apparent on MRI.

In summary, antiretroviral treatment, particularly HAART, when initiated in children or adults with clinical signs of HIV encephalopathy, is frequently followed by regression of white matter abnormalities, high signal abnormalities in gray matter structures, and/or cerebral atrophy. Further research is needed to define more clearly the time course and sequence of these changes, to determine the duration of these ameliorating effects, to determine to what extent complete resolution of structural damage can be achieved, and to explain individual differences in treatment response. As noted above, questions also remain about brain structural effects of the treatments themselves, particularly when continued over longer periods of time. For example, Schweinsburg et al. (2005) found reduced n-acetyl aspartate (NAA), an indicator of neuronal integrity, on MR spectroscopic imaging that seemed to be associated with treatment of dideoxynucleocides. Langford et al. (2002) described the neuropathology associated with a severe form of HIV-related leukoencephalopathy, which appeared on imaging before death as extensive white matter abnormality. The authors noted that these cases seemed to have a more severe leukoencephalopathy than cases examined before the advent of HAART. They speculated that perivascular infiltration by HIV-infected monocytes, perhaps stimulated by HAART-associated immune restoration, may have lead to injury of brain endothelial cells and subsequent myelin loss, axonal damage, and astrogliosis. Further studies will be needed to elucidate the complex interactions between HIV-related neurodegenerative mechanisms and potent antiretroviral treatments.

DIFFUSION IMAGING

While structural MRI, particularly when combined with quantitative measurement techniques, has been useful in describing the CNS complications of HIV infection, the potential limitations of the technique for early detection and diagnosis are also clear. While their sensitivity to the prevalent and diagnostically important white matter abnormalities of the disorder are a major advantage, such changes are relatively nonspecific, and the differentiation of different causes for the abnormalities is difficult with conventional structural MRI. Diffusion imaging techniques, such as diffusion tensor imaging (DTI), have made it possible to examine the structural integrity of white matter and individual fiber tracts. DTI measures the motion associated with diffusion of water molecules in tissues, and diffusion is influenced by the tissue microstructure. In CSF, water molecules diffuse randomly and freely in all directions, thus diffusion in ventricles and sulci is high and isotropic. In gray and white matter, more water molecules are bound within the tissue, so diffusion is lower. However, while the direction of diffusion in gray matter is, like in CSF, relatively random (or isotropic), diffusion in the fiber bundles of the white matter exhibits anisotropy, presumably because there is less restriction of diffusion along the long axis of the fiber bundles than perpendicular to them. With DTI, degree of diffusion anisotropy can be mapped, and the tensor data can be further analyzed to distinguish specific fiber tracts and to detect alterations of the degree of diffusivity or pattern of anisotropy that may occur due to demyelination or axonal damage.

In an early DTI study of HIV, Pomara and his associates (2001) studied six HIV+ individuals and a matched group of nine HIV- controls. Four of the six HIV+ subjects met criteria for AIDS and five of the six were receiving HAART (the remaining subject was receiving no antiretroviral treatment). All subjects were living independently and none carried a neurological diagnosis. Although this was a small study, it was carefully conducted. Estimates of fractional anisotropy (FA) were obtained from specific regions of interest in cerebral white matter and no areas of visible hyperintensity were included. Although there were no group differences in calculated proton density or T2 values, nor in mean diffusivity, FA was significantly decreased in frontal lobe white matter and increased in the genu of the internal capsule in HIV+ subjects relative to controls. The decreased FA in the frontal lobe is consistent with other reports of frontal lobe damage. Increased FA has been observed in regions of crossing fibers when the fiber tracts are damaged selectively. Based on secondary analyses, the authors speculated that the increased FA in internal capsule may result from selective damage to fibers from the posterior limb of the internal capsule. Whatever the explanation of these findings, they suggest that DTI measures of diffusion anisotropy may be more sensitive to HIV-related white matter damage than other MRI methods.

At nearly the same time as the previous study was published, Filippi and colleagues (2001) reported a DTI study of ten HIV+ subjects. The HIV+ subjects of this study were all referred for imaging because of complaints of headaches or other neurological symptoms. However, individuals in whom imaging revealed white matter abnormality were excluded. Six of the ten patients were receiving HAART. Filippi et al. (2001) measured diffusion anisotropy with UA_{SURP}, reportedly a more sensitive measure of anisotropy in fiber tracts than FA as used in the Pomara et al. study (2001), as well as average diffusion. Both measures were obtained in multiple locations throughout the white matter. Comparisons were made across three groups with different viral load levels (<400, 10,000-20,000, and >400,000 copes/mm^3); although no matched controls were examined concurrently with the patients of this study, values were compared to control values obtained in a previous study. The individuals with low viral loads had relatively normal average diffusion and anisotropy values, whereas the individuals within the higher viral load groups demonstrated reduced anisotropy and increased average diffusion. In this early study it appeared that both increasing diffusion and decreasing anisotropy in the genu and splenium of the corpus callosum may index disease progression in the CNS, even without visible lesions in the white matter.

A number of studies have now reported that FA is significantly lower in HIV+ participants in frontal brain regions (Filippi, et al., 2001; Gongvatana et al., 2009; Pomara, et al., 2001; Ragin, Storey, Cohen, Edelman, & Epstein, 2004; Ragin, Storey, Cohen, Epstein, & Edelman, 2004). Cloak et al. (2004) reported that an increase in the apparent diffusion coefficient in frontal white matter was associated with increases in the MR spectroscopy glial marker myoinositol (MI) and worse cognitive performance. Thus, increased diffusion and decreased fractional anisotropy may reflect glial activation or inflammation, which may contribute directly to cognitive deficits.

Two recent DTI studies have focused on effects of HIV-infection on corpus callosum. Wu et al. (2006) compared FA and mean diffusivity in 11 HIV+ and 11 HIV- participants and reported that FA was decreased and diffusivity increased in the splenium of the HIV+ individuals. They also observed that the severity of the abnormalities was associated with severity of cognitive impairment. In a larger recent study of 21 HIV+ and 19 HIV- participants (Muller-Oehring, Schulte, Rosenbloom, Pfefferbaum, & Sullivan, 2010), DTI parameters revealed loss of integrity in callosal fiber tracts, worse in posterior than in anterior segments. The severity and spatial pattern of callosal diffusion alterations were related to performance variability on a visuospatial task requiring local-global feature integration.

Chen et al. (2009) used DTI to perform a more global analysis of diffusion parameters in cerebral white matter. They compared results from 21 nondemented and 8 demented HIV+ individuals to 18 seronegative controls. Both HIV+ groups exhibited widespread increases in diffusivity and decreases in FA relative to controls, though the alterations in the demented group were more severe, particularly in parietal areas. Disproportionate effects on radial (transverse) diffusivity relative to axial (longitudinal) diffusivity were noted. This pattern has in some contexts been associated with dysmyelination, and may signal that loss of myelin plays a role in HIV-related white matter damage. Our group also recently reported that increased diffusivity and decreased FA in internal capsule, superior longitudinal fasciculus, and optic radiation was linked to the presence of neurocognitive impairment within HIV+ individuals (Gongvatana et al., 2009). Tate et al. (2010) used global tractography to measure FA values in 23 HIV+ and 20 HIV- participants and related these to cognitive performance. Although the results did not demonstrate large differences between the groups, within the HIV+ group global FA measures correlated with 8 of the 12 cognitive domains tested. Reduced global FA values were associated with poorer performance on tests of tapping, switching, verbal interference, and mazes.

The largest and most comprehensive DTI study to date was reported by Pfefferbaum et al. (2009). They performed tractography to measure diffusion parameters in each of 17 major brain fiber tracts, and examined 42 HIV+ and 88 HIV- participants. Their results revealed few group differences on tract FA values, but increased diffusivity was observed in many tracts, including posterior sectors of the corpus callosum, internal and external capsules, and superior cingulate bundles. AIDS patients had prominent increases in axial (longitudinal) diffusivity in posterior callosum, fornix, and superior cingulate, a pattern considered to be indicative of axonal damage. Unmedicated patients had more prominent increases in radial (transverse) diffusivity in occipital forceps, inferior cingulate, and superior longitudinal fasciculus, suggesting dysmyelination.

In summary, the findings in DTI studies confirm and extend those in earlier morphometry studies that indicate prominent white matter damage in HIV+ individuals. They suggest that effects on brain fiber tracts are widespread, and that in some patients axonal function may be compromised as the disease progresses. There is also evidence that dysmyelination may be present, perhaps particularly in unmedicated patients.

AGING IN HIV-INFECTED INDIVIDUALS

A few studies have begun to examine the effects of aging in HIV+ individuals. In a recent study (Jernigan et al., 2005), we found evidence for a significant age-by-HIV interaction within statistical models predicting total cortex, frontal cortex, and temporal cortex volumes. Our first impression was that these effects were probably attributable to the association of age with disease progression. That is, since neurodegenerative changes are likely to accelerate during later stages of the illness, and older subjects are more likely to have reached that stage, the interactions could reflect accelerating changes in individuals with more advanced disease. This would be consistent with our earlier longitudinal study of HIV-related brain volume loss in which greater volume loss over time was seen in CDC-C stage participants than in those in CDC-A and -B stages (Stout et al., 1998). We conducted post-hoc analyses to determine whether the age-by-HIV interactions were mediated by the presence of more advanced disease in the older HIV+ individuals. Two measures of disease progression were examined: the current CD4 cell measure and an estimate of years HIV positive at the time of study. Of these, the latter was significantly correlated with age within the HIV+ participants. However, addition of these variables as covariates did not diminish the magnitude of the interaction. Surprisingly, although there was a modest association between estimated years of infection and age within the HIV+ participants, there was no evidence that more years of infection was associated with more cortical atrophy. The magnitude of the interaction effect was not reduced appreciably by the inclusion of this estimate of disease duration in the models predicting total, frontal, or temporal cortex. Greater reduction in CD4 cells was not related to increased age, and inclusion of this covariate also did not reduce the magnitude of the interaction effects. However, there was evidence of an independent effect of lower CD4 cells associated with lower cortical volumes. The age-by-HIV interaction effects remained significant in these models, leaving open the possibility that they represent genuine interactions, such that alterations present in the older brain potentiate the effects of HIV.

We have also examined the relationship between increases in signal abnormalities (areas of elevated T2 signal on MRI) in the white matter during normal aging and the prevalence of these abnormalities in HIV+ individuals by comparing our findings (using the same morphometry methods) in these two populations. Figure 9.2.4 illustrates the distinction graphically. There is clear evidence that HIV+ individuals exhibit increased prevalence of white matter abnormality at a much earlier age than do HIV- individuals. In fact, the distribution of values in the HIV+ individuals in their 30s and 40s resembles the distribution in HIV- individuals in their 60s and 70s.

Interestingly, Chang et al. (2008) recently reported that increases in diffusivity in the corpus callosum of HIV+ individuals over a one-year period significantly exceeded those in seronegative controls. Furthermore, diffusion changes over time were linked to deteriorating cognitive performance within the HIV+ individuals. These findings are consistent with the morphometry results in suggesting that HIV-related neurodegeneration may accelerate the effects of aging.

CHALLENGES IN NEUROIMAGING RESEARCH

As the foregoing review implies, the evaluation of CNS effects of HIV, including brain structural effects, has become increasingly complicated by variability due to the treatment status and treatment history of the patients. Some therapies in some patients clearly seem to act to prevent and/or reverse the progression of degenerative changes; however, there is also evidence that progression or relapse can occur even while receiving the most potent treatments available. This implies that, at the least, results of assessments of brain structure must be presented with accompanying information about the treatment history of the participants.

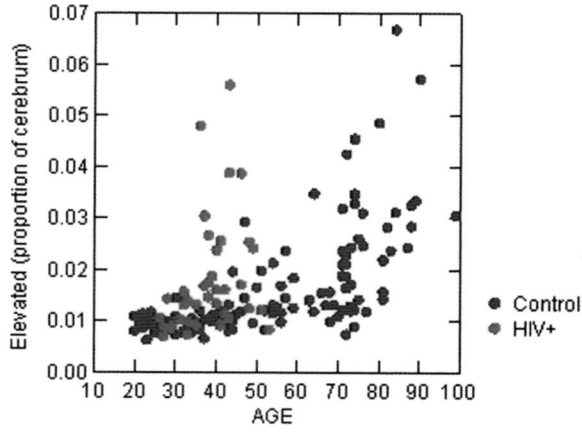

Figure 9.2.4 Plotted against the age of the participants is the volume of white matter tissue with elevated T2 values (indicative of white matter abnormality), expressed as a proportion of the cerebral cranial vault. Values for HIV- participants are shown in blue, HIV+ in red. HIV+ individuals in their 40s demonstrate white matter abnormalities not typically seen in uninfected controls until their 60s.

A number of putative mechanisms for HIV-related neurodegeneration have emerged. It is likely that a combination of these account for the observed effects. In a review focusing on the role of neuroimaging, Avison et al. (2002) drew attention to the distinction between mechanisms associated with inflammatory processes and noninflammatory, or neurotoxic, mechanisms. As these authors explained, it is very likely that these processes lead to different patterns and degrees of brain structural abnormality. Individuals may be disproportionately vulnerable to one or the other of these neurodegenerative processes, and this may account for some of the inter-individual variation. One process may dominate at different levels of immunosuppression, or at different viral levels. Different treatments may abate one process more effectively than the other. Avison et al. (2002) suggested that inflammatory pathways may lead to more prominent spectroscopic abnormalities in choline and *myo*-inositol concentrations, while noninflammatory pathways may disproportionately decrease N-acetyl aspartate levels. This is an intriguing possibility. But it is also possible that these different pathways lead to different MRI findings. For example, gliosis may produce a particular pattern of signal alteration in white matter and may be associated with tissue hypertrophy in some cases, while neurotoxicity and neurodegeneration may produce the prominent gray and white matter volume loss often observed. These and other questions remain unanswered.

Most neuroimaging investigators make the assumption that the changes they will observe will be in a predictable direction. That is, they expect that brain tissue volumes will tend to decrease, CSF volumes will therefore increase, and signal abnormality in white matter will become more extensive, as progression of the illness occurs. In some cases this may not be strictly true. Some of the signal alteration in white matter, for example, may be due to immune processes that are attenuated later in the illness when immunosuppression is more severe. This could lead to apparent regression of the structural abnormalities in a progressing illness. Such apparent waxing and waning of abnormalities presents significant interpretative challenges in neuroimaging research.

The goals of neuroimaging research in the study of HIV infection are to provide information relevant to an understanding of the neuropathological processes, and to contribute added sensitivity and specificity to diagnosis and treatment of CNS complications. It seems clear that these MRI methods, particularly in combination with other imaging techniques, such as spectroscopy and perfusion imaging, will play an important role in achieving these goals. However, the complexity of this protracted illness demands intense research efforts. Perhaps what is most needed are additional longitudinal studies of HIV+ individuals at varying stages of the illness, with careful clinical characterization and sequential, multimodality imaging examinations. At least one cohort of HIV+ individuals should be studied with such examinations at closer follow-up intervals than have been reported to date if we are to link dynamic changes in viral levels and immune function, as well as treatment status and host factors to specific neuropathological effects of HIV.

ACKNOWLEDGMENTS

This chapter was supported by the following grants from the National Institutes of Health: P30-MH62512, N01-MH22005, R01-MH79752, P01-DA12065, and P50-DA026306.

REFERENCES

Archibald, S. L., Masliah, E., Fennema-Notestine, C., Marcotte, T. D., Ellis, R. J., McCutchan, J. A., et al. (2004). Correlation of in vivo neuroimaging abnormalities with postmortem human immunodeficiency virus encephalitis and dendritic loss. *Arch Neurol, 61*(3), 369–376.

Avison, M. J., Nath, A., & Berger, J. R. (2002). Understanding pathogenesis and treatment of HIV dementia: a role for magnetic resonance? *Trends Neurosci, 25*(9), 468–473.

Aylward, E. H., Brettschneider, P. D., McArthur, J. C., Harris, G. J., Schlaepfer, T. E., Henderer, J. D., et al. (1995). Magnetic resonance imaging measurement of gray matter volume reductions in HIV dementia. *Am J Psychiatry, 152*(7), 987–994.

Aylward, E. H., Henderer, J. D., McArthur, J. C., Brettschneider, P. D., Harris, G. J., Barta, P. E., et al. (1993). Reduced basal ganglia volume in HIV-1-associated dementia: results from quantitative neuroimaging. *Neurology, 43*(10), 2099–2104.

Bornstein, R. A., Chakeres, D., Brogan, M., Nasrallah, H. A., Fass, R. J., Para, M., et al. (1992). Magnetic resonance imaging of white matter lesions in HIV infection. *J Neuropsychiatry Clin Neurosci, 4*(2), 174–178.

Cardenas, V., Meyerhoff, D., Studholme, C., Kornak, J., Rothlind, J., Lampiris, H., et al. (2009). Evidence for ongoing brain injury in human immunodeficiency virus-positive patients treated with antiretroviral therapy. *J Neurovirol,* 1–10.

Castelo, J. M., Courtney, M. G., Melrose, R. J., & Stern, C. E. (2007). Putamen hypertrophy in nondemented patients with human immunodeficiency virus infection and cognitive compromise. *Arch Neurol, 64*(9), 1275–1280.

Chang, L., Wang, G. J., Volkow, N. D., Ernst, T., Telang, F., Logan, J., et al. (2008). Decreased brain dopamine transporters are related to cognitive deficits in HIV patients with or without cocaine abuse. *Neuroimage, 42*(2), 869–878.

Chen, Y., An, H., Zhu, H., Stone, T., Smith, J. K., Hall, C., et al. (2009). White matter abnormalities revealed by diffusion tensor imaging in non-demented and demented HIV+ patients. *Neuroimage, 47*(4), 1154–1162.

Clements, J. E., Li, M., Gama, L., Bullock, B., Carruth, L. M., Mankowski, J. L., et al. (2005). The central nervous system is a viral reservoir in simian immunodeficiency virus—infected macaques on combined antiretroviral therapy: a model for human immunodeficiency virus patients on highly active antiretroviral therapy. *J Neurovirol, 11*(2), 180–189.

Cloak, C. C., Chang, L., & Ernst, T. (2004). Increased frontal white matter diffusion is associated with glial metabolites and psychomotor slowing in HIV. *J Neuroimmunol, 157*(1-2), 147–152.

Cohen, R. A., Harezlak, J., Schifitto, G., Hana, G., Clark, U., Gongvatana, A., et al. (2010). Effects of nadir CD4 count and duration of human immunodeficiency virus infection on brain volumes in the highly active antiretroviral therapy era. *J Neurovirol, 16*(1), 25–32.

d'Arminio Monforte, A., Cinque, P., Mocroft, A., Goebel, F. D., Antunes, F., Katlama, C., et al. (2004). Changing incidence of central nervous system diseases in the EuroSIDA cohort. *Ann Neurol, 55*(3), 320–328.

DeCarli, C., Civitello, L. A., Brouwers, P., & Pizzo, P. A. (1993). The prevalence of computed tomographic abnormalities of the cerebrum in 100 consecutive children symptomatic with the human immune deficiency virus. *Ann Neurol, 34*(2), 198–205.

DeCarli, C., Fugate, L., Falloon, J., Eddy, J., Katz, D. A., Friedland, R. P., et al. (1991). Brain growth and cognitive improvement in children with human immunodeficiency virus-induced encephalopathy after 6 months of continuous infusion zidovudine therapy. *J Acquir Immune Defic Syndr*, *4*(6), 585–592.

Elovaara, I., Poutiainen, E., Raininko, R., Valanne, L., Virta, A., Valle, S. L., et al. (1990). Mild brain atrophy in early HIV infection: the lack of association with cognitive deficits and HIV-specific intrathecal immune response. *J Neurol Sci*, *99*(2-3), 121–136.

Ferrando, S. J., Rabkin, J. G., van Gorp, W., Lin, S. H., & McElhiney, M. (2003). Longitudinal improvement in psychomotor processing speed is associated with potent combination antiretroviral therapy in HIV-1 infection. *J Neuropsychiatry Clin Neurosci*, *15*(2), 208–214.

Filippi, C. G., Sze, G., Farber, S. J., Shahmanesh, M., & Selwyn, P. A. (1998). Regression of HIV encephalopathy and basal ganglia signal intensity abnormality at MR imaging in patients with AIDS after the initiation of protease inhibitor therapy. *Radiology*, *206*(2), 491–498.

Filippi, C. G., Ulug, A. M., Ryan, E., Ferrando, S. J., & van Gorp, W. (2001). Diffusion tensor imaging of patients with HIV and normal-appearing white matter on MR images of the brain. *AJNR Am J Neuroradiol*, *22*(2), 277–283.

Flowers, C. H., Mafee, M. F., Crowell, R., Raofi, B., Arnold, P., Dobben, G., et al. (1990). Encephalopathy in AIDS patients: Evaluation with MR imaging. *AJNR Am J Neuroradiol*, *11*(6), 1235–1245.

Gelman, B. B., & Guinto, F. C., Jr. (1992). Morphometry, histopathology, and tomography of cerebral atrophy in the acquired immunodeficiency syndrome. *Ann Neurol*, *32*(1), 31–40.

Gongvatana, A., Schweinsburg, B. C., Taylor, M. J., Theilmann, R. J., Letendre, S. L., Alhassoon, O. M., et al. (2009). White matter tract injury and cognitive impairment in human immunodeficiency virus-infected individuals. *J Neurovirol*, *15*(2), 187–195.

Hestad, K., McArthur, J. H., Dal Pan, G. J., Selnes, O. A., Nance-Sproson, T. E., Aylward, E., et al. (1993). Regional brain atrophy in HIV-1 infection: Association with specific neuropsychological test performance. *Acta Neurol Scand*, *88*(2), 112–118.

Jernigan, T. L., Archibald, S., Hesselink, J. R., Atkinson, J. H., Velin, R. A., McCutchan, J. A., et al. (1993). Magnetic resonance imaging morphometric analysis of cerebral volume loss in human immunodeficiency virus infection. The HNRC Group. *Arch Neurol*, *50*(3), 250–255.

Jernigan, T. L., Gamst, A. C., Archibald, S. L., Fennema-Notestine, C., Mindt, M. R., Marcotte, T. D., et al. (2005). Effects of methamphetamine dependence and HIV infection on cerebral morphology. *Am J Psychiatry*, *162*(8), 1461–1472.

Jernigan, T. L., Archibald, S. L., Fennema-Notestine, C., Taylor, M. J., Theilmann, R. J., Julaton, M. D., . . . Grant, I., (2011). Clinical factors related to brain structure in HIV: the CHARTER study. *J Neurovirol*, *17*(3), 248–257.

Johann-Liang, R., Lin, K., Cervia, J., Stavola, J., & Noel, G. (1998). Neuroimaging findings in children perinatally infected with the human immunodeficiency virus. *Pediatr Infect Dis J*, *17*(8), 753–754.

Klunder, A. D., Chiang, M. C., Dutton, R. A., Lee, S. E., Toga, A. W., Lopez, O. L., et al. (2008). Mapping cerebellar degeneration in HIV/AIDS. *Neuroreport*, *19*(17), 1655–1659.

Langford, T. D., Letendre, S. L., Marcotte, T. D., Ellis, R. J., McCutchan, J. A., Grant, I., et al. (2002). Severe, demyelinating leukoencephalopathy in AIDS patients on antiretroviral therapy. *AIDS*, *16*(7), 1019–1029.

Letendre, S., Marquie-Beck, J., Capparelli, E., Best, B., Clifford, D., Collier, A. C., et al. (2008). Validation of the CNS Penetration-Effectiveness rank for quantifying antiretroviral penetration into the central nervous system. *Arch Neurol*, *65*(1), 65–70.

Levin, H. S., Williams, D. H., Borucki, M. J., Hillman, G. R., Williams, J. B., Guinto, F. C., Jr., et al. (1990). Magnetic resonance imaging and neuropsychological findings in human immunodeficiency virus infection. *J Acquir Immune Defic Syndr*, *3*(8), 757–762.

Levy, R. M., Bredesen, D. E., & Rosenblum, M. L. (1988). Opportunistic central nervous system pathology in patients with AIDS. *Ann Neurol*, *23 Suppl*, S7–12.

Levy, R. M., Rosenbloom, S., & Perrett, L. V. (1986). Neuroradiologic findings in AIDS: A review of 200 cases. *AJR Am J Roentgenol*, *147*(5), 977–983.

Maschke, M., Kastrup, O., Esser, S., Ross, B., Hengge, U., & Hufnagel, A. (2000). Incidence and prevalence of neurological disorders associated with HIV since the introduction of highly active antiretroviral therapy (HAART). *J Neurol Neurosurg Psychiatry*, *69*(3), 376–380.

Miller, R. F., Lucas, S. B., Hall-Craggs, M. A., Brink, N. S., Scaravilli, F., Chinn, R. J., et al. (1997). Comparison of magnetic resonance imaging with neuropathological findings in the diagnosis of HIV and CMV associated CNS disease in AIDS. *J Neurol Neurosurg Psychiatry*, *62*(4), 346–351.

Moeller, A. A., & Backmund, H. C. (1990). Ventricle brain ratio in the clinical course of HIV infection. *Acta Neurol Scand*, *81*(6), 512–515.

Muller-Oehring, E. M., Schulte, T., Rosenbloom, M. J., Pfefferbaum, A., & Sullivan, E. V. (2010). Callosal degradation in HIV-1 infection predicts hierarchical perception: A DTI study. *Neuropsychologia*, *48*(4), 1133–1143.

Olsen, W. L., Longo, F. M., Mills, C. M., & Norman, D. (1988). White matter disease in AIDS: Findings at MR imaging. *Radiology*, *169*(2), 445–448.

Pfefferbaum, A., Rosenbloom, M. J., Rohlfing, T., Kemper, C. A., Deresinski, S., & Sullivan, E. V. (2009). Frontostriatal fiber bundle compromise in HIV infection without dementia. *AIDS*, *23*(15), 1977–1985.

Pomara, N., Crandall, D. T., Choi, S. J., Johnson, G., & Lim, K. O. (2001). White matter abnormalities in HIV-1 infection: A diffusion tensor imaging study. *Psychiatry Res*, *106*(1), 15–24.

Post, M. J., Berger, J. R., & Quencer, R. M. (1991). Asymptomatic and neurologically symptomatic HIV-seropositive individuals: Prospective evaluation with cranial MR imaging. *Radiology*, *178*(1), 131–139.

Post, M. J., Levin, B. E., Berger, J. R., Duncan, R., Quencer, R. M., & Calabro, G. (1992). Sequential cranial MR findings of asymptomatic and neurologically symptomatic HIV+ subjects. *AJNR Am J Neuroradiol*, *13*(1), 359–370.

Post, M. J., Sheldon, J. J., Hensley, G. T., Soila, K., Tobias, J. A., Chan, J. C., et al. (1986). Central nervous system disease in acquired immunodeficiency syndrome: Prospective correlation using CT, MR imaging, and pathologic studies. *Radiology*, *158*(1), 141–148.

Price, D. B., Inglese, C. M., Jacobs, J., Haller, J. O., Kramer, J., Hotson, G. C., et al. (1988). Pediatric AIDS. Neuroradiologic and neurodevelopmental findings. *Pediatr Radiol*, *18*(6), 445–448.

Ragin, A. B., Storey, P., Cohen, B. A., Edelman, R. R., & Epstein, L. G. (2004). Disease burden in HIV-associated cognitive impairment: A study of whole-brain imaging measures. *Neurology*, *63*(12), 2293–2297.

Ragin, A. B., Storey, P., Cohen, B. A., Epstein, L. G., & Edelman, R. R. (2004). Whole brain diffusion tensor imaging in HIV-associated cognitive impairment. *AJNR Am J Neuroradiol*, *25*(2), 195–200.

Rottenberg, D. A., Sidtis, J. J., Strother, S. C., Schaper, K. A., Anderson, J. R., Nelson, M. J., et al. (1996). Abnormal cerebral glucose metabolism in HIV-1 seropositive subjects with and without dementia. *J Nucl Med*, *37*(7), 1133–1141.

Sacktor, N., Lyles, R. H., Skolasky, R., Kleeberger, C., Selnes, O. A., Miller, E. N., et al. (2001). HIV-associated neurologic disease incidence changes: Multicenter AIDS Cohort Study, 1990-1998. *Neurology*, *56*(2), 257–260.

Schweinsburg, B. C., Taylor, M. J., Alhassoon, O. M., Gonzalez, R., Brown, G. G., Ellis, R. J., et al. (2005). Brain mitochondrial injury in human immunodeficiency virus-seropositive (HIV+) individuals taking nucleoside reverse transcriptase inhibitors. *J Neurovirol*, *11*(4), 356–364.

Sibtain, N. A. & Chinn, R. J. S. . (2002). Imaging of the central nervous system in HIV infection. *Imaging*, *14*, 48–59.

Sibtain, N. A., Butt, S., & Connor, S. E. (2007). Imaging features of central nervous system haemangiopericytomas. *Eur Radiol*, *17*(7), 1685–1693.

Stout, J. C., Ellis, R. J., Jernigan, T. L., Archibald, S. L., Abramson, I., Wolfson, T., et al. (1998). Progressive cerebral volume loss in human immunodeficiency virus infection: A longitudinal volumetric magnetic resonance imaging study. HIV Neurobehavioral Research Center Group. *Arch Neurol*, *55*(2), 161–168.

Strazielle, N., & Ghersi-Egea, J. F. (2005). Factors affecting delivery of antiviral drugs to the brain. *Rev Med Virol*, *15*(2), 105–133.

Tate, D. F., Conley, J., Paul, R. H., Coop, K., Zhang, S., Zhou, W., et al. (2010). Quantitative diffusion tensor imaging tractography metrics are associated with cognitive performance among HIV-infected patients. *Brain Imaging Behav, 4*(1), 68–79.

Tepper, V. J., Farley, J. J., Rothman, M. I., Houck, D. L., Davis, K. F., Collins-Jones, T. L., et al. (1998). Neurodevelopmental/neuroradiologic recovery of a child infected with HIV after treatment with combination antiretroviral therapy using the HIV-specific protease inhibitor ritonavir. *Pediatrics, 101*(3), E7.

Thompson, P. M., Dutton, R. A., Hayashi, K. M., Toga, A. W., Lopez, O. L., Aizenstein, H. J., et al. (2005). Thinning of the cerebral cortex visualized in HIV/AIDS reflects CD4+ T lymphocyte decline. *Proc Natl Acad Sci U S A, 102*(43), 15647–15652.

Thurnher, M. M., Schindler, E. G., Thurnher, S. A., Pernerstorfer-Schon, H., Kleibl-Popov, C., & Rieger, A. (2000). Highly active antiretroviral therapy for patients with AIDS dementia complex: Effect on MR imaging findings and clinical course. *AJNR Am J Neuroradiol, 21*(4), 670–678.

Tozzi, V., Balestra, P., Salvatori, M. F., Vlassi, C., Liuzzi, G., Giancola, M. L., et al. (2009). Changes in cognition during antiretroviral therapy: Comparison of 2 different ranking systems to measure antiretroviral drug efficacy on HIV-associated neurocognitive disorders. *J Acquir Immune Defic Syndr, 52*(1), 56–63.

Tozzi, V., Narciso, P., Galgani, S., Sette, P., Balestra, P., Gerace, C., et al. (1993). Effects of zidovudine in 30 patients with mild to end-stage AIDS dementia complex. *AIDS, 7*(5), 683–692.

Wu, Y., Storey, P., Cohen, B. A., Epstein, L. G., Edelman, R. R., & Ragin, A. B. (2006). Diffusion alterations in corpus callosum of patients with HIV. *AJNR Am J Neuroradiol, 27*(3), 656–660.

9.3

PSYCHOLOGICAL EVALUATIONS

Jordan Elizabeth Cattie, Steven Paul Woods, and Igor Grant

Neuropsychology, an applied neuroscience broadly concerned with the behavioral manifestations of brain dysfunction, provides a valuable window into the central nervous system effects of HIV. Neuropsychological testing can directly inform the evaluation, management, and treatment of patients infected with HIV. Ideally, all HIV-infected patients would receive a comprehensive baseline neuropsychological evaluation upon diagnosis to facilitate detection of emergent neurobehavioral changes. Although such testing rarely occurs, largely due to cost considerations, routine brief baseline neuropsychological assessment has been adopted in other settings (e.g., in athletes at risk for head injuries). This approach may provide a model for HIV care as recognition of the prevalence and impact of HAND continues to grow among physicians who treat HIV. This chapter discusses a wide range of topics relevant to neuropsychological testing in the HIV population.

INTRODUCTION: WHAT IS CLINICAL NEUROPSYCHOLOGY?

Neuropsychology is an applied neuroscience that is broadly concerned with the behavioral manifestations of brain dysfunction. This formal subdiscipline of psychology first emerged in the 1940s, when casualties of World War II created an acute demand for psychologists to assess and rehabilitate brain-injured veterans. In the following years, a trend toward the objective measurement of mental abilities (e.g., intelligence) spurred the development of the performance-based tests and interpretive approaches (e.g., demographically adjusted normative standards) that are commonly used in the modern practice of neuropsychology (Morgan & Ricker, 2008). Today, neuropsychology is a method of objectively evaluating brain function by studying cognitive, behavioral, and emotional phenomena in order to inform, operationalize, and evaluate patient care (Lezak et al., 2004). Although neuropsychology overlaps with the fields of neuropsychiatry and behavioral neurology, the principal clinical methods and therapies of these approaches remain largely distinct. The latter disciplines are primarily focused on understanding the neurobiological underpinnings of brain dysfunction (Mendez et al., 1995), whereas neuropsychology places relatively greater emphasis on 1) the performance-based, objective assessment of higher-level cognitive abilities (e.g., memory and executive functions); 2) the role of cognitive, behavioral, and emotional

factors on everyday functioning outcomes (e.g., employment, automobile driving, and household management); and 3) delineation of patterns of strengths and weaknesses from which to optimize rehabilitation efforts (Beaumont, 2008).

WHAT IS THE ROLE OF NEUROPSYCHOLOGY IN THE MANAGEMENT OF HIV?

Neuropsychology can directly inform the evaluation, management, and treatment of patients infected with HIV. Neurocognitive disorders, including frank dementia, have been observed in HIV-infected individuals since the early years of the epidemic (Perry & Jacobsen, 1986; Snider et al., 1983). In 1987, Grant and colleagues published the first comprehensive neuropsychological study of HIV infection, in which prominent executive dysfunction, bradyphrenia, episodic memory deficits, and abnormal magnetic resonance (MR) imaging findings were observed even in medically asymptomatic individuals. While the prevalence of severe forms of HIV-associated neurocognitive disorders (HAND) has decreased since the use of combination antiretroviral therapies (cART) became widespread in the late 1990s, the prevalence and incidence of less severe forms of HAND remains a significant public health concern (Ances & Clifford, 2008). Today, approximately 30% of medically asymptomatic individuals and as many as 40–50% of symptomatic individuals exhibit neurocognitive impairment (Baldewicz et al., 2005; Heaton et al., 2009). Moreover, the functional impact of cognitive decrements in persons infected with HIV is well documented, with approximately 30–50% of individuals with HIV-associated neurocognitive impairment experiencing related functional problems in their everyday lives (Heaton et al., 2004). Specifically, neurocognitively impaired individuals often have significant vocational difficulties (e.g., van Gorp et al., 1999), increased dependence in their instrumental activities of daily living (IADLs; Heaton et al., 2004), poorer adherence to cART (Waldrop-Valverde et al., 2006), greater risk of automobile driving accidents (Marcotte et al., 2004), and lower health-related quality of life (Rosenbloom et al., 2007). For a more detailed review of these topics, the reader is referred to excellent recent papers on the epidemiology (Grant, this volume), cognitive profiles (Woods et al., 2009), and functional impact (Gorman et al., 2009) of HAND.

HIV is a lentivirus that exerts pathogenic effects in both the immune and central nervous systems. The virus infiltrates the central nervous system (CNS) early in the course of the disease (Grant et al., 1987), and although HIV does not productively infect neurons, HIV-related changes can be observed widely throughout the neocortex, white matter, and deep grey matter (e.g., Ellis et al., 2009). Although HIV-associated neuropathologies are evident in a broad array of brain regions (e.g., hippocampus, parietal cortex), the fronto-striatal-thalamo-cortical circuits are among the most commonly affected regions (e.g., Aylward et al., 1993). Consequently, HIV is associated with a profile of neurocognitive deficits similar to other disorders that affect these fronto-striatal pathways, such as Huntington's and Parkinson's diseases (see Tröster & Woods, 2010). At the group level, HIV is associated with generally mild-to-moderate deficits in speeded information processing (e.g., Heaton et al., 1995), fine-motor coordination (e.g., Carey et al., 2004b), attention/working memory (e.g., Martin et al., 2001), executive functions (e.g., Martin et al., 2004), and memory (Delis et al., 1995). In contrast, deficits in cognitive abilities typically associated with the posterior neocortex, such as constructional praxis, receptive language, and basic visuoperception, are less common in HIV-infected individuals (e.g., Heaton et al., 1995).

Given the prevalence and functional implications of neurocognitive impairment in HIV-positive individuals, a comprehensive neuropsychological evaluation may be important to diagnosing and treating neuroAIDS. Specifically, a neuropsychological evaluation is a useful method for: 1) detecting the nature and extent of cognitive deficits; 2) differential diagnosis of neurocognitive disorders, especially when the evaluation is accompanied by neuroimaging and a comprehensive neuromedical evaluation; 3) delineating a profile of absolute and relative neuropsychological strengths and weaknesses, for use in selecting compensatory strategies to lessen the impact of cognitive deficits on everyday functioning; 4) monitoring changes in neurocognitive status related to treatment and/or disease progression; 5) evaluating patients whose suspected disease has not been detected by standard neurodiagnostic methods; 6) determining the appropriateness and practicality of certain medical interventions for a patient (e.g., adherence to a complicated medication regimen); 7) assessing the individual's capacity to provide informed consent to treatment; and 8) guiding decisions related to competence and planning for future financial, legal, and living arrangements (Lezak et al., 2004; Tröster & Woods, 2003; Morgan & Ricker, 2008). Most evaluations serve several of these purposes, so it is often important to integrate assessment strategies in order to obtain the necessary information about a particular patient (Lezak et al., 2004). Prior to requesting neuropsychological testing, these listed purposes should be used to determine whether neuropsychological assessment is appropriate to address the specific question(s) raised by the patient, clinician, and/or other care providers.

As such, it would be ideal for every HIV-infected patient to receive a baseline neuropsychological evaluation upon diagnosis in order to more easily detect emergent neurobehavioral changes. This is especially true because of the various premorbid CNS confounds that are risk factors for HIV transmission (e.g., substance abuse) that can make interpretation of the etiology of cognitive deficits difficult. However, baseline assessment rarely occurs, largely due to cost considerations. While uncommon in early stage HIV infection, routine brief baseline neuropsychological assessments have been adopted in other settings (e.g., athletes at risk for head injuries; Maroon et al., 2000), which may be emulated as recognition of the prevalence and impact of HAND continues to grow among physicians treating HIV.

APPROACHES TO NEUROPSYCHOLOGICAL EVALUATION

Individual components and the overall length of neuropsychological evaluations will vary widely across different clinical and research settings for HIV-infected individuals. Under ideal circumstances, the neuropsychological evaluation should include each of the following components: 1) a clinical interview with the patient and knowledgeable informants, such as family members; 2) a review of medical records to investigate the patient's medical, psychiatric, and social history; 3) informal observations regarding the patient's behavior, cognition, sensory-perceptual abilities, basic motor functions, and affect; 4) the administration of objective, performance-based psychometric tests to measure current neurocognitive functions (e.g., intelligence, attention, executive functions, language, information processing speed, learning and memory, visuospatial abilities, praxis, motor skills, and sensory-perception); 5) the self-report and performance-based assessment of key areas of everyday functioning, such as employment, household chores, and medication adherence; 6) administration of standardized questionnaires designed to assess mood state, quality of life/coping, and personality characteristics; 7) complementary neuromedical and/or psychiatric evaluation, perhaps to include neuroimaging; and 8) in many clinical and research settings, the provision of integrated verbal and/or written recommendations to the referral source, patient, family, and health care providers (Tröster & Woods, 2003).

CLINICAL INTERVIEW AND COGNITIVE COMPLAINTS

As mentioned above, information on cognitive functioning is derived both from the initial patient history (i.e., self- and other-report) as well as from direct neuropsychological examination. After a careful and thorough patient history, persons with HIV infection should be questioned closely on the incidence, course, and severity of any complaints related to perceived declines in attention/concentration, mental efficiency and speed, recall of recent and remote events, language, motor coordination, sensory-perception, and executive functions (such as planning, multitasking, and problem-solving). Cognitive complaints and affective distress can be assessed through a careful clinical interview, a review of medical records, and/or standardized self- and other-report questionnaires, including the Patient's Assessment of Own Functioning (PAOFI; Chelune et al., 1986) the Bewilderment/ Confusion subscale of the Profile of Mood States (POMS; McNair et al., 1981), and the Prospective and Retrospective Memory Questionnaire (PRMQ; Crawford et al., 2003).

Unfortunately, the value of self-reported information depends heavily on subjective factors that are not always easy for the clinician to evaluate. For instance, patients may interpret terms such as "memory" or "attention/concentration" quite differently from the way they are used professionally. Additionally, some HIV-infected patients may be unaware of changes in their cognitive functioning (i.e., mild anosognosia), whereas others may tend to amplify cognitive complaints. For all of these reasons, self-reported cognitive difficulties do not correlate strongly with more objective indications of brain functioning derived from neuropsychological, neurological, and neuroimaging examinations. Instead, cognitive complaints tend to be associated with greater levels of fatigue, anxiety, and depression (e.g., Rourke et al., 1999). For example, Rourke and colleagues demonstrated that, although there was a modest relationship between self-reported and performance-based cognitive deficits, mood disturbance was nevertheless the strongest predictor of cognitive complaints (Rourke et al., 1999). Accordingly, it is imperative to exercise caution when interpreting data obtained from self-report, particularly among individuals with possible mood disorders. When possible, it is advisable to gather information from other persons who are familiar with the patient's history and current functioning, including significant others, friends, family members, and health care professionals. Most importantly, these data suggest that self-reported cognitive deficits are not sufficient for diagnosis of HAND in the absence of supportive neurocognitive and psychiatric data (see Antinori et al., 2007).

MOOD

Given the profound effects of affective distress on cognitive complaints (e.g., Rourke et al., 1999) and everyday functioning outcomes (e.g., Heaton et al., 2004), it is important to assess current mood state and history of mood disorders when evaluating patients for HAND. The prevalence of MDD, for example, is significantly elevated as compared to general population rates (Ciesla & Roberts, 2001), with estimates generally varying between approximately 35% (Wolff et al., 2010) and almost 50% (Dew et al., 1997). Depression has been associated with medication nonadherence (Walkup et al., 2008), poorer health-related quality of life (de Boer-van der Kolk et al., 2010), and risk of mortality (Ickovics et al., 2001). Other mood states, such as anxiety (Owe-Larsson et al., 2009) and fatigue (Millikin et al., 2003), are also common in HIV, and warrant examination due to their implications for everyday functioning outcomes. Assessment may involve focused self-report measures such as the Beck Depression Inventory (BDI-II; Beck et al., 1996), Beck Anxiety Inventory (BAI; Beck et al., 1988), or State-Trait

Anxiety Inventory (STAI; Gaudry et al., 1975). Alternatively, more comprehensive measures such as the Profile of Mood States (McNair et al., 1981) or Minnesota Multiphasic Personality Inventory-II (Butcher et al., 1989) might be used when a broader assessment of mood is indicated. It is important to note, however, that the interpretation of mood questionnaires may change when physical symptoms are present due to possible confounds of constitutional symptoms (e.g., fatigue and appetite changes; Perkins et al., 1995). Formal diagnosis of mood disorders can be obtained using structured clinical interviews, such as the Composite International Diagnostic Interview (CIDI; World Health Organization, 1997) or the Structured Clinical Interview for DSM-IV (SCID; First et al., 1996).

BEHAVIORAL OBSERVATIONS

Informal clinical observations of patient behavior are critical to the interpretation of neuropsychological data. If test stimuli or instructions are not perceived or manipulated in the standard fashion, test results may not be valid or interpretable. For example, the presence of peripheral impairments (e.g., gross sensory abnormalities) may preclude one from attributing deficits on neuropsychological tests to brain dysfunction. It is also important to note other qualitative features of an individual's performance, such as whether they are easily distracted by extraneous factors (e.g., noises outside the testing room), appear aware of their strengths and weaknesses during testing, or otherwise approach tasks in a nontypical way. In particular, notes detailing the patient's approach to solving problems during testing (e.g., relying upon verbal strategies when solving nonverbal problems) can enrich the interpretation of neuropsychological findings and guide dispositional planning. Also of importance are observations regarding the patient's level of orientation, gross sensory (e.g., visual acuity, hearing) and cognitive functioning (e.g., attention, language, and memory), affect, motivation, frustration tolerance, concern about performance, and social skills, all of which can provide valuable supplemental information that will aid the clinician in the interpretation of objective psychometric testing.

NEUROPSYCHOLOGICAL TESTS

The bulk of the examination itself will typically focus on formal assessment of cognitive functioning, as the newly updated diagnostic criteria for HAND have given greater weight to this aspect of the disorder (Antinori et al., 2007). Although information provided by self-report and informal clinical observation is valuable in its own right, it is essential that the patient is examined by standardized normative cognitive assessment procedures with published normative standards and documented validity and reliability. A comprehensive neuropsychological evaluation is preferable in this regard, but other procedures such as structured mental status examinations or cognitive screening procedures can also be used in certain instances (as further described below). A working knowledge of the psychometric properties and clinical implications of each test is necessary for competent selection, administration, and interpretation of neuropsychological tests. Readers seeking more comprehensive information should refer to the online supplement accompanying the most recent update to the nosology of HAND (Antinori et al., 2007).

Neuropsychological tests may be viewed as probes of different cognitive abilities, such as learning, attention, or perceptual motor skills. However, it is important to remember that a single neuropsychological test often measures multiple or overlapping ability areas, and there is no single perfect test corresponding exactly to a putative cognitive ability. Neuropsychological tests also vary in the degree to which they are affected by person-specific characteristics, such as effort, age, education, and cultural background. Accordingly, a single neuropsychological test abnormality should not be reflexively interpreted to indicate neurocognitive impairment. Individuals may have difficulties with a particular neuropsychological test for many reasons, including non-neurological factors (e.g., hearing loss). Therefore, a clinical diagnosis cannot usually be based on a single test, or on a small grouping of tests that may not properly assess all relevant ability areas. For this reason, it is important to assess multiple cognitive ability domains, utilizing at least two tests of each domain to ensure proper coverage. A diagnosis of HAND can be confirmed by assessing multiple areas of cognitive function that have demonstrated effects of HIV infection. These domains should include executive functions, episodic memory, information processing speed, attention and working memory, motor skills, language, and sensoriperception (Woods et al., 2009).

TEST BATTERY SELECTION

Careful selection of an appropriate neuropsychological test battery is critical in that one must be able to detect and delineate the cognitive sequelae of HIV-related changes in the central nervous system (CNS). A recommended list of neuropsychological tests in each domain is provided by Antinori et al. (2007). Ideally, tests will have demonstrated adequate psychometric properties, including temporal stability, specificity, sensitivity, and predictive validity along with minimal measurement error (Strauss et al., 2006). Depending on the purpose of testing, the length and components of a neuropsychological battery will vary. For example, a comprehensive neuropsychological test battery will likely be required if the purpose of testing is to determine whether an asymptomatic airline pilot is able to perform his/her job duties safely, whereas a more focused screening battery might be used to rule out a suspected HIV-associated dementia (HAD) diagnosis in a psychiatric inpatient. Clinicians and research protocol designers must carefully weigh the advantages and disadvantages of the numerous available tests and test batteries available for their purposes.

EXTENDED NEUROPSYCHOLOGICAL BATTERIES

Extended neuropsychological batteries were initially adopted to meet the need for comprehensive and exploratory data in early phases of research on neuropsychological sequelae of HIV infection. As such, a 1990 National Institute of Mental Health (NIMH) workgroup originally recommended an extended (i.e., 7–9 hour) neuropsychological test battery to assess HIV effects on a broad range of cognitive domains. The rationale was that neuropsychological assessment is most sensitive when multiple, overlapping procedures are incorporated to cover a broad array of cognitive functions (Alexander & Stuss, 2000). As compared to the performance of individual measures in describing cognitive impairments, the battery approach improved the overall classification accuracy of neuropsychological assessment techniques in HIV (Heaton et al., 1995). The comprehensive battery approach includes coverage of all domains of interest, and has the ability to detect deficits with maximal sensitivity. Consequently, comprehensive batteries are particularly useful for complex clinical cases, as well as investigation of research questions in populations and subpopulations that are largely exploratory. However, this approach is quite time consuming and requires more resources than is feasible in many clinical and research settings.

FOCUSED NEUROPSYCHOLOGICAL BATTERIES

As clinicians and researchers have become increasingly knowledgeable about the cognitive effects of HIV, it has become a common practice to select a focused battery of tests that is tailored to specific research or clinical hypotheses. Most neuropsychological studies today incorporate a 2–3 hour battery of tests (e.g., Waldrop-Valverde et al., 2010), which still allows adequate coverage of the domains of interest. Reasonably brief, focused neuropsychological batteries are potentially more cost-effective and assist in minimizing the risk of Type I error (false positives) due to multiple statistical comparisons across tests. Nevertheless, this approach still requires substantial investment of time, expense, and expertise in administering, scoring, and interpretation of test data. As a result, it may not be feasible in all settings.

BRIEF COGNITIVE SCREENING TESTS

Several brief cognitive screening techniques are available in the event that a comprehensive or focused neuropsychological evaluation is not indicated or cannot be achieved. Although not ideal, Antinori et al. (2007) allow for diagnosis of HAND using brief cognitive tests in settings in which a comprehensive battery is not feasible. Cognitive screenings vary in length and complexity, but can generally be completed in less than 10 minutes either at the patient's bedside or in the clinician's office. Although they are cursory by design, screening tests can provide valuable information for the purposes of staging dementia and/or determining whether a clinician should refer the patient elsewhere for a more comprehensive neuropsychological evaluation. Standardized and familiar tests, such as Folstein's MMSE (Folstein et al., 1975) or the Mattis Dementia Rating Scale (Mattis, 1988), are not particularly useful for screening for HIV-related cognitive impairment, even in HAD. This is because such tests have ceiling effects and tend to focus on "cortical" cognitive functions, such as basic expressive language. Tests such as these are less sensitive to the "frontostriatal" aspects of cognitive functioning shown to be impaired in persons with HIV-related neurocognitive disorders (e.g., executive dysfunction).

In an effort to address this notable limitation of existing cognitive screening tests, Power and colleagues (Power et al., 1995) developed the HIV Dementia Scale (HDS). The HDS is a modification of the MMSE that is specifically intended for use in outpatient settings as a rapid screening tool. This 5-minute test instrument includes a measure of mental flexibility, an antisaccades test, timed alphabet test, timed construction test, and a brief memory exam (i.e., a four-item recall). The HDS shows superior sensitivity relative to the MMSE (Power et al., 1995), and it can be easily administered as a screening battery in settings such as HIV clinics to provide baseline and follow-up cognitive data. More recently, demographically adjusted normative standards for the HDS were developed and validated. This was necessary due to the high rate of false negatives (Smith et al., 2003), making the test less sensitive to mild cognitive impairments as well as observed effects of age and education. For example, a highly educated person with mild cognitive decline was more likely to be classified as normal when compared to the general population than when compared to individuals of similar age and educational attainment. The application of these norms (adjusted for age and education) improved classification accuracy overall, most notably raising sensitivity from 17.2% to 70.7%, and improved classification accuracy overall. The odds ratio was increased from 3 to approximately 6 when using norms versus raw scores for identifying participants with HAND, meaning that an individual with an impaired HDS score was six times more likely to be diagnosed with HAND (Morgan et al., 2008).

MEASURES OF EVERYDAY FUNCTIONING

Of individuals receiving diagnoses of HAND, up to 50% may experience significant interference with everyday functioning (Heaton et al., 2004). For this reason, it is essential to evaluate patients using both self-report and laboratory-based tasks that approximate instrumental activities of daily living (IADLs) to assess the real-world implications of neuropsychological impairment. Standardized laboratory measures include tests of shopping, cooking, driving, financial management, medication management, and vocational abilities. For example, the Direct Assessment of Functional Status instrument (DAFS; Lowenstein & Bates, 1992) includes functional measures (e.g., shopping, financial skills) designed for the assessment of dementia, and the Medication Management Test (MMT; Albert et al., 1999) assesses an individual's ability to dispense medications and adhere to a hypothetical prescription regimen. Caveats to this approach include low external validity for specific individuals, the lack

of demographically adjusted normative data for these tasks, and, finally, concerns regarding long administration times and feasibility. Consequently, most clinicians and researchers use self-report measures (e.g. IADL scale, Lawton & Brody, 1969) to assess the extent to which patients independently function across domains. The IADL scale (Lawton & Brody, 1969) is commonly used in HIV patients, and is designed to identify the extent of assistance needed to complete activities such as grocery shopping, preparing meals, and managing money. Other self-report measures are also informative in determining the functional impact of HIV. The Medical Outcomes Study HIV Health Survey (MOS-HIV) is a commonly used measure of health-related quality of life (HRQoL) in HIV, and can be administered in just 5 minutes. The MOS-HIV assesses health perceptions, pain, physical, role, social and cognitive functioning, mental health, energy, health distress and quality of life (Wu et al., 1997).

EXPERIMENTAL COGNITIVE NEUROPSYCHOLOGY

Although all clinical cases and many research questions call for the use of standardized and well-validated neuropsychological tests, some research efforts will be enhanced by using experimental methods derived from cognitive neuropsychology. Novel assessment techniques and alternative data interpretation approaches rooted in cognitive science have been used in order to test and better characterize mechanisms and associated neural systems underlying the cognitive deficits in persons infected with HIV (see Woods et al., 2009 for a review). In recent years, researchers have used this approach to expand our knowledge of working memory (Martin et al., 2001), executive functions (Martin et al., 2004), attention (Levine et al., 2006), and memory (Carey et al., 2006). Such approaches may augment the discriminant validity and specificity of neuropsychological measures, as well as improve their diagnostic usefulness in identifying HIV-related neurocognitive disorders (Woods et al., 2009). Novel cognitive tasks may also improve the prediction and assessment of everyday functioning (e.g., nonadherence; Woods et al., 2009), and therefore better inform dispositional planning.

INTERPRETATION OF NEUROPSYCHOLOGICAL DATA

Methods of data interpretation (e.g., clinical ratings versus mean group comparisons) can significantly influence the conclusions drawn from a neuropsychological study. Here we review several different methodologies for interpreting neuropsychological findings that are commonly used in neuroAIDS research.

MEAN GROUP DIFFERENCES ON RAW SCORES

Assessment of the neuropsychological deficits in HIV has typically involved between-groups comparisons of mean test scores on individual measures. This mean group difference approach is generally easy to apply, and has fairly consistently demonstrated neuropsychological differences between HIV-infected samples and demographically similar seronegative comparison groups (e.g., Bornstein et al., 1993). This approach is especially useful for studies in which the neuropsychological measures do not have available norms, for example, in studies that use experimental measures. However, this approach increases the likelihood that any unusual performances (i.e., significantly above average), even in a minority of participants, will prevent detection of neuropsychological impairment at the group level. This approach may be insensitive in detecting neuropsychological deficits, particularly in medically asymptomatic groups who tend to demonstrate more subtle cognitive impairment. These impairments are often inconsistent across cognitive ability domains, vary across individuals, and may affect only a minority of individuals (Heaton et al., 1994). Finally, the mean group difference approach carries with it the potential to increase the risk of Type I errors (i.e., false positives) due to multiple statistical comparisons (Ingraham & Aiken, 1996). For this reason, the American Psychological Association Task Force on Statistical Inference (1999) recommends the inclusion of effect sizes as complementary statistics in order to better estimate the magnitude of the observed effects (Zakzanis, 2001).

NORMATIVE STANDARDS

In neuropsychology, normative standards ("norms") are used to compare an individual's performance to that of neurologically healthy persons of similar age, education level, sex, and cultural identity, thereby providing an estimation of the individual's functioning relative to the abilities of their peers. This relativistic definition of normality is used to infer whether the individual evidences impairment in cognitive function, which might be suggestive of a decline from premorbid levels. Norms should be used when the following criteria are met: 1) available normative data represent an unbiased, representative sample of the population of interest; 2) the individual of interest is analogous to the comparison group; and 3) demographic variables known to significantly impact test performance have been adequately considered (Heaton et al., 2009). Such variables may include age, education, socioeconomic status, ethnic group, independent living status, current or past illnesses, drug and alcohol use, and psychiatric diagnoses. Broadly representative groups (representing as much of the general population as possible) may be used for comparison, or an investigator may choose to use more specific norms that are stratified or otherwise corrected by relevant variables (Strauss et al., 2006). The use of appropriate norms can minimize the risk of Type I and Type II error, resulting in more accurate diagnoses of impairment.

MEAN STANDARD SCORES

Though comparisons of individual raw scores can be informative, composite scores (e.g., z-scores) can provide a valuable index with which to summarize an individual's current level of functioning across domains and at a global level. Standard normative scores tend to have a good distribution and range of scores, which can be used to encompass the full range of performance on neuropsychological tests. This allows the detection of returns to normal ranges as well as returns to personal best levels of functioning (Cysique et al., 2009), both of which are indicators that may be important for longitudinal questions (e.g. Iudicello et al., 2010). For example, investigations using this technique have suggested that severity of neurocognitive impairment at the initiation of cART remains an important predictor of persistent neuropsychological deficits (e.g., Tozzi et al., 2007). One notable limitation of this approach, however, is that comparisons of standard scores do not emphasize impairment, so they may not be sensitive to HAND in some instances.

GLOBAL DEFICIT SCORES (GDS)

One of the most widely used approaches for summarizing neurocognitive function is the Global Deficit Score (GDS; Carey et al., 2004a; Heaton et al., 1995). The GDS is derived directly from T-scores by weighing the number and severity of deficits more heavily than any superior and average performances in an individual's neuropsychological profile. Specifically, demographically corrected t-scores on individual neuropsychological tests are transformed into deficit scores ranging from zero (within normal limits) to five (severely impaired), then averaged to create the GDS (e.g., Heaton et al., 1995). The GDS is strongly related to clinical ratings, and provides comparable classification accuracy rates (Carey et al., 2004a). Perhaps most importantly, the GDS shows considerable construct validity and is associated with functional impairment (Heaton et al., 2004), microstructural white matter abnormalities (e.g., Chang et al., 2008), neuronal damage (Chana et al., 2006), and is sensitive to the positive effects of antiretroviral therapy (Letendre et al., 2004). In light of these findings as well as prior research, the GDS is recommended as a useful method of assessing neuropsychological functioning in HIV infected populations. However, several important caveats of the GDS should be considered, including its limited range of values, its insensitivity to variability in normal range, possible ceiling effects, and the fact that the cut point for GDS impairment does not require impairment in two domains, as outlined in the Frascati diagnostic criteria (Antinori et al., 2007).

CLINICAL RATINGS

Clinical ratings were previously recommended as a "gold standard" for HAND because they were believed to be uniquely sensitive to the mild and unique patterns of impairment often observed in HIV+ individuals (Heaton et al., 1995). To derive these ratings after a battery is administered and scored, the neuropsychological tests are grouped by domain of functioning (e.g., attention/working memory and executive function) and raw scores are converted to demographically corrected t-scores. Using these T-scores, clinical ratings are assigned to each domain of functioning assessed using a nine-point scale that ranges from one (above average performance) to nine (severely impaired performance). The cutoff score of five indicates definite mild impairment, while a score of four is borderline. Next, based on the clinical ratings in each ability area, a rating of global neuropsychological status is generated. As mentioned above, participants must exhibit impaired ratings in two or more cognitive domains in order to be classified as globally neuropsychologically impaired.

One unique aspect of clinical ratings is that raters are able to afford an appropriate weight to diverse patterns of mild deficits. Prior research reveals that clinical ratings are highly sensitive to the relatively mild and inconsistent pattern of cognitive deficits associated with HIV infection, especially those in asymptomatic patients (Heaton et al., 1994). Blind clinical ratings of neuropsychological test performance has been used by Heaton (1995) to demonstrate NP impairment in HIV+ individuals that is not better explained by findings from medical, neurological, neuroimaging, and psychiatric examinations. However, though inter-rater reliabilities for clinical ratings are excellent for identifying the presence and severity of neuropsychological impairment (Woods et al., 2004), limitations of the clinical ratings approach include their limited range, skewed distributions, and the significant investments of time, expense, and expertise required to obtain these values.

ASSESSING COGNITION OVER TIME

The chronic nature of HIV disease in the cART era has brought to the forefront numerous important clinical research (e.g., cognitive improvement with effective cART) and clinical (e.g., identifying incident HAND) issues that require longitudinal cognitive assessments. Unfortunately, the repeated administration of neuropsychological tests is fraught with methodological, statistical, and interpretive complications. Several factors unrelated to brain functioning may explain changes in neuropsychological test performance over repeated administrations (Temkin et al., 1999). One of the most common problems is that individuals can demonstrate better scores on repeated administration, simply due to the effects of practice. The magnitude of such "practice effects" is variable across cognitive domains (and specific tests), but they tend to be greatest on the second administration of tasks of problem solving and memory. Parallel (or alternate) test forms and/or a dual (repeated) baseline approach should be used whenever possible in order to minimize the potential effects of practice (Duff et al., 2001). In addition, a variety of statistical procedures are available to assess the reliability of changes in neuropsychological test performance. For example, regression-based prediction formulas use initial test performance and demographic characteristics to calculate predicted performance, then compare predicted and observed follow-up test performance to determine the significance of change (Cysique et al., 2009; Duff et al., 2008). Reliable change indices provide a user-friendly means of classifying individual test scores as having improved or declined by utilizing confidence intervals around expected practice effects (e.g., Basso et al., 1999). Assessing global cognitive change may be accomplished by grouping tests by domain (e.g., declines/improvements in two or more

cognitive domains), using a battery-based z-score approach (e.g., Woods et al., 2006), or examining summary scores, such as the GDS (e.g., Carey et al., 2004a).

APPLICATION OF NEUROPSYCHOLOGY IN HIV

As depicted in Figure 9.3.1, a multitude of biological, social, and psychiatric factors can impact neuropsychological test performance. In addition, vast differences in the presentation of HIV (e.g., disease characteristics, treatment duration and methods) as well as many common comorbidities complicate the interpretation of neuropsychological findings. Demographic factors such as age, education, sex, and ethnicity also affect neuropsychological performance independently, and data should be interpreted cautiously when tasks have not been validated in the samples of administration. Moreover, the influence of premorbid and comorbid conditions, including histories of CNS disease (e.g., seizure disorder) and trauma (e.g., closed head injury), hepatitis C, psychoactive medications, learning disabilities, psychiatric conditions (e.g., bipolar disorder), substance abuse, vascular risks and systemic illnesses (e.g., liver disease) need to be considered carefully when interpreting results from neuropsychological testing.

HIV DISEASE CHARACTERISTICS

Although cART has drastically improved survival rates and decreased the incidence of HAD in the past decade, the prevalence of milder HAND has not declined, and continues to be a major public health concern (McArthur et al., 2004). Neuropsychological findings have been shown to vary according to several viral, immune, and neurological factors as well as Centers for Disease Control (CDC) clinical staging, disease histories, and current antiretroviral medication regimens. For example, studies show that severity of neurocognitive impairment can vary with disease progression, with relatively small effect sizes for neuropsychological performance (relative to seronegatives) across domains for asymptomatic patients (0.05-0.21), small-to-moderate effect sizes for symptomatic HIV+ patients (0.18-0.65), and medium-to-large effect sizes in patients with AIDS (.42-.82; Reger et al., 2002). Therefore, clinicians and investigators seeking to gain understanding of an individual's risk for HIV-related cognitive impairment are encouraged to collect detailed information related to these markers. When possible, research designs should incorporate important HIV disease characteristics and match (or stratify) HIV samples on these characteristics.

In the pre-cART era, a patient's neurocognitive functioning was reliably associated with their current CD4 count, viral load, and the presence of any opportunistic infections (e.g., Valcour et al., 2006). However, as cART has become more widespread, cognitive impairments are still evident in individuals with well-managed HIV disease (e.g., high CD4 counts, undetectable viral loads; Robinson-Papp et al., 2009). In the CHARTER study of 1555 cases followed in University

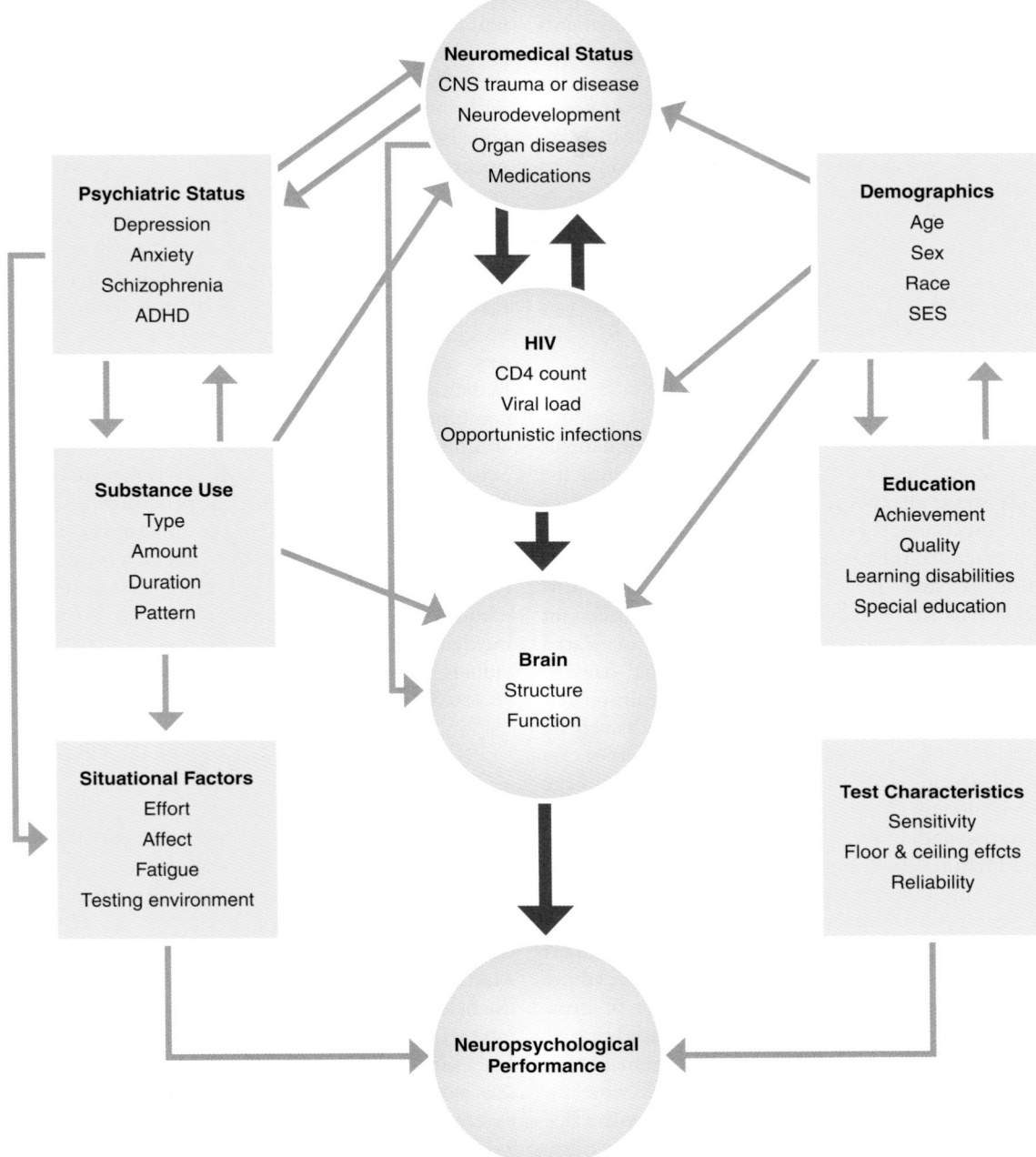

Figure 9.3.1 Flow chart depicting the relationships between neuromedical, psychiatric, environmental, person-specific, and test characteristics on neuropsychological test performance. SES, Socioeconomic status; ADHD, attention-deficit hyperactivity disorder. (Adapted from Grant et al., 1987)

clinics about half manifested some degree of neurocognitive impairment, despite the majority receiving combination ART (Heaton, et al, 2010). In fact, autopsy evidence shows that rates of neuropathology in HIV-infected patients may have actually increased over time (Neuenburg et al., 2002). These changes in prevalence may be indicative of a shift from florid replication of HIV in the brain to more diverse and indirect mechanisms of neuronal injury and loss (Everall et al., 2009). For all of these reasons, nadir CD4 counts may be more informative for estimating cognitive functioning than current CD4

levels (Tozzi et al., 2005). A variety of mechanisms of HIV-induced brain pathology have been proposed, including microglial and glial activation, possibly mediated by oxidative stress to cause neuronal apoptosis and axonal injury (Gray et al., 2001), neuroinflammation (Everall et al., 2005), and vasculopathy (Brilla et al., 1999). To this end, HAND has been linked to a variety of biomarkers of neuronal injury and protection, including tau, a protein associated with neuroaxonal damage (Brew et al., 2005), monocyte chemoattractant protein-1 (MCP-1), representing protective macrophage activation (Eugenin et al., 2003), erythropoietin, a neuroprotectant (Keswani et al., 2004), beta-amyloid, protein fragments that reduce synaptic plasticity (Green et al., 2005) and S100β, representing astrocytosis (Pemberton & Brew, 2001). Research continues in order to identify objective biomarkers for use in diagnosing and predicting the presence and severity of HIV-associated brain disease, as well as distinguishing the impact of HIV from that of other confounding conditions (Brew & Letendre, 2009).

DEMOGRAPHIC INFLUENCES ON NEUROPSYCHOLOGICAL TESTS

AGE AND VASCULAR RISK

The CDC estimates that by 2015, one-half of all individuals living with HIV/AIDS in the United States will be over the age of 50 (Johnson et al., 2009). This statistic reflects a shift in the epidemic, precipitated by the widespread use of cART, which greatly extended the life expectancy of individuals with HIV infection. As such, HIV-infected individuals are now more vulnerable to the well-documented normal effects of aging on the brain, as well as the numerous age-associated comorbidities that can confer additional neuronal damage and subsequent structural and functional brain-related impairments. For example, older HIV-infected adults may be at risk for cerebrovascular disease and elevated markers of cardiovascular risk (Monsuez et al., 2009), which may damage cerebral vessels directly (McMurtray et al., 2007) or increase immune activation and, in turn, cause additional neural injury and loss of function (Tan, Nath, & Hoke, 2010). In fact, recent cardiac computed tomography data suggest that vascular age is increased by approximately 15 years over chronological age in HIV (Guaraldi et al., 2009). In addition, brain pathology and neuroimaging studies indicate that older adults with HIV have, for example, increased accumulation of intra-neuronal amyloid beta (Achim et al., 2009), decreased frontal lobe volumes (McMurtray et al., 2007), and functional brain demands equivalent to HIV-negative individuals who are 15–20 years older (Ances et al., 2010). Older adults with HIV exhibit greater prevalence and severity of deficits in a variety of specific cognitive abilities, including attention, psychomotor speed, memory, executive functions, and motor skills (Becker, 1997; Hinkin et al., 1999; Hardy et al., 2004; Valcour et al., 2004). They are also three times more likely to receive neurocognitive diagnoses, including HAD (e.g., Valcour et al., 2004). Nevertheless, important questions remain regarding biological mechanisms (e.g., vascular and metabolic), cognitive profiles (e.g., increased rates of forgetting), and everyday functioning effects (e.g., driving) of HAND in older adults.

EDUCATION

Effects of education on cognitive performance should guide test selection and interpretation, particularly on tasks of higher-order cognitive functions (e.g., intelligence, memory, and executive functions such as problem solving). In highly educated groups, "easy" tests such as serial 7s or the MMSE will likely not detect differences between controls and seropositive individuals who have MND, while difficult tests (e.g., the PASAT) may not detect differences in seropositive adults with lower levels of education because control participants will also perform poorly. For this reason, education-corrected norms are offered by many normative datasets for neuropsychological tasks (Strauss et al., 2006). Another influential conceptualization of the impact of education on neuropsychological outcomes is labeled "cognitive reserve," and attempts to explain individual differences in cognitive performance despite similar levels of brain pathology (Stern, 2009). Specifically, the ability to recruit alternate networks or adopt new cognitive strategies in HIV is thought to be influenced by behavioral variables, and is often operationalized using a combination of years of education, a measure of occupational attainment, and an estimate of premorbid functioning. Seropositive individuals with low cognitive reserve scores have lower neuropsychological performance overall (Pereda et al., 2000) and show more early neuropsychological impairments, while seropositive individuals with greater cognitive reserve may exhibit fewer clinical effects of underlying neuropathologic processes (Stern et al., 1996). Overall, reduced incidence of neurocognitive decline is observed among individuals with higher reserve IQ, regardless of disease status (Basso & Bornstein, 1999).

SEX

While more men than women are HIV+ across all ethnic groups in the United States, the global proportion of women infected with HIV has been approximately 50% since the 1990s. Unfortunately, women have been underrepresented in studies, and most work examining HIV-related impairments has taken place in predominantly male samples (Maki & Martin-Thormeyer, 2009). Despite limited investigation in the field, several studies have detected different neuropsychological impairment patterns in HIV-infected men and women. For example, Failde-Garrido et al., (2008) report that men showed the greatest impairment in visual memory, attention, psychomotor speed and abstract reasoning, while HIV+ women exhibited more impaired attention, psychomotor speed and verbal memory. HIV-infected women may also be at increased risk for cognitive decline due to the higher prevalence of mental health and psychosocial problems, fewer years of education, and higher age reported on average (Maki & Martin-Thormeyer, 2009). Research on gender differences in neuropsychological performance is mixed and limited by small sample sizes, and no studies have yet examined the effects of female-specific characteristics (e.g., ovarian hormones) or highly comorbid factors (e.g., posttraumatic stress), both of which have known effects on cognitive function (Maki & Martin-Thormeyer, 2009). Research continues in order to clarify the mechanisms by which hormones and hormonal birth control may affect susceptibility or progression of HIV disease. Notably, estrogens (17beta-estradiol) have exhibited neuroprotective effects by reducing neuronal apoptosis in rats (Corasaniti et al. 2005). Though the etiologies by which differences emerge are not yet clear, sex-based normative corrections are widely available for commonly used neuropsychological tests, and are strongly recommended to minimize the potential influence of sex on neuropsychological test results. In addition, research designs that use neuropsychological tests should match groups of interest on sex in order to control for possible disparities.

ETHNICITY AND LANGUAGE

The possible impact of ethnicity and culture on neuropsychological test performance must be carefully considered when interpreting neuropsychological data. Differences have been reported between Caucasians and other ethnic groups (e.g., African-Americans and Hispanics) on measures of verbal and nonverbal cognitive abilities, though both reliability and validity of tests are threatened when applied to cultural and linguistic groups that are not adequately represented in the standardization sample (Padilla & Medina, 1996). Ethnicity differences are most often observed in favor of the majority group, and care must be taken to ensure that differences from majority groups are not reflexively interpreted as pathological (Padilla & Medina, 1996). Recent studies show that differences in neuropsychological test results between ethnicities may be partially due to discrepancies between years of schooling and educational attainment, which are more common in Hispanic and African-American individuals than in non-Hispanic white individuals (e.g., Ryan et al., 2005). Ethnicity-corrected normative adjustments are nevertheless recommended to minimize the risk of misclassifying individuals from diverse backgrounds as cognitively impaired. Research groups should be matched on ethnicity whenever possible.

As the HIV epidemic includes individuals of varied cultural backgrounds, it is important to consider the roles of associated important variables. Language is a powerful determinant of performance, especially in more verbal measures of neuropsychological performance. Literal translation is not advisable, as poor wording, inappropriate item content, or inaccurate translation may introduce item bias. Once translated, items may sample different domains and have significantly different meanings as well as psychometric properties (Lezak et al., 2004). Further, language is important even when a measure is not translated, and it is important to establish linguistic equivalence of the measure for ethnic minority individuals (Allen & Walsh, 2000). Although the language of administration may be the same, words or phrases may hold systematically different meanings for members of certain minority or cultural groups. Just as verbal tasks are translated between languages, functional assessments (e.g., medication management, cooking, finances) are also translated with minor modifications to ensure that they are culturally relevant and appropriate (Mindt et al., 2003).

HEPATITIS C VIRUS

Possibly due to the shared risk factors for transmission, a high proportion (approximately 15–50%) of HIV-infected persons are also infected with the hepatitis C virus (HCV). HCV is a neurotropic virus that is associated with neuroimaging abnormalities (Thannoun & Quinn, 1996) and increased risk for neurocognitive impairment (Garrido et al., 2009), which may in turn affect everyday functioning (Vigil et al., 2008). HCV is most common in individuals who have injected drugs, been homeless in the last year, and currently exhibit more severe depressive symptoms (Hall et al., 2004). Currently, millions of people worldwide are co-infected with HIV and HCV (Gonzales et al., 2010). Both HIV and HCV adversely affect neuropsychological performance across domains and suggest frontal-subcortical dysfunction (Hilsabeck et al., 2003). Though coinfection may affect the nature and course of neurocognitive functioning, the precise etiologies are not known (Gonzalez & Cherner, 2008). Thus far, literature on the CNS effects of co-infection shows a pattern of mixed findings, with some studies showing higher rates of global impairment (e.g., Hinkin et al., 2008) and some studies reporting null findings (e.g., Clifford et al., 2009). Thus, whether and how HCV alters the nature and course of HAND remains unknown, but is an important direction for future research. Efforts are complicated by differences in sample characteristics on other important variables affecting cognition in HCV such as disease severity (Perry et al., 2005), injection drug use (Hilsabeck et al., 2003), psychiatric comorbidities (Douaihy et al., 2008), psychosocial variables (Grassi et al., 2002), methamphetamine dependence (Letendre et al., 2005), fatigue symptoms (Weissenborn et al., 2005), history of alcohol consumption (Fontana et al., 2005), and obesity (Shepard et al., 2005).

MOOD

Rates of major depression and other mood disorders are elevated in HIV+ persons. Prevalence estimates vary, but a recent large-scale study of 1125 HIV-positive individuals reported that 39% of patients presented with a current mood disorder (Pence et al., 2006). For this reason, mood diagnoses should be an important consideration in both research designs and data interpretation for individual patients. Seronegative patients with major depressive disorder (MDD) may exhibit impairment in the areas of attention, memory, executive functions, and psychomotor speed (e.g., Goggin et al., 1997). However, the preponderance of studies in HIV-infected individuals shows that depression does not increase the risk of HAND (e.g., Grant et al., 1993; Cysique et al., 2007). Although self-reported symptoms of depression correlate weakly with some cognitive domains (e.g., Castellon et al., 2006), diagnoses of (current or lifetime) MDD do not appear to have additive effects on neurocognitive impairment in HIV-infected persons. Cysique and colleagues (2007), for example, found no neuropsychological performance differences with either lifetime or incident major depression, and no increased rates of cognitive worsening among individuals with incident major depression. Nevertheless, mood symptoms may affect risk-taking (e.g., Bouseman et al., 2009) and everyday functioning (Heaton et al. 2004). Future research should examine the combined effects of HIV and psychiatric conditions with known cognitive effects, such as bipolar disorder (e.g., Moore et al., 2005).

SUBSTANCE USE

Perhaps because of well-documented lifestyle risks and modes of HIV infection related to substance use (Norman et al., 2009), persons infected with HIV have notably high (typically between 40% and 75%) rates of comorbid substance abuse and dependence (Pence et al., 2006). Substances such as methamphetamine, alcohol, cocaine, and marijuana are also among the most frequently abused (e.g., Chander et al., 2006). Given the known impact of various licit (e.g., alcohol) and illicit (e.g., methamphetamine, cocaine) substances on the CNS and cognitive functioning, substance use disorders represent a potentially significant factor for the development and maintenance of HAND. Substance abuse may also exacerbate existing neuropsychological dysfunction (e.g., Carey et al., 2006) and compromise adherence to treatment (Reback et al., 2003), as well as exert residual cognitive impairments in the case of prior drug abuse/dependence in HIV-positive individuals (Basso & Bornstein, 2003). Methamphetamine, for example, is associated with more severe loss of interneurons (Chana et al., 2006) and increased risk for neurocognitive impairment (Rippeth et al., 2004), especially in advanced disease (Carey et al., 2006). Further study is needed in order to better understand the effects of substance abuse on the progression of HIV-related cognitive decline. However, current studies can contribute to these efforts by confirming that toxicology does not reflect current substance abuse prior to neuropsychological testing, by gathering detailed information regarding patients' history of substance abuse (e.g., type, duration, frequency, and amount), and by including detailed exclusionary and inclusionary criteria.

OTHER COMORBID FACTORS

Persons with HIV disease, at least those in Western settings, tend to experience more CNS insults and injuries that may contribute in independent, additive, or multiplicative ways to neurocognitive impairment. For example, their higher risk lifestyles may increase likelihood of incurring head injuries, and there is some evidence that HIV+ persons with such histories have more neurocognitive impairment, and also evidence of neuronal dysfunction based on magnetic resonance spectroscopy ascertained reduction in the neuronal marker N acetyl aspartarte (Lin, et al., 2011). Other comorbidities that can contribute to neurocognitive impairment include history of learning disability or attention deficit hyperactivity disorder. In the CHARTER Study, it was noted that rates of neurocognitive impairment increased from about 40% in those with minimal comobidities, to about 80% in those with major comorbidities (Heaton, et al., 2010). Thus, careful documentation of such comorbidities is important in the attribution of any neurocognitive decrement to HIV, or factors that may independently, or additively contribute to such impairment.

SUMMARY

Neuropsychological testing provides a valuable window into CNS effects of HIV. Such testing has revealed that neurocognitive impairment remains prevalent in the cART era, affecting 30–50% of persons with HIV. The use of neuropsychological tests should involve selection of approaches that broadly assess the many cognitive domains that can be affected by HIV, while emphasizing those which test ability areas most likely to be impacted (e.g., frontostriatal functions that include executive and memory disturbances). Selection of tests for which normative data exist to adjust for the effects of age, education, and other demographic influences is important. In addition, the possible role of cofactors (e.g., drug abuse, hepatitis C) must be considered in evaluating the specific effects of HIV, or its treatment, on neurocognition.

ACKNOWLEDGMENTS

This chapter was supported by grant P30-MH62512 from the National Institute of Mental Health and grant P50-DA026306 from the National Institute on Drug Abuse.

REFERENCES

Achim, C. L., Adame, A., Dumaop, W., Everall, I. P., & Masliah, E. (2009). Increased accumulation of intraneuronal amyloid beta in HIV-infected patients. *Journal of Neuroimmune Pharmacology*, 4, 190–199.

Albert, S. M., Weber, C. M., Todak, G., Polanco, C., Clouse, R., McElhiney, M. ... Marder, K. (1999). An observed performance test of medication management ability in HIV: Relation to neuropsychological status and medication adherence outcomes. *AIDS and Behavior*, 3, 121–128.

Alexander, M. P. & Stuss, D. T. (2000). Disorders of frontal lobe functioning. *Seminars in Neurology*, 20, 427–437.

Allen, J. & Walsh, J. A. (2000). A construct-based approach to equivalence: Methodologies for cross-cultural/multicultural personality assessment research. In R. H. Dana, (Ed.), *Handbook of cross-cultural and multicultural personality assessment* (pp. 63–85). Mahwah, NJ: Lawrence Erlbaum Associates, Inc.

Ances, B. M. & Clifford, D. B. (2008). HIV-associated neurocognitive disorders and the impact of combination antiretroviral therapies. *Current Neurology and Neuroscience Reports*, 8, 455–461.

Ances, B. M., Vaida, F., Yeh, M. J., et al. (2010). HIV infection and aging independently affect brain function as measured by functional magnetic resonance imaging. *The Journal of Infectious Diseases*, 201, 336–340.

Antinori, A., Arendt, G., Becker, J., et al. (2007). Updated research nosology for HIV-associated neurocognitive disorders. *Neurology*, 69, 1789–1799.

Aylward, E. H., Henderer, J. D., McArthur, J. D., et al. (1993). Reduced basal ganglia volume in HIV-1-associated dementia: Results from quantitative neuroimaging. *Neurology*, 43, 2099–2104.

Baldewicz, T., Leserman, J., Silva, S., et al. (2005). Changes in neuropsychological functioning with progression of HIV-1 infection: Results of an 8-year longitudinal investigation. *AIDS and Behavior*, 8, 345–355.

Basso, M. R. & Bornstein, R. A. (2003). Effects of past noninjection drug abuse upon executive function and working memory in HIV infection. *Journal of Clinical and Experimental Neuropsychology*, 25, 893–903.

Basso, M. R., Bornstein, R. A., & Lang, J. M. (1999). Practice effects on commonly used measures of executive function across twelve months. *Clinical Neuropsychologist*, 13, 283–292.

Beaumont, J. G. (2008). *Introduction to neuropsychology: Second Edition.* New York, NY: The Guilford Press.

Beck, A. T., Epstein, N., Brown, G., & Steer, R. A. (1988). An inventory for measuring clinical anxiety: Psychometric properties. *Journal of Consulting and Clinical Psychology, 56,* 893–897.

Beck, A. T., Steer, R. A., & Brown, G. K. (1996). *Manual for Beck Depression Inventory II* (BDI-II). San Antonio, TX: Psychology Corporation.

Becker, J. T., Sanchez, J., Dew, M. A., Lopez, O. L., Dorst, S. K., & Banks, G. (1997). Neuropsychological abnormalities among HIV-infected individuals in a community-based sample. *Neuropsychology, 11,* 592–601.

Bousman, C. A., Cherner, M., Ake, C., et al. (2009). Negative mood and sexual behavior among non-monogamous men who have sex with men in the context of methamphetamine and HIV. *Journal of Affective Disorders, 119,* 84–91.

Brew, B. & Letendre, S. (2009). Biomarkers of HIV-related central nervous system disease. In Paul, Sacktor, Valcour, & Tashima, (Eds.), *HIV and the brain.* Boston, MA: Humana Press.

Brew, B. J., Pemberton, L., Blennow, K., Wallin, A., & Hagberg, L. (2005). CSF amyloid beta42 and tau levels correlate with AIDS dementia complex. *Neurology, 65,* 1490–1492.

Brilla, R., Nabavi, D. G., Schulte-Altedorneburg, G., et al. (1999). Cerebral vasculopathy in HIV infection revealed by transcranial Doppler - A pilot study. *Stroke, 30,* 811–813.

Butcher, J., Dahlstrom, W., Graham, J., Tellegen, A., & Kreammer, B. (1989). *The Minnesota Multiphasic Personality Inventory-2 (MMPI-2) Manual for Administration and Scoring.* Minneapolis, MN: University of Minneapolis Press.

Bornstein, R. A., Nasrallah, H. A., Para, M. F., Whitacre, C. C., Rosenberger, P., & Fass, R. J. (1993). Neuropsychological performance in symptomatic and asymptomatic HIV infection. *AIDS, 7,* 519–524.

Carey, C. L., Woods, S. P., Gonzalez, R., et al. (2004a). Predictive validity of global deficit scores in detecting neuropsychological impairment in HIV infection. *Journal of Clinical and Experimental Neuropsychology, 26,* 307–19.

Carey, C. L., Woods, S. P., Gonzalez, R., et al. (2004b). Initial validation of a screening battery for the detection of HIV-associated cognitive impairment. *The Clinical Neuropsychologist, 18,* 234–248.

Carey, C. L., Woods, S. P., Rippeth, J. D., et al. (2006). Additive deleterious effects of methamphetamine dependence and immunosuppression on neuropsychological functioning in HIV infection. *AIDS and Behavior, 10,* 185–190.

Castellon, S. A., Hardy, D. J., Hinkin, C. H., et al. (2006). Components of depression in HIV-1 infection: Their differential relationship to neurocognitive performance. *Journal of Clinical and Experimental Neuropsychology, 28* (3), 420–437.

Chana, G., Everall, I. P., Crew, L., et al. (2006). Cognitive deficits and degeneration of interneurons in HIV+ methamphetamine users. *Neurology, 67,* 1486–1489.

Chang, L., Wong, V., Nakama, H., et al. (2008). Greater than age-related changes in brain diffusion in HIV patients after 1 year. *Journal of Neuroimmune Pharmacology, 3,* 265–274.

Chander, G., Himelhoch, S., & Moore, R. D. (2006). Substance abuse and psychiatric disorders in HIV-positive patients: Epidemiology and impact on antiretroviral therapy. *Drugs, 66,* 769–789.

Chelune, G. J., Heaton, R. K., & Lehman, R. A. (1986). Neuropsychological and personality correlates of patients' complaints of disability. In G. Goldstein & R. E. Tarter (Eds.), *Advances in clinical neuropsychology, 3rd Ed.* (pp. 95–126). New York: Plenum Press.

Clifford, D. B., Smurzynski, M., Park, L. S., et al. (2009). Effects of active HCV replication on neurologic status in HIV RNA virally suppressed patients. *Neurology, 73,* 309–314.

Ciesla, J. A. & Roberts, J. E. (2001). Meta-analysis of the relationship between HIV infection and risk for depressive disorders. *American Journal of Psychiatry, 158,* 725–730.

Corasaniti, M. T., Amantea, D., Russo, R., et al. (2005). 17 beta-estradiol reduces neuronal apoptosis induced by HIV-1 gp120 in the neocortex of rat. *Neurotoxicology, 26,* 893–903.

Crawford, J. R., Smith, G., Maylor, E. A., Della Sala, S., & Logie, R. H. (2003). The prospective and retrospective memory questionnaire (PRMQ): Normative data and latent structure in a large non-clinical sample. *Memory, 11,* 261–275.

Cysique, L. A., Deutsch, R., Atkinson, J. H. et al. (2007). Incident major depression does not affect neuropsychological functioning in HIV-infected men. *Journal of the International Neuropsychological Society, 13,* 1–11.

Cysique, L. A., Vaida, F., Letendre, S., et al. (2009). Dynamics of cognitive change in impaired HIV-positive patients initiating antiretroviral therapy. *Neurology, 73,* 342–348.

Dawes, S., Suarez, P., Casey, C. Y., et al. (2008). Variable patterns of neuropsychological performance in HIV-1 infection. *Journal of Clinical and Experimental Neuropsychology, 30,* 613–626.

de Boer-van der Kolk, M., Sprangers, M., Prins, I., Smit, C., de Wolf, F., & Nieuwkerk, P. T. (2010). Health-related quality of life and survival among HIV-infected patients receiving highly active antiretroviral therapy: A study of patients in the AIDS therapy evaluation in the Netherlands (ATHENA) cohort. *Clinical Infectious Diseases, 50,* 255–263.

Delis, D. C., Peavy, G., Heaton, R., et al. (1995). Do patients with HIV-associated minor cognitive/motor disorder exhibit a "subcortical" memory profile? Evidence using the California Verbal Learning Task. *Assessment, 2,* 151–165.

Dew, M. A., Becker, J. T., Sanchez, J., et al. (1997). Prevalence and predictors of depressive, anxiety and substance use disorders in HIV-infected and uninfected men: A longitudinal evaluation. *Psychological Medicine, 27,* 395–409.

Douaihy, A., Hilsabeck, R. C., Azzam, P., Jain, A., & Daley, D. C. (2008). Neuropsychiatric aspects of coinfection with HIV and hepatitis C virus. *AIDS Reader, 18,* 425–436.

Duff, K., Schoenberg, M. R., Patton, D. E., Mold, J. W., Scott, J. G., & Adams, R. L. (2008). Predicting cognitive change across 3 years in community-dwelling elders. *Archives of Clinical Neuropsychology, 22,* 651–661.

Duff, K., Westervelt, H. J., McCaffrey, R. J., & Haase, R. F. (2001). Practice effects, test-retest stability, and dual baseline assessments with the California Verbal Learning Test in an HIV sample. *Archives of Clinical Neuropsychology, 16,* 461–476.

Ellis, R. J., Calero, P., & Stockin, M. D. (2009). HIV infection and the central nervous system: A primer. *Neuropsychology Review, 19,* 144–151.

Eugenin, E. A., Branes, M. C., Berman, J. W., & Saez, J. C. (2003). TNF-alpha plus IFN-gamma induce connexin43 expression and formation of gap junctions between human monocytes/macrophages that enhance physiological responses. *Journal of Immunology, 170,* 1320–1328.

Everall, I. P., Hansen, L. A., & Masliah, E. (2005). The shifting patterns of HIV encephalitis neuropathology. *Neurotoxicity Research, 8,* 51–61.

Everall, I., Vaida, F., Khanlou, N., et al. (2009). Cliniconeuropathologic correlates of human immunodeficiency virus in the era of antiretroviral therapy. *Journal of Neurovirology, iFirst,* 1–11.

Failde-Garrido, J. M., Alvarez, M. R., & Simon-Lopez, M. A. (2008). Neuropsychological impairment and gender differences in HIV-1 infection. *Psychiatry and Clinical Neurosciences, 62,* 494–502.

First, M. B., Spitzer, R. L., Gibbon, M., & Williams, J. B. (1996). *Structured clinical interview for DSM-IV Axis I Disorders-Patient Edition* (SCID-I/P, Version 2.0). New York: NY State Psychiatric Institute.

Folstein, M. F., Folstein, S. E., & McHugh, P. R. (1975). "Mini-Mental State": A practical method for grading the cognitive state of patients for the clinician. *Journal of Psychiatric Research, 12,* 189–198.

Fontana, R. J., Bieliauskas, L., Back-Madruga, C., et al. (2005). Cognitive function in hepatitis C patients with advanced fibrosis enrolled in the HALT-C trial. *Journal of Hepatology, 43,* 614–622.

Garrido, J. M.F., Alvarez, M. R., Castro, J. L., & Lopez MAS (2009). Neuropsychological performance in patients with human inmunodeficiency (HIV) and hepatitis C virus (HCV) coinfection. *Neurologia, 24,* 154–159.

Gaudry, E., Vagg, P., & Spielberger, C. D. (1975). Validation of the state-trait distinction in anxiety research. *Multivariate Behavioral Research*, *10*, 331–341.

Gonzalez, R. & Cherner, M. (2008). Co-factors in HIV neurobehavioural disturbances: Substance abuse, hepatitis C and aging. *International Review of Psychiatry*, *20*, 49–60.

Gonzalez, V. D., Landay, A. L., & Sandberg, J. K. (2010). Innate immunity and chronic immune activation in HCV/HIV-1 co-infection. *Clinical Immunology*, *135*, 12–25.

Goggin, K. J., Zisook, S., Heaton, R. K., et al. (1997). Neuropsychological performance of HIV-1 infected men with major depression. *Journal of the International Neuropsychological Society*, *3*, 457–464.

Gorman, A. A., Foley, J. M., Ettenhofer, M. L., Hinkin, C. H., & van Gorp, W. G. (2009). Functional consequences of HIV-associated neuropsychological impairment. *Neuropsychology Review*, *19*, 186–203.

Grant, I., Atkinson, J. H., Hesselink, et al. (1987). Evidence for early central nervous system involvement in the acquired immunodeficiency syndrome (AIDS) and other human immunodeficiency virus (HIV) infections. *Annals of Internal Medicine*, *107*, 828–836.

Grant, I., Olshen, R. A., Atkinson, J. H., et al. (1993). Depressed mood does not explain neuropsychological deficits in HIV-infected persons. *Neuropsychology*, *7*, 53–61.

Grassi, L., Satriano, J., Serra, A., et al. (2002). Emotional stress, psychosocial variables and coping associated with hepatitis C virus and human immunodeficiency virus infections in intravenous drug users. *Psychotherapy and Psychosomatics*, *71*, 342–349.

Gray, F., Adle-Biassette, H., Chretien, F., de la Grandmaison, G. L., & Force, G. (2001). Neuropathology and neurodegeneration in human immunodeficiency virus infection—Pathogenesis of HIV-induced lesions of the brain, correlations with HIV-associated disorders and modifications according to treatments. *Clinical Neuropathology*, *20*, 146–155.

Green, D. A., Masliah, E., Vinters, H. V., Beizai, P., Moore, D. J., & Achim, C. L. (2005). Brain deposition of beta-amyloid is a common pathologic feature in HIV positive patients. *AIDS*, *19*, 407–411.

Guaraldi, G., Zona, S., Alexopoulos, N., et al. (2009). Coronary aging in HIV-infected patients. *Clinical Infectious Diseases*, *49*, 1756–1762.

Hall, C. S., Charlebois, E. D., Hahn, J. A., Moss, A. R., & Bangsberg, D. R. (2004). Hepatitis C virus infection in San Francisco's HIV-infected urban poor: High prevalence but low treatment rates. *Journal of General Internal Medicine*, *19*, 357–365.

Hardy, D. J., Castellon, S. A., & Hinkin, C. H. (2004). Perceptual span deficits in adults with HIV. *Journal of the International Neuropsychological Society*, *10*, 135–140.

Heaton, R., Grant, I., Butters, N., et al. (1995). The HNRC 500–Neuropsychology of HIV infection at different disease stages. *Journal of the International Neuropsychological Society*, *1*, 231–251.

Heaton, R., Marcotte, T. D., Mindt, M. R., et al. (2004). The impact of HIV-associated neuropsychological impairment on everyday functioning. *Journal of the International Neuropsychological Society*, *10*, 317–331.

Heaton, R., Ryan, L., & Grant, I. (2009). Demographic influences and use of demographically corrected norms in neuropsychological assessment. In Grant & Adams (Eds.) *Neuropsychological assessment of neuropsychiatric and neuromedical disorders*. New York, NY: Oxford University Press, Inc.

Heaton, R., Velin, R. A., McCutchan, J. A., et al. (1994). Neuropsychological impairment in human immunodeficiency virus infection: Implications for employment. *Psychosomatic Medicine*, *56*, 8–17.

Heaton RK, Clifford DB, Franklin Jr DR, Woods SP, Ake C, Vaida F, Ellis RJ, Letendre SL, Marcotte TD, Atkinson JH, Rivera-Mindt M, Vigil OR, Taylor MJ, Collier AC, Marra CM, Gelman BB, McArthur JC, Morgello S, Simpson DM, McCutchan JA, Abramson I, Gamst A, Fennema-Notestine C, Jernigan TL, Wong J, Grant I, the CHARTER Group. (2010). HIV-associated neurocognitive disorders persist in the era of potent antiretroviral therapy. *Neurology*, *75*, 2087–2096 .

Hilsabeck, R. C., Hassanein, T. I., Carlson, M. D., Ziegler, E. A., & Perry, W. (2003). Cognitive functioning and psychiatric symptomatology in patients with chronic hepatitis C. *Journal of the International Neuropsychological Society*, *9*, 847–854.

Hinkin, C. H., Castellon, S. A., Hardy, D. J., Granholm, E., & Siegle, G. (1999). Computerized and traditional stroop task dysfunction in HIV-1 infection. *Neuropsychology*, *13*, 306–316.

Hinkin, C. H., Castellon, S. A., Levine, A. J., Barclay, T. R., & Singer, E. J. (2008). Neurocognition in individuals co-infected with HIV and hepatitis C. *Journal of Addictive Diseases*, *27*, 11–17.

Ickovics, J. R., Hamburger, M. E., Vlahov, D., et al. (2001). Mortality, CD4 cell count decline, and depressive symptoms among HIV-seropositive women. *Journal of the American Medical Association*, *285*, 1466–1474.

Ingraham, L. J. & Aiken, C. B. (1996). An empirical approach to determining criteria for abnormality in test batteries with multiple measures. *Neuropsychology*, *10*, 120–124.

Iudicello, J. E., Woods, S. P., Vigil, O., et al. (2010). Longer term improvement in neurocognitive functioning and affective distress among methamphetamine users who achieve stable abstinence. *Journal of Clinical and Experimental Neuropsychology*, *2*, 1–15.

Johnson, C. J., Heckman, T. G., Hansen, N. B., Kochman, A., & Sikkema, K. J. (2009). Adherence to antiretroviral medication in older adults living with HIV/AIDS: A comparison of alternative models. *AIDS Care*, *21*, 541–551.

Keswani, S. C., Leitz, G. J., & Hoke, A. (2004). Erythropoietin is neuroprotective in models of HIV sensory neuropathy. *Neuroscience Letters*, *371*, 102–105.

Lawton, M. P. & Brody, E. M. (1969). Assessment of older people: Self-maintaining and instrumental activities of daily living. *The Gerontologist*, *9*, 179–186.

Letendre, S. L., Cherner, M., Ellis, R. J., et al. (2005). The effects of hepatitis C, HIV, and methamphetamine dependence on neuropsychological performance: Biological correlates of disease. *AIDS*, *19*, S72–S78.

Letendre, S. L., McCutchan, J. A., Childers, M. E., et al. (2004). Enhancing antiretroviral therapy for human immunodeficiency virus cognitive disorders. *Annals of Neurology*, *56*, 416–423.

Levine, A., Hardy, D., Miller, E., Castellon, S., Longshore, D., & Hinkin, C. (2006). The effect of recent stimulant use on sustained attention in HIV-infected adults. *Journal of Clinical and Experimental Neuropsychology*, *28*, 29–42.

Lezak, M., Howieson, D., & Loring, D. (2004). *Neuropsychological assessment*. New York: Oxford University Press.

Lin K, Taylor MJ, Heaton RK, Franklin D, Jernigan TL, Fennema-Notestine C, McCutchan A, Atkinson JH, McArthur J, Morgello Simpson D, Collier A, Marra C, Gelman B, Clifford D, Grant I, for the CHARTER Group. (2011). Effects of traumatic brain injury on cognitive functioning and cerebral metabolites in HIV infected individuals. *Journal of Clinical and Experimental Neuropsychology*, *33*, 326–334.

Lowenstein, D. A. & Bates, B. C. (1992). *Manual for administration and scoring the Direct Assessment of Functional Status scale for older adults (DAFS)*. Miami Beach, FL: Mount Sinai Medical Center.

Maki, P. M. & Martin-Thormeyer, E. (2009). HIV, cognition and women. *Neuropsychology Review*, *19*, 204–214.

Marcotte, T. D., Wolfson, T., Rosenthal, T. J., et al. (2004). A multimodal assessment of driving performance in HIV infection. *Neurology*, *63*, 1417–1422.

Maroon, J. C., Lovell, M. R., Norwig, J., Podell, K., Powell, J. W., & Hartl, A (2000). Cerebral concussion in athletes: Evaluation and neuropsychological testing. *Neurosurgery*, *47*, 659–669.

Martin, E., Pitrak, D., Weddington, W., et al. (2004). Cognitive impulsivity and HIV serostatus in substance dependent males. *Journal of the International Neuropsychological Society*, *10*, 931–938.

Martin, E., Sullivan, S., Reed, R., et al. (2001). Auditory working memory in HIV-1 infection. *Journal of the International Neuropsychological Society*, *7*, 20–26.

Mattis, S. (1988). *Dementia Rating Scale: Professional manual*. Odessa, FL: Psychological Assessment Resources.

McArthur, J. C., McDermott, M. P., McClernon, D., et al. (2004). Attenuated central nervous system infection in advanced HIV/AIDS with combination antiretroviral therapy. *Archives of Neurology, 61,* 1687–1696.

McMurtray, A., Nakamoto, B., Shikuma, C., & Valcour, V. (2007). Small-vessel vascular disease in human immunodeficiency virus infection: The Hawaii aging with HIV cohort study. *Cerebrovascular Diseases, 24,* 236–241.

McNair, D. M., Lorr, M., & Droppleman, L. F. (1981). *Manual for the profile of mood states.* San Diego: Educational and Industrial Testing Service.

Mendez, M., van Gorp, W., & Cummings, J. (1995). Neuropsychiatry, neuropsychology, and behavioral neurology: A critical comparison. *Neuropsychiatry, Neuropsychology and Behavioral Neurology, 8,* 297–302.

Millikin, C. P., Rourke, S. B., Halman, M. H., & Power, C. (2003). Fatigue in HIV/AIDS is associated with depression and subjective neurocognitive complaints but not neuropsychological functioning. *Journal of Clinical and Experimental Neuropsychology, 25,* 201–215.

Mindt, M. R., Cherner, M., Marcotte, T. D., et al. (2003). The functional impact of HIV-associated neuropsychological impairment in Spanish-Speaking adults: A pilot study. *Journal of Clinical and Experimental Neuropsychology, 25* (1), 122–132.

Monsuez, J. J., Goujon, C., Wyplosz, B., Couzigou, C., Escaut, L., & Vittecoq, D. (2009). Cerebrovascular diseases in HIV-infected patients. *Current HIV Research, 7,* 475–480.

Moore, D. J., Atkinson, J. H., Akiskal, H., Gonzalez, R., Wolfson, T., & Grant, I. (2005). Temperament and risky behaviors: A pathway to HIV? *Journal of Affective Disorders, 85,* 191–200.

Morgan, E. E., Woods, S. P., Scott, J. C., et al. (2008). Predictive validity of demographically adjusted normative standards for the HIV Dementia Scale. *Journal of Clinical and Experimental Neuropsychology, 30,* 83–90.

Morgan, J. E. & Ricker, J. H. (2008). *Textbook of clinical neuropsychology.* Taylor & Francis: Oxford, U.K.

Neuenburg, J., Brodt, H., Herndier, B., et al. (2002). HIV-related neuropathology, 1985 to 1999: Rising prevalence of HIV encephalopathy in the era of highly active antiretroviral therapy. *Journal of Acquired Immune Deficiency Syndromes, 31,* 171–177.

Norman, L. R., Basso, M., Kumar, A., & Malow, R. (2009). Neuropsychological consequences of HIV and substance abuse: A literature review and implications for treatment and future research. *Current Drug Abuse Reviews, 2,* 143–156.

Owe-Larsson, B., Sall, L., Salamon, E., & Allgulander, C. (2009). HIV infection and psychiatric illness. *African Journal of Psychiatry, 12,* 115–128.

Padilla, A. M. & Medina, A. (1996). Cross-cultural sensitivity in assessment. In L. S. Suzuki, P. J. Meller, & J. G. Ponterotto (Eds.), *Handbook of multicultural assessment: Clinical, psychological, and educational applications* (pp. 3–28). San Francisco: Jossey-Bass.

Peavy, G., Jacobs, D., Salmon, D., et al. (1994). Verbal memory performance of patients with human immunodeficiency virus infection: Evidence of subcortical dysfunction. *Journal of Clinical and Experimental Neuropsychology, 16,* 508–523.

Pemberton, L. A. & Brew, B. J. (2001). Cerebrospinal fluid S-100beta and its relationship with AIDS dementia complex. *Journal of Clinical Virology, 22* (3), 249–253.

Pence, B., Miller, W. C., Whetten, K., Eron, J. J., & Gaynes, B. N. (2006). Prevalence of DSM-IV-defined mood, anxiety, and substance use disorders in an HIV clinic in the southeastern United States. *Journal of Acquired Immunodeficiency Syndromes, 42,* 298–306.

Pereda, M., Ayuso-Mateos, J. L., Del Barrio, A. G., et al. (2000). Factors associated with neuropsychological performance in HIV-seropositive subjects without AIDS. *Psychological Medicine, 30,* 205–217.

Perkins, D., Leserman, J., Stern, R., et al. (1995). Somatic symptoms and HIV infection: Relationship to depressive symptoms and indicators of HIV disease. *American Journal of Psychiatry, 152,* 1776–1781.

Perry, W., Carlson, M. D., Barakat, F., et al. (2005). Neuropsychological test performance in patients co-infected with hepatitis C virus and HIV. *AIDS, 19,* S79–S84.

Perry, S. & Jacobsen, P (1986). Neuropsychiatric manifestations of AIDS-spectrum disorders. *Hospital and Community Psychiatry, 37,* 135–142.

Power, C., Selnes, O. A., Grim, J. A., & McArthur, J. C. (1995). HIV Dementia Scale: A rapid screening test. *Journal of Acquired Immune Deficiency Syndromes and Human Retrovirology, 8,* 273–278.

Reback, C. J., Larkins, S., & Shoptaw, S. (2003). Methamphetamine abuse as a barrier to HIV medication adherence among gay and bisexual men. *AIDS Care-Psychological and Socio-Medical Aspects of AIDS/HIV, 15,* 775–785.

Reger, M., Welsh, R., Razani, J., Martin, D. J., & Boone, K. B. (2002). A meta-analysis of the neuropsychological sequelae of HIV infection. *Journal of the International Neuropsychological Society, 8,* 410–424.

Rippeth, J. D., Heaton, R. K., Carey, C. L., et al. (2004). Methamphetamine dependence increases risk of neuropsychological impairment in HIV infected persons. *Journal of the International Neuropsychological Society, 10,* 1–14.

Robinson-Papp, J., Elliott, K. J., & Simpson, D. M. (2009). HIV-related neurocognitive impairment in the HAART era. *Current HIV/AIDS Reports, 6,* 146–152.

Rosenbloom, M. J., Sullivan, E. V., Sassoon, S. A., et al. (2007). Alcoholism, HIV infection, and their comorbidity: Factors affecting self-rated health-related quality of life. *Journal of Studies on Alcohol and Drugs, 68,* 115–125.

Rourke, S. B., Halman, M. H., & Bassel, C. (1999). Neurocognitive complaints in HIV-infection and their relationship to depressive symptoms and neuropsychological functioning. *Journal of Clinical and Experimental Neuropsychology, 21,* 737–756.

Ryan, E. L., Baird, R., Mindt, M. R., Byrd, D., Monzones, J., & Morgello, S. (2005). Neuropsychological impairment in racial/ethnic minorities with HIV infection and low literacy levels: Effects of education and reading level in participant characterization. *Journal of the International Neuropsychological Society, 11,* 889–898.

Shepard, C. W., Finelli, L., & Alter, M. (2005). Global epidemiology of hepatitis C virus infection. *Lancet Infectious Diseases, 5,* 558–567.

Smith, C. A., van Gorp, W. G., Ryan, E. R., Ferrando, S. J., & Rabkin, T. (2003). Screening subtle HIV-related cognitive dysfunction: The clinical utility of the HIV dementia scale. *Journal of Acquired Immune Deficiency Syndromes, 33,* 116–118.

Snider, W. D., Simpson, D. M., Nielsen, S., Gold, J., Metroka, C. E., & Posner, J. B. (1983). Neurological complications of acquired immune deficiency syndrome: Analysis of 50 patients. *Annals of Neurology, 14,* 403–418.

Stern, Y. (2009). Cognitive reserve. *Neuropsychologia, 47* (10), 2015–2028.

Stern, R. A., Silva, S. G., Chaisson, N., & Evans, D. L. (1996). Influence of cognitive reserve on neuropsychological functioning in asymptomatic human immunodeficiency virus-1 infection. *Archives of Neurology, 53,* 148–153.

Strauss, E., Sherman, E., & Spreen, O. (2006). *A compendium of neuropsychological tests: administration, norms, and commentary: Third Edition.* Oxford University Press: New York.

Tan, K., Nath, A., & Hoke, A. (2010). HIV Infection and the PNS. In O. Meucci (Ed.), *Chemokine Receptors and NeuroAIDS* (pp. 51–85): Springer New York.

Temkin, N. R., Heaton, R. K., Grant, I., & Dikmen, S. S. (1999). Detecting significant change in neuropsychological test performance: a comparison of four models. *Journal of the International Neuropsychological Society, 5,* 357–369.

Thannoun, A. S. & Quinn, P. G. (1996). Reversible neurologic deficit and residual magnetic resonance imaging (MRI) abnormalities led to diagnosis of chronic hepatitis C viral (HCV) infection. *Gastroenterology, 110,* A1344–A1344.

Tozzi, V., Balestra, P., Bellagamba, R., Salvatori, M. C., Visco-Comandini, U., & Vlassi, C. (2007). Persistence of neuropsychologic deficits despite long-term highly active antiretroviral therapy in patients with HIV-related neurocognitive impairment: Prevalence and risk factors. *Journal of Acquired Immune Deficiency Syndromes, 1,* 174–182.

Tozzi, V., Balestra, P., Lorenzini, et al. (2005). Prevalence and risk factors for human immunodeficiency virus-associated neurocognitive impairment, 1996 to 2002: Results from an urban observational cohort. *Journal of Neurovirology, 11*, 265–273.

Tröster, A. & Woods, S. P. (2003). Neuropsychological aspects of Parkinson's disease and parkinsonian symptoms. In R. Pahwa, K. Lyons, & W. Koller (Eds.), *Handbook of Parkinson's disease, Third Edition*. New York, NY: Marcel Dekker, Inc.

Tröster, A. & Woods, S. P. (2010). Neuropsychology of movement disorders and motor neuron disease. In C. Armstrong (Ed.), *Handbook of medical neuropsychology: Applications of cognitive neuroscience*, pp. 315–334. New York: Springer.

Valcour, V. & Paul, R. (2006). HIV infection and dementia in older adults. *Clinical Infectious Diseases, 42*, 1449–1454.

Valcour, V., Shikuma, C., Shiramizu, B., et al. (2004). Age, apolipoprotein E4, and the risk of HIV dementia: the Hawaii Aging with HIV Cohort. *Journal of Neuroimmunology, 157*, 197–202.

van Gorp, W. G., Baerwald, J. P., Ferrando, S. J., McElhiney, M. C., & Rabkin, J. G. (1999). The relationship between employment and neuropsychological impairment in HIV infection. *Journal of the International Neuropsychological Society, 5*, 534–539.

Vigil, O., Posada, C., Woods, S. P., et al. (2008). Impairments in fine-motor coordination and speed of information processing predict declines in everyday functioning in hepatitis C infection. *Journal of Clinical and Experimental Neuropsychology, 30*, 805–815.

Walker, A. J., Batchelor, J., & Shores, A. (2009). Effects of education and cultural background on performance on WAIS-III, WMS-III, WAIS-R, and WMS-R measures: Systematic review. *Australian Psychologist, 44*, 216–223.

Walkup, J., Wei, W., Sambamoorthi, U., & Crystal, S. (2008). Antidepressant treatment and adherence to combination antiretroviral therapy among patients with AIDS and diagnosed depression. *Psychiatry Quarterly, 79*, 43–53.

Waldrop-Valverde, D., Jones, D., Weiss, S., Kumar, M., & Metsch, L. (2010). The effects of low literacy and cognitive impairment on medication adherence in HIV-positive injecting drug users. *AIDS Care, 20*, 1202–1210.

Waldrop-Valverde, D., Ownby, R., Wilkie, F., Mack, A., Kumar, M., & Metsch, L. (2006). Neurocognitive aspects of medication adherence in HIV-positive injecting drug users. *AIDS and Behavior, 10*, 287–297.

Weissenborn, K., Bokemeyer, M., Krause, J., Ennen, J., & An, B. (2005). Neurological and neuropsychiatric syndromes associated with liver disease. *AIDS, 19*, S93–S98.

Wolff, L., Alvarado, M., & Wolff, R. (2010). Depression in HIV infection: Prevalence, risk factors and management. *Revista Chilena de Infectología, 27*, 65–74.

Woods, S. P., Childers, M., Ellis, R. J., Guaman, S., Grant, I., & Heaton, R. K (2006). A battery approach for measuring neuropsychological change. *Archives of Clinical Neuropsychology, 21*, 83–89.

Woods, S., Dawson, M., Weber, E., Gibson, S., Grant, I., & Atkinson, J. (2009). Timing is everything: Antiretroviral nonadherence is associated with impairment in time-based prospective memory. *Journal of the International Neuropsychological Society, 15*, 45–52.

Woods, S. P., Moore, D. J., Weber, E., & Grant, I. (2009). Cognitive neuropsychology of HIV-associated neurocognitive disorders. *Neuropsychology Review, 19*, 152–168.

Woods, S. P., Rippeth, J. D., Frol, A. B., et al. (2004). Interrater reliability of clinical ratings and neurocognitive diagnoses in HIV. *Journal of Clinical and Experimental Neuropsychology, 26*, 759–778.

World Health Organization. (1997). *Composite International Diagnostic Interview* (CIDI) 2.1. Geneva, Switzerland.

Wu, A. W., Revicki, D. A., Jacobson, D., & Malitz, F. E. (1997). Evidence for reliability, validity and usefulness of the Medical Outcomes Study HIV Health Survey (MOS-HIV). *Quality of Life Research, 6*, 481–493.

Zakzanis, K. K. (2001). Statistics to tell the truth, the whole truth, and nothing but the truth: Formulae, illustrative numerical examples, and heuristic interpretation of effect size analyses for neuropsychological researchers. *Archives of Clinical Neuropsychology, 16*, 653–667.

9.4

VIRAL AND CELLULAR BIOMARKERS DURING ANTIRETROVIRAL THERAPY

Scott L. Letendre and Ronald J. Ellis

The persistence of HIV-associated neurocognitive disorders (HAND) in patients who seem to be effectively treated with antiretroviral therapy is a subject of active investigation. This chapter examines the effects of antiretroviral therapy on viral and host biomarkers, drawing particular attention to data indicating that antiretroviral treatment may not be fully adequate with respect to the central nervous system. The chapter's focus is limited to biomarkers in cerebrospinal fluid, which is commonly used as surrogates for pathologic and therapeutic events in the brain. In constructing this review, we performed several PubMed keyword searches and selected those publications that contained data relevant to the effects of antiretroviral therapy on a viral or host biomarker. We then review these publications and attempt to identify informative patterns in the data that might link changes in different biomarkers in CSF to antiretroviral therapy and disease characteristics.

INTRODUCTION

Potent antiretroviral therapy has improved the survival of people infected with HIV by reducing HIV replication and improving immune function. These benefits have led to reductions in the incidence of many HIV-related complications, including HIV-associated neurocognitive disorders (HAND; e.g., Sacktor et al., 2001). Because people with HIV are living longer and because antiretroviral therapy does not reverse HAND in all individuals (Cysique et al., 2009), HAND has remained common (Robertson et al., 2007; Simioni et al., 2010; Heaton et al., 2010, In press) and may be even more common in people in the earlier stages of disease (Heaton et al., 2010, in press). The persistence of HAND in people who seem to be effectively treated is an area of active investigation and may have several overlapping explanations, including shifts over the past decade in the demographics, comorbidities, and behaviors of people living with HIV disease; the adverse effects of immune recovery and persistent immune activation; accelerated aging; and incomplete activity and neurotoxicity of antiretroviral therapy in the nervous system.

This chapter will focus on this last aspect of this complex scenario: the impact of antiretroviral therapy on the nervous system. In particular, the chapter will review evidence of the effects of antiretroviral therapy on viral and host biomarkers, with a specific focus on data indicating that treatment may not completely treat the nervous system. We limited the review to biomarkers in cerebrospinal fluid (CSF), which is a well accepted surrogate—albeit an imperfect one—for pathologic and therapeutic events in the brain. To accomplish this, we performed a PubMed search for publications with the keywords "antiretroviral" and "cerebrospinal fluid." This search identified 392 references, which we reviewed to identify those that contained the data of interest (i.e., evidence of the effects of ART on a viral or host biomarker). This list was augmented with additional biomarker-specific searches, for example, for "β2 microglobulin," "cerebrospinal fluid," and "HIV." This chapter will not address topics reviewed by other chapters, including the effects of antiretrovirals on neuropsychological, neuroimaging, or autopsy findings; the effects of antiretrovirals on opportunistic infections of the central nervous system (CNS); and differences in antiretroviral distribution into the nervous system.

ANTIRETROVIRAL THERAPY AND VIRAL BIOMARKERS IN CEREBROSPINAL FLUID

VIRAL MARKERS BEFORE THE COMMERCIAL AVAILABILITY OF HIV RNA ASSAYS

Antiretrovirals exert their primary therapeutic effect by reducing HIV replication. Before HIV replication could be quantified by measuring viral RNA, other methods were used to estimate antiretroviral effectiveness. The first part of this section will focus on two of these: measurement of p24, an HIV-encoded core protein; and cell culture of CSF. After commercial viral load assays were widely available, effectiveness was estimated by measuring HIV RNA, either with reverse transcription polymerase chain reaction (RT-PCR), branched DNA (bDNA), or nucleic acid sequence-based amplification (NASBA). The second part of this section will discuss antiretroviral-induced changes in quantitative RT-PCR. A discussion of changes in HIV genotype or phenotype is beyond the chapter's scope.

The use of HIV-encoded proteins to estimate disease activity generally coincided with the use of single and dual therapy, which is less effective than current therapy that combines at least three drugs. Despite this limitation, most studies demonstrated reduction of these proteins in CSF. For example, in a cross-sectional analysis, Royal and colleagues

(Royal et al., 1994) detected p24 less frequently in the CSF of demented patients taking antiretrovirals than in that of those who did not. Longitudinal studies confirmed this finding. For example, McKinney et al. (1991) showed that 24 weeks of zidovudine monotherapy reduced p24 concentrations in the CSF of 88 children with AIDS. In another pediatric study, Laverda et al. (1994) confirmed that p24 was more frequently detected in the CSF of children with progressive encephalopathy than in asymptomatic children (66% versus 12%) and that zidovudine induced its "disappearance." Unfortunately, some studies did not measure p24 before initiating therapy. This is important since p24 is not detectable in the CSF of all untreated patients (Foudraine et al., 2001), raising concerns about the actual effectiveness of monotherapy.

In addition to their p24 findings, McKinney et al. (1991) showed that zidovudine reduced the proportion of CSF cell cultures from which HIV was isolated. More recently, Andersson and colleagues (2000) compared CSF samples from subjects who either were or were not taking antiretroviral therapy and found that the rate of cell culture positivity declined from 45% (137 of 303) to 28% (39 of 140). HIV virions were recovered most frequently from cell cultures of CSF specimens that had more than 5,000 HIV RNA copies/mL.

VIRAL MARKERS FOLLOWING THE COMMERCIAL AVAILABILITY OF HIV RNA ASSAYS

CROSS-SECTIONAL STUDIES OR LONGITUDINAL STUDIES WITH SPARSE SAMPLING

Since 1996, antiretroviral effectiveness in CSF has been estimated by measuring HIV RNA instead of p24. Table 9.4.1 summarizes the findings of relevant cross-sectional and longitudinal studies. Important considerations when considering the results include the potency of the antiretrovirals used, the duration of therapy, and the sensitivity of the assay. The earliest HIV RNA studies, for example, sampled individuals who received less potent mono- or dual-therapy (instead of the more effective triple combination therapy commonly used today) and used less sensitive assays than more recent reports.

Table 9.4.1 REPORTS THAT ALLOWED CONCLUSIONS ABOUT THE RELATIONSHIP BETWEEN ANTIRETROVIRAL USE AND HIV RNA LEVELS IN CSF

FIRST AUTHOR	YEAR	LOCATION	HIV RNA LLQ	SAMPLE SIZE	PROPORTION USING ART	ART DURATION ESTIMATE	DETECTABLE HIV RNA IN ART+
Cross-Sectional							
Gisslen (Gisslen, Norkrans et al., 1997)	1997	Sweden	200	10	100%	4.6 months	0%
McArthur (McArthur, McClernon et al., 1997)	1997	USA	100	207	53%	< or ≥ 3 months	a
Cameron (Cameron, Japour et al., 1999)	1999	Canada	400	15	100%	48 weeks	7%
Garcia (Garcia, Romeu et al., 1999)	1999	Spain	20	8	100%	52 weeks	0%
Kravcik (Kravcik, Gallicano et al., 1999)	1999	Canada	80	24	100%	-	0%
Krivine (Krivine, Force et al., 1999)	1999	France	200	22	14%	-	33%
Martin (Martin, Sonnerborg et al., 1999)	1999	Sweden	50	25	100%	12 months	20%
Moyle (Moyle, Sadler et al., 1999)	1999	UK	2000	5	100%	> 3 months	60%
Tashima (Tashima, Caliendo et al., 1999)	1999	USA	400	9	100%	26 weeks	0%
Gisslen (Gisslen, Svennerholm et al., 2000)	2000	Sweden	20	45	100%	-	31%
Corti (Corti, Villafane et al., 2001)	2001	Argentina	-	18	100%	-	22%
Gunthard (Gunthard, Havlir et al., 2001)	2001	Switzerland	50	13	100%	2 years	0%
Lafeuillade (Lafeuillade, Solas et al., 2002)	2002	France	50	40	100%	> 6 months	13%
Solas (Solas, Lafeuillade et al., 2003)	2003	France	50	41	100%	> 6 months	13%
McArthur (McArthur, McDermott et al., 2004)	2004	USA	80	371	71%	-	b
Cysique (Cysique, Brew et al., 2005)	2005	Australia	100	78	100%	> 8 weeks	47%
Spudich (Spudich, Nilsson et al., 2005)	2005	USA	20	100	54%	-	c
von Giesen (von Giesen, Adams et al., 2005)	2005	Germany	50	71	73%	40 months	> 75%
Spudich (Spudich, Lollo et al., 2006)	2006	USA	2.5	139	59%	29 months	28%
Yilmaz (Yilmaz, Svennerholm et al., 2006)	2006	Sweden	2	13	100%	34 months	0%

(Continued)

Table 9.4.1 (CONTINUED)

FIRST AUTHOR	YEAR	LOCATION	HIV RNA LLQ	SAMPLE SIZE	PROPORTION USING ART	ART DURATION ESTIMATE	DETECTABLE HIV RNA IN ART+
Arendt (Arendt, Nolting et al., 2007)	2007	Germany	50	109	71%	-	16%
Letendre (Letendre, Marquie-Beck et al., 2008)	2008	USA	50	467	100%	≥ 3 months	17%
Yilmaz (Yilmaz, Price et al., 2008)	2008	Sweden	50	134	100%	2 years	12%
Yilmaz (Yilmaz, Price et al., 2008)	2008	Sweden	2.5	64	100%	~2 years	45%
Letendre (Letendre, McClernon et al., 2009)	2009	USA	2	300	100%	~16 months	41%
Longitudinal-Sparse							
Gisslen (Gisslen, Norkrans et al. 1997),	1997	Sweden	200	21	100%	8.9 months	69%
Foudraine (Foudraine, Hoetelmans et al., 1998)	1998	Netherlands	1000	22	100%	12 weeks	0%
Eggers (Eggers, van Lunzen et al., 1999)	1999	Germany	200	15	100%	14 days	60%
Garcia (Garcia, Alonso et al., 2000)	2000	Spain	200	10	100%	52 weeks	0%
Gisolf (Gisolf, Enting et al., 2000)	2000	Netherlands	400	26	100%	12 weeks	19%
Gisolf (a) (Gisolf, van Praag et al., 2000)	2000	Netherlands	50	27	100%	12 weeks	41%
Gisolf (b) (Gisolf, van Praag et al., 2000)	2000	Netherlands	50	12	100%	48 weeks	25%
Cinque (Cinque, Presi et al., 2001)	2001	Italy	400	15	100%	6 weeks	60%
Enting (Enting, Prins et al., 2001)	2001	Netherlands	40	6	100%	48 weeks	17%
Foudraine (Foudraine, Jurriaans et al., 2001)	2001	Netherlands	50	33	100%	48 weeks	0%
Sabri (Sabri, De Milito et al., 2001)	2001	Sweden	50	7	100%	4 months	14%
Abdulle (a) (Abdulle, Hagberg et al., 2002)	2002	Sweden	50	21	100%	1 year	10%
Abdulle (b) (Abdulle, Hagberg et al., 2002)	2002	Sweden	50	11	100%	2 years	0%
Antinori (Antinori, Giancola et al., 2002)	2002	Italy	80	29	100%	77 days	24%
DeLuca (De Luca, Ciancio et al., 2002)	2002	Italy	100	50	100%	7 weeks	58%
Podzamczer (Podzamczer, Ferrer et al., 2002)	2002	Spain	200	17	100%	12 months	0%
Chang (Chang, Ernst et al., 2003)	2003	USA	-	33	100%	3 months	18%
Eggers (Eggers, Hertogs et al., 2003)	2003	Germany	20-50	40	100%	~3 weeks	14%
Polis (Polis, Suzman et al., 2003)	2003	USA	50	22	100%	12 months	0%
Bestetti (Bestetti, Presi et al., 2004)	2004	Italy	400	18	100%	≥ 9 months	28%
Chang (Chang, Ernst et al., 2004)	2004	USA	50	24	100%	3 months	29%
Cinque (Cinque, Nebuloni et al., 2004)	2004	Italy	400	16	100%	12 weeks	10%
Letendre (Letendre, McCutchan et al., 2004)	2004	USA	50	31	100%	15 weeks	45%
Robertson (Robertson, Robertson et al., 2004)	2004	USA	50	48	100%	6 months	d
Sevigny (Sevigny, Albert et al., 2004)	2004	USA	80	203	73%	21 months	52%
Yilmaz (a) (Yilmaz, Stahle et al., 2004)	2004	Sweden	50	11	100%	3 months	18%
Yilmaz (b) (Yilmaz, Stahle et al., 2004)	2004	Sweden	50	7	100%	12 months	0%
Mellgren (Mellgren, Antinori et al., 2005)	2005	Sweden	50	74	100%	3 months	24%
Yilmaz (Yilmaz, Fuchs et al., 2006)	2006	Sweden	50	8	100%	48 weeks	29%
Letendre (Letendre, van den Brande et al., 2007)	2007	USA	50	8	100%	24 weeks	0%
Vernazza (Vernazza, Daneel et al., 2007)	2007	Switzerland	50	20	100%	24 weeks	15%
Marra (Marra, Zhao et al., 2009)	2009	USA	50	79	100%	52 weeks	0%
Canestri (Canestri, Lescure et al., 2010)	2010	France	200	11	100%	> 6 months	100%

The duration of ART and lower limit of quantitation (LLQ) could not be determined for all reports. LLQ = Lower limit of quantitation, ART = Antiretroviral therapy
a - HIV RNA levels in CSF were independent of antiretroviral use
b - Among those taking antiretrovirals, people with HAD had higher HIV RNA levels in CSF
c - 11% had higher HIV RNA levels in CSF than in plasma
d - Levels declined from mean 2.7 to 1.4 log10 c/mL

Differences in drug distribution across the blood-brain barrier may also affect the effectiveness of antiretroviral therapy in the nervous system and this topic is reviewed in a separate chapter.

Early studies demonstrated that nucleoside analog reverse transcriptase inhibitors (NRTIs) alone reduced HIV RNA below quantitation in antiretroviral-naive individuals, although the assays used had relatively high lower limits of quantitation compared with next generation assays. For example, Gisslen et al. (1997) reported that HIV RNA was below 200 copies/mL in the CSF of 10 individuals who had taken ART for a mean of 4.6 months. Later, this group published a more detailed report that zidovudine reduced HIV RNA in CSF but didanosine did not (Gisslen et al., 1997). Similar to these findings for didanosine, McArthur et al. (1997) found in a larger group that HIV RNA levels in CSF were independent of antiretroviral exposure. However, by combining just two NRTIs (lamivudine and either zidovudine or stavudine), Foudraine et al. (1998) were able to suppress HIV RNA below 400 copies/mL in all 22 participants after 12 weeks.

Similar to the data on NRTI monotherapy, early findings support that monotherapy with first-generation protease inhibitors does not consistently suppress HIV RNA levels in CSF. For example, in a cross-sectional study, Kravcik and colleagues (1999) found that saquinavir and ritonavir reduced HIV RNA levels in CSF below 80 copies/mL when it also did so in plasma. When subjects failed therapy, however, HIV RNA levels in CSF were relatively higher than plasma levels, suggesting that failure may have occurred in CSF first. Consistent with the limited effectiveness of protease inhibitors in CSF, a larger, randomized, clinical trial showed that 12 weeks of saquinavir and ritonavir failed to reduce HIV RNA levels below 400 copies/mL in 71% (10/14) of participants. The addition of a single NRTI, stavudine, resulted in viral suppression in CSF in 92% of participants (Gisolf et al., 2000). More recent studies of later generation protease inhibitors, such as lopinavir (Yeh et al., 2007) and atazanavir (Vernazza et al., 2007), have since confirmed that ritonavir-boosted protease inhibitors alone suppress HIV RNA in CSF in most—but not all—individuals.

Treatment with at least three drugs seems to be a better option for the nervous system. For example, Krivine et al. (1999) reported that subjects taking at least three antiretrovirals had lower HIV RNA levels in CSF, although 1 of 3 taking combination therapy still had an HIV RNA level in CSF above 200 copies/mL. When Garcia et al. (2000) compared the effectiveness of dual versus triple therapy in 94 individuals, all 10 subjects who underwent lumbar puncture reduced their HIV RNA levels below 20 copies/mL at 52 weeks (Garcia et al. 2000). In a pediatric study, McCoig et al. (2002) had similar results in comparing dual versus triple therapy in 23 children, although 10% still had measurable HIV RNA in CSF after 48 weeks of therapy. Gisslen et al. (2000) also confirmed that HIV RNA in CSF was less frequently detectable in subjects taking three antiretrovirals than in those taking fewer drugs.

As mono- and dual-therapy use declined, subsequent studies focused on the effectiveness of specific regimens in parent clinical trials or regimens that contained a specific drug of interest. For example, Martin et al. (1999) found that indinavir-containing regimens reduced HIV RNA in CSF to below 50 copies/mL in most subjects, although 20% remained detectable. Gunthard et al. (2001) found that up to 2.5 years of treatment with zidovudine–lamivudine–indinavir reduced HIV RNA in CSF below 50 copies/mL in all 13 participants. While indinavir is the best penetrating drug in its class, even regimens that contain two NRTIs and a highly protein-bound drug, such as the non-nucleoside reverse transcriptase inhibitor efavirenz, can uniformly reduce HIV RNA in CSF to below 400 copies/mL (Tashima et al., 1999).

Instead of administering a uniform regimen, our group studied the effects of individualized antiretroviral therapy on HIV RNA levels in antiretroviral experienced individuals. Combination therapy reduced HIV RNA in CSF in 17 of 31 (55%) individuals after a mean of 15 weeks ((Letendre, McCutchan et al., 2004). Importantly, half of these reductions occurred even in the absence of substantial reductions in plasma HIV RNA. Antinori et al. (2002),) found that a mean of 11 weeks of individualized therapy reduced CSF HIV RNA levels by approximately 1 $\log_{10}$ copies/mL and to below 80 copies/mL in 22 of 29 participants (76%). HIV RNA reductions in CSF were associated with reductions of HIV RNA in plasma and the duration of therapy, findings that have been confirmed by others. In another observational cohort ($N = 50$), De Luca et al. (2002) found that a median of 7 weeks of individualized therapy reduced HIV RNA in CSF by 0.19 to 1.00 log10 copies/mL. In this study, CSF HIV RNA reductions were associated with higher CD4 counts at baseline (> 100/μL) and the use of at least three drugs classified as CNS "penetrating."

Others have also studied the antiviral response in CSF in special populations, such as individuals who have very recently been infected by HIV. For example, in individuals with acute or early HIV infection, Pilcher et al. (2001) found that: (1) HIV RNA levels in the CSF of five subjects with early HIV infection were higher than those of historical, chronically infected controls; and (2) 24 weeks of didanosine–stavudine–nevirapine reduced HIV RNA levels in CSF below 50 copies/mL in all five. Similarly, Enting et al. (2001) evaluated six subjects with acute or early HIV infection and found that treatment with five drugs (zidovudine–lamivudine–abacavir–nevirapine–indinavir) reduced HIV RNA levels in CSF, after both 8 and 48 weeks. In comparison, in two patients with severe HIV-associated dementia, Iftimovici et al. (1998) found that combination antiretroviral therapy reduced HIV RNA in plasma below 400 copies/mL, but failed to do so in CSF. Thus, the stage of HIV disease and the complications of HIV disease may influence the antiviral response in the nervous system.

LONGITUDINAL STUDIES WITH MORE INTENSIVE SAMPLING

The longitudinal studies described thus far employed relatively sparse sampling to demonstrate antiviral effectiveness. Several more labor-intensive studies have used even more frequent sampling to estimate the dynamics of viral decay in CSF. For example, as early as 1997, Stellbrink et al. (1997) reported that antiretroviral therapy reduced HIV RNA in CSF after just 8–24 days. By utilizing more frequent sampling in 13 subjects, Staprans et al. (1999) showed that during the first 11 days of therapy, the crude HIV RNA half-life was longer and the decay rate slower in CSF than in plasma. Interestingly, subjects who had lower pre-treatment blood CD4+ lymphocyte counts also demonstrated slower decay in CSF. Eggers et al. (2000) multiply sampled ventricular CSF in one individual and identified a longer elimination half-life (4.2 days) in CSF than in plasma (2.3 days) in response to zidovudine-lamivudine-saquinavir-ritonavir. Ellis et al (2000) confirmed and extended these findings by multiply sampling 12 individuals. Specifically, they found that HIV RNA levels in CSF (1) declined at a rate similar to plasma in subjects with earlier HIV disease (CD4+ lymphocyte counts ≥ 400/μl) or with a pleocytosis (CSF leukocytes ≥ 5/μl); (2) declined more slowly than plasma in subjects with advanced HIV disease (CD4+ lymphocyte counts < 400/μl) and without a pleocytosis (CSF leukocytes < 5/μl); and (3) failed to decline substantially in subjects with HIV-associated dementia (HAD), even after up to 6 weeks of therapy. These viral response groups are typical of other reports and examples are shown graphically in Figure 9.4.1.

Haas et al. (2000; 2003) used even more intensive "continuous" sampling in four subjects. Their unique sampling method obtained CSF via an indwelling lumbar intrathecal catheter, a peristaltic pump, and an automatic fraction collector, yielding 288 mL of CSF per procedure. Their first manuscript (Haas et al., 2000) reported viral decay during the first 48 hours of therapy with stavudine-lamivudine-nelfinavir and their second manuscript (Haas et al. 2003) reported viral decay over a later 48 hours that began 72 hours after initiating therapy. The first 48 hours of therapy saw consistent declines in HIV RNA levels in plasma but more variable declines in HIV RNA levels in CSF ranging from -0.38 to -1.18 $\log_{10}$ copies/mL. Of the four subjects, one had more rapid decay of HIV RNA in CSF than in plasma and one had substantially slower decay in CSF than in plasma. Of note, only higher antiretroviral concentrations correlated with more rapid HIV RNA decay in CSF. The 2003 report aimed to identify whether viral decay in CSF had a second phase, reflecting HIV deriving from longer-lived cells, such as brain macrophages. To accomplish this, HIV RNA levels were measured from 17 aliquots obtained over 48 hours, beginning on the fourth day after initiating therapy. Slopes of regression lines for days 4 and 5 ranged from -0.061 to -0.231 $\log_{10}$ copies/mL per day, which corresponded to viral decay half-lives of 1.3 to 4.9 days. Estimates of viral decay half-lives during the first 3 days of therapy ranged from 0.9 to 2.8 days. Thus, this unique, intensive study strongly supports that viral decay in CSF has two phases and that some individuals (1 of 4 in this analysis) may have much slower decay in CSF than in plasma.

Eggers et al (2003) extended these findings further by evaluating a larger number of adults (N = 40), 25% of whom had HAND. Subjects who had HAND had slower viral decay in CSF and a higher degree of compartmental discordance than those without HAND. In this analysis, slower viral decay in CSF was not associated with lower CD4+ cell counts or HIV disease stage. More recently, Schnell et al. (2009) confirmed the association between HAND and slower viral decay in CSF, although this was not universal. HIV decayed as rapidly in CSF as in blood in about half of the individuals with neurologic disease but more slowly in the other half. The distinction between these two groups may have been in their disease stage: Subjects who had lower CD4+ cell counts (as well as lower CSF leukocyte counts) had slower viral decay in CSF than in plasma. Differences in viral decay between CSF and plasma are summarized in Figure 9.4.2. Based on this and earlier animal findings from their group (Harrington et al., 2005), the authors concluded that infiltrating macrophages may replace CD4+ T-cells as the primary source of productive viral replication in the CNS of people with HAND, particularly those with more advanced immune suppression.

Intensive sampling methods can also be used to identify associations between HIV RNA changes and changes in other biomarkers. For example, because monocyte chemotactic

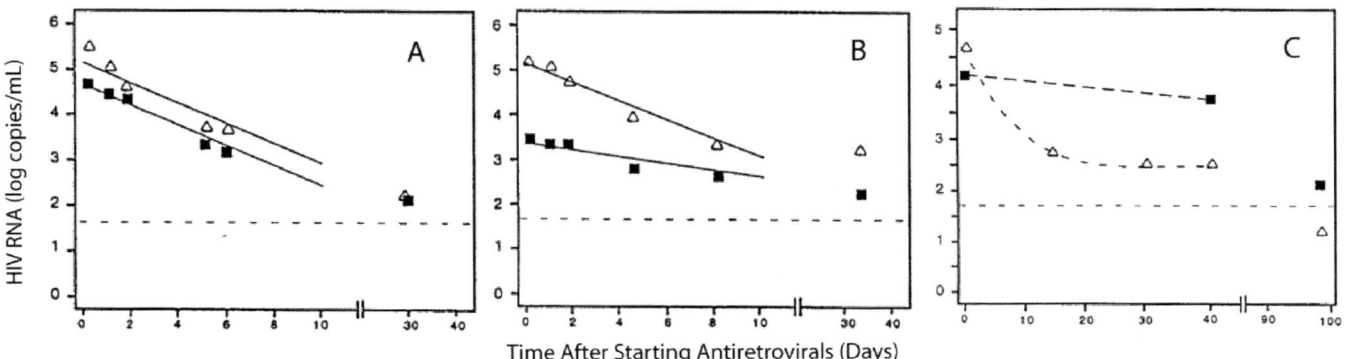

Figure 9.4.1 HIV reductions in plasma and CSF following initiation of antiretroviral therapy. Ellis et al. found that HIV RNA in CSF: (a) declined at a similar rate to plasma in subjects with earlier HIV disease (CD4 ≥ 400/μl) or with a pleocytosis (CSF leukocytes ≥ 5/μl); (b) declined more slowly than plasma in subjects with advanced HIV disease (CD4 < 400/μl) and without a pleocytosis (i.e., CSF leukocytes were less than 5/μL); or (c) failed to decline substantially in subjects with HIV-associated dementia, even after up to 6 weeks of therapy (Ellis et al., 2000). Graphics used with author's permission.

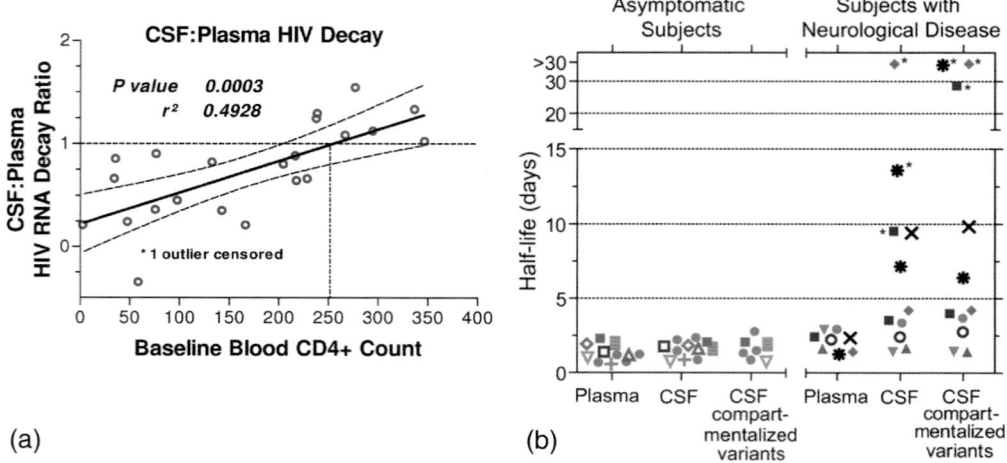

Figure 9.4.2 The relationship between viral decay in CSF and disease characteristics. Several studies that intensively sampled CSF identified that viral decay was slower in CSF than in plasma as CD4+ cell counts in blood declined (A, e.g., Spudich et al., 2005) or as neurocognitive disease occurred (B, e.g., Schnell et al., 2009). Graphics used with permission of the authors.

protein (MCP)-1 has been strongly implicated in HAND, Monteiro de Almeida et al. (2005) compared antiretroviral-induced changes in HIV RNA in CSF and plasma to changes in MCP-1 in seven adults. Substantial variability existed in this small sample but the study identified that MCP-1 levels are higher in CSF than in plasma (confirming prior reports) and that different populations may exist in terms of MCP-1 responsiveness to antiretroviral-induced declines in HIV RNA. In some individuals, MCP-1 levels fell in parallel with HIV RNA levels. Others, however, maintained high levels of MCP-1 in CSF despite declines in HIV RNA. Six of the subjects also interrupted therapy and were again intensively sampled. While substantial inter-individual variability was again present with rises in MCP-1 preceding rises in HIV RNA in CSF in some individuals but following them in others. Overall, the analyses supported that HIV RNA and MCP-1 levels in CSF were linked in many individuals and that MCP-1 levels may remain elevated even after HIV RNA levels decline below reliable quantitation. In a follow-up analysis, Monteiro de Almeida et al. (2006) identified that increases in MCP-1 in CSF following treatment interruption preceded increases in CSF leukocyte counts, which have been linked to HIV RNA levels in CSF (Marra et al. 2007).

Other studies of viral dynamics in CSF following treatment interruption by Eggers et al. (1999) and Price et al. (2001; Price & Deeks, 2004) preceded this work. Eggers et al. identified a close relationship between the rise of HIV RNA in CSF and the appearance of leukocytes in CSF—but not albumin—supporting that HIV was replicating in migrating leukocytes, not appearing from passive influx across a leaky blood-CSF barrier. The Price et al. work confirmed the link between higher HIV RNA levels and higher CSF leukocyte counts and identified that HIV RNA levels increased more rapidly in CSF than in plasma. Smith et al. (2009) subsequently used clonal *env* sequences from paired CSF and plasma specimens to identify that people who have pleocytosis (i.e., abnormally elevated leukocyte counts in CSF) have

more closely related viral populations in these fluids, suggesting that migration of leukocytes across the blood-brain and blood-CSF barriers disrupts compartmentalization. These findings mirrored earlier findings using *pol* sequences and phenotypes from Price et al. (2001): In individuals with pleocytosis who interrupted therapy, the predominant HIV quasispecies shifted simultaneously in CSF and plasma from a drug-resistant to a more drug-susceptible phenotype with identical and simultaneous changes in genotypes associated with drug resistance. Table 9.4.2 summarizes studies that estimated viral decay in CSF.

Many other projects have investigated the adaptation of HIV to the cells of the nervous system by genotyping *env* (e.g., Pillai et al., 2006) or *pol* (e.g., Strain et al., 2005; Hightower et al., 2009). These projects have identified that, for example, individuals who are taking antiretroviral therapy but have detectable HIV RNA levels are more likely to have drug resistance mutations that are present in CSF but absent from plasma. A detailed summary of these genotype-focused projects is beyond the scope of this review.

In summary, these data support several important conclusions.

- First, HIV RNA in CSF derives from a mixture of blood and nervous system cells and the relative contribution from nervous system cells expands as CD4+ cell counts decline.

- Second, combination antiretroviral therapy that includes at least one nucleoside analog reduces HIV RNA in the CSF of almost all individuals, especially if it suppresses replication in plasma.

- Third, in some patients, antiretrovirals reduce HIV RNA in CSF even when they fail to do so in plasma. This suggests that HIV in the nervous system may retain antiretroviral susceptibility longer than in plasma because of the different cellular sources of HIV, the generally lower levels of HIV, and the lower concentrations

Table 9.4.2 REPORTS THAT ESTIMATED VIRAL DECAY IN CSF

FIRST AUTHOR	YEAR	LOCATION	HIV RNA LLQ	SAMPLE SIZE	ART DURATION	VIRAL DECAY $T_{1/2}$ (DAYS)	
						CSF ESTIMATE	PLASMA ESTIMATE
Staprans (Staprans, Marlowe et al., 1999)	1999	USA	50	13	14.2 weeks	3.2	2.4
Eggers (Eggers, Stuerenburg et al., 2000)	2000	Germany	50	1	27 days	4.2	2.3
Ellis (Ellis, Gamst et al., 2000)	2000	USA	50	5	~40 days	3.4	1.3
Haas (Haas, Clough et al., 2000)	2000	USA	50	4	2 days	1.3-4.0	*
Haas (Haas, Johnson et al., 2003)	2003	USA	50	4	5 days	1.3-4.9	*
Eggers (Eggers, Hertogs et al., 2003)	2003	Germany	50	40	~3 weeks	*	*
Harrington (Harrington, Haas et al., 2005)	2005	USA	50	4	3-5 days	0.8-3.7	*
Spudich (Spudich, Huang et al., 2005)	2005	USA	20	28	11 days	*	*
Schnell (Schnell, Spudich et al., 2009)	2009	USA	50	15	~14 weeks	1.6-9.8	0.6-2.9

Following initiation of antiretroviral therapy, at least two phases of viral decay can occur, similar to plasma. In some individuals, such as those with HAND or with lower CD4+ cell counts, the slower phase of viral decay can predominate.
* Did not calculate viral decay half-lives, LLQ = Lower limit of quantitation, ART = Antiretroviral therapy

of antiretrovirals. Studies have also linked these discordant responses to immune activation: HIV RNA in CSF remains suppressed as long as HIV RNA levels in plasma are maintained below their pre-treatment setpoint along and low levels of immune activation. Once immune activation and HIV RNA levels rise in plasma rise and CD4+ cell counts in blood decline, HIV tends to reappear in CSF. These findings also suggest that continuing antiretroviral therapy that is failing in plasma may have benefits for the nervous system. Choosing to continue failing antiretroviral therapy, however, must be considered carefully because of its unproven benefit, the continued risk of adverse events, and the risk of selection of drug resistance-associated mutations.

• Fourth, antiretrovirals reduce HIV RNA more slowly in CSF than in plasma in some individuals. Specifically, viral decay in CSF may be slower in individuals with lower CD4$^+$ lymphocyte counts or in patients with HAND. Considering recent findings linking lower nadir CD4+ cell counts and greater risk of HAND (Muñoz-Moreno et al., 2008; Ellis et al., 2010), determining whether slower relative decay rates in CSF are reversed with immune recovery will be important. Together, these data suggest that CNS-targeted treatment may be needed to completely suppress HIV replication in the nervous system of patients with AIDS or with HAND.

ANTIRETROVIRAL THERAPY AND HOST BIOMARKERS IN CEREBROSPINAL FLUID

Similar to studies of viral biomarkers, research on host biomarkers has expanded markedly in recent years. This expansion is due in part to advances in HIV pathogenesis,

multiplex technologies, and discovery-driven science. Both viral and host biomarkers provide important insights into HIV neuropathogenesis since both viral proteins and immune-mediated mechanisms can injure the nervous system. Conceptual models of HIV pathogenesis in the nervous system vary but common elements typically include a viral component, an immune-mediated or neurotoxin component, and a neuronal injury component (Ellis et al., 2007). In keeping with these models, experts have proposed a combination of biomarkers that might include a viral biomarker, an immune activation biomarker, and a neuronal injury biomarker (Price et al., 2007). The hope is that such a combination could better assist with the diagnosis of HAND, the identification of individuals with reversible HAND, the selection of optimum therapy, and the estimation of prognosis. Unfortunately, the field is still far from this ideal. Understanding the impact of antiretroviral therapy on the two host biomarkers in this ideal combination is also critically important and it seems likely that different combinations of biomarkers may be needed for individuals with HAND who are taking antiretroviral therapy and those who are not.

Markers of monocyte and microglial activation were among the first host biomarkers investigated, because patients dying with HIV encephalitis had evidence of microglial nodules and perivascular infiltrates with monocyte-derived macrophages. For example, many early studies focused on β-2 microglobulin (β2M) and neopterin, two relatively nonspecific markers of monocyte proliferation. Other early studies did focus on a more specific pathway, neuronal excitotoxicity via the *N*-methyl-D-aspartate (NMDA) receptor, by measuring CSF concentrations of quinolinic acid.

More recent studies have either identified other markers of immune activation, such as soluble CD14 and soluble tumor necrosis factor (TNF) receptors, or have focused on other mechanisms or signs of HIV-induced brain injury.

For example, the discovery that chemokine receptors are coreceptors for HIV cell entry led to investigations into their role, and that of their ligands, in neuropathogenesis. The observation that the blood-brain barrier (BBB) is damaged in many HIV-infected individuals led to investigations of mediators of BBB injury, such as matrix metalloproteases (MMPs). The recognition that the most numerous cells in the brain, astrocytes, can also contribute to brain injury led to investigations of proteins produced by these cells, such as monocyte chemotactic protein-1 (MCP-1) and S100β. While all these investigations add to the current state of knowledge of HIV neuropathogenesis, this review of host biomarkers will focus on those for which data exist regarding the impact of antiretrovirals, similar to the preceding section. Table 9.4.3 summarizes published reports that evaluated whether biomarkers in CSF differed between users and non-users of antiretrovirals in cross-sectional analyses or whether initiation or interruption of antiretroviral therapy led to changes in biomarker concentrations in longitudinal analyses.

BIOMARKERS OF MACROPHAGE AND MICROGLIAL ACTIVATION

Many cross-sectional studies established consistent links between HAND and elevated CSF concentrations of two markers of macrophage activation and turnover, β2M and neopterin (Elovaara et al., 1989; Fuchs et al., 1989; Sonnerborg et al., 1989; Imberciadori et al., 1990; Lucey et al., 1991; Perrella et al., 1991; Peter et al., 1991; Bogner et al., 1992; Carrieri et al., 1992; Lazzarin et al., 1992; McArthur et al., 1992; Hagberg et al., 1993). β2M is a small polypeptide that is expressed on the surface of many nucleated cells, including monocytes and microglia. It forms the light chain of the class I histocompatibility complex antigen molecule and is released by cell destruction or membrane turnover (Ravel, 1995). Like β2M, neopterin is also derived from monocytes. Unlike β2M, neopterin is a component of another pathway, biopterin synthesis, and is an indirect indicator of the activity of T cells and interferon-α (Ravel, 1995). Therefore, while both biomarkers are considered relatively "nonspecific" indicators of macrophage activation, they each reflect different mechanisms in this process.

Several longitudinal studies extended these cross-sectional findings, showing that markers of macrophage activation increased with advancing HIV disease. For example, over up to 4 years of follow-up, Elovaara et al. (Elovaara & Muller, 1993) reported that β2M concentrations in CSF increased in seven of nine patients who developed new or progressive neurological disease. In 19 individuals followed for up to 6 years, Gisslen et al. (1994) reported that CSF β2M and neopterin concentrations increased while CD4 counts dropped. In a study of incident neurocognitive impairment, Brew and colleagues (1996) evaluated 35 neurologically asymptomatic participants, 17 of whom progressed to at least AIDS dementia complex (ADC) stage 1 during follow-up. Univariate analyses supported that CSF concentrations of β2M and neopterin were associated with

incident impairment. In a multivariate analysis, CSF β2M concentrations greater than 5 mg/L conferred a remarkable 17-fold increased risk of ADC (Brew et al., 1996). This compares with a cut-off of 3.8 mg/L suggested earlier by McArthur et al. (1992) that had a sensitivity of 44%, specificity of 90%, and a positive predictive value of 88% for the diagnosis of HIV dementia. These findings provided important insights into HIV neuropathogenesis but most did not assess the effects of antiretroviral therapy on β2M and neopterin. Several subsequent studies did.

For example, as early as 1990, Brew reported that neopterin declined in the CSF of patients with AIDS dementia complex who improved with zidovudine monotherapy (Brew et al., 1990). Two years later, Hagberg et al. (1991) confirmed that 5 months of zidovudine monotherapy reduced neopterin and β2M in CSF in two patients with HIV-associated neurological complications. The following year, Brew reported similar findings in a larger cohort of 78 zidovudine-treated subjects who had at least borderline neurocognitive impairment at entry (Brew et al., 1992). These improvements were not restricted to those with neurocognitive complications: Zidovudine also reduced β2M in the CSF of neurologically normal individuals (Hagberg et al., 1992). Monotherapy-associated β2M reductions were also reported for lamivudine (van Leeuwen et al., 1995) and didanosine (Gisslen et al., 1997). One study, however, did report that zidovudine reduced CSF β2M more effectively than didanosine (Hagberg et al., 1996). Given these findings with monotherapy, the observation that dual therapy also reduced CSF β2M concentrations was not unexpected.

With zidovudine monotherapy, CSF β2M seems to decline after as little as 6 weeks (Elovaara et al., 1994) or as much as 12 months (Gisslen et al., 1994). In a cohort of 145 subjects, Gulevich et al. (1993) identified that maximal β2M and neopterin reductions occurred when zidovudine was administered for intermediate durations (46–365 days), compared with shorter or longer periods. These data support that nucleoside analogs consistently reduce β2M and neopterin in CSF over a relatively brief duration.

The benefits of combination therapy may be more durable. For example, in a small primary HIV infection study of treatment with at least five antiretroviral drugs, Enting et al. (2001) showed that elevated CSF β2M levels normalized by 8 weeks and remained durably normalized after 48 weeks of therapy. A year later, Abdulle et al. (2002) reported that up to 2 years of individualized combination antiretroviral therapy (primarily zidovudine–lamivudine–indinavir) also normalized CSF β2M in all 30 participants. One important aspect of this study is that only 55% of the participants normalized their CSF neopterin concentrations after 2 years. This raises concern that even combination therapy may not durably suppress macrophage activation completely, a theory supported by other findings (Gisolf, van Praag et al., 2000).

More recent studies have investigated another marker of macrophage activation, soluble CD14. CD14 is found principally on human monocytes and exists in both membrane and soluble forms. Soluble CD14 (sCD14) is released by stimulated monocytes in vitro (Landmann et al., 2000) and

Table 9.4.3 REPORTS THAT ALLOWED CONCLUSIONS ABOUT THE RELATIONSHIP BETWEEN ANTIRETROVIRAL USE AND HOST BIOMARKERS IN CSF

FIRST AUTHOR	YEAR	LOCATION	BIOMARKER	DESIGN	SAMPLE SIZE	PROPORTION USING ART	ART DURATION ESTIMATE	FINDINGS
Macrophage-Microglial Activation, Albumin, and IgG								
Brew (Brew, Bhalla et al., 1990)	1990	USA	Neopterin	L	9	100%	8 weeks	Levels declined with ZDV
Hagberg (Hagberg, Andersson et al., 1991)	1991	Sweden	β2M, Neopterin	L	2	100%	5 months	Levels declined with ZDV
Brew (Brew, Bhalla et al., 1992)	1992	USA	β2M	L	10	100%	8 weeks	Levels declined with ZDV in 90%
Elovaara (Elovaara, Poutiainen et al., 1994)	1994	Finland	β2M, IgG	L	14	100%	12 months	β2M declined with ZDV but IgG did not
Gisslen (Gisslen, Chiodi et al., 1994)	1994	Sweden	β2M, Neopterin	L	8	100%	3–12 months	Levels declined with ZDV
Gulevich (Gulevich, McCutchan et al., 1993)	1994	USA	β2M, Neopterin	C-S	145	100%	Variable	Lower levels with 46–365 days of ZDV vs. shorter or longer durations
Hagberg (Hagberg, Norkrans et al., 1996)	1996	Sweden	Neopterin	L	17	100%	3–12 months	Lower neopterin levels with ZDV but not ddI
Gisslen (Gisslen, Norkrans et al., 1997)	1997	Sweden	β2M, Neopterin	L	21	100%	3–13 months	Lower neopterin levels with ZDV but not ddI
Gendelman (Gendelman, Zheng et al., 1998)	1998	USA	sCD14	L	1	100%	6 weeks	Levels declined with ART
Enting (Enting, Foudraine et al. 2000)	2000	Netherlands	β2M	L	16	100%	12 weeks	Levels declined with ART
Ryan (Ryan, Zheng et al., 2001)	2001	USA	sCD14	C-S	28	100%	1–35 months	Levels unrelated to ART duration
Abdulle (Abdulle, Hagberg et al., 2002)	2002	Sweden	β2M, neopterin	L	30	100%	2 years	β2M normalized in 100% and neopterin in 55%
Yilmaz (Yilmaz, Stahle et al., 2004)	2004	Sweden	β2M, Neopterin	L	11	100%	3–12 months	Levels declined with ART
Abdulle (Abdulle, Hagberg et al., 2005)	2005	Sweden	Albumin, IgG	L	38	100%	2 years	Albumin normal in 100%, IgG index abnormal in 41%
Cysique (Cysique, Brew et al., 2005)	2005	Australia	β2M	L	76	100%	12 weeks	Elevated levels in 43%
Spudich (Spudich, Lollo et al., 2006)	2006	USA	Neopterin	C-S	139	59%	29 months	Lower levels with successful ART vs. off ART or failing ART
Yilmaz (Yilmaz, Fuchs et al., 2006)	2006	Sweden	β2M, IgG	C-S	13	100%	34 months	β2M abnormal in 23%, IgG abnormal in 46%
Yilmaz (Yilmaz, Fuchs et al., 2006)	2006	Sweden	β2M, Neopterin, IgG	L	8	100%	48 weeks	Neopterin (86%) and IgG (71%) remained abnormal
Eden (Eden, Price et al., 2007)	2007	Sweden	Neopterin, IgG	L	16	100%	4 years	Abnormal levels in 60%
Yilmaz (Yilmaz, Price et al., 2008)	2008	Sweden	Neopterin	C-S	350	45%	~2 years	Lower levels with ART
MCP-1								
Enting (Enting, Foudraine et al., 2000)	2000	Netherlands	MCP-1	L	16	100%	12 weeks	Levels did not change during ART
Gisolf (Gisolf, van Praag et al., 2000)	2000	Netherlands	MCP-1	L	23	100%	48 weeks	Levels rose during ART
DeLuca (DeLuca, Ciancio et al., 2002)	2002	Italy	MCP-1	C-S	56	20%	7 weeks	Similar levels with & without ART
Chang (Chang, Ernst et al., 2004)	2004	USA	MCP-1	L	24	100%	3 months	Lower levels with ART but remained higher in those with HAND

(*Continued*)

Table 9.4.3 (CONTINUED)

FIRST AUTHOR	YEAR	LOCATION	BIOMARKER	DESIGN	SAMPLE SIZE	PROPORTION USING ART	ART DURATION ESTIMATE	FINDINGS
McArthur (McArthur, McDermott et al., 2004)	2004	USA	MCP-1	C-S	371	71%	-	Levels did not differ across HAND-ART groups
Sevigny (Sevigny, Albert et al., 2004)	2004	USA	MCP-1	L	203	90%	21 months	Higher CSF levels associated with shorter times to HAND
Monteiro (Monteiro de Almeida, Letendre et al., 2005)	2005	USA	MCP-1	L	97	100%	90 days	Changes in CSF linked to changes in HIV RNA
Arendt (Arendt, Nolting et al., 2007)	2007	Germany	MCP-1	C-S	109	71%	-	Higher levels with ART and detectable HIV RNA in CSF
Cytokines & Chemokines Other than MCP-1								
Gendelman (Gendelman, Zheng et al., 1998)	1998	USA	TNF-α	L	1	100%	6 weeks	Levels declined with ART
Krivine (Krivine, Force et al., 1999)	1999	France	IFN-α	C-S	22	14%	-	Undetectable in all on ART
Enting (Enting, Foudraine et al., 2000)	2000	Netherlands	sTNFR-I, sTNFR-II	L	16	100%	12 weeks	Levels did not change during ART
Gisolf (Gisolf, van Praag et al., 2000)	2000	Netherlands	IP-10, sTNFR-II	L	23	100%	48 weeks	Levels rose in a subgroup on ART with suppressed HIV RNA
Ryan (Ryan, Zheng et al., 2001)	2001	USA	TNF-α, sTNFR-II	C-S	28	100%	1-35 months	Lower levels of sTNFR-II with longer ART durations
Sporer (Sporer, Kastenbauer et al., 2003)	2003	Germany	Fractalkine	L	1	100%	-	Levels decreased with ART
McArthur (McArthur, McDermott et al., 2004)	2004	USA	TNF-α	C-S	371	71%	-	Lower levels in plasma but not CSF with ART
Sevigny (Sevigny, Albert et al., 2004)	2004	USA	TNF-α	L	203	90%	21 months	Higher plasma levels associated with shorter times to HAND
Cinque (Cinque, Bestetti et al., 2005)	2005	Italy	IP-10	L	33	91%	12 weeks	Lower levels with ART with rises after interruption
Neurofilament-Light								
Gisslen (Gisslen, Rosengren et al., 2005)	2005	Sweden	NF-L	L	8	100%	-	Levels rose in 38% after ART interruption
Abdulle (Abdulle, Mellgren et al., 2007)	2007	Sweden	NF-L	L	4	100%	1-3 years	Levels declined with ART with neurocognitive improvement
Mellgren (Mellgren, Price et al., 2007)	2007	Sweden	NF-L	L	21	100%	1 year	Abnormal levels in 52% after 3 months of ART; 25% after 1 year

CSF Leukocytes

Reference	Year	Country	Biomarker	C-S/L	N	%	Duration	Finding
Neuenberg (Neuenberg, Furlan et al., 2005)	2005	USA	CD16+ Monocytes	C-S	76	100%	-	Highest levels in CSF with ART, especially with protease inhibitors
Neuenberg (Neuenberg, Cho et al., 2005)	2005	USA	CD38/HLA-DR CD45RA/CD62L	C-S	57	70%	-	Lower levels on ART but higher than seronegatives
Marra (Marra, Maxwell et al., 2007)	2007	USA	Leukocyte Count	L	50	66%	-	Abnormal levels were less common in ART users
Sinclair (Sinclair, Ronquillo et al., 2008)	2008	USA	CD8+ TC activation	C-S	123	57%	> 3 months	Lower levels with successful ART vs. failing ART or no ART

Other

Reference	Year	Country	Biomarker	C-S/L	N	%	Duration	Finding
Gulevich (Gulevich, McCutchan et al., 1993)	1994	USA	Quinolinic acid	C-S	145	100%	Variable	Similar levels with 46-365 days of ZDV vs. shorter or longer durations
Gendelman (Gendelman, Zheng et al., 1998)	1998	USA	Quinolinic acid	L	1	100%	6 weeks	Levels declined with ART
Valle (Valle, Price et al., 2004)	2004	USA	Quinolinic Acid	L	20	100%	< 1 year	Levels declined with ART with neurocognitive improvement
Pemberton (Pemberton & Brew, 2001)	2001	Australia	S100β	C-S	49	100%	-	High levels with more severe HAND despite ART
Woods (Woods, Iudicello et al., 2010)	2009	USA	S100β	C-S	74	74%	-	Higher levels with worse action fluency
Cinque (Cinque, Nebuloni et al., 2004)	2004	Italy	uPA, uPAR	L	16	100%	12 weeks	Declined with ART but did not normalize in all
Sporer (Sporer, Koedel et al., 2005)	2005	Germany	uPA, PdPA	L	1	100%	1 year	Declined with ART
Vittecoq (Vittecoq, Jardel et al., 2002)	2002	France	Lactate	C-S	6	100%	Variable	Abnormal levels in 67%
Arendt (Arendt, Nolting et al., 2007)	2007	Germany	Lactate, Gal3	C-S	109	71%	-	Higher Gal3 levels with ART and detectable HIV RNA in CSF
McArthur (McArthur, McDermott et al., 2004)	2004	USA	M-CSF	C-S	371	71%	-	Lower levels with ART & HAND
Sevigny (Sevigny, Albert et al., 2004)	2004	USA	M-CSF, MMP-2	L	203	90%	21 months	Not associated with time to HAND
Gisslen (Gisslen, Chiodi et al., 1994)	1994	Sweden	Tryptophan	L	14	100%	3-30 months	Levels rose with ART and decreases in neopterin
Ferrarese (Ferrarese, Aliprandi et al., 2001)	2001	Italy	Glutamate, Aspartate	C-S	30	-	-	Glutamate, but not aspartate, lower with ART
Sabri (Sabri, De Milito et al., 2001)	2001	Sweden	sFas, FasL	L	7	100%	3-5 months	Lower sFas levels with ART but FasL increased in 43%
Sporer (Sporer, Koedel et al., 2004)	2004	Germany	VEGF	L	2	100%	-	Declined with ART in serum but not CSF
Burdo (Burdo, Ellis et al., 2008)	2008	USA	Osteopontin	C-S	95	84%	-	Higher plasma levels with HAND

Host biomarkers varied in their response to antiretroviral therapy with some biomarkers normalizing with effective therapy but others either remaining elevated or rising later in therapy following an initial decline. The proportion using ART and the duration of ART could not be determined for all reports. L = Longitudinal, C-S = Cross-sectional, ART = Antiretroviral therapy elevations in serum are associated with HIV disease progression in vivo (Nockher, Bergmann et al., 1994; Lien, Aukrust et al., 1998). An important distinction compared with other markers of macrophage activation may be that, in the CNS, sCD14 may derive primarily from trafficking lymphocytes and monocytes, rather than native microglia (Cauwels, Frei et al., 1999). The importance of sCD14 has risen in recent years with the realization that HIV severely injures gut-associated lymphoid tissue, allowing bacteria to more easily enter the bloodstream (Brenchley et al., 2006). Bacterial products, such as lipopolysaccharides, bind to CD14 and are potent immune stimulants. Lipopolysaccharide concentrations in blood correlate with soluble CD14 concentrations and have been linked to HAND (Ancuta, Kamat et al., 2008).

In a study of neuropsychological performance, Ryan et al. (2001) reported that sCD14 concentrations were higher in plasma in impaired subjects taking combination antiretroviral therapy compared with unimpaired subjects who were also taking antiretrovirals. Since all subjects took antiretrovirals, the study estimated their effect on sCD14 concentrations by using the duration of antiretroviral use, identifying no relationship between longer durations of ART and lower sCD14 concentrations. In a cross-sectional analysis, we measured sCD14 in plasma and CSF specimens from subjects enrolled in a study of the effects of HIV and methamphetamine on neuropsychological performance. sCD14 was detectable in all HIV-infected participants and CSF concentrations (median, 5.13; interquartile range (IQR), 5.01–5.25 log10 pg/mL) were approximately 1 $\log_{10}$ lower than plasma (median, 6.26; IQR, 6.19–6.32 log10 pg/mL). In this cohort, antiretroviral therapy was not associated with lower sCD14 concentrations in CSF (5.11 versus 5.16; $p = 0.11$) or plasma (6.26 versus 6.24; $p = 0.71$) (unpublished data). In contrast, Gendelman et al. (1998) did find that combination therapy reduced sCD14 levels in plasma and CSF in an incident case of severe HAND.

Soluble CD14 may also have relevance to a theory of HIV neuropathogenesis that links HAND to subsets of activated monocytes, designated CD14[+]/CD16[+] and CD14[+]/CD69[+], that: originate in the bone marrow; expand with HIV infection (Thieblemont et al., 1995); are found in higher percentages in the peripheral blood of impaired individuals (Pulliam, Gascon et al., 1997); and may be more likely to migrate into the CNS (Gartner & Liu, 2002). In one study of subjects who were not neurocognitively characterized, those treated with antiretroviral therapy reduced the proportion of circulating CD16-expressing monocytes compared with untreated subjects (Amirayan-Chevillard et al., 2000). In another study, antiretroviral therapy reduced percentages of circulating CD14[+]/CD69[+] monocytes in subjects with HAND, compared with: (1) HIV-infected, antiretroviral-treated, nondemented subjects; and (2) HIV-infected, untreated subjects (Kusdra et al.,2002). These direct measurements of an activated population of circulating monocytes may be even more important than those of sCD14, an indirect measure.

CYTOKINES AND CHEMOKINES

Cytokines constitute a group of small proteins that have diverse pro-inflammatory and anti-inflammatory effects and are produced by many types of cells (Holland, 2001). Many cytokines have been implicated in neuroinflammatory disorders, including HIV encephalitis. We will focus on two groups of cytokines: tumor necrosis factor (TNF) super-family-related proteins (primarily TNF-α and soluble TNF receptors) and chemotactic cytokines (or chemokines) (primarily CC chemokines, such as MCP-1, macrophage inflammatory protein (MIP)-1 α and β, and RANTES (regulated upon activation, normal T-cell expressed and secreted).

Many of these proteins are produced by monocyte-derived cells ("monokines"), and so could also be considered markers of macrophage activation (Verani, Scarlatti et al., 1997). We chose to classify them separately for two reasons: (1) they function via pathways distinct from β2M, neopterin, and sCD14 and (2) they have a special role in HIV pathogenesis, particularly the chemokines. The overall scope of this section will again be limited by the chapter's focus on the effects of antiretrovirals.

TNF-α is a pro-inflammatory cytokine that is produced by activated macrophages and microglia and plays a central role in several disease processes, including HAND. For example, TNF-α's mRNA expression in brain and concentrations in CSF are elevated in subjects with HAD (Mastroianni et al., 1990; Mastroianni et al., 1992; Perrella et al., 1992; Achim et al., 1993; Ciardi et al., 1993; Wesselingh et al., 1994). This may be linked to TNF-α's ability to upregulate HIV replication (Zoumpourlis et al. 1992). However, in blood, TNF-α is rapidly cleared and so may be difficult to measure in this, and other, body fluids. The soluble TNF receptors, p55 (TNFR-I) and p75 (TNFR-II), are more easily measured than TNF-α itself (Hober et al., 1996) and their expression is linked to TNF-α. TNF receptors are expressed by microglia and oligodendrocytes and this expression is upregulated in the brains of AIDS patients (Sippy et al., 1995). Like TNF-α, soluble TNF receptor levels in CSF are also increased in subjects with HAD (Vullo et al., 1995).

Many studies have investigated the relationships between TNF-related proteins and HAND but far fewer have assessed the effects of antiretrovirals on these relationships. Two studies noted that either dual (Nokta et al., 1997) or combination therapy (Franco et al., 1999) reduced TNF-α and sTNFR-II concentrations in serum or plasma. We recently measured TNF-α and sTNFR-II in CSF and plasma from subjects enrolled in a study of the effects of HIV and methamphetamine on neuropsychological performance. As expected, most (143 of 197, 72%) CSF concentrations of TNF-α, but not sTNFR-II (eight of 197, 4%), were below the sensitivity of our assays. In a cross-sectional analysis, neither TNF-α nor sTNFR-II concentrations in CSF differed between those who reported antiretroviral use and those who did not. However, the CSF-to-plasma ratio of TNF-α was higher in those who took antiretrovirals, indicating that therapy may reduce plasma concentrations out of proportion to CSF concentrations.

No other studies have assessed the effect of antiretrovirals on TNF-α concentrations in CSF but some have assessed their effect on soluble TNF receptors. For example, in the same study in which Enting found that two NRTIs reduced β2M concentrations in CSF, they reported that treatment did not reduce sTNFR-II concentrations in CSF but they were below detection in most participants at baseline (Enting, Foudraine et al., 2000). In contrast, another study reported that 48 weeks of antiretroviral therapy may have reduced sTNFR-II concentrations in CSF below detectable (15 of 26 (58%) before treatment versus 11 of 13 (85%) after treatment; $p = 0.09$; one-sided Fisher's Exact Test; Gisolf, van Praag et al., 2000). This report also noted that, in one participant, CSF sTNFR-II levels increased between weeks 12 and 48, even while HIV RNA in CSF and sTNFR-II in serum were undetectable. This is a very important finding since it indicates that monocyte-derived cells may reactivate in the CNS despite otherwise successful therapy.

Other TNF-related markers have been implicated in HIV neuropathogenesis. For example, HAND is associated with two apoptosis-inducing proteins, Fas ligand (FasL) and TRAIL (TNF-related apoptosis-inducing ligand). FasL is upregulated in brain tissue from HIV-infected individuals (Elovaara et al., 1999) and may play a critical role in astrocyte death (Saas et al., 1997). However, in a murine model, TRAIL was associated with neuronal apoptosis but FasL was not ((Miura et al., 2003). Data on TRAIL in CSF are sparse but FasL is elevated in CSF (Sporer et al., 2000; Towfighi et al., 2004) and correlates with HIV RNA levels in CSF (Sabri et al., 2001) in HIV-infected, cognitively impaired subjects. Sporer noted that 26 of 56 (46%) subjects took antiretrovirals but did not report whether treatment was associated with a difference in FasL concentrations. However, Sabri reported that FasL concentrations declined, in parallel with HIV RNA, in the CSF of seven subjects following 3–5 months of antiretroviral therapy.

Chemokines are cytokines that have the specific function of attracting cells towards their signal (chemotaxis). Chemokines assumed particular importance when their receptors, primarily CCR5 and CXCR4, were shown to be used by HIV for cell entry. CCR5 is expressed on several cell types, including lymphocytes, monocytes, and microglia, and is used by monocyte-tropic HIV strains. CXCR4 is also expressed on several cell types, including lymphocytes and neurons, and is used by T cell-tropic HIV strains. Chemokine pathways seem to be instrumental in neural development and have been implicated in other neuroinflammatory disease processes.

We measured concentrations of the CCR5 ligands, MIP-1α, MIP-1β, and RANTES in 73 neurocognitively characterized subjects. All three were elevated in the CSF of subjects with HAND but did not seem to be affected by current antiretroviral use (Letendre, Lanier et al., 1999). Kelder et al. (1998) confirmed that RANTES was elevated in the CSF of subjects with dementia and showed that MCP-1 was selectively increased in the CSF of demented individuals, compared with those diagnosed with other neuroinflammatory disorders. Antiretroviral use was not explicitly addressed in this report, though.

In contrast to these retrospective cohort-based studies, we prospectively analyzed the effects of 12 weeks of individualized antiretroviral therapy on immune marker changes in 12 neurocognitively impaired individuals. We found that: MIP-1β clearly declined in CSF in response to 12 weeks of therapy (mean difference, −69 pg/mL; $p = 0.009$; matched pairs 2-way t-test); RANTES in CSF may have declined (mean difference, −13 pg/mL; $p = 0.09$); but MIP-1α and MCP-1 did not. Using more intensive sampling over a shorter period of time, we recently showed that antiretrovirals do reduce MCP-1 levels in CSF and that this decline seems to be linked to reductions in HIV RNA (Monteiro de Almeida et al., 2005).

Two studies previously cited in this review also reported on antiretroviral therapy and MCP-1 levels. Enting et al. (2000) found that MCP-1 levels in CSF did not change in response to dual therapy. However, MCP-1 levels in cases were similar to controls, indicating that MCP-1 levels may not have been elevated at baseline. Gisolf et al. (2000) also found that MCP-1 levels in CSF were similar to those in controls at baseline but showed that levels declined during the first 8 weeks of treatment. By 48 weeks, however, MCP-1 increased in the CSF of almost all participants, even when HIV RNA remained suppressed. De Luca et al. (2002) recently confirmed this finding when they found that elevated MCP-1 levels in the CSF of subjects with neurological disorders were not reduced by antiretrovirals. In fact, MCP-1 levels greater than 1 ng/mL at baseline were independently associated with failure to reduce HIV RNA below 100 copies/mL at follow-up, suggesting that high levels of neuroinflammation may reduce antiretroviral effectiveness in the CNS. Since MCP-1 seems to be strongly associated with HIV-associated dementia (Gonzalez et al., 2002), the failure of antiretroviral therapy to normalize MCP-1 concentrations in CSF has important implications.

Many other chemokines have been implicated in HIV neuropathogenesis, including fractalkine (Pereira et al., 2001; Cotter et al., 2002) and the CXC chemokines, SDF-1 (Kaul & Lipton, 1999) and IP-10 (Sanders et al., 1998; Kolb et al., 1999). In contrast to TNF-α and MCP-1, few studies have reported CSF concentrations of these chemokines and fewer still have reported the effects of antiretroviral therapy. Sporer et al. (2003) did report that fractalkine declined in CSF, but not in serum, following initiation of antiretrovirals in one demented patient. Gisolf's study also reported that, similarly to MCP-1, IP-10 seemed to increase in CSF after 48 weeks of therapy.

NEUROFILAMENT-LIGHT

As discussed above, a panel of biomarkers consisting of a viral biomarker, an immune activation biomarker, and a neuronal biomarker may be needed to diagnose HAND. The light subunit of the neurofilament protein—or neurofilament-light (NF-L)—is a major structural component of myelinated axons, is a leading candidate for a neuronal biomarker in HAND. NF-L concentrations in CSF may be a sensitive marker of axonal damage in ischemic and neurodegenerative conditions (Gisslen, Rosengren et al., 2005). Neuronal damage from acute ischemia is evident as a leakage of NF-L into the CSF proportional to the severity of the injury (Rosen et al., 2004). NF-L is also elevated in chronic disorders with white matter injury, such as multiple sclerosis (Malmestrom et al., 2003). Vascular dementia is also associated with moderately elevated NF-L levels in CSF (Rosengren et al., 1999).

The Sahlgrenska group with their colleagues in San Francisco, Milan, and Sydney has performed the NF-L work in HIV disease thus far, showing that higher NF-L levels are higher in individuals with HAND than in neuroasymptomatic controls. They have also shown a dose effect, with higher concentrations in individuals with more severe HAND compared to individuals with mild HAND. They also demonstrated that antiretroviral therapy reduces NF-L concentrations and that these reductions correlate with neurocognitive improvement (Abdulle, Mellgren et al., 2007; Mellgren, Price et al., 2007). Finally, they identified that NF-L levels rose with interruption of antiretroviral therapy (Gisslen et al., 2005). This high standard of evidence for association has been met by few if any other biomarkers, although the research ideally should be confirmed by an independent source before NF-L can be recommended as a biomarker with potential clinical utility.

EXCITOTOXINS

In 1995, Lipton and Gendelman published a seminal overview of AIDS neuropathogenesis (Lipton & Gendelman, 1995). In this review, the authors speculated that the final common pathway of neuronal injury in AIDS involved the overactivation of two kinds of calcium ion channels: voltage-dependent channels and NMDA receptors. NMDA receptors are a subtype of the glutamate receptors that mediate excitatory neurotransmission in the brain. Toxins synthesized by activated macrophages overstimulate these receptors, causing increased levels of intraneuronal calcium. As a result, the cell releases glutamate. Glutamate then overexcites neighboring neurons, further increasing the concentration of intracellular calcium. This, in turn, produces neuronal injury and leads to the release of more glutamate. To assess excitotoxic stimuli in vivo, investigators have measured glutamate or quinolinic acid in CSF. Quinolinic acid is an endogenous NMDA receptor agonist that is synthesized from L-tryptophan via the kynurenine pathway and may mediate excitotoxic neuronal injury.

Ferrarese et al. (1997) first reported that glutamate concentrations were elevated in the CSF of patients with HAND. Contrary evidence from our center was published later that year by Espey et al. (1999). Despite this conflicting report, Ferrarese later confirmed that glutamate concentrations were elevated five-fold in patients with HAND, compared with normal subjects, those with Alzheimer's dementia, or those

with other neurological disorders (Ferrarese et al., 2001). In this report, Ferrarese also reported lower CSF glutamate levels in subjects who were taking antiretrovirals, primarily mono- or dual-therapy.

Even earlier than these reports of glutamate, Heyes et al. (Heyes, Brew et al., 1991; Heyes, Lackner et al., 1991) reported that HIV-infected individuals had high concentrations of quinolinic acid in CSF. In this early study, CSF concentrations of quinolinic acid correlated with those of β2M and neopterin, linking this excitotoxin to macrophage activation. Quinolinic acid concentrations are also elevated in brain tissue from patients dying with AIDS (Achim, Heyes et al., 1993) and correlate with HIV RNA levels in CSF (Staprans et al., 1999; Heyes et al., 2001). In 1994, our group did not find a cross-sectional association between quinolinic acid levels in CSF and the use of zidovudine (Gulevich, McCutchan et al., 1993). Brouwers et al. (1993) confirmed that quinolinic acid was also elevated in children with HIV encephalopathy and, in a longitudinal analysis, found that zidovudine reduced quinolinic acid in CSF. In a well-documented case of incident dementia, Gendelman et al. (1998) documented a substantial decline in quinolinic acid in CSF and plasma following 6 weeks of combined antiretroviral and anti-inflammatory therapies. Finally, Valle et al. (2004) performed cross-sectional (N = 62) and longitudinal (N = 20) analyses of quinolinic acid levels, with kinetic modeling of quinolinic acid changes in those starting antiretroviral therapy in the longitudinal component. The kinetic modeling identified that antiretroviral therapy reduced quinolinic acid levels and that these reductions were linked more strongly to reductions in HIV RNA levels in CSF than to reductions in quinolinic acid levels in blood. In a subset of three individuals with HAND, declines in quinolinic acid also paralleled improvements in neurocognitive performance.

Together, these findings support the hypothesis that antiretrovirals reduce excitotoxins in CSF, which is not surprising since they may be linked to HIV replication and macrophage activation, which are also reduced by antiretroviral treatment.

BLOOD–BRAIN BARRIER INTEGRITY AND ENDOTHELIAL ACTIVATION

The best known measure of BBB integrity is CSF albumin, commonly operationalized as a ratio to serum albumin concentrations or a gradient that accounts for immunoglobulin G (IgG) concentrations. CSF and serum albumin concentrations have also been used as a method of standardizing concentrations of other biomarkers. Most reports that assessed CSF albumin levels in people with HAND preceded the widespread availability of potent antiretroviral therapy. For example, Elovaara et al. (1987) reported that the albumin ratio was slightly increased in patients with neurological "deficits." In 1991, Marshall et al. reported that the albumin ratio increased over time in a cohort of 124 neuroasymptomatic individuals (Marshall et al., 1991). The following year, Hall et al. (1992) reported that "disturbances" in the albumin ratio in 30% of 59 subjects were greater in those with more advanced HIV disease. Singer et al. (1994) confirmed this finding in 139 subjects. In 2001, Andersson et al. (2001) reported increased albumin ratios in only 15% of 110 neurosymptomatic, HIV-infected subjects but none of the subjects were taking antiretrovirals. Four years later, Abdulle et al (2005) reported that CSF albumin concentrations were normal in 38 neuroasymptomatic individuals after 2 years of antiretroviral therapy, although IgG concentrations remained abnormal in 41%.

Matrix metalloproteinases (MMPs) are a family of neutral proteases that are important in normal development and have been implicated in many pathological processes, including neuroinflammation. In the CNS, MMPs can degrade components of the basal lamina, leading to disruption of the BBB (Rosenberg, 2002). Sporer et al. (1998) found that active MMP-9 was detected more frequently in HIV-infected subjects with neurological deficits or CNS opportunistic infections and was associated with higher CSF-to-serum albumin ratios. Conant et al. (1999) confirmed that MMP-9 (along with MMP-2) activity was more frequently detectable in the CSF of subjects with HIV dementia (9/16), compared with nondemented seropositive (2/11) or seronegative (0/11) controls. Liuzzi et al. (2000) reconfirmed this finding more recently in 138 HIV-infected individuals. None of these studies explicitly addressed the effects of antiretrovirals on MMPs, however.

HIV gp120 and pro-inflammatory cytokines can upregulate adhesion molecules on the luminal surface of brain microvascular endothelial cells ((Huang & Jong, 2001)). One such molecule is intercellular adhesion molecule (ICAM)-1. Rieckmann et al. (1993) measured a soluble form of ICAM-1 (sICAM-1) in CSF, finding that levels were higher in patients with bacterial meningitis or multiple sclerosis than in HIV seropositive subjects and were associated with a damaged BBB. Heidenreich et al. (1994) compared sICAM-1 levels in HIV seropositive patients to a different group (HIV seronegative patients without neuroinflammatory disorders) and found that CSF levels were, in fact, higher among HIV seropositive patients. The highest levels were found in serum from patients with "HIV encephalopathy." Neither report specifically addressed the effects of antiretrovirals on sICAM-1 levels in CSF, but Wolf et al. (2002) reported that combination antiretroviral treatment reduced plasma markers of endothelial activation, including sICAM-1.

OTHER SELECTED MARKERS

Many other pathways have been implicated in HIV neuropathogenesis by basic neuroscience experiments and animal studies. As a result, clinical investigators have measured other biomarkers in patient-derived specimens in an attempt to validate these findings. Similar to other biomarkers, though, most studies have focused on the relationships between each biomarker and the CNS rather than on the effects of antiretroviral therapy on the biomarker.

S100β

Astrocytes are the most abundant cell type in the CNS and have many functions, including neuronal support and maintenance of the BBB (Brack-Werner, 1999). Astrocytes have high concentrations of S100β, a low molecular weight acidic calcium-binding protein that is associated with neurodegenerative disorders. Green et al. (1999) found that patients with CNS infections, but not HAND, had higher S100β concentrations in CSF than HIV-uninfected controls but did not explicitly address the antiretroviral effect. Pemberton and Brew (2001) reported that S100β levels in CSF were higher in HIV-infected individuals with either more advanced or more rapidly progressive HAND. Unfortunately, the authors could not comment on a treatment effect since all participants were taking antiretrovirals. In a recent study from our group (Woods et al., 2010), we also did not report the impact of antiretroviral therapy on S100β levels. Performing a post-hoc cross-sectional analysis, though, identifies that individuals who took antiretrovirals (n = 53) had similar S100β concentrations in CSF as those who did not (n = 18) (mean 1.05 vs. 0.98 pg/mL, p = 0.65).

INTERFERONS

Early studies identified that concentrations of interferon (IFN)-γ in CSF were higher in HIV-infected than -uninfected controls (Fuchs et al., 1990; Griffin et al., 1991). Later, Rho et al. (1995) reported that IFN-α was elevated in individuals with HAND, compared with HIV-infected individuals without HAND and HIV-uninfected controls. This was subsequently confirmed by Krivine et al. (1999) and Perrella et al. (2001). In the Krivine study, all subjects taking antiretroviral therapy had undetectable IFN-α concentrations in CSF (0/3) compared with 42% (8/19) of subjects taking no therapy or less potent regimens ($p = 0.16$; Pearson chi square).

OXIDATIVE STRESS

Interferon-γ can induce the expression of nitric oxide synthase (NOS) and the subsequent production of nitric oxide (NO) by astrocytes. Superoxide anions react with NO to yield neurotoxic substances, such as peroxynitrite (Lipton & Gendelman, 1995). Two studies identified high levels of inducible nitric oxide synthase in brain tissue from patients dying with AIDS dementia (Rostasy, Monti et al., 1999), particularly those with rapidly progressive disease (Adamson, McArthur et al., 1999). Giovannoni et al. (1998) measured nitrate and nitrite in CSF, finding higher levels in 24 AIDS patients with CNS complications, compared to HIV-uninfected individuals with neuroinflammatory disorders. In the previously cited case of incident HAND, Gendelman et al. (1998) found that antiretroviral therapy reduced NO levels in CSF, along with TNF-α and quinolinic acid. Finally, Murr et al. (2002) hypothesized that neopterin may be a marker of reactive oxygen species. Since antiretrovirals frequently lower neopterin levels, they may also reduce oxidative stress.

PLATELET-ACTIVATING FACTOR

IFN-γ can also induce a variety of cells to produce platelet-activating factor (PAF), a phospholipid that modulates several CNS processes (Maclennan, Smith et al., 1996). Experimental data support the importance of PAF in HIV neuropathogenesis (Nottet et al., 1995; Nishida et al., 1996; Perry et al., 1998; Pulliam, Zhou et al., 1998; Persidsky, Limoges et al., 2001; Smith et al., 2001). In vivo, Gelbard et al. (1994) found that immunosuppressed patients with CNS "dysfunction" had high levels of PAF in CSF. Combined, these findings were compelling enough to lead to a clinical trial of a PAF antagonist, lexipafant, which seemed to improve neuropsychological test scores (Schifitto et al., 1999). No studies have investigated the effect of antiretrovirals on PAF concentrations, but Khovidhunkit et al. (Khovidhunkit, Memon et al., 1999) did report that initiation of a new antiretroviral regimen did not reduce PAF activity in plasma, despite successful suppression of HIV RNA.

SUMMARY AND CONCLUSIONS

Integrating the findings of such a large number of diverse studies is challenging. In general, though, the data are reasonably consistent: effective antiretroviral therapy reduces viral and host biomarkers in the CSF of most individuals. This is especially true when antiretroviral therapy is effective (i.e., when it suppresses HIV replication below the detection limit of commercial assays) in individuals who have early-stage disease and normal neurocognitive performance.

Unfortunately, antiretroviral therapy does not durably reduce all viral and host biomarkers in all individuals. For example, on the basis of information presented in this review, we might conclude the following.

- Didanosine reduces HIV replication in the CNS less effectively than zidovudine.

- Combining two nucleoside reverse transcriptase inhibitors reduces HIV replication below detection in most, if not all, individuals.

- Poorly penetrating protease inhibitors reduce HIV replication in the CNS more slowly than nucleoside reverse transcriptase inhibitors.

- A small proportion of antiretroviral-treated individuals will have HIV RNA levels above the lower limit of quantitation in CSF when they are below the lower limit of quantitation in plasma.

- Antiretrovirals may reduce HIV replication in the CNS less effectively in individuals with worse immune suppression or with HAND.

- Antiretrovirals may continue to suppress HIV RNA in CSF even when they fail to do so in plasma.

- Effective antiretroviral therapy may not consistently normalize markers of macrophage activation (e.g. as measured by neopterin or soluble TNF receptors).

- Even when effective therapy initially reduces neuroinflammation (e.g. as measured by IP-10 or MCP-1), it may recur again months later, possibly reflecting low-level HIV replication in the brain or mild immune recovery disease.

The primary research implication of these conclusions is that future patient-based studies of HIV neuropathogenesis should carefully control for antiretroviral use since it can have potent effects on HIV replication and cellular activation in people living with HIV. Extensive antiretroviral use among study participants may broadly reduce viral and host biomarkers, which may adversely affect a study's power. In fact, concentrations of some host biomarkers seem to be lower among recent study cohorts compared with earlier reports. For example, in a pre-HAART cohort, Brew et al. (1996) found that β2M concentrations greater than 5 mg/L were associated with a 17-fold increased risk of HAND. However, participants in Schifitto et al.'s (1999) study of lexipafant had much lower concentrations than this (mean ~2.3 mg/L). Similarly, in a study of the investigational drug CPI-1189, we found that neurocognitively impaired participants had lower than expected concentrations of several inflammatory markers. Another important observation from this trial, with implications for research, is the retrospective identification of imbalances at baseline between treatment arms in concentrations of host biomarkers in CSF (Clifford et al., 2002). Such imbalances between treatment arms in neuroinflammation, or antiretroviral use, could bias the findings of HAND-focused clinical trials. Future clinical trials of the effectiveness of neuroprotective or anti-inflammatory therapies in people with HAND should consider incorporating at least two biomarker-focused elements into their designs. First, trials should make additional efforts to ensure balanced antiretroviral use and viral and host biomarker concentrations between arms (e.g., adaptive randomization). Second, at enrollment, trials may want to ensure that participants have abnormal levels of the biomarkers that are linked to the pathways modulated by the study drug (e.g., elevated levels of oxidative stress biomarkers in a trial of an antioxidant).

The primary clinical implication of these conclusions is that measurement of viral and host biomarkers may have a role in determining risk for and treatment of HAND. For example, higher than expected levels of HIV RNA, MCP-1, neopterin, and NF-L in CSF in a neuroasymptomatic individual may indicate an increased risk for incident HAND, which may then dictate increased surveillance and perhaps preventive therapy. For the time being, the only preventive therapy appears to treatment with antiretrovirals that reach therapeutic concentrations in the CNS. Once an at-risk patient is treated with antiretrovirals, continued or recurrent elevations of neuroinflammatory or neurodegenerative biomarkers in CSF may indicate a need for antiretroviral intensification or anti-inflammatory or neuroprotective therapy. For patients with neurocognitive impairment without evidence of inflammation, other etiologies may be sought (e.g., comorbidities, such as recreational drug or alcohol use), which may then indicate the need for other interventions.

ACKNOWLEDGMENTS

This chapter was supported by the following grants: P30-MH62512 from the National Institute of Mental Health, U01-MH83506 from the National Institute of Mental Health, and N01-MH22005 from the National Institute of Mental Health (NIMH) and National Institute of Neurological Disorders and Stroke (NINDS).

REFERENCES

Abdulle, S., Hagberg, L., et al. (2005). Effects of antiretroviral treatment on blood-brain barrier integrity and intrathecal immunoglobulin production in neuroasymptomatic HIV-1-infected patients. *HIV Med, 6*(3), 164–169.

Abdulle, S., Hagberg, L., et al. (2002). Continuing intrathecal immunoactivation despite two years of effective antiretroviral therapy against HIV-1 infection. *AIDS, 16*(16), 2145–2149.

Abdulle, S., Mellgren, A., et al. (2007). CSF neurofilament protein (NFL)—a marker of active HIV-related neurodegeneration. *J Neurol, 254*(8), 1026–1032.

Achim, C. L., Heyes, M. P., et al. (1993). Quantitation of human immunodeficiency virus, immune activation factors, and quinolinic acid in AIDS brains. *J Clin Invest, 91*(6), 2769–2775.

Adamson, D. C., McArthur, J. C., et al. (1999). Rate and severity of HIV-associated dementia (HAD): Correlations with Gp41 and iNOS. *Mol Med, 5*(2), 98–109.

Amirayan-Chevillard, N., Tissot-Dupont, H., et al. (2000). Impact of highly active anti-retroviral therapy (HAART) on cytokine production and monocyte subsets in HIV-infected patients. *Clin Exp Immunol, 120*(1), 107–112.

Ancuta, P., Kamat, A., et al. (2008). Microbial translocation is associated with increased monocyte activation and dementia in AIDS patients. *PLoS One, 3*(6), e2516.

Andersson, L. M., Hagberg, L., et al. (2001). Increased blood-brain barrier permeability in neuro-asymptomatic HIV-1-infected individuals—correlation with cerebrospinal fluid HIV-1 RNA and neopterin levels. *J Neurovirol, 7*(6), 542–547.

Andersson, L. M., Svennerholm, B., et al. (2000). Higher HIV-1 RNA cutoff level required in cerebrospinal fluid than in blood to predict positive HIV-1 isolation. *J Med Virol, 62*(1), 9–13.

Antinori, A., Giancola, M. L., et al. (2002). Factors influencing virological response to antiretroviral drugs in cerebrospinal fluid of advanced HIV-1-infected patients. *AIDS, 16*(14), 1867–1876.

Arendt, G., Nolting, T., et al. (2007). Intrathecal viral replication and cerebral deficits in different stages of human immunodeficiency virus disease. *J Neurovirol, 13*(3), 225–232.

Bestetti, A., Presi, S., et al. (2004). Long-term virological effect of highly active antiretroviral therapy on cerebrospinal fluid and relationship with genotypic resistance. *J Neurovirol, 10* Suppl 1, 52–57.

Bogner, J. R., Junge-Hulsing, B., et al. (1992). Expansion of neopterin and beta 2-microglobulin in cerebrospinal fluid reaches maximum levels early and late in the course of human immunodeficiency virus infection. *Clin Investig, 70*(8), 665–669.

Brack-Werner, R. (1999). Astrocytes: HIV cellular reservoirs and important participants in neuropathogenesis. *AIDS, 13*(1), 1–22.

Brenchley, J. M., Price, D. A., et al. (2006). Microbial translocation is a cause of systemic immune activation in chronic HIV infection. *Nat Med, 12*(12). 1365–1371.

Brew, B. J., Bhalla, R. B., et al. (1990). Cerebrospinal fluid neopterin in human immunodeficiency virus type 1 infection. *Ann Neurol, 28*(4), 556–560.

Brew, B. J., Bhalla, R. B., et al. (1992). Cerebrospinal fluid beta 2-microglobulin in patients with AIDS dementia complex: An expanded series including response to zidovudine treatment. *AIDS, 6*(5), 461–465.

Brew, B. J., Dunbar, N., et al. (1996). Predictive markers of AIDS dementia complex: CD4 cell count and cerebrospinal fluid concentrations of beta 2-microglobulin and neopterin. *J Infect Dis, 174*(2), 294–298.

Brouwers, P., Heyes, M. P., et al. (1993). Quinolinic acid in the cerebrospinal fluid of children with symptomatic human immunodeficiency virus type 1 disease: Relationships to clinical status and therapeutic response. *J Infect Dis, 168*(6), 1380–1386.

Burdo, T. H., Ellis, R. J., et al. (2008). Osteopontin is increased in HIV-associated dementia. *J Infect Dis, 198*(5), 715–722.

Cameron, D. W., Japour, A. J., et al. (1999). Ritonavir and saquinavir combination therapy for the treatment of HIV infection. *AIDS, 13*(2), 213–224.

Canestri, A., Lescure, F. X., et al. (2010). Discordance between cerebral spinal fluid and plasma HIV replication in patients with neurological symptoms who are receiving suppressive antiretroviral therapy. *Clin Infect Dis, 50*(5), 773–778.

Carrieri, P. B., Indaco, A., et al. (1992). Cerebrospinal fluid beta-2-microglobulin in multiple sclerosis and AIDS dementia complex. *Neurol Res, 14*(3), 282–283.

Cauwels, A., Frei, K., et al. (1999). The origin and function of soluble CD14 in experimental bacterial meningitis. *J Immunol, 162*(8), 4762–4772.

Chang, L., Ernst, T., et al. (2004). Antiretroviral treatment alters relationship between MCP-1 and neurometabolites in HIV patients. *Antivir Ther, 9*(3), 431–440.

Chang, L., Ernst, T., et al. (2003). Persistent brain abnormalities in antiretroviral-naive HIV patients 3 months after HAART. *Antivir Ther, 8*(1), 17–26.

Ciardi, M., Sharief, M. K., et al. (1993). Intrathecal synthesis of interleukin-2 and soluble IL-2 receptor in asymptomatic HIV-1 seropositive individuals. Correlation with local production of specific IgM and IgG antibodies. *J Neurol Sci, 115*(1), 117–122.

Cinque, P., Bestetti, A., et al. (2005). Cerebrospinal fluid interferon-gamma-inducible protein 10 (IP-10, CXCL10) in HIV-1 infection. *J Neuroimmunol, 168*(1-2), 154–163.

Cinque, P., Nebuloni, M., et al. (2004). The urokinase receptor is overexpressed in the AIDS dementia complex and other neurological manifestations. *Ann Neurol, 55*(5), 687–694.

Cinque, P., Presi, S., et al. (2001). Effect of genotypic resistance on the virological response to highly active antiretroviral therapy in cerebrospinal fluid. *AIDS Res Hum Retroviruses, 17*(5), 377–383.

Conant, K., McArthur, J. C., et al. (1999). Cerebrospinal fluid levels of MMP-2, 7, and 9 are elevated in association with human immunodeficiency virus dementia. *Ann Neurol, 46*(3), 391–398.

Corti, M. E., Villafane, M. F., et al. (2001). [Cerebrospinal fluid viral load in HIV-1 positive hemophilic patients treated with HAART]. *Medicina (B Aires), 61*(6), 821–824.

Cotter, R., Williams, C., et al. (2002). Fractalkine (CX3CL1) and brain inflammation: Implications for HIV-1-associated dementia. *J Neurovirol, 8*(6), 585–598.

Cysique, L. A., Brew, B. J., et al. (2005). Undetectable cerebrospinal fluid HIV RNA and beta-2 microglobulin do not indicate inactive AIDS dementia complex in highly active antiretroviral therapy-treated patients. *J Acquir Immune Defic Syndr, 39*(4), 426–429.

Cysique, L. A., Vaida, F., et al. (2009). Dynamics of cognitive change in impaired HIV-positive patients initiating antiretroviral therapy. *Neurology, 73*(5), 342–348.

De Luca, A., Ciancio, B. C., et al. (2002). Correlates of independent HIV-1 replication in the CNS and of its control by antiretrovirals. *Neurology, 59*(3), 342–347.

Eden, A., Price, R. W., et al. (2007). Immune activation of the central nervous system is still present after >4 years of effective highly active antiretroviral therapy. *J Infect Dis, 196*(12), 1779–1783.

Eggers, C., Hertogs, K., et al. (2003). Delayed central nervous system virus suppression during highly active antiretroviral therapy is associated with HIV encephalopathy, but not with viral drug resistance or poor central nervous system drug penetration. *AIDS, 17*(13), 1897–1906.

Eggers, C., Stellbrink, H. J., et al. (1999). Quantification of JC virus DNA in the cerebrospinal fluid of patients with human immunodeficiency virus-associated progressive multifocal leukoencephalopathy—a longitudinal study. *J Infect Dis, 180*(5), 1690–1694.

Eggers, C., Stuerenburg, H. J., et al. (2000). Rapid clearance of human immunodeficiency virus type 1 from ventricular cerebrospinal fluid during antiretroviral treatment. *Ann Neurol, 47*(6), 816–819.

Eggers, C. C., van Lunzen, J., et al. (1999). HIV infection of the central nervous system is characterized by rapid turnover of viral RNA in cerebrospinal fluid. *J Acquir Immune Defic Syndr Hum Retrovirol, 20*(3), 259–264.

Ellis, R., Langford, T. D., et al. (2007). HIV and antiretroviral therapy in the brain: Neuronal injury and repair. *Nat Rev Neurosci, 8*, 33–44.

Ellis, R. J., Gamst, A. C., et al. (2000). Cerebrospinal fluid HIV RNA originates from both local CNS and systemic sources. *Neurology, 54*(4), 927–936.

Elovaara, I., Iivanainen, M., et al. (1989). CSF and serum beta-2-microglobulin in HIV infection related to neurological dysfunction. *Acta Neurol Scand, 79*(2), 81–87.

Elovaara, I., Iivanainen, M., et al. (1987). CSF protein and cellular profiles in various stages of HIV infection related to neurological manifestations. *J Neurol Sci, 78*(3), 331–342.

Elovaara, I. & Muller, K. M. (1993). Cytoimmunological abnormalities in cerebrospinal fluid in early stages of HIV-1 infection often precede changes in blood. *J Neuroimmunol, 44*(2), 199–204.

Elovaara, I., Poutiainen, E., et al. (1994). Zidovudine reduces intrathecal immunoactivation in patients with early human immunodeficiency virus type 1 infection. *Arch Neurol, 51*(9), 943–950.

Elovaara, I., Sabri, F., et al. (1999). Upregulated expression of Fas and Fas ligand in brain through the spectrum of HIV-1 infection. *Acta Neuropathol, 98*(4), 355–362.

Enting, R. H., Foudraine, N. A., et al. (2000). Cerebrospinal fluid beta2-microglobulin, monocyte chemotactic protein-1, and soluble tumour necrosis factor alpha receptors before and after treatment with lamivudine plus zidovudine or stavudine. *J Neuroimmunol, 102*(2), 216–221.

Enting, R. H., Prins, J. M., et al. (2001). Concentrations of human immunodeficiency virus type 1 (HIV-1) RNA in cerebrospinal fluid after antiretroviral treatment initiated during primary HIV-1 infection. *Clin Infect Dis, 32*(7), 1095–1099.

Espey, M. G., Ellis, R. J., et al. (1999). Relevance of glutamate levels in the CSF of patients with HIV-1-associated dementia complex. *Neurology, 53*(5), 1144–1145.

Ferrarese, C., Aliprandi, A., et al. (2001). Increased glutamate in CSF and plasma of patients with HIV dementia. *Neurology, 57*(4), 671–675.

Ferrarese, C., Riva, R., et al. (1997). Elevated glutamate in the cerebrospinal fluid of patients with HIV dementia. *JAMA, 277*(8), 630.

Foudraine, N. A., Hoetelmans, R. M., et al. (1998). Cerebrospinal-fluid HIV-1 RNA and drug concentrations after treatment with lamivudine plus zidovudine or stavudine. *Lancet, 351*(9115), 1547–1551.

Foudraine, N. A., Jurriaans, S. et al. (2001). Durable HIV-1 suppression with indinavir after failing lamivudine-containing double nucleoside therapy: A randomized controlled trial. *Antivir Ther, 6*(1), 55–62.

Franco, J. M., Rubio, A., et al. (1999). Reduction of immune system activation in HIV-1-infected patients undergoing highly active antiretroviral therapy. *Eur J Clin Microbiol Infect Dis, 18*(10), 733–736.

Fuchs, D., Chiodi, F., et al. (1989). Neopterin concentrations in cerebrospinal fluid and serum of individuals infected with HIV-1. *AIDS, 3*(5), 285–288.

Fuchs, D., Forsman, A., et al. (1990). Immune activation and decreased tryptophan in patients with HIV-1 infection. *J Interferon Res, 10*(6), 599–603.

Garcia, F., Alonso, M. M., et al. (2000). Comparison of immunologic restoration and virologic response in plasma, tonsillar tissue, and cerebrospinal fluid in HIV-1-infected patients treated with double versus triple antiretroviral therapy in very early stages: The Spanish EARTH-2 Study. Early Anti-Retroviral Therapy Study. *J Acquir Immune Defic Syndr, 25*(1), 26–35.

Garcia, F., Romeu, J., et al. (1999). A randomized study comparing triple versus double antiretroviral therapy or no treatment in HIV-1-infected patients in very early stage disease: The Spanish Earth-1 study. *AIDS, 13*(17), 2377–2388.

Gartner, S. & Liu, Y. (2002). Insights into the role of immune activation in HIV neuropathogenesis. *J Neurovirol, 8*(2), 69–75.

Gelbard, H. A., Nottet, H. S., et al. (1994). Platelet-activating factor: a candidate human immunodeficiency virus type 1-induced neurotoxin. *J Virol, 68*(7), 4628–4635.

Gendelman, H. E., Zheng, J., et al. (1998). Suppression of inflammatory neurotoxins by highly active antiretroviral therapy in human immunodeficiency virus-associated dementia. *J Infect Dis, 178*(4), 1000–1007.

Giovannoni, G., Miller, R. F., et al. (1998). Elevated cerebrospinal fluid and serum nitrate and nitrite levels in patients with central nervous system complications of HIV-1 infection: A correlation with blood-brain-barrier dysfunction. *J Neurol Sci, 156*(1), 53–58.

Gisolf, E. H., Enting, R. H., et al. (2000). Cerebrospinal fluid HIV-1 RNA during treatment with ritonavir/saquinavir or ritonavir/saquinavir/stavudine. *AIDS, 14*(11) 1583–1589.

Gisolf, E. H., van Praag, R. M., et al. (2000). Increasing cerebrospinal fluid chemokine concentrations despite undetectable cerebrospinal fluid HIV RNA in HIV-1-infected patients receiving antiretroviral therapy. *J Acquir Immune Defic Syndr, 25*(5), 426–433.

Gisslen, M., Chiodi, F., et al. (1994). Markers of immune stimulation in the cerebrospinal fluid during HIV infection: A longitudinal study. *Scand J Infect Dis, 26*(5), 523–533.

Gisslen, M., Hagberg, L., et al. (1997). HIV-1 RNA is not detectable in the cerebrospinal fluid during antiretroviral combination therapy. *AIDS, 11*(9) 1194.

Gisslen, M., Norkrans, G., et al. (1997). The effect on human immunodeficiency virus type 1 RNA levels in cerebrospinal fluid after initiation of zidovudine or didanosine. *J Infect Dis, 175*(2), 434–437.

Gisslen, M., Rosengren, L., et al. (2005). Cerebrospinal fluid signs of neuronal damage after antiretroviral treatment interruption in HIV-1 infection. *AIDS Res Ther, 2*, 6.

Gisslen, M., Svennerholm, B., et al. (2000). Cerebrospinal fluid and plasma viral load in HIV-1-infected patients with various anti-retroviral treatment regimens. *Scand J Infect Dis, 32*(4), 365–369.

Gonzalez, E., Rovin, B. H., et al. (2002). HIV-1 infection and AIDS dementia are influenced by a mutant MCP-1 allele linked to increased monocyte infiltration of tissues and MCP-1 levels. *Proc Natl Acad Sci U S A, 99*(21), 13795–13800.

Green, A. J., Giovannoni, G., et al. (1999). Cerebrospinal fluid S-100b concentrations in patients with HIV infection. *AIDS, 13*(1), 139–140.

Griffin, D. E., McArthur, J. C., et al. (1991). Neopterin and interferon-gamma in serum and cerebrospinal fluid of patients with HIV-associated neurologic disease. *Neurology, 41*(1), 69–74.

Gulevich, S. J., McCutchan, J. A., et al. (1993). Effect of antiretroviral therapy on the cerebrospinal fluid of patients seropositive for the human immunodeficiency virus. *J Acquir Immune Defic Syndr, 6*(9), 1002–1007.

Gunthard, H. F., Havlir, D. V., et al. (2001). Residual human immunodeficiency virus (HIV) Type 1 RNA and DNA in lymph nodes and HIV RNA in genital secretions and in cerebrospinal fluid after suppression of viremia for 2 years. *J Infect Dis, 183*(9), 1318–1327.

Haas, D. W., Clough, L. A., et al. (2000). Evidence of a source of HIV type 1 within the central nervous system by ultraintensive sampling of cerebrospinal fluid and plasma. *AIDS Res Hum Retroviruses, 16*(15), 1491–1502.

Haas, D. W., Johnson, B. W., et al. (2003). Two phases of HIV RNA decay in CSF during initial days of multidrug therapy. *Neurology, 61*(10), 1391–1396.

Hagberg, L., Andersson, M., et al. (1991). Effect of zidovudine on cerebrospinal fluid in patients with HIV infection and acute neurological disease. *Scand J Infect Dis, 23*(6), 681–685.

Hagberg, L., L. Dotevall, et al. (1993). Cerebrospinal fluid neopterin concentrations in central nervous system infection. *J Infect Dis, 168*(5), 1285–1288.

Hagberg, L., Norkrans, G., et al. (1992). Cerebrospinal fluid neopterin and beta 2-microglobulin levels in neurologically asymptomatic HIV-infected patients before and after initiation of zidovudine treatment. *Infection, 20*(6), 313–315.

Hagberg, L., Norkrans, G., et al. (1996). Intrathecal immunoactivation in patients with HIV-1 infection is reduced by zidovudine but not by didanosine. *Scand J Infect Dis, 28*(4), 329–333.

Hall, C. D., Snyder, C. R., et al. (1992). Cerebrospinal fluid analysis in human immunodeficiency virus infection. *Ann Clin Lab Sci, 22*(3), 139–143.

Harrington, P. R., D. W. Haas, et al. (2005). Compartmentalized human immunodeficiency virus type 1 present in cerebrospinal fluid is produced by short-lived cells. *J Virol, 79*(13), 7959–7966.

Heaton, R. K., Clifford, D. B., et al. (2010 (In Press)). HIV-associated neurocognitive disorders persist in the era of potent antiretroviral therapy. *Neurology*.

Heaton, R. K., Franklin, D. R., et al. (2010 (In Press)). HIV-associated neurocognitive disorders before and during the era of combination antiretroviral therapy: Differences in rates, nature and predictors. *J Neurovirol*.

Heidenreich, F., Arendt, G., et al. (1994). Serum and cerebrospinal fluid levels of soluble intercellular adhesion molecule 1 (sICAM-1) in patients with HIV-1 associated neurological diseases. *J Neuroimmunol, 52*(2), 117–126.

Heyes, M. P., Brew, B., et al. (1991). Cerebrospinal fluid quinolinic acid concentrations are increased in acquired immune deficiency syndrome. *Adv Exp Med Biol, 294*, 687–690.

Heyes, M. P., Ellis, R. J. et al. (2001). Elevated cerebrospinal fluid quinolinic acid levels are associated with region-specific cerebral volume loss in HIV infection. *Brain, 124*(Pt 5), 1033–1042.

Heyes, M. P., Lackner, A., et al. (1991). Cerebrospinal fluid and serum neopterin and biopterin in D-retrovirus-infected rhesus macaques (Macaca mulatta): Relationship to clinical and viral status. *AIDS, 5*(5), 555–560.

Hightower, G. K., Letendre, S. L., et al. (2009). Select resistance-associated mutations in blood are associated with lower CSF viral loads and better neuropsychological performance. *Virology, 394*(2), 243–248.

Hober, D., Benyoucef, S., et al. (1996). High plasma level of soluble tumor necrosis factor receptor type II (sTNFRII) in asymptomatic HIV-1-infected patients. *Infection, 24*(3), 213–217.

Holland, S. M. (2001). Cytokine therapeutics in infectious diseases. Philadelphia, Pennsylvania: Lippincott Williams and Wilkins.

Huang, S. H. & Jong, A. Y. (2001). Cellular mechanisms of microbial proteins contributing to invasion of the blood-brain barrier. *Cell Microbiol, 3*(5), 277–287.

Iftimovici, E., Rabian, C., et al. (1998). Longitudinal comparison of HIV-1 RNA burden in plasma and cerebrospinal fluid in two patients starting triple combination antiretroviral therapy. *AIDS, 12*(5), 535–537.

Imberciadori, G., Piersantelli, N., et al. (1990). Study of beta-2 microglobulin and neopterin in serum and cerebrospinal fluid of HIV-infected patients. *Acta Neurol (Napoli), 12*(1), 58–61.

Kaul, M. & Lipton, S. A. (1999). Chemokines and activated macrophages in HIV gp120-induced neuronal apoptosis. *Proc Natl Acad Sci U S A, 96*(14), 8212–8216.

Kelder, W., McArthur, J. C., et al. (1998). Beta-chemokines MCP-1 and RANTES are selectively increased in cerebrospinal fluid of patients with human immunodeficiency virus-associated dementia. *Ann Neurol, 44*(5), 831–835.

Khovidhunkit, W., Memon, R. A., et al. (1999). Plasma platelet-activating factor acetylhydrolase activity in human immunodeficiency virus infection and the acquired immunodeficiency syndrome. *Metabolism, 48*(12), 1524–1531.

Kolb, S. A., Sporer, B., et al. (1999). Identification of a T cell chemotactic factor in the cerebrospinal fluid of HIV-1-infected individuals as interferon-gamma inducible protein 10. *J Neuroimmunol, 93*(1-2), 172–181.

Kravcik, S., Gallicano, K., et al. (1999). Cerebrospinal fluid HIV RNA and drug levels with combination ritonavir and saquinavir. *J Acquir Immune Defic Syndr, 21*(5), 371–375.

Krivine, A., Force, G., et al. (1999). Measuring HIV-1 RNA and interferon-alpha in the cerebrospinal fluid of AIDS patients: Insights into the pathogenesis of AIDS dementia complex. *J Neurovirol, 5*(5), 500–506.

Kusdra, L., McGuire, D., et al. (2002). Changes in monocyte/macrophage neurotoxicity in the era of HAART: Implications for HIV-associated dementia. *AIDS, 16*(1), 31–38.

Lafeuillade, A., Solas, C., et al. (2002). Differences in the detection of three HIV-1 protease inhibitors in non-blood compartments: Clinical correlations. *HIV Clin Trials, 3*(1), 27–35.

Landmann, R., Muller, B., et al. (2000). CD14, new aspects of ligand and signal diversity. *Microbes Infect, 2*(3), 295–304.

Laverda, A. M., Gallo, P., et al. (1994). Cerebrospinal fluid analysis in HIV-1-infected children: Immunological and virological findings before and after AZT therapy. *Acta Paediatr, 83*(10), 1038–1042.

Lazzarin, A., Castagna, A., et al. (1992). Cerebrospinal fluid beta 2-microglobulin in AIDS related central nervous system involvement. *J Clin Lab Immunol, 38*(4), 175–186.

Letendre, S., Marquie-Beck, J., et al. (2008). Validation of the CNS penetration-effectiveness rank for quantifying antiretroviral penetration into the central nervous system. *Arch Neurol, 65*(1), 65–70.

Letendre, S., McClernon, D. et al. (2009). Persistent HIV in the central nervous system during treatment is associated with worse antiretroviral therapy penetration and cognitive impairment. 16th Conference on Retroviruses and Opportunistic Infections, Montreal, Quebec.

Letendre, S. L., Lanier, E. R., et al. (1999). Cerebrospinal fluid beta chemokine concentrations in neurocognitively impaired individuals infected with human immunodeficiency virus type 1. *J Infect Dis, 180*(2), 310–319.

Letendre, S. L., McCutchan, J. A., et al. (2004). Enhancing antiretroviral therapy for human immunodeficiency virus cognitive disorders. *Ann Neurol, 56*(3), 416–423.

Letendre, S. L., van den Brande, G., et al. (2007). Lopinavir with Ritonavir Reduces the HIV RNA Level in Cerebrospinal Fluid. *Clin Infect Dis, 45*(11).

Lien, E., Aukrust, P., et al. (1998). Elevated levels of serum-soluble CD14 in human immunodeficiency virus type 1 (HIV-1) infection: Correlation to disease progression and clinical events. *Blood, 92*(6), 2084–2092.

Lipton, S. A. & Gendelman, H. E. (1995). Seminars in medicine of the Beth Israel Hospital, Boston. Dementia associated with the acquired immunodeficiency syndrome. *N Engl J Med, 332*(14), 934–940.

Liuzzi, G. M., Mastroianni, C. M., et al. (2000). Increased activity of matrix metalloproteinases in the cerebrospinal fluid of patients with HIV-associated neurological diseases. *J Neurovirol, 6*(2), 156–163.

Lucey, D. R., McGuire, S. A., et al. (1991). Comparison of spinal fluid beta 2-microglobulin levels with CD4+ T cell count, in vitro T helper cell function, and spinal fluid IgG parameters in 163 neurologically normal adults infected with the human immunodeficiency virus type 1. *J Infect Dis, 163*(5), 971–975.

Maclennan, K. M., Smith, P. F., et al. (1996). Platelet-activating factor in the CNS. *Prog Neurobiol, 50*(5-6), 585–596.

Malmestrom, C., Haghighi, S., et al. (2003). Neurofilament light protein and glial fibrillary acidic protein as biological markers in MS. *Neurology, 61*(12), 1720–1725.

Marra, C. M., Maxwell, C. L., et al. (2007). Interpreting cerebrospinal fluid pleocytosis in HIV in the era of potent antiretroviral therapy. *BMC Infect Dis, 7*, 37.

Marra, C. M., Zhao, Y., et al. (2009). Impact of combination antiretroviral therapy on cerebrospinal fluid HIV RNA and neurocognitive performance. *AIDS, 23*(11) 1359–1366.

Marshall, D. W., Brey, R. L., et al. (1991). CSF changes in a longitudinal study of 124 neurologically normal HIV-1-infected U.S. Air Force personnel. *J Acquir Immune Defic Syndr,4*(8), 777–781.

Martin, C., Sonnerborg, A., et al. (1999). Indinavir-based treatment of HIV-1 infected patients: Efficacy in the central nervous system. *AIDS, 13*(10), 1227–1232.

Mastroianni, C. M., Paoletti, F., et al. (1990). Elevated levels of tumor necrosis factor (TNF) in the cerebrospinal fluid from patients with HIV-associated neurological disorders. *Acta Neurol (Napoli), 12*(1), 66–67.

Mastroianni, C. M., Paoletti, F., et al. (1992). Tumour necrosis factor (TNF-alpha) and neurological disorders in HIV infection. *J Neurol Neurosurg Psychiatry, 55*(3), 219–221.

McArthur, J. C., McClernon, D. R., et al. (1997). Relationship between human immunodeficiency virus-associated dementia and viral load in cerebrospinal fluid and brain. *Ann Neurol, 42*(5), 689–698.

McArthur, J. C., McDermott, M. P., et al. (2004). Attenuated central nervous system infection in advanced HIV/AIDS with combination antiretroviral therapy. *Arch Neurol, 61*(11), 1687–1696.

McArthur, J. C., Nance-Sproson, T. E., et al. (1992). The diagnostic utility of elevation in cerebrospinal fluid beta 2-microglobulin in HIV-1 dementia. Multicenter AIDS Cohort Study. *Neurology, 42*(9), 1707–1712.

McCoig, C., Castrejon, M. M., et al. (2002). Effect of combination antiretroviral therapy on cerebrospinal fluid HIV RNA, HIV resistance, and clinical manifestations of encephalopathy. *J Pediatr, 141*(1), 36–44.

McKinney, R. E., Jr., Maha, M. A., et al. (1991). A multicenter trial of oral zidovudine in children with advanced human immunodeficiency virus disease. The Protocol 043 Study Group. *N Engl J Med, 324*(15), 1018–1025.

Mellgren, A., Antinori, A., et al. (2005). Cerebrospinal fluid HIV-1 infection usually responds well to antiretroviral treatment. *Antivir Ther, 10*(6), 701–707.

Mellgren, A., Price, R. W., et al. (2007). Antiretroviral treatment reduces increased CSF neurofilament protein (NFL) in HIV-1 infection. *Neurology, 69*(15), 1536–1541.

Miura, Y., Misawa, N., et al. (2003). Tumor necrosis factor-related apoptosis-inducing ligand induces neuronal death in a murine model of HIV central nervous system infection. *Proc Natl Acad Sci U S A, 100*(5), 2777–2782.

Monteiro de Almeida, S., Letendre, S., et al. (2006). Relationship of CSF leukocytosis to compartmentalized changes in MCP-1/CCL2 in the CSF of HIV-infected patients undergoing interruption of antiretroviral therapy. *J Neuroimmunol, 179*(1-2), 180–185.

Monteiro de Almeida, S., Letendre, S., et al. (2005). Dynamics of monocyte chemoattractant protein type one (MCP-1) and HIV viral load in human cerebrospinal fluid and plasma. *J Neuroimmunol, 169*(1-2), 144–152.

Moyle, G. J., Sadler, M., et al. (1999). Plasma and cerebrospinal fluid saquinavir concentrations in patients receiving combination antiretroviral therapy. *Clin Infect Dis, 28*(2), 403–404.

Murr, C., Widner, B., et al. (2002). Neopterin as a marker for immune system activation. *Curr Drug Metab, 3*(2), 175–187.

Neuenburg, J. K., Cho, T. A., et al. (2005). T-cell activation and memory phenotypes in cerebrospinal fluid during HIV infection. *J Acquir Immune Defic Syndr, 39*(1). 16–22.

Neuenburg, J. K., Furlan, S., et al. (2005). Enrichment of activated monocytes in cerebrospinal fluid during antiretroviral therapy. *AIDS, 19*(13), 1351–1359.

Nishida, K., Markey, S. P., et al. (1996). Increased brain levels of platelet-activating factor in a murine acquired immune deficiency syndrome are NMDA receptor-mediated. *J Neurochem, 66*(1), 433–435.

Nockher, W. A., Bergmann, L., et al. (1994). Increased soluble CD14 serum levels and altered CD14 expression of peripheral blood monocytes in HIV-infected patients. *Clin Exp Immunol,98*(3), 369–374.

Nokta, M., Rossero, R., et al. (1997). Kinetics of tumor necrosis factor alpha and soluble TNFRII in HIV-infected patients treated with a triple combination of stavudine, didanosine, and hydroxyurea. *AIDS Res Hum Retroviruses, 13*(18), 1633–1638.

Nottet, H. S., Jett, M., et al. (1995). A regulatory role for astrocytes in HIV-1 encephalitis. An overexpression of eicosanoids, platelet-activating factor, and tumor necrosis factor-alpha by activated HIV-1-infected monocytes is attenuated by primary human astrocytes. *J Immunol, 154*(7), 3567–3581.

Pemberton, L. A. & Brew, B. J. (2001). Cerebrospinal fluid S-100beta and its relationship with AIDS dementia complex. *J Clin Virol, 22*(3), 249–253.

Pereira, C. F., Middel, J., et al. (2001). Enhanced expression of fractalkine in HIV-1 associated dementia. *J Neuroimmunol, 115*(1-2), 168–175.

Perrella, O., Carreiri, P. B., et al. (2001). Transforming growth factor beta-1 and interferon-alpha in the AIDS dementia complex (ADC): Possible relationship with cerebral viral load? *Eur Cytokine Netw, 12*(1), 51–55.

Perrella, O., Carrieri, P. B., et al. (1992). Cerebrospinal fluid cytokines in AIDS dementia complex. *J Neurol, 239*(7), 387–388.

Perrella, O., Carrieri, P. B., et al. (1991). Cerebrospinal fluid beta-2-microglobulin in HIV-1 infection, as a marker of neurological involvement. *Neurol Res, 13*(2), 131–132.

Perry, S. W., Hamilton, J. A., et al. (1998). Platelet-activating factor receptor activation. An initiator step in HIV-1 neuropathogenesis. *J Biol Chem, 273*(28), 17660–17664.

Persidsky, Y., Limoges, J., et al. (2001). Reduction in glial immunity and neuropathology by a PAF antagonist and an MMP and TNFalpha inhibitor in SCID mice with HIV-1 encephalitis. *J Neuroimmunol, 114*(1-2), 57–68.

Peter, J. B., McKeown, K. L., et al. (1991). Neopterin and beta 2-microglobulin and the assessment of intra-blood-brain-barrier synthesis of HIV-specific and total IgG. *J Clin Lab Anal, 5*(5), 317–320.

Pilcher, C. D., Shugars, D. C., et al. (2001). HIV in body fluids during primary HIV infection: implications for pathogenesis, treatment and public health. *AIDS, 15*(7), 837–845.

Pillai, S. K., Pond, S. L., et al. (2006). Genetic attributes of cerebrospinal fluid-derived HIV-1 env. *Brain, 129*(Pt 7), 1872–1883.

Podzamczer, D., Ferrer, E., et al. (2002). A randomized clinical trial comparing nelfinavir or nevirapine associated to zidovudine/lamivudine in HIV-infected naive patients (the Combine Study). *Antivir Ther, 7*(2), 81–90.

Polis, M. A., Suzman, D. L., et al. (2003). Suppression of cerebrospinal fluid HIV burden in antiretroviral naive patients on a potent four-drug antiretroviral regimen. *AIDS, 17*(8), 1167–1172.

Price, R. W. & Deeks, S. G. (2004). Antiretroviral drug treatment interruption in human immunodeficiency virus-infected adults: Clinical and pathogenetic implications for the central nervous system. *J Neurovirol, 10* Suppl 1, 44–51.

Price, R. W., Epstein, L. G., et al. (2007). Biomarkers of HIV-1 CNS infection and injury. *Neurology, 69*(18), 1781–1788.

Price, R. W., Paxinos, E. E., et al. (2001). Cerebrospinal fluid response to structured treatment interruption after virological failure. *AIDS, 15*(10), 1251–1259.

Pulliam, L., Gascon, R., et al. (1997). Unique monocyte subset in patients with AIDS dementia. *Lancet, 349*(9053), 692–695.

Pulliam, L., Zhou, M., et al. (1998). Differential modulation of cell death proteins in human brain cells by tumor necrosis factor alpha and platelet activating factor. *J Neurosci Res, 54*(4), 530–538.

Ravel, R. (1995). Clinical laboratory medicine: Clinical application of laboratory data. St Louis, Missouri: Mosby-Year Book, Inc.

Rho, M. B., Wesselingh, S., et al. (1995). A potential role for interferon-alpha in the pathogenesis of HIV-associated dementia. *Brain Behav Immun, 9*(4), 366–377.

Rieckmann, P., Nunke, K., et al. (1993). Soluble intercellular adhesion molecule-1 in cerebrospinal fluid: An indicator for the inflammatory impairment of the blood-cerebrospinal fluid barrier. *J Neuroimmunol, 47*(2), 133–140.

Robertson, K. R., Nakasujja, N., et al. (2007). Pattern of neuropsychological performance among HIV positive patients in Uganda. *BMC Neurol, 7*, 8.

Robertson, K. R., Robertson, W. T., et al. (2004). Highly active antiretroviral therapy improves neurocognitive functioning. *J Acquir Immune Defic Syndr*, 36(1), 562–566.

Rosen, H., Karlsson, J. E., et al. (2004). CSF levels of neurofilament is a valuable predictor of long-term outcome after cardiac arrest. *J Neurol Sci*, 221(1–2), 19–24.

Rosenberg, G. A. (2002). Matrix metalloproteinases in neuroinflammation. *Glia*, 39(3), 279–291.

Rosengren, L. E., Karlsson, J. E., et al. (1999). Neurofilament protein levels in CSF are increased in dementia. *Neurology*, 52(5), 1090–1093.

Rostasy, K., Monti, L., et al. (1999). Human immunodeficiency virus infection, inducible nitric oxide synthase expression, and microglial activation: Pathogenetic relationship to the acquired immunodeficiency syndrome dementia complex. *Ann Neurol*, 46(2), 207–216.

Royal, W., 3rd, Selnes, O. A., et al. (1994). Cerebrospinal fluid human immunodeficiency virus type 1 (HIV-1) p24 antigen levels in HIV-1-related dementia. *Ann Neurol*, 36(1), 32–39.

Ryan, L. A., Zheng, J., et al. (2001). Plasma levels of soluble CD14 and tumor necrosis factor-alpha type II receptor correlate with cognitive dysfunction during human immunodeficiency virus type 1 infection. *J Infect Dis*, 184(6), 699–706.

Saas, P., Walker, P. R., et al. (1997). Fas ligand expression by astrocytoma in vivo: Maintaining immune privilege in the brain? *J Clin Invest*, 99(6), 1173–1178.

Sabri, F., De Milito, A., et al. (2001). Elevated levels of soluble Fas and Fas ligand in cerebrospinal fluid of patients with AIDS dementia complex. *J Neuroimmunol*, 114(1-2), 197–206.

Sacktor, N., Tarwater, P. M., et al. (2001). CSF antiretroviral drug penetrance and the treatment of HIV-associated psychomotor slowing. *Neurology*, 57(3), 542–544.

Sanders, V. J., Pittman, C. A., et al. (1998). Chemokines and receptors in HIV encephalitis. *AIDS*, 12(9), 1021–1026.

Schifitto, G., Sacktor, N., et al. (1999). Randomized trial of the platelet-activating factor antagonist lexipafant in HIV-associated cognitive impairment. Neurological AIDS Research Consortium. *Neurology*, 53(2), 391–396.

Schnell, G., Spudich, S., et al. (2009). Compartmentalized human immunodeficiency virus type 1 originates from long-lived cells in some subjects with HIV-1-associated dementia. *PLoS Pathog*, 5(4), e1000395.

Sevigny, J. J., Albert, S. M., et al. (2004). Evaluation of HIV RNA and markers of immune activation as predictors of HIV-associated dementia. *Neurology*, 63(11), 2084–2090.

Simioni, S., Cavassini, M., et al. (2010). Cognitive dysfunction in HIV patients despite long-standing suppression of viremia. *AIDS*, 24(9), 1243–1250.

Sinclair, E., Ronquillo, R., et al. (2008). Antiretroviral treatment effect on immune activation reduces cerebrospinal fluid HIV-1 infection. *J Acquir Immune Defic Syndr*, 47(5), 544–552.

Singer, E. J., Syndulko, K., et al. (1994). Intrathecal IgG synthesis and albumin leakage are increased in subjects with HIV-1 neurologic disease. *J Acquir Immune Defic Syndr*, 7(3), 265–271.

Sippy, B. D., Hofman, F. M., et al. (1995). Increased expression of tumor necrosis factor-alpha receptors in the brains of patients with AIDS. *J Acquir Immune Defic Syndr Hum Retrovirol*, 10(5), 511–521.

Smith, D. G., Guillemin, G. J., et al. (2001). Quinolinic acid is produced by macrophages stimulated by platelet activating factor, Nef and Tat. *J Neurovirol*, 7(1), 56–60.

Smith, D. M., Zarate, S., et al. (2009). Pleocytosis is associated with disruption of HIV compartmentalization between blood and cerebral spinal fluid viral populations. *Virology*, 385(1), 204–208.

Solas, C., Lafeuillade, A., et al. (2003). Discrepancies between protease inhibitor concentrations and viral load in reservoirs and sanctuary sites in human immunodeficiency virus-infected patients. *Antimicrob Agents Chemother*, 47(1), 238–243.

Sonnerborg, A. B., von Stedingk, L. V., et al. (1989). Elevated neopterin and beta 2-microglobulin levels in blood and cerebrospinal fluid occur early in HIV-1 infection. *AIDS*, 3(5), 277–283.

Sporer, B., Kastenbauer, S., et al. (2003). Increased intrathecal release of soluble fractalkine in HIV-infected patients. *AIDS Res Hum Retroviruses*, 19(2), 111–116.

Sporer, B., Koedel, U., et al. (2000). Increased levels of soluble Fas receptor and Fas ligand in the cerebrospinal fluid of HIV-infected patients. *AIDS Res Hum Retroviruses*, 16(3), 221–226.

Sporer, B., Koedel, U., et al. (2004). Vascular endothelial growth factor (VEGF) is increased in serum, but not in cerebrospinal fluid in HIV associated CNS diseases. *J Neurol Neurosurg Psychiatry*, 75(2), 298–300.

Sporer, B., Koedel, U., et al. (2005). Evaluation of cerebrospinal fluid uPA, PAI-1, and soluble uPAR levels in HIV-infected patients. *J Neuroimmunol*, 163(1-2), 190–194.

Sporer, B., Paul, R., et al. (1998). Presence of matrix metalloproteinase-9 activity in the cerebrospinal fluid of human immunodeficiency virus-infected patients. *J Infect Dis*, 178(3), 854–857.

Spudich, S., Lollo, N., et al. (2006). Treatment benefit on cerebrospinal fluid HIV-1 levels in the setting of systemic virological suppression and failure. *J Infect Dis*, 194(12), 1686–1696.

Spudich, S. S., Huang, W., et al. (2005). HIV-1 chemokine coreceptor utilization in paired cerebrospinal fluid and plasma samples: A survey of subjects with viremia. *J Infect Dis*, 191(6), 890–898.

Spudich, S. S., Nilsson, A. C., et al. (2005). Cerebrospinal fluid HIV infection and pleocytosis: Relation to systemic infection and antiretroviral treatment. *BMC Infect Dis*, 5, 98.

Staprans, S., Marlowe, N., et al. (1999). Time course of cerebrospinal fluid responses to antiretroviral therapy: Evidence for variable compartmentalization of infection. *AIDS*, 13(9), 1051–1061.

Stellbrink, H. J., Eggers, C., et al. (1997). Rapid decay of HIV RNA in the cerebrospinal fluid during antiretroviral combination therapy. *AIDS*, 11(13), 1655–1657.

Strain, M. C., Letendre, S., et al. (2005). Genetic composition of human immunodeficiency virus type 1 in cerebrospinal fluid and blood without treatment and during failing antiretroviral therapy. *J Virol*, 79(3), 1772–1788.

Tashima, K. T., Caliendo, A. M., et al. (1999). Cerebrospinal fluid human immunodeficiency virus type 1 (HIV-1) suppression and efavirenz drug concentrations in HIV-1-infected patients receiving combination therapy. *J Infect Dis*, 180(3), 862–864.

Thieblemont, N., Weiss, L., et al. (1995). CD14lowCD16high: A cytokine-producing monocyte subset which expands during human immunodeficiency virus infection. *Eur J Immunol*, 25(12), 3418–3424.

Towfighi, A., Skolasky, R. L., et al. (2004). CSF soluble Fas correlates with the severity of HIV-associated dementia. *Neurology*, 62(4), 654–656.

Valle, M., Price, R. W., et al. (2004). CSF quinolinic acid levels are determined by local HIV infection: Cross-sectional analysis and modelling of dynamics following antiretroviral therapy. *Brain*, 127(Pt 5), 1047–1060.

van Leeuwen, R., Katlama, C., et al. (1995). Evaluation of safety and efficacy of 3TC (lamivudine) in patients with asymptomatic or mildly symptomatic human immunodeficiency virus infection: A phase I/II study. *J Infect Dis*, 171(5), 1166–1171.

Verani, A., Scarlatti, G., et al. (1997). C-C chemokines released by lipopolysaccharide (LPS)-stimulated human macrophages suppress HIV-1 infection in both macrophages and T cells. *J Exp Med*, 185(5), 805–816.

Vernazza, P., Daneel, S., et al. (2007). The role of compartment penetration in PI-monotherapy: the Atazanavir-Ritonavir Monomaintenance (ATARITMO) Trial. *AIDS*, 21(10), 1309–1315.

Vittecoq, D., Jardel, C., et al. (2002). Mitochondrial damage associated with long-term antiretroviral treatment: Associated alteration or causal disorder?" *J Acquir Immune Defic Syndr*, 31(3), 299–308.

von Giesen, H. J., Adams, O., et al. (2005). Cerebrospinal fluid HIV viral load in different phases of HIV-associated brain disease. *J Neurol*, 252(7), 801–807.

Vullo, V., Mastroianni, C. M., et al. (1995). Increased cerebrospinal fluid levels of soluble receptors for tumour necrosis factor in HIV-infected patients with neurological diseases. *AIDS*, 9(9) 1099–1100.

Wesselingh, S. L., Glass, J., et al. (1994). Cytokine dysregulation in HIV-associated neurological disease. *Adv Neuroimmunol, 4*(3), 199–206.

Wolf, K., Schulz, C., et al. (2002). "=Tumour necrosis factor-alpha induced CD70 and interleukin-7R mRNA expression in BEAS-2B cells. *Eur Respir J, 20*(2), 369–375.

Woods, S. P., Iudicello, J. E., et al. (2010). HIV-associated deficits in action (verb) generation may reflect astrocytosis. *J Clin Exp Neuropsychol, 32*(5), 522–527.

Yeh, R. F., Letendre, S., et al. (2007). Single Agent Therapy with Lopinavir/ritonavir Controls HIV-1 Replication in the Central Nervous System. 14th Conference on Retroviruses and Opportunistic Infections, Los Angeles, California.

Yilmaz, A., Fuchs, D., et al. (2006). Cerebrospinal fluid HIV-1 RNA, intrathecal immunoactivation, and drug concentrations after treatment with a combination of saquinavir, nelfinavir, and two nucleoside analogues: The M61022 study. *BMC Infect Dis, 6,* 63.

Yilmaz, A., Price, R. W., et al. (2008). Persistent intrathecal immune activation in HIV-1-infected individuals on antiretroviral therapy. *J Acquir Immune Defic Syndr, 47*(2), 168–173.

Yilmaz, A., Stahle, L., et al. (2004). Cerebrospinal fluid and plasma HIV-1 RNA levels and lopinavir concentrations following lopinavir/ritonavir regimen. *Scand J Infect Dis, 36*(11–12), 823–828.

Yilmaz, A., Svennerholm, B., et al. (2006). Cerebrospinal fluid viral loads reach less than 2 copies/ml in HIV-1-infected patients with effective antiretroviral therapy. *Antivir Ther, 11*(7), 833–837.

Zoumpourlis, V., Eliopoulos, A. G., et al. (1992). Transcriptional activation of the human immunodeficiency virus long terminal repeat sequences by tumor necrosis factor. *Anticancer Res, 12*(6B), 2065–2068.

9.5

VIRAL DYNAMICS

Davey M. Smith and Ronald J. Ellis

The central nervous system (CNS) possesses specific physiologic and anatomic characteristics that can contribute to the genetic evolution of HIV both in the CNS and systemically. The CNS can function as a reservoir, a compartment, and a drug sanctuary. A viral "reservoir" harbors replication-competent virus, making it possible for the virus to re-emerge after a period of suppression. A viral "compartment" refers to a situation wherein viral movement is restricted between anatomic sites or tissues, such as between the brain and blood. In the CNS, this restricted movement can ultimately lead to a divergence of genetic sequences between compartments. A "drug sanctuary" refers to a restriction of access of medication. As a drug sanctuary, the CNS can create an environment that facilitates additional genetic divergence between the viral populations in blood and CNS. These divergences can have clinical consequences in terms of the selection for antiretroviral resistance. This chapter reviews the evidence and clinical consequences of HIV-1 evolution and dynamics associated with the specialized tissues of the CNS.

INTRODUCTION

HIV can inflict neurologic damage sufficient to cause dementia and other CNS disorders, and unique physiologic and anatomic characteristics of the CNS are important in shaping the evolution of HIV locally and systemically. Thus, the CNS can function as a reservoir, a compartment, and a drug sanctuary. A reservoir is a cell population or tissue that harbors replication-competent virus. Such cellular and tissue reservoirs permit the virus to re-emerge even after long periods of suppression by immune or pharmacologic mechanisms. For example, macrophages and microglia, which can become infected with HIV, most likely serve as the long-lived viral reservoir in the CNS. Such reservoirs represent a major obstacle to eradicating HIV within hosts, because currently available antiretroviral agents work principally by interfering with the generation of new virions, but do not eliminate the virus from already infected cells (Chun, 1997; Finzi, 1999; Perelson, 2002; Ramratnam, 2000; Wong et al., 1997). Viral compartmentalization refers to the restriction of virus movement between anatomic sites or tissues such as the brain and blood. This genetic isolation, or restriction of gene flow between two viral populations, can ultimately lead to divergence of genetic sequences between the two compartments (Figure 9.5.1). Changes in viral genetics over time may occur due to

genetic drift, genetic shift, recombination, and mutation. Neuroadaptation can occur when there is selection of virus that can replicate better in the CNS. This increase in replication capacity in the local environment is known as increased viral fitness. Finally, the CNS can serve as a drug sanctuary due to restriction of access of antiretroviral medications to the viral populations in the CNS. As a drug sanctuary, the CNS can create an environment for further differences in the genetics between the viral populations in blood and CNS, and these differences can have clinical consequences in terms of the selection for antiretroviral resistance. In this chapter, we will review the evidence and clinical consequences of HIV-1 evolution and dynamics that can occur in the specialized tissues of the CNS.

VIRAL ENTRY AND EXPANSION IN THE CNS

Soon after the transmission of HIV, there is a period of rapid viral replication in the absence of specific immune defenses, resulting in very high viral titers in the blood (Daar, Moudgil, Meyer, & Ho, 1991; Little, McLean, Spina, Richman, & Havlir, 1999; Schacker, Collier, Hughes, Shea, & Corey, 1996). These high levels of HIV disseminate throughout the body and within days to weeks all tissues have been seeded, including anatomic compartments like the CNS (An, Groves, Gray, & Scaravilli, 1999; Chiodi et al., 1992; Davis et al., 1992; Gray et al., 1992). Entry of the virus into the CNS probably occurs through a Trojan horse mechanism via trafficking of infected mononuclear cells (Gartner, 2000). During acute infection, the CNS viral population in the CNS is genetically homogeneous and is typically dependent upon persistent re-seeding from the blood (Ritola et al., 2004). Eventually, a small CNS "reservoir" of latent provirus in macrophages, microglia is established (Lackner et al., 1991), and the initial viral genetic diversity is relatively low because of the small number of "founder" virus species (Keele et al., 2008). As CNS virus replicates, the population diversifies, gradually accumulating a large amount of genetic variation through processes described below. Diversification occurs simultaneously in the blood and other compartments under somewhat different selection pressures. Continued genotypic diversification and expansion of cellular reservoirs occurs in the CNS, and CNS-adapted variants often arise and proliferate. These neuroadapted viral variants can give rise to CNS

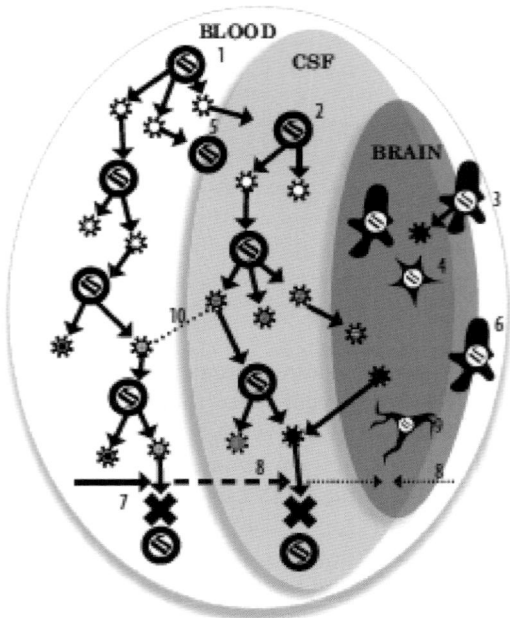

Figure 9.5.1 Schematic representation of HIV compartmentalization and trafficking blood, CSF, and brain. Active viral replication occurs in a subset of productivity infected lymphocytes in blood(1) and cerebrospinal fluid(2), and can also occur in brain tissue macrophages(3) and microglia(4). Additionally, proviral DNA exists in a different subset of latently infected cells (lymphocytes, monocytes/macrophages, and microglia), which serve as viral reservoirs. Lymphocytes and macrophages and associated HIV viral particles can traffic between blood and CSF(5), blood and brain(6), and brain and CSF. Antiretroviral drugs(7) block infection of new lymphocytes and monocytes/macrophages. However, because drug penetration into the brain and CSF(8) is reduced relative to blood, the CNS can serve as a protected "drug sanctuary." Infected and uninfected activated macrophages and microglia in brain tissue produce neurotoxins that injure neurons(9) as "bystanders." A variety of viral species arises over time. The relative proportions of different species in the brain, CSF, and blood may become quite divergent(10) when viral and cellular trafficking is limited or absent.

disease (Harrington et al., 2009; Pillai et al., 2006; Strain, Little et al., 2005).

ANATOMIC AND PHYSIOLOGIC BASIS OF VIRAL COMPARTMENTALIZATION IN THE CNS

The CNS, comprising cerebrospinal fluid (CSF), spinal cord, and brain tissue, is separated from blood by anatomical and physiological barriers. Importantly, not all distinct anatomic compartments or organs demonstrate viral compartmentalization. For example, the spleen is an anatomic compartment with specialized tissues, but the virus seen there is not usually different from what is seen contemporaneously in the blood. The CNS serves as both an anatomic compartment and a viral compartment, since the anatomic and physiologic barriers that separate the CNS from other tissues can restrict virus flow (Clarke, White, & Weber, 2000; Nickle et al., 2003; Smith, Kingery et al., 2004).

The blood-brain barrier (BBB) is comprised of capillary endothelial cells joined by tight junctions, a capillary basement membrane, and astrocyte foot processes. Together, these components regulate the outflow of macromolecules from the capillary lumen into brain tissue. Further, the capillaries for the brain's blood supply differ from capillaries in other organs with less pinocytotic vesicles, stronger tight junctions, and more mitochondria. Transport across blood capillary barriers is active and not passive. The blood-cerebrospinal fluid barrier (BCB) is similar to the BBB with a few differences in its specialized ependymal cells, which overlie the capillary endothelium. Observed increases in blood-derived protein concentrations in CSF in neurological diseases also may be explained by a reduced CSF flow rate and volume exchange, resulting in increased molecular net flux into CSF without changes in permeability coefficients (Reiber, 1994).

Additional differences between the CNS and other tissues include immunological surveillance and cytokine milieu. The CNS, like several other anatomical sites (testes, eyes), exhibits "immune privilege." One component of CNS immune privilege is the brain's lack of direct connection to the blood through an organized lymphatic drainage system. This is important because lymphatic systems transport immune cells (B and T lymphocytes, natural killer (NK) cells, neutrophils, monocytes) to and from lymphoid tissues where adaptive immune responses can be activated. Instead, a fraction of extracellular fluid from the brain parenchyma drains into the CSF space, eventually emptying into cervical lymph nodes (Cashion, Banks, Bost, & Kastin, 1999). Because of this, the CNS has few cells that constitutively express major histocompatibility complex (MHC) class I antigen and almost none that express class II, although these can be increased during periods of immune activation (An, et al., 1996). Also, professional antigen-presenting cells are rare (Hickey & Kimura, 1988; Pope, Vanderlugt, Rahbe, Lipton, & Miller, 1998), and normally there is little immunoglobulin or complement in CSF (Zwahlen, Nydegger, Vaudaux, Lambert, & Waldvogel, 1982). The CNS has its own resident antigen-presenting cells, microglia (Hickey, 2001), that are supplemented by perivascular macrophages from the periphery in episodes of CNS inflammation (Flaris, Densmore, Molleston, & Hickey, 1993; Williams & Hickey, 2002). Such macrophages and microglia locally produce a number of cytokines and chemokines that govern inflammatory responses.

CEREBROSPINAL FLUID AS A WINDOW TO THE BRAIN

Direct assessment of viral variants from brain parenchyma in living patients (e.g., via brain biopsy) is rarely feasible, but CSF virus may sometimes be an informative surrogate. This is because the brain extracellular fluid space communicates directly with the CSF via the ependyma lining the ventricles, the pial-glial membrane adjacent to the subarachnoid space and within Virchow-Robin spaces surrounding cerebral vessels. Because the choroid plexus secretes an additional fraction of CSF, there is some uncertainty about the sources of virus found in CSF. Despite these limitations, viral populations in CSF are likely to be reflective of virus in CNS parenchyma (Oldendorf & Davson, 1967).

HIV BURDEN IN THE CNS

HIV-1 RNA and DNA are readily detectable and have been measured directly in brain tissues from autopsy in several reports of relatively small case series (Langford et al., 2006; McClernon et al., 2001). Although it is likely that viral levels change substantially over the course of disease in brain tissue, this has been difficult to demonstrate empirically since most autopsy tissues are derived from individuals who had very advanced HIV disease. HIV RNA levels (viral loads) in CSF can be readily measured also. As noted above, CSF virus may reflect mixed populations originating from both local CNS and systemic sources.

Whereas systemically HIV mainly infects activated CD4 T lymphocytes, in the CNS the principal target cells are microglia and monocyte-derived macrophages (Pratt et al., 1996; Schrager & D'Souza, 1998; Strizki et al., 1996). In untreated individuals during the asymptomatic period of chronic HIV infection, blood viral loads are typically quite stable (approximately $\pm$ 0.5 $\log_{10}$ copies/mL) (Deeks et al., 1997; Raboud et al., 1996), but these levels differ substantially between individuals, reflecting patient-specific viral "set points" (Deeks et al., 1997; Henrard et al., 1995; Mellors et al., 1995). These viral levels and set points can reliably predict progression to AIDS and death (Mellors et al., 1996). CSF viral loads also demonstrate patient-specific set points, with similar variability over time in untreated individuals ($\pm$ 0.5 $\log_{10}$ HIV RNA copies/ml) over several years (Ellis et al., 2003). Many inter-related factors can influence CSF viral loads, including viral loads in the blood, levels of CNS immune activation, other co-infections, and antiretroviral therapy (Ellis et al., 1997). CSF viral loads are typically lower than blood, except for occasional instances in which they are equal or higher (Ellis et al., 2003; Smith et al., 2009). The clinical significance of these instances remains unclear. In untreated individuals, increasing CSF viral load has been associated with a greater risk of HIV-associated neurocognitive disorders (HAND), addressed elsewhere in this volume.

METHODS TO ASSESS HIV DIVERSITY AND COMPARTMENTALIZATION

Viral genetic diversity in HIV infection arises for three principal reasons. First, HIV replicates prolifically, producing 10–100 billion new virions each day (Perelson, Neumann, Markowitz, Leonard, & Ho, 1996). Second, HIV-1 reverse transcriptase shows low fidelity in proof-reading transcription errors (Mansky & Temin, 1995). Third, viral recombination occurs readily among virions dually infecting target cells, thereby contributing to the development of sequence heterogeneity. Thus, sequence diversity accumulates over time

(Duffy, Shackelton, & Holmes, 2008; Perelson et al., 1996). In association with these forces, evolutionary mechanisms like purifying and diversifying selection, stochastic and founder effects, and genetic drift shape the changes observed in viral diversity and population dynamics (Neher & Leitner, 2010).

Viral population diversity is characterized genotypically by sequencing cell-free HIV RNA or proviral HIV DNA. These two methods provide different views of the genetic diversity of an infecting viral population. Specifically, since HIV DNA provirus most often represents archived and latent virus that can persist in resting cells for months to years, the sequences generated from HIV DNA provide a "historical" perspective on viral evolution (Fujimura et al., 1997). By contrast, HIV RNA sequences provide a perspective on concurrent and actively replicating viral populations. Viral variants can also be characterized with respect to their phenotypic characteristics. Important viral phenotypic attributes include differential affinities for target cell surface chemokine receptors or ability to replicate in specific cell types.

Anatomic-specific segregation of viral variants provides direct evidence for compartmentalization of HIV infection. To study CNS compartmentalization in HIV, researchers must combine clinical, molecular biology, and phylogenetic methods. First, adequate clinical samples must be obtained. This often involves precise study designs that allow for complete characterization of study participants. Examples of clinical questions that need to be answered to design appropriate compartmentalization studies include: Should the study design be cross-over, case-control, or randomized intervention; should the subjects be sampled cross-sectionally or longitudinally; what anatomic compartments are being compared; how are samples collected and stored to evaluate HIV RNA or HIV DNA, and so on. Also important in these studies is the determination of which HIV coding region will be sampled, for example, *pol, env, tat,* and so on, and the development and validation of suitable molecular techniques to sample the viral populations of interest. Clonal sequencing has been the industry standard where viral genomes are transfected into commercially available bacterial platforms so as to ensure individual sampling of genomes. Terminal dilution polymerase reaction sampling followed by Sanger sequencing methods (aka single genome sequencing) also has its proponents and is used widely (Butler, Pacold, Jordan, Richman, & Smith, 2009). Both of these methods are more expensive and labor intensive than standard population-based sequencing, but population-based sequencing only evaluates the viral population as a whole and is not sufficient for determining the presence or prevalence of minority viral variants. Another powerful technique in the characterization of viral compartmentalization is the heteroduplex tracking assay, which can characterize complex viral populations by evaluating patterns of generated heteroduplexes in polyacrylamide gels, and has been used effectively to demonstrate that viral compartmentalization in the CSF is associated with HIV-associated dementia, giving evidence of neuroadaptation and damage (Harrington et al., 2009; Resch, Parkin, Stuelke, Watkins, & Swanstrom, 2001). Other methods, like length polymorphism analysis (Smith, Wong et al., 2004) and base pair mixture analysis (Poon et al., 2007) are other potential less costly tools to evaluate compartmentalization. Recently, the use of ultradeep sequencing, or pyrosequencing, has been proposed (Wang, Mitsuya, Gharizadeh, Ronaghi, & Shafer, 2007). This method has the ability to sample and sequence a viral population hundreds of thousands of times, far exceeding the capacity of either clonal or single genome sequencing. Based on a per-base cost, this method has enormous potential to be the least costly and the most robust; however, continued validation must be performed for this method to be a viable technique to investigate compartmental evolution.

The next important consideration in investigating viral compartmentalization is how the data are analyzed. Phylogenetic analytical techniques are used to determine the relatedness of sampled sequences. Although these methods are continually being improved, they are the mainstay of sequence analysis. Broadly, phylogenetic methods comprise a variety of techniques for evaluating the relatedness of viral populations in different tissues by comparing their genetic sequences. These analyses are inferential statistical methods that reconstruct relationships between observed sequences, usually depicted as phylogenetic or "family" tree (Figure 9.5.2). In these trees, the evolutionary relatedness of viral sequences is encoded in the distances between nodes or branches on the tree. Sequences that share a common ancestry are represented closer on a tree, while those that are more divergent are farther away in the tree. The relatedness of these sequences, that is,

branches in the topology, can be statistically evaluated by either bootstrapping or maximum likelihood methods. Other phylogenetic methods allow for the deduction of ancestral sequences, the timing of evolutionary changes, the positive and negative selection occurring at genetic sites, and so forth. There are also specialized phylogenetic methods that can estimate and statistically measure the restriction of gene flow between compartments, that is, viral compartmentalization and sub-compartmentalization. The two most common forms of these analyses are the Slatkin-Maddison and Fst tests. A good review of the utility of these measures can be found by Zarate, Pond, Shapshak, and Frost (2007). Other methods, such as supervised learning methods, have also been used to investigate sequence characteristics or genetic motifs that are conserved during compartmentalization or disease states (Pillai et al., 2005; Pillai et al., 2006). Understanding which genetic motifs are associated with which disease state may be very important in understanding the pathogenic mechanisms of HIV in the CNS.

EVIDENCE OF VIRAL COMPARTMENTALIZATION IN THE CNS

Selection pressures on local viral populations can result in viral variants uniquely adapted to the local environment. Such pressures include CNS-specific immune responses,

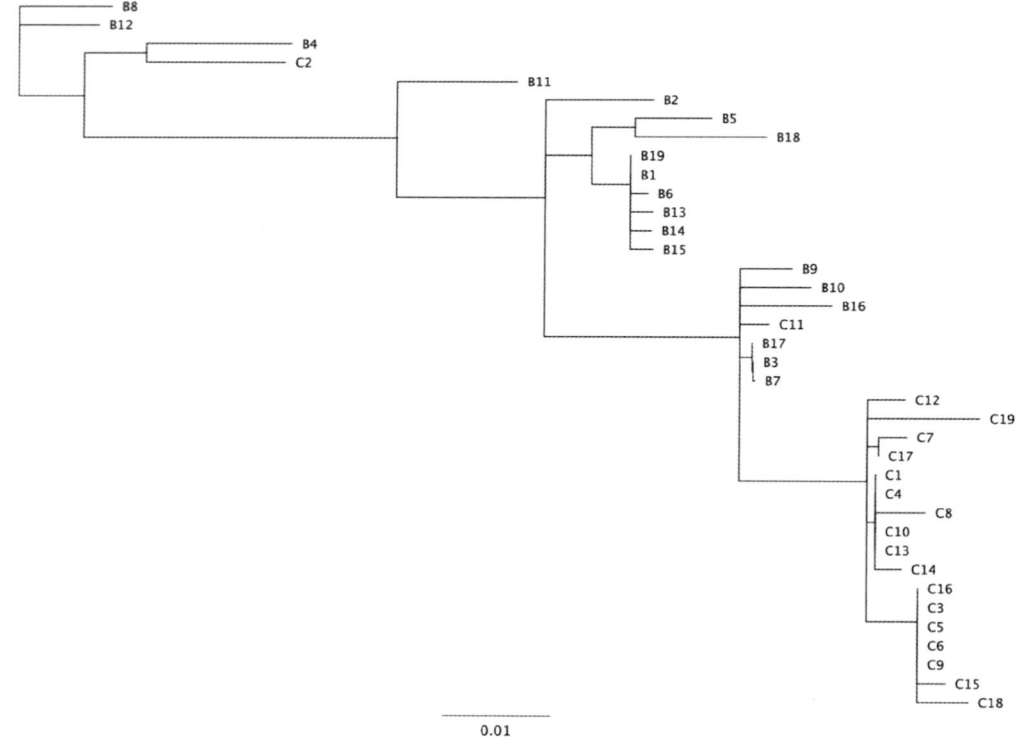

Figure 9.5.2 Maximum likelihood cladogram based on *env* sequences derived from HIV RNA extracted from paired blood (B) and CSF (C) samples. The *env* phylogram revealed significant compartmentalization between viral populations in blood and CSF (Slatkin Maddison Test p<0.01), that is, blood and CSF viral sequences largely clustered separately. Notice that two viral clones from the CSF (C2 and C11) can be found with the viral clones derived from the blood and not with other CSF clones. Even though viral compartmentalization was statistically significant, this demonstrates that compartmentalization is often not absolute.

target cell characteristics, or antiretroviral drug pressures. These variants may be the basis of at least some of the neurocognitive dysfunction observed during HIV infection and AIDS (Harrington et al., 2009; Pillai et al., 2006). The properties of degree of compartmentalization, relative gene flow between compartments, and replicative activity (latent vs. highly active replication) are not absolute and often fluctuate. They are also relative since they are measured by comparing snapshots, such as HIV RNA from CSF versus HIV DNA from peripheral blood mononuclear cells (PBMC) versus HIV RNA in blood plasma. In individual patients, viral populations can show a marked degree of heterogeneity, and the trends of viral diversity tend to increase over the course of HIV infection (Markham et al., 1998). Within larger anatomic compartments there can also be sub-compartments, which represent specialized cell types or tissues. For example, virus found in the brain parenchyma could be different than virus found in CSF and virus in the prostate may be different than virus in seminal plasma, and all of these viral populations may be distinct from virus circulating in the blood.

The complex combination of factors that lead to compartmentalization creates an environment in which immunologic, pharmacologic, and biologic selective forces can act upon the viral population to favor variants with an advantageous traits, that is, phenotypes, in particular niches. The relationship between virus and host changes over the course of infection, and may depend on a number of factors. At time of initial infection these factors may include route of infection, size, and diversity of initial viral inoculum, viral phenotype that is transmitted, stage of infection, and treatment status of source partner. For the new host, viral evolution and diversity are influenced by these and other factors, such as use of antiretroviral therapy, viral, bacterial, and fungal co-infections or comorbid illnesses, immune activation status, HLA haplotype, neutralizing antibody response, and many other factors. Although the complexity of these interactions might be daunting, the genetic variation that makes HIV such a problem for the immune system and antiretroviral therapy also affords a window into its pathogenic mechanisms. Analysis of viral genetic information during the course of infection allows for better understanding of the interactions between virus and host and the evolutionary forces that are at work. These analyses are based on a battery of phylogenetic methods that can be helpful tools to analyze the mechanisms of HIV neuropathogenesis and are described below.

For example, in an HIV-infected individual harboring some variants that use the CCR5 co-receptor and other variants that use the CXCR4 co-receptor to infect target cells, CCR5-using variants almost always predominate in the CNS as compared to the blood (Pratt et al., 1996; Schrager & D'Souza, 1998). During serial passage of virus in cell culture, HIV can evolve to use the CCR5 co-receptor and replicate efficiently in microglia and monocyte-derived macrophages (Strizki et al., 1996). Further, viral isolates from the brain parenchyma of patients who had severe HIV-associated dementia most often used the CCR5 chemokine receptor to infect target cells (Albright et al., 1999; He et al., 1997).

VIRAL MIGRATION AND PLEOCYTOSIS

When sampling the viral populations in blood and CNS, viral compartmentalization is not always demonstrated. Additionally, compartmentalization of viral populations can fluctuate over time such that a given individual may demonstrate compartmentalization between blood and CNS at one time but not another. One of the factors that may influence the extent of compartmentalization is viral migration, which can occur through a variety of mechanisms. For example, activation of lymphocytes and other immune cells in the periphery increases their propensity to traffic into the CNS (Persidsky & Poluektova, 2006; Price et al., 2001). Upon entering the CNS, these activated cells—some of which may be infected—then either produce virus or activate local infected cells to produce HIV RNA. Alternatively, increases in CSF viral replication, such as occurs after the discontinuation of antiretroviral therapy, increase CNS inflammation, and blood-derived lymphocytes then traffic into CNS in response. To determine how CNS inflammation can change the viral dynamics in the CNS, studies were conducted among patients who developed pleocytosis (Smith et al., 2009). Pleocytosis is the appearance of leukocytes in the CSF (>5 cells/mm^3), and is used clinically as a marker of meningeal inflammation. Pleocytosis occurs intermittently during HIV-1 infection, reflecting meningeal inflammation due to a wide variety of bacterial, fungal, parasitic, and viral pathogens, including HIV itself.

These investigations found that during episodes of pleocytosis there was a disruption of viral compartmentalization between the CNS and blood. Although these studies did not clarify if inflammation in the CNS "pulled" the pleocytosis cells from the blood into the CSF or if inflammation in the blood "pushed" activated cells into the CSF, the studies did show that viral populations in blood and CSF converged genetically during pleocytosis (Smith et al., 2009). Over time, instances of inflammation marked by pleocytosis may increase viral genetic diversity in the CNS and potentially provide greater genotypic variation to fuel viral neuroadaptation and associated neuropathogenicity. Increased viral trafficking and increased viral burdens would increase the concentration of viral proteins in the CNS, which may directly or indirectly mediate neurotoxic effects without genetic changes in the local virus. Alternatively, pleocytosis and associated disruption of viral compartmentalization may have no effect on HAND, but may only serve as a marker of the true cause of HAND—CNS inflammation. Because of the small number of participants in this study, HAND was not assessed in relation to pleocytosis or viral compartmentalization; therefore, it remains unclear to what degree HAND is associated with persistent or intermittent inflammation and to what extent CNS inflammation is the mechanism underlying HAND. Also, given the small nature of our study, we were unable to assess other important processes, like stochastic and founder effects and host immune responses that are likely to influence the entire gamut of the inter-related factors of pleocytosis, compartmentalization, intra-host evolution, neuroadaptation, and neurovirulence; therefore, future studies such as these are needed to further delineate the mechanisms of HIV-mediated neuropathogenesis.

Chemokines and cytokines are soluble factors that can be secreted by a variety of cells, including cells in the CNS, such as macrophages, microglia, astrocytes, and endothelial cells (Conant et al., 1998) (Huang et al., 2000; Ransohoff, 2002; Conant et al. 1998). The CC- or beta-chemokines, which include monocyte chemoattractant protein-1 (MCP-1), macrophage inflammatory protein 1 alpha and 1 beta (MIP-1a, MIP-1b), and the natural CCR5 ligand, RANTES, are particularly important in the CNS by dictating immune activation and cellular trafficking (Gonzalez et al., 2002) (Gu et al., 1999; Lu et al., 1998). These factors most likely play roles that can both disrupt viral compartmentalization by signaling immune cell trafficking into the CNS (Monteiro de Almeida et al., 2006) and re-enforce compartmentalization by recruiting specialized monocytes to the CNS that support infection by unique viral variants. Although these factors have been associated with the presence of HAND (Kelder, McArthur, Nance-Sproson, McClernon, & Griffin, 1998), it is not known whether the damage is caused by the change in viral dynamics in the CNS or whether the inflammatory response in the CNS itself is a harmful process.

CNS AS A SANCTUARY

The goal of modern antiretroviral therapy regimens is to suppress viral replication as low as possible, often to levels that are undetectable to modern diagnostic assays, so as to allow the immune system to recover. In clinical practice, the effectiveness of this therapy viral replication is measured as the viral burden or "viral loads" in the blood. For the CNS, we can measure similar viral loads in the CSF, and in individuals naïve to antiretroviral therapy, the levels of these viral loads in the CSF are associated with the amount of neurologic damage from HIV infection (Ellis et al., 1997). Therefore, a current goal in the clinical treatment of HIV is to also suppress viral replication in all anatomic compartments, including the CNS, as well as the blood. This requires agents that are able to penetrate these anatomic sanctuaries to sufficient levels so as to suppress viral replication (Letendre et al., 2004). Even though current antiretroviral therapies can suppress viral replication and improve quality and length of life, HAND persists even during the era of widespread use of highly active antiretroviral therapy drug combinations (Heaton et al., 2010). The mechanisms of this neurologic damage are unclear, as correlations between HAND and CSF viral load have diminished or disappeared during the current era (Sevigny et al., 2004). Hypotheses for these observations include that current combination therapies improve neuropsychological performance in some individuals (Sacktor et al., 1999), but impairment may persist in some individuals who even attain CSF virologic suppression (Heaton et al., 2010; Starace et al., 2002). Studies are currently ongoing to investigate if early treatment can thwart some of these long-lasting neurologic effects.

Similarly to the way the CNS can restrict viral gene flow, it also can restrict antiretroviral agents from entering the CNS, providing a kind of pharmacologic sanctuary for the virus. The differential penetration of antiretroviral drugs into CNS tissues is based on their physical and chemical characteristics and interaction with the blood-brain and blood-CSF barriers. The specific mechanisms of restriction include physical characteristics of antiretrovirals (e.g., molecular size, lipophilicity, charge, and protein binding), as well as their affinity as substrates for molecular pumps such as p-glycoprotein (Enting, 1998; Wynn, Brundage, & Fletcher, 2002). Differential drug penetration into the CNS is documented in both animal and human clinical studies (Antinori et al., 2002; Cunningham, Smith, Satchell, Cooper, & Brew, 2000; Limoges et al., 2001; McCoig et al., 2002). The extent of restriction varies according to the specific antiretroviral agent.

When antiretroviral drug concentrations are not sufficient to fully suppress viral replication, then the selection of antiretroviral resistant variants can occur (Richman, 2001). HIV strains isolated from CNS tissues at autopsy or from CSF during life can differ in *pol* sequences compared with those from other tissues (Smit et al., 2004; Strain, Letendre et al., 2005). Differences in *pol* between CNS and blood viral populations may have important clinical consequences, as they can promote the selection of resistance-associated mutations (Kepler & Perelson, 1998). For example, if the antiretrovirals penetrate poorly into the CNS and therefore there are sub-therapeutic drug concentrations, the development of resistant strains may be accelerated in the CNS. Once antiretroviral resistance develops, even in a sanctuary, it can theoretically "spill" into the blood and other compartments so as to prevent the maximal effectiveness of antiretroviral therapy.

On the other hand, the development of resistance-associated mutations often comes at cost to the resistant viruses. Although these resistant viruses may be able to replicate better in the presence of antiretroviral drugs, they often cannot replicate to the same high levels as viruses that do not contain these resistant mutations. Thus, these variants with resistance-associated mutations can exhibit reduced replication capacity and result in lower viral loads in blood (Deeks et al., 2001). This reduced replication capacity or "fitness" can result in improved clinical outcome, including neurocognitive functioning (Hightower et al., 2009).

Similar to the problems of sampling viral populations, it is not practical in humans to measure brain parenchymal concentrations of antiretroviral drugs in vivo, or to assess their effect in brain tissue directly; therefore, CSF measurements have been used as a surrogate. Many antiretroviral drugs can be measured in CSF, and data on CSF pharmacokinetics demonstrate that antiretroviral agents penetrate into the CNS differently (Haas et al., 2000; Letendre et al., 2009; Letendre, Capparelli, Ellis, & McCutchan, 2000). Concentrations of antiretroviral agents in the CSF may over- or under-estimate drug concentrations in the brain parenchyma (Enting et al., 2001; Groothuis & Levy, 1997; Yazdanian, 1999), but CSF levels of antiretroviral agents in the brain, measured at autopsy, were closer, but not equivalent, to levels in the CSF than to levels in the blood (Brewster et al., 1997).

SUMMARY AND CONCLUSIONS

Although most knowledge of the natural history of HIV infection is based on the study of viral populations in blood, and to a lesser extent lymphoid tissue (e.g., spleen, lymph nodes, gut-associated lymphoid tissue), HIV also infects and replicates in cells in other anatomic sites. Because these anatomic and cellular compartments differ in the relative abundance and composition of specific HIV target-cells, host immune surveillance, antiretroviral drug penetration, and other factors, virus populations in blood may poorly reflect virus populations in other anatomic tissues, like the CNS.

Studies of viral dynamics and genetics demonstrate that viral compartmentalization is governed by cellular, anatomical, and physiological properties that separate the CNS from other tissues, and may present special challenges to the medical management of HIV. Further, the reaching of the "Holy Grail" of eradication of HIV by antiretroviral or immune therapies may require special attention to sites, such as the CNS, which can function as: (i) viral compartments with independent viral replication and evolution, (ii) reservoirs which can harbor replication competent virus for long periods and are not eradicated by currently available therapies, and (iii) drug sanctuaries that can restrict the concentrations of various antiretroviral agents, yielding resistant strains that may reseed the periphery.

ACKNOWLEDGMENTS

We would like to thank George Hightower for his art work and phylogenetic expertise. This work was supported by National Institutes of Health grants MH58076, MH59745, MH62512, DA12065, MH22005, MH083552, AI077304, AI69432, DA024654-01, MH62512, AI27670, AI38858, AI43638, AI43752, AI047745, NS51132, UCSD Centers for AIDS Research (AI36214), AI29164, AI47745, AI57167, and the Research Center for AIDS and HIV Infection of the San Diego Veterans Affairs Healthcare System (10-92-035).

REFERENCES

Albright, A. V., Shieh, J. T., Itoh, T., Lee, B., Pleasure, D., O'Connor, M. J., et al. (1999). Microglia express CCR5, CXCR4, and CCR3, but of these, CCR5 is the principal coreceptor for human immunodeficiency virus type 1 dementia isolates. *J Virol*, 73(1), 205–213.

An, S. F., Ciardi, A., Giometto, B., Scaravilli, T., Gray, F., & Scaravilli, F. (1996). Investigation on the expression of major histocompatibility complex class II and cytokines and detection of HIV-1 DNA within brains of asymptomatic and symptomatic HIV-1-positive patients. *Acta Neuropathol*, 91(5), 494–503.

An, S. F., Groves, M., Gray, F., & Scaravilli, F. (1999). Early entry and widespread cellular involvement of HIV-1 DNA in brains of HIV-1 positive asymptomatic individuals. *J Neuropathol Exp Neurol*, 58(11), 1156–1162.

Antinori, A., Giancola, M. L., Grisetti, S., Soldani, F., Alba, L., Liuzzi, G., et al. (2002). Factors influencing virological response to antiretroviral drugs in cerebrospinal fluid of advanced HIV-1-infected patients. *AIDS*, 16(14), 1867–1876.

Brewster, M. E., Anderson, W. R., Webb, A. I., Pablo, L. M., Meinsma, D., Moreno, D., et al. (1997). Evaluation of a brain-targeting zidovudine chemical delivery system in dogs. *Antimicrob Agents Chemother*, 41(1), 122–128.

Butler, D. M., Pacold, M. E., Jordan, P. S., Richman, D. D., & Smith, D. M. (2009). The efficiency of single genome amplification and sequencing is improved by quantitation and use of a bioinformatics tool. *J Virol Methods*, 162(1-2), 280–283.

Cashion, M. F., Banks, W. A., Bost, K. L., & Kastin, A. J. (1999). Transmission routes of HIV-1 gp120 from brain to lymphoid tissues. *Brain Res*, 822(1-2), 26–33.

Chiodi, F., Keys, B., Albert, J., Hagberg, L., Lundeberg, J., Uhlen, M., et al. (1992). Human immunodeficiency virus type 1 is present in the cerebrospinal fluid of a majority of infected individuals. *J Clin Microbiol*, 30(7), 1768–1771.

Chun, T. W. (1997). Presence of an inducible HIV-1 latent reservoir during highly active antiretroviral therapy. *Proc.Natl Acad.Sci.USA*, 94, 13193–13197.

Clarke, J. R., White, N. C., & Weber, J. N. (2000). HIV compartmentalization: Pathogenesis and clinical implications. *AIDS Rev*, 2, 15–22.

Conant, K., Garzino-Demo, A., Nath, A., McArthur, J. C., Halliday, W., Power, C., et al. (1998). Induction of monocyte chemoattractant protein-1 in HIV-1 Tat-stimulated astrocytes and elevation in AIDS dementia 1. *Proc Natl Acad Sci USA*, 95(6), 3117–3121.

Cunningham, P. H., Smith, D. G., Satchell, C., Cooper, D. A., & Brew, B. (2000). Evidence for independent development of resistance to HIV-1 reverse transcriptase inhibitors in the cerebrospinal fluid. *AIDS*, 14(13), 1949–1954.

Daar, E. S., Moudgil, T., Meyer, R. D., & Ho, D. D. (1991). Transient high levels of viremia in patients with primary human immunodeficiency virus type 1 infection. *N Engl J Med*, 324(14), 961–964.

Davis, L. E., Hjelle, B. L., Miller, V. E., Palmer, D. L., Llewellyn, A. L., Merlin, T. L., et al. (1992). Early viral brain invasion in iatrogenic human immunodeficiency virus infection. *Neurology*, 42(9), 1736–1739.

Deeks, S. G., Coleman, R. L., White, R., Pachl, C., Schambelan, M., Chernoff, D. N., et al. (1997). Variance of plasma human immunodeficiency virus type 1 RNA levels measured by branched DNA within and between days. *J Infect Dis*, 176(2), 514–517.

Deeks, S. G., Wrin, T., Liegler, T., Hoh, R., Hayden, M., Barbour, J. D., et al. (2001). Virologic and immunologic consequences of discontinuing combination antiretroviral-drug therapy in HIV-infected patients with detectable viremia. *N Engl J Med*, 344(7), 472–480.

Duffy, S., Shackelton, L. A., & Holmes, E. C. (2008). Rates of evolutionary change in viruses: Patterns and determinants. *Nat Rev Genet*, 9(4), 267–276.

Ellis, R. J., Childers, M. E., Zimmerman, J. D., Frost, S. D., Deutsch, R., & McCutchan, J. A. (2003). Human immunodeficiency virus-1 RNA levels in cerebrospinal fluid exhibit a set point in clinically stable patients not receiving antiretroviral therapy. *J Infect Dis*, 187(11), 1818–1821.

Ellis, R. J., Hsia, K., Spector, S. A., Nelson, J. A., Heaton, R. K., Wallace, M. R., et al. (1997). Cerebrospinal fluid human immunodeficiency virus type 1 RNA levels are elevated in neurocognitively impaired individuals with acquired immunodeficiency syndrome. HIV Neurobehavioral Research Center Group. *Ann Neurol*, 42(5), 679–688.

Enting, R. H. (1998). Antiretroviral drugs and the central nervous system. *AIDS*, 12, 1941–1955.

Enting, R. H., Prins, J. M., Jurriaans, S., Brinkman, K., Portegies, P., & Lange, J. M. (2001). Concentrations of human immunodeficiency virus type 1 (HIV-1) RNA in cerebrospinal fluid after antiretroviral treatment initiated during primary HIV-1 infection. *Clin Infect Dis*, 32(7), 1095–1099.

Finzi, D. (1999). Latent infection of CD4+ T cells provides a mechanism for lifelong persistence of HIV-1, even in patients on effective combination therapy. *Nature Med.*, 5, 512–517.

Flaris, N. A., Densmore, T. L., Molleston, M. C., & Hickey, W. F. (1993). Characterization of microglia and macrophages in the central nervous system of rats: definition of the differential expression of molecules using standard and novel monoclonal antibodies in normal CNS and in four models of parenchymal reaction. *Glia*, 7(1), 34–40.

Fujimura, R. K., Goodkin, K., Petito, C. K., Douyon, R., Feaster, D. J., Concha, M., et al. (1997). HIV-1 proviral DNA load across neuroanatomic regions of individuals with evidence for HIV-1-associated dementia. *J Acquir Immune Defic Syndr Hum Retrovirol*, 16(3), 146–152.

Gartner, S. (2000). HIV infection and dementia. *Science*, 287(5453), 602–604.

Gonzalez, E., Rovin, B. H., Sen, L., Cooke, G., Dhanda, R., Mummidi, S., et al. (2002). HIV-1 infection and AIDS dementia are influenced by a mutant MCP-1 allele linked to increased monocyte infiltration of tissues and MCP-1 levels. *Proc Natl Acad Sci U S A*, 99(21), 13795–13800.

Gray, F., Lescs, M. C., Keohane, C., Paraire, F., Marc, B., Durigon, M., et al. (1992). Early brain changes in HIV infection: Neuropathological study of 11 HIV seropositive, non-AIDS cases. *J Neuropathol Exp Neurol*, 51(2), 177–185.

Groothuis, D. R. & Levy, R. M. (1997). The entry of antiviral and antiretroviral drugs into the central nervous system. *J Neurovirol*, 3(6), 387–400.

Gu L, Tseng SC, Rollins BJ. (1999) Monocyte chemoattractant protein-1. *Chem Immunol*;72:7–29.

Haas, D. W., Stone, J., Clough, L. A., Johnson, B., Spearman, P., Harris, V. L., et al. (2000). Steady-state pharmacokinetics of indinavir in cerebrospinal fluid and plasma among adults with human immunodeficiency virus type 1 infection. *Clin Pharmacol Ther*, 68(4), 367–374.

Harrington, P. R., Schnell, G., Letendre, S. L., Ritola, K., Robertson, K., Hall, C., et al. (2009). Cross-sectional characterization of HIV-1 env compartmentalization in cerebrospinal fluid over the full disease course. *AIDS*, 23(8), 907–915.

He, J., Chen, Y., Farzan, M., Choe, H., Ohagen, A., Gartner, S., et al. (1997). CCR3 and CCR5 are co-receptors for HIV-1 infection of microglia. *Nature*, 385(6617), 645–649.

Heaton, R. K., Clifford, D. B., Franklin Jr, D. R., Woods, S. P., Ake, C., Vaida, F., et al. (2010). HIV-associated neurocognitive disorders persist in the era of potent antiretroviral therapy. *Neurology*, 75(23), 2087–96.

Henrard, D. R., Daar, E., Farzadegan, H., Clark, S. J., Phillips, J., Shaw, G. M., et al. (1995). Virologic and immunologic characterization of symptomatic and asymptomatic primary HIV-1 infection. *J Acquir Immune Defic Syndr Hum Retrovirol*, 9(3), 305–310.

Hickey, W. F. (2001). Basic principles of immunological surveillance of the normal central nervous system. *Glia*, 36(2), 118–124.

Hickey, W. F. & Kimura, H. (1988). Perivascular microglial cells of the CNS are bone marrow-derived and present antigen in vivo. *Science*, 239(4837), 290–292.

Hightower, G. K., Letendre, S. L., Cherner, M., Gibson, S. A., Ellis, R. J., Wolfson, T. J., et al. (2009). Select resistance-associated mutations in blood are associated with lower CSF viral loads and better neuropsychological performance. *Virology*.

Huang D, Han Y, Rani MR, Glabinski A, Trebst C, Sorensen T, Tani M, Wang J, Chien P, O'Bryan S, Bielecki B, Zhou ZL, Majumder S, Ransohoff RM. (2000). Chemokines and chemokine receptors in inflammation of the nervous system: manifold roles and exquisite regulation. *Immunol Rev*;177:52–67.

Keele, B. F., Giorgi, E. E., Salazar-Gonzalez, J. F., Decker, J. M., Pham, K. T., Salazar, M. G., et al. (2008). Identification and characterization of transmitted and early founder virus envelopes in primary HIV-1 infection. *Proc Natl Acad Sci U S A*, 105(21), 7552–7557.

Kelder, W., McArthur, J. C., Nance-Sproson, T., McClernon, D., & Griffin, D. E. (1998). Beta-chemokines MCP-1 and RANTES are selectively increased in cerebrospinal fluid of patients with human immunodeficiency virus-associated dementia. *Ann Neurol*, 44(5), 831–835.

Kepler, T. B. & Perelson, A. S. (1998). Drug concentration heterogeneity facilitates the evolution of drug resistance. *Proc Natl Acad Sci U S A*, 95(20), 11514–11519.

Lackner, A. A., Smith, M. O., Munn, R. J., Martfeld, D. J., Gardner, M. B., Marx, P. A., et al. (1991). Localization of simian immunodeficiency

virus in the central nervous system of rhesus monkeys. *Am J Pathol*, 139(3), 609–621.

Langford, D., Marquie-Beck, J., de Almeida, S., Lazzaretto, D., Letendre, S., Grant, I., et al. (2006). Relationship of antiretroviral treatment to postmortem brain tissue viral load in human immunodeficiency virus-infected patients. *J Neurovirol*, 12(2), 100–107.

Letendre S, Ellis RJ, Best BB, Bhatt A, Marquie-Beck J, LeBlanc S, Rossi S, Capparelli E and McCutchan JA. (2009) Penetration and Effectiveness of Antiretroviral Therapy in the Central Nervous System. *Anti-Inflammatory & Anti-Allergy Agents in Medicinal Chemistr*, 8, 169–183.

Letendre, S. L., Capparelli, E. V., Ellis, R. J., & McCutchan, J. A. (2000). Indinavir population pharmacokinetics in plasma and cerebrospinal fluid. The HIV Neurobehavioral Research Center Group. *Antimicrob Agents Chemother*, 44(8), 2173–2175.

Letendre, S. L., McCutchan, J. A., Childers, M. E., Woods, S. P., Lazzaretto, D., Heaton, R. K., et al. (2004). Enhancing antiretroviral therapy for human immunodeficiency virus cognitive disorders. *Ann Neurol*, 56(3), 416–423.

Limoges, J., Poluektova, L., Ratanasuwan, W., Rasmussen, J., Zelivyanskaya, M., McClernon, D. R., et al. (2001). The efficacy of potent antiretroviral drug combinations tested in a murine model of HIV-1 encephalitis. *Virology*, 281(1), 21–34.

Little, S. J., McLean, A. R., Spina, C. A., Richman, D. D., & Havlir, D. V. (1999). Viral dynamics of acute HIV-1 infection. *J Exp Med*, 190(6), 841–850.

Lu B, Rutledge BJ, Gu L, Fiorillo J, Lukacs NW, Kunkel SL, North R, Gerard C, Rollins BJ.(1998). Abnormalities in monocyte recruitment and cytokine expression in monocyte chemoattractant protein 1-deficient mice. *J Exp Med*, 16;187(4):601–8.

Mansky, L. M. & Temin, H. M. (1995). Lower in vivo mutation rate of human immunodeficiency virus type 1 than that predicted from the fidelity of purified reverse transcriptase. *The Journal of Virology*, 69(8), 5087–5094.

Markham, R. B., Wang, W. C., Weisstein, A. E., Wang, Z., Munoz, A., Templeton, A., et al. (1998). Patterns of HIV-1 evolution in individuals with differing rates of CD4 T cell decline. *Proc Natl Acad Sci U S A*, 95(21), 12568–12573.

McClernon, D. R., Lanier, R., Gartner, S., Feaster, P., Pardo, C. A., St Clair, M., et al. (2001). HIV in the brain: RNA levels and patterns of zidovudine resistance. *Neurology*, 57(8), 1396–1401.

McCoig, C., Castrejon, M. M., Castano, E., De Suman, O., Baez, C., Redondo, W., et al. (2002). Effect of combination antiretroviral therapy on cerebrospinal fluid HIV RNA, HIV resistance, and clinical manifestations of encephalopathy. *J Pediatr*, 141(1), 36–44.

Mellors, J. W., Kingsley, L. A., Rinaldo, C. R., Jr., Todd, J. A., Hoo, B. S., Kokka, R. P., et al. (1995). Quantitation of HIV-1 RNA in plasma predicts outcome after seroconversion. *Ann Intern Med*, 122(8), 573–579.

Mellors, J. W., Rinaldo, C. R., Gupta, P., White, R. M., Todd, J. A., & Kingsley, L. A. (1996). Prognosis in HIV-1 infection predicted by the quantity of virus in plasma. *Science*, 272(5265), 1167–1170.

Monteiro de Almeida, S., Letendre, S., Zimmerman, J., Kolakowski, S., Lazzaretto, D., McCutchan, J. A., et al. (2006). Relationship of CSF leukocytosis to compartmentalized changes in MCP-1/CCL2 in the CSF of HIV-infected patients undergoing interruption of antiretroviral therapy. *J Neuroimmunol*, 179(1-2), 180–185.

Neher, R. A. & Leitner, T. (2010). Recombination rate and selection strength in HIV intra-patient evolution. *PLoS Comput Biol*, 6(1), e1000660.

Nickle, D. C., Jensen, M. A., Shriner, D., Brodie, S. J., Frenkel, L. M., Mittler, J. E., et al. (2003). Evolutionary indicators of human immunodeficiency virus type 1 reservoirs and compartments. *J Virol*, 77(9), 5540–5546.

Oldendorf, W. H. & Davson, H. (1967). Brain extracellular space and the sink action of cerebrospinal fluid. *Trans Am Neurol Assoc*, 92, 123–127.

Perelson, A. S. (2002). Modelling viral and immune system dynamics. *Nat Rev Immunol*, 2(1), 28–36.

Perelson, A. S., Neumann, A. U., Markowitz, M., Leonard, J. M., & Ho, D. D. (1996). HIV-1 dynamics in vivo: Virion clearance rate, infected cell life-span, and viral generation time 1. *Science, 271*(5255), 1582–1586.

Persidsky, Y. & Poluektova, L. (2006). Immune privilege and HIV-1 persistence in the CNS. *Immunol Rev, 213,* 180–194.

Pillai, S. K., Good, B., Pond, S. K., Wong, J. K., Strain, M. C., Richman, D. D., et al. (2005). Semen-specific genetic characteristics of human immunodeficiency virus type 1 env. *J Virol, 79*(3), 1734–1742.

Pillai, S. K., Pond, S. L. K., Liu, Y., Good, B. M., Strain, M. C., Ellis, R. J., et al. (2006). Genetic attributes of cerebrospinal fluid-derived HIV-1 env. *Brain, 129,* 1872–1883.

Poon, A. F., Kosakovsky Pond, S. L., Bennett, P., Richman, D. D., Leigh Brown, A. J., & Frost, S. D. (2007). Adaptation to human populations is revealed by within-host polymorphisms in HIV-1 and hepatitis C virus. *PLoS Pathog, 3*(3), e45.

Pope, J. G., Vanderlugt, C. L., Rahbe, S. M., Lipton, H. L., & Miller, S. D. (1998). Characterization of and functional antigen presentation by central nervous system mononuclear cells from mice infected with Theiler's murine encephalomyelitis virus. *J Virol, 72*(10), 7762–7771.

Pratt, R. D., Nichols, S., McKinney, N., Kwok, S., Dankner, W. M., & Spector, S. A. (1996). Virologic markers of human immunodeficiency virus type 1 in cerebrospinal fluid of infected children. *J Infect Dis, 174*(2), 288–293.

Price, R. W., Paxinos, E. E., Grant, R. M., Drews, B., Nilsson, A., Hoh, R., et al. (2001). Cerebrospinal fluid response to structured treatment interruption after virological failure. *AIDS, 15*(10), 1251–1259.

Raboud, J. M., Montaner, J. S., Conway, B., Haley, L., Sherlock, C., O'Shaughnessy, M. V., et al. (1996). Variation in plasma RNA levels, CD4 cell counts, and p24 antigen levels in clinically stable men with human immunodeficiency virus infection. *J Infect Dis, 174*(1), 191–194.

Ramratnam, B. (2000). The decay of the latent reservoir of replication-competent HIV-1 is inversely correlated with the extent of residual viral replication during prolonged anti-retroviral therapy. *Nature Med., 6,* 82–85.

Ransohoff RM. (2002). The chemokine system in neuroinflammation: an update. *J Infect Dis, 1;*186 Suppl 2:S152–6.

Reiber, H. (1994). Flow rate of cerebrospinal fluid (CSF)—a concept common to normal blood-CSF barrier function and to dysfunction in neurological diseases. *J Neurol Sci, 122*(2), 189–203.

Resch, W., Parkin, N., Stuelke, E. L., Watkins, T., & Swanstrom, R. (2001). A multiple-site-specific heteroduplex tracking assay as a tool for the study of viral population dynamics. *Proceedings of the National Academy of Sciences of the United States of America, 98,* 176–181.

Richman, D. D. (2001). HIV chemotherapy. *Nature, 410*(6831), 995–1001.

Ritola, K., Pilcher, C. D., Fiscus, S. A., Hoffman, N. G., Nelson, J. A., Kitrinos, K. M., et al. (2004). Multiple V1/V2 env variants are frequently present during primary infection with human immunodeficiency virus type 1. *J Virol, 78*(20), 11208–11218.

Sacktor, N. C., Lyles, R. H., Skolasky, R. L., Anderson, D. E., McArthur, J. C., McFarlane, G., et al. (1999). Combination antiretroviral therapy improves psychomotor speed performance in HIV-seropositive homosexual men. Multicenter AIDS Cohort Study (MACS). *Neurology, 52*(8), 1640–1647.

Schacker, T., Collier, A. C., Hughes, J., Shea, T., & Corey, L. (1996). Clinical and epidemiologic features of primary HIV infection. *Annals of Internal Medicine, 125*(4), 257–264.

Schrager, L. K. & D'Souza, M. P. (1998). Cellular and anatomical reservoirs of HIV-1 in patients receiving potent antiretroviral combination therapy. *JAMA, 280*(1), 67–71.

Sevigny, J. J., Albert, S. M., McDermott, M. P., McArthur, J. C., Sacktor, N., Conant, K., et al. (2004). Evaluation of HIV RNA and markers of immune activation as predictors of HIV-associated dementia. *Neurology, 63*(11), 2084–2090.

Smit, T. K., Brew, B. J., Tourtellotte, W., Morgello, S., Gelman, B. B., & Saksena, N. K. (2004). Independent evolution of human immunodeficiency virus (HIV) drug resistance mutations in diverse areas of the brain in HIV-infected patients, with and without dementia, on antiretroviral treatment. *J Virol, 78*(18), 10133–10148.

Smith, D. M., Kingery, J. D., Wong, J. K., Ignacio, C. C., Richman, D. D., & Little, S. J. (2004). The prostate as a reservoir for HIV-1. *AIDS, 18*(11), 1600–1602.

Smith, D. M., Wong, J. K., Hightower, G. K., Ignacio, C. C., Koelsch, K. K., Daar, E. S., et al. (2004). Incidence of HIV superinfection following primary infection. *JAMA, 292*(10), 1177–1178.

Smith, D. M., Zarate, S., Shao, H., Pillai, S. K., Letendre, S. L., Wong, J. K., et al. (2009). Pleocytosis is associated with disruption of HIV compartmentalization between blood and cerebral spinal fluid viral populations. *Virology, 385*(1), 204–208.

Starace, F., Bartoli, L., Aloisi, M. S., Antinori, A., Narciso, P., Ippolito, G., et al. (2002). Cognitive and affective disorders associated to HIV infection in the HAART era: Findings from the NeuroICONA study. Cognitive impairment and depression in HIV/AIDS. The NeuroICONA study. *Acta Psychiatr Scand, 106*(1), 20–26.

Strain, M. C., Letendre, S., Pillai, S. K., Russell, T., Ignacio, C. C., Gunthard, H. F., et al. (2005). Genetic composition of human immunodeficiency virus type 1 in cerebrospinal fluid and blood without treatment and during failing antiretroviral therapy. *J Virol, 79*(3), 1772–1788.

Strain, M. C., Little, S. J., Daar, E. S., Havlir, D. V., Gunthard, H. F., Lam, R. Y., et al. (2005). Effect of treatment, during primary infection, on establishment and clearance of cellular reservoirs of HIV-1. *J Infect Dis, 191*(9), 1410–1418.

Strizki, J. M., Albright, A. V., Sheng, H., O'Connor, M., Perrin, L., & Gonzalez-Scarano, F. (1996). Infection of primary human microglia and monocyte-derived macrophages with human immunodeficiency virus type 1 isolates: Evidence of differential tropism. *J Virol, 70*(11), 7654–7662.

Wang, C., Mitsuya, Y., Gharizadeh, B., Ronaghi, M., & Shafer, R. W. (2007). Characterization of mutation spectra with ultra-deep pyrosequencing: Application to HIV-1 drug resistance. *Genome Res, 17*(8), 1195–1201.

Williams, K. C. & Hickey, W. F. (2002). Central nervous system damage, monocytes and macrophages, and neurological disorders in AIDS. *Annu Rev Neurosci, 25,* 537–562.

Wong, J. K., Hezareh, M., Gunthard, H. F., Havlir, D. V., Ignacio, C. C., Spina, C. A., et al. (1997). Recovery of replication-competent HIV despite prolonged suppression of plasma viremia. *Science, 278*(5341), 1291–1295.

Wynn, H. E., Brundage, R. C., & Fletcher, C. V. (2002). Clinical implications of CNS penetration of antiretroviral drugs. *CNS Drugs, 16*(9), 595–609.

Yazdanian, M. (1999). Blood-brain barrier properties of human immunodeficiency virus antiretrovirals. *J Pharm Sci, 88*(10), 950–954.

Zarate, S., Pond, S. L., Shapshak, P., & Frost, S. D. (2007). Comparative study of methods for detecting sequence compartmentalization in human immunodeficiency virus type 1. *J Virol, 81*(12), 6643–6651.

Zwahlen, A., Nydegger, U. E., Vaudaux, P., Lambert, P. H., & Waldvogel, F. A. (1982). Complement-mediated opsonic activity in normal and infected human cerebrospinal fluid: Early response during bacterial meningitis. *J Infect Dis, 145*(5), 635–646.

9.6

VIRAL CLADES
ROLE IN HIV NEUROPATHOGENESIS

Wenxue Li and Avindra Nath

Despite the rapid transglobal spread of HIV-1 infection, the has emerged as distinct subtypes or clades in different geographical regions. This sequence diversity seems to have profound effects in the spread of the virus, its ability to infect various cells types, the efficiency of viral replication, the propensity to develop drug resistance, and its ability to cause neurocognitive disorders. While clade B virus is still the best studied, it is becoming evident that clade D-infected individuals have higher rates of neurocognitive disorders, while the converse may be true for clade C-infected individuals. This chapter reviews the evidence and the molecular basis for these clade differences.

INTRODUCTION

HIV-1 infection continues to spread despite the use of combination anti-retroviral therapy (cART). One of the challenges in eradication of HIV-1 infection is the remarkable diversity of the HIV-1 genome. There are three classes of HIV-1 worldwide: M (major), O (outlier), and N (non-major and non-outlier) (Gao et al., 1999; Hahn et al., 2000). The M group is the predominant form of HIV-1 in circulation, with over 90% coverage of all the HIV-1 cases. According to its envelope diversity, group M can be further subclassified into nine major subtypes or clades: A, B, C, D, F, G, H, J, and K (Hemelaar et al., 2006). Additionally, there are circulating recombinant forms (CRFs) and unique recombinant forms (URFs) of HIV-1. HIV-1 clades and CRFs have distinctive geographical distributions (reviewed in Liner et al., 2007, see chapter 11.6). Clade C infects the largest population of HIV-1 patients, and is predominant in Southern and Eastern Africa, China, and India (Figure 9.6.1). Clade A and A/G recombinant variants predominate in West and Central Africa while Clade D predominates in East and Central Africa. Clade B is the predominant HIV-1 species infecting the Americas, Europe, and Australia. It is the best studied HIV-1 clade, although the population infected by clade B is comparatively small. Other clades and recombinant variants combined infect a small population, and are limited mainly to Central, Eastern, and Western Africa, and small patches of other areas. However, the HIV-1 genome continues to evolve. New HIV-1 strains are constantly being identified. Frequent immigration and globalization are continuously changing the geographical spread of HIV-1 infection (Kousiappa et al., 2009).

There are multiple factors contributing to the wide variation of HIV-1 genomes. The intrinsic cause is the lack of proofreading function of HIV-1 reverse transcriptase (RT). Normally, the DNA transcriptase possesses the 3' to 5' exonuclease activity, which can correct mismatch errors during DNA synthesis. But HIV-1 RT lacks this capacity, resulting in an error rate of approximately 3.4×10^{-5} mismatches per base pair in each replication cycle (Preston et al., 1988; Ji & Loeb, 1992). In addition, HIV-1 genome has a high replication rate, which further contributes to the rapid accumulation of genetic mutations. To make thing worse, the HIV-1 genome also has a high propensity for recombination. When an individual is infected by two or more different HIV-1 strains, recombination of the viral genome may occur in co-infected cells (Robertson et al., 1995; Blackard et al., 2002), leading to further viral diversification. Adding to these factors, host genetics, nutrition, environmental and therapeutic selection, and drugs of abuse may also drive the overall evolution of HIV-1.

EFFECTS OF HIV-1 CLADES ON DISEASE PROGRESSION

The role of the differences in HIV-1 clades on disease progression is not clear. Some researchers believe that HIV-1 genomic variation alone is not sufficient to cause significant differences in disease transmission and progression (Hu et al., 1999; Kandathil et al., 2005). Studies found that although clade B and A/E recombinants were introduced in Thailand at about the same time, new cases of infection by A/E subtype were significantly more than that by clade B (Hu et al., 1999). The researchers attributed this to a founder effect, meaning that A/E recombinant was introduced earlier than clade B and the time window allowed A/E to establish its domination. Another study in Thailand attributed the disease progression to viral load but not other significant factors (Kilmarx et al., 2000).

However, other studies suggest that there are disparities in transmission and pathogenecity among different HIV-1 subtypes. A prospective study of registered female sex workers in Senegal compared the transmission and disease progression of HIV-1 clades A, C, D, and G (Kanki et al., 1999).

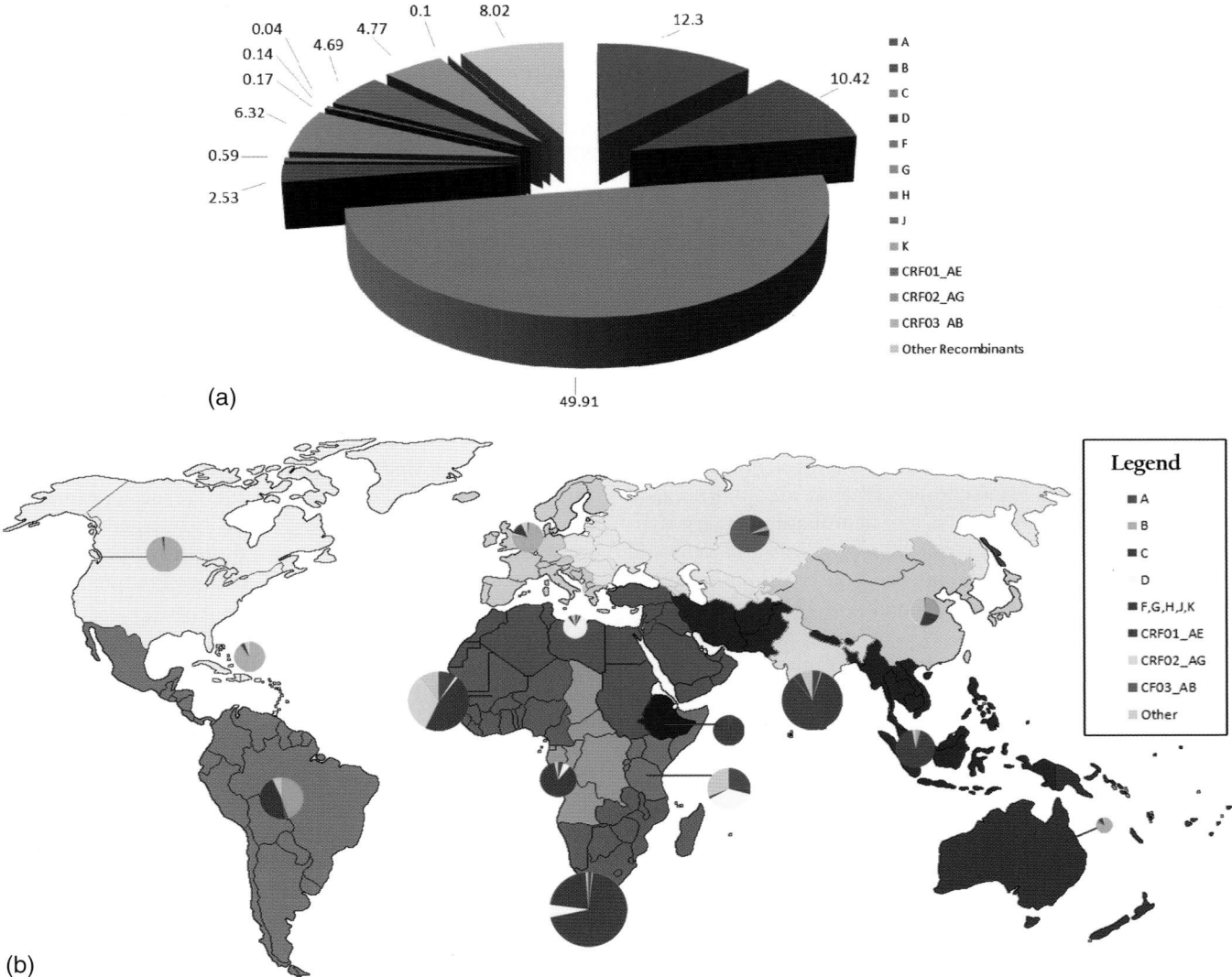

(a)

(b)

Figure 9.6.1 (a) Frequent immigration and globalization are continuously changing the geographical spread of HIV-1 infection (Kousiappa et al., 2009). (b) Global and regional distribution of HIV-1 clades and recombinants. From WHO/UNAIDS report titled "Global and reginal distribution of HIV-1 genetic subtypes and recombinants in 2004" by (Hemelaar et al., 2006).

The researchers found that women infected with non-A clades were eight times more likely to develop AIDS than were those infected with clade A. In addition, women with clade A infection have longer AIDS-free survival time than those with non-A clades. In Uganda, studies showed an increased rate of disease progression among clade D-infected patients compared to those with clade A infection (Kaleebu et al., 2002; Kiwanuka et al., 2008). A study from Kenya showed that mortality rate is higher among patients infected with clade D than those infected with clade A or C (Baeten et al., 2007). The decline of CD4+ cell count was faster in patients with clade D infection. In Tanzania, clade D was found to be more pathogenic than clade A, followed by clade C and recombinant viruses (Vasan et al., 2006). Clade D HIV-1 was associated with highest risk of death. Importantly, all clades of HIV probably display similar sensitivity to antiviral drugs. However, viruses from some subtypes and/or geographical regions may

have a greater propensity to develop resistance against certain drugs than do other viral variants (Spira et al., 2003).

IMPACT OF HIV-1 CLADES ON NEUROPATHOGENESIS

To date, the research on clade-specific differences in the progression of neurocognitive disorder is sparse. A recent study in Uganda found that 31% of HIV-infected patients met the criteria of HIV-associated dementia (HAD), while another 47% patients fell into the category of mild cognitive impairment on neuropsychological testing (Wong et al., 2007). In Uganda, clades A and D are predominant. However, in Ethiopia where clade C is predominant, no neurocoginitive impairment was found in HIV-positive individuals (Clifford et al., 2007). These studies raised the possibility that different HIV subtypes could cause differences in HIV-associated neurological disease (HAND). In addition, it has been noted that HAD affected about 15–30% of infected Americans before the era of CART (McArthur et al., 1993). However, in India, where clade C is predominant, the prevalence of severe form of HAD is significantly lower (2–4%) in CART-naïve HIV-infected patients, although milder forms of dementia have also been reported (Satishchandra et al., 2000; Gupta et al., 2007). A recent study evaluated the effects of different HIV-1 clades on HAND in Uganda (Sacktor et al., 2009). In the study, gag and gp41 regions of HIV-1 from 60 infected individuals were subtyped and their neuropsychological scores were assessed. It was found that patients infected with clade D had higher frequency of dementia compared to patients with clade A infection. In a mouse model, it was found that mice exposed to clade C HIV-1 isolate had less memory impairment than mice exposed to clade B HIV-1 isolate (Rao et al., 2008). Clade C HIV-1 isolate also showed less neuropathogenicity than clade B HIV-1 isolate in terms of astrogliosis and neuronal loss (Rao et al., 2008). Although these observations indicated the clade-specific neuropathogenicity of HIV-1, its mechanism is largely unexplored. HIV clade D found in Africa is highly virulent. Tat protein from this clade is a very potent transactivator of HIV replication and these functional changes are attributed to mutation in amino acids 61 S/G, 63 T/Q, and 67 S/D. These changes result in binding to TAR with higher affinity and prevent inactivation by a protein kinase called PKR. PKR can phosphorylate Tat and inhibit its binding to TAR (McMillan et al., 1995; Peloponese et al., 1999). Nuclear magnetic resonance structure shows that the major difference between clade B and D is the presence of a short alpha helix in clade D-Tat in region V, which is replaced by two beta turns in clade B-Tat (Gregoire et al., 2001).

CO-RECEPTOR USAGE BY HIV CLADES AND NEUROPATHOGENESIS

Clade D virus has a propensity to exhibit dual tropism compared to other clades (Huang et al., 2007; Kaleebu et al., 2007), and may favor the CXCR4 co-receptor primarily observed in T-cells (Zhang et al., 1996; Tscherning et al., 1998). Clades A and C tend to use CCR5 co-receptor, which is non-syncitium inducing, and are associated with slower viral growth and replication (Tscherning et al., 1998; Abebe et al., 1999; Peeters et al., 1999). This could explain why clade D HIV-1 appears to be more pathogenic than other clades. However, CCR5 is the principal chemokine receptor present on microglia and macrophages (Albright et al., 1999) and are essential for viral entry into these cells types (He et al., 1997). Studies with clade B virus suggest that these cells are the major target for HIV infection in the brain, and further viral isolates from the brain are predominantly CCR5 tropic. In a study conducted in Southern India, viruses from 40 HIV-positive, asymptomatic or symptomatic individuals in India were isolated. Of 40 isolates, 39 used CCR5. Thirty-three isolates were subtype C,

three isolates were subtype A, and four isolates were HIV-2. Only 1 HIV-2 isolate, from a symptomatic individual, was dual tropic. Therefore, a majority of isolates from India belonged to subtype C and all the isolates utilized CCR5 exclusively, irrespective of HIV disease status (Cecilia et al., 2000). Similar analysis of the co-receptor usage of clade C isolates from Ethiopia and Botswana supports the usage of the CCR5 co-receptor by HIV-1 clade C strains. No Ethiopian or Botswanian isolates exclusively used the CXCR4 co-receptor (Loemba et al., 2002). Previous studies have shown that brain isolates from HIV clade B infections are predominantly CCR5 tropic even when peripheral blood and lymph node isolates from the same patients are CXCR4 tropic (Shieh et al., 1998). One would then predict that there might be early and increased viral infection of the brain with clade C virus. However, viral tropism in the brain and its effects have yet to be characterized with clades other than clade B virus. In lymphocytes, clade B Tat, but not clade C Tat, increases CXCR4 surface expression on resting CD4+ T cells through a CCR2b-dependent mechanism that does not involve de novo protein synthesis, increasing the susceptibility of resting T cells to get infected with HIV-1 (Campbell et al., 2010).

ROLES OF HIV-1 TAT PROTEIN IN THE NEUROPATHOGENESIS OF HIV-1 CLADES

The neuropathogenesis of HAND, characterized by neurodegeneration and glial cell activation, is not fully understood. It has been recognized that HIV-1 protein Tat plays a critical role in the pathogenesis of HAND, by causing direct neurotoxicity and indirectly via activation of astrocytes and microglia. Tat can cause calcium dysregulation and lead to neuronal death (Haughey et al., 1999; Haughey & Mattson, 2002). The excessive calcium influx induced by Tat can be blocked by antagonists of NMDA glutamate receptor (Bonavia et al., 2001). Our recent study using HEK 293 cell model further demonstrated that Tat directly binds to NMDA receptor and causes cell death (Li et al., 2008). We also found that clade C Tat is significantly less toxic than clade B Tat proteins This difference could be attributable to the Cys31Ser polymorphism in clade C Tat (see Figure 9.6.2), while other clades of Tat have a conserved dicysteine motif (Cys30Cys31). Mutagenesis experiments confirmed that Cys31 could be an important determinant of Tat neurotoxicity (Kigozi et al., 2008). Our results are consistent with recent report in that clade C Tat is less toxic to human primary neurons than clade B Tat (Mishra et al., 2008). Compared to clade B Tat, clade C Tat-induced neuronal damage, including alteration of decrease of mitochondrial function, oxidative stress, and activation of caspase-3, are considerably lower (Mishra et al., 2008).

The ability of Tat to activate glial cells and induce cytokines/chemokines is also clade dependent. For instance, clade C Tat induces less monocyte chemoattractant protein-1/CCL-2 from human astrocytes than clade B Tat (Mishra et al., 2008; Rao et al., 2008). In one study, the cysteine to serine mutation at position 31, found in clade C Tat protein,

```
                    10        20        30        40        50        60        70        80        90       100
           ....|....|....|....|....|....|....|....|....|....|....|....|....|....|....|....|....|....|....|....|  ..
Consensus  MEPVDPNLEPWNHPGSQPKTACNKCYCKKCCYHCQVCFLKKGLGISYGRKKRRQRRRAPQSSKDHQNPIPKQPLSQTRGDPTGPEESKKKVESKTETDPF D$
Clade_A1   .D...........T.P.S..................N...........GT.............IP..Q.VS............A...R. .$
Clade_A2   .....K........................N.............P..GPS..N..........S.P..QRVS.......E....A...R. .$
Clade_B    ......R....K.......TN.....F.....IT..........D.QT..VSLS...A..P......K.......RE.....V .$
Clade_C    ...................H.S...L....QT..........S..P..E.......S...P.......S............$
Clade_D    .D...........R.P..........IT.............P..GGQA..D......S..P......K.$------------- --
Clade_F1   ..L....D.....T.P.T.....R.F...W..TT..........H.T....QI..D.V.......A..N....K....E....AK...C .$
Clade_F2   ..V...K.D.....E.P.......F...L..TR..........T....EI..D.V.......K.............K..L .$
Clade_G    .D...............M..W.....N..........KH..G.......V....PT..N............$
Clade_H    .D.....Q..........N..........L...........S...GT.A.LQ..........R.......K.$------------- --
```

Figure 9.6.2 Consensus sequence of different clades of Tat. Made from HIV sequence database (http://www.hiv.lanl.gov/).

was found to result in a marked decrease in IL-10 production in monocytes compared with clade B Tat due to its inability to induce intracellular calcium flux through L-type calcium channels (Wong et al., 2010). However, in another study, IL-4 and IL-10 were found to be higher in clade C Tat compared to clade B Tat-treated monocytes (Gandhi et al., 2009). A differential effect of clade B and C Tat on the kynurenic acid pathway in astrocytes has also been shown (Samikkannuet al., 2009).

The differential effects of the clades on Tat-induced transactivation of the HIV-1 long terminal repeat (LTR) has also been studied. Tat proteins derived from HIV-1 clades C and E are strong transactivators of LTR activity; Tat E also has a longer half-life than the other Tat proteins and interacts more efficiently with the stem-loop TAR element. Chimeric Tat proteins harboring the Tat E activation domain are also strong transactivators of LTR. The unique lysine residue at position 40 of Tat E contributes to the interaction with cyclin T1 and to the higher affinity of Tat E for cyclin T1 than that of Tat C which is critical for LTR transactivation (Desfosses et al., 2005).

Once the virus enters the brain it may continue to evolve, acquiring sequence heterogeneity different from that in lymphoid organs due to the different selective pressures in the brain. Thus far, only a limited number of studies have looked at viral sequences from brain tissue and fewer have tried to make any functional correlation of the viral sequences. However, available evidence tends to suggest that brain-derived viral sequences tend to favor its establishment as a reservoir, for example, brain derived *tat* sequences from HIV-demented patients are poor transactivators of the HIV-LTR, which permits the virus to stay latent and thus escape the immune system (Johnston et al., 2001). At the same time, they acquire more neurotoxic properties and both Tat and gp120 sequences from HIV-demented patients show increased neurotoxic potential (Power et al., 1998; Johnston et al., 2001).

In summary, HIV-1 clade differences can have profound effects on its geographical distribution, transmission, and disease pathogenesis. Molecular studies clearly show that the molecular diversity in co-receptor usage and that of HIV-1 Tat protein can significantly impact the neuropathogenesis of HIV-1 infection. However, further studies are necessary to determine the role of the other HIV-1 genes in the molecular pathogenesis of HIV-1 infection.

REFERENCES

Abebe, A., Demissie, D., et al. (1999). HIV-1 subtype C syncytium- and non-syncytium-inducing phenotypes and coreceptor usage among Ethiopian patients with AIDS. *AIDS*, *13*(11), 1305–1311.

Albright, A. V., Shieh, J. T. C., et al. (1999). Microglia express CCR5, CXCR4, and CCR3, but of these, CCR5 is the principal coreceptor for human immunodeficiency virus type 1 dementia isolates. *J Virol*, *73*(1), 205–213.

Baeten, J. M., Chohan, B., et al. (2007). HIV-1 subtype D infection is associated with faster disease progression than subtype A in spite of similar plasma HIV-1 loads. *J Infect Dis*, *195*(8), 1177–1180.

Blackard, J. T., Cohen, D. E., et al. (2002). Human immunodeficiency virus superinfection and recombination: Current state of knowledge and potential clinical consequences. *Clin Infect Dis*, *34*(8), 1108–1114.

Bonavia, R., Bajetto, A., et al. (2001). HIV-1 Tat causes apoptotic death and calcium homeostasis alterations in rat neurons. *Biochem Biophys Res Commun*, *288*(2), 301–308.

Campbell, G. R., Loret, E. P., et al. (2010). HIV-1 clade B Tat, but not clade C Tat, increases X4 HIV-1 entry into resting but not activated CD4+ T cells. *J Biol Chem*, *285*(3), 1681–1691.

Cecilia, D., Kulkarni, S. S., et al. (2000). Absence of coreceptor switch with disease progression in human immunodeficiency virus infections in India. *Virology*, *271*(2), 253–258.

Clifford, D. B., Mitike, M. T., et al. (2007). Neurological evaluation of untreated human immunodeficiency virus infected adults in Ethiopia. *J Neurovirol*, *13*(1), 67–72.

Desfosses, Y., Solis, M., et al. (2005). Regulation of human immunodeficiency virus type 1 gene expression by clade-specific Tat proteins. *J Virol*, *79*(14), 9180–9191.

Gandhi, N., Saiyed, Z., et al. (2009). Differential effects of HIV type 1 clade B and clade C Tat protein on expression of proinflammatory and antiinflammatory cytokines by primary monocytes. *AIDS Res Hum Retroviruses*, *25*(7), 691–699.

Gao, F., Bailes, E., et al. (1999). Origin of HIV-1 in the chimpanzee Pan troglodytes troglodytes. *Nature*, *397*(6718), 436–441.

Gregoire, C., Peloponese, Jr., J. M., et al. (2001). Homonuclear (1)H-NMR assignment and structural characterization of human immunodeficiency virus type 1 Tat Mal protein. *Biopolymers*, *62*(6), 324–335.

Gupta, J. D., Satishchandra, P., et al. (2007). Neuropsychological deficits in human immunodeficiency virus type 1 clade C-seropositive adults from South India. *J Neurovirol*, *13*(3), 195–202.

Hahn, B. H., Shaw, G. M., et al. (2000). AIDS as a zoonosis: Scientific and public health implications. *Science*, *287*(5453), 607–614.

Haughey, N. J., Holden, C. P., et al. (1999). Involvement of inositol 1,4,5-trisphosphate-regulated stores of intracellular calcium in calcium dysregulation and neuron cell death caused by HIV-1 protein tat. *J Neurochem*, *73*(4), 1363–1374.

Haughey, N. J. & Mattson, M. P. (2002). Calcium dysregulation and neuronal apoptosis by the HIV-1 proteins Tat and gp120. *J Acquir Immune Defic Syndr*, *31*Suppl 2, S55–61.

He, J., Chen, Y., et al. (1997). CCR3 and CCR5 are co-receptors for HIV-1 infection of microglia. *Nature*, *385*(6617), 645–649.

Hemelaar, J., Gouws, E., et al. (2006). "=Global and regional distribution of HIV-1 genetic subtypes and recombinants in 2004. *AIDS*, *20*(16), W13–23.

Hu, D. J., Buve, A., et al. (1999). What role does HIV-1 subtype play in transmission and pathogenesis? An epidemiological perspective. *AIDS*, *13*(8), 873–881.

Huang, W., Eshleman, S. H., et al. (2007). Coreceptor tropism in human immunodeficiency virus type 1 subtype D: High prevalence of CXCR4 tropism and heterogeneous composition of viral populations. *J Virol*, *81*(15), 7885–7893.

Ji, J. P. & Loeb, L. A. (1992). Fidelity of HIV-1 reverse transcriptase copying RNA in vitro. *Biochemistry*, *31*(4), 954–958.

Johnston, J. B., Zhang, K., et al. (2001). HIV-1 Tat neurotoxicity is prevented by matrix metalloproteinase inhibitors. *Ann Neurol*, *49*(2), 230–241.

Kaleebu, P., French, N., et al. (2002). Effect of human immunodeficiency virus (HIV) type 1 envelope subtypes A and D on disease progression in a large cohort of HIV-1-positive persons in Uganda. *J Infect Dis*, *185*(9), 1244–1250.

Kaleebu, P., Nankya, I. L., et al. (2007). Relation between chemokine receptor use, disease stage, and HIV-1 subtypes A and D: Results from a rural Ugandan cohort. *J Acquir Immune Defic Syndr*, *45*(1), 28–33.

Kandathil, A. J., Ramalingam, S., et al. (2005). Molecular epidemiology of HIV. *Indian J Med Res*, *121*(4), 333–344.

Kanki, P. J., Hamel, D. J., et al. (1999). Human immunodeficiency virus type 1 subtypes differ in disease progression. *J Infect Dis*, *179*(1), 68–73.

Kilmarx, P. H., Limpakarnjanarat, K., et al. (2000). Disease progression and survival with human immunodeficiency virus type 1 subtype E infection among female sex workers in Thailand. *J Infect Dis*, *181*(5), 1598–606.

Kiwanuka, N., Laeyendecker, O., et al. (2008). Effect of human immunodeficiency virus Type 1 (HIV-1) subtype on disease progression in persons from Rakai, Uganda, with incident HIV-1 infection. *J Infect Dis*, *197*(5), 707–713.

Kousiappa, I., Van De Vijver, D. A., et al. (2009). Near full-length genetic analysis of HIV sequences derived from Cyprus: Evidence of a highly polyphyletic and evolving infection. *AIDS Res Hum Retroviruses*, *25*(8), 727–740.

Li, W., Huang, Y., Reid, R., Steiner, J., Malpica-Llanos, T., Darden, T.A., et al. (2008). NMDA receptor activation by HIV-Tat protein is clade dependent. *J Neuroscience*, *28*, 12190–8.

Liner, K. J., 2nd, Hall, C. D., et al. (2007). Impact of human immunodeficiency virus (HIV) subtypes on HIV-associated neurological disease. *J Neurovirol*, *13*(4), 291–304.

Loemba, H., Brenner, B., et al. (2002). Co-receptor usage and HIV-1 intraclade C polymorphisms in the protease and reverse transcriptase genes of HIV-1 isolates from Ethiopia and Botswana. *Antivir Ther*, *7*(2), 141–148.

McArthur, J. C., Hoover, D. R., et al. (1993). Dementia in AIDS patients: Incidence and risk factors. Multicenter AIDS Cohort Study. *Neurology*, *43*(11), 2245–2252.

McMillan, N. A., Chun, R. F., et al. (1995). HIV-1 Tat directly interacts with the interferon-induced, double-stranded RNA-dependent kinase, PKR. *Virology*, *213*(2), 413–424.

Mishra, M., Vetrivel, S., et al. (2008). Clade-specific differences in neurotoxicity of human immunodeficiency virus-1 B and C Tat of human neurons: Significance of dicysteine C30C31 motif. *Ann Neurol*, *63*(3), 366–376.

Peeters, M., Vincent, R., et al. (1999). Evidence for differences in MT2 cell tropism according to genetic subtypes of HIV-1: Syncytium-inducing variants seem rare among subtype C HIV-1 viruses. *J Acquir Immune Defic Syndr Hum Retrovirol*, *20*(2), 115–121.

Peloponese, J. M., Jr., Collette, Y., et al. (1999). Full peptide synthesis, purification, and characterization of six Tat variants. Differences observed between HIV-1 isolates from Africa and other continents. *J Biol Chem*, *274*(17), 11473–11478.

Power, C., McArthur, J. C., et al. (1998). Neuronal death induced by brain-derived human immunodeficiency virus type 1 envelope genes differs between demented and nondemented AIDS patients. *J Virol*, *72*(11), 9045–9053.

Preston, B. D., Poiesz, B. J., et al. (1988). Fidelity of HIV-1 reverse transcriptase. *Science*, *242*(4882), 1168–1171.

Rao, V. R., Sas, A. R., et al. (2008). HIV-1 clade-specific differences in the induction of neuropathogenesis. *J Neurosci*, *28*(40), 10010–10016.

Robertson, D. L., Sharp, P. M., et al. (1995). Recombination in HIV-1. *Nature*, *374*(6518), 124–126.

Sacktor, N., Nakasujja, N., et al. (2009). HIV subtype D is associated with dementia, compared with subtype A, in immunosuppressed individuals at risk of cognitive impairment in Kampala, Uganda. *Clin Infect Dis*, *49*(5), 780–786.

Samikkannu, T., Saiyed, Z. M., et al. (2009). Differential regulation of indoleamine-2,3-dioxygenase (IDO) by HIV type 1 clade B and C Tat protein. *AIDS Res Hum Retroviruses*, *25*(3), 329–335.

Satishchandra, P., Nalini, A., et al. (2000). Profile of neurologic disorders associated with HIV/AIDS from Bangalore, south India (1989-96). *Indian J Med Res*, *111*, 14–23.

Shieh, J. T., Albright, A. V., et al. (1998). Chemokine receptor utilization by human immunodeficiency virus type 1 isolates that replicate in microglia. *J Virol*, *72*(5), 4243–4249.

Spira, S., Wainberg, M. A., et al. (2003). Impact of clade diversity on HIV-1 virulence, antiretroviral drug sensitivity and drug resistance. *J Antimicrob Chemother*, *51*(2), 229–240.

Tscherning, C., Alaeus, A., et al. (1998). Differences in chemokine coreceptor usage between genetic subtypes of HIV-1. *Virology*, *241*(2), 181–188.

Vasan, A., Renjifo, B., et al. (2006). Different rates of disease progression of HIV type 1 infection in Tanzania based on infecting subtype. *Clin Infect Dis*, *42*(6), 843–852.

Wong, J. K., Campbell, G. R., et al. (2010). Differential induction of interleukin-10 in monocytes by HIV-1 Clade B and Clade C Tat proteins. *J Biol Chem*.

Wong, M. H., Robertson, K., et al. (2007). Frequency of and risk factors for HIV dementia in an HIV clinic in sub-Saharan Africa. *Neurology*, *68*(5), 350–355.

Zhang, L., Huang, Y., et al. (1996). HIV-1 subtype and second-receptor use. *Nature*, *383*(6603), 768.

9.7

PROTEOMICS AND BIOMARKERS

Gwenael Pottiez, Jayme Wiederin, and Pawel Ciborowski

Proteome, a term that was created from the combination of "protein" and "genome," refers to the entire set of proteins expressed by a genome, cell, or tissue under a specified set of conditions. Just as genomics refers to the study of genes or genomes, so proteomics refers to the study of proteins or proteomes. More specifically, proteomics is the global study of the expression, localizations, functions, and interactions of proteins in any biological system. Proteomics emerged in the mid-1990s as a separate scientific field due to a rapid advancement in analytical technologies that made possible the reliable identification of multiple proteins simultaneously from the same biological sample. A biomarker, broadly defined, is any identifiable feature that reflects quantitative changes in a biological system. Biomarkers can indicate changes relevant to any aspect of a biological process or disease. This chapter explores the use of proteins, identified through proteomic methods, as biomarkers in the study and clinical management of HIV-associated disease. The particular focus is HIV-associated central nervous system disease.

INTRODUCTION

A broad definition of biomarker is any feature reflecting quantitative alterations in the status of a biological system. Taking this definition one step further, biomarkers can be classified into many groups which have a more focused characteristic and many biomarkers will likely belong to more than one group. Classifying biomarkers as predictive, prognostic, or diagnostic is simple and useful in clinical proteomics. For example, a diagnostic biomarker which is characterized by high sensitivity and specificity can be also classified as disease biomarker. The latter classification might be informative about molecular mechanisms underlying disease, but may not meet the criteria for qualifying as a diagnostic biomarker. On the other hand, biomarkers of developmental processes may be informative about initiation of, for example, differentiation or growth; however, may not inform about the final outcome of such process. Therefore, each type of biomarker has different purposes and must meet specific criteria of its application.

A biomarker does not necessarily need to be a biomolecule (molecular marker or signature molecule), but it can be a specific characteristic, feature, indicator, or alteration in any biological structure objectively measuring changes. Because proteomics is a global study of the expression, localizations,

functions, and interactions of proteins in any biological system, its focus is on proteins as biomarkers.

The term proteomics originated from genetic studies as a complement of proteins expressed by genome. The field of proteomics emerged in mid-1990s as a separate scientific field (Wilkins et al., 1996) due to the rapid advancement in analytical technologies that allowed using profiling methods with high confidence in reproducibility. One prominent example is how two-dimensional polyacrylamide gel electrophoresis (2D SDS-PAGE), originally developed in late '70s (O'Farrell, 1975; Barritault et al., 1976), was elevated as a profiling technique with the introduction of immobilized pH gradient (IPG strips) gels (Gelfi & Reghetti, 1983).

Protein microarrays, which emerged during the last 5 to 10 years, added yet another powerful tool in global screening of gene products in complex biological systems. Growth of all kinds of databases, and new and improved algorithms for database searches, opened the door for high throughput experiments with substantially increased quality of protein identification and quantitative measurements (Vigil, Davies, & Feigner, 2010; Haab, 2001).

Proteomic experiments are relative comparisons of protein expression representing two or more different conditions. They can be performed using various systems and samples such as cell culture, cell organelles, tissue from surgery, or biological fluids. Regardless which experimental system or profiling platform is used, proteomic analyses require samples containing sufficient initial amount of protein, which in contrast to nucleic acids, cannot be amplified. Therefore, each experiment will have specific limitations such as sample availability and quality, processing method, nature of protein subset and methods of profiling and detection. In some instances, such as investigation of cytokines, a profiling experiment can be performed much more effectively using methods other than typical proteomic profiling.

Clinical proteomics utilize mostly body fluids and tissues, and to lesser extent primary cells isolated from patients. Limitation of the latter approach is the small initial quantity of protein from isolated cells, which does not allow performing detailed investigation of medium to low abundant proteins in an unbiased type of experiment. In neurological disorders, we face an added challenge of available clinical material. Cerebrospinal fluid (CSF) contains 10 to 100 times less protein than plasma and a more limited volume of CSF can be drawn from patients. Use of brain tissue samples, which can be obtained only post-mortem from rapid autopsy programs, sparks controversy about the protein quality and stability, considering rapid molecular changes, for example, hypoxia, in the brain after death. Whether plasma can specifically reflect changes undergoing in the central nervous system (CNS) or will remain as a source of surrogate biomarkers is still not clear.

CSF is an attractive material for clinical proteomics of neurodegenerative disorders because it has direct contact with the CNS; however, there are also a number of limitations to using CSF for clinical proteomics. Besides limitation of quantity, another one is that lumbar puncture is an invasive and sometimes uncomfortable procedure to which some patients may not consent. Proteomic experiments, in spite of advanced technologies, need relatively large amounts of proteins to perform analyses and determine possible biomarkers and usually CSF samples contain too-low levels of proteins. Blood, plasma, and serum samples can be obtained much more easily than CSF; however, exchange of proteins between blood and brain is regulated by the blood-brain barrier (BBB). Due to the selective nature of the BBB, this poses a limitation of using plasma for biomarker discovery in neurodegenerative diseases.

BIOMARKERS OF HIV-ASSOCIATED NEUROCOGNITIVE DISORDER (HAND)– WHAT ARE WE LOOKING FOR?

Despite of many years of research, we still do not have solid biomarkers of HAND. Meanwhile, complications from HIV infection of the brain also may have undergone change due to new and improved therapies. The incidence of HIV-associated dementia (HAD) has declined, while the rate of less severe cognitive impairments remains about the same (Ances & Ellis, 2007; Wiederin et al., 2009). This raises not only the question of why do we not have biomarkers or whether evolution of cognitive impairments make them obsolete, but also what will biomarkers be or what do we expect them to be. What kind of biomarkers are we looking for in plasma/serum that will reflect ongoing disease of the CNS? This is not a question specific for HAND but also for other neurodegenerative disorders such as Alzheimer's, Parkinson's diseases, and so forth. It is quite obvious that proteomics is expected to discover new proteinaceous biomarkers. Will "biomarker of HAND" consist of a set of viral products, proteins, and nucleic acids; set of deregulated hosts' proteins of immune system; set of proteins reflecting neuronal death; or some unique combination of all categories? The following paragraphs will try to address these questions, although there is not one simple answer.

PROTEOMIC PLATFORMS

Proteomic experiments can be approached in two different ways. One is a global and unbiased approach in which compounding factors are minimized and the expected outcome is changes in protein expression between two or more groups.

Such experiments ask an open-ended question and the results generated identify many proteins that are not necessarily associated with a specific and known molecular mechanism relevant to HAND or other disease of interest. The second approach is directed or biased proteomics in which experiments are designed to address a more specific question related to changes of specific group of proteins, for example, proteins from the complement system, redox proteins, glycosylated or phosphorylated proteins.

In the subsequent sections, the general term "body fluids" will specifically refer to plasma, serum, and/or CSF samples, which are the most relevant fluids for discovery of biomarkers of HAND.

PROTEOMIC PLATFORMS IN CLINICAL APPLICATIONS

A major concern of proteomic analysis of body fluids is the high dynamic range in protein concentration where 14 proteins constitute approximately 95% of total protein. At the same time, it is hypothesized that biomarkers of disease will be of medium-to-low abundance proteins. Due to limitation of proteomic technologies to deal with high dynamic range of concentrations, the presence of highly abundant proteins masks the presence of the lower abundant proteins. Therefore, these high-abundant proteins need to be removed from body fluids prior to profiling. Several technologies have been developed; however, immunodepletion has been shown to be the most effective at this time. Immunodepletion does present some controversy, as there may be some nonspecific binding of proteins, resulting in the unintended removal of lower-abundant proteins which may provide important insights to biomarkers for disease state and changes. However, the immunodepletion strategy is the best way to prepare body fluids for proteomic analysis and has been used in many studies related to the discovery of biomarkers of HIV-associated neurological diseases (Pendyala et al., 2007; Rozek et al., 2007; Rozek et al., 2008). Common proteins to immunodeplete from clinical samples are serum albumin, α_1-antitrypsin, IgM, haptoglobin, fibrinogen, orosomucoid, apolipoprotein A-I and A-II, apolipoprotein B, IgG, IgA, transferrin, α_2-macroglobulin, and complement C3, which correspond to 95% of the proteins. A controversy remains: What is the optimal number of proteins to be immunodepleted? Our experience shows that 14 (listed above) to 18 would be the most appropriate.

Proteomic profiling of body fluids is limited to two experimental methods: analysis of intact proteins or protein-derived peptides. Peptides are fragments of proteins usually resulting from proteolytic digestion with trypsin. Fig. 9.7.1 provides an overview of these two approaches. Two-dimensional electrophoresis (2-DE) is an example of protein-based profiling, which compares differential expression of intact proteins that are separated by isoelectric focusing in first dimension followed by separation by mass in the second dimension (Table 9.7.1). A peptide-based approach is to make an in-solution enzymatic digestion of sample of interest (plasma, CSF, sera)

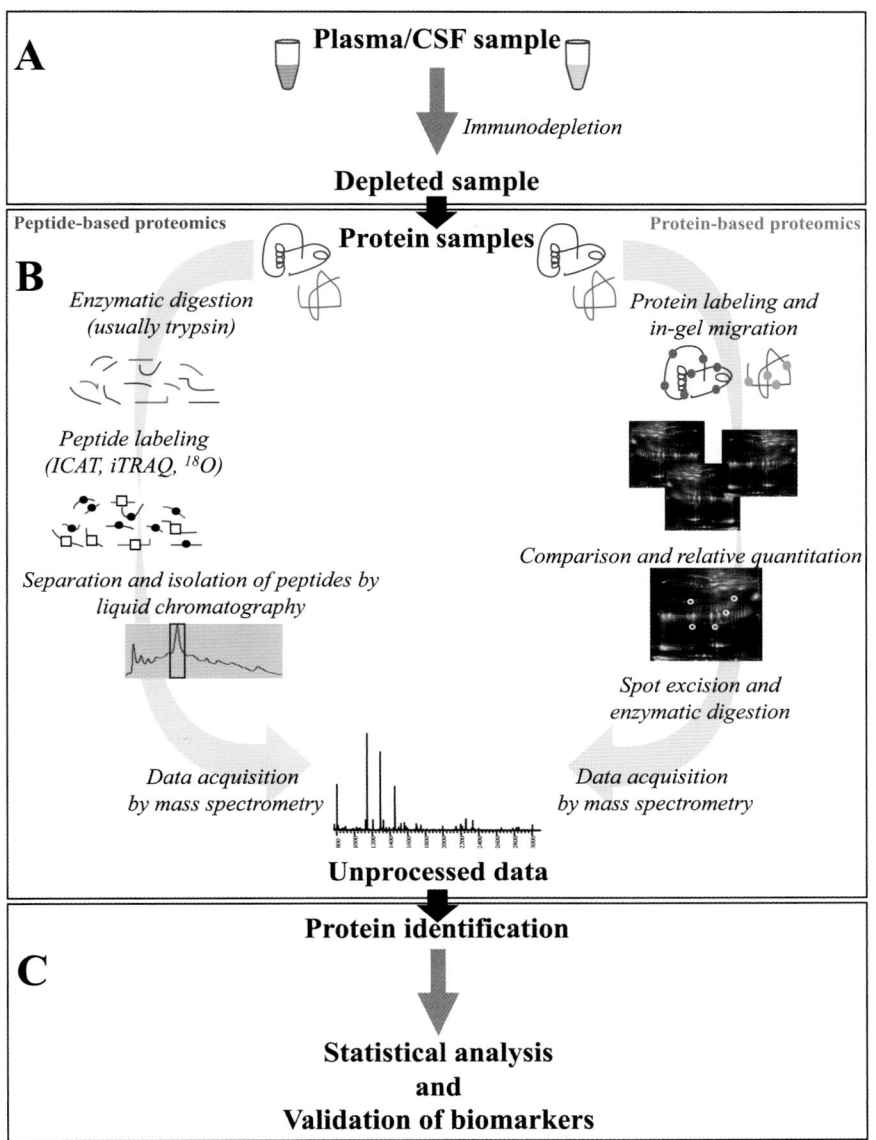

Figure 9.7.1 *Experimental design for biomarker discovery using proteomic platforms.* Proteomic analysis comprises three steps: (A) High abundant proteins from clinical samples mask the presence of low abundant proteins, therefore reducing potential biomarker information gained from proteomic studies; hence, the first step of a clinical proteomic study is the immunodepletion of the high abundant proteins from samples of interest. (B) The second step may be performed according to two strategies: protein-based and peptide-based proteomics platforms. Protein-based proteomics begins with labeling and separation of full-length proteins, which are detectable as spots in a gel. Quantification is performed by the comparing the intensity of the spots of interest, which are subsequently excised from the gel, digested using trypsin, and identified by mass spectrometry. Peptide-based proteomics starts with an enzymatic digestion (usually trypsin) of the proteins resulting in fragments called peptides. Peptides are labeled and used for the relative quantification of proteins. Finally, the identification and quantification of the proteins is made by mass spectrometry. (C) Computer software is used to identify proteins for possible biomarkers, followed by statistical analysis and validation.

using trypsin, followed by chemically labeling peptides with iTRAQ (isobaric tagging for absolute and relative quantification) and subsequently performing LC-MS/MS for peptide quantitation and protein identification. Alternatively, ICAT (isotope-coded affinity tag) or O^{18} labeling can be used for quantitation analysis of peptides. Both gel-based and mass-spectrometry-based techniques, as well as some existing alternatives, are discussed in further detail in this section.

Increased reproducibility of 2-DE resulted from the development of immobilized pH gradient (IPG) strips.

Another development that reduced variability between 2-DE gels was differential in-gel electrophoresis (DIGE), which adds another step to the in-gel separation where fluorescent molecules (Cy3, Cy5) are covalently linked to the proteins (Unlu, Morgan, & Minden, 1997). Since these fluorescent molecules have different excitation and emission wavelengths, two different samples of interest can be combined and separated in the same gel. This allows for a more sensitive detection and quantitation of protein spots using a scanner able to image gels of fluorescent-labeled proteins

Table 9.7.1 SUMMARY OF THE MOST FREQUENTLY USED PROTEOMIC TECHNIQUES

NAME (ABBREVIATION)	DESCRIPTION	ADVANTAGES	DRAWBACKS	REFERENCES
1-Dimensional Electrophoresis (1-DE)	Proteins are separated according to their mass.	Widely used technique, fast, easy to set up and inexpensive.	Low resolution, for fractionation of medium to low complexity samples. One band contains multiple proteins, thus utility as quantitative method is limited unless combined with western blot analysis.	Pendyala et al., 2007; Laspiur et al., 2007; Ciborowski et al., 2007
2-Dimensional Electrophoresis (2-DE)	Proteins are separated according to their pI (global charge) and then according to their mass.	Excellent technique for profiling of complex mixtures of whole proteins. Gives more information about protein isoforms and post-translational modifications	Limitation due to the pI of the proteins. Limitation due to the absence in the gel of the high and low mass proteins. Variations between gels induced by the migrations.	Unlu, Morgan, & Minden, 1997
2-Differential In-Gel Electrophoresis (2-D DIGE)	Proteins are labeled with fluorescent dyes for more precise quantification.	Fluorescence is more sensitive and more suitable for samples with high dynamic range of protein concentration.	First limitations of this technique are those ones from the 2-DE technique. Moreover, some differences exist between fluorescent dye labeling.	Rozek et al., 2008; Rozek et al., 2007
Mass Spectrometric Label Free Quantitation	Protein samples are digested and generated peptides are separated and analyzed by mass spectrometry. Relative quantification is obtained by comparison of MS spectrum.	No chemical modification is needed. Fragmentation of proteins (enzymatic digestion) is the only manipulation step in sample preparation.	Peak intensity for a peptide in mass spectrometry is highly associated to the sample composition. Then, the comparison of the peak intensity between spectra from different samples may be a limitation. No information available about the complete protein or post-translational modifications.	Wiener et al., 2004
Isotope Coded Affinity Tag (ICAT)	Proteins or peptides are labeled at cysteine residues with normal biotin (^{12}C) or biotin containing six ^{13}C. Labeled samples undergo affinity purification. Relative quantification is performed by comparison of ^{12}C and ^{13}C levels.	Using biotin for labeling allows for affinity purification of the proteins or after digest, purification of peptides reducing sample complexity.	3% of proteins do not contain cysteine. Moreover, this amino acid has a low level of expression within protein. This reduces the information and the quantification capability. No information available about the complete protein or post-translational modifications.	Gygi et al., 1999
Isobaric Tag for Relative and Absolute Quantification (iTRAQ)	Proteins are usually enzymatically digested, then, peptides are labeled with isobaric tags. Proteins are identified based on peptide sequencing and quantified based on relative comparisons of tags.	As proteins are digested protein's mass or pI are not limitations in this technique. Labels are added to N-terminal and lysine, after tryptic digest all peptides generated have a free N-terminal extremity. Moreover, lysine residue has a high level of expression in proteins. Thus, quantification is not limited.	No information is provided about the complete protein or about the post-translational modifications. Chemical labeling step variability.	Ross et al. 2004;
^{18}O labeling of peptides	Proteins are digested in the presence of H$_2$^{18}O water. Then, during digestion, ^{18}O is integrated to generated peptides, which allows quantification by comparison of peak intensity between peptides with ^{16}O and peptides with ^{18}O.	Enzymatic digestion is responsible for the labeling removing variability of chemical labeling. Quantification is performed during mass spectrometry analysis by comparison in one spectrum of the peak intensity of ^{16}O and ^{18}O.	Protein samples should be digested in 100% pure H$_2$^{18}O. The C-terminal peptides are not labeled.	Yao et al., 2001

(Continued)

Table 9.7.1 (CONTINUED)

NAME (ABBREVIATION)	DESCRIPTION	ADVANTAGES	DRAWBACKS	REFERENCES
Stable Isotope Labeling with Amino acid in Cell culture (SILAC)	Amino acids containing natural and stable heavy isotopes, such as ^{13}C and/or ^{15}N replace normal amino acids during culture to synthesize new proteins.	Samples with proteins containing normal amino acids–"light" - and those containing isotope amino acids -"heavy" - are pooled, digested and analyzed by mass spectrometry. Quantification is based on relative comparison of peak intensity (light to heavy).	Because of metabolic labeling nature of this method, its applicability is limited to cell cultures and cannot be applied to clinical samples, such as plasma or CSF. No information is provided about the complete protein or post-translational modifications.	Ong et al., 2002
Surface-Enhanced Laser Desorption/ Ionization (SELDI)	Protein samples are simplified using functionalized surfaces. Then, bound proteins are analyzed using mass spectrometry. The relative comparison is performed between spectra using peak intensity.	Fractionation of sample is performed directly on mass spectrometry target (chip). Fast data acquisition and analysis. Information is provided for full-length proteins.	The only information obtained from this technique is the relative abundance of "feature." Requires additional experimental steps for protein identification.	Cazares et al., 1999; Pendyala et al., 2007; Kadiu et al., 2007; Laspiur et al., 2007; Ciborowski et al., 2007; Agrawal et al., 2006; Rozek et al. 2008

based on different excitation and emission wavelengths. Nevertheless, a single study includes many gels that require alignment and the protein spots from all gels should be compared to relatively quantify the proteins. This step is executed through dedicated software which compares spots according to their position on the gel and evaluates the relative intensity of each spot. This analysis is time consuming and requires a human validation of the results.

One approach we present for mass spectrometry-based quantitation of peptides is iTRAQ, which was developed in 2004 (Ross et al., 2004). For this technique, proteins are digested in-solution and peptides are labeled using distinct tags with different isoforms of the same molecule. This technique allows the quantitation of up to eight distinct samples using eight distinct tags in the same experiment.

Along with constant development of technology for clinical proteomics, the role of some proteomic profiling platforms is diminishing. Surface-enhanced laser desorption ionization time-of-flight (SELDI-TOF) was developed in early 1990s (Hutchens & Yip, 1993) and commercialized by Ciphergen, Inc. in 1997 with the hope of fast discovery of many proteinaceous biomarkers. This platform is based on analysis of undigested proteins which are selectively bound to a chip surface based on such chemical characteristics as positive/negative charge at any given pH or hydrophobicity/hydrophilicity, and so forth. SELDI-TOF enables the comparison of peak intensity from mass spectra revealing relative differences in protein abundances for any given mass to charge ratio (m/z). Since this method does not provide identification of proteins, it therefore must be complemented with other approaches (Pendyala et al., 2007; Toro-Nieves et al., 2009). Wiederin et al. (2009) analyzed serum proteins initially by immunodepleting, using IgY-12 affinity chromatography to remove the twelve most abundant proteins, fractionated depleted samples on weak cation exchange (WCX)

high performance liquid chromatograpy (HPLC), followed by 1-dimensional electrophoresis (1-DE) to identify biomarker candidates of HAD. This platform was also used to investigate cytosolic proteins comparing proteomes of macrophages isolated from HIV-infected nondemented or demented individuals (Kadiu et al., 2007). Likewise, Laspiur et al. (2007) compared CSF samples from patients with normal cognition and cognitive impairment by simplifying the samples using reverse phase (RP) liquid chromatography, analyzing fractions with SELDL-TOF and 1-DE methods to determine a possible biomarker of cognitive impairment. Biomarkers revealed with those studies are discussed later in this chapter.

Another gel-based complementary technique is 1-DE, which is performed by separating proteins as bands according to their molecular weight. However, 1-DE bands usually contain a mix of proteins and before protein identification each band of proteins must be trypsin-digested in gel and the peptides generated need to be separated by liquid chromatography. Thus, this method is used for samples of lower complexity, while samples of high complexity such as body fluids need to be pre-fractionated by other means. However, this is a good approach to profile secreted proteins of cells obtained from diseased people. For example, when applied to investigation of immune cells from patients, this strategy reveals information about proteins released by these cells (Ciborowski et al., 2007). Accordingly, once proteins are identified, the study can be directed to body fluid samples to validate putative biomarkers.

CELL-BASED PROTEOMICS

All of the proteomic techniques described above can also be used in cell-based proteomics. However, one technique, stable isotope labeling with amino acids in cell culture (SILAC), cannot be used to study proteomes of body fluids. In this method, labels are natural isotopes, ^{13}C and ^{15}N incorporated into amino acids (Ong et al., 2002), which are added to cell culture. In consequence, new proteins made by cells will contain labeled "heavy" amino acids incorporated during natural metabolic process. Comparisons of two conditions, one non-labeled and the other one labeled with "heavy" amino acids, allows quantitation of differences in proteins on a broad scale. One caveat is that in such experiments, cells should be labeled with "heavy" amino acids at the 100% rate, which cannot be accomplished with nondividing cells, such as monocyte-derived macrophages. This can be overcome by adding additional controls measuring rate of incorporation without affecting the system (Kraft-Terry et al., 2011). This approach is currently used in several laboratories to study interactions between cells of the CNS (Wang et al., 2008; Wang et al., 2008; Sun et al., 2008; Liu et al., 2009; Hinkin et al., 2008).

Several other cell-based proteomic studies aiming at discovery of biomarkers for HAND have been conducted (Ricardo-Dukelow et al., 2007; Barroga et al., 1997; Ragin et al., 2006; Wojna et al., 2004). Another biased profiling approach is to use cells which are targets of HIV, such as mononuclear phagocytes and T lymphocytes, that are obtained from patients (primary cells) and experimentally infected *in vitro* (Ciborowski et al., 2007; Wojna et al., 2004). In this case, we can investigate the secretome of infected macrophages and cross-validate the results with clinical material such as CSF and plasma.

PROFILING OF CEREBROSPINAL FLUID

Profiling of CSF is almost as old as the field of proteomics itself and still carries the hope for discovery of new biomarkers of neurodegenerative diseases, including HAND (Unlu et al., 2000). Shortage of proteins due to the nature and availability of CSF was and still is a challenge of all these studies. For a general map of proteins present in CSF, samples can be pooled and such a strategy was used in early studies (Yuan, Russell, Wood, & Desiderio, 2002). Because of limitations of 2DE, the SELDI-TOF platform was an attractive alternative for quick discovery of biomarkers in CSF; however, lack of direct translation from observed molecular weight of protein and its identification, and issues related to reproducibility reduced greatly enthusiasm for this approach. Eventually, only a small number of studies were published, including those that attempted to use this platform for biomarker discovery of HAND (Luciano-Montalvo et al., 2008; Pendyala et al., 2007; Rozek et al., 2007; Berger et al., 2005).

Further studies suggested that proteins such as MIF, SOD-1, and cystatin C, amongst others, might be involved in cognitive impairment (Agrawal et al., 2006; Ciborowski et al., 2007). Another study based on 2D-DIGE analysis highlighted vitamin D binding protein, complement C3, cystatin C, procollagen C–endopeptidase enhancer, clusterin, and gelsolin as possible CSF biomarkers of HAD (Rozek et al., 2007). Among these biomarkers candidates, MIF is related to the viral replication while SOD-1 is an enzyme involved in antioxidant processes and is linked to neuronal protection

against apoptosis induced by HIV-1 gp120 (Louboutin et al., 2007; Louboutin et al., 2009; Agrawal et al., 2010) and Tat (Agrawal, Louboutin, & Strayer, 2007). Finally, cystatin C, whose levels are increased in plasma during HIV infection, has been linked to highly active antiretroviral therapy (HAART); level of cystatin C decreases with HAART treatment and increases when such therapy is discontinued (Jaroszewicz et al., 2006; Mocroft et al., 2009;). A summary of these data is presented in Table 9.7.2.

Recent proteomic studies showed identification of 1,500 unique proteins in CSF (Waybright et al., 2010). Although this study reflects unquestionable progress in proteomics of CSF, quantitative comparisons that meet criteria of diagnostic biomarkers remain an obstacle. Also, other methods such as iTRAQ are used to investigate proteome of CSF (Abdi et al., 2006; Ogata et al., 2007). These methods are now being used to further explore biomarkers of HAND in CSF and plasma (Ciborowski et al., unpublished). In conclusion, proteomic profiling of CSF for biomarkers of HAND is still in its early stages and limited to the unbiased approach. Biased proteomic profiling waits to be explored.

PROFILING OF SERUM/PLASMA

Blood (plasma, serum) remains in the center of the biomarker discovery effort. Blood can be easily obtained with minimally invasive intervention of the venipuncture. Nevertheless, the main question remains open whether plasma/serum can be a source of biomarkers for neurodegenerative disorders including HAND. As mentioned above, the blood-brain barrier regulates the exchange of proteins and metabolites between the CNS and blood; thus, we may expect that proteins can only "leak" from the CNS to blood and their concentration will likely be under limits of detection using even the most sensitive analytical techniques. On the other hand, we also expect that exchange of proteins and metabolites between CNS and blood is a form of exchange of "information" that can be captured. Another caveat is that protein identification requires usually less material than reliable quantitation of such protein within the milieu of complex mixture and high dynamic range. Despite these limitations, several studies have been performed in our and other laboratories trying to find such "information" also in the form of surrogate biomarkers. Wiederin et al. (2009) show the distribution of three potential biomarkers: ceruloplasmin, afamin, and gelsolin, between HIV-infected patients with or without HAD (Fig. 9.7.2). This study was limited to discovery phase and validation based on very small cohort of samples; therefore, it is premature to conclude about potential utility of these proteins as biomarkers with diagnostic or prognostic value. This study also shows the presence of outliers; however, the sample cohort does not provide any further information about whether these samples do not fit because of imperfect clinical classification or other external factors such as drug and/or alcohol use. Interestingly, one of those biomarkers, afamin, was also identified in another study using monkey plasma to show the factors involved in the pathogenicity of

PROTEIN NAME	ANALYZED BODY FLUID	FUNCTION	REFERENCES
Afamin	Plasma	Member of albumin family, postulated to be a transporter of yet unknown ligand. Differential expression associated with HAND, however mechanism unknown.	Pendyala et al., 2007; Torres-Munoz et al., 2001; Wiederin et al., 2009
Ceruloplasmin	Plasma	Copper binding and transporter of iron across cell membrane. Differential expression associated with HAND, however mechanism unknown.	Pendyala et al., 2007; Torres-Munoz et al., 2001; Wiederin et al., 2009
Clusterin	CSF	Clusterin produced in the brain by astrocytes may have a neuroprotective effect during HIV infection.	Irani et al., 2006
Complement C3	CSF Plasma	Plays central role in the activation of the complement system which is important for host innate immunity response to infection. Mechanism of correlation with HAND unclear.	Torres-Munoz et al. 2001
Cystatin C	CSF Plasma	Plasma level increases during HIV infection, decreases with antiretroviral therapy (HAART). An interruption of antiretroviral therapy results in an increase in cystatin C.	Rozek et al. 2007; Ciborowski et al., 2007; Mocroft et al., 2009;
Gelsolin	CSF Plasma	Associated with several inflammatory disorders and neurological disorders. Differential expression associated with HAND, however mechanism unknown.	Pendyala et al., 2007; Ross et al., 2004; Kulakowski et al., 2008; Velazquez et al., 2009; DiNublie 2008; Wiederin et al., 2009
Macrophage migration inhibitor factor (MIF)	CSF	May activate macrophage thus leading to pro-inflammatory responses.	Rozek et al., 2007
Procollagen C–endopeptidase enhancer	CSF	Involved in activation of collagen proteins, biological significance during HIV infection to be determined.	Rozek et al., 2007
Superoxide dismutase (SOD-1)	CSF	Involved in antioxidant processes and is linked to the neuronal protection against apoptosis induced by HIV-1 gp120 and Tat.	Ciborowski et al., 2007; Agrawal et al., 2007; Jaroszewicz et al., 2006;
Vitamin D binding protein (DBP)	CSF Plasma	Multifunctional protein which carries vitamin D but unclear link between DBP and HIV infection	Rozek et al 2007; Ciborowski et al., 2007

SIV (Pendyala et al., 2010). This serves as an example that an effort to discover new biomarkers must come from various directions and that lower-than-expected number of new potential biomarkers resulting from proteomic study must come from integration of animal models, cell based models, clinical studies, and technology, not technology alone.

Several of our studies showed differential expression of proteins belonging to complement cascade which were associated with various stages of HIV infection. Our observations were also made in samples of SIV-infected rhesus macaques (unpublished study). These observations are not surprising because the complement inflammatory cascade is part of the innate immune response bridging with acquired immunity by enhancing antibody responses and immunologic memory, lysing foreign cells and clearing immune complexes and apoptotic cells, all of which are important during retroviral infection. Complement cascade, regardless of how initiated, meet in a "hub" point of C3 component. Importantly, C3 modulates adaptive immunity at various levels, including T-cell proliferation, regulatory T-cell development and B-cell activation and differentiation (Morgan et al., 2005; Kemper & Atkinson, 2007; Carroll, 2004). Therefore, differential expression of complement C3 and other factors such as C4, C5, and so

forth, will reflect ongoing inflammatory process; however, it is difficult to separate neuroinflammation from inflammation on the periphery during HIV infection based only on measurements of these factors in plasma. Moreover, validation of each component is a challenging task. One solution that we have postulated would be measuring a-40 chain, a polypeptide fragment derived from C3 after final processing. This would be a measure of complete processing of C3 and could be compared to intact precursor. This hypothesis, however, needs to be further tested.

Regardless, whether these proteins will be validated in further studies or not, our results demonstrate that neurodegenerative diseases will require a set of changes as combined biomarkers to add a molecular component to clinical diagnosis based on neurocognitive evaluation. Moreover, changes in potential biomarkers must be validated by our understanding the molecular mechanism underlying HAND and other neurodegenerative diseases to eliminate confounding effect. A protein can have different properties, as circulating free in blood or being in a complex with other molecules. For example, it is known that gelsolin binds lipophosphatidic acid (LPA) at very high affinity; however, the biological meaning of this interaction is not known. One hypothesis is

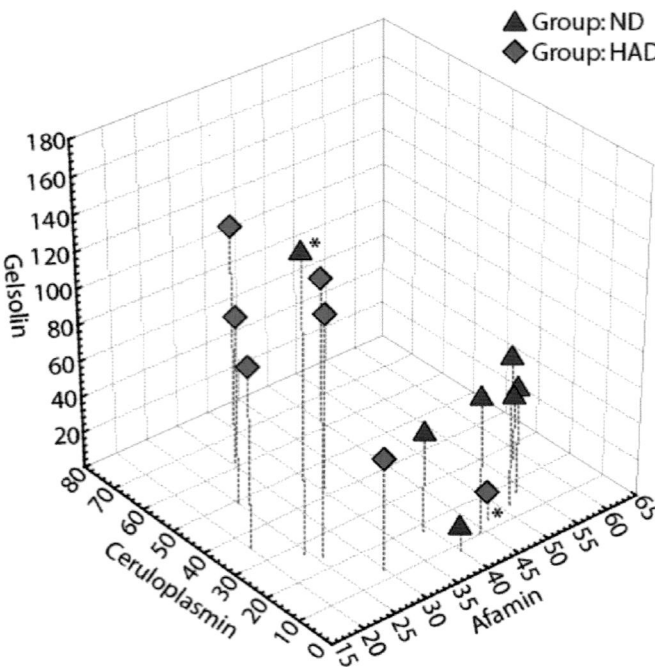

Group: ND
Group: HAD

Figure 9.7.2 *Sample Classification.* Classification of ND and HAD samples based on levels of afamin, ceruloplasmin and gelsolin as determined by densitometry measurements of Western blot films. Samples marked with an asterisk represent outliers. ND-non-demented; HAD-demented.

that LPA bound to gelsolin acquires new functional properties; however, there is no study showing the effect of such interactions on the functions of gelsolin.

PROFILING OF VIRAL PROTEINS

Viral proteins as potential diagnostic biomarkers have been in the center of interest because they affect the CNS in many ways, including neurotoxicity and toxicity to the BBB (King, Eugenin, Buckner, & Berman, 2006). Multiple studies have shown direct and indirect effect of viral proteins on neuronal injury (reviewed by Kaul et al., 2005). Furthermore, genetic studies postulate the existence of *env* genotypes associated with neurotropism and neurovirulence (Korber et al., 1994; Kuiken et al., 1995; Power et al., 1994; Di Stefano et al., 1996), although other studies have questioned this hypothesis (Ohagen et al., 2003; Reddy, & Dalmasso, 2003). Regardless of the conclusions of these studies, we have learned about genetic segregation of HIV between CSF and blood and its implication for therapy monitoring (Strain et al., 2005; Bottiggi et al., 2007).

HIV gp120 plays a critical role in virus entry into the target cells and contributes to neuronal death via various mechanisms (Nath & Sacktor, 2006; Nath et al., 2008; Wojna et al., 2006; Jurado et al., 1999). However, mutations and evolving glycosylation impair antibody-based neutralization. Subsequent studies using computational analysis of gp120C2-V3 loop led to the hypothesis of existence of "hot loops" in the viral genome, which have been suggested as

markers of future treatment strategies (Reddy et al., 1996). On the other hand, the level of gp120 as well as other viral structural proteins in patients treated with HAART is very low and often undetectable (Notermans et al., 1998; Cavert et al., 1997), although some patients show symptoms of neurocognitive impairment (Alvarez et al., 2006). This raises two important questions, one technical and one biological in nature. First, is whether sensitivity of protein analytical chemistry is sufficient for meaningful profiling. Second, is how these proteins can contribute to neurotoxicity at the borderline detection level. Here we discuss the first of these two questions.

The newest generation of mass spectrometers interfaced with liquid chromatography systems are sensitive enough to make it possible to derive peptide sequence from fragmented precursor ion at the high attomolar level if such peptide is efficiently ionized. If peptides are ionized less efficiently, femto- and pico-molar amount is necessary. Considering multistep manipulation during sample preparation, where every step causes some loss of protein, the initial amount of viral proteins needs to be much higher and very often in the high picomolar (100 pmoles of gp120 is equivalent of 12 ug of pure protein). To obtain such amounts of viral protein from a limited amount of CSF is difficult at best, if it is even possible. Therefore, mass spectrometry analysis will be limited to very few peptides, undermining the idea of comprehensive profiling. Another difficulty in profiling gp120 is high level of structurally diverse and extended N-linked glycans that are synthesized by host's cell glycosylation system. In most instances of our proteomic analyses of CSF, only one unique peptide per viral protein has been detected. Gp120 protein was represented by only a few peptides; however, the identified peptides were from conserved regions (Kristiansen et al., 2010). Therefore, it is unlikely that proteomic profiling of viral proteins directly in *ex vivo* specimen will provide useful information unless viral proteins are isolated by affinity chromatography. Gene sequencing of viral isolates, which can be amplified in *in vitro* cultures, seems to be a much more effective approach.

DATA ANALYSIS: BIOINFORMATICS, STATISTICS, AND VALIDATION

In the first step of proteomic data analysis, we use bioinformatic tools, such as protein database search algorithms for protein identification, often combined with modules that perform quantitative comparisons based on differences in amounts of peptides derived from protein (iTRAQ, see Fig. 9.7.1), or at the level of intact protein prior to protein identification (2DE DIGE, see Fig. 9.7.1) (Kirchner et al., 2010; Anderson et al., 2007). Such software packages also contain modules for statistical analysis. Nevertheless, critical steps need to be taken during the experimental design phase to secure all required data for proper downstream statistical analysis (Krogh et al., 2007; Kang et al., 2009). For example, if an experiment uses chemical labelling with a molecular tag such as a Cy dye or iTRAQ label, the experimental design should include a "scrambling" scheme that one sample type such as "visit 1" is labelled with all tags used in such an experiment. This will remove tag bias that may occur during chemical reaction. Bioinformatic analysis of proteomic approaches, as in all other "-omics" (i.e., genomic, metabolomic) approaches, generates large data sets showing many differences in protein expression regardless of platform used. Therefore, a major goal of statistical analysis is to remove from such data sets variability introduced during experimental design; for example, assembly of a patient's cohort and execution of a profiling experiment, and narrow differences to those which are meaningful and relevant to biology.

The decision about number of technical and biological replicates is another step required prior to execution of an experiment. An example of technical replicates is the multiple labeling (also called reciprocal labeling) of the same sample with the purpose of control of a technical process. A properly executed experiment by a well-trained person should have minimal variation, thus reducing the need for technical replicates. A biological replicate means performing the experiments with samples derived from independent sources, such as multiple cultures of one cell line, multiple cell lines, biopsies, or individuals enrolled in the study. Biological replicates are essential for linking observed change with a biological effect of an experiment as well as for validation. Therefore, biological replicates are more informative than technical replicates and factors such as variability originating from genetic background of enrolled patients cannot be assessed based on technical replicates only. However, quality of biological replicates is essential.

Once bioinformatic and statistical analysis is performed and a number of proteins show differential expression under investigated conditions, a cohort of samples and methods need to be selected for validation. The general rule of validation is that it should be performed using different experimental means than were used during discovery phase and usually involves a larger separate cohort of samples. Validation, which is a targeted type of experiment, requires much less material; therefore, availability of limited samples such as CSF is more widely available for validation than for performing full unbiased proteomic profiling. There is a variety of validation methods to choose from; however, the most popular are quantitative Western blot and ELISA assays. Another validation method, which has been known for many years, but is gaining recent attention in proteomics, is multiple reaction monitoring (MRM) (Yocum & Chinnaiyan, 2009). This method of validation is independent of antibodies, thus eliminating the problem of availability and specificity of antibodies, and measures directly the quantity of peptides belonging to the protein of interest. Moreover, multiple proteins can be measured in one analytical run, which takes approximately 2 hours. Because MRM uses a defined precursor ion and matches fragment ions generated in collision chamber of mass spectrometer, this approach uses, in a sense, the mass spectrometer as a "secondary antibody" that has absolute structural specificity. MRM is also an excellent analytical tool to investigate concurrent changes in levels of multiple proteins, aiding in data interpretation.

Statistical analysis is a parallel step to translate validated data to utility of a candidate as useful diagnostic biomarker. Statistical analysis addresses three questions: sensitivity, specificity, and correlation (or lack of) with other parameters in a blinded study. Many biomarker candidates fail to show their utility when used to discriminate between diseased and control patients, regardless of careful and thorough up-stream analysis. Complement C3 can be used as one example. This protein shows differential expression in many proteomic profiling experiments; however, these differences did not translate when other means of analytical measure were used. Consultation of experimental design with professional statisticians prior to initiation of the discovery phase will help identify at which point a candidate fails as a biomarker and thus will reduce costs and effort in subsequent experiments.

CONCLUSION

In its young lifetime, proteomics has already evolved from the initial fascination with ability to identify high numbers of proteins in a single experiment. Proteomics has also evolved in the sense that quantitation is now widely available and quantitative mass spectrometry of proteins has become a standard method in proteomics laboratories along with 2D SDS-PAGE. Bioinformatic tools are much more advanced and tremendous progress has been made in how proteomic data need to be analyzed, resulting in constantly increasing their quality. At the same time, proteomics did not deliver hundreds of new biomarkers, which was the initial expectation. This paradox taught us that technology itself is not sufficient and a strong biological foundation of proteomic experiments is crucial. If a subtle change at the protein level may have a profound biological effect, how do we differentiate between biologically important changes and natural variation among populations of patients? Discovering new biomarkers of HAND is even more challenging. ART therapy successfully reduced the number of more severe dementias; however, the percentage of patients suffering from milder neurocognitive impairment has not changed, and differences between various stages of HAND are much more subtle. It becomes quite obvious that understanding functions of complex biological systems will require coordinated monitoring of a large number of parameters at the same time and well-designed proteomics, genomics, transcriptomics, metabolomics, as well as neuro-imaging experiments. Once we know how to integrate these data, new molecular biomarkers will emerge.

REFERENCES

Abdi, F., Quinn, J. F., Jankovic, J., McIntosh, M., Leverenz, J. B., Peskind, E., et al. (2006). Detection of biomarkers with a multiplex quantitative proteomic platform in cerebrospinal fluid of patients with neurodegenerative disorders. *J Alzheimers Dis, 9*, 293–348.

Agrawal, L., Louboutin, J. P., Marusich, E., Reyes, B. A., Van Bockstaele, E. J., & Strayer, D. S. (2010). Dopaminergic neurotoxicity of HIV-1 gp120: Reactive oxygen species as signaling intermediates. *Brain Res, 1306*, 116–130.

Agrawal, L., Louboutin, J. P., Reyes, B. A., Van Bockstaele, E. J., & Strayer, D. S. (2006). Antioxidant enzyme gene delivery to protect from HIV-1 gp120-induced neuronal apoptosis. *Gene Ther*, 13, 1645–1656.

Agrawal, L., Louboutin, J. P., & Strayer, D. S. (2007). Preventing HIV-1 Tat-induced neuronal apoptosis using antioxidant enzymes: mechanistic and therapeutic implications. *Virology*, 363, 462–472.

Alvarez, S., Jimenez, J. L., Serramia, M. J., Gonzalez, M., Canto-Nogues, C., & Munoz-Fernandez, M. A. (2006). Lack of association of HIV-1 biological or molecular properties with neurotropism for brain cells. *J Mol Neurosci*, 29, 131–144.

Ances, B. M. & Ellis. R. J. (2007). Dementia and neurocognitive disorders due to HIV-1 infection. *Semin Neurol*, 27, 86–92.

Anderson, T. J., Tchernyshyov, I., Diez, R., Cole, R. N., Geman, D., Dang, C. V., et al. (2007). Discovering robust protein biomarkers for disease from relative expression reversals in 2-D DIGE data. *Proteomics*, 7, 1197–1207.

Barritault, D., Expert-Bezancon, A., Milet, M., & Hayes, D. H. (1976). Inexpensive and easily built small scale 2D electrophoresis equipment. *Anal Biochem*, 70,600–611.

Barroga, C. F., Ellis, R., Nelson, J., Heaton, R. K., Atkinson, J. H., McCutchan, J. A., et al. (1997). HIV-1 neurocognitive disorders and chemokine receptors. *AIDS*, 11, 1651–1652.

Berger, J. R., Avison, M., Mootoor, Y., & Beach, C. (2005). Cerebrospinal fluid proteomics and human immunodeficiency virus dementia: Preliminary observations. *J Neurovirol*, 11, 557–562.

Bottiggi, K. A., Chang, J. J., Schmitt, F. A., Avison, M. J., Mootoor, Y., Nath, A., et al. (2007). The HIV Dementia Scale: Predictive power in mild dementia and HAART. *J Neurol Sci*, 260, 11–15.

Carroll, M. C. (2004). The complement system in regulation of adaptive immunity. *Nat Immunol*, 5, 981–986.

Cavert, W., Notermans, D. W., Staskus, K., Wietgrefe, S. W., Zupancic, M., Gebhard, K., et al. (1997). Kinetics of response in lymphoid tissues to antiretroviral therapy of HIV-1 infection. *Science*, 276, 960–964.

Ciborowski, P., Kadiu, I., Rozek, W., Smith, L., Bernhardt, K., Fladseth, M., et al. (2007). Investigating the human immunodeficiency virus type 1-infected monocyte-derived macrophage secretome. *Virology*, 363, 198–209.

DiNubile, M. J. (2008). Plasma gelsolin as a biomarker of inflammation. *Arthritis Res Ther*, 10, 124.

Di Stefano, M., Wilt, S., Gray, F., Dubois-Dalcq, M., & Chiodi, F. (1996). HIV type 1 V3 sequences and the development of dementia during AIDS, *AIDS Res Hum Retroviruses*, 12, 471–476.

Jr, G. W., Cazares, L. H., Leung, S. M., Nasim, S., Adam, B. L., Yip, T. T., et al. (1999). Proteinchip(R) surface enhanced laser desorption/ionization (SELDI) mass spectrometry: A novel protein biochip technology for detection of prostate cancer biomarkers in complex protein mixtures. *Prostate Cancer Prostatic Dis*, 2, 264–276.

Gelfi, C. & Righetti, P. G. (1983). Preparative isoelectric focusing in immobilized pH gradients. II. A case report. *J Biochem Biophys Methods*, 8, 157–172.

Gygi, S. P., Rist, B., Gerber, S. A., Turecek, F., Gelb, M. H., & Aebersold, R. (1999). Quantitative analysis of complex protein mixtures using isotope-coded affinity tags. *Nat Biotechnol*, 17, 994–999.

Haab, B. B. (2001). Advances in protein microarray technology for protein expression and interaction profiling. *Curr Opin Drug Discov Devel*, 4,116–123.

Hinkin, C. H., Castellon, S. A., Levine, A. J., Barclay, T. R., & Singer, E. J. (2008). Neurocognition in individuals co-infected with HIV and hepatitis C. *J Addict Dis*, 27, 11–17.

Hutchens, T. & Yip, T. (1993). New desorption strategies for the mass spectrometric analysis of macromolecules. *Rapid Communications in Mass Spectrometry*, 7, 576–580.

Irani, D. N., Anderson, C., Gundry, R., Cotter, R., Moore, S., Kerr, D. A., et al. (2006). Cleavage of cystatin C in the cerebrospinal fluid of patients with multiple sclerosis. *Ann Neurol*, 59, 237–247.

Jaroszewicz, J., Wiercinska-Drapalo, A., Lapinski, T. W., Prokopowicz, D., Rogalska, M., & Parfieniuk, A. (2006). Does HAART improve renal function? An association between serum cystatin C concentration, HIV viral load and HAART duration. *Antivir Ther*, 11, 641–645.

Jurado, A., Rahimi-Moghaddam, P., Bar-Jurado, S., Richardson, J. S., Jurado, M., & Shuaib, A. (1999). Genetic markers on HIV-1 gp120 C2-V3 region associated with the expression or absence of cognitive motor complex in HIV/AIDS. *J NeuroAIDS*, 2, 15–28.

Kadiu, I., Ricardo-Dukelow, M., Ciborowski, P., & Gendelman, H. E. (2007). Cytoskeletal protein transformation in HIV-1-infected macrophage giant cells. *J Immunol*, 178, 6404–6415.

Kang, Y., T., Techanukul, A., Mantalaris, & Nagy, J. M. (2009). Comparison of three commercially available DIGE analysis software packages: Minimal user intervention in gel-based proteomics. *J Proteome Res*, 8, 1077–1084.

Kaul, M., Zheng, J., Okamoto, S., Gendelman, H. E., & Lipton, S. A. (2005). HIV-1 infection and AIDS: Consequences for the central nervous system. *Cell Death Differ*, 12 Suppl 1, 878–892.

Kemper, C. & Atkinson, J. P. (2007). T-cell regulation: With complements from innate immunity. *Nat Rev Immunol*, 7, 9–18.

King, J. E., Eugenin, E. A., Buckner, C. M., & Berman, J. W. (2006). HIV tat and neurotoxicity. *Microbes Infect*, 8, 1347–1357.

Kirchner, M., Renard, B. Y., Kothe, U., Pappin, D. J., Hamprecht, F. A., Steen, H., et al. (2010). Computational protein profile similarity screening for quantitative mass spectrometry experiments. *Bioinformatics*, 26, 77–83.

Korber, B. T., Kunstman, K. J., Patterson, B. K., Furtado, M., McEvilly, M. M., Levy, R., et al. (1994). Genetic differences between blood- and brain-derived viral sequences from human immunodeficiency virus type 1-infected patients: Evidence of conserved elements in the V3 region of the envelope protein of brain-derived sequences. *J Virol*, 68, 7467–7481.

Kraft-Terry, S. D., Engebretsen, I. L., Bastola, D. K.., Fox, H. S., Ciborowski, P., & Gendelman, H. E. (2011). http://www.ncbi.nlm.nih.gov/pubmed/21500866" Pulsed Stable Isotope Labeling of Amino Acids in Cell Culture Uncovers the Dynamic Interactions between HIV-1 and the Monocyte-Derived Macrophage. *J Proteome Res*, 3, 2852–2862.

Kristiansen, L. C., Jacobsen, S., Jessen, F., & Jorgensen, B. M. (2010) Using a cross-model loadings plot to identify protein spots causing 2-DE gels to become outliers in PCA. *Proteomics*,

Krogh, M., Liu, Y., Waldemarson, S., Valastro, B., & James, P. (2007). Analysis of DIGE data using a linear mixed model allowing for protein-specific dye effects. *Proteomics*, 7, 4235–4244.

Kuiken, C. L., Goudsmit, J., Weiller, G. F., Armstrong, J. S., Hartman, S., Portegies, P., et al. (1995). Differences in human immunodeficiency virus type 1 V3 sequences from patients with and without AIDS dementia complex. *J Gen Virol*, 76 (Pt 1), 175–180.

Kulakowska, A., Drozdowski, W., Sadzynski, A., Bucki, R., & Janmey, P. A. (2008). Gelsolin concentration in cerebrospinal fluid from patients with multiple sclerosis and other neurological disorders. *Eur J Neurol*, 15, 584–588.

Laspiur, J. P., Anderson, E. R., Ciborowski, P., Wojna, V., Rozek, W., Duan, F., et al. (2007). CSF proteomic fingerprints for HIV-associated cognitive impairment. *J Neuroimmunol*, 192, 157–170.

Liu, J., Gong, N., Huang, X., Reynolds, A. D., Mosley, R. L., & Gendelman, H. E. (2009). Neuromodulatory activities of CD4+CD25+ regulatory T cells in a murine model of HIV-1-associated neurodegeneration. *J Immunol*, 182, 3855–3865.

Louboutin, J. P., Agrawal, L., Reyes, B. A., Van Bockstaele, E. J., & Strayer, D. S. (2007). Protecting neurons from HIV-1 gp120-induced oxidant stress using both localized intracerebral and generalized intraventricular administration of antioxidant enzymes delivered by SV40-derived vectors. *Gene Ther*, 14, 1650–1661.

Louboutin, J. P., Agrawal, L., Reyes, B. A., Van Bockstaele, E. J., & Strayer, D. S. (2009). HIV-1 gp120 neurotoxicity proximally and at a distance from the point of exposure: Protection by rSV40 delivery of antioxidant enzymes. *Neurobiol Dis*, 34, 462–476.

Luciano-Montalvo, C., Ciborowski, P., Duan, F., Gendelman, H. E., & Melendez, L. M. (2008). Proteomic analyses associate cystatin B with restricted HIV-1 replication in placental macrophages. *Placenta*, 29, 1016–1023.

Mocroft, A., Wyatt, C., Szczech, L., Neuhaus, J., El-Sadr, W., Tracy, R., et al. (2009). Interruption of antiretroviral therapy is associated with increased plasma cystatin C. *AIDS*, 23, 71–82.

Morgan, B. P., Marchbank, K. J., Longhi, M. P., Harris, C. L., & Gallimore, A. M. (2005). Complement: Central to innate immunity and bridging to adaptive responses. *Immunol Lett, 97*, 171–179.

Nath, A. & Sacktor, N. (2006). Influence of highly active antiretroviral therapy on persistence of HIV in the central nervous system. *Curr Opin Neurol, 19*, 358–361.

Nath, A., Schiess, N., Venkatesan, A., Rumbaugh, J., Sacktor, N., & McArthur, J. (2008). Evolution of HIV dementia with HIV infection. *Int Rev Psychiatry, 20*, 25–31.

Notermans, D. W., Jurriaans, S., de Wolf, F., Foudraine, N. A., de Jong, J. J., Cavert, W., et al. (1998). Decrease of HIV-1 RNA levels in lymphoid tissue and peripheral blood during treatment with ritonavir, lamivudine and zidovudine. Ritonavir/3TC/ZDV Study Group. *AIDS 12*, 167–173.

O'Farrell, P. H. (1975). High resolution two-dimensional electrophoresis of proteins. *J Biol Chem, 250*, 4007–4021.

Ogata, Y., Charlesworth, M. C., Higgins, L., Keegan, B. M., Vernino, S., & Muddiman, D. C. (2007). Differential protein expression in male and female human lumbar cerebrospinal fluid using iTRAQ reagents after abundant protein depletion. *Proteomics, 7*, 3726–3734.

Ohagen, A., Devitt, A., Kunstman, K. J., Gorry, P. R., Rose, P. P., Korber, B., et al. (2003). Genetic and functional analysis of full-length human immunodeficiency virus type 1 env genes derived from brain and blood of patients with AIDS. *J Virol, 77*, 12336–12345.

Ong, S. E., Blagoev, B., Kratchmarova, I., Kristensen, D. B., Steen, H., Pandey, A., et al. (2002). Stable isotope labeling by amino acids in cell culture, SILAC, as a simple and accurate approach to expression proteomics. *Mol Cell Proteomics, 1*, 376–386.

Pendyala, G., Trauger, S. A., Siuzdak, G., & Fox, H. S. (2010) Quantitative plasma proteomic profiling identifies the vitamin E binding protein afamin as a potential pathogenic factor in SIV induced CNS disease. *J Proteome Res, 9*, 352–358.

Pendyala, G., Want, E. J., Webb, W., Siuzdak, W., & Fox, H. S. (2007). Biomarkers for neuroAIDS: The widening scope of metabolomics. *J Neuroimmune Pharmacol, 2*, 72–80.

Power, C., McArthur, J. C., Johnson, R. T., Griffin, D. E., Glass, J. D., Perryman, S., et al. (1994). Demented and nondemented patients with AIDS differ in brain-derived human immunodeficiency virus type 1 envelope sequences. *J Virol, 68*, 4643–4649.

Ragin, A. B., Wu, Y., Storey, P., Cohen, B. A., Edelman, R. R., & Epstein, L. G. (2006). Monocyte chemoattractant protein-1 correlates with subcortical brain injury in HIV infection. *Neurology, 66*, 1255–1257.

Reddy, R. T., Achim, C. L., Sirko, D. A., Tehranchi, S., Kraus, F. G., Wong-Staal, F., et al. (1996). Sequence analysis of the V3 loop in brain and spleen of patients with HIV encephalitis. *AIDS Res Hum Retroviruses, 12*, 477–482.

Reddy, G. & Dalmasso, E. A. (2003). SELDI ProteinChip(R) array technology: Protein-based predictive medicine and drug discovery applications. *J Biomed Biotechnol*, (no journal number), 237–241.

Ricardo-Dukelow, M., Kadiu, I., Rozek, W., Schlautman, J., Persidsky, Y., Ciborowski, P., et al. (2007). HIV-1 infected monocyte-derived macrophages affect the human brain microvascular endothelial cell proteome: New insights into blood-brain barrier dysfunction for HIV-1-associated dementia. *J Neuroimmunol, 185*, 37–46.

Ross, P. L., Huang, Y. N., Marchese, J. N., Williamson, B., Parker, K., Hattan, S., et al. (2004). Multiplexed protein quantitation in Saccharomyces cerevisiae using amine-reactive isobaric tagging reagents. *Mol Cell Proteomics, 3*, 1154–1169.

Rozek, W., Horning, J., Anderson, J., & Ciborowski, P. (2008). Sera proteomic biomarker profiling in HIV-1 infected subjects with cognitive impairment. *Proteomics - Clinical Applications, 2*, 1484–1507.

Rozek, W., Ricardo-Dukelow, M., Holloway, S., Gendelman, H. E., Wojna, V., L. Melendez, M., et al. (2007). Cerebrospinal fluid proteomic profiling of HIV-1-infected patients with cognitive impairment. *J Proteome Res, 6*, 4189–4199.

Strain, M. C., Letendre, S., Pillai, S. K., Russell, T., Ignacio, C. C., Gunthard, H. F., et al. (2005). Genetic composition of human immunodeficiency virus type 1 in cerebrospinal fluid and blood without treatment and during failing antiretroviral therapy. *J Virol, 79*, 1772–1788.

Sun, J., Zheng, J. H., Zhao, M., Lee, S., & Goldstein, H. (2008). Increased in vivo activation of microglia and astrocytes in the brains of mice transgenic for an infectious R5 human immunodeficiency virus type 1 provirus and for CD4-specific expression of human cyclin T1 in response to stimulation by lipopolysaccharides. *J Virol, 82*, 5562–5572.

Toro-Nieves, D. M., Rodriguez, Y., Plaud, M., Ciborowski, P., Duan, F., Perez Laspiur, J., et al. (2009). Proteomic analyses of monocyte-derived macrophages infected with human immunodeficiency virus type 1 primary isolates from Hispanic women with and without cognitive impairment. *J Neurovirol, 15*, 36–50.

Torres-Munoz, J. E., Redondo, M., Czeisler, C., Roberts, B., Tacoronte, N., & Petito, C. K. (2001). Upregulation of glial clustering in brains of patients with AIDs. *Brain Res, 888*, 297–301.

Unlu, M., de Lange, R. P., de Silva, R., Kalaria, R., & St Clair, D. (2000). Detection of complement factor B in the cerebrospinal fluid of patients with cerebral autosomal dominant arteriopathy with subcortical infarcts and leukoencephalopathy disease using two-dimensional gel electrophoresis and mass spectrometry. *Neurosci Lett, 282*, 149–152.

Unlu, M., Morgan, M. E., & Minden, J. S. (1997). Difference gel electrophoresis: A single gel method for detecting changes in protein extracts. *Electrophoresis, 18*, 2071–2077.

Velazquez, I., Plaud, M., Wojna, V., Skolasky, R., Laspiur, J. P., & Melendez, L. M. (2009). Antioxidant enzyme dysfunction in monocytes and CSF of Hispanic women with HIV-associated cognitive impairment. *J Neuroimmunol, 206*, 106–111.

Vigil, A. D., Davies, H., & Felgner, P. L. (2010) Defining the humoral immune response to infectious agents using high-density protein microarrays. *Future Microbiol, 5, 241–251*.

Wang, T., Gong, N., Liu, J., Kadiu, I., Kraft-Terry, S. D., Mosley, R. L., et al. (2008). Proteomic modeling for HIV-1 infected microglia-astrocyte crosstalk. *PLoS One, 3*, e2507.

Wang, T., Gong, N., Liu, J., Kadiu, I., Kraft-Terry, S. D., Schlautman, J. D., et al. (2008). HIV-1-infected astrocytes and the microglial proteome. *J Neuroimmune Pharmacol, 3*, 173–186

Waybright, T., Avellino, A. M., Ellenbogen, R. G., Hollinger, B. J., Veenstra, T. D., & Morrison, R. S. (2010). Characterization of the human ventricular cerebrospinal fluid proteome obtained from hydrocephalic patients. *J Proteomics*.

Wiederin, J., Rozek, W., Duan, F., & Ciborowski, P. (2009). Biomarkers of HIV-1 associated dementia: Proteomic investigation of sera. *Proteome Sci, 7*, 8.

Wiener, M. C., Sachs, J. R., Deyanova, E. G., & Yates, N. A. (2004). Differential mass spectrometry: A label-free LC-MS method for finding significant differences in complex peptide and protein mixtures. *Anal Chem, 76*, 6085–6096.

Wilkins, M. R., Pasquali, C., Appel, R. D., Ou, K., Golaz, O., Sanchez, J. C., et al. (1996). From proteins to proteomes: Large scale protein identification by two-dimensional electrophoresis and amino acid analysis. *Biotechnology, 14*, 61–65.

Wojna, V., Carlson, K. A., Luo, X., Mayo, R., Melendez, L. M., Kraiselburd, E., et al. (2004). Proteomic fingerprinting of human immunodeficiency virus type 1-associated dementia from patient monocyte-derived macrophages: A case study. *J Neurovirol, 10* Suppl 1, 74–81.

Wojna, V., Skolasky, R. L., Hechavarria, R., Mayo, R., Selnes, O., McArthur, J. C., et al. (2006). Prevalence of human immunodeficiency virus-associated cognitive impairment in a group of Hispanic women at risk for neurological impairment. *J Neurovirol, 12*, 356–364.

Yao, X., Freas, A., Ramirez, J., Demirev, P. A., & Fenselau, C. (2001). Proteolytic 18O labeling for comparative proteomics: Model studies with two serotypes of adenovirus. *Anal Chem, 73*, 2836–2842.

Yocum, A. K. & Chinnaiyan, A. M. (2009). Current affairs in quantitative targeted proteomics: Multiple reaction monitoring-mass spectrometry. *Brief Funct Genomic Proteomic, 8*, 145–157.

Yuan, X., Russell, T., Wood, G., & Desiderio, D. M. (2002). Analysis of the human lumbar cerebrospinal fluid proteome. *Electrophoresis, 23*, 1185–1196.

SECTION 10

CHILDREN AND ADOLESCENTS

Stuart A. Lipton

10.1

CLINICAL AND PATHOLOGICAL FEATURES OF HIV-1 ENCEPHALOPATHY IN CHILDREN AND ADOLESCENTS

Mark Mintz, Leroy R. Sharer, and Lucy A. Civitello

With the advent of effective antiretroviral drugs administered to HIV-infected women, the incidence of mother-to-child transmission of HIV-1 infection has been dramatically reduced. However, there are many parts of the world where there is inadequate accessibility or compliance with protocols to disrupt perinatal HIV-1 infection, or there remains a prevalence of horizontal modes of infection, and thus, HIV-1 infection in children continues to be an important international public health crisis, particularly in sub-Saharan Africa. A defining clinical feature of acquired immunodeficiency syndrome (AIDS), HIV-1-associated progressive encephalopathy (PE) can cause impairment of brain development and growth, leading to significant motor dysfunction, neurodevelopmental regression, and neurocognitive impairment. From the direct and indirect effects of HIV-1 infection, as well as drug toxicities, the central and peripheral nervous systems (CNS/PNS) are also susceptible to stroke, seizures, opportunistic infections, CNS lymphomas, myelopathies, myopathies, neuropathies, and neuropsychiatric disorders. Neuropathological studies have led to a better understanding of the neuropathogenesis of HIV-1 infection and associated complications. Combination antiretroviral drug therapies are crucial in combating PE, and have led to a marked reduction in the incidence and prevalence of PE.

EPIDEMIOLOGY AND TRANSMISSION

Human immunodeficiency virus type 1 (HIV-1) infection has created a devastating international public health crisis for children (Association Francois-Xavier Bagnoud; Centers for Disease Control and Prevention, 1994). The Joint United Nations Programme on HIV/AIDS (UNAIDS) has estimated that there were 2.1 million children (under 15 years of age) living with HIV-1 throughout the world—9 out of 10 from sub-Saharan Africa—with 430,000 new infections per year (www.unaids.org, 2009). One in seven of the two million people who died of AIDS in 2008 were children, approximating that 31 children die every hour from AIDS (www. unaids.org, 2009). Furthermore, parental deaths from AIDS have left over 15 million children orphaned, 77% of them in sub-Saharan Africa, and many of these orphans are also

HIVinfected (Association Francois Bagnoud; www.unaids. org, 2009; Shah, 2008). In some countries, children have accounted for the majority of HIV-1 infection (Mintz et al., 1995). Thus, the prevention, identification, and treatment of pediatric HIV-1 is an important component of the battle against HIV/AIDS, with increases in long-term survival and decreases in overall morbidities that have correlated to advances in therapeutic interventions (Selik & Lindegren, 2003; Gibb et al., 2003; McConnell et al., 2005; Judd et al., 2007).

HIV-1-associated neurological disease in children, most commonly referred to as HIV-1-associated progressive encephalopathy (PE), is the clinical corollary of the direct and indirect effects of central nervous system (CNS) and/or systemic HIV-1 infection, and is analogous to what is termed in adults as AIDS dementia complex (ADC), or more recently nosology of HIV-associated neurocognitive disorder (HAND) with subtypes of asymptomatic neurocognitive impairment, minor neurocognitive impairment, and HIV-associated dementia (Mintz et al., 1989; Epstein et al., 1986; Sharer et al., 1986; Belman et al., 1988; Sharer & Mintz, 1993; Mintz & Epstein, 1992; Working Group of the AAN AIDS Task Force, 1991; Scott et al., 1989; Janssen, 1992; Janssen et al., 1992; Mintz, 1994; Schwartz & Major, 2006; Singer et al., 2010) (see Table 10.1.1). PE has been reported to be an initial presenting clinical manifestation of the acquired immunodeficiency syndrome (AIDS) in up to 18% of children and adolescents, and the overall incidence of PE has been previously reported to range from 30% up to 90% of HIV-1-infected children (Belman et al., 1988; Mintz & Epstein, 1992; Janssen, 1992; Janssen et al., 1992). However, the practice of earlier institution of effective antiretroviral (ART) regimens, particularly highly active ART drug therapies (HAART), have contributed to over a 50% decline in the incidence of PE in children, translating to a present rate of 5.1 cases per 1,000 person-years (Mintz & Epstein, 1992; Working Group of the AAN AIDS Task Force, 1991; Scott et al., 1989; Janssen,1992; Janssen et al., 1992; Mintz, 1994; Sullivan et al., 2001; Blanche et al., 1997; The European Collaborative Study,1990; Lobato et al., 1995; Tardieu et al., 2000; Chiriboga et al., 2005; Patel et al., 2008; Patel et al., 2009; Stromme et al., 2008).

Table 10.1.1 COMPARISON OF CLINICAL FEATURES OF NEUROAIDS: ADULTS VERSUS CHILDREN (ADAPTED FROM MINTZ 1999)*

ADULTS	CHILDREN
Horizontally acquired primary infection	Vertically acquired primary infection
Long latency from primary infection to symptoms	Rapidity to symptoms after primary infection
Deterioration of a mature CNS	Impairment of growth of an immature CNS
CNS Ol frequent	CNS Ol infrequent
PNS involved often	PNS rarely involved
CSF non-specific for ADC	CSF non-specific for PE
Aseptic meningitis at time of seroconversion	Aseptic meningitis ill-defined
Seizures common	Seizures infrequent
Psychiatric complications Common	Learning/attentional disorders common
Brain 'atrophy'	Impaired brain growth
Motor deterioration/cognitive decline/dementia	Progressive motor dysfunction/ neurodevelopmental decline
Vacuolar myelopathy observed	Vacuolar myelopathy rare
Cerebrovascular disease/stroke Occurs	Cerebrovascular disease/stroke occurs rarely
Usually associated with immune deficiency	Usually associated with immune deficiency

*CNS, central nervous system; PNS, peripheral nervous system; ADC, AIDS dementia complex; PE. HIV-associated progressive encephalopathy; Ol, opportunistic infections; CSF. cerebrospinal fluid

Similar to the distribution of other AIDS-defining illnesses, progressive neurologic disease in perinatallyinfected children has three clinical presentations: an "early" aggressive and progressive form clinically recognized during the first 1–2 years of life, frequently an isolated or presenting symptom of AIDS; a "late" onset that can occur many years after perinatal infection; and a salutatory clinical course, with, relative stability or improvement interspersed with deterioration (Epstein et al. 1986; Belman et al., 1988; Mintz & Epstein, 1992; Mintz, 1994; Tardieu et al., 2000; Mintz, 1999; Blanche et al., 1990). Early onset PE has been reported to be more prevalent than ADC (approximating 10% in the first year and 4% in the second year, compared to less than 0.5% in adults), with late onset correlating more closely to the incidence of ADC in adults (less than 1% per year in both children and adults), resulting in an overall cumulative incidence of HIV-1-associated encephalopathy in children greater than ADC/HAND in the adult population (Scott et al.,1989; Tardieu et al., 2000; Grubman et al., 1995; Nozyce et al., 1994; Mintz, 1999; Cooper et al., 1998; Blanche et al., 1990). (see chapter 7.2) This phenomenon, as well as the different clinical presentations and disease progression in infants and children as compared to adults, may be in part a result of primary HIVinfection, or neurotoxic effects of neuroinflammatory substances or neurotoxins arising from HIV-1 infection of other brain cells or regions, of neural progenitor cells (phenotypically restricted but mitotically active products of neural stem cells), due to developmental differences in distribution and functions of these cells, as well as susceptibility to infection and indirect neurotoxic effects (Schwartz & Major, 2006). However, with the advent of widespread use of HAART, the epidemiology of PE and ADC/HAND are

changing, and it is unclear if these statistical differences between children and adults remain valid. Additionally, the introduction of ART in the second and third trimester to HIV-1-infected mothers has greatly reduced the incidence of perinatally infected infants, although there is the occasional infant who escapes the preventative benefits of pre- and perinatally administered ART and who may not necessarily be protected against the early development of HIV-1-associated encephalopathy (Tardieu et al., 2000; Mofenson, 1999; American Academy of Pediatrics, 2008; Centers for Disease Control and Prevention, 2006).

In the United States, in contradistinction to the adult population, infants and children born to mothers infected with HIV-1 acquire infection predominantly via mother-to-child vertical transmission: either transplacentally during fetal development; peri/intrapartum as the fetus traverses through the birth canal; or rarely post-natally by means of contaminated breast milk or the feeding of premasticated food to infants (Scott et al., 1989; Blanche et al., 1990; Douglas & King, 1992; Oxtoby, 1994; Lyman et al., 1990; Gaur et al., 2009). There are extraordinary reports of HIV-1-infected infants passing infection to an uninfected mother via breast-feeding.The utilization of ART during pregnancy has markedly reduced perinatal transmission rates (Mofenson, 1999; Connor et al., 1994; Jackson et al., 2003). Vigilant screening of the blood supply and heat treatment of factor VIII compounds has greatly reduced the risk of horizontal transmission from contaminated blood products (Oxtoby, 1994; Cohen et al., 1991). Unfortunately, in much of the world, because of a lack of resources, extensive reuse of needles and syringes not adequately sterilized, coupled with a paucity of oral medications, has led to a high incidence of nosocomial pediatric HIV-1 infection by means of horizontal transmission, in some countries occurring at a greater rate than in adults (Mintz et al., 1995; Hersh et al., 1991). Nevertheless, with the ongoing international epidemic of HIV infection, vertical perinatal transmission remains predominant and prevalent throughout the world, particularly in countries with limited availability of ART drugs for prevention of mother-to-child transmission, even when there are partnerships between governmental and nongovernmental agencies (Adams & Palumbo,2007). In adolescents, infection is acquired as in adults—that is, via sexual relations, reuse of contaminated needles or syringes in drug users, or via tainted blood products (predominantly in the hemophiliac population prior to efficient decontamination of factor VIII) (Brookmeyer, 1991; Hein et al., 1995; D'Angelo, 1994; Futterman & Hein, 1994). However, as treatment regimens improve, there is a growing population of perinatally infected "long-term survivors" thriving into adolescence and beyond (Sullivan, 2001; Grubman et al., 1995; Gortmaker et al., 2001). It is not clear as yet if latent infection of the CNS, successfully suppressed by HAART regimens, could lead to clinical neurological disease in long-term survivors due to reactivation of latent infection as HAART regimens lose effectiveness or resistance develops over the longterm (Lambotte et al., 2003).

Thus, vertical transmission of HIV-1 exposes the developing and immature fetal and neonatal central nervous system (CNS) to potential detrimental pathogenic processes, which is in contradistinction to the situation of exposure of a mature nervous system to virus by horizontal modes of infection, the predominant mode of transmission in adults and adolescents (Lyman et al., 1990; Schwartz & Major, 2006). Infection of the brain at immature stages of development may account for the earlier and more rapid clinical presentations of HIV-1-associated neurological disease seen in young children, more prominently observed and reported before the widespread utilization of ART drugs in pregnant women and earlier combination HAART therapies with good CNS penetration in infants and children, as compared with the long latency often seen prior to the onset of neurological disease in adults (Blanche et al., 1997; Blanche et al., 1990; Price et al., 1988; Brouwers et al., 1995; Chiappini et al., 2007). Treatment of HIV-infected pregnant females is crucial for disrupting mother-to-child HIV-1 transmission, and may alter the severity of disease in those infants who unfortunately fail to escape fetal or perinatal infection (American Academy of Pediatrics, 2008). Timing of infection (fetal versus intrapartum), virulence of the acquired viral strain, and other poorly understood immune factors may account for variations in the clinical rapidity and bimodal expression of clinical symptomatology that is often observed in infants (Tardieu et al., 2000; Blanche et al., 1990; Schwartz & Major, 2006; Llorente et al., 2006). In areas of the world where horizontal infection of children predominates, and in studies of neonates and hemophiliacs infected via blood transfusions or contaminated factor VIII, the incidence of HIV-1-associated neurological disease is much lower or more latent, adding further credence to the hypothesis that the CNS is more susceptible to virulent infection during fetal and neonatal development (Mintz et al.,

1995; Cohen et al., 1991; Hersh et al., 1991; Whitt et al., 1993; Schwartz & Major, 2006). However, there exist subpopulations of children with perinatally acquired HIV-1 infection who also have a prolonged asymptomatic phase prior to the onset of AIDS symptomatology or encephalopathy, although this situation is changing with the use of combination HAART in infants and young children (Persaud et al., 1992; Chiappini et al., 2007; Shanbhag et al., 2005; Lindsey et al., 2007; Sanchez-Ramon et al., 2003; Chiriboga et al., 2005).

Progressive encephalopathy can be the defining clinical symptom of AIDS, and may be the initial presenting clinical manifestation, seen much more frequently in the first year of life. Prior to the HAART era, up to 56% in infants developing AIDS less than one year old, and 32% of older children, compared to 9% of adults, developed neurological manifestations of HIV infection, but now such a presentation has been much reduced and delayed with the advent of widespread and earlier institution of ART and combination HAART in infected mothers, infants, and young children (Blanche et al., 1997; Tardieu et al., 2000; Cooper et al., 1998; Blanche et al., 1990; Benhammou et al., 2007; Lindsey et al., 2007; Shanbhag et al., 2005; Chiappini et al., 2007; Patel et al., 2009). (see chapter 10.2) PE usually manifests at a time of severe immune deficiency and concomitant systemic complications of AIDS (Mintz, 1994,1999). Systemic infection, medical complications, and/or medication toxicities may play a role in causing neurodevelopmental difficulties (Pollack et al., 1997; Benhammou et al., 2007; Blanche et al., 2006; Blanche et al., 1999).

DIAGNOSIS OF PEDIATRIC HIV INFECTION

The diagnosis of HIV-1 infection in infants and children can be difficult, but in areas with accessible laboratories and testing resources, it can now be identified as early as the newborn period in the vast majority of infected infants (Panel on Antiretroviral Therapy and Medical Management of HIV-Infected Children, 2010; Working Group, 1999). Because earlier treatment is more effective in controlling HIV-1 infection and preventing the onset of AIDS symptomatology, it is vital to identify infection in those infants known to have been exposed to HIV in utero, during labor, or the postpartum period, and in other infants and children at risk. In those infants that have been HIV-1 exposed, viral diagnostic testing is recommended at 14–21 days of age, repeated at 1–2 months and at 4–6 months (Panel on Antiretroviral Therapy and Medical Management of HIV-Infected Children, 2010). Viral diagnostic testing should be considered in the newborn at high risk for HIV-1 infection, such as those with HIV-1-infected mothers who did not receive prenatal care or prenatal ART, or offspring of mothers with HIV viral loads >1,000 copies/mL close to the time of delivery (Panel on Antiretroviral Therapy and Medical Management of HIV-Infected Children, 2010). Virologic tests, such as HIV DNA PCR or quantitative and qualitative HIV RNA assays, are preferable to antibody tests because of the transplacental transfer of maternal antibodies; HIV culture, although very specific, is not used as a routine

HIV diagnostic test (Schneider et al., 2008; Panel on Antiretroviral Therapy and Medical Management of HIV-Infected Children, 2010; Havens & Mofenson, 2009). In those HIV-exposed infants and children greater than six months of age who have no clinical or virologic evidence of HIV infection and no hypogammaglobulinemia, two or more negative HIV antibody tests definitively excludes HIV infection (Panel on Antiretroviral Therapy and Medical Management of HIV-Infected Children, 2010). With rare exception, children older than 18 months of age can be considered HIV infected with an HIV positive antibody test and confirmatory Western blot or immunofluorescence assay (IFA) (Panel on Antiretroviral Therapy and Medical Management of HIV-Infected Children, 2010; Sohn et al., 2009).

Thus, strategies for determining and identifying perinatal HIV-1 exposure are necessary, such as counseling and offering voluntary HIV testing early in pregnancy (with consent and an opt-out approach), repeating HIV testing in the third trimester for women with early negative HIV antibody tests but who remain at high risk of HIV infection (Panel on Antiretroviral Therapy and Medical Management of HIV-Infected Children, 2010; Centers for Disease Control and Prevention, 2001; Mofenson, 2000; American College of Obstetricians and Gynecologists, 1997; CDC, 2006; Centers for Disease Control and Prevention, 2002; U.S. Preventive Task Force, 2005). Since ART chemoprophylaxis should be administered quickly after birth to prevent mother-to-child transmission, use of a rapid HIV antibody assay or an expedited ELISA test is crucial for those infants born to mothers who have not been tested for HIV infection during pregnancy or labor.

NEUROLOGICAL DISORDERS

In children, the direct and indirect effects of CNS and systemic HIV-1 infection can adversely impact neurological, neurodevelopmental, and neuropsychiatric functioning (Mintz, 1994; Mintz, 1999; Pollack et al., 1997; Panel on Antiretroviral Therapy, 2010)[see Table 10.1.2]. There are many additional environmental and prenatal confounders impacting on psychometric testing and neurological function, including prenatal exposure to drugs of abuse or ART, complications of maternal HIV-1 infection, other prenatal and perinatal insults, genetic predisposition to cognitive difficulties or behavioral problems, psychosocial and socioeconomic difficulties, and poor compliance with treatment regimens (Wilkins et al., 1990; Satz et al., 1993; Mellins et al., 2003; Bachanas et al., 2001; Forsyth et al., 1996; Lois, 2000; Hochhauser et al., 2008; Bagenda et al., 2006).

PROGRESSIVE ENCEPHALOPATHY

Clinical Findings

The debilitating syndromes of PE and ADC/HAND result in an insidious and severe clinical and pathologic neurological deterioration (see Table 10.1.1). Since there exists additional

Table 10.1.2 CLINICAL NEUROLOGICAL FINDINGS ASSOCIATED WITH HIV-1 INFECTION IN CHILDREN

COMMON FINDINGS

Impaired brain growth
  Loss of velocity of increase of serial head circumference measurements
  progressive 'atrophy' on serial neuroimaging studies

Progressive motor dysfuntion
  Loss of fine and gross motor function
  'Spasticity'
  Extrapyramidal syndromes

Loss, plateau, or an inadequate rate of neurodevelopmental milestone acquisition

OCCASIONAL FINDINGS

Focal neurological signs
  Consider focal CNS lesion (mass, stroke, OI)
Seizures
  Consider infectious process
  Consider focal CNS lesion (mass, stroke, OI)

UNCOMMON FINDINGS

Bulbar(cranical nerve) deficits
  Consider infiltrating neoplastic or infectious processes

Symptoms or signs of myelopathies
  Consider infectious processes/OI

Symptoms or signs of neuropathy/mypathy
  Consider infectious process/OI
  Consider drug toxicity

systemic immune deficiency, combined with the intrinsic diminished immune surveillance of the CNS, the CNS becomes susceptible to various opportunistic infections (OI) and oncological processes. Such OI add further morbidity and mortality, and in some cases may also be a co-factor or primary instigator producing neurological symptoms (Mintz, 1992; Clifford & Campbell, 1992; Saito et al., 1994; Epstein et al., 1988)[see chapter 8.5].

The predominant clinical neurological findings of PE seen in the pediatric population with HIV-1 infection represent a well-defined triad: 1) impaired brain growth, determined by serial head circumference measurements (in children less than two years old) or by progressive brain parenchymal volume loss on serial neuroimaging studies ("atrophy"); 2) progressive and symmetric motor dysfunction (abnormalities of strength, tone, and reflexes; ataxia or gait disturbance); and 3) loss, plateau, or an inadequate rate of acquisition of neurodevelopmental milestones (verified by standardized developmental scales or neuropsychological tests) (Epstein et al., 1986; Belman et al., 1988; Mintz & Epstein, 1992; Mintz, 1992; Brouwers et al., 1994; Schneider et al., 2008; Centers for Disease Control and Prevention, 1994) (Figure 10.1.1; Table 10.1.2, 10.1.3). Not all three findings necessarily occur in all children with PE, but in the neurologically normal child at baseline, progression in one of the three areas, or in the neurologically abnormal child at baseline progression in two of the three areas, is utilized to make a clinical diagnosis of PE (Working Group of the American Academy of Neurology AIDS Task Force, 1991; Panel on Antiretroviral Therapy, 2010; Working Group, 1999; Schneider et al., 2008; Centers for Disease Control and Prevention, 1994) (Table 10.1.3).

These neurological findings should not be explainable by other clinical phenomena, concurrent illness, or disease except HIV infection. It is important to define the progressive and persistent nature of these symptoms, by utilizing a carefully taken medical and neurodevelopmental history and clinical examination. Serial neuroimaging studies and psychometric testing can also assist in defining progression (Brouwers et al., 1995; States et al., 1997; Stout et al., 1998). Overall, the clinical manifestations are the clinical correlate of the neuropathological findings of HIV-1 infection (see below).

HIV-1-infected children with PE may present with fulminant neurological symptoms and signs, or they can proceed along a variable and nonlinear course, with periods of spontaneous improvement and stabilization, although the overall long-term natural history of PE is a stepwise deterioration or relentless downhill progression; PE is associated with poor survival, although HAART may be tempering the outcomes (Lobato et al., 1995; Mintz, 1999; Cooper et al., 1998; Brouwers et al., 1994; Chiriboga et al., 2005; Panel on Antiretroviral Therapy and Medical Management of HIV-Infected Children, 2010; Patel et al., 2009; Lindsey et al., 2007). (see chapter 10.2). Also parallel to the adult situation, PE is often associated with immune deficiency, but is not directly correlated with CD4 lymphocyte surrogate markers, although there is a relationship to viral burden (Brouwers et al., 1994; Epstein et al., 1987; Mintz, 1993; Brouwers et al., 1994; Brouwers et al., 1995; Pratt et al., 1996). However, PE may develop even in the face of immune competence (Tardieu et al., 2000). CSF and brain viral burden can be relatively low compared to plasma in children with severe PE, and although prenatal ART medications can markedly reduce perinatal

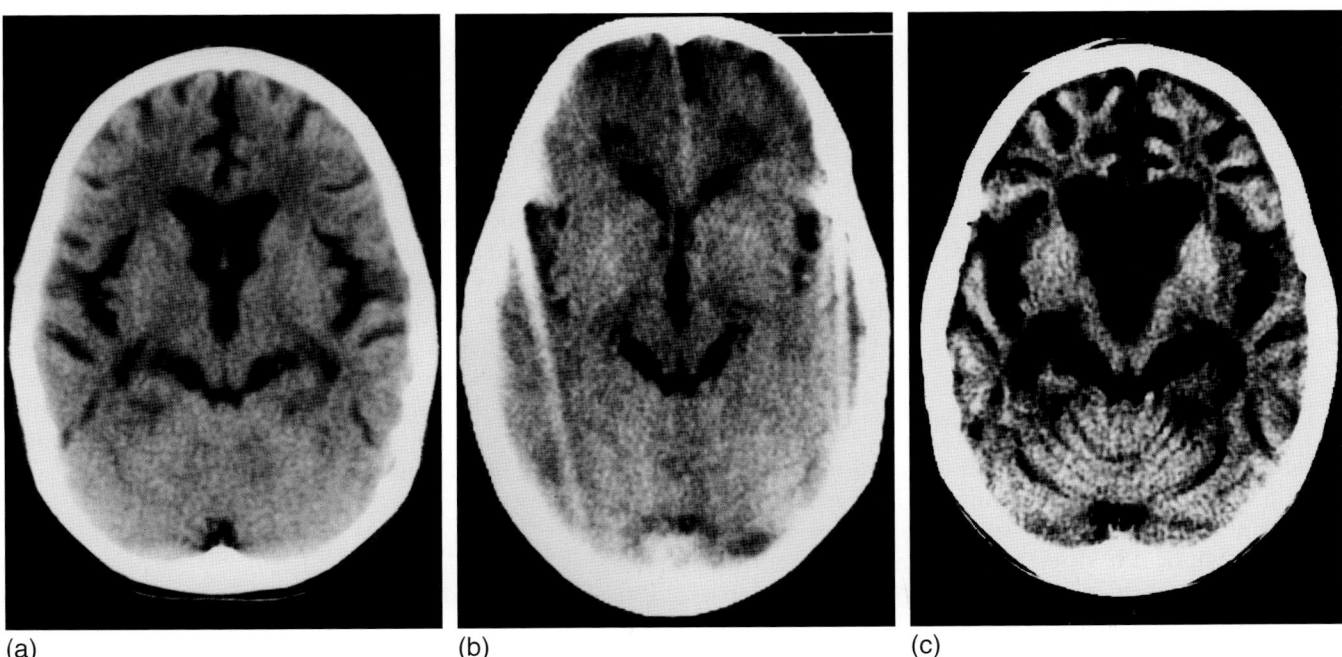

(a) (b) (c)

Figure 10.1.1 a) CT scan revealing moderate 'atrophy' in a child with PE. b) Radiological and associated clinical improvement after 6 months of AZT. c) Severe cerebral destruction and neurological dysfunction 2 years later, despite receiving AZT and alternative antiretroviral agents. (Reprinted with permission from Mintz, 1993).

Table 10.1.3 NEURODEVELOPMENTAL CRITERIA FOR CNS DISEASE PROGRESSION (WORKING GROUP ON ANTIRETROVIRAL THERAPY AND MEDICAL MANAGEMENT OF INFANTS, CHILDREN AND ADOLESCENTS WITH HIV INFECTION, 1998)

Human immunodeficiency virus type 1 (HIV-1)-associated neurological disease. Progression, in the absence of alternative explanations, can be defined by meeting the following criteria in (I) or (II).

I For the child who is neurologically normal at baseline, meeting the criteria in one of the following major domains: (A); (B); or (C)

II For the child who possesses neurologically or development abnormalities at baseline, meeting the criteria in two of the following major domains: (A); (B); or (C)

A Impairment of brain growth, in the absence of alternative etiologies, document by eight (1), (2), (3), or (4) and should be *persistent or progressive as documented by 2 measure separated by at least 2 months*

  1 For infants < 1 year of age, failure to attain above the fifth percentile head circumference growth curve (National Center for Health Statistics growth curves; Hamill *et al.* 1979), with neither an alternative explanation nor a diagnosis of congenital microcephaly

  2 For infants < 3 year of age, crossing 2 major growth curve percentiles from a baseline measurement, without alternative explanation (Hamill *et al.* 1979). Consider neuroimaging correlation

  3 For any age, falling below the fifth percentile without an alternative explanation. Consider neuroimaging correlation

  4 For any age, serial neuroimaging studies, performed under the same conditions and reviewed/compared simultaneously, documenting progressive and significant loss of cerebral parenchymal volume ('atrophy'), without other cause

B Decline of cognitive function, documented by psychometric testing persistent on at least *2 individual valid assessments separated by at least 1 month*

  1 For infants from birth to 3 year, fall of 2 standard deviations (SD) on a standardized, non-screening developmental assessment (for example, the mental develoment index (MDI) of the Bayley Scales of Infant development[*†]

  2 For children > 3 years, a fall of > 1SD on a standardized test of intelligence[†]

  3 At any age, loss of previously attained cognitive or language milestones, without alternative explanation, and confirmed by standardized testing[*†]

C Clinical motor dysfunction, without alternative explanation, documented to be progressive on 2 *individual examinations separated by at least 1 month* in:

  1 loss or significant deterioration of previously attained motor skills or in any two of the following subcriteria (2), (3), or (4);

  2 diffuse and symmetric loss or deterioration in power or strenght that is not the result of a systemic, nutritional, or metabolic complication;

  3 diffuse and symmetric abnormalities of tone, including, but not limited to, hypotonia, hypertonia, or rigidity;

  4 diffuse symmetric, and pathologicallly increased deep tendon reflexes.

[*] Scores corrected for prematurity may lead to factitious results. Thus, consider utilizing uncorrected scores for prematures.
[†] For children who start with developmental deley, or for those children transitioning to a different standardized test, consult a psychologist to determine change over time.

HIV-1 transmission to the fetus, they do not necessarily prevent the early development of PE (Tardieu et al., 2000; Connor et al., 1994). This suggests that PE which develops early after perinatal infection may be the result of factors other than the HIV-1 burden within the CNS, including: coexisting fetal viral infections, the timing of fetal brain infection, or poorly understood immune or genetic factors (Blanche et al., 1997; Tardieu et al., 2000; Scarmato et al., 1996; Llorente et al., 2006; Shiramizu et al., 2006).

Impaired Brain Growth

Children with PE often experience an impairment of brain growth, which is observed clinically and has been confirmed in various neuropathological studies (Sharer et al., 1986; Sharer & Mintz, 1993)(see below). Since the rapid head growth velocity seen in infancy results from expansion of brain volume, a plateau or decrease in the velocity of head circumference on serial measurements is a reflection of impaired brain growth in children under two years of age. In the older child with closed skull sutures, the velocity of increasing head circumference has slowed, and, therefore, an

inordinately prolonged interval is necessary to detect any change or plateau in velocity. Consequently, in this older age group, serial computed tomograms (CT) or magnetic resonance images (MRI) can be utilized to detect progressive loss of brain parenchymal volume (Figure 10.1.2). For infants of HIV-1-infected mothers, a reduction of birth head circumference is suggestive of in utero CNS HIV-1 infection, and suggests a high risk for the development of PE in the first 1–2 years of life, although such previous reports may be tempered with the changes in treatment approaches to pediatric HIV infection and the earlier initiation of HAART (Tardieu et al.,2000; Panel on Antiretroviral Therapy and Medical Management of HIV-Infected Children, 2010).

Progressive Motor Dysfunction

Progressive motor dysfunction should be carefully delineated from the nonprogressive motor deficits seen in static encephalopathies (SE). Motor deficits usually result in impairment of fine motor function and eventually, gross motor skills. Gait disturbances are observed primarily from pyramidal or extrapyramidal dysfunction rather than from cerebellar

Table 10.1.4 RECOMMENDED SCHEDULE OF NEUROLOGICAL/PSYCHOMETRIC TESTING FOR CHILDREN WITH HIV INFECTION (ADAPTED FROM WORKING GROUP ON ANTIRETROVIRAL THERAPY AND MEDICAL MANAGEMENT OF INFANTS, CHILDREN AND ADOLESCENTS WITH HIV INFECTION 1998)

| Test* | Baseline | SCHEDULE OF TESTING FOR CHILDREN AT AGE (YEARS) | | | |
		<1	1-3	3-10	>10
Psychometric[†]	Yes	Every 3–4 months	Every 6 months[§]	Yearly[§]	Every 2 years[§]
			Every 3–4 months[¶]	Every 4–6 months[¶]	Every 4–6 months[¶]
Neurological[‡]	Yes	Every 3–4 months	Every 6 months[§]	Yearly[+]	Every 2 years[§]
			Every 3–4 months[¶]	Every 4–6 months[¶]	Every 4-6 months[¶]
MRI/CT	Consider[‖]	Consider[‖]	Consider[‖]	Consider[‖]	Consider[‖]
CSF	**	**	**	**	**

* MRI, magnetic resonance imaging: CT, computerized tomography; CSR, cerebrospinal fluid.
[†] Use standardized psychometric tests of global mental ability with reliable age norms; testing should be administered by a licensed psychologist. Declines of > 2 standard deviation (SD) units (< 3 years old) or >1 SD unit (> 3 years old) should be confirmed with repeat testing in 1 month.
[‡] Clinical neurological examinations should focus on measures of head circumference (< 3 years old) and motor function. Significant decreases in head circumference velocity or loss of Parenchymal volume on serial neuroimaging should be confirmed with repeat measures/studies in 2 months. Clinical motor dysfunction should be confirmed in 1 month.
[§] Neurologically/neurodevelopmentally normal or static/non-progressive deficits.
[¶] Neurologically/neurodevelopmentally abnormal with progressive deficits.
[‖] Particularly useful if there is a decrease in head circumference velocity, significant motor abnormalities, focality on clinical neurological examination, or a deterioration in cognitive or behavioral function. The interval of repeat neuroimaging studies will depend upon the individual clinical situation, but can be helpful in making treatment decisions.
** No specific recommendations can be offered at this time, but there is growing evidence that HIV PCR of the CSF may be a useful adjunctive surrogate marker of neurological drug efficacy and/or neurological disease progression/improvement.

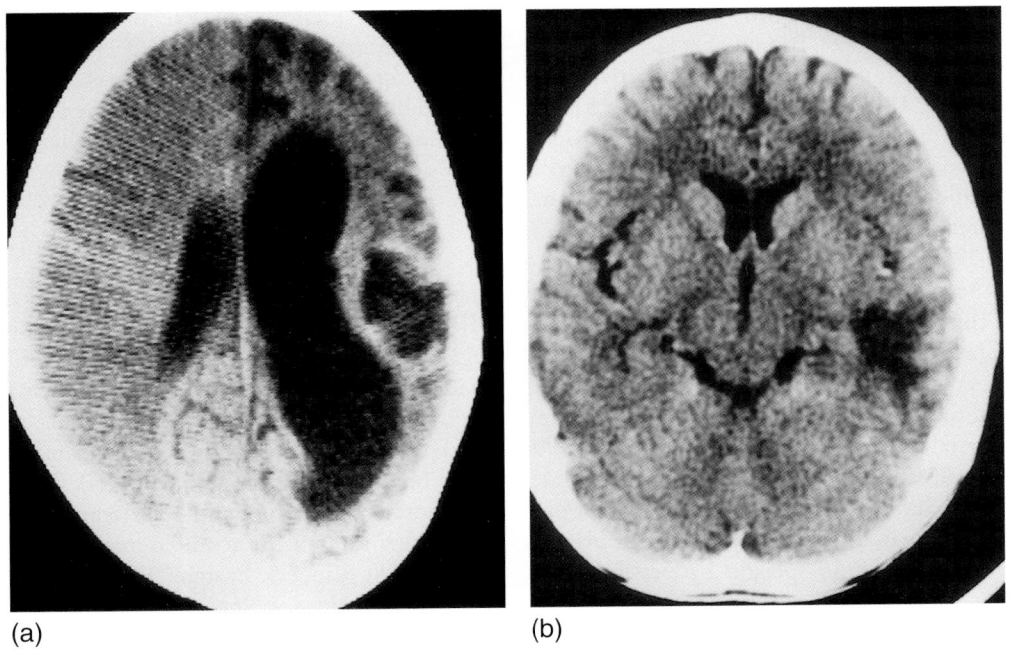

(a)　　　　　　　　　　　　(b)

Figure 10.1.2 CT scans of a) a 9-year-old boy with an acute infarction involving the entire right anterior circulation with evidence of a previous massive stroke of the entire left anterior circulation and b) a 12-year-old boy with an (old) embolic stroke involving a branch of the left middle cerebral artery. (Reprinted with permission from Mintz, 1998).

involvement (Mintz et al., 1996; Lord et al., 1995). Hyper- or hypotonia is manifest, and spasticity is common. Significant motor milestones are not achieved or, if previously attained, are lost. In severe cases, previously ambulatory and functional children become spastic, and nonambulatory, requiring assistance in activities of daily living. Some children with PE can display elements of an extrapyramidal syndrome (EPS) manifesting as rigidity, dysarthria with drooling, hypomimetic facies, and gait disturbances (Mintz et al., 1996; Pressman, 1992).

Motor deficits are usually symmetric. The onset of focality, even if superimposed on a background of spasticity, should raise suspicions of a structural cerebral lesion, such as a mass lesion or infarct (Mintz, 1999; Epstein et al., 1988; Park et al., 1990; Kugler et al., 1991; Frank et al., 1989). Interestingly, cranial nerves and brainstem nuclei are usually spared, despite the fact that HIV-1 is often identified within the brainstem at postmortem; clinical brainstem syndromes have been rarely reported (Raphael et al., 1989). Involvement of the cranial nerves should raise the suspicion of infiltrating neoplastic or infectious processes. Nevertheless, oromotor dysphagia and dysarthria often accompanies severe disease, likely due to a "pseudobulbar"-type palsy resulting from frontal lobe or extrapyramidal dysfunction (Mintz et al., 1996; Pressman, 1992).

Neurodevelopmental Decline

A frequent concomitant to clinical neurological decline or symptomatic systemic disease is a plateau in the acquisition, or a frank regression, of neurodevelopmental milestones and achievement in psychometric measures (Mintz, 1996a, 1996b). Developmental problems are often multifactorial, and environmental, pyschosocial, and nutritional factors may have an important influence on neurodevelopmental outcome and testing (Mintz, 1996b). Formal developmental testing of HIV-1-infected infants has yielded conflicting results, with abnormalities in age-appropriate testing of motor skills or pre-linguistic abilities predominating (Brouwers et al., 1995; Nozyce et al., 1994; Fennell, 1993; Brouwers et al., 1990). The school-age child is at risk for impairment of cognitive functioning (Brouwers et al., 1994; Brouwers et al., 1992; Hanna & Mintz, 1995). Psychometric testing has proven very useful in determining developmental disabilities and identifying "at risk" school-age children so that appropriate educational placement and intervention can proceed (Fennell, 1993; Hanna & Mintz, 1995).

Neurodevelopmental testing in infants and children should be correlated with clinical neurological assessments and laboratory investigations, and should be an integral part of the care of the HIV-infected pediatric patient, especially those with neurological abnormalities or receiving antiretroviral therapy (Panel on Antiretroviral Therapy, 2010; Working Group, 1999; Kairam, 1993; Mitchell et al., 1997) (Table 10.1.3 and 10.1.4). It would be of utility to have a neuropsychometric marker presaging neurological disease in otherwise asymptomatic HIV-1-infected children, but as yet no specific battery has been predictive of PE in otherwise asymptomatic children. Mild cognitive impairment may also be attributable to HIV-1 infection, but can have a multitude of other etiologies in this complex population, and often is undiagnosed (Willen, 2006; Singer et al., 2010). In studies that have examined the impact of HAART regimens with varying degrees of CNS penetration, there was a marked survival benefit in those receiving CNS-penetrating HAART regimens, but no major benefit in reducing PE compared to nonpenetrating regimens (Patel et al., 2009). This survival phenomenon may be in part the result of more effective treatment of undiagnosed milder

forms of HIV-associated encephalopathy (Brew, 2009). This is in contradistinction to adults, where milder forms of neurocognitive deficit do not respond to HAART (Cysique et al., 2004).

Neurodevelopmental and/or neurocognitive decline can also be indicative of ART treatment failure, but other considerations are warranted, including immune reconstitution inflammatory syndrome (Panel on Antiretroviral Therapy and Medical Management of HIV-Infected Children, 2010). The latter can sometimes be differentiated by the timing of occurrence, usually within 4–8 weeks of starting ART in individuals with significant immune compromise at initiation of therapy, or those with active or subclinical CNS opportunistic infections (OI) (Panel on Antiretroviral Therapy and Medical Management of HIV-Infected Children, 2010; Riedel et al., 2006; Singer et al., 2010).

A dilemma occurs with the infant who presents with developmental delay but not regression: a condition that can often precede a frank developmental decline, be persistent, or spontaneously improve with time. However, in an infant of a HIV-1-infected mother who presents with significant neurodevelopmental delays, there should be a high suspicion that this may represent the beginning of HIV-1-related neurologic disease, such as PE. Children born to HIV-1-infected mothers who are observed to be developmentally delayed should be assessed for evidence of HIV-1 infection (although it is now standard in many countries to routinely assess for laboratory evidence of HIV-1 infection in all children born to HIV-infected mothers) and if HIV-1 positive should be treated for HIV-1 infection as per standard guidelines, and should be followed carefully over time for signs of PE (Panel on Antiretroviral Therapy and Medical Management of HIV-Infected Children, 2010).

STATIC ENCEPHALOPATHIES

Static encephalopathies (SE) can also occur in children with HIV-1 infection, and represent fixed, nonprogressive neurologic or neurodevelopmental deficits, often etiologically related to identifiable historical insults, such as prematurity, intrauterine exposure to toxins or infectious agents, genetic factors, or head trauma. These children may manifest developmental delay, but not regression; static motor deficits, but not progressive motor dysfunction; and microcephaly vera ("true" microcephaly), but rarely the acquired microcephaly of PE (Belman et al., 1988; Mintz & Epstein, 1992; Mintz ,1999; Brouwers et al., 1994; Mintz, 1996b). It is unclear if HIV-1 infection of the CNS is the primary causative or contributing factor to SE, or whether SE is solely resulting from non-HIV-1-related neurological insults or genetic factors. Prior to the HAART era, children with HIV-1 infection and SE may spontaneously improve with time, may follow a static course, or may evidence neurological decline and PE (with a latency of up to five years) (Epstein et al., 1986; Belman et al., 1988; Mintz & Epstein, 1992). Thus, care must be taken not to mistake a child with SE who very slowly improves, but increasingly deviates from normal development, and falsely interpret this as PE.

OTHER NEUROLOGICAL MANIFESTATIONS

There are other noteworthy neurological disorders that occur in association with HIV-1 infection. It is incumbent to differentiate those that are a result of the direct or indirect effects of HIV-1 infection such as associated immune deficiency and OI, other organ system dysfunction, versus etiologies unrelated to HIV-1 infection.

Seizures

Seizures occur more frequently than would be expected in a general pediatric population, but are usually symptomatic of an underlying provocation, as is often seen in adults (Mintz, 1994; Mintz, 1999; Wong et al., 1990, (Table 10.1.2). Seizures, particularly those of partial/focal onset, raise particular concerns of underlying focal cerebral pathology, such as a mass lesion, infarction/stroke, or infectious process, or may be a surrogate marker of underlying ART drug toxicity from mitochondrial dysfunction (Blanche et al., 2006; Wilmshurst et al., 2006). If a seizure is manifest, a neuroimaging study is indicated to identify any focal neurological pathology or concomitant evidence of PE. If a CNS inflammatory or infectious process is suspected, and there are no contraindications to performing a lumbar puncture, examination of the cerebrospinal fluid (CSF) may be useful (Roos, 2002).

Complex partial seizures (CPS), common in the HIV-1-infected population who experience seizures, can often mimic psychiatric syndromes, particularly if arising from the temporal or frontal lobe regions (Working Group of the American Academy of Neurology AIDS Task Force, 1991; Mintz, 1996a). Behaviors of "anger," "rage," disinhibited behavior, or in some cases psychotic-like episodes may result from, or be associated with, underlying epileptic discharges in the brain. Further history or observation revealing evidence of an "aura"; impairment or clouding of consciousness during the behavioral change; automatisms; poor memory for the behavioral episode; recurrent staring spells; or tiredness/somnolence following the episode may help to define CPS. The electroencephalogram (EEG) may reveal epileptiform cortical discharges, but the cause and effect relationship of a cortical electrical disturbance with a certain behavioral pattern may be difficult (Tinuper et al., 1990). In some cases, long-term (24–72 hours) ambulatory or video EEG monitoring may be helpful in establishing an electroclinical correlation. Alternatively, an empirical therapeutic trial of antiepileptic medication may be considered.

Cerebrovascular Disease/Stroke

Strokes have been reported, surprisingly less often than might be expected considering the extensive HIV-related cerebrovascular pathology that is uncovered at autopsy (Sharer & Mintz, 1993; Mintz, 1994; Park et al., 1990; Kugler et al., 1991; Frank et al., 1989,(Figure 10.1.2). Consideration of inflammatory or infectious processes leading to local vasculitis is important (Frank et al., 1989). Cardiomyopathic states, a common finding in pediatric AIDS, could theoretically lead to ischemic CNS events (Mintz, 1995). Extensive investigation of stroke events is necessary to differentiate processes not resulting directly from HIV-1 infection, especially concomitant cardiogenic or CNS infectious, inflammatory, oncologic, hematologic, or metabolic mechanisms. A syndrome of "reversible occipital parietal encephalopathy" has also been reported, possibly a result of underlying vascular pathology (Frank et al., 1998). Wernicke's encephalopathy is a rare complication, and may be the result of or exacerbated by unknown effects of HIV-1, but more likely is a result of thiamine deficiency (Mintz et al., 1993, (Figure 10.1.3).

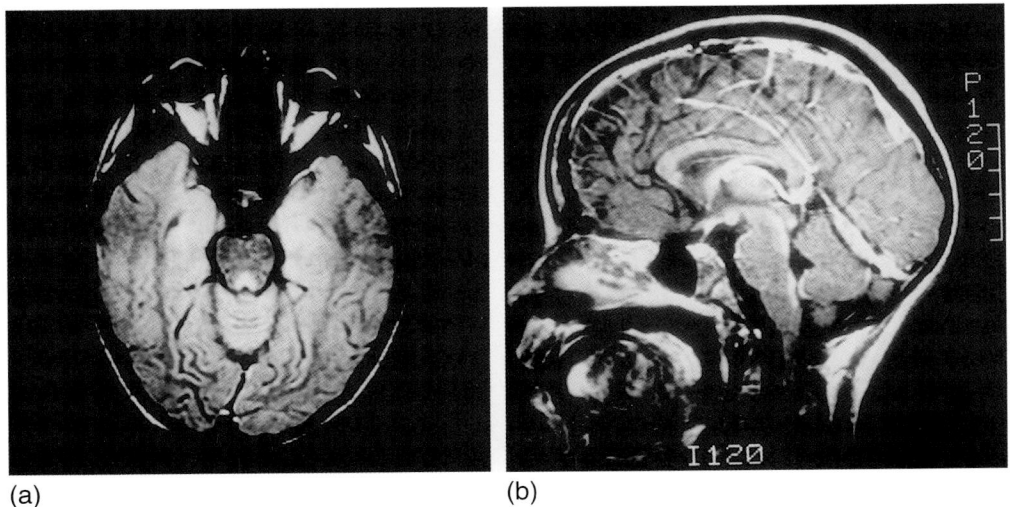

(a)   (b)

Figure 10.1.3 MRI scans of an 11-year-old girl with an acute Wernicke's encephalopathy syndrome. a) Axial proton density (TR, 2500 ms; TE, 30 ms) MRI revealing increased signal intensity in the dorsal midbrain. b) Gadolinium-enhanced midsagittal T1-weighted (TR, 550 ms; TE, 33 ms) image revealing contrast enhancement of the floor of the fourth ventricle, dorsal midbrain, inferior colliculus, and mammillary body. Gadolinium enhancement was also observed in the dorsal-medial thalamus (not shown). (Reprinted with permission from Mintz, 1998).

Myelopathies

Vacuolar myelopathies and other spinal cord pathologies are found in up to 30% of adult post-mortem specimens, but are rarely uncovered clinically in children, and often result from a reactivated infection such as measles or cytomegalovirus (CMV) (Sharer & Mintz, 1993; Sharer et al,. 1992; Petito et al., 1985; Sharer et al., 1990; Dickson et al., 1989; Wilmshurst et al., 2006). Neoplasms involving the spinal cord have also been reported (Wilmshurst et al., 2006). Spinal cord syndromes can be evident clinically, but on occasion spinal cord pathology is discovered only at post-mortem examination (Sharer & Mintz, 1993; Sharer et al., 1992; Petito et al., 1985; Sharer et al., 1990; Dickson et al., 1989) (see below).

Neuromuscular Disorders

HIV-1-associated painful neuropathies are a major source of morbidity in the adult, but are very rare in children, although it may be an under-recognized phenomena due to the difficulty in diagnosing neuropathic conditions in children (Jay & Dalakas, 1994; Floeter et al., 1997). However, neuropathies can be manifest as a complication of nucleoside analogue therapy (particularly dideoxyinosine [ddI], dideoxycytosine [ddC], or stavudine [d4T]), or from OI such as CMV (Working Group, 1998; Jay & Dalakas, 1994; Floeter et al., 1997). Relief usually occurs with cessation or dose reduction of the drug, but pain may continue for weeks after discontinuing the offending nucleoside analogue because of the "coasting" phenomena. Severe generalized flaccid paralysis associated with absent nerve conduction velocities has also been reported (Wilmshurst et al., 2006).

Mitochondrial toxicities induced by various ART drugs have become an increasingly recognized and problematic clinical dilemma, including central and peripheral nervous system dysfunction (Benhammou et al., 2007; Blanche et al., 2006; Blanche et al., 1999; Panel on Antiretroviral Therapy and Medical Management of HIV-Infected Children, 2010; Van Dyke et al., 2008; Aurpibul et al., 2007). Initially, zidovudine (ZDV)-associated myopathy has been reported in children (Walter et al., 1991). This entity has been shown to result from mitochondrial dysfunction/pathology, and laboratory evidence suggests that carnitine supplementation can amelioratein vitro findings (Mintz, 1995; Dalakas et al., 1990; Semino-Mora et al., 1994). Cardiomyopathy is present in 30% of children diagnosed with PE, compared to only 2% of children without PE; thus, careful cardiac investigation is indicated in all children diagnosed with PE (Cooper et al., 1998). This suggests a possible common pathogenic mechanism for PE and HIV-associated cardiomyopathy (such as mitochondrial dysfunction).

OPPORTUNISTIC INFECTIONS

Acute or chronic CNS OI or neoplasms (particularly primary CNS lymphoma) are rare in infants and young children with HIV-1 infection unless there is an active or reactivated congenital OI, but are more prevalent in older children and adolescents (Scott et al., 1989; Mintz, 1994; Epstein et al., 1988; Cohen-Addad et al., 1988; Centers for Disease Control and Prevention, 2009b)(see chapter 8.5). Furthermore, the introduction of HAART has further reduced the incidence of pediatric OI (Gona et al., 2006). Because of the insidious clinical presentation of these infections, an OI should always be considered in cases of acute or chronic behavioral or mental status changes, overall neurologic deterioration, chronic headache syndromes, in children with focal or asymmetric neurologic findings, or in the immune reconstitution inflammatory syndrome (Report of the Quality Standards Subcommittee of the American Academy of Neurology, 1998; Panel on Antiretroviral Therapy and Medical Management of HIV-Infected Children, 2010; U.S. Preventive Task Force,2005). Non-congenital CNS OI and primary CNS lymphoma are invariably associated with significant systemic immune deficiency as measured by age-adjusted CD4 markers (Panel on Antiretroviral Therapy, 2010; USPHS/IDSA, 1997; Denny et al., 1992; European Collaborative Study,1992,(Table 4).

Fungal CNS OI, such as cryptococcal meningitis, usually presents initially with pernicious manifestations of chronic headache, malaise, and fever, but can explosively appear with an altered mental status and precipitous CNS decline (Panel on Antiretroviral Therapy, 2010; Clifford & Campbell, 1992; Leggiadro et al., 1991). Parasitic lesions such as *Toxoplasma gondii* abcesses (congenital or acquired) or oncologic processes such as primary CNS lymphomas (these lymphomas are not strictly an OI, but have been associated with Epstein-Barr virus and are usually seen in cases of severe immune deficiency), can present with headache or focal neurologic signs; depending on the CNS location, organic behavioral changes can also be a manifestation (Epstein et al., 1988; Cohen-Addad et al., 1988; Porter & Sande, 1992; Kingma et al., 1999, Figures 10.1.4 and 10.1.5). Viral OI, such as herpes simplex or CMV encephalitis, can manifest as insidious bizarre or disinhibited behavior (Jue & Whitley, 1994; Arribas et al., 1996). Additionally, CMV encephalitis can mimic PE, as well as cause "unexplained" psychotic symptomatology (Hernandez & Barros,1994). As discussed above, CMV may also cause a progressive myelopathy, and may predispose to PE (Sharer et al., 1992; Kovacs et al., 1999). Reactivation or primary acquisition of measles can present as a subacute encephalomyelitis (Sharer & Mintz, 1993; Sharer et al., 1992). Progressive multifocal leukoencephalopathy (PML)—caused by the JC virus of the PAPOVA family—may cause a "subcortical" dementing process often accompanied by focal neurologic motor signs, as well as psychiatric symptomatology; PML is rare in children (Report of the Quality Standards Subcommittee of the American Academy of Neurology, 1998; Vandersteenhoven et al., 1992; Morriss et al., 1997; Wilmshurst et al., 2006). In cases of behavioral or personality changes, reactivation of neurosyphilis requires consideration in adults, but, unless acquired congenitally or through sexual abuse, is quite rare in children (Marra, 1992). Although HAART has been associated with a reduced incidence and prevalence of OI, such infections

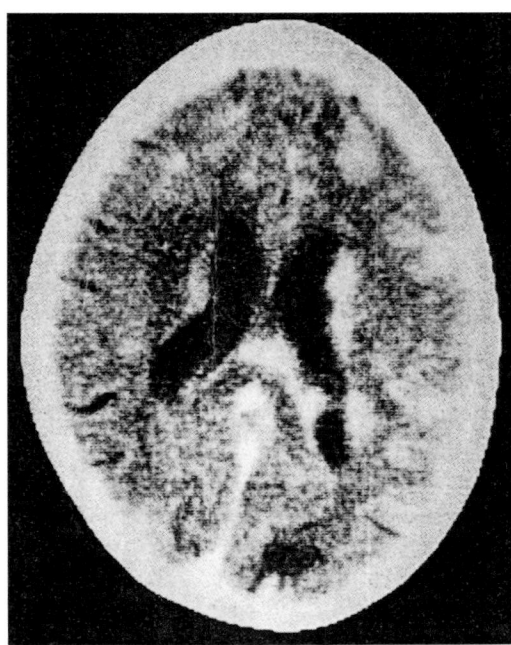

Figure 10.1.4 CT scan utilizing a double dose of contrast with a 1 hour delay revealing multifocal, contrast-enhancing lesions histologically proven to be a primary CNS B-Cell lymphoma in a 10-year-old boy. (Reprinted with permission from Epstein et al., 1988).

continue to be problematic in many HIV-infected children (Chiappini et al., 2007; Gona et al., 2006).

Interestingly, important systemic OI that leads to major morbidity and mortality, such as *Pneumocystis carinii or Mycobacterium avium intracellulare*, are not important pathogens in the CNS (Oleske et al., 1994). However, although not considered a classic OI, with the rise of *Mycobacterium tuberculosis* (TB) infection in HIV-1-infected children, particularly multiply drug-resistant TB, TB meningitis may become an important factor in overall CNS morbidity and mortality (Panel on Antiretroviral Therapy, 2010; Working Group, 1999; Gutman et al., 1994, Figure 10.1.6). Severe systemic bacterial infections continue at high rates, and can affect/infect the CNS as well (Chiappini et al., 2007).

Obviously, it is important to identify a CNS OI or oncology, as some may be treatable and reversible (Centers for Disease Control and Prevention, 2009b). As a general rule (with exceptions), the majority of noncongenital CNS OI are manifest in individuals greater than 6 years old with severely depressed immune function, characterized by absolute CD4 lymphocyte counts of <200, and especially susceptible in ranges of <50-100. Although noncongenital CNS OI are rare in infants and young children less than 6 years old, these secondary infections need consideration in the proper clinical setting, particularly if CD4 lymphocyte counts are below age adjusted norms(see Table 10.1.5). However, it is common for congenitally acquired CNS OI to reactivate in infancy (particularly toxoplasmosis or CMV), and primary CNS lymphoma has also been identified in this age group (Epstein et al., 1988; Cohen-Addad et al., 1988; Kovacs et al., 1999).

Prior to acute therapy for CNS OI, it is useful to establish a definitive diagnosis, although such an approach is neither always possible nor feasible. Depending on the clinical scenario; neuroimaging studies; examination of the serum and/or CSF including serologic, microbiologic, or immunologic parameters; and—in rare instances—brain biopsy, may be of use. In the instance of suspected CNS toxoplasmosis, the neuroradiologic response to an empirical trial of anti-toxoplasma therapy often obviates the need for more invasive procedures (Report of the Quality Standards Subcommittee of the American Academy of Neurology,1998). In addition, "routine" bacterial, viral, fungal, and parasitic causes of meningitis and encephalitis need to be considered as potential etiologic agents of an abnormal CNS presentation. Treatments of such infections are handled with appropriate standard of care infectious disease recommendations. Some clinicians utilize intravenous immunoglobulin (IVIG) to reduce the risk of recurrent serious bacterial infections; it is unknown if such an approach impacts neurological disease (Panel on Antiretroviral Therapy, 2010). If there is immune function, certain vaccines, such as measles, may help to protect against contracting an encephalitis (Panel on Antiretroviral Therapy and Medical Management of HIV-Infected Children, 2010).

The overall approach to prevent opportunistic and recurrent serious bacterial infections in immune-compromised children requires avoidance of exposure to the pathogen, systematic monitoring of immunologic and virologic status, appropriate administration of vaccinations, selective use of immunoglobulin replacement therapy, utilization of prophylactic antimicrobials when indicated, and to provide prophylaxis against recurrent disease after a bout of acute OI disease (USPHS/IDSA, 1997). Because of a lack of efficacious prophylactic regimens for many important CNS OI, acute and recurrent CNS OI still remain an important source of morbidity and mortality, particularly in the older child and adolescent. Treatment of adolescents with CNS OI should be managed according to guidelines established for adults (Centers for Disease Control and Prevention, 2009a; USPHS/IDSA, 1997). After acute treatment for established CNS OI, particularly fungal and parasitic infections and certain viral entities, lifelong maintenance/suppressive therapy is usually indicated (Panel on Antiretroviral Therapy, 2010). Without such a chronic approach, reactivation of these ubiquitous pathogens often occurs. However, as immune systems are reconstituted by more effective antiretroviral therapies, possibly there may be guidelines in the future for the cessation of maintenance therapy.

Controversy surrounds a standard approach to CNS OI surveillance in children. When acute or subclinical CNS OI is suspected, neuroimaging is usually indicated. Some clinicians utilize screening protocols for CMV infection (antibody analysis, urine culture, retinitis, recovery from a tissue biopsy) when the absolute CD4 lymphocyte counts drop below acceptable thresholds, and may institute prophylaxis prior to actual CMV disease; it is not known if such an approach prevents CMV encephalitis.In adult and adolescent patients with CD4 counts <50/ul, there has been

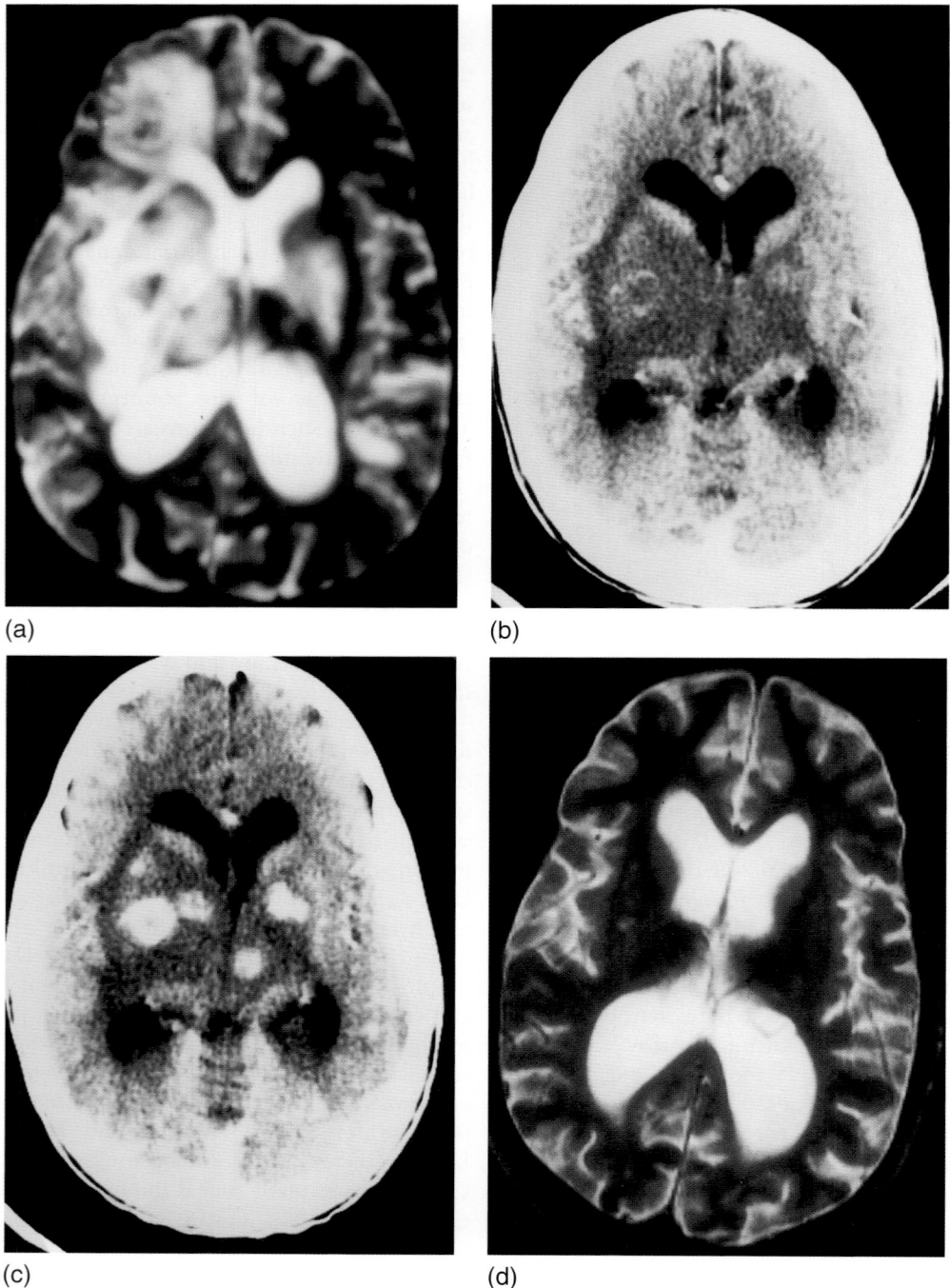

Figure 10.1.5 16-year-old HIV-1-infected female with onset of left hemiparesis. a) MRI T2-weighted image reveals increase in signal throughout the right hemisphere. b) CT with a double dose contrast and immediate scanning shows the vague outline of contrast-enhancing lesions. c) CT performed 1 hour after the double dose contrast reveals multiple contrast-enhancing lesions. d) T2-weighted MRI after anti-toxoplasma therapy displays a complete resolution of lesions. (Reprinted with permission from Mintz, 1992).

evidence that antimicrobial prophylaxis may prevent crypto-coccal disease; however, because of the low incidence of cryptococcal meningitis in young children and infants, there are no recommended specific screening protocols for crypto-coccal serum antigen, nor for prophylactic regimens in infants and children. Prophylaxis against common OI, such as *Pneumocystis carinii* pneumonia (PCP), has greatly

impacted on the survival and quality of life of HIV-1-infected individuals (Panel on Antiretroviral Therapy, 2010; Centers for Disease Control and Prevention, 2009a). Prophylaxis of PCP often protects the CNS against toxo-plasmosis; however, in children receiving prophylaxis with agents other than TMP/SMX, serologic screening may be of use to identify those children requiring additional

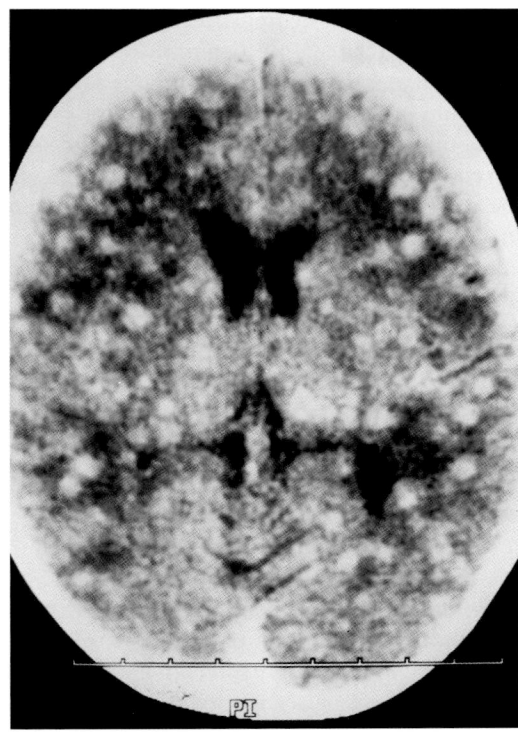

Figure 10.1.6 CT scan with contrast of a young HIV-1-infected child with multiple-drug-resistant pulmonary tuberculosis that disseminated to the CNS. (Reprinted with permission from Mintz, 1998).

prophylaxis against *Toxoplasma* (Panel on Antiretroviral Therapy, 2010; Centers for Disease Control and Prevention, 2009a).

CLINICAL AND LABORATORY EXAMINATIONS AND INVESTIGATIONS

CLINICAL EXAMINATIONS

Serial clinical neurological examinations can help to establish a diagnosis of PE or SE(Table 10.1.3 and 10.1.4). The clinical parameters most sensitive to change over time from the effects of HIV-1 or antiretroviral therapies include items in the domain of motor function: 1) fine motor slowing; 2) gross motor transformations; 3) alterations of tone, with pathologic findings, separately or in combination, of hypertonia, hypotonia, or extrapyramidal dystonia/rigidity; and 4) accentuation/disinhibition of deep tendon reflexes (DTR). [Table 2, 3 and 5] (Working Group of the American Academy of Neurology AIDS Task Force, 1991; Panel on Antiretroviral Therapy, 2010; Denckla, 1985). Additionally, in children under 2 years, a decrease in the velocity of head growth determined by serial measurements of head circumference indicates impaired brain growth. Abnormalities of cranial nerve function are often indicative of inflammation at the base of the brain, and should prompt investigations for CNS OI or acute/chronic infection, vasculitic mechanisms, infiltrating CNS neoplastic processes, or brainstem pathology. Disorders of posture and balance, in the absence of CNS OI, are usually manifestations of extrapyramidal or pyramidal dysfunction related to HIV-1 infection, or to secondary complications, such as stroke or OI. Motor dysfunction, particularly if discrepant in the lower extremities, coupled with a distinct sensory level and/or bowel/bladder involvement, suggests a myelopathy (Sharer et al., 1992).

Clinical neurological examinations have historically been subjective and difficult to standardize. There have been attempts to quantify and standardize such tests (Fennell, 1993; Kairam, 1993; Denckla, 1985; Fletcher et al., 1991). A more "scoreable" quantitative and reliable clinical neurological examination battery would be a useful tool in clinical trials of drug efficacy, and for establishing more accurate research definitions of PE (Kairam, 1993; AIDS Clinical Trials Group).

Neurocognitive dysfunction or decline is a hallmark of the direct and indirect effects of HIV-1 infection of the CNS. Such testing is important as part of a baseline assessment. Serial cognitive evaluations are important surrogate markers for determining the efficacy of treatment interventions, identifying treatment failures, or as surrogate markers of comorbid CNS pathological processes, such as insidious OI (Tardieu et al., 1995; Shanbhag et al., 2005; Hochhauser et al., 2008; Bagenda et al., 2006; Willen, 2006; Jeremy et al., 2005).

Table 10.1.5 1994 REVISED HUMAN IMMUNODEFICIENCY VIRUS PEDIATRIC CLASSIFICATION SYSTEM: IMMUNE CATEGORIES BASED ON AGE-SPECIFIC CD4+T CELL COUNT AND PERCENTAGE (MODIFIED FROM CENTERS FOR DISEASE CONTROL 1994B)

IMMUNE CATEGORY	CD4+ T CELL COUNT (PERCENTAGE) AT AGE		
	< 12 MONTHS NO./MM³ (%)	1–5 YRS NO./MM³ (%)	6–12 YRS NO./MM³ (%)
Category 1: No suppression	≥ 1500 (≥ 25)	≥ 1000 (≥ 25)	≥ 500 (≥ 25)
Category 2: Moderate suppression	750–1499 (15–24)	500–999 (15–24)	200–499 (15–24)
Category 3: Severe suppression	< 750 (< 15)	< 500 (< 15)	< 200 (< 15)

NEURORADIOLOGIC EXAMINATIONS

Serial CT or MRI studies can be employed to evaluate the many neuropathologic changes that occur in PE, such as cerebral parenchymal volume loss affecting primarily the subcortical white matter and basal ganglia regions ("central atrophy" and/or ventriculomegaly "ex-vacuo") or basal ganglia/periventricular frontal white matter mineralizations ("calcifications") (Scarmato et al., 1996; DeCarli et al.,1993; Belman et al., 1986; Wolters et al., 1995, Figure 10.1.1; Table 10.1.3. Language dysfunction and progressive motor and developmental/cognitive impairments have been shown to correlate with CT abnormalities (Brouwers et al., 1995). Neuroimaging is an important modality to identify CNS mass lesions and inflammatory processes (Singer et al., 2010).

Previously, quantitative measures of cortical atrophy on CT scans have been shown to correlate to CSF viral load, suggesting that neuroimaging can be a potential surrogate marker of HIV activity in the CNS (Civitello et al., 1999). To assess for CNS OI or mass lesions, CT scan with contrast (particularly the technique of double-dose contrast with a one-hour delay) or MRI with gadolinium contrast are the most sensitive (Mintz, 1999) (Figure 10.1.5). Improvements in quantification and standardization of cerebral parenchymal loss with quantitative MRI or CT would allow the use of neuroimaging studies as important surrogate markers of disease progression or drug efficacy (Civitello et al.,1999; Jernigan et al., 1993). Modalities such as magnetic resonance spectroscopy (MRS) or positron emission tomography (PET) may emerge as possible important tools in providing an early surrogate marker of PE, as well as providing an additional objective measure of drug efficacy (Pavlakis et al., 1998).

BLOOD AND CEREBROSPINAL FLUID

The cerebrospinal fluid (CSF) profile is rather nonspecific, even in the face of florid clinical PE, except in instances of acute or chronic CNS infection; however, if there is severe systemic immunodeficiency, an inflammatory response may not be mounted (Epstein et al., 1987). The CSF may reveal a mild pleocytosis or increased protein, or can prove to be normal. The aseptic meningitis, which is often observed in adults at the time of seroconversion, has not been well characterized in children, as most children acquire primary CNS infection perinatally.Identification of HIV-1 (by quantitative microculture, p24 antigen, or polymerase chain reaction [PCR]) or intrathecally synthesized anti-HIV-1 IgG can be found in the CSF in PE, but not necessarily in all cases (Panel on Antiretroviral Therapy, 2010; Working Group, 1999; Pratt et al., 1996; Zaknun et al., 1997). In fact, perinatally infected infants may show low or undetectable levels of CSF HIV-RNA despite clinical PE (Tardieu et al., 2000). However, CSF HIV-1 culture positivity is associated with a higher incidence of a very mild pleocytosis (Pratt et al., 1996). Overall, the finding of HIV-1 in the CSF confirms CNS infection, but does not necessarily predict the clinical state.

HIV-1 RNA viral load may be a more accurate predictive virologic CSF measure.When ART drugs were first shown to be effective for PE, ZDV demonstrated the ability to sterilize the CSF of HIV-1 after only 6 months or less of therapy (McKinney et al., 1991). Markers of immune activation in the CSF and serum—such as tumor necrosis factor (TNF), beta-2-microglobulin, neopterin, and quinolinic acid—have correlated well to ADC and PE, suggesting that secondary cytotoxic messengers may play a role in neuropathogenesis (Zaknun et al., 1997; Mintz et al., 1989; Perrella et al., 1992; Wesselingh et al., 1993; McArthur et al., 1992; Heyes et al., 1991; Grimaldi et al., 1991; Brew et al., 1990). Low counts of blood CD8(+) lymphocytes and high amounts of circulating monocytes may have a predictive value forPE (Sanchez-Ramon et al., 2003). Further study is required in determining how to utilize these virologic and cytokine surrogate markers in neurologic treatment decisions. However, assessment of viral isolates from the CSF for resistance to ART drugs can be very useful, since there may be different resistance patterns between the CSF and plasma compartments (Antinori et al., 2005).

In cases of primary CNS lymphoma, the CSF can reveal a hypoglycoracchia and elevated protein, but this can also be seen in cases of CNS tuberculosis and other infections (Epstein et al., 1988). CSF may also be useful in diagnosing certain cases of OI by detecting cryptococcal antigen, anti-toxoplasma antibodies, and the utilization of PCR for various OI, such as CMV. However, a lumbar puncture is relatively contraindicated in instances of intracranial mass lesions associated with increased intracranial pressure.

NEUROPHYSIOLOGIC STUDIES

Event-related potentials and EEG records may show changes that may correlate to PE or ADC (Frank et al., 1992; Arendt et al., 1993; Tinuper et al., 1990; Romero et al., 2007). However, these parameters require further study and standardization to be of clinical utility in HIV-1 infection. EEG is an important tool for identification of underlying epileptic processes. In patients with behavior patterns suggestive of frontal or temporal lobe dysfunction—particularly in cases of fluctuating symptomatology, alterations of consciousness, or with post-ictal states—EEG monitoring, especially long-term ambulatory or video-EEG, may assist in establishing an electroclinical correlation of an epileptic condition to the behavioral aberration. In such cases, treatments directed against the symptomatic epilepsy may cause behavioral improvements. Additionally, subclinical spikes can be associated with neuropsychological dysfunction (Mintz et al., 2009).

PSYCHIATRIC AND BEHAVIORAL MANIFESTATIONS

Not surprisingly, there are a significant array of neurobehavioral aberrations and educational difficulties observed in HIV-1-infected children (Mintz, 1999; Wolters & Brouwers, 1998; Hernandez & Barros, 1994; Spiegel & Mayers, 1991; Cohen et al., 1994; Perrin & Gerrity, 1984; Klindworth et al.,1989;

Krener & Miller, 1989; Stuber, 1990; Haiken et al., 1991; Tardieu et al., 1995; Misdrahi et al., 2004). Surprisingly, recent studies have found no major difference between HIV-positive versus HIV-negative youth in terms of mental health, sexual and substance use risk behavior, and family variables (Flisher & Dawes, 2009). Although there may not be major differences in psychopathology in these groups, when comparing HIV-positive to HIV-negative children who were HIV exposed or live with family members who are HIV infected, psychopathology is in increased in both groups (Gadow et al., 2010). Nevertheless, overt neuropsychiatric symptoms are often attributable to organic pathology of the CNS, particularly if associated with clinically diagnosed PE or a concomitant CNS OI. However, a significant portion of conspicuous psychiatric symptoms may also result from reaction to chronic illness; environmental and social issues; familial or genetic predisposition; drug toxicities; or immune reconstitution inflammatory syndrome (Panel on Antiretroviral Therapy and Medical Management of HIV-Infected Children, 2010; Hatherlil & Flisher, 2009; Benhammou et al., 2007; Blanche et al., 2006). Psychotic symptoms or primary depression are rarely described in children, but may be under-reported (Hernandez & Barros, 1994). Language and communication impairments can be significant in children with PE (Wolters & Brouwers, 1998). Emotional and behavioral manifestations of preschool and school children center predominantly around disorders of attention and impulse control, particularly attention deficit/hyperactivity disorder (ADHD), but also may include depression, anxiety, adjustment disorders, and learning disabilities, and may not necessarily be a result of HIV-1 infection or treatment side effects; uninfected siblings often have similar behavioral problems (Mellins et al., 2003; Mellins et al., 1994; Forsyth et al., 1996). The stress of coping with their own chronic illness, and often that of family members as well, adds additional emotional and behavioral burdens to the child's life (Rotheram-Borus et al., 1998). Not only are these problems a concern for the mental health and quality of life of a child, but emotional issues may even impact upon immune functioning (Howland et al., 2000).

ACUTE PSYCHOSES AND MENTAL STATUS CHANGES

Although frequent in adult HIV-1-infected populations, acute psychoses and organic brain syndromes are rarely reported in children (Hernandez & Barros, 1994; Spiegel & Mayers, 1991; Pao et al., 2000). Increasingly, there is a subgroup of perinatally infected children surviving for prolonged periods—the so-called "long-term survivors" (Grubman et al., 1995; Pao et al., 2000). Many of these children manifest a multitude of HIV-associated complications and require an array of chronic and toxic medications. Although rare, acute psychoses in these children can often complicate the end-stages of disease, often associated with PE, or result from nutritional deficiencies or intercurrent infections (such as CMV encephalitis); complex partial seizures may also mimic an acute psychosis (Mintz, 1996b; Mintz et al., 1993). Alternatively, CNS OI may be the precipitating cause of

the psychotic symptoms (Mintz, 1996a). Acute psychotic symptoms observed in children, long-term survivors, and adolescents have included the sudden onset of confusion, agitation, delerium, mania, and catatonia (Hernandez & Barros, 1994).

Any acute change in behavior or mental status—particularly if accompanied by lethargy, headache, or seizures—raises issues of metabolic derangements, toxic substances, nutritional deficiencies, increased intracranial pressure from mass lesions or other causes, infectious complications/OI that may be affecting the CNS, or a side effect of ART from the immune reconstitution inflammatory syndrome (Hatherlil & Flisher, 2009). Of course, one must examine for signs of meningismus or headache suggestive of meningeal irritation from inflammation or infection, but in the immune-deficient state often accompanying HIV-1 infection, the lack of an appropriate inflammatory response to a CNS pathogen may mask the classic clinical signs of meningitis or meningoencephalitis. Neuroimaging studies and lumbar puncture (if not contraindicated by mass lesion) may assist in establishing the presence of a CNS inflammatory process.

In addition to systemic consequences of poor nutrition, inadequate nutrition can lead to various CNS consequences, including acute changes in mental status. Wernicke's encephalopathy, associated with inadequate thiamine (vitamin B-1) intake, has been reported in adults and children with HIV-1 infection, even without major CNS or systemic symptomatology (Mintz et al., 1993; Butterworth et al., 1991, Figure 10.1.3). Furthermore, disruptions in systemic electrolyte homeostasis can cause abrupt changes in mental status or precipitate seizures. Substance abuse needs to be considered in adolescents. Toxic ingestion should be regarded as a differential diagnostic possibility in children who may have accidentally ingested poisons or be at risk for exposure to environmental toxins, such as lead.

DEPRESSION

In children with HIV-1 infection, major depression has not been as well defined as in the adult population, and many older children and adolescents suffer from depression that may be reactive to their situation of chronic illness and frequently associated family dysfunction or illness (Esposito et al., 1999; Havens et al., 1996). It is not clear in children whether CNS HIV-1 infection may be contributing to an organic depression, or if the incidence of depression and affective illness is any higher in HIV-infected children (Moss et al., 1998; Campbell, 1997).

As in any chronic illness affecting children, a depressed mood may occur, especially if in addition multiple family members are suffering from AIDS (Perrin & Gerrity, 1984). Apathy, social withdrawal, and anorexia are part of the manifestations of depression in chronic illness, but at times may be difficult to separate from the organic effects of HIV-1 or OI. Reactive depression may also occur from prolonged hospitalization. In the child and adolescent who can comprehend a medically deteriorating situation, apathy and a feeling of helplessness may cause an affective withdrawal leading to noncompliance with medications and other medically necessary regimens, which can worsen their condition (Mellins et al., 2003; Rabkin & Chesney, 1998). In assessing a child with a marked depressive affect, unless a psychosocial precipitant or CNS organic etiology can be identified there should be a careful assessment of nutritional needs and consideration of metabolic or endocrine disturbances, particularly thyroid dysfunction (Brouwers et al., 1995).

DISORDERS OF ATTENTION

Although there have been a number of reports citing a high incidence of ADHD in HIV-1-infected children, when proper control groups are utilized there may not be an association of ADHD with HIV disease (Mellins et al., 2003,). In otherwise neurologically asymptomatic children, it is unclear the causal relationship of HIV-1 to an attentional deficit, as other identifiable historical risk factors in the prenatal/perinatal/family/environmental history, or external factors such as lead poisoning or treatment regimens adversely effecting the CNS, may be more contributory. Large cohorts have demonstrated similar rates of ADHD between infected and uninfected siblings, even when controlled for maternal drug use (Mellins et al., 2003). However, in frank PE, ADHD may result from structural changes within the white matter (Brouwers et al., 1995). With more advanced CNS disease, the traits of ADHD may actually diminish, possibly because the child is less able to motorically respond (Brouwers et al., 1995).

LEARNING DISORDERS/EDUCATIONAL ISSUES

The reasons and contributors to academic difficulties of HIV-1-infected children are multifactorial and often include genetic, familial, and environmental issues not directly related to HIV-1 (Misdrahi et al., 2004; Hochhauser et al., 2008). Children with HIV-1 infection, particularly those with PE, SE, or significant systemic illness, display an inordinately high percentage of learning disorders (LD), educational difficulties, and ADHD, adding alarmingly to the burden of limited special educational services, although for inner city youth there may not be a significant difference for stable HIV-infected youth from their uninfected peers (Task Force on Pediatric AIDS,1991; Lindsey et al., 2007).

If an LD is suspected, identifiable etiologies should first be sought from the history, such as fetal drug or alcohol exposure, or a family history of an LD. A physical examination should assess for dysmorphic disorders or other non-HIV-1-related neurologic disorders, which may be an "organic" cause of an LD. As with all children with LD, assessment of vision and hearing is essential, but is particularly important with symptomatic HIV-1 disease as recurrent otitis media or OI (CMV) may cause dysfunction of these senses. In addition, the child should be assessed for PE, SE, ADHD, or underlying emotional contributors. Poor school performance may result from many missed school days from illness/hospitalization and not necessarily from an intrinsic LD. When appropriate, a child should be offered homebound instruction, treatment for ADHD, or be assessed for special educational services (Katz, 1994; Chanock & Simonds, 1994).

Children with HIV-1 infection have a moral and legal right to a full education in the mainstream classroom to the extent that their health permits and behavior remains compatible with classroom attendance (Katz, 1994; Chanock & Simonds, 1994; Shirley & Ross, 1989; American Academy of Pediatrics, 1987). Children with HIV-1 infection and developmental disabilities can receive public education unless they display exclusionary and specific aggressive behavior patterns that increase transmission risk, such as biting, or possess uncoverable, open skin lesions, diarrhea from infectious agents, or pulmonary tuberculosis (although pulmonary tuberculosis is not very infectious in young children) (Shirley & Ross, 1989; American Academy of Pediatrics, 1987). In case of an accident, schools should be prepared to handle bodily fluids or blood, utilizing universal precautions.

The secrecy that often surrounds disclosure issues encompassing the diagnosis of HIV-1 infection can cause additional stress, poor self-esteem, and impaired peer interactions, and lead to academic difficulties (Brady et al., 1996). However, most HIV-1 infected school age children perceive themselves as adequately well-adjusted to their social network. Additionally, in the child open about his/her diagnosis, social stigmatization can occur, although this has been lessened in recent years with many celebrated and publicized cases, as well as community education concerning the lack of transmission risk with casual contact.

NUTRITIONAL DEFICIENCIES

Malnutrition is the most common worldwide cause of immunodeficiency and plays a major role in childhood mortality (Mintz, 1996b). Likewise, the CNS and PNS are susceptible to nutritional deficiencies of protein/calories, vitamin cofactors, and other micronutrients (Mintz,1996b; Chopra & Sharma, 1992). Children with HIV-1 infection are prone to inadequate nutrition as a result of inadequate intake, dietary imbalances, intestinal malabsorption, intercurrent or concomitant infectious complications (with their accompanying increase in metabolic demands), drug therapies, and psychiatric disorders or emotional deprivation (Mintz, 1996b; Laue & Cutler, 1994). Conversely, adverse neurological toxicities can result from overzealous utilization of alternative therapies that include vitamin/co-factor supplementation or animal/plant/environmental toxins. Pathologic CNS and PNS effects of nutritional deficiencies are often subtle and difficult to differentiate from clinical or psychiatric manifestations of HIV-1 infection, OI, environmental toxins, or substance abuse (in adolescents). Furthermore, there is scant data concerning specific nutrient deficiencies and PE. Therefore, it is important to control for the child's nutritional background when assessing for HIV-1-associated CNS and PNS disorders.

PROTEIN-CALORIE MALNUTRITION

Protein deficiency can be identified in HIV-infected children, even prior to the onset of AIDS. Although previously suggested as a potential mechanism of PE, no specific clinical correlations to protein status and HIV-1-associated neurological disease has been forthcoming (Mintz, 1996b). It is usually very difficult to differentiate the rather nonspecific clinical neurological signs of protein-calorie malnutrition from the often concomitant findings of vitamin deficiencies, infectious complications, environmental toxins, drug toxicities, or lack of appropriate social stimulation (Chopra & Sharma, 1992).

VITAMIN/CO-FACTOR DEFICIENCIES

Altered nutritional status is defined by poor weight growth velocity, loss of lean body mass, low weight for height, or a low serum albumin (Panel on Antiretroviral Therapy, 2010). In the HIV-1-infected child not achieving appropriate growth milestones, vitamin/micronutrient deficiencies should also be suspected, particularly vitamins of the A, B, D, and E classes, iron, selenium, zinc, and L-carnitine. Wernicke's encephalopathy has been reported in HIV-1-infected adults and children (Mintz et al., 1993; Butterworth et al., 1991, Figure 10.1.3). Although likely a result of thiamine deficiency, there may exist an enhanced susceptibility secondary to HIV-1 infection, subsequent immune deficiency, or drug therapies. Peripheral neuropathies are also a known complication of thiamine deficiency, although not reported in children with HIV-1 infection.

Although B12 deficiency has been postulated as a possible cause of AIDS dementia complex (ADC) or vacuolar myelopathy, other B-vitamin deficiencies have not been specifically correlated to neurologic disease in the pediatric HIV-infected population (Beach et al., 1992; Dowling et al., 1993). In fact, routine B12 screening of pediatric participants in early antiretroviral drug trials failed to reveal any consistent B12 deficiency (Walter et al., 1991). Vitamins A and E have been linked to aspects of morbidity, mortality, and transmission of HIV-1 infection, but have not been correlated to any specific neurologic difficulties (Periquet et al., 1995; Anonymous, 1994; Semba et al., 1993).

There is increasing evidence that patients with HIV-1 infection have an alteration of lipid and fatty acid metabolism, which may be related to cytokine dysregulation, and thus, would have an important theoretical impact on PE (Chang et al., 1990; Begin et al., 1989). L-carnitine plays an important role in fatty acid and mitochondrial metabolism, has been found to be deficient in HIV-1-infected patients, and appears to be an important factor in AZT-induced myopathies (Mintz, 1995). Since L-carnitine has been shown to modulate cytokine production, it can by hypothesized that L-carnitine may be involved in neuropathogenic mechanisms of HIV-1 infection—particularly in patients receiving nucleoside drug therapy—although direct evidence linking L-carnitine and PE is lacking. L-carnitine may be able to reverse some of the effects of mitochondrial dysfunction in

HIV-associated cardiomyopathies and AZT-induced myopathies (Semino-Mora et al., 1994).

PATHOLOGY

INTRODUCTION

Many of the neuropathological features of HIV-1 infection in children are similar to those that occur in infected adults, but there are some important differences as well. Our own findings recapitulated in this chapter are based on neuropathological examination of 80 children with HIV-1 infection who came to autopsy, with much of this information detailed in previous publications (Sharer et al., 1986; Sharer & Cho, 1989, 1997), and with most of the cases from before the era of highly active antiretroviral therapy (HAART). Little new autopsy information from HIV-1-infected children has emerged recently in the US, largely because of the success in preventing vertical transmission from HIV-1-infected mothers to their offspring and also because of successful treatment of children with antiretroviral agents. This greatly improved situation in children in the US and the developed world has yet to occur in much of the developing world, where there are still large numbers of children with HIV-1 infection, as noted elsewhere in this book.

OPPORTUNISTIC INFECTIONS AND RELATED CONDITIONS

An important aspect of the pathology in this group of pediatric cases, compared with many series of adults with AIDS, is the low incidence of opportunistic or reactivated, latent infections. Several adult series from the pre-HAART era reported that up to 50% of cases coming to post-mortem examination had either opportunistic infections or primary lymphoma in the CNS (Petito et al., 1986; Anders et al., 1986), while the incidence in our group of children was less than 15% for these complications (Sharer & Cho, 1989, 1997). The reasons for the low incidence of these lesions are not entirely clear, but they almost certainly are related, in part, to a lower rate of exposure to offending agents in subjects with a shorter life span. This explanation holds best for such common pathogens as *Toxoplasma gondii, Cryptococcus neoformans*, and JC virus, the causative agent of progressive multifocal leukoencephalopathy (PML). By contrast, cytomegalovirus (CMV), which is highly prevalent in children (Yow et al., 1987), and human herpes virus type 6 (HHV-6), which is a nearly universal infection in children before the age of 2 years (Hall et al., 1994), might be expected to be more prevalent infections in the CNS in children with AIDS, and this is, in fact, the case. The most common opportunistic pathogen in the CNS in our series of children dying of AIDS has been CMV (Sharer & Cho, 1997), and we have also found evidence of latent HHV-6 infection in many of our cases (Saito et al., 1995). We have seen no cases of histologically verified CNS toxoplasmosis in our autopsy series, other than a newborn with congenital toxoplasmosis, the offspring of a mother who died with AIDS and CNS toxoplasmosis (Cohen-Addad et al., 1988). Over 20 years ago we suggested that a mass lesion in the brain of a child with HIV-1 infection and AIDS should not be treated for toxoplasmosis but should be biopsied emergently, since it was more likely to be lymphoma than toxoplasmosis (Epstein et al., 1988a). Our experience since that time has borne this out, since we have seen several cases of brain lymphoma, usually at biopsy, but still no cases of toxoplasmosis in children.

HIV-1 ENCEPHALITIS IN CHILDREN

Study of AIDS in children, in which there are few confounding opportunistic infections compared with adults, has provided support for the hypothesis that HIV-1 is directly related to progressive encephalopathy, by either direct or indirect means, and it has also afforded evidence that cofactors are not necessary for the neuropathogenesis of HIV-1 infection.

An early consensus report gave the following working definition for the pathology of HIV-1 encephalitis: The lesions are characterized by multiple disseminated foci of microglia, macrophages, and multinucleated giant cells; if giant cells are not found, demonstration of the presence of HIV-1 antigens or specific nucleic acid sequences is also required (Budka et al., 1991). Using this definition, particularly with regard to the presence of multinucleated giant cells in the central nervous system (CNS), we found an incidence of HIV-1 encephalitis of approximately 60% in young children (Sharer & Cho, 1997; Kozlowksi, 1990).

In children, HIV-1 encephalitis roughly correlates with the presence of clinical encephalopathy. As with adults, however, some children with progressive encephalopathy have little or no evidence of HIV-1 encephalitis, although generally these cases have had neuropathological abnormalities of some sort. Indeed, less than 10% of the brains in our series of children with AIDS were completely normal on neuropathological examination. In general, there has been a better correlation of encephalitis and encephalopathy in children than in adults, with fewer exceptions.

An important feature of HIV-1 encephalitis, in both children and adults, is monocyte/macrophage activation associated with inflammatory cell infiltrates that consist of infected microglia and macrophages admixed with reactive astrocytes, lymphocytes, and occasional plasma cells. Often the inflammatory cell infiltrates have multinucleated giant cells within them, but in many cases they may be devoid of these larger cells (Figure 10.1.7). Conversely, multinucleated giant cells can in some instances be seen in isolation, often about or near blood vessels. In Figure 10.1.8, the multinucleated giant cells themselves can be considered to be a form of monocyte/macrophage pathology, since they arise by fusion of cells of this type (Michaels et al., 1988). Multinucleated giant cellsvary greatly in size and appearance, from cells with clusters of nuclei and minimal amounts of visible cytoplasm, to large, or true, "giant" cells measuring up to 70 microns or more in diameter, with copious cytoplasm and varying cytological features (Sharer & Cho, 1997; Sharer et al., 1985; Gray et al., 1988). The microglial responses are reminiscent

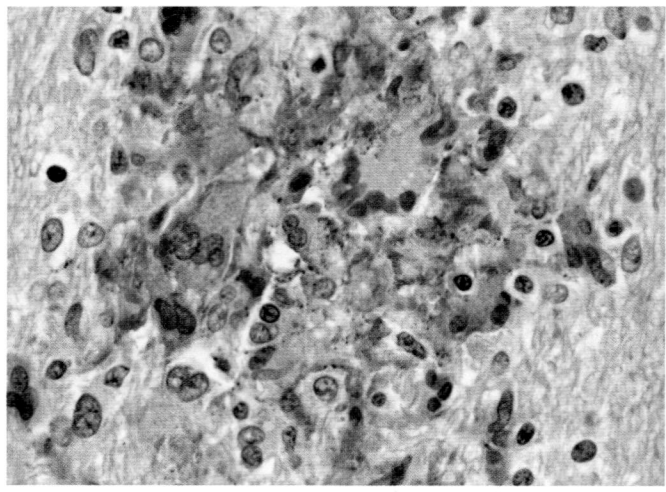

Figure 10.1.7 Inflammatory cell lesion including multinucleated giant cells, cerebral white matter from a 12-year-old girl with HIV-1 infection, AIDS, and HIV-1 encephalitis. Several positive cells, with one negative multinucleated giant cell as well. Immunohistochemistry on formalin-fixed, paraffin embedded section, using an antibody to p24 core protein of HIV-1 (Dako), diaminobenzidine with light hematoxylin counterstain, 10X objective.

of classical glial-microglial nodules, a hallmark of virus infection of the CNS. The HIV-1-related lesions tend to be less dense and more diffuse than the typically "tight" microglial nodules of virus encephalitis; and in gray matter they are usually unassociated with neuronophagia, which rarely occurs in HIV-1 encephalitis. The cell infiltrates may be accompanied by pallor and mild microcystic change as well as by local extension into the leptomeninges, and they may rarely include small foci of necrosis (Sharer et al., 1997).

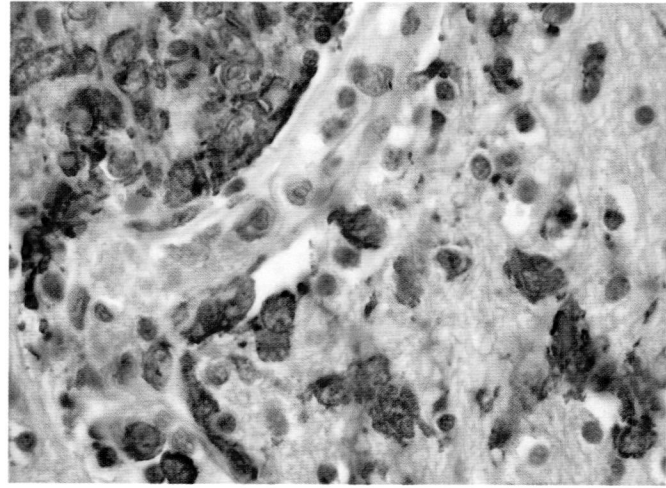

Figure 10.1.8 Perivascular inflammatory cell infiltrate, including multinucleated cells, cerebral white matter from a 12-year-old girl with HIV-1 infection, AIDS and HIV-1 encephalitis. Immunohistochemistry on formalin-fixed, paraffin embedded section, using an antibody to the monocyte/macrophage/microglial marker Iba-1 (Wako, Japan), diaminobenzidine with light hematoxylin counterstain, 25X objective.

Both types of lesions, that is, multinucleated giant cells and inflammatory cell infiltrates, have a predilection for certain regions of the CNS, including the deep gray structures, especially the basal ganglia, and also the central white matter of the cerebral hemispheres and the brainstem, particularly the basis pontis. However, these lesions can be encountered in any part of the CNS in a child with HIV-1 infection, from the cerebral cortex to the gray and white matter of the spinal cord. We have not observed multinucleated giant cells in the subarachnoid space or leptomeninges in any of our cases, although this has been reported to occur in adults (Budka & Gray, 1993). Similarly, we have not identified such cells in the stroma or elsewhere in the choroid plexus, although this structure may be inflamed and may contain virus-infected cells (Falangola et al., 1995).

In addition to multinucleated cells and infiltrates of infected inflammatory cells, there are other important features of HIV-1 encephalitis in children, many of them shared with the pathology seen in adults with AIDS. The most common among them is white matter pathology, most often manifest as diffuse pallor of the myelin when viewed at low magnification on various histological stains. The central white matter of the cerebral hemispheres, that is, the centrum semiovale, is the location where this myelin change can be most readily recognized and indeed where it is usually most severe, but it may also be apparent in the deep cerebellar white matter (corpus medullaris). This white matter or myelin pallor is usually accompanied by reactive astrocytosis, which can be detected with techniques for demonstrating astrocytes, of which the most commonly used is immunohistochemistry for glial fibrillary acidic protein (GFAP). Indeed, white matter astrocytosis is often much less apparent with routine hematoxylin and eosin staining, while it is usually striking with GFAP. In occasional cases there are true foci of demyelination in the white matter, with patchy, sharply delimited zones of myelin loss. However, this picture is highly unusual, despite the mistaken belief of some that HIV-1 encephalitis is a demyelinating disease. Even rarer is the gross appearance of white matter pallor in the brain of a young child, suggesting hypomyelination (Sharer et al., 1986; Epstein et al., 1988b). Microscopical white matter pathology, consisting of either pallor, astrocytosis, or, as is generally the case, both together, is quite common in the brains of children who have come to post-mortem examination with HIV-1 infection, occurring in about 75% of the cases in our series.

The term "HIV leukoencephalopathy" has been used by some observers to indicate the presence of the combination of HIV-related inflammation and white matter pallor (Budka, 1991). Many cases of HIV-1 encephalitis in children exhibit these two features together and, indeed, almost all cases that have inflammatory cell infiltrates and multinucleated giant cells in the cerebral white matter also exhibit diffuse white matter pallor histologically. However, the obverse is not always the case, since white matter pallor can be present without any inflammatory changes, as can also be seen in the brains of adults.

A striking finding in the brains of children with AIDS is the presence of mineralizations, which are generally basophilic and which are usually most prominent in the basal ganglia (putamen and globus pallidus) and the deep cerebral white matter. These mineralizations vary from small, extracellular, basophilic, or occasionally eosinophilic deposits adjacent to small blood vessels, to large extracellular nodules that the examiner may even palpate on gross examination, where the cut surface of the basal ganglia may have a gritty texture. By various histochemical techniques, they have been found to consist of calcium salts, with other minerals also present, particularly iron (Sharer et al., 1986). In occasional cases, the walls of larger vessels, which may also be inflamed, may become mineralized within the basal ganglia (Sharer et al., 1986). However, the small vessels about which many of the mineralizations are located did not exhibit HIV-1 p25 gag protein immunoreactivity on immunohistochemical examination of frozen sections using monoclonal antibodies to p25. The pathogenesis of the juxtavascular mineralizations is unknown, but we have postulated that they arise because of local disruption of the blood-brain barrier, which is probably a transient phenomenon (Epstein et al., 1987). We have also noted extensive juxtavascular mineralizations in the cerebral cortex in a few of our cases (Sharer & Mintz, 1993).

In our autopsy series, mineralization has been the single most frequent histopathological change in the CNS of children who die with HIV-1 infection, occurring in over 90% of cases. This change, when it is severe, is readily detected ante mortem on computerized tomographic (CT) imaging of the brain (Belman et al., 1986; DeCarli et al., 1993), a sensitive diagnostic modality for increased tissue density. The incidence, on the order of 10–25% of radiographically demonstrable calcifications in the brains of children with AIDS, is much lower than that detected by histopathology, since many of the mineralizations are microscopical and hence beyond the resolution of the CT scan. It has been suggested that mineralizations are more common in the brains of children who have acquired HIV-1 infection from the mother either in utero or during the perinatal period rather than after birth, for example, through transfusion of infected blood products (DeCarli et al., 1993). Our own observations indicate that they can also occur in cases with postnatal transmission of virus, although it should be noted that we have not had a large number cases of postnatal transmission. Mineralization of vessels in the basal ganglia occurs in many uninfected, normal, older (over 60 years of age) people, unassociated with CNS dysfunction, presumably as a consequence of normal aging. We have occasionally noted this change in younger (under 40 years of age) adults with HIV-1 infection coming to post-mortem examination, but it is usually much less striking and less extensive than it has been in our childhood cases.

Another feature of HIV-1 encephalitis in children that is not a usual feature of the disorder in adults is inflammation (Sharer & Cho, 1989) of blood vessel walls producing a vasculitic-like picture, usually without fibrinoid necrosis. It is less common than the changes described above, occurring in 25–30% of our childhood AIDS cases. The vascular lesions consist of cuffing and infiltration of the walls of small- and medium-sized parenchymal vessels by lymphocytes, monocytes, and occasional multinucleated giant cells, most often involving vessels in the hemispheric white matter and the basal ganglia. The vessels do not contain thrombi, and there usually are no infarcts or ischemic lesions in the nearby parenchyma.

INFECTION OF CELLS IN THE CNS IN CHILDREN WITH HIV-1

There is abundant evidence for direct, productive HIV-1 infection in the CNS of cells of monocyte/macrophage origin, in both adults and children, based on observations of various sorts. Studies supporting this view have come from immunohistochemistry, electron microscopy, and molecular methods (in situ hybridization and, in situ DNA amplification by polymerase chain reaction [PCR] and detection, referred to as in situ PCR). From time to time, papers have appeared that have claimed that there is infection of neuroectodermally derived cells, including astrocytes, oligodendrocytes, and neurons. We and others have documented HIV-1 infection of astrocytes, in both children (Saito et al., 1994; Tornatore et al., 1994a) and adults (Ranki et al., 1995). Astrocyte infection had previously been classified as latent or restricted (Tornatore et al., 1994b). Accordingly, we elected to determine if there was similar restricted infection in brain tissue, and we studied the early regulatory gene product nef. Our results indicated overexpression of nef sequences in the brains of children who had severe HIV-1 encephalitis (Saito et al., 1994). We postulated that failure to detect this type of infection in the past by in situ hybridization had resulted, at least in part, from the use of probes that did not include the overexpressed early regulatory HIV-1 gene sequences. The studies of Tornatore et al. (1994a) in children and Ranki et al. (1995) in adults have supported these findings. While this astrocytic infection appears to be nonproductive, it is not unreasonable to assume that this would result in some perturbation of astrocytic function (Oldstone et al., 1982), as has been suggested from in vitro studies of astrocyte cultures, in which HIV-1-infected astrocytes demonstrated decreased glutamate uptake (Wang et al., 2004).

Infection of neurons, whether latent, restricted, or productive, has been a more controversial subject, with at least two groups claiming, on the basis of in situ PCR studies, that there is extensive, presumably latent, infection of these cells (Nuovo et al., 1994; Bagasra et al., 1996). Our own studies (Sharer et al., 1996) in children and those of Takahashi and co-workers (1996) in adults, also using in situ PCR, have not supported these observations. It is uncertain why a discrepancy exists between these studies. Both our study and that of Takahashi and co-workers used formalin-fixed, paraffin-embedded tissues, while the study of Bagasra et al. (1996) employed frozen tissue, with the possibility of decreased sensitivity of the fixed specimens. More recently, we have investigated this issue in a different manner, using laser capture microdissection of cells from formalin-fixed, paraffin-embedded brain specimens from children with AIDS, with localization of HIV-1 sequences by PCR in cells of monocyte-macrophage origin, astrocytes, and neurons

(Trillo-Pazos, 2003). It should be pointed out that the relevance of latent neuronal infection to the pathogenesis of HIV-associated encephalopathy has been questioned (Wiley, 1996).

TREATMENT

The cornerstone of treating children with HIV-1 infection is to reduce the overall viral burden and preserving or reconstituting immune function while simultaneously optimizing nutrition, providing appropriate antimicrobial prophylaxis against OI, administering indicated immunizations, minimizing pain, and treating acute complications (Panel on Antiretroviral Therapy and Medical Management of HIV-Infected Children, 2010). The ecumenical goal of improving the child's quality of life must be tempered against the potentially severe toxicities and side effects of complex medication regimens (Oleske & Czarniecki, 1999; Van Dyke et al., 2008; Aurpibul et al., 2007; Delaugerre et al., 2009). However, it is now clear that the benefits of early, combination drug therapies outweigh their risks in most cases, although often requiring lifelong treatment to maintain viral suppression (Panel on Antiretroviral Therapy and Medical Management of HIV-Infected Children, 2010; Saitoh et al., 2002).

In the approach to treating a child with a chronic infection and a disease fraught with psychosocial implications and complications, one should establish reasonable outcome goals and expectations. ART drug failures are usually the result of drug resistance (minimized with combination therapies using drugs from multiple classes), medication intolerance, poor adherence, individual and developmental differences in pharmacokinetics, or an incomplete virologic, immunologic, or clinical response to a prescribed ART regimen. Specific antiretroviral therapies (ART), particularly HAART, coupled with OI/antibacterial prophylaxis has revolutionized the treatment of HIV-1-infected children, markedly prolonging survival (Panel on Antiretroviral Therapy and Medical Management of HIV-Infected Children, 2010; Viani et al., 2004; Brady et al., 2010; Judd et al., 2007; Palladino et al., 2009). Previously, the use of ART monotherapy, after an initial response, was often associated with CNS deterioration despite continuation or alterations of antiretroviral treatment regimens, mostly due to the development of ART drug resistance that more readily occurs with monotherapy (Mintz et al., 1990; Tudor-Williams et al., 1992) [Figure 10.1.1]. The use of HAART has reduced the incidence of CNS relapse, reduced the incidence of PE, and tempered the severity of PE, although the development of drug resistance continues to be a problem (Raskino et al., 1999; Lindsey et al., 2007; Mitchell, 2006). However, PE still exists, particularly in areas of the world with limited access to HAART or drugs in general, and therefore a necessary aim for the future is to develop adjunctive CNS-specific therapies that are complementary to antiretroviral drugs. (see chapter 11.6) Such therapies should be designed to attack the many proffered neuropathogenic mechanisms by either reducing upregulated cytokine production, preventing neuronal apoptosis, blocking cytotoxic effects of excitatory neurotransmitters, or disrupting/correcting aberrant biochemical pathways.

TREATMENT FOR CNS/PNS COMPLICATIONS

Antiretroviral Drugs

The cornerstone of reducing HIV-1 viral load, both systemically and within the CNS, is the use of antiretroviral drugs, which disrupt the replication and life cycle of the virus. Antiretroviral drugs fall into a number of major drug classes, including nucleoside and nucleotide analogue reverse transcriptase inhibitors (NRTI, NtRTI), non-nucleoside reverse transcriptase inhibitors (NNRTI), protease inhibitors (PI), entry inhibitors, and integrase inhibitors. Additionally, neurodevelopmental deterioration or signs of PE are one of a number of surrogate markers utilized in considering a change in a child's antiretroviral regimen (Panel on Antiretroviral Therapy and Medical Management of HIV-Infected Children, 2010; Working Group, 1999, Table 10.1.3). Early strategies for treating symptomatic HIV-1-infected patients with a single antiretroviral agent has now shifted to presently recommended initial therapeutic regimens that consist of a combination of antiretroviral agents, started as soon as HIV-1 infection is identified or suspected, particularly under 12 months, whether symptomatic or asymptomatic and regardless of immune status or viral load (Panel on Antiretroviral Therapy and Medical Management of HIV-Infected Children, 2010; Faye et al., 2004). The philosophy behind such an aggressive approach provides for the best opportunity to preserve immune function, suppress viral replication and viral spread to uninfected organs, to delay or suspend disease progression, and avoid drug resistance. However, such an approach is not without potential risk. Nevertheless, although aggressive and early therapy can enhance the opportunities for drug side effects, ART monotherapy is no longer considered a viable option for HIV-1-infected children and adolescents (Panel on Antiretroviral Therapy and Medical Management of HIV-Infected Children, 2010). If a child is older than one year and remains ART naïve, ART can still be very useful and is indicated in most instances, but can be deferred if there is immune competence and no or mild symptoms (Panel on Antiretroviral Therapy and Medical Management of HIV-Infected Children, 2010). There are recommendations for initial combination ART therapies in children who are ARTnaïve, with references to using a three-drug regimen that includes a non-nucleoside/nucleotide reverse transcriptase inhibitor or protease inhibitor, plus a dual nucleoside/nucleotide analogue reverse transcriptase inhibitor "backbone" (Panel on Antiretroviral Therapy and Medical Management of HIV-Infected Children, 2010). There are certain combinations that should not be given to HIV-infected children, including monotherapy, two NRTIs alone, dual-NNRTI combinations, and others, some with exceptions (Panel on Antiretroviral Therapy and Medical Management of HIV-Infected Children, 2010). Treatment endpoints and goals should be elimination of clinical symptoms known to be amenable to ART, suppression of viral load to the limits of assay quantitation, and preservation or normalization of immune status. Children receiving ART should be closely monitored, including clinical status, complete blood counts with differentials, chemistries, lipids, CD4 cell count/percentage, HIV RNA viral loads, and assessment of adherence (Panel on Antiretroviral Therapy and Medical Management of HIV-Infected Children, 2010).

Despite the early optimism brought about by HAART, there were early reports in adults suggesting that the CNS may be a more problematic compartment for antiretroviral drugs to penetrate and suppress HIV-1 replication within the CNS, correlating to a rise in ADC-related illnesses despite HAART (Brodt et al., 1997). However, these fears have been largely overcome with newer ART agents that have better CNS penetration, leading to better, although not dramatically improved, effectiveness of CNS-penetrating HAART regimens in combating HIV infection and PE. Thus, it is generally suggested to utilize HAART regimens with good CNS penetration, particularly if there are clinical signs or symptoms of PE (Patel et al., 2009; Letendre et al., 2008)(Table 10.1.3 and 10.1.6). In children, HAART regimens with good CNS penetration have

Table 10.1.6 CENTRAL NERVOUS SYSTEM PENETRATION SCALE FOR ANTIRETROVIRAL DRUGS

1(LOWEST PENETRATION)	2(MEDIUMPENETRATION)	3(HIGHEST PENETRATION)
Didanosine(ddI)	Emtricitabine(FTC)	Abacavir(ABC)
Tenofovir (TFV)	Lamivudine(3TC)	Zidovudine(ZDV)
Zalcitabine(ddC)	Stavudine(d4T)	Delavirdine(DLV)
Nelfinavir(NFV)	Efavirenz(EFV)	Nevirapine(NVP)
Ritonavir(RTV)	Amprenavir (APV)	Amprenavir/ritonavir(APV-r)
Saquinavir(SQV)	Atazanavir(ATV)	Atazanavir/ritonavir(ATV-r)
Saquinavir/ritonavir(SQV-r)	Fosamprenavir(f-APV)	Fosamprenavir/ritonavir(f-APV-r)
Tipranavir/ritonavir(TPV-r)	Indinavir(IDV)	Indinavir/ritonavir(IDV-r)
Enfuvirtide(T-20)		Lopinavir/ritonavir(LPV-r)

From Patel/Ming: With permission.

been shown to improve survival over HAART regimens with less CNS penetration, although the reasons for this observation are not known (Patel et al., 2009; Brew, 2009). However, there is evidence that perinatally infected children remain at long-term risk of neurological dysfunction despite HAART regimens (Tardieu, 2009; Wood et al., 2009; Bagenda et al., 2006). There is ongoing concern that as drug regimens are more effective in suppressing systemic HIV-1 infection, the incidence and prevalence of HIV-1-associated neurologic disease may rise again in the future, as the CNS can act as a harbor for latent viruses (Tardieu, 2009).

Rehabilitation

Many of the children with PE require extensive physical and occupational therapy. Patients presenting with extrapyramidal symptoms (EPS) may benefit from levodopa therapy (Mintz et al., 1996). With the use of levodopa, children with EPS can often exhibit improvements in ambulation, rigidity, activity levels, facial expression, swallowing, and a cessation of drooling. In cases of severe spasticity with tendon contractures not amenable to physical therapy or splinting alone, pharmacological anti-spastic agents can be of use (such as benzodiazepines or baclofen), local injection of botulitum toxin, and on occasion, ethanol nerve blocks or surgical tendon lengthenings may also be beneficial. Speech pathologists can assist in patients with feeding difficulties or dysarthria; children with language deficits can benefit from speech and language therapies (Pressman, 1992; Wolters et al., 1995). Hearing loss, especially in those children with recurrent/chronic otitis media, should be investigated as a cause of language dysfunction. Sign language or communication boards can provide useful communication adjuncts in children with significant expressive language deficits. Infants and children with fine and gross motor impairments can benefit from physical and occupational therapy (Lord et al., 1995; Parks, 1994).

Many children with HIV-1 infection will require specific developmental rehabilitation services (Crocker, 1989, 1992). In children with cognitive impairment, evaluation for alternative classroom settings or special educational services should proceed; in infants and young children, evaluation for early intervention or preschool disability programs may be appropriate. Home tutoring or home-based educational programs deny proper socialization experiences, and should be reserved for those children unable to attend school or day care. Day care can be encouraged; many regions have established day care programs specifically designed for HIV-1-infected children. However, aggressive or biting behaviors, or uncovered secreting lesions, may preclude a child's attendance (American Academy of Pediatrics, 1987; Hirschfeld et al., 1996).

Pain

The prevalence of pain in hospitalized HIV-infected children has been estimated at 88%, with up to 59% of ambulatory patients reporting that pain is having a negative impact on their lives (Panel on Antiretroviral Therapy and Medical Management of HIV-Infected Children, 2010; Hirschfeld et al., 1996; Gaughan et al., 2002). Children with HIV-1 infection can experience pain from various medical procedures (particularly needle sticks and lumbar punctures); somatic pain (such as myalgias/arthralgias); visceral pain; neuropathic pain; or headache. In addition to the obvious humane aspects of pain relief, attention to aspects of analgesia for procedural or chronic pain will allow for better compliance with diagnostic procedures or therapeutic regimens, behavioral improvement, and a more realistic framework in which to measure behavioral, cognitive, or neurological dysfunction. For the patient with chronic, severe pain failing non-narcotic medications, narcotics (particularly opioids) are often necessary and should not be avoided. In patients with severe or unpredictable pain, consistent analgesic regimens are preferred to avoid breakthrough pain. Anticipation and anxiety of situational pain, such as occurs on a periodic clinic visit, can lead to oppositional and noncompliant behavior patterns. For procedural pain, such as needle sticks or lumbar punctures, nonpharmacologic cognitive-behavioral techniques such as distraction or guided imagery have proven to be successful; often, this approach can be enhanced with the use of cutaneous topical anesthesia (French et al., 1994; Walco et al., 1992; Czarniecki et al., 1993; Miser et al., 1994). Guidelines for the management of pain in HIV-1-infected children are published (Panel on Antiretro-viral Therapy and Medical Management of HIV-Infected Children, 2010; Varni et al., 1989).

Nutritional/Metabolic Therapies

General experience of the effects of malnutrition on the CNS dictates that children with HIV-1 infection should receive adequate and optimal protein-calorie nutrition (Isaranurug & Chompikul, 2009). Furthermore, malnutrition can lead to a worsening of immune function, which could impact the CNS by increasing the susceptibility to CNS OI, and possibly enhance neuropathogenic pathways. Optimal nutrition should be an integral part of the HIV-1-infected child's overall medical care. Underlying gastrointestinal or infectious diseases that may be causing nutritional deficiencies should be identified and treated. When oral intake is inadequate, tube or parenteral feeding may be necessary. Vitamin, co-factor, and other essential micronutrient supplementation should be provided as is clinically indicated. There is little data concerning the clinical efficacy of specific vitamin/co-factor supplements on ameliorating PE; anecdotal reports concerning the neurocognitive benefits of B12 in adults have not been observed in children (Herzlich & Schiano, 1993). Additionally, various drug therapies can precipitate pathologic deficiencies of important nutrients, and supplements may be useful in such situations (Mintz, 1996b; Mintz, 1995; Semino-Mora et al., 1994).

Disruption of the metabolic pathways involving folate-dependent methyl-group transfer has also been regarded by some authors to be a potential pathogenic mechanism of neurologic dysfunction in HIV-1-infected children (Smith et al., 1987; Bottiglieri & Hyland, 1994; Castagna et al., 1995). Low levels of S-adenosylmethionine (SAM), 5-methyltetrahydrofolate, methionine, and glutathione have been found to be deficient in serum and CSF of both children and adults with HIV-1-related neurologic disorders (Castagna et al., 1995). Administration of methyl group donors such as SAMe and GSH can reverse identifiable deficiencies within the CSF, and therefore are of theoretical use, but no clinical data exists concerning reversal or prevention of PE.

Carnitine supplementation may be useful in augmenting fatty acid metabolism, especially if a child is receiving a nucleoside analogue drug, but direct clinical evidence for its use in HIV-1-infected children is lacking (Mintz, 1995; Periquet et al., 1995). Carnitine supplementation may be useful for AZT-induced muscle disease (Semino-Mora et al., 1994).

Care must be taken in the administration of micronutrients, particularly if a precise deficiency has not been identified, as many vitamins, minerals, and other co-factors/supplements can be CNS and/or systemically toxic in excess. Nevertheless, there is a strong rationale and need for further research in the area of nutritional supplementation and its relationship to the amelioration and prevention of HIV-1 related CNS or PNS disease (Mintz, 1996b).

Immunomodulatory Therapy

At least in countries with available drug resources, it is clear that virtually all children with HIV-1 infection will be receiving anti-RV therapies, and many will be taking various combinations of drugs (Working Group, 1999). However, the efficacy of these drugs in ameliorating or protecting against PE are limited, and it may be necessary to develop adjunctive drug therapies directed at the indirect, neuropathogenic effects of HIV-1 infection within the CNS (see chapter 11.6).

Certain extracts of fish oils, such as omega-3 and omega-6 polyunsaturated fatty acids, may have a hypothetical use in PE, as these compounds have been shown in some autoimmune diseases to inhibit arachidonic acid metabolites and tumor necrosis factor (possible cofactors in the neuropathogenesis of PE); however, no specific data exists to directly support this notion (DeCaterina et al., 1994). In PE, there is anecdotal evidence of steroid efficacy, although controlled studies are lacking (Stiehm et al., 1992). Steroids markedly reduce the production and release of cytokines produced from macrophage/MGC activation, and proffer hypothetical promise. However, side effects may limit their use.

Overall, there has been a growing interest in alternative and adjunctive therapies which can either "boost" and reconstitute a compromised immune system, enhance intrinsic immune defenses directed against HIV-1, or modulate secondary cytotoxic pathways precipitated by HIV-1, but without specific data in pediatrics (Amman & Duliege, 1994; Spector, 1991).

Vaccines may be useful not only in immunizing against HIV-1 infection in uninfected individuals, but may also assist in providing a "boost" to the immune system in established HIV-1 infection. However, many of the vaccines presently being studied utilize parts of the HIV-1 envelope, such as gp120/160. These glycoproteins may be putative cytotoxic mediators, and it is unknown if these vaccines may be CNS

toxic (Lipton, 1993). Unfortunately, most clinical vaccine trials are not assessing for potential neurological dysfunction.

TREATMENT OF PSYCHIATRIC AND NEUROBEHAVIORAL COMPLICATIONS

Mental health concerns have not been sufficiently addressed in the HIV-1-infected and uninfected pediatric population (Mellins et al., 2003; Havens et al., 1997; Kotchick & Forehand, 1999; Flisher & Dawes, 2009; King et al., 2009; Letwaba & Minde, 2010). The need for neurobehavioral support mechanisms is quite evident given the high incidence of neurobehavioral problems in HIV-1-infected children as well as their uninfected siblings (Gadow et al., 2010). Psychotherapy, often in conjunction with pharmacological approaches, is useful in the approach to affective and other neurobehavioral/neuropsychiatric disorders. The clinician should always be alert for suicidal tendencies in older children, adolescents, and adults, and implement crisis intervention if indicated.

Little has been reported about specific psychotherapy in the HIV-infected pediatric population, but paradigms previously developed for populations with developmental disabilities and chronic illness can be employed (Spiegel & Mayers, 1991; Havens et al., 1997). Short-term psychotherapy is indicated in assisting children and adolescents deal with psychological traumas such as family death or sexual abuse, and long-term therapies may be necessary for children to deal with issues of chronic illness and societal stigmas of HIV-1 infection. Combinations of individual and family therapies may be necessary. In nonverbal children, or in those with significant neurological impairments, functional analyses of behavior coupled with behavioral modification therapies may be more useful.

Appropriate laboratory, clinical, and psychological monitoring should occur in children and adolescents receiving psychoactive drugs. Apart from stimulant medications, the majority of psychoactive medications are not specifically approved for use in the pediatric population, but there is a literature to support the "off label" use in children of a number of compounds. It is usually necessary to provide adjunctive and concomitant psycho- or behavioral therapies when administering these drugs to maximize their benefit.

Certain drugs administered for reasons other than PE may have significant CNS side effects, particularly on behavior. For example, the anti-epileptic agent phenobarbital may precipitate or exacerbate hyperactive behavior patterns, and some anti-epileptic medications may potentially increase suicidality.

In children with depression, there may be benefit from selective serotonin reuptake inhibitors (SSRI), tricyclic antidepressants, or other antidepressants if there is no medical contraindication to their use. Neuroleptics, SSRI, anti-epileptics, other mood stabilizers, or anti-anxiety agents may be helpful in PE, as it can be in any child who is developmentally disabled or braininjured, if severe maladaptive or dysregulated behaviors exist. Acute psychoses may respond to neuroleptic treatment. A precaution is that the population possessing PE or ADC may be somewhat more susceptible to neuroleptic side effects (Hriso et al., 1991).

In conjunction with behavioral and educational approaches, psychostimulants such as methylphenidate or mixed amphetamine salts are very useful in addressing attentional deficits with or without hyperactivity/impulsivity, and often are efficacious in low doses. Appetite suppression with stimulants can be an undesirable side effect, particularly in the patients with poor weight gain. Adolescents with clinical depression and a lack of energy or psychomotor slowing may respond to stimulant therapy (Holmes et al., 1989). Newly released nonstimulant medications (selective norepinephrine reuptake inhibitors: atomoxetine) have not been specifically studied in HIV infection. Alpha-2 adrenergic agonists can be useful in tempering impulsivity and other ADHD symptoms, and/or the physiological responses to anxiety.

PREVENTION OF HIV-1 INFECTION

Clearly, the best form of "treatment" of a chronic infectious disease is prevention of primary infection and of further spread. Vertical transmission of HIV-1 infection can be significantly reduced if ART drugs are given to HIV-1-infected pregnant females (Mofenson, 1999; Mofenson & Fowler, 1999). HAART does not alter neurodevelopment or behavior in fetuses exposed to HAART who are ultimately HIV-negative. However, if a child born to an HIV-infected mother receiving prenatal ART is ultimately infected, the incidence of PE is unchanged in infancy, suggesting that there are other neuropathogenic mechanisms causing PE in infants not directly related to viral burden, or that resistant, neurovirulent viral forms are being selected for (Tardieu et al., 2000). The vigilant screening of the blood supply and heat treatment of Factor VIII compounds has markedly reduced the risk of "horizontal" transmission from contaminated blood products. Unfortunately, in much of the world, because of a lack of resources, extensive reuse of needles and syringes not adequately sterilized within health care institutions, coupled with an inadequate supply of oral medications, has led to a high incidence of nosocomial pediatric HIV-1 infection by means of horizontal transmission, in some countries occurring at a greater rate in children than adults (Mintz et al., 1995; Hersh et al., 1991). Needle exchange programs may be a useful alternative for intravenous drug-using populations, as they have been shown to reduce the spread of infection in these groups.

Adolescents at high risk for HIV infection include drug-using adolescents, runaways, gay and bisexual youth, individuals with sexually transmitted diseases, and sexually abused individuals (Hein et al., 1995; D'Angelo, 1994). However, many HIV-1-infected youth do not possess the "classical" transmission risk factors. Possibly, all sexually active adolescents should be considered at "high-risk" of acquiring or transmitting HIV-1 infection. Unfortunately, AIDS- related knowledge does not necessarily reduce the risk of sexual transmission in adolescents (Keller et al., 1991). Dissemination of "safe sex" practices and other aspects of HIV-1 prevention represent the best means of prevention available, and should be targeted to all adolescents regardless of their or society's perception of risk. HIV-1-infected youth require intensive education regarding the potential for spread of infection, and uninfected youth need advice on primary prevention. Instruction on latex condom use (particularly in conjunction with nonoxynol-9 spermicide) and/or sexual abstention or delay should be directed to all adolescents regardless of "risk" status. The adverse cognitive effects and psychomotor slowing of PE or ADC add additional difficulties in counseling and managing high-risk behaviors, and can lead to noncompliance and poor adherence with treatment regimens (Panel on Antiretroviral Therapy and Medical Management of HIV-Infected Children, 2010).

In young children, casual contact is not an important means of HIV-1 transmission. Children are encouraged to attend day care and school, but in children who manifest biting or excessively aggressive behaviors, attendance in a group setting is not advised or allowed (Task Force on Pediatric AIDS,1991; Katz, 1994; Chanock & Simonds, 1994). Attempts at behavioral modification to alter these behavior patterns are often successful, sometimes in conjunction with psychopharmacological therapy.

SUMMARY

HIV-1 infection is presently a worldwide pandemic. In the United States, pediatric infection is usually acquired in a "vertical" fashion from mother-to-child, although the utilization of ART drugs during pregnancy has markedly reduced the incidence of transmission. Nevertheless, "horizontal" transmission (via contaminated blood products, needles, or syringes; or by sexual contact) exists, and can be a concerning mode of transmission in parts of the world. In addition to severe immune deficiency and multi-organ dysfunction, the CNS is a major target of HIV-1 infection. Infants and children are uniquely at risk for the encephalopathic effects of HIV-1, resulting from infection of an immature nervous system. There is a wide spectrum of neurological and behavioral manifestations of PE, but underlying non-HIV-1-related etiologic precipitants should be eliminated. PE is a clinical diagnosis that may be supported by neurodiagnostic and laboratory studies. Furthermore, although rare in infants and young children, CNS OI can also precipitate neurological or psychiatric dysfunction, or may mimic or confuse the diagnosis of PE.

Efficacious treatments for children with HIV-1 infection are available, but should be utilized pragmatically with an overall goal of improving the quality of life. Combinations of antiretroviral drugs from various classes are essential in suppressing viral replication, preserving or reconstituting immune function, and treating clinical complications of infection, including PE, but require lifelong use with careful clinical and laboratory monitoring of potential side effects. In addition, many infants, children, and adolescents require OI prophylaxis/treatment, attention to maximization of motor and language function, alleviation of pain, mainstreaming in the educational setting when possible, and the institution of psychotherapy and/or psychoactive medications when needed. Adverse behavioral patterns may respond to combinations of behavioral management protocols with drug therapies; underlying treatable mechanisms of maladaptive behaviors should be explored. Uninfected siblings may have similar rates of behavioral problems, reinforcing the "family" nature of HIV disease. Correction of nutritional deficiencies, and in certain instances supplementation, is essential. Nevertheless, new horizons have yet to be conquered in providing innovative adjunctive therapies directed at specific neuropathogenic pathways. As the pendulum of the HIV epidemic has swung from dying with AIDS to living with HIV infection, diagnostic studies and therapeutic interventions must be carefully tempered with maximization of a child's quality of life.

REFERENCES

Adams, L. V. & Palumbo, P. (2007).The time to treat the children is now. *The Journal of Infectious Diseases*, 195, 1396–1398.

AIDS Clinical Trials Group, National Institutes of Health, Washington, D.C.; Protocol #188.

AIDS Epidemic Update 2009; Joint United Nations Programme on HIV/AIDS (UNAIDS), www.unaids.org

Alimenti, A., Forbes, J. C., Oberlander, T. F., et al. (2006).A prospective controlled study of neurodevelopment in HIV-uninfected children exposed to combination antiretroviral drugs in pregnancy. *Pediatrics*, 118, e1139–e1145.

American Academy of Pediatrics Committee on Infectious Diseases. (1987). Health guidelines for the attendance in day-care and foster care settings of children infected with human immunodeficiency virus. *Pediatrics*, 79, 466.

American Academy of Pediatrics Committee on Pediatric AIDS. (2008). HIV testing and prophylaxis to prevent mother-to-child transmission in the United States. *Pediatrics*, 122(5), 1127–1134.

American College of Obstetricians and Gynecologists. (1997). Human immunodeficiency virus infections in pregnancy. *International Journal of Gynecology & Obstetrics*, 57(1), 73–80.

Amman, A. J. & Duliege, A-M.S. (1994). Biologic and immunomodulating factors in treatment of pediatric AIDS. In C. M. Wilfert & P. A. Pizzo, (Eds.). *Pediatric AIDS: The challenge of HIV infection in infants, children, and adolescents*, pp. 689–713. Baltimore: Williams and Wilkins.

Anders, K. H., Guerra, W. F., Tomiyasu, U., Verity, M. A. & Vinters, H. V. (1986). The neuropathology of AIDS. UCLA experience and review. *American Journal of Pathology*, 124, 537–558.

Anonymous. (1994). Maternal vitamin A deficiency is associated with increased mother-to-child transmission of the human immunodeficiency virus (HIV). *Nutrition Review*, 52, 281–282.

Antinori, A., Perno, C. F., Giancola, M. L., et al. (2005). Efficacy of cerebrospinal fluid (CSF)-penetrating antiretroviral drugs against HIV in the neurological compartment: Different patterns of phenotypic resistance in CSF and plasma. *Clinical Infectious Diseases*, 41(12), 1787–1793.

Arendt, G., Hefter, H., & Jablonowski, H. (1993). Acoustically evoked event-related potentials in HIV-associated dementia. *Electroencephalography and Clinical Neurophysiology*, 86, 152–160.

Arribas, J. R., Storch, G. A., Clifford, D. B., & Tselis, A. C. (1996). Cytomegalovirus encephalitis. *Annals of Internal Medicine*, 125, 577–587.

Association Francois-Xavier Bagnoud; http://www.fxb.org

Aurpibul, L., Puthanakit, T., Lee, B., et al. (2007). Lipodystrophy and metabolic changes in HIV-infected children on non-nucleoside reverse transcriptase inhibitor-based antiretroviral therapy. *Antiviral Therapy*, 12(8), 1247–1254.

Bachanas, P. J., Kullgren, K., Suzman, S. K., et al. (2001). Predictors of psychological adjustment in school-age children infected with HIV. *Journal of Pediatric Psychology*, 26, 343–352.

Bagasra, O., Lavi, E., Bobroski, L., et al. (1996).Cellular reservoirs of HIV-1 in the central nervous system of infected individuals: Identification by the combination of in situ polymerase chain reaction and immunohistochemistry. *AIDS*, 10, 573–585.

Bagenda, D., Nassali, A., Kalyesubula, I., et al. (2006). Health, neurologic and cognitive status of HIV-infected, long surviving and antiretroviral naive Ugandan children. *Pediatrics*, 117, 729–740.

Beach, R. S., Morhan, R., Wilkie, F. et al. (1992). Plasma vitamin B12 level as a potential cofactor in studies of human immunodeficiency virus type 1-related cognitive changes. *Archives of Neurology*, 49, 501–506.

Begin, M. E., Manku, M. S., & Horrobin, D. F.(1989). Plasma fatty acid levels in patients with acquired immune deficiency syndrome and in controls. *Prostaglandins Leukotrienes Essential Fatty Acids*, 37, 135–137.

Belman, A.L., Diamond, G., Dickson, D., et al. (1988). Pediatric acquired immunodeficiency syndrome: Neurologic syndromes. *American Journal of Diseases of Children*, 142(1), 29–35.

Belman, A. L., Lantos, G., Horoupian, D. C., et al. (1986). AIDS: Calcification of the basal ganglia in infants and children. *Neurology*, 36, 1192–1199.

Benhammou, V., Tardieu, M., Warszawski, J., Rustin, P. & Blanche, S. (2007). Clinical mitochondrial dysfunction in uninfected children born to HIV-infected mothers following perinatal exposure to nucleoside analogues. *Environmental & Molecular Mutagenesis*, 48(3–4), 173–178.

Blanche, S., Newell, M. L., Mayaux, M-J.,et al. (1997). Morbidity and mortality in European children vertically infected by HIV-1: The French Pediatric HIV Infection Study Group and European Collaborative Study.*J AIDS and Human Retrovirology*, 14, 442–450.

Blanche, S., Tardieu, M., Benhammou, V., Warszawski, J., & Rustin, P. (2006). Mitochondrial dysfunction following perinatal exposure to nucleoside analogues. *AIDS*, 20, 1685–1690.

Blanche, S., Tardieu, M., Duliege, A. M., et al. (1990). Longitudinal study of 94 symptomatic infants with perinatally acquired human immunodeficiency virus infection: Evidence for a bimodal expression of clinical and biological symptoms. *American Journal of Diseases of Children*, 144, 1210–1215.

Blanche, S., Tardieu, M., Rustin, P., et al. (1999). Persistent mitochondrial dysfunction and perinatal exposure to antiretroviral nucleoside analogues. *Lancet*, 354, 1084–1089.

Bottiglieri, T. & Hyland, K. (1994). S-adenosylmethionine levels in psychiatric and neurological disorders: A review. *Acta Neurologica Scandinavica*, 154(suppl), 19–26.

Brackis-Cott, E., Kang, E., Dolezal, C., Abrams, E. J., & Mellins, C. A. (2009). Brief report: Language ability and school functioning of youth perintally infected with HIV. *J Pediatric Health Care*, 23, 158–164.

Brady, M. T., Clark, C., Weedy, C., et al. (1996). Disclosure of HIV diagnosis to children in AIDS Clinical Trials (ACTG) 219. Presented at the XI International AIDS Conference on AIDS, Vancouver, Canaza.

Brady, M. T., Oleske, J. M., Williams, P. L., et al. (2010). Declines in mortality rates and changes in causes of death in HIV-1-infected children during the HAART era. *Journal of Acquired Immune Deficiency Syndrome*, 53(1), 86–94.

Brew, B. J. (2009). HIV, the brain, children, HAART and "neuro-HAART": A complex mix. *AIDS*, 23, 1909–1910.

Brew, B. J., Bhalla, R. B., Paul, M., et al. (1990). Cerebrospinal fluid neopterin in human immunodeficiency virus type 1 infection. *Ann Neurology*, 28, 556–560.

Brodt, H. R., Kamps, B. S., Gute, P., et al. (1997). Changing incidence of AIDS-defining illnesses in theera of antiretroviral combination therapy. *AIDS*, 11, 1731–1738.

Brookmeyer, R. (1991). Reconstruction and future trends of the AIDS epidemic in the United States. *Science*, 253, 37–42.

Brouwers, P., Belman, A. L., & Epstein, L. (1994). Central nervous system involvement: Manifestations, evaluation, and pathogenesis. In C. M. Wilfert & P. A. Pizzo, (Eds.). *Pediatric AIDS: The Challenge of HIV infection in infants, children, and adolescents*, pp.443–456. Baltimore: Williams and Wilkins.

Brouwers, P., DeCarli, C., Tudor-Williams, G., Civitello, L., Moss, H., & Pizzo, P. (1994). Interrelations among patterns of change in neurocognitive, CT brain imaging, and CD4 measures associated with antiretroviral therapy in children with symptomatic HIV infection. *Advances in Neuroimmunology, 4,* 223–231.

Brouwers, P., DeCarli, D., Civitello, L., Moss, H., Wolters, P. & Pizzo, P. (1995). Correlation between computed tomographic brain scan abnormalities and neuropsychological function in children with symptomatic human immunodeficiency virus disease. *Archives of Neurology, 53,* 39–44.

Brouwers, P., Moss, H., Wolters, P., et al. (1990). Effect of continuous-infusion zidovudine therapy on neuropsychologic functioning in children with symptomatic human immunodeficiency virus infection. *Journal of Pediatrics, 117,* 980–985.

Brouwers, P., Moss, H., Wolters, P., El-Amin, D., Tassone, E., & Pizzo, P. A.(1992). Neurobehavioral typology of school-age children with symptomatic HIV disease [abstract]. *Journal of Clinical and Experimental Neuropsychology, 14,* 113.

Brouwers, P., Tudor-Williams, G., DeCarli, C., et al. (1995). Relation between stage of disease and neurobehavioral measures in children with symptomatic HIV disease. *AIDS, 9,* 713–720.

Brouwers, P., van derVlugt, H., Moss, H., Wolters, P. & Pizzo, P. (1995). White matter changes on CT brain scan are associated with neurobehavioral dysfunction in children with symptomatic HIV disease. *Child Neuropsychology, 1,* 93–105.

Budka, H. (1991). Neuropathology of human immunodeficiency virus infection.*Brain Pathology, 1,* 163–175.

Budka, H. & Gray, F. (1993). HIV-induced central nervous system pathology. In FGray, ed. *Atlas of the neuropathology of HIV infection,* pp. 1–46. Oxford University Press, Oxford.

Budk, H., Wiley, C. A., Kleihues, P., et al. (1991). HIV-associated disease of the nervous system: Review of nomenclature and proposal for neuropathology-based terminology. *Brain Pathology, 1,* 143–152.

Butterworth, R. F., Gaudreau, C., Vincelette, J., Bourgault, A-M., Lamonthe, F. & NutiniA-M. (1991). Thiamine deficiency and Wernicke's encephalopathy in AIDS. *Metabolic Brain Disease, 6,* 207–212.

Campbell, T. (1997). A review of the psychological effects of vertically acquired HIV infection in infants and children. *British Journal of Health Psychology, 2,* 1–13.

Castagna, A., LeGrazie, C., Accordini, A., et al. (1995). Cerebrospinal fluid S-adenosylmethionine (SAMe) and glutathione concentrations in HIV infection: Effect of parenteral treatment with SAMe. *Neurology, 45,* 1678–1683.

Centers for Disease Control (CDC). (2006). Revised recommendations for HIV testing of adults, adolescents, and pregnant women in health care settings. *MMWR, 55*(No. RR–14).

Centers for Disease Control and Prevention (CDC). (1994a). 1994 revised classification system for human immunodeficiency virus infection in children less than 13 years of age. *MMWR, 43*(RR-12), 1–10.

Centers for Disease Control and Prevention. (1994b). Recommendations of the U.S. Public Health Service Task Force on the use of zidovudine to reduce perinatal transmission of human immunodeficiency virus. *MMWR, 43,* 1–20.

Centers for Disease Control and Prevention. (2001). Revised guidelines for HIV counseling, testing, and referral and revised recommendations for HIV screening of pregnant women. *MMWR, 50*(RR-19), 1–110.

Centers for Disease Control and Prevention (CDC). (2002). HIV testing among pregnant women—United States and Canada, 1998-2001. *MMWR, 51*(45), 1013–1016.

Centers for Disease Control and Prevention. (2006). Reduction in perinatal transmission of HIV infection—United States, 1985-2005. *MMWR, 55*(21), 592–597.

Centers for Disease Control and Prevention. (2009a). Guidelines for the prevention and treatment of opportunistic infections in HIV-infected adults and adolescents. *MMWR, 58*(RR-4), 1–216.

Centers for Disease Control and Prevention. (2009b). Guidelines for the prevention and treatment of opportunistic infections in HIV-exposed and HIV-infected children. *MMWR, 58*(RR-11), 1–176.

Centers for Disease Control (CDC), (1987). Revision of the CDC surveillance case definition for acquired immunodeficiency syndrome. *MMWR, 36* (1S Suppl), 3S–15S.

Chang, J., Basit, A., Fordyce-Baum, M. K., et al. (1990). Plasma fatty acids in early HIV-1 infection (abstract).*FASEB Journal, 4,* A796.

Chanock, S. & Simonds, R. J. (1994). Medical issues related to provision of care for HIV-infected children in hospital, home, day care, school, and community. In C. M. Wilfert & P. A. Pizzo, eds. *Pediatric AIDS: The challenge of HIV infection in infants, children, and adolescents,* pp. 907–921. Baltimore: Williams and Wilkins

Chiao, S. K., Romero, D. L., & Johnson, D. E. (2009). Current HIV therapeutics: Mechanistic and chemical determinants of toxicity. *Current Opinion in Drug Discovery & Development, 12,* 53–60.

Chiappini, E., Galli, L., Tovo, P. A., et al. (2007). Changing patterns of clinical events in perinatally HIV-1-infected children during the era of HAART. *AIDS, 21,* 1607–1615.

Chiriboga, C. A., Fleishman, S., Champion, S., Gaye-Robinson, L. & Abrams, E. J. (2005). Incidence and prevalence of HIV encephalopathy in children with HIV infection receiving highly active antiretroviral therapy (HAART). *Journal of Pediatrics, 146,* 402–407.

Chopra, J. S. & Sharma, A. (1992).Protein energy malnutrition and the nervous system. *Journal of the Neurological Sciences, 110,* 8–20.

Civitello, L., Brouwers, P., DeCarli, C., Wolters, P., & Sei, S. (1999). Relation between neuroimaging abnormalities and cerebrospinal fluid viral load in children with human immunodeficiency virus disease. *Annals of Neurology, 46,* 521.

Clifford, D. B. (1998). Neurologic complications of human immunodeficiency virus infection. *Neurologist, 4,* 54–65.

Clifford, D. B. & Campbell, J. W. (1992). Management of neurologic opportunistic disorders in human immunodeficiency virus infection. *Seminars in Neurology, 12,* 28–33.

Cohen-Addad, N., Joshi, V., & Sharer, L. (1988). Congenital acquired immunodeficiency syndrome and congenital toxoplasmosis: Pathologic support for a chronology of events. *Journal of Perinatology, 3,* 328–331.

Cohen, S. E., Mundy, T., Karassik, B., et al. (1991). Neuropsychological functioning in human immunodeficiency virus type 1 sepositive children infected through neonatal blood transfusion. *Pediatrics, 88,* 58–68.

Cohen, H. J., Papola, P. & Alvarez, M. (1994). Neurodevelopmental abnormalities in school-age children with HIV infection. *Journal of School Health, 64,* 11–13.

Connor, E. M., Sperling, R. S., Gelber, R., et al. (1994). Reduction of maternal-infant transmission of immunodeficiency virus type 1 with zidovudine treatment. *New Engl J Med, 331,* 1173–1180.

Cooper, E. R., Hanson, C., Diaz, C., et al. (1998). Encephalopathy and progression of human immunodeficiency virus disease in a cohort of children with perinatally acquired human immunodeficiency virus infection. Women and Infants Transmission Study Group. *J Pediatrics, 132,* 808–812.

Crocker, A. C.(1989). Developmental services for children with HIV infection. *Mental Retardation, 27,* 223–225.

Crocker, A. C. (1992). Summary of policy recommendations. In A. C. Crocker, H. J. Cohen, & T. A. Kastner, eds. *HIV infection and developmental disabilities,* pp. (Ch. 30). Baltimore: Paul H. Brookes Publishing Co.

Cysique, L.A., Maruff, P., & Brew, B. J. (2004). Prevalence and pattern of neuropsychological impairment in HIV/AIDS infection across pre-HAART and HAART eras: A combined study of 2 cohorts. *Journal of Neurovirology, 10,* 350–357.

Czarniecki, L., Boland, M., & Oleske, J. (1993). Pain in children with HIV infection. *Journal of the Physicians for AIDS Care, 1,* 492.

D'Angelo, L. J. (1994). HIV infections and AIDS in adolescents. In C. M. Wilfert & P. A. Pizzo, eds. *Pediatric AIDS: The challenge of HIV infection in infants, children, and adolescents,* pp. 71–82. Baltimore: Williams and Wilkins.

Dalakas, M. C., Illa, I., Pezeshkpour, G. H., et al. (1990). Mitochondrial myopathy caused by long-term zidovudine therapy. *New England Journal of Medicine, 322,* 1098–1105.

DeCarli, C., Civitello, L., Brouwers, P. & Pizzo, P. A. (1993). The prevalence of computed tomographic abnormalities of the cerebrum in 100 consecutive children symptomatic with the human immunodeficiency virus. *Annals of Neurology, 34*, 198–205.

DeCaterina, R., Endres, S., Kristensen, S. D., & Schmidt, E. B. (1994). N-3 fatty acids and renal diseases. *American Journal of Kidney Diseases, 24*, 397–415.

Delaugerre. C., Chaix, M. L., Blanche, S., et al. (2009). Perinatal acquisition of drug-resistant HIV-1 infection: Mechanisms and long-term outcome. *Retrovirology, 6*, 85.

Denckla, M. B. (1985). Revised neurological examination for subtle signs. *Psychopharmacology Bulletin, 21*, 773–775.

Denny, T., Yogev, R., Gelman, R., et al. (1992). Lymphocyte subsets in healthy children during the first 5 years of life. *JAMA, 267*, 2484–2488.

Dickson, D. W., Belman, A. L., Kim, T. S., et al. (1989). Spinal cord pathology in pediatric acquired immunodeficiency syndrome. *Neurology, 39*, 227–235.

Douglas, G. C. & King, B. F. (1992). Maternal-fetal transmission of human immunodeficiency virus: A review of possible routes and cellular mechanisms of infection. *Clinical Infectious Diseases, 15*, 678–691.

Dowling, S., Lambe, J., & Mulcahy, F. (1993).Vitamin B12 and folate status in human immunodeficiency virus infection. *European Journal of Clinical Nutrition, 47*, 803–807.

Epstein, L. G., Berman, C. Z., Sharer, L. R., Khademi, M. & Desposito, F. 1987). Unilateral calcification and contrast enhancement of the basal ganglia in a child with AIDS encephalopathy. *American Journal of Neuroradiology, 8*, 163–165.

Epstein, L. G., DiCarlo, F. J., Joshi, V. V., et al. (1988a). Primary lymphoma of the central nervous system in children with acquired immunodeficiency syndrome. *Pediatrics, 82*, 355–363.

Epstein, L. G., Sharer, L. R. & Goudsmit, J. (1988b). Neurological and neuropathological features of human immunodeficiency virus infection in children. *Annals of Neurology, 23*(suppl.), S19–23.

Epstein, L. G., Goudsmit, J., Paul, D. A., et al. (1987). Expression of human immunodeficiency virus in cerebrospinal fluid of children with progressive encephalopathy. *Annals of Neurology, 21*, 397–401.

Epstein, L. G., Sharer, L. R., Oleske, J. M., et al. (1986). Neurologic manifestations of HIV infection in children. *Pediatrics, 78*, 678–687.

Esposito, S., Musetti, L., Musetti, M. C., et al. (1999). Behavioral and psychological disorders in uninfected children aged 6 to 11 years born to human immunodeficiency virus-seropositive mothers. *Journal of Developmental & Behavioral Pediatrics, 20*, 411–417.

The European Collaborative Study. (1990). Neurologic signs in young children with human immunodeficiency virus infection. *Pediatric Infectious Disease Journal, 9*, 402–406.

European Collaborative Study. (1992). Age-related standards for T lymphocyte subsets based on uninfected children born to human immunodeficiency virus infected women. *Pediatric Infectious Disease Journal, 11*, 1018–1026.

Falangola, M. F., Hanly, A., Galvao-Castro, B. & Petito, C. K. (1995). HIV infection of human choroid plexus: A possible mechanism of viral entry into the CNS. *Journal of Neuropathology & Experimental Neurology, 54*, 497–503.

Faye, A., LeChenadec, J., Dollfus, C., et al. (2004). Early versus deferred antiviral multidrug therapy in infants infected with HIV. *Clinical Infectious Diseases, 39*,1692–1698.

Fennell, E. B. (1993). Assessing neurobehavioral changes in HIV+ infants and children. *Annals of the New York Academy of Sciences, 693*, 141.

Fletcher, J. M., Francis, D. J., Pequegnat, W., et al. (1991). Neurobehavioral outcomes in diseases of childhood.*American Psychologist, 46*, 1267–1277.

Flisher, A. J. & Dawes, A. (2009). Synergistic Opportunities: Mental Health and HIV/AIDS. *Journal of the American Academy of Child and Adolescent Psychiatry, 48*(8), 780–781.

Floeter, M. K., Civitello, L. A., Everett, C. R., Dambrosia, J., & Luciano, C. A. (1997). Peripheral neuropathy in children with HIV infection. *Neurology, 49*, 207–212.

Forsyth, B. W., Damour, L., Nagler, S. & Adnopoz, J. (1996). The psychological effects of parental human immunodeficiency virus infection on uninfected children. *Archives of Pediatrics & Adolescent Medicine, 150*, 1015–1020.

Frank, Y., Lim, W., Kahn, E., et al. (1989). Multiple ischemic infarcts in a child with AIDS, varicella zoster infection, and cerebral vasculitis. *Pediatric Neurology, 5*, 64–67.

Frank, Y., Pavlakis, S., Black, K. & Bakshi, S.Reversible occipital parietal encephalopathy syndrome in AIDS. *Neurology, 51*, 915–916.

Frank, Y., Vishnubhakat, S. M., & Pahwa, S. (1992). Brainstem auditory evoked responses in infants and children with AIDS. *Pediatric Neurology, 8*, 262–266.

French, M. D., Gina, M., Painter, E. C, & Coury, D. (1994). Blowing away shot pain; a technique for pain management during immunization. *Pediatrics, 93*(3), 384–388.

Futterman, D. & Hein, K. (1994). Medical management of adolescents with HIV infection. In C. M. Wilfert & P. A. Pizzo, eds. *Pediatric AIDS: The challenge of HIV infection in infants, children, and adolescents*, pp. 757–772. Baltimore :Williams and Wilkins.

Gadow, K. D., Chernoff, M., Williams, P. L., et al. (2010). Co-occurring psychiatric symptoms in children perinatally infected with HIV and peer comparison sample. *Journal of Developmental & Behavioral Pediatrics, 31*, 116–128.

Garrabou, G., Moren, C., Gallego-Escuredo, J. M., et al. (2009). Genetic and functional mitochondrial assessment of HIV-infected patients developing HAART-related hyperlactatemia. *Journal of Acquired Immune Deficiency Syndrome, 52*(4), 443–451.

Gaughan, D. M., Hughes, M. D., Seage, G. R., et al. for the PACTG219 Team. (2002). The prevalence of pain in pediatric HIV/AIDS as reported by participants in the Pediatric Late Outcomes Study (PACTG 219). *Pediatrics, 109*, 1144–1152.

Gaur, A. H., Dominguez, K. L., Kalish, M. L., Rivera-Hernandez, D., Donohoe, M., Brooks, J. T.et al. (2009). Practice offeeding premasticated food to infants: A potential risk factor for HIV transmission. *Pediatrics, 124*, 658–666. Originally published online Jul 20, 2009; DOI: 10.1542/peds.2008-3614.

Gibb, D. M., Duong, T., Tookey, P. A., et al. (2003). National study of HIV in pregnancy and childhood collaborative HIV pediatric study. Decline in mortality, AIDS, and hospital admissions in perinatally HIV-1 infected children in the United Kingdom and Ireland. *BMJ, 327*(7422), 1019.

Gona, P., vanDyke, R., Williams, P. L., et al. (2006). Incidence of opportunistic and other infections in HIV-infected children in the HAART era.*JAMA, 296*(3), 292–300.

Gortmaker, S. L., Hughes, M., Cervia, J., et al. (2001). Effect of combination therapy including protease inhibitors on mortality among children and adolescents infected with HIV-1. *New England Journal of Medicine, 345*, 1522–1528.

Gray, F., Gherardi, R., & Scaravilli, F. (1988). The neuropathology of the acquired immune deficiency syndrome (AIDS). A review. *Brain, 111*(Pt. 2), 245–266.

Grimaldi, L. M., Martino, G. V., Franciotta, D. M., et al. (1991). Elevated alpha-tumor necrosis factor levels in spinal fluid from HIV-1-infected patients with central nervous system involvement. *Annals of Neurology, 29*, 21–25.

Grubman, S., Gross, E., Lerner-Weiss, N., et al. (1995). Older children and adolescents living with perinatally acquired human immunodeficiency virus infection. *Pediatrics, 95*, 657–663.

Gutman, L. T., Moye, J., Zimmer, B., & Tian, C. (1994). Tuberculosis in human immunodeficiency virus-exposed or infected United States children. *The Pediatric Infectious Disease Journal, 13*, 963–968.

Haiken, H., Hernandez, M., & Mintz, M. (1991). School-aged HIV-infected children and access to education. *Pediatric AIDS and HIV Infection, 2*, 74–79.

Hall, C. B., Long, C. E., Schnabel, K. C., et al. (1994). Human herpesvirus-6 infection in children.A prospective study of complications and reactivation. *New England Journal of Medicine, 331*, 432–438.

Hanna, J. & Mintz, M. (1995). Neurological and neurodevelopmental functioning in pediatric HIV infection. In N. Boyd-Franklin,

G. L. Steiner, & M. Boland, eds. *Children, families and HIV/AIDS: Psychosocial and psychotherapeutic issues*, pp. 30–50. New York: Guilford Press.

Hatherlil, S. & Flisher, A. (2009). Delirium in children with HIV/AIDS. *Journal of Child Neurology, 24*, 879–883.

Havens, J. F., Mellins, C. A., & Pilowsky, D. (1996). Mental health issues in HIV-affected women and children. *International Review of Psychiatry, 8*, 217–225.

Havens, J. F., Mellins, C. A., & Ryan, S. (1997). The mental health treatment of children and families affected by HIV-AIDS. In L. Wicks, ed. *AIDS and psychotherapy*, pp. 101–114. Washington, DC: Taylor and Francis.

Havens, P.L.&Mofenson, L.M.(2009). Evaluation and management of the infant exposed to HIV-1 in the United States. *Pediatrics, 123*(1), 175–187.

Hein, K., Dell, R., Futterman, D., Rotheram-Borus, M.J.,&Shaffer, N.(1995). Comparison of HIV+ and HIV- adolescents: Risk factors and psychosocial determinants. *Pediatrics, 95*, 96–104.

Hernandez, M. & Barros, J. (1994). A new challenge in children with HIV: Psychosis [abstract], Presented at the Seventh Annual Conference of the Association of Nurses in AIDS Care, Nashville, Tennessee, November 10–12, 1994.

Hersh, B. S., Popovici, F., Apetrei, R. C., et al. (1991). Acquired immunodeficiency syndrome in Romania. *Lancet, 338*, 645–649.

Herzlich, B. C. & Schiano, T. D. (1993). Reversal of apparent AIDS dementia complex following treatment with vitamin B12. *Journal of Internal Medicine, 233*, 495–497.

Heyes, M.P., Brew, B.J., Martin, A., et al. (1991). Quinolinic acid in cerebrospinal fluid and serum in HIV-1 infection: Relationship to clinical and neurological status. *Annals of Neurology, 29*, 202–209.

Hirschfeld, S., Laue, L., Cutler, G.B.,&Pizzo, P.A.(1996).Hypothyroidism in pediatric HIV infection. *Journal of Pediatrics, 128*, 70–74.

Hirschfeld, S., Moss, H., Dragisic, K., Smith, W., & Pizzo, P. (1996). Pain in pediatric human immunodeficiency virus infection: Incidence and characteristics in a single-institution pilot study. *Pediatrics, 98*, 449–452.

Hochhauser, C. J., Gaur, S., Marone, R., & Lewis, M. (2008). The impact of environmental risk factors on HIV-associated cognitive decline in children. *AIDS Care, 20*(6), 692–699.

Holmes, V. F., Fernandez, F., & Levy, J. K. (1989). Psychostimulant responses in AIDS-related complex patients. *Journal of Clinical Psychiatry, 50*, 5.

Howland, L. C., Gortmaker, S. L., Mofenson, L. M., et al. (2000). Effects of negative life events on immune suppression in children and youth infected with human immunodeficiency virus type-1. *Pediatrics, 106*, 540–546.

Hriso, E., Kuhn, T., Masdeu, J. C., & Grundman, M. (1991). Extrapyramidal symptoms due to dopamine-blocking agents in patients with AIDS encephalopathy. *American Journal of Psychiatry, 148*, 1558–1561.

Isaranurug, S. & Chompikul, J. (2009). Emotional Development and Nutritional Status of HIV/AIDS Orphaned Children Aged 6-12 Years Old in Thailand. *Maternal and Child Health Journal, 13*, 138–143.

Jackson, J. B., Musoke, P., Fleming, T., et al. (2003). Intra- partum and neonatal single-dose nevirapine compared with zidovudine for prevention of mother-to-child transmission of HIV-1 in Kampala, Uganda: 18-month follow-up of the HIVNET 012 randomised trial. *Lancet, 362*, 859–868.

Janssen, R. S. (1992). Epidemiology of human immunodeficiency virus infection and the neurologic complications of the infection. *Seminars in Neurology, 12*, 10–17.

Janssen, R. S., Nwanyanwu, O. C., Selik, R. M., & Stehr-Green, J. (1992). Epidemiology of human immunodeficiency virus encephalopathy in the United States. *Neurology, 42*, 1472–1476.

Jay, C. & Dalakas, M. C. (1994). Myopathies and neuropathies in HIV-infected adults and children. In C. M. Wilfert & P. A. Pizzo, eds. *Pediatric AIDS: The challenge of HIV infection ininfants, children, and adolescents*, pp. 559–575. Baltimore :Williams and Wilkins.

Jeremy, R. J., Kim, S., Nozyce, M., et al. (2005). Neuropsychological functioning and viral load in stable antiretroviral therapy-experienced HIV-infected children. *Pediatrics, 115*, 380–387.

Jernigan, T. L., Archilbald, S., Hesselink, J. R., et al. (1993). Magnetic resonance imaging morphometric analysis of cerebral volume loss in human immunodeficiency virus infection. *Archives of Neurology, 50*, 250–255.

Judd, A., Doerholt, K., Tookey, P. A., et al. (2007). Morbidity, mortality, and response to treatment by children in the United Kingdom and Ireland with perinatally acquired HIV infection during 1996–2006: Planning for teenage and adult care. *Clinical Infectious Diseases, 45*(7), 918–924.

Jue, S. & Whitley, R. J. (1994). Herpes virus infections in children with human immunodeficiency virus. In C. M. Wilfert & P. A. Pizzo, eds. *Pediatric AIDS: The challenge of HIV infection ininfants, children, and adolescents*, pp. 348–364. Baltimore :Williams and Wilkins.

Kairam, R. (1993). Reliability of neurologic assessment in a collaborative study of HIV infection in children. *Annals of the New York Academy of Sciences, 693*, 123–140.

Katz, D. L. (1994). Legal issues relevant to HIV-infected children in home, day care, school, and community. In C. M. Wilfert & P. A. Pizzo, eds. *Pediatric AIDS: The challenge of HIV infection in infants, children, and adolescents*, pp. 907–923. Baltimore:Williams and Wilkins.

Keller, S. E., Bartlett, J. A., Schleifer, S. J., et al. (1991). HIV-relevant sexual behavior among a healthy inner-city heterosexual adolescent population in an endemic area of HIV. *Journal of Adolescent Health Care, 12*, 44–48.

King, E., DeSilva, M., Stein, A., & Patel, V. (2009). Interventions for improving the psychosocial well-being of children affected by HIV and AIDS. *Cochrane Database of Systematic Reviews, 2*, CD006733.

Kingma, D. W., Mueller, B. U., Frekko, K., et al. (1999). Low-grade monoclonal Epstein-Barr virus-associated lymphoproliferative disorder of the brain presenting as human immunodeficiency virus-associated encephalopathy in a child with acquired immunodeficiency syndrome. *Archives of Pathology & Laboratory Medicine, 123*, 83–87.

Klindworth, L. M., Dokecki, P. R., Baumeister, A. A., & Kupstas, F.D. (1989). Pediatric AIDS, developmental disabilities, and education: Areview. *AIDS and Education and Prevention, 1*, 291–302.

Kotchick, B. A. & Forehand, R. (1999). The family health project: A longitudinal investigation of children whose mother are HIV-infected. Presented at the NIMH conference "The Role of Families in Preventing and Adapting to HIV-infection and AIDS," July 1999, Philadelphia, PA.

Kovacs, A., Schluchter, M., Easley, K., et al. (1999). Cytomegalovirus infection and HIV-1 disease progression in infants born to HIV-1 infected women. *New England Journal of Medicine, 341*, 77–84.

Kozlowski, P. B., Brudkowska, J., Kraszpulski, M., et al. (1997). Microencephaly in children congenitally infected with human immunodeficiency virus-a gross-anatomical morphometric study. *Acta Neuropathologica, 93*, 136–145.

Kozlowski, P. B., Sher, J. H., Dickson, D. W., et al. (1990). Central nervous system in pediatric HIV infection: Experience from a multicenter study. In P. B. Kozlowski, D. A. Snider, P. M. Vietze, & H. M. Wisniewski, (Eds.). *Brain in pediatric AIDS*, pp. 132–146. Karger, Basel.

Krener, P. & Miller, F. B. (1989). Psychiatric response to HIV spectrum disease in children and adolescents. *Journal of the American Academy of Child and Adolescent Psychiatry, 28*, 596.

Kugler, S. L., Barzilai, A., Hodes, D. S., et al. (1991). Acute hemiplegia associated with HIV infection. *Pediatric Neurology, 7*, 207–210.

Lambotte, O., Deiva, K., & Tardieu, M. (2003). HIV-1 Persistence, Viral Reservoir, and the Central Nervous System in the HAART Era. *Brain Pathology, 13*, 95–103.

Laue, L. & Cutler, G. B. (1994). Abnormalities in growth and development. In C. M. Wilfert and P. A. Pizzo, eds. *Pediatric AIDS: The challenge of HIV infection in infants, Children, and adolescents*, pp. 541–545. Baltimore :Williams and Wilkins.

Leggiadro, R. J., Kline, M. W., & Hughes, W. T. (1991). Extrapulmonary cryptococcosis in children with AIDS. *The Pediatric Infectious Disease Journal, 10*, 658–662.

Letendre, S., Marquie-Beck, J., Capparelli, E., et al. (2008). Validation of the CNS penetration-effectiveness rank for quantifying antiretroviral penetration into the central nervous system. *Archives of Neurology, 65*, 65–70.

Letwaba, R. & Minde, K. (2010). Maintaining Effective Psychosocial Treatment Strategies for Children With HIV/AIDS in Africa: An ongoing challenge. *World Perspectives, 31*(1), 50–53.

Lindsey, J. C., Malee, K. M., Brouwers, P., & Hughes, M. D. (2007). Neurodevelopmental functioning in HIV-infected infants and young children before and after the introduction of protease inhibitor-based highly active antiretroviral therapy. *Pediatrics, 119,* e681–e693.

Lipton, S. A. (1993). Human immunodeficiency virus-infected macrophages, gp 120 and N-methyl-D-aspartate neurotoxicity. *Annals of Neurology, 33,* 227–228.

Lobato, M. N., Caldwell, M. B., Ng, P., Oxtoby, M. J., Consortium PSoDC. (1995). Encephalopathy in children with perinatally acquired human immunodeficiency virus infection. *Journal of Pediatrics., 26,* 710–715.

Howland, L. C. (2000). Effects of negative life events on immune suppression in children and youth infected with human immunodeficiency virus type 1. *Pediatrics, 106*(3), 540–546.

Llorente, A., Brouwers, P., Thompson, B., et al. (2006). Effects of polymorphisms of chemokine receptors on neurodevelopment and the onset of encephalopathy in children with perinatal HIV-1 infection.*Applied Neuropsychology, 13*(3), 180–189.

Lord, D., Danoff, J., & Smith, M. (1995). Motor assessment of infants with human immunodeficiency virus infection: A retrospective review of multiple cases. *Pediatric Physical Therapy, 7,* 9–13.

Lyman, W. D., Kress, Y., Kure, K., et al. (1990). Detection of HIV in fetal central nervous system tissue. *AIDS, 4,* 917–920.

Marra, C. M. (1992). Syphilis and human immunodeficiency virus infection. *Seminars in Neurology, 12,* 43–50.

McArthur, J. C., Nance-Sproson, T. E., Griffin, D. E., et al. (1992). The diagnostic utility of elevation in cerebrospinal fluid beta-2-microglobulin in HIV-1 dementia. *Neurology, 42,* 1707–1712.

McConnell, M. S., Byers, R. H., Frederick, T., et al. (2005). Trends in antiretroviral therapy use and survival rates for a large cohort of HIV-infected children and adolescents in the United States, 1989-2001. *Journal of Acquired Immune Deficiency Syndrome, 38*(4), 488–494.

McKinney, R. E., Maha, M. A., Connor, E. M., et al. (1991). A multicenter trial of oral zidovudine in children with advanced human immunodeficiency virus disease. *New England Journal of Medicine, 324,* 1018–1025.

Mellins, C. A., Levenson, R. L., Zawadzki, R., Kairam, R., & Weston, M. (1994). Effects of pediatric HIV infection and prenatal drug exposure on mental and psychomotor development. *Journal of Pediatric Psychology, 19,* 617–628.

Mellins, C. A., Smith, R., O'Driscoll, P., et al. (2003). High rates of behavioral problems in perinatally HIV-infected children are not linked to HIV disease. *Pediatrics, 111,* 384–393.

Michaels, J., Price, R. W., & Rosenblum, M. K. (1988). Microglia in the giant cell encephalitis of acquired immune deficiency syndrome: Proliferation, infection and fusion. *Acta Neuropathologica, 76,* 373–379.

Mintz, M.(1992). R. Yogev & E. M. Connor,(Eds.). Neurologic abnormalities. In *Management of HIV infection ininfants and children [First Edition],* pp. 247–285. St. Louis: Mosby-Year Book Inc,.

Mintz, M. (1993). Neurological manifestations and the results of treatment of pediatric HIV infection. In N. Fejerman & N. A. Chamoles, (Eds.). *New trends in pediatric neurology,* pp. 161–168. Amsterdam: Excerpta Medical, Elsevier Science Publishers BV.

Mintz, M. (1994). Clinical comparison of adult and pediatric NeuroAIDS. *Advances in Neuroimmunology, 4,* 207–221.

Mintz, M.(1995). Carnitine in HIV/AIDS.*Journal of Child Neurology, 10*(supplement No. 2), S40–S44.

Mintz, M. (1996a). Neurobehavioral manifestations of pediatric AIDS. In Y. Frank, ed. *Pediatric behavioral neurology,* pp. 335–365. Boca Raton: CRC Press.

Mintz, M.(1996b). Neurological and developmental problems in pediatric HIV infection. *Journal ofNutrition, 126,* S2663–S2673.

Mintz, M. (1998). Clinical features of HIV infection in children. In H.E. Gendelman, S. Lipton, L. Epstein, and S.Y. Swindells, eds. *The Neurology of AIDS,* pp. 385-407. Chapman and Hall/International Thomson Publishing, New York.

Mintz, M. (1999). Clinical features and treatment interventions for human immunodeficiency virus-associated neurologic disease in children. *Seminal Neurology, 19,* 165–176.

Mintz, M., Boland, M., O'Hara, M-J.,et al. (1995). Pediatric HIV infection in Elista, Russia: Interventional strategies. *American Journal of Public Health, 85,* 586–588.

Mintz, M., Connor, E. M., Oleske, J. M., et al. (1990) AIDS Clinical Trials Group Protocol #043: Neurologic deterioration in children on long-term zidovudine therapy. (Presented at the Ninth AIDS Clinical Trials Group Meeting, Bethesda, Maryland, July 10-13, 1990.)

Mintz, M., Epstein, L. G., & Koenigsberger, M. R. (1989). Neurological manifestations of acquired immunodeficiency syndrome in children. International Pediatrics, 4, 161–171.

Mintz, M. & Epstein, L. G. (1992). Neurologic manifestations of pediatric acquired immunodeficiency syndrome: Clinical features and therapeutic approaches. *Seminars in Neurology, 12,* 51–56.

Mintz, M., LeGoff, D., Scornaienchi, J., et al. (2009). The under- recognized epilepsy spectrum: The effects of levetiracetam on neuropsychological functioning in relation to subclinical spike production. *Journal of Child Neurology, 24*(7), 807–815. Pre-published February 2, 2009, doi:10.1177/0883073808330762

Mintz, M., McSherry, G., Hoyt, L. G., et al. (1993). Wernicke's encephalopathy in a child with HIV infection. *Clinical Neuropathology, 12,* S25.

Mintz, M., Rapaport, T. R., Oleske, J. M., et al. (1989). Elevated serum levels of tumor necrosis factor are associated with progressive encephalopathy in children with acquired immunodeficiency syndrome. *American Journal of Diseases of Children, 143,* 771–774.

Mintz, M., Tardieu, M., Hoyt, L., McSherry, G., Mendelson, J., & Oleske, J. M. (1996). Levodopa therapy improves motor function in HIV-infected children. *Neurology, 47,* 1583–1585.

Misdrahi, D., Vila, G., Funk-Brentano, I., Tardieu, M., Blanche, S., & Mouren-Simeoni, M. C. (2004). DSM-IV mental disorders and neurological complications in children and adolescents with human immunodeficiency virus type 1 infection (HIV-1). *European Psychiatry, 19*(3), 182–184.

Miser, A. W., Goh, T. S., Dose, A. M., et al. (1994). Trial of a topically administered local anesthetic (EMLA cream) for pain relief during central venous port accesses in children with cancer. *Journal of Pain and Symptom Management, 9,* 259–264.

Mitchell, C. D. (2006). HIV-1 Encephalopathy among perinatally infected children: Neuropathogenesis and response to highly active antiretroviral therapy. *Mental Retardation and Developmental Disabilities Research Reviews, 12,* 216–222.

Mitchell, W. G., Lynn, H., Bale, J. F., et al. (1997). Longitudinal neurological follow-up of a group of HIV-seropositive and HIV-seronegative hemophiliacs: Results from the Hemophilia growth and development study. *Pediatrics, 100*(5), 817–824.

Mofenson, L. M. (1999). Interruption of maternal-fetal transmission. *AIDS, 13*(Supplement):S205–14.

Mofenson, L. M. (2000). Technical report: Perinatal human immunodeficiency virus testing and prevention of transmission. Committee on Pediatric Aids. *Pediatrics, 106*(6), E88.

Mofenson, L. M. & Fowler, M. G. for the Pediatric AIDS Clinical Trials Group and Protocol 076/185/219 teams(1999). Interruption of maternal-fetal transmission. *AIDS, 13*(suppl), S205–214.

Morriss, M. C., Rutstein, R. M., Rudy, B., Desrochers, C., Hunter, J. V., & Zimmerman, R. A. (1997). Progressive multifocal leukoencephalopathy in an HIV-infected child. *Neuroradiology, 39,* 142–144.

Moss, H. A., Bose, S., Wolters, P., & Brouwers, P. A. (1998). Preliminary study of factors associated with psychological adjustment and disease course in school-age children infected with human immunodeficiency virus. *Journal of Developmental & Behavioral Pediatrics, 19,* 18–25.

Nozyce, M., Hittelman, J., Muenz, L., Durako, S. J., Fischer, M. L., & Willoughby, A. (1994). Effect of perinatally acquired human immunodeficiency virus infection on neurodevelopment in children during the first two years of life. *Pediatrics, 94,* 883–891.

Nuovo, G. J., Gallery, F., MacConnell, P., & Braun, A. (1994). In situ detection of polymerase chain reaction-amplified HIV-1 nucleic acids and tumor necrosis factor-alpha RNA in the central nervous system. *American Journal of Pathology, 144,* 659–666.

Oldstone, M. B., Sinha, Y. N., Blount, P., et al. (1982). Virus-induced alterations in homeostasis: Alteration in differentiated functions. *Science, 218,* 1125–1127.

Oleske, J. M. & Czarniecki, L. (1999). Continuum of palliative care: Lessons from caring for children infected with HIV-1. *Lancet, 354,* 1287–1291.

Oleske, J., Mofenson, L., Lenderking, W., et al. (1994). PCP prophylaxis (PRO) among children followed in ACTG Pediatric Long-term Protocol 219. *Clinical Infectious Diseases, 19,* 611.

Oxtoby, M. J. (1994). Vertically acquired HIV infection in the United States. In C. M. Wilfert & P. A. Pizzo, eds. *Pediatric AIDS: The challenge of HIV infection in infants, children, and adolescents,* pp. 1–20. Williams and Wilkins, Baltimore.

Palladino, C., Bellón, J. M., Inmaculada, J., et al. (2009). Impact of Highly Active Antiretroviral Therapy (HAART) on AIDS and death in a cohort of vertically HIV type 1-infected children: 1980–2006. *AIDS Research and Human Retroviruses, 25*(11), 1091–1097.

Panel on Antiretroviral Therapy and Medical Management of HIV-Infected Children.(2010). Guidelines for the Use of Antiretroviral Agents in Pediatric HIV Infection. August 16, 2010; pp 1–219. Availableathttp://aidsinfo.nih.gov/ContentFiles/PediatricGuidelines. pdf. Accessed September 26, 2010.

Pao, M., Lyon, M., D'Angelo, L, Schuman, W., Tipnis, T., & Mrazek, D. (2000). Psychiatric diagnoses in adolescents seropositive for the human immunodeficiency virus. *Archives of Pediatrics & Adolescent Medicine, 154,* 240–244.

Park, Y. D., Belman, A. L., Kim, T-S., et al. (1990). Stroke in pediatric acquired immunodeficiency syndrome. *Annals of Neurology, 28,* 303–311.

Parks, R. A.(1994). Occupational therapy with children who are HIV positive. In *Developmental disabilities,* pp. (4)5–6. Rockville, MD: American Occupational Therapy Association.

Patel, K., Hernán, M. A., Williams, P. L., et al. (2008). Long-term effectiveness of highly active anti-retroviral therapy on the survival of children and adolescents infected with HIV-1: A ten-year follow-up study. *Clinical Infectious Diseases, 46,* 507–515.

Patel, K., Ming, X., Williams, P. L., et al. (2009). Impact of HAART and CNS-penetrating antiretroviral regimens on HIV encephalopathy among perinatally infected children and adolescents. *AIDS, 23*(14), 1893–901.

Pavlakis, S. G., Lu, D., Frank, Y., et al. (1998). Brain lactate and N-acetylaspartate in pediatric AIDS encephalopathy. *American Journal of Neuroradiology, 19,* 383–385.

Periquet, B. A., Jammes, N. M., Lambert, W. E., et al. (1995). Micronutrient levels in HIV-1 infected children. *AIDS, 9,* 887–893.

Perrella, O., Carrieri, P. B., Guarnaccia, D., & Soscia, M. (1992). Cerebrospinal fluid cytokines in AIDS dementia complex. *Journal of Neurology, 239,* 387–388.

Perrin, E. C.&Gerrity, P. S. (1984). Development of children with a chronic illness. *Pediatric Clinics of North America, 31,* 19–31.

Persaud, D., Sulachni, C., Rigaud, M., et al. (1992). Delayed recognition of human immunodeficiency virus infection in preadolescent children. *Pediatrics, 90,* 688–691.

Petito, C. K., Cho, E. S., Lemann, W., Navia, B. A., & Price, R. W. (1986). Neuropathology of acquired immunodeficiency syndrome (AIDS): An autopsy review. *Journal of Neuropathology & Experimental Neurology, 45,* 635–646.

Petito, C. K., Navia, B. A., Cho, E-S., et al. (1985). Vacuolar myelopathy pathologically resembling subacute combined degeneration in patients with the acquired immunodeficiency syndrome. *New England Journal of Medicine, 312,* 874–879.

Pollack, H., Glasberg, H., Lee, E., et al. (1997). Impaired early growth of infants perinatally infected with human immunodeficiency virus: Correlation with viral load. *Journal of Pediatrics, 130,* 915–922.

Porter, S. B. & Sande, M. A. (1992). Toxoplasmosis of the central nervous system in the acquired immunodeficiency syndrome. *New England Journal of Medicine, 327,* 1643.

Pratt, R. D., Nichols, S., McKinney, N., Kwok, S., Dankner, W. M., & Spector, S. A. (1996). Virologic markers of human immunodeficiency virus type 1 in cerebrospinal fluid of infected children. *The Journal of Infectious Diseases, 174,* 288–293.

Pressman, H. (1992). Communication Disorders and Dysphagia in Pediatric AIDS. *ASHA, 34*(1), 45–47.

Price, R. W., Brew, B., Sidtis, J., et al. (1988). The brain in AIDS: Central nervous system HIV-1 infection and AIDS dementia complex. *Science, 239,* 586–592.

Rabkin, C. and Chesney, M. A. (1998). Adhering to complex regimens for HIV. *GMHC Treatment Issue, 12,* 8–11.

Ranki, A., Nyberg, M., Ovod, V.,et al. (1995).Abundant expression of HIV Nef and Rev proteins in brain astrocytes in vivo is associated with dementia. *AIDS, 9,* 1001–1008.

Raphael, S. A., deLeon, G., & Sapin, J. (1989).Symptomatic primary human immunodeficiency virus infection of the brain stem in a child. (letter) *Pediatric Infectious Disease Journal, 8,* 654–656.

Raskino, C., Pearson, D. A., Baker, C. J., et al. (1999). Neurologic, neurocognitive, and brain growth outcomes in human immunodeficiency virus-infected children receiving different nucleoside antiretroviral regimens. *Pediatrics, 104,* e32 (http://www.pediatrics.org/cgi/content/full/104/3/e32).

Reportof the Quality Standards Subcommittee of the American Academy of Neurology. (1998). Evaluation and management of intracranial mass lesions in AIDS. *Neurology, 50,* 21–26.

Riedel, D. J., Pardo, C. A., McArthur, J., et al. (2006). Therapy insight: CNS manifestations of HIV-associated immune reconstitution inflammatory syndrome. *Nature Clinical Practice Neurology, 2,* 557–565.

Rogers, M. G., White, C. R., Sander, R., et al. (1991). Lack of transmission of human immunodeficiency virus from infected children to their household contacts. *Pediatrics, 85,* 210.

Romero, A., Pelegrina, R. M., & Mayor, R. J. (2007). Cognitive slowing in cognitive-motor disorder associated to type 1 human immunodeficiency virus: TR and P300. *Actas Espanolas de Psiquiatria, 35,* 221–228.

Roos, K. L. (2002). What I have learned about infectious diseases with my sleeves rolled up. *Seminars in Neurology, 22,* 9–15.

Rotheram-Borus, M. J., Robin, L., Reid, H. M., & Draimin, B. (1998). Parent-adolescent conflict and stress when parents are living with AIDS. *Family Process,* 37, 83–94.

Saito, Y., Sharer, L. R., Dewhurst, S., Blumberg, B., Hall, C. B., & Epstein, L. G. (1994). Cellular localization of human herpesvirus-6 in the brains of children with AIDS encephalopathy. (abstract) *Neuroscience of HIV Infection: Basic and Clinical Frontiers.* Vancouver, Canada. .

Saito, Y., Sharer, L. R., Epstein, L. G., et al. (1994). Overexpression of nef as a marker for restricted HIV-1 infection of astrocytes in postmortem pediatric central nervous tissues. *Neurology, 44,* 474–481.

Saito, Y., Sharer, L. R., Dewhurst, S., Blumberg, B. M., Hall, C. B., & Epstein, L. G. (1995). Cellular localization of human herpesvirus-6 in the brains of children with AIDS encephalopathy. *Journal of Neurovirology, 1,* 30–39.

Saitoh, A., Hsia, K., Fenton, T., et al. (2002). Persistence of human immunodeficiency virus (HIV) type 1 DNA in peripheral blood despite prolonged suppression of plasma HIV-1 RNA in children. *Journal of Infectious Diseases, 185*(10), 1409–1416.

Sanchez-Ramon, S., Bellon, J.M., Resino, S., et al. (2003). Low blood CD8(+) T-lymphocytes and high circulating monocytes are predictors of HIV-1-associated progressive encephalopathy in children. *Pediatrics, 111,* E168–175.

Sanchez-Ramon, S., Resino, S., BellonCano, J. M., Ramos, J. T., Gurbindo, D., & Munoz-Fernandez, A. (2003). Neuroprotective effects of early antiretrovirals in vertical HIV infection. *Pediatric Neurology, 29*(3), 218–221.

Satz, P., Morgenstern, H., Miller, E. N., et al. (1993). Low education as a possible risk factor for cognitive abnormalities in HIV-1: Findings from the multicenter AIDS Cohort Study (MACS). *Journal of the Acquired Immune Deficiency Syndrome, 6,* 503–511.

Scarmato, V., Frank, Y., Rozenstein, A., et al. (1996). Central brain atrophy in childhood AIDS encephalopathy. *AIDS,* 10, 1227–1231.

Schneider, E., Whitmore, S., Glynn, K. M., et al. (2008). Revised surveillance case definitions for HIV infection among adults, adolescents, and children aged <18 months and for HIV infection and AIDS among children aged 18 months to <13 years—United States, 2008. *MMWR*, 57(RR–10), 1–12.

Schwartz, L. & Major, E. O. (2006). Neural progenitors and HIV-1- associated central nervous system disease in adults and children. *Current HIV Research, 4*, 319–327.

Scott, G. B., Hutto, C., Makuch, R. W., et al. (1989). Survival in children with perinatally acquired human immunodeficiency virus type 1 infection. *New England Journal of Medicine, 321*, 1791–1796.

Selik, R. M. & Lindegren, M. L. (2003).Changes in deaths reported with human immunodeficiency virus infection among United States children less than thirteen years old, 1987 through 1999. *Pediatric Infectious Disease Journal, 22*(7), 635–641.

Semba, R. D., Graham, N. M., Caiaffa, W. T., Margolick, J. B., Clement, L., & Vlahov, D. Increased mortality associated with vitamin A deficiency during human immunodeficiency virus type 1 infection. *Archives of Internal Medicine, 153*, 2149–2154.

Semino-Mora, M. C., Leon-Monzon, M. E., & Dalakas, M. C. (1994). Effect of L-carnitine on the zidovudine-induced destruction of human myotubes; Part I: L-Carnitine prevents the myotoxicity of AZT in vitro. *Laboratory Investigation, 71*, 102–112.

Singer, E. J., Valdes-Sueiras, M., Commins, D., & Levine, A. (2010). Neurologic presentations of AIDS. *Neurologic Clinics, 28*, 253–275.

Shah, I. (2008). Prevalence of orphans among HIV infected children—a preliminary study from a pediatric HIV centre in Western India. *Journal of Tropical Pediatrics, 54*(4), 258–260.

Shanbhag, M. C., Rutstein, R. M., Zaoutis, T., Zhao, H., Chao, D., & Radcliffe, J. (2005). Neurocognitive functioning in pediatric immunodeficiency virus infection: Effect of combined therapy. *Archives of Pediatric & Adolescent Medicine, 159*, 651–656.

Sharer, L. R. (1992). Pathology of HIV-1 infection of the central nervous system. A review. *Journal of Neuropathology & Experimental Neurology, 51*, 3–11.

Sharer, L. R., Cho, E. S., & Epstein, L. G. (1985). Multinucleated giant cells and HTLV-III in AIDS encephalopathy. *Human Pathology, 16*, 760.

Sharer, L. R. & Cho, E. S. (1989). Neuropathology of HIV infection: Adults versus children. *Progress in AIDS Pathology, 1*, 131–141.

Sharer, L. R. & Cho, E. S. (1997). Central nervous system. In C. Moran & F. G. Mullick, eds. *Systemic pathology of HIV infection and AIDS in children*, pp 267–293. Washington, DC: Armed Forces Institute of Pathology.

Sharer, L. R., Dowling, P. C., Michaels, J., et al. (1990). Spinal cord disease in children with HIV-1 infection: A combined molecular biological and neuropathological study. *Neuropathology and Applied Neurobiology, 16*, 317–331.

Sharer, L. R., Epstein, L. G., Cho, E. S., et al. (1986). Pathologic features of AIDS encephalopathy in children: Evidence for LAV/HTLV-III infection of brain. *Human Pathology, 17*, 271–284.

Sharer, L. R., Mintz, M., Vinters, H. V., & Epstein, L. G. (1992). Vacuolar myelopathy in children with AIDS. Presented to the IV International Conference on Neuroscience of HIV Infection: Basic and Clinical Frontiers 1992. Amsterdam, Holland: July 15, 1992.

Sharer, L. R. & Mintz, M. (1993). Neuropathology of AIDS in children. In F. Scaravilli, ed. *AIDS—The pathology of the nervous system*, pp. 201–214. Berlin: Springer Verlag.

Sharer, L. R., Saito, Y., DaCunha, A., et al.(1996). In situ amplification and detection of HIV-1 DNA in fixed pediatric AIDS brain tissue. *Human Pathology, 27*, 614–617.

Sharer, L. R., Saito, Y., & Blumberg, B. M. (1997). Neuropathology of HIV-1 infection of the brain. In J. Berger & R. Levy, eds. *AIDS and the nervous system, second edition*, pp. 461–479. Philadelphia: Lippincott-Raven.

Shiramizu, B., Lau, E., Tamamoto, A., Uniatowski, J., & Troelstrup, D. (2006). Feasibility assessment of cerebrospinal fluid from HIV-1-infected children for HIV-1 proviral DNA and monocyte chemoattractant protein 1 alleles. *Journal of Investigative Medicine, 54*, 468–472.

Shirley, L. R. & Ross, S. A. (1989). Risk of transmission of human immunodeficiency virus by bite of an infected toddler. *Journal of Pediatrics, 114*, 425.

Smith, I., Howells, D. W., Knedall, B., Levinsky, R., & Hyland, K. (1987). Folate deficiency and demyelination in AIDS (lett). *Lancet, 2*, 215.

Sohn, A. H., Thanh, T. C., Thinh le, Q., et al. (2009). Failure of human immunodeficiency virus enzyme immunoassay to rule out infection among polymerase chain reaction-negative Vietnamese infants at 12 months of age. *Pediatric Infectious Disease Journal, 28*(4), 273–276.

Spector, S. (1991). Immunotherapy for HIV infection. *The AIDS Reader, 5*, 26.

Spiegel, L. & Mayers, A. (1991). Psychosocial aspects of AIDS in children and adolescents. *Pediatric Clinics of North America, 38*, 153–167.

States, L. J., Zimmerman, R. A., & Rutstein, R. M. (1997). Imaging of pediatric central nervous system HIV infection. *Neuroimaging Clinics of North America, 7*(2), 321–339.

Stiehm, E. R., Bryson, Y. J., Frenkel, L. M., et al. (1992). Prednisone improves human immunodeficiency virus encephalopathy in children. *Pediatric Infectious Disease Journal, 11*, 49.

Stout, J., Ellis, R. J., Jernigan, J., et al.(1998). Progressive cerebral volume loss in human immunodeficiency virus infection: A longitudinal volumetric magnetic resonance imaging study. *JAMA, 55*, 161–168.

Stromme, P., Magnus, P., Kanavin, Q. J., Rootweit, T., Woldseth, B., & Abdelnoor, M. (2008). Mortality in childhood progressive encephalopathy from 1985 to 2004 in Oslo, Norway: A population-based study. *Acta Paediatrica, 97*, 35–40.

Stuber, M. L. (1990). Psychiatric consultation issues in pediatric HIV and AIDS. *Journal of the American Academy of Child and Adolescent Psychiatry, 29*, 463–467.

Sullivan, J. L., et al. (2001). The changing face of Pediatric HIV-1 infection. *New England Journal of Medicine, 344*(21), 1568–1569.

Takahashi, K., Wesselingh, S. L., Griffin, D. E., McArthur, J. C., Johnson, R. T., & Glass, J. D. (1996). Localization of HIV-1 in human brain using polymerase chain reaction/in situ hybridization and immunocytochemistry. *Annals of Neurology, 39*, 705–711.

Tardieu, M. (1998). HIV-1 and the developing central nervous system. *Developmental Medicine and Child Neurology, 40*, 843–846.

Tardieu, M. (2009). The risk of very long-term brain dysfunction in treated adolescents with perinatally acquired HIV-1 infection. *AIDS, 23*(14), 1891–1892.

Tardieu, M., LeChenadec, J., Persoz, A., et al. (2000). HIV-1-related encephalopathy in infants compared to children and adults. *Neurology, 54*, 1089–1095.

Tardieu, M., Mayaux, M. J., Seibel, N., et al. (1995). Cognitive assessment of school-age children infected with maternally transmitted human immunodeficiency virus type 1. *Journal of Pediatrics, 126*, 375–379.

Task Force on Pediatric AIDS. (1991). Education of children with human immunodeficiency virus infection. *Pediatrics, 88*(3), 645–648.

Tinuper, P., deCarolis, P., Galeotti, M., et al. (1990). Electroencephalogram and HIV infection: A prospective study in 100 patients. *Clinical Electroencephalography, 21*, 145–150.

Tornatore, C., Chandra, R., Berger, J. R., & Major, E. O. (1994a). HIV-1 infection of subcortical astrocytes in the pediatric central nervous system. *Neurology, 44*, 481–487.

Tornatore, C., Meyers, K., Atwood, W., Conant, K., & Major, E. (1994b). Temporal patterns of human immunodeficiency virus type 1 transcripts in human fetal astrocytes. *Journal of Virology, 68*, 93–102.

Trillo-Pazos, G., Diamanturos, A., Rislove, L., et al. (2003). Detection of HIV-1 DNA in microglia/macrophages, astrocytes and neurons isolated from brain tissue with HIV-1 encephalitis by laser capture microdissection. *Brain Pathology, 13*, 144–154.

Tudor-Williams, G., St.Clair, M., McKinney, R.E., et al. (1992). HIV-1 sensitivity to zidovudine and clinical outcome in children.*Lancet, 339*, 15–19.

U. S. Preventive Task Force (2005). Screening for HIV: Recommendation statement. *Annals of Internal Medicine, 143*(1), 32–37.

USPHS/IDSA (1997). 1997 report on the prevention of opportunistic infections in persons infected with human immunodeficiency virus. *MMWR, 46*(No. RR–12).

VanDyke, R. B., Wang, L., & Williams, P. L. (2008). Toxicities associated with dual nucleoside reverse-transcriptase inhibitor regimens in HIV-infected children. *Journal of Infectious Diseases, 198*(11), 1599–1608.

VanRie, A., Mupuala, A., & Dow, A. (2008). Impact of the HIV/AIDS epidemic on the neurodevelopment of preschool-aged children in Kinshasa, Democratic Republic of Congo. *Pediatrics, 122*, e123–e128.

Vandersteenhoven, J. J., Dhaibo, G., Boyko, O. B., et al. (1992). Progressive Multifocal leukoencephalopathy in pediatric acquired immunodeficiency syndrome. *Pediatric Infectious Disease Journal, 11*, 232–237.

Varni, J. W., Walco, G. A., & Katz, E. R. (1989). Assessment and management of chronic and recurrent pain in children with chronic diseases. *Pediatrician, 16*, 56.

Viani, R. M., Araneta, M. R., Deville, J. G., et al. (2004). Decrease in hospitalization and mortality rates among children with perinatally acquired HIV type 1 infection receiving highly active antiretroviral therapy. *Clinical Infectious Diseases, 39*(5), 725–731.

Walco, G. A., Varni, J. W., and Ilowite, N. T. (1992). Cognitive-behavioral pain management in children with juvenile rheumatoid arthritis. *Pediatrics, 89*, 1075.

Walter, E. B., Drucker, R. P., McKinney, R. E., & Wilfert, C. M. (1991). Myopathy in human immunodeficiency virus-infected children receiving long-term zidovudine therapy. *Journal of Pediatrics, 119*, 152–155.

Wang, Z., Trillo-Pazos, G., Kim, S.Y., et al. (2004). Effects of human immunodeficiency virus type 1 on astrocyte gene expression and function: Potential role in neuropathogenesis. *Journal of Neurovirology, 10*(Suppl), 1, 25–32.

Wesselingh, S. L., Power, C., Glass, J. D., et al. (1993). Intracerebral cytokine messenger RNA expression in acquired immunodeficiency syndrome dementia. *Annals of Neurology, 33*, 576–582.

Whitt, J. K., Hooper, S. R., Tennison, M. B., et al. (1993). Neuropsychologic functioning of human immunodeficiency virus-infected children with hemophilia. *Journal of Pediatrics, 122*, 52–59.

Wiley, C. A. (1996). Polymerase chain reaction in situ hybridization-opening Pandora's box? *Annals of Neurology, 39*, 691–692.

Wilkins, J. W., Robertson, K. R., van derHorst, C., et al. (1990). The importance of confounding factors in the evaluation of neuropsychological changes in patients infected with human immunodeficiency virus. *Journal of Acquired Immune Deficiency Syndrome, 3*, 938–942.

Willen, E. J. (2006). Neurocognitive Outcomes in Pediatric HIV. *Mental Retardation and Developmental Disabilities Research Reviews, 12*, 223–228.

Wilmshurst, J. M., Burgess, J., Hartley, P., & Eley, B. (2006). Specific neurologic complications of Human Immunodeficiency Virus Type 1 (HIV-1) infection in children. *Journal of Child Neurology, 21*, 788–794.

Wolters, P. L., Brouwers, P., Moss, H. A., & Pizzo, P. A. (1995). Differential receptive and expressive language functioning of children with symptomatic HIV disease and relation to CT scan brain abnormalities. *Pediatrics, 95*(1), 112–119.

Wolters, P. L. & Brouwers, P. (1998). Evaluation of neurodevelopmental deficits in children with HIV infection. In H. E. Gendelman, S. Lipton, L. Epstein, and S. Y. Swindells, (Eds.). *The neurology of AIDS*, pp. 425–442. New York: Chapman and Hall/International Thomson Publishing.

Wong, M. C., Suite, N. D., & Labar, D. R. (1990). Seizures in human immunodeficiency virus infection. *Archives of Neurology, 47*, 640–642.

Wood, S. M., Shah, S. S., Steenhoff, A. P., & Rustein, R. M. (2009). The impact of AIDS diagnoses on long-term neurocogitive and psychiatric outcome of surviving adolescents with perinatally-acquired HIV. *AIDS, 23*, 1859–1865.

Working Group of the American Academy of Neurology AIDS Task Force (1991). Nomenclature and research case definitions for neurologic manifestations of human immunodeficiency virus-type 1 (HIV-1) infection. *Neurology, 41*, 778–785.

Working Group on Antiretroviral Therapy and Medical Management of HIV-Infected Children (1999). Guidelines for the use of antiretroviral agents in pediatric HIV infection. *Journal of the International Association of Physicians in AIDS Care, 5*(suppl), 4–20. [www.iapac.org]

Yow, M. D., White, N. H., Tabe,rL. H., et al. (1987). Acquisition of cytomegalovirus infection from birth to 10 years: A longitudinal serologic study. *Journal of Pediatrics, 110*, 37–42.

Zaknun, D., Orav, J., Kornegay, J., et al. (1997). Correlation of ribonucleic acid polymerase chain reaction, acid dissociated p24 antigen, and neopterin with progression of disease: A retrospective, longitudinal study of vertically acquired human immunodeficiency virus type 1 infection in children. *The Journal of Pediatrics, 130*, 898–905.

10.2

INFANTS, CHILDREN, AND ADOLESCENTS

NERVOUS SYSTEM DISEASE IN THE ERA OF COMBINATION ANTIRETROVIRAL THERAPY

Annelies Van Rie and Anna Dow

In children, HIV infection is associated with a wide range of neurodevelopmental delays and neuropsychiatric complications, as well as an increased risk of central nervous system (CNS) infections, neoplasms, and cerebrovascular complications. Highly active antiretroviral therapy (HAART) has resulted in a dramatic decrease in severe presentations of HIV infection (such as HIV encephalopathy), but milder forms of neurodevelopmental delay and behavioral problems are likely to continue occurring in HIV-infected children, even those who are clinically and immunologically stable. This chapter summarizes current knowledge about CNS disease manifestations in HIV-positive children infected by mother-to-child transmission. The chapter discusses both developed and developing countries and emphasizes knowledge relevant to the era of antiretroviral treatment.

INTRODUCTION

Infection with the human immunodeficiency virus (HIV) is associated with central nervous system (CNS) disorders in children, including HIV encephalopathy, opportunistic CNS infections, CNS neoplasms, and cerebrovascular disorders. Prior to the availability of antiretroviral treatment (ART), CNS disorders were a common manifestation of pediatric HIV infection. The presentation of HIV encephalopathy ranged from severe global deficits in cognitive, motor, language, and behavioral functions to mild impairments in selective domains, reflecting the wide range of factors that influence the impact of the HIV virus on the developing brain in an individual child, including mode of infection, timing of infection, age at HIV diagnosis, access to HIV care and treatment, and the quality of the child's environment. Determination of the extent of HIV-associated neurodevelopmental and neurobehavioral manifestations therefore requires comprehensive assessment of the different domains using age and culturally appropriate tools and interpreting the findings in the broader context of the child.

In the US and Europe, highly active antiretroviral therapy (HAART) has significantly decreased the incidence of severe pediatric HIV encephalopathy, but mild forms of neurodevelopmental deficits remain frequent, especially in school-aged children. While HAART can thus arrest and reverse neurodevelopmental delay, the magnitude of this effect is variable and has not been well defined in children, making it difficult to determine the prognosis for normal brain capacity into adulthood for HAART-treated, perinatally infected children. Unfortunately, most of our knowledge on pediatric CNS manifestations is based on reports from the US and Europe, even though virtually all new pediatric HIV infections occur in the developing world. It is highly unlikely that the US and European data are directly applicable to children in the developing world, due to the high level of substance abuse in HIV-infected women in the US; the high level of malnutrition in sub-Saharan African children; the vast difference in childrearing environment; and the difference in care, with most children in Africa being diagnosed late in the disease process. Few studies have documented CNS manifestations of HIV-infected children in Africa, where over 80% of children living with HIV reside, and data on neurodevelopment in HIV-infected African children receiving ART have only recently emerged. This chapter summarizes the current knowledge about CNS manifestations in children infected with HIV via mother-to-child transmission in both developed and developing countries, with an emphasis on knowledge relevant to the antiretroviral treatment era.

PATHOGENESIS OF HIV-ASSOCIATED CNS DISORDERS IN CHILDREN

HIV ENCEPHALOPATHY

Human immunodeficiency virus (HIV)-associated neurodevelopmental delay is a consequence of the central nervous system (CNS) invasion of the virus. HIV enters the CNS early in infection and persists in the CNS compartment over the entire course of infection (An et al., 1999). In 1987, Epstein et al. identified HIV-specific antibodies in the cerebrospinal fluid (CSF) of HIV-infected children with encephalopathy, indicating active CNS infection with HIV (Epstein et al., 1987). Based on findings of PCR and in situ hybridization of CNS tissue of aborted fetuses from HIV-positive women,

Lyman et al. demonstrated that HIV can infect human CNS tissue very early after infection (Lyman et al., 1990).

The mechanisms of HIV-1 neuropathogenesis are not fully understood in children. Mechanisms are, however, likely to be similar to those in adults, except for the important difference that HIV causes devastating neurological insults to an immature brain in children, whereas the virus causes damage to a fully developed CNS in adults. In adults, HIV invades the CNS primarily via HIV-infected CD4+ T lymphocytes and macrophages that cross the blood-brain barrier, thereby transporting the virus into the nervous system in a Trojan horse manner (Boisse et al., 2008). Macrophages and microglia are the major cell types in the brain that express both CD4 and chemokine co-receptors necessary for productive HIV-1 infection. HIV-1 may also infect astrocytes in a CD4-independent, nonproductive fashion, and infected astrocytes may act as a latent HIV reservoir (Kramer-Hammerle et al., 2005). HIV exerts its neurovirulence through two processes: direct neurotoxic effects of HIV-encoded proteins such as gp120, Vpr, and Tat; and release of neurotoxic chemicals, proinflammatory cytokines, and other chemo-attractants by activated or infected macrophages, microglia, and astrocytes in response to infection (Kaulet al., 2001; Albright et al., 2003; Kramer-Hammerle et al., 2005; Boisse et al., 2008).

The neuropathological correlates of HIV infection have been assessed in autopsy studies of HIV-infected children and were found to be comprised of microglial nodules, multinucleated giant cells, monocytoid cell infiltration, reactive astrocytosis, myelin pallor, and neuronal apoptosis (Dicksonet al., 1989; Gelbard et al., 1995; Gendelman et al., 2004). These processes lead to the observation that atrophy, symmetrical ventriculomegaly, basal ganglia calcifications, and periventricular white matter lesions are the commonest findings of neuroimaging studies in HIV-infected children. Because central atrophy is more prominent than cortical atrophy (which is usually in the frontal lobes), ventriculomegaly is typically disproportionate to the degree of cortical atrophy (DeCarliet al., 1993; Kieck & Andronikou, 2004).

OTHER HIV-ASSOCIATED CNS MANIFESTATIONS

CNS manifestations other than HIV encephalopathy are rare in HIV-infected children in the developed world. With increasing numbers of HIV-infected children surviving beyond the first year of life in developing countries, the prevalence of CNS manifestations other than HIV encephalopathy is likely to increase (Wilmshurst et al., 2006). These include other CNS infections such as tuberculous (TB) meningitis, cerebral malaria, bacterial meningitis, neoplasms, cerebrovascular complications, and CNS manifestations of the immune reconstitution inflammatory syndrome (IRIS). Recognition of these disorders is important as their presentation and therapeutic approach is different from that for HIV encephalopathy.

Bacterial meningitis is ten times more common in developing than in developed countries. A study of 598 Malawian children demonstrated poorer outcomes of bacterial meningitis in ART-naïve, HIV-infected children, with significantly higher case fatality rate (65% in HIV-infected versus 36% in HIV-uninfected children), and significantly lower rates of full recovery (15% in HIV-infected versus 30% in HIV-uninfected children). The rate of sequelae was similar in both groups. HIV-infected children were also at higher risk of recurrent episodes of bacterial meningitis (relative risk 6.4, 95% CI: 3.5–11.1) (Molyneux, 2005). It is unclear whether the risk of bacterial meningitis remains elevated in children receiving HAART.

Plasmodium falciparum (*P. falciparum*) and HIV infect many children in sub-Saharan Africa. Both pathogens affect the CNS, with HIV penetrating the brain parenchyma and *P. falciparum* sequestering within the deep vascular beds of the white and gray matter of the brain. Following cerebral malaria, an estimated 11% of children develop neurological deficits, most of which improve within two years after the insult, and about one in four (24%) children may have neurocognitive impairments (Newton, 2005). Malaria and HIV co-infection could worsen neurodevelopmental impairments, but as yet, there is no data on the effect of HIV on the neurocognitive outcome of children with severe malaria or the effect of malaria on the neurocognitive trajectory of HIV-infected children.

The HIV epidemic has resulted in a dramatic increase in the incidence of active tuberculosis, especially in sub-Saharan Africa. The incidence of TB in HIV-infected children is high, especially among those with immunodeficiency (Elenga et al., 2005). The outcome of TB meningitis in the pre-ART era was significantly worse in children with HIV co-infection. In a study in South Africa, HIV-infected children with TB meningitis were more likely than HIV-negative children to die (30% versus 0%), and were more likely to have moderate (30% versus 24%) or severe (30% versus 19%) neurological sequelae (Topleyet al., 1998).

The prevalence of cerebrovascular disease in children with HIV/AIDS is estimated at 1.3–2.6%, but not all children with cerebrovascular manifestations are symptomatic (Shah et al., 1996; Patsalideset al., 2002). The vascular abnormalities in children with HIV could be due to viral agents such as HIV and varicella zoster, as well as due to the effect of toxic cytokines produced as a result of the HIV infection. This leads to a pan-arteritis with ischemic damage to the vasa vasorum resulting in aneurysmal dilation or stenosis. These abnormalities are seen most often in young, vertically infected children due to the susceptibility of the immature vessels to these toxic agents. HIV vasculopathy occurs with end-stage disease and is associated with a poor prognosis (Georgeet al., 2009).

CNS lymphoma, progressive multifocal leukoencephalopathy (PML), and cryptococal meningitis (CM) are rare in HIV-infected children but have a very high case fatality rate. Burkitt's lymphoma, which is associated with Epstein-Barr infection, was estimated to be 1,000 times more common among adults living with HIV than the general population, but experience with CNS lymphoma in children is limited to a few case reports (Beral et al., 1991; Falloet al., 2005).

Case reports of PML in children have documented altered speech, hemiplegia, facial palsy, and cerebellar dysfunction as presenting symptoms. Neuroimaging reveals that multiple bilateral areas of white matter demyelination without contrast enhancement or mass effect are typical findings (Oberdorferet al., 2009). CM in children can present acutely or subacutely, with headache, nuchal rigidity, vomiting, impaired mental status, convulsions, and focal neurologic signs (Gumbo et al., 2002; Kauret al., 2003).

Immune reconstitution inflammatory syndrome (IRIS) is a paradoxical worsening of a patient's clinical condition that is attributable to the recovery of the immune system that develops after initiation of HAART. In adults, pathogens associated with IRIS include PML, varicella-zoster virus, cytomegalovirus, Epstein-Barr virus, tuberculosis, cryptococcus, candida, and toxoplasmosis (Johnson & Nath). Information on pediatric CNS IRIS is limited to a few case reports of PML in HIV-infected child associated with ART initiation (Nuttall et al., 2004; Oberdorferet al., 2009), and acute demyelinating encephalomyelitis, cryptococcal reactivation, and disseminated herpes simplex in an HIV-infected child following HAART (van Toornet al., 2005).

CLASSIFICATION OF NEURODEVELOPMENTAL DISORDERS IN HIV-INFECTED CHILDREN

In the pre-ART era, the classic triad of pediatric HIV-related encephalopathy included developmental delay, acquired microcephaly, and pyramidal tract motor deficits (Belmanet al., 1988). Pediatric encephalopathy was traditionally classified as subacute progressive encephalopathy, characterized by progressive global deterioration and loss of previously acquired skills or abilities; plateau course progressive encephalopathy, where the acquisition of new skills significantly slows or stops, but previously acquired milestones are not lost; or static encephalopathy, where the child continues to gain new skills and abilities but at a slower rate than normal (Belman et al., 1988). This classification is based on longitudinal follow-up of children naïve to antiretroviral therapy, an approach no longer clinically or ethically acceptable. In 1991, the Working Group of the American Academy of Neurology AIDS Task Force published the nomenclature and research case definitions for neurologic manifestations of HIV infection. In this document, CNS disorders were classified as HIV encephalopathy, CNS compromise, or apparently normal (1991). While the classification of research nosology for HIV-associated neurocognitive disorders in adults was revised in 2007 to critically review the adequacy and utility of the 1991 definitional criteria and to identify aspects that require updating, particularly since the advent of ART, this process was unfortunately not performed for pediatric HIV-associated neurocognitive disorders (Antinori et al., 2007). One of the important changes was the addition of the term "asymptomatic neurocognitive impairment" for individuals with subclinical impairment. We propose to introduce a similar category of subclinical neurodevelopmental delay for

pediatric HIV. Criteria for the revised classification are listed in Table 10.2.1. Because of the key importance of cognitive development (schooling, future life prospects), special emphasis in the classification is placed on the child's cognitive development. The criteria are developed such that they can be used for initial and follow-up assessments.

In cases of HIV-encephalopathy, children have severe delay in their cognitive development and in at least one other developmental domain. The CNS structures are severely compromised, resulting in global deficits of cognitive, language, motor, and daily living skills. In children of school-going age, the cognitive impairment interferes markedly with their academic achievement. This severe presentation has become less frequent and is now mainly seen in children presenting late in the HIV disease process. HIV encephalopathy is classified by the World Health Organization as a clinical stage 4 of HIV/AIDS in infants and children (WHO, 2006). All children with HIV encephalopathy are thus eligible for ART, independent of their level of immunodeficiency as measured by CD4 absolute count or CD4 percentage. Overall cognitive functioning that is borderline delayed and impacts mildly on academic achievement in school-going children characterizes HIV-related CNS compromise. The mild cognitive delay can be associated with impairments below the average range in other neurodevelopmental domains. Children with subclinical neurodevelopmental delay have overall cognitive functioning within the normal range and normal neurological exam, but scored below the average for selective neurodevelopmental functions such as expressive language, attention, visual spatial processing, executive function, or memory (Bisiacchi et al., 2000; Blanchette et al., 2002; Koekkoek et al., 2007). This form is often observed in school-aged children on ART and ART-naïve, long-term survivors, both in the developed (Tardieu et al., 1995; Blanchette et al., 2002; Martin et al., 2006; Koekkoek et al., 2007; Wood et al., 2009) and developing world (Bagenda et al., 2006).

In case of evidence of another HIV-associated cause for the neurodevelopmental delay (e.g., sequelae of bacterial meningitis, cerebral malaria, tuberculous meningitis) it will often not be possible to distinguish whether HIV is the direct or indirect cause of the severe neurodevelopmental delay.

EPIDEMIOLOGY OF HIV-ENCEPHALOPATHY

BURDEN OF ENCEPHALOPATHY BEFORE THE INTRODUCTION OF HAART

Early reports from the pre-ART era in the US and Europe estimated that between 50–90% of children infected with HIV via mother-to-child transmission had encephalopathy (Epstein et al., 1986; Belman et al., 1988). These observations were most likely biased as they were based on case series of young children presenting with advanced AIDS. Subsequent estimates in the pre-ART era suggested that between 13–35% of children with HIV infection and 35–50% of children diagnosed with AIDS developed HIV encephalopathy, with

Table 10.2.1 CLASSIFICATION OF NEURODEVELOPMENTAL DISORDERS IN HIV-INFECTED CHILDREN

HIV-ENCEPHALOPATHY (SEVERE DELAY)

Neurodevelopmental scores in the delayed range for cognitive functioning and at least one other domain.

- Delayed development is defined as ≥ 2 standard deviations below the age-appropriate mean in the normative population or control group on standardized neuropsychological tests.
- Typically the impairment is in multiple domains, including cognitive, language, defective attention/concentration, and motor development.
- Neurodevelopmental delay can be accompanied by abnormal neurologic exam such as significant increased or decreased tone, abnormal reflexes, cerebellar, gait, or movement abnormalities
- Neurodevelopmental delay may also be accompanied by brain-imaging abnormalities, including the hallmark findings of HIV-associated encephalopathy: symmetrical ventricular enlargement, cortical atrophy, white matter attenuation, and basal ganglion calcification.
- In children of school-going age, the cognitive impairment produces marked interference with academic achievement.

CNS COMPROMISE (MILD TO MODERATE NEURODEVELOPMENTAL DELAY)

- Neurodevelopmental scores in the borderline range for cognitive functioning and delayed or borderline score in at least one other domain
- Borderline delay is defined as performance ≥ 1 but < 2 standard deviation below the age-appropriate mean in the normative population or control group on standardized neuropsychological tests.
- Cognitive delay can be associated with delayed or borderline motor, language, or behavioral functioning.
- Neurodevelopmental delay can be accompanied by abnormal neurologic findings but these do not significantly affect daily function.
- In children of school-going age, the cognitive impairment interferes mildly with academic achievement.

HIV-ASSOCIATED SUBCLINICAL NEURODEVELOPMENTAL DELAY (ASYMPTOMATIC NEURODEVELOPMENTAL DELAY)

- Neurodevelopmental scores in the normal range for overall cognitive functioning but delay in one or more specific sub-domains of cognitive functioning such as attention, memory, abstraction and executive functions, speed of information processing, sensory-perceptual, visual motor and visual spatial processing, visual motor speed and coordination, language, or behavioral functioning.
- Normal score is defined as a score within 1 standard deviation of the age-appropriate mean in the normative population or control group on standardized neuropsychological tests
- Borderline delay is defined as performance ≥ 1 but < 2 standard deviation below the age-appropriate mean in the normative population or control group on standardized neuropsychological tests.
- Neurodevelopmental delay cannot be accompanied by abnormal neurologic findings.
- In children of school-going age, the impairment observed on neurodevelopmental assessment does not interfere with academic achievement.

NORMAL NEURODEVELOPMENT

- Neurodevelopmental scores in the normal range for overall cognitive, motor, and language functioning
- Normal score is defined as a score within 1 standard deviation of the age-appropriate mean in the normative population or control group on standardized neuropsychological tests.
- At a minimum, overall cognitive, motor and language functioning needs to be assessed to classify a child as having normal development. In countries where standardized tests for language development do not exist, simple screening tests for language development can be used. Ideally, comprehensive assessment of sub-domains is also performed, especially in older children.

higher rates among children presenting with symptomatic disease at a very early age (Gabuzda & Hirsch, 1987, 1990; Gay et al., 1995; Lobato et al., 1995; Englund et al., 1996; Blanche et al., 1997; Cooper et al., 1998; Tardieu et al., 2000). The highest incidence rate of HIV-related CNS manifestations occurs in the first two years of life, with incidence rates of 9.9% in the first year of life, 4.2% in the second, and less than 1% in the third year of life and thereafter (Tardieu et al., 2000). The wide ranges in reported rates of HIV encephalopathy arise, at least in part, from the mixture of assessment tools used, diversity in number of domains assessed, and the different ages at which the children were assessed. Studies of ART-naïve, sub-Saharan African children similarly reported high proportions of HIV-infected children with severe delay in their development, with estimates of 50–90%

developmental delay among children with advanced pediatric AIDS (Baillieu & Potterton, 2008; Van Rie et al., 2008), and 15–30% prevalence of neurodevelopmental delay when children with less severe immunosuppression or asymptomatic HIV infection were included in the study population (Msellati et al., 1993; Drotar et al., 1997). Limited studies from Latin America (Bruck et al., 2001; Czornyj, 2006) and Asia (Sanmaneechai et al., 2005; Hamidet al., 2008) have reported comparable findings.

FACTORS ASSOCIATED WITH RISK AND SEVERITY OF HIV ENCEPHALOPATHY

The large variation in severity of HIV-associated neurodevelopmental delay has been associated with the timing and mode of infection, the severity of immunosuppression in mother and child, viral and host factors, and environmental factors. Timing of infection plays a critical role. Children who acquired HIV infection in utero have earlier and more rapid progression of HIV disease and more severe disease (Newell, 1998). Similarly, the onset of neurodevelopmental delay in children infected in the last weeks of pregnancy, a period of rapid brain growth, is earlier and characterized by more rapid progression of HIV-related encephalopathy, an observation that has been made both in developed and developing countries (Pollack et al., 1996; Smith et al., 2000; Tardieu et al., 2000; McGrath et al., 2006). Infection through breastfeeding, transfusion of blood, or blood products is associated with lower incidence rates and less severe HIV-associated CNS disease (Cohen et al., 1991). Adolescents infected with HIV through sexual transmission also appear to have severe CNS disease (Mitchell, 2001).

Severity of HIV disease in infant and mother is another important risk factor. The risk of encephalopathy is higher in HIV-infected children born to mothers with more advanced disease, as measured by maternal CD4 cell count and viral load at the time of delivery (Blanche et al., 1994). A higher plasma viral load in infancy has also been associated with an increased risk of encephalopathy, although it is not predictive of the age at onset of CNS manifestations (Pollack, Kuchuk et al., 1996; Cooper et al., 1998; Lindsey et al., 2000). Children with more advanced disease early in life (lower CD4 percentage) or higher levels of immune activation early in life (percentage CD8(+)HLA-DR(+) cells at age 1 or 2 months), have poorer psychomotor and mental development in the first years of life (Blanche et al., 1994; Brouwers et al., 1995; Lobato et al., 1995; Cooper et al., 1998; Mekmullica et al., 2009). A history of an AIDS-defining illness increases the risk of encephalopathy during the preschool and early school age years, whereas children without a history of class C event tend to perform as well as uninfected children in measures of general cognitive ability (Smith et al., 2006).

Viral and host genetics may also determine the risk and severity of HIV-associated CNS disease. Viral subtype impacts HIV disease progression in adults, with individuals infected with subtype D virus having a faster progression to AIDS and a higher mortality rate than do individuals infected with HIV subtype A (Kiwanuka et al., 2008). HIV subtypes also have a different biological impact on neurological complications of HIV infection, with HIV dementia being more common among subtype D–infected persons than among subtype A–infected persons (Sacktor et al., 2009). In contrast, Boivin et al. reported that HIV subtype A may be associated with poorer neuropsychological performance compared with subtype D in ART-naïve long-term survivors (age 6 to 12). This difference was only statistically significant (after adjustment for confounders and multiple comparisons) for simultaneous processing. The proportion of children classified as impaired (defined as ≥ 2 SD below the mean in the control group) did not differ between subtype (19% for subtype A and 17% for subtype D). There was also no difference in motor score by HIV-subtype (Boivin et al., 2010). The potential mechanisms for a differential rate of neurovirulence by subtype is still unclear but may relate to differential neurotoxicity of Tat by HIV subtype, or to viral envelope diversity (Sacktor et al., 2009).

Besides genetic viral factors, an increasing body of data supports host genetic factors as an important determinant of HIV disease progression. Variants in genes encoding chemokine receptors for cell binding and entry and their natural ligands have been shown to modify the risk for infection and disease progression, with individuals heterozygous for CCR5 wild type/delta 32 being less likely to be infected with HIV-1 and showing a slower rate of disease progression (Singh & Spector, 2009). In a study of over 1,000 HIV-infected children, those with the CCR5-wt/delta32 genotype at study entry had higher mean CD4 lymphocyte counts or CD4 percentages, higher cognitive scores, and lower plasma HIV RNA levels than those with the wt/wt genotype. Moreover, children with the CCR5- wt/delta32 genotype were less likely to be severely impaired at baseline or experience CNS impairment during follow-up than those with the homozygous wild type (Singh et al., 2003).

Finally, environmental factors play an important role in the neurodevelopmental outcome of HIV-infected children. Children who are at high risk of HIV infection are often also at risk for environmental factors that can negatively affect their development. These factors include maternal drug abuse, lack of prenatal care, shorter duration of breastfeeding, repeated periods of hospitalization of the child, parental illness or death, poor home environment, and lack of normal interaction with peers due to stigma. The impact of environmental risk factors on HIV-associated cognitive decline in children has recently been reviewed and studied by Hochhauser et al. (Hochhauser et al., 2008). Children with higher numbers of environmental risk factors have lower scores on measures of cognitive performance. Several pathways have been suggested, including families preoccupied with life crises being less able to provide the stimulating and varied experiences that foster cognitive growth, decreases in emotional support in conditions of chronic poverty, or increases in endogenous glucocorticoids in response to stress, which can lead to temporally related declines in cognitive functioning (Hochhauser et al., 2008). HIV and environmental stressors have independent deleterious consequences for cognitive functioning, and also have a robust relationship with each other. This interrelationship has been assessed in two studies. In a longitudinal study of 618 HIV-positive children, Howland et al. observed that those children exposed to at least two negative life-events had a significantly greater risk of developing immune suppression (as measured by CD4%) after one year than did those who had not experienced any (Howland et al., 2000). Hochhauser et al. documented that immunosuppression was associated with poorer cognitive outcome in the high environmental risk children, but not among those with lower levels of environmental risk (Hochhauser et al., 2008). The impact of environmental factors on the neurodevelopment of HIV-infected children has also been assessed through comparisons of the development of HIV-infected children with HIV-exposed, uninfected children. These studies have resulted in conflicting results, with some indicating normal neurodevelopment in HIV-exposed, uninfected children (Msellati et al., 1993; Drotar et al., 1997), whereas others found higher rates of delayed development in these children when compared to relevant controls (Boivin et al., 1995; Van Rie et al., 2008). These apparently contradictory results may be the consequence of a selection bias in recruitment of HIV-uninfected children. If exposed, uninfected children are of low environmental risk (not affected by HIV), then these children may develop similarly to controls, whereas exposed, uninfected children growing up as orphans or with mothers who are bedridden due to AIDS (children affected by HIV) are more likely to suffer from a suboptimal home environment (Van Rie et al., 2008).

THE EFFECT OF ANTIRETROVIRAL TREATMENT AND HAART

Antiretroviral treatment reduces HIV replication, which results in a reduction of activated circulating monocytes, and in turn leads to a reduction of HIV-infected macrophages entering the CNS. The reduction of HIV viral load and activated monocytes in the CNS reduces the HIV-associated neuroinflammation and production of neurotoxins, thus reducing the neurotoxic effects of HIV infection (Cysique et al., 2009). Pizzo and Brouwers first demonstrated the effect of antiretroviral drugs on pediatric CNS manifestations. In their landmark randomized control trial (RCT) of children age 6 months to 12 years with symptomatic HIV infection, they documented highly significant and sustained improvements in neuropsychologic function as well as reversal of radiological abnormalities on neuroimaging in response to continuous intravenous zidovudine monotherapy (Pizzo et al., 1988; Brouwers et al., 1990). Subsequently, Raskino et al. demonstrated in a large cohort of symptomatic HIV-infected children (age 3 months to 18 years) that combination therapy with ZDV and didanosine was more effective against HIV-associated CNS manifestations than either drug in monotherapy, with statistically significant mean improvements from baseline for cognitive scores and head circumference growth, less progressive cortical atrophy, and a reduction in the proportion of children with motor dysfunction (Raskino et al., 1999).

The effect of HAART on the morbidity and mortality of HIV-infected children has been dramatic, with similar improvements in clinical, immunological, and virologic outcomes observed in developed and developing countries (Sutcliffe et al., 2008). Several studies in the US have demonstrated that ART also significantly reduces the burden of HIV encephalopathy. A cohort study observed a decrease in the prevalence of HIV encephalopathy from 40.7% in 113 children born before 1996 to 18.2% among the 33 children born after 1996 (Shanbhag et al., 2005). Among 126 vertically infected children, of which 60% were on HAART, the prevalence of active progressive HIV encephalopathy dropped from 31% in 1992 to 1.6% in 2000, leading the authors to conclude that encephalopathy in the HAART era was an infrequent and reversible complication of HIV infection that responds well to effective antiretroviral control (Chiriboga

et al., 2005). In a large multicenter cohort of 2,398 perinatally HIV-infected children enrolled in the pre- HAART and HAART eras, HAART use was associated with a tenfold decrease in the incidence of HIV encephalopathy (Patel et al., 2009), similar to the tenfold decrease in CNS disease observed in adults (d'Arminio Monforte et al., 2004). Another publication on the same cohort (PACTG 219) reported that the overall incidence rate of HIV encephalopathy during follow-up (mean 59 months) was low: 0.38 per 100 person years (95% CI, 0.3-0.5), and showed a statistically significant decrease between 2001 and 2006, from 1.15 per 100 person years in 2001 to 0.07 per 100 person years in 2006 (Nachman et al., 2009). No data have been published on the population-level impact of HAART on the burden of HIV encephalopathy in developing world countries.

There are few longitudinal studies on neurodevelopmental outcomes following the initiation of HAART in ART-naïve children in the US and Europe. The impact of HAART on neurodevelopment in children in the US was mostly studied cross-sectionally, in children born before 1997 who initiated HAART after receiving single or double agent antiretroviral treatment. Most of these studies demonstrated improvements in neurodevelopment upon HAART initiation. For example, Chiriboga et al. found that all children with encephalopathy substantially improved with a change in antiretroviral therapy, with improvement in cognitive functions and head size often preceding that of motor function (Chiriboga et al., 2005). McCoig et al. randomly assigned 23 children who had failed on AZT monotherapy to ABC/3TC/ZDV or 3TC/ZDV. Initiation of either antiretroviral regimen decreased CSF HIV RNA and improved both neurologic and neuropsychologic outcome (McCoig et al., 2002). Shanbhag et al. found that the neurocognitive functioning of children who started HAART when neurologically healthy at baseline was preserved over time (Shanbhag et al., 2005). In a cross-sectional study of children on HAART for at least a year, Martin et al. found that the mean cognitive scores were in the normal range (within one standard deviation of the normative mean), but a subgroup of children characterized by lower CD4 counts and brain scan abnormalities had below average cognitive functioning (Martin et al., 2006). More details on the domain-specific impacts of HAART are noted in the next section of this chapter.

In contrast to the beneficial effects of non-nucleoside reverse transcriptase inhibitors (NNRTI) containing HAART, effects of protease inhibitor (PI)-based HAART on neurodevelopment among ARV-experienced children have been disappointing. Tamula et al. reported on four cases of children who exhibited immunologic, virologic, and clinical stability while on a PI-containing HAART, yet demonstrated significant cognitive decline (Tamula et al., 2003). Lindsey et al. observed only limited improvements in neurodevelopmental functioning upon initiation of PI-based HAART initiation in young children (Lindsey et al., 2007). Jeremy et al. reported that clinically and immunologically stable children with mild cognitive and fine motor impairments who failed their antiretroviral treatment (as shown by detectable viral load), showed only limited improvement following the change to a PI-based

HAART therapy (Jeremy et al., 2005). Similarly, no significant change in mean intelligence quotient was found between baseline and follow-up, and no change was found in the mean rating of CT brain scan abnormalities among ARV-experienced children who started ritonavir-based HAART (Hazra et al., 2007). The limited effect of PI-based HAART on neurodevelopment in children could be explained by lower CNS penetration of many PIs, except for lopinavir, indinavir, and amprenavir (McCoig et al., 2002; Koopmans et al., 2009). In adults, it has been shown that individuals on regimens containing greater numbers of CSF-penetrating drugs showed significantly greater reduction in CSF viral load, and those attaining CSF virological suppression demonstrated greater neuropsychological improvement than those who did not (Letendre et al., 2004). The only study to date that assessed impact of CNS-penetrating ART on HIV encephalopathy among children and adolescents did not find a statistically significant association between high CNS-penetrating regimens and lower incidence of HIV encephalopathy, but did observe a significant survival benefit of using high CNS-penetrating regimens after diagnosis of HIV encephalopathy (Patel et al., 2009).

Data on neurodevelopmental outcomes in the ART era in developing world are limited to a few studies. A study followed 39 South African children (mean age 7 years) for 6 months after initiation of an NNRTI (48.7%) or PI-based (51.3%) HAART regimen found that even though the speech and motor deficits were frequent at baseline, the prevalence and extent of deficits did not change significantly in response to HAART (Smith et al., 2008). In contrast, a study in the Democratic Republic of Congo found that after one year of entry into care, HIV-infected children experienced accelerated motor development but similar gains in cognitive development compared with control children (Van Rie et al., 2009).

Among adults, several studies have shown that HAART has led to a dramatic decline in the incidence of HIV-associated dementia, but the prevalence of milder HIV-associated neurocognitive disorders has remained similar (Brew, 2004). It is unclear whether these mild or subclinical forms of neurodevelopmental and neurobehavioral disorders are due to continued slow replication of HIV in the CNS because of compartmentalization, treatment with poorly CNS penetrating antiretrovirals, poor adherence, or environmental factors (Koopmans et al., 2009). Milder forms of neurodevelopmental disorders in children on HAART in the US and Europe, especially older children stable on ART, have also been described (Nozyce et al., 2006; Koekkoek et al., 2007). Data on the prevalence of mild neurodevelopmental delays in children on HAART in developing countries is lacking.

children without delay at baseline are at risk of developing neurodevelopmental delay while receiving HAART.

In the pre-HAART era, the effects of ART on neurodevelopment were shown to be the largest during the first 6 months of treatment, in children younger than 30 months of age, and in children with severe delay prior to start of ART (Raskino et al., 1999). In the HAART era, the risk of developing encephalopathy has been associated with the plasma viral load on HAART at time of diagnosis of encephalopathy, but not plasma viral load at time of HAART initiation (Chiriboga et al., 2005). Viral load in the CNS has also been associated with the impact of HAART on CNS manifestations. McCoig et al. observed that a reduction in the proportion of children with measurable HIV viral load in the CSF was accompanied by a decrease in the proportion of children with neurological abnormalities (McCoig et al., 2002). Severity of disease is another factor associated with severity of neurodevelopment on HAART. Among 41 vertically-infected children (mean age 11.2 years) of whom 75% had global cognitive functioning in the average range and who and had been treated with HAART for at least one year, those with minimal to moderate CT brain scan abnormalities had significantly lower cognitive functioning than children with normal scans, and children with worse immune status (CD4+ counts ≤ 500) scored lower on subtests measuring processing speed. Viral load in this study was unrelated to cognitive test scores (Martin et al., 2006). Data from developing countries are limited to an exploratory analysis which suggested that younger children and those presenting earlier in the disease process may experience accelerated greater gains in development following initiation of HIV care (Van Rie et al., 2009).

Timing of ART initiation could be another important determining factor. Early HIV diagnosis and early treatment initiation with HAART have been shown to significantly improve clinical outcome, reducing early infant mortality by 76% and HIV progression by 75% (Violari et al., 2008). Given these results and the devastating effects of HIV on brain development, it can be hypothesized that early treatment with HAART will also improve neurological outcomes. A study from France suggested that early-onset severe HIV disease with encephalopathy might be prevented by the initiation of HAART before the age of 6 months (Faye et al. 2004). While it is not possible to conclude from this observational study that early HAART treatment would result in normal cognitive and behavioral development, it is tempting to do so. Studies are currently underway in South Africa and Malawi to assess the effect of early HAART treatment on neurodevelopmental outcomes.

FACTORS ASSOCIATED WITH THE EFFECT OF HAART ON NEURODEVELOPMENT

Little has been published on the demographic, clinical, laboratory, and treatment factors associated with neurodevelopmental trajectory in children initiating HAART. An understanding of these factors is important to predict which children with pre-existing neurodevelopmental delay are more likely to improve or deteriorate on HAART, and which

DOMAINS OF NEURODEVELOPMENTAL, NEUROBEHAVIORAL, AND NEUROPSYCHOLOGICAL IMPAIRMENTS

COGNITIVE

Detrimental effects of HIV infection on cognitive development were frequent in the pre-HAART era in both the developed (Brouwers et al., 1990; Nozyce et al., 1994; Wolters et al., 1994; Chase et al., 1995) and developing (Drotar et al., 1997; Drotar et al., 1999) world, especially in young children (Nozyce et al., 1994; Drotar et al., 1997; Knight et al., 2000; Bruck et al., 2001; Lindsey et al., 2007; Baillieu & Potterton, 2008; Van Rie et al., 2008). In contrast, assessments of cognitive development in older ART-naïve Ugandan children age 6 to 12 years did not differ significantly from age- and gender-matched HIV-exposed, uninfected children and HIV-unexposed controls. The authors hypothesized that this may reflect a survivor bias, as children in this setting with more advanced disease would likely have died before reaching school-going age (Bagenda et al., 2006).

Cognitive delay has been associated with severe HIV disease, defined either by higher viral load (Jeremy et al., 2005), presence of an AIDS defining illness (Nozyce et al., 1994), or other markers of severe disease (Foster et al., 2006; Martin et al., 2006; Smith et al., 2006). In addition to direct effects of HIV, environmental factors also contribute to the cognitive delays seen in infected children as HIV- exposed, uninfected children also lag behind in their cognitive development when compared to control children (Puthanakit et al., 2010; Van Rie et al., 2009). General cognitive functioning has also been shown to correlate well with other assessments of CNS functioning, including brain imaging (Brouwers et al., 1995) and CSF analysis (Sei et al., 1996).

The effect of antiretroviral treatment on cognitive development in children is not entirely clear, in part because the treatment regimens have changed drastically over the past two decades. Raskino et al. found patients receiving zidovudine monotherapy and zizdovudine plus ddI combination therapy showed significant improvement with cognitive function compared with ddI monotherapy. While the effect of zidovudine monotherapy was not sustained, combination therapy was associated with improvement in cognitive scores, even at 96 weeks after initiation of therapy (Raskino et al., 1999). A study of the impact of PI-based HAART found a positive but limited impact of HAART on cognitive scores in the first three years of life (Lindsey et al., 2007), while another study found improvement in only the vocabulary score (Jeremy et al., 2005). In the Democratic Republic of Congo, initiation of medical care, including antiretrovirals for eligible children, resulted in improvement in cognitive functioning, especially among younger children (Van Rie et al., 2009).

Studies of school-aged children in the antiretroviral treatment era in the US have found that global cognitive functioning may be similar to that seen in uninfected peers. In contrast, a study in Thailand of children 6–12 years of age found that the proportion of children with average intelligence (based on the WISC-III) was only 21% among HIV-infected children (87% on ART), compared with 49% in HIV-exposed, uninfected children and 76% in controls (Puthanakit et al.). Even though global cognitive functioning in developing world countries is often within normal limits, delays frequently exist in subtests such as processing speed, working memory, vocabulary, attentional deficit, and tasks involving executive function. Cognitive delay in children on treatment occurred most often in children with higher levels of immune suppression or abnormal CT findings (Bisiacchi et al., 2000; Blanchette et al., 2002; Martin et al., 2006; Koekkoek et al., 2007). Martin et al. suggested that low scores on global or subtest for cognitive functioning may be a result of ongoing viral replication in the CNS despite systemic virologic control, or residual effects of static HIV-related CNS disease (Martin et al., 2006).

MOTOR

In treatment-naïve children living in developed and developing countries, motor impairment often presented early in infection and as one of the most adversely affected areas of neurodevelopment (Epstein et al., 1985; Msellati et al., 1993; Boivin et al., 1995; Chase et al., 1995; Drotar et al., 1997; Knight et al., 2000; Jeremy et al., 2005; McGrath et al., 2006; Lindsey et al., 2007; Van Rie et al., 2007). In infants and young children, abnormal muscle tone, decreased muscle strength, delayed motor development, and even loss of acquired motor milestones were commonly reported (Belman et al., 1988; Lord et al., 1995; Raskino et al., 1999). Delays in fine and gross motor development can occur as early as four months, and can increase over time, as greater deceleration in the rate of motor development has been documented compared with HIV-exposed, uninfected infants and unexposed infants (Chase et al., 1995; Drotar et al., 1997; Drotar et al., 1999; McGrath et al., 2006). Prevalence rates of motor delay in young children have varied from 30% among one-year-old children in Uganda to more than 80% in children less than 30 months of age in both South Africa and the Democratic Republic of Congo (Baillieu & Potterton, 2008; Van Rie et al., 2008). In South African children 18 to 30 months of age, mean motor development was 9.65 months delayed (Baillieu & Potterton, 2008). Some studies have found motor delay to be worse in younger children. In a study in the US, the proportion of children with at least one motor function abnormality decreased with age, from 44% in children less than one year of age to 22% in children 12 to 29 months and 8% in children 30 months to 18 years of age (Raskino et al., 1999). Motor problems in long-term surviving treatment-naïve school-aged children may be less severe, and may range from subtle perceptual-motor difficulties (Epstein et al., 1986; Parks & Danoff, 1999) and weaknesses in fine motor strength and speed (Blanchette et al., 2002), to disturbances of gross motor functions affecting running agility and speed (Parks & Danoff, 1999). As has been seen in other areas of neurodevelopment, motor delay is associated with advanced HIV disease (Msellati et al., 1993; Nozyce et al., 1994; Foster et al., 2006; Lindsey et al., 2007).

Combination antiretroviral treatment has the potential to reverse motor impairment in young children. Raskino et al. observed a statistically significant decline in the proportion of children with abnormal motor function in the first 24 weeks of treatment among children receiving ZDV plus ddI but not in children on ZDV or ddI monotherapy arms (Raskino et al., 1999). Experiences with PI-based HAART are mixed. Initiation of a PI-based regimen in previously treated children 3.5 to 17 years of age did not result in improvement of fine-motor functioning (Jeremy et al., 2005), while another study found treatment with a PI-based regimen tended to improve motor scores among children started on treatment at the mean age of 20.4 months (Lindsey et al., 2007). In a developing world context, entrance into care resulted in improvements in motor function in children 18 to 29 months of age. After one year of care (including HAART for those eligible), the motor development of HIV- infected children was similar to that of HIV-exposed, uninfected children (Van Rie et al., 2009). Gross motor delay may be partially due to decreased muscle strength as a result of the chronic HIV disease, poor nutrition, or other environmental factors, particularly in a developing world setting. Referral to physical therapy may be indicated when these children enter care (Parks & Danoff, 1999; Baillieu & Potterton, 2008).

LANGUAGE

In the pre-ART era, HIV infection was associated with delay of acquisition of language milestones and increasing language deficits as children grew older (Condini et al., 1991; Coplan et al., 1998). The detrimental effects of HIV on language were more pronounced in expressive language than in receptive language, and were sometimes seen before declines in general cognitive function (Wolters et al., 1997; Coplan et al., 1998). Language delay is also frequently seen in HIV-infected children in the developing world. An early study from Rwanda found that infected children scored significantly lower than both exposed, uninfected children and control children on tests of language acquisition (Msellati et al., 1993). Global language delay was detected in 82.5% of treatment-naïve South African children age 18–30 months (Baillieu & Potterton, 2008). In the Democratic Republic of Congo, 85% of ART-naïve children 18–71 months of age demonstrated delays in language expression, and 77% had delays in language comprehension, a significantly higher proportion compared to HIV-negative controls (Van Rie et al., 2008). Due to limited data, the association with severity of disease is not clear.

Antiretroviral treatment other than HAART may affect language development less compared to motor and cognitive development. Wolters at al. observed a short-lived period of protection where language skills did not deteriorate for six months, but following this period receptive and expressive language skills declined significantly despite antiretroviral therapy, even in children whose overall cognitive function remained stable (Wolters et al., 1997).

Assessment of receptive language of HIV-infected school-aged children and adolescents (9–16 years), 84% of whom were receiving antiretroviral treatment, found that 62% scored below average and 39% scored below the 10th percentile. HIV-exposed, uninfected children also scored poorly on the same assessment, although they scored significantly better than the infected children. None of the health variables examined, including CD4 and VL, were significantly associated with performance on the assessment. Thirty-seven percent of the HIV-infected children in this study had been held back at some point, and 52% had ever attended a special education class, indicating that these children were experiencing challenges in the academic setting (Brackis-Cott et al., 2009).

BEHAVIORAL AND PSYCHIATRIC PROBLEMS

Prior to the availability of antiretroviral treatment, children with HIV exhibited a high prevalence of behavioral and psychiatric problems, especially attention deficit disorders (Moss et al., 1994). The direct contribution of HIV is unclear, as many HIV-infected children are exposed to other known risk factors for behavioral and psychiatric disorders, including genetic and environmental factors, such as prenatal drug exposure and loss of a parent. For example, while case reports indicated high rates of attention deficit disorders among treatment-naïve HIV-infected children, a study to determine the relationship between HIV infection and disruptive behavior disorders in treatment-naïve children in the context of prenatal drug exposure found similarly high rates of behavioral and psychiatric morbidity in school-age children with HIV infection, HIV exposed, uninfected children, and non-HIV-exposed children (Havens et al., 1994). Data from this and other studies suggest that while there may be neurotoxicity directly due to the virus, the high prevalence of behavioral and psychological issues is likely a result of environmental issues, including family disruption, exposure to poverty, and trauma (Bachanas et al, 2001; Mellins et al., 2003; Jeremy et al., 2005; Chernoff et al., 2009).

Moss at al. demonstrated that behavioral problems in children with severe HIV encephalopathy improve on ART (Moss et al., 1994). There is also evidence that, even in the presence of effective treatment, HIV-infected children continue to have high rates of behavioral and psychiatric problems, again likely due to environmental factors. In a study of clinically and immunologically stable, antiretroviral-experienced, HIV-infected children, parents reported high rates of behavioral problems including psychosomatic (28%), hyperactivity (20%) and impulsive-hyperactive (19%), conduct (16%), and anxiety (85%) problems, rates that are higher than established childhood norms (Nozyce et al., 2006). A study based on youth- and caregiver-reported psychiatric disorders in children 9–16 years of age, 84% of whom were receiving antiretroviral treatment, found that 61% of children were reported to have a psychiatric disorder of some type, 49% were reported to have an anxiety disorder, and 18% were reported to have attention deficit hyperactivity disorder (ADHD). Compared with exposed, uninfected children, HIV-infected children were more likely to have any psychiatric disorder (OR 1.59, 95% CI 1.03-2.47) and ADHD (OR 2.45, 95% CI 1.20-4.99) (Mellins et al., 2009). Another study of HIV-infected adolescents, the majority of whom were being treated, found that 48% had a diagnosed psychiatric illness, with children with more advanced HIV disease being more likely to have a history of psychiatric diagnosis, psychiatric hospitalization, or a learning disorder (Woods et al., 2009). A study of children <15 years of age found that the incidence of psychiatric hospitalization was higher in HIV-infected children compared to the general pediatric population (relative risk 3.62, 95% CI 2.11-5.8).

The median age of psychiatric hospitalization was 11 years, and the most frequent diagnoses were depression and behavioral disorders (Gaughan et al., 2004).

Published data on behavioral and psychiatric disorders in HIV-infected children in the developing world are not yet available.

NEURODEVELOPMENT AND IN UTERO EXPOSURE TO ANTIRETROVIRAL DRUGS IN HIV-EXPOSED UNINFECTED CHILDREN

Antiretroviral drugs effectively prevent the transmission of HIV from mother to child, and have reduced mother-to-child transmission of HIV to less than 2% in the United States. Prevention of mother-to-child transmission programs are now implemented widely across the globe, making in utero ARV exposure and its potential consequences a global issue. As many ARV drugs cross the placenta and some have demonstrated mutagenic and carcinogenic effects in animal studies, concern has been raised regarding possible adverse consequences of prenatal ARV exposure, including neurologic toxicity (Walker & Poirier, 2007). Several cases of persistent mitochondrial dysfunction with neurologic symptoms were reported in HIV-uninfected children perinatally exposed to zidovudine (Barret et al., 2003), and a small neuroimaging study demonstrated abnormalities including hyperintensity in the central white matter and in the pontine tegmentum in children with antiretroviral-induced mitochondrial dysfunction, similar to those observed in congenital mitochondrial diseases (Tardieu et al., 2005). More recently, a large study provided reassurance regarding the safety of in utero ARV exposure. After controlling for important confounders, the Mental Developmental Index and Psychomotor Developmental Index scores at 2 years of age were not lower among 1,694 exposed to ARV in utero compared to 146 children not exposed to ARV in utero (Williams et al., 2010).

NEURODEVELOPMENTAL AND NEUROPSYCHOLOGICAL ASSESSMENT

NEED FOR COMPREHENSIVE NEURODEVELOPMENTAL AND NEUROPSYCHOLOGICAL ASSESSMENT INTEGRATED INTO ROUTINE PEDIATRIC HIV CARE

Neurodevelopmental assessment is a critical but difficult part of the comprehensive evaluation of HIV-infected children. It is critical because of the high rates of neurodevelopmental and neuropsychological disorders in these children, even in the ART era. It is difficult for several reasons. Evaluations need to take a developmental approach, which requires different tools for different ages. The broad range of domains that can be affected requires a comprehensive assessment. Simple screening tests or even global assessments without specific

subtests may provide an oversimplified or misleading picture and not be sensitive enough to detect milder forms of CNS disorders, especially for cognitive development among older children and children stable on ART (Martin et al., 2006). Most neurodevelopmental assessment tools, especially those assessing cognitive development in older children, have not been validated for use in settings outside the US and Europe. Qualified practitioners to perform neurodevelopmental assessments in developing countries are also scarce. Finally, HIV-infected children are exposed to various environmental factors that can contribute to the neurodevelopmental and behavioral disorders, making it difficult to distinguish the direct effect of HIV infection from other medical and environmental factors that also affect children's growth. This renders it difficult for the caregiver to predict the degree of improvement that can be expected upon initiation of care and treatment.

Neurodevelopmental and neuropsychological assessments need to be performed throughout the lifespan of HIV-infected children. The assessment at time of HIV diagnosis aims to determine the areas and degree of neurodevelopmental delay as well as behavioral problems present at baseline. This is crucial as HIV encephalopathy can be the first symptom of HIV and poor neurodevelopmental scores can predict later disease progression independent of immunological and virological markers (Llorente et al., 2003). Furthermore, HIV encephalopathy is classified as a World Health Organization (WHO) clinical stage 4 HIV disorder, making all children with encephalopathy eligible for HAART (WHO, 2006). The results of the neurodevelopmental and neuropsychological assessments should thus be integrated with the results from other evaluations, including general medical exam; neurological exam; immunological, bacteriological, and other laboratory assessments; brain imaging studies; and nutritional assessment, to determine the best care and treatment plan for the individual child. Unfortunately, while assessment for HIV- encephalopathy is well integrated into the care of HIV-infected children in the US and Europe, such evaluation is rarely performed as part of routine care in developing countries. Consequently, even children with severe neurodevelopmental delay are not initiated on HAART if they are not eligible based on CD4 criteria or presence of other stage 4 disease markers.

Following baseline assessment, repeated evaluations are needed to assess the effectiveness of HAART and other interventions on neurodevelopmental delay and behavioral disorders. The frequency and timing of assessments needs to balance the need for timely identification of improvements or deterioration, the human resources available, and methodological issues of practice effects and the age restrictions for individual assessment tools.

In addition to performing psychometric test assessments, it is important to observe the behavior of the child during the test session and to allow the parent or primary caregiver to describe the child's behavior in the home environment since children often behave differently in the assessment setting than at home. It is also essential for the assessor to make sure children are generally well at time of assessment, to allow children to establish a rapport with the person administering the assessment before starting formal assessment, to respond when children become fatigued or bored, and to be sensitive to children with behavioral difficulties (Wolters & Brouwers, 2005).

SELECTION OF APPROPRIATE ASSESSMENT TOOL

All children will show developmental growth over time. The critical issue is thus to determine whether the rate of growth in HIV-infected children is the same, greater, or smaller than what is expected based on normally occurring developmental growth. Validated and standardized tests allow comparison with the rate of growth in a normative group reflecting the socioeconomics of the population. The optimal assessment tool assesses a wide range of abilities (including cognitive function, receptive and expressive language, fine and gross motor skills, executive function, attention, memory, and adaptive behavior) and facilitates analysis of results across domains (Wolters & Brouwers, 2005). Table 10.2.2 lists some of the assessment tools that have been used in the evaluation of HIV-infected children.

Table 10.2.2 PSYCHOMETRIC TOOLS USED FOR ASSESSMENT OF HIV-INFECTED CHILDREN

PSYCHOMETRIC TEST	DOMAIN	AGE RANGE	EXAMPLES OF COUNTRIES WHERE TEST HAS BEEN USED
Bayley Scales of Infant Development (BSID)–original and updated versions (Bayley, 2006)	Cognitive, motor, language, social-emotional, adaptive behavior	1– 42 months	US (Nozyce et al., 1994; Chase et al., 1995; Raskino et al., 1999; Knight et al., 2000; Smith et al., 2000; Jeremy et al., 2005; McGrath et al., 2006; Lindsey et al., 2007), UK (Foster et al., 2006), Democratic Republic of Congo (Van Rie et al., 2008), South Africa (Baillieu & Potterton, 2008), Uganda (Drotar et al., 1997)
Clinical Adaptive Test/Clinical Linguistic and Auditory Milestone Scale (CAT/CLAMS) (Wachtel et al., 1994)	Language acquisition, visual-motor problem-solving	1–36 months	Brazil (Bruck et al., 2001)
Clinical Evaluation of Language Fundamentals Revised (CELF-R) (Semel et al., 1987)	Evaluates language disorders by assessing content, form and memory	5–16 years	US (Wolters et al., 1997)
Conners' Parent Rating Scale (Conners, 1989)	Behavioral and emotional problems	3–17 years	US (Mellins et al., 2003)
Denver Developmental Screening Test (Frankenburg et al., 1981)	Language, person-social, fine motor-adaptive and gross motor	1–72 months	Brazil (Bruck et al., 2001), Rwanda (Msellati et al., 1993)
Fagan Test of Infant Intelligence (Fagan & Detterman, 1992)	Information-processing ability	6–12 months	Uganda (Drotar et al., 1997)
Griffiths Mental Development Scale (Huntley, 1996)	Cognitive development	2–6 years	UK (Foster et al., 2006)
Kaufmann Assessment Battery for Children (Kaufman & Kaufman, 1983)	Sequential-processing scale, simultaneous-processing scale, achievement scale, nonverbal scale	2.5–12.5 years	Uganda (Bagenda et al., 2006)
McCarthy Scales of Children's Abilities (McCarthy, 1972)	Verbal, perceptual-performance, quantitative, memory, motor	2.5–8.5 years	US (Raskino et al., 1999; Smith et al., 2006), UK (Foster et al., 2006)
Peabody Developmental Motor Scales (Folio & Fewell, 1983)	Motor development	Birth through 5 years	Democratic Republic of Congo (Van Rie et al., 2007)
Peabody Picture Vocabulary Test (Dunn & Dunn, 1997)	Receptive language	≥ 2.5 years	US (Brackis-Cott et al., 2009)
Snijders-Oomen Non-verbal Intelligence Test (SON-R) (Tellegen & Laros, 1993)	Cognitive development	2.5–17 years	Democratic Republic of Congo (Van Rie et al., 2007), The Netherlands (Koekkoek et al., 2007)
Wechsler Preschool and Primary Scale of Intelligence- Revised (Wechsler, 2002)	Cognitive/Intelligence	3.5–6 years	US (Jeremy, Kim et al. 2005), UK (Fishkin, Armstrong et al. 2000)
Wechsler Intelligence Scale for Children–Revised (WISC-R) (Wechsler, 2003)	Cognitive/Intelligence	6–17 years	US (Nozyce et al., 1994; Raskino et al., 1999; Jeremy et al., 2005; Martin et al., 2006)
Wide Range Achievement (WRAT-III) (Wilkinson, 1993)	Basic skills needed for reading, spelling and arithmetic	≥5 years	Uganda (Bagenda et al., 2006), US (Brackis-Cott et al., 2009)

Situations exist where age-appropriate, standardized tests are not valid. This can occur when a child has a physical or sensory impairment that limits their ability to respond to test items; when the functioning of a child is significantly lower than their chronological age which decreases the ability to score enough points in the test battery; or when the standard tests have not been validated in the population of interest (Wolters & Brouwers, 2005). For assessment of cognitive functioning in children with physical or sensory impairments, tests for blind, hearing impaired, or physically impaired children, or assessment procedures not relying on verbal, motor, or visual responses can be used. For children not fluent in the language for which the test was standardized and validated, nonverbal tests or interpreters can be used.

NEURODEVELOPMENTAL AND NEUROPSYCHOLOGICAL ASSESSMENT IN A DEVELOPING WORLD SETTING

Performing neurodevelopmental assessment is especially difficult in developing countries, as most psychometric tests originate from the US and Europe and were designed to for the culture, language, and socioeconomic status of these populations. It is unlikely that the standards obtained in the normative groups in the US or Europe are applicable to children residing in sub-Saharan Africa or other regions of the world because of differences in cultural norms and values, socioeconomic circumstances, culture, child-rearing practices, exposure to manufactured toys, and schooling (Jukes & Grigorenko, 2010; Nampijja et al., 2010). Performance on neurodevelopmental tests may differ between populations because of a genuine difference between populations, for example because of different levels of schooling, or because of a testing bias, when the difficulty of a test item differs between individuals of identical cognitive ability, for example because of differences in language structure (Jukes & Grigorenko, 2010). The difficulty in evaluating whether an observed difference is genuine or biased leads to difficulties in interpretation of scores, especially in older children, and is likely to affect cognitive and adaptive behavior more strongly than motor function.

Different approaches have been used to address this issue including translation of existing tests and collection of normative data, cultural adaptation of existing tests followed by validation, and development of new tests. Translation means that an already existing test is administered in the local language but otherwise the original test content is left almost intact. Translation of psychometric tests should be done in line with published guidelines (Van de Vijver & Hambleton, 1996). Test adaptation involves translation of the original test and modification of it as much as is required to suit the culture, education, and socio-economic diversity of the target population. The degree of transformation needed will depend on the differences between the population of origin and the population for which it is adapted (Nampijja et al., 2010). Test adaptation should be performed according to published guidelines (Hambleton, 1994). Adaptation involves trying out new test items for unfamiliar ones, construction of new

norms, examining the validity and reliability of the new version, and standardizing the new scores on the target population. Psychometric properties important to assess are distribution of the scores, sensitivity to the effect of age, and other important determinants factors such as schooling, internal and test-retest reliability, and associations between measures within and across domains.

Translation and adaptation has been shown to be a realistic and worthwhile strategy for obtaining valid and reliable measures in a resource-limited setting. A study in Uganda aimed at translating and adapting Western measures of working memory, general cognitive ability, attention, executive function, and motor ability in order to obtain a cognitive instrument suitable for assessing 5-year-old children (Nampijja et al., 2010). Measures were selected, translated, and modified to suit the local culture, education, and socioeconomic background of the target population. Analysis of validity and reliability characteristics showed that 8 (at least 1 from each domain) out of the 11 measures were successfully adapted on the basis that they showed adequate task comprehension, optimum levels of difficulty to demonstrate individual and group differences in abilities, sensitivity to effects of age and education, and good internal as well as test-retest reliability.

Once a test has been translated and administered to a population with different background characteristics than the normative population, the original normative data can no longer be used to determine which children have normal (within on SD), borderline (between 1 and 2 SD below the mean), or delayed (score 2 or more SD below the mean) development. Translation of existing tests should thus be followed by collection of normative data. A study in Cameroon collected normative data on psychometric tests to assess the executive functions and memory of school-aged children. Criteria for tests inclusions were simplicity of administration, few verbal demands, and broad cross-cultural applicability. With the exception of the Block Design test (WISC-IV) and a Verbal Phonemic Fluency test, results among 125 healthy children demonstrated that the battery of 14 cognitive tests was appropriate for neuropsychological evaluation in Cameroon (Ruffieux et al., 2010). Alternative to the collection of new norms (z-scores), one can compare scores within one individual to assess the impact of an intervention, or compare means between populations. This allows comparison within individuals or between groups but does not allow classification of scores as normal, borderline, or delayed. An example of this approach is a study in which the effect of access to HIV care for HIV-infected children was assessed by comparing the 1-year trajectory of development of HIV-infected children with that of HIV-exposed, uninfected, and HIV-unexposed children (Van Rie et al., 2009).

A third approach consists of the development of new psychometric test instruments. An example of this is the Kilifi Developmental Inventory for assessment of psychomotor development of children 6 to 35 months and the Kilifi Developmental Checklist, which assessed four developmental domains in Kenyan children from 12 months to school age (Abubakar et al., 2008). Based on the developers' experiences, these tools are reliable, reflect maturational changes, and can identify children with developmental delay. It is unclear how they perform against standard psychometric tests and how they perform outside of the specific context in which they were developed.

Besides the lack of validated standardized psychometric tests, another important challenge to successful neurodevelopmental assessment of HIV-infected children in developing countries is the scarcity not only of experienced health care workers in general but also health professionals experienced in neurodevelopmental and behavioral assessment. A screening tool that could be used by a variety of health professionals would be a more feasible method to screen large numbers of children, identify at an early stage those who need to be further evaluated, and allow implementation of early interventions to mitigate neurodevelopmental impairments. Validated screening tests including the Denver Developmental Screening Test for ages 0 to 6 years, one of the most widely used screening test for developmental problems in children, and the Bayley III screening test for ages 1 to 42 months. The Denver Developmental Screening Test has been successfully used for assessment of treatment-naïve HIV-infected children in the pre-HAART era in Brazil and Rwanda (Msellati et al., 1993; Bruck et al., 2001). Because of the relatively low sensitivity of the screening test, it is unclear how well this test can identify milder forms of neurodevelopmental delay in the HAART era.

Similar to comprehensive psychometric tests, screening tests have also been translated, adapted, or newly developed for use in developing world settings. For example, Khan et al. developed the Rapid Neurodevelopmental Assessment tool for children aged 0 to 24 months, which screens for primitive reflexes, gross motor, fine motor, vision, hearing, speech, cognition, behavior, and seizures. The reliability was determined for 50 children and validity in 30 children by simultaneous administration of the adapted Bayley Scales of Infant Development II as the gold standard. The investigators found good validity and discriminatory validity for

neurodevelopmental impairment in most functional domains, and demonstrated that the tool can be used by professionals from a range of backgrounds (Khan et al., 2010).

TIMING OF LONGITUDINAL ASSESSMENTS

The frequency and timing of assessments needs to reflect a balance in the need to identify improvements or deterioration in a timely manner and the amount of practice effect generated by repeated assessments. The interval between tests to observe changes in neurodevelopment in HIV-infected children will depend on the rate of progression expected in the child, which is mainly determined by the child's age, the severity of clinical and radiological CNS disease at baseline, the severity of immunodeficiency, and the duration of ART. The magnitude of possible practice effects is associated with the child's rate of development, comparative level of functioning, health status, and the potential for latent learning (Wolters & Brouwers, 2005). Practice effects are smaller for younger children and for children with lower intelligence quotients. A possible schedule for serial assessment of children in the HAART era is presented in Table 10.2.3.

INTERPRETATION AND COMMUNICATION OF TEST RESULTS

The interpretation of neurodevelopmental test results can be complicated by the complex interaction between biological and socio-environmental factors, the need for test transitions as the child gets older, and the lack of normative data in many populations.

Disentangling direct effects of HIV and HIV treatment from powerful indirect and environmental effects such as genetic, health, disease, poverty, and psychosocial factors, is complex but important to determine the correct treatment plan and to estimate the potential effect of HAART (Van Rie et al., 2007). A detailed history of cognitive abilities of parents and siblings, and detailed information on the child's

Table 10.2.3 SCHEDULE FOR SERIAL NEURODEVELOPMENTAL ASSESSMENT FOR HIV-INFECTED CHILDREN

AGE OF THE CHILD	ART STATUS	SERIAL ASSESSMENT SCHEDULE	ASSESSMENT
≤ 12 month of age	All children should receive ART	Evaluate at HIV diagnosis, start of ART and 6 months after start of ART.	General cognitive, motor, language, and behavioral assessment
1 to 2 years	Not on ART*	At HIV diagnosis and every 3 months thereafter due to high risk of developing neurodevelopmental deficits	General cognitive, motor, language, and behavioral assessment
	On ART	Every 6 months	
2 to 5 years	Not on ART	At HIV diagnosis and every 6 months thereafter	General cognitive, motor, language, and behavioral assessment
	On ART	Annually	
≥ 6 years	Not on ART	Annually	General cognitive plus subtests of executive functioning, verbal fluency, processing speed, working memory, and attention (Martin et al., 2006)
	On ART	Every 2 to 3 years if stable on ART and age-appropriate school performance, annually otherwise	

* In some countries, guidelines may recommend ART for all children age 1-2 years

medical history, including complications during pregnancy or birth, preterm birth, and prior CNS infections such as bacterial meningitis or severe malaria, are important to determine potential other causes of delay in individual children (Wolters & Brouwers, 2005). Neuro-imaging, immunological (CD4 count or percentage), and virological (viral load) markers of disease severity can also provide clues as these markers have been associated with the neurodevelopmental trajectory in individual children (Brouwers et al., 1995; Martin et al. 2006). The inclusion of control groups such as HIV-exposed, uninfected children living in similar home environment conditions as HIV-infected children can help in determining the direct effects of HIV on a population level (Van Rie et al., 2009).

Another difficulty in interpreting test results can occur when a change in psychometric instrument is needed as the child gets older. In clinical practice, it is recommended that, when a child with stable functioning reaches the appropriate age to transfer to a test for an older age group, the change should be made as soon as possible. When deterioration in functioning is suspected following test transition, the test that was previously administered should be given again if possible or the new test needs to be repeated as soon as repeat testing is valid (i.e., in 6 months). For a child with significant developmental delays, the transfer to a test for an older age group may be postponed if the test for the younger age group can be expected to more appropriately assess the development. In research setting, the child should be kept on the same test as long as possible in order to obtain consistent methodology (Wolters & Brouwers, 2005).

A third important difficulty of test result interpretation arises when normative data for a standardized test are not available for the population of interest. As discussed in the previous section, several approaches have been suggested to address this issue, including translation and cultural adaptation of existing tests and development of new tests. Unless normative data exist for the population of interest, the use of a demographically relevant control group is necessary to interpret the scores obtained in the HIV-infected population.

Careful communication of test results to the parents or primary caregiver is important. Test results should be discussed in the broader context of the disease, the child, and the child's environment. It is important to acknowledge parental fears and expectations and to help alleviate concerns by explaining what is currently known about HIV, how treatment can reverse developmental deficits, and how HAART can protect the CNS. It should further be emphasized that predicting any trajectory of infection or neurodevelopment in an individual child with certainty is difficult (Wolters & Brouwers, 2005). When the child is found to have developmental deficits, the family should be informed about available and culturally appropriate interventions, which can be administered by professional health care workers or by the caregiver at home (World Health Organization, 1997; Potterton et al., 2009). Sharing of the findings of psychometric tests with the school should also be discussed with the parents of school-aged children.

CONCLUSION

HIV infection is associated with a wide range of neurodevelopmental delays, neuropsychiatric complications, and increased risk of CNS infections, neoplasms, and cerebrovascular complications. HAART has resulted in a dramatic decrease in severe presentations (HIV encephalopathy), but milder forms of neurodevelopmental delay and behavioral problems are likely to occur in HIV-infected children, even those who are clinically and immunologically stable. As most studies assessing the impact of HAART have been performed in US or European treatment-experienced children, it is difficult to predict the long-term outcome of treatment-naïve children initiating HAART, especially those who start HAART very early in life (first 6 months of life), as is currently recommended by the WHO.

Comprehensive neurodevelopmental assessment of HIV-infected children at diagnosis and during follow-up is critical but difficult, especially in developing countries, due to the lack of standardized and validated psychometric assessment tools for use outside of the US and Europe, and because of the lack of capacity for neurodevelopmental assessment in those countries where the burden of pediatric HIV is the highest. Development of appropriate tools and human resources are thus urgently needed.

Important questions for future research are the effect of HAART initiation in children age < 6 months of age on neurodevelopment, the role of HIV compartmentalization in the CNS of children stable on HAART, and the relative penetration of different antiretroviral drugs in young children. Another important question in the HAART era is whether mild developmental delay and cognitive impairment are due to the neurotoxic effects of HIV or environmental factors. Answers to these questions will provide the evidence required to determine the optimal HAART regimen for young children.

ACKNOWLEDGMENTS

Support for this chapter was provided by the Eunice Kennedy Shriver National Institute of Child Health and Human Development (NICHD), National Institutes of Health (NIH) grant R01HD053216, awarded to the University of North Carolina at Chapel Hill, North Carolina, USA and Malawi Liverpool Welcome Trust in Blantyre, Malawi.

REFERENCES

(1990). Neurologic signs in young children with human immunodeficiency virus infection. The European Collaborative Study. *Pediatr Infect Dis J, 9*(6), 402–406.

(1991). Nomenclature and research case definitions for neurologic manifestations of human immunodeficiency virus-type 1 (HIV-1) infection. Report of a Working Group of the American Academy of Neurology AIDS Task Force. *Neurology, 41*(6), 778–785.

Abubakar, A., Holding, P., et al. (2008). Monitoring psychomotor development in a resource-limited setting: An evaluation of the Kilifi Developmental Inventory, *Ann Trop Paediatr, 28*(3), 217–226.

Albright, A. V., Soldan, S. S., et al. (2003). Pathogenesis of human immunodeficiency virus-induced neurological disease. *J Neurovirol, 9*(2), 222–227.

An, S. F., Groves, M., et al. (1999). Early entry and widespread cellular involvement of HIV-1 DNA in brains of HIV-1 positive asymptomatic individuals. *J Neuropathol Exp Neurol, 58*(11), 1156–1162.

Antinori, A., Arendt, G., et al. (2007). Updated research nosology for HIV-associated neurocognitive disorders. *Neurology, 69*(18), 1789–1799.

Bachanas, P. J., Kullgren, K. A., et al. (2001). Predictors of psychological adjustment in school-age children infected with HIV. *J Pediatr Psychol, 26*(6), 343–352.

Bagenda, D., Nassali, A., et al. (2006). Health, neurologic, and cognitive status of HIV-infected, long-surviving, and antiretroviral-naive Ugandan children. *Pediatrics, 117*(3), 729–740.

Baillieu, N. & Potterton, J. (2008). The extent of delay of language, motor, and cognitive development in HIV-positive infants. *J Neurol Phys Ther, 32*(3), 118–121.

Barret, B., Tardieu, M., et al. (2003). Persistent mitochondrial dysfunction in HIV-1-exposed but uninfected infants: Clinical screening in a large prospective cohort. *AIDS, 17*(12). 1769–1785.

Bayley, N. (2006). Bayley Scales of Infant Development. San Antonio, TX: Psychological Corporation.

Belman, A. L., Diamond, G., et al. (1988). Pediatric acquired immunodeficiency syndrome. Neurologic syndromes. *Am J Dis Child 142*(1). 29–35.

Beral, V., Peterman, T., et al. (1991). AIDS-associated non-Hodgkin lymphoma. *Lancet, 337*(8745). 805–809.

Bisiacchi, P. S., Suppiej, A., et al. (2000). Neuropsychological evaluation of neurologically asymptomatic HIV-infected children. *Brain Cogn, 43*(1-3), 49–52.

Blanche, S., Mayaux, J., et al. (1994). Relation of the course of HIV infection in children to the severity of the disease in their mothers at delivery. *N Engl J Med, 330*(5), 308–312.

Blanche, S., Newell, M. L., et al. (1997). Morbidity and mortality in European children vertically infected by HIV-1. The French Pediatric HIV Infection Study Group and European Collaborative Study. *J Acquir Immune Defic Syndr Hum Retrovirol, 14*(5), 442–450.

Blanchette, N., Smith, M. L., et al. (2002). Cognitive development in school-age children with vertically transmitted HIV infection. *Dev Neuropsychol, 21*(3), 223–241.

Boisse, L., Gill, M. J., et al. (2008). HIV infection of the central nervous system: Clinical features and neuropathogenesis. *Neurol Clin, 26*(3), 799–819.

Boivin, M. J., Green, S. D., et al. (1995). A preliminary evaluation of the cognitive and motor effects of pediatric HIV infection in Zairian children. *Health Psychol, 14*(1), 13–21.

Boivin, M. J., Ruel, T. D., et al. HIV-subtype A is associated with poorer neuropsychological performance compared with subtype D in antiretroviral therapy-naive Ugandan children. *AIDS, 24*(8), 1163–1170.

Brackis-Cott, E., Kang, E., et al. (2009). The impact of perinatal HIV infection on older school-aged children's and adolescents' receptive language and word recognition skills. *AIDS Patient Care STDS, 23*(6), 415–421.

Brew, B. J. (2004). Evidence for a change in AIDS dementia complex in the era of highly active antiretroviral therapy and the possibility of new forms of AIDS dementia complex. *AIDS, 18* Suppl 1, S75–78.

Brouwers, P., DeCarli, C., et al. (1995). Correlation between computed tomographic brain scan abnormalities and neuropsychological function in children with symptomatic human immunodeficiency virus disease. *Arch Neurol, 52*(1), 39–44.

Brouwers, P., Moss, H., et al. (1990). Effect of continuous-infusion zidovudine therapy on neuropsychologic functioning in children with symptomatic human immunodeficiency virus infection. *J Pediatr, 117*(6), 980–985.

Brouwers, P., Tudor-Williams, G., et al. (1995). Relation between stage of disease and neurobehavioral measures in children with symptomatic HIV disease. *AIDS, 9*(7), 713–720.

Bruck, I., Tahan, T. T., et al. (2001). Developmental milestones of vertically HIV-infected and seroreverters children: Follow up of 83 children. *Arq Neuropsiquiat,r 59*(3-B), 691–695.

Chase, C., Vibbert, M., et al. (1995). Early neurodevelopmental growth in children with vertically transmitted human immunodeficiency virus infection. *Arch Pediatr Adolesc Med, 149*(8), 850–855.

Chernoff, M., Nachman S., et al. (2009). Mental health treatment patterns in perinatally HIV-infected youth and controls. *Pediatrics, 124*(2), 627–636.

Chiriboga, C. A., Fleishman, S., et al. (2005). Incidence and prevalence of HIV encephalopathy in children with HIV infection receiving highly active anti-retroviral therapy (HAART). *J Pediatr, 146*(3), 402–407.

Cohen, S. E., Mundy, T., et al. (1991). Neuropsychological functioning in human immunodeficiency virus type 1 seropositive children infected through neonatal blood transfusion. *Pediatrics, 88*(1), 58–68.

Condini, A., Axia, G., et al. (1991). Development of language in 18–30-month-old HIV-1-infected but not ill children. *AIDS, 5*(6), 735–739.

Conners, C. (1989). Conners' Rating Scales. North Tonawanda, NY: Multi-Health Systems.

Cooper, E. R., Hanson, C., et al. (1998). Encephalopathy and progression of human immunodeficiency virus disease in a cohort of children with perinatally acquired human immunodeficiency virus infection. Women and Infants Transmission Study Group. *J Pediatr, 132*(5), 808–812.

Coplan, J., Contello, K. A., et al. (1998). Early language development in children exposed to or infected with human immunodeficiency virus. *Pediatrics, 102*(1), e8.

Cysique, L. A., Vaida, F., et al. (2009). Dynamics of cognitive change in impaired HIV-positive patients initiating antiretroviral therapy. *Neurology, 73*(5), 342–348.

Czornyj, L. A. (2006). Encephalopathy in children infected by vertically transmitted human immunodeficiency virus. *Rev Neurol, 42*(12), 743–753.

d'Arminio Monforte, A., Cinque, P., et al. (2004). Changing incidence of central nervous system diseases in the EuroSIDA cohort. *Ann Neurol, 55*(3), 320–328.

DeCarli, C., Civitello, L. A., et al. (1993). The prevalence of computed tomographic abnormalities of the cerebrum in 100 consecutive children symptomatic with the human immune deficiency virus. *Ann Neurol, 34*(2), 198–205.

Dickson, D. W., Belman, A. L., et al. (1989). Central nervous system pathology in pediatric AIDS: An autopsy study. *APMIS, Suppl 8*, 40–57.

Drotar, D., Olness, K., et al. (1997). Neurodevelopmental outcomes of Ugandan infants with human immunodeficiency virus type 1 infection. *Pediatrics, 100*(1), E5.

Drotar, D., Olness, K., et al. (1999). Neurodevelopmental outcomes of Ugandan infants with HIV infection: An application of growth curve analysis. *Health Psychol, 18*(2), 114–121.

Dunn, L. M. & Dunn, L. M. (1997). Peabody Picture Vocabulary Test. Circle Pines, MN: American Guidance Service.

Elenga, N., Kouakoussui, K. A., et al. (2005). Diagnosed tuberculosis during the follow-up of a cohort of human immunodeficiency virus-infected children in Abidjan, Cote d'Ivoire: ANRS 1278 study. *Pediatr Infect Dis J, 24*(12), 1077–1082.

Englund, J. A., Baker, C. J., et al. (1996). Clinical and laboratory characteristics of a large cohort of symptomatic, human immunodeficiency virus-infected infants and children. AIDS Clinical Trials Group Protocol 152 Study Team. *Pediatr Infect Dis J 15*(11), 1025–1036.

Epstein, L. G., Goudsmit, J., et al. (1987). Expression of human immunodeficiency virus in cerebrospinal fluid of children with progressive encephalopathy. *Ann Neurol, 21*(4), 397–401.

Epstein, L. G., Sharer, L. R., et al. (1985). Progressive encephalopathy in children with acquired immune deficiency syndrome. *Ann Neurol, 17*(5), 488–496.

Epstein, L. G., Sharer, L. R., et al. (1986). Neurologic manifestations of human immunodeficiency virus infection in children. *Pediatrics, 78*(4), 678–687.

Fagan, J. F. & Detterman, D. (1992). The Fagan Test of Infant Intelligence: A technical summary. *Journal of Applied Developmental Psychology, 13,* 73–193.

Fallo, A., De Matteo, E., et al. (2005). Epstein-Barr virus associated with primary CNS lymphoma and disseminated BCG infection in a child with AIDS. *Int J Infect Dis, 9*(2), 96–103.

Faye, A., Le Chenadec, J., et al. (2004). Early versus deferred antiretroviral multidrug therapy in infants infected with HIV type 1. *Clin Infect Dis, 39*(11), 1692–1698.

Fishkin, P. E., Armstrong, F. D., et al. (2000). Brief report: Relationship between HIV infection and WPPSI-R performance in preschool-age children. *J Pediatr Psychol, 25*(5), 347–351.

Folio, M. & Fewell, R. (1983). Peabody Developmental Motor Scales and Activity Cards. Chicago, IL: Riverside.

Foster, C. J., Biggs, R. L., et al. (2006). Neurodevelopmental outcomes in children with HIV infection under 3 years of age. *Dev Med Child Neurol, 48*(8), 677–682.

Frankenburg, W. K., Fandal, A. W., et al. (1981). The newly abbreviated and revised Denver Developmental Screening Test. *J Pediatr, 99*(6), 995–999.

Gabuzda, D. H. & Hirsch, M. S. (1987). Neurologic manifestations of infection with human immunodeficiency virus. Clinical features and pathogenesis. *Ann Intern Med, 107*(3), 383–391.

Gaughan, D. M., Hughes, M. D., et al. (2004). Psychiatric hospitalizations among children and youths with human immunodeficiency virus infection. *Pediatrics, 113*(6), e544–551.

Gay, C. L., Armstrong, F. D., et al. (1995). The effects of HIV on cognitive and motor development in children born to HIV-seropositive women with no reported drug use: Birth to 24 months. *Pediatrics 96*(6), 1078–1082.

Gelbard, H. A., Jame, H. J., et al. (1995). Apoptotic neurons in brains from paediatric patients with HIV-1 encephalitis and progressive encephalopathy. *Neuropathol Appl Neurobiol, 21*(3), 208–217.

Gendelman, H. E., Diesing, S., et al. (2004). The neuropathogenesis of HIV infection. In G. P. Wormser (Ed.). *AIDS and other manifestations of HIV infection,* pp. 95–115. Amsterdam: Elsevier.

George, R., Andronikou, S., et al. (2009). Central nervous system manifestations of HIV infection in children. *Pediatr Radiol, 39*(6), 575–585.

Gumbo, T., Kadzirange, G., et al. (2002). *Cryptococcus neoformans* meningoencephalitis in African children with acquired immunodeficiency syndrome. *Pediatr Infect Dis J, 21*(1), 54–56.

Hambleton, R. K. (1994). Guidelines for adapting educational and pscyhological tests: A progress report. *European Journal of Psychological Assessment, 10,* 16.

Hamid, M. Z., Aziz, N. A., et al. (2008). Clinical features and risk factors for HIV encephalopathy in children. *Southeast Asian J Trop Med Public Health, 39*(2), 266–272.

Havens, J. F., Whitaker, A. H., et al. (1994). Psychiatric morbidity in school-age children with congenital human immunodeficiency virus infection: A pilot study. *J Dev Behav Pediatr, 15*(3 Suppl), S18–25.

Hazra, R., Jankelevich, S., et al. (2007). Immunologic, virologic, and neuropsychologic responses in human immunodeficiency virus-infected children receiving their first highly active antiretroviral therapy regimen. *Viral Immunol, 20*(1), 131–141.

Hochhauser, C. J., Gaur, S., et al. (2008). The impact of environmental risk factors on HIV-associated cognitive decline in children. *AIDS Care, 20*(6), 692–699.

Howland, L. C., Gortmaker, S. L., et al. (2000). Effects of negative life events on immune suppression in children and youth infected with human immunodeficiency virus type 1. *Pediatrics, 106*(3), 540–546.

Huntley, M. (1996). The Griffiths Mental Development Scales. Oxon: The Test Agency Ltd.

Jeremy, R. J., Kim, S., et al. (2005). Neuropsychological functioning and viral load in stable antiretroviral therapy-experienced HIV-infected children. *Pediatrics, 115*(2), 380–387.

Johnson, T. & Nath, A. (2010). Neurological complications of immune reconstitution in HIV-infected populations. *Ann N Y Acad Sci, 1184,* 106–120.

Jukes, M. C. H. & Grigorenko, E. L. (2010). Assessment of cognitive abilities in multiethnic countries: The case of the Wolof and Mandika in Gambia. *British Journal of Educational Psychology, 80,* 20.

Kaufman, A. S. & Kaufman, N. L. (1983). Kaufman Assessment Battery for Children: Administration and Scoring Manual. Circle Pines, MN: American Guidance Services Inc.

Kaul, M., Garden, G. A., et al. (2001). Pathways to neuronal injury and apoptosis in HIV-associated dementia. *Nature, 410*(6831), 988–994.

Kaur, R., Rawat, D., et al. (2003). Cryptococcal meningitis in pediatric AIDS. *J Trop Pediatr, 49*(2),124–125.

Khan, N. Z., Muslima, H., et al. (2010). Validation of rapid neurodevelopmental assessment instrument for under-two-year-old children in Bangladesh. *Pediatrics, 125*(4), e755–762.

Kieck, J. R. & Andronikou, S. (2004). Usefulness of neuro-imaging for the diagnosis of HIV encephalopathy in children. *S Afr Med J, 94*(8), 628–630.

Kiwanuka, N., Laeyendecker, O., et al. (2008). Effect of human immunodeficiency virus Type 1 (HIV-1) subtype on disease progression in persons from Rakai, Uganda, with incident HIV-1 infection. *J Infect Dis, 197*(5), 707–713.

Knight, W. G., Mellins, C. A., et al. (2000). Brief report: Effects of pediatric HIV infection on mental and psychomotor development. *J Pediatr Psychol, 25*(8), 583–587.

Koekkoek, S., de Sonneville, L. M., et al. (2008). Neurocognitive function profile in HIV-infected school-age children. *Eur J Paediatr Neurol,* 2008;12(4):290–7.

Koopmans, P. P., Ellis, R., et al. (2009). Should antiretroviral therapy for HIV infection be tailored for intracerebral penetration? *Neth J Med, 67*(6), 206–211.

Kramer-Hammerle, Rothenaigner, S., I., et al. (2005). Cells of the central nervous system as targets and reservoirs of the human immunodeficiency virus. *Virus Res, 111*(2), 194–213.

Letendre, S. L., McCutchan, J. A., et al. (2004). Enhancing antiretroviral therapy for human immunodeficiency virus cognitive disorders. *Ann Neurol, 56*(3), 416–423.

Lindsey, J. C., Hughes, M. D., et al. (2000). Treatment-mediated changes in human immunodeficiency virus (HIV) type 1 RNA and CD4 cell counts as predictors of weight growth failure, cognitive decline, and survival in HIV-infected children. *J Infect Dis, 182*(5), 1385–1393.

Lindsey, J. C., Malee, K. M., et al. (2007). Neurodevelopmental functioning in HIV-infected infants and young children before and after the introduction of protease inhibitor-based highly active antiretroviral therapy. *Pediatrics, 119*(3), e681–693.

Llorente, A., Brouwers, P., et al. (2003). Early neurodevelopmental markers predictive of mortality in infants infected with HIV-1. *Dev Med Child Neurol, 45*(2), 76–84.

Lobato, M. N., Caldwell, M. B., et al. (1995). Encephalopathy in children with perinatally acquired human immunodeficiency virus infection. Pediatric Spectrum of Disease Clinical Consortium. *J Pediatr, 126*(5 Pt 1), 710–715.

Lord, D., Danoff, J., et al. (1995). Motor assessment of infants with human immunodeficiency virus: A retrospective review of multiple cases. *Pedatr. Phys. Ther, 7,* 9–13.

Lyman, W. D., Kress, Y., et al. (1990). Detection of HIV in fetal central nervous system tissue. *Aids, 4*(9), 917–920.

Martin, S. C., Wolters, P. L., et al. (2006). Cognitive functioning in school-aged children with vertically acquired HIV infection being treated with Highly Active Antiretroviral Therapy (HAART). *Dev Neuropsychol, 30*(2), 633–657.

McCarthy, D. (1972). McCarthy Scales of Children's Abilities. San Antonio, TX: Psychological Corporation.

McCoig, C., Castrejon, M. M., et al. (2002). Effect of combination antiretroviral therapy on cerebrospinal fluid HIV RNA, HIV resistance, and clinical manifestations of encephalopathy. *J Pediatr, 141*(1), 36–44.

McGrath, N., Bellinger, D., et al. (2006). Effect of maternal multivitamin supplementation on the mental and psychomotor development of children who are born to HIV-1-infected mothers in Tanzania. *Pediatrics, 117*(2), e216–225.

McGrath, N., Fawzi, W. W., et al. (2006). The timing of mother-to-child transmission of human immunodeficiency virus infection and the neurodevelopment of children in Tanzania. *Pediatr Infect Dis J, 25*(1), 47–52.

Mekmullica, J., Brouwers, P., et al. (2009). Early immunological predictors of neurodevelopmental outcomes in HIV-infected children. *Clin Infect Dis, 48*(3), 338–346.

Mellins, C. A., Brackis-Cott, E., et al. (2009). Rates and types of psychiatric disorders in perinatally human immunodeficiency virus-infected youth and seroreverters. *J Child Psychol Psychiatry, 50*(9), 1131–1138.

Mellins, C. A., Smith, R., et al. (2003). High rates of behavioral problems in perinatally HIV-infected children are not linked to HIV disease. *Pediatrics, 111*(2), 384–393.

Mitchell, W. (2001). Neurological and developmental effects of HIV and AIDS in children and adolescents. *Ment Retard Dev Disabil Res Rev, 7*(3), 211–216.

Molyneux, E. (2005). Human immunodeficiency virus infection and pediatric bacterial meningitis in developing countries. *J Neurovirol, 11* Suppl 3, 6–10.

Moss, H. A., Brouwers, P., et al. (1994). The development of a Q-sort behavioral rating procedure for pediatric HIV patients. *J Pediatr Psychol, 19*(1), 27–46.

Msellati, P., Lepage, P., et al. (1993). Neurodevelopmental testing of children born to human immunodeficiency virus type 1 seropositive and seronegative mothers: A prospective cohort study in Kigali, Rwanda. *Pediatrics, 92*(6), 843–848.

Nachman, S. A., Chernoff, M., et al. (2009). Incidence of noninfectious conditions in perinatally HIV-infected children and adolescents in the HAART era. *Arch Pediatr Adolesc Med, 163*(2), 164–171.

Nampijja, M., Apule, B., et al. (2010). Adaptation of Western measures of cognition for assessing 5-year-old semi-urban Ugandan children. *Br J Educ Psychol, 80*(Pt 1), 15–30.

Newell, M. L. (1998). Mechanisms and timing of mother-to-child transmission of HIV-1. *AIDS, 12*(8), 831–837.

Newton, C. R. (2005). Interaction between *Plasmodium falciparum* and human immunodeficiency virus type 1 on the central nervous system of African children. *J Neurovirol, 11* Suppl 3, 45–51.

Nozyce, M., Hittelman, J., et al. (1994). Effect of perinatally acquired human immunodeficiency virus infection on neurodevelopment in children during the first two years of life. *Pediatrics, 94*(6 Pt 1), 883–891.

Nozyce, M. L., Lee, S. S., et al. (2006). A behavioral and cognitive profile of clinically stable HIV-infected children. *Pediatrics, 117*(3), 763–770.

Nuttall, J. J., Wilmshurst, J. M., et al. (2004). Progressive multifocal leukoencephalopathy after initiation of highly active antiretroviral therapy in a child with advanced human immunodeficiency virus infection: A case of immune reconstitution inflammatory syndrome. *Pediatr Infect Dis J, 23*(7), 683–685.

Oberdorfer, P., Washington, C. H., et al. (2009). Progressive multifocal leukoencephalopathy in HIV-infected children: A case report and literature review. *Int J Pediatr, 2009,* 348507.

Parks, R. A. & Danoff, J. V. (1999). Motor performance changes in children testing positive for HIV over 2 years. *Am J Occup Ther, 53*(5), 524–528.

Patel, K., Ming, X., et al. (2009). Impact of HAART and CNS-penetrating antiretroviral regimens on HIV encephalopathy among perinatally infected children and adolescents. *AIDS, 23*(14), 1893–1901.

Patsalides, A. D., Wood, L. V., et al. (2002). Cerebrovascular disease in HIV-infected pediatric patients: Neuroimaging findings. *AJR Am J Roentgenol, 179*(4), 999–1003.

Pizzo, P. A., Eddy, J., et al. (1988). Effect of continuous intravenous infusion of zidovudine (AZT) in children with symptomatic HIV infection. *N Engl J Med, 319*(14), 889–896.

Pollack, H., Kuchuk, A., et al. (1996). Neurodevelopment, growth, and viral load in HIV-infected infants. *Brain Behav Immun, 10*(3), 298–312.

Potterton, J., Stewart, A., et al. (2010). The effect of a basic home stimulation programme on the development of young children infected with HIV. *Dev Med Child Neurol, 52*(6), 547–51.

Puthanakit, T., Aurpibul, L., et al. (2010). Poor cognitive functioning of school-aged children in Thailand with perinatally acquired HIV infection taking antiretroviral therapy. *AIDS Patient Care STDS, 24*(3), 141–146.

Raskino, C., Pearson, D. A., et al. (1999). Neurologic, neurocognitive, and brain growth outcomes in human immunodeficiency virus-infected children receiving different nucleoside antiretroviral regimens. Pediatric AIDS Clinical Trials Group 152 Study Team. *Pediatrics, 104*(3), e32.

Ruffieux, N., Njamnshi, A. K., et al. (2010). Neuropsychology in Cameroon: First normative data for cognitive tests among school-aged children. *Child Neuropsychol, 16*(1), 1–19.

Sacktor, N., Nakasujja, N., et al. (2009). HIV subtype D is associated with dementia, compared with subtype A, in immunosuppressed individuals at risk of cognitive impairment in Kampala, Uganda. *Clin Infect Dis, 49*(5), 780–786.

Sanmaneechai, O., Puthanakit, T., et al. (2005). Growth, developmental, and behavioral outcomes of HIV-affected preschool children in Thailand. *J Med Assoc Thai, 88*(12), 1873–1879.

Sei, S., Stewart, S. K., et al. (1996). Evaluation of human immunodeficiency virus (HIV) type 1 RNA levels in cerebrospinal fluid and viral resistance to zidovudine in children with HIV encephalopathy. *J Infect Dis, 174*(6), 1200–1206.

Semel, E., Wiig, E., et al. (1987). Clinical Evaluation of Language Fundamentals-Revised. San Antonio: Psychological Corporation.

Shah, S. S., Zimmerman, R. A., et al. (1996). Cerebrovascular complications of HIV in children. *AJNR Am J Neuroradiol, 17*(10), 1913–1917.

Shanbhag, M. C., Rutstein, R. M., et al. (2005). Neurocognitive functioning in pediatric human immunodeficiency virus infection: Effects of combined therapy. *Arch Pediatr Adolesc Med, 159*(7), 651–656.

Singh, K. K., Barroga, C. F., et al. (2003). Genetic influence of CCR5, CCR2, and SDF1 variants on human immunodeficiency virus 1 (HIV-1)-related disease progression and neurological impairment, in children with symptomatic HIV-1 infection. *J Infect Dis, 188*(10), 1461–1472.

Singh, K. K. & Spector, S. A. (2009). Host genetic determinants of human immunodeficiency virus infection and disease progression in children. *Pediatr Res 65,*(5 Pt 2), 55R–63R.

Smith, L., Adnams, C., et al. (2008). Neurological and neurocognitive function of HIV-infected children commenced on antiretroviral therapy. *South African Journal of Child Health, 2*(3).

Smith, R., Malee, K., et al. (2000). Timing of perinatal human immunodeficiency virus type 1 infection and rate of neurodevelopment. The Women and Infant Transmission Study Group. *Pediatr Infect Dis J, 19*(9), 862–871.

Smith, R., Malee, K., et al. (2006). Effects of perinatal HIV infection and associated risk factors on cognitive development among young children. *Pediatrics, 117*(3), 851–862.

Sutcliffe, C. G., van Dijk, J. H., et al. (2008). Effectiveness of antiretroviral therapy among HIV-infected children in sub-Saharan Africa. *Lancet Infect Dis, 8*(8), 477–489.

Tamula, M. A., Wolters, P. L., et al. (2003). Cognitive decline with immunologic and virologic stability in four children with human immunodeficiency virus disease. *Pediatrics, 112*(3 Pt 1), 679–684.

Tardieu, M., Brunelle, F., et al. (2005). Cerebral MR imaging in uninfected children born to HIV-seropositive mothers and perinatally exposed to zidovudine. *AJNR Am J Neuroradiol, 26*(4), 695–701.

Tardieu, M., Le Chenadec, J., et al. (2000). HIV-1-related encephalopathy in infants compared with children and adults. French Pediatric HIV Infection Study and the SEROCO Group. *Neurology, 54*(5), 1089–1095.

Tardieu, M., Mayaux, M. J., et al. (1995). Cognitive assessment of school-age children infected with maternally transmitted human immunodeficiency virus type 1. *J Pediatr, 126*(3), 375–379.

Tellegen, P. & Laros, J. (1993). The construction and validation of a non-verbal test of intelligence: The revision of the Snijders-Oomens tests. *Eur J Psychol Assess, 9*, 147–157.

Topley, J. M., Bamber, S., et al. (1998). Tuberculous meningitis and co-infection with HIV. *Ann Trop Paediatr, 18*(4), 261–266.

Van de Vijver, F. J. R. & Hambleton, R. K. (1996). Translating tests: Some practical guidelines. *European Psychologist, 1*, 2.

Van Rie, A., Dow, A., et al. (2009). Neurodevelopmental trajectory of HIV-infected children accessing care in Kinshasa, Democratic Republic of Congo. *J Acquir Immune Defic Syndr, 52*(5), 636–642.

Van Rie, A., Harrington, P. R., et al. (2007). Neurologic and neurodevelopmental manifestations of pediatric HIV/AIDS: A global perspective. *Eur J Paediatr Neurol, 11*(1), 1–9.

Van Rie, A., Mupuala, A., et al. (2008). Impact of the HIV/AIDS epidemic on the neurodevelopment of preschool-aged children in Kinshasa, Democratic Republic of the Congo. *Pediatrics, 122*(1), e123–128.

van Toorn, R., Kritzinger, F., et al. (2005). Acute demyelinating encephalomyelitis (ADEM), cryptococcal reactivation and disseminated Herpes simplex in an HIV infected child following HAART. *Eur J Paediatr Neurol, 9*(5), 355–359.

Violari, A., Cotton, M. F., et al. (2008). Early antiretroviral therapy and mortality among HIV-infected infants. *N Engl J Med, 359*(21), 2233–2244.

Wachtel, R. C., Shapiro, B. K., et al. (1994). CAT/CLAMS. A tool for the pediatric evaluation of infants and young children with developmental delay. Clinical Adaptive Test/Clinical Linguistic and Auditory Milestone Scale. *Clin Pediatr (Phila), 33*(7), 410–415.

Walker, V. E. & Poirier, M. C. (2007). Special issue on health risks of perinatal exposure to nucleoside reverse transcriptase inhibitors. *Environ Mol Mutagen, 48*(3–4), 159–165.

Wechsler, D. (2002). Wechsler Preschool and Primary Scale of Intelligence. San Antonio, TX: Psychological Corporation.

Wechsler, D. (2003). Wechsler Intelligence Scale for Children. San Antonio, TX: Psychological Corporation.

WHO, (1997). *Improving mother/child interaction to promote better psychosocial development in children.* Programme on Mental Health. International Child Development Programmes.

WHO (2006). *Antiretroviral therapy of HIV infection in infants and children: Towards universal access. Recommendations for a public health approach.* Geneva: World Health Organization.

Wilkinson, G. S. (1993). Wide Range Achievement Test. Lutz, FL: Psychological Assessment Resources, Inc.

Williams, P. L., Marino, M., et al. (2010). Neurodevelopment and in utero antiretroviral exposure of HIV-exposed uninfected infants. *Pediatrics, 125*(2), e250–60.

Wilmshurst, J. M., Burgess, J., et al. (2006). Specific neurologic complications of human immunodeficiency virus type 1 (HIV-1) infection in children. *J Child Neurol, 21*(9), 788–794.

Wolters, P. & Brouwers, P. (2005). Evaluation of neurodevelopmental deficits in children with HIV-1 infection. In H. E. Gendelman, I. Gtant, I. P. Everall, S. A. Lipton, & S. Swindels, (Eds.). *The neurology of AIDS.* Oxford: Oxford University Press.

Wolters, P. L., Brouwers, P., et al. (1997). Receptive and expressive language function of children with symptomatic HIV infection and relationship with disease parameters: A longitudinal 24-month follow-up study. *AIDS, 11*(9), 1135–1144.

Wolters, P. L., Brouwers, P., et al. (1994). Adaptive behavior of children with symptomatic HIV infection before and after zidovudine therapy. *J Pediatr Psychol, 19*(1), 47–61.

Wood, S. M., Shah, S. S., et al. (2009). The impact of AIDS diagnoses on long-term neurocognitive and psychiatric outcomes of surviving adolescents with perinatally acquired HIV. *AIDS, 23*(14), 1859–1865.

Woods, S. P., Moore, D. J., et al. (2009). Cognitive neuropsychology of HIV-associated neurocognitive disorders. *Neuropsychol Rev, 19*(2), 152–168.

10.3

PSYCHOSOCIAL ASPECTS OF NEUROLOGICAL IMPAIRMENT IN CHILDREN WITH AIDS

Lori Wiener and Claude Mellins

Despite HAART, children with perinatally acquired HIV-1 infection remain at risk of brain dysfunction. The entire spectrum of the clinician's skills is required when working with these young patients and their families. Diagnostic skills are required to address the indirect and direct effects of the virus on multiple family members. Clinical skills are essential for designing individual, family, and group therapeutic modalities that address overall health and development as well as the specific neuropsychological effects of HIV. Advocacy skills benefit patients and families by linking them with invaluable psychological, social support, educational, and concrete services. For the clinician, working with these young patients and their families can become highly personal, as the clinician becomes an important part of the child's and family's life. This chapter considers the psychosocial impact of neurological impairment on the HIV-infected child. In particular, the chapter focuses on 1) the prevalence of impairment, 2) the nature of the developmental challenges, and 3) interventions that can best meet the psychosocial, educational, and therapeutic needs of these children and their families.

INTRODUCTION

Neurological, neurocognitive, and neurodevelopmental impairment has been associated with the natural history of pediatric HIV infection since the disease was first identified in children. In general, the severity of neurological and neuropsychological compromise increases with the severity of HIV-related illness (Jeremy et al., 2005; Nozyce et al., 2006). The trajectory of deficits, however, is not typically linear, nor does it affect children in uniform patterns. Neurocognitive dysfunction can present at any point across the developmental spectrum and in disparate patterns of behavior, affecting cognitive and psychosocial as well as emotional functions (Willen, 2006). Although not all are affected, neurodevelopmental deterioration is one of the most disconcerting and devastating manifestations of HIV infection to witness in perinatally HIV-infected children. As the child who once was verbally adept and cheerful begins to search for words, forget meaningful conversations, or have a general change in personality, the clinician grieves along with the family. Fortunately, with the advent of ART, children with perinatally acquired HIV infection have shown markedly improved immune function and long-term survival along with a decline in the incidence of progressive encephalopathy (Shanbhag et al., 2005). Yet, neurological impairments associated with HIV infection in childhood, some of which can be subtle, can continue to present a significant challenge to the overall quality of life of affected children and their families. Helping families cope and adjust to these neurological manifestations requires more than providing medical information and changing medications. The child's deviation from a normative developmental course will create perturbations in the child and family's interface with society as well as internally within the family. Clinicians must help families explore the implications of their child's problems within a developmental context, help families adjust to the special needs of their child, and provide assistance accessing needed community services. In examining the psychosocial impact of neurological impairment on the HIV-infected child, this chapter will cover the 1) prevalence of impairment, 2) developmental challenges, and 3) interventions that can be utilized to best meet the psychosocial, educational, and therapeutic needs of these children and their families.

PREVALENCE

Early estimates of AIDS-related neurologic impairment that reported a prevalence of 50–62% (Belman, 1990, 1992) were based on retrospective studies and clinical trials that included children who were more likely to be severely compromised. Other studies that have incorporated asymptomatic, mildly compromised children, and children who have benefited from earlier and more effective medical interventions associated with successes in treatment development, all have led to lower prevalence rates (16–19%) (Chiriboga, Fleishman, Champion, Gaye-Robinson, & Abrams, 2005). Accurate estimates of the prevalence of neurological impairment among children with AIDS are difficult to obtain or to disentangle from other concurrent biomedical or maternal behavioral characteristics that are known to also affect neuropsychological outcomes in infants and children.

HIV can enter the central nervous system (CNS), but the specific neurological consequences of HIV infection in any given individual are dependent upon multiple factors, including viral burden and CD4 cell count, as well as whether the insult was the result of an acute event or a chronic process (Mintz, 1999; Mitchell, 2001), the age of the child at the time of the assessment, the expected developmental milestones associated with that point in time (Coscia et al., 2001; Armstrong et al., 1993), and the age at which the child began HAART therapy (Mintz, 1999). Early reports indicated that ART had the potential to ameliorate the development and progression of HIV-related CNS compromise (Mintz, 1994; Brouwers, Belman, & Epstein, 1990; McKinney et al., 1991; Pizzo, 1989). More recently, in a study of the neurobehavioral outcomes in 126 children perinatally infected with HIV, the rate of HIV encephalopathy was 1.6% (Chiriboga et al., 2005) compared to 24–35% in the era prior to HAART (Cooper et al., 1998; Cooper et al., 1998; Chiriboga et al., 2005; Tardieu et al., 2000; Lobato, Caldwell, Ng, & Oxtoby, 1995). Yet, in spite of better prognostic factors, CNS compromise can occur without substantial immunosuppression (Jeremy et al., 2005) and children who experienced progressive encephalopathy continue to show higher rates of residual, neurological, cognitive, and academic difficulties along with more subtle neuropsychological outcomes (e.g., vocabulary) even with a treatment-associated significantly reduced HIV RNA viral load (Chiriboga et al., 2005). Furthermore, recent studies in the US with larger samples of older HIV-infected children, most of whom had some experience with HAART, generally report cognitive delays and deficits when comparing HIV-infected children to population norms (Nozyce et al., 2006; Smith et al., 2006).

As noted, several important methodological issues present challenges to assessing true prevalence of neuropsychological deficits in perinatally HIV-infected children. The first challenge is finding appropriate comparison or control groups. Background characteristics also known to affect neuro-psychological outcomes such as prenatal drug use, poverty, exposure to violence, and other environmental and sociocultural factors are often present in families affected by HIV. In both US and international studies, some investigators have failed to find significant neurological or cognitive differences between the HIV-infected and comparison groups or HIV-infected ART-naïve children, with gender matched HIV-exposed, but uninfected or HIV-unexposed children (Bagenda et al., 2006), presumably because both groups are affected by these other factors. However, others have reported differences in IQ between HIV-infected school age children and controls (Sanmaneechai, Puthanakit, Louthrenoo, & Sirisanthana, 2005 ; Smith et al., 2006). Despite the differences in IQ between the groups, progression to AIDS has been consistently associated with poorer neuropsychological outcomes (Smith et al., 2006 ; Nozyce et al., 2006).

Next, discordance in prevalence rates across studies of HIV-infected children can result from lack of consistent measurement and diagnostic criteria for identifying neurological impairments. Researchers and clinicians have alternatively identified neurological impairments through neurological exams, various forms of psychometric testing, and neuroimaging studies. These methods identify different numbers of children with impairments and show questionable agreement across specific children.

Prevalence data also mask the age effects observed. The prevalence of HIV-associated neurological impairment is not equally distributed across age. The greatest prevalence falls during infancy (Wolters et al., 2005). It has been cautiously suggested that if a child survives to the age of 4–5 years of life without neurological impairment that they are less likely to develop severe neurological impairments later (Belman, 1992). Despite the methodological constraints, consistent throughout all studies is severity of illness as a variable negatively affecting neuropsychological outcomes. (Nozyce et al., 2006; Smith et al., 2006).

NEUROLOGICAL MANIFESTATIONS

HIV-related neurologic impairment in the pediatric population has been fairly common and has not mirrored the better-defined AIDS dementia described in the adult population. Prior to the widespread use of ART, two patterns of neurodevelopment were described in HIV-infected infants and children. Acute courses of neurological impairment, also known as HIV-associated progressive encephalopathy of childhood, are characterized by a loss of previously acquired skills or a failure to acquire new skills (Wolters et al., 2005) although children may remain relatively stable for extended time periods (Simpson et al., 1996; Willen, 2006). Static encephalopathy, another form of encephalopathy in children with HIV, is characterized by nonprogressive delays or deficits in cognitive, motor, adaptive, and/or language function, with skills ranging from low average to markedly impaired (Brouwers, Suppiej, & Laverda, 1994). A subset of children infected with HIV display relatively mild and subtle neurocognitive deficits in the areas of attention, expressive language, social skills, memory (Bisiacchi et al., 2000), and affect (Ultmann et al., 1987), and can also have deficits associated with non-HIV risk factors (Havens, Whitaker, Feldman, & Ehrhardt, 2008). In extreme forms, HIV-related neurologic impairment has been associated with spastic diplegia, quadriparesis, and blindness (Epstein et al., 1986). Prior to ART, HIV-associated CNS dysfunction was often one of the earliest sign of the disease process in infants and children and considered a poor prognostic marker (Pizzo et al., 1988). However, many children are living into young adulthood and the neurocognitive profiles in HIV-infected older adolescents and young adults are only now emerging,

Even with treatment, susceptibility to developing HIV CNS disease remains a concern throughout development. Adherence to HAART regimens plays a key role as suboptimal drug levels in the CSF may lead to the emergence of drug resistant virus in the CNS (Gissen et al., 2001). Moreover, the CNS may be a key anatomical reservoir for persistent HIV-1 replication (Enting et al., 2001; Schrager et al., 1998; Sonza et al., 2001) since many antiretroviral agents, including protease inhibitors (PIs), have poor CNS penetration (Aweeka et al., 1999; Swindells, Zheng, & Gendelman, 1999). Frontal cortical thinning has been strongly linked with cognitive impairment and may underlie the commonly observed HIV-related decline in frontal lobe functions such as attention, executive function, and working memory in survivors (Thompson et al., 2005). These cognitive impairments could significantly affect academic success in HIV-infected long-term survivors.

NEUROPSYCHIATRIC MANIFESTATIONS

More recent attention has been given to the possible association between HIV CNS disease and psychiatric manifestations. Throughout the epidemic, clinical reports have indicated high rates of mental health problems (Havens et al., 2008). However, research studies of psychiatric disorders in pediatric HIV/AIDS have been limited by small and diverse demographic samples, lack of consistent testing measurements, frequent subthreshold DSM-IV diagnoses, lack of appropriate control groups, pre-HAART exposure, and a paucity of available child and adolescent AIDS psychiatrists (Lourie, Pao, Brown, & Hunter, 2005). A few studies suggest that DSM-defined psychiatric diagnoses in pediatric HIV/AIDS can be substantial. One review reported prevalence rates of attention deficit hyperactivity disorder at 28.6%, anxiety disorders at 24.3%, and depression at 25% (Scharko, 2006). In one study of HIV-infected youth ages 6–15, higher rates of depression (47%) and attentional disorders (29%) were found, with and the data suggesting depression likely to be associated with encephalopathy and worsening immune function (Misdrahi et al., 2004). A small report of HIV-infected adolescents with sexually acquired HIV found high rates of mood disorder and substance abuse (Pao et al., 2000), while a more recent study of adolescents with perinatally acquired HIV, using the Diagnostic Interview Schedule for Children (DISC-IV), reported higher rates of anxiety and other disorders (Mellins, Brackis-Cott, Dolezal, & Abrams, 2006) than had been cited in earlier reports. Along with psychiatric symptoms and disorders, a higher rate of psychotropic medication use and of psychiatric hospitalizations in HIV-infected children compared with HIV-uninfected controls has also been reported (Gaughan et al., 2004) with psychostimulants and antidepressants being most commonly prescribed (Wiener, Battles, Ryder, & Pao, 2006a). In a recent study by Wood and colleagues (2009) designed to explore the association between previous severe HIV disease, defined as past CDC class C diagnosis, and neurocognitive and psychiatric outcomes in long-term survivors of perinatally acquired HIV, a distant history of AIDS diagnosis was associated with an increased risk of both neurocognitive and psychiatric impairment (Wood, Shah, Steenhoff, & Rutstein, 2009). The authors found 48% had a diagnosed psychiatric illness, with 18% having multiple psychiatric comorbidities confirming the overall high rates of behavioral disorders, ADHD, and psychiatric hospitalization within the HIV-infected adolescent population. Further research is clearly needed to delineate whether early treatment, possibly soon after birth and definitely prior to AIDS diagnosis, might lead to improved CNS outcomes.

Considering the potential neurocognitive consequences of HIV infection, serial neurodevelopmental assessments are recommended: 1) every 6 months for children under 2 years due to a higher risk of developing CNS disease, 2) once a year for children between the ages of 2–8 years (unless they exhibit neurodevelopmental deficits), and 3) every 2 years for children over 8 years who exhibit stable functioning in the average range (Wolters et al., 2005). The significant long-term behavioral, psychiatric, and educational needs of these youth suggest that mental health evaluations and services should remain available for all HIV positive youth as they transition to adulthood.

DEVELOPMENTAL CONSIDERATIONS

When considering the psychosocial aspects of neurologic impairment in children with AIDS, it is necessary to utilize a developmental framework. The impact of neurological impairment will differ for the child and family depending on the age of the child, the child's developmental history prior to the onset of neurological problems, and the course of the neuropathological process. When neurological impairments interfere with the attainment or timing of social-developmental tasks, psychosocial conflicts are likely to be precipitated.

INFANCY

A primary task of infancy is the development of relationships with others (particularly the caregiver). The successful completion of this task is dependent on the quality of the interactions between the infant and caregiver. Feeding, clothing, changing, cuddling, eye contact, soothing, and playing with an infant are the basis for the development of a mutually rewarding relationship between a caregiver and infant. Early manifestations of HIV-associated neurological disease in infancy include floppy muscle tone, irritability or passivity, and/or exaggerated primitive reflexes, or may not be easily apparent. Later in infancy, spastic diplegia or quadriparesis may develop. Either a passive or an irritable infant may lead a caregiver to feel rejected or frustrated. Abnormalities in muscle tone and/or aberrant reflexes may interfere with the enjoyment of cuddling of either the infant or caregiver and increase the infant's general irritability. As a result, challenges to parent-infant bonding may occur, which in turn can negatively affect parent-child relationship factors (e.g., attachment, communication) and overall child behavior. Other factors (e.g., prenatal drug exposure, environment, biomedical, or genetic factors) may also cause developmental delays, so HIV causality is often difficult to determine. With highly active antiretroviral therapy, many of the severe neurological manifestations of HIV have been diminished. Yet, some studies find cognitive effects persist, suggesting that psychosocial challenges in parent-infant bonding should continue to be considered and evaluated throughout development.

PRESCHOOL

As children move out of infancy, our expectations are for them to expand their physical and social world from one that is almost totally dependent on their caregivers to one that is characterized by increased freedom of movement, social contact, cognitive and linguistic skills, and generally increased autonomy. This movement toward autonomy is predicated on the successful development of motor and cognitive skills and abilities. In addition, toddlers and preschoolers need to develop a level of social competence as they move into more varied and complex relationships outside the family. Any and all of these prerequisites to autonomy may be delayed or disrupted by AIDS-related static, progressive encephalopathies, or even mild, sub-clinical impairments.

On the more severe end of the continuum, and very rarely seen, preschool-aged children with AIDS-related encephalopathies may fail to roll, sit up, stand, walk, and/or develop language. In this extreme course, the child will remain indefinitely infant-like, and families need to come to terms with a vastly different developmental course than which is normally expected.

Children with static encephalopathies are likely to follow a qualitatively normal developmental course, but in a delayed timeframe. In this scenario, families have the opportunity to see developmental progress in their child and to participate and find joy in this natural process. However, no family lives in a vacuum. Invariably, parents will become aware of their child's delays. Frequently other parents with unaffected children will make comments about when their child sat up, walked, said, "ma ma," and so forth, which serve to highlight the delayed developmental course of the preschooler with static encephalopathy. Adjusting to a child's developmental delays is an extremely emotional and personal experience. Social exchanges, however well intentioned, that emphasize a child's dissimilarity may result in parents or caregivers becoming hurt, defensive or withdrawing socially while others reach out for much needed support and guidance.

When preschoolers develop a progressive encephalopathy, it is typically a difficult or sometimes devastating psychosocial event for the family and child. The specific neurological complications are usually compounded by a general systemic decline in the child's fight with AIDS. In this scenario, the child's prior pattern of normal development is disrupted by failure to obtain new skills or an actual loss of previously obtained milestones. Affective blunting and social withdrawal may occur. Frequently, children will become clingy and insecure, demanding the constant presence of their caregiver. The onset of a progressive encephalopathy must be viewed as a catastrophic psychosocial event for a family. It may mark a turning point in the child's disease process, leading to a relatively rapid demise or, particularly now with new treatments, signal a move into a chronic course of disability with plateaus, recoveries, and losses.

SCHOOL-AGE

Within the "school-aged" grouping, we are including children spanning latency age into adolescence. There are clear qualitative differences in the social and academic environments of early elementary school and the later elementary years and middle or junior high school. Subtle neurological deficits in early elementary school children may not be picked up as quickly or prove as disruptive to their daily routines. As the

degree of impairment increases, the child's ability to participate successfully at school, in the community, and at home becomes more challenged. Greater accommodations from the child and family as well as schools and people in the community become necessary to enable successful participation.

School-aged children who are experiencing HIV-related neurological impairments are likely to fall into two groups. The first group is composed of children that have experienced relatively long-term static encephalopathies. These children will have had a history of developmental delays that may or may not be fully attributable to HIV and in most cases they will either be involved in special education or at the least will be receiving special attention within the regular education system. The second group includes those who have previously functioned without impairment or with minimal impairment, but at a certain point in later childhood or adolescence develop neurological problems.

School-aged children with extended histories of developmental delay are likely to have similar experiences as same-age children without HIV who have learning disabilities or some degree of mental retardation. In order to have successful school experiences, most of these children will require some degree of special educational services or other modifications within the regular education system. Children with developmental delays are likely to have difficulty in developing age-appropriate social relationships. Caregivers frequently become concerned with their children becoming involved with students who will take advantage of them. As children with HIV-associated neurological impairments reach early adolescence, concerns about emerging sexuality arise. These concerns are more frequently directed toward the possibility of the child being taken advantage of sexually by older or higher-functioning children. Attention also needs to be paid to the child's own emerging curiosity and interest.

When a previously asymptomatic school-aged child experiences the onset of a progressive neurological impairment, their change in status is likely to be met with a significant upheaval. The degree of upheaval will depend on the extent to which the neurological manifestations interfere with the child's previously established routines and level of functioning as well as the family's previous expectations of the child. Children may experience hyperactivity and attention problems that interfere with their schoolwork. In fact, several studies have suggested increased rates of attention deficit hyperactivity disorder in this population (Mellins et al., 2009). Affective blunting and social withdrawal can also disrupt social relationships as well as schoolwork. Most manifestations that interfere with a child's functioning will serve to reduce their independence and increase their need to be sheltered by their caregivers. Older children who become neurologically compromised may manifest it in idiosyncratic and highly aberrant (psychotic-like) behavior. Other manifestations of dramatic deterioration may result in muteness, losses of motor function which disrupt all aspects of the child's prior routines, resulting in a withdrawal from school and community involvement.

An acute neurological impairment may become an ongoing stressful event, not only for the child and family, but also for the entire classroom, school, and/or neighborhood. Depending on the nature of the child's relationships with other children and adults at school and in the community, the child's deteriorating health may be met with an outpouring of support, an awkward distancing, or in the worst case, rejection. After the early elementary years, the social stigma of HIV/AIDS is likely to add tension to the child's relationship with peers and school staff. Although it cannot be assumed that the reaction will be negative, it is a distinct possibility that families must consider. Regardless of whether the family discloses the diagnosis, friends and others will be very curious and ask questions concerning the child's illness. Helping both the child and caregivers to be prepared for such questions is a service often greatly appreciated. Teaching about the types of neuropsychological deficits that can present in children living with HIV allows caregivers to help distinguish the indirect effects of the disease from the direct ones.

ADOLESCENCE

Adolescence is a developmental stage that poses many challenges for youth without chronic health conditions including separation and individuation from parents, peer and romantic relationships, academic and vocational development, and issues related to independent living and adult roles (Hamburg, 1990). HIV seriously complicates the normal developmental challenges of this stage, including puberty, sexuality, and the desire to "fit in."

When delivering a diagnosis, reviewing treatment options, or talking to a family about disclosure-related issues, youth cognitive impairment must be considered (Wiener et al., 2006b). While positive outcomes associated with disclosure, including the promotion of trust, improved adherence, enhanced support services, open family communication, and better long-term health and emotional well-being, have been reported (Lipson, 1994; Funck-Brentano, 1997; 1999, Wiener, Battles, & Heilman, 1998; Mellins et al., 2002; Wiener, Battles, & Wood, 2007) a youth's HIV CNS disease can impact a parent's decision about diagnosis disclosure. A youngster with neurological impairment may not be able to keep the diagnosis to him or herself and an impulsive disclosure of HIV/AIDS could have disastrous effects on the family. These youth may have difficulty understanding the importance of adherence to medications. The potential negative individual and public health risks of nonadherence and risky sexual behavior substantively add a sense of urgency to the issue of disclosure of HIV status.

As noted earlier, cognitive impairment can manifest with specific problems associated with processing speed, memory, and other measures of executive planning and judgment. Neurologically, as children age, their physical and cognitive abilities become increasingly complex and adult-like. Consequently, their schoolwork and social interactions become increasingly demanding. As the level of social, cognitive, and physical demands placed on the adolescent increases, the higher the likelihood that subtle neurological problems will prove disruptive to their daily functioning. Therefore, a youngster who has "done well" to this point, may benefit from educational intervention and adaptations.

Many perinatally infected youth have delays in physical development, including the onset of puberty. These delays, as well as the potential for a negative self-image posed by having a chronic health condition, present a risk factor for emotional distress. Adolescence is a time of increasing interest in body image and a link between poor body image with mental health and sexual risk outcomes in both boys and girls has been described (Benjet et al., 2001; Wingood, Diclemente, Harrington, & Davies, 2002). This makes decisions around sexual behavior even more critical at this juncture. Furthermore, threats to cognitive development, particularly executive function and frontal lobe activities can seriously impair judgment and ability to manage the emotional regulation needed for decisions about the onset of sex and safe-sex behavior. As many of these youth were not expected to live until adolescence, their caregivers and providers have not necessarily engaged them in conversations about sexual health and sexual risk behavior. Perinatally infected youth will require significant support in managing the complex issues of integrating healthy sexual development with their HIV infection. Open and honest communication around patterns of sexual behavior, disclosure to sexual partners and strategies for the prevention of the spread of HIV are essential. Secondary prevention among HIV-infected youth must be addressed, so that these youth do not re-expose themselves or infect others (Havens et al., 2008).

Similarly, lack of developed executive function, including judgment and ability to understand ART can result in poor or inconsistent adherence to ART. Unfortunately, ART requires near perfect adherence (Havens et al., 2008; Smith, 2006; Garcia de Olalla et al., 2002), something adolescents across chronic conditions have had considerable difficulty with (Smith et al., 2005). Parents often assume youth can manage their medications once they reach a certain age. However, neurological effects of HIV-infected youth in addition to normative developmental challenges indicate that parents may need to stay involved in medication management. Nonadherence has not only individual health consequences (e.g., development of drug-resistant strains of HIV, poor immune function), but also public health consequences, given the possibility of transmission of drug-resistant strains of the virus to potential partners (Rice, Batterham, & Rotheram-Borus, 2006 ; Wiener, Mellins, Marhefka, & Battles, 2007).

Finally, another task of normative adolescence is separation and individuation from parents. For developmentally delayed or cognitively impaired youth, this may be extremely challenging for both youth and caregivers. When the adolescent ages toward young adulthood, and transition to adult care is being considered, the adolescent may not have the skills needed to independently communicate information, keep up with appointments, remain adherent, or make health care decisions. Observations of adolescent CNS compromise, impairment of executive abilities, combined with notation of poor social or psychological function should point to the need for careful consideration pertaining to earlier disclosure and transition to adult care (Armstrong, Seidel, & Swales, 2002).

DIFFERENTIAL DIAGNOSIS: INDIRECT VERSUS DIRECT EFFECTS OF HIV ON BEHAVIOR AND AFFECT

It is not uncommon for a caregiver to report a change in the HIV-infected child's behavior and/or affect. The need to help the family and health care team differentiate between the direct and indirect effects of HIV-infection is one of the most frequent challenges facing the clinician. Direct effects refer to organic changes produced by the virus impairing the CNS, whereas indirect effects consist of psychogenic reactions associated with being infected with HIV or other environmental/ contextual causes such as trauma, violence in the environment, changes in family, or economic stressors (Moss et al., 1994, Moss, Wolters, Brouwers, Hendricks, & Pizzo, 1996). The psychological impact of HIV on the child is tremendous and often staggering. Many children find themselves worrying about an ill parent(s); lying to neighbors, friends, and schoolmates about both their disease status and frequent school absences; and becoming frightened about medical procedures and hospitalizations; while simultaneously experiencing fears associated with a parent's death, their own death, and the uncertainties of the future. Belman, Brouwers, and Moss (1992) classified the stress associated with HIV infection into three primary categories: (1) medical factors (e.g., medical procedures and hospitalizations, recurring interfering medical symptoms, loss of abilities, pain, and discomfort); (2) psychological stressors (secrecy, fear of ostracism, death, guilt, uncertainties of future, inhibited sexual activity [adolescents], need to alter future perspectives); and (3) social stressors (ostracism by school community and extended family; underachievement due to absenteeism). The authors describe some of these stressors as omnipresent, whereas others are transient or modulated by prevailing medical and psychosocial conditions and by the developmental status of the child. These categories are still present today and are very helpful in deciphering changes in the child's behavior and affect and should be incorporated into a comprehensive psychosocial assessment.

Psychosocial assessments, along with neuropsychological evaluations, are best obtained as soon after the family presents to the medical center as possible. The assessment should include information about the child's personality; his or her relationship with parents, siblings, and peers; functioning in school and play; coping abilities; prior losses; knowledge and reaction to the diagnosis; and energy level and mood (Wiener, & Taylor-Brown, 2010; Pao et al., 2008). While noting all behavioral changes at home, school, and play, the assessment should take into consideration any recent disclosure of diagnosis to extended family members, peers, neighbors, or school; changes in parental health; and/or whether or not the child has recently learned about the death of someone he or she knew well. Fear of rejection and fears associated with separation and death can precipitate an anxiety or depressive reaction. In order to develop a treatment plan, it is essential for the clinician to work closely with the health care team in sorting out the direct and indirect effects of HIV. Changes in antiretroviral agents are often indicated when the changes in the child's behavior are the result of the direct effects of the virus.

Psychotherapeutic interventions such as counseling techniques, behavioral and stress management approaches, or pharmacologic tools are often indicated to address the potentially significant indirect effects of HIV on the child and family. Differentiating between the contribution of HIV infection and of prenatal drug exposure to neurobehavioral dysfunction is equally complex and therefore incorporating the presence of in utero exposure to drugs is essential as well. Finally, it is important to keep in mind that developmental stage interacts with neurobehavioral dysfunction and that assessments need to be repeated as children age.

The epidemiology of HIV creates a unique challenge when both child and parent present with neurological manifestations of the disease. Ongoing neuropsychological assessments which include evaluation of the child and the environment, pre-existing and emerging risk and protective factors, the social supports available, and the influence of neurological deterioration on the parent's parenting ability are essential (Watkins, Brouwers, & Huntzinger, 1992). Assisting HIV-positive parents in early permanency planning is always encouraged and should be done as early as possible. This includes legal interventions to prospectively plan for the child's health care and custody arrangements. Actively working with the parents to identify future care providers reaffirms their control over the family situation and reassures their children about who will raise them (Taylor-Brown et al., 1993). Although difficult, early planning is easier than when HIV-infected parents have deteriorated in health or neuropsychiatric function.

IMPLICATIONS FOR INTERVENTIONS

Two levels of intervention for children affected by AIDS-related neurological impairment and their families are described in the following section: within the family system and beyond the family system. Interventions that occur within the child/family system include child and family therapy, the introduction of behavioral techniques, support groups for caregivers, and support for other children in the family. Interventions that occur beyond the family system include assisting families with advocating for daycare and school placements that can accommodate the varying neuropsychological needs of affected children, as well as case management to deal with concrete service needs such as appropriate, housing, and when indicated, obtaining proper equipment such as a wheelchair.

WITHIN CHILD/FAMILY SYSTEM

Developmentally Sensitive Approach to the Child and Family

Infants experiencing neurological impairments can be unusually challenging to their caregivers. Oftentimes, professionals experienced in the needs and care of developmentally delayed infants can assist caregivers with fostering more mutually satisfying interactions with their infant. Teaching caregivers ways to manage irritability or cope with infant delays in reaching milestones, or strategies for special positioning needs for low- and high-tone babies, early reflexes, and physical therapy exercises and interventions that they can do with their infant can provide new ways for caregivers to interact with and help their baby as well as improve caregiver-infant bonding. Although their baby may not become "age-appropriate," helping their child develop a new skill is a deeply rewarding opportunity for parenting and relationship building.

Preschoolers and school-aged children with neurological impairments may benefit from services such as physical and occupational therapy, speech and language therapies, as well as special education, depending upon the nature of the impairment. Caregivers may need assistance developing realistic expectations and in measuring progress. Often, caregivers desire concrete information and training that will assist them in meeting the specialized needs of their child.

Although ART has significantly improved the health and well-being of children living with HIV in countries with adequate resources, there are still children with significant CNS impairment and poor health outcomes. The care needs of severely impaired children can seriously stress the financial, physical, and emotional resources of caregivers. Caregivers of an older severely impaired child may require assistance completing daily living tasks such as bathing, changing, and transporting. Home health, hospice, and respite care agencies may be able to provide such needed services. Caregivers may need to be encouraged to take advantage of these services since many caregivers are reluctant to leave their child under the care of others. Many find themselves being their child's "nurse" and wanting very much to return to the role of "parent." This is a hard cycle to break once the child has become accustomed to their caregiver providing all these services. As part of the comprehensive and complex services needed, providing tips on parenting skills which incorporates the changing needs of the child as well as their own feelings of grief and loss are essential as well. At other times, children, as well as their caregivers, need and can benefit from more intensive psychotherapeutic interventions.

PSYCHOTHERAPEUTIC SERVICES

As traditional therapeutic goals of family counseling work toward open and honest communication, the same goals apply when addressing neuropsychological changes. Children, regardless of age, recognize changes within themselves and often find adaptive ways to adjust to such changes. The anxiety produced by these changes is significantly higher, however, when they are not being openly discussed. Children will be better able to cope with their illness and all of its complexities when the family can honestly discuss disease progression, treatments, and tests required while reassuring the child that he or she will not be alone or in pain and will continued to be loved.

Play therapy, art therapy and verbal psychotherapeutic techniques can be quite helpful and powerful. For the young child, play therapy is a useful tool in creating an environment where he or she can express feelings and fears of isolation, separation, and bodily changes. For children who are nonverbal or suffer from neurological deterioration, what cannot be "told" can possibly be played out or depicted in drawing or paintings (Wiener et al., 1998). In fact, most children express very little about the emotional consequences of their illness. As described earlier, clinical symptoms can easily be perceived as emotional reactions. Drawings represent a form of communication that reveals the inner world of the child and provides children with the opportunity to psychologically master situations in their life that feel insurmountable. They could also allow children to communicate to those around them about their individual symptoms. In this regard, an illuminating open-ended question "What does HIV look like inside your body?" has been both revealing and useful in terms of understanding the child's concern and diagnosing medical problems (see Fig. 10.3.1). B.P., the only child to draw disease only in his head, was later found to have an aneurysm, which eventually took his life.

Incomplete stories is a verbal technique which has been very useful with HIV-infected children (Wiener et al., 1998). When the clinician questions the child about what he or she is thinking, a one-word answer is often produced. Incomplete sentences such as "I wonder if. ..." allows a child to express the thoughts they wonder, worry, and are concerned about in a nonthreatening style. The clinician then has the opportunity to help the child elaborate on selected topics. For example, when two children seen together responded to "I wonder if. ..." with 'if all these thoughts going through my head will ever stop,' the clinician drew a picture of a head and had the two children 'fill the head' with the thoughts (see Fig. 10.3.2).

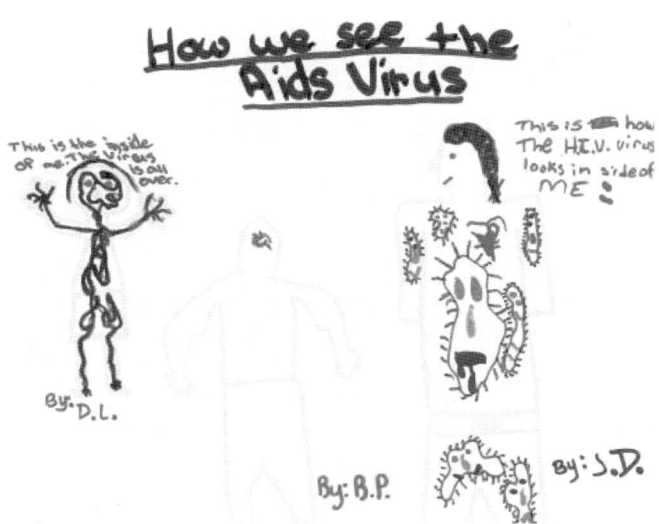

Figure 10.3.1 The external shapes of the bodies are all drawn in yellow. This choice of color as an outline versus the rich colors and much more detailed drawing used in depicting the AIDS virus shows how visible these children feel the AIDS virus is and how exposed (transparency of color of their bodies) they feel. Lack of detail to their physical bodies contrasted to the detail given to the virus shows the feelings of helplessness these children live with facing something over which they have no control. DL, age 10; BP, age 10; JD, age 12.

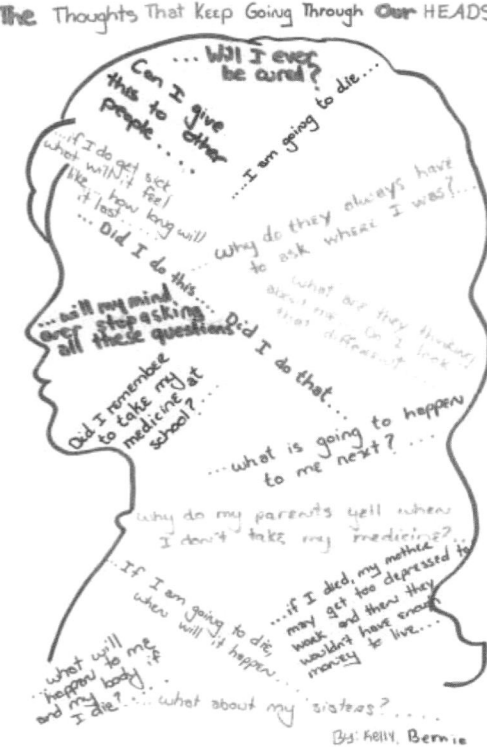

The Thoughts That Keep Going Through Our HEADS

...Will I ever be cured?...

Can I give this to other people...

...I am going to die...

...if I do get sick what will it feel like, how long will it last?...

Did I do this...

why do they always have to ask where I was?...

...what are they thinking... am I a lot different, I think?...

...will my mind ever stop asking all these questions...

Did I do that...

Did I remember to take my medicine at school?...

...what is going to happen to me next?...

why do my parents yell when I don't take my medicine?...

...If I am going to die, when will it happen...

...if I died, my mother may get too depressed to work and then they wouldn't have enough money to live...

what will happen to my body, and my? I die?...

...what about my sisters?...

By: Kelly, Bernie

Figure 10.3.2 Many children find it difficult to verbalize their fears, hopes, or worries. A symbolic silhouette allows children to externalize their inner thoughts—an important step in understanding the concerns that burden them and in beginning the process of communicating about topics which previously felt too frightening to address.

One child, quite concerned about forgetting things, prompted neuropsychological testing and later, a change in therapy.

HIV-infected children have been found to experience separation anxiety (Wiener, Battles, & Riekert, 1999; Riekert, Wiener, & Battles, 1999; Havens et al., 1994). Most frequently, caregivers report their child's difficulties exacerbated at bedtime, specifically in terms of falling asleep. For the more active child, lying down to go to sleep is a time when they begin to reflect on their own disease status, fears associated with not waking up, or the death of a parent. Such periods of anxieties and tension can become associated with bedtime to the point of severe insomnia (Dahl, 1994). These children are usually excellent candidates for several short-term psychotherapy modalities, which can help identify the sources of anxiety and help the child to channel their anxiety in more adaptive ways. Specific interventions will need to be tailormade while taking into consideration the child's age, developmental stage, family circumstances, disease status, the degree of pain or discomfort the child is experiencing, and the caregiver's ability to provide limit-setting and nurturance. Helpful modalities have included more traditional psychodynamic approaches supported with creative interventions at home such as child-made worry boxes, visual imagery, relaxation and hypnosis techniques, and biofeedback. Helping the parent maintain consistent medication and bedtime rituals is also quite helpful. An appropriate differential diagnostic

assessment is a prerequisite to appropriate treatment planning. For those children who experience persistent insomnia, a more comprehensive evaluation for depression is needed. For clinically depressed children or children with other neuropsychiatric problems that influence affect regulation or reality testing, pharmacological support is often indicated. Psychopharmacologic agents must be considered in the context of other signs or symptoms related to manifestations of HIV disease or side effects from antiretroviral therapy. Close monitoring of the child's mood, thought processes, and emotional concerns is essential to a favorable outcome. The potential coexistence of psychopathological and neurological manifestations of HIV can complicate a diagnosis and appropriate treatment decisions, as the following clinical vignette illustrates.

M., a 14-year-old girl with transfusion-acquired HIV, presented to her medical team with frequent crying, withdrawal from peers, poor personal hygiene, notes expressing suicidal ideation, and a refusal to attend school. In response to a significant drop in her absolute T4 cell count, M. had been taken off AZT only two months prior to the development of these symptoms in order to begin a new antiretroviral therapy.

Despite attempts by her physician and psychologist to understand the etiology of M.'s apparent depression, M. continued to refuse to talk about her feelings. It was only after being "bullied" by her mother did M. blurt out "Wait until you see my next MRI. I bet the virus is in my brain."

M. had suffered many recent losses. Her father had recently died of HIV complications. During the final months of his life, he experienced considerable dementia. For several years M. has been part of a peer group consisting of HIV-infected girls at her community hospital. One of the girls had recently died. Another friend had begun refusing to take her medications and had also expressed suicidal thoughts. M. frequently commented, "I feel like my friends and I are all cars on the train and I'm the last one."

Cognitive tests were administered and were found to be unchanged from earlier studies. Computerized tomography (CT) studies revealed no positive findings. M. was diagnosed with clinical depression and psychopharmacological treatment and psychotherapy was begun. While the acute symptoms associated with M.'s depression have lifted, she continues to struggle with the meaning of her life. She requires and receives tremendous support from her family, medical team, school, and community.

SUPPORT GROUPS FOR CAREGIVERS

Almost all caregivers of HIV-infected children have the strong need to talk to others faced with the same life situation. This is especially true for those whose children are neurologically compromised. In addition to general issues related to stigma, disclosure, adherence, and parenting (particularly balancing promoting independence with overprotectiveness), feelings of helplessness, sadness, anger, and anticipatory mourning, along with the impact that the child's increased dependency has on caregivers, are topics frequently addressed in support groups. Within the groups, practical advice regarding specialized services, community resources, national organizations, insurance, and discussion about ways to become actively involved in the child's medical care is common. Caregivers often share telephone numbers and addresses and become available to each other on an as-needed basis. They also share in the joy of a child's improved neurological status and grieve together when deterioration is observed. While group support is not helpful for everyone, and many do not have the time or resources to attend a support group, those who do often report mutual support to be the most useful modality throughout their child's illness.

SUPPORT FOR OTHER CHILDREN IN FAMILIES

The significant effects on the well children in the household have been reported elsewhere. Good psychosocial management takes into account the impact of the HIV-infected child's illness on the well child. Whether or not the diagnosis is revealed to the healthy children in the family, open communication about neurological changes taking place is of great importance. Caregivers should be encouraged at an early stage to acknowledge to their children that the ill child's condition will last forever, though periods of good health and normal family life can be anticipated. If the HIV-infected child should begin to demonstrate behavioral and/or personality changes, including increased hyperactivity or social withdrawal, these need to be honestly discussed as well. Too often, the well children in the family perceive a change in the ill-child's behavior as merely means for additional attention. These children frequently feel "neglected," as they perceive their own needs pale in comparison to those of the rest of the "infected household." They are often burdened with jealousy and, subsequently, experience guilt for escaping the affliction. (Fanos et al., 1994) While some well children wish that they too could be infected and therefore not have to go on living after their parent(s) and sibling(s) die, many others worry that they too will develop neurological symptomatology, such as loss of memory, and then die as a result. The anxiety, guilt, fears, and sadness that these children live with can be overwhelming and the opportunity to express these feelings is essential. The clinician should explore and tap into community-based support groups for children experiencing loss. Several bereavement camp programs include HIV-positive as well as affected family members. Both support groups and camp programs help counteract the loneliness and isolation that these children experience while living under the shadow of their ill family member(s) illness. Moreover, many uninfected siblings were exposed to the same pre- and post-natal environmental stressors that effect cognitive function as their infected siblings. Consequently, they also may be at risk for poor neuropsychiatric outcomes, yet their needs are often ignored or unidentified by services systems (Mellins et al., 2009, 2008).

BEYOND FAMILY SYSTEM

Young children with neurological impairments are likely to have need of specialized services which may not be available in traditional home or day-care settings and which necessitate involvement with a new and confusing array of professional child service providers. This may involve physical and occupational therapy, social work, special education, and other specialties. With the implementation of Public Law 99-457 part H (now housed within the Individual with Disabilities Education Act—IDEA) throughout the United States, most communities have organized systems dedicated to the coordination of special services for infants and toddlers with, or at risk for, disabilities (birth to three years). Caregivers often need assistance accessing this system and obtaining effective advocacy to ensure that their child receives the services that they need in a timely fashion. They may also need assistance in navigating complex bureaucracies in order to obtain necessary services, benefits, or equipment. Approaches that can prove helpful include persistent correspondence with health insurance companies as well as detailed documentation of need. Families should also consider applying to the federal and state programs through their local health department as well as private organizations such as the Shriners and Civitans.

Children and adolescents experiencing static and progressive impairments require attention from the schools. From a curricular standpoint, their needs for individualized education plans may be accommodated through the relatively well-developed special education system within the public schools in the United States. As with all parents with children experiencing academic problems in school, finding the right fit or program at school is typically a high priority. Advocacy from physicians, psychologists, or social workers is often helpful in the process of getting local schools to accommodate the special needs of children.

Children with HIV-associated neurological impairment may need concrete assistance in developing effective social skills and in finding safe opportunities to socialize with peers. Many schools and community mental health agencies offer social skills training programs for children and adolescents. Most areas also have recreation programs and camps that can provide opportunities for socialization with adult supervision. Clinicians should work to develop linkages with these agencies and organizations.

CONCLUSION

Within the pediatric population, developmental delays, loss of milestones, and behavioral/affective changes are often the most concrete and disturbing expression of HIV disease with which families are confronted. Despite HAART, children with perinatally acquired HIV1 infection remain at risk of subsequent brain dysfunction (Tardieu, 2009). The entire spectrum of clinician's skills is required when working within this field. Assessment skills are needed for understanding the family's social, environmental, emotional, and financial history. Diagnostic skills are required for sorting out the indirect and direct effects of the virus on multiple family members. Furthermore, the population of HIV-infected children are typically from impoverished, disenfranchised families who must cope with many other significant environmental stressors and traumas as well as genetic influences that have affected multiple generations that also effect psychosocial function. These children often come from families that have fallen through the safety net of care systems for years, given multigenerational patterns of substance use, poverty, and even mental health problems. Clinical skills are essential for designing individual, family, and group therapeutic modalities that address overall health and development as well as the specific neuropsychological effects of HIV. Families benefit tremendously from the clinician's advocacy skills, especially in terms of linking them with the psychological, social support, educational, and concrete services that the child requires to enhance his or her quality of life.

One cannot underestimate the significant effect that a child's neurocognitive deterioration has on the health care provider. It is not uncommon for providers to feel overwhelmed by the psychosocial, medical, educational, and dependency needs of the families. Gradual changes in a child's appearance or cognitive acuity are difficult to witness, especially when the family is turning to you to "make things better." This work is as existentially challenging as it is emotionally volatile. We inevitably become a very important part of each child and family's life. Despite the inherent sadness and anxiety-provoking nature of this work, it is nevertheless about living and about affirming life (Winiarski, 1991). As every child and family has unique struggles to overcome, each one will teach us a new lesson about ways to live. These are gifts, which are easy to miss amidst the numerous losses. It is up to us to find ways to renew our own strength and energy, so that we can give to each child and family, as we gave to the ones before them. For those who have lost their battle with AIDS, what they were able to do in their short time here will never be forgotten.

REFERENCES

American Academy of Pediatrics (1999). Disclosure of illness status to children and adolescents with HIV infection. American Academy of Pediatrics Committee on Pediatrics AIDS. *Pediatrics, 103,* 164–166.

Armstrong, D., Levy, J., Briery, B., Vazquez, E., Jensen, M., Miloslavich, K., et al. (2002). Merging of neuroscience, psychosocial functioning, and bioethics in pediatric HIV. 110th Annual American Psychological Association, Chicago.

Armstrong, F. D., Seidel, J. F., & Swales, T. P. (1993). Pediatric HIV infection: A neuropsychological and educational challenge. *J Learn Disabil, 26,* 92–103.

Aweeka, F., Jayewardene, A., Staprans, S., Bellibas, S. E., Kearney, B., Lizak, P., et al. (1999). Failure to detect nelfinavir in the cerebrospinal fluid of HIV-1—infected patients with and without AIDS dementia complex. *J Acquir Immune Defic Syndr Hum Retrovirol, 20,* 39–43.

Bagenda, D., Nassali, A., Kalyesubula, I., Sherman, B., Drotar, D., Boivin, M. J., et al. (2006). Health, neurologic, and cognitive status of HIV-infected, long-surviving, and antiretroviral-naive Ugandan children. *Pediatrics, 117,* 729–40.

Belman, A. L. (1990). AIDS and pediatric neurology. *Neurol Clin, 8,* 571–603.

Belman, A. L. (1992). Acquired immunodeficiency syndrome and the child's central nervous system. *Pediatr Clin North Am, 39,* 691–714.

Benjet, C. & Hernandez-Guzman, L. (2001). Gender differences in psychological well-being of Mexican early adolescents. *Adolescence, 36,* 47–65.

Bisiacchi, P. S., Suppiej, A., & Laverda, A. (2000). Neuropsychological evaluation of neurologically asymptomatic HIV-infected children. *Brain Cogn, 43,* 49–52.

Brouwers, P., Belman, A., & Epstein, L. (1994). CNS involvement: Manifestations, evaluation, and pathogenesis. In, P. Pizzo& C. Wilfeet, (Eds.). *Pediatric AIDS: The challenge of HIV infection in infants, children, and adolescents,* 2nd ed. Baltimore: Williams and Wilkins.

Brouwers, P., Moss, H., Wolters, P., Eddy, J., Balis, F., Poplack, D. G., et al. (1990). Effect of continuous-infusion zidovudine therapy on neuropsychologic functioning in children with symptomatic human immunodeficiency virus infection. *J Pediatr, 117,* 980–985.

Chiriboga, C. A, Fleishman, S., Champion, S., Gaye-Robinson, L., & Abrams, E. J.(2005). Incidence and prevalence of HIV encephalopathy in children with HIV infection receiving highly active anti-retroviral therapy (HAART). *J Pediatr, 146,* 402–407.

Cooper, D. A. & Emery, S. (1998). Therapeutic strategies for HIV infection—time to think hard. *N Engl J Med, 339,* 1319–1321.

Cooper, E. R., Hanson, C., Diaz, C., Mendez, H., Abboud, R., Nugent, R., et al. (1998). Encephalopathy and progression of human immunodeficiency virus disease in a cohort of children with perinatally acquired human immunodeficiency virus infection. Women and Infants Transmission Study Group. *J Pediatr, 132,* 808–812.

Coscia, J. M., Christensen, B. K., Henry, R. R., Wallston, K., Radcliffe, J., & Rutstein, R. (2001). Effects of home environment, socioeconomic status, and health status on cognitive functioning in children with HIV-1 infection. *J Pediatr Psychol, 26,* 321–329.

Dahl, R. (1994). Child and adolescent sleep disorders. In D. M. Kaufman, G. E. Solomon, & C. Pfeffer, (Eds.). *Child and adolescent neurology for psychiatrists.* Baltimore: Williams & Wilkins.

Enting, R. H., Prins, J. M., Jurriaans, S., Brinkman, K., Portegies, P., & Lange, J. M. (2001). Concentrations of human immunodeficiency virus type 1 (HIV-1) RNA in cerebrospinal fluid after antiretroviral treatment initiated during primary HIV-1 infection. *Clin Infect Dis, 32,* 1095–1099.

Epstein, L. G., Sharer, L.R., Oleske, J. M., Connor, E. M., Goudsmit, J., Bagdon, L., et al. (1986). Neurologic manifestations of human immunodeficiency virus infection in children. *Pediatrics, 78,* 678–687.

Fanos, J. H. & Wiener, L.(1994). Tomorrow's survivors: Siblings of human immunodeficiency virus-infected children. *J Dev Behav Pediatr, 15,* S43–48.

Funck-Brentano, I. E. A. (1997). Patterns of disclsoure and perceptons of the Human Immunodeficiency Virus in infected elementary school-aged children. *Archives of Pediatric and Adolescent Medicine, 151,* 978–985.

Garcia De Olalla, P., Knobel, H., Carmona, A., Guelar, A., Lopez-Colomes, J. L., & Cayla J. A. (2002). Impact of adherence and highly active antiretroviral therapy on survival in HIV-infected patients. *J Acquir Immune Defic Syndr, 30,* 105–110.

Gaughan, D. M., Hughes, M. D., Oleske, J. M., Malee, K., Gore, C. A., & Nachman, S. (2004). Psychiatric hospitalizations among children and youths with human immunodeficiency virus infection. *Pediatrics, 113,* e544–551.

Gissen, M. & Hagberg. (2001). Antiretroviral treatment of central nervous system HIV-1 infection: A review. *HIV Medicine, 2,* 97–104.

Hamburg, B. A. (1990). *Life skills training: Preventive interventions for young adolescents.* New York: Carnegie Corporation.

Havens, J. F. & Mellins, C. A. (2008). Psychiatric aspects of HIV/AIDS in childhood and adolescence. In M. Rutter, & E. Taylor, (Eds.). *Child and adolescent psychiatry.* 5th ed. Oxford, UK: Blackwell.

Havens, J. F., Whitaker, A. H., Feldman, J. F., & Ehrhardt, A. A. (1994). Psychiatric morbidity in school-age children with congenital human immunodeficiency virus infection: A pilot study. *J Dev Behav Pediatr,* S18–25.

Jeremy, R. J., Kim, S., Nozyce, M., Nachman, S., Mcintosh, K., Pelton, S. I., et al. (2005). Neuropsychological functioning and viral load in stable antiretroviral therapy-experienced HIV-infected children. *Pediatrics, 115*, 380–387.

Lipson, M. (1994). Disclosure of diagnosis to children with human immunodeficiency virus or acquired immunodeficiency syndrome. *J Dev Behav Pediatr, 15*, S61–65.

Lobato, M. N., Caldwell, M. B., Ng, P., & Oxtoby, M. J. (1995). Encephalopathy in children with perinatally acquired human immunodeficiency virus infection. Pediatric Spectrum of Disease Clinical Consortium. *J Pediatr, 126*, 710–715.

Lourie, K. J., Pao, M., Brown, L. K., & Hunter, H. (2005). Psychiatric issues in pediatric HIV/AIDS. In K. Citron, M. J. Brouillette, & A. Beckett (Eds.). *HIV and psychiatry. A training and resource manual.* 2nd ed. Cambridge: Cambridge University Press.

Mckinney, R. E., Jr., Maha, M. A., Connor, E. M., Feinberg, J., Scott, G. B., Wulfsohn, M., et al. (1991). A multicenter trial of oral zidovudine in children with advanced human immunodeficiency virus disease. The Protocol 043 Study Group. *N Engl J Med, 324*, 1018–1025.

Mellins, C., Brackis-Cott, E., Dolezal, C., Richards, A., Nicholas, S. W., & Abrams, E. J. (2002). Patterns of HIV status disclosure to perinatally HIV-infected children and subsequent mental health outcomes. *Clinical Child Psycholgy and Psychiatry, 7*, 101–114.

Mellins, C. A., Brackis-Cott, E., Dolezal, C., & Abrams, E. J. .(2006). Psychiatric disorders in youth with perinatally acquired human immunodeficiency virus infection. *Pediatr Infect Dis J, 25*, 432–437.

Mellins, C. A., Brackis-Cott, E., Dolezal, C., Leu, C. S., Valentin, C., & Meyer-Bahlburg, H. F. (2008). Mental health of early adolescents from high-risk neighborhoods: The role of maternal HIV and other contextual, self-regulation, and family factors. *J Pediatr Psychol, 33*, 1065–1075.

Mellins, C. A., Brackis-Cott, E., Leu, C. S., Elkington, K. S., Dolezal, C., Wiznia, A., et al. (2009). Rates and types of psychiatric disorders in perinatally human immunodeficiency virus-infected youth and seroreverters. *J Child Psychol Psychiatry, 50*, 1131–1138.

Mintz, M. (1994). Clinical comparison of adult and pediatric NeuroAIDS. *Adv Neuroimmunol, 4*, 207–221.

Mintz, M. (1999). Clinical features and treatment interventions for human immunodeficiency virus-associated neurologic disease in children. *Semin Neurol, 19*, 165–176.

Misdrahi, D., Vila, G., Funk-Brentano, I., Tardieu, M., Blanche, S., & Mouren-Simeoni, M. C. (2004). DSM-IV mental disorders and neurological complications in children and adolescents with human immunodeficiency virus type 1 infection (HIV-1). *Eur Psychiatry, 19*, 182–184.

Mitchell, W. (2001). Neurological and developmental effects of HIV and AIDS in children and adolescents. *Ment Retard Dev Disabil Res Rev, 7*, 211–216.

Moss, H. A., Brouwers, P., Wolters, P. L., Wiener, L., Hersh, S., & Pizzo, P. A. (1994). The development of a Q-sort behavioral rating procedure for pediatric HIV patients. *J Pediatr Psychol, 19*, 27–46.

Moss, H. A., Wolters, P. L., Brouwers, P., Hendricks, M. L., & Pizzo, P. A. (1996). Impairment of expressive behavior in pediatric HIV-infected patients with evidence of CNS disease. *J Pediatr Psychol, 21*, 379–400.

Nozyce, M. L., Lee, S. S., Wiznia, A., Nachman, S., Mofenson, L. M., Smith, M. E., et al. (2006). A behavioral and cognitive profile of clinically stable HIV-infected children. *Pediatrics, 117*, 763–770.

Pao, M., Lyon, M., D'Angelo, L. J., Schuman, W. B., Tipnis, T., & Mrazek, D. A. (2000). Psychiatric diagnoses in adolescents seropositive for the human immunodeficiency virus. *Arch Pediatr Adolesc Med, 154*, 240–244.

Pao, M. & Wiener, L. (2008). Children and Adolescents. In M. A. Cohen & J. M. Gorman (Eds.). *Comprehensive textbook of AIDS psychiatry.* New York: Oxford University Press.

Pizzo, P. A. (1989). Emerging concepts in the treatment of HIV infection in children. *Jama, 262*, 1989–1992.

Pizzo, P. A., Eddy, J., Falloon, J., Balis, F. M., Murphy, R. F., Moss, H., et al. (1988). Effect of continuous intravenous infusion of zidovudine (AZT) in children with symptomatic HIV infection. *N Engl J Med, 319*, 889–896.

Rice, E., Batterham, P., & Rotheram-Borus, M. J. (2006). Unprotected sex among youth living with HIV before and after the advent of highly active antiretroviral therapy. *Perspect Sex Reprod Health, 38*, 162–167.

Riekert, K., Wiener, L., & Battles, H. (1999). Prediction of psychological distress in school-age children with HIV. *Children's Health Care, 28* (3), 201–220.

Sanmaneechai, O., Puthanakit, T., Louthrenoo, O., & Sirisanthana, V. (2005). Growth, developmental, and behavioral outcomes of HIV-affected preschool children in Thailand. *J Med Assoc Thai, 88*, 1873–1879.

Scharko, A. M. (2006). DSM psychiatric disorders in the context of pediatric HIV/AIDS. *AIDS Care, 18*, 441–445.

Schrager, L. K. & D'souza, M. P. (1998). Cellular and anatomical reservoirs of HIV-1 in patients receiving potent antiretroviral combination therapy. *Jama, 280*, 67–71.

Shanbhag, M. C., Rutstein, R. M., Zaoutis, T., Zhao, H., Chao, D., & Radcliffe, J. (2005). Neurocognitive functioning in pediatric human immunodeficiency virus infection: Effects of combined therapy. *Arch Pediatr Adolesc Med, 159*, 651–656.

Simpson, D. M. & Berger, J. R. (1996). Neurologic manifestations of HIV infection. *Med Clin North Am, 80*, 1363–1394.

Smith, B. A. & Shuchman, M. (2005). Problem of nonadherence in chronically ill adolescents: Strategies for assessment and intervention. *Current Opinion In Pediatrics, 17*, 613–618.

Smith, R., Malee, K., Leighty, R., Brouwers, P., Mellins, C., Hittelman, J., et al. (2006). Effects of perinatal HIV infection and associated risk factors on cognitive development among young children. *Pediatrics, 117*, 851–862.

Smith, R. J. (2006). Adherence to antiretroviral HIV drugs: How many doses can you miss before resistance emerges?. *Proc Biol Sci, 273*, 617–624.

Sonza, S. & Crowe, S. M. (2001). Reservoirs for HIV infection and their persistence in the face of undetectable viral load. *AIDS Patient Care STDS, 15*, 511–518.

Swindells, S., Zheng, J., & Gendelman, H. E. (1999). HIV-associated dementia: New insights into disease pathogenesis and therapeutic interventions. *AIDS Patient Care STDS, 13*, 153–163.

Tardieu, M. (2009). The risk of very long-term brain dysfunction in treated adolescents with perinatally acquired HIV-1 infection. *Aids, 23*, 1891–1892.

Tardieu, M., Le Chenadec, J., Persoz, A., Meyer, L., Blanche, S., & Mayaux, M. J. (2000). HIV-1-related encephalopathy in infants compared with children and adults. French Pediatric HIV Infection Study and the SEROCO Group. *Neurology, 54*, 1089–1095.

Taylor-Brown, S. & Wiener, L. (1993). Making Videotapes of HIV-Infected women for their children. *Families in Society, 74*, 468–480.

Thompson, P. M., Dutton, R. A., Hayashi, K. M., Toga, A. W., Lopez, O. L., Aizenstein, H. J., et al. (2005). Thinning of the cerebral cortex visualized in HIV/AIDS reflects CD4+ T lymphocyte decline. *Proc Natl Acad Sci U S A, 102*, 15647–15652.

Ultmann, M. H., Diamond, G. W., Ruff, H. A., Belman, A. L., Novick, B. E., Rubinstein, A., et al. (1987). Developmental abnormalities in children with acquired immunodeficiency syndrome (AIDS): A follow-up study. *Int J Neurosci, 32*, 661–667.

Watkins, J. M., Brouwers, P., & Huntzinger, R. (1992). Neuropsychological Assessmen. In M. Stuber, (Ed.). *Children and AIDS*. Washington, DC: American Psychiatric Press.

Wiener, L., Battles, H., Ryder, C., & Pao, M. (2006a). Psychotropic medication use in HIV-infected youth receiving treatment at a single institution. *Journal of Child and Adolescent Psychopharmacology, 16*(6), 747–753.

Wiener, L., Battles, & Riekert, K. A. (1999). Longitudinal study of psychological distress symptoms in HIV-infected, school-aged children. *Journal of HIV/AIDS Prevention and Education for Adolescents and Children, 3*, 13–36.

Wiener, L. & Figueroa, V. (1998). Children speaking with children and families about HIV infection. In P. A. Pizzo & C. M. Wilfert (Eds.). *Pediatric AIDS: The challenge of HIV infection in infants, children, and adolescents*. 3rd ed. Baltimore: Williams & Wilkins.

Wiener, L. & Lyons, M. (2006b). HIV Disclosure: Who knows? Who needs to know? Clinical and ethical considerations. In L. D'Angelo & M. Lyons (Eds.). (no city) *Teenagers and AIDS*.

Wiener, L., Mellins, C. A., Marhefka, S., & Battles, H. B. (2007). Disclosure of an HIV diagnosis to children: History, current research, and future directions. *J Dev Behav Pediatr, 28*, 155–166.

Wiener, L. & Taylor-Brown, S. (2010). The impact of HIV on children and adolescents. Inn C. C. Poindexter (Ed.). *Handbook of HIV and social work*. Hoboken: John Wiley & Sons.

Wiener, L. S., Battles, H. B., & Heilman, N. E. (1998). Factors associated with parents' decision to disclose their HIV diagnosis to their children. *Child Welfare, 77*, 115–135.

Wiener, L. S., Battles, H. B., & Wood, L. V. (2007). A longitudinal study of adolescents with perinatally or transfusion acquired HIV infection: Sexual knowledge, risk reduction self-efficacy and sexual behavior. *AIDS Behav, 11*, 471–478.

Willen, E. J. (2006). Neurocognitive outcomes in pediatric HIV. *Ment Retard Dev Disabil Res Rev, 12*, 223–228.

Wingood, G. M., Diclemente, R. J., Harrington, K., & Davies, S. L. (2002). Body image and African American females' sexual health. *J Womens Health Gend Based Med, 11*, 433–439.

Winiarski, M. (1991). *AIDS Related psychotherapy*, New York: Pergamon Press.

Wolters, P. & Brouwers, P. (2005). Neurobehavioral function and assessment of children and adolescents with HIV-1 infection. In S. Zeichner & J. S. Read (Eds.). *Textbook of pediatric care*. Cambridge: Cambridge University Press.

Wood, S. M., Shah, S. S., Steenhoff, A. P., & Rutstein, R. M. (2009). The impact of AIDS diagnoses on long-term neurocognitive and psychiatric outcomes of surviving adolescents with perinatally acquired HIV. *AIDS, 23*, 1859–1865.

10.4

GROWING UP WITH HIV DISEASE

Shirley F. Delair, Leslie K. Serchuck, and Lynnae Schwartz

In the US and other resource-rich countries, there are two distinct populations of HIV-1-infected youths: those who grew up with the disease after having been infected through maternal-to-child transmission and adolescents newly infected through participation in high-risk behaviors. Each of these groups faces unique challenges, as well as the shared burden of struggling to mature into fully independent and productive adults in the face of a serious disease. Of major concern for both groups is the cumulative central nervous system effects of HIV-1 in the brain, the possibly disease-amplifying effects of stress that are inherent in living with HIV, adverse reactions to medications, and the burdens of chronic illness. This chapter focuses on challenges confronting these young people, highlighting what is known about how HIV-1 disease impacts the individual's transition into full adulthood.

INTRODUCTION

Pediatric HIV-1 infection acquired through maternal-to-child transmission (MTCT) is a global health concern posing unique challenges to young patients, their families, and society. In the US and other resource-rich countries, there are now two distinct populations of HIV-1-infected youths: aging-up vertically infected through maternal-to-child transmission (MTCT), and adolescents newly infected through adult high-risk behaviors. Despite overlapping ages (adolescence to early adulthood), each group faces unique challenges incurred by their HIV status, as well as the shared burdens of maturing into fully independent and productive adulthood. Of major concern for both groups are the cumulative central nervous system (CNS) effects of HIV-1 in the brain, the possibly disease-amplifying negative effects of stress inherent in living with HIV, adverse reactions to medications, and the burdens of chronic illness.

MTCT-infected children with disease responsive to combination antiretroviral therapies (cART) are entering adolescence and early adulthood after what may be a lifetime exposure to multiple potent medications. Although HAART and CNS-penetrating antiretroviral regimens have dramatically reduced the incidence of HIV-encephalopathy (Patel et al., 2009), the developmental, neurocognitive, and psychiatric consequences of sustained CNS and immune system exposure to cART are incompletely understood. It is also

likely that HIV entry into the CNS occurs with initial infection. It is doubtful that this early wave of CNS virus is fully cleared from the CNS by immune mechanisms, and accumulating evidence from SIV (simian immunodeficiency virus) models and human cohorts suggests that a predominantly latent infection of brain microglia and astrocytes is established, with low-grade, chronically upregulated expression of multiple proinflammatory molecules (Zink et al., 2010). This, more so than cART exposure, may exert a significant negative effect on neurocognition, attentional capacity, mood and affect that, in combination or alone, compromises the maturing youth's capacity to thrive as a fully independent adult.

Although the duration of exposure to cART and the effects of CNS viral entry are considerably shorter for adolescents who are HIV+ through adult behaviors, neural network maturation is not yet complete. The consequences of HIV-associated inflammation, cART, and CNS viral load in youths at this stage of brain development are incompletely understood, but are unlikely to be nil. Demographic studies suggest that the majority of newly infected youth are infected through men who have sex with men (MSM) in the context of additional risk behaviors, including the use of illicit substances, for example, club drugs, and sex with multiple partners (Jennings et al., 2009; Barnes et al., 2010; Sill, Constantine, Wilson, & Peralta, 2010). This set of behaviors may increase the risk of acquiring resistant disease, and amplify adverse CNS responses to infection.

Finally, both MTCT youths and adolescents with adult high-risk behavior acquired HIV-1 disease are confronted with the responsibilities and burdens imposed by their diagnosis. The goal of this chapter is to review the challenges confronting these youths, highlighting what is known about how HIV-1 disease impacts their transition into full adulthood. A comprehensive review of the medical challenges facing youths growing up with HIV has recently been published (Hazra, Siberry, & Mofenson, 2010).

EPIDEMIOLOGY

According to UNAIDS, at the end of 2007 an estimated 2 million children under age 15 were infected and living with HIV/AIDS throughout the world, with 370,000 newly infected each year and 270,000 annual pediatric deaths due to AIDS (Joint United Nations Program on HIV/AIDS, 2008).

The advent of effective cART in pregnant women and revised standards for prenatal HIV testing (opt-out versus opt-in) has dramatically reduced the risk and incidence of new perinatal infection in resource-rich countries (Patel et al., 2008; Foster et al., 2009; Brady et al., 2010), although the residual risk is not zero. Centers for Disease Control (CDC) data for the US through 2008 suggest that the identified number of new cases of vertically acquired HIV-1 infection is 150 cases per year or less (34 in 2008) (CDC, 2011). Contrariwise, larger numbers of newly infected adolescents and youths under 24 years of age are being identified, especially through venue-based rapid testing (Barnes et al., 2010).

In the US, as of the end of 2007, approximately 15,500 adolescents between the ages of 13–19 years old (34 states reporting) were living with a diagnosis of HIV or AIDS, including an estimated 8,500 vertically infected youths progressing through adolescence and young adulthood (Hazra et al., 2010).

QUALITY OF LIFE

The quality of life of children with chronic diseases and that of their families/primary caregivers is unavoidably affected by their health condition, even if optimally stabilized with the best available care and social supports. This may be especially true for HIV-affected families in urban America confronting multiple major life stressors (Mellins & Ehrhardt, 1994).

Pediatric AIDS Clinical Trials Group (PACTG) 219C data through 2003, reported in 2006, suggest that primary caregiver perceptions of quality of life for HIV+ infected children up to 11 years of age was lower in HIV+ than for HIV uninfected. Perinatally exposed and HIV+ infected adolescents not on antiretroviral therapies (ART) were judged by the caregivers to have poorer health status than those on ART (Lee, Gortmaker, McIntosh, Hughes, & Oleske, 2006). The children and adolescents themselves were not queried in this survey, but they were in pain data reported from PAGTG 1055. In the HIV+ cohort, primary caregivers perceived their child to have less pain affecting activities of daily life than the youths themselves reported (Serchuck et al., 2010). Key to interpreting this data is an appreciation that "pain" can be a representational construct, symbolizing for the patient or caregiver an impression as to how life in a more general way is experienced. Taken together, these reports and the larger literature on pain and coping in pediatric patients with chronic disease (Boekaerts & Röder, 1999) suggest that living with HIV-1 disease impinges on quality of life for the infected youths to an extent that may be underestimated by their primary caregivers. That noted, there are also data to suggest that HIV+ youths and their families exhibit psychosocial resilience and stability (New, Lee, & Elliott, 2007) exceeding that of uninfected comparison cohorts (Bachanas et al., 2001; Serchuck et al., 2010).

COMPLIANCE WITH MEDICAL MANAGEMENT

Adherence is a challenge in the management of pediatric HIV. Infants and the younger child depend on parents for administration of their medication. Parents themselves must be reliable and stable in order to manage multiple medications and overcome the poor palatability of current pediatric formulation of cART. For aging-up youth, multiple factors affect patient compliance with recommended medical management regimens to control HIV-1 disease, especially in youths coping with the many challenges and turbulences of adolescence. While transitioning more responsibility for medication and health maintenance to the maturing young person is the goal, the most effective time and way to do this for HIV+ youth has not been defined.

Additionally, fatigue and declining health amongst aging primary caregivers who stepped in to care for the young child after the biological parents were unable to do so due to HIV-related and other illness and death may severely limit their ability to assure compliance in the now maturing youth striving for independence and testing boundaries. This burden of care is even more so for aging caregivers of youths with neurocognitive or psychiatric issues, as the caregivers face the reality that their now maturing child will need ongoing support for far longer than initially anticipated.

Demographic factors in particular need to be considered for youths newly infected in adolescence through adult behaviors, where parental ties may be deeply strained, especially for youths infected through MSM. The youth may effectively be an emancipated minor, living outside of parental control and/or parental capacity to assure compliance with any aspect of medical management or recommendations concerning risk mitigation. Mental health and behavioral issues may limit the youth's willingness or capacity to utilize social and mental health services regardless of outreach initiatives and efforts to maximize access (Marhefka et al., 2009). Data from the Adolescent Trials Network for HIV/AIDS Interventions suggest that HIV+ youths with concomitant emotional distress report significantly less adherence to cART, and more substance abuse and unprotected sex (Nugent et al., 2010). Much research is needed to determine optimal ways to reach and support these young people. To that end, reports on the experience of community-based centers of care targeting this vulnerable population of youths are very much needed.

Economic constraints are an additional and critical factor in compliance, as limited state and federal resources may be insufficient to cover the costs of medications, clinic care, supportive social services, and other fundamentals of stable living essential for compliance with medical regimens of some complexity.

THE ETHICS AND CHALLENGE OF DISCLOSURE

HIV status disclosure is perhaps the most challenging dilemma for aging-up as well as newly infected youths, their primary caretakers, family members, and health care providers. It is a topic that provokes much controversy and emotion. The consequences of disclosure are feared, even though the risks of nondisclosure to the health of the HIV+ youth and others (e.g., if the HIV+ adolescent indulges in unsafe behaviors) are clear and fearful unto themselves. For adolescents, the dilemma of disclosure epitomizes their developmental position pivoting between the burdens of responsible adulthood and a still-maturing capacity for complex decision-making and impulse control.

In most instances in which conflict occurs, the problem is not simply resolved by amassing objective evidence of the "right" medical choice for the child. Rather, the conflict is generally a result of differing values and perceptions of what is in the best interests of that child. Family dynamics including cultural and religious differences and fear of stigmatization and discrimination may further complicate the issue. Research has shown that parents' decisions to disclose are affected by their fears about the emotional consequences of disclosure for the child, as well as their fears about the child's anger towards the parent, and the potential social consequences associated with the child sharing the diagnosis with others, including ostracism; negative reactions from family, friends, and school; and lack of community support (Waugh, 2003; Klitzman, Marhefka, Mellins, & Wiener, 2008). There are also issues of "super confidentiality," because HIV+ status disclosure for a child vertically infected necessarily discloses maternal infection with HIV.

The perspective of U.S. health care providers may differ considerably from that of primary caregivers and family members of the HIV+ youth, based in part on the health care provider's perspective that children of advancing age and mental competence have the capacity to participate in decisions central to their health, and should therefore be given age-appropriate information about their disease and treatments. Some would even question the ethics of withholding information concerning the youth's diagnosis, feeling that withholding such information unfairly hinders the aging-up child's ability to make sense of their illness-related experiences. For children in clinical trials where the minimum age of assent is 7 years, these ethical concerns extend to the completeness of consent to participate in research that is nontherapeutic (Barfield & Kane, 2008).

Support for this point of view amongst health care providers comes from broadly accepted paradigms of normal human development, including the rule of sevens, which has served as a legal criterion for centuries and is instantiated in the practices of religions and current assent and consent practices in medicine and research. The rule of sevens divides a young person's life into three sections: birth to seven, seven to fourteen, and fourteen to twenty-one years old. Prior to about seven years old, children lack the cognitive development required for autonomous decision making. At the age of seven, children are considered to have the capacity to distinguish right from wrong. Fourteen is the age at which adolescents are considered accountable for their actions: both legally and socially. But in MTCT HIV disease, the subtle but nevertheless potentially capacity-changing consequences

of long-standing CNS exposure to HIV -1 and/or CNS-penetrating cART have to be taken into account (Hazra et al., 2010), as does mental health status which may or may not be directly linked to HIV-1 disease (Mellins et al., 2003; Mellins et al., 2009; Chernoff et al., 2009; Gadow 2010; Williams et al., 2010).

There are currently no laws in any US state that make it punishable for a clinician to disclose the disease status to an HIV+ infected patient, including a minor. However, disclosure to a minor of his/her infection status without parental permission may damage the relationship between the parent/legal guardian and the child, parent and physician, and potentially physician and child (LaFleur, 2008). A related question is whether or not a parent/legal guardian has the legal right to withhold their child's HIV infection status from him or her. On the whole, the law assumes that parents will act in the best interests of the child and thus laws may be interpreted to support a parent's decision regarding disclosure. The Supreme Court of the United States has established that the Due Process Clause of the Fourteenth Amendment protects "the fundamental right of parents to make decisions concerning the care, custody, and control of their children" (*Troxel v Granville*, 2000). Supported by this decision, parents have the right to make decisions regarding the care of their children, including medical care and diagnosis disclosure, as long as the decision made is informed and in the child's best interest, even if others might take exception to how "best interest" is defined.

The potential conflict over disclosure between parents and caregivers may be particularly heightened for HIV+ youth infected through adult acquired behaviors, and for aging-up vertically infected with loosening ties to their primary caregiver, but who are still less than 18 years of age. Some may qualify for status as an "emancipated minor," defined as those who are 1) self-supporting and/or not living at home; 2) married; 3) pregnant or a parent; 4) in the military; or 5) declared to be emancipated by a court. Additionally, many states give decision-making authority (without the need for parental involvement) to some minors who are otherwise unemancipated but who have decision-making capacity ("mature minors") or who are seeking treatment for certain medical conditions, such as sexually transmitted diseases, pregnancy, and drug or alcohol abuse. The situations in which minors are deemed to be totally or partially emancipated are defined by statute and case law and may vary from state to state. These are situations that pertain to some numbers of aging-up vertically infected and adolescents with behavior-acquired disease.

A recommendation favoring age-appropriate disclosure was issued by the American Academy of Pediatrics based on limited studies suggesting that children informed of their diagnosis had higher self-esteem, and parents who disclosed had less depression (Committee on Pediatric AIDS, 1999). The impact of disclosure of HIV+ status on perception of health, physical and social functioning, psychological status, and symptom distress was examined in 395 subjects enrolled in PACTG 219C. The study population used in the analysis was restricted to perinatally

HIV+ children at least 5 years of age participating in PACTG 219C between September 2000 and December 2005; the median age of disclosure was 11 years of age. Subjects were followed for 36 months prior to and after disclosure. Interestingly, no statistically significant difference was noted for any of the quality of life domains other than a post-disclosure decline in physical functioning, which likely reflected advancing disease in an aging cohort (Butler et al., 2009).

Data supportive of disclosure comes from a pilot study cohort of HIV+ youth in Puerto Rico, which showed that youths informed of their diagnosis had improved feelings of normalcy and better adherence to recommended therapies compared to their pre-disclosure status (Blasini et al., 2004). A retrospective study of Romanian youth identified an increased association between CD4 decline and death in children unaware of their diagnosis compared to those informed of their status (Ferris et al., 2007). The consensus of opinion amongst physicians and health care providers working with HIV+ youth appears to favor age-appropriate disclosure despite the confounding concerns, including concomitant disclosure of maternal HIV+ status in MTCT.

SEXUALITY, RISKS, AND PREGNANCY

Questions of sexual identity, risk tolerance, and social acceptance loom large for both perinatally infected youths aging-up into adolescence and early adulthood and those infected through adult behaviors. In contrast to their uninfected peers, these issues are unavoidably linked to risk imposed on others, including sexual partners and, with pregnancy, the resultant infant. A failure to act responsibly, regardless of whether the risky behavior is a result of HIV effects on neurocognitive and psychological functioning or not, carries potentially life-changing and even deadly consequences for others unlike any imposed by chronic diseases such as cancer or diabetes in aging-up youth. A confounding factor is the fact that many youths whose behaviors place their sexual and drug-sharing partners at higher risk of infection appear to be unengaged with traditional health care, social service, and mental health outreach venues, and even if engaged, risk-engendered behaviors may not be curtailed.

Fears that the incidence of pregnancy in adolescent and young adult women HIV+ through vertical transmission are rising, are based on CDC statistics for risk behaviors and sexual activity amongst adolescents participating in anonymized surveys and abstracted medical records data (Jennings et al., 2009; Koenig et al., 2010). Analysis of data from PACTG 219C yielded first pregnancy rates amongst perinatally infected adolescent females in that cohort of 18.8 per 1000 person-years, with additional pregnancies in 7 of 38 (Brogly et al., 2007). The actual U.S. incidence of pregnancy in MTCT adolescents is unknown because reporting such pregnancies to a central registry (http://www.apregistry.com/patient.htm) is voluntary.

ACADEMIC CHALLENGES AND PRODUCTIVE INDEPENDENT LIVING

Although cART has dramatically reduced the incidence of acute progressive HIV encephalopathy in all populations of HIV+ children and young adults, there remains a deep concern, supported to some extent by both the clinical and basic science literature, that the maturing CNS is nevertheless at risk for neuronal loss with decrements in neurocognitive capacity, especially for children who received a Class C (AIDS) diagnosis earlier in life prior to disease stabilization on cART (Wood, Shah, Steenhoff, & Rutstein, 2009). There are also data to suggest that HIV+ children with stable disease have lower developmental and cognitive scores than established age- and gender-matched childhood normative values (Nozyce et al., 2006). If confirmed in longitudinal cohort studies, these findings identify a critically important area of concern and potential obstacle to full independence.

A related question is whether functional neurocognitive domains in aging-up vertically infected youths differ from their HIV-negative community peers. Concisely summarizing an extensive literature more fully reviewed elsewhere in this set of chapters, for younger children the answer may be that cognitive performance does not appear to differ significantly between the three groups: HIV exposed but uninfected, HIV negative and never exposed, and HIV+ living in similar communities with otherwise comparable life circumstances. It remains to be determined if this holds true through adolescence and young adulthood, where academics and the need to acquire independent life management skills converge to demand more sophisticated memory acquisition, comprehension, and computational ability. Research in this area is critically needed.

CONCLUSIONS

Youths HIV+ from MTCT or through adult high-risk behaviors face many challenges in their transition towards adulthood, made all the more difficult because of HIV-1-associated CNS effects on the maturing brain, social and economic pressures, and the complex demands of managing a chronic illness safely.

REFERENCES

http://www.cdc.gov/hiv/topics/surveillance/basic.htm#hivest

Bachanas, P. J., Kullgren, K. A., Schwartz, K. S., Lanier, B., McDaniel, J. S., Smith, J., et al. (2001). Predictors of psychological adjustment in school-age children infected with HIV. J Pediatric Psychology, 26(6), 343–352.

Barfield, R. C. & Kane, J. R. (2008). Balancing disclosure of diagnosis and assent for research in children with HIV. JAMA, 300(5), 576–578.

Barnes, W., D'Angelo, L., Yamazaki, M., Belzer, M., Schroeder, S., Palmer-Castor, J., et al. (2010). Identification of HIV-infected 12–24 year old men and women in 15 US cities through venue-based testing. Archives Pediatric Adolescent Medicine, 164(3), 273–276.

Blasini, I., Chantry, C., Cruz, C., Ortiz, L., Salabarria, I., Sacalley, N., et al. (2004). Disclosure model for pediatric patients living with HIV in Puerto Rico. *Journal of Developmental and Behavioral Pediatrics*, 25(3), 181–189.

Boekaerts, M. & Röder, I. (1999). Stress, coping, and adjustment in children with a chronic disease: A review of the literature. *Disability and Rehabilitation*, 21(7), 311–337.

Brady, M.T., Oleske, J. M., Williams, P. L., Elgie, C., Mofenson, L. M., Danker, W. M., et al. For the Pediatric AIDS Clinical Trials Group 219/219C Team. (2010). Declines in mortality rates and changes in causes of death in HIV-1-infected children during the HAART era. *J Acquired Immune Deficiency Syndromes*, 53(1), 86–94.

Brogly, S. B., Watts, D. H., Ylitalo, N., Franco, E. L., Seage, G. R. 3rd, Oleske, J., et al. (2007). Reproductive health of adolescent girls perinatally infected with HIV. *American J Public Health*, 97(6), 1047–1052.

Butler, A. M., Williams, P. L., Howland, L. C., Storm, D., Hutton, N., & Seage, G. R., 3rd for the Pediatric AIDS Clinical Trials Group 219C Study Team. (2009). Impact of disclosure of HIV infection on health-related quality of life among children and adolescents with HIV infection. *Pediatrics*, 123 (3), 935–943.

Centers for Disease Control and Prevention. HIV/AIDS Surveillance in Adolescents and Young Adults (through 2007) slide set. http://www.cdc.gov/hiv/topics/surveillance/resources/slides/adolescents/index.htm

Centers for Disease Control and Prevention. *HIV Surveillance Report, 2009*; vol. 21. http://www.cdc.gov/hiv/topics/surveillance/resources/reports/. Published February 2011. Accessed March 28, 2011.

Chernoff, M., Nachman, S., Williams, P., Brouwers, P., Heston, J., Hodge, J., et al. for the IMPAACT P1055 Study Team. (2009). Mental health treatment patterns in perinatally HIV-infected youth and controls. *Pediatrics*, 124(2), 627–636.

Committee on Pediatric AIDS, America Academy of Pediatrics. (1999). Disclosure of illness status to children and adolescents with HIV infection. *Pediatrics*, 103(1), 164–166.

Federal Interagency Forum on Child and Family Statistics. (2008). *America's children in brief: Key national indicators of well-being, (2008)*. Available at: http://www.childstats.gov/americaschildren/

Ferris, M., Burau, K., Schweitzer, A. M., Mihale, S., Murray, N., Preda, A., et al. (2007). The influence of disclosure of HIV diagnosis on time to disease progression in a cohort of Romanian children and teens. *AIDS Care*, 19(9), 1088–1094.

Flanagan-Klygis, E., Ross, L. F., Lantos, J., Frader, J., & Yogev, R. (2001). Disclosing the diagnosis of HIV in pediatrics. *J Clinical Ethics*, 12(2), 150–157.

Foster, C., Judd, A., Tookey, P., Tudor-Williams, G., Dunn, D., Shingadia D, et al. on behalf of the Collaborative HIV Paediatric Study (CHIPS). (2009). Young people in the United Kingdom and Ireland with perinatally acquired HIV: The pediatric legacy for adult services. *AIDS Patient Care and STDs*, 23(3), 159–166.

Funck-Bretano, I., Costagliola, D., Seibel, N., Straub, E., Tardieu, M., & Blanche, S. (1997). Patterns of disclosure and perceptions of the human immunodeficiency virus in infected elementary school-age children. *Archives Pediatric Adolescent Medicine*, 151(10), 978–985.

Gadow, K. D., Chernoff, M., Williams, P. L., Brouwers, P., Morse, E., Heston, J., et al. (2010). Co-occuring psychiatric symptoms in children perinatally infected with HIV and peer comparison sample. *J Developmental Behavioral Pediatrics*, 31(2), 116–128.

Hazra, R., Siberry, G. K., & Mofenson, L. M. (2010). Growing up with HIV: Children, adolescents, and young adults with perinatally acquired HIV infection. *Annual Review of Medicine*, 61, 169–185.

Jennings, J. M., Ellen, J. M., Deeds, B. G., Harris, R., Muenz, L. R., Barnes, W., et al. for the Adolescent Trials Network for HIV/AIDS Interventions. (2009). Youth living with HIV and partner-specific risk for the secondary transmission of HIV. *Sexually Transmitted Diseases*, 36(7), 439–444.

Joint United Nations Programme on HIV/AIDS. (2008). *Report on the global AIDS epidemic*. UNAIDS, Geneva: p33. http://www.unaids.org/en/KnowledgeCentre/HIVData/GlobalReport/(2008)/(2008)_Global_report.asp

Klitzman, R., Marhefka, S., Mellins, C., & Wiener, L. (2008). Ethical issues concerning disclosures of HIV diagnoses to perinatally infected children and adolescents. *J Clinical Ethics*, 19(1), 31–42.

Koenig, L. J., Pais, S. L., Chandwani, S., Hodge, K., Abramowitz, S., Barnes, W., et al. (2010). Sexual transmission risk behavior of adolescents with HIV acquired perinatally or -through risky behaviors. *J Acquired Immune Deficiency Diseases*, 55(3), 380–90.

LaFleur, S. (2008). Legal questions can arise when treating HIV-infected minors. *HIV Clinician*, 20(3), 7–8.

Lee, G. M., Gortmaker, S. L., McIntosh, K., Hughes, M. D., & Oleske, J. M. for the Pediatrics AIDS Clinical Trials Group Protocol 219C Team. (2006). Quality of life for children and adolescents: Impact of HIV infection and antiretroviral treatment. *Pediatrics*, 117(2), 273–283.

Lipson, M. (1993).What do you say to a child with AIDS? *Hastings Center Report*, 23(2), 6–12.

Lipson, M. (1994). Disclosure of diagnosis to children with human immunodeficiency virus or acquired immunodeficiency syndrome. *J Developmental Behavioral Pediatrics*, 15(3), S61–S65.

Mellins, C. A. & Ehthardt, A. A. (1994). Families affected by pediatric acquired immunodeficiency syndrome: Sources of stress and coping. *Journal of Developmental Behavioral Pediatrics*, 15(3), S54–S60.

Mellins, C. A., Smith, R., O'Driscoll, P., Magder, L. S., Brouwers, P., Chase, C., et al. for the Women and Infant Transmission Study Group (2003). High rates of behavioral problems in perinatally HIV-infected children are not linked to HIV disease. *Pediatrics*, 111(2), 384–393.

Mellins, C. A., Brackis-Cott, E., Leu, C-S., Elkington, K. S., Dolezal, C., Wiznia, A, et al. (2009). Rates and types of psychiatric disorders in perinatally human immunodeficiency virus-infected youth and seroreverters. *J Child Psychology Psychiatry*, 50(9), 1131–1138.

Marhefka, S. L., Lyon, M., Koenig, L. J., Orban, L., Stein, R., Lewis, J., et al. (2009). Emotional and behavioral problems and mental health service utilization of youth living with HIV acquired perinatally or later in life. *AIDS Care*, 21(11), 1447–1454.

New, M. J., Lee, S. S., & Elliott, B. M. (2007). Psychological adjustment in children and families living with HIV. *J Pediatric Psychology*, 32(2), 123–131.

Nozyce, M. L., Lee, S. S., Wiznia, A., Nachman, S., Mofenson, L. M., Smith, M. .E, et al. (2006). A behavioral and cognitive profile of clinically stable HIV-infected children. *Pediatrics*, 117(3), 763–770.

Nugent, N. R., Brown, L. K., Belzer, M., Harper, G.W., Nachman, S., & Naar-King, S. for the Adolescent Trials Network for HIV/AIDS Interventions. (2010). Youth living with HIV and problem substance use: Elevated distress is associated with nonadherence and sexual risk. *J International Association Physicians AIDS Care*, 9(2), 113–115.

Patel, K., Hernan, M. A., Williams, P. L., Seeger, J. D., McIntosh, K., Van Dyke, R. B., et al., for the Pediatric AIDS Clinical Trials Group 219/219C Study Team. (2008). Long-term effectiveness of highly active antiretroviral therapy on the survival of children and adolescents with HIV infection: A 10-year follow-up study. *Clinical Infectious Diseases*, 46, 507–515.

Patel, K., Ming, X., Williams, P. L., Robertson, K. R., Oleske, J. M., & Seage,G.R. 3rd and the International Maternal Pediatric Adolescent AIDS Clinical Trials 219/219C Study Team. (2009). Impact of HAART and CNS-penetrating antiretroviral regimens on HIV encephalopathy among perinatally infected children and adolescents. *AIDS*, 23(14), 1893–1901.

Serchuck, L. K., Williams, P. L., Nachman, S., Gadow, K. D., Chernoff, M., & Schwartz, L. for the IMPAACT 1055 Team. (2010). Prevalence of pain and association with psychiatric symptom severity in perinatally HIV-infected children as compared to controls living in HIV-affected households. *AIDS Care*, 22(5), 640–648.

Sill, A. M., Constantine, N. T., Wilson, C. M., & Peralta, L. for the Adolescent Trials Network for HIV/AIDS Interventions. (2010). Demographic profiles of newly acquired HIV infections among adolescents and young adults in the US. *J Adolescent Health*, 46, 93–96.

Smith, R., Malee, K., Leighty, R., Brouwers, R., Mellins, C., Hittleman, J., et al. for the Women and Infants Transmission Study Group. (2006). Effects of perinatal HIV infection and the associated risk factors on cognitive development among young children. *Pediatrics, 117*(3), 851–862.

Troxel v. *Granville*, (2000). 530 U.S. 57, 66, 120 S.Ct. 2054, 2060.

Waugh, S. (2003). Parental views on disclosure of diagnosis to their HIV-positive children. *AIDS Care, 15*(2), 169–176.

Williams, P. L., Marino, M., Malee, K., Brogly, S., Hughes, M. D., & Mofenson, L. M. for the PACTG 219C Team. (2010). Neurodevelopment and in utero antiretroviral exposure of HIV-exposed uninfected infants. *Pediatrics, 125*(2), e250–e260. DOI: 10.1542/peds.2009-1112.

Williams, P. L., Leister, E., Chernoff, M., Nachman, S., Morse, E., Di Poalo, V., et al. for IMPAACT 1055 Team. (2010). Substance use and its association with psychiatric symptoms in perinatally HIV-infected and HIV-affected adolescents. *AIDS Behavior, 14*(5), 1072–82.

Wood, S. M., Shah, S. S., Steenhoff, A. P., & Rutstein, R. M. (2009). The impact of AIDS diagnosis on long-term neurocognitive and psychiatric outcomes of surviving adolescents with perinatally acquired HIV. *AIDS, 23*, 1859–1865.

Zink, M. C., Brice, A. K., Kelly, K. M., Queen, S. E., Gama, L., Li, M., et al. (2010). Simian Immunodeficiency Virus-infected macaques treated with highly active antiretroviral therapy have reduced central nervous system viral replication and inflammation but persistence of viral DNA. *J Infectious Diseases, 202*(1), 161–170.

SECTION 11

ANTIRETROVIRAL AND ADJUNCTIVE THERAPIES

Susan Swindells

11.1

CURRENT CONCEPTS IN THE TREATMENT OF HIV INFECTION WITH FOCUS ON BRAIN DISEASE

Susan Swindells and Uriel Sandkovsky

Over the last few years, guidelines for initiation of antiretroviral therapy (ART) have evolved with a trend towards starting therapy at earlier stages of disease and initiation of therapy is now recommended for all patients with CD4 counts of less than 350 cells/mm³ by the World Health Organization and less than 500 cells/mm³ by US guideline committees. This change was largely driven by results of randomized and observational clinical trials demonstrating benefit from early initiation of therapy, the availability of newer and more tolerable drugs, and a marked decrease in pill burden. HIV viremia of > 100,000 copies/mL and a decrease of more than 100 CD4 cell counts in one year are also included in the consideration to start therapy earlier. The presence of hepatitis B and C co-infections, high risk for cardiovascular disease, and/or the presence of HIV-associated nephropathy also warrant special attention since controlling HIV replication improves outcomes. Specialist expertise is recommended to assess the potential risks and benefits of specific decisions about the management of HIV diseases, preferably in the context of a multidisciplinary team.

Current principles of treatment are outlined in this chapter, with particular emphasis on issues relevant to nervous system disease. For additional information and updates, readers are referred to the HIV/AIDS Treatment Information Service at http://www.aidsinfo.nih.gov/.

EVALUATION OF THE HIV-INFECTED PATIENT

The laboratory diagnosis of HIV infection is made by demonstration of antibodies against HIV. In addition to the conventional serum enzyme-linked immunoabsorbent assay (ELISA), there are now several rapid diagnostic tests available that can be performed on blood or oral fluids and some can also be performed on fingerstick samples. A positive screening test must be confirmed by a Western blot, indirect immunofluorescence assay or a second rapid test using different methodology. During the initial visit, a comprehensive medical history that includes detailed HIV-related information and a complete physical examination should be obtained, including an assessment for ongoing depression or other psychiatric disorder. The best approach to patient care is attained with a multidisciplinary team that includes social workers, case managers, nurses, and

physicians among others. Recommended baseline laboratory tests include a complete blood count; full chemistry profile including fasting glucose; liver function tests; lipid profile; and hepatitis A, B, and C and syphilis serology. Consider also testing for antibodies to *Toxoplasma gondii*. Each patient should be assessed for possible *Mycobacterium tuberculosis* (MTB) infection by either a tuberculin skin test or an interferon-γ release assay. Screening for the presence of other sexually transmitted diseases (STDs) should also be done.

The evaluation required to guide decisions regarding antiretroviral therapy (ARV) includes assessment of the clinical, virological, and immunological status of the patient. A baseline neurological examination should also include assessment of cognitive function, described elsewhere in this textbook. Monitoring CD4+ T cell counts and plasma HIV RNA (viral load) provide essential information about risk of disease progression and should be performed at the time of diagnosis and at least every 3 to 6 months thereafter.

Testing for resistance to antiretroviral agents is now considered an essential tool to guide antiretroviral therapy. Current guidelines recommend resistance testing at baseline, either during acute HIV infection or at the time of diagnosis, and in the event of virologic failure or suboptimal suppression of plasma viremia on therapy (Panel on Antiretroviral Guidelines for Adults and Adolescents, 2011; Hirsch et al., 2008). Clinical trials have shown benefit when resistance testing was used to guide antiretroviral drug selection, especially when compared to clinical judgment alone (Meynard et al., 2002; Vray et al., 2003; Palella et al., 2009).

Resistance may be assessed by genotyping assays, which detect key mutations in HIV reverse transcriptase, protease, and more recently integrase genes, or by phenotyping, which quantitates the ability of a patient's virus to grow in different concentrations of antiretroviral drugs. A tropism assay to assess whether the virus uses CCR5 or CXCR4 co-receptors or both (dual-tropic virus) to enter the cells is also available and recommended before using CCR5 receptor antagonists.

Currently available resistance-testing assays are not always readily available and are expensive. The usual turnaround time is about 1–2 weeks for genotype and 3 weeks for phenotype, tropism, or integrase assays (Panel on Antiretroviral Guidelines for Adults and Adolescents, 2011; Hirsch et al., 2008; Kuritzkes et al., 2008; Little et al., 2002; Weinstock et al., 2004; Whitcomb et al., 2007; Fransen et al., 2008).

Relevant evaluations to assess patients for risk of opportunistic diseases and other comorbid conditions should also be performed and chemoprophylaxis initiated when appropriate (Kaplan et al., 2009). Female patients should undergo gynecological examination including Papanicolaou smear at least annually and mammography after age 50 (Aberg et al., 2009). Males should be screened for hypogonadism if there is evidence of bone mineral loss or when symptoms of fatigue, weight loss, and decreased libido are present. Bone mineral density should be assessed in women 65 years or older, or any patient male or female over 50 years old who has one or more risk factors for premature bone loss. All patients should undergo screening for colon cancer after the age of 50.

WHEN SHOULD ANTIRETROVIRAL THERAPY BE INITIATED?

The goals of ART are maximal and durable suppression of viral load, restoration and/or preservation of immune function, improvement in quality of life, reduction in morbidity and mortality, and prevention of HIV transmission (Panel on Antiretroviral Guidelines for Adults and Adolescents, 2011). Preservation of future treatment options should also be considered when making decisions about when to start therapy and in choosing a regimen. Decisions regarding starting therapy are largely based on CD4+ T cell count thresholds, although higher viral load has been shown to increase risk of disease progression and should be considered, especially when the level exceeds 100,000 copies/mL (Panel on Antiretroviral Guidelines for Adults and Adolescents, 2011; Thompson et al., 2010; Egger et al., 2002; When To Start Consortium

et al., 2009). Although some cohort studies have shown that plasma viremia tends to be lower in women than in men with early HIV disease, rates of disease progression do not differ by gender and there are no gender-specific recommendations (Farzadegan et al., 1998; Collazos, Asensi, & Carton, 2007).

Current guidelines recommend treatment for all patients with symptomatic HIV disease or acquired immunodeficiency syndrome (AIDS), and for asymptomatic patients with CD4+ T cell counts < 350 cells/mm^3 (Table 11.1.1). There is strong evidence to support improved survival and delay of disease progression when therapy is started with CD4 counts < 200 cells/mm^3. The CIPRA HT-001 trial conducted in Haiti was stopped prematurely when higher mortality and more incident tuberculosis were observed among patients who deferred therapy to CD4 counts < 200 cells/mm^3 or developed an AIDS-defining condition, compared with patients with treatment at CD4 count of 200–350 cells/mm^3. A subgroup analysis of 249 participants in the SMART study also showed a trend to lower risk of serious AIDS- and non-AIDS-related events in individuals who initiated ART immediately, compared with those who deferred therapy until the CD4 count dropped to < 250 cells/mm^3. Death was four times more common in the latter group; however, the number of events was small (6 and 21 respectively) (Strategies for Management of Antiretroviral Therapy (SMART) Study Group et al., 2006; Severe, Pape, & Fitzgerald, 2009). The ART cohort collaboration (ART-CC) showed a 1.4 times increased risk of death for patients initiating ART at CD4 counts between 200–350 compared to those who initiated therapy at CD4 > 350 cells/mm^3 (May et al., 2007). These and other studies have led to the recommendation to start ART at higher CD4 levels (WHO ART Guideline Groups and Committee, 2009; Panel on

Table 11.1.1 RECOMMENDATIONS FOR INITIATION OF ANTIRETROVIRAL THERAPY IN CHRONICALLY INFECTED PATIENTS

CLINICAL CATEGORY	CD4+ T-CELL COUNT	PLASMA HIV RNA	DHHS 2011	IAS USA 2010	WHO 2009
Symptomatic	Any	Any	Treat	Treat	Treat
Asymptomatic	< 200/mm^3	Any	Treat	Treat	Treat
Asymptomatic	200–350/mm^3	Any	Treat	Treat	Treat
Asymptomatic	350–500/mm^3	Any	Treat	Treat	Not included
Asymptomatic	> 500/mm^3	Any	Optional	Consider	Not included
Asymptomatic	Any	>100,000 copies/mL	Treat	Treat	Not included
Asymptomatic	CD4 decline rate > 100/cells per year	Any	Treat	Treat	Not included
Hepatitis B co-infection	Any CD4	Any	Treat	Treat	Treat
HIVAN	Any CD4	Any	Treat	Treat	Not Included
Pregnancy	Any CD4	Any	Treat	Treat	Treat
Tuberculosis co-infection	<200/mm^3 200–350/mm^3 >350/mm^3	Any	Start within 2 weeks Start after 8 weeks Start after 8–24 weeks	Not included	Treat Treat Treat but limited data to support

HIVAN: HIV-associated nephropathy.

Antiretroviral Guidelines for Adults and Adolescents, 2011; Thompson et al., 2010).

Current DHHS guidelines have divided recommendations on initiating ART when the CD4 count is above 350 CD4 cells/mm³. Initiation of therapy at CD4 counts between 350–500 cells/mm³ was strongly supported by more than half of the panel and moderately supported by the rest. Current IAS-USA 2010 guidelines recommend starting therapy at these CD4 count levels. There are currently no data from prospective randomized studies to address this question. Nevertheless, there are several observational studies that provide accumulating evidence to support the initiation of ART with CD4 counts > 350 cells/mm³. Deferring therapy until the 251 to 350 cells/mm³ range is associated with a higher rate of progression to AIDS and mortality when compared with initiating therapy in the 351 to 450 cells/mm³ range (When To Start Consortium et al., 2009; May et al., 2007). In the North American cohort study (NA-ACCORD), there was an increased risk of death in patients who deferred therapy until CD4 count < 350 cells/mm³ compared with patients who initiated therapy with CD4 count between 351 and 500 cells/mm³. The NA-ACCORD study also showed increased mortality in patients who deferred therapy to CD4 levels below 500 cells/mm³ in contrast to findings from the ART-CC (Kitahata et al., 2009).

The neurological complications that may accompany uncontrolled HIV replication and CD4 depletion suggest a potential benefit of earlier initiation of ART. In the CASCADE cohort, there was a marked decline in the incidence of HIV-associated dementia when the periods before and after the use of potent ART were compared. The lowest risk for development of HIV-associated dementia was observed in patients whose CD4 counts were above 350 cells/mm³ (Bhaskaran et al., 2008; Hardy & Vance, 2009; Ellis et al., 2010). Additional clinical data are needed to better define the relative roles of ongoing HIV replication, potential neurotoxicity of antiretroviral agents and importance of CSF penetrance in the development of HIV-related nervous system disease.

Previous concerns about the negative impact of ART on quality of life, accompanying serious adverse effects, and the risk of development of viral resistance have decreased since the availability of tolerable regimens with significantly lower pill burden. Although the guidelines outline preferred and alternative treatment regimens, treatment should always be individualized based on such factors as immune status, viral load, baseline resistance testing, potential toxicities and risk factors for their development, comorbid conditions, concomitant medications, and psychosocial factors such as the patients' commitment and potential to adhere to therapy. Potential risks and benefits of early versus late initiation of ART are outlined in Table 11.1.2.

OTHER INDICATIONS FOR ANTIRETROVIRAL THERAPY

In addition to chronic HIV disease, ART is indicated for patients with hepatitis B co-infection and HIV-associated nephropathy (HIVAN), and during pregnancy to decrease risk of mother-to-child transmission (MTCT) (Perinatal HIV Guidelines Working Group, 2009). Patients with hepatitis C co-infection are at risk of accelerated progression to liver fibrosis and cirrhosis with CD4 counts < 350 cells/mm³; restoring immune function with earlier initiation of antiretroviral therapy may slow this process. Current guidelines recommend starting ART in HIV/HCV co-infection according to the recommendation for ART-naïve patients (Panel on Antiretroviral Guidelines for Adults and Adolescents, 2011). Management of HIV-infected pregnant women is outside the scope of this chapter, but current guidelines can be found at http://aidsinfo.nih.gov/ContentFiles/PerinatalGL.pdf. ART plays an important role in post-exposure prophylaxis; recommendations can also be found at the Department of Health and Human Services (DHHS) website and include algorithms for risk assessment for both occupational and non-occupational settings. A one-month course of combination ART is generally recommended for high-risk exposures. Emerging data also support the use of antiretroviral agents for pre-exposure prophylaxis in high-risk populations (Brown et al., 2010; Baeten et al., 2010). An intravaginal gel

Table 11.1.2 POTENTIAL RISKS AND BENEFITS OF EARLY VERSUS LATE INITIATION OF ANTIRETROVIRAL THERAPY

EARLY		LATE	
Benefits	*Risks*	*Benefits*	*Risks*
Control of viral replication easier to achieve/maintain	Drug-related reduction in quality of life	Avoid negative impact on quality of life	Possible greater difficulty in suppressing viral replication
Delay or prevention of immunodeficiency	Greater cumulative drug-related adverse events including metabolic and cardiovascular disease	Avoid drug-related adverse events	Possible risk of immune system depletion and persistent immune activation
Lower risk of drug resistance	Increased cost, development of drug resistance	Delay in development of drug resistance	
Decreased risk of HIV transmission	Non-adherence to therapy and limitation of future treatment options	Preserve maximum number of options when risk of disease progression is highest	Possible increased risk of HIV transmission

formulation of tenofovir used with sexual activity conferred 39% protection in unifected women in a recent randomized clinical trial in South Africa, discussed in more detail below (Abdool Karim Q et al., 2010). Similar levels of protection were seen in a trial of uninfected men who have sex with men and took oral tenofovir daily (Grant et al., 2010). This strategy is further being evaluated with several ongoing trials worldwide. There strategies may facilitate "treatment as prevention," a new concept with the aim of treating high risk populations in order to decrease the transmission of HIV (Panel on Antiretroviral Guidelines for Adults and Adolescents, 2011). Management considerations for HIV-infected children are discussed elsewhere in this book.

ACUTE HIV INFECTION

At least 50%, and perhaps as much as 90%, of persons will experience symptoms several days to several weeks after primary infection. Often overlooked by patients and clinicians, when diagnosed correctly, patients will benefit from a correct diagnosis during this stage of HIV disease. As HIV-1 invades the CNS soon after infection, symptoms may also appear that are consistent with aseptic meningitis. Typically monophasic and self-limiting, such symptoms include headache, fever, malaise, lymphadenopathy, pharyngitis, and rash (Kinloch-de Loes et al., 1993). Acute myopathy, neuritis or neuropathy, Bell's palsy, and Guillain-Barre syndrome have been described. HIV-antibody testing may be negative or indeterminate; therefore, plasma HIV RNA is the preferred method of diagnosis (Aberg et al., 2009). Data from clinical trials to inform decisions about treatment of primary HIV disease are limited and inconclusive. Theoretically, early intervention may decrease the severity of acute disease, potentially alter the viral set point, preserve immune function, and decrease the risk of transmission (Lafeuillade et al., 1997; Lillo et al., 1999; Malhotra et al., 2000; Smith et al., 2004). Recommendations for specific regimens are similar to those for established infection with the caveat that clinically significant resistance to protease inhibitors (PI) is less common than resistance to NNRTIs in naïve patients; therefore, a PI-based regimen is preferred until drug-resistance test results are available. The duration of therapy is more controversial in the setting of acute HIV infection and patients should be counseled on the potential need for lifelong treatment.

CHOICE OF INITIAL THERAPY

DHHS guidelines outline preferred, alternative, and acceptable regimens, which are for the most part based on data obtained from randomized clinical trials. Standard care includes combination therapy with at least three agents, and multiple combinations are possible. The choice of specific drugs should be individualized, taking into account tolerability, adverse effect profiles, dosing intervals, food requirements, and potential drug-drug interactions. Preferred regimens include two nucleoside reverse transcriptase inhibitors (NRTI) with a protease inhibitor (PI) or nonnucleoside reverse transcriptase inhibitors (NNRTI) or an integrase strand transfer inhibitor (INSTI). Table 11.1.3 outlines currently licensed antiretroviral agents with preferred and alternative regimens, and compares DHHS, International Antiviral Society (IAS)-USA, and World Health Organization (WHO) guidelines. Triple NRTI therapy is virologically inferior and is not recommended, especially for patients with viral loads in excess of 100,000 copies/mL or more advanced disease (Gulick et al., 2004).

Characteristics of specific agents are listed in Table 11.1.4. Adherence to therapy is a critical factor for treatment success (Paterson et al., 2000). Several studies have shown that less frequent dosing intervals are associated with better adherence, and once-daily dosing of antiretroviral agents has now become common practice (Panel on Antiretroviral Guidelines for Adults and Adolescents, 2011; Stone et al., 2001; Rosenbach, Allison, & Nadler, 2002; Nilsson Schonnesson et al., 2007). Fixed dose combinations of NRTIs are widely available. In 2006, the first fixed dose combination antiretroviral tablet containing tenofovir, emtricitabine, and efavirenz was licensed in the United States, permitting triple therapy with one pill once a day (Abramowicz, 2006). The use of ritonavir to pharmacologically enhance (boost) other protease inhibitors by inhibition of cytochrome p450 enzymes has allowed less frequent dosing of currently used protease inhibitors, also decreasing gastrointestinal side effects (Murphy et al., 2001; Flexner, 2000; Gathe et al., 2009; Mills et al., 2009). Special food requirements may be minimized by this strategy. Novel antiretroviral boosters without antiviral activity against HIV are in development and will be potential alternatives to the use of ritonavir (Mathias et al., 2010).

SHOULD CNS PENETRANCE BE CONSIDERED?

Since the early days of the AIDS epidemic, HIV has been identified in the brain parenchyma and was quickly assumed to be the cause of the AIDS dementia complex. Widespread use of potent combination ART has resulted in marked declines in the incidence and prevalence of neurological complications of HIV disease (Schmitt et al., 1988; Ferrando et al., 1998; Sacktor et al., 1999; Robertson et al., 2004). However, there are patients in whom neurologic impairment continues despite successful viral suppression, suggesting ongoing neuronal injury (Kaul, 2009; Boisse, Gill, & Power, 2008; Liner, Hall, & Robertson, 2008; Letendre et al., 2004; Robertson et al., 2007; Simioni et al., 2009). Some investigators believe that antiretroviral drugs with better CSF penetration might be more effective for the prevention and treatment of HIV-associated cognitive dysfunction (McArthur, Sacktor, & Selnes, 1999; Letendre et al., 2008; Koopmans et al., 2009). Observational data showed equivalent benefits on the reversal of neurocognitive deficits for antiretroviral regimens with different predicted CSF penetration (Sacktor et al., 2001). However, improvement in HIV-related brain disease has been demonstrated from antiretroviral regimens with poor CSF

Table 11.1.3 COMPARISON OF ANTIRETROVIRAL REGIMENS RECOMMENDATIONS AMONG DHHS, IAS-USA, AND WHO (*FOR COMPLETE RECOMMENDATIONS, READERS ARE REFERRED TO THE SOURCE DOCUMENTS.*)

	DHHS 2011	IAS-USA 2010	WHO 2009
Preferred	TDF/FTC plus one of the following: EFV ATV/r DRV/r RAL Pregnant women: ZDV/3TC + LPV/r	TDF/FTC plus one of the following: EFV DRV/r ATV/r RAL	TDF or ZDV + FTC or 3TC plus one of the following: EFV or NVP
Alternative	(ABC or ZDV)/3TC + EFV ZDV/3TC + NVP ATV/r + (ABC or ZDV)/3TC FPV/r + TDF/FTC FPV/r + (ZDV or ABC)/3TC LPV/r + (ABC or ZDV)/3TC LPV/r + TDF/FTC	ABC/3TC Plus EFV or DRV/r or ATV/r or LPV/r or FPV/r or MVC	2 NRTI (as in preferred regimens) Plus LPV/r or ATV/r
Acceptable	EFV + ddI + (FTC or 3TC) ATV or DRV/r + (ABC or ZDV)/3TC RAL + (ABC or ZDV)/3TC MVC + ZDV/3TC MVC + TDF/FTC or ABC/3TC	ZDV/3TC/ABC + TDF in special circumstances.	
Not recommended	ZDV/3TC/ABC ZDV/3TC/ABC + TDF	Maraviroc-based PI monotherapy	

ZDV: zidovudine; 3TC: lamivudine; FTC: emtricitabine; TDF: tenofovir disoproxil fumarate; ABC: abacavir; ddI: didanosine; EFV: efavirenz; NVP: nevirapine; ATV: atazanavir; DRV: darunavir; FPV: fosamprenavir; LPV: lopinavir; MVC: maraviroc; SQV: saquinavir; RAL: raltegravir. (r) = ritonavir used as a pharmacologic booster. In the United States TDF/FTC: Truvada®; ABC/3TC: Epzicom®; ZDV/3TC: Combivir®; TDF/FTC and ZDV/3TC are available as generic drugs in some developing countries.
PI: protease inhibitor.

Table 11.1.4 CHARACTERISTICS OF ANTIRETROVIRAL AGENTS

NUCLEOSIDE/NUCLEOTIDE REVERSE TRANSCRIPTASE INHIBITORS (NRTIs)

Generic/Brand Name	How Supplied	Usual Adult Dose	Food Effect	Elimination
Abacavir (ABC)/ Ziagen	300 mg tablets or 20 mg/ mL oral solution	300 mg b.i.d. or 600 mg daily	None	Metabolized by alcohol dehydrogenase and glucuronyl transferase; 82% renal excretion of metabolites
Atripla (TDF/FTC/ EFV)	Combination tablet	1 tablet at or before bedtime	Take on an empty stomach to reduce side effects	As for individual ingredients
Combivir (ZDV/3TC)	Fixed-dose combination tablet	1 b.i.d.	None	As for individual ingredients
Didanosine (ddI)/ Videx-EC (enteric coated capsules) [Buffered tablets are no longer available]	125 mg, 200 mg, 250 mg, or 400 mg enteric coated capsules 10 mg/mL oral solution	Body weight ≥ 60 kg: 400 mg once daily*; with TDF, 250 mg once daily Body weight < 60 kg: 250 mg once daily*; with TDF, 200 mg once daily *Preferred dosing with oral solution is b.i.d.	Take 1/2 hour before or 2 hours after meals	Renal excretion, 50%
Emtricitabine (FTC) / Emtriva	200 mg hard gelatin capsule or 10 mg/mL oral solution	200 mg capsule once daily or 240 mg (24 mL) oral solution once daily	None	Renal excretion 86%. Adjustment necessary in renal failure.
Epzicom (ABC/3TC)	Fixed-dose combination tablet	1 daily	None	As for individual ingredients

(*Continues*)

Table 11.1.4 CHARACTERISTICS OF ANTIRETROVIRAL AGENTS (CONTINUED)

NUCLEOSIDE/NUCLEOTIDE REVERSE TRANSCRIPTASE INHIBITORS (NRTIS)

Generic/Brand Name	How Supplied	Usual Adult Dose	Food Effect	Elimination
Lamivudine(3TC)/ Epivir	150, 300 mg tablets or 10 mg/mL oral solution	150 mg b.i.d. Or 300 mg daily	None	Renal excretion 70% unchanged
Stavudine (d4T)/Zerit	15, 20, 30, 40 mg capsules or 1 mg/mL oral solution	Body weight ≥60 kg: 40 mg b.i.d. Body weight <60 kg: 30 mg b.i.d.* *WHO recommends 30 mg b.i.d. regardless of body weight	None	Renal excretion, 50%
Tenofovir disoproxil fumarate (TDF)/Viread	300 mg tablets	300 mg daily	Increased bioavailability when taken with food	Renal excretion
Trizivir (ZDV/3TC/ ABC)	Fixed-dose combination tablet	1 b.i.d.	None	As for individual ingredients
Truvada (TDF/FTC)	Fixed-dose combination tablet	1 daily	None	As for individual ingredients
Zidovudine (ZDV) or azidothymidine (AZT)/ Retrovir	100 mg capsules, 300 mg tablets or 10 mg/ mL intravenous solution	200 mg t.i.d. or 300 mg b.i.d.	None	Metabolized to azidothymidine glucuronide; renal excretion of glucuronide

NONNUCLEOSIDE REVERSE TRANSCRIPTASE INHIBITORS (NNRTIS)

Generic/Brand Name	How Supplied for Adults	Usual Adult Dose	Food Effect	Elimination
Delavirdine (DLV) Rescriptor	100 mg tablets or 200 mg tablets	400 mg t.i.d.	None	Metabolized by cytochrome P450 (3A4 substrate and inhibitor); 51% excreted in urine, 44% in feces
Efavirenz (EFV)/ Sustiva	50 mg, 200 mg capsules or 600 mg tablets	600 mg qhs	Take on an empty stomach	Metabolized by CYPs 2B6 and 3A4 CYP3A4 mixed inducer/ inhibitor (more an inducer than an inhibitor) 14–34% excreted in urine, 16–61% in feces
Rilpivirine (TMC278)/ Edurant.	25 mg tablets	25 mg daily Take with food	Metabolized by CYP3A4 85% excreted in feces.	6% urine
Etravirine (ETR)/ Intelence	100 or 200 mg tablets	200 mg b.i.d	Take following a meal	CYP3A4, 2C9, and 2C19 substrate 3A4 inducer; 2C9 and 2C19 inhibitor
Nevirapine (NVP)/ Viramune	200 mg tablets or 50 mg/ 5 mL of oral suspension	200 mg q day for 14 days then 200 mg b.i.d.	None	Metabolized by cytochrome P450 and 3A inducer; 80% excreted in urine (glucuronidated metabolites, <5% unchanged); 10% in feces

PROTEASE INHIBITORS (PIs)

Generic/Brand Name	How Supplied for Adults	Usual Adult Dose	Food Effect	Elimination
Atazanavir (ATV)/ Reyataz	100, 150, 200, 300 mg capsules	ARV-naïve patients: 400 mg once daily or ATV 300 mg + RTV 100 mg once daily. With TDF or for ARV-experienced patients: ATV 300 mg + RTV 100 mg once daily. With EFV in treatment-naïve patients: ATV 400 mg + RTV 100 mg once daily		CYP3A4 inhibitor and substrate Dosage adjustment in hepatic insufficiency recommended

(Continues)

Table 11.1.4 (CONTINUED)

PROTEASE INHIBITORS (PIS)

Generic/Brand Name	How Supplied for Adults	Usual Adult Dose	Food Effect	Elimination
Darunavir (DRV)/ Prezista	75, 150, 400, 600 mg tablets	ARV-naïve patients: DRV 800 mg + RTV 100 mg daily ARV-experienced patients: DRV 600 mg + RTV 100 mg b.i.d Unboosted DRV is **not** recommended	Take without regard to meals.	Cytochrome P450 (3A4 inhibitor and substrate)
Fosamprenavir (FPV)/ Lexiva	700 mg tablet or 50 mg/ mL oral suspension	FPV 1,400 mg b.i.d. or FPV 1,400 mg + RTV 100–200 mg once daily FPV 700 mg + RTV 100 mg b.i.d. Once-daily dosing **not** recommended for PI-experienced pts With EFV: FPV 700 mg + RTV 100 mg BID or FPV 1,400 mg + RTV 300 mg	May be taken with or without food	Cytochrome P450 3A4 substrate, inducer and inhibitor
Indinavir (IDV)/ Crixivan	200 mg, 333 mg, 400 mg capsules	800 mg q 8 hours With RTV: IDV 800 mg + RTV 100–200 mg b.i.d.	Take 1 hour before or 2 hours after meals With RTV: without regard to meals	Cytochrome P450 (3A4 inhibitor and substrate) Dosage adjustment in hepatic insufficiency
Lopinavir + ritonavir (LPV/r)/Kaletra	LPV 200 mg + RTV 50 mg or LPV 100 mg + RTV 25 mg tablets Oral solution: 5 mL contains LPV 400 mg + RTV 100 mg (contains 42% alcohol)	400 mg LPV + 100 mg RTV b.i.d. or 800 mg LPV/200 mg RTV daily (4 tablets). Once daily only for PI-naïve, not for PI-experienced, pregnant women, or patients receiving NNRTIs With EFV or NVP: LPV/r 500 mg/125 mg tablets b.i.d. (use a combination of two LPV/r 200 mg/50 mg tablets + one LPV/r 100 mg/25 mg tablet to make a total dose of LPV/r 500 mg/125 mg) or LPV/r 533 mg/133 mg oral solution b.i.d.	Tablet: Take without regard to meals Oral solution: Take with food	Cytochrome P450 3A4 inhibitor and substrate
Nelfinavir (NFV)/ Viracept	250 mg, 625 mg tablets or 50 mg/g oral powder	750 mg t.i.d. or 1250 mg b.i.d.	Take with food	Cytochrome P450 CYP2C19 and 3A4 substrate metabolized to active M8 metabolite; 3A4 inhibitor
Ritonavir (RTV)/ Norvir	100 mg capsules or tablets 80 mg/mL oralsolution	As pharmacokinetic booster for other PIs: 100–400 mg per day in 1–2 divided doses	Take with food	Cytochrome P450 3A4 >2D6; potent 3A4, 2D6 inhibitor
Saquinavir (SQV)/ Invirase	500 mg tablets or 200 mg capsules	(SQV 1,000 mg + RTV 100 mg) b.i.d Unboosted SQV is **not** recommended.	Take within 2 hours after a meal	Cytochrome P450 3A4 inhibitor and substrate
Tipranavir (TPV)/ Aptivus	250 mg capsules or 100 mg/mL oral solution	TPV 500 mg + RTV 200 mg PO b.i.d. Unboosted TPV is **not** recommended.	Take without regard to meals	Cytochrome P450 3A4 inducer and substrate Net effect when combined with RTV: CYP 3A4, 2D6 inhibitor

(*Continues*)

Table 11.1.4 CHARACTERISTICS OF ANTIRETROVIRAL AGENTS (CONTINUED)

FUSION INHIBITORS

Generic/Brand Name	How Supplied for Adults	Usual Adult Dose	Food Effect	Elimination
Enfuvirtide (T20)/ Fuzeon	Injectable, supplied as lyophilized powder. Approximately 90 mg/mL when reconstituted	90 mg (1 mL) subcutaneously b.i.d.	Not applicable	Catabolism to its constituent amino acids, with subsequent recycling of the amino acids in the body

CCR5 INHIBITORS

Maraviroc (MVC)/ Selzentry	150, 300 mg tablets	150 mg b.i.d. when given with strong CYP3A inhibitors (with or without CYP3A inducers) including PIs (except TPV/r) 300 mg b.i.d. when given with NRTIs, T-20, TPV/r, NVP, and other drugs that are not strong CYP3A inhibitors or inducers 600 mg b.i.d. when given with CYP3A inducers, including EFV, ETR, etc.	Take without regard to meals	Cytochrome P450 3A4 substrate

INSTIS (INTEGRASE STRAND TRANSFER INHIBITORS)

Raltegravir (RAL)/ Isentress	400 mg tablets	400 mg b.i.d. With rifampin: 800 mg b.i.d.	Take without regard to meals	UGT1A1-mediated glucuronidation

penetrance, suggesting that antiretroviral effects in the periphery, for example, on monocyte trafficking or levels of pro-inflammatory cytokines, may be key issues in the treatment of HIV-associated neurological complications (Gendelman et al., 1998; Ryan et al., 2001; Fischer-Smith et al., 2008; Yadav & Collman, 2009). More recent observational data derived from the National NeuroAIDS Tissue Consortium (NNTC) showed the same prevalence of parenchymal brain disease among patients that were treated with NRTIs and PIs; however, the risk of parenchymal brain pathology was halved in patients exposed to NNRTIs (Everall et al., 2009).

The physiology of antiretroviral penetration in the CSF is complex and depends on several factors such as the molecular characteristics of the drugs, characteristics of the blood-brain barrier (BBB), and the presence of active drug transporters that limit the availability of certain drugs (Varatharajan & Thomas, 2009). In general, PIs including ritonavir are highly plasma-protein-bound and have poor penetration into CSF, with the exception of atazanavir, lopinavir, and fosamprenavir that have intermediate penetration. Enfuvirtide does not penetrate due to its large molecular weight, although this is not the case for NRTIs; for example, zidovudine has excellent penetration but tenofovir does not, possibly due to active efflux transporters (Anthonypillai, Gibbs, & Thomas, 2006). Newer agents appear to have CSF penetrance to varying degrees, such as darunavir, maraviroc, and possibly raltegravir (although drug levels vary and may be limited by efflux transporters for the latter) (Yilmaz et al., 2009a; Yilmaz et al., 2009b; Yilmaz et al., 2009c). Darunavir and etravirine are present in CSF exceed wild-type IC_{50}; etravirine concentrations in CSF were higher than expected in a recent 9 patient study (Best et al., 2011). The clinical relevance of these findings is unclear, but limited data suggest that drugs with poor CSF penetration are less likely to fully suppress HIV replication in the CSF, and in turn, patients who achieve undetectable viral load in the CSF show higher rates of neurocognitive improvement (Letendre et al., 2004; Foudraine et al., 1998; Tashima et al., 1999; Kravcik et al., 1999; Gisolf et al., 2000). The development of nanoformulated antiretroviral agents may prove an effective way of bypassing the BBB, enhancing drug concentrations in the CNS, and achieving higher rates of virologic control in that compartment, although this has yet to be tested (Nowacek & Gendelman, 2009). Inadequately treated virus in the CNS may lead to virological escape and/or promote the development of resistance (Antinori et al., 2003; Antinori et al., 2005). Overall, the importance of CSF penetration of antiretroviral agents remains controversial and randomized prospective clinical trial data are lacking. This issue is reviewed in detail in Chapter 10.3.

NEW AGENTS, NEW STRATEGIES

Major improvements in available antiretroviral agents and their formulations have led to simpler and better-tolerated regimens with greater efficacy. Despite these advances, options other than life-long triple combination therapy are still needed. Development of new agents and/or strategies for the management of HIV-1 disease focuses on regimens that include novel targets and which are simpler, better tolerated, and with decreased or altered potential for the development of viral resistance. The identification of the critical role of medication adherence in the success of the regimen has focused attention on decreasing the complexity of currently available regimens (Paterson et al., 2000). Novel inhibitors of reverse transcriptase and HIV protease continue to be developed, some of which offer different resistance profiles with less cross-resistance, for example, etravirine and riplivirine (Panel on Antiretroviral Guidelines for Adults and Adolescents, 2011; Azijn et al., 2010; Fulco & McNicholl, 2009). New classes of anti-HIV drugs include the CCR5-receptor antagonists, for example maraviroc, and the integrase strand transfer inhibitors such as raltegravir (Hicks & Gulick, 2009; MacArthur & Novak, 2008). There have been several candidates for immune-based therapy (e.g., interleukin-7, cyclosporine) but recent trials have shown no clinical benefit despite increases in CD4 T-cell count levels (INSIGHT-ESPRIT Study Group et al., 2009; Markowitz et al., 2010; Tavel et al., 2010). Interest persists in development of strategies with potential to eliminate viral reservoirs. Thus far, addition of immunomodulating or additional antiretroviral agents to intensify therapy has failed to demonstrate sustained decreases in low-level plasma viremia (Archin et al., 2010; Dinoso et al., 2009; McMahon et al., 2010).

Several trials have addressed the safety and efficacy of intermittent therapy, most using CD4-guided treatment interruptions. The SMART study enrolled 5,472 participants with CD4 cell counts above 350 cells/mm³, randomized to continuous or episodic therapy (Strategies for Management of Antiretroviral Therapy (SMART) Study Group et al., 2006). Interrupting therapy was associated with an increased risk of opportunistic infections, disease progression, or death compared with the continuous antiretroviral therapy arm. The TRIVACAN study performed in Côte d'Ivoire also showed that interruption was an inferior strategy and morbidity, mainly invasive bacterial infections, led to premature closing of the study (Danel et al., 2006). These and other studies together have led to the conclusion that intermittent therapy cannot be recommended because of a greater risk of CD4 decline, morbidity, and mortality.

On the other hand, after viral suppression with a triple therapy regimen, simplified maintenance therapy with a boosted protease inhibitor maintains virologic suppression in most patients (McKinnon, Mellors, & Swindells, 2009). In those experiencing virologic failure, drug resistance has been rare and resumption of NRTI has generally resulted in resuppression of viremia. However, potential disadvantages of boosted PI maintenance therapy include poor penetration into sanctuary sites, such as the central nervous system, raising concern about the selection of resistant variants and the development of central nervous system (CNS) disease (Wynn, Brundage, & Fletcher, 2002).

Antiretroviral drugs are usually administered in fixed standard doses to HIV-infected adults. This results in large variations in systemic exposure as a result of the inter-individual variations in pharmacokinetics. Significant correlations have been found between protease inhibitor (PI) or non-nucleoside reverse transcriptase inhibitors (NNRTI) plasma concentrations and virological outcome or toxicity (Acosta et al., 1999; Acosta, Gerber, & Adult Pharmacology Committee of the AIDS Clinical Trials Group, 2002; Descamps et al., 2000;

Gatti et al., 1999; Marzolini et al., 2001). A recent retrospective study demonstrated that patients who had therapeutic drug concentrations of either PIs or NNRTIs achieved virologic control more frequently than those who had subtherapeutic levels (Fabbiani et al., 2009). This has led to interest in therapeutic drug monitoring (TDM) as a potential management tool. Appropriate therapeutic drug concentrations that will predict therapeutic response and/or limit toxicities are not well defined. Moreover, availability of the testing is another limiting factor (Panel on Antiretroviral Guidelines for Adults and Adolescents, 2011; Burger et al., 2003; Fletcher et al., 2002; Panel de expertos de Gesida y Plan Nacional sobre el Sida, 2009). Potential scenarios when TDM might be appropriate include patients whose pharmacokinetics are difficult to predict; for example, pregnant women, heavily treatment-experienced patients, adjusting antiretroviral dosing in patients with organ dysfunction, when toxicity might be related to higher drug concentrations, and when alternative dosing regimens are used (Panel on Antiretroviral Guidelines for Adults and Adolescents, 2011). Many antiretroviral agents are metabolized in the liver by the p450 system and this, in turn, is influenced by genetic diversity that leads to individual differences in drug metabolism (Motsinger et al., 2006; Haas et al., 2009). Ultimately, regimens may be able to be tailored even more precisely using genomic information.

ART also plays a key role in preventing HIV transmission. It is clear that lower plasma viral loads are associated with lower concentrations of virus in genital secretions, although there is evidence of persistent HIV replication in genital secretions of patients with viral loads below the limit of detection (Sheth et al., 2009). A study conducted in Rwanda and Zambia among 2,993 serodiscordant couples showed substantial reduction of transmission to the HIV-negative person if their partner was taking ART; less high-risk sexual behaviors were recorded in those on ART, and both ART and change in behavior independently reduced HIV transmission (Sullivan et al., 2009). Despite accumulating evidence to support treatment to reduce HIV virus transmission, this approach requires further investigation and is not currently recommended.

"Test and Treat" is a potential strategy supported by mathematical modeling, demonstrating that universal HIV testing with early antiretroviral treatment, coupled with current prevention approaches, could dramatically decrease the number of HIV infections and potentially create a so-called "elimination phase" (Granich et al., 2009). Although this is an appealing strategy, cost, patient's readiness to start therapy, adherence, potential drug toxicities, and development of resistance are all major obstacles that may preclude success (Blower, Kahn, & Okano, 2010). Interventional trials to test this are underway in the US and other countries.

TREATMENT FAILURE

A regimen may fail for several interrelated reasons including inadequate adherence, intolerance, impaired drug absorption and/or metabolism, pharmacokinetic interactions, the potency of the regimen, and viral resistance. Careful assessment of contributing factors is essential before changing therapy. In the case of drug intolerance, a substitution for the offending agent should be made, ideally with a drug from the same class but with a different toxicity profile. Dosing modifications may be needed to correct for drug interactions when using certain combination of NNRTIs and/or PIs (Panel on Antiretroviral Guidelines for Adults and Adolescents, 2011). Identification of potential adherence problems and targeted interventions, such as treatment of mental illness, can enhance response to therapy (Stenzel et al., 2001). If viral resistance is suspected, testing for mutations is helpful in choosing subsequent regimens and has been shown to improve virological outcomes when compared to clinical judgment alone (Meynard et al., 2002; Vray et al., 2003). Criteria for selection of alternative options should include the potency and tolerability of the regimen with a view to maximizing patient adherence. It is recommended that at least two, but preferably three, fully active agents be added to an already failing regimen; with few exceptions, adding only one drug to a failing regimen is not recommended. The advent of new antiretroviral agents and new classes now often allows patients failing therapy to achieve the goal of undetectable viremia(Panel on Antiretroviral Guidelines for Adults and Adolescents, 2011; Thompson et al., 2010).

ADHERENCE

Adherence to the regimen has been identified as a critical factor in determining the success or failure of antiretroviral therapy (Paterson et al., 2000). Previously identified predictors of suboptimal adherence include active substance abuse, mental illness (including depression), neurocognitive decline and dementia, complex antiretroviral regimens, adverse effects of drugs, treatment fatigue, lack of patient education and/or trust, and limited access to medical care (Panel on Antiretroviral Guidelines for Adults and Adolescents,2011). It is widely acknowledged that simplification of the regimen, decreased frequency of dosing, and minimizing side effects and drug-drug interactions have helped to address this challenging problem (McKinnon, Mellors, & Swindells, 2009).

One of the most important ways to maximize adherence success is to utilize a multidisciplinary team approach including nurses, social workers, pharmacists, and medication managers. This facilitates assessment of patients' readiness to start therapy, provision of detailed and culturally appropriate patient education, simplifying access to care, and building trusting relationships between patients and providers. Ongoing monitoring of adherence at every clinic visit is also recommended, although it should be acknowledged that patient self-report predictably overestimates adherence (Arnsten et al., 2001). Some behavioral interventions designed to improve adherence have been successful but may be difficult to replicate in clinical practice (Chesney, 2006). Directly observed therapy (DOT) has proven effective for intravenous drug users in one randomized trial (Altice et al., 2007), but a recent meta-analysis showed no benefit when compared to self-administered treatment in the general population (Ford et al., 2009; Gross et al., 2009). DOT is also labor-intensive, expensive, intrusive, and programmatically complex to implement (Lucas, Flexner, & Moore, 2002).

Cognitive impairment is also a contributor to reduced adherence and has been shown to have significant impact (Lovejoy & Suhr, 2009; Ettenhofer et al., 2009). Moreover, several recommended strategies to improve adherence rely on adequate comprehension, memory, and literacy. Simply forgetting is one of the most common reasons cited by surveyed patients about why doses were missed (Ickovics & Meisler, 1997). It is therefore reasonable to speculate that cognitive dysfunction adversely influences medication compliance and affected patients may respond poorly to conventional approaches. Education of family and friends and their recruitment as participants may be helpful in this setting.

COMPLICATIONS

Increased longevity of HIV-infected persons has shifted the focus of management from prevention of disease progression to a chronic disease model. As a result, dealing with the complications of antiretroviral therapy now represents a significant challenge for investigators, clinicians and patients. Commonly reported adverse effects are summarized in Table 11.1.5, with special emphasis on those related to the nervous system. Acute or short-term adverse effects can be troublesome and have been shown to negatively impact adherence (d'Arminio Monforte et al., 2000). The incidence of treatment-limiting toxicities has decreased with the advent of newer antiretroviral agents; for example, lactic acidosis and progressive ascending neuromuscular syndrome are rarely seen. However, chronic or long-term toxicities that develop after months or years of therapy are still problematic. Among the most distressing are peripheral neuropathy (discussed in Chapter 7.9), and metabolic complications (Wohl et al., 2006). The latter include disorders of fat distribution (lipoatrophy and fat accumulation), dyslipidemia, glucose intolerance and diabetes, and bone disorders (osteopenia, osteoporosis, and osteonecrosis). In addition, conditions that are classically associated with the normal aging process appear to be occurring at earlier ages in HIV-infected persons. NRTIs and PIs are chronologically associated with the development of peripheral lipoatrophy and central fat accumulation, which in turn are associated with insulin resistance. The underlying mechanism causing lipoatrophy is thought to be mitochondrial toxicity, particularly from thymidine analog NRTIs such as stavudine and zidovudine. Insulin resistance may also be due to mitochondrial toxicity in muscle caused by NRTIs or impairment of insulin-mediated glucose uptake by adipocytes via inhibition of Glut-4 receptors (Murata, Hruz, & Mueckler, 2000). Cardiovascular disease is now a major cause of mortality in HIV-infected persons, and some studies have shown increased risk with prolonged exposure to ART (DAD Study Group et al., 2007). PIs may also induce hyperlipidemia by increasing hepatic VLDL production and it has been shown that PIs inhibit proteosomal degradation of nascent

Table 11.1.5 ADVERSE EFFECTS OF LICENSED ANTIRETROVIRAL AGENTS

DRUG	GENERAL EFFECTS	NERVOUS SYSTEM EFFECTS
Abacavir	Hypersensitivity reaction symptoms may include fever, rash, nausea, vomiting, malaise or fatigue, or respiratory symptoms such as sore throat, cough, or shortness of breath, lactic acidosis with hepatic steatosis (rare) Possible increased risk of MI with recent or current use of ABC	
Atazanavir	Indirect hyperbilirubinemia, nephrolithiasis, prolonged PR interval—first degree symptomatic AV block in some patients, use with caution in patients with underlying conduction defects or on concomitant medications that can cause PR prolongation Hyperglycemia Fat maldistribution Possible increased bleeding episodes in patients with hemophilia	
Darunavir	Skin rash; Stevens-Johnson syndrome and erythrema multiforme have been reported Transaminase elevation Hepatotoxicity, diarrhea, nausea Metabolic complications Possible increased bleeding in patients with hemophilia	Headache
Delavirdine	Rash, increased transaminases	Headache
Didanosine	Pancreatitis, nausea, diarrhea, lactic acidosis with hepatic steatosis (rare) Potential association with noncirrhotic portal hypertension	Peripheral neuropathy
Efavirenz	Rash, increased transaminases Teratogenic in nonhuman primate and potentially teratogenic in humans False-positive results reported with some cannabinoid and benzodiazepine screening assays	CNS effects including dizziness, somnolence, insomnia, abnormal dreams, confusion, impaired concentration and memory, agitation, depersonalization, hallucinations, euphoria
Emtricitabine	Neutropenia, lactic acidosis with hepatic steatosis (rare) Hyperpigmentation/skin discoloration Severe acute exacerbation of hepatitis may occur in HBV-coinfected patients who discontinue FTC	
Enfuvirtide	Local injection site reactions in almost all patients (pain, erythema, induration, nodules and cysts, pruritus, ecchymosis) Increased bacterial pneumonia Hypersensitivity reaction (rare), symptoms may include rash, fever, nausea, vomiting, chills, rigors, hypotension, or elevated serum transaminases; rechallenge is **not** recommended	
Etravirine	Rash, nausea Hypersensitivity reactions have been reported, characterized by rash, constitutional findings, and sometimes organ dysfunction, including hepatic failure (uncommon)	
Fosamprenavir	GI intolerance, diarrhea, nausea, vomiting, increased transaminases, metabolic complications Skin rash, mephrolithiasis Possible increased bleeding episodes in patients with hemophilia	Headache
Indinavir	Nephrolithiasis, GI intolerance, indirect hyperbilirubinemia, alopecia, metabolic complications, rash, metallic taste, thrombocytopenia, and hemolytic anemia Possible increased bleeding episodes in patients with hemophilia	Headache, asthenia, blurred vision, dizziness
Lamivudine	Neutropenia, lactic acidosis with hepatic steatosis (rare) Severe acute exacerbation of hepatitis may occur in HBV-coinfected patients who discontinue 3TC	
Lopinavir	GI intolerance: nausea, vomiting, diarrhea, increased transaminases, metabolic complications PR interval prolongation, QT interval prolongation and torsade de pointes Possible increased bleeding episodes in patients with hemophilia	Asthenia
Maraviroc	Abdominal pain, cough, musculoskeletal symptoms, pyrexia, rash, upper respiratory tract infections, hepatotoxicity, orthostatic hypotension	Dizziness
Nelfinavir	Diarrhea, metabolic complications	
Nevirapine	Rash including Stevens-Johnson syndrome, hepatitis including fatal hepatic necrosis	
Raltegravir	Nausea, diarrhea, pyrexia, CPK elevation, rash	Headache

(Continued)

Table 11.1.5 ADVERSE EFFECTS OF LICENSED ANTIRETROVIRAL AGENTS (CONTINUED)

DRUG	GENERAL EFFECTS	NERVOUS SYSTEM EFFECTS
Rilpivirine	Rash, nausea, vomiting, abdominal pain.	Depression, insomnia, headache.
Ritonavir	GI intolerance, nausea, vomiting, diarrhea, hepatitis, pancreatitis, metabolic complications Possible increased bleeding episodes in patients with hemophilia	Circumoral and extremity paresthesias Asthenia Taste perversion
Saquinavir	GI intolerance, diarrhea, increased transaminases, metabolic complications Possible increased bleeding episodes in patients with hemophilia	Headache
Stavudine	Pancreatitis, lactic acidosis with hepatic steatosis (rare) Lipoatrophy, Hyperlipidemia	Peripheral neuropathy Rapidly progressive ascending neuromuscular weakness (rare)*
Tenofovir	Diarrhea, nausea, vomiting, and flatulence Renal insufficiency, Fanconi syndrome Osteomalacia Potential for decrease in bone mineral density Lactic acidosis with hepatic steatosis (rare) Severe acute exacerbation of hepatitis may occur in HBV-coinfected patients who discontinue TDF	Headache, asthenia
Tipranavir	Hepatotoxicity: clinical hepatitis, hepatic decompensation and hepatitis-associated fatalities (uncommon) Rash Metabolic complications Possible increased bleeding episodes in patients with hemophilia	Fatal and nonfatal intracranial hemorrhages (rare). Most patients had underlying comorbidity, such as brain lesion, head trauma, recent neurosurgery, coagulopathy, hypertension, or alcoholism or were on medication with increased risk of bleeding (uncommon).
Zidovudine	Gastrointestinal intolerance Nail pigmentation Bone marrow suppression, gastrointestinal intolerance, lactic acidosis with hepatic steatosis (rare but potentially life-threatening toxicity)	Headache, insomnia, asthenia

*The neuromuscular weakness syndrome is defined as new onset of limb weakness in an HIV-infected individual, with or without sensory involvement, in the absence of potentially confounding medical illnesses. This can be either acute (1–2 weeks) or subacute (> 2 weeks) and affect either lower or both lower and upper extremities.

apolipoprotein B (Liang et al., 2001). Impairment of endothelial function has been implicated as an underlying mechanism for increased cardiovascular events (Hsue et al., 2009). Continuing efforts are needed to address potentially modifiable risk factors for cardiovascular disease, including interventions for cigarette smoking, optimal management of dyslipidemia, and the correct timing and choice of drugs for antiretroviral therapy. The initiation of ART is associated with mild to moderate bone loss, which tends to stabilize over time. In the SMART study, continuous exposure to antiretrovirals was associated with greater loss of bone density (Grund et al., 2009). Tenofovir was implicated as the cause of decreased bone mineral density of the lumbar spine in the Gilead 903 trial, but the clinical significance in patients remains unclear (Gallant et al., 2004). Overall, management of metabolic complications follows treatment guidelines for uninfected patients. Treatment for some conditions can be complicated by drug-drug interactions, particularly the management of dyslipidemia.

Although rare, immediate life-threatening toxicities associated with antiretroviral therapy are of particular concern. These include abacavir hypersensitivity, pancreatitis, lactic acidosis, hepatitis, and Stevens-Johnson syndrome. Some adverse events are predictable and can be prevented; for example, not prescribing nevirapine to female patients with CD4 counts > 250 cells/mm³ or 400 cells/mm³ in men, to decrease the risk

of hypersensitivity syndrome and hepatonecrosis. Screening for the HLA-B*5701 MHC class I allele before administering abacavir significantly decreases risk of hypersensitivity reactions (Mallal et al., 2008).

IMMUNE RECONSTITUTION INFLAMMATORY SYNDROME

Atypical inflammatory disorders associated with immune recovery may manifest as immune reconstitution inflammatory syndromes (IRIS). IRIS appearing after the introduction of ART in the setting of infectious processes can be caused by an inflammatory reaction against pathogen-specific antigens (paradoxical reaction), or unmasking of an unrecognized silent or subtle opportunistic infection (French, Price, & Stone, 2004; French, 2009). The differential diagnosis also includes treatment failure or adverse drug reactions. *Mycobacterium tuberculosis, Mycobacterium avium*, and *Cryptococcus neoformans* are among the most common pathogens associated with IRIS; with *Cryptococcus*, progressive multifocal leukoencephalopathy (PML), and toxoplasmosis being the most common pathogens associated with IRIS involving the CNS. Cryptococcal immune reconstitution can manifest as early as three days or up to almost one year after initiation of therapy. Risk factors include early initiation of antiretroviral therapy after diagnosis, high fungal burden (fungemia), or high cryptococcal antigen levels at presentation (Shelburne et al., 2005). IRIS in the setting of PML has been reported to occur within the first weeks to months of therapy. Presentation may include unmasking of previously silent lesions or deterioration of known lesions. Some patients exhibit atypical features including surrounding edema and mass effect of the lesions or contrast enhancement on MRI. Rarely, brain inflammation with herniation may complicate the picture (Vendrely et al., 2005). Although there have been suggestions of IRIS due to cerebral toxoplasmosis, a clear association remains to be demonstrated (Pfeffer et al., 2009). Only a few cases of IRIS complicating HIV-associated dementia and HIV encephalitis have been reported (Miller et al., 2004). Corticosteroids, hydroxychloroquine, thalidomide, and other drugs have been used to try to ameliorate the inflammatory response, but a clear benefit to support their routine use has not been established.

CONCLUSIONS

Remarkable progress has been achieved in developing effective antiretroviral therapy, and access to treatment in resource-limited countries is much improved, although still falls short of covering all those who need treatment. New, simpler, and more tolerable regimens have become available in the last several years. Antiretroviral agents including drugs with improved resistance profiles and from new classes with novel mechanisms of action have been developed. Neurological complications of HIV disease still lack specific therapies and the significance of CSF penetrance of ART remains controversial. The trend toward earlier initiation of antiretroviral therapy has the potential to prevent HIV-associated brain disease, but this has yet to be conclusively proven.

REFERENCES

Abdool Karim, Q., Abdool Karim, S. S., Frohlich, J. A., Grobler, A. C., Baxter, C., Mansoor, L. E., et al. (2010). Effectiveness and safety of tenofovir gel, an antiretroviral microbicide, for the prevention of HIV infection in women. Science, 329 (5996) (Sep 3), 1168–1174.

Abramowicz, M. (2006). A once-daily combination tablet (Atripla) for HIV. Med Letter, 48(1244), 78–79.

Aberg, J. A., Kaplan, J. E., Libman, H., Emmanuel, P., Anderson, J. R., Stone, V. E., et al., & HIV Medicine Association of the Infectious Diseases Society of America. (2009). Primary care guidelines for the management of persons infected with human immunodeficiency virus: 2009 update by the HIV Medicine Association of the Infectious Diseases Society of America. CID, 49(5), 651–681.

Acosta, E. P., Gerber, J. G., & Adult Pharmacology Committee of the AIDS Clinical Trials Group. (2002. Position paper on therapeutic drug monitoring of antiretroviral agents. AIDS Res Hum Retroviruses, 18(12), 825–834.

Acosta, E. P., Henry, K., Baken, L., Page, L. M., & Fletcher, C. V. (1999). Indinavir concentrations and antiviral effect. Pharmacotherapy, 19(6), 708–712.

Altice, F. L., Maru, D. S., Bruce, R. D., Springer, S. A., & Friedland, G. H. (2007). Superiority of directly administered antiretroviral therapy over self-administered therapy among HIV-infected drug users: A prospective, randomized, controlled trial. CID, 45(6), 770–778.

Anthonypillai, C., Gibbs, J. E., & Thomas, S. A. (2006). The distribution of the anti-HIV drug, tenofovir (PMPA), into the brain, CSF and choroid plexuses. Cerebrospinal Fluid Res, 3,1.

Antinori, A., Cingolani, A., Giancola, M. L., Forbici, F., De Luca, A., & Perno, C. F. (2003). Clinical implications of HIV-1 drug resistance in the neurological compartment. Scand J Infect Dis Suppl, 106, 41–44.

Antinori, A., Perno, C. F., Giancola, M. L., Forbici,F., Ippolito, G., Hoetelmans, R. M., et al. (2005). Efficacy of cerebrospinal fluid (CSF)-penetrating antiretroviral drugs against HIV in the neurological compartment: Different patterns of phenotypic resistance in CSF and plasma. CID, 41(12),1787–1793.

Archin, N. M., Cheema, M., Parker, D., Wiegand, A., Bosch, R. J., Coffin, J. M., et al. (2010). Antiretroviral intensification and valproic acid lack sustained effect on residual HIV-1 viremia or resting CD4+ cell infection. PloS One, 5(2), (Feb 23): e9390.

Arnsten, J. H., Demas, P. A., Farzadegan, H., Grant, R. W., Gourevitch, M. N., Chang, C. J., et al. 2001. Antiretroviral therapy adherence and viral suppression in HIV-infected drug users: Comparison of self-report and electronic monitoring. CID, 33(8),1417–1423.

Azijn, H., Tirry, I., Vingerhoets, J., de Bethune, M. P., Kraus, G., Boven, K., et al. (2010). TMC278, a next-generation nonnucleoside reverse transcriptase inhibitor (NNRTI), active against wild-type and NNRTI-resistant HIV-1. Antimicrob Agents Chemother, 54(2), 718–727.

Baeten, J., Ndase, P., Mugo, N., Donnell,D., Mujugira, A., Kidoguchi, L., et al. (2010). Demographic, behavioral, and clinical characteristics of HIV-1 serodiscordant couples enrolled into an efficacy trial of pre-exposure prophylaxis. Abstract 959. 17th Conference on Retroviruses and Opportunistic Infections, San Francisco, California, February 16–19, 2010.

Best, B. M., Letendre, S., Croteau, D., Capparelli, E., Clifford, D., Gelman, B., et al. (2010). Therapeutic Darunavir and Etravirine Concentrations in Cerebrospinal Fluid. Abstract 643. 18th Conference on Retroviruses and Opportunistic Infections, Boston, Massachusetts, February 27th – March 2nd, 2011.

Bhaskaran, K., Mussini, C. Antinori, A. Walker, A. S. Dorrucci, M. Sabin, C. et al. & CASCADE Collaboration.(2008). Changes in the incidence and predictors of human immunodeficiency virus-associated dementia in the era of highly active antiretroviral therapy. Ann Neurol, 63(2), 213–221.

Blower, S., Kahn, J., & Okano, J. (2010). A "Test and Treat" strategy in South Africa is likely to lead to a self-sustaining epidemic composed of only NNRTI-resistant strains. Abstract 966. 17th Conference on Retroviruses and Opportunistic Infections, San Francisco, California, February 16–19, 2010.

Boisse, L., Gill, M. J., & Power, C. (2008). HIV infection of the central nervous system: Clinical features and neuropathogenesis. Neurol Clin, 26(3), 799–819.

Brown, K., Patterson, K., Malone, S., Shaheen, N., Prince, H., Dumond, J., et al. (2010). Antiretrovirals for prevention: Maraviroc exposure in the semen and rectal tissue of healthy male volunteers after single and multiple dosing. Abstract 85. 17th Conference on Retroviruses and Opportunistic Infections, San Francisco, California, February 16–19, 2010.

Burger, D., Hugen, P., Reiss, P., Gyssens, I., Schneider, M., Kroon, F., et al. (2003). Therapeutic drug monitoring of nelfinavir and indinavir in treatment-naive HIV-1-infected individuals. AIDS, 17(8), 1157–1165.

Chesney, M. A. (2006). The elusive gold standard. Future perspectives for HIV adherence assessment and intervention. J Acquir Immune Defic Syndr (1999), 43 Suppl 1, S149–55.

Collazos, J., Asensi,V., & Carton, J. A. (2007). Sex differences in the clinical, immunological and virological parameters of HIV-infected patients treated with HAART. AIDS, 21 (7), 835–843.

D:A:D Study Group, Sabin, C. A., Worm, S. W., Weber, R., Reiss, P. El-Sadr, W. et al. (2008). Use of nucleoside reverse transcriptase inhibitors and risk of myocardial infarction in HIV-infected patients enrolled in the D:A:D study: A multi-cohort collaboration. Lancet, 371(9622), 1417–1426.

DAD Study Group, Friis-Moller, N., Reiss, P. Sabin, C. A., Weber, R. Monforte, A. et al. (2007). Class of antiretroviral drugs and the risk of myocardial infarction. *N Engl J Med*, 356(17), 1723–1735.

Danel, C., Moh, R., Minga, A., Anzian, A., Ba-Gomis, O., Kanga, C. et al. (2006). CD4-guided structured antiretroviral treatment interruption strategy in HIV-infected adults in West Africa (Trivacan ANRS 1269 trial): A randomised trial. *Lancet*, 367(9527), 1981–1989.

d'Arminio Monforte, A., Lepri, A. C., Rezza, G., Pezzotti, P., Antinori, A. A., Phillips, N., et al. (2000). Insights into the reasons for discontinuation of the first highly active antiretroviral therapy (HAART) regimen in a cohort of antiretroviral naive patients. *AIDS*, 14(5), 499–507.

Descamps, D., Flandre, P., Calvez, V., Peytavin, G., Meiffredy,V., Collin, G., et al. (2000). Mechanisms of virologic failure in previously untreated HIV-infected patients from a trial of induction-maintenance therapy. *JAMA*, 283(2), 205–211.

Dinoso, J. B., Kim, S. Y., Wiegand, A. M., Palmer, S. E., Gange, S. J., Cranmer, L., et al. (2009). Treatment intensification does not reduce residual HIV-1 viremia in patients on highly active antiretroviral therapy. *Proc Natl Acad Sci USA*, 106(23), 9403–9408.

Egger, M., May, M., Chene, G., Phillips, A. N., Ledergerber, B., Dabis, F., et al. (2002). Prognosis of HIV-1-infected patients starting highly active antiretroviral therapy: A collaborative analysis of prospective studies. *Lancet*, 360(9327), 119–129.

Ellis, R., Heaton, R., Letendre, S., et al. (2010). Higher CD4 nadir is associated with reduced rates of HIV-associated neurocognitive disorders in the CHARTER study: Potential implications for early treatment initiation. Abstract 429. 17th Conference on Retroviruses and Opportunistic Infections, San Francisco, California, February 16–19, 2010.

Ettenhofer, M. L., Hinkin, C. H., Castellon, S. A, Durvasula,R., Ullman, J., Lam, M. et al. (2009). Aging, neurocognition, and medication adherence in HIV infection. *Am J Geriatr Psychiatry*, 17(4), 281–290.

Everall, I., Vaida, F., Khanlou, N., Lazzaretto, D., Achim, C., Letendre, et al. (2009). Cliniconeuropathologic correlates of human immunodeficiency virus in the era of antiretroviral therapy. *J Neurovirol*, 15(5–6), 360–370.

Fabbiani, M., Di Giambenedetto, S., Bracciale, L., Bacarelli, A., Ragazzoni, E., Cauda, R. et al. (2009). Pharmacokinetic variability of antiretroviral drugs and correlation with virological outcome: 2 years of experience in routine clinical practice. *J Antimicrob Chemother*, 64(1), 109–117.

Farzadegan, H., Hoover, D. R., Astemborski, J., Lyles, C. M., Margolick, J. B., Markham, R. B., et al. (1998). Sex differences in HIV-1 viral load and progression to AIDS. *Lancet* 352(9139), 1510–1514.

Ferrando, S., van Gorp, W., McElhiney, M., Goggin, K., Sewell, M., & Rabkin, J. (1998). Highly active antiretroviral treatment in HIV infection: Benefits for neuropsychological function. *AIDS*, 12(8), F65–70.

Fischer-Smith, T., Bell, C., Croul, S., Lewis, M., & Rappaport, J. (2008). Monocyte/macrophage trafficking in acquired immunodeficiency syndrome encephalitis: Lessons from human and nonhuman primate studies. *J Neurovirol*, 14(4), 318–326.

Fletcher, C. V., Anderson, P. L., Kakuda,T. N., Schacker, T. W., Henry, K., Gross, C. R., et al. (2002). Concentration-controlled compared with conventional antiretroviral therapy for HIV infection. *AIDS*, 16(4), 551–560.

Flexner, C. (2000). Dual protease inhibitor therapy in HIV-infected patients: Pharmacologic rationale and clinical benefits. *Annu Rev Pharmacol Toxicol*, 40, 649–674.

Ford, N., Nachega, J. B., Engel, M. E., & Mills, E. J. (2009). Directly observed antiretroviral therapy: A systematic review and meta-analysis of randomised clinical trials. *Lancet*, 374(9707), 2064–2071.

Foudraine, N. A., Hoetelmans, R. M., Lange, J. M., de Wolf, F., van Benthem, B. H., Maas, J. J., Keet, I. P., & Portegies, P. (1998). Cerebrospinal-fluid HIV-1 RNA and drug concentrations after treatment with lamivudine plus zidovudine or stavudine. *Lancet*, 351(9115), 1547–1551.

Fransen, S., Gupta, S., Huang, W., et al. (2008). Performance characteristics and validation of the PhenoSense® integrase assay. Poster 1214. 48th Annual Interscience Conference on Antimicrobial Agents and Chemotherapy (ICAAC)/46th Annual Meeting of the Infectious Diseases Society of America (IDSA), Washington, DC, October 25–28, 2008.

French, M. A. (2009). HIV/AIDS: Immune reconstitution inflammatory syndrome: A reappraisal. *CID*, 48(1), 101–107.

French, M. A., Price, P., & Stone, S. F. (2004). Immune restoration disease after antiretroviral therapy. *AIDS*, 18(12), 1615–1627.

Fulco, P. P. & McNicholl, I. R. (2009). Etravirine and rilpivirine: Nonnucleoside reverse transcriptase inhibitors with activity against human immunodeficiency virus type 1 strains resistant to previous nonnucleoside agents. *Pharmacotherapy*, 29(3), 281–294.

Gallant, J. E., Staszewski, S., Pozniak, A. L., DeJesus, E., J. Suleiman, M., Miller, M. D., et al. (2004). Efficacy and safety of tenofovir DF vs stavudine in combination therapy in antiretroviral-naive patients: A 3-year randomized trial. *JAMA*, 292(2), 191–201.

Gathe, J., da Silva, B. A., Cohen, D. E., Loutfy, M. R., Podzamczer, D., Rubio, R., et al. (2009). A once-daily lopinavir/ritonavir-based regimen is noninferior to twice-daily dosing and results in similar safety and tolerability in antiretroviral-naive subjects through 48 weeks. *J Acquir Immune Defic Syndr*, 50(5), 474–481.

Gatti, G., Di Biagio, A., Casazza, R., De Pascalis, C., Bassetti, M., Cruciani, M. et al. (1999). The relationship between ritonavir plasma levels and side-effects: Implications for therapeutic drug monitoring. *AIDS*, 13(15), 2083–2089.

Gendelman, H. E., Zheng, J., Coulter, C. L., Ghorpade, A., Che, M., Thylin, M., et al. (1998). Suppression of inflammatory neurotoxins by highly active antiretroviral therapy in human immunodeficiency virus-associated dementia. *JID*, 178(4), 1000–1007.

Gisolf, E. H., Enting, R. H., Jurriaans, S., de Wolf, F., van der Ende, M. E., Hoetelmans, R. M., et al. (2000). Cerebrospinal fluid HIV-1 RNA during treatment with ritonavir/saquinavir or ritonavir/saquinavir/stavudine. *AIDS*, 14(11), 1583–1589.

Granich, R. M., Gilks, F., Dye, C., De Cock, M., & Williams, B. G. (2009). Universal voluntary HIV testing with immediate antiretroviral therapy as a strategy for elimination of HIV transmission: A mathematical model. *Lancet*, 373(9657), 48–57.

Grant, R. M., Lama, J. R., Anderson, P. L., McMahan, V., Liu, A. Y., Vargas, L., et al. (2010). Preexposure chemoprophylaxis for HIV prevention in men who have sex with men. *N Engl J Med*, 363(27), 2578–99.

Gross, R., Tierney, C., Andrade, A., Lalama, C. Rosenkranz, S., Eshleman, H., et al.(2009). Modified directly observed antiretroviral therapy compared with self-administered therapy in treatment-naive HIV-1-infected patients: A randomized trial. *Arch Int Med*, 169(13), 1224–1232.

Grund, B., Peng, G., Gibert, C. L., Hoy, J. F., Isaksson, R. L., Shlay, J. C., et al. (2009). Continuous antiretroviral therapy decreases bone mineral density. *AIDS*, 23(12), 1519–1529.

Gulick, R. M., Ribaudo, H. J., Shikuma, C. M., Lustgarten, S., Squires, K. E., Meyer 3rd, W. A. E., et al. (2004). Triple-nucleoside regimens versus efavirenz-containing regimens for the initial treatment of HIV-1 infection. *N Engl J Med*, 350(18), 1850–1861.

Haas, D. W., Gebretsadik, T., Mayo, G., Menon, U. N., Acosta, E. P., Shintani, A. et al. (2009). Associations between CYP2B6 polymorphisms and pharmacokinetics after a single dose of nevirapine or efavirenz in African Americans. *JID*, 199(6), 872–880.

Hardy, D. J. & Vance. E. (2009). The neuropsychology of HIV/AIDS in older adults. *Neuropsychology Review*, 19(2), 263–272.

Hicks, C. & Gulick, R. M. (2009). Raltegravir: The first HIV type 1 integrase inhibitor. *CID*, 48(7), 931–939.

Hirsch, M. S., Gunthard, H. F., Schapiro, J. M., Brun-Vezinet, F., Clotet, B., Hammer, S. M., et al. (2008). Antiretroviral drug resistance testing in adult HIV-1 infection: 2008 recommendations of an international AIDS society-USA panel. *CID*, 47(2), 266–285.

Hsue, P. Y., Hunt, P. W., Wu, Y., Schnell, A., Ho, J. E., Hatano, H., et al. (2009). Association of abacavir and impaired endothelial function in treated and suppressed HIV-infected patients. *AIDS*, 23(15), 2021–2027.

Ickovics, J. R. & Meisler, A. W. (1997). Adherence in AIDS clinical trials: A framework for clinical research and clinical care. *J Clin Epidemiol*, 50(4), 385–391.

INSIGHT-ESPRIT Study Group, SILCAAT Scientific Committee, Abrams, D., Levy, Y., Losso, M. H., Babiker, A., et al. (2009). Interleukin-2 therapy in patients with HIV infection. *N Engl J Med*, *361*(16), 1548–1559.

Kaplan, J. E., Benson, C., Holmes, K. H., Brooks, J. T., Pau, A., Masur, H., et al. (2009). Guidelines for prevention and treatment of opportunistic infections in HIV-infected adults and adolescents: Recommendations from CDC, the National Institutes of Health, and HIV Medicine Association of the Infectious Diseases Society of America. *MMWR Morb Mortal Wkly Rep*, 58(RR-4),1,207; quiz CE1–4.

Kaul, M. (2009). HIV-1 associated dementia: Update on pathological mechanisms and therapeutic approaches. *Curr Opin Neurol*, *22*(3), 315–320.

Kinloch-de Loes, S., de Saussure, P., Saurat, J. H., Stalder, H., Hirschel, B., & Perrin, L. H. (1993). Symptomatic primary infection due to human immunodeficiency virus type 1: Review of 31 cases. *CID*, *17*(1), 59–65.

Kitahata, M. M., Gange, S. J., Abraham, A. G., Merriman, B., Saag, M. S., Justice, A. C., et al. (2009). Effect of early versus deferred antiretroviral therapy for HIV on survival. *N Engl J Med*, *360*(18), 1815–1826.

Koopmans, P. P., Ellis, R., Best, B. M., & Letendre, S. (2009). Should antiretroviral therapy for HIV infection be tailored for intracerebral penetration? *Neth J Med*, *67*(6), 206–211.

Kravcik, S., Gallicano, K., Roth, V., Cassol, S., Hawley-Foss, N., Badley, A., et al. (1999). Cerebrospinal fluid HIV RNA and drug levels with combination ritonavir and saquinavir. *J Acquir Immune Defic Syndr*, *21*(5), 371–375.

Kuritzkes, D. R., Lalama, C. M., Ribaudo, H. J., Marcial, M., Meyer 3rd, W. A., Shikuma, C., et al. (2008). Preexisting resistance to nonnucleoside reverse-transcriptase inhibitors predicts virologic failure of an efavirenz-based regimen in treatment-naive HIV-1-infected subjects. *JID 197*(6), 867–870.

Lafeuillade, A., Poggi, C., Tamalet, C., Profizi, N., Tourres, C., & Costes, O. (1997). Effects of a combination of zidovudine, didanosine, and lamivudine on primary human immunodeficiency virus type 1 infection. *JID*, *175*(5), 1051–1055.

Letendre, S. L., McCutchan, J. A., Childers, M. E., Woods, S. P., Lazzaretto, D., Heaton R. K., et al. (2004). Enhancing antiretroviral therapy for human immunodeficiency virus cognitive disorders. *Ann Neurol*, *56*(3), 416–423.

Letendre, S., Marquie-Beck, J., Capparelli, E., Best, B., Clifford, D., Collier, A. C., et al. (2008). Validation of the CNS penetration-effectiveness rank for quantifying antiretroviral penetration into the central nervous system. *Arch Neurol*, *65*(1), 65–70.

Liang, J. S., Distler, O., Cooper, D. A., Jamil, H., Deckelbaum, R. J., Ginsberg, H. N., et al. (2001). HIV protease inhibitors protect apolipoprotein B from degradation by the proteasome: A potential mechanism for protease inhibitor-induced hyperlipidemia. *Nature Med*, *7*(12),1327–1331.

Lillo, F. B., Ciuffreda, D., Veglia, F., Capiluppi, B., Mastrorilli, E., Vergani, B., et al. (1999). Viral load and burden modification following early antiretroviral therapy of primary HIV-1 infection. *AIDS*, *13*(7), 791–796.

Liner, K. J., 2nd, Hall, C. D., & Robertson, K. R. (2008). Effects of antiretroviral therapy on cognitive impairment. *Current HIV/AIDS Reports*, *5*(2), 64–71.

Little, S. J., Holte, S., Routy, J. P., Daar, E. S., Markowitz, M., Collier, A. C., et al. (2002). Antiretroviral-drug resistance among patients recently infected with HIV. *N Engl J Med*, *347*(6), 385–394.

Lovejoy, T. I. & Suhr, J. A. (2009). The relationship between neuropsychological functioning and HAART adherence in HIV-positive adults: A systematic review. *J Behav Med*, *32*(5), 389–405.

Lucas, G. M., Flexner, C. W., & Moore, R. D. (2002). Directly administered antiretroviral therapy in the treatment of HIV infection: Benefit or burden? *AIDS Patient Care STDs*, *16*(11), 527–535.

MacArthur, R. D. & Novak, R. M. (2008). Reviews of anti-infective agents: Maraviroc: The first of a new class of antiretroviral agents. *CID*, *47*(2), 236–241.

Malhotra, U., Berrey, M. M., Huang, Y., Markee, J., Brown, D. J., Ap, S., et al. (2000). Effect of combination antiretroviral therapy on T-cell immunity in acute human immunodeficiency virus type 1 infection. *JID*, *181*(1), 121–131.

Mallal, S., Phillips, E., Carosi, G., Molina, J. M., Workman, C., Tomazic, J., et al. (2008). HLA-B*5701 screening for hypersensitivity to abacavir. *N Engl J Med*, *358*(6), 568–579.

Markowitz, M., Vaida, F., Hare, C. B., Boden, D., Mohri, H., Hecht, F. M., et al. 2010. The virologic and immunologic effects of cyclosporine as an adjunct to antiretroviral therapy in patients treated during acute and early HIV-1 infection. *JID*, *201*(9), 1298–1302.

Marzolini, C., Telenti, A., Decosterd, L. A., Greub, G., Biollaz, J., & Buclin, T.(2001). Efavirenz plasma levels can predict treatment failure and central nervous system side effects in HIV-1-infected patients. *AIDS*, *15*(1), 71–75.

Mathias, A. A., German, P., Murray, B. P., Wei, L., Jain, A., West, S., et al. (2010). Pharmacokinetics and pharmacodynamics of GS-9350: A novel pharmacokinetic enhancer without anti-HIV activity. *Clin Pharmacol Ther*, *87*(3), 322–329.

May, M., Sterne, J. A., Sabin, C., Costagliola, D., Justice, A. C., Thiebaut, R., et al.(2007). Prognosis of HIV-1-infected patients up to 5 years after initiation of HAART: Collaborative analysis of prospective studies. *AIDS*, *21*(9), 1185–1197.

McArthur, J. C., Sacktor, N., & Selnes, O. (1999). Human immunodeficiency virus-associated dementia. *Seminars Neurol*, *19*(2),129–150.

McKinnon, J. E., Mellors, J. W., & Swindells, S. (2009). Simplification strategies to reduce antiretroviral drug exposure: Progress and prospects. *Antiviral Therapy*, *14*(1), 1–12.

McMahon, D., Jones, J., Wiegand, A., Gange, S. J., Kearney, M., Palmer, S., et al. (2010). Short-course raltegravir intensification does not reduce persistent low-level viremia in patients with HIV-1 suppression during receipt of combination antiretroviral therapy. *CID*, *50*(6), 912–919.

Meynard, J. L., Vray, M., Morand-Joubert, L., Race, E., Descamps, D., Peytavin, G., et al. (2002). Phenotypic or genotypic resistance testing for choosing antiretroviral therapy after treatment failure: A randomized trial. *AIDS*, *16*(5), 727–736.

Miller, R. F., Isaacson, P. G., Hall-Craggs, M., Lucas, S., Gray, F., Scaravilli, F., et al. (2004). Cerebral CD8+ lymphocytosis in HIV-1 infected patients with immune restoration induced by HAART. *Acta Neuropathol*, *108*(1), 17–23.

Mills, A. M., Nelson, M., Jayaweera, D., Ruxrungtham, K., Cassetti, I., Girard, P. M., et al. (2009). Once-daily darunavir/ritonavir vs. lopinavir/ritonavir in treatment-naive, HIV-1-infected patients: 96-week analysis. *AIDS*, *23*(13), 1679–1688.

Motsinger, A. A., Ritchie, M. D., Shafer, R. W., Robbins, G. K., Morse, G. D., Labbe, L., et al. (2006). Multilocus genetic interactions and response to efavirenz-containing regimens: An adult AIDS clinical trials group study. *Pharmacogenetics and Genomics, 16*(11), 837–845.

Murata, H., Hruz, P. W., & Mueckler, M. (2000). The mechanism of insulin resistance caused by HIV protease inhibitor therapy. *J Biol Chem*, *275*(27), 20251–20254.

Murphy, R. L., Brun, S., Hicks, C., Eron, J. J., Gulick, R., King, M., et al. (2001). ABT-378/ritonavir plus stavudine and lamivudine for the treatment of antiretroviral-naive adults with HIV-1 infection: 48-week results. *AIDS*, *15*(1), F1–9.

Nilsson Schonnesson, L., Williams, M. L., Ross, M. W., Bratt, G., & Keel, B. (2007). Factors associated with suboptimal antiretroviral therapy adherence to dose, schedule, and dietary instructions. *AIDS and Behavior*, *11*(2), 175–183.

Nowacek, A. & Gendelman, H. E. (2009). NanoART, neuroAIDS and CNS drug delivery. *Nanomedicine*, *4*(5), 557–574.

Palella, F. J., Jr, Armon, C., Buchacz, K., Cole, S. R., Chmiel, J. S., Novak, R. M., et al. (2009). The association of HIV susceptibility testing with survival among HIV-infected patients receiving antiretroviral therapy: A cohort study. *Ann Intern Med*, *151*(2), 73–84.

Panel de expertos de Gesida y Plan Nacional sobre el Sida. (2009). Recommendations from the GESIDA/Spanish AIDS plan regarding antiretroviral treatment in adults with human immunodeficiency virus infection (update February 2009). *Enfermedades Infecciosas y Microbiologia Clinica*, *27*(4), 222–235.

Panel on Antiretroviral Guidelines for Adults and Adolescents. (2011). *Guidelines for the use of antiretroviral agents in HIV-1-infected adults and adolescents.* Department of Health and Human Services. January 10, 2011; 1–166. In DHHS [database online]. 2009 [cited March, 30th 2011]. Available from http://www.aidsinfo.nih.gov.library1.unmc.edu:2048/ContentFiles/AdultandAdolescentGL.pdf.

Paterson, D. L., Swindells, S., Mohr, J., Brester, M., Vergis, E. N., Squier, C., et al. (2000). Adherence to protease inhibitor therapy and outcomes in patients with HIV infection. *Ann Intern Med, 133*(1), 21–30.

Perinatal HIV Guidelines Working Group. (2009). Perinatal HIV Guidelines Working Group. Public Health Service Task Force recommendations for use of antiretroviral drugs in pregnant HIV-infected women for maternal health and interventions to reduce perinatal HIV transmission in the United States. http://aidsinfo.nih.gov.library1.unmc.edu:2048/contentfiles/PerinatalGL.pdf. *DHHS*, (April 29, 2009).

Pfeffer, G., Prout A., Hooge, J., & Maguire, J. (2009). Biopsy-proven immune reconstitution syndrome in a patient with AIDS and cerebral toxoplasmosis. *Neurology, 73*(4), 321–322.

Robertson, K. R., Robertson, W. T., Ford, S., Watson, D., Fiscus, S., Harp, A. G., et al. (2004). Highly active antiretroviral therapy improves neurocognitive functioning. *J Acquir Immune Defic Syndr, 36*(1), 562–566.

Robertson, K. R., Smurzynski, M., Parsons, T. D., Wu, K., Bosch, R. J., Wu, J., et al. (2007). The prevalence and incidence of neurocognitive impairment in the HAART era. *AIDS, 21*(14),1915–1921.

Rosenbach, K. A., Allison, R., & Nadler, J. P. (2002). Daily dosing of highly active antiretroviral therapy. *CID, 34*(5), 686–692.

Ryan, L. A., Zheng, J., Brester, M., Bohac, D., Hahn, F., Anderson, J., et al. (2001). Plasma levels of soluble CD14 and tumor necrosis factor-alpha type II receptor correlate with cognitive dysfunction during human immunodeficiency virus type 1 infection. *JID, 184*(6), 699–706.

Sacktor, N., Tarwater, P. M., Skolasky, R. L., McArthur, J. C., Selnes, O. A., Becker, J., et al. (2001). CSF antiretroviral drug penetrance and the treatment of HIV-associated psychomotor slowing. *Neurology, 57*(3), 542–544.

Sacktor, N. C., Lyles, R. H., Skolasky, R. L., Anderson, D. E., McArthur, J. C., McFarlane, G., et al. (1999). Combination antiretroviral therapy improves psychomotor speed performance in HIV-seropositive homosexual men. multicenter AIDS cohort study (MACS). *Neurology, 52*(8),1640–1647.

Schmitt, F. A., Bigley, J. W., McKinnis, R., Logue, P. E., Evans, R. W., & Drucker, J. L. (1988). Neuropsychological outcome of zidovudine (AZT) treatment of patients with AIDS and AIDS-related complex. *N Engl J Med, 319*(24), 1573–1578.

Severe, P., Pape, J., & Fitzgerald, D. W. (2009). A randomized clinical trial of early versus standard antiretroviral therapy for HIV-infected patients with a CD4 T cell count of 200–350 cells/mL (CIPRAHT001). Abstract H-1230c. *49th Interscience Conference on Antimicrobial Agents and Chemotherapy*, San Francisco, California, September 12–15, 2009.

Shelburne, S. A.,3rd, Darcourt, J., White Jr, A. C., Greenberg, S. B., Hamill, R. J., Atmar, R. L., et al. (2005). The role of immune reconstitution inflammatory syndrome in AIDS-related cryptococcus neoformans disease in the era of highly active antiretroviral therapy. *CID, 40*(7), 1049–1052.

Sheth, P. M., Kovacs, C., Kemal, K. S., Jones, R. B., Raboud, J. M., Pilon, R., et al. (2009). Persistent HIV RNA shedding in semen despite effective antiretroviral therapy. *AIDS, 23*(15), 2050–2054.

Simioni, S., Cavassini, M., Annoni, J. M., Rimbault Abraham, A., Bourquin, I., Schiffer, V., et al. (2009). Cognitive dysfunction in HIV patients despite long-standing suppression of viremia. *AIDS*, (Dec 7).

Smith, D. E., Walker, B. D., Cooper, D. A., Rosenberg, E. S., & Kaldor, J. M. (2004). Is antiretroviral treatment of primary HIV infection clinically justified on the basis of current evidence? *AIDS, 18*(5), 709–718.

Stenzel, M. S., McKenzie, M., Mitty, J. A., & Flanigan, T. P. (2001). Enhancing adherence to HAART: A pilot program of modified directly observed therapy. *The AIDS Reader, 11*(6), 324–328.

Stone, V. E., Hogan, J. W., Schuman, P., Rompalo, A. M., Howard, A. A., Korkontzelou, C. (2001). Antiretroviral regimen complexity, self-reported adherence, and HIV patients' understanding of their regimens: Survey of women in the HER study. *J Acquir Immune Defic Syndr, 28*(2), 124–131.

Strategies for Management of Antiretroviral Therapy (SMART) Study Group, El-Sadr, W. M., Lundgren, J. D., Neaton, J. D., Gordin, F., Abrams, D., et al. (2006). CD4+ count-guided interruption of antiretroviral treatment. *N Engl J Med, 355*(22), 2283–2296.

Strategies for Management of Anti-Retroviral Therapy/INSIGHT & DAD Study Groups. (2008). Use of nucleoside reverse transcriptase inhibitors and risk of myocardial infarction in HIV-infected patients. *AIDS, 22*(14), F17–24.

Sullivan, P., Kayitenkore, K., Chomba, E., Karita, E., Mwananyanda, L., Vwalika, C., et al. (2009). Reduction of HIV transmission risk and high risk sex while prescribed ART: Results from discordant couples in Rwanda and Zambia. Abstract 52bLB. 16th Conference on Retroviruses and Opportunistic Infection, Montreal, Canada, February 8–11, 2009.

Tashima, K. T., Caliendo, A. M., Ahmad, M., Gormley, J. M., Fiske, W. D., Brennan, J. M., et al. (1999). Cerebrospinal fluid human immunodeficiency virus type 1 (HIV-1) suppression and efavirenz drug concentrations in HIV-1-infected patients receiving combination therapy. *JID, 180*(3), 862–864.

Tavel, J. A., INSIGHT STALWART Study Group, Babiker, A., Fox, L., Gey, D., Lopardo, G., et al. (2010). Effects of intermittent IL-2 alone or with peri-cycle antiretroviral therapy in early HIV infection: The STALWART study. *PloS One* 5, (2) (Feb 23): e9334.

Thompson, M. A., Aberg, J. A., Cahn, P., Montaner, J. S., Rizzardini, G., Telenti, A., et al.(2010). Antiretroviral treatment of adult HIV infection: 2010 recommendations of the International AIDS Society-USA panel. *JAMA, 304*(3), 321–333.

Varatharajan, L. & Thomas, S. A. (2009). The transport of anti-HIV drugs across blood-CNS interfaces: Summary of current knowledge and recommendations for further research. *Antiviral Res, 82*(2), A99–109.

Vendrely, A., Bienvenu, B., Gasnault, J., Thiebault, J. B., Salmon, D., & Gray, F. (2005). Fulminant inflammatory leukoencephalopathy associated with HAART-induced immune restoration in AIDS-related progressive multifocal leukoencephalopathy. *Acta Neuropathol, 109*(4), 449–455.

Vray, M., Meynard, J. L., Dalban, C., Morand-Joubert, L., Clavel, F., Brun-Vezinet, F., et al. (2003). Predictors of the virological response to a change in the antiretroviral treatment regimen in HIV-1-infected patients enrolled in a randomized trial comparing genotyping, phenotyping and standard of care (Narval Trial, ANRS 088). *Antiviral Therapy, 8*(5), 427–434.

Weinstock, H. S., Zaidi, I., Heneine, W., Bennett, D., Garcia-Lerma, J. G., Douglas Jr, J. M., et al. (2004). The epidemiology of antiretroviral drug resistance among drug-naive HIV-1-infected persons in 10 US cities. *JID, 189*(12), 2174–2180.

When To Start Consortium, Sterne, J. A., May, M., Costagliola, D., de Wolf, F., Phillips, A. N., et al. (2009). Timing of initiation of antiretroviral therapy in AIDS-free HIV-1-infected patients: A collaborative analysis of 18 HIV cohort studies. *Lancet, 373*(9672), 1352–1363.

Whitcomb, J. M., Huang, W., Fransen, S., Limoli, K., Toma, J., Wrin, T., et al. (2007). Development and characterization of a novel single-cycle recombinant-virus assay to determine human immunodeficiency virus type 1 coreceptor tropism. *Antimicrob Agents Chemother, 51*(2), 566–575.

WHO ART Guideline Groups and Committee. (2009). *Rapid advice: Antiretroviral therapy for HIV infection in adults and adolescents -November 2009 [electronic version].* http://www.who.int/hiv/pub/arv/rapid_advice_art.pdf. http://www.who.int/hiv/pub/arv/advice/en/index.html (accessed December 1st, 2009).

Wohl, D. A., McComsey, G., Tebas, P., Brown, T. T., Glesby, M. J., Reeds, D., et al. (2006). Current concepts in the diagnosis and management of metabolic complications of HIV infection and its therapy. *CID, 43*(5), 645–653.

Wynn, H. E., Brundage, R. C., & Fletcher, C. V. (2002). Clinical implications of CNS penetration of antiretroviral drugs. *CNS Drugs, 16*(9), 595–609.

Yadav, A. & Collman, R. G. (2009). CNS inflammation and macrophage/microglial biology associated with HIV-1 infection. *J Neuroimmune Pharmacol, 4*(4), 430–447.

Yilmaz, A., Gisslen, M., Spudich, S., Lee, E., Jayewardene, A., Aweeka, F., et al. (2009a). Raltegravir cerebrospinal fluid concentrations in HIV-1 infection. *PloS One, 4*(9), (Sep 1): e6877.

Yilmaz, A., Izadkhashti, A., Price, R. W., Mallon, P. W., De Meulder, M., Timmerman, P., et al. (2009b). Darunavir concentrations in cerebrospinal fluid and blood in HIV-1-infected individuals. *AIDS Res Hum Retroviruses, 25*(4), 457–461.

Yilmaz, A., Watson, V., Else, L., & Gisslen, M.(2009c). Cerebrospinal fluid maraviroc concentrations in HIV-1 infected patients. *AIDS, 23*(18), 2537–2540.

11.2

PHARMACOLOGY OF ANTIRETROVIRAL THERAPIES

Scott L. Letendre, J. Allen McCutchan, Ronald J. Ellis,
Brookie M. Best, and Edmund V. Capparelli

After more than a decade of widespread use, combination antiretroviral therapy has not reduced the prevalence of HIV-associated neurocognitive disorders (HAND). Low drug concentrations in the brain, due to poor drug penetration of the blood-brain barrier by many antiretroviral therapies (ART), may partially explain why HAND persists or develops in treated patients. In this chapter, we review the relevant pharmacology of ART and accumulating evidence that the use of antiretrovirals that reach therapeutic concentrations in the central nervous system (CNS) are the best options to prevent and treat HIV-induced brain injury. Topics covered include an overview of the problem, pharmacokinetics of ART in the CNS, determinants of CNS penetration by ART, means of estimating CNS penetration by ART, pharmacodynamics of ART in the CNS, and the development of a clinically useful metric for the CNS effectiveness of antiretroviral drugs.

OVERVIEW OF PHARMACOLOGICAL ISSUES OF ANTIRETROVIRALS IN THE CENTRAL NERVOUS SYSTEM

Widespread use of combination antiretroviral therapy (ART) has not reduced the prevalence of HIV-associated neurocognitive disorders (HAND) after more than a decade. Incomplete suppression of HIV in the nervous system by some antiretroviral drugs could contribute to this persisting high prevalence. Because HAND decreases medication adherence, quality of life, and survival, optimizing prevention and treatment of HAND is an important goal of therapy.

Optimal treatment of the CNS appears to be limited for some patients by poor penetration of the blood-brain barrier (BBB) by many antiretroviral drugs. Low drug concentrations in the brain may partially explain why HAND persists or develops in treated patients. In this chapter we review the relevant pharmacology of antiretrovirals and accumulating evidence that the use of drugs that reach therapeutic concentrations in the CNS are the best options to prevent and treat HIV-induced brain injury.

In spite of the importance of healthy cognition to the quality of patients' lives, consensus treatment guidelines for HAND have yet to be formulated. Formulating recommendations for CNS-optimized treatment strategies requires a level of clinical evidence that is not yet available, but observational studies provide interim guidance and controlled interventional studies are underway.

PERSISTENCE OF HAND IN THE ERA OF COMBINATION ANTIRETROVIRAL THERAPY

Antiretroviral therapy (ART) has markedly reduced morbidity and mortality from HIV infection (Dore et al., 1999; Deutsch et al., 2001; Cysique, Maruff, & Brew, 2004), but the prevalence of HIV-associated neurocognitive disorders (HAND) has risen to an estimated 30–55% (Tozzi et al., 2001; Tozzi et al., 2004). Several factors may contribute to this high prevalence of cognitive impairment. First, ART-enabled improvements in survival have allowed longer duration of HIV infection and aging of the HIV-infected population (Valcour & Paul, 2006), both of which increase risk for HAND. Interactions between HIV-induced brain damage and age-related neurodegenerative diseases such as Alzheimer's and Parkinson's diseases are an active area of investigation. Second, HAND and especially milder forms like mild neurocognitive disorder (MND) occur in persons with higher CD4+ cell counts than in the pre-highly active antiretroviral therapy (HAART) era (Sacktor et al., 1999; Maschke et al., 2000). Third, ART does not completely reverse HAND in all individuals (Ferrando, Rabkin, van Gorp, Lin, & McElhiney, 2003). Neurocognitive impairment persists in nearly a quarter of ART-treated patients and may develop for the first time in another fifth (Robertson et al., 2007; McCutchan et al., 2007). Since HAND contributes to lower quality of life, impaired vocational functioning, poor medication adherence, difficulty with activities of daily living, and shorter survival (Sevigny et al., 2007; Ellis et al., 1997), optimizing prevention and treatment of neurocognitive functioning should be an important goal of ART.

MEASURING CONCENTRATIONS OF ANTIRETROVIRALS IN THE CENTRAL NERVOUS SYSTEM

Measurement of antiretroviral concentrations in the brain of living humans (e.g., by brain biopsy) is not currently feasible, so measurement in cerebrospinal fluid (CSF) has been used as a surrogate to understand antiretroviral pharmacology in the CNS. Several reviews have addressed the relationships between plasma, CSF, and brain concentrations of antiretrovirals (Enting et al., 1998; Yazdanian, 1999; Groothuis & Levy, 1997). For some antibacterials, CSF and brain drug levels by microdialysis are essentially equivalent (Granero et al., 1995), while for other drugs, they may differ markedly (Jarurtanasirikul et al., 1996). Drug concentrations in CSF may either over- or under-estimate brain parenchymal concentrations. In one study, for example, zidovudine concentrations in CSF actually exceeded those in brain tissue. Despite this, concentrations in CSF are better correlated with those in the brain than with concentrations in blood Brewster et al., 1997).

In favor of the validity of measuring drug concentrations in CSF is the observation that drugs appear to behave similarly at the BBB (within the endothelium of the brain capillaries) and the blood-CSF barrier (BCSFB) (within the choroid plexus). Moreover, CSF is composed, in part, of brain interstitial fluid which crosses the relatively permeable brain-CSF interface formed of ependymal cells. Thus, even though drug concentrations in brain parenchyma in humans are difficult to measure, CSF concentrations are considered an acceptable surrogate for brain levels of many drugs.

Several assay methods are available for measuring drug concentrations in CSF. In general the limits of detection for the analysis of drugs in CSF are lower than in plasma due to the less complex assemblage of lipoprotein constituents in cerebrospinal fluid, which translates into better analyte recovery and reduced matrix interference for CSF assays. Highly sensitive assays utilizing high performance liquid chromatography (HPLC) with ultraviolet detection and liquid chromatography/mass spectrometry (LC/MS) can detect concentrations of approximately 10–100 ng/ml (0.01–0.1µg/mL) (Aannoutse et al., 2001). Tandem mass spectrometry methods assays typically offer tenfold or greater sensitivity than HPLC methods and may be necessary to measure the very low concentrations of some drugs in CSF. Immunoassays with sensitivities ranging from 5–10 ng/mL have been used for some antiretrovirals, such as nucleotide reverse transcriptase inhibitors (NRTIs). Since most assays measure the total concentration of both protein-bound and unbound (free) drug, additional assays are necessary to measure only the active (unbound) form of the drug. Because CSF contains much lower levels of drug-binding proteins than plasma, higher proportions of drugs in the CSF are free and active. Thus, comparisons of levels of highly protein-bound drugs in plasma and CSF should take into account the greater fraction of unbound, active drug in CSF.

PHARMACOKINETICS OF ANTIRETROVIRAL DRUGS IN THE CENTRAL NERVOUS SYSTEM

Even though normal cognition is essential to maintaining excellent quality of life, consensus guidelines for treating and preventing HIV-associated neurocognitive disorders have yet to be formulated after more than 25 years. In part, this is because optimized antiretroviral treatment of the CNS requires a standard of evidence that is not yet available. Specifically, randomized, controlled clinical trials have not yet demonstrated that better penetrating antiretroviral regimens better treat HAND.

ART effects in the CNS are limited, in part, by variation among antiretrovirals in penetration of the BBB, which reduces concentrations of antiretrovirals in the CNS compared to the blood (Huisman et al., 2000; Wijnholds et al., 2000; Wu, Clement, & Pardridge, 1998; Brewster et al., 1997). Thus, differences among antiretrovirals in crossing the BBB and, by implication, in penetrating the brain may explain differences in their capacity to prevent or reverse HAND.

In addition to being a distinct pharmacologic compartment, the CNS is a virologic compartment. HIV in the CSF and brain reflects the cumulative effects of HIV trafficking from the blood, "autonomous" HIV replication in glia, and local selection by distinct cellular tropisms, immune responses, and drugs. HIV in the brain and CSF can replicate and evolve distinctly from HIV in other organ systems. In the brain, HIV primarily replicates in long-lived macrophages and microglia (Ellis et al., 1997; Staprans et al., 1999), rather than lymphocytes. HIV compartmentalization in the CNS is more common in advanced stages of disease (Ellis et al., 1997; Price, 2000). The mechanism for the segregation of the CNS from other compartments in advanced disease is unclear. Even without therapy, selective pressures on HIV in the CNS differ sufficiently from those in the blood and lymphatic compartment that HIV cloned at autopsy from the brain and CSF are genetically similar to each other, but distinct from those in the spleen. Such genetic segregation implies very limited trafficking of HIV between the blood and CNS. HIV in the CNS can have differing resistance patterns than HIV in the blood, probably because of compartmentalization and sub-therapeutic antiretroviral concentrations in the CNS (Canestri et al., 2010).

Attention to these issues is particularly important in people with AIDS since they are at greatest risk for virologic compartmentalization and for the clinical syndromes that comprise HAND (Heaton et al., 1995). This chapter will review the CSF pharmacology of antiretrovirals and accumulating evidence that the use of drugs that reach therapeutic concentrations in the CNS are the best options to prevent and treat HIV-induced brain injury.

DETERMINANTS OF CENTRAL NERVOUS SYSTEM PENETRATION BY ANTIRETROVIRALS

To reach the CNS, drugs must penetrate the BBB, which is composed of a) endothelial cells joined by tight junctions, b) astrocyte foot processes, and c) several pumps that selectively counteract diffusion across the endothelium. A similar BCSFB shields the CSF from some blood components. The determinants of CNS penetration by antiretrovirals include a number of nonspecific physicochemical factors related to diffusion across the blood-CNS barriers (Taylor & Pereira, 2000), as well as specific mechanisms for drug transport.

Nonspecific physicochemical factors affecting penetration include (1) protein binding (less is better); (2) molecular size (smaller is better); (3) lipophilicity (more is better); (4) pH and degree of ionization (neutral is better); and (5) increased barrier permeability, which can be caused by various conditions, including systemic or CNS inflammation. Table 11.2.1 summarizes physiochemical characteristics of most currently available antiretrovirals.

Protein binding is particularly important since only the unbound fraction of drugs is diffusible across the BBB. Drug-binding proteins, such as alpha-1-acid glycoprotein (AAG) and albumin, are too large to penetrate the BBB (Sadler et al., 2001; Anderson et al., 2000). The importance of drug-binding proteins can be demonstrated by comparing the effective concentrations (EC) of antiretroviral drugs to growth of HIV in tissue culture with or without serum. Highly bound drugs have markedly increased EC_{50} values (concentration needed for 50% inhibition of replication) if serum or AAG is added (Zhang, Schooley, & Gerber, 1999). Highly bound antiretrovirals like ritonavir (> 98% bound) have 20–40-fold increases in EC_{50} values while a less bound drug, indinavir (~60% bound), has only 2–3-fold increases.

A measure of a drug's lipophilicity is the octanol-water partition coefficient (LogP), which is the ratio, in a two-phase system at equilibrium, of a drug's concentration in the octanol (lipophilic) phase to its concentration in the aqueous (hydrophilic) phase. Hydrophilic drugs such as tenofovir are predicted to have poor CNS penetration, since they are relatively insoluble in the lipid-rich membrane components of the BBB. A drug's dissociation constant (pKa) provides an indirect measure of ionization state at a given pH and aids in estimating whether molecules are uncharged (neutral) at physiologic pH.

Table 11.2.1 PHYSICOCHEMICAL CHARACTERISTICS OF ANTIRETROVIRALS

	MOLECULAR WEIGHT (G/MOL)	PROTEIN BINDING (%)	UNBOUND FRACTION (%)	OCTANOL-WATER PARTITION COEFFICIENT (LogP)		DISSOCIATION CONSTANT (pKa)
				MDL QSAR	KOWWIN	
Nucleoside/Nucleotide Reverse Transcriptase Inhibitors						
Abacavir	286.34	49	51	1.08	1.62	0.4, 5.1
Didanosine	236.23	< 5	> 95	-0.8	-1.11	9.1
Emtricitabine	247.25	< 4	> 96	0.18	-2.56	2.6
Lamivudine	229.26	< 36	> 64	0.34	-2.62	4.3
Stavudine	224.22	"negligible"	~100	-0.06	-0.79	10
Tenofovir	287.22	1	99	-1.19	-1.57	3.8
Zalcitabine	211.22	< 4	> 96	-0.11	-1.72	4.4
Zidovudine	267.24	34–38	62–66	-0.7	-7.05	9.7
Non-Nucleoside Reverse Transcriptase Inhibitors						
Delavirdine	456.57	98	2	3.97	2.34	4.3–4.6
Efavirenz	315.68	99.5	0.5	4.79	4.69	10.2
Nevirapine	266.3	60	40	1.28	3.89	2.8
Etravirine	435.28	99.9	0.1	3.52	4.02	*
Protease Inhibitors						
Fosamprenavir	505.63	90	10	1.82	2.25	1.9
Atazanavir	704.86	86	14	6.98	2.88	*
Darunavir	628.81	98–99	1	5.71	5.94	*
Indinavir	613.8	60	40	2.39	1.91	6.2
Lopinavir	720.96	98–99	1	6.63	6.27	2.8
Nelfinavir	585.61	90	10	-0.46	2.17	*
Ritonavir	567.79	> 98	< 2	5.33	5.53	6.0, 11.1
Saquinavir	670.85	98	2	6.16	2.55	1.1, 7.1
Tipranavir	547.67	95	5	2.23	1.88	*
Fusion/Entry Inhibitors						
Enfuvirtide	4491.92	92	8	-0.875	*	4.3
Maraviroc	513.67	76	24	5.9	5.8	*
Integrase Inhibitors						
Raltegravir	444	83	17	0.49	*	*

* No data available

DRUG EFFLUX PUMPS AFFECTING CENTRAL NERVOUS SYSTEM PENETRATION

While concentrations of a drug in the CNS can be estimated by physical factors, marked deviations from these predictions can occur because of active transport of the drug out of the brain by efflux pumps (de Lange & Danhof, 2002). At least three classes of drug transporters can limit ART drug penetration at the BBB: a) P glycoprotein pumps (P-gp), b) multidrug resistance proteins (MRP), and c) organic anion transporters (OAT). These families of molecular pumps are expressed on the luminal surface of brain microvascular endothelial cells and can pump substrates back into the vascular lumen, interfering with their diffusion into the CNS. For example, NRTIs, although not highly protein-bound, can have poorer CSF penetration than would be expected based on their physico-chemical properties. NRTIs are partly blocked at the BBB and BCSFB by the mrp-1 pump that may be identical to that which removes benzylpenicillins (Masereeuw et al., 1994; Enting et al., 1998).

Protease inhibitors and integrase inhibitors are substrates for P-glycoprotein, an ATP-dependent efflux transporter of the ATP-binding cassette family (Lee et al., 1998; Rao et al., 1999), which markedly reduces CNS tissue concentrations (Enting et al., 1998). This pump both acts on and is inhibited by some PIs (Bousquet et al., 2008; Olson et al., 2002).

Cytochrome P-450 isozymes are a critical determinant of plasma levels of many drugs through effects on drug metabolism at the gastrointestinal epithelium and in the liver and are present in the CNS. While they markedly alter antiretroviral concentrations in blood, P-450 isozymes do not appear to directly influence CNS drug concentrations through local metabolism or transport. The metabolism of many PIs is markedly inhibited by the effect of ritonavir on the 3A4 P-450 isoenzyme. For this reason, low doses of ritonavir are combined with many other PIs (e.g., atazanavir, lopinavir, darunavir) to increase their blood concentrations. Ritonavir may enhance PI penetration into the CNS by inhibiting P-gp on the surface of brain endothelial cells (Huisman, et al., 2001).

ESTIMATING ANTIRETROVIRAL PENETRATION INTO THE CENTRAL NERVOUS SYSTEM

A simple method to estimate the CNS penetration of a drug is the ratio of its concentration in CSF to its concentration in blood plasma, the CSF-to-plasma ratio or fractional penetrance. However, the interpretation of these ratios is complicated by pharmacokinetic differences in the CSF compartment compared to blood Many antiretrovirals are absorbed into and eliminated from the systemic circulation relatively rapidly, whereas drug influx to or efflux from the CNS can be much slower. Thus, after a dose, CSF drug levels are often slower to reach peak and are lower, but persist for longer. Under these conditions, the CSF-to-plasma ratio can vary markedly as a function of blood and CSF collection times relative to the dosing time (see Figure 11.2.1). Marked differences in absorption, distribution, metabolism, and elimination of drugs from both the systemic and CSF compartments

lead to high variability of drug levels between patients, further complicating the interpretation of isolated CSF-to-plasma ratios.

Pharmacokinetic approaches to modeling drug concentrations in CSF and blood are more reliable for studying CNS penetration than are ratios of drug concentrations in both fluids. In classical pharmacokinetic studies, small numbers of individuals are sampled at multiple points in the dosing interval either by repeated lumbar punctures or through an indwelling subarachnoid cannula. The latter technique is relatively demanding of patients and investigators, but allows frequent sampling (Haas, Stone, et al., 2000; Haas, Clough, et al., 2000). Repeated concentration measurements in CSF allow determination of the drug area under concentration time curve (AUC) in CSF. The ratio of the CSF-to-plasma AUC ratio provides an overall time-averaged estimate of penetration that avoids the influence of collection time seen with individual sample assessments of the CSF-to-plasma ratio.

An alternate approach, population pharmacokinetics, infers pharmacokinetic parameters from a single or a few samples collected at a variety of times during the typical dosing interval from many individuals. This method has important advantages, such as enabling analyses of drug concentrations from difficult-to-access body fluids from larger numbers of subjects and providing information about inter-individual variability in relative and absolute CSF concentrations. Population analysis of combined plasma and CSF concentrations can estimate the pharmacokinetic parameters in each compartment and the expected inter-subject variation.

Measures of drug exposure such as a) peak, b) trough, c) mean concentrations, or d) areas under the time-concentration curves can be estimated for both plasma and CSF drug levels by either the classical or population approach. These models can also estimate the inter-compartmental drug transfer between the plasma and the CSF. Which of these measures of exposure best correlates with the effects of antiretrovirals in the CNS remains unclear.

Two examples of population pharmacokinetic models are shown in Figure 11.2.1. In Figure 11.2.1a, plasma levels of abacavir exceed those in CSF early in the dosing interval, whereas CSF levels exceed those in plasma at the end of the interval (Capparelli et al., 2005). This pattern is typical of several NRTIs. Figure 11.2.1b is an example of the different relationship that is common among PIs: CSF levels of indinavir are nearly constant during the dosing interval even though plasma levels markedly vary (Letendre et al., 2000). In both situations, CSF-to-plasma ratios dramatically vary over the dosing interval. Thus, the informative value of the CSF-to-plasma ratio at a single time is very limited without data from pharmacokinetic analysis on the expected levels throughout the dosing interval.

PHARMACODYNAMICS OF ANTIRETROVIRAL DRUGS IN THE CENTRAL NERVOUS SYSTEM

Pharmacodynamics describes the relationships between drug exposure and therapeutic or toxic effects. For antiretroviral drugs, pharmacodynamics in the systemic compartment usually refers to their antiviral (decline in HIV RNA levels in blood or CSF) or immunologic (increase in CD4+

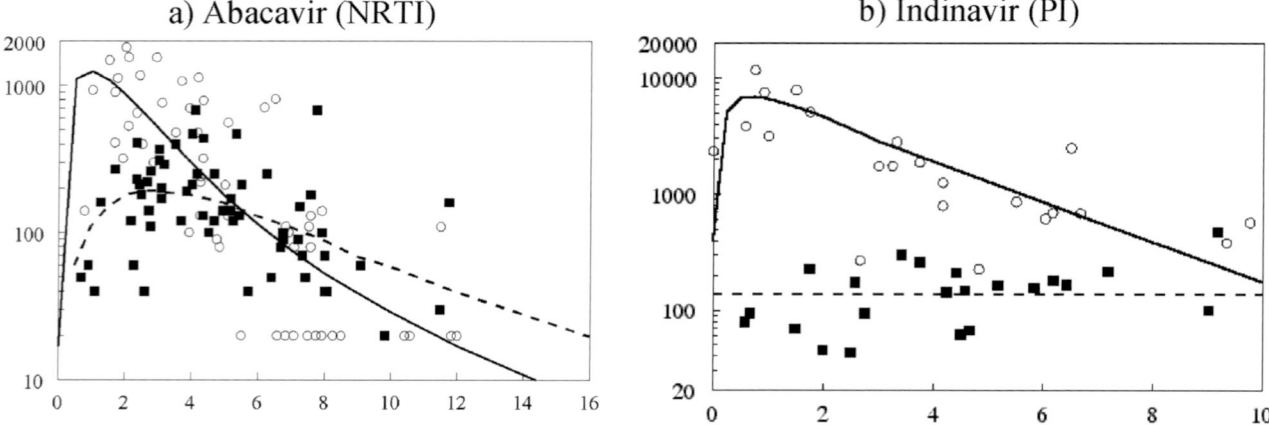

Figure 11.2.1 *Examples of Population Pharmacokinetic Modeling in CSF.* Both figures graph concentrations in CSF and blood of many HIV-infected volunteers without active CNS infections (log scale on vertical axis) by the time (in hours after dose on the horizontal axis). a) CSF values for an nucleoside reverse transcriptase inhibitor (NRTI), abacavir are shown in blue triangles and their average in the blue line. Blood plasma values are shown in red circles and average in the red line. Concentrations and CSF-to-plasma ratio varies markedly over the dosing interval. The areas under the time-concentration curves (AUC) for abacavir was 36% indicating that penetration into the CSF is more than a third of that in plasma. b) CSF concentrations of a protease inhibitor (PI), indinavir, (black squares and dashed line) were much lower than those in blood (open circles and solid line), but exceeded the IC_{50} (not shown). The slope of the time-concentration curve in the CSF for indinavir is zero, indicating that it does not vary over the dosing interval, which is similar to most other PIs.

lymphocyte counts) efficacy (Chaillou et al., 2002; Descamps et al., 2000; Burger et al., 2001; Burger et al., 1998; Back et al., 2002; Marzolini et al., 2001; Marzolini, Telenti, et al., 2001; Fletcher et al., 2000; Powderly et al., 1999; Yasuda et al., 2004). Numerous studies have linked lower PI concentrations in blood to virologic failure in blood. For example, in ACTG 343, individuals who had lower indinavir trough concentrations (C_{min}) were more likely to fail therapy within 24 weeks than those who had higher indinavir C_{min} values (Acosta, Havlir, & Richman, 2000). Low antiretroviral concentrations lead to failure of suppression by allowing evolution of resistant HIV strains (i.e., replication under selective pressure). In contrast, very high drug levels in blood can increase the risk for many toxicities (Burger et al., 2001; Marzolini et al., 2001; Best et al., 2004; Gonzalez de Requena et al., 2003).

The relationships among drug concentrations, HIV drug resistance, and other factors (e.g., adherence, host genetics) are complex and still being defined (Miller et al., 2003; Bangsberg, Moss, & Deeks, 2004; Bangsberg et al., 2004; King et al., 2003). Nevertheless, inter-patient differences in absorption, distribution, and elimination of antiretrovirals result in different pharmacokinetic profiles in the components of their ARV regimens, which can influence efficacy and/or toxicity. Thus, the individual components of ARV regimens may be either too low or too high, supporting the concept of a therapeutic window.

MEASURES OF HIV DRUG SUSCEPTIBILITY AND RESISTANCE

Susceptibility to an anti-infective drug is often summarized by the concentrations required to inhibit degrees of replication or growth of the pathogen in vitro. For viruses, including HIV, the drug concentrations required to inhibit 50% (IC_{50}) or 90% (IC_{90}) of viral replication are common metrics. Inhibitory concentrations for drug-sensitive (wild-type) virus can then

be compared to the concentrations required to inhibit replication of drug-resistant virus and their ratio, or fold-difference, is an indicator of the reduced susceptibility of the resistant virus relative to the susceptible virus. For example, a resistant virus with an IC_{50} of 8 µg/mL has a 4-fold reduced susceptibility compared to a wild-type virus that has an IC_{50} of 2 µg/mL. Modest reductions in susceptibility can sometimes be overcome by increasing doses or decreasing metabolism of the drug. Some drug-resistance mutations produce such large reductions in susceptibility (>100 fold), however, that they cannot be clinically overcome.

The effect of a drug on HIV in the blood and CSF requires attention to both levels of drugs and inhibitory concentrations of the drug for HIV. The standard metric for this purpose is the inhibitory quotient (IQ) or the ratio of the drug concentration in a body fluid over the concentration required to inhibit the pathogen (e.g., IC_{50}). Thus, if the trough level of drug in blood or CSF does not exceed the IC_{50}, the drug would not be expected to completely suppress viral replication in that compartment for the entire dosing interval. The accuracy of IQ-derived measures has been extensively investigated in the systemic compartment (represented by blood) (e.g., Shulman et al., 2002), but not for other compartments such as the CNS. Despite this important limitation, comparing antiretroviral concentrations in CSF to HIV inhibitory concentrations can provide important insights into differences between drugs in effectiveness in the nervous system.

COMPARISONS OF LEVELS AND IN VITRO ACTIVITY OF AVAILABLE ANTIRETROVIRAL DRUGS

Table 11.2.2 summarizes the concentrations in CSF and blood of most of the antiretrovirals approved by the U. S. Food and Drug Administration (FDA) along with ranges of

50% inhibitory concentrations (IC_{50}). Values were derived from published studies, conference abstracts, package inserts, and drug references. For many drugs, the trough (lowest) drug concentrations in CSF were lower than the highest IC_{50} values in the range, suggesting that in some patients CNS replication could occur when concentrations in CSF reach their trough. Because the methods to determine drug and inhibitory concentrations varied between studies, the values in this table are only estimates for comparing the relative likelihood that different drugs will achieve inhibitory concentrations in CSF.

Several factors other than pharmacokinetics influence the pharmacodynamics of antiretroviral drugs. First, their sites of action are within human cells. The two major determinants of intracellular penetration of antiretrovirals are protein binding, since only the unbound fraction is available to enter the cell, and intracellular activation, since some drugs must be altered to their active form within the cell. For example, before they can inhibit reverse transcriptase, NRTIs must be phosphorylated, the efficiency of which can vary with the type and activation state of the target cell (St. Clair et al., 1987).

Second, antiretroviral drugs may also differ in their ability to suppress HIV replication in specific classes of CNS cells. Replication of HIV in the CNS occurs primarily in macrophages and microglia, rather than astrocytes, oligodendrocytes, or neurons, which can be damaged without replicating HIV. Thus, although peripheral blood mononuclear cells (lymphocytes and monocytes = PBMCs) or purified lymphocytes are commonly used for in vitro assays of antiretroviral efficacy, cultures of monocytes or macrophages (M/Ms) may be more relevant to studies of efficacy in the CNS.

This distinction is important since antiretroviral efficacy may substantially differ between M/Ms and PBMCs for some antiretrovirals, particularly NRTIs (Richman, Kornbluth, & Carson, 1987; Aquaro et al., 1997; Perno et al., 1998; Rusconi, Merrill, & Hirsch, 1994). For example, levels of dNTPs (2'-deoxy-nucleoside triphosphates), which compete with NRTIs for intracellular phosphorylation, are 7–40-fold lower in M/Ms than lymphocytes. This suggests that lower intracellular concentrations of NRTIs could effectively compete against endogenous dNTPs for intracellular phosphorylation, and therefore be incorporated into extending HIV DNA chains, resulting in greater inhibition of HIV replication in M/M than in lymphocytes. Since non-nucleoside reverse transcriptase inhibitors (NNRTIs) do not require phosphorylation for their antiviral effect, differences in their activity between M/M and lymphocytes are not expected. The CNS effectiveness of PIs may be reduced by the high concentrations required to inhibit replication in chronically infected M/M. Other factors, such as the cellular activation state and lymphocyte drug transporters, could also influence susceptibility of HIV-infected cells to antiretroviral drugs.

PHARMACODYNAMICS OF ARV DRUGS ON CNS HIV LEVELS AND BRAIN FUNCTION

Virologic Effects of ART in the CNS

Figure 11.2.2 shows examples of common patterns of virologic responses to ART of HIV in CSF and blood. Most patients with sensitive HIV suppress their virion levels below the limits of quantitation in both compartments within 12 to

Table 11.2.2 SUMMARY OF PUBLISHED DATA ON ANTIRETROVIRAL CONCENTRATIONS IN CSF AND IC_{50} RANGES

	CONCENTRATION RANGE IN CSF	IC_{50} RANGE	CSF-TO-IC_{50} RATIO		
			MEDIAN	LOW	HIGH
Nucleoside Reverse Transcriptase Inhibitors					
Abacavir	0.5–1.83	0.24–1.49	4	0.34	7.6
Didanosine	0.17–0.51	2.53–15.84	0.11	0.01	0.2
Lamivudine	0.05–1.14	0.78–4.90	0.74	0.01	1.5
Stavudine	0.20–0.36	0.34–2.12	0.58	0.09	1.1
Zidovudine	0.12–0.41	0.01–0.04	22	3	41
Non-Nucleoside Reverse Transcriptase Inhibitors					
Efavirenz	0.006–0.09	0.008–0.052	5.7	0.12	11
Nevirapine	1.3–10.9	0.023–0.142	241	8.9	474
Protease Inhibitors					
Amprenavir	BLQ - 0.36	0.0046–0.0289	39	BLQ	78
Indinavir	0.03–0.66	0.0031–0.0195	108	1.5	213
Lopinavir	0.006–0.042	0.0019–0.0475	11	0.13	22
Nelfinavir	BLQ - 0.36	0.0014–0.0088	4.3	BLQ	8.6
Ritonavir	BLQ - 0.032	0.0049–0.0308	3.3	BLQ	6.5
Saquinavir	BLQ - 0.008	0.001–0.006	4	BLQ	4

Letendre, S., Ellis, R., Grant, I., & McCutchan, J. (2001) .The CSF Concentration/IC50 Ratio: A Predictor of CNS Antiretroviral (ARV) Efficacy (Abstract 614) In 8th Conference on Retroviruses and Opportunistic Infections, Chicago, 2001.

24 weeks, as illustrated in Figure 11.2.2a. Others respond in CSF alone (Figure 11.2.2b) or in neither compartment (not shown) (Spudich et al., 2006; Letendre, Ellis, & McCutchan, 2000). ART response in blood, but not in CSF (Figure 11.2.2c), is uncommon but occurs primarily in advanced HIV disease or with severe HAND (dementia) (Ellis et al., 2000). Discordant responses in which HIV persists in the CSF after complete suppression in the blood requires autonomous HIV replication in the CNS because measurable levels of virions are no longer entering the CNS from the blood. This situation could arise from drug-resistant HIV in the CNS, sub-therapeutic antiretroviral concentrations in the CNS, or possibly other reasons.

Clinical evidence for the importance of penetration to suppression of HIV in CSF comes from small studies that administered PIs only, NRTIs only, or combinations of NRTIs and NNRTIs. Two studies demonstrated good suppression of HIV in CSF with combinations of NRTIs alone or with an NNRTI, all of which penetrate the CNS reasonably well. Foudraine et al., for example, treated patients with lamivudine and either zidovudine or stavudine and found that ARV-naive patients responded in the CSF if their blood RNA levels responded (Foudraine et al., 1998). Similarly, Tashima reported that efavirenz-containing regimens suppressed HIV in CSF if they also suppressed HIV in blood(Tashima et al., 1999). However, this study administered EFV, which is approximately 99.5% bound by plasma proteins, simultaneously with two drugs with known CNS efficacy, zidovudine and lamivudine, and did not measure pre-treatment HIV RNA levels in CSF. Overall, though, regimens that reduce HIV in blood generally reduce HIV in CSF, also.

In contrast, two studies administered the dual-PI regimen, ritonavir and saquinavir, neither of which penetrates into CSF well. Both studies found that HIV in CSF was often not suppressed (Kravcik et al., 1999; Kravcik, 2001; Gisolf et al., 2000). Kravcik found that five patients failing combination therapy had a reversal of the usual ratio of plasma to HIV RNA levels in CSF (from approximately 40 to 0.3). Higher levels in CSF at the time of failure suggested that the CNS

remained untreated or escaped control earlier than the plasma. In the second study, among six patients beginning therapy with ritonavir and saquinavir, all had detectable HIV RNA levels in CSF after 12 weeks of treatment. These studies identified that antiretrovirals that poorly penetrate into the CNS can fail to suppress HIV in CSF.

In addition to methodological inconsistencies, other limitations affect interpretation of these data. First, some studies did not measure HIV RNA levels in CSF prior to initiating therapy. Since some patients demonstrate only low levels of HIV replication in CSF, failure to clearly exclude them biases the results. Second, multiple drugs were typically started simultaneously. While this is appropriate in clinical practice, it hampers attribution to a single drug of effectiveness in the CNS. Third, many studies did not confirm that the participants' HIV strains were susceptible to the study drugs or did not clearly exclude antiretroviral-experienced patients, who may harbor resistant mutants. Fourth, most did not enroll individuals with lower CD4 counts, the group at greatest risk for neurocognitive complications and in whom CNS penetration is most critical. Instead, many studies predominantly enrolled individuals who had higher CD4 counts, in whom HIV RNA in CSF often originates primarily from blood. The applicability of the findings of these studies to patients with more advanced disease is unclear. Finally, when antiretroviral concentrations were measured, many studies were not designed to control for post-dose sampling times well enough to allow population pharmacokinetic modeling. Instead, such studies relied on calculation of a limited range of CSF-to-plasma concentration ratios, providing little insight into whether CSF concentrations reached therapeutic levels.

Clinical Effects of ART in the CNS

As summarized in Table 11.2.3, numerous studies have addressed the role of penetration of ART regimens into the CNS as a determinant of treatment or prophylaxis of HAND. Many of the studies were limited by their small, observational, and cross-sectional designs. In addition, the studies

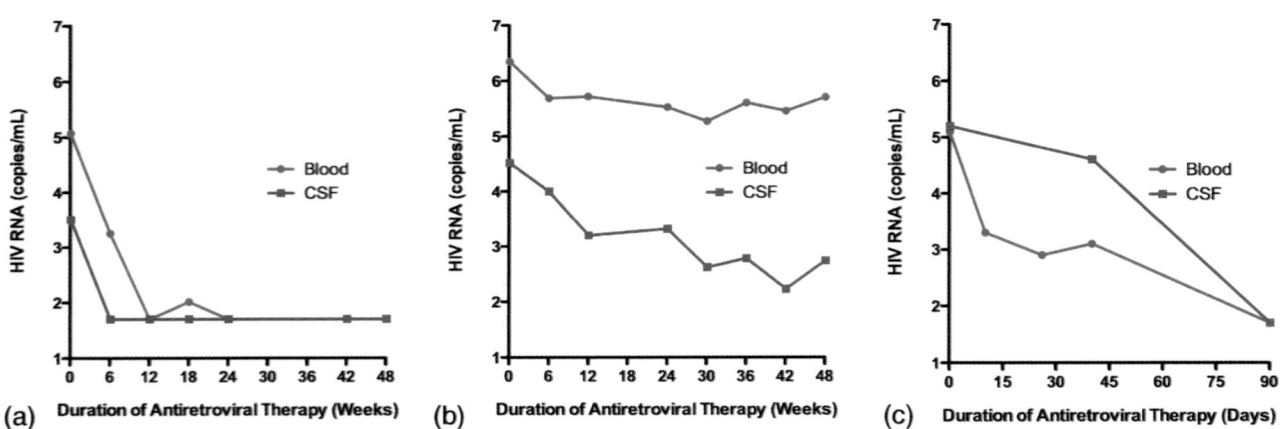

Figure 11.2.2 *Patterns of HIV RNA Response in CSF and Blood to ART.* a) Concordant response in CSF and blood, b) Discordant response: HIV RNA reductions in CSF but not blood, c) Discordant response: substantially delayed response in CSF compared with blood.

varied in target populations, measures of CNS penetration, and measures of neuropsychological outcome, making comparisons difficult. For example, to assess penetration, some studies focused on individual drugs (e.g., zidovudine or indinavir), some utilized an additive penetration "score" for the entire regimen, and others directly measured antiretroviral concentrations in CSF.

Measures of clinical outcome in these studies were even more diverse, and included clinical staging (e.g., Memorial Sloan-Kettering AIDS Dementia Complex staging), neuropsychological testing (either brief or comprehensive batteries), neuroimaging, or evoked potentials. Even when studies were prospectively accrued, they either lacked comparison groups or CNS response was only a secondary objective. Not surprisingly, these varying methods have yielded inconsistent results and failed to consistently define the importance of CNS penetration. Larger, prospective, controlled trials are needed to adequately address if better penetration produces better neurovirologic or neurocognitive outcomes.

DEVELOPMENT OF A CLINICALLY USEFUL CNS EFFECTIVENESS METRIC FOR ANTIRETROVIRAL DRUGS

APPROACH

Standardized measures of the relative CNS effectiveness of antiretroviral regimens are required for optimal prevention or treatment of neurocognitive impairment. Since CNS penetration seems important for optimization of therapy, we have attempted to both estimate penetration and study its role in pharmacodynamics. While several approaches to estimating penetration or effectiveness have been described, they often failed to adequately justify their methods. Because these approaches used varying definitions of CNS penetration and varying outcomes, direct comparisons between the studies was difficult.

Using the information described earlier in this chapter (physicochemical characteristics, pharmacokinetics, pharmacodynamics), we undertook an approach that was based on hierarchical valuation of evidence and was designed to (1) include all commercially available antiretrovirals; (2) accommodate new drugs as they are introduced; and (3) provide a method for combining the penetration of the multiple drugs in antiretroviral regimens. Since no single metric is universally accepted as a valid index of CNS penetration or effectiveness, the proposed system considered data available in peer-reviewed manuscripts, conference abstracts, package inserts, and drug references. Also, because the quality and type of evidence about CNS effectiveness varies greatly among drugs, our approach describes not only the predicted CNS effectiveness, but also identifies and weights the quality of the evidence supporting predictions. This multi-dimensional approach provides a relative, rather than an absolute, scale of CNS penetration for drugs and regimens.

An extensive literature review was conducted on all currently available antiretrovirals. Drugs such as zalcitabine and

Table 11.2.3 STUDIES COMPARING THE PHARMACODYNAMICS OF CNS-PENETRATING VERSUS NON-PENETRATING ANTIRETROVIRAL DRUGS ON EITHER HIV RNA LEVELS IN CSF OR NEUROCOGNITIVE FUNCTIONING. FUNCTIONAL STUDIES VARIED IN MEASURES OF OUTCOMES FROM CLINICAL STAGING TO MOTOR TESTING TO COMPREHENSIVE NP TESTING

AUTHOR	YEAR	DESIGN	N	PENETRATION MEASURE	EFFECT
HIV RNA in CSF					
Cysique [102]	2004	P	37	CPE	Lower
Marra [101]	2009	P	79	CPE	Lower
Antinori [81]	2005	C-S	63	No. of penetrators	Lower
von Giesen [82]	2005	C-S	71	ZDV, d4T	Similar
Letendre [83]	2004	P	31	No. of penetrators	Lower
Eggers [84]	2003	P	40	Multiple	Similar
Solas [85]	2003	C-S	41	IDV	Similar
Marra [86]	2003	P	25	ZDV, IDV	Similar
Lafeuillade [87]	2002	C-S	41	IDV vs. LPV-r or NFV	Similar
Robertson [88]	2002	C-S	98	No. of penetrators	Similar
Antinori (a) [89]	2002	C-S	75	IDV	Lower
Antinori (b) [89]	2002	P	29	≥ 3 Penetrators	Lower
DeLuca (a)[90]	2002	C-S	134	No. of penetrators	Similar
DeLuca (b)[90]	2002	P	50	No. of penetrators	Lower
Letendre[80]	2001	C-S	1239	NNRTI- vs. PI-based	Lower
Gisolf[91]	2000	P*	27	SQV-r+d4T vs. SQV-r	Lower
Murphy[92]	2000	P*	27	APV-ZDV-3TC vs. APV	Lower

(Continues)

Table 11.2.3 (CONTINUED)

AUTHOR	YEAR	DESIGN	N	PENETRATION MEASURE	EFFECT
Measures of Brain Injury					
Simioni [105]	2010	C-S	200	CPE	Trend
Ellis [104]	2009	P	2,636	CPE	**Better**
Tozzi [103]	2009	P	185	CPE	**Better**
Cysique [102]	2009	P	37	CPE	**Better**
Marra [101]	2009	P	26	CPE	**Less Improvement**
von Giesen[82]	2005	C-S	71	ZDV, d4T	Similar
Letendre[83]	2004	P	31	No. of penetrators	Similar
Antinori[93]	2004	C-S	165	No. of penetrators	Similar
Cysique[94]	2004	P	97	≥ 3 Penetrators	**Better**
Evers (a)[95]	2004	C-S	306	Multiple	**Better**
Evers (b)[95]	2004	P	110	Multiple	Similar
Robertson[96]	2004	P	29	No. of penetrators	Similar
Sevigny[97]	2004	P	395	No. of penetrators	Similar
Marra[86]	2003	P	25	ZDV, IDV	**Better**
Chang[98]	2003	P	33	≥ 2 Penetrators	Similar
Dougherty[99]	2002	P	96	Single vs. Multiple	Similar
von Giesen[82]	2002	P	104	NVP vs. EFV	**Better**
Sacktor[100]	2001	P	73	Single vs. Multiple	Similar

C-S = Cross-Sectional; P = Prospective, longitudinal; VL = Viral Load; NP = Neuropsychological; *Controlled Prospective Studies.

delavirdine were omitted from consideration since they are no longer prescribed due to toxic side-effects or limited potency. Also, because the HIV protease inhibitor ritonavir is routinely prescribed in lower, pharmacologic-boosting doses, rather than higher therapeutic doses, it was considered as a boosting agent only. Since some drugs, such as atazanavir, are given with or without ritonavir boosting, we independently considered data for boosted and unboosted formulations. Tables 11.2.1, 11.2.2, and 11.2.3 summarize a selection of the three different types of data that we summarized and considered hierarchically (physicochemical characteristics < pharmacokinetics < pharmacodynamics) in creating CNS penetration rankings.

Descriptive statistics characterizing CSF drug concentrations (e.g., median or mean and range) were compiled from the literature as published in primary reports. When only plasma concentrations and CSF-to-plasma ratios were reported, CSF concentrations were back-calculated using the available data. Other studies reported area-under-the-curve (AUC) estimates, rather than point concentrations. To estimate point concentrations comparable to those reported in the majority of studies, back-calculations again were performed. Since dosage and dosing interval varied between studies for some drugs, this information was also compiled to allow its consideration in rankings. To account for PK interactions between drugs, co-administration of other antiretrovirals was noted. Studies in which HIV protease inhibitors were boosted by the addition of low-dose ritonavir were clearly specified.

Data for each drug were summarized in a standardized format, as illustrated in Table 11.2.4 for nevirapine. If no direct CSF concentration measurements were available, the minimum concentration of the drug in plasma over the dosing interval (C_{min}) for PIs and NNRTIs or its average (C_{ave}) for NRTIs was multiplied by the unbound fraction to estimate CNS drug exposure. CSF PK estimates were interpreted by comparison to IC_{50} estimates for wild-type HIV strains. When available, IC_{50} values were taken from the median population values of the Monogram Biosciences PhenoSense assay (Parkin et al., 2004) to standardize experimental conditions. CSF PK values that exceeded the IC_{50} were interpreted as predicting at least fair CNS efficacy.

The general approach to rating the data was similar to that used to generate clinical guidelines. Two independent dimensions were considered: the estimated CNS effectiveness and the quality of the evidence. The CNS penetration score (CPE) or "effectiveness" for each drug was ranked at three levels, from best (1.0) through worst (0.0). Evidence was considered to be "Limited" if it derived only from physicochemical characteristics (molecular weight, protein binding, lipid solubility, charge). Evidence quality was considered "Moderate" when PK data were available (i.e., measured drug concentrations in CSF). Evidence was considered "Strong" if pharmacodynamic data such as changes in CSF HIV levels or neurocognitive function were reported.

Physicochemical data that were considered included unbound fraction, molecular weight, electrical charge at

Table 11.2.4 EXAMPLE OF DATA COMPILATION. NEVIRAPINE LEVELS IN CSF EXCEEDED THE WILD-TYPE IC_{50} BY UP TO 116-FOLD (10.4 μM/0.09 μM).

FIRST AUTHOR	JOURNAL OR CONFERENCE	YEAR	SAMPLE SIZE	DOSE (MG)	IC_{50} (μM)	CSF MEDIAN OR MEAN (μM)	CSF LOWEST (μM)	CSF HIGHEST (μM)	CSF-TO-PLASMA RATIO	PLASMA RNAGE (μM)	PLASMA CMIN (μM)	PLASMA CMAX (μM)	AUC_{24} (μM·H)
Kearny	CROI	1999	6	200 qD	-	1.45	1.26	10.4	AUC ratio 29%	3.33–44.4	-	-	-
van Praag	AAC	2002	9	200 bid	-	3.49	0.82	6.89	-	-	6.1–25.7	18–35.4	196–713
Antinori	CID	2005	16	-	-	-	-	-	41–77%	-	-	-	-
Antinori	CROI	2002	-	-	-	-	-	-	63%	-	-	-	-
Parkin	AAC	2004	-	-	0.09	-	-	-	-	-	-	-	-
	Summary				0.09	2.47	0.82	10.4	63% (median)	3.33–44.4	13.89	18–35.4	196–713
									29–77% (range)				

physiologic pH, and lipid solubility. For PIs and NNRTIs, protein binding was considered to be the principal determinant of CNS penetration, while for NRTIs, which are active intracellularly, lipid solubility and molecular weight were considered principal determinants.

0.0–Physicochemical characteristics were below average compared to other drugs in its class

0.5–Physicochemical characteristics were average compared to other drugs in its class

1.0–Physicochemical characteristics were above average compared to other drugs in its class

For example, the protease inhibitor darunavir would be assigned a score of 1.0 based on an intermediate molecular weight in its class (548 g/mol), a relatively high unbound fraction for its class (5%), and relatively high lipophilicity (LogP 2.23). This relativistic rating approach has uncertain validity but allows for estimation of CNS penetration before PK or PD data are available, an approach that is particularly valuable for investigational or recently approved antiretrovirals.

Ranking was specific to each drug class, taking into account distinctive pharmacological characteristics of the agents in each class. For example, because the NRTIs require intracellular activation through phosphorylation and because the intracellular NRTI-triphosphate has slower elimination than the unphosphorylated NRTI in plasma, trough plasma concentrations (C_{min}) are a poor surrogate for activity. Because of the more rapid clearance of extracellular NRTIs, little or no drug remains in plasma at the end of the dosing interval. As a result, the dosing intervals for many NRTIs have been lengthened without loss of activity. For this reason, we considered the average plasma concentration of NRTIs over the dosing interval (C_{ave}) as a more appropriate surrogate for CNS activity.

Since fractional protein binding of NRTIs is generally lower than that for protease inhibitors or NNRTIs (for most NRTIs, at least 30% of drug is unbound) and is of uncertain significance for a drug that can accumulate intracellularly, rankings for NRTIs were less dependent on protein binding. Because lipophilicity varies greatly within the NRTI class, octanol water coefficients were given greater weight in ranking the NRTIs relative to one another. Since rankings are relative within each drug class, a rank of 1.0 for a protease inhibitor may not be similar to a rank of 1.0 for an NNRTI or NRTI.

To compare pharmacokinetic data between drugs (and estimate effectiveness), drug concentrations were compared to inhibitory concentrations. The ratio of the drugs concentrations in CSF to the median population IC_{50} value for wild-type HIV using the PhenoSense assay was used in this rating system. Because the absolute minimum ratio to achieve consistent CNS effectiveness is not defined, a within-class relative definition was again used.

0.0–Fewer than 25% of drug concentrations in CSF exceed the IC_{50} or the median CSF-to-IC_{50} ratio is less than 1.

0.5–Between 25% and 75% of drug concentrations in CSF are above the IC_{50} or the median CSF-to-IC_{50} ratio is between 1- and 5-fold.

1.0–More than 75% of drug concentrations in CSF are above the IC_{50} and the median CSF-to-IC_{50} ratio exceeds 5-fold.

For example, for nevirapine, all drug concentrations reported in CSF exceed the IC_{50} (0.09 µM) with the approximate mean (2.47 µM) exceeding it by 27-fold. These data support a rank of 1.0 for nevirapine (Table 11.2.4).

Assessment of pharmacodynamics is particularly challenging since the methods of pharmacodynamic studies vary so greatly. For this reason, a relativistic approach was again used. The fundamental question was, "When used by itself or in a manner that allowed assessment of its independent therapeutic effect, how well did the drug of interest perform relative to historical data for drugs in its class?" The scarcity of pharmacodynamic data limits standardization of criteria, making the pharmacodynamic standard even more qualitative than the others. One example of a quantitative criterion based on our review of the data is:

0.0–More than 20% of HIV RNA levels in CSF were above 50 copies/mL after at least 12 weeks of therapy.

0.5–Between 10 and 20% of HIV RNA levels in CSF were above 50 copies/mL after at least 12 weeks of therapy.

1.0–Fewer than 10% of HIV RNA levels in CSF were above 50 copies/mL after at least 12 weeks of therapy.

For example, in a study of boosted lopinavir, HIV RNA levels in CSF were above 50 copies/mL in 1 of 11 (9%) cases (Yeh et al., 2007), supporting a rank of 1.0, compared with a study of boosted atazanavir, in which HIV RNA levels in CSF were above 50 copies/mL in 3 of 20 (15%) of cases (Vernazza et al., 2007), supporting a rank of 0.5.

VALIDATION OF THE CPE RANKING SYSTEM

Table 11.2.5 lists the CNS penetration-effectiveness (CPE) ranks and the strength of the evidence for currently available antiretrovirals in the United States. A substantial proportion of these has scores less than 1.0, suggesting suboptimal penetration. To evaluate the clinical validity of this hierarchical ranking system, we compared the sum of the drug-specific CPE ranks for all drugs regimens in 467 volunteers in the CHARTER (CNS HIV AntiRetroviral Therapy Effects Research) study to their current HIV RNA levels in CSF (Letendre et al., 2008).

CHARTER is a multicenter, prospective, observational study was designed to recruit a cohort that was similar to the U.S. population of HIV-infected individuals and to determine the effects of ART on the nervous system. Data from baseline evaluations that occurred between October 2003 and January 2006 were included in this cross-sectional analysis. Of 833

Table 11.2.5 COMPILATION TABLE FOR PHYSICOCHEMICAL (PC), PHARMACOKINETIC (PK), AND PHARMACODYNAMIC (PD) DATA RATINGS

	PC SCORE	PK SCORE	PD SCORE	FINAL SCORE	STRENGTH OF EVIDENCE
NRTIs					
Abacavir	0.5	1.0	1.0	1.0	Strong
Didanosine	1.0	0.0	0.0	0.0	Strong
Emtricitabine	0.5	1.0	*	1.0	Moderate
Lamivudine	0.5	0.5	*	0.5	Moderate
Stavudine	0.5	0.5	*	0.5	Moderate
Tenofovir	0.0	0.0	*	0.0	Moderate
Zidovudine	0.5	1.0	1.0	1.0	Strong
NNRTIs					
Efavirenz	0.5	0.0–1.0	*	0.5	Moderate
Etravirine	0.0	0.0	*	0.0	Limited
Nevirapine	1.0	1.0	*	1.0	Moderate
Protease Inhibitors					
Atazanavir	1.0	0.5	0.5	0.5	Strong
Atazanavir-rtv	1.0	0.5	0.5	0.5	Strong
Darunavir	1.0	1.0	*	1.0	Moderate
Lopinavir-rtv	0.5	1.0	1.0	1.0	Strong
Tipranavir-rtv	0.0	*	*	0.0	Limited
Indinavir	1.0	1.0	*	1.0	Moderate
Indinavir-rtv	1.0	1.0	*	1.0	Moderate
Fosamprenavir	1.0	0.5	*	0.5	Moderate
Fosamprenavir-rtv	1.0	0.5	*	0.5	Moderate
Nelfinavir	0.5	0.0	0.0	0.0	Strong
Saquinavir-rtv	0.5	0.0	0.0	0.0	Strong
Entry or Fusion Inhibitors					
Maraviroc	0.5	0.5	*	0.5	Moderate
Enfuvirtide	0.0	0.0	0.0	0.0	Strong
Integrase Inhibitor					
Raltegravir	0.5	1.0	*	1.0	1.0

HIV+ volunteers enrolled in the CHARTER study, venipuncture and lumbar puncture were successfully performed on 659 (79%). Of these, 467 (71%) met eligibility criteria for this analysis by reporting current ART use and having HIV RNA measured in both CSF and blood. This analysis used the initial version of the CPE scoring system in which 1 was better, 0.5 intermediate, and 0 was worse for each drug.

In this cohort, the median CPE score for each regimen was 1.5 (interquartile range 1–2) (Figure 11.2.3a). Lower CPE scores, indicating worse estimated ART penetration into the CNS, correlated with higher HIV RNA levels in CSF (Spearman's Rho = −0.12, p = 0.008) (Figure 11.2.3b). In addition, CPE scores less than or equal to the median were associated with an 88% increase in the odds of a detectable HIV RNA level in CSF (i.e., above 50 copies/mL). In multivariate regression, lower CPE scores were associated with detectable HIV RNA levels in CSF even after adjusting for total number of antiretrovirals, medication adherence, HIV RNA levels in blood, duration and type of the current ART regimen, and current CD4 count. In the best regression model, each unit decrease in CPE score was associated with a nearly 2.5-fold increase in the odds of having detectable HIV RNA in CSF (adjusted OR = 2.43, 95% CI 1.56–3.93). In an alternate model, CPE scores below 2.0 were associated with more than a 3-fold increase in the odds of having detectable HIV RNA in CSF (OR = 3.32, 95% CI 1.62–6.71).

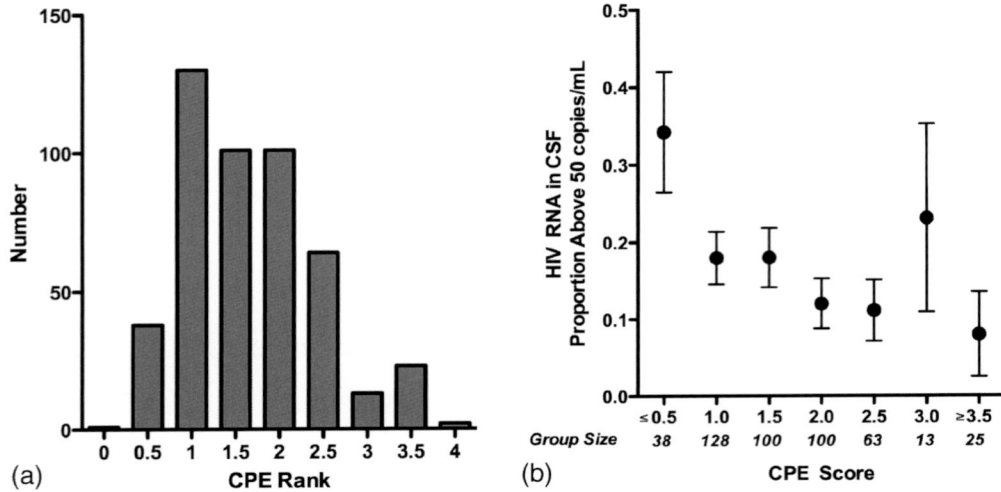

Figure 11.2.3 Distribution of CPE Scores (a) and their relation to HIV RNA levels in CSF (b). Total CPE scores for 467 regimens varied widely over a range form 0 to 4. After adjusting for other important covariates, each unit decrease in CPE score was associated with a nearly 2.5-fold increase in the odds of detectable HIV RNA in CSF.

Since this analysis was published, other groups have evaluated the CPE ranking system. For example, Tozzi and colleagues identified that higher CPE ranks were associated with better neuropsychological performance in a cohort study after a mean of 1.5 years of ART (Tozzi et al., 2009). Using ante-mortem and autopsy data from 392 volunteers in the U.S. National NeuroAIDS Tissue Consortium, Everall and colleagues identified that higher CPE ranks during the period of observation prior to death were associated with a lower prevalence of typical HIV-associated brain pathology at autopsy (Everall et al., 2008). Further analysis identified that the ART association with brain pathology was particularly strong for NNRTIs. Using data from the French Hospital Database on HIV, Gasnault and colleagues found that use of ART with higher CPE ranks was associated with better survival among people with AIDS who were diagnosed with progressive multifocal leukoencephalopathy (PML) Gasnault et al., 2008). Finally, using data from our Center from a study other than CHARTER, we identified that better CPE ranks were associated with greater improvements in neuropsychological performance among people diagnosed with HAND and initiating a new ART regimen (Letendre et al., 2008).

Together, these findings support the validity of this standardized approach to assessing the penetration and effectiveness of antiretrovirals in the CNS. CPE influences reduction in HIV RNA levels in the CNS, prevention and treatment of HAND, and treatment of some CNS opportunistic infections. The approach we have outlined is evidence based, can evolve as new data become available, is easy-to-adopt by practicing clinicians, and could be incorporated into treatment guidelines to encourage clinicians to optimally protect the brain when selecting a new ART regimen.

Acceptance of the CPE scoring system is limited by the fact that supporting data are mostly observational and cross-sectional. CPE has not yet been validated by a prospective, controlled trial (Ellis, 2007). For this reason, we have undertaken a randomized, strategy trial of CNS-targeted ART (May

et al., 2007; Ellis et al.). As of early 2010, this trial was enrolling in Baltimore, St. Louis, and San Diego, with new sites opening in San Francisco and New York in later in 2010. The study compares cognitive improvement in patients with impairment at baseline who are treated with regimens that are chosen to be a) systemically effective and b) randomly selected to be either maximally or minimally CNS penetrating. The results should provide more compelling evidence for or against the need to consider CNS penetration in selection of ART regimens.

ACKNOWLEDGMENTS

The authors gratefully acknowledge research support from the National Institutes of Health (R01 MH58076, P30 MH62512), Abbott Laboratories, GlaxoSmithKline, Merck & Co., and Tibotec, Inc.

REFERENCES

Aamnoutse, R. E., Verweij-van Wissen, C. P., Underberg, W. J., Kleinnijenhuis, J., Hekster, Y. A., & Burger, D. M. (2001). High-performance liquid chromatography of HIV protease inhibitors in human biological matrices. *J Chromatogr B Biomed Sci Appl, 764*(1–2), 363–384.

Acosta, E., Havlir, D. V., & Richman, D. D. (2000). In Pharmacodynamics (PD) of indinavir (IDV) in protease-naive HIV-infected patients receiving ZDV and 3TC, 7th Conference on Retroviruses and Opportunistic Infections, San Francisco, CA, January 30-February 2; San Francisco, CA, 2000.

Anderson, P. L., Brundage, R. C., Bushman, L., Kakuda, T. N. Remmel, R. P., & Fletcher, C. V. (2000) Indinavir plasma protein binding in HIV-1-infected adults. *AIDS (London, England)* 2000, *14*(15), 2293–2297.

Antinori, A., Giancola, M. L., Grisetti, S., Soldani, F., Alba, L., Liuzzi, G., et al. (2002). Factors influencing virological response to antiretroviral drugs in cerebrospinal fluid of advanced HIV-1-infected patients. *AIDS (London, England),16*(14), 1867–1876.

Antinori, A., Larussa, D., Cingolani, A., Lorenzini, P., Bossolasco, S., Finazzi, M. G., et al. (2004). Prevalence, associated factors, and prognostic determinants of AIDS-related toxoplasmic encephalitis in the era of advanced highly active antiretroviral therapy. *Clin Infect Dis*, *39*(11), 1681–1691.

Antinori, A., Perno, C. F., Giancola, M. L., Forbici, F., Ippolito, G., Hoetelmans, R. M., et al. (2005). Efficacy of cerebrospinal fluid (CSF)-penetrating antiretroviral drugs against HIV in the neurological compartment: Different patterns of phenotypic resistance in CSF and plasma. *Clin Infect Dis*, *41*(12), 1787–1793.

Aquaro, S., Perno, C. F., Balestra, E., Balzarini, J., Cenci, A., Francesconi, M., et al. (1997). Inhibition of replication of HIV in primary monocyte/macrophages by different antiviral drugs and comparative efficacy in lymphocytes. *J Leukoc Biol*, *62*(1), 138–143.

Back, D., Gatti, G., Fletcher, C., Garaffo, R., Haubrich, R., Hoetelmans, R., et al. (2002). Therapeutic drug monitoring in HIV infection: Current status and future directions. *AIDS (London, England,)* 16 Suppl 1, S5–37.

Bangsberg, D. R., Moss, A. R., & Deeks, S. G. (2004). Paradoxes of adherence and drug resistance to HIV antiretroviral therapy. *J Antimicrob Chemother*, *53*(5), 696–699.

Bangsberg, D. R., Porco, T. C., Kagay, C., Charlebois, E. D., Deeks, S. G., Guzman, D., et al. (2004). Modeling the HIV protease inhibitor adherence-resistance curve by use of empirically derived estimates. *The Journal of Infectious Diseases*, *190*(1), 162–165.

Best, B., May, S., Witt, M., Kemper, C., Larsen, R., Diamond, C., et al. (2004). In *Relationship between lopinavir (LPV) concentration and changes in lipid levels at 24 weeks*, 11th Conference on Retroviruses and Opportunistic Infections, San Francisco, CA, February 8–11; San Francisco, CA, 2004.

Brewster, M. E., Anderson, W. R., Webb, A. I., Pablo, L. M., Meinsma, D., Moreno, D., et al. (1997). Evaluation of a brain-targeting zidovudine chemical delivery system in dogs. *Antimicrobial Agents and Chemotherapy*, *41*(1), 122–128.

Burger, D., Felderhof, M., Phanupak, P., Duncombe, C., Mahanontharit, A., Yeamwanichnun, W., et al. (2001). In *Both short-term virological efficacy and drug-associated nephrotoxicity are related to indinavir (IDV) pharmacokinetics (PK) in HIV-1-infected Thai patients*, 8th Conference on Retroviruses and Opportunistic Infections, Chicago, IL, February 4–8; Chicago, IL, 2001; p 264.

Burger, D. M., Hoetelmans, R. M., Hugen, P. W., Mulder, J. W., Meenhorst, P. L., Koopmans, P. P., et al. (1998). Low plasma concentrations of indinavir are related to virological treatment failure in HIV-1-infected patients on indinavir-containing triple therapy. *Antiviral Therapy*, *3*(4), 215–220.

Canestri, A., et al. (2010). Discordance between cerebral spinal fluid and plasma HIV replication in patients with neurological symptoms who are receiving suppressive antiretroviral therapy. *Clin Infect Dis*, 50, 773–8.

Capparelli, E. V., Letendre, S. L., Ellis, R. J., Patel, P., Holland, D., & McCutchan, J. A., (2005). Population pharmacokinetics of abacavir in plasma and cerebrospinal fluid. *Antimicrobial Agents and Chemotherapy*, *49*(6), 2504–2506.

Chaillou, S., Durant, J., Garraffo, R., Georgenthum, E., Roptin, C., Clevenbergh, P., et al. (2002). Intracellular concentration of protease inhibitors in HIV-1-infected patients: Correlation with MDR-1 gene expression and low dose of ritonavir. *HIV Clinical Trials,* *3*(6), 493–501.

Chang, L., Ernst, T., Witt, M. D., Ames, N., Walot, I., Jovicich, J., et al. (2003). Persistent brain abnormalities in antiretroviral-naive HIV patients 3 months after HAART. *Antiviral Therapy*, *8*(1), 17–26.

Cysique, L. A., Maruff, P., & Brew, B. J. (2004). Antiretroviral therapy in HIV infection: Are neurologically active drugs important? *Archives of Neurology*, *61*(11), 1699–1704.

Cysique, L. A., Maruff, P., & Brew, B. J. (2004). Prevalence and pattern of neuropsychological impairment in human immunodeficiency virus-infected/acquired immunodeficiency syndrome (HIV/AIDS) patients across pre- and post-highly active antiretroviral therapy eras: A combined study of two cohorts. *Journal of Neurovirology*, *10*(6), 350–357.

Cysique, L. A., Vaida, F., Letendre, S., Gibson, S., Cherner, M., Woods, S. P., et al. (2009). Dynamics of cognitive change in impaired

HIV-positive patients initiating antiretroviral therapy. *Neurology*, Aug 4;*73*(5), 342–348.

de Lange, E. C. & Danhof, M. (2002). Considerations in the use of cerebrospinal fluid pharmacokinetics to predict brain target concentrations in the clinical setting: Implications of the barriers between blood and brain. *Clin Pharmacokinet*, *41*(10), 691–703.

De Luca, A., Ciancio, B. C., Larussa, D., Murri, R., Cingolani, A., Rizzo, M. G., et al. (2002). Correlates of independent HIV-1 replication in the CNS and of its control by antiretrovirals. *Neurology*, *59*(3), 342–347.

Descamps, D., Flandre, P., Calvez, V., Peytavin, G., Meiffredy, V., Collin, G., et al. (2000). Mechanisms of virologic failure in previously untreated HIV-infected patients from a trial of induction-maintenance therapy. *JAMA*, *283*(2), 205–211.

Deutsch, R., Ellis, R. J., McCutchan, J. A., Marcotte, T. D., Letendre, S., & Grant, I., (2001). AIDS-associated mild neurocognitive impairment is delayed in the era of highly active antiretroviral therapy. *AIDS*, *15*(14), 1898–1899.

Dore, G. J., Correll, P. K., Li, Y., Kaldor, J. M., Cooper, D. A., & Brew, B. J., (1999). Changes to AIDS dementia complex in the era of highly active antiretroviral therapy. *AIDS*, *13*(10), 1249–1253.

Dougherty, R. H., Skolasky, R. L., Jr., & McArthur, J. C. (2002). Progression of HIV-associated dementia treated with HAART. *The AIDS Reader*, *12*(2), 69–74.

Eggers, C., Hertogs, K., Sturenburg, H. J., van Lunzen, J., & Stellbrink, H. J. (2003). Delayed central nervous system virus suppression during highly active antiretroviral therapy is associated with HIV encephalopathy, but not with viral drug resistance or poor central nervous system drug penetration. *AIDS (London, England)*, *17*(13), 1897–1906.

Ellis, R. J. (2007). Clinical trials in HIV CNS disease and treatment management. *J Neuroimmune Pharmacol*, *2*(1), 20–25.

Ellis, R. J., Gamst, A. C., Capparelli, E., Spector, S. A., Hsia, K., Wolfson, T., et al. (2000). Cerebrospinal fluid HIV RNA originates from both local CNS and systemic sources. *Neurology*, *54*(4), 927–936.

Ellis, R. J., Hsia, K., Spector, S. A., Nelson, J. A., Heaton, R. K., Wallace, M. R., (1997). Cerebrospinal fluid human immunodeficiency virus type 1 RNA levels are elevated in neurocognitively impaired individuals with acquired immunodeficiency syndrome. HIV Neurobehavioral Research Center Group. *Ann Neurol*, *42*(5), 679–688.

Ellis, R., Letendre, S., Clifford, D., Sacktor, N., & McCutchan, J. Cognitive Intervention Trial 2 (ClinicalTrials.gov identifier NCT00624195). http://clinicaltrials.gov/ct2/show/NCT00624195.

Ellis, R.J., Smurzynski, M., Wu, K., Bosch, R.J., Robertson, K., Evans, S., et al. (2009)., Effects of CNS Antiretroviral (ARV) Distribution on Neurocognitive (NC) Impairment in the AIDS Clinical Trials Group (ACTG) Longitudinal Linked Randomized Trials (ALLRT) Study. Annual Meeting American Neurological Association, 2009, Abstract T-107.

Enting, R. H., Hoetelmans, R. M., Lange, J. M., Burger, D. M., Beijnen, J. H., & Portegies, P. (1998). Antiretroviral drugs and the central nervous system. *AIDS (London, England)*, *12*(15), 1941–1955.

Everall, I. P., Vaida, F., Letendre, S., Lazzaretto, D., Gelman, B. B., Morgello, S., et al. (2008). Reducing the prevalence of primary HIV brain pathology by antiretrovirals (Abstract 67). In *15th Conference on Retroviruses and Opportunistic Infections*.

Evers, S., Rahmann, A., Schwaag, S., Frese, A., Reichelt, D., & Husstedt, I. W. (2004). Prevention of AIDS dementia by HAART does not depend on cerebrospinal fluid drug penetrance. *AIDS Research and Human Retroviruses*, *20*(5), 483–491.

Ferrando, S. J., Rabkin, J. G., van Gorp, W., Lin, S. H., & McElhiney, M. (2003). Longitudinal improvement in psychomotor processing speed is associated with potent combination antiretroviral therapy in HIV-1 infection. *J Neuropsychiatry Clin Neurosci*, *15*(2), 208–214.

Fletcher, C. V., Kawle, S. P., Kakuda, T. N., Anderson, P. L., Weller, D., Bushman, L. R., et al. (2000). Zidovudine triphosphate and lamivudine triphosphate concentration-response relationships in HIV-infected persons. *AIDS (London, England)*,*14*(14), 2137–2144.

Foudraine, N. A., Hoetelmans, R. M., Lange, J. M., de Wolf, F., van Benthem, B. H., Maas, J. J., et al. (1998). Cerebrospinal-fluid HIV-1

RNA and drug concentrations after treatment with lamivudine plus zidovudine or stavudine. *Lancet, 351*(9115), 1547–1551.

Gasnault, J., Lanoy, E., Bentata, M., Guiguet, M., Costagliola, D. (2008). Intracerebral penetrating ART are more efficient on survival of HIV+ patients with progressive multifocal leucoencephalopathy (ANRS CO4 - FHDH) (Abstract 386). In *15th Conference on Retroviruses and Opportunistic Infections*, Boston.

Gisolf, E. H., Enting, R. H., Jurriaans, S., de Wolf, F., van der Ende, M. E., Hoetelmans, R. M., et al. (2000). Cerebrospinal fluid HIV-1 RNA during treatment with ritonavir/saquinavir or ritonavir/saquinavir/ stavudine. *AIDS (London, England), 14*(11), 1583–1589.

Gisolf, E. H., van Praag, R. M., Jurriaans, S., Portegies, P., Goudsmit, J., Danner, S. A., et al. (2000). Increasing cerebrospinal fluid chemokine concentrations despite undetectable cerebrospinal fluid HIV RNA in HIV-1-infected patients receiving antiretroviral therapy. *J Acquir Immune Defic Syndr, 25*(5), 426–433.

Gonzalez de Requena, D., Blanco, F., Garcia-Benayas, T., Jimenez-Nacher, I., Gonzalez-Lahoz, J., & Soriano, V. (2003). Correlation between lopinavir plasma levels and lipid abnormalities in patients taking lopinavir/ritonavir. *AIDS Patient Care STDS, 1*(9), 443–445.

Granero, L., Santiago, M., Cano, J., Machado, A.,& Peris, J. E. (1995). Analysis of ceftriaxone and ceftazidime distribution in cerebrospinal fluid of and cerebral extracellular space in awake rats by in vivo microdialysis. *Antimicrobial Agents and Chemotherapy, 39*(12), 2728–2731.

Groothuis, D. R. & Levy, R. M. (1997). The entry of antiviral and antiretroviral drugs into the central nervous system. *Journal of Neurovirology, 3*(6), 387–400.

Haas, D. W., Clough, L. A., Johnson, B. W., Harris, V. L., Spearman, P., Wilkinson, G. R., et al. (2000). Evidence of a source of HIV type 1 within the central nervous system by ultraintensive sampling of cerebrospinal fluid and plasma. *AIDS Research and Human Retroviruses, 16*(15), 1491–1502.

Haas, D. W., Stone, J., Clough, L. A., Johnson, B., P., S., Harris, V. L., et al. (2000). Steady state pharmacokinetics of indinavir in cerebrospinal fluid and plasma among adults with human immunodeficiency virus type 1 infection. *Clinical Pharmacology and Therapeutics, 68*(4), 367–374.

Heaton, R. K., Grant, I., Butters, N., White, D. A., Kirson, D., Atkinson, J. H., et al. (1995). The HNRC 500—neuropsychology of HIV infection at different disease stages. HIV Neurobehavioral Research Center. *J Int Neuropsychol Soc, 1*(3), 231–251.

Huisman, M. T., Smit, J. W., Hoetelmans, R. M., Wiltshire, H. R., Beijnen, J. H., Schinkel, A. H. (2000). In *The role of P-glycoprotein in oral bioavailability, brain and fetal penetration of the HIV protease inhibitor saquinavir*, Fifth International Congress on Drug Therapy in HIV Infection, Glasgow, United Kingdom: (publisher?).

Huisman, M. T., Smit, J. W., Wiltshire, H. R., Hoetelmans, R. M., Beijnen, J. H.,& Schinkel, A. H. (2001). P-glycoprotein limits oral availability, brain, and fetal penetration of saquinavir even with high doses of ritonavir. *Mol Pharmacol, 59*(4), 806–813.

Jaruratanasirikul, S., Hortiwakul, R., Tantisarasart, T., Phuenpathom, N., & Tussanasunthornwong, S. (1996). Distribution of azithromycin into brain tissue, cerebrospinal fluid, and aqueous humor of the eye. *Antimicrobial Agents and Chemotherapy, 40*(3), 825–826.

King, M., Brun, S., Tschampa, J., Moseley, J., & Kempf, D. (2003) Relationship between adherence and the development of viral resistance in antiretroviral-naive patients treated with lopinavir/ritonavir (lpv/r) or nelfinavir (nfv). *Antiviral Therapy, 8*(Suppl 1), S408.

Kravcik, S. (2001). Pharmacology and clinical experience with saquinavir. *Expert Opin Pharmacother, 2*(2), 303–315.

Kravcik, S., Gallicano, K., Roth, V., Cassol, S., Hawley-Foss, N., Badley, A., et al. (1999). Cerebrospinal fluid HIV RNA and drug levels with combination ritonavir and saquinavir. *J Acquir Immune Defic Syndr, 21*(5), 371–375.

Lafeuillade, A., Solas, C., Halfon, P., Chadapaud, S., Hittinger, G.,& Lacarelle, B. (2002). Differences in the detection of three HIV-1 protease inhibitors in non-blood compartments: Clinical correlations. *HIV Clinical Trials, 3*(1) 27–35.

Lee, C. G., Gottesman, M. M., Cardarelli, C. O., Ramachandra, M., Jeang, K. T., Ambudkar, S. V., et al. (1998). HIV-1 protease inhibitors are substrates for the MDR1 multidrug transporter. *Biochemistry, 37*(11), 3594–3601.

Letendre, S., Ellis, R., Cysique, L. A., Cherner, M., Gibson, S., Heaton, R., et al. (2008). Low-grade immune restoration disease may limit recovery from HIV-associated neurocognitive impairment (Abstract 68). In *15th Conference on Retroviruses and Opportunistic Infections*, Boston.

Letendre, S. L., Capparelli, E. V., Ellis, R. J., & McCutchan, J. A. (2000). Indinavir population pharmacokinetics in plasma and cerebrospinal fluid. The HIV Neurobehavioral Research Center Group. *Antimicrobial Agents and Chemotherapy, 44*(8), 2173–2175.

Letendre, S., Ellis, R., Grant, I., & McCutchan, J. (2001). The CSF Concentration/IC50 Ratio: A Predictor of CNS Antiretroviral (ARV) Efficacy (Abstract 614) In *8th Conference on Retroviruses and Opportunistic Infections*, Chicago, 2001.

Letendre, S., Ellis, R., & McCutchan, J. (2000). Frequent Dissociation of Plasma and CSF HIV RNA Responses During Antiretroviral Therapy (Abstract 305). In *7th Conference on Retroviruses and Opportunistic Infections*, San Francisco, 2000.

Letendre, S., Marquie-Beck, J., Capparelli, E., Best, B., Clifford, D., Collier, A. C., et al. (2008). Validation of the CNS Penetration-Effectiveness rank for quantifying antiretroviral penetration into the central nervous system. *Archives of, 65*(1), 65–70.

Letendre, S. L., McCutchan, J. A., Childers, M. E., Woods, S. P., Lazzaretto, D., Heaton, R. K., et al. (2004). Enhancing antiretroviral therapy for human immunodeficiency virus cognitive disorders. *Ann Neurol, 56*(3), 416–423.

Marra, C. M., Lockhart, D., Zunt, J. R., Perrin, M. Coombs, R. W.,& Collier, A. C. (2003). Changes in CSF and plasma HIV-1 RNA and cognition after starting potent antiretroviral therapy. *Neurology, 60*(8), 1388–1390.

Marra, C. M., Zhao, Y., Clifford, D. B., Letendre, S., Evans, S., Henry, K., et al. (2009). AIDS Clinical Trials Group 736 Study Team. Impact of combination antiretroviral therapy on cerebrospinal fluid HIV RNA and neurocognitive performance. *AIDS, 23*(11), 1359–1366.

Marzolini, C., Greub, G., Decosterd, L., Biollaz, J., Telenti, A., & Buclin, T.(2001). In Routine antiretroviral plasma levels of NNRTIs and PIs correlate with viral suppression and adverse events, 8th Conference on Retroviruses and Opportunistic Infections, Chicago, IL, February 4–8; Chicago, IL, 2001; p 266.

Marzolini, C., Telenti, A., Decosterd, L. A., Greub, G., Biollaz, J., & Buclin, T. (2001). Efavirenz plasma levels can predict treatment failure and central nervous system side effects in HIV-1-infected patients. *AIDS (London, England),15*(1), 71–75.

Maschke, M., Kastrup, O., Esser, S., Ross, B., Hengge, U., & Hufnagel, A. (2000). Incidence and prevalence of neurological disorders associated with HIV since the introduction of highly active antiretroviral therapy (HAART). *J Neurol Neurosurg Psychiatry, 69*(3), 376–380.

Masereeuw, R., Jaehde, U., Langemeijer, M. W., de Boer, A. G., & Breimer, D. D. (1994). In vitro and in vivo transport of zidovudine (AZT) across the blood-brain barrier and the effect of transport inhibitors. *Pharm Res, 11*(2), 324–330.

May, S., Letendre, S., Haubrich, R., McCutchan, J. A., Heaton, R., Capparelli, E., et al. (2007). Meeting practical challenges of a trial involving a multitude of treatment regimens: An example of a multicenter randomized controlled clinical trial in neuroAIDS. *J Neuroimmune Pharmacol, 2*(1), 97–104.

McCutchan, J. A., Wu, J. W., Robertson, K., Koletar, S. L., Ellis, R. J., Cohn, S., et al. (2007). HIV suppression by HAART preserves cognitive function in advanced, immune-reconstituted AIDS patients. *AIDS (London, England), 21*(9), 1109–1117.

Miller, L., McCutchan, J. A, Keiser, P., Kemper, C., Witt, M., Leedom, J., et al. (2003). Accumulation of antiretroviral resistance in treatment-experienced patients: The impact of medication adherence. *Antiviral Therapy, 8*(Suppl 1), S418.

Murphy. In *Antiviral Activity and Pharmacokinetics of Amprenavir with or without Zidovudine/3TC in the Cerebral Spinal Fluid of HIV-Infected Adults*, 7th CROI, San Fransisco, CA, San Fransisco, CA, 2000.

Parkin, N. T., Hellmann, N. S., Whitcomb, J. M., Kiss, L., Chappey, C., & Petropoulos, C. J. (2004). Natural variation of drug susceptibility in wild-type human immunodeficiency virus type 1. *Antimicrobial Agents and Chemotherapy*, 48(2), 437–443.

Perno, C. F., Newcomb, F. M., Davis, D. A., Aquaro, S., Humphrey, R. W., Calio, R., et al. (1998). Relative potency of protease inhibitors in monocytes/macrophages acutely and chronically infected with human immunodeficiency virus. *The Journal of Infectious Diseases*, 178(2), 413–422.

Powderly, W. G., Saag, M. S., Chapman, S., Yu, G., Quart, B., & N.J. (1999). Predictors of optimal virological response to potent antiretroviral therapy. *AIDS (London, England)*, (13), 1873–1880.

Price, R. W. (2000). The two faces of HIV infection of cerebrospinal fluid. *Trends Microbiol, 8*(9), 387–391.

Rao, V. V., Dahlheimer, J. L., Bardgett, M. E., Snyder, A. Z., Finch, R. A., Sartorelli, A. C., et al. (1999). Choroid plexus epithelial expression of MDR1 P glycoprotein and multidrug resistance-associated protein contribute to the blood-cerebrospinal-fluid drug-permeability barrier. *Proceedings of the National Academy of Sciences of the United States of America*, 96 (7), 3900–3905.

Richman, D. D., Kornbluth, R. S., & Carson, D. A. (1987). Failure of dideoxynucleosides to inhibit human immunodeficiency virus replication in cultured human macrophages. *J Exp Med*, 166 (4), 1144–1149.

Robertson, K. R., Fiscus, S., Robertson, W. T., Meeker, R., & Hall, C. D. (2002) In *CSF HIV RNA and CNS Penetrating Antiretroviral Regimens*, 9th Conference on Retroviruses and Opportunistec Infections, University of North Carolina, Chapel Hill, University of North Carolina, Chapel Hill, 2002.

Robertson, K. R., Robertson, W. T., Ford, S., Watson, D., Fiscus, S., Harp, A. G., et al. (2004). Highly active antiretroviral therapy improves neurocognitive functioning. *J Acquir Immune Defic Syndr*, 36(1), 562–566.

Robertson, K. R. Smurzynski, M., Parsons, T. D., Wu, K., Bosch, R. J., Wu, J., et al. (2007). The prevalence and incidence of neurocognitive impairment in the HAART era. *AIDS (London, England)*, 21(14), 1915–1921.

Rusconi, S., Merrill, D. P., & Hirsch, M. S. (1994). Inhibition of human immunodeficiency virus type 1 replication in cytokine-stimulated monocytes/macrophages by combination therapy. *The Journal of Infectious Diseases*, 170(6), 1361–1366.

Sacktor, N., Lyles, R. H., Skolasky, R. L., Anderson, D. E., McArthur, J. C., McFarlane, G., et al. (1999). Combination antiretroviral therapy improves psychomotor speed performance in HIV-seropositive homosexual men: Multicenter AIDS Cohort Study (MACS). *Neurology*, (52), 1640–1647.

Sacktor, N., Tarwater, P. M., Skolasky, R. L., McArthur, J. C., Selnes, O. A., Becker, J., et al. (2001). CSF antiretroviral drug penetrance and the treatment of HIV-associated psychomotor slowing. *Neurology*, 57(3), 542–544.

Sadler, B. M., Gillotin, C., Lou, Y., & Stein, D. S. (2001). In vivo effect of alpha(1)-acid glycoprotein on pharmacokinetics of amprenavir, a human immunodeficiency virus protease inhibitor. *Antimicrobial Agents andCchemotherapyy*, 45(3), 852–856.

Sevigny, J. J., Albert, S. M., McDermott, M. P., McArthur, J. C., Sacktor, N., Conant, K., et al. (2004). Evaluation of HIV RNA and markers of immune activation as predictors of HIV-associated dementia. *Neurology*, 63(11), 2084–2090.

Sevigny, J. J., Albert, S. M., McDermott, M. P., Schifitto, G., McArthur, J. C., Sacktor, N., et al. (2007). An evaluation of neurocognitive status and markers of immune activation as predictors of time to death in advanced HIV infection. *Archives of Neurology*, 64(1), 97–102.

Shulman, N., Zolopa, A., Havlir, D., Hsu, A., Renz, C., Boller, S., et al. (2002). Virtual inhibitory quotient predicts response to ritonavir boosting of indinavir-based therapy in human immunodeficiency virus-infected patients with ongoing viremia. *Antimicrobial Agents and Chemotherapy*, 46(12), 3907–3916.

Simioni, S., Cavassini, M., Annoni, J. M., Rimbault Abraham, A., Bourquin, I., et al. (2010). Cognitive dysfunction in HIV patients despite long-standing suppression of viremia. *AIDS*, 24(9), 1243–1250.

Solas, C., Lafeuillade, A., Halfon, P., Chadapaud, S., Hittinger, G., & Lacarelle, B. (2003). Discrepancies between protease inhibitor concentrations and viral load in reservoirs and sanctuary sites in human immunodeficiency virus-infected patients. *Antimicrobial Agents and Chemotherapy*, 47(1), 238–243.

Spudich, S., Lollo, N., Liegler, T., Deeks, S. G., & Price, R. W. (2006). Treatment benefit on cerebrospinal fluid HIV-1 levels in the setting of systemic virological suppression and failure. *The Journal of Infectious Diseases*, 194(12), 1686–1696.

St Clair, M. H., Richards, C. A., Spector, T.,Weinhold, K. J., Miller, W. H., Langlois, A. J., et al. (1987). 3'-Azido-3'-deoxythymidine triphosphate as an inhibitor and substrate of purified human immunodeficiency virus reverse transcriptase. *Antimicrobial Agents and Chemotherapy*, 31(12), 1972–1977.

Staprans, S., Marlowe, N., Glidden, D., Novakovic-Agopian, T., Grant, R. M., Heyes, M., et al. (1999). Time course of cerebrospinal fluid responses to antiretroviral therapy: Evidence for variable compartmentalization of infection. *AIDS (London, England)*, 13(9), 1051–1061.

Tashima, K. T., Caliendo, A. M., Ahmad, M., Gormley, J. M., Fiske, W. D., Brennan, J. M., et al. (1999). Cerebrospinal fluid human immunodeficiency virus type 1 (HIV-1) suppression and efavirenz drug concentrations in HIV-1-infected patients receiving combination therapy. *The Journal of Infectious Diseases*, 180(3), 862–864.

Taylor, S. & Pereira, A. (2000). Penetration of HIV-1 protease inhibitors into CSF and semen. *HIV Medicine, 1 Suppl 2*, 18–22.

Tozzi, V., Balestra, P., Salvatori, M. F., Vlassi, C., Liuzzi, G., Giancola, M., et al. (2009). Changes in cognition during antiretroviral therapy: Comparison of 2 different ranking systems to measure antiretroviral drug efficacy on HIV-associated neurocognitive disorders. *J Acquir Immune Defic Syndr*, 52(1), 56–63.

Tozzi, V., Balestra, P., Galgani, S., Narciso, P., Sampaolesi, A., Antinori, Aet al. (2001). Changes in neurocognitive performance in a cohort of patients treated with HAART for 3 years. *J Acquir Immune Defic Syndr*, 28(1), 19–27.

Tozzi, V., Balestra, P., Murri, R., Galgani, S., Bellagamba, R., Narciso, P., et al. (2004). Neurocognitive impairment influences quality of life in HIV-infected patients receiving HAART. *Int J STD AIDS*, 15(4), 254–259.

Tozzi, V., Balestra, P., Salvatori, M., Vlassi, C., Liuzzi, G., Menichetti, S., et al. (2009). Changes in cognition during HAART: Comparison of 2 different scoring systems to measure antiretroviral drug efficacy on HIV dementia. *J Acquir Immune Defic Syndr*, 52(1), 56–63.

Valcour, V. & Paul, R. (2006). HIV infection and dementia in older adults. *Clin Infect Dis*, 42(10), 1449–1454.

von Giesen, H. J., Adams, O., Koller, H., & Arendt, G. (2005). Cerebrospinal HIV viral load in different phases of HIV-associated brain disease. *Journal of Neurology*, 252(7), 801–807.

Wijnholds, J., deLange, E. C., Scheffer, G. L., van den Berg, D. J., Mol, C. A., van der Valk, M., et al. (2000). Multidrug resistance protein 1 protects the choroid plexus epithelium and contributes to the blood-cerebrospinal fluid barrier. *J Clin Invest*, 105(3), 279–285.

Wu, D., Clement, J. G., & Pardridge, W. M. (1998). Low blood-brain barrier permeability to azidothymidine (AZT), 3TC, and thymidine in the rat. *Brain Research*, 791(1–2), 313–316.

Yasuda, J. M., Miller, C., Currier, J. S., Forthal, D. N, Kemper, C. A., Beall, G. N., et al. (2004). The correlation between plasma concentrations of protease inhibitors, medication adherence and virological outcome in HIV-infected patients. *Antiviral Therapy*, 9(5), 753–761.

Yazdanian, M. (1999). Blood-brain barrier properties of human immunodeficiency virus antiretrovirals. *Journal of Pharmaceutical Sciences*, 88(10), 950–954.

Zhang, X. Q., Schooley, R. T., & Gerber, J. G. (1999). The effect of increasing alpha1-acid glycoprotein concentration on the antiviral efficacy of human immunodeficiency virus protease inhibitors. *The Journal of Infectious Diseases*, 180(6), 1833–1837.

11.3

TREATMENT OF OPPORTUNISTIC INFECTIONS ASSOCIATED WITH HUMAN IMMUNODEFICIENCY VIRUS INFECTION

David B. Clifford

The advent of HIV challenges clinicians to enhance their understanding of opportunistic infections (OIs) that were encountered only rarely in the pre-HIV era. This chapter discusses the treatment of those OIs of the nervous system that are uniquely increased in the setting of HIV. The chapter focuses specifically on those infections that are most common in the developed world; some less common infections are not considered. In thinking about these OIs, it must be remembered that HIV-infected patients are subject to the full range of complications and illnesses, not only those that are uniquely prevalent among HIV patients. Therefore, restricting the differential diagnosis to uniquely HIV-associated complications is inappropriate. Furthermore, in the immunosuppressed population, it is common for several complications to occur simultaneously. Thus, unlike in the assessment of the non-immunosuppressed patient, seeking a single parsimonious diagnosis without equally searching for two or more simultaneously occurring complications is to invite error.

INTRODUCTION

The physician caring for patients with human immunodeficiency virus (HIV) infection will encounter patients requiring treatment of opportunistic infections that were very rare in the era prior to HIV, but are routinely encountered in practices of immunodeficient patients. The advent of HIV has brought both a challenge and an opportunity to enhance our understanding of these infections, and to improve therapeutic approaches to them. In this chapter, the major opportunistic infections of the nervous system that are uniquely increased in the setting of HIV will be addressed. However, the astute clinician must never forget that HIV-infected patients are subject to any complication or illness, so restriction of the differential to the uniquely HIV-associated conditions is inappropriate. Furthermore, in contrast to most experience in medicine, several complications occur simultaneously in the vulnerable, immunosuppressed population. Thus, it is an invitation to error, if one approaches the HIV-infected patient thinking only of the set of complications addressed in this monograph, or seeking only a single best diagnosis.

Infections that have been particularly prominent in HIV-infected patients, and will be addressed, include toxoplasma encephalitis, cryptococcal meningitis, progressive multifocal leukoencephalopathy, cytomegalovirus encephalitis, radiculomyelitis and neuropathy, and neurosyphilis. Clearly, these do not represent a comprehensive panel of infections, but they do represent the most important and treatable of the unusual infectious complications encountered in neuroAIDS in the developed world. Since several of these are caused by reactivation of latent pathogens, in some cases prophylactic therapy is part of patient management. Similarly, in many cases successful therapy only arrests the clinical conditions, but does not clear the organism from the body, making ongoing suppressive therapy critical. Successful reconstitution of the immune system with antiretroviral therapy has resulted in opportunities to safely discontinue such suppressive therapy in some cases. Appropriate parameters for prophylaxis, treatment, and suppression continue to evolve, but current understanding will be reviewed in this chapter.

TOXOPLASMA ENCEPHALITIS

The intracellular parasite *Toxoplasma gondii* ascended rapidly from a very rare complication of immune deficiency states, to one of the most common complications of HIV infection in the 1980s, as the AIDS epidemic took hold. Therapeutic plans derive from the fact that this is almost always a re-activation of latent prior infection. The segment of HIV population at greatest risk can be identified by detection of serum IgG antibodies to toxoplasma early in the course of caring for an individual. Part of sound HIV patient management is to determine toxoplasma exposure status early in the infection and be ready to treat this complication should it occur. This also identifies a population for whom prophylactic therapy is appropriate if the immune status declines. Finally, treatment cannot realistically rid the body of this organism, necessitating post-treatment maintenance therapy until immune reconstitution is accomplished.

ACUTE TOXOPLASMA ENCEPHALITIS

Toxoplasma encephalitis (TE) is a subacute, progressive encephalitis producing diffuse or multifocal symptoms that

978

typically worsen on a time course of days to a few weeks. Prompt therapy is critical and generally rewarding. Optimal therapy (Table 11.3.1) employs pyrimethamine and sulfadiazine. Folinic acid (leucovorin) is given as a folate supplement to protect the bone marrow from pyrimethamine toxicity which is otherwise dose limiting. A loading dose of 200 mg pyrimethamine orally followed by 75 mg daily is used. While these standard doses of pyrimethamine are generally adequate, inter-patient serum levels are variable, and measuring plasma concentrations when therapy is failing should be considered (Klinker, Langmann, & Richter, 1996). Sulfadiazine, 2–8 grams daily in divided doses, has been found to be highly effective when used with pyrimethamine (Leport et al., 1988). Special care to assure optimal hydration is required as crystalluria may occur. Folinic acid is also administered and generally 5–10 mg by mouth daily is sufficient. In sulfa allergic patients, clindamycin 600 mg per day IV (and eventually orally) in four divided doses may be substituted for sulfadiazine. The efficacy of clindamycin or sulfadiazine-based therapies appears roughly similar, at least when the first three weeks of clindamycin is given intravenously, with toxicities dictating which should be used in any particular patient (Dannemann et al., 1992; Katlama, 1991; Katlama, 1996). Skin rashes are the most common toxicities of both of these treatment regimens. Clindamycin has substantial gastrointestinal (GI) toxicity (nausea, vomiting, diarrhea, liver function test abnormalities) and hematologic toxicity is often encountered in these patients (neutropenia, leukopenia). The sulfa-based group had similar complaints, but also in rare cases had flank pain and crystalluria. When sulfadiazine is believed to be the optimal therapy, but sulfa allergy precludes its use, a majority of subjects can be desensitized by gradually increasing oral doses of sulfadiazine at 3-hourly intervals over 5 days (Tenant-Flowers et al., 1991). Alternative therapies include trimethoprim-sulfamethoxazole, atovaquone, clarithromycin, or azithromycin-based combinations (Katlama et al., 1996; Lacassin et al., 1995; Fernandez-Martin et al., 1991; Torre et al., 1998).

In general, the acute course of therapy should be at least 6 weeks, but this should be adjusted dependent on severity and clinical status. Thereafter, suppressive therapy is required

Table 11.3.1 **TOXOPLASMA THERAPY**

Prophylaxis: IgG positive subjects with CD4 < 200 cells/μL

Sulfamethoxazole/trimethoprim

Acute toxoplasma encephalitis:

Pyrimethamine 200 mg po loading dose, then 75 mg PO qd

Sulfadiazine 1.5 grams q 6 h

Folinic acid 5–10 mg qd PO

Alternative for sulfadiazine: Clindamycin 150–300 mg q6h IV/PO

Other therapies with activity: Atovaquone, azithromycin, clarithromycin

Maintenance: Pyrimethamine 25–50 mg qd, sulfadiazine 500 mg PO qid, folinic acid 5–10 mg qd.

Discontinue: If CD4 > 200 μL for > 3 months for prophylaxis and > 6 months for maintenance.

until immune reconstitution can be achieved to >200 CD4 lymphocytes/mm³. Suppressive therapies typically continue agents used in acute therapy at half the dose (St. Georgiev, 1994). However, less aggressive maintenance may be successful, including pyrimethamine 50 mg daily alone (de Gans et al., 1992) and atovaquone (Katlama et al., 1996). Alternatively, combined therapies either twice or thrice weekly may be sufficient for maintenance therapy after TE (Schurmann et al., 2001; Podzamczer et al., 2000). Single therapy regimens have not been successful for acute therapy, as suggested by the failure of trimetrexate to achieve lasting suppression of TE (Masur et al., 1993)). The high cost of standard therapy has encouraged substitution of trimethoprim-sulfamethoxazole regimens, particularly in the developing world. This treatment is supported by one small clinical trial but should be demonstrated with an adequately powered clinical trial in the developing world (Torre et al., 1998).

The rate of clinical response is important in this disorder since treatment is often the most rapid diagnostic tool practically available to the clinician. In successful therapy, more than 80% of responders demonstrated clinical improvement in the first week of therapy and more than 90% with response improved with respect to at least half of clinical abnormalities in the first 14 days of therapy (Luft et al., 1993). Radiologic response may also be appreciated relatively early, although radiologic improvement lags behind the clinical improvement. Overall response to therapy varies, with over half of patients showing complete or good recovery of neurological function, while some are left with substantial fixed neurological deficits.

These observations mean that rapid initiation of effective toxoplasma therapy when this diagnosis is considered may demonstrate improvement in a matter of days. Further deterioration of the neurological condition while on therapy dictates reconsideration of the diagnosis and further invasive measures, including brain biopsy, to determine the appropriate diagnosis. For valid interpretation of clinical response to a diagnostic treatment challenge for possible TE, it is important to avoid the use of corticosteroids, as these may give transient, nonspecific clinical improvements blurring the interpretation of a response with initiation of TE antibiotic therapy. However, if a patient's condition is deemed critical due to brain swelling associated with possible TE, corticosteroids may contribute to an even more rapid, and potentially life-saving, response, so clinical judgment is required to decide if it is safe to perform a therapeutic diagnostic challenge without use of corticosteroids.

Since toxoplasma encephalitis generally presents in untreated HIV-infected patients, the appropriate timing for initiation of antiretroviral therapy (ART) must also be considered. No large studies of this specific question are available, but in general, it is now recommended to start ART as soon as convenient after establishing successful treatment for the opportunistic complication (Zolopa et al., 2009). In contrast to several other opportunistic CNS diseases, immune reconstitution syndrome (IRIS) has generally not been a serious complication, although rare cases of IRIS have been described with TE (Pfeffer et al., 2009).

Clearly, it is better to avoid TE entirely if possible. This is generally accomplished when prophylactic therapy is initiated (Ribera et al., 1999; Weigel et al., 1997). Virtually all subjects at risk for TE may be identified by screening for toxoplasma antibodies. When the CD4 count drops below 200 CD4 lymphocytes/mm³, prophylaxis is recommended. This range overlaps with similar treatment clinically indicated as prophylactic therapy for pneumocystis pneumonia (Ribera et al., 1999; Weigel et al., 1997; Antinori et al., 1995). Most commonly, TE is now encountered in subjects not taking any prophylactic medication, or on aerosolized pentamidine (due to sulfa allergy).

In the current era of highly active antiretroviral therapy (HAART), improvement in immune status accompanies viral suppression. This reduces the risk of TE activation, and permits safe discontinuation of either primary prophylactic therapies or maintenance therapy. Current recommendations are for discontinuation of primary prophylactic therapy after CD4 counts exceed 200 cells/mm³ for three months (Furrer et al., 2000; Centers for Disease Control, 2002). It also seems safe, based primarily on substantial cohort experiences to cautiously discontinue maintenance therapy after six months of successful HIV viral suppression and elevation of CD4 > 200 cells/mm³ (CDC, 2002; Soriano et al., 2000).

CRYPTOCOCCAL MENINGITIS

While cryptococcal meningitis (CM) was also a relatively common infection prior to the era of HIV, it has become a very frequent complication of HIV, for which therapy has advanced considerably. This complication generally has a subacute onset, but in immunodeficient hosts it may progress rapidly. Outcomes have substantially improved in the era of effective HIV therapy, with one report suggesting mortality rate of 63.8 (95% CI 53–75) in the pre-HAART era falling to 15.3 (CI 12–18%) post-HAART (Lortholary et al., 2006). Thus, immediate treatment is required. Induction therapy (Table 11.3.2) with amphotericin B (with or without flucytosine which may be poorly tolerated due to marrow toxicity) is suggested based on earlier sterilization of CSF and slightly lower mortality rates in the early stage of treatment (Saag et al., 2002). Amphotericin B is used at 0.5–0.7 mg/kg/day in D5W solution. Flucytosine dosing is 100–150 mg/kg/day in four doses if tolerated by marrow toxicity. Often advanced HIV disease and other marrow-toxic therapy precludes use of flucytosine. Given the expense and difficulty of this therapy in developing world sites where HIV-associated CM is common, formal evaluation of higher dose fluconazole therapy is under investigation. A small study supported combinations of 1200 mg/day fluconazole with flucytosine as an alternative to amphotericin B based therapy (Milefchik et al., 2008; Nussbaum et al., 2010). After induction therapy, fluconazole has become standard therapy with consolidation for 8–10 weeks at 400 mg/d and maintenance therapy at 200 mg/d thereafter. Long-term requirements for suppressive therapy depend on the response to ART. Timing for optimal initiation of ART has not yet been systematically studied. In one report

with 35 cases of CM comparing early to late initiation of ART, early initiation was supported since there was less AIDS progression/death in this arm with no increase in adverse events of loss of virologic response compared to deferred ART. Others, however, report rather common and potentially clinically serious IRIS in CM, suggesting that some delay to achieve early control of CM might be advisable. However, long-term prognosis is dependent on successful HIV control, so unnecessary delay in immune reconstitution only invites other complications and potential morbidity. After > 6 months of full suppression of HIV with ART, with CSF sterile and with CD4 > 200 cells/μl, it appears safe to discontinue suppressive fluconazole therapy (CDC. 2002).

Amphotericin B therapy must be administered intravenously, preferably through a central catheter. A standard initiation of this drug includes a test dose of 1 mg in 20 ml of D5W given over 15–20 minutes. The patient should be closely monitored for 4 hours, then a dose of 0.3 mg/kg IV may be given over 2–6 hours. This is followed by a standard dose of 0.7 mg/kg. Systemic reaction with rigors is sometimes encountered and may be ameliorated by pretreatment with meperidine (15–20 mg intravenously) and phenergan (25 mg intravenous) (Harrison & McArthur, 1996). Since renal toxicity is the most serious toxicity of amphotericin therapy, monitoring must include creatinine, potassium, and electrolytes several times a week. Reduction in doses of amphotericin are required if creatinine levels rise substantially. Flucytosine is toxic to the bone marrow, and this drug should be discontinued if leucopenia or progressive anemia occurs during therapy, and the patient monitored with regular complete blood counts. Liposomal preparations of amphotericin have the advantage of being better tolerated and less renal toxic, although they are substantially more expensive (Leenders et al., 1997).

Elevated intracranial pressure is one of the most serious signs of severe disease with guarded prognosis. Repeated lumbar punctures are recommended if the patient is clinically not improving or is deteriorating. Transient improvement in intracranial pressure may be obtained by repeat spinal taps, but when the pressure remains elevated, and particularly when signs of cranial nerve impairment are notable, consideration of shunting (e.g. lumboperitoneal) or Ommaya reservoir

Table 11.3.2 CRYPTOCOCCAL MENINGITIS THERAPY

Prophylaxis: not indicated

Acute cryptococcal meningitis:

Initial therapy (~3 weeks):

Amphotericin B 0.7 mg/kg per day IV (adjusted for renal status)

± Flucytosine 25 mg/kg q 6 h PO (during induction if tolerated)

Consolidation therapy:

Fluconazole 400 mg/d PO

Maintenance:

Fluconazole 200 mg/d PO

Discontinue: If CD4 > 200 cells/μL for > 6 months

placement should be entertained. The role of corticosteroids in control of pathologically increased ICP remains controversial, but is often employed when increased pressure is causing progressive neurological deterioration.

Milder presentations of cryptococcal meningitis can probably be safely treated with oral fluconazole therapy from the outset. This is generally better tolerated, and avoids the requirement of ongoing venous access. Its long half-life allows once daily dosing. Clinical trials are underway to explore higher doses of fluconazole from 1200–2000 mg/day as a means of augmenting the potency of this therapy, but at present they have not been compared to amphotericin-based therapy (Nussbaum et al., 2010). Monitoring of liver function tests is appropriate with fluconazole.

The time to sterilizing the CSF measured with quantitative fungal cultures is currently being used as a surrogate marker for progress in therapy. However, improvement of the clinical signs of meningitis is the most critical way to judge response to therapy. Since sterilizing the CSF is an important marker of success as well, a final lumbar puncture documenting sterile CSF represents careful and appropriate management for CM. It should be noted that the cryptococcal antigen titers that are often followed frequently do not become negative, even after long periods of complete control of the infection. Titers are a concern if they rise, but the rate and degree to which they decline should not be a major goal of therapy.

PROGRESSIVE MULTIFOCAL LEUKOENCEPHALOPATHY

Progressive multifocal leukoencephalopathy (PML) is a serious disease that was quite rare prior to the HIV epidemic, but became an important cause for mortality amongst AIDS patients. It is estimated that as many as 5% of AIDS deaths in some areas are due to this opportunistic brain infection by the JC virus. The rarity of the disease prior to HIV had resulted in a paucity of systematic investigation of treatment for PML. In the current era, the quest to demonstrate effective therapy has been frustrated by the fact that the disease is often so aggressively lethal, that there is insufficient time to make a firm diagnoses and to inaugurate specific therapies. Until recently, a brain biopsy was required to make this diagnosis. At present, progress in making the diagnosis of PML has resulted in generally reliable criteria, allowing the diagnosis to be rapidly achieved (Cinque, Koralnik, & Clifford, 2003). The fundamentals of making this diagnosis include recognition of a progressive, focal neurological disease in an immunodeficient patient, demonstrating symptoms referable to MR-identified lesions in white matter of the brain and detecting JC virus DNA in the CSF by polymerase chain reaction (PCR). When these criteria are met, the diagnosis is secure enough to include positive subjects in research trials, and to be used for clinical decision making and counselling. In the HAART era, PML cases are generally either in patients off of therapy with severe immunodeficiency, or occur in the first few months of therapy. Diagnosis of the early treatment cases is challenging, since it is more common in these patients

that CSF JC viral loads are low, and are more often beneath the level of detection. Since the cases come to light as the immune system is regenerating, these cases may also be associated with significant immune reconstitution inflammatory syndrome (IRIS) and the MR lesions may have both contrast enhancement and mass effect. In patients who have no detectable JC DNA in the cerebrospinal fluid, brain biopsy may still be necessary to confirm this diagnosis, although often repeat CSF samples over a few weeks' time allows the diagnosis with CSF PCR.

Anecdotal reports of treating this disease, as well as in vitro studies (Hou & Major, 1998; Major et al., 1992), suggest that cytosine arabinoside might be beneficial for PML. Some clinicians continue to use this therapy, although no clinical trial supports its use, and the drug is known to have very poor penetration of the brain, making it very unlikely that it has a useful place in therapeutics for PML (Major et al., 1992). Since the Neurologic AIDS Research Consortium/ACTG study of cytosine arabinoside, this treatment has largely been abandoned (Hall et al., 1998).

Cidofovir has also been widely tried in treatment of PML, based on anecdotal data suggested that it might have in vivo activity against PML. An open label toxicity trial organized by the Neurologic AIDS Research Consortium in the United States demonstrated reasonable tolerability, but disappointing outcomes, with use of cidofovir in conjunction with ART (Marra et al., 2002). A large meta-analysis of six data sets in which cidofovir was tested demonstrated no useful activity for this disease (DeLuca et al., 2008).

Improvement of the immune status of HIV-infected patients undergoing successful ART has significantly changed the course of PML. Consequently it appears that optimal HIV therapy is the most important thing that should be offered subjects with PML. A group of subjects followed in the early period of HAART therapy showed prolonged survival exceeding 40 weeks (compared with 12–14 weeks prior to HAART) (Clifford et al., 1999; Cinque, Casari, & Bertelli, 1998; Giudici et al., 2000; Antinori et al., 2001; Taoufik, Delfraissy, & Gasnault, 2000; Gasnault et al., 1999; Miralles et al., 1998; Inui et al., 1999; Dworkin et al., 1999; Tassie et al., 1999). In the best of cases, clinical and radiologic progression from PML is arrested and in some cases some improvement in function and brain lesions may be documented. However, most patients are left with fixed deficits that do not improve, and typically it takes several months for the initiation or refinement of ART to cause this beneficial change. Sadly, not all PML patients respond to improvement in HIV therapy. There are probably several causes for failure. Rapidly progressing PML sometimes causes fatal neurological lesions before immune constitution occurs, representing a group of patients for whom a direct antiviral therapy for the JC virus could be critical. In others immune reconstitution cannot be achieved either due to HIV resistance to therapy, issues with compliance, or advanced unresponsive immunosuppression. With the evolution of HIV therapy including new classes of potent antiretroviral agents, this population is becoming much smaller. It is curious that ART is less successful in blocking development of PML than many of the other opportunistic complications.

For instance, cytomegalovirus encephalitis is now rarely encountered in treated patients, whereas there is a continued presentation of PML patients (Clifford et al., 1999). The treatment onset PML makes it even plausible that immune activation poses a period of higher risk for PML that is not seen with other opportunistic diseases. An additional concern that may result in suboptimal outcomes has been raised concerning ART for PML in that there may be a harmful excessive immune activation, exacerbating symptoms and perhaps even causing additional neurological damage. IRIS reactions are extremely common in association with PML, and are sometimes severe and may be life threatening (Tan et al., 2009; Vendrely et al., 2005). Case reports of substantial inflammatory response in this setting certainly suggest this in PML (Miralles et al., 2001). Increasing reports of contrast enhancement in brain-imaging studies in the HAART era are also consistent with this if one assumes that the enhancement reflects increased inflammatory response and breakdown of the blood-brain barrier (Port et al., 1999; Wheeler et al., 1993; Kotecha et al., 1998). While it is appropriate to be concerned about immunosuppression with corticosteroids when a lethal secondary viral disease is occurring, it is almost certainly appropriate to use corticosteroid therapy in this setting. Studies of series of cases have associated better outcomes with earlier and more aggressive corticosteroid use, consistent with the concept that in the setting of IRIS it becomes the most dangerous contributor to mortality (Tan et al., 2009; Cinque et al., 2001). However, the need for urgent immune reconstitution given the rapidly progressive natural history of PML appears to leave little room for less-than-optimal HIV therapy until a directly active therapy is available for the JC virus itself.

Efforts continue to identify an effective and tolerable therapy for PML. An interesting effort comes as the result of a high throughput drug screen project evaluating potential drugs in an astrocyte JC infection model in vitro. From a group of 2,000 drugs, mefloquine was identified as a candidate compound that is known to achieve appropriate drug levels in the brain, limit JC infection in vitro, and have a reasonable safety profile for use in humans (Brickelmaier et al., 2009). An international clinical trial was performed to determine if the in vitro activity can be appreciated in patients with PML (Clifford et al., 2009). Sadly, this clinical trial failed to support efficacy of mefloquine. (Clifford et al, 2011).

Another alternative therapy that has received consideration has been interferon-α. Again, retrospective studies undertaken during the era when HAART was first introduced suggested that this agent might have useful activity (Huang et al., 1998). However, more careful analysis of the effects of the interferon as opposed to the likely effects of ART suggests that in fact most of the benefit was derived from the ART (Geschwind, Skolasky, Royal, & McArthur, 2001). The possibility that interferon-β might harbor activity for PML was further deflated by the reports of PML emerging in the setting of natalizumab therapy with interferon-β (Kleinschmidt-DeMasters & Tyler, 2005; Langer-Gould et al., 2005). While concern that interferon-β therapy was associated with increased risk of PML has proved unlikely with emergence of natalizumab-associated cases without this drug, it is clear that even pretreatment did not prevent emergence and progression of PML in this setting.

Recent reports of the utilization of a specific serotonin receptor (5HT2a) for cell entry by JC virus has led to the hypothesis that blockade of these receptors might have activity against this infection (Elphick et al., 2004). In vitro data support this mechanism, but drugs selective for the receptor appear not to block the spread of established infection in vitro, making the in vivo efficacy less likely. Nevertheless, widespread use of mirtazapine, which is a well-tolerated antidepressant drug binding the 5HT2a receptor, has occurred. Without controlled studies, it is difficult to determine if some degree of activity exists, although extensive retrospective collections fail to provide much hope that this is active (Marzocchetti et al., 2009). Given the relatively benign nature of the drug, it remains widely tried when other approaches are failing.

An additional aspect of treatment of PML stems from the increasing recognition of seizures associated with this disease (Lima, Drislane, & Koralnik, 2006). This is surprising, since PML is a white matter disease, while seizures are generally associated with gray matter diseases. Recognition of seizures as part of the clinical spectrum of PML has largely emerged during the era when immune reconstitution has been more routinely achieved. It appears that PML with IRIS may be the setting in which seizures and other paroxysmal events are most commonly seen. Since it is emerging that the PML cases seen in the setting of monoclonal therapies such as natalizumab are often quite inflammatory, it comes as no surprise that seizures have been presenting symptoms, and not rare significant clinical events in the course of PML, and require active anticonvulsant therapy.

CYTOMEGALOVIRUS NEUROLOGIC MANIFESTATIONS

Very advanced HIV disease is associated with frequent neurological complications due to cytomegalovirus (CMV) (Cinque & McCabe, 1997; Arribas et al., 1996). The most intensively studied of these complications is CMV retinitis, one of the most serious and troubling complications of untreated or inadequately treated AIDS (Jacobson, 1997). This complication, along with CMV encephalitis, CMV radiculomyelitis, and CMV neuropathy, represent the primary spectrum of neurologic disease associated with this virus in immunosuppressed subjects. Prior to HAART therapy, almost 25% of AIDS patients had CMV encephalitis (CE) at death. CE presents as a progressive encephalopathy that can be confused with AIDS dementia complex, but is more rapidly progressive. It is often associated with other CMV end-organ disease complications such as retinitis, adrenal gland involvement, GI and pulmonary CMV disease. Diagnosis is made by noting the progressive non-focal encephalopathy associated with positive CMV DNA detection by PCR in the CSF (Arribas et al., 1995; Shinkai & Spector, 1995).

Through experience in treating CMV retinitis, three parenteral active drugs were approved that could control CMV retinitis. Ganciclovir, foscarnet, and cidofovir are successfully used for retinitis, and actively employed for the other neurological complications (Table 11.3.3). All must be given intravenously. Ganciclovir is the easiest of the three to use, with primary toxicity being bone-marrow suppression most commonly involving leucopenia and thrombocytopenia (Crumpacker, 1996). However, the CNS penetrance of ganciclovir is not ideal, and often CMV encephalitis develops in subjects already treated with ganciclovir for retinitis either because of developing viral resistance or because of the limited levels achieved in the CNS. Foscarnet is a nephrotoxic drug, and requires closer monitoring and more cautious infusion than ganciclovir. However, it probably penetrates the CSF compartment and by extension the CNS better than ganciclovir (Raffi et al., 1993). Sadly, outcomes were not demonstrably better with foscarnet than with ganciclovir (Holida et al., 1995). Thus, just prior to introduction of HAART, experienced clinicians were attempting the difficult task of using both ganciclovir and foscanet (Studies of Ocular Complications of AIDS Research Group, 1994) to treat aggressive CMV infections, including encephalitis (Enting et al., 1992; Van Droogenbroeck et al., 1998). Limited observations collected prior to the decline in CMV complications with HAART suggested better outcomes when this approach was used (Katlama et al., 1995). Cidofovir, the last of the three drugs introduced for CMV, has been used in fewer cases and its efficacy relative to foscarnet or combination ganciclovir and foscarnet is unknown (Sadler et al., 1997). It is nephrotoxic, and use requires pre-treatment with probenecid, which often causes allergic reactions in sulfa-allergic patients. Other toxicities include iritis, uveitis and ocular hypotony, making careful ophthalmologic monitoring necessary. The place of the oral prodrug valganciclovir, which is widely used when CMV viremia is detected and clearly is active, has not been exposed to widespread use for active nervous system complications because these have been infrequent since HAART was introduced (Kaplan et al., 2009).

Table 11.3.3 CYTOMEGALOVIRUS ENCEPHALITIS THERAPY

Prophylaxis: optimal HIV therapy

Acute CMV encephalitis:

Loading: Ganciclovir 5 mg/kg q 12 h IV x 2 weeks

± Foscarnet 60 mg/kg q8h IV x 2 weeks (adjusted for renal function)

Alternative therapy:

Cidofovir 5 mg/kg IV weekly x 2

Probenecid 2 g PO 3 h before, 1 g 2 & 8 h after dose

Hydration before dosing, adjust for renal function

Maintenance: Ganciclovir 5 mg/kg/d, 5 days per week

± Foscarnet 90 mg/kg/d IV

or

Cidofovir 5 mg/kg IV q 2 weeks with probenecid pretreatment

Discontinue maintenance treatment: If CD4 > 100–150 cells/μL for > 6 months

---

Another unique presentation of CMV is the radiculomyelitis syndrome. This presents as a subacute progressive paraplegia with pain radiating to the lower extremity (LE) and saddle-area anesthesia. This CMV-related syndrome is unique in that it is most often associated with a substantial polymorphonuclear reaction in the CSF, as well as having very high CMV DNA loads in the CSF. This CSF formula contrasts with the CE syndrome that may have a rather unremarkable CSF. The radiculomyelitis syndrome responds to effective and prompt CMV therapy, although the clinical response may be delayed and partial (Anders & Goebel, 1998; Cohen et al., 1993; Kim & Hollander, 1993). Without treatment this condition is rapidly fatal. Its response may be better than that of the encephalitis because of greater breakdown of the blood-brain barrier associated with the inflammatory response and elevated CSF protein that typifies this complication. However, when radiculomyelitis develops in patients already on therapy, more aggressive treatment with ganciclovir and foscarnet is probably warranted (Karmochkine et al., 1994; Jacobson et al., 1988; de Gans et al., 1990; Tokumoto & Hollander, 1993). The neuropathy of CMV presents as mononeuritis multiplex in very advanced patients. Successful therapy for CMV is rational and may result in arrest of the disease but with extremely advanced disease (Said et al., 1991; Roullet et al., 1994) it may be difficult to reverse this complication.

Decline in the prominence of CMV complications in HIV has been remarkable in the HAART era, changing a frequent lethal complication to an uncommon challenge only seen in advanced untreated patients. An immune reconstitution inflammatory syndrome (IRIS) is clearly possible when ARV treatment is started during active CMV disease, but reports of its management make it clear that it generally is self-limited if ART is continued, so the place of corticosteroids remains speculative for this disorder.

NEUROSYPHILIS

Historically, syphilis was recognized for its multiple neurological manifestations and the complexity of the differential it could mimic. It is ironic that HIV has taken its place in the modern neurologist's challenges, but these conditions now coincidentally intersect in their clinical presentations. Diagnosis remains somewhat challenging, as CNS manifestation of syphilis take many forms. Neurosyphilis is not likely unless there is some evidence of a reactive spinal fluid with some measure of either increased cells or protein. Presence of CSF VDRL titers is diagnostic, but not sensitive to neurosyhilis. Serum titers of RPR greater than 1:32 have proven highly suggestive for neurosyphilis (Marra et al., 2004). Since HIV and syphilis are both sexually transmitted diseases, they share a population at risk, and co-infection is not rare. It is possible that the development of neurosyphilis is accelerated or made more frequent by concurrent HIV infection, and treatment may be more difficult (Gordon et al., 1994). This problem has been reinforced by apparent treatment failures in HIV-infected patients even after use of intramuscular ceftriaxone therapy. A recently reported study sought to compare 10-day treatments with penicillin G 4 MU IV every four hours versus ceftriaxone 2.0 grams IV daily. The study was not definitive, and possible treatment failures make it necessary to follow up whatever therapy is employed with great care. In this study with 30 subjects, no difference between the groups was demonstrated for CSF WBC, CSF protein concentration, or CSF-VDRL titers. However, serum RPR titers improved more commonly in the ceftriaxone-treated subjects. The once-daily dosing of ceftriaxone makes this regimen easier to administer in most circumstances. In any case, when concomitant neurosyphilis could explain the CSF and clinical findings in an HIV-infected patient, aggressive therapy with IV penicillin or ceftriaxone should probably be given, followed by careful post-therapy evaluation (Marra et al., 2000). Management of penicillin-allergic patients is an additional challenge since one cannot assume that cross-reacting allergies for cephalosporins will not be present. Consideration of penicillin de-sensitization is still recommended for this situation since alternative treatments are not demonstrated to be effective treatment for neurosyphilis.

REFERENCES

Anders, H-J. & Goebel, F-D. (1998). Cytomegalovirus polyradiculopathy in patients with AIDS. *Clin Infect Dis*, 27, 345–52.

Antinori, A., Ammassari, A., Giancola, M. L., Cingolani, A., Grisetti, S., Murri, R., et al. (2001). Epidemiology and prognosis of AIDS-associated progressive multifocal leukoencephalopathy in the HAART era. *J Neurovirol*, 7(4), 323–8.

Antinori, A., Murri, R., Ammassari, A., De Luca, A., Linzalone, A., Cingolani, A., et al. (1995). Aerosolized pentamidine, cotrimoxazole and dapsone-pyrimethamine for primary prophylaxis of *Pneumocystis carinii* pneumonia and toxoplasma encephalitis. *AIDS*, 9, 1343–50.

Arribas, J. R., Clifford, D. B., Fichtenbaum, C. J., Powderly, W. G., & Storch, G. A. (1995). Levels of cytomegalovirus (CMV) DNA in cerebrospinal fluid of patients with AIDS and CMV infection of the central nervous system. *J Infect Dis*, 172, 527–31.

Arribas, J. R., Storch, G. A., Clifford, D. B., & Tselis, A. C. (1996). Cytomegalovirus encephalitis. *Ann Intern Med*, 125, 577–87.

Brickelmaier, M., Lugovskoy, A., Kartikeyan, R., Reviriego-Mendoza, M. M., Allaire, N., Simon, K., et al. (2009). Identification and characterization of mefloquine efficacy against JC virus in vitro. *Antimicrobial Agents and Chemotherapy*, 53(5), 1840–9.

Centers for Disease Control. (2002). Guidelines for preventing opportunistic infections among HIV-infected persons—2002. *Morbidity and Mortality Weekly Report*, 51, 1–27.

Cinque, P. & McCabe, K. (1997). Cytomegalovirus infections of the central nervous system. *Intervirology*, 40, 85–97.

Cinque, P., Casari, S., & Bertelli, D. (1998). Progressive multifocal leukoencephalopathy, HIV and highly active antiretroviral therapy. *N Engl J Med*, 848–9.

Cinque, P., Koralnik, I. J., & Clifford, D. B. (2003). The evolving face of human immunodeficiency virus-related progressive multifocal leukoencephalopathy: Defining a consensus terminology. *Journal of Neurovirology*, 9, 88–92.

Cinque, P., Pierotti, C., Vigano, M. G., Bestetti, A., Fausti, C., Bertelli, D., et al. (2001). The good and evil of HAART in HIV-related progressive multifocal leukoencephalopathy. *J Neurovirol*, 7(4), 358–63.

Clifford, D., Brew, B., Cinque, P., Gorelik, L., Bennett, D., Panzara, M., et al. (2009). Design of a clinical trial of mefloquine in patients with progressive multifocal leukoencephalopathy. *Multiple Sclerosis*, 15, S87. Ref Type: Abstract

Clifford, D. B., Yiannoutsos, C., Glicksman, M., Simpson, D. M., Singer, E. J., Piliero, P. J., et al. (1999). HAART improves prognosis in HIV-associated progressive multifocal leukoencephalopathy. *Neurology*, 52, 623–5.

Clifford, D, Nath, A, Cinque, P, Brew, B, Workman, A, Lorelik, L, Zhao, J, Duda, P. (2011). Mefloquine Treatment in Patients with Progressive Multifocal Leukoencephalopathy. *Neurology*, 76, A28.

Cohen, B. A., McArthur, J. C., Grohman, S., Patterson, B., & Glass, J. D. (1993). Neurologic prognosis of cytomegalovirus polyradiculomyelopathy in AIDS. *Neurology*, 43, 493–9.

Crumpacker, C. S. (1996). Ganciclovir. *N Engl J Med*, 335, 721–9.

Dannemann, B., McCutchan, J. A., Israelski, D., Antoniskis, D., Leport, C., Luft, B., et al. (1992). Treatment of toxoplasmic encephalitis in patients with AIDS—A randomized trial comparing Pyrimethamine plus Clindamycin to Pyrimethamine plus Sulfadiazine. *Ann Intern Med 116*, 33–43.

de Gans, J., Portegies, P., Reiss, P., Troost, D., van Gool, T., & Lange, J. M. A. (1992). Pyrimethamine alone as maintenance therapy for central nervous system toxoplasmosis in 38 patients with AIDS. *Journal of Acquired Immune Deficiency Syndromes*, 5, 137–42.

de Gans, J., Portegies, P., Tiessens, G., Troost, D., Danner, S. A., & Lange, J. M. A. (1990). Therapy for cytomegalovirus polyradiculomyelitis in patients with AIDS: Treatment with ganciclovir. *AIDS*, 4, 421–5.

De Luca, A., Ammassari, A., Pezzotti, P., Cinque, P., Gasnault, J., Berenguer, J., et al. (2008). Cidofovir in addition to antiretroviral treatment is not effective for AIDS-associated progressive multifocal leukoencephalopathy: A multicohort analysis. *AIDS*, 22, 1759–67.

Dworkin, M. S., Wan, P. T., Hanson, D. L., Jones, J. L., for Adult & Adolescent Spectrum of HIV Disease Project. (1999). Progressive multifocal leukoencephalopathy: Improved survival of human immunodeficiency virus-infected patients in the protease inhibitor era. *Journal of Infectious Diseases*, 180, 621–5.

Elphick, G. F., Querbes, W., Jordan, J. A., Gee, G. V., Eash, S., Manley, K., et al. (2004). The human polyomavirus, JCV, uses serotonin receptors to infect cells. *Science*, 306, 1380–3.

Enting, R., de Gans, J., Reiss, P., Jansen, C., & Portegies, P. (1992). Ganciclovir/foscarnet for cytomegalovirus meningoencephalitis in AIDS. *Lancet*, 340, 559.

Fernandez-Martin, J., Leport, C., Morlat, P., Meyohas, M. C., Chauvin, J. P., & Vilde, J. L. (1991). Pyrimethamine-clarithromycin combination for therapy of acute toxoplasma encephalitis in patients with AIDS. *Antimicrobial Agents and Chemotherapy*, 35, 2049–52.

Furrer, H., Opravil, M., Bernasconi, E., Telenti, A., Egger, M., for the Swiss HIV Cohort Study. (2000). Stopping primary prophylaxis in HIV-1-infected patients at high risk of toxoplasma encephalitis. *Lancet*, 355, 2217–8.

Gasnault, J., Taoufik, Y., Goujard, C., Kousignian, P., Abbed, K., Boué, F., et al. (1999). Prolonged survival without neurological improvement in patients with AIDS-related progressive multifocal leukoencephalopathy on potent combined antiretroviral therapy. *Journal of Neurovirology*, 5, 421–9.

Geschwind, M. D., Skolasky, R. I., Royal, W. S., & McArthur, J. C. (2001). The relative contributions of HAART and alpha-interferon for therapy of progressive multifocal leukoencephalopathy in AIDS. *J Neurovirol*, 7(4), 353–7.

Giudici, B., Vaz, B., Bossolasco, S., Casari, S., Brambilla, A. M., Lüke, W., et al. (2000). Highly active antiretroviral therapy and progressive multifocal leukoencephalopathy: Effects on cerebrospinal fluid markers of JC virus replication and immune response. *Clinical Infectious Diseases*, 30, 95–9.

Gordon, S. M., Eaton, M. E., George, R., Larsen, S., Lukehart, S. A., Kuypers, J., et al. (1994). The response of symptomatic neurosyphilis to high-dose intravenous penicillin G in patients with human immunodeficiency virus infection. *N Engl J Med*, 331, 1469–73.

Hall, C. D., Dafni, U., Simpson, D., Clifford, D. B., Wetherill, P. E., Cohen, B., et al. (1998). Failure of cytarabine in progressive multifocal leukoencephalopathy associated with human immunodeficiency virus infection. *N Engl J Med*, 338, 1345–51.

Harrison, M. J. G. & McArthur, J. C. (1996). *AIDS and neurology*. Edinburgh: Churchill Livingstone.

Holida, M. D., Trigg, M. E., Rumelhart, S. L., Lee, N. F., Kook, H., & Peters, C. (1995). Cytomegalovirus encephalitis resistant to anti-cytomegalovirus therapy. *AIDS, 9*, 531–2.

Hou, J. & Major, E. O. (1998). The efficacy of nucleoside analogs against JC virus multiplication in a persistently infected human fetal brain cell line. *Journal of Neurovirology, 4*, 451–6.

Huang, S. S., Skolasky, R. L., Dal Pan, G. J., Royal, W., III, & McArthur, J. C. (1998). Survival prolongation in HIV-associated progressive multifocal leukoencephalopathy treated with alpha-Interferon: An observational study. *J Neurovirol, 4*, 324–32.

Inui, K., Miyagawa, H., Sashihara, J., Miyoshi, H., Tanaka-Taya, K., Nishigaki, T., et al. (1999). Remission of progressive multifocal leukoencephalopathy following highly active antiretroviral therapy in a patient with HIV infection. *Brain & Development, 21*, 416–9.

Jacobson, M. A. (1997). Treatment of cytomegalovirus retinitis in patients with the acquired immunodeficiency syndrome. *N Engl J Med, 337*, 105–14.

Jacobson, M. A., Mills, J., Rush, J., O'Donnell, J. J., Miller, R. G., Greco, C., et al. (1988). Failure of antiviral therapy for acquired immunodeficiency syndrome-related cytomegalovirus myelitis. *Arch Neurol, 45*, 1090–2.

Kaplan, J. E., Benson, C., Holmes, K. K., Brooks, J. T., Pau, A., & Masur, H. (2009). Centers for Disease Control and Prevention: Guidelines for prevention and treatment of opportunistic infections in HIV-infected adults and adolescents. *Morbidity and Mortality Weekly Report (MMWR), 58*(RR-4), 1–210.

Karmochkine, M., Molina, J. M., Scieux, C., Welker, Y., Morinet, F., Decazes, J. M., et al. (1994). Combined therapy with ganciclovir and foscarnet for cytomegalovirus polyradiculomyelitis in patients with AIDS. *American Journal of Medicine, 97*, 196–7.

Katlama, C. (1991). Evaluation of the efficacy and safety of clindamycin plus pyrimethamine for induction and maintenance therapy of toxoplasmic encephalitis in AIDS. *Eur J Clin Microbiol Infect Dis, 10*, 189–91.

Katlama, C. (1996). Diagnosis and treatment of toxoplasmosis of the CNS in patients with AIDS. *CNS Drugs, 5*, 331–43.

Katlama, C., Anduze-Faris, B., Fillet, A-M., Boukli, N., Gasnault, J., Gostagliola, D., et al. (1995). A controlled study of foscarnet-ganciclovir combination for central nervous system (CNS) infection with cytomegalovirus (CMV) in HIV patients. *Abstracts of the 5th Conference on Retroviruses and Opportunistic Infection, 128*. Ref Type: Abstract.

Katlama, C., Mouthon, B., Gourdon, D., Lapierre, D., Rousseau, F., & Atovaquone Expanded Access Group. (1996). Atovaquone as long-term suppressive therapy for toxoplasmic encephalitis in patients with AIDS and multiple drug intolerance. *AIDS, 10*, 1107–12.

Kim, Y. S. & Hollander, H. (1993). Polyradiculopathy due to cytomegalovirus: Report of two cases in which improvement occurred after prolonged therapy and review of the literature. *Clin Infect Dis, 17*, 32–7.

Kleinschmidt-DeMasters, B. K. & Tyler, K. L. (2005). Progressive multifocal leukoencephalopathy complicating treatment with natalizumab and interferon beta-1a for multiple sclerosis. *New England Journal of Medicine, 353*, 369–74.

Klinker, H., Langmann, P., & Richter, E. (1996). Plasma pyrimethamine concentrations during long-term treatment for cerebral toxoplasmosis in patients with AIDS. *Antimicrobial Agents and Chemotherapy, 40*, 1623–7.

Kotecha, N., George, M. J., Smith, T. W., Corvi, F., & Litofsky, N. S. (1998). Enhancing progressive multifocal leukoencephalopathy: An indicator of improved immune status. *Am J Med, 105*, 541–3.

Lacassin, F., Schaffo, D., Perronne, C., Longuet, P., Leport, C., & Vilde, J. L. (1995). Clarithromycin-minocycline combination as salvage therapy for toxoplasmosis in patients infected with human immunodeficiency virus. *Antimicrobial Agents and Chemotherapy, 39*, 276–7.

Langer-Gould, A., Atlas, S. W., Bollen, A. W., & Pelletier, D. (2005). Progressive multifocal leukoencephalopathy in a patient treated with natalizumab. *New England Journal of Medicine, 353*, 375–81.

Leenders, A. C., Reiss, P., Portegies, P., Clezy, K., Hop, W. C., Hoy, J., et al. (1997). Liposomal amphotericin B (AmBisome) compared with amphotericin B both followed by oral fluconazole in the treatment of AIDS-associated cryptococcal meningitis. *AIDS, 11*, 1463–71.

Leport, C., Raffi, F., Matheron, S., Katlama, C., Regnier, B., Saimot, A. G., et al. (1988). Treatment of central nervous system toxoplasmosis with pyrimethamine/sulfadiazine combination in 35 patients with the acquired immunodeficiency syndrome. *American Journal of Medicine, 84*, 94–100.

Lima, M. A., Drislane, F. W., & Koralnik, I. J. (2006). Seizures and their outcome in progressive multifocal leukoencephalopathy. *Neurology, 66*, 262–4.

Lortholary, O., Poizat, G., Zeller, V., Neuville, S., Boibieux, A., Alvarez, M., et al. (2006). Long-term outcome of AIDS-associated cryptococcosis in the era of combination antiretroviral therapy. *AIDS, 20*, 2183–91.

Luft, B. L., Hafner, R., Korzun, A. H., Leport, C., Antoniskis, D., Bosler, E. M., et al. (1993). Toxoplasmic encephalitis in patients with the acquired immunodeficiency syndrome. *N Engl J Med, 329*, 995–1000.

Major, E. O., Amemiya, K., Tornatore, C. S., Houff, S. A., & Berger, J. R. (1992). Pathogenesis and molecular biology of progressive multifocal leukoencephalopathy, the JC virus-induced demyelinating disease of the human brain. *Clinical Microbiology Reviews, 5*, 49–73.

Marra, C. M., Boutin, P., McArthur, J. C., Hurwitz, S., Simpson, P. A., Haslett, J. A., et al. (2000). A pilot study evaluating ceftriaxone and penicillin G as treatment agents for neurosyphilis in human immunodeficiency virus-infected individuals. *Clin Infect Dis, 30*, 540–4.

Marra, C. M., Maxwell, C. L., Smith, S. L., Lukehart, S. A., Rompalo, A. M., Eaton, M., et al. (2004). Cerebrospinal fluid abnormalities in patients with syphilis: Association with clinical and laboratory features. *Journal of Infectious Diseases, 189*, 369–76.

Marra, C. M., Rajicic, N., Barker, D. E., Cohen, B. A., Clifford, D., Post, M. J. D., et al. (2002). A pilot study of cidofovir for progressive multifocal leukoencephalopathy in AIDS. *AIDS, 16*, 1–7.

Marzocchetti, A., Tompkins, T., Clifford, D. B., Gandhi, R. T., Kesari, S., Berger, J. R., et al. (2009). Determinants of survival in progressive multifocal leukoencephalopathy. *Neurology, 73*, 1551–8.

Masur, H., Polis, M. A., Tuazon, C. U., Ogata-Arakaki, D., Kovacs, J. A., Katz, D., et al. (1993). Salvage trial of trimetrexate-leucovorin for the treatment of cerebral toxoplasmosis in patients with AIDS. *Journal of Infectious Diseases, 167*, 1422–6.

Milefchik, E., Leal, M. A., Haubrich, R., Bozzette, S. A., Tilles, J. G., Leedom, J. M., et al. (2008). Fluconazole alone or combined with flucytosine for the treatment of AIDS-associated cryptococcal meningitis. *Medical Mycology, 46*, 393–5.

Miralles, P., Berenguer, J., García de Viedma, D., Padilla, B., Cosin, J., Lopez-Bernaldo de Quirós, J. C., et al. (1998). Treatment of AIDS-associated progressive multifocal leukoencephalopathy with highly active antiretroviral therapy. *AIDS, 12*, 2467–72.

Miralles, P., Berenguer, J., Lacruz, C., Cosin, J., Lopez, J. C., Padilla, B., et al. (2001). Inflammatory reactions in progressive multifocal leukoencephalopathy after highly active antiretroviral therapy. *AIDS, 15*, 1900–2.

Nussbaum, J. C., Jackson, A., Namarika, D., Phulusa, J., Kenala, J., Kanyemba, C., et al. (2010). Combination flucytosine and high-dose fluconazole compared with fluconazole monotherapy for the treatment of cryptococcal meningitis: A randomized trial in Malawi. *Clinical Infectious Diseases, 50*, 338–44.

Pfeffer, G., Prout, A., Hooge, J., & Maguire, J. (2009). Biopsy-proven immune reconstitution syndrome in a patient with AIDS and cerebral toxoplasmosis. *Neurology, 73*, 321–2.

Podzamczer, D., Miro, J. M., Ferrer, E., Gatell, J. M., Ramón, J. M., Ribera, E., et al. (2000). Thrice-weekly sulfadiazine-pyrimethamine for maintenance therapy of toxoplasmic encephalitis in HIV-infected patients. *Eur J Clin Microbiol Infect Dis, 19*, 89–95.

Port, J. D., Miseljic, S., Lee, R. R., Ali, S. Z., Nicol, T. L., Royal, S., III, et al. (1999). Progressive multifocal leukoencephalopathy demonstrating contrast enhancement on MRI and uptake of thallium-201: A case report. *Neuroradiology*, *41*, 895–8.

Raffi, F., Taburet, A. M., Ghaleh, B., Huart, A., & Singlas, E. (1993). Penetration of foscarnet into cerebrospinal fluid of AIDS patients. *Antimicrob Agents Chemother*, *37*, 1777–80.

Ribera, E., Fernandez-Sola, A., Juste, C., Rovira, A., Romero, F. J., Armadans-Gil, L., et al. (1999). Comparison of high and low doses of trimethoprim-sulfamethoxazole for primary prevention of toxoplasmic encephalitis in human immunodeficiency virus-infected patients. *Clinical Infectious Diseases*, *29*, 1461–6.

Roullet, E., Assuerus, V., Gozlan, J., Ropert, A., Said, G., Baudrimont, M., et al. (1994). Cytomegalovirus multifocal neuropathy in AIDS: Analysis of 15 consecutive cases. *Neurology*, *44*, 2174–82.

Saag, M. S., Powderly, W. G., Cloud, G. A., Robinson, P., Grieco, M. H., Sharkey, P. K., et al. (2002). Comparison of amphotericin B with fluconazole in the treatment of acute AIDS-associated cryptococcal meningitis. *N Engl J Med*, *326*, 83–9.

Sadler, M., Morris-Jones, S., Nelson, M., & Gazzard, B. G. (1997). Successful treatment of cytomegalovirus encephalitis in an AIDS patient using cidofovir (letter). *AIDS*, *11*, 1293–4.

Said, G., Lacroix, C., Chemouilli, P., Goulon-Goeau, C., Roullet, E., Penaud, D., et al. (1991). Cytomegalovirus neuropathy in acquired immunodeficiency syndrome: A clinical and pathological study. *Ann Neurol*, *29*, 139–46.

Schürmann, D., Bergmann, F., Albrecht, H., Padberg, J., Grünewald, T., Behnsch, M., et al. (2001). Twice-weekly pyrimethamine-sulfadoxine effectively prevents Pneumocystis carinii pneumonia relapse and toxoplasmic encephalitis in patients with AIDS. *Journal of Infection*, *42*, 8–15.

Shinkai, M. & Spector, S. A. (1995). Quantitation of human cytomegalovirus (HCMV) DNA in cerebrospinal fluid by competitive PCR in AIDS patients with different HCMV central nervous system diseases. *Scand J Infect Dis*, *27*, 559–61.

Soriano, V., Dona, C., Rodríguez-Rosado, R., Barreiro, P., & González-Lahoz, J. (2000). Discontinuation of secondary prophylaxis for opportunistic infections in HIV-infected patients receiving highly active antiretroviral therapy. *AIDS*, *14*, 383–6.

St Georgiev, V. (1994). Management of toxoplasmosis. *Drugs*, *48*, 179–88.

Studies of Ocular Complications of AIDS Research Group in collaboration with the AIDS Clinical Trials Group. (1994). Foscarnet-Ganciclovir cytomegalovirus retinitis trial. 4. Visual outcomes. *Ophthalmology*, *101*, 1250–61.

Tan, K., Roda, R., Ostrow, L., McArthur, J., & Nath, A. (2009). PML-IRIS in patients with HIV infection. Clinical manifestations and treatment with steroids. *Neurology*, *72*, 1458–64.

Tassie, J. M., Gasnault, J., Bentata, M., Deloumeaux, J., Boué, F., Billaud, E., et al. (1999). Survival improvement of AIDS-related progressive multifocal leukoencephalopathy in the era of protease inhibitors. *AIDS*, *13*, 1881–7.

Taoufik, Y., Delfraissy, J. F., & Gasnault, J. (2000). Highly active antiretroviral therapy does not improve survival of patients with high JC virus load in the cerebrospinal fluid at progressive multifocal leukoencephalopathy diagnosis. *AIDS*, *14*, 758–9.

Tenant-Flowers, M., Boyle, M. J., Carey, D., Marriott, D. J., Harkness, J. L., Penny, R., et al. (1991). Sulphadiazine desensitization in patients with AIDS and cerebral toxoplasmosis. *AIDS*, *5*, 311–5.

Tokumoto, J. I. N. & Hollander, H. (1993). Cytomegalovirus polyradiculopathy caused by a ganciclovir-resistant strain. *Clin Infect Dis*, *17*, 854–6.

Torre, D., Casari, S., Speranza, F., Donisi, A., Gregis, G., Poggio, A. et al. (1998). Randomized trial of Trimethoprim-Sulfamethoxazole versus Pyrimethamine-Sulfadiazine for therapy of toxoplasmic encephalitis in patients with AIDS. *Antimicrob Agents Chemother*, *42*, 1346–9.

Van Droogenbroeck, J., De Ceuninck, M., Snoeck, H. W., Schroyens, W., & Berneman, Z. (1998). Successful treatment of cytomegalovirus encephalitis in a patient with Hodgkin's disease in remission. *Ann Hematol*, *76*, 179–81.

Vendrely, A., Bienvenu, B., Gasnault, J., Thiebault, J. B., Salmon, D., & Gray, F. (2005). Fulminant inflammatory leukoencephalopathy associated with HAART-induced immune restoration in AIDS-related progressive multifocal leukoencephalopathy. *Acta Neuropathol*, *109*, 449–55.

Weigel, H. M., De Vries, E., Regez, R. M., Henrichs, J. H., Ten Velden, J. J. A. M., Frissen, P. H. J., et al. (1997). Cotrimoxazole is effective as primary prophylaxis for toxoplasmic encephalitis in HIV-infected patients: A case control study. *Scand J Infect Dis*, *29*, 499–502.

Wheeler, A. L., Truwit, C. L., Kleinschmidt-DeMasters, B. K., Byrne, W. R., & Hannon, R. N. (1993). Progressive multifocal leukoencephalopathy: Contrast enhancement on CT scans and MR images. *AJR*, *161*, 1049–51.

Zolopa, A. R., Andersen, J., Komarow, L., Sanne, I., Sanchez, A., Hogg, E., et al. (2009). Early antiretroviral therapy reduces AIDS progression/death in individuals with acute opportunistic infections: A multicenter randomized strategy trial. *PLoS ONE*, *4*(5), e5575.

11.4

NANOFORMULATED MEDICINES

Upal Roy, Shantanu Balkundi, JoEllyn McMillan, and Howard E. Gendelman

Nanomaterials can antiretroviral efficacy, pharmacokinetics, and patient compliance. Importantly, such materials may also be used for bioimaging to effect disease diagnosis and therapeutic monitoring. The targeted objectives are to attenuate human immunodeficiency virus (HIV) infection and positively affect the disease course in the infected human host. We posit that antiretroviral therapy delivery can be realized for human use by formulating or encapsulating drugs with surfactants. Such nanoformulated drugs are readily taken up by the reticuloendothelial system (RES), the natural target for HIV. Recent works have explored the development of cell-based delivery systems using macrophages as drug carriers. This scheme has been shown to enhance nervous system RES delivery, as macrophages are actively phagocytic cells and readily cross tissue barriers. Another major advantage of using cells as drug carriers is the potential to deliver a broad range of medicines with different biochemical properties to disease sites. This chapter discusses the potentials and perils for nanoformulated drug developments, with a focus on antiretroviral agents.

INTRODUCTION

HUMAN IMMUNODEFICIENCY VIRUS TYPE ONE (HIV-1) INFECTION OF THE CENTRAL NERVOUS SYSTEM (CNS)

HIV-1 infection is characterized by prolonged clinical latency, progressive viral replication with selective loss of CD4+ T lymphocytes, and immune dysfunction. Within end-organ tissues such as the CNS, HIV-1 infection occurs predominantly in mononuclear phagocytes (MP; blood-borne macrophages, dendritic cells, and microglia), which serve as a viral reservoir (Alexaki, Liu. & Wigdahl, 2008; Rao, Ghorpade, & Labhasetwar, 2009; Dahl, Josefsson, & Palmer, 2010). With disease, progressive histopathological features include but are not limited to cerebral atrophy, ventricular enlargement, and chronic inflammatory responses (reviewed by Pittella, 2009; Wohlschlaeger, Wenger, Mehraein, & Weis, 2009). Associated with the most severe form of HIV-associated neurocognitive disorders (HAND), namely HIV-1-associated dementia (or HAD), a multinucleated giant cell encephalitis ensues that is characterized by viral infection within MP lineage cells, astrogliosis, neuronal loss (predominantly in the frontal cortex and basal ganglia), myelin pallor, and microglial nodules (Moore et al., 2006; Antinori et al., 2007; Gongvatana et al., 2009).

Underlying the tempo and progression of disease, the number of immune-competent MPs best correlates with cognitive impairment in the infected host. MPs are carried into the brain as a consequence of ongoing and chronic neuroinflammatory reactions orchestrated by interleukin-6 (IL-6) secretion from endothelial cells in the blood-brain barrier (BBB) (Chaudhuri, Yang, Gendelman, Persidsky, & Kanmogne, 2008) and perpetuated through macrophage chemoattractant protein-1 (MCP-1) secretion by MPs and astrocytes (Peng et al., 2008; Kraft-Terry, Buch, Fox, & Gendelman, 2009). In HIV-1 infected patients, the infected monocytes readily cross the BBB and release virus into the brain parenchyma. The virus can accumulate in perivascular macrophages and microglia, leading to a range of neurological disorders, collectively termed HAND.

HIV-1, THE BLOOD-BRAIN BARRIER (BBB), AND CNS DRUG DELIVERY

Barriers to CNS drug delivery are posed by CNS structure, function, and physiology. Structural barriers include the BBB, the blood-cerebrospinal fluid barrier (BCB), and the cerebrospinal fluid (CSF)-brain barrier (CSFB) (Taylor & Pereira, 2000; Pardridge, 2005; McGee, Smith, & Aweeka, 2006). To enter into extravascular compartments, drug molecules must cross the endothelial cell lining of the microvasculature. The presence of tight junctions between endothelial cells and the lack of intracellular clefts and fenestrae in brain capillaries in the BBB and BCB greatly restricts drug transfer across the endothelial cell layer at these sites. The loosely linked ependymal cells of the CSFB, however, allow diffusion of dissolved compounds in both directions between the blood and CSF (McGee et al., 2006). The BBB plays an important role in regulating drug concentration, including antiretroviral therapeutics (ART), in the CNS (Ivey, MacLean, & Lackner, 2009; Varatharajan & Thomas, 2009; Zastre et al., 2009). It is composed of cellular and extracellular components, including brain microvascular endothelial cells (BMVEC); perivascular elements such as astrocytes, pericytes, and leptomeningeal cells; the endothelial basement membrane; and the parenchymal covering (Miller, Bauer, & Hartz, 2008). Under physiologic conditions, this vascular barrier selectively regulates intracellular and paracellular exchange of macromolecules and cells between the blood and the CNS, although not all the factors that regulate drug entry into the brain across the BBB are understood. Tight junctions between BMVECs formed by the interaction of various transmembrane proteins effectively prevent drug entry into the CNS (McGee et al., 2006). Thus, despite an extremely large capillary surface area, permeability of many drugs, including ART, through the BBB is very low (Liu & Chen, 2005; Liu, Chen, & Smith, 2008a).

The physical and chemical characteristics of drugs and their interaction with BBB components will affect their CNS bioavailability. In order to facilitate drug ingress into the CNS, clinical strategies have been explored to disrupt the BBB, including chemical, osmotic, biochemical, and ultrasound disruption (Nowacek & Gendelman, 2009). However, disruption of the BBB could compromise the integrity of the CNS by allowing entry of unwanted blood components into the brain parenchyma. Thus, understanding the barriers to drug penetrance into the CNS and sustaining drug levels in viral sanctuaries remains critical in designing new therapeutic strategies for HAND.

The limited diffusion of drugs across the BBB is attributed not only to its anatomical structure, but also to the expression of selective efflux transporters and drug-metabolizing enzymes. Adenosine triphosphate (ATP)-binding cassette (ABC) transporters are very crucial in this respect. ABC transporters were first recognized in cancer cells and observed to affect cell entry of chemotherapeutic agents (Kuo, 2009). More recently, these transporters have been found to play a key role in the lack of efficacy of ART. Specifically, the efflux of protease inhibitors (PIs) and nucleoside reverse transcriptase inhibitors (NRTIs) by ABC transporters has been identified in the maintenance of viral reservoirs, including the CNS, in HIV-1-infected patients (Ronaldson & Bendayan, 2006). Among the ABC transporters, P-glycoprotein (Pgp) is present on the luminal side of the BBB and has broad substrate specificity, which includes many ART drugs (Bachmeier, Spitzenberger, Elmquist, & Miller, 2005; Zastre et al., 2009). Because of its abundance and broad range of substrates it may be the most important membrane transporter in regard to biodistribution of ART. Other transporters that contribute to ART efflux and limit drug penetration into the CNS are the breast cancer resistance protein (BCRP) and the multidrug-resistance associated proteins (MRPs) (Loscher & Potschka, 2005). BCRP has a cellular distribution in the BBB similar to that of Pgp. While the ART drugs ritonavir, saquinavir, and nelfinavir are not substrates for this transporter, they can inhibit the transport of other drugs, such as atazanavir (Wang & Baba, 2005). The MRPs are also localized on the luminal side of the BBB. The protease inhibitors saquinavir, ritonavir, and lopinavir are substrates for mainly MRP-1 and -2, while minor activity is observed with MRP-4 and -5 (Eilers, Roy, & Mondal, 2008).

In addition to the presence of efflux transporters, the BBB contains drug metabolism capability. The activity of certain enzymes such as γ-glutamyl transpeptidase, alkaline phosphatase, and aromatic acid decarboxylase, which can contribute to metabolism and activation of exogenous compounds, is elevated within BMVECs (Varatharajan & Thomas, 2009). Plasma protein binding of drugs can also limit drug transport across the BBB. ART drugs bind extensively to plasma proteins, which restricts their access to the CNS (McGee et al., 2006; Alexaki et al., 2008).

The BCB, with tight junctions between epithelial cells of the choroid plexus, acts as a barrier between the blood and CSF for the metabolism and efflux that occurs within the tissue itself. Despite the presence of tight junctions, the BCB is leakier than the BBB; its leakiness could account for the small amount of albumin in the CSF and may have functional consequences (Varatharajan & Thomas, 2009). The molecular and structural composition of the BCB is much different than the BBB and the distribution of drug transporters is different between the two barrier systems, suggesting the need for separate studies of the BCB. Importantly, drug penetration across the BCB does not guarantee transport through the BBB because of the diffusion distance between CSF and the brain interstitial fluid.

Development of ways to overcome the barriers to CNS drug delivery is of great clinical interest and relevance. Delivery of drugs by nanocarrier systems is one important strategy that could overcome several barriers to CNS drug delivery, including poor BBB penetration, extensive binding to plasma proteins, and the presence of drug efflux pumps at the BBB that diminish drug levels in the CNS parenchyma (das Neves, Amiji, Bahia, & Sarmento, 2009).

HARNESSING NANOMEDICINES FOR HIV/AIDS

NANOMEDICINE

Nanotechnology-based systems have been developed with some success to overcome the barriers to drug delivery to viral sanctuary sites such as the CNS (Begley, 2004; Tiwari & Amiji, 2006; das Neves et al., 2009). For example, in rodents, zalcitabine-loaded liposomes can be retained in the CNS (Kim, Scheerer, Geyer, & Howell, 1990). However, in these studies, drug was administered by intraventricular injection, limiting translatability to the clinical setting. Kuo et al. (Kuo & Chen, 2006; Kuo & Su, 2007; Kuo & Chen, 2009) tested various nanocarriers, including polybutylcyanoacrylate nanoparticles (NPs), methylmethacrylate-sulfopropyl-methacrylate NPs, and cationic solid lipid NPs (CSLNs), to permeate into in vitro models of the BBB based on brain-microvascular endothelial cells. Vyas et al. prepared nanoemulsion formulations containing [^{3}H]-saquinavir and observed higher plasma and brain concentrations of the drug in mice following oral administration of the nanoemulsion formulation as compared to an aqueous suspension of the drug (Vyas et al., 2008). However, when the same formulation was given by intravenous injection and the pharmacokinetic analyses of both studies were compared, it was concluded that the increased enteric absorption and brain concentrations of the drug were due to preferential uptake of polyunsaturated essential fatty acids in the emulsions and Pgp inhibition by the co-surfactant (Vyas, Shahiwala, & Amiji, 2008; das Neves et al., 2009).

Various properties of nanomaterials can be utilized to combat viral mechanisms, including viral infection and growth (reviewed by Nowacek & Gendelman, 2009). Gold and silver NPs have been used in bioimaging, in various bioassays, and in therapeutics (Jennings & Strouse, 2007; Gasparyan, 2009). Gold NPs are easy to fabricate and molecules of interest can be conjugated to the surface of the NPs. The possibility of using gold NPs for treatment of HIV infection has recently been explored (Bowman et al., 2008). Gold NPs were conjugated to SDC-1721, a fragment of the potent HIV inhibitor TAK-779, which acts by allosteric inhibition of the CCR5 receptor. This group observed that SDC-1721-conjugated gold NPs showed antiviral activity and, importantly, that free SDC-1721 did not inhibit HIV infection. These studies also demonstrated that gold NPs are effective in converting normally inactive drugs into active antiviral agents. Silver NPs have also been shown to be effective HIV inhibitors *in vitro*. Selective inhibition based on the size of the silver NPs was observed (Elechiguerra et al., 2005). Silver NPs in the size range of 1–10 nm attached to the virus. The inhibition was drug free and occurred through preferential binding to HIV-1 gp120 glycoprotein knobs. Another example of NPs used in ART is the development of indinavir NPs fabricated with disteroyl phoshatidylcholine and methyl polyethylene glycol-disteroyl phosphatidylethanolamine (Hockett et al., 1999; Brodie et al., 2000). These NPs were designed to attack the residual virus that is present in the lymphoid tissues of patients undergoing ART.

One of the problems faced in antiretroviral therapy is that many ART drugs are metabolized rapidly and eliminated from circulation, requiring at least daily oral administration. Long-acting parenteral formulations of ART could be of potential benefit in this regard. Nanoformulated versions of rilpivirine and indinavir have been developed that have provided extended drug levels and antiviral activity for weeks following in vivo administration in animal and human studies. NPs of rilpivirine, a poorly water-soluble NNRTI, coated with poloxamer 338 or E-α-tocopheryl polyethylene glycol 1000 succinate surfactants have been manufactured by wet milling (Baert et al., 2009). After a single subcutaneous administration of the nanoformulation, plasma drug levels in dogs were constant at 25 ng/mL for 20 days and then declined to 1–3 ng/mL after 3 months (Baert et al., 2009; van 't Klooster et al., 2010). Indinavir-NPs have been used to develop a bone-marrow-derived macrophage (BMM) ART-NP delivery system by Dou et al. (2009). The small size of the NPs and their stable nature allowed them to be packaged within macrophages for subsequent systemic trafficking and sustained drug distribution. In these studies, an indinavir nanosuspension was loaded into BMMs and administered intravenously into naive mice. A single administration of indinavir-NP-loaded BMMs after HIV infection showed sustained antiretroviral therapeutic responses with concomitant immune reconstitution up to 14 days. These results together have shown successful application of NPs in long-term ART drug delivery. Indeed, the development of antiretroviral NPs opens up new and promising opportunities for antiretroviral therapy.

DRUG CARRIER SYSTEMS

Nanotechnology can be used to develop nanopharmaceuticals that can be designed specifically for various drugs to improve drug delivery for CNS disorders (Figure 11.4.1). Several nano drug-delivery systems have been developed; however, they need further improvement to optimize drug bioavailability and therapeutic index (Kabanov & Alakhov, 2002). Hurdles must be overcome in several related areas pertaining to (a) the time that the active ingredient remains in the body in bioavailable form, (b) the pattern and rate of drug degradation and elimination, (c) selection of vehicles that can effectively carry the drug, including across relevant membranes and barriers, and (d) identification of drug effects on sites other than those specifically targeted. New emerging technologies have focused on the physical characteristics of the drug to increase the stability and improve the bioavailability of poorly soluble drugs (Kabanov & Alakhov, 2002). Synthetic polymers are being used in the pharmaceutical industry because of their ability to overcome some of the biological barriers in a drug-delivery system, due to their high molecular mass compared to the drug (Langer, 1998). These polymers can help to increase the overall effectiveness of the drugs and can help to maintain drug bioavailability by combining with drug molecules.

MICELLAR DRUG CARRIERS

Micellar drug carriers have been a popular choice and have been explored using various polymeric micelles. Many reports have described the use of polymeric micelles to deliver poorly soluble drugs that have high bioavailability. Batz et al. showed that block polymers can be used for drug delivery by conjugating one segment of the polymers to a hydrophobic drug and keeping the water-soluble segment unmodified (Batz et al., 1977). These block polymers further self-assemble into micelles. Various amphiphilic molecules can be used for self-assembly into the micelles. The concentration at which these amphiphilic molecules form micelles is called the critical micelle concentration (CMC) (Jones & Leroux, 1999). Micelles have an anisotropic water distribution within their structure. Such a system has a corona formed by the hydrophilic part of the molecule and a core that is made up of the hydrophobic block and the conjugated drug (Jones & Leroux, 1999). The special position of the solubilized drug in a micellar system will depend on the polarity of the drug. The nonpolar molecules are solubilized in the micellar core, and substances that have intermediate polarity are distributed along the surfactant molecules in certain intermediate positions. Amphiphilic block polymers and polymeric micelles have been extensively used in drug-delivery systems for poorly soluble drugs. Kabanov et al. demonstrated that micelles formed using polymeric block polymers that had non-covalently bound drug in their cores were delivered in vivo to the CNS (Kabanov & Alakhov, 2002). Brain-specific antibodies assisted in the targeted delivery of the micelle-incorporated drug. The hydrophobic core is used to store and transport the drug in the system. These carrier systems are referred to as "micellar nanocontainers," since the micelles are

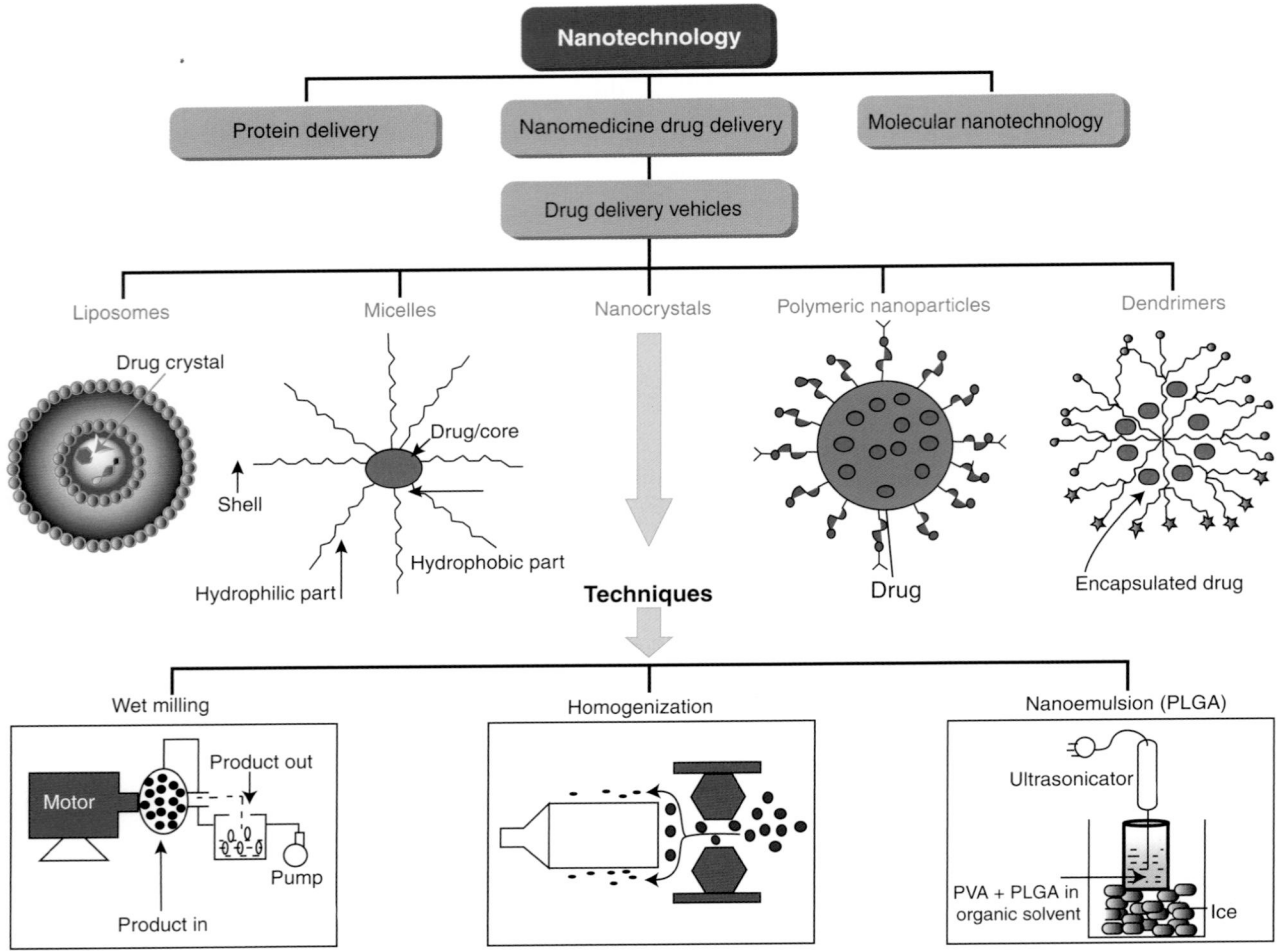

Figure 11.4.1 Nanomedicine and drug delivery. Nanotechnology has been applied for protein and drug delivery and molecular assemblies. Several nanodrug delivery systems were developed to optimize drug bioavailability and to achieve targeted delivery. These include liposomes, made up of vesicles of one or more phospholipid layers used to load drugs for targeted delivery. Block copolymers conjugate one segment of the polymers with a hydrophobic drug and keep the water-soluble segment unmodified. The block polymers further self-assemble into micelles. The hydrophobic core is used to store and transport the drug in the system. These are referred to as "micellar nanocontainers." Polymeric NPs can also be fabricated by dissolving or encapsulating drugs to obtain nanospheres or nanocapsules. In some cases, the drug molecules are attached to the surface of the NPs. Dendrimers are star shaped polymers that may also be used for drug delivery. Possible sites for covalent attachment of drugs, solubilizing groups, targeting groups and encapsulated drug are shown. The illustration also shows techniques to produce nanocrystals. Wet milling uses grinding media to grind drug crystals and various surfactants while the homogenizer uses high pressure to produce NPs that are coated with surfactants. An ultrasonicator can also be used to incorporate drug crystals in poly(lactide-co-glycolide) particles by the water-in-oil-in-water emulsion solvent diffusion method is shown.

in the nanoscale range (Kabanov & Alakhov, 2002). The cargo space created by the hydrophobic part of the micelles has been shown to be useful in increasing the bioavailability of the active component and also in modifying the pharmacokinetic profile and biodistribution of the incorporated drug (Torchilin, 2007) and helps to maintain the micelles in a dispersed phase. The encapsulation of the drug in the hydrophobic core also helps to reduce undesirable drug interactions with cells and plasma proteins. The core also protects the active ingredient being transported from metabolic degradation in a physiological system. One of the most important advantages of such a system is the ability of the micellar formulations to be used in applications involving drug delivery

across the BBB, since the micellar formulations are able to transport the active agents into body compartments where the free drug alone cannot penetrate. They also have a low CMC value and a slow rate of dissociation that allows the loaded drugs to remain in the system for a longer period of time and provides greater drug delivery to the target site. Pluronic block copolymers are important in pharmaceutical applications because of their intrinsic properties that enhance drug performance. A pluronic-based formulation of an anticancer drug has been used in a Phase I clinical trial (Kabanov & Alakhov, 2002). The formulation was used to increase the effectiveness of doxorubicin in a multiple-drug resistant tumor.

POLYMERIC NANOPARTICLES

Polymeric NPs are prepared using a variety of polymers. Drugs of interest can either be dissolved or encapsulated to obtain nanospheres or nanocapsules. Alternatively, polymeric NPs can be formulated by attaching the drug to the surface of the NP. Nanocapsules are fabricated by confining the drug to a cavity surrounded by a polymer membrane; nanospheres are matrix systems formed by a uniform dispersion of the drug. In recent years, the development of biodegradable polymers and their use for various drug-delivery applications have been described (Patel, Goyal, Bhadada, Bhatt, & Amin, 2009; Tan, Choong, & Dass, 2009; Ishihara & Mizushima, 2010; Ishihara, Takahashi, Higaki, Mizushima, & Mizushima, 2010; Kumari, Yadav, & Yadav, 2010). Natural polymers that have been used extensively in drug delivery include chitosan, sodium alginate, gelatins A and B, and albumin. Common chemically inert, nontoxic polymeric materials that have been used for pharmaceutical applications include polyvinyl alcohol (PVA), polyacrylic acid (PAA), polyacrylamide, polyethylene glycol (PEG), and biodegradable polymers such as polylactides (PLA), polyglycolides (PGA), poly(lactide-co-glycolides) (PLGA), and polycaprolactone. These polymers are broken down into biologically acceptable molecules that are easily metabolized. Use of polymeric NPs for drug delivery to the brain has been described (Chen, Dalwadi, & Benson, 2004). Some of the advantages of using polymeric NPs for drug uptake by the brain are enhanced retention in the brain-blood capillaries, leading to a high concentration gradient across the BBB; passage through tight junctions; and transcytosis of NPs through the endothelium. Improvement in the brain bioavailability of encapsulated drugs by coating the NPs with polysorbate-80 has been reported. Polysorbate-80 has been shown to be effective in increasing the uptake of drugs into BMVECs (Chen et al., 2004). Some of the proposed mechanisms by which this can be achieved include increased BMVEC membrane fluidization, facilitated endocytosis, and inhibition of the Pgp efflux system. Two common polymeric NPs that have been used to increase delivery of ART drugs to the CNS are polybutylcyanoacrylate (PBCA) and methylmethacrylate-sulfopropylmethacrylate. PBCA was shown to be better than methylmethacrylate-sulfopropylmethacrylate for transporting zidovudine, lamivudine, delavirdine, and saquinavir across BMVECs (Kuo & Chen, 2006). These studies demonstrate that polymeric NPs are a good choice for increasing delivery of ART across the BBB. Although there are many advantages to using polymeric NPs for drug delivery, there are also a few disadvantages. These include residual contamination from the production process by organic solvents, polymer initiation, large polymer aggregates, toxic monomers, and toxic degradation products (Kante et al., 1982; Kaur, Bhandari, Bhandari, & Kakkar, 2008c). The production of these NPs is also expensive and there has been no development in producing them on a large scale (Muller, Mader, & Gohla, 2000; Gohla & Dingler, 2001). Since the polymeric NPs are able to pass through the BBB but have toxicity and stability issues, recent studies have focused on another suitable option for drug delivery application for the brain, namely, solid lipid NPs (SLNs).

LIPID-BASED NANOCARRIERS

Lipid-based nanocarriers have shown promise for delivery of ART drugs to the CNS (Polt et al., 1994). There is a vast amount of literature available on use of physiological lipids and phospholipids for nanocarriers (Wong, Chattopadhyay, Wu, & Bendayan, 2010). The lipid-based formulations have been shown to be clinically safe and they are easily available. One of the properties that make lipid-based carriers useful for CNS drug delivery is their natural tendency to target the BBB. This makes lipid-based carriers a popular choice for CNS delivery of ART drugs. The various lipid-based carriers that are available are SLNs, micro- or nanoemulsions, and liposomes. SLNs have been used in drug delivery as effective colloidal drug carrier systems (Polt et al., 1994). They are spherical lipid particles in the nanometer range that are dispersed in water or an aqueous surfactant solution. The NPs usually consist of a solid hydrophobic core and are coated with a phospholipid monolayer. The hydrophobic core can be used to dissolve lipophilic drugs. This forms a carrier system that helps to achieve targeted delivery. SLNs that are smaller than 200 nm are not taken up by the RES (Chen et al., 2004), thus avoiding uptake by the liver Kupffer cells. This also helps to achieve controlled and sustained drug release for weeks, production of high drug payloads, and increased biocompatibility of biodegradable carrier lipids (zur Muhlen, Schwarz, & Mehnert, 1998; Muller et al., 2000). SLN formulations have been shown to be stable for three years as compared to a much shorter shelf life of other colloidal carrier systems (Kaur et al., 2008c). High-pressure homogenization can be used to cost-effectively produce them (Gohla & Dingler, 2001). As compared to the polymeric NPs, where large-scale production is not feasible, SLNs can be processed on a large scale and can also be sterilized (Kaur et al., 2008c).

The use of SLNs to deliver hydrophilic drugs such as diminazine and other lipophilic drugs including paclitaxel, vinblastine, camptothecin, etoposide, and cyclosporine has been described (Yang, Zhu, Lu, Liang, & Yang, 1999; Cavalli, Caputo, & Gasco, 2000; Chen, Yang, Lu, & Zhang, 2001; Kaur et al., 2008c). The lipophilic nature of the drug and the size of the NPs make it easy for the carriers to enter the blood. They are also easily recognized and phagocytosed by cells of the RES, Kupffer cells of the liver, and splenic macrophages. Various methods have been explored to overcome these limitations. Surface coatings with hydrophilic polymers or surfactants have been used to prevent recognition by the RES and to increase their availability at the target site. The size of the SLNs was reduced to below 200 nm to increase blood circulation time, making it possible for the drug to be in contact with the BBB for a longer time (Gohla & Dingler, 2001; Chen et al., 2004; Oyewumi, Yokel, Jay, Coakley, & Mumper, 2004). The use of ligands has also been reported in order to increase retention of the SLNs at the BBB and leading to an increase in the concentration of the NPs at the surface of the BBB (Lockman et al., 2003). Thole and coworkers have reported the use of antibodies that can act as Trojan horses for delivery of NPs (Thole, Nobmann, Huwyler, Bartmann, & Fricker, 2002). Peptidomimetic antibodies that bind to BBB transcytosis receptors have also been proposed by Harris et al. to achieve delivery of entrapped active compounds into the brain parenchyma without inducing alteration in the BBB permeability (Harris & Chess, 2003). Various combination carrier systems that have a nanoparticulate drug carrier system combined with the novel targeting principles of "differential protein adsorption" for drug delivery to the brain have also been reported (Muller & Keck, 2004).

MICROEMULSIONS AND NANOEMULSIONS AS DRUG CARRIERS

This class of nanocarriers usually involves oil-in-water formulations. The oil phase is highly dispersed to submicron-sized droplets and various surfactants and co-surfactants are used to stabilize these formulations (Vyas et al., 2008). This type of carrier system is suitable for highly lipophilic ART drugs. Administration to mice of a saquinavir nanoemulsion with an average droplet diameter of 100–200 nm resulted in a three-fold increase in the concentration of drug in the systemic circulation as compared to the free drug. The increase in the area under the curve (AUC) was about fivefold for Balb/C mice. It was proposed that in addition to improving BBB permeability, this type of carrier system, due to the size of the carriers, might be used to penetrate other barriers, such as the gastrointestinal tract when used as oral formulations (Vyas et al., 2008).

LIPOSOMES AS DRUG CARRIERS

Liposomes are vesicles made of one or more phospholipid bilayers (Webb, Rebstein, Lamson, & Bally, 2007; Gershkovich, Wasan, & Barta, 2008; Sawant & Dodiya, 2008). Various liposomal systems have been developed and evaluated for the treatment of cerebral ischemia, using citicoline (Fresta, Puglisi, Di Giacomo, & Russo, 1994), and epilepsy, using phenytoin (Mori et al., 1995). Compared to drug alone, increased CNS drug levels were observed following liposomal drug treatment (Garg, Asthana, Agashe, Agrawal, & Jain, 2006; Wong et al., 2010). Liposomal formulations have not been explored to a great extent for delivery of ART drugs for treating CNS disease. Wong and coworkers have reported a few liposomal formulations for delivery of antiviral and antifungal drugs (Dusserre et al., 1995; Zhang, Xie, Li, Wang, & Hou, 2003; Wong et al., 2010). Examples include liposomal formulations made with foscarnet and amphotericin B. Liposomal foscarnet was able to increase the drug level in rat brains by 13-fold when compared to free foscarnet solution. Free amphotericin B shows toxicities and limited BBB penetrance. Importantly, liposomal amphotericin B (L-AMB or AmBisome) reaches higher concentrations in plasma, remains longer in circulation, and concentrates in the RES providing sustained delivery to areas of infection. Most importantly, L-AMB attains high concentrations in brain tissue. Improvements in the use of liposomes are actively being investigated. Amphotericin B combined with brain-targeting peptides significantly increases its drug transport across an artificial BBB (Zhang et al., 2003; Wong et al., 2010). Liposomes have the potential to be used for effective treatment of HIV-associated CNS complications.

INTRACELLULAR DRUG DISTRIBUTION

Nanotechnology-based carrier systems are helpful in targeting several types of immune cells that are involved in the pathogenesis of HIV. Macrophages are an integral part of the RES and also are responsible for the uptake and clearance of administered-drug-loaded NPs (das Neves et al., 2009). The rate of uptake of NPs by macrophages is dependent on the physical and chemical properties of the NPs, namely, their composition, size, and surface charge (Schafer et al., 1992; das Neves et al., 2009). Enhanced NP uptake by macrophages that were infected with HIV was observed when polymethylmethacrylate-based and albumin-based NPs loaded with zidovudine were presented to macrophages in vitro (Bender, von Briesen, Kreuter, Duncan, & Rubsamen-Waigmann, 1994; das Neves et al., 2009). Propylcyclohexylamine PCHA NPs were also effective for increasing phagocytosis and antiviral activity of saquinavir and zalcitabine in HIV-infected monocyte/macrophages cultures (Bender et al., 1996; das Neves et al., 2009). Amiji et al. showed that poly (ethylene oxide)-modified poly (epsilon-caprolactone) (PEO-PCL) NPs can target macrophages without potentially compromising prolonged drug bioavailability in vivo (Shah & Amiji, 2006). Dou et al. observed significant uptake in HIV-infected macrophages with the use of indinavir-loaded lipid-based NPs (Dou et al., 2007). Poly(ethyleneimine) (PEI) nanogels were tested by Vinogradov and coworkers to deliver zidovudine triphosphate (Vinogradov, Kohli, & Zeman, 2005; das Neves et al., 2009) to the interior of cells. They observed that the higher affinity of the developed cationic nanogels for cell membranes enhanced their uptake by two cancer cell lines and resulted in increased intracellular levels of zidovudine triphosphate.

LYMPHOID SYSTEM DRUG DELIVERY

HIV-1 susceptible cells are predominantly in the lymphoid organs and RES. This fact has been used to target ART drugs to these sites in investigations of alternate systems for anti-HIV therapy. Löbenberg et al. have demonstrated that the normal uptake of NPs by macrophages present in the RES can be used to target cells in the lymphoid organs (Lobenberg & Kreuter, 1996; Lobenberg, Araujo, von Briesen, Rodgers, & Kreuter, 1998b; das Neves et al., 2009). After intravenous administration of [¹⁴C]-zidovudine-loaded PHCA NPs in a rat model, drug levels in the tissues of the RES were 18-fold higher than when drug alone was administered in an aqueous solution. Radioluminography confirmed accumulation of zidovudine-loaded NPs in macrophage-rich organs, mostly the gastrointestinal tract and the liver (Lobenberg et al., 1998a). Similar effects were observed following oral administration of the zidovudine-NPs (Lobenberg, Maas, & Kreuter, 1998b). These observations were supported by another study in which zidovudine-loaded poly (iso-hexylcyanoacrylate) NPs were orally administered to rats (Dembri, Montisci, Gantier, Chacun, & Ponchel, 2001). Drug accumulation in the intestinal mucosa was observed after direct gastrointestinal administration. The concentration of zidovudine in Peyer's patches was around four times higher following drug-NP delivery than for delivery of the free drug. The tissue concentrations (30–45μM) exceeded the IC_{50} (0.06–1.36μM) for anti-viral activity (Dembri et al., 2001; das Neves et al., 2009). It was thus shown that zidovudine concentrations were higher in the gastrointestinal tract and gut-associated lymphoid tissue, which are important sites for HIV replication and perpetuation (das Neves et al., 2009). Jin et al. have investigated self-assembled drug-delivery systems based on amphiphilic drug-cholesteryl conjugates (Jin, Ai, Xin, & Chen, 2008b). This system has adequate physical-chemical characteristics, including a narrow submicron size distribution, prolonged shelf life after freeze-drying, and is stable after sterilization. These characteristics make this system suitable for parenteral administration of nucleoside analogues (Jin et al., 2008b; Jin, Xin, Ai, & Chen, 2008a). The cholesteryl derivatives self-arrange in various nanosized structures. This was demonstrated by *in vivo* studies done with cholesteryl-succinyl didanosine nanotubes that showed preferential distribution of the drug conjugates towards the spleen, liver, and lungs after intravenous injection to rats (das Neves et al., 2009; Jin et al., 2009). Higher indinavir levels in lymph nodes of HIV2$_{287}$-infected pig-tailed macaques were observed following subcutaneous administration of indinavir-loaded liposomes than when an aqueous indinavir suspension was used (Kinman et al., 2003; das Neves et al., 2009). Snedecor et al. showed, using mathematical models, that concomitant use of PEGylated indinavir-loaded liposomes and conventional indinavir regimens could extend drug half-life before experiencing any resistance (Snedecor, Sullivan, & Ho, 2006; das Neves et al., 2009). Active drug targeting is another interesting approach used for delivering antiretroviral drugs to lymphoid organs. Gagne et al. used anti-HLA-DR immunoglobulin-modified liposomes to enhance the indinavir delivery to lymphoid tissues in mice and were successful in maintaining anti-HIV activity of the drug in vitro (Gagne, Desormeaux, Perron, Tremblay, & Bergeron, 2002). In vivo mouse studies involving solid lipid indinavir-NPs have shown that administration of NP-loaded monocyte-macrophages resulted in therapeutic drug concentrations in lymphoid and nonlymphoid tissues for at least 14 days. This resulted in a reduced number of virus-infected cells in plasma, lymph nodes, spleen, liver, and lungs and promoted CD4+ T cell protection in an HIV-1-infected humanized immunodeficient rodent model (Dou et al., 2006; Gorantla et al., 2006).

TRANSDERMAL DRUG DELIVERY

Transdermal delivery of ART drugs using liposomes has also been described (Jain, Tiwary, & Jain, 2006; Jain, Tiwary, Sapra, & Jain, 2007; Jain, Tiwary, & Jain, 2008; das Neves et al., 2009). Following topical administration of zidovudine-loaded liposomes to rats, plasma levels were 12-fold greater than when the drug was formulated as a hydrophilic ointment. There was also preferential drug distribution to the spleen and lymph nodes (RES organs) when liposomal formulations were used (Jain et al., 2006, 2008). Further studies are required to assess the amounts of drug needed to achieve therapeutic levels using transdermal delivery systems.

RECEPTOR-MEDIATED DRUG TARGETING

Active drug targeting has also been explored. Kreuter et al. have used transferrin receptors present in the luminal membrane of BMVECs as preferred targets for enhanced ART drug delivery to the CNS using nanocarrier systems (Kreuter, 2001). Zidovudine-loaded PEGylated albumin NPs were developed and administered intravenously to rats by Mishra et al. (2006). CNS uptake of zidovudine was enhanced by anchoring transferrin to the PEGylated NPs. An increase in distribution of drug to the brain was observed for the NP system as compared to the free drug (Mishra et al., 2006). In other studies, ritonavir-loaded PLGA NPs were conjugated with HIV-1 transactivating transcriptor (Tat) peptide to overcome the BBB and the efflux action of Pgp (Rao, Reddy, Horning, & Labhasetwar, 2008; das Neves et al., 2009). Following intravenous injection of Tat-NPs, drug levels in the CNS were up to 800 times higher after 2 weeks compared to administration of the drug in an aqueous solution (Rao et al., 2008). Thus, along with enhanced CNS drug delivery, sustained levels of ritonavir in the brain were observed using this targeted delivery system.

BARRIER PENETRATION AND CELLULAR DRUG CARRIERS

Brain cells and associated neurons are especially sensitive to environmental changes, which may cause brain or neuronal tissue damage. BMVECs and the BBB provide protection for the CNS from circulating endogenous and exogenous compounds. The BBB restricts the entry of unwanted molecules and selectively transports desired substances to make a regulatory barrier between the CNS and the systemic circulation. However, the BBB does not completely prevent all molecules from passing into the brain. Certain small and large hydrophilic molecules can enter the brain by active transport. In addition, a few receptor-mediated transport systems act to shuttle macromolecules into the brain, the most well-known of which is the transferrin receptor (Rubin & Staddon, 1999).

The use of drug carriers to improve drug delivery and antiviral efficacy has been the focus of many studies over the last decade. Modifications in drug design and carriers have been developed in an effort to decrease metabolism, improve cellular endocytosis, and avoid drug efflux transport in the BBB. In recent years, the development of drug nanocarriers has been described (Dou et al., 2006; Vyas, Shah, & Amiji, 2006; Dou et al., 2009; Nowacek et al., 2009; Nowacek et al., 2010). In nanocarrier-based drug delivery, drugs are packaged within delivery systems that are less than 1,000 nm in diameter (most commonly 100–500 nm). Nanocarriers offer numerous advantages over other conventional systems because of their small particle size, narrow size distribution, large surface area, and insulation properties for drugs encapsulated in the carrier. Depending on the particle size and surface charges, nanocarriers can also be used to regulate the biodistribution of ART drugs (Vyas et al., 2006).

While optimizing nanocarrier-based drug delivery, it is important to consider the ability of the drug carrier to enter into the CNS. A cell-based delivery system may be able to overcome the barriers to drug entry posed by the BBB. Macrophages offer many advantages as cell-based carriers for nanoformulated drugs to the brain. They have been shown to uptake liposomes, dendrimers, solid lipid nanoparticles (NPs) (SLNs), cationic SLNs (CSLNs), and polymeric gelatin NPs (Kuo, 2005; Kuo & Chen, 2006; Chattopadhyay, Zastre, Wong, Wu, & Bendayan, 2008). In this way, they can carry drugs across the BBB and deliver them to the site of disease or injury. Another major advantage of using macrophages as carriers is that macrophages can deliver a broad range of drugs with different biochemical properties to sites of CNS disease. Of significance, many neurodegenerative diseases, including HIV encephalitis (HIVE), have an inflammatory component that can attract macrophages (Kadiu, Glanzer, Kipnis, Gendelman, & Thomas, 2005; Vestweber, 2007; Liu et al., 2008b) across the BBB. The macrophages can release phagocytosed particles and cytotoxic mediators by exocytosis, further strengthening the utility of these cells as delivery agents of drugs to the CNS.

NANOFORMULATED ANTIRETROVIRAL DRUG THERAPIES (NANOART)

Nanomedicine is being used to develop HIV and neuroAIDS therapeutics. Although current ART has proven to be very effective in controlling viral burdens, persistent viral replication in the CNS remains a concern. ART targeting viral replication remains the mainstay of interdictive efforts to combat HIV disease (Dou et al., 2009). The potential value of nanoART is based on the notion that treatment of HAND may be limited by drug penetration into the CNS as well as by compliance and viral resistance patterns. The properties of nanomaterials can be utilized to combat viral mechanisms, including CNS infection and viral replication (reviewed by Nowacek & Gendelman, 2009). For HIV-1-infected patients, ART delivery to the CNS can be increased by attaching the drugs to NPs or by encapsulating them within surfactants. Such NPs can be readily taken up by the RES (Kaur et al., 2008b) and can improve CNS drug delivery (Chen et al., 2004).

Macrophage targeting is one way to enhance CNS drug delivery of ART. The fact that these cells are abundant and can migrate to the CNS makes macrophage-based drug delivery an attractive strategy for nanoART. Studies by Kaur et al. support this strategy (Kaur, Nahar, & Jain, 2008a). Following subcutaneous injections for didanosine-loaded, mannan-coated gelatin NPs to rats, drug levels were 12.4 times higher in brain tissue as compared to treatment with didanosine in aqueous solution (Kaur, Jain, & Tiwary, 2008a). In addition, Dou et al. have shown that indinavir levels are higher in mouse brain following intravenous administration of mouse BMM loaded with lipid-based indinavir-loaded NPs (Dou et al., 2009) than when indinavir-NPs are administered alone or when free drug is administered. Further studies are needed to demonstrate the significance of macrophage-mediated transport of ART drug-loaded nanosystems to the CNS for achieving higher brain levels of ART drugs. The development of macrophages as carriers of nanoART formulations has been a central focus of the Gendelman laboratory. This group has developed a range of nanoART formulations that can be taken up by macrophages and remain inside the cells for an extended period of time (Nowacek & Gendelman, 2009). These nanoART formulations were manufactured by high-pressure homogenization, wet milling, or sonication of crystalline drug with various surfactants. Surfactant coatings of poloxamer 188 (p188), PVA, mPEG, and PLGA were used to encapsulate crystalline particles of indinavir, ritonavir, atazanavir, and efavirenz. The nanoART formulations were efficiently taken up by human monocyte-derived macrophages (MDM) in an ex vivo system in 30 min. Uptake was dependent on both size and charge of the NPs and the surfactant coating. Drug was retained inside the cells for up to 14 days and was able to inhibit HIV-1 replication in infected macrophages in a dose-dependent manner. Of particular interest, when multiple nanoART formulations (of atazanavir, ritonavir, and efavirenz) were presented to MDM in combination, uptake of each was independent of the presence of the others (Nowacek et al., 2010). Dramatic improvement in antiviral activity was observed in infected macrophages when the combination nanoART was given as opposed to administration of the individual nanoART formulations. These studies are an important step in the development of a cell-based delivery system for ART drugs.

For nanoART to be developed as a potential treatment for HIV infection in vivo, potential hurdles need to be overcome. One question is whether nanoparticle-laden macrophages can retain nanoART in vivo and release it in therapeutically effective amounts. Studies using indinavir nanosuspensions demonstrated that mouse BMM loaded ex vivo with nanoART and administered to HIV-1-infected mice can travel to the sites of HIV infection and release the drug to inhibit viral replication for a period of up to 2 weeks (Dou et al., 2006; Dou et al., 2007; Dou et al., 2009).

An additional hurdle is whether nanoART-laden macrophages can cross the BBB and release drug at the site of infection in the CNS. Dou et al. have demonstrated that while the majority of nanoART carrying macrophages localize in the spleen, liver, and lungs of mice, a significant portion do reach the brain and target to a site of HIV-1 infection (Dou et al., 2009). Once there, the cells persist and release drug for an extended period of time.

These studies demonstrated that nanoART-loaded macrophages can deliver nanoART to sites of HIV-1 infection in the brain. However, a practical method for applying this work is still under development. The above studies exposed the macrophages to nanoART ex vivo and then adoptively transferred the nanoART-laden macrophages into a test animal. However, ex vivo exposure of cells followed by transfer of these cells into the target organism is not a clinically relevant method for drug delivery. The development of nanoART formulations that can specifically target and be taken up by monocytes/macrophages in vivo is necessary. Various routes of delivery of nanoART, including oral and intramuscular injection methods, are currently being explored.

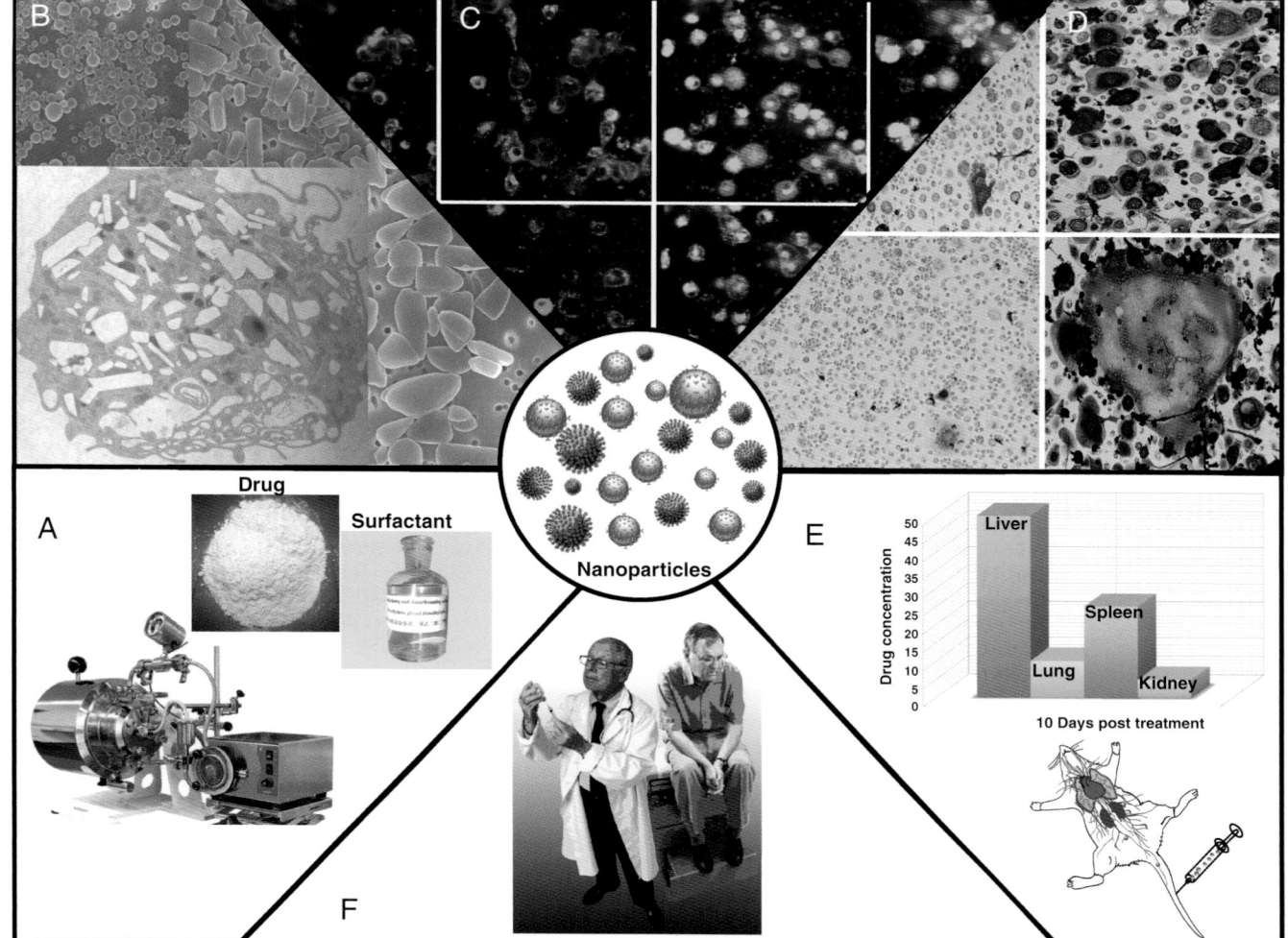

Figure 11.4.2 Interdisciplinary development of nanoART. Modalities that are site-specific hold considerable promise for human use and their development are illustrated herein. (A) Neuroprotective, anti-inflammatory, anti-apoptotic, or anti-microbial agents are packaged into NPs with surfactant and protein coats that target circulating immunocytes or diseased regions within the CNS. (B) The particles are developed in size, shape, charge, and coating to facilitate their uptake into circulating monocytes. (C) The cells that are circulating in the body will scavenge the particles into endocytic vesicles as a delivery vehicle. Laboratory tests can measure uptake and release of the fluorescently tagged drug-laden particles from monocytes and macrophages. (D) In the case of HIV-1 infections, for example, the drug-laden NPs not housed within macrophages would release antiretroviral drugs leading to inhibition of viral replication, measured by the absence of multinucleated giant cells and HIV-1 p24 protein expression. (E) Such formulations can then be tested in animals demonstrating sustained drug levels for an extended period. (F) Final therapeutic use in humans will be dependent upon toxicity measures, pharmacokinetic responses and untoward side-effects. (Adapted from *Nanomedicine*, 2009, 4(5):557–74, with permission from Future Medicine Ltd).

A clinically practical method embodying the above concepts can, for clarity, be described as a series of discrete steps. (Figure 11.4.2). First, the drug is packaged with a surfactant and protein coating that can target the immunocyte or the area of disease. Second, the size, shape, charge, and coating are optimized to enhance uptake by circulating monocytes. Third, following the introduction of the optimized, packaged drug into the organism, circulating monocytes can scavenge the NPs and carry them in secretory vesicles to sites of disease. Fourth, drug released from the monocytes/macrophages can inhibit the disease process, for example, viral replication in HIV-1 infection. Uptake and release processes can be tested using cultured monocytes and monocyte-derived macrophages. Fifth, laboratory animal tests can determine sustained drug levels following in vivo administration of the nanoformulated drug. Finally, sustained therapeutic efficacy in humans can be observed using formulations that have been demonstrated in animal models to have favorable pharmacokinetics and no untoward side effects.

REFERENCES

Alexaki, A., Liu. Y., & Wigdahl, B. (2008). Cellular reservoirs of HIV-1 and their role in viral persistence. *Curr HIV Res*, 6, 388–400.

Antinori, A., et al. (2007). Updated research nosology for HIV-associated neurocognitive disorders. *Neurology*, 69, 1789–1799.

Bachmeier, C. J., Spitzenberger, T. J., Elmquist, W. F., & Miller, D. W. (2005). Quantitative assessment of HIV-1 protease inhibitor interactions with drug efflux transporters in the blood-brain barrier. *Pharm Res*, 22, 1259–1268.

Baert, L., van't Klooster, G., Dries, W., Francois, M., Wouters, A., Basstanie, E., et al. (2009). Development of a long-acting injectable formulation with nanoparticles of rilpivirine (TMC278) for HIV treatment. *Eur J Pharm Biopharm, 72,* 502–508.

Batz, H. G., Daniel, H., Franzmann, G., Koldehoff, J., Merz, H., Ringsdorf, H., et al. (1977). [Pharmacologically active polymers. 9th communication: Retard forms of morphine antagonists (author's transl)]. *Arzneimittelforschung, 27,* 1884–1888.

Begley, D. J. (2004). Delivery of therapeutic agents to the central nervous system: The problems and the possibilities. *Pharmacol Ther, 104,* 29–45.

Bender, A., Schfer, V., Steffan, A. M., Royer, C., Kreuter, J., Rubsamen-Waigmann, H., et al.(1994). Inhibition of HIV in vitro by antiviral drug-targeting using nanoparticles. *Res Virol, 145,* 215–220.

Bender, A. R., von Briesen, H., Kreuter, J., Duncan, I. B., & Rubsamen-Waigmann, H. (1996). Efficiency of nanoparticles as a carrier system for antiviral agents in human immunodeficiency virus-infected human monocytes/macrophages in vitro. *Antimicrob Agents Chemother, 40,* 1467–1471.

Bowman, M. C., Ballard, T. E., Ackerson, C. J., Feldheim, D. L., Margolis, D. M., & Melander, C. (2008). Inhibition of HIV fusion with multivalent gold nanoparticles. *J Am Chem Soc, 130,* 6896–6897.

Brodie, S. J., Patterson, B. K., Lewinsohn, D. A., Diem, K., Spach, D., Greenberg, P. D., et al. (2000). HIV-specific cytotoxic T lymphocytes traffic to lymph nodes and localize at sites of HIV replication and cell death. *J Clin Invest, 105,* 1407–1417.

Cavalli, R., Caputo, O., & Gasco, M. R. (2000). Preparation and characterization of solid lipid nanospheres containing paclitaxel. *Eur J Pharm Sci, 10,* 305–309.

Chattopadhyay, N., Zastre, J., Wong, H. L., Wu, X. Y., & Bendayan, R. (2008). Solid lipid nanoparticles enhance the delivery of the HIV protease inhibitor, atazanavir, by a human brain endothelial cell line. *Pharm Res, 25,* 2262–2271.

Chaudhuri, A., Yang, B., Gendelman, H. E., Persidsky, Y., & Kanmogne, G. D. (2008). STAT1 signaling modulates HIV-1-induced inflammatory responses and leukocyte transmigration across the blood-brain barrier. *Blood, 111,* 2062–2072.

Chen, D. B., Yang, T. Z., Lu, W. L., & Zhang, Q. (2001). In vitro and in vivo study of two types of long-circulating solid lipid nanoparticles containing paclitaxel. *Chem Pharm Bull (Tokyo), 49,* 1444–1447.

Chen, Y., Dalwadi, G., & Benson, H. A. (2004). Drug delivery across the blood-brain barrier. *Curr Drug Deliv, 1,* 361–376.

Dahl, V., Josefsson, L., & Palmer, S. (2010). HIV reservoirs, latency, and reactivation: Prospects for eradication. *Antiviral Res, 85,* 286–294.

das Neves, J., Amiji, M. M., Bahia, M. F., & Sarmento, B. (2009). Nanotechnology-based systems for the treatment and prevention of HIV/AIDS. *Adv Drug Deliv Rev, 62,* 458–477.

Dembri, A., Montisci, M. J., Gantier, J. C., Chacun, H., & Ponchel, G. (2001). Targeting of 3'-azido 3'-deoxythymidine (AZT)-loaded poly(isohexylcyanoacrylate) nanospheres to the gastrointestinal mucosa and associated lymphoid tissues. *Pharm Res, 18,* 467–473.

Dou, H., Grotepas, C. B., McMillan, J. M., Destache, C. J., Chaubal, M., Werling, J., et al. (2009). Macrophage delivery of nanoformulated antiretroviral drug to the brain in a murine model of neuroAIDS. *J Immunol, 183,* 661–669.

Dou, H., Morehead, J., Destache, C. J., Kingsley, J. D., Shlyakhtenko, L., Zhou, Y., et al. (2007). Laboratory investigations for the morphologic, pharmacokinetic, and anti-retroviral properties of indinavir nanoparticles in human monocyte-derived macrophages. *Virology, 358,* 148–158.

Dou, H., Destache, C. J., Morehead, J. R., Mosley, R. L., Boska, M. D., Kingsley, J., et al. (2006). Development of a macrophage-based nanoparticle platform for antiretroviral drug delivery. *Blood, 108,* 2827–2835.

Dusserre, N., Lessard, C., Paquette, N., Perron, S., Poulin, L., Tremblay, M., et al. (1995). Encapsulation of foscarnet in liposomes modifies drug intracellular accumulation, in vitro anti-HIV-1 activity, tissue distribution and pharmacokinetics. *AIDS, 9,* 833–841.

Eilers, M., Roy, U., & Mondal, D. (2008). MRP (ABCC) transporters-mediated efflux of anti-HIV drugs, saquinavir and zidovudine, from human endothelial cells. *Exp Biol Med (Maywood), 233,* 1149–1160.

Elechiguerra, J. L., Burt, J. L., Morones, J. R., Camacho-Bragado, A., Gao, X., Lara, H. H., et al. (2005). Interaction of silver nanoparticles with HIV-1. *J Nanobiotechnology, 3,* 6.

Fresta, M., Puglisi, G., Di Giacomo, C., & Russo, A. (1994). Liposomes as in-vivo carriers for citicoline: Effects on rat cerebral post-ischaemic reperfusion. *J Pharm Pharmacol, 46,* 974–981.

Gagne, J. F., Desormeaux, A., Perron, S., Tremblay, M. J., & Bergeron, M. G. (2002). Targeted delivery of indinavir to HIV-1 primary reservoirs with immunoliposomes. *Biochim Biophys Acta, 1558,* 198–210.

Garg, M., Asthana, A., Agashe, H. B., Agrawal, G. P., & Jain, N. K. (2006). Stavudine-loaded mannosylated liposomes: in vitro anti-HIV-I activity, tissue distribution and pharmacokinetics. *J Pharm Pharmacol, 58,* 605–616.

Gasparyan, V. K. (2009). Gold and silver nanoparticles in bioassay, cell visualization and therapy. *Curr Clin Pharmacol, 4,* 159–163.

Gershkovich, P., Wasan, K. M., & Barta, C. A. (2008). A review of the application of lipid-based systems in systemic, dermal/transdermal, and ocular drug delivery. *Crit Rev Ther Drug Carrier Syst, 25,* 545–584.

Gohla, S. H. & Dingler, A. (2001). Scaling up feasibility of the production of solid lipid nanoparticles (SLN). *Pharmazie, 56,* 61–63.

Gongvatana, A., Schweinsburg, B. C., Taylor, M. J., Theilmann, R. J., Letendre, S. L., Alhassoon, O. M., et al (2009). White matter tract injury and cognitive impairment in human immunodeficiency virus-infected individuals. *J Neurovirol, 15,* 187–195.

Gorantla, S., Dou, H., Boska, M., Destache, C. J., Nelson, J., Poluektova, L., et al. (2006). Quantitative magnetic resonance and SPECT imaging for macrophage tissue migration and nanoformulated drug delivery. *J Leukoc Biol, 80,* 1165–1174.

Harris, J. M. & Chess, R. B. (2003). Effect of pegylation on pharmaceuticals. *Nat Rev Drug Discov, 2,* 214–221.

Hockett, R. D., Kilby, J. M., Derdeyn, C. A., Saag, M. S., Sillers, M., Squires, K., et al. (1999). Constant mean viral copy number per infected cell in tissues regardless of high, low, or undetectable plasma HIV RNA. *J Exp Med, 189,* 1545–1554.

Ishihara, T. & Mizushima, T. (2010). Techniques for efficient entrapment of pharmaceuticals in biodegradable solid micro/nanoparticles. *Expert Opin Drug Deliv, 7,* 565–575.

Ishihara, T., Takahashi, M., Higaki, M., Mizushima, Y., & Mizushima, T. (2010). Preparation and characterization of a nanoparticulate formulation composed of PEG-PLA and PLA as anti-inflammatory agents. *Int J Pharm, 385,* 170–175.

Ivey, N. S., MacLean, A. G., & Lackner, A. A. (2009). Acquired immunodeficiency syndrome and the blood-brain barrier. *J Neurovirol, 15,* 111–122.

Jain, S., Tiwary, A. K., & Jain, N. K. (2006). Sustained and targeted delivery of an anti-HIV agent using elastic liposomal formulation: Mechanism of action. *Curr Drug Deliv, 3,* 157–166.

Jain, S., Tiwary, A. K., & Jain, N. K. (2008). PEGylated elastic liposomal formulation for lymphatic targeting of zidovudine. *Curr Drug Deliv, 5,* 275–281.

Jain, S., Tiwary, A. K., Sapra, B., & Jain, N. K. (2007). Formulation and evaluation of ethosomes for transdermal delivery of lamivudine. *AAPS PharmSciTech, 8,* E111.

Jennings, T. & Strouse, G. (2007). Past, present, and future of gold nanoparticles. *Adv Exp Med Biol, 620,* 34–47.

Jin, Y., Xin, R., Ai, P., & Chen, D. (2008a). Self-assembled drug delivery systems 2. Cholesteryl derivatives of antiviral nucleoside analogues: Synthesis, properties and the vesicle formation. *Int J Pharm, 350,* 330–337.

Jin, Y., Ai, P., Xin, R., & Chen, D. (2008b). Morphological transformation of self-assembled nanostructures prepared from cholesteryl acyl didanosine and the optimal formulation of nanoparticulate systems:

Effects of solvents, acyl chain length and poloxamer 188. *J Colloid Interface Sci*, 326, 275–282.

Jin, Y., Ai, P., Xin, R., Tian, Y., Dong, J., Chen, D., et al. (2009). Self-assembled drug delivery systems: Part 3. In vitro/in vivo studies of the self-assembled nanoparticulates of cholesteryl acyl didanosine. *Int J Pharm*, 368, 207–214.

Jones, M. & Leroux, J. (1999). Polymeric micelles—a new generation of colloidal drug carriers. *Eur J Pharm Biopharm*, 48, 101–111.

Kabanov, A. V. & Alakhov, V. Y. (2002). Pluronic block copolymers in drug delivery: From micellar nanocontainers to biological response modifiers. *Crit Rev Ther Drug Carrier Syst*, 19, 1–72.

Kadiu, I., Glanzer, J. G., Kipnis, J., Gendelman, H. E., & Thomas, M. P. (2005). Mononuclear phagocytes in the pathogenesis of neurodegenerative diseases. *Neurotox Res*, 8, 25–50.

Kante, B., Couvreur, P., Dubois-Krack, G., De Meester, C., Guiot, P., Roland, M., et al. (1982). Toxicity of polyalkylcyanoacrylate nanoparticles I: Free nanoparticles. *J Pharm Sci*, 71, 786–790.

Kaur, A., Jain, S., & Tiwary, A. K. (2008a). Mannan-coated gelatin nanoparticles for sustained and targeted delivery of didanosine: in vitro and in vivo evaluation. *Acta Pharm*, 58, 61–74.

Kaur, C. D., Nahar, M., & Jain, N. K. (2008b). Lymphatic targeting of zidovudine using surface-engineered liposomes. *J Drug Target*, 16, 798–805.

Kaur, I. P., Bhandari, R., Bhandari, S., & Kakkar, V. (2008c). Potential of solid lipid nanoparticles in brain targeting. *J Control Release*, 127, 97–109.

Kim, S., Scheerer, S., Geyer, M. A., & Howell, S. B. (1990). Direct cerebrospinal fluid delivery of an antiretroviral agent using multivesicular liposomes. *J Infect Dis*, 162, 750–752.

Kinman, L., Brodie, S. J., Tsai, C. C., Bui, T., Larsen, K., Schmidt, A., et al. (2003). Lipid-drug association enhanced HIV-1 protease inhibitor indinavir localization in lymphoid tissues and viral load reduction: A proof of concept study in HIV-2287-infected macaques. *J Acquir Immune Defic Syndr*, 34, 387–397.

Kraft-Terry, S. D., Buch, S. J., Fox, H. S., & Gendelman, H. E. (2009). A coat of many colors: Neuroimmune crosstalk in human immunodeficiency virus infection. *Neuron*, 64, 133–145.

Kreuter, J. (2001). Nanoparticulate systems for brain delivery of drugs. *Adv Drug Deliv Rev*, 47, 65–81.

Kumari, A., Yadav, S. K., & Yadav, S. C. (2010). Biodegradable polymeric nanoparticles based drug delivery systems. *Colloids Surf B Biointerfaces*, 75, 1–18.

Kuo, M. T. (2009). Redox regulation of multidrug resistance in cancer chemotherapy: Molecular mechanisms and therapeutic opportunities. *Antioxid Redox Signal*, 11, 99–133.

Kuo, Y. C. (2005). Loading efficiency of stavudine on polybutylcyanoacrylate and methylmethacrylate-sulfopropylmethacrylate copolymer nanoparticles. *Int J Pharm*, 290, 161–172.

Kuo, Y. C. & Chen, H. H. (2006). Effect of nanoparticulate polybutylcyanoacrylate and methylmethacrylate-sulfopropylmethacrylate on the permeability of zidovudine and lamivudine across the in vitro blood-brain barrier. *Int J Pharm*, 327, 160–169.

Kuo, Y. C. & Su, F. L. (2007). Transport of stavudine, delavirdine, and saquinavir across the blood-brain barrier by polybutylcyanoacrylate, methylmethacrylate-sulfopropylmethacrylate, and solid lipid nanoparticles. *Int J Pharm*, 340, 143–152.

Kuo, Y. C. & Chen, H. H. (2009). Entrapment and release of saquinavir using novel cationic solid lipid nanoparticles. *Int J Pharm*, 365, 206–213.

Langer, R. (1998). Drug delivery and targeting. *Nature*, 392, 5–10.

Liu, X. & Chen, C. (2005). Strategies to optimize brain penetration in drug discovery. *Curr Opin Drug Discov Devel*, 8, 505–512.

Liu, X., Chen, C., & Smith, B. J. (2008a). Progress in brain penetration evaluation in drug discovery and development. *J Pharmacol Exp Ther*, 325, 349–356.

Liu, Y., Uberti, M. G., Dou, H., Banerjee, R., Grotepas, C. B., Stone, D. K., et al. (2008b). Ingress of blood-borne macrophages across the blood-brain barrier in murine HIV-1 encephalitis. *J Neuroimmunol*, 200, 41–52.

Lobenberg, R. & Kreuter, J. (1996). Macrophage targeting of azidothymidine: A promising strategy for AIDS therapy. *AIDS Res Hum Retroviruses*, 12, 1709–1715.

Lobenberg, R., Maas, J., & Kreuter, J. (1998a). Improved body distribution of 14C-labelled AZT bound to nanoparticles in rats determined by radioluminography. *J Drug Target*, 5, 171–179.

Lobenberg, R., Araujo, L., von Briesen, H., Rodgers, E., & Kreuter, J. (1998b). Body distribution of azidothymidine bound to hexyl-cyanoacrylate nanoparticles after i.v. injection to rats. *J Control Release*, 50, 21–30.

Lockman, P. R., Oyewumi, M. O., Koziara, J. M., Roder, K. E., Mumper, R. J., & Allen, D. D. (2003). Brain uptake of thiamine-coated nanoparticles. *J Control Release*, 93, 271–282.

Loscher, W. & Potschka, H. (2005). Blood-brain barrier active efflux transporters: ATP-binding cassette gene family. *NeuroRx*, 2, 86–98.

McGee, B., Smith, N., & Aweeka, F. (2006). HIV pharmacology: Barriers to the eradication of HIV from the CNS. *HIV Clin Trials*, 7, 142–153.

Miller, D. S., Bauer, B., & Hartz, A. M. (2008). Modulation of P-glycoprotein at the blood-brain barrier: opportunities to improve central nervous system pharmacotherapy. *Pharmacol Rev*, 60, 196–209.

Mishra, V., Mahor, S., Rawat, A., Gupta, P. N., Dubey, P., Khatri, K., et al. (2006). Targeted brain delivery of AZT via transferrin anchored pegylated albumin nanoparticles. *J Drug Target*, 14, 45–53.

Moore, D. J., Masliah, E., Rippeth, J. D., Gonzalez, R., Carey, C. L., Cherner, M., et al. (2006). Cortical and subcortical neurodegeneration is associated with HIV neurocognitive impairment. *AIDS*, 20, 879–887.

Mori, N., Kurokouchi, A., Osonoe, K., Saitoh, H., Ariga, K., Suzuki, K., et al. (1995). Liposome-entrapped phenytoin locally suppresses amygdaloid epileptogenic focus created by db-cAMP/EDTA in rats. *Brain Res*, 703, 184–190.

Muller, R. H. & Keck, C. M. (2004). Challenges and solutions for the delivery of biotech drugs—a review of drug nanocrystal technology and lipid nanoparticles. *J Biotechnol*, 113, 151–170.

Muller, R. H., Mader, K., & Gohla, S. (2000). Solid lipid nanoparticles (SLN) for controlled drug delivery - a review of the state of the art. *Eur J Pharm Biopharm*, 50, 161–177.

Nowacek, A. & Gendelman, H. E. (2009). NanoART, neuroAIDS and CNS drug delivery. *Nanomedicine (Lond)*, 4, 557–574.

Nowacek, A. S., McMillan, J., Miller, R., Anderson, A., Rabinow, B., & Gendelman, H. E. (2010). Nanoformulated Antiretroviral Drug Combinations Extend Drug Release and Antiretroviral Responses in HIV-1-Infected Macrophages: Implications for NeuroAIDS Therapeutics. *J Neuroimmune Pharmacol*, In Press.

Nowacek, A. S., Miller, R. L., McMillan, J., Kanmogne, G., Kanmogne, M., Mosley, R. L., et al. (2009). NanoART synthesis, characterization, uptake, release and toxicology for human monocyte-macrophage drug delivery. *Nanomedicine (Lond)*, 4, 903–917.

Oyewumi, M. O., Yokel, R. A., Jay, M., Coakley, T., & Mumper, R. J. (2004). Comparison of cell uptake, biodistribution and tumor retention of folate-coated and PEG-coated gadolinium nanoparticles in tumor-bearing mice. *J Control Release*, 95, 613–626.

Pardridge, W. M. (2005). The blood-brain barrier: Bottleneck in brain drug development. *NeuroRx*, 2, 3–14.

Patel, M. M., Goyal, B. R., Bhadada, S. V., Bhatt, J. S., & Amin, A. F. (2009). Getting into the brain: Approaches to enhance brain drug delivery. *CNS Drugs*, 23, 35–58.

Peng, F., Dhillon, N. K., Yao, H., Zhu, X., Williams, R., & Buch, S. (2008). Mechanisms of platelet-derived growth factor-mediated neuroprotection—implications in HIV dementia. *Eur J Neurosci*, 28, 1255–1264.

Pittella, J. E. (2009). Central nervous system involvement in Chagas disease: A hundred-year-old history. *Trans R Soc Trop Med Hyg*, 103, 973–978.

Polt, R., Porreca, F., Szabo, L. Z., Bilsky, E. J., Davis, P., Abbruscato, T. J., et al. (1994). Glycopeptide enkephalin analogues produce analgesia in mice: Evidence for penetration of the blood-brain barrier. *Proc Natl Acad Sci USA, 91*, 7114–7118.

Rao, K. S., Ghorpade, A., & Labhasetwar, V. (2009). Targeting anti-HIV drugs to the CNS. *Expert Opin Drug Deliv, 6*, 771–784.

Rao, K. S., Reddy, M. K., Horning, J. L., & Labhasetwar, V. (2008). TAT-conjugated nanoparticles for the CNS delivery of anti-HIV drugs. *Biomaterials, 29*, 4429–4438.

Ronaldson, P. T. & Bendayan, R. (2006). HIV-1 viral envelope glycoprotein gp120 triggers an inflammatory response in cultured rat astrocytes and regulates the functional expression of P-glycoprotein. *Mol Pharmacol, 70*, 1087–1098.

Rubin, L. L. & Staddon, J. M. (1999). The cell biology of the blood-brain barrier. *Annu Rev Neurosci, 22*, 11–28.

Sawant, K. K. & Dodiya, S. S. (2008). Recent advances and patents on solid lipid nanoparticles. *Recent Pat Drug Deliv Formul, 2*, 120–135.

Schafer, V., von Briesen, H., Andreesen, R., Steffan, A. M., Royer, C., Troster, S., et al. (1992). Phagocytosis of nanoparticles by human immunodeficiency virus (HIV)-infected macrophages: a possibility for antiviral drug targeting. *Pharm Res, 9*, 541–546.

Shah, L. K. & Amiji, M. M. (2006). Intracellular delivery of saquinavir in biodegradable polymeric nanoparticles for HIV/AIDS. *Pharm Res, 23*, 2638–2645.

Snedecor, S. J., Sullivan, S. M., & Ho, R. J. (2006). Feasibility of weekly HIV drug delivery to enhance drug localization in lymphoid tissues based on pharmacokinetic models of lipid-associated indinavir. *Pharm Res, 23*, 1750–1755.

Tan, M. L., Choong, P. F., & Dass, C. R. (2009). Review: Doxorubicin delivery systems based on chitosan for cancer therapy. *J Pharm Pharmacol, 61*, 131–142.

Taylor, S. & Pereira, A. (2000). Penetration of HIV-1 protease inhibitors into CSF and semen. *HIV Med, 1* Suppl 2, 18–22.

Thole, M., Nobmann, S., Huwyler, J., Bartmann, A., & Fricker, G. (2002). Uptake of cationzied albumin coupled liposomes by cultured porcine brain microvessel endothelial cells and intact brain capillaries. *J Drug Target, 10*, 337–344.

Tiwari, S. B. & Amiji, M. M. (2006). A review of nanocarrier-based CNS delivery systems. *Curr Drug Deliv, 3*, 219–232.

Torchilin, V. P. (2007). Micellar nanocarriers: Pharmaceutical perspectives. *Pharm Res, 24*, 1–16.

van't Klooster, G., Hoeben, E., Borghys, H., Looszova, A., Bouche, M. P., van Velsen, F., et al. (2010). Pharmacokinetics and disposition of rilpivirine (TMC278) nanosuspension as a long-acting injectable anti-retroviral formulation. *Antimicrob Agents Chemother, 54*, 2042–2050.

Varatharajan, L. & Thomas, S. A. (2009). The transport of anti-HIV drugs across blood-CNS interfaces: Summary of current knowledge and recommendations for further research. *Antiviral Res, 82*, A99–109.

Vestweber, D. (2007). Molecular mechanisms that control leukocyte extravasation through endothelial cell contacts. *Ernst Schering Found Symp Proc*, 151–167.

Vinogradov, S. V., Kohli, E., & Zeman, A. D. (2005). Cross-linked polymeric nanogel formulations of 5'-triphosphates of nucleoside analogues: Role of the cellular membrane in drug release. *Mol Pharm, 2*, 449–461.

Vyas, T. K., Shah, L., & Amiji, M. M. (2006). Nanoparticulate drug carriers for delivery of HIV/AIDS therapy to viral reservoir sites. *Expert Opin Drug Deliv, 3*, 613–628.

Vyas, T. K., Shahiwala, A., & Amiji, M. M. (2008). Improved oral bioavailability and brain transport of Saquinavir upon administration in novel nanoemulsion formulations. *Int J Pharm, 347*, 93–101.

Wang, X. & Baba, M. (2005). The role of breast cancer resistance protein (BCRP/ABCG2) in cellular resistance to HIV-1 nucleoside reverse transcriptase inhibitors. *Antivir Chem Chemother, 16*, 213–216.

Webb, M. S., Rebstein, P., Lamson, W., & Bally, M. B. (2007). Liposomal drug delivery: Recent patents and emerging opportunities. *Recent Pat Drug Deliv Formul, 1*, 185–194.

Wohlschlaeger, J., Wenger, E., Mehraein, P., & Weis, S. (2009). White matter changes in HIV-1 infected brains: A combined gross anatomical and ultrastructural morphometric investigation of the corpus callosum. *Clin Neurol Neurosurg, 111*, 422–429.

Wong, H. L., Chattopadhyay, N., Wu, X. Y., & Bendayan, R. (2010). Nanotechnology applications for improved delivery of antiretroviral drugs to the brain. *Adv Drug Deliv Rev, 62*, 503–517.

Yang, S., Zhu, J., Lu, Y., Liang, B., & Yang, C. (1999). Body distribution of camptothecin solid lipid nanoparticles after oral administration. *Pharm Res, 16*, 751–757.

Zastre, J. A., Chan, G. N., Ronaldson, P. T., Ramaswamy, M., Couraud, P. O., Romero, I. A., et al. (2009). Up-regulation of P-glycoprotein by HIV protease inhibitors in a human brain microvessel endothelial cell line. *J Neurosci Res, 87*, 1023–1036.

Zhang, X., Xie, J., Li, S., Wang, X., & Hou, X. (2003). The study on brain targeting of the amphotericin B liposomes. *J Drug Target, 11*, 117–122.

zur Muhlen, A., Schwarz, C., & Mehnert, W. (1998). Solid lipid nanoparticles (SLN) for controlled drug delivery—drug release and release mechanism. *Eur J Pharm Biopharm, 45*, 149–155.

11.5

ANTIRETROVIRAL NANOTHERAPIES

Madhavan P. N. Nair and Zainulabedin M. Saiyed

Although highly active antiretroviral therapy (HAART) has significantly reduced the severity of HIV disease, complete eradication of virus from hard-to-access reservoirs in the HIV-infected patient remains a major challenge. The central nervous system (CNS), protected by its blood-brain barrier (BBB), represents one of the major anatomical reservoirs for HIV-1. Nanotechnology-based drug-delivery systems have shown tremendous potential for penetrating the BBB and targeting antiretroviral drugs to the brain. This review highlights selected nanotechnology-based drug-delivery systems that hold the potential for future effective treatment of HIV-associated neurocognitive disorders (HAND). Results from our laboratory on the use of magnetically guided nanocarrier-based drug-delivery systems for targeting active forms of antiretroviral drugs to the brain are discussed.

INTRODUCTION

The global burden of the HIV epidemic is staggering, with more than 30 million people infected with HIV-1 (UNAIDS, 2009). Currently, there are over 20 different antiretroviral drugs approved in the United States that are classified into nucleoside reverse transcriptase inhibitors (NRTI), nonnucleoside reverse transcriptase inhibitors (NNRTI), protease inhibitors (PI), fusion inhibitors (FI) and integrase strand transfer inhibitors (ISTI) (Thompson et al., 2010; Vyas, Shahiwala, & Amiji, 2008). Introduction of highly active antiretroviral therapy has significantly reduced the disease severity; however, complete eradication of virus from hidden reservoirs in the HIV-infected subject still remains as a big challenge (Vyas, Shah, & Amiji, 2006). In addition to T-lymphocytes, macrophages, lymph nodes, bone marrow, spleen, and lungs, the central nervous system represents one of the major anatomical reservoirs for HIV-1. The progressive HIV-1 replication in the brain leads to a range of neurological disorders which is collectively known as HIV-associated neurocognitive disorders (Antinori et al., 2007). One of the major limiting factors in treatment of HAND is impermeability of the BBB to HAART (Kulkovsky & Bray, 2006). In recent years, nanotechnology-based drug delivery systems have shown tremendous potential for targeting antiretroviral drugs to the brain. This review highlights selected nanotechnology-based drug-delivery systems that have potential for future effective treatment of HAND. Further, results from our laboratory on the use of magnetically guided nanocarrier-based drug delivery for targeting active forms of antiretroviral drugs to the brain are briefly discussed.

HIV-ASSOCIATED NEUROCOGNITIVE DISORDERS

Human immunodeficiency virus (HIV-1) is known to harbor in the brain as indicated by the presence of large quantities of unintegrated viral DNA in the brains of HIV-infected individuals (Pang et al., 1990). The mechanism of virus entry into the brain is not clearly elucidated; however, the resulting infection leads to a number of CNS disorders collectively known as HAND. HAND is characterized by development of cognitive, motor, or behavioral abnormalities that are linked to progressive virus infection and immune deterioration (Ikezu, 2009). One of the characteristics of the disease is the transmigration of HIV-harboring mononuclear cells, especially monocytes/macrophages, across the BBB, resulting in dissemination of virus to the brain. Continuous virus replication in the brain leads to formation of multinucleated giant cells (MGC), which are the hallmark of HIV-1 encephalitis (HIVE). Pathologically, HIVE is characterized by diffuse myelin damage (spongy myelinopathy, gliosis), neuronal loss, vascular damage, microglial nodules, and lymphocytic infiltrates (Bell, Brettle, Chiswick, & Simmonds, 1998).

Although HAART has greatly reduced the disease severity, thereby improving survival and quality of life, individual patient responses are still quite variable, and the prevalence of neurological complications remains high (Robertson & Hall, 2007; Murri et al., 2006). Currently, no effective treatment exists for HAND, which is mainly attributed to poor penetrability of HAART across the BBB. The selective permeability of the BBB is due to the distinct morphology and enzymatic properties of endothelial cells that enable them to form complex tight junctions with minimal endocytic activity. This provides a physiological barrier that limits the transport of many blood-borne elements, such as macromolecules and circulating leukocytes to the brain (Lesniak & Brem, 2004). Previous studies report that delivery of antiretroviral therapy (ART) to the brain is limited, especially due to the physical structure of the BBB, presence of efflux pumps, and higher expression of metabolizing enzymes, which makes the BBB an effective barrier against many antiretroviral drugs (Nowacek & Gendelman, 2009). In order to increase the efficacy of ART, novel approaches to deliver antiretroviral drugs to the brain are warranted.

NANOTECHNOLOGY AND DRUG DELIVERY ACROSS THE BLOOD-BRAIN BARRIER

It is well established that 100% of large molecule drugs (such as peptides, recombinant proteins, monoclonal antibodies, nucleic-acid-based drugs) and more than 98% of small drug molecules do not cross the BBB (Pardridge, 2007). The existing approaches to deliver drugs to the brain include: (1) transcranial drug delivery, (2) transnasal drug delivery, (3) transient disruption of BBB using hyperosomotic solutions, and (4) lipidization of small molecules. Some of the technologies available now make use of endogenous BBB transporters to piggyback drugs across the BBB (Pardridge, 2007). In recent years, advent of nanotechnology has stimulated the development of innovative systems for the delivery of drugs and diagnostic agents (Suri, Fenniri, & Singh, 2007). It is now possible to synthesize, characterize, and specifically tailor the functional properties of nanoparticles for various clinical as well as diagnostic applications. Additionally, nanoformulations of small drugs delivered systemically are more efficacious and may be less toxic than the same drug delivered in free form. This effectiveness of nanoparticle-based drug-delivery systems is attributed to their small size, controlled time release of the drug, and modification of drug pharmacokinetics and biodistribution profile (Suri, Fenniri, & Singh., 2007; Sarin, 2009). Researchers have explored various nanocarrier systems such as liposomes, micelles, nanoparticles, nanocontainers, nanoemulsion, dendrimers, and others for delivery of therapeutic agents to the brain (Silva, 2007; Ojewole, Mackraj, Naidoo, & Govender, 2008). Concisely, there is a considerable and impressive amount of basic and preclinical studies demonstrating the potential of nanoparticles-based delivery systems to target drugs to the brain (Silva, 2007).

NANOMEDICINE AND TARGETED DELIVERY OF ANTI-HIV DRUGS

Nanoparticle drug-delivery systems have been increasingly used to improve the efficacy of antiretroviral drugs. Lipid indinavir nanoparticles were effectively targeted to the lymphoid tissue of HIV-infected macaques with sixfold higher indinavir concentrations (Kinman et al., 2006). Another study performed in C3H mice reported 126 times higher indinavir concentration in lymphoid tissue using anti-HLA-DR immunoliposomes (Gagne, Desormeaux, & Perron, 2002). In ex vivo cellular uptake study, didanosine encapsulated in mannosylated gelatin nanoparticles have shown 18 times enhanced uptake of drugs by alveolar macrophages compared to free drug (Jain et al., 2008). Mainardes and coworkers (2009) reported that in vitro uptake of azidothymidine loaded poly(lactic acid)-poly(ethylene glycol) nanoparticles by polymorphonuclear cells is dependent on the concentration of PEG and its ratio in the polymer. More recently, a combination of antiretroviral drugs that included ritonavir, lopinavir, and efavirenz was loaded in a poly-(lactic-co-glycolic-acid) (PLGA) nanoparticles and a sustained release of these drugs until 28 days was observed in in vitro peripheral blood mononuclear cell (PBMC) cultures (Destache et al., 2009).

In case of CNS drug delivery of anti-HIV drugs, nanoformulations of stavudine (D4T), delavirdine (DLV), and saquinavir (SQV) with polybutylcyanoacrylate (PBCA), methylmethacrylate-sulfoproprylmethacrylate (MMA-SPM), and solid lipid nanoparticles (SLN) were prepared and their efficiency to cross the in vitro BBB model was reported. An enhanced permeability was observed for D4T, DLV, and SQV by about 12–16 folds on PBCA, 3–7 folds on MMA-SPM, and 4–11 folds in SLN, respectively (Kuo & Su, 2007). In the recent paper, Kuo and Kuo (2008) showed the impact of electromagnetic field on the enhanced permeability of saquinavir (SQV) across the in vitro BBB model. Rao and coworkers (2008) showed that trans-activating transcriptor (TAT) peptide conjugated nanoparticles bypasses the efflux action of P-glycoprotein and increases the transport of the encapsulated ritonavir across the BBB. Further, solid lipid nanoparticles of atazanavir (~167 nm) were efficiently taken up by in vitro human brain microvascular endothelial cell line (hCMEC/D3), supporting the potential of these nanoparticles to deliver atazanavir to the brain (Chattopadhyay et al., 2008). Thus, the development of nanomedicine-based therapy for HAND has immense potential.

MONOCYTES/MACROPHAGE-BASED NANOFORMULATION DELIVERY OF ANTI-HIV DRUGS

Previous studies have also attempted to use monocytes/macrophage-based drug carrier for targeted delivery to the brain (Jain et al., 2003; Dou et al., 2006, 2009). Such an approach utilizes the ability of phagocytes to cross the BBB and migrate towards inflammatory site via the process known as diapedesis and chemotaxis. Also, studies report that monocytes/macrophages can cross an intact BBB under normal physiological condition (Perry, Anthony, Bolton, & Brown, 1997). Likewise, Dou et al. developed a bone-marrow-derived macrophage (BMM) pharmacological nanoparticle delivery system (nanoART) for antiretroviral drugs. In this case, nanoparticle indinavir (NP-IDV) formulation packaged BMM showed sustained antiretroviral responses for 14 days (Dou et al., 2006). This research demonstrated that macrophages can deliver drugs to sites of viral infection and show sustained antiretroviral activities. More recently, the same group also reported successful targeting of NP-IDV-BMM to the brain in a severe combined immunodeficient (SCID) model of HIVE, indicating the therapeutic potential of macrophage-based nanoparticles platform for HAND (Dou et al., 2009).

TARGETED DRUG DELIVERY USING MAGNETIC NANOPARTICLES

One type of nanoparticle that has gained increasing interest in recent years for biomedical applications is the magnetic nanoparticle, or magnetic fluid, which mainly consists of nano-sized iron-oxide particles (Fe_3O_4 or γFe_2O_3) suspended in a carrier liquid. Magnetic nanoparticles have been increasingly used as carrier for binding proteins, enzymes, or drugs (Saiyed, Telang, & Ramchand, 2003; Pankhurst, Connolly, Jones, & Dobson, 2003). Drug-loaded magnetic nanocarriers offer advantages in terms of site-specific targeting (by application of an external magnetic field), tissue retention, and sustained release of drugs. Magnetically guided drug delivery systems have been successfully used to increase the efficacy and reduce the toxic side effects associated with chemotherapy (Ito, Shinkai, Honda, & Kobayashi, 2005). Previous study in rodent model has shown successful delivery of anticancer drugs bound to magnetic nanoparticles to treat brain carcinomas (Chertok et al., 2008). Further, magnetic nanoparticles have been used as an imaging agent in the brain for diagnostic purposes (Riviere et al., 2007). We and others have also previously reported successful immobilization of several clinically and biotechnologically important proteins and enzymes onto magnetic nanoparticles (Saiyed et al., 2007). However, site-specific targeting of active NRTIs bound to magnetic nanocarriers has not been reported.

Delivery of active phosphorylated form of NRTIs offers an advantage because NRTIs per se have low intracellular ability to convert to active nucleoside 5′-triphosphate (NTP) form due to inefficiency of enzyme thymidylate kinase in human cells (Lavie et al., 1997). This leads to the development of drug resistance, toxicity, and insufficient effective drug levels in virus target tissue (Nuesch et al., 2005; Doualla-Bell et al., 2004; Adachi, Reid, & Schuetz, 2002; Fellay et al., 2001; Benbrik, 1997). However, delivery of active NRTIs poses a challenge in terms of protecting the NTPs from cellular phosphatases and neutralizing the electronegative charge of NTP. We reported for the first time that 3′-Azido-3′-Deoxythymidine-5′-triphosphate (AZTTP; an active form of AZT) can be directly bound to magnetic nanoparticles by ionic interaction and provide an effective magnetically guided nanoformulation that can inhibit HIV-1 replication (Saiyed, Gandhi, & Nair, 2009). The mechanism of direct adsorption of AZTTP was attributed to the strong interaction of triphosphate groups of AZTTP with the Fe_3O_4 nanoparticles. This ionic interaction may help to neutralize the electronegative charge of AZTTP and make their mass transport easier across the cellular barriers. Our results showed that magnetic nanoparticles (MP)-bound AZTTP (MP-AZTTP) completely retained its biological activity as assessed by inhibition of HIV-1 replication in PBMCs.

MAGNETIC NANOCARRIER DELIVERY OF AZTTP ACROSS THE BLOOD-BRAIN BARRIER

Over the last decade, the hybrid systems made of magnetic nanoparticles and liposomes, that is, magnetoliposomes, have attracted more attention for various biological and medical applications. Magnetoliposomes are magnetic derivatives of liposomes and are prepared by entrapment of ferrofluids within the core of liposomes. Magnetoliposome have been investigated as new tools for hyperthermia, as contrast agent for magnetic resonance imaging (MRI), magnetic drug targeting or delivery, and for cell sorting (reviewed by Saiyed, Telang, & Ramchand ., 2003; Pankhurst, Connolly, Jones, & Dobson., 2003; Ito, Shinkai, Honda, & Kobayashi ., 2005). Therefore, we further developed a magnetic nanocarrier by encapsulation of MP-AZTTP in the liposomes, followed by transmigration of MP-AZTTP liposomes across the in vitro BBB model system in presence of an external magnetic field (Saiyed, Gandhi, & Nair, 2010). The schematic representation of the magnetic nanocarrier is shown in Figure 11.5.1.

Transmission electron microscopic examination of MP-AZTTP liposomes revealed the mean size ~ 150 nm (Figure 11.5.2). The MP-AZTTP liposome was found to be effective inhibitor of HIV-1 in nanomolar concentration range. The anti-HIV activity was comparable to free AZTTP at various doses tested at day 7 post HIV-infection in PBMCs. However, on day 14 post infection p24 antigen levels were found to be slightly lower (although not significant) in MP-AZTTP liposome-treated cultures compared to free AZTTP cultures (Figure 11.5.3). This observation indicates a possible sustained release effect of AZTTP due to higher retention time in liposomes. Similar effect was reported earlier where 2,′ 3′-dideoxycytidine-5′-triphosphate (ddCTP) was encapsulated in liposomes and it remained stable for days (Szebeni et al., 1990). Thus, the encapsulation of MP-AZTTP in liposomes would increase their efficacy, biocompatibility, and also protect the active NRTIs from degradation by cellular phosphatases. Previous few studies have shown increased drug activity and reduced cytotoxicity of 5′-triphosphates of NRTI encapsulated within the nanogel carriers or erythrocytes (Vinogradov, Kohli, & Zeman, 2005; Magnani et al., 1994).

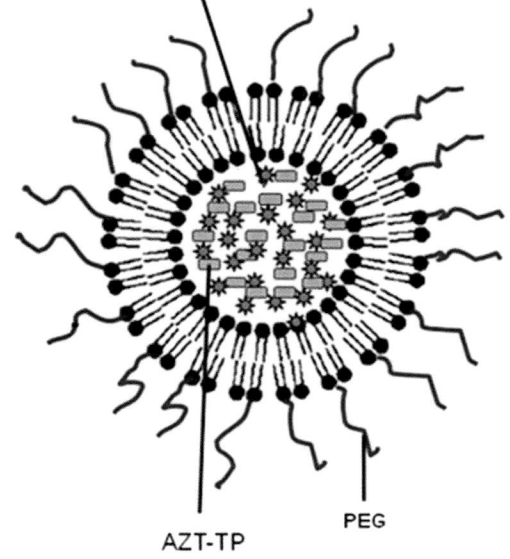

Figure 11.5.1 Schematic of magnetic nanocarrier for antiretroviral drug delivery to the brain.

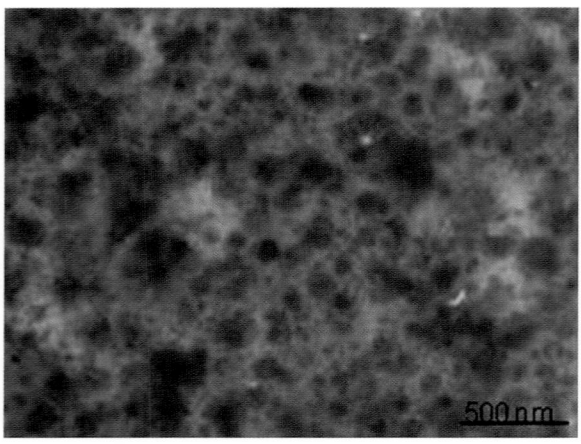

Figure 11.5.2 TEM micrograph of MP-AZTTP liposomes stained with uranyl acetate dye (negative stain).

It has been reported that under normal circumstances AZTTP is unable to cross the blood-brain barrier (BBB) (Vinogradov, 2007). On the contrary, AZT itself (non-phosphorylated form) is able to cross the BBB; however, its antiviral efficacy is limited due to poor intracellular phosphorylation to active form AZTTP, which acts as a chain terminator during reverse transcription of the viral RNA genome. AZT is converted to AZTTP by the action of three enzymes: thymidine kinase (TK), thymidylate kinase (TMPK), and nucleoside diphosphate kinase. However, the rate-limiting step is the phosphorylation of AZT monophosphate (AZTMP) to AZT

diphosphate (AZTDP) catalysed by the enzyme thymidylate kinase (TMPK), which is inefficient in human cells (Lavie et al., 1997). Therefore, we evaluated the transport of MP-AZTTP liposomes across the in vitro BBB model under the influence of an external magnetic field. The BBB model consisted of two-compartment wells in a culture plate with human brain microvascular endothelial cells (BMVEC) grown to confluency on the upper side, whereas the confluent layer of human astrocytes were grown on the underside. The result showed that the apparent permeability of AZZTP was three-fold higher in magnetic nanoformulation compared to free AZTTP (Figure 11.5.4). This indicates that transmigration ability of AZTTP across the BBB increased significantly on binding to magnetic nanoparticles followed by transport under the influence of an external magnetic field. Thus, brain-specific delivery of active NRTIs through an effective carrier would provide significant therapeutic benefits for treatment of HAND.

Several studies have evaluated monocytes/macrophage-based nanocarrier drug-delivery systems for targeting ART to the brain (Dou et al., 2006; 2009). In our studies, we also observed an efficient uptake of rhodamine labeled MP-AZTTP liposomes by monocytes. Most importantly, the phagocytosis of magnetic nanoparticles/liposomes by monocytes makes them magnetic cells that respond to an external magnetic field. Our results indicated that MP-AZTTP liposomes-loaded monocytes showed enhanced migration across the BBB model in response to an external magnetic force. Similarly, Muthana and co-workers (2008) have demonstrated increased migration of magnetic monocytes across a human endothelial cell layer into a tumor spheroid, indicating the potential of magnetic approach for gene and drug delivery. Also, RGD-anchored magnetic liposomes loaded with anti-inflammatory drug diclofenac have been successfully targeted to the brain via monocyte/neutrophil-mediated transport (Jain et al., 2003). Thus, we envisage that this magnetic liposomal drug

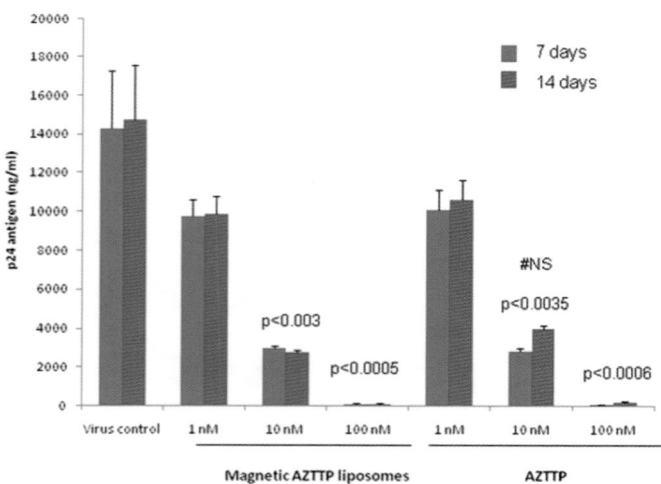

Figure 11.5.3 Magnetic AZTTP liposomes inhibit HIV-1 p24 production. PBMCs (1X10[6] cells/ml) obtained from normal subjects were infected with native HIV-1 IIIB (NIH AIDS Research and Reference Reagent Program Cat# 398) at a concentration of 10[3.0] TCID$_{50}$/ml cells for 3 h and washed 3 times with Hank's balanced salt solution (GIBCO-BRL, Grand Island, NY) before being returned to culture with and without free AZTTP or magnetic AZTTP liposomes (1–100 nM) for 7 and 14 days. The culture supernatants were quantitated for HIV-1 p24 antigen using a p24 ELISA kit (ZeptoMetrix Corporation, Buffalo, NY). The data represents the average of 3 independent experiments and is expressed as ng/ml. Statistical analysis was done using Student's t-test.

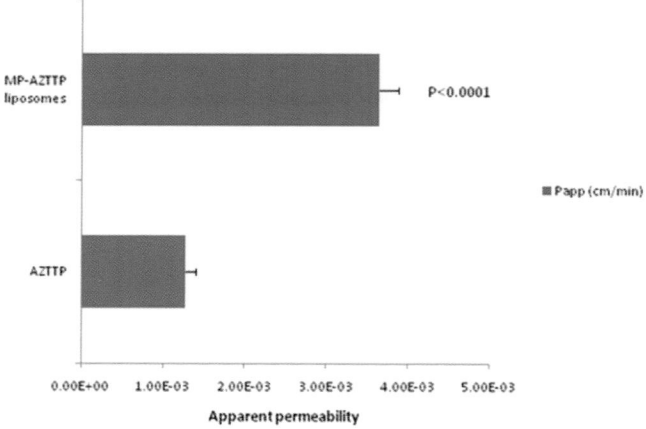

Figure 11.5.4 Transmigration of MP-AZTTP liposomes across the in vitro BBB model. Apparent permeability coefficients (Papp) of AZTTP transport across the BBB model as free and in magnetic liposomes. The data represents the mean ± SE of 3 independent experiments and is expressed as cm/min. Statistical analysis was performed using Student's t-test.

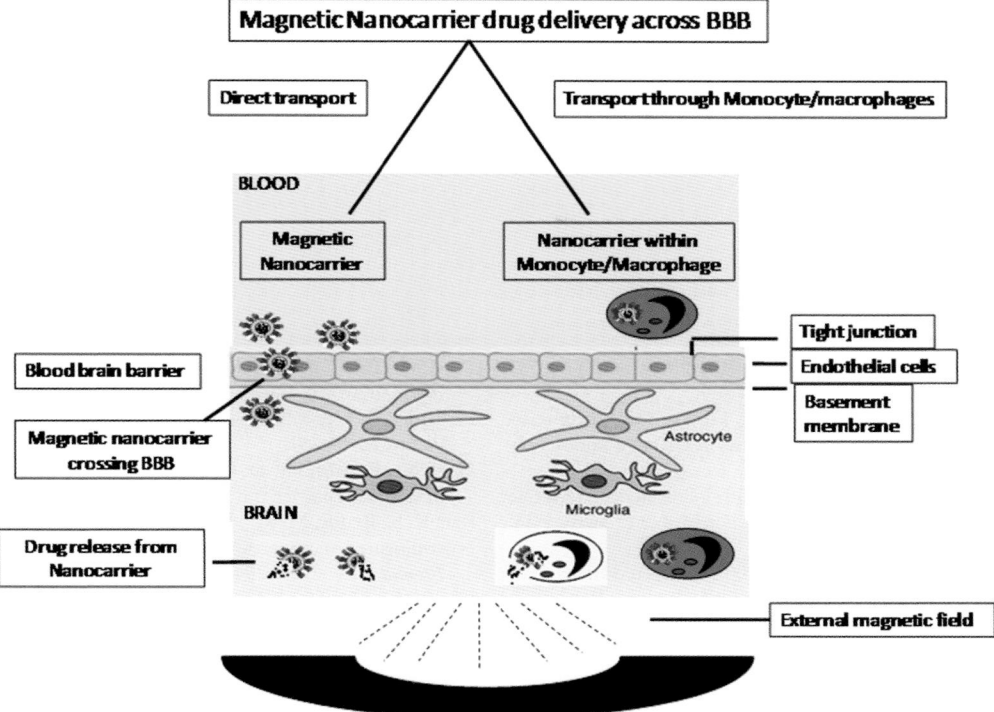

Figure 11.5.5 Hypothetical model of magnetic nanocarrier mediated drug delivery across the BBB.

delivery could also provide a viable approach to overcome the problem of poor BBB penetration of several antiretroviral agents. Also, the transport of magnetic nanoformulation across the BBB occurs by two routes: (1) direct delivery of magnetic nanoformulation under the influence of an external magnetic field, and (2) uptake of these nanoformulations by circulating monocytes/macrophages, which can then tranverse the BBB. A hypothetical model depicting the delivery of magnetic AZTTP nanoformulation across the BBB is presented in Figure 11.5.5.

In our studies of specific drug-targeting to the brain to eliminate the remaining HIV-1 reservoirs, we have developed a magnetic AZTTP liposomal nanoformulation for the first time and shown that it effectively inhibits HIV-1 replication in an in vitro model of infection. In addition, our results indicate that magnetic AZTTP nanoformulations migrate across an established BBB model via direct and monocyte-mediated transport by application of an external magnetic field (Saiyed, Gandhi, & Nair., 2010). Therefore, the delivery of AZTTP using magnetic liposomes is expected to be more therapeutic and may reduce the risk of developing drug-resistant viral strains and further reduce the clinical toxicities associated with the use of high doses of NRTIs.

CONCLUSIONS

Despite significant advances in understanding the immunopathogenesis and neuropathogenesis of HIV infection and impact of HAART, the search for optimal treatment approach

for HAND still remains a major challenge. Results presented in this paper indicate that nanotechnology-based drug-delivery systems offer a promising approach to overcome many challenges associated with ART. Therefore, development of novel strategies to improve the ART bioavailability and increase the permeability across the BBB could be of therapeutic significance in eliminating the hidden virus reservoirs and affecting the clinical outcome of HAND.

ACKNOWLEDGMENTS

This work was supported in part by National Institutes of Health grants R37DA025576, R01DA021537, RO1DA027049, and R01DA085259.

REFERENCES

Adachi, M., Reid, G., & Schuetz, J. D. (2002). Therapeutic and biological importance of getting nucleotides out of cells: A case for the ABC transporters, MRP4 and 5. *Adv Drug Deliv Rev*, 54(10), 1333–1342.

Antinori, A., Arendt, G., Becker, J. T., et al. (2007). Updated research nosology for HIV-associated neurocognitive disorders. *Neurology, 69*, 1789–1799.

Bell, J. E., Brettle, R. P., Chiswick, A., & Simmonds, P. (1998). HIV encephalitis, proviral load and dementia in drug users and homosexuals with AIDS Effect of neocortical involvement. *Brain, 121*, 2043–2052.

Benbrik, E., Chariot, P., & Bonavaud, S., et al. (1997). Cellular and mitochondrial toxicity of zidovudine (AZT), didanosine (ddI) and zalcitabine (ddC) on cultured human muscle cells. *J Neurol Sci, 149*, 19–25.

Chattopadhyay, N., Zastre, J., Wong, H., et al. (2008). Solid lipid nanoparticles enhance the delivery of the HIV protease inhibitor, atazanavir, by a human brain endothelial cell line. *Pharm Res 25*(10), 2262–2271.

Chertok, B., Moffat, B. A., David, A. E., et al. (2008). Iron oxide nanoparticles as a drug delivery vehicle for MRI monitored magnetic targeting of brain tumors. *Biomaterials, 29*(4), 487–496.

Destache, C. J., Belgum, T., Christensen, K., et al. (2009). Combination antiretroviral drugs in PLGA nanoparticle for HIV-1. *BMC Infect Dis, 9*, 198.

Dou, H., Destache, C. J., Morehead, J. R., et al. (2006). Development of a macrophage-based nanoparticle platform for antiretroviral drug delivery. *Blood 108*, 2827–2835.

Dou, H., Grotepas, C. B., McMillan, J. M., et al. (2009). Macrophage delivery of nanoformulated antiretroviral drug to the brain in a murine model of neuroAIDS. *J Immunol, 183*, 661–669.

Doualla-Bell, F., Turner, D., Loemba, H., et al. (2004). HIV drug resistance and optimization of antiviral treatment in resource-poor countries. *Med Sci, 20*, 882–886.

Fellay, J., Boubaker, K., Ledergerber, B., et al. (2001). Prevalence of adverse events associated with potent antiretroviral treatment: Swiss HIV Cohort Study. *Lancet, 358*, 1322–7.

Gagne, J. F., Desormeaux, A., & Perron, S. (2002). Targeted delivery of indinavir to HIV-1 primary reservoirs with immunoliposomes. *Biochim Biophys Acta, 1558*, 198–210.

Ikezu, T. (2009). The aging of human-immunodeficiency-virus associated neurocognitive disorders. *J Neuroimmune Pharmacol, 4*, 161–162.

Ito, A., Shinkai, M., Honda, H., & Kobayashi, T. (2005). Medical application of functionalized magnetic nanoparticles. *J Biosci Bioeng, 100*, 1–11.

Jain, S., Mishra, V., Singh, P., et al. (2003). RGD-anchored magnetic liposomes for monocytes/neutrophils-mediated brain targeting. *Int J Pharm, 261*, 43–55.

Jain, S. K., Gupta, Y., Jain, A., et al. (2008). Mannosylated gelatin nanoparticles bearing an anti-HIV drug didanosine for site-specific delivery. *Nanomed, 4*, 41–48.

Kinman, L., Bui, T., Larsen, K., et al. (2006). Optimization of lipid-indinavir complexes for localization in lymphoid tissues of HIV-infected macaques. *J Acquir Immune Defic Syndr, 42*(2), 155–161.

Kulkovsky, J. & Bray, S. (2006). HAART-persistent HIV-1 latent reservoirs their origin, mechanisms of stability, and potential strategies for eradication. *Curr HIV Res. 4*, 199–208.

Kuo, Y. & Kuo, C. (2008). Electromagnetic interference in the permeability of saquinavir across the blood-brain barrier using nanoparticulate carriers. *Int J Pharm, 351*, 271–281.

Kuo, Y. C. & Su, F. (2007). Transport of stavudine, delavirdine, and saquinavir across the blood-brain barrier by polybutylcyanoacrylate, methylmethacrylate-sulfopropylmethacrylate, and solid lipid nanoparticles. *Int J Pharm, 340*, 143–152.

Lavie, A., Schlichting, I., Vetter, I. R., et al. (1997). The bottleneck in AZT activation. *Nat Med 3*, 922–924.

Lesniak, M. S. & Brem, H. (2004). Targeted therapy for brain tumors. *Nat Rev Drug Discov, 3*(6), 499–508.

Magnani, M., Rossi, L., Fraternale, A., et al. (1994). Feline immunodeficiency virus infection of macrophages: in vitro and in vivo inhibition by dideoxycytidine-5'-triphosphate-loaded erythrocytes. *AIDS Res Hum Retrovir, 10*, 1179–1186.

Mainardes, R. M., Gremiao, M. P., Brunetti, I. L., et al. (2009). Zidovudine-loaded PLA and PLA-PEG blend nanoparticles: Influence of polymer type on phagocytic uptake by polymorphonuclear cells. *J Pharm Sci, 98*, 257–267.

Murri, R., Lepri, A. C., Paola, C., et al. (2006). Is moderate HIV viremia associated with a higher risk of clinical progression in HIV-infected people treated with highly active antiretroviral therapy: Evidence from the Italian Cohort of Antiretroviral-Naïve Patients Study. *J Acquir Immune Defic Syndr, 41*, 23–30.

Muthana, M., Scott, S. D., Farrow, N., et al. (2008). A novel magnetic approach to enhance the efficacy of cell-based gene therapies. *Gene Therapy, 15*, 902–910.

Nowacek, A. & Gendelman, H. E. (2009). NanoART, neuroAIDS and CNS drug delivery. *Nanomed, 4*(5), 557–574.

Nuesch, R., Ananworanich, J., Sirivichayakul, S., et al. (2005). Development of HIV with drug resistance after CD4 cell count–guided structured treatment interruptions in patients treated with highly active antiretroviral therapy after dual–nucleoside analogue treatment. *Clin Infect Dis, 40*, 728–734.

Ojewole, E., Mackraj, I., Naidoo, P., & Govender, T. (2008). Exploring the use of novel drug delivery systems for antiretroviral drugs. *Eur J Pharm Biopharm, 70*, 697–710.

Pang, S., Koyangi, Y., Miles, S., et al. (1990). High levels of unintegrated HIV-1 DNA in brain tissue of AIDS dementia patients. *Nature, 34*, 85–89.

Pankhurst, Q. A., Connolly, J., Jones, S. K., & Dobson, J. (2003). Applications of magnetic nanoparticles in biomedicine. *J Phys D–Appl Phys, 36*(13), 167–181.

Pardridge, W. M. (2007). Blood-brain barrier delivery. *Drug Discovery Today, 12*, 54–61.

Perry, V. H., Anthony, D. C., Bolton, S. J., & Brown, H. C. (1997). The blood-brain barrier and inflammatory response. *Mol Med, 3*, 335–341.

Rao, K. S., Reddy, M. K., Horning, J. L., & Labhasetwar, V. (2008). TAT-conjugated nanoparticles for the CNS delivery of anti-HIV drugs. *Biomaterials, 29*, 4429–4438.

Riviere, C., Martina, M. S., Riviere, C., et al. (2007). Magneting targeting of nanometric magnetic fluid loaded liposomes to specific brain intravascular areas: A dynamic imaging study in mice. *Radiology, 244*, 439–448.

Robertson, K. R. & Hall, C. D. (2007). Assessment of neuroAIDS in the international setting. *J Neuroimmune Pharmacol, 2*, 105–111.

Saiyed, Z. M., Gandhi, N. H., & Nair, M. P. N. (2009). AZT 5'-triphosphate nanoformulation suppresses HIV-1 replication in peripheral blood mononuclear cells. *J Neurovirol, 15*, 343–347.

Saiyed, Z. M., Gandhi, N. H., & Nair, M. P. N. (2010). Magnetic nanoformulation of azidothymidine 5'-triphosphate for targeted delivery across the blood-brain barrier. *Int J Nanomed, 5*, 157–166.

Saiyed, Z. M., Telang, S. D., & Ramchand, C. N. (2003). Application of magnetic techniques in the field of drug discovery and biomedicine. *BioMagn Res Technol, 1*, 1–8.

Saiyed, Z. M., Sharma, S., Godawat, R., et al. (2007). Activity and stability of alkaline phosphatase (ALP) immobilized onto magnetic nanoparticles. *J Biotechnol, 131*, 240–244.

Sarin, H. (2009). Recent progress towards the development of effective systemic chemotherapy for the treatment of malignant brain tumors. *J Transl Med, 7*, 77.

Silva, G. A. (2007). Nanotechnology approaches for drug and small molecule delivery across the blood-brain barrier. *Nanotechnol, 67*, 113–116.

Suri, S. S., Fenniri, H., & Singh, B. (2007). Nanotechnology-based drug delivery systems. *J Occupational Med Toxicol, 2*, 16.

Szebeni, J., Wahl, S. M., Betageri, G. V., et al. (1990). Inhibition of HIV-1 in monocyte/macrophage cultures by 2,' 3'-dideoxycytidine-5'-triphosphate, free and in liposomes. *AIDS Res Hum Retroviruses, 6*, 691–702.

Thompson, M. A., Aberg, J. A., Cahn, P., et al. (2010). Antiretroviral treatment of adult HIV infection: 2010 recommendations of the international AIDS society—USA panel. *JAMA, 304*(3), 321–333.

UNAIDS, WHO: (2009). AIDS epidemic update: December 2009. UNAIDS 2009. UNAIDS/09.36E. JC1700E.ISBN 9789291738328

Vinogradov, S. V., Kohli, E., & Zeman, A. D. (2005). Crosslinked polymeric nanogel formulation of 5'-triphosphates of nucleoside analogs: Role of the cellular membrane in drug release. *Mol Pharm, 2*, 449–461.

Vinogradov, S. V. (2007). Polymeric nanogel formulations of nucleoside analogs. *Expert Opin Drug Deliv, 4*(1), 5–17.

Vyas, T. K., Shah, L., & Amiji, M. M. (2006). Nanoparticulate drug carriers for delivery of HIV/AIDS therapy to viral reservoir sites. *Expert Opin Drug Deliv, 3*, 613–628.

Vyas, T. K., Shahiwala, A., & Amiji, M. M. (2008). Improved oral bioavailability and brain transport of saquinavir upon administration in novel nanoemulsion formulations. *Int J Pharm, 347*, 93–101.

11.6

ADJUNCTIVE MEDICINES

Harris A. Gelbard and Stuart A. Lipton

Antiretroviral drugs are the only therapy currently in general use for the treatment of HIV-associated neurocognitive disorders (HAND), but the treatment response to these agents may be unsatisfactory or short lived. One reason for this unsatisfactory response may be that the pathophysiology of HAND is initiated by the virus but involves a cascade of ongoing inflammation mediated by peripheral and central immune effector cells, viral neurotoxins, pro-inflammatory cellular metabolites, and by a reduction in normal levels of trophic factors in the central nervous system. Steps in this inflammatory cascade may provide useful targets for adjunctive therapies for HAND. There is a similar need for adjunctive therapies for HIV-associated peripheral neuropathy. This chapter discusses the design of clinical trials for these therapies as well as particular targets and drugs.

ISSUES IN THE DESIGN OF CLINICAL TRIALS FOR HIV-ASSOCIATED NEUROLOGIC DISEASE

Although cognitive impairment has been recognized as a major complication of HIV infection, it has been difficult to perform clinical trials for HIV-associated neurocognitive disease (HAND), which encompasses the most severe form of neurologic disease, HIV-1 associated dementia (HAD). The first published double-blind, placebo-controlled multicenter trial for HAD was started more than 23 years ago and reported the benefit of high dose zidovudine (formerly called AZT) in patients with established HAD. This trial of approximately 30 patients was significantly smaller than planned and took a longer time than expected to reach this level of enrollment. Subsequent clinical trials planned by the AIDS Clinical Trial Group (ACTG) and other multicenter organizations have found recruitment of patients to therapeutic trials slow and difficult. Part of the difficulty has been in achieving a consensus about the prevalence and importance of HAND as an ongoing disease in a population that has had relatively stable management of HIV-1 with combination antiretroviral therapy (cART). Because of the lack of fully vetted biomarkers for HAND that can be routinely sampled, and the expense and logistical hurdles of newer neuroimaging modalities, people with HAND must be willing to tolerate the fairly rigorous neuropsychological assessments that have become standard elements of these trials. From a historical perspective, the early trials focused on the effect of antiviral treatment, and by the time the trial was in progress, antiviral treatment standards often had shifted. Perhaps the most dramatic change in therapy has occurred after the introduction and refinement of protease inhibitors. The widespread administration of combination antiretroviral therapy (cART) to patients with AIDS has shifted the time course and clinical presentation of neurologic disease. Although patients that are not naïve to cART may still present with dementia as an AIDS-defining illness (Welch & Morse, 2002), patients are living longer and exhibiting minor cognitive and minor motor deficits that comprise the majority of HAND earlier in the course of their illness (Geraci & Simpson, 2001). On a cautionary note, HAND actually appears to be increasing in prevalence (Neuenburg et al., 2002), suggesting that cART may not be efficacious in preventing direct effects on neuronal and glial function in the central nervous system (CNS). This also appears to be true outside the CNS, because the prevalence of peripheral neuropathy persists in patients with HIV-1 (Sacktor, 2002). Since the last edition of this textbook, clinical trials of adjunctive therapies have largely used "off-the-shelf" drugs developed for the treatment of other neurologic diseases while allowing concurrent best standard antiviral treatment (for the rationale of this approach, see below). A successfully completed multicenter, placebo-controlled, randomized phase II trial of an adjunctive therapy, memantine, a drug that blocks the ion channel associated with the N-methyl-D-aspartate (NMDA) subtype of glutamate receptor in the brain, is highlighted below and illustrates some of the difficulties in achieving clinically significant neuroprotection in the CNS of patients with HAND.

Equally problematic for successful clinical trials focused on neuroprotection has been convincing the greater scientific community committed to treatment options for HIV-1 that HAND represents a significant source of morbidity despite the success of cART in changing HIV-1 into a chronic, medically manageable disease. Within the past year, the Neurological AIDS Research Consortium (NARC) came to the conclusion that consortium investigators needed to reformulate their goals and approach to therapeutic intervention because trials of commercially available adjunctive therapies had not resulted in efficacious neuroprotection against HAND, outside of the introduction of new antiretroviral agents that comprise cART. Indeed, in a recent meta-analysis, Uthman and Abdulmalik (2008) reported that ten Phase 1 studies of adjunctive therapies to cART did not establish efficacy for the symptoms of HAND. However, this in no way diminishes the importance of the NARC in building the infrastructure and designing analytical tools to conduct clinical trials research. Historically, since the advent of cART, the NARC, in conjunction with the AIDS Clinical Trials Group (ACTG) of the National Institutes of Health, had adopted the policy of conducting relatively small (30–40 patients) Phase 1 pilot clinical trials to evaluate compounds for safety and tolerability, with the secondary goal of obtaining neuropsychologic, and where possible neuroimaging, or other measures of efficacy. Subjects were enrolled in these 10–12 week trials and were randomized in a double-blinded fashion to placebo or treatment intervention. Initially, subjects in a Phase 1A trial receiving cART—the adjunctive agent—were evaluated for increases in viral load and indices of cART drug metabolism that would reflect potential adverse pharmacokinetic interactions. If no such adverse interactions occurred, subjects would enroll in a Phase 1B trial to determine tolerability and safety of cART regimens with the adjunctive agent under study. Once compounds were screened in this fashion, particularly safe and potentially effective compounds could then be more thoroughly investigated in larger (80–120 patients followed for 16–24 weeks) clinical trials aimed at determining the therapeutic efficacy of the intervention. This staged procedure also allowed the protocols of clinical trials to be responsive to changes in antiviral treatments. A longer-term goal was to assess potential interventions in more prolonged studies to determine if such medications were also efficacious in preventing the onset of cognitive impairment. Such trials would probably require hundreds patients with relatively advanced HIV disease followed for 1–2 years—an economic hurdle that would clearly require a level of fiscal support beyond NIH or foundation budgets. Additional logistical hurdles to be addressed included large enough enrollment populations to validate therapeutic endpoints in HAND, where different subsets of neuropsychologic parameters can fluctuate between follow-up visits, and the lack of a neuroimaging biomarker that directly correlates with single or aggregate (i.e., Z-score) neuropsychologic parameters.

There continues to be some debate about the best operational definition of HAND for inclusion in clinical trials. Patients who meet the full diagnostic criteria for HIV-associated dementia are often too systemically ill with HIV infection or cognitively impaired to participate in a clinical trial lasting for more than a few weeks. Patients with neuropsychological test abnormalities (e.g., two test results that are one standard deviation below the mean) have been another way of defining cognitive impairment for inclusion in trials, but such patients may never go on to develop the full spectrum of dementia. These issues of the definition of cognitive impairment and the clinical criteria for inclusion in a study, the difficulties in achieving consensus on either biomarkers or neuroimaging parameters as surrogate measures of changes in HAND, and the lack of demonstrated efficacy of "off-the-shelf" pharmacologic agents for HAND have contributed to the perception that multicenter clinical trials to assess new drugs for HAND need to be completely revamped and better integrated with ongoing studies conducted under the auspices of the ACTG.

To test drugs in patients with HAND, most clinical trials use not only the clinical neurologic examination but also a standard battery of neuropsychological tests originally developed by John J. Sidtis and Richard W. Price (see chapters by Richard Price and Igor Grant, this volume). In this manner, we can quantitatively follow the severity of the cognitive dysfunction. In early clinical trials it was found that the antiretroviral drug zidovudine is effective for dementia for about 12 weeks and then patients level off and get worse. This provided the initial impetus to develop an adjunctive drug to better treat the cognitive changes more persistently. Also, clinical trials of adjunctive drugs for HAND, if given with current regimens of cART, should include patients who have been on cART for at least 8–12 weeks to allow for the full effect of cART on viral replication and immunologic indices. However, the sophistication of current cART regimens bears no resemblance to the therapeutic arsenal available to clinicians in 2005. For example, in the last edition, we discussed the nucleoside analogs didanosine (ddI), zalcitabine (ddC), stavudine (d4T), and lamivudine (3TC) and the available protease inhibitors (saquinavir, ritonavir, indinavir), and noted there was either poor penetration of the blood-brain barrier in adults or this information was not yet known. We also mentioned that there is limited information on the efficacy of didanosine or zalcitabine to treat HIV-1 dementia (Yarchoan et al., 1990). In marked contrast, a survey of the ACTG progress report during the 2009/2010 time period (Andrade et al.,2010)describes no fewer than three trials with the HIV integrase inhibitor raltegravir, including A5248, a prospective, open-label, multicenter protocol to estimate the first phase of viral decay in ART-naïve subjects receiving raltegravir with emtricitabine/tenofovir (Truvada, a combination of a nucleoside reverse transcriptase inhibitor with a nucleotide reverse transcriptase inhibitor) (Arribas et al., 2010). Since newer combinations of protease inhibitors such as darunavir and ritonavir have proved equally efficacious to the same treatment with two nucleoside reverse transcriptase inhibitors in terms of viral load reduction <50 copies/ml; A5262 is investigating the combination of raltegravir with darunavir/ritonavir in treatment-naïve patients (Ellis et al., 2010). Additionally, there are multiple immunomodulatory trials such as NWCS 283R, which examines the ability of PEG-interferon α-mediated suppression of HIV-1 in chronically infected individuals (Andrade et al). A5212 is a double-blind, Phase II study to determine whether multiple doses of recombinant human keratinocyte growth factor can increase CD4+ levels in individuals with low viral load but inadequate T cell indices (Andrade et al).

Despite the sophistication and complexity of ACTG trials in the search for eradication of infection, our concern that HIV-1 would be able to maintain sanctuary reservoirs in the CNS that would evade cART and continue to contribute to the pathogenesis of HAND has proven dismayingly accurate. Ongoing studies such as CNS HIV Anti-Retroviral Therapy Effects Research (CHARTER) in this country as well as studies in Canada and Switzerland have demonstrated that between 50–69% of people living with HIV-1 have some type of HAND (Power, Boissé, Rourke, & Gill, 2009; Simioni et al., 2010; Giulian, Wendt, Vaca, & Noonan, 1993).

RATIONALE FOR ADJUNCTIVE THERAPIES IN HAND

Antiretroviral agents are the only therapy currently in general use for treatment of HAND, but treatment response may be unsatisfactory or short lived. The duration of treatment response is not clear but is thought to be relatively short lived. One reason for the unsatisfactory response to anti-retroviral agents may be that the pathophysiology of HIV-related cognitive impairment is initiated by the virus but involves a complicated cascade that involves ongoing inflammation mediated by peripheral and central immune effector cells, viral neurotoxins, pro-inflammatory cellular metabolites and a reduction in normal levels of trophic factors in the CNS. Thus, effective therapy may then need to focus on these other indirect mechanisms of neuronal injury.

The number of HIV-infected cells in the brain is relatively small, consisting predominantly of macrophages and microglia, and therefore the question of how relatively few cells can produce so much dysfunction of uninfected neurons has lead to our understanding that neurologic disease occurs in part because of exposure to viral neurotoxins, alterations in homeostatic levels of cellular pro-inflammatory cytokines and chemokines, and disruption of normal immune effector cell function in the CNS. Many molecules that may be neurotoxic are released by HIV-infected or activated macrophages/microglia or by dysfunctional astrocytes, may play a role in the generation of the clinical dementia syndrome (Lipton & Gendelman, 1995; Kaul & Lipton, 1999).

EXCITOTOXIC DAMAGE TO NEURONS: THE PRIME MOVER FOR EARLY CLINICAL TRIALS FOR HAND

Potential factors include: (i) HIV-1 proteins gp120 and Tat (both of which may activate macrophages and microglia); (ii) excitatory amino acids such as quinolinate, cysteine, and glutamate; (iii) cytokines, including tumor necrosis factor-alpha (TNF-α), interleukin-1 beta (IL-1β), and interleukin-6 (IL-6); (iv) lipid species including arachidonic acid and platelet-activating factor (PAF); (v) free radical species such as superoxide anion ($O_2^{\cdot-}$) and nitric oxide (NO$\cdot$); (vi) chemokines such as SDF-1α[15]; and (vii) other factors that remain to be identified from macrophages or microglia. Additionally, lack of normal neurotrophic factors could contribute to the neuronal injury as well (Kaul & Lipton, 1999; Kaul & Lipton, 2000; Lipton & Rosenberg, 1994). There is a common denominator implicated in this form of neuronal injury in HIV-associated dementia as well as in other neurodegenerative disorders. Many of these small molecules act directly or indirectly as "excitotoxins," causing damage via over-stimulation of nerve cell activity which produces excessive increases in intracellular Ca^{2+} levels, with subsequent free radical production and caspase activation (Garden et al., 2002; Bonfoco, Krainc, Ankarcrona, Nicotera, & Lipton, 1995). In HIV-associated dementia the type of "excitotoxic" process proceeds relatively slowly, apparently resulting in synaptic damage, followed by apoptosis rather than necrosis (Petito & Roberts, 1995;

Garden et al., 2002). Apoptosis is a process of cell involution with chromatin condensation and may be associated with a cascades of intracellular signal transduction that are still being elucidated, but, at least in the case of gp120-induced neuronal injury, appears to involve a p38 mitogen-activated protein kinase (MAPK) pathway and caspase activation (Kaul & Lipton, 1999; . Dreyer, Kaiser, Offermann, & Lipton, 1990). An important caveat to note is that apoptotic cell death of vulnerable neurons proceeds in the setting of chronic neuroinflammation, which is likely to be a greater determinant of clinically significant neurologic disease.

In both tissue culture and animal models, neuronal damage can be largely inhibited by antagonists of the N-methyl-D-aspartate (NMDA) subtype of glutamate receptor (Lipton & Gendelman, 1995; Lipton et al., 1990; Giulian, Vaca, & Noonan, 1990; Lipton, Sucher, Kaiser, & Dreyer, 1991; Savio & Levi, 1993; Dawson, Dawson, Uhl, & Snyder, 1993; Toggas, Masliah, & Mucke, 1996; Lei, Zhang, Abele, & Lipton, 1992). For these reasons, studies in AIDS patients with dementia of a clinically tolerated NMDA antagonist as an adjunctive agent to antiretroviral therapy was approved by the ACTG (see below). In addition, under some conditions, antagonists of voltage-dependent calcium channels (another mode of entry of Ca^{2+} into neurons) can alleviate neuronal damage due to excessive activation of NMDA receptors, occurring, for example, with exposure to gp120 (Lipton et al., 1990; Dawson et al., 1991). For this reason, calcium channel antagonists have been studied by the ACTG in published trials for HIV-associated dementia (see below).

Free radicals, including nitric oxide and superoxide anion, have been shown to be generated by the excitotoxic processes in neurons as well as by activated- or HIV-infected macrophages (Kaul & Lipton, 1999; Garden et al., 2002; Toggas, Masliah, & Mucke, 1996; Lafon-Cazal, Pietri, Culcasi, & Bockaert, 1993; Bukrinsky et al., 1995; Beckman et al., 1990). Nitric oxide (NO$\cdot$) and superoxide anion ($O_2^{\cdot-}$) can react to form a highly neurotoxic species, peroxynitrite (ONOO$^-$) (Lipton et al., 1993; Coyle & Puttfarken, 1993). Reactive oxygen species in the absence of NO$\cdot$ may also play a role as they have been implicated in the pathogenesis of neurodegenerative diseases and glutamate neurotoxicity has been suggested to be mediated, at least in part, by free radicals (Gelbard et al., 1995). Reactive oxygen species or peroxynitrite can attack proteins, deoxynucleic acid, and lipid membranes, resulting in the disruption of cellular function and integrity. The carbon radicals generated by oxygen radical attack, particularly those formed within polyunsaturated fatty acids, undergo molecular arrangement, which, in turn, undergo lipid peroxidation to form additional organic peroxy radicals. The peroxy radicals extract hydrogen from adjacent fatty acids and thereby propagate the lipid peroxidation process. Peroxynitrite can also contribute to lipid peroxidation or nitration of tyrosine residues, resulting in protein dysfunction. In mild to moderate amounts, both reactive oxygen species and peroxynitrite appear to be able to precipitate neuronal apoptosis (Gelbard et al., 1995), similar to findings demonstrated in cerebral cortex and basal ganglia of patients with HIV-1 encephalitis (Garden et al., 2002). Thus, drugs or molecular interventions, such as expression of the anti-apoptotic bcl-2 gene, inhibition of caspases, inhibition of the p38 MAPK pathway, or scavengers that decrease radical species, might be considered as adjunctive therapies for HAND.

INVOLVEMENT OF THE KINOME IN THE PATHOGENESIS OF HAND: A RATIONALE FOR CURRENT AND FUTURE THERAPIES

Since the last edition of this chapter, considerable progress has been made in understanding the importance of the kinome and its role in contributing to the neuropathogenesis of HAND. In particular, the cumulative evidence that mixed lineage kinase type 3 (MLK3), which is pathologically activated in models of neurodegeneration for HAND, Alzheimer's disease (AD), and Parkinson's disease (PD), might be such a target has been of considerable interest to the field. Preclinical studies of Cephalon's "first generation" MLK inhibitor, CEP1347, have shown that this agent can protect neurons against a considerable range of insults, including exposure to the Alzheimer's peptide, Aß (Saporito, Thomas, & Scott, 2000). Studies using the 1-methyl-4-phenyl-1,2,3,6-tetrahydropyridine (MPTP) model of Parkinsonism have demonstrated the efficacy of CEP1347 in treating motor deficits and neuronal degeneration (Lotharius et al., 2005), and CEP1347-mediated neuroprotection has also been observed in an in vitro model for Parkinson's disease, using methamphetamine-exposed human mesencephalic-derived neurons (Lotharius et al., 2005). Because HAND can present with dopaminergic dysfunction, these data suggested to us that CEP1347 might also be protective in the context of HAND. In fact, Bodner et al.(Bodner et al., 2002; Bodner, Toth & Miller, 2004) have shown that CEP1347 can protect primary rat hippocampal neurons as well as dorsal root ganglion neurons from the otherwise neurotoxic effects of exposure to HIV-1 gp120. Sui et al. (2006) demonstrated that Tat and gp120 induced autophosphorylation of MLK3 in primary rat neurons and this effect was abolished by the addition of CEP1347. While the physiological roles for MLKs remain unclear (Eggert et al., 2009), these studies suggest that MLK3 activity is increased by HIV-1 neurotoxins, resulting in downstream signaling events that trigger neuronal death and damage, along with monocyte activation (accompanied by release of inflammatory cytokines). Most recently, CEP1347 was demonstrated to be neuroprotective in an in vivo model of HIV-1 infection, reversing microglial activation and restoring normal synaptic architecture, as well as restoring macrophage secretory profiles to a trophic versus toxic phenotype in response to HIV-1 infection (Eggert et al., 2010).

Integrating a working model of HIV-1 neuropathogenesis based on the clinical phenotype of HAND and current functional neuroimaging data with the signal transduction pathways that subserve MLK3 activation has been extraordinarily complicated because MLK3 transduces multiple inflammatory signals in mononuclear phagocytes and glia as well as pro-apoptotic signals in vulnerable neurons (Bodner et al., 2004; Gallo & Johnson, 2002; Eggert et al., 2010). Glial and immune effector cell pathways downstream of MLK3 include chemokine production (CCL2, CXCL8) from astrocytes (Zheng et al., 2008; El-Hage et al., 2006), as well as monocyte chemotaxis in response to CCL2 (Conant et al, 1998). The significance of CCL2 upregulation resulting from pathologic activation of MLK3 is underscored by neuropathologic studies demonstrating CCL2 elevation in brain tissue from patients with a premortem diagnosis of HIV-1 dementia (Bisson et al, 2008). Despite the fact that targeted deletion of MLKs 1, 2 and 3 results in apparently normal neurologic phenotypes (Brancho et al, 2005; New et al., 1998), deletion of MLK3 results in a selective reduction in tumor necrosis factor (TNF)-stimulated c-Jun NH_2-terminal kinase (JNK) activity (New et al., 1998). TNF-α mediates a significant part of Tat-mediated toxicity in models of HAND (Asami et al., 2006), and inhibition of this pathway by CEP-1347 may account for the reduction in neuroinflammation we observed in our models of HAND (Eggert et al., 2010).

However, there is another equally important aspect to the role of MLK3 inhibition as a potential therapeutic strategy for HAND: trophic factor (i.e., brain-derived neurotrophic factor, e.g., BDNF) withdrawal from microglia may occur in response to infiltrating, inflammatory leukocytes (Batchelor et al, 1999; Lai & Todd, 2008; Najajima et al., 2001; Roux et al., 2002), and for synaptic architecture to survive and remain functional in this setting, there may be an additional requirement for activation of the phosphatidylinositol 3-kinase (PI3-kinase) pathway (Wang, Paden, & Johnson, 2005; Wang et al., 2008). This is germane to neurons that express the TrkB receptor for BDNF because MLK3 inhibition, while increasing TrkB expression, does not result in sustained activation of TrkB and the downstream PI3-kinase-Akt-GSK3β pathway without the presence of BDNF (Liu et al., 2009). Indeed, restoration of adaptive immunity in an in vivo model of HAND is associated with neuroprotection of synaptic architecture and upregulation of BDNF (Wang & Johnson, 2008). A critical caveat here is that BDNF signaling through TrkB receptors results in activation-dependent downregulation of TrkB; thus, both MLK3 inhibition and activation of the PI3-kinase pathway, either through BDNF or GSK-3β inhibition may be necessary for long-term survival of synaptic architecture. Whether MLK inhibitors will prove to be efficacious in human clinical trials for HAND, however, remains to be determined.

CLINICAL TRIALS OF L-TYPE CALCIUM CHANNEL ANTAGONISTS FOR HAND

Based on the evidence cited above regarding excitotoxic mechanisms of neuronal injury, a phase I-II clinical trial with the L-type calcium channel antagonist nimodipine was completed by the ACTG in years past. This small pilot study of 38 patients lacked sufficient power to prove efficacy. However, it did show that oral nimodipine was well tolerated without significant side effects at both at high and low dosages (60 mg five times per day and 30 mg three times per day, respectively). Moreover, a trend toward improvement on high dose nimodipine was noted on quantitative neuropsychological testing compared to placebo. Also, a trend toward less painful peripheral neuropathy was noted by objective and subjective criteria for either low or high dose nimodipine compared to placebo (p = 0.07). These findings indicated that a trial with a larger number of patients may be warranted (Lipton, 1993).

CLINICAL TRIALS OF NMDA ANTAGONISTS FOR HAND

To build on the findings with calcium channel antagonists and to more directly address the role of calcium entry via NMDA-receptor operated channels, the ACTG more recently completed a clinical trial with the NMDA receptor antagonist memantine. As detailed elsewhere (Lipton & Rosenberg, 1994; Lipton, 1992), many NMDA receptor antagonists are not clinically tolerated, while memantine appears to be tolerated by humans at concentrations that are effective neuroprotectants. Several NMDA antagonists have been found to prevent neuronal injury associated with HIV-infected macrophages, gp120-activated macrophages, or potential toxins, including platelet-activating factor, cysteine, or quinolinate (Lipton & Gendelman, 1995; Giulan et al., 1990; Lipton et al., 1991; Savio & Levi, 1993; Dawson et al., 1993; Toggas et al., 1996; Lipton, 1992a, Muller et al., 1992; Lipton, 1992b; Lipton, 1993; Chen et al., 1992). Among these, a promising drug because of its long experience in patients with other diseases, is memantine, which has been approved for the treatment of moderate-to-severe Alzheimer's disease by the U. S., Food and Drug Administration (FDA). Memantine blocks the NMDA receptor-associated ion channel only when it is excessively (i.e., pathologically) open. Unlike other NMDA open-channel blockers, such as dizocilpine (MK-801), memantine does not remain in the channel for an excessively long time, and this kinetic parameter (relatively fast "off rate" contributing to its low affinity of binding in the channel) correlates with its safe use in humans for many decades in Europe as a treatment for Parkinson's disease and more recently Alzheimer's disease (Lipton & Rosenberg, 1994; Lipton & Jenson, 1992). Increasing concentrations of glutamate or other NMDA agonists cause NMDA channels to remain open on average for a greater fraction of time. Under such conditions, an open-channel blocking drug such as memantine has a better chance to enter the channel and block it. Because of this mechanism of action, termed uncompetitive inhibition, the untoward effects of greater (pathologic) concentrations of glutamate are prevented to a greater extent than the effects of lower (physiologic) concentrations (Lipton, 1992a). This combination of attributes afforded to memantine, *U*ncompetitive inhibition coupled with a relatively *F*ast *O*ff-rate, has led to the term "UFO" mechanism of action to describe the clinically tolerated mode of antagonism of memantine (Lipton, 2007, Lindl et al., 2010). Moreover, in both in vitro and in vivo model systems memantine can ameliorate gp120-associated neuronal injury (Lei et al., 1992; Muller et al., 1992; Lipton, 1992b; Schiffitto et al., 2007). A phase II double-blind, randomized, placebo-controlled,

multicenter trial of memantine (plus best antiretroviral therapy) has been completed in patients with HIV-1 associated neurologic disease. The results were significant in the primary analysis of magnetic resonance spectroscopy (MRS) data as well as in a last-observation-carry-forward analysis of neurocognitive testing lasting into the washout period of drug therapy (20 weeks), although the primary analysis just missed significance after 16 weeks of therapy (p = 0.054) (Zhao et al., 2010). A major lesson from this trial was that treatment periods should last at least 20 weeks in order to see the full benefit of a potentially neuroprotective drug. Interestingly, this was the first clinical study of HAND in which surrogate markers (magnetic resonance spectroscopy [MRS] in this case) were validated with clinical presentation, as quantified by neurocognitive testing, and in which the surrogate markers appeared to be more sensitive than neuropsychologic testing or neurologic examination. MRS was used to quantify N-acetylaspartate (NAA), a metabolite that is chiefly found in neurons in the adult brain. The ratio of NAA to creatine (Cr) can be used as an index of neuronal function and viability. Significant increases in NAA/Cr were observed in the multivariate analysis among individuals receiving memantine compared to placebo in the frontal white matter and the parietal cortex (p = 0.04 and 0.023, respectively). Since the last edition of this chapter, the ACTG 301 study was extended to up to a 60-week open-label phase, following the 20-week double-blind, placebo-controlled trial (Le & Lipton, 2001). While participants randomized to memantine (vs. placebo) in the initial 12-week open-label phase had a statistically significant improvement in an aggregate neuropsychological score (NPZ-8), no significant changes were noted during the 48-week extension phase. Thus, the results of this study raise the question of whether initial alterations in MRS parameters are ultimately predictive of neuropsychologic outcomes. During the last decade, based on phase III clinical trial results, memantine was approved by the European Union and more recently in the US for the treatment of Alzheimer's disease (The Dana Consortium, 1997). While newer derivatives of memantine may hold even greater promise in the future (The Dana Consortium, 1997; Lipton, 2007, Lindl et al., 2010), the lack of long-term improvement in HAND with 11 months of memantine as an adjunctive therapy suggests that additional approaches are likely to be necessary, particularly with respect to reversing or preventing the effects of chronic neuroinflammation.

DRUGS THAT AMELIORATE THE DOWNSTREAM EFFECTS OF EXCESSIVE GLUTAMATE RECEPTOR ACTIVATION— ANTI-OXIDANTS

During the past five years, several clinical trials have investigated the potential impact of antioxidant medications in the treatment of HIV-1 dementia. Trials with OPC-14117, a vitamin-E-like analog with excellent CNS penetration, were completed. OPC-14117 tolerability profile was no different from placebo and was not associated with any severe adverse experiences

(Kagan et al., 1992). Patients treated with OPC-14117 had a significant improvement in the global impression score compared to placebo-treated patients, and there were trends towards improvement in the Rey Auditory Verbal Learning and timed gait test favoring the OPC group. These results suggested that OPC-14117 was a potential candidate for further study in treatment of HIV-related neurologic disease. Another study investigated alpha-lipoic acid (thioctic acid), a naturally occurring enzymatic cofactor for pyruvate dehydrogenase and, in conjunction with its oxidation-reduction partner dihydrolipoic acid, a potent scavenger of reactive oxygen species. Lipoic acid also enhances the free radical scavenging mechanisms of vitamin E and the glutathione system (Tang & Aizenman, 1993). Depletion of glutathione in AIDS patients has been noted to contribute to an abnormal redox state, and lipoic acid may possibly offset this problem. Additionally, lipoic acid can also limit excessive NMDA receptor activity by oxidizing the redox modulatory site of the receptor (Kim & Lipton, 1994). In this study, thioctic acid was paired with selegiline, a marketed mono-amine oxidase inhibitor (deprenyl) that has trophic effects on injured neurons in low doses, possibly by a mechanism of stimulation of anti-apoptotic factors. Specifically, selegiline may upregulate bcl-2, which may block TNF-induced neuronal apoptosis (The Dana Consortium, 1998). This randomized, double-blind, placebo-controlled, parallel group study used a 2 X 2 factorial design such that the patients were assigned to placebo, thioctic acid alone, selegiline alone, or the combination of thioctic acid and selegiline. A total of 36 patients were randomized and re-evaluated 2, 4, and 10 weeks after randomization. Both selegiline and thioctic acid were well tolerated with few adverse events. The most common adverse events in the selegiline group (18 subjects either alone or combined) were headache ($n = 2$) and nausea ($n = 2$). Six of the 18 subjects on selegiline had clinically insignificant increases in blood levels of phosphate (compared to one subject not on selegiline). Patients receiving selegiline demonstrated significant improvement on tests of verbal memory and psychomotor speed, compared to subjects not receiving selegiline, but the trend for patients receiving thioctic acid was toward worse performance (Sacktor et al., 2000). These data and results from a subsequent pilot study (Evans et al., 2007), lead to a larger study of selegiline for HIV-associated dementia funded by the AIDS Clinical Trials Group (ACTG) and the Neurological AIDS Research Consortium (NARC) ("Phase II, placebo-controlled, double-blind study of the selegiline transdermal system in the treatment of HIV-1-associated cognitive impairment," ACTG 5090). Ultimately, the authors concluded that selegiline was ineffective in ameliorating brain metabolism parameters, CSF protein carbonyl concentration (as a marker of oxidative stress) or neuropsychologic indices (Schifitto et al., 2009; Clifford et al., 2002).

The antioxidant CP-1189, an agent that is able to ameliorate TNF-α-induced neurotoxicity in in vitro models, was investigated in Phase I trials (Schifitto et al., 1999). Although well tolerated, no demonstrable improvements in neuropsychological indices were noted in HIV-infected subjects with cognitive-motor impairments.

ADJUNCTIVE DRUGS THAT AFFECT G PROTEIN-COUPLED RECEPTORS

An early trial of adjunctive therapy used lexipafant, a platelet-activating factor (PAF) receptor antagonist (Gelbard et al., 1994). PAF is an evanescent phospholipid mediator that can be released from postsynaptic neurons after excessive NMDA receptor activation, as well as from HIV-1-infected mononuclear phagocytes that have been antigenically stimulated. Once released, it can promote increased presynaptic glutamate release and was shown to mediate, at least in part, HIV-related neuronal damage (Perry et al., 1998). PAF has also been implicated as a mediator capable of inducing other inflammatory HIV-1 neurotoxins, including TNF-α.[88] Lexipafant was extremely well tolerated, with 88% of patients in the active treatment group versus 93% in the placebo group completing the study. Trends toward improved cognitive performance, especially with respect to verbal memory, were observed in the lexipafant group, but discontinuation of manufacture for the drug prevented follow-up studies.

ADJUNCTIVE DRUGS WITH EFFECTS ON THE KINOME: GLYCOGEN SYNTHASE KINASE 3β

Phase I trials for patients with HAND have been completed using the anticonvulsant and mood-stabilizing drug sodium valproate, as well as lithium (Schifitto et al., 2009; Maggirwar et al., 1999). The rationale for this was based on sodium valproate and lithium's ability, among other properties, to inhibit glycogen synthase kinase 3-beta (GSK-3β), an enzyme complex that when over-activated by HIV-1 neurotoxins Tat and PAF, can induce neuronal apoptosis (Tong et al., 2001; Wang et al., 2007). Both drugs were safe and well tolerated as adjunctive therapeutic agents; in particular, patients receiving valproate as adjunctive therapy showed trends in improvement of neuropsychological performance and brain metabolism.

IMMUNOMODULATORY THERAPIES

A recent Phase 1 randomized, placebo-controlled, double-blind study (NCT00428519), "Effects of Treatment With Aprepitant (Emend®) in HIV-Infected Individuals," has been completed and data analyses are underway. The trial was based on in vitro data demonstrating that treatment with neurokinin-1 receptor antagonists such as aprepitant decreases CCR5 expression in macrophages and lymphocytes, as well as infection with primary R5 strains of HIV (McGrath & Hadlock, 2007). Because aprepitant penetrates the CNS, it is hoped that this type of therapy will decrease viral infection in the CNS and neuroinflammation with clinical improvement of HAND.

Another approach has been to use mitoguazone, a polyamine inhibitor that selectively depletes CD16+ cells containing HIV-1 DNA and preventing CNS infiltration. While mitoguazone was originally developed as an anticancer drug, this type of treatment is aimed at eradicating CD16+ cells as a viral reservoir for HIV-1 (McGrath and Hadlock, 2007).

Finally, in an approach as yet untested in CNS models of HAND, investigators have screened for a small molecule, RN-18, that antagonizes the HIV-1 protein Vif, which targets the DNA-editing enzyme, APOBEC3G. Indeed, RN-18 reduces HIV infectivity by increasing APOBEC3G incorporation into virions, suggesting that it holds promise for augmenting innate immunity against HIV-1 (Nathan et al., 2008).

ANTI-INFLAMMATORY THERAPIES WITH EFFECTS ON THE KINOME

Based on promising early work in a model of SIV encephalitis that demonstrated a reduction in the severity of CNS inflammation, p38 activation, and lower CNS viral replication with the tetracycline antibiotic minocycline (Follsteadt, Barber, & Zink, 2008), a 24-week randomized, placebo-controlled, double-blind trial with minocycline with an optional 24-week open-label phase for subjects with a CD4 count in the 251–350 range was initiated for Ugandan patients with HAND (NCT00855062) under the auspices of the NARC. Unfortunately, the trial was halted because of lack of a therapeutic response. While this trial provides a cautionary note for the complexities of pharmacologic treatment of the kinome, particularly in the CNS, another very promising effort is currently investigating a series of lead compounds with far more selective activity against mixed lineage kinases, and MLK3 in particular, that have excellent CNS penetration profiles, as well as anti-inflammatory and neuroprotective activities in both in vitro and in vivo models of HAND (Gelbard, Dewhurst, & Goodfellow, 2010).

Additionally, other clinical trials for HIV-associated dementia are being discussed that would test caspase inhibitors, p38 MAPK antagonists, α-chemokine receptor antagonists, and various neurotrophic or neuroprotective factors for the reasons outlined above. One of the most intriguing examples of potential therapy involves erythropoietin (EPO), a cytokine drug commonly used to treat anemia in patients AIDS and chronic renal failure. Recently, EPO was discovered to be present not only in the kidney, but also in the brain. Moreover, the neuroprotective and potentially neurogenic properties of EPO have recently been characterized (Kang et al., 2010). EPO, when combined with insulin-like growth factor I (IGF-I), stimulates in a synergistic manner at least two neuroprotective pathways. These include the phosphokinase/transcription factor cascades associated with phosphoinositide 3-kinase (PI3-K)/Akt (protein kinase B) and Janus kinase-2 (Jak2)/nuclear factor kappa B (NF-kB) (Kang et al., 2010; Digicaylioglu & Lipton, 2001). Moreover, EPO and IGF-I have been shown to ameliorate neuronal injury engendered by HIV/gp120 in recent in vitro experiments as well as in in vivo rodent models of HAND when administered transnasally (Kang et al., 2010). As alluded to above when NMDA receptor antagonists were discussed, most drugs tested in the brain have failed in advanced clinical trials not because they are not effective as neuroprotectants, but because they have intolerable side effects. Since both EPO and IGF-I are already FDA approved and well tolerated, these agents may be potential candidates for adjunctive therapy for HAND.

DESIGN OF CLINICAL TRIALS AND RATIONALE FOR ADJUNCTIVE THERAPY FOR THE PAINFUL NEUROPATHY ASSOCIATED WITH AIDS

Distal sensory polyneuropathy is one of most common complications of AIDS. The clinical syndrome is very similar to the neuropathy associated with diabetes mellitus or alcohol abuse. The cause of the neuropathy associated with HIV-1 infection is as yet unknown although some evidence suggests that HIV-1 DNA may be expressed in dorsal root ganglion cells (Apostolski et al., 1993). There is also evidence that the gp120 protein binds to sensory ganglia neurons (Schiffitto et al., 2006). Thus, as in HIV-associated dementia, constituents of HIV-1 may have a direct role in the pathogenesis of the painful neuropathies associated with AIDS. In addition, increased levels of interleukin-6 in dorsal root ganglia suggest a possible role for HIV-induced cytotoxicity in neuropathogenesis (Apostolski et al., 1993). Interestingly, calcium channel antagonists, NMDA antagonists, and inhibitors of nitric oxide synthase can ameliorate painful neuropathies of diverse etiologies. For this reason, several of the HIV-associated dementia trials that investigated these agents also monitor painful neuropathy, but results have not demonstrated any efficacy for these agents (Ellis et al., 2010).

Several nucleoside analog drugs used to treat AIDS can also cause peripheral neuropathy and can thus be confused with the neuropathy associated with HIV-1 itself. Both didanosine and zalcitabine were recognized in early clinical trials to cause a dose-dependent peripheral neuropathy. Other nucleoside analogs introduced more recently have also been associated with the development or exacerbation of peripheral neuropathy. Since the last chapter of this textbook, a cross-sectional analyses of patients from the CHARTER study demonstrated that HIV-associated sensory neuropathy (HIV-SN; 57% of patients) and neuropathic pain (38% of patients) due to this condition in the cART era remain prevalent, causing substantial disability despite successful cART (Kieburtz et al., 1998). The risk factors for HIV-SN included increasing age, lower CD4 nadir, current cART use, and past use of specific dideoxynucleoside analogue antiretrovirals ("D-drugs") and risk factors for neuropathic pain included past D-drug use and higher CD4 nadir.

Therapeutic interventions for peripheral neuropathy to date have been more limited than previous trials for HAND. One placebo-controlled, randomized study evaluated peptide T at a dosage of 6 mg per day given intranasally. Eighty patients were randomized to either treatment or placebo control groups and followed for 12 weeks. There was no significant difference in pain scores or nerve conduction studies between the two groups. The ACTG sponsored a study designed to assess symptomatic pain relief in HIV-related neuropathy involving amitriptyline, mexiletine, or placebo. The study assessed short-term safety and effectiveness of these interventions in reducing neuropathic pain; however, the drugs were not particularly effective (Kieburtz et al., 1998).

More recently, ACTG Study 291 assessed the relative efficacy of treatment with recombinant human nerve growth factor (rh-NGF) to ameliorate distal sensory neuropathy (DSP) in patients with HIV-1 (Schifitto et al., 2001). Importantly, administration of rh-NGF was safe and well tolerated, and diminished pain associated with DSP. However, no significant improvement in the severity of DSP was observed, as adjudged by neurologic exam, quantitative sensory testing, and epidermal nerve fiber density. Clearly, additional therapies warrant testing for HIV-associated neuropathic pain.

CONCLUSIONS

The last five years have lead to an explosion of new preclinical studies relating to the neuropathogenesis and identification of molecular targets for intervention in HAND and the painful neuropathy associated with HIV infection. Despite the lack of progress in identifying or creating new agents for the efficacious treatment of HAND and sensory neuropathy, the recognition that both these conditions are widely prevalent in the population living with HIV-1 has forced us to redouble our efforts to develop new therapies. We believe this is an achievable goal that is best integrated within the framework of the ACTG, as well as new partnerships between the NIH, academia, and industry. It is noteworthy that our progress toward achieving efficacious therapies for HAND and sensory neuropathy has encountered the same stumbling blocks that have confronted efforts to develop successful therapies for other crippling neurodegenerative diseases such as Alzheimer's and Parkinson's disease. Fortunately, these have been timely lessons for the scientific community involved in developing new therapeutics for neuroAIDS.

ACKNOWLEDGMENTS

Disclosure Statement: Harris Gelbard is the holder of an international patent application for novel inhibitors of MLK3 for the use of neurodegenerative conditions, including HAND. This patent is assigned to the University of Rochester Medical Center. Stuart Lipton is the holder of multiple worldwide patents for the use of memantine in neurodegenerative conditions, including HIV-associated dementia and HAND. These patents are assigned to his former institution, where the initial work was performed (Harvard Medical School/Children's Hospital, Boston), and have been sublicensed to Forest Laboratories in New York City. Concerning the licensure of the memantine patents, Dr. Lipton participates in a royalty-sharing plan that is administered through the Harvard-affiliated hospitals.

REFERENCES

Andrade, A., Rosenkranz, S., Daar, E., Jacobson, J., Acosta, E., Lederman, M., et al. Longer Phase I Viral Decay in Treatment-naïve Patients Receiving Raltegravir-based ART: Preliminary Results from ACTG 5248. Paper . 263 17th Conference on Retroviruses and Opportunistic Infections, CROI 2010, San Francisco, CA.

Apostolski, S., McAlarney, T., Quattrini, A., et al. (1993). The gp120 glycoprotein of human immunodeficiency virus type 1 binds to sensory ganglion neurons. *Ann Neurol, 34*, 855–863.

Arribas, J. R., Horban, A., Gerstoft, J., Fätkenheuer, G., Nelson, M., Clumeck, N., et al. (2010). The MONET trial: Darunavir/ritonavir with or without nucleoside analogues, for patients with HIV RNA below 50 copies/ml. *AIDS, 24*(2), 223–30. PMID: 20010070.

Asami, T., et al. (2006). Autocrine activation of cultured macrophages by brain-derived neurotrophic factor. *Biochem Biophys Res Commun, 344*(3), 941–7.

Batchelor, P. E., et al. (1999). Activated macrophages and microglia induce dopaminergic sprouting in the injured striatum and express brain-derived neurotrophic factor and glial cell line-derived neurotrophic factor. *J Neurosci, 19*(5), 1708–16.

Beckman, J. S., Beckman, T. W., Chen, J., Marshall, P. A., & Freeman, B. A. (1990). Apparent hydroxyl radical production by peroxynitrite: Implications for endothelial injury from nitric oxide and superoxide. *Proc Natl Acad Sci USA, 87*, 1620–1624.

Bisson, N., et al., (2008). Mice lacking both mixed-lineage kinase genes Mlk1 and Mlk2 retain a wild type phenotype. *Cell Cycle, 7*(7), 909–16.

Bodner, A., et al., (2002). Mixed lineage kinase 3 mediates gp120IIIB-induced neurotoxicity. *J Neurochem, 82*(6), 1424–34.

Bodner, A., Toth, P. T., & Miller, R. J, (2004). Activation of c-Jun N-terminal kinase mediates gp120IIIB- and nucleoside analogue-induced sensory neuron toxicity. *Exp Neurol, 188*(2). 246–53.

Bonfoco, E., Krainc, D., Ankarcrona, M., Nicotera, P., & Lipton, S. A. (1995). Apoptosis and necrosis: Two distinct events induced respectively by mild and intense insults with NMDA or nitric oxide/superoxide in cortical cell cultures. *Proc Natl Acad Sci USA, 92*, 7162–7166.

Bozyczko-Coyne, D., et al. (2001). CEP-1347/KT-7515, an inhibitor of SAPK/JNK pathway activation, promotes survival and blocks multiple events associated with a beta-induced cortical neuron apoptosis. *J Neurochem, 77*(3), 849–63.

Brancho, D., et al. (2005). Role of MLK3 in the regulation of mitogen-activated protein kinase signaling cascades. *Mol Cell Biol, 25*(9) 3670–81.

Bukrinsky, M. I., Nottet, H. S. L. M., Schmidtmayerova, H., et al. (1995). Regulation of nitric oxide synthase activity in human immunodeficiency virus type 1 (HIV-1)-infected monocytes: Implications for HIV-associated neurological disease. *J Exp Med, 181*, 735–745.

Chen, H-S. V., Pellegrini, J. W., Aggarwal, S. K., et al. (1992). Open-channel block of NMDA responses by memantine: Therapeutic advantage against NMDA receptor-mediated neurotoxicity. *J Neurosci, 12*, 4427–4436.

Clifford, D. B., McArthur, J. C., Schifitto, G., Kieburtz, K., McDermott, M. P., Letendre, S/, et al. Neurologic AIDS Research Consortium. (2002). A randomized clinical trial of CPI-1189 for HIV-associated cognitive-motor impairment. *Neurology, 59*, 1568–1573.

Conant, K., et al., (1998). Induction of monocyte chemoattractant protein-1 in HIV-1 Tat-stimulated astrocytes and elevation in AIDS dementia. *Proc Natl Acad Sci U S A, 95*(6) 3117–21.

Coyle, J. T. & Puttfarken, P. (1993). Oxidative stress, glutamate and neurodegenerative disorders. *Science, 262*, 689–695.

Dawson, V. L., Dawson, T. M., London, E. D., Bredt, D. S., & Snyder, S. H. (1991). Nitric oxide mediates glutamate neurotoxicity in primary cortical cultures. *Proc Natl Acad Sci USA, 88*, 6368–6371.

Dawson, V. L., Dawson, T. M., Uhl, G. R., & Snyder, S. H. (1993). Human immunodeficiency virus-1 coat protein neurotoxicity mediated by nitric oxide in primary cortical cultures. *Proc Natl Acad Sci USA, 90*, 3256–3259.

Digicaylioglu, M. & Lipton, S. A. (2001). Erythropoietsin mediated neuroprotection involves cross-talk between Jak2 and NF-κB signalling cascades. *Nature, 412*, 641–647.

Dreyer, E. B., Kaiser, P. K., Offermann, J. T., & Lipton, S. A. (1990). HIV-1 coat protein neurotoxicity prevented by calcium channel antagonists. *Science, 248*, 364–367.

Eggert, D., et al. (2009). Neuroprotective activities of CEP-1347 in models of neuroAIDS. *J Immunol.*

El-Hage, N., et al. (2006). HIV-1 Tat and opiate-induced changes in astrocytes promote chemotaxis of microglia through the expression of MCP-1 and alternative chemokines. *Glia, 53*(2) 132–46.

Ellis, R., Heaton, R., Letendre, S., Badiee, J., Munoz-Moreno, J., Vaida, F., et al. and the CHARTER group. (2010). Higher CD4 Nadir Is Associated with Reduced Rates of HIV-associated Neurocognitive Disorders in the CHARTER Study: Potential Implications for Early Treatment Initiation. Paper. 429, The 17th Conference on Retroviruses and Opportunistic Infections, 2010 CROI, San Francisco, CA.

Ellis, R. J., Rosario, D., Clifford, D. B., McArthur, J. C., Simpson, D., Alexander, T., et al.; CHARTER Study Group. (2010). Continued high prevalence and adverse clinical impact of human immunodeficiency virus-associated sensory neuropathy in the era of combination antiretroviral therapy: The CHARTER Study. *Arch Neurol, 67*(5), 552–8. PMID: 20457954.

Evans, S. R., Yeh, T. M., Sacktor, N., Clifford, D. B., Simpson, D., Miller, E. N., et al.; AIDS Clinical Trials Group and the Neurologic AIDS Research Consortium. (2007). Selegiline transdermal system (STS) for HIV-associated cognitive impairment: Open-label report of ACTG 5090. *HIV Clin Trials, 8*(6), 437–46. PMID: 18042509.

Follstaedt, S. C., Barber, S. A., & Zink, M. C. (2008). Mechanisms of minocycline-induced suppression of simian immunodeficiency virus encephalitis: Inhibition of apoptosis signal-regulating kinase 1. *J Neurovirol, 14*(5), 376–88. Epub 2008 Nov 12. PMID: 19003592.

Gallo, K. A. & Johnson, G. L. (2002). Mixed-lineage kinase control of JNK and p38 MAPK pathways. *Nat Rev Mol Cell Biol, 3*(9), 663–72.

Gao, Y. J., et al. (2009). JNK-induced MCP-1 production in spinal cord astrocytes contributes to central sensitization and neuropathic pain. *J Neurosci, 29*(13), 4096–108.

Garden, G., Budd, S. L.,. Tsai, E., Hanson, L., Kaul, M., D'Emilia, D. M., et al. (2002). Caspase cascades in HIV-associated neurodegeneration. *J Neurosci, 22*, 4015–4024.

Gelbard, H. A., Dewhurst, S., & Goodfellow, V. S. MLK inhibitors and methods of use. Composition of matter, attorney docket: URMC0001–101-US. International Patent Publication No. WO 2010/068483 A2.

Gelbard, H. A., James, H., Sharer, L., et al. (1995). Identification of apoptotic neurons in post-mortem brain tissue with HIV-1 encephalitis and progressive encephalopathy. *Neuropathol Appl Neurobiol, 21*, 208–217.

Gelbard, H. A., Nottet, H. S. L. M., Swindells, S., Jett, M., Dzenko, K. A., Genis, P., et al. (1994). Platelet-activating factor: A candidate human immunodeficiency virus type 1-induced neurotoxin. *J Virol, 68*, 4628–4635.

Geraci, A. P. & Simpson, D. M. (2001). Neurological manifestations of HIV-1 infection in the HAART era. *Compr Ther, 27*, 232–241.

Giulian, D., Vaca, K., & Noonan, C. A. (1990). Secretion of neurotoxins by mononuclear phagocytes infected with HIV-1. *Science, 250*, 1593–1596.

Giulian, D., Wendt, E., Vaca, K., & Noonan, C. A. (1993). The envelope glycoprotein of human immunodeficiency virus type 1 stimulates release of neurotoxins from monocytes. *Proc Natl Acad Sci USA, 90*, 2769–2773.

Kagan, V. E., Shvedova, A., Serbinova, E., et al. (1992). Dihydrolipoic acid—a universal antioxidant both in the membrane and in the aqueous phase. Reduction of peroxyl, ascorbyl and chromanoxyl radicals. *Biochem Pharmacol, 44*, 1637–1649.

Kang, Y. J., Digicaylioglu, M., Russo, R., Kaul, M., Achim, C. L., Fletcher, L., et al. (2010). Erythropoietin plus insulin-like growth factor-I protects against neuronal damage in a murine model of human immunodeficiency virus-associated neurocognitive disorders. *Ann Neurol, 68*, 342–352.

Kaul, M. & Lipton, S. A. (1999). Chemokines and activated macrophages in gp120-induced neuronal apoptosis. *Proc Natl Acad Sci USA, 96*, 8212–8216.

Kaul, M. & Lipton, S. A. (2000). The NMDA receptor—its role in neuronal apoptosis and HIV-associated dementia. *Science Online: NeuroAIDS, 3*, 1–5.

Kaul, M., Garden, G. A., & Lipton, S. A. (2001). Pathways to neuronal injury and apoptosis in HIV-associated dementia. *Nature, 410*, 988–994.

Kieburtz, K., Simpson, D., Yiannoutsos, C., Max, M. B., Hall, C. D., Ellis, R. J., et al. (1998). A randomized trial of amitriptyline and mexiletine for painful neuropathy in HIV infection. AIDS Clinical Trial Group 242 Protocol Team. *Neurology, 51*, 1682–1688.

Kim, W-K. & Lipton, S. A. (1994). Lipoic acid- and dihydrolipoic acid-mediated modulation of NMDA evoked Ca2+ responses in cortical neurons. *Soc Neurosci Abstr, 20*.

Lafon-Cazal, M., Pietri, S., Culcasi, M., & Bockaert, J. (1993). NMDA-dependent superoxide production and neurotoxicity. *Nature, 364*, 535–537.

Lai, A. Y. & Todd, K. G, (2008). Differential regulation of trophic and proinflammatory microglial effectors is dependent on severity of neuronal injury. *Glia, 56*(3), 259–70.

Le, D. & Lipton, S. A. (2001). Potential and current use of N-methyl-D-aspartate (NMDA) receptor antagonists in diseases of aging. *Drugs & Aging, 18*, 717–724.

Lei, S. Z., Zhang, D., Abele, A. E., & Lipton, S. A. (1992). Blockade of NMDA receptor-mediated mobilization of intracellular Ca2+ prevents neurotoxicity. *Brain Res, 598*, 196–202.

Lindl, D. A., Marks, D. R., Kolson, D. L., & Jordan-Sciutto, K. L. (2010). HIV-associated neurocognitive disorder: Pathogenesis and therapeutic opportunities. *J Neuroimmune Pharmacol, 5*, 294–309.

Lipton, S. A. (1992a). Memantine prevents HIV coat protein-induced neuronal injury in vitro. *Neurology, 42*, 1403–1405.

Lipton, S. A. (1992b). Models of neuronal injury in AIDS: Another role for the NMDA receptor? *Trends Neurosci, 15*, 75–79.

Lipton, S. A. (1992c). 7-Chlorokynurenate ameliorates neuronal injury mediated by HIV envelope protein gp120 in retinal cultures. *Eur J Neurosci, 4*, 1411–1415.

Lipton, S. A. (1993a). Human immunodeficiency virus-infected macrophages, gp120, and N-methyl-D-aspartate receptor-mediated neurotoxicity. *Ann Neurol, 33*, 227–228.

Lipton, S. A. (1993b). Prospects for clinically tolerated NMDA antagonists: Open-channel blockers and alternative redox states of nitric oxide. *Trends Neurosci, 16*, 527–532.

Lipton, S. A. (2006). Paradigm shift in neuroprotection by NMDA receptor blockade: Memantine and beyond. *Nat Rev Drug Dev, 5*, 160–170.

Lipton, S. A. (2007). Pathologically activated therapeutics for neuroprotection. *Nature Rev Neurosci, 8*, 803–808.

Lipton, S. A. & Gendelman, H. E. (1995). The dementia associated with the acquired immunodeficiency syndrome. *N Engl J Med, 332*, 934–940.

Lipton, S. A. & Jensen, F. E. (1992). Memantine, a clinically-tolerated NMDA open-channel blocker, prevents HIV coat protein-induced neuronal injury in vitro and in vivo. *Soc Neurosci Abstr, 18*, 757.

Lipton, S. A. & Rosenberg, P. A. (1994). Mechanisms of disease: Excitatory amino acids as a final common pathway for neurologic disorders. *N Engl J Med, 330*, 613–622.

Lipton, S. A., Choi, Y-B., Pan, Z-H., et al. (1993). A redox-based mechanism for the neuroprotective and neurodestructive effects of nitric oxide and related nitroso-compounds. *Nature, 364*, 626–632.

Lipton, S. A., Kaiser, P. K., Sucher, N. J., Dreyer, E. B., & Offermann, J. T. (1990). AIDS virus coat protein sensitizes neurons to NMDA receptor-mediated toxicity. *Soc Neurosci Abstr, 16*, 289.

Lipton, S. A., Sucher, N. J., Kaiser, P. K., & Dreyer, E. B. (1991). Synergistic effects of HIV coat protein and NMDA receptor-mediated neurotoxicity. *Neuron, 7*, 111–118.

Liu, J., et al., (2009). Neuromodulatory activities of CD4+CD25+ regulatory T cells in a murine model of HIV-1-associated neurodegeneration. *J Immunol, 182*(6), 3855–65.

Lotharius, J., et al., (2005). Progressive degeneration of human mesencephalic neuron-derived cells triggered by dopamine-dependent oxidative stress is dependent on the mixed-lineage kinase pathway. *J Neurosci, 25*(27), 6329–42.

Maggirwar, S. B., Tong, N., Ramirez, S., Gelbard, H. A., & Dewhurst, S. (1999). HIV-1 Tat-mediated activation of glycogen synthase kinase-3 beta contributed to Tat-mediated neurotoxicity. *J Neurochem, 73*, 578–586.

McGrath, M. S. & Hadlock, K. G. (WO/2007/035957) Methods for treating viral infections using polyamine analogs.

Müller, W. E. G., Schröder, H. C., Ushijima, H., Dapper, J., & Bormann, J. (1992). gp120 of HIV-1 induces apoptosis in rat cortical cell cultures: prevention by memantine. *Eur J Pharmacol—Molec Pharm Sect, 226*, 209–214.

Nakajima, K., et al., (2001). Neurotrophin secretion from cultured microglia. *J Neurosci Res, 65*(4), 322–31.

Nathans, R., Cao, H., Sharova, N., Ali, A., Sharkey, M., Stranska, R., et al. (2008). Small-molecule inhibition of HIV-1 Vif. *Nat Biotechnol, 26*(10), 1187–92. Epub 2008 Sep 21. PMID: 18806783.

Navia, B. A., Dafni, R., Simpson, D., Tucker, T., Singer, E., McArthur, J. C., et al. (1998). A phase I/II trial of nimodipine for HIV-related neurological complications. *Neurology, 51*, 221–228.

Neuenburg, J. K., Brodt, H. R., Herndier, B. G., Bickel, M., Bacchetti, P., Price, R. W., et al. HIV-related neuropathology, 1985 to 1999: Rising prevalence of HIV encephalopathy in the era of highly active antiretroviral therapy. *J Acquir Immune Defic Syndr, 31*, 171–177.

New, D. R., et al. (1998). HIV-1 Tat induces neuronal death via tumor necrosis factor-alpha and activation of non-N-methyl-D-aspartate receptors by a NFkappaB-independent mechanism. *J Biol Chem, 273*(28), 17852–8.

Perry, S. W., Dbaibo, G., Dzenko, K. A., Epstein, L. G., Hannan, Y., Whittaker, J. S., et al. (1998). PAF receptor activation: An initiator step in HIV-1 neuropathogenesis. *J Biol Chem, 273*, 17660–17664.

Petito, C. K. & Roberts, B. (1995). Evidence of apoptotic cell death in HIV encephalitis. *Am J Pathol, 146*, 1121–1130.

Power, C., Boissé, L., Rourke, S., & Gill, M. J. (2009). NeuroAIDS: An evolving epidemic. *Can J Neurol Sci, 36*(3), 285–95. PMID: 19534327.

Roux, P. P., et al. (2002). K252a and CEP1347 are neuroprotective compounds that inhibit mixed-lineage kinase-3 and induce activation of Akt and ERK. *J Biol Chem, 277*(51), 49473–80.

Sacktor, N. (2002). The epidemiology of human immunodeficiency virus-associated neurological disease in the era of highly active antiretroviral therapy. *J Neurovirol, 8*(Suppl 2), 115–121.

Sacktor, N., Schifitto, G., McDermott, M. P., Marder, K., McArthur, J. C., & Kieburtz, K. (2000). Transdermal selegiline in HIV-associated cognitive impairment: Pilot placebo-controlled study. *Neurology, 54*, 233–235.

Saporito, M. S., Thomas, B. A., & Scott, R. W, (2000). MPTP activates c-Jun NH(2)-terminal kinase (JNK) and its upstream regulatory kinase MKK 4 in nigrostriatal neurons in vivo. *J Neurochem, 75*(3), 1200–8.

Savio, T. & Levi, G. (1993). Neurotoxicity of HIV coat protein gp120, NMDA receptors, and protein kinase C: A study with rat cerebellar granule cell cultures. *J Neurosci Res, 34*, 265–272.

Schifitto, G., Navia, G. A., Yiannoustsos, C. T., Marra, C. M., Chang, L., Ernst, T., et al. (2007). Memantine and HIV-associated cognitive impairment: A neuropsychological and proton magnetic resonance spectroscopy study. *AIDS, 21*, 1877–1886.

Schifitto, G., Peterson, D. R., Zhong, J., Ni, H., Cruttenden, K., Gaugh, M., et al. (2006). Valproic acid adjunctive therapy for HIV-associated cognitive impairment: A first report. *Neurology, 66*(6), 919–21. Epub 2006 Mar 1. PMID: 16510768.

Schifitto, G., Sacktor, N., Marder, K., McDermott, M. P., McArthur, J. C., Kieburtz, K., et al., Neurological AIDS Research Consortium. (1999). Randomized trial of the platelet-activating factor antagonist lexipafant in HIV-associated cognitive impairment. *Neurol, 53*, 391–396.

Schifitto, G., Yiannoutsos, C. T., Ernst, T., Navia, B. A., Nath, A., Sacktor, N., et al.; ACTG 5114 Team. (2009). Selegiline and oxidative stress in HIV-associated cognitive impairment. *Neurology, 73*(23), 1975–81. Epub 2009 Nov 4. PMID: 19890073.

Schifitto, G., Yiannoutsos, C., Simpson, D. M., Adornato, B. T., Singer, E. J., Hollander, H., et al. The AIDS Clinical Trials Group Team 291. (2001). Long-term treatment with recombinant nerve growth factor for HIV-associated sensory neuropathy. *Neurology, 57*, 1313–1316.

Schifitto, G., Yiannoutsos, C. T., Simpson, D. M., Marra, C. M., Singer, E. J., Kolson, D. L., et al.; Adult AIDS Clinical Trials Group (ACTG) 301 tEAM. (2006). A placebo-controlled study of memantine for the treatment of human immunodeficiency virus-associated sensory neuropathy. *J Neurovirol, 12*(4), 328–31. PMID: 16966223

Schifitto, G., Zhong, J., Gill, D., Peterson, D. R., Gaugh, M. D., Zhu, T., et al. (2009). Lithium therapy for human immunodeficiency virus type 1-associated neurocognitive impairment. *J Neurovirol, 15*(2), 176–86.

Simioni, S., Cavassini, M., Annoni, J. M., Rimbault, A. A., Bourquin, I., et al. (2010). Cognitive dysfunction in HIV patients despite long-standing suppression of viremia. *AIDS, 24*(9), 1243–50. PMID: 19996937.

Sui, Z., et al. (2006). Inhibition of mixed lineage kinase 3 prevents HIV-1 Tat-mediated neurotoxicity and monocyte activation. *J Immunol, 177*(1), 702–11.

Talley, A., Dewhurst, S., Perry, S., et al. (1995). Tumor necrosis factor alpha induces apoptosis in human neuronal cells: Protection by the antioxidant N-acetylcysteine and the genes bcl 2 and crmA. *Mol Cell Biol, 15*, 2359–2366.

Tang, L. H. & Aizenman, E. (1993). Allosteric modulation of the NMDA receptor by dihydrolipoic and lipoic acid in rat cortical neurons in vitro. *Neuron, 11*, 857–863.

The Dana Consortium. (1997). Safety and tolerability of the antioxidant OPC-14117 in HIV-associated cognitive impairment. *Neurology, 49*, 142–146.

The Dana Consortium on Therapy for HIV Dementia and Related Cognitive Disorders. (1998). A randomized, double-blind, placebo-controlled trial of deprenyl and thioctic acid in human immunodeficiency virus-associated cognitive impairment. *Neurology, 50*, 645–651.

Toggas, S. M., Masliah, E., & Mucke, L. (1996). Prevention of HIV-1 gp120-induced neuronal damage in the central nervous system of transgenic mice by the NMDA receptor antagonist memantine. *Brain Res, 706*, 303–307.

Tong, N., Sanchez, J. F., Maggirwar, S. B., Ramirez, S., Dewhurst, S., & Gelbard, H. A. (2001). Activation of glycogen synthase kinase 3 beta (GSK-3β) by platelet activating factor mediates migration and cell death in cerebellar granule neurons. *Eur J Neurosci, 13*, 1913–1922.

Uthman, O. A. & J. O. Abdulmalik. (2008). Adjunctive therapies for AIDS dementia complex. *Cochrane Database Syst Rev*, (3), p. CD006496.

Wang, L. H. & Johnson, E. M. Jr., (2008). Mixed lineage kinase inhibitor CEP-1347 fails to delay disability in early Parkinson disease. *Neurology, 71*(6), 462; author reply 462–3.

Wang, L. H., Paden, A. J., & Johnson, E. M. Jr. (2005). Mixed-lineage kinase inhibitors require the activation of Trk receptors to maintain long-term neuronal trophism and survival. *J Pharmacol Exp Ther, 312*(3), 1007–19.

Wang, T., et al., (2008). HIV-1-infected astrocytes and the microglial proteome. *J Neuroimmune Pharmacol, 3*(3), 173–86.

Wang, X., Douglas, S. D., Song, L., Wang, Y. J., & Ho, W. Z. (2007). Neurokinin-1 receptor antagonist (aprepitant) suppresses HIV-1 infection of microglia/macrophages. *J Neuroimmune Pharmacol, 2*(1), 42–8. Epub 2007 Jan 12. PMID: 18040825.

Welch, K. & Morse, A. (2002). The clinical profile of end-stage AIDS in the era of highly active antiretroviral therapy. *AIDS Patient Care STDS, 16*, 75–81.

Yarchoan, R., Pluda, J. M., Thomas, R. V., et al. (1990). Long-term toxicity/activity profile of 2, 3 -dideoxyinosine in AIDS and AIDS-related complex. *Lancet, 336*, 526–529.

Yoshioka, M., Shapshak, P., Srivastava, A. K., et al. (1994). Expression of HIV-1 and interleukin-6 in lumbosacral dorsal root ganglia in patients with AIDS. *Neurology, 44*, 1120–1130.

Zhao, Y., Navia, B. A., Marra, C. M., Singer, E. J., Chang, L., Berger, J., et al.; Adult Aids Clinical Trial Group (ACTG) 301 Team. (2010). Memantine for AIDS dementia complex: Open-label report of ACTG 301. *HIV Clin Trials, 11*(1), 59–67. PMID: 20400412.

Zheng, J. C., et al. (2008). HIV-1-infected and/or immune-activated macrophages regulate astrocyte CXCL8 production through IL-1beta and TNF-alpha: Involvement of mitogen-activated protein kinases and protein kinase R. *J Neuroimmunol, 200*(1–2), 100–10.

Zink, M. C., Uhrlaub, J., DeWitt, J., Voelker, T., Bullock, B., Mankowski, J., et al. (2005). Neuroprotective and anti-human immunodeficiency virus activity of minocycline. *JAMA, 293*(16), 2003–11. PMID: 15855434.

SECTION 12

PSYCHIATRY AND PSYCHOBIOLOGY

Ian Paul Everall

12.1

PSYCHIATRIC DISORDERS

J. Hampton Atkinson, Nichole A. Duarte, and Glenn J. Treisman

This chapter reviews the epidemiology, clinical course, impact, and treatment of the most prevalent behavioral and psychiatric syndromes associated with HIV infection. These psychiatric conditions can broadly be classified either as primary, meaning the syndrome preceded the date of infection, or secondary, suggesting that the condition is directly or indirectly attributable to HIV itself, to cofactors associated with HIV infection, or to HIV treatments. The most prevalent primary disorders are mood disorders (major depression and bipolar disorder), alcohol and substance abuse (particularly abuse of injection drugs and stimulants), schizophrenia, and personality disorders. The most prevalent secondary conditions are mood syndromes (either depressive or manic) and deliria. Primary disorders may be associated with increased risk of infection, whereas both primary and secondary disorders may impact life quality, functioning, medical compliance, and perhaps survival.

INTRODUCTION

The intersection of behavioral disorders—psychiatric disorders and substance abuse—and HIV is a major challenge to clinicians, researchers, and policy makers. This convergence has been termed a "syndemic," to describe a state in which two or more linked conditions interact synergistically and contribute to excess burden of disease in a population (Walkup & Blank, 2008). On the one hand, behavioral disorders may help drive the acquisition, transmission, and progression of HIV illness; on the other hand, it is likely that viral-induced dysregulation in functioning of neural networks, along with drug abuse, may precipitate or accentuate psychiatric syndromes in certain individuals, based on evidence that substances of abuse and mediators of both psychopathology and HIV-neuropathogenesis share common neural pathways and receptor systems. This chapter reviews the epidemiology, clinical course, impact, and treatment of the most prevalent behavioral and psychiatric syndromes associated with HIV infection. These psychiatric conditions can broadly be classified either as primary, meaning the syndrome preceded date of infection, or secondary, suggesting the condition is directly or indirectly attributable to HIV itself, to cofactors associated with HIV infection, or to HIV treatments. The most prevalent psychiatric disorders in HIV populations are mood disorders (major depression and bipolar disorder), alcohol and substance abuse or dependence (particularly injection drugs

and stimulants), schizophrenia, and personality disorders, and as primary disorders they may be associated with increased risk of infection. Mood syndromes (either depressive or manic), and deliria are probably the most prevalent secondary conditions. Both primary and secondary disorders may impact life quality, everyday functioning, adherence to medical care, and perhaps survival.

ESTIMATING PREVALENCE OF PSYCHIATRIC AND SUBSTANCE DISORDERS IN HIV

The worldwide standard for estimating the prevalence of psychiatric disorders is large scale study of the population based on assessments of a randomly selected sample (usually numbering in the tens of thousands of individuals) living in the community, who are examined by an interviewer using a standardized psychiatric instrument. The result yields estimates of lifetime and more recent (e.g., within the last 12 months) occurrence of specific psychiatric disorders, diagnosed using widely accepted criteria, like the International Classification of Diseases (ICD-10) or Diagnostic and Statistical Manual-IV (DSM-IV). Prime recent examples of this approach are the World Health Organization-sponsored World Mental Health Survey (World Health Organization, 1997), the United States (U.S.) National Comorbidity Survey (Kessler et al., 1994), the U.S. National Epidemiological Survey on Alcohol and Related Conditions (Grant et al., 2003), and the New Zealand Mental Health Survey (Wells et al., 2006). The nature of the AIDS epidemic and the expense of such research make this approach impractical for HIV, leaving us with sample frequency estimates based primarily on a relatively small number of individuals. Even accurate estimates of the sample frequency remain elusive, primarily because methodological issues have led to widely varying reports of the proportion of "cases" (Rabkin, 2008). One methodological limitation is sampling. Some estimates are based on case studies (Deuchar, 1984) and series derived from hospitalized or clinic samples referred for psychiatric evaluation (Dilley et al., 1985; Perry & Tross, 1984). This bias likely overstates the association of HIV with psychiatric conditions, and sampling from community volunteers usually reflects lower estimates (Rabkin, 2008). Beyond the distinction between clinic and community is the changing nature of the HIV epidemic itself. Initial research, in North America and

Europe, studied an index population of urban, generally more affluent, gay men; more recently, the epidemic in the developed world has centered on injection drug users (Rabkin, 2008). These populations are only partially overlapping, and substance abuse is by itself associated with psychiatric comorbidity. One more sampling issue is the stage of HIV disease studied. This is important because current rates of substance abuse and mood disorder, for example, may differ between early and late stage disease: Compared to asymptomatic HIV infection, frank AIDS appears to be associated with greater risk of mood disorder but lower likelihood of substance abuse (Atkinson et al., 2008). Finally, it should also be noted that many studies of association of psychopathology and HIV fail to include an HIV-negative control group from the same "risk" category (e.g., homosexual men or injection drug users). When this is done, rates of disorders are often similar between infected and uninfected individuals.

Other methodological issues include criterion variance in case definition (Rabkin, 2008). Psychiatric diagnosis requires specific diagnostic criteria be met. These criteria consist of sets of specific symptoms or behaviors, along with evidence that the syndrome has an impact on everyday function. Different studies use different diagnostic schemes. This adds variation since there are differences between ICD-10 and DSM-IV criteria. The forthcoming edition of the Diagnostic and Statistical Manual, DSM-V, will include revised criteria for various disorders, which may add additional variability. Researchers likewise use different measurement methods. Two main types of diagnostic instruments have been used in the HIV psychiatric research literature. Some measures (e.g., Diagnostic Interview Schedule, DIS; Robins et al., 1995; Composite International Diagnostic Instrument, CIDI; World Health Organization, 1997) are for use by nonclinicians. These measures are fully structured, meaning that every question is asked verbatim and each response is pre-specified (usually in "yes-no" format). No interviewer "judgment" is involved as to whether the criterion symptom meets the threshold for being clinically "meaningful." Their concordance with clinician-based measures is moderate to good, particularly for major depression and substance use disorder (e.g., concordance 0.6–0.9; Haro et al., 2006), but is less than acceptable for other important conditions like bipolar disorder (which is over-estimated) and schizophrenia (under-estimated, Whittchen, 1998).

Research using instruments requiring clinician interviewers are generally considered the gold standard. In this approach, clinicians use all available data, and render a clinical judgment on whether each criterion symptom is present and whether the "package" of symptoms and interference with function meets criteria for a clinical diagnosis. Among these measures, the Structured Clinical Interview for DSM-IV (SCID; First et al., 1994) is most widely used in the literature. The expense of clinical personnel, plus the work of training and maintaining multiple interviewers to a criterion inter-rater reliability makes use of these instruments less feasible for larger scale studies.

Perhaps most impacting on frequency estimates is the confusion generated by use of self-report measures to identify diagnoses like "depression" or "drug abuse" when what is actually detected may be "depressed or distressed mood" or an index of "drug use" rather than a syndromic disorder (e.g., Rabkin, 2008). Although there is evidence for some correspondence of self-report scores and clinician diagnosis, there is variability, and studies often employ different self-report measures and different cut-scores to define cases. The usual result is an overestimation of frequency of clinical diagnoses. Another methodological issue is information variance, or what the patient reports to the interviewer (e.g., recall bias). This may affect estimates of frequency in patients with HIV-associated neurocognitive impairment, who may fail to recall episodes of mood or substance use disorders. Few studies report on the neurocognitive characteristics of the sample. Finally there are some important gaps in the literature that impact any discussion of "prevalence" of psychiatric disorder in HIV. There is still little data on women (see Morrison et al., 2002), as well as on African-American and Hispanic populations. The relevance of such gaps is that, for example, and independent of HIV, women as a group appear to be at elevated risk for certain psychiatric disorders (e.g., major depression) compared to men (Robbins & Regier, 1991). Consistent with this observation, recent reports suggest HIV-infected women may have higher rates of mood disorders than do infected men (Morrison et al., 2002). Moreover, the impact or expression of psychiatric disorders may vary across cultural groups (Hough et al., 1987). Perhaps most important is that most data are obtained from samples in North America and northwest Europe, despite the fact that the majority of infected individuals live in Africa, China, and India. It is likely that the psychiatric profiles of these populations will differ from each other and from the Western world.

MOOD DISORDERS

Major depression and bipolar disorder are the most prevalent primary mood disorders in HIV. Diagnosis of a primary mood disorder implies that its onset preceded HIV infection or that the episode does not appear to be physiologically related to HIV illness. The diagnosis of a primary mood disorder also implies the syndrome is not due to intoxication or withdrawal from substances of abuse (e.g., alcohol, CNS depressants, cocaine, amphetamines) and is not due to medications used to treat HIV or it associated conditions. Secondary mood disorders are diagnosed if the disturbance in mood is thought to be due to the physiological effects of medical illness or to medications or substances of abuse. The subtypes are (a) with depressive features (if full criteria for major depression or mania are not met); (b) with major depression-like episode (if full criteria for major depression are evident); (c) with manic features (if mood is euphoric); and (d) with mixed features (if symptoms of depression and mania are present but neither predominates). Simply because a mood disturbance occurs after the point of HIV infection does not mean that the disorder is "secondary" to HIV. Current data suggests that most mood disorders in HIV are the result of disorders commencing before HIV, or whose "first onset" is after HIV but which do not appear to be physiologically related to HIV. There is emerging evidence that advanced HIV disease may be associated with a secondary major depression, and strong clinical evidence that later-stage HIV disease is associated with a 'secondary' manic syndrome (e.g., Triesman et al., 1998; Lyketsos et al., 1993). It is likely, however, that the most prevalent secondary mood disorders in HIV-infected populations are substance-induced (due to intoxication withdrawal from alcohol, cocaine, or methamphetamine). These distinctions are relevant in framing a research agenda and in selecting treatment strategies.

MAJOR DEPRESSION

Epidemiology

Population-based community epidemiologic surveys indicate a lifetime prevalence of major depressive disorder among men at 3–19% and for women at 5–21% (e.g., Robbins et al., 1991; Kessler et al., 1994; Kessler et al., 2005 Grant et al., 2003Wells et al., 2006;). Twelve-month prevalence ranges from 4–10% (Robbins et al., 1991; Kessler et al., 1994; Kessler et al., 2005; Wells et al., 2006; Grant et al., 2003). This is compared to studies of men at highest risk for HIV (homosexual or IDU men), where lifetime frequency is estimated to range between 25% and 35% (Atkinson et al., 1988; Williams et al., 1991; Perkins et al., 1994; Rosenberg et al., 1992; Bing et al., 2001; Evans et al., 2002). Most studies in HIV also report current (last 30 days) prevalence of major depression: The rates have generally been in the range of 5–20% for seropositive homosexual/bisexual or IDU individuals (Williams et al., 1991; Evans et al., 2005). This upper limit is reflected in recent clinic samples using rigorous diagnostic evaluation (e.g., 21%, Gaynes et al., 2008). Perhaps the most representative survey, the U.S. national HIV Cost and Utilization Study, examined over 2,800 HIV+ individuals receiving medical care (Frankel et al., 1999). Patients were screened for mood disorders, and were then examined with a psychodiagnostic interview if the screener was positive. The current prevalence of major depression was 22% (Hayes et al., 2000).

Women may be at even higher risk: Those who are IDUs or partners of IDUs have lifetime rates approaching 40% (e.g., 33%). One study of women without substance use disorders found almost 20% had current major depression compared 5% among HIV-negative women (Morrison et al., 2002); another study noted frequency of 15% in HIV+ women, compared to 10% in sociodemographically matched seronegative controls (Evans et al. 2002). Other studies of non-substance-using women have shown current rates around 2% (e.g., 34%).

Whether HIV+ individuals have higher current or lifetime occurrence of major depression compared to HIV-negative individuals drawn from the same risk group is unclear (Rabkin, 2008. Most cross-sectional surveys find no difference in frequencies (Rabkin, 2008); one meta-analysis noted higher rates for infected individuals (Ciesla & Roberts, 2001; Rabkin, 2008). In a related fashion it is uncertain if disease stage heightens risk of major depression. Most cross-sectional surveys do not feature comparisons across carefully diagnosed disease stages, and instead treat all seropositive individuals as a single group. Some studies do find no differences between rigorously staged medically asymptomatic (e.g., Centers for Disease Control [CDC] Stage A) and symptomatic stages (Stages B and C; e.g., Atkinson et al., 1988) in cross-sectional rates of current (last 30 days) major depression. On the other hand, one 2-year follow-up study suggested an annual 20% risk of a major depressive episode in patients with medically symptomatic disease, which was about double the risk of medically asymptomatic individuals, whose rates were equivalent to uninfected risk-group controls (Atkinson et al., 2008). Apart from research findings, the general clinical impression is that advanced illness elevates risk of mood disorder.

In summary, individuals from groups at highest risk for HIV infection appear to have elevated rates of major depression that preceded infection; after infection, their risk of major depression is at least in line with, and may exceed, the frequency in samples of other chronic medical and neurological illness (e.g., stroke, multiple sclerosis, Alzheimer's disease, Huntington's disease, Parkinson's disease; Cummings & Trimble, 1995). Women may be particularly vulnerable to major depression (Morrison et al., 2002).

Etiology

The etiology of depressive disorders involves social, behavioral, and neurobiological factors (Whetten et al., 2008). Separately, each of these by itself is the subject of comprehensive reviews and texts (e.g., Brown & Harris, 1978a; Green & Pope, 2000; Nestler et al., 2002). In the context of HIV, primary major depression can spontaneously occur before HIV, after infection, or at any stage of illness due to the interplay of any or all of these factors. Adverse life events common to HIV (e.g., bereavement, loss of job) can result in major depressive episodes (e.g., see Moore et al., 1999). A history of physical and sexual abuse is highly prevalent (30–50%) in both HIV+ men and women (Whetten et al., 2008) and may be a background or predisposing factor. Social stigma and discrimination against gay and bisexual individuals is widespread, as is bias towards those infected with HIV (Whetten et al., 2008). Women may bear this burden disproportionally (Hader et al., 2001). Although most studies suggest that in about 50% of cases of major depression in HIV the first episode preceded the date of seroconversion (e.g., Atkinson et al., 1988), *secondary* depressive mood disorders may be ascribed to neurobiological factors directly associated with HIV. For example, one recent autopsy study of individuals dying of advanced HIV found evidence that altered somatostatin gene expression in the brain was associated with a history of recent pre-mortem depressive illness when compared to those dying without mood disorder (Everall et al., 2006). It is tempting to speculate that such changes in gene expression underlie the observation that risk of major depression increases in later-stage HIV. Other factors associated with secondary depression include substance-induced depression and depressive episodes due to medications, alcohol, or drugs. There is some concern, but little evidence, that protease inhibitors induce major depressive episodes. On the other hand, it is clear that treatment of comorbid hepatitis with interferon alpha induces a depressive mood disorder (Valentine, 1998). Heavy alcohol consumption (drinking to the point of intoxication throughout the day for 30 days) is associated with a depressive mood disorder, which remits after about one month of sobriety (Brown & Schuckit, 1998). Binges of cocaine or methamphetamine use (repeated daily use for 3–5 days) are associated with a depressive syndrome after cessation (a withdrawal syndrome). These stimulant-induced disorders spontaneously remit in less than a week.

Diagnosis

The DSM-IV diagnosis of major depression requires that five (or more) of nine symptoms are present nearly every day for the same 2-week period. At least one of these symptoms must be (a) depressed mood or (b) loss of interest or pleasure in usually pleasurable activity. The symptom complex must cause meaningful distress or impairment in daily activities, including social or occupational obligations, and not be the product of medications, drug or alcohol use, or medical illness.

The nine criterion symptoms are (a) subjective report of depressed mood, or observation by other (tearfulness); (b) diminished interest or pleasure in almost all activities; (c) unintended weight loss or gain (> 5% of body weight in a month) or diminished appetite; (d) insomnia or hypersomnia; (e) observable psychomotor retardation or agitation; (f) fatigue or loss of energy; (g) feelings of absolute worthlessness or excessive guilt (not simply self-reproach or guilt about being ill); (h) diminished ability to think, concentrate, or be decisive; and (i) recurrent thought of death (not just fear of dying), or suicidal ideation or plans. The differential diagnosis includes primary major depression, major depression-like syndromes due to HIV illness or treatment of its comorbid conditions, and substance-induced mood disorders due to intoxication or withdrawal. In most cases the differential is rather straightforward. A diagnosis of major depression secondary to HIV is at present generally restricted to cases in which the only reportable antecedent to the mood episode is a clear worsening of HIV disease with a contemporaneous and sudden decline in mood. Diagnosis of a substance-induced disorder depends on history of recent introduction of a medication (e.g., prednisone) or detection of substance abuse.

Course

There are few longer-term prospective studies, and most of these evaluate depression symptoms rather than major depressive episodes. Chronic depressive symptoms seem to characterize a substantial minority of HIV+ individuals. For example, the multisite, seven-year Women's Interagency HIV Study (WIHS) reported that about one-third of the cohort experienced clinically significant depressive symptoms on 75% of their semi-annual follow-up visits (Cook et al., 2004).

According to the HIV Epidemiology Research Study, 42% of the cohort reported clinically significant depressive symptoms on at least 75% of their bi-annual follow-up visits (Ickovics et al., 2001). The Multicenter AIDS Cohort Study reported an average 45% increase in depressive symptoms among participants at two-year follow-up; the most pronounced increase in depressive symptomology occurred in those participants who subsequently developed AIDS (Lyketsos et al., 1996).

There is some variation in risk over time, likely due to variations in sampling. One study reported the cumulative two-year incidence of major depressive episode ranged from 20% in physically asymptomatic CDC stages to almost 40% in those with medically symptomatic disease (Atkinson et al., 2008). Most of these two-year incident cases were recurrent mood disorder rather than new onset, as might be expected given the high lifetime base rates in certain high-risk groups (e.g., homosexual/bisexual men, IDUs; Atkinson & Grant, 1994). The course of individual depressive episodes is variable. Individuals may have infrequent depressive episodes spaced widely apart, whereas a few individuals have more frequent episodes (two or more annually). In some cases, a more chronic course ensues (Atkinson & Grant, 1994). Whether major depression is more severe or intractable in the neurocognitively impaired person is unknown.

Impact

The practical importance of major depression is that it impacts everyday function, including adherence to antiretroviral treatment, and perhaps affects progression of HIV disease. A focus of current research is the important role that depression plays in the progression and prognosis of HIV illness. A recent study reports that seropositive women with depression had significantly higher activated CD8 T lymphocyte counts and significantly lower natural killer cell activity than seropositive women without depression (Evans et al., 2002b). In addition, mortality from AIDS was doubled among women with chronic depressive symptoms compared to women without depressive symptoms (Ickovics et al., 2001).

Treatment

Regardless of whether the depressive disorder is primary or secondary to HIV, medications, or substances of abuse, the greatest barrier to treatment is under-diagnosis: Data from the HIV Costs and Service Utilization Study (HCSUS) found that 45% of those with a diagnosis of major depression did not have this documented in the medical record (Whetten et al., 2008; Asch et al., 2003). Except for the substance-induced conditions, in which definitive treatment is removal of the offending agent, antidepressant pharmacotherapy is the mainstay of treatment for major depression. Cognitive-behavioral therapy can be effective for mild-to-moderately severe cases of depression (Safren et al., 2008). Several randomized clinical trials have demonstrated the efficacy of different classes of antidepressants (e.g. Rabkin et al., 1994a; Rabkin et al., 1994b; Rabkin, 1994c; Zisook et al., 1998).

The patients with the best chance of improvement are those who adhere to the medication regimen. For example, in homeless, substance-abusing, and difficult-to-reach populations, patients receiving directly observed therapy with antidepressants have better outcomes than those referred to standard psychiatric clinics (Bangsberg et al., 2006), and the same is true for patients whose antidepressant treatment is closely monitored by nurse care managers (Pyne et al., 2005). Because adverse effects are a leading cause of discontinuing treatment, most clinicians select agents based on minimizing side-effect profiles or using side effects to therapeutic advantage. For example, if insomnia is a prominent problem, a sedating antidepressant may be employed. In addition, if the patient has chronic diarrhea, it would be prudent to use an agent with few gastrointestinal effects. Side effects should be assessed at every visit. Independent treatment of severe persistent side effects may preserve adherence and switching medication regimens to a more tolerable agent may be necessary. The antidepressant class of choice by consensus panels is the serotonin-selective reuptake inhibitors (SSRIs) based on their more favorable side-effect profile, followed by the serotonin-noradrenaline reuptake inhibitors (SNRIs; Freudenreich et al., 2010). Among the SSRIs, the standard initial choices are citalopram or escitalopram, based on tolerability. Although tricyclic antidepressants have equivalent efficacy, they may be less well tolerated in patients with HIV, particularly due to anticholinergic side effects (Repetto et al., 2003). In medically ill HIV patients it is prudent to use the dictum of geriatric psychiatry, "start low and go slow," meaning to start antidepressants at the lowest starting dose and titrate slowly upwards to the expected therapeutic dose. An adequate trial at a particular dose is six weeks. If the initial trial fails, the modern approach is either to select another agent from the same class (e.g., another SSRI. like sertraline),

or to switch to another class of antidepressant medication (e.g., an SNRI, like duloxetine). Outcomes are generally equivalent with either strategy, at least in non-HIV populations (e.g., Fava et al., 2003). Referral for psychiatric consultation is probably warranted after the first or second trial failure, since combination treatment with two or more antidepressants or augmenting agents or very high dosages may be needed. Among the most common causes of treatment "resistance" is the presence of undetected substance use disorders. After the initial introduction of modern antiretroviral agents there were concerns about drug-drug interactions with many standard antidepressants, based on effects on common metabolic pathways (e.g., Cytochrome P450; see Sandson et al., 2005). In practice, these potential interactions appear to be clinically relevant only in selected instances in either direction (i.e., antiretrovirals altering antidepressant concentrations, or antidepressants altering antiretroviral levels). Table 12.1.1 summarizes the antidepressants whose plasma concentrations are reported to be most likely to be affected, the direction of the effect, and specific antiretroviral agents involved. Tricyclic antidepressants are particularly affected. For example amitriptyline, nortriptyline, imipramine concentrations may be increased by regimens employing ritonavir, and desipramine concentrations may be increased by nelfinavir and ritonavir-containing therapies. Of the SSRIs, paroxetine concentrations may be decreased by darunavir and fosamprenavir, and sertraline concentrations reduced by darunavir. Trazodone is an antidepressant with serotonin reuptake inhibitor properties, and is most often used as a hypnotic for insomnia. Its concentration is increased by darunavir, indinavir, lopinavir/ritonaivr and ritonavir. Levels of bupropion, an antidepressant with noradrenaline and dopamine reuptake inhibition, are decreased by efavirenz, lopinavir/ritonavir, and tipranavir. If antidepressants in Table 12.1.1

Table 12.1.1 OVERVIEW OF ANTIDEPRESSANTS USED FOR MAJOR DEPRESSION IN HIV ILLNESS

DRUG	START DOSE	USUAL THERAPEUTIC DOSE	INTERACTIONS WITH HIV MEDICINES
Nortriptyline (Pamelor)	10–25 mg q hs	50–150 mg q hs	*Increase nortriptyline levels* Fluconazole, Lopinavir/Ritonavir, Ritonavir
Desipramine (Norpramin)	10–25 mg q hs	50–200 mg q hs	*Increase desipramine levels* Lopinavir/Ritonavir, Ritonavir
Imipramine (Tofranil)	10–25 mg q hs	100–300 mg q hs	*Increase imipramine levels* Lopinavir/Ritonavir, Ritonavir
Amitriptyline (Elavil)	10–25 mg q hs	100–300 mg q hs	*Increase amitriptyline levels* Lopinavir/Ritonavir, Ritonavir
Clomipramine (Anafranil)	25 mg q hs	100–200 mg q hs	*Increase clomipramine levels* Lopinavir/Ritonavir, Ritonavir
Doxepin (Sinequan)	10–25 mg q hs	150–250 mg q hs	*Increase doxepin levels* Lopinavir/Ritonavir, Ritonavir
Trazodone (Desyrel)	50–100 mg q hs	50–150 mg q hs for sleep; 200–600 mg q hs for depression	*Increases trazodone levels* Lopinavir/Ritonavir, Ritonavir
Sertraline (Zoloft)	25-50 mg q hs or am	100-200 mg q hs or am	*Decreases sertraline levels* Darunavir
Bupropion (Wellbutrin)	100 mg q am	150–400 mg/d in divided doses	*Decrease bupropion levels* Efavirenz, Lopinavir/ritonavir, Tipranavir

are employed close monitoring may be necessary to achieve therapeutic benefits and avoid and adverse side effects.

MANIA AND BIPOLAR DISORDERS

Epidemiology

Population-based surveys suggest bipolar disorder type I, a mood disorder with at least one manic episode in its course, has a lifetime prevalence of 2% (Grant et al., 2004). Bipolar disorder II, which consists of hypomanic episodes and recurrent major depressive episodes, has a lifetime community prevalence of about 0.5% (Judd & Akiskal, 2003). Because both mania and hypomania may be characterized by risk taking, impaired judgment, activation, heightened sexual drive, and concurrent substance abuse, patients with bipolar disorder are at increased risk of HIV infection (Meade et al., 2008). By some estimates, the prevalence of bipolar disorder in HIV outpatient psychiatric populations is around 8% (Beyer et al., 2007; Cruess et al., 2003). As described below, manic episodes can be due to HIV disease itself (secondary disorder). There are no formal studies of the prevalence of manic episodes caused by HIV. Before the era of modern combination antiretroviral treatment, clinic samples of convenience cited a prevalence of around 1% (Schmidt & Miller, 1988), but with current treatment regimens secondary mania has virtually disappeared in North American and European settings.

Etiology

The etiology of bipolar disorder is unknown but it is thought to involve genetic, personal, and social factors (Hilty et al., 1999). HIV is not thought to be a causative factor in bipolar disorder (i.e., HIV disease itself does not universally cause manic or hypomanic episodes and recurrent major depression); however, it is clear that HIV can precipitate what is termed a "secondary" manic episode. Secondary mania ("AIDS mania") appears to be a consequence of late-stage HIV disease and co-occurring neurocognitive impairment (Mijch et al., 1999). In a case series conducted prior to the introduction of potent combination antiretrovirals, patients whose first manic episode occurred late in their HIV course, when their CD4 count was below 200, were compared with patients whose first manic episode came earlier, when their CD4 count was above 200. The patients whose first manic episodes occurred later were less likely to have a personal or a family history of mania or any mood disorder, suggesting they were less likely to have underlying bipolar disorder or a genetic predisposition to mania. Patients whose first manic episode occurred later were also more likely to have dementia or other cognitive impairment indicating brain damage (Lyketsos et al., 1997; Ellen et al., 1999). Secondary mania is presently most often observed in the developing world (e.g., Africa), where the absence of early diagnosis and modern antiretroviral treatment means that patients are likely to present with advanced disease (Nakamuli-Mpungu et al., 2006).

Diagnosis

The diagnosis of idiopathic bipolar mania using DSM-IV criteria requires at least a one-week period of an abnormally elevated, expansive, or irritable mood (or of any duration if hospitalization is required because of the mood abnormality). At least three of the following symptoms (four if the mood is irritable but not elevated) must be concurrent: (a) highly inflated self-esteem or grandiosity; (b) diminished need for sleep (e.g., feels rested after only two or three hours sleep); (c) increased talkativeness; (d) subjective sense of racing thoughts or rapid shifting from thought to thought (flight of ideas); (e) distractibility; (f) increased activity (either aimless agitation or in goal-directed work, school, social, or sexual activity); and (g) excessive involvement in pleasurable activity at high risk for adverse consequences (e.g., buying sprees, sexual sprees).

AIDS mania seems to have a somewhat different clinical profile than mania associated with idiopathic bipolar disorder. Patients with AIDS mania tend to have more cognitive impairment and in some cases are likely to be irritable, aggressive, paranoid, and to have auditory and visual hallucinations (Nakamuli-Mpungu et al., 2006). Without a previous dementia diagnosis it may be difficult to ascertain AIDS mania in the midst of an acute manic episode. History usually reveals progressive cognitive decline prior to the onset of mania. Prominent psychomotor slowing that sometimes accompanies the cognitive slowing of AIDS dementia may replace the expected hyperactivity of mania, which complicates the differential diagnosis. A delirium with hyperactive features must be considered in the differential diagnosis. Delirium is associated with rapidly shifting attention and hypervigilance, though this may be initially difficult to distinguish from the activated state in mania. Also included in the differential diagnosis should be mania precipitated by the treatment of comorbid conditions, including the treatment of chronic hepatitis C (HCV) infection with pegylated interferon (Onyike et al., 2009) as well as other frequently used substances like steroids, isoniazid, dopaminergic agents, triazolobenzodiazepines (e.g., triazolam, Halcion[R]), and cimedtidine.

Course

Clinical experience suggests that AIDS mania is usually quite severe in its presentation and malignant in its course. According to a study conducted by Lyketsos et al. (1997), late-onset patients (i.e., secondary mania) had a greater total number of manic symptoms than early-onset patients (i.e., primary mania). Patients exhibiting secondary mania were also more commonly irritable and less commonly hyper-talkative compared to patients who exhibited primary mania. AIDS mania is characterized by a more chronic course (as opposed to episodic) and remission is often spontaneous and infrequent with symptoms usually remerging with the cessation of treatment. In part due to their cognitive deficits, which are likely confounded by severe manic symptomology, patients who exhibit AIDS mania are less able to pursue treatment independently or consistently (Lyketsos et al., 1997). One clinically described presentation of mania, either primary or secondary, is the delusional belief that one has discovered a cure for HIV, or has been cured. While this may serve to boost the mood of otherwise demoralized and depressed patients, it may also result in the resumption of high-risk behavior and lead to the spread of HIV and exposure to other infectious entities. When euphoria is a prominent symptom in otherwise debilitated late-stage patients, caregivers may wistfully question the humaneness of robbing patients of the illusion of happiness. It is the clearly impairing, often devastating effects of the other symptoms of mania that tips the balance of the risk/benefit equation towards treatment.

Treatment

The treatment of mania in early-stage HIV infection is not substantially different than the standard treatment of bipolar disorder. It relies on the use of mood-stabilizing medications such as lithium salts, and valproic acid, as well as antipsychotic agents, now more commonly atypical agents. These medications decrease manic symptoms and may prevent recurrence of manic episodes.

As HIV infection advances and the patient has a lower CD4 count, more medical illness, increasing CNS involvement, and is at greater overall physiologic vulnerability, treatment strategies may be somewhat different. While treatment with traditional mood-stabilizing medications may be preferred, this can be very difficult in patients with advanced disease. Patients experiencing AIDS mania may respond to treatment with antipsychotic medications alone. In general, late-stage patients are far more sensitive to the therapeutic effects, but even more so to the toxic side effects, of antipsychotic agents. In late-stage disease the dose of antipsychotic needed may be much lower than customarily used for mania in other settings. The more advanced the patients' HIV and/or dementia, the more sensitive they are to dosage changes that might otherwise seem trivial. These patients can develop extrapyramidal symptoms, but will also prove very sensitive to the side effects, especially delirium, of anticholinergic agents. Drug-drug interactions between antipsychotics and antiretrovirals appear to be limited. For example olanzapine concentrations may be decreased by ritonaivr.

Atypical antipsychotics, such as quetiapine (Seroquel), risperidone (Risperdal), olanzapine (Zyprexa), ziprasidone (Geodon), and aripiprazole (Abilify) have mostly replaced older medications (Fruedenreich et al., 2010). These agents may have fewer side effects than traditional antipsychotics, but have liabilities (e.g., high risk of metabolic syndrome with olanzapine; hyperprolactinemia with risperidone). Due to their more favorable side-effect profile, these medications are now often first-line, and may be primary treatment in most advanced cases. Starting doses should be low and titrated to a level that is effective. Total daily doses of risperidone may be as low as 1–3 mg; for olanzepine the dose may be as low as 2–10 mg daily. There has been considerable experience with traditional mood-stabilizing agents in selected AIDS mania patients, but with relatively sparse documentation. Lithium use has been problematic for several reasons,

including high rates of associated delirium and cognitive difficulty, gastrointestinal symptoms including nausea and diarrhea, the likelihood of renal insufficiency in this population, and polyuria resulting in dehydration. Lithium is also rarely associated with the development of diabetes insipidus. The major problem with lithium in patients with advanced disease has been rapid fluctuations in blood level, occurring even in the hospital on previously stable doses, causing lithium toxicity. Valproic acid has been used with success, titrating to the usual therapeutic serum levels of 50–100 mg/dl. Enteric-coated formulations (Depakote) are better tolerated in most patients. Use is sometimes limited by side effects, or because of concerns of hepatotoxicity in cases where patients have comorbid chronic viral hepatitis; in these cases monitoring of liver function tests is necessary, but hepatic toxicity is not often a problem. In cases of severe hepatic mycobacterium avium complex (MAC) infiltration (e.g., with portal hypertension), valproic acid should likely be avoided. Valproate can also inhibit hematopoeitic function so white blood cell and platelet counts must be monitored. Carbamazepine may also be effective, but can be poorly tolerated because of sedation, and has a potential for synergistic bone marrow suppression in combination with antiretroviral medications and HIV itself. Anticonvulsants such as gabapentin (Neurontin) and lamotrigine (Lamictal) may be effective, but there is little data on their use. Electroconvulsive therapy has been successfully used in AIDS mania patients who did not tolerate conventional therapy (Ferrando & Nims, 2006).

PSYCHOTIC DISORDERS

Psychosis refers to severe mental illness which impairs everyday function, perceptions, thinking, and in some instances, basic neurocognitive abilities. Schizophrenia, the most prevalent primary psychotic illness, is associated with high rates of HIV infection, ranging from 4% and 19% in large urban centers of the AIDS pandemic (Cournos et al., 1991), and with high rates of co-morbid HCV infection (Cournos & McKinnon, 2005). Part of this vulnerability to infection is due to high rates of concurrent substance abuse. And although many individuals with schizophrenia are not sexually active, those who are active are at high risk because psychosis is marked by poor impulse control, difficulty planning, and limited abilities in judging and evaluating the consequences of one's actions. This makes them likely to engage in unprotected sex, have multiple sex partners, and to trade sex for money or other goods, and to engage in sex while intoxicated (Cournos et al., 1994). Women with schizophrenia are thought to be especially vulnerable and at higher risk for HIV. Further, there is evidence that patients with more positive symptoms and impulse control problems are at increased risk for high-risk sexual behavior despite demonstration of adequate knowledge of HIV risk factors (McKinnon et al., 1996). Practitioners who see patients with schizophrenia should screen carefully for risk behaviors in addition to inquiring about knowledge of HIV risks. One screening tool, the Risk Behaviors

Questionnaire (RBQ), consists of 13 questions and has been validated for use in psychiatric patients (Volavka et al., 1992).

In terms of secondary mental disorders, it appears that in late stage disease, HIV itself is associated with a "new-onset" psychosis. The term psychosis in this context probably represents mostly undiagnosed delirium, but may additionally include both schizophreniform and affective psychosis.

Epidemiology

The community prevalence of schizophrenia is 1–2% (Robbins & Regier, 1991). In some urban centers, up to 5–10% of persons with schizophrenia admitted to psychiatric hospitals may be infected with HIV (Cournos et al., 1991). Most studies of new-onset HIV psychosis were conducted before the HAART era. These chart or clinic reviews suggest frequencies ranging from 0.2% to 15% in persons without other known causes of psychotic symptoms (e.g., delirium) (Harris et al., 1991; Sewell, 1996). Any estimates of the frequency of "HIV psychosis" must take into account that new-onset delusions and hallucinations in patients with HIV are just as likely to be a delirium: In one series of first-onset psychotic symptoms, 42% of patients had delirium, 50% of the sample had evidence of opportunistic cerebral infection or metabolic encephalopathy (Alieiati, 2001).

Etiology

Schizophrenia is a chronic neurodevelopmental illness attributed to complex interactions of genetic and environmental factors. It has been described as a "two-hit" illness, with some neurocognitive impairment observed early in life before onset of clinical symptoms, then further decline after psychotic symptoms commence in late adolescence or early adulthood (Twamley et al., 2003). The neurocognitive difficulties seen in schizophrenia and HIV are somewhat similar, with impairments in learning, executive function, speeded information processing, and motor function (Twamley et al., 2003). In HIV psychosis, the etiology is unknown but has been attributed to direct effects of HIV on subcortical structures, opportunistic infection, or the interaction of HIV and other CNS viruses such as cytomegalovirus or herpes simplex virus (Harris et al., 1991), and high levels of intracellular free calcium, leading to inappropriate neurotransmitter release (Dolder et al., 2004). Separately, psychotic symptoms or psychotic syndromes can occur in HIV-infected patients due to alcohol or drug abuse, or to treatment with antiretrovirals (e.g., efavirenz) or treatment with interferon for comorbid hepatitis C infection (Hoffman et al., 2003; Poulsen & Lublin, 2003).

Diagnosis

Diagnosis begins with distinguishing the presence of psychotic symptoms (i.e., delusions and hallucinations) from psychotic syndromes or disorders. The core concept of a psychotic syndrome defined in the DSM-IV is the presence of delusions, hallucinations, disorganized speech, thought, or behavior. Delusions are falsely held beliefs that cannot be influenced by reason or contradictory evidence. Disorganized speech implies statements are not logically connected and whose content makes no sense; loose associations and incoherence are examples of disorganized speech (and presumably thought). Disorganized behavior is random, disconnected, or odd behavior (Fauman, 1994). When isolated psychotic symptoms like paranoia or auditory hallucinations develop in the course of HIV-associated dementia (HAD), the initial diagnosis might be "HAD with delusions (or hallucinations)." The clinician should watch for evolution of a delirium. If psychotic symptoms result from exposure to medication or drug of abuse (e.g., methamphetamine), the DSM-IV designates the picture as a "substance-induced psychotic disorder." For a florid psychotic syndrome attributable to physiology of HIV illness the classification "psychotic disorder due to HIV" would be appropriate.

The clinical presentation in new-onset psychotic disorder due to HIV is variable. Delusions are prevalent (occurring in almost 90% of cases in some series) with persecutory, grandiose, or somatic components. The content usually is not as complex and bizarre as with schizophrenia. Nevertheless, persecutory themes can be quite involved; similarly, somatic delusions may be elaborate (pain due to "lasers" emitted from veiled powers). Delusions of thoughts being inserted into one's mind by outside forces, thought broadcasting (one's thoughts being audible to others), and of one's physical acts being controlled by others are also described. Most case studies also report looseness of associations or frankly disorganized thinking. Visual hallucinations are often evident but auditory hallucinations, like hearing a running commentary on one's actions, may occur (Harris et al., 1991; De Ronchi et al., 2006).

Some studies find that disturbances of mood often accompany HIV-associated psychosis, with anxiety being the most prevalent symptom, followed by depressed mood, euphoria, or irritability, and mixed depressed and euphoric states (Sewell et al., 1994a). Lability, flatness, and inappropriate laughter or anger are also described (Harris et al., 1991). Other studies report that paranoid delusions are prominent and affective symptoms uncommon, especially when compared to first-onset psychosis in HIV-negative controls (De Ronchi et al., 2006).

Reflecting the association of psychotic disorders with late-stage disease, neurological examination shows impairment in memory or other cognitive functions in up to one-third of patients with psychosis (Sewell et al., 1994a, De Ronchi et al., 2006). Neurological findings are nonspecific, usually consisting of ataxia, mild increases in motor tone, hyperreflexia, and tremor. Cerebrospinal fluid is generally unremarkable. Electroencephalography often shows diffuse cortical slowing. Brain computed tomography and magnetic resonance imaging reveal increased central volume in many cases. Focal neurologic abnormalities suggest a specific etiology (e.g., tumor, opportunistic infection, or vascular insult).

Course

There is no evidence that the course of schizophrenia itself differs in HIV-infected and uninfected individuals, although worse overall outcomes in individuals infected with HIV might be expected, for several reasons. Schizophrenia is generally associated with inattention to medical illness and poor self-care across a wide range of conditions. Part of this may be attributable to underlying psychotic processes, as well as to the fundamental neurocognitive impairments associated with this illness. Comorbid substance abuse is prevalent and further compromises self-care. Although the seriously mentally ill are generally thought to have good access to antiretrovirals (Blank et al., 2002), adherence to treatment may be severely impacted by the "triple hit" of substance abuse, and the neurocognitive impairments due both to HIV and to schizophrenia itself. To this must be added problems of poverty and homelessness, which further interfere with self-care.

The course of HIV psychosis is distinctly less favorable. Before the advent of combination antiretroviral therapy, HIV psychosis, and particularly psychotic symptoms coexisting with HIV dementia (HAD with delusions or hallucinations), indicated a very poor prognosis, with death in six months or less (Sewell et al., 1994a). Modern therapy probably improves the prognosis, but there is little published data. Individuals with psychosis in the context of mild neurocognitive abnormalities historically have had a more favorable (Sewell et al., 1994a) outlook.

Treatment

The principles of treatment for HIV-infected patients with schizophrenia follow the same basic principles as any other patient with schizophrenia, namely control of symptoms with medications and psychosocial support and rehabilitation. In these cases, however, close ties with HIV providers are strongly suggested, so that HIV treatment can be coordinated and monitored.

New onset psychotic symptoms attributable to HIV respond to neuroleptics. Randomized studies of first generation antipsychotics indicated high-potency (e.g., haloperidol [Haldol®]) and low-potency agents (thioridazine [Mellaril®]) were equally effective in ameliorating symptoms (Sewell et al., 1994b). The usual therapeutic dose is one-tenth to one-third that used for primary psychoses like schizophrenia (Sewell et al., 1994b). The time course of response is similar to that observed in schizophrenia, with the majority of improvement occurring within the first six weeks of therapy. It is unclear why such low-dose regimens are adequate but it may be related to pharmacokinetic changes associated with chronic disease, or to HIV-associated damage to subcortical limbic or basal ganglia structures. HIV patients with new-onset psychosis are often very sensitive to medication-induced extrapyramidal side effects (Sewell et al., 1994b; Hriso et al., 1991). This has led most current authorities (e.g., Freudenreich et al., 2010) to favor low-dose treatment with second generation or atypical neuroleptics described above (e.g., risperidone, olanzepine, quetiapine, ziprasidone, and aripiprozole). Quetiapine is often favored because it is not usually associated with extrapyramidal side effects even in diseases like HIV which affect the basal ganglia. Since olanzapine is the atypical most associated with metabolic syndrome, and risperidone most associated with

hyperprolactinemia, some clinicians commence treatment with other agents.

Extrapyramidal side effects can be managed with low doses of benztropine mesylate (Cogentin®), 1–3 mg daily, but amantadine (Symmetrel®) 50–100 mg twice daily can be used instead to avoid the "deliriogenic" anticholinergic effects of benztropine mesylate. Neuroleptic malignant syndrome is thought to be a particular risk for patients with HIV-associated dementia. Antipsychotics are associated with increased risk of mortality in patients with dementia and second-generation agents are associated with risk of metabolic syndrome (highest risk for olanzepine, lowest risk for aripiprozole and ziprasidone; Freudenreich et al., 2010).

PSYCHOACTIVE SUBSTANCE USE DISORDERS

The importance of substance use disorders to the acquisition and transmission of HIV worldwide cannot be overstated. Alcohol or substance use disorders may be associated with high-risk sexual behavior; transmission may also occur by sharing of infected needles or contaminated "works" used for intranasal application. Psychoactive substance use disorders reduce adherence to HIV treatment (Chandler et al., 2006). Substance use disorders frequently are comorbid with schizophrenia, bipolar disorder, and antisocial personality disorder.

Epidemiology

The upcoming revision of the DSM (DSM-V) is anticipated to classify substance abuse and dependence under the single entity of "substance use disorder." Nevertheless, a review of epidemiologic data using DSM-IV criteria is instructive for describing the scope of the problem. For this purpose we will also use data from U.S. prevalence surveys (e.g., Kessler et al., 2005). The prevalence of an alcohol use disorder is highest among young adults (18–29), as are new infection rates of HIV. Rates of high-risk behavior (unplanned and unprotected sex) for HIV infection also appear to be 1.5 to 2 times higher among individuals who got drunk for the first time at a younger age (before age 13) than those who do not begin drinking until age 19 or older (Hingson et al., 2003). Lifetime rates of alcohol dependence in the age range of 18–44 years are around 17% for men compared to 8% for women (Hasin et al., 2007). Among homosexual/bisexual men and injection drug-using (IDU) men and women, the lifetime rates of alcohol use disorders are two to four times higher than in the general population (i.e., 20 to 40% in gay men). Comorbidity, the presence of two or more substance use disorders, is common among individuals infected with HIV. For example, in HIV-infected samples with methamphetamine dependence, rates of lifetime alcohol use disorders exceed 25% (Atkinson et al., 2003).

The overall general population rate in the United States for lifetime drug abuse or dependence is around 14% for men and 7% for women (Compton et al., 2007). Methamphetamine and amphetamine, cocaine, and heroin are the major substances of abuse relevant to HIV. Worldwide there are more regular users of amphetamine and methamphetamine (35 million) than any other street drug, with the exception of cannabis; next come cocaine (15 million) and heroin (10 million; United Nations Office on Drugs and Crime, 2010). There is considerable geographic variation regarding substance of choice. HIV infection related to use of these substances varies according. For example, HIV infection due to heroin is prominent in many major eastern United States cities, China, and parts of Southeast Asia; amphetamine is the substance most widely associated with HIV in the western and mid-western United States and some Southeast Asian nations.

Etiology

Psychoactive substance use disorders are conceptualized as the result of a process culminating in loss of control over use of the substance. This process involves an interaction of antecedent and consequent factors. Antecedents include overarching social factors (availability of the substance, peer group pressures) and individual factors (genetic vulnerability, early learning, mood states). As an example, the relative risk for developing severe alcohol problems is fourfold higher in close family members of an alcoholic and in twins who are adopted away (Schuckit, 2000). Genetically transmitted differences in the reinforcing and toxic effects of alcohol or substances may explain this finding (Jaffe, 2000). Nevertheless, dependence seems solely related to environmental circumstances in some families. The etiology of substance abuse in those at risk for HIV infection illustrates the complexity of this issue. It has been speculated that at least among homosexual/bisexual individuals, the developmental stresses of establishing an alternate sexual identity, and of negotiating this within the context of family expectations and stigmatization by society, may contribute to substance use. The disinhibiting characteristics of alcohol and other drugs have long been associated with conflicted sex acts. Further, there has been a longstanding practice to use amyl nitrate and amphetamines (or other stimulants) to assist erection and greater frequency of sex. The stress of HIV infection does not appear to increase risk of developing an alcohol or non-alcohol substance use disorder.

Diagnosis

The nosology of DSM-V intends to combine abuse and dependence into one disorder (substance use disorder), classify its severity according to the number of positive diagnostic criteria, and to add a specifier describing whether tolerance or withdrawal is present. The fundamental criterion, a maladaptive pattern of substance use leading to clinically significant impairment or distress, remains unchanged from DSM-IV criteria. Two or more of the following must be present within a 12-month period: (a) failure to fulfil a major role obligation (e.g., poor work performance or absences; neglect of children or household; school expulsion); (b) recurrent use in situations involving physical hazard (e.g., driving an automobile); (c) substance-related legal problems (e.g., arrest); (d) continued use despite social problems resulting from use (e.g., arguments with spouse about intoxication, physical fights); (e) intake of substance in larger amounts for longer periods than was intended; (f) desire to cut down or control use; (g) a great deal of time is taken up obtaining the substance, using it or recovering from its effects; (h) reduction in usual social, occupational, or recreational activities; (i) continued use despite presence of persistent or recurrent physical or psychological problem due to the substance; and (j) craving or a strong desire to use. Tolerance (need for markedly increased amounts to achieve effects or markedly decreased effect at the same level of use) is an additional criterion, as is evidence of a withdrawal syndrome. If two to three criteria are met, severity is "moderate," if four or more are positive, the disorder is classified as "severe."

Diagnosis depends on a high index of suspicion based either on current findings (e.g., unexplained deterioration in work or relationships; intermittent hypertension [due to alcohol and stimulant use]; positive urine toxicology; elevated GGT [from alcohol]); or on eliciting a past history of abuse or dependence, and noting relapse has likely occurred. Direct inquiry about criterion symptoms can lead to diagnosis; often the patient underestimates the impact of abuse or dependence on everyday life. More valid data may come from interviewing significant others.

Course

The course of psychoactive substance use disorders is one of relapse and remission. In general, one-year follow-up studies of treated psychoactive substance use patients who are not infected with HIV showed only 40 to 60% remain completely abstinent, while 15 to 30% resume heavy use (O'Brien & McLellan, 1996). HIV infection does not appear to be a common stimulus of new-onset substance use disorder. Studies of HIV-seropositive homosexual/bisexual individuals (with follow-up of 2 years' duration) suggest that incident alcohol and non-alcohol substance use disorders represent relapses of disorders whose original onset preceded likely date of seroconversion (Atkinson et al., 2008). Emphasis on health promotion and education about the adverse health consequences of alcohol and other substances of abuse may be having a positive effect, but much remains to be done. Some studies note that for infected methamphetamine-dependent individuals, rates of relapse exceed 30% annually and are comparable in HIV-infected and non-infected groups; rates are equivalent in those who have progressed to frank AIDS (Atkinson et al., 2003). Such data suggest that one should not dismiss the possibility of relapse simply because the patient has advanced HIV disease; on grounds that medical illness reduces motivation or capacity to find and use substances.

Independently, both HIV and abuse of alcohol and other substances are associated with neurocognitive impairment. Their combined effects are now being evaluated. It may be that HIV-infected individuals who have a comorbid psychoactive substance use disorder are at increased risk of adverse neurological effects. For example, one study examining HIV-infected men who had lifetime (but not current) methamphetamine dependence showed significant additive adverse effects of methamphetamine and HIV on neurocognitive function (Rippeth et al., 2004). The mechanisms and neural pathways by which HIV and methamphetamine exert their combined effects are under investigation, and may involve drug interaction with HIV proteins (e.g., gp120, gp41, Tat, Vpr) and caspase-dependent pathways and neuronal apoptosis (Cadet & Krssnova, 2007).

Treatment

Treatment of substance use disorders is always complex, particularly in the HIV context, where there is an intersection of serious medical illness and the need to adhere to life-long antiretroviral therapy along with a high likelihood of co-occurring psychiatric disorder. "Harm reduction" rather than abstinence is the usual goal. The overall aim is to limit the serious or prolonged bouts of alcohol or substance use, while keeping the patient in regular contact with his or her physician, on antiretroviral therapy, and in stable housing. A "combined" treatment model is advocated, in which alcohol or drug treatment is co-located with social services, and with medical care providing access to antiretrovirals and preventive strategies for opportunistic infections, all delivered at one site, if possible (Altice et al., 2006). Mainstays of substance abuse treatment include self-help groups (e.g., Alcoholics Anonymous, Narcotics Anonymous); professionally led group or individual programs using cognitive-behavioral or motivational interviewing therapies are also used. Cognitive-behavioral programs typically educate individuals about antecedents and consequences of alcohol and substance use, train patients to recognize and manage urges to drink or use, and teach skills for resisting social pressures and organizing life around activities other than drinking or using. Motivational therapies focus on restoring a sense of control over substance use and identifying powerful motivations for sobriety. Medical evaluation involves individualizing treatment for HIV to minimize the impact of antiretroviral treatment on everyday life and promote adherence. Assessment for comorbid psychiatric disorders (e.g., major depression), which if undetected can thwart rehabilitation, is also included. Social services involve help with housing, childcare, transportation, and food or legal assistance. Training in HIV prevention to reduce risk of transmission may also be offered.

DELIRIUM

Epidemiology

Delirium is generally considered one of the most frequent complications in hospitalized HIV-infected patients, and some estimate a frequency of over 50% of AIDS patients develop this condition (Dilley et al., 1985). Delirium is likely to be as under diagnosed and undertreated in HIV populations as in general medical or surgical patients. Given that deliria may be the "presenting sign" of emergent, life-threatening illness, prompt detection and therapy is essential.

Etiology

Delirium is the syndrome that results from global cerebral dysfunction and it has the cardinal features of a change in the level of consciousness (alertness), a waxing and waning mental state, and an impairment of attention. This state is more common in patients with brain disease or who have compromised metabolic function, or patients who are taking multiple medications or have systemic illness; all of these factors are likely present in HIV patients.

The cause of delirium should be aggressively investigated via intensive medical examination. Vital signs and oxygen saturation, careful history and physical examination, laboratory tests, EKG, radiological exams, and critical review of all medications are essential to the workup. Possible etiologies include toxic (poisonings, substances and new, recently changed or interacting medications, especially medications with potent anticholinergic activity), metabolic (electrolyte disturbances), infectious (CNS infections or sepsis), endocrine (especially thyroid and adrenal axes), neoplastic (especially CNS), cardiovascular (myocardial infarction, arrhythmia), neurological (seizure, stroke), pulmonary (hypoxia, hypercapnea), and traumatic (head injury, burns) causes. Most deliria in HIV probably represent a combination of factors: systemic illness, underlying neurocognitive impairment, and treatment regimens that include multiple medications with CNS effects. Search for etiology should be prioritized to diagnose conditions that are life threatening, or might result in irreversible brain injury if not reversed. These would include Wernicke's aphasia, hypertensive encephalopathy, hypoglycemia, hyperperfusion of the CNS, hypoxemia (e.g., *Pneumocystis corinii* pneumonia can be complicated by hypoxemia), meningitis or encephalitis (bacterial, fungal, viral, or parasitic), or intracranial bleed (Slavney, 1998). Other causes of delirium in late-stage AIDS include severe nutritional deficiencies (e.g., vitamin B12) and electrolyte imbalance (e.g., hyponatremia). Therapeutic agents associated with delirium include antihistamines, benzodiazepines, and agents with anticholinergic properties, such as amitriptyline (Elavil®, prescribed for neuropathic pain) and opioids.

Diagnosis

DSM diagnostic criteria identify two cardinal symptoms: (a) the defining problem is reduced clarity of awareness of the environment (abnormality of level of alertness) and there is also reduced ability to focus, shift, or sustain attention; and (b) a change in cognition (e.g., memory deficit, disorientation, language disturbance or perceptual disturbances like misinterpretations, illusions, hallucinations) not better explained by dementia. The disturbance rapidly evolves and fluctuates. Deliria can be classified as hyper-alert/hyper-active, hypo-alert/hypo-active, or mixed (Adams, 1988). In most settings, the hyper-alert (hypervigilant) type is the most frequent, but perhaps detection bias plays a role, since quiet or hypoactive deliria are often difficult to detect (Schwartz & Masand, 2002). Diagnosis begins with a high index of suspicion, since deliria can present in both outpatient and inpatient settings.

Course

The course of deliria in HIV is similar to that of deliria in other illnesses: a brief prodromal phase, an acute phase during which the diagnosis is made, and then either resolution or a more persisting subacute phase, with persisting symptomology, which lasts for weeks or longer. This latter phase is termed intermediate duration cognitive disorder. Delirium associated with HIV dementia typically has a poor prognosis (Sewell et al., 1994a).

Treatment

Treatment consists of detection and therapy of the underlying etiology. Reorienting the patient within the environment has also proven beneficial. This may include orienting materials such as calendars and clocks, window views, and active reassurance and reorientation by family and staff. If at all possible, the maintenance of normal diurnal rhythm is helpful. Symptoms of hyperalert-hyperaroused delirium (e.g., agitation, anxiety, aggressiveness, paranoia, hallucinations) respond to standard treatment (Adams, 1988): low doses of high-potency neuroleptics such as haloperidol (Haldol®), 0.25–5 mg one to three times daily has been the standard for years. Atypical neuroleptics are also widely used. Risperidone is usually dosed at 0.25 mg to 1 mg, one to four times daily; the usual upper dose limit is 4–5 mg due to extrapyramidal effects. Olanzepine 2.5 mg to 20 mg at bedtime is also effective; some experts note that higher doses do not lead to better efficacy. Quetiapine is often dosed at 25–50 mg twice daily, with an upper dose of 600 mg daily (Schwartz & Massand, 2002). The hypoalert-hypoaroused form of delirium is thought to be less responsive to treatment. Extrapyramidal symptoms are associated with high-potency agents in advanced HIV illness (e.g., haloperidol, or higher dose risperidone). Patients with underlying HIV-associated dementia appear to be at highest risk. For patients who do not respond to low-dose oral therapy, intravenous haloperidol should be given in individual doses from 1 to 10 mg every hour. Although risk of extrapyramidal symptoms may be lower for intravenous treatment compared to oral routes, up to one-half of patients treated intravenously may still have extrapyramidal symptoms (Adams, 1988). Benzodiazepines alone (e.g., lorazepam) may worsen confusion and even cause acute disinhibition (Breitbart, 1994); however, these agents are effective in treating alcohol withdrawal or benzodiazepine- withdrawal delirium.

PERSONALITY DISORDERS

Personality is defined by the emotional and behavioral characteristics or traits that constitute stable and predictable ways that an individual relates to, perceives, and thinks about the environment and the self (Livesley, 2001; Rutter, 1987).

Personality traits are not positive or negative; they are adaptive in one setting and maladaptive in another. Individuals vary in the degree to which they possess a given trait and in the way it influences their behavior. *Personality disorder* is usually diagnosed when the severity of a trait exerts enough of an impact on the behavior of an individual to cause dysfunction (Paris, 1996).

The persistence of modifiable risk factors among persons who are HIV infected, or who are at risk for infection, has been an area of intense research. A subset of HIV-infected substance users (Latkin et al., 2009), patients presenting at HIV primary care clinics for medical treatment (Beyer et al., 2007), and HIV-infected men who have sex with other men (Fox et al., 2009) all have been shown to continue risky behaviors despite educational interventions and substantial awareness of risk. Risk behaviors in general are associated with certain characteristics of personality. The fact that knowledge of HIV and its transmission is insufficient to deter these individuals from engaging in HIV risk behaviors suggests that certain personality characteristics may be related to HIV transmission.

Traditional approaches in risk-reduction counseling emphasize the avoidance of negative consequences in the future, such as condom use during sexual intercourse to prevent STDs. Such educational approaches have proved ineffective for individuals with certain personality characteristics (Kalichman et al., 1996; Trobst et al., 2000). Effective prevention and treatment programs for HIV-infected individuals must consider specific personality factors that render this population vulnerable to practicing risky behaviors that further endanger their health as well as the health of others.

Supporting the contention that personality contributes to HIV risk is the high rate of personality disorders found in HIV-infected patients. Prevalence rates of personality disorders among HIV-infected patients (19%–36%) and individuals at risk for HIV (15%–20%) (Hansen et al., 2009) are high and significantly exceed rates found in the general population (10%, Johnson et al., 1995). The most common personality disorders among HIV-infected patients are antisocial and borderline types (Bennett et al., 2009). Antisocial personality disorder is the most commonly diagnosed Axis II disorder among HIV-infected individuals (Perkins et al., 1993) and it has been shown to be a risk factor for HIV infection (Weissman, 1993). Individuals with personality disorder, particularly antisocial personality disorder, have high rates of substance abuse and are more likely to inject drugs and share needles compared with those without an Axis II diagnosis (Hansen et al., 2009). A confound for this finding is that approximately half of substance abusers meet criteria for a diagnosis of antisocial personality disorder; however, this may be an artifact of the criteria used for defining antisocial personality. Less confounding is the fact that individuals with antisocial personality disorder also have higher numbers of lifetime sexual partners, engage in unprotected anal sex, and contract more STDs compared with individuals without antisocial personality disorder (Ladd et al., 2003).

Dimensional Nature of Personality

Patients have personality features that are continuous rather than categorical, and may have less or more of a particular trait. Many personality experts find the idea of dimensional traits more useful than categories when describing patients. A diagnosis of antisocial or borderline personality disorder can be stigmatizing in health care settings. A classification system based on a continuum approach may be a better predictor of HIV risk behavior than are DSM-IV-TR Axis II categories (American Psychiatric Association, 2000; Tourian et al., 1997).

Models of personality traits can describe individuals along dimensions of extroversion-introversion and stability-instability (Jung, 1923; Costa at al., 1994). The dimension of extroversion-introversion refers to the individual's basic tendency to respond to stimuli with either excitation or inhibition. Individuals who are extroverted are 1) present oriented; 2) feeling directed; and 3) reward seeking (Eysenck, 1990; Lucas et al., 2000). Their chief focus is their immediate and emotional experience. Feelings dominate thoughts, and the primary motivation is immediate gratification or relief from discomfort. Extroverts are sociable, crave excitement, take risks, and act impulsively. They tend to be carefree, inconsistent, and optimistic. By contrast, introverted individuals are 1) future and past oriented; 2) cognition directed; and 3) consequence avoidant. Logic and function predominate over feelings. Introverts are motivated by appraisal of past experience and avoidance of future adverse consequences. They will not engage in a pleasurable activity if it might pose a threat in the future. Introverted individuals are quiet, dislike excitement, and distrust the impulse of the moment. They tend to be orderly, reliable, and rather pessimistic.

The second personality dimension, stability-instability, defines the degree of emotionality or lability. The emotions of stable individuals are aroused slowly and minimally, and return quickly to baseline. By contrast, unstable individuals have intense, mercurial emotions that are easily aroused and return slowly to baseline. If these two personality dimensions are juxtaposed, four personality types emerge: stable introvert, stable extrovert, unstable introvert, and unstable extrovert.

Personality traits influence a variety of sexual risk behaviors, yet there is relatively little research on sexual risk taking from the major personality models. On the Eysenck Personality Questionnaire (EPQ), extroversion is associated with sexual promiscuity, desire for sexual novelty, multiple sex partners (Eysenck, 1976; McCown, 1991; McCown, 1993), and overall sexual risk taking (modest effective size in quantitative review). Neuroticism (instability) is related to unprotected anal sex. Psychoticism is a trait not discussed above, but is sometimes described as a lack of conscience, and is associated with number of sexual partners and unprotected sex in several studies. On the Neuroticism-Extraversion-Orientation (NEO) personality inventory, Neuroticism (instability) is associated with unprotected sex and to a lesser extent, sex with multiple partners. Low conscientiousness is also associated with unprotected sex. Low openness to experience is associated with the denial of risk of HIV infection. One study uses a questionnaire that defines Novelty Seeking, and finds that it is associated with unprotected sex, while a different questionnaire shows that a trait defined as Sensation Seeking predicts number of sex partners, unprotected sex, and high-risk sex encounters, such as sex with a stranger, across a variety of populations (Zuckerman, 1984).

Research on personality traits has shown links between Extroversion and Neuroticism to drug and alcohol addiction (Lodhi & Thakur, 1993). On the EPQ, Psychoticism, and to a lesser extent Neuroticism, have been linked prospectively to alcohol dependence in a six-year study. Impulsive sensation seeking (on the Zuckerman Kuhlman Personality Questionnaire) is consistently associated with addiction severity as well as amount and variety of illegal substance use. While there is no specific "alcoholic" or "drug-using" personality, there appears to be a modest link between substance abuse and either impulsivity/high novelty seeking or high on Neuroticism/negative emotionality. Individuals with *both* these traits may be at the greatest risk of addiction.

Treatment Implications

Psychiatric and medical treatment of patients with extroverted and/or emotionally unstable personalities is challenging. Such patients are often baffling or frustrating for physicians and other medical providers because they engage in high-risk sex and substance use behaviors in spite of knowing the risks, or fail to adhere to treatment regimens for HIV infection in spite of knowing the consequences. Personality traits reflect relatively stable, lifelong modes of responding; thus, direct efforts to change these traits are unlikely to be successful. It is possible, however, to modify the behavior that is an expression of the trait. By recognizing individual differences in risk-related personality characteristics, interventions can be better targeted and their impact maximized. Although treatment of personality disorders is beyond the scope of this chapter, effective treatment involves psychotherapy that focuses on behavior rather than psychological insight. Successful outcomes require firm limits, reliable treatment contracts, and clinicians experienced in the care of patients with personality disorders.

HIV, AGING, AND PSYCHIATRIC DISORDER

Antiretroviral therapy has prolonged life such that individuals who became infected in their twenties or thirties might expect a near-normal life span. General population surveys suggest the prevalence of psychiatric disorders decreases with age (Rabkin et al., 2003). It is unknown whether this will be true in the HIV context. There is concern that older HIV-infected men and women may have elevated rates of distress or psychiatric disorder because of the additive burden of HIV and non-HIV illness, likelihood of repeated personal losses over time, diminished financial resources due to the combination of limited employability and health care costs, and stigmatization due to HIV infection (Rabkin et al., 2003;

Nokes et al., 2000). On the other hand, some studies suggest that the elderly are better able to cope and are more resilient than younger individuals (Klapow et al., 2002). One troubling finding is that although the prevalence of mental disorders may decrease with age, rates of suicide increase, at least in men.

SUICIDE

Before combination antiretroviral treatment was available, individuals with advanced HIV disease were thought to have up to a 30-fold risk of committing suicide compared with seronegative men matched for age and social position (Kizer et al., 1988; Marzuk et al., 1988). These rates exceeded even the heightened risk for suicide in other neurological diseases, such as Huntington's disease, and were attributed to the dismal prognosis of HIV infection. With the introduction of more effective treatment in 1996, these rates were expected to fall. Indeed a recent 20-year population-based study covering the era from 1988 to 2008, the Swiss Cohort Study, reported that suicide decreased significantly in both men and women after the introduction of combination treatment, with a steeper decline in men (Keiser et al., 2010). The correlation of declining CD4 cell counts with increasing suicide rates supported the notion that effective therapies were likely responsible for this reduction in completed suicide. Nevertheless, suicide rates in the HIV-infected populations were over threefold higher in men and almost six fold higher in women compared to the general population. Among HIV-infected individuals, risk of suicide was higher in men, in older individuals, and in those with histories of injection drug use and psychiatric disorder.

Despite advances in treatment, suicide is still more likely in HIV disease than in other life-threatening conditions like cancer, end-stage renal disease, and multiple sclerosis (Keiser et al., 2010). Moreover, recent studies in several U.S. cities indicate almost 20% of HIV-infected individuals reported suicidal ideation within the preceding week (Carrico et al., 2007). What can explain these high rates of suicidality? Life expectancy is shortened by HIV, and even with improved therapy the burden of illness remains considerable. Perhaps as important are the stigmatization of HIV and of homosexuality, discrimination, resulting social isolation, and the psychiatric "background" of populations at risk for HIV. Substance abuse is a risk factor for suicide, and independently for HIV; likewise, mood disorders are prevalent in populations at risk for HIV, and advancing HIV disease itself is associated with first-onset mood disorder. It may be that mental disorder is becoming relatively more important in suicidality than disease progression (Keiser et al., 2010).

Suicide attempt and suicidal ideation are associated with major depressive disorder, bipolar disorders, schizophrenia, and/or substance use disorders. These suicidal behaviors generally commence before likely date of seroconversion (McKegney & O'Dowd, 1992). Women may be at elevated risk for suicidal ideation (Brown & Rundell, 1989, 1990). Thus, although debate over the distinction between suicide and the right to choose death or to refuse unwanted treatment are important issues, it is imperative that individuals expressing suicidal behaviors or ideas should be examined for a major psychiatric disorder and be offered appropriate treatment.

CONCLUSION

Major depression, psychoactive substance use disorders, schizophrenia, and bipolar disorder are the most prevalent primary and secondary psychiatric disorders associated with HIV and AIDS. These conditions may increase risk of acquisition or transmission of HIV, or complicate its treatment. All may have important effects on life quality. Effective treatments already are available for each of these conditions, and active research is investigating improved methods for their diagnosis and therapy. The complex interaction between these syndromes and HIV offers many opportunities for collaboration between scientists and clinicians working at the interfaces of biomedicine, public health, and neuropsychiatry.

ACKNOWLEDGMENTS

This work was supported by Grant P50 MH45294 from the National Institute of Mental Health and by the Department of Veterans Affairs.

REFERENCES

Adams, F. (1988). Emergency intravenous sedation of the delirious, medically ill patient. *Journal of Clinical Psychiatry*, *49*(Suppl 1), 22–27.

Aliciati, A. (2001). New-onset delusions and hallucinations in patients infected with HIV. *Journal of Psychiatry and Neuroscience*, *26*, 229–234.

Altice, F. L., Sullivan, L. E., et al. (2006). The potential role of buprenorphine in the treatment of opioid dependence in HIV-infected individuals and in HIV infection prevention. *Clinical Infectious Diseases Journal*, *43*(Suppl 4) S178–S183.

American Psychiatric Association. (2000). *Diagnostic and statistical manual of mental disorders, 4th edition, Text Revision*. Washington, DC: American Psychiatric Association.

Asch, S. M., Kilbourne, A. M., Gifford, A. L., Burnam, M. A., Turner, B., Shapiro, M. F., et al. (2003). For the SCSUS Consortium. Underdiagnosis of depression in HIV: Who are we missing? *Journal of General Internal Medicine*, *18*, 450–560.

Atkinson, J. H., Grant, I., Kennedy, C. J., Richman, D. D., Spector, S A., & McCutchan, J. A. (1988). Prevalence of psychiatric disorders among men infected with human immunodeficiency virus. *Archives of General Psychiatry*, *45*(9), 859–864.

Atkinson, J. H. & Grant, I. (1994). Natural history of neuropsychiatric manifestations of HIV disease. *Psychiatric Clinics of North America*, *17*, 17–33.

Atkinson, J. H., Young, C., Cherner, M., Heaton, R., Marcotte, T., & Grant, I. (2003). Prevalence and one-year course of psychiatric disorder in HIV-infected, methamphetamine dependent individuals. Presented at the American Psychosomatic Society Annual Meeting, March 8, 2003, Phoenix, AZ.

Atkinson, J. H., Heaton, R. K., Patterson, T. L., et al. (2008). Two-year prospective study of major depressive disorder in HIV-infected men. *Journal of Affective Disorders*, *108*(3), 225–234.

Bangsberg, D. R., Acosta, E. P., Gupta, R., et al. (2006). Adherence-resistance relationships for protease and non-nucleoside reverse transcriptase inhibitors explained by virological fitness. *AIDS*, *20*(2), 223–231.

Bennett, W. R., Joesch, J. M., Mazur, M., et al. (2009). Characteristics of HIV-positive patients treated in a psychiatric emergency department. *Psychiatric Services*, *60*, 398–401.

Beyer, J. L., Taylor, L., Gersing, K. R., et al. (2007). Prevalence of HIV infection in a general psychiatric outpatient population. *Psychosomatics*, *48*, 31–37.

Bing, E. G., Burnam, M. A., Longshore, D., et al. (2001). Psychiatric disorders and drug use among human immunodeficiency virus-infected adults in the United States. *Archives of General Psychiatry*, *58*, 721–728.

Blank, M. B., Mandell, D. S., Aiken, L., & Hadley, T. R. (2002). Co-occurrence of HIV and serious mental illness among Medicaid recipients. *Psychiatric Services*, *53*, 868–873.

Breitbart, W. (1994). Psycho-oncology: Depression, anxiety, delirium. *Seminars in Oncology Nursing*, *21*, 754–769.

Brown, G. W. & Harris, T. O. (1978). *Social origins of depression. A study of psychiatric disorders in women*. London: Tavistock.

Brown, O. R. & Rundell, J. R. (1989). Suicidal tendencies in women with human immunodeficiency virus infection. *American Journal of Psychiatry*, *146*, 556–557.

Brown, O. R. & Rundell, J. R. (1990). Prospective study of psychiatric morbidity in HIV-seropositive women without AIDS. *General Hospital Psychiatry*, *12*, 30–35.

Brown, S. A. & Schuckit, M. A. (1998). Changes in depression among abstinent alcoholics. *Journal of Studies on Alcohol*, *49*, 412–417.

Cadet, J. L. & Krssnova, I. N. (2007). Interactions of HIV and methamphetamine: Cellular and molecular mechanisms of toxicity potentiation. *Neurotoxicity Research*, *12*, 181–204.

Compton, W. M., Thomas, Y. F., Stinson, F. S, & Grant, B. F. (2007). Prevalence, correlates, disability, and comorbidiity of DSM-IV drug abuse and dependence in the United States: Results from the national epidemiologic survey on alcohol related conditions. *Archives of General Psychiatry*, *64*(5), 566–576.

Carrico, A. W., Johnson, M. O., Morin, S. F., et al. (2007). Correlates of suicidal ideation among HIV-positive persons. *AIDS*, *21*, 1199–1203.

Chandler, G. S., Himelhoch, S., & Moore, R. D (2006). Substance abuse and psychiatric disorders in HIV-positive patients: Epidemiology and impact on antiretroviral therapy. *Drugs*, *66*, 769–789.

Ciesla, J. A. & Roberts, J. E. (2001). Meta-analysis of the relationship between HIV infection and risk for depressive disorders. *American Journal of Psychiatry*, *158*, 725–730.

Cook, J. A., Grey, D., Burke, J. et al. (2004). Depressive symptoms and AIDS-related mortality among a multisite cohort of HIV+ women. *American Journal of Public Health*, *94*, 1133–1140.

Costa, P. T. Jr. & Widiger, T.A. (Eds.). (1994). *Personality disorders and the five-factor model of personality*. Washington DC: American Psychological Association.

Cournos, F., Empfield, M., Horwath, E., et al. (1991). HIV seroprevalence among patients admitted to two psychiatric hospitals. *American Journal of Psychiatry*, *148*, 1225–1230.

Cournos, F., Guido, J. R., Coomaraswamy, S., Meyer-Bahlburg, H., Sugden, R., & Horwath, E. (1994). Sexual activity and risk of HIV infection among patients with schizophrenia. *America Journal of Psychiatry*, *151*, 228–232.

Cournos, F. & McKinnon, K. (2005). Schizophrenia and comorbid human immunodeficiency virus and hepatitis C virus. *Journal of Clinical Psychiatry*, *66*(6), 27–33.

Cruess, D. G., Evans, D. L., Repetto, M. J., et al. (2003). Prevalence, diagnosis, and pharmacological treatment of mood disorders in HIV disease. *Biological Psychiatry*, *54*(3), 307–316.

Cummings, J. L. & Trimble, M. R. (1995). *Concise guide to neuropsychiatry and behavioral neurology*. Washington, DC: American Psychiatric Association Press.

De Ronchi, D., Bellini, F., & Cremante, G. (2006). *AIDS Care*, *18*, 872–878.

Deuchar, N. (1984). AIDS in New York City with particular reference to the psycho-social aspects. *British Journal of Psychiatry*, *145*, 612–619.

Dilley, J. W., Ochitill, H. N., Perl, M., & Volberding, P. (1985). Findings in psychiatric consultations with patients with acquired immunodeficiency syndrome and related disorders. *American Journal of Psychiatry*, *142*, 82–86.

Dolder, C. R., Patterson, T. L., & Jeste, D. V. (2004). HIV, psychosis and again: Past, present, and future. *AIDS*, *18*(Suppl 1), S35–S42.

Ellen, S. R., Judd, F. K., Mijch, A. M., & Cockram, A. (1999). Secondary mania in patients with HIV infection. *Australian and New Zealand Journal of Psychiatry*, *33*, 353–360.

Evans, D. L., Mason, K., Bauer, R., Leserman, J., & Petitto, J. (2002a). Neuropsychiatric manifestations of HIV-1 infection and Aids. In: D. Charney, J. Coyle, K. Davis, & C. Nemeroff, (Eds.). *Psychopharmacology: The fifth generation of progress*, pp. 1281–00. New York: NY Raven Press.

Evans, D. L., Ten Have, T. R., Douglas, S. D., et al. (2002b). Association of depression with viral load, CD8T lymphocytes, and natural killer cells in women with HIV infection. *American Journal of Psychiatry*, *159*, 1752–1759.

Evans, D. L., Charney, D. S., Lewis, L., et al. (2005). Disorders in the medically ill: Scientific review and recommendations. *Biological Psychiatry*, *58*, 175–189.

Everall, I. P., Salaria, S., Atkinson, J. H., et al. (2006). Diminished somatostatin gene expression in individuals with HIA and major depressive disorder. *Neurology*, *67*, 1867–1896.

Eysenck, J. H. (1976). *Sex and personality*, London: Open Books.

Eysenck, H. J. (1990). Genetic and environmental contributions to individual differences: The three major dimensions of personality. *Journal of Personality and Social Psychology*, *58*, 245–261.

Fauman, M. A. (1994). *Study Guide to DSM-IV*. Washington, DC: American Psychiatric Press.

Fava, M., Rush, A. J., Trivedi, M. H., et al. (2003). Background and rationale for the Sequenced Treatment Alternatives to Relieve Depression (STAR*D) Study. *Psychiatric Clinics of North America*, *26*, 457–494.

Ferrando, S. J. & Nims, C. (2006). HIV-associated mania treated with electroconvulsive therapy and highly active antiretroviral therapy. *Psychosomatics*, *47*, 170–174.

First, M. B., Spitzer, R. L., Gibbon, M., & Williams, J. B. W. (1994). *Structured clinical interview for Axis I DSM-IV disorders—patient edition (SCID-I/P, version 2.0)*. New York: Biometrics Research Department, New York State Psychiatric Institute.

Fox, J., White, P. J., Macdonald, N., et al. (2009). Reductions in HIV transmission risk behavior following diagnosis of primary HIV infection: A cohort of high-risk men who have sex with men. *HIV Medicine*, *10*, 432–438.

Frankel, M. R., Shapiro, M. F., Duan, N., et al. (1999). National probability samples in studies of low-prevalence diseases. Part II: Designing and implementing the HIV cost and services utilization study sample. *Health Services Research*, *34*(5 Pt 1), 969–992.

Freudenreich, O., Goforth, H. W., Cozza, K. L., Mimiage, M. J., Safren, S. A., Bachman G., & Cohen, M. A. (2010). Psychiatric treatment of persons with HIV/AIDS: An HIV-psychiatry consensus survey of current practices. *Psychosomatics*, *51*(6), 480–488.

Gaynes, B. N., Rush, A. J., Trivedi, M. H., et al. (2008). Primary versus specialty care outcomes for depressed outpatients managed with measurement-based care: Results from Star*D. *Journal of General Internal Medicine*, *23*(5), 551–560.

Grant, B. F., Moore, T. C., Shepard, J., & Kaplan, K. (2003). *Source and accuracy statement: Wave 1 National Epidemiologic Survey on Alcohol and Related Conditions (NESARC)*. Bethesda, MD: National Institute on Alcohol Abuse and Alcoholism.

Grant, B. F., Stinson, F. S., Dawson, D. A., et al. (2004). Prevalence and co-occurrence of substance use disorders and independent mood and anxiety disorders. *Archives of General Psychiatry*, *61*(8), 807–816.

Green, C. A. & Pope, C. R. (2000) Depressive symptoms, health promotion, and health risk behaviors. *American Journal of Health Promotion*, *15*, 29–34.

Hader, S. L., Smith, D. K., Moore, J. S., & Holmberg, S. D. (2001). HIV infection in women in the United States: Status at the millennium. *Journal of the American Medical Association, 285,* 1186–1192.

Hansen, N. B., Cavanaugh, C. E., Vaughan, E. L., et al. (2009). The influence of personality disorder indication, social support, and grief on alcohol and cocaine use among HIV-positive adults coping with AIDS-related bereavement. *AIDS and Behavior, 13,* 375–384.

Haro, J. M., Arbabsadeh-Bouchez, S., Brugha, S., et al. (2006). Concordance of the Composite International Diagnostic Interview version 3.0 (CIDI 3.0) with standardized clinical assessments in the WHO World Mental Health surveys. *International Journal of Methods in Psychiatric Research, 15(4),* 167–180.

Harris, J., Jeste, D. V., Gleghorn, A., & Sewell, D. D. (1991). New-onset psychosis in HIV-infected patients. *Journal of Clinical Psychiatry, 52,* 369–376.

Hasin, D. S., Stinson, F. S., Ogburn, E., & Grant, B. F. (2007). Prevalence, correlates, disability, and comorbidiity of DSM-IV alcohol abuse and dependence in the United States: Results from the national epidemiologic survey on alcohol related conditions. *Archives of General Psychiatry, 64(7),* 830–842.

Hays, R. D., Cunningham, W. E., Sherbourne, C. D., et al. (2000). Health-related quality of life in patients with human immunodeficiency virus infection in the United States: Results from the HIV cost and services utilization study. *The American Journal of Medicine, 108(9),* 714–722.

Hilty, D. M., Brady, K. T., & Hales, R. E. (1999). A Review of bipolar disorder among adults. *Psychiatric Services, 50,* 201–213.

Hingson, R., Heeren, T., Winter, M. R., & Wechsler, H. (2003). Early age of drunkenness as a factor in college students' unplanned and unprotected sex attributable to drinking. *Pediatrics, 111(1),* 34–41.

Hoffman, R. G., Chan, M. A., Alfonso, C. A., et al. (2003). Treatment of interferon-induced psychosis in patients with comorbid hepatitis C and HIV. *Psychosomatics, 44,* 417–420.

Hough, R. L., Landsverk, J. A., Karno, M., et al. (1987). Utilization of health and mental health services by Los Angeles Mexican Americans and non-Hispanic whites. *Archives of General Psychiatry, 44,* 702–709.

Hriso, E., Kuhn, T., Masdeu, J. C., Grundman, M. (1991). Extrapyramidal symptoms due to dopamine-blocking agents in patients with AIDS encephalopathy. *American Journal of Psychiatry, 148,* 1558–1561.

Ickovics, J. R., Hamburger, M. E., Vlahov, D., et al. (2001). Mortality, CD4 cell count decline, and depressive symptoms among HIV-seropositive women. *Journal of the American Medical Association, 285,* 1466–1474.

Jaffe, J. H. (2000). Substance-related disorders. In B. J. Sadock & V. A. Sadock, (Eds.). *Comprehensive textbook of psychiatry, seventh edition,* pp 924–52. Philadelphia: Lippincott, Williams & Wilkins.

Johnson, J. G., Williams, J. B. W., Rabkin, J. G., et al. (1995). Axis I psychiatric symptomatology associated with HIV infection and personality disorder. *American Journal of Psychiatry, 152,* 551–554.

Judd, L. L. & Akiskal, H. S. (2003). The prevalence and disability of bipolar spectrum disorders in the U.S. population: Re-analyses of the ECA database taking into account subthreshold cases. *Journal of Affective Disorders, 73,* 123–131.

Jung, C. (1923). *Psychological types.* New York: Harcourt Brace.

Kalichman, S. C., Heckkman, T., Kelly, J. A. (1996). Sensation-seeking as an explanation for the association between substance use and HIV-related risky sexual behavior. *Archives of Sexual Behavior, 25,* 141–154.

Keiser, O., Spoerri, A., & Brinkhof, M. W. G., (2010). Suicide in HIV-infected individuals and the general population in Switzerland, 1988–2008. *American Journal of Psychiatry, 167,* 143–140.

Kessler, R., McGonagle, K., Zhao, S., et al. (1994). Lifetime and 12-month prevalence of DSM-III-R psychiatric disorders in the United States: Results from the National Comorbidity Survey. *Archives of General Psychiatry, 5 1,* 8–19.

Kessler, R. C., Chiu, W. T., Demler, O., & Walters, E. E. (2005). Prevalence, severity, and comorbidity of twelve-month DSM-IV disorders in the National Comorbidity Survey Replication (NCS-R). *Archives of General Psychiatry, 6,* 617–627.

Kizer, K., Green, W., & Perkins, M. (1988). AIDS and suicide in California. *Journal of the American Medical Association, 259,* 1333–1337.

Klapow, J., Kroenke, K., Horton, T., Schmidt, S., Spitzer, R., & Williams, J. B. W. (2002). Psychological disorders and distress in older primary care patients: A comparison of older and younger samples. *Psychosomatic Medicine, 64,* 635–643.

Ladd, G. T. & Petry, N. M. (2009). Antisocial personality in treatment-seeking cocaine abusers: Psychosocial functioning and HIV risk. *Journal of Substance Abuse Treatment, 24(4),* 323–330.

Latkin, C. A., Kuramoto, S. J., Davey-Rothwell, M. A., et al. (2009). Social norms, social networks, and HIV risk behavior among injection drug users. *AIDS Behavior, 14,* 1159–1168.

Livesley, W. J. (2001). Conceptual and taxonomic issues. In: W. J. Livesley (ed.). *Handbook of personality disorders,* pp. 3–38. New York: Guilford Press.

Lodhi, P. H. & Thakur, S. (1993). Personality of drug addicts: Eysenckian analysis. *Personality and Individual Differences, 15,* 121–128.

Lucas, R. E., Diener, E., Grob, A., Suh, E. M., & Shao, L. (2000). Cross-cultural evidence for the fundamental features of extraversion. *Journal of Personality and Social Psychology, 79,* 452–468.

Lyketsos, C. G., Hanson, A. L., Fishman, M., Rosenblatt, A., McHugh, P. R., & Treisman, G. J. (1993). Manic syndrome early and late in the course of HIV. *American Journal of Psychiatry, 150,* 326–327.

Lyketsos, G. C. et al. (1996). Changes in depressive symptoms as AIDS develops. *American Journal of Psychiatry, 153,* 1420–1437.

Lyketsos, C. G., Schwartz, J., Fishman, M., Treisman, G. (1997). AIDS mania. *Neuropsychiatry and Clinical Neurosciences, 9,* 277–279.

Marzuk, P. M., Tierney, H., Tardiff, K., et al. (1988). Increased risk of suicide in persons with AIDS. *Journal of the American Medical Association, 259,* 1333–1337.

McCown, W. (1991). Contributions of the EPN paradigm to HIV prevention: A preliminary study. *Personality and Individual Differences, 12,* 1301–1303.

McCown, W. (1993). Personality factors predicting failure to practice safer sex by HIV-positive males. *Personality and Individual Differences, 14,* 613–615.

McKegney, F. P. & O'Dowd, M. A. (1992). Suicidality and HIV status. *American Journal of Psychiatry, 149,* 396–398.

McKinnon, K., Cournos, F., Sugden, R., Guido, J. R., & Herman, R. (1996). The relative contributions of psychiatric symptoms and AIDS knowledge to HIV risk behaviors among people with severe mental illness. *Journal of Clinical Psychiatry, 57,* 506–13.

Meade, C. S., Graff, F. S., Griffin, M. L., & Weiss, R. D. (2008). HIV risk behavior among patients with co-occurring bipolar and substance use disorders: Associations with mania and drug abuse. *Drug and Alcohol Dependence, 92(1–3),* 296–300.

Mich, A. M., Judd, F.K., Lyketsos, C.G., Ellen, S., & Cockram, A. (1999). Secondary mania in patients with HIV infection: are antiretrovirals protective? *Journal of Neuropsychiatry and Clinical Neuroscience, 11(4),* 475–480.

Moore, J., Schuman, P., Schoenbaum, E., Boland, B., Solomon, L., & Smith, D. (1999). Severe adverse life events and depressive symptoms among women with or at risk for HIV infection in four cities in the United States of America. *AIDS, 13,* 2459–2468.

Morrison, M., Petitto, J., Ten Have, T., et al. (2002). Depressive and anxiety disorders in women with HIV infection. *American Journal of Psychiatry, 5,* 789–796.

Nakamuli-Mpungu, E., Musisi, S., Mpungu, S. K., & Katabira, E. (2006). Primary mania versus HIV-related secondary mania in Uganda. *American Journal of Psychiatry, 163,* 1349–1354.

Nestler, E. J., Barrot, M., DiLeone, R. J., Eisch, A. J., Gold, S. J., & Monteggia, L. M. (2002). Neurobiology of depression. *Neuron, 34(1),* 13–25.

Nokes, K., Holzemer, W., Corless, I., et al. (2000). Health-related quality of life in persons younger and older than 50 who are living with HIV/AIDS. *Research on Aging, 22,* 290–310.

O'Brien, C. P. & McLellan, A. T. (1996). Myths about the treatment of addiction. *Lancet, 347(8996),* 237–240.

Onyike, C U., Bonner, J. O., Lyketsos, C. G., Treisman, G. J. (2009). Mania during treatment of chronic hepatitis C infection with pegylated interferon and ribavirin. *American Journal of Psychiatry, 161*, 429–435.

Paris, J. (1996). *Social factors in the personality disorders: A biopsychosocial approach to etiology and treatment.* Cambridge, England: Cambridge University Press.

Perkins, D. O., Davidson, E. J., Leserman, J., et al. (1993). Personality disorder in patients infected with HIV: A controlled study with implications for clinical care. *American Journal of Psychiatry, 150*, 309–315.

Perkins, D., Stern, R., Golden, R., Murphy, C., Naftolowitz, D., & Evans, D. (1994). Mood disorders in HIV infection: Prevalence and risk factors in a non-epicenter of the AIDS epidemic. *American Journal of Psychiatry, 151*, 233–236.

Perry, S. W. & Tross, S. (1984). Psychiatric problems of AIDS inpatients at the New York Hospital: Preliminary report. *Public Health Report, 99*, 200–205.

Poulsen, H. D. & Lublin, H. K. F. (2003). Efavirenz-induced psychosis leading to involuntary detention. *AIDS, 17*, 451–455.

Pyne, J. M., Rost, K. M., Farahati, F., et al. (2005). One size fits some: The impact of patient treatment attitudes on the cost-effectiveness of a depression primary care intervention. *Psychological Medicine, 35*(6), 839–854.

Rabkin, J. G., Wagner, G., Rabkin, R. (1994a). Effects of sertraline on mood and immune status in patients with major depression and HIV illness: An open trial. *Journal of Clinical Psychiatry, 55*, 433–439.

Rabkin, J. G., Rabkin, R., Harrison, W., & Wagner, G. (1994b). Effect of imipramine on mood and enumerative measures of immune status in depressed patients with HIV illness. *American Journal of Psychiatry, 151*, 516–523.

Rabkin, J. G., Rabkin, R., & Wagner, G. (1994c). Effects of fluoxetine on mood and immune status in depressed patients with HIV illness. *Journal of Clinical Psychiatry, 55*, 92–97.

Rabkin, J. G., Wagner, G. J., & Rabkin, R. (1999). Fluoxetine treatment for depression in patients with HIV and AIDS: A randomized, placebo-controlled trial. *American Journal of Psychiatry, 156*, 101–107.

Rabkin, J., McElhiney, M., Ferrando, S., & Williams, J. B. W. (2003). Assessment and prevalence of psychopathology in HIV/AIDS. Presented at the NIMH Conference on HIV and Aging, April 22–23, 2003.

Rabkin, J.G. (2008). HIV and depression: 2008 review and update. *Current HIV/AIDS Report, 5*(4), 163–171.

Repetto, M. J., Evans, D. L., Cruess, D. G., Gettes, D. R., Douglas, S. D., & Petitto, J. M. (2003). Neuropsychopharmacologic treatment of depression and other neuropsychiatric disorders in HIV-infected individuals. *CNS Spectrums, 1*, 59–63.

Rippeth, J. D., Heaton, R. K., Carey, C. L., et al. (2004). Methamphetamine dependence increases risk of risk of neuropsychological impairment in HIV infected persons. *Journal of the International Neuropsychological Society, 10*(1), 1–14.

Robbins, L. N., Regier, D. A., (eds.). (1991). *Psychiatric disorders in America.* New York: The Free Press.

Robins, L. N., Cottler, L., Bucholz, K., et al. (1995). *The Diagnostic interview schedule, version IV.* St. Louis, MO: Washington University.

Rosenberger, P., Bornstein, R., Nasrallah, H., et al. (1992). Psychopathology in HIV infection: Lifetime and current assessment. *Comprehensive Psychiatry, 34*, 150–158.

Rutter, M. (1987). Temperament, personality and personality disorder. *British Journal of Psychiatry, 150*, 443–458.

Safren, S. A., Gonzalez, J. S., & Soroudi, N. (2008). *CBT for depression and adherence in individuals with chronic illness: Therapist guide (treatments that work).* New York: Oxford University Press.

Sandson, N. B., Armstrong, S. C., & Cozza, K. L. (2007). An overview of psychotropic drug-drug interactions. *Psychosomatics, 46*(5), 464–494.

Schmidt, U. & Miller, D. (1988). Two cases of hypomania in AIDS. *British Journal of Psychiatry, 52*, 839–842.

Schuckit, M. (2000). Alcohol use disorders. In B. J. Sadock & V. A. Sadock, (eds.). *Comprehensive textbook of psychiatry, seventh edition,* pp. 953–70. Philadelphia: Lippincott, Williams & Wilkins.

Schwartz, T. L. & Masand, P. S. (2002). The role of atypical antipsychotics in the treatment of delirium. *Psychosomatics, 43*, 171–174.

Sewell, D. D., Jeste, D. V., Atkinson, J. H., et al. (1994a). HIV-associated psychosis: A prospective, study of 20 cases. San Diego HIV Neurobehavioral Research Center Group. *American Journal of Psychiatry, 151*, 237–242.

Sewell, D. D., Jeste, D. V., McAdams, L. A., et al. (1994b). Neuroleptic treatment of HIV-associated psychosis. HNRC Group. *Neuropsychopharmacology, 10*(4), 223–229.

Slavney, P. R. (1998). Delirium. *Psychiatric dimensions of medical practice,* pp.9–62. Baltimore, MD: Johns Hopkins University Press.

Tourian, K., Alterman, A., Metzger, D., et al. (1997). Validity of three measures of antisociality in predicting HIV risk behaviors in methadone-maintenance patients. *Drug Alcohol Dependence, 47*, 99–107.

Treisman, G., Fishman, M., Schwartz, J., Hutton, H., & Lyketsos, C. (1998). Mood disorders in HIV infection. *Depression and Anxiety, 7*, 178–187.

Trobst, K. K., Wiggins, J. S., Costa Jr., P. T., Herbst, J. H., McCrae, R. R., & Masters III, H. L. (2000). Personality psychology and problem behaviors: HIV risk and the five-factor model. *Journal of Personality, 68*, 1232–1252.

Twamley, E. W., Jeste, D. V., & Bellack, A. S. (2003). A review of cognitive training in schizophrenia. *Oxford Journals of Medicine, 29*(2), 359–382.

United Nations Office on Drugs and Crime (2010). World Drug Report. Geneva: United Nations Publications.

Valentine, A. D., Meyers, C. A., Kling, M. A., Richelson, E., & Hauser, P. (1998). Mood and cognitive side effects of interferon-alpha therapy. *Seminars in Oncology, 25*(Suppl 1), 39–47.

Volavka, J., Convit, A., O'Donnell, J., Douyon, R., Evangelista, C., & Czobor, P. (1992). Assessment of risk factors for HIV infection among psychiatric inpatients. *Hospital and Community Psychiatry, 43*, 482–485.

Walkup, J. & Blank, M. B. (2008). The impact of mental health and substance abuse factors on HIV prevention and treatment. *Journal of Acquired Immune Deficiency Syndrome, 47*(Suppl 1), S15–S19.

Weissman, M. M. (1993). The epidemiology of personality disorders: A 1990 update. *Journal of Personality Disorders, 7*(Suppl 1), 44–62.

Wells, J. E., Oakley Brown, M. A., Scott, K. M., et al. (2006). Prevalence, interference with life and severity of 12 month DSM-IV disorders in Te Rau Hinengaro: The New Zealand Mental Health Survey, *Australian and New Zealand Journal of Psychiatry, 40*(10), 845–854.

Whetten, K., Reif, S., Whetten, R., & Murphy-McMillan, L. K. (2008). Trauma, mental health, distrust, and stigma among HIV-positive persons: Implications for effective care. *Psychosomatic Medicine, 70*, 531–538.

Williams, J., Rabkin, J., Remien, R., Gorman, J., & Ehrhardt, A. (1991). Multidisciplinary baseline assessment of homosexual men with and without HIV infection: Standardized clinical assessment of current and lifetime psychopathology. *Archives of General Psychiatry, 48*, 124–130.

Wittchen, H. U. (1998). Reliability and validity studies of the WHO Composite International Diagnostic Interview (CIDI): A critical review. *Journal of Psychiatric Research, 28* (Suppl 1), 57–84.

World Health Organization. (1997). *Composite International Diagnostic Interview (CIDI) 2.1,* Geneva, Switzerland.

Zisook, S., Peterkin, J., Goggin, K. J., Sledge, P., Atkinson, J. H., & Grant, I. (1998). Treatment of major depression in HIV-seropositive men. HIV Neurobehavioral Research Center Group. *Journal of Clinical Psychiatry, 59*, 217–224.

Zuckerman, M. (1984). Sensation seeking: A comparative approach to a human trait. *Behavioral and Brain Sciences, 7*, 413–471.

12.2

NEUROCOGNITION IN HIV AND SUBSTANCE USE DISORDERS

Andrew J. Levine, Raul Gonzalez, and Eileen M. Martin

This chapter summarizes neurocognitive research on HIV-seropositive individuals who have past or current substance abuse disorders. The work focuses on studies conducted since the introduction of combination antiretroviral therapy. Neuropathological and neurocognitive consequences of HIV disease are described in detail elsewhere in this volume and as such we now focus on neurocognitive correlates of specific drugs of abuse; placing special emphasis on the independent and additive effects of these drugs on the brain and cognition and on implications for clinical management. Finally, we describe promising strategies for treating this vulnerable population, with a specific focus on cognition.

INTRODUCTION

The frequency of substance use disorders (SUDs) among HIV+ individuals often makes it difficult to distinguish substance-related neuropathological and cognitive effects from those effects due to HIV-associated neurocognitive disorder (HAND). Detecting the presence of HAND in individuals with a concurrent SUD is further complicated by multiple SUD-associated comorbid conditions, including head injury, psychiatric illness, cerebrovascular risk, and attention deficit/hyperactivity disorder (Martin-Thormeyer & Paul, 2009) Neurocognitive impairment, whether secondary to HIV, substance abuse, or both, complicates clinical management, increases high-risk sexual and injection practices with exacerbation in the risk of HIV transmission and superinfection, and limits capacity for successful treatment adherence and ability to function independently. Additionally, clinical management of HIV+ substance-dependent individuals is further complicated by psychosocial consequences such as chaotic living environments, homelessness, and risk of incarceration. Therefore, understanding the complex relationship between SUD and HAND is critical in both the clinical and research milieu.

In this chapter, we summarize relevant neurocognitive research among HIV+ individuals with past or current SUDs. We focus our review on studies conducted since the introduction of combination antiretroviral therapy (cART). Neuropathological and neurocognitive consequences of HIV disease are described extensively elsewhere in this volume; therefore, we focus our review on neurocognitive correlates of specific drugs of abuse among HIV+ persons with special emphasis on their independent and additive effects on brain and cognition and their translational implications for clinical management. Finally, we describe promising strategies for treating this vulnerable population, with specific focus on neurocognitive factors.

The objectives of this chapter are as follows;

- Briefly summarize the neuropathological effects of both HIV and SUDs in order to provide a foundation for understanding their additive neurocognitive sequelae.

- Provide a concise review of post-cART literature describing the neurocognitive consequences of commonly abused substances in the context of HIV. When addressing substances that have not been studied in the context of HIV, we summarize and extrapolate literature regarding their neurocognitive effects among HIV-seronegative individuals.

- List common comorbid factors that can further contribute to or increase the risk of neurocognitive complications in HIV+ substance-using individuals (SUIs).

- Describe treatment-related issues especially germane to HIV+ SUIs. This includes cART adherence and a summary of evidence-based treatment options.

CELLULAR AND NEUROANATOMICAL ASPECTS OF HIV AND SUBSTANCES OF ABUSE

The neuropathological substrates of HAND, sometimes termed HIV encephalitis (HIVE) or HIV leukoencephalopathy, is associated with persistent HIV infection and inflammation. Prior to the advent of cART, HIVE was found in between 20–50% of cases, with greater prevalence in SUIs (Bell et al., 1996; Martinez et al., 1995). Also prior to widespread cART use, HIVE was characterized by disruption of the blood-brain barrier, neuronal loss, myelin pallor, reactive astrocytosis (monocytes, microglial nodules, and multinucleated giant cells), and identification of p24 and other viral antigens in the brain by immunohistochemistry (Budka, 1991). However, in the post-cART era, immunoactivation resulting in neuroinflammation may be the primary cause of HAND neuropathogenesis (Anthony & Bell, 2008). In addition, there are more indications of age-associated neurodegenerative disease in the HIV+ brain, such as excessive beta amyloid, tau and phosphorylated tau, alpha synuclein, and ubiquitin deposits, as well as increased levels of synaptodendritic damage (Brew, Crowe, Landay, Cysique, & Guillemin, 2009; Gelman & Nguyen, 2009; Gelman & Schuenke, 2004; Gelman, Spencer, Holzer, & Soukup, 2006; Green et al., 2005; Khanlou et al., 2009).

A range of substances of abuse, including opiates, cocaine, methamphetamine, MDMA (ecstasy), and alcohol are all known to increase immunosuppression and enhance viral replication (e.g., Dhillon, 2007; Liang et al., 2008) Interactions between viral proteins such as gp120 and tat and substances of abuse facilitate breakdown of the blood-brain barrier, release of TNF-α and other pro-inflammatory cytokines, upregulate CCR5 expression, and increase oxidative stress (Hauser, 2006; Khurdayan et al., 2004; Liang et al., 2008; Flora et al., 2003, 2005; Flores & McCord, 1998). Further, methamphetamine acts via dopamine receptors on perivascular macrophages (Gaskill et al., 2009) and increases HIV infection of these cells (Liang et al., 2008). Together, these findings point to the additive effects of drug abuse and HIV on neuropathogenesis.

Anatomically, HIV has historically been associated with morphologic and functional changes in the basal ganglia nuclei, frontal lobes, and white matter tracts connecting these regions (Berger & Nath, 1997; Dal Pan et al., 1992; Itoh, Mehraein, & Weis, 2000; Power et al., 1993). However, more recent findings in the cART era have increasingly shown pathology in other cortical regions, the cerebellum, and the hippocampus (Chiang et al., 2007; Klunder et al., 2008; Thompson et al., 2006; Wang et al., 2010). Drugs of abuse can act on a wide range of neuroanatomic regions, but there is considerable overlap between regions affected by HIV and drug use. For example, like HIV, stimulants such as cocaine and methamphetamine preferentially affect the fronto-striatal system of the brain, including the basal ganglia and prefrontal cortex (Ernst, Chang, Leonido-Yee, & Speck, 2000; Goldstein & Volkow, 2002) and have a deleterious effect on dopaminergic (DA) neurons and functioning (Berger, Kumar, Kumar, Fernandez, & Levin, 1994; Berman, O'Neill, Fears, Bartzokis, & London, 2008; Engelmayer et al., 2001; Jones, Olafson, Del Bigio, Peeling, & Nath, 1998; Larsson, Hagberg, Forsman, & Norkrans, 1991; Sardar, Czudek, & Reynolds, 1996). Further, chronic methamphetamine use and HIV additively result in neuronal injury and glial activation, as shown in a MRS study (Chang, Ernst, Speck, & Grob, 2005).

In summary, this brief sampling of studies demonstrates the biological and anatomical foundation for additive neurocognitive sequelae of HIV and substance abuse. We refer the readers to chapters 4.5, 4.6, 4.7, and 4.8 in this volume for more detailed and comprehensive reviews.

NEUROCOGNITIVE DEFICITS IN HIV+ SUBSTANCE USERS

Drug-using individuals who participated in the earliest studies of neurocognitive effects of HIV consisted almost exclusively of injection drug users (IDUs), primarily opiate addicts. The current literature on substance abuse and HIV encompasses a much more diverse patient population with a broader range of age, education, ethnic characteristics, and clinical care needs and a wider range of substances of abuse that are not necessarily injected, and these are the studies discussed now.

This section reviews post-cART neurocognitive studies of HIV+ individuals that have specifically targeted the effects of comorbid substance dependence or abuse, with particular attention to their potentially additive or synergistic effects. For convenience, these studies are grouped according to the primary substance targeted for study; however, very few individuals abuse single substances; as such, acute effects of specific drugs or drug classes on neurocognitive performance can be characterized to some degree, but inferences regarding chronic use are considerably more limited.

ALCOHOL

Comorbid alcohol dependence in HIV+ persons can disrupt multiple cognitive functions, most evident among those with chronic heavy drinking. A recent study by Rothlind and colleagues (2005) compared the neurocognitive functioning of groups of HIV+ and HIV- "light" and "heavy" drinkers using a battery of neuropsychological tests. Heavy drinking was defined by self-reported average consumption of at least 100 (80 for women) standard alcoholic drinks per month for the prior three years, with active drinking at time of study. The authors reported that both heavy alcohol use and a positive HIV serostatus were individually associated with poorer neurocognitive test scores. Further, patients with both a positive HIV serostatus and heavy alcohol use showed even greater deficits on tasks requiring speeded information processing, suggesting an additive relationship between alcohol and HIV. Importantly, better neurocognitive functioning was observed in the seropositive group taking cART and with lower viral load, regardless of level of alcohol consumption, suggesting that neurocognitive impairment can be attenuated with adequate antiretroviral treatment among alcohol users. In another study, Green et al. (2004) administered a comprehensive battery of neurocognitive tests to demographically similar groups of HIV+ and HIV- men with and without a positive history of alcohol use disorder. Compared with non-alcoholic HIV+ subjects, the alcoholic HIV+ men had slowed information processing and impaired verbal reasoning; however, no differences in neurocognitive performance were observed between HIV- alcoholic and nonalcoholic participants, suggesting an interactive effect between HIV and alcohol. A larger study by Durvasula et al. of HIV and alcohol effects on neurocognition (2006) among 497 African-American males reported that motor and mental slowing were prominent among HIV+ men but only those who had used alcohol during the year leading up to testing. Additional evidence of additive or synergistic effects of alcohol and HIV have been reported in recent years, including greater impairment on measures of immediate episodic memory (Fama, Rosenbloom, Nichols, Pfefferbaum, & Sullivan, 2009), psychomotor speed, sustained attention, and associative learning (Sassoon et al., 2007). Importantly, in both studies, no deficits were detected in either single-risk group (HIV+ or alcoholism).

These studies have demonstrated consistently that there is a greater risk of neurocognitive impairment among HIV+ individuals with heavy alcohol use, particularly among heavy drinkers who have consumed alcohol within the past 12 months and who have poorer viral suppression. It is also inferred that some degree of cognitive impairment could persist for up to 12 months, following cessation of drinking, with most prominent disruption of the patient's capacity for speeded information processing. However, since psychomotor slowing is a prominent neurocognitive deficit among HIV+ individuals, (see Woods et al., this volume) it may be difficult to distinguish alcohol effects from those of HIV.

CANNABIS

Despite a growing trend to facilitate access to cannabis for medicinal purposes among those with HIV, there have been few studies examining how cannabis use may affect neurocognitive functioning among those with HIV. Among this population, cannabis use has been most consistently associated with memory problems (Ranganathan & D'Souza, 2006; Gonzalez, 2007), which appear to improve with abstinence (Pope, 2001). There have been competing theories on whether cannabis may be neuroprotective or neurotoxic in the context of HIV. However, the little evidence available to date suggests that cannabis use is detrimental to brain functioning among those with HIV, although the exact mechanisms remain unclear.

To date, only two published studies have specifically examined the effects of cannabis use on the brain functioning of HIV+ individuals. Both suggest that cannabis use may be harmful under some conditions, but the evidence is somewhat equivocal. Cristiani, Pukey-Martin, and Bornstein (2004) compared the neuropsychological performance of healthy controls and participants with HIV, stratified by history of marijuana use and HIV disease stage. They found that symptomatic HIV+ individuals that used marijuana frequently performed more poorly on a global measure of neuropsychological functioning compared to those with history of minimal or no marijuana use. In contrast, Chang, Cloak, Yakupov, and Ernst (2006) found that use of marijuana did not affect neuropsychological performance among their HIV+ subjects, as they reported no significant interactions between HIV serostatus and history of marijuana use. However, when they compared brain metabolite levels across groups using magnetic resonance spectroscopy (MRS), they found evidence of negative additive effects of marijuana use and HIV for some (but not all) metabolites in the basal ganglia and thalamus.

Clearly, the neurocognitive effect of cannabis use among those with HIV is an area in need of extensive study. It may be that controlled administration of cannabinergic drugs may be useful for management of some symptoms associated with HIV infection, but the current literature is equivocal regarding detrimental neurocognitive effects of cannabis. If these are present, the question of clinical tolerability, as with other drugs (e.g., opiates and benzodiazepines) remains to be determined.

COCAINE

Use of crack or powder cocaine is common among HIV+ drug users, but surprisingly few studies have evaluated their neurocognitive effects. A study of 237 HIV+ and HIV-African-American males reported that a positive HIV serostatus or cocaine history were each associated with increased risk for slowed mental processing speed, but that vulnerability to neurocognitive impairment was not compounded among those with both risk factors (Durvasula et al., 2000). Levine et al. (2006a) studied the integrity of sustained attention/vigilance in a group of 17 HIV+ individuals that abused stimulants (primarily cocaine) and 23 HIV+ persons with no history of substance use disorder but well matched otherwise with the stimulant using group. Groups were tested on the Continuous Performance Test (Conners, 2000), a standardized and widely used measure of sustained attention, and on a battery of clinical neurocognitive tasks. HIV+ persons with stimulant abuse performed the attention test more erratically than those who had not abused stimulants. Interestingly, the groups did not differ on other measures of attention, indicating a selective effect on sustained attention due to stimulant use.

Combining neuroimaging with neurocognitive assessment, Chang and colleagues (2008) conducted a PET study with two groups of HIV+ individuals (with or without a history of cocaine use) and a group of HIV-seronegative controls using C^{11}-labeled receptor imaging. They found abnormally decreased dopamine transporter (DAT) in the putamen among both HIV+ groups, and in the caudate only among the HIV+ cocaine users. Importantly, decreased DAT functioning was associated with poorer overall neuropsychological functioning regardless of cocaine use or HIV status (Chang et al., 2008). As such, while this study did find evidence for increased neurophysiological alterations in HIV+ cocaine users, no clinical correlation was detected with the neurocognitive tests used by the investigators.

At the time of this writing, more detailed studies are needed to determine what factors are associated with neurocognitive deficits among HIV+ users of cocaine. As one example, current evidence has raised the question of increased vulnerability to neurocognitive impairment among HIV+ female crack users (e.g., Maki & Martin-Thormeyer, 2009). The literature on gender differences in drug dependence has shown that compared with men, women are more highly responsive to cocaine/crack effects and that crack use is highly predictive of high-risk sexual behavior among women but not men (Lejuez, Bornovalova, Reynolds, Daughters, & Curtin, 2007). Cook and colleagues (2008) reviewed data on drug abuse and HIV disease progression among a sample of 1,686 HIV+ women enrolled in a longitudinal study of HIV disease progression. They reported that compared with women with no or non-crack drug abuse history, persistent crack users had significantly lower CD4 counts and higher HIV RNA levels; further, persistent users were three times as likely to die from AIDS-related causes.

METHAMPHETAMINE

Neurotoxic effects of methamphetamine use have been well documented (Chang, Alicata, Ernst, & Volkow, 2007; Nordahl, Salo, & Leamon, 2003). In a series of publications, investigators at the University of California, San Diego have reported clear evidence of additive and synergistic effects of HIV and methamphetamine use on neurocognition and biochemical, structural, and functional brain imaging. In an initial study, Rippeth et al. (2004) administered a comprehensive battery of neurocognitive tests to methamphetamine users and nonusers with and without a positive HIV serostatus. Each of these risk factors was associated with cognitive impairment, with the highest rate among HIV+ methamphetamine users (Rippeth et al., 2004). Carey and colleagues (2006) evaluated neurocognitive functioning among a group of HIV+ methamphetamine users to address the potential influence of HIV disease severity on methamphetamine-associated neurocognitive impairment. They found that neurocognitive impairment was significantly higher among HIV+ methamphetamine users with advanced disease compared with subjects without significant disease progression (Carey et al., 2006). Providing clinicopathological correlation, this group reported that global neurocognitive impairment and memory scores were significant predictors of severity of neuronal damage, which was significantly more extensive for HIV+ methamphetamine users with HIV encephalitis compared with methamphetamine users without HIV encephalitis and with HIV+ non-methamphetamine users without HIV encephalitis (Chana et al., 2006) The question of whether or not methamphetamine use and HIV infection have a synergistic impact on brain functioning was recently examined by Ances et al (2011). The researchers found a trend for decreased baseline cerebral blood flow (CBF) among HIV+ individuals as compared to HIV-negative controls, and statistically significant CBF changes among HIV-negative former methamphetamine dependent individuals as compared to HIV-negative individuals without history of methamphetamine dependence. Both groups (HIV+/non-methamphetamine and HIV-/amphetamine) also showed statistically significant CBF changes during a motor task as compared to their comparison groups. However, no interaction was observed between HIV serostatus and history of methamphetamine dependence, suggesting that HIV and methamphetamines effects on cerebral blood flow would be additive, not synergistic.

Interestingly, this group recently reported that comorbid HIV and methamphetamine dependence did not increase the likelihood of complaints about problems with everyday functions, such as driving and managing finances, beyond that found with either HIV or methamphetamine dependence alone (Sadek, Vigil, Grant, & Heaton, 2007).

While assessment of everyday functions was obtained with self-report questionnaires, the results suggest that the neurocognitive deficits detected in the aforementioned studies may not necessarily translate to everyday functioning.

NICOTINE

Rates of cigarette smoking have been estimated at up to 88% among individuals in substance abuse treatment (Richter et al., 2002) and HIV+ individuals are three times as likely to smoke as the general population (Webb, Vanable, Carey, & Blair, 2007). However, there are minimal data regarding neurocognitive consequences of nicotine use among HIV+ smokers. Durazzo and colleagues (Durazzo et al., 2007) investigated the effects of chronic cigarette smoking and alcohol use using structural MRI and neurocognitive studies of HIV+ heavy drinkers and healthy controls. They found that compared with controls, the nonsmoking HIV+ persons with heavy alcohol use showed significantly smaller volume in prefrontal cortex; however, scans of HIV+ persons with both chronic cigarette use and heavy drinking showed significantly lower volumes in frontal, temporal, and parietal cortex. In addition, this group performed significantly more poorly on tests of memory and learning as compared to the HIV+ nonsmoking heavy drinkers. These findings illustrate the need to address history of nicotine dependence as a source of additional neurocognitive and neurobiological burden among HIV+ subjects with alcohol dependence.

A recent study of women (Wojna et al., 2007) illustrates the complexity of potential neurocognitive effects of cigarette smoking and HIV serostatus. They reported that current cigarette smoking was associated with higher plasma viral burden and greater immunosuppression; however, they did not find any significant associations between neurocognitive functioning and either current or past history of smoking. Additionally, when analyses were restricted to the HIV+ women, individuals with a history of smoking performed significantly higher on measures of frontal/executive functioning. While this finding may seem counterintuitive, it is consistent with reports from animal studies that nicotine has protective effects (Gonzalez-Lira et al., 2006). Currently, the mixed findings regarding nicotine use and neurocognitive functioning in HIV make it impossible to make conclusions regarding nicotine use in HIV. However, considering the multiple health hazards associated with cigarette smoking, cessation programs are likely to be beneficial for HIV+ persons.

CLUB DRUGS

"Club drugs" are those that have traditionally been used at dance clubs and raves, and include 3,4-methylene-dioxymethamphetamine (MDMA, or "ecstasy"), ketamine ("Special K"), and gamma-hydroxybutyrate (GHB). Club drug use is more prevalent among men who have sex with men (MSM) (Cochran, Ackerman, Mays, & Ross, 2004) as compared to the general population. For example, 12% of a population-based sample of MSM reported MDMA use during the previous 6 months. Twenty-five percent of MSM attending gay circuit-parties reported GHB use, while 43% reported ketamine use (Lee, Galanter, Dermatis, & McDowell, 2003). Surprisingly, despite the high rate of club-drug use among MSM, there are no published studies that examine the cognitive effects of these substances in the context of neuroAIDS. Here we draw on the current literature on the neurocognitive effects of club-drug (primarily MDMA) use in general, and in the context of neuroAIDS where available.

MDMA has both stimulant and hallucinogenic properties and has been termed "enactogenic" (Parrott, 2001); use is associated with feelings of euphoria, heightened empathy, and well-being (Parrott, 1996). As such, it is prone to abuse. MDMA use is a risk factor for unsafe sexual practices among young adults (Sterk, Klein, & Elifson, 2008) and risky sexual lifestyles among MSM (Klitzman, Greenberg, Pollack, & Dolezal, 2002; Lee et al., 2003). As such MDMA use is a risk factor for exposure to HIV as well as neurocognitive impairment. Further, fatalities among HIV+ MDMA users who are taking the protease inhibitor ritonavir have been reported (Mirken, 1997).

There are no neuropsychological studies of MDMA effects among HIV+ individuals published as of the date of this volume. Even among non-HIV samples, the existing literature of the neurocognitive sequelae of MDMA use is largely focused on the residual effects of its recent use. Studies using meta-analysis do report deficits across a range of cognitive domains (primarily in memory) in MDMA users when compared to controls (Kalechstein, De La Garza, Mahoney, Fantegrossi, & Newton, 2007; Verbaten, 2003), although some deficits may be worsened considerably by concurrent marijuana use (Verbaten, 2003). However, it is important to note that many of the studies included in these two meta-analyses were influenced by multiple comorbid factors that potentially confound the results: polysubstance use, unknown MDMA content in substances sold as ecstasy, and various psychiatric and medical comorbidities. Halpern et al (2004) reported on neurocognitive performance among a unique sample of individuals with a wide range of lifetime MDMA use, but minimal use of other substances (Halpern et al., 2004). They reported that the raw test scores for the MDMA users were generally lower compared to non-using controls, but very few comparisons resulted in statistically significant group differences. Neurocognitive functioning among mild-to-moderate MDMA users was not significantly different from controls, findings replicated in a later study (Hanson & Luciana, 2010). However, lifetime MDMA users (60–450 lifetime uses), did perform significantly poorer on measures of processing speed and executive function. Both of these neurocognitive functions are prominently affected among HIV+ persons, which raises the question of potential additive effects in these domains.

Ketamine resembles phencyclidine in chemical structure. It is typically used as a veterinary tranquilizer, but when used in humans has powerful hallucinogenic and euphoric effects. Importantly, while ketamine can be smoked or taken orally, it is frequently injected and as such may indirectly affect HIV risk. Ketamine use is associated with lasting memory deficits, executive functioning, and visuospatial impairment among frequent users (>4 uses per week) (Morgan, Monaghan, & Curran, 2004). Ketamine use is also associated with higher incidence of psychotic symptoms that may persist long after cessation of use (Morgan, Muetzelfeldt, & Curran, 2009). However, studies indicate that cognitive functioning between ex-users and non-users is similar, suggesting behavioral improvement with increased periods of abstinence. It remains to be determined if the pattern and timeline of neurocognitive deficits due to ketamine use will be similar in the context of HIV.

GHB is a naturally occurring metabolite found in the human brain that binds to both GHB and g-aminobutyric acid (GABA) receptors, modulating arousal and memory functioning (Teter & Guthrie, 2001). Synthetic GHB is a popular club drug that produces euphoria, thus making it prone to abuse. There is evidence that GHB may also modulate striatal dopamine levels (Hechler et al., 1993), suggesting potential for interaction in those with HIV due to the virus' effects on dopamine functioning (Kumar et al., 2009). There are essentially no studies of long-term effects of GHB on neurocognition in humans. Animal studies show that repeated low-dose GHB administration, in theory comparable to that taken by recreational drug users, results in marked neuronal loss in the CA1 region of the hippocampus and in the prefrontal cortex (Pedraza, Garcia, & Navarro, 2009). Because these two areas are involved in a variety of cognitive functions and are affected by HIV, the relevance to HIV+ humans is clear.

In sum, evidence of neurocognitive deficits among club-drug users is determined by multiple factors, including concurrent use of other substances and duration of abstinence. However, there is currently no information on the effect of these drugs among HIV+ persons

TREATMENT ISSUES IN HIV+ SUBSTANCE USERS

HIV+ individuals with comorbid SUD are a treatment challenge. HIV+ individuals with untreated SUD are less likely to receive cART therapy or achieve viral suppression even when cART is prescribed (Lucas, Cheever, Chaisson, & Moore, 2001). Such individuals often face a difficult road; the dual stigma of HIV and substance abuse makes access to treatment more difficult (Reif, Geonnotti, & Whetten, 2006), and the lack of effective and consistent medical care may make abstinence more difficult. Further, both researchers and clinicians must contend with direct and indirect medical consequences of drug abuse, such as head injury, stroke, and malnutrition. Additionally, SUDs are frequently accompanied by a spectrum of neuropsychiatric conditions, including mood disorders, anxiety disorders such as PTSD and social phobia, ADHD and learning disabilities, and personality disorders, adding to the complexities and challenges in treatment (Biederman, Wilens, Mick, Faraone, & Spencer, 1998; Chilcoat & Breslau, 1998; Grant et al., 2004; Grant et al., 2004b). Finally, personality traits prevalent among SUIs, such as sensation-seeking and antisociality influence both neurocognitive function and risk behavior (Vassileva, Gonzalez, Bechara, & Martin, 2007; Vassileva, Petkova, et al., 2007; Zuckerman, 1996; Zuckerman & Kuhlman, 2000). As such, clinicians should be mindful of comorbid conditions and make appropriate referrals to substance use clinics and mental health professionals (see Table 12.2.1).

ADHERENCE

In most individuals, viral suppression requires optimal adherence to cART. Optimal adherence varies across studies, but usually requires that at least 80% of scheduled doses be taken (Malta, Strathdee, Magnanini, & Bastos, 2008). Adherence rates among active substance users have consistently been found to be suboptimal in studies utilizing electronic monitoring, with rates often in the range of 50–65% (Arnsten et al., 2001; Arnsten et al., 2002; Hinkin et al., 2007; Levine et al., 2005; McNabb et al., 2001). Levine et al. (2005) utilized cluster analysis to determine weekly adherence patterns among 222 HIV+ individuals monitored with an electronic monitoring system. Five adherence patterns were found, with the group identified as the poorest adherers having the highest rate of substance abusers. This group's adherence rates quickly dropped to below 20% during the one-month observational period. Fortunately, abstinent drug users or individuals with access to substance use and mental health treatment have better adherence rates (Crystal, Sambamoorthi, Moynihan, & McSpiritt, 2001; Hinkin et al., 2007). Examining factors associated with cART nonadherence in HIV+ substance users, Malta et al. (2008) conducted a review of 41 studies

Table 12.2.1 COMORBID FACTORS THAT MAY CONTRIBUTE TO NEUROCOGNITIVE DYSFUNCTION IN HIV+ SUIs

FACTOR OR ILLNESS	REFERENCES
Head Injury	(Jaffe, O'Neill, Vandergoot, Gordon, & Small, 2000)
Cerebrovascular Risk	(Becker et al., 2009; Foley et al., 2010; Martin-Schild et al., 2010)
ADHD or other developmental disorder	
Psychiatric Illness	(Levine et al., 2009; Wardle et al., 2011)
Hepatitis C	(Cherner et al., 2005; Hinkin, Castellon, Levine, Barclay, & Singer, 2008; Martin et al., 2004; Parsons et al., 2006; Richardson et al., 2005)
Risk-Taking Personality	(Hardy, Hinkin, Levine, Castellon, & Lam, 2006; Martin et al., 2004; Gonzalez et al., 2005;)
Poor cART Adherence	(Ettenhofer, Foley, Castellon, & Hinkin, 2010; Hinkin et al., 2007; Hinkin et al., 2002; Levine et al., 2005)

that included over 15,000 patients (Malta et al., 2008). While active substance use was associated with poorer adherence, various treatments improved this. For example, higher adherences rates were found among individuals receiving care in structured settings, as well as those in drug substitution therapy (e.g., methadone treatment). Additional factors resulting in poor adherence included poor self-esteem (Liu et al., 2006), recent incarceration (Kerr, Marsh, Li, Montaner, & Wood, 2005), and negative outcome expectations (Kerr et al., 2004). Studies examining the interaction between neurocognitive impairment and adherence in substance users have shown executive functioning and psychomotor speed to be associated with poor adherence among substance-using cohorts (Hinkin et al., 2004; Waldrop-Valverde et al., 2006). Findings from such studies have led to remediation and compensatory programs, as discussed in the following section.

OVERCOMING NEUROCOGNITIVE DEFICITS IN THE TREATMENT OF HIV SUIs

Fortunately, there has been considerable interest in treatment for SUDs in HIV+ individuals, including those with neurocognitive deficits. Recently, Norman et al. (2009) outlined ways in which neurocognitive deficits common to HIV may have a detrimental effect upon HIV-preventative behavior (Norman, Basso, Kumar, & Malow, 2009). For example, cognitive-behavioral techniques commonly used with substance abusers might be difficult to remember and implement in the face of learning and executive deficits experienced by HIV+ individuals. To counter this, they suggest cognitive remediation strategies. These strategies could include the frequent use of multimodal presentation of materials in order to facilitate learning and consistent training in a distraction-free environment to overcome impairments in retention and attention. Norman et al. recommend that patients be assessed frequently so that they have opportunity to evaluate the efficacy of their treatment strategies. Further, such feedback is crucial in maintaining motivation. In order to facilitate the application of skills in day-to-day life, Norman et al. suggest that treatment should include real-world scenarios and situations. Assistance from the patients' social support network and other health care providers may also improve the chance of success. In fact, group treatment may be the preferred treatment modality for neurocognitively impaired HIV+ SUIs, as this context encourages and strengthens prosocial behaviors. Group treatment could also reduce feelings of isolation and provide interpersonal support from peers with similar backgrounds.

From a medical standpoint, perhaps the most important aspect of HIV treatment is maintaining strict adherence to cART. Therefore, thorough knowledge of potential obstacles could improve treatment outcomes. Woods et al. (2008) undertook a substantive review in order to summarize evidence regarding barriers and facilitators to cART adherence among IDUs, which can also be applied to SUIs in general (Wood, Kerr, Tyndall, & Montaner, 2008). In their review, they describe the best evidence for the optimal HIV treatment among substance users. They identified decreased access to treatment and poor adherence to treatment as existing challenges. Within each of these are socio-political, individual, and provider-based barriers. For example, adherence to medication among SUIs includes socio-political barriers such as incarceration and financial constraints, individual barriers such as fear of side effects and psychiatric illness, and provider-based barriers such as physicians' belief that SUIs will not be able to adhere to their regimen. In the context of this chapter, cognitive deficits would fall under individual barriers. A number of evidence-based interventions have been developed that are aimed at reducing these specific barriers to treatment. Examples of strategies aimed at addressing socio-political barriers include outreach programs and meeting SUIs on their own terms (e.g., through needle exchange programs). Examples of strategies that address individual-based concerns include increased efforts to improve health insurance coverage and free access to medical care, utilizing HIV-experienced physicians in order to improve the treatment relationship, and providing substance abuse treatment and housing support in order to reduce physicians' reluctance to prescribe cART. The recommendations put forth by Norman et al. (2009), described above, can also be considered individual-based strategies. Finally, provider-related strategies include modifications of clinics in order to improve uptake and adherence to cART by being highly flexible, comprehensive, and interdisciplinary. Key features of such programs include on-site pharmacists, HIV specialist nurses, drop-in services, geographic proximity, and case management services. A final important strategy mentioned by Woods et al. is the linking of addiction treatment (e.g., substitution therapy) with cART. Such "directly administered therapy programs," which also provide daily supervision of antiretroviral intake, are associated with improved adherence. Note, however, that there are potential difficulties with substitution therapies. For example, concurrent psychoactive medication and opioid substitution therapies such as methadone have been associated with impaired cognitive performance (Mintzer & Stitzer, 2002). Further, pharmacokinetic studies of various ARTs and methadone or buprenorphine indicate that, when taken together, there are alterations in metabolic concentrations of both drug classes that may have adverse consequences on HIV disease status and opioid-therapy effectiveness (Bruce et al., 2006; McCance-Katz et al., 2007). However, recent findings from a 5-year longitudinal study provide a more sanguine outlook, indicating that consistent opioid substitution therapy is predictive of virologic suppression (Roux et al., 2009). For a further review of treatment, readers are referred to a recent review by Bruce and colleagues (Bruce, Kresina, & McCance-Katz, 2010). Clinicians' awareness of such research will help facilitate its application and development.

Finally, integrated behavioral and medical interventions have been successfully applied to HIV+ substance users, although the optimal structure remains unclear. For example, variations in ease of communication between health care providers, availability of office space, professional autonomy, and available services exist between integrated HIV clinics/ substance use treatment centers and those that are simply co-located (Lombard, Proescholdbell, Cooper, Musselwhite, & Quinlivan, 2009). However, some essential features emerge from the literature, including the need for both conditions to be treated simultaneously by health care with proper experience/training, minimizing the stigma associated with either condition, installing valid methods for detecting the presence of either condition, and providing other key services for clients within a single location.

SUMMARY

The studies reviewed in this chapter largely describe the putative additive risk of substance abuse on neurocognitive functioning in those with HIV. However, the interaction between substance abuse and HAND has not been well detailed among numerous commonly abused drugs. Indeed, despite their high prevalence among those with HIV, drugs such as marijuana, cocaine, and the class collectively known as "club drugs" have received relatively little attention. Further, the conflicting results found among studies examining the interaction of nicotine use and HIV emphasizes the need to elucidate the complex relationships between addictive substances and HIV. Research across different substance types among HIV+ individuals has not been balanced; most post-cART studies focus on stimulants such as methamphetamine. This is likely due to the high use of this drug among HIV+ persons (Stall et al., 2001), and its serious impact on neurologic functioning. However, this imbalance is shifting, as funding agencies such as the National Institute of Drug Abuse begin to encourage studies involving as-of-yet understudied substances. In addition, studies examining drug combinations with synergistic neurotoxic effects (e.g., alcohol and cocaine) are necessary. Finally, available literature indicates the importance of additional studies of sex differences in neuroAIDS and substance use, which have potentially critical implications for clinical practice and treatment.

Continued research into evidence-based treatment strategies must occur in tandem with the investigation of mechanisms of HAND neuropathogenesis among SUIs. The treatment hurdles associated with each condition alone are difficult to overcome; individuals with comorbid SUD and HAND represent an especially difficult population. However, identifying the individual barriers to treatment make it possible to address each simultaneously and effectively.

REFERENCES

Ances, B. M., Vaida, F., Cherner, M., Yeh, M. J., Liang, C. L., Gardner, C., et al. Grant I, Ellis RJ, (2011). HIV and chronic methamphetamine dependence affect cerebral blood flow. *J Neuroimmune Pharmacol*, [Epub ahead of print]

Anthony, I. C. & Bell, J. E. (2008). The neuropathology of HIV/AIDS. *Int Rev Psychiatry*, 20(1), 15–24.

Arnsten, J. H., Demas, P. A., Farzadegan, H., Grant, R. W., Gourevitch, M. N., Chang, C. J., et al. (2001). Antiretroviral therapy adherence and viral suppression in HIV-infected drug users: Comparison of self-report and electronic monitoring. *Clin Infect Dis*, *33*(8), 1417–1423.

Arnsten, J. H., Demas, P. A., Grant, R. W., Gourevitch, M. N., Farzadegan, H., Howard, A. A., et al. (2002). Impact of active drug use on antiretroviral therapy adherence and viral suppression in HIV-infected drug users. *J Gen Intern Med*, *17*(5), 377–381.

Becker, J. T., Kingsley, L., Mullen, J., Cohen, B., Martin, E., Miller, E. N., et al. (2009). Vascular risk factors, HIV serostatus, and cognitive dysfunction in gay and bisexual men. *Neurology*, *73*(16), 1292–1299.

Bell, J. E., Donaldson, Y. K., Lowrie, S., McKenzie, C. A., Elton, R. A., Chiswick, A., et al. (1996). Influence of risk group and zidovudine therapy on the development of HIV encephalitis and cognitive impairment in AIDS patients. *AIDS*, *10*(5), 493–499.

Berger, J. R., Kumar, M., Kumar, A., Fernandez, J. B., & Levin, B. (1994). Cerebrospinal fluid dopamine in HIV-1 infection. *AIDS*, *8*(1), 67–71.

Berger, J. R. & Nath, A. (1997). HIV dementia and the basal ganglia. *Intervirology*, *40*(2–3), 122–131.

Berman, S., O'Neill, J., Fears, S., Bartzokis, G., & London, E. D. (2008). Abuse of amphetamines and structural abnormalities in the brain. *Ann N Y Acad Sci*, *1141*, 195–220.

Biederman, J., Wilens, T. E., Mick, E., Faraone, S. V., & Spencer, T. (1998). Does attention-deficit hyperactivity disorder impact the developmental course of drug and alcohol abuse and dependence? *Biological Psychiatry*, *44*(4), 269–273.

Brew, B. J., Crowe, S. M., Landay, A., Cysique, L. A., & Guillemin, G. (2009). Neurodegeneration and ageing in the HAART era. *J Neuroimmune Pharmacol*, *4*(2), 163–174.

Bruce, R.D., Altice, F.L., Gourevitch, M.N., & Friedland, G.H. (2006). Pharmacokinetic drug interactions between opioid agonist therapy and antiretroviral medications: implications and management for clinical practice. *J Acquir Immune Defic Syndr*, *41*(5), 563–72.

Bruce, R. D., Kresina, T. F., & McCance-Katz, E. F. (2010). Medication-assisted treatment and HIV/AIDS: Aspects in treating HIV-infected drug users. *AIDS*, *24*(3), 331–340.

Budka, H. (1991). Neuropathology of human immunodeficiency virus infection. *Brain Pathol*, *1*(3), 163–175.

Carey, C. L., Woods, S. P., Rippeth, J. D., Gonzalez, R., Heaton, R. K., & Grant, I. (2006). Additive deleterious effects of methamphetamine dependence and immunosuppression on neuropsychological functioning in HIV infection. *AIDS Behav*, *10*(2), 185–190.

Chana, G., Everall, I. P., Crews, L., Langford, D., Adame, A., Grant, I., et al. (2006). Cognitive deficits and degeneration of interneurons in HIV+ methamphetamine users. *Neurology*, *67*(8), 1486–1489.

Chang, L., Alicata, D., Ernst, T., & Volkow, N. (2007). Structural and metabolic brain changes in the striatum associated with methamphetamine abuse. *Addiction*, *102* Suppl 1, 16–32.

Chang, L., Ernst, T., Speck, O., & Grob, C. S. (2005). Additive effects of HIV and chronic methamphetamine use on brain metabolite abnormalities. *Am J Psychiatry*, *162*(2), 361–369.

Chang, L., Wang, G. J., Volkow, N. D., Ernst, T., Telang, F., Logan, J., et al. (2008). Decreased brain dopamine transporters are related to cognitive deficits in HIV patients with or without cocaine abuse. *Neuroimage*, *42*(2), 869–878.

Cherner, M., Letendre, S., Heaton, R. K., Durelle, J., Marquie-Beck, J., Gragg, B., et al. (2005). Hepatitis C augments cognitive deficits associated with HIV infection and methamphetamine. *Neurology*, *64*(8), 1343–1347.

Chiang, M. C., Dutton, R. A., Hayashi, K. M., Lopez, O. L., Aizenstein, H. J., Toga, A. W., et al. (2007). 3D pattern of brain atrophy in HIV/AIDS visualized using tensor-based morphometry. *Neuroimage*, *34*(1), 44–60.

Chilcoat, H. D. & Breslau, N. (1998). Posttraumatic stress disorder and drug disorders: Testing causal pathways. *Arch Gen Psychiatry*, *55*(10), 913–917.

Cochran, S. D., Ackerman, D., Mays, V. M., & Ross, M. W. (2004). Prevalence of non-medical drug use and dependence among homosexually active men and women in the US population. *Addiction*, *99*(8), 989–998.

Conners, C. (2000). *Conners' Continuous Performance Test II. Technical Guide and Software Manual.* Canada.: Multi-Health Systems, Inc.

Cook, J. A., Burke-Miller, J. K., Cohen, M. H., Cook, R. L., Vlahov, D., Wilson, T. E., et al. (2008). Crack cocaine, disease progression, and mortality in a multicenter cohort of HIV-1 positive women. *AIDS*, *22*(11), 1355–1363.

Cristiani, S. A., Pukay-Martin, N. D., & Bornstein, R. A. (2004). Marijuana use and cognitive function in HIV-infected people. *J Neuropsychiatry Clin Neurosci*, *16*, 330–335.

Crystal, S., Sambamoorthi, U., Moynihan, P. J., & McSpiritt, E. (2001). Initiation and continuation of newer antiretroviral treatments among Medicaid recipients with AIDS. *J Gen Intern Med*, *16*(12), 850–859.

Dal Pan, G. J., McArthur, J. H., Aylward, E., Selnes, O. A., Nance-Sproson, T. E., Kumar, A. J., et al. (1992). Patterns of cerebral atrophy in HIV-1-infected individuals: Results of a quantitative MRI analysis. *Neurology*, *42*(11), 2125–2130.

Dhillon, N. K., Williams, R., Peng, F., Tsai, Y., Dhillon, S., Nicolay, B., et al. (2007). Cocaine mediated enhancement of virus replication in macrophages: Implications for human immunodeficiency virus-associated dementia *Journal of Neurovirology*, *13*, 483–495 (2007).

Durazzo, T., Rothlind, J., Cardenas, V., Studholme, C., Weiner, M., & Meyerhoff, D. (2007). Chronic cigarette smoking and heavy drinking in human immunodeficiency virus: Consequences for neurocognition and brain morphology. *Alcohol*, *41*, 489–501 (2007).

Durvasula, R. S., Myers, H. F., Mason, K., & Hinkin, C. (2006). Relationship between alcohol use/abuse, HIV infection and neuropsychological performance in African American men. *J Clin Exp Neuropsychol*, *28*(3), 383–404.

Durvasula, R. S., Myers, H. F., Satz, P., Miller, E. N., Morgenstern, H., Richardson, M. A., et al. (2000). HIV-1, cocaine, and neuropsychological performance in African American men. *J Int Neuropsychol Soc*, *6*(3), 322–335.

Engelmayer, J., Larsson, M., Lee, A., Lee, M., Cox, W. I., Steinman, R. M., et al. (2001). Mature dendritic cells infected with canarypox virus elicit strong anti-human immunodeficiency virus CD8+ and CD4+ T-cell responses from chronically infected individuals. *J Virol*, *75*(5), 2142–2153.

Ernst, T., Chang, L., Leonido-Yee, M., & Speck, O. (2000). Evidence for long-term neurotoxicity associated with methamphetamine abuse: A 1H MRS study. *Neurology*, *54*(6), 1344–1349.

Ettenhofer, M. L., Foley, J., Castellon, S. A., & Hinkin, C. H. (2010) Reciprocal prediction of medication adherence and neurocognition in HIV/AIDS. *Neurology*, *74*(15), 1217–1222.

Fama, R., Rosenbloom, M. J., Nichols, B. N., Pfefferbaum, A., & Sullivan, E. V. (2009). Working and episodic memory in HIV infection, alcoholism, and their comorbidity: Baseline and 1-year follow-up examinations. *Alcohol Clin Exp Res*, *33*(10), 1815–1824.

Flora, G., Lee, Y. W., Nath, A., Hennig, B., Maragos, W., & Toborek, M. (2003). Methamphetamine potentiates HIV-1 tat protein mediated activation of redox sensitive pathways in discrete regions of the brain. *Experimental Neurology*, *179*, 60–70.

Flora, G., Pu, H., Lee, Y. W., Ravikumar, R., Nath, A., Hennig, B., et al. (2005). Proinflammatory synergism of ethanol and HIV-1 tat protein in brain tissue. *Experimental Neurology*, *191*, 2–12.

Flores, S. C. & McCord, J. M. (1998). Oxidative stress and human immunodeficiency virus. *Advances in Molecular and Cell Biology*, *25*, 71–94.

Foley, J., Ettenhofer, M., Wright, M. J., Siddiqi, I., Choi, M., Thames, A. D., et al. (2010) Neurocognitive functioning in HIV-1 infection: effects of cerebrovascular risk factors and age. *Clin Neuropsychol*, *24*(2), 265–285.

Gaskill, P. J., Calderon, T. M., Luers, A. J., Eugenin, E. A., Javitch, J. A., & Berman, J. W. (2009). Human immunodeficiency virus (HIV) infection of human macrophages is increased by dopamine: a bridge between HIV-associated neurologic disorders and drug abuse. *Am J Pathol*, *175*(3), 1148–1159.

Gelman, B. B. & Nguyen, T. P. (2009). Synaptic proteins linked to HIV-1 infection and immunoproteasome induction: Proteomic analysis of human synaptosomes. *J Neuroimmune Pharmacol*.

Gelman, B. B. & Schuenke, K. (2004). Brain aging in acquired immunodeficiency syndrome: Increased ubiquitin-protein conjugate is correlated with decreased synaptic protein but not amyloid plaque accumulation. *J Neurovirol*, 10(2), 98–108.

Gelman, B. B., Spencer, J. A., Holzer, C. E., 3rd, & Soukup, V. M. (2006). Abnormal striatal dopaminergic synapses in National NeuroAIDS Tissue Consortium subjects with HIV encephalitis. *J Neuroimmune Pharmacol*, 1(4), 410–420.

Goldstein, R. Z. & Volkow, N. D. (2002). Drug addiction and its underlying neurobiological basis: neuroimaging evidence for the involvement of the frontal cortex. *Am J Psychiatry*, 159(10), 1642–1652.

Gonzalez, R. (2007). Acute and non-acute effects of cannabis on brain functioning and neuropsychological performance. *Neuropsychology Review*, 347–361.

Gonzalez, R., Vassileva, J., Bechara, A., Grbesic, S., Sworowski, L., Novak, R. M., et al., (2005). The influence of executive functions, sensation seeking, and HIV serostatus on the risky sexual practices of substance-dependent individuals. *J Intl Neuropsychol Soc*, 11, 121–131.

Gonzalez-Lira, B., Rueda-Orozco, P. E., Galicia, O., Montes-Rodriguez, C. J., Guzman, K., Guevara-Martinez, M., et al. (2006). Nicotine prevents HIVgp120-caused electrophysiological and motor disturbances in rats. *Neurosci Lett*, 394(2), 136–139.

Grant, B. F., Stinson, F. S., Dawson, D. A., Chou, S. P., Dufour, M. C., Compton, W., et al. (2004a). Prevalence and co-occurrence of substance use disorders and independent mood and anxiety disorders. *Arch Gen Psychiatry*, 61, 807–816.

Grant, B. F., Stinson, F. S., Dawson, D. A., Chou, S. P., Ruan, J., & Pickering, R. P. (2004b). Co-occurrence of 12-month alcohol and drug use disorders and personality disorders in the United States. *Arch Gen Psychiatry*, 61, 361–368.

Green, D. A., Masliah, E., Vinters, H. V., Beizai, P., Moore, D. J., & Achim, C. L. (2005). Brain deposition of beta-amyloid is a common pathologic feature in HIV positive patients. *AIDS*, 19(4), 407–411.

Green, J. E., Saveanu, R. V., & Bornstein, R. A. (2004). The effect of previous alcohol abuse on cognitive function in HIV infection. *Am J Psychiatry*, 161(2), 249–254.

Halpern, J. H., Pope, H. G., Jr., Sherwood, A. R., Barry, S., Hudson, J. I., & Yurgelun-Todd, D. (2004). Residual neuropsychological effects of illicit 3,4-methylenedioxymethamphetamine (MDMA) in individuals with minimal exposure to other drugs. *Drug Alcohol Depend*, 75(2), 135–147.

Hanson, K. L. & Luciana, M. (2010) Neurocognitive impairments in MDMA and other drug users: MDMA alone may not be a cognitive risk factor. *J Clin Exp Neuropsychol*, 32(4), 337–349.

Hardy, D. J., Hinkin, C. H., Levine, A. J., Castellon, S. A., & Lam, M. N. (2006). Risky decision making assessed with the gambling task in adults with HIV. *Neuropsychology*, 20(3), 355–360.

Hauser, K. F., El-Hage, N., Buch, S., Nath, A., Tyor, W.R., Bruce-Keller, et al. (2006). Impact of opiate-HIV-1 interactions on neurotoxic signaling. *Journal of Neuroimmune Pharmacology*, 1, 98–105.

Hechler, V., Peter, P., Gobaille, S., Bourguignon, J. J., Schmitt, M., Ehrhardt, J. D., et al. (1993). gamma-Hydroxybutyrate ligands possess antidopaminergic and neuroleptic-like activities. *J Pharmacol Exp Ther*, 264(3), 1406–1414.

Hinkin, C. H., Barclay, T. R., Castellon, S. A., Levine, A. J., Durvasula, R. S., Marion, S. D., et al. (2007). Drug use and medication adherence among HIV-1 infected individuals. *AIDS Behav*, 11(2), 185–194.

Hinkin, C. H., Castellon, S. A., Durvasula, R. S., Hardy, D. J., Lam, M. N., Mason, K. I., et al. (2002). Medication adherence among HIV+ adults: Effects of cognitive dysfunction and regimen complexity. *Neurology*, 59(12), 1944–1950.

Hinkin, C. H., Castellon, S. A., Levine, A. J., Barclay, T. R., & Singer, E. J. (2008). Neurocognition in individuals co-infected with HIV and hepatitis C. *J Addict Dis*, 27(2), 11–17.

Hinkin, C. H., Hardy, D. J., Mason, K. I., Castellon, S. A., Durvasula, R. S., Lam, M. N., et al. (2004). Medication adherence in HIV-infected

adults: Effect of patient age, cognitive status, and substance abuse. *AIDS*, 18 Suppl 1, S19–25.

Itoh, K., Mehraein, P., & Weis, S. (2000). Neuronal damage of the substantia nigra in HIV-1 infected brains. *Acta Neuropathol (Berl)*, 99(4), 376–384.

Jaffe, M. P., O'Neill, J., Vandergoot, D., Gordon, W. A., & Small, B. (2000). The unveiling of traumatic brain injury in an HIV/AIDS population. *Brain Inj*, 14(1), 35–44.

Jones, M., Olafson, K., Del Bigio, M. R., Peeling, J., & Nath, A. (1998). Intraventricular injection of human immunodeficiency virus type 1 (HIV-1) tat protein causes inflammation, gliosis, apoptosis, and ventricular enlargement. *J Neuropathol Exp Neurol*, 57(6), 563–570.

Kalechstein, A. D., De La Garza, R., Mahoney, J. J., Fantegrossi, W. E., & Newton, T. F. (2007). MDMA use and neurocognition: A meta-analytic review. *Psychopharmacology (Berl)*, 189(4), 531–537.

Kerr, T., Marsh, D., Li, K., Montaner, J., & Wood, E. (2005). Factors associated with methadone maintenance therapy use among a cohort of polysubstance using injection drug users in Vancouver. *Drug Alcohol Depend*, 80(3), 329–335.

Kerr, T., Palepu, A., Barness, G., Walsh, J., Hogg, R., Montaner, J., et al. (2004). Psychosocial determinants of adherence to highly active antiretroviral therapy among injection drug users in Vancouver. *Antivir Ther*, 9(3), 407–414.

Khanlou, N., Moore, D. J., Chana, G., Cherner, M., Lazzaretto, D., Dawes, S., et al. (2009). Increased frequency of alpha-synuclein in the substantia nigra in human immunodeficiency virus infection. *J Neurovirol*, 15(2), 131–138.

Khurdayan, V. K., Buch, S., El Hage, N., Lutz, S. E., Goebel, S. M., Singh, I. N., et al. (2004). Preferential vulnerability of astroglia and glial precursors to combined opioid and HIV-1 Tat exposure in vitro. *Eur J Neurosci.*, 19(12), 3171–3182.

Klitzman, R. L., Greenberg, J. D., Pollack, L. M., & Dolezal, C. (2002). MDMA ("ecstasy") use, and its association with high risk behaviors, mental health, and other factors among gay/bisexual men in New York City. *Drug Alcohol Depend*, 66(2), 115–125.

Klunder, A. D., Chiang, M. C., Dutton, R. A., Lee, S. E., Toga, A. W., Lopez, O. L., et al. (2008). Mapping cerebellar degeneration in HIV/AIDS. *Neuroreport*, 19(17), 1655–1659.

Kumar, A. M., Fernandez, J., Singer, E. J., Commins, D., Waldrop-Valverde, D., Ownby, R. L., et al. (2009). Human immunodeficiency virus type 1 in the central nervous system leads to decreased dopamine in different regions of postmortem human brains. *J Neurovirol*, 1–18.

Larsson, M., Hagberg, L., Forsman, A., & Norkrans, G. (1991). Cerebrospinal fluid catecholamine metabolites in HIV-infected patients. *J Neurosci Res*, 28(3), 406–409.

Lee, S. J., Galanter, M., Dermatis, H., & McDowell, D. (2003). Circuit parties and patterns of drug use in a subset of gay men. *J Addict Dis*, 22(4), 47–60.

Lejuez, C. W., Bornovalova, M. A., Reynolds, E. K., Daughters, S. B., & Curtin, J. J. (2007). Risk factors in the relationship between gender and crack/cocaine. *Experimental and Clinical Psychopharmacology*, 15(2), 165–175.

Levine, A. J., Hardy, D. J., Miller, E., Castellon, S. A., Longshore, D., & Hinkin, C. H. (2006a). The effect of recent stimulant use on sustained attention in HIV-infected adults. *J Clin. Exp. Neuropsychol.*, 28(1), 29–42.

Levine, A. J., Hinkin, C. H., Castellon, S. A., Mason, K. I., Lam, M. N., Perkins, A., et al. (2005). Variations in patterns of highly active antiretroviral therapy (HAART) adherence. *AIDS Behav*, 9(3), 355–362.

Levine, A. J., Singer, E. J., Sinsheimer, J. S, Hinkin, C. H., Papp, J., Dandekar, S., et al. (2009). CCL3 genotype and current depression increase risk of HIV-associated dementia. *Neurobehavioral HIV Medicine*, 1, 1–7.

Liang, H., Wang, X., Chen, H., Song, L., Ye, L., Wang, S. H., et al. (2008). Methamphetamine enhances HIV infection of macrophages. *Am J Pathol*, 172(6), 1617–1624.

Liu, H., Longshore, D., Williams, J. K., Rivkin, I., Loeb, T., Warda, U. S., et al. (2006). Substance abuse and medication adherence among

HIV-positive women with histories of child sexual abuse. *AIDS Behav*, 10(3), 279–286.

Lombard, F., Proescholdbell, R. J., Cooper, K., Musselwhite, L., & Quinlivan, E. B. (2009). Adaptations across clinical sites of an integrated treatment model for persons with HIV and substance abuse. *AIDS Patient Care STDS*, 23(8), 631–638.

Lucas, G. M., Cheever, L. W., Chaisson, R. E., & Moore, R. D. (2001). Detrimental effects of continued illicit drug use on the treatment of HIV-1 infection. *J Acquir Immune Defic Syndr*, 27(3), 251–259.

Maki, P. M., & Martin-Thormeyer, E. M. (2009). HIV, cognition and women. Neuropsychology Review, 19, 204–214.

Malta, M., Strathdee, S. A., Magnanini, M. M., & Bastos, F. I. (2008). Adherence to antiretroviral therapy for human immunodeficiency virus/acquired immune deficiency syndrome among drug users: A systematic review. *Addiction*, 103(8), 1242–1257.

Martin, E. M., Novak, R. M., Fendrich, M., Vassileva, J., Gonzalez, R., Grbesic, S., et al. (2004). Stroop performance in drug users classified by HIV and hepatitis C virus serostatus. *Journal of the International Neuropsychological Society*, 10, 298–300.

Martin, E. M., Pitrak, D. L., Weddington, W., Rains, N. A., Nunnally, G., Nixon, H., et al. (2004). Cognitive impulsivity and HIV serostatus in substance dependent males. *Journal of the International Neuropsychological Society*, 10, 931–938.

Martin-Schild, S., Albright, K. C., Hallevi, H., Barreto, A. D., Philip, M., Misra, V., et al. (2010) Intracerebral hemorrhage in cocaine users. *Stroke*, 41(4), 680–684.

Martin-Thormeyer, E. M., & Paul, R. H. (2009) Drug abuse and hepatitis C infection as comorbid features of HIV associated neurocognitive disorder: Neurocognitive and neuroimaging features. *Neuropsychology Review*, 19, 215–231

Martinez, A. J., Sell, M., Mitrovics, T., Stoltenburg-Didinger, G., Iglesias-Rozas, J. R., Giraldo-Velasquez, M. A., et al. (1995). The neuropathology and epidemiology of AIDS. A Berlin experience. A review of 200 cases. *Pathol Res Pract*, 191(5), 427–443.

McCance-Katz, E. F., Moody, D. E., Morse, G. D., Ma, Q., DiFrancesco, R., Friedland, G., et al. (2007). Interaction between buprenorphine and atazanavir or atazanavir/ritonavir. *Drug Alcohol Depend*, 91(2-3), 269–78.

McNabb, J., Ross, J. W., Abriola, K., Turley, C., Nightingale, C. H., & Nicolau, D. P. (2001). Adherence to highly active antiretroviral therapy predicts virologic outcome at an inner-city human immunodeficiency virus clinic. *Clin Infect Dis*, 33(5), 700–705.

Mintzer, M. Z., & Stitzer, M. L. (2002). Cognitive impairment in methadone maintenance patients. *Drug Alcohol Depend*, 67(1), 41–51.

Mirken, B. (1997). Danger: Possibly fatal interactions between ritonavir and "ecstasy," some other psychoactive drugs. *AIDS Treat News* (No 265), 5.

Morgan, C. J., Monaghan, L., & Curran, H. V. (2004). Beyond the K-hole: A 3-year longitudinal investigation of the cognitive and subjective effects of ketamine in recreational users who have substantially reduced their use of the drug. *Addiction*, 99(11), 1450–1461.

Morgan, C. J., Muetzelfeldt, L., & Curran, H. V. (2009). Ketamine use, cognition and psychological wellbeing: A comparison of frequent, infrequent and ex-users with polydrug and non-using controls. *Addiction*, 104(1), 77–87.

Nordahl, T. E., Salo, R., & Leamon, M. (2003). Neuropsychological effects of chronic methamphetamine use on neurotransmitters and cognition: a review. *J Neuropsychiatry Clin Neurosci*, 15(3), 317–325.

Norman, L. R., Basso, M., Kumar, A., & Malow, R. (2009). Neuro psychological consequences of HIV and substance abuse: A literature review and implications for treatment and future research. *Curr Drug Abuse Rev*, 2(2), 143–156.

Parrott, A. C. (1996). Ecstasy (MDMA): Mood effects in recreational polydrug users. *European Neuropsychopharmacology*, 6(Supplement 3), 45–45.

Parrott, A. C. (2001). Human psychopharmacology of Ecstasy (MDMA): A review of 15 years of empirical research. *Hum Psychopharmacol*, 16(8), 557–577.

Parsons, T. D., Tucker, K. A., Hall, C. D., Robertson, W. T., Eron, J. J., Fried, M. W., et al. (2006). Neurocognitive functioning and HAART in HIV and hepatitis C virus co-infection. *AIDS*, 20(12), 1591–1595.

Pedraza, C., Garcia, F. B., & Navarro, J. F. (2009). Neurotoxic effects induced by gammahydroxybutyric acid (GHB) in male rats. *Int J Neuropsychopharmacol*, 12(9), 1165–1177.

Pope, H. G., Gruber, A. J., Hudson, J. I., Huestis, M. A., & Yurgelun-Todd, D. (2001). Neuropsychological performance in long-term cannabis users. *Archives of General Psychiatry*, 58(10), 909–915

Power, C., Kong, P. A., Crawford, T. O., Wesselingh, S., Glass, J. D., McArthur, J. C., et al. (1993). Cerebral white matter changes in acquired immunodeficiency syndrome dementia: Alterations of the blood-brain barrier. *Ann Neurol*, 34(3), 339–350.

Ranganathan, M., & D'Souza, D. C. (2006). The acute effects of cannabinoids on memory in humans: A review. *Psychopharmacology (Berl)*, 188(4), 425–444.

Reif, S., Geonnotti, K. L., & Whetten, K. (2006). HIV infection and AIDS in the Deep South. *Am J Public Health*, 96(6), 970–973.

Richardson, J. L., Nowicki, M., Danley, K., Martin, E. M., Cohen, M. H., Gonzalez, R., et al. (2005). Neuropsychological functioning in a cohort of HIV- and hepatitis C virus-infected women. *AIDS*, 19(15), 1659–1667.

Richter, K. P., Ahluwalia, H. K., Mosier, M. C., Nazir, N., & Ahluwalia, J. S. (2002). A population-based study of cigarette smoking among illicit drug users in the United States. *Addiction*, 97(7), 861–9.

Rippeth, J. D., Heaton, R. K., Carey, C. L., Marcotte, T. D., Moore, D. J., Gonzalez, R., et al. (2004). Methamphetamine dependence increases risk of neuropsychological impairment in HIV infected persons. *J Int Neuropsychol Soc*, 10(1), 1–14.

Rothlind, J. C., Greenfield, T. M., Bruce, A. V., Meyerhoff, D. J., Flenniken, D. L., Lindgren, J. A., et al. (2005). Heavy alcohol consumption in individuals with HIV infection: Effects on neuropsychological performance. *J Int. Neuropsychol. Soc.*, 11(1), 70–83.

Roux, P., Carrieri, M. P., Cohen, J., Ravaux, I., Poizot-Martin, I., Dellamonica, P., et al. (2009). Retention in opioid substitution treatment: A major predictor of long-term virological success for HIV-infected injection drug users receiving antiretroviral treatment. *Clin Infect Dis*, 49(9), 1433–1440.

Sadek, J. R., Vigil, O., Grant, I., & Heaton, R. K. (2007). The impact of neuropsychological functioning and depressed mood on functional complaints in HIV-1 infection and methamphetamine dependence. *J Clin Exp Neuropsychol*, 29(3), 266–276.

Sardar, A. M., Czudek, C., & Reynolds, G. P. (1996). Dopamine deficits in the brain: The neurochemical basis of parkinsonian symptoms in AIDS. *Neuroreport*, 7(4), 910–912.

Sassoon, S. A., Fama, R., Rosenbloom, M. J., O'Reilly, A., Pfefferbaum, A., & Sullivan, E. V. (2007). Component cognitive and motor processes of the digit symbol test: Differential deficits in alcoholism, HIV infection, and their comorbidity. *Alcohol Clin Exp Res*, 31(8), 1315–1324.

Stall, R., Paul, J. P., Greenwood, G., Pollack, L. M., Bein, E., Crosby, G. M., et al. (2001). Alcohol use, drug use and alcohol-related problems among men who have sex with men: The Urban Men's Health Study. *Addiction*, 96(11), 1589–1601.

Sterk, C. E., Klein, H., & Elifson, K. W. (2008). Young adult ecstasy users and multiple sexual partners: Understanding the factors underlying this HIV risk practice. *J Psychoactive Drugs*, 40(3), 237–244.

Teter, C. J. & Guthrie, S. K. (2001). A comprehensive review of MDMA and GHB: Two common club drugs. *Pharmacotherapy*, 21(12), 1486–1513.

Thompson, P. M., Dutton, R. A., Hayashi, K. M., Lu, A., Lee, S. E., Lee, J. Y., et al. (2006). 3D mapping of ventricular and corpus callosum abnormalities in HIV/AIDS. *Neuroimage*, 31(1), 12–23.

Vassileva, J., Gonzalez, R., Bechara, A., & Martin, E. M. (2007). Are all drug addicts impulsive? Effects of antisociality and extent of multidrug use on cognitive and motor impulsivity. *Addict. Behav*, 32(12), 3071–3076.

Vassileva, J., Petkova, P., Georgiev, S., Martin, E. M., Tersiyski, R., Raycheva, M., et al. (2007). Impaired decision-making in psychopathic heroin addicts. *Drug Alcohol Depend, 86*(2–3), 287–289.

Verbaten, M. N. (2003). Specific memory deficits in ecstasy users? The results of a meta-analysis. *Hum Psychopharmacol, 18*(4), 281–290.

Waldrop-Valverde, D., Ownby, R. L., Wilkie, F. L., Mack, A., Kumar, M., & Metsch, L. (2006). Neurocognitive aspects of medication adherence in HIV-positive injecting drug users. *AIDS Behav, 10*(3), 287–297.

Wang, Y., Zhang, J., Gutman, B., Chan, T. F., Becker, J. T., Aizenstein, H. J., et al. (2010). Multivariate tensor-based morphometry on surfaces: Application to mapping ventricular abnormalities in HIV/AIDS. *Neuroimage, 49*(3), 2141–2157.

Wardle, M. C., Gonzalez, R., Bechara, A., & Martin-Thormeyer, E. M. (2010). Iowa Gambling Task performance and emotional distress interact to predict risky sexual behavior in individuals with dual substance and HIV diagnoses. *J Clin Exp Neuropsychology, 32*, 1110–1121.

Webb, M. S., Vanable, P. A., Carey, M. P., & Blair, D. C. (2007). Cigarette smoking among HIV+ men and women: Examining health, substance use, and psychosocial correlates across the smoking spectrum. *Journal of Behavioral Medicine, 30*(5), 371–383.

Wojna, V., Robles, L., Skolasky, R. L., Mayo, R., Selnes, O., de la Torre, T., et al. (2007). Associations of cigarette smoking with viral immune and cognitive function in human immunodeficiency virus-seropositive women. *J Neurovirol, 13*(6), 561–568.

Wood, E., Kerr, T., Tyndall, M. W., & Montaner, J. S. (2008). A review of barriers and facilitators of HIV treatment among injection drug users. *AIDS, 22*(11), 1247–1256.

Zuckerman, M. (1996). The psychobiological model for impulsive unsocialized sensation seeking: A comparative approach. *Neuropsychobiology, 34*, 125–129.

Zuckerman, M. & Kuhlman, D. M. (2000). Personality and risk-taking: Common biosocial factors. *J Pers, 68*(6), 999–1029.

12.3

PSYCHOBIOLOGY OF RISK BEHAVIOR

David G. Ostrow

Among the various risk-taking behaviors engaged in by persons at high risk of becoming infected with HIV or transmitting HIV, we know the most about drug abuse behavior and sexual behavior. This chapter focuses on those two types of risk-taking behavior, and on their inter-relationships. We discuss the neurobiological basis of sexual risk-taking and drug-related risk taking in order to uncover their similarities, overlaps, and congruencies. We conclude with several hypotheses about how interactions may have arisen among sexual risk-taking behavior, drug risk-taking behavior, and HIV transmission, and we consider the implications of these interactions for effective HIV prevention interventions.

INTRODUCTION

Scientists have been trying for over 50 years to understand risk-taking behavior in rational decision-making terms, so that it can ultimately be reduced to specific CNS regional activities (e.g., neurotransmitter and other "rational" determinants of neuronal communication). However, since prehistoric times, humans have sought out and tactically used inebriants to reduce or abolish the rational, inhibitory neuronal signals that restrain risk-taking behaviors. Thus, to understand the psychobiology of risk-taking behaviors, one must look at the interactions between the brain, sexual organs and motivations, and "sex-drugs" (defined as drugs taken specifically to prolong or intensify sexual performance and pleasure), often by suppressing the behavioral control areas of the brain (long referred to as the "ego" in Freudian psychoanalytical terms) in order to unleash the pleasure/reward centers of the brain (or the "id" in Freudian terms). Thus this chapter is organized along understanding the complex interplay of psychological, neurophysiological, and environmental factors that result in risky sexual and drug-use behaviors, and to provide an overall integrative model that illustrates these interactions on both developmental and salient experiential timelines. In this way we hope to disentangle the dual epidemics of HIV and drug use that continue to threaten the health of sexually active men who have sex with men (MSM) (Stall & Purcell, 2000) and develop effective integrated interventions.

Since we know the most about drug and sexual risk-taking among persons at risk of becoming infected or transmitting HIV, we will concentrate on those two types of behaviors and their inter-relationships in determining the relationships between psychobiological processes and HIV transmission.

Thus we begin this chapter with a discussion of the neurobiological basis of sexual and drug abuse in order to see their similarities, overlaps, and congruencies in risk-taking behavior that creates the psychobiological milieu for efficient HIV and other STI transmission. We conclude this chapter with several hypotheses about how these specific sex-drug and HIV transmission interactions may have arisen and their implications for effective HIV prevention interventions for sex-drug using persons.

Finally, since this is a text on HIV and the CNS, we would be remiss if we didn't at least mention that HIV itself can alter the functioning of many of the brain regions and neurotransmitter systems involved in regulating risky behavior. For further information on the HIV-compromised brain, the reader is referred to other chapters in this book, and Martin et al. (2004). In addition, recent *in vitro* and *in vivo* research has shown that the HIV virus itself can disrupt both mucosal epithelial membrane barrier functions and neuronal and renal processes involved in synaptic transmission and blood filtering, respectively (Nazli et al., 2010; Kim, Martemyanov, & Thayer, 2008; Fischer et al., 2010). For our purposes, we concentrate on the physically uncompromised brain and leave it to others to describe how the effects of HIV infection or HIV disease may alter the structure and workings of the brain to make risk-taking behaviors more or less likely.

THE CENTRAL NERVOUS SYSTEM AND SEXUAL AND DRUG GRATIFICATION

The most obvious connections between sexual and drug-use gratification systems at the neurotransmitter (NT) and cellular tract levels are the fact that dopamine (DA) appears to be a final common pathway for both systems, so that anything that changes the kinetics of DA release, binding to post-synaptic receptors, and its removal through active re-uptake and pre-synaptic metabolism will change the "tone" of this potent "reward" NT in both sexual and drug-use behaviors. Perturbations of DA tone in the areas of the brain responsible for experiencing an orgasm or drug-induced euphoria (see Fig. 12.3.1 A-C) can be the result of innate genetic differences (such as the reduced affinity of the 5HT re-uptake transporter seen in the brains of some persons with high levels of sensation seeking and reward dependency), be acquired through age and accompanying insult to the DA-producing neurons of the striatum (as seen in Parkinson's disease), or be transitory due to the ingestion of compounds, such as cocaine, that reversibly "poison" the 5HT re-uptake system while blocking retrograde inhibition of pre-synaptic DA. Other mental disorders seem to arise, at least in part, from altered sensitivity of the main post-synaptic DA receptors, such as seen in some forms of schizophrenia. When these highly sensitive DA receptors are blocked by DA antagonists (such as antipsychotic drugs), there can also be reduced feedback via post-synaptic "auto-receptors" that normally turn on or off the production of DA by the pre-synaptic neurons. In addition, there can be a proliferation of post-synaptic DA receptors, some with altered affinity for DA, as an adaptation to the long-term use of antipsychotic drugs—such a mechanism is thought to contribute to the development of movement disorders, such as tardive dyskinesia, among individuals with schizophrenia chronically treated with typical antipsychotics. (Figure 12.3.1, Panel B).

PERSONALITY TRAITS AND THE PSYCHOBIOLOGY OF RISK-TAKING IN MEN WHO HAVE SEX WITH MEN

SEXUAL-SENSATION SEEKING, THE TPQ PERSONALITY INDEX (TPI), AND THE GENETICS OF DOPAMINE AND 5HT ACTIVITY

Many studies, reviewed by Zuckerman (2006), the originator of the Sensation-Seeking Scale (SSS), demonstrate a high level of genetic heritability of high SSS scores, thus making it one of the most strongly biologically derived of all personality traits studied, with twin study correlations often at the high end of such patterns (r-squares of .45–.60). Thus, a concise review of the genetically and biologically determined aspects of sexual sensation seeking (SSS) among humans, particularly men and their sexually relevant components of SSS, such as low inhibition, desire for sensation and impulsivity/aggressiveness, can be a useful approach to those same factors that might underlie sexual sensation seeking and hence sexual and drug risk-taking behavior, among MSM at risk for HIV infection or transmission.

In terms of the molecular genetics of CNS neurotransmitters, it has been shown, in both human and animal studies, that sexual sensation seeking correlates strongly with specific neurotransmitter activity genes of both the dopamine (DA) and serotonin (5HT) systems and that the direction of these correlations support the putative mechanistic models described above for the reinforcement of sexual and drug risk behaviors. Specifically, a longer allele (7 repeats of a specific section) of the DA D_4 receptor gene, DDR_4, has high correlations with both the SSS and the Novelty Seeking (NS) Scale of Cloninger's TPQ personality inventory (2005). The SSS and Cloninger NS scales are highly inter-correlated in the one study that has performed both measures (r = .68); and the seeking of novel forms of sexual expression is a key component of the Sexual Sensation Seeking subscale of the Men's Attitude Survey (Ostrow et al., 2008). There is also an interaction between DDR_4 and the 5HT re-uptake transporter gene's shorter alleles; since all of these behaviors have a significant genetic component, the presence of one or more variant genes presumably act as risk factors for these behaviors.

Since the primary neurotransmitter of the reward pathway is dopamine (see Fig. 12.3.1A), genes for dopamine synthesis, degradation, receptors, and transporters are reasonable candidates. However, serotonin, norepinephrine, GABA, opioid, and cannabinoid neurons all modify dopamine metabolism and dopamine neurons. It has been proposed that defects in various combinations of the genes for these neurotransmitters result in a reward deficiency syndrome (RDS) and that such individuals are at risk for abuse of the unnatural rewards. Because of its importance, the gene for the dopamine D_2 receptor was a major candidate gene. Studies in the past decade have shown that in various subject groups the Taq I A1 allele of the DRD_2 gene is associated with alcoholism, drug abuse, smoking, obesity, compulsive gambling, and several personality traits. Ebstein and Auerbach (2002) summarize their findings as being

> "consistent with both human and animal studies that activation of DA pathways promotes exploratory and impulsive behaviors, whereas serotonergic pathways are generally inhibitory and advance avoidance behavior."

SEXUAL COMPULSIVITY, COMPULSIVE BEHAVIOR IN GENERAL, AND NEUROTRANSMITTER SYSTEMS

Sexual compulsivity (also known as sexual addiction or compulsive sexual behavior) has been shown in a variety of cross-sectional samples to be associated not only with increased frequency of unprotected anal sex but also combining sex with drug or alcohol use, "barebacker" identification, intentions to bareback, and various sexual fetishes that might increase the transmission of HIV through sexual risk-taking (Grov, Parsons, & Bimbi, 2009), as well as increased likelihood of a sexually transmitted infection (STI) in the past year (Dilley et al., 2008). Thus, it appears to function as a common underlying vulnerability to risk-taking behavior, at least in MSM samples, similar to the proposed role of sexual sensation seeking among gay/bisexual men (Kalichman, Greenberg, & Abel, 1995). However, much less is known about the putative genetic or neurotransmitter system connections between sexual compulsivity and risk-taking behavior, which has mostly been studied using innovative scales developed specifically for at-risk MSM and not directly linked to specific personality types or traits (Kalichman, Greenberg, & Abel, 1997).

Comings and Blum (2000) have suggested that since all compulsive behaviors have a significant genetic component, the presence of one or more variant genes presumably acts as risk factors for these behaviors. As indicated above, genes for dopamine synthesis, degradation, receptors, and transporters are the most probable candidates. However, specific studies of DA receptor or other NT systems in sexual compulsivity or risk taking among MSM are lacking in the literature. Therefore, unlike the situation with sexual sensation seeking, where we

A

The brain's natural pleasure/reward system

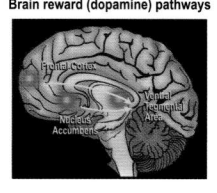

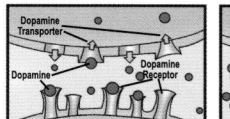

Brain reward (dopamine) pathways

These brain circuits are important for natural rewards such as food, music, and art.

Many drugs of abuse increase dopamine in specific brain synapses.

SEX

METH, COCAINE, CRACK

Typically, dopamine increases in response to natural rewards such as food. When stimulants are taken, dopamine synthesis and release increase while inactivation (reuptake) is blocked.

Drug
Effects

B

Stimulants, such as cocaine or methamphetamine, hijack the brain's main reward system leading to addiction to drug and sex.

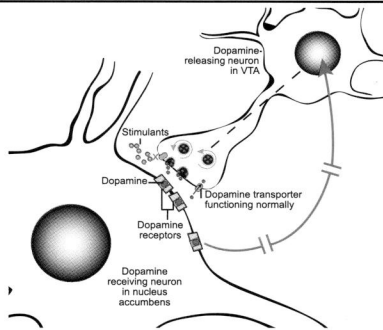

Stimulants (meth, coke, crack, X)

⬆ DA/NE in brain reward centers

⬆ Pulse, heart rate

⬇ Re-uptake metabolism of DA/NE

C

The brain, at ejaculation, turns off vigilance center (the amygdala).

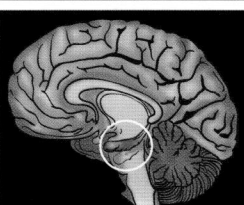

Stimulants
-Prolong/Retard Ejaculation
-Suppress Cortical Inputs
-Flood Reward Center

EDD's
- Prolonged and repeated orgasms
- In combination with poppers, can cause severe ⬇ BP → further suppression of cortical/thalamic inhibitions and stroke (rare)

Poppers
-CNS "Rush" to further ⬇ behavioral inhibitions/judgment
-Blindness (rare), blue-tinted vision (infrequent)
-In combination with EDD's, can cause severe ⬇ BP → further suppression of cortical/thalamic inhibitions & stroke (rare)

D

The penis becomes erect through <u>vasodilation</u>. EDD's* increase potency by inhibiting the enzyme that inactivates the intracellular messenger that causes vasodilation in the penis.

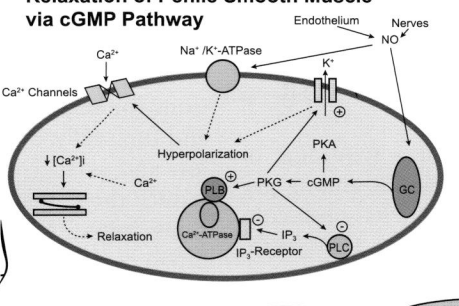

Relaxation of Penile Smooth Muscle via cGMP Pathway

Stimulants
-Inhibit erectile function "Crystal Dick"
-Increase penile sensitivity

Poppers
-Increase blood flow to penis
➡ Overcome erectile problems can facilitate orgasmic response

EDD's
-Inhibit PDE-5, ⬆ cGMP levels ➡
-Prolong erection ⬇ blood pressure

E

The receptive sexual orifice (anus in men; vagina and anus in women) has smooth muscle to maintain continence. Inhaled nitrates ("poppers") relax these muscles, making entry of erect penis easier, more pleasurable and less painful.

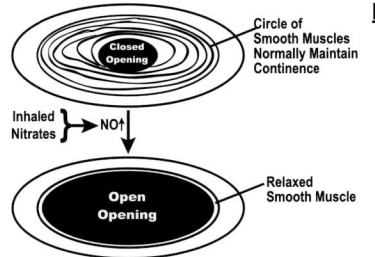

Poppers
⬆ NO concentration in smooth muscle of anus/vagina ➡ expansion
➡ Facilitates "rough" intercourse ➡⬆ permeability of genital mucosal membranes to HIV.

Stimulants
-If applied to anus ("booty bump"), ⬆ pleasure of receptive intercourse ⬇ pain.
- Can cause irritation, ulceration and eventual perforation of anal canal.

Figure 12.3.1 *Biological Mechanisms of Behavioral Risk-Taking in Humans: From the Brain's Reward/Pleasure Centers to The End-Organs of Sexual Intercourse in MSM* 1A: Brain Reward/Addiction Pathways 1B: Brain on Stimulants 1C: Male Brain at Ejaculation 1D: End Organ—The Effects of Drugs on Penis 1E: End Organ—The Effects of Drugs on Anus, Panel 12.3.1 C shows what happens within the brain during sexual intercourse that includes ejaculation and orgasm, while Figure 12.3.1 B shows what happens when a person is using a stimulant drug of abuse, such as methamphetamine, cocaine, or crack, to get high. Obvious DA signaling similarities in both of these situations indicate the potential for synergy between the addiction to sexual risk-taking and the addiction to stimulant drugs, again making the case for a synergy of biological processes favoring risk-taking over risk-reducing behaviors among sex-drug using MSM. In addition, several intra-individual vulnerabilities with biological substrata have been identified as being associated with increased sexual and drug risk-taking among MSM; their psychobiological underpinnings are described next.

can correlate levels of sexual and drug risk-taking behavior with specific genetic contributions to NT activity within the brain, the most we can say at this time is that sexual compulsivity is associated with a variety of risk-taking behaviors among MSM and that a portion of that association is possibly determined by genetically determined differences in the same DA and other neurotransmitter pathways that are observed for sexual sensation seeking among gay/bisexual men.

In a qualitative study of compulsive sexuality attributions among 183 gay/bisexual men in NYC (Parsons et al., 2008), the men attributed both intrinsic and extrinsic sources for the development of sexual compulsivity (SC). Some participants endorsed a belief in a predisposition toward sexually compulsive behavior, whereas others identified factors such as emotional neglect, sexual abuse, or the availability and accessibility of sexual partners. Whatever the underlying genetic, NT, or environmental influences on the development of SC among MSM, there is at least one cognitive-behavioral intervention study (Dilley et al., 2008) that demonstrated that HIV-negative MSM in the highest quartile of SC scores on the Kalichman index were near-significantly (p<.06) more likely to show reduced levels of unprotected anal sex (UAS)with serodiscordant partners (post-intervention) than men in the other three quartiles. Again, this finding is consistent with the general belief that SC is a component of addictive sexual behavior that may be amenable to treatments—cognitive-behavioral, biological, or combinations—already in clinical use for other addictive behaviors.

SEX-DRUG USE AND RISK BEHAVIOR

Since the beginning of the recognition of a syndrome of immune destruction and opportunistic diseases among gay men and intravenous drug users (IDUs), there has been considerable interest in how non-IDU may enhance HIV transmission both directly and indirectly (Ostrow, 1994). This has been a particularly productive approach when applied to long-term longitudinal studies that include high-risk, but HIV-negative, men, such as the Multicenter AIDS Cohort Study (or MACS), that allow direct biological confirmation of self-reported behavioral data through the observation of HIV-seroconversion rates associated with those behavioral patterns during prospective observation.

Most recently, we have examined the role that specific combinations of drugs of choice for sexual enhancement have had on the risk of HIV infection as well as their causal attribution to the overall rates of HIV seroconversion among the cohort at-large (Plankey et al., 2008; Ostrow. Plankey et al., 2009). This work has allowed us to definitively demonstrate that three specific categories of sex-drugs, namely stimulants, poppers, and erectile dysfunction drugs (EDDs), are tightly linked to the majority of new HIV infections observed over the past 8–9 years (see Figures 12.3.2 & 12.3.3, below, as well as the right hand summaries of these drugs' effects in Figure 12.3.1 above). These findings have several important implications for the design of HIV-prevention interventions

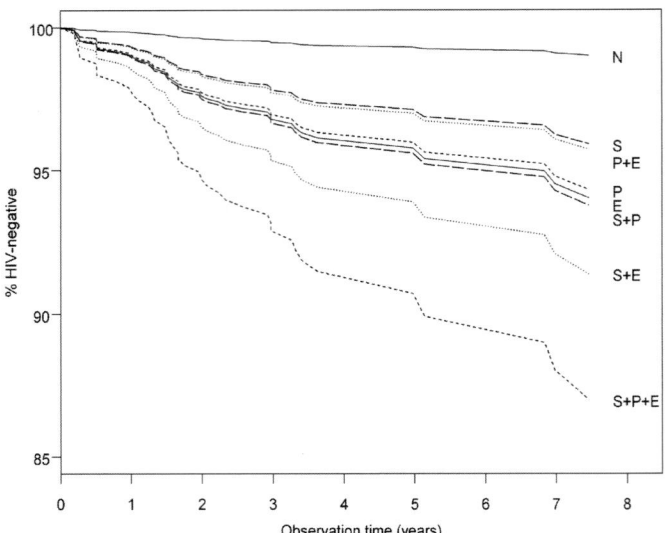

Figure 12.3.2 *Survival Curves for Remaining HIV-Uninfected for the Combo* Drug Use Subgroups. Legend: N= No sex-drug use; S= Stimulant-only use; P= Popper-only use; E= Erectile dysfunction drug (EDD) only use.   From Ostrow, D. G., Plankey, M. W., et al., *AIDS*, 2009.

for drug-using MSM and other non-IDU populations. Most important, in our opinion, is the clear re-demonstration that the most at-risk MSM are polydrug users and that their specific choice of drugs are those that work synergistically to enhance their sexual pleasure and endurance, and that these same drug combinations act to facilitate both sexual disinhibition and HIV transmission. This means that any interventions for such men must target their polydrug use directly and forcefully, as it is an integral part of their sexual behaviors and partner-selection patterns that must be changed to reduce the rising rates of HIV/HCV and other STI infections among MSM, particularly drug-using men in major urban centers of the US.

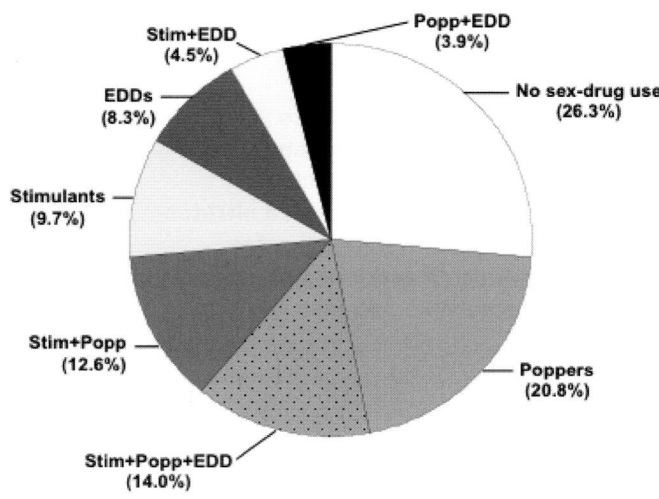

Figure 12.3.3 *HIV Seroconversion (%) Attributable to Sex-Drug Use.* From Ostrow, D. G., Plankey, M. W., et al., *AIDS*, 2009.

A MODEL THAT INTEGRATES BIOLOGICAL, CNS, ORGANISMAL, AND PSYCHOSOCIAL DETERMINANTS OF RISK-TAKING AND HIV PREVENTION IMPLICATIONS FOR DRUG-USING MSM

The interacting and synergistic effects of innate vulnerabilities and strengths, developmental patterns, antagonistic neural and neurotransmitter pathways, and the strategically applied use of sex-drugs to tip the balance between rational decision making and risky pleasure seeking as depicted in Figure 12.3.1 and described in this chapter may make the reader's mind feel like they are encountering an Escherian Mobius strip of infinite variety and without a beginning or an end; what many in the field have referred to as a conundrum of inseparable, interlocked, or intertwining factors that resists scientific analysis of its component parts and the development of targeted interventions to prevent the spread of HIV among drug-using MSM. However, it is hoped that by separately describing the component parts of this complicated amalgam of paths from intact cognition to what may seem irrational behavior, we have provided the reader of this chapter with a guide to specific places for potential interventions. When such targeted interventions are applied systematically and in combination to the problem behaviors that result in the transmission of HIV and other STIs among drug using MSM, the result could be practical and effective intervention systems. Along with techniques to unmask and fortify innate strengths that have kept the majority of MSM from engaging in sex-drug-fueled risk behaviors that contribute to the majority of current HIV infections, such multilevel and developmental intervention systems could help vulnerable men avoid or recover from sex-drug use and HIV risk-taking. (Lim et al., 2010). Thus, the final part of this chapter is to lay out the multidimensional biological-social-psychological components of adult sexual risk-taking that can serve as a "road map" for anyone wanting to pursue HIV prevention among sex-drug using MSM and other vulnerable sex-drug using subpopulations.

CONCLUSIONS

This model (Figure 12.3.4) raises the question of why a particular set of drugs, all of which have both CNS and end-organ vasoactive signaling properties, have become the "drug cocktail" of choice for MSM seeking both maximal behavioral disinhibition and more intense and prolonged sexual pleasure. We hypothesize that the combination of underlying

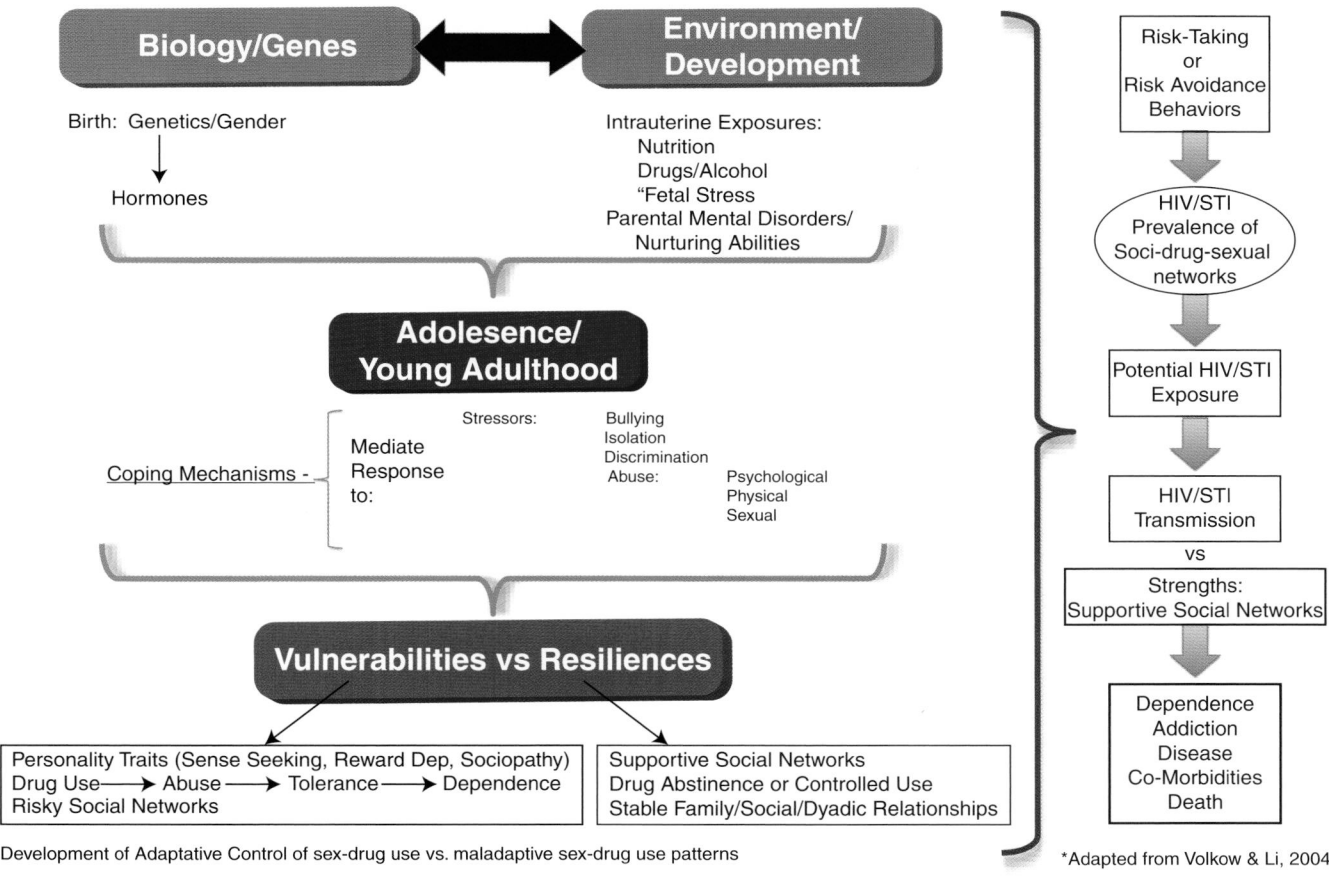

Figure 12.3.4 *An Integrated Psychobiological Model of Behavioral Risk-Taking Among Drug-Using MSM*

"syndemic" vulnerabilities combined with the ease of sexual hook-ups and spread of information in the Internet post-HAART era of decreased concern about HIV/AIDS has selected for (exerted selective pressure on MSM seeking intense sexual gratification) the choice of this particular drug cocktail. Conversely, the combined properties of sex-drugs preferred by the highest risk MSM enhance pleasure and minimize cognitive control to the point that marathon/group sex/poly-drug-fueled orgiastic sexual experiences have become normative in the lives of these riskiest MSM (Semple, Zians, Strathdee, & Patterson, 2008).

Given the recent report by Nazli et al. (2010) on the damage that HIV itself can cause to anorectal mucosa, thus completing the cycle of HIV—increased vulnerability combined with drug use that causes increased trauma to rectum—leads to increased infectivity for both insertive and receptive partners. This study lends further support to our need for effective rectal (and vaginal) microbicides that will stop HIV in situ before it makes contact with rectal or vaginal mucosa, given Nazli et al.'s finding that HIV triggers inflammatory cytokines/chemokines, thus compromising the mucosal/epithelial lining, allowing HIV, as well as other viruses and bacteria, to gain entry, leading directly to transepithelial infection.

Thus, we conclude with another hypothesis—namely that the HIV virus itself may have adapted, through selective transmission of mutations with the ability to disrupt cellular junctions of the target genital epithelium, to take advantage of the preference of sex-drug using MSM to engage in a particular type of risk-taking, namely unprotected anal intercourse in the context of vasoactive drugs that themselves increase the vulnerability of rectal and penile mucosal membranes. This would explain both the relative inability of HIV transmission to occur through the oral ingestion of semen (Ostrow, DiFranceisco, Chmiel, Wagstaff, & Wesch, 1995), as well as the relatively rapid saturation of HIV infection among groups of "barebackers," or men who prefer unprotected anal sex (Halkitis et al., 2005). If this hypothesis turns out to be true, then the current arguments over whether to utilize biological or behavioral prevention methods will, in the end, turn out to be moot. Since risk taking is the combined result of biological, environmental, developmental, social, and behavioral processes that both maximize sexual gratification and promote infection by a virus that appears to be unique in its ability to mutate to take advantage of the resulting optimal conditions for its transmission, it will take a combination of biological, social, environmental, and behavioral interventions to ultimately reduce its sexual spread.

ACKNOWLEDGMENTS

The author would like to acknowledge the excellent graphic assistance of Ms. Judy Konig (Figures 12.3.2 & 12.3.3) of CAMACS, and of Robin Taylor and Bill Wassom (Figures 12.3.1 and 12.3.4) of the University of Nebraska Medical Center for their efforts in turning my ideas into concrete illustrations.

I would also like to thank my long-term colleague, Ronald C Stall, PhD, of the University of Pittsburgh, for his very helpful review and suggestions on an earlier draft of this chapter.

REFERENCES

Cloninger, C. R. (2005). Measurement of personality and its disorders. In J. M. Oldham, A. E. Skodol, & D. S. Bender (Eds.). *The American psychiatric publishing textbook of personality disorders*, (pp. 143–153). Washington DC: American Psychiatric Publishing.

Comings, D. E. & Blum, K. (2000). Reward deficiency syndrome: Genetic aspects of behavioral disorders. *Progress in Brain Research, 126,* 325–341.

Dilley, J. W., Loeb, L., Marson, K., Chen, S., Schwarcz, S., Paul, J., et al. (2008). Sexual compulsiveness and change in unprotected anal intercourse: Unexpected results from a randomized controlled HIV counseling intervention study. *J AIDS, 48,* 113–114.

Ebstein, R. P., & Auerbach, J. G. (2002). Dopamine D4 receptor and serotonin transporter promoter polymorphisms and temperament in early childhood. In J. Benjamin, R. P. Ebstein, & R. H. Belmaker (Eds.). *Molecular Genetics and the Human Personality*, (pp. 143–153). Washington DC: American Psychiatric Publishing.

Fischer, M. J., Wyatt, C. M., Gordon, K., Gibert, C. L., Brown, S. T., Rimland, D., et al. (2010). Hepatitis C and the risk of kidney disease and mortality in Veterans with HIV. *J AIDS, 53,* 222–226.

Grov, C., Parsons, J. T., & Bimbi, D. S. (2009). Sexual compulsivity and sexual risk in gay and bisexual men. *Arch Sex Behav.* Online.

Halkitis, P., N., Wilton, L., Wolitski, R. J., Parsons, J. T., Hoff, C. C., Bimbi, D. S. (2005). Barebacking identity among HIV-positive gay and bisexual men: Demographic, psychological, and behavioral correlates. *AIDS, 19,* S27–S35.

Howe, S., Cole, S. R., Ostrow, D. G., & Mehta, Kirk. (2010). A prospective study of alcohol consumption and HIV acquisition among injection drug users (ALIVE). Manuscript in preparation.

Kalichman S. C., Greenberg, J., & Abel, G. G. (1997). HIV-seropositive men who engage in high-risk sexual behavior: Psychological characteristics and implications for prevention. *AIDS Care, 9* (4): 441–450.

Kalichman, S. C. & David, R. (1995). Sexual sensation seeking and sexual compulsivity scales: Validity, and predicting HIV risk behavior. *J Personality Assessment, 65,* 586–601.

Kim, H. J., Martemyanov, K. A., & Thayer S. A. (2008). Human immunodeficiency virus protein tat induces synapse loss via a reversible process that is distinct from cell death. *J Neurosci, 28,* 12604–12613.

Lim, S. H., H, A., Guadamuz, T., Kao, K., Plankey, M., Ostrow, D. G., et al. (2010). Childhood sexual abuse, gay-related victimization, HIV infection, and syndemic productions among men who have sex with men (MSM): Findings from the Multicenter AIDS Cohort Study (MACS). Oral presentation at the XVIII International AIDS Conference, Vienna, July 21, 2010.

Martin, E. M., Pitrak, D., Weddington, W., Rains, N. A., Nunnally, G., Nixon, H., et al. (2004). Cognitive impulsivity and HIV serostatus in substance dependent males. *J Intern Neuropsych Soc, 10,* 931–938.

Nazli, A., Chan, O., Dobson-Belaire, W. N., Ouellet, M., Tremblay, M. J., Gray-Owen, S. D., et al. (2010). Exposure to HIV-1 directly impairs mucosal epithelial barrier integrity allowing microbial translocation. *PLoS Pathogens,* 6:e10000852.

Ostrow, D. G. (2000). The role of drugs in the sexual lives of men who have sex with men: Continuing barriers to researching this question. *AIDS & Behavior, 4,* 205–219.

Ostrow, D. G. (1994). Substance use and HIV-transmitting behaviors among gay and bisexual men. In R. J. Battjes, A. Sloboda, & W. C. Grace (Eds.). *The context of HIV risk among drug users and their sexual partners*, NIDA Research Monograph 143, pp. 88–113. Rockville, MD: USDHHS.

Ostrow, D. G., DiFranceisco, W., Chmiel, J. S., Wagstaff, D., & Wesch, J. (1995). A case-control study of HIV-1 seroconversion and risk-related behaviors in the Chicago MACS/CCS cohort, 1984–1992. *Am J Epi 142*, 875–883.

Ostrow, D. G., Plankey, M. W., Cox, C., Li, X., Shoptaw, S., Jacobson, L. P., et al. (2009). Specific sex-drug combinations contribute to the majority of recent HIV seroconversions among MSM in the MACS. *J AIDS*, 349–355.

Ostrow, D. G., Silverberg, M., Cook, R. C., Chmiel, J. S., Johnson, L., Li, Xuihoung, et al. (2008). A prospective study of attitudinal and relationship factors as predictors of sexual risk in the MACS. *AIDS & Behavior, 12*, 127–138.

Parsons, J. T., Kelly, B. C., Bimbi, D. S., DiMarie, L., Wainberg, M. W., & Morgenstern, J. (2008). Explanations for the origins of sexual compulsivity among gay and bisexual men. *Arch Sex* Behav, *37*, 817–826.

Sander, P., Cole, S. R., Ostrow, D. G., et al. (2010). A prospective study of alcohol consumption and HIV acquisition among men who have sex with men (MACS). Manuscript in preparation.

Semple, S. J., Zians, J., Strathdee, S. A., & Patterson, T. L. (2008). Sexual marathons and methamphetamine use among HIV-positive men who have sex with men. *Arch Sex Behavior, 38*,583–590.

Stall, R. & Purcell, D. W (2000). Intertwining epidemics: A review of research on substance use among men who have sex with men and its connection to the AIDS epidemic. *AIDS & Behavior, 4*, 181–192.

Volkow, N. D. & Li, T. K. (2004). Drug addiction: The neurobiology of behavior gone awry. *Nat Rev Neurosci, 5*, 963–970.

Zuckerman, M. (2006). Biosocial bases of sensation seeking. In T. Canli (Ed.). *Biology of personality and individual differences*, pp. 37–58. New York: Guilford Press.

12.4

EVERYDAY IMPACT OF HIV-ASSOCIATED NEUROCOGNITIVE DISORDERS

Thomas D. Marcotte, J. Cobb Scott, Charles H. Hinkin, and Robert K. Heaton

Rates of HIV-associated neurocognitive disorders (HAND) are not markedly different now from what they were during the pre-HAART era, though the most severe form of HAND, dementia, is less common now than previously and, overall, there has been a shift within the HAND spectrum towards mild-to-moderate impairments. There is now substantial evidence that HIV-associated neurocognitive impairments less severe than dementia can significantly affect daily functioning. In this chapter, we detail research regarding the effects of HAND on survival, quality of life, instrumental activities of daily living, medication adherence, vocational functioning, automobile driving, and other specific cognitive aspects of everyday functioning. We conclude with recommendations for future research.

Despite significant advances in pharmacological treatments for HIV, and concomitant reductions in morbidity and mortality, HIV-related neuropsychological impairments remain common. For example, in a recent study based upon baseline evaluations in CHARTER (a six-site study in the US), 52% of 1,565 HIV+ individuals evidenced at least a mild degree of global neurocognitive impairment (Heaton et al., 2010). A 40% impairment rate was found even in those individuals with minimal comorbidities. These findings, surprisingly, are not substantially different from those reported in the pre-HAART era (Heaton et al., 2011), in which rates ranged from 30% in individuals in the early, medically asymptomatic phase of the disease (Bornstein et al., 1992; Heaton et al., 1995; Stern et al., 1991; White, Heaton, & Monsch, 1995) to 55% in persons with an AIDS-defining opportunistic condition (Heaton et al., 1995). It does appear, however, that severe dementia is less common in the HAART era and that impairments are more frequently in the mild-to-moderate range.

Over the years, various groups have sought to operationally define HIV-related neurocognitive/neurologic conditions. Although specifics have varied, important components of these schemas have been determination of 1) the presence of neuropsychological impairment and 2) whether these impairments impact everyday activities (American Academy of Neurology AIDS Task Force, 1991; Antinori et al., 2007; Grant & Atkinson, 1995b).

Based upon apparent changes in the phenomenology of HIV-related cognitive dysfunction as well as a desire to further refine the criteria, the National Institute of Mental Health and National Institute of Neurological Disorders and Stroke tasked a workgroup to revisit the AAN criteria (Antinori et al., 2007). The workgroup adopted a revised nosology (the "Frascati criteria") that was consistent with schema proposed earlier by Grant and Atkinson (1995a), emphasizing the *neurocognitive* complications of HIV and excluding the motor, social/personality, and emotional abnormalities that were part of the AAN criteria. Importantly, the revised nosology also classifies cases in which there may be objective cognitive impairment but no evidence that it is affecting everyday functioning, as studies have suggested that these milder impairments may still reflect brain pathology (Cherner et al., 2007) and predict mortality (Ellis et al., 1997). As such, it is believed to be important to monitor individuals with milder impairments more closely and adapt treatment strategies appropriately.

In brief, the revised criteria (Antinori et al., 2007) are as follows (for each diagnosis, it is required that the cognitive impairment cannot be explained by other comorbidities, nor can it be the result of a delirium):

Asymptomatic Neurocognitive Impairment (ANI). Performance is at least one standard deviation (SD) below the mean of demographically adjusted normative scores in at least two cognitive domains (attention-information processing, language, abstraction-executive, complex perceptual motor skills, memory [including learning and recall], simple motor skills, *or* sensory perceptual abilities). At least five cognitive domains need to be assessed.

Minor Neurocognitive Disorder (MND). MND meets the ANI criteria above. In addition, the neurocognitive abnormality must result in at least mildly impaired everyday functioning and cannot meet criteria for dementia. Indicators of mild functional decline include needing increased assistance with at least two instrumental activities of daily living (IADLs; e.g., medication management, driving), inability to perform some aspects of a previous job, reduced efficiency or productivity, problems with ≥ 2 aspects of cognition in daily life, or performing >1 SD below an appropriate normative mean on at least one performance-based, standardized functional test.

HIV-Associated Dementia (HAD). HAD requires a) acquired moderate-to-severe cognitive impairment (at least 2 SD below demographically corrected normative means in at least two different cognitive areas [see above]), and b) marked difficulty in everyday functioning due to the cognitive impairment. Major functional decline requires two or more of the following: unable to maintain former employment, requires substantially greater assistance with more than two IADLs, significantly greater difficulty with ≥ 4 aspects of cognition, or scores >2 SD below an appropriate normative mean on at least one performance-based standardized functional task or > 1 SD below the mean on at least two tasks.

In addition, there is now a classification for "in remission," based upon indications that neurocognitive impairment can have a waxing/waning course in some HIV+ individuals.

Functional status is clearly important in both patient care and research, and there is now considerable evidence that HIV-associated neurocognitive impairments short of dementia can significantly affect daily functioning. In the following sections we detail research to date regarding the effects of HAND on survival, quality of life, instrumental activities of daily living, medication adherence, vocational functioning, automobile driving, and specific cognitive aspects of everyday functioning that are not included in the prior sections, and conclude with recommendations for future research.

It should be noted that there are many different approaches to examining real-world performance. Some of the following studies examine "manifest functioning," or indicators of how the individual does in the real world (employment status, driving crashes). Oftentimes, however, real-world performance is examined via self-report, which can be significantly affected by mood, such that depressed individuals tend to over-report deficits that are not objectively apparent (Hinkin et al., 1996; Rourke, Halman, & Bassel, 1999; van Gorp et al., 1991; Wilkins et al., 1991). In addition, real-world performance can be affected by many other factors, such as motivation, physical conditions, environment, disability status, and so forth (Marcotte, Scott, Kamat, & Heaton, 2009c). Thus, in an attempt to minimize the influence of these factors, a number of investigations have utilized objective, laboratory-based measures of functional capacity, often tools that closely approximate the components of real world tasks.

NEUROPSYCHOLOGICAL PERFORMANCE AS A PREDICTOR OF SURVIVAL

Since the early years of the HIV epidemic, a handful of studies have indicated that HAND is associated with increased mortality. This was particularly true of patients with severe dementia, who in the pre-HAART era survived a median of six months following a dementia diagnosis (McArthur et al., 1993), although patients without an AIDS diagnosis still died more rapidly than cognitively normal subjects (Mayeux et al., 1993). In a study of participants without HIV-associated dementia from the HIV Neurobehavioral Research Center (HNRC), the highest mortality rate was found for those

subjects with minor neurocognitive disorder. Participants with asymptomatic impairment had a lower mortality rate than those with MND, but it was still higher than neuropsychologically (NP) normal participants, even after controlling for medical status (Ellis et al., 1997). With a different cohort, Sacktor and colleagues (1996) reported that a sustained decline (over two or more visits) in psychomotor performance was the strongest neuropsychological predictor of death during the follow-up period.

A limited number of studies have examined this issue in the HAART era. Tozzi and colleagues (2005) followed 412 HIV+ participants for a median of 32.4 months. As would be expected, virologic response was strongly associated with subsequent mortality. In addition, though, patients with neurocognitive impairment were more likely to experience failure of virologic suppression. Most importantly, while the presence of HAND did not affect survival in those with on-going viral suppression, in those patients who experienced virologic failure there was a threefold increase in mortality in patients with HAND, even after controlling for age, HIV transmission modality, hepatitis C, Centers for Disease Control (CDC) stage, and baseline CD4 cell count and viral load (Tozzi et al., 2005).

Despite these relatively consistent findings, the reasons for the relationship between HAND and mortality are not fully understood. It could be that cognitively impaired individuals are less likely to be adherent to antiretroviral (ARV) medications (Hinkin et al., 2004), and future studies may show that the increasing simplicity of HIV medication regimens (e.g., single daily dosages) improves survival in impaired cohorts. Furthermore, it is possible that the central nervous system (CNS) might serve as an additional reservoir for HIV replication, as studies have demonstrated differing viral evolution in the cerebrospinal fluid (CSF). Lastly, individuals with HAND may have less capacity to utilize resources (e.g., support groups, meal services, in-home care providers) to manage their disease, and such reduced utilization may contribute to declining health.

Regardless of the mechanism(s), the continued finding that HAND predicts reduced survival argues for the importance of monitoring cognitive status (and perhaps CSF viral levels) in patients with HIV (Tozzi et al., 2005).

QUALITY OF LIFE

Numerous studies have shown that advanced HIV disease stage and related medical symptoms (Revicki, Wu, & Murray, 1995), as well as comorbid substance abuse and psychiatric disorders (Liu et al., 2006; Sherbourne et al., 2000), are associated with worse quality of life. In addition, a number of studies has indicated that HAND can significantly affect quality of life, even after controlling for medical factors (Kaplan et al., 1995; Kaplan et al., 1997; Parsons, Braaten, Hall, & Robertson, 2006; Revicki et al., 1995; Tozzi et al., 2004; Trepanier et al., 2005). For example, among a sample of approximately 500 HIV+ subjects drawn from the HNRC in the pre-HAART era, quality of life diminished as the severity of cognitive impairment increased, even after controlling for relevant medical factors (Kaplan et al., 1995). Lowest quality of life was evident in individuals with syndromic impairment (MND, HAD) (Kaplan, Mausbach, Marcotte, & Patterson, 2009). Similar findings have been reported in a small sample of HIV-infected women (Osowiecki et al., 2000). In the HAART era, using an Italian translation of the Medical Outcomes Study (MOS)–HIV instrument with 111 patients, cognitively impaired individuals reported poorer quality of life across all domains—physical health summary score, mental health summary score, pain, physical functioning, role functioning, social functioning, mental health, energy, health distress, cognitive functioning, general health perceptions, and quality of life (Tozzi et al., 2004). Similar to previous studies in the pre-HAART era, quality of life was lower in those with higher levels of cognitive impairment.

ACTIVITIES OF DAILY LIVING

The inability of HIV-infected individuals to perform basic activities of daily living, such as grooming, dressing, and bathing, is typically the result of advanced physical symptoms; only in the case of severe dementia do cognitive impairments affect these types of activities (Boccellari et al., 1994). More complex activities, though, such as money management, meal preparation, medication management, and job-related skills (i.e., IADLs) may be affected by more subtle cognitive impairments. Given the ongoing high prevalence of such impairments, assessing complex IADL functioning has added importance.

One of the most comprehensive studies of everyday functioning in HIV was carried out by Heaton and colleagues (2004), who examined 267 HIV-infected individuals (58% with an AIDS diagnosis) with a comprehensive functional battery, including standardized instruments assessing grocery shopping, cooking, financial management, medication management, and vocational functioning. Participants performed the tasks using mock scenarios and items, as though they were performing the activity in daily life. For example, the Shopping task, adapted from the Direct Assessment of Functional Status (DAFS; Loewenstein & Bates, 1992), required subjects to select items off a shelf from a previously presented grocery list, while Cooking required participants to follow recipes and coordinate the timing of a meal, using simulated items, a microwave, and hotplate. The Finances assessment included the Financial Skills (calculating currency) subtest from the DAFS, as well as a new task that required individuals to pay bills and balance their checkbook while maintaining a minimum balance of $100 (to allow for emergency or other unforeseen needs). Medication Management was a modification of the Medication Management Test designed by Albert and colleagues (Albert et al., 1999). Lastly, Vocational Skills were evaluated using standardized work samples (MESA SF2, Valpar International Corporation, 1986) and vocational assessment software (COMPASS, Valpar International Corporation, 1992).

Compared to cognitively intact HIV+ participants, the group with neuropsychological impairment performed significantly worse on all functional measures. A global measure (Functional Deficit Score; FDS) derived from test results on the entire functional battery proved to be the most sensitive measure to cognitive difficulties. Similar findings have been reported in a Spanish-speaking cohort (Mindt et al., 2003). The largest group differences were found on Vocational Skills, followed by Finances and Medication Management. Impairments in executive functioning, learning, verbal abilities, and attention/working memory were most predictive of performance on the functional measures.

Of note, both neuropsychological and functional scores were independent predictors of "real world" functional status (i.e., self-reported cognitive difficulties, level of dependence in IADLs, and employment status) in this study. Thus, a) even mild-to-moderate levels of cognitive dysfunction can impact everyday functioning; and b) neuropsychological evaluations may not completely assess the abilities needed to successfully execute these tasks in real life. In the assessment of HIV-infected individuals, as well as other conditions with neurologic compromise, functional tests that more directly assess capacity may prove useful in predicting everyday outcomes (Marcotte & Grant, 2009a).

It is important to note that depressed mood was also a significant predictor of both self-reported dependence and cognitive complaints, so it remains important to consider affective status when assessing functional capacity and predicting functioning outside of the laboratory.

MEDICATION MANAGEMENT

The advent of HAART significantly decreased the morbidity and mortality associated with HIV infection. However, it is vital that patients adhere to their prescribed regimens, since deviations from the recommended dosing and dietary instructions decrease drug concentrations, lower the likelihood of viral suppression, and increase the risk for progression to AIDS (Bangsberg et al., 2001; Chesney et al., 2000). Poor adherence may lead to the emergence of drug-resistant viral mutations, resulting in reduced effectiveness of the specific, and pharmacologically related, medication regimens. Previous studies indicate that adherence rates should approximate 90–95% of prescribed doses in order to avoid negative clinical virologic outcomes (Bangsberg, 2006; Haubrich et al., 1999), although there are indications that lower adherence rates may be adequate for newer regimens. Unfortunately, studies using various methodologies to assess adherence indicate that up to 40% of individuals fail to take medications in accordance with dosage, time, and dietary instructions (Chesney et al., 2000; Hinkin et al., 2004; Maher et al., 1999; Nieuwkerk et al., 2001; Singh et al., 1996). Adherence to any medication regimen is challenging when, as in HIV, the duration of treatment is long, patients are often asymptomatic, treatment is designed to prevent rather than cure, and side effects are common. Moreover, HIV-associated neurocognitive impairments make medication management, already a challenging task, even more difficult.

As with other instrumental activities of daily living, one of the challenges in understanding the contributors, and barriers, to medication adherence is establishing a "gold standard" regarding measurement of medication adherence.

Self-report, or simply asking participants via interviews or questionnaires the degree to which they have been adherent to their prescribed regimen, is the most commonly used method. However, there are reasons to be concerned that participants may overestimate actual adherence rates, particularly in individuals with cognitive impairment. For example, when compared to electronic monitoring results (see below), participants who openly admit poor adherence tend to be accurate, while those who report perfect to near-perfect adherence may overestimate their rates by 10–20% (Arnsten et al., 2001; Levine et al., 2005). Self-report also appears to be affected by the time interval that is being estimated, as individuals have been shown to be more accurate over shorter time frames (Levine et al., 2006). Despite the decided limitations inherent in self-report, because of its ease and simplicity of use virtually all clinicians and many, if not most, researchers rely upon this approach.

Pill counts involve counting the number of pills remaining in a patient's pillbox and comparing this to the number of pills the individual should have ingested based upon his/her prescription. Excess doses are assumed to represent doses not taken as prescribed. Limitations to this approach include the assumption that pills not in the container were taken (and not lost or discarded), as well as an inability to determine whether the pills were taken as scheduled (Gorman, Foley, Ettenhofer, Hinkin, & van Gorp, 2009). In addition, patients may remove extra doses in anticipation of the upcoming pill count and thus appear more adherent than they actually are. A modified approach is the "unannounced pill count," in which staff go to patient residences without warning in order to assess adherence. This approach has correlated well with biologic outcomes such as HIV viral load (Bangsberg et al., 2001), but can be cost- and time-prohibitive. Yet another variant is "unannounced telephone pill counts" (Kalichman et al., 2008). Using this approach, patients are telephoned and asked to count out their remaining pills, which again theoretically minimizes their opportunity to quickly calculate the "correct" number of remaining pills. This reduces the economic costs associated with home visits while still maintaining reasonable correlation with biologic outcomes.

Pharmacy refill records are another objective measure of estimated adherence levels. If patients are refilling their prescriptions as scheduled, it is assumed with this method that they are likely to be taking their medications as prescribed. Since this method is less obtrusive, it may be less prone to participants manipulating their pill counts to have higher adherence estimates. Unfortunately, this approach has shortcomings similar to those seen with pill counts and lacks granularity in terms of tracking adherence over short timeframes (Gorman et al., 2009). This approach works best in settings with centralized computerized pharmacy records (e.g., V.A. Medical Centers); it is more cumbersome when patients utilize different pharmacies.

Electronic measuring devices, such as the Medication Event Monitoring System (MEMS; Aprex Corp, Union City, CA), may be particularly helpful in assessing adherence in individuals with cognitive impairment, since they may have difficulty remembering whether or not they took their medications as prescribed. Such systems use a computer chip in the top of the pill bottle that records the date, time, and duration of pill bottle opening, data which can later be downloaded by the investigator. It appears that this method may be more accurate than pill counts or self-report. For example, MEMS data is more closely related to viral suppression than self-report (Arnsten et al., 2001). However, one limitation with this approach is the bulkiness of the MEMS bottle, which may make it cumbersome to carry around inconspicuously, and may result in "pocket-dosing," or patients taking out an extra dose for use at a later time point (Hinkin et al., 2004).

Performance-based measures have been utilized by a limited number of investigators. Theoretically, this approach enables the assessment of one's capacity to perform the various medication-related tasks and can perhaps identify those who are at increased risk for poor adherence. One measure designed with this purpose is the Medication Management Test (MMT) (Albert et al., 1999). Respondents are scored according to their ability to interpret prescription label and medication insert information ("medication inference" component) and to dispense five medications from pre-specified prescription medication bottles ("pill dispensing" component). Items in the medication inference component require respondents to perform simple calculations to determine how many days a prescription will last and whether they have missed a dose of medicine based on a pill count. Other items ask respondents to identify particular dosing instructions (i.e., to determine, based on label information, which of the five medicines should be taken with food or may cause drowsiness). In the pill component, subjects are scored on their ability to transfer "pills" from prescription bottles to a medication organizer, a box designed to hold a week's supply of pills. The original test and its modification are reliable measures of medication management skill and have been validated against cognitive status in a number of HIV patient samples (Albert et al., 1999; Heaton et al., 2004).

In a study of three different patient samples, Albert and colleagues (1999) found that patients with low scores in executive function and psychomotor skills were less able to follow label information and correctly pour different medicines. People scoring one or more standard deviations below age- and education-adjusted norms correctly poured only three of the five medicines, on average, while respondents with better cognitive performance correctly poured four of the five medicines. Thus, mild cognitive impairment was associated with an increased risk of one additional error in medication management.

Heaton and colleagues (2004) adapted the MMT by reordering test items by ascending order of difficulty, rewording some test items and the mock medication insert, and reducing the number of fictitious medications (from 5 to 3) and inference items (from 15 to 7). This revised MMT requires approximately 10 minutes to administer and has been shown to correlate with neuropsychological deficits in executive function and memory in HIV-infected individuals (Heaton et al., 2004).

Given the inherent limitations in each of the above-described assessment approaches, there is a general consensus that a multi-modal approach to assessing adherence—using self-report and objectives measures—provides the best estimate of adherence in this (and most) populations.

PREDICTORS OF ADHERENCE

Various studies have identified a number of consistent non-cognitive predictors of poor adherence, including adverse side effects of drugs (Mocroft et al., 2005), negative health beliefs regarding treatment (Horne et al., 2004), comorbid psychiatric disorders (Starace et al., 2002), comorbid substance abuse (Hinkin et al., 2007), and younger age (Hinkin et al., 2004).

With respect to cognitive factors, it appears that impairments in memory, executive function, and psychomotor functioning are associated with significant difficulties with medication management. In a series of studies, Hinkin and colleagues (Ettenhofer, Foley, Castellon, & Hinkin, 2010; Hinkin et al., 2007; Hinkin et al., 2002; Hinkin et al., 2004; Levine et al., 2006) examined adherence to HIV medication regimens using MEMS caps. Impairments in attention, memory, executive functioning, and psychomotor speed were associated with lower adherence rates across all age groups. However, the impact of cognitive impairment was most significant in those individuals with complex medication regimens (three or more doses per day). Contrary to expectations, older participants (ages 50–69) were far more adherent than younger subjects (53% of older participants achieved a 95% adherence rate vs. 26% of younger participants). Possible explanations for this finding are that taking medication impacts the lifestyle of older individuals less, or that it is easier for older individuals to accommodate pill taking into their daily activities. In addition, older adults are more likely to have prior experiences taking daily medications for other age-related illnesses. Of note, further analyses indicated that while there was little difference in cognitive performance between the two younger groups and the older adherers, the older participants who were poor adherers had much worse cognitive functioning.

Most likely, the relationship between cognition and adherence in HIV is bi-directional. Individuals who fail to adhere are most likely to experience increased viral load and disease progression, increasing the risk for the development of cognitive impairment, while impaired individuals are also more likely to be nonadherent.

Investigators have begun to develop new interventions to improve adherence. Andrade and colleagues (2005) used the Disease Management Assistance System, a simple auditory reminding device that notified individuals of the timing and dosing of their medications, in a randomized clinical trial. Although adherence rates after treatment did not significantly differ between the treatment (80%) and control groups (65%), an analysis of individuals with memory impairment revealed significantly greater adherence in the treatment group (77%) when compared to the control subjects (57%). However, the use of such a reminding program may have unintended

consequences, including reductions in quality of life for some individuals (Wu et al., 2006). Psychosocial and educational interventions are also being developed to improve adherence by adjusting health beliefs and providing problem solving skills and support for overcoming barriers such as psychiatric symptoms (Golin et al., 2006; Wagner et al., 2006), although the outcome of such interventions awaits further study.

VOCATIONAL FUNCTIONING

Although there is certainly an "aging" of patients with HIV, it is still a condition primarily of the young-to-middle aged segment of society, a group with many years of potential work life ahead of them. In the mid 1990s, as a consequence of new medications, many HIV-infected individuals experienced a "second life" (Rabkin & Ferrando, 1997), with the possibility that they might be able to return to work (Martin, Arns, Batterham, Afifi, & Steckart, 2006). More recently, with the continued advances in treatment options, the lifespan of individuals with HIV infection has approached that of the uninfected population. However, the constellation of symptoms associated with HIV, including cognitive impairment, may still result in work-related disability. It has been estimated that the productivity loss due to HIV infection may cost as much as $22,000 per person-year (Liu, Guo, & Smith, 2004), providing another reason to examine the factors that contribute to vocational decline, as well as successful return to work.

In the pre-HAART era, individuals with AIDS were 2.7 times more likely to lose full-time employment over a 6-month follow-up period than demographically similar HIV-negative individuals (Kass, Munoz, Chen, Zucconi, & Bing, 1994). With respect to HIV-related neurocognitive impairments, one study (Heaton et al., 1994) found that unemployment was almost three times higher in HIV-seropositive individuals with cognitive impairment than neuropsychologically normal HIV+ individuals (26.9% vs. 9.7%). Similar results were seen even after removing subjects having disabling medical conditions (17.5% vs. 7.9%). Among those who were working, cognitive impairment was associated with a higher reported rate of difficulty performing jobs compared to those who were cognitively normal (29.6% vs. 5.9%, respectively). Even participants classified as having mild impairment were more likely to be unemployed (22% vs. 10%) and more likely to complain of decreased work ability (28% vs. 6%) compared to cognitively normal subjects.

In a different study (Albert et al., 1995), medically asymptomatic HIV+ participants who were employed at baseline and followed for up to 4.5 years had a relative risk of work disability of 2.76 when compared to HIV-seronegative participants. This was primarily driven by a much higher risk (RR, 8.47) for the subset of participants who developed severe cognitive impairment; those HIV+ participants without impairment at follow-up did not have an elevated disability risk (RR, 2.21). A study of individuals with advanced HIV disease (van Gorp, Baerwald, Ferrando, McElhiney, & Rabkin, 1999) similarly found that unemployed participants were twice as likely to be impaired as those who were employed

(22% vs. 11%). Even after controlling for age, CD4 cell count, and level of physical limitations, unemployed participants were still found to perform more poorly on tasks of learning and memory (CVLT total), response inhibition (Stroop Color-Word), and cognitive flexibility (Trails B). Physical disabilities and performance on Trails B were significant predictors of employment status, with modest accuracy in identifying unemployed (77%) and employed (55%) subjects.

One of the limitations of studies examining manifest vocational functioning (e.g., real world employment status) is that they do not necessarily provide information as to whether individuals have the cognitive capability to work. The employability of an HIV+ person may be affected by physical declines or disability eligibility (which may also impact access to insurance/medications), among other factors. One way to address this limitation would be to have participants complete a performance-based assessment of their vocational capacity (i.e., objective tests of their abilities), that can be administered within the lab or clinic.

Heaton and colleagues took this approach in a series of studies examining the vocational impact of HIV-related neuropsychological impairments (Heaton et al., 2004; Heaton et al., 1996). Participants completed a standardized battery of vocation-related tasks (Valpar International Corporation, 1986, 1992) that consisted of both manual (e.g., placing wires through loops) and computerized tasks (assessing abilities such as shape discrimination and tracking). This multi-modal, criterion-referenced vocational battery provided ability estimates of 13 job abilities identified by the U.S. Department of Labor (U.S. Department of Labor, 1991). Since most jobs within the U.S. economy have been classified by the Department of Labor as to the level of performance on each ability that is needed to adequately perform the job functions, this enabled a comparison of current performance (on the work sample battery) with previous ability as demonstrated by the jobs that individuals held throughout their work history.

Three groups—HIV-negative, HIV+ neuropsychological normal, and HIV+ neuropsychologically impaired—were matched according to their prior work history (indicating similar premorbid vocational levels). The HIV+ NP-impaired subjects performed more poorly across most objectively assessed work ability areas, suggesting that they had suffered the greatest decline in vocational functioning. This was confirmed by a direct comparison of current functioning and work history: the two neuropsychologically normal groups demonstrated higher current functioning than expected given their work history (since a person's work often doesn't require his/her highest ability levels), whereas the HIV+ cognitively impaired group had reduced abilities compared to their prior work history, suggesting a decline from previous functioning.

Similar results were found in a larger cohort from the HAART era, with the discrepancy between prior work ability and current vocational functioning being almost three times greater in the NP-impaired group (Heaton et al., 2004). An AIDS diagnosis, depressive symptomatology, and NP deficits in abstraction/executive functioning, verbal function, and attention/working memory abilities were the strongest predictors of work sample performance.

HAART holds the promise of potentially giving unemployed HIV+ individuals an opportunity to return to work. However, while HAART increases the probability of HIV+ individuals remaining employed (Goldman & Bao, 2004), numerous studies have reported that only a small proportion of individuals who were unemployed at baseline became employed at follow-up (Martin et al., 2006; Rabkin, McElhiney, Ferrando, van Gorp, & Lin, 2004). There have thus been attempts to identify predictors for those HIV+ persons who can become productively employed. In these latter studies, the most robust predictors of employment and hours worked were the receipt of disability payments (those receiving payments were less likely to return to work), as well as past or current diagnosis of depressive disorder, physical limitations, and worse performance on neuropsychological measures. These findings are consistent with the notion that the most significant barriers to returning to work for individuals infected with HIV were the potential loss of disability benefits and publicly funded health insurance (Brooks, Martin, Ortiz, & Veniegas, 2004), and the fear that benefits may not be reinstated once taken away, even with worsening health (Razzano, Hamilton, & Perloff, 2006). Another potential barrier is that HIV+ individuals may enter the workforce after many years of unemployment and thus may be more likely to be offered low-wage or part-time positions, which may provide inadequate or minimal health insurance (Lem et al., 2005).

On the other hand, one study found that 52% of individuals unemployed at baseline found some sort of employment during two years of follow-up (van Gorp et al., 2007). The investigators sought to identify neuropsychological predictors of return to work. Only performance on a measure of learning (California Verbal Learning Test) predicted finding employment. Older age, presence of an AIDS diagnosis, and length of unemployment were reported as barriers to finding work.

Few studies have examined the effectiveness of an occupational rehabilitation program with HIV-infected individuals. One program combined psychoeducation with occupational therapy services and addressed a range of physical, psychosocial, and environmental issues (Kielhofner et al., 2004). Of the 90 participants who completed the program, 60 (66.7%) returned to work. A recent study examined the degree to which neuropsychological test performance predicted outcomes in a controlled trial of a vocational rehabilitation program (Chernoff, Martin, Schrock, & Huy, 2010). Although executive functioning was statistically significant in predicting employment status at the end of the study, the effect was small, and in general the neuropsychological test results were not predictive of steps taken towards achieving employment. The authors cautioned that, despite this cohort reporting being ready to return to work, other factors, such as self-efficacy and sense of purpose, might be more predictive of success than cognitive functioning. Clearly, more prospective studies in this area are needed, especially since increasing numbers of individuals may be participating in vocational rehabilitation or assistance programs (McGinn, Gahagan, & Gibson, 2005).

AUTOMOBILE DRIVING

Driving an automobile is a complex task requiring intact perception, attention, tracking, choice reaction, sequential movements, and judgment and planning. As with employment, driving an automobile is an activity that HIV+ individuals would be expected to undertake frequently. Surprisingly, there has been limited research on the impact that HIV-associated neurocognitive disorders may have on driving ability. While assessment of driving abilities is challenging since there is currently no clear standard for the concept of "impaired driving skills" (Marcotte & Scott, 2004a), there is evidence, via a number of methodologies, that a subset of HIV-infected individuals with cognitive impairment experience an overall reduction in driving abilities.

In a sample of 146 HIV-infected participants surveyed at the HIV Neurobehavioral Research Center, 29% reported a decline in their driving ability since becoming infected (Marcotte et al., 2000). Cognitively impaired individuals were much less likely to be driving than NP-intact individuals (OR = 2.9, p = .02), even after controlling for CDC stage and employment status. However, participants did not necessarily attribute their reduction in driving abilities to cognitive difficulties, so it is unclear whether this represents an appropriate adaptive response to impaired driving skills.

As with medication adherence, one of the challenges in determining the impact of HIV-related impairments on everyday functioning is identifying a methodology that can serve as the "gold standard" for driving impairments. Approaches include reviewing driving history, assessing performance on a laboratory-based driving simulator, and evaluating abilities based upon an on-road drive.

Traffic ticket and crash history have the advantage of providing one with an extended sample of behavior, which may offer the most realistic impression of how individuals perform under conditions in which they actually drive. However, this information can be biased. Not all crashes are reported to authorities, and participants, particularly those with cognitive impairment, may not have accurate recall of their driving history. Participants may also be biased towards reporting results that cast them in the best light. In addition, crashes and tickets are both rare occurrences that may not capture reductions in driving ability, especially since a crash may be avoided because of the defensive behavior of other drivers (or alternatively could be the fault of other drivers). Acknowledging these limitations, we examined self-reported driving history in 105 HIV+ individuals at the HNRC who had recently driven an automobile (Marcotte et al., 2000). Twenty-five of the subjects were classified as cognitively impaired. The two groups were similar with respect to demographic and medical characteristics, as well as driving history (e.g., miles driven in the prior year, proportion admitting to driving while intoxicated). Compared to NP-normal subjects, NP-impaired subjects were more likely to have a moving violation (33% vs. 10%) in the prior year, with a trend toward having a higher crash rate (33% vs. 18%).

Objective, laboratory-based assessments overcome some of the limitations in using crash/ticket history. Driving simulators enable one to examine driving behavior under controlled conditions. They ensure that all subjects undergo a similar driving experience, and facilitate examination of performance during critical incidents, such as emergency (e.g., pedestrian walking into the roadway) or novel (e.g., fog) situations that cannot be ethically or feasibly recreated during on-road driving. These situations are important, since driving can in some ways be equated to flying a plane—under most conditions the task is relatively routine and involves overlearned behaviors, though there are rare, but critical, events (e.g., crash avoidance, or in-flight emergency) that require intact higher-level and integrated skills.

Utilizing an interactive, computer-based driving simulator, our group (Marcotte et al., 1999) studied 68 HIV-infected individuals at varying disease stages, assessing lane tracking, divided attention, driving in traffic, and crash avoidance. Cognitively impaired individuals demonstrated greater "swerving" within their lane, resulting in a five times higher likelihood of failing the lane-tracking task based upon previously developed criteria. Cognitively impaired participants also displayed a significantly higher number of simulator crashes on a city driving simulation compared to cognitively intact individuals (2.3 crashes versus 1.5 crashes); those diagnosed with MND had the highest number of crashes. Impairments in the domains of abstraction/executive functioning and attention/speed of information processing were most often associated with poor performance on the simulations.

Despite dramatic improvements in graphics and computing capabilities, simulators still do not fully recreate the multisensory driving experience (3-D environment, sounds, feel of the roadway, number of typical cars in the road). And even though participants take the testing seriously, they are still aware that in a crash there will be no property damage or bodily injury.

On-road driving evaluations overcome these limitations, and are most often considered the gold standard for identifying impaired drivers. Participants typically drive a standardized route and are scored by driving instructors on tasks such as scanning the environment, maintaining safe distances, and whether they make dangerous maneuvers. Importantly, reliability of scoring is good when structured evaluations are used (Hunt et al., 1997; Marcotte et al., 2004b; Odenheimer et al., 1994).

We thus sought to extend our previous findings by implementing a multi-modal assessment that included a 35 minute on-road driving evaluation, computer-based simulations that emulated city driving and assessed navigation skills, and neuropsychological testing (Marcotte et al., 2004b). The structured on-road evaluation included both residential and highway driving, and ratings were completed by two examiners. The simulations were designed to capture abilities not normally assessed in driving evaluations (quick decision-making [i.e., in emergency or novel situations] and the ability to effectively navigate using a map).

We assessed 40 HIV+ and 20 HIV-negative control participants. The HIV+ NP-impaired participants, in contrast to the HIV- and HIV+ NP-normal groups, were classified as unsafe in the on-road evaluation at a higher rate

(36% versus 6%), had more crashes on simulated routine and emergency driving tasks, and made almost three times the number of navigational errors as the other groups. The HIV- and HIV+ NP-normal participants, on the other hand, performed similarly on all evaluations. We concluded that HIV seropositivity alone does not increase the risk for driving impairment, but rather it is the cognitive changes that might occur in the presence of HIV. Importantly, performance on the neuropsychological tests, number of crashes on city driving, and route efficiency on the navigation task were all independent predictors of on-road performance, indicating that data from a direct assessment of driving skills (e.g., via simulator) yields data relevant to real-world performance above and beyond NP data alone. Impairment in executive functioning was the strongest predictor of failing the on-road evaluation. Notably, some of the individuals who failed the on-road driving test lacked awareness of their performance which indicates that clinicians should be cautious when relying on a patient's self-report of driving ability. These individuals had impairments that were generally greater than mild, particularly in executive functioning and learning.

Simulators may only be available in select clinics and labs, and so we sought to determine whether other measures might be useful in extending the utility of common neuropsychological tests in predicting at-risk drivers. We focused on visual attention, which is widely believed to be an important component of safe driving (Marcotte & Scott, 2009b). The study (Marcotte et al., 2006) utilized the Useful Field of View (UFOV, Visual Resources, 1998) task, which has shown particular success in identifying older at-risk drivers (e.g., Ball, Owsley, Sloane, Roenker, & Bruni, 1993; Myers, Ball, Kalina, Roth, & Goode, 2000; Owsley et al., 1998). This computerized measure assesses the amount of time it takes an individual to accurately acquire both central and peripheral visual information without head or eye movements. In this study, HIV+ participants performed significantly worse on the UFOV compared to HIV-seronegative participants, particularly on a subtest emphasizing divided attention. This was not solely the result of advancing disease nor high levels of general cognitive impairment, as individuals impaired on the UFOV covered the spectrum of disease stages and severity of cognitive impairment, suggesting a process occurring at least partially independent of disease progression, as well as a cognitive deficit not entirely captured by conventional neuropsychological tests. The subset of HIV+ individuals classified as "high risk" on the UFOV had a significantly greater number of on-road crashes in the previous year compared to those who were not at high risk. A classification of NP impaired *and* "high risk" on the UFOV yielded a positive predictive value of 75% and a negative predictive value of 95% for crashes in the past year, suggesting that UFOV impairment may be most risky in the presence of other cognitive impairments. Perhaps such individuals may not be able to compensate for visual attention deficits using other cognitive skills, such as deciding on an appropriate driving action (i.e., using executive skills in deciding to slow down in a high-risk situation) or executing an appropriate (i.e., quick and efficient) motor response (i.e., braking).

In summary, these studies suggest that HIV alone does not add to the risk of driving deficits, but rather it is the cognitive impairment that may accompany HIV infection in some individuals that is responsible for the increased risk. In addition, it is only a subset of cognitively impaired individuals who appear to have impaired driving abilities. Identifying which specific individuals are impaired drivers remains a challenge, although evolving technologies, such as a "naturalistic driving" approach (in which unobtrusive monitors and cameras are placed in a participant's own car) (Neale, Dingus, Klauer, Sudweeks, & Goodman, 2005) hold promise for improving our understanding of the factors affecting driving ability in this population.

OTHER COMPONENTS OF EVERYDAY FUNCTIONING

PROSPECTIVE MEMORY

One construct receiving increasing attention in the HIV literature in recent years is prospective memory, which denotes the ability to successfully execute a future intention (or more simply, "remember to remember") in the absence of explicit cues. Examples of prospective memory in daily life include remembering to take a medication after a meal or remembering to mail a letter on the way home from work. Prospective memory is essential to independent living and has been hypothesized to be a stronger contributor to the independent performance of several IADLs (e.g., medication adherence) than retrospective memory (Park & Kidder, 1996). Prospective memory is also dependent on the integrity of frontostriatal circuits (Simons, Scholvinck, Gilbert, Frith, & Burgess, 2006), which are commonly affected by HIV, lending credence to the relevance of this construct in HIV disease. Supporting its importance, the most commonly reported reason that HIV+ persons give for missing medication doses is simply "forgetting" (Chesney et al., 2000).

Studies have suggested that HIV infection is associated with a breakdown in the strategic (i.e., executive) encoding and retrieval aspects of prospective memory. HIV-infected individuals report more frequent prospective memory failures than seronegative individuals, particularly in aspects of daily functioning that require self-initiated cue monitoring and retrieval (i.e., when no salient, external cue is available) (Woods et al., 2007). Moreover, individuals with HIV infection demonstrate impairment on performance-based measures of prospective memory that are characterized by deficient performance when the task demands involve self-initiated retrieval but normal performance when retrieval demands are minimized with a recognition post-test (Carey, Woods, Rippeth, Heaton, & Grant, 2006). Studies have also indicated that HIV-associated prospective memory impairment is correlated with worse performance on measures of strategic verbal encoding, verbal working memory, and executive functions, attesting to its construct validity in HIV (Carey et al., 2006; Martin et al., 2007).

Importantly, emerging evidence also points to the ecological relevance of prospective memory in HIV infection.

Prospective memory has been associated with increased risk of dependence in self-reported IADL functioning (e.g., financial management) in an HIV-infected sample, over and above that which was explained by retrospective memory impairment and affective status (Woods et al., 2008a). Interestingly, despite low correlations between self-reported complaints of prospective memory and objective performance on a measure of prospective memory, Woods and colleagues found that both variables accurately predicted IADL status in this study, indicating that they may assess distinct aspects of daily functioning. Furthermore, prospective memory has been reported to be a significant, independent predictor of both subjective (Woods et al., 2008b) and objective (Woods et al., 2009) medication adherence in persons living with HIV. In the latter study by Woods and colleagues, individuals with HIV-associated prospective memory impairment at baseline were almost six times more likely to be classified as "non-adherent" (based on MEMS data) at 5-week follow-up than participants whose prospective memory performance fell within normal limits. Studies have also shown prospective memory impairment to be associated with high-risk behaviors in HIV seropositive polysubstance users, including medication non-adherence (Contardo, Black, Beauvais, Dieckhaus, & Rosen, 2009) and risky sexual and injection-drug-use behaviors (Martin et al., 2007). Taken together, these studies suggest that prospective memory is a unique and ecologically important aspect of cognitive functioning that, although not captured by traditional neuropsychological assessment techniques, may be essential to assess in HIV disease. A useful avenue for future study might be to examine the influence of prospective memory on the ability of individuals with HIV to maintain their health and reduce risky behavior. As Martin and colleagues (2007) have posited, the capacity to maintain drug abstinence, safe sexual practices, and adherence may depend not only on one's ability to plan and remember appropriate risk reduction and medication management strategies but also on one's ability to "remember to remember" such strategies.

MULTITASKING

While the performance-based functional tests mentioned in sections above (i.e., medication management test) are reasonably sensitive to HIV-associated declines in IADL, questions remain regarding the extent to which these tests' highly structured nature fully captures the various cognitive abilities involved in successful everyday functioning, including the environmental demands and complexities of daily life. In other words, most individuals do not carry out activities of daily living by following specific instructions in a tightly controlled environment, but instead operate in open-ended situations with multiple competing demands (Burgess et al., 2006). Thus, measuring an individual's ability to prioritize, organize, and structure a course of action in the face of competing alternatives (i.e., multitask) may be of particular importance in assessing IADL functioning, although this skill is not readily measured by standard neurocognitive or functional tests.

A recent study investigated the potential relevance of multitasking ability in HIV+ individuals and its relationship to self-reported IADL independence (Scott et al., 2011). In this study, a standardized measure of multitasking was developed that involved balancing the demands of four interconnected performance-based functional tasks (i.e., financial management, cooking, medication management, and telephone communication). HIV-seropositive individuals demonstrated significantly worse overall performance, an elevated number of errors, and fewer attempts at performing tasks simultaneously on the multitasking test as compared to an HIV-seronegative group. More importantly, multitasking deficits were uniquely predictive of IADL dependence in the HIV+ sample beyond the effects of depression and global neurocognitive impairment. Thus, multitasking ability may play an important role in successful everyday functioning in HIV+ individuals, although this possibility awaits further confirmation.

DECISION MAKING

In recent years, studies of cognitive and behavioral outcomes in HIV have also examined additional areas of everyday functioning that are relevant to the management and prevention of the disease. Given that infection with HIV has long been associated with high-risk behaviors, including unprotected sex, promiscuity, and intravenous drug use (Wolitski, Valdiserri, Denning, & Levine, 2001), an emergent research direction has focused on decision-making and the prediction of risky behaviors in individuals with HIV. Studies that elucidate the factors influencing risk behaviors are critical to preventing high-risk sexual behavior that may facilitate the spread of HIV as well as endanger already infected individuals by potentially exposing them to drug-resistant strains of the virus. In addition, risky decision making can result in increased substance use, leading to poorer everyday outcomes and increasing the likelihood of transmitting HIV through injection drug use, which currently accounts for approximately 20% of new HIV cases in the US (Centers for Disease Control and Prevention, 2006).

A number of factors have been associated with increased risk behaviors in HIV-infected samples, including demographic variables such as ethnicity (Lemp et al., 1994), education (Semple, Zians, Grant, & Patterson, 2006), and age (Mansergh & Marks, 1998); drug abuse (Rhodes et al., 1999); beliefs about HIV and its treatment (Dilley, Woods, & McFarland, 1997); and mental health status (Otto-Salaj & Stevenson, 2001). Recent studies, however, have also investigated the cognitive and personality factors associated with HIV and drug-use risk behavior. Some studies have utilized cognitive tests of decision making, such as the Iowa Gambling Task (IGT), to investigate whether cognitive impulsivity or poor decision making is more prevalent in HIV-infected individuals. The IGT, created by Bechara and colleagues (1997), assesses various cognitive components of decision making and involves selecting cards from four decks that have different contingencies for monetary rewards and losses, with the overall goal of making as much money as possible. Prudent decision makers come to realize that some decks will, over time, result in a net loss, while other decks eventually result in a net gain. Using the IGT, Martin and colleagues (2004) reported that HIV+ substance-dependent individuals made significantly more disadvantageous choices on the IGT and did not learn to avoid the disadvantageous decks over time when compared to a group of substance-dependent HIV-seronegative individuals, indicating that HIV infection may be associated with an increased level of cognitive impulsivity. Hardy et al. (2006) reported similar results, finding that HIV+ participants had an increased likelihood of selecting cards from the disadvantageous decks compared to an HIV- group. In addition, selection of these cards was associated with measures of inhibitory processing and delayed recall in exploratory analyses, suggesting that individuals who frequently chose from these decks might have had difficulty inhibiting more risky selections and remembering the previous losses due to their infrequency.

Other studies indicate that personality traits may also be relevant in predicting engagement in risky behaviors. In other words, longstanding traits, which may predate active substance use or HIV disease, may influence how individuals make and react to decisions. A number of studies has reported that the dispositional trait of sensation seeking, defined as the need to maintain a high level of arousal accompanied by a willingness to take risks to reach that arousal state (Zuckerman, Bone, Neary, Mangelsdorff, & Brustman, 1972), is associated with risky sexual practices among individuals with HIV (Crawford et al., 2003; Kalichman, Heckman, & Kelly, 1996). Gonzalez and colleagues (2005) attempted to distinguish between the influence of executive functions, HIV serostatus, and sensation seeking on risky sexual practices in polysubstance abusers. Sensation seeking, but not executive functions, was associated with risky sexual practices in the previous six months in both HIV-infected and HIV-seronegative groups, but this relationship was primarily driven by the association between the two within the HIV-infected group. Interestingly, one study has suggested that HIV+ individuals with high levels of sensation seeking evidence enhancement in certain aspects of selective attention (Hardy, Castellon, Hinkin, Levine, & Lam, 2008), although the implications of these findings for functional outcomes are unclear. Based on the results of these and similar studies (Moore et al., 2005), it seems important to consider both decision making and temperamental characteristics in assessing risk behavior patterns in HIV-infected individuals, especially when taking into account the actions that an individual might undertake in the real world, such as driving.

SUMMARY AND DIRECTIONS FOR FUTURE RESEARCH

There is now substantial research demonstrating that HIV-associated neurocognitive disorders significantly impact everyday functioning, including various activities of daily living, medication management, vocational abilities, and driving skills. This research spans the pre-HAART, early HAART, and current treatment eras. Such impairments incur large societal costs in terms of care, reduced workforce, and, with respect to risky behaviors and nonadherence, the increased likelihood of spreading drug-resistant HIV strains. Given the apparent decline of severe dementia in the HAART era, it is even more incumbent upon researchers and clinicians to understand the mechanisms whereby functional abilities are impacted in order to identify individuals before their quality of life is significantly affected.

There are many factors that may contribute to success or failure at daily tasks, including physical impairments, psychiatric conditions (e.g., depression), substance use, comorbid medical conditions (e.g., hepatitis C), motivational levels, experience, and compensatory strategies (Marcotte et al., 2009c). Despite these contributors, neurocognitive status remains a relatively robust predictor of real-world functioning. The predictive power of neuropsychological testing appears to be enhanced by the addition of performance-based measures of everyday functioning—laboratory/clinic based measures that mimic components of real-world tasks (e.g., driving simulators, medication management tasks). Such tools have great promise for providing the clinician with information regarding the person's capacity to carry out a task. These aforementioned other factors may help explain discrepancies between this laboratory-based assessment of capacity and the degree to which the person actually performs the activity in the real world. Thus, attending to psychiatric and motivational issues will likely prove important in preventing disability and negative functional outcomes (Rosenbloom et al., 2007; Sadek, Vigil, Grant, & Heaton, 2007).

While many everyday tasks are universal, they can also differ substantially from culture to culture. Most research on the neurocognitive aspects of HIV has been done in western countries and with primarily English-speaking cohorts, where clade B virus is predominant. However, clade C is the most common viral subtype worldwide, and many other variants abound. In order to determine the effects of diseases and brain dysfunction across cultures it would be ideal to standardize instruments as much as possible, but this may be neither easy nor appropriate. Similar to the application of western neuropsychological tests to other populations, the field may need to develop culture-specific norms for everyday functioning measures, even within different segments of societies. For example, Spanish speakers in the U.S. may have different approaches to money management and cooking than native English speakers. In some cases, particularly when individuals have very little or no education, measures of functional ability may prove to be the best way to determine whether cognitive decline has occurred.

As the HIV+ population continues to age, concerns mount regarding the possible impact that aging with HIV may have on cognition and functional outcomes. Various comorbidities associated with aging may affect everyday performance (e.g., neurovascular risk factors), and it will be important to ensure we have functional batteries that assess these skills and are sensitive to any additive or interactive effects.

Over the past decade, greater importance has been placed on the question of whether behavioral or pharmaceutical interventions significantly improve one's real world functioning and quality of life. A key area that has been lacking in many trials of neurotherapeutics for HIV-related cognitive problems is careful examination of the impact that these medications have (or do not have) on real-world functioning, as neuropsychological measures do not necessarily completely meet the spirit of the requirement to assess functional outcomes. For example, is significant improvement in Trails B time important if it fails to translate into a functional change in daily life? To this end, the United States Food and Drug Administration now requires clinical trials for the treatment of Alzheimer's disease (Laughren, 2001) and schizophrenia (Buchanan et al., 2005) to have co-primary measures that assess a clinically meaningful/relevant functional outcome. Ecologically-oriented measures would be an important addition to such clinical trials in HIV disease.

Most studies of HIV and everyday functioning involve null hypothesis significance testing in order to determine if there is a statistically significant difference between groups with and without a given brain condition. However, in order to be clinically useful, such measures should be designed to help clinicians and researchers identify individuals at risk for impaired real-world functioning. Investigators should thus report classification accuracy statistics such as sensitivity, specificity, and overall accuracy (hit rate), and the even more clinically relevant measures such as the positive predictive value (PPV; chances that someone who is impaired on a laboratory-based test also has impaired everyday functioning), negative predictive value (NPV; chance that if someone was unimpaired on the laboratory-based measure that he/she is also unimpaired in real world functioning), and risk ratios (e.g., likelihood and odds ratios) (Woods, Weinborn, & Lovejoy, 2003). Such information would help us better understand the utility, and universality, of different approaches.

Lastly, given the now clearly long-term survivability with HIV, it must be asked to what degree are HIV-associated neurocognitive disorders and HIV-associated deficits in everyday functioning remediable? A handful of studies have been conducted addressing this question, but clearly the future calls for additional evaluations as to whether cognitive rehabilitation (e.g., processing speed training) might ultimately help individuals regain, or retain, their ability to successfully function across a myriad of daily tasks.

REFERENCES

Albert, S. M., Marder, K., Dooneief, G., Bell, K., Sano, M., & Todak, G. (1995). Neuropsychologic impairment in early HIV infection. A risk factor for work disability. *Arch Neurol*, 52(5), 525–530.

Albert, S. M., Weber, C. M., Todak, G., Polanco, C., Clouse, R., & McElhiney, M. (1999). An observed performance test of medication management ability in HIV: Relation to neuropsychological status and medication adherence outcomes. *AIDS and Behavior*, 3(2), 121–128.

American Academy of Neurology AIDS Task Force. (1991). Nomenclature and research case definitions for neurologic manifestations of human immunodeficiency virus-type 1 (HIV-1) infection. *Neurology*, 41, 778–785.

Andrade, A. S., McGruder, H. F., Wu, A. W., Celano, S. A., Skolasky, R. L., Jr., & Selnes, O. A. (2005). A programmable prompting device improves adherence to highly active antiretroviral therapy in HIV-infected subjects with memory impairment. *Clin Infect Dis*, 41(6), 875–882.

Antinori, A., Arendt, G., Becker, J. T., Brew, B. J., Byrd, D. A., & Cherner, M. (2007). Updated research nosology for HIV-associated neurocognitive disorders. *Neurology*, 69(18), 1789–1799.

Arnsten, J. H., Demas, P. A., Farzadegan, H., Grant, R. W., Gourevitch, M. N., & Chang, C. J. (2001). Antiretroviral therapy adherence and viral suppression in HIV-infected drug users: Comparison of self-report and electronic monitoring. *Clin Infect Dis*, 33(8), 1417–1423.

Ball, K., Owsley, C., Sloane, M. E., Roenker, D. L., & Bruni, J. R. (1993). Visual attention problems as a predictor of vehicle crashes in older drivers. *Investigational Ophthalmology and Visual Science*, 34(11), 3110–3123.

Bangsberg, D. R. (2006). Less than 95% adherence to nonnucleoside reverse-transcriptase inhibitor therapy can lead to viral suppression. *Clin Infect Dis*, 43(7), 939–941.

Bangsberg, D. R., Perry, S., Charlebois, E. D., Clark, R. A., Roberston, M., & Zolopa, A. R. (2001). Non-adherence to highly active antiretroviral therapy predicts progression to AIDS. *AIDS*, 15(9), 1181–1183.

Bechara, A., Damasio, H., Tranel, D., & Damasio, A. R. (1997). Deciding advantageously before knowing the advantageous strategy. *Science*, 275(5304), 1293–1295.

Boccellari, A. & Zeifert, P. (1994). Management of neurobehavioral impairment in HIV-1 infection. *Psychiatric Clinics of North America*, 17(1), 183–203.

Bornstein, R. A., Nasrallah, H. A., Para, M. F., Whitacre, C. C., Rosenberger, P., & Fass, R. J. (1992). Neuropsychological performance in asymptomatic HIV infection. *J Neuropsychiatry Clin Neurosci*, 4, 386–394.

Brooks, R. A., Martin, D. J., Ortiz, D. J., & Veniegas, R. C. (2004). Perceived barriers to employment among persons living with HIV/AIDS. *AIDS Care*, 16(6), 756–766.

Buchanan, R. W., Davis, M., Goff, D., Green, M. F., Keefe, R. S., & Leon, A. C. (2005). A summary of the FDA-NIMH-MATRICS workshop on clinical trial design for neurocognitive drugs for schizophrenia. *Schizophr Bull*, 31(1), 5–19.

Burgess, P. W., Alderman, N., Forbes, C., Costello, A., Coates, L. M., & Dawson, D. R. (2006). The case for the development and use of "ecologically valid" measures of executive function in experimental and clinical neuropsychology. *J Int Neuropsychol Soc*, 12(2), 194–209.

Carey, C. L., Woods, S. P., Rippeth, J. D., Heaton, R. K., & Grant, I. (2006). Prospective memory in HIV-1 infection. *J Clin Exp Neuropsychol*, 28(4), 536–548.

Centers for Disease Control and Prevention. (2006). *HIV/AIDS surveillance report, 2005* (Vol. 17). Atlanta, GA: U.S. Department of Health and Human Services, Centers for Disease Control and Prevention.

Cherner, M., Cysique, L., Heaton, R. K., Marcotte, T. D., Ellis, R. J., & Masliah, E. (2007). Neuropathologic confirmation of definitional criteria for human immunodeficiency virus-associated neurocognitive disorders. *J Neurovirol*, 13(1), 23–28.

Chernoff, R. A., Martin, D. J., Schrock, D. A., & Huy, M. P. (2010). Neuropsychological functioning as a predictor of employment activity in a longitudinal study of HIV-infected adults contemplating workforce reentry. *J Int Neuropsychol Soc*, 16(1), 38–48.

Chesney, M. A., Ickovics, J. R., Chambers, D. B., Gifford, A. L., Neidig, J., & Zwickl, B. (2000). Self-reported adherence to antiretroviral medications among participants in HIV clinical trials: The AACTG adherence instruments. Patient Care Committee & Adherence Working Group of the Outcomes Committee of the Adult AIDS Clinical Trials Group (AACTG). *AIDS Care*, 12(3), 255–266.

Contardo, C., Black, A. C., Beauvais, J., Dieckhaus, K., & Rosen, M. I. (2009). Relationship of prospective memory to neuropsychological function and antiretroviral adherence. *Arch Clin Neuropsychol*, 24(6), 547–554.

Crawford, I., Hammack, P. L., McKirnan, D. J., Ostrow, D., Zamboni, B. D., & Robinson, B. (2003). Sexual sensation seeking, reduced concern about HIV, and sexual risk behaviour among gay men in primary relationships. *AIDS Care*, 15(4), 513–524.

Dilley, J. W., Woods, W. J., & McFarland, W. (1997). Are advances in treatment changing views about high-risk sex? *N Engl J Med*, 337(7), 501–502.

Ellis, R. J., Deutsch, R., Heaton, R. K., Marcotte, T. D., McCutchan, J. A., & Nelson, J. A., . . . (1997). Neurocognitive impairment is an independent risk factor for death in HIV infection. *Arch Neurol*, *54*(4), 416–424.

Ettenhofer, M. L., Foley, J., Castellon, S. A., & Hinkin, C. H. (2010). Reciprocal prediction of medication adherence and neurocognition in HIV/AIDS. *Neurology*, *74*(15), 1217–1222.

Goldman, D. P. & Bao, Y. (2004). Effective HIV treatment and the employment of HIV(+) adults. *Health Serv Res*, *39*(6 Pt 1), 1691–1712.

Golin, C. E., Earp, J., Tien, H. C., Stewart, P., Porter, C., & Howie, L. (2006). A 2-arm, randomized, controlled trial of a motivational interviewing-based intervention to improve adherence to antiretroviral therapy (ART) among patients failing or initiating ART. *J Acquir Immune Defic Syndr*, *42*(1), 42–51.

Gonzalez, R., Vassileva, J., Bechara, A., Grbesic, S., Sworowski, L., & Novak, R. M. (2005). The influence of executive functions, sensation seeking, and HIV serostatus on the risky sexual practices of substance-dependent individuals. *J Int Neuropsychol Soc*, *11*(2), 121–131.

Gorman, A. A., Foley, J. M., Ettenhofer, M. L., Hinkin, C. H., & van Gorp, W. G. (2009). Functional consequences of HIV-associated neuropsychological impairment. *Neuropsychol Rev*, *19*(2), 186–203.

Grant, I. & Atkinson, J. H. (1995a). Psychiatric aspects of acquired immune deficiency syndrome. In H. I. Kaplan & B. J. Sadock (Eds.). *Comprehensive textbook of psychiatry/VI* (Vol. 2, Sect. 29.2), pp. 1644–1669. Baltimore: Williams and Wilkins.

Grant, I. & Atkinson, J. H. (1995b). Psychobiology of HIV infection. In H. I. Kaplan & B. J. Sadock (Eds.). *Comprehensive textbook of psychiatry/VI* (Vol. VI). Baltimore: Williams & Wilkins.

Hardy, D. J., Castellon, S. A., Hinkin, C. H., Levine, A. J., & Lam, M. N. (2008). Sensation seeking and visual selective attention in adults with HIV/AIDS. *AIDS Behav*, *12*(6), 930–934.

Hardy, D. J., Hinkin, C. H., Levine, A. J., Castellon, S. A., & Lam, M. N. (2006). Risky decision making assessed with the gambling task in adults with HIV. *Neuropsychology*, *20*(3), 355–360.

Haubrich, R. H., Little, S. J., Currier, J. S., Forthal, D. N., Kemper, C. A., & Beall, G. N. (1999). The value of patient-reported adherence to antiretroviral therapy in predicting virologic and immunologic response. California Collaborative Treatment Group. *AIDS*, *13*(9), 1099–1107.

Heaton, R. K., Clifford, D. B., Franklin, D. R., Jr., Woods, S. P., Ake, C., Vaida, F., Ellis, R. J., Letendre, S. L., Marcotte, T. D., Atkinson, J. H., Rivera-Mindt, M., Vigil, O. R., Taylor, M. J., Collier, A. C., Marra, C. M., Gelman, B. B., McArthur, J. C., Morgello, S., Simpson, D. M., McCutchan, J. A., Abramson, I., Gamst, A., Fennema-Notestine, C., Jernigan, T. L., Wong, J., Grant, I., the CHARTER Group. (2010). HIV-associated neurocognitive disorders persist in the era of potent antiretroviral therapy. *Neurology*, *75*(23), 2087–96.

Heaton, R. K., Franklin, D. R., Ellis, R. J., McCutchan, J. A., Letendre, S. L., Leblanc, S., Corkran, S. H., Duarte, N. A., Clifford, D. B., Woods, S. P., Collier, A. C., Marra, C. M., Morgello, S., Mindt, M. R., Taylor, M. J., Marcotte, T. D., Atkinson, J. H., Wolfson, T., Gelman, B. B., McArthur, J. C., Simpson, D. M., Abramson, I., Gamst, A., Fennema-Notestine, C., Jernigan, T. L., Wong, J., Grant I., the CHARTER Group, and the HNRC Group. (2011). HIV-associated neurocognitive disorders before and during the era of combination antiretroviral therapy: differences in rates, nature, and predictors. *Journal of Neurovirology*, *17*(1), 3–16.

HNRC 500: Heaton, R. K., Grant, I., Butters, N., White, D. A., Kirson, D., Atkinson, J. H., . . . The HNRC Group (1995). The HNRC 500—Neuropsychology of HIV infection at different disease stages. *Journal of the International Neuropsychological Society*, *1*, 231–251.

Heaton, R. K., Marcotte, T. D., Mindt, M. R., Sadek, J., Moore, D. J., & Bentley, H., . . . The HNRC group (2004). The impact of HIV-associated neuropsychological impairment on everyday functioning. *J Int Neuropsychol Soc*, *10*(3), 317–331.

Heaton, R. K., Marcotte, T. D., White, D. A., Ross, D., Meredith, K., & Taylor, M. J. (1996). Nature and vocational significance of neuropsychological impairment associated with HIV infection. *The Clinical Neuropsychologist*, *10*(1), 1–14.

Heaton, R. K., Velin, R. A., McCutchan, J. A., Gulevich, S. J., Atkinson, J. H., & Wallace, M. R., . . . The HNRC Group (1994). Neuropsychological impairment in human immunodeficiency virus-infection: Implications for employment. *Psychosomatic Medicine*, *56*(1), 8–17.

Hinkin, C. H., Barclay, T. R., Castellon, S. A., Levine, A. J., Durvasula, R. S., & Marion, S. D. (2007). Drug use and medication adherence among HIV-1 infected individuals. *AIDS Behav*, *11*(2), 185–194.

Hinkin, C. H., Castellon, S. A., Durvasula, R. S., Hardy, D. J., Lam, M. N., & Mason, K. I. (2002). Medication adherence among HIV+ adults: Effects of cognitive dysfunction and regimen complexity. *Neurology*, *59*(12), 1944–1950.

Hinkin, C. H., Hardy, D. J., Mason, K. I., Castellon, S. A., Durvasula, R. S., & Lam, M. N. (2004). Medication adherence in HIV-infected adults: Effect of patient age, cognitive status, and substance abuse. *AIDS*, *18* Suppl 1, S19–25.

Hinkin, C. H., van Gorp, W. G., Satz, P., Marcotte, T., Durvasula, R. S., & Wood, S. (1996). Actual versus self-reported cognitive dysfunction in HIV-1 infection: Memory-metamemory dissociations. *J Clin Exp Neuropsychol*, *18*(3), 431–443.

Horne, R., Buick, D., Fisher, M., Leake, H., Cooper, V., & Weinman, J. (2004). Doubts about necessity and concerns about adverse effects: Identifying the types of beliefs that are associated with non-adherence to HAART. *Int J STD AIDS*, *15*(1), 38–44.

Hunt, L. A., Murphy, C. F., Carr, D., Duchek, J. M., Buckles, V., & Morris, J. C. (1997). Reliability of the Washington University Road Test. A performance-based assessment for drivers with dementia of the Alzheimer type. *Arch Neurol*, *54*(6), 707–712.

Kalichman, S. C., Amaral, C. M., Cherry, C., Flanagan, J., Pope, H., & Eaton, L. (2008). Monitoring medication adherence by unannounced pill counts conducted by telephone: Reliability and criterion-related validity. *HIV Clin Trials*, *9*(5), 298–308.

Kalichman, S. C., Heckman, T., & Kelly, J. A. (1996). Sensation seeking as an explanation for the association between substance use and HIV-related risky sexual behavior. *Arch Sex Behav*, *25*(2), 141–154.

Kaplan, R. M., Anderson, J. P., Patterson, T. L., McCutchan, J. A., Weinrich, J. D., & Heaton, R. K. (1995). Validity of the Quality of Well-Being Scale for persons with human immunodeficiency virus infection. *Psychosom Med*, *57*(2), 138–147.

Kaplan, R. M., Mausbach, B. T., Marcotte, T. D., & Patterson, T. L. (2009). The impact of cognitive impairment on health-related quality of life. In T. D. Marcotte & I. Grant (Eds.), *Neuropsychology of everyday functioning*. New York: Guilford Press.

Kaplan, R. M., Patterson, T. L., Kerner, D. N., Atkinson, J. H., Heaton, R. K., & Grant, I., and the HNRC Group (1997). The Quality of Well-Being scale in asymptomatic HIV-infected patients. HNRC Group. HIV Neural Behavioral Research Center. *Qual Life Res*, *6*(6), 507–514.

Kass, N. E., Munoz, A., Chen, B., Zucconi, S. L., & Bing, E. G. (1994). Changes in employment, insurance, and income in relation to HIV status and disease progression. The Multicenter AIDS Cohort Study. *J Acquir Immune Defic Syndr*, *7*(1), 86–91.

Kielhofner, G., Braveman, B., Finlayson, M., Paul-Ward, A., Goldbaum, L., & Goldstein, K. (2004). Outcomes of a vocational program for persons with AIDS. *Am J Occup Ther*, *58*(1), 64–72.

Laughren, T. (2001). A regulatory perspective on psychiatric syndromes in Alzheimer disease. *Am J Geriatr Psychiatry*, *9*(4), 340–345.

Lem, M., Moore, D., Marion, S., Bonner, S., Chan, K., & O'Connell, J. (2005). Back to work: Correlates of employment among persons receiving highly active antiretroviral therapy. *AIDS Care*, *17*(6), 740–746.

Lemp, G. F., Hirozawa, A. M., Givertz, D., Nieri, G. N., Anderson, L., & Lindegren, M. L. (1994). Seroprevalence of HIV and risk behaviors among young homosexual and bisexual men. The San Francisco/Berkeley Young Men's Survey. *JAMA*, *272*(6), 449–454.

Levine, A. J., Hinkin, C. H., Castellon, S. A., Mason, K. I., Lam, M. N., & Perkins, A. (2005). Variations in patterns of highly active antiretroviral therapy (HAART) adherence. *AIDS Behav*, *9*(3), 355–362.

Levine, A. J., Hinkin, C. H., Marion, S., Keuning, A., Castellon, S. A., Lam, M. M. (2006). Adherence to antiretroviral medications in HIV: Differences in data collected via self-report and electronic monitoring. *Health Psychol*, *25*(3), 329–335.

Liu, C., Ostrow, D., Detels, R., Hu, Z., Johnson, L., Kingsley, L. (2006). Impacts of HIV infection and HAART use on quality of life. *Qual Life Res, 15*(6), 941–949.

Liu, G. G., Guo, J. J., & Smith, S. R. (2004). Economic costs to business of the HIV/AIDS epidemic. *Pharmacoeconomics, 22*(18), 1181–1194.

Loewenstein, D. A. & Bates, B. C. (1992). *Manual for administration and scoring the Direct Assessment of Functional Status scale for older adults (DAFS)*. Miami Beach, FL: Mount Sinai Medical Center.

Maher, K., Klimas, N., Fletcher, M. A., Cohen, V., Maggio, C. M., & Triplett, J. (1999). Disease progression, adherence, and response to protease inhibitor therapy for HIV infection in an Urban Veterans Affairs Medical Center. *J Acquir Immune Defic Syndr, 22*(4), 358–363.

Mansergh, G. & Marks, G. (1998). Age and risk of HIV infection in men who have sex with men. *AIDS, 12*(10), 1119–1128.

Marcotte, T. D. & Grant, I. (2009a). Future directions in the assessment of everyday functioning. In T. D. Marcotte & I. Grant (Eds.). *Neuropsychology of everyday functioning*. New York: Guilford Press.

Marcotte, T. D., Heaton, R. K., Reicks, C., Gonzalez, R., Grant, I., & the HNRC Group. (2000). HIV-related neuropsychological impairment and automobile driving. *Journal of the International Neuropsychological Society, 6*(2), 233 [Abstract].

Marcotte, T. D., Heaton, R. K., Wolfson, T., Taylor, M. J., Alhassoon, O., & Arfaa, K.,Grant, I., and HNRC Group (1999). The impact of HIV-related neuropsychological dysfunction on driving behavior. The HNRC Group. *J Int Neuropsychol Soc, 5*(7), 579–592.

Marcotte, T. D., Lazzaretto, D., Scott, J. C., Roberts, E., Woods, S. P., & Letendre, S., and the HNRC Group (2006). Visual attention deficits are associated with driving accidents in cognitively-impaired HIV-infected individuals. *Journal of Clinical and Experimental Neuropsychology, 28*(1), 13–28.

Marcotte, T. D. & Scott, J. C. (2004a). The assessment of driving abilities. *Advances in Transportation Studies: An International Journal*, 79–90.

Marcotte, T. D. & Scott, J. C. (2009b). Neuropsychological performance and the assessment of driving behavior. In I. Grant & K. M. Adams (Eds.). *Neuropsychological assessment of neuropsychiatric disorders* (3rd ed.). New York, NY: Oxford University Press.

Marcotte, T. D., Scott, J. C., Kamat, R., & Heaton, R. K. (2009c). Neuropsychology and the prediction of everyday functioning. In T. D. Marcotte & I. Grant (Eds.). *Neuropsychology of Everyday Functioning*. New York: Guilford Press.

Marcotte, T. D., Wolfson, T., Rosenthal, T. J., Heaton, R. K., Gonzalez, R., & Ellis, R. J. (2004b). A multimodal assessment of driving performance in HIV infection. *Neurology, 63*(8), 1417–1422.

Martin, D. J., Arns, P. G., Batterham, P. J., Afifi, A. A., & Steckart, M. J. (2006). Workforce reentry for people with HIV/AIDS: Intervention effects and predictors of success. *Work, 27*(3), 221–233.

Martin, E. M., Nixon, H., Pitrak, D. L., Weddington, W., Rains, N. A., & Nunnally, G. (2007). Characteristics of prospective memory deficits in HIV-seropositive substance-dependent individuals: Preliminary observations. *J Clin Exp Neuropsychol, 29*(5), 496–504.

Martin, E. M., Pitrak, D. L., Weddington, W., Rains, N. A., Nunnally, G., & Nixon, H. (2004). Cognitive impulsivity and HIV serostatus in substance dependent males. *J Int Neuropsychol Soc, 10*(7), 931–938.

Mayeux, R., Stern, Y., Tang, M.-X., Todak, G., Marder, K., & Sano, J. (1993). Mortality risks in gay men with human immunodeficiency virus infection and cognitive impairment. *Neurology, 43*, 176–182.

McArthur, J. C., Hoover, D. R., Bacellar, H., Miller, E. N., Cohen, B. A., & Becker, J. T. (1993). Dementia in AIDS patients: Incidence and risk factors. *Neurology, 43*, 2245–2252.

McGinn, F., Gahagan, J., & Gibson, E. (2005). Back to work: Vocational issues and strategies for Canadians living with HIV/AIDS. *Work, 25*(2), 163–171.

Mindt, M., Cherner, M., Marcotte, T., Moore, D., Bentley, H., & Esquivel, M. (2003). The Functional impact of HIV-associated neuropsychological impairment in Spanish-speaking adults: A pilot study. *J Clin Exp Neuropsychol, 25*(1), 122–132.

Mocroft, A., Phillips, A. N., Soriano, V., Rockstroh, J., Blaxhult, A., & Katlama, C. (2005). Reasons for stopping antiretrovirals used in an initial highly active antiretroviral regimen: Increased incidence of stopping due to toxicity or patient/physician choice in patients with hepatitis C co-infection. *AIDS Res Hum Retroviruses, 21*(6), 527–536.

Moore, D. J., Atkinson, J. H., Akiskal, H., Gonzalez, R., Wolfson, T., & Grant, I. (2005). Temperament and risky behaviors: A pathway to HIV? *J Affect Disord, 85*(1–2), 191–200.

Myers, R. S., Ball, K. K., Kalina, T. D., Roth, D. L., & Goode, K. T. (2000). Relation of useful field of view and other screening tests to on-road driving performance. *Perceptual and Motor Skills, 91*(1), 279–290.

Neale, V. L., Dingus, T. A., Klauer, S. G., Sudweeks, J., & Goodman, M. (2005). *An overview of the 100-Car Naturalistic Study and findings*. Washington, D.C.: National Highway Traffic Safety Administration.

Nieuwkerk, P. T., Sprangers, M. A., Burger, D. M., Hoetelmans, R. M., Hugen, P. W., & Danner, S. A. (2001). Limited patient adherence to highly active antiretroviral therapy for HIV-1 infection in an observational cohort study. *Arch Intern Med, 161*(16), 1962–1968.

Odenheimer, G. L., Beaudet, M., Jette, A. M., Albert, M. S., Grande, L., & Minaker, K. L. (1994). Performance-based driving evaluation of the elderly driver: Safety, reliability, and validity. *J Gerontol, 49*(4), M153–159.

Osowiecki, D. M., Cohen, R. A., Morrow, K. M., Paul, R. H., Carpenter, C. C., & Flanigan, T. (2000). Neurocognitive and psychological contributions to quality of life in HIV-1-infected women. *AIDS, 14*(10), 1327–1332.

Otto-Salaj, L. L. & Stevenson, L. Y. (2001). Influence of psychiatric diagnoses and symptoms on HIV risk behavior in adults with serious mental illness. *AIDS Read, 11*(4), 197–204, 206–198.

Owsley, C., Ball, K., McGwin, G., Jr., Sloane, M. E., Roenker, D. L., & White, M. (1998). Visual processing impairment and risk of motor vehicle crash among older adults. *JAMA, 279*(14), 1083–1088.

Park, D. C. & Kidder, D. P. (1996). Prospective memory and medication adherence. In M. Brandimonte, G. O. Einstein, & M. A. McDaniel (Eds.). *Prospective memory: Theory and applications*, pp. 369–390. Mahwah, NJ: Erlbaum.

Parsons, T. D., Braaten, A. J., Hall, C. D., & Robertson, K. R. (2006). Better quality of life with neuropsychological improvement on HAART. *Health Qual Life Outcomes, 4*, 11.

Rabkin, J. G. & Ferrando, S. (1997). A "second life" agenda. Psychiatric research issues raised by protease inhibitor treatments for people with the human immunodeficiency virus or the acquired immunodeficiency syndrome. *Archives of General Psychiatry, 54*(11), 1049–1053.

Rabkin, J. G., McElhiney, M., Ferrando, S. J., Van Gorp, W., & Lin, S. H. (2004). Predictors of employment of men with HIV/AIDS: A longitudinal study. *Psychosom Med, 66*(1), 72–78.

Razzano, L. A., Hamilton, M. M., & Perloff, J. K. (2006). Work status, benefits, and financial resources among people with HIV/AIDS. *Work, 27*(3), 235–245.

Revicki, D. A., Wu, A. W., & Murray, M. I. (1995). Change in clinical status, health status, and health utility outcomes in HIV-infected patients. *Med Care, 33*(4 Suppl), AS173–182.

Rhodes, F., Deren, S., Wood, M. M., Shedlin, M. G., Carlson, R. G., & Lambert, E. Y. (1999). Understanding HIV risks of chronic drug-using men who have sex with men. *AIDS Care, 11*(6), 629–648.

Rosenbloom, M. J., Sullivan, E. V., Sassoon, S. A., O'Reilly, A., Fama, R., & Kemper, C. A. (2007). Alcoholism, HIV infection, and their comorbidity: Factors affecting self-rated health-related quality of life. *J Stud Alcohol Drugs, 68*(1), 115–125.

Rourke, S. B., Halman, M. H., & Bassel, C. (1999). Neuropsychiatric correlates of memory-metamemory dissociations in HIV-infection. *J Clin Exp Neuropsychol, 21*(6), 757–768.

Sacktor, N. C., Bacellar, H., Hoover, D. R., Nance-Sproson, T. E., Selnes, O. A., & Miller, E. N. (1996). Psychomotor slowing in HIV infection: A predictor of dementia, AIDS and death. *J Neurovirol, 2*(6), 404–410.

Sadek, J. R., Vigil, O., Grant, I., & Heaton, R. K. (2007). The impact of neuropsychological functioning and depressed mood on functional complaints in HIV-1 infection and methamphetamine dependence. *J Clin Exp Neuropsychol, 29*(3), 266–276.

Scott, J. C., Woods, S. P., Vigil, O., Heaton, R. K., Schweinsburg, B. C., Ellis, R. J., Grant, I., & Marcotte, T. D. (2011). A neuropsychological investigation of multitasking in HIV infection: Implications for everyday functioning. *Neuropsychology*, 25, 511–519.

Semple, S. J., Zians, J., Grant, I., & Patterson, T. L. (2006). Methamphetamine use, impulsivity, and sexual risk behavior among HIV-positive men who have sex with men. *J Addict Dis*, 25(4), 105–114.

Sherbourne, C. D., Hays, R. D., Fleishman, J. A., Vitiello, B., Magruder, K. M., & Bing, E. G. (2000). Impact of psychiatric conditions on health-related quality of life in persons with HIV infection. *Am J Psychiatry*, 157(2), 248–254.

Simons, J. S., Scholvinck, M. L., Gilbert, S. J., Frith, C. D., & Burgess, P. W. (2006). Differential components of prospective memory? Evidence from fMRI. *Neuropsychologia*, 44(8), 1388–1397.

Singh, N., Squier, C., Sivek, C., Wagener, M., Nguyen, M. H., & Yu, V. L. (1996). Determinants of compliance with antiretroviral therapy in patients with human immunodeficiency virus: Prospective assessment with implications for enhancing compliance. *AIDS Care*, 8(3), 261–269.

Starace, F., Ammassari, A., Trotta, M. P., Murri, R., De Longis, P., & Izzo, C. (2002). Depression is a risk factor for suboptimal adherence to highly active antiretroviral therapy. *J Acquir Immune Defic Syndr*, 31 Suppl 3, S136–139.

Stern, Y., Marder, K., Bell, K., Chen, J., Dooneief, G., & Goldstein, S. (1991). Multidisciplinary assessment of homosexual men with and without human immunodeficiency virus infection. III. Neurologic and neuropsychological findings. *Archives of General Psychiatry*, 48, 131–138.

Tozzi, V., Balestra, P., Murri, R., Galgani, S., Bellagamba, R., & Narciso, P. (2004). Neurocognitive impairment influences quality of life in HIV-infected patients receiving HAART. *Int J STD AIDS*, 15(4), 254–259.

Tozzi, V., Balestra, P., Serraino, D., Bellagamba, R., Corpolongo, A., & Piselli, P. (2005). Neurocognitive impairment and survival in a cohort of HIV-infected patients treated with HAART. *AIDS Res Hum Retroviruses*, 21(8), 706–713.

Trepanier, L. L., Rourke, S. B., Bayoumi, A. M., Halman, M. H., Krzyzanowski, S., & Power, C. (2005). The impact of neuropsychological impairment and depression on health-related quality of life in HIV-infection. *J Clin Exp Neuropsychol*, 27(1), 1–15.

U.S. Department of Labor. (1991). *Dictionary of occupational titles* (4th ed.). Washington, D.C.: U.S. Government Printing Office.

Valpar International Corporation. (1986). *Microcomputer Evaluation and Screening Assessment (MESA) Short Form 2*. Tucson, AZ: Valpar International Corporation.

Valpar International Corporation. (1992). *Computerized Assessment (COMPASS)*. Tucson, AZ: Valpar International Corporation.

Van Gorp, W., Satz, P., Hinkin, C., Selnes, O., Miller, E., & McArthur, J. (1991). Metacognition in HIV-1 seropositive asymptomatic individuals: Self-ratings versus objective neuropsychological performance. *J Clin Exp Neuropsychol*, 13, 812–819.

van Gorp, W. G., Baerwald, J. P., Ferrando, S. J., McElhiney, M. C., & Rabkin, J. G. (1999). The relationship between employment and neuropsychological impairment in HIV infection. *J Int Neuropsychol Soc*, 5(6), 534–539.

van Gorp, W. G., Rabkin, J. G., Ferrando, S. J., Mintz, J., Ryan, E., & Borkowski, T. (2007). Neuropsychiatric predictors of return to work in HIV/AIDS. *J Int Neuropsychol Soc*, 13(1), 80–89.

Visual Resources, I. (1998). *UFOV Useful Field of View Manual*. Chicago, IL: The Psychological Corporation.

Wagner, G. J., Kanouse, D. E., Golinelli, D., Miller, L. G., Daar, E. S., & Witt, M. D. (2006). Cognitive-behavioral intervention to enhance adherence to antiretroviral therapy: A randomized controlled trial (CCTG 578). *AIDS*, 20(9), 1295–1302.

White, D. A., Heaton, R. K., & Monsch, A. U. (1995). Neuropsychological studies of asymptomatic Human Immunodeficiency Virus-Type 1-infected individuals. *J Int Neuropsychol Soc*, 1, 304–315.

Wilkins, J. W., Robertson, K. R., Snyder, C. R., Robertson, W. K., van der Horst, C., & Hall, C. D. (1991). Implications of self-reported cognitive and motor dysfunction in HIV-positive patients. *American Journal of Psychiatry*, 148, 641–643.

Wolitski, R. J., Valdiserri, R. O., Denning, P. H., & Levine, W. C. (2001). Are we headed for a resurgence of the HIV epidemic among men who have sex with men? *Am J Public Health*, 91(6), 883–888.

Woods, S. P., Carey, C. L., Moran, L. M., Dawson, M. S., Letendre, S. L., & Grant, I., and the HIV Neurobehavioral Research Center (HNRC) Group (2007). Frequency and predictors of self-reported prospective memory complaints in individuals infected with HIV. *Arch Clin Neuropsychol*, 22(2), 187–195.

Woods, S. P., Dawson, M. S., Weber, E., Gibson, S., Grant, I., & Atkinson, J. H., and the HIV Neurobehavioral Research Center (HNRC) Group (2009). Timing is everything: Antiretroviral nonadherence is associated with impairment in time-based prospective memory. *J Int Neuropsychol Soc*, 15(1), 42–52.

Woods, S. P., Iudicello, J. E., Moran, L. M., Carey, C. L., Dawson, M. S., & Grant, I. and the HIV Neurobehavioral Research Center (HNRC) Group (2008a). HIV-associated prospective memory impairment increases risk of dependence in everyday functioning. *Neuropsychology*, 22(1), 110–117.

Woods, S. P., Moran, L. M., Carey, C. L., Dawson, M. S., Iudicello, J. E., & Gibson, S. . . . and The HIV Neurobehavioral Research Center (HNRC) Group (2008b). Prospective memory in HIV infection: Is "remembering to remember" a unique predictor of self-reported medication management? *Arch Clin Neuropsychol*, 23(3), 257–270.

Woods, S. P., Weinborn, M., & Lovejoy, D. W. (2003). Are classification accuracy statistics underused in neuropsychological research? *J Clin Exp Neuropsychol*, 25(3), 431–439.

Wu, A. W., Snyder, C. F., Huang, I. C., Skolasky, R., McGruder, H. F., & Celano, S. A. (2006). A randomized trial of the impact of a programmable medication reminder device on quality of life in patients with AIDS. *AIDS Patient Care STDS*, 20(11), 773–781.

Zuckerman, M., Bone, R. N., Neary, R., Mangelsdorff, D., & Brustman, B. (1972). What is the sensation seeker? Personality trait and experience correlates of the Sensation-Seeking Scales. *J Consult Clin Psychol*, 39(2), 308–321.

12.5

FACING LEGAL AND ETHICAL CHALLENGES IN THE TREATMENT OF AIDS

Warren B. Treisman and Glenn J. Treisman

Physicians who manage people living with HIV sometimes must grapple with issues that are not strictly medical in nature. One such important area, which is the focus of this chapter, pertains to the legal implications of treatment decisions and the need for the physician to avoid legal liability. In this chapter, we consider three issues that can be of particular relevance to physicians treating HIV-positive patients: weighing patient confidentiality against the need to inform endangered third parties of possible harm, questions pertaining to physician-assisted suicide, and the challenge of obtaining informed consent in the setting of cognitive impairment. This chapter can provide valuable background on these important issues. Nonetheless, legal questions such as these have state- and country-specific legal analyses, so the at-risk practitioner is strongly advised to explore the applicable statutes and case law.

Doctors are asked to reconcile many conflicting issues when caring for patients. Resolution of these problems involves the simultaneous applications of ethical thought, standards of care, legal considerations, and clinical reasoning. Health care providers should think clinically first, and when unable to resolve a conflict between legal, ethical, and moral considerations, try to do what is best for the patient, and in the best interests of the patient. In this setting, consultation with ethics committees, lawyers, and psychiatrists are common.

Much has been written on the quartet of autonomy, beneficence, nonmaleficence, and justice as the ethical pillars of medical treatment. The proper balance of these principles in the care of patients generally, as well as in individual cases, has been frequently debated; the appropriate role of the provider in the application of these pillars has also been a source of controversy. Specialized lawyers are often consulted about the legal considerations in particular cases. Such attorneys can contribute to an understanding of both the written law and the practicality of liability imposed by the legal system. Psychiatrists can sometimes answer the questions of patients' capacity to understand and make decisions that are competent and reasonable, and can be of assistance in documenting impairments, disordered thinking, and emotional vulnerabilities that can impair patients' decision-making capabilities.

The doctor-patient relationship is complex and based in part on an inequality of power between the two: The patient is sick, vulnerable, and likely at a disadvantage regarding medical knowledge. The doctor is allowed access to the patient's private thoughts and private bodily parts and functions. No one expects a physician to share similar intimacies with patients. While the patient may get sicker or even die, the doctor not only continues to live in health, but gets remunerated for whatever services have been provided. The imbalance in this relationship heightens the responsibility of the doctor to act unwaveringly in the patient's best interest. The doctor is constrained by the relationship not to take advantage of patients and their circumstances. Issues of confidentiality, informed consent, and the requirement that a doctor be certain that the patient is capable of making an informed decision are considered primary duties of the physician directly as a result of this special relationship.

One contentious issue is that of autonomy as opposed to beneficence. Patients may request treatment that is directly harmful, such as the patient with the delusional belief that there are parasites in his or her arm who requests an amputation. This would not be the appropriate treatment even if such a parasite were present, and yet in some conditions, such as delusional parasitosis, there may be no other obvious sign of mental illness, and the patient may appear competent to request the treatment. The same issue is raised much more subtly in the case of the 21-year-old woman who requests breast augmentation surgery so that she can work as an exotic dancer. The patient in such a situation may not be able to appreciate the fact that the long-term health risks posed by such a procedure may well outweigh any potential financial benefits in the shorter term. Patients who are weary of the burden and thus wish to stop taking medications may not be able to appreciate fully the additional burdens they may face as a result: the escalation of their illnesses.

Medical providers have an obligation to consider risks and benefits of treatments, the certainty of the diagnosis and prognosis, and the risks of alternative or non-treatment when deciding what courses of treatment it is reasonable to offer. The courts have frequently sided with the injured patients when clinicians have allowed themselves to provide harmful treatments at the request of patients. Ultimately, patients have the right to obtain care elsewhere if they disagree with their clinicians, and only under the most unusual of circumstances can they be compelled to take treatment that they wish to refuse.

Physicians managing people living with the HIV must grapple with several nonmedical issues. Aside from the goal of balancing the ethical dilemmas presented in the care of this population, practitioners must also consider the legal implications in treatment decisions in order to avoid potential liability. Many of the issues faced in HIV clinics have received attention in the literature from other medical settings, such as geriatrics, oncology, neonatal care, psychiatry, and general medicine. We will discuss and attempt to offer some clarity concerning two common problems more specific to the HIV care setting that have been particularly difficult. The ethical, moral, and standard-of-care issues will only be mentioned in passing as they inform the legal issues, which are the focus of this chapter. Each issue has a state- and country-specific legal analysis, so the practitioner is strongly advised to explore the applicable statutes and case law regarding these topics.[1]

CONFIDENTIALITY WEIGHED AGAINST FORESEEABLE INJURY TO THIRD PARTIES

State statutes define the legal level of confidentiality owed to a patient. In general, the physician owes a patient privacy in care. However, when the physician learns from a patient of a foreseeable and credible risk of serious harm to a third party, potential liability may attach if the physician fails to discharge appropriately the duty to disclose the threat. This duty to disclose is frequently referred to as a "Tarasoff" duty. Tarasoff is the name of the plaintiffs who sought damages for the murder of their daughter by a psychiatric patient. The patient had revealed his intention to kill the victim to his psychologist, but the psychologist had not disclosed the danger to the eventual victim. The psychologist's attorney argued that there was no duty to warn a third party because of the required confidentiality, and also because there was no legally recognized "special relationship" between the psychologist and the third-party victim. The California Supreme Court identified the physician's dilemma of maintaining the privacy of the patient, but determined that the protection of the safety of the public must outweigh the patient's privacy rights.

> "We conclude that the public policy favoring protection of the confidential character of patient-psychotherapist communications must yield to the extent to which disclosure is essential to avert danger

to others. The protective privilege ends where the public peril begins."[2]

The court found that the "special relationship" existed through the patient.

Although the California Supreme Court's decision in *Tarasoff* was quite controversial at the time, the holding was later codified in California statutes. [3] The statute specifically requires that the patient make a serious threat of physical violence against a reasonably identifiable victim. Only in that circumstance must the psychotherapist identify the threat to the victim and the police. Various state statutes identify specific criteria to be used in determining whether the patient's threat meets the triggering threshold of the danger. Other laws outline the various ways the physician's duty may be discharged.[4] The statutes generally afford doctors legal protection from liability for disclosure of patients' confidential statements.

The physician managing an individual with HIV may be presented with a comparable quandary. A patient may disclose to her physician that she is engaging in unprotected sex with a specific partner, or that she is sharing needles for IV drug use with specific contacts. The Tarasoff concerns are present, in that the physician is aware of a serious and foreseeable risk of harm to a specific person or group.[5] However, the California Legislature chose not to attach legal liability based on a failure to warn under these circumstances. California law provides the physician the authority to disclose the information to a "person reasonably believed to be the spouse, or to a person reasonably believed to be a sexual partner or a person with whom the patient has shared the use

---

2. *Tarasoff v. Regents of University of California* (1976) 17 Cal.3d 425, 442 [131 Cal.Rptr. 14, 551 P.2d 334].

3. California Civil Code § 43.92. states:
   (a) There shall be no monetary liability on the part of, and no cause of action shall arise against, any person who is a psychotherapist as defined in Section 1010 of the Evidence Code in failing to warn of and protect from a patient's threatened violent behavior or failing to predict and warn and protect from a patient's violent behavior except where the patient has communicated to the psychotherapist a serious threat of physical violence against a reasonably identifiable victim or victims.
   (b) If there is a duty to warn and protect under the limited circumstances specified above, the duty shall be discharged by the psychotherapist making reasonable efforts to communicate the threat to the victim or victims and to a law enforcement agency.

4. For a text that outlines the various state approaches to the Tarasoff duty, please see *Ethics in HIV-Related Psychotherapy: Clinical Decision Making in Complex Cases*, John R. Anderson and Robert Barret, eds. (American Psychological Association 2001).

5. Though the risk of harm is present for an HIV patient's contacts, *Tarasoff* involved a risk of harm to a third party who was not engaging in participatory conduct of any sort. The risk to an entirely unsuspecting third party, as in *Tarasoff*, seems fundamentally different than the risk associated with IV drug use or consensual sexual encounters. In both examples, the participants are already aware that they are using drugs or having unprotected sex and that there are potential life-threatening risks associated with those behaviors. Thus, a warning regarding a partner's actual HIV infection would only serve to more specifically quantify the risk of which the third-party participant was already generally aware. On the other hand, Tatiana Tarasoff had no reason whatsoever to suspect the risk to which her murderer's psychologist was privy. Therefore, attaching tort liability for a physician's failure to warn third parties in the HIV setting is a much farther stretch than that of the *Tarasoff* case.

---

1. There are texts that outline the statutory scheme of each state regarding HIV and AIDS. As the law is in constant motion on these issues, you should look at the statutes and, if possible, see how the state appellate courts interpret the statutes in the case law. "State statutes dealing with HIV and AIDS: A comprehensive state-by-state summary" (1999 ed.) *Law & Sexuality*, Annual 1998, v.8. There is also considerable variation in different countries as regards HIV and AIDS. These have been constantly changing as well. The adoption of any universal legal standards is unlikely in the near future.

of hypodermic needles" after either obtaining permission from the patient, or if that permission is denied, then without it.[6] Section C of the statute specifically identifies that such notice is permissive and the physician has no duty to make such a disclosure.[7] Additionally, if the disclosure is made by the physician, the disclosure cannot include the identity of the patient.[8]

In reality, California physicians are unlikely to take the risk of disclosure when there is no legal duty to do so. There is a counterincentive to such disclosure, as there are specific prerequisites to disclosure that a patient might later claim were not entirely achieved. The cautious practitioner will not take the risk. Nevertheless, many states have adopted this permissive approach.

There is a movement in some states toward compelling the physician to disclose positive HIV test data to State Departments of Health and allowing the agency the ability to disclose the information to people who appear to be at risk. New York has adopted an approach that allows the doctor to notify the public health officer that there are "contacts" at risk and the public health officer then makes the notification. The patient is afforded counseling regarding the doctor's intention to notify the contact or the public health officer.[9]

---

6. California Health & Safety Code § 121015 states:
(a) Notwithstanding Section 120980 or any other provision of law, no physician and surgeon who has the results of a confirmed positive test to detect HIV infection of a patient under his or her care shall be held criminally or civilly liable for disclosing to a person reasonably believed to be the spouse, or to a person reasonably believed to be a sexual partner or a person with whom the patient has shared the use of hypodermic needles, or to the local health officer, that the patient has tested positive on a test to detect HIV infection, except that no physician and surgeon shall disclose any identifying information about the individual believed to be infected, except as required in Section 121022.
(b) No physician and surgeon shall disclose the information described in subdivision (a) unless he or she has first discussed the test results with the patient and has offered the patient appropriate educational and psychological counseling, that shall include information on the risks of transmitting the human immunodeficiency virus to other people and methods of avoiding those risks, and has attempted to obtain the patient's voluntary consent for notification of his or her contacts. The physician and surgeon shall notify the patient of his or her intent to notify the patient's contacts prior to any notification. When the information is disclosed to a person reasonably believed to be a spouse, or to a person reasonably believed to be a sexual partner, or a person with whom the patient has shared the use of hypodermic needles, the physician and surgeon shall refer that person for appropriate care, counseling, and follow-up. This section shall not apply to disclosures made other than for the purpose of diagnosis, care, and treatment of persons notified pursuant to this section, or for the purpose of interrupting the chain of transmission.
(c) This section is permissive on the part of the attending physician, and all requirements and other authorization for the disclosure of test results to detect HIV infection are limited to the provisions contained in this chapter, Chapter 10 (commencing with Section 121075) and Sections 1603.1 and 1603.3. No physician has a duty to notify any person of the fact that a patient is reasonably believed to be infected with HIV, except as required by Section 121022.
(d) The local health officer may alert any persons reasonably believed to be a spouse, sexual partner, or partner of shared needles of an individual who has tested positive on an HIV test about their exposure, without disclosing any identifying information about the individual believed to be infected or the physician making the report, and shall refer any person to whom a disclosure is made pursuant to this subdivision for appropriate care and follow-up. Upon completion of the local health officer's efforts to contact any person pursuant to this subdivision, all records regarding that person maintained by the local health officer pursuant to this subdivision, including, but not limited to, any individual identifying information, shall be expunged by the local health officer.
(e) The local health officer shall keep confidential the identity and the seropositivity status of the individual tested and the identities of the persons contacted, as long as records of contacts are maintained.
(f) Except as provided in Section 1603.1, 1603.3, or 121022, no person shall be compelled in any state, county, city, or local civil, criminal, administrative, legislative, or other proceedings to identify or provide identifying characteristics that would identify any individual reported or person contacted pursuant to this section.

7. California Health & Safety Code § 121015, subsection (c).

8. California Health & Safety Code § 121015, subsection (d).

9. N.Y. Pub. Health Law § 2782, subsections 4 and 5, provide:
4. (a) A physician may disclose confidential HIV-related information under the following conditions:
(1) disclosure is made to a contact, to a public health officer for the purpose of making the disclosure to said contact and pursuant to section twenty-one hundred thirty of this chapter; or
(2) the physician believes disclosure is medically appropriate and there is a significant risk of infection to the contact; and
(3) the physician has counseled the protected individual regarding the need to notify the contact; and
(4) the physician has informed the protected individual of his or her intent to make such disclosure to a contact, the physician's responsibility to report the infected individual's case pursuant to section twenty-one hundred thirty of this chapter and has given the protected individual the opportunity to express a preference as to whether disclosure should be made by the physician directly or to a public health officer for the purpose of said disclosure. If the protected individual expresses a preference for disclosure by a public health officer, the physician shall honor such preference.
(5) If a physician chooses to make a notification pursuant to this section, he or she shall report to the municipal health commissioner of district health officer on his or her efforts to notify the contacts of the protected individual. Such report shall be in a manner and on forms prescribed by the commissioner and shall include the identity of the protected individual and any contacts as well as information as to whether the contacts were successfully notified.
(6) Within a reasonable time of receiving a report that a physician or his or her designated agent did not notify or verify notification of contacts provided by the protected individual, the health commissioner or district health officer of the municipality from which the report originates shall take reasonable measures to notify such contacts and otherwise comply with the provisions of this chapter.
(b) When making such disclosures to the contact, the physician or public health officer shall provide or make referrals for the provision of the appropriate medical advice and counseling for coping with the emotional consequences of learning the information and for changing behavior to prevent transmission or contraction of HIV infection. The physician or public health officer shall not disclose the identity of the protected individual or the identity of any other contact. A physician or public health officer making a notification pursuant to this subdivision shall make such disclosure in person, except where circumstances reasonably prevent doing so.
(c) A physician or public health officer shall have no obligation to identify or locate any contact except as provided pursuant to title three of article twenty-one of this chapter.
(d) A physician may, upon the consent of a parent or guardian, disclose confidential HIV-related information to a state, county, or local health officer for the purpose of reviewing the medical history of a child to determine the fitness of the child to attend school.
(e) A physician may disclose confidential HIV-related information pertaining to a protected individual to a person (known to the physician) authorized pursuant to law to consent to health care for a protected individual when the physician reasonably believes that:
(1) disclosure is medically necessary in order to provide timely care and treatment for the protected individual; and
(2) after appropriate counseling as to the need for such disclosure, the protected individual will not inform a person authorized by law to consent to health care; provided, however, that the physician shall not make such disclosure if, in the judgment of the physician:
(A) the disclosure would not be in the best interest of the protected individual; or
(B) the protected individual is authorized pursuant to law to consent to such care and treatment.
Any decision or action by a physician under this paragraph, and the basis therefore, shall be recorded in the protected individual's medical record.
5. (a) Whenever disclosure of confidential HIV-related information is made pursuant to this article, except for disclosures made pursuant to paragraph (a) of subdivision one of this section or paragraph (a) or (e) of subdivision four of this section, such disclosure shall be accompanied or followed by a statement in writing which includes the following or substantially similar language: "This

The patient may elect to have the public health officer make the communication. The New York legislation is unusual in that it compels notification by the public health officer in cases where the risk "merits contact tracing in order to protect the public health."[10]

States such as Michigan impose a duty on the treating physician to take action to warn when the physician is aware of a risk of transmission.[11] The duty is easy to discharge by

referring the patient to the local public health office to complete a survey of potential third parties that may be harmed.

A medical provider may, with reasonable confidence, counsel a patient that beyond the health aspects of exposing another person to HIV, there is also potential criminal and civil liability for exposing another person to HIV. Criminal liability for intent to expose does not require actual transmission of the illness.[12]

A direct cause of action has been established for liability to third parties for the physician's failure to inform adequately the patient about his illness and its potential for communication. In *Reisner v. Regents of the University of California*, a minor patient had contracted HIV infection through a transfusion. Her physician's failure to warn her and her parents about the dangers of the HIV

---

information has been disclosed to you from confidential records which are protected by state law. State law prohibits you from making any further disclosure of this information without the specific written consent of the person to whom it pertains, or as otherwise permitted by law. Any unauthorized further disclosure in violation of state law may result in a fine or jail sentence or both. A general authorization for the release of medical or other information is NOT sufficient authorization for further disclosure." An oral disclosure shall be accompanied or followed by such a notice within ten days.

(b) Except for disclosures made pursuant to paragraph (c) of subdivision one of this section, or to persons reviewing information or records in the ordinary course of ensuring that a health facility is in compliance with applicable quality of care standards or any other authorized program evaluation, program monitoring or service review, or to governmental agents requiring information necessary for payments to be made on behalf of patients or clients pursuant to contract or in accordance to law, a notation of all such disclosures shall be placed in the medical record of a protected individual, who shall be informed of such disclosures upon request; provided, however, that for disclosures made to insurance institutions such a notation need only be entered at the time the disclosure is first made.

10. N.Y. Pub. Health Law § 2133. Contact tracing of cases of AIDS, HIV-related illness, or HIV infection.
   1. Every municipal health commissioner or the department's district health officer, upon determination that such reported case or, any other known case of HIV infection merits contact tracing in order to protect the public health, shall personally or through their qualified representatives notify the known contacts of the protected individual. Such contact tracing shall be done consistent with protocols developed pursuant to section twenty-one hundred thirty-seven of this title.
   2. Such contact shall also be informed of (a) the nature of HIV, (b) the known routes of transmission of the virus, (c) as circumstances may require, the risks of prenatal and perinatal transmission, (d) actions he or she can take to limit further transmission of the virus, (e) other facilities or community based organizations which are accessible to the person that provide counseling, medical care and treatment, further information or other appropriate services for persons infected with HIV.
   3. In notifying any contact identified in the course of any investigation conducted pursuant to this section, the physician or public health officer shall not disclose the identity of the protected individual or the identify of any other contact.
   4. A physician or public health officer making a notification to a contact pursuant to this section shall make such notification in person except where circumstances reasonably prevent doing so.

11. Michigan Compiled Laws § 333.5131, subsections 1 and 5 provide:
   (1) All reports, records, and data pertaining to testing, care, treatment, reporting, and research, and information pertaining to partner notification under section 5114a, that are associated with the serious communicable diseases or infections of HIV infection and acquired immunodeficiency syndrome are confidential. A person shall release reports, records, data, and information described in this subsection only pursuant to this section.
   (5) Subject to subsection (7), subsection (1) does not apply to the following:
   (a) Information pertaining to an individual who is HIV infected or has been diagnosed as having acquired immunodeficiency syndrome, if the information is disclosed to the department, a local health department, or other health care provider for 1 or more of the following purposes:
   (i) To protect the health of an individual.
   (ii) To prevent further transmission of HIV.
   (iii) To diagnose and care for a patient.
   (b) Information pertaining to an individual who is HIV infected or has been diagnosed as having acquired immunodeficiency syndrome, if the information is disclosed by a physician or local health officer to an individual who is known by the physician or local health officer to be a contact of the individual who is HIV infected or has been diagnosed as having acquired immunodeficiency syndrome, if the physician or local health officer determines that the disclosure of the information is necessary to prevent a reasonably foreseeable risk of further

transmission of HIV. This subdivision imposes an affirmative duty upon a physician or local health officer to disclose information pertaining to an individual who is HIV infected or has been diagnosed as having acquired immunodeficiency syndrome to an individual who is known by the physician or local health officer to be a contact of the individual who is HIV infected or has been diagnosed as having acquired immunodeficiency syndrome. A physician or local health officer may discharge the affirmative duty imposed under this subdivision by referring the individual who is HIV infected or has been diagnosed as having acquired immunodeficiency syndrome to the appropriate local health department for assistance with partner notification under section 5114a. The physician or local health officer shall include as part of the referral the name and, if available, address and telephone number of each individual known by the physician or local health officer to be a contact of the individual who is HIV infected or has been diagnosed as having acquired immunodeficiency syndrome.
   (c) Information pertaining to an individual who is HIV infected or has been diagnosed as having acquired immunodeficiency syndrome, if the information is disclosed by an authorized representative of the department or by a local health officer to an employee of a school district, and if the department representative or local health officer determines that the disclosure is necessary to prevent a reasonably foreseeable risk of transmission of HIV to pupils in the school district. An employee of a school district to whom information is disclosed under this subdivision is subject to subsection (1).
   (d) Information pertaining to an individual who is HIV infected or has been diagnosed as having acquired immunodeficiency syndrome, if the disclosure is expressly authorized in writing by the individual. This subdivision applies only if the written authorization is specific to HIV infection or acquired immunodeficiency syndrome. If the individual is a minor or incapacitated, the written authorization may be executed by the parent or legal guardian of the individual.
   (e) Information disclosed under section 5114, 5114a, 5119(3), 5129, 5204, or 20191 or information disclosed as required by rule promulgated under section 5111(1)(b) or (i).
   (f) Information pertaining to an individual who is HIV infected or has been diagnosed as having acquired immunodeficiency syndrome, if the information is part of a report required under the child protection law, 1975 PA 238, MCL 722.621 to 722.636.
   (g) Information pertaining to an individual who is HIV infected or has been diagnosed as having acquired immunodeficiency syndrome, if the information is disclosed by the department of social services, the department of mental health, the probate court, or a child placing agency in order to care for a minor and to place the minor with a child care organization licensed under 1973 PA 116, MCL 722.111 to 722.128. The person disclosing the information shall disclose it only to the director of the child care organization or, if the childcare organization is a private home, to the individual who holds the license for the child care organization. An individual to whom information is disclosed under this subdivision is subject to subsection (1). As used in this subdivision, "child care organization" and "child placing agency" mean those terms as defined in section 1 of 1973 PA 116, MCL 722.111. (emphasis added)

12. For an overview of state criminal laws regarding HIV exposure, please see "State Criminal Statutes on HIV Exposure," http://www.lambdalegal.org/our-work/publications/general/state-criminal-statutes-hiv.html, See also "State Criminal Statutes on HIV Transmission" (2008), http://www.aclu.org/lgbt-rights_hiv-aids/state-criminal-statutes-hiv-transmission

infection and its contagion to others gave rise to liability on the part of the physician to the patient's subsequently infected boyfriend.[13] From a psychiatric standpoint, infecting a loved one with HIV can be seen as harmful to the patient himself. Therefore, another source of potential liability for the clinician is the possible *post facto* interpretation that she had a duty to violate confidentiality and warn potential infectees, not, in this instance, for the sake of those potential infectees, but rather in order to protect the emotional health of the patient himself.

Clinicians are advised to document clearly their clinical reasoning for the decisions they have made regarding these issues of confidentiality and warning. Documentation of facts such as that there are no clear potential victims, that the patient has agreed to take precautions or inform his partner(s), or that reports have already been made to appropriate persons or officials are all useful. Knowledge of the individual state requirements regarding Tarasoff-type laws, HIV partner notification and Health Department reporting, and special duties to report have been seen by courts as part of the standard of care.

SUICIDE, ASSISTED SUICIDE, AND NATURAL DEATH WITHOUT MEDICAL INTERRUPTION

HIV-infected patients have seen a dramatic decrease in mortality throughout the world since the advent of effective antiviral treatment. HIV is now seen by most as a chronic illness. This does not mean that patients do not die, nor does it mean that they are not significantly burdened by HIV and associated conditions, treatments, and their side effects. In fact, patients with a variety of conditions (particularly major depression), and in a variety of circumstances, may find death preferable to their current lives. Although most clinicians see the wish to die as the outcome of thinking affected by a psychiatric disturbance, many have found circumstances where they wished to help patients end their life either by euthanasia, assisted suicide, or by withdrawal of treatment.

Arguments have been advanced for preventing medical providers from actively being involved in ending lives. Although there is a relief of suffering, some argue that helping to hasten death simply is not an appropriate role for the physician. Certainly such a responsibility has not generally been handled well by the medical profession. (See the discussion Footnote 15 & 17) Further complicating any ethical analysis of this issue is the fact that many patients (such as those with depression or inadequately treated pain) may well feel differently with the passage of time or with improved treatment.

The legal battles surrounding assisted suicide have laid a framework for discussion that narrows the issues considerably. This is a changing area of law, so research of your current state or country statutes on this area of law is highly recommended.[14]

Most states now have some legislation that codifies the early court decisions regarding the distinction between refusal of life sustaining care and suicide. The longstanding distinction was recognized again by the United States Supreme Court in *Vacco v. Quill*[15] and in *Washington v. Glucksberg*.[16] Both cases represented an attempt to establish a fundamental right to control one's own death by challenging a state's ability to make physician-assisted suicide illegal. The high court refused to find such a right. The Court found that common law established a distinction, however subtle,

---

13. *Reisner v. Regents of University of California* (1995) 31 Cal.App. 4th 1195, 37 Cal.Rptr.2d 518.

14. A summary of state laws regarding assisted suicide and an outline of the various state statutes outlawing the practice are contained in *The Right to Die*, Meisel and Cerminara (Aspen Law & Business, 2002).

15. In *Vacco v. Quill* 521 U.S. 793 (1997) the Court stated:
Unlike the Court of Appeals, we think the distinction between assisting suicide and withdrawing life-sustaining treatment, a distinction widely recognized and endorsed in the medical profession and in our legal traditions, is both important and logical; it is certainly rational. ... The distinction comports with fundamental legal principles of causation and intent. First, when a patient refuses life-sustaining medical treatment, he dies from an underlying fatal disease or pathology; but if a patient ingests lethal medication prescribed by a physician, he is killed by that medication. See, e.g., People v. Kevorkian, 447 Mich. 436, 470–472, 527 N.W.2d 714, 728 (1994), *cert. denied*, 514 U.S. 1083 (1995); Matter of Conroy, 98 N.J. 321, 355, 486 A.2d 1209, 1226 (1985) (when feeding tube is removed, death "result[s]... from [the patient's] underlying medical condition"); In re Colyer, 99 Wash.2d 114, 123, 660 P.2d 738, 743 (1983) ("[D]eath which occurs after the removal of life sustaining systems is from natural causes"); American Medical Association, Council on Ethical and Judicial Affairs, Physician-Assisted Suicide, 10 Issues in Law & Medicine 91, 92 (1994) ("When a life-sustaining treatment is declined, the patient dies primarily because of an underlying disease"). Furthermore, a physician who withdraws, or honors a patient's refusal to begin, life-sustaining medical treatment purposefully intends, or may so intend, only to respect his patient's wishes and "to cease doing useless and futile or degrading things to the patient when [the patient] no longer stands to benefit from them." Assisted Suicide in the United States, Hearing before the Subcommittee on the Constitution of the House Committee on the Judiciary, 104th Cong., 2d Sess., 368 (1996) (testimony of Dr. Leon R. Kass). The same is true when a doctor provides aggressive palliative care; in some cases, painkilling drugs may hasten a patient's death, but the physician's purpose and intent is, or may be, only to ease his patient's pain. A doctor who assists a suicide, however, "must, necessarily and indubitably, intend primarily that the patient be made dead." *Id.*, at 367. Similarly, a patient who commits suicide with a doctor's aid necessarily has the specific intent to end his or her own life, while a patient who refuses or discontinues treatment might not. See, for example, Matter of Conroy, *supra*, at 351, 486 A.2d at 1224 (patients who refuse life-sustaining treatment "may not harbor a specific intent to die" and may instead "fervently wish to live, but to do so free of unwanted medical technology, surgery, or drugs"); Superintendent of Belchertown State School v. Saikewicz, 373 Mass. 728, 743, n. 11, 370 N.E.2d 417, 426, n. 11 (1977) ("[I]n refusing treatment the patient may not have the specific intent to die"). The law has long used actors' intent or purpose to distinguish between two acts that may have the same result. *See, e.g.*, United States v. Bailey, 444 U.S. 394, 403–406 (1980) ("[T]he... common law of homicide often distinguishes... between a person who knows that another person will be killed as the result of his conduct and a person who acts with the specific purpose of taking another's life"); Morissette v. United States, 342 U.S. 246, 250 (1952) (distinctions based on intent are "universal and persistent in mature systems of law"); M. Hale, 1 Pleas of the Crown 412 (1847) ("If A., with an intent to prevent gangrene beginning in his hand doth without any advice cut off his hand, by which he dies, he is not thereby felo de se for tho it was a voluntary act, yet it was not with an intent to kill himself"). Put differently, the law distinguishes actions taken "because of" a given end from actions taken "in spite of" their unintended but foreseen consequences. Feeney, 442 U. S., at 279; Compassion in Dying v. Washington, 79 F.3d 790, 858 (9th Cir. 1996) (Kleinfeld, J., dissenting) ("When General Eisenhower ordered American soldiers onto the beaches of Normandy, he knew that he was sending many American soldiers to certain death. ... His purpose, though, was to... liberate Europe from the Nazis")."
521 U.S. at 800 to 803.

16. 521 U.S. 702 (1997).

between the refusal of care and suicide. The patient has the right to refuse care, even if such refusal will result in death. The patient may express the wish to refuse or have life-sustaining care withdrawn in testamentary or other legal documents or through a surrogate who has been either appointed or identified through a power of attorney. Jurisdictions differ as to the standard of proof required to establish the incompetent patient's intent to have care discontinued. On the other hand, in these two cases, the U.S. Supreme Court noted that suicide is abhorrent and generally prohibited.[17]

The Court found that a patient has no Constitutional right to assisted suicide in the *Quill* and *Glucksberg* cases. In those cases, the Court examined the laws of the States of New York and Washington that prohibited assisted suicide

17. The Supreme Court reviewed the legal background regarding suicide in Glucksberg:
In almost every State—indeed, in almost every western democracy—it is a crime to assist a suicide. The States' assisted-suicide bans are not innovations. Rather, they are longstanding expressions of the States' commitment to the protection and preservation of all human life. ... [S]ee Stanford v. Kentucky, 492 U.S. 361, 373 (1989) ("[T]he primary and most reliable indication of [a national] consensus is... the pattern of enacted laws"). Indeed, opposition to and condemnation of suicide—and, therefore, of assisting suicide—are consistent and enduring themes of our philosophical, legal, and cultural heritages. *See generally*, Marzen, O'Dowd, Crone & Balch, Suicide: A Constitutional Right?, 24 Duquesne L. Rev. 1, 17–56 (1985) (hereinafter Marzen); New York State Task Force on Life and the Law, When Death is Sought: Assisted Suicide and Euthanasia in the Medical Context 77–82 (May 1994) (hereinafter New York Task Force). More specifically, for over 700 years, the Anglo-American common-law tradition has punished or otherwise disapproved of both suicide and assisting suicide. ... In the 13th century, Henry de Bracton, one of the first legal-treatise writers, observed that "[j]ust as a man may commit felony by slaying another so may he do so by slaying himself." 2 Bracton on Laws and Customs of England 423 (f. 150) (G. Woodbine ed., S. Thorne transl., 1968). The real and personal property of one who killed himself to avoid conviction and punishment for a crime were forfeit to the king; however, thought Bracton, "if a man slays himself in weariness of life or because he is unwilling to endure further bodily pain... [only] his movable goods [were] confiscated." *Id.*, at 423–424 (f. 150). Thus, "[t]he principle that suicide of a sane person, for whatever reason, was a punishable felony was... introduced into English common law." Centuries later, Sir William Blackstone, whose Commentaries on the Laws of England not only provided a definitive summary of the common law but was also a primary legal authority for 18th and 19th century American lawyers, referred to suicide as "self-murder" and "the pretended heroism, but real cowardice, of the Stoic philosophers, who destroyed themselves to avoid those ills which they had not the fortitude to endure. ..." 4 W. Blackstone, Commentaries *189. Blackstone emphasized that "the law has... ranked [suicide] among the highest crimes," *ibid*, although, anticipating later developments, he conceded that the harsh and shameful punishments imposed for suicide "borde[r] a little upon severity." *Id.*, at *190. For the most part, the early American colonies adopted the common-law approach. For example, the legislators of the Providence Plantations, which would later become Rhode Island, declared in 1647, that "[s]elf-murder is by all agreed to be the most unnatural, and it is by this present Assembly declared, to be that, wherein he that doth it, kills himself out of a premeditated hatred against his own life or other humor:... his goods and chattels are the king's custom, but not his debts nor lands; but in case he be an infant, a lunatic, mad or distracted man, he forfeits nothing." The Earliest Acts and Laws of the Colony of Rhode Island and Providence Plantations 1647–1719, p. 19 (J. Cushing ed. 1977). Virginia also required ignominious burial for suicides, and their estates were forfeit to the crown. A. Scott, Criminal Law in Colonial Virginia 108, and n. 93, 198, and n. 15 (1930). Over time, however, the American colonies abolished these harsh common-law penalties. William Penn abandoned the criminal-forfeiture sanction in Pennsylvania in 1701, and the other colonies (and later, the other States) eventually followed this example. ... Zephaniah Swift, who would later become Chief Justice of Connecticut, wrote in 1796 that "[t]here can be no act more contemptible, than to attempt to punish an offender for a crime, by exercising a mean act of revenge upon lifeless clay, that is insensible of the punishment. There can be no greater cruelty, than the inflicting [of] a punishment, as the forfeiture of goods, which must fall solely on the innocent offspring of the offender. ... [Suicide] is so abhorrent to the feelings of mankind, and that strong love of life which is implanted in the human heart, that it cannot be so frequently committed, as to become dangerous to society. There can of course be no necessity of any punishment." 2 Z. Swift, A System of the Laws of the State of Connecticut 304 (1796).
This statement makes it clear, however, that the movement away from the common law's harsh sanctions did not represent an acceptance of suicide; rather, as Chief

Justice Swift observed, this change reflected the growing consensus that it was unfair to punish the suicide's family for his wrongdoing. ... Nonetheless, although states moved away from Blackstone's treatment of suicide, courts continued to condemn it as a grave public wrong. See, for example, Bigelow v. Berkshire Life Ins. Co., 93 U.S. 284, 286 (1876) (suicide is "an act of criminal self-destruction"); Von Holden v. Chapman, 87 App. Div. 2d 66, 70–71, 450 N. Y. S. 2d 623, 626–627 (1982); Blackwood v. Jones, 111 Fla. 528, 532, 149 So. 600, 601 (1933) ("No sophistry is tolerated... which seek[s] to justify self-destruction as commendable or even a matter of personal right").
That suicide remained a grievous, though nonfelonious, wrong is confirmed by the fact that colonial and early state legislatures and courts did not retreat from prohibiting assisting suicide. Swift, in his early 19th century treatise on the laws of Connecticut, stated that "[i]f one counsels another to commit suicide, and the other by reason of the advice kills himself, the advisor is guilty of murder as principal." 2 Z. Swift, A Digest of the Laws of the State of Connecticut 270 (1823). This was the well-established common-law view, *see* In re Joseph G., 34 Cal.3d 429, 434–435, 667 P.2d 1176, 1179 (1983); Commonwealth v. Mink, 123 Mass. 422, 428 (1877) ("'Now if the murder of one's self is felony, the accessory is equally guilty as if he had aided and abetted in the murder'") (quoting Chief Justice Parker's charge to the jury in Commonwealth v. Bowen, 13 Mass. 356 (1816)), as was the similar principle that the consent of a homicide victim is "wholly immaterial to the guilt of the person who cause[d] [his death]," 3 J. Stephen, A History of the Criminal Law of England 16 (1883); see 1 F. Wharton, Criminal Law Section(s) 451–452 (9th ed. 1885); Martin v. Commonwealth, 184 Va. 1009, 1018–1019, 37 S. E. 2d 43, 47 (1946) ("'The right to life and to personal security is not only sacred in the estimation of the common law, but it is inalienable'"). And the prohibitions against assisting suicide never contained exceptions for those who were near death. Rather, "[t]he life of those to whom life ha[d] become a burden of those who [were] hopelessly diseased or fatally wounded—nay, even the lives of criminals condemned to death, [were] under the protection of law, equally as the lives of those who [were] in the full tide of life's enjoyment, and anxious to continue to live." Blackburn v. State, 23 Ohio St. 146, 163 (1872).
The earliest American statute explicitly to outlaw assisting suicide was enacted in New York in 1828, Act of Dec. 10, 1828, ch. 20, Section(s) 4, 1828 N. Y. Laws 19 (codified at 2 N. Y. Rev. Stat. pt. 4, ch. 1, tit. 2, art. 1, Section(s) 7, p. 661 (1829)), and many of the new States and Territories followed New York's example. Marzen 73–74. Between 1857 and 1865, a New York commission led by Dudley Field drafted a criminal code that prohibited "aiding" a suicide and, specifically, "furnish[ing] another person with any deadly weapon or poisonous drug, knowing that such person intends to use such weapon or drug in taking his own life." *Id.*, at 76–77. By the time the Fourteenth Amendment was ratified, it was a crime in most States to assist a suicide. ... The Field Penal Code was adopted in the Dakota Territory in 1877, in New York in 1881, and its language served as a model for several other western states' statutes in the late 19th and early 20th centuries. Marzen 76–77, 205–206, 212–213. California, for example, codified its assisted-suicide prohibition in 1874, using language similar to the Field Code's. In this century, the Model Penal Code also prohibited "aiding" suicide, prompting many states to enact or revise their assisted-suicide bans. The Code's drafters observed that "the interests in the sanctity of life that are represented by the criminal homicide laws are threatened by one who expresses a willingness to participate in taking the life of another, even though the act may be accomplished with the consent, or at the request, of the suicide victim." American Law Institute, Model Penal Code Section(s) 210.5, Comment 5, p. 100 (Official Draft and Revised Comments 1980).
Though deeply rooted, the States' assisted-suicide bans have in recent years been reexamined and, generally, reaffirmed. Because of advances in medicine and technology, Americans today are increasingly likely to die in institutions, from chronic illnesses. President's Commission for the Study of Ethical Problems in Medicine and Biomedical and Behavioral Research, Deciding to Forego Life-Sustaining Treatment 16–18 (1983). Public concern and democratic action are therefore sharply focused on how best to protect dignity and independence at the end of life, with the result that there have been many significant changes in state laws and in the attitudes these laws reflect. Many states, for example, now permit "living wills," surrogate health-care decision making, and the withdrawal or refusal of life-sustaining medical treatment. See... People v. Kevorkian, 447 Mich. 436, 478–480, and nn. 53–56, 527 N.W. 2d 714, 731–732... (1994). At the same time, however, voters and legislators continue for the most part to reaffirm their States' prohibitions on assisting suicide.
521 U.S. 710 to 716.

in order to determine whether a legitimate state interest was served by the law. The *Glucksberg* opinion provided a detailed list of interests served by the anti-assisted-suicide statute: preservation of human life;[18] protection of vulnerable groups from the major public health problem of suicide;[19] protecting those who are depressed and in pain from suicide when treatment for pain and depression could afford them relief;[20] maintaining the integrity of the medical profession and avoiding having the patient's trust undermined by a notion that the physician's goal is not to heal the patient, but rather to encourage suicide;[21] protecting the vulnerable ill from the potential for coercion and overreaching due to financial interests of family or insurance companies;[22] and finally, avoiding a move of the legal paradigm in the direction of voluntary and involuntary euthanasia. The court reflected on the statistics in the Netherlands showing that the practice of euthanasia was not restricted to competent, terminally ill adults and may extend in practice to nonconsenting parties.[23]

The Court did point out that pain management through medication, even if it hastened the process that would lead to the patient's death, was appropriate under the laws of both Washington and New York. There is a movement in medicine to provide more and better training in effective pain management. Such training and implementation is especially important when considered in connection with the compelling reports that patients who initially opted for assisted suicide, and then obtained appropriate supportive medication and care for their depression, abandoned their desire to hasten death.

Despite the various ethical tribulations, assisted suicide is now legal in three States: Oregon, Washington, and Montana.[24] Oregon's statute allowing assisted suicide[25] has

18. "First, Washington has an unqualified interest in the preservation of human life. ... The State's prohibition on assisted suicide, like all homicide laws, both reflects and advances its commitment to this interest. ... This interest is symbolic and aspirational as well as practical...." 521 U.S. 728 to 729.

19. "Relatedly, all admit that suicide is a serious public-health problem, especially among persons in otherwise vulnerable groups. See Washington State Dept. of Health, Annual Summary of Vital Statistics 1991, pp. 29–30 (Oct. 1992) (suicide is a leading cause of death in Washington of those between the ages of 14 and 54). ... The State has an interest in preventing suicide, and in studying, identifying, and treating its causes. " 521 U.S. at 730.

20. "Those who attempt suicide—terminally ill or not—often suffer from depression or other mental disorders. ... Physician-Assisted Suicide and Euthanasia in the Netherlands: A Report of Chairman Charles T. Canady to the Subcommittee on the Constitution of the House Committee on the Judiciary, 104th Cong., 2d Sess., 10–11 (Comm. Print 1996); cf. Back, Wallace, Starks, & Pearlman, Physician-Assisted Suicide and Euthanasia in Washington State, 275 JAMA 919, 924 (1996) ('[I]ntolerable physical symptoms are not the reason most patients request physician-assisted suicide or euthanasia'). Research indicates, however, that many people who request physician-assisted suicide withdraw that request if their depression and pain are treated. H. Hendin, Seduced by Death: Doctors, Patients and the Dutch Cure 24–25 (1997). ... [L]egal physician-assisted suicide could make it more difficult for the State to protect depressed or mentally ill persons, or those who are suffering from untreated pain, from suicidal impulses." 521 U.S. at 730–731.

21. "The State also has an interest in protecting the integrity and ethics of the medical profession. ... [T]he American Medical Association, like many other medical and physicians' groups, has concluded that "[p]hysician-assisted suicide is fundamentally incompatible with the physician's role as healer." American Medical Association, Code of Ethics Section(s) 2.211 (1994); *see* Council on Ethical and Judicial Affairs, Decisions Near the End of Life, 267 JAMA 2229, 2233 (1992). ... And physician-assisted suicide could, it is argued, undermine the trust that is essential to the doctor-patient relationship by blurring the time-honored line between healing and harming." 521 U.S. at 731.

22. "Next, the State has an interest in protecting vulnerable groups-including the poor, the elderly, and disabled persons-from abuse, neglect, and mistakes. The Court of Appeals dismissed the State's concern that disadvantaged persons might be pressured into physician-assisted suicide as 'ludicrous on its face.' ... We have recognized, however, the real risk of subtle coercion and undue influence in end-of-life situations. ... If physician-assisted suicide were permitted, many might resort to it to spare their families the substantial financial burden of end-of-life health-care costs.
The State's interest here goes beyond protecting the vulnerable from coercion; it extends to protecting disabled and terminally ill people from prejudice, negative and inaccurate stereotypes, and "societal indifference."... The State's assisted-suicide ban reflects and reinforces its policy that the lives of terminally ill, disabled, and elderly people must be no less valued than the lives of the young and healthy, and that a seriously disabled person's suicidal impulses should be interpreted and treated the same way as anyone else's." 521 U.S. at 731 to 732.

23. "Finally, the State may fear that permitting assisted suicide will start it down the path to voluntary and perhaps even involuntary euthanasia. The Court of Appeals struck down Washington's assisted-suicide ban only as applied to competent, terminally ill adults who wish to hasten their deaths by obtaining medication prescribed by their doctors. ... Washington insists, however, that the impact of the court's decision will not and cannot be so limited. Brief for Petitioners 44–47. ... Thus, it turns out that what is couched as a limited right to 'physician-assisted suicide' is likely, in effect, a much broader license, which could prove extremely difficult to police and contain. Washington's ban on assisting suicide prevents such erosion.
This concern is further supported by evidence about the practice of euthanasia in the Netherlands. The Dutch government's own study revealed that in 1990, there were 2,300 cases of voluntary euthanasia (defined as "the deliberate termination of another's life at his request"), 400 cases of assisted suicide, and more than 1,000 cases of euthanasia without an explicit request. In addition to these latter 1,000 cases, the study found an additional 4,941 cases where physicians administered lethal morphine overdoses without the patients' explicit consent. Physician-Assisted Suicide and Euthanasia in the Netherlands: A Report of Chairman Charles T. Canady, at 12–13 (citing Dutch study). This study suggests that, despite the existence of various reporting procedures, euthanasia in the Netherlands has not been limited to competent, terminally ill adults who are enduring physical suffering, and that regulation of the practice may not have prevented abuses in cases involving vulnerable persons, including severely disabled neonates and elderly persons suffering from dementia. *Id.*, at 16–21; *see generally* C. Gomez, Regulating Death: Euthanasia and the Case of the Netherlands (1991); H. Hendin, Seduced by Death: Doctors, Patients, and the Dutch Cure (1997). ... Washington, like most other States, reasonably ensures against this risk by banning, rather than regulating, assisting suicide. 521 U.S. at 732 to 735.

24. In Oregon by statute ("Oregon Death with Dignity Act"), in Washington by public initiative, and in Montana by the Montana Supreme Court's interpretation of Montana law in Baxter v. Montana, DA 09–0051, MT 449, decided Dec. 31, 2009. The Montana Supreme Court found that a terminally ill patient's consent to physician aid in dying constitutes a statutory defense to a charge of homicide against the aiding physician when no other consent exceptions apply.

25. Oregon Revised Statutes 127.815 §3.01. Attending physician responsibilities.
(1) The attending physician shall:
 (a) Make the initial determination of whether a patient has a terminal disease, is capable, and has made the request voluntarily;
 (b) Request that the patient demonstrate Oregon residency pursuant to ORS 127.860;
 (c) To ensure that the patient is making an informed decision, inform the patient of:
 (A) His or her medical diagnosis;
 (B) His or her prognosis;
 (C) The potential risks associated with taking the medication to be prescribed;
 (D) The probable result of taking the medication to be prescribed; and
 (E) The feasible alternatives, including, but not limited to, comfort care, hospice care and pain control;
 (d) Refer the patient to a consulting physician for medical confirmation of the diagnosis, and for a determination that the patient is capable and acting voluntarily;
 (e) Refer the patient for counseling if appropriate pursuant to ORS 127.825;
 (f) Recommend that the patient notify next of kin;

been legally challenged several times[26] and was reinstated by popular initiative. The law is in force and as of the 2008 report by the State of Oregon, about 401 people had been assisted in dying based upon the law.[27] There appears to be a growing public interest in and acceptance of physician-assisted suicide.[28]

Nevertheless, the battle over physician-assisted suicide may not be entirely over. The Oregon law was challenged on a federal level by then Attorney General John Ashcroft and later by his successor, Alberto Gonzales, through enforcement of the federal Controlled Substance Act (CSA). Initially,

---

(g) Counsel the patient about the importance of having another person present when the patient takes the medication prescribed pursuant to ORS 127.800 to 127.897 and of not taking the medication in a public place;

(h) Inform the patient that he or she has an opportunity to rescind the request at any time and in any manner, and offer the patient an opportunity to rescind at the end of the 15 day waiting period pursuant to ORS 127.840;

(i) Verify, immediately prior to writing the prescription for medication under ORS 127.800 to 127.897, that the patient is making an informed decision;

(j) Fulfill the medical record documentation requirements of ORS 127.855;

(k) Ensure that all appropriate steps are carried out in accordance with ORS 127.800 to 127.897 prior to writing a prescription for medication to enable a qualified patient to end his or her life in a humane and dignified manner; and

(*l*) (A) Dispense medications directly, including ancillary medications intended to facilitate the desired effect to minimize the patient's discomfort, provided the attending physician is registered as a dispensing physician with the Board of Medical Examiners, has a current Drug Enforcement Administration certificate and complies with any applicable administrative rule; or

(B) With the patient's written consent:

(i) Contact a pharmacist and inform the pharmacist of the prescription; and

(ii) Deliver the written prescription personally or by mail to the pharmacist, who will dispense the medications to either the patient, the attending physician or an expressly identified agent of the patient.

(2) Notwithstanding any other provision of law, the attending physician may sign the patient's death certificate. [1995 c.3 §3.01; 1999 c.423 §3]

26. Lee v. State of Oregon, 869 F.Supp. 1491 (D. Or. 1994) (order granting preliminary injunction), the district court granted summary judgment for plaintiffs on their Equal Protection claim and issued a permanent injunction against the Act's enforcement on August 3, 1995; Lee v. State of Oregon, 891 F. Supp. 1439 (D. Or. 1995) (declaratory judgment and permanent injunction); Lee v. State of Oregon, 891 F.Supp. 1429 (D. Or. 1995) (equal protection opinion). Essentially, the district court found that the Act violated the Equal Protection Clause because it provided insufficient safeguards to prevent against an incompetent (i.e., depressed) terminally-ill adult from committing suicide, thereby irrationally depriving terminally-ill adults of the safeguards against suicide that are provided to adults who are not terminally ill. The district court did not address plaintiffs' other claims for relief. Lee v. Oregon, 107 F.3d 1382 (9th Cir. 1997).

27. Gov. John Kitzhaber, who is a physician, signed the law into effect in 1998. The State of Oregon tracks the use of assisted suicide in an annual report. *See* http://www.oregon.gov/DHS/ph/pas/ar-index.shtml.

28. "Polls have repeatedly shown that a large majority of Americans—sometimes nearing 90%—fully endorse recent legal changes granting terminally ill patients, and sometimes their families, the prerogative to accelerate their death by refusing or terminating treatment. ...Other polls indicate that a majority of Americans favor doctor-assisted suicide for the terminally ill. In April, 1990, the Roper Report found that 64% of Americans believed that the terminally ill should have the right to request and receive physician aid-in-dying. ... Another national poll, conducted in October 1991, shows that 'nearly two out of three Americans favor doctor-assisted suicide and euthanasia for terminally ill patients who request it.'... A 1994 Harris poll found 73% of Americans favor legalizing physician-assisted suicide. ... Three States have held referenda on proposals to allow physicians to help terminally ill, competent adults commit suicide with somewhat mixed results. In Oregon, voters approved the carefully-crafted referendum by a margin of 51 to 49 percent in November of 1994. ... In Washington and California where the measures contained far fewer practical safeguards, they narrowly failed to pass, each drawing 46 percent of the vote. ... As such referenda indicate, there is unquestionably growing popular support for permitting doctors to provide assistance to terminally ill patients who wish to hasten their deaths." Compassion v. Washington, 79 F.3d 790, 810 (9th Cir. 1996), Washington v. Glucksberg, 521 U.S. 702 (1997).

Ashcroft issued a directive stating that assisting suicide was not a "legitimate medical purpose," and therefore prescribing, dispensing, or administering federally controlled substances to assist suicide violated the CSA. This was a reversal of the position taken in June 1998 by Ashcroft's predecessor, Attorney General Janet Reno. Oregon's Federal District Court did not favor Ashcroft's interpretation and enjoined the application of the directive.

On final appeal, in *Gonzales v. Oregon*,[29] the United States Supreme Court did not support the use of the CSA to undermine a state's own determination of an appropriate medical purpose. The Court found that "[t]he CSA explicitly contemplates a role for the States in regulating controlled substances, as evidenced by its pre-emption provision." The Court made the injunction against Ashcroft's original directive permanent.

It does not appear that the current Democratic administration will attempt to attack the legislation, but this writer believes that future conservative administrations may well renew the effort to undo the Oregon law and those like it in other states. Though there appears to be a strong public opinion favoring allowing people to control their destinies on end-of-life issues, there is also a very strong opposing opinion that suicide, in any form, is immoral and should be illegal.

Guidelines for application of the Oregon law have been developed, but are still being debated and assessed.[30] Additionally, standards for consent, both for physician-assisted suicide and also for passive withdrawal of life-sustaining care, are also being developed.[31] Anticipate a good deal of further discussion in the future on the topic of how best to manage terminally ill patients.

INFORMED CONSENT, DEMENTIA, AND MEDICAL GUIDANCE

The term "informed consent" suggests, perhaps erroneously, that the patient is making an affirmative choice in her care. The reality is often that the patient is merely acquiescing to the treatment choice of the physician after being informed of the nature of the care being offered and, perhaps, some alternatives to it. The patient comes to the doctor ill, vulnerable, and outside of their normal milieu. The doctor is in a superior position of power in the relationship, being in possession of a special body of knowledge and experience relative to the patient's illness that far exceeds the average patient's understanding of her condition. In this setting, the doctor has the responsibility to direct the patient's care so that it is in the patient's best interest, making consent an

---

29. 546 U.S. 243 (2005). See also *Oregon v. Ashcroft*, 368 F.3d 1118 (9th Cir. 2004), which is the same case at the federal appellate level.

30. Caplan, Snyder and Faber-Langendoen, "The Role of Guidelines in the Practice of Physician-Assisted Suicide," *Assisted Suicide: Finding a Common Ground* (Indiana University Press, 2002).

31. Whiting, Raymond, *A Natural Right to Die: Twenty-Three Centuries of Debate*, (Greenwood Press, 2002).

almost foregone conclusion for most situations. This is a critical test for trust in the doctor's relationship with the patient.

In attempting to represent the best interest of the patient, the physician will often encounter competing interests. Certain types of care may be in the best interest of the patient, but may require a greater exertion of effort than the physician is willing or able to provide. Certain types of care or medication may be too costly or time consuming for the doctor, facility, or insurance company, while nevertheless being undeniably the correct approach for the patient. The physician may have personal beliefs that conflict with the goals of treatment, such as the belief that the patient would be better off dead, or that a certain treatment is immoral or provides too little benefit to justify the expenditure of resources required. It is under these circumstances that the patient must be able to rely on the physician to provide the utmost fidelity in the goal of healing the patient.

The term "competence" is often used in the description of the process of informed consent. A person, if competent, may make a particular decision or perform a certain task, such as consenting to a particular procedure. The ability to consent to different procedures and treatments requires different levels of competence. Although the legal definitions vary in different jurisdictions, in medical terms, competence to provide informed consent to care consists of the ability to understand the condition being treated, the risks and benefits of treatment, the alternative treatments, the potential consequences of each course of action, the ability to consider the choices rationally, and the ability to participate in the treatment. The patient may be seriously limited and incompetent for other purposes, but still competent to provide informed consent for care.

The assessment of competency to consent to care is quite different from the general level of competence necessary to enter into other types of contracts, execute a will or trust, convey property, or marry. The State of California, as an example, has developed a structure of legislation that characterizes the differing standards between legal competence and competence to provide informed consent to medical care. The legislation creates a rebuttable presumption[32] that people have capacity and the fact that they have a disease that will cause the deterioration of their mental function, alone, does not make them incompetent.[33,34] The California Legislature

specifically defined the capacity necessary for informed consent to medical care in a separate section.[35] The patient must understand the nature and seriousness of his illness and the nature of the treatment being proposed; he must be able to participate rationally in the treatment decision; and must have

---

(a) A determination that a person is of unsound mind or lacks the capacity to make a decision or do a certain act, including, but not limited to, the incapacity to contract, to make a conveyance, to marry, to make medical decisions, to execute wills, or to execute trusts, shall be supported by evidence of a deficit in at least one of the following mental functions, subject to subdivision (b), and evidence of a correlation between the deficit or deficits and the decision or acts in question:
(1) Alertness and attention, including, but not limited to, the following:
(A) Level of arousal or consciousness.
(B) Orientation to time, place, person, and situation.
(C) Ability to attend and concentrate.
(2) Information processing, including, but not limited to, the following:
(A) Short- and long-term memory, including immediate recall.
(B) Ability to understand or communicate with others, either verbally or otherwise.
(C) Recognition of familiar objects and familiar persons.
(D) Ability to understand and appreciate quantities.
(E) Ability to reason using abstract concepts.
(F) Ability to plan, organize, and carry out actions in one's own rational self-interest.
(G) Ability to reason logically.
(3) Thought processes. Deficits in these functions may be demonstrated by the presence of the following:
(A) Severely disorganized thinking.
(B) Hallucinations.
(C) Delusions.
(D) Uncontrollable, repetitive, or intrusive thoughts.
(4) Ability to modulate mood and affect. Deficits in this ability may be demonstrated by the presence of a pervasive and persistent or recurrent state of euphoria, anger, anxiety, fear, panic, depression, hopelessness or despair, helplessness, apathy or indifference, that is inappropriate in degree to the individual's circumstances.
(b) A deficit in the mental functions listed above may be considered only if the deficit, by itself or in combination with one or more other mental function deficits, significantly impairs the person's ability to understand and appreciate the consequences of his or her actions with regard to the type of act or decision in question.
(c) In determining whether a person suffers from a deficit in mental function so substantial that the person lacks the capacity to do a certain act, the court may take into consideration the frequency, severity, and duration of periods of impairment.
(d) The mere diagnosis of a mental or physical disorder shall not be sufficient in and of itself to support a determination that a person is of unsound mind or lacks the capacity to do a certain act.
(e) This part applies only to the evidence that is presented to, and the findings that are made by, a court determining the capacity of a person to do a certain act or make a decision, including, but not limited to, making medical decisions. Nothing in this part shall affect the decision making process set forth in Section 1418.8 of the Health and Safety Code, nor increase or decrease the burdens of documentation on, or potential liability of, health care providers who, outside the judicial context, determine the capacity of patients to make a medical decision.
812. Except where otherwise provided by law, including, but not limited to, Section 813 and the statutory and decisional law of testamentary capacity, a person lacks the capacity to make a decision unless the person has the ability to communicate verbally, or by any other means, the decision, and to understand and appreciate, to the extent relevant, all of the following:
(a) The rights, duties, and responsibilities created by, or affected by the decision.
(b) The probable consequences for the decision maker and, where appropriate, the persons affected by the decision.
(c) The significant risks, benefits, and reasonable alternatives involved in the decision.

35. California Probate Code § 813 provides:
813.
(a) For purposes of a judicial determination, a person has the capacity to give informed consent to a proposed medical treatment if the person is able to do all of the following:
(1) Respond knowingly and intelligently to queries about that medical treatment.
(2) Participate in that treatment decision by means of a rational thought process.

---

32. "Rebuttable presumption" is a legal term meaning that the fact is assumed to be true until the opponent presents evidence to the contrary.

33. California Probate Code § 810 provides:
The Legislature finds and declares the following:
(a) For purposes of this part, there shall exist a rebuttable presumption affecting the burden of proof that all persons have the capacity to make decisions and to be responsible for their acts or decisions.
(b) A person who has a mental or physical disorder may still be capable of contracting, conveying, marrying, making medical decisions, executing wills or trusts, and performing other actions.
(c) A judicial determination that a person is totally without understanding, or is of unsound mind, or suffers from one or more mental deficits so substantial that, under the circumstances, the person should be deemed to lack the legal capacity to perform a specific act, should be based on evidence of a deficit in one or more of the person's mental functions rather than on a diagnosis of a person's mental or physical disorder.

34. California Probate Code §§ 811 and 812 provide:
811.

an understanding of the duration, risks, benefits, and alternatives to the care. The statute specifically points out that a person having capacity to consent to medical care also has the capacity to refuse care.

There is a significant legal risk involved in the determination of capacity to provide informed consent. The physician should test and document the ability of the patient to comprehend the requisite issues described above and to reason through treatment options. Maintaining documentation showing that the patient understands the risks and benefits of the proposed treatment and alternatives is a standard of care. In a situation where there may be doubt regarding capacity to consent, a physician should clearly document her assessment of the capacity of the patient. If there is a reasonable doubt as to the patient's capacity, the physician should bring in an expert for a consultation on that issue. If the patient lacks capacity to provide informed consent and treatment is rendered despite that lack, the treatment is considered to have been rendered against the will of the patient. In this situation, there must be adequate documentation as to the reasons the treatment was rendered without consent, or why substituted consent was obtained. In most states, urgent care can be provided with substituted consent, and life-threatening conditions can be treated on an emergency basis without consent, provided a good faith effort to obtain consent was made, or the situation was too dire to allow time for this effort. Documentation of the rationale for such treatment is critical. Treatment rendered without consent is battery and may subject the physician to liability for damages, including punitive damages, even in the absence of proof of a specific injury.

The patient has the right to consent to care or refuse care, and the physician has the obligation to secure consent and make certain that the patient is competent to give consent. The U.S. Supreme Court has supported a competent patient's right to refuse care even if it will lead to his death.[36]

A competent patient may also establish a surrogate who has the power to consent to care or to refuse care for the patient according to the patient's written instruction establishing the surrogate. Clinicians may wish to encourage the selection of a substitute decision-maker or surrogate in conditions or treatments where the patient is likely to be incompetent at some point, such as dementia, treatments that provoke delirium or unconsciousness, or during brain surgery. The directions to the surrogate should specifically identify the interests of the patient. The patient should indicate if he desires to participate in experimental care, as well.

The surrogate may be restricted from consenting to the patient's participation in studies or experimental care if the instrument does not specifically provide the surrogate with that power. Cautious consideration is required in making advance directives and electing surrogate care. The patient may never have experienced the very states about which he is being asked to make decisions. Under the influence of the disturbing image of infirmity, combined with public opinion against the artificial extension of life, many patients initially state that they never want to be artificially ventilated, only to find their minds changed radically when they experience air hunger and severe cough.

As cognitive change is a continuing process, the physician has the challenge and obligation to identify the ongoing competency of the patient. Poor judgment on the patient's part can be an important issue and is a gray zone of law and medicine. Consider the circumstance in which the patient is clearly cognitively able to give informed consent, but is impaired in her ability to do so by factors such as personality difficulty, addiction, immaturity, discomfort, or poor insight. In a life-threatening circumstance, it is crucial that consultation be sought to determine whether the patient is competency-impaired and thus unable to make a reasonable decision. A case example is the patient with a life-threatening disorder who nevertheless wishes to leave the hospital, in opposition to the physician's advice. If the patient dies, it could be challenging to prove later that the poor judgment the patient exhibited was not a result of a psychiatric disorder that was overlooked (particularly if the patient has had a lifetime pattern of self-destructive behavior). The choice between respect for a patient's autonomy and allowing that patient to die of a treatable condition is, of course, difficult. Determining the cause of self-destructive decisions involves a thorough psychiatric evaluation, an examination of life-long patterns of behavior and beliefs, and contact with one or more third parties to provide outside information about the patient. Given a choice between wrongful death and an allegation of battery for a beneficial treatment, it would be harder for the patient's attorney to convince a jury to provide an award for the battery.

The issue of capacity to consent is particularly challenging when the physician determines that the patient does have proper capacity in regards to the informed medical consent, but it is obvious to outside observers that the patient does not have other legal capacity or is limited in some obvious way. Obtaining substituted, or surrogate, consent that agrees with the patient's decision is an easy solution when possible.

Capacity may depend on the moment the patient's evaluation is performed. A doctor assessing a patient suffering from dementia during a particularly lucid moment may conclude that the patient has capacity to provide informed consent, while another physician may make the same type of assessment later in the day and come to the opposite conclusion. It is likely that the doctor under the former circumstances will have trouble establishing in court that actual informed consent was obtained. While complete immunization from liability in this area is impossible, the consistent documentation of capacity and the liberal employment of

---

(3) Understand all of the following items of minimum basic medical treatment information with respect to that treatment:
(A) The nature and seriousness of the illness, disorder, or defect that the person has.
(B) The nature of the medical treatment that is being recommended by the person's health care providers.
(C) The probable degree and duration of any benefits and risks of any medical intervention that is being recommended by the person's health care providers, and the consequences of lack of treatment.
(D) The nature, risks, and benefits of any reasonable alternatives.
(b) A person who has the capacity to give informed consent to a proposed medical treatment also has the capacity to refuse consent to that treatment.

36. Vacco v. Quill, 521 U.S. 793 (1997); Washington v. Glucksberg, 521 U.S. 702 (1997).

consultants to verify capacity certainly will reduce the chances that the physician will have a problem.

CONCLUSION

The medical practitioner must stay abreast of her local state's position on these issues. The laws are in a state of flux. It appears that the law regarding liability to third parties for failure to warn of the potential for HIV transmission is moving toward becoming more physician friendly. The future of the law relating to assisted suicide is unclear, but the trend towards legalization appears to be expanding. The Federal Courts afford the states a high level of deference for the control of local medical interests. As legal notions shift on the issue of physician-assisted suicide, the role of physicians in that process must be carefully evaluated to assure the highest level of public trust and accountability.

12.6

NEUROPSYCHOLOGICAL TESTING

Kevin R. Robertson, Kevin J. Liner, Michelle Ro, and Robert K. Heaton

Neuropsychological testing of HIV-infected individuals has an important role to play in the diagnosis and management of HIV-associated neurocognitive disorders. The value of such testing may be particularly great in resource-limited settings, especially internationally, where non-behavioral diagnostic modalities such as neuroimaging are limited or nonexistent. This chapter, which discusses neuropsychological testing in resource-limited settings, may be particularly relevant to geographic areas where the disease burden is high, such as sub-Saharan Africa and South Asia. This chapter discusses the goals, current status, and challenges associated with neuropsychological assessment and interpretation in resource-limited settings.

INTRODUCTION

Since the introduction of combination antiretroviral therapy (cART) in developed nations, there has been a significant decrease in HIV-associated dementia (HAD), the severest form of HIV-associated neurocognitive disorders (HAND). However, the milder forms of HAND, mild neurocognitive disorder (MND), and asymptomatic neurocognitive impairment (ANI), continue to persist despite treatment, most likely due to residual viral replication in the brain combined with increased longevity (Antinori et al., 2007; Robertson et al., 2007b). Though HIV impacts populations all across the world, research has been focused in western, developed countries. Recent efforts in assessing the neuropsychological (NP) impact of HIV internationally have yielded some preliminary results on the pattern and progression of HAND in resource-limited settings (RLS) (Robertson et al., 2009; Heaton et al., 2008; Cysique et al., 2010). Further studies should be conducted to better understand HAND globally.

Neuropsychological assessments are essential to diagnosing HAND and the impact of cART on cognition. They are especially useful measures in RLS, where technologies for non-behavioral methods of diagnosis, such as neuroimaging, are unavailable. With the right normative standards, valid and reliable NP assessments can detect mild forms of cognitive impairment and may predict functional manifestations. Characterization of HAND pattern and progression through NP testing is important for proper diagnosis and monitoring of treatment outcomes. The present chapter discusses the goals, current status, and challenges associated with NP assessment and interpretation in RLS.

GLOBAL EPIDEMIOLOGY OF HIV/HAND

HIV infection is a global epidemic which involves various viral subtypes and impacts vastly different populations. It affects approximately 33 million people world-wide, with only about 6% concentrated in North America, Western and Central Europe, and Oceania, where the disease has been most extensively researched (WHO/UNAIDS, 2008). In contrast, according to the 2008 UNAIDS report on the global AIDS epidemic, sub-Saharan Africa alone accounted for about 67% of individuals living with HIV, 75% of AIDS deaths, and 1.9 million of the 2.7 million new infections in 2007. Asia represents about 15% (5 million) of the total HIV population, with the epidemic growing rapidly particularly in Indonesia, Pakistan, and Vietnam. Central Asia and Eastern Europe are estimated to have about 4.5% (1.5 million) of the people living with HIV, mostly in the Russian Federation and Ukraine. Latin America accounts for approximately 5% (1.7 million) of the global HIV population. The disease also affects people in the Middle East, North Africa, and the Caribbean, with comparatively smaller numbers (WHO/UNAIDS, 2008).

Due to the rapid evolution of the virus, HIV presents numerous subtypes which are concentrated in different areas around the world. Generally, subtype B predominates in North America, Western Europe, Oceania, the Caribbean, and parts of Latin America. In areas like West Central Africa, numerous subtypes are represented, including the nine major subtypes of HIV-1 Group M (A–D, F–H, J, and K), subtypes of HIV-1 N and O, and HIV-2. In South and Southeast Asia, subtype CFRO1_AE tends to predominate. In India and Southern Africa, clade C is the most common. This large variety of viral strains creates challenges in understanding the profile, progression, and optimal treatment of HIV and HAND. Neuropsychological assessments are important tools in understanding the impact of viral clade on the cognitive characteristics of HIV world-wide. However, the impact of culture, education, and socioeconomic status on NP performance still needs to be better understood before accurate comparisons can be made.

PURPOSE OF NEUROPSYCHOLOGICAL (NP) ASSESSMENTS

When approaching NP assessments of HIV-infected populations, there are several aims to consider:

1. Determining the presence of neurocognitive impairment directly associated with HIV

2. Assessing whether or not neurocognitive impairment is related to other comorbid factors, such as co-infections (e.g., with hepatitis C virus) or psychiatric conditions (affective or substance use disorders)

3. Understanding associations between neurocognitive impairment and HIV disease variables, such as viral load, current and nadir CD4 count, and neuropathogenic biomarkers

4. Exploring the impact HAND has on typical activities of daily living, which can have very different cognitive requirements for different populations

5. Determining optimal treatment parameters, including time of treatment initiation, ART regimen CNS penetration, and factors which facilitate medication adherence

6. Offering feedback reports on disease progression and treatment response to patients and clinicians (Robertson et al., 2009).

However, there are numerous challenges in achieving each of these aims. One of the major impediments to assessing neurocognitive impairment in individuals with HIV is the presence of other comorbid conditions. A study conducted in the United States found that less than 10% of HAND-presenting subjects had no other comorbidities, while most patients had 2 to 3 potentially contributing conditions (Heaton et al., 2009). The choice not to include patients with comorbidities in HAND research may demonstrate more precisely the direct influence of HIV, but it may also result in a less representative sample. This is especially the case in RLS, where malnutrition and a variety of other diseases, such as highly prevalent exposures to malaria and hepatitis C, may affect the majority of the population. In these situations, researchers should differentiate between neurocognitive deficits related to comorbidities and those attributable to HIV to the best of their ability (Robertson et al., 2009). Due to the NP impairment associated with various combinations of comorbid conditions, it can be difficult to understand the characteristics of cognitive impairment that are attributable to HIV alone.

Though efforts have been made to provide guidelines for rating NP impact of certain co-morbidities within the context of HIV, further clinical research should be conducted in developed and developing countries to better validate these guidelines (Antinori et al., 2007). Two areas that require investigation are the impact of comorbidities on rate of NP impairment in HIV, as well as their impact on potential relationships between NP impairment and HIV disease variables, such as nadir CD4

count, treatment effects, viral loads, and biomarkers of inflammation (Robertson et al., 2009). A recent study revealed that in the era of combination ART, nadir rather than current CD4 counts predict risk of HAND, with higher nadir CD4 counts related to decreased risk of HAND (Ellis et al., 2010). Some comorbidities, such as co-infection with the hepatitis C virus (HCV), have been shown to influence cognition independently while also compounding the deficits associated with HIV. A study conducted in HCV-infected individuals with comorbid HIV or methamphetamine dependence revealed that HCV serostatus was a significant predictor of global NP impairment and deficits in the areas of learning, motor skills, and abstraction (Cherner et al., 2005).

Though neuropsychiatric conditions, such as depression, have also been assumed to influence cognition, studies indicate that depression typically does not affect NP performance in HIV-infected patients (Cysique et al., 2007; Goggin et al., 1997). A study conducted in HIV-infected men did not reveal any significant difference in NP impairment between HIV groups with and without major depressive disorder or incident major depressive episodes (Cysique et al., 2007). Similar results were found in an earlier cross-sectional study of depressed and non-depressed HIV subjects, in which no correlations were found between depression severity and neurocognitive impairment (Goggin et al., 1997). However, a recent study reveals that depression may impact medication adherence, either directly through lack of motivation or indirectly through decreased social support (Bangsberg et al., 2010). Interruptions in medication adherence could impact the progression of cognitive deficits through higher viral loads in plasma and CNS. Further research should also be conducted on the possible cognitive influence of other comorbid NP conditions found with HIV, such as mania and other conditions associated with psychosis (Dube, Benton, Cruess, & Evans, 2005).

Another challenge is to understand the impact of HAND on activities of daily living (ADLs), especially in different populations. Neurocognitive deficits which typically impact everyday life in a western, developed society may be less likely to impact daily functioning in a rural, agrarian population to the same degree (Robertson, Liner, & Heaton, 2009). Therefore, though not every population can be canvassed, researchers should attempt to classify difficulty with ADLs in a manner that best fits each culture. The effects of HAND on daily function have mostly been researched in western, developed countries. Studies have shown that HAND can impede daily activities such as shopping, driving, financial management, and medication adherence. In addition, deficits in the areas of executive functioning, memory, and learning have also been associated with unemployment (Gorman, Foley, Ettenhofer, Hinkin, & van Gorp, 2009). To better understand how HAND may interfere with daily functioning in RLS, different tools or questionnaires which involve less complex (or at least different) activities may be required to elucidate the relevant effects. The Bolton Functional Assessment developed for use in Uganda is a good example.

In addition to cultural differences, the process of collecting information concerning daily function through self-report introduces several potentially confounding factors, including the patient's degree of insight and level of complexity in his/her daily activities. Depression may also bias self-report, and may hinder clear determination of the impact of other comorbidities on HIV disease. HIV-positive individuals experiencing depression are often prone to report an increased rate of cognitive complaints in comparison to their non-depressed counterparts, even without any objective evidence of cognitive impairment (Cysique et al., 2007; Rourke, Halman, & Bassel, 1999). As a result, complaints concerning difficulty with daily activities issued by depressed HIV subjects should also be supported by an independent informant or other secondary measures. Despite these possible confounding factors, the cognitive complaints of depressed HIV subjects have been associated with actual functional decline, demonstrating that the complaints should not be entirely dismissed on the basis of neuropsychiatric conditions (Sadek, Vigil, Grant, & Heaton, 2007).

Subjective self-reports concerning activities of daily living may complicate the NP impairment classification process, possibly resulting in distinct cognitive conditions receiving the same label or the same condition receiving different labels. At the Frascati conference, steps were made in agreeing to classify HAND without any detection of difficulty in ADLs as "asymptomatic neurocognitive impairment," in order to distinguish between asymptomatic and symptomatic conditions (Antinori et al., 2007; Cherner et al., 2007). Until the problems with functional assessments are worked out, it may be more valuable to focus on the nature of impairment based on NP test performance with less emphasis on ADLs, especially in studying cross-cultural comparisons.

Another area of contention is determining optimal treatment parameters that both reduce viral load and benefit cognition. Though the significance of beginning antiretroviral treatment at CD4 cell counts $\leq 200/\mu L$ has been well documented, recent evidence indicates that initiating at higher counts may be more beneficial (Sterne et al., 2009; Kitahata et al., 2009). In 2009, the United States Department of Health and Human Services updated cART treatment guidelines, strongly recommending that all patients with CD4 cell counts < 350 cells/mm3 start treatment (Panel on Antiretroviral Guidelines for Adults and Adolescents. Guidelines for the use of antiretroviral agents in HIV-1-infected adults and adolescents. http://www.aidsinfo.nih.gov/ContentFiles/AdultandAdolescentGL.pdf.). Treatment is also strongly recommended for patients who have a history of an AIDS-defining illness or any of the following conditions: pregnancy, HIV-associated nephropathy, or hepatitis B co-infection with evidence of HepB treatment. The recent study which indicates that higher nadir CD4 levels are associated with reduced risk of HAND supports initiation at higher CD4 counts (Ellis et al., 2010). Treatment initiation for patients with CD4 counts > 350 may help prevent cognitive decline by preserving higher CD4 levels. Unfortunately, in resource-limited settings, limited access to health care providers and optimal antiretroviral medication often hinders initiation at higher CD4 counts and could increase the risk of developing HAND.

There is also a debate concerning the impact of antiretroviral CNS penetration on cognition. Recent evidence from developed countries suggests that cART regimens with higher penetration correlate with cognitive improvement in HIV-positive subjects (Tozzi et al., 2009; Ellis et al., 2009; Patel et al., 2009). However, at least one study found that higher ranking regimens were related to poorer neurocognitive performance, suggesting that cART may also have neurotoxic effects (Marra et al., 2009). The influence of cART CNS penetration on cognition has yet to be assessed in RLS.

NEUROCOGNITIVE STUDIES IN RESOURCE-LIMITED SETTINGS

Information on the prevalence and profile of HAND in RLS is still limited. In western, developed settings, the initiation of cART and protease inhibitors (PIs) dramatically reduced HIV-associated dementia (HAD) and the prevalence of CNS opportunistic diseases, including cryptococcal meningitis, primary CNS lymphoma, cerebral toxoplasmosis, and progressive multifocal leukoencephalopathy (d'Arminio Monforte et al., 2004). In RLS, however, CNS opportunistic diseases and infections are still common, and continue to complicate diagnosis and management of CNS disease that is more directly attributable to HIV. Though numerous studies have been conducted, variations in assessment methodology, test administration, definition of NP deficits, and other environmental or cultural factors have made it difficult to make cross-comparisons on the prevalence and presentation of HAND.

Several different NP testing batteries have been applied internationally with varying results. The World Health Organization (WHO) conducted one of the earliest international studies assessing HIV-associated cognitive impairment. Objective clinical assessments, ratings of performance in daily function, and additional neurological examinations were included as well. Results revealed HIV-related NP impairment at approximately 19.1% in Zaire, 18.4% in Thailand, 15.3% in Kenya, and 13.0% in Brazil. Neurological examinations revealed higher deficit percentages of about 66% in Thailand, 54% in Brazil, 41% in Zaire, and 40% in Kenya (Maj et al., 1994). A brief testing battery that is currently in use is the International HIV Dementia Scale (IHDS), which is used as a screening battery to identify individuals at risk for dementia. It is composed of three subtests: timed fingertapping, a timed alternating hand sequence test, and recall of four words at 2 minutes (Sacktor et al., 2005). One study applying the IHDS in a rural setting in Ethiopia did not detect cognitive differences between HIV-positive and -negative individuals (Clifford et al., 2007), but other studies have reported the utility of the IHDS in distinguishing the two groups, as well as HIV-positive individuals at risk for dementia (Robertson et al., 2009). Studies employing detailed NP test batteries have reported cognitive impairment prevalence rates of 56%, 34%, and 31% in India, China, and Uganda, respectively (Heaton et al., 2008; Robertson et al., 2007; Yepthomi et al., 2006). The differences in impairment rates may be attributable to variations in HIV clade, environmental factors, cultural nuances, or neuropsychological methods. Identifying the testing strategy that can best be applied across various international settings is important in being able to compare the prevalence and pattern of HAND in different settings. Though longer, more involved batteries may have the advantage of sensitivity, they may also introduce more challenges in terms of translation and interpretation of tests across populations with different cultural, linguistic, and educational backgrounds. Shorter batteries may lack a certain degree of sensitivity but could be easier to transfer internationally.

Among studies conducted in sub-Saharan Africa, HAND prevalence rates have been reported to be as low as 3% or as high as 54% (Belec et al., 1989; Howlett, Nkya, Mmuni, & Missalek, 1989). Recent on-going studies in this region using the International HIV Dementia Scale (IHDS) have shown HAND prevalence rates to be about 21.1% in Cameroon, 33% in Zambia, and 38% in Botswana (Robertson et al., 2010). As these and other studies progress, more information will be revealed concerning the state of HAND in sub-Saharan Africa. A recent study in Uganda on HIV+ subjects demonstrated neurocognitive improvement following the initiation of Stavudine-based therapy, particularly in the areas of verbal memory and fluency, motor performance, psychomotor speed, and executive functioning (Sacktor et al., 2009). HIV-negative individuals were assessed as a control group. NP assessments were conducted using the IHDS and a full neuropsychological testing battery. The subjects also experienced functional improvement, which was measured by the Karnofsky scale. Despite these apparent benefits, approximately 31–38% of the participants developed peripheral neuropathy symptoms, indicating that less toxic antiretroviral regimens should be pursued.

Recent studies in Asia have also begun to reveal the international presence and pattern of HAND. Research conducted on cohorts in China and the United States reported that the Chinese subjects demonstrated deficits in the areas of processing speed, abstraction/executive function, and learning, similar to their American counterparts (Cysique et al., 2007). The study also ascertained that significant country effects were found only in the domains of verbal fluency and processing speed. Depression had an insignificant effect on NP performance, though it did relate to increased cognitive complaints and unemployment. To assess cognitive deficits, the researchers translated and slightly adapted the neuropsychological battery from the U.S. version to better fit the Chinese population. The NP testing battery included measures assessing verbal fluency, attention/working memory, speed of information processing, executive functioning, learning/memory, and motor functions (Cysique et al., 2007). In addition to revealing the pattern of HAND in China, the study also demonstrated the potential transferability of western tests to other cultures after making appropriate adaptations. Building on these results, a study assessing HIV and HCV co-infected individuals in rural China revealed NP impairment in about 37% of both HIV-monoinfected subjects and HIV/HCV co-infected subjects, although there was a significant HCV effect among HIV participants (impairment rates of 23.3% vs. 12.5% in controls uninfected with either virus) (Heaton et al., 2008).

Another study in Thailand attempted to ascertain the possible impact of immunologic and virologic factors on NP performance in first-time initiators of HAART (Valcour et al., 2009). The researchers discovered that baseline monocyte HIV DNA levels significantly predicted HAD symptoms, with HIV DNA counts surpassing 3.5 log10 copies/106 monocytes at baseline, discriminating all HAD from non-HAD cases. Further studies should continue to explore possible relationships between cognition and virologic factors for diagnostic and treatment purposes.

Data are also being accumulated on the influence of HIV clades on HAND patterns, though this research is still in its beginning stages. A study on HIV-positive subjects in Uganda set out to determine differences in dementia state or severity relative to viral subtypes A, C, or D (Sacktor et al., 2009). The study assessed 60 ART-naive HIV-infected subjects who underwent analysis of the gag and gp41 regions in order to ascertain HIV subtype. HAND diagnosis was made using the IHDS and a detailed NP test battery. The Karnofsky scale was used to assess functional impairment. The results revealed that 89% of the individuals with subtype D exhibited HAND in comparison to 24% of those with subtype A, indicating that subtype D individuals may be more prone to CNS dysfunction (Sacktor et al., 2009). These results are consistent with studies that suggest subtype D progresses more rapidly to AIDS and death than subtype A (Laeyendecker et al., 2006).

In addition, studies have shown the presence of HAND in clade C cohorts in South Africa and HIV-infected individuals in Zambia, where clade C accounts for about 95% of the variants. HIV-infected clade C subjects in South Africa demonstrated significant deficits in Color Trails 2, Animal Fluency, Stroop Color-Word interference, and Digit Symbol (Joska et al., 2010). In Zambia, the HIV Neurobehavioral Research Center (NHRC) International neuropsychological test battery was used to diagnose HAND in approximately 33% of the HIV+ subjects (Grant et al., 2010). These studies support previous results from research in South India on clade C individuals, which reported mild to moderate neurocognitive impairment in about 60.5% of the HIV-seropositive subjects, particularly in the areas of fluency, working memory, and learning (Gupta et al., 2007).

Addressing the lack of cross-cultural studies using a standardized testing battery, a current international study (ACTG 5199) has been conducting assessments in Brazil, India, Malawi, Peru, South Africa, Thailand, and Zimbabwe to further understand the prevalence of HAND and NP response to cART internationally (Robertson et al., 2009). The brief testing battery, which included grooved pegboard, timed gait, semantic verbal fluency, and fingertapping, was administered every 24 weeks after cART initiation to all 293 participants. The participants were randomized to treatment with didanosine enteric-coated (ddI) + emtricitabine (FTC) + atazanavir (ATV) in the AIDS Clinical Trials Group (ACTG) Study A5175 (PEARLS), and did not include groups on alternate treatment regimens or untreated control groups for comparison. The preliminary results demonstrated that HIV subjects experienced cognitive improvement after initiating CART, though the magnitude of improvement differed by country.

The source of this variation is still unclear, but may be mediated by differences in culture and test administration or possibly differences in pathogenesis between HIV clades. Further international studies should be conducted using demographically matched and country-specific HIV-negative controls.

The studies outlined in this section provide evidence for the existence of HAND in RLS, despite differences in culture or HIV clade. However, it is difficult to draw conclusions concerning the impact of country, culture, or clade on HAND prevalence or pattern based on the studies available. Differences in inclusion/exclusion criteria, test instruments, normative standards, and definitional systems of NP impairment introduce numerous barriers to making accurate cross-study comparisons (Robertson et al., 2009). Though the Frascati guidelines have set definitions for HAND based on NP performance, daily function, and presence of comorbidities, further work should be pursued in achieving consistency across international studies (Antinori et al., 2007). In addition, many of the studies lack HIV-negative or untreated control groups due to the pressure of limited time and resources. Despite these challenges, researchers should make it a priority to include control groups in order to draw accurate conclusions concerning HAND. As future efforts are pursued, it is important to understand which neurocognitive tests are the most internationally viable and which factors may influence the applicability and generalizability of norms. Steps should continue to be taken towards establishing greater consistency in testing methods and instruments in order to enable accurate cross-cultural comparisons.

ISSUES IN PERFORMING NEUROPSYCHOLOGICAL ASSESSMENTS IN RESOURCE-LIMITED SETTINGS

Numerous factors can hinder successful administration of NP assessments in RLS, some of which include limitations in health care infrastructure and staff, geographical impediments, overwhelming disease burden, and lack of neuropsychological expertise.

Some of the greatest challenges facing NP assessments in RLS are the dearth of access to clinics and treatment, inadequate staffing, and socioeconomic hindrances to study retention. In developing countries, the hospitals and clinics tend to be concentrated in the more urban areas, making it difficult for those in remote areas to obtain proper care. In addition, unpaved roads and lack of transportation options often compound the situation. For study participants, being involved with an assessment may involve giving up a day of work to travel and be evaluated or treated. A recent study conducted in rural Uganda demonstrates that compensating for transportation costs may help to increase study retention and medication adherence (Emenyonu et al., 2010). Food insecurity is another factor that may hinder assessment retention and medication adherence. One study shows that some patients in Uganda discontinued medication or routine care due to the competing demand of obtaining food (Tsai et al., 2010). Nutritional support may be a necessary supplement to ART

therapy in RLS. As a result of these factors and more, NP assessments in RLS can be challenging to manage due to study drop-out rates and difficulty with recruitment.

In addition to patient poverty and limited medical resources, the overwhelming disease burden present in most RLS adds to the challenge. It is reported that an estimated 25 million people in sub-Saharan Africa live with HIV, with numbers reaching up to 30% of the population in certain areas (WHO/UNAIDS, 2008). Numerous other life-threatening diseases, such as tuberculosis and malaria, also demand the urgent attention of health care personnel. Many of these diseases can impact the CNS as well, making it more challenging to understand the neurocognitive deficits associated with HIV alone. Additionally, many people are suffering from the direct and perhaps more life-threatening symptoms of the diseases, which require immediate treatment and take priority over neurocognitive assessment. This can create problems in initiating and carrying out NP studies, especially in areas where funds are already limited.

Another obstacle in RLS is the lack of neuropsychological expertise available to administer, score, and interpret assessment results. As a result, specialists are often acquired from other countries to train clinical personnel or conduct studies themselves. Formal training in performing neurological and neuropsychological examinations is an important component of research, as standardized and consistent methods of assessment administration are imperative to obtaining accurate data. Though such training is harder to achieve in RLS, it can be enabled by designating study sites used for training, providing access to training media outlining neurological examinations and NP instruments, creating on-line certification programs, and coordinating periodic follow-up with the examiners at each site (Robertson et al., 2009). A continuously updated review of NP examination methodology and instruments should also be established between the study investigators and site examiners. The practice of formal training and strengthening examination infrastructure will help further neuroAIDS research while also benefitting health care fields in RLS.

ISSUES IN INTERPRETATION OF NEUROPSYCHOLOGICAL ASSESSMENTS IN RESOURCE-LIMITED SETTINGS

Interpreting assessments in international settings can be more challenging than conducting them. Determining the psychometric properties (reliability and validity) of western tests is a difficult task even within the numerous ethnic groups of the United States (Pedraza et al., 2008). Researchers have encountered challenges in adapting tests for Spanish-speaking subgroups, for example, due to the great cultural diversity of people emigrating from or residing in Spanish-speaking countries, and varying levels of acculturation in the US. (Wilkie et al., 2004). Taking the western tests and trying to apply them abroad in RLS introduces additional, potentially confounding factors, some of which were discussed in the previous section. Though the effectiveness of these testing batteries has been proven in the United States and other western countries, the validity and reliability of many instruments in other countries have yet to be established. Assessment validity deals with whether or not the test, question, or skill has the same meaning to both the test-maker and test-taker. Assessment reliability refers to whether or not test results show consistency for an individual or group over separate administrations or within the same administration. Several factors challenge assessment validity and reliability in RLS, including distinguishing which cognitive tasks or abilities cannot be considered "pan-human" (e.g., speed of information processing is likely to be less important in the lives of many people in RLS). Also, determining population norms is important for interpreting test results, especially in individual people (vs. matched research groups). Such norms do not exist in most RLS, and generalizability from one such setting to another cannot be assumed.

Even when the skills assessed by NP tests may be considered "pan-human," differences in educational, cultural, and linguistic backgrounds can influence those abilities. Several studies assessing normal populations in various cultures using standardized tests have reported different levels of cognitive performance between ethnic groups. The WHO-Neurobehavioral Core Test Battery (WHO-NCTB) study revealed significant differences in performance between western countries and different populations on seven neurobehavioral measures: Digit Symbol, Digit Span, Benton Visual Memory Test/ Recognition Form, Santa Ana Dexterity Test, Simple Reaction Time, Pursuit Aiming II, and Profile of Mood States (Anger et al., 2000). Several other studies support the presence of NP performance differences across populations in a wide variety of domains, including the areas of language (Llorente, Turcich, & Lawrence, 2004), verbal memory and fluency (Razani, Burciaga, Madore, & Wong, 2007), simple attention (Anger et al., 1993), simple visual attention (Paul et al., 2007), information processing speed (Llorente et al., 2004; Anger et al., 1993), spatial based tests (Mayes, Jahoda, & Neilson, 1988; Holding et al., 2004; Jahoda, 1979; Rosselli & Ardila, 2003), timed and sustained performance tasks (Anger et al., 1993; Agranovich & Puente, 2007; Byrd, Touradji, Tang, & Manly, 2004; Chung et al., 2003), digit based tests (Hedden et al., 2002), and perception (Nisbett & Miyamoto, 2005). On the other hand, similar NP performance has been described in different populations on tests of nonverbal skills (Hsieh & Tori, 2007; Razani, Murcia, Tabares, & Wong, 2007), simple reaction time and visual retention (Anger et al., 1993), simple attention (Paul et al., 2007), counting and summation (Hsieh & Tori, 2007), a visuo-spatial measure of processing speed (Hedden et al., 2002), and motor-based skills (Parsons, Rogers, Hall, & Robertson, 2007). When group differences exist, it can be difficult to determine whether or not the tests are appropriate or if the results simply reflect a need for separate norms. The existence of group differences does not necessarily imply that a test is invalid. For example, significantly different results in NP performance between groups of individuals in their 20s and 60s should be expected and indicate the need for distinct normative standards applied to each group, rather than indicating any group difference in test validity.

Group differences on NP tests, especially between cultures and international populations, may also be influenced by numerous biases, which have been classified into three categories: construct bias, method bias, and item bias (de Klerk, 2008). Construct bias refers to differences in the definition of the construct being assessed from one group to another. Different definitions of HIV neurocognitive deficits, especially in international studies, often make cross-comparisons difficult to achieve. Method bias results from variations in test construction or administration, including confounds introduced by the instruments themselves. For example, one assessment may measure quality of life through the Karnofsky scale while another uses the Zubrod scale, introducing differences which complicate comparison. Administrative method bias may be present in situations where the test administrator is not fluent in the target language, perhaps hindering the optimal performance of that population in comparison to others. Item bias occurs when the test content is interpreted differently by people in different groups. For example, a test item depicting an escalator could be interpreted as a staircase in areas less familiar with technology. In the process of transferring tests to new populations, each of these biases should be accounted for as much as possible.

Language differences also account for some of the difficulty in successful transfer of western tests to RLS. Even if the tests are professionally translated, problems can surface in the wording of the tasks. Standard instructions which may seem straight-forward to western audiences may require modifications to fit the idioms and common language of the target population in order to convey the same meaning. There are instances in which no word is available in the target language to directly translate from the original, which can inadvertently alter the difficulty level of word lists or passages. Despite these potential difficulties, western tests will eventually have to be translated for use in developing countries. It is important that translations are carried out by a professional who is fluent in the target language, in concert with a neuropsychologist who understands what the test is intended to measure and what information the standard English instructions are intended to convey. As an extra precaution, the tests may also have to be re-translated into the original language by an independent translator who is not familiar with the testing measures (Cysique et al., 2007). Another option is to have the test translated by a committee of professionals knowledgeable in various areas, such as the target language and culture or psychology (de Klerk, 2008). Though these precautions may not guarantee the complete absence of linguistic or cultural inconsistencies, they should be applied to achieve the closest and most effective possible translations. Once translated, the tests should be administered by a neuropsychologist or trained professional who is fluent in the target language, so that any remaining confusions can be clarified and progress encouraged through informal rapport. It is also helpful to run a pilot study of the newly translated assessment with the target population in order to gauge comprehension (Robertson et al., 2009; Cysique et al., 2007). In one particular attempt to alter western NP tests for another culture, researchers at the University of Miami reworked the word lists and phrases in six verbal learning, memory, and fluency measures to make them viable for Hispanic populations (Wilkie et al., 2004). In order to achieve close translations of each test, the researchers employed a panel of professionals representing various Hispanic countries who were knowledgeable in neuropsychology and the Spanish language or culture.

The existence of culturally distinct subgroups and language dialects in certain countries makes it even more difficult to translate tests and generate normative data. This is the case in India, Indonesia, and several African countries, such as Zambia and Nigeria. Recently, the Eighth Schedule of the Constitution of India reported 22 official languages, an increase from the previous 14 documented in "The Official Languages Act, 1963" (The Constitution of India: The Official Languages Act, 1963). Overall, approximately 400 individual mother tongues are used in India alone. In order to administer and gather normative data for NP tests across the country, researchers will need to go beyond the main Hindi dialects and translate the tests into the other official languages, according to the dominant language in each area assessed. This process of translating and adapting tests to each region requires a meticulous, time-consuming, and expensive process.

In addition to translation, several points should be addressed in order to facilitate accurate interpretation. Visual and auditory stimuli familiar only to those in western populations, such as certain technologies, foods, or even animals, should either be adapted to fit the culture or excluded. Substituting tasks which do not require knowledge of language or letters for those that do (for example, the Color Trails Test for the Trail Making Test) may be necessary and more valid in some areas (i.e., drastically different education or symbol-based writing) (Robertson et al., 2009). Even if these criteria are met, there is evidence that culture may have an impact on nonverbal assessments as well, such as in tests involving processing speed (Rosselli & Ardila, 2003). Additionally, lack of familiarity with computers, writing instruments, or test-taking itself can influence NP testing outcomes for subjects in RLS. Therefore, even nonverbal assessments may need to be constructed with sensitivity to cultural differences.

The concept of "test-wiseness" refers to test-taking skills that are acquired incidentally through exposure to formal academic systems instead of through direct education and training (Rosselli & Ardila, 2003). In classrooms in western settings, children are taught to sit still, work quickly and accurately, take notes, listen to and follow instructions, and perform other behaviors which are important in successfully completing NP assessments. Generally, 9 to 12 years of formal education provides enough experience to acquire and practice these test-taking skills. However, in RLS, students often do not receive the same training in test-wiseness due to high teacher-to-pupil ratios, scarcity of school supplies, and other factors which may result in less stringent or formal testing procedures. Therefore, western tests created for those who are experienced in quick and accurate test-taking may be received differently in RLS. For example, the Trail-Making Test B requires the test-taker to connect randomly placed letter and number sequences in order while alternating back and forth between the two sequences. In western countries, people with nine or more years of education (the vast majority of the U.S. population) are able to perform this task with relative ease. For semi-literate or non-western populations who have less experience manipulating numbers and letters, performance on the task is likely to be significantly lower (Mitrushina, Boone, Razani, & Elia, 2005; Spreen & Strauss, 1991). Although they may know the correct order, these populations typically take longer to retrieve the sequences before connecting them, which could be misinterpreted as a cognitive deficit in executive functioning. In addition to lack of literacy, as noted above, other cultures may not share the western test-taking priorities which emphasize speed coupled with accuracy. In some cultures, being cautious and thoughtful is a much more prized quality, resulting in slower, more meticulous test taking approaches. In the framework of a western timed test, the lagging, careful approach could be reported inaccurately as a cognitive deficit. Several studies have supported such cultural effects on time of performance in testing tasks. In one particular study, a normal group of monolingual English-speaking Anglo-Americans completed the Trail Making Test Part B and Stroop Tests B and C significantly faster than an ethnically diverse normal group (Razani et al., 2007). Another study reported that Zairian children took longer to complete the Tactual Performance Test than American and Canadian children (Boivin, Giordani, & Bornefeld, 1995). Researchers also found a significant culture effect between US and Russian normal adults on the timed Color Trails and Ruff Figural Fluency tests, with results in favor of the American adults (Agranovich & Puente, 2007).

When cultural or educational differences exist, different sets of normative or control data are necessary to interpret and compare the results accurately. Despite differences in performance across international populations, tests assessing processing speed and other abilities tapped by western NP test batteries appear to be sensitive to HIV deficits in both the developing and developed world (Heaton et al., 2008; Robertson et al., 2007; Cysique et al., 2007). Other cultures may not prioritize processing speed as much as western settings, but we should not assume that it is an irrelevant or noninfluential factor in RLS.

Gathering normative data for NP tests in RLS can be an especially daunting task due to difficulties in subject recruitment and study management. Hundreds of normal subjects are required to establish truly adequate normative standards. Recruiting and keeping track of such a large group of subjects in RLS can be a challenge in itself. Studies show that larger program sizes can be associated with greater loss-to-follow-up, which may be associated with loss of care in relating to individual participants, or even to administrative errors (Myer et al., 2010). Lack of documented medical histories and presence of psychiatric, medical, and neurological confounds often further complicate the recruitment process. Additionally, as noted above, a variety of essential demographic factors need to be addressed in the process of developing norms. Urban versus rural settings, ethnicity, and additional socioeconomic factors may also need to be examined. The ultimate goal is to be able to correct for all demographic influences on test performance in order to establish usable normative standards for expected, normal performances in individual participants. Due to the obstacles involved with controlling for demographic factors and attaining sizable normative samples, the task of collecting normative data often is an especially resource-intensive enterprise. As a result, funding agencies and the private sector have been reluctant to support these basic normative data studies. Therefore, many researchers opt for recruiting smaller local control groups instead of running large-scale normative studies. The downsides of these control groups are inadequate sample sizes to fully represent (control for) the important demographic characteristics of the population as a whole. As such, the data may be insufficient to develop normative standards for characterizing HAND in the region being assessed (Robertson et al., 2009).

Since developing normative standards for every population or subculture in the world cannot be achieved with available resources, future studies should focus on the generalizability of norms which have already been established. Existing norms and NP assessments in the US have been employed in other western countries with comparable validity (Paul et al., 2007; Bornstein et al., 1993; Portegies et al., 1993; Tozzi et al., 2005; Wright et al., 2008), indicating that generalizability may be possible in areas which share similar cultural experiences and backgrounds. Norms developed in one RLS therefore may be applicable to others sharing similar characteristics. The cultural, education, linguistic, or socioeconomic factors that influence generalizability across populations should be further assessed for future application.

SUMMARY

In conclusion, there is still much more work to be done in understanding HAND as a global condition. Since a majority of the HIV-infected population resides in RLS, further efforts should be focused on administering and adapting tests for areas such as sub-Saharan Africa and South Asia. To achieve these goals, numerous challenges will have to be addressed, including, but not limited to, overwhelming disease burden, limited neuropsychological expertise, infrastructural deficiencies, cultural differences, and the need for appropriate normative standards in target populations. Though some western tests may not be culturally relevant in RLS, researchers have applied these tests to ascertain HIV-associated cognitive deficits in international studies with relative sensitivity. For future studies, the cultural and socioeconomic factors that influence the relevance of western tests to non-western settings should be better characterized in order to enable cross-study comparisons.

REFERENCES

The Constitution of India: The Official Languages Act. (1963). Government of India Ministry of Law and Justice. Panel on Antiretroviral Guidelines for Adults and Adolescents. *Guidelines for the use of antiretroviral agents in HIV-1-infected adults and adolescents.* http://www.aidsinfo.nih.gov/ContentFiles/AdultandAdolescentGL.pdf.

Agranovich, A. V. & Puente, A. E. (2007). Do Russian and American normal adults perform similarly on neuropsychological tests? Preliminary findings on the relationship between culture and test performance. *Arch Clin Neuropsychol, 22*(3), 273–282.

Anger, W. K., Cassitto, M. G., Liang, Y. X., Amador, R., Hooisma, J., Chrislip, D. W., et al. (1993). Comparison of performance from three continents on the WHO-Recommended Neurobehavioral Core Test Battery. *Environ Res, 62*(1), 125–147.

Anger, W. K., Liang, Y. X., Nell, V., Kang, S. K., Cole, D., Bazylewicz-Walczak, B., et al. (2000). Lessons learned—15 years of the WHO-NCTB: A review. *Neurotoxicology, 21*(5), 837–846.

Antinori, A., Arendt, G., Becker, J. T., Brew, B. J., Byrd, D. A., Cherner, M., et al. (2007). Updated research nosology for HIV-associated neurocognitive disorders. *Neurology, 69*(18), 1789–1799.

Bangsberg, D. R., Tsai, A. C., Weiser, S., Emenyonu, N., Mwebesa, B., Bajunirwe, F., C., et al. (2010). Depression Symptom Severity is Associated with Missed Doses, Treatment Interruptions, and Viral Failure among HIV+ ART-Treated Individuals in Rural Uganda. Paper read at 17th Conference on Retroviruses and Opportunistic Infections, at San Francisco, CA.

Belec, L., Martin, P. M., Vohito, M. D., Gresenguet, G., Tabo, A., & Georges, A. J. (1989). Low prevalence of neuro-psychiatric clinical manifestations in central African patients with acquired immune deficiency syndrome. *Transactions of the Royal Society of Tropical Medicine and Hygiene, 83*(6), 844–846.

Boivin, M. J., Giordani, B., & Bornefeld, B. (1995). Use of the Tactual Performance Test for cognitive ability testing with African children. *Neuropsychology, 9*(3), 409–417.

Bornstein, R. A., Nasrallah, H. A., Para, M. F., Whitacre, C. C., Rosenberger, P., & Fass, R. J. (1993). Neuropsychological performance in symptomatic and asymptomatic HIV infection. *AIDS, 7*(4), 519–524.

Byrd, D. A., Touradji, P., Tang, M. X., & Manly, J. J. (2004). Cancellation test performance in African American, Hispanic, and White elderly. *J Int Neuropsychol Soc, 10*(3), 401–411.

Cherner, M., Cysique, L., Heaton, R. K., Marcotte, T. D., Ellis, R. J., Masliah, E., et al. (2007). Neuropathologic confirmation of definitional criteria for human immunodeficiency virus-associated neurocognitive disorders. *J Neurovirol, 13*(1), 23–28.

Cherner, M., Letendre, S., Heaton, R. K., Durelle, J., Marquie-Beck, J., Gragg, B., et al. (2005). Hepatitis C augments cognitive deficits associated with HIV infection and methamphetamine. *Neurology, 64*(8), 1343–1347.

Chung, J. H., Sakong, J., Kang, P. S., Kim, C. Y., Lee, K. S., Jeon, M. J., et al. (2003). Cross-cultural comparison of neurobehavioral performance in Asian workers. *Neurotoxicology, 24*(4–5):533–540.

Clifford, D. B., Mitike, M. T., Mekonnen, Y., Zhang, J., Zenebe, G., Melaku, Z., et al. (2007). Neurological evaluation of untreated human immunodeficiency virus infected adults in Ethiopia. *J Neurovirol, 13*(1), 67–72.

Cysique, L. A., Deutsch, R., Atkinson, J. H., Young, C., Marcotte, T. D., Dawson, L., et al. (2007). Incident major depression does not affect neuropsychological functioning in HIV-infected men. *J Int Neuropsychol Soc, 13*(1), 1–11.

Cysique, L. A., Jin, H., Franklin, Jr., D. R., Morgan, E. E., Shi, C., Yu, X., et al. (2007). Neurobehavioral effects of HIV-1 infection in China and the United States: A pilot study. *J Int Neuropsychol Soc, 13*(5), 781–790.

Cysique, L. A., Letendre, S. L., Ake, C., Jin, H., Franklin, D. R., Gupta, S., et al. (2010). Incidence and nature of cognitive decline over 1 year among HIV-infected former plasma donors in China. *AIDS, 24*(7), 983–990.

d'Arminio Monforte, A., Cinque, P., Mocroft, A., Goebel, F. D., Antunes, F., Katlama, C., et al. (2004). Changing incidence of central nervous system diseases in the EuroSIDA cohort. *Ann Neurol, 55*(3), 320–328.

de Klerk, G. (2008). Cross-cultural testing. In M. Born, C. D. Foxcroft, & R. Butter (Eds.). Online Readings in Testing and Assessment,

International Test Commission, http://www.intestcom.org/Publications/ORTA/cross+cultural+testing.php.

Dube, B., Benton, T., Cruess, D. G., & Evans, D. L. (2005). Neuropsychiatric manifestations of HIV infection and AIDS. *J. Psychiatry Neurosci*, 30(4), 237–246.

Ellis, R. (2009). Effects of CNS Antiretroviral Distribution on neurocognitive impairment in the AIDS Clinical Trials Group (ACTG) Longitudinal Linked Randomized Trials (ALLRT) Study. Paper read at 134th Annual Meeting of the American Neurological Association, at Baltimore, MD.

Ellis, R. J., Heaton, R. K., Letendre, S., Badiee, J., Munoz-Moreno, J. A., Vaida, F., et al. (2010). Higher CD4 Nadir is Associated with Reduced Rates of HIV-Associated Neurocognitive Disorders in the CHARTER Study: Potential Implications for Early Treatment Initiation. Paper read at 17th Conference on Retroviruses and Opportunistic Infections, at San Francisco, CA.

Emenyonu, N. I., Muyindike, W., Habyarimana, J., Pops-Eleches, C., Thirumurthy, H. Ragland, K., et al. (2010). Cash Transfers to Cover Clinic Transportation Costs Improve Adherence and Retention in Care in a HIV Treatment Program in Rural Uganda. Paper read at 17th Conference on Retroviruses and Opportunistic Infections, at San Francisco, CA.

Goggin, K. J., Zisook, S., Heaton, R. K., Atkinson, J. H., Marshall, S., McCutchan, J. A., et al. (1997). Neuropsychological performance of HIV-1 infected men with major depression. HNRC Group. HIV Neurobehavioral Research Center. *J Int Neuropsychol Soc*, 3(5): 457–464.

Gorman, A. A., Foley, J. M., Ettenhofer, M. L., Hinkin, C. H., & van Gorp, W. G. (2009). Functional consequences of HIV-associated neuropsychological impairment. *Neuropsychol, Rev 19*(2), 186–203.

Grant, I., Menon, A., Hestad, K., Imasiku, M., Shilalukey Ngoma, M., Kalima, K., et al. (2010). NeuroAIDS in Zambia: Pilot Project. Presented at NeuroAIDS in Africa, at Cape Town, South Africa.

Gupta, J. D., Satishchandra, P., Gopukumar, K., Wilkie, F., Waldrop-Valverde, D., Ellis, R., et al. (2007). Neuropsychological deficits in human immunodeficiency virus type 1 clade C-seropositive adults from South India. *J Neurovirol*, 13(3), 195–202.

Heaton, R., Franklin, D., Clifford, D., Woods, S., Rivera Mindt, M., Vigil, O., et al. (2009). HIV-associated Neurocognitive Impairment Remains Prevalent in the Era of Combination ART: The CHARTER Study. Paper read at 16th Conference on Retroviruses and Opportunistic Infections, at Montreal.

Heaton, R. K., Cysique, L. A., Jin, H., Shi, C., Yu, X., Letendre, S., et al. (2008). Neurobehavioral effects of human immunodeficiency virus infection among former plasma donors in rural China. *J Neurovirol*, 1–14.

Hedden, T., Park, D. C., Nisbett, R., Ji, L. J., Jing, Q., & Jiao, S. (2002). Cultural variation in verbal versus spatial neuropsychological function across the life span. *Neuropsychology*, 16(1), 65–73.

Holding, P. A., Taylor, H. G., Kazungu, S. D., Mkala, T., Gona, J., Mwamuye, B., et al. (2004). Assessing cognitive outcomes in a rural African population: Development of a neuropsychological battery in Kilifi District, Kenya. *J Int Neuropsychol Soc*, 10(2), 246–260.

Howlett, W. P., Nkya, W. M., Mmuni, K. A., & Missalek, W. R. (1989). Neurological disorders in aids and HIV disease in the northern zone of Tanzania. *AIDS*, 3(5), 289–296.

Hsieh, S. L. & Tori, C. D. (2007). Normative data on cross-cultural neuropsychological tests obtained from Mandarin-speaking adults across the life span. *Arch Clin Neuropsychol*, 22(3), 283–296.

Jahoda, G. (1979). On the nature of difficulties in spatial-perceptual tasks: Ethnic and sex differences. *Br J Psychol*, 70(3), 351–363.

Joska, J. A., Thomas, K. G., Stein, D. J., Seedat, S., Carey, P. D., Laidlaw, D., et al. (2010). Neuropsychological profile of patients commencing HAART in Cape Town, South Africa–Preliminary Findings. Presented at NeuroAIDS in Africa, at Cape Town, South Africa.

Kitahata, M. M., Gange, S. J., Abraham, A. G., Merriman, B., Saag, M. S., Justice, A. C., et al. (2009). Effect of early versus deferred antiretroviral therapy for HIV on survival. *N Engl J Med*, 360(18), 1815–1826.

Laeyendecker, O., Li, X., Arroyo, M., McCutchan, F., et al. (2006). The effect of HIV subtype on rapid disease progression in Rakai, Uganda.

13th Conference on Retroviruses and Opportunistic Infections. Denver, CO.

Llorente, A. M., Turcich, M., & Lawrence, K. A. (2004). Differences in neuropsychological performance associated with ethnicity in children with HIV-1 infection: Preliminary findings. *Appl Neuropsychol*, 11(1), 47–53.

Maj, M., Satz, P., Janssen, R., Zaudig, M., Starace, F., D'Elia, L., et al. (1994). WHO Neuropsychiatric AIDS study, cross-sectional phase II. Neuropsychological and neurological findings. *Arch Gen Psychiatry*, 51(1), 51–61.

Marra, C. M., Zhao, Y., Clifford, D. B., Letendre, S., Evans, S., Henry, K., et al. (2009). Impact of combination antiretroviral therapy on cerebrospinal fluid HIV RNA and neurocognitive performance. *AIDS*, 23(11), 1359–1366.

Mayes, J. T., Jahoda, G., & Neilson, I. (1988). Patterns of visual-spatial performance and "spatial ability": Dissociation of ethnic and sex differences. *Br J Psychol*, 79(Pt 1), 105–119.

Mitrushina, M., Boone, K., Razani, J., & Elia, L. D. (2005). Handbook of normative data for neuropsychological assessment. 2 ed. New York: Oxford University Press, USA.

Myer, L., Grimsrud, A., Cornell, M., Fairall, L., Przesky, H., van Cutsem, G., et al. (2010). Impact of antiretroviral therapy programme size on loss-to-follow-up: The leDEA-SA collaboration. Paper read at 17th Conference on retroviruses and opportunistic infections, at San Francisco, CA.

Nisbett, R. E. & Miyamoto, Y. (2005). The influence of culture: Holistic versus analytic perception. *Trends Cogn Sci*, 9(10), 467–473.

Parsons, T. D., Rogers, S., Hall, C., & Robertson, K. (2007). Motor based assessment of neurocognitive functioning in resource-limited international settings. *J Clin Exp Neuropsychol*, 29(1), 59–66.

Patel, K., Ming, X., Williams, P. L., Robertson, K. R., Oleske, J. M., & Seage, 3rd, G. R. (2009). Impact of HAART and CNS-penetrating antiretroviral regimens on HIV encephalopathy among perinatally infected children and adolescents. *AIDS*, 23(14), 1893–1901.

Paul, R. H., Gunstad, J., Cooper, N., Williams, L. M., Clark, C. R., Cohen, R. A., et al. (2007). Cross-cultural assessment of neuropsychological performance and electrical brain function measures: Additional validation of an international brain database. *Int J Neurosci*, 117(4), 549–568.

Pedraza, O. & Mungas, D. (2008). Measurement in cross-cultural neuropsychology. *Neuropsychol Rev*, 18(3), 184–193.

Portegies, P., Enting, R. H., de Gans, J., Algra, P. R., Derix, M. M., Lange, J. M., et al. (1993). Presentation and course of AIDS dementia complex: 10 years of follow-up in Amsterdam, The Netherlands. *AIDS*, 7(5), 669–675.

Razani, J., Burciaga, J., Madore, M., & Wong, J. (2007a). Effects of acculturation on tests of attention and information processing in an ethnically diverse group. *Arch Clin Neuropsychol*, 22(3), 333–341.

Razani, J., Murcia, G., Tabares, J., & Wong, J. (2007b). The effects of culture on WASI test performance in ethnically diverse individuals. *Clin Neuropsychol*, 21(5), 776–788.

Robertson, K., Liner, J., & Heaton, R. (2009). Neuropsychological assessment of HIV-infected populations in international settings. *Neuropsychol Rev*, 19(2), 232–249.

Robertson, K. R., Jiang, H., Tripathy, S., Santos, B., Silva, M. T., Montano, S., et al. (2009). Improved Neuropsychological Function during HAART in Diverse Resource-limited Settings: AIDS Clinical Trials Group Study A 5199, the International Neurological Study. Paper read at 16th Conference on Retroviruses and Opportunistic Infections, at Montreal.

Robertson, K. R., Liner, J., Hakim, J., Sankalé, J. L., Grant, I., Letendre, S., et al. (2010). NeuroAIDS in Africa. *Journal of Neurovirology*, 16(3), e–pub ahead of print.

Robertson, K. R., Nakasujja, N., Wong, M., Musisi, S., Katabira, E., Parsons, T. D., et al. (2007a). Pattern of neuropsychological performance among HIV-positive patients in Uganda. *BMC Neurol*, 7, 8.

Robertson, K. R., Smurzynski, M., Parsons, T. D., Wu, K., Bosch, R. J., Wu, J., et al. (2007b). The prevalence and incidence of neurocognitive impairment in the HAART era. *AIDS*, 21(14), 1915–1921.

Rosselli, M. & Ardila, A. (2003). The impact of culture and education on non-verbal neuropsychological measurements: A critical review. *Brain Cogn 52*(3), 326–333.

Rourke, S. B., Halman, M. H., & Bassel, C. (1999). Neurocognitive complaints in HIV-infection and their relationship to depressive symptoms and neuropsychological functioning. *J Clin Exp Neuropsychol, 21*(6), 737–756.

Sacktor, N. C., Wong, M., Nakasujja, N., Skolasky, R. L., Selnes, O. A., Musisi, S., et al. (2005). The International HIV Dementia Scale: A new rapid screening test for HIV dementia. *AIDS, 19*(13), 1367–1374.

Sacktor, N., Nakasujja, N., Skolasky, R. L., Rezapour, M., Robertson, K., Musisi, S., et al. (2009). HIV subtype D is associated with dementia, compared with subtype A, in immunosuppressed individuals at risk of cognitive impairment in Kampala, Uganda. *Clin Infect Dis, 49*(5), 780–786.

Sacktor, N., Nakasujja, N., Skolasky, R. L., Robertson, K., Musisi, S., Ronald, A., et al. (2009). Benefits and risks of stavudine therapy for HIV-associated neurologic complications in Uganda. *Neurology, 72*(2), 165–170.

Sadek, J. R., Vigil, O., Grant, I., & Heaton, R. K. (2007). The impact of neuropsychological functioning and depressed mood on functional complaints in HIV-1 infection and methamphetamine dependence. *J Clin Exp Neuropsychol, 29*(3), 266–276.

Spreen, O. & Strauss, E. (1991). A compendium of neuropsychological tests: Administration, norms, and commentary. 2 ed. New York: Oxford University Press.

Sterne, J. A., May, M., Costagliola, D., de Wolf, F., Phillips, A. N., Harris, R., et al. (2009). Timing of initiation of antiretroviral therapy in AIDS-free HIV-1-infected patients: a collaborative analysis of 18 HIV cohort studies. *Lancet, 373*(9672), 1352–1363.

Tozzi, V., Balestra, P., Salvatori, M. F., Vlassi, C., Liuzzi, G., Giancola, M. L., et al. (2009). Changes in cognition during antiretroviral therapy: Comparison of 2 different ranking systems to measure antiretroviral drug efficacy on HIV-associated neurocognitive disorders. *J Acquir Immune Defic Syndr, 52*(1), 56–63.

Tozzi, V., Balestra, P., Serraino, D., Bellagamba, R., Corpolongo, A., Piselli, P., et al. (2005). Neurocognitive impairment and survival in a cohort of HIV-infected patients treated with HAART. *AIDS Res Hum Retroviruses, 21*(8), 706–713.

Tsai, A. C., Bangsberg, D. R., Senkungu, J., Frongillo, E., Emenyonu, N., Kawuma, A., et al. (2010). Food Insecurity, Competing Demands, and Health Care Utilization among HIV+ Adults in Uganda. Paper read at 17th Conference on Retroviruses and Opportunistic Infections, at San Francisco, CA.

Valcour, V. G., Shiramizu, B. T., Sithinamsuwan, P., Nidhinandana, S., Ratto-Kim, S., Ananworanich, J., et al. (2009). HIV DNA and cognition in a Thai longitudinal HAART initiation cohort: The SEARCH 001 Cohort Study. *Neurology, 72*(11), 992–998.

WHO/UNAIDS. (2008). 2008 Report on the global AIDS epidemic.

Wilkie, F. L., Goodkin, K., Ardila, A., Concha, M., Lee, D., Lecusay, R., et al. (2004). HUMANS: An English and Spanish neuropsychological test battery for assessing HIV-1-infected individuals—initial report. *Appl Neuropsychol, 11*(3), 121–33.

Wright, E., Brew, B., Arayawichanont, A., Robertson, K., Samintharapanya, K., Kongsaengdao, S., et al. (2008). Neurologic disorders are prevalent in HIV-positive outpatients in the Asia-Pacific region. *Neurology, 71*(1), 50–56.

Yepthomi, T., Paul, R., Vallabhaneni, S., Kumarasamy, N., Tate, D. F., Solomon, S., et al. (2006). Neurocognitive consequences of HIV in southern India: A preliminary study of clade C virus. *J Int Neuropsychol Soc, 12*(3), 424–430.

12.7

THE IMPACT OF HIV SUBTYPE AND CULTURAL AND SOCIODEMOGRAPHIC FACTORS ON HIV-1 INFECTION AND ASSOCIATED NEUROPATHOGENESIS IN AFRICA

Adelina Holguin, Damien C. Tully, and Charles Wood

Although home to just over 10% of the world's population, sub-Saharan Africa recently accounted for 71% of the world's HIV infections. At roughly the same time, it was estimated that 22.4 million Africans were living with HIV, 1.9 million became newly infected with HIV, and an estimated 1.4 million AIDS-related deaths occurred in sub-Saharan Africa. This chapter discusses HIV-1 infection in Africa, with particular emphasis on three topics: diversity of viral subtype, African culture, and sociodemographic influences. These topics are explored both as they affect and are affected by the HIV-1 epidemic. Understanding these complex relationships is important for a variety of reasons, including policy, clinical care, and the construction of appropriate research protocols.

INTRODUCTION

HIV-1 has now emerged as one of the greatest modern pandemics with an estimated 33.4 million people currently infected worldwide (WHO, 2009). The greatest impediment to producing an HIV-1 vaccine and for the development of effective anti-viral drugs is the high rate of HIV's evolution (Rambaut, Posada, Crandall, & Holmes, 2004). This ability of HIV-1 to change leads directly to high levels of sequence diversity both within and between infected individuals and in the pandemic (Archer & Robertson, 2007). Sub-Saharan Africa, with its dissimilar topography and diverse culture, is also a region where surmountable efforts are concentrated to control the HIV/AIDS epidemic. The efforts to subside the HIV-1 epidemic in sub-Sahara are hindered due to the wide diversity of HIV strains across the African continent. Consequently, health concerns are a top priority at a global level and these concerns span from HIV transmission, to disease progression and pathogenesis. All of these facets of HIV-1 affect the development of HIV-associated neuropathogenesis, which then lead to the development of neurocognitive disorders. A cycle manifests from disease progression on an individual's culture, socioeconomic status, and health status and that in turn results in fueling HIV-1 transmission, disease progression, pathogenesis, and neuropathogenesis. HIV-1 subtype diversity, culture, and sociodemographic factors are three important themes to explore, as they are critical factors that may influence clinical research on HIV-1 transmission, disease progression, pathogenesis, and neuropathogenesis.

HIV/AIDS IN AFRICA

Although home to only just over 10% of the world's population, sub-Saharan Africa accounts for 71% of the world's HIV infections (WHO, 2009). In 2008, it was estimated that 22.4 million Africans were living with HIV, 1.9 million became newly infected with HIV, and an estimated 1.4 million AIDS-related deaths occurred in sub-Saharan Africa (WHO, 2009). A substantial amount of evidence now suggests that HIV may have originated from the African continent in the early 1900s through zoonotic heuristics from nonhuman primates to human, and throughout the period the virus has evolved and spread to other regions of the world. The second feature of the African HIV epidemic is the subtypes or clades of HIV found distributed across African countries. Both HIV-1 and HIV-2 can be found in Africa, with HIV-2 found mostly in West African countries such as Cameroon. Even among HIV-1, a mixture of different subtypes is found in different regions of the continent. It is possible that this is due to the early introduction and subsequent diversity of HIV-1 in the continent. Nevertheless, it is possible that there are biological differences among these different subgroups that may affect disease progression, transmission, pathogenesis, and neuropathogenesis in the infected individual. Therefore, it is important to first have a better understanding of the HIV-1 subtypes in Africa.

The position that Africa plays in the worldwide HIV/AIDS epidemic is critical as the 19 countries worldwide with the highest prevalence of reported infections are all African countries (WHO, 2009). The HIV-1 prevalence rates of the most adversely affected African countries range from the highest infection rate of 26% of adults in Swaziland to the lowest rate of infection in Northern Africa where HIV-1 prevalence is under 1% of the adult population (WHO, 2009).

The primary mode of HIV-1 transmission in Africa is through heterosexual contact, thus explaining the large numbers of women as well as men infected. In recent years, information on men who have sex with men has become available in sub-Saharan Africa (Smith, Tapsoba, Peshu, Sanders, & Jaffe, 2009). Same-sex HIV-1 transmission is gaining attention as a component of many national epidemics though the subject is considered taboo in Africa where strict laws are instituted prohibiting same-sex activity (Ottosson, 2009). Another mode of transmission less extensively studied than others is injecting drug users in sub-Saharan Africa. While some studies have found that injecting drug use is increasing in some countries, such as Kenya where it accounted for an estimated 3.8% of new infections in 2006 (Gelmon, Kenya, Oguya, Cheluget, & Girmay, 2009), it still remains rarer than in other regions of the world. A final mode of transmission that accounts for a substantial although decreasing portion of HIV-1 infections in many African countries is mother-to-child transmission. All of these modes of transmission can be influenced by HIV-1 strain and virulence of strain.

THE IMPACT AND EXTENT OF HIV-1 DIVERSITY

Genetic heterogeneity is key to HIV-1 diversity that has manifested into the classification of four distantly related groups: Main group (M), Outlier group (O) (Charneau et al., 1994; Gurtler et al., 1994), non-M or -O group (N) (Simon et al., 1998), and the most recently discovered, designated alphabetically, P group (Plantier et al., 2009). These viruses have been transmitted to humans on at least four occasions as the group phylogenetic branches are interspersed with those of various simian immunodeficiency virus (SIV) strains indicating that HIV-1 subtypes arose from independent crossover events (Gao et al., 1999; Rambaut, Robertson, Pybus, Peeters, & Holmes, 2001). The distribution and prevalence of the four HIV-1 groups are distinct: group N strains are very rare epidemiologically with cases only isolated from individuals in Cameroon (Ayouba et al., 2000; Bodelle et al., 2004), group O strains while more widespread are restricted to western central Africa (Gurtler et al., 1994; Peeters et al., 1997), and group P is a new HIV-1 group described from a single Cameroonian patient residing in France (Plantier et al., 2009). The M group has a global distribution and dominates the AIDS pandemic accounting for more than 90% of reported HIV-1 infections. The diversity within this group has led to a further subdivision into different lineages or clades termed subtypes and are composed of a total of nine subtypes A–D, F–H, J, and K (Robertson et al., 2000). Different HIV-1 subtypes display as much as 20–30% variation in their *env* sequences while other genes such as *gag* and *pol* display less diversity since they encode the viral structural proteins and the three crucial enzymes (protease, reverse transcriptase, and integrase) (Hemelaar, Gouws, Ghys, & Osmanov, 2006). Remarkably, even within subtypes there is significant amount of diversity with subtypes A and F further subdivided into another level termed subtypes A1–A5 (Gao et al., 2001; Meloni et al., 2004; Vidal et al., 2006; Vidal et al., 2009) and F1–F2 (Triques et al., 1999; Triques et al., 2000), respectively. Former subtypes "E" and "I" have now

been reclassified as circulating recombinant forms (CRFs) (Carr et al., 1996; Gao et al., 1998; Paraskevis, Magiorkinis, Vandamme, Kostrikis, & Hatzakis, 2001) and are designated as CRF01_AE and CRF04_cpx of which over 40 CRFs have been designated (LANL HIV Sequence Database, http://hiv-web.lanl.gov). These CRFs are generated by recombination between distinct subtypes and/or other CRFs and are spreading at epidemic rates in various parts of the world. But by far, the most important recombinants in the pandemic are the first two: CRF01_AE and CRF02_AG.

DISTRIBUTION OF HIV-1 SUBTYPES IN AFRICA

The severity and nature of the HIV-1 epidemic differs by subregion and by country with distinct geographic subtype patterns seen within Africa (see Figure 12.7.1). The greatest diversity and highest prevalence of HIV-1 is in sub-Saharan Africa. The oldest epidemic of HIV-1 in the world is in West Central Africa where diversity is at its highest with all known subtypes, many CRFs, and a variety of unique strains that circulate in this region (Vidal, Bazepeo, Mulanga, Delaporte, & Peeters, 2000; Yang et al., 2005). Despite this abundance of genetic diversity, one form, CRF02_AG, predominates (Howard, Olaylele, & Rasheed, 1994). CRF02_AG is a recombinant derived from subtype A and G and is the major strain in West and West Central Africa and has caused at least 9 million infections worldwide (McCutchan, 2000). One explanation for the high prevalence of this strain in Africa may be in part due to its long presence in the epidemic, with some

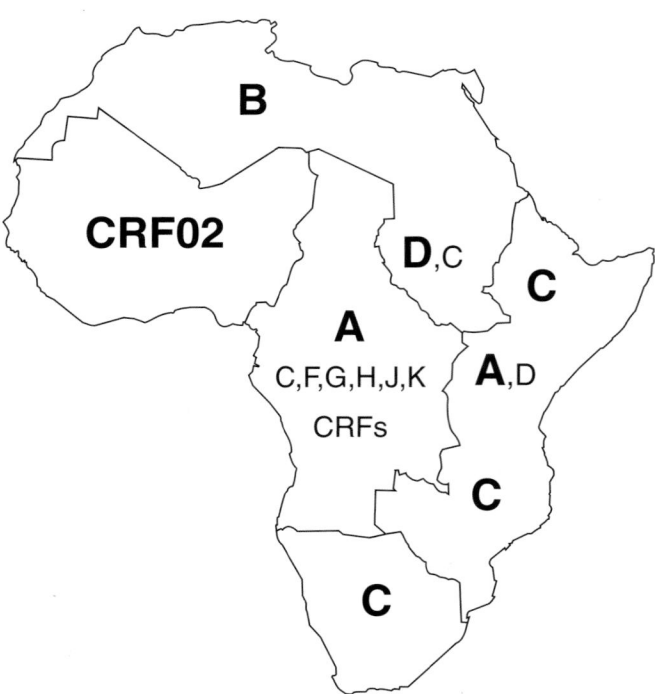

Figure 12.7.1 Prevalence of HIV-1 subtypes circulating among the main regions (East, West, North, South, and Central) in Africa. The primary subtype circulating within a region is designated in a larger font size and marked in bold.

suggesting that CRF02 may be as old as the pure subtypes (Carr et al., 1998). Recent evidence from Cameroon suggests that this strain is becoming more genetically homogenous in both the South and West regions (Powell, Barengolts, Mayr, & Nyambi, 2010). If this is indeed true, it is particularly encouraging with respect to vaccine design and development. However, considering that nearly every known HIV-1 type, group, subtype, and recombinant form can still be identified in the infected population, it remains a public health issue. A clear example of this dynamic diversity is the identification of a recent HIV-1 lineage, designated group P (Plantier et al., 2009). This new viral strain was reported in a Cameroonian woman living in France where its viral sequence forms a phylogenetic cluster with SIV sequences from western gorillas (SIVgor), suggesting that this HIV-1 group originated from gorillas (Plantier et al., 2009). Another case from an infected male in Yaoundé, Cameroon has confirmed the circulation of this strain in Cameroon, although the actual prevalence of this group remains to be determined (Vallari et al., 2010). Although Cameroon and the Democratic Republic of Congo (DRC) have likely seeded the entire HIV-1 pandemic, recombinant form CRF02_AG does not represent the majority of strains in the DRC, where HIV-1 diversity is unprecedented and exceeds that of all other nations combined (Kita et al., 2004; Niama et al., 2006; Vidal et al., 2000; Yang et al., 2005). Subtype distribution in the DRC mirrors quite well to the distribution of subtypes in West, South, and East Africa. Kinshasa, the capital and largest city of the DRC is a "diversity hotspot" where a mixture of subtypes and recombinants predominate, similar to the diversity observed in Western African nations (Yang et al., 2005). In contrast, in the southeastern city of Lubumbashi, subtype C predominates, while in Likasi, intersubtype recombinants are found at a higher rate than reported in other regions of the country (Kita et al., 2004). Meanwhile, in the eastern part of the country subtype A prevails in Kisangani and in East African countries. In the Central African Republic a very high and increasing diversity of strains circulate with a number of complex recombinant forms outweighing other subtypes (Marechal et al., 2006; Matsika-Claquin et al., 2004; Punzi et al., 2005).

West Africa shares a similar epidemiological pattern as that of Central Africa with regard to CRF02_AG (Agwale et al., 2002; Fischetti et al., 2004; Nkengasong et al., 2000; Peeters et al., 2000) with prevalence rates as high as 59% in Ghana and neighboring countries (Fischetti et al., 2004). Other subtypes including A, C, D, G, J, and K also circulate in West Africa. One complex recombinant form designated as CRF06_cpx comprised of subtypes A, G, K, and J has emerged in this region and is spreading within Nigeria, Mali, Ivory Coast, Niger, and Burkina Faso (Montavon et al., 2002).

In East Africa, subtypes A and D dominate the epidemic although they differ in frequency between regions. Subtype A is the primary form in Kenya (Khamadi et al., 2005; Khamadi et al., 2009; Khoja et al., 2008; Lihana et al., 2009; Steain et al., 2005), while subtype D accounts for the majority of the circulating viruses in Uganda (Collinson-Streng et al., 2009; Harris et al., 2002; Herbeck et al., 2007; Hu et al., 2000). The epidemic in Kenya is heterogeneous in nature with a continual

spread of subtype A in Nairobi followed by subtypes D, C, and G (Khoja et al., 2008). A worrying trend for Kenya is the emergence of recombinant, most of which harbor subtype A genomic fragments (Lihana et al., 2009). The presence of recombinant viruses in this population suggests that subtype A is slowly evolving with time and diverging into new strains. For instance, CRF10 was first identified in western Kenya (Songok et al., 2003). In the Rakai district of Uganda, where AIDS was first identified in East Africa (Serwadda et al., 1985), subtype distribution varied by geographic region with significantly more subtype D variants in the southern-most communities and significantly more subtype A infections in northern community clusters (Collinson-Streng et al., 2009). This is in agreement with phylodynamic analyses of the Ugandan viruses where it was shown that type A variants were introduced earlier than subtype D variants (Gray et al., 2009). Another report confirmed that in Uganda subtypes A and D are transmitted without geographic constraints and are not associated with significantly different transmission rates (Herbeck et al., 2007).

Tanzania is among the sub-Saharan Africa countries most affected by the HIV-1 pandemic (WHO, 2009). Molecular epidemiological studies conducted in the Kagera and Kilimanjaro regions identified that subtypes A and C predominate, followed by subtype D (Nyombi, Kristiansen, Bjune, Muller, & Holm-Hansen, 2008a; Nyombi et al., 2008b). Such studies indicate that subtypes A and D were the first to circulate in equal proportions during the initial phase of the epidemic in Tanzania. Since 2000/01, the prevalence of subtype C has increased while subtype A has remained relatively stable and the rate of subtype D infections has declined (Nyombi et al., 2008a). However, CRF10 has emerged (Koulinska et al., 2001). The differences in diversity between regions in northern Tanzania, specifically in Kagera and Kilimanjaro, may be the result of the influence of neighboring epidemics in Uganda and Kenya.

The epidemic in the eastern tip of Africa, north of Kenya and in Djibouti, is dominated by subtype C (Maslin et al., 2005). Similarly, subtype C accounts for almost all infections in Ethiopia where two genetically distinct groups have been reported, with only very sporadic cases of infections with types A and D (Abebe et al., 1997; Abebe et al., 2001; Hussein et al., 2000).

In Southern Africa the epidemic is dominated by subtype C that encompasses the region from Tanzania to South Africa. Countries with dominant HIV-1 subtype C are Zambia, Botswana, Mozambique, Malawi, and South Africa (Candotti et al., 2001; Lahuerta et al., 2008; McCormack et al., 2002; Parreira et al., 2006; zur Megede et al., 2002). Angola, unlike other regional countries, is mainly a region where subtypes D and G prevail (De Baar et al., 2000), similar to its neighboring countries to the north.

Northern Africa remains one of the only regions where HIV-1 infection rates are still very low. However, the limited literature available suggests that subtype B may be the predominant circulating subtype. In Algeria, a single molecular epidemiology study revealed a high diversity of strains with subtype B dominating, particularly in the northern part of the country, but a number of inter-CRF recombinants was found, particularly in the southern part of Algeria that borders sub-Saharan Africa (Bouzeghoub et al., 2006; Bouzeghoub et al., 2008). In Egypt, a prevalence of subtype B infections was found consequently from an HIV-1 infection outbreak among renal dialysis patients (El Sayed et al., 2000). Studies from Morocco and Tunisia have indicated that subtype B is present (Ben Halima et al., 2001; Elharti et al., 1997). Molecular characterization of sequences from nosocomial transmission in Libya found that all the patients were infected with the monophyletic recombinant form CRF02_AG (Ben Halima et al., 2001; Yerly et al., 2001). In Sudan, which borders nine other African countries, there is an intermixing of subtypes with a predominance of subtypes C and D with other strains such as subtypes A and B (Hierholzer et al., 2002). It is clear from the literature that HIV-1 subtype distribution is complex and dynamic in the continent of Africa. Given the breadth of genetic diversity among the HIV-1 subtypes, one might expect significant biological differences between the clades. However, it is understandable that after a quarter of a century since the discovery of HIV-1, the development of a vaccine remains unattainable and research progress has been slow and challenging, especially in the area of HIV-1 disease progression, transmission, pathogenesis, and neuropathogenesis in the continent of Africa.

TRANSMISSION, PATHOGENESIS, AND DISEASE PROGRESSION

The impact of HIV-1 transmission, virulence, and disease progression between subtypes is highly influenced by geographical, socioeconomic, and epidemiological factors. In addition, the interplay of interactions between the human host and HIV-1 may influence transmission and disease progression. These known differences include HLA class I types which may vary according to the infecting subtype (Nguyen et al., 2004). Other factors such as high-risk behaviors that increase the probability of re-infection or super infection (van der Kuyl & Cornelissen, 2007), or even non-immune host factors such as male circumcision, may all act as co-factors that will influence the transmission of HIV (Hu, Buve, Baggs, van der Groen, & Dondero, 1999). It has been suggested that the chemokine co-receptor differs between subtypes, with viruses utilizing the CCR5 (R5) co-receptor more frequently transmitted than strains using the CXCR4 (X4 viruses) phenotype. In terms of pathogenicity, X4 viruses are associated with more rapid progression to AIDS for individuals infected with subtype B. The frequency of X4 viruses is lower in subtype C than in subtype B but may be on the rise (Cilliers et al., 2003). Although all subtypes can use both co-receptors, subtype D may be dual-tropic (R5X4 virus) in most cases (Huang et al., 2007). Disease progression may be influenced by the host immune response to HIV-1 infection, such as altered CXCR4 function that decreases the viral ligand-receptor interactions (Munerato et al., 2003).

There are suggestions that subtypes may affect transmission efficiency, but a consistent subtype-associated difference in transmissibility remains to be demonstrated. A study in Tanzania found that subtypes A, C, and recombinant viruses are more likely to be perinatally transmitted than subtype D (Renjifo et al., 2001) and a subsequent report suggested that subtype C seems to be more frequently transmitted in utero than subtype B (Renjifo et al., 2004). In Kenya, it was reported that a high propensity of vertical transmission in utero was in those mostly infected with subtype D than those infected with subtype A (Yang et al., 2003). Another Kenyan study demonstrated that women infected with subtype C were more likely to shed infected vaginal cells than those infected with subtypes A or D (John-Stewart et al., 2005). These disparate findings from different countries show that subtype fitness can be influenced by mode of transmission and subtype, notwithstanding the effects on disease progression.

Although there have been several prospective studies performed on subtype-specific differences in disease progression, the results were controversial. For example, no differences in disease progression were found between patients infected with subtypes B and C in Israel (Weisman et al., 1999) or among a large Swedish study of patients infected with subtypes A, B, C, and D (Weisman et al., 1999). Similarly, a multicenter study of 335 patients from Senegal and Cameroon did not show any significant differences in survival or clinical disease progression for people infected with CRF02_AG strains and those infected with other CRFs or subtypes (Laurent et al., 2002). However, a number of studies have found subtype-specific disease progression patterns. In Uganda, a cohort of 1,045 patients provided compelling evidence that infection with subtype A progresses more slowly than subtype D or recombinants (Kaleebu et al., 2002). This was more recently confirmed in another study from the Rakai district, where it was found that faster disease progression led to death in those infected with subtype D and recombinants compared to those primarily infected with subtype A (Kiwanuka et al., 2008). Furthermore, an earlier study reported that female sex workers in Senegal infected with non-A subtypes were eight times more likely to develop AIDS compared to those infected with subtype A (Kanki et al., 1999). Taken together, a consensus can be reached that some viral strains are more virulent and this virulence can affect the progression of the disease. However, the intricacies of the virus-host interactions provoking the underlying pathogenesis are still to be teased apart, though it's challenging due to this high subtype variability and virulence. Even more so challenging is to understand viral strain and fitness in HIV-1 associated neuropathogenesis.

IMPACT OF HIV-1 VARIANTS ON NEUROPATHOGENESIS

What is known about the effects of HIV-1 on neurocognitive decline in both children and adults is mostly attributed to research done in the developed/industrialized countries (Belman et al., 1988; Copper & Hanson, 1988; Epstein, Sharer, & Gajdusek, 1986; Heaton & Miller, 2004; Lobato, 1995; McArthur et al., 1993; McArthur, Brew, & Nath, 2005; Navia, Jordan, & Price, 1986; Smith et al., 2006). Although considerable progress has been made in developing countries, understanding the effects of HIV-1 on cognitive impairment in these regions continues to be a major focus of research efforts, particularly with the hope of identifying similar or disparate patterns of neurocognitive decline, depending on the clade of the virus in a specific region and its unique neuropathogenesis. Although Africa is an ideal setting to examine issues related to subtype and the risk of HIV-1 dementia, the existing literature is small and not cohesively interpreted across African countries. The first evidence that HIV-1 subtypes may differ in terms of neurocognitive pathogenesis was reported by Sacktor et al. (2009). The investigators examined the severity of HIV-1-associated cognitive impairment among individuals initiating antiretroviral therapy in a single clinic in Uganda (Sacktor et al., 2009). These results suggest that HIV-1 dementia may be more common among adults infected with subtype D than in those infected with subtype A, and suggested that subtype D effects on neuropsychological performance was similar to that of subtype B (Sacktor et al., 2009). More recently, a study investigated the neuropsychological impact of subtypes A and D on HIV-1-infected antiretroviral-therapy-naïve Ugandan children (Boivin et al., 2010). In contrast to the findings of Sacktor et al. (2009), the cross-sectional study demonstrated that children infected with subtype A had poorer neurocognitive performance than those with subtype D. This stark difference in subtype association may be due to a number of factors. One such difference between the two studies is that Sacktor et al. (2009) included adults at a more advanced disease stage who qualified for antiretroviral therapy (ART) while the latter study enrolled children who were at an earlier stage of disease and had lesser degrees of clinically defined manifestations. Unlike adults, the neuropathology manifested in children is classified primarily as an HIV-1 encephalopathy. The manifestation of HIV-1 encephalopathy can occur at different developmental stages with varying degrees of severity (Epstein et al., 1986; Mintz, 1996). The neurological impairment due to HIV-1 encephalopathy at an early age can continue throughout the development of a child. Therefore, children's neuropsychological functioning is primarily manifested by failure to achieve developmental milestones, plateaus in the traditional developmental trajectory, and/or regression of those abilities that have already been acquired (Belman et al., 1988). Areas of neurodevelopment that show particular vulnerability to the effects of HIV-1 when the disease has progressed to AIDS are those of executive function, attention, memory, language, and motor abilities (Smith et al., 2006). Executive function appears to be affected by HIV-1 early on in the progression of disease (Bisiacchi, Suppiej, & Laverda, 2000). These studies are valuable in diagnosing children infected with HIV-1, though the usefulness of this information may not necessarily be applicable in developing countries due to cultural, socioeconomic, and geographic regional differences.

Although epidemiological trends show subtype C is rapidly increasing and most prevalent in Africa, very little is known about the cognitive deficits in HIV-1 subtype C infection. The pattern of neuropsychological performance in a sample of untreated HIV-1 positive patients from Ethiopia, predominant HIV-1 subtype C region, revealed that motor speed was significantly slower in HIV-infected individuals compared to match controls; however, since no significant differences were found in all other tasks, there was no clear evidence for HIV-associated neurocognitive impairment (Clifford et al., 2007). A study from South Africa, a middle-resource country, found that HIV-associated neurocognitive disorders were present in 23.5% of a sample of 536 HIV-1-infected individuals (Joska, Fincham, Stein, Paul, & Seedat, 2009). Furthermore, the neurocognitive impairment was associated with post-traumatic stress and alcohol abuse. Although all three studies took place in regions were subtype C is predominant, the findings were not consistent. Due to the geographical distribution of these three countries, other factors such as sociodemographic parameters need to be considered. The challenge to compare neurocognitive impairment across the African continent becomes more difficult when not only geography and economic status is factored in, but also HIV subtype.

Neuropsychological studies normally include a series of sociodemographic factors that include, but are not limited to, gender, marital status, and occupation. However, the number and type of sociodemographic parameters can vary from study to study. Culture and sociodemographics are explored more in depth in the following sections with the objective to provide some background and awareness of how these factors may be inadvertently influenced by HIV-1 transmission and disease progression and/or vice versa. This is important to be considered in research design as these factors may affect interpretation of findings in studies related to neuropathogenesis.

IMPACT ON HIV-1 INFECTION, DISEASE PROGRESSION AND NEUROPATHOGENESIS AT THE CULTURAL LEVEL

FAMILY STRUCTURE

One of the prominent cultural alterations caused by HIV-1 has been the African family structure. One major disruption in the family structure in the African setting was the care of children of deceased parents. It was customary for children of deceased parents to be taken care of by a close family member (sisters, grandmothers, etc.) (Majumdar & Mazaleni, 2010). This family structure has mostly been disrupted with the increasing death toll attributed to the HIV-1 epidemic, and now it has become more cumbersome for families to care for those children (Appleton, 2000). According to UNICEF, it is estimated that 14 million children have been left orphaned due to the HIV-1 epidemic (Smith, 2002). Currently, in Africa, there are a multitude of orphanages with many of those children testing positive for HIV-1 and it is estimated that over 2 million children will become orphaned by the end of 2010 (Cluver, Gardner, & Operario, 2007). The increase in orphanages puts a greater strain on the economic burden of many African countries, leaving the orphan organizations to heavily rely on donations to stay afloat. Consequently, the education of these children suffer, making it difficult to cover school fees, purchase necessary school supplies, and meet basic needs (Murray, 2010). Although it is known that the well-being of a child is negatively affected by the loss of parents and that affects the performance of a child in school, the neuropsychological impact of these children is not known. This is mainly a consequence of unavailable resources and trained professionals in the clinical practice. Another constraint is the difficulty to include children from orphanages in neuropsychological studies due to the lack of a legal guardian that can consent to a minor's participation. Therefore, a growing number of children with a high probability of testing positive for HIV-1 are not accounted for, leaving them out of the reach of research, hence, not adequately represented in the outcome of findings.

GENDER

The prevalence of HIV-1 infections in Africa is higher in women (WHO, 2009). In many African countries, women' rights continue to be suppressed, with mostly patriarchal systems in place. Women may be shunted from their home or left by their husband once their HIV-1 status is known (Smith, 2002). In Uganda, for example, HIV-1-infected women have been known to be restricted to move around on their bicycles. Restriction of movement poses a tremendous health risk as well as risk to the livelihood of an individual if attempting to seek out monetary means or reach medical sites, and even to participation in research projects. In some regions, women are expected to share their roles as wives with other relatives of the husband. These practices expose these women to higher probabilities of HIV-1 transmission. In this respect, HIV-1 has further negatively impacted progress in women rights in the African setting. Violence towards women is an existing domestic issue in Africa that has now been exacerbated by the HIV-1 epidemic. Violence can pertain to rape, battery, homicide, incest, psychological abuse, forced prostitution, trafficking of women, and sexual harassment. Any of these characteristics of violence are risks of HIV-1 transmission. The laws regarding ownership of land in Africa have also been impacted by the HIV-1 epidemic. For example, in bordering regions shared by Malawi, Zambia, and Tanzania, it was found that if a husband dies, the brother of the husband has the authority to dictate if the wife of the deceased is to remain on the premise and assume ownership of the land. With the HIV-1 epidemic, many families have been left stranded following what has been coined "land grabbing" by relatives of the deceased (Mbaya, 2002; Seeley, 2004 #2). Few studies have investigated the effects of HIV-1 between genders, with conflicting reports, whereby some conclude no gender differences (Bouwman et al., 1998; Chiesi et al., 1996; Everall et al., 2009; Robertson et al., 2004), others suggest that there is a higher risk for females in acquiring AIDS dementia complex (Chiesi et al., 1996), or that women manifest neurologic symptoms earlier than men (Marder et al., 1995). If HIV-1 can affect female and males differentially then this becomes a critical issue for the development of therapeutics. Future investigations should closely examine the effects of ARV treatment between genders.

FAITH AND COMMON BELIEFS

Beliefs have shown to be a critical factor surrounding the epidemic of HIV-1. For instance, in Ethiopia some individuals continue to believe that HIV is a punishment as a consequence of immoral behavior (Heike, 2007). A study performed in Ghana that explored relationships between religion, HIV/AIDS, and sexual practices of men, found that among the three major religions present, Christian, Muslim, and traditional, those affiliated with Christianity and Islam reported higher rates of circumcised men compared to those affiliated with traditional beliefs, with percentage rates of 95.61%, 97.86%, and 73.36%, respectively (Gyimah, Tenkorang, Takyi, Adjei, & Fosu, 2010). Religion has a strong influence on decisions that pertain to medical practices such as circumcision. Due to the high rate of HIV-1 transmission and recent reports that uncircumcised men can have a higher risk of infection (Bailey et al., 2007; Gray et al., 2007), circumcision has become a top priority in health care. It is unlikely that a person will accept this type of scientific claim if it goes against his/her accepted beliefs. It is worth noting that findings by Gyimah et al. (2010) have shown that religion did not dictate sexual behaviors alone, but its role could be influenced by other sociodemographic factors, especially by education. This is consistent with other reports that have found that Christians tend to have more education than other religious affiliations in Africa (Garner, 2000) and tend to have a higher probability of risky sexual behaviors than those of other belief systems (Gyimah et al., 2010). These beliefs and occurrence of risky behaviors have had an impact on HIV-1 transmission in the region.

Research efforts focused on AIDS awareness have had some successes with collaborations with religious institutions. These successes are primarily attributed to female participation. The downside of involving religious institutions in AIDS awareness is a gender disparity that leaves HIV-1-infected men without proper information and education. Furthermore, it is not uncommon for sermons to include issues related to sexual behavior that can impact social norms within a specific culture. However, in the face of an epidemic as that of HIV-1, discouraging condom use, objecting to sex education, and/or supporting ideas that viral transmission is a form of punishment counteracts all of the efforts invested in HIV awareness and, most importantly, in HIV prevention (Gyimah et al., 2010). Beliefs vary in both prevalence and denomination across Africa. For example, in Cameroon, there are just as many different religions and ethnic groups as there are HIV-1 subtypes. In contrast, several tribal groups exist in Zambia with two dominating tribes and greater than 90% of the population is Christian, yet only HIV-1 C subtype predominates. Therefore, study design should reflect these proportions in their sample population to generate a better comprehensive profile of the effects of HIV-1 in the African setting.

Practices such as witchcraft can also influence how effective HIV-1 studies may be conducted in the African setting when medical examinations are pertinent for clinical evaluations, especially in neuropsychological assessment. In many cases, when witchcraft is highly intermeshed with the culture, it is difficult to perform necessary medical procedures such as collecting blood specimens (Heike, 2007). Such is the case when blood specimens are necessary, especially during clinical trials related to HIV, where it is necessary to obtain serological measures (full blood counts), immunological levels (CD4 counts), or viral loads. HIV continues to be highly stigmatized in Africa and that prevents people from freely expressing their medical needs and seeking medical attention. With the HIV-1 epidemic, these beliefs have become more rigid, with people highly reluctant to provide a blood sample when requested to assess HIV serostatus. Furthermore, the idea that the person's health condition is caused by factors other than through viral infection can influence an infected individual's decision to seek medical attention and/or adhere to treatment or participation in research studies.

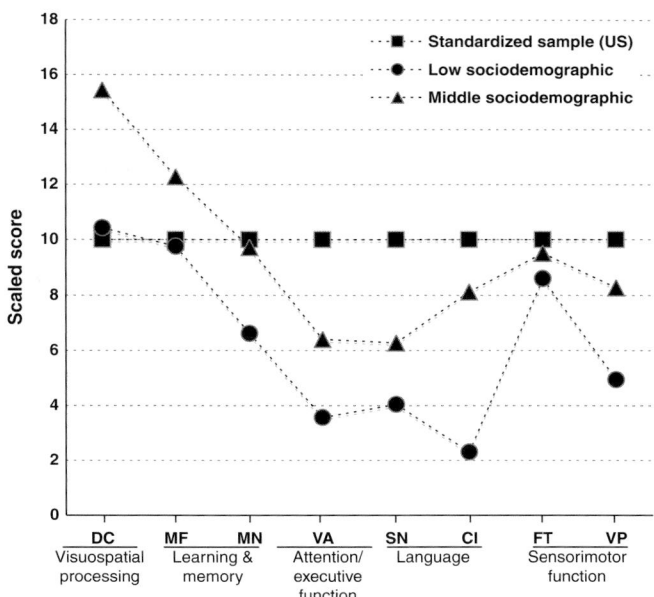

Figure 12.7.2 Neuropsychological performance differences on the NEPSY test of Zambian children with an average age of 9 years old compared to standardized US norms. Children (n = 19) from a low sociodemographic background and children (n = 25) from a middle sociodemographic background* neuropsychological performance is plotted along with the NEPSY standardized US norms+. The children' assessment included tasks from all five NEPSY domains: Design copying (DC) (Visuospatial Processing), Comprehension of Instruction (CI) and Speeded Naming (SN) (Language), Memory for Faces (MF) and Memory for Names (MN) (Memory and Learning), Visual Attention (VA) (Attention and Executive Function), and Finger Tapping (FT) and Visuomotor Precision (VP) (Sensorimotor Function). The trend in performance reveals that children of middle class background with better education perform better compared to those children that are of low resources and low education although both groups are from Lusaka (urban area) Zambia. + NEPSY norms with a mean of 10 and standard deviation of 3. *Data of Zambian children was adapted from Mulenga, K., Ahonen, T., and Aro, M., (2001), Performance of Zambian children on the NEPSY: A pilot study. *Developmental Neuropsychology*, 20(1), 375–383.

IMPACT OF HIV-1 INFECTION AND DISEASE MANIFESTATION AT THE SOCIODEMOGRAPHIC LEVEL

EDUCATION

The impact of education on HIV-1 infection and disease manifestation is another major issue. It is well accepted that the level and quality of education can be a major factor, especially in studies that assess neuropsychological status. This is pertinent when performing investigations to assess effects of HIV-1 on neurocognitive function. A small pilot study recently completed in Zambia, in which children were recruited from families living significantly below the poverty line even by the Zambian guidelines, revealed poor performance on a series of neuropsychological examinations using a standardized neuropsychological assessment for children (NEPSY) (Korkman & Kemp, 1998). When comparing the children from this cohort to that of another cohort which was comprised of children from a middle class status, though both cohorts of children were from the same urban area in Zambia, a marked difference in performance was observed (Figure 12.7.2). A worthy note is that extrinsic factors can also interplay in a child's performance. Children from low-resource countries are at increased risk for abnormal cognitive development due to the high rates of malnutrition, high rates of maternal deaths, poor medical care, lack of adequate educational system, and high risk of HIV-1 infection and other sub-tropical diseases (Ministry of Health [Zambia], 2006). Also, deaths in the family also affect the children, shown by a study done in Swaziland that children's performance was negatively impacted when a child lost his or her caretaker to HIV-1 infection and that, in turn, affected the child's physical, emotional, and mental welfare (Barnett, 2001).

IMPACT OF HIV-1 ON HEALTH CARE

In Africa, the lack of resources, especially in the medical field, is severe. Additionally, trained personnel are highly lacking and with the HIV-1 epidemic manpower has become more scarce. For instance, in Zambia, the first report that showed

HIV-1 prevalence in this low-resource country found that rates of HIV-1 infections were higher in the more educated/professionals such as doctors and nurses (Melbye et al., 1986). Over the years, many of the infected died, leaving a substantial void in the medical field, from which the country has not recovered. Now, after a quarter of a century, with the country still dealing with the HIV-1 epidemic, Zambia is ranked as one of the poorest countries (2009) with limited manpower in the medical profession and with HIV-1 prevalence rates of 14% (Ministry of Health [Zambia], 2006) in a population estimated at 12 million (CSO, 2009). The country is now in a state of an over-burdened health care system and an economy near collapse. The lack of adequate diagnostic equipment and services for proper diagnosis is also a huge health concern as it leads to premature deaths that could otherwise be prevented. The lack of proper diagnostic tools have also affected and limited investigations, especially those focused on the pathogenesis of HIV-1, and those that need the involvement of local health care facilities. This scenario is not exclusive to Zambia, but it is reminiscent of many other African countries

(HIV/AIDS, 2002; Nabyonga-Orem, Bazeyo, Okema, Karamagi, & Walker, 2008).

A major constraint in investigations performed in low-resource countries of Africa is the lack of trained personnel that are necessary to carry out a project. Studies that require personnel from the same cultural background, such as neuropsychological studies, require extensive on-ground training. Though this has shown to be successful from a small study in Zambia, time and monetary investment is tremendous, and requires the assurance that the trained personnel will stay through the completion of the project. Projects in neuropsychological testing require a trained clinical psychologist and a full-course training can take several months. Furthermore, the probability of having less healthy controls may be higher in low-resource countries where malnutrition and/or other endemics are common comorbid factors. These are some of the many challenges that arise when conducting research in low-resource countries, especially in HIV-1 neuropathogenesis investigations.

MARITAL STATUS

Marital status (single, married, divorced, separated, or widowed) is a factor that is normally included as part of sociodemographic parameters and is one that is highly impacted by the HIV-1 epidemic. A high incidence of widows has been reported in HIV-1-positive individuals in Africa. Furthermore, it is revealed that high-risk sexual activity is consistently reported to be higher in single, divorced, or widowed individuals as compared to those who are married (Kuate et al., 2009; Nabyonga-Orem et al., 2008). A case study that alludes to the conundrum of HIV-1 transmission is the recently discovered HIV-1 group P variant from a Cameroonian woman (Plantier et al., 2009). The woman was 63 years old when she tested positive for HIV-1 after falling ill in France. She was reported to have no HIV infection in her immediate family,

that is, children. Her husband died from stroke, though HIV serostatus was not known. She did, however, report that after she was widowed she had sexual partners in Cameroon. Individuals that are widowed are at a high risk of contracting HIV and in support of this sociodemographic data from a small study from Zambia revealed that 14% of the HIV-infected individuals were widowed, whereas in the uninfected controls none were widowed (Table 12.7.1). These differences were independent of income and education level. It is clear that demographics can be changed due to HIV and in turn, this change can result in further transmission of infection. An important note as new HIV-1 subtypes are found, more investigations are required to determine the pathology of new strains and how these strains may affect the neuropathology of HIV-1 as compared to other strains. This is important in the development of therapeutics as viral-host interactions are different between strains, as mentioned earlier.

LABOR

It is well recognized that HIV-1 has a tremendous effect on an economy, mostly with the decline in labor force. One of the most vulnerable groups for HIV-1 infection is individuals between the ages of 15 to 45 (WHO, 2009). This group comprises the greater bulk of the workforce in many African countries and it is the most reproductive/child-bearing period. However, the high vulnerability to HIV-1 in individuals between the ages of 15 to 45 has resulted in loss of labor due to inability to perform occupational tasks, leaving an occupation to care for a sick family member, or dying from AIDS. This has created a vicious cycle which has hindered the economic development of these countries, which in turn has affected the ability of governments to provide health care for HIV-1-infected individuals, resulting in disease progressions and deaths. According to the Food and Agricultural Organization (FAO), an estimated 7 million agricultural

Table 12.7.1 SOCIODEMOGRAPHIC PARAMETERS FOR HIV SERONEGATIVES AND SEROPOSITIVES DERIVED FROM A SMALL SAMPLE STUDY FROM ZAMBIA. THE VARIABLES INCLUDE SEX, AGE, EDUCATION, DEPENDENTS, AND MARITAL STATUS. MEAN, STANDARD ERROR OF THE MEAN (SEM), PERCENTAGES AND RANGES ARE PROVIDED WHERE APPROPRIATE

VARIABLES	HIV- MEAN (SEM)	PERCENT [RANGE]	HIV+ MEAN (SEM)	PERCENT [RANGE]
Sex (M/F)-Number	16/11		32/51	
Age-years	31 (1.5)	[18–55]	34 (0.8)	[18–57]
Education-years	9 (0.4)	[5–14]	9 (0.2)	[2–16]
Dependents	5 (0.5)	[0–12]	3 (3.0)	[0–9]
Marital status				
Single	7	(26%)	17	(21%)
Married	17	(63%)	37	(45%)
Separated	0	(0%)	2	(2%)
Divorced	2	(7%)	3	(4%)
Widowed	0	(0%)	12	(14%)
Unknown	1	(4%)	12	(14%)

workers suffered AIDS-related deaths in the last 25 years in the most affected sub-Saharan countries. Loss of labor as well as salary due to attending funerals also contributes to the decline in production and the income of an individual. A study that focused on household welfare in Uganda, reported that up to 77% who missed work was due to HIV-1-related issues compared to only 32% of those that were not HIV-1 infected. Furthermore, of those 77%, over three-quarters of them were absent for over a month (Nabyonga-Orem et al., 2008). In Zimbabwe, as much as 10% loss of salary was attributable to leaving work to attend a funeral (HIV/AIDS, 2002). It is predicted that the HIV-1 epidemic will inflict more AIDS-related deaths, estimated at 16 million by 2020 (HIV/AIDS, 2002). Agriculture is a sector that has been devastatingly affected by the epidemic, leaving countries with scarce food resources, and with the growing spread of HIV-1, the future is grim for affected African countries that rely heavily on agriculture. In summary, HIV-1 has disrupted the production and function of economies in settings where poverty is already rampant and also compounded by other endemics.

CONCLUSIONS

The geographic distribution of HIV-1 subtypes is not random and varies widely across the globe, with different regional prevalence for specific subtypes; for example, in North America subtype B predominates with almost 99% of cases, whereas the same subtype accounts for only 0.2% of infections in Southern Africa. The epidemiology of HIV-1 is dynamic over time, with strains constantly evolving and new strains emerging. For example, in sub-Saharan Africa, subtype C has outgrown other subtypes, practically to extinction, such as subtypes B and D, which were common in that region in the early 1980s. The sheer magnitude of the different HIV-1 types places a severe constraint on diagnostics and development of treatment and vaccine strategies. The role that HIV-1 diversity plays on transmission, pathogenesis, disease progression, and neuropathogenesis still needs to be fully evaluated in order to understand the complete significance of viral subtypes.

There is no disagreement that HIV-1 with its intricate genetic variability has challenged not only the scientific community, but has also disrupted cultural norms, altered socioeconomic dynamics, and shaken belief systems. Over the last twenty years, researchers have made some progress in understanding the effects of HIV-1 from a medical perspective by assessing general health and neurological disorders, as well as neuropsychological impairment. This progress is pertinent along with pushing forward for the availability of ART treatment in sub-Saharan Africa to ameliorate the devastation HIV-1 has had in the developing setting. However, the breadth of research, especially of the effect of HIV-1 on neuropathology effects on infected individuals, is limited by the extent of available resources in the region where the study is taking place. Additionally, as depicted in this review, HIV-1 subtype, culture, and sociodemographics are all important factors that interplay in study design and outcome of studies being carried out in the African settings, especially those that study neuropsychological function in HIV-infected individuals. More recent studies are already incorporating the same neuropsychological tools and this has improved the ability to compare findings from one study to another. Therefore, a standardized sociodemographic format with similar information is necessary not only to obtain a better insight to the patterns of HIV disease related to neuropathogenesis from the different African regions, but also needed for better comparative analysis between studies derived across Africa. In doing so, the research community would benefit from better understanding the challenges of one country to that of another when conducting neuropathogenesis studies.

ACKNOWLEDGMENTS

We like to thank the support of PHS grants R21-MH080612, RO1 CA75903, TW01492, T32 AI060547 and P20 RR15635 to CW. AH is supported by the Fogarty ARRA Supplement for U.S. Global Health Postdoctoral Scientist Support.

REFERENCES

Abebe, A., Kuiken, C. L., Goudsmit, J. et al. (1997). HIV type 1 subtype C in Addis Ababa, Ethiopia. *AIDS Res Hum Retroviruses*, 13, 1071–5.

Abebe, A., Lukashov, V. V., Pollakis, G., Kliphuis, A., Fontanet, A. L., Goudsmit, J., et al. (2001). Timing of the HIV-1 subtype C epidemic in Ethiopia based on early virus strains and subsequent virus diversification. *AIDS*, 15, 1555–61.

Agwale, S. M., Zeh, C., Robbins, K. E., et al. (2002). Molecular surveillance of HIV-1 field strains in Nigeria in preparation for vaccine trials. *Vaccine*, 20, 2131–9.

Appleton, J. (2000). "At my age I should be sitting under that tree": The impact of AIDS on Tanzanian lakeshore communities. *Gend Dev*, 8, 19–27.

Archer, J. & Robertson, D. L. (2007). Understanding the diversification of HIV-1 groups M and O. *AIDS*, 21, 1693–700.

Ayouba, A., Souquieres, S., Njinku, B., et al. (2000). HIV-1 group N among HIV-1-seropositive individuals in Cameroon. *AIDS*, 14, 2623–5.

Bailey, R. C., Moses, S., Parker, C. B., Agot, K., Maclean, I., Krieger, J. N., et al. (2007). Male circumcision for HIV prevention in young men in Kisumu, Kenya: A randomised controlled trial. *Lancet*, 369, 643–56.

Barnett, T., Whiteside, A., Desmond, C. (2001). The Social and economic impact of HIV/AIDS in poor countries: a review of studies and lessons. Progress in developmental studies 1, 2, 151–170.

Belman, A. L., Diamond, G., Dickson, D., Horoupian, D., Llena, J., Lantos, G., et al. (1988). Pediatric acquired immunodeficiency syndrome. Neurologic syndromes. *Am J Dis Child*, 142, 29–35.

Ben Halima, M., Pasquier, C., Slim, A., Ben Chaabane, T., Arrouji, Z., Puel, J., et al. (2001). First molecular characterization of HIV-1 Tunisian strains. *J Acquir Immune Defic Syndr*, 28, 94–6.

Bisiacchi, P. S., Suppiej, A., & Laverda, A. (2000). Neuropsychological evaluation of neurologically asymptomatic HIV-infected children. *Brain Cogn*, 43, 49–52.

Bodelle, P., Vallari, A., Coffey, R., McArthur, C. P., Beyeme, M., Devare, S. G., et al. (2004). Identification and genomic sequence of an HIV type 1 group N isolate from Cameroon. *AIDS Res Hum Retroviruses*, 20, 902–8.

Boivin, M. J., Ruel, T. D., Boal, H. E., et al. (2010). HIV-subtype A is associated with poorer neuropsychological performance compared with subtype D in antiretroviral therapy-naive Ugandan children. *AIDS*, 24, 1163–70.

Bouwman, F. H., Skolasky, R. L., Hes, D., Selnes, O. A., Glass, J. D., Nance-Sproson, T. E., et al. (1998). Variable progression of HIV-associated dementia. *Neurology*, 50, 1814–20.

Bouzeghoub, S., Jauvin, V., Recordon-Pinson, P., Garrigue, I., Amrane, A., Belabbes el, H., et al. (2006). High diversity of HIV type 1 in Algeria. *AIDS Res Hum Retroviruses*, 22, 367–72.

Bouzeghoub, S., Jauvin, V., Pinson, P., Schrive, M. H., Jeannot, A. C., Amrane, A., et al. (2008). First observation of HIV type 1 drug resistance mutations in Algeria. *AIDS Res Hum Retroviruses*, 24, 1467–73.

Candotti, D., Mundy, C., Kadewele, G., Nkhoma, W., Bates, I., & Allain, J. P. (2001). Serological and molecular screening for viruses in blood donors from Ntcheu, Malawi: High prevalence of HIV-1 subtype C and of markers of hepatitis B and C viruses. *J Med Virol*, 65, 1–5.

Carr, J. K., Salminen, M. O., Koch, C., Gotte, D., Artenstein, A. W., Hegerich, P. A., et al. (1996). Full-length sequence and mosaic structure of a human immunodeficiency virus type 1 isolate from Thailand. *J Virol*, 70, 5935–43.

Carr, J. K., Salminen, M. O., Albert, J., Sanders-Buell, E., Gotte, D., Birx, D. L., et al. (1998). Full genome sequences of human immunodeficiency virus type 1 subtypes G and A/G intersubtype recombinants. *Virology*, 247, 22–31.

Charneau, P., Borman, A. M., Quillent, C., Guetard, D., Chamaret, S., Cohen, J., et al. (1994). Isolation and envelope sequence of a highly divergent HIV-1 isolate: Definition of a new HIV-1 group. *Virology*, 205, 247–53.

Chiesi, A., Vella, S., Dally, L. G., et al. (1996). Epidemiology of AIDS dementia complex in Europe. AIDS in Europe Study Group. *J Acquir Immune Defic Syndr Hum Retrovirol*, 11, 39–44.

Cilliers, T., Nhlapo, J., Coetzer, M., Orlovic, D., Ketas, T., Olson, W. C., et al. (2003). The CCR5 and CXCR4 coreceptors are both used by human immunodeficiency virus type 1 primary isolates from subtype C. *J Virol*, 77, 4449–56.

Clifford, D. B., Mitike, M. T., Mekonnen, Y., et al. (2007). Neurological evaluation of untreated human immunodeficiency virus infected adults in Ethiopia. *J Neurovirol*, 13, 67–72.

Cluver, L., Gardner, F., & Operario, D. (2007). Psychological distress amongst AIDS-orphaned children in urban South Africa. *J Child Psychol Psychiatry*, 48, 755–63.

Collinson-Streng, A. N., Redd, A. D., Sewankambo, N. K., et al. (2009). Geographic HIV type 1 subtype distribution in Rakai district, Uganda. *AIDS Res Hum Retroviruses*, 25, 1045–8.

Copper, E. & Hanson, C. (1988). Encephalopathy and progression of human immunodeficiency virus disease in a cohort of children with perinatally acquired human immunodeficiency virus infection. *J Pediatrics*, 132, 808–09.

Central Statistics Office of Zambia (2009). Zambia Demographic and Health Survey 2007. Edited by T. D. R. C. T. Ministry of Health (MOH), University of Zambia, and Macro International Inc.: Calverton, Maryland, USA: Central Statistics Office of Zambia and Macro International Inc.

De Baar, M. P., De Ronde, A., Berkhout, B., Cornelissen, M., Van Der Horn, K. H., Van Der Schoot, A. M., et al. (2000). Subtype-specific sequence variation of the HIV type 1 long terminal repeat and primer-binding site. *AIDS Res Hum Retroviruses*, 16, 499–504.

El Sayed, N. M., Gomatos, P. J., Beck-Sague, C. M., et al. (2000). Epidemic transmission of human immunodeficiency virus in renal dialysis centers in Egypt. *J Infect Dis*, 181, 91–7.

Elharti, E., Elaouad, R., Amzazi, S., Himmich, H., Elhachimi, Z., Apetrei, C., et al. (1997). HIV-1 diversity in Morocco. *AIDS*, 11, 1781–3.

Epstein, L. G., Sharer, L. R., & Gajdusek, D. C. (1986). Hypothesis: AIDS encephalopathy is due to primary and persistent infection of the brain with a human retrovirus of the lentivirus subfamily. *Med Hypotheses*, 21, 87–96.

Everall, I., Vaida, F., Khanlou, N., et al. (2009). Cliniconeuropathologic correlates of human immunodeficiency virus in the era of antiretroviral therapy. *J Neurovirol*, 1–11.

Fischetti, L., Opare-Sem, O., Candotti, D., Sarkodie, F., Lee, H., & Allain, J. P. (2004). Molecular epidemiology of HIV in Ghana: Dominance of CRF02_AG. *J Med Virol*, 73, 158–66.

Gao, F., Robertson, D. L., Carruthers, C. D., et al. (1998). An isolate of human immunodeficiency virus type 1 originally classified as subtype I represents a complex mosaic comprising three different group M subtypes (A, G, and I). *J Virol*, 72, 10234–41.

Gao, F., Bailes, E., Robertson, D. L., et al. (1999). Origin of HIV-1 in the chimpanzee Pan troglodytes troglodytes. *Nature*, 397, 436–41.

Gao, F., Vidal, N., Li, Y., et al. (2001). Evidence of two distinct sub-subtypes within the HIV-1 subtype A radiation. *AIDS Res Hum Retroviruses*, 17, 675–88.

Garner, R. C. (2000). Safe sects? Dynamic religion and AIDS in South Africa. *J Mod Afr Stud*, 38, 41–69.

Gelmon, L., Kenya, P., Oguya, F., Cheluget, B., & Girmay, H. (2009). *Kenya: HIV prevention response and modes of transmission analysis.* Nairobi, Kenya: National AIDS Control Council.

Gray, R. H., Kigozi, G., Serwadda, D., et al. (2007). Male circumcision for HIV prevention in men in Rakai, Uganda: A randomised trial. *Lancet*, 369, 657–66.

Gray, R. R., Tatem, A. J., Lamers, S., et al. (2009). Spatial phylodynamics of HIV-1 epidemic emergence in east Africa. *AIDS*, 23, F9–F17.

Gurtler, L. G., Hauser, P. H., Eberle, J., von Brunn, A., Knapp, S., Zekeng, L., et al. (1994). A new subtype of human immunodeficiency virus type 1 (MVP-5180) from Cameroon. *J Virol*, 68, 1581–5.

Gyimah, S. O., Tenkorang, E. Y., Takyi, B. K., Adjei, J., & Fosu, G. (2010). Religion, HIV/AIDS and sexual risk-taking among men in Ghana. *J Biosoc Sci*, 1–17.

Harris, M. E., Serwadda, D., Sewankambo, N., et al. (2002). Among 46 near full length HIV type 1 genome sequences from Rakai District, Uganda, subtype D and AD recombinants predominate. *AIDS Res Hum Retroviruses*, 18, 1281–90.

Heaton, R. & Miller, S. (2004). Revised comprehensive norms for an expanded Halstead-Reitan Battery: Demographically adjusted neuropsychological norms for African American and Caucasian adults (HRB). Odessa, FL: Psychological Assessment Resources.

Heike, B. (2007). The rise of occult powers, AIDS and the Roman Catholic Church in Western Uganda. *Journal of Religion in Africa*, 37, 41–58.

Hemelaar, J., Gouws, E., Ghys, P. D., & Osmanov, S. (2006). Global and regional distribution of HIV-1 genetic subtypes and recombinants in 2004. *AIDS*, 20, W13–23.

Herbeck, J. T., Lyagoba, F., Moore, S. W., Shindo, N., Biryahwaho, B., Kaleebu, P., et al. (2007). Prevalence and genetic diversity of HIV type 1 subtypes A and D in women attending antenatal clinics in Uganda. *AIDS Res Hum Retroviruses*, 23, 755–60.

Hierholzer, M., Graham, R. R., El Khidir, I., et al. (2002). HIV type 1 strains from East and West Africa are intermixed in Sudan. *AIDS Res Hum Retroviruses*, 18, 1163–6.

HIV/AIDS (2002). *Impact of HIV/AIDS: Guidelines for studies of the social and economic impact.* Edited by UNAIDS, data.unaids.org/Publications/IRC-pub01/JC326-Guidelines.

Howard, T. M., Olaylele, D. O., & Rasheed, S. (1994). Sequence analysis of the glycoprotein 120 coding region of a new HIV type 1 subtype A strain (HIV-1IbNg) from Nigeria. *AIDS Res Hum Retroviruses*, 10, 1755–7.

Hu, D. J., Buve, A., Baggs, J., van der Groen, G., & Dondero, T. J. (1999). What role does HIV-1 subtype play in transmission and pathogenesis? An epidemiological perspective. *AIDS*, 13, 873–81.

Hu, D. J., Baggs, J., Downing, R. G., et al. (2000). Predominance of HIV-1 subtype A and D infections in Uganda. *Emerg Infect Dis*, 6, 609–15.

Huang, W., Eshleman, S. H., Toma, J., et al. (2007). Co-receptor tropism in human immunodeficiency virus type 1 subtype D: High prevalence of CXCR4 tropism and heterogeneous composition of viral populations. *J Virol*, 81, 7885–93.

Human Development Reports. (2009). Statistics. | Human Development Reports (HDR) | United Nations Development Programme (UNDP).

Hussein, M., Abebe, A., Pollakis, G., Brouwer, M., Petros, B., Fontanet, A. L., et al. (2000). HIV-1 subtype C in commercial sex workers in Addis Ababa, Ethiopia. *J Acquir Immune Defic Syndr*, 23, 120–7.

John-Stewart, G. C., Nduati, R. W., Rousseau, C. M., Mbori-Ngacha, D. A., Richardson, B. A., Rainwater, S., et al. (2005). Subtype C Is associated with increased vaginal shedding of HIV-1. *J Infect Dis*, 192, 492–6.

Joska, J. A., Fincham, D. S., Stein, D. J., Paul, R. H., & Seedat, S. (2009). Clinical correlates of HIV-associated neurocognitive disorders in South Africa. *AIDS Behavior*.

Kaleebu, P., French, N., Mahe, C., et al. (2002). Effect of human immunodeficiency virus (HIV) type 1 envelope subtypes A and D on disease progression in a large cohort of HIV-1-positive persons in Uganda. *J Infect Dis*, 185, 1244–50.

Kanki, P. J., Hamel, D. J., Sankale, J. L., et al. (1999). Human immunodeficiency virus type 1 subtypes differ in disease progression. *J Infect Dis*, 179, 68–73.

Khamadi, S. A., Ochieng, W., Lihana, R. W., et al. (2005). HIV type 1 subtypes in circulation in northern Kenya. *AIDS Res Hum Retroviruses*, 21, 810–4.

Khamadi, S. A., Lihana, R. W., Osman, S., et al. (2009). Genetic diversity of HIV type 1 along the coastal strip of Kenya. *AIDS Res Hum Retroviruses*, 25, 919–23.

Khoja, S., Ojwang, P., Khan, S., Okinda, N., Harania, R., & Ali, S. (2008). Genetic analysis of HIV-1 subtypes in Nairobi, Kenya. *PLoS One*, 3, e3191.

Kita, K., Ndembi, N., Ekwalanga, M., et al. (2004). Genetic diversity of HIV type 1 in Likasi, southeast of the Democratic Republic of Congo. *AIDS Res Hum Retroviruses*, 20, 1352–7.

Kiwanuka, N., Laeyendecker, O., Robb, M., et al. (2008). Effect of human immunodeficiency virus Type 1 (HIV-1) subtype on disease progression in persons from Rakai, Uganda, with incident HIV-1 infection. *J Infect Dis*, 197, 707–13.

Korkman, M. & Kemp, S. (1998). *NEPSY: A developmental neuropsychological assessment. Manual.* San Antonio, TX: Harcourt Brace.

Koulinska, I. N., Ndung'u, T., Mwakagile, D., Msamanga, G., Kagoma, C., Fawzi, W., et al. (2001). A new human immunodeficiency virus type 1 circulating recombinant form from Tanzania. *AIDS Res Hum Retroviruses*, 17, 423–31.

Kuate, S., Mikolajczyk, R. T., Forgwei, G. W., Tih, P. M., Welty, T. K., & Kretzschmar, M. (2009). Time trends and regional differences in the prevalence of HIV infection among women attending antenatal clinics in two provinces in Cameroon. *J Acquir Immune Defic Syndr*, 52, 258–64.

Lahuerta, M., Aparicio, E., Bardaji, A., et al. (2008). Rapid spread and genetic diversification of HIV type 1 subtype C in a rural area of southern Mozambique. *AIDS Res Hum Retroviruses*, 24, 327–35.

Laurent, C., Bourgeois, A., Faye, M. A., et al. (2002). No difference in clinical progression between patients infected with the predominant human immunodeficiency virus type 1 circulating recombinant form (CRF) 02_AG strain and patients not infected with CRF02_AG, in Western and West-Central Africa: A four-year prospective multicenter study. *J Infect Dis*, 186, 486–92.

Lihana, R. W., Khamadi, S. A., Lwembe, R. M., et al. (2009). The changing trend of HIV type 1 subtypes in Nairobi. *AIDS Res Hum Retroviruses*, 25, 337–42.

Lobato, M. N. (1995). Encephalopathy in children with perinatally acquired human immunodeficiency virus infection. Pediatric Spectrum of Disease Clinical Consortium. *Journal of Pediatrics*, 126, 710–5.

Majumdar, B. & Mazaleni, N. (2010). The experiences of people living with HIV/AIDS and of their direct informal caregivers in a resource-poor setting. *Journal of the International AIDS Society*, 13.

Marder, K., Liu, X., Stern, Y., et al. (1995). Risk of human immunodeficiency virus type 1-related neurologic disease in a cohort of intravenous drug users. *Arch Neurol*, 52, 1174–82.

Marechal, V., Jauvin, V., Selekon, B., et al. (2006). Increasing HIV type 1 polymorphic diversity but no resistance to antiretroviral drugs in untreated patients from Central African Republic: A 2005 study. *AIDS Res Hum Retroviruses*, 22, 1036–44.

Maslin, J., Rogier, C., Berger, F., Khamil, M. A., Mattera, D., Grandadam, M., et al. (2005). Epidemiology and genetic characterization of HIV-1 isolates in the general population of Djibouti (Horn of Africa). *J Acquir Immune Defic Syndr*, 39, 129–32.

Matsika-Claquin, M. D., Massanga, M., Menard, D., Mazi-Nzapako, J., Tenegbia, J. P., Mandeng, M. J., et al. (2004). HIV epidemic in Central African Republic: High prevalence rates in both rural and urban areas. *J Med Virol*, 72, 358–62.

Mbaya, S. (2002). HIV/AIDS and is impact on land issues in Malawi. In FAO/SAR PN Workshop on HIV/AIDS and Land, Pretoria.

McArthur, J. C., Hoover, D. R., Bacellar, H., et al. (1993). Dementia in AIDS patients: Incidence and risk factors. Multicenter AIDS Cohort Study. *Neurology*, 43, 2245–52.

McArthur, J. C., Brew, B. J., & Nath, A. (2005). Neurological complications of HIV infection. *Lancet Neurol*, 4, 543–55.

McCormack, G. P., Glynn, J. R., Crampin, A. C., et al. (2002). Early evolution of the human immunodeficiency virus type 1 subtype C epidemic in rural Malawi. *J Virol*, 76, 12890–9.

McCutchan, F. E. (2000). Understanding the genetic diversity of HIV-1. *AIDS*, 14 Suppl 3, S31–44.

Melbye, M., Njelesani, E. K., Bayley, A., et al (1986). Evidence for heterosexual transmission and clinical manifestations of human immunodeficiency virus infection and related conditions in Lusaka, Zambia. *Lancet*, 2, 1113–5.

Meloni, S. T., Sankale, J. L., Hamel, D. J., Eisen, G., Gueye-Ndiaye, A., Mboup, S., et al. (2004). Molecular epidemiology of human immunodeficiency virus type 1 sub-subtype A3 in Senegal from 1988 to 2001. *J Virol*, 78, 12455–61.

Ministry of Health [Zambia], Central Statistics Office [Zambia], and ORC Macro (2006). Zambia HIV/AIDS Service Provision Assessment Survey 2005. Calverton, Maryland, USA: Ministry of Health, Central Statistical Office, and ORC Macro.

Mintz, M. (1996). Neurological and developmental problems in pediatric HIV infection. *J Nutr*, 126, 2663S–73S.

Montavon, C., Toure-Kane, C., Nkengasong, J. N., Vergne, L., Hertogs, K., Mboup, S., et al. (2002). CRF06-cpx: A new circulating recombinant form of HIV-1 in West Africa involving subtypes A, G, K, and J. *J Acquir Immune Defic Syndr*, 29, 522–30.

Mulenga, K., Ahonen, T., & Aro, M., (2001), Performance of Zambian children on the NEPSY: A pilot study. *Developmental Neuropsychology*, 20(1), 375–383

Munerato, P., Azevedo, M. L., Sucupira, M. C., Pardini, R., Pinto, G. H., et al. (2003). Frequency of polymorphisms of genes coding for HIV-1 co-receptors CCR5 and CCR2 in a Brazilian population. *Braz J Infect Dis*, 7, 236–40.

Murray, C. J. (2010). Collaborative community-based care for South African children orphaned by HIV/AIDS. *J Spec Pediatr Nurs*, 15, 88–92.

Nabyonga-Orem, J., Bazeyo, W., Okema, A., Karamagi, H., & Walker, O. (2008). Effect of HIV/AIDS on household welfare in Uganda rural communities: A review. *East Afr Med, J* 85, 187–96.

Navia, B. A., Jordan, B. D., & Price, R. W. (1986). The AIDS dementia complex: I. Clinical features. *Ann Neurol*, 19, 517–24.

Nguyen, L., Chaowanachan, T., Vanichseni, S., et al (2004). Frequent human leukocyte antigen class I alleles are associated with higher viral load among HIV type 1 seroconverters in Thailand. *J Acquir Immune Defic Syndr*, 37, 1318–23.

Niama, F. R., Toure-Kane, C., Vidal, N., et al (2006). HIV-1 subtypes and recombinants in the Republic of Congo. *Infect Genet Evol*, 6, 337–43.

Nkengasong, J. N., Luo, C. C., Abouya, L., et al. (2000). Distribution of HIV-1 subtypes among HIV-seropositive patients in the interior of Cote d'Ivoire. *J Acquir Immune Defic Syndr*, 23, 430–6.

Nyombi, B. M., Kristiansen, K. I., Bjune, G., Muller, F., & Holm-Hansen, C. (2008a). Diversity of human immunodeficiency virus type 1 subtypes in Kagera and Kilimanjaro regions, Tanzania. *AIDS Res Hum Retroviruses*, 24, 761–9.

Nyombi, B. M., Nkya, W., Barongo, L., Bjune, G., Kristiansen, K. I., Muller, F., et al. (2008b). Evolution of human immunodeficiency virus type 1 serotypes in northern Tanzania: A retrospective study. *APMIS*, 116, 507–14.

Ottosson, D. (2009). *State-sponsored homophobia: A world survey of laws prohibiting same sex activity between consenting adults.* Brussels: International Lesbian, Gay, Bisexual, Trans and Intersex Association.

Paraskevis, D., Magiorkinis, M., Vandamme, A. M., Kostrikis, L. G., & Hatzakis, A. (2001). Re-analysis of human immunodeficiency virus type 1 isolates from Cyprus and Greece, initially designated "subtype I," reveals a unique complex A/G/H/K/? mosaic pattern. *J Gen Virol*, 82, 575–80.

Parreira, R., Piedade, J., Domingues, A., et al. (2006). Genetic characterization of human immunodeficiency virus type 1 from Beira, Mozambique. *Microbes Infect*, 8, 2442–51.

Peeters, M., Gueye, A., Mboup, S., et al (1997). Geographical distribution of HIV-1 group O viruses in Africa. *AIDS*, 11, 493–8.

Peeters, M., Esu-Williams, E., Vergne, L., et al. (2000). Predominance of subtype A and G HIV type 1 in Nigeria, with geographical differences in their distribution. *AIDS Res Hum Retroviruses*, 16, 315–25.

Plantier, J. C., Leoz, M., Dickerson, J. E., De Oliveira, F., Cordonnier, F., Lemee, V., et al. (2009). A new human immunodeficiency virus derived from gorillas. *Nat Med*, 15, 871–2.

Powell, R., Barengolts, D., Mayr, L., & Nyambi, P. (2010). The evolution of HIV-1 diversity in rural Cameroon and its implications in vaccine design and trials. *VIRUSES*, 2, 639–54.

Punzi, G., Saracino, A., Brindicci, G., Scarabaggio, T., Lagioia, A., Angarano, G., et al. (2005). HIV infection and protease genetic diversity in a rural area of the Southern Central African Republic. *J Med Virol*, 77, 457–9.

Rambaut, A., Robertson, D. L., Pybus, O. G., Peeters, M., & Holmes, E. C. (2001). Human immunodeficiency virus. Phylogeny and the origin of HIV-1. *Nature*, 410, 1047–8.

Rambaut, A., Posada, D., Crandall, K. A., & Holmes, E. C. (2004). The causes and consequences of HIV evolution. *Nat Rev Genet*, 5, 52–61.

Renjifo, B., Fawzi, W., Mwakagile, D., et al (2001). Differences in perinatal transmission among human immunodeficiency virus type 1 genotypes. *J Hum Virol*, 4, 16–25.

Renjifo, B., Gilbert, P., Chaplin, B., Msamanga, G., Mwakagile, D., Fawzi, W., et al. (2004). Preferential in-utero transmission of HIV-1 subtype C as compared to HIV-1 subtype A or D. *AIDS*, 18, 1629–36.

Robertson, D. L., Anderson, J. P., Bradac, J. A., et al. (2000). HIV-1 nomenclature proposal. *Science*, 288, 55–6.

Robertson, K. R., Kapoor, C., Robertson, W. T., Fiscus, S., Ford, S., & Hall, C. D. (2004). No gender differences in the progression of nervous system disease in HIV infection. *J Acquir Immune Defic Syndr*, 36, 817–22.

Sacktor, N., Nakasujja, N., Skolasky, R. L., et al (2009). HIV subtype D is associated with dementia, compared with subtype A, in immunosuppressed individuals at risk of cognitive impairment in Kampala, Uganda. *Clin Infect Dis*, 49, 780–6.

Serwadda, D., Mugerwa, R. D., Sewankambo, N. K., et al (1985). Slim disease: A new disease in Uganda and its association with HTLV-III infection. *Lancet*, 2, 849–52.

Simon, F., Mauclere, P., Roques, P., Loussert-Ajaka, I., Muller-Trutwin, M. C., Saragosti, S., et al. (1998). Identification of a new human immunodeficiency virus type 1 distinct from group M and group O. *Nat Med*, 4, 1032–7.

Smith, A. D., Tapsoba, P., Peshu, N., Sanders, E. J., & Jaffe, H. W. (2009). Men who have sex with men and HIV/AIDS in sub-Saharan Africa. *Lancet*, 374, 416–22.

Smith, M. K. (2002). Gender, poverty and intergenerational vulnerability to HIV/AIDS. *Gender and Development*, 10, 63–70.

Smith, R., Malee, K., Leighty, R., Brouwers, P., Mellins, C., Hittelman, J., Chase, C., et al. (2006). Effects of perinatal HIV infection and associated risk factors on cognitive development among young children. *Pediatrics*, 117, 851–62.

Songok, E. M., Lihana, R. W., Kiptoo, M. K., et al. (2003). Identification of env CRF-10 among HIV variants circulating in rural western Kenya. *AIDS Res Hum Retroviruses*, 19, 161–5.

Steain, M. C., Wang, B., Yang, C., Shi, Y. P., Nahlen, B., Lal, R. B., et al. (2005). HIV type 1 sequence diversity and dual infections in Kenya. *AIDS Res Hum Retroviruses*, 21, 882–5.

Triques, K., Bourgeois, A., Saragosti, S., et al. (1999). High diversity of HIV-1 subtype F strains in Central Africa. *Virology*, 259, 99–109.

Triques, K., Bourgeois, A., Vidal, N., et al. (2000). Near-full-length genome sequencing of divergent African HIV type 1 subtype F viruses leads to the identification of a new HIV type 1 subtype designated K. *AIDS Res Hum Retroviruses*, 16, 139–51.

Vallari, A., Yamaguchi, J., Holzmayer, V., et al. (2010). HIV-1 Group P: Confirmation of Group P in Cameroon. In 17th Conference on Retroviruses and Opportunistic Infections. San Francisco.

van der Kuyl, A. C. & Cornelissen, M. (2007). Identifying HIV-1 dual infections. *Retrovirology*, 4, 67.

Vidal, N., Peeters, M., Mulanga-Kabeya, C., et al. (2000). Unprecedented degree of human immunodeficiency virus type 1 (HIV-1) group M genetic diversity in the Democratic Republic of Congo suggests that the HIV-1 pandemic originated in Central Africa. *J Virol*, 74, 10498–507.

Vidal, N., Mulanga, C., Bazepeo, S. E., Lepira, F., Delaporte, E., & Peeters, M. (2006). Identification and molecular characterization of sub-subtype A4 in central Africa. *AIDS Res Hum Retroviruses*, 22, 182–7.

Vidal, N., Bazepeo, S. E., Mulanga, C., Delaporte, E., & Peeters, M. (2009). Genetic characterization of eight full-length HIV type 1 genomes from the Democratic Republic of Congo (DRC) reveal a new sub-subtype, A5, in the A radiation that predominates in the recombinant structure of CRF26_A5U. *AIDS Res Hum Retroviruses*, 25, 823–32.

Weisman, Z., Kalinkovich, A., Borkow, G., Stein, M., Greenberg, Z., & Bentwich, Z. (1999). Infection by different HIV-1 subtypes (B and C) results in a similar immune activation profile despite distinct immune backgrounds. *J Acquir Immune Defic Syndr*, 21, 157–63.

WHO (2009). World Health Organization: (http://www.aidsetc.org/aidsetc?page=cm-105_disease).

Yang, C., Li, M., Newman, R. D., et al. (2003). Genetic diversity of HIV-1 in western Kenya: Subtype-specific differences in mother-to-child transmission. *AIDS*, 17, 1667–74.

Yang, C., Li, M., Mokili, J. L., et al. (2005). Genetic diversification and recombination of HIV type 1 group M in Kinshasa, Democratic Republic of Congo. *AIDS Res Hum Retroviruses*, 21, 661–6.

Yerly, S., Quadri, R., Negro, F., Barbe, K. P., Cheseaux, J. J., Burgisser, P., et al. (2001). Nosocomial outbreak of multiple blood-borne viral infections. *J Infect Dis*, 184, 369–72.

zur Megede, J., Engelbrecht, S., de Oliveira, T., Cassol, S., Scriba, T. J., van Rensburg, E. J., et al. (2002). Novel evolutionary analyses of full-length HIV type 1 subtype C molecular clones from Cape Town, South Africa. *AIDS Res Hum Retroviruses*, 18, 1327–32.

INDEX

Page numbers followed by "*f*", "*t*", or "*n*" denote figures, tables, or notes, respectively